2026

ICD-10-CM
FOR PHYSICIANS

Jackie L. Koesterman, CPC
Coding and Reimbursement Specialist
JDK Medical Coding EDU
Grand Forks, North Dakota

BUCK'S

INCLUDES
NETTER'S
ANATOMY
ART

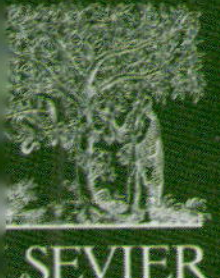

Elsevier
3251 Riverport Lane
St. Louis, Missouri 63043

BUCK'S 2026 ICD-10-CM FOR PHYSICIANS

ISBN: 978-0-443-38078-5

Senior Content Strategist: Luke Held
Content Development Manager: Danielle Frazier
Senior Content Development Specialist: Joshua S. Rapplean
Publishing Services Manager: Deepthi Unni
Project Manager: Nayagi Anandan
Senior Book Designer: Maggie Reid

Printed in Canada

Last digit is the print number: 9 8 7 6 5 4 3 2 1

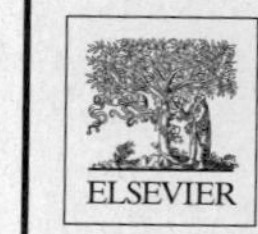
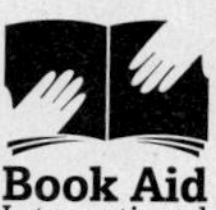

DEDICATION

To all who require of themselves the highest level of accuracy, integrity, and professionalism. You enhance our profession and are a tremendous asset to health care. May this manual be of assistance to you.

With Greatest Admiration.

Carol J. Buck, MS

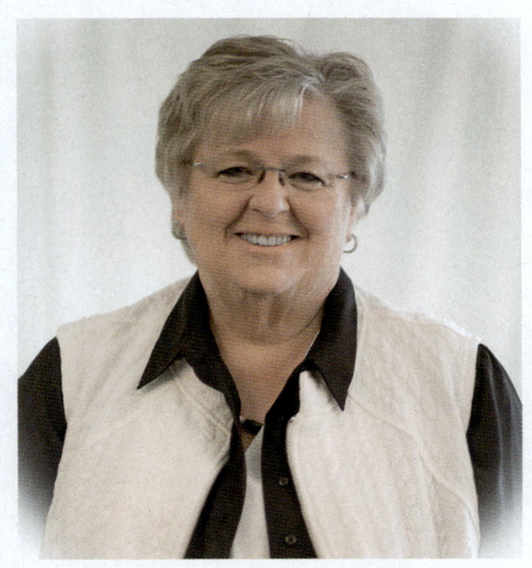

DEVELOPMENT OF THIS EDITION

Lead Technical Collaborator

Jackie L. Koesterman, CPC
Coding and Reimbursement Specialist
JDK Medical Coding EDU
Grand Forks, North Dakota

Query Team

**Robin Linker, CHCA, CHCAS, CPC-I,
   COC, CCS-P, CPC-P, MCS-P, CHC**
AAPC Approved Instructor
CEO, Robin Linker & Education Associates, Inc.; and
Association of Health Care Auditors and Educators
Aurora, Colorado

CONTENTS

GUIDE TO USING THE 2026 ICD-10-CM FOR PHYSICIANS

Medical coding has long been a part of the health care profession. Through the years medical coding systems have become more complex and extensive. Today, medical coding is an intricate and immense process that is present in every health care setting. The increased use of electronic submissions for health care services only increases the need for coders who understand the coding process.

2026 ICD-10-CM for Physicians, Professional Edition was developed to help meet the needs of coding professionals at all levels by offering a comprehensive coding text at a reasonable price.

All material strictly adheres to the latest government versions available at the time of publication. Updates from the *Definitions of Medicare Code Edits* (MCE) will be posted to the companion website (www.codingupdates.com) when available.

Illustrations and Items

The ICD-10-CM Tabular List contains illustrations, pictures, and items to assist you in understanding difficult terminology, diseases/conditions, or coding in a specific category. Items are always shaded with ▓▓▓▓▓ ink so that the added material is not mistaken for official notations or instructions. ▓▓▓▓ shading is used for other annotations in the text. Your ideas on what other descriptions or illustrations should be in future editions of this text are always appreciated.

Instructional Notations

Includes Notes

Includes

The word "Includes" appears immediately under certain categories to further define, or give examples of, the content of the category.

Excludes Notes

The ICD-10-CM has two types of excludes notes. Each note has a different definition for use, but they are both similar in that they indicate that codes excluded from each other are independent of each other.

Excludes1

A type 1 Excludes note is a pure excludes. It means "NOT CODED HERE!" An Excludes1 note indicates that the code excluded should never be used at the same time as the code above the Excludes1 note. An Excludes1 is for use when two conditions cannot occur together, such as a congenital form versus an acquired form of the same condition.

Excludes2

A type 2 Excludes note represents "NOT INCLUDED HERE." An Excludes2 note indicates that the condition excluded is not part of the condition it is excluded from, but a patient may have both conditions at the same time. When an Excludes2 note appears under a code, it is acceptable to use both the code and the excluded code together.

Code First/Use Additional Code notes (etiology/manifestation paired codes)

Certain conditions have both an underlying etiology and multiple body system manifestations due to the underlying etiology. For such conditions the ICD-10-CM has a coding convention that requires the underlying condition be sequenced first, followed by the manifestation. Wherever such a combination exists, there is a "use additional code" note at the etiology code, and a "code first" note at the manifestation code. These instructional notes indicate the proper sequencing order of the codes, etiology followed by manifestation.

In most cases the manifestation codes will have in the code title, "in diseases classified elsewhere." Codes with this title are a component of the etiology/manifestation convention. The code title indicates that it is a manifestation code. "In diseases classified elsewhere" codes are never permitted to be used as first-listed or principal diagnosis codes. They must be used in conjunction with an underlying condition code, and they must be listed following the underlying condition.

Use additional

The words indicate an instructional note that another code may be needed.

Code first

The words indicate an instructional note that directs the coder to sequence the underlying condition before the manifestation.

Code also

A "code also" note instructs that two codes may be required to fully describe a condition, but the sequencing of the two codes is discretionary, depending on the severity of the conditions and the reason for the encounter.

7th characters and placeholder X

For codes less than 6 characters that require a 7th character, a placeholder X should be assigned for all characters less than 6. The 7th character must always be the 7th character of a code.

Annotated

Throughout the manual, revisions, additions, and deleted codes or words are indicated by the following symbols:

➡   **Revised:** Revisions within the line or code from the previous edition are indicated by the arrow.

▶   **New:** Additions to the previous edition are indicated by the triangle.

~~deleted~~   **Deleted:** Deletions from the previous edition are struck through.

ICD-10-CM Tabular List Symbols

●   **Use Additional Character(s):** The red stop sign cautions that the code requires additional character(s) to ensure the greatest specificity.

X   For codes less than 6 characters that require a 7th character, a placeholder X should be assigned for all characters less than 6. The 7th character must always be the 7th character of a code.

OGCR   The *Official Guidelines for Coding and Reporting* symbol includes the placement of a portion of a guideline as that guideline pertains to the code by which it is located. The complete OGCR are located in Part I.

🅷🅲🅲   The **Hierarchical condition category (HCC)** was initiated in 2004 for the reimbursement for patients with Medicare Advantage plans (Medicare Part C). HCC is based on a list of chronic or severity of illness diagnosis codes that CMS uses to determine reimbursements to Medicare Advantage plans. The HCC risk adjustment factor data is calculated for an entire year for encounters of the patient's care.

▸   **Manifestation Code:** Describes the manifestation of an underlying disease, not the disease itself, and therefore should not be assigned as a principal diagnosis, according to the *Definitions of Medicare Code Edits* (MCE).

Age conflict: The *Definitions of Medicare Code Edits* (MCE) detects inconsistencies between a patient's age and diagnosis. For example, a 5-year-old patient with benign prostatic hypertrophy or a 78-year-old pregnant female.

The diagnosis is clinically and virtually impossible in a patient of the stated age. Therefore, either the diagnosis or the age is presumed to be incorrect. There are four age categories for diagnoses in the *Definitions of Medicare Code Edits* (MCE):

N   • Newborn. Age of 0 years; a subset of diagnoses intended only for newborns and neonates (e.g., fetal distress, perinatal jaundice).

P   • Pediatric. Age range is 0-17 years inclusive (e.g., Reye's syndrome, routine child health exam).

M   • Maternity. Age range is 9-64 years inclusive (e.g., diabetes in pregnancy, antepartum pulmonary complication).

A   • Adult. Age range is 15-124 years inclusive (e.g., senile delirium, mature cataract).

♀♂   **Sex conflict:** *Definitions of Medicare Code Edits* (MCE) detects inconsistencies between a patient's sex and any diagnosis or procedure on the patient's record. For example, a male patient with cervical cancer (diagnosis) or a female patient with a prostatectomy (procedure). In both instances, the indicated diagnosis or the procedure conflicts with the stated sex of the patient. Therefore, either the patient's diagnosis, procedure, or sex is presumed to be incorrect.

Key words

Highlight identifies key words within similar code descriptions in a particular category.

Coding Clinic Identifies the year, quarter, and page number that presents information about an ICD-10-CM code in the American Hospital Association's *Coding Clinic®* for ICD-10-CM.

Visit codingupdates.com for the full list of *2026* Present on Admission codes.

SYMBOLS AND CONVENTIONS

ICD-10-CM Tabular

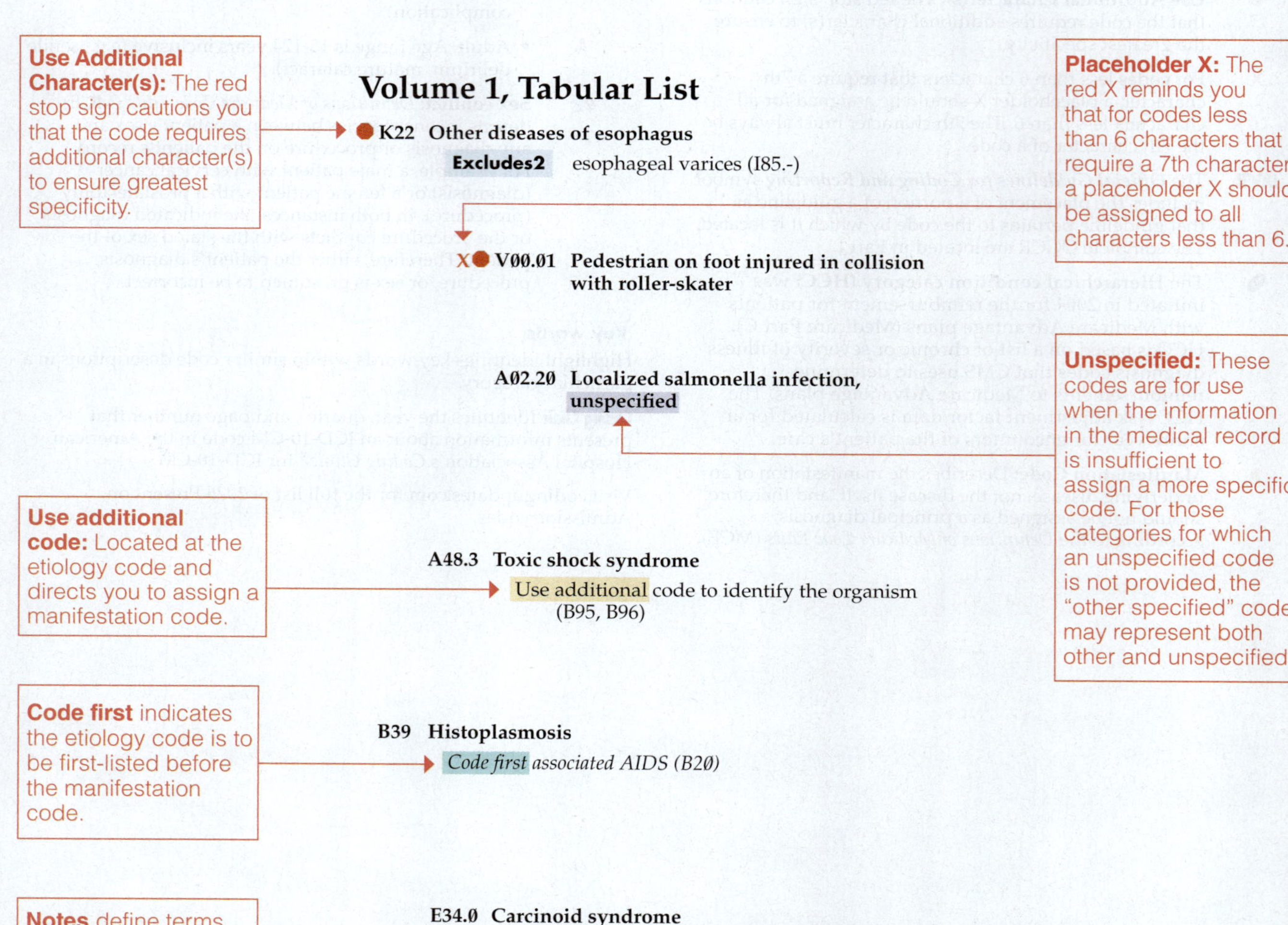

Volume 1, Tabular List

Use Additional Character(s): The red stop sign cautions you that the code requires additional character(s) to ensure greatest specificity.

● **K22   Other diseases of esophagus**

Excludes2   esophageal varices (I85.-)

Placeholder X: The red X reminds you that for codes less than 6 characters that require a 7th character, a placeholder X should be assigned to all characters less than 6.

X ● **V00.01   Pedestrian on foot injured in collision with roller-skater**

A02.20   Localized salmonella infection, unspecified

Unspecified: These codes are for use when the information in the medical record is insufficient to assign a more specific code. For those categories for which an unspecified code is not provided, the "other specified" code may represent both other and unspecified.

Use additional code: Located at the etiology code and directs you to assign a manifestation code.

A48.3   Toxic shock syndrome

Use additional code to identify the organism (B95, B96)

Code first indicates the etiology code is to be first-listed before the manifestation code.

B39   Histoplasmosis

Code first associated AIDS (B20)

Notes define terms or give coding instructions.

E34.0   Carcinoid syndrome

Note: May be used as an additional code to identify functional activity associated with a carcinoid tumor.

Codes or index entries are for purposes of illustration only and may not be current.

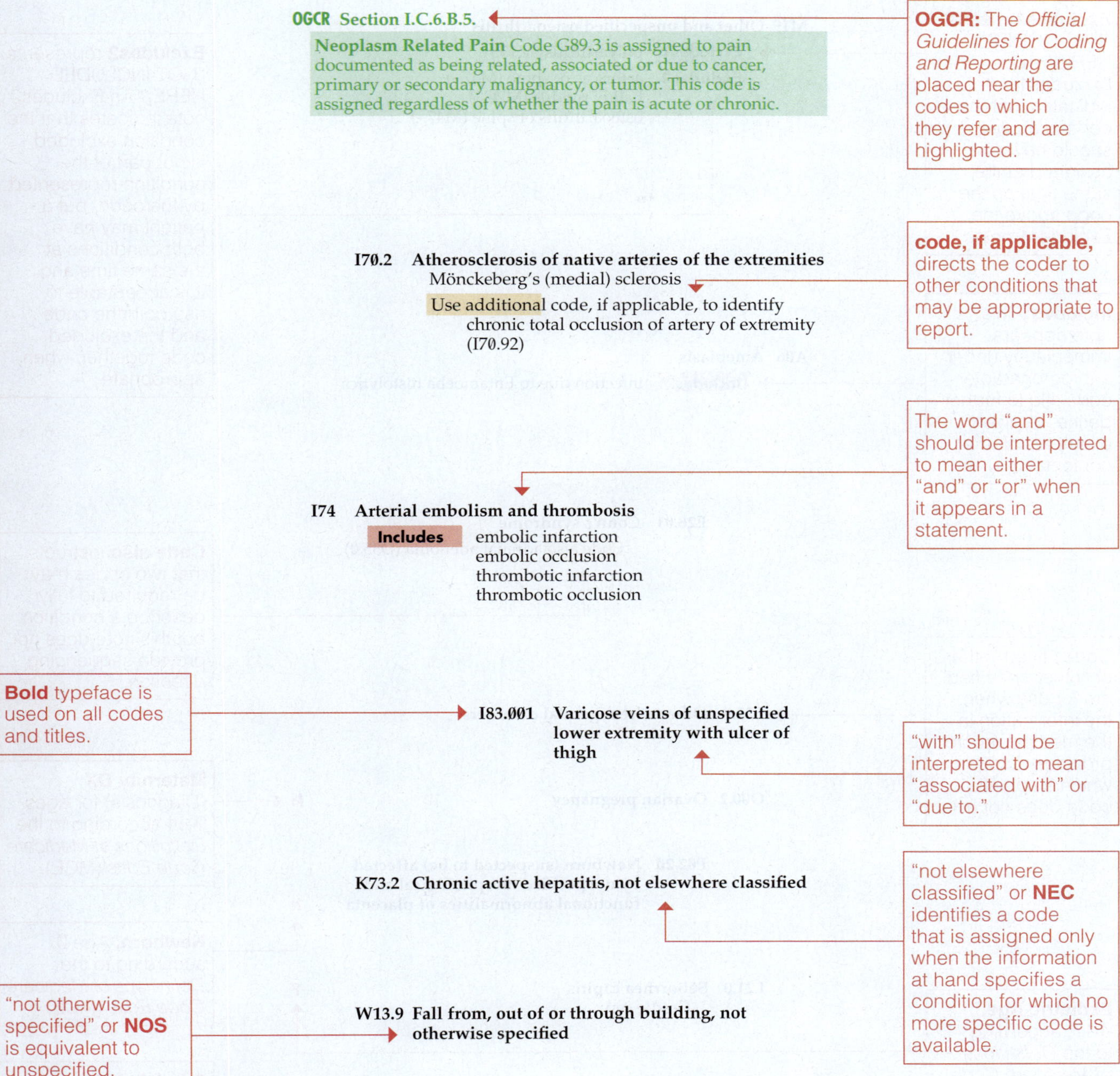

Codes or index entries are for purposes of illustration only and may not be current.

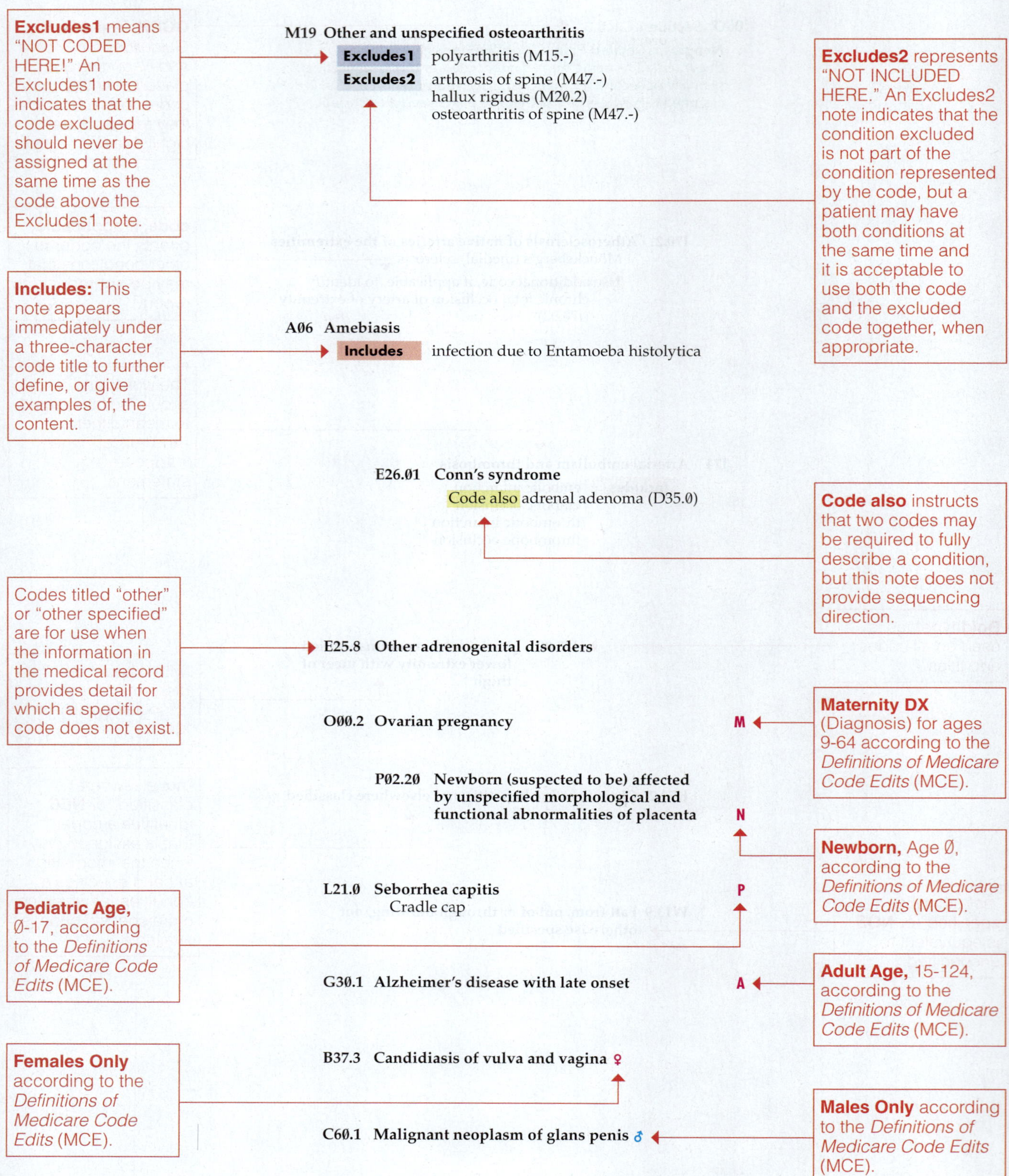

Codes or index entries are for purposes of illustration only and may not be current.

Manifestation according to the *Definitions of Medicare Code Edits* (MCE).

H22 *Disorders of iris and ciliary body in diseases classified elsewhere*

Code first underlying disease, such as:
gout (M1A-, M10.-)

Key Term Highlight identifies key words within similar code descriptions in a particular category.

F10.21   Alcohol dependence, **in remission**

Coding Clinic identifies the year, quarter, and page number that presents information about an ICD-10-PCS code in the American Hospital Association's *Coding Clinic®*.

B96.5   Pseudomonas (aeruginosa) (mallei) (pseudomallei) as the cause of diseases classified elsewhere
Coding Clinic: 2015, Q1, P18

Codes or index entries are for purposes of illustration only and may not be current.

Alphabetic Index

Main terms are in **bold** typeface.

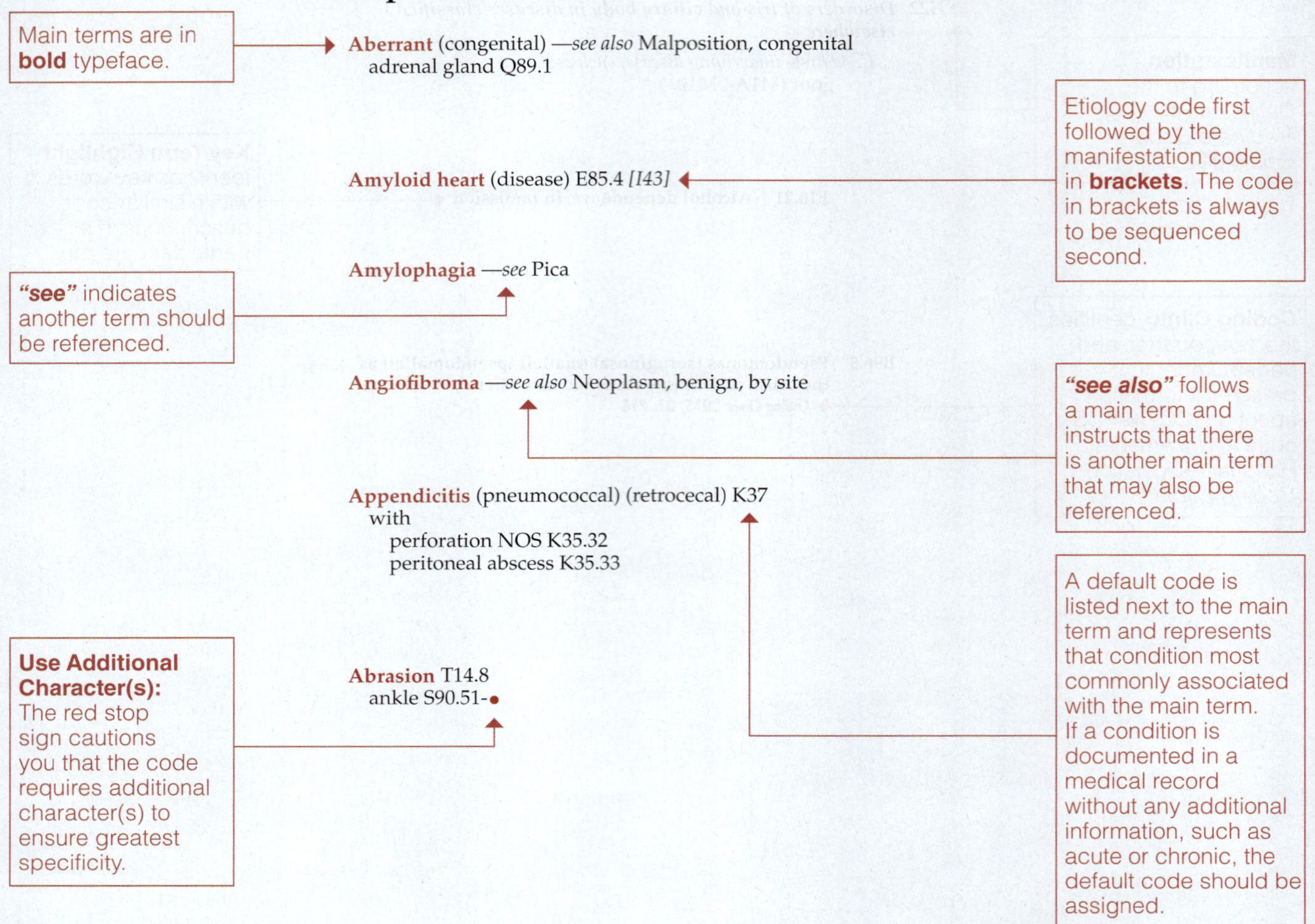

Etiology code first followed by the manifestation code in **brackets**. The code in brackets is always to be sequenced second.

"**see**" indicates another term should be referenced.

"**see also**" follows a main term and instructs that there is another main term that may also be referenced.

Use Additional Character(s): The red stop sign cautions you that the code requires additional character(s) to ensure greatest specificity.

A default code is listed next to the main term and represents that condition most commonly associated with the main term. If a condition is documented in a medical record without any additional information, such as acute or chronic, the default code should be assigned.

Codes or index entries are for purposes of illustration only and may not be current.

GUIDE TO THE 2026 ICD-1O-CM UPDATES

No Change		**CHAPTER 1**
No Change		**CERTAIN INFECTIOUS AND PARASITIC DISEASES (A00-B99)**

<u>**VIRAL HEPATITIS (B15-B19)**</u>

No Change	**B18**	**Chronic viral hepatitis**
Add		Use Additional code, if applicable, for ascites (R18.8)

<u>**PEDICULOSIS, ACARIASIS AND OTHER INFESTATIONS (B85-B89)**</u>

No Change	**B88**	**Other infestations**
No Change		**B88.0** **Other acariasis**
Delete		Acarine dermatitis
Delete		Dermatitis due to Demodex species
Delete		Dermatitis due to Dermanyssus gallinae
Delete		Dermatitis due to Liponyssoides sanguineus
Delete		Trombiculosis
Add		**B88.01** **Infestation by Demodex mites**
Add		Demodex brevis infestation
Add		Demodex folliculorum infestation
Add		Code also, if applicable, eyelid inflammation (H01.8-)
Add		**B88.09** **Other acariasis**
Add		Acarine dermatitis
Add		Dermatitis due to Dermanyssus gallinae
Add		Dermatitis due to Liponyssoides sanguineus
Add		Trombiculosis

<u>**BACTERIAL AND VIRAL INFECTIOUS AGENTS (B95-B97)**</u>

No Change	**B96**	**Other bacterial agents as the cause of diseases classified elsewhere**
No Change		**B96.2** **Escherichia coli [E. coli] as the cause of diseases classified elsewhere**
No Change		**B96.21** **Shiga toxin-producing Escherichia coli [E. coli] [STEC] O157 as the cause of diseases classified elsewhere**
Revise from		O157:H7 Escherichia coli [E.coli] with or without confirmation of Shiga toxin-production
Revise to		O157:H7 Escherichia coli [E. coli] with or without confirmation of Shiga toxin-production
Revise from		Shiga toxin-producing Escherichia coli [E.coli] O157:H7 with or without confirmation of Shiga toxin-production
Revise to		Shiga toxin-producing Escherichia coli [E. coli] O157:H7 with or without confirmation of Shiga toxin-production
No Change		**B96.22** **Other specified Shiga toxin-producing Escherichia coli [E. coli] [STEC] as the cause of diseases classified elsewhere**
Revise from		Non-O157 Shiga toxin-producing Escherichia coli [E.coli]
Revise to		Non-O157 Shiga toxin-producing Escherichia coli [E. coli]
Revise from		Non-O157 Shiga toxin-producing Escherichia coli [E.coli] with known O group
Revise to		Non-O157 Shiga toxin-producing Escherichia coli [E. coli] with known O group

No Change		**CHAPTER 2**
No Change		**NEOPLASMS (C00-D49)**

<u>**MALIGNANT NEOPLASMS OF BREAST (C50)**</u>

No Change	**C50**	**Malignant neoplasm of breast**
Add		**C50.A** **Malignant inflammatory neoplasm of breast**
		Inflammatory breast cancer (IBC)
Add		**C50.A0** **Malignant inflammatory neoplasm of unspecified breast**
Add		**C50.A1** **Malignant inflammatory neoplasm of right breast**
Add		**C50.A2** **Malignant inflammatory neoplasm of left breast**

<u>**SECONDARY NEUROENDOCRINE TUMORS (C7B)**</u>

No Change	**C7B**	**Secondary neuroendocrine tumors**
No Change		**C7B.0** **Secondary carcinoid tumors**
		C7B.04 **Secondary carcinoid tumors of peritoneum**
Revise from		Mesentary metastasis of carcinoid tumor
Revise to		Mesentery metastasis of carcinoid tumor

<u>**MALIGNANT NEOPLASMS OF ILL-DEFINED, OTHER SECONDARY AND UNSPECIFIED SITES (C76-C80)**</u>

No Change	**C77**	**Secondary and unspecified malignant neoplasm of lymph nodes**
No Change		**Excludes1**
Revise from		mesentary metastasis of carcinoid tumor (C7B.04)
Revise to		mesentery metastasis of carcinoid tumor (C7B.04)

<u>**BENIGN NEOPLASMS, EXCEPT BENIGN NEUROENDOCRINE TUMORS (D10-D36)**</u>

No Change	**D12**	**Benign neoplasm of colon, rectum, anus and anal canal**
No Change		**D12.6** **Benign neoplasm of colon, unspecified**
Delete		**Excludes1** inflammatory polyp of colon (K51.4-)
Add		**Excludes2** inflammatory polyp of colon (K51.4-)

<u>**NEOPLASMS OF UNCERTAIN BEHAVIOR, POLYCYTHEMIA VERA AND MYELODYSPLASTIC SYNDROMES (D37-D48)**</u>

No Change	**D48**	**Neoplasm of uncertain behavior of other and unspecified sites**
No Change		**D48.1** **Neoplasm of uncertain behavior of connective and other soft tissue**
No Change		**D48.11** **Desmoid tumor**
Add		Aggressive fibromatosis

No Change

CHAPTER 3

No Change

DISEASES OF THE BLOOD AND BLOOD-FORMING ORGANS AND CERTAIN DISORDERS INVOLVING THE IMMUNE MECHANISM (D50-D89)

No Change

NUTRITIONAL ANEMIAS (D50-D53)

No Change **D53   Other nutritional anemias**

No Change   **D53.8   Other specified nutritional anemias**

Delete   **Excludes1**   nutritional deficiencies without anemia, such as:

Delete   copper deficiency NOS (E61.0)

Delete   molybdenum deficiency NOS (E61.5)

Delete   zinc deficiency NOS (E60)

Add   **Excludes2**   nutritional deficiencies without anemia, such as:

Add   copper deficiency NOS (E61.0)

Add   molybdenum deficiency NOS (E61.5)

Add   zinc deficiency NOS (E60)

No Change

COAGULATION DEFECTS, PURPURA AND OTHER HEMORRHAGIC CONDITIONS (D65-D69)

No Change **D68   Other coagulation defects**

No Change   **D68.3   Hemorrhagic disorder due to circulating anticoagulants**

No Change   **D68.31   Hemorrhagic disorder due to intrinsic circulating anticoagulants, antibodies, or inhibitors**

No Change   **D68.312   Antiphospholipid antibody with hemorrhagic disorder**

Delete   **Excludes1**   antiphospholipid antibody syndrome (D68.61)

Delete   antiphospholipid antibody with hypercoagulable state (D68.61)

Delete   lupus anticoagulant (LAC) with hypercoagulable state (D68.62)

Delete   systemic lupus erythematosus [SLE] inhibitor with hypercoagulable state (D68.62)

Add   **Excludes2**   antiphospholipid antibody syndrome (D68.61)

Add   antiphospholipid antibody with hypercoagulable state (D68.61)

Add   lupus anticoagulant (LAC) with hypercoagulable state (D68.62)

Add   systemic lupus erythematosus [SLE] inhibitor with hypercoagulable state (D68.62)

No Change   **D68.6   Other thrombophilia**

No Change   **D68.61   Antiphospholipid syndrome**

Delete   **Excludes1**   anti-phospholipid antibody with hemorrhagic disorder (D68.312)

Delete   lupus anticoagulant syndrome (D68.62)

Add   **Excludes2**   anti-phospholipid antibody with hemorrhagic disorder (D68.312)

Add   lupus anticoagulant syndrome (D68.62)

No Change   **D68.62   Lupus anticoagulant syndrome**

Delete   **Excludes1**   anticardiolipin syndrome (D68.61)

Delete   antiphospholipid syndrome (D68.61)

Delete   lupus anticoagulant (LAC) with hemorrhagic disorder (D68.312)

Add   **Excludes2**   anticardiolipin syndrome (D68.61)

Add   antiphospholipid syndrome (D68.61)

Add   lupus anticoagulant (LAC) with hemorrhagic disorder (D68.312)

No Change

OTHER DISORDERS OF BLOOD AND BLOOD-FORMING ORGANS (D70-D77)

No Change **D71   Functional disorders of polymorphonuclear neutrophils**

Delete   Cell membrane receptor complex [CR3] defect

Delete   Chronic (childhood) granulomatous disease

Delete   Congenital dysphagocytosis

Delete   Progressive septic granulomatosis

Add   **D71.1   Leukocyte adhesion deficiency**

Add   LAD-I

Add   LAD-II

Add   LAD-III

Add   Leukocyte adhesion deficiency type I

Add   Leukocyte adhesion deficiency type II

Add   Leukocyte adhesion deficiency type III

Add   **D71.8   Other functional disorders of polymorphonuclear neutrophils**

Add   Cell membrane receptor complex [CR3] defect

Add   Chronic (childhood) granulomatous disease

Add   Congenital dysphagocytosis

Add   Progressive septic granulomatosis

Add   **D71.9   Functional disorders of polymorphonuclear neutrophils, unspecified**

No Change

CERTAIN DISORDERS INVOLVING THE IMMUNE MECHANISM (D80-D89)

No Change   **Excludes1**

Revise from   functional disorders of polymorphonuclear neutrophils (D71)

Revise to   functional disorders of polymorphonuclear neutrophils (D71-)

No Change   **CHAPTER 4**

No Change   **ENDOCRINE, NUTRITIONAL AND METABOLIC DISEASES (E00-E89)**

No Change   **DIABETES MELLITUS (E08-E13)**

No Change E11   **Type 2 diabetes mellitus**
No Change   **E11.9   Type 2 diabetes mellitus without complications**
Add   **Excludes1**   type 2 diabetes mellitus, without complications in remission (E11.A)

Add   **E11.A   Type 2 diabetes mellitus without complications in remission**
Add   **Excludes1**   type 2 diabetes mellitus, with complications (E11.0-E11.8)
Add   type 2 diabetes mellitus, without complications not in remission (E11.9)

No Change   **DISORDERS OF OTHER ENDOCRINE GLANDS (E20-E35)**

No Change E27   **Other disorders of adrenal gland**
No Change   **E27.5   Adrenomedullary hyperfunction**
Add   **Code also,** if applicable:
Add   malignant pheochromocytoma (C74.1-)
Add   pheochromocytoma (benign) (D35.0-)
Add   secondary hypertension (I15.2)

No Change   **METABOLIC DISORDERS (E70-E88)**

No Change E71   **Disorders of branched-chain amino-acid metabolism and fatty-acid metabolism**
No Change   **E71.5   Peroxisomal disorders**
No Change   **E71.54   Other peroxisomal disorders**
No Change   **E71.540   Rhizomelic chondrodysplasia punctata**
Delete   **Excludes1**   chondrodysplasia punctata NOS (Q77.3)

No Change E72   **Other disorders of amino-acid metabolism**
No Change   **E72.5   Disorders of glycine metabolism**
No Change   **E72.53   Primary hyperoxaluria**
Add   **Excludes1**   secondary hyperoxaluria (E72.54-)
Add   **E72.530   Primary hyperoxaluria, type 1**
Add   **E72.538   Other specified primary hyperoxaluria**
Add   Primary hyperoxaluria, type 2
Add   Primary hyperoxaluria, type 3
Add   **E72.539   Primary hyperoxaluria, unspecified**
Add   **E72.54   Secondary hyperoxaluria**
Add   **Excludes1**   primary hyperoxaluria (E72.53-)
Add   **E72.540   Dietary hyperoxaluria**
Add   **E72.541   Enteric hyperoxaluria**
Add   **E72.548   Other secondary hyperoxaluria**
Add   **E72.549   Secondary hyperoxaluria, unspecified**

No Change E78   **Disorders of lipoprotein metabolism and other lipidemias**
No Change   **E78.0   Pure hypercholesterolemia**
No Change   **E78.01   Familial hypercholesterolemia**
Add   **E78.010   Homozygous familial hypercholesterolemia [HoFH]**

Add   **E78.011   Heterozygous familial hypercholesterolemia [HeFH]**
Add   **E78.019   Familial hypercholesterolemia, unspecified**
Add   Familial hypercholesterolemia NOS

No Change E83   **Disorders of mineral metabolism**
No Change   **E83.3   Disorders of phosphorus metabolism and phosphatases**
Add   **Excludes2**   disorders of pyrophosphate metabolism (E83.82-)
No Change   **E83.8   Other disorders of mineral metabolism**
Add   **E83.82   Disorders of pyrophosphate metabolism**
Add   **E83.820   Generalized arterial calcification of infancy with unspecified genetic causality**
Add   **Code also,** if applicable, associated conditions such as:
Add   heart failure (I50.-)
Add   other secondary hypertension (I15.8)
Add   **E83.821   ENPP1 deficiency causing generalized arterial calcification of infancy**
Add   **Code also,** if applicable, associated conditions such as:
Add   heart failure (I50.-)
Add   other secondary hypertension (I15.8)
Add   **E83.822   ENPP1 deficiency causing autosomal recessive hypophosphatemic rickets type 2**
Add   **E83.823   ABCC6 deficiency causing generalized arterial calcification of infancy**
Add   **Code also,** if applicable, associated conditions such as:
Add   heart failure (I50.-)
Add   other secondary hypertension (I15.8)
Add   **E83.824   ABCC6 deficiency causing pseudoxanthoma elasticum**
Add   **E83.825   CD73 deficiency causing arterial calcification**

No Change E88   **Other and unspecified metabolic disorders**
No Change   **E88.0   Disorders of plasma-protein metabolism, not elsewhere classified**
No Change   **E88.02   Plasminogen deficiency**
No Change   **Code also,**
Revise from   , if applicable, ligneous conjunctivitis (H10.51)
Revise to   , if applicable, ligneous conjunctivitis (H10.51-)
No Change   **E88.1   Lipodystrophy, not elsewhere classified**
Lipodystrophy NOS
Add   **E88.10   Lipodystrophy, unspecified**
Add   Lipodystrophy NOS
Add   **E88.11   Partial lipodystrophy**
Add   Acquired partial lipodystrophy (APL)
Add   Barraquer-Simons lipodystrophy
Add   Familial partial lipodystrophy (FPLD)
Add   **E88.12   Generalized lipodystrophy**
Add   Acquired generalized lipodystrophy (AGL)
Add   Berardinelli-Siep syndrome
Add   Congenital generalized lipodystrophy (CGL)
Add   Lawrence syndrome

Add		E88.13	**Localized lipodystrophy**
Add			Injection lipodystrophy
Add			Insulin lipodystrophy
Add		E88.14	**HIV-associated lipodystrophy**
Add			*Code first* any human immunodeficiency virus [HIV] disease (B20)
Add			Use Additional code for adverse effect, if applicable, to identify drug (T37.5X5-)
Add		E88.19	**Other lipodystrophy, not elsewhere classified**

No Change E88.4 **Mitochondrial metabolism disorders**

No Change		E88.43	**Disorders of mitochondrial tRNA synthetases**
Add			ARS2-related mitochondrial disorders
Add			LBSL
Add			Leukoencephalopathy with brainstem - spinal cord involvement - lactate elevation
Add			Leukoencephalopathy with thalamus - brainstem involvement - high lactate
Add			LTBL
Add			Mitochondrial aminoacyl-tRNA synthetase disorders
Add			*Code also*, if applicable, associated condition such as:
Add			leukoencephalopathy (G93.49)

No Change # CHAPTER 5

No Change # MENTAL, BEHAVIORAL AND NEURODEVELOPMENTAL DISORDERS (F01-F99)

No Change **MENTAL DISORDERS DUE TO KNOWN PHYSIOLOGICAL CONDITIONS (F01-F09)**

No Change	F02	**Dementia in other diseases classified elsewhere**
No Change		*Code first*
Revise from		multiple sclerosis (G35)
Revise to		multiple sclerosis (G35.-)

No Change **ANXIETY, DISSOCIATIVE, STRESS-RELATED, SOMATOFORM AND OTHER NONPSYCHOTIC MENTAL DISORDERS (F40-F48)**

No Change	F42	**Obsessive-compulsive disorder**
No Change		**Excludes2**
Revise from		obsessive-compulsive symptoms occurring in depression (F32-F33)
Revise to		obsessive-compulsive symptoms occurring in depression (F32.-, F33.3)

No Change	F48	**Other nonpsychotic mental disorders**
No Change	F48.2	**Pseudobulbar affect**
No Change		*Code first*
Revise from		multiple sclerosis (G35)
Revise to		multiple sclerosis (G35-)

No Change **DISORDERS OF ADULT PERSONALITY AND BEHAVIOR (F60-F69)**

No Change	F63	**Impulse disorders**
No Change	F63.2	**Kleptomania**
No Change		**Excludes2**
Revise from		depressive disorder with stealing (F31-F33)
Revise to		depressive disorder with stealing (F31.-, F32.-, F33.-)

No Change # CHAPTER 6

No Change # DISEASES OF THE NERVOUS SYSTEM (G00-G99)

No Change **INFLAMMATORY DISEASES OF THE CENTRAL NERVOUS SYSTEM (G00-G09)**

No Change	G00		**Bacterial meningitis, not elsewhere classified**
No Change		G00.1	**Pneumococcal meningitis**
Revise from			Meningtitis due to Streptococcal pneumoniae
Revise to			Meningitis due to Streptococcal pneumoniae

No Change	G04		**Encephalitis, myelitis and encephalomyelitis**
No Change			**Excludes2**
Revise from			multiple sclerosis (G35)
Revise to			multiple sclerosis (G35-)

No Change **EXTRAPYRAMIDAL AND MOVEMENT DISORDERS (G20-G26)**

No Change	G23		**Other degenerative diseases of basal ganglia**
No Change		G23.3	**Hypomyelination with atrophy of the basal ganglia and cerebellum**
Add			TUBB4A-related neurologic disorders

No Change **OTHER DEGENERATIVE DISEASES OF THE NERVOUS SYSTEM (G30-G32)**

No Change	G31		**Other degenerative diseases of nervous system, not elsewhere classified**
No Change		G31.8	**Other specified degenerative diseases of nervous system**
Add		G31.87	**Primary progressive apraxia of speech**

No Change **DEMYELINATING DISEASES OF THE CENTRAL NERVOUS SYSTEM (G35-G37)**

No Change	G35		**Multiple sclerosis**
Delete			Disseminated multiple sclerosis
Delete			Generalized multiple sclerosis
Delete			Multiple sclerosis NOS
Delete			Multiple sclerosis of brain stem
Delete			Multiple sclerosis of cord
Add		G35.A	**Relapsing-remitting multiple sclerosis**
Add			**Excludes1** demyelinating disease of central nervous system, unspecified (G37.9)
Add		G35.B	**Primary progressive multiple sclerosis**
Add		G35.B0	**Primary progressive multiple sclerosis, unspecified**
Add		G35.B1	**Active primary progressive multiple sclerosis**
Add			Primary progressive multiple sclerosis with evidence of inflammatory disease activity
Add		G35.B2	**Non-active primary progressive multiple sclerosis**
Add			Primary progressive multiple sclerosis without evidence of inflammatory disease activity
Add		G35.C	**Secondary progressive multiple sclerosis**
Add		G35.C0	**Secondary progressive multiple sclerosis, unspecified**
Add		G35.C1	**Active secondary progressive multiple sclerosis**
Add			Secondary progressive multiple sclerosis with evidence of inflammatory disease activity
Add		G35.C2	**Non-active secondary progressive multiple sclerosis**
Add			Secondary progressive multiple sclerosis without evidence of inflammatory disease activity
Add		G35.D	**Multiple sclerosis, unspecified**
Add			Disseminated multiple sclerosis
Add			Generalized multiple sclerosis
Add			Multiple sclerosis NOS
Add			Multiple sclerosis of brain stem
Add			Multiple sclerosis of cord

No Change	G37	Other demyelinating diseases of central nervous system
No Change		G37.3	Acute transverse myelitis in demyelinating disease of central nervous system
No Change		**Excludes1**
Revise from			multiple sclerosis (G35)
Revise to			multiple sclerosis (G35-)
No Change		G37.9	Demyelinating disease of central nervous system, unspecified
Add			Clinically isolated syndromes

DISEASES OF MYONEURAL JUNCTION AND MUSCLE (G70-G73)

No Change	G71	**Primary disorders of muscles**
No Change		G71.0	**Muscular dystrophy**
No Change			G71.03	**Limb girdle muscular dystrophies**
Add				G71.036	Limb girdle muscular dystrophy due to fukutin related protein dysfunction
Add					LGMD R9 FKRP-related
Add					Limb girdle muscular dystrophy due to FKRP deficiency
Add					Limb girdle muscular dystrophy type 2I
No Change				G71.038	Other limb girdle muscular dystrophy
Add					LGMD R9 FKRP-related
Add					Limb girdle muscular dystrophy due to fukutin related protein dysfunction
Add					Limb girdle muscular dystrophy type 2I

OTHER DISORDERS OF THE NERVOUS SYSTEM (G89-G99)

No Change	G89	**Pain, not elsewhere classified**
No Change		**Excludes2**
Revise from		pelvic and perineal pain (R10.2)
Revise to		pelvic and perineal pain (R10.2-)

No Change
CHAPTER 7

No Change
DISEASES OF THE EYE AND ADNEXA (H00-H59)

No Change
DISORDERS OF EYELID, LACRIMAL SYSTEM AND ORBIT (H00-H05)

No Change	H01	**Other inflammation of eyelid**
No Change		H01.8	**Other specified inflammations of eyelid**
Add			Code also, if applicable, infestation by Demodex mites (B88.01)
Add		H01.81	Other specified inflammation of right upper eyelid
Add		H01.82	Other specified inflammation of right lower eyelid
Add		H01.83	Other specified inflammation of right eye, unspecified eyelid
Add		H01.84	Other specified inflammation of left upper eyelid
Add		H01.85	Other specified inflammation of left lower eyelid
Add		H01.86	Other specified inflammation of left eye, unspecified eyelid
Add		H01.89	Other specified inflammation of unspecified eye, unspecified eyelid
Add		H01.8A	Other specified inflammation of right eye, upper and lower eyelids
Add		H01.8B	Other specified inflammation of left eye, upper and lower eyelids

No Change	H05	**Disorders of orbit**
No Change		H05.8	**Other disorders of orbit**
Add			H05.83	Thyroid orbitopathy
Add				Graves' ophthalmopathy
Add				Graves' orbitopathy
Add				Thyroid eye disease
Add				Code also, if applicable, any associated conditions such as:
Add				autoimmune thyroiditis (E06.3)
Add				thyrotoxicosis with diffuse goiter (E05.0-)
Add			H05.831	Thyroid orbitopathy, right orbit
Add			H05.832	Thyroid orbitopathy, left orbit
Add			H05.833	Thyroid orbitopathy, bilateral
Add			H05.839	Thyroid orbitopathy, unspecified orbit

DISORDERS OF CHOROID AND RETINA (H30-H36)

No Change	H33	**Retinal detachments and breaks**
No Change		H33.3	**Retinal breaks without detachment**
Delete			**Excludes1**	peripheral retinal degeneration without break (H35.4-)
Add			**Excludes2**	peripheral retinal degeneration without break (H35.4-)
No Change	H35	**Other retinal disorders**
No Change		H35.4	**Peripheral retinal degeneration**
Delete			**Excludes1**	peripheral retinal degeneration with retinal break (H33.3-)
Add			**Excludes2**	peripheral retinal degeneration with retinal break (H33.3-)

GLAUCOMA (H40-H42)

No Change	H40	**Glaucoma**
No Change		H40.8	**Other glaucoma**
Add			H40.84	Neovascular secondary angle closure glaucoma
Add				Code first the underlying condition such as:
Add				central retinal vein occlusion (H34.81)
Add				diabetes mellitus (E08.39, E09.39, E10.39, E11.39, E13.39)
Add				retinal ischemia (H35.82)
Add			H40.841	Neovascular secondary angle closure glaucoma, right eye
Add			H40.842	Neovascular secondary angle closure glaucoma, left eye
Add			H40.843	Neovascular secondary angle closure glaucoma, bilateral
Add			H40.849	Neovascular secondary angle closure glaucoma, unspecified eye
No Change	H42	**Glaucoma in diseases classified elsewhere**
		Excludes1	neovascular secondary angle closure glaucoma (H40.84-)
Add			

VISUAL DISTURBANCES AND BLINDNESS (H53-H54)

No Change	H53	**Visual disturbances**
No Change		H53.0	**Amblyopia ex anopsia**
No Change			H53.03	**Strabismic amblyopia**
Delete			**Excludes1**	amblyopia due to vitamin A deficiency (E50.5)
Add			**Excludes2**	strabismus (H50-)

No Change   **CHAPTER 9**

No Change   **DISEASES OF THE CIRCULATORY SYSTEM (I00-I99)**

No Change   **PULMONARY HEART DISEASE AND DISEASES OF PULMONARY CIRCULATION (I26-I28)**

No Change I27   Other pulmonary heart diseases
No Change   I27.8   Other specified pulmonary heart diseases
Add   I27.84   Fontan related circulation
Add   I27.840   Fontan-associated liver disease [FALD]
Add   I27.841   Fontan-associated lymphatic dysfunction
Add   Code also associated conditions such as:
Add   chylothorax (J94.0)
Add   Fontan associated protein-losing enteropathy (K90.89)
Add   plastic (obstructive) bronchitis (J44.89)
Add   I27.848   Other Fontan-associated condition
Add   Use Additional code to specify the Fontan associated condition
Add   I27.849   Fontan related circulation, unspecified

No Change   **OTHER FORMS OF HEART DISEASE (I30-I5A)**

No Change I51   Complications and ill-defined descriptions of heart disease
Delete   Excludes1   any condition in I51.4-I51.9 due to hypertension (I11.-)
Delete   any condition in I51.4-I51.9 due to hypertension and chronic kidney disease (I13.-)
Delete   heart disease specified as rheumatic (I00-I09)
Add   Excludes2   heart disease specified as rheumatic (I00-I09)
No Change   I51.5   Myocardial degeneration
Add   Excludes1   myocardial degeneration due to hypertension (I11.-)
Add   myocardial degeneration due to hypertension and chronic kidney disease (I13.-)
No Change   I51.7   Cardiomegaly
Add   Excludes1   cardiomegaly due to hypertension (I11.-)
Add   cardiomegaly due to hypertension and chronic kidney disease (I13.-)

No Change   **DISEASES OF ARTERIES, ARTERIOLES AND CAPILLARIES (I70-I79)**

No Change I70   Atherosclerosis
No Change   I70.9   Other and unspecified atherosclerosis
Add   Excludes2   disorders of pyrophosphate metabolism (E83.82-)

No Change   **DISEASES OF VEINS, LYMPHATIC VESSELS AND LYMPH NODES, NOT ELSEWHERE CLASSIFIED (I80-I89)**

No Change I80   Phlebitis and thrombophlebitis
No Change   Code first
Revise from   phlebitis and thrombophlebitis complicating abortion, ectopic or molar pregnancy (O00-O07, O08.7)
Revise to   , if applicable: phlebitis and thrombophlebitis complicating abortion, ectopic or molar pregnancy (O00-O07, O08.7)

No Change   **CHAPTER 10**

No Change   **DISEASES OF THE RESPIRATORY SYSTEM (J00-J99)**

No Change   **OTHER ACUTE LOWER RESPIRATORY INFECTIONS (J20-J22)**

No Change J20   Acute bronchitis
No Change   Excludes2
Revise from   allergic bronchitis NOS (J45.909-)
Revise to   allergic bronchitis NOS (J45.909)

No Change   **CHRONIC LOWER RESPIRATORY DISEASES (J40-J4A)**

No Change J40   Bronchitis, not specified as acute or chronic
No Change   Excludes1
Revise from   allergic bronchitis NOS (J45.909-)
Revise to   allergic bronchitis NOS (J45.909)

No Change J43   Emphysema
Revise from   Excludes1   emphysema due to inhalation of chemicals, gases, fumes or vapors (J68.4)
Revise to   Excludes2   emphysema due to inhalation of chemicals, gases, fumes or vapors (J68.4)

No Change J44   Other chronic obstructive pulmonary disease
Delete   Excludes1   chronic bronchitis NOS (J42)
Delete   chronic simple and mucopurulent bronchitis (J41.-)
Delete   chronic tracheitis (J42)
Delete   chronic tracheobronchitis (J42)
Add   Excludes2   chronic bronchitis NOS (J42)
Add   chronic simple and mucopurulent bronchitis (J41.-)
Add   chronic tracheitis (J42)
Add   chronic tracheobronchitis (J42)

No Change   **OTHER RESPIRATORY DISEASES PRINCIPALLY AFFECTING THE INTERSTITIUM (J80-J84)**

No Change J84   Other interstitial pulmonary diseases
No Change   J84.1   Other interstitial pulmonary diseases with fibrosis
Add   Code also, if applicable, pulmonary fibrosis (chronic) due to inhalation of chemicals, gases, fumes or vapors (J68.4)
Delete   Excludes1   pulmonary fibrosis (chronic) due to inhalation of chemicals, gases, fumes or vapors (J68.4)

No Change   **CHAPTER 11**

No Change   **DISEASES OF THE DIGESTIVE SYSTEM (K00-K95)**

No Change   **DISEASES OF LIVER (K70-K77)**

No Change K75   Other inflammatory liver diseases
No Change   K75.8   Other specified inflammatory liver diseases
No Change   K75.81   Nonalcoholic steatohepatitis (NASH)
Add   Metabolic dysfunction-associated steatohepatitis (MASH)

No Change K76   Other diseases of liver
No Change   K76.0   Fatty (change of) liver, not elsewhere classified
Add   Metabolic dysfunction-associated steatotic liver disease (MASLD)

No Change	**CHAPTER 12**		
No Change	**DISEASES OF THE SKIN AND SUBCUTANEOUS TISSUE (L00–L99)**		
No Change	**INFECTIONS OF THE SKIN AND SUBCUTANEOUS TISSUE (L00–L08)**		
No Change	**L02**	Cutaneous abscess, furuncle and carbuncle	
No Change		**L02.2** Cutaneous abscess, furuncle and carbuncle of trunk	
No Change			**L02.21** Cutaneous abscess of trunk
Revise from			**L02.212** Cutaneous abscess of back [any part, except buttock]
Revise from			**L02.212** Cutaneous abscess of back [any part, except buttock and flank]
No Change			**L02.217** Cutaneous abscess of flank
No Change		**L02.22** Furuncle of trunk	
Revise from			**L02.222** Furuncle of back [any part, except buttock]
Revise to			**L02.222** Furuncle of back [any part, except buttock and flank]
No Change			**L02.227** Furuncle of flank
No Change	**L03**	Cellulitis and acute lymphangitis	
No Change		**L03.3** Cellulitis and acute lymphangitis of trunk	
No Change		**L03.31** Cellulitis of trunk	
Add			**L03.31A** Cellulitis of flank
No Change		**L03.32** Acute lymphangitis of trunk	
Add			**L03.32A** Acute lymphangitis of flank

DERMATITIS AND ECZEMA (L20–L30)

No Change		
No Change	**Excludes2**	
Revise from		chronic (childhood) granulomatous disease (D71)
Revise to		chronic (childhood) granulomatous disease (D71-)

URTICARIA AND ERYTHEMA (L49–L54)

No Change	**L51**	Erythema multiforme
No Change	**Use additional**	
Revise from		inflammation of eyelid (H01.8)
Revise to		inflammation of eyelid (H01.8-)

OTHER DISORDERS OF THE SKIN AND SUBCUTANEOUS TISSUE (L80–L99)

No Change	**L97**	Non-pressure chronic ulcer of lower limb, not elsewhere classified	
No Change		**L97.2** Non-pressure chronic ulcer of calf	
Add		Non-pressure chronic ulcer of shin	
No Change	**L98**	Other disorders of skin and subcutaneous tissue, not elsewhere classified	
No Change		**L98.4** Non-pressure chronic ulcer of skin, not elsewhere classified	
Add		**L98.43** Non-pressure chronic ulcer of abdomen	
Add			**L98.431** Non-pressure chronic ulcer of abdomen limited to breakdown of skin
Add			**L98.432** Non-pressure chronic ulcer of abdomen with fat layer exposed
Add			**L98.433** Non-pressure chronic ulcer of abdomen with necrosis of muscle
Add			**L98.434** Non-pressure chronic ulcer of abdomen with necrosis of bone
Add			**L98.435** Non-pressure chronic ulcer of abdomen with muscle involvement without evidence of necrosis
Add			**L98.436** Non-pressure chronic ulcer of abdomen with bone involvement without evidence of necrosis
Add			**L98.438** Non-pressure chronic ulcer of abdomen with other specified severity
Add			**L98.439** Non-pressure chronic ulcer of abdomen with unspecified severity
Add		**L98.44** Non-pressure chronic ulcer of chest	
Add			**L98.441** Non-pressure chronic ulcer of chest limited to breakdown of skin
Add			**L98.442** Non-pressure chronic ulcer of chest with fat layer exposed
Add			**L98.443** Non-pressure chronic ulcer of chest with necrosis of muscle
Add			**L98.444** Non-pressure chronic ulcer of chest with necrosis of bone
Add			**L98.445** Non-pressure chronic ulcer of chest with muscle involvement without evidence of necrosis
Add			**L98.446** Non-pressure chronic ulcer of chest with bone involvement without evidence of necrosis
Add			**L98.448** Non-pressure chronic ulcer of chest with other specified severity
Add			**L98.449** Non-pressure chronic ulcer of chest with unspecified severity
Add		**L98.45** Non-pressure chronic ulcer of neck	
Add			**L98.451** Non-pressure chronic ulcer of neck limited to breakdown of skin
Add			**L98.452** Non-pressure chronic ulcer of neck with fat layer exposed
Add			**L98.453** Non-pressure chronic ulcer of neck with necrosis of muscle
Add			**L98.454** Non-pressure chronic ulcer of neck with necrosis of bone
Add			**L98.455** Non-pressure chronic ulcer of neck with muscle involvement without evidence of necrosis
Add			**L98.456** Non-pressure chronic ulcer of neck with bone involvement without evidence of necrosis
Add			**L98.458** Non-pressure chronic ulcer of neck with other specified severity
Add			**L98.459** Non-pressure chronic ulcer of neck with unspecified severity
Add		**L98.46** Non-pressure chronic ulcer of face	
Add			**L98.461** Non-pressure chronic ulcer of face limited to breakdown of skin
Add			**L98.462** Non-pressure chronic ulcer of face with fat layer exposed
Add			**L98.463** Non-pressure chronic ulcer of face with necrosis of muscle
Add			**L98.464** Non-pressure chronic ulcer of face with necrosis of bone
Add			**L98.465** Non-pressure chronic ulcer of face with muscle involvement without evidence of necrosis
Add			**L98.466** Non-pressure chronic ulcer of face with bone involvement without evidence of necrosis
Add			**L98.468** Non-pressure chronic ulcer of face with other specified severity
Add			**L98.469** Non-pressure chronic ulcer of face with unspecified severity

Add	L98.47	Non-pressure chronic ulcer of groin
Add	L98.471	Non-pressure chronic ulcer of groin limited to breakdown of skin
Add	L98.472	Non-pressure chronic ulcer of groin with fat layer exposed
Add	L98.473	Non-pressure chronic ulcer of groin with necrosis of muscle
Add	L98.474	Non-pressure chronic ulcer of groin with necrosis of bone
Add	L98.475	Non-pressure chronic ulcer of groin with muscle involvement without evidence of necrosis
Add	L98.476	Non-pressure chronic ulcer of groin with bone involvement without evidence of necrosis
Add	L98.478	Non-pressure chronic ulcer of groin with other specified severity
Add	L98.479	Non-pressure chronic ulcer of groin with unspecified severity
Add	L98.A	Non-pressure chronic ulcer of upper limb, not elsewhere classified
Add		Chronic ulcer of upper limb NOS
Add		Non-healing ulcer of upper limb
Add		Ulcer of upper limb NEC
Add	**Excludes2**	gangrene (I96)
Add		pressure ulcer (pressure area) (L89.-)
Add		skin infections (L00-L08)
Add		specific infections classified to A00-B99
Add		ulcer of lower limb NEC (L97.-)
Add		varicose ulcer (I83.0-I83.93)
Add	L98.A1	Non-pressure chronic ulcer of upper arm
Add		Non-pressure chronic ulcer of axilla
Add	L98.A11	Non-pressure chronic ulcer of right upper arm
Add	L98.A111	Non-pressure chronic ulcer of right upper arm limited to breakdown of skin
Add	L98.A112	Non-pressure chronic ulcer of right upper arm with fat layer exposed
Add	L98.A113	Non-pressure chronic ulcer of right upper arm with necrosis of muscle
Add	L98.A114	Non-pressure chronic ulcer of right upper arm with necrosis of bone
Add	L98.A115	Non-pressure chronic ulcer of right upper arm with muscle involvement without evidence of necrosis
Add	L98.A116	Non-pressure chronic ulcer of right upper arm with bone involvement without evidence of necrosis
Add	L98.A118	Non-pressure chronic ulcer of right upper arm with other specified severity
Add	L98.A119	Non-pressure chronic ulcer of right upper arm with unspecified severity
Add	L98.A12	Non-pressure chronic ulcer of left upper arm
Add	L98.A121	Non-pressure chronic ulcer of left upper arm limited to breakdown of skin
Add	L98.A122	Non-pressure chronic ulcer of left upper arm with fat layer exposed
Add	L98.A123	Non-pressure chronic ulcer of left upper arm with necrosis of muscle
Add	L98.A124	Non-pressure chronic ulcer of left upper arm with necrosis of bone
Add	L98.A125	Non-pressure chronic ulcer of left upper arm with muscle involvement without evidence of necrosis
Add	L98.A126	Non-pressure chronic ulcer of left upper arm with bone involvement without evidence of necrosis
Add	L98.A128	Non-pressure chronic ulcer of left upper arm with other specified severity
Add	L98.A129	Non-pressure chronic ulcer of left upper arm with unspecified severity
Add	L98.A19	Non-pressure chronic ulcer of unspecified upper arm
Add	L98.A191	Non-pressure chronic ulcer of unspecified upper arm limited to breakdown of skin
Add	L98.A192	Non-pressure chronic ulcer of unspecified upper arm with fat layer exposed
Add	L98.A193	Non-pressure chronic ulcer of unspecified upper arm with necrosis of muscle
Add	L98.A194	Non-pressure chronic ulcer of unspecified upper arm with necrosis of bone

Add   L98.A195 Non-pressure chronic ulcer of unspecified upper arm with muscle involvement without evidence of necrosis

Add   L98.A196 Non-pressure chronic ulcer of unspecified upper arm with bone involvement without evidence of necrosis

Add   L98.A198 Non-pressure chronic ulcer of unspecified upper arm with other specified severity

Add   L98.A199 Non-pressure chronic ulcer of unspecified upper arm with unspecified severity

Add   L98.A2 Non-pressure chronic ulcer of forearm

Add   L98.A21 Non-pressure chronic ulcer of right forearm

Add   L98.A211 Non-pressure chronic ulcer of right forearm limited to breakdown of skin

Add   L98.A212 Non-pressure chronic ulcer of right forearm with fat layer exposed

Add   L98.A213 Non-pressure chronic ulcer of right forearm with necrosis of muscle

Add   L98.A214 Non-pressure chronic ulcer of right forearm with necrosis of bone

Add   L98.A215 Non-pressure chronic ulcer of right forearm with muscle involvement without evidence of necrosis

Add   L98.A216 Non-pressure chronic ulcer of right forearm with bone involvement without evidence of necrosis

Add   L98.A218 Non-pressure chronic ulcer of right forearm with other specified severity

Add   L98.A219 Non-pressure chronic ulcer of right forearm with unspecified severity

Add   L98.A22 Non-pressure chronic ulcer of left forearm

Add   L98.A221 Non-pressure chronic ulcer of left forearm limited to breakdown of skin

Add   L98.A222 Non-pressure chronic ulcer of left forearm with fat layer exposed

Add   L98.A223 Non-pressure chronic ulcer of left forearm with necrosis of muscle

Add   L98.A224 Non-pressure chronic ulcer of left forearm with necrosis of bone

Add   L98.A225 Non-pressure chronic ulcer of left forearm with muscle involvement without evidence of necrosis

Add   L98.A226 Non-pressure chronic ulcer of left forearm with bone involvement without evidence of necrosis

Add   L98.A228 Non-pressure chronic ulcer of left forearm with other specified severity

Add   L98.A229 Non-pressure chronic ulcer of left forearm with unspecified severity

Add   L98.A29 Non-pressure chronic ulcer of unspecified forearm

Add   L98.A291 Non-pressure chronic ulcer of unspecified forearm limited to breakdown of skin

Add   L98.A292 Non-pressure chronic ulcer of unspecified forearm with fat layer exposed

Add   L98.A293 Non-pressure chronic ulcer of unspecified forearm with necrosis of muscle

Add   L98.A294 Non-pressure chronic ulcer of unspecified forearm with Necrosis of bone

Add   L98.A295 Non-pressure chronic ulcer of unspecified forearm with Muscle involvement without evidence of necrosis

Add   L98.A296 Non-pressure chronic ulcer of unspecified forearm with bone involvement without evidence of necrosis

Add   L98.A298 Non-pressure chronic ulcer of unspecified forearm with other specified severity

Add   L98.A299 Non-pressure chronic ulcer of unspecified forearm with unspecified severity

Add	L98.A3	Non-pressure chronic ulcer of hand
Add	L98.A31	Non-pressure chronic ulcer of right hand
Add	L98.A311	Non-pressure chronic ulcer of right hand limited to breakdown of skin
Add	L98.A312	Non-pressure chronic ulcer of right hand with fat layer exposed
Add	L98.A313	Non-pressure chronic ulcer of right hand with necrosis of muscle
Add	L98.A314	Non-pressure chronic ulcer of right hand with necrosis of bone
Add	L98.A315	Non-pressure chronic ulcer of right hand with muscle involvement without evidence of necrosis
Add	L98.A316	Non-pressure chronic ulcer of right hand with bone involvement without evidence of necrosis
Add	L98.A318	Non-pressure chronic ulcer of right hand with other specified severity
Add	L98.A319	Non-pressure chronic ulcer of right hand with unspecified severity
Add	L98.A32	Non-pressure chronic ulcer of left hand
Add	L98.A321	Non-pressure chronic ulcer of left hand limited to breakdown of skin
Add	L98.A322	Non-pressure chronic ulcer of left hand with fat layer exposed
Add	L98.A323	Non-pressure chronic ulcer of left hand with necrosis of muscle
Add	L98.A324	Non-pressure chronic ulcer of left hand with necrosis of bone
Add	L98.A325	Non-pressure chronic ulcer of left hand with muscle involvement without evidence of necrosis
Add	L98.A326	Non-pressure chronic ulcer of left hand with bone involvement without evidence of necrosis
Add	L98.A328	Non-pressure chronic ulcer of left hand with other specified severity
Add	L98.A329	Non-pressure chronic ulcer of left hand with unspecified severity
Add	L98.A39	Non-pressure chronic ulcer of unspecified hand
Add	L98.A391	Non-pressure chronic ulcer of unspecified hand limited to breakdown of skin
Add	L98.A392	Non-pressure chronic ulcer of unspecified hand with fat layer exposed
Add	L98.A393	Non-pressure chronic ulcer of unspecified hand with necrosis of muscle
Add	L98.A394	Non-pressure chronic ulcer of unspecified hand with necrosis of bone
Add	L98.A395	Non-pressure chronic ulcer of unspecified hand with muscle involvement without evidence of necrosis
Add	L98.A396	Non-pressure chronic ulcer of unspecified hand with bone involvement without evidence of necrosis
Add	L98.A398	Non-pressure chronic ulcer of unspecified hand with other specified severity
Add	L98.A399	Non-pressure chronic ulcer of unspecified hand with Unspecified severity

No Change

CHAPTER 13

No Change

DISEASES OF THE MUSCULOSKELETAL SYSTEM AND CONNECTIVE TISSUE (M00-M99)

No Change

INFLAMMATORY POLYARTHROPATHIES (M05-M14)

No Change	M05	Rheumatoid arthritis with rheumatoid factor
Add	M05.A	Abnormal rheumatoid factor and anti-citrullinated protein antibody with rheumatoid arthritis
Add		*Code first rheumatoid arthritis with rheumatoid factor by site, if known (M05.00 to M05.8A)*

OTHER JOINT DISORDERS (M20-M25)

No Change **M21** Other acquired deformities of limbs

No Change **M21.1** Varus deformity, not elsewhere classified

No Change **M21.15** Varus deformity, not elsewhere classified, hip

Revise from M21.159 Varus deformity, not elsewhere classified, unspecified

Revise to **M21.159** Varus deformity, not elsewhere classified, unspecified hip

No Change **M24** Other specific joint derangements

No Change **M24.0** Loose body in joint

No Change **M24.07** Loose body in ankle and toe joints

Revise from M24.076 Loose body in unspecified toe joints

Revise to **M24.076** Loose body in unspecified toe joint(s)

SYSTEMIC CONNECTIVE TISSUE DISORDERS (M30-M36)

No Change **M36** Systemic disorders of connective tissue in diseases classified elsewhere

No Change **M36.3** Arthropathy in other blood disorders

Add *Code first* underlying disease, such as:

Add disease of blood and blood-forming organs, unspecified (D75.9)

Add other hemoglobinopathies (D58.2)

Add thalassemia (D56.-)

DISORDERS OF MUSCLES (M60-M63)

No Change **M61** Calcification and ossification of muscle

No Change **M61.1** Myositis ossificans progressiva

No Change **M61.12** Myositis ossificans progressiva, upper arm

Revise from M61.129 Myositis ossificans progressiva, unspecified arm

Revise to **M61.129** Myositis ossificans progressiva, unspecified upper arm

No Change

CHAPTER 14

No Change

DISEASES OF THE GENITOURINARY SYSTEM (N00-N99)

GLOMERULAR DISEASES (N00-N08)

No Change **N00** Acute nephritic syndrome

No Change **N00.5** Acute nephritic syndrome with diffuse mesangiocapillary glomerulonephritis

Delete Acute nephritic syndrome with membranoproliferative glomerulonephritis, types 1 and 3, or NOS

Add **N00.B** Acute nephritic syndrome with immune complex membranoproliferative glomerulonephritis

Add **N00.B1** Acute nephritic syndrome with idiopathic immune complex membranoproliferative glomerulonephritis (IC-MPGN)

Add **N00.B2** Acute nephritic syndrome with secondary immune complex membranoproliferative glomerulonephritis (IC-MPGN)

No Change **N04** Nephrotic syndrome

No Change **N04.5** Nephrotic syndrome with diffuse mesangiocapillary glomerulonephritis

Delete Nephrotic syndrome with membranoproliferative glomerulonephritis, types 1 and 3, or NOS

Add **N04.B** Nephrotic syndrome with immune complex membranoproliferative glomerulonephritis (IC-MPGN)

Add **N04.B1** Nephrotic syndrome with idiopathic immune complex membranoproliferative glomerulonephritis (IC-MPGN)

Add **N04.B2** Nephrotic syndrome with secondary immune complex membranoproliferative glomerulonephritis (IC-MPGN)

No Change **N07** Hereditary nephropathy, not elsewhere classified

Add **N07.B** Hereditary nephropathy, not elsewhere classified with APOL1-mediated kidney disease [AMKD]

Add AMKD (with glomerulonephritis)

Add AMKD (with glomerulosclerosis)

DISORDERS OF BREAST (N60-N65)

No Change **N61** Inflammatory disorders of breast

No Change **Excludes1**

Revise from inflammatory carcinoma of breast (C50.9)

Revise from inflammatory carcinoma of breast (C50.A-)

NONINFLAMMATORY DISORDERS OF FEMALE GENITAL TRACT (N80-N98)

Add

Add **N85** Other noninflammatory disorders of uterus, except cervix

Add **N85.A** Isthmocele

No Change Code also

Revise from pelvic and perineal pain (R10.2)

Revise from pelvic and perineal pain (R10.2-)

No Change

CHAPTER 15

No Change

PREGNANCY, CHILDBIRTH AND THE PUERPERIUM (O00-O9A)

COMPLICATIONS OF LABOR AND DELIVERY (O60-O77)

No Change **O70** Perineal laceration during delivery

No Change **O70.1** Second degree perineal laceration during delivery

No Change **Excludes1**

Revise from perineal laceration involving anal sphincter (O70.2)

Revise to perineal laceration involving anal sphincter (O70.2-)

No Change **O70.4** Anal sphincter tear complicating delivery, not associated with third degree laceration

No Change **Excludes1**

Revise from anal sphincter tear with third degree perineal laceration (O70.2)

Revise to anal sphincter tear with third degree perineal laceration (O70.2-)

COMPLICATIONS PREDOMINANTLY RELATED TO THE PUERPERIUM (O85-O92)

No Change **O90** Complications of the puerperium, not elsewhere classified

No Change **O90.4** Postpartum acute kidney failure

No Change **Excludes1**

Revise from non-anuria and oliguria (R34)

Revise to anuria and oliguria (R34)

No Change **CHAPTER 16**

No Change **CERTAIN CONDITIONS ORIGINATING IN THE PERINATAL PERIOD (P00-P96)**

No Change **ABNORMAL FINDINGS ON NEONATAL SCREENING (P09)**

No Change **P09** Abnormal findings on neonatal screening

Revise from P09.6 Abnormal findings on neonatal screening for neonatal hearing loss

Revise to P09.6 Abnormal findings on neonatal hearing screening

No Change **CHAPTER 17**

Revise from **CONGENITAL MALFORMATIONS, DEFORMATIONS AND CHROMOSOMAL ABNORMALITIES (Q00-Q99)**

Revise to **CONGENITAL MALFORMATIONS, DEFORMATIONS, CHROMOSOMAL ABNORMALITIES, AND GENETIC DISORDERS (Q00- QA0)**

No Change This chapter contains the following blocks:

Add QA0   Genetic disorders, not elsewhere classified

No Change **CONGENITAL MALFORMATIONS OF THE CIRCULATORY SYSTEM (Q20-Q28)**

No Change **Q28** Other congenital malformations of circulatory system

No Change Q28.8 Other specified congenital malformations of circulatory system

Add **Excludes2** disorders of pyrophosphate metabolism (E83.82-)

No Change **CONGENITAL MALFORMATIONS AND DEFORMATIONS OF THE MUSCULOSKELETAL SYSTEM (Q65-Q79)**

No Change **Q75** Other congenital malformations of skull and face bones

No Change Q75.0 Craniosynostosis

Revise from Q75.00 Craniosynostosis unspecified

Revise to Q75.00 Craniosynostosis, unspecified

Revise from Q75.001 Craniosynostosis unspecified, unilateral

Revise to Q75.001 Craniosynostosis, unspecified type, unilateral

Revise from Q75.002 Craniosynostosis unspecified, bilateral

Revise to Q75.002 Craniosynostosis, unspecified type, bilateral

Revise from Q75.009 Craniosynostosis unspecified

Revise to Q75.009 Craniosynostosis, unspecified

Q75.02 Coronal craniosynostosis
Non-deformational anterior plagiocephaly

Revise from Q75.021 Coronal craniosynostosis unilateral

Revise to Q75.021 Coronal craniosynostosis, unilateral

Revise from Q75.022 Coronal craniosynostosis bilateral

Revise to Q75.022 Coronal craniosynostosis, bilateral

Revise from Q75.029 Coronal craniosynostosis unspecified

Revise to Q75.029 Coronal craniosynostosis, unspecified

No Change **Q77** Osteochondrodysplasia with defects of growth of tubular bones and spine

No Change Q77.3 Chondrodysplasia punctata

No Change **Excludes1**

Revise from Rhizomelic chondrodysplasia punctata (E71.43)

Revise to Rhizomelic chondrodysplasia punctata (E71.540)

No Change **OTHER CONGENITAL MALFORMATIONS (Q80-Q89)**

No Change **Q82** Other congenital malformations of skin

No Change Q82.8 Other specified congenital malformations of skin

Add **Excludes2** disorders of pyrophosphate metabolism (E83.82-)

No Change **Q87** Other specified congenital malformation syndromes affecting multiple systems

No Change Q87.8 Other specified congenital malformation syndromes, not elsewhere classified

Add Q87.87 Hao-Fountain Syndrome
Add HAFOUS
Add Use Additional code, if applicable, for associated conditions such as:
Add autism spectrum disorder (F84.0)
Add developmental speech disorder (F80.-)
Add epilepsy, by specific type (G40.-)
Add intellectual disabilities (F70-F79)
Add pervasive developmental disorders (F84.-)

Add Q87.88 CTNNB1 syndrome
Add Use Additional code, if applicable, for associated conditions such as:
Add cerebral palsy (G80.-)
Add congenital heart malformations (Q20.0-Q24.9)
Add developmental disorder of speech and language (F80.-)
Add exudative retinopathy (H35.02-)
Add intellectual disability (F70-F79)
Add microcephaly (Q02)

No Change **Q89** Other congenital malformations, not elsewhere classified

No Change Q89.8 Other specified congenital malformations

Add Q89.81 Kabuki syndrome
Add Kabuki syndrome, type 1, due to KMT2D mutation
Add Kabuki syndrome, type 2, due to KDM6A mutation
Add Niikawa-Kuroki syndrome

Add Q89.89 Other specified congenital malformations

No Change **CHROMOSOMAL ABNORMALITIES, NOT ELSEWHERE CLASSIFIED (Q90-Q99)**

No Change **Q99** Other chromosome abnormalities, not elsewhere classified

No Change Q99.8 Other specified chromosome abnormalities

Add Q99.81 Usher syndrome
Add Use Additional code to identify any auditory and visual manifestations
Add Q99.811 Usher syndrome, type 1
Add Q99.812 Usher syndrome, type 2
Add Q99.813 Usher syndrome, type 3
Add Q99.818 Other Usher syndrome
Add Usher syndrome, type 4
Add Q99.819 Usher syndrome, unspecified
Add Q99.89 Other specified chromosome abnormalities

Add **GENETIC DISORDERS, NOT ELSEWHERE CLASSIFIED (QA0)**

Add **QA0 Neurodevelopmental disorders related to specific genetic pathogenic variants**

Add Code also, if applicable, any associated conditions, such as:

Add attention-deficit hyperactivity disorders (F90.-)
Add autism spectrum disorder (F84.0)
Add developmental and epileptic encephalopathy (G93.45)
Add epilepsy, by specific type (G40.-)
Add intellectual disabilities (F70-F79)
Add pervasive developmental disorders (F84.-)

Add **QA0.0 Neurodevelopmental disorders related to pathogenic variants in specific genes**

Add **QA0.01 Neurodevelopmental disorders related to pathogenic variants in certain specific genes**

Add **QA0.010 Neurodevelopmental disorders, related to pathogenic variants in ion channel genes**

Add **QA0.0101 SCN2A-related neurodevelopmental disorder**

Add **QA0.0102 CACNA1A-related neurodevelopmental disorder**

Add **QA0.0109 Neurodevelopmental disorder related to pathogenic variant in other ion channel gene**
SCN8A-related neurodevelopmental disorder

Add **QA0.011 Neurodevelopmental disorders, related to pathogenic variants in glutamate receptor genes**

Add **QA0.012 Neurodevelopmental disorders, related to pathogenic variants in other receptor genes**

Add **QA0.013 Neurodevelopmental disorders, related to pathogenic variants in other transporter and solute carrier genes**

Add **QA0.0131 SLC6A1-related disorder**
GABA transporter 1 deficiency

Add **QA0.0139 Neurodevelopmental disorder, related to pathogenic variant in other transporter or solute carrier gene**

Add **QA0.014 Neurodevelopmental disorders, related to pathogenic variants in synapserelated genes**

Add **QA0.0141 Syntaxin-binding protein 1-related disorder**
STXBP1-related disorders

Add **QA0.0142 DLG4-related synaptopathy**

Add **QA0.0149 Neurodevelopmental disorder, related to pathogenic variant in other synapse related gene**
Other genetic synaptopathy

Add **QA0.015 Neurodevelopmental disorders, related to genes associated with transcription and gene expression**

Add **QA0.0151 FOXG1 syndrome**
FOXG1-related disorder
FOXG1-related encephalopathy
FOXG1-related neurodevelopmental disorder

Add **QA0.0159 Neurodevelopmental disorder, related to other genes associated with transcription and gene expression**

Add **QA0.8 Other neurodevelopmental disorders related to pathogenic variants in other specific genes**

No Change **CHAPTER 18**

No Change **SYMPTOMS, SIGNS AND ABNORMAL CLINICAL AND LABORATORY FINDINGS, NOT ELSEWHERE CLASSIFIED (R00-R99)**

No Change **SYMPTOMS AND SIGNS INVOLVING THE DIGESTIVE SYSTEM AND ABDOMEN (R10-R19)**

No Change **R10 Abdominal and pelvic pain**
Add **Excludes2** costovertebral (angle) tenderness (R39.85)
No Change **R10.1 Pain localized to upper abdomen**
Add **Excludes2** pain localized to flank (R10.A-)
Add pelvic and perineal pain (R10.2-)
No Change **R10.2 Pelvic and perineal pain**
Add **Excludes2** pain localized to other parts of lower abdomen (R10.3-)
Add pain localized to upper abdomen (R10.1-)
Add **R10.20 Pelvic and perineal pain unspecified side**
Add **R10.21 Pelvic and perineal pain right side**
Add **R10.22 Pelvic and perineal pain left side**
Add **R10.23 Pelvic and perineal pain bilateral**
Add **R10.24 Suprapubic pain**
No Change **R10.3 Pain localized to other parts of lower abdomen**
Add **Excludes2** pain localized to flank (R10.A-)
pelvic and perineal pain (R10.2-)
No Change **R10.8 Other abdominal pain**
No Change **R10.81 Abdominal tenderness**
Add **Excludes2** pain localized to other parts of lower abdomen (R10.3-)
Add pain localized to upper abdomen (R10.1-)
No Change **R10.82 Rebound abdominal tenderness**
Add **Excludes2** pain localized to other parts of lower abdomen (R10.3-)
Add pain localized to upper abdomen (R10.1-)

Add		R10.85	Abdominal pain of multiple sites
Add		**Excludes1**	abdominal rigidity NOS (R19.3)
Add			generalized abdominal pain associated with acute abdomen (R10.0)
Add			generalized abdominal pain NOS (R10.84)
Add			localized abdominal pain (R10.1-R10.4-)
Add		R10.8A	Flank tenderness
Add		R10.8A1	Right flank tenderness
Add		R10.8A2	Left flank tenderness
Add		R10.8A3	Suprapubic tenderness
Add		R10.8A9	Flank tenderness, unspecified
			Flank tenderness NOS
Add	R10.A		Pain localized to flank
Add			Lateral abdomen pain
Add			Lateral flank pain
			Latus region pain
Add		**Excludes2**	pain localized to other parts of lower abdomen (R10.3-)
Add			pain localized to upper abdomen (R10.1-)
Add		R10.A0	Flank pain, unspecified side
Add		R10.A1	Flank pain, right side
Add		R10.A2	Flank pain, left side
Add		R10.A3	Flank pain, bilateral
No Change R11			Nausea and vomiting
No Change	R11.1		Vomiting
Add		R11.16	Cannabis hyperemesis syndrome
Add			Cannabinoid hyperemesis syndrome
Add			Code also
Add			cannabis abuse (F12.1-)
Add			cannabis dependence (F12.2-)
Add			cannabis use, unspecified (F12.92-, F12.93, F12.95-, F12.98-, F12.99)
Add			manifestations, such as:
Add			dehydration (E86.0)
Add			electrolyte imbalance (E87.8)
No Change R15			Fecal incontinence
No Change	R15.0		Incomplete defecation
Delete		**Excludes1**	constipation (K59.0-)
Delete			fecal impaction (K56.41)
Add		**Excludes2**	constipation (K59.0-)
Add			fecal impaction (K56.41)

No Change

SYMPTOMS AND SIGNS INVOLVING THE GENITOURINARY SYSTEM (R30-R39)

No Change R39			Other and unspecified symptoms and signs involving the genitourinary system
No Change	R39.1		Other difficulties with micturition
No Change		R39.12	Poor urinary stream
Revise from			Weak urinary steam
Revise to			Weak urinary stream
No Change	R39.8		Other symptoms and signs involving the genitourinary system
Add		R39.85	Costovertebral (angle) tenderness
Add		**Excludes2**	abdominal and pelvic pain (R10.-)
Add		R39.851	Costovertebral (angle) tenderness, right side
Add		R39.852	Costovertebral (angle) tenderness, left side
Add		R39.853	Costovertebral (angle) tenderness, bilateral
Add		R39.859	Costovertebral (angle) tenderness, unspecified side

No Change			**SYMPTOMS AND SIGNS INVOLVING COGNITION, PERCEPTION, EMOTIONAL STATE AND BEHAVIOR (R40-R46)**
No Change R40			Somnolence, stupor and coma
No Change	R40.1		Stupor
No Change		**Excludes1**	
Revise from			depressive stupor (F31-F33)
Revise to			depressive stupor (F31.-, F32.-, F33.-)
No Change	R40.2		Coma
No Change		R40.2A	Nontraumatic coma due to underlying condition
Add		**Excludes1**	coma scale, best motor response (R40.24.-)
Add			coma scale, best verbal response (R40.22.-)
Add			coma scale, eyes open (R40.21.-)
Add			Glasgow coma scale, total score (R40.23.-)

No Change

GENERAL SYMPTOMS AND SIGNS (R50-R69)

No Change R52			Pain, unspecified
No Change		**Excludes1**	
Revise from			pelvic and perineal pain (R10.2)
Revise to			pelvic and perineal pain (R10.2-)
No Change R53			Malaise and fatigue
No Change	R53.8		Other malaise and fatigue
No Change		**Excludes1**	
Revise from			exhaustion and fatigue due to recurrent depressive episode (F33)
Revise to			exhaustion and fatigue due to recurrent depressive episode (F33-)
No Change R62			Lack of expected normal physiological development in childhood and adults
No Change	R62.5		Other and unspecified lack of expected normal physiological development in childhood
No Change		R62.51	Failure to thrive (child)
Add			Faltering growth
No Change R65			Symptoms and signs specifically associated with systemic inflammation and infection
No Change	R65.2		Severe sepsis
No Change		R65.21	Severe sepsis with septic shock
Add		**Excludes1**	postprocedural septic shock (T81.12-)
No Change R69			Illness, unspecified
Add			Unknown and unspecified cases of morbidity
Add			Unknown and unspecified causes of morbidity

No Change

ABNORMAL FINDINGS ON EXAMINATION OF BLOOD, WITHOUT DIAGNOSIS (R70-R79)

No Change R76			Other abnormal immunological findings in serum
No Change	R76.8		Other specified abnormal immunological findings in serum
Delete			Raised level of immunoglobulins NOS
Add		R76.81	Abnormal rheumatoid factor and anti-citrullinated protein antibody without rheumatoid arthritis
Add			Abnormal anti-CCP
Add			Abnormal anti-cyclic citrullinated protein antibody and rheumatoid factor
Add		**Excludes1**	rheumatoid arthritis with rheumatoid factor (M05.-)
Add		R76.89	Other specified abnormal immunological findings in serum
Add			Raised level of immunoglobulins NOS

No Change | **ABNORMAL FINDINGS ON EXAMINATION OF URINE, WITHOUT DIAGNOSIS (R80-R82)**

No Change R82 Other and unspecified abnormal findings in urine

No Change   R82.9 Other and unspecified abnormal findings in urine

No Change   R82.99 Other abnormal findings in urine

No Change   R82.992 Hyperoxaluria

No Change   **Excludes1**

Delete   Primary hyperoxaluria (E72.53)

Add   primary hyperoxaluria (E72.53-)

Add   secondary hyperoxaluria (E72.54-)

No Change | **ABNORMAL FINDINGS ON EXAMINATION OF OTHER BODY FLUIDS, SUBSTANCES AND TISSUES, WITHOUT DIAGNOSIS (R83-R89)**

No Change R87 Abnormal findings in specimens from female genital organs

No Change   R87.6 Abnormal cytological findings in specimens from female genital organs

No Change   R87.61 Abnormal cytological findings in specimens from cervix uteri

No Change   R87.619 Unspecified abnormal cytological findings in specimens from cervix uteri

Revise from   Atypical endocervial cells of cervix NOS

Revise to   Atypical endocervical cells of cervix NOS

No Change

CHAPTER 19

No Change

INJURY, POISONING AND CERTAIN OTHER CONSEQUENCES OF EXTERNAL CAUSES (S00-T88)

No Change | **INJURIES TO THE NECK (S10-S19)**

No Change S12 Fracture of cervical vertebra and other parts of neck

No Change   S12.8 Fracture of other parts of neck

Revise from   Hyoid bone

Revise to   Fracture of hyoid bone

Revise from   Larynx

Revise to   Fracture of larynx

Revise from   Thyroid cartilage

Revise to   Fracture of thyroid cartilage

Revise from   Trachea

Revise to   Fracture of trachea

No Change | **INJURIES TO THE ABDOMEN, LOWER BACK, LUMBAR SPINE PELVIS AND EXTERNAL GENITALS (S30-S39)**

No Change S30 Superficial injury of abdomen, lower back, pelvis and external genitals

No Change   S30.1 Contusion of abdominal wall

Delete   Contusion of flank

Delete   Contusion of groin

Add   S30.11 Contusion of abdominal wall

Add   S30.12 Contusion of groin

Add   S30.13 Contusion of flank (latus) region

No Change   S30.8 Other superficial injuries of abdomen, lower back, pelvis and external genitals

No Change   S30.81 Abrasion of abdomen, lower back, pelvis and external genitals

Add   S30.81A Abrasion of flank

No Change   S30.82 Blister (nonthermal) of abdomen, lower back, pelvis and external genitals

Add   S30.82A Blister (nonthermal) of flank

No Change   S30.84 External constriction of abdomen, lower back, pelvis and external genitals

Add   S30.84A External constriction of flank

No Change   S30.85 Superficial foreign body of abdomen, lower back, pelvis and external genitals

Add   S30.85A Superficial foreign body of flank

No Change   S30.86 Insect bite (nonvenomous) of abdomen, lower back, pelvis and external genitals

Add   S30.86A Insect bite (nonvenomous) of flank

No Change   S30.87 Other superficial bite of abdomen, lower back, pelvis and external genitals

Add   S30.87A Other superficial bite of flank

No Change   S30.9 Unspecified superficial injury of abdomen, lower back, pelvis and external genitals

Add   S30.9A Unspecified superficial injury of flank

No Change S31 Open wound of abdomen, lower back, pelvis and external genitals

No Change   S31.1 Open wound of abdominal wall without penetration into peritoneal cavity

No Change   S31.10 Unspecified open wound of abdominal wall without penetration into peritoneal cavity

Add   S31.106 Unspecified open wound of abdominal wall, right flank without penetration into peritoneal cavity

Add   S31.107 Unspecified open wound of abdominal wall, left flank without penetration into peritoneal cavity

Add   S31.10A Unspecified open wound of abdominal wall, unspecified flank without penetration into peritoneal cavity

Add   Open wound of abdominal wall of flank NOS without penetration into peritoneal cavity

No Change   S31.11 Laceration without foreign body of abdominal wall without penetration into peritoneal cavity

Add   S31.116 Laceration without foreign body of abdominal wall, right flank without penetration into peritoneal cavity

Add   S31.117 Laceration without foreign body of abdominal wall, left flank without penetration into peritoneal cavity

Add   S31.11A Laceration without foreign body of abdominal wall, unspecified flank without penetration into peritoneal cavity

Add   Laceration without foreign body of flank NOS without penetration into peritoneal cavity

No Change   S31.12 Laceration with foreign body of abdominal wall without penetration into peritoneal cavity

Add   S31.126 Laceration with foreign body of abdominal wall, right flank without penetration into peritoneal cavity

Add   S31.127 Laceration with foreign body of abdominal wall, left flank without penetration into peritoneal cavity

Add	S31.12A	Laceration with foreign body of abdominal wall unspecified flank without penetration into peritoneal cavity
Add		Laceration with foreign body of abdominal wall of flank NOS without penetration into peritoneal cavity
No Change	S31.13	Puncture wound of abdominal wall without foreign body without penetration into peritoneal cavity
Add	S31.136	Puncture wound of abdominal wall without foreign body, right flank without penetration into peritoneal cavity
Add	S31.137	Puncture wound of abdominal wall without foreign body, left flank without penetration into peritoneal cavity
Add	S31.13A	Puncture wound of abdominal wall without foreign body, unspecified flank without penetration into peritoneal cavity
Add		Puncture wound of abdominal wall of flank NOS without foreign body
No Change	S31.14	Puncture wound of abdominal wall with foreign body without penetration into peritoneal cavity
Add	S31.146	Puncture wound of abdominal wall with foreign body, right flank without penetration into peritoneal cavity
Add	S31.147	Puncture wound of abdominal wall with foreign body, left flank without penetration into peritoneal cavity
Add	S31.14A	Puncture wound of abdominal wall with foreign body, unspecified flank without penetration into peritoneal cavity
Add		Puncture wound of abdominal wall with foreign body of flank NOS without penetration into peritoneal cavity
No Change	S31.15	Open bite of abdominal wall without penetration into peritoneal cavity
Add	S31.156	Open bite of abdominal wall, right flank without penetration into peritoneal cavity
Add	S31.157	Open bite of abdominal wall, left flank without penetration into peritoneal cavity
Add	S31.15A	Open bite of abdominal wall, unspecified flank without penetration into peritoneal cavity
Add		Open bite of abdominal wall of flank NOS without penetration into peritoneal cavity
No Change	S31.6	Open wound of abdominal wall with penetration into peritoneal cavity
No Change	S31.60	Unspecified open wound of abdominal wall with penetration into peritoneal cavity
Add	S31.606	Unspecified open wound of abdominal wall, right flank with penetration into peritoneal cavity
Add	S31.607	Unspecified open wound of abdominal wall, left flank with penetration into peritoneal cavity
Add	S31.60A	Unspecified open wound of abdominal wall, unspecified flank with penetration into peritoneal cavity
Add		Unspecified open wound of abdominal wall of flank NOS, with penetration into peritoneal cavity
No Change	S31.61	Laceration without foreign body of abdominal wall with penetration into peritoneal cavity
Add	S31.616	Laceration without foreign body of abdominal wall, right flank with penetration into peritoneal cavity
Add	S31.617	Laceration without foreign body of abdominal wall, left flank with penetration into peritoneal cavity
Add	S31.61A	Laceration without foreign body of abdominal wall, unspecified flank with penetration into peritoneal cavity
Add		Laceration without foreign body of abdominal wall of flank NOS, with penetration into peritoneal cavity
No Change	S31.62	Laceration with foreign body of abdominal wall with penetration into peritoneal cavity
Add	S31.626	Laceration with foreign body of abdominal wall, right flank with penetration into peritoneal cavity
Add	S31.627	Laceration with foreign body of abdominal wall, left flank with penetration into peritoneal cavity
Add	S31.62A	Laceration with foreign body of abdominal wall, unspecified flank with penetration into peritoneal cavity
Add		Laceration with foreign body of abdominal wall, flank NOS, with penetration into peritoneal cavity
No Change	S31.63	Puncture wound without foreign body of abdominal wall with penetration into peritoneal cavity
Add	S31.636	Puncture wound of abdominal wall without foreign body, right flank with penetration into peritoneal cavity

Add		S31.637	Puncture wound of abdominal wall without foreign body, left flank with penetration into peritoneal cavity
Add		S31.63A	Puncture wound of abdominal wall without foreign body, unspecified flank with penetration into peritoneal cavity
Add			Puncture wound of abdominal wall without foreign body, flank NOS, with penetration into peritoneal cavity
No Change		S31.64	Puncture wound with foreign body of abdominal wall with penetration into peritoneal cavity
Add		S31.646	Puncture wound of abdominal wall with foreign body, right flank with penetration into peritoneal cavity
Add		S31.647	Puncture wound of abdominal wall with foreign body, left flank with penetration into peritoneal cavity
Add		S31.64A	Puncture wound of abdominal wall with foreign body, unspecified flank with penetration into peritoneal cavity
Add			Puncture wound of abdominal wall with foreign body, flank NOS, with penetration into peritoneal cavity
No Change		S31.65	Open bite of abdominal wall with penetration into peritoneal cavity
Add		S31.656	Open bite of abdominal wall, right flank with penetration into peritoneal cavity
Add		S31.657	Open bite of abdominal wall, left flank with penetration into peritoneal cavity
Add		S31.65A	Open bite of abdominal wall, unspecified flank with penetration into peritoneal cavity
Add			Open bite of abdominal wall, flank NOS, with penetration into peritoneal cavity
No Change	S37	Injury of urinary and pelvic organs	
No Change	S37.6	Injury of uterus	
Delete		**Excludes1**	injury to gravid uterus (O9A.2-)

No Change	S62	Fracture at wrist and hand level	
Revise from	S62.9	Unspecified fracture of wrist and hand	
Revise to	S62.9	Unspecified fracture of hand	
Revise from		S62.90	Unspecified fracture of unspecified wrist and hand
Revise to		S62.90	Unspecified fracture of unspecified hand
Revise from		S62.91	Unspecified fracture of right wrist and hand
Revise to		S62.91	Unspecified fracture of right hand
Revise from		S62.92	Unspecified fracture of left wrist and hand
Revise to		S62.92	Unspecified fracture of left hand

No Change	S74	Injury of nerves at hip and thigh level	
No Change		S74.2	Injury of cutaneous sensory nerve at hip and thigh level
Revise from		S74.21	Injury of cutaneous sensory nerve at hip and high level, right leg
Revise to		S74.21	Injury of cutaneous sensory nerve at hip and thigh level, right leg

No Change	T36	Poisoning by, adverse effect of and underdosing of systemic antibiotics	
Add		T36.A	Poisoning by, adverse effect of and underdosing of fluoroquinolone antibiotics
Add		T36.AX	Poisoning by, adverse effect of and underdosing of fluoroquinolone antibiotics
Add		T36.AX1	Poisoning by fluoroquinolone antibiotics, accidental (unintentional)
Add			Poisoning by fluoroquinolone antibiotics NOS
Add		T36.AX2	Poisoning by fluoroquinolone antibiotics, intentional self-harm
Add		T36.AX3	Poisoning by fluoroquinolone antibiotics, assault
Add		T36.AX4	Poisoning by fluoroquinolone antibiotics, undetermined
Add		T36.AX5	Adverse effect of fluoroquinolone antibiotics
Add		T36.AX6	Underdosing of fluoroquinolone antibiotics

No Change	T65	Toxic effect of other and unspecified substances	
No Change		T65.8	Toxic effect of other specified substances
Add		T65.84	Toxic effect of xylazine
Add			Use Additional code(s) for all associated manifestations, such as:
Add			cellulitis and acute lymphangitis (L03.-)
Add			cutaneous abscess, furuncle and carbuncle (L02.-)
Add			non-pressure chronic ulcer of lower limb, not elsewhere classified (L97.-)
Add			non-pressure chronic ulcer of skin, not elsewhere classified (L98.4-)
Add		T65.841	Toxic effect of xylazine, accidental (unintentional)
			Toxic effect of xylazine NOS
Add		T65.842	Toxic effect of xylazine, intentional self-harm
Add		T65.843	Toxic effect of xylazine, assault
Add		T65.844	Toxic effect of xylazine, undetermined

No Change	T75	Other and unspecified effects of other external causes	
No Change		T75.8	Other specified effects of external causes
Add		T75.83	Effects of war theater
Add			Use Additional code to identify associated manifestations
Add		T75.830	Gulf war illness
Add			Gulf war syndrome
Add		T75.838	Effects of other war theater

No Change	**T78**		**Adverse effects, not elsewhere classified**
No Change		**T78.0**	**Anaphylactic reaction due to food**
No Change			**T78.07** **Anaphylactic reaction due to milk and dairy products**
Add			**T78.070** **Anaphylactic reaction due to milk and dairy products with tolerance to baked milk**
Add			**Excludes1** Anaphylactic reaction due to milk and dairy products with reactivity to baked milk (T78.071)
Add			**T78.071** **Anaphylactic reaction due to milk and dairy products with reactivity to baked milk**
Add			**Excludes1** Anaphylactic reaction due to milk and dairy products with tolerance to baked milk (T78.070)
Add			**T78.079** **Anaphylactic reaction due to milk and dairy products, unspecified**
No Change			**T78.08** **Anaphylactic reaction due to eggs**
Add			**T78.080** **Anaphylactic reaction due to egg with tolerance to baked egg**
Add			**Excludes1** Anaphylactic reaction due to egg with reactivity to baked egg (T78.081)
Add			**T78.081** **Anaphylactic reaction due to egg with reactivity to baked egg**
Add			**Excludes1** Anaphylactic reaction due to egg with tolerance to baked egg (T78.080)
Add			**T78.089** **Anaphylactic reaction due to eggs, unspecified**
No Change		**T78.1**	**Other adverse food reactions, not elsewhere classified**
Add			**T78.11** **Other adverse food reactions due to milk and dairy products**
Add			**T78.110** **Other adverse food reactions due to milk and dairy products with tolerance to baked milk**
Add			**Excludes1** Other adverse food reaction due to milk and dairy products with reactivity to baked milk (T78.111)
Add			**T78.111** **Other adverse food reaction due to milk and dairy products with reactivity to baked milk**
Add			**Excludes1** Other adverse food reaction due to milk and dairy products with tolerance to baked milk (T78.110)
Add			**T78.119** **Other adverse food reaction due to milk and dairy products with baked milk tolerance/reactivity, unspecified**
Add			**T78.12** **Other adverse food reaction due to eggs**
Add			**T78.120** **Other adverse food reaction due to egg with tolerance to baked egg**
Add			**Excludes1** Other adverse food reaction due to egg with reactivity to baked egg (T78.121)
Add			**T78.121** **Other adverse food reaction due to egg with reactivity to baked egg**
Add			**Excludes1** Other adverse food reaction due to egg with tolerance to baked egg (T78.120)
Add			**T78.129** **Other adverse food reaction due to egg with baked egg tolerance/reactivity, unspecified**
Add			**T78.19** **Other adverse food reactions, not elsewhere classified**

No Change

CHAPTER 20

No Change

EXTERNAL CAUSES OF MORBIDITY (V00-Y99)

No Change

PEDESTRIAN INJURED IN TRANSPORT ACCIDENT (V00-V09)

No Change	**V06**		**Pedestrian injured in collision with other nonmotor vehicle**
No Change		**V06.9**	**Pedestrian injured in collision with other nonmotor vehicle, unspecified whether traffic or nontraffic accident**
No Change		**V06.93**	**Pedestrian on standing micro-mobility pedestrian conveyance injured in collision with other nonmotor vehicle, unspecified whether traffic or nontraffic accident**
No Change		**V06.938**	**Pedestrian on other standing micro-mobility pedestrian conveyance injured in collision with other nonmotor vehicle, unspecified whether traffic or nontraffic accident**
Revise from			Pedestrian on hoverboard injured in collision with other nonmotor, unspecified whether traffic or nontraffic accident
Revise to			Pedestrian on hoverboard injured in collision with other nonmotor vehicle, unspecified whether traffic or nontraffic accident

No Change		**EXPOSURE TO INANIMATE MECHANICAL FORCES (W20-W49)**
No Change	W44	Foreign body entering into or through a natural orifice
No Change	W44.A	Battery entering into or through a natural orifice
No Change		W44.A9 Other batteries entering into or through a natural orifice
Revise from		Cylindrical battery
Revise to		Cylindrical battery entering into or through a natural orifice
No Change		W44.H Other sharp object entering into or through a natural orifice
Add		W44.H9 Other sharp object entering into or through a natural orifice
Add		Shard pottery entering into or through a natural orifice
No Change	W45	Foreign body or object entering through skin
Add		W45.3 Fishing hook entering through skin

No Change		**ASSAULT (X92-Y09)**
No Change	Y07	Perpetrator of assault, maltreatment and neglect
No Change	Y07.4	Other family member, perpetrator of maltreatment and neglect
No Change		Y07.43 Stepparent or stepsibling, perpetrator of maltreatment and neglect
Revise from		Y07.435 Stepbrother, perpetrator or maltreatment and neglect
Revise to		Y07.435 Stepbrother, perpetrator of maltreatment and neglect

No Change		**LEGAL INTERVENTION, OPERATIONS OF WAR, MILITARY OPERATIONS, AND TERRORISM (Y35-Y38)**
No Change	Y36	Operations of war
Add		Y36.A Blast overpressure in war operations
Add		Code also type of explosive, if known
Add		accidental detonation of on board munitions (Y36.140)
Add		explosion of grenade (Y36.290)
Add		explosion of torpedo (Y36.040)
Add		improvised explosive device (Y36.230)
Add		Y36.A1 Low level blast overpressure in war operations
Add		LLB overpressure in war operations
Add		Low level blast overpressure due to explosion in war operations
Add		Y36.A2 High level blast overpressure in war operations
Add		High level blast overpressure due to explosion in war operations
Add		HLB overpressure in war operations
No Change	Y37	Military operations
Add		Y37.A Blast overpressure in military operations
Add		Code also type of explosive, if known
Add		accidental detonation of on board munitions (Y37.140)
Add		explosion of grenade (Y37.290)
Add		explosion of torpedo (Y37.040)
Add		improvised explosive device (Y37.230)
Add		Y37.A1 Low level blast overpressure in military operations
Add		LLB overpressure in military operations
Add		Low level blast overpressure due to explosion in military operations
Add		Y37.A2 High level blast overpressure in military operations
Add		High level blast overpressure due to explosion in military operations
Add		HLB overpressure in military operations

No Change		**SUPPLEMENTARY FACTORS RELATED TO CAUSES OF MORBIDITY CLASSIFIED ELSEWHERE (Y90-Y99)**
No Change	Y93	Activity codes
Add		Note: Y93.L Other outdoor activity
Add		Y93.L Other outdoor activity
Add		Y93.L1 Activity, splitting wood
Add		Y93.L9 Activity, other outdoor activity

No Change   **CHAPTER 21**

No Change   **FACTORS INFLUENCING HEALTH STATUS AND CONTACT WITH HEALTH SERVICES (Z00-Z99)**

No Change		**PERSONS ENCOUNTERING HEALTH SERVICES FOR EXAMINATIONS (Z00-Z13)**
Delete		**Excludes1** examinations related to pregnancy and reproduction (Z30-Z36, Z39.-)
Add		**Excludes2** examinations related to pregnancy and reproduction (Z30-Z36, Z39.-)
No Change	Z01	Encounter for other special examination without complaint, suspected or reported diagnosis
Delete		**Excludes1** encounter for laboratory and radiologic examinations as a component of general medical examinations (Z00.0-)
Add		**Excludes2** encounter for laboratory and radiologic examinations as a component of general medical examinations (Z00.0-)

No Change		**GENETIC CARRIER AND GENETIC SUSCEPTIBILITY TO DISEASE (Z14-Z15)**
No Change	Z15	Genetic susceptibility to disease
No Change		Z15.0 Genetic susceptibility to malignant neoplasm
Add		Z15.05 Genetic susceptibility to malignant neoplasm of fallopian tube(s)
Add		Z15.06 Genetic susceptibility to malignant neoplasm of digestive system
Add		Z15.060 Genetic susceptibility to colorectal cancer
Add		Z15.068 Genetic susceptibility to other malignant neoplasm of digestive system
Add		Genetic susceptibility to biliary tract cancer
Add		Genetic susceptibility to gastric cancer
Add		Genetic susceptibility to pancreatic cancer
Add		Genetic susceptibility to small bowel cancer
Add		Z15.07 Genetic susceptibility to malignant neoplasm of urinary tract
Add		Z15.3 Genetic susceptibility to kidney disease
Add		Code also, if applicable, hypertension (I10-I1A)

No Change		**ENCOUNTERS FOR OTHER SPECIFIC HEALTH CARE (Z40-Z53)**
No Change	Z40	Encounter for prophylactic surgery
No Change		Z40.0 Encounter for prophylactic surgery for risk factors related to malignant neoplasms
No Change		Use additional
Revise from		code to identify risk factor
Revise to		code to identify risk factor, such as genetic susceptibility to malignant neoplasm Z15.-
No Change		Z40.02 Encounter for prophylactic removal of ovary(s)
Delete		Encounter for prophylactic removal of ovary(s) and fallopian tube(s)

No Change		Z40.8	Encounter for other prophylactic surgery
Add		Z40.81	Encounter for prophylactic surgery for removal of ovary(s) for persons without known genetic/familial risk factors
Add			Encounter for prophylactic oophorectomy for persons without known genetic/ familial risk factors
Add		Z40.82	Encounter for prophylactic surgery for removal of fallopian tube(s) for persons without known genetic/familial risk factors
Add			Encounter for prophylactic salpingectomy for persons without known genetic/familial risk factors
Add			Opportunistic salpingectomy
Add		Z40.89	Encounter for other prophylactic surgery

PERSONS WITH POTENTIAL HEALTH HAZARDS RELATED TO SOCIOECONOMIC AND PSYCHOSOCIAL CIRCUMSTANCES (Z55-Z65)

No Change

No Change Z56			Problems related to employment and unemployment
No Change	Z56.6		Other physical and mental strain related to work
Add			Workplace stress
No Change	Z56.8		Other problems related to employment
No Change		Z56.89	Other problems related to employment
Add			Furloughed
Add			Underemployed
No Change Z59			Problems related to housing and economic circumstances
No Change	Z59.0		Homelessness
No Change		Z59.02	Unsheltered homelessness
Add			Lives in a homeless encampment
No Change	Z59.1		Inadequate housing
No Change		Z59.12	Inadequate housing utilities
Add		**Excludes2**	financial insecurity, difficulty paying for utilities (Z59.861)
No Change		Z59.19	Other inadequate housing
Add			Poor housing weatherization
No Change	Z59.8		Other problems related to housing and economic circumstances
No Change		Z59.81	Housing instability, housed
No Change		Z59.819	Housing instability, housed unspecified
No Change		**Excludes2**	
Revise from			financial insecurity (Z59.86)
Revise to			financial insecurity (Z59.86-)
No Change		Z59.86	Financial insecurity
Delete			Bankruptcy
Add		Z59.861	Financial insecurity, difficulty paying for utilities
Add			Difficulty paying for electricity
Add			Difficulty paying for heat
Add			Difficulty paying for oil
Add			Difficulty paying water bill
Add			Utility disconnect notice due to inability to pay
Add		**Excludes2**	inadequate housing utilities (Z59.12)
Add		Z59.868	Other specified financial insecurity
Add			Bankruptcy
Add		Z59.869	Financial insecurity, unspecified

No Change		Z59.87	Material hardship due to limited financial resources, not elsewhere classified
Delete			Unable to obtain adequate utilities due to limited financial resources
No Change		**Excludes2**	
Revise from			financial insecurity, not elsewhere classified (Z59.86)
Revise to			financial insecurity, not elsewhere classified (Z59.86-)

PERSONS WITH POTENTIAL HEALTH HAZARDS RELATED TO FAMILY AND PERSONAL HISTORY AND CERTAIN CONDITIONS INFLUENCING HEALTH STATUS (Z77-Z99)

No Change

No Change Z77			Other contact with and (suspected) exposures hazardous to health
Add		Z77.3	Contact with and (suspected) exposure to war theater
Add		Z77.31	Contact with and (suspected) exposure to Gulf War theater
Add			Contact with and (suspected) exposure to Persian Gulf War theater
Add		Z77.39	Contact with and (suspected) exposure to other war theater
Add			Agent Orange exposure
No Change Z80			Family history of primary malignant neoplasm
No Change		Z80.4	Family history of malignant neoplasm of genital organs
Add		Z80.44	Family history of malignant neoplasm of fallopian tube(s)
No Change Z83			Family history of other specific disorders
No Change		Z83.7	Family history of diseases of the digestive system
No Change		Z83.71	Family history of colonic polyps
Revise from		Z83.718	Other family history of colon polyps
Revise to		Z83.718	Family history of other colon polyps
No Change Z84			Family history of other conditions
No Change		Z84.1	Family history of disorders of kidney and ureter
Add		Z84.11	Family history of APOL1-mediated kidney disease [AMKD]
Add		Z84.19	Family history of other disorders of kidney and ureter
Add		Z84.A	Family history of exposure to diethylstilbestrol
Add			DES granddaughter or grandson
Add			Family history of DES exposure
Add			Third generation DES exposure
No Change Z85			Personal history of malignant neoplasm
No Change		Z85.4	Personal history of malignant neoplasm of genital organs
Add		Z85.4A	Personal history of malignant neoplasm of fallopian tube(s)
No Change Z86			Personal history of certain other diseases
No Change		Z86.0	Personal history of in-situ and benign neoplasms and neoplasms of uncertain behavior
No Change		Z86.00	Personal history of in-situ neoplasm
Add		Z86.00A	Personal history of in-situ neoplasm of the fallopian tube(s)

No Change **Z87**		Personal history of other diseases and conditions		
No Change	**Z87.4**		Personal history of diseases of genitourinary system	
No Change		**Z87.41**	Personal history of dysplasia of the female genital tract	
No Change			**Excludes1**	
Revise from				personal history of intraepithelial neoplasia III of female genital tract (Z86.001, Z86.008)
Revise to				personal history of intraepithelial neoplasia III of female genital tract (Z86.001, Z86.008, Z86.00A)
Revise from				personal history of malignant neoplasm of female genital tract (Z85.40-Z85.44)
Revise to				personal history of malignant neoplasm of female genital tract (Z85.40-Z85.44, Z85.4A)
No Change **Z91**		Personal risk factors, not elsewhere classified		
No Change	**Z91.0**		Allergy status, other than to drugs and biological substances	
No Change		**Z91.01**	Food allergy status	
No Change			**Z91.011** Allergy to milk products	
Add				**Z91.0110** Allergy to milk products, unspecified
Add				**Z91.0111** Allergy to milk products with tolerance to baked milk
Add				**Excludes1**
				Allergy to milk products with re-activity to baked milk (Z91.0112)
Add				**Z91.0112** Allergy to milk products with reactivity to baked milk
Add				**Excludes1**
				Allergy to milk products with toler-ance to baked milk (Z91.0111)

No Change		**Z91.012** Allergy to eggs		
Add				**Z91.0120** Allergy to eggs, unspecified
Add				**Z91.0121** Allergy to eggs with tolerance to baked egg
Add				**Excludes1**
				Allergy to eggs with reactivity to baked egg (Z91.0122)
Add				**Z91.0122** Allergy to eggs with reactivity to baked egg
Add				**Excludes1**
				Allergy to egg with tolerance to baked egg (Z91.0121)
Add		**Z91.B**	Personal risk factor of exposure to diethylstilbestrol	
Add			DES daughter or son	
Add			Personal risk factor of exposure to DES	
Add			Personal risk factor of exposure to DES in utero	
Add			Second generation DES exposure	
Add			Code also, associated conditions, such as:	
Add			conditions classifiable to C50.-	
Add			osteoporosis (M80.-)	
Add			premature menopause (E28.31-)	
No Change **Z98**		Other postprocedural states		
Add		**Excludes2** Fontan related circulation (I27.84-)		
No Change **Z99**		Dependence on enabling machines and devices, not elsewhere classified		
No Change	**Z99.1**		Dependence on respirator	
No Change		**Z99.11**	Dependence on respirator [ventilator] status	
Add			Ventilator status	

PART I

Introduction

ICD-10-CM Official Guidelines for Coding and Reporting FY2026 (October 1, 2025 - September 30, 2026)

Narrative changes appear in **bold** text
Items <u>underlined</u> have been moved within the guidelines since the 2025 version
Italics are used to indicate revisions to heading changes

The Centers for Medicare and Medicaid Services (CMS) and the National Center for Health Statistics (NCHS), two departments within the U.S. Federal Government's Department of Health and Human Services (DHHS), provide the following guidelines for coding and reporting using the International Classification of Diseases, 10th Revision, Clinical Modification (ICD-10-CM). These guidelines should be used as a companion document to the official version of the ICD-10-CM as published on the NCHS website. The ICD-10-CM is a morbidity classification published by the United States for classifying diagnoses and reason for visits in all health care settings. The ICD-10-CM is based on the ICD-10, the statistical classification of disease published by the World Health Organization (WHO).

These guidelines have been approved by the four organizations that make up the Cooperating Parties for the ICD-10-CM: the American Hospital Association (AHA), the American Health Information Management Association (AHIMA), CMS, and NCHS.

These guidelines are a set of rules that have been developed to accompany and complement the official conventions and instructions provided within the ICD-10-CM itself. The instructions and conventions of the classification take precedence over guidelines. These guidelines are based on the coding and sequencing instructions in the Tabular List and Alphabetic Index of ICD-10-CM, but provide additional instruction. Adherence to these guidelines when assigning ICD-10-CM diagnosis codes is required under the Health Insurance Portability and Accountability Act (HIPAA). The diagnosis codes (Tabular List and Alphabetic Index) have been adopted under HIPAA for all health care settings. A joint effort between the health care provider and the coder is essential to achieve complete and accurate documentation, code assignment, and reporting of diagnoses and procedures. These guidelines have been developed to assist both the health care provider and the coder in identifying those diagnoses that are to be reported. The importance of consistent, complete documentation in the medical record cannot be overemphasized. Without such documentation accurate coding cannot be achieved. The entire record should be reviewed to determine the specific reason for the encounter and the conditions treated.

The term "encounter" is used for all settings, including hospital admissions. In the context of these guidelines, the term "provider" is used throughout the guidelines to mean physician or any qualified health care practitioner who is legally accountable for establishing the patient's diagnosis. Only this set of guidelines, approved by the Cooperating Parties, is official.

The guidelines are organized into sections. Section I includes the structure and conventions of the classification and general guidelines that apply to the entire classification, and chapter-specific guidelines that correspond to the chapters as they are arranged in the classification. Section II includes guidelines for selection of principal diagnosis for non-outpatient settings. Section III includes guidelines for reporting additional diagnoses in non-outpatient settings. Section IV is for outpatient coding and reporting. It is necessary to review all sections of the guidelines to fully understand all of the rules and instructions needed to code properly.

ICD-10-CM Official Guidelines for Coding and Reporting

GUIDELINES (ICD-10-CM)

21. Chapter 21: Factors Influencing Health Status and Contact with Health Services (Z00-Z99)
    a. Use of Z Codes in Any Healthcare Setting
    b. Z Codes Indicate a Reason for an Encounter or Provide Additional Information about a Patient Encounter
    c. Categories of Z Codes
22. Chapter 22: Codes for Special Purposes (U00-U85)

Section II. Selection of Principal Diagnosis

A. Codes for symptoms, signs, and ill-defined conditions
B. Two or more interrelated conditions, each potentially meeting the definition for principal diagnosis
C. Two or more diagnoses that equally meet the definition for principal diagnosis
D. Two or more comparative or contrasting conditions
E. A symptom(s) followed by contrasting/comparative diagnoses
F. Original treatment plan not carried out
G. Complications of surgery and other medical care
H. Uncertain Diagnosis
I. Admission from Observation Unit
    1. Admission Following Medical Observation
    2. Admission Following Post-Operative Observation
J. Admission from Outpatient Surgery
K. Admissions/Encounters for Rehabilitation

Section III. Reporting Additional Diagnoses

A. Previous conditions
B. Abnormal findings
C. Uncertain Diagnosis

Section IV. Diagnostic Coding and Reporting Guidelines for Outpatient Services

A. Selection of first-listed condition
    1. Outpatient Surgery
    2. Observation Stay
B. Codes from A00.0 through T88.9, Z00-Z99, U00-U85
C. Accurate reporting of ICD-10-CM diagnosis codes
D. Codes that describe symptoms and signs
E. Encounters for circumstances other than a disease or injury
F. Level of Detail in Coding
    1. ICD-10-CM codes with 3, 4, 5, 6, or 7 characters
    2. Use of full number of characters required for a code
    3. Highest level of specificity
G. ICD-10-CM code for the diagnosis, condition, problem, or other reason for encounter/visit
H. Uncertain diagnosis
I. Chronic diseases
J. Code all documented conditions that coexist
K. Patients receiving diagnostic services only
L. Patients receiving therapeutic services only
M. Patients receiving preoperative evaluations only
N. Ambulatory surgery
O. Routine outpatient prenatal visits
P. Encounters for general medical examinations with abnormal findings
Q. Encounters for routine health screenings

Appendix I: Present on Admission Reporting Guidelines

Section I. Conventions, General Coding Guidelines, and Chapter Specific Guidelines

The conventions, general guidelines, and chapter-specific guidelines are applicable to all health care settings unless otherwise indicated. The conventions and instructions of the classification take precedence over guidelines.

A. Conventions for the ICD-10-CM

The conventions for the ICD-10-CM are the general rules for use of the classification independent of the guidelines. These conventions are incorporated within the Alphabetic Index and Tabular List of the ICD-10-CM as instructional notes.

1. **The Alphabetic Index and Tabular List**

    The ICD-10-CM is divided into the Alphabetic Index, an alphabetical list of terms and their corresponding code, and the Tabular List, a structured list of codes divided into chapters based on body system or condition. The Alphabetic Index consists of the following parts: the Index of Diseases and Injury, the Index of External Causes of Injury, the Table of Neoplasms, and the Table of Drugs and Chemicals.

    See Section I.C.2. **Neoplasms**
    See Section I.C.19. Adverse effects, poisoning, underdosing and toxic effects

2. **Format and Structure:**

    The ICD-10-CM Tabular List contains categories, subcategories and codes. Characters for categories, subcategories and codes may be either a letter or a number. All categories are 3 characters. A 3-character category that has no further subdivision is equivalent to a code. Subcategories are either 4 or 5 characters. Codes may be 3, 4, 5, 6 or 7 characters. That is, each level of subdivision after a category is a subcategory. The final level of subdivision is a code. Codes that have applicable 7th characters are still referred to as codes, not subcategories. A code that has an applicable 7th character is considered invalid without the 7th character.

    The ICD-10-CM uses an indented format for ease in reference

3. **Use of codes for reporting purposes**

    For reporting purposes only codes are permissible, not categories or subcategories, and any applicable 7th character is required.

4. **Placeholder character**

    The ICD-10-CM utilizes a placeholder character "X". The "X" is used as a placeholder at certain codes to allow for future expansion. An example of this is at the poisoning, adverse effect and underdosing codes, categories T36-T50. Where a placeholder exists, the X must be used in order for the code to be considered a valid code.

5. **7th Characters**

    Certain ICD-10-CM categories have applicable 7th characters. The applicable 7th character is required for all codes within the category, or as the notes in the Tabular List instruct. The 7th character must always be the 7th character in the data field. If a code that requires a 7th character is not 6 characters, a placeholder X must be used to fill in the empty characters.

6. Abbreviations

a. Alphabetic Index abbreviations

NEC "Not elsewhere classifiable"
This abbreviation in the Alphabetic Index represents "other specified". When a specific code is not available for a condition the Alphabetic Index directs the coder to the "other specified" code in the Tabular List.

NOS "Not otherwise specified"
This abbreviation is the equivalent of unspecified.

b. Tabular List abbreviations

NEC "Not elsewhere classifiable"
This abbreviation in the Tabular List represents "other specified". When a specific code is not available for a condition, the Tabular List includes an NEC entry under a code to identify the code as the "other specified" code.

NOS "Not otherwise specified"
This abbreviation is the equivalent of unspecified.

7. Punctuation

[ ] Brackets are used in the Tabular List to enclose synonyms, alternative wording or explanatory phrases. Brackets are used in the Alphabetic Index to identify manifestation codes.

( ) Parentheses are used in both the Alphabetic Index and Tabular List to enclose supplementary words that may be present or absent in the statement of a disease or procedure without affecting the code number to which it is assigned. The terms within the parentheses are referred to as nonessential modifiers. The nonessential modifiers in the Alphabetic Index to Diseases apply to subterms following a main term except when a nonessential modifier and a subentry are mutually exclusive, the subentry takes precedence. For example, in the ICD-10-CM Alphabetic Index under the main term Enteritis, "acute" is a nonessential modifier and "chronic" is a subentry. In this case, the nonessential modifier "acute" does not apply to the subentry "chronic".

: Colons are used in the Tabular List after an incomplete term which needs one or more of the modifiers following the colon to make it assignable to a given category.

, Commas are used in the Alphabetic Index and have different meanings based on the context of the Index entry, including alternate verbiage, modifier (essential and nonessential), or alternative for "and/or."

8. Use of "and".

See Section I.A.14. Use of the term "And"

9. Other and Unspecified codes

a. "Other" codes
Codes titled "other" or "other specified" are for use when the information in the medical record provides detail for which a specific code does not exist. Alphabetic Index entries with NEC in the line designate "other" codes in the Tabular List. These Alphabetic Index entries represent specific disease entities for which no specific code exists so the term is included within an "other" code.

b. "Unspecified" codes
Codes titled "unspecified" are for use when the information in the medical record is insufficient to assign a more specific code. For those categories for which an unspecified code is not provided, the "other specified" code may represent both other and unspecified.
See Section I.B.18 Use of signs/symptoms/unspecified codes

10. Includes Notes
This note appears immediately under a 3-character code title to further define, or give examples of, the content of the category.

11. Inclusion terms
List of terms is included under some codes. These terms are the conditions for which that code is to be used. The terms may be synonyms of the code title, or, in the case of "other specified" codes, the terms are a list of the various conditions assigned to that code. The inclusion terms are not necessarily exhaustive. Additional terms found only in the Alphabetic Index may also be assigned to a code.

12. Excludes Notes
The ICD-10-CM has two types of excludes notes. Each type of note has a different definition for use, but they are all similar in that they indicate that codes excluded from each other are independent of each other.

a. Excludes1
A type 1 Excludes note is a pure excludes note. It means "NOT CODED HERE!" An Excludes1 note indicates that the code excluded should never be used at the same time as the code above the Excludes1 note. An Excludes1 is used when two conditions cannot occur together, such as a congenital form versus an acquired form of the same condition.

An exception to the Excludes1 definition is the circumstance when the two conditions are unrelated to each other. If it is not clear whether the two conditions involving an Excludes1 note are related or not, query the provider. For example, code F45.8, Other somatoform disorders, has an Excludes1 note for "sleep related teeth grinding (G47.63)" because "teeth grinding" is an inclusion term under F45.8. Only one of these two codes should be assigned for teeth grinding. However, psychogenic dysmenorrhea is also an inclusion term under F45.8, and a patient could have both this condition and sleep-related teeth grinding. In this case, the two conditions are clearly unrelated to each other, and so it would be appropriate to report F45.8 and G47.63 together.

b. Excludes2

A Type 2 Excludes note represents "Not included here." An excludes2 note indicates that the condition excluded is not part of the condition represented by the code, but a patient may have both conditions at the same time. When an Excludes2 note appears under a code, it is acceptable to use both the code and the excluded code together, when appropriate.

13. Etiology/manifestation convention ("code first", "use additional code" and "in diseases classified elsewhere" notes)

Certain conditions have both an underlying etiology and multiple body system manifestations due to the underlying etiology. For such conditions, the ICD-10-CM has a coding convention that requires the underlying condition be sequenced first, if applicable, followed by the manifestation. Wherever such a combination exists, there is a "use additional code" note at the etiology code, and a "code first" note at the manifestation code. These instructional notes indicate the proper sequencing order of the codes, etiology followed by manifestation.

In most cases the manifestation codes will have in the code title, "in diseases classified elsewhere." Codes with this title are a component of the etiology/manifestation convention. The code title indicates that it is a manifestation code. "In diseases classified elsewhere" codes are never permitted to be used as first-listed or principal diagnosis codes. They must be used in conjunction with an underlying condition code and they must be listed following the underlying condition. See category F02, Dementia in other diseases classified elsewhere, for an example of this convention.

There are manifestation codes that do not have "in diseases classified elsewhere" in the title. For such codes, there is a "use additional code" note at the etiology code and a "code first" note at the manifestation code and the rules for sequencing apply.

In addition to the notes in the Tabular List, these conditions also have a specific Alphabetic Index entry structure. In the Alphabetic Index both conditions are listed together with the etiology code first followed by the manifestation codes in brackets. The code in brackets is always to be sequenced second.

An example of the etiology/manifestation convention is dementia with Parkinson's disease. In the Alphabetic Index, **a** code **from category** G20 is listed first, followed by code F02.80 or F02.81 in brackets. A code from category G20- represents the underlying etiology, Parkinson's disease, and must be sequenced first, whereas *codes* F02.80 and F02.81 represent the manifestation of dementia in diseases classified elsewhere, with or without behavioral disturbance.

"Code first" and "Use additional code" notes are also used as sequencing rules in the classification for certain codes that are not part of an etiology/manifestation combination.

See Section I.B.7. Multiple coding for a single condition.

14. "And"

The word "and" should be interpreted to mean either "and" or "or" when it appears in a title.

For example, cases of "tuberculosis of bones", "tuberculosis of joints" and "tuberculosis of bones and joints" are classified to subcategory A18.0, Tuberculosis of bones and joints.

15. "With"

The word "with" or "in" should be interpreted to mean "associated with" or "due to" when it appears in a code title, the Alphabetic Index, (either under a main term or subterm) or an instructional note in the Tabular List. The classification presumes a causal relationship between the two conditions linked by these terms in the Alphabetic Index or Tabular List. These conditions should be coded as related even in the absence of provider documentation explicitly linking them, unless the documentation clearly states the conditions are unrelated or when another guideline exists that specifically requires a documented linkage between two conditions (e.g., sepsis guideline for "acute organ dysfunction that is not clearly associated with the sepsis").

For conditions not specifically linked by these relational terms in the classification or when a guideline requires that a linkage between two conditions be explicitly documented provider documentation must link the conditions in order to code them as related.

The word "with" in the Alphabetic Index is sequenced immediately following the main term or subterm, not in alphabetical order.

16. "See" and "See Also"

The "see" instruction following a main term in the Alphabetic Index indicates that another term should be referenced. It is necessary to go to the main term referenced with the "see" note to locate the correct code.

A "see also" instruction following a main term in the Alphabetic Index instructs that there is another main term that may also be referenced that may provide additional Alphabetic Index entries that may be useful. It is not necessary to follow the "see also" note when the original main term provides the necessary code.

17. "Code also" note

A "code also" note instructs that two codes may be required to fully describe a condition, but this note does not provide sequencing direction. The sequencing depends on the circumstances of the encounter.

18. Default codes

A code listed next to a main term in the ICD-10-CM Alphabetic Index is referred to as a default code. The default code represents that condition that is most commonly associated with the main term, or is the unspecified code for the condition. If a condition is documented in a medical record (for example, appendicitis) without any additional information, such as acute or chronic, the default code should be assigned.

19. Code assignment and Clinical Criteria
The assignment of a diagnosis code is based on the provider's diagnostic statement that the condition exists. The provider's statement that the patient has a particular condition is sufficient. Code assignment is not based on clinical criteria used by the provider to establish the diagnosis. **If there is conflicting medical record documentation, query the provider.**

B. General Coding Guidelines

1. Locating a code in the ICD-10-CM
To select a code in the classification that corresponds to a diagnosis or reason for visit documented in a medical record, first locate the term in the Alphabetic Index, and then verify the code in the Tabular List. Read and be guided by instructional notations that appear in both the Alphabetic Index and the Tabular List.

It is essential to use both the Alphabetic Index and Tabular List when locating and assigning a code. The Alphabetic Index does not always provide the full code. Selection of the full code, including laterality and any applicable 7th character can only be done in the Tabular List. A dash (-) at the end of an Alphabetic Index entry indicates that additional characters are required. Even if a dash is not included at the Alphabetic Index entry, it is necessary to refer to the Tabular List to verify that no 7th character is required.

2. Level of Detail in Coding
Diagnosis codes are to be used and reported at their highest number of characters available and to the highest level of specificity documented in the medical record.

ICD-10-CM diagnosis codes are composed of codes with 3, 4, 5, 6, or 7 characters. Codes with three characters are included in ICD-10-CM as the heading of a category of codes that may be further subdivided by the use of 4th and/or 5th characters and/or 6th characters, which provide greater detail.

A 3-character code is to be used only if it is not further subdivided. A code is invalid if it has not been coded to the full number of characters required for that code, including the 7th character, if applicable.

3. Code or codes from A00.0 through T88.9, Z00-Z99.8, U00-U85
The appropriate code or codes from A00.0 through T88.9, Z00-Z99.8 and U00-U85 must be used to identify diagnoses, symptoms, conditions, problems, complaints or other reason(s) for the encounter/visit.

4. Signs and symptoms
Codes that describe symptoms and signs, as opposed to diagnoses, are acceptable for reporting purposes when a related definitive diagnosis has not been established (confirmed) by the provider. Chapter 18 of ICD-10-CM, Symptoms, Signs, and Abnormal Clinical and Laboratory Findings, Not Elsewhere Classified (codes R00.0 - R99) contains many, but not all codes for symptoms.

See Section I.B.18 Use of signs/symptoms/ unspecified codes

5. Conditions that are an integral part of a disease process
Signs and symptoms that are associated routinely with a disease process should not be assigned as additional codes, unless otherwise instructed by the classification.

6. Conditions that are not an integral part of a disease process
Additional signs and symptoms that may not be associated routinely with a disease process should be coded when present.

7. Multiple coding for a single condition
In addition to the etiology/manifestation convention that requires two codes to fully describe a single condition that affects multiple body systems, there are other single conditions that also require more than one code. "Use additional code" notes are found in the Tabular List at codes that are not part of an etiology/manifestation pair where a secondary code is useful to fully describe a condition. The sequencing rule is the same as the etiology/manifestation pair, "use additional code" indicates that a secondary code should be added, if known.

For example, for bacterial infections that are not included in Chapter 1, a secondary code from category B95, Streptococcus, Staphylococcus, and Enterococcus, as the cause of diseases classified elsewhere, or B96, Other bacterial agents as the cause of diseases classified elsewhere, may be required to identify the bacterial organism causing the infection. A "use additional code" note will normally be found at the infectious disease code, indicating a need for the organism code to be added as a secondary code.

"Code first" notes are also under certain codes that are not specifically manifestation codes but may be due to an underlying cause. When there is a "code first" note and an underlying condition is present, the underlying condition should be sequenced first, if known.

"Code, if applicable, any causal condition first," notes indicate that this code may be assigned as a principal diagnosis when the causal condition is unknown or not applicable. If a causal condition is known, then the code for that condition should be sequenced as the principal or first-listed diagnosis.

Multiple codes may be needed for sequela, complication codes and obstetric codes to more fully describe a condition. See the specific guidelines for these conditions for further instruction.

8. Acute and Chronic Conditions
If the same condition is described as both acute (subacute) and chronic, and separate subentries exist in the Alphabetic Index at the same indentation level, code both and sequence the acute (subacute) code first.

9. Combination Code

A combination code is a single code used to classify:

Two diagnoses, or

A diagnosis with an associated secondary process (manifestation)

A diagnosis with an associated complication

Combination codes are identified by referring to subterm entries in the Alphabetic Index and by reading the inclusion and exclusion notes in the Tabular List.

Assign only the combination code when that code fully identifies the diagnostic conditions involved or when the Alphabetic Index so directs. Multiple coding should not be used when the classification provides a combination code that clearly identifies all of the elements documented in the diagnosis. When the combination code lacks necessary specificity in describing the manifestation or complication, an additional code should be used as a secondary code.

10. Sequela (Late Effects)

A sequela is the residual effect (condition produced) after the acute phase of an illness or injury has terminated. There is no time limit on when a sequela code can be used. The residual may be apparent early, such as in cerebral infarction, or it may occur months or years later, such as that due to a previous injury. Examples of sequela include: scar formation resulting from a burn, deviated septum due to a nasal fracture, and infertility due to tubal occlusion from old tuberculosis. Coding of sequela generally requires two codes sequenced in the following order: the condition or nature of the sequela is sequenced first. The sequela code is sequenced second.

An exception to the above guidelines are those instances where the code for the sequela is followed by a manifestation code identified in the Tabular List and title, or the sequela code has been expanded (at the 4th, 5th, or 6th character levels) to include the manifestation(s). The code for the acute phase of an illness or injury that led to the sequela is never used with a code for the late effect.

See Section I.C.9. Sequelae of cerebrovascular disease

See Section I.C.15. Sequelae of complication of pregnancy, childbirth and the puerperium

See Section I.C.19. Application of 7th characters for Chapter 19

11. Impending or Threatened Condition

Code any condition described at the time of discharge as "impending" or "threatened" as follows:

If it did occur, code as confirmed diagnosis.

If it did not occur, reference the Alphabetic Index to determine if the condition has a subentry term for "impending" or "threatened" and also reference main term entries for "Impending" and for "Threatened."

If the subterms are listed, assign the given code.

If the subterms are not listed, code the existing underlying condition(s) and not the condition described as impending or threatened.

12. Reporting Same Diagnosis Code More Than Once

Each unique ICD-10-CM diagnosis code may be reported only once for an encounter. This applies to bilateral conditions when there are no distinct codes identifying laterality or two different conditions classified to the same ICD-10-CM diagnosis code.

13. Laterality

Some ICD-10-CM codes indicate laterality, specifying whether the condition occurs on the left, right or is bilateral. If no bilateral code is provided and the condition is bilateral, assign separate codes for both the left and right side. If the side is not identified in the medical record, assign the code for the unspecified side.

When a patient has a bilateral condition and each side is treated during separate encounters, assign the "bilateral" code (as the condition still exists on both sides), including for the encounter to treat the first side. For the second encounter for treatment after one side has previously been treated and the condition no longer exists on that side, assign the appropriate unilateral code for the side where the condition still exists (e.g., cataract surgery performed on each eye in separate encounters). The bilateral code would not be assigned for the subsequent encounter, as the patient no longer has the condition in the previously-treated site. If the treatment on the first side did not completely resolve the condition, then the bilateral code would still be appropriate.

When laterality is not documented by the patient's provider, code assignment for the affected side may be based on medical record documentation from other clinicians. If there is conflicting medical record documentation regarding the affected side, the patient's provider should be queried for clarification. Codes for "unspecified" side should rarely be used, such as when the documentation in the record is insufficient to determine the affected side and it is not possible to obtain clarification.

14. Documentation by Clinicians Other than the Patient's Provider

Code assignment is based on the documentation by the patient's provider (i.e., physician or other qualified healthcare practitioner legally accountable for establishing the patient's diagnosis). There are a few exceptions when code assignment may be based on medical record documentation from clinicians who are not the patient's provider (i.e., physician or other qualified healthcare practitioner legally accountable for establishing the patient's diagnosis).

In this context, "clinicians" other than the patient's provider refer to healthcare professionals permitted, based on regulatory or accreditation requirements or internal hospital policies, to document in a patient's official medical record.

These exceptions include codes for:

- Body Mass Index (BMI)
- Depth of non-pressure chronic ulcers
- Pressure ulcer stage

- Coma scale
- NIH stroke scale (NIHSS)
- Social determinants of health (SDOH) **classified to Chapter 21**
- Laterality
- Blood alcohol level
- Firearm injury intent

This information is typically, **or may be,** documented by other clinicians involved in the care of the patient (e.g., a dietitian often documents the BMI, a nurse often documents the pressure ulcer stages, and an emergency medical technician often documents the coma scale). However, the associated diagnosis (such as overweight, obesity, acute stroke, pressure ulcer, or a condition classifiable to category F10, Alcohol related disorders) must be documented by the patient's provider. If there is conflicting medical record documentation, either from the same clinician or different clinicians, the patient's provider should be queried for clarification.

The BMI, coma scale, and NIHSS blood alcohol level codes**,** codes for social determinants of health **and underimmunization status** should only be reported as secondary diagnoses.

See Section I.C.21.c.17 for additional information regarding coding social determinants of health.

15. Syndromes
Follow the Alphabetic Index guidance when coding syndromes. In the absence of Alphabetic Index guidance, assign codes for the documented manifestations of the syndrome. Additional codes for manifestations that are not an integral part of the disease process may also be assigned when the condition does not have a unique code.

16. Documentation of Complications of Care
Code assignment is based on the provider's documentation of the relationship between the condition and the care or procedure, unless otherwise instructed by the classification. The guideline extends to any complications of care, regardless of the chapter the code is located in. It is important to note that not all conditions that occur during or following medical care or surgery are classified as complications. There must be a cause-and-effect relationship between the care provided and the condition, and **the documentation must support that the condition is clinically significant. It is not necessary for the provider to explicitly document the term "complication." For example, if the condition alters the course of the surgery as documented in the operative report, then it is would be appropriate to report a complication code.** Query the provider for clarification **if the documentation is not clear as to the relationship between the condition and the care or procedure.**

17. Borderline Diagnosis
If the provider documents a "borderline" diagnosis at the time of discharge, the diagnosis is coded as confirmed, unless the classification provides a specific entry (e.g., borderline diabetes). If a borderline condition has a specific index entry in ICD-10-CM, it should be coded as such. Since borderline conditions are not uncertain diagnoses, no distinction is made between the care setting (inpatient versus outpatient). Whenever the documentation is unclear regarding a borderline condition, coders are encouraged to query for clarification.

18. Use of Sign/Symptom/Unspecified Codes
Sign/symptom and "unspecified" codes have acceptable, even necessary, uses. While specific diagnosis codes should be reported when they are supported by the available medical record documentation and clinical knowledge of the patient's health condition, there are instances when signs/symptoms or unspecified codes are the best choices for accurately reflecting the healthcare encounter. Each healthcare encounter should be coded to the level of certainty known for that encounter.

As stated in the introductory section of these official coding guidelines, a joint effort between the healthcare provider and the coder is essential to achieve complete and accurate documentation, code assignment, and reporting of diagnoses and procedures. The importance of consistent, complete documentation in the medical record cannot be overemphasized. Without such documentation accurate coding cannot be achieved. The entire record should be reviewed to determine the specific reason for the encounter and the conditions treated.

If a definitive diagnosis has not been established by the end of the encounter, it is appropriate to report codes for sign(s) and/or symptom(s) in lieu of a definitive diagnosis. When sufficient clinical information isn't known or available about a particular health condition to assign a more specific code, it is acceptable to report the appropriate "unspecified" code (e.g., a diagnosis of pneumonia has been determined, but not the specific type). Unspecified codes should be reported when they are the codes that most accurately reflect what is known about the patient's condition at the time of that particular encounter. It would be inappropriate to select a specific code that is not supported by the medical record documentation or conduct medically unnecessary diagnostic testing in order to determine a more specific code.

19. Coding for Healthcare Encounters in Hurricane Aftermath

a. Use of External Cause of Morbidity Codes
An external cause of morbidity code should be assigned to identify the cause of the injury(ies) incurred as a result of the hurricane. The use of external cause of morbidity codes is supplemental to the application of ICD-10-CM codes. External cause of morbidity codes are never to be recorded as a principal diagnosis (first-listed in non-inpatient settings). The appropriate injury code should be sequenced before any external cause codes. The external cause of morbidity codes capture how the injury or health condition happened (cause), the intent (unintentional or

accidental; or intentional, such as suicide or assault), the place where the event occurred, the activity of the patient at the time of the event, and the person's status (e.g., civilian, military). They should not be assigned for encounters to treat hurricane victims' medical conditions when no injury, adverse effect or poisoning is involved. External cause of morbidity codes should be assigned for each encounter for care and treatment of the injury. External cause of morbidity codes may be assigned in all health care settings. For the purpose of capturing complete and accurate ICD-10-CM data in the aftermath of the hurricane, a healthcare setting should be considered as any location where medical care is provided by licensed healthcare professionals.

b. Sequencing of External Causes of Morbidity Codes

Codes for cataclysmic events, such as a hurricane, take priority over all other external cause codes except child and adult abuse and terrorism and should be sequenced before other external cause of injury codes. Assign as many external cause of morbidity codes as necessary to fully explain each cause. For example, if an injury occurs as a result of a building collapse during the hurricane, external cause codes for both the hurricane and the building collapse should be assigned, with the external causes code for hurricane being sequenced as the first external cause code. For injuries incurred as a direct result of the hurricane, assign the appropriate code(s) for the injuries, followed by the code X37.0-, Hurricane (with the appropriate 7th character), and any other applicable external cause of injury codes. Code X37.0- also should be assigned when an injury is incurred as a result of flooding caused by a levee breaking related to the hurricane. Code X38.-, Flood (with the appropriate 7th character), should be assigned when an injury is from flooding resulting directly from the storm. Code X36.0-, Collapse of dam or man-made structure, should not be assigned when the cause of the collapse is due to the hurricane. Use of code X36.0- is limited to collapses of man-made structures due to earth surface movements, not due to storm surges directly from a hurricane.

c. Other External Causes of Morbidity Code Issues

For injuries that are not a direct result of the hurricane, such as an evacuee that has incurred an injury as a result of a motor vehicle accident, assign the appropriate external cause of morbidity code(s) to describe the cause of the injury, but do not assign code X37.0-, Hurricane. If it is not clear whether the injury was a direct result of the hurricane, assume the injury is due to the hurricane and assign code X37.0-, Hurricane, as well as any other applicable external cause of morbidity codes. In addition to code X37.0-, Hurricane, other possible applicable external cause of morbidity codes include:

X30-	Exposure to excessive natural heat
X31-	Exposure to excessive natural cold
X38-	Flood

d. Use of Z codes

Z codes (other reasons for healthcare encounters) may be assigned as appropriate to further explain the reasons for presenting for healthcare services, including transfers between healthcare facilities or provide additional information relevant to a patient encounter. The ICD-10-CM Official Guidelines for Coding and Reporting identify which codes maybe assigned as principal or first-listed diagnosis only, secondary diagnosis only, or principal/first-listed or secondary (depending on the circumstances). Possible applicable Z codes include:

Z59.0-	Homelessness
Z59.1	Inadequate housing
Z59.5	Extreme poverty
Z75.1	Person awaiting admission to adequate facility elsewhere
Z75.3	Unavailability and inaccessibility of health-care facilities
Z75.4	Unavailability and inaccessibility of other helping agencies
Z76.2	Encounter for health supervision and care of other healthy infant and child
Z99.12	Encounter for respirator [ventilator] dependence during power failure

The external cause of morbidity codes and the Z codes listed above are not an all-inclusive list. Other codes may be applicable to the encounter based upon the documentation. Assign as many codes as necessary to fully explain each healthcare encounter. Since patient history information may be very limited, use any available documentation to assign the appropriate external cause of morbidity and Z codes.

20. Multiple Sites Coding

The classification defines "multiple" as involving two or more sites. Follow chapter specific guidelines for assigning codes for "multiple sites." In the absence of chapter specific guidelines, assign codes describing specified sites individually when documented. When the specified site(s) are not documented, assign the appropriate code for "multiple sites."

C. Chapter-Specific Coding Guidelines

In addition to general coding guidelines, there are guidelines for specific diagnoses and/or conditions in the classification. Unless otherwise indicated, these guidelines apply to all health care settings. Please refer to Section II for guidelines on the selection of principal diagnosis.

1. Chapter 1: Certain Infectious and Parasitic Diseases (A00-B99, U07.1, U09.9)

a. Human Immunodeficiency Virus (HIV) Infections

1) Code only confirmed cases

Code only confirmed cases of HIV infection/illness. This is an exception to the hospital inpatient guideline Section II, H.

In this context, "confirmation" does not require documentation of positive serology or culture for HIV; the provider's diagnostic statement that the patient is HIV positive, or has an HIV-related illness is sufficient.

2) Selection and sequencing of HIV codes

(a) HIV disease

If the term "AIDS" or "HIV disease" is documented or if the patient is treated for any HIV-related illness or is described as having any condition(s) resulting from the patient's HIV positive status; code B20, Human immunodeficiency virus [HIV], should be assigned.

(b) Patient admitted for HIV-related condition

If a patient is admitted for an HIV-related condition, the principal diagnosis should be B20, Human immunodeficiency virus [HIV] disease followed by additional diagnosis codes for all reported HIV-related conditions.

An exception to this guideline is if the reason for admission is hemolytic-uremic syndrome associated with HIV disease. Assign code D59.31, Infection-associated hemolytic-uremic syndrome, followed by code B20, Human immunodeficiency virus [HIV] disease.

(c) Patient with HIV disease admitted for unrelated condition

If a patient with HIV disease is admitted for an unrelated condition (such as a traumatic injury), the code for the unrelated condition (e.g., the nature of injury code) should be the principal diagnosis. Code B20 would be reported as a secondary diagnosis. Codes for other documented conditions should also be reported as secondary diagnoses.

(d) Patient newly diagnosed with HIV disease

Whether the patient is newly diagnosed or has had previous admissions/encounters for HIV conditions is irrelevant to the sequencing decision.

(e) Asymptomatic human immunodeficiency virus

When "HIV positive," "HIV test positive," or similar terminology is documented, and there is no documentation of symptoms or HIV-related illness, code Z21, Asymptomatic human immunodeficiency virus [HIV] infection status, should be assigned.

(f) Inconclusive HIV serology

Patients with documentation of inconclusive HIV serology, may be assigned code R75, Inconclusive laboratory evidence of human immunodeficiency virus [HIV].

(g) Previously diagnosed HIV-related illness

Patients with documentation of a prior diagnosis of an HIV-related illness should be coded to B20. Once an HIV-related illness has developed, code B20 should always be assigned on every subsequent admission/encounter. Patients previously diagnosed with any HIV illness (B20) should never be assigned to R75, Inconclusive laboratory evidence of human immunodeficiency virus [HIV] or Z21, Asymptomatic human immunodeficiency virus [HIV] infection status.

(h) HIV Infection in Pregnancy, Childbirth and the Puerperium

When a patient presents during pregnancy, childbirth or the puerperium, with documented symptomatic HIV disease or an HIV- related illness, assign a code from subcategory O98.7-, Human immunodeficiency [HIV] disease complicating pregnancy, childbirth and the puerperium, followed by code B20 and additional code(s) for any HIV-related illness(es).

Codes from Chapter 15 always take sequencing priority.

When a patient presents during pregnancy, childbirth, or the puerperium with documented asymptomatic HIV infection status or is HIV-positive, assign a code from subcategory O98.7- followed by code Z21.

(i) Encounters for HIV testing for HIV

If a patient without signs or symptoms is tested for HIV, assign code Z11.4, Encounter for screening for human immunodeficiency virus [HIV]. Use additional codes for any associated high-risk behavior, if applicable.

If a patient with signs or symptoms of HIV presents for HIV testing, code the signs and symptoms. An additional counseling code Z71.7, Human immunodeficiency virus [HIV] counseling, may be assigned if counseling is provided during the encounter for the test. Code Z11.4, Encounter for screening for human immunodeficiency virus [HIV], should not be assigned if HIV signs or symptoms are present.

When a patient presents for follow up regarding their HIV test results and the test result is negative, assign code Z71.7, Human immunodeficiency virus [HIV] counseling.

If the results are positive, see previous guidelines and assign codes as appropriate.

(j) HIV disease or HIV positive status managed by antiretroviral medication

If a patient with documented HIV disease, HIV-related illness or AIDS is currently managed on antiretroviral medications, assign code B20, Human immunodeficiency virus [HIV] disease.

If a patient with documented HIV positive status is currently managed on antiretroviral medication, assign code Z21, Asymptomatic human immunodeficiency virus [HIV] infection status, in the absence of any additional documentation of HIV disease, HIV-related illness or AIDS.

Code Z79.899, Other long term (current) drug therapy, may be assigned as an additional code to identify the long-term (current) use of antiretroviral medications.

(k) Encounter for HIV Prophylaxis Measures

When a patient presents for administration of pre-exposure prophylaxis medication for HIV, assign code Z29.81, Encounter for HIV pre-exposure prophylaxis. Pre-exposure prophylaxis (PrEP) is intended to prevent infection in people who are at risk for getting HIV through sex or injection drug use. Any risk factors for HIV should also be coded.

b. Infectious agents as the cause of diseases classified to other chapters

Certain infections are classified in chapters other than Chapter 1 and no organism is identified as part of the infection code. In these instances, it is necessary to use an additional code from Chapter 1 to identify the organism. A code from category B95, Streptococcus, Staphylococcus, and Enterococcus as the cause of diseases classified to other chapters, B96, Other bacterial agents as the cause of diseases classified to other chapters, or B97, Viral agents as the cause of diseases classified to other chapters, is to be used as an additional code to identify the organism. An instructional note will be found at the infection code advising that an additional organism code is required.

c. Infections resistant to antibiotics

Many bacterial infections are resistant to current antibiotics. It is necessary to identify all infections documented as antibiotic resistant. Assign a code from category Z16, Resistance to antimicrobial drugs, following the infection code only if the infection code does not identify drug resistance.

d. Sepsis, Severe Sepsis, and Septic Shock

1) Coding of Sepsis and Severe Sepsis

(a) Sepsis

For a diagnosis of sepsis, assign the appropriate code for the underlying systemic infection. If the type of infection or causal organism is not further specified, assign code A41.9, Sepsis, unspecified organism.

A code from subcategory R65.2, Severe sepsis, should not be assigned unless severe sepsis or an associated acute organ dysfunction is documented.

(i) Negative or inconclusive blood cultures and sepsis
Negative or inconclusive blood cultures do not preclude a diagnosis of sepsis in patients with clinical evidence of the condition, however, the provider should be queried.

(ii) Urosepsis
The term urosepsis is a nonspecific term. It is not to be considered synonymous with sepsis. It has no default code in the Alphabetic Index. Should a provider use this term, he/she must be queried for clarification.

(iii) Sepsis with organ dysfunction
If a patient has sepsis and associated acute organ dysfunction or multiple organ dysfunction (MOD), follow the instructions for coding severe sepsis.

(iv) Acute organ dysfunction that is not clearly associated with the sepsis
If a patient has sepsis and an acute organ dysfunction, but the medical record documentation indicates that the acute organ dysfunction is related to a medical condition other than the sepsis, do not assign a code from subcategory R65.2, Severe sepsis. An acute organ dysfunction must be associated with the sepsis in order to assign the severe sepsis code. If the documentation is not clear as to whether an acute organ dysfunction is related to the sepsis or another medical condition, query the provider.

(b) Severe sepsis

The coding of severe sepsis requires a minimum of 2 codes: first a code for the underlying systemic infection, followed by a code from subcategory R65.2, Severe sepsis. If the causal organism is not documented, assign code A41.9, Sepsis, unspecified organism, for the infection. Additional code(s) for the associated acute organ dysfunction are also required.

Due to the complex nature of severe sepsis, some cases may require querying the provider prior to assignment of the codes.

2) Septic shock

(a) Septic shock generally refers to circulatory failure associated with severe sepsis, and therefore, it represents a type of acute organ dysfunction.

For all cases of septic shock, the code for the systemic infection should be sequenced first, followed by code R65.21, Severe sepsis with septic shock or code T81.12, Postprocedural septic shock. Any additional codes for the other acute organ dysfunctions should also be assigned. As noted in the sequencing instructions in the Tabular List, the code for septic shock cannot be assigned as a principal diagnosis.

3) Sequencing of severe sepsis

If severe sepsis is present on admission, and meets the definition of principal diagnosis, the underlying systemic infection should be assigned as principal diagnosis followed by the appropriate code from subcategory R65.2 as required by the sequencing rules in the Tabular List. A code from subcategory R65.2 can never be assigned as a principal diagnosis.

When severe sepsis develops during an encounter (it was not present on admission) the underlying systemic infection and the appropriate code from subcategory R65.2 should be assigned as secondary diagnoses.

Severe sepsis may be present on admission but the diagnosis may not be confirmed until sometime after admission. If the documentation is not clear whether severe sepsis was present on admission, the provider should be queried.

For infection-associated hemolytic-uremic syndrome with severe sepsis, see guideline I.C.1.d.9.

4) Sepsis or severe sepsis with a localized infection

If the reason for admission is sepsis or severe sepsis and a localized infection, such as pneumonia or cellulitis, a code(s) for the underlying systemic infection should be assigned first and the code for the localized infection should be assigned as a secondary diagnosis. If the patient has severe sepsis, a code from subcategory R65.2 should also be assigned as a secondary diagnosis. If the patient is admitted with a localized infection, such as pneumonia, and sepsis/severe sepsis doesn't develop until after admission, the localized infection should be assigned first, followed by the appropriate sepsis/severe sepsis codes.

For hemolytic-uremic syndrome associated with sepsis, see guideline I.C.1.d.9.

5) Sepsis due to a postprocedural infection

(a) Documentation of causal relationship

As with all postprocedural complications, code assignment is based on the provider's documentation of the relationship between the infection and the procedure.

(b) Sepsis due to a postprocedural infection

For **sepsis** following a **postprocedural wound (surgical site) infection**, a code from **T81.41** to T81.43, Infection following a procedure, or a code from O86.00 to O86.03, Infection of obstetric surgical wound, that identifies the site of the infection should be **sequenced** first, if known. Assign an additional code for sepsis following a procedure (T81.44) or sepsis following an obstetrical procedure (O86.04). Use an additional code to identify the infectious agent. If the patient has severe sepsis the appropriate code from subcategory R65.2 should also be assigned with the additional code(s) for any acute organ dysfunction.

For infections following infusion, transfusion, therapeutic injection, or immunization, a code from subcategory T80.2, Infections following infusion, transfusion, and therapeutic injection, or code T88.0-, Infection following immunization, should be coded first, followed by the code for the specific infection. If the patient has severe sepsis, the appropriate code from subcategory R65.2 should also be assigned, with the additional codes(s) for any acute organ dysfunction.

(c) Postprocedural infection and postprocedural septic shock

If a postprocedural infection has resulted in postprocedural septic shock, assign the codes indicated above for sepsis due to a postprocedural infection, followed by code T81.12-, Postprocedural septic shock. Do not assign code R65.21, Severe sepsis with septic shock. Additional code(s) should be assigned for any acute organ dysfunction.

6) Sepsis and severe sepsis associated with a noninfectious process (condition)

In some cases a noninfectious process (condition), such as trauma, may lead to an infection which can result in sepsis or severe sepsis. If sepsis or severe sepsis is documented as associated with a noninfectious condition, such as a burn or serious injury, and this condition meets the definition for principal diagnosis, the code for the noninfectious condition should be sequenced first, followed by the code for the resulting infection. If severe sepsis is present, a code from subcategory R65.2 should also be assigned with any associated organ dysfunction(s) codes. It is not necessary to assign a code from subcategory R65.1, Systemic inflammatory response syndrome (SIRS) of non-infectious origin, for these cases.

If the infection meets the definition of principal diagnosis it should be sequenced before the non-infectious condition. When both the associated non-infectious condition and the infection meet the definition of principal diagnosis either may be assigned as principal diagnosis.

Only one code from category R65, Symptoms and signs specifically associated with systemic inflammation and infection, should be assigned. Therefore, when a non-infectious condition leads to an infection resulting in severe sepsis, assign the appropriate code from subcategory R65.2, Severe sepsis. Do not additionally assign a code from subcategory R65.1, Systemic inflammatory response syndrome (SIRS) of non-infectious origin.

See Section I.C.18. SIRS due to non-infectious process

7) Sepsis and septic shock complicating abortion, pregnancy, childbirth, and the puerperium

See Section I.C.15. Sepsis and septic shock complicating abortion, pregnancy, childbirth and the puerperium

8) Newborn sepsis

See Section I.C.16. f. Bacterial sepsis of Newborn

9) Hemolytic-uremic syndrome associated with sepsis

If the reason for admission is hemolytic-uremic syndrome that is associated with sepsis, assign code D59.31, Infection-associated hemolytic-uremic syndrome, as the principal diagnosis. Codes for the underlying systemic infection and any other conditions (such as severe sepsis) should be assigned as secondary diagnoses.

e. Methicillin Resistant Staphylococcus aureus (MRSA) Conditions

1) Selection and sequencing of MRSA codes

(a) Combination codes for MRSA infection

When a patient is diagnosed with an infection that is due to methicillin resistant Staphylococcus aureus (MRSA), and that infection has a combination code that includes the causal organism (e.g., sepsis, pneumonia) assign the appropriate combination code for the condition (e.g., code A41.02, Sepsis due to Methicillin resistant Staphylococcus aureus or code J15.212, Pneumonia due to Methicillin resistant Staphylococcus aureus). Do not assign code B95.62, Methicillin resistant Staphylococcus aureus infection as the cause of diseases classified elsewhere, as an additional code because the combination code includes the type of infection and the MRSA organism. Do not assign a code from subcategory Z16.11, Resistance to penicillins, as an additional diagnosis.

See Section C.1. for instructions on coding and sequencing of sepsis and severe sepsis.

(b) Other codes for MRSA infection

When there is documentation of a current infection (e.g., wound infection, stitch abscess, urinary tract infection) due to MRSA, and that infection does not have a combination code that includes the causal organism, assign the appropriate code to identify the condition along with code B95.62, Methicillin resistant Staphylococcus aureus infection as the cause of diseases classified elsewhere for the MRSA infection. Do not assign a code from subcategory Z16.11, Resistance to penicillins.

(c) Methicillin susceptible Staphylococcus aureus (MSSA) and MRSA colonization

The condition or state of being colonized or carrying MSSA or MRSA is called colonization or carriage, while an individual person is described as being colonized or being a carrier. Colonization means that MSSA or MSRA is present on or in the body without necessarily causing illness. A positive MRSA colonization test might be documented by the provider as "MRSA screen positive" or "MRSA nasal swab positive".

Assign code Z22.322, Carrier or suspected carrier of Methicillin resistant Staphylococcus aureus, for patients documented as having MRSA colonization. Assign code Z22.321, Carrier or suspected carrier of Methicillin susceptible Staphylococcus aureus, for patients documented as having MSSA colonization. Colonization is not necessarily indicative of a disease process or as the cause of a specific condition the patient may have unless documented as such by the provider.

(d) MRSA colonization and infection

If a patient is documented as having both MRSA colonization and infection during a hospital admission, code Z22.322, Carrier or suspected carrier of Methicillin resistant Staphylococcus aureus, and a code for the MRSA infection may both be assigned.

f. Zika virus infections

1) Code only confirmed cases

Code only a confirmed diagnosis of Zika virus (A92.5, Zika virus disease) as documented by the provider. This is an exception to the hospital inpatient guideline Section II, H.

In this context, "confirmation" does not require documentation of the type of test performed; the provider's diagnostic statement that the condition is confirmed is sufficient. This code should be assigned regardless of the stated mode of transmission.

If the provider documents "suspected", "possible" or "probable" Zika, do not assign code A92.5. Assign a code(s) explaining the reason for encounter (such as fever, rash, or joint pain) or Z20.821, Contact with and (suspected) exposure to Zika virus.

g. Coronavirus infections

1) COVID-19 infection (infection due to SARS-CoV-2)

(a) Code only confirmed cases

Code only a confirmed diagnosis of the 2019 novel coronavirus disease (COVID-19) as documented by the provider. For a confirmed diagnosis, assign code U07.1, COVID-19. This is an exception to the hospital inpatient guideline Section II, H. In this context, "confirmation" does not require documentation of a positive test result for COVID-19; the provider's documentation that the individual has COVID-19 is sufficient.

If the provider documents "suspected," "possible," "probable," or "inconclusive" COVID-19, do not assign code U07.1. Instead, code the signs and symptoms reported. *See guideline I.C.1.g.1.g.*

(b) Sequencing of codes

When COVID-19 meets the definition of principal diagnosis, code U07.1, COVID-19, should be sequenced first, followed by the appropriate codes for associated manifestations, except when another guideline requires that certain codes be sequenced first, such as obstetrics, sepsis, or transplant complications.

For a COVID-19 infection that progresses to sepsis, see Section I.C.1.d. Sepsis, Severe Sepsis, and Septic Shock

See Section I.C.15.s. for COVID-19 infection in pregnancy, childbirth, and the puerperium

See Section I.C.16.h. for COVID-19 infection in newborn

For a COVID-19 infection in a lung transplant patient, see Section I.C.19.g.3.a. Transplant complications other than kidney.

(c) Acute respiratory manifestations of COVID-19

When the reason for the encounter/admission is a respiratory manifestation of COVID-19, assign code U07.1, COVID-19, as the principal/first-listed diagnosis and assign code(s) for the respiratory manifestation(s) as additional diagnoses.

The following conditions are examples of common respiratory manifestations of COVID-19.

(i) Pneumonia

For a patient with pneumonia confirmed as due to COVID-19, assign codes U07.1, COVID-19, and J12.89, Other viral pneumonia.

(ii) Acute bronchitis
For a patient with acute bronchitis confirmed as due to COVID-19, assign codes U07.1, and J20.8, Acute bronchitis due to other specified organisms.

Bronchitis not otherwise specified (NOS) due to COVID-19 should be coded using code U07.1 and J40, Bronchitis, not specified as acute or chronic.

(iii) Lower respiratory infection
If the COVID-19 is documented as being associated with a lower respiratory infection, not otherwise specified (NOS), or an acute respiratory infection, NOS, codes U07.1 and J22, Unspecified acute lower respiratory infection, should be assigned.

If the COVID-19 is documented as being associated with a respiratory infection, NOS, codes U07.1 and J98.8, Other specified respiratory disorders, should be assigned.

(iv) Acute respiratory distress syndrome
For acute respiratory distress syndrome (ARDS) due to COVID-19, assign codes U07.1, and J80, Acute respiratory distress syndrome.

(v) Acute respiratory failure
For acute respiratory failure due to COVID-19, assign code U07.1, and code J96.0-, Acute respiratory failure.

(d) Non-respiratory manifestations of COVID-19
When the reason for the encounter/admission is a **nonrespiratory** manifestation (e.g., viral enteritis) of COVID-19, assign code U07.1, COVID-19, as the principal/first-listed diagnosis and assign code(s) for the manifestation(s) as additional diagnoses.

(e) Exposure to COVID-19
For asymptomatic individuals with actual or suspected exposure to COVID-19, assign code Z20.828, Contact with and (suspected) exposure to other viral communicable diseases.

For symptomatic individuals with actual or suspected exposure to COVID-19 and the infection has been ruled out, or test results are inconclusive or unknown, assign code Z20.828, Contact with and (suspected) exposure to other viral communicable diseases. See guideline I.C.21.c.1, Contact/Exposure, for additional guidance regarding the use of category Z20 codes.

If COVID-19 is confirmed, see guideline I.C.1.g.1.a.

(f) Screening for COVID-19
For screening for COVID-19, including preoperative testing, assign code Z11.52, Encounter for screening for COVID-19.

(g) Signs and symptoms without definitive diagnosis of **COVID19**
For patients presenting with any signs/symptoms associated with COVID-19 (such as fever, etc.) but a definitive diagnosis has not been established, assign the appropriate code(s) for each of the presenting signs and symptoms such as:
- R05.1, Acute cough, or R05.9, Cough, unspecified
- R06.02 Shortness of breath
- R50.9 Fever, unspecified

If a patient with signs/symptoms associated with COVID-19 also has an actual or suspected contact with or exposure to COVID-19, assign Z20.828, Contact with and (suspected) exposure to other viral communicable diseases, as an additional code.

(h) Asymptomatic individuals who test positive for COVID-19
For asymptomatic individuals who test positive for COVID-19, and there is no provider documentation of a diagnosis of COVID-19, query the provider as to whether or not the individual has COVID-19. A false positive laboratory test is possible, and it is the provider's responsibility to confirm the diagnosis and document accordingly.

(i) Personal history of COVID-19
For patients with a history of COVID-19, assign code Z86.19, Personal history of other infectious and parasitic diseases.

(j) Follow-up visits after COVID-19 infection has resolved
For individuals who previously had COVID-19 without residual symptom(s) or condition(s), and are being seen for follow-up evaluation, and COVID-19 test results are negative, assign codes Z09, Encounter for follow-up examination after completed treatment for conditions other than malignant neoplasm, and Z86.19, Personal history of other infectious and parasitic diseases.

For follow-up visits for individuals with symptom(s) or condition(s) related to a previous COVID-19 infection, see guideline I.C.1.g.1.m.
See Section I.C.21.c.8, Factors influencing health states and contact with health services, Follow-up

(k) Encounter for antibody testing
For an encounter for antibody testing that is not being performed to confirm a current COVID-19 infection, nor is a follow-up test after resolution of COVID-19, assign Z01.84, Encounter for antibody response examination.

Follow the applicable guidelines above if the individual is being tested to confirm a current COVID-19 infection.

For follow-up testing after a COVID-19 infection, see guideline I.C.1.g.1.j.

(l) Multisystem Inflammatory Syndrome
For individuals with multisystem inflammatory syndrome (MIS) and COVID-19, assign code U07.1, COVID-19, as the principal/first-listed diagnosis and assign code M35.81, Multisystem inflammatory syndrome, as an additional diagnosis.

If an individual with a history of COVID-19 develops MIS, assign codes M35.81, Multisystem inflammatory syndrome, and U09.9, Post COVID-19 condition, unspecified.

If an individual with a known or suspected exposure to COVID-19, and no current COVID-19 infection or history of COVID-19, develops MIS, assign codes M35.81, Multisystem inflammatory syndrome, and Z20.822, Contact with and (suspected) exposure to COVID-19.

Additional codes should be assigned for any associated complications of MIS.

(m) Post COVID-19 Condition
For sequela of COVID-19, or associated symptoms or conditions that develop following a previous COVID-19 infection, assign a code(s) for the specific symptom(s) or condition(s) related to the previous COVID-19 infection, if known, and code U09.9, Post COVID-19 condition, unspecified.

Code U09.9 should not be assigned for manifestations of an active (current) COVID-19 infection.

If a patient has a condition(s) associated with a previous COVID-19 infection and develops a new active (current) COVID-19 infection, code U09.9 may be assigned in conjunction with code U07.1, COVID-19, to identify that the patient also has a condition(s) associated with a previous COVID-19 infection. Code(s) for the specific condition(s) associated with the previous COVID-19 infection and code(s) for manifestation(s) of the new active (current) COVID-19 infection should also be assigned.

(n) Underimmunization for COVID-19 Status CodeZ28.310, Unvaccinated for COVID-19, may be assigned when the patient has not received a COVID-19 vaccine of any type. Code Z28.311, Partially vaccinated for COVID-19, may be assigned when the patient has been partially vaccinated for COVID-19 as per the recommendations of the Centers for Disease Control and Prevention (CDC) in place at the time of the encounter. For information, visit the CDC's website
https://www.cdc.gov/covidschedule.
See Section I.B.14. for underimmunization documentation by clinicians other than patient's provider.

2. **Chapter 2: Neoplasms (C00-D49)**
   General guidelines
Chapter 2 of the ICD-10-CM contains the codes for most benign and all malignant neoplasms. Certain benign neoplasms, such as prostatic adenomas, may be found in the specific body system chapters. To properly code a neoplasm it is necessary to determine from the record if the neoplasm is benign, in-situ, malignant, or of uncertain histologic behavior. If malignant, any secondary (metastatic) sites should also be determined.

Primary malignant neoplasms overlapping site boundaries
A primary malignant neoplasm that overlaps two or more contiguous (next to each other) sites should be classified to the subcategory/code .8 ("overlapping lesion"), unless the combination is specifically indexed elsewhere. For multiple neoplasms of the same site that are not contiguous such as tumors in different quadrants of the same breast, codes for each site should be assigned.

Malignant neoplasm of ectopic tissue
Malignant neoplasms of ectopic tissue are to be coded to the site of origin mentioned (e.g., ectopic pancreatic malignant neoplasms involving the stomach are coded to malignant neoplasm of pancreas, unspecified) (C25.9).

The neoplasm table in the Alphabetic Index should be referenced first. However, if the histological term is documented, that term should be referenced first, rather than going immediately to the Neoplasm Table, in order to determine which column in the Neoplasm Table is appropriate. For example, if the documentation indicates "adenoma," refer to the term in the Alphabetic Index to review the entries under this term and the instructional note to "see also neoplasm, by site, benign." The table provides the proper code based on the type of neoplasm and the site. It is important to select the proper column in the table that corresponds to the type of neoplasm. The Tabular List should then be referenced to verify that the correct code has been selected from the table and that a more specific site code does not exist.

See Section I.C.21. Factors influencing health status and contact with health services, Status, for information regarding Z15.0, codes for genetic susceptibility to cancer.

a. *Admission/Encounter for treatment of primary site*
If the **malignancy is chiefly responsible for occasioning the patient admission/encounter and treatment is directed at the primary site,** designate the **primary** malignancy as the principal **/first-listed** diagnosis.

The only exception to this guideline is if the administration of chemotherapy, immunotherapy or external beam radiation therapy **is chiefly responsible for occasioning the admission/ encounter. In that case,** assign the appropriate Z51.— code as the first-listed or principal diagnosis, and the **underlying** diagnosis or problem for which the service is being performed as a secondary diagnosis.

b. *Admission/Encounter for* **treatment of secondary site**
When a patient is admitted because of a primary neoplasm with metastasis and treatment is directed toward the secondary site only, the secondary

neoplasm is designated as the principal diagnosis even though the primary malignancy is still present.

c. Coding and sequencing of complications

Coding and sequencing of complications associated with the malignancies or with the therapy thereof are subject to the following guidelines:

1) Anemia associated with malignancy

When admission/encounter is for management of an anemia associated with the malignancy, and the treatment is only for anemia, the appropriate code for the malignancy is sequenced as the principal or first-listed diagnosis followed by the appropriate code for the anemia (such as code D63.0, Anemia in neoplastic disease).

2) Anemia associated with chemotherapy, immunotherapy and radiation therapy

When the admission/encounter is for management of an anemia associated with an adverse effect of the administration of chemotherapy or immunotherapy and the only treatment is for the anemia, the anemia code is sequenced first followed by the appropriate codes for the neoplasm and the adverse effect (T45.1X5, Adverse effect of antineoplastic and immunosuppressive drugs).

When the admission/encounter is for management of an anemia associated with an adverse effect of radiotherapy, the anemia code should be sequenced first, followed by the appropriate neoplasm code and code Y84.2, Radiological procedure and radiotherapy as the cause of abnormal reaction of the patient, or of later complication, without mention of misadventure at the time of the procedure.

3) Management of dehydration due to the malignancy

When the admission/encounter is for management of dehydration due to the malignancy and only the dehydration is being treated (intravenous rehydration), the dehydration is sequenced first, followed by the code(s) for the malignancy.

4) Treatment of a complication resulting from a surgical procedure

When the admission/encounter is for treatment of a complication resulting from a surgical procedure, designate the complication as the principal or first-listed diagnosis if treatment is directed at resolving the complication.

d. Primary malignancy previously excised

When a primary malignancy has been previously excised or eradicated from its site and there is no further treatment directed to that site and there is no evidence of any existing primary malignancy, at that site a code from category Z85, Personal history of malignant neoplasm, should be used to indicate the former site of the malignancy. Any mention of extension, invasion, or metastasis to another site is coded as a secondary malignant neoplasm to that site. The secondary site may be the principal or first-listed diagnosis with the Z85 code used as a secondary code.

See section I.C.2.t. Secondary malignant neoplasm of lymphoid tissue.

e. Admissions/Encounters involving *antineoplastic* chemotherapy, immunotherapy and radiation therapy

1) Episode of care involves surgical removal of neoplasm

When an episode of care involves the surgical removal of a neoplasm, primary or secondary site, followed by adjunct chemotherapy or radiation treatment during the same episode of care, the code for the neoplasm should be assigned as principal or first-listed diagnosis.

2) Patient admission/encounter chiefly for administration of *antineoplastic* chemotherapy, immunotherapy and radiation therapy

If a patient admission/encounter is **chiefly** for the administration of chemotherapy, immunotherapy or external beam radiation therapy for the treatment of a neoplasm, assign code Z51.0, Encounter for antineoplastic radiation therapy, or Z51.11, Encounter for antineoplastic chemotherapy, or Z51.12, Encounter for antineoplastic immunotherapy as the first-listed or principal diagnosis. If the reason for the encounter is more than one type of antineoplastic therapy, code Z51.0 and codes from subcategory Z51.1 may be assigned together, in which case one of these codes would be reported as a secondary diagnosis.

The malignancy for which the therapy is being administered should be assigned as a secondary diagnosis.

If a patient admission/encounter is for the insertion or implantation of radioactive elements (e.g., brachytherapy) the appropriate code for the malignancy is sequenced as the principal or first-listed diagnosis. Code Z51.0 should not be assigned.

3) Patient admitted for radiation therapy, chemotherapy or immunotherapy and develops complications

When a patient is admitted for the purpose of external beam radiotherapy, immunotherapy or chemotherapy and develops complications such as uncontrolled nausea and vomiting or dehydration, the principal or first-listed diagnosis is Z51.0, Encounter for antineoplastic radiation therapy, or Z51.11, Encounter for antineoplastic chemotherapy, or Z51.12, Encounter for antineoplastic immunotherapy followed by any codes for the complications.

When a patient is admitted for the purpose of insertion or implantation of radioactive elements (e.g., brachytherapy) and develops complications such as uncontrolled nausea and vomiting or dehydration, the principal or first-listed diagnosis is the appropriate code for the malignancy followed by any codes for the complications.

f. Admission/encounter to determine extent of malignancy

When the reason for admission/encounter is to determine the extent of the malignancy, or for a procedure such as paracentesis or thoracentesis, the primary malignancy or appropriate metastatic site is designated as the principal or first-listed diagnosis, even though chemotherapy or radiotherapy is administered.

g. Symptoms, signs, and abnormal findings listed in Chapter 18 associated with neoplasms

Symptoms, signs, and ill-defined conditions listed in Chapter 18 characteristic of, or associated with, an existing primary or secondary site malignancy cannot be used to replace the malignancy as principal or first-listed diagnosis, regardless of the number of admissions or encounters for treatment and care of the neoplasm.

See Section I.C.21. Factors influencing health status and contact with health services, Encounter for prophylactic organ removal.

h. Admission/encounter for pain control/management

See Section I.C.6. for information on coding admission/encounter for pain control/management.

i. Malignancy in two or more noncontiguous sites

A patient may have more than one malignant tumor in the same organ. These tumors may represent different primaries or metastatic disease, depending on the site. Should the documentation be unclear, the provider should be queried as to the status of each tumor so that the correct codes can be assigned.

j. Disseminated malignant neoplasm, unspecified

Code C80.0, Disseminated malignant neoplasm, unspecified, is for use only in those cases where the patient has advanced metastatic disease and no known primary or secondary sites are specified. It should not be used in place of assigning codes for the primary site and all known secondary sites.

k. Malignant neoplasm without specification of site

Code C80.1, Malignant (primary) neoplasm, unspecified, equates to Cancer, unspecified. This code should only be used when no determination can be made as to the primary site of a malignancy. This code should rarely be used in the inpatient setting.

l. Sequencing of neoplasm codes

1) Encounter for treatment of primary malignancy

If the reason for the encounter is for treatment of a primary malignancy, assign the malignancy as the principal/first-listed diagnosis. The primary site is to be sequenced first, followed by any metastatic sites.

2) Encounter for treatment of secondary malignancy

When an encounter is for a primary malignancy with metastasis and treatment is directed toward the metastatic (secondary) site(s) only, the metastatic site(s) is designated as the principal/first-listed diagnosis. The primary malignancy is coded as an additional code.

3) Malignant neoplasm in a pregnant patient

When a pregnant patient has a malignant neoplasm, a code from subcategory O9A.1-,

Malignant neoplasm complicating pregnancy, childbirth, and the puerperium, should be sequenced first, followed by the appropriate code from Chapter 2 to indicate the type of neoplasm.

4) Encounter for complication associated with a neoplasm

When an encounter is for management of a complication associated with a neoplasm, such as dehydration, and the treatment is only for the complication, the complication is coded first, followed by the appropriate code(s) for the neoplasm.

The exception to this guideline is anemia. When the admission/encounter is for management of an anemia associated with the malignancy, and the treatment is only for anemia, the appropriate code for the malignancy is sequenced as the principal or first-listed diagnosis followed by code D63.0, Anemia in neoplastic disease.

5) Complication from surgical procedure for treatment of a neoplasm

When an encounter is for treatment of a complication resulting from a surgical procedure performed for the treatment of the neoplasm, designate the complication as the principal/first-listed diagnosis. See the guideline regarding the coding of a current malignancy versus personal history to determine if the code for the neoplasm should also be assigned.

6) Pathologic fracture due to a neoplasm

When an encounter is for a pathological fracture due to a neoplasm, and the focus of treatment is the fracture, a code from subcategory M84.5, Pathological fracture in neoplastic disease, should be sequenced first, followed by the code for the neoplasm.

If the focus of treatment is the neoplasm with an associated pathological fracture, the neoplasm code should be sequenced first, followed by a code from M84.5 for the pathological fracture.

m. Current malignancy versus personal history of malignancy

When a primary malignancy has been excised but further treatment, such as an additional surgery for the malignancy, radiation therapy or chemotherapy is directed to that site, the primary malignancy code should be used until treatment is completed.

When a primary malignancy has been previously excised or eradicated from its site, there is no further treatment (of the malignancy) directed to that site, and there is no evidence of any existing primary malignancy at that site, a code from category Z85, Personal history of malignant neoplasm, should be used to indicate the former site of the malignancy.

Codes from subcategories Z85.0 – Z85.85 should only be assigned for the former site of a primary malignancy, not the site of a secondary malignancy. Code Z85.89, may be assigned for the former site(s) of either a primary or secondary malignancy.

See Section I.C.21. Factors influencing health status and contact with health services, History (of)

n. Leukemia, Multiple Myeloma, and Malignant Plasma Cell Neoplasms in remission versus personal history

The categories for leukemia, and category C90, Multiple myeloma and malignant plasma cell neoplasms, have codes indicating whether or not the leukemia has achieved remission. There are also codes Z85.6, Personal history of leukemia, and Z85.79, Personal history of other malignant neoplasms of lymphoid, hematopoietic and related tissues. If the documentation is unclear, as to whether the leukemia has achieved remission, the provider should be queried.

See Section I.C.21. Factors influencing health status and contact with health services, History (of)

o. Aftercare following surgery for neoplasm

See Section I.C.21. Factors influencing health status and contact with health services, Aftercare

p. Follow-up care for completed treatment of a malignancy

See Section I.C.21. Factors influencing health status and contact with health services, Follow-up

q. Prophylactic organ removal for prevention of malignancy

See Section I.C. 21, Factors influencing health status and contact with health services, Prophylactic organ removal

r. Malignant neoplasm associated with transplanted organ

A malignant neoplasm of a transplanted organ should be coded as a transplant complication. Assign first the appropriate code from category T86.-, Complications of transplanted organs and tissue, followed by code C80.2, Malignant neoplasm associated with transplanted organ. Use an additional code for the specific malignancy.

s. Breast Implant Associated Anaplastic Large Cell Lymphoma

Breast implant associated anaplastic large cell lymphoma (BIA-ALCL) is a type of lymphoma that can develop around breast implants. Assign code C84.7A, Anaplastic large cell lymphoma, ALK-negative, breast, for BIA-ALCL or C84.7B, Anaplastic large cell lymphoma, ALK-negative, in remission, for BIA-ALCL in remission. Do not assign a complication code from chapter 19.

t. Secondary malignant neoplasm of lymphoid tissue

When a malignant neoplasm of lymphoid tissue metastasizes beyond the lymph nodes, a code from categories C81-C85 with a final character identifying "extranodal and solid organ sites" should be assigned rather than a code for the secondary neoplasm of the affected solid organ. For example, for metastasis of diffuse large B-cell lymphoma to the lung, brain and left adrenal gland, assign code C83.398, Diffuse large B-cell lymphoma of other extranodal and solid organ sites.

3. **Chapter 3: Disease of the blood and blood-forming organs and certain disorders involving the immune mechanism (D50-D89)**

Reserved for future guideline expansion

4. **Chapter 4: Endocrine, Nutritional, and Metabolic Diseases (E00-E89)**

a. Diabetes mellitus

The diabetes mellitus codes are combination codes that include the type of diabetes mellitus, the body system affected, and the complications affecting that body system. As many codes within a particular category as are necessary to describe all of the complications of the disease may be used. They should be sequenced based on the reason for a particular encounter. Assign as many codes from categories E08 – E13 as needed to identify all of the associated conditions that the patient has.

1) Type of diabetes

The age of a patient is not the sole determining factor, though most type 1 diabetics develop the condition before reaching puberty. For this reason type 1 diabetes mellitus is also referred to as juvenile diabetes.

(a) Presymptomatic Type 1 Diabetes Mellitus Codes E10.A-, Type 1 diabetes mellitus, presymptomatic, are assigned for early-stage type 1 diabetes that predates the onset of symptoms.

(b) Type 2 diabetes mellitus in remission Code E11.A, Type 2 diabetes mellitus without complications in remission, is assigned based on provider documentation that the diabetes mellitus is in remission. If the documentation is unclear as to whether the Type 2 diabetes mellitus has achieved remission, the provider should be queried. For example, the term "resolved" is not synonymous with remission.

2) Type of diabetes mellitus not documented

If the type of diabetes mellitus is not documented in the medical record the default is E11.-, Type 2 diabetes mellitus.

3) Diabetes mellitus and the use of insulin, oral hypoglycemics, and injectable non-insulin drugs

If the documentation in a medical record does not indicate the type of diabetes but does indicate that the patient uses insulin, code E11, Type 2 diabetes mellitus, should be assigned. Additional code(s) should be assigned from category Z79 to identify the long-term (current) use of insulin or oral hypoglycemic drugs, or injectable non-insulin antidiabetic, as follows: If the patient is treated with both oral **hypoglycemic drugs** and insulin, both code Z79.4, Long term (current) use of insulin, and code Z79.84, Long term (current) use of oral hypoglycemic drugs, should be assigned. If the patient is treated with both insulin and an injectable non-insulin antidiabetic drug, assign codes Z79.4, Long-term (current) use of insulin, and **Z79.85, Long-term (current) use of injectable non-insulin antidiabetic drugs.** If the patient is treated with both oral hypoglycemic drugs and an injectable non-insulin antidiabetic drug, assign codes Z79.84, Long-term (current) use of oral hypoglycemic drugs, and **Z79.85, Long-term (current) use of injectable non-insulin antidiabetic drugs.** Code Z79.4 should not be assigned if insulin is given temporarily to bring a type 2 patient's blood sugar under control during an encounter.

4) Diabetes mellitus in pregnancy and gestational diabetes

See Section I.C.15. Diabetes mellitus in pregnancy. See Section I.C.15. Gestational (pregnancy induced) diabetes

5) Complications due to insulin pump malfunction

(a) Underdose of insulin due to insulin pump failure

An underdose of insulin due to an insulin pump failure should be assigned to a code from subcategory T85.6, Mechanical complication of other specified internal and external prosthetic devices, implants and grafts, that specifies the type of pump malfunction, as the principal or first-listed code, followed by code T38.3X6-, Underdosing of insulin and oral hypoglycemic [antidiabetic] drugs. Additional codes for the type of diabetes mellitus and any associated complications due to the underdosing should also be assigned.

(b) Overdose of insulin due to insulin pump failure

The principal or first-listed code for an encounter due to an insulin pump malfunction resulting in an overdose of insulin, should also be T85.6-, Mechanical complication of other specified internal and external prosthetic devices, implants and grafts, followed by code T38.3X1-, Poisoning by insulin and oral hypoglycemic [antidiabetic] drugs, accidental (unintentional).

6) Secondary diabetes mellitus

Codes under categories E08, Diabetes mellitus due to underlying condition, E09, Drug or chemical induced diabetes mellitus and E13, Other specified diabetes mellitus, identify complications/ manifestations associated with secondary diabetes mellitus. Secondary diabetes is always caused by another condition or event (e.g., cystic fibrosis, malignant neoplasm of pancreas, pancreatectomy, adverse effect of drug, or poisoning).

(a) Secondary diabetes mellitus and the use of insulin or hypoglycemic drugs

For patients with secondary diabetes mellitus who routinely use insulin or oral hypoglycemic drugs, or injectable non-insulin drugs, an additional code(s) from category Z79 should be assigned to identify the long-term (current) use of insulin or oral hypoglycemic drugs, or non-injectable non-insulin drugs as follows: If the patient is treated with both oral **hypoglycemic drugs** and insulin, both code Z79.4, Long term (current) use of insulin, and code Z79.84, Long term (current) use of oral hypoglycemic drugs, should be assigned. If the patient is treated with both insulin and an injectable non-insulin antidiabetic drug, assign codes Z79.4,

Long- term (current) use of insulin, and **Z79.85, Long-term (current) use of injectable non-insulin antidiabetic drugs.** If the patient is treated with both oral hypoglycemic drugs and an injectable non-insulin antidiabetic drug, assign codes Z79.84, Long-term (current) use of oral hypoglycemic drugs, and **Z79.85, Long-term (current) use of injectable non-insulin antidiabetic drugs.** Code Z79.4 should not be assigned if insulin is given temporarily to bring a type 2 patient's blood sugar under control during an encounter.

(b) Assigning and sequencing secondary diabetes codes and its causes

The sequencing of the secondary diabetes codes in relationship to codes for the cause of the diabetes is based on the Tabular List instructions for categories E08, E09 and E13.

(i) Secondary diabetes mellitus due to pancreatectomy
For postpancreatectomy diabetes mellitus (lack of insulin due to the surgical removal of all or part of the pancreas), assign code E89.1, Postprocedural hypoinsulinemia. Assign a code from category E13 as the principal or firstlisted diagnosis and a code from subcategory Z90.41-, Acquired absence of pancreas, as additional codes.

(ii) Secondary diabetes due to drugs
Secondary diabetes may be caused by an adverse effect of correctly administered medications, poisoning or sequela of poisoning.

See Section I.C.19.e for coding of adverse effects and poisoning, and Section I.C.20 for external cause code reporting.

b. Obesity

The obesity codes in category E66, Overweight and obesity, include codes related to the cause of obesity, such as drug-induced obesity (E66.1), and codes related to effects of obesity, such as code E66.2, Morbid (severe) obesity with alveolar hypoventilation. There are other codes related to obesity in other categories of the classification, such as E88.82, Obesity due to disruption of MC4R pathway; and codes in fifth character subcategory O99.21, Obesity complicating pregnancy, childbirth, and the puerperium.

1) Obesity class

The obesity class codes in subcategory E66.81, Obesity class, require a fifth character to convey the severity of obesity. The obesity class should be documented in the medical record by the provider for these codes to be assigned. The obesity class codes can be reported with other obesity codes in the classification found in Chapters 4 and 15 to fully describe the condition. However, if both class 3 obesity and morbid obesity are documented, only a code for class 3 obesity should be assigned as it is more specific.

5. **Chapter 5: Mental, Behavioral and Neurodevelopmental disorders (F01 – F99)**

   a. Pain disorders related to psychological factors

   Assign code F45.41, for pain that is exclusively related to psychological disorders. As indicated by the Excludes1 note under category G89, a code from category G89 should not be assigned with code F45.41

   Code F45.42, Pain disorders with related psychological factors, should be used with a code from category G89, Pain, not elsewhere classified, if there is documentation of a psychological component for a patient with acute or chronic pain.
   See Section I.C.6. Pain

   b. Mental and behavioral disorders due to psychoactive substance use

   1) In Remission

   Selection of codes **describing** "in remission" for categories F10-F19, Mental and behavioral disorders due to psychoactive substance use (categories F10-F19 with -11, -.21, **-91**) requires the provider's clinical judgment **and** are assigned only on the basis of provider documentation (as defined in the Official Guidelines for Coding and Reporting), unless otherwise instructed by the classification.

   Mild substance use disorders in early or sustained remission are classified to the appropriate codes for substance abuse in remission, and moderate or severe substance use disorders in early or sustained remission are classified to the appropriate codes for substance dependence in remission.

   2) Psychoactive Substance Use, Abuse and Dependence

   When the provider documentation refers to use, abuse and dependence of the same substance (e.g., alcohol, opioid, cannabis, etc.), only one code should be assigned to identify the pattern of use based on the following hierarchy:

   - If both use and abuse are documented, assign only the code for abuse
   - If both abuse and dependence are documented, assign only the code for dependence
   - If use, abuse and dependence are all documented, assign only the code for dependence
   - If both use and dependence are documented, assign only the code for dependence.

   3) Psychoactive Substance Use, Unspecified

   As with all other unspecified diagnoses, the codes for unspecified psychoactive substance use disorders (F10.9-, F11.9-, F12.9-, F13.9-, F14.9-, F15.9-, F16.9-, F18.9-, F19.9-) should only be assigned based on provider documentation and when they meet the definition of a reportable diagnosis (see Section III, Reporting Additional Diagnoses). These codes are to be used only when the psychoactive substance use is associated 1with a substance related disorder (chapter 5 such as sexual dysfunction and sleep disorder, or a mental or behavioral disorder) or medical condition, and such a relationship is documented by the provider.

   4) Medical Conditions Due to Psychoactive Substance Use, Abuse and Dependence

   Medical conditions due to substance use, abuse, and dependence are not classified as substance-induced disorders. Assign the diagnosis code for the medical condition as directed by the Alphabetical Index along with the appropriate psychoactive substance use, abuse or dependence code. For example, for alcoholic pancreatitis due to alcohol dependence, assign the appropriate code from subcategory K85.2, Alcohol induced acute pancreatitis, and the appropriate code from subcategory F10.2, such as code F10.20, Alcohol dependence, uncomplicated. It would not be appropriate to assign code F10.288, Alcohol dependence with other alcohol-induced disorder.

   5) Blood Alcohol Level

   A code from category Y90, Evidence of alcohol involvement determined by blood alcohol level, may be assigned when this information is documented and the patient's provider has documented a condition classifiable to category F10, Alcohol related disorders. The blood alcohol level does not need to be documented by the patient's provider in order for it to be coded.

   See Section I.B.14. for blood alcohol level documentation by clinicians other than patient's provider.

   c. Factitious Disorder

   Factitious disorder imposed on self or Munchausen's syndrome is a disorder in which a person falsely reports or causes his or her own physical or psychological signs or symptoms. For patients with documented factitious disorder on self or Munchausen's syndrome, assign the appropriate code from subcategory F68.1-, Factitious disorder imposed on self.

   Munchausen's syndrome by proxy (MSBP) is a disorder in which a caregiver (perpetrator) falsely reports or causes an illness or injury in another person (victim) under his or her care, such as a child, an elderly adult, or a person who has a disability. The condition is also referred to as "factitious disorder imposed on another" or "factitious disorder by proxy." The perpetrator, not the victim, receives this diagnosis. Assign code F68.A, Factitious disorder imposed on another, to the perpetrator's record. For the victim of a patient suffering from MSBP, assign the appropriate code from categories T74, Adult and child abuse, neglect and other maltreatment, confirmed, or T76, Adult and child abuse, neglect and other maltreatment, suspected.

   See Section I.C.19.f. Adult and child abuse, neglect and other maltreatment

   d. Dementia

   The ICD-10-CM classifies dementia (categories F01, F02, and F03) on the basis of the etiology and severity (unspecified, mild, moderate or severe). Selection of the appropriate severity level requires the provider's clinical judgment and codes should be assigned only on the basis of provider documentation (as defined in the

Official Guidelines for Coding and Reporting), **unless otherwise instructed by the classification. If the documentation does not provide information about the severity of the dementia, assign the appropriate code for unspecified severity.**

If a patient is admitted to an inpatient acute care hospital or other inpatient facility setting with dementia at one severity level and it progresses to a higher severity level, assign one code for the highest severity level reported during the stay.

6. **Chapter 6: Diseases of the Nervous System (G00-G99)**

   a. **Dominant/nondominant side**

   Codes from category G81, Hemiplegia and hemiparesis, and subcategories, G83.1, Monoplegia of lower limb, G83.2, Monoplegia of upper limb, and G83.3, Monoplegia, unspecified, identify whether the dominant or nondominant side is affected. Should the affected side be documented, but not specified as dominant or nondominant, and the classification system does not indicate a default, code selection is as follows:

   - For ambidextrous patients, the default should be dominant.
   - If the left side is affected, the default is non-dominant.
   - If the right side is affected, the default is dominant.

   b. **Pain - Category G89**

   1) **General coding information**

   Codes in category G89, Pain, not elsewhere classified, may be used in conjunction with codes from other categories and chapters to provide more detail about acute or chronic pain and neoplasm-related pain, unless otherwise indicated below.

   If the pain is not specified as acute or chronic, post-thoracotomy, postprocedural, or neoplasm-related, do not assign codes from category G89.

   A code from category G89 should not be assigned if the underlying (definitive) diagnosis is known, unless the reason for the encounter is pain control/management and not management of the underlying condition.

   When an admission or encounter is for a procedure aimed at treating the underlying condition (e.g., spinal fusion, kyphoplasty), a code for the underlying condition (e.g., vertebral fracture, spinal stenosis) should be assigned as the principal diagnosis. No code from category G89 should be assigned.

   (a) **Category G89 Codes as Principal or First-Listed Diagnosis**

   Category G89 codes are acceptable as principal diagnosis or the first-listed code:

   - When pain control or pain management is the reason for the admission/encounter (e.g., a patient with displaced intervertebral disc, nerve impingement and severe back pain presents for injection of steroid into the spinal canal). The underlying cause of the pain should be reported as an additional diagnosis, if known.

   - When a patient is admitted for the insertion of a neurostimulator for pain control, assign the appropriate pain code as the principal or first-listed diagnosis. When an admission or encounter is for a procedure aimed at treating the underlying condition and a neurostimulator is inserted for pain control during the same admission/encounter, a code for the underlying condition should be assigned as the principal diagnosis and the appropriate pain code should be assigned as a secondary diagnosis.

   (b) **Use of Category G89 Codes in Conjunction with Site-Specific Pain Codes**

   (i) **Assigning Category G89 and Site-Specific Pain Codes**

   Codes from category G89 may be used in conjunction with codes that identify the site of pain (including codes from Chapter 18) if the category G89 code provides additional information. For example, if the code describes the site of the pain, but does not fully describe whether the pain is acute or chronic, then both codes should be assigned.

   (ii) **Sequencing of Category G89 Codes with Site-Specific Pain Codes**

   The sequencing of category G89 codes with site-specific pain codes (including Chapter 18 codes), is dependent on the circumstances of the encounter/admission as follows:

   - If the encounter is for pain control or pain management, assign the code from category G89 followed by the code identifying the specific site of pain (e.g., encounter for pain management for acute neck pain from trauma is assigned code G89.11, Acute pain due to trauma, followed by code M54.2, Cervicalgia, to identify the site of pain).
   - If the encounter is for any other reason except pain control or pain management, and a related definitive diagnosis has not been established (confirmed) by the provider, assign the code for the specific site of pain first, followed by the appropriate code from category G89.

   2) **Pain due to devices, implants and grafts**
   See Section I.C.19. Pain due to medical devices

   3) **Postoperative Pain**
   The provider's documentation should be used to guide the coding of postoperative pain, as well as Section III. Reporting Additional Diagnoses and Section IV. Diagnostic Coding and Reporting in the Outpatient Setting.

   The default for post-thoracotomy and other postoperative pain not specified as acute or chronic is the code for the acute form.

   Routine or expected postoperative pain immediately after surgery should not be coded.

(a) Postoperative pain not associated with specific postoperative complication

Postoperative pain not associated with a specific postoperative complication is assigned to the appropriate postoperative pain code in category G89.

(b) Postoperative pain associated with specific postoperative complication

Postoperative pain associated with a specific postoperative complication (such as painful wire sutures) is assigned to the appropriate code(s) found in Chapter 19, Injury, poisoning, and certain other consequences of external causes. If appropriate, use additional code(s) from category G89 to identify acute or chronic pain (G89.18 or G89.28).

4) Chronic pain

Chronic pain is classified to subcategory G89.2. There is no time frame defining when pain becomes chronic pain. The provider's documentation should be used to guide use of these codes.

5) Neoplasm Related Pain

Code G89.3 is assigned to pain documented as being related, associated or due to cancer, primary or secondary malignancy, or tumor. This code is assigned regardless of whether the pain is acute or chronic.

This code may be assigned as the principal or first-listed code when the stated reason for the admission/encounter is documented as pain control/pain management. The underlying neoplasm should be reported as an additional diagnosis.

When the reason for the admission/encounter is management of the neoplasm and the pain associated with the neoplasm is also documented, code G89.3 may be assigned as an additional diagnosis. It is not necessary to assign an additional code for the site of the pain.

See Section I.C.2 for instructions on the sequencing of neoplasms for all other stated reasons for the admission/encounter (except for pain control/pain management).

6) Chronic pain syndrome

Central pain syndrome (G89.0) and chronic pain syndrome (G89.4) are different than the term "chronic pain," and therefore codes should only be used when the provider has specifically documented this condition.

See Section I.C.5. Pain disorders related to psychological factors

7. Chapter 7: Diseases of the Eye and Adnexa (H00-H59)

a. Glaucoma

1) Assigning Glaucoma Codes

Assign as many codes from category H40, Glaucoma, as needed to identify the type of glaucoma, the affected eye, and the glaucoma stage.

2) Bilateral glaucoma with same type and stage

When a patient has bilateral glaucoma and both eyes are documented as being the same type and stage, and there is a code for bilateral glaucoma, report only the code for the type of glaucoma, bilateral, with the seventh character for the stage.

When a patient has bilateral glaucoma and both eyes are documented as being the same type and stage, and the classification does not provide a code for bilateral glaucoma (i.e., subcategories H40.10, H40.11 and H40.20) report only one code for the type of glaucoma with the appropriate seventh character for the stage.

3) Bilateral glaucoma stage with different types or stages

When a patient has bilateral glaucoma and each eye is documented as having a different type or stage, and the classification distinguishes laterality, assign the appropriate code for each eye rather than the code for bilateral glaucoma.

When a patient has bilateral glaucoma and each eye is documented as having a different type, and the classification does not distinguish laterality (i.e., subcategories H40.10, H40.11 and H40.20), assign one code for each type of glaucoma with the appropriate 7th character for the stage.

When a patient has bilateral glaucoma and each eye is documented as having the same type, but different stage, and the classification does not distinguish laterality (i.e., subcategories H40.10, H40.11 and H40.20), assign a code for the type of glaucoma for each eye with the 7th character for the specific glaucoma stage documented for each eye.

4) Patient admitted with glaucoma and stage evolves during the admission

If a patient is admitted with glaucoma and the stage progresses during the admission, assign the code for highest stage documented.

5) Indeterminate stage glaucoma

Assignment of the 7th character "4" for "indeterminate stage" should be based on the clinical documentation. The 7th character "4" is used for glaucomas whose stage cannot be clinically determined. This 7th character should not be confused with the 7th character "0", unspecified, which should be assigned when there is no documentation regarding the stage of the glaucoma.

b. Blindness

If "blindness" or "low vision" of both eyes is documented but the visual impairment category is not documented, assign code H54.3, Unqualified visual loss, both eyes. If "blindness" or "low vision" in one eye is documented but the visual impairment category is not documented, assign a code from H54.6-, Unqualified visual loss, one eye. If "blindness" or "visual loss" is documented without any information about whether one or both eyes are affected, assign code H54.7, Unspecified visual loss.

8. Chapter 8: Diseases of the Ear and Mastoid Process (H60-H95)

Reserved for future guideline expansion

9. Chapter 9: Diseases of the Circulatory System (I00-I99)

a. Hypertension

The classification presumes a causal relationship between hypertension and heart involvement and between hypertension and kidney involvement, as the two conditions are linked by the term "with" in the Alphabetic Index. These conditions should be coded as related even in the absence of provider documentation explicitly linking them, unless the documentation clearly states the conditions are unrelated.

For hypertension and conditions not specifically linked by relational terms such as "with," "associated with" or "due to" in the classification, provider documentation must link the conditions in order to code them as related.

1) Hypertension with Heart Disease

Hypertension with heart conditions classified to I50.-, Heart failure, I51.4-, Myocarditis, unspecified, I51.89, Other ill-defined heart diseases, and I51.9, Heart disease, unspecified, is assigned to a code from category I11, Hypertensive heart disease. Use additional code(s) from category I50, Heart failure, or I51, Complications and ill-defined descriptions of heart disease, to identify the heart condition.

Hypertension with heart conditions classified to I51.5, Myocardial degeneration, or I51.7, Cardiomegaly, is assigned to a code from category I11, Hypertensive heart disease. No additional code is assigned to identify the specific heart condition.

The same heart conditions (I50.-, I51.4-I51.7, I51.89, I51.9) with hypertension are coded separately if the provider has documented they are unrelated to the hypertension. The applicable hypertension code I10, Essential (primary) hypertension, or a code from category I15, Secondary hypertension, should be assigned. Sequence according to the circumstances of the admission/encounter.

2) Hypertensive Chronic Kidney Disease

Assign codes from category I12, Hypertensive chronic kidney disease, when both hypertension and a condition classifiable to category N18, Chronic kidney disease (CKD), are present. CKD should not be coded as hypertensive if the provider indicates the CKD is not related to the hypertension.

The appropriate code from category N18 should be used as a secondary code with a code from category I12 to identify the stage of chronic kidney disease.

See Section I.C.14. Chronic kidney disease.

If a patient has hypertensive chronic kidney disease and acute renal failure, the acute renal failure should also be coded. Sequence according to the circumstances of the admission/encounter.

3) Hypertensive Heart and Chronic Kidney Disease

Assign codes from combination category I13, Hypertensive heart and chronic kidney disease, when there is hypertension with both heart and chronic kidney disease. If heart failure is present,

assign an additional code from category I50 to identify the type of heart failure.

The appropriate code from category N18, Chronic kidney disease, should be used as a secondary code with a code from category I13 to identify the stage of chronic kidney disease.

See Section I.C.14. Chronic kidney disease.

The codes in category I13, Hypertensive heart and chronic kidney disease, are combination codes that include hypertension, heart disease and chronic kidney disease. The Includes note at I13 specifies that the conditions included at I11 and I12 are included together in I13. If a patient has hypertension, heart disease and chronic kidney disease then a code from I13 should be used, not codes from I11 or I12.

For patients with both acute renal failure and chronic kidney disease the acute renal failure should also be coded. Sequence according to the circumstances of the admission/encounter.

4) Hypertensive Cerebrovascular Disease

For hypertensive cerebrovascular disease, first assign the appropriate code from categories I60-I69, followed by the appropriate hypertension code.

5) Hypertensive Retinopathy

Subcategory H35.0, Background retinopathy and retinal vascular changes, should be used with a code from category I10 – I15, Hypertensive disease to include the systemic hypertension. The sequencing is based on the reason for the encounter.

6) Hypertension, Secondary

Secondary hypertension is due to an underlying condition. Two codes are required: one to identify the underlying etiology and one from category I15 to identify the hypertension. Sequencing of codes is determined by the reason for admission/encounter.

7) Hypertension, Transient

Assign code R03.0, Elevated blood pressure reading without diagnosis of hypertension, unless patient has an established diagnosis of hypertension. Assign code O13.-, Gestational [pregnancy-induced] hypertension without significant proteinuria, or O14.-, Pre-eclampsia, for transient hypertension of pregnancy.

8) Hypertension, Controlled

This diagnostic statement usually refers to an existing state of hypertension under control by therapy. Assign the appropriate code from categories I10-I15, Hypertensive diseases.

9) Hypertension, Uncontrolled

Uncontrolled hypertension may refer to untreated hypertension or hypertension not responding to current therapeutic regimen. In either case, assign the appropriate code from categories I10-I15, Hypertensive diseases.

10) Hypertensive Crisis

Assign a code from category I16, Hypertensive crisis, for documented hypertensive urgency, hypertensive emergency or unspecified hypertensive crisis. Code also any identified hypertensive disease (I10-I15). The sequencing is based on the reason for the encounter.

11) Pulmonary Hypertension

Pulmonary hypertension is classified to category I27, Other pulmonary heart diseases. For secondary pulmonary hypertension (I27.1, I27.2-), code also any associated conditions or adverse effects of drugs or toxins. The sequencing is based on the reason for the encounter, except for adverse effects of drugs.

See Section I.C.19.e

12) Hypertension, Resistant

Resistant hypertension refers to blood pressure of a patient with hypertension that remains above goal in spite of the use of antihypertensive medications. Assign code I1A.Ø, Resistant hypertension, as an additional code when apparent treatment resistant hypertension, treatment resistant hypertension, or true resistant hypertension is documented by the provider. A code for the specific type of existing hypertension is sequenced first, if known.

b. Atherosclerotic Coronary Artery Disease and Angina

ICD-10-CM has combination codes for atherosclerotic heart disease with angina pectoris. The subcategories for these codes are I25.11, Atherosclerotic heart disease of native coronary artery with angina pectoris and I25.7, Atherosclerosis of coronary artery bypass graft(s) and coronary artery of transplanted heart with angina pectoris.

When using one of these combination codes it is not necessary to use an additional code for angina pectoris. A causal relationship can be assumed in a patient with both atherosclerosis and angina pectoris, unless the documentation indicates the angina is due to something other than the atherosclerosis.

If a patient with coronary artery disease is admitted due to an acute myocardial infarction (AMI), the AMI should be sequenced before the coronary artery disease.

See Section I.C.9. Acute myocardial infarction (AMI)

c. Intraoperative and Postprocedural Cerebrovascular Accident

Medical record documentation should clearly specify the cause-and-effect relationship between the medical intervention and the cerebrovascular accident in order to assign a code for intraoperative or postprocedural cerebrovascular accident.

Proper code assignment depends on whether it was an infarction or hemorrhage and whether it occurred intraoperatively or postoperatively. If it was a cerebral hemorrhage, code assignment depends on the type of procedure performed.

d. Sequelae of Cerebrovascular Disease

1) Category I69, Sequelae of Cerebrovascular disease

Category I69 is used to indicate conditions classifiable to categories I60-I67 as the causes of sequela (neurologic deficits), themselves classified elsewhere. These "late effects" include neurologic deficits that persist after initial onset of conditions classifiable to categories I60-I67. The neurologic deficits caused by cerebrovascular disease may be present from the onset or may arise at any time after the onset of the condition classifiable to categories I60-I67.

Codes from category I69, Sequelae of cerebrovascular disease, that specify hemiplegia, hemiparesis and monoplegia identify whether the dominant or nondominant side is affected. Should the affected side be documented, but not specified as dominant or nondominant, and the classification system does not indicate a default, code selection is as follows:

- For ambidextrous patients, the default should be dominant.
- If the left side is affected, the default is non-dominant.
- If the right side is affected, the default is dominant.

2) Codes from category I69 with codes from I60-I67

Codes from category I69 may be assigned on a health care record with codes from I60-I67, if the patient has a current cerebrovascular disease and deficits from an old cerebrovascular disease.

3) Codes from category I69 and Personal history of transient ischemic attack (TIA) and cerebral infarction (Z86.73)

Codes from category I69 should not be assigned if the patient does not have neurologic deficits.

See Section I.C.21. 4. History (of) for use of personal history codes

e. Acute myocardial infarction (AMI)

1) Type 1 ST elevation myocardial infarction (STEMI) and non ST elevation myocardial infarction (NSTEMI)

The ICD-10-CM codes for type 1 acute myocardial infarction (AMI) identify the site, such as anterolateral wall or true posterior wall. Subcategories I21.0-I21.2 and code I21.3 are used for type 1 ST elevation myocardial infarction (STEMI). Code I21.4, Non-ST elevation (NSTEMI) myocardial infarction, is used for type 1 non ST elevation myocardial infarction (NSTEMI) and nontransmural MIs.

If a type 1 NSTEMI evolves to STEMI, assign the STEMI code. If a type 1 STEMI converts to NSTEMI due to thrombolytic therapy, it is still coded as STEMI.

For encounters occurring while the myocardial infarction is equal to, or less than, 4 weeks old, including transfers to another acute setting or a postacute setting, and the myocardial infarction meets the definition for "other diagnoses" (see Section III, Reporting Additional Diagnoses), codes from category I21 may continue to be reported. For encounters after the 4 week time frame and the patient is still receiving care related to the myocardial infarction, the appropriate aftercare code should be assigned, rather than a code from category I21. For old or healed myocardial infarctions not requiring further care, code I25.2, Old myocardial infarction, may be assigned.

2) Acute myocardial infarction, unspecified

Code I21.9, Acute myocardial infarction, unspecified, is the default for unspecified acute myocardial infarction or unspecified type. If only type 1 STEMI or transmural MI without the site is documented, assign code I21.3, ST elevation (STEMI) myocardial infarction of unspecified site.

3) AMI documented as nontransmural or subendocardial but site provided

If an AMI is documented as nontransmural or subendocardial, but the site is provided, it is still coded as a subendocardial AMI.

See Section I.C.21.3 for information on coding status post administration of tPA in a different facility within the last 24 hours.

4) Subsequent acute myocardial infarction

A code from category I22, Subsequent ST elevation (STEMI) and non ST elevation (NSTEMI) myocardial infarction, is to be used when a patient who has suffered a type 1 or unspecified AMI has a new AMI within the 4 week time frame of the initial AMI. A code from category I22 must be used in conjunction with a code from category I21. The sequencing of the I22 and I21 codes depends on the circumstances of the encounter.

Do not assign code I22 for subsequent myocardial infarctions other than type 1 or unspecified. For subsequent type 2 AMI assign only code I21.A1. For subsequent type 4 or type 5 AMI, assign only code I21.A9.

If a subsequent myocardial infarction of one type occurs within 4 weeks of a myocardial infarction of a different type, assign the appropriate codes from category I21 to identify each type. Do not assign a code from I22. Codes from category I22 should only be assigned if both the initial and subsequent myocardial infarctions are type 1 or unspecified.

5) Other Types of Myocardial Infarction

The ICD-10-CM provides codes for different types of myocardial infarction. Type 1 myocardial infarctions are assigned to codes I21.0-I21.4.

Type 2 myocardial infarction (myocardial infarction due to demand ischemia or secondary to ischemic imbalance) is assigned to code I21.A1, Myocardial infarction type 2 with the underlying cause coded first, if applicable. Do not assign code I24.8, Other forms of acute ischemic heart disease, for the demand ischemia. If a type 2 AMI is described as NSTEMI or STEMI, only assign code I21.A1. Codes I21.01-I21.4 should only be assigned for type 1 AMIs.

Acute myocardial infarctions type 3, 4a, 4b, 4c, and 5 are assigned to code I21.A9, Other myocardial infarction type.

The "Code also" and "Code first" notes should be followed related to complications, and for coding of postprocedural myocardial infarctions during or following cardiac surgery.

6) Myocardial Infarction with Coronary Microvascular Dysfunction

Coronary microvascular dysfunction (CMD) is a condition that impacts the microvasculature by restricting microvascular flow and increasing microvascular resistance. Code I21.B, Myocardial infarction with coronary microvascular dysfunction, is assigned for myocardial infarction with coronary microvascular disease, myocardial infarction with coronary microvascular dysfunction, and myocardial infarction with non-obstructive coronary arteries (MINOCA) with microvascular disease.

10. Chapter 10: Diseases of the Respiratory System (J00-J99, U07.1)

a. Chronic Obstructive Pulmonary Disease [COPD] and Asthma

1) Acute exacerbation of chronic obstructive bronchitis and asthma

The codes in categories J44 and J45 distinguish between uncomplicated cases and those in acute exacerbation. An acute exacerbation is a worsening or a decompensation of a chronic condition. An acute exacerbation is not equivalent to an infection superimposed on a chronic condition, though an exacerbation may be triggered by an infection.

b. Acute Respiratory Failure

1) Acute respiratory failure as principal diagnosis

A code from subcategory J96.0, Acute respiratory failure, or subcategory J96.2, Acute and chronic respiratory failure, may be assigned as a principal diagnosis when it is the condition established after study to be chiefly responsible for occasioning the admission to the hospital, and the selection is supported by the Alphabetic Index and Tabular List. However, chapter-specific coding guidelines (such as obstetrics, poisoning, HIV, newborn) that provide sequencing direction take precedence.

2) Acute respiratory failure as secondary diagnosis

Respiratory failure may be listed as a secondary diagnosis if it occurs after admission, or if it is present on admission, but does not meet the definition of principal diagnosis.

3) Sequencing of acute respiratory failure and another acute condition

When a patient is admitted with respiratory failure and another acute condition (e.g., myocardial infarction, cerebrovascular accident, aspiration pneumonia), the principal diagnosis will not be the same in every situation. This applies whether the other acute condition is a respiratory or nonrespiratory condition. Selection of the principal diagnosis will be dependent on the circumstances of admission. If both the respiratory failure and the other acute condition are equally responsible for occasioning the admission to the hospital, and there are no chapter-specific sequencing rules, the guideline regarding two or more diagnoses that equally meet the definition for principal diagnosis (Section II, C.) may be applied in these situations.

If the documentation is not clear as to whether acute respiratory failure and another condition are equally responsible for occasioning the admission, query the provider for clarification.

c. Influenza due to certain identified influenza viruses

Code only confirmed cases of influenza due to certain identified influenza viruses (category J09), and due to other identified influenza virus (category J10). This is an exception to the hospital inpatient guideline Section II, H. (Uncertain Diagnosis).

In this context, "confirmation" does not require documentation of positive laboratory testing specific for avian or other novel influenza A or other identified influenza virus. However, coding should be based on the provider's diagnostic statement that the patient has avian influenza, or other novel influenza A, for category J09, or has another particular identified strain of influenza, such as H1N1 or H3N2, but not identified as novel or variant, for category J10.

If the provider records "suspected" or "possible" or "probable" avian influenza, or novel influenza, or other identified influenza, then the appropriate influenza code from category J11, Influenza due to unidentified influenza virus, should be assigned. A code from category J09, Influenza due to certain identified influenza viruses, should not be assigned nor should a code from category J10, Influenza due to other identified influenza virus.

d. Ventilator associated Pneumonia

1) Documentation of Ventilator associated Pneumonia

As with all procedural or postprocedural complications, code assignment is based on the provider's documentation of the relationship between the condition and the procedure.

Code J95.851, Ventilator associated pneumonia, should be assigned only when the provider has documented ventilator associated pneumonia (VAP). An additional code to identify the organism (e.g., Pseudomonas aeruginosa, code B96.5) should also be assigned. Do not assign an additional code from categories J12-J18 to identify the type of pneumonia.

Code J95.851 should not be assigned for cases where the patient has pneumonia and is on a mechanical ventilator and the provider has not specifically stated that the pneumonia is ventilator-associated pneumonia. If the documentation is unclear as to whether the patient has a pneumonia that is a complication attributable to the mechanical ventilator, query the provider.

2) Ventilator associated Pneumonia Develops after Admission

A patient may be admitted with one type of pneumonia (e.g., code J13, Pneumonia due to Streptococcus pneumonia) and subsequently develop VAP. In this instance, the principal diagnosis would be the appropriate code from categories J12-J18 for the pneumonia diagnosed at the time of admission. Code J95.851, Ventilator associated pneumonia, would be assigned as an additional diagnosis when the provider has also documented the presence of ventilator associated pneumonia.

e. Vaping-related disorders

For patients presenting with condition(s) related to vaping, assign code U07.0, Vaping-related disorder, as the principal diagnosis. For lung injury due to vaping, assign only code U07.0. Assign additional codes for other manifestations, such as acute respiratory failure (subcategory J96.0-) or pneumonitis (code J68.0).

Associated respiratory signs and symptoms due to vaping, such as cough, shortness of breath, etc., are not coded separately, when a definitive diagnosis has been established. However, it would be appropriate to code separately any gastrointestinal symptoms, such as diarrhea and abdominal pain.

11. Chapter 11: Diseases of the Digestive System (K00-K95)

Reserved for future guideline expansion

12. Chapter 12: Diseases of the Skin and Subcutaneous Tissue (L00-L99)

a. Pressure ulcer stage codes

1) Pressure ulcer stages

Codes in category L89, Pressure ulcer, identify the site and stage of the pressure ulcer.

The ICD-10-CM classifies pressure ulcer stages based on severity, which is designated by stages 1-4, deep tissue pressure injury, unspecified stage, and unstageable.

Assign as many codes from category L89 as needed to identify all the pressure ulcers the patient has, if applicable.

See Section I.B.14 for pressure ulcer stage documentation by clinicians other than patient's provider

2) Unstageable pressure ulcers

Assignment of the code for unstageable pressure ulcer (L89.--0) should be based on the clinical documentation. These codes are used for pressure ulcers whose stage cannot be clinically determined (e.g., the ulcer is covered by eschar or has been treated with a skin or muscle graft). This code should not be confused with the codes for unspecified stage (L89.--9). When there is no documentation regarding the stage of the pressure ulcer, assign the appropriate code for unspecified stage (L89.9).

If during an encounter, the stage of an unstageable pressure ulcer is revealed after debridement, assign only the code for the stage revealed following debridement.

3) Documented pressure ulcer stage

Assignment of the pressure ulcer stage code should be guided by clinical documentation of the stage or documentation of the terms found in the Alphabetic Index. For clinical terms describing the stage that are not found in the Alphabetic Index, and there is no documentation of the stage, the provider should be queried.

4) Patients admitted with pressure ulcers documented as healed

No code is assigned if the documentation states that the pressure ulcer is completely healed at the time of admission.

5) Pressure ulcers documented as healing

Pressure ulcers described as healing should be assigned the appropriate pressure ulcer stage code based on the documentation in the medical record. If the documentation does not provide information about the stage of the healing pressure ulcer, assign the appropriate code for unspecified stage.

If the documentation is unclear as to whether the patient has a current (new) pressure ulcer or if the patient is being treated for a healing pressure ulcer, query the provider.

For ulcers that were present on admission but healed at the time of discharge, assign the code for the site and stage of the pressure ulcer at the time of admission.

6) Patient admitted with pressure ulcer evolving into another stage during the admission

If a patient is admitted to an inpatient hospital with a pressure ulcer at one stage and it progresses to a higher stage, two separate codes should be assigned: one code for the site and stage of the ulcer on admission and a second code for the same ulcer site and the highest stage reported during the stay.

7) Pressure-induced deep tissue damage

For pressure-induced deep tissue damage or deep tissue pressure injury, assign only the appropriate code for pressure-induced deep tissue damage (L89.--6).

b. Non-Pressure Chronic Ulcers

1) Patients admitted with non-pressure ulcers documented as healed

No code is assigned if the documentation states that the non-pressure ulcer is completely healed at the time of admission.

2) Non-pressure ulcers documented as healing

Non-pressure ulcers described as healing should be assigned the appropriate non-pressure ulcer code based on the documentation in the medical record. If the documentation does not provide information about the severity of the healing non-pressure ulcer, assign the appropriate code for unspecified severity.

If the documentation is unclear as to whether the patient has a current (new) non-pressure ulcer or if the patient is being treated for a healing non-pressure ulcer, query the provider.

For ulcers that were present on admission but healed at the time of discharge, assign the code for the site and severity of the non-pressure ulcer at the time of admission.

3) Patient admitted with non-pressure ulcer that progresses to another severity level during the admission

If a patient is admitted to an inpatient hospital with a non-pressure ulcer at one severity level and it progresses to a higher severity level, two separate codes should be assigned: one code for the site and severity level of the ulcer on admission and a second code for the same ulcer site and the highest severity level reported during the stay.

See Section I.B.14 for pressure ulcer stage documentation by clinicians other than patient's provider

13. Chapter 13: Diseases of the Musculoskeletal System and Connective Tissue (M00-M99)

a. Site and laterality

Most of the codes within Chapter 13 have site and laterality designations. The site represents the bone, joint or the muscle involved.

1) Bone versus joint

For certain conditions, the bone may be affected at the upper or lower end (e.g., avascular necrosis of bone, M87, Osteoporosis, M80, M81). Though the portion of the bone affected may be at the joint, the site designation will be the bone, not the joint.

2) Multiple sites

Codes describing specified sites are assigned individually by site when documented. When the specified site(s) are not documented, assign the appropriate code for "multiple sites."

b. Acute traumatic versus chronic or recurrent musculoskeletal conditions

Many musculoskeletal conditions are a result of previous injury or trauma to a site, or are recurrent conditions. Bone, joint or muscle conditions that are the result of a healed injury are usually found in Chapter 13. Recurrent bone, joint or muscle conditions are also usually found in Chapter 13. Any current, acute injury should be coded to the appropriate injury code from Chapter 19. Chronic or recurrent conditions should generally be coded with a code from Chapter 13. If it is difficult to determine from the documentation in the record which code is best to describe a condition, query the provider.

c. Coding of Pathologic Fractures

Seventh character A is for use as long as the patient is receiving active treatment for the fracture. While the patient may be seen by a new or different provider over the course of treatment for a pathological fracture, assignment of the 7th character is based on whether the patient is undergoing active treatment and not whether the provider is seeing the patient for the first time.

Seventh character, D is to be used for encounters after the patient has completed active treatment for the fracture and is receiving routine care for the fracture during the healing or recovery phase. The other 7th characters, listed under each subcategory in the Tabular List, are to be used for subsequent encounters for treatment of problems associated with the healing, such as malunions, nonunions, and sequelae.

Care for complications of surgical treatment for fracture repairs during the healing or recovery phase should be coded with the appropriate complication codes.

See Section I.C.19. Coding of traumatic fractures

d. Osteoporosis

Osteoporosis is a systemic condition, meaning that all bones of the musculoskeletal system are affected. Therefore, site is not a component of the codes under category M81, Osteoporosis without current pathological fracture. The site codes under category M80, Osteoporosis with current pathological fracture, identify the site of the fracture, not the osteoporosis.

1) Osteoporosis without pathological fracture

Category M81, Osteoporosis without current pathological fracture, is for use for patients with osteoporosis who do not currently have a pathologic fracture due to the osteoporosis, even if they have had a fracture in the past. For patients with a history of osteoporosis fractures, status code Z87.310, Personal history of (healed) osteoporosis fracture, should follow the code from M81.

2) Osteoporosis with current pathological fracture

Category M80, Osteoporosis with current pathological fracture, is for patients who have a current pathologic fracture at the time of an encounter. The codes under M80 identify the site of the fracture. A code from category M80, not a traumatic fracture code, should be used for any patient with known osteoporosis who suffers a fracture, even if the patient had a minor fall or trauma, if that fall or trauma would not usually break a normal, healthy bone.

e. Multisystem Inflammatory Syndrome

See Section I.C.1.g.1.l for Multisystem Inflammatory Syndrome

14. Chapter 14: Diseases of Genitourinary System (N00-N99)

a. Chronic kidney disease

1) Stages of chronic kidney disease (CKD)

The ICD-10-CM classifies CKD based on severity. The severity of CKD is designated by stages 1-5. Stage 2, code N18.2, equates to mild CKD; stage 3, codes N18.30-N18.32, equate to moderate CKD; and stage 4, code N18.4, equates to severe CKD. Code N18.6, End stage renal disease (ESRD), is assigned when the provider has documented end-stage-renal disease (ESRD).

If both a stage of CKD and ESRD are documented, assign code N18.6 only.

2) Chronic kidney disease and kidney transplant status

Patients who have undergone kidney transplant may still have some form of chronic kidney disease (CKD) because the kidney transplant may not fully restore kidney function. Therefore, the presence of CKD alone does not constitute a transplant complication. Assign the appropriate N18 code for the patient's stage of CKD and code Z94.0, Kidney transplant status. If a transplant complication such as failure or rejection or other transplant complication is documented, see Section I.C.19.g for information on coding complications of a kidney transplant. If the documentation is unclear as to whether the patient has a complication of the transplant, query the provider.

3) Chronic kidney disease with other conditions

Patients with CKD may also suffer from other serious conditions, most commonly diabetes mellitus and hypertension. The sequencing of the CKD code in relationship to codes for other contributing conditions is based on the conventions in the Tabular List.

See I.C.9. Hypertensive chronic kidney disease.
See I.C.19. Chronic kidney disease and kidney transplant complications.

15. Chapter 15: Pregnancy, Childbirth, and the Puerperium (O00-O9A)

a. General Rules for Obstetric Cases

1) Codes from chapter 15 and sequencing priority

Obstetric cases require codes from chapter 15, codes in the range O00-O9A, Pregnancy, Childbirth, and the Puerperium. Chapter 15 codes have sequencing priority over codes from other chapters. Additional codes from other chapters may be used in conjunction with chapter 15 codes to further specify conditions. Should the provider document that the pregnancy is incidental to the encounter, then code Z33.1, Pregnant state, incidental, should be used in place of any chapter 15 codes. It is the provider's responsibility to state that the condition being treated is not affecting the pregnancy.

2) Chapter 15 codes used only on the maternal record

Chapter 15 codes are to be used only on the maternal record, never on the record of the newborn.

3) Final character for trimester

The majority of codes in Chapter 15 have a final character indicating the trimester of pregnancy. The timeframes for the trimesters are indicated at the beginning of the chapter. If trimester is not a component of a code it is because the condition always occurs in a specific trimester, or the concept of trimester of pregnancy is not applicable. Certain codes have characters for only certain trimesters because the condition does not occur in all trimesters, but it may occur in more than just one.

Assignment of the final character for trimester should be based on the provider's documentation of the trimester (or number of weeks) for the current admission/encounter. This applies to the assignment of trimester for pre-existing conditions as well as those that develop during or are due to the pregnancy. The provider's documentation of the number of weeks may be used to assign the appropriate code identifying the trimester.

Whenever delivery occurs during the current admission, and there is an "in childbirth" option for the obstetric complication being coded, the "in childbirth" code should be assigned.

When the classification does not provide an obstetric code with an "in childbirth" option, it is appropriate to assign a code describing the current trimester.

4) Selection of trimester for inpatient admissions that encompass more than one trimester

In instances when a patient is admitted to a hospital for complications of pregnancy during one trimester and remains in the hospital into a subsequent trimester, the trimester character for the antepartum complication code should be assigned on the basis of the trimester when the complication developed, not the trimester of the discharge. If the condition developed prior to the current admission/encounter or represents a pre-existing condition, the trimester character for the trimester at the time of the admission/encounter should be assigned.

5) Unspecified trimester

Each category that includes codes for trimester has a code for "unspecified trimester." The "unspecified trimester" code should rarely be used, such as when the documentation in the record is insufficient to determine the trimester and it is not possible to obtain clarification.

6) 7th character for fetus identification

Where applicable, a 7th character is to be assigned for certain categories (O31, O32, O33.3 - O33.6, O35, O36, O40, O41, O60.1, O60.2, O64, and O69) to identify the fetus for which the complication code applies.

Assign 7th character "0":
- For single gestations
- When the documentation in the record is insufficient to determine the fetus affected and it is not possible to obtain clarification.
- When it is not possible to clinically determine which fetus is affected.

7) Completed weeks of gestation

In ICD-10-CM, "completed" weeks of gestation refers to full weeks. For example, if the provider documents gestation at 39 weeks and 6 days, the code for 39 weeks of gestation should be assigned, as the patient has not yet reached 40 completed weeks.

b. Selection of OB Principal or First-listed Diagnosis

1) Routine outpatient prenatal visits

For routine outpatient prenatal visits when no complications are present, a code from category Z34, Encounter for supervision of normal pregnancy, should be used as the first-listed diagnosis. These codes should not be used in conjunction with chapter 15 codes.

2) Supervision of High-Risk Pregnancy

Codes from category O09, Supervision of high-risk pregnancy, are intended for use only during the prenatal period. For complications during the labor or delivery episode as a result of a high-risk pregnancy, assign the applicable complication codes from chapter 15. If there are no complications during the labor or delivery episode, assign code O80, Encounter for full-term uncomplicated delivery.

For routine prenatal outpatient visits for patients with high-risk pregnancies, a code from category O09, Supervision of high-risk pregnancy, should be used as the first-listed diagnosis. Secondary Chapter 15 codes may be used in conjunction with these codes if appropriate.

3) Episodes when no delivery occurs

In episodes when no delivery occurs, the principal diagnosis should correspond to the principal complication of the pregnancy which necessitated the encounter. Should more than one complication exist, all of which are treated or monitored, any of the complication codes may be sequenced first.

4) When a delivery occurs

When an obstetric patient is admitted and delivers during that admission, the condition that prompted the admission should be sequenced as the principal diagnosis. If multiple conditions prompted the admission, sequence the one most related to the delivery as the principal diagnosis. A code for any complication of the delivery should be assigned as an additional diagnosis. In cases of cesarean delivery, if the patient was admitted with a condition that resulted in the performance of a cesarean procedure, that condition should be selected as the principal diagnosis. If the reason for the admission was unrelated to the condition resulting in the cesarean delivery, the condition related to the reason for the admission should be selected as the principal diagnosis.

5) Outcome of delivery

A code from category Z37, Outcome of delivery, should be included on every maternal record when a delivery has occurred. These codes are not to be used on subsequent records or on the newborn record.

c. Pre-existing conditions versus conditions due to the pregnancy

Certain categories in Chapter 15 distinguish between conditions of the mother that existed prior to pregnancy (pre-existing) and those that are a direct result of pregnancy. When assigning codes from Chapter 15, it is important to assess if a condition was pre-existing prior to pregnancy or developed during or due to the pregnancy in order to assign the correct code.

Categories that do not distinguish between pre-existing and pregnancy-related conditions may be used for either. It is acceptable to use codes specifically for the puerperium with codes complicating pregnancy and childbirth if a condition arises postpartum during the delivery encounter.

d. Pre-existing hypertension in pregnancy

Category O10, Pre-existing hypertension complicating pregnancy, childbirth and the puerperium, includes codes for hypertensive heart and hypertensive chronic kidney disease. When assigning one of the O10 codes that includes hypertensive heart disease or hypertensive chronic kidney disease, it is necessary to add a secondary code from the appropriate hypertension category to specify the type of heart failure or chronic kidney disease.

See Section I.C.9. Hypertension.

e. Fetal Conditions Affecting the Management of the Mother

1) Codes from categories O35 and O36

Codes from categories O35, Maternal care for known or suspected fetal abnormality and damage, and O36, Maternal care for other fetal problems, are assigned only when the fetal condition is actually responsible for modifying the management of the mother, i.e., by requiring diagnostic studies, additional observation, special care, or termination of pregnancy. The fact that the fetal condition exists does not justify assigning a code from this series to the mother's record.

2) In utero surgery

In cases when surgery is performed on the fetus, a diagnosis code from category O35, Maternal care for known or suspected fetal abnormality and damage, should be assigned identifying the fetal condition. Assign the appropriate procedure code for the procedure performed.

No code from Chapter 16, the perinatal codes, should be used on the mother's record to identify fetal conditions. Surgery performed in utero on a fetus is still to be coded as an obstetric encounter.

f. HIV Infection in Pregnancy, Childbirth and the Puerperium

During pregnancy, childbirth or the puerperium, a patient admitted because of an HIV-related illness should receive a principal diagnosis from subcategory O98.7-, Human immunodeficiency [HIV] disease complicating pregnancy, childbirth and the puerperium, followed by the code(s) for the HIV-related illness(es).

Patients with asymptomatic HIV infection status admitted during pregnancy, childbirth, or the puerperium should receive codes of O98.7- and Z21, Asymptomatic human immunodeficiency virus [HIV] infection status.

g. Diabetes mellitus in pregnancy

Diabetes mellitus is a significant complicating factor in pregnancy. Pregnant patients who are diabetic should be assigned a code from category O24, Diabetes mellitus in pregnancy, childbirth, and the puerperium, first, followed by the appropriate diabetes code(s) (E08-E13) from Chapter 4.

h. Longterm use of insulin and oral hypoglycemics

See section I.C.4.a.3 for information on the longterm use of insulin and oral hypoglycemics.

i. Gestational (pregnancy induced) diabetes

Gestational (pregnancy induced) diabetes can occur during the second and third trimester of pregnancy in patients who were not diabetic prior to pregnancy. Gestational diabetes can cause complications in the pregnancy similar to those of pre-existing diabetes mellitus. It also puts the patient at greater risk of developing diabetes after the pregnancy. Codes for gestational diabetes are in subcategory O24.4, Gestational diabetes mellitus. No other code from category O24, Diabetes mellitus in pregnancy, childbirth, and the puerperium, should be used with a code from O24.4.

The codes under subcategory O24.4 include diet controlled, insulin controlled, and controlled by oral hypoglycemic drugs. If a patient with gestational diabetes is treated with both diet and insulin, only the code for insulin-controlled is required. If a patient with gestational diabetes is treated with both diet and oral hypoglycemic medications, only the code for "controlled by oral hypoglycemic drugs" is required. Codes Z79.4, Long-term (current) use of insulin, Z79.84, Long-term (current) use of oral hypoglycemic drugs, **and Z79.85, Long-term (current) use of injectable non-insulin antidiabetic drugs,** should not be assigned with codes from subcategory O24.4.

An abnormal glucose tolerance in pregnancy is assigned a code from subcategory O99.81, Abnormal glucose complicating pregnancy, childbirth, and the puerperium.

j. Sepsis and septic shock complicating abortion, pregnancy, childbirth and the puerperium

When assigning a chapter 15 code for sepsis complicating abortion, pregnancy, childbirth, and the puerperium, a code for the specific type of infection should be assigned as an additional diagnosis. If severe sepsis is present, a code from subcategory R65.2, Severe sepsis, and code(s) for associated organ dysfunction(s) should also be assigned as additional diagnoses.

k. Puerperal sepsis

Code O85, Puerperal sepsis, should be assigned with a secondary code to identify the causal organism (e.g., for a bacterial infection, assign a code from category B95-B96, Bacterial infections in conditions classified elsewhere). A code from category A40, Streptococcal sepsis, or A41, Other sepsis, should not be used for puerperal sepsis. If applicable, use additional codes to identify severe sepsis (R65.2-) and any associated acute organ dysfunction.

Code O85 should not be assigned for sepsis following an obstetrical procedure (See Section I.C.1.d.5.b., Sepsis due to a postprocedural infection).

l. Alcohol, tobacco and drug use during pregnancy, childbirth and the puerperium

1) Alcohol use during pregnancy, childbirth and the puerperium

Codes under subcategory O99.31, Alcohol use complicating pregnancy, childbirth, and the puerperium, should be assigned for any pregnancy case when a patient uses alcohol during the pregnancy or postpartum. A secondary code from category F10, Alcohol related disorders, should also be assigned to identify manifestations of the alcohol use.

2) Tobacco use during pregnancy, childbirth and the puerperium

Codes under subcategory O99.33, Smoking (tobacco) complicating pregnancy, childbirth, and the puerperium, should be assigned for any pregnancy case when a patient uses any type of tobacco product during the pregnancy or postpartum. A secondary code from category F17, Nicotine dependence, should also be assigned to identify the type of nicotine dependence.

3) Drug use during pregnancy, childbirth and the puerperium

Codes under subcategory O99.32, Drug use complicating pregnancy, childbirth, and the puerperium, should be assigned for any pregnancy case when a patient uses drugs during the pregnancy or postpartum. This can involve illegal drugs, or inappropriate use or abuse of prescription drugs. Secondary code(s) from categories F11-F16 and F18-F19 should also be assigned to identify manifestations of the drug use.

m. Poisoning, toxic effects, adverse effects and underdosing in a pregnant patient

A code from subcategory O9A.2, Injury, poisoning and certain other consequences of external causes complicating pregnancy, childbirth, and the puerperium, should be sequenced first, followed by the appropriate injury, poisoning, toxic effect, adverse effect or underdosing code, and then the additional code(s) that specifies the condition caused by the poisoning, toxic effect, adverse effect or underdosing.

See Section I.C.19. Adverse effects, poisoning, underdosing and toxic effects.

n. Normal Delivery, Code O80

1) Encounter for full term uncomplicated delivery

Code O80 should be assigned when a patient is admitted for a full-term normal delivery and delivers a single, healthy infant without any complications antepartum, during the delivery, or postpartum during the delivery episode. Code O80 is always a principal diagnosis. It is not to be used if any other code from chapter 15 is needed to describe a current complication of the antenatal, delivery, or postnatal period. Additional codes from other chapters may be used with code O80 if they are not related to or are in any way complicating the pregnancy.

2) Uncomplicated delivery with resolved antepartum complication

Code O80 may be used if the patient had a complication at some point during the pregnancy, but the complication is not present at the time of the admission for delivery.

3) Outcome of delivery for O80

Z37.0, Single live birth, is the only outcome of delivery code appropriate for use with O80.

o. The Peripartum and Postpartum Periods

1) Peripartum and Postpartum periods

The postpartum period begins immediately after delivery and continues for six weeks following delivery. The peripartum period is defined as the last month of pregnancy to five months postpartum.

2) Peripartum and postpartum complication

A postpartum complication is any complication occurring within the six week period.

3) Pregnancy-related complications after 6-week period

Chapter 15 codes may also be used to describe pregnancy-related complications after the peripartum or postpartum period if the provider documents that a condition is pregnancy related.

4) Admission for routine postpartum care following delivery outside hospital

When the mother delivers outside the hospital prior to admission and is admitted for routine postpartum care and no complications are noted, code Z39.0, Encounter for care and examination of mother immediately after delivery, should be assigned as the principal diagnosis.

5) Pregnancy associated cardiomyopathy

Pregnancy associated cardiomyopathy, code O90.3, is unique in that it may be diagnosed in the third trimester of pregnancy but may continue to progress months after delivery. For this reason, it is referred to as peripartum cardiomyopathy. Code O90.3 is only for use when the cardiomyopathy develops as a result of pregnancy in a patient who did not have pre-existing heart disease.

p. Code O94, Sequelae of complication of pregnancy, childbirth, and the puerperium

1) Code O94

Code O94, Sequelae of complication of pregnancy, childbirth, and the puerperium, is for use in those cases when an initial complication of a pregnancy develops a sequela or sequelae requiring care or treatment at a future date.

2) After the initial postpartum period

This code may be used at any time after the initial postpartum period.

3) Sequencing of Code O94

This code, like all sequela codes, is to be sequenced following the code describing the sequelae of the complication.

q. Termination of Pregnancy and Spontaneous abortions

1) Abortion with Liveborn Fetus

When an attempted termination of pregnancy results in a liveborn fetus assign code Z33.2, Encounter for elective termination of pregnancy and a code from category Z37, Outcome of Delivery.

2) Retained Products of Conception following an abortion

Subsequent encounters for retained products of conception following a spontaneous abortion or elective termination of pregnancy, without complications are assigned O03.4, Incomplete spontaneous abortion without complication or code O07.4, Failed attempted termination of pregnancy without complication. This advice is appropriate even when the patient was discharged previously with a discharge diagnosis of complete abortion. If the patient has a specific complication associated with the spontaneous abortion or elective termination of pregnancy in addition to retained products of conception, assign the appropriate complication code (e.g., O03.-, O04.-, O07.-) instead of code O03.4 or O07.4

3) Complications leading to abortion

Codes from chapter 15 may be used as additional codes to identify any documented complications of the pregnancy in conjunction with codes in categories in O04, O07 and O08.

4) Hemorrhage following elective abortion
For hemorrhage post elective abortion, assign code O04.6, Delayed or excessive hemorrhage following (induced) termination of pregnancy. Do not assign code O72.1, Other immediate postpartum hemorrhage, as this code should not be assigned for post abortion conditions.

r. Abuse in a pregnant patient
For suspected or confirmed cases of abuse of a pregnant patient, a code(s) from subcategories O9A.3, Physical abuse complicating pregnancy, childbirth, and the puerperium, O9A.4, Sexual abuse complicating pregnancy, childbirth, and the puerperium, and O9A.5, Psychological abuse complicating pregnancy, childbirth, and the puerperium, should be sequenced first, followed by the appropriate codes (if applicable) to identify any associated current injury due to physical abuse, sexual abuse, and the perpetrator of abuse.

See Section I.C.19. Adult and child abuse, neglect and other maltreatment.

s. COVID-19 infection in pregnancy, childbirth, and the puerperium
During pregnancy, childbirth or the puerperium, when COVID-19 is the reason for admission/encounter, code O98.5-, Other viral diseases complicating pregnancy, childbirth and the puerperium, should be sequenced as the principal/first-listed diagnosis, and code U07.1, COVID-19, and the appropriate codes for associated manifestation(s) should be assigned as additional diagnoses. Codes from Chapter 15 always take sequencing priority.

If the reason for admission/encounter is unrelated to COVID-19 but the patient has been diagnosed with COVID-19 during the admission/encounter, the appropriate code for the reason for admission/encounter should be sequenced as the principal/first-listed diagnosis, and codes O98.5- and U07.1, as well as the appropriate codes for associated COVID-19 manifestations, should be assigned as additional diagnoses.

16. Chapter 16: Certain Conditions Originating in the Perinatal Period (P00-P96)
For coding and reporting purposes the perinatal period is defined as before birth through the 28th day following birth. The following guidelines are provided for reporting purposes

a. General Perinatal Rules

1) Use of Chapter 16 Codes
Codes in this chapter are never for use on the maternal record. Codes from Chapter 15, the obstetric chapter, are never permitted on the newborn record. Chapter 16 codes may be used throughout the life of the patient if the condition is still present.

2) Principal Diagnosis for Birth Record
When coding the birth episode in a newborn record, assign a code from category Z38, Liveborn infants according to place of birth and type of delivery, as the principal diagnosis. A code from category Z38 is assigned only once, to a newborn at the time of birth. If a newborn is transferred to another institution, a code from category Z38 should not be used at the receiving hospital.

A code from category Z38 is used only on the newborn record, not on the mother's record.

3) Use of Codes from other Chapters with Codes from Chapter 16
Codes from other chapters may be used with codes from chapter 16 if the codes from the other chapters provide more specific detail. Codes for signs and symptoms may be assigned when a definitive diagnosis has not been established. If the reason for the encounter is a perinatal condition, the code from chapter 16 should be sequenced first.

4) Use of Chapter 16 Codes after the Perinatal Period
Should a condition originate in the perinatal period, and continue throughout the life of the patient, the perinatal code should continue to be used regardless of the patient's age.

5) Birth process or community acquired conditions
If a newborn has a condition that may be either due to the birth process or community acquired and the documentation does not indicate which it is, the default is due to the birth process and the code from Chapter 16 should be used. If the condition is community-acquired, a code from Chapter 16 should not be assigned.

For COVID-19 infection in a newborn, see guideline I.C.16.h.

6) Code all clinically significant conditions
All clinically significant conditions noted on routine newborn examination should be coded. A condition is clinically significant if it requires:
- clinical evaluation; or
- therapeutic treatment; or
- diagnostic procedures; or
- extended length of hospital stay; or
- increased nursing care and/or monitoring; or
- has implications for future health care needs

Note: The perinatal guidelines listed above are the same as the general coding guidelines for "additional diagnoses," except for the final point regarding implications for future health care needs. Codes should be assigned for conditions that have been specified by the provider as having implications for future health care needs.

b. Observation and Evaluation of Newborns for Suspected Conditions not Found

1) Use of Z05 codes
Assign a code from category Z05, Observation and evaluation of newborn for suspected **diseases and** conditions ruled out, to identify those instances when a healthy newborn is evaluated for a suspected condition/**disease** that is determined after study not to be present. Do not use a code

from category Z05 when the patient **is documented to have** signs or symptoms of a suspected problem; in such cases code the sign or symptom.

2) Z05 on other than the birth record
A code from category Z05 may also be assigned as a principal or firstlisted code for readmissions or encounters when the code from category Z38 code no longer applies. Codes from category Z05 are for use only for healthy newborns and infants for which no condition after study is found to be present.

3) Z05 on a birth record
A code from category Z05 is to be used as a secondary code after the code from category Z38, Liveborn infants according to place of birth and type of delivery.

c. Coding Additional Perinatal Diagnoses

1) Assigning codes for conditions that require treatment
Assign codes for conditions that require treatment or further investigation, prolong the length of stay, or require resource utilization.

2) Codes for conditions specified as having implications for future health care needs
Assign codes for conditions that have been specified by the provider as having implications for future health care needs.

Note: This guideline should not be used for adult patients.

d. Prematurity and Fetal Growth Retardation
Providers utilize different criteria in determining prematurity. A code for prematurity should not be assigned unless it is documented. Assignment of codes in categories P05, Disorders of newborn related to slow fetal growth and fetal malnutrition, and P07, Disorders of newborn related to short gestation and low birth weight, not elsewhere classified, should be based on the recorded birth weight and estimated gestational age.

When both birth weight and gestational age are available, two codes from category P07 should be assigned, with the code for birth weight sequenced before the code for gestational age.

e. Low birth weight and immaturity status
Codes from category P07, Disorders of newborn related to short gestation and low birth weight, not elsewhere classified, are for use for a child or adult who was premature or had a low birth weight as a newborn and this is affecting the patient's current health status.

See Section I.C.21. Factors influencing health status and contact with health services, Status.

f. Bacterial Sepsis of Newborn
Category P36, Bacterial sepsis of newborn, includes congenital sepsis. If a perinate is documented as having sepsis without documentation of congenital or community acquired, the default is congenital and a code from category P36 should be assigned. If the P36 code includes the causal organism, an additional code from category B95, Streptococcus, Staphylococcus, and Enterococcus as the cause of diseases classified elsewhere, or B96, Other bacterial

agents as the cause of diseases classified elsewhere, should not be assigned. If the P36 code does not include the causal organism, assign an additional code from category B96. If applicable, use additional codes to identify severe sepsis (R65.2-) and any associated acute organ dysfunction.

g. Stillbirth
Code P95, Stillbirth, is only for use in institutions that maintain separate records for stillbirths. No other code should be used with P95. Code P95 should not be used on the mother's record.

h. COVID-19 Infection in Newborn
For a newborn that tests positive for COVID-19, assign code U07.1, COVID-19, and the appropriate codes for associated manifestation(s) in neonates/newborns in the absence of documentation indicating a specific type of transmission. For a newborn that tests positive for COVID-19 and the provider documents the condition was contracted in utero or during the birth process, assign codes P35.8, Other congenital viral diseases, and U07.1, COVID-19. When coding the birth episode in a newborn record, the appropriate code from category Z38, Liveborn infants according to place of birth and type of delivery, should be assigned as the principal diagnosis.

17. Chapter 17: Congenital malformations, deformations, and chromosomal abnormalities (Q00-QA0)
Assign an appropriate code(s) from categories Q00-QA0, Congenital malformations, deformations, and chromosomal abnormalities when a malformation/deformation or chromosomal abnormality is documented. A malformation/deformation/or chromosomal abnormality may be the principal/first-listed diagnosis on a record or a secondary diagnosis.

When a malformation/deformation/or chromosomal abnormality does not have a unique code assignment, assign additional code(s) for any manifestations that may be present.

When the code assignment specifically identifies the malformation/deformation/or chromosomal abnormality, manifestations that are an inherent component of the anomaly should not be coded separately. Additional codes should be assigned for manifestations that are not an inherent component.

Codes from Chapter 17 may be used throughout the life of the patient. If a congenital malformation or deformity has been corrected, a personal history code should be used to identify the history of the malformation or deformity. Although present at birth, a malformation/deformation/or chromosomal abnormality may not be identified until later in life. Whenever the condition is diagnosed by the provider, it is appropriate to assign a code from codes Q00-QA0.

For the birth admission, the appropriate code from category Z38, Liveborn infants, according to place of birth and type of delivery, should be sequenced as the principal diagnosis, followed by any congenital anomaly codes, Q00-QA0.

18. Chapter 18: Symptoms, signs, and abnormal clinical and laboratory findings, not elsewhere classified (R00-R99)

Chapter 18 includes symptoms, signs, abnormal results of clinical or other investigative procedures, and ill-defined conditions regarding which no diagnosis classifiable elsewhere is recorded. Signs and symptoms that point to a specific diagnosis have been assigned to a category in other chapters of the classification.

a. Use of symptom codes

Codes that describe symptoms and signs are acceptable for reporting purposes when a related definitive diagnosis has not been established (confirmed) by the provider.

b. Use of a symptom code with a definitive diagnosis code

Codes for signs and symptoms may be reported in addition to a related definitive diagnosis when the sign or symptom is not routinely associated with that diagnosis, such as the various signs and symptoms associated with complex syndromes. The definitive diagnosis code should be sequenced before the symptom code.

Signs or symptoms that are associated routinely with a disease process should not be assigned as additional codes, unless otherwise instructed by the classification.

c. Combination codes that include symptoms

ICD-10-CM contains a number of combination codes that identify both the definitive diagnosis and common symptoms of that diagnosis. When using one of these combination codes, an additional code should not be assigned for the symptom.

d. Repeated falls

Code R29.6, Repeated falls, is for use for encounters when a patient has recently fallen and the reason for the fall is being investigated.

Code Z91.81, History of falling, is for use when a patient has fallen in the past and is at risk for future falls. When appropriate, both codes R29.6 and Z91.81 may be assigned together.

e. Coma

Code R40.20, Unspecified coma, should be assigned when the underlying cause of the coma is not known, or the cause is a traumatic brain injury and the coma scale is not documented in the medical record.

Do not report codes for unspecified coma, individual or total Glasgow coma scale scores for a patient with a medically induced coma or a sedated patient.

1) Coma Scale

The coma scale codes (R40.21- to R40.24-) can be used in conjunction with traumatic brain injury codes. These codes cannot be used with code R40.2A, Nontraumatic coma due to underlying condition. They are primarily for use by trauma registries, but they may be used in any setting where this information is collected. The coma scale codes should be sequenced after the diagnosis code(s).

These codes, one from each subcategory, are needed to complete the scale. The 7th character indicates when the scale was recorded. The 7th character should match for all three codes.

At a minimum, report the initial score documented on presentation at your facility. This may be a score from the emergency medicine technician (EMT) or in the emergency department. If desired, a facility may choose to capture multiple coma scale scores.

Assign code R40.24-, Glasgow coma scale, total score, when only the total score is documented in the medical record and not the individual score(s).

If multiple coma scores are captured within the first 24 hours after hospital admission, assign only the code for the score at the time of admission. ICD-10-CM does not classify coma scores that are reported after admission but less than 24 hours later.

See Section I.B.14. for coma scale documentation by clinicians other than patient's provider

f. Functional quadriplegia

GUIDELINE HAS BEEN DELETED EFFECTIVE OCTOBER 1, 2017

g. SIRS due to Non-Infectious Process

The systemic inflammatory response syndrome (SIRS) can develop as a result of certain non-infectious disease processes, such as trauma, malignant neoplasm, or pancreatitis. When SIRS is documented with a noninfectious condition, and no subsequent infection is documented, the code for the underlying condition, such as an injury, should be assigned, followed by code R65.10, Systemic inflammatory response syndrome (SIRS) of non-infectious origin without acute organ dysfunction, or code R65.11, Systemic inflammatory response syndrome (SIRS) of non-infectious origin with acute organ dysfunction. If an associated acute organ dysfunction is documented, the appropriate code(s) for the specific type of organ dysfunction(s) should be assigned in addition to code R65.11. If acute organ dysfunction is documented, but it cannot be determined if the acute organ dysfunction is associated with SIRS or due to another condition (e.g., directly due to the trauma), the provider should be queried.

h. Death NOS

Code R99, Ill-defined and unknown cause of mortality, is only for use in the very limited circumstance when a patient who has already died is brought into an emergency department or other healthcare facility and is pronounced dead upon arrival. It does not represent the discharge disposition of death.

i. NIHSS Stroke Scale

The NIH stroke scale (NIHSS) codes (R29.7- -) can be used in conjunction with acute stroke codes (I60-I63) to identify the patient's neurological status and the severity of the stroke. The stroke scale codes should be sequenced after the acute stroke diagnosis code(s).

At a minimum, report the initial score documented. If desired, a facility may choose to capture multiple stroke scale scores.

See Section I.B.14 for NIHSS stroke scale documentation by clinicians other than patient's provider

19. **Chapter 19: Injury, poisoning, and certain other consequences of external causes (S00-T88)**

   a. **Application of 7th Characters in Chapter 19**

   Most categories in chapter 19 have a 7th character requirement for each applicable code. Most categories in this chapter have three 7th character values (with the exception of fractures): A, initial encounter, D, subsequent encounter and S, sequela. Categories for traumatic fractures have additional 7th character values. While the patient may be seen by a new or different provider over the course of treatment for an injury, assignment of the 7th character is based on whether the patient is undergoing active treatment and not whether the provider is seeing the patient for the first time.

   For complication codes, active treatment refers to treatment for the condition described by the code, even though it may be related to an earlier precipitating problem. For example, code T84.50XA, Infection and inflammatory reaction due to unspecified internal joint prosthesis, initial encounter, is used when active treatment is provided for the infection, even though the condition relates to the prosthetic device, implant or graft that was placed at a previous encounter.

   7th character "A", initial encounter is used for each encounter where the patient is receiving active treatment for the condition.

   7th character "D" subsequent encounter is used for encounters after the patient has completed active treatment of the condition and is receiving routine care for the condition during the healing or recovery phase.

   The aftercare Z codes should not be used for aftercare for conditions such as injuries or poisonings, where 7th characters are provided to identify subsequent care. For example, for aftercare of an injury, assign the acute injury code with the 7th character "D" (subsequent encounter).

   7th character "S", sequela, is for use for complications or conditions that arise as a direct result of a condition, such as scar formation after a burn. The scars are sequelae of the burn. When using 7th character "S", it is necessary to use both the injury code that precipitated the sequela and the code for the sequela itself. The "S" is added only to the injury code, not the sequela code. The 7th character "S" identifies the injury responsible for the sequela. The specific type of sequela (e.g., scar) is sequenced first, followed by the injury code.

   See Section I.B.10. Sequelae, (Late Effects)

   b. **Coding of Injuries**

   When coding injuries, assign separate codes for each injury unless a combination code is provided, in which case the combination code is assigned. Codes from category T07, Unspecified multiple injuries should not be assigned in the inpatient setting unless information for a more specific code is not available. Traumatic injury codes (S00-T14.9) are not to be used for normal, healing surgical wounds or to identify complications of surgical wounds.

   The code for the most serious injury, as determined by the provider and the focus of treatment, is sequenced first.

   1) **Superficial injuries**

   Superficial injuries such as abrasions or contusions are not coded when associated with more severe injuries of the same site.

   2) **Primary injury with damage to nerves/ blood vessels**

   When a primary injury results in minor damage to peripheral nerves or blood vessels, the primary injury is sequenced first with additional code(s) for injuries to nerves and spinal cord (such as category S04), and/or injury to blood vessels (such as category S15). When the primary injury is to the blood vessels or nerves, that injury should be sequenced first.

   3) **Iatrogenic injuries**

   Injury codes from Chapter 19 should not be assigned for injuries that occur during, or as a result of, a medical intervention. Assign the appropriate complication code(s).

   c. **Coding of Traumatic Fractures**

   The principles of multiple coding of injuries should be followed in coding fractures. Fractures of specified sites are coded individually by site in accordance with both the provisions within categories S02, S12, S22, S32, S42, S49, S52, S59, S62, S72, S79, S82, S89, S92 and the level of detail furnished by medical record content.

   A fracture not indicated as open or closed should be coded to closed. A fracture not indicated whether displaced or not displaced should be coded to displaced.

   More specific guidelines are as follows:

   1) **Initial vs. subsequent encounter for fractures**

   Traumatic fractures are coded using the appropriate 7th character for initial encounter (A, B, C) for each encounter where the patient is receiving active treatment for the fracture. The appropriate 7th character for initial encounter should also be assigned for a patient who delayed seeking treatment for the fracture or nonunion.

   Fractures are coded using the appropriate 7th character for subsequent care for encounters after the patient has completed active treatment of the fracture and is receiving routine care for the fracture during the healing or recovery phase.

   Care for complications of surgical treatment for fracture repairs during the healing or recovery phase should be coded with the appropriate complication codes.

   Care of complications of fractures, such as malunion and nonunion, should be reported with the appropriate 7th character for subsequent care with nonunion (K, M, N,) or subsequent care with malunion (P, Q, R).

Malunion/nonunion: The appropriate 7th character for initial encounter should also be assigned for a patient who delayed seeking treatment for the fracture or nonunion.

The open fracture designations in the assignment of the 7th character for fractures of the forearm, femur and lower leg, including ankle are based on the Gustilo open fracture classification. When the Gustilo classification type is not specified for an open fracture, the 7th character for open fracture type I or II should be assigned (B, E, H, M, Q).

A code from category M80, not a traumatic fracture code, should be used for any patient with known osteoporosis who suffers a fracture, even if the patient had a minor fall or trauma, if that fall or trauma would not usually break a normal, healthy bone.

See Section I.C.13. Osteoporosis.

The aftercare Z codes should not be used for aftercare for traumatic fractures. For aftercare of a traumatic fracture, assign the acute fracture code with the appropriate 7th character.

2) Multiple fractures sequencing

Multiple fractures are sequenced in accordance with the severity of the fracture.

3) Physeal fractures

For physeal fractures, assign only the code identifying the type of physeal fracture. Do not assign a separate code to identify the specific bone that is fractured.

d. Coding of Burns and Corrosions

The ICD-10-CM makes a distinction between burns and corrosions. The burn codes are for thermal burns, except sunburns, that come from a heat source, such as a fire or hot appliance. The burn codes are also for burns resulting from electricity and radiation. Corrosions are burns due to chemicals. The guidelines are the same for burns and corrosions.

Current burns (T20-T25) are classified by depth, extent and by agent (X code). Burns are classified by depth as first degree (erythema), second degree (blistering), and third degree (full-thickness involvement). Burns of the eye and internal organs (T26-T28) are classified by site, but not by degree.

1) Sequencing of burn and related condition codes

Sequence first the code that reflects the highest degree of burn when more than one burn is present.

  a. When the reason for the admission or encounter is for treatment of external multiple burns, sequence first the code that reflects the burn of the highest degree.

  b. When a patient has both internal and external burns, the circumstances of admission govern the selection of the principal diagnosis or first-listed diagnosis.

  c. When a patient is admitted for burn injuries and other related conditions such as smoke inhalation and/or respiratory failure, the circumstances of admission govern the selection of the principal or first-listed diagnosis.

2) Burns of the same anatomic site

Classify burns of the same anatomic site and on the same side but of different degrees to the subcategory identifying the highest degree recorded in the diagnosis (e.g., for second and third degree burns of right thigh, assign only code T24.311-).

3) Non-healing burns

Non-healing burns are coded as acute burns. Necrosis of burned skin should be coded as a non-healed burn.

4) Infected burn

For any documented infected burn site, use an additional code for the infection.

5) Assign separate codes for each burn site

When coding burns, assign separate codes for each burn site. Category T30, Burn and corrosion, body region unspecified is extremely vague and should rarely be used.

Codes for burns of "multiple sites" should only be assigned when the medical record documentation does not specify the individual sites.

6) Burns and corrosions classified according to extent of body surface involved

Assign codes from category T31, Burns classified according to extent of body surface involved, or T32, Corrosions classified according to extent of body surface involved, for acute burns or corrosions when the site of the burn or corrosion is not specified or when there is a need for additional data. It is advisable to use category T31 as additional coding when needed to provide data for evaluating burn mortality, such as that needed by burn units. It is also advisable to use category T31 as an additional code for reporting purposes when there is mention of a thirddegree burn involving 20 percent or more of the body surface. Codes from categories T31 and T32 should not be used for sequelae of burns or corrosions.

Categories T31 and T32 are based on the classic "rule of nines" in estimating body surface involved: head and neck are assigned nine percent, each arm nine percent, each leg 18 percent, the anterior trunk 18 percent, posterior trunk 18 percent, and genitalia one percent. Providers may change these percentage assignments where necessary to accommodate infants and children who have proportionately larger heads than adults, and patients who have large buttocks, thighs, or abdomen that involve burns.

7) Encounters for treatment of sequela of burns

Encounters for the treatment of the late effects of burns or corrosions (i.e., scars or joint contractures) should be coded with a burn or corrosion code with the 7th character "S" for sequela.

8) Sequelae with a late effect code and current burn

When appropriate, both a code for a current burn or corrosion with 7th character "A" or "D" and a burn or corrosion code with 7th character "S" may be assigned on the same record (when both a current burn and sequelae of an old burn exist). Burns and corrosions do not heal at the same rate and a current healing wound may still exist with sequela of a healed burn or corrosion.

See Section I.B.10. Sequela, (Late Effects)

9) Use of an external cause code with burns and corrosions

An external cause code should be used with burns and corrosions to identify the source and intent of the burn, as well as the place where it occurred.

e. Adverse Effects, Poisoning, Underdosing and Toxic Effects

Codes in categories T36-T65 are combination codes that include the substance that was taken as well as the intent. No additional external cause code is required for poisonings, toxic effects, adverse effects and underdosing codes.

1) Do not code directly from the Table of Drugs

Do not code directly from the Table of Drugs and Chemicals. Always refer back to the Tabular List.

2) Use as many codes as necessary to describe

Use as many codes as necessary to describe completely all drugs, medicinal or biological substances.

3) If the same code would describe the causative agent

If the same code would describe the causative agent for more than one adverse reaction, poisoning, toxic effect or underdosing, assign the code only once.

4) If two or more drugs, medicinal or biological substances

If two or more drugs, medicinal or biological substances are taken, code each individually unless a combination code is listed in the Table of Drugs and Chemicals.

If multiple unspecified drugs, medicinal or biological substances were taken, assign the appropriate code from subcategory T50.91, Poisoning by, adverse effect of and underdosing of multiple unspecified drugs, medicaments and biological substances.

5) The occurrence of drug toxicity is classified in ICD-10-CM as follows:

(a) Adverse Effect

When coding an adverse effect of a drug that has been correctly prescribed and properly administered, assign the appropriate code for the nature of the adverse effect followed by the appropriate code for the adverse effect of the drug (T36-T50). The code for the drug should have a 5th or 6th character "5" (for example T36.0X5-) Examples of the nature of an adverse effect are tachycardia, delirium, gastrointestinal hemorrhaging, vomiting, hypokalemia, hepatitis, renal failure, or respiratory failure.

(b) Poisoning

When coding a poisoning or reaction to the improper use of a medication (e.g., overdose, wrong substance given or taken in error, wrong route of administration), first assign the appropriate code from categories T36-T50. The poisoning codes have an associated intent as their 5th or 6th character (accidental, intentional self-harm, assault and undetermined). If the intent of the poisoning is unknown or unspecified, code the intent as accidental intent. The undetermined intent is only for use if the documentation

in the record specifies that the intent cannot be determined. Use additional code(s) for all manifestations of poisonings.

If there is also a diagnosis of abuse or dependence of the substance, the abuse or dependence is assigned as an additional code.

Examples of poisoning include:

(i) Error was made in drug prescription Errors made in drug prescription or in the administration of the drug by provider, nurse, patient, or other person.

(ii) Overdose of a drug intentionally taken If an overdose of a drug was intentionally taken or administered and resulted in drug toxicity, it would be coded as a poisoning.

(iii) Nonprescribed drug taken with correctly prescribed and properly administered drug.

If a nonprescribed drug or medicinal agent was taken in combination with a correctly prescribed and properly administered drug, any drug toxicity or other reaction resulting from the interaction of the two drugs would be classified as a poisoning.

(iv) Interaction of drug(s) and alcohol. When a reaction results from the interaction of a drug(s) and alcohol, this would be classified as poisoning.

See Section I.C.4. if poisoning is the result of insulin pump malfunctions.

For Sequela (Late Effects) see Section I.B.10.

(c) Underdosing

Underdosing refers to taking less of a medication than is prescribed by a provider or a manufacturer's instruction. Discontinuing the use of a prescribed medication on the patient's own initiative (not directed by the patient's provider) is also classified as an underdosing. For underdosing, assign the code from categories T36-T50 (fifth or sixth character "6").

Documentation of a change in the patient's condition is not required in order to assign an underdosing code.

Documentation that the patient is taking less of a medication than is prescribed or discontinued the prescribed medication is sufficient for code assignment.

Codes for underdosing should never be assigned as principal or first-listed codes. If a patient has a relapse or exacerbation of the medical condition for which the drug is prescribed because of the reduction in dose, then the medical condition itself should be coded.

Noncompliance (Z91.12-, Z91.13-, **Z91.14-** and **Z91.A4-**) or complication of care (Y63.6-Y63.9) codes are to be used with an underdosing code to indicate intent, if known.

(d) Toxic Effects

When a harmful substance is ingested or comes in contact with a person, this is classified as a toxic effect. The toxic effect codes are in categories T51-T65. **When coding a toxic effect, assign the toxic effect code first, followed by codes for all associated manifestations of the toxic effect.**

Toxic effect codes have an associated intent: accidental, intentional self-harm, assault and undetermined.

For Sequela (Late Effects) see Section I.B.10. Sequela

f. Adult and child abuse, neglect and other maltreatment

Sequence first the appropriate code from categories T74, Adult and child abuse, neglect and other maltreatment, confirmed, or T76, Adult and child abuse, neglect and other maltreatment, suspected, for abuse, neglect and other maltreatment, followed by any accompanying mental health or injury code(s).

If the documentation in the medical record states abuse or neglect it is coded as confirmed (T74.-). It is coded as suspected if it is documented as suspected (T76.-).

For cases of confirmed abuse or neglect an external cause code from the assault section (X92-Y09) should be added to identify the cause of any physical injuries. A perpetrator code (Y07) should be added when the perpetrator of the abuse is known. For suspected cases of abuse or neglect, do not report external cause or perpetrator code.

If a suspected case of abuse, neglect or mistreatment is ruled out during an encounter code Z04.71, Encounter for examination and observation following alleged physical adult abuse, ruled out, or code Z04.72, Encounter for examination and observation following alleged child physical abuse, ruled out, should be used, not a code from T76.

If a suspected case of alleged rape or sexual abuse is ruled out during an encounter code Z04.41, Encounter for examination and observation following alleged adult rape or code Z04.42, Encounter for examination and observation following alleged child rape, should be used, not a code from T76.

If a suspected case of forced sexual exploitation or forced labor exploitation is ruled out during an encounter, code Z04.81, Encounter for examination and observation of victim following forced sexual exploitation, or code Z04.82, Encounter for examination and observation of victim following forced labor exploitation, should be used, not a code from T76.

See Section I.C.15. Abuse in a pregnant patient.

g. Complications of care

1) General guidelines for complications of care

(a) Documentation of complications of care

See Section I.B.16. for information on documentation of complications of care.

2) Pain due to medical devices

Pain associated with devices, implants or grafts left in a surgical site (for example painful hip prosthesis) is assigned to the appropriate code(s) found in Chapter 19, Injury, poisoning, and certain other consequences of external causes. Specific codes for pain due to medical devices are found in the T code section of the ICD-10-CM. Use additional code(s) from category G89 to identify acute or chronic pain due to presence of the device, implant or graft (G89.18 or G89.28).

3) Transplant complications

(a) Transplant complications other than kidney

Codes under category T86, Complications of transplanted organs and tissues, are for use for both complications and rejection of transplanted organs. A transplant complication code is only assigned if the complication affects the function of the transplanted organ. Two codes are required to fully describe a transplant complication: the appropriate code from category T86 and a secondary code that identifies the complication.

Pre-existing conditions or conditions that develop after the transplant are not coded as complications unless they affect the function of the transplanted organs.

See Section I.C.21. for transplant organ removal status
See Section I.C.2. for malignant neoplasm associated with transplanted organ.

See I.C.1.d.4. for sequencing of sepsis due to infection in transplanted organ

(b) Kidney transplant complications

Patients who have undergone kidney transplant may still have some form of chronic kidney disease (CKD) because the kidney transplant may not fully restore kidney function. Code T86.1- should be assigned for documented complications of a kidney transplant, such as transplant failure or rejection or other transplant complication. Code T86.1- should not be assigned for post kidney transplant patients who have chronic kidney (CKD) unless a transplant complication such as transplant failure or rejection is documented. If the documentation is unclear as to whether the patient has a complication of the transplant, query the provider.

Conditions that affect the function of the transplanted kidney, other than CKD, should be assigned a code from subcategory T86.1, Complications of transplanted organ, Kidney, and a secondary code that identifies the complication.

For patients with CKD following a kidney transplant, but who do not have a complication such as failure or rejection, *see Section I.C.14. Chronic kidney disease and kidney transplant status.*

See I.C.1.d.4. for sequencing of sepsis due to infection in transplanted organ

4) Complication codes that include the external cause

As with certain other T codes, some of the complications of care codes have the external cause included in the code. The code includes the nature of the complication as well as the type of procedure that caused the complication. No external cause code indicating the type of procedure is necessary for these codes.

5) Complications of care codes within the body system chapters

Intraoperative and postprocedural complication codes are found within the body system chapters with codes specific to the organs and structures of that body system. These codes should be sequenced first, followed by a code(s) for the specific complication, if applicable.

Complication codes from the body system chapters should be assigned for intraoperative and postprocedural complications (e.g., the appropriate complication code from chapter 9 would be assigned for a vascular intraoperative or postprocedural complication) unless the complication is specifically indexed to a T code in chapter 19.

20. Chapter 20: External Causes of Morbidity (V00-Y99)

The external causes of morbidity codes should never be sequenced as the first-listed or principal diagnosis.

External cause codes are intended to provide data for injury research and evaluation of injury prevention strategies. These codes capture how the injury or health condition happened (cause), the intent (unintentional or accidental; or intentional, such as suicide or assault), the place where the event occurred the activity of the patient at the time of the event, and the person's status (e.g., civilian, military).

There is no national requirement for mandatory ICD-10-CM external cause code reporting. Unless a provider is subject to a state-based external cause code reporting mandate or these codes are required by a particular payer, reporting of ICD-10-CM codes in Chapter 20, External Causes of Morbidity, is not required. In the absence of a mandatory reporting requirement, providers are encouraged to voluntarily report external cause codes, as they provide valuable data for injury research and evaluation of injury prevention strategies.

a. General External Cause Coding Guidelines

1) Used with any code in the range of A00.0-T88.9, Z00-Z99

An external cause code may be used with any code in the range of A00.0-T88.9, Z00-Z99, classification that represents a health condition due to an external cause. Though they are most applicable to injuries, they are also valid for use with such things as infections or diseases due to an external source, and other health conditions, such as a heart attack that occurs during strenuous physical activity.

2) External cause code used for length of treatment

Assign the external cause code, with the appropriate 7th character (initial encounter, subsequent encounter or sequela) for each encounter for which the injury or condition is being treated.

Most categories in Chapter 20 have a 7th character requirement for each applicable code. Most categories in this chapter have three 7th character values: A, initial encounter, D, subsequent encounter and S, sequela. While the patient may be seen by a new or different provider over the course of treatment for an injury or condition, assignment of the 7th character for external cause should match the 7th character of the code assigned for the associated injury or condition for the encounter.

3) Use the full range of external cause codes

Use the full range of external cause codes to completely describe the cause, the intent, the place of occurrence, and if applicable, the activity of the patient at the time of the event, and the patient's status, for all injuries, and other health conditions due to an external cause.

4) Assign as many external cause codes as necessary

Assign as many external cause codes as necessary to fully explain each cause. If only one external code can be recorded, assign the code most related to the principal diagnosis.

5) The selection of the appropriate external cause code

The selection of the appropriate external cause code is guided by the Alphabetic Index of External Causes and by Inclusion and Exclusion notes in the Tabular List.

6) External cause code can never be a principal diagnosis

An external cause code can never be a principal (first-listed) diagnosis.

7) Combination external cause codes

Certain of the external cause codes are combination codes that identify sequential events that result in an injury, such as a fall which results in striking against an object. The injury may be due to either event or both. The combination external cause code used should correspond to the sequence of events regardless of which caused the most serious injury.

8) No external cause code needed in certain circumstances

No external cause code from Chapter 20 is needed if the external cause and intent are included in a code from another chapter (e.g., T36.0X1- Poisoning by penicillins, accidental (unintentional)).

b. Place of Occurrence Guideline

Codes from category Y92, Place of occurrence of the external cause, are secondary codes for use after other external cause codes to identify the location of the patient at the time of injury or other condition.

Generally, a place of occurrence code is assigned only once, at the initial encounter for treatment. However, in the rare instance that a new injury occurs during hospitalization, an additional place of occurrence code may be assigned. No 7th characters are used for Y92.

Do not use place of occurrence code Y92.9 if the place is not stated or is not applicable.

c. Activity Code

Assign a code from category Y93, Activity code, to describe the activity of the patient at the time the injury or other health condition occurred.

An activity code is used only once, at the initial encounter for treatment. Only one code from Y93 should be recorded on a medical record.

The activity codes are not applicable to poisonings, adverse effects, misadventures or sequela.

Do not assign Y93.9, Unspecified activity, if the activity is not stated.

A code from category Y93 is appropriate for use with external cause and intent codes if identifying the activity provides additional information about the event.

d. Place of Occurrence, Activity, and Status Codes Used with other External Cause Code

When applicable, place of occurrence, activity, and external cause status codes are sequenced after the main external cause code(s). Regardless of the number of external cause codes assigned, generally there should be only one place of occurrence code, one activity code, and one external cause status code assigned to an encounter. However, in the rare instance that a new injury occurs during hospitalization, an additional place of occurrence code may be assigned.

e. If the Reporting Format Limits the Number of External Cause Codes

If the reporting format limits the number of external cause codes that can be used in reporting clinical data, report the code for the cause/intent most related to the principal diagnosis. If the format permits capture of additional external cause codes, the cause/intent, including medical misadventures, of the additional events should be reported rather than the codes for place, activity, or external status.

f. Multiple External Cause Coding Guidelines

More than one external cause code is required to fully describe the external cause of an illness or injury. The assignment of external cause codes should be sequenced in the following priority:

If two or more events cause separate injuries, an external cause code should be assigned for each cause. The first-listed external cause code will be selected in the following order:

External codes for child and adult abuse take priority over all other external cause codes.

See Section I.C.19., Child and Adult abuse guidelines.

External cause codes for terrorism events take priority over all other external cause codes except child and adult abuse.

External cause codes for cataclysmic events take priority over all other external cause codes except child and adult abuse and terrorism.

External cause codes for transport accidents take priority over all other external cause codes except cataclysmic events, child and adult abuse and terrorism.

Activity and external cause status codes are assigned following all causal (intent) external cause codes.

The first-listed external cause code should correspond to the cause of the most serious diagnosis due to an assault, accident, or self-harm, following the order of hierarchy listed above.

g. Child and Adult Abuse Guideline

Adult and child abuse, neglect and maltreatment are classified as assault. Any of the assault codes may be used to indicate the external cause of any injury resulting from the confirmed abuse.

For confirmed cases of abuse, neglect and maltreatment, when the perpetrator is known, a code from Y07, Perpetrator of maltreatment and neglect, should accompany any other assault codes.

See Section I.C.19. Adult and child abuse, neglect and other maltreatment

h. Unknown or Undetermined Intent Guideline

If the intent (accident, self-harm, assault) of the cause of an injury or other condition is unknown or unspecified, code the intent as accidental intent. All transport accident categories assume accidental intent.

1) Use of undetermined intent

External cause codes for events of undetermined intent are only for use if the documentation in the record specifies that the intent cannot be determined.

i. Sequelae (Late Effects) of External Cause Guidelines

1) Sequelae external cause codes

Sequela are reported using the external cause code with the 7th character "S" for sequela. These codes should be used with any report of a late effect or sequela resulting from a previous injury.

See Section I.B.10. Sequela (Late Effects)

2) Sequela external cause code with a related current injury

A sequela external cause code should never be used with a related current nature of injury code.

3) Use of sequela external cause codes for subsequent visits

Use a late effect external cause code for subsequent visits when a late effect of the initial injury is being treated. Do not use a late effect external cause code for subsequent visits for follow-up care (e.g., to assess healing, to receive rehabilitative therapy) of the injury when no late effect of the injury has been documented.

j. Terrorism Guidelines

1) Cause of injury identified by the Federal Government (FBI) as terrorism

When the cause of an injury is identified by the Federal Government (FBI) as terrorism, the first-listed external cause code should be a code from category Y38, Terrorism. The definition of terrorism employed by the FBI is found at the inclusion note at the beginning of category Y38. Use additional code for place of occurrence (Y92.-). More than one

Y38 code may be assigned if the injury is the result of more than one mechanism of terrorism.

2) Cause of an injury is suspected to be the result of terrorism

When the cause of an injury is suspected to be the result of terrorism a code from category Y38 should not be assigned. Suspected cases should be classified as assault.

3) Code Y38.9, Terrorism, secondary effects

Assign code Y38.9, Terrorism, secondary effects, for conditions occurring subsequent to the terrorist event. This code should not be assigned for conditions that are due to the initial terrorist act.

It is acceptable to assign code Y38.9 with another code from Y38 if there is an injury due to the initial terrorist event and an injury that is a subsequent result of the terrorist event.

k. External Cause Status

A code from category Y99, External cause status, should be assigned whenever any other external cause code is assigned for an encounter, including an Activity code, except for the events noted below. Assign a code from category Y99, External cause status, to indicate the work status of the person at the time the event occurred. The status code indicates whether the event occurred during military activity, whether a non-military person was at work, whether an individual including a student or volunteer was involved in a non-work activity at the time of the causal event.

A code from Y99, External cause status, should be assigned, when applicable, with other external cause codes, such as transport accidents and falls. The external cause status codes are not applicable to poisonings, adverse effects, misadventures or late effects.

Do not assign a code from category Y99 if no other external cause codes (cause, activity) are applicable for the encounter.

An external cause status code is used only once, at the initial encounter for treatment. Only one code from Y99 should be recorded on a medical record.

Do not assign code Y99.9, Unspecified external cause status, if the status is not stated.

21. Chapter 21: Factors influencing health status and contact with health services (Z00-Z99)

Note: The chapter-specific guidelines provide additional information about the use of Z codes for specified encounters.

a. Use of Z Codes in Any Healthcare Setting

Z codes are for use in any healthcare setting. Z codes may be used as either a first-listed (principal diagnosis code in the inpatient setting) or secondary code, depending on the circumstances of the encounter. Certain Z codes may only be used as first-listed or principal diagnosis.

b. Z Codes Indicate a Reason for an Encounter
or Provide Additional Information about a Patient Encounter

Z codes are not procedure codes. A corresponding procedure code must accompany a Z code to describe any procedure performed.

c. Categories of Z Codes
1) Contact/Exposure

Category Z20 indicates contact with, and suspected exposure to, communicable diseases. These codes are for patients who are suspected to have been exposed to a disease by close personal contact with an infected individual or are in an area where a disease is epidemic.

Category Z77, Other contact with and (suspected) exposures hazardous to health, indicates contact with and suspected exposures hazardous to health.

Contact/exposure codes may be used as a first-listed code to explain an encounter for testing, or, more commonly, as a secondary code to identify a potential risk.

2) Inoculations and vaccinations

Code Z23 is for encounters for inoculations and vaccinations. It indicates that a patient is being seen to receive a prophylactic inoculation against a disease. Procedure codes are required to identify the actual administration of the injection and the type(s) of immunizations given. Code Z23 may be used as a secondary code if the inoculation is given as a routine part of preventive health care, such as a well-baby visit.

3) Status

Status codes indicate that a patient is either a carrier of a disease or has the sequelae or residual of a past disease or condition. This includes such things as the presence of prosthetic or mechanical devices resulting from past treatment. A status code is informative, because the status may affect the course of treatment and its outcome. A status code is distinct from a history code. The history code indicates that the patient no longer has the condition.

A status code should not be used with a diagnosis code from one of the body system chapters, if the diagnosis code includes the information provided by the status code. For example, code Z94.1, Heart transplant status, should not be used with a code from subcategory T86.2, Complications of heart transplant. The status code does not provide additional information. The complication code indicates that the patient is a heart transplant patient.

For encounters for weaning from a mechanical ventilator, assign a code from subcategory J96.1, Chronic respiratory failure, followed by code Z99.11, Dependence on respirator [ventilator] status.

The status Z codes/categories are:

Z14   Genetic carrier

Genetic carrier status indicates that a person carries a gene, associated with a particular disease, which may be passed to offspring who may develop that disease. The person does not have the disease and is not at risk of developing the disease.

Z15   Genetic susceptibility to disease Genetic susceptibility indicates that a person has a gene that increases the risk of that person developing the disease.

Codes from category Z15 should generally not be used as principal or first-listed codes. If the patient has the condition to which he/she is susceptible, and that condition is the reason for the encounter, the code for the current condition should be sequenced first. If the patient is being seen for follow-up after completed treatment for this condition, and the condition no longer exists, a follow-up code should be sequenced first, followed by the appropriate personal history and genetic susceptibility codes. If the purpose of the encounter is genetic counseling associated with procreative management, code Z31.5, Encounter for genetic counseling, should be assigned as the first-listed code, followed by a code from category Z15. Additional codes should be assigned for any applicable family or personal history.

Z16   Resistance to antimicrobial drugs
        This category indicates that a patient has a condition that is resistant to antimicrobial drug treatment. Sequence the infection code first.

Z17   Estrogen, and other hormones and factors receptor status

Z18   Retained foreign body fragments

Z19   Hormone sensitivity malignancy status

Z21   Asymptomatic HIV infection status This code indicates that a patient has tested positive for HIV but has manifested no signs or symptoms of the disease.

Z22   Carrier of infectious disease Carrier status indicates that a person harbors the specific organisms of a disease without manifest symptoms and is capable of transmitting the infection.

Z28.3   Underimmunization status

See Section I.B.14. for underimmunization documentation by clinicians other than the patient's provider.

Z33.1   Pregnant state, incidental This code is a secondary code only for use when the pregnancy is in no way complicating the reason for visit. Otherwise, a code from the obstetric chapter is required.

Z66   Do not resuscitate
This code may be used when it is documented by the provider that a patient is on do not resuscitate status at any time during the stay.

Z67   Blood type

Z68   Body mass index (BMI)
        BMI codes should only be assigned when there is an associated reportable diagnosis (such as obesity or anorexia) documented by the patient's provider. When the documentation reflects fluctuating BMI values during the current encounter for an associated reportable condition, assign a code for the most severe value.

See Section I.B.14 for BMI documentation by clinicians other than the patient's provider.

Z74.01   Bed confinement status

Z76.82   Awaiting organ transplant status

Z78   Other specified health status
Code Z78.1, Physical restraint status, may be used when it is documented by the provider that a patient has been put in restraints during the current encounter. Please note that this code should not be reported when it is documented by the provider that a patient is temporarily restrained during a procedure.

Z79   Long-term (current) drug therapy
Codes from this category indicate a patient's continuous use of a prescribed drug (including such things as aspirin therapy) for the long-term treatment of a condition or for prophylactic use. It is not for use for patients who have addictions to drugs. This subcategory is not for use of medications for detoxification or maintenance programs to prevent withdrawal symptoms (e.g., methadone maintenance for opiate dependence). Assign the appropriate code for the drug use, abuse, or dependence instead.

Assign a code from Z79 if the patient is receiving a medication for an extended period as a prophylactic measure (such as for the prevention of deep vein thrombosis) or as treatment of a chronic condition (such as arthritis) or a disease requiring a lengthy course of treatment (such as cancer). Do not assign a code from category Z79 for medication being administered for a brief period of time to treat an acute illness or injury (such as a course of antibiotics to treat acute bronchitis).

Z88   Allergy status to drugs, medicaments and biological substances Except: Z88.9, Allergy status to unspecified drugs, medicaments and biological substances status

Z89   Acquired absence of limb

Z90   Acquired absence of organs, not elsewhere classified

Z91.0-   Allergy status, other than to drugs and biological substances

Z92.82   Status post administration of tPA (rtPA) in a different facility within the last 24 hours prior to admission to a current facility Assign code Z92.82, Status post administration of tPA (rtPA) in a different facility within the last 24 hours prior to admission to current facility, as a secondary diagnosis when a patient is received by transfer into a facility and documentation indicates they were administered tissue plasminogen activator (tPA) within the last 24 hours prior to admission to the current facility. This guideline applies even if the patient is still receiving the tPA at the time they are received into the current facility. The appropriate code for the condition for which the tPA was administered (such as cerebrovascular disease or myocardial infarction) should be assigned first. Code Z92.82 is only applicable to the receiving facility record and not to the transferring facility record.

Z93	Artificial opening status
Z94	Transplanted organ and tissue status
Z95	Presence of cardiac and vascular implants and grafts
Z96	Presence of other functional implants
Z97	Presence of other devices
Z98	Other postprocedural states

Assign code Z98.85, Transplanted organ removal status, to indicate that a transplanted organ has been previously removed. This code should not be assigned for the encounter in which the transplanted organ is removed. The complication necessitating removal of the transplant organ should be assigned for that encounter.

See Section I.C.19. for information on the coding of organ transplant complications.

| Z99 | Dependence on enabling machines and devices, not elsewhere classified |

Note: Categories Z89-Z90 and Z93-Z99 are for use only if there are no complications or malfunctions of the organ or tissue replaced, the amputation site or the equipment on which the patient is dependent.

4) History (of)

There are two types of history Z codes, personal and family. Personal history codes explain a patient's past medical condition that no longer exists and is not receiving any treatment, but that has the potential for recurrence, and therefore may require continued monitoring.

Family history codes are for use when a patient has a family member(s) who has had a particular disease that causes the patient to be at higher risk of also contracting the disease.

Personal history codes may be used in conjunction with follow-up codes and family history codes may be used in conjunction with screening codes to explain the need for a test or procedure. History codes are also acceptable on any medical record regardless of the reason for visit. A history of an illness, even if no longer present, is important information that may alter the type of treatment ordered.

The reason for the encounter (for example, screening or counseling) should be sequenced first and the appropriate personal and/or family history code(s) should be assigned as additional diagnos(es).

The history Z code categories are:

Z80	Family history of primary malignant neoplasm
Z81	Family history of mental and behavioral disorders
Z82	Family history of certain disabilities and chronic diseases (leading to disablement)
Z83	Family history of other specific disorders
Z84	Family history of other conditions
Z85	Personal history of malignant neoplasm
Z86	Personal history of certain other diseases
Z87	Personal history of other diseases and conditions
Z91.4-	Personal history of psychological trauma, not elsewhere classified
Z91.5	Personal history of self-harm
Z91.81	History of falling
Z91.82	Personal history of military deployment
Z91.85	**Personal history of military service**
Z92	Personal history of medical treatment Except: Z92.0, Personal history of contraception Except: Z92.82, Status post administration of tPA (rtPA) in a different facility within the last 24 hours prior to admission to a current facility

5) Screening

Screening is the testing for disease or disease precursors in seemingly well individuals so that early detection and treatment can be provided for those who test positive for the disease (e.g., screening mammogram).

The testing of a person to rule out or confirm a suspected diagnosis because the patient has some sign or symptom is a diagnostic examination, not a screening. In these cases, the sign or symptom is used to explain the reason for the test.

A screening code may be a first-listed code if the reason for the visit is specifically the screening exam. It may also be used as an additional code if the screening is done during an office visit for other health problems. A screening code is not necessary if the screening is inherent to a routine examination, such as a pap smear done during a routine pelvic examination.

Should a condition be discovered during the screening then the code for the condition may be assigned as an additional diagnosis.

The Z code indicates that a screening exam is planned. A procedure code is required to confirm that the screening was performed.

The screening Z codes/categories:

Z11	Encounter for screening for infectious and parasitic diseases
Z12	Encounter for screening for malignant neoplasms
Z13	Encounter for screening for other diseases and disorders Except: Z13.9, Encounter for screening, unspecified
Z36	Encounter for antenatal screening for mother

6) Observation

There are three observation Z code categories. They are for use in very limited circumstances when a person is being observed for a suspected condition that is ruled out. The observation codes are not for use if an injury or illness or any signs or symptoms related to the suspected condition are present. In such cases the diagnosis/symptom code is used with the corresponding external cause code.

The observation codes are primarily to be used as a principal/first-listed diagnosis. An observation code may be assigned as a secondary diagnosis code when the patient is being observed for a condition that is ruled out and is unrelated to the principal/first-listed diagnosis. Also, when the principal diagnosis is required to be a code from category Z38, Liveborn infants according to place of birth and type of delivery, then a code from category Z05, Encounter for observation and evaluation of newborn for suspected diseases and conditions ruled out, is sequenced after the Z38 code. Additional codes may be used in addition to the observation code, but only if they are unrelated to the suspected condition being observed.

Codes from subcategory Z03.7, Encounter for suspected maternal and fetal conditions ruled out, may either be used as a first-listed or as an additional code assignment depending on the case. They are for use in very limited circumstances on a maternal record when an encounter is for a suspected maternal or fetal condition that is ruled out during that encounter (for example, a maternal or fetal condition may be suspected due to an abnormal test result). These codes should not be used when the condition is confirmed. In those cases, the confirmed condition should be coded. In addition, these codes are not for use if an illness or any signs or symptoms related to the suspected condition or problem are present. In such cases the diagnosis/symptom code is used.

Additional codes may be used in addition to the code from subcategory Z03.7, but only if they are unrelated to the suspected condition being evaluated.

Codes from subcategory Z03.7, may not be used for encounters for antenatal screening of mother. *See Section I.C.21. Screening.*

For encounters for suspected fetal condition that are inconclusive following testing and evaluation, assign the appropriate code from category O35, O36, O40 or O41.

The observation Z code categories:

Z03	Encounter for medical observation for suspected diseases and conditions ruled out
Z04	Encounter for examination and observation for other reasons Except: Z04.9, Encounter for examination and observation for unspecified reason
Z05	Encounter for observation and evaluation of newborn for suspected diseases and conditions ruled out

7) Aftercare

Aftercare visit codes cover situations when the initial treatment of a disease has been performed and the patient requires continued care during the healing or recovery phase, or for the long-term consequences of the disease. The aftercare Z code should not be used if treatment is directed at a current, acute disease. The diagnosis code is to be used in these cases.

The aftercare Z codes should also not be used for aftercare for injuries. For aftercare of an injury, assign the acute injury code with the appropriate 7th character (for subsequent encounter).

The aftercare codes are generally first-listed to explain the specific reason for the encounter. An aftercare code may be reported as an additional code when a specific type of aftercare is provided in addition to the reason for the encounter. An example of this would be the closure of a colostomy during an encounter for treatment of another condition.

Aftercare codes should be used in conjunction with other aftercare codes or diagnosis codes to provide better detail on the specifics of an aftercare encounter visit, unless otherwise directed by the classification. The sequencing of multiple aftercare codes depends on the circumstances of the encounter.

Certain aftercare Z code categories need a secondary diagnosis code to describe the resolving condition or sequelae. For others, the condition is included in the code title.

Additional Z code aftercare category terms include fitting and adjustment, and attention to artificial openings.

Status Z codes may be used with aftercare Z codes to indicate the nature of the aftercare. For example code Z95.1, Presence of aortocoronary bypass graft, may be used with code Z48.812, Encounter for surgical aftercare following surgery on the circulatory system, to indicate the surgery for which the aftercare is being performed. A status code should not be used when the aftercare code indicates the type of status, such as using Z43.0, Encounter for attention to tracheostomy, with Z93.0, Tracheostomy status.

The aftercare codes are generally found in the following categories:

Z42	Encounter for plastic and reconstructive surgery following medical procedure or healed injury
Z43	Encounter for attention to artificial openings
Z44	Encounter for fitting and adjustment of external prosthetic device
Z45	Encounter for adjustment and management of implanted device
Z46	Encounter for fitting and adjustment of other devices
Z47	Orthopedic aftercare
Z48	Encounter for other postprocedural aftercare
Z49	Encounter for care involving renal dialysis
Z51	Encounter for other aftercare and medical care

8) Follow-up

The follow-up codes are used to explain continuing surveillance following completed treatment of a disease, condition, or injury. They imply that the condition has been fully treated and no longer exists. They should not be confused with aftercare codes, or injury codes with a 7th character for subsequent encounter, that explain ongoing care of a healing condition or its sequelae. Follow-up codes may be used in conjunction with history codes to provide the full picture of the healed condition and its treatment. The follow-up code is sequenced first, followed by the history code.

A follow-up code may be used to explain multiple visits. Should a condition be found to have recurred on the follow-up visit, then the diagnosis code for the condition should be assigned in place of the follow-up code.

The follow-up Z **codes**/categories:

Z08   Encounter for follow-up examination after completed treatment for malignant neoplasm

Z09   Encounter for follow-up examination after completed treatment for conditions other than malignant neoplasm

Codes Z08, Encounter for follow-up examination after completed treatment for malignant neoplasm, and Z09, Encounter for follow up examination after completed treatment for conditions other than malignant neoplasm, may be assigned following any type of completed treatment modality (including both medical and surgical treatments).

Z39   Encounter for maternal postpartum care and examination

9) Donor

Codes in category Z52, Donors of organs and tissues, are used for living individuals who are donating blood or other body tissue. These codes are for individuals donating for others, as well as for self-donations. They are not used to identify cadaveric donations.

10) Counseling

Counseling Z codes are used when a patient or family member receives assistance in the aftermath of an illness or injury, or when support is required in coping with family or social problems.

The counseling Z codes/categories:

Z30.0-   Encounter for general counseling and advice on contraception

Z31.5   Encounter for procreative genetic counseling

Z31.6-   Encounter for general counseling and advice on procreation

Z32.2   Encounter for childbirth instruction

Z32.3   Encounter for childcare instruction

Z69   Encounter for mental health services for victim and perpetrator of abuse

Z70   Counseling related to sexual attitude, behavior and orientation

Z71   Persons encountering health services for other counseling and medical advice, not elsewhere classified

Note: Code Z71.84, Encounter for health counseling related to travel, is to be used for health risk and safety counseling for future travel purposes.

Code Z71.85, Encounter for immunization safety counseling, is to be used for counseling of the patient or caregiver regarding the safety of a vaccine. This code should not be used for the provision of general information regarding risks and potential side effects during routine encounters for the administration of vaccines.

Code Z71.87, Encounter for pediatric-to-adult transition counseling, should be assigned when pediatric-to-adult transition counseling is the sole reason for the encounter or when this counseling is provided in addition to other services, such as treatment of a chronic condition. If both transition counseling and treatment of a medical condition are provided during the same encounter, the code(s) for the medical condition(s) treated and code Z71.87 should be assigned, with sequencing depending on the circumstances of the encounter.

Z76.81   Expectant mother prebirth pediatrician visit

11) Encounters for Obstetrical and Reproductive Services

See Section I.C.15. Pregnancy, Childbirth, and the Puerperium, for further instruction on the use of these codes.

Z codes for pregnancy are for use in those circumstances when none of the problems or complications included in the codes from the Obstetrics chapter exist (a routine prenatal visit or postpartum care). Codes in category Z34, Encounter for supervision of normal pregnancy, are always first listed and are not to be used with any other code from the OB chapter.

Codes in category Z3A, Weeks of gestation, may be assigned to provide additional information about the pregnancy. Category Z3A codes should not be assigned for pregnancies with abortive outcomes (categories O00-O08), elective termination of pregnancy (code Z33.2), nor for postpartum conditions, as category Z3A is not applicable to these conditions. The date of the admission should be used to determine weeks of gestation for inpatient admissions that encompass more than one gestational week.

The outcome of delivery, category Z37, should be included on all maternal delivery records. It is always a secondary code. Codes in category Z37 should not be used on the newborn record.

Z codes for family planning (contraceptive) or procreative management and counseling should be included on an obstetric record either during the pregnancy or the postpartum stage, if applicable.

Z codes/categories for obstetrical and reproductive services:

Z30   Encounter for contraceptive management

Z31   Encounter for procreative management

Z32.2   Encounter for childbirth instruction

Z32.3   Encounter for childcare instruction

Z33   Pregnant state

Z34 Encounter for supervision of normal pregnancy

Z36 Encounter for antenatal screening of mother

Z3A Weeks of gestation

Z37 Outcome of delivery

Z39 Encounter for maternal postpartum care and examination

Z76.81 Expectant mother prebirth pediatrician visit

12) Routine and Administrative Examinations

The Z codes allow for the description of encounters for routine examinations, such as, a general check-up, or, examinations for administrative purposes, such as, a pre-employment physical. The codes are not to be used if the examination is for diagnosis of a suspected condition or for treatment purposes. In such cases the diagnosis code is used. During a routine exam, should a diagnosis or condition be discovered, it should be coded as an additional code. Pre-existing and chronic conditions and history codes may also be included as additional codes as long as the examination is for administrative purposes and not focused on any particular condition.

Some of the codes for routine health examinations distinguish between "with" and "without" abnormal findings. Code assignment depends on the information that is known at the time the encounter is being coded. For example, if no abnormal findings were found during the examination, but the encounter is being coded before test results are back, it is acceptable to assign the code for "without abnormal findings." When assigning a code for "with abnormal findings," additional code(s) should be assigned to identify the specific abnormal finding(s).

Pre-operative examination and pre-procedural laboratory examination Z codes are for use only in those situations when a patient is being cleared for a procedure or surgery and no treatment is given.

The Z codes/categories for routine and administrative examinations:

Z00 Encounter for general examination without complaint, suspected or reported diagnosis

Z01 Encounter for other special examination without complaint, suspected or reported diagnosis

Z02 Encounter for administrative examination
Except: Z02.9, Encounter for administrative examinations, unspecified

Z32.0- Encounter for pregnancy test

13) Miscellaneous Z Codes

The miscellaneous Z codes capture a number of other health care encounters that do not fall into one of the other categories. Some of these codes identify the reason for the encounter; others are for use as additional codes that provide useful information on circumstances that may affect a patient's care and treatment.

Prophylactic Organ Removal

For encounters specifically for prophylactic removal of an organ (such as prophylactic removal of breasts due to a genetic susceptibility to cancer or a family history of cancer), the principal or first-listed code should be a code from subcategory Z40.0, Encounter for prophylactic surgery for risk factors related to malignant neoplasms, or subcategory Z40.8, Encounter for other prophylactic surgery. If applicable, assign additional code(s) to identify any associated risk factor (such as genetic susceptibility or family history).

If the patient has a malignancy of one site and is having prophylactic removal at another site to prevent either a new primary malignancy or metastatic disease, a code for the malignancy should also be assigned in addition to a code from subcategory Z40.0, Encounter for prophylactic surgery for risk factors related to malignant neoplasms. A Z40.0 code should not be assigned if the patient is having organ removal for treatment of a malignancy, such as the removal of the testes for the treatment of prostate cancer.

Miscellaneous Z codes/subcategories/categories:

Z28 Immunization not carried out
Except: Z28.3, Underimmunization status

Z29 Encounter for other prophylactic measures

Z40 Encounter for prophylactic surgery

Z41 Encounter for procedures for purposes other than remedying health state
Except: Z41.9, Encounter for procedure for purposes other than remedying health state, unspecified

Z72 Problems related to lifestyle
Note: These codes should be assigned only when the documentation specifies that the patient has an associated problem

Z73 Problems related to life management difficulty
Note: These codes should be assigned only when the documentation specifies that the patient has an associated problem.

Z74 Problems related to care provider dependency Except: Z74.01, Bed confinement status

Z75 Problems related to medical facilities and other health care

Z76.0 Encounter for issue of repeat prescription

Z76.3 Healthy person accompanying sick person

Z76.4 Other boarder to healthcare facility

Z76.5 Malingerer [conscious simulation]

Z91.1- Patient's noncompliance with medical treatment and regimen

Z91.A- Caregiver's noncompliance with patient's medical treatment and regimen

Z91.B Personal risk factor of exposure to diethylstilbestrol

Z91.83 Wandering in diseases classified elsewhere
Z91.84- Oral health risk factors
Z91.89 Other specified personal risk factors, not elsewhere classified

See Section I.B.14 for Z55-Z65 Persons with potential health hazards related to socioeconomic and psychosocial circumstances, documentation by clinicians other than the patient's provider

14) Nonspecific Z Codes

Certain Z codes are so non-specific, or potentially redundant with other codes in the classification, that there can be little justification for their use in the inpatient setting. Their use in the outpatient setting should be limited to those instances when there is no further documentation to permit more precise coding. Otherwise, any sign or symptom or any other reason for visit that is captured in another code should be used.

Nonspecific Z codes/categories:

Z02.9 Encounter for administrative examinations, unspecified
Z04.9 Encounter for examination and observation for unspecified reason
Z13.9 Encounter for screening, unspecified
Z41.9 Encounter for procedure for purposes other than remedying health state, unspecified
Z52.9 Donor of unspecified organ or tissue
Z86.59 Personal history of other mental and behavioral disorders
Z88.9 Allergy status to unspecified drugs, medicaments and biological substances status
Z92.0 Personal history of contraception

15) Z Codes That May Only be Principal/First-Listed Diagnosis

The following Z codes/subcategories/categories may only be reported as the principal/first-listed diagnosis, except when there are multiple encounters on the same day and the medical records for the encounters are combined:

Z00 Encounter for general examination without complaint, suspected or reported diagnosis
 Except: Z00.6
Z01 Encounter for other special examination without complaint, suspected or reported diagnosis
Z02 Encounter for administrative examination
Z04 Encounter for examination and observation for other reasons
Z33.2 Encounter for elective termination of pregnancy
Z31.81 Encounter for male factor infertility in female patient
Z31.83 Encounter for assisted reproductive fertility procedure cycle
Z31.84 Encounter for fertility preservation procedure

Z34 Encounter for supervision of normal pregnancy
Z39 Encounter for maternal postpartum care and examination
Z38 Liveborn infants according to place of birth and type of delivery
Z40 Encounter for prophylactic surgery
Z42 Encounter for plastic and reconstructive surgery following medical procedure or healed injury
Z51.0 Encounter for antineoplastic radiation therapy
Z51.1- Encounter for antineoplastic chemotherapy and immunotherapy
Z52 Donors of organs and tissues Except: Z52.9, Donor of unspecified organ or tissue
Z76.1 Encounter for health supervision and care of foundling
Z76.2 Encounter for health supervision and care of other healthy infant and child
Z99.12 Encounter for respirator [ventilator] dependence during power failure

16) Newborns and Infants

See Section I.C.16. Newborn (Perinatal) Guidelines, for further instruction on the use of these codes.

Newborn Z codes/subcategories/categories:

Z76.1 Encounter for health supervision and care of foundling
Z00.1- Encounter for routine child health examination
Z38 Liveborn infants according to place of birth and type of delivery

17) Social Determinants of Health

Social determinants of health (SDOH) codes describing social problems, conditions, or risk factors that influence a patient's health should be assigned when this information is documented in the patient's medical record. Assign as many SDOH codes as are necessary to describe all of the social problems, conditions, or risk factors documented during the current episode of care. For example, a patient who lives alone may suffer an acute injury temporarily impacting their ability to perform routine activities of daily living. When documented as such, this would support assignment of code Z60.2, Problems related to living alone. However, merely living alone, without documentation of a risk or unmet need for assistance at home, would not support assignment of code Z60.2. Documentation by a clinician (or patient-reported information that is signed off by a clinician) that the patient expressed concerns with access and availability of food would support assignment of code Z59.41, Food insecurity. Similarly, medical record documentation indicating the patient is experiencing homelessness would support assignment of a code from subcategory Z59.0-, Homelessness.

For social determinants of health classified to chapter 21, such as information found in categories Z55-Z65, Persons with potential health hazards related to socioeconomic and psychosocial circumstances, code assignment may be based on medical record documentation from clinicians involved in the care of the patient who are not the patient's provider since this information represents social information, rather than medical diagnoses.

For example, coding professionals may utilize documentation of social information from social workers, community health workers, case managers, or nurses, if their documentation is included in the official medical record.

Patient self-reported documentation may be used to assign codes for social determinants of health, as long as the patient self-reported information is signed-off by and incorporated into the medical record by either a clinician or provider.

Social determinants of health codes are located primarily in these Z code categories:

Z55	Problems related to education and literacy
Z56	Problems related to employment and unemployment
Z57	Occupational exposure to risk factors
Z58	Problems related to physical environment
Z59	Problems related to housing and economic circumstances
Z60	Problems related to social environment
Z62	Problems related to upbringing
Z63	Other problems related to primary support group, including family circumstances
Z64	Problems related to certain psychosocial circumstances
Z65	Problems related to other psychosocial circumstances

See Section I.B.14. Documentation by Clinicians Other than the Patient's Provider.

22. **Chapter 22: Codes for Special Purposes (U00-U85)**

U07.0	Vaping-related disorder (see Section I.C.10.e., Vaping-related disorders)
U07.1	COVID-19 (see Section I.C.1.g.1., COVID-19 infection)
U09.9	Post COVID-19 condition, unspecified (see Section I.C.1.g.1.m)

Section II. Selection of Principal Diagnosis

The circumstances of inpatient admission always govern the selection of principal diagnosis. The principal diagnosis is defined in the Uniform Hospital Discharge Data Set (UHDDS) as "that condition established after study to be chiefly responsible for occasioning the admission of the patient to the hospital for care."

The UHDDS definitions are used by hospitals to report inpatient data elements in a standardized manner. These data elements and their definitions can be found in the July 31, 1985, Federal Register (Vol. 50, No, 147), pp. 31038-40.

Since that time, the application of the UHDDS definitions has been expanded to include all nonoutpatient settings (acute care, short term, long-term care and psychiatric hospitals; home health agencies;

rehab facilities; nursing homes, etc. . .). The UHDDS definitions also apply to hospice services (all levels of care).

In determining principal diagnosis, coding conventions in the ICD-10-CM, the Tabular List and Alphabetic Index take precedence over these official coding guidelines. *(See Section I.A., Conventions for the ICD-10-CM)*

The importance of consistent, complete documentation in the medical record cannot be overemphasized. Without such documentation the application of all coding guidelines is a difficult, if not impossible, task.

A. **Codes for symptoms, signs, and ill-defined conditions**

Codes for symptoms, signs, and ill-defined conditions from Chapter 18 are not to be used as principal diagnosis when a related definitive diagnosis has been established.

B. **Two or more interrelated conditions, each potentially meeting the definition for principal diagnosis**

When there are two or more interrelated conditions (such as diseases in the same ICD-10-CM chapter or manifestations characteristically associated with a certain disease) potentially meeting the definition of principal diagnosis, either condition may be sequenced first, unless the circumstances of the admission, the therapy provided, the Tabular List, or the Alphabetic Index indicate otherwise.

C. **Two or more diagnoses that equally meet the definition for principal diagnosis**

In the unusual instance when two or more diagnoses equally meet the criteria for principal diagnosis as determined by the circumstances of admission, diagnostic workup and/or therapy provided, and the Alphabetic Index, Tabular List, or another coding guidelines does not provide sequencing direction, any one of the diagnoses may be sequenced first.

D. **Two or more comparative or contrasting conditions.**

In those rare instances when two or more contrasting or comparative diagnoses are documented as "either/or" (or similar terminology), they are coded as if the diagnoses were confirmed and the diagnoses are sequenced according to the circumstances of the admission. If no further determination can be made as to which diagnosis should be principal, either diagnosis may be sequenced first

E. **A symptom(s) followed by contrasting/comparative diagnoses**

GUIDELINE HAS BEEN DELETED EFFECTIVE OCTOBER 1, 2014

F. **Original treatment plan not carried out**

Sequence as the principal diagnosis the condition, which after study occasioned the admission to the hospital, even though treatment may not have been carried out due to unforeseen circumstances.

G. **Complications of surgery and other medical care**

When the admission is for treatment of a complication resulting from surgery or other medical care, the complication code is sequenced as the principal diagnosis. If the complication is classified to the T80-T88 series and the code lacks the necessary specificity in describing the complication, an additional code for the specific complication should be assigned.

H. Uncertain Diagnosis

If the diagnosis documented at the time of discharge is qualified as "probable," "suspected," "likely," "questionable," "possible," or "still to be ruled out," "compatible with," "consistent with," or other similar terms indicating uncertainty, code the condition as if it existed or was established. The bases for these guidelines are the diagnostic workup, arrangements for further workup or observation, and initial therapeutic approach that correspond most closely with the established diagnosis.

Note: This guideline is applicable only to inpatient admissions to short-term, acute, long-term care and psychiatric hospitals.

I. Admission from Observation Unit

1. Admission Following Medical Observation

When a patient is admitted to an observation unit for a medical condition, which either worsens or does not improve, and is subsequently admitted as an inpatient of the same hospital for this same medical condition, the principal diagnosis would be the medical condition which led to the hospital admission.

2. Admission Following Post-Operative Observation

When a patient is admitted to an observation unit to monitor a condition (or complication) that develops following outpatient surgery, and then is subsequently admitted as an inpatient of the same hospital, hospitals should apply the Uniform Hospital Discharge Data Set (UHDDS) definition of principal diagnosis as "that condition established after study to be chiefly responsible for occasioning the admission of the patient to the hospital for care."

J. Admission from Outpatient Surgery

When a patient receives surgery in the hospital's outpatient surgery department and is subsequently admitted for continuing inpatient care at the same hospital, the following guidelines should be followed in selecting the principal diagnosis for the inpatient admission:

- If the reason for the inpatient admission is a complication, assign the complication as the principal diagnosis.
- If no complication, or other condition, is documented as the reason for the inpatient admission, assign the reason for the outpatient surgery as the principal diagnosis.
- If the reason for the inpatient admission is another condition unrelated to the surgery, assign the unrelated condition as the principal diagnosis.

K. Admissions/Encounters for Rehabilitation

When the purpose for the admission/encounter is rehabilitation, sequence first the code for the condition for which the service is being performed. For example, for an admission/encounter for rehabilitation for right-sided dominant hemiplegia following a cerebrovascular infarction, report code I69.351, Hemiplegia and hemiparesis following cerebral infarction affecting right dominant side, as the first-listed or principal diagnosis.

If the condition for which the rehabilitation service is being provided is no longer present, report the appropriate aftercare code as the first-listed or principal diagnosis, unless the rehabilitation service is being provided following an injury. For rehabilitation services following active treatment of an injury, assign the injury code with the appropriate seventh character for subsequent encounter as the first-listed or principal diagnosis. For example, if a patient with severe degenerative osteoarthritis of the hip, underwent hip replacement and the current encounter/admission is for rehabilitation, report code Z47.1, Aftercare following joint replacement surgery, as the first-listed or principal diagnosis. If the patient requires rehabilitation post hip replacement for right intertrochanteric femur fracture, report code S72.141D, Displaced intertrochanteric fracture of right femur, subsequent encounter for closed fracture with routine healing, as the first-listed or principal diagnosis.

See Section I.C.21.c.7., Factors influencing health states and contact with health services, Aftercare.

See Section I.C.19.a., for additional information about the use of 7th characters for injury codes.

Section III. Reporting Additional Diagnoses

GENERAL RULES FOR OTHER (ADDITIONAL) DIAGNOSES

For reporting purposes the definition for "other diagnoses" is interpreted as additional **clinically significant** conditions that affect patient care in terms of requiring:

    clinical evaluation; or

    therapeutic treatment; or

    diagnostic procedures; or

    extended length of hospital stay; or

    increased nursing care and/or monitoring.

The UHDDS item #11-b defines Other Diagnoses as "all conditions that coexist at the time of admission, that develop subsequently, or that affect the treatment received and/or the length of stay. Diagnoses that relate to an earlier episode which have no bearing on the current hospital stay are to be excluded." UHDDS definitions apply to inpatients in acute care, short-term, long term care and psychiatric hospital setting. The UHDDS definitions are used by acute care short-term hospitals to report inpatient data elements in a standardized manner. These data elements and their definitions can be found in the July 31, 1985, Federal Register (Vol. 50, No, 147), pp. 31038-40.

Since that time, the application of the UHDDS definitions has been expanded to include all non-outpatient settings (acute care, short term, long term care and psychiatric hospitals; home health agencies; rehab facilities; nursing homes, etc. . .). The UHDDS definitions also apply to hospice services (all levels of care).

The following guidelines are to be applied in designating "other diagnoses" when neither the Alphabetic Index nor the Tabular List in ICD-10-CM provide direction. The listing of the diagnoses in the patient record is the responsibility of the provider.

A. Previous conditions

If the provider has included a diagnosis in the final diagnostic statement, such as the discharge summary or the face sheet, it should ordinarily be coded. Some providers include in the diagnostic statement resolved conditions or diagnoses and status-post procedures from previous admissions that have no bearing on the current stay. Such conditions are not to be reported and are coded only if required by hospital policy.

However, history codes (categories Z80-Z87) may be used as secondary codes if the historical condition or family history has an impact on current care or influences treatment.

B. Abnormal findings

Abnormal findings (laboratory, x-ray, pathologic, and other diagnostic results) are not coded and reported unless the provider indicates their clinical significance. If the findings are outside the normal range and the provider has ordered other tests to evaluate the condition or prescribed treatment, it is appropriate to ask the provider whether the abnormal finding should be added.

Please note: This differs from the coding practices in the outpatient setting for coding encounters for diagnostic tests that have been interpreted by a provider.

C. Uncertain Diagnosis

If the diagnosis documented at the time of discharge is qualified as "probable," "suspected," "likely," "questionable," "possible," or "still to be ruled out," "compatible with," "consistent with," or other similar terms indicating uncertainty, code the condition as if it existed or was established. The bases for these guidelines are the diagnostic workup, arrangements for further workup or observation, and initial therapeutic approach that correspond most closely with the established diagnosis.

Note: This guideline is applicable only to inpatient admissions to short-term, acute, long-term care and psychiatric hospitals.

Section IV. Diagnostic Coding and Reporting Guidelines for Outpatient Services

These coding guidelines for outpatient diagnoses have been approved for use by hospitals/ providers in coding and reporting hospital-based outpatient services and provider-based office visits. Guidelines in Section I, Conventions, general coding guidelines and chapter-specific guidelines, should also be applied for outpatient services and office visits.

Information about the use of certain abbreviations, punctuation, symbols, and other conventions used in the ICD-10-CM Tabular List (code numbers and titles), can be found in Section IA of these guidelines, under "Conventions Used in the Tabular List." Section I.B. contains general guidelines that apply to the entire classification. Section I.C. contains chapter-specific guidelines that correspond to the chapters as they are arranged in the classification. Information about the correct sequence to use in finding a code is also described in Section I.

The terms encounter and visit are often used interchangeably in describing outpatient service contacts and, therefore, appear together in these guidelines without distinguishing one from the other.

Though the conventions and general guidelines apply to all settings, coding guidelines for outpatient and provider reporting of diagnoses will vary in a number of instances from those for inpatient diagnoses, recognizing that:

The Uniform Hospital Discharge Data Set (UHDDS) definition of principal diagnosis does not apply to hospital-based outpatient services and provider-based office visits.

Coding guidelines for inconclusive diagnoses (probable, suspected, rule out, etc.) were developed for inpatient reporting and do not apply to outpatients.

A. Selection of first-listed condition

In the outpatient setting, the term first-listed diagnosis is used in lieu of principal diagnosis.

In determining the first-listed diagnosis the coding conventions of ICD-10-CM, as well as the general and disease specific guidelines take precedence over the outpatient guidelines.

Diagnoses often are not established at the time of the initial encounter/visit. It may take two or more visits before the diagnosis is confirmed.

The most critical rule involves beginning the search for the correct code assignment through the Alphabetic Index. Never begin searching initially in the Tabular List as this will lead to coding errors.

1. Outpatient Surgery

When a patient presents for outpatient surgery (same day surgery), code the reason for the surgery as the first-listed diagnosis (reason for the encounter), even if the surgery is not performed due to a contraindication.

2. Observation Stay

When a patient is admitted for observation for a medical condition, assign a code for the medical condition as the first-listed diagnosis.

When a patient presents for outpatient surgery and develops complications requiring admission to observation, code the reason for the surgery as the first reported diagnosis (reason for the encounter), followed by codes for the complications as secondary diagnoses.

B. Codes from A00.0 through T88.9, Z00-Z99, U00-U85

The appropriate code(s) from A00.0 through T88.9, Z00-Z99, and U00-U85 must be used to identify diagnoses, symptoms, conditions, problems, complaints, or other reason(s) for the encounter/visit.

C. Accurate reporting of ICD-10-CM diagnosis codes
For accurate reporting of ICD-10-CM diagnosis codes, the documentation should describe the patient's condition, using terminology which includes specific diagnoses as well as symptoms, problems, or reasons for the encounter. There are ICD-10-CM codes to describe all of these.

D. Codes that describe symptoms and signs
Codes that describe symptoms and signs, as opposed to diagnoses, are acceptable for reporting purposes when a diagnosis has not been established (confirmed) by the provider. Chapter 18 of ICD-10-CM, Symptoms, Signs, and Abnormal Clinical and Laboratory Findings Not Elsewhere Classified (codes R00-R99) contains many, but not all codes for symptoms.

E. Encounters for circumstances other than a disease or injury
ICD-10-CM provides codes to deal with encounters for circumstances other than a disease or injury. The Factors Influencing Health Status and Contact with Health Services codes (Z00-Z99) are provided to deal with occasions when circumstances other than a disease or injury are recorded as diagnosis or problems.
See Section I.C.21., Factors influencing health status and contact with health services.

F. Level of Detail in Coding
1. ICD-10-CM codes with 3, 4, 5, 6 or 7 characters
ICD-10-CM is composed of codes with 3, 4, 5, 6 or 7 characters. Codes with three characters are included in ICD-10-CM as the heading of a category of codes that may be further subdivided by the use of fourth, fifth, sixth or seventh characters to provide greater specificity.
2. Use of full number of characters required for a code
A 3-character code is to be used only if it is not further subdivided. A code is invalid if it has not been coded to the full number of characters required for that code, including the 7th character, if applicable.
3. Highest level of specificity
Code to the highest level of specificity when supported by the medical record documentation.

G. ICD-10-CM code for the diagnosis, condition, problem, or other reason for encounter/visit
List first the ICD-10-CM code for the diagnosis, condition, problem, or other reason for encounter/visit shown in the medical record to be chiefly responsible for the services provided. List additional codes that describe any coexisting conditions. In some cases the first-listed diagnosis may be a symptom when a diagnosis has not been established (confirmed) by the provider.

H. Uncertain diagnosis
Do not code diagnoses documented as "probable," "suspected," "questionable," "rule out," "compatible with," "consistent with," or "working diagnosis" or other similar terms indicating uncertainty. Rather, code the condition(s) to the highest degree of certainty for that encounter/visit, such as symptoms, signs, abnormal test results, or other reason for the visit.
Please note: This differs from the coding practices used by short-term, acute care, long-term care and psychiatric hospitals.

I. Chronic diseases
Chronic diseases treated on an ongoing basis may be coded and reported as many times as the patient receives treatment and care for the condition(s)

J. Code all documented conditions that coexist
Code all documented conditions that coexist at the time of the encounter/visit, and that require or affect patient care treatment or management. Do not code conditions that were previously treated and no longer exist. However, history codes (categories Z80-Z87) may be used as secondary codes if the historical condition or family history has an impact on current care or influences treatment.

K. Patients receiving diagnostic services only
For patients receiving diagnostic services only during an encounter/visit, sequence first the diagnosis, condition, problem, or other reason for encounter/visit shown in the medical record to be chiefly responsible for the outpatient services provided during the encounter/visit. Codes for other diagnoses (e.g., chronic conditions) may be sequenced as additional diagnoses.

For encounters for routine laboratory/radiology testing in the absence of any signs, symptoms, or associated diagnosis, assign Z01.89, Encounter for other specified special examinations. If routine testing is performed during the same encounter as a test to evaluate a sign, symptom, or diagnosis, it is appropriate to assign both the Z code and the code describing the reason for the non-routine test.

For outpatient encounters for diagnostic tests that have been interpreted by a physician, and the final report is available at the time of coding, code any confirmed or definitive diagnosis(es) documented in the interpretation. Do not code related signs and symptoms as additional diagnoses.
Please note: This differs from the coding practice in the hospital inpatient setting regarding abnormal findings on test results.

L. Patients receiving therapeutic services only
For patients receiving therapeutic services only during an encounter/visit, sequence first the diagnosis, condition, problem, or other reason for encounter/visit shown in the medical record to be chiefly responsible for the outpatient services provided during the encounter/visit. Codes for other diagnoses (e.g., chronic conditions) may be sequenced as additional diagnoses.

The only exception to this rule is that when the primary reason for the admission/encounter is chemotherapy or radiation therapy, the appropriate Z code for the service is listed first, and the diagnosis or problem for which the service is being performed listed second.

M. Patients receiving preoperative evaluations only

For patients receiving preoperative evaluations only, sequence first a code from subcategory Z01.81, Encounter for pre-procedural examinations, to describe the pre-op consultations. Assign a code for the condition to describe the reason for the surgery as an additional diagnosis. Code also any findings related to the pre-op evaluation.

N. Ambulatory surgery

For ambulatory surgery, code the diagnosis for which the surgery was performed. If the postoperative diagnosis is known to be different from the preoperative diagnosis at the time the diagnosis is confirmed, select the postoperative diagnosis for coding, since it is the most definitive.

O. Routine outpatient prenatal visits

See Section I.C.15., Routine outpatient prenatal visits.

P. Encounters for general medical examinations with abnormal findings

The subcategories for encounters for general medical examinations, Z00.0- and encounter for routine child health examination, Z00.12-, provide codes for with and without abnormal findings. Should a general medical examination result in an abnormal finding, the code for general medical examination with abnormal finding should be assigned as the first-listed diagnosis. An examination with abnormal findings refers to a condition/diagnosis that is newly identified or a change in severity of a chronic condition (such as uncontrolled hypertension, or an acute exacerbation of chronic obstructive pulmonary disease) during a routine physical examination. A secondary code for the abnormal finding should also be coded.

Q. Encounters for routine health screenings

See Section I.C.21., Factors influencing health status and contact with health services, Screening

Appendix I
Present on Admission Reporting Guidelines

Introduction

These guidelines are to be used as a supplement to the ICD-10-CM Official Guidelines for Coding and Reporting to facilitate the assignment of the Present on Admission (POA) indicator for each diagnosis and external cause of injury code reported on claim forms (UB-04 and 837 Institutional).

These guidelines are not intended to replace any guidelines in the main body of the ICD-10-CM Official Guidelines for Coding and Reporting. The POA guidelines are not intended to provide guidance on when a condition should be coded, but rather, how to apply the POA indicator to the final set of diagnosis codes that have been assigned in accordance with Sections I, II, and III of the official coding guidelines. Subsequent to the assignment of the ICD-10-CM codes, the POA indicator should then be assigned to those conditions that have been coded.

As stated in the Introduction to the ICD-10-CM Official Guidelines for Coding and Reporting, a joint effort between the healthcare provider and the coder is essential to achieve complete and accurate documentation, code assignment, and reporting of diagnoses and procedures. The importance of consistent, complete documentation in the medical record cannot be overemphasized. Medical record documentation from any provider involved in the care and treatment of the patient may be used to support the determination of whether a condition was present on admission or not. In the context of the official coding guidelines, the term "provider" means a physician or any qualified healthcare practitioner who is legally accountable for establishing the patient's diagnosis.

These guidelines are not a substitute for the provider's clinical judgment as to the determination of whether a condition was/was not present on admission. The provider should be queried regarding issues related to the linking of signs/symptoms, timing of test results, and the timing of findings.

Please see the CDC website for the detailed list of ICD-10-CM codes that do not require the use of a POA indicator (https://www.cdc.gov/nchs/icd/icd-10-cm/files.html). The codes and categories on this exempt list are for circumstances regarding the healthcare encounter or factors influencing health status that do not represent a current disease or injury or that describe conditions that are always present on admission.

General Reporting Requirements

All claims involving inpatient admissions to general acute care hospitals or other facilities that are subject to a law or regulation mandating collection of present on admission information.

Present on admission is defined as present at the time the order for inpatient admission occurs—conditions that develop during an outpatient encounter, including emergency department, observation, or outpatient surgery, are considered as present on admission.

POA indicator is assigned to principal and secondary diagnoses (as defined in Section II of the Official Guidelines for Coding and Reporting) and the external cause of injury codes.

Issues related to inconsistent, missing, conflicting or unclear documentation must still be resolved by the provider.

If a condition would not be coded and reported based on UHDDS definitions and current official coding guidelines, then the POA indicator would not be reported.

Reporting Options

Y - Yes

N - No

U - Unknown

W - Clinically undetermined

Unreported/Not used - (Exempt from POA reporting)

Reporting Definitions

Y = present at the time of inpatient admission

N = not present at the time of inpatient admission

U = documentation is insufficient to determine if condition is present on admission

W = provider is unable to clinically determine whether condition was present on admission or not

Timeframe for POA Identification and Documentation

There is no required timeframe as to when a provider (per the definition of "provider" used in these guidelines) must identify or document a condition to be present on admission. In some clinical situations, it may not be possible for a provider to make a definitive diagnosis (or a condition may not be recognized or reported by the patient) for a period of time after admission. In some cases it may be several days before the provider arrives at a definitive diagnosis. This does not mean that the condition was not present on admission. Determination of whether the condition was present on admission or not will be based on the applicable POA guideline as identified in this document, or on the provider's best clinical judgment.

If at the time of code assignment the documentation is unclear as to whether a condition was present on admission or not, it is appropriate to query the provider for clarification.

Assigning the POA Indicator

Condition is on the "Exempt from Reporting" list

Leave the "present on admission" field blank if the condition is on the list of ICD-10-CM codes for which this field is not applicable. This is the only circumstance in which the field may be left blank.

POA Explicitly Documented

Assign "Y" for any condition the provider explicitly documents as being present on admission.

Assign "N" for any condition the provider explicitly documents as not present at the time of admission.

Conditions diagnosed prior to inpatient admission

Assign "Y" for conditions that were diagnosed prior to admission (example: hypertension, diabetes mellitus, asthma)

Conditions diagnosed during the admission but clearly present before admission

Assign "Y" for conditions diagnosed during the admission that were clearly present but not diagnosed until after admission occurred.

Diagnoses subsequently confirmed after admission are considered present on admission if at the time of admission they are documented as suspected, possible, rule out, differential diagnosis, or constitute an underlying cause of a symptom that is present at the time of admission.

Condition develops during outpatient encounter prior to inpatient admission

Assign "Y" for any condition that develops during an outpatient encounter prior to a written order for inpatient admission.

Documentation does not indicate whether condition was present on admission

Assign "U" when the medical record documentation is unclear as to whether the condition was present on admission. "U" should not be routinely assigned and used only in very limited circumstances. Coders are encouraged to query the providers when the documentation is unclear.

Documentation states that it cannot be determined whether the condition was or was not present on admission

Assign "W" when the medical record documentation indicates that it cannot be clinically determined whether or not the condition was present on admission.

Chronic condition with acute exacerbation during the admission

If a single code identifies both the chronic condition and the acute exacerbation, see POA guidelines pertaining to codes that contain multiple clinical concepts.

If a single code only identifies the chronic condition and not the acute exacerbation (e.g., acute exacerbation of chronic leukemia), assign "Y."

Conditions documented as possible, probable, suspected, or rule out at the time of discharge

If the final diagnosis contains a possible, probable, suspected, or rule out diagnosis, and this diagnosis was based on signs, symptoms or clinical findings suspected at the time of inpatient admission, assign "Y."

If the final diagnosis contains a possible, probable, suspected, or rule out diagnosis, and this diagnosis was based on signs, symptoms or clinical findings that were not present on admission, assign "N".

Conditions documented as impending or threatened at the time of discharge

If the final diagnosis contains an impending or threatened diagnosis, and this diagnosis is based on symptoms or clinical findings that were present on admission, assign "Y".

If the final diagnosis contains an impending or threatened diagnosis, and this diagnosis is based on symptoms or clinical findings that were not present on admission, assign "N".

Acute and Chronic Conditions

Assign "Y" for acute conditions that are present at time of admission and "N" for acute conditions that are not present at time of admission.

Assign "Y" for chronic conditions, even though the condition may not be diagnosed until after admission.

If a single code identifies both an acute and chronic condition, see the POA guidelines for codes that contain multiple clinical concepts.

Codes That Contain Multiple Clinical Concepts

Assign "N" if at least one of the clinical concepts included in the code was not present on admission (e.g., COPD with acute exacerbation and the exacerbation was not present on admission; gastric ulcer that does not start bleeding until after admission; asthma patient develops status asthmaticus after admission).

Assign "Y" if all of the clinical concepts included in the code were present on admission (e.g., duodenal ulcer that perforates prior to admission).

For infection codes that include the causal organism, assign "Y" if the infection (or signs of the infection) were present on admission, even though the culture results may not be known until after admission (e.g., patient is admitted with pneumonia and the provider documents Pseudomonas as the causal organism a few days later).

Same Diagnosis Code for Two or More Conditions

When the same ICD-10-CM diagnosis code applies to two or more conditions during the same encounter (e.g., two separate conditions classified to the same ICD-10-CM diagnosis code):

Assign "Y" if all conditions represented by the single ICD-10-CM code were present on admission (e.g., bilateral unspecified age-related cataracts).

Assign "N" if any of the conditions represented by the single ICD-10-CM code was not present on admission (e.g., traumatic secondary and recurrent hemorrhage and seroma is assigned to a single code T79.2, but only one of the conditions was present on admission).

Obstetrical conditions

Whether or not the patient delivers during the current hospitalization does not affect assignment of the POA indicator. The determining factor for POA assignment is whether the pregnancy complication or obstetrical condition described by the code was present at the time of admission or not.

If the pregnancy complication or obstetrical condition was present on admission (e.g., patient admitted in preterm labor), assign "Y".

If the pregnancy complication or obstetrical condition was not present on admission (e.g., 2nd degree laceration during delivery, postpartum hemorrhage that occurred during current hospitalization, fetal distress develops after admission), assign "N".

If the obstetrical code includes more than one diagnosis and any of the diagnoses identified by the code were not present on admission assign "N".

(e.g., Category O11, Pre-existing hypertension with pre-eclampsia)

Perinatal conditions

Newborns are not considered to be admitted until after birth. Therefore, any condition present at birth or that developed in utero is considered present at admission and should be assigned "Y". This includes conditions that occur during delivery (e.g., injury during delivery, meconium aspiration, exposure to streptococcus B in the vaginal canal).

Congenital conditions and anomalies

Assign "Y" for congenital conditions and anomalies except for categories Q00-Q99, Congenital anomalies, which are on the exempt list. Congenital conditions are always considered present on admission.

External cause of injury codes

Assign "Y" for any external cause code representing an external cause of morbidity that occurred prior to inpatient admission (e.g., patient fell out of bed at home, patient fell out of bed in emergency room prior to admission).

Assign "N" for any external cause code representing an external cause of morbidity that occurred during inpatient hospitalization (e.g., patient fell out of hospital bed during hospital stay, patient experienced an adverse reaction to a medication administered after inpatient admission).

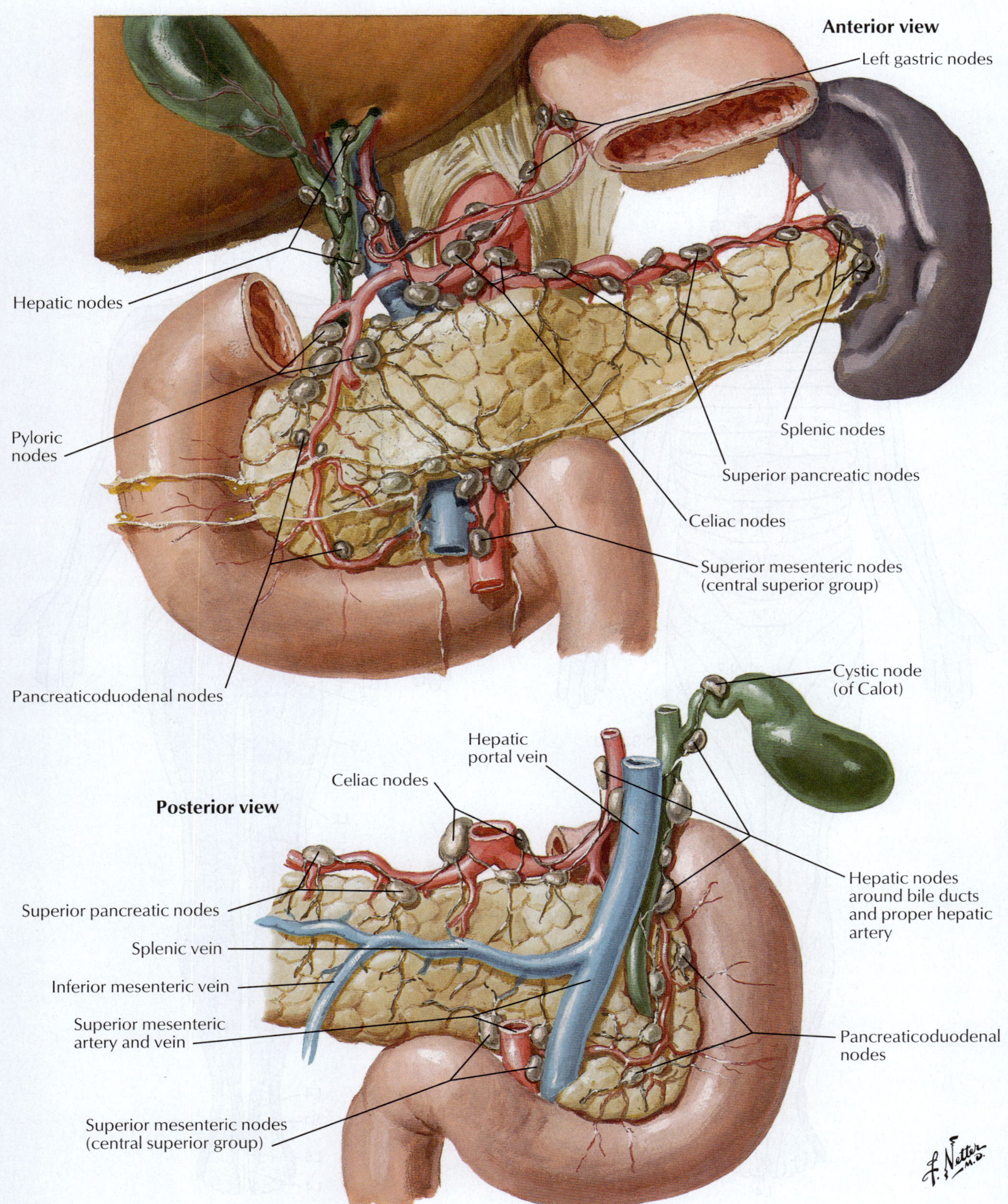

Plate 1 Lymph Vessels and Nodes of Pancreas. (Copyright 2025 Elsevier Inc. All rights reserved. www.netterimages.com. Image ID: 4420)

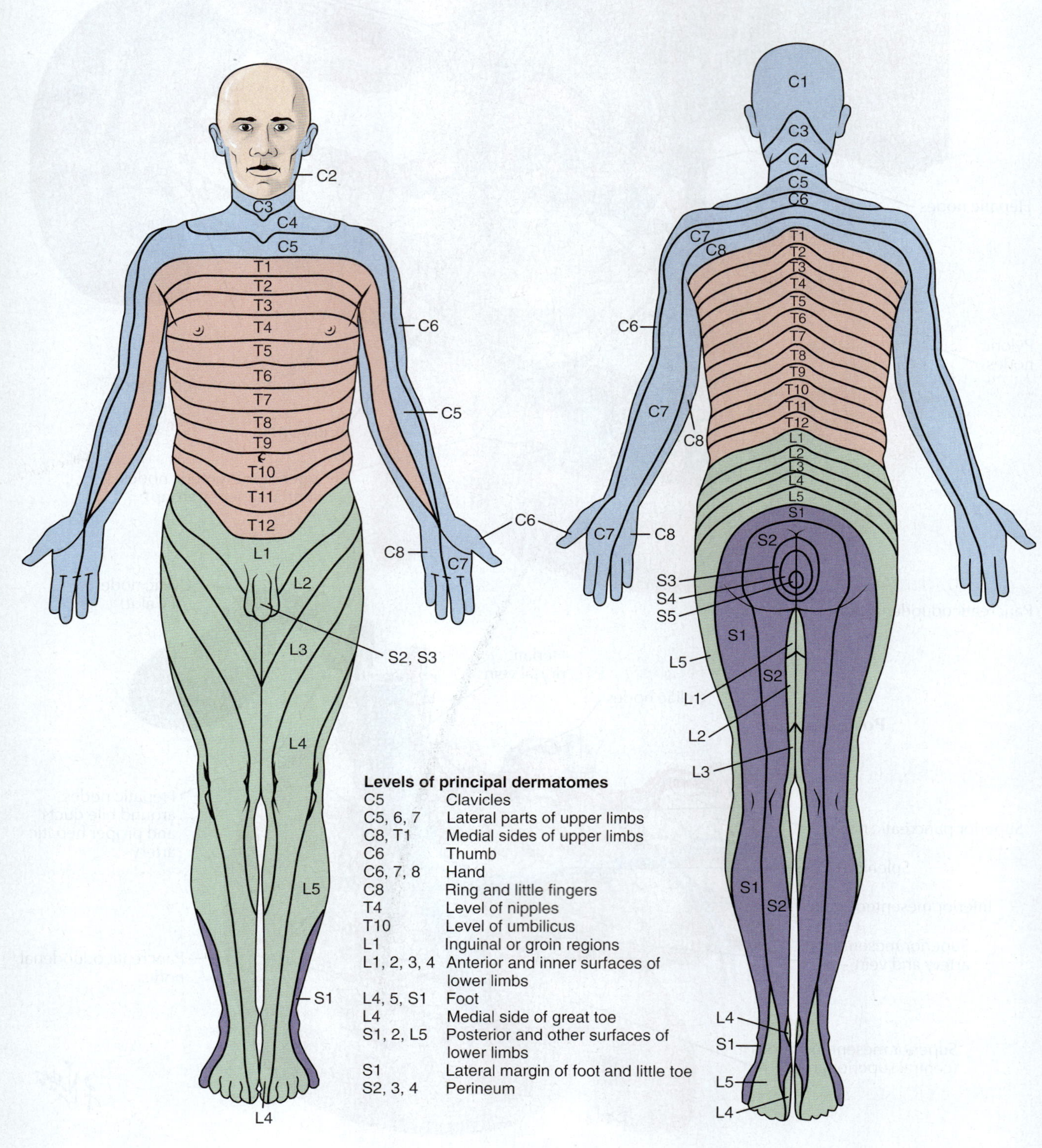

Levels of principal dermatomes

C5	Clavicles
C5, 6, 7	Lateral parts of upper limbs
C8, T1	Medial sides of upper limbs
C6	Thumb
C6, 7, 8	Hand
C8	Ring and little fingers
T4	Level of nipples
T10	Level of umbilicus
L1	Inguinal or groin regions
L1, 2, 3, 4	Anterior and inner surfaces of lower limbs
L4, 5, S1	Foot
L4	Medial side of great toe
S1, 2, L5	Posterior and other surfaces of lower limbs
S1	Lateral margin of foot and little toe
S2, 3, 4	Perineum

Plate 2 Schematic demarcation of Dermatomes. (Miller MD, Hart JA, MacKnight JM: Essential Orthopaedics, ed 2, Philadelphia, 2020, Elsevier.)

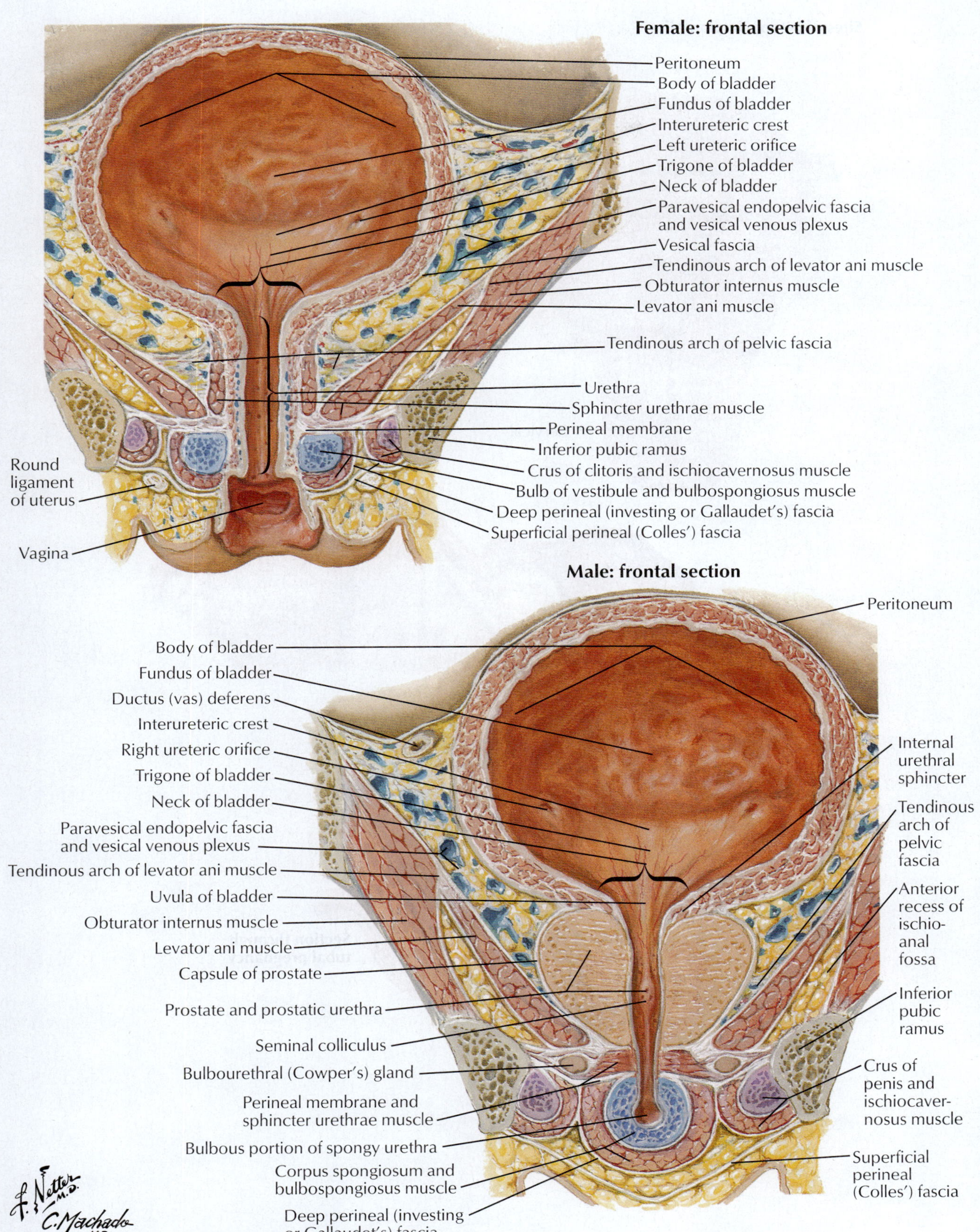

Plate 3 Urinary Bladder: Female and Male. (Copyright 2025 Elsevier Inc. All rights reserved. www.netterimages.com. Image ID: 4714)

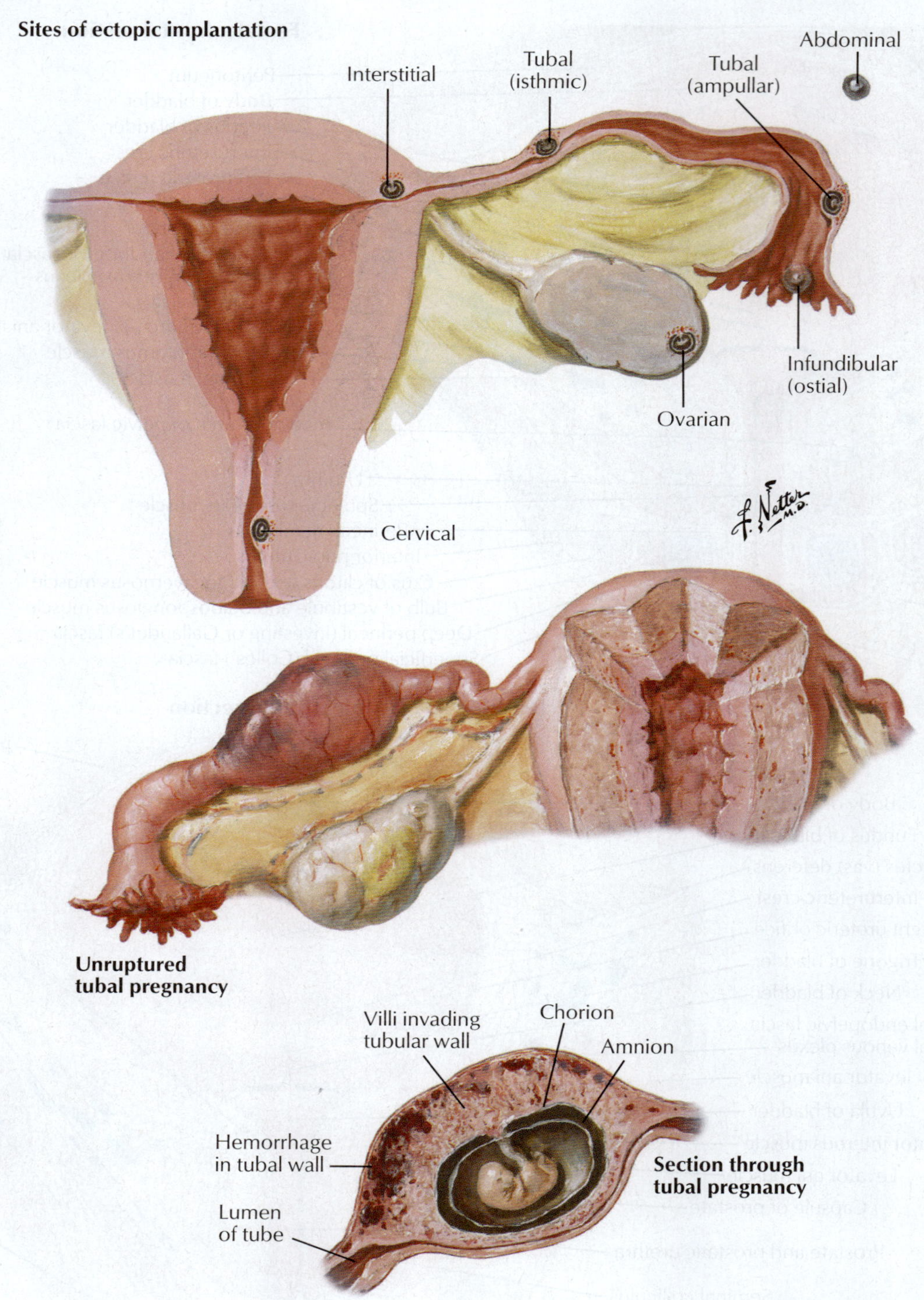

Plate 4 Ectopic Pregnancy. (Copyright 2025 Elsevier Inc. All rights reserved. www.netterimages.com. Image ID: 5148)

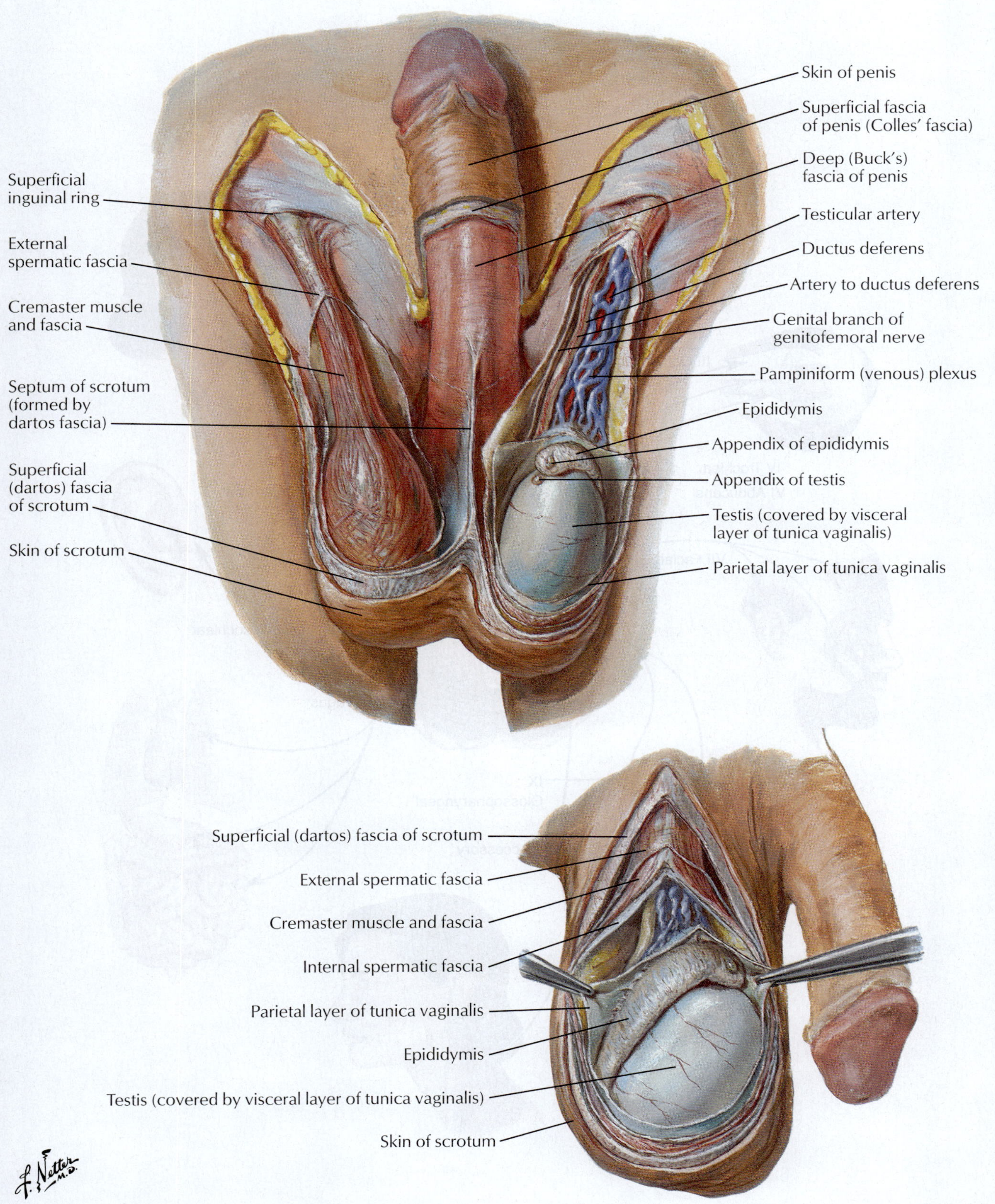

Plate 5 Scrotum and Contents. (Copyright 2025 Elsevier Inc. All rights reserved. www.netterimages.com. Image ID: 4686)

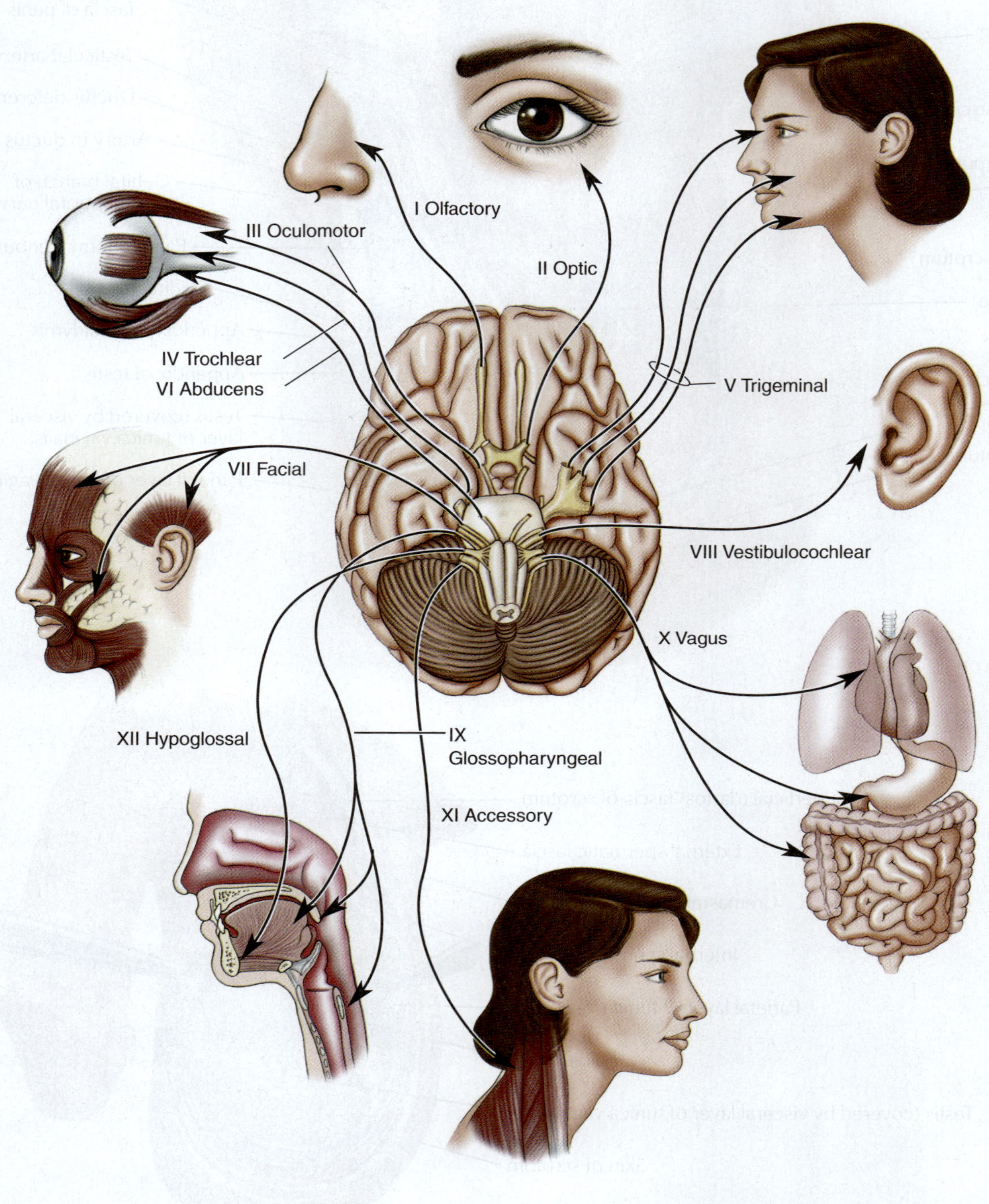

Plate 6 Cranial Nerves (12 pairs) are known by their numbers (Roman numerals) and names. (Herlihy BL: The Human Body in Health and Illness, ed 6, St. Louis, 2018, Elsevier.)

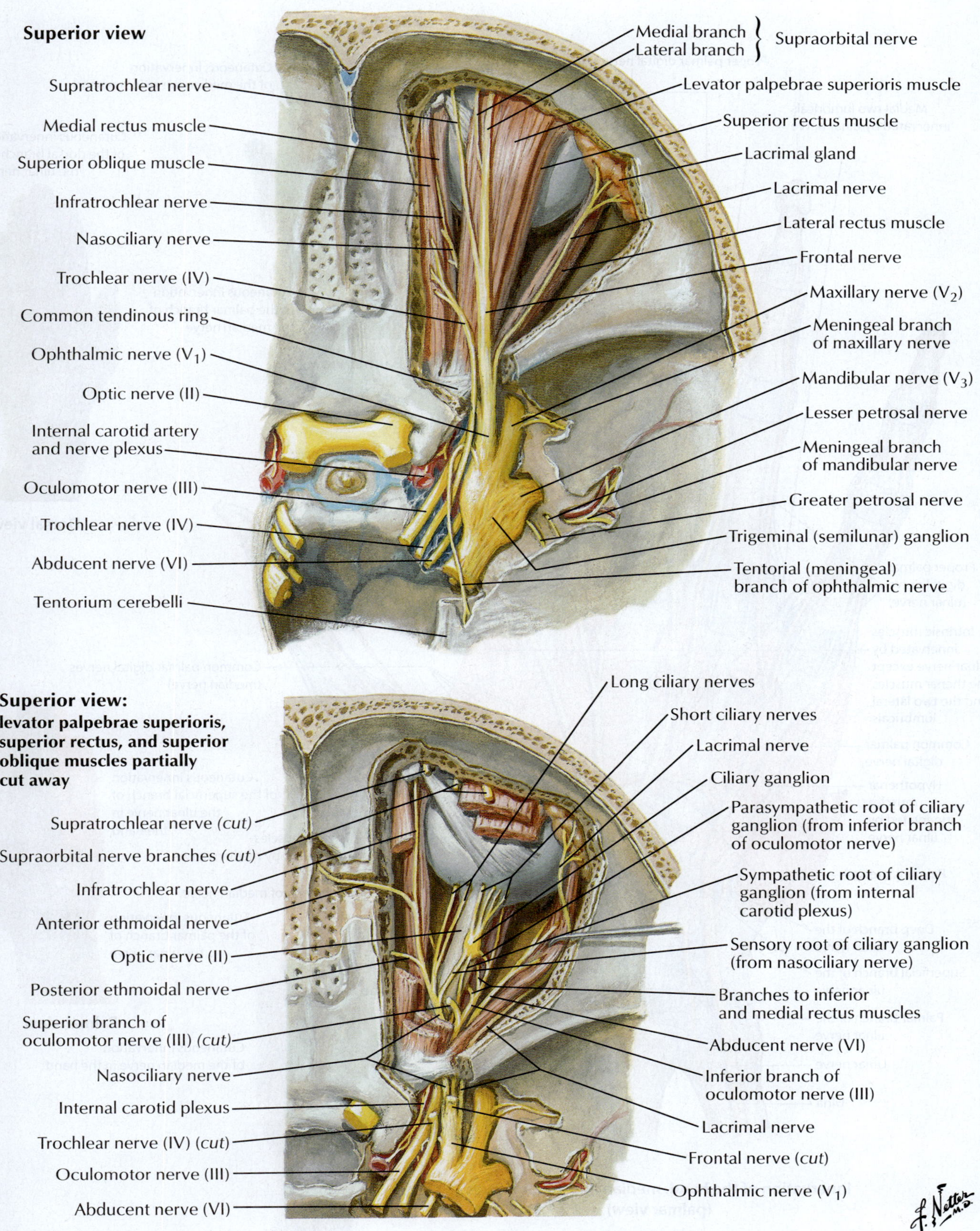

ANATOMY ILLUSTRATIONS

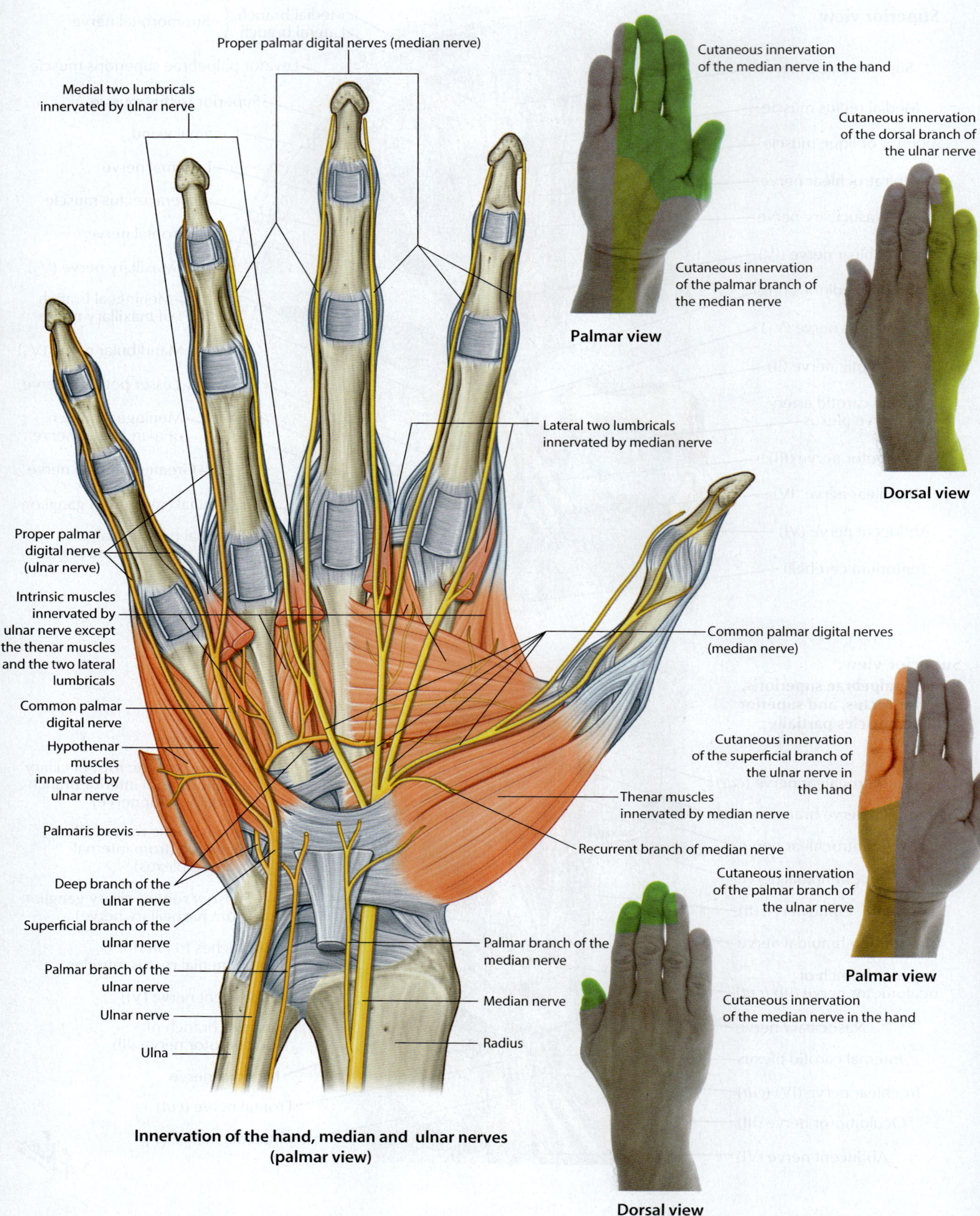

Innervation of the hand, median and ulnar nerves (palmar view)

Plate 8   Innervation of the Hand: Median and Ulnar Nerves (From Drake RL, Vogl AW, Mitchell AWM, Tibbitts RM, Richardson PE: Gray's Atlas of Anatomy, ed 2, Philadelphia, 2015, Churchill Livingstone.)

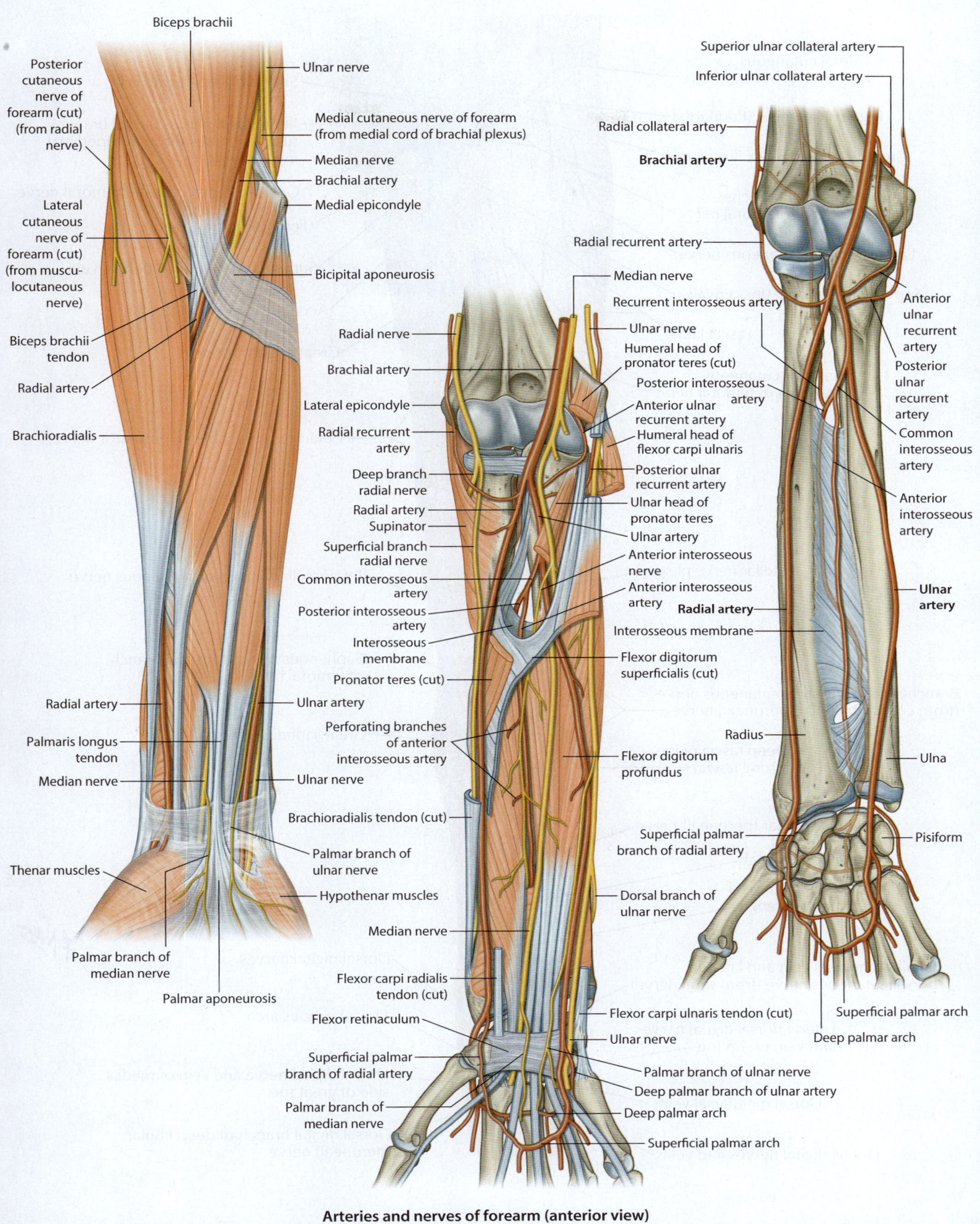

Plate 9 Arteries and Nerves of the Forearm (Anterior View) (From Drake RL, Vogl AW, Mitchell AWM, Tibbitts RM, Richardson PE: Gray's Atlas of Anatomy, ed 2, Philadelphia, 2015, Churchill Livingstone.)

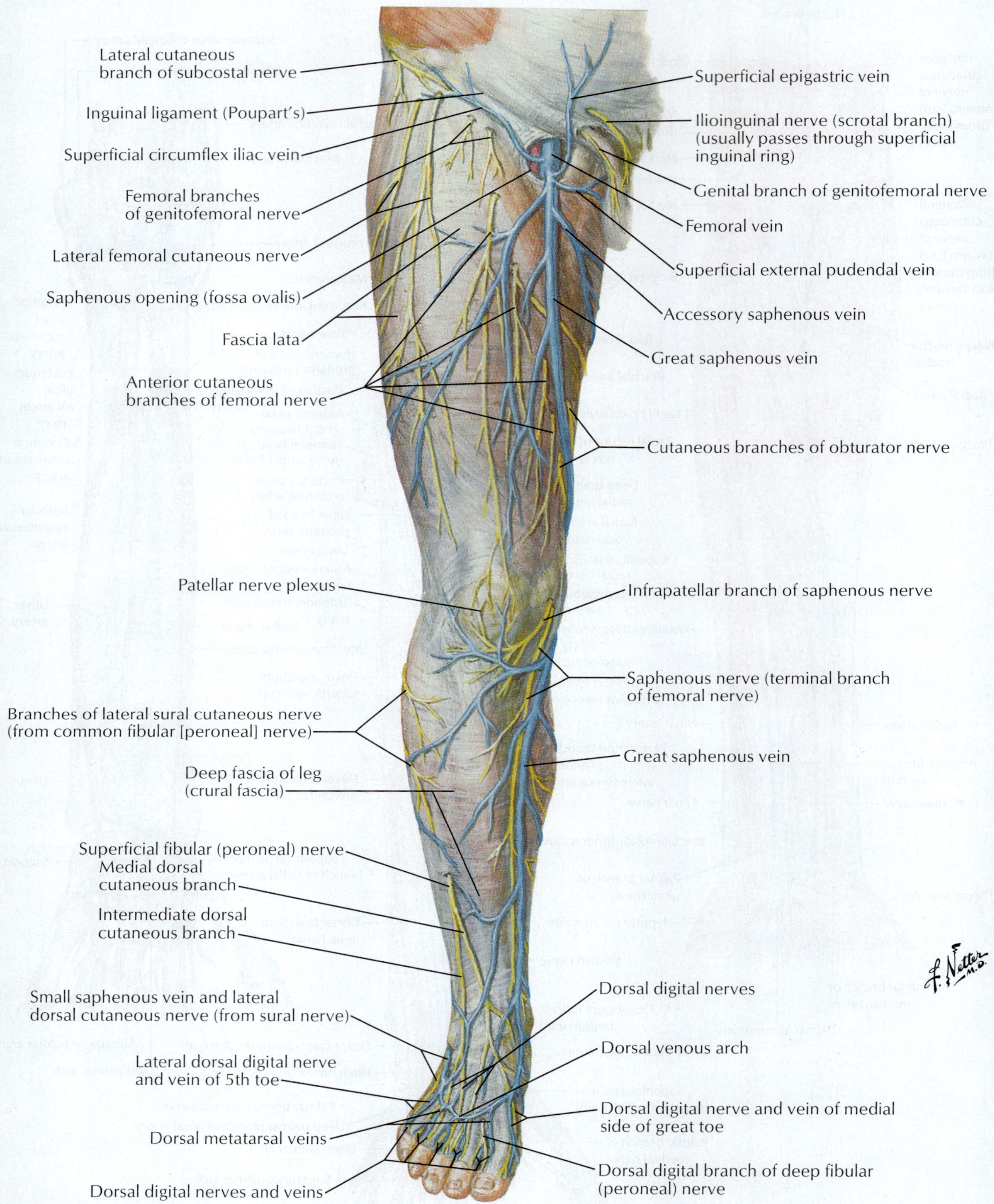

Plate 10 Superficial Nerves and Veins of Lower Limb: Anterior View. (Copyright 2025 Elsevier Inc. All rights reserved. www.netterimages.com. Image ID: 4846)

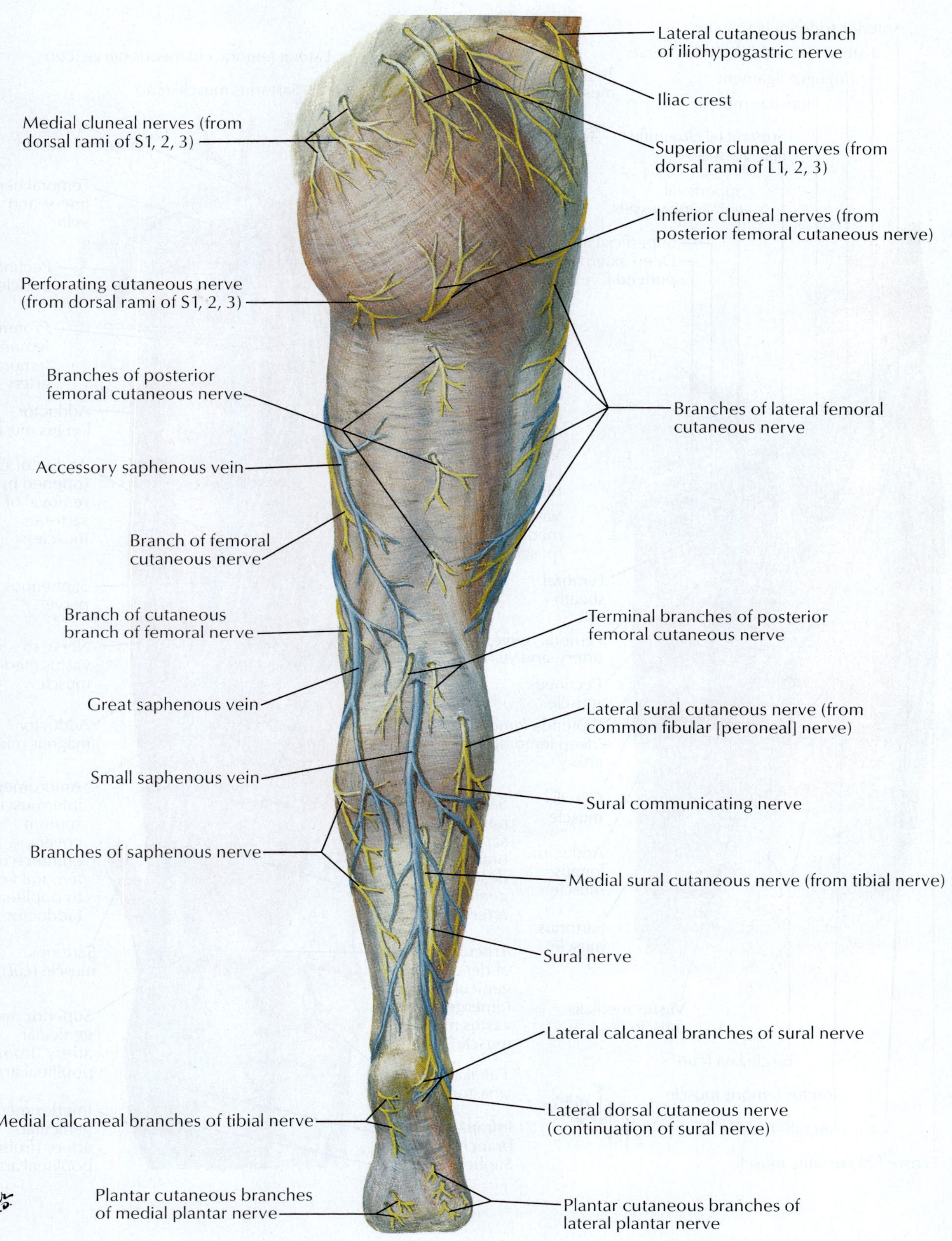

Lateral cutaneous branch of iliohypogastric nerve
Iliac crest
Superior cluneal nerves (from dorsal rami of L1, 2, 3)
Medial cluneal nerves (from dorsal rami of S1, 2, 3)
Inferior cluneal nerves (from posterior femoral cutaneous nerve)
Perforating cutaneous nerve (from dorsal rami of S1, 2, 3)
Branches of posterior femoral cutaneous nerve
Branches of lateral femoral cutaneous nerve
Accessory saphenous vein
Branch of femoral cutaneous nerve
Branch of cutaneous branch of femoral nerve
Terminal branches of posterior femoral cutaneous nerve
Great saphenous vein
Lateral sural cutaneous nerve (from common fibular [peroneal] nerve)
Small saphenous vein
Sural communicating nerve
Branches of saphenous nerve
Medial sural cutaneous nerve (from tibial nerve)
Sural nerve
Lateral calcaneal branches of sural nerve
Medial calcaneal branches of tibial nerve
Lateral dorsal cutaneous nerve (continuation of sural nerve)
Plantar cutaneous branches of medial plantar nerve
Plantar cutaneous branches of lateral plantar nerve
F. Netter M.D.

Superficial dissections

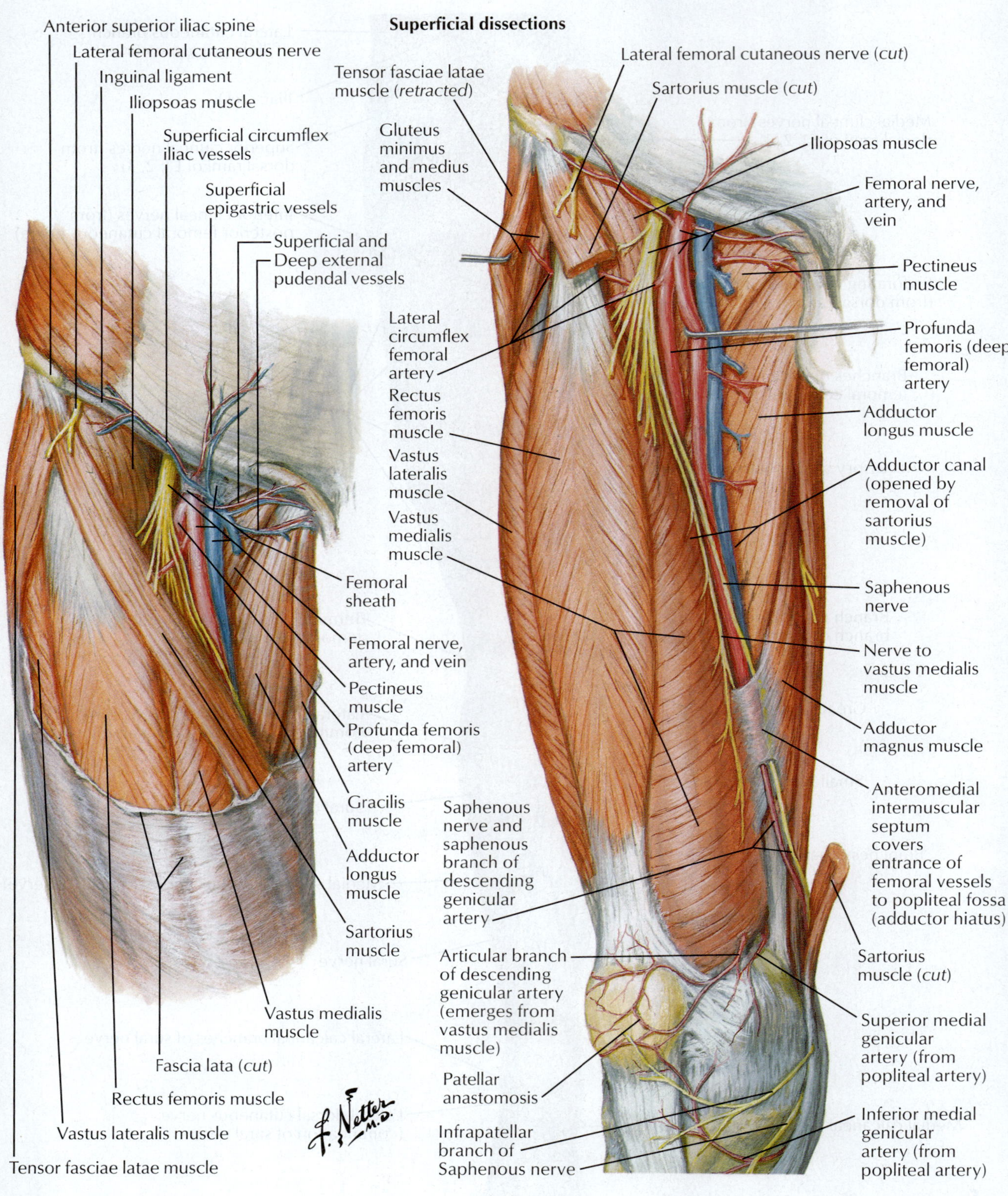

Plate 12 Arteries and Nerves of Thigh: Anterior Views. (Copyright 2025 Elsevier Inc. All rights reserved. www.netterimages.com. Image ID: 4475)

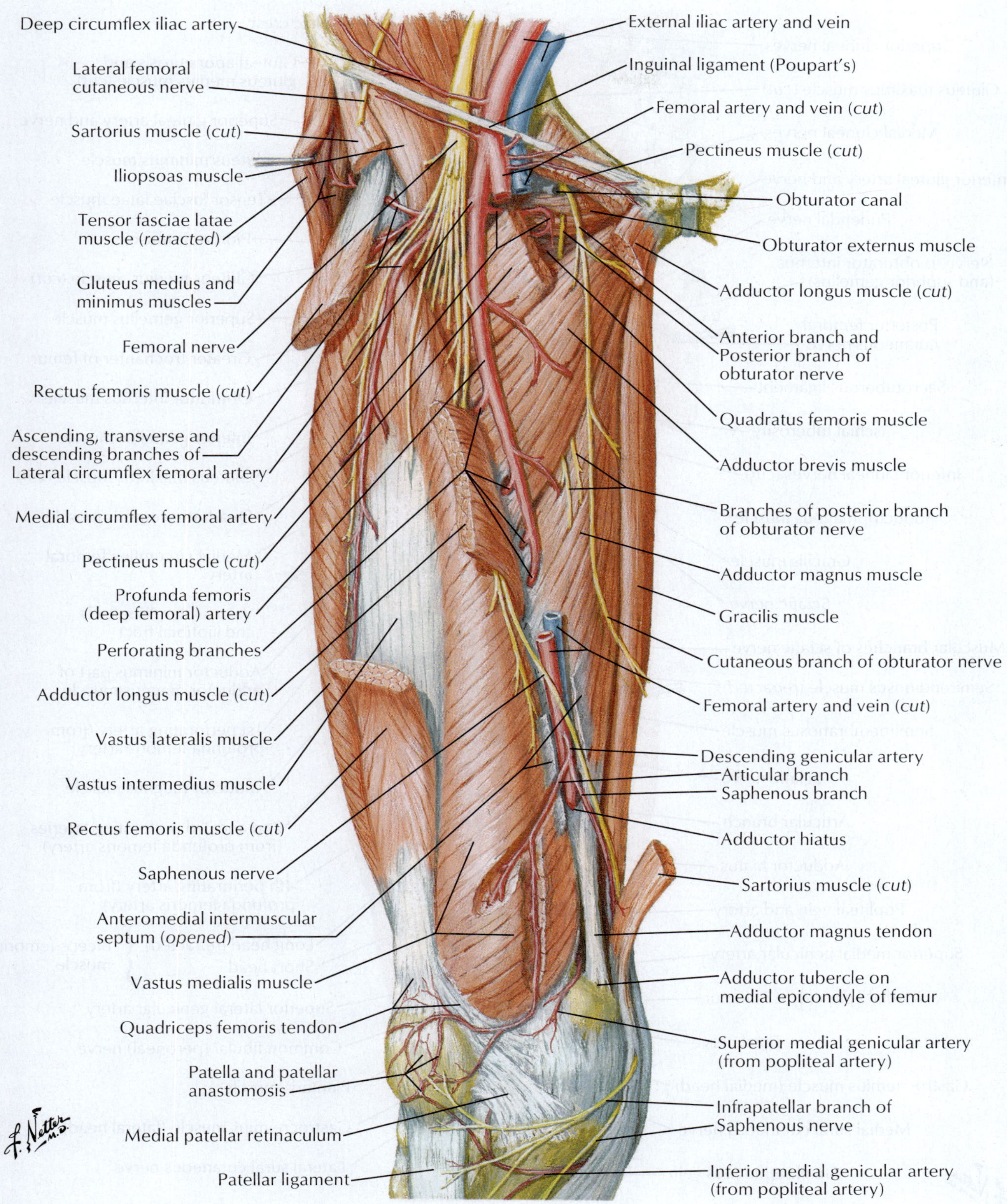

ANATOMY ILLUSTRATIONS

Deep dissection

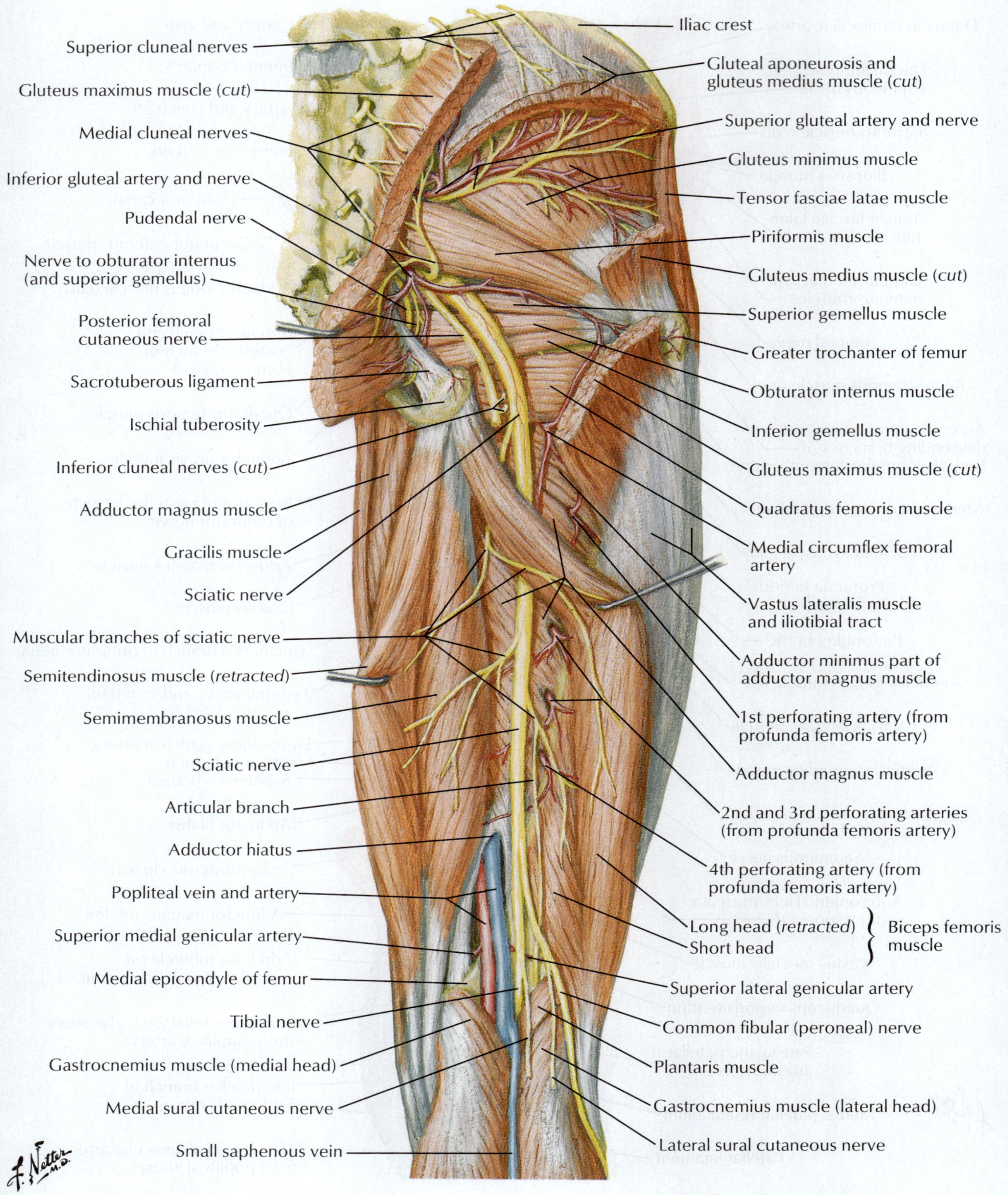

Plate 14 Arteries and Nerves of Thigh: Posterior View. (Copyright 2025 Elsevier Inc. All rights reserved. www.netterimages.com. Image ID: 49317)

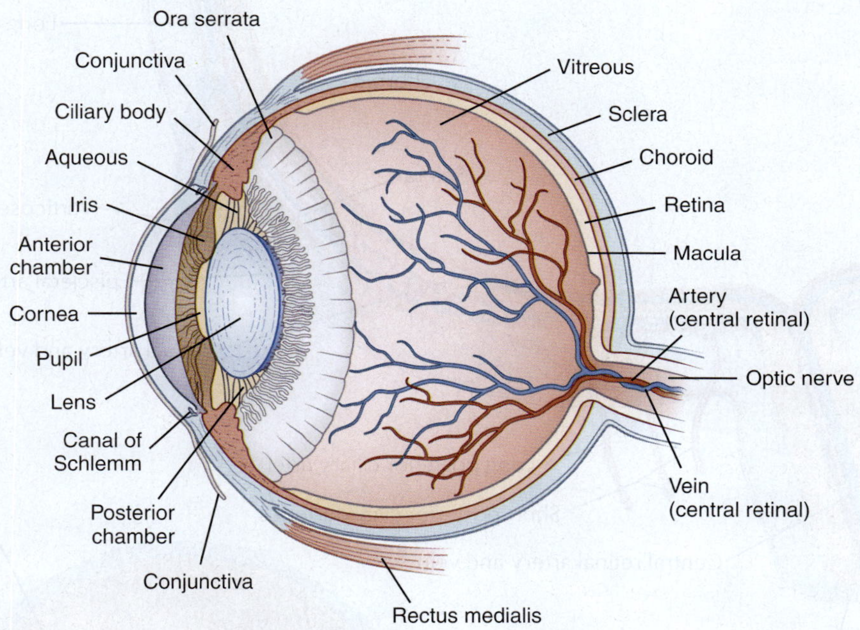

Plate 15 Anatomy of the eye. (Dehn RW, Asprey DP: Essential Clinical Procedures, ed 3, Philadelphia, 2013, Saunders.)

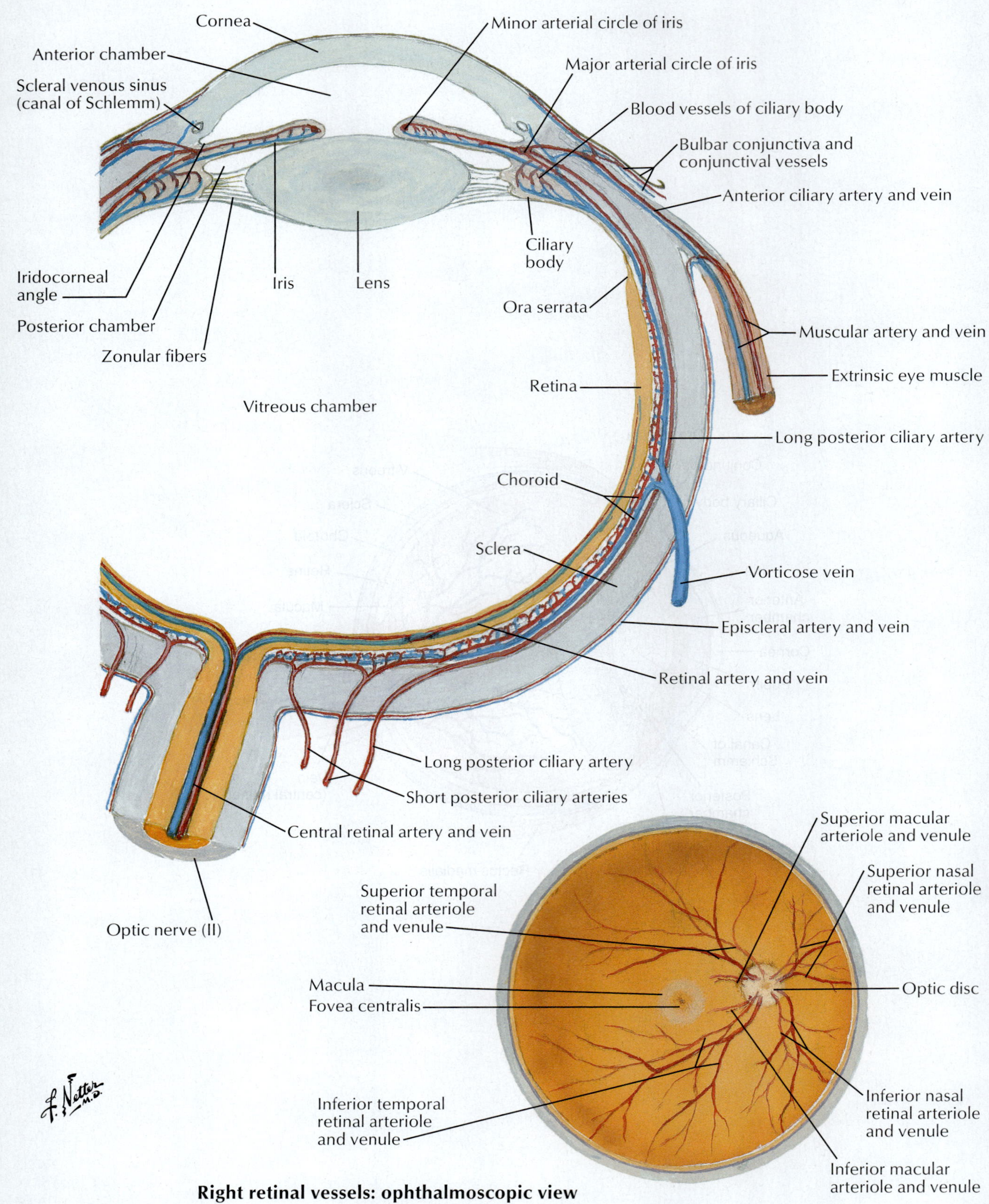

Right retinal vessels: ophthalmoscopic view

Plate 16 Intrinsic Arteries and Veins of Eye. (Copyright 2025 Elsevier Inc. All rights reserved. www.netterimages.com. Image ID: 49107)

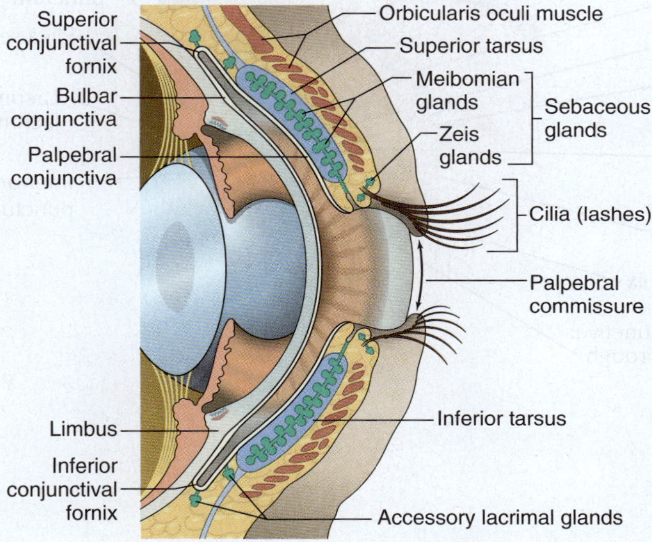

Plate 17   Anatomy of the conjunctiva and eyelids. (Kumar V, Abbas AK, Aster JC: Robbins and Cotran Pathologic Basis of Disease, ed 9, Philadelphia, 2015, Saunders.)

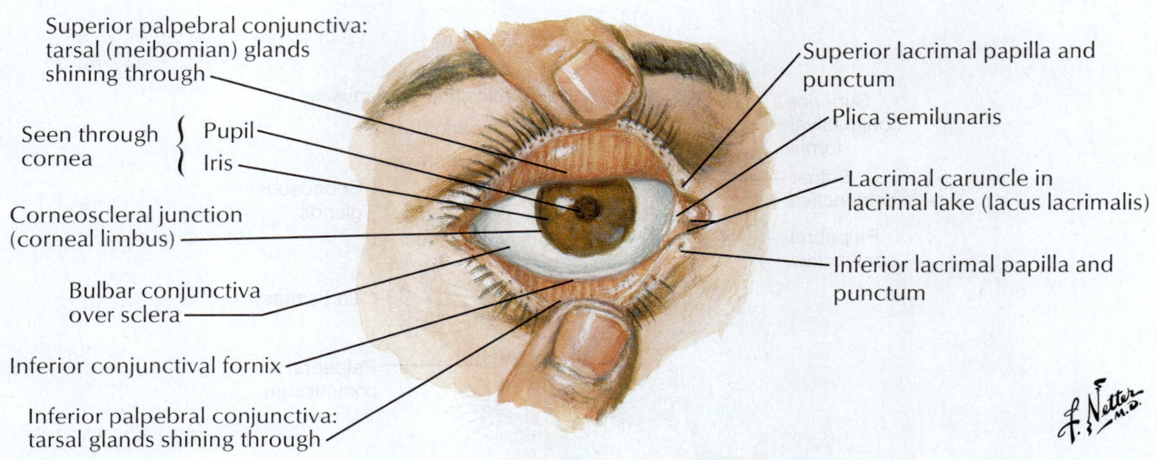

Plate 18 Eyelid. (Copyright 2025 Elsevier Inc. All rights reserved. www.netterimages.com. Image ID: 4557)

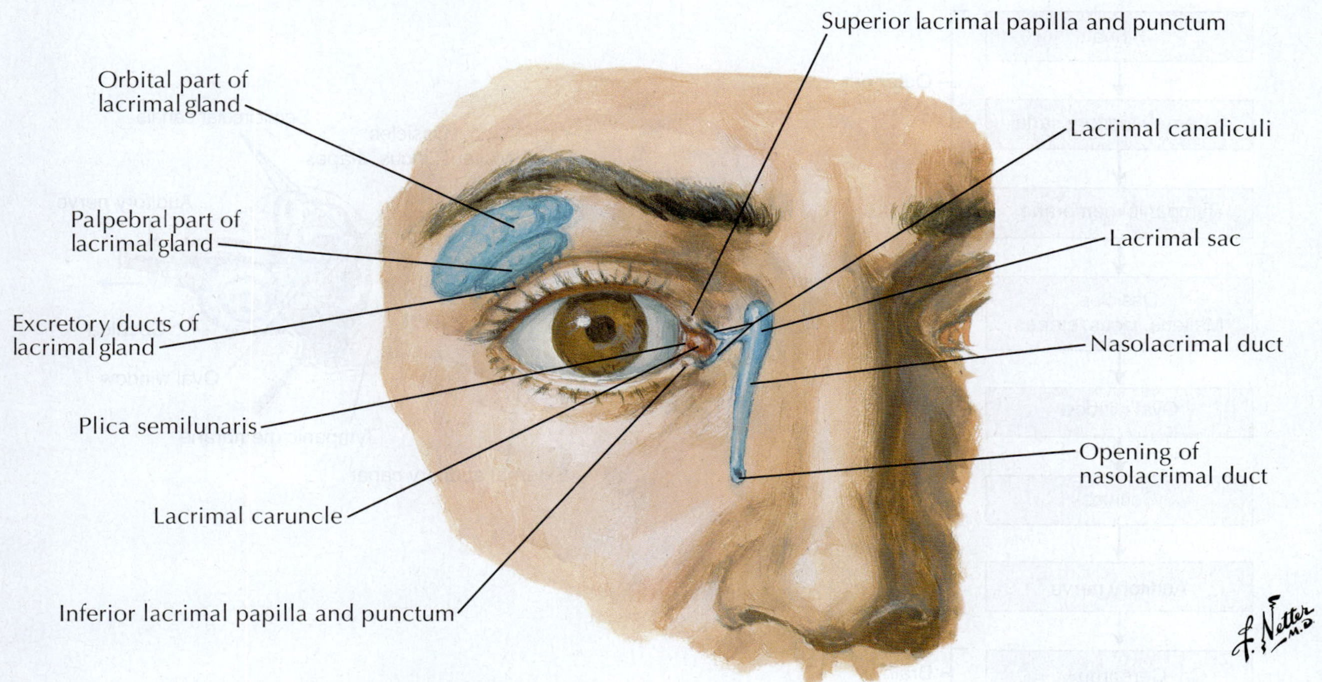

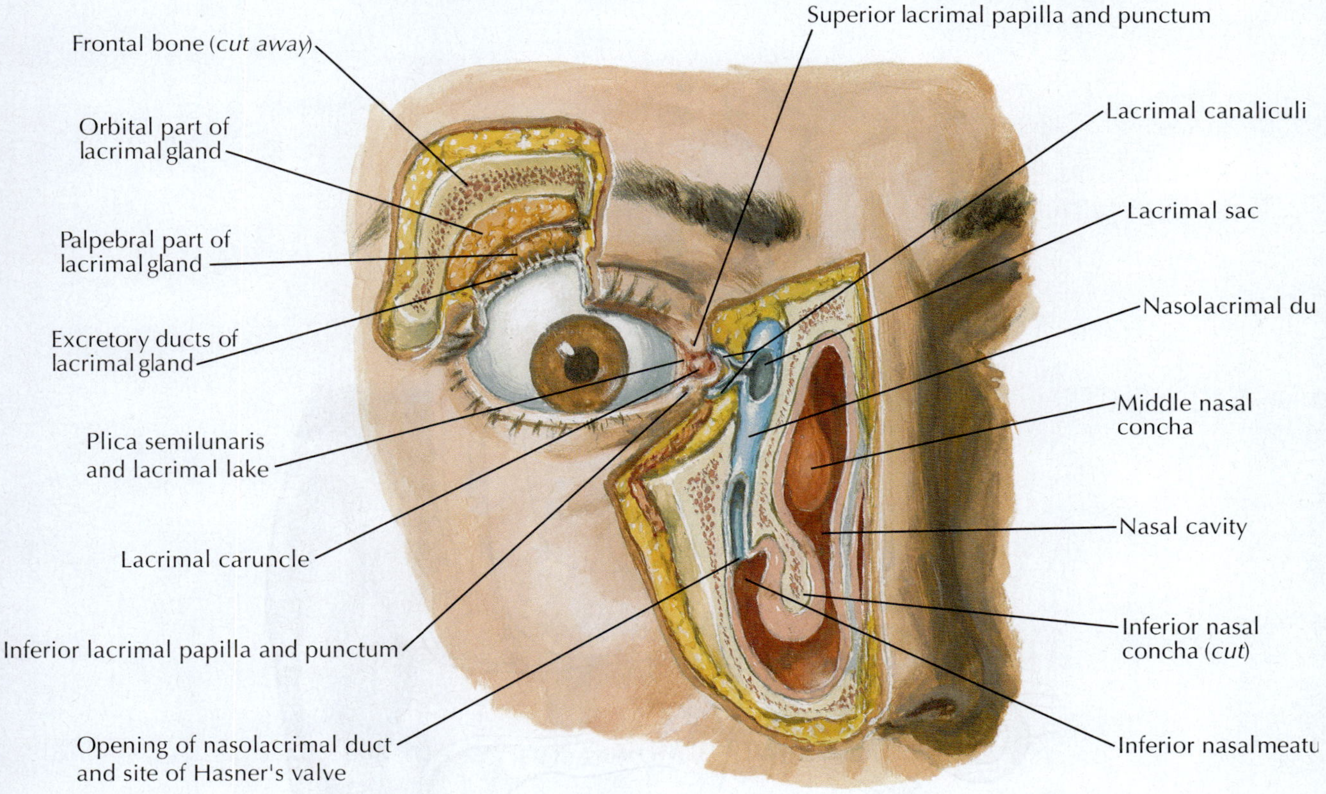

Superior lacrimal papilla and punctum
Orbital part of lacrimal gland
Lacrimal canaliculi
Palpebral part of lacrimal gland
Lacrimal sac
Excretory ducts of lacrimal gland
Nasolacrimal duct
Plica semilunaris
Opening of nasolacrimal duct
Lacrimal caruncle
Inferior lacrimal papilla and punctum

Superior lacrimal papilla and punctum
Frontal bone (*cut away*)
Lacrimal canaliculi
Orbital part of lacrimal gland
Lacrimal sac
Palpebral part of lacrimal gland
Nasolacrimal du
Excretory ducts of lacrimal gland
Middle nasal concha
Plica semilunaris and lacrimal lake
Nasal cavity
Lacrimal caruncle
Inferior nasal concha (*cut*)
Inferior lacrimal papilla and punctum
Inferior nasalmeatu
Opening of nasolacrimal duct and site of Hasner's valve

Plate 19 Lacrimal Apparatus.

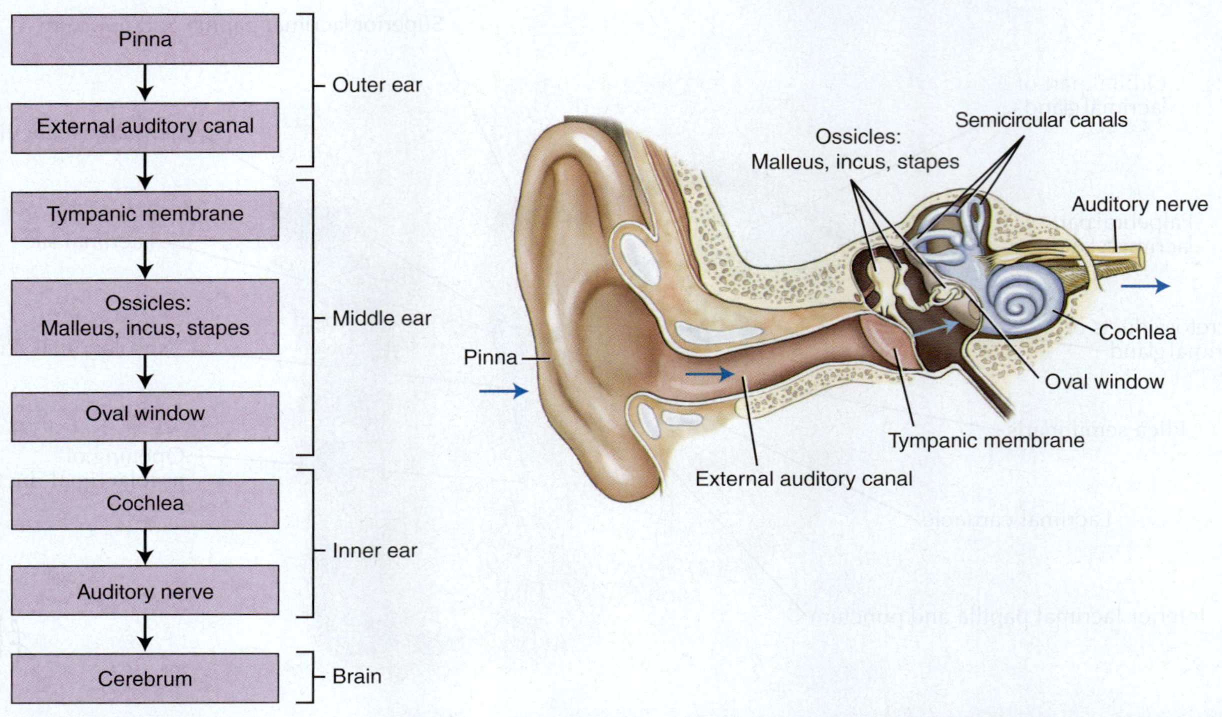

Plate 20   Pathway of Sound. (LaFleur Brooks D, LaFleur Brooks M: Basic Medical Language, ed 4, St. Louis, 2013, Mosby.)

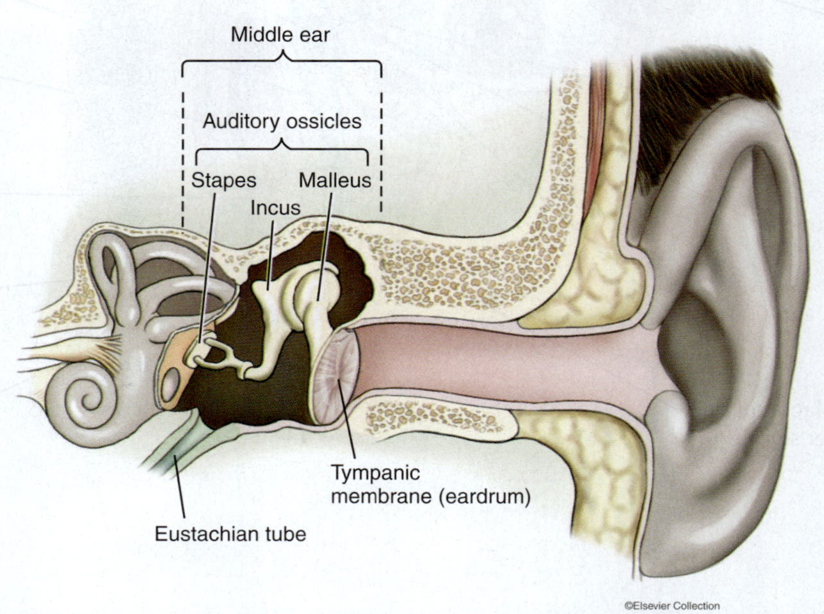

Plate 21   Middle ear structures. (©Elsevier Collection.)

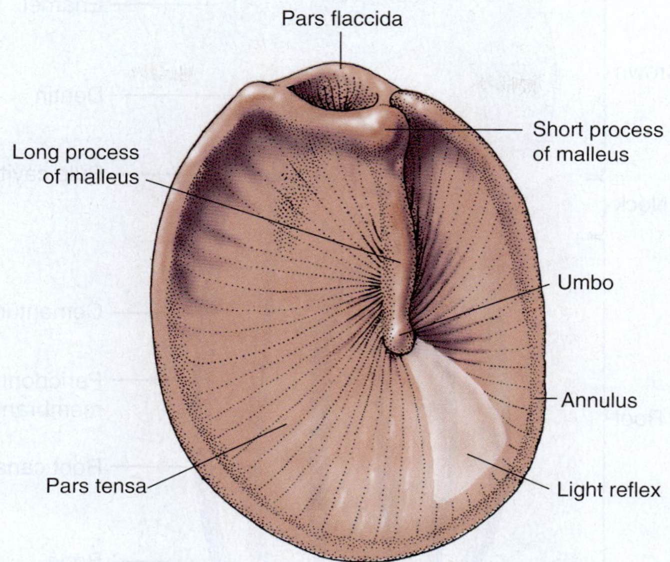

Plate 22   Structural landmarks of tympanic membrane. (Ignatavicius DD, Workman ML: Medical-Surgical Nursing: Patient-Centered Collaborative Care, ed 7, St. Louis, 2013, Saunders.)

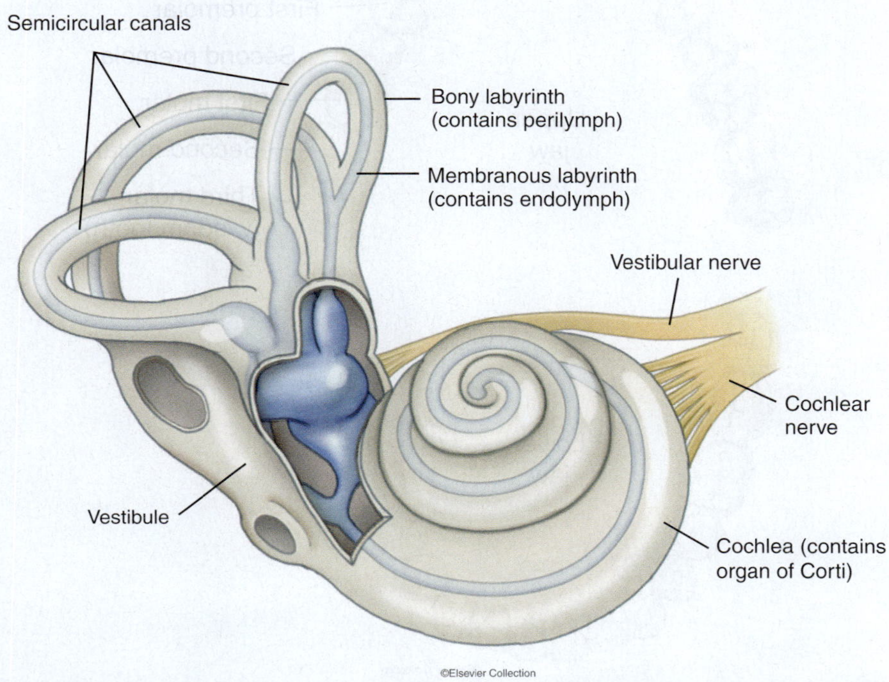

Plate 23   Inner ear structures. (©Elsevier Collection.)

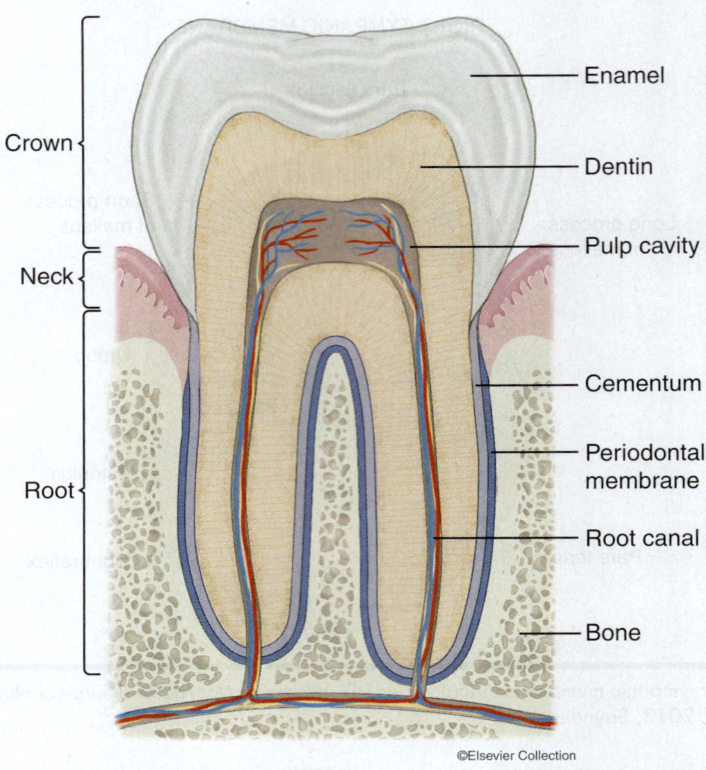

Plate 24 The Tooth. (©Elsevier Collection).

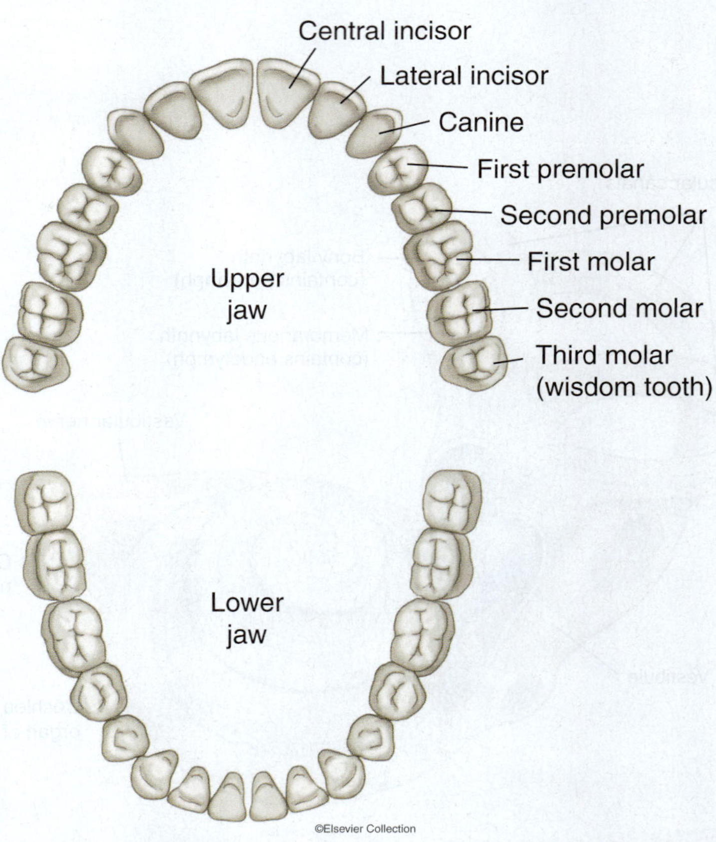

Plate 25 Adult Teeth. (©Elsevier Collection).

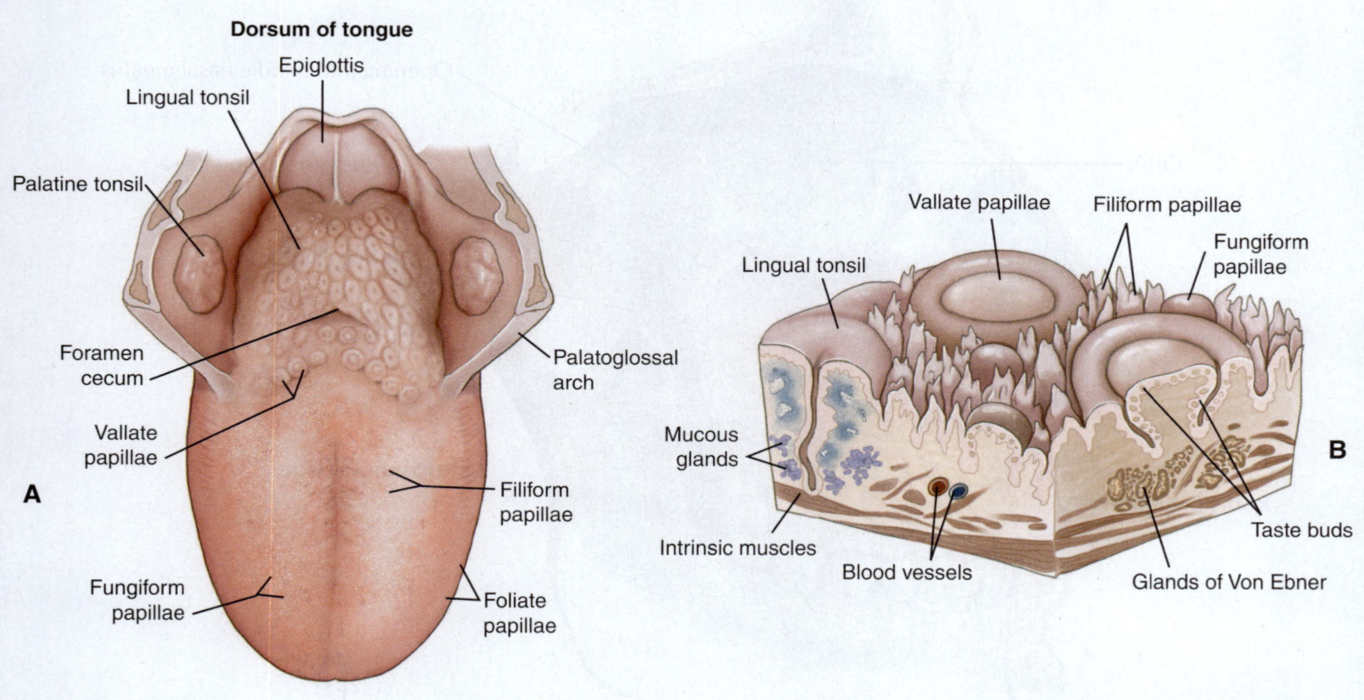

Plate 26   A, Dorsal view of tongue showing the roughened large lingual tonsils on the posterior of the tongue and the foliate papillae on the side. B, Section of dorsal of the tongue showing a cutaway through lingual papillae and showing von Ebner's glands at the base of the vallate papilla. (Brand RW, Isselhard DE: *Anatomy of Orofacial Structures: A Comprehensive Approach*, ed 8, St. Louis, 2019, Elsevier.)

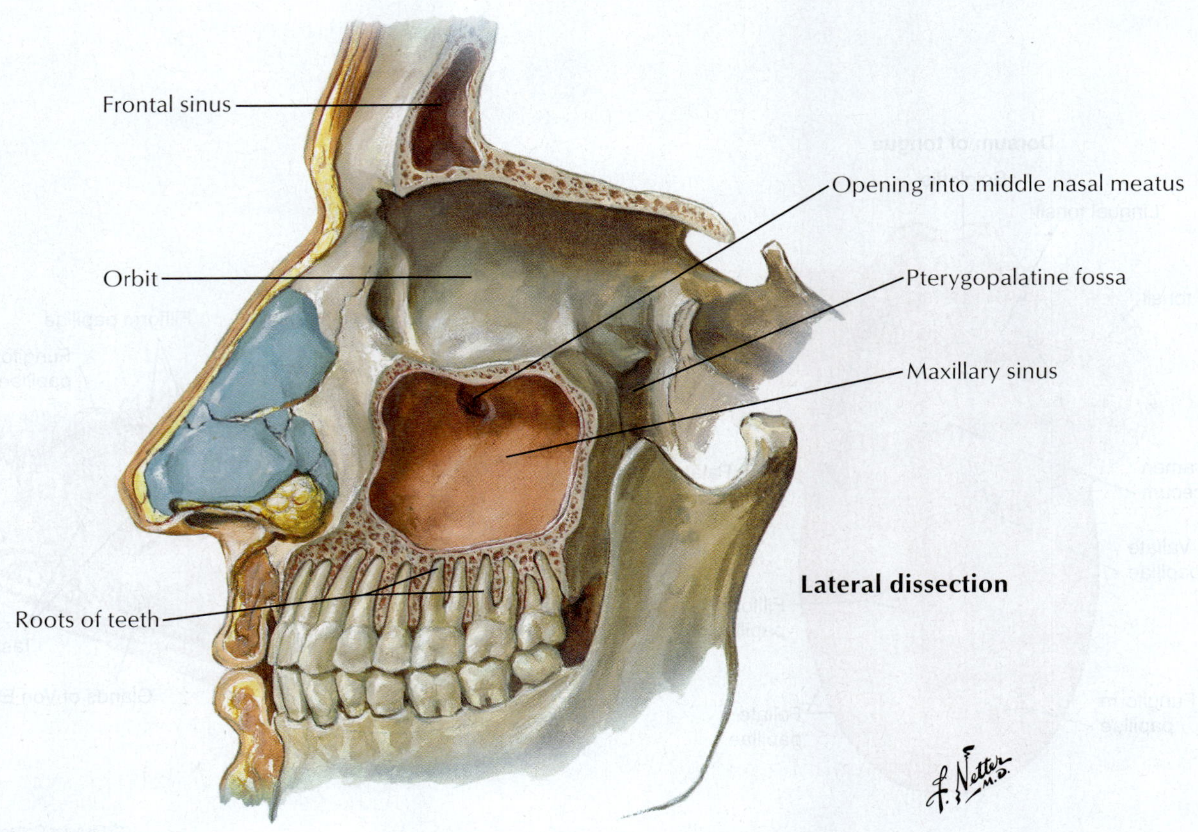

Plate 27   Paranasal Sinuses. (Copyright 2025 Elsevier Inc. All rights reserved. www.netterimages.com. Image ID: 8427)

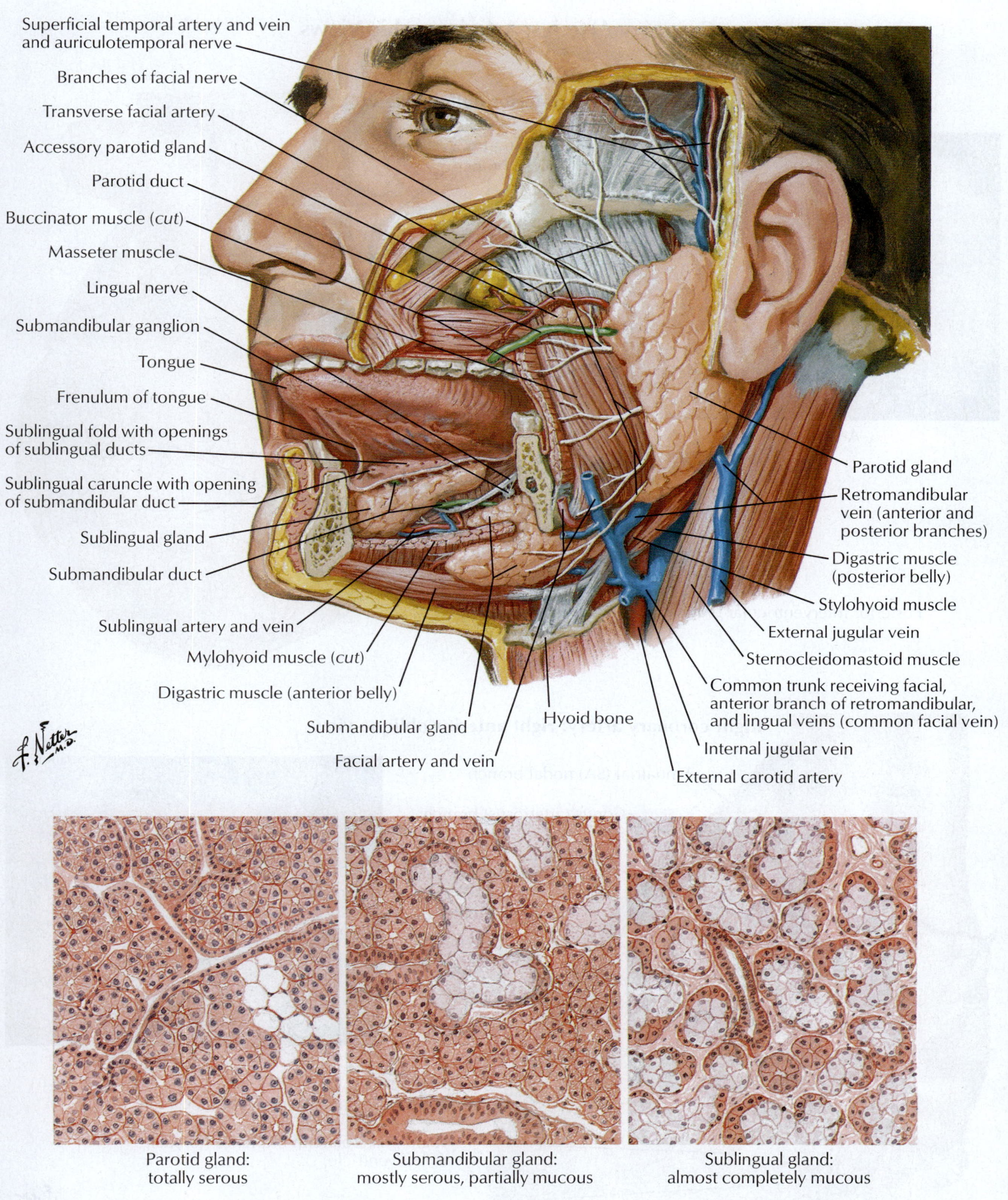

ANATOMY ILLUSTRATIONS

Plate 28 Salivary Glands. (Copyright 2025 Elsevier Inc. All rights reserved. www.netterimages.com. Image ID: 4396)

Coronary Arteries: Arteriographic Views

Right coronary artery: left anterior oblique view

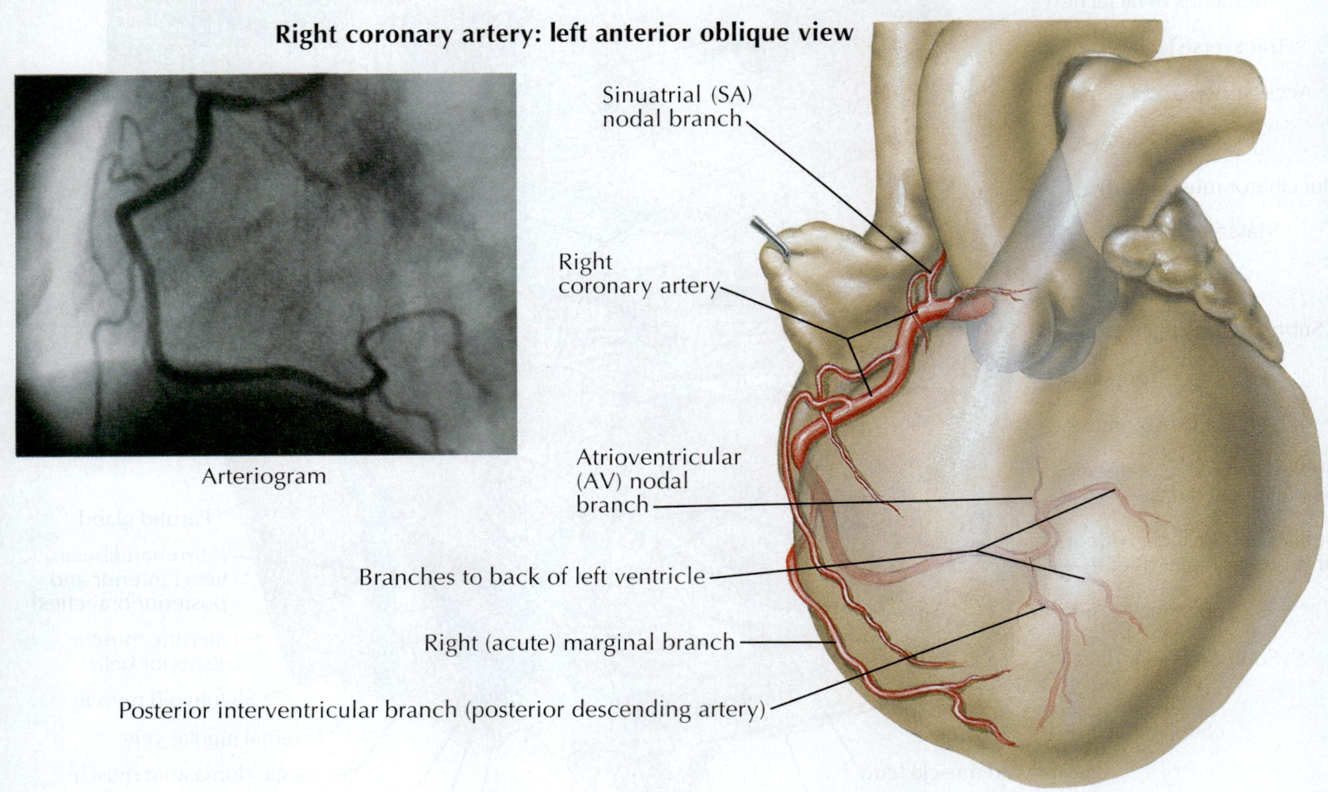

Right coronary artery: right anterior oblique view

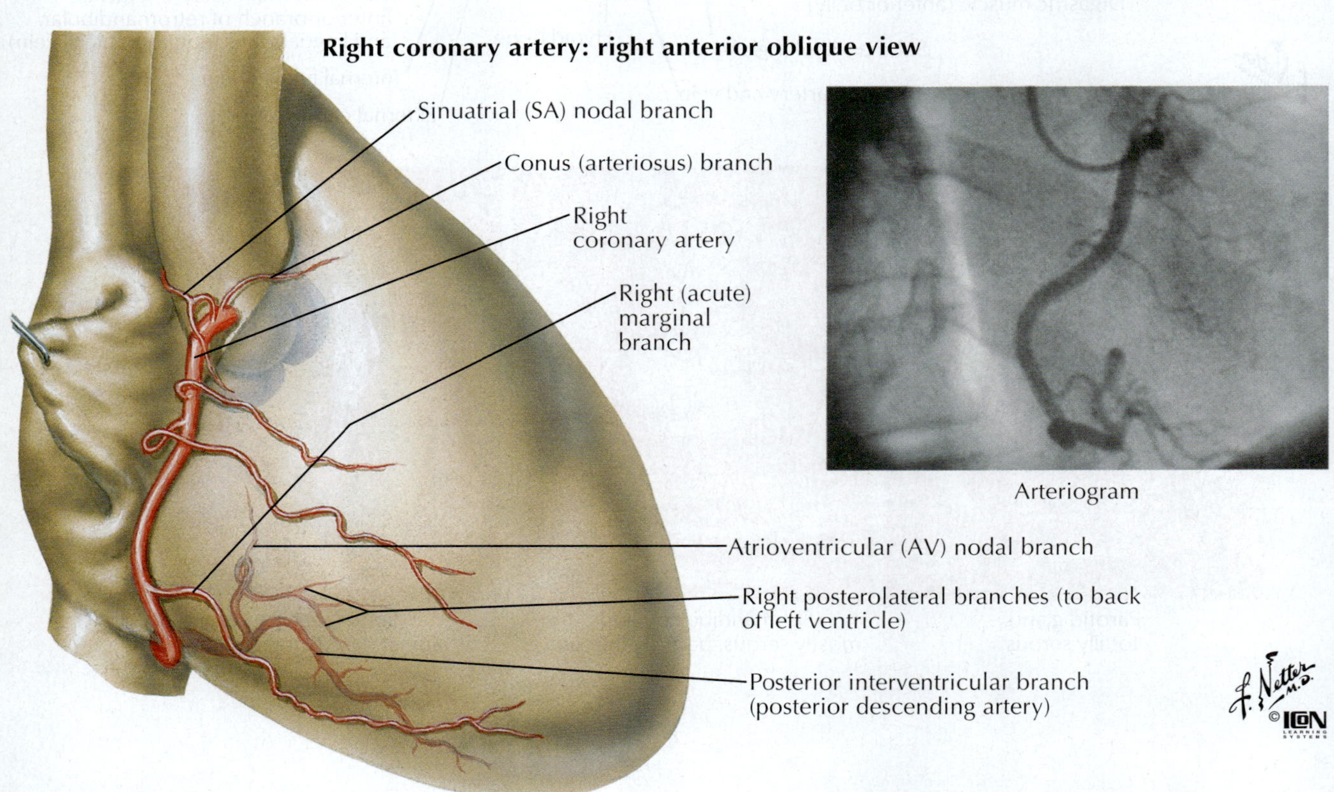

Plate 29 Coronary Arteries: Arteriographic Views. (Copyright 2025 Elsevier Inc. All rights reserved. www.netterimages.com. Image ID: 4725)

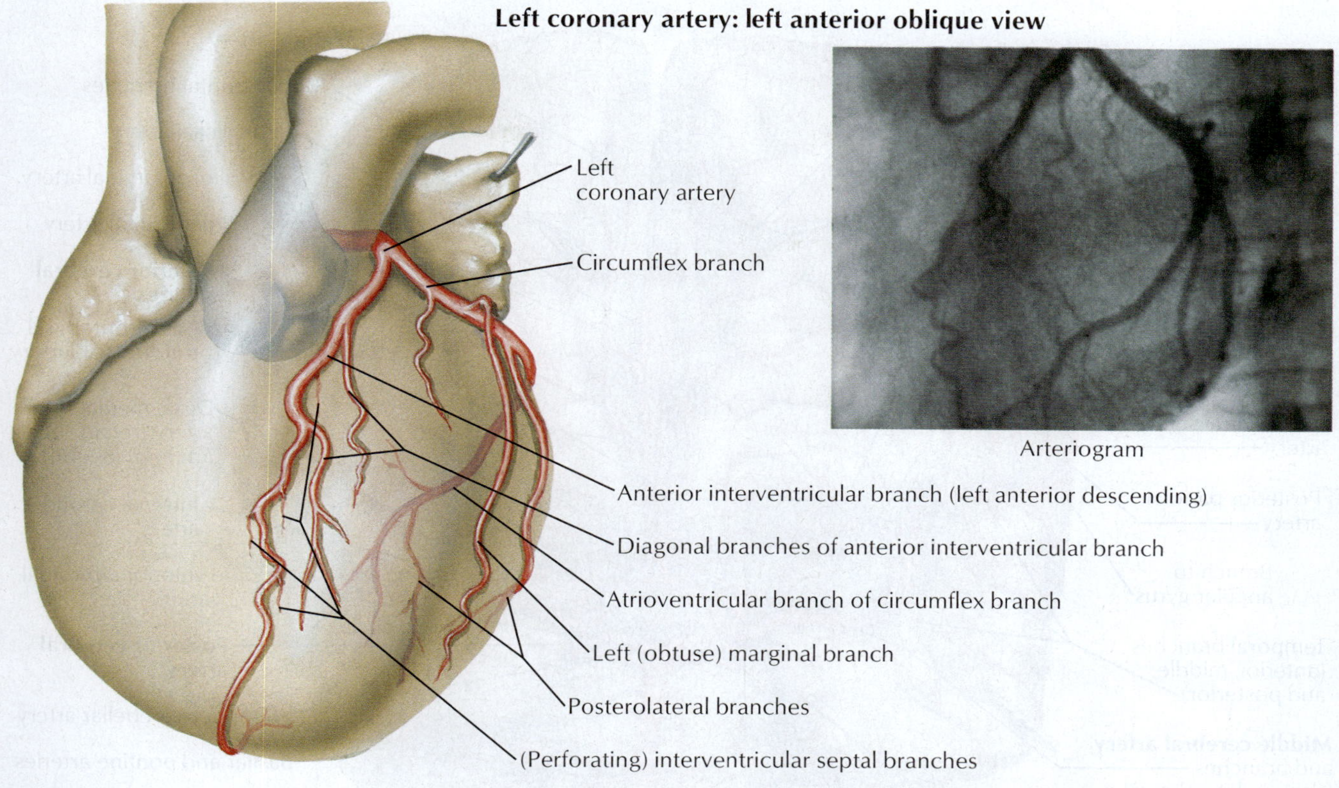

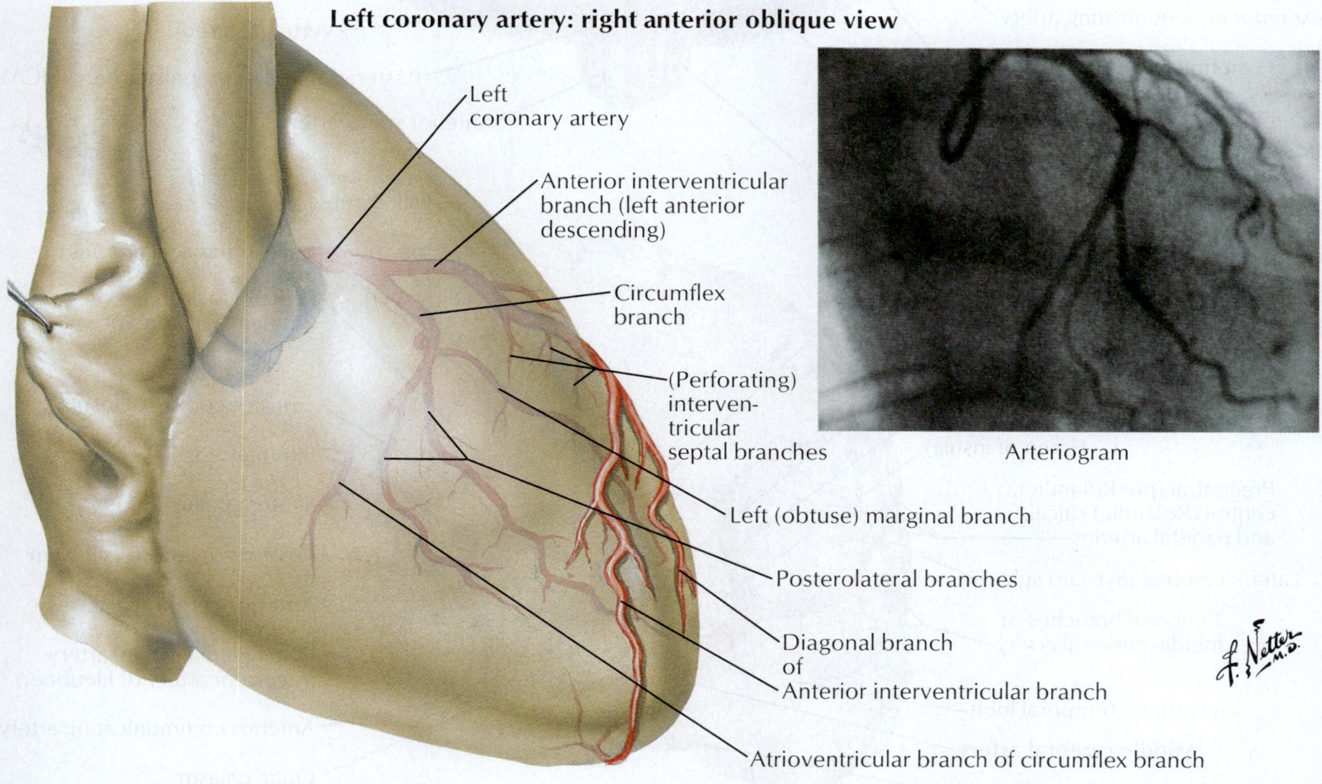

Plate 30 Coronary Arteries: Arteriographic Views. (Copyright 2025 Elsevier Inc. All rights reserved. www.netterimages.com. Image ID: 4542)

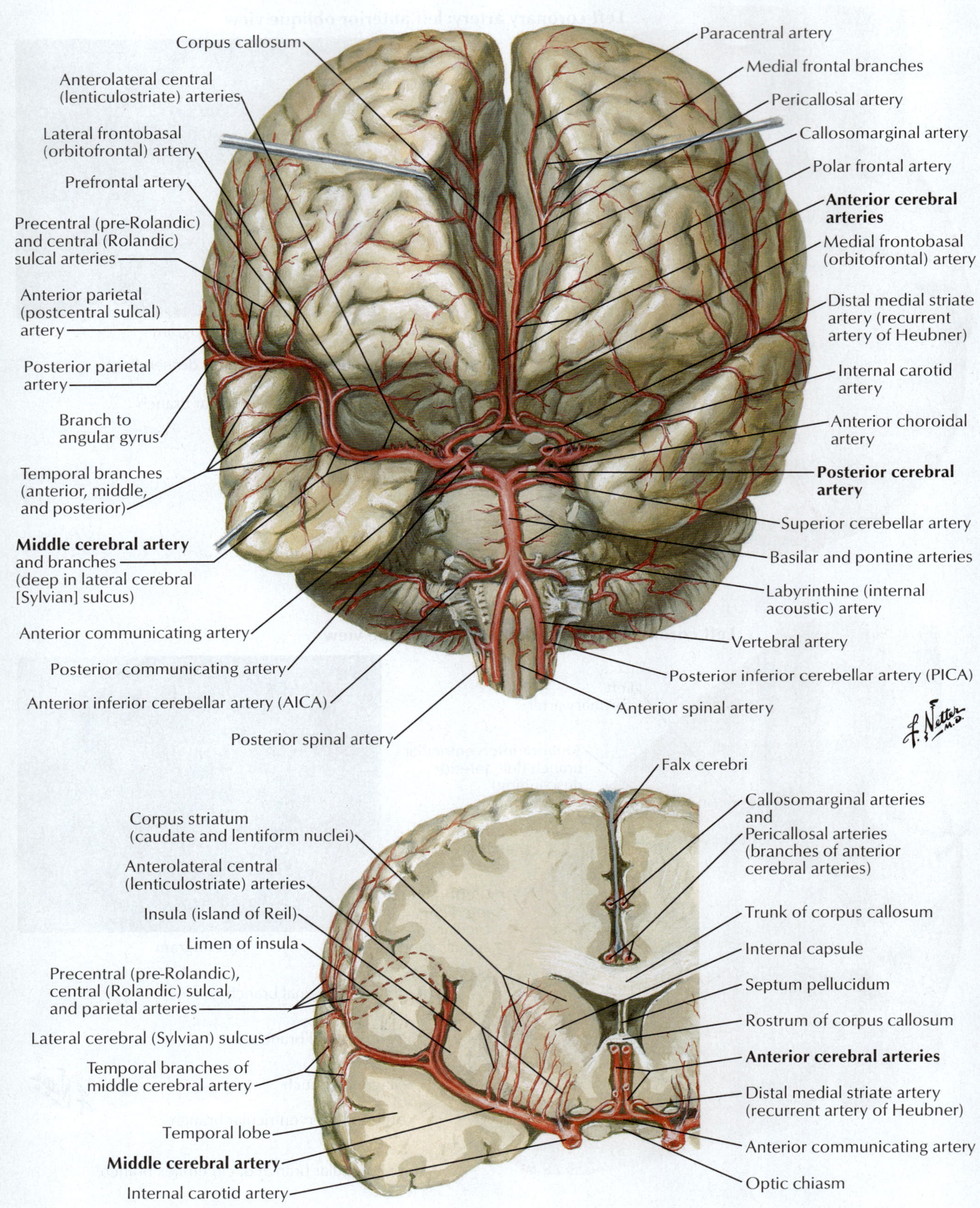

Plate 31 Arteries of Brain: Frontal View and Section. (Copyright 2025 Elsevier Inc. All rights reserved. www.netterimages.com. Image ID: 4588)

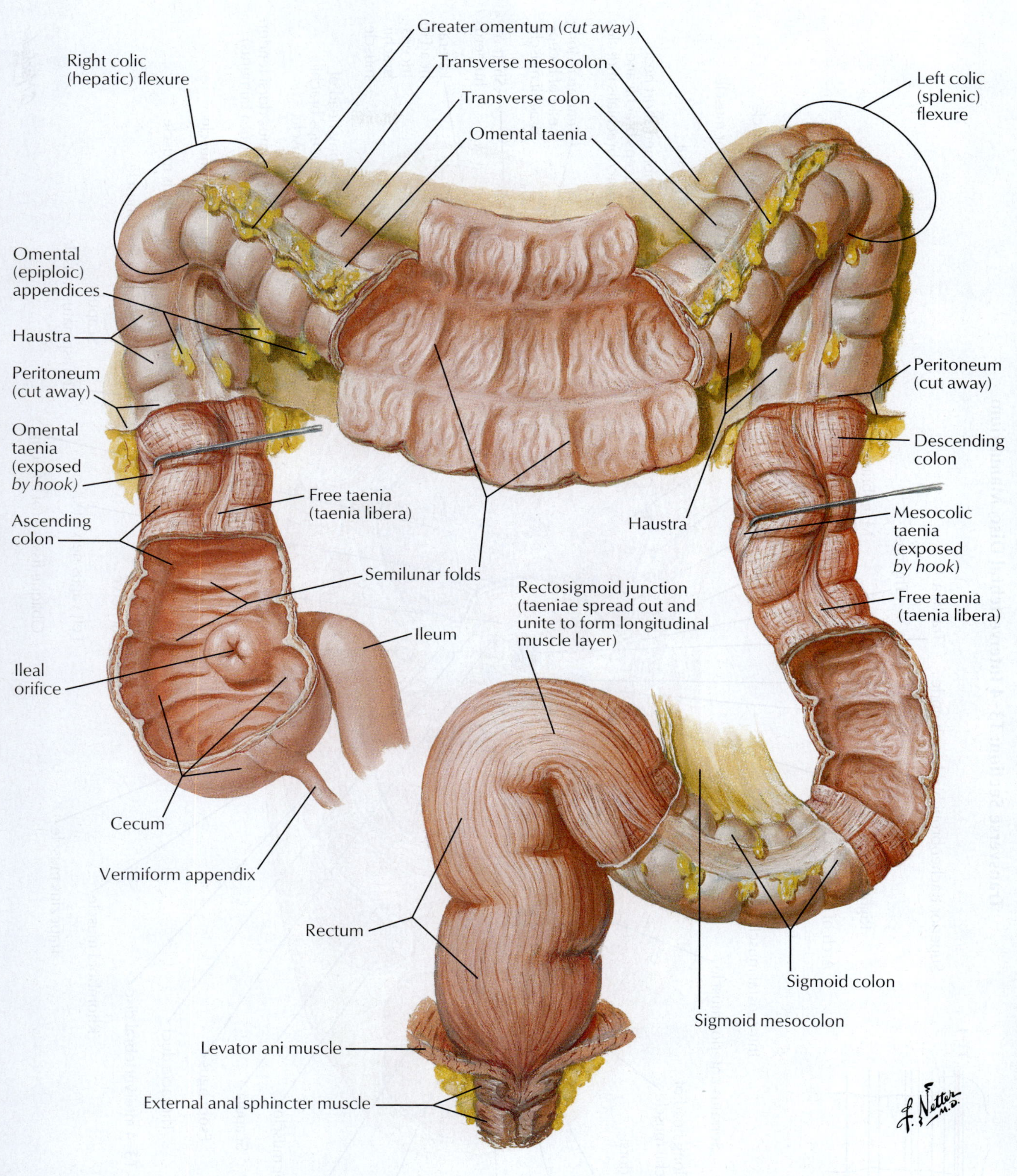

Plate 32 Mucosa and Musculature of Large Intestine. (Copyright 2025 Elsevier Inc. All rights reserved. www.netterimages.com. Image ID: 4778)

Transverse Section: T3–4 Intervertebral Disc, Manubrium

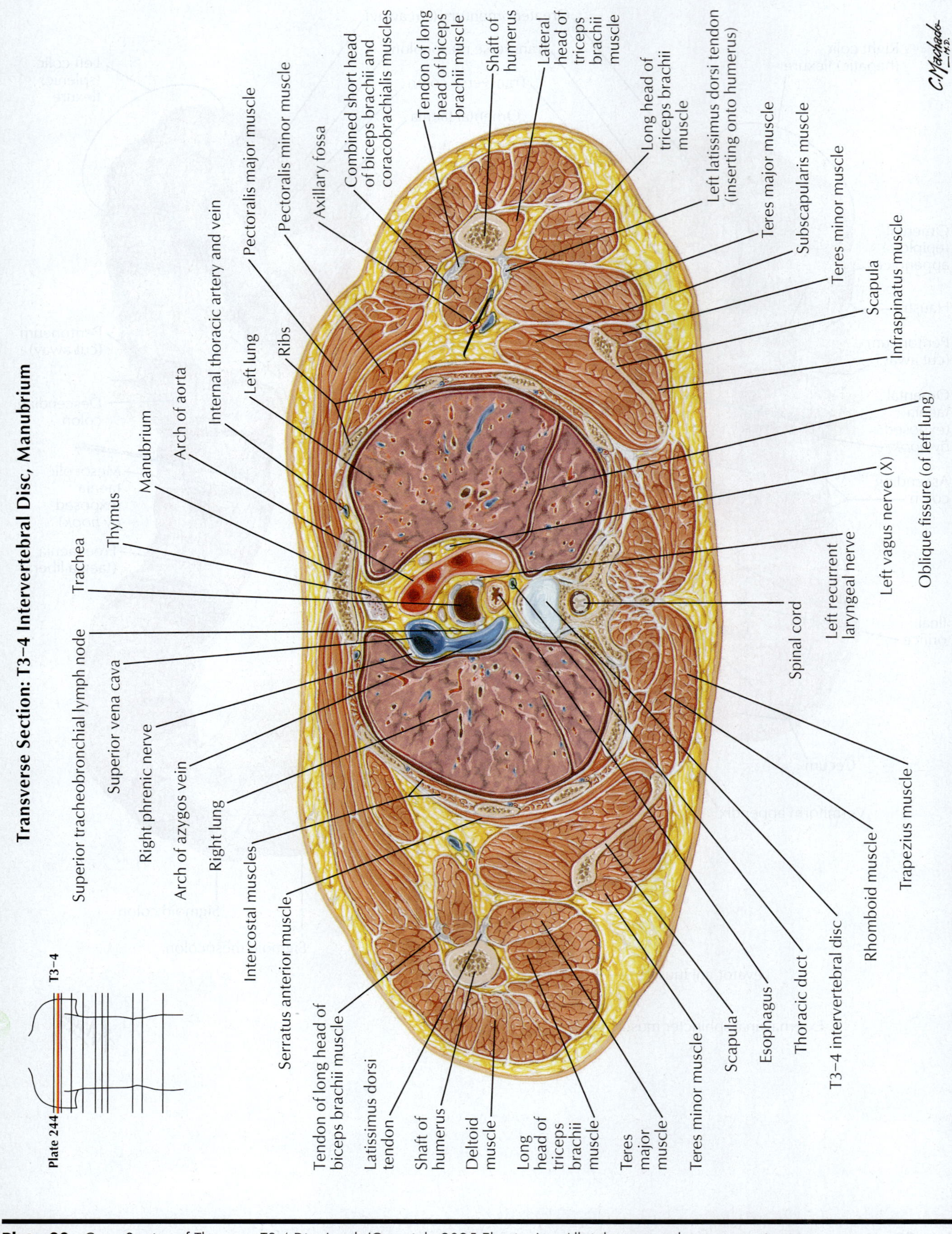

Plate 33 Cross Section of Thorax at T3-4 Disc Level. (Copyright 2025 Elsevier Inc. All rights reserved. www.netterimages.com. Image ID: 4880)

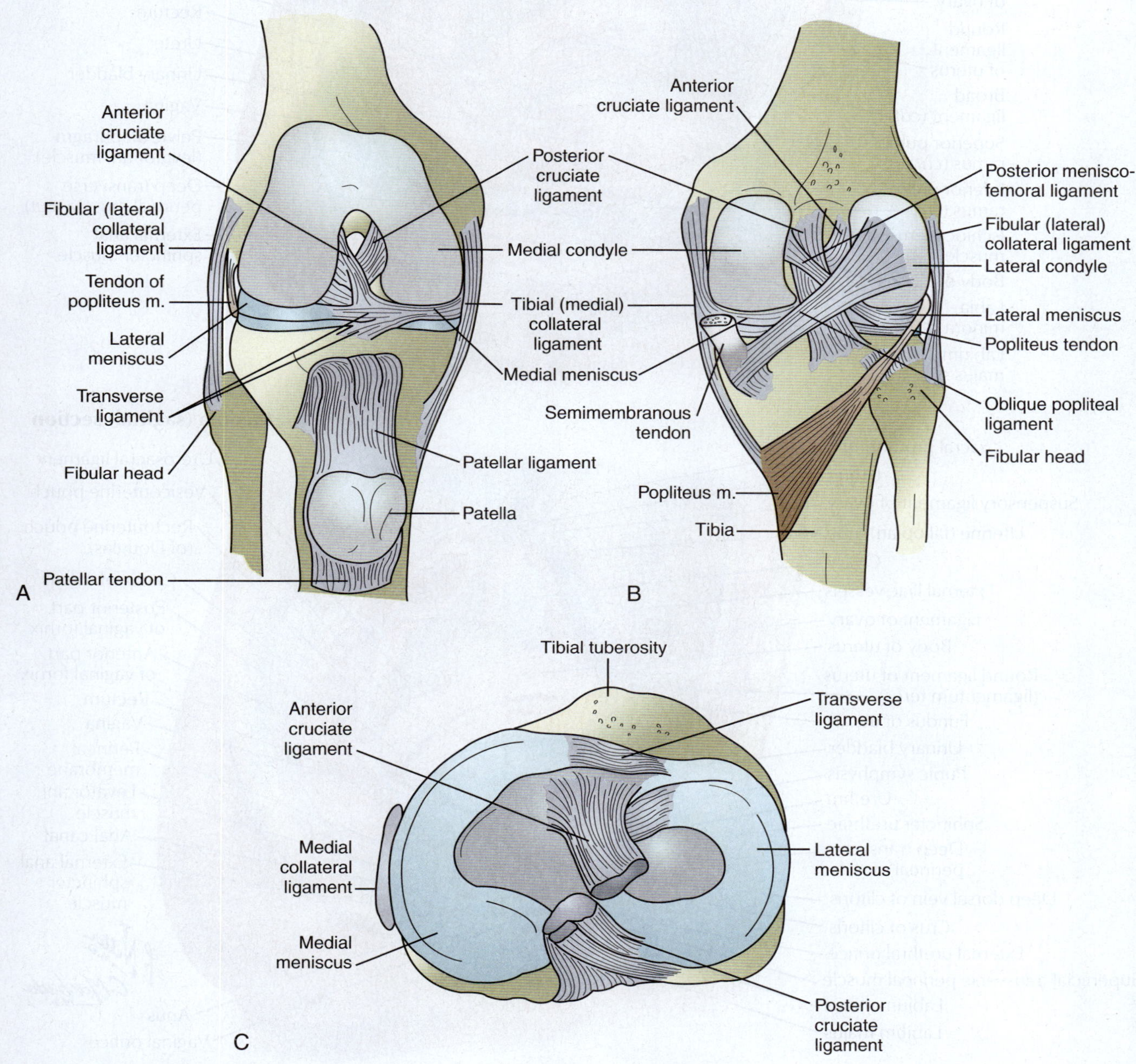

Plate 34 Knee joint opened; anterior, posterior, and proximal views. A, Anterior view of the knee joint, opened by folding the patella and patellar ligament inferiorly. On the lateral side is the fibular collateral ligament, separated by the popliteal tendon from the lateral meniscus. On the medial side, the tibial collateral ligament is attached to the medial meniscus. The anterior and posterior cruciate ligaments are seen between the femoral condyles. B, Posterior view of the opened knee joint with a more complete view of the posterior cruciate ligament. C, The femur is removed, showing the proximal (articular) end of the right tibia. On the medial side is the gently curved medial meniscus; on the lateral side is the more tightly curved lateral meniscus. The anterior end of the medial meniscus is anchored to the surface of the tibia by the transverse ligament. The cut ends of the anterior and posterior cruciate ligaments are shown, as well as the meniscofemoral ligament. (Fritz S: Mosby's Essential Sciences for Therapeutic Massage: Anatomy, Physiology, Biomechanics, and Pathology, ed 5, St. Louis, 2017, Elsevier.)

Paramedian (sagittal) dissection

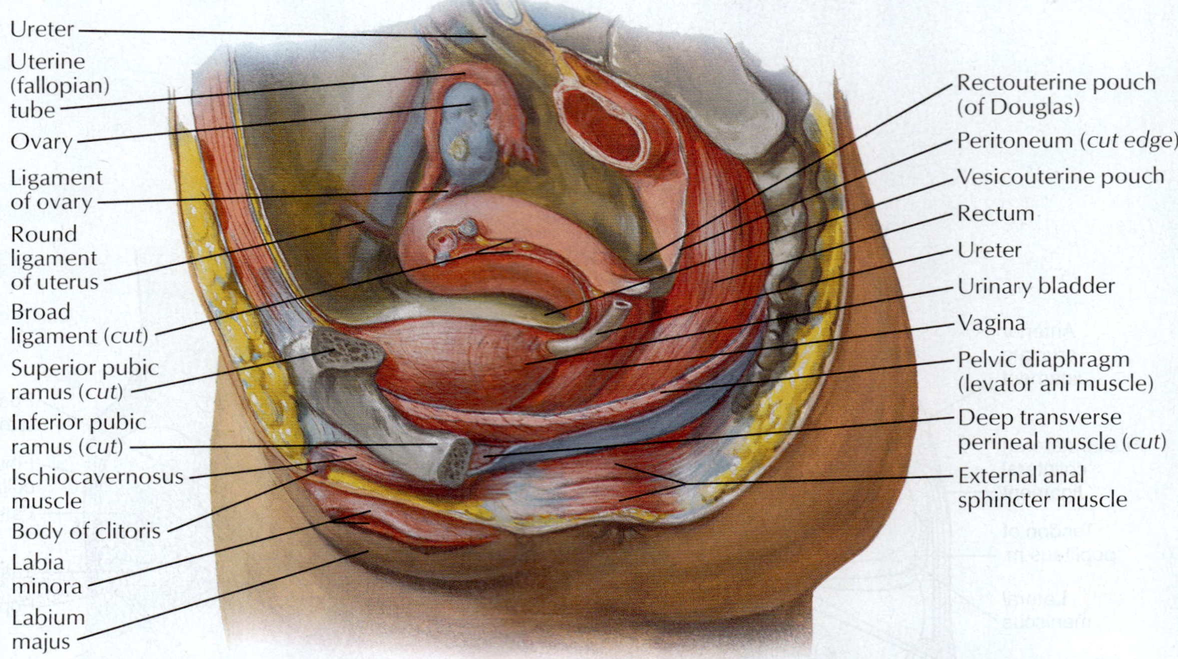

Median (sagittal) section

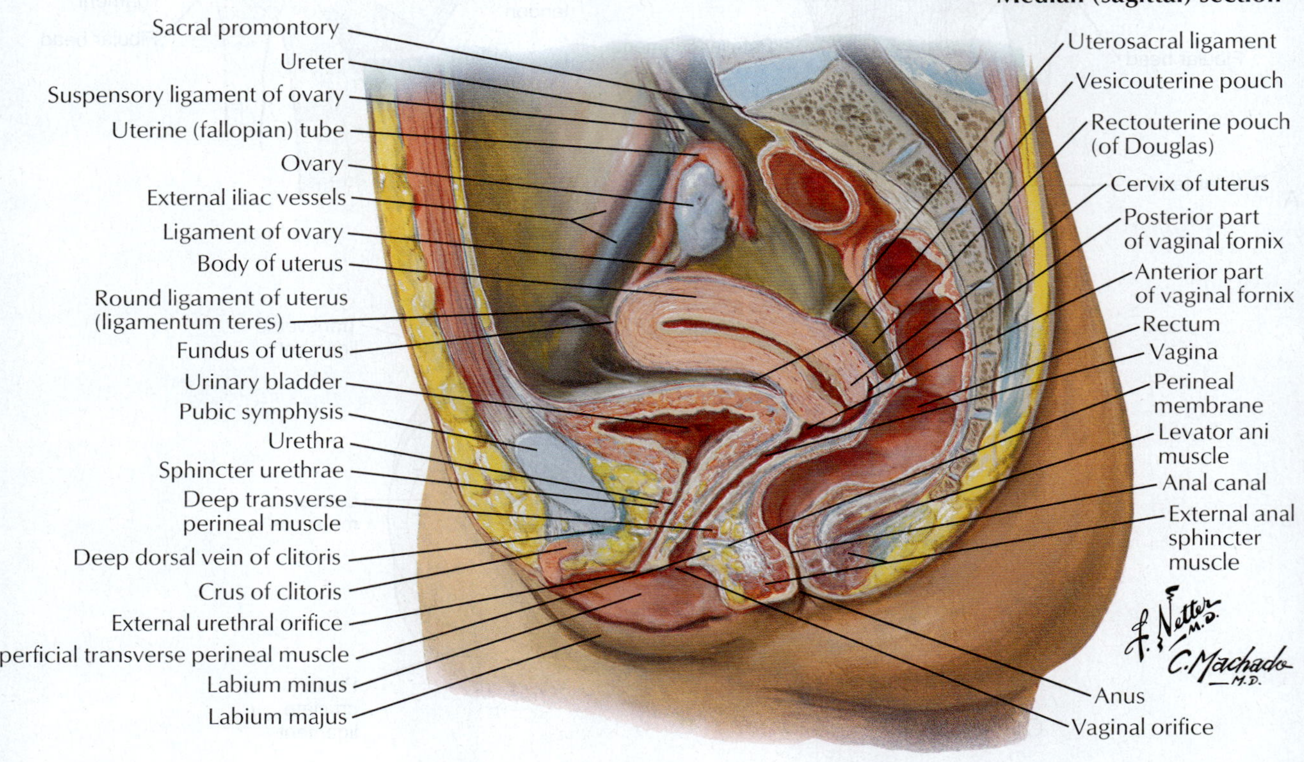

PART II

Alphabetic Index

A

Aarskog's syndrome Q87.19
Abandonment —*see* Maltreatment
Abasia (-astasia) (hysterical) F44.4
Abderhalden-Kaufmann-Lignac syndrome (cystinosis) E72.04
Abdomen, abdominal —*see also* condition
  acute R10.0
  angina K55.1
  muscle deficiency syndrome Q79.4
Abdominalgia —*see* Pain, abdominal
Abduction contracture, hip or other joint —*see* Contraction, joint
Aberrant (congenital) —*see also* Malposition, congenital
  adrenal gland Q89.1
  artery (peripheral) Q27.8
    basilar NEC Q28.1
    cerebral Q28.3
    coronary Q24.5
    digestive system Q27.8
    eye Q15.8
    lower limb Q27.8
    precerebral Q28.1
    pulmonary Q25.79
    renal Q27.2
    retina Q14.1
    specified site NEC Q27.8
    subclavian Q27.8
    upper limb Q27.8
    vertebral Q28.1
  breast Q83.8
  endocrine gland NEC Q89.2
  hepatic duct Q44.5
  pancreas Q45.3
  parathyroid gland Q89.2
  pituitary gland Q89.2
  sebaceous glands, mucous membrane, mouth, congenital Q38.6
  spleen Q89.09
  subclavian artery Q27.8
  thymus (gland) Q89.2
  thyroid gland Q89.2
  vein (peripheral) NEC Q27.8
    cerebral Q28.3
    digestive system Q27.8
    lower limb Q27.8
    precerebral Q28.1
    specified site NEC Q27.8
    upper limb Q27.8
Aberration
  distantial —*see* Disturbance, visual
  mental F99
Abetalipoproteinemia E78.6
Abiotrophy R68.89
Ablatio, ablation
  retinae —*see* Detachment, retina
Ablepharia, ablepharon Q10.3
Abnormal, abnormality, abnormalities —*see also* Anomaly
  acid-base balance (mixed) E87.4
  albumin R77.0
  alphafetoprotein R77.2
  alveolar ridge K08.9
  anatomical relationship Q89.9
  ▶ anti-cyclic citrullinated protein antibody and rheumatoid factor R76.81
  ▶ anti-CCP (cyclic citrullinated protein) R76.81
  apertures, congenital, diaphragm Q79.1
  atrial septal, specified NEC Q21.19
  auditory perception H93.29- ●
    diplacusis —*see* Diplacusis
    hyperacusis —*see* Hyperacusis
    recruitment —*see* Recruitment, auditory
    threshold shift —*see* Shift, auditory threshold
  autosomes Q99.9
    fragile site Q95.5
  basal metabolic rate R94.8
  biosynthesis, testicular androgen E29.1
  bleeding time R79.1
  blood amino-acid level R79.83
  blood level (of)
    cobalt R79.0
    copper R79.0
    iron R79.0
    lithium R78.89
    magnesium R79.0
    mineral NEC R79.0
    zinc R79.0

Abnormal, abnormality, abnormalities (Continued)
  blood pressure
    elevated R03.0
    low reading (nonspecific) R03.1
  blood sugar R73.09
  blood-gas level R79.81
  bowel sounds R19.15
    absent R19.11
    hyperactive R19.12
  brain scan R94.02
  breathing R06.9
  caloric test R94.138
  cerebrospinal fluid R83.9
    cytology R83.6
    drug level R83.2
    enzyme level R83.0
    hormones R83.1
    immunology R83.4
    microbiology R83.5
    nonmedicinal level R83.3
    specified type NEC R83.8
  chemistry, blood R79.9
    C-reactive protein R79.82
    drugs —*see* Findings, abnormal, in blood
    gas level R79.81
    minerals R79.0
    pancytopenia D61.818
    PTT R79.1
    specified NEC R79.89
    toxins —*see* Findings, abnormal, in blood
  chest sounds (friction) (rales) R09.89
  chromosome, chromosomal Q99.9
    with more than three X chromosomes, female Q97.1
    analysis result R89.8
      bronchial washings R84.8
      cerebrospinal fluid R83.8
      cervix uteri NEC R87.89
      nasal secretions R84.8
      nipple discharge R89.8
      peritoneal fluid R85.89
      pleural fluid R84.8
      prostatic secretions R86.8
      saliva R85.89
      seminal fluid R86.8
      sputum R84.8
      synovial fluid R89.8
      throat scrapings R84.8
      vagina R87.89
      vulva R87.89
      wound secretions R89.8
    dicentric replacement Q93.2
    ring replacement Q93.2
    sex Q99.8
      female phenotype Q97.9
        specified NEC Q97.8
      male phenotype Q98.9
        specified NEC Q98.8
      structural male Q98.6
    specified NEC Q99.8
  clinical findings NEC R68.89
  coagulation D68.9
    newborn, transient P61.6
    profile R79.1
    time R79.1
  communication —*see* Fistula
  conjunctiva, vascular H11.41- ●
  coronary artery Q24.5
  cortisol-binding globulin E27.8
  course, eustachian tube Q17.8
  creatinine clearance R94.4
  cytology
    anus R85.619
      atypical squamous cells cannot exclude high grade squamous intraepithelial lesion (ASC-H) R85.611
      atypical squamous cells of undetermined significance (ASC-US) R85.610
      cytologic evidence of malignancy R85.614
      high grade squamous intraepithelial lesion (HGSIL) R85.613
      human papillomavirus (HPV) DNA test high risk positive R85.81
        ~~low risk positive R85.82~~
      ▶ low risk positive R85.82
      inadequate smear R85.615
      low grade squamous intraepithelial lesion (LGSIL) R85.612

Abnormal, abnormality, abnormalities (Continued)
  cytology (Continued)
    anus (Continued)
      satisfactory anal smear but lacking transformation zone R85.616
      specified NEC R85.618
      unsatisfactory smear R85.615
    female genital organs —*see* Abnormal, Papanicolaou (smear)
  dark adaptation curve H53.61
  dentofacial NEC —*see* Anomaly, dentofacial
  development, developmental Q89.9
    central nervous system Q07.9
  diagnostic imaging
    abdomen, abdominal region NEC R93.5
    biliary tract R93.2
    bladder R93.41
    breast R92.8
    central nervous system NEC R90.89
    cerebrovascular NEC R90.89
    coronary circulation R93.1
    digestive tract NEC R93.3
    gastrointestinal (tract) R93.3
    genitourinary organs R93.89
    head R93.0
    heart R93.1
    intrathoracic organ NEC R93.89
    kidney R93.42- ●
    limbs R93.6
    liver R93.2
    lung (field) R91.8
    musculoskeletal system NEC R93.7
    renal pelvis R93.41
    retroperitoneum R93.5
    site specified NEC R93.89
    skin and subcutaneous tissue R93.89
    skull R93.0
    testis R93.81- ●
    urinary organs specified NEC R93.49
    ureter R93.41
  direction, teeth, fully erupted M26.30
  ear ossicles, acquired NEC H74.39- ●
    ankylosis —*see* Ankylosis, ear ossicles
    discontinuity —*see* Discontinuity, ossicles, ear
    partial loss —*see* Loss, ossicles, ear (partial)
  Ebstein Q22.5
  echocardiogram R93.1
  echoencephalogram R90.81
  echogram —*see* Abnormal, diagnostic imaging
  electrocardiogram [ECG] [EKG] R94.31
  electroencephalogram [EEG] R94.01
  electrolyte —*see* Imbalance, electrolyte
  electromyogram [EMG] R94.131
  electro-oculogram [EOG] R94.110
  electrophysiological intracardiac studies R94.39
  electroretinogram [ERG] R94.111
  erythrocytes
    congenital, with perinatal jaundice D58.9
  feces (color) (contents) (mucus) R19.5
  finding —*see* Findings, abnormal, without diagnosis
  fluid
    amniotic —*see* Abnormal, specimen, specified
    cerebrospinal —*see* Abnormal, cerebrospinal fluid
    peritoneal —*see* Abnormal, specimen, digestive organs
    pleural —*see* Abnormal, specimen, respiratory organs
    synovial —*see* Abnormal, specimen, specified
    thorax (bronchial washings) (pleural fluid) — *see* Abnormal, specimen, respiratory organs
    vaginal —*see* Abnormal, specimen, female genital organs
  form
    teeth K00.2
    uterus —*see* Anomaly, uterus
  function studies
    auditory R94.120
    bladder R94.8
    brain R94.09
    cardiovascular R94.30
    ear R94.128
    endocrine NEC R94.7
    eye NEC R94.118
    kidney R94.4
    liver R94.5
    nervous system
      central NEC R94.09
      peripheral NEC R94.138

▶ New ⇒ Revised ~~deleted~~ Deleted ● Use Additional Character(s)

A

Abnormal, abnormality, abnormalities (Continued)
  specimen (Continued)
    respiratory organs (Continued)
      hormones R84.1
      immunology R84.4
      microbiology R84.5
      nonmedicinal level R84.3
      specified type NEC R84.8
    specified organ, system and tissue NOS R89.9
      cytology R89.6
      drug level R89.2
      enzyme level R89.0
      histology R89.7
      hormones R89.1
      immunology R89.4
      microbiology R89.5
      nonmedicinal level R89.3
      specified type NEC R89.8
    synovial fluid —see Abnormal, specimen,
      specified
    thorax (bronchial washings) (pleural fluids) —
      see Abnormal, specimen, respiratory
      organs
    vagina (secretion) (smear) R87.629
    vulva (secretion) (smear) R87.69
    wound secretion —see Abnormal, specimen,
      specified
  spermatozoa —see Abnormal, specimen, male
    genital organs
  sputum (amount) (color) (odor) R09.3
  stool (color) (contents) (mucus) R19.5
    bloody K92.1
    guaiac positive R19.5
  synchondrosis Q78.8
  thermography —see also Abnormal, diagnostic
    imaging R93.89
  thyroid-binding globulin E07.89
  tooth, teeth (form) (size) K00.2
  toxicology (findings) R78.9
  transport protein E88.09
  tumor marker NEC R97.8
  ultrasound results —see Abnormal, diagnostic
    imaging
  umbilical cord complicating delivery O69.9
  urination NEC R39.198
  urine (constituents) R82.90
    bile R82.2
    cytological examination R82.89
    drugs R82.5
    fat R82.0
    glucose R81
    heavy metals R82.6
    hemoglobin R82.3
    histological examination R82.89
    ketones R82.4
    microbiological examination (culture) R82.79
    myoglobin R82.1
    positive culture R82.79
    protein —see Proteinuria
    specified substance NEC R82.998
      chromoabnormality NEC R82.91
    substances nonmedical R82.6
  uterine hemorrhage —see Hemorrhage, uterus
  vectorcardiogram R94.39
  visually evoked potential (VEP) R94.112
  white blood cells D72.9
    specified NEC D72.89
  X-ray examination —see Abnormal, diagnostic
    imaging

Abnormity (any organ or part) —see Anomaly

Abocclusion M26.29
  hemolytic disease (newborn) P55.1
  incompatibility reaction ABO —see
    Complication(s), transfusion,
    incompatibility reaction, ABO

Abolition, language R48.8

Aborter, habitual or recurrent —see Loss (of),
  pregnancy, recurrent

Abortion (complete) (spontaneous) O03.9
  with
    retained products of conception —see
      Abortion, incomplete
  attempted (elective) (failed) O07.4
    complicated by O07.30
      afibrinogenemia O07.1
      cardiac arrest O07.36
      chemical damage of pelvic organ(s) O07.34
      circulatory collapse O07.31
      cystitis O07.38
      defibrination syndrome O07.1
      electrolyte imbalance O07.33

Abortion (Continued)
  attempted (Continued)
    complicated by (Continued)
      embolism (air) (amniotic fluid) (blood clot)
        (fat) (pulmonary) (septic) (soap) O07.2
      endometritis O07.0
      genital tract and pelvic infection O07.0
      hemolysis O07.1
      hemorrhage (delayed) (excessive) O07.1
      infection
        genital tract or pelvic O07.0
        urinary tract O07.38
      intravascular coagulation O07.1
      laceration of pelvic organ(s) O07.34
      metabolic disorder O07.33
      oliguria O07.32
      oophoritis O07.0
      parametritis O07.0
      pelvic peritonitis O07.0
      perforation of pelvic organ(s) O07.34
      renal failure or shutdown O07.32
      salpingitis or salpingo-oophoritis O07.0
      sepsis O07.37
      shock O07.31
      specified condition NEC O07.39
      tubular necrosis (renal) O07.32
      uremia O07.32
      urinary tract infection O07.38
      venous complication NEC O07.35
        embolism (air) (amniotic fluid) (blood
         clot) (fat) (pulmonary) (septic)
         (soap) O07.2
  complicated (by) (following) O03.80
    afibrinogenemia O03.6
    cardiac arrest O03.86
    chemical damage of pelvic organ(s) O03.84
    circulatory collapse O03.81
    cystitis O03.88
    defibrination syndrome O03.6
    electrolyte imbalance O03.83
    embolism (air) (amniotic fluid) (blood clot)
      (fat) (pulmonary) (septic) (soap) O03.7
    endometritis O03.5
    genital tract and pelvic infection O03.5
    hemolysis O03.6
    hemorrhage (delayed) (excessive) O03.6
    infection
      genital tract or pelvic O03.5
      urinary tract O03.88
    intravascular coagulation O03.6
    laceration of pelvic organ(s) O03.84
    metabolic disorder O03.83
    oliguria O03.82
    oophoritis O03.5
    parametritis O03.5
    pelvic peritonitis O03.5
    perforation of pelvic organ(s) O03.84
    renal failure or shutdown O03.82
    salpingitis or salpingo-oophoritis O03.5
    sepsis O03.87
    shock O03.81
    specified condition NEC O03.89
    tubular necrosis (renal) O03.82
    uremia O03.82
    urinary tract infection O03.88
    venous complication NEC O03.85
      embolism (air) (amniotic fluid) (blood clot)
        (fat) (pulmonary) (septic) (soap) O03.7
  failed —see Abortion, attempted
  habitual or recurrent N96
    with current abortion —see categories O03-O04
    without current pregnancy N96
    care in current pregnancy O26.2-•
  incomplete (spontaneous) O03.4
    complicated (by) (following) O03.30
      afibrinogenemia O03.1
      cardiac arrest O03.36
      chemical damage of pelvic organ(s) O03.34
      circulatory collapse O03.31
      cystitis O03.38
      defibrination syndrome O03.1
      electrolyte imbalance O03.33
      embolism (air) (amniotic fluid) (blood clot)
        (fat) (pulmonary) (septic) (soap) O03.2
      endometritis O03.0
      genital tract and pelvic infection O03.0
      hemolysis O03.1
      hemorrhage (delayed) (excessive) O03.1
      infection
        genital tract or pelvic O03.0
        urinary tract O03.38

Abortion (Continued)
  incomplete (Continued)
    complicated (Continued)
      intravascular coagulation O03.1
      laceration of pelvic organ(s) O03.34
      metabolic disorder O03.33
      oliguria O03.32
      oophoritis O03.0
      parametritis O03.0
      pelvic peritonitis O03.0
      perforation of pelvic organ(s) O03.34
      renal failure or shutdown O03.32
      salpingitis or salpingo-oophoritis O03.0
      sepsis O03.37
      shock O03.31
      specified condition NEC O03.39
      tubular necrosis (renal) O03.32
      uremia O03.32
      urinary infection O03.38
      venous complication NEC O03.35
        embolism (air) (amniotic fluid) (blood
         clot) (fat) (pulmonary) (septic)
         (soap) O03.2
  induced (encounter for) Z33.2
    complicated by O04.80
      afibrinogenemia O04.6
      cardiac arrest O04.86
      chemical damage of pelvic organ(s) O04.84
      circulatory collapse O04.81
      cystitis O04.88
      defibrination syndrome O04.6
      electrolyte imbalance O04.83
      embolism (air) (amniotic fluid) (blood clot)
        (fat) (pulmonary) (septic) (soap) O04.7
      endometritis O04.5
      genital tract and pelvic infection O04.5
      hemolysis O04.6
      hemorrhage (delayed) (excessive) O04.6
      infection
        genital tract or pelvic O04.5
        urinary tract O04.88
      intravascular coagulation O04.6
      laceration of pelvic organ(s) O04.84
      metabolic disorder O04.83
      oliguria O04.82
      oophoritis O04.5
      parametritis O04.5
      pelvic peritonitis O04.5
      perforation of pelvic organ(s) O04.84
      renal failure or shutdown O04.82
      salpingitis or salpingo-oophoritis O04.5
      sepsis O04.87
      shock O04.81
      specified condition NEC O04.89
      tubular necrosis (renal) O04.82
      uremia O04.82
      urinary tract infection O04.88
      venous complication NEC O04.85
        embolism (air) (amniotic fluid) (blood
         clot) (fat) (pulmonary) (septic)
         (soap) O04.7
  inevitable O03.4
  missed O02.1
  spontaneous —see Abortion (complete)
    (spontaneous)
    threatened O20.0
  threatened (spontaneous) O20.0
  tubal O00.10-•
    with intrauterine pregnancy O00.11-

Abortus fever A23.1

Aboulomania F60.7

Abrami's disease D59.8

Abramov-Fiedler myocarditis (acute isolated
  myocarditis) I40.1

Abrasion T14.8
  abdomen, abdominal (wall) S30.811
  alveolar process S00.512
  ankle S90.51-•
  antecubital space —see Abrasion, elbow
  anus S30.817
  arm (upper) S40.81-•
  auditory canal —see Abrasion, ear
  auricle —see Abrasion, ear
  axilla —see Abrasion, arm
  back, lower S30.810
  breast S20.11-•
  brow S00.81
  buttock S30.810
  calf —see Abrasion, leg
  canthus —see Abrasion, eyelid
  cheek S00.81
    internal S00.512

  ▶ New   ⇨ Revised   ~~deleted~~ Deleted   • Use Additional Character(s)

A

▶ New   ➡ Revised   ~~deleted~~ Deleted   ● Use Additional Character(s)

Abscess *(Continued)*
  peritoneum, peritoneal (perforated) (ruptured) K65.1
    with appendicitis (*see also* Appendicitis) K35.33
    pelvic
      female —*see* Peritonitis, pelvic, female
      male K65.1
    postoperative T81.43
    puerperal, postpartum, childbirth O85
    tuberculous A18.31
  peritonsillar J36
  perityphlic K35.33
  periureteral N28.89
  periurethral N34.0
    gonococcal (accessory gland) (periurethral) A54.1
  periuterine —*see also* Disease, pelvis, inflammatory N73.2
  perivesical —*see* Cystitis, specified type NEC
  petrous bone —*see* Petrositis
  phagedenic NOS L02.91
    chancroid A57
  pharynx, pharyngeal (lateral) J39.1
  pilonidal L05.01
  pituitary (gland) E23.6
  pleura J86.9
    with fistula J86.0
  popliteal —*see* Abscess, lower limb
  postcecal K35.33
  postlaryngeal J38.7
  postnasal J34.0
  postoperative (any site) (*see also* Infection, postoperative wound) T81.49
    retroperitoneal K68.11
  postpharyngeal J39.0
  posttonsillar J36
  post-typhoid A01.09
  pouch of Douglas —*see* Peritonitis, pelvic, female
  premammary —*see* Abscess, breast
  prepatellar —*see* Abscess, lower limb
  presacral K68.19
  prostate N41.2
    gonococcal (acute) (chronic) A54.22
  psoas muscle K68.12
  puerperal - code by site under Puerperal, abscess
  pulmonary —*see* Abscess, lung
  pulp, pulpal (dental) K04.01
    irreversible K04.02
    reversible K04.01
  rectovaginal septum K63.0
  rectovesical —*see* Cystitis, specified type NEC
  rectum K61.1
  renal —*see* Abscess, kidney
  retina —*see* Inflammation, chorioretinal
  retrobulbar —*see* Abscess, orbit
  retrocecal K65.1
  retrolaryngeal J38.7
  retromammary —*see* Abscess, breast
  retroperitoneal NEC K68.19
    postprocedural K68.11
  retropharyngeal J39.0
  retrouterine —*see* Peritonitis, pelvic, female
  retrovesical —*see* Cystitis, specified type NEC
  root, tooth K04.7
    with sinus (alveolar) K04.6
  round ligament —*see also* Disease, pelvis, inflammatory N73.2
  rupture (spontaneous) NOS L02.91
  sacrum (tuberculous)
    nontuberculous M46.28
  salivary (duct) (gland) K11.3
  scalp (any part) L02.811
  scapular —*see* Osteomyelitis, specified type NEC
  sclera —*see* Scleritis
  scrofulous (tuberculous) A18.2
  scrotum N49.2
  seminal vesicle N49.0
  septal, dental K04.7
    with sinus (alveolar) K04.6
  serous —*see* Periostitis
  shoulder (region) —*see* Abscess, upper limb
  sigmoid K63.0
  sinus (accessory) (chronic) (nasal) —*see also* Sinusitis
    intracranial venous (any) G06.0
  Skene's duct or gland N34.0
  skin —*see* Abscess, by site
  specified site NEC L02.818
  spermatic cord N49.1
  sphenoidal (sinus) (chronic) J32.3
  spinal cord (any part) (staphylococcal) G06.1
    tuberculous A17.81

Abscess *(Continued)*
  spine (column) (tuberculous) A18.01
    epidural G06.1
    nontuberculous —*see* Osteomyelitis, vertebra
  spleen D73.3
    amebic A06.89
  stitch T81.41
    following an obstetrical procedure O86.01
  subarachnoid G06.2
    brain G06.0
    spinal cord G06.1
  subareolar —*see* Abscess, breast
  subcecal K35.33
  subcutaneous —*see also* Abscess, by site
    following procedure T81.41
      obstetrical O86.01
    pheomycotic (chromomycotic) B43.2
  subdiaphragmatic K65.1
  subdural G06.2
    brain G06.0
      sequelae G09
    spinal cord G06.1
  sub-fascial, following an obstetrical procedure O86.02
  subgaleal L02.811
  subhepatic K65.1
  sublingual K12.2
    gland K11.3
  submammary —*see* Abscess, breast
  submandibular (region) (space) (triangle) K12.2
    gland K11.3
  submaxillary (region) L02.01
    gland K11.3
  submental L02.01
    gland K11.3
  subperiosteal —*see* Osteomyelitis, specified type NEC
  subphrenic K65.1
    following an obstetrical procedure O86.03
    postoperative T81.43
  suburethral N34.0
  sudoriparous L75.8
  supraclavicular (fossa) —*see* Abscess, upper limb
  supralevator K61.5
  suprapelvic, acute N73.0
  suprarenal (capsule) (gland) E27.8
  sweat gland L74.8
  tear duct —*see* Inflammation, lacrimal, passages, acute
  temple L02.01
  temporal region L02.01
  temporosphenoidal G06.0
  tendon (sheath) M65.00
    ankle M65.07-●
    foot M65.07-●
    forearm M65.03-●
    hand M65.04-●
    lower leg M65.06-●
    pelvic region M65.05-●
    shoulder region M65.01-●
    specified site NEC M65.08
    thigh M65.05-●
    upper arm M65.02-●
  testis N45.4
  thigh —*see* Abscess, lower limb
  thorax J86.9
    with fistula J86.0
  throat J39.1
  thumb —*see also* Abscess, hand
    nail —*see* Cellulitis, finger
  thymus (gland) E32.1
  thyroid (gland) E06.0
  toe (any) —*see also* Abscess, foot
    nail —*see* Cellulitis, toe
  tongue (staphylococcal) K14.0
  tonsil(s) (lingual) J36
  tonsillopharyngeal J36
  tooth, teeth (root) K04.7
    with sinus (alveolar) K04.6
    supporting structures NEC —*see* Periodontitis, aggressive, localized
  trachea J39.8
  trunk L02.219
    abdominal wall L02.211
    back L02.212
    chest wall L02.213
    groin L02.214
    perineum L02.215
    umbilicus L02.216
  tubal —*see* Salpingitis
  tuberculous —*see* Tuberculosis, abscess
  tubo-ovarian —*see* Salpingo-oophoritis

Abscess *(Continued)*
  tunica vaginalis N49.1
  umbilicus L02.216
  upper
    limb L02.41-●
    respiratory J39.8
  urethral (gland) N34.0
  urinary N34.0
  uterus, uterine (wall) —*see also* Endometritis
    ligament —*see also* Disease, pelvis, inflammatory N73.2
    neck —*see* Cervicitis
  uvula K12.2
  vagina (wall) —*see* Vaginitis
  vaginorectal —*see* Vaginitis
  vas deferens N49.1
  vermiform appendix K35.33
  vertebra (column) (tuberculous) A18.01
    nontuberculous —*see* Osteomyelitis, vertebra
  vesical —*see* Cystitis, specified type NEC
  vesico-uterine pouch —*see* Peritonitis, pelvic, female
  vitreous (humor) —*see* Endophthalmitis, purulent
  vocal cord J38.3
  von Bezold's —*see* Mastoiditis, acute
  vulva N76.4
  vulvovaginal gland N75.1
  web space —*see* Abscess, hand
  wound T81.49
  wrist —*see* Abscess, upper limb
Absence (of) (organ or part) (complete or partial)
  adrenal (gland) (congenital) Q89.1
    acquired E89.6
  albumin in blood E88.09
  alimentary tract (congenital) Q45.8
    upper Q40.8
  alveolar process (acquired) —*see* Anomaly, alveolar
  ankle (acquired) Z89.44-●
  anus (congenital) Q42.3
    with fistula Q42.2
  aorta (congenital) Q25.41
  appendix, congenital Q42.8
  arm (acquired) Z89.20-●
    above elbow Z89.22-●
      congenital (with hand present) —*see* Agenesis, arm, with hand present and hand —*see* Agenesis, forearm, and hand
    below elbow Z89.21-●
      congenital (with hand present) —*see* Agenesis, arm, with hand present and hand —*see* Agenesis, forearm, and hand
    congenital —*see* Defect, reduction, upper limb
    shoulder (following explantation of shoulder joint prosthesis) (joint) (with or without presence of antibiotic-impregnated cement spacer) Z89.23-●
      congenital (with hand present) —*see* Agenesis, arm, with hand present
  artery (congenital) (peripheral) Q27.8
    brain Q28.3
    coronary Q24.5
    pulmonary Q25.79
    specified NEC Q27.8
    umbilical Q27.0
  atrial septum (congenital) Q21.19
  auditory canal (congenital) (external) Q16.1
  auricle (ear), congenital Q16.0
  bile, biliary duct, congenital Q44.5
  bladder (acquired) Z90.6
    congenital Q64.5
  bowel sounds R19.11
  brain Q00.0
    part of Q04.3
  breast(s) (and nipple(s)) (acquired) Z90.1-●
    congenital Q83.8
  broad ligament Q50.6
  bronchus (congenital) Q32.4
  canaliculus lacrimalis, congenital Q10.4
  cerebellum (vermis) —Q04.3
  cervix (acquired) (with uterus) Z90.710
    with remaining uterus Z90.712
    congenital Q51.5
  chin, congenital Q18.8
  cilia (congenital) Q10.3
    acquired —*see* Madarosis
  clitoris (congenital) Q52.6
  coccyx, congenital Q76.49
  cold sense R20.8

▶ New   ⬛ Revised   ~~deleted~~ Deleted   ● Use Additional Character(s)

Absence *(Continued)*
  thumb (acquired) Z89.01-●
    congenital —*see* Agenesis, hand
  thymus gland Q89.2
  thyroid (gland) (acquired) E89.0
    cartilage, congenital Q31.8
    congenital E03.1
  toe(s) (acquired) Z89.42-●
    with foot —*see* Absence, foot and ankle
    congenital —*see* Agenesis, foot
    great Z89.41-●
  tongue, congenital Q38.3
  trachea (cartilage), congenital Q32.1
  transverse aortic arch, congenital Q25.49
  tricuspid valve Q22.4
  umbilical artery, congenital Q27.0
  upper arm and forearm with hand present,
    congenital —*see* Agenesis, arm, with hand
    present
  ureter (congenital) Q62.4
    acquired Z90.6
  urethra, congenital Q64.5
  uterus (acquired) Z90.710
    with cervix Z90.710
    with remaining cervical stump Z90.711
    congenital Q51.0
  uvula, congenital Q38.5
  vagina, congenital Q52.0
  vas deferens (congenital) Q55.4
    acquired Z90.79
  vein (peripheral) congenital NEC Q27.8
    cerebral Q28.3
    digestive system Q27.8
    great Q26.8
    lower limb Q27.8
    portal Q26.5
    precerebral Q28.1
    specified site NEC Q27.8
    upper limb Q27.8
  vena cava (inferior) (superior), congenital Q26.8
  ventricular septum Q20.4
  vertebra, congenital Q76.49
  von Willebrand factor, complete (near) (see also
    Disease, von Willebrand) D68.03
  vulva, congenital Q52.71
  wrist (acquired) Z89.12-●
Absorbent system disease I87.8
Absorption
  carbohydrate, disturbance K90.49
  chemical —*see* Table of Drugs and Chemicals
    through placenta (newborn) P04.9
      environmental substance P04.6
      nutritional substance P04.5
      obstetric anesthetic or analgesic drug P04.0
  drug NEC —*see* Table of Drugs and Chemicals
    addictive
      through placenta (newborn) (*see also*
        Newborn, affected by, maternal,
        use of) P04.40
        cocaine P04.41
        hallucinogens P04.42
        specified drug NEC P04.49
    medicinal
      through placenta (newborn) P04.19
    through placenta (newborn) P04.19
      obstetric anesthetic or analgesic drug P04.0
  fat, disturbance K90.49
    pancreatic K90.3
  noxious substance —*see* Table of Drugs and
    Chemicals
  protein, disturbance K90.49
  starch, disturbance K90.49
  toxic substance —*see* Table of Drugs and Chemicals
  uremic —*see* Uremia
Abstinence symptoms, syndrome
  alcohol F10.239
    with delirium F10.231
  cocaine F14.23
  neonatal P96.1
  nicotine —*see* Dependence, drug, nicotine, with,
    withdrawal
  opioid F11.93
    with dependence F11.23
  psychoactive NEC F19.939
    with
      delirium F19.931
      dependence F19.239
        with
          delirium F19.231
          perceptual disturbance F19.232
        uncomplicated F19.230
      perceptual disturbance F19.932
    uncomplicated F19.930

Abstinence symptoms, syndrome *(Continued)*
  sedative F13.939
    with
      delirium F13.931
      dependence F13.239
        with
          delirium F13.231
          perceptual disturbance F13.232
        uncomplicated F13.230
      perceptual disturbance F13.932
    uncomplicated F13.930
  stimulant NEC F15.93
    with dependence F15.23
Abulia R68.89
Abulomania F60.7
Abuse
  adult —*see* Maltreatment, adult
    as reason for
      couple seeking advice (including offender)
        Z63.0
  alcohol (non-dependent) F10.10
    with
      anxiety disorder F10.180
      intoxication F10.129
        with delirium F10.121
        uncomplicated F10.120
      mood disorder F10.14
      other specified disorder F10.188
      psychosis F10.159
        delusions F10.150
        hallucinations F10.151
      sexual dysfunction F10.181
      sleep disorder F10.182
      unspecified disorder F10.19
      withdrawal F10.139
        with
          perceptual disturbance F10.132
        delirium F10.131
        uncomplicated F10.130
    counseling and surveillance Z71.41
    in remission (early) (sustained) F10.11
  amphetamine (or related substance) —*see also*
    Abuse, drug, stimulant NEC
    stimulant NEC F15.10
      with
        anxiety disorder F15.180
        intoxication F15.129
          with
            delirium F15.121
            perceptual disturbance F15.122
        withdrawal F15.13
  analgesics (non-prescribed) (over the counter)
    F55.8
  antacids F55.0
  antidepressants —*see* Abuse, drug, psychoactive
    NEC
  anxiolytic —*see* Abuse, drug, sedative
  barbiturates —*see* Abuse, drug, sedative
  caffeine —*see* Abuse, drug, stimulant NEC
  cannabis, cannabinoids —*see* Abuse, drug,
    cannabis
  child —*see* Maltreatment, child
  cocaine —*see* Abuse, drug, cocaine
  drug NEC (non-dependent) F19.10
    with sleep disorder F19.182
    amphetamine type —*see* Abuse, drug,
      stimulant NEC
    analgesics (non-prescribed) (over the counter)
      F55.8
    antacids F55.0
    antidepressants —*see* Abuse, drug,
      psychoactive NEC
    anxiolytics —*see* Abuse, drug, sedative
    barbiturates —*see* Abuse, drug, sedative
    caffeine —*see* Abuse, drug, stimulant
      NEC
    cannabis F12.10
      with
        anxiety disorder F12.180
        intoxication F12.129
          with
            delirium F12.121
            perceptual disturbance F12.122
          uncomplicated F12.120
        other specified disorder F12.188
        psychosis F12.159
          delusions F12.150
          hallucinations F12.151
        unspecified disorder F12.19
        withdrawal F12.13
      in remission (early) (sustained) F12.11

Abuse *(Continued)*
  drug NEC *(Continued)*
    cocaine F14.10
      with
        anxiety disorder F14.180
        intoxication F14.129
          with
            delirium F14.121
            perceptual disturbance
              F14.122
          uncomplicated F14.120
        mood disorder F14.14
        other specified disorder F14.188
        psychosis F14.159
          delusions F14.150
          hallucinations F14.151
        sexual dysfunction F14.181
        sleep disorder F14.182
        unspecified disorder F14.19
        withdrawal F14.13
      in remission (early) (sustained)
        F14.11
    counseling and surveillance Z71.51
    hallucinogen F16.10
      with
        anxiety disorder F16.180
        flashbacks F16.183
        intoxication F16.129
          with
            delirium F16.121
            perceptual disturbance
              F16.122
          uncomplicated F16.120
        mood disorder F16.14
        other specified disorder F16.188
        perception disorder, persisting F16.183
        psychosis F16.159
          delusions F16.150
          hallucinations F16.151
        unspecified disorder F16.19
      in remission (early) (sustained) F16.11
    hashish —*see* Abuse, drug, cannabis
    herbal or folk remedies F55.1
    hormones F55.3
    hypnotics —*see* Abuse, drug, sedative
    inhalant F18.10
      with
        anxiety disorder F18.180
        dementia, persisting F18.17
        intoxication F18.129
          with delirium F18.121
          uncomplicated F18.120
        mood disorder F18.14
        other specified disorder F18.188
        psychosis F18.159
          delusions F18.150
          hallucinations F18.151
        unspecified disorder F18.19
      in remission (early) (sustained) F18.11
    in remission (early) (sustained) F19.11
    laxatives F55.2
    LSD —*see* Abuse, drug, hallucinogen
    marihuana —*see* Abuse, drug, cannabis
    morphine type (opioids) —*see* Abuse, drug,
      opioid
    opioid F11.10
      with
        intoxication F11.129
          with
            delirium F11.121
            perceptual disturbance F11.122
          uncomplicated F11.120
        mood disorder F11.14
        opioid-associated amnestic syndrome
          F11.188
        other specified disorder F11.188
        psychosis F11.159
          delusions F11.150
          hallucinations F11.151
        sexual dysfunction F11.181
        sleep disorder F11.182
        unspecified disorder F11.19
        withdrawal F11.13
      in remission (early) (sustained) F11.11
    PCP (phencyclidine) (or related substance) —
      see Abuse, drug, hallucinogen
    psychoactive NEC F19.10
      with
        amnestic disorder F19.16
        anxiety disorder F19.180
        dementia F19.17

▶ New   ⇒ Revised   ~~deleted~~ Deleted   ● Use Additional Character(s)

Adenoma *(Continued)*
- basophil-acidophil, mixed
  - specified site —*see* Neoplasm, benign, by site
  - unspecified site D35.2
- beta-cell
  - pancreas D13.7
  - specified site NEC —*see* Neoplasm, benign, by site
  - unspecified site D13.7
- bile duct D13.4
  - common D13.5
  - extrahepatic D13.5
  - intrahepatic D13.4
  - specified site NEC —*see* Neoplasm, benign, by site
  - unspecified site D13.4
- black D35.00
- bronchial D38.1
  - cylindroid type —*see* Neoplasm, lung, malignant
- ceruminous D23.2-●
- chief cell D35.1
- chromophobe
  - specified site —*see* Neoplasm, benign, by site
  - unspecified site D35.2
- colloid
  - specified site —*see* Neoplasm, benign, by site
  - unspecified site D34
- eccrine, papillary —*see* Neoplasm, skin, benign
- endocrine, multiple
  - single specified site —*see* Neoplasm, uncertain behavior, by site
  - two or more specified sites D44-●
  - unspecified site D44.9
- endometrioid —*see also* Neoplasm, benign
  - borderline malignancy —*see* Neoplasm, uncertain behavior, by site
- eosinophil
  - specified site —*see* Neoplasm, malignant, by site
  - unspecified site D35.2
- fetal
  - specified site —*see* Neoplasm, benign, by site
  - unspecified site D34
- follicular
  - specified site —*see* Neoplasm, benign, by site
  - unspecified site D34
- hepatocellular D13.4
- Hurthle cell D34
- islet cell
  - pancreas D13.7
  - specified site NEC —*see* Neoplasm, benign, by site
  - unspecified site D13.7
- liver cell D13.4
- macrofollicular
  - specified site —*see* Neoplasm, benign, by site
  - unspecified site D34
- malignant, malignum —*see* Neoplasm, malignant, by site
- microcystic
  - pancreas D13.6
  - specified site NEC —*see* Neoplasm, benign, by site
  - unspecified site D13.6
- microfollicular
  - specified site —*see* Neoplasm, benign, by site
  - unspecified site D34
- mucoid cell
  - specified site —*see* Neoplasm, benign, by site
  - unspecified site D35.2
- multiple endocrine
  - single specified site —*see* Neoplasm, uncertain behavior, by site
  - two or more specified sites D44-●
  - unspecified site D44.9
- nipple D24-●
- papillary —*see also* Neoplasm, benign, by site
  - eccrine —*see* Neoplasm, skin, benign, by site
- Pick's tubular
  - specified site —*see* Neoplasm, benign, by site
  - unspecified site
    - female D27.9
    - male D29.20
- pleomorphic
  - carcinoma in —*see* Neoplasm, salivary gland, malignant
  - specified site —*see* Neoplasm, malignant, by site
  - unspecified site C08.9

Adenoma *(Continued)*
- polypoid —*see also* Neoplasm, benign
  - adenocarcinoma in —*see* Neoplasm, malignant, by site
  - adenocarcinoma in situ —*see* Neoplasm, in situ, by site
- prostate —*see* Neoplasm, prostate, benign
- rete cell D29.20
- sebaceous —*see* Neoplasm, skin, benign
- Sertoli cell
  - specified site —*see* Neoplasm, benign, by site
  - unspecified site
    - female D27.9
    - male D29.20
- skin appendage —*see* Neoplasm, skin, benign
- sudoriferous gland —*see* Neoplasm, skin, benign
- sweat gland —*see* Neoplasm, skin, benign
- testicular
  - specified site —*see* Neoplasm, benign, by site
  - unspecified site
    - female D27.9
    - male D29.20
- tubular —*see also* Neoplasm, benign, by site
  - adenocarcinoma in —*see* Neoplasm, malignant, by site
  - adenocarcinoma in situ —*see* Neoplasm, in situ, by site
  - Pick's
    - specified site —*see* Neoplasm, benign
    - unspecified site
      - female D27.9
      - male D29.20
- tubulovillous —*see also* Neoplasm, benign, by site
  - adenocarcinoma in —*see* Neoplasm, malignant, by site
  - adenocarcinoma in situ —*see* Neoplasm, in situ, by site
- villous —*see* Neoplasm, uncertain behavior, by site
  - adenocarcinoma in —*see* Neoplasm, malignant, by site
  - adenocarcinoma in situ —*see* Neoplasm, in situ, by site
- water-clear cell D35.1

Adenomatosis
- endocrine (multiple) E31.20
  - single specified site —*see* Neoplasm, uncertain behavior, by site
- erosive of nipple D24-●
- pluriendocrine —*see* Adenomatosis, endocrine
- pulmonary D38.1
  - malignant —*see* Neoplasm, lung, malignant
- specified site —*see* Neoplasm, benign, by site
- unspecified site D12.6

Adenomatous
- goiter (nontoxic) E04.9
  - with hyperthyroidism —*see* Hyperthyroidism, with, goiter, nodular
  - toxic —*see* Hyperthyroidism, with, goiter, nodular

Adenomyoma —*see also* Neoplasm, benign, by site
- prostate —*see* Enlarged, prostate

Adenomyometritis N80.00

Adenomyosis (uterus) N80.03

Adenopathy (lymph gland) R59.9
- generalized R59.1
- inguinal R59.0
- localized R59.0
- mediastinal R59.0
- mesentery R59.0
- syphilitic (secondary) A51.49
- tracheobronchial R59.0
  - tuberculous A15.4
    - primary (progressive) A15.7
- tuberculous —*see also* Tuberculosis, lymph gland
  - tracheobronchial A15.4
    - primary (progressive) A15.7

Adenosalpingitis —*see* Salpingitis

Adenosarcoma —*see* Neoplasm, malignant, by site

Adenosclerosis I88.8

Adenosis (sclerosing) **breast** —*see* Fibroadenosis, breast

Adenovirus, as cause of disease classified elsewhere B97.0

Adentia (complete) (partial) —*see* Absence, teeth

Adherent —*see also* Adhesions
- labia (minora) N90.89
- pericardium (nonrheumatic) I31.0
  - rheumatic I09.2

Adherent *(Continued)*
- placenta (with hemorrhage) O72.0
  - without hemorrhage O73.0
- prepuce, newborn N47.0
- scar (skin) L90.5
- tendon in scar L90.5

Adhesions, adhesive (postinfective) K66.0
- with intestinal obstruction K56.50
  - complete K56.52
  - incomplete K56.51
  - partial K56.51
- abdominal (wall) —*see* Adhesions, peritoneum
- appendix K38.8
- bile duct (common) (hepatic) K83.8
- bladder (sphincter) N32.89
- bowel —*see* Adhesions, peritoneum
- cardiac I31.0
  - rheumatic I09.2
- cecum —*see* Adhesions, peritoneum
- cervicovaginal N88.1
  - congenital Q52.8
  - postpartal O90.89
  - old N88.1
- cervix N88.1
- ciliary body NEC —*see* Adhesions, iris
- clitoris N90.89
- colon —*see* Adhesions, peritoneum
- common duct K83.8
- congenital —*see also* Anomaly, by site
  - fingers —*see* Syndactylism, complex, fingers
  - omental, anomalous Q43.3
  - peritoneal Q43.3
  - tongue (to gum or roof of mouth) Q38.3
- conjunctiva (acquired) H11.21-●
  - congenital Q15.8
- cystic duct K82.8
- diaphragm —*see* Adhesions, peritoneum
- due to foreign body —*see* Foreign body
- duodenum —*see* Adhesions, peritoneum
- ear
  - middle H74.1-●
- epididymis N50.89
- epidural —*see* Adhesions, meninges
- epiglottis J38.7
- eyelid H02.59
- female pelvis N73.6
- gallbladder K82.8
- globe H44.89
- heart I31.0
  - rheumatic I09.2
- ileocecal (coil) —*see* Adhesions, peritoneum
- ileum —*see* Adhesions, peritoneum
- intestine —*see also* Adhesions, peritoneum
  - with obstruction K56.50
    - complete K56.52
    - incomplete K56.51
    - partial K56.51
- intra-abdominal —*see* Adhesions, peritoneum
- iris H21.50-●
  - anterior H21.51-●
  - goniosynechiae H21.52-●
  - posterior H21.54-●
  - to corneal graft T85.898
- joint —*see* Ankylosis
  - knee M23.8X
  - temporomandibular M26.61-●
- labium (majus) (minus), congenital Q52.5
- liver —*see* Adhesions, peritoneum
- lung J98.4
- mediastinum J98.59
- meninges (cerebral) (spinal) G96.12
  - congenital Q07.8
  - tuberculous (cerebral) (spinal) A17.0
- mesenteric —*see* Adhesions, peritoneum
- nasal (septum) (to turbinates) J34.89
- ocular muscle —*see* Strabismus, mechanical
- omentum —*see* Adhesions, peritoneum
- ovary N73.6
  - congenital (to cecum, kidney or omentum) Q50.39
- paraovarian N73.6
- pelvic (peritoneal)
  - female N73.6
    - postprocedural N99.4
  - male —*see* Adhesions, peritoneum
  - postpartal (old) N73.6
  - tuberculous A18.17
- penis to scrotum (congenital) Q55.8
- periappendiceal —*see also* Adhesions, peritoneum

New   Revised   ~~deleted~~ Deleted   • Use Additional Character(s)

Admission (Continued)
  fitting (Continued)
    cystostomy device Z46.6
    dental prosthesis Z46.3
    dentures Z46.3
    device NEC
      abdominal Z46.89
      nervous system Z46.2
        implanted —see Admission, adjustment,
          device, implanted, nervous system
      orthodontic Z46.4
      prosthetic Z44.9
        breast Z44.3
        dental Z46.3
        eye Z44.2- ●
      substitution
        auditory Z46.2
          implanted —see Admission,
            adjustment, device, implanted,
            hearing device
        nervous system Z46.2
          implanted —see Admission,
            adjustment, device, implanted,
            nervous system
        visual Z46.2
          implanted Z45.31
    hearing aid Z46.1
    ileostomy device Z46.89
    intestinal appliance or device NEC Z46.89
    neuropacemaker (brain) (peripheral nerve)
      (spinal cord) Z46.2
      implanted Z45.42
    orthodontic device Z46.4
    orthopedic device (brace) (cast) (shoes) Z46.89
    prosthesis Z44.9
      arm —see Admission, adjustment, artificial,
        arm
      breast Z44.3
      dental Z46.3
      eye Z44.2- ●
      leg —see Admission, adjustment, artificial, leg
      specified type NEC Z44.8
    spectacles Z46.0
  follow-up examination Z09
  intrauterine device management Z30.431
    initial prescription Z30.014
  mental health evaluation Z00.8
    requested by authority Z04.6
  observation —see Observation
  Papanicolaou smear, cervix Z12.4
    for suspected malignant neoplasm Z12.4
  plastic and reconstructive surgery following
    medical procedure or healed injury NEC
    Z42.8
  plastic surgery, cosmetic NEC Z41.1
  postpartum observation
    immediately after delivery Z39.0
    routine follow-up Z39.2
  poststerilization (for restoration) Z31.0
    aftercare Z31.42
  procreative management Z31.9
  prophylactic (measure) —see also Encounter,
    prophylactic measures
  ▶ oophorectomy for persons without known
      genetic/ familial risk factors Z40.81
    organ removal Z40.00
      breast Z40.01
      fallopian tube(s) Z40.03
        with ovary(s) Z40.02
      ▶ for persons without known genetic/
        familial risk factors Z40.82
      ovary(s) Z40.02
      ▶ for persons without known genetic/
        familial risk factors Z40.81
      specified organ NEC Z40.09
      testes Z40.09
  ▶ salpingectomy for persons without known
      genetic/ familial risk factors Z40.82
    vaccination Z23
  psychiatric examination (general) Z00.8
    requested by authority Z04.6
  radiation therapy (antineoplastic) Z51.0
  reconstructive surgery following medical
    procedure or healed injury NEC Z42.8
  removal of
    cystostomy catheter Z43.5
    drains Z48.03
    dressing (nonsurgical) Z48.00
    implantable subdermal contraceptive Z30.46
    intrauterine contraceptive device Z30.432
    neuropacemaker (brain) (peripheral nerve)
      (spinal cord) Z46.2
      implanted Z45.42

Admission (Continued)
  removal of (Continued)
    staples Z48.02
    surgical dressing Z48.01
    sutures Z48.02
    ureteral stent Z46.6
  respirator [ventilator] use during power failure
    Z99.12
  restoration of organ continuity (poststerilization)
    Z31.0
    aftercare Z31.42
  sensitivity test —see also Test, skin
    allergy NEC Z01.82
    Mantoux Z11.1
  tuboplasty following previous sterilization Z31.0
    aftercare Z31.42
  vasoplasty following previous sterilization Z31.0
    aftercare Z31.42
  vision examination Z01.00
    with abnormal findings Z01.01
      following failed vision screening Z01.020
        with abnormal findings Z01.021
    infant or child (over 28 days old) Z00.129
      with abnormal findings Z00.121
  waiting period for admission to other facility Z75.1
Adnexitis (suppurative) —see Salpingo-oophoritis
Adolescent X-linked adrenoleukodystrophy
  E71.521
Adrenal (gland) —see condition
Adrenalism, tuberculous A18.7
Adrenalitis, adrenitis E27.8
  autoimmune E27.1
  meningococcal, hemorrhagic A39.1
Adrenarche, premature E27.0
Adrenocortical syndrome —see Cushing's,
  syndrome
Adrenogenital syndrome E25.9
  acquired E25.8
  congenital E25.0
  salt loss E25.0
Adrenogenitalism, congenital E25.0
Adrenoleukodystrophy E71.529
  neonatal E71.511
  X-linked E71.529
    Addison only phenotype E71.528
    Addison-Schilder E71.528
    adolescent E71.521
    adrenomyeloneuropathy E71.522
    childhood cerebral E71.520
    other specified E71.528
Adrenomyeloneuropathy E71.522
Adventitious bursa —see Bursopathy, specified
  type NEC
Adverse effect —see Table of Drugs and Chemicals,
  categories T36-T50, with 6th character 5
Advice —see Counseling
Adynamia (episodica) (hereditary) (periodic) G72.3
Aeration lung imperfect, newborn —see Atelectasis
Aerobullosis T70.3
Aerocele —see Embolism, air
Aerodermectasia
  subcutaneous (traumatic) T79.7
Aerodontalgia T70.29
Aeroembolism T70.3
Aerogenes capsulatus infection A48.0
Aero-otitis media T70.0
Aerophagy, aerophagia (psychogenic) F45.8
Aerophobia F40.228
Aerosinusitis T70.1
Aerotitis T70.0
Affection —see Disease
Afibrinogenemia —see also Defect, coagulation D68.8
  acquired D65
  congenital D68.2
  following ectopic or molar pregnancy O08.1
  in abortion —see Abortion, by type, complicated
    by, afibrinogenemia
  puerperal O72.3
African
  sleeping sickness B56.9
  tick fever A68.1
  trypanosomiasis B56.9
    gambian B56.0
    rhodesian B56.1
Aftercare —see also Care Z51.89
  following surgery (for) (on)
    amputation Z47.81
    attention to
      drains Z48.03
      dressings (nonsurgical) Z48.00
        surgical Z48.01
      sutures Z48.02

Aftercare (Continued)
  following surgery (Continued)
    circulatory system Z48.812
    delayed (planned) wound closure Z48.1
    digestive system Z48.815
    explantation of joint prosthesis (staged
      procedure)
      hip Z47.32
      knee Z47.33
      shoulder Z47.31
    genitourinary system Z48.816
    joint replacement Z47.1
    neoplasm Z48.3
    nervous system Z48.811
    oral cavity Z48.814
    organ transplant
      bone marrow Z48.290
      heart Z48.21
      heart-lung Z48.280
      kidney Z48.22
      liver Z48.23
      lung Z48.24
      multiple organs NEC Z48.288
      specified NEC Z48.298
    orthopedic NEC Z47.89
    planned wound closure Z48.1
    removal of internal fixation device Z47.2
    respiratory system Z48.813
    scoliosis Z47.82
    sense organs Z48.810
    skin and subcutaneous tissue Z48.817
    specified body system
      circulatory Z48.812
      digestive Z48.815
      genitourinary Z48.816
      nervous Z48.811
      oral cavity Z48.814
      respiratory Z48.813
      sense organs Z48.810
      skin and subcutaneous tissue Z48.817
      teeth Z48.814
    specified NEC Z48.89
    spinal Z47.89
    teeth Z48.814
  fracture — code to fracture with seventh
    character D
  involving
    removal of
      drains Z48.03
      dressings (nonsurgical) Z48.00
      staples Z48.02
      surgical dressings Z48.01
      sutures Z48.02
  neuropacemaker (brain) (peripheral nerve)
    (spinal cord) Z46.2
    implanted Z45.42
  orthopedic NEC Z47.89
  postprocedural —see Aftercare, following surgery
After-cataract —see Cataract, secondary
Agalactia (primary) O92.3
  elective, secondary or therapeutic O92.5
Agammaglobulinemia (acquired (secondary))
  (nonfamilial) D80.1
  with
    immunoglobulin-bearing B-lymphocytes D80.1
    lymphopenia D81.9
  autosomal recessive (Swiss type) D80.0
  Bruton's X-linked D80.0
  common variable (CVAgamma) D80.1
  congenital sex-linked D80.0
  hereditary D80.0
  lymphopenic D81.9
  Swiss type (autosomal recessive) D80.0
  X-linked (with growth hormone deficiency)
    (Bruton) D80.0
Aganglionosis (bowel) (colon) Q43.1
Age (old) —see Senility
Agenesis
  adrenal (gland) Q89.1
  alimentary tract (complete) (partial) NEC Q45.8
    upper Q40.8
  anus, anal (canal) Q42.3
    with fistula Q42.2
  aorta Q25.41
  appendix Q42.8
  arm (complete) Q71.0- ●
    with hand present Q71.1- ●
  artery (peripheral) Q27.9
    brain Q28.3
    coronary Q24.5
    pulmonary Q25.79
    specified NEC Q27.8
    umbilical Q27.0

Agenesis *(Continued)*
  auditory (canal) (external) Q16.1
  auricle (ear) Q16.0
  bile duct or passage Q44.5
  bladder Q64.5
  bone Q79.9
  brain Q00.0
    part of Q04.3
  breast (with nipple present) Q83.8
    with absent nipple Q83.0
  bronchus Q32.4
  canaliculus lacrimalis Q10.4
  carpus —*see* Agenesis, hand
  cartilage Q79.9
  cecum Q42.8
  cerebellum Q04.3
  cervix Q51.5
  chin Q18.8
  cilia Q10.3
  circulatory system, part NOS Q28.9
  clavicle Q74.0
  clitoris Q52.6
  coccyx Q76.49
  colon Q42.9
    specified NEC Q42.8
  corpus callosum Q04.0
  cricoid cartilage Q31.8
  diaphragm (with hernia) Q79.1
  digestive organ(s) or tract (complete) (partial)
      NEC Q45.8
    upper Q40.8
  ductus arteriosus Q28.8
  duodenum Q41.0
  ear Q16.9
    auricle Q16.0
    lobe Q17.8
  ejaculatory duct Q55.4
  endocrine (gland) NEC Q89.2
  epiglottis Q31.8
  esophagus Q39.8
  eustachian tube Q16.2
  eye Q11.1
    adnexa Q15.8
  eyelid (fold) Q10.3
  face
    bones NEC Q75.8
    specified part NEC Q18.8
  fallopian tube Q50.6
  femur —*see* Defect, reduction, lower limb,
      longitudinal, femur
  fibula —*see* Defect, reduction, lower limb,
      longitudinal, fibula
  finger (complete) (partial) —*see* Agenesis, hand
  foot (and toes) (complete) (partial) Q72.3-●
  forearm (with hand present) —*see* Agenesis, arm,
      with hand present
    and hand Q71.2-●
  gallbladder Q44.0
  gastric Q40.2
  genitalia, genital (organ(s))
    female Q52.8
      external Q52.71
      internal NEC Q52.8
    male Q55.8
  glottis Q31.8
  hair Q84.0
  hand (and fingers) (complete) (partial) Q71.3-●
  heart Q24.8
    valve NEC Q24.8
      pulmonary Q22.0
  hepatic Q44.79
  humerus —*see* Defect, reduction, upper limb
  hymen Q52.4
  ileum Q41.2
  incus Q16.3
  intestine (small) Q41.9
    large Q42.9
      specified NEC Q42.8
  iris (dilator fibers) Q13.1
  jaw M26.09
  jejunum Q41.1
  kidney(s) (partial) Q60.2
    bilateral Q60.1
    unilateral Q60.0
  labium (majus) (minus) Q52.71
  labyrinth, membranous Q16.5
  lacrimal apparatus Q10.4
  larynx Q31.8
  leg (complete) Q72.0-●
    with foot present Q72.1-●
    lower leg (with foot present) —*see* Agenesis,
      leg, with foot present
      and foot Q72.2-●

Agenesis *(Continued)*
  lens Q12.3
  limb (complete) Q73.0
    lower —*see* Agenesis, leg
    upper —*see* Agenesis, arm
  lip Q38.0
  liver Q44.79
  lung (fissure) (lobe) (bilateral) (unilateral)
      Q33.3
  mandible, maxilla M26.09
  metacarpus —*see* Agenesis, hand
  metatarsus —*see* Agenesis, foot
  muscle Q79.8
    eyelid Q10.3
    ocular Q15.8
  musculoskeletal system NEC Q79.8
  nail(s) Q84.3
  neck, part Q18.8
  nerve Q07.8
  nervous system, part NEC Q07.8
  nipple Q83.2
  nose Q30.1
  nuclear Q07.8
  organ
    of Corti Q16.5
    or site not listed —*see* Anomaly, by site
  osseous meatus (ear) Q16.1
  ovary
    bilateral Q50.02
    unilateral Q50.01
  oviduct Q50.6
  pancreas Q45.0
  parathyroid (gland) Q89.2
  parotid gland(s) Q38.4
  patella Q74.1
  pelvic girdle (complete) (partial) Q74.2
  penis Q55.5
  pericardium Q24.8
  pituitary (gland) Q89.2
  prostate Q55.4
  punctum lacrimale Q10.4
  radioulnar —*see* Defect, reduction, upper limb
  radius —*see* Defect, reduction, upper limb,
      longitudinal, radius
  rectum Q42.1
    with fistula Q42.0
  renal Q60.2
    bilateral Q60.1
    unilateral Q60.0
  respiratory organ NEC Q34.8
  rib Q76.6
  roof of orbit Q75.8
  round ligament Q52.8
  sacrum Q76.49
  salivary gland Q38.4
  scapula Q74.0
  scrotum Q55.29
  seminal vesicles Q55.4
  septum
    atrial Q21.19
    between aorta and pulmonary artery Q21.4
    ventricular Q20.4
  shoulder girdle (complete) (partial) Q74.0
  skull (bone) Q75.8
    with
      anencephaly Q00.0
      encephalocele —*see* Encephalocele
      hydrocephalus Q03.9
        with spina bifida —*see* Spina bifida, by
          site, with hydrocephalus
      microcephaly Q02
  spermatic cord Q55.4
  spinal cord Q06.0
  spine Q76.49
  spleen Q89.01
  sternum Q76.7
  stomach Q40.2
  submaxillary gland(s) (congenital) Q38.4
  tarsus —*see* Agenesis, foot
  tendon Q79.8
  testicle Q55.0
  thymus (gland) Q89.2
  thyroid (gland) E03.1
    cartilage Q31.8
  tibia —*see* Defect, reduction, lower limb,
      longitudinal, tibia
  tibiofibular —*see* Defect, reduction, lower limb,
      specified type NEC
  toe (and foot) (complete) (partial) —*see* Agenesis,
      foot
  tongue Q38.3
  trachea (cartilage) Q32.1

Agenesis *(Continued)*
  ulna —*see* Defect, reduction, upper limb,
      longitudinal, ulna
  upper limb —*see* Agenesis, arm
  ureter Q62.4
  urethra Q64.5
  urinary tract NEC Q64.8
  uterus Q51.0
  uvula Q38.5
  vagina Q52.0
  vas deferens Q55.4
  vein(s) (peripheral) Q27.9
    brain Q28.3
    great NEC Q26.8
    portal Q26.5
  vena cava (inferior) (superior) Q26.8
  vermis of cerebellum Q04.3
  vertebra Q76.49
  vulva Q52.71
Ageusia R43.2
Agitated —*see* condition
Agitation R45.1
▶ **AGL (acquired generalized lipodystrophy)** E88.12
Aglossia (congenital) Q38.3
Aglossia-adactylia syndrome Q87.0
Aglycogenosis E74.00
Agnosia (body image) (other senses) (tactile) R48.1
  developmental F88
  verbal R48.1
    auditory R48.1
      developmental F80.2
    developmental F80.2
  visual (object) R48.3
Agoraphobia F40.00
  with panic disorder F40.01
  without panic disorder F40.02
Agrammatism R48.8
Agranulocytopenia —*see* Agranulocytosis
Agranulocytosis (chronic) (cyclical) (genetic)
    (infantile) (periodic) (pernicious) (*see also*
    Neutropenia) D70.9
  congenital D70.0
  cytoreductive cancer chemotherapy sequela D70.1
  drug-induced D70.2
    due to cytoreductive cancer chemotherapy
      D70.1
  due to infection D70.3
  secondary D70.4
    drug-induced D70.2
      due to cytoreductive cancer chemotherapy
        D70.1
Agraphia (absolute) R48.8
  with alexia R48.0
  developmental F81.81
Ague (dumb) —*see* Malaria
Agyria Q04.3
Ahumada-del Castillo syndrome E23.0
Aichomophobia F40.298
AIDS (related complex) B20
Ailment heart —*see* Disease, heart
Ailurophobia F40.218
Ainhum (disease) L94.6
AIN —*see* Neoplasia, intraepithelial, anal
AIPHI (acute idiopathic pulmonary hemorrhage in
    infants (over 28 days old)) R04.81
Air
  anterior mediastinum J98.2
  compressed, disease T70.3
  conditioner lung or pneumonitis J67.7
  embolism (artery) (cerebral) (any site) T79.0
    with ectopic or molar pregnancy O08.2
    due to implanted device NEC —*see*
      Complications, by site and type,
      specified NEC
    following
      abortion —*see* Abortion by type,
        complicated by, embolism
      ectopic or molar pregnancy O08.2
      infusion, therapeutic injection or
        transfusion T80.0
    in pregnancy, childbirth or puerperium —*see*
      Embolism, obstetric
    traumatic T79.0
  hunger, psychogenic F45.8
  rarefied, effects of —*see* Effect, adverse, high
      altitude
  sickness T75.3
Airplane sickness T75.3
Akathisia (drug-induced) (treatment- induced)
    G25.71
  neuroleptic induced (acute) G25.71
  tardive G25.71

▶ New　　⇒ Revised　　~~deleted~~ Deleted　　● Use Additional Character(s)

▶ New   ▶ Revised   ~~deleted~~ Deleted   ● Use Additional Character(s)

Amputation *(Continued)*
traumatic *(Continued)*
forearm (complete) S58.91-●
at elbow level (complete) S58.01-●
partial S58.02-●
between elbow and wrist (complete) S58.11-●
partial S58.12-●
partial S58.92-●
genital organ(s) (external)
female (complete) S38.211
partial S38.212
male
penis (complete) S38.221
partial S38.222
scrotum (complete) S38.231
partial S38.232
testes (complete) S38.231
partial S38.232
hand (complete) (wrist level) S68.41-●
finger(s) alone —*see* Amputation, traumatic, finger
partial S68.42-●
thumb alone —*see* Amputation, traumatic, thumb
transmetacarpal (complete) S68.71-●
partial S68.72-●
head
ear —*see* Amputation, traumatic, ear
nose (partial) S08.812
complete S08.811
part S08.89
scalp S08.0
hip (and thigh) (complete) S78.91-●
at hip joint (complete) S78.01-●
partial S78.02-●
between hip and knee (complete) S78.11-●
partial S78.12-●
partial S78.92-●
labium (majus) (minus) (complete) S38.21-●
partial S38.21-●
leg (lower) S88.91-●
at knee level S88.01-●
partial S88.02-●
between knee and ankle S88.11-●
partial S88.12-●
partial S88.92-●
nose (partial) S08.812
complete S08.811
penis (complete) S38.221
partial S38.222
scrotum (complete) S38.231
partial S38.232
shoulder —*see* Amputation, traumatic, arm
at shoulder joint —*see* Amputation, traumatic, arm, at shoulder joint
testes (complete) S38.231
partial S38.232
thigh —*see* Amputation, traumatic, hip
thorax, part of S28.1
breast —*see* Amputation, traumatic, breast
thumb (complete) (metacarpophalangeal) S68.01-●
partial S68.02-●
transphalangeal (complete) S68.51-●
partial S68.52-●
toe (lesser) S98.13-●
great S98.11-●
partial S98.12-●
more than one S98.21-●
partial S98.22-●
partial S98.14-●
vulva (complete) S38.211
partial S38.212
Amputee (bilateral) (old) Z89.9
Amsterdam dwarfism Q87.19
Amusia R48.8
developmental F80.89
Amyelencephalus, amyelencephaly Q00.0
Amyelia Q06.0
Amygdalitis —*see* Tonsillitis
Amygdalolith J35.8
Amyloid heart (disease) E85.4 [I43]
Amyloidosis (generalized) (primary) E85.9
with lung involvement E85.4 [J99]
familial E85.2
genetic E85.2
heart E85.4 [I43]
hemodialysis-associated E85.3
light chain (AL) E85.81
liver E85.4 [K77]
localized E85.4
neuropathic heredofamilial E85.1

Amyloidosis *(Continued)*
non-neuropathic heredofamilial E85.0
organ limited E85.4
Portuguese E85.1
pulmonary E85.4 [J99]
secondary systemic E85.3
senile systemic (SSA) E85.82
skin (lichen) (macular) E85.4 [L99]
specified NEC E85.89
subglottic E85.4 [J99]
wild-type transthyretin-related (ATTR) E85.82
Amylopectinosis (brancher enzyme deficiency) E74.03
Amylophagia —*see* Pica
Amyoplasia congenita Q79.8
Amyotonia M62.89
congenita G70.2
Amyotrophia, amyotrophy, amyotrophic G71.8
congenita Q79.8
diabetic —*see* Diabetes, amyotrophy
lateral sclerosis G12.21
neuralgic G54.5
spinal progressive G12.25
Anacidity, gastric K31.83
psychogenic F45.8
Anaerosis of newborn P28.89
Analbuminemia E88.09
Analgesia —*see* Anesthesia
Analphalipoproteinemia E78.6
Anaphylactic
purpura D69.0
shock or reaction —*see* Shock, anaphylactic
Anaphylactoid shock or reaction —*see* Shock, anaphylactic
Anaphylactoid syndrome of pregnancy O88.01-●
Anaphylaxis —*see* Shock, anaphylactic
Anaplasia cervix —*see also* Dysplasia, cervix N87.9
Anaplasmosis [A. phagocytophilum] (transfusion transmitted) A79.82
human A77.49
Anarthria R47.1
Anasarca R60.1
cardiac —*see* Failure, heart, congestive
lung J18.2
newborn P83.2
nutritional E43
pulmonary J18.2
renal N04.9
Anastomosis
aneurysmal —*see* Aneurysm
arteriovenous ruptured brain I60.8
intestinal K63.89
complicated NEC K91.89
involving urinary tract N99.89
intracerebral I61.8
intraparenchymal I61.8
intraventricular I61.5
retinal and choroidal vessels (congenital) Q14.8
subarachnoid I60.8
Anatomical narrow angle H40.03-●
Ancylostoma, ancylostomiasis (braziliense) (caninum) (ceylanicum) (duodenale) B76.0
Necator americanus B76.1
Andersen's disease (glycogen storage) E74.09
Anderson-Fabry disease E75.21
Andes disease T70.29
Andrews' disease (bacterid) L08.89
Androblastoma
benign
specified site —*see* Neoplasm, benign, by site
unspecified site
female D27.9
male D29.20
malignant
specified site —*see* Neoplasm, malignant, by site
unspecified site
female C56.9
male C62.90
specified site —*see* Neoplasm, uncertain behavior, by site
tubular
with lipid storage
specified site —*see* Neoplasm, benign, by site
unspecified site
female D27.9
male D29.20
specified site —*see* Neoplasm, benign, by site
unspecified site
female D27.9
male D29.20

Androblastoma *(Continued)*
unspecified site
female D39.10
male D40.10
Androgen insensitivity syndrome —*see also* Syndrome, androgen insensitivity E34.50
Androgen resistance syndrome —*see also* Syndrome, androgen insensitivity E34.50
Android pelvis Q74.2
with disproportion (fetopelvic) O33.3
causing obstructed labor O65.3
Androphobia F40.290
Anectasis, pulmonary (newborn) —*see* Atelectasis
Anemia (essential) (general) (hemoglobin deficiency) (infantile) (primary) (profound) D64.9
with (due to) (in)
disorder of
anaerobic glycolysis D55.29
pentose phosphate pathway D55.1
koilonychia D50.9
achlorhydric D50.8
achrestic D53.1
Addison (-Biermer) (pernicious) D51.0
agranulocytic —*see* Agranulocytosis
amino-acid-deficiency D53.0
aplastic D61.9
congenital D61.09
drug-induced D61.1
due to
drugs D61.1
external agents NEC D61.2
infection D61.2
radiation D61.2
idiopathic D61.3
red cell (pure) D60.9
chronic D60.0
congenital D61.01
specified type NEC D60.8
transient D60.1
specified type NEC D61.89
toxic D61.2
aregenerative
congenital D61.09
asiderotic D50.9
atypical (primary) D64.9
Baghdad spring D55.0
Balantidium coli A07.0
Biermer's (pernicious) D51.0
blood loss (chronic) D50.0
acute D62
bothriocephalus B70.0 [D63.8]
brickmaker's B76.9 [D63.8]
cerebral I67.89
childhood D58.9
chlorotic D50.8
chronic
blood loss D50.0
hemolytic D58.9
idiopathic D59.9
simple D53.9
chronica congenita aregenerativa D61.09
combined system disease NEC D51.0 [G32.0]
due to dietary vitamin B12 deficiency D51.3 [G32.0]
complicating pregnancy, childbirth or puerperium —*see* Pregnancy, complicated by (management affected by), anemia
congenital P61.4
aplastic D61.09
due to isoimmunization NOS P55.9
dyserythropoietic, dyshematopoietic D64.4
following fetal blood loss P61.3
Heinz body D58.2
hereditary hemolytic NOS D58.9
pernicious D51.0
spherocytic D58.0
Cooley's (erythroblastic) D56.1
cytogenic D51.0
deficiency D53.9
2, 3 diphosphoglycurate mutase D55.29
2, 3 PG D55.29
6 phosphogluconate dehydrogenase D55.1
6-PGD D55.1
amino-acid D53.0
combined B12 and folate D53.1
enzyme D55.9
drug-induced (hemolytic) D59.2
glucose-6-phosphate dehydrogenase (G6PD) D55.0
glycolytic D55.29
nucleotide metabolism D55.3

▶ New ◆ Revised ~~deleted~~ Deleted ● Use Additional Character(s)

Anemia *(Continued)*
  osteosclerotic D64.89
  ovalocytosis (hereditary) —*see* Elliptocytosis
  paludal —*see also* Malaria B54 *[D63.8]*
  pernicious (congenital) (malignant) (progressive)
    D51.0
  pleochromic D64.89
    of sprue D52.8
  posthemorrhagic (chronic) D50.0
    acute D62
    newborn P61.3
  postoperative (postprocedural)
    due to (acute) blood loss D62
      chronic blood loss D50.0
    specified NEC D64.89
  postpartum O90.81
  pressure D64.89
  progressive D64.9
    malignant D51.0
    pernicious D51.0
  protein-deficiency D53.0
  pseudoleukemica infantum D64.89
  pure red cell D60.9
    congenital D61.01
  pyridoxine-responsive D64.3
  pyruvate kinase deficiency D55.21
  refractory D46.4
    with
      excess of blasts D46.20
        1 (RAEB 1) D46.21
        2 (RAEB 2) D46.22
        in transformation (RAEB T) —*see*
          Leukemia, acute myeloblastic
      hemochromatosis D46.1
      sideroblasts (ring) (RARS) D46.1
    without ring sideroblasts, so stated D46.0
    without sideroblasts without excess of blasts
      D46.0
    megaloblastic D53.1
    sideroblastic D46.1
    sideropenic D50.9
  Rietti-Greppi-Micheli D56.9
  scorbutic D53.2
  secondary to
    blood loss (chronic) D50.0
      acute D62
    hemorrhage (chronic) D50.0
      acute D62
  semiplastic D61.89
  sickle-cell —*see* Disease, sickle-cell
  sideroblastic D64.3
    hereditary D64.0
    hypochromic, sex-linked D64.0
    pyridoxine-responsive NEC D64.3
    refractory D46.1
    secondary (due to)
      disease D64.1
      drugs and toxins D64.2
    specified type NEC D64.3
  sideropenic (refractory) D50.9
    due to blood loss (chronic) D50.0
      acute D62
  simple chronic D53.9
  specified type NEC D64.89
  spherocytic (hereditary) —*see* Spherocytosis
  splenic D64.89
  splenomegalic D64.89
  stomatocytosis D58.8
  syphilitic (acquired) (late) A52.79 *[D63.8]*
  target cell D64.89
  thalassemia D56.9
  thrombocytopenic —*see* Thrombocytopenia
  toxic D61.2
  tropical B76.9 *[D63.8]*
    macrocytic D52.8
  tuberculous A18.89 *[D63.8]*
  vegan D51.3
  vitamin
    B6-responsive D64.3
    B12 deficiency (dietary) pernicious D51.0
  von Jaksch's D64.89
  Witts' (achlorhydric anemia) D50.8
Anemophobia F40.228
Anencephalus, anencephaly Q00.0
Anergasia —*see* Psychosis, organic
Anesthesia, anesthetic R20.0
  complication or reaction NEC —*see also*
    Complications, anesthesia T88.59
    due to
      correct substance properly administered —
        see Table of Drugs and Chemicals, by
        drug, adverse effect

Anesthesia, anesthetic *(Continued)*
  complication or reaction NEC *(Continued)*
    due to *(Continued)*
      overdose or wrong substance given —*see*
        Table of Drugs and Chemicals, by
        drug, poisoning
      unintended awareness under general
        anesthesia during procedure T88.53
        personal history of Z92.84
  cornea H18.81-•
  dissociative F44.6
  functional (hysterical) F44.6
  hyperesthetic, thalamic G89.0
  hysterical F44.6
  local skin lesion R20.0
  sexual (psychogenic) F52.1
  shock (due to) T88.2
  skin R20.0
  testicular N50.9
Anetoderma (maculosum) (of) L90.8
  Jadassohn-Pellizzari L90.2
  Schweninger-Buzzi L90.1
Aneurin deficiency E51.9
Aneurysm (anastomotic) (artery) (cirsoid) (diffuse)
  (false) (fusiform) (multiple) (saccular) I72.9
  abdominal (aorta) I71.40
    infrarenal I71.43
      ruptured I71.33
    juxtarenal I71.42
      ruptured I71.32
    pararenal I71.41
      ruptured I71.31
    ruptured I71.30
    syphilitic A52.01
  aorta, aortic (nonsyphilitic) I71.9
    abdominal I71.40
      dissecting —*see* Dissection, aorta, abdominal
      ruptured I71.30
    arch I71.22
      ruptured I71.12
    arteriosclerotic I71.9
      ruptured I71.8
    ascending I71.21
      ruptured I71.11
    congenital Q25.43
    descending I71.9
      abdominal I71.40
        ruptured I71.30
      ruptured I71.8
      thoracic I71.23
        ruptured I71.13
    dissecting —*see* Dissection, aorta
    root Q25.43
    ruptured I71.8
    sinus, congenital Q25.43
    syphilitic A52.01
    thoracic I71.20
      ruptured I71.10
    thoracoabdominal I71.60
      paravisceral I71.62
        ruptured I71.52
      ruptured I71.50
      supraceliac I71.61
        ruptured I71.51
    thorax, thoracic I71.20
      arch I71.22
        ruptured I71.12
      ascending I71.21
        ruptured I71.11
      descending I71.23
        ruptured I71.13
      ruptured I71.10
        arch I71.12
        ascending I71.11
        descending I71.13
    transverse I71.22
      ruptured I71.12
    valve (heart) —*see also* Endocarditis, aortic
      I35.8
  arteriosclerotic I72.9
    cerebral I67.1
      ruptured —*see* Hemorrhage, intracranial,
        subarachnoid
  arteriovenous (congenital) —*see also*
    Malformation, arteriovenous
    acquired I77.0
      brain I67.1
        ruptured —*see* Aneurysm,
          arteriorvenous, brain, ruptured
      coronary I25.41
      pulmonary I28.0
    brain Q28.2

Aneurysm *(Continued)*
  arteriovenous *(Continued)*
    acquired *(Continued)*
      ruptured I60.8
        intracerebral I61.8
        intraparenchymal I61.8
        intraventricular I61.5
        subarachnoid I60.8
    peripheral —*see* Malformation, arteriovenous,
      peripheral
    precerebral vessels Q28.0
    specified site NEC —*see also* Malformation,
      arteriovenous
    acquired I77.0
  basal —*see* Aneurysm, brain
  basilar (trunk) I72.5
  berry (congenital) (nonruptured) I67.1
    ruptured I60.7
  brain I67.1
    arteriosclerotic I67.1
      ruptured —*see* Hemorrhage, intracranial,
        subarachnoid
    arteriovenous (congenital) (nonruptured) Q28.2
      acquired I67.1
        ruptured —*see* Aneurysm,
          arteriorvenous, brain, ruptured
      ruptured —*see* Aneurysm, arteriorvenous,
        brain, ruptured
    berry (congenital) (nonruptured) I67.1
      ruptured —*see also* Hemorrhage,
        intracranial, subarachnoid I60.7
    congenital Q28.3
      aorta (root) (sinus) Q25.43
      ruptured I60.7
    meninges I67.1
      ruptured I60.8
    miliary (congenital) (nonruptured) I67.1
      ruptured —*see also* Hemorrhage,
        intracranial, subarachnoid I60.7
    mycotic I67.1
      with endocarditis - *see also* Endocarditis
      ruptured —*see* Hemorrhage, intracranial,
        subarachnoid
    syphilitic (hemorrhage) A52.05
  cardiac (false) —*see also* Aneurysm, heart I25.3
  carotid artery (common) (external) I72.0
    internal (intracranial) I67.1
      extracranial portion I72.0
    ruptured into brain I60.0-•
    syphilitic A52.09
      intracranial A52.05
  cavernous sinus I67.1
    arteriovenous (congenital) (nonruptured)
      Q28.3
      ruptured I60.8
  celiac I72.8
  central nervous system, syphilitic A52.05
  cerebral —*see* Aneurysm, brain
  chest —*see* Aneurysm, thorax
  circle of Willis I67.1
    congenital Q28.3
      ruptured I60.6
    ruptured I60.6
  common iliac artery I72.3
  congenital (peripheral) Q27.8
    aorta (root) (sinus) Q25.43
    brain Q28.3
      ruptured I60.7
    coronary Q24.5
    digestive system Q27.8
    lower limb Q27.8
    pulmonary Q25.79
    retina Q14.1
    specified site NEC Q27.8
    upper limb Q27.8
  conjunctiva —*see* Abnormality, conjunctiva,
    vascular
  conus arteriosus —*see* Aneurysm, heart
  coronary (arteriosclerotic) (artery) I25.41
    arteriovenous, congenital Q24.5
    congenital Q24.5
    ruptured —*see* Infarct, myocardium
    syphilitic A52.06
    vein I25.89
  cylindroid (aorta) I71.9
    ruptured I71.8
    syphilitic A52.01
  ductus arteriosus Q25.0
  endocardial, infective (any valve) I33.0
  femoral (artery) (ruptured) I72.4
  gastroduodenal I72.8
  gastroepiploic I72.8

Aneurysm *(Continued)*
  heart (wall) (chronic or with a stated duration of over 4 weeks) I25.3
    valve —*see* Endocarditis
  hepatic I72.8
  iliac (common) (artery) (ruptured) I72.3
  infective I72.9
    endocardial (any valve) I33.0
  innominate (nonsyphilitic) I72.8
    syphilitic A52.09
  interauricular septum —*see* Aneurysm, heart
  interventricular septum —*see* Aneurysm, heart
  intrathoracic (nonsyphilitic) (*see also* Aneurysm, aorta, thorax) I71.20
    ruptured (*see also* Aneurysm, aorta, thorax, ruptured) I71.10
    syphilitic A52.01
  lower limb I72.4
  lung (pulmonary artery) I28.1
  mediastinal (nonsyphilitic) I72.8
    syphilitic A52.09
  miliary (congenital) I67.1
    ruptured —*see* Hemorrhage, intracerebral, subarachnoid, intracranial
  mitral (heart) (valve) I34.89
  mural —*see* Aneurysm, heart
  mycotic I72.9
    endocardial (any valve) I33.0
    ruptured, brain —*see* Hemorrhage, intracerebral, subarachnoid
  myocardium —*see* Aneurysm, heart
  neck I72.0
  pancreaticoduodenal I72.8
  patent ductus arteriosus Q25.0
  peripheral NEC I72.8
    congenital Q27.8
      digestive system Q27.8
      lower limb Q27.8
      specified site NEC Q27.8
      upper limb Q27.8
  popliteal (artery) (ruptured) I72.4
  precerebral
    congenital (nonruptured) Q28.1
    specified site, NEC I72.5
  pulmonary I28.1
    arteriovenous Q25.72
      acquired I28.0
    syphilitic A52.09
    valve (heart) —*see* Endocarditis, pulmonary
  racemose (peripheral) I72.9
    congenital —*see* Aneurysm, congenital
  radial I72.1
  Rasmussen NEC A15.0
  renal (artery) I72.2
  retina —*see also* Disorder, retina, microaneurysms
    congenital Q14.1
    diabetic —*see* E08-E13 with .3-●
  sinus of Valsalva Q25.43
  specified NEC I72.8
  spinal (cord) I72.8
    syphilitic (hemorrhage) A52.09
  splenic I72.8
  subclavian (artery) (ruptured) I72.8
    syphilitic A52.09
  superior mesenteric I72.8
  syphilitic (aorta) A52.01
    central nervous system A52.05
    congenital (late) A50.54 *[I79.0]*
    spine, spinal A52.09
  thoracoabdominal (aorta) I71.60
    ruptured I71.50
    syphilitic A52.01
  thorax, thoracic (aorta) (arch) (nonsyphilitic) — *see* Aneurysm, aorta, thorax
    ruptured —*see* Aneurysm, aorta, thorax, ruptured
    syphilitic A52.01
  traumatic (complication) (early), specified site — *see* Injury, blood vessel
  tricuspid (heart) (valve) I07.8
  ulnar I72.1
  upper limb (ruptured) I72.1
  valve, valvular —*see* Endocarditis
  visceral NEC I72.8
  venous —*see also* Varix I86.8
    congenital Q27.8
      digestive system Q27.8
      lower limb Q27.8
      specified site NEC Q27.8
      upper limb Q27.8
  ventricle —*see* Aneurysm, heart
  vertebral artery I72.6
  visceral NEC I72.8

Angelman syndrome Q93.51
Anger R45.4
Angiectasis, angiectopia I99.8
Angiitis I77.6
  allergic granulomatous M30.1
  hypersensitivity M31.0
  necrotizing M31.9
    specified NEC M31.8
  nervous system, granulomatous I67.7
Angina (attack) (cardiac) (chest) (heart) (pectoris) (syndrome) (vasomotor) I20.9
  with
    atherosclerotic heart disease —*see* Arteriosclerosis, coronary (artery)
    coronary microvascular disease I20.81
    coronary microvascular dysfunction I20.81
    documented spasm I20.1
  abdominal K55.1
  accelerated —*see* Angina, unstable
  agranulocytic —*see* Agranulocytosis
  angiospastic —*see* Angina, with documented spasm
  aphthous B08.5
  crescendo —*see* Angina, unstable
  croupous J05.0
  cruris I73.9
  de novo effort —*see* Angina, unstable
  diphtheritic, membranous A36.0
  equivalent I20.89
  exudative, chronic J37.0
  following acute myocardial infarction I23.7
  gangrenous diphtheritic A36.0
  intestinal K55.1
  Ludovici K12.2
  Ludwig's K12.2
  malignant diphtheritic A36.0
  membranous J05.0
    diphtheritic A36.0
    Vincent's A69.1
  mesenteric K55.1
  monocytic —*see* Mononucleosis, infectious
  of effort —*see* Angina, specified NEC
  phlegmonous J36
    diphtheritic A36.0
  post-infarctional I23.7
  pre-infarctional —*see* Angina, unstable
  Prinzmetal —*see* Angina, with documented spasm
  progressive —*see* Angina, unstable
  pseudomembranous A69.1
  pultaceous, diphtheritic A36.0
  refractory I20.2
  spasm-induced —*see* Angina, with documented spasm
  specified NEC I20.89
  stable I20.89
  stenocardia —*see* Angina, specified NEC
  stridulous, diphtheritic A36.2
  tonsil J36
  trachealis J05.0
  unstable I20.0
  variant —*see* Angina, with documented spasm
  Vincent's A69.1
  worsening effort —*see* Angina, unstable
Angioblastoma —*see* Neoplasm, connective tissue, uncertain behavior
Angiocholecystitis —*see* Cholecystitis, acute
Angiocholitis —*see also* Cholecystitis, acute K83.09
Angiodysgenesis spinalis G95.19
Angiodysplasia (cecum) (colon) K55.20
  with bleeding K55.21
  duodenum (and stomach) K31.819
    with bleeding K31.811
  stomach (and duodenum) K31.819
    with bleeding K31.811
Angioedema (allergic) (any site) (with urticaria) T78.3
  episodic, with eosinophilia D72.118
  hereditary D84.1
Angioendothelioma —*see* Neoplasm, uncertain behavior, by site
  benign D18.00
    intra-abdominal D18.03
    intracranial D18.02
    skin D18.01
    specified site NEC D18.09
  bone —*see* Neoplasm, bone, malignant
  Ewing's —*see* Neoplasm, bone, malignant
Angioendotheliomatosis C85.8-●
Angiofibroma —*see also* Neoplasm, benign, by site
  juvenile
    specified site —*see* Neoplasm, benign, by site
    unspecified site D10.6

Angiohemophilia (A) (B) —*see* Disease, von Willebrand
Angioid streaks (choroid) (macula) (retina) H35.33
Angiokeratoma —*see* Neoplasm, skin, benign
  corporis diffusum E75.21
Angioleiomyoma —*see* Neoplasm, connective tissue, benign
Angiolipoma —*see also* Lipoma
  infiltrating —*see* Lipoma
Angioma —*see also* Hemangioma, by site
  capillary I78.1
  hemorrhagicum hereditaria I78.0
  intra-abdominal D18.03
  intracranial D18.02
  malignant —*see* Neoplasm, connective tissue, malignant
  plexiform D18.00
    intra-abdominal D18.03
    intracranial D18.02
    skin D18.01
    specified site NEC D18.09
  senile I78.1
  serpiginosum L81.7
  skin D18.01
  specified site NEC D18.09
  spider I78.1
  stellate I78.1
  venous Q28.3
Angiomatosis Q82.8
  bacillary A79.89
  encephalotrigeminal Q85.89
  hemorrhagic familial I78.0
  hereditary familial I78.0
  liver K76.4
Angiomyolipoma —*see* Lipoma
Angiomyoliposarcoma —*see* Neoplasm, connective tissue, malignant
Angiomyoma —*see* Neoplasm, connective tissue, benign
Angiomyosarcoma —*see* Neoplasm, connective tissue, malignant
Angiomyxoma —*see* Neoplasm, connective tissue, uncertain behavior
Angioneurosis F45.8
Angioneurotic edema (allergic) (any site) (with urticaria) T78.3
  hereditary D84.1
Angiopathia, angiopathy I99.9
  cerebral I67.9
    amyloid E85.4 *[I68.0]*
  diabetic (peripheral) —*see* Diabetes, angiopathy
  peripheral I73.9
    diabetic —*see* Diabetes, angiopathy
    specified type NEC I73.89
  retinae syphilitica A52.05
  retinalis (juvenilis)
    diabetic —*see* Diabetes, retinopathy
    proliferative —*see* Retinopathy, proliferative
Angiosarcoma —*see also* Neoplasm, connective tissue, malignant
  liver C22.3
Angiosclerosis —*see* Arteriosclerosis
Angiospasm (peripheral) (traumatic) (vessel) (*see also* Vasospasm) I73.9
  brachial plexus G54.0
  cerebral G45.9
  cervical plexus G54.2
  nerve
    arm —*see* Mononeuropathy, upper limb
      axillary G54.0
      median —*see* Lesion, nerve, median
      ulnar —*see* Lesion, nerve, ulnar
    axillary G54.0
    leg —*see* Mononeuropathy, lower limb
    median —*see* Lesion, nerve, median
    plantar —*see* Lesion, nerve, plantar
    ulnar —*see* Lesion, nerve, ulnar
Angiospastic disease or edema I73.9
Angiostrongyliasis
  due to
    Parastrongylus
      cantonensis B83.2
      costaricensis B81.3
  intestinal B81.3
Anguillulosis —*see* Strongyloidiasis
Angulation
  cecum —*see* Obstruction, intestine
  coccyx (acquired) M43.8X8
    congenital NEC Q76.49
  femur (acquired) —*see also* Deformity, limb, specified type NEC, thigh
    congenital Q74.2

▶ New   ➡ Revised   ~~deleted~~ Deleted   ● Use Additional Character(s)

▶ New   ⇨ Revised   ~~deleted~~ Deleted   • Use Additional Character(s)

Antibody
anticardiolipin R76.0
  with
    hemorrhagic disorder D68.312
    hypercoagulable state D68.61
antiphosphatidylglycerol R76.0
  with
    hemorrhagic disorder D68.312
    hypercoagulable state D68.61
antiphosphatidylinositol R76.0
  with
    hemorrhagic disorder D68.312
    hypercoagulable state D68.61
antiphosphatidylserine R76.0
  with
    hemorrhagic disorder D68.312
    hypercoagulable state D68.61
antiphospholipid R76.0
  with
    hemorrhagic disorder D68.312
    hypercoagulable state D68.61
Anticardiolipin syndrome D68.61
Anticoagulant, circulating (intrinsic) —*see also* -
  Disorder, hemorrhagic D68.318
drug-induced (extrinsic) —*see also* - Disorder,
  hemorrhagic D68.32
iatrogenic D68.32
Antidiuretic hormone syndrome E22.2
Antimonial cholera —*see* Poisoning, antimony
Antiphospholipid
antibody
  with hemorrhagic disorder D68.312
  syndrome D68.61
Antisocial personality F60.2
Antithrombinemia —*see* Circulating
  anticoagulants
Antithromboplastinemia D68.318
Antithromboplastinogenemia D68.318
Antitoxin complication or reaction —*see*
  Complications, vaccination
Antlophobia F40.228
Antritis J32.0
maxilla J32.0
  acute J01.00
    recurrent J01.01
stomach K29.50
  with bleeding K29.51
Antrum, antral —*see* condition
Anuria R34
calculous (impacted) (recurrent) —*see also*
  Calculus, urinary N20.9
following
  abortion —*see* Abortion by type complicated
    by, renal failure
  ectopic or molar pregnancy O08.4
newborn P96.0
postprocedural N99.0
postrenal N13.8
puerperal O90.49
traumatic (following crushing) T79.5
Anus, anal —*see* condition
Anusitis K62.89
Anxiety F41.9
depression F41.8
episodic paroxysmal F41.0
generalized F41.1
hysteria F41.8
neurosis F41.1
panic type F41.0
reaction F41.1
separation, abnormal (of childhood) F93.0
specified NEC F41.8
state F41.1
Aorta, aortic —*see* condition
Aortectasia —*see* Ectasia, aorta
with aneurysm —*see* Aneurysm, aorta
Aortitis (nonsyphilitic) (calcific) I77.6
arteriosclerotic I70.0
Doehle-Heller A52.02
luetic A52.02
rheumatic —*see* Endocarditis, acute, rheumatic
specific (syphilitic) A52.02
syphilitic A52.02
  congenital A50.54 [I79.1]
Apathetic thyroid storm —*see* Thyrotoxicosis
Apathy R45.3
Apeirophobia F40.228
Apepsia K30
psychogenic F45.8
Aperistalsis, esophagus K22.0
Apertognathia M26.29
Apert's syndrome Q87.0

Aphagia R13.0
psychogenic F50.9
Aphakia (acquired) (postoperative) H27.0-•
congenital Q12.3
Aphasia (amnestic) (global) (nominal) (semantic)
  (syntactic) R47.01
acquired, with epilepsy (Landau-Kleffner
  syndrome) —*see* Epilepsy, specified NEC
auditory (developmental) F80.2
developmental (receptive type) F80.2
  expressive type F80.1
  Wernicke's F80.2
following
  cerebrovascular disease I69.920
    cerebral infarction I69.320
    intracerebral hemorrhage I69.120
    nontraumatic intracranial hemorrhage NEC
      I69.220
    specified disease NEC I69.820
    subarachnoid hemorrhage I69.020
primary progressive (*see also* Dementia, in,
  diseases specified elsewhere) G31.01 [F02.80]
  with behavioral disturbance (*see also*
    Dementia, in, diseases specified
    elsewhere) G31.01 [F02.81-•]
progressive isolated (*see also* Dementia, in,
  diseases specified elsewhere) G31.01 [F02.80]
  with behavioral disturbance (*see also*
    Dementia, in, diseases specified
    elsewhere) G31.01 [F02.81-•]
sensory F80.2
syphilis, tertiary A52.19
Wernicke's (developmental) F80.2
Aphonia (organic) R49.1
hysterical F44.4
psychogenic F44.4
Aphthae, aphthous —*see also* condition
Bednar's K12.0
cachectic K14.0
epizootic B08.8
fever B08.8
oral (recurrent) K12.0
stomatitis (major) (minor) K12.0
thrush B37.0
ulcer (oral) (recurrent) K12.0
  genital organ(s) NEC
    female N76.6
    male N50.89
  larynx J38.7
Apical —*see* condition
Apiphobia F40.218
▶ **APL (acquired partial lipodystrophy)** E88.11
Aplasia —*see also* Agenesis
abdominal muscle syndrome Q79.4
alveolar process (acquired) —*see* Anomaly, alveolar
  congenital Q38.6
aorta (congenital) Q25.41
axialis extracorticalis (congenita) E75.29
bone marrow (myeloid) D61.9
  congenital D61.01
brain Q00.0
  part of Q04.3
bronchus Q32.4
cementum K00.4
cerebellum Q04.3
cervix (congenital) Q51.5
congenital pure red cell D61.01
corpus callosum Q04.0
cutis congenita Q84.8
erythrocyte congenital D61.01
extracortical axial E75.29
eye Q11.1
fovea centralis (congenital) Q14.1
gallbladder, congenital Q44.0
iris Q13.1
labyrinth, membranous Q16.5
limb (congenital) Q73.8
  lower —*see* Defect, reduction, lower limb
  upper —*see* Agenesis, arm
lung, congenital (bilateral) (unilateral) Q33.3
pancreas Q45.0
parathyroid-thymic D82.1
Pelizaeus-Merzbacher E75.27
penis Q55.5
prostate Q55.4
red cell (with thymoma) D60.9
  acquired D60.9
    due to drugs D60.9
  adult D60.9
  chronic D60.0
  congenital D61.01
  constitutional D61.01

Aplasia (Continued)
red cell (Continued)
  due to drugs D60.9
  hereditary D61.01
  of infants D61.01
  primary D61.01
  pure D61.01
    due to drugs D60.9
  specified type NEC D60.8
  transient D60.1
round ligament Q52.8
skin Q84.8
spermatic cord Q55.4
spleen Q89.01
testicle Q55.0
thymic, with immunodeficiency D82.1
thyroid (congenital) (with myxedema) E03.1
uterus Q51.0
ventral horn cell Q06.1
Apnea, apneic (of) (spells) R06.81
newborn P28.40
  central P28.41
  mixed P28.43
  obstructive P28.42
  sleep
    primary P28.30
      central P28.31
      mixed P28.33
      obstructive P28.32
      specified NEC P28.39
  specified NEC P28.49
prematurity P28.49
sleep G47.30
  central (primary) G47.31
    idiopathic G47.31
    in conditions classified elsewhere G47.37
  obstructive (adult) (pediatric) G47.33
    hypopnea G47.33
  primary central G47.31
  specified NEC G47.39
Apneumatosis, newborn P28.0
Apocrine metaplasia (breast) —*see* Dysplasia,
  mammary, specified type NEC
Apophysitis (bone) —*see also* Osteochondropathy
calcaneus M92.6
juvenile M92.9
Apoplectiform convulsions (cerebral ischemia) I67.82
Apoplexia, apoplexy, apoplectic
adrenal A39.1
heart (auricle) (ventricle) —*see* Infarct, myocardium
heat T67.01
hemorrhagic (stroke) —*see* Hemorrhage,
  intracranial
meninges, hemorrhagic —*see* Hemorrhage,
  intracranial, subarachnoid
uremic N18.9 [I68.8]
Appearance
bizarre R46.1
specified NEC R46.89
very low level of personal hygiene R46.0
Appendage
epididymal (organ of Morgagni) Q55.4
intestine (epiploic) Q43.8
preauricular Q17.0
testicular (organ of Morgagni) Q55.29
Appendicitis (pneumococcal) (retrocecal) K37
with
  gangrene K35.891
    with localized peritonitis K35.31
  perforation NOS K35.32
  peritoneal abscess K35.33
  peritonitis NEC K35.33
    generalized K35.209
      with
        abscess K35.219
          with perforation or rupture K35.211
          following rupture or perforation of
            appendix NOS K35.211
          without perforation or rupture
            K35.210
        perforation or rupture K35.201
        following rupture or perforation of
          appendix NOS K35.201
        without rupture or perforation of
          appendix K35.200
    localized K35.30
      with
        gangrene K35.32
        perforation K35.32
          and abscess K35.33
      ruptured NOS (with localized peritonitis)
        K35.32

▶ New   ➡ Revised   ~~deleted~~ Deleted   • Use Additional Character(s)

Appendicitis *(Continued)*
  acute (catarrhal) (fulminating) (obstructive)
      (retrocecal) (suppurative) K35.80
    with
      gangrene K35.891
      peritoneal abscess K35.33
      peritonitis NEC K35.33
        generalized K35.209
          with
            abscess K35.219
              with perforation or rupture
                  K35.211
              following rupture or perforation
                  of appendix NOS K35.211
              without perforation or rupture
                  K35.210
              perforation or rupture K35.201
            following rupture or perforation of
                appendix NOS K35.201
            without rupture or perforation of
                appendix K35.200
        localized K35.30
          with
            gangrene K35.32
            perforation K35.32
            and abscess K35.33
      specified NEC K35.890
        with gangrene K35.891
      with localized peritonitis K35.31
    amebic A06.89
    chronic (recurrent) K36
    exacerbation —*see* Appendicitis, with, gangrene
    gangrenous —*see* Appendicitis, acute
    healed (obliterative) K36
    interval K36
    neurogenic K36
    obstructive K36
    recurrent K36
    relapsing K36
      ruptured NOS (with localized peritonitis) K35.32
    subacute (adhesive) K36
    subsiding K36
    suppurative —*see* Appendicitis, acute
    tuberculous A18.32
Appendicopathia oxyurica B80
Appendix, appendicular —*see also* condition
    epididymis Q55.4
    Morgagni
      female Q50.5
      male (epididymal) Q55.4
        testicular Q55.29
    testis Q55.29
Appetite
    depraved —*see* Pica
    excessive R63.2
    lack or loss —*see also* Anorexia R63.0
      nonorganic origin F50.89
      psychogenic F50.89
    perverted (hysterical) —*see* Pica
Apple peel syndrome Q41.1
Apprehension state F41.1
Apprehensiveness, abnormal F41.9
Approximal wear K03.0
Apraxia (classic) (ideational) (ideokinetic)
      (ideomotor) (motor) (verbal) R48.2
    following
      cerebrovascular disease I69.990
        cerebral infarction I69.390
        intracerebral hemorrhage I69.190
        nontraumatic intracranial hemorrhage NEC
            I69.290
        specified disease NEC I69.890
        subarachnoid hemorrhage I69.090
    oculomotor, congenital H51.8
▶ primary progressive, of speech G31.87
Aptyalism K11.7
Apudoma —*see* Neoplasm, uncertain behavior,
      by site
Aqueous misdirection H40.83-●
Arabicum elephantiasis —*see* Infestation, filarial
Arachnitis —*see* Meningitis
Arachnodactyly —*see* Syndrome, Marfan
Arachnoiditis (acute) (adhesive) (basal) (brain)
      (cerebrospinal) —*see* Meningitis
Arachnophobia F40.210
Arboencephalitis, Australian A83.4
Arborization block (heart) I45.5
ARC (AIDS-related complex) B20
Arch
    aortic Q25.49
    bovine Q25.49
Arches —*see* condition
Arcuate uterus Q51.810

Arcuatus uterus Q51.810
Arcus (cornea) **senilis** —*see* Degeneration, cornea,
      senile
Arc-welder's lung J63.4
Areflexia R29.2
Areola —*see* condition
Argentaffinoma —*see also* Neoplasm, uncertain
      behavior, by site
    malignant —*see* Neoplasm, malignant, by site
    syndrome E34.09
Argininemia E72.21
Arginosuccinic aciduria E72.22
Argyll Robertson phenomenon, pupil or
    syndrome (syphilitic) A52.19
    atypical H57.09
    nonsyphilitic H57.09
Argyria, argyriasis
    conjunctival H11.13-●
    from drug or medicament —*see* Table of Drugs
      and Chemicals, by substance
Argyrosis, conjunctival H11.13-●
Arhinencephaly Q04.1
Ariboflavinosis E53.0
Arm —*see* condition
Arnold-Chiari disease, obstruction or syndrome
      (type II) Q07.00
    with
      hydrocephalus Q07.02
        with spina bifida Q07.03
      spina bifida Q07.01
        with hydrocephalus Q07.03
    type III —*see* Encephalocele
    type IV Q04.8
Aromatic amino-acid metabolism disorder E70.9
    specified NEC E70.89
Arousals, confusional G47.51
Arrest, arrested
    cardiac I46.9
      complicating
        abortion —*see* Abortion, by type,
            complicated by, cardiac arrest
        anesthesia (general) (local) or other
            sedation —*see* Table of Drugs and
            Chemicals, by drug
          in labor and delivery O74.2
          in pregnancy O29.11-●
            postpartum, puerperal O89.1
        delivery (cesarean) (instrumental) O75.4
      due to
        cardiac condition I46.2
        specified condition NEC I46.8
      intraoperative I97.71-●
      newborn P29.81
      personal history, successfully resuscitated Z86.74
      postprocedural I97.12-●
        obstetric procedure O75.4
    cardiorespiratory —*see* Arrest, cardiac
    circulatory —*see* Arrest, cardiac
    deep transverse O64.0
    development or growth
      bone —*see* Disorder, bone, development or
          growth
      child R62.50
      tracheal rings Q32.1
    epiphyseal
      complete
        femur M89.15-●
        humerus M89.12-●
        tibia M89.16-●
        ulna M89.13-●
      forearm M89.13-●
        specified NEC M89.13-●
      ulna —*see* Arrest, epiphyseal, by type, ulna
      lower leg M89.16-●
        specified NEC M89.168
      tibia —*see* Arrest, epiphyseal, by type, tibia
      partial
        femur M89.15-●
        humerus M89.12-●
        tibia M89.16-●
        ulna M89.13-●
      specified NEC M89.18
    granulopoiesis —*see* Agranulocytosis
    growth plate —*see* Arrest, epiphyseal
    heart —*see* Arrest, cardiac
    legal, anxiety concerning Z65.3
    physeal —*see* Arrest, epiphyseal
    respiratory R09.2
      newborn P28.81
    sinus I45.5
    spermatogenesis (complete) —*see* Azoospermia
      incomplete —*see* Oligospermia
    transverse (deep) O64.0

Arrhenoblastoma
    benign
      specified site —*see* Neoplasm, benign, by site
      unspecified site
        female D27.9
        male D29.20
    malignant
      specified site —*see* Neoplasm, malignant, by site
      unspecified site
        female C56.9
        male C62.90
    specified site —*see* Neoplasm, uncertain
        behavior, by site
    unspecified site
      female D39.10
      male D40.10
Arrhythmia (auricle)(cardiac) (juvenile)(nodal)
      (reflex)(supraventricular)(transitory)
      (ventricle) I49.9
    block I45.9
    extrasystolic I49.49
    newborn
      bradycardia P29.12
      occurring before birth P03.819
        before onset of labor P03.810
        during labor P03.811
      tachycardia P29.11
    psychogenic F45.8
    sinus I49.8
    specified NEC I49.8
    vagal R55
    ventricular re-entry I47.0
Arrillaga-Ayerza syndrome (pulmonary sclerosis
      with pulmonary hypertension) I27.0
Arsenical pigmentation L81.8
    from drug or medicament —*see* Table of Drugs
      and Chemicals
Arsenism —*see* Poisoning, arsenic
Arterial —*see* condition
Arteriofibrosis —*see* Arteriosclerosis
Arteriolar sclerosis —*see* Arteriosclerosis
Arteriolith —*see* Arteriosclerosis
Arteriolitis I77.6
    necrotizing, kidney I77.5
    renal —*see* Hypertension, kidney
Arteriolosclerosis —*see* Arteriosclerosis
Arterionephrosclerosis —*see* Hypertension, kidney
Arteriopathy I77.9
    cerebral autosomal dominant, with subcortical
        infarcts and leukoencephalopathy
        (CADASIL) I67.850
Arteriosclerosis, arteriosclerotic (diffuse)
      (obliterans) (of) (senile) (with calcification)
      I70.90
    with
      chronic limb-threatening ischemia —*see*
          Arteriosclerosis, with critical limb
          ischemia
      critical limb ischemia
        bypass graft I70.329
          autologous vein graft I70.429
            leg I70.429
              with
                gangrene (and intermittent
                    claudication, rest pain, and
                    ulcer) I70.469
                rest pain (and intermittent
                    claudication) I70.429
            bilateral I70.423
              with
                gangrene (and intermittent
                    claudication, rest pain,
                    and ulcer) I70.463
                rest pain (and intermittent
                    claudication) I70.423
            left I70.422
              with
                gangrene (and intermittent
                    claudication, rest pain,
                    and ulcer) I70.462
                rest pain (and intermittent
                    claudication) I70.422
                ulceration (and intermittent
                    claudication and rest
                    pain) I70.449
                ankle I70.443
                calf I70.442
                foot site NEC I70.445
                heel I70.444
                lower leg NEC I70.448
                mid foot I70.444
                thigh I70.441

Arteriosclerosis, arteriosclerotic *(Continued)*
  with *(Continued)*
    critical limb ischemia *(Continued)*
      bypass graft *(Continued)*
        autologous vein graft *(Continued)*
          leg *(Continued)*
            right I70.421
              with
                gangrene (and intermittent
                    claudication, rest pain,
                    and ulcer) I70.461
                rest pain (and intermittent
                    claudication) I70.421
                ulceration (and intermittent
                    claudication and rest
                    pain) I70.439
                  ankle I70.433
                  calf I70.432
                  foot site NEC I70.435
                  heel I70.434
                  lower leg NEC I70.438
                  midfoot I70.434
                  thigh I70.431
          leg I70.329
            with
              gangrene (and intermittent
                  claudication, rest pain, and
                  ulcer) I70.369
              rest pain (and intermittent
                  claudication) I70.329
            bilateral I70.323
              with
                gangrene (and intermittent
                    claudication, rest pain, and
                    ulcer) I70.363
                rest pain (and intermittent
                    claudication) I70.323
            left I70.322
              with
                rest pain (and intermittent
                    claudication) I70.322
                ulceration (and intermittent
                    claudication and rest pain)
                    I70.349
                  ankle I70.343
                  calf I70.342
                  foot site NEC I70.345
                  heel I70.344
                  lower leg NEC I70.348
                  midfoot I70.344
                  thigh I70.341
            right I70.321
              with
                gangrene (and intermittent
                    claudication, rest pain, and
                    ulcer) I70.361
                rest pain (and intermittent
                    claudication) I70.321
                ulceration (and intermittent
                    claudication and rest pain)
                    I70.339
                  ankle I70.333
                  calf I70.332
                  foot site NEC I70.335
                  heel I70.334
                  lower leg NEC I70.338
                  midfoot I70.334
                  thigh I70.331
        nonautologous biological graft
            I70.529
          leg I70.529
            with
              gangrene (and intermittent
                  claudication, rest pain, and
                  ulcer) I70.569
              rest pain (and intermittent
                  claudication) I70.529
            bilateral I70.523
              with
                gangrene (and intermittent
                    claudication, rest pain,
                    and ulcer) I70.563
                rest pain (and intermittent
                    claudication) I70.523
            left I70.522
              with
                gangrene (and intermittent
                    claudication, rest pain,
                    and ulcer) I70.562
                rest pain (and intermittent
                    claudication) I70.522

Arteriosclerosis, arteriosclerotic *(Continued)*
  with *(Continued)*
    critical limb ischemia *(Continued)*
      bypass graft *(Continued)*
        nonautologous biological graft
            (Continued)
          leg *(Continued)*
            left *(Continued)*
              with *(Continued)*
                ulceration (and intermittent
                    claudication and rest
                    pain) I70.549
                  ankle I70.543
                  calf I70.542
                  foot site NEC I70.545
                  heel I70.544
                  lower leg NEC I70.548
                  midfoot I70.544
                  thigh I70.541
            right I70.521
              with
                gangrene (and intermittent
                    claudication, rest pain,
                    and ulcer) I70.561
                rest pain (and intermittent
                    claudication) I70.521
                ulceration (and intermittent
                    claudication and rest
                    pain) I70.539
                  ankle I70.533
                  calf I70.532
                  foot site NEC I70.535
                  heel I70.534
                  lower leg NEC I70.538
                  midfoot I70.534
                  thigh I70.531
        nonbiological graft I70.629
          leg I70.629
            with
              gangrene (and intermittent
                  claudication, rest pain, and
                  ulcer) I70.669
              rest pain (and intermittent
                  claudication) I70.629
            bilateral I70.623
              with
                gangrene (and intermittent
                    claudication, rest pain,
                    and ulcer) I70.663
                rest pain (and intermittent
                    claudication) I70.623
            left I70.622
              with
                gangrene (and intermittent
                    claudication, rest pain,
                    and ulcer) I70.662
                rest pain (and intermittent
                    claudication) I70.622
                ulceration (and intermittent
                    claudication and rest
                    pain) I70.649
                  ankle I70.643
                  calf I70.642
                  foot site NEC I70.645
                  heel I70.644
                  lower leg NEC I70.648
                  midfoot I70.644
                  thigh I70.641
            right I70.621
              with
                gangrene (and intermittent
                    claudication, rest pain,
                    and ulcer) I70.661
                rest pain (and intermittent
                    claudication) I70.621
                ulceration (and intermittent
                    claudication and rest
                    pain) I70.639
                  ankle I70.633
                  calf I70.632
                  foot site NEC I70.635
                  heel I70.634
                  lower leg NEC I70.638
                  midfoot I70.634
                  thigh I70.631
        specified graft NEC I70.729
          leg I70.729
            with
              gangrene (and intermittent
                  claudication, rest pain, and
                  ulcer) I70.769

Arteriosclerosis, arteriosclerotic *(Continued)*
  with *(Continued)*
    critical limb ischemia *(Continued)*
      bypass graft *(Continued)*
        specified graft NEC *(Continued)*
          leg *(Continued)*
            with *(Continued)*
              rest pain (and intermittent
                  claudication) I70.729
            bilateral I70.723
              with
                gangrene (and intermittent
                    claudication, rest pain,
                    and ulcer) I70.763
                rest pain (and intermittent
                    claudication)
                    I70.723
            left I70.722
              with
                gangrene (and intermittent
                    claudication, rest pain,
                    and ulcer) I70.762
                rest pain (and intermittent
                    claudication)
                    I70.722
                ulceration (and intermittent
                    claudication and rest
                    pain) I70.749
                  ankle I70.743
                  calf I70.742
                  foot site NEC I70.745
                  heel I70.744
                  lower leg NEC I70.748
                  midfoot I70.744
                  thigh I70.741
            right I70.721
              with
                gangrene (and intermittent
                    claudication, rest pain,
                    and ulcer) I70.761
                rest pain (and intermittent
                    claudication) I70.721
                ulceration (and intermittent
                    claudication and rest
                    pain) I70.739
                  ankle I70.733
                  calf I70.732
                  foot site NEC I70.735
                  heel I70.734
                  lower leg NEC I70.738
                  midfoot I70.734
                  thigh I70.731
          leg I70.229
            with
              gangrene (and intermittent
                  claudication, rest pain, and ulcer)
                  I70.269
              rest pain (and intermittent
                  claudication) I70.229
            bilateral I70.223
              with
                gangrene (and intermittent
                    claudication, rest pain, and
                    ulcer) I70.263
                rest pain (and intermittent
                    claudication) I70.223
            left I70.222
              with
                gangrene (and intermittent
                    claudication, rest pain, and
                    ulcer) I70.262
                rest pain (and intermittent
                    claudication) I70.222
                ulceration (and intermittent
                    claudication and rest pain)
                    I70.249
                  ankle I70.243
                  calf I70.242
                  foot site NEC I70.245
                  heel I70.244
                  lower leg NEC I70.248
                  midfoot I70.244
                  thigh I70.241
            right I70.221
              with
                gangrene (and intermittent
                    claudication, rest pain, and
                    ulcer) I70.261
                rest pain (and intermittent
                    claudication)
                    I70.221

▶ New   ➡ Revised   ~~deleted~~ Deleted   ● Use Additional Character(s)

▶ New   ➞ Revised   ~~deleted~~ Deleted   ● Use Additional Character(s)

Asthma, asthmatic (*Continued*)
Rostan's I50.1
sandblaster's J62.8
sequoiosis J67.8
severe persistent J45.50
with
exacerbation (acute) J45.51
status asthmaticus J45.52
specified NEC J45.998
stonemason's J62.8
thymic E32.8
tuberculous —*see* Tuberculosis, pulmonary
Wichmann's (laryngismus stridulus) J38.5
wood J67.8
Astigmatism (compound) (congenital) H52.20-●
irregular H52.21-●
regular H52.22-●
Astraphobia F40.220
Astroblastoma
specified site —*see* Neoplasm, malignant,
by site
unspecified site C71.9
Astrocytoma (cystic)
anaplastic
specified site —*see* Neoplasm, malignant, by
site
unspecified site C71.9
fibrillary
specified site —*see* Neoplasm, malignant, by
site
unspecified site C71.9
fibrous
specified site —*see* Neoplasm, malignant, by
site
unspecified site C71.9
gemistocytic
specified site —*see* Neoplasm, malignant, by
site
unspecified site C71.9
juvenile
specified site —*see* Neoplasm, malignant, by
site
unspecified site C71.9
pilocytic
specified site —*see* Neoplasm, malignant, by
site
unspecified site C71.9
piloid
specified site —*see* Neoplasm, malignant, by
site
unspecified site C71.9
protoplasmic
specified site —*see* Neoplasm, malignant, by
site
unspecified site C71.9
specified site NEC —*see* Neoplasm, malignant,
by site
subependymal D43.2
giant cell
specified site —*see* Neoplasm, uncertain
behavior, by site
unspecified site D43.2
specified site —*see* Neoplasm, uncertain
behavior, by site
unspecified site D43.2
unspecified site C71.9
Astroglioma
specified site —*see* Neoplasm, malignant, by
site
unspecified site C71.9
Asymbolia R48.8
Asymmetry —*see also* Distortion
between native and reconstructed breast
N65.1
face Q67.0
jaw (lower) —*see* Anomaly, dentofacial, jaw-
cranial base relationship, asymmetry
Asynergia, asynergy R27.8
ventricular I51.89
Asystole (heart) —*see* Arrest, cardiac
At risk
for
dental caries Z91.849
high Z91.843
low Z91.841
moderate Z91.842
falling Z91.81
feeling loneliness Z65.8
social isolation Z91.89
Ataxia, ataxy, ataxic R27.0
acute R27.8
autosomal recessive Friedreich G11.11

Ataxia, ataxy, ataxic (*Continued*)
brain (hereditary) G11.9
cerebellar (hereditary) G11.9
with defective DNA repair G11.3
alcoholic G31.2
early-onset G11.10
with
essential tremor G11.19
myoclonus [Hunt's ataxia] G11.19
retained tendon reflexes G11.19
in
alcoholism G31.2
myxedema E03.9 [*G13.2*]
neoplastic disease —*see also* Neoplasm
D49.9 [*G32.81*]
specified disease NEC G32.81
late-onset (Marie's) G11.2
cerebral (hereditary) G11.9
congenital nonprogressive G11.0
family, familial —*see* Ataxia, hereditary
following
cerebrovascular disease I69.993
cerebral infarction I69.393
intracerebral hemorrhage I69.193
nontraumatic intracranial hemorrhage NEC
I69.293
specified disease NEC I69.893
subarachnoid hemorrhage I69.093
Friedreich's (heredofamilial) (cerebellar) (spinal)
G11.11
gait R26.0
hysterical F44.4
general R27.8
gluten M35.9 [*G32.81*]
with celiac disease K90.0 [*G32.81*]
hereditary G11.9
with neuropathy G60.2
cerebellar —*see* Ataxia, cerebellar
spastic G11.4
specified NEC G11.8
spinal (Friedreich's) G11.11
heredofamilial —*see* Ataxia, hereditary
Hunt's G11.19
hysterical F44.4
locomotor (progressive) (syphilitic) (partial)
(spastic) A52.11
diabetic —*see* Diabetes, ataxia
Marie's (cerebellar) (heredofamilial) (late- onset)
G11.2
nonorganic origin F44.4
nonprogressive, congenital G11.0
psychogenic F44.4
Roussy-Lévy G60.0
Sanger-Brown's (hereditary) G11.2
spastic hereditary G11.4
spinal
hereditary (Friedreich's) G11.11
progressive (syphilitic) A52.11
spinocerebellar, X-linked recessive G11.19
telangiectasia (Louis-Bar) G11.3
Ataxia-telangiectasia (Louis-Bar) G11.3
Atelectasis (massive) (partial) (pressure)
(pulmonary) J98.11
newborn P28.10
due to resorption P28.11
partial P28.19
primary P28.0
secondary P28.19
primary (newborn) P28.0
tuberculous —*see* Tuberculosis, pulmonary
Atelocardia Q24.9
Atelomyelia Q06.1
Atheroembolism
of
extremities
lower I75.02-●
upper I75.01-●
kidney I75.81
specified NEC I75.89
Atheroma, atheromatous —*see also* Arteriosclerosis
I70.90
aorta, aortic I70.0
valve —*see also* Endocarditis, aortic I35.8
aorto-iliac I70.0
artery —*see* Arteriosclerosis
basilar (artery) I67.2
carotid (artery) (common) (internal) I67.2
cerebral (arteries) I67.2
coronary (artery) I25.10
with angina pectoris —*see* Arteriosclerosis,
coronary (artery)

Atheroma, atheromatous (*Continued*)
degeneration —*see* Arteriosclerosis
heart, cardiac —*see* Disease, heart, ischemic,
atherosclerotic
mitral (valve) I34.89
myocardium, myocardial —*see* Disease, heart,
ischemic, atherosclerotic
pulmonary valve (heart) —*see also* Endocarditis,
pulmonary I37.8
tricuspid (heart) (valve) I36.8
valve, valvular —*see* Endocarditis
vertebral (artery) I67.2
Atheromatosis —*see* Arteriosclerosis
Atherosclerosis —*see also* Arteriosclerosis
coronary
artery I25.10
with angina pectoris —*see* Arteriosclerosis,
coronary (artery),
due to
calcified coronary lesion (severely)
I25.84
lipid rich plaque I25.83
transplanted heart I25.811
bypass graft I25.812
with angina pectoris —*see* Arteriosclerosis,
coronary (artery)
native coronary artery I25.811
with angina pectoris —*see* Arteriosclerosis,
coronary (artery)
Athetosis (acquired) R25.8
bilateral (congenital) G80.3
congenital (bilateral) (double) G80.3
double (congenital) G80.3
unilateral R25.8
Athlete's
foot B35.3
heart I51.7
Athrepsia E41
Athyrea (acquired) —*see also* Hypothyroidism
congenital E03.1
Atonia, atony, atonic
bladder (sphincter) (neurogenic) N31.2
capillary I78.8
cecum K59.89
psychogenic F45.8
colon —*see* Atony, intestine
congenital P94.2
esophagus K22.89
intestine K59.89
psychogenic F45.8
stomach K31.89
neurotic or psychogenic F45.8
uterus (during labor) O62.2
with hemorrhage (postpartum) O72.1
postpartum (with hemorrhage) O72.1
without hemorrhage O75.89
Atopy —*see* History, allergy
Atransferrinemia, congenital E88.09
Atresia, atretic
alimentary organ or tract NEC Q45.8
upper Q40.8
ani, anus, anal (canal) Q42.3
with fistula Q42.2
aorta (ring) Q25.29
aortic (orifice) (valve) Q23.0
arch Q25.21
congenital with hypoplasia of ascending
aorta and defective development of
left ventricle (with mitral stenosis)
Q23.4
in hypoplastic left heart syndrome Q23.4
aqueduct of Sylvius Q03.0
with spina bifida —*see* Spina bifida, with
hydrocephalus
artery NEC Q27.8
cerebral Q28.3
coronary Q24.5
digestive system Q27.8
eye Q15.8
lower limb Q27.8
pulmonary Q25.5
specified site NEC Q27.8
umbilical Q27.0
upper limb Q27.8
auditory canal (external) Q16.1
bile duct (common) (congenital) (hepatic)
Q44.2
acquired —*see* Obstruction, bile duct
bladder (neck) Q64.39
obstruction Q64.31
bronchus Q32.4
cecum Q42.8

▶ New　　⇨ Revised　　~~deleted~~ Deleted　　● Use Additional Character(s)

Atrophy, atrophic *(Continued)*
- muscle, muscular *(Continued)*
  - myelopathic —*see* Atrophy, muscle, spinal
  - myotonic G71.11
  - neuritic G58.9
  - neuropathic (peroneal) (progressive) G60.0
  - pelvic (disuse) N81.84
  - peroneal G60.0
  - progressive (bulbar) G12.21
    - adult G12.1
    - infantile (spinal) G12.0
    - spinal G12.25
      - adult G12.1
      - infantile G12.0
  - pseudohypertrophic G71.02
  - shoulder region M62.51-●
  - specified site NEC M62.58
  - spinal G12.9
    - adult form G12.1
    - Aran-Duchenne G12.21
    - childhood form, type II G12.1
    - distal G12.1
    - hereditary NEC G12.1
    - infantile, type I (Werdnig-Hoffmann) G12.0
    - juvenile form, type III (Kugelberg-Welander) G12.1
    - progressive G12.25
    - scapuloperoneal form G12.1
    - specified NEC G12.8
  - syphilitic A52.78
  - thigh M62.55-●
  - upper arm M62.52-●
- myocardium —*see* Degeneration, myocardial
- myometrium (senile) N85.8
  - cervix N88.8
- myopathic NEC —*see* Atrophy, muscle
- myotonia G71.11
- nail L60.3
- nasopharynx J31.1
- nerve —*see also* Disorder, nerve
  - abducens —*see* Strabismus, paralytic, sixth nerve
  - accessory G52.8
  - acoustic or auditory —*see* subcategory H93.3
  - cranial G52.9
    - eighth (auditory) —*see* subcategory H93.3
    - eleventh (accessory) G52.8
    - fifth (trigeminal) G50.8
    - first (olfactory) G52.0
    - fourth (trochlear) —*see* Strabismus, paralytic, fourth nerve
    - second (optic) H47.20
    - sixth (abducens) —*see* Strabismus, paralytic, sixth nerve
    - tenth (pneumogastric) (vagus) G52.2
    - third (oculomotor) —*see* Strabismus, paralytic, third nerve
    - twelfth (hypoglossal) G52.3
  - hypoglossal G52.3
  - oculomotor —*see* Strabismus, paralytic, third nerve
  - olfactory G52.0
  - optic (papillomacular bundle)
    - syphilitic (late) A52.15
      - congenital A50.44
  - pneumogastric G52.2
  - trigeminal G50.8
  - trochlear —*see* Strabismus, paralytic, fourth nerve
  - vagus (pneumogastric) G52.2
- neurogenic, bone, tabetic A52.11
- nutritional E43
  - with marasmus E41
- old age R54
- olivopontocerebellar G23.8
- optic (nerve) H47.20
  - glaucomatous H47.23-●
  - hereditary H47.22
  - primary H47.21-●
  - specified type NEC H47.29-●
  - syphilitic (late) A52.15
    - congenital A50.44
- orbit H05.31-●
- ovary (senile) N83.31-●
  - with fallopian tube N83.33-●
- oviduct (senile) —*see* Atrophy, fallopian tube
- palsy, diffuse (progressive) G12.22
- pancreas (duct) (senile) K86.89
- parotid gland K11.0
- pelvic muscle N81.84
- penis N48.89

Atrophy, atrophic *(Continued)*
- pharynx J39.2
- pluriglandular E31.8
  - autoimmune E31.0
- polyarthritis M15.9
- prostate N42.89
- pseudohypertrophic (muscle) G71.02
- renal —*see also* Sclerosis, renal N26.1
- retina, retinal (postinfectional) H35.89
- rhinitis J31.0
- salivary gland K11.0
- scar L90.5
- sclerosis, lobar (of brain) (*see also* Dementia, in, diseases specified elsewhere) G31.09 [F02.80]
  - with behavioral disturbance (*see also* Dementia, in, diseases specified elsewhere) G31.09 [F02.81-●]
- scrotum N50.89
- seminal vesicle N50.89
- senile R54
  - due to radiation (nonionizing) (solar) L57.8
- skin (patches) (spots) L90.9
  - degenerative (senile) L90.8
  - due to radiation (nonionizing) (solar) L57.8
  - senile L90.8
- spermatic cord N50.89
- spinal (acute) (cord) G95.89
  - muscular —*see* Atrophy, muscle, spinal
  - paralysis G12.20
    - acute —*see* Poliomyelitis, paralytic
    - meaning progressive muscular atrophy G12.25
- spine (column) —*see* Spondylopathy, specified NEC
- spleen (senile) D73.0
- stomach K29.40
  - with bleeding K29.41
- striate (skin) L90.6
  - syphilitic A52.79
- subcutaneous L90.9
- sublingual gland K11.0
- submandibular gland K11.0
- submaxillary gland K11.0
- Sudeck's —*see* Algoneurodystrophy
- suprarenal (capsule) (gland) E27.49
  - primary E27.1
- systemic affecting central nervous system in
  - myxedema E03.9 [G13.2]
  - neoplastic disease —*see also* Neoplasm D49.9 [G13.1]
  - specified disease NEC G13.8
- tarso-orbital fascia, congenital Q10.3
- testis N50.0
- thenar, partial —*see* Syndrome, carpal tunnel
- thymus (fatty) E32.8
- thyroid (gland) (acquired) E03.4
  - with cretinism E03.1
  - congenital (with myxedema) E03.1
- tongue (senile) K14.8
  - papillae K14.4
- trachea J39.8
- tunica vaginalis N50.89
- turbinate J34.89
- tympanic membrane (nonflaccid) H73.82-●
  - flaccid H73.81-●
- upper respiratory tract J39.8
- uterus, uterine (senile) N85.8
  - cervix N88.8
  - due to radiation (intended effect) N85.8
    - adverse effect or misadventure N99.89
- vagina (senile) N95.2
- vas deferens N50.89
- vascular I99.8
- vertebra (senile) —*see* Spondylopathy, specified NEC
- vulva (senile) N90.5
- Werdnig-Hoffmann G12.0
- yellow —*see* Failure, hepatic

Attack, attacks
- with alteration of consciousness (with automatisms) —*see* Epilepsy, localization-related, symptomatic, with complex partial seizures
- without alteration of consciousness —*see* Epilepsy, localization-related, symptomatic, with simple partial seizures
- Adams-Stokes I45.9
- akinetic —*see* Epilepsy, generalized, specified NEC

Attack, attacks *(Continued)*
- angina —*see* Angina
- atonic —*see* Epilepsy, generalized, specified NEC
- benign shuddering G25.83
- cataleptic —*see* Catalepsy
- coronary —*see* Infarct, myocardium
- cyanotic, newborn P28.2
- drop NEC R55
- epileptic —*see* Epilepsy
- heart —*see* Infarct, myocardium
- hysterical F44.9
- jacksonian —*see* Epilepsy, localization-related, symptomatic, with simple partial seizures
- myocardium, myocardial —*see* Infarct, myocardium
- myoclonic —*see* Epilepsy, generalized, specified NEC
- panic F41.0
- psychomotor —*see* Epilepsy, localization-related, symptomatic, with complex partial seizures
- salaam —*see* Epilepsy, spasms
- schizophreniform, brief F23
- shuddering, benign G25.83
- Stokes-Adams I45.9
- syncope R55
- transient ischemic (TIA) G45.9
  - specified NEC G45.8
- unconsciousness R55
  - hysterical F44.89
- vasomotor R55
- vasovagal (paroxysmal) (idiopathic) R55

Attention (to)
- artificial
  - opening (of) Z43.9
    - digestive tract NEC Z43.4
      - colon Z43.3
      - ilium Z43.2
      - stomach Z43.1
    - specified NEC Z43.8
    - trachea Z43.0
    - urinary tract NEC Z43.6
      - cystostomy Z43.5
      - nephrostomy Z43.6
      - ureterostomy Z43.6
      - urethrostomy Z43.6
    - vagina Z43.7
- colostomy Z43.3
- cystostomy Z43.5
- deficit disorder or syndrome F98.8
  - with hyperactivity —*see* Disorder, attention-deficit hyperactivity
- gastrostomy Z43.1
- ileostomy Z43.2
- jejunostomy Z43.4
- nephrostomy Z43.6
- surgical dressings Z48.01
- sutures Z48.02
- tracheostomy Z43.0
- ureterostomy Z43.6
- urethrostomy Z43.6

Attrition
- gum —*see* Recession, gingival
- tooth, teeth (excessive) (hard tissues) K03.0

Atypical, atypism —*see also* condition
- cells (on cytolgocial smear) (endocervical) (endometrial) (glandular)
  - cervix R87.619
  - vagina R87.629
- cervical N87.9
- endometrium N85.9
  - hyperplasia N85.00
- parenting situation Z62.9

Auditory —*see* condition
Aujeszky's disease B33.8
Aurantiasis, cutis E67.1
Auricle, auricular —*see also* condition
- cervical Q18.2
Auriculotemporal syndrome G50.8
Austin Flint murmur (aortic insufficiency) I35.1
Australian
- Q fever A78
- X disease A83.4
Autism, autistic (childhood) (infantile) F84.0
- atypical F84.9
- spectrum disorder F84.0
Autoantibodies, multiple confirmed islet, with normoglycemia E10.A1
Autodigestion R68.89
Autoerythrocyte sensitization (syndrome) D69.2
Autographism L50.3

Autoimmune
  disease (systemic) M35.9
  inhibitors to clotting factors D68.311
  lymphoproliferative syndrome [ALPS] D89.82
  thyroiditis E06.3
Autoimmunity, confirmed islet, with dysglycemia
  E10.A2
Autointoxication R68.89
Automatism G93.89
  with temporal sclerosis G93.81
  epileptic —*see* Epilepsy, localization- related,
    symptomatic, with complex partial
    seizures
  paroxysmal, idiopathic —*see* Epilepsy,
    localization-related, symptomatic, with
    complex partial seizures
Autonomic, autonomous
  bladder (neurogenic) N31.2
  hysteria seizure F44.5
Autosensitivity, erythrocyte D69.2
Autosensitization, cutaneous L30.2
Autosome —*see* condition by chromosome
  involved
Autotopagnosia R48.1
Autotoxemia R68.89
Autumn —*see* condition
Avellis' syndrome G46.8
Aversion
  oral R63.39
    ➡ newborn P92.8
    nonorganic origin F98.2
  sexual F52.1
Aviator's
  disease or sickness —*see* Effect, adverse, high
    altitude
  ear T70.0
Avitaminosis (multiple) —*see also* Deficiency,
    vitamin E56.9
  B E53.9
    with
      beriberi E51.11
      pellagra E52
  B2 E53.0
  B6 E53.1
  B12 E53.8
  D E55.9
    with rickets E55.0
  G E53.0
  K E56.1
  nicotinic acid E52
AVNRT (atrioventricular nodal re-entrant
    tachycardia) I47.19
AVRT (atrioventricular nodal re-entrant
    tachycardia) I47.19
Avulsion (traumatic)
  blood vessel —*see* Injury, blood vessel
  bone —*see* Fracture, by site
  cartilage —*see also* Dislocation, by site
    symphyseal (inner), complicating delivery
      O71.6
  external site other than limb —*see* Wound, open,
    by site
  eye S05.7- ●
  head (intracranial)
    external site NEC S08.89
    scalp S08.0
  internal organ or site —*see* Injury, by site
  joint —*see also* Dislocation, by site
    capsule —*see* Sprain, by site
  kidney S37.06- ●
  ligament —*see* Sprain, by site
  limb —*see also* Amputation, traumatic, by site
    skin and subcutaneous tissue —*see* Wound,
      open, by site
  muscle —*see* Injury, muscle
  nerve (root) —*see* Injury, nerve
  scalp S08.0
  skin and subcutaneous tissue —*see* Wound,
    open, by site
  spleen S36.032
  symphyseal cartilage (inner), complicating
    delivery O71.6
  tendon —*see* Injury, muscle
  tooth S03.2
Awareness of heart beat R00.2
Axenfeld's
  anomaly or syndrome Q15.0
  degeneration (calcareous) Q13.4
Axilla, axillary —*see also* condition
  breast Q83.1
Axonotmesis —*see* Injury, nerve

Ayerza's disease or syndrome (pulmonary artery
    sclerosis with pulmonary hypertension) I27.0
Azoospermia (organic) N46.01
  due to
    drug therapy N46.021
    efferent duct obstruction N46.023
    infection N46.022
    radiation N46.024
    specified cause NEC N46.029
    systemic disease N46.025
Azotemia R79.89
  meaning uremia N19
Aztec ear Q17.3
Azygos
  continuation inferior vena cava Q26.8
  lobe (lung) Q33.1

B

Baastrup's disease —*see* Kissing spine
Babesiosis B60.00
  due to
    Babesia
      divergens B60.03
      duncani B60.02
      KO-1 B60.09
      microti B60.01
      MO-1 B60.03
      species
        unspecified B60.00
      venatorum B60.09
    specified NEC B60.09
Babington's disease (familial hemorrhagic
    telangiectasia) I78.0
Babinski's syndrome A52.79
Baby
  crying constantly R68.11
  floppy (syndrome) P94.2
Bacillary —*see* condition
Bacilluria R82.71
Bacillus —*see also* Infection, bacillus
  abortus infection A23.1
  anthracis infection A22.9
  coli infection —*see also* Escherichia coli B96.20
  Flexner's A03.1
  mallei infection A24.0
  Shiga's A03.0
  suipestifer infection —*see* Infection, salmonella
Back —*see* condition
Backache (postural) M54.9
  sacroiliac M53.3
  specified NEC M54.89
Backflow —*see* Reflux
Backward reading (dyslexia) F81.0
Bacteremia R78.81
  with sepsis —*see* Sepsis
Bactericholia —*see* Cholecystitis, acute
Bacterid, bacteride (pustular) L40.3
Bacterium, bacteria, bacterial
  agent NEC, as cause of disease classified
    elsewhere B96.89
  in blood —*see* Bacteremia
  in urine —*see* Bacteriuria
Bacteriuria, bacteruria (asymptomatic) R82.71
Bacteroides
  fragilis, as cause of disease classified elsewhere
    B96.6
Bad
  heart —*see* Disease, heart
  trip
    due to drug abuse —*see* Abuse, drug,
      hallucinogen
    due to drug dependence —*see* Dependence,
      drug, hallucinogen
Baelz's disease (cheilitis glandularis apostematosa)
    K13.0
Baerensprung's disease (eczema marginatum)
    B35.6
Bagasse disease or pneumonitis J67.1
Bagassosis J67.1
Baker's cyst —*see* Cyst, Baker's
Bakwin-Krida syndrome (metaphyseal dysplasia)
    Q78.5
Balancing side interference M26.56
Balanitis (circinata) (erosiva) (gangrenosa)
    (phagedenic) (vulgaris) N48.1
  amebic A06.82
  candidal B37.42

Balanitis (*Continued*)
  due to Haemophilus ducreyi A57
  gonococcal (acute) (chronic) A54.23
  xerotica obliterans N48.0
Balanoposthitis N47.6
  gonococcal (acute) (chronic) A54.23
  ulcerative (specific) A63.8
Balanorrhagia —*see* Balanitis
Balantidiasis, balantidiosis A07.0
Bald tongue K14.4
Baldness —*see also* Alopecia
  male-pattern —*see* Alopecia, androgenic
Balkan grippe A78
Balloon disease —*see* Effect, adverse, high altitude
Balo's disease (concentric sclerosis) G37.5
Bamberger-Marie disease —*see* Osteoarthropathy,
    hypertrophic, specified type NEC
Bancroft's filariasis B74.0
Band(s)
  adhesive —*see* Adhesions, peritoneum
  anomalous or congenital —*see also* Anomaly,
    by site
    heart (atrial) (ventricular) Q24.8
    intestine Q43.3
    omentum Q43.3
  cervix N88.1
  constricting, congenital Q79.8
  gallbladder (congenital) Q44.1
  intestinal (adhesive) —*see* Adhesions,
    peritoneum
  obstructive
    intestine K56.50
      complete K56.52
      incomplete K56.51
      partial K56.51
    peritoneum K56.50
      complete K56.52
      incomplete K56.51
      partial K56.51
  periappendiceal, congenital Q43.3
  peritoneal (adhesive) —*see* Adhesions,
    peritoneum
  uterus N73.6
    internal N85.6
  vagina N89.5
Bandemia D72.825
Bandl's ring (contraction), **complicating delivery**
    O62.4
Bangkok hemorrhagic fever A91
Bang's disease (brucella abortus) A23.1
➡ **Bankruptcy** (anxiety concerning) Z59.868
Bannister's disease T78.3
  hereditary D84.1
Banti's disease or syndrome (with cirrhosis) (with
    portal hypertension) K76.6
Bar, median, prostate —*see* Enlargement, enlarged,
    prostate
Barcoo disease or rot —*see* Ulcer, skin
Barlow's disease E54
Barodontalgia T70.29
Baron Münchausen syndrome —*see* Disorder,
    factitious
Barosinusitis T70.1
Barotitis T70.0
Barotrauma T70.29
  odontalgia T70.29
  otitic T70.0
  sinus T70.1
➡ **Barraquer** (-Simons) **disease or syndrome**
    (progressive lipodystrophy) E88.11
Barré-Guillain disease or syndrome G61.0
Barré-Liéou syndrome (posterior cervical
    sympathetic) M53.0
Barrel chest M95.4
Barrett's
  disease —*see* Barrett's, esophagus
  esophagus K22.70
    with dysplasia K22.719
      high grade K22.711
      low grade K22.710
    without dysplasia K22.70
  syndrome —*see* Barrett's, esophagus
  ulcer K22.10
    with bleeding K22.11
    without bleeding K22.10
Barth syndrome E78.71
Bársony (-Polgár) (-Teschendorf) **syndrome**
    (corkscrew esophagus) K22.4
Bartholinitis (suppurating) N75.8
  gonococcal (acute) (chronic) (with abscess)
    A54.1

▶ New   ➡ Revised   ~~deleted~~ Deleted   ● Use Additional Character(s)

▶ New ⇒ Revised ~~deleted~~ Deleted ● Use Additional Character(s)

▶ New   ⟹ Revised   ~~deleted~~ Deleted   ● Use Additional Character(s)

▶ New ➡ Revised ~~deleted~~ Deleted ● Use Additional Character(s)

Bronchitis (diffuse) (fibrinous) (hypostatic) (infective) (membranous) J40
with
  influenza, flu or grippe —*see* Influenza, with, respiratory manifestations NEC
  obstruction (airway) (lung) J44.89
  tracheitis (15 years of age and above) J40
    acute or subacute J20.9
    chronic J42
    under 15 years of age J20.9
acute or subacute (with bronchospasm or obstruction) J20.9
  with
    bronchiectasis J47.0
    chronic obstructive pulmonary disease J44.0
  chemical (due to gases, fumes or vapors) J68.0
  due to
    fumes or vapors J68.0
    Haemophilus influenzae J20.1
    Mycoplasma pneumoniae J20.0
    radiation J70.0
    specified organism NEC J20.8
    Streptococcus J20.2
    virus
      coxsackie J20.3
      echovirus J20.7
      parainfluenzae J20.4
      respiratory syncytial (RSV) J20.5
      rhinovirus J20.6
  viral NEC J20.8
allergic (acute) J45.909
  with
    exacerbation (acute) J45.901
    status asthmaticus J45.902
arachidic T17.528
aspiration (due to food and vomit) J69.0
asthmatic J45.9
  chronic J44.89
    with
      acute lower respiratory infection J44.0
      exacerbation (acute) J44.1
capillary —*see* Pneumonia, broncho
caseous (tuberculous) A15.5
Castellani's A69.8
catarrhal (15 years of age and above) J40
  acute —*see* Bronchitis, acute
  chronic J41.0
  under 15 years of age J20.9
chemical (acute) (subacute) J68.0
  chronic (*see also* Disease, respiratory, chronic, due to chemicals, gases, fumes or vapors) J42
  due to fumes or vapors (*see also* Disease, respiratory, chronic, due to chemicals, gases, fumes or vapors) J42
    chronic J68.4
chronic J42
  with
    airways obstruction J44.89
    tracheitis (chronic) J42
  asthmatic (obstructive) J44.89
  catarrhal J41.0
  chemical (due to fumes or vapors) (*see also* Disease, respiratory, chronic, due to chemicals, gases, fumes or vapors) J42
  due to
    chemicals, gases, fumes or vapors (inhalation) (*see also* Disease, respiratory, chronic, due to chemicals, gases, fumes or vapors) J42
    radiation J70.1
    tobacco smoking J41.0
  emphysematous J44.89
  mucopurulent J41.1
  non-obstructive J41.0
  obliterans —*see* Bronchiolitis, obliterans
  obstructive J44.89
  purulent J41.1
  simple J41.0
croupous —*see* Bronchitis, acute
due to gases, fumes or vapors (chemical) J68.0
emphysematous (obstructive) J44.89
exudative —*see* Bronchitis, acute
fetid J41.1
grippal —*see* Influenza, with, respiratory manifestations NEC
in those under 15 years age —*see* Bronchitis, acute
  chronic —*see* Bronchitis, chronic
influenzal —*see* Influenza, with, respiratory manifestations NEC

Bronchitis *(Continued)*
mixed simple and mucopurulent J41.8
moulder's J62.8
mucopurulent (chronic) (recurrent) J41.1
  acute or subacute J20.9
  simple (mixed) J41.8
obliterans (chronic) —*see* Bronchiolitis, obliterans
obstructive (chronic) (diffuse) J44.89
pituitous J41.1
pneumococcal, acute or subacute J20.2
pseudomembranous, acute or subacute —*see* Bronchitis, acute
purulent (chronic) (recurrent) J41.1
  acute or subacute —*see* Bronchitis, acute
putrid J41.1
senile (chronic) J42
simple and mucopurulent (mixed) J41.8
smokers' J41.0
spirochetal NEC A69.8
subacute —*see* Bronchitis, acute
suppurative (chronic) J41.1
  acute or subacute —*see* Bronchitis, acute
tuberculous A15.5
under 15 years of age —*see* Bronchitis, acute
  chronic —*see* Bronchitis, chronic
viral NEC, acute or subacute —*see also* Bronchitis, acute J20.8
Bronchoalveolitis J18.0
Bronchoaspergillosis B44.1
Bronchocele meaning goiter E04.0
Broncholithiasis J98.09
  tuberculous NEC A15.5
Bronchomalacia J98.09
  congenital Q32.2
Bronchomycosis NOS B49 *[J99]*
  candidal B37.1
Bronchopleuropneumonia —*see* Pneumonia, broncho
Bronchopneumonia —*see* Pneumonia, broncho
Bronchopneumonitis —*see* Pneumonia, broncho
Bronchopulmonary —*see* condition
Bronchopulmonitis —*see* Pneumonia, broncho
Bronchorrhagia (*see* Hemoptysis)
Bronchorrhea J98.09
  acute J20.9
  chronic (infective) (purulent) J42
Bronchospasm (acute) J98.01
  with
    bronchiolitis, acute J21.9
    bronchitis, acute (conditions in J20) —*see* Bronchitis, acute
  due to external agent —*see* condition, respiratory, acute, due to
  exercise induced J45.990
Bronchospirochetosis A69.8
  Castellani A69.8
Bronchostenosis J98.09
Bronchus —*see* condition
Brontophobia F40.220
Bronze baby syndrome P83.88
Brooke's tumor —*see* Neoplasm, skin, benign
Brown enamel of teeth (hereditary) K00.5
Brown's sheath syndrome H50.61-•
Brown-Séquard disease, paralysis or syndrome G83.81
Bruce sepsis A23.0
Brucellosis (infection) A23.9
  abortus A23.1
  canis A23.3
  dermatitis A23.9
  melitensis A23.0
  mixed A23.8
  sepsis A23.9
    melitensis A23.0
    specified NEC A23.8
  suis A23.2
Bruck-de Lange disease Q87.19
Bruck's disease —*see* Deformity, limb
BRUE (brief resolved unexplained event) R68.13
Brugsch's syndrome Q82.8
Bruise (skin surface intact) —*see also* Contusion
with
  open wound —*see* Wound, open
  internal organ —*see* Injury, by site
  newborn P54.5
  scalp, due to birth injury, newborn P12.3
  umbilical cord O69.5
Bruit (arterial) R09.89
  cardiac R01.1
Brush burn —*see* Abrasion, by site

Bruton's X-linked agammaglobulinemia D80.0
Bruxism
  psychogenic F45.8
  sleep related G47.63
Bubbly lung syndrome P27.0
Bubo I88.8
  blennorrhagic (gonococcal) A54.89
  chancroidal A57
  climatic A55
  due to Haemophilus ducreyi A57
  gonococcal A54.89
  indolent (nonspecific) I88.8
  inguinal (nonspecific) I88.8
    chancroidal A57
    climatic A55
    due to H. ducreyi A57
    infective I88.8
  scrofulous (tuberculous) A18.2
  soft chancre A57
  suppurating —*see* Lymphadenitis, acute
  syphilitic (primary) A51.0
    congenital A50.07
  tropical A55
  virulent (chancroidal) A57
Bubonic plague A20.0
Bubonocele —*see* Hernia, inguinal
Buccal —*see* condition
Buchanan's disease or osteochondrosis M91.0
Buchem's syndrome (hyperostosis corticalis) M85.2
Bucket-handle fracture or tear (semilunar cartilage) —*see* Tear, meniscus
Budd-Chiari syndrome (hepatic vein thrombosis) I82.0
Budgerigar fancier's disease or lung J67.2
Buds
  breast E30.1
    in newborn P96.89
Buerger's disease (thromboangiitis obliterans) I73.1
Bulbar —*see* condition
Bulbus cordis (left ventricle) (persistent) Q21.8
Bulimia (nervosa) F50.2-•
  atypical F50.9
  normal weight F50.9
Bulky
  stools R19.5
  uterus N85.2
Bulla (e) R23.8
  lung (emphysematous) (solitary) J43.9
    newborn P25.8
Bullet wound —*see also* Puncture
  fracture - code as Fracture, by site
  internal organ —*see* Injury, by site
Bundle
  branch block (complete) (false) (incomplete) — *see* Block, bundle-branch
  of His —*see* condition
Bunion M21.61-•
  tailor's M21.62-•
Bunionette M21.62-•
Buphthalmia, buphthalmos (congenital) Q15.0
Burdwan fever B55.0
Bürger-Grütz disease or syndrome E78.3
Buried
  penis (congenital) Q55.64
    acquired N48.83
  roots K08.3
Burke's syndrome K86.89
Burkholderia
  cepacia A49.8
  mallei A24.0
  pseudomallei —*see* Melioidosis
Burkitt
  cell leukemia C91.0-•
  lymphoma (malignant) C83.7-•
    small noncleaved, diffuse C83.7-•
    spleen C83.77
    undifferentiated C83.7-•
  tumor C83.7-•
  type
    acute lymphoblastic leukemia C91.0-•
    undifferentiated C83.7-•
Burn (electricity) (flame) (hot gas, liquid or hot object) (radiation) (steam) (thermal) T30.0
  abdomen, abdominal (muscle) (wall) T21.02
    first degree T21.12
    second degree T21.22
    third degree T21.32

▶ New　　➡ Revised　　~~deleted~~ Deleted　　● Use Additional Character(s)

▶ New   ➡ Revised   ~~deleted~~ Deleted   ● Use Additional Character(s)

▶ New   ➡ Revised   ~~deleted~~ Deleted   • Use Additional Character(s)

Cardialgia —*see* Pain, precordial
Cardiectasis —*see* Hypertrophy, cardiac
Cardiochalasia K21.9
Cardiomalacia I51.5
Cardiomegalia glycogenica diffusa E74.02 *[I43]*
Cardiomegaly —*see also* Hypertrophy, cardiac
  congenital Q24.8
  glycogen E74.02 *[I43]*
  idiopathic I51.7
Cardiomyoliposis I51.5
Cardiomyopathy (familial) (idiopathic) I42.9
  alcoholic I42.6
  amyloid E85.4 *[I43]*
    transthyretin-related (ATTR) familial E85.4
      [I43]
  arteriosclerotic —*see* Disease, heart, ischemic,
    atherosclerotic
  beriberi E51.12
  cobalt-beer I42.6
  congenital I42.4
  congestive I42.0
  constrictive NOS I42.5
  dilated I42.0
  due to
    alcohol I42.6
    beriberi E51.12
    cardiac glycogenosis E74.02 *[I43]*
    drugs I42.7
    external agents NEC I42.7
    Friedreich's ataxia G11.11
    myotonia atrophica G71.11 *[I43]*
    progressive muscular dystrophy (*see also*
      Dystrophy, muscular, by type) G71.09
      [I43]
  glycogen storage E74.02 *[I43]*
  hypertensive —*see* Hypertension, heart
  hypertrophic (nonobstructive) I42.2
    obstructive I42.1
      congenital Q24.8
  in
    Chagas' disease (chronic) B57.2
      acute B57.0
    sarcoidosis D86.85
  ischemic I25.5
  metabolic E88.9 *[I43]*
    thyrotoxic E05.90 *[I43]*
      with thyroid storm E05.91 *[I43]*
  newborn I42.8
    congenital I42.4
  non-ischemic (*see also* by cause) I42.8
  nutritional E63.9 *[I43]*
    beriberi E51.12
  obscure of Africa I42.8
  peripartum O90.3
  postpartum O90.3
  restrictive NEC I42.5
  rheumatic I09.0
  secondary I42.9
  specified NEC I42.8
  stress induced I51.81
  takotsubo I51.81
  thyrotoxic E05.90 *[I43]*
    with thyroid storm E05.91 *[I43]*
  toxic NEC I42.7
  transthyretin-related (ATTR) familial amyloid
    E85.4
  tuberculous A18.84
  viral B33.24
Cardionephritis —*see* Hypertension,
  cardiorenal
Cardionephropathy —*see* Hypertension,
  cardiorenal
Cardionephrosis —*see* Hypertension, cardiorenal
Cardiopathia nigra I27.0
Cardiopathy —*see also* Disease, heart I51.9
  idiopathic I42.9
  mucopolysaccharidosis E76.3 *[I52]*
Cardiopericarditis —*see* Pericarditis
Cardiophobia F45.29
Cardiorenal —*see* condition
Cardiorrhexis —*see* Infarct, myocardium
Cardiosclerosis —*see* Disease, heart, ischemic,
  atherosclerotic
Cardiosis —*see* Disease, heart
Cardiospasm (esophagus) (reflex) (stomach)
  K22.0
  congenital Q39.5
    with megaesophagus Q39.5
Cardiostenosis —*see* Disease, heart
Cardiosymphysis I31.0
Cardiovascular —*see* condition

Carditis (acute) (bacterial) (chronic) (subacute)
  I51.89
  meningococcal A39.50
  rheumatic —*see* Disease, heart, rheumatic
  rheumatoid —*see* Rheumatoid, carditis
  viral B33.20
Care (of) (for) (following)
  child (routine) Z76.2
  family member (handicapped) (sick)
    creating problem for family Z63.6
    provided away from home for holiday relief
      Z75.5
    unavailable, due to
      absence (person rendering care) (sufferer)
        Z74.2
      inability (any reason) of person rendering
        care Z74.2
  foundling Z76.1
  holiday relief Z75.5
  improper —*see* Maltreatment
  lack of (at or after birth) (infant) —*see*
    Maltreatment, child, neglect
  lactating mother Z39.1
  palliative Z51.5
  postpartum
    immediately after delivery Z39.0
    routine follow-up Z39.2
  respite Z75.5
  unavailable, due to
    absence of person rendering care Z74.2
    inability (any reason) of person rendering
      care Z74.2
  well-baby Z76.2
Caries
  bone NEC A18.03
  dental (dentino enamel junction)
    (early childhood) (of dentine)
    (pre-eruptive) (recurrent) (to the pulp)
    K02.9
    arrested (coronal) (root) K02.3
    chewing surface
      limited to enamel K02.51
      penetrating into dentin K02.52
      penetrating into pulp K02.53
    coronal surface
      chewing surface
        limited to enamel K02.51
        penetrating into dentin K02.52
        penetrating into pulp K02.53
      pit and fissure surface
        limited to enamel K02.51
        penetrating into dentin K02.52
        penetrating into pulp K02.53
      smooth surface
        limited to enamel K02.61
        penetrating into dentin K02.62
        penetrating into pulp K02.63
    pit and fissure surface
      limited to enamel K02.51
      penetrating into dentin K02.52
      penetrating into pulp K02.53
    primary, cervical origin K02.52
    root K02.7
    smooth surface
      limited to enamel K02.61
      penetrating into dentin K02.62
      penetrating into pulp K02.63
  external meatus —*see* Disorder, ear, external,
    specified type NEC
  hip (tuberculous) A18.02
  initial (tooth)
    chewing surface K02.51
    pit and fissure surface K02.51
    smooth surface K02.61
  knee (tuberculous) A18.02
  labyrinth —*see* subcategory H83.8
  limb NEC (tuberculous) A18.03
  mastoid process (chronic) —*see* Mastoiditis,
    chronic
    tuberculous A18.03
  middle ear —*see* subcategory H74.8
  nose (tuberculous) A18.03
  orbit (tuberculous) A18.03
  ossicles, ear —*see* Abnormal, ear ossicles
  petrous bone —*see* Petrositis
  root (dental) (tooth) K02.7
  sacrum (tuberculous) A18.01
  spine, spinal (column) (tuberculous)
    A18.01
  syphilitic A52.77
    congenital (early) A50.02 *[M90.80]*

Caries (*Continued*)
  tooth, teeth —*see* Caries, dental
  tuberculous A18.03
  vertebra (column) (tuberculous) A18.01
Carious teeth —*see* Caries, dental
Carneous mole O02.0
Carnitine insufficiency E71.40
Carotenemia (dietary) E67.1
Carotenosis (cutis) (skin) E67.1
Carotid body or sinus syndrome G90.01
Carotidynia G90.01
Carpal tunnel syndrome —*see* Syndrome, carpal
  tunnel
Carpenter's syndrome Q87.0
Carpopedal spasm —*see* Tetany
Carr-Barr-Plunkett syndrome Q97.1
Carrier (suspected) of
  Acinetobacter baumannii Z22.349
    carbapenem-resistant Z22.340
    carbapenem-sensitive Z22.341
  amebiasis Z22.1
  bacterial disease NEC Z22.39
    diphtheria Z22.2
    intestinal infectious NEC Z22.1
    typhoid Z22.0
    meningococcal Z22.31
    sexually transmitted Z22.4
    specified NEC Z22.39
    staphylococcal (Methicillin susceptible)
      Z22.321
      Methicillin resistant Z22.322
    streptococcal Z22.338
      group B Z22.330
        complicating pregnancy or delivery
          O99.82- ●
    typhoid Z22.0
  cholera Z22.1
  diphtheria Z22.2
  E. coli (Escherichia coli) Z22.35-
  Enterobacterales Z22.359
    carbapenem-resistant Z22.350
    carbapenem-sensitive Z22.358
    Enterobacterales, specified type NEC Z22.358
    ESBL-producing Z22.358
    extended-spectrum beta-lactamase producing
      Z22.358
  gastrointestinal pathogens NEC Z22.1
  genetic Z14.8
    cystic fibrosis Z14.1
    hemophilia A (asymptomatic) Z14.01
      symptomatic Z14.02
  gestational, pregnant Z33.1
  gonorrhea Z22.4
  HAA (hepatitis Australian-antigen) B18.8
  HB (c)(s)-AG B18.1
  hepatitis (viral) B18.9
    Australia-antigen (HAA) B18.8
    B surface antigen (HBsAg) B18.1
      with acute delta- (super)infection B17.0
    C B18.2
    specified NEC B18.8
  human T-cell lymphotropic virus type-1 (HTLV-
    1) infection Z22.6
  infectious organism Z22.9
    specified NEC Z22.8
  K. pneumoniae (Klebsiella pneumoniae) Z22.35-
  meningococci Z22.31
  Salmonella typhosa Z22.0
  serum hepatitis —*see* Carrier, hepatitis
  staphylococci (Methicillin susceptible) Z22.321
    Methicillin resistant Z22.322
  streptococci Z22.338
    group B Z22.330
      complicating pregnancy or delivery
        O99.82- ●
  syphilis Z22.4
  typhoid Z22.0
  venereal disease NEC Z22.4
Carrion's disease A44.0
Carter's relapsing fever (Asiatic) A68.1
Cartilage —*see* condition
Caruncle (inflamed)
  conjunctiva (acute) —*see* Conjunctivitis, acute
  labium (majus) (minus) N90.89
  lacrimal —*see* Inflammation, lacrimal, passages
  myrtiform N89.8
  urethral (benign) N36.2
Cascade stomach K31.2
Caseation lymphatic gland (tuberculous) A18.2
Cassidy (-Scholte) **syndrome** (malignant carcinoid)
  E34.09

▶ New   ⇨ Revised   ~~deleted~~ Deleted   ● Use Additional Character(s)

▶ New　⇒ Revised　~~deleted~~ Deleted　● Use Additional Character(s)

Closure *(Continued)*
  of artificial opening —*see* Attention to, artificial,
    opening
  primary angle, without glaucoma damage
    H40.06-●
  vagina N89.5
  valve —*see* Endocarditis
  vulva N90.5
Clot (blood) —*see also* Embolism
  artery (obstruction) (occlusion) —*see* Embolism
  bladder N32.89
  brain (intradural or extradural) —*see* Occlusion,
    artery, cerebral
  circulation I74.9
  heart —*see also* Infarct, myocardium
    not resulting in infarction I51.3
  vein —*see* Thrombosis
Clouded state R40.1
  epileptic —*see* Epilepsy, specified NEC
  paroxysmal —*see* Epilepsy, specified NEC
Cloudy antrum, antra J32.0
Clouston's (hidrotic) **ectodermal dysplasia**
  Q82.4
Cloverleaf skull Q75.051
Clubbed nail pachydermoperiostosis M89.40
  [L62]
Clubbing of finger(s) (nails) R68.3
Clubfinger R68.3
  congenital Q68.1
Clubfoot (congenital) Q66.89
  acquired —*see* Deformity, limb, clubfoot
  equinovarus Q66.0-●
  paralytic —*see* Deformity, limb, clubfoot
Clubhand (congenital) (radial) Q71.4-●
  acquired —*see* Deformity, limb, clubhand
Clubnail R68.3
  congenital Q84.6
Clump, kidney Q63.1
Clumsiness, clumsy child syndrome F82
Cluttering F98.81
Clutton's joints A50.51 [M12.80]
Coagulation, intravascular (diffuse)
  (disseminated) —*see also* Defibrination
  syndrome
  complicating abortion —*see* Abortion, by type,
    complicated by, intravascular coagulation
  COVID-19 associated (see also COVID-19)
    D65
  following ectopic or molar pregnancy O08.1
Coagulopathy —*see also* Defect, coagulation
  consumption D65
  intravascular D65
    newborn P60
Coalition
  calcaneo-scaphoid Q66.89
  tarsal Q66.89
Coalminer's
  elbow —*see* Bursitis, elbow, olecranon
  lung or pneumoconiosis J60
Coalworker's lung or pneumoconiosis J60
Coarctation
  aorta (preductal) (postductal) Q25.1
  pulmonary artery Q25.71
Coated tongue K14.3
Coats' disease (exudative retinopathy) —*see*
  Retinopathy, exudative
Cocaine-induced
  anxiety disorder F14.980
  bipolar and related disorder F14.94
  depressive disorder F14.94
  obsessive-compulsive and related disorder
    F14.988
  psychotic disorder F14.959
  sleep disorder F14.982
  sexual dysfunction F14.981
Cocainism —*see* Disorder, cocaine use
Coccidioidomycosis B38.9
  cutaneous B38.3
  disseminated B38.7
  generalized B38.7
  meninges B38.4
  prostate B38.81
  pulmonary B38.2
    acute B38.0
    chronic B38.1
  skin B38.3
  specified NEC B38.89
Coccidioidosis —*see* Coccidioidomycosis
Coccidiosis (intestinal) A07.3
Coccydynia, coccygodynia M53.3
Coccyx —*see* condition
Cochin-China diarrhea K90.1

Cockayne's syndrome Q87.19
Cocked up toe —*see* Deformity, toe, specified NEC
Cock's peculiar tumor L72.3
Codman's tumor —*see* Neoplasm, bone, benign
Coenurosis B71.8
Coffee-worker's lung J67.8
Cogan's syndrome H16.32-●
  oculomotor apraxia H51.8
Coitus, painful (female) N94.10
  male N53.12
  psychogenic F52.6
Cold J00
  with influenza, flu, or grippe —*see* Influenza,
    with, respiratory manifestations NEC
  agglutinin disease or hemoglobinuria (chronic)
    D59.12
  bronchial —*see* Bronchitis
  chest —*see* Bronchitis
  common (head) J00
  effects of T69.9
    specified effect NEC T69.8
  excessive, effects of T69.9
    specified effect NEC T69.8
  exhaustion from T69.8
  exposure to T69.9
    specified effect NEC T69.8
  head J00
  injury syndrome (newborn) P80.0
  on lung —*see* Bronchitis
  rose J30.1
  sensitivity, auto-immune D59.12
  symptoms J00
  virus J00
Coldsore B00.1
Colibacillosis A49.8
  as the cause of other disease (see also Escherichia
    coli) B96.20
  generalized (see also Sepsis, Escherichia coli)
    A41.50
Colic (bilious) (infantile) (intestinal) (recurrent)
  (spasmodic) R10.83
  abdomen R10.83
    psychogenic F45.8
  appendix, appendicular K38.8
  bile duct —*see* Calculus, bile duct
  biliary —*see* Calculus, bile duct
  common duct —*see* Calculus, bile duct
  cystic duct —*see* Calculus, gallbladder
  Devonshire NEC —*see* Poisoning, lead
  gallbladder —*see* Calculus, gallbladder
  gallstone —*see* Calculus, gallbladder
    gallbladder or cystic duct —*see* Calculus,
      gallbladder
  hepatic (duct) —*see* Calculus, bile duct
  hysterical F45.8
  kidney N23
  lead NEC —*see* Poisoning, lead
  mucous K58.9
    with diarrhea K58.0
    psychogenic F54
  nephritic N23
  painter's NEC —*see* Poisoning, lead
  pancreas K86.89
  psychogenic F45.8
  renal N23
  saturnine NEC —*see* Poisoning, lead
  ureter N23
  urethral N36.8
    due to calculus N21.1
  uterus NEC N94.89
    menstrual —*see* Dysmenorrhea
  worm NOS B83.9
Colicystitis —*see* Cystitis
Colitis (acute) (catarrhal) (chronic) (noninfective)
  (hemorrhagic) (see also Enteritis) K52.9
  allergic K52.29
    with
      food protein-induced enterocolitis
        syndrome K52.21
      proctocolitis K52.29
  amebic (acute) —*see also* Amebiasis A06.0
    nondysenteric A06.2
  anthrax A22.2
  bacillary —*see* Infection, Shigella
  balantidial A07.0
  Clostridioides difficile
    not specified as recurrent A04.72
    recurrent A04.71
  Clostridium difficile
    not specified as recurrent A04.72
    recurrent A04.71
  coccidial A07.3

Colitis *(Continued)*
  collagenous K52.831
  cystica superficialis K52.89
  dietary counseling and surveillance (for)
    Z71.3
  dietetic —*see also* Colitis, allergic K52.29
  drug-induced K52.1
  due to radiation K52.0
  eosinophilic K52.82
  food hypersensitivity —*see also* Colitis, allergic
    K52.29
  giardial A07.1
  granulomatous —*see* Enteritis, regional, large
    intestine
  infectious —*see* Enteritis, infectious
  indeterminate, so stated K52.3
  ischemic K55.9
    acute (subacute) —*see also* Ischemia, intestine,
      acute K55.039
    chronic K55.1
    due to mesenteric artery insufficiency
      K55.1
    fulminant (acute) —*see also* Ischemia, intestine,
      acute K55.039
  left sided K51.50
    with
      abscess K51.514
      complication K51.519
        specified NEC K51.518
      fistula K51.513
      obstruction K51.512
      rectal bleeding K51.511
  lymphocytic K52.832
  membranous
    psychogenic F54
  microscopic K52.839
    specified NEC K52.838
  mucous —*see* Syndrome, irritable, bowel
    psychogenic F54
  noninfective K52.9
    specified NEC K52.89
  polyposa —*see* Polyp, colon, inflammatory
  protozoal A07.9
  pseudomembranous
    not specified as recurrent A04.72
    recurrent A04.71
  pseudomucinous —*see* Syndrome, irritable,
    bowel
  regional —*see* Enteritis, regional, large intestine
    infectious A09
  segmental —*see* Enteritis, regional, large
    intestine
  septic —*see* Enteritis, infectious
  spastic K58.9
    with diarrhea K58.0
    psychogenic F54
  staphylococcal A04.8
    foodborne A05.0
  subacute ischemic —*see also* Ischemia, intestine,
    acute K55.039
  thromboulcerative —*see also* Ischemia, intestine,
    acute K55.039
  toxic NEC K52.1
    due to
      Clostridioides difficile
        not specified as recurrent A04.72
        recurrent A04.71
      Clostridium difficile
        not specified as recurrent A04.72
        recurrent A04.71
  transmural —*see* Enteritis, regional, large
    intestine
  trichomonal A07.8
  tuberculous (ulcerative) A18.32
  ulcerative (chronic) K51.90
    with
      complication K51.919
        abscess K51.914
        fistula K51.913
        obstruction K51.912
        rectal bleeding K51.911
        specified complication NEC K51.918
    enterocolitis —*see* Enterocolitis, ulcerative
    ileocolitis —*see* Ileocolitis, ulcerative
    mucosal proctocolitis —*see* Proctocolitis,
      mucosal
    proctitis —*see* Proctitis, ulcerative
    pseudopolyposis —*see* Polyp, colon,
      inflammatory
    psychogenic F54
    rectosigmoiditis —*see* Rectosigmoiditis,
      ulcerative

▶ New   ⇒ Revised   ~~deleted~~ Deleted   ● Use Additional Character(s)

▶ New   ➡ Revised   ~~deleted~~ Deleted   ● Use Additional Character(s)

New   Revised   ~~deleted~~ Deleted   ● Use Additional Character(s)

Complication *(Continued)*
fixation device, internal *(Continued)*
  mechanical *(Continued)*
    displacement *(Continued)*
      limb *(Continued)*
        radius T84.12-●
        tarsal T84.223
        tibia T84.12-●
        ulna T84.12-●
      specified bone NEC T84.228
      spine T84.226
    malposition —*see* Complications, fixation
      device, internal, mechanical,
      displacement
    obstruction —*see* Complications, fixation
      device, internal, mechanical, specified
      type NEC
    perforation —*see* Complications, fixation
      device, internal, mechanical, specified
      type NEC
    protrusion —*see* Complications, fixation
      device, internal, mechanical, specified
      type NEC
    specified type NEC
      limb T84.199
        carpal T84.290
        femur T84.19-●
        fibula T84.19-●
        humerus T84.19-●
        metacarpal T84.290
        metatarsal T84.293
        phalanx
          foot T84.293
          hand T84.290
        radius T84.19-●
        tarsal T84.293
        tibia T84.19-●
        ulna T84.19-●
      specified bone NEC T84.298
      vertebra T84.296
  specified type NEC T84.89
    embolism T84.81
    fibrosis T84.82
    hemorrhage T84.83
    pain T84.84
    specified complication NEC T84.89
    stenosis T84.85
    thrombosis T84.86
following
  acute myocardial infarction NEC
    I23.8
  aneurysm (false) (of cardiac wall) (of heart
    wall) (ruptured) I23.3
  angina I23.7
  atrial
    septal defect I23.1
    thrombosis I23.6
  cardiac wall rupture I23.3
  chordae tendinae rupture I23.4
  defect
    septal
      atrial (heart) I23.1
      ventricular (heart) I23.2
  hemopericardium I23.0
  papillary muscle rupture I23.5
  rupture
    cardiac wall I23.3
      with hemopericardium I23.0
    chordae tendineae I23.4
    papillary muscle I23.5
  specified NEC I23.8
  thrombosis
    atrium I23.6
    auricular appendage I23.6
    ventricle (heart) I23.6
  ventricular
    septal defect I23.2
    thrombosis I23.6
ectopic or molar pregnancy O08.9
  cardiac arrest O08.81
  sepsis O08.82
  specified type NEC O08.89
  urinary tract infection O08.83
termination of pregnancy —*see*
  Abortion
gastrointestinal K92.9
  bile duct prosthesis —*see* Complications, bile
    duct implant
  esophageal anti-reflux device —*see*
    Complications, esophageal anti-reflux
    device

Complication *(Continued)*
gastrointestinal *(Continued)*
  postoperative
    colostomy —*see* Complications, colostomy
    dumping syndrome K91.1
    enterostomy —*see* Complications,
      enterostomy
    gastrostomy —*see* Complications,
      gastrostomy
    malabsorption NEC K91.2
    obstruction —*see also* Obstruction, intestine,
      postoperative K91.30
    postcholecystectomy syndrome K91.5
    specified NEC K91.89
    vomiting after GI surgery K91.0
  prosthetic device or implant
    bile duct prosthesis —*see* Complications,
      bile duct implant
    esophageal anti-reflux device —*see*
      Complications, esophageal
      anti-reflux device
    specified type NEC
      embolism T85.818
      fibrosis T85.828
      hemorrhage T85.838
      mechanical
        breakdown T85.518
        displacement T85.528
        malfunction T85.518
        malposition T85.528
        obstruction T85.598
        perforation T85.598
        protrusion T85.598
        specified NEC T85.598
      pain T85.848
      specified complication NEC T85.898
      stenosis T85.858
      thrombosis T85.868
  gastrostomy (stoma) K94.20
    hemorrhage K94.21
    infection K94.22
    malfunction K94.23
    mechanical K94.23
    specified complication NEC K94.29
  genitourinary
    device or implant T83.9
      genital tract T83.9
        infection or inflammation T83.69
        intrauterine contraceptive device —*see*
          Complications, intrauterine,
          contraceptive device
        mechanical —*see* Complications, by
          device, mechanical
        mesh —*see* Complications, prosthetic
          device or implant, mesh
        penile prosthesis —*see* Complications,
          prosthetic device, penile
        specified type NEC T83.89
          embolism T83.81
          fibrosis T83.82
          hemorrhage T83.83
          pain T83.84
          specified complication NEC T83.89
          stenosis T83.85
          thrombosis T83.86
        vaginal mesh —*see* Complications,
          prosthetic device or implant, mesh
      urinary system T83.9
        cystostomy catheter —*see* Complication,
          catheter, cystostomy
        electronic stimulator —*see*
          Complications, electronic stimulator
          device, urinary
        indwelling urethral catheter —*see*
          Complications, catheter, urethral,
          indwelling
        infection or inflammation T83.598
          indwelling urethral catheter T83.511
        kidney transplant —*see* Complication,
          transplant, kidney
        organ graft —*see* Complication, graft,
          urinary organ
        specified type NEC T83.89
          embolism T83.81
          fibrosis T83.82
          hemorrhage T83.83
          mechanical T83.198
            breakdown T83.118
            displacement T83.128
            malfunction T83.118
            malposition T83.128

Complication *(Continued)*
gastrointestinal *(Continued)*
  device or implant *(Continued)*
    urinary system *(Continued)*
      specified type NEC *(Continued)*
        mechanical *(Continued)*
          obstruction T83.198
          perforation T83.198
          protrusion T83.198
          specified NEC T83.198
      sphincter, implanted T83.191
      stent (ileal conduit) (nephroureteral)
        T83.193
      ureteral indwelling T83.192
        pain T83.84
        specified complication NEC T83.89
        stenosis T83.85
        thrombosis T83.86
      sphincter implant —*see* Complications,
        implant, urinary sphincter
  postprocedural
    pelvic peritoneal adhesions N99.4
    renal failure N99.0
    specified NEC N99.89
    stoma —*see* Complications, stoma, urinary
      tract
    urethral stricture —*see* Stricture, urethra,
      postprocedural
    vaginal
      adhesions N99.2
      vault prolapse N99.3
graft (bypass) (patch) —*see also* Complications,
  prosthetic device or implant
  aorta —*see* Complications, graft, vascular
  arterial —*see* Complication, graft, vascular
  bone T86.839
    failure T86.831
    infection T86.832
    mechanical T84.318
      breakdown T84.318
      displacement T84.328
      protrusion T84.398
      specified type NEC T84.398
    rejection T86.830
    specified type NEC T86.838
  carotid artery —*see* Complications, graft,
    vascular
  cornea T86.849-
    failure T86.841-
    infection T86.842-
    mechanical T85.398
      breakdown T85.318
      displacement T85.328
      protrusion T85.398
      specified type NEC T85.398
    rejection T86.840-
    retroprosthetic membrane T85.398
    specified type NEC T86.848-
  femoral artery (bypass) —*see* Complication,
    extremity artery (bypass) graft
  genital organ or tract —*see* Complications,
    genitourinary, device or implant, genital
    tract
  muscle T84.9
    breakdown T84.410
    displacement T84.420
    embolism T84.81
    fibrosis T84.82
    hemorrhage T84.83
    infection and inflammation T84.7
    mechanical NEC T84.490
    pain T84.84
    specified type NEC T84.89
    stenosis T84.85
    thrombosis T84.86
  nerve —*see* Complication, prosthetic device or
    implant, specified NEC
  skin —*see* Complications, prosthetic device or
    implant, skin graft
  tendon T84.9
    breakdown T84.410
    displacement T84.420
    embolism T84.81
    fibrosis T84.82
    hemorrhage T84.83
    infection and inflammation T84.7
    mechanical NEC T84.490
    pain T84.84
    specified type NEC T84.89
    stenosis T84.85
    thrombosis T84.86

Complication (*Continued*)
  graft (*Continued*)
    urinary organ T83.9
      embolism T83.81
      fibrosis T83.82
      hemorrhage T83.83
      infection and inflammation T83.598
        indwelling urethral catheter T83.511
      mechanical
        breakdown T83.21
        displacement T83.22
        erosion T83.24
        exposure T83.25
        leakage T83.23
        malposition T83.22
        obstruction T83.29
        perforation T83.29
        protrusion T83.29
        specified NEC T83.29
      pain T83.84
      specified type NEC T83.89
      stenosis T83.85
      thrombosis T83.86
    vascular T82.9
      embolism T82.818
      femoral artery —*see* Complication,
        extremity artery (bypass) graft
      fibrosis T82.828
      hemorrhage T82.838
      mechanical
        breakdown T82.319
          aorta (bifurcation) T82.310
          carotid artery T82.311
          specified vessel NEC T82.318
        displacement T82.329
          aorta (bifurcation) T82.320
          carotid artery T82.321
          specified vessel NEC T82.328
        leakage T82.339
          aorta (bifurcation) T82.330
          carotid artery T82.331
          specified vessel NEC T82.338
        malposition T82.329
          aorta (bifurcation) T82.320
          carotid artery T82.321
          specified vessel NEC T82.328
        obstruction T82.399
          aorta (bifurcation) T82.390
          carotid artery T82.391
          specified vessel NEC T82.398
        perforation T82.399
          aorta (bifurcation) T82.390
          carotid artery T82.391
          specified vessel NEC T82.398
        protrusion T82.399
          aorta (bifurcation) T82.390
          carotid artery T82.391
          specified vessel NEC T82.398
      pain T82.848
      specified complication NEC T82.898
      stenosis T82.858
      thrombosis T82.868
  heart I51.9
    assist device
      infection and inflammation T82.7
    following acute myocardial infarction —
      see Complications, following, acute
      myocardial infarction
    postoperative —*see* Complications, circulatory
      system
    transplant —*see* Complication, transplant, heart
      and lung(s) —*see* Complications, transplant,
      heart, with lung
    valve
      graft (biological) T82.9
        embolism T82.817
        fibrosis T82.827
        hemorrhage T82.837
        infection and inflammation T82.7
        mechanical T82.228
          breakdown T82.221
          displacement T82.222
          leakage T82.223
          malposition T82.222
          obstruction T82.228
          perforation T82.228
          protrusion T82.228
        pain T82.847
        specified type NEC T82.897
        stenosis T82.857
        thrombosis T82.867

Complication (*Continued*)
  heart (*Continued*)
    valve (*Continued*)
      prosthesis T82.9
        embolism T82.817
        fibrosis T82.827
        hemorrhage T82.837
        infection or inflammation T82.6
        mechanical T82.09
          breakdown T82.01
          displacement T82.02
          leakage T82.03
          malposition T82.02
          obstruction T82.09
          perforation T82.09
          protrusion T82.09
        pain T82.847
        specified type NEC T82.897
          mechanical T82.09
        stenosis T82.857
        thrombosis T82.867
  hematoma
    intraoperative —*see* Complication,
      intraoperative, hemorrhage
    postprocedural —*see* Complication,
      postprocedural, hematoma
  hemodialysis —*see* Complications, dialysis
  hemorrhage
    intraoperative —*see* Complication,
      intraoperative, hemorrhage
    postprocedural —*see* Complication,
      postprocedural, hemorrhage
  IEC (immune effector cellular) therapy T80.82
  ileostomy (stoma) —*see* Complications,
    enterostomy
  immune effector cellular (IEC) therapy T80.82
  immunization (procedure) —*see* Complications,
    vaccination
  implant —*see also* Complications, by site and type
    urinary sphincter T83.9
      embolism T83.81
      fibrosis T83.82
      hemorrhage T83.83
      infection and inflammation T83.591
      mechanical
        breakdown T83.111
        displacement T83.121
        leakage T83.191
        malposition T83.121
        obstruction T83.191
        perforation T83.191
        protrusion T83.191
        specified NEC T83.191
      pain T83.84
      specified type NEC T83.89
      stenosis T83.85
      thrombosis T83.86
  infusion (procedure) T80.90
    air embolism T80.0
    blood —*see* Complications, transfusion
    catheter —*see* Complications, catheter
    infection T80.29
    pump —*see* Complications, cardiovascular,
      device or implant
    sepsis T80.29
    serum reaction —*see also* Reaction, serum T80.69
      anaphylactic shock —*see also* Shock,
        anaphylactic T80.59
    specified type NEC T80.89
  inhalation therapy NEC T81.81
  injection (procedure) T80.90
    drug reaction —*see* Reaction, drug
    infection T80.29
    sepsis T80.29
    serum (prophylactic) (therapeutic) —*see*
      Complications, vaccination
    specified type NEC T80.89
    vaccine (any) —*see* Complications, vaccination
  inoculation (any) —*see* Complications,
    vaccination
  insulin pump
    infection and inflammation T85.72
    mechanical
      breakdown T85.614
      displacement T85.624
      leakage T85.633
      malposition T85.624
      obstruction T85.694
      perforation T85.694
      protrusion T85.694
      specified NEC T85.694

Complication (*Continued*)
  intestinal pouch NEC K91.858
  intraocular lens (prosthetic) T85.9
    embolism T85.818
    fibrosis T85.828
    hemorrhage T85.838
    infection and inflammation T85.79
    mechanical
      breakdown T85.21
      displacement T85.22
      malposition T85.22
      obstruction T85.29
      perforation T85.29
      protrusion T85.29
      specified NEC T85.29
    pain T85.848
    specified type NEC T85.898
    stenosis T85.858
    thrombosis T85.868
  intraoperative (intraprocedural)
    cardiac arrest —*see also* Infarct, myocardium,
      associated with revascularization
      procedure
      during cardiac surgery I97.710
      during other surgery I97.711
    cardiac functional disturbance NEC —*see also*
      Infarct, myocardium, associated with
      revascularization procedure
      during cardiac surgery I97.790
      during other surgery I97.791
    hemorrhage (hematoma) (of)
      circulatory system organ or structure
        during cardiac bypass I97.411
        during cardiac catheterization I97.410
        during other circulatory system
          procedure I97.418
        during other procedure I97.42
      digestive system organ
        during procedure on digestive system
          K91.61
        during procedure on other organ K91.62
      ear
        during procedure on ear and mastoid
          process H95.21
        during procedure on other organ H95.22
      endocrine system organ or structure
        during procedure on endocrine system
          organ or structure E36.01
        during procedure on other organ E36.02
      eye and adnexa
        during ophthalmic procedure H59.11- ●
        during other procedure H59.12- ●
      genitourinary organ or structure
        during procedure on genitourinary
          organ or structure N99.61
        during procedure on other organ N99.62
      mastoid process
        during procedure on ear and mastoid
          process H95.21
        during procedure on other organ H95.22
      musculoskeletal structure
        during musculoskeletal surgery
          M96.810
        during non-orthopedic surgery M96.811
        during orthopedic surgery M96.810
      nervous system
        during a nervous system procedure
          G97.31
        during other procedure G97.32
      respiratory system
        during other procedure J95.62
        during procedure on respiratory system
          organ or structure J95.61
      skin and subcutaneous tissue
        during a dermatologic procedure L76.01
        during a procedure on other organ
          L76.02
      spleen
        during a procedure on other organ
          D78.02
        during a procedure on the spleen D78.01
    puncture or laceration (accidental)
      (unintentional) (of)
      brain
        during a nervous system procedure
          G97.48
        during other procedure G97.49
      circulatory system organ or structure
        during circulatory system procedure
          I97.51
        during other procedure I97.52

▶ New   ⇒ Revised   ~~deleted~~ Deleted   ● Use Additional Character(s)

Complication *(Continued)*
  intraoperative *(Continued)*
    puncture or laceration (accidental) digestive system *(Continued)*
      circulatory system organ or structure *(Continued)*
        during procedure on digestive system K91.71
        during procedure on other organ K91.72
      ear
        during procedure on ear and mastoid process H95.31
        during procedure on other organ H95.32
      endocrine system organ or structure
        during procedure on endocrine system organ or structure E36.11
        during procedure on other organ E36.12
      eye and adnexa
        during ophthalmic procedure H59.21-●
        during other procedure H59.22-●
      genitourinary organ or structure
        during procedure on genitourinary organ or structure N99.71
        during procedure on other organ N99.72
      mastoid process
        during procedure on ear and mastoid process H95.31
        during procedure on other organ H95.32
      musculoskeletal structure
        during musculoskeletal surgery M96.820
        during non-orthopedic surgery M96.821
        during orthopedic surgery M96.820
      nervous system
        during a nervous system procedure G97.48
        during other procedure G97.49
      respiratory system
        during other procedure J95.72
        during procedure on respiratory system organ or structure J95.71
      skin and subcutaneous tissue
        during a dermatologic procedure L76.11
        during a procedure on other organ L76.12
      spleen
        during a procedure on other organ D78.12
        during a procedure on the spleen D78.11
    specified NEC
      circulatory system I97.88
      digestive system K91.81
      ear H95.88
      endocrine system E36.8
      eye and adnexa H59.88
      genitourinary system N99.81
      mastoid process H95.88
      musculoskeletal structure M96.89
      nervous system G97.81
      respiratory system J95.88
      skin and subcutaneous tissue L76.81
      spleen D78.81
  intraperitoneal catheter (dialysis) (infusion) —*see* Complication(s), catheter, intraperitoneal dialysis
  intrathecal infusion pump
    infection and inflammation T85.738
    mechanical
      breakdown T85.615
      displacement T85.625
      leakage T85.635
      malfunction T85.695
      malposition T85.625
      obstruction T85.695
      perforation T85.695
      protrusion T85.695
      specified NEC T85.695
  intrauterine
    contraceptive device
      embolism T83.81
      fibrosis T83.82
      hemorrhage T83.83
      infection and inflammation T83.69
      mechanical
        breakdown T83.31
        displacement T83.32
        malposition T83.32
        obstruction T83.39
        perforation T83.39
        protrusion T83.39
        specified NEC T83.39
      pain T83.84
      specified type NEC T83.89
      stenosis T83.85
      thrombosis T83.86
    procedure (fetal), to newborn P96.5

Complication *(Continued)*
  jejunostomy (stoma) —*see* Complications, enterostomy
  joint prosthesis, internal T84.9
    breakage (fracture) T84.01-●
    dislocation T84.02-●
    displacement T84.02-●
    fracture T84.01-●
    infection or inflammation T84.50
      hip T84.5-●
      knee T84.5-●
      specified joint NEC T84.59
    instability T84.02-●
    malposition —*see* Complications, joint prosthesis, mechanical, displacement
    mechanical
      breakage, broken T84.01-●
      dislocation T84.02-●
      fracture T84.01-●
      instability T84.02-●
      leakage —*see* Complications, joint prosthesis, mechanical, specified NEC
      loosening T84.039
        hip T84.03-●
        knee T84.03-●
        specified joint NEC T84.038
      obstruction —*see* Complications, joint prosthesis, mechanical, specified NEC
      osteolysis T84.059
        hip T84.05-●
        knee T84.05-●
      perforation —*see* Complications, joint prosthesis, mechanical, specified NEC
        osteolysis T84.059
        other specified joint T84.058
      periprosthetic osteolysis, by site T84.05-●
      protrusion —*see* Complications, joint prosthesis, mechanical, specified NEC
      specified complication NEC T84.099
        hip T84.09-●
        knee T84.09-●
        other specified joint T84.098
      subluxation T84.02-●
      wear of articular bearing surface T84.069
        hip T84.06-●
        knee T84.06-●
        other specified joint T84.068
    specified joint NEC T84.89
      embolism T84.81
      fibrosis T84.82
      hemorrhage T84.83
      pain T84.84
      specified complication NEC T84.89
      stenosis T84.85
      thrombosis T84.86
    subluxation T84.02-●
  kidney transplant —*see* Complications, transplant, kidney
  labor O75.9
    specified NEC O75.89
  liver transplant (immune or nonimmune) —*see* Complications, transplant, liver
  lumbar puncture G97.1
    cerebrospinal fluid leak G97.0
    headache or reaction G97.1
  lung transplant —*see* Complications, transplant, lung
    and heart —*see* Complications, transplant, lung, with heart
  male genital N50.9
    device, implant or graft —*see* Complications, genitourinary, device or implant, genital tract
    postprocedural or postoperative —*see* Complications, genitourinary, postprocedural
      specified NEC N99.89
  mastoid (process) procedure
    intraoperative H95.88-●
      hematoma —*see* Complications, intraoperative, hemorrhage (hematoma) (of), mastoid process
      hemorrhage —*see* Complications, intraoperative, hemorrhage (hematoma) (of), mastoid process
      laceration —*see* Complications, intraoperative, puncture or laceration..., mastoid process
      specified NEC H95.88-●
    postmastoidectomy —*see* Complications, postmastoidectomy

Complication *(Continued)*
  mastoid (process) procedure *(Continued)*
    postoperative H95.89-●
      external ear canal stenosis H95.81-●
      hematoma —*see* Complications..., postprocedural, hematoma (of), mastoid process
      hemorrhage —*see* Complications..., postprocedural, hemorrhage (of), mastoid process
      postmastoidectomy —*see* Complications, postmastoidectomy
      seroma —*see* Complications, postprocedural, seroma (of), mastoid process
      specified NEC H95.89-●
  mastoidectomy cavity —*see* Complications, postmastoidectomy
  mechanical —*see* Complications, by site and type, mechanical
  medical procedures (*see also* Complication(s), intraoperative) T88.9
  metabolic E88.9
    postoperative E89.89
    specified NEC E89.89
  molar pregnancy NOS O08.9
    damage to pelvic organs O08.6
    embolism O08.2
    genital infection O08.0
    hemorrhage (delayed) (excessive) O08.1
    metabolic disorder O08.5
    renal failure O08.4
    shock O08.3
    specified type NEC O08.0
    venous complication NEC O08.7
  musculoskeletal system —*see also* Complication, intraoperative (intraprocedural), by site
    device, implant or graft NEC —*see* Complications, orthopedic, device or implant
    internal fixation (nail) (plate) (rod) —*see* Complications, fixation device, internal
    joint prosthesis —*see* Complications, joint prosthesis
    postoperative (postprocedural) M96.89
      with Osteoporosis —*see* Osteoporosis
      fracture following insertion of device — *see* Fracture, following insertion of orthopedic implant, joint prosthesis or bone plate
      joint instability after prosthesis removal M96.89
      lordosis M96.4
      postlaminectomy syndrome NEC M96.1
        kyphosis M96.2
      pseudarthrosis M96.0
      specified complication NEC M96.89
    post radiation M96.89
      kyphosis M96.3
      scoliosis M96.5
      specified complication NEC M96.89
  nephrostomy (stoma) —*see* Complications, stoma, urinary tract, external NEC
  nervous system G98.8
    central G96.9
    device, implant or graft —*see also* Complication, prosthetic device or implant, specified NEC
      electronic stimulator (electrode(s)) —*see* Complications, electronic stimulator device
      specified NEC
        infection and inflammation T85.738
        mechanical T85.695
          breakdown T85.615
          displacement T85.625
          leakage T85.635
          malfunction T85.695
          malposition T85.625
          obstruction T85.695
          perforation T85.695
          protrusion T85.695
          specified NEC T85.695
      ventricular shunt —*see* Complications, ventricular shunt
    electronic stimulator (electrode(s)) —*see* Complications, electronic stimulator device
    postprocedural G97.82
      intracranial hypotension G97.2
      specified NEC G97.82
      spinal fluid leak G97.0

Complication (*Continued*)
newborn, due to intrauterine (fetal) procedure
    P96.5
nonabsorbable (permanent) sutures —*see*
    Complication, sutures, permanent
obstetric O75.9
    procedure (instrumental) (manual) (surgical)
        specified NEC O75.4
    specified NEC O75.89
    surgical wound NEC O90.89
        hematoma O90.2
        infection O86.00
ocular lens implant —*see* Complications,
    intraocular lens
ophthalmologic
    postprocedural bleb —*see* Blebitis
orbital prosthesis T85.9
    embolism T85.818
    fibrosis T85.828
    hemorrhage T85.838
    infection and inflammation T85.79
    mechanical
        breakdown T85.31-●
        displacement T85.32-●
        malposition T85.32-●
        obstruction T85.39-●
        perforation T85.39-●
        protrusion T85.39-●
        specified NEC T85.39-●
    pain T85.848
    specified type NEC T85.898
    stenosis T85.858
    thrombosis T85.868
organ or tissue transplant (partial) (total) —*see*
    Complications, transplant
orthopedic —*see also* Disorder, soft tissue
    device or implant T84.9
        bone
            device or implant —*see* Complication,
                bone, device NEC
            graft —*see* Complication, graft, bone
        breakdown T84.418
        displacement T84.428
        electronic bone stimulator —*see*
            Complications, electronic stimulator
            device, bone
        embolism T84.81
        fibrosis T84.82
        fixation device —*see* Complication, fixation
            device, internal
        hemorrhage T84.83
        infection or inflammation T84.7
        joint prosthesis —*see* Complication, joint
            prosthesis, internal
        malfunction T84.418
        malposition T84.428
        mechanical NEC T84.498
        muscle graft —*see* Complications, graft,
            muscle
        obstruction T84.498
        pain T84.84
        perforation T84.498
        protrusion T84.498
        specified complication NEC T84.89
        stenosis T84.85
        tendon graft —*see* Complications, graft,
            tendon
        thrombosis T84.86
    fracture (following insertion of device) —
       see Fracture, following insertion of
       orthopedic implant, joint prosthesis or
       bone plate
    postprocedural M96.89
        fracture —*see* Fracture, following insertion
            of orthopedic implant, joint prosthesis
            or bone plate
        postlaminectomy syndrome NEC M96.1
            kyphosis M96.3
            lordosis M96.4
        postradiation
            kyphosis M96.2
            scoliosis M96.5
        pseudarthrosis post-fusion M96.0
        specified type NEC M96.89
pacemaker (cardiac) —*see* Complications,
    cardiovascular device or implant, electronic
pancreas transplant —*see* Complications,
    transplant, pancreas
penile prosthesis (implant) —*see* Complications,
    prosthetic device, penile
perfusion NEC T80.90

Complication (*Continued*)
perineal repair (obstetrical) NEC O90.89
    disruption O90.1
    hematoma O90.2
    infection (following delivery) O86.09
phototherapy T88.9
    specified NEC T88.8
postmastoidectomy NEC H95.19-●
    cyst, mucosal H95.13-●
    granulation H95.12-●
    inflammation, chronic H95.11-●
    recurrent cholesteatoma H95.0-●
postoperative —*see* Complications,
    postprocedural
    circulatory —*see* Complications, circulatory
        system
    ear —*see* Complications, ear
    endocrine —*see* Complications, endocrine
    eye —*see* Complications, eye
    lumbar puncture G97.1
        cerebrospinal fluid leak G97.0
    nervous system (central) (peripheral) —*see*
        Complications, nervous system
    respiratory system —*see* Complications,
        respiratory system
postprocedural —*see also* Complications, surgical
    procedure
    cardiac arrest —*see also* Infarct, myocardium,
        associated with revascularization
        procedure
        following cardiac surgery I97.120
        following other surgery I97.121
    cardiac functional disturbance NEC —*see also*
        Infarct, myocardium, associated with
        revascularization procedure
        following cardiac surgery I97.190
        following other surgery I97.191
    cardiac insufficiency
        following cardiac surgery I97.110
        following other surgery I97.111
    chorioretinal scars following retinal surgery
        H59.81-●
    following cataract surgery
        cataract (lens) fragments H59.02-●
        cystoid macular edema H59.03-●
        specified NEC H59.09-●
        vitreous (touch) syndrome H59.01-●
    heart failure
        following cardiac surgery I97.130
        following other surgery I97.131
    hematoma (of)
        circulatory system organ or structure
            following cardiac bypass I97.631
            following cardiac catheterization
                I97.630
            following other circulatory system
                procedure I97.638
            following other procedure I97.621
        digestive system
            following procedure on digestive system
                K91.870
            following procedure on other organ
                K91.871
        ear
            following other procedure H95.52
            following procedure on ear and mastoid
                process H95.51
        endocrine system
            following endocrine system procedure
                E89.820
            following other procedure E89.821
        eye and adnexa
            following ophthalmic procedure
                H59.33-●
            following other procedure H59.34-●
        genitourinary organ or structure
            following procedure on genitourinary
                organ or structure N99.840
            following procedure on other organ
                N99.841
        mastoid process
            following other procedure H95.52
            following procedure on ear and mastoid
                process H95.51
        musculoskeletal structure
            following musculoskeletal surgery
                M96.840
            following non-orthopedic surgery
                M96.841
            following orthopedic surgery
                M96.840

Complication (*Continued*)
postprocedural (*Continued*)
    hematoma (*Continued*)
        nervous system
            following nervous system procedure
                G97.61
            following other procedure G97.62
        respiratory system
            following other procedure J95.861
            following procedure on respiratory
                system organ or structure J95.860
        skin and subcutaneous tissue
            following dermatologic procedure L76.31
            following procedure on other organ
                L76.32
        spleen
            following procedure on other organ
                D78.32
            following procedure on the spleen D78.31
    hemorrhage (of)
        circulatory system organ or structure
            following cardiac bypass I97.611
            following cardiac catheterization I97.610
            following other circulatory system
                procedure I97.618
            following other procedure I97.620
        digestive system
            following procedure on digestive system
                K91.840
            following procedure on other organ
                K91.841
        ear
            following other procedure H95.42
            following procedure on ear and mastoid
                process H95.41
        endocrine system
            following endocrine system procedure
                E89.810
            following other procedure E89.811
        eye and adnexa
            following ophthalmic procedure
                H59.31-●
            following other procedure H59.32-●
        genitourinary organ or structure
            following procedure on genitourinary
                organ or structure N99.820
            following procedure on other organ
                N99.821
        mastoid process
            following other procedure H95.42
            following procedure on ear and mastoid
                process H95.41
        musculoskeletal structure
            following musculoskeletal surgery
                M96.830
            following non-orthopedic surgery
                M96.831
            following orthopedic surgery M96.830
        nervous system
            following nervous system procedure
                G97.51
            following other procedure G97.52
        respiratory system
            following other procedure J95.831
            following procedure on respiratory
                system organ or structure J95.830
        skin and subcutaneous tissue
            following dermatologic procedure L76.21
            following a procedure on other organ
                L76.22
        spleen
            following procedure on other organ
                D78.22
            following procedure on the spleen
                D78.21
    seroma (of)
        circulatory system organ or structure
            following cardiac bypass I97.641
            following cardiac catheterization I97.640
            following other circulatory system
                procedure I97.648
            following other procedure I97.622
        digestive system
            following procedure on digestive system
                K91.872
            following procedure on other organ
                K91.873
        ear
            following other procedure H95.54
            following procedure on ear and mastoid
                process H95.53

▶ New   ➡ Revised   ~~deleted~~ Deleted   ● Use Additional Character(s)

Complication (Continued)
  postprocedural (Continued)
    seroma (Continued)
      endocrine system
        following endocrine system procedure
          E89.822
        following other procedure E89.823
      eye and adnexa
        following ophthalmic procedure
          H59.35-●
        following other procedure H59.36-●
      genitourinary organ or structure
        following procedure on genitourinary
          organ or structure N99.842
        following procedure on other organ
          N99.843
      mastoid process
        following other procedure H95.54
        following procedure on ear and mastoid
          process H95.53
      musculoskeletal structure
        following musculoskeletal surgery
          M96.842
        following non-orthopedic surgery M96.843
        following orthopedic surgery M96.842
      nervous system
        following nervous system procedure
          G97.63
        following other procedure G97.64
      respiratory system
        following other procedure J95.863
        following procedure on respiratory
          system organ or structure J95.862
      skin and subcutaneous tissue
        following dermatologic procedure L76.33
        following procedure on other organ L76.34
      spleen
        following procedure on other organ
          D78.34
        following procedure on the spleen D78.33
   specified NEC
      circulatory system I97.89
      digestive K91.89
      ear H95.89
      endocrine E89.89
      eye and adnexa H59.89
      genitourinary N99.89
      mastoid process H95.89
      metabolic E89.89
      musculoskeletal structure M96.89
      nervous system G97.82
      respiratory system J95.89
      skin and subcutaneous tissue L76.82
      spleen D78.89
  pregnancy NEC —*see* Pregnancy, complicated by
  prosthetic device or implant T85.9
    bile duct —*see* Complications, bile duct
      implant
    breast —*see* Complications, breast implant
    bulking agent
      ureteral
        erosion T83.714
        exposure T83.724
      urethral
        erosion T83.713
        exposure T83.723
    cardiac and vascular NEC —*see*
      Complications, cardiovascular device or
      implant
    corneal transplant —*see* Complications, graft,
      cornea
    electronic nervous system stimulator —*see*
      Complications, electronic stimulator
      device
    epidural infusion catheter —*see*
      Complications, catheter, epidural
    esophageal anti-reflux device —*see*
      Complications, esophageal anti-reflux
      device
    genital organ or tract —*see* Complications,
      genitourinary, device or implant, genital
      tract
      specified NEC T83.79
    heart valve —*see* Complications, heart, valve,
      prosthesis
    infection or inflammation T85.79
      intestine transplant T86.852
      liver transplant T86.43
      lung transplant T86.812
      pancreas transplant T86.892
      skin graft T86.822

Complication (Continued)
  prosthetic device or implant (Continued)
    intraocular lens —*see* Complications,
      intraocular lens
    intraperitoneal (dialysis) catheter —*see*
      Complication(s), catheter, intraperitoneal
      dialysis
    joint —*see* Complications, joint prosthesis,
      internal
    mechanical NEC T85.698
      dialysis catheter (vascular) —*see also*
        Complication, catheter, dialysis,
        mechanical
        peritoneal —*see* Complication(s),
          catheter, intraperitoneal
          dialysis
      gastrointestinal device T85.598
      ocular device T85.398
      subdural (infusion) catheter T85.690
      suture, permanent T85.692
        that for bone repair —*see* Complications,
          fixation device, internal
          (orthopedic), mechanical
      ventricular shunt
        breakdown T85.01
        displacement T85.02
        leakage T85.03
        malposition T85.02
        obstruction T85.09
        perforation T85.09
        protrusion T85.09
        specified NEC T85.09
  mesh
    erosion (to surrounding organ or tissue)
      T83.718
      urethral (into pelvic floor muscles)
        T83.712
      vaginal (into pelvic floor muscles)
        T83.711
    exposure (into surrounding organ or tissue)
      T83.728
      urethral (through urethral wall) T83.722
      vaginal (into vagina) (through vaginal
        wall) T83.721
  orbital —*see* Complications, orbital prosthesis
  penile T83.9
    embolism T83.81
    fibrosis T83.82
    hemorrhage T83.83
    infection and inflammation T83.61
    mechanical
      breakdown T83.410
      displacement T83.420
      leakage T83.490
      malposition T83.420
      obstruction T83.490
      perforation T83.490
      protrusion T83.490
      specified NEC T83.490
    pain T83.84
    specified type NEC T83.89
    stenosis T83.85
    thrombosis T83.86
  prosthetic materials NEC
    erosion (to surrounding organ or tissue)
      T83.718
    exposure (into surrounding organ or tissue)
      T83.728
  skin graft T86.829
    artificial skin or decellularized allodermis
      embolism T85.818
      fibrosis T85.828
      hemorrhage T85.838
      infection and inflammation T85.79
      mechanical
        breakdown T85.613
        displacement T85.623
        malfunction T85.613
        malposition T85.623
        obstruction T85.693
        perforation T85.693
        protrusion T85.693
        specified NEC T85.693
      pain T85.848
      specified type NEC T85.898
      stenosis T85.858
      thrombosis T85.868
    failure T86.821
    infection T86.822
    rejection T86.820
    specified NEC T86.828

Complication (Continued)
  prosthetic device or implant (Continued)
    sling
      urethral (female) (male)
        erosion T83.712
        exposure T83.722
    specified NEC T85.9
      embolism T85.818
      fibrosis T85.828
      hemorrhage T85.838
      infection and inflammation T85.79
      mechanical
        breakdown T85.618
        displacement T85.628
        leakage T85.638
        malfunction T85.618
        malposition T85.628
        obstruction T85.698
        perforation T85.698
        protrusion T85.698
        specified NEC T85.698
      pain T85.848
      specified type NEC T85.898
      stenosis T85.858
      thrombosis T85.868
    subdural infusion catheter —*see*
      Complications, catheter, subdural
    sutures —*see* Complications, sutures
    urinary organ or tract NEC —*see*
      Complications, genitourinary, device or
      implant, urinary system
    vascular —*see* Complications, cardiovascular
      device, graft or implant
    ventricular shunt —*see* Complications,
      ventricular shunt (device)
  puerperium —*see* Puerperal
  puncture, spinal G97.1
    cerebrospinal fluid leak G97.0
    headache or reaction G97.1
  pyelogram N99.89
  radiation
    kyphosis M96.2
    scoliosis M96.5
  reattached
    extremity (infection) (rejection)
      lower T87.1X-●
      upper T87.0X-●
    specified body part NEC T87.2
  reconstructed breast
    asymmetry between native and reconstructed
      breast N65.1
    deformity N65.0
    disproportion between native and
      reconstructed breast N65.1
    excess tissue N65.0
    misshappen N65.0
  reimplant NEC —*see also* Complications,
    prosthetic device or implant
    limb (infection) (rejection) —*see*
      Complications, reattached, extremity
    organ (partial) (total) —*see* Complications,
      transplant
    prosthetic device NEC —*see* Complications,
      prosthetic device
  renal N28.9
    allograft —*see* Complications, transplant,
      kidney
    dialysis —*see* Complications, dialysis
  respirator
    mechanical J95.850
      specified NEC J95.859
  respiratory system J98.9
    device, implant or graft —*see* Complication,
      prosthetic device or implant, specified
      NEC
    lung transplant —*see* Complications,
      prosthetic device or implant, lung
      transplant
    postoperative J95.89
      air leak J95.812
      Mendelson's syndrome (chemical
        pneumonitis) J95.4
      pneumothorax J95.811
      pulmonary insufficiency (acute) (after
        nonthoracic surgery) J95.2
        chronic J95.3
        following thoracic surgery J95.1
      respiratory failure (acute) J95.821
        acute and chronic J95.822
      specified NEC J95.89

▶ New ⬛ Revised ~~deleted~~ Deleted ● Use Additional Character(s)

▶ New   ➡ Revised   ~~deleted~~ Deleted   ● Use Additional Character(s)

▶ New   ⇨ Revised   ~~deleted~~ Deleted   ● Use Additional Character(s)

Corrosion *(Continued)*
  ear (auricle) (external) (canal) T20.41
    drum T28.91
    first degree T20.51
    second degree T20.61
    third degree T20.71
  elbow T22.429
    first degree T22.529
    left T22.422
      first degree T22.522
      second degree T22.622
      third degree T22.722
    right T22.421
      first degree T22.521
      second degree T22.621
      third degree T22.721
    second degree T22.629
    third degree T22.729
  entire body —*see* Corrosion, multiple body
    regions
  epidermal loss - code as Corrosion, second
    degree, by site
  epiglottis T27.4
  erythema, erythematous - code as Corrosion,
    first degree, by site
  esophagus T28.6
  extent (percentage of body surface)
    less than 10 percent T32.0
    10-19 percent (0-9 percent third degree) T32.10
      with 10-19 percent third degree T32.11
    20-29 percent (0-9 percent third degree) T32.20
      with
        10-19 percent third degree T32.21
        20-29 percent third degree T32.22
    30-39 percent (0-9 percent third degree) T32.30
      with
        10-19 percent third degree T32.31
        20-29 percent third degree T32.32
        30-39 percent third degree T32.33
    40-49 percent (0-9 percent third degree) T32.40
      with
        10-19 percent third degree T32.41
        20-29 percent third degree T32.42
        30-39 percent third degree T32.43
        40-49 percent third degree T32.44
    50-59 percent (0-9 percent third degree) T32.50
      with
        10-19 percent third degree T32.51
        20-29 percent third degree T32.52
        30-39 percent third degree T32.53
        40-49 percent third degree T32.54
        50-59 percent third degree T32.55
    60-69 percent (0-9 percent third degree) T32.60
      with
        10-19 percent third degree T32.61
        20-29 percent third degree T32.62
        30-39 percent third degree T32.63
        40-49 percent third degree T32.64
        50-59 percent third degree T32.65
        60-69 percent third degree T32.66
    70-79 percent (0-9 percent third degree) T32.70
      with
        10-19 percent third degree T32.71
        20-29 percent third degree T32.72
        30-39 percent third degree T32.73
        40-49 percent third degree T32.74
        50-59 percent third degree T32.75
        60-69 percent third degree T32.76
        70-79 percent third degree T32.77
    80-89 percent (0-9 percent third degree) T32.80
      with
        10-19 percent third degree T32.81
        20-29 percent third degree T32.82
        30-39 percent third degree T32.83
        40-49 percent third degree T32.84
        50-59 percent third degree T32.85
        60-69 percent third degree T32.86
        70-79 percent third degree T32.87
        80-89 percent third degree T32.88
    90 percent or more (0-9 percent third degree)
      T32.90
      with
        10-19 percent third degree T32.91
        20-29 percent third degree T32.92
        30-39 percent third degree T32.93
        40-49 percent third degree T32.94
        50-59 percent third degree T32.95
        60-69 percent third degree T32.96
        70-79 percent third degree T32.97
        80-89 percent third degree T32.98
        90-99 percent third degree T32.99

Corrosion *(Continued)*
  extremity —*see* Corrosion, limb
  eye(s) and adnexa T26.9-•
    with resulting rupture and destruction of
      eyeball T26.7-•
    conjunctival sac —*see* Corrosion, cornea
    cornea —*see* Corrosion, cornea
    lid —*see* Corrosion, eyelid
    periocular area —*see* Corrosion eyelid
    specified site NEC T26.8-•
  eyeball —*see* Corrosion, eye
  eyelid(s) T26.5-•
  face —*see* Corrosion, head
  finger T23.429
    first degree T23.529
    left T23.422
      first degree T23.522
      second degree T23.622
      third degree T23.722
    multiple sites (without thumb) T23.439
      with thumb T23.449
        first degree T23.549
        left T23.442
          first degree T23.542
          second degree T23.642
          third degree T23.742
        right T23.441
          first degree T23.541
          second degree T23.641
          third degree T23.741
        second degree T23.649
        third degree T23.749
      first degree T23.539
      left T23.432
        first degree T23.532
        second degree T23.632
        third degree T23.732
      right T23.431
        first degree T23.531
        second degree T23.631
        third degree T23.731
      second degree T23.639
      third degree T23.739
    right T23.421
      first degree T23.521
      second degree T23.621
      third degree T23.721
    second degree T23.629
    third degree T23.729
  flank —*see* Corrosion, abdomen
  foot T25.429
    first degree T25.529
    left T25.422
      first degree T25.522
      second degree T25.622
      third degree T25.722
    multiple with ankle —*see* Corrosion, lower,
      limb, multiple, ankle and foot
    right T25.421
      first degree T25.521
      second degree T25.621
      third degree T25.721
    second degree T25.629
    third degree T25.729
  forearm T22.419
    first degree T22.519
    left T22.412
      first degree T22.512
      second degree T22.612
      third degree T22.712
    right T22.411
      first degree T22.511
      second degree T22.611
      third degree T22.711
    second degree T22.619
    third degree T22.719
  forehead T20.46
    first degree T20.56
    second degree T20.66
    third degree T20.76
  fourth degree - code as Corrosion, third degree,
    by site
  full thickness skin loss - code as Corrosion, third
    degree, by site
  gastrointestinal tract NEC T28.7
  genital organs
    external
      female T21.47
        first degree T21.57
        second degree T21.67
        third degree T21.77

Corrosion *(Continued)*
  genital organs *(Continued)*
    external *(Continued)*
      male T21.46
        first degree T21.56
        second degree T21.66
        third degree T21.76
    internal T28.8
  groin —*see* Corrosion, abdominal wall
  hand(s) T23.409
    back —*see* Corrosion, dorsum of hand
    finger —*see* Corrosion, finger
    first degree T23.509
    left T23.402
      first degree T23.502
      second degree T23.602
      third degree T23.702
    multiple sites with wrist T23.499
      first degree T23.599
      left T23.492
        first degree T23.592
        second degree T23.692
        third degree T23.792
      right T23.491
        first degree T23.591
        second degree T23.691
        third degree T23.791
      second degree T23.699
      third degree T23.799
    palm —*see* Corrosion, palm
    right T23.401
      first degree T23.501
      second degree T23.601
      third degree T23.701
    second degree T23.609
    third degree T23.709
    thumb —*see* Corrosion, thumb
  head (and face) (and neck) T20.40
    cheek —*see* Corrosion, cheek
    chin —*see* Corrosion, chin
    ear —*see* Corrosion, ear
    eye(s) only —*see* Corrosion, eye
    first degree T20.50
    forehead —*see* Corrosion, forehead
    lip —*see* Corrosion, lip
    multiple sites T20.49
      first degree T20.59
      second degree T20.69
      third degree T20.79
    neck —*see* Corrosion, neck
    nose —*see* Corrosion, nose
    scalp —*see* Corrosion, scalp
    second degree T20.60
    third degree T20.70
  hip(s) —*see* Corrosion, lower, limb
  inhalation —*see* Corrosion, respiratory tract
  internal organ(s) (*see also* Corrosion, by site)
    T28.90
    alimentary tract T28.7
      esophagus T28.6
    esophagus T28.6
    genitourinary T28.8
    mouth T28.5
    pharynx T28.5
    specified organ NEC T28.99
  interscapular region —*see* Corrosion, back, upper
  intestine (large) (small) T28.7
  knee T24.429
    first degree T24.529
    left T24.422
      first degree T24.522
      second degree T24.622
      third degree T24.722
    right T24.421
      first degree T24.521
      second degree T24.621
      third degree T24.721
    second degree T24.629
    third degree T24.729
  labium (majus) (minus) —*see* Corrosion, genital
    organs, external, female
  lacrimal apparatus, duct, gland or sac —
    see Corrosion, eye, specified site
    NEC
  larynx T27.4
    with lung T27.5
  leg(s) (meaning lower limb(s)) —*see* Corrosion,
    lower limb
  limb(s)
    lower —*see* Corrosion, lower, limb
    upper —*see* Corrosion, upper limb

▶ New   ➡ Revised   ~~deleted~~ Deleted   • Use Additional Character(s)

▶ New   ⇨ Revised   ~~deleted~~ Deleted   ● Use Additional Character(s)

▶ New   ⇥ Revised   ~~deleted~~ Deleted   ● Use Additional Character(s)

Cystadenofibroma
  clear cell —*see* Neoplasm, benign, by site
  endometrioid D27.9
    borderline malignancy D39.1-●
    malignant C56.-●
  mucinous
    specified site —*see* Neoplasm, benign, by site
    unspecified site D27.9
  serous
    specified site —*see* Neoplasm, benign, by site
    unspecified site D27.9
  specified site —*see* Neoplasm, benign, by site
  unspecified site D27.9
Cystadenoma —*see also* Neoplasm, benign, by site
  bile duct D13.4
  endometrioid —*see* Neoplasm, benign, by site
    borderline malignancy —*see* Neoplasm,
      uncertain behavior, by site
  malignant —*see* Neoplasm, malignant, by site
  mucinous
    borderline malignancy
      ovary C56.-●
      specified site NEC —*see* Neoplasm,
        uncertain behavior, by site
      unspecified site C56.9
    papillary
      borderline malignancy
        ovary C56.-●
        specified site NEC —*see* Neoplasm,
          uncertain behavior, by site
        unspecified site C56.9
      specified site —*see* Neoplasm, benign, by site
      unspecified site D27.9
    specified site —*see* Neoplasm, benign, by site
    unspecified site D27.9
  papillary
    borderline malignancy
      ovary C56.-●
      specified site NEC —*see* Neoplasm,
        uncertain behavior, by site
      unspecified site C56.9
    lymphomatosum
      specified site —*see* Neoplasm, benign, by
        site
      unspecified site D11.9
    mucinous
      borderline malignancy
        ovary C56.-●
        specified site NEC —*see* Neoplasm,
          uncertain behavior, by site
        unspecified site C56.9
      specified site —*see* Neoplasm, benign, by
        site
      unspecified site D27.9
    pseudomucinous
      borderline malignancy
        ovary C56.-●
        specified site NEC —*see* Neoplasm,
          uncertain behavior, by site
        unspecified site C56.9
      specified site —*see* Neoplasm, benign, by
        site
      unspecified site D27.9
  serous
    borderline malignancy
      ovary C56.-●
      specified site NEC —*see* Neoplasm,
        uncertain behavior, by site
      unspecified site C56.9
      specified site —*see* Neoplasm, benign, by
        site
      unspecified site D27.9
    specified site —*see* Neoplasm, benign, by site
    unspecified site D27.9
  pseudomucinous
    borderline malignancy
      ovary C56.-●
      specified site NEC —*see* Neoplasm,
        uncertain behavior, by site
      unspecified site C56.9
    papillary
      borderline malignancy
        ovary C56.-●
        specified site NEC —*see* Neoplasm,
          uncertain behavior, by site
        unspecified site C56.9
      specified site —*see* Neoplasm, benign, by
        site
      unspecified site D27.9
  specified site —*see* Neoplasm, benign, by site
  unspecified site D27.9

Cystadenoma *(Continued)*
  serous
    borderline malignancy
      ovary C56.-●
      specified site NEC —*see* Neoplasm,
        uncertain behavior, by site
      unspecified site C56.9
    papillary
      borderline malignancy
        ovary C56.-●
        specified site NEC —*see* Neoplasm,
          uncertain behavior, by site
        unspecified site C56.9
      specified site —*see* Neoplasm, benign, by
        site
      unspecified site D27.9
    specified site —*see* Neoplasm, benign, by site
    unspecified site D27.9
Cystathionine synthase deficiency E72.11
Cystathioninemia E72.19
Cystathioninuria E72.19
Cystic —*see also* condition
  breast (chronic) —*see* Mastopathy, cystic
  corpora lutea (hemorrhagic) N83.1-●
  duct —*see* condition
  eyeball (congenital) Q11.0
  fibrosis —*see* Fibrosis, cystic
  kidney (congenital) Q61.9
    adult type Q61.2
    infantile type NEC Q61.19
      collecting duct dilatation Q61.11
    medullary Q61.5
  liver, congenital Q44.6
  lung disease J98.4
    congenital Q33.0
  mastitis, chronic —*see* Mastopathy, cystic
  medullary, kidney Q61.5
  meniscus —*see* Derangement, knee, meniscus,
    cystic
  ovary N83.20-●
Cysticercosis, cysticerciasis B69.9
  with
    epileptiform fits B69.0
    myositis B69.81
  brain B69.0
  central nervous system B69.0
  cerebral B69.0
  ocular B69.1
  specified NEC B69.89
Cysticercus cellulose infestation —*see*
  Cysticercosis
Cystinosis (malignant) E72.04
Cystinuria E72.01
Cystitis (exudative) (hemorrhagic) (septic)
  (suppurative) N30.90
  with
    fibrosis —*see* Cystitis, chronic, interstitial
    hematuria N30.91
    leukoplakia —*see* Cystitis, chronic, interstitial
    malakoplakia —*see* Cystitis, chronic,
      interstitial
    metaplasia —*see* Cystitis, chronic, interstitial
    prostatitis N41.3
  acute N30.00
    with hematuria N30.01
    of trigone N30.30
      with hematuria N30.31
  allergic —*see* Cystitis, specified type NEC
  amebic A06.81
  bilharzial B65.9 [N33]
  blennorrhagic (gonococcal) A54.01
  bullous —*see* Cystitis, specified type NEC
  calculous N21.0
  chlamydial A56.01
  chronic N30.20
    with hematuria N30.21
    interstitial N30.10
      with hematuria N30.11
    of trigone N30.30
      with hematuria N30.31
    specified NEC N30.20
      with hematuria N30.21
  cystic (a) —*see* Cystitis, specified type NEC
  diphtheritic A36.85
  echinococcal
    granulosus B67.39
    multilocularis B67.69
  emphysematous —*see* Cystitis, specified type
    NEC
  encysted —*see* Cystitis, specified type NEC
  eosinophilic —*see* Cystitis, specified type NEC

Cystitis *(Continued)*
  follicular —*see* Cystitis, of trigone
  gangrenous —*see* Cystitis, specified type NEC
  glandularis —*see* Cystitis, specified type NEC
  gonococcal A54.01
  incrusted —*see* Cystitis, specified type NEC
  interstitial (chronic) —*see* Cystitis, chronic,
    interstitial
  irradiation N30.40
    with hematuria N30.41
  irritation —*see* Cystitis, specified type NEC
  malignant —*see* Cystitis, specified type NEC
  of trigone N30.30
    with hematuria N30.31
  panmural —*see* Cystitis, chronic, interstitial
  polyposa —*see* Cystitis, specified type NEC
  prostatic N41.3
  puerperal (postpartum) O86.22
  radiation —*see* Cystitis, irradiation
  specified type NEC N30.80
    with hematuria N30.81
  subacute —*see* Cystitis, chronic
  submucous —*see* Cystitis, chronic, interstitial
  syphilitic (late) A52.76
  trichomonal A59.03
  tuberculous A18.12
  ulcerative —*see* Cystitis, chronic, interstitial
Cystocele (-urethrocele)
  female N81.10
    with prolapse of uterus —*see* Prolapse, uterus
    lateral N81.12
    midline N81.11
    paravaginal N81.12
  in pregnancy or childbirth O34.8-●
    causing obstructed labor O65.5
  male N32.89
Cystolithiasis N21.0
Cystoma —*see also* Neoplasm, benign, by site
  endometrial, ovary N80.10-●
  mucinous
    specified site —*see* Neoplasm, benign, by site
    unspecified site D27.9
  serous
    specified site —*see* Neoplasm, benign, by site
    unspecified site D27.9
  simple (ovary) N83.29-●
Cystoplegia N31.2
Cystoptosis N32.89
Cystopyelitis —*see* Pyelonephritis
Cystorrhagia N32.89
Cystosarcoma phyllodes D48.6-●
  benign D24-●
  malignant —*see* Neoplasm, breast, malignant
Cystostomy
  attention to Z43.5
  complication —*see* Complications, cystostomy
  status Z93.50
    appendico-vesicostomy Z93.52
    cutaneous Z93.51
    specified NEC Z93.59
Cystourethritis —*see* Urethritis
Cystourethrocele —*see also* Cystocele
  female N81.10
    with uterine prolapse —*see* Prolapse, uterus
    lateral N81.12
    midline N81.11
    paravaginal N81.12
  male N32.89
Cytomegalic inclusion disease
  congenital P35.1
Cytomegalovirus infection B25.9
Cytomycosis (reticuloendothelial) B39.4
Cytopenia D75.9
  refractory
    with multilineage dysplasia D46.A
      and ring sideroblasts (RCMD RS) D46.B
Czerny's disease (periodic hydrarthrosis of the
  knee) —*see* Effusion, joint, knee

—————— **D** ——————

Daae (-Finsen) **disease** (epidemic pleurodynia)
  B33.0
Dabney's grip B33.0
Da Costa's syndrome F45.8
Dacryoadenitis, dacryadenitis H04.00-●
  acute H04.01-●
  chronic H04.02-●

▶ New   ➡ Revised   ~~deleted~~ Deleted   ● Use Additional Character(s)

  ▶ New   ➡ Revised   ~~deleted~~ Deleted   ● Use Additional Character(s)

► New   ➡ Revised   ~~deleted~~ Deleted   ● Use Additional Character(s)

▶ New　　➡ Revised　　~~deleted~~ Deleted　　● Use Additional Character(s)

▶ New   ⇨ Revised   ~~deleted~~ Deleted   ● Use Additional Character(s)

▶ New   ➡ Revised   ~~deleted~~ Deleted   ● Use Additional Character(s)

Dermatitis *(Continued)*
pruriginosa L13.0
pruritic NEC L30.8
psychogenic F54
purulent L08.0
pustular
contagious B08.02
subcorneal L13.1
pyococcal L08.0
pyogenica L08.0
repens L40.2
Ritter's (exfoliativa) L00
Schamberg's L81.7
schistosome B65.3
seasonal bullous L30.8
seborrheic L21.9
infantile L21.1
specified NEC L21.8
sensitization NOS L23.9
septic L08.0
solare L57.8
specified NEC L30.8
stasis I87.2
with
varicose ulcer —*see* Varix, leg, with ulcer,
with inflammation
varicose veins —*see* Varix, leg, with,
inflammation
due to postthrombotic syndrome —*see*
Syndrome, postthrombotic
suppurative L08.0
traumatic NEC L30.4
trophoneurotica L13.0
ultraviolet (sun) (chronic exposure) L57.8
acute L56.8
varicose —*see* Varix, leg, with, inflammation
vegetans L10.1
verrucosa B43.0
vesicular, herpesviral B00.1
Dermatoarthritis, lipoid E78.81
Dermatochalasis, eyelid H02.839
left H02.836
lower H02.835
upper H02.834
right H02.833
lower H02.832
upper H02.831
Dermatofibroma (lenticulare) —*see* Neoplasm,
skin, benign
protuberans —*see* Neoplasm, skin, uncertain
behavior
Dermatofibrosarcoma (pigmented) (protuberans)
—*see* Neoplasm, skin, malignant
Dermatographia L50.3
Dermatolysis (exfoliativa) (congenital) Q82.8
acquired L57.4
eyelids —*see* Blepharochalasis
palpebrarum —*see* Blepharochalasis
senile L57.4
Dermatomegaly NEC Q82.8
Dermatomucosomyositis (*see also*
Dermatomyositis) M33.10
with
myopathy M33.12
respiratory involvement M33.11
specified organ involvement NEC M33.19
Dermatomycosis B36.9
furfuracea B36.0
specified type NEC B36.8
Dermatomyositis (acute) (chronic) —*see also*
Dermatopolymyositis
adult —*see also* Dermatomyositis, specified NEC
M33.10
in (due to) neoplastic disease —*see also*
Neoplasm D49.9 [M36.0]
juvenile M33.00
with
myopathy M33.02
respiratory involvement M33.01
specified organ involvement NEC M33.09
amyopathic M33.03
without myopathy M33.03
specified NEC M33.10
with
myopathy M33.12
respiratory involvement M33.11
specified organ involvement NEC M33.19
amyopathic M33.13
without myopathy M33.13
Dermatoneuritis of children —*see* Poisoning,
mercury

Dermatophilosis A48.8
Dermatophytid L30.2
Dermatophytide —*see* Dermatophytosis
Dermatophytosis (epidermophyton) (infection)
(Microsporum) (tinea) (Trichophyton) B35.9
beard B35.0
body B35.4
capitis B35.0
corporis B35.4
deep-seated B35.8
disseminated B35.8
foot B35.3
granulomatous B35.8
groin B35.6
hand B35.2
nail B35.1
perianal (area) B35.6
scalp B35.0
specified NEC B35.8
Dermatopolymyositis M33.90
with
myopathy M33.92
respiratory involvement M33.91
specified organ involvement NEC M33.99
amyopathic M33.93
in neoplastic disease —*see also* Neoplasm D49.9
[M36.0]
juvenile M33.00
with
myopathy M33.02
respiratory involvement M33.01
specified organ involvement NEC M33.09
amyopathic M33.03
without myopathy M33.03
specified NEC M33.10
myopathy M33.12
respiratory involvement M33.11
specified organ involvement NEC M33.19
amyopathic M33.13
without myopathy M33.13
without myopathy M33.93
Dermatopolyneuritis —*see* Poisoning, mercury
Dermatorrhexis (*see also* Syndrome, Ehlers-Danlos)
Q79.60
acquired L57.4
Dermatosclerosis —*see also* Scleroderma
localized L94.0
Dermatosis L98.9
Andrews' L08.89
Bowen's —*see* Neoplasm, skin, in situ
bullous L13.9
specified NEC L13.8
exfoliativa L26
eyelid (noninfectious) (*see also* Dermatitis, eyelid)
H01.9
discoid lupus erythematosus —*see* Lupus,
erythematosus, eyelid
xeroderma —*see* Xeroderma, acquired, eyelid
factitial L98.1
febrile neutrophilic L98.2
gonococcal A54.89
herpetiformis L13.0
juvenile L12.2
linear IgA L13.8
menstrual NEC L98.8
neutrophilic, febrile L98.2
occupational —*see* Dermatitis, contact
papulosa nigra L82.1
pigmentary L81.9
progressive L81.7
Schamberg's L81.7
psychogenic F54
purpuric, pigmented L81.7
pustular, subcorneal L13.1
transient acantholytic L11.1
Dermographia, dermographism L50.3
Dermoid (cyst) —~~*see also* Neoplasm, benign, by site~~
with malignant transformation C56-
due to radiation (nonionizing) L57.8
Dermopathy
infiltrative with thyrotoxicosis —*see*
Thyrotoxicosis
nephrogenic fibrosing L90.8
Dermophytosis —*see* Dermatophytosis
▶ **DES**
▶ child (daughter) (son) Z91.B
▶ grandchild (granddaughter) (grandson) Z84.A
▶ second generation Z91.B
▶ third generation Z84.A
Descemetocele H18.73-
Descemet's membrane —*see* condition

Descending —*see* condition
Descensus uteri —*see* Prolapse, uterus
Desert
rheumatism B38.0
sore —*see* Ulcer, skin
Desertion (newborn) —*see* Maltreatment
Desmoid (extra-abdominal) (tumor) —*see*
Neoplasm, connective tissue, uncertain
behavior
abdominal wall D48.113
back D48.117
buttock D48.116
chest wall D48.111
extremity
lower D48.116
upper D48.115
head and neck D48.110
intraabdominal D48.114
intrathoracic D48.112
pelvic cavity D48.114
pelvic girdle D48.116
peritoneal D48.114
retroperitoneal D48.114
shoulder girdle D48.115
site unspecified D48.119
specified site NEC D48.118
Despondency F32.A
Desquamation, skin R23.4
Destruction, destructive —*see also* Damage
articular facet —*see also* Derangement, joint,
specified type NEC
knee M23.8X-
vertebra —*see* Spondylosis
bone —*see also* Disorder, bone, specified type NEC
syphilitic A52.77
joint —*see also* Derangement, joint, specified
type NEC
sacroiliac M53.3
rectal sphincter K62.89
septum (nasal) J34.89
tuberculous NEC —*see* Tuberculosis
tympanum, tympanic membrane
(nontraumatic) —*see* Disorder, tympanic
membrane, specified NEC
vertebral disc —*see* Degeneration, intervertebral
disc
Destructiveness —*see also* Disorder, conduct
adjustment reaction —*see* Disorder, adjustment
Desultory labor O62.2
Detachment
cartilage —*see* Sprain
cervix, annular N88.8
complicating delivery O71.3
choroid (old) (postinfectional) (simple)
(spontaneous) H31.40-
hemorrhagic H31.41-
serous H31.42-
ligament —*see* Sprain
meniscus (knee) —*see also* Derangement, knee,
meniscus, specified NEC
current injury —*see* Tear, meniscus
due to old tear or injury —*see* Derangement,
knee, meniscus, due to old tear
retina (without retinal break) (serous) H33.2-
with retinal:
break H33.00-
giant H33.03-
multiple H33.02-
single H33.01-
dialysis H33.04-
pigment epithelium —*see* Degeneration,
retina, separation of layers, pigment
epithelium detachment
rhegmatogenous —*see* Detachment, retina,
with retinal, break
specified NEC H33.8
total H33.05-
traction H33.4-
vitreous (body) H43.81
Detergent asthma J69.8
Deterioration
epileptic F06.8
general physical R53.81
heart, cardiac —*see* Degeneration, myocardial
mental —*see* Psychosis
myocardial, myocardium —*see* Degeneration,
myocardial
senile (simple) R54
Deuteranomaly (anomalous trichromat)
H53.53
Deuteranopia (complete) (incomplete) H53.53

Development
  abnormal, bone Q79.9
  arrested R62.50
    bone —*see* Arrest, development or growth, bone
    child R62.50
    due to malnutrition E45
  defective, congenital —*see also* Anomaly, by site
    cauda equina Q06.3
    left ventricle Q24.8
      in hypoplastic left heart syndrome Q23.4
    valve Q24.8
      pulmonary Q22.3
  delayed (*see also* Delay, development) R62.50
    arithmetical skills F81.2
    language (skills) (expressive) F80.1
    learning skill F81.9
    mixed skills F88
    motor coordination F82
    reading F81.0
    specified learning skill NEC F81.89
    speech F80.9
    spelling F81.81
    written expression F81.81
  imperfect, congenital —*see also* Anomaly, by site
    heart Q24.9
    lungs Q33.6
  incomplete
    bronchial tree Q32.4
    organ or site not listed —*see* Hypoplasia, by site
    respiratory system Q34.9
  sexual, precocious NEC E30.1
  tardy, mental (*see also* Disability, intellectual) F79
Developmental —*see* condition
  testing, infant or child —*see* Examination, child
Devergie's disease (pityriasis rubra pilaris) L44.0
Deviation (in)
  conjugate palsy (eye) (spastic) H51.0
  esophagus (acquired) K22.89
  eye, skew H51.8
  midline (jaw) (teeth) (dental arch) M26.29
    specified site NEC —*see* Malposition
  nasal septum J34.2
    congenital Q67.4
  opening and closing of the mandible M26.53
  organ or site, congenital NEC —*see* Malposition, congenital
  septum (nasal) (acquired) J34.2
    congenital Q67.4
  sexual F65.9
    bestiality F65.89
    erotomania F52.8
    exhibitionism F65.2
    fetishism, fetishistic F65.0
      transvestism F65.1
    frotteurism F65.81
    masochism F65.51
    multiple F65.89
    necrophilia F65.89
    nymphomania F52.8
    pederosis F65.4
    pedophilia F65.4
    sadism, sadomasochism F65.52
    satyriasis F52.8
    specified type NEC F65.89
    transvestism F64.1
    voyeurism F65.3
  teeth, midline M26.29
  trachea J39.8
  ureter, congenital Q62.61
Device
  cerebral ventricle (communicating) in situ Z98.2
  contraceptive —*see* Contraceptive, device
  drainage, cerebrospinal fluid, in situ Z98.2
Devic's disease G36.0
Devil's
  grip B33.0
  pinches (purpura simplex) D69.2
Devitalized tooth K04.99
Devonshire colic —*see* Poisoning, lead
Dextraposition, aorta Q20.3
  in tetralogy of Fallot Q21.3
Dextrinosis, limit (debrancher enzyme deficiency) E74.03
Dextrocardia (true) Q24.0
  with
    complete transposition of viscera Q89.3
    situs inversus Q89.3

Dextrotransposition, aorta Q20.3
d-glycericacidemia E72.59
Dhat syndrome F48.8
Dhobi itch B35.6
Di George's syndrome D82.1
Di Guglielmo's disease C94.0- ●
Diabetes, diabetic (mellitus) (sugar) E11.9
  with
    amyotrophy E11.44
    arthropathy NEC E11.618
    autonomic (poly)neuropathy E11.43
    cataract E11.36
    Charcot's joints E11.610
    chronic kidney disease E11.22
    circulatory complication NEC E11.59
    coma due to
      hyperosmolarity E11.01
      hypoglycemia E11.641
      ketoacidosis E11.11
    complication E11.8
      specified NEC E11.69
    dermatitis E11.620
    foot ulcer E11.621
    gangrene E11.52
    gastroparalysis E11.43
    gastroparesis E11.43
    glomerulonephrosis, intracapillary E11.21
    glomerulosclerosis, intercapillary E11.21
    hyperglycemia E11.65
    hyperosmolarity E11.00
      with coma E11.01
    hypoglycemia E11.649
      with coma E11.641
    ketoacidosis E11.10
      with coma E11.11
    kidney complications NEC E11.29
    Kimmelstiel-Wilson disease E11.21
    loss of protective sensation (LOPS) —*see* Diabetes, by type, with neuropathy
    mononeuropathy E11.41
    myasthenia E11.44
    necrobiosis lipoidica E11.620
    nephropathy E11.21
    neuralgia E11.42
    neurologic complication NEC E11.49
    neuropathic arthropathy E11.610
    neuropathy E11.40
    ophthalmic complication NEC E11.39
    oral complication NEC E11.638
    osteomyelitis E11.69
    periodontal disease E11.630
    peripheral angiopathy E11.51
      with gangrene E11.52
    polyneuropathy E11.42
    renal complication NEC E11.29
    renal tubular degeneration E11.29
    retinopathy E11.319
      with macular edema E11.311
        resolved following treatment E11.37
      nonproliferative E11.329
        with macular edema E11.321
        mild E11.329
          with macular edema E11.321
        moderate E11.339
          with macular edema E11.331
        severe E11.349
          with macular edema E11.341
      proliferative E11.359
        with
          combined traction retinal detachment and rhegmatogenous retinal detachment E11.354
          macular edema E11.351
          stable proliferative diabetic retinopathy E11.355
          traction retinal detachment involving the macula E11.352
          traction retinal detachment not involving the macula E11.353
    skin complication NEC E11.628
    skin ulcer NEC E11.622
  brittle —*see* Diabetes, type 1
  bronzed E83.110
  complicating pregnancy —*see* Pregnancy, complicated by, diabetes
  dietary counseling and surveillance Z71.3
  due to
    autoimmune process —*see* Diabetes, type 1
    immune mediated pancreatic islet beta-cell destruction —*see* Diabetes, type 1

Diabetes, diabetic (*Continued*)
  due to drug or chemical E09.9
    with
      amyotrophy E09.44
      arthropathy NEC E09.618
      autonomic (poly)neuropathy E09.43
      cataract E09.36
      Charcot's joints E09.610
      chronic kidney disease E09.22
      circulatory complication NEC E09.59
      complication E09.8
        specified NEC E09.69
      dermatitis E09.620
      foot ulcer E09.621
      gangrene E09.52
      gastroparalysis E09.43
      gastroparesis E09.43
      glomerulonephrosis, intracapillary E09.21
      glomerulosclerosis, intercapillary E09.21
      hyperglycemia E09.65
      hyperosmolarity E09.00
        with coma E09.01
      hypoglycemia E09.649
        with coma E09.641
      ketoacidosis E09.10
        with coma E09.11
      kidney complications NEC E09.29
      Kimmelstiel-Wilson disease E09.21
      mononeuropathy E09.41
      myasthenia E09.44
      necrobiosis lipoidica E09.620
      nephropathy E09.21
      neuralgia E09.42
      neurologic complication NEC E09.49
      neuropathic arthropathy E09.610
      neuropathy E09.40
      ophthalmic complication NEC E09.39
      oral complication NEC E09.638
      periodontal disease E09.630
      peripheral angiopathy E09.51
        with gangrene E09.52
      polyneuropathy E09.42
      renal complication NEC E09.29
      renal tubular degeneration E09.29
    ▶ retinal, hemorrhage E09.39
      retinopathy E09.319
        with macular edema E09.311
          resolved following treatment E09.37
        nonproliferative E09.329
          with macular edema E09.321
          mild E09.329
            with macular edema E09.321
          moderate E09.339
            with macular edema E09.331
          severe E09.349
            with macular edema E09.341
        proliferative E09.359
          with
            combined traction retinal detachment and rhegmatogenous retinal detachment E09.354
            macular edema E09.351
            stable proliferative diabetic retinopathy E09.355
            traction retinal detachment involving the macula E09.352
            traction retinal detachment not involving the macula E09.353
      skin complication NEC E09.628
      skin ulcer NEC E09.622
  due to underlying condition E08.9
    with
      amyotrophy E08.44
      arthropathy NEC E08.618
      autonomic (poly)neuropathy E08.43
      cataract E08.36
      Charcot's joints E08.610
      chronic kidney disease E08.22
      circulatory complication NEC E08.59
      complication E08.8
        specified NEC E08.69
      dermatitis E08.620
      foot ulcer E08.621
      gangrene E08.52
      gastroparalysis E08.43
      gastroparesis E08.43
      glomerulonephrosis, intracapillary E08.21
      glomerulosclerosis, intercapillary E08.21
      hyperglycemia E08.69

  ▶ New   ➡ Revised   ~~deleted~~ Deleted   ● Use Additional Character(s)

Diabetes, diabetic *(Continued)*
  type 2 *(Continued)*
    with *(Continued)*
      ketoacidosis E11.10
        with coma E11.11
      kidney complications NEC E11.29
      Kimmelstiel-Wilson disease E11.21
      mononeuropathy E11.41
      myasthenia E11.44
      necrobiosis lipoidica E11.620
      nephropathy E11.21
      neuralgia E11.42
      neurologic complication NEC E11.49
      neuropathic arthropathy E11.610
      neuropathy E11.40
      ophthalmic complication NEC E11.39
      oral complication NEC E11.638
      osteomyelitis E11.69
      periodontal disease E11.630
      peripheral angiopathy E11.51
        with gangrene E11.52
      polyneuropathy E11.42
      renal complication NEC E11.29
      renal tubular degeneration E11.29
      ▶ retinal, hemorrhage E09.39
      retinopathy E11.319
        with macular edema E11.311
          resolved following treatment E11.37
        nonproliferative E11.329
          with macular edema E11.321
          mild E11.329
            with macular edema E11.321
          moderate E11.339
            with macular edema E11.331
          severe E11.349
            with macular edema E11.341
        proliferative E11.359
          with
            combined traction retinal
              detachment and
              rhegmatogenous retinal
              detachment E11.354
            macular edema E11.351
            stable proliferative diabetic
              retinopathy E11.355
            traction retinal detachment
              involving the macula E11.352
            traction retinal detachment not
              involving the macula E11.353
      skin complication NEC E11.628
      skin ulcer NEC E11.622
    ▶ without complications in remission E11.A
    uncontrolled
      meaning
        hyperglycemia —*see* Diabetes, by type,
          with, hyperglycemia
        hypoglycemia —*see* Diabetes, by type, with,
          hypoglycemia
  ▶ without complications in remission E11.A
Diacyclothrombopathia D69.1
Diagnosis deferred R69
Dialysis (intermittent) (treatment)
  noncompliance (with) Z91.158
    due to financial hardship Z91.151
  renal (hemodialysis) (peritoneal), status Z99.2
  retina, retinal —*see* Detachment, retina, with
    retinal, dialysis
Diamond-Blackfan anemia (congenital
  hypoplastic) D61.01
Diamond-Gardener syndrome (autoerythrocyte
  sensitization) D69.2
Diaper rash L22
Diaphoresis (excessive) R61
Diaphragm —*see* condition
Diaphragmalgia R07.1
Diaphragmatitis, diaphragmitis J98.6
Diaphysial aclasis Q78.6
Diaphysitis —*see* Osteomyelitis, specified type NEC
Diarrhea, diarrheal (disease) (infantile)
  (inflammatory) R19.7
  achlorhydric K31.83
  allergic K52.29
    due to
      colitis —*see* Colitis, allergic
      enteritis —*see* Enteritis, allergic
  ambeic —*see also* Amebiasis A06.0
    with abscess —*see* Abscess, amebic
    acute A06.0
    chronic A06.1
    nondysenteric A06.2
  bacillary —*see* Dysentery, bacillary
  balantidial A07.0

Diarrhea, diarrheal *(Continued)*
  cachectic NEC K52.89
  Chilomastix A07.8
  choleriformis A00.1
  chronic (noninfectious) K52.9
  coccidial A07.3
  Cochin-China K90.1
    strongyloidiasis B78.0
  Dientamoeba A07.8
  dietetic —*see also* Diarrhea, allergic K52.29
  drug-induced K52.1
  due to
    bacteria A04.9
      specified NEC A04.8
    Campylobacter A04.5
    Capillaria philippinensis B81.1
    Clostridium difficile
      not specified as recurrent A04.72
      recurrent A04.71
    Clostridium perfringens (C) (F) A04.8
    Cryptosporidium A07.2
    drugs K52.1
    Escherichia coli A04.4
      enteroaggregative A04.4
      enterohemorrhagic A04.3
      enteroinvasive A04.2
      enteropathogenic A04.0
      enterotoxigenic A04.1
      specified NEC A04.4
    food hypersensitivity —*see also* Diarrhea,
      allergic K52.29
    Necator americanus B76.1
    S. japonicum B65.2
    specified organism NEC A08.8
      bacterial A04.8
      viral A08.39
    Staphylococcus A04.8
    Trichuris trichiuria B79
    virus —*see* Enteritis, viral
    Yersinia enterocolitica A04.6
  dysenteric A09
  endemic A09
  epidemic A09
  flagellate A07.9
  Flexner's (ulcerative) A03.1
  functional K59.1
    following gastrointestinal surgery K91.89
    psychogenic F45.8
  Giardia lamblia A07.1
  giardial A07.1
  hill K90.1
  infectious A09
  malarial —*see* Malaria
  ➡ mite B88.09
  mycotic NEC B49
  neonatal (noninfectious) P78.3
  nervous F45.8
  neurogenic K59.1
  noninfectious K52.9
  postgastrectomy K91.1
  postvagotomy K91.1
  protozoal A07.9
    specified NEC A07.8
  psychogenic F45.8
  specified
    bacterium NEC A04.8
    virus NEC A08.39
  strongyloidiasis B78.0
  toxic K52.1
  trichomonal A07.8
  tropical K90.1
  tuberculous A18.32
  viral —*see* Enteritis, viral
Diastasis
  cranial bones M84.88
    congenital NEC Q75.8
  joint (traumatic) —*see* Dislocation
  muscle M62.00
    ankle M62.07-●
    congenital Q79.8
    foot M62.07-●
    forearm M62.03-●
    hand M62.04-●
    lower leg M62.06-●
    pelvic region M62.05-●
    shoulder region M62.01-●
    specified site NEC M62.08
    thigh M62.05-●
    upper arm M62.02-●
  recti (abdomen)
    complicating delivery O71.89
    congenital Q79.59

Diastema, tooth, teeth, fully erupted M26.32
Diastematomyelia Q06.2
Diataxia, cerebral G80.4
Diathesis
  allergic —*see* History, allergy
  bleeding (familial) D69.9
  cystine (familial) E72.00
  gouty —*see* Gout
  hemorrhagic (familial) D69.9
    newborn NEC P53
  spasmophilic R29.0
Diaz's disease or osteochondrosis (juvenile)
  (talus) —*see* Osteochondrosis, juvenile, tarsus
Dibothriocephalus, dibothriocephaliasis (latus)
  (infection) (infestation) B70.0
  larval B70.1
Dicephalus, dicephaly Q89.4
Dichotomy, teeth K00.2
Dichromat, dichromatopsia (congenital) —*see*
  Deficiency, color vision
Dichuchwa A65
Dicroceliasis B66.2
Didelphia, didelphys —*see* Double uterus
Didymytis N45.1
  with orchitis N45.3
Dietary
  inadequacy or deficiency E63.9
  surveillance and counseling Z71.3
Dietl's crisis N13.8
Dieulafoy lesion (hemorrhagic)
  duodenum K31.82
  esophagus K22.89
  intestine (colon) K63.81
  stomach K31.82
Difficult, difficulty (in)
  acculturation Z60.3
  feeding R63.30
    elderly R63.39
    infant NOS R63.39
    newborn P92.9
      breast P92.5
      specified NEC P92.8
    nonorganic (infant or child) F98.29
    specified NEC R63.39
  intubation, in anesthesia T88.4
  mechanical, gastroduodenal stoma
    K91.89
    causing obstruction —*see also* Obstruction,
      intestine, postoperative K91.30
  micturition
    need to immediately re-void R39.191
    position dependent R39.192
    specified NEC R39.198
  reading (developmental) F81.0
    secondary to emotional disorders F93.9
  spelling (specific) F81.81
    with reading disorder F81.89
    due to inadequate teaching Z55.8
  swallowing —*see* Dysphagia
  understanding
    health related information Z55.6
    medication instructions Z55.6
  walking R26.2
  work
    conditions NEC Z56.5
    schedule Z56.3
Diffuse —*see* condition
DiGeorge's syndrome (thymic hypoplasia)
  D82.1
Digestive —*see* condition
Dihydropyrimidine dehydrogenase disease
  (DPD) E88.89
Diktyoma —*see* Neoplasm, malignant, by site
Dilaceration, tooth K00.4
Dilatation
  anus K59.89
    venule —*see* Hemorrhoids
  aorta (focal) (general) —*see* Ectasia, aorta
    with aneurysm —*see* Aneurysm, aorta
    congenital Q25.44
  artery —*see* Aneurysm
  bladder (sphincter) N32.89
    congenital Q64.79
  blood vessel I99.8
  bronchial J47.9
    with
      exacerbation (acute) J47.1
      lower respiratory infection J47.0
  calyx N28.89
    due to obstruction —*see* Hydronephosis
  capillaries I78.8

▶ New   ➡ Revised   ~~deleted~~ Deleted   ● Use Additional Character(s)

► New ⇨ Revised ~~deleted~~ Deleted ● Use Additional Character(s)

Disease, diseased *(Continued)*
 parasitic *(Continued)*
  mouth B37.0
  skin NOS B88.9
  specified type —*see* Infestation
  tongue B37.0
 parathyroid (gland) E21.5
  specified NEC E21.4
 Parkinson's G20.A1
  with dyskinesia
   with
    fluctuations G20.B2
    OFF episodes G20.B2
   without mention of
    fluctuations G20.B1
    OFF episodes G20.B1
  without dyskinesia
   with
    fluctuations G20.A2
    OFF episodes G20.A2
   without mention of
    fluctuations G20.A1
    OFF episodes G20.A1
 parodontal K05.6
 Parrot's (syphilitic osteochondritis) A50.02
 Parry's (exophthalmic goiter) —*see*
  Hyperthyroidism, with, goiter (diffuse)
 Parson's (exophthalmic goiter) —*see*
  Hyperthyroidism, with, goiter (diffuse)
 Paxton's (white piedra) B36.2
 pearl-worker's —*see* Osteomyelitis, specified
  type NEC
 Pellegrini-Stieda (calcification, knee joint) —*see*
  Bursitis, tibial collateral
 pelvis, pelvic
  female NOS N94.9
   specified NEC N94.89
  gonococcal (acute) (chronic) A54.24
  inflammatory (female) N73.9
   acute N73.0
   chlamydial A56.11
   chronic N73.1
   specified NEC N73.8
   syphilitic (secondary) A51.42
    late A52.76
   tuberculous A18.17
  organ, female N94.9
  peritoneum, female NEC N94.89
 penis N48.9
  inflammatory N48.29
   abscess N48.21
   cellulitis N48.22
  specified NEC N48.89
 periapical tissues NOS K04.90
 periodontal K05.6
  specified NEC K05.5
 periosteum —*see* Disorder, bone, specified type
  NEC
 peripheral
  arterial I73.9
  autonomic nervous system G90.9
  nerves —*see* Polyneuropathy
  vascular NOS I73.9
   in diabetes mellitus —*see* Diabetes, by type,
    with peripheral angiopathy
 peritoneum K66.9
  pelvic, female NEC N94.89
  specified NEC K66.8
 persistent mucosal (middle ear) H66.20
  left H66.22
   with right H66.23
  right H66.21
   with left H66.23
 Petit's —*see* Hernia, abdomen, specified site NEC
 pharynx J39.2
  specified NEC J39.2
 Phocas' —*see* Mastopathy, cystic
 photochromogenic (acid-fast bacilli)
  (pulmonary) A31.0
  nonpulmonary A31.9
 Pick's (*see also* Dementia, in, diseases specified
  elsewhere) G31.01 [*F02.80*]
  with behavioral disturbance (*see also*
   Dementia, in, diseases specified
   elsewhere) G31.01 [*F02.81-●*]
  brain (*see also* Dementia, in, diseases specified
   elsewhere) G31.01 [*F02.80*]
   with behavioral disturbance (*see also*
    Dementia, in, diseases specified
    elsewhere) G31.01 [*F02.81-●*]
  of pericardium (pericardial pseudocirrhosis of
   liver) I31.1

Disease, diseased *(Continued)*
 pigeon fancier's J67.2
 pineal gland E34.8
 pink —*see* Poisoning, mercury
 Pinkus' (lichen nitidus) L44.1
 pinworm B80
 Piry virus A93.8
 pituitary (gland) E23.7
 pituitary-snuff-taker's J67.8
 pleura (cavity) J94.9
  specified NEC J94.8
 pneumatic drill (hammer) T75.21
 Pollitzer's (hidradenitis suppurativa) L73.2
 polycystic
  kidney or renal Q61.3
   adult type Q61.2
   childhood type NEC Q61.19
    collecting duct dilatation Q61.11
  liver or hepatic Q44.6
  lung or pulmonary J98.4
   congenital Q33.0
  ovary, ovaries E28.2
  spleen Q89.09
 polyethylene T84.05-●
 Pompe's (glycogenosis II) E74.02
 Posadas-Wernicke B38.9
 Potain's (pulmonary edema) —*see* Edema, lung
 prepuce N47.8
  inflammatory N47.7
   balanoposthitis N47.6
 Pringle's (tuberous sclerosis) Q85.1
 prion, central nervous system A81.9
  specified NEC A81.89
 prostate N42.9
  specified NEC N42.89
 protozoal B64
  acanthamebiasis —*see* Acanthamebiasis
  African trypanosomiasis —*see* African
   trypanosomiasis
  babesiosis —(*see also* Babesiosis)
   B60.00
  Chagas disease —*see* Chagas disease
  intestine, intestinal A07.9
  leishmaniasis —*see* Leishmaniasis
  malaria —*see* Malaria
  naegleriasis B60.2
  pneumocystosis B59
  specified organism NEC B60.8
  toxoplasmosis —*see* Toxoplasmosis
 pseudo-Hurler's E77.0
 psychiatric F99
 psychotic —*see* Psychosis
 Puente's (simple glandular cheilitis) K13.0
 puerperal —*see also* Puerperal O90.89
 pulmonary —*see also* Disease, lung
  artery I28.9
  chronic obstructive J44.9
   with
    acute bronchitis J44.0
    exacerbation (acute) J44.1
    lower respiratory infection (acute)
     J44.0
   decompensated J44.1
    with
     exacerbation (acute) J44.1
  heart I27.9
   specified NEC I27.89
  hypertensive (vascular) —*see also*
   Hypertension, pulmonary I27.20
   primary (idiopathic) I27.0
  valve I37.9
   rheumatic I09.89
 pulp (dental) NOS K04.90
 pulseless M31.4
 Putnam's (subacute combined sclerosis with
  pernicious anemia) D51.0
 Pyle (-Cohn) (metaphyseal dysplasia) Q78.5
 ragpicker's or ragsorter's A22.1
 Raynaud's —*see* Raynaud's disease
 reactive airway —*see* Asthma
 Reclus' (cystic) —*see* Mastopathy, cystic
 rectum K62.9
  specified NEC K62.89
 Refsum's (heredopathia atactica
  polyneuritiformis) G60.1
 renal (functional) (pelvis) —*see also* Disease,
  kidney N28.9
  with
   edema —*see* Nephrosis
   glomerular lesion —*see* Glomerulonephritis
    with edema —*see* Nephrosis
   interstitial nephritis N12

Disease, diseased *(Continued)*
 renal *(Continued)*
  acute N28.9
  chronic —*see also* Disease, kidney, chronic
   N18.9
  cystic, congenital Q61.9
  diabetic —*see* E08-E13 with .22
  end-stage (failure) N18.6
   due to hypertension I12.0
  fibrocystic (congenital) Q61.8
  hypertensive —*see* Hypertension, kidney
  lupus M32.14
  phosphate-losing (tubular) N25.0
  polycystic (congenital) Q61.3
   adult type Q61.2
   childhood type NEC Q61.19
    collecting duct dilatation Q61.11
  rapidly progressive N01.9
  subacute N01.9
 Rendu-Osler-Weber (familial hemorrhagic
  telangiectasia) I78.0
 renovascular (arteriosclerotic) —*see*
  Hypertension, kidney
 respiratory (tract) J98.9
  acute or subacute NOS J06.9
   due to
    chemicals, gases, fumes or vapors
     (inhalation) J68.3
    external agent J70.9
     specified NEC J70.8
    radiation J70.0
    smoke inhalation J70.5
   noninfectious J39.8
  chronic NOS J98.9
   due to
    chemicals, gases, fumes or vapors J68.4
    external agent J70.9
     specified NEC J70.8
    radiation J70.1
   newborn P27.9
    specified NEC P27.8
  due to
   chemicals, gases, fumes or vapors J68.9
    acute or subacute NEC J68.3
    chronic J68.4
   external agent J70.9
    specified NEC J70.8
  newborn P28.9
   specified type NEC P28.89
  upper J39.9
   acute or subacute J06.9
   noninfectious NEC J39.8
   specified NEC J39.8
   streptococcal J06.9
 retina, retinal H35.9
  Batten's or Batten-Mayou E75.4 [*H36.89*]
  specified NEC H35.89
 rheumatoid —*see* Arthritis, rheumatoid
 rickettsial NOS A79.9
  specified type NEC A79.89
 Riga (-Fede) (cachectic aphthae) K14.0
 Riggs' (compound periodontitis) —*see*
  Periodontitis
 Ritter's L00
 Rivalta's (cervicofacial actinomycosis) A42.2
 rod body G71.21
 Robles' (onchocerciasis) B73.01
 Roger's (congenital interventricular septal
  defect) Q21.0
 Rosenthal's (factor XI deficiency) D68.1
 Ross River B33.1
 Rossbach's (hyperchlorhydria) K31.89
  psychogenic F45.8
 Rotes Quérol —*see* Hyperostosis, ankylosing
 Roth (-Bernhardt) —*see* Mononeuropathy, lower
  limb, meralgia paresthetica
 Runeberg's (progressive pernicious anemia)
  D51.0
 sacroiliac NEC M53.3
 salivary gland or duct K11.9
  inclusion B25.9
  specified NEC K11.8
  virus B25.9
 sandworm B76.9
 Schimmelbusch's —*see* Mastopathy, cystic
 Schmorl's —*see* Schmorl's disease or nodes
 Schönlein (-Henoch) (purpura rheumatica)
  D69.0
 Schottmüller's —*see* Fever, paratyphoid
 Schultz's (agranulocytosis) —*see*
  Agranulocytosis
 Schwalbe-Ziehen-Oppenheim G24.1

▶ New   ⇒ Revised   ~~deleted~~ Deleted   ● Use Additional Character(s)

Disorder *(Continued)*
  adrenogenital *(see also* Adrenogenital syndrome)
      E25.9
    drug-induced E25.8
    iatrogenic E25.8
    idiopathic E25.8
  adult personality (and behavior) F69
    specified NEC F68.8
  affective (mood) —*see* Disorder, mood
  aggressive, unsocialized F91.1
  alcohol-related F10.99
    with
      amnestic disorder, persisting F10.96
      anxiety disorder F10.980
      dementia, persisting F10.97
      intoxication F10.929
        with delirium F10.921
        uncomplicated F10.920
      mood disorder F10.94
      other specified F10.988
      psychotic disorder F10.959
        with
          delusions F10.950
          hallucinations F10.951
      sexual dysfunction F10.981
      sleep disorder F10.982
  alcohol use
    mild F10.10
      with
        alcohol-induced
          anxiety disorder F10.180
          bipolar and related disorder F10.14
          depressive disorder F10.14
          psychotic disorder F10.159
          sexual dysfunction F10.181
          sleep disorder F10.182
        alcohol intoxication F10.129
          delirium F10.121
      in remission (early) (sustained) F10.11
    moderate or severe F10.20
      with
        alcohol-induced
          anxiety disorder F10.280
          bipolar and related disorder F10.24
          depressive disorder F10.24
          major neurocognitive disorder,
              amnestic-confabulatory type
              F10.26
          major neurocognitive disorder,
              nonamnestic-confabulatory type
              F10.27
          mild neurocognitive disorder F10.288
          psychotic disorder F10.259
          sexual dysfunction F10.281
          sleep disorder F10.282
        alcohol intoxication F10.229
          delirium F10.221
      in remission (early) (sustained) F10.21
  allergic —*see* Allergy
  alveolar NEC J84.09
  amino-acid
    cystathioninuria E72.19
    cystinosis E72.04
    cystinuria E72.01
    glycinuria E72.09
    homocystinuria E72.11
    metabolism —*see* Disturbance,
        metabolism, amino-acid
      specified NEC E72.89
    neonatal, transitory P74.8
    renal transport NEC E72.09
    transport NEC E72.09
  amnesic, amnestic
    alcohol-induced F10.96
      with dependence F10.26
    due to (secondary to) general medical
        condition F04
    psychoactive NEC-induced F19.96
      with
        abuse F19.16
        dependence F19.26
    sedative, hypnotic or anxiolytic-•
        induced F13.96
      with dependence F13.26
  amphetamine-type substance use
    mild F15.10
      in remission (early) (sustained) F15.11
    moderate F15.20
      in remission (early) (sustained) F15.21
    severe F15.20
      in remission (early) (sustained) F15.21

Disorder *(Continued)*
  amphetamine (or other stimulant) use
    mild
      with
        amphetamine (or other stimulant)
            -induced
          anxiety disorder F15.180
          bipolar and related disorder F15.14
          depressive disorder F15.14
          obsessive-compulsive and related
              disorder F15.188
          psychotic disorder F15.159
          sexual dysfunction F15.181
        amphetamine, cocaine, or other
            stimulant intoxication
          with perceptual disturbances F15.122
          without perceptual disturbances F15.129
        intoxication delirium F15.121
    moderate or severe
      with
        amphetamine (or other stimulant)
            -induced
          anxiety disorder F15.280
          obsessive-compulsive and related
              disorder F15.288
          sexual dysfunction F15.281
          bipolar and related disorder F15.24
          depressive disorder F15.24
          psychotic disorder F15.259
        amphetamine, cocaine, or other
            stimulant intoxication
          with perceptual disturbances F15.222
          without perceptual disturbances
              F15.229
        intoxication delirium F15.221
  anaerobic glycolysis with anemia D55.29
  anxiety F41.9
    due to (secondary to)
      alcohol F10.980
        in
          abuse F10.180
          dependence F10.280
      amphetamine F15.980
        in
          abuse F15.180
          dependence F15.280
      anxiolytic F13.980
        in
          abuse F13.180
          dependence F13.280
      caffeine F15.980
        in
          abuse F15.180
          dependence F15.280
      cannabis F12.980
        in
          abuse F12.180
          dependence F12.280
      cocaine F14.980
        in
          abuse F14.180
          dependence F14.180
      general medical condition F06.4
      hallucinogen F16.980
        in
          abuse F16.180
          dependence F16.280
      hypnotic F13.980
        in
          abuse F13.180
          dependence F13.280
      inhalant F18.980
        in
          abuse F18.180
          dependence F18.280
      phencyclidine F16.980
        in
          abuse F16.180
          dependence F16.280
      psychoactive substance NEC F19.980
        in
          abuse F19.180
          dependence F19.280
      sedative F13.980
        in
          abuse F13.180
          dependence F13.280
      volatile solvents F18.980
        in
          abuse F18.180
          dependence F18.280

Disorder *(Continued)*
  anxiety *(Continued)*
    generalized F41.1
    illness F45.21
    mixed
      with depression (mild) F41.8
      specified NEC F41.3
    organic F06.4
    phobic F40.9
      of childhood F40.8
    specified NEC F41.8
  aortic valve —*see* Endocarditis, aortic
  aromatic amino-acid metabolism E70.9
    specified NEC E70.89
  arteriole NEC I77.89
  artery NEC I77.89
  articulation —*see* Disorder, joint
  attachment (childhood)
    disinhibited F94.2
    reactive F94.1
  attention-deficit hyperactivity (adolescent)
      (adult) (child) F98.8
    combined
      presentation F90.2
      type F90.2
    hyperactive
      impulsive presentation F90.1
      type F90.1
    inattentive
      presentation F90.0
      type F90.0
    specified type NEC F90.8
  attention-deficit without hyperactivity
      (adolescent) (adult) (child) F90.0
  auditory processing (central) H93.25
  autism spectrum F84.0
  autistic F84.0
  autoimmune D89.89
  autonomic nervous system G90.9
    specified NEC G90.89
  avoidant
    child or adolescent F40.10
    restrictive food intake F50.82
  balance
    acid-base E87.8
      mixed E87.4
    electrolyte E87.8
    fluid NEC E87.8
  behavioral (disruptive) —*see* Disorder, conduct
  bereavement, persistent complex F43.81
  beta-amino-acid metabolism E72.89
  bile acid and cholesterol metabolism E78.70
    Barth syndrome E78.71
    other specified E78.79
    Smith-Lemli-Opitz syndrome E78.72
  bilirubin excretion E80.6
  binge eating F50.81-•
  binocular
    movement H51.9
      convergence
        excess H51.12
        insufficiency H51.11
      internuclear ophthalmoplegia —*see*
          Ophthalmoplegia, internuclear
      palsy of conjugate gaze H51.0
      specified type NEC H51.8
    vision NEC —*see* Disorder, vision, binocular
  bipolar (I) (seasonal) (type 1) F31.9
    and related due to a known physiological
        condition
      with
        manic features F06.33
        manic- or hypomanic-like episodes F06.33
        mixed features F06.34
    current (or most recent) episode
      depressed F31.9
        with psychotic features F31.5
        without psychotic features F31.30
          mild F31.31
          moderate F31.32
          severe (without psychotic features)
              F31.4
            with psychotic features F31.5
      hypomanic F31.0
      manic F31.9
        with psychotic features F31.2
        without psychotic features F31.10
          mild F31.11
          moderate F31.12
          severe (without psychotic features)
              F31.13
            with psychotic features F31.2

▶ New   ⇥ Revised   ~~deleted~~ Deleted   ● Use Additional Character(s)

▶ New   ➡ Revised   ~~deleted~~ Deleted   • Use Additional Character(s)

▶ New   ⇨ Revised   ~~deleted~~ Deleted   • Use Additional Character(s)

▶ New   ⬛ Revised   ~~deleted~~ Deleted   • Use Additional Character(s)

Distortion *(Continued)*
    bladder Q64.79
    brain Q04.9
    cervix (uteri) Q51.9
    chest (wall) Q67.8
        bones Q76.8
    clavicle Q74.0
    clitoris Q52.6
    coccyx Q76.49
    common duct Q44.5
    coronary Q24.5
    cystic duct Q44.5
    ear (auricle) (external) Q17.3
        inner Q16.5
        middle Q16.4
            ossicles Q16.3
    endocrine NEC Q89.2
    eustachian tube Q17.8
    eye (adnexa) Q15.8
    face bone(s) NEC Q75.8
    fallopian tube Q50.6
    femur NEC Q68.8
    fibula NEC Q68.8
    finger(s) Q68.1
    foot Q66.9- ●
    genitalia, genital organ(s)
        female Q52.8
            external Q52.79
            internal NEC Q52.8
    gyri Q04.8
    hand bone(s) Q68.1
    heart (auricle) (ventricle) Q24.8
        valve (cusp) Q24.8
    hepatic duct Q44.5
    humerus NEC Q68.8
    hymen Q52.4
    intrafamilial communications Z63.8
    jaw NEC M26.89
    labium (majus) (minus) Q52.79
    leg NEC Q68.8
    lens Q12.8
    liver Q44.79
    lumbar spine Q76.49
        with disproportion O33.8
            causing obstructed labor O65.0
    lumbosacral (joint) (region) Q76.49
        kyphosis —*see* Kyphosis, congenital
        lordosis —*see* Lordosis, congenital
    nerve Q07.8
    nose Q30.8
    organ
        of Corti Q16.5
        or site not listed —*see* Anomaly, by site
            ossicles, ear Q16.3
    oviduct Q50.6
    pancreas Q45.3
    parathyroid (gland) Q89.2
    pituitary (gland) Q89.2
    radius NEC Q68.8
    sacroiliac joint Q74.2
    sacrum Q76.49
    scapula Q74.0
    shoulder girdle Q74.0
    skull bone(s) NEC Q75.8
        with
            anencephalus Q00.0
            encephalocele —*see* Encephalocele
            hydrocephalus Q03.9
                with spina bifida —*see* Spina bifida, with
                    hydrocephalus
            microcephaly Q02
    spinal cord Q06.8
    spine Q76.49
        kyphosis —*see* Kyphosis, congenital
        lordosis —*see* Lordosis, congenital
    spleen Q89.09
    sternum NEC Q76.7
    thorax (wall) Q67.8
        bony Q76.8
    thymus (gland) Q89.2
    thyroid (gland) Q89.2
    tibia NEC Q68.8
    toe(s) Q66.9- ●
    tongue Q38.3
    trachea (cartilage) Q32.1
    ulna NEC Q68.8
    ureter Q62.8
    urethra Q64.79
        causing obstruction Q64.39
    uterus Q51.9
    vagina Q52.4

Distortion *(Continued)*
    vertebra Q76.49
        kyphosis —*see* Kyphosis, congenital
        lordosis —*see* Lordosis, congenital
    visual —*see also* Disturbance, vision
        shape and size H53.15
    vulva Q52.79
    wrist (bones) (joint) Q68.8
Distress
    abdomen —*see* Pain, abdominal
    acute respiratory R06.03
        syndrome (adult) (child) J80
    epigastric R10.13
    fetal P84
        complicating pregnancy —*see* Stress, fetal
    gastrointestinal (functional) K30
        psychogenic F45.8
    intestinal (functional) NOS K59.9
        psychogenic F45.8
    maternal, during labor and delivery O75.0
    relationship, with spouse or intimate partner
        Z63.0
    respiratory (adult) (child) R06.03
        newborn P22.9
            specified NEC P22.8
        orthopnea R06.01
        psychogenic F45.8
        shortness of breath R06.02
        specified type NEC R06.09
Distribution vessel, atypical Q27.9
    coronary artery Q24.5
    precerebral Q28.1
Districhiasis L68.8
Disturbance(s) —*see also* Disease
    absorption K90.9
        calcium E58
        carbohydrate K90.49
        fat K90.49
            pancreatic K90.3
        protein K90.49
        starch K90.49
        vitamin —*see* Deficiency, vitamin
    acid-base equilibrium E87.8
        mixed E87.4
    activity and attention (with hyperkinesis) —*see*
        Disorder, attention-deficit hyperactivity
    amino acid transport E72.00
    assimilation, food K90.9
    auditory nerve, except deafness —*see*
        subcategory H93.3
    behavior —*see* Disorder, conduct
    blood clotting (mechanism) —*see also* Defect,
        coagulation D68.9
    cerebral
        nerve —*see* Disorder, nerve, cranial
        status, newborn P91.9
            specified NEC P91.88
    circulatory I99.9
    conduct —*see also* Disorder, conduct F91.9
        adjustment reaction —*see* Disorder,
            adjustment
        compulsive F63.9
        disruptive F91.9
        hyperkinetic —*see* Disorder, attention-deficit
            hyperactivity
        socialized F91.2
        specified NEC F91.8
        unsocialized F91.1
    coordination R27.8
    cranial nerve —*see* Disorder, nerve, cranial
    deep sensibility —*see* Disturbance, sensation
    digestive K30
        psychogenic F45.8
    electrolyte —*see also* Imbalance, electrolyte
        newborn, transitory P74.49
            hyperammonemia P74.6
            hyperchloremia P74.421
            hyperchloremic metabolic acidosis P74.421
            hypochloremia P74.422
            potassium balance
                hyperkalemia P74.31
                hypokalemia P74.32
            sodium balance
                hypernatremia P74.21
                hyponatremia P74.22
            specified type NEC P74.49
    emotions specific to childhood and adolescence
        F93.9
        with
            anxiety and fearfulness NEC F93.8
            elective mutism F94.0

Disturbance *(Continued)*
    emotions specific to childhood and adolescence
        (Continued)
        with *(Continued)*
            oppositional disorder F91.3
            sensitivity (withdrawal) F40.10
            shyness F40.10
            social withdrawal F40.10
        involving relationship problems F93.8
        mixed F93.8
        specified NEC F93.8
    endocrine (gland) E34.9
        neonatal, transitory P72.9
            specified NEC P72.8
    equilibrium R42
    fructose metabolism E74.10
    gait —*see* Gait
        hysterical F44.4
        psychogenic F44.4
    gastrointestinal (functional) K30
        psychogenic F45.8
    habit, child F98.9
    hearing, except deafness and tinnitus —*see*
        Abnormal, auditory perception
    heart, functional (conditions in I44-I50)
        due to presence of (cardiac) prosthesis
            I97.19- ●
        ▶other surgery I97.191
        postoperative I97.89
            cardiac surgery —*see also* Infarct,
                myocardium, associated with
                ▸revascularization procedure I97.190 - ●
    hormones E34.9
    innervation uterus (parasympathetic)
        (sympathetic) N85.8
    keratinization NEC
        gingiva K05.10
            nonplaque induced K05.11
            plaque induced K05.10
        lip K13.0
        oral (mucosa) (soft tissue) K13.29
        tongue K13.29
    learning (specific) —*see* Disorder, learning
    memory —*see* Amnesia
        mild, following organic brain damage F06.8
    mental F99
        associated with diseases classified elsewhere
            F54
    metabolism E88.9
        with
            abortion —*see* Abortion, by type with other
                specified complication
            ectopic pregnancy O08.5
            molar pregnancy O08.5
        amino-acid E72.9
            aromatic E70.9
            branched-chain E71.2
            straight-chain E72.89
            sulfur-bearing E72.10
        ammonia E72.20
        arginine E72.21
        arginosuccinic acid E72.22
        carbohydrate E74.9
        cholesterol E78.9
        citrulline E72.23
        cystathionine E72.19
        general E88.9
        glutamine E72.89
        histidine E70.40
        homocystine E72.19
        hydroxylysine E72.3
        in labor or delivery O75.89
        iron E83.10
        lipoid E78.9
        lysine E72.3
        methionine E72.19
        neonatal, transitory P74.9
            calcium and magnesium P71.9
                specified type NEC P71.8
            carbohydrate metabolism P70.9
                specified type NEC P70.8
            specified NEC P74.8
        ornithine E72.4
        phosphate E83.39
        sodium NEC E87.8
        threonine E72.89
        tryptophan E70.5
        tyrosine E70.20
        urea cycle E72.20
    motor R29.2
    nervous, functional R45.0

Disturbance *(Continued)*
- neuromuscular mechanism (eye), due to syphilis A52.15
- nutritional E63.9
  - nail L60.3
- ocular motion H51.9
  - psychogenic F45.8
- oculogyric H51.8
  - psychogenic F45.8
- oculomotor H51.9
  - psychogenic F45.8
- olfactory nerve R43.1
- optic nerve NEC —*see* Disorder, nerve, optic
- oral epithelium, including tongue NEC K13.29
- perceptual due to
  - alcohol withdrawal F10.232
  - amphetamine intoxication F15.922
    - in
      - abuse F15.122
      - dependence F15.222
  - anxiolytic withdrawal F13.232
  - cannabis intoxication (acute) F12.922
    - in
      - abuse F12.122
      - dependence F12.222
  - cocaine intoxication (acute) F14.922
    - in
      - abuse F14.122
      - dependence F14.222
  - hypnotic withdrawal F13.232
  - opioid intoxication (acute) F11.922
    - in
      - abuse F11.122
      - dependence F11.222
  - phencyclidine intoxication (acute) F16.122
  - sedative withdrawal F13.232
- personality (pattern) (trait) —*see also* Disorder, personality F60.9
- following organic brain damage F07.9
- polyglandular E31.9
  - specified NEC E31.8
- potassium balance, newborn
  - hyperkalemia P74.31
  - hypokalemia P74.32
- psychogenic F45.9
- psychomotor F44.4
- psychophysical visual H53.16
- pupillary —*see* Anomaly, pupil, function
- reflex R29.2
- rhythm, heart I49.9
- salivary secretion K11.7
- sensation (cold) (heat) (localization) (tactile discrimination) (texture) (vibratory) NEC R20.9
  - hysterical F44.6
  - skin R20.9
    - anesthesia R20.0
    - hyperesthesia R20.3
    - hypoesthesia R20.1
    - paresthesia R20.2
    - specified type NEC R20.8
  - smell R43.9
    - and taste (mixed) R43.8
    - anosmia R43.0
    - parosmia R43.1
    - specified NEC R43.8
  - taste R43.9
    - and smell (mixed) R43.8
    - parageusia R43.2
    - specified NEC R43.8
- sensory —*see* Disturbance, sensation
- situational (transient) —*see also* Disorder, adjustment
  - acute F43.0
- sleep G47.9
  - nonorganic origin F51.9
- smell —*see* Disturbance, sensation, smell
- sociopathic F60.2
- sodium balance, newborn
  - hypernatremia P74.21
  - hyponatremia P74.22
- speech R47.9
  - developmental F80.9
  - specified NEC R47.89
- stomach (functional) K31.9
- sympathetic (nerve) G90.9
- taste —*see* Disturbance, sensation, taste
- temperature
  - regulation, newborn P81.9
    - specified NEC P81.8
  - sense R20.8
    - hysterical F44.6

Disturbance *(Continued)*
- tooth
  - eruption K00.6
  - formation K00.4
  - structure, hereditary NEC K00.5
- touch —*see* Disturbance, sensation
- vascular I99.9
  - arteriosclerotic —*see* Arteriosclerosis
- vasomotor I73.9
- vasospastic I73.9
- vision, visual H53.9
  - following
    - cerebral infarction I69.398
    - cerebrovascular disease I69.998
      - specified NEC I69.898
    - intracerebral hemorrhage I69.198
    - nontraumatic intracranial hemorrhage NEC I69.298
    - specified disease NEC I69.898
    - subarachnoid hemorrhage I69.098
  - psychophysical H53.16
  - specified NEC H53.8
  - subjective H53.10
    - day blindness H53.11
    - discomfort H53.14-●
    - distortions of shape and size H53.15
    - loss
      - sudden H53.13-●
      - transient H53.12-●
    - specified type NEC H53.19
- voice R49.9
  - psychogenic F44.4
  - specified NEC R49.8

Diuresis R35.89
Diver's palsy, paralysis or squeeze T70.3
Diverticulitis (acute) K57.92
- bladder —*see* Cystitis
- ileum —*see* Diverticulitis, intestine, small
- intestine K57.92
  - with
    - abscess, perforation K57.80
      - with bleeding K57.81
    - bleeding K57.93
  - congenital Q43.8
  - large K57.32
    - with
      - abscess, perforation K57.20
        - with bleeding K57.21
      - bleeding K57.33
      - small intestine K57.52
        - with
          - abscess, perforation K57.40
            - with bleeding K57.41
          - bleeding K57.53
  - small K57.12
    - with
      - abscess, perforation K57.00
        - with bleeding K57.01
      - bleeding K57.13
      - large intestine K57.52
        - with
          - abscess, perforation K57.40
            - with bleeding K57.41
          - bleeding K57.53

Diverticulosis K57.90
- with bleeding K57.91
- large intestine K57.30
  - with
    - bleeding K57.31
    - small intestine K57.50
      - with bleeding K57.51
- small intestine K57.10
  - with
    - bleeding K57.11
    - large intestine K57.50
      - with bleeding K57.51

Diverticulum, diverticula (multiple) K57.90
- appendix (noninflammatory) K38.2
- bladder (sphincter) N32.3
  - congenital Q64.6
- bronchus (congenital) Q32.4
  - acquired J98.09
- calyx, calyceal (kidney) N28.89
- cardia (stomach) K31.4
- cecum —*see* Diverticulosis, intestine, large
  - congenital Q43.8
- colon —*see* Diverticulosis, intestine, large
  - congenital Q43.8
- duodenum —*see* Diverticulosis, intestine, small
  - congenital Q43.8
- epiphrenic (esophagus) K22.5

Diverticulum, diverticula *(Continued)*
- esophagus (congenital) Q39.6
  - acquired (epiphrenic) (pulsion) (traction) K22.5
- eustachian tube —*see* Disorder, eustachian tube, specified NEC
- fallopian tube N83.8
- gastric K31.4
- heart (congenital) Q24.8
- ileum —*see* Diverticulosis, intestine, small
- jejunum —*see* Diverticulosis, intestine, small
- kidney (pelvis) (calyces) N28.89
  - with calculus —*see* Calculus, kidney
- Meckel's (displaced) (hypertrophic) Q43.0
  - malignant —*see* Table of Neoplasms, small intestine, malignant
- midthoracic K22.5
- organ or site, congenital NEC —*see* Distortion
- pericardium (congenital) (cyst) Q24.8
  - acquired I31.8
- pharyngoesophageal (congenital) Q39.6
  - acquired K22.5
- pharynx (congenital) Q38.7
- rectosigmoid —*see* Diverticulosis, intestine, large
  - congenital Q43.8
- rectum —*see* Diverticulosis, intestine, large
- Rokitansky's K22.5
- seminal vesicle N50.89
- sigmoid —*see* Diverticulosis, intestine, large
  - congenital Q43.8
- stomach (acquired) K31.4
  - congenital Q40.2
- trachea (acquired) J39.8
- ureter (acquired) N28.89
  - congenital Q62.8
- ureterovesical orifice N28.89
- urethra (acquired) N36.1
  - congenital Q64.79
- ventricle, left (congenital) Q24.8
- vesical N32.3
  - congenital Q64.6
- Zenker's (esophagus) K22.5

Division
- cervix uteri (acquired) N88.8
- glans penis Q55.69
- labia minora (congenital) Q52.79
- ligament (partial or complete) (current) —*see also* Sprain
  - with open wound —*see* Wound, open
- muscle (partial or complete) (current) —*see also* Injury, muscle
  - with open wound —*see* Wound, open
- nerve (traumatic) —*see* Injury, nerve
- spinal cord —*see* Injury, spinal cord, by region
- vein I87.8

Divorce, causing family disruption Z63.5
Dix-Hallpike neurolabyrinthitis —*see* Neuronitis, vestibular
Dizziness R42
- hysterical F44.89
- psychogenic F45.8
DMAC (disseminated mycobacterium avium-intracellulare complex) A31.2
DNR (do not resuscitate) Z66
Doan-Wiseman syndrome (primary splenic neutropenia) —*see* Agranulocytosis
Doehle-Heller aortitis A52.02
Dog bite —*see* Bite
Dohle body panmyelopathic syndrome D72.0
Dolichocephaly Q67.2
- non-deformational Q75.01
Dolichocolon Q43.8
Dolichostenomelia —*see* Syndrome, Marfan
Donohue's syndrome E34.8
Donor (organ or tissue) Z52.9
- blood (whole) Z52.000
  - autologous Z52.010
  - specified component (lymphocytes) (platelets) NEC Z52.008
    - autologous Z52.018
    - specified donor NEC Z52.098
  - specified donor NEC Z52.090
  - stem cells Z52.001
    - autologous Z52.011
    - specified donor NEC Z52.091
- bone Z52.20
  - autologous Z52.21
  - marrow Z52.3
  - specified type NEC Z52.29
- cornea Z52.5

▶ New   ⏵ Revised   ~~deleted~~ Deleted   ● Use Additional Character(s)

Dysbetalipoproteinemia (familial) E78.2
Dyscalculia R48.8
  developmental F81.2
Dyschezia K59.00
Dyschondroplasia (with hemangiomata) Q78.4
Dyschromia (skin) L81.9
Dyscollagenosis M35.9
Dyscranio-pygo-phalangy Q87.0
Dyscrasia
  blood (with) D75.9
    antepartum hemorrhage —*see* Hemorrhage,
      antepartum, with coagulation defect
    intrapartum hemorrhage O67.0
    newborn P61.9
      specified type NEC P61.8
    puerperal, postpartum O72.3
  polyglandular, pluriglandular E31.9
Dysendocrinism E34.9
Dysentery, dysenteric (catarrhal) (diarrhea)
    (epidemic) (hemorrhagic) (infectious)
    (sporadic) (tropical) A09
  abscess, liver A06.4
  amebic —*see also* Amebiasis A06.0
    with abscess —*see* Abscess, amebic
    acute A06.0
    chronic A06.1
  arthritis —*see also* category M01 A09
    bacillary —*see also* category M01 A03.9
  bacillary A03.9
    arthritis —*see also* category M01 A03.9
    Boyd A03.2
    Flexner A03.1
    Schmitz (-Stutzer) A03.0
    Shiga (-Kruse) A03.0
    Shigella A03.9
      boydii A03.2
      dysenteriae A03.0
      flexneri A03.1
      group A A03.0
      group B A03.1
      group C A03.2
      group D A03.3
      sonnei A03.3
      specified type NEC A03.8
    Sonne A03.3
    specified type NEC A03.8
  balantidial A07.0
  Balantidium coli A07.0
  Boyd's A03.2
  candidal B37.82
  Chilomastix A07.8
  Chinese A03.9
  coccidial A07.3
  Dientamoeba (fragilis) A07.8
  Embadomonas A07.8
  Entamoeba, entamebic —*see* Dysentery, amebic
  Flexner-Boyd A03.2
  Flexner's A03.1
  Giardia lamblia A07.1
  Hiss-Russell A03.1
  Lamblia A07.1
  leishmanial B55.0
  malarial —*see* Malaria
  metazoal B82.0
  monilial B37.82
  protozoal A07.9
  Salmonella A02.0
  schistosomal B65.1
  Schmitz (-Stutzer) A03.0
  Shiga (-Kruse) A03.0
  Shigella NOS —*see* Dysentery, bacillary
  Sonne A03.3
  strongyloidiasis B78.0
  trichomonal A07.8
  viral —*see also* Enteritis, viral A08.4
Dysequilibrium R42
Dysesthesia R20.8
  hysterical F44.6
Dysferlinopathy G71.033
Dysfibrinogenemia (congenital) D68.2
Dysfunction
  adrenal E27.9
    hyperfunction E27.0
  autonomic
    due to alcohol G31.2
    somatoform F45.8
  bladder N31.9
    neurogenic NOS —*see* Dysfunction, bladder,
      neuromuscular
    neuromuscular NOS N31.9
      atonic (motor) (sensory) N31.2
      autonomous N31.2
      flaccid N31.2

Dysfunction (Continued)
  bladder N31.9 (Continued)
    neuromuscular NOS (Continued)
      nonreflex N31.2
      reflex N31.1
      specified NEC N31.8
      uninhibited N31.0
  bleeding, uterus N93.8
  cerebral G93.89
  chronic
    coronary microvascular I25.85
    lung allograft J4A.9
      mixed J4A.0
      specified NEC J4A.8
  colon K59.9
    psychogenic F45.8
  colostomy K94.03
  coronary microvascular I25.85
    with
      angina pectoris I20.81
      myocardial infarction I21.B
    acute I24.81
    chronic I25.85
  cystic duct K82.8
  cystostomy (stoma) —*see* Complications,
    cystostomy
  ejaculatory N53.19
    anejaculatory orgasm N53.13
    painful N53.12
    premature F52.4
    retarded N53.11
  endocrine NOS E34.9
  endometrium N85.8
  enterostomy K94.13
  erectile —*see* Dysfunction, sexual, male, erectile
  feeding, pediatric
    acute R63.31
    chronic R63.32
  gallbladder K82.8
  gastrostomy (stoma) K94.23
  gland, glandular NOS E34.9
    meibomian, of eyelid —*see* Dysfunction,
      meibomian gland
  heart I51.89
  hemoglobin D75.89
  hepatic K76.89
  hypophysis E23.7
  hypothalamic NEC E23.3
  ileostomy (stoma) K94.13
  jejunostomy (stoma) K94.13
  kidney —*see* Disease, renal
  labyrinthine —*see* subcategory H83.2
  left ventricular, following sudden emotional
    stress I51.81
  liver K76.89
  ► lymphatic
    ► Fontan-associated I27.841
  male —*see* Dysfunction, sexual, male
  meibomian gland, of eyelid H02.889
    left H02.886
      lower H02.885
      upper H02.884
      upper and lower eyelids H02.88B
    right H02.883
      lower H02.882
      upper H02.881
      upper and lower eyelids H02.88A
  multifidus muscles, lumbar region M62.85
  orgasmic (female) F52.31
    male F52.32
  ovary E28.9
    specified NEC E28.8
  papillary muscle I51.89
  parathyroid E21.4
  physiological NEC R68.89
    psychogenic F59
  pineal gland E34.8
  pituitary (gland) E23.3
  platelets D69.1
  polyglandular E31.9
    specified NEC E31.8
  psychophysiologic F59
  psychosexual F52.9
    with
      dyspareunia F52.6
      premature ejaculation F52.4
      vaginismus F52.5
  pylorus K31.9
  rectum K59.9
    psychogenic F45.8
  reflex (sympathetic) —*see* Syndrome, pain,
    complex regional I

Dysfunction (Continued)
  segmental —*see* Dysfunction, somatic
  senile R54
  sexual (due to) R37
    alcohol F10.981
    amphetamine F15.981
      in
        abuse F15.181
        dependence F15.281
    anxiolytic F13.981
      in
        abuse F13.181
        dependence F13.281
    cocaine F14.981
      in
        abuse F14.181
        dependence F14.281
    excessive sexual drive F52.8
    failure of genital response (male) F52.21
    female F52.22
    female N94.9
      aversion F52.1
      dyspareunia N94.10
        psychogenic F52.6
      frigidity F52.22
      nymphomania F52.8
      orgasmic F52.31
      psychogenic F52.9
        aversion F52.1
        dyspareunia F52.6
        frigidity F52.22
        nymphomania F52.8
        orgasmic F52.31
        vaginismus F52.5
      vaginismus N94.2
        psychogenic F52.5
    hypnotic F13.981
      in
        abuse F13.181
        dependence F13.281
    inhibited orgasm (female) F52.31
      male F52.32
    lack
      of sexual enjoyment F52.1
      or loss of sexual desire F52.0
    male N53.9
      anejaculatory orgasm N53.13
      ejaculatory N53.19
        painful N53.12
        premature F52.4
        retarded N53.11
      erectile N52.9
        drug induced N52.2
        due to
          disease classified elsewhere N52.1
          drug N52.2
        postoperative (postprocedural) N52.39
          following
            cryotherapy N52.37
            interstitial seed therapy N52.36
            prostate ablative therapy N52.37
            prostatectomy N52.34
              radical N52.31
            radiation therapy N52.35
            radical cystectomy N52.32
            ultrasound ablative therapy
              N52.37
            urethral surgery N52.33
        psychogenic F52.21
        specified cause NEC N52.8
        vasculogenic
          arterial insufficiency N52.01
            with corporo-venous occlusive
              N52.03
          corporo-venous occlusive N52.02
            with arterial insufficiency N52.03
      impotence —*see* Dysfunction, sexual, male,
        erectile
      psychogenic F52.9
        aversion F52.1
        erectile F52.21
        orgasmic F52.32
        premature ejaculation F52.4
        satyriasis F52.8
        specified type NEC F52.8
      specified type NEC N53.8
    nonorganic F52.9
      specified NEC F52.8
    opioid F11.981
      in
        abuse F11.181
        dependence F11.281

▶ New   ⇒ Revised   ~~deleted~~ Deleted   ● Use Additional Character(s)

▶ New   ➡ Revised   ~~deleted~~ Deleted   • Use Additional Character(s)

▶ New　　⇨ Revised　　~~deleted~~ Deleted　　● Use Additional Character(s)

▶ New ⟹ Revised ~~deleted~~ Deleted ● Use Additional Character(s)

Encounter (Continued)
  observation (for) (ruled out)
    alarm, without findings
      apnea Z03.83
      bradycardia Z03.83
      oximeter Z03.83
    condition suspected related to home
      physiologic monitoring device
      Z03.83
    newborn Z05.81
      apnea alarm Z05.81
      bradycardia alarm Z05.81
      malfunction of home cardiorespiratory
        monitor Z05.81
      non-specific findings home physiologic
        monitoring device Z05.81
      pulse oximeter alarm without findings
        Z05.81
    exposure to (suspected)
      anthrax Z03.810
      biological agent NEC Z03.818
    malfunction of home cardiorespiratory
      monitor Z03.83
    non-specific findings home physiologic
      monitoring device Z03.83
  palliative care Z51.5
  pediatrician visit, by expectant parent(s)
    (adoptive) Z76.81
  placental sample (taken vaginally) —*see*
    also Encounter, antenatal screening
    Z36.9
  plastic and reconstructive surgery following
    medical procedure or healed injury NEC
    Z42.8
  postoperative —*see* Aftercare
  pregnancy
    supervision of —*see* Pregnancy, supervision of
    test Z32.00
      result negative Z32.02
      result positive Z32.01
  procreative management and counseling for
    gestational carrier Z31.7
  prophylactic measures Z29.9
    antivenin Z29.12
    fluoride administration Z29.3
    HIV pre-exposure Z29.81
    immunotherapy for respiratory syncytial
      virus (RSV) Z29.11
    rabies immune globin Z29.14
    Rho (D) immune globulin Z29.13
    specified NEC Z29.89
  radiation therapy (antineoplastic) Z51.0
  radiological (as part of a general medical
    examination) Z00.00
    with abnormal findings Z00.01
  reconstructive surgery following medical
    procedure or healed injury NEC Z42.8
  removal (of) —*see also* Removal
    artificial
      arm Z44.00-●
        complete Z44.01-●
        partial Z44.02-●
      eye Z44.2-●
      leg Z44.10-●
        complete Z44.11-●
        partial Z44.12-●
    breast implant Z45.81
      tissue expander (with or without
        synchronous insertion of permanent
        implant) Z45.81
    device Z46.9
      specified NEC Z46.89
    external
      fixation device — code to fracture with
        seventh character D
      prosthesis, prosthetic device Z44.9
        breast Z44.3-●
        specified NEC Z44.8
    implanted device NEC Z45.89
    insulin pump Z46.81
    internal fixation device Z47.2
    myringotomy device (stent) (tube) Z45.82
    nervous system device NEC Z46.2
      brain neuropacemaker Z46.2
      visual substitution device Z46.2
        implanted Z45.31
    non-vascular catheter Z46.82
    orthodontic device Z46.4
    stent
      ureteral Z46.6
    urinary device Z46.6

Encounter (Continued)
  repeat cervical smear to confirm findings of
    recent normal smear following initial
    abnormal smear Z01.42
  respirator [ventilator] use during power failure
    (Z99.12)
  Rh typing Z01.83
  screening —*see* Screening
  specified NEC Z76.89
  sterilization Z30.2
  suspected condition, ruled out
    amniotic cavity and membrane Z03.71
    cervical shortening Z03.75
    fetal anomaly Z03.73
    fetal growth Z03.74
    maternal and fetal conditions NEC Z03.79
    oligohydramnios Z03.71
    placental problem Z03.72
    polyhydramnios Z03.71
  suspected exposure (to), ruled out
    anthrax Z03.810
    biological agents NEC Z03.818
  termination of pregnancy, elective Z33.2
  testing —*see* Test
  therapeutic drug level monitoring Z51.81
  titration, insulin pump Z46.81
  to determine fetal viability of pregnancy O36.80
  training
    insulin pump Z46.81
  X-ray of chest (as part of a general medical
    examination) Z00.00
    with abnormal findings Z00.01

Encystment —*see* Cyst
Endarteritis (bacterial, subacute) (infective) I77.6
  brain I67.7
  cerebral or cerebrospinal I67.7
  deformans —*see* Arteriosclerosis
  embolic —*see* Embolism
  obliterans —*see also* Arteriosclerosis
    pulmonary I28.8
  pulmonary I28.8
  retina —*see* Vasculitis, retina
  senile —*see* Arteriosclerosis
  syphilitic A52.09
    brain or cerebral A52.04
    congenital A50.54 [I79.8]
  tuberculous A18.89
Endemic —*see* condition
Endocarditis (chronic) (marantic) (nonbacterial)
    (thrombotic) (valvular) I38
  with rheumatic fever (conditions in I00)
    active —*see* Endocarditis, acute, rheumatic
    inactive or quiescent (with chorea) I09.1
  acute or subacute I33.9
    infective I33.0
    rheumatic (aortic) (mitral) (pulmonary)
      (tricuspid) I01.1
      with chorea (acute) (rheumatic)
        (Sydenham's) I02.0
  aortic (heart) (nonrheumatic) (valve) I35.8
    with
      mitral disease I08.0
        with tricuspid (valve) disease I08.3
        active or acute I01.1
          with chorea (acute) (rheumatic)
            (Sydenham's) I02.0
      rheumatic fever (conditions in I00)
        active —*see* Endocarditis, acute, rheumatic
        inactive or quiescent (with chorea) I06.9
      tricuspid (valve) disease I08.2
        with mitral (valve) disease I08.3
    acute or subacute I33.9
    arteriosclerotic I35.8
    rheumatic I06.9
      with mitral disease I08.0
        with tricuspid (valve) disease I08.3
        active or acute I01.1
          with chorea (acute) (rheumatic)
            (Sydenham's) I02.0
      active or acute I01.1
        with chorea (acute) (rheumatic)
          (Sydenham's) I02.0
      specified NEC I06.8
    specified cause NEC I35.8
    syphilitic A52.03
  arteriosclerotic I38
  atypical verrucous (Libman-Sacks) M32.11
  bacterial (acute) (any valve) (subacute) I33.0
  candidal B37.6
  congenital Q24.8
  constrictive I33.0

Endocarditis (Continued)
  Coxiella burnetii A78 [I39]
  Coxsackie B33.21
  due to
    prosthetic cardiac valve T82.6
    Q fever A78 [I39]
    Serratia marcescens I33.0
    typhoid (fever) A01.02
  gonococcal A54.83
  infectious or infective (acute) (any valve)
    (subacute) I33.0
  lenta (acute) (any valve) (subacute) I33.0
  Libman-Sacks M32.11
  listerial A32.82
  Löffler's I42.3
  malignant (acute) (any valve) (subacute) I33.0
  meningococcal A39.51
  mitral (chronic) (double) (fibroid) (heart)
    (inactive) (valve) (with chorea) I05.9
    with
      aortic (valve) disease I08.0
        with tricuspid (valve) disease I08.3
        active or acute I01.1
          with chorea (acute) (rheumatic)
            (Sydenham's) I02.0
        rheumatic fever (conditions in I00)
          active —*see* Endocarditis, acute,
            rheumatic
          inactive or quiescent (with chorea) I05.9
      tricuspid (valve) disease I08.1
        with aortic (valve) disease I08.3
    active or acute I01.1
      with chorea (acute) (rheumatic)
        (Sydenham's) I02.0
      bacterial I33.0
    arteriosclerotic I34.89
    nonrheumatic I34.89
      acute or subacute I33.9
    specified NEC I05.8
  monilial B37.6
  multiple valves I08.9
    specified disorders I08.8
  mycotic (acute) (any valve) (subacute) I33.0
  pneumococcal (acute) (any valve) (subacute) I33.0
  pulmonary (chronic) (heart) (valve) I37.8
    with rheumatic fever (conditions in I00)
      active —*see* Endocarditis, acute, rheumatic
      inactive or quiescent (with chorea) I09.89
        with aortic, mitral or tricuspid disease
          I08.8
    acute or subacute I33.9
      rheumatic I01.1
        with chorea (acute) (rheumatic)
          (Sydenham's) I02.0
    arteriosclerotic I37.8
    congenital Q22.2
    rheumatic (chronic) (inactive) (with chorea)
      I09.89
      active or acute I01.1
        with chorea (acute) (rheumatic)
          (Sydenham's) I02.0
    syphilitic A52.03
  purulent (acute) (any valve) (subacute) I33.0
  Q fever A78 [I39]
  rheumatic (chronic) (inactive) (with chorea) I09.1
    active or acute (aortic) (mitral) (pulmonary)
      (tricuspid) I01.1
      with chorea (acute) (rheumatic)
        (Sydenham's) I02.0
  rheumatoid —*see* Rheumatoid, carditis
  septic (acute) (any valve) (subacute) I33.0
  streptococcal (acute) (any valve) (subacute)
    I33.0
  subacute —*see* Endocarditis, acute
  suppurative (acute) (any valve) (subacute) I33.0
  syphilitic A52.03
  toxic I33.9
  tricuspid (chronic) (heart) (inactive) (rheumatic)
    (valve) (with chorea) I07.9
    with
      aortic (valve) disease I08.2
        mitral (valve) disease I08.3
      mitral (valve) disease I08.1
        aortic (valve) disease I08.3
      rheumatic fever (conditions in I00)
        active —*see* Endocarditis, acute,
          rheumatic
        inactive or quiescent (with chorea) I07.8
    active or acute I01.1
      with chorea (acute) (rheumatic)
        (Sydenham's) I02.0

▶ New   ➡ Revised   ~~deleted~~ Deleted   ● Use Additional Character(s)

▶ New   ⇨ Revised   ~~deleted~~ Deleted   ● Use Additional Character(s)

Note: the following terms are to be considered
equivalent to intractable: pharmacoresistant
(pharmacologically resistant), treatment
resistant, refractory (medically) and poorly
controlled

▶ New   ➡ Revised   ~~deleted~~ Deleted   ● Use Additional Character(s)

Exposure *(Continued)*
    mold (toxic) Z77.120
    nickel dust Z77.018
    noise Z77.122
    occupational
        air contaminants NEC Z57.39
        dust Z57.2
        environmental tobacco smoke Z57.31
        extreme temperature Z57.6
        noise Z57.0
        radiation Z57.1
        risk factors Z57.9
            specified NEC Z57.8
        toxic agents (gases) (liquids) (solids) (vapors)
            in agriculture Z57.4
        toxic agents (gases) (liquids) (solids) (vapors)
            in industry NEC Z57.5
        vibration Z57.7
    parasitic disease NEC Z20.7
    pediculosis Z20.7
    persecution Z60.5
    pfiesteria piscicida Z77.121
    poliomyelitis Z20.89
    pollution
        air Z77.110
        environmental NEC Z77.118
        soil Z77.112
        water Z77.111
    polycyclic aromatic hydrocarbons Z77.028
    prenatal (drugs) (toxic chemicals) —see
        Newborn, affected by, noxious substances
        transmitted via placenta or breast milk
    rabies Z20.3
    radiation, naturally occurring NEC Z77.123
    radon Z77.123
    red tide (Florida) Z77.121
▶ risk factor, personal, to diethylstibestrol (DES)
        (in utero) Z91.B
    rubella Z20.4
    second hand tobacco smoke (acute) (chronic)
        Z77.22
        in the perinatal period P96.81
    sexually-transmitted disease Z20.2
    smallpox (laboratory) Z20.89
    syphilis Z20.2
    terrorism Z65.4
    torture Z65.4
    tuberculosis Z20.1
    uranium Z77.012
    varicella Z20.820
    venereal disease Z20.2
    viral disease NEC Z20.828
    war Z65.5
    water pollution Z77.111
        Zika virus Z20.821
Exsanguination —*see* Hemorrhage
Exstrophy
    abdominal contents Q45.8
    bladder Q64.10
        cloacal Q64.12
        specified type NEC Q64.19
        supravesical fissure Q64.11
Extensive —*see* condition
Extra —*see also* Accessory
    marker chromosomes (normal individual) Q92.61
        in abnormal individual Q92.62
    rib Q76.6
        cervical Q76.5
Extrasystoles (supraventricular) I49.49
    atrial I49.1
    auricular I49.1
    junctional I49.2
    ventricular I49.3
Extrauterine gestation or pregnancy —*see*
    Pregnancy, by site
Extravasation
    blood R58
    chyle into mesentery I89.8
    pelvicalyceal N13.8
    pyelosinus N13.8
    urine (from ureter) R39.0
    vesicant agent
        antineoplastic chemotherapy T80.810
        other agent NEC T80.818
Extremity —*see* condition, limb
Extrophy —*see* Exstrophy
Extroversion
    bladder Q64.19
    uterus N81.4
        complicating delivery O71.2
        postpartal (old) N81.4

Extruded tooth (teeth) M26.34
Extrusion
    breast implant (prosthetic) T85.42
    eye implant (globe) (ball) T85.328
    intervertebral disc —*see* Displacement,
        intervertebral disc
    ocular lens implant (prosthetic) —*see*
        Complications, intraocular lens
    vitreous —*see* Prolapse, vitreous
Exudate
    causing irritant dermatitis L24.A9
    pleural —*see* Effusion, pleura
    retina H35.89
    wound fluids causing irritant dermatitis L24.A9
Exudative —*see* condition
Eye, eyeball, eyelid —*see* condition
Eyestrain —*see* Disturbance, vision, subjective
Eyeworm disease of Africa B74.3

F

Faber's syndrome (achlorhydric anemia) D50.9
Fabry (-Anderson) **disease** E75.21
Facet syndrome M47.89-●
Faciocephalalgia, autonomic —*see also*
    Neuropathy, peripheral, autonomic G90.09
Factor(s)
    psychic, associated with diseases classified
        elsewhere F54
    psychological
        affecting physical conditions F54
        or behavioral
            affecting general medical condition F54
            associated with disorders or diseases
                classified elsewhere F54
Fahr disease (of brain) G23.8
Fahr Volhard disease (of kidney) I12.-●
Failure, failed
    abortion —*see* Abortion, attempted
    aortic (valve) I35.8
        rheumatic I06.8
    attempted abortion —*see* Abortion, attempted
    biventricular I50.82
        due to left heart failure I50.814
    bone marrow —*see* Anemia, aplastic
    cardiac —*see* Failure, heart
    cardiorenal (chronic) —*see also* Failure, renal,
        and Failure, heart I50.9
        hypertensive I13.2
    cardiorespiratory (*see also* Failure, heart) R09.2
    cardiovascular (chronic) —*see* Failure, heart
    cerebrovascular I67.9
    cervical dilatation in labor O62.0
    circulation, circulatory (peripheral) R57.9
        newborn P29.89
    compensation —*see* Disease, heart
    compliance with medical treatment or
        regimen —*see* Noncompliance
    congestive —*see* Failure, heart, congestive
    dental implant (endosseous) M27.69
        due to
            failure of dental prosthesis M27.63
            lack of attached gingiva M27.62
            occlusal trauma (poor prosthetic design)
                M27.62
            parafunctional habits M27.62
            periodontal infection (peri-implantitis) M27.62
            poor oral hygiene M27.62
        osseointegration M27.61
            due to
                complications of systemic disease M27.61
                poor bone quality M27.61
            iatrogenic M27.61
        post-osseointegration
            biological M27.62
            due to complications of systemic disease
                M27.62
            iatrogenic M27.62
            mechanical M27.63
        pre-integration M27.61
        pre-osseointegration M27.61
        specified NEC M27.69
    descent of head (at term) of pregnancy (mother)
        O32.4
    endosseous dental implant —*see* Failure, dental
        implant
    engagement of head (term of pregnancy)
        (mother) O32.4

Failure, failed *(Continued)*
    erection (penile) —*see also* Dysfunction, sexual,
        male, erectile N52.9
        nonorganic F52.21
    examination(s), anxiety concerning Z55.2
    expansion terminal respiratory units (newborn)
        (primary) P28.0
    forceps NOS (with subsequent cesarean
        delivery) O66.5
    gain weight (child over 28 days old) R62.51
        adult R62.7
        newborn P92.6
    genital response (male) F52.21
        female F52.22
    heart (acute) (senile) (sudden) I50.9
        with
            acute pulmonary edema —*see* Failure,
                ventricular, left
            decompensation I50.9
                with
                    normal ejection fraction I50.33
                    preserved ejection fraction I50.33
                    reduced ejection fraction I50.23
                        with diastolic dysfunction I50.43
                    combined systolic and diastolic
                        I50.43
                    diastolic I50.33
                    right I50.813
                    systolic I50.23
        dilatation —*see* Disease, heart
        hypertension —*see* Hypertension, heart
        normal ejection fraction —*see* Failure, heart,
            diastolic
        preserved ejection fraction —*see* Failure,
            heart, diastolic
        reduced ejection fraction —*see* Failure,
            heart, systolic
    arteriosclerotic I70.90
    biventricular I50.82
        due to left heart failure I50.814
    combined left-right sided I50.82
        due to left heart failure I50.814
    compensated —*see also* Failure, heart, by type
        as diastolic or systolic, chronic
        I50.9
    complicating
        anesthesia (general) (local) or other
            sedation
            in labor and delivery O74.2
            in pregnancy O29.12-●
            postpartum, puerperal O89.1
        delivery (cesarean) (instrumental) O75.4
    congestive I50.9
        with rheumatic fever (conditions in I00)
            active I01.8
            inactive or quiescent (with chorea) I09.81
        newborn P29.0
        rheumatic (chronic) (inactive) (with chorea)
            I09.81
            active or acute I01.8
                with chorea I02.0
    decompensated —*see also* Failure, heart, by
        type as diastolic or systolic, acute and
        chronic I50.9
    degenerative —*see* Degeneration, myocardial
    diastolic (congestive) (left ventricular) I50.30
        acute (congestive) I50.31
            and (on) chronic (congestive) I50.33
        chronic (congestive) I50.32
            and (on) acute (congestive) I50.33
        combined with systolic (congestive) I50.40
            acute (congestive) I50.41
                and (on) chronic (congestive) I50.43
            chronic (congestive) I50.42
                and (on) acute (congestive) I50.43
    due to presence of cardiac prosthesis I97.13-●
    end stage —*see also* Failure, heart, by type as
        diastolic or systolic, chronic I50.84
▶ following cardiac surgery I97.130
▶ following other surgery I97.131
    high output NOS I50.83
    hypertensive —*see* Hypertension, heart
    left (ventricular) —*see also* Failure, ventricular,
        left
        combined diastolic and systolic —*see*
            Failure, heart, diastolic, combined
            with systolic
        diastolic —*see* Failure, heart, diastolic
        systolic —*see* Failure, heart, systolic
    low output (syndrome) NOS I50.9
    newborn P29.0

▶ New   ⇒ Revised   ~~deleted~~ Deleted   ● Use Additional Character(s)

▶ New   ➡ Revised   ~~deleted~~ Deleted   ● Use Additional Character(s)

▶ New   ➡ Revised   ~~deleted~~ Deleted   • Use Additional Character(s)

Fistula *(Continued)*
pancreatic K86.89
pancreaticoduodenal K86.89
parotid (gland) K11.4
  region K12.2
penis N48.89
perianal K60.30
pericardium (pleura) (sac) —*see* Pericarditis
pericecal K63.2
perineorectal K60.40
perineosigmoidal K63.2
perineum, perineal (with urethral involvement)
    NEC N36.0
  tuberculous A18.13
  ureter N28.89
perirectal K60.40
  tuberculous A18.32
peritoneum K65.9
pharyngoesophageal J39.2
pharynx J39.2
  branchial cleft (congenital) Q18.0
pilonidal (infected) (rectum) —*see* Sinus, pilonidal
pleura, pleural, pleurocutaneous,
    pleuroperitoneal J86.0
  tuberculous NEC A15.6
pleuropericardial I31.8
portal vein-hepatic artery, congenital Q26.6
postauricular H70.81- •
postoperative, persistent T81.83
  specified site —*see* Fistula, by site
preauricular (congenital) Q18.1
prostate N42.89
pulmonary J86.0
  arteriovenous I28.0
    congenital Q25.72
  tuberculous —*see* Tuberculosis, pulmonary
pulmonoperitoneal J86.0
rectal (infectional) K60.40
  complex K60.429
    chronic K60.422
    initial K60.421
    new K60.421
    occurring following complete healing
      K60.423
    persistent K60.422
    recurrent K60.423
  extrasphincteric K60.42- •
  high intersphincteric K60.42- •
  low intersphincteric K60.41- •
  simple K60.419
    chronic K60.412
    initial K60.411
    new K60.411
    occurring following complete healing
      K60.413
    persistent K60.412
    recurrent K60.413
  superficial K60.41- •
  suprasphincteric K60.42- •
  transsphincteric K60.42- •
rectolabial N82.4
rectosigmoid (intercommunicating) K63.2
rectoureteral N28.89
rectourethral N36.0
  congenital Q64.73
rectouterine N82.4
  congenital Q51.7
rectovaginal N82.3
  congenital Q52.2
  tuberculous A18.18
rectovesical N32.1
  congenital Q64.79
rectovesicovaginal N82.3
rectovulval N82.4
  congenital Q52.79
rectum (to skin) K60.40
  congenital Q43.6
    with absence, atresia and stenosis Q42.0
  tuberculous A18.32
renal N28.89
retroauricular —*see* Fistula, postauricular
salivary duct or gland (any) K11.4
  congenital Q38.4
scrotum (urinary) N50.89
  tuberculous A18.15
semicircular canals —*see* subcategory H83.1
sigmoid K63.2
  to bladder N32.1
sinus —*see* Sinusitis
skin L98.8
  to genital tract (female) N82.5

Fistula *(Continued)*
splenocolic D73.89
stercoral K63.2
stomach K31.6
sublingual gland K11.4
submandibular gland K11.4
submaxillary (gland) K11.4
  region K12.2
thoracic J86.0
  duct I89.8
thoracoabdominal J86.0
thoracogastric J86.0
thoracointestinal J86.0
thorax J86.0
thyroglossal duct Q89.2
thyroid E07.89
trachea, congenital (external) (internal)
    Q32.1
tracheoesophageal J86.0
  congenital Q39.2
    with atresia of esophagus Q39.1
  following tracheostomy J95.04
traumatic arteriovenous —*see* Injury, blood
    vessel, by site
tuberculous - code by site under Tuberculosis
typhoid A01.09
umbilicourinary Q64.8
urachus, congenital Q64.4
ureter (persistent) N28.89
ureteroabdominal N28.89
ureterorectal N28.89
ureterosigmoido-abdominal N28.89
ureterovaginal N82.1
ureterovesical N32.2
urethra N36.0
  congenital Q64.79
  tuberculous A18.13
urethroperineal N36.0
urethroperineovesical N32.2
urethrorectal N36.0
  congenital Q64.73
urethroscrotal N50.89
urethrovaginal N82.1
urethrovesical N32.2
urinary (tract) (persistent) (recurrent) N36.0
uteroabdominal N82.5
  congenital Q51.7
uteroenteric, uterointestinal N82.4
  congenital Q51.7
uterorectal N82.4
  congenital Q51.7
uteroureteric N82.1
uterourethral Q51.7
uterovaginal N82.8
uterovesical N82.1
  congenital Q51.7
uterus N82.8
vagina (postpartal) (wall) N82.8
vaginocutaneous (postpartal) N82.5
vaginointestinal NEC N82.4
    large intestine N82.3
    small intestine N82.2
vaginoperineal N82.5
vasocutaneous, congenital Q55.7
vesical NEC N32.2
vesicoabdominal N32.2
vesicocervicovaginal N82.1
vesicocolic N32.1
vesicocutaneous N32.2
vesicoenteric N32.1
vesicointestinal N32.1
vesicometrorectal N82.4
vesicoperineal N32.2
vesicorectal N32.1
  congenital Q64.79
vesicosigmoidal N32.1
vesicosigmoidovaginal N82.3
vesicoureteral N32.2
vesicoureterovaginal N82.1
vesicourethral N32.2
vesicourethrorectal N32.1
vesicouterine N82.1
  congenital Q51.7
vesicovaginal N82.0
vulvorectal N82.4
  congenital Q52.79

Fit R56.9
epileptic —*see* Epilepsy
fainting R55
hysterical F44.5
newborn P90

Fitting (and adjustment) (of)
artificial
  arm —*see* Admission, adjustment, artificial, arm
  breast Z44.3
  eye Z44.2- •
  leg —*see* Admission, adjustment, artificial, leg
automatic implantable cardiac defibrillator (with
    synchronous cardiac pacemaker) Z45.02
brain neuropacemaker Z46.2
  implanted Z45.42
cardiac defibrillator —*see* Fitting (and
    adjustment) (of), automatic implantable
    cardiac defibrillator
catheter, non-vascular Z46.82
colostomy belt Z46.89
contact lenses Z46.0
CRT-D (resynchronization therapy defibrillator)
    Z45.02
CRT-P (cardiac resynchronization therapy
    pacemaker) Z45.018
  pulse generator Z45.010
cystostomy device Z46.6
defibrillator, cardiac —*see* Fitting (and
    adjustment) (of), automatic implantable
    cardiac defibrillator
dentures Z46.3
device NOS Z46.9
  abdominal Z46.89
  gastrointestinal NEC Z46.59
  implanted NEC Z45.89
  nervous system Z46.2
    implanted —*see* Admission, adjustment,
      device, implanted, nervous system
  orthodontic Z46.4
  orthoptic Z46.0
  orthotic Z46.89
  prosthetic (external) Z44.9
    breast Z44.3
    dental Z46.3
    eye Z44.2- •
    specified NEC Z44.8
  specified NEC Z46.89
  substitution
    auditory Z46.2
      implanted —*see* Admission, adjustment,
        device, implanted, hearing device
    nervous system Z46.2
      implanted —*see* Admission, adjustment,
        device, implanted, nervous system
    visual Z46.2
      implanted Z45.31
  urinary Z46.6
gastric lap band Z46.51
gastrointestinal appliance NEC Z46.59
glasses (reading) Z46.0
hearing aid Z46.1
ileostomy device Z46.89
insulin pump Z46.81
intestinal appliance NEC Z46.89
myringotomy device (stent) (tube) Z45.82
neuropacemaker Z46.2
  implanted Z45.42
non-vascular catheter Z46.82
orthodontic device Z46.4
orthopedic device (brace) (cast) (corset) (shoes)
    Z46.89
pacemaker (cardiac) (cardiac resynchronization
    therapy (CRT-P)) Z45.018
  nervous system (brain) (peripheral nerve)
    (spinal cord) Z46.2
    implanted Z45.42
  pulse generator Z45.010
portacath (port-a-cath) Z45.2
prosthesis (external) Z44.9
  arm —*see* Admission, adjustment, artificial,
    arm
  breast Z44.3
  dental Z46.3
  eye Z44.2- •
  leg —*see* Admission, adjustment, artificial, leg
  specified NEC Z44.8
spectacles Z46.0
wheelchair Z46.89

Fitzhugh-Curtis syndrome
due to
  Chlamydia trachomatis A74.81
  Neisseria gonorrhea (gonococcal peritonitis)
    A54.85

Fitz's syndrome (acute hemorrhagic
    pancreatitis) —*see also* Pancreatitis,
    acute K85.80

▶ New　　➡ Revised　　~~deleted~~ Deleted　　● Use Additional Character(s)

▶ New   ⇨ Revised   ~~deleted~~ Deleted   ● Use Additional Character(s)

► New ⇒ Revised ~~deleted~~ Deleted • Use Additional Character(s)

▶ New   ➡ Revised   ~~deleted~~ Deleted   ● Use Additional Character(s)

F

▶ New   ➡ Revised   ~~deleted~~ Deleted   ● Use Additional Character(s)

▶ New   ➡ Revised   ~~deleted~~ Deleted   ● Use Additional Character(s)

▶ New   ➡ Revised   ~~deleted~~ Deleted   ● Use Additional Character(s)

▶ New　　➡ Revised　　~~deleted~~ Deleted　　● Use Additional Character(s)

▶ New ⇒ Revised ~~deleted~~ Deleted ● Use Additional Character(s)

▶ New   ➡ Revised   ~~deleted~~ Deleted   ● Use Additional Character(s)

▶ New   ➡ Revised   ~~deleted~~ Deleted   ● Use Additional Character(s)

► New ➡ Revised ~~deleted~~ Deleted ● Use Additional Character(s)

▶ New   ⬆ Revised   ~~deleted~~ Deleted   ● Use Additional Character(s)

— **I** —

▶ New   ⬛ Revised   ~~deleted~~ Deleted   • Use Additional Character(s)

Infarct, infarction (Continued)
cerebral (Continued)
  due to (Continued)
    embolism
      cerebral arteries I63.4- ●
      precerebral arteries I63.1- ●
    occlusion NEC
      cerebral arteries I63.5- ●
      precerebral arteries I63.2- ●
      small artery I63.81
    stenosis NEC
      cerebral arteries I63.5- ●
      precerebral arteries I63.2- ●
      small artery I63.81
    thrombosis
      cerebral artery I63.3- ●
      precerebral artery I63.0- ●
  intraoperative
    during cardiac surgery I97.810
    during other surgery I97.811
  neonatal P91.82- ●
  perinatal (arterial ischemic) P91.82- ●
  postprocedural
    following cardiac surgery I97.820
    following other surgery I97.821
  specified NEC I63.89
colon (acute) (agnogenic) (embolic)
  (hemorrhagic) (nonocclusive)
  (nonthrombotic) (occlusive) (segmental)
  (thrombotic) (with gangrene) —see also
  Infarct, intestine K55.049
coronary artery —see Infarct, myocardium
embolic —see Embolism
fallopian tube N83.8
gallbladder K82.8
heart —see Infarct, myocardium
hepatic K76.3
hypophysis (anterior lobe) E23.6
impending (myocardium) I20.0
intestine (acute) (agnogenic) (embolic)
  (hemorrhagic) (nonocclusive)
  (nonthrombotic) (occlusive) (thrombotic)
  (with gangrene) K55.069
  diffuse K55.062
  focal K55.061
  large K55.049
    diffuse K55.042
    focal K55.041
  small K55.029
    diffuse K55.022
    focal K55.021
kidney N28.0
lacunar I63.81
liver K76.3
lung (embolic) (thrombotic) —see Embolism,
  pulmonary
lymph node I89.8
mesentery, mesenteric (embolic) (thrombotic)
  (with gangrene) —see also Infarct, intestine
  K55.069
muscle (ischemic) M62.20
  ankle M62.27- ●
  foot M62.27- ●
  forearm M62.23- ●
  hand M62.24- ●
  lower leg M62.26- ●
  pelvic region M62.25- ●
  shoulder region M62.21- ●
  specified site NEC M62.28
  thigh M62.25- ●
  upper arm M62.22- ●
myocardium, myocardial (acute) (with stated
  duration of 4 weeks or less) I21.9
  with
    coronary microvascular disease I21.B
    coronary microvascular dysfunction I21.B
    nonobstructive coronary arteries
      [MINOCA] with microvascular
      disease I21.B
  associated with revascularization procedure
    I21.A9
  diagnosed on ECG, but presenting no
    symptoms I25.2
  due to
    demand ischemia I21.A1
    ischemic imbalance I21.A1
  healed or old I25.2
  intraoperative —see also Infarct, myocardium,
    associated with revascularization
    procedure
    during cardiac surgery I97.790
    during other surgery I97.791

Infarct, infarction (Continued)
myocardium, myocardial (Continued)
  non-Q wave I21.4
  non-ST elevation (NSTEMI) I21.4
    subsequent I22.2
  nontransmural I21.4
  past (diagnosed on ECG or other
    investigation, but currently presenting
    no symptoms) I25.2
  postprocedural —see also Infarct, myocardium,
    associated with revascularization
    procedure
    following cardiac surgery —see also Infarct,
      myocardium, type 4 or type 5 I97.190
    following other surgery I97.191
  Q wave —see also Infarct, myocardium, ST
    elevation, by site I21.3
  secondary to
    demand ischemia I21.A1
    ischemic imbalance I21.A1
  ST elevation (STEMI) I21.3
    anterior (anteroapical) (anterolateral)
      (anteroseptal) (Q wave) (wall) I21.09
      subsequent I22.0
    inferior (diaphragmatic) (inferolateral)
      (inferoposterior) (wall) NEC I21.19
      subsequent I22.1
    inferoposterior transmural (Q wave) I21.11
    involving
      coronary artery of anterior wall NEC
        I21.09
      coronary artery of inferior wall NEC
        I21.19
      diagonal coronary artery I21.02
      left anterior descending coronary artery
        I21.02
      left circumflex coronary artery I21.21
      left main coronary artery I21.01
      oblique marginal coronary artery
        I21.21
      right coronary artery I21.11
    lateral (apical-lateral) (basal-lateral) (high)
      I21.29
      subsequent I22.8
    posterior (posterobasal) (posterolateral)
      (posteroseptal) (true) I21.29
      subsequent I22.8
    septal I21.29
      subsequent I22.8
    specified NEC I21.29
      subsequent I22.8
    subsequent I22.9
  subsequent (recurrent) (reinfarction) I22.9
    anterior (anteroapical) (anterolateral)
      (anteroseptal) (wall) I22.0
    diaphragmatic (wall) I22.1
    inferior (diaphragmatic) (inferolateral)
      (inferoposterior) (wall) I22.1
    lateral (apical-lateral) (basal-lateral) (high)
      I22.8
    non-ST elevation (NSTEMI) I22.2
    posterior (posterobasal) (posterolateral)
      (posteroseptal) (true) I22.8
    septal I22.8
    specified NEC I22.8
    ST elevation I22.9
      anterior (anteroapical) (anterolateral)
        (anteroseptal) (wall) I22.0
      inferior (diaphragmatic) (inferolateral)
        (inferoposterior) (wall) I22.1
      specified NEC I22.8
    subendocardial I22.2
    transmural I22.9
      anterior (anteroapical) (anterolateral)
        (anteroseptal) (wall) I22.0
      diaphragmatic (wall) I22.1
      inferior (diaphragmatic) (inferolateral)
        (inferoposterior) (wall) I22.1
      lateral (apical-lateral) (basal-lateral)
        (high) I22.8
      posterior (posterobasal) (posterolateral)
        (posteroseptal) (true) I22.8
      specified NEC I22.8
    type 1 —see also Infarction, myocardial,
      subsequent, by site, or by ST elevation
      or non-ST elevation I22.9
    type 2 I21.A1
    type 3 I21.A9
    type 4 I21.A9
    type 5 I21.A9
  syphilitic A52.06

Infarct, infarction (Continued)
myocardium, myocardial (Continued)
  transmural (see also, Infarct, myocardium, ST
    elevation, by site) I21.3
    anterior (anteroapical) (anterolateral)
      (anteroseptal) (Q wave) (wall) NEC
      I21.09
    inferior (diaphragmatic) (inferolateral)
      (inferoposterior) (Q wave) (wall) NEC
      I21.19
    inferoposterior (Q wave) I21.11
    lateral (apical-lateral) (basal-lateral) (high)
      NEC I21.29
    posterior (posterobasal) (posterolateral)
      (posteroseptal) (true) NEC I21.29
    septal NEC I21.29
    specified NEC I21.29
  type 1 —see also Infarction, myocardial,
    by site, or by ST elevation or non-ST
    elevation I21.9
  type 2 I21.A1
  type 3 I21.A9
  type 4 (a) (b) (c) I21.A9
  type 5 I21.A9
  nontransmural I21.4
omentum —see also Infarct, intestine K55.069
ovary N83.8
pancreas K86.89
papillary muscle —see Infarct, myocardium
parathyroid gland E21.4
pituitary (gland) E23.6
placenta O43.81- ●
prostate N42.89
pulmonary (artery) (vein) (hemorrhagic) —see
  Embolism, pulmonary
renal (embolic) (thrombotic) N28.0
retina, retinal (artery) —see Occlusion, artery,
  retina
spinal (cord) (acute) (embolic) (nonembolic)
  G95.11
spleen D73.5
  embolic or thrombotic I74.8
subendocardial (acute) (nontransmural) I21.4
suprarenal (capsule) (gland) E27.49
testis N50.1
thrombotic —see also Thrombosis
  artery, arterial —see Embolism
thyroid (gland) E07.89
ventricle (heart) —see Infarct, myocardium
Infecting —see condition
Infection, infected, infective (opportunistic) B99.9
  with
    drug resistant organism —see Resistance (to),
      drug —see also specific organism
    lymphangitis —see Lymphangitis
    organ dysfunction (acute) R65.20
      with septic shock R65.21
  abscess (skin) - code by site under Abscess
  Absidia —see Mucormycosis
  Acanthamoeba —see Acanthamebiasis
  Acanthocheilonema (perstans) (streptocerca)
    B74.4
  accessory sinus (chronic) —see Sinusitis
  achorion —see Dermatophytosis
  Acinetobacter baumannii, as cause of disease
    classified elsewhere B96.83
  Acremonium falciforme B47.0
  acromioclavicular M00.9
  Actinobacillus (actinomycetem-comitans) A28.8
    mallei A24.0
    muris A25.1
  Actinomadura B47.1
  Actinomyces (israelii) —see also Actinomycosis
    A42.9
  Actinomycetales —see Actinomycosis
  actinomycotic NOS —see Actinomycosis
  adenoid (and tonsil) J03.90
    chronic J35.02
  adenovirus NEC
    as cause of disease classified elsewhere B97.0
    unspecified nature or site B34.0
  aerogenes capsulatus A48.0
  aertrycke —see Infection, salmonella
  alimentary canal NOS —see Enteritis, infectious
  Allescheria boydii B48.2
  Alternaria B48.8
  alveolus, alveolar (process) K04.7
  Ameba, amebic (histolytica) —see Amebiasis
  amniotic fluid, sac or cavity O41.10- ●
    chorioamnionitis O41.12- ●
    placentitis O41.14- ●

▶ New   ➡ Revised   ~~deleted~~ Deleted   ● Use Additional Character(s)

▶ New   ➔ Revised   ~~deleted~~ Deleted   • Use Additional Character(s)

▶ New   ➡ Revised   ~~deleted~~ Deleted   ● Use Additional Character(s)

Injury (*Continued*)
anus —*see* Injury, abdomen
aorta (thoracic) S25.00
  abdominal S35.00
    laceration (minor) (superficial) S35.01
      major S35.02
    specified type NEC S35.09
  laceration (minor) (superficial) S25.01
    major S25.02
  specified type NEC S25.09
arm (upper) S49.9-●
  blood vessel —*see* Injury, blood vessel,
    arm
  contusion —*see* Contusion, arm, upper
  fracture —*see* Fracture, humerus
  lower —*see* Injury, forearm
  muscle —*see* Injury, muscle, shoulder
  nerve —*see* Injury, nerve, arm
  open —*see* Wound, open, arm
  specified type NEC S49.8-●
  superficial —*see* Injury, superficial, arm
artery (complicating trauma) —*see also* Injury,
  blood vessel, by site
  cerebral or meningeal —*see* Injury, intracranial
auditory canal (external) (meatus) S09.91
auricle, auris, ear S09.91
axilla —*see* Injury, shoulder
back —*see* Injury, back, lower
bile duct S36.13
birth —*see also* Birth, injury P15.9
bladder (sphincter) S37.20
  at delivery O71.5
  contusion S37.22
  laceration S37.23
  obstetrical trauma O71.5
  specified type NEC S37.29
blast (air) (hydraulic) (immersion) (underwater)
  NEC T14.8
  acoustic nerve trauma —*see* Injury, nerve,
    acoustic
  bladder —*see* Injury, bladder
  brain —*see* Concussion
    primary, specified NEC S06.8A-●
  colon —*see* Injury, intestine, large, blast
    injury
  ear (primary) S09.31-●
    secondary S09.39-●
  generalized T70.8
  lung —*see* Injury, intrathoracic, lung, blast
    injury
  multiple body organs T70.8
  peritoneum S36.81
  rectum S36.61
  retroperitoneum S36.898
  small intestine S36.419
    duodenum S36.410
    specified site NEC S36.418
  specified
    intra-abdominal organ NEC S36.898
    pelvic organ NEC S37.899
blood vessel NEC T14.8
  abdomen S35.9-●
    aorta —*see* Injury, aorta, abdominal
    celiac artery —*see* Injury, blood vessel,
      celiac artery
    iliac vessel —*see* Injury, blood vessel, iliac
    laceration S35.91
    mesenteric vessel —*see* Injury, mesenteric
    portal vein —*see* Injury, blood vessel, portal
      vein
    renal vessel —*see* Injury, blood vessel,
      renal
    specified vessel NEC S35.8X-●
    splenic vessel —*see* Injury, blood vessel,
      splenic
    vena cava —*see* Injury, vena cava, inferior
  ankle —*see* Injury, blood vessel, foot
  aorta (abdominal) (thoracic) —*see* Injury,
    aorta
  arm (upper) NEC S45.90-●
    forearm —*see* Injury, blood vessel,
      forearm
    laceration S45.91-●
    specified
      site NEC S45.80-●
        laceration S45.81-●
        specified type NEC S45.89-●
      type NEC S45.99-●
    superficial vein S45.30-●
      laceration S45.31-●
      specified type NEC S45.39-●

Injury (*Continued*)
blood vessel NEC (*Continued*)
  axillary
    artery S45.00-●
      laceration S45.01-●
      specified type NEC S45.09-●
    vein S45.20-●
      laceration S45.21-●
      specified type NEC S45.29-●
  azygos vein —*see* Injury, blood vessel,
    thoracic, specified site NEC
  brachial
    artery S45.10-●
      laceration S45.11-●
      specified type NEC S45.19-●
    vein S45.20-●
      laceration S45.219
      specified type NEC S45.29-●
  carotid artery (common) (external) (internal,
    extracranial) S15.00-●
    internal, intracranial S06.8-●
    laceration (minor) (superficial) S15.01-●
      major S15.02-●
    specified type NEC S15.09-●
  celiac artery S35.219
    branch S35.299
      laceration (minor) (superficial)
        S35.291
        major S35.292
      specified NEC S35.298
    laceration (minor) (superficial) S35.211
      major S35.212
    specified type NEC S35.218
  cerebral —*see* Injury, intracranial
  deep plantar —*see* Injury, blood vessel, plantar
    artery
  digital (hand) —*see* Injury, blood vessel,
    finger
  dorsal
    artery (foot) S95.00-●
      laceration S95.01-●
      specified type NEC S95.09-●
    vein (foot) S95.20-●
      laceration S95.21-●
      specified type NEC S95.29-●
  due to accidental laceration during
    procedure —*see* Laceration, accidental
    complicating surgery
  extremity —*see* Injury, blood vessel, limb
  femoral
    artery (common) (superficial) S75.00-●
      laceration (minor) (superficial)
        S75.01-●
        major S75.02-●
      specified type NEC S75.09-●
    vein (hip level) (thigh level) S75.10-●
      laceration (minor) (superficial)
        S75.11-●
        major S75.12-●
      specified type NEC S75.19-●
  finger S65.50-●
    index S65.50-●
      laceration S65.51-●
      specified type NEC S65.59-●
    laceration S65.51-●
    little S65.50-●
      laceration S65.51-●
      specified type NEC S65.59-●
    middle S65.50-●
      laceration S65.51-●
      specified type NEC S65.59-●
    specified type NEC S65.59-●
    thumb —*see* Injury, blood vessel, thumb
  foot S95.90-●
    dorsal
      artery —*see* Injury, blood vessel, dorsal,
        artery
      vein —*see* Injury, blood vessel, dorsal,
        vein
    laceration S95.91-●
    plantar artery —*see* Injury, blood vessel,
      plantar artery
    specified
      site NEC S95.80-●
        laceration S95.81-●
        specified type NEC S95.89-●
      specified type NEC S95.99-●
  forearm S55.90-●
    laceration S55.91-●
    radial artery —*see* Injury, blood vessel,
      radial artery

Injury (*Continued*)
blood vessel NEC (*Continued*)
  forearm (*Continued*)
    specified
      site NEC S55.80-●
        laceration S55.81-●
        specified type NEC S55.89-●
      type NEC S55.99-●
    ulnar artery —*see* Injury, blood vessel, ulnar
      artery
    vein S55.20-●
      laceration S55.21-●
      specified type NEC S55.29-●
  gastric
    artery —*see* Injury, mesenteric, artery,
      branch
    vein —*see* Injury, blood vessel, abdomen
  gastroduodenal artery —*see* Injury,
    mesenteric, artery, branch
  greater saphenous vein (lower leg level)
    S85.30-●
    hip (and thigh) level S75.20-●
      laceration (minor) (superficial)
        S75.21-●
        major S75.22-●
      specified type NEC S75.29-●
    laceration S85.31-●
    specified type NEC S85.39-●
  hand (level) S65.90-●
    finger —*see* Injury, blood vessel, finger
    laceration S65.91-●
    palmar arch —*see* Injury, blood vessel,
      palmar arch
    radial artery —*see* Injury, blood vessel,
      radial artery, hand
    specified
      site NEC S65.80-●
        laceration S65.81-●
        specified type NEC S65.89-●
      type NEC S65.99-●
    thumb —*see* Injury, blood vessel, thumb
    ulnar artery —*see* Injury, blood vessel, ulnar
      artery, hand
  head S09.0
    intracranial —*see* Injury, intracranial
    multiple S09.0
  hepatic
    artery —*see* Injury, mesenteric, artery
    vein —*see* Injury, vena cava, inferior
  hip S75.90-●
    femoral artery —*see* Injury, blood vessel,
      femoral, artery
    femoral vein —*see* Injury, blood vessel,
      femoral, vein
    greater saphenous vein —*see* Injury, blood
      vessel, greater saphenous, hip level
    laceration S75.91-●
    specified
      site NEC S75.80-●
        laceration S75.81-●
        specified type NEC S75.89-●
      type NEC S75.99-●
  hypogastric (artery) (vein) —*see* Injury, blood
    vessel, iliac
  iliac S35.5-●
    artery S35.51-●
    specified vessel NEC S35.5-●
    uterine vessel —*see* Injury, blood vessel,
      uterine
    vein S35.51-●
  innominate —*see* Injury, blood vessel, thoracic,
    innominate
  intercostal (artery) (vein) —*see* Injury, blood
    vessel, thoracic, intercostal
  jugular vein (external) S15.20-●
    internal S15.30-●
      laceration (minor) (superficial)
        S15.31-●
        major S15.32-●
      specified type NEC S15.39-●
    laceration (minor) (superficial) S15.21-●
      major S15.22-●
    specified type NEC S15.29-●
  leg (level) (lower) S85.90-●
    greater saphenous —*see* Injury, blood
      vessel, greater saphenous
    laceration S85.91-●
    lesser saphenous —*see* Injury, blood vessel,
      lesser saphenous
    peroneal artery —*see* Injury, blood vessel,
      peroneal artery

  ▶ New   ⇒ Revised   ~~deleted~~ Deleted   ● Use Additional Character(s)

Injury (Continued)
epididymis S39.94
epigastric region S39.91
epiglottis NEC S19.89
esophageal plexus —*see* Injury, nerve, thorax, sympathetic
esophagus (thoracic part) —*see also* Injury, intrathoracic, esophagus
  cervical NEC S19.85
eustachian tube S09.30-●
eye S05.9-●
  avulsion S05.7-●
  ball —*see* Injury, eyeball
  conjunctiva S05.0-●
  cornea
    abrasion S05.0-●
    laceration S05.3-●
      with prolapse S05.2-●
  lacrimal apparatus S05.8X-●
  orbit penetration S05.4-●
  specified site NEC S05.8X-●
eyeball S05.8X-●
  contusion S05.1-●
  penetrating S05.6-●
    with
      foreign body S05.5-●
      prolapse or loss of intraocular tissue S05.2-●
      without prolapse or loss of intraocular tissue S05.3-●
  specified type NEC S05.8-●
eyebrow S09.93
eyelid S09.93
  abrasion —*see* Abrasion, eyelid
  contusion —*see* Contusion, eyelid
  open —*see* Wound, open, eyelid
face S09.93
fallopian tube S37.509
  bilateral S37.502
    blast injury S37.512
    contusion S37.522
    laceration S37.532
    specified type NEC S37.592
  blast injury (primary) S37.519
    bilateral S37.512
    secondary —*see* Injury, fallopian tube, specified type NEC
    unilateral S37.511
  contusion S37.529
    bilateral S37.522
    unilateral S37.521
  laceration S37.539
    bilateral S37.532
    unilateral S37.531
  specified type NEC S37.599
    bilateral S37.592
    unilateral S37.591
  unilateral S37.501
    blast injury S37.511
    contusion S37.521
    laceration S37.531
    specified type NEC S37.591
fascia —*see* Injury, muscle
fifth cranial nerve (trigeminal) —*see* Injury, nerve, trigeminal
finger (nail) S69.9-●
  blood vessel —*see* Injury, blood vessel, finger
  contusion —*see* Contusion, finger
  dislocation —*see* Dislocation, finger
  fracture —*see* Fracture, finger
  muscle —*see* Injury, muscle, finger
  nerve —*see* Injury, nerve, digital, finger
  open —*see* Wound, open, finger
  specified NEC S69.8-●
  sprain —*see* Sprain, finger
  superficial —*see* Injury, superficial, finger
first cranial nerve (olfactory) —*see* Injury, nerve, olfactory
flank —*see* Injury, abdomen
foot S99.92-●
  blood vessel —*see* Injury, blood vessel, foot
  contusion —*see* Contusion, foot
  dislocation —*see* Dislocation, foot
  fracture —*see* Fracture, foot
  muscle —*see* Injury, muscle, foot
  open —*see* Wound, open, foot
  specified type NEC S99.82-●
  sprain —*see* Sprain, foot
  superficial —*see* Injury, superficial, foot
forceps NOS P15.9

Injury (Continued)
forearm S59.91-●
  blood vessel —*see* Injury, blood vessel, forearm
  contusion —*see* Contusion, forearm
  fracture —*see* Fracture, forearm
  muscle —*see* Injury, muscle, forearm
  nerve —*see* Injury, nerve, forearm
  open —*see* Wound, open, forearm
  specified NEC S59.81-●
  superficial —*see* Injury, superficial, forearm
forehead S09.90
fourth cranial nerve (trochlear) —*see* Injury, nerve, trochlear
gallbladder S36.129
  contusion S36.122
  laceration S36.123
  specified NEC S36.128
ganglion
  celiac, coeliac —*see* Injury, nerve, lumbosacral, sympathetic
  gasserian —*see* Injury, nerve, trigeminal
  stellate —*see* Injury, nerve, thorax, sympathetic
  thoracic sympathetic —*see* Injury, nerve, thorax, sympathetic
gasserian ganglion —*see* Injury, nerve, trigeminal
gastric artery —*see* Injury, blood vessel, celiac artery, branch
gastroduodenal artery —*see* Injury, blood vessel, celiac artery, branch
gastrointestinal tract —*see* Injury, intra-abdominal
  with open wound into abdominal cavity —*see* Wound, open, with penetration into peritoneal cavity
  colon —*see* Injury, intestine, large
  rectum —*see* Injury, intestine, large, rectum
    with open wound into abdominal cavity S36.61
  small intestine —*see* Injury, intestine, small
  specified site NEC —*see* Injury, intra-abdominal, specified, site NEC
  stomach —*see* Injury, stomach
genital organ(s)
  external S39.94
    specified NEC S39.848
  internal S37.90
    fallopian tube —*see* Injury, fallopian tube
    ovary —*see* Injury, ovary
    prostate —*see* Injury, prostate
    seminal vesicle —*see* Injury, pelvis, organ, specified site NEC
    uterus —*see* Injury, uterus
    vas deferens —*see* Injury, pelvis, organ, specified site NEC
  obstetrical trauma O71.9
gland
  lacrimal laceration —*see* Injury, eye, specified site NEC
  salivary S09.93
  thyroid NEC S19.84
globe (eye) S05.90
  specified NEC S05.8X-●
groin —*see* Injury, abdomen
gum S09.90
hand S69.9-●
  blood vessel —*see* Injury, blood vessel, hand
  contusion —*see* Contusion, hand
  fracture —*see* Fracture, hand
  muscle —*see* Injury, muscle, hand
  nerve —*see* Injury, nerve, hand
  open —*see* Wound, open, hand
  specified NEC S69.8-●
  sprain —*see* Sprain, hand
  superficial —*see* Injury, superficial, hand
head S09.90
  with loss of consciousness S06.9-●
  specified NEC S09.8-●
heart (traumatic) S26.90
  with hemopericardium S26.00
    contusion S26.01
    laceration (mild) S26.020
      major S26.022
      moderate S26.021
    specified type NEC S26.09
  without hemopericardium S26.10
    contusion S26.11
    laceration S26.12
    specified type NEC S26.19

Injury (Continued)
heart (Continued)
  contusion S26.91
  laceration S26.92
  non-traumatic (acute) (chronic) (non-ischemic) I5A
  specified type NEC S26.99
heel —*see* Injury, foot
hepatic
  artery —*see* Injury, blood vessel, celiac artery, branch
  duct —*see* Injury, liver
  vein —*see* Injury, vena cava, inferior
hip S79.91-●
  blood vessel —*see* Injury, blood vessel, hip
  contusion —*see* Contusion, hip
  dislocation —*see* Dislocation, hip
  fracture —*see* Fracture, femur, neck
  muscle —*see* Injury, muscle, hip
  nerve —*see* Injury, nerve, hip
  open —*see* Wound, open, hip
  specified NEC S79.81-●
  sprain —*see* Sprain, hip
  superficial —*see* Injury, superficial, hip
hymen S39.94
hypogastric
  blood vessel —*see* Injury, blood vessel, iliac
  plexus —*see* Injury, nerve, lumbosacral, sympathetic
ileum —*see* Injury, intestine, small
iliac region S39.91
instrumental (during surgery) —*see* Laceration, accidental complicating surgery
  birth injury —*see* Birth, injury
  nonsurgical —*see* Injury, by site
  obstetrical O71.9
    bladder O71.5.
    cervix O71.3
    high vaginal O71.4
    perineal NOS O70.9
    urethra O71.5
    uterus O71.5
      with rupture or perforation O71.1
internal T14.8
  aorta —*see* Injury, aorta
  bladder (sphincter) —*see* Injury, bladder
    with
      ectopic or molar pregnancy O08.6
    following ectopic or molar pregnancy O08.6
    obstetrical trauma O71.5
  bronchus, bronchi —*see* Injury, intrathoracic, bronchus
  cecum —*see* Injury, intestine, large
  cervix (uteri) —*see also* Injury, uterus
    with ectopic or molar pregnancy O08.6
    following ectopic or molar pregnancy O08.6
    obstetrical trauma O71.3
  chest —*see* Injury, intrathoracic
  gastrointestinal tract —*see* Injury, intra-abdominal
  heart —*see* Injury, heart
  intestine NEC —*see* Injury, intestine
  intrauterine —*see* Injury, uterus
  mesentery —*see* Injury, intra-abdominal, specified, site NEC
  pelvis, pelvic (organ) S37.92
    following ectopic or molar pregnancy (subsequent episode) O08.6
    obstetrical trauma NEC O71.5
    rupture or perforation O71.1
    specified NEC S39.83
  rectum —*see* Injury, intestine, large, rectum
  stomach —*see* Injury, stomach
  ureter —*see* Injury, ureter
  urethra (sphincter) following ectopic or molar pregnancy O08.6
  uterus —*see* Injury, uterus
interscapular area —*see* Injury, thorax
intestine
  large S36.509
    ascending (right) S36.500
      blast injury (primary) S36.510
        secondary S36.590
      contusion S36.520
      laceration S36.530
      specified type NEC S36.590
    blast injury (primary) S36.519
      ascending (right) S36.510
      descending (left) S36.512
      rectum S36.61

▶ New   ➡ Revised   ~~deleted~~ Deleted   ● Use Additional Character(s)

▶ New ▶ Revised ~~deleted~~ Deleted • Use Additional Character(s)

Injury (Continued)
nerve NEC (Continued)
  hand S64.9-●
    median —see Injury, nerve, median, hand
    radial —see Injury, nerve, radial, hand
    specified NEC —see subcategory S64.8
    ulnar —see Injury, nerve, ulnar, hand
  hip (level) S74.9-●
    cutaneous sensory —see Injury, nerve,
      cutaneous sensory, hip
    femoral —see Injury, nerve, femoral
    sciatic —see Injury, nerve, sciatic
    specified site NEC —see subcategory S74.8
  hypoglossal S04.89-●
    specified type NEC S04.89-●
  lateral plantar S94.0-●
  leg (lower) S84.9-●
    cutaneous sensory —see Injury, nerve,
      cutaneous sensory, leg
    peroneal —see Injury, nerve, peroneal
    specified site NEC —see subcategory S84.8
    tibial —see Injury, nerve, tibial
    upper —see Injury, nerve, thigh
  lower
    back —see Injury, nerve, abdomen, specified
      site NEC
      peripheral —see Injury, nerve, abdomen,
        peripheral
    limb —see Injury, nerve, leg
  lumbar plexus —see Injury, nerve,
    lumbosacral, sympathetic
  lumbar spinal —see Injury, spinal, lumbar
  peripheral S34.6
    root S34.21
    sympathetic S34.5
  lumbosacral
    plexus —see Injury, nerve, lumbosacral,
      sympathetic
    sympathetic S34.5
  medial plantar S94.1-●
  median (forearm level) S54.1-●
    hand (level) S64.1-●
    upper arm (level) S44.1-●
    wrist (level) —see Injury, nerve, median,
      hand
  musculocutaneous S44.4-●
  musculospiral (upper arm level) —see Injury,
    nerve, radial, upper arm
  neck S14.9
    peripheral S14.4
    specified site NEC S14.8
    sympathetic S14.5
  ninth cranial (glossopharyngeal) —see Injury,
    nerve, glossopharyngeal
  oculomotor S04.1-●
    contusion S04.1-●
    laceration S04.1-●
    specified type NEC S04.1-●
  olfactory S04.81-●
    specified type NEC S04.81-●
  optic S04.01-●
    contusion S04.01-●
    laceration S04.01-●
    specified type NEC S04.01-●
  pelvic girdle —see Injury, nerve, hip
  pelvis —see Injury, nerve, abdomen, specified
    site NEC
    peripheral —see Injury, nerve, abdomen,
      peripheral
  peripheral NEC T14.8
    abdomen —see Injury, nerve, abdomen,
      peripheral
    lower back —see Injury, nerve, abdomen,
      peripheral
    neck —see Injury, nerve, neck, peripheral
    pelvis —see Injury, nerve, abdomen,
      peripheral
    specified NEC T14.8
  peroneal (lower leg level) S84.1-●
    foot S94.2-●
  plexus
    brachial —see Injury, brachial plexus
    celiac, coeliac —see Injury, nerve,
      lumbosacral, sympathetic
    mesenteric, inferior —see Injury, nerve,
      lumbosacral, sympathetic
    sacral —see Injury, lumbosacral plexus
    spinal
      brachial —see Injury, brachial plexus
      lumbosacral —see Injury, lumbosacral
        plexus

Injury (Continued)
nerve NEC (Continued)
  pneumogastric —see Injury, nerve, vagus
  radial (forearm level) S54.2-●
    hand (level) S64.2-●
    upper arm (level) S44.2-●
    wrist (level) —see Injury, nerve, radial, hand
  root —see Injury, nerve, spinal, root
  sacral plexus —see Injury, lumbosacral plexus
  sacral spinal —see Injury, spinal, sacral
  peripheral S34.6
    root S34.22
    sympathetic S34.5
  sciatic (hip level) (thigh level) S74.0-●
  second cranial (optic) —see Injury, nerve, optic
  self-inflicted, without suicidal intent R45.88
  seventh cranial (facial) —see Injury, nerve,
    facial
  shoulder —see Injury, nerve, arm
  sixth cranial (abducent) —see Injury, nerve,
    abducens
  spinal
    plexus —see Injury, nerve, plexus, spinal
    root
      cervical S14.2
      dorsal S24.2
      lumbar S34.21
      sacral S34.22
      thoracic —see Injury, nerve, spinal, root,
        dorsal
  splanchnic —see Injury, nerve, spinal,
    sympathetic
  sympathetic NEC —see Injury, nerve,
    lumbosacral, sympathetic
    cervical —see Injury, nerve, cervical
      sympathetic
  tenth cranial (pneumogastric or vagus) —see
    Injury, nerve, vagus
  thigh (level) —see Injury, nerve, hip
    cutaneous sensory —see Injury, nerve,
      cutaneous sensory, hip
    femoral —see Injury, nerve, femoral
    sciatic —see Injury, nerve, sciatic
    specified NEC —see Injury, nerve, hip
  third cranial (oculomotor) —see Injury, nerve,
    oculomotor
  thorax S24.9
    peripheral S24.3
    specified site NEC S24.8
    sympathetic S24.4
  thumb, digital —see Injury, nerve, digital,
    thumb
  tibial (lower leg level) (posterior) S84.0-●
  toe —see Injury, nerve, ankle
  trigeminal S04.3-●
    contusion S04.3-●
    laceration S04.3-●
    specified type NEC S04.3-●
  trochlear S04.2-●
    contusion S04.2-●
    laceration S04.2-●
    specified type NEC S04.2-●
  twelfth cranial (hypoglossal) —see Injury,
    nerve, hypoglossal
  ulnar (forearm level) S54.0-●
    arm (upper) (level) S44.0-●
    hand (level) S64.0-●
    wrist (level) —see Injury, nerve, ulnar, hand
  vagus S04.89-●
    specified type NEC S04.89-●
  wrist (level) —see Injury, nerve, hand
  ninth cranial nerve (glossopharyngeal) —see
    Injury, nerve, glossopharyngeal
nose (septum) S09.92
obstetrical O71.9
  specified NEC O71.89
occipital (region) (scalp) S09.90
  lobe —see Injury, intracranial
optic chiasm S04.02
optic radiation S04.03-●
optic tract and pathways S04.03-●
orbit, orbital (region) —see Injury, eye
  penetrating (with foreign body) —see Injury,
    eye, orbit, penetrating
  specified NEC —see Injury, eye, specified site
    NEC
ovary, ovarian S37.409
  bilateral S37.402
    contusion S37.422
    laceration S37.432
    specified type NEC S37.492

Injury (Continued)
ovary, ovarian (Continued)
  blood vessel —see Injury, blood vessel, ovarian
  contusion S37.429
    bilateral S37.422
    unilateral S37.421
  laceration S37.439
    bilateral S37.432
    unilateral S37.431
  specified type NEC S37.499
    bilateral S37.492
    unilateral S37.491
  unilateral S37.401
    contusion S37.421
    laceration S37.431
    specified type NEC S37.491
palate (hard) (soft) S09.93
pancreas S36.209
  body S36.201
    contusion S36.221
    laceration S36.231
      major S36.261
      minor S36.241
      moderate S36.251
    specified type NEC S36.291
  contusion S36.229
  head S36.200
    contusion S36.220
    laceration S36.230
      major S36.260
      minor S36.240
      moderate S36.250
    specified type NEC S36.290
  laceration S36.239
    major S36.269
    minor S36.249
    moderate S36.259
  specified type NEC S36.299
  tail S36.202
    contusion S36.222
    laceration S36.232
      major S36.262
      minor S36.242
      moderate S36.252
    specified type NEC S36.292
parietal (region) (scalp) S09.90
  lobe —see Injury, intracranial
patellar ligament (tendon) S76.10-●
  laceration S76.12-●
  specified NEC S76.19-●
  strain S76.11-●
pelvis, pelvic (floor) S39.93
  complicating delivery O70.1
  joint or ligament, complicating delivery O71.6
  organ S37.90
    with ectopic or molar pregnancy
      O08.6
    complication of abortion —see Abortion
    contusion S37.92
    following ectopic or molar pregnancy
      O08.6
    laceration S37.93
    obstetrical trauma NEC O71.5
    specified
      site NEC S37.899
        contusion S37.892
        laceration S37.893
        specified type NEC S37.898
      type NEC S37.99
  specified NEC S39.83
penis S39.94
perineum S39.94
peritoneum S36.81
  laceration S36.893
periurethral tissue —see Injury, urethra
  complicating delivery O71.82
phalanges
  foot —see Injury, foot
  hand —see Injury, hand
pharynx NEC S19.85
pleura —see Injury, intrathoracic, pleura
plexus
  brachial —see Injury, brachial plexus
  cardiac —see Injury, nerve, thorax,
    sympathetic
  celiac, coeliac —see Injury, nerve, lumbosacral,
    sympathetic
  esophageal —see Injury, nerve, thorax,
    sympathetic
  hypogastric —see Injury, nerve, lumbosacral,
    sympathetic

▶ New　➡ Revised　~~deleted~~ Deleted　● Use Additional Character(s)

▶ New   ⇒ Revised   ~~deleted~~ Deleted   • Use Additional Character(s)

    ▶ New   ⇒ Revised   ~~deleted~~ Deleted   ● Use Additional Character(s)

▶ New   ▶ Revised   ~~deleted~~ Deleted   • Use Additional Character(s)

L

▶ New　　⇨ Revised　　~~deleted~~ Deleted　　● Use Additional Character(s)

▶ New　⇒ Revised　~~deleted~~ Deleted　● Use Additional Character(s)

Leontiasis
  ossium M85.2
  syphilitic (late) A52.78
    congenital A50.59
Lepothrix A48.8
Lepra —*see* Leprosy
Leprechaunism E34.8
Leprosy A30.-●
  with muscle disorder A30.9 [M63.80]
    ankle A30.9 [M63.87-●]
    foot A30.9 [M63.87-●]
    forearm A30.9 [M63.83-●]
    hand A30.9 [M63.84-●]
    lower leg A30.9 [M63.86-●]
    multiple sites A30.9 [M63.89]
    pelvic region A30.9 [M63.85-●]
    shoulder region A30.9 [M63.81-●]
    specified site NEC A30.9 [M63.88]
    thigh A30.9 [M63.85-●]
    upper arm A30.9 [M63.82-●]
  anesthetic A30.9
  BB A30.3
  BL A30.4
  borderline (infiltrated) (neuritic) A30.3
    lepromatous A30.4
    tuberculoid A30.2
  BT A30.2
  dimorphous (infiltrated) (neuritic) A30.3
  I A30.0
  indeterminate (macular) (neuritic) A30.0
  lepromatous (diffuse) (infiltrated) (macular)
    (neuritic) (nodular) A30.5
  LL A30.5
  macular (early) (neuritic) (simple) A30.9
  maculoanesthetic A30.9
  mixed A30.3
  neural A30.9
  nodular A30.5
  primary neuritic A30.3
  specified type NEC A30.8
  TT A30.1
  tuberculoid (major) (minor) A30.1
Leptocytosis, hereditary D56.9
Leptomeningitis (chronic) (circumscribed)
  (hemorrhagic) (nonsuppurative) —*see*
  Meningitis
Leptomeningopathy G96.198
Leptospiral —*see* condition
Leptospirochetal —*see* condition
Leptospirosis A27.9
  canicola A27.89
  due to Leptospira interrogans serovar
    icterohaemorrhagiae A27.0
  icterohemorrhagica A27.0
  pomona A27.89
  Weil's disease A27.0
Leptus dermatitis B88.09
Leriche's syndrome (aortic bifurcation occlusion)
  I74.09
Leri's pleonosteosis Q78.8
Leri-Weill syndrome Q77.8
Lermoyez' syndrome —*see* Vertigo, peripheral
  NEC
Lesch-Nyhan syndrome E79.1
Leser-Trélat disease L82.1
  inflamed L82.0
Lesion(s) (nontraumatic)
  abducens nerve —*see* Strabismus, paralytic, sixth
    nerve
  alveolar process K08.9
  angiocentric immunoproliferative
    D47.Z9
  anorectal K62.9
  aortic (valve) I35.9
  auditory nerve —*see* subcategory
    H93.3
  basal ganglion G25.9
  bile duct —*see* Disease, bile duct
  biomechanical M99.9
    specified type NEC M99.89
      abdomen M99.89
      acromioclavicular M99.87
      cervical region M99.81
      cervicothoracic M99.81
      costochondral M99.88
      costovertebral M99.88
      head region M99.80
      hip M99.85
      lower extremity M99.86
      lumbar region M99.83

Lesion (Continued)
  biomechanical (Continued)
    specified type NEC (Continued)
      lumbosacral M99.83
      occipitocervical M99.80
      pelvic region M99.85
      pubic M99.85
      rib cage M99.88
      sacral region M99.84
      sacrococcygeal M99.84
      sacroiliac M99.84
      specified NEC M99.89
      sternochondral M99.88
      sternoclavicular M99.87
      thoracic region M99.82
      thoracolumbar M99.82
      upper extremity M99.87
  bladder N32.9
  bone —*see* Disorder, bone
  brachial plexus G54.0
  brain G93.9
    congenital Q04.9
    vascular I67.9
      degenerative I67.9
      hypertensive I67.4
  buccal cavity K13.79
  calcified —*see* Calcification
  cameron —*see* Ulcer, stomach
  canthus —*see* Disorder, eyelid
  carate —*see* Pinta, lesions
  cardia K31.9
  cardiac —*see also* Disease, heart I51.9
    congenital Q24.9
    valvular —*see* Endocarditis
  cauda equina G83.4
  cecum K63.9
  cerebral —*see* Lesion, brain
  cerebrovascular I67.9
    degenerative I67.9
    hypertensive I67.4
  cervical (nerve) root NEC G54.2
  chiasmal —*see* Disorder, optic, chiasm
  chorda tympani G51.8
  coin, lung R91.1
  colon K63.9
  combined periodontic - endodontic K05.5
  congenital —*see* Anomaly, by site
  conjunctiva H11.9
  conus medullaris —*see* Injury, conus medullaris
  coronary artery —*see* Ischemia, heart
  cranial nerve G52.9
    eighth —*see* Disorder, ear
    eleventh G52.9
    fifth G50.9
    first G52.0
    fourth —*see* Strabismus, paralytic, fourth
      nerve
    seventh G51.9
    sixth —*see* Strabismus, paralytic, sixth nerve
    tenth G52.2
    twelfth G52.3
  cystic —*see* Cyst
  degenerative —*see* Degeneration
  duodenum K31.9
  edentulous (alveolar) ridge, associated with
    trauma, due to traumatic occlusion K06.2
  en coup de sabre L94.1
  eyelid —*see* Disorder, eyelid
  gasserian ganglion G50.8
  gastric K31.9
  gastroduodenal K31.9
  gastrointestinal K63.9
  gingiva, associated with trauma K06.2
  glomerular
    focal and segmental —*see also* N00-N07 with
      fourth character .1 N05.1
    minimal change —*see also* N00-N07 with
      fourth character .0 N05.0
  heart (organic) —*see* Disease, heart
  hyperchromic, due to pinta (carate) A67.1
  hyperkeratotic —*see* Hyperkeratosis
  hypothalamic E23.7
  ileocecal K63.9
  ileum K63.9
  iliohypogastric nerve G57.8-●
  inflammatory —*see* Inflammation
  intestine K63.9
  intracerebral —*see* Lesion, brain
  intrachiasmal (optic) —*see* Disorder, optic,
    chiasm

Lesion (Continued)
  intracranial, space-occupying R90.0
  joint —*see* Disorder, joint
    sacroiliac (old) M53.3
  keratotic —*see* Keratosis
  kidney —*see* Disease, renal
  laryngeal nerve (recurrent) G52.2
  lip K13.0
  liver K76.9
  lumbosacral
    plexus G54.1
    root (nerve) NEC G54.4
  lung (coin) R91.1
  maxillary sinus J32.0
  mitral I05.9
  Morel-Lavallée —*see* Hematoma,
    by site
  motor cortex NEC G93.89
  mouth K13.79
  nerve G58.9
    femoral G57.2-●
    median G56.1-●
      carpal tunnel syndrome —*see* Syndrome,
        carpal tunnel
    plantar G57.6-●
    popliteal (lateral) G57.3-●
      medial G57.4-●
    radial G56.3-●
    sciatic G57.0-●
    spinal —*see* Injury, nerve, spinal
    ulnar G56.2-●
  nervous system, congenital Q07.9
  nonallopathic —*see* Lesion, biomechanical
  nose (internal) J34.89
  obstructive —*see* Obstruction
  obturator nerve G57.8-●
  oral mucosa K13.70
  organ or site NEC —*see* Disease, by site
  osteolytic —*see* Osteolysis
  peptic K27.9
  periodontal, due to traumatic occlusion K05.5
  pharynx J39.2
  pigment, pigmented (skin) L81.9
  pinta —*see* Pinta, lesions
  polypoid —*see* Polyp
  prechiasmal (optic) —*see* Disorder, optic, chiasm
  primary —*see also* Syphilis, primary A51.0
    carate A67.0
    pinta A67.0
    yaws A66.0
  pulmonary J98.4
    valve I37.9
  pylorus K31.9
  rectosigmoid K63.9
  retina, retinal H35.9
  sacroiliac (joint) (old) M53.3
  salivary gland K11.9
    benign lymphoepithelial K11.8
  saphenous nerve G57.8-●
  sciatic nerve G57.0-●
  secondary —*see* Syphilis, secondary
  shoulder (region) M75.9-●
    specified NEC M75.8-●
  sigmoid K63.9
  sinus (accessory) (nasal) J34.89
  skin L98.9
    suppurative L08.0
  SLAP S43.43-●
  spinal cord G95.9
    congenital Q06.9
  spleen D73.89
  stomach K31.9
  superior glenoid labrum S43.43-●
  syphilitic —*see* Syphilis
  tertiary —*see* Syphilis, tertiary
  thoracic root (nerve) NEC G54.3
  tonsillar fossa J35.9
  tooth, teeth K08.9
    white spot
      chewing surface K02.51
      pit and fissure surface K02.51
      smooth surface K02.61
  traumatic —*see* specific type of injury by site
  tricuspid (valve) I07.9
    nonrheumatic I36.9
  trigeminal nerve G50.9
  ulcerated or ulcerative —*see* Ulcer, skin
  uterus N85.9
  vagina N89.8
  vulva N90.89

Lesion *(Continued)*
  vagus nerve G52.2
  valvular —*see* Endocarditis
  vascular I99.9
    affecting central nervous system I67.9
    following trauma NEC T14.8
    umbilical cord, complicating delivery O69.5
  warty —*see* Verruca
  white spot (tooth)
    chewing surface K02.51
    pit and fissure surface K02.51
    smooth surface K02.61
Less than a high school diploma Z55.5
Lethargic —*see* condition
Lethargy R53.83
Letterer-Siwe's disease C96.0
Leukemia, leukemic C95.9-●
  acute basophilic C94.8-●
  acute bilineal C95.0-●
  acute erythroid C94.0-●
  acute lymphoblastic C91.0-●
  acute megakaryoblastic C94.2-●
  acute megakaryocytic C94.2-●
  acute mixed lineage C95.0-●
  acute monoblastic (monoblastic/monocytic)
    C93.0-●
  acute monocytic (monoblastic/monocytic)
    C93.0-●
  acute myeloblastic (minimal differentiation)
    (with maturation) C92.0-●
  acute myeloid, NOS C92.0-●
    with
      11q23-abnormality C92.6-●
      dysplasia of remaining hematopoiesis and/
        or myelodysplastic disease in its
        history C92.A-●
      multilineage dysplasia C92.A-●
      variation of MLL-gene C92.6-●
      M6 (a)(b) C94.0-●
      M7 C94.2-●
  acute myelomonocytic C92.5-●
  acute promyelocytic C92.4-●
  adult T-cell (HTLV-1-associated) (acute variant)
    (chronic variant) (lymphomatoid variant)
    (smouldering variant) C91.5-●
  aggressive NK-cell C94.8-●
  AML (1/ETO) (M0) (M1) (M2) (without a FAB
    classification) C92.0-●
  AML M3 C92.4-●
  AML M4 (Eo with inv(16) or t(16;16)) C92.5-●
  AML M5 C93.0-●
  AML M5a C93.0-●
  AML M5b C93.0-●
  AML Me with t (15;17) and variants C92.4-●
  atypical chronic myeloid, BCR/ABL-negative
    C92.2-●
  biphenotypic acute C95.0-●
  blast cell C95.0-●
  Burkitt-type, mature B-cell C91.A-●
  chronic eosinophilic (*see also* Syndrome,
    hypereosinophilic, myeloid) C94.8-●
  chronic lymphocytic, of B-cell type C91.1-●
  chronic monocytic C93.1-●
  chronic myelogenous (Philadelphia chromosome
    (Ph1) positive) (t(9;22)) (q34;q11) (with
    crisis of blast cells) C92.1-●
  chronic myeloid, BCR/ABL-positive C92.1-●
    atypical, BCR/ABL-negative C92.2-●
  chronic myelomonocytic C93.1-●
  chronic neutrophilic D47.1
  CMML (-1) (-2) (with eosinophilia) C93.1-●
  granulocytic —*see also* Category C92 C92.9-●
  hairy-cell C91.4-●
  juvenile myelomonocytic C93.3-●
  lymphoid C91.9-●
    specified NEC C91.Z-●
  mast cell C94.3-●
  mature B-cell, Burkitt-type C91.A-●
  monocytic (subacute) C93.9-●
    specified NEC C93.Z-●
  myelogenous —*see also* Category C92 C92.9-●
  myeloid C92.9-●
    specified NEC C92.Z-●
  plasma cell C90.1-●
  plasmacytic C90.1-●
  prolymphocytic
    of B-cell type C91.3-●
    of T-cell type C91.6-●
  specified NEC C94.8-●
  stem cell, of unclear lineage C95.0-●
  subacute lymphocytic C91.9-●

Leukemia, leukemic *(Continued)*
  T-cell large granular lymphocytic C91.Z-●
  unspecified cell type C95.9-●
    acute C95.0-●
    chronic C95.1-●
Leukemoid reaction —*see also* Reaction, leukemoid
  D72.823-●
Leukoaraiosis (hypertensive) I67.81
Leukoariosis —*see* Leukoaraiosis
Leukocoria —*see* Disorder, globe, degenerated
  condition, leucocoria
Leukocytopenia D72.819
Leukocytosis D72.829
  eosinophilic D72.19
Leukoderma, leukodermia NEC L81.5
  syphilitic A51.39
  late A52.79
Leukodystrophy G31.80
Leukoedema, oral epithelium K13.29
Leukoencephalitis G04.81
  with vanishing white matter disease G11.6
  acute (subacute) hemorrhagic G36.1
    postimmunization or postvaccinal G04.02
  LMNB1-related autosomal dominant G90.B
  metachromatic E75.25
  pol III-related G11.5
  postinfectious G04.01
  subacute sclerosing A81.1
  van Bogaert's (sclerosing) A81.1
Leukoencephalopathy —*see also* Encephalopathy
  G93.49
  ~~with calcifications and cysts G93.43~~
  ▶with
    ▶brainstem - spinal cord involvement - lactate
      elevation E88.43
    ▶calcifications and cysts G93.43
    ▶thalamus - brainstem involvement - high
      lactate E88.43
  adult-onset, with axonal spheroids (and
    pigmented glia) G93.44
  Binswanger's I67.3
  heroin vapor G92.8
  megalencephalic, with subcortical cysts
    G93.42
  metachromatic E75.25
  multifocal (progressive) A81.2
  postimmunization and postvaccinal G04.02
  progressive multifocal A81.2
  reversible, posterior G93.6
  van Bogaert's (sclerosing) A81.1
  vascular, progressive I67.3
Leukoerythroblastosis D75.9
Leukokeratosis —*see also* Leukoplakia
  mouth K13.21
  nicotina palati K13.24
  oral mucosa K13.21
  tongue K13.21
  vocal cord J38.3
Leukokraurosis vulva (e) N90.4
Leukoma (cornea) —*see also* Opacity, cornea
  adherent H17.0-●
  interfering with central vision —*see* Opacity,
    cornea, central
Leukomalacia, cerebral, newborn P91.2
  periventricular P91.2
Leukomelanopathy, hereditary D72.0
Leukonychia (punctata) (striata) L60.8
  congenital Q84.4
Leukopathia unguium L60.8
  congenital Q84.4
Leukopenia D72.819
  basophilic D72.818
  chemotherapy (cancer) induced D70.1
  congenital D70.0
  cyclic D70.0
  drug induced NEC D70.2
    due to cytoreductive cancer chemotherapy D70.1
  eosinophilic D72.818
  familial D70.0
  infantile genetic D70.0
  malignant D70.9
  periodic D70.0
  transitory neonatal P61.5
Leukopenic —*see* condition
Leukoplakia
  anus K62.89
  bladder (postinfectional) N32.89
  buccal K13.21
  cervix (uteri) N88.0
  esophagus K22.89
  gingiva K13.21

Leukoplakia *(Continued)*
  hairy (oral mucosa) (tongue) K13.3
  kidney (pelvis) N28.89
  larynx J38.7
  lip K13.21
  mouth K13.21
  oral epithelium, including tongue (mucosa) K13.21
  palate K13.21
  pelvis (kidney) N28.89
  penis (infectional) N48.0
  rectum K62.89
  syphilitic (late) A52.79
  tongue K13.21
  ureter (postinfectional) N28.89
  urethra (postinfectional) N36.8
  uterus N85.8
  vagina N89.4
  vocal cord J38.3
  vulva N90.4
Leukorrhea N89.8
  due to Trichomonas (vaginalis) A59.00
  trichomonal A59.00
Leukosarcoma C85.9
Levocardia (isolated) Q24.1
  with situs inversus Q89.3
Levotransposition Q20.5
Lev's disease or syndrome (acquired complete
  heart block) I44.2
Levulosuria —*see* Fructosuria
Levurid L30.2
Lewy body (ies) (disease) G31.83
Leyden-Möbius dystrophy —*see* Dystrophy,
  Leyden-Möbius
Leydig cell
  carcinoma
    specified site —*see* Neoplasm, malignant, by
      site
    unspecified site
      female C56.9-●
      male C62.9-●
  tumor
    benign
      specified site —*see* Neoplasm, benign, by
        site
      unspecified site
        female D27.-●
        male D29.2-●
    malignant
      specified site —*see* Neoplasm, malignant,
        by site
      unspecified site
        female C56.-●
        male C62.9-●
    specified site —*see* Neoplasm, uncertain
      behavior, by site
    unspecified site
      female D39.1-●
      male D40.1-●
Leydig-Sertoli cell tumor
  specified site —*see* Neoplasm, benign, by site
  unspecified site
    female D27.-●
    male D29.2-●
LGMD —*see* Dystrophy, muscular, limb-girdle
LGSIL (Low grade squamous intraepithelial lesion
  on cytologic smear of)
  anus R85.612
  cervix R87.612
  vagina R87.622
Liar, pathologic F60.2
Libido
  decreased R68.82
Libman-Sacks disease M32.11
Lice (infestation) B85.2
  body (Pediculus corporis) B85.1
  crab B85.3
  head (Pediculus capitis) B85.0
  mixed (classifiable to more than one of the titles
    B85.0-B85.3) B85.4
  pubic (Phthirus pubis) B85.3
Lichen L28.0
  albus L90.0
    penis N48.0
    vulva N90.4
  amyloidosis E85.4 *[L99]*
  atrophicus L90.0
    penis N48.0
    vulva N90.4
  congenital Q82.8
  myxedematosus L98.5
  nitidus L44.1

▶ New   ⇨ Revised   ~~deleted~~ Deleted   ● Use Additional Character(s)

▶ New   ⇒ Revised   ~~deleted~~ Deleted   ● Use Additional Character(s)

M

▶ New   ⇒ Revised   ~~deleted~~ Deleted   ● Use Additional Character(s)

▶ New ⇒ Revised ~~deleted~~ Deleted ● Use Additional Character(s)

  ▶ New   ⇨ Revised   ~~deleted~~ Deleted   ● Use Additional Character(s)

▶ New   ➡ Revised   ~~deleted~~ Deleted   ● Use Additional Character(s)

Meningitis (Continued)
  H. influenzae G00.0
  in (due to)
    adenovirus A87.1
    African trypanosomiasis B56.9 [G02]
    anthrax A22.8
    bacterial disease NEC A48.8 [G01]
    Chagas' disease (chronic) B57.41
    chickenpox B01.0
    coccidioidomycosis B38.4
    Diplococcus pneumoniae G00.1
    enterovirus A87.0
    herpes (simplex) virus B00.3
      zoster B02.1
    infectious mononucleosis B27.92
    leptospirosis A27.81
    Listeria monocytogenes A32.11
    Lyme disease A69.21
    measles B05.1
    mumps (virus) B26.1
    neurosyphilis (late) A52.13
    parasitic disease NEC B89 [G02]
    poliovirus A80.9 [G02]
    preventive immunization, inoculation or
      vaccination G03.8
    rubella B06.02
    Salmonella infection A02.21
    specified cause NEC G03.8
    Streptococcal pneumoniae G00.1
    typhoid fever A01.01
    varicella B01.0
    viral disease NEC A87.8
    whooping cough A37.90
    zoster B02.1
  infectious G00.9
  influenzal (H. influenzae) G00.0
  Klebsiella G00.8
  leptospiral (aseptic) A27.81
  lymphocytic (acute) (benign) (serous)
    A87.2
  meningococcal A39.0
  Mima polymorpha G00.8
  Mollaret (benign recurrent) G03.2
  monilial B37.5
  mycotic NEC B49 [G02]
  Neisseria A39.0
  nonbacterial G03.9
  nonpyogenic NEC G03.0
  ossificans G96.198
  pneumococcal streptococcus pneumoniae
    G00.1
  poliovirus A80.9 [G02]
  postmeasles B05.1
  purulent G00.9
    specified organism NEC G00.8
  pyogenic G00.9
    specified organism NEC G00.8
  Salmonella (arizonae) (Cholerae-Suis)
    (enteritidis) (typhimurium) A02.21
  septic G00.9
    specified organism NEC G00.8
  serosa circumscripta NEC G03.0
  serous NEC G93.2
  specified organism NEC G00.8
  sporotrichosis B42.81
  staphylococcal G00.3
  sterile G03.0
  Streptococcal (acute) G00.2
    pneumoniae G00.1
  suppurative G00.9
    specified organism NEC G00.8
  syphilitic (late) (tertiary) A52.13
    acute A51.41
    congenital A50.41
    secondary A51.41
  Torula histolytica (cryptococcal) B45.1
  traumatic (complication of injury) T79.8
  tuberculous A17.0
  typhoid A01.01
  viral NEC A87.9
  Yersinia pestis A20.3
Meningocele (spinal) —*see also* Spina bifida
  with hydrocephalus —*see* Spina bifida, by site,
    with hydrocephalus
  acquired (traumatic) G96.198
  cerebral —*see* Encephalocele
Meningocerebritis —*see* Meningoencephalitis
Meningococcemia A39.4
  acute A39.2
  chronic A39.3

Meningococcus, meningococcal —*see also*
  condition A39.9
  adrenalitis, hemorrhagic A39.1
  carrier (suspected) of Z22.31
  meningitis (cerebrospinal) A39.0
Meningoencephalitis —*see also* Encephalitis
  G04.90
  acute NEC —*see also* Encephalitis, viral A86
  bacterial NEC G04.2
  California A83.5
  diphasic A84.1
  eosinophilic B83.2
  epidemic A39.81
  herpesviral, herpetic B00.4
    due to herpesvirus 6 B10.01
    due to herpesvirus 7 B10.09
    specified NEC B10.09
  in (due to)
    blastomycosis NEC B40.81
    diseases classified elsewhere G05.3
    free-living amebae B60.2
    Hemophilus influenzae (H. influenzae)
      G00.0
    herpes B00.4
      due to herpesvirus 6 B10.01
      due to herpesvirus 7 B10.09
      specified NEC B10.09
    H. influenzae G00.0
    Lyme disease A69.22
    mercury —*see* subcategory T56.1
    mumps B26.2
    Naegleria (amebae) (organisms) (fowleri)
      B60.2
    Parastrongylus cantonensis B83.2
    toxoplasmosis (acquired) B58.2
      congenital P37.1
  infectious (acute) (viral) A86
  influenzal (H. influenzae) G00.0
  Listeria monocytogenes A32.12
  lymphocytic (serous) A87.2
  mumps B26.2
  parasitic NEC B89 [G05.3]
  pneumococcal G04.2
  primary amebic B60.2
  specific (syphilitic) A52.14
  specified organism NEC G04.81
  staphylococcal G04.2
  streptococcal G04.2
  syphilitic A52.14
  toxic NEC G92.8
    due to mercury —*see* subcategory
      T56.1
  tuberculous A17.82
  virus NEC A86
Meningoencephalocele —*see also* Encephalocele
  syphilitic A52.19
    congenital A50.49
Meningoencephalomyelitis —*see also*
  Meningoencephalitis
  acute NEC (viral) A86
    disseminated G04.00
      postimmunization or postvaccination
        G04.02
      postinfectious G04.01
    due to
      actinomycosis A42.82
      Torula B45.1
      Toxoplasma or toxoplasmosis (acquired)
        B58.2
        congenital P37.1
    postimmunization or postvaccination
      G04.02
Meningoencephalomyelopathy G96.9
Meningoencephalopathy G96.9
Meningomyelitis —*see also* Meningoencephalitis
  bacterial NEC G04.2
  blastomycotic NEC B40.81
  cryptococcal B45.1
  in diseases classified elsewhere G05.4
  meningococcal A39.81
  syphilitic A52.14
  tuberculous A17.82
Meningomyelocele —*see also* Spina bifida
  syphilitic A52.19
Meningomyeloneuritis —*see* Meningoencephalitis
Meningoradiculitis —*see* Meningitis
Meningovascular —*see* condition
Menkes' disease or syndrome E83.09
  meaning maple-syrup-urine disease E71.0
Menometrorrhagia N92.1

Menopause, menopausal (asymptomatic) (state)
  Z78.0
  arthritis (any site) NEC —*see* Arthritis, specified
    form NEC
  bleeding N92.4
  depression (single episode) F32.89
    agitated (single episode) F32.2
      recurrent episode F33.9
    psychotic (single episode) F32.89
      zrecurrent episode F33.8
    recurrent episode F33.9
    melancholia (single episode) F32.89
      recurrent episode F33.8
  paranoid state F22
  postirradiation (postprocedural)
    asymptomatic E89.40
    symptomatic E89.41
  premature E28.319
    asymptomatic E28.319
      postirradiation E89.40
      postsurgical E89.40
    symptomatic E28.310
      postirradiation E89.41
      postsurgical E89.41
  psychosis NEC F28
  symptomatic N95.1
  toxic polyarthritis NEC —*see* Arthritis, specified
    form NEC
Menorrhagia (primary) N92.0
  climacteric N92.4
    menopausal N92.4
  menopausal N92.4
  perimenopausal N92.4
  postclimacteric N95.0
  postmenopausal N95.0
  preclimacteric or premenopausal N92.4
  pubertal (menses retained) N92.2
Menostaxis N92.0
Menses, retention N94.89
Menstrual —*see* Menstruation
Menstruation
  absent —*see* Amenorrhea
  anovulatory N97.0
  cycle, irregular N92.6
  delayed N91.0
  disorder N93.9
    psychogenic F45.8
  during pregnancy O20.8
  excessive (with regular cycle) N92.0
    with irregular cycle N92.1
    at puberty N92.2
  frequent N92.0
  infrequent —*see* Oligomenorrhea
  irregular N92.6
    specified NEC N92.5
  latent N92.5
  membranous N92.5
  painful —*see also* Dysmenorrhea N94.6
    primary N94.4
    psychogenic F45.8
    secondary N94.5
  passage of clots N92.0
  precocious E30.1
  protracted N92.5
  rare —*see* Oligomenorrhea
  retained N94.89
  retrograde N92.5
  scanty —*see* Oligomenorrhea
  suppression N94.89
  vicarious (nasal) N94.89
Mental —*see also* condition
  deficiency —*see* Disability, intellectual
  deterioration —*see* Psychosis
  disorder —*see* Disorder, mental
  exhaustion F48.8
  insufficiency (congenital) —*see* Disability,
    intellectual
  observation without need for further medical
    care Z03.89
  retardation —*see* Disability, intellectual
  subnormality —*see* Disability, intellectual
  upset —*see* Disorder, mental
Meralgia paresthetica G57.1-●
Mercurial —*see* condition
Mercurialism —*see* subcategory T56.1
MERRF syndrome (myoclonic epilepsy
  associated with ragged-red fiber)
  E88.42
Merkel cell tumor —*see* Carcinoma, Merkel cell
Merocele —*see* Hernia, femoral

M

▶ New   ⇛ Revised   ~~deleted~~ Deleted   ● Use Additional Character(s)

M

▶ New   ⇨ Revised   ~~deleted~~ Deleted   ● Use Additional Character(s)

▶ New   ➡ Revised   ~~deleted~~ Deleted   ● Use Additional Character(s)

▶ New   ⇨ Revised   ~~deleted~~ Deleted   ● Use Additional Character(s)

▶ New   ⇒ Revised   ~~deleted~~ Deleted   ● Use Additional Character(s)

▶ New   ➡ Revised   ~~deleted~~ Deleted   • Use Additional Character(s)

▶ New   ⇒ Revised   ~~deleted~~ Deleted   ● Use Additional Character(s)

▶ New   ⇒ Revised   ~~deleted~~ Deleted   ● Use Additional Character(s)

▶ New   ⇒ Revised   ~~deleted~~ Deleted   ● Use Additional Character(s)

▶ New   ➡ Revised   ~~deleted~~ Deleted   ● Use Additional Character(s)

Osteolysis (Continued)
  scapula M89.51-●
  skull M89.58
  tarsus M89.57-●
  tibia M89.56-●
  toe M89.57-●
  ulna M89.53-●
  vertebra M89.58
Osteoma —see also Neoplasm, bone, benign
  osteoid —see also Neoplasm, bone, benign
    giant —see Neoplasm, bone, benign
Osteomalacia M83.9
  adult M83.9
    drug-induced NEC M83.5
    due to
      malabsorption (postsurgical) M83.2
      malnutrition M83.3
    specified NEC M83.8
  aluminium-induced M83.4
  infantile —see Rickets
  juvenile —see Rickets
  oncogenic E83.89
  pelvis M83.8
  puerperal M83.0
  senile M83.1
  vitamin-D-resistant in adults E83.31 [M90.8-●]
    carpus E83.31 [M90.84-●]
    clavicle E83.31 [M90.81-●]
    femur E83.31 [M90.85-●]
    fibula E83.31 [M90.86-●]
    finger E83.31 [M90.84-●]
    humerus E83.31 [M90.82-●]
    ilium E83.31 [M90.88]
    ischium E83.31 [M90.88]
    metacarpus E83.31 [M90.84-●]
    metatarsus E83.31 [M90.87-●]
    multiple sites E83.31 [M90.89]
    neck E83.31 [M90.88]
    ▶ pubic ramus [pubis] E83.31 [M90.88]
    radius E83.31 [M90.83-●]
    rib E83.31 [M90.88]
    scapula E83.31 [M90.819]
    skull E83.31 [M90.88]
    tarsus E83.31 [M90.879]
    tibia E83.31 [M90.869]
    toe E83.31 [M90.879]
    ulna E83.31 [M90.839]
    vertebra E83.31 [M90.88]
Osteomyelitis (general) (infective) (localized)
  (neonatal) (purulent) (septic) (staphylococcal)
  (streptococcal) (suppurative) (with periostitis)
  M86.9
  acute M86.10
    carpus M86.14-●
    clavicle M86.11-●
    femur M86.15-●
    fibula M86.16-●
    finger M86.14-●
    hematogenous M86.00
      carpus M86.04-●
      clavicle M86.01-●
      femur M86.05-●
      fibula M86.06-●
      finger M86.04-●
      humerus M86.02-●
      ilium M86.08
      ischium M86.08
      mandible M27.2
      metacarpus M86.04-●
      metatarsus M86.07-●
      multiple sites M86.09
      neck M86.08
      orbit H05.02-●
      petrous bone —see Petrositis
      radius M86.03-●
      rib M86.08
      scapula M86.01-●
      skull M86.08
      tarsus M86.07-●
      tibia M86.06-●
      toe M86.07-●
      ulna M86.03-●
      vertebra —see Osteomyelitis, vertebra
    humerus M86.12-●
    ilium M86.18
    ischium M86.18
    mandible M27.2
    metacarpus M86.14-●
    metatarsus M86.17-●
    multiple sites M86.19

Osteomyelitis (Continued)
  acute (Continued)
    neck M86.18
    orbit H05.02-●
    petrous bone —see Petrositis
    radius M86.13-●
    rib M86.18
    scapula M86.11-●
    skull M86.18
    tarsus M86.17-●
    tibia M86.16-●
    toe M86.17-●
    ulna M86.13-●
    vertebra —see Osteomyelitis, vertebra
  chronic (or old) M86.60
    with draining sinus M86.40
      carpus M86.44-●
      clavicle M86.41-●
      femur M86.45-●
      fibula M86.46-●
      finger M86.44-●
      humerus M86.42-●
      ilium M86.48
      ischium M86.48
      mandible M27.2
      metacarpus M86.44-●
      metatarsus M86.47-●
      multiple sites M86.49
      neck M86.48
      orbit H05.02-●
      petrous bone —see Petrositis
      ➡ pubic ramus [pubis] M86.48
      radius M86.43-●
      rib M86.48
      scapula M86.41-●
      skull M86.48
      tarsus M86.47-●
      tibia M86.46-●
      toe M86.47-●
      ulna M86.43-●
      vertebra —see Osteomyelitis, vertebra
    carpus M86.64-●
    clavicle M86.61-●
    femur M86.65-●
    fibula M86.66-●
    finger M86.64-●
    hematogenous NEC M86.50
      carpus M86.54-●
      clavicle M86.51-●
      femur M86.55-●
      fibula M86.56-●
      finger M86.54-●
      humerus M86.52-●
      ilium M86.58
      ischium M86.58
      mandible M27.2
      metacarpus M86.54-●
      metatarsus M86.57-●
      multifocal M86.30
        carpus M86.34-●
        clavicle M86.31-●
        femur M86.35-●
        fibula M86.36-●
        finger M86.34-●
        humerus M86.32-●
        ilium M86.38
        ischium M86.38
        metacarpus M86.34-●
        metatarsus M86.37-●
        multiple sites M86.39
        neck M86.38
        ➡ pubic ramus [pubis] M86.38
        radius M86.33-●
        rib M86.38
        scapula M86.31-●
        skull M86.38
        tarsus M86.37-●
        tibia M86.36-●
        toe M86.37-●
        ulna M86.33-●
        vertebra —see Osteomyelitis, vertebra
      multiple sites M86.59
      neck M86.58
      orbit H05.02-●
      petrous bone —see Petrositis
      ➡ pubic ramus [pubis] M86.58
      radius M86.53-●
      rib M86.58
      scapula M86.51-●
      skull M86.58

Osteomyelitis (Continued)
  chronic (Continued)
    with draining sinus (Continued)
      tarsus M86.57-●
      tibia M86.56-●
      toe M86.57-●
      ulna M86.53-●
      vertebra —see Osteomyelitis,
        vertebra
    humerus M86.62-●
    ilium M86.659
    ischium M86.659
    mandible M27.2
    metacarpus M86.64-●
    metatarsus M86.67-●
    multifocal —see Osteomyelitis, chronic,
      hematogenous, multifocal
    multiple sites M86.69
    neck M86.68
    orbit H05.02-●
    petrous bone —see Petrositis
    radius M86.63-●
    rib M86.68
    scapula M86.61-●
    skull M86.68
    tarsus M86.67-●
    tibia M86.66-●
    toe M86.67-●
    ulna M86.63-●
    vertebra —see Osteomyelitis, vertebra
  echinococcal B67.2
  Garré's —see Osteomyelitis, specified type
    NEC
  in diabetes mellitus —see E08-E13 with .69
  jaw (acute) (chronic) (lower) (neonatal)
    (suppurative) (upper) M27.2
  nonsuppurating —see Osteomyelitis, specified
    type NEC
  orbit H05.02-●
  petrous bone —see Petrositis
  Salmonella (arizonae) (cholerae-suis) (enteritidis)
    (typhimurium) A02.24
  sclerosing, nonsuppurative —see Osteomyelitis,
    specified type NEC
  specified type NEC —see also subcategory
    M86.8X-●
    mandible M27.2
    orbit H05.02-●
    petrous bone —see Petrositis
    vertebra —see Osteomyelitis, vertebra
  subacute M86.20
    carpus M86.24-●
    clavicle M86.21-●
    femur M86.25-●
    fibula M86.26-●
    finger M86.24-●
    humerus M86.22-●
    mandible M27.2
    metacarpus M86.24-●
    metatarsus M86.27-●
    multiple sites M86.29
    neck M86.28
    orbit H05.02-●
    petrous bone —see Petrositis
    radius M86.23-●
    rib M86.28
    scapula M86.21-●
    skull M86.28
    tarsus M86.27-●
    tibia M86.26-●
    toe M86.27-●
    ulna M86.23-●
    vertebra —see Osteomyelitis,
      vertebra
  syphilitic A52.77
    congenital (early) A50.02 [M90.80]
  tuberculous —see Tuberculosis, bone
  typhoid A01.05
  vertebra M46.20
    cervical region M46.22
    cervicothoracic region M46.23
    lumbar region M46.26
    lumbosacral region M46.27
    occipito-atlanto-axial region
      M46.21
    sacrococcygeal region M46.28
    thoracic region M46.24
    thoracolumbar region M46.25
Osteomyelofibrosis D47.4
Osteomyelosclerosis D75.89

Osteonecrosis M87.9
  due to
    drugs —*see* Osteonecrosis, secondary, due to, drugs
    trauma —*see* Osteonecrosis, secondary, due to, trauma
  idiopathic aseptic M87.00
    ankle M87.07-●
    carpus M87.03-●
    clavicle M87.01-●
    femur M87.05-●
    fibula M87.06-●
    finger M87.04-●
    humerus M87.02-●
    ilium M87.050
    ischium M87.050
    metacarpus M87.04-●
    metatarsus M87.07-●
    multiple sites M87.09
    neck M87.08
    pelvis M87.050
    pubic ramus [pubis] M87.050
    radius M87.03-●
    rib M87.08
    scapula M87.01-●
    skull M87.08
    tarsus M87.07-●
    tibia M87.06-●
    toe M87.07-●
    ulna M87.03-●
    vertebra M87.08
  secondary NEC M87.30
    carpus M87.33-●
    clavicle M87.31-●
    due to
      drugs M87.10
        carpus M87.13-●
        clavicle M87.11-●
        femur M87.15-●
        fibula M87.16-●
        finger M87.14-●
        humerus M87.12-●
        ilium M87.150
        ischium M87.150
        jaw M87.180
        metacarpus M87.14-●
        metatarsus M87.17-●
        multiple sites M87.19
        neck M87.188
        pubic ramus [pubis] M87.150
        radius M87.13-●
        rib M87.188
        scapula M87.11-●
        skull M87.188
        tarsus M87.17-●
        tibia M87.16-●
        toe M87.17-●
        ulna M87.13-●
        vertebra M87.188
      hemoglobinopathy NEC D58.2 [M90.50]
        carpus D58.2 [M90.54-●]
        clavicle D58.2 [M90.51-●]
        femur D58.2 [M90.55-●]
        fibula D58.2 [M90.56-●]
        finger D58.2 [M90.54-●]
        humerus D58.2 [M90.52-●]
        ilium D58.2 [M90.58]
        ischium D58.2 [M90.58]
        metacarpus D58.2 [M90.54-●]
        metatarsus D58.2 [M90.57-●]
        multiple sites D58.2 [M90.59]
        neck D58.2 [M90.58]
        pubic ramus [pubis] D58.2 [M90.58]
        radius D58.2 [M90.53-●]
        rib D58.2 [M90.58]
        scapula D58.2 [M90.51-●]
        skull D58.2 [M90.58]
        specified NEC D58.2 [M90.58]
        tarsus D58.2 [M90.57-●]
        tibia D58.2 [M90.56-●]
        toe D58.2 [M90.57-●]
        ulna D58.2 [M90.53-●]
        vertebra D58.2 [M90.58]
      trauma (previous) M87.20
        carpus M87.23-●
        clavicle M87.21-●
        femur M87.25-●
        fibula M87.26-●
        finger M87.24-●
        humerus M87.22-●
        ilium M87.25-●

Osteonecrosis (Continued)
  due to (Continued)
    due to (Continued)
      trauma (Continued)
        ischium M87.250
        metacarpus M87.250
        metatarsus M87.27-●
        multiple sites M87.29
        neck M87.28
        pubic ramus [pubis] M87.250
        radius M87.23-●
        rib M87.28
        scapula M87.21-●
        skull M87.28
        tarsus M87.27-●
        tibia M87.26-●
        toe M87.27-●
        ulna M87.23-●
        vertebra M87.28
    femur M87.35-●
    fibula M87.36-●
    finger M87.34-●
    humerus M87.32
    ilium M87.350
  in
    caisson disease T70.3 [M90.50]
      carpus T70.3 [M90.54-●]
      clavicle T70.3 [M90.51-●]
      femur T70.3 [M90.55-●]
      fibula T70.3 [M90.56-●]
      finger T70.3 [M90.54-●]
      humerus T70.3 [M90.52-●]
      ilium T70.3 [M90.58]
      ischium T70.3 [M90.58]
      metacarpus T70.3 [M90.54-●]
      metatarsus T70.3 [M90.57-●]
      multiple sites T70.3 [M90.59]
      neck T70.3 [M90.58]
      pubic ramus [pubis] T70.3 [M90.58]
      radius T70.3 [M90.53-●]
      rib T70.3 [M90.58]
      scapula T70.3 [M90.51-●]
      skull T70.3 [M90.58]
      tarsus T70.3 [M90.57-●]
      tibia T70.3 [M90.56-●]
      toe T70.3 [M90.57-●]
      ulna T70.3 [M90.53-●]
      vertebra T70.3 [M90.58]
    ischium M87.350
    metacarpus M87.34-●
    metatarsus M87.37-●
    multiple site M87.39
    neck M87.38
    pubic ramus [pubis] M87.350
    radius M87.33-●
    rib M87.38
    scapula M87.319
    skull M87.38
    tarsus M87.379
    tibia M87.366
    toe M87.379
    ulna M87.33-●
    vertebra M87.38
  specified type NEC M87.80
    carpus M87.83-●
    clavicle M87.81-●
    femur M87.85-●
    fibula M87.86-●
    finger M87.84-●
    humerus M87.82-●
    ilium M87.850
    ischium M87.850
    metacarpus M87.84-●
    metatarsus M87.87-●
    multiple sites M87.89
    neck M87.88
    pubic ramus [pubis] M87.850
    radius M87.83-●
    rib M87.88
    scapula M87.81-●
    skull M87.88
    tarsus M87.87-●
    tibia M87.86-●
    toe M87.87-●
    ulna M87.83-●
    vertebra M87.88

Osteo-onycho-arthro-dysplasia Q87.2
Osteo-onychodysplasia, hereditary Q87.2
Osteopathia condensans disseminata Q78.8

Osteopathy —*see also* Osteomyelitis, Osteonecrosis, Osteoporosis
  after poliomyelitis M89.60
    carpus M89.64-●
    clavicle M89.61-●
    femur M89.65-●
    fibula M89.66-●
    finger M89.64-●
    humerus M89.62-●
    ilium M89.68
    ischium M89.68
    metacarpus M89.64-●
    metatarsus M89.67-●
    multiple sites M89.69
    neck M89.68
    pubic ramus [pubis] M89.68
    radius M89.63-●
    rib M89.68
    scapula M89.61-●
    skull M89.68
    tarsus M89.67-●
    tibia M89.66-●
    toe M89.67-●
    ulna M89.63-●
    vertebra M89.68
  in (due to)
    renal osteodystrophy N25.0
    specified diseases classified elsewhere —*see* subcategory M90.8
Osteopenia M85.8-●
  borderline M85.8-●
Osteoperiostitis —*see* Osteomyelitis, specified type NEC
Osteopetrosis (familial) Q78.2
Osteophyte M25.70
  ankle M25.77-●
  elbow M25.72-●
  foot joint M25.77-●
  hand joint M25.74-●
  hip M25.75-●
  knee M25.76-●
  shoulder M25.71-●
  spine M25.78
  vertebrae M25.78
  wrist M25.73-●
Osteopoikilosis Q78.8
Osteoporosis (female) (male) M81.0
  with current pathological fracture M80.00
  age-related M81.0
    with current pathologic fracture M80.00
      carpus M80.04-●
      clavicle M80.01-●
      femur M80.05-●
      fibula M80.06-●
      finger M80.04-●
      hip M80.05-●
      humerus M80.02-●
      ilium M80.0B-●
      ischium M80.0B-●
      metacarpus M80.04-●
      metatarsus M80.07-●
      pelvis M80.0B-●
      pubic ramus [pubis] M80.0B-●
      radius M80.03-●
      rib(s) M80.0A
      scapula M80.01-●
      site specified NEC M80.0A
      tarsus M80.07-●
      tibia M80.06-●
      toe M80.07-●
      ulna M80.03-●
      vertebra M80.08
  disuse M81.8
    with current pathological fracture M80.80
      carpus M80.84-●
      clavicle M80.81-●
      fibula M80.86-●
      finger M80.84-●
      humerus M80.82-●
      ilium M80.0B-●
      ischium M80.0B-●
      metacarpus M80.84-●
      metatarsus M80.87-●
      pelvis M80.0B-●
      pubic ramus [pubis] M80.0B-●
      radius M80.83-●
      scapula M80.81-●
      site specified NEC M80.8A
      tarsus M80.87-●
      tibia M80.86-●

▶ New　　⇨ Revised　　~~deleted~~ Deleted　　● Use Additional Character(s)

Osteoporosis (Continued)
  disuse (Continued)
    with current pathological fracture (Continued)
      toe M80.87-●
      ulna M80.83-●
      vertebra M80.88
  drug-induced —see Osteoporosis, specified type
    NEC
  idiopathic —see Osteoporosis, specified type NEC
  involutional —see Osteoporosis, age-related
  Lequesne M81.6
  localized M81.6
  postmenopausal M81.0
    with pathological fracture M80.00
      carpus M80.04-●
      clavicle M80.01-●
      femur M80.85-●
      fibula M80.06-●
      finger M80.04-●
      hip M80.85-●
      humerus M80.02-●
      ilium M80.0A
      ischium M80.0A
      metacarpus M80.04-●
      metatarsus M80.07-●
      pelvis M80.0B-●
      ▶ pubic ramus [pubis] M80.0B-●
      radius M80.03-●
      scapula M80.01-●
      site specified NEC M80.0A
      tarsus M80.07-●
      tibia M80.06-●
      toe M80.07-●
      ulna M80.03-●
      vertebra M80.08
  postoophorectomy —see Osteoporosis, specified
    type NEC
  postsurgical malabsorption —see Osteoporosis,
    specified type NEC
  post-traumatic —see Osteoporosis, specified type
    NEC
  senile —see Osteoporosis, age-related
  specified type NEC M81.8
    with pathological fracture M80.80
      carpus M80.84-●
      clavicle M80.81-●
      femur M80.85-●
      fibula M80.86-●
      finger M80.84-●
      hip M80.85-●
      humerus M80.82-●
      ⇒ ilium M80.8B-●
      ⇒ ischium M80.8B-●
      metacarpus M80.84-●
      metatarsus M80.87-●
      ⇒ pelvis M80.8B-●
      radius M80.83-●
      ▶ pubic ramus [pubis] M80.8B-●
      scapula M80.81-●
      site specified NEC M80.8A
      tarsus M80.87-●
      tibia M80.86-●
      toe M80.87-●
      ulna M80.83-●
      vertebra M80.88

Osteopsathyrosis (idiopathica) Q78.0
Osteoradionecrosis, jaw (acute) (chronic) (lower)
  (suppurative) (upper) M27.2
Osteosarcoma (any form) —see Neoplasm, bone,
  malignant
Osteosclerosis Q78.2
  acquired M85.8-●
  congenita Q77.4
  fragilitas (generalisata) Q78.2
  myelofibrosis D75.81
Osteosclerotic anemia D64.89
Osteosis
  cutis L94.2
  renal fibrocystic N25.0
Österreicher-Turner syndrome Q87.2
Ostium
  atrioventriculare commune Q21.23
  primum (arteriosum) (defect) (persistent) Q21.20
  secundum (arteriosum) (defect) (patent)
    (persistent) Q21.11
Ostrum-Furst syndrome Q75.8
Otalgia —see subcategory H92.0
Otitis (acute) H66.90
  with effusion —see also Otitis, media,
    nonsuppurative
    purulent —see Otitis, media, suppurative

Otitis (Continued)
  adhesive —see subcategory H74.1
  chronic —see also Otitis, media, chronic
    with effusion —see also Otitis, media,
      nonsuppurative, chronic
  externa H60.9-●—
    abscess —see Abscess, ear, external
    acute (noninfective) H60.50-●
      actinic H60.51-●
      chemical H60.52-●
      contact H60.53-●
      eczematoid H60.54-●
      infective —see Otitis, externa, infective
      reactive H60.55-●
      specified NEC H60.59-●
    cellulitis —see Cellulitis, ear
    chronic H60.6-●
    diffuse —see Otitis, externa, infective, diffuse
    hemorrhagic —see Otitis, externa, infective,
      hemorrhagic
    in (due to)
      aspergillosis B44.89
      candidiasis B37.84
    ⇒   erysipelas A46 [H62.4-●]
      herpes (simplex) virus infection B00.1
      zoster B02.8
    ⇒   impetigo L01.00 [H62.4-●]
    ⇒   infectious disease NEC B99 [H62.4-●]
    ⇒   mycosis NEC B36.9 [H62.4-●]
    ⇒   parasitic disease NEC B89 [H62.4-●]
    ⇒   viral disease NEC B34.9 [H62.4-●]
      zoster B02.8
    infective NEC H60.39-●
      abscess —see Abscess, ear, external
      cellulitis —see Cellulitis, ear
      diffuse H60.31-●
      hemorrhagic H60.32-●
      swimmer's ear —see Swimmer's, ear
    malignant H60.2-●
  ⇒ mycotic NEC B36.9 [H62.4-●]
    in
      aspergillosis B44.89
      candidiasis B37.84
      moniliasis B37.84
    necrotizing —see Otitis, externa,
      malignant
    Pseudomonas aeruginosa —see Otitis, externa,
      malignant
    reactive —see Otitis, externa, acute,
      reactive
    specified NEC —see subcategory H60.8
  ⇒ tropical NEC B36.9 H62.4-●
    in
      aspergillosis B44.89
      candidiasis B37.84
      moniliasis B37.84
  insidiosa —see Otosclerosis
  interna —see subcategory H83.0
  media (hemorrhagic) (staphylococcal)
    (streptococcal) H66.9-●
    with effusion (nonpurulent) —see Otitis,
      media, nonsuppurative
    acute, subacute H66.90
      allergic —see Otitis, media, nonsuppurative,
        acute, allergic
      exudative —see Otitis, media, suppurative,
        acute
      mucoid —see Otitis, media,
        nonsuppurative, acute
      necrotizing —see also Otitis, media,
        suppurative, acute
        in
          measles B05.3
          scarlet fever A38.0
      nonsuppurative NEC —see Otitis, media,
        nonsuppurative, acute
      purulent —see Otitis, media, suppurative,
        acute
      sanguinous —see Otitis, media,
        nonsuppurative, acute
      secretory —see Otitis, media,
        nonsuppurative, acute, serous
      seromucinous —see Otitis, media,
        nonsuppurative, acute
      serous —see Otitis, media, nonsuppurative,
        acute, serous
      suppurative —see Otitis, media,
        suppurative, acute
      allergic —see Otitis, media,
        nonsuppurative
      catarrhal —see Otitis, media, nonsuppurative

Otitis (Continued)
  media (Continued)
    chronic H66.90
      with effusion (nonpurulent) —see Otitis,
        media, nonsuppurative, chronic
      allergic —see Otitis, media, nonsuppurative,
        chronic, allergic
      benign suppurative —see Otitis, media,
        suppurative, chronic, tubotympanic
      catarrhal —see Otitis, media,
        nonsuppurative, chronic, serous
      exudative —see Otitis, media, suppurative,
        chronic
      mucinous —see Otitis, media,
        nonsuppurative, chronic, mucoid
      mucoid —see Otitis, media,
        nonsuppurative, chronic, mucoid
      nonsuppurative NEC —see Otitis, media,
        nonsuppurative, chronic
      purulent —see Otitis, media, suppurative,
        chronic
      secretory —see Otitis, media,
        nonsuppurative, chronic, mucoid
      seromucinous —see Otitis, media,
        nonsuppurative, chronic
      serous —see Otitis, media, nonsuppurative,
        chronic, serous
      suppurative —see Otitis, media,
        suppurative, chronic
      transudative —see Otitis, media,
        nonsuppurative, chronic, mucoid
    exudative —see Otitis, media,
      nonsuppurative
    in (due to) (with)
      influenza —see Influenza, with, otitis
        media
      measles B05.3
      scarlet fever A38.0
      tuberculosis A18.6
      viral disease NEC B34.- ● [H67.- ●]
    mucoid —see Otitis, media,
      nonsuppurative
    nonsuppurative H65.9-●
      acute or subacute NEC H65.19-●
        allergic H65.11-●
          recurrent H65.11-●
        recurrent H65.19-●
        secretory —see Otitis, media,
          nonsuppurative, serous
        serous H65.0-●
          recurrent H65.0-●
      chronic H65.49-●
        allergic H65.41-●
        mucoid H65.3-●
        serous H65.2-●
    postmeasles B05.3
    purulent —see Otitis, media, suppurative
    secretory —see Otitis, media,
      nonsuppurative
    seromucinous —see Otitis, media,
      nonsuppurative
    serous —see Otitis, media, nonsuppurative
    suppurative H66.4-●
      acute H66.00-●
        with rupture of ear drum H66.01-●
        recurrent H66.00-●
          with rupture of ear drum H66.01-●
      chronic —see also subcategory H66.3
        atticoantral H66.2-●
        benign —see Otitis, media, suppurative,
          chronic, tubotympanic
        tubotympanic H66.1-●
    transudative —see Otitis, media,
      nonsuppurative
    tuberculous A18.6
Otocephaly Q18.2
Otolith syndrome —see subcategory H81.8
⇒ **Otomycosis** (diffuse) NEC B36.9 [H62.4-●]
  in
    aspergillosis B44.89
    candidiasis B37.84
    moniliasis B37.84
Otoporosis —see Otosclerosis
Otorrhagia (nontraumatic) H92.2-●
  traumatic - code by Type of injury
Otorrhea H92.1-●
  cerebrospinal (fluid) G96.01
    postoperative G96.08
    specified NEC G96.08
    spontaneous G96.01
    traumatic G96.08

▶ New　　➡ Revised　　~~deleted~~ Deleted　　● Use Additional Character(s)

Paraganglioma *(Continued)*
  extra-adrenal *(Continued)*
    specified site —*see* Neoplasm, uncertain
      behavior, by site
    unspecified site D44.7
  gangliocytic D13.2
    specified site —*see* Neoplasm, benign, by site
    unspecified site D13.2
  glomus jugulare D44.7
    malignant C75.5
  jugular D44.7
  malignant C75.5
    specified site —*see* Neoplasm, malignant, by
      site
    unspecified site C75.5
  nonchromaffin D44.7
    malignant C75.5
      specified site —*see* Neoplasm, malignant,
        by site
      unspecified site C75.5
    specified site —*see* Neoplasm, uncertain
      behavior, by site
    unspecified site D44.7
  parasympathetic D44.7
    specified site —*see* Neoplasm, uncertain
      behavior, by site
    unspecified site D44.7
  specified site —*see* Neoplasm, uncertain
    behavior, by site
  sympathetic D44.7
    specified site —*see* Neoplasm, uncertain
      behavior, by site
    unspecified site D44.7
  unspecified site D44.7
Parageusia R43.2
  psychogenic F45.8
Paragonimiasis B66.4
Paragranuloma, Hodgkin —*see* Lymphoma,
  Hodgkin, specified NEC
Parahemophilia —*see also* Defect, coagulation
  D68.2
Parakeratosis R23.4
  variegata L41.0
Paralysis, paralytic (complete) (incomplete) G83.9
  with
    syphilis A52.17
  abducens, abducent (nerve) —*see* Strabismus,
    paralytic, sixth nerve
  abductor, lower extremity G57.9-●
  accessory nerve G52.8
  accommodation —*see also* Paresis, of
    accommodation
    hysterical F44.89
  acoustic nerve (except Deafness) —*see*
    subcategory H93.3
  agitans —*see also* Parkinsonism G20.C
    arteriosclerotic G21.4
  alternating (oculomotor) G83.89
  amyotrophic G12.21
  ankle G57.9-●
  anus (sphincter) K62.89
  arm —*see* Monoplegia, upper limb
  ascending (spinal), acute G61.0
  association G12.29
  asthenic bulbar G70.00
    with exacerbation (acute) G70.01
    in crisis G70.01
  ataxic (hereditary) G11.9
    general (syphilitic) A52.17
  atrophic G58.9
    infantile, acute —*see* Poliomyelitis, paralytic
    progressive G12.22
    spinal (acute) —*see* Poliomyelitis, paralytic
  axillary G54.0
  Babinski-Nageotte's G83.89
  Bell's G51.0
    newborn P11.3
  Benedikt's G46.3
  birth injury P14.9
    spinal cord P11.5
  bladder (neurogenic) (sphincter) N31.2
  bowel, colon or intestine K56.0
  brachial plexus G54.0
    birth injury P14.3
    newborn (birth injury) P14.3
  brain G83.9
    diplegia G83.0
    triplegia G83.89
  bronchial J98.09
  Brown-Séquard G83.81

Paralysis, paralytic *(Continued)*
  bulbar (chronic) (progressive) G12.22
    infantile —*see* Poliomyelitis, paralytic
    poliomyelitic —*see* Poliomyelitis, paralytic
    pseudo G12.29
  bulbospinal G70.00
    with exacerbation (acute) G70.01
    in crisis G70.01
  cardiac —*see also* Failure, heart I50.9
  cerebrocerebellar, diplegic G80.1
  cervical
    plexus G54.2
    sympathetic G90.09
  Céstan-Chenais G46.3
  Charcot-Marie-Tooth type G60.0
  Clark's G80.9
  colon K56.0
  compressed air T70.3
  compression
    arm G56.9-●
    leg G57.9-●
    lower extremity G57.9-●
    upper extremity G56.9-●
  congenital (cerebral) —*see* Palsy, cerebral
  conjugate movement (gaze) (of eye) H51.0
    cortical (nuclear) (supranuclear) H51.0
  cordis —*see* Failure, heart
  cranial or cerebral nerve G52.9
  creeping G12.22
  crossed leg G83.89
  crutch —*see* Injury, brachial plexus
  deglutition R13.0
    hysterical F44.4
  dementia A52.17
  descending (spinal) NEC G12.29
  diaphragm (flaccid) J98.6
    due to accidental dissection of phrenic nerve
      during procedure —*see* Puncture,
      accidental complicating surgery
  digestive organs NEC K59.89
  diplegic —*see* Diplegia
  divergence (nuclear) H51.8
  diver's T70.3
  Duchenne's
    birth injury P14.0
    due to or associated with
      motor neuron disease G12.22
      muscular dystrophy G71.01
  due to intracranial or spinal birth injury —*see*
    Palsy, cerebral
  embolic (current episode) I63.4-●
  Erb (-Duchenne) (birth) (newborn) P14.0
  Erb's syphilitic spastic spinal A52.17
  esophagus K22.89
  eye muscle (extrinsic) H49.9
    intrinsic —*see also* Paresis, of accommodation
  facial (nerve) G51.0
    birth injury P11.3
    congenital P11.3
    following operation NEC —*see* Puncture,
      accidental complicating surgery
    newborn (birth injury) P11.3
  familial (recurrent) (periodic) G72.3
    spastic G11.4
  fauces J39.2
  finger G56.9-●
  gait R26.1
  gastric nerve (nondiabetic) G52.2
  gaze, conjugate H51.0
  general (progressive) (syphilitic) A52.17
    juvenile A50.45
  glottis J38.00
    bilateral J38.02
    unilateral J38.01
  gluteal G54.1
  Gubler (-Millard) G46.3
  hand —*see* Monoplegia, upper limb
  heart —*see* Arrest, cardiac
  hemiplegic —*see* Hemiplegia
  hyperkalemic periodic (familial) G72.3
  hypoglossal (nerve) G52.3
  hypokalemic periodic G72.3
  hysterical F44.4
  ileus K56.0
  infantile —*see also* Poliomyelitis, paralytic A80.30
    bulbar —*see* Poliomyelitis, paralytic
    cerebral —*see* Palsy, cerebral
    spastic —*see* Palsy, cerebral, spastic
  infective —*see* Poliomyelitis, paralytic
  inferior nuclear G83.9
  internuclear —*see* Ophthalmoplegia, internuclear

Paralysis, paralytic *(Continued)*
  intestine K56.0
  iris H57.09
    due to diphtheria (toxin) A36.89
  ischemic, Volkmann's (complicating trauma)
    T79.6
  Jackson's G83.89
  jake —*see* Poisoning, food, noxious, plant
  Jamaica ginger (jake) G62.2
  juvenile general A50.45
  Klumpke (-Déjérine) (birth) (newborn) P14.1
  labioglossal (laryngeal) (pharyngeal) G12.29
  Landry's G61.0
  laryngeal nerve (recurrent) (superior) (unilateral)
    J38.00
    bilateral J38.02
    unilateral J38.01
  larynx J38.00
    bilateral J38.02
    due to diphtheria (toxin) A36.2
    unilateral J38.01
  lateral G12.23
  lead —*see* subcategory T56.0
  left side —*see* Hemiplegia
  leg G83.1-●
    both —*see* Paraplegia
    crossed G83.89
    hysterical F44.4
    psychogenic F44.4
    transient or transitory R29.818
      traumatic NEC —*see* Injury, nerve, leg
  levator palpebrae superioris —*see*
      Blepharoptosis, paralytic
  limb —*see* Monoplegia
  lip K13.0
  Lissauer's A52.17
  lower limb —*see* Monoplegia, lower limb
    both —*see* Paraplegia
  lung J98.4
  median nerve G56.1-●
  medullary (tegmental) G83.89
  mesencephalic NEC G83.89
    tegmental G83.89
  middle alternating G83.89
  Millard-Gubler-Foville G46.3
  monoplegic —*see* Monoplegia
  motor G83.9
  muscle, muscular NEC G72.89
    due to nerve lesion G58.9
    eye (extrinsic) H49.9
      intrinsic —*see* Paresis, of accommodation
      oblique —*see* Strabismus, paralytic, fourth
        nerve
    iris sphincter H21.9
    ischemic (Volkmann's) (complicating trauma)
      T79.6
    progressive G12.21
    progressive, spinal G12.25
    pseudohypertrophic G71.02
    spinal progressive G12.25
  musculocutaneous nerve G56.9-●
  musculospiral G56.9-●
  nerve —*see also* Disorder, nerve
    abducent —*see* Strabismus, paralytic, sixth
      nerve
    accessory G52.8
    auditory (except Deafness) —*see* subcategory
      H93.3
    birth injury P14.9
    cranial or cerebral G52.9
    facial G51.0
      birth injury P11.3
      congenital P11.3
      newborn (birth injury) P11.3
    fourth or trochlear —*see* Strabismus, paralytic,
      fourth nerve
    newborn (birth injury) P14.9
    oculomotor —*see* Strabismus, paralytic, third
      nerve
    phrenic (birth injury) P14.2
    radial G56.3-●
    seventh or facial G51.0
      newborn (birth injury) P11.3
    sixth or abducent —*see* Strabismus, paralytic,
      sixth nerve
    syphilitic A52.15
    third or oculomotor —*see* Strabismus,
      paralytic, third nerve
    trigeminal G50.9
    trochlear —*see* Strabismus, paralytic, fourth
      nerve
    ulnar G56.2-●

► New   ⇒ Revised   ~~deleted~~ Deleted   ● Use Additional Character(s)

Perforation, perforated *(Continued)*
  broad ligament N83.8
    with or following ectopic or molar pregnancy O08.6
    obstetrical trauma O71.6
  by
    device, implant or graft —*see also* Complications, by site and type, mechanical T85.628
      arterial graft NEC —*see* Complication, cardiovascular device, mechanical, vascular
      breast (implant) T85.49
      catheter NEC T85.698
        cystostomy T83.090
        dialysis (renal) T82.49
          intraperitoneal T85.691
        infusion NEC T82.594
          spinal (epidural) (subdural) T85.690
        urinary —*see also* Complications, catheter, urinary T83.098
      electronic (electrode) (pulse generator) (stimulator)
        bone T84.390
        cardiac T82.199
          electrode T82.190
          pulse generator T82.191
          specified type NEC T82.198
        nervous system —*see* Complication, prosthetic device, mechanical, electronic nervous system stimulator
        urinary —*see* Complication, genitourinary, device, urinary, mechanical
      fixation, internal (orthopedic) NEC —*see* Complication, fixation device, mechanical
      gastrointestinal —*see* Complications, prosthetic device, mechanical, gastrointestinal device
      genital NEC T83.498
        intrauterine contraceptive device T83.39
        penile prosthesis T83.490
      heart NEC —*see* Complication, cardiovascular device, mechanical
      joint prosthesis —*see* Complications, joint prosthesis, mechanical, specified NEC, by site
      ocular NEC —*see* Complications, prosthetic device, mechanical, ocular device
      orthopedic NEC —*see* Complication, orthopedic, device, mechanical
      specified NEC T85.628
      urinary NEC —*see also* Complication, genitourinary, device, urinary, mechanical
        graft T83.29
      vascular NEC —*see* Complication, cardiovascular device, mechanical
      ventricular intracranial shunt T85.09
    foreign body left accidentally in operative wound T81.539
    instrument (any) during a procedure, accidental —*see* Puncture, accidental complicating surgery
  cecum K35.22
    with localized peritonitis K35.32
  cervix (uteri) N88.8
    with or following ectopic or molar pregnancy O08.6
    obstetrical trauma O71.3
  colon K63.1
    newborn P78.0
    obstetrical trauma O71.5
    traumatic —*see* Laceration, intestine, large
  common duct (bile) K83.2
  cornea (due to ulceration) —*see* Ulcer, cornea, perforated
  cystic duct K82.2
  diverticulum (intestine) K57.80
    with bleeding K57.81
    large intestine K57.20
      with
        bleeding K57.21
        small intestine K57.40
          with bleeding K57.41
    small intestine K57.00
      with
        bleeding K57.01
        large intestine K57.40
          with bleeding K57.41

Perforation, perforated *(Continued)*
  ear drum —*see* Perforation, tympanum
  esophagus K22.3
  ethmoidal sinus —*see* Sinusitis, ethmoidal
  frontal sinus —*see* Sinusitis, frontal
  gallbladder K82.2
  heart valve —*see* Endocarditis
  ileum K63.1
    newborn P78.0
    obstetrical trauma O71.5
    traumatic —*see* Laceration, intestine, small
  instrumental, surgical (accidental) (blood vessel) (nerve) (organ) —*see* Puncture, accidental complicating surgery
  intestine NEC K63.1
    with ectopic or molar pregnancy O08.6
    newborn P78.0
    obstetrical trauma O71.5
    traumatic —*see* Laceration, intestine
    ulcerative NEC K63.1
      newborn P78.0
  jejunum, jejunal K63.1
    obstetrical trauma O71.5
    traumatic —*see* Laceration, intestine, small
    ulcer —*see* Ulcer, gastrojejunal, with perforation
  joint prosthesis —*see* Complications, joint prosthesis, mechanical, specified NEC, by site
  mastoid (antrum) (cell) —*see* Disorder, mastoid, specified NEC
  maxillary sinus —*see* Sinusitis, maxillary
  membrana tympani —*see* Perforation, tympanum
  nasal
    septum J34.89
      congenital Q30.3
      syphilitic A52.73
    sinus J34.89
      congenital Q30.8
      due to sinusitis —*see* Sinusitis
  palate —*see also* Cleft, palate Q35.9
    syphilitic A52.79
  palatine vault —*see also* Cleft, palate, hard Q35.1
    syphilitic A52.79
    congenital A50.59
  pars flaccida (ear drum) —*see* Perforation, tympanum, attic
  pelvic
    floor S31.030
      with
        ectopic or molar pregnancy O08.6
        penetration into retroperitoneal space S31.031
        retained foreign body S31.040
          with penetration into retroperitoneal space S31.041
      following ectopic or molar pregnancy O08.6
      obstetrical trauma O70.1
    organ S37.99
      adrenal gland S37.818
      bladder —*see* Perforation, bladder
      fallopian tube S37.599
        bilateral S37.592
        unilateral S37.591
      kidney S37.09-•
      obstetrical trauma O71.5
      ovary S37.499
        bilateral S37.492
        unilateral S37.491
      prostate S37.828
      specified organ NEC S37.898
      ureter —*see* Perforation, ureter
      urethra —*see* Perforation, urethra
      uterus —*see* Perforation, uterus
  perineum —*see* Laceration, perineum
  pharynx J39.2
  rectum K63.1
    newborn P78.0
    obstetrical trauma O71.5
    traumatic S36.63
  root canal space due to endodontic treatment M27.51
  sigmoid K63.1
    newborn P78.0
    obstetrical trauma O71.5
    traumatic S36.533
  sinus (accessory) (chronic) (nasal) J34.89
  sphenoidal sinus —*see* Sinusitis, sphenoidal

Perforation, perforated *(Continued)*
  surgical (accidental) (by instrument) (blood vessel) (nerve) (organ) —*see* Puncture, accidental complicating surgery
  traumatic
    external —*see* Puncture
    eye —*see* Puncture, eyeball
    internal organ —*see* Injury, by site
  tympanum, tympanic (membrane) (persistent post-traumatic) (postinflammatory) H72.9-•
    attic H72.1-•
      multiple —*see* Perforation, tympanum, multiple
      total —*see* Perforation, tympanum, total
    central H72.0-•
      multiple —*see* Perforation, tympanum, multiple
      total —*see* Perforation, tympanum, total
    marginal NEC —*see* subcategory H72.2
    multiple H72.81-•
    pars flaccida —*see* Perforation, tympanum, attic
    total H72.82-•
    traumatic, current episode S09.2-•
  typhoid, gastrointestinal —*see* Typhoid
  ulcer —*see* Ulcer, by site, with perforation
  ureter N28.89
    traumatic S37.19
  urethra N36.8
    with ectopic or molar pregnancy O08.6
    following ectopic or molar pregnancy O08.6
    obstetrical trauma O71.5
    traumatic S37.39
      at delivery O71.5
  uterus
    with ectopic or molar pregnancy O08.6
    by intrauterine contraceptive device T83.39
    following ectopic or molar pregnancy O08.6
    obstetrical trauma O71.1
    traumatic S37.69
      obstetric O71.1
  uvula K13.79
    syphilitic A52.79
  vagina
    obstetrical trauma O71.4
    other trauma - *see* Puncture, vagina

Periadenitis mucosa necrotica recurrens K12.0
Periappendicitis (acute) —*see* Appendicitis
Periarteritis nodosa (disseminated) (infectious) (necrotizing) M30.0
Periarthritis (joint) —*see also* Enthesopathy
  Duplay's M75.0-•
  gonococcal A54.42
  humeroscapularis —*see* Capsulitis, adhesive
  scapulohumeral —*see* Capsulitis, adhesive
  shoulder —*see* Capsulitis, adhesive
  wrist M77.2-•
Periarthrosis (angioneural) —*see* Enthesopathy
Pericapsulitis, adhesive (shoulder) —*see* Capsulitis, adhesive
Pericarditis (with decompensation) (with effusion) I31.9
  with rheumatic fever (conditions in I00)
    active —*see* Pericarditis, rheumatic
    inactive or quiescent I09.2
  acute (hemorrhagic) (nonrheumatic) (Sicca) I30.9
    with chorea (acute) (rheumatic) (Sydenham's) I02.0
    benign I30.8
    nonspecific I30.0
    rheumatic I01.0
      with chorea (acute) (Sydenham's) I02.0
  adhesive or adherent (chronic) (external) (internal) I31.0
    acute —*see* Pericarditis, acute
    rheumatic I09.2
  bacterial (acute) (subacute) (with serous or seropurulent effusion) I30.1
  calcareous I31.1
  cholesterol (chronic) I31.8
    acute I30.9
  chronic (nonrheumatic) I31.9
    rheumatic I09.2
  constrictive (chronic) I31.1
  coxsackie B33.23
  fibrinocaseous (tuberculous) A18.84
  fibrinopurulent I30.1
  fibrinous I30.8
  fibrous I31.0

▶ New   ⬛ Revised   ~~deleted~~ Deleted   • Use Additional Character(s)

▶ New   ⇨ Revised   ~~deleted~~ Deleted   ● Use Additional Character(s)

▶ New   ⇨ Revised   ~~deleted~~ Deleted   ● Use Additional Character(s)

▶ New ➡ Revised ~~deleted~~ Deleted ● Use Additional Character(s)

▶ New   ⇒ Revised   ~~deleted~~ Deleted   ● Use Additional Character(s)

▶ New   ⮕ Revised   ~~deleted~~ Deleted   ● Use Additional Character(s)

► New   ⇒ Revised   ~~deleted~~ Deleted   • Use Additional Character(s)

▶ New   ➡ Revised   ~~deleted~~ Deleted   ● Use Additional Character(s)

▶ New ⬛ Revised ~~deleted~~ Deleted • Use Additional Character(s)

▶ New   ➡ Revised   ~~deleted~~ Deleted   ● Use Additional Character(s)

Purpura *(Continued)*
  cryoglobulinemic D89.1
  Devil's pinches D69.2
  fibrinolytic —*see* Fibrinolysis
  fulminans, fulminous D65
  gangrenous D65
  hemorrhagic, hemorrhagica D69.3
    not due to thrombocytopenia D69.0
  Henoch (-Schönlein) (allergic) D69.0
  hypergammaglobulinemic (benign)
      (Waldenström's) D89.0
  idiopathic (thrombocytopenic) D69.3
    nonthrombocytopenic D69.0
  immune thrombocytopenic D69.3
  infectious D69.0
  malignant D69.0
  neonatorum P54.5
  nervosa D69.0
  newborn P54.5
  nonthrombocytopenic D69.2
    hemorrhagic D69.0
    idiopathic D69.0
  nonthrombopenic D69.2
  peliosis rheumatica D69.0
  posttransfusion (post-transfusion) (from (fresh)
      whole blood or blood products) D69.51
  primary D69.49
  red cell membrane sensitivity D69.2
  rheumatica D69.0
  Schönlein (-Henoch) (allergic) D69.0
  scorbutic E54 [D77]
  senile D69.2
  simplex D69.2
  symptomatica D69.0
  telangiectasia annularis L81.7
  thrombocytopenic D69.49
    congenital D69.42
    hemorrhagic D69.3
    hereditary D69.42
    idiopathic D69.3
    immune D69.3
    neonatal, transitory P61.0
    thrombotic M31.19
  thrombohemolytic —*see* Fibrinolysis
  thrombolytic —*see* Fibrinolysis
  thrombopenic D69.49
  thrombotic, thrombocytopenic M31.19
  toxic D69.0
  vascular D69.0
  visceral symptoms D69.0
Purpuric spots R23.3
Purulent —*see* condition
Pus
  in
    stool R19.5
    urine N39.0
  tube (rupture) —*see* Salpingo-oophoritis
Pustular rash L08.0
Pustule (nonmalignant) L08.9
  malignant A22.0
Pustulosis palmaris et plantaris L40.3
Putnam (-Dana) disease or syndrome —*see*
    Degeneration, combined
Putrescent pulp (dental) K04.1
Pyarthritis, pyarthrosis —*see* Arthritis, pyogenic
    or pyemic
  tuberculous —*see* Tuberculosis, joint
Pyelectasis —*see* Hydronephrosis
Pyelitis (congenital) (uremic) —*see also*
    Pyelonephritis
  with
    calculus —*see* category N20
      with hydronephrosis N13.6
    contracted kidney N11.9
  acute N10
  chronic N11.9
    with calculus —*see* category N20
      with hydronephrosis N13.6
  cystica N28.84
  puerperal (postpartum) O86.21
  tuberculous A18.11
Pyelocystitis —*see* Pyelonephritis
Pyelonephritis —*see also* Nephritis,
    tubulo-interstitial
  with
    calculus —*see* category N20
      with hydronephrosis N13.6
    contracted kidney N11.9
  acute N10
  calculous —*see* category N20
      with hydronephrosis N13.6

Pyelonephritis *(Continued)*
  chronic N11.9
    with calculus —*see* category N20
      with hydronephrosis N13.6
    associated with ureteral obstruction or
        stricture N11.1
    nonobstructive N11.8
      with reflux (vesicoureteral) N11.0
    obstructive N11.1
    specified NEC N11.8
  in (due to)
    brucellosis A23.9 [N16]
    cryoglobulinemia (mixed) D89.1 [N16]
    cystinosis E72.04
    diphtheria A36.84
    glycogen storage disease E74.09 [N16]
    leukemia NEC C95.9-● [N16]
    lymphoma NEC C85.90 [N16]
    multiple myeloma C90.0-● [N16]
    obstruction N11.1
    Salmonella infection A02.25
    sarcoidosis D86.84
    sepsis A41.9 [N16]
    Sjögren's disease M35.04
    toxoplasmosis B58.83
    transplant rejection T86.91 [N16]
    Wilson's disease E83.01 [N16]
  nonobstructive N12
    with reflux (vesicoureteral) N11.0
    chronic N11.8
  syphilitic A52.75
Pyelonephrosis (obstructive) N11.1
  chronic N11.9
Pyelophlebitis I80.8
Pyeloureteritis cystica N28.85
Pyemia, pyemic (fever) (infection) (purulent) —*see*
    also Sepsis
  joint —*see* Arthritis, pyogenic or pyemic
  liver K75.1
  pneumococcal A40.3
  portal K75.1
  postvaccinal T88.0
  puerperal, postpartum, childbirth O85
  specified organism NEC A41.89
  tuberculous —*see* Tuberculosis, miliary
Pygopagus Q89.4
Pyknoepilepsy (idiopathic) —*see* Pyknolepsy
Pyknolepsy G40.A09
  intractable G40.A19
    with status epilepticus G40.A11
    without status epilepticus G40.A19
  not intractable G40.A09
    with status epilepticus G40.A01
    without status epilepticus G40.A09
Pylephlebitis K75.1
Pyle's syndrome Q78.5
Pylethrombophlebitis K75.1
Pylethrombosis K75.1
Pyloritis K29.90
  with bleeding K29.91
Pylorospasm (reflex) NEC K31.3
  congenital or infantile Q40.0
  neurotic F45.8
  newborn Q40.0
  psychogenic F45.8
Pylorus, pyloric —*see* condition
Pyoarthrosis —*see* Arthritis, pyogenic or pyemic
Pyocele
  mastoid —*see* Mastoiditis, acute
  sinus (accessory) —*see* Sinusitis
  turbinate (bone) J32.9
  urethra —*see also* Urethritis N34.0
Pyocolpos —*see* Vaginitis
Pyocystitis N30.80
  with hematuria N30.81
Pyoderma, pyodermia L08.0
  gangrenosum L88
  newborn P39.4
  phagedenic L88
  vegetans L08.81
Pyodermatitis L08.0
  vegetans L08.81
Pyogenic —*see* condition
Pyohydronephrosis N13.6
Pyometra, pyometrium, pyometritis —*see*
    Endometritis
Pyomyositis (tropical) —*see* Myositis, infective
Pyonephritis N12
Pyonephrosis N13.6
  tuberculous A18.11

Pyo-oophoritis —*see* Salpingo-oophoritis
Pyo-ovarium —*see* Salpingo-oophoritis
Pyopericarditis, pyopericardium I30.1
Pyophlebitis —*see* Phlebitis
Pyopneumopericardium I30.1
Pyopneumothorax (infective) J86.9
  with fistula J86.0
  tuberculous NEC A15.6
Pyosalpinx, pyosalpingitis —*see also*
    Salpingo-oophoritis
Pyothorax J86.9
  with fistula J86.0
  tuberculous NEC A15.6
Pyoureter N28.89
  tuberculous A18.11
Pyramidopallidonigral syndrome G20.C
Pyrexia (of unknown origin) R50.9
  atmospheric T67.01
  during labor NEC O75.2
  heat T67.01
  newborn P81.9
    environmentally-induced P81.0
  persistent R50.9
  puerperal O86.4
Pyroglobulinemia NEC E88.09
Pyromania F63.1
Pyrosis R12
Pyuria (bacterial) R82.81

Q

Q fever A78
  with pneumonia A78
Quadricuspid aortic valve Q23.88
Quadrilateral fever A78
Quadriparesis —*see* Quadriplegia
  meaning muscle weakness M62.81
Quadriplegia G82.50-●
  complete
    C1-C4 level G82.51
    C5-C7 level G82.53
  congenital (cerebral) (spinal) G80.8
    spastic G80.0
  embolic (current episode) I63.4-●
  functional R53.2
  incomplete
    C1-C4 level G82.52
    C5-C7 level G82.54
  thrombotic (current episode) I63.3-●
  traumatic — code to injury with seventh
      character S
    current episode —*see* Injury, spinal (cord),
        cervical
Quadruplet, pregnancy —*see* Pregnancy,
    quadruplet
Quarrelsomeness F60.3
Queensland fever A77.3
Quervain's disease M65.4
  thyroid E06.1
Queyrat's erythroplasia D07.4
  penis D07.4
  specified site —*see* Neoplasm, skin, in situ
  unspecified site D07.4
Quincke's disease or edema T78.3
  hereditary D84.1
Quinsy (gangrenous) J36
Quintan fever A79.0
Quintuplet, pregnancy —*see* Pregnancy, quintuplet

R

Rabbit fever —*see* Tularemia
Rabies A82.9
  contact Z20.3
  exposure to Z20.3
  inoculation reaction —*see* Complications,
      vaccination
  sylvatic A82.0
  urban A82.1
Rachischisis —*see* Spina bifida
Rachitic —*see also* condition
  deformities of spine (late effect) (sequelae) E64.3
  pelvis (late effect) (sequelae) E64.3
    with disproportion (fetopelvic) O33.0
      causing obstructed labor O65.0

Reaction (Continued)
  serum (Continued)
    specified reaction NEC
      due to
        administration of blood and blood
          products T80.61
        immunization T80.62
        serum specified NEC T80.69
        vaccination T80.62
  situational —*see* Disorder, adjustment
  somatization —*see* Disorder, somatoform
  spinal puncture G97.1
    dural G97.1
  stress (severe) F43.9
    acute (agitation) ("daze") (disorientation)
      (disturbance of consciousness) (flight
      reaction) (fugue) F43.0
    specified NEC F43.89
  surgical procedure —*see* Complications, surgical
    procedure
  tetanus antitoxin —*see* Complications,
    vaccination
  toxic, to local anesthesia T81.59
    in labor and delivery O74.4
    in pregnancy O29.3X-●
    postpartum, puerperal O89.3
  toxin-antitoxin —*see* Complications, vaccination
  transfusion (blood) (bone marrow)
    (lymphocytes) (allergic) —*see*
    Complications, transfusion
  tuberculin skin test, abnormal R76.11
  vaccination (any) —*see* Complications,
    vaccination
  withdrawing, child or adolescent F93.8
Reactive airway disease —*see* Asthma
Reactive depression —*see* Reaction, depressive
Rearrangement
  chromosomal
    balanced (in) Q95.9
      abnormal individual (autosomal) Q95.2
        non-sex (autosomal) chromosomes Q95.2
        sex/non-sex chromosomes Q95.3
      specified NEC Q95.8
Recalcitrant patient —*see* Noncompliance
Recanalization, thrombus —*see* Thrombosis
Recession, receding
  chamber angle (eye) H21.55-●
  chin M26.09
  gingival (postinfective) (postoperative)
    generalized K06.020
      minimal K06.021
      moderate K06.022
      severe K06.023
    localized K06.010
      minimal K06.011
      moderate K06.012
      severe K06.013
Recklinghausen's disease Q85.01
  bones E21.0
Reclus' disease (cystic) —*see* Mastopathy, cystic
Recrudescence
  deficit
    cerebral infarction - see Sequelae, infarction,
      cerebral
    stroke - see Sequelae, infarction, cerebral
  sequelae
    cerebral infarction - see Sequelae, infarction,
      cerebral
    stroke - see Sequelae, infarction, cerebral
Recrudescent typhus (fever) A75.1
Recruitment, auditory H93.21-●
Rectalgia K62.89
Rectitis K62.89
Rectocele
  female (without uterine prolapse) N81.6
    with uterine prolapse N81.4
      complete N81.3
      incomplete N81.2
  in pregnancy —*see* Pregnancy, complicated by,
    abnormal, pelvic organs or tissues NEC
  male K62.3
Rectosigmoid junction —*see* condition
Rectosigmoiditis K63.89
  ulcerative (chronic) K51.30
    with
      complication K51.319
        abscess K51.314
        fistula K51.313
        obstruction K51.312
        rectal bleeding K51.311
        specified NEC K51.318

Rectourethral —*see* condition
Rectovaginal —*see* condition
Rectovesical —*see* condition
Rectum, rectal —*see* condition
Recurrent —*see* condition
  pregnancy loss —*see* Loss (of), pregnancy,
    recurrent
Red bugs B88.09
Red-cedar lung or pneumonitis J67.8
Red tide —*see also* Table of Drugs and Chemicals
  T65.82-●
Reduced
  mobility Z74.09
  ventilatory or vital capacity R94.2
Redundant, redundancy
  anus (congenital) Q43.8
  clitoris N90.89
  colon (congenital) Q43.8
  foreskin (congenital) N47.8
  intestine (congenital) Q43.8
  labia N90.69
  organ or site, congenital NEC —*see* Accessory
  panniculus (abdominal) E65
  prepuce (congenital) N47.8
  pylorus K31.89
  rectum (congenital) Q43.8
  scrotum N50.89
  sigmoid (congenital) Q43.8
  skin L98.7
    and subcutaneous tissue L98.7
    of face L57.4
    eyelids —*see* Blepharochalasis
  stomach K31.89
Reduplication —*see* Duplication
Reflex R29.2
  hyperactive gag J39.2
  pupillary, abnormal —*see* Anomaly, pupil,
    function
  vasoconstriction I73.9
  vasovagal R55
Reflux K21.9
  acid K21.9
  esophageal K21.9
    with esophagitis (without bleeding) K21.00
      with bleeding K21.01
    newborn P78.83
  gastroesophageal K21.9
    with esophagitis (without bleeding)
      K21.00
      with bleeding K21.01
  mitral —*see* Insufficiency, mitral
  ureteral —*see* Reflux, vesicoureteral
  vesicoureteral (with scarring) N13.70
    with
      nephropathy N13.729
        with hydroureter N13.739
          bilateral N13.732
          unilateral N13.731
        without hydroureter N13.729
          bilateral N13.722
          unilateral N13.721
      bilateral N13.722
      unilateral N13.721
      pyelonephritis (chronic) N11.0
    without nephropathy N13.71
    congenital Q62.7
Reforming, artificial openings —*see* Attention to,
  artificial, opening
Refractive error —*see* Disorder, refraction
Refsum's disease or syndrome G60.1
Refusal of
  food, psychogenic F50.89
  treatment (because of) Z53.20
    left against medical advice (AMA) Z53.29
    left without being seen Z53.21
    patient's decision NEC Z53.29
    reasons of belief or group pressure Z53.1
Regional —*see* condition
Regurgitation R11.10
  aortic (valve) —*see* Insufficiency, aortic
  food —*see also* Vomiting
    with reswallowing —*see* Rumination
    newborn P92.1
  gastric contents —*see* Vomiting
  heart —*see* Endocarditis
  mitral (valve) —*see* Insufficiency, mitral
    congenital Q23.3
  myocardial —*see* Endocarditis
  pulmonary (valve) (heart) I37.1
    congenital Q22.2
    syphilitic A52.03

Regurgitation (Continued)
  tricuspid —*see* Insufficiency, tricuspid
  valve, valvular —*see* Endocarditis
    congenital Q24.8
  vesicoureteral —*see* Reflux, vesicoureteral
Reichmann's disease or syndrome K31.89
Reifenstein syndrome E34.52
Reinsertion
  implantable subdermal contraceptive Z30.46
  intrauterine contraceptive device Z30.433
Reiter's disease, syndrome, or urethritis
  M02.30
  ankle M02.37-●
  elbow M02.32-●
  foot joint M02.37-●
  hand joint M02.34-●
  hip M02.35-●
  knee M02.36-●
  multiple site M02.39
  shoulder M02.31-●
  vertebra M02.38
  wrist M02.33-●
Rejection
  food, psychogenic F50.89
  transplant T86.91
    bone T86.830
      marrow T86.01
    cornea T86.840-●
    heart T86.21
      with lung(s) T86.31
    intestine T86.850
    kidney T86.11
    liver T86.41
    lung(s) T86.810
      with heart T86.31
    organ (immune or nonimmune cause) T86.91
    pancreas T86.890
    skin (allograft) (autograft) T86.820
    specified NEC T86.890
    stem cell (peripheral blood) (umbilical cord)
      T86.5
Relapsing fever A68.9
  Carter's (Asiatic) A68.1
  Dutton's (West African) A68.1
  Koch's A68.9
  louse-borne (epidemic) A68.0
  Novy's (American) A68.1
  ~~Obermeyers's (European) A68.0~~
  ▶ Obermeyer's (European) A68.0
  Spirillum A68.9
  tick-borne (endemic) A68.1
Relationship
  occlusal
    open anterior M26.220
    open posterior M26.221
Relaxation
  anus (sphincter) K62.89
    psychogenic F45.8
  arch (foot) —*see also* Deformity, limb, flat foot
  back ligaments —*see* Instability, joint, spine
  bladder (sphincter) N31.2
  cardioesophageal K21.9
  cervix —*see* Incompetency, cervix
  diaphragm J98.6
  joint (capsule) (ligament) (paralytic) —*see* Flail,
    joint
    congenital NEC Q74.8
  lumbosacral (joint) —*see* subcategory M53.2
  pelvic floor N81.89
  perineum N81.89
  posture R29.3
  rectum (sphincter) K62.89
  sacroiliac (joint) —*see* subcategory M53.2
  scrotum N50.89
  urethra (sphincter) N36.44
  vesical N31.2
Release from prison, anxiety concerning Z65.2
Remains
  canal of Cloquet Q14.0
  capsule (opaque) Q14.8
Remittent fever (malarial) B54
Remnant
  canal of Cloquet Q14.0
  capsule (opaque) Q14.8
  cervix, cervical stump (acquired) (postoperative)
    N88.8
  cystic duct, postcholecystectomy K91.5
  fingernail L60.8
    congenital Q84.6
  meniscus, knee —*see* Derangement, knee,
    meniscus, specified NEC
  thyroglossal duct Q89.2

▶ New   ⇨ Revised   ~~deleted~~ Deleted   ● Use Additional Character(s)

▶ New   ⇨ Revised   ~~deleted~~ Deleted   ● Use Additional Character(s)

S

Sarcoma *(Continued)*
  melanotic —*see* Melanoma
  meningeal —*see* Neoplasm, meninges, malignant
  meningothelial —*see* Neoplasm, meninges, malignant
  mesenchymal —*see also* Neoplasm, connective tissue, malignant
    mixed —*see* Neoplasm, connective tissue, malignant
  mesothelial —*see* Mesothelioma
  monstrocellular
    specified site —*see* Neoplasm, malignant, by site
    unspecified site C71.9
  myeloid C92.3-●
  neurogenic —*see* Neoplasm, nerve, malignant
  odontogenic C41.1
    upper jaw (bone) C41.0
  osteoblastic —*see* Neoplasm, bone, malignant
  osteogenic —*see also* Neoplasm, bone, malignant
    juxtacortical —*see* Neoplasm, bone, malignant
    periosteal —*see* Neoplasm, bone, malignant
  periosteal —*see also* Neoplasm, bone, malignant
    osteogenic —*see* Neoplasm, bone, malignant
  pleomorphic cell —*see* Neoplasm, connective tissue, malignant
  reticulum cell (diffuse) —*see* Lymphoma, diffuse large cell
    nodular —*see* Lymphoma, follicular
    pleomorphic cell type —*see* Lymphoma, diffuse large cell
  rhabdoid —*see* Neoplasm, malignant, by site
  round cell —*see* Neoplasm, connective tissue, malignant
  small cell —*see* Neoplasm, connective tissue, malignant
  soft tissue —*see* Neoplasm, connective tissue, malignant
  spindle cell —*see* Neoplasm, connective tissue, malignant
  stromal (endometrial) C54.1
    isthmus C54.0
  synovial —*see also* Neoplasm, connective tissue, malignant
    biphasic —*see* Neoplasm, connective tissue, malignant
    epithelioid cell —*see* Neoplasm, connective tissue, malignant
    spindle cell —*see* Neoplasm, connective tissue, malignant
Sarcomatosis
  meningeal —*see* Neoplasm, meninges, malignant
  specified site NEC —*see* Neoplasm, connective tissue, malignant
  unspecified site C80.1
Sarcopenia (age-related) M62.84
Sarcosinemia E72.59
Sarcosporidiosis (intestinal) A07.8
SARS-CoV-2 —*see also* COVID-19
  sequelae (post acute) U09.9
Satiety, early R68.81
Saturnine —*see* condition
Saturnism
  overdose or wrong substance given or taken — *see* Table of Drugs and Chemicals, by drug, poisoning
Satyriasis F52.8
Sauriasis —*see* Ichthyosis
SBE (subacute bacterial endocarditis) I33.0
Scabies (any site) B86
Scabs R23.4
Scaglietti-Dagnini syndrome E22.0
Scald —*see* Burn
Scalenus anticus (anterior) **syndrome** G54.0
Scales R23.4
Scaling, skin R23.4
Scalp —*see* condition
Scapegoating affecting child Z62.3
Scaphocephaly, non-deformational Q75.01
Scapulalgia M89.8X1
Scapulohumeral myopathy G71.02
Scar, scarring —*see also* Cicatrix L90.5
  adherent L90.5
  atrophic L90.5
  cervix
    in pregnancy or childbirth —*see* Pregnancy, complicated by, abnormal cervix
  cheloid L91.0

Scar, scarring *(Continued)*
  chorioretinal H31.00-●
    posterior pole macula H31.01-●
    postsurgical H59.81-●
    solar retinopathy H31.02-●
    specified type NEC H31.09-●
  choroid —*see* Scar, chorioretinal
  conjunctiva H11.24-●
  cornea H17.9
    xerophthalmic —*see also* Opacity, cornea
      vitamin A deficiency E50.6
  defect (isthmocele) O34.22
  duodenum, obstructive K31.5
  hypertrophic L91.0
  keloid L91.0
  labia N90.89
  lung (base) J98.4
  macula —*see* Scar, chorioretinal, posterior pole
  muscle M62.89
  myocardium, myocardial I25.2
  painful L90.5
  posterior pole (eye) —*see* Scar, chorioretinal, posterior pole
  retina —*see* Scar, chorioretinal
  trachea J39.8
  transmural uterine, in pregnancy O34.29
  uterus N85.8
    in pregnancy O34.29
  vagina N89.8
    postoperative N99.2
  vulva N90.89
Scarabiasis B88.2
Scarlatina (anginosa) (maligna) A38.9
  myocarditis (acute) A38.1
    old —*see* Myocarditis
  otitis media A38.0
  ulcerosa A38.8
Scarlet fever (albuminuria) (angina) A38.9
Schamberg's disease (progressive pigmentary dermatosis) L81.7
Schatzki's ring (acquired) (esophagus) (lower) K22.2
  congenital Q39.3
Schaufenster krankheit I20.89
Schaumann's
  benign lymphogranulomatosis D86.1
  disease or syndrome —*see* Sarcoidosis
Scheie's syndrome E76.03
Schenck's disease B42.1
Scheuermann's disease or osteochondrosis —*see* Osteochondrosis, juvenile, spine
Schilder (-Flatau) **disease** G37.0
Schilling-type monocytic leukemia C93.0-●
Schimmelbusch's disease, cystic mastitis, or hyperplasia —*see* Mastopathy, cystic
Schistosoma infestation —*see* Infestation, Schistosoma
Schistosomiasis B65.9
  with muscle disorder B65.9 *[M63.80]*
    ankle B65.9 *[M63.87-●]*
    foot B65.9 *[M63.87-●]*
    forearm B65.9 *[M63.83-●]*
    hand B65.9 *[M63.84-●]*
    lower leg B65.9 *[M63.86-●]*
    multiple sites B65.9 *[M63.89]*
    pelvic region B65.9 *[M63.85-●]*
    shoulder region B65.9 *[M63.81-●]*
    specified site NEC B65.9 *[M63.88]*
    thigh B65.9 *[M63.85-●]*
    upper arm B65.9 *[M63.82-●]*
  Asiatic B65.2
  bladder B65.0
  chestermani B65.8
  colon B65.1
  cutaneous B65.3
  due to
    S. haematobium B65.0
    S. japonicum B65.2
    S. mansoni B65.1
    S. mattheii B65.8
  Eastern B65.2
  genitourinary tract B65.0
  intestinal B65.1
  lung NEC B65.9 *[J99]*
    pneumonia B65.9 *[J17]*
  Manson's (intestinal) B65.1
  oriental B65.2
  pulmonary NEC B65.9 *[J99]*
    pneumonia B65.9
  Schistosoma
    haematobium B65.0
    japonicum B65.2
    mansoni B65.1

Schistosomiasis *(Continued)*
  specified type NEC B65.8
  urinary B65.0
  vesical B65.0
Schizencephaly Q04.6
Schizoaffective psychosis F25.9
Schizodontia K00.2
Schizoid personality F60.1
Schizophrenia, schizophrenic F20.9
  acute (brief) (undifferentiated) F23
  atypical (form) F20.3
  borderline F21
  catalepsy F20.2
  catatonic (type) (excited) (withdrawn) F20.2
  cenesthopathic, cenesthesiopathic F20.89
  childhood type F20.9
  chronic undifferentiated F20.9
  cyclic F25.0
  disorganized (type) F20.1
  flexibilitas cerea F20.2
  hebephrenic (type) F20.1
  incipient F21
  latent F21
  negative type F20.5
  paranoid (type) F20.0
  paraphrenic F20.0
  post-psychotic depression F32.89
  prepsychotic F21
  prodromal F21
  pseudoneurotic F21
  pseudopsychopathic F21
  reaction F23
  residual (state) (type) F20.5
  restzustand F20.5
  schizoaffective (type) —*see* Psychosis, schizoaffective
  simple (type) F20.89
  simplex F20.89
  specified type NEC F20.89
  spectrum and other psychotic disorder F29
    specified NEC F28
  stupor F20.2
  syndrome of childhood F84.5
  undifferentiated (type) F20.3
  ➡ chronic F20.9
Schizothymia (persistent) F60.1
Schlatter-Osgood disease or osteochondrosis M92.52-●
Schlatter's tibia —*see* Osteochondrosis, juvenile, tibia
Schmidt's syndrome (polyglandular, autoimmune) E31.0
Schmincke's carcinoma or tumor —*see* Neoplasm, nasopharynx, malignant
Schmitz (-Stutzer) **dysentery** A03.0
Schmorl's disease or nodes
  lumbar region M51.46
  lumbosacral region M51.47
  sacrococcygeal region M53.3
  thoracic region M51.44
  thoracolumbar region M51.45
Schneiderian
  papilloma —*see* Neoplasm, nasopharynx benign
    specified site —*see* Neoplasm, benign, by site
    unspecified site D14.0
  specified site —*see* Neoplasm, malignant, by site
    unspecified site C30.0
Scholte's syndrome (malignant carcinoid) E34.09
Scholz (-Bielchowsky-Henneberg) **disease or syndrome** E75.25
Schönlein (-Henoch) **disease or purpura** (primary) (rheumatic) D69.0
Schottmuller's disease A01.4
Schroeder's syndrome (endocrine hypertensive) E27.0
Schüller-Christian disease or syndrome C96.5
Schultze's type acroparesthesia, simple I73.89
Schultz's disease or syndrome —*see* Agranulocytosis
Schwalbe-Ziehen-Oppenheim disease G24.1
Schwannoma —*see also* Neoplasm, nerve, benign
  malignant —*see also* Neoplasm, nerve, malignant
    with rhabdomyoblastic differentiation —*see* Neoplasm, nerve, malignant
  melanocytic —*see* Neoplasm, nerve, benign
  pigmented —*see* Neoplasm, nerve, benign
Schwannomatosis Q85.03
Schwartz (-Jampel) **syndrome** G71.13
Schwartz-Bartter syndrome E22.2
Schweninger-Buzzi anetoderma L90.1

  ▶ New   ⬤ Revised   ~~deleted~~ Deleted   • Use Additional Character(s)

▶ New   ⇒ Revised   ~~deleted~~ Deleted   ● Use Additional Character(s)

▶ New   ➡ Revised   ~~deleted~~ Deleted   ● Use Additional Character(s)

▶ New   ⇨ Revised   ~~deleted~~ Deleted   ● Use Additional Character(s)

▶ New   ➡ Revised   ~~deleted~~ Deleted   ● Use Additional Character(s)

New Revised ~~deleted~~ Deleted • Use Additional Character(s)

Stricture *(Continued)*
- nasolacrimal duct —*see also* Stenosis, lacrimal, duct
  - congenital Q10.5
- nasopharynx J39.2
  - syphilitic A52.73
- nose J34.89
  - congenital Q30.0
- nostril (anterior) (posterior) J34.89
  - congenital Q30.0
  - syphilitic A52.73
    - congenital A50.59 [J99]
- organ or site, congenital NEC —*see* Atresia, by site
- os uteri —*see* Stricture, cervix
- osseous meatus (ear) (congenital) Q16.1
  - acquired —*see* Stricture, auditory canal, acquired
- oviduct —*see* Stricture, fallopian tube
- pelviureteric junction (congenital) Q62.11
  - acquired, with hydronephrosis N13.0
- penis, by foreign body T19.4
- pharynx J39.2
- prostate N42.89
- pulmonary, pulmonic
  - artery (congenital) Q25.6
    - acquired I28.8
    - noncongenital I28.8
  - infundibulum (congenital) Q24.3
  - valve I37.0
    - congenital Q22.1
  - vein, acquired I28.8
  - vessel NEC I28.8
- punctum lacrimale —*see also* Stenosis, lacrimal, punctum
  - congenital Q10.5
- pylorus (hypertrophic) K31.1
  - adult K31.1
  - congenital Q40.0
  - infantile Q40.0
- rectosigmoid —*see also* Obstruction, intestine, specified NEC K56.699
- rectum (sphincter) K62.4
  - congenital Q42.1
    - with fistula Q42.0
  - due to
    - chlamydial lymphogranuloma A55
    - irradiation K91.89
    - lymphogranuloma venereum A55
  - gonococcal A54.6
  - inflammatory (chlamydial) A55
  - syphilitic A52.74
  - tuberculous A18.32
- renal artery I70.1
  - congenital Q27.1
- salivary duct or gland (any) K11.8
- sigmoid (flexure) —*see* Obstruction, intestine
- spermatic cord N50.89
- stoma (following) (of)
  - colostomy K94.03
  - enterostomy K94.13
  - gastrostomy K94.23
  - ileostomy K94.13
  - tracheostomy J95.03
- stomach K31.89
  - congenital Q40.2
  - hourglass K31.2
- subaortic Q24.4
  - hypertrophic (acquired) (idiopathic) I42.1
- subglottic J38.6
- syphilitic NEC A52.79
- trachea J39.8
  - congenital Q32.1
  - syphilitic A52.73
  - tuberculous NEC A15.5
- tracheostomy J95.03
- tricuspid (valve) —*see* Stenosis, tricuspid
- tunica vaginalis N50.89
- ureter (postoperative) N13.5
  - with
    - hydronephrosis N13.1
      - with infection N13.6
    - pyelonephritis (chronic) N11.1
  - congenital —*see* Atresia, ureter
  - tuberculous A18.11
- ureteropelvic junction (congenital) Q62.11
  - acquired, with hydronephrosis N13.0
- ureterovesical orifice N13.5
  - with infection N13.6

Stricture *(Continued)*
- urethra (organic) (spasmodic) (see also Stricture, urethra, male N35.919)
  - associated with schistosomiasis B65.0 [N37]
  - congenital Q64.39
    - valvular (posterior) Q64.2
  - due to
    - infection —*see* Stricture, urethra, postinfective
    - trauma —*see* Stricture, urethra, post-traumatic
  - female N35.92
  - gonococcal, gonorrheal A54.01
  - infective NEC —*see* Stricture, urethra, postinfective
  - late effect (sequelae) of injury —*see* Stricture, urethra, post-traumatic
  - male N35.919
    - anterior urethra N35.914
    - bulbous urethra N35.912
    - meatal N35.911
    - membranous urethra N35.913
    - overlapping sites N35.916
  - postcatheterization —*see* Stricture, urethra, postprocedural
  - postinfective NEC
    - female N35.12
    - male N35.119
      - anterior urethra N35.114
      - bulbous urethra N35.112
      - meatal N35.111
      - membranous urethra N35.113
      - overlapping sites N35.116
  - postobstetric N35.021
  - postoperative —*see* Stricture, urethra, postprocedural
  - postprocedural
    - female N99.12
    - male N99.114
      - anterior bulbous urethra N99.113
      - bulbous urethra N99.111
      - fossa navicularis N99.115
      - meatal N99.110
      - membranous urethra N99.112
      - overlapping sites N35.116
  - post-traumatic
    - female N35.028
      - due to childbirth N35.021
    - male N35.014
      - anterior urethra N35.013
      - bulbous urethra N35.011
      - meatal N35.010
      - membranous urethra N35.012
      - overlapping sites N35.016
  - sequela (late effect) of
    - childbirth N35.021
    - injury —*see* Stricture, urethra, post-traumatic
  - specified cause NEC
    - female N35.82
    - male N35.819
      - anterior urethra N35.814
      - bulbous urethra N35.812
      - meatal N35.811
      - membranous urethra N35.813
      - overlapping sites N35.816
  - syphilitic A52.76
  - traumatic —*see* Stricture, urethra, post-traumatic
  - valvular (posterior), congenital Q64.2
- urinary meatus —*see* Stricture, urethra
- uterus, uterine (synechiae) N85.6
  - os (external) (internal) —*see* Stricture, cervix
- vagina (outlet) —*see* Stenosis, vagina
- valve (cardiac) (heart) —*see also* Endocarditis
  - congenital
    - aortic Q23.0
    - mitral Q23.2
    - pulmonary Q22.1
    - tricuspid Q22.4
- vas deferens N50.89
  - congenital Q55.4
- vein I87.1
- vena cava (inferior) (superior) NEC I87.1
  - congenital Q26.0
- vesicourethral orifice N32.0
  - congenital Q64.31
- vulva (acquired) N90.5

Stridor R06.1
- congenital (larynx) P28.89

Stridulous —*see* condition

Stroke (apoplectic) (brain) (ischemic) (paralytic) I63.9
- cerebral, perinatal P91.82-●
- cerebrovascular (ischemic) I63.9
  - chronic (old) (remote) (imaging) (without sequelae) Z86.73
    - with residual defects - see Sequelae, disease, cerebrovascular
  - embolic I63.-●
    - thrombolic I63.-●
- cryptogenic —*see also* infarction, cerebral I63.9
- epileptic —*see* Epilepsy
- heat T67.01
  - exertional T67.02
  - specified NEC T67.09
- in evolution I63.9
- intraoperative
  - during cardiac surgery I97.810
  - during other surgery I97.811
- ischemic, perinatal arterial P91.82-●
- lightning —*see* Lightning
- meaning
  - cerebral hemorrhage — code to Hemorrhage, intracranial
  - cerebral infarction — code to Infarction, cerebral
- neonatal P91.82-●
- postprocedural
  - following cardiac surgery I97.820
  - following other surgery I97.821
- sun T67.01
  - specified NEC T67.09
- unspecified (NOS) I63.9

Stromatosis, endometrial D39.0
Strongyloidiasis, strongyloidosis B78.9
- cutaneous B78.1
- disseminated B78.7
- intestinal B78.0
Strophulus pruriginosus L28.2
Struck by lightning —*see* Lightning
Struma —*see also* Goiter
- Hashimoto E06.3
- lymphomatosa E06.3
- nodosa (simplex) E04.9
  - endemic E01.2
    - multinodular E01.1
  - multinodular E04.2
    - iodine-deficiency related E01.1
  - toxic or with hyperthyroidism E05.20
    - with thyroid storm E05.21
    - multinodular E05.20
      - with thyroid storm E05.21
    - uninodular E05.10
      - with thyroid storm E05.11
  - toxicosa E05.20
    - with thyroid storm E05.21
    - multinodular E05.20
      - with thyroid storm E05.21
    - uninodular E05.10
      - with thyroid storm E05.11
  - uninodular E04.1
- ovarii D27.-●
- Riedel's E06.5
Strumipriva cachexia E03.4
Strümpell-Marie spine —*see* Spondylitis, ankylosing
Strümpell-Westphal pseudosclerosis E83.01
Stuart deficiency disease (factor X) D68.2
Stuart-Prower factor deficiency (factor X) D68.2
Student's elbow —*see* Bursitis, elbow, olecranon
Stump —*see* Amputation
Stunting, nutritional E45
Stupor (catatonic) R40.1
- depressive (single episode) F32.89
  - recurrent episode F33.8
- dissociative F44.2
- manic F30.2
- manic-depressive F31.89
- psychogenic (anergic) F44.2
- reaction to exceptional stress (transient) F43.0
Sturge (-Weber) (-Dimitri) (-Kalischer) disease or syndrome Q85.89
Stuttering F80.81
- adult onset F98.5
- childhood onset F80.81
- following cerebrovascular disease —*see* Disorder, fluency, following cerebrovascular disease
- in conditions classified elsewhere R47.82
Sty, stye (external) (internal) (meibomian) (zeisian) —*see* Hordeolum
Subacidity, gastric K31.89
- psychogenic F45.8

▶ New   ⇨ Revised   ~~deleted~~ Deleted   ● Use Additional Character(s)

Syndrome (*Continued*)
due to abnormality
chromosomal Q99.9
sex
female phenotype Q97.9
male phenotype Q98.9
specified NEC Q99.8
dumping (postgastrectomy) K91.1
nonsurgical K31.89
Dupré's (meningism) R29.1
dysmetabolic X E88.810
dyspraxia, developmental F82
Eagle-Barrett Q79.4
Eaton-Lambert —*see* Syndrome, Lambert-Eaton
Ebstein's Q22.5
ectopic ACTH E24.3
eczema-thrombocytopenia D82.0
Eddowes' Q78.0
effort (psychogenic) F45.8
Ehlers-Danlos Q79.60
classical (cEDS) (classical EDS) Q79.61
hypermobile (hEDS) (hypermobile EDS) Q79.62
specified NEC Q79.69
vascular (vascular EDS) (vEDS) Q79.63
Eisenmenger's I27.83
Ekman's Q78.0
electric feet E53.8
Ellis-van Creveld Q77.6
empty nest Z60.0
endocrine-hypertensive E27.0
entrapment —*see* Neuropathy, entrapment
eosinophilia-myalgia M35.89
epileptic —*see also* Epilepsy, by type
absence G40.A09
intractable G40.A19
with status epilepticus G40.A11
without status epilepticus G40.A19
not intractable G40.A09
with status epilepticus G40.A01
without status epilepticus G40.A09
Erdheim-Chester (ECD) E88.89
Erdheim's E22.0
erythrocyte fragmentation D59.4
Evans D69.41
exhaustion F48.8
extrapyramidal G25.9
specified NEC G25.89
eye retraction —*see* Strabismus
eyelid-malar-mandible Q87.0
Faber's D50.9
facet M47.89-•
facet joint (*see also* Spondylosis) M47.819
facial pain, paroxysmal G50.0
Fallot's Q21.3
familial cold autoinflammatory M04.2
familial eczema-thrombocytopenia (Wiskott-
Aldrich) D82.0
Fanconi (-de Toni) (-Debré) E72.09
with cystinosis E72.04
fatigue
chronic G93.32
postviral G93.31
psychogenic F48.8
faulty bowel habit K59.39
Feil-Klippel (brevicollis) Q76.1
Felty's —*see* Felty's syndrome
fertile eunuch E23.0
fetal
alcohol (dysmorphic) Q86.0
hydantoin Q86.1
Fiedler's I40.1
first arch Q87.0
fish odor E72.89
Fisher's G61.0
Fitzhugh-Curtis
due to
Chlamydia trachomatis A74.81
Neisseria gonorrhea (gonococcal
peritonitis) A54.85
Fitz's —*see also* Pancreatitis, acute K85.80
Flajani (-Basedow) E05.00
with thyroid storm E05.01
flatback —*see* Flatback syndrome
floppy
baby P94.2
iris (intraoperative) (IFIS) H21.81
mitral valve I34.1
flush E34.09
Foix-Alajouanine G95.19
Fong's Q87.2
food protein-induced enterocolitis (FPIES)
K52.21

Syndrome (*Continued*)
foramen magnum G93.5
Foster-Kennedy H47.14-•
Foville's (peduncular) G46.3
▶ FOXG1 QA0.0151
fragile X Q99.2
Franceschetti Q75.4
Frey's
auriculotemporal G50.8
hyperhidrosis L74.52
Friderichsen-Waterhouse A39.1
Froin's G95.89
frontal lobe F07.0
Fukuhara E88.49
functional
bowel K59.9
prepubertal castrate E29.1
Gaisböck's D75.1
ganglion (basal ganglia brain) G25.9
geniculi G51.1
Gardner-Diamond D69.2
gastroesophageal
junction K22.0
laceration-hemorrhage K22.6
gastrojejunal loop obstruction K91.89
Gee-Herter-Heubner K90.0
Gelineau's G47.419
with cataplexy G47.411
genito-anorectal A55
Gerstmann-Sträussler-Scheinker (GSS) A81.82
Gianotti-Crosti L44.4
giant platelet (Bernard-Soulier) D69.1
Gilles de la Tourette's F95.2
Glass Q87.89
Gleich's D72.118
goiter-deafness E07.1
▌Goldberg Q89.89
Goldberg-Maxwell E34.51
Good's D83.8
▌Gopalan's (burning feet) E53.8
Gorlin's Q87.89
Gougerot-Blum L81.7
Gouley's I31.1
Gower's R55
gray or grey (newborn) P93.0
platelet D69.1
Gubler-Millard G46.3
Guillain-Barré (-Strohl) G61.0
▶ Gulf war T75.830
gustatory sweating G50.8
Hadfield-Clarke K86.89
hair tourniquet —*see* Constriction, external, by
site
Hamman's J98.19
hand-foot L27.1
hand-shoulder G90.89
hantavirus (cardio)-pulmonary (HPS) (HCPS)
B33.4
▶ Hao-Fountain (HAFOUS) Q87.87
happy puppet Q93.51
Harada's H30.81-•
Hayem-Faber D50.9
headache NEC G44.89
complicated NEC G44.59
Heberden's I20.89
Hedinger's E34.01
Hegglin's D72.0
HELLP (hemolysis, elevated liver enzymes and
low platelet count) O14.2-•
complicating
childbirth O14.24
puerperium O14.25
hemolytic-uremic D59.30
atypical D59.39
genetic D59.32
hereditary D59.32
infection-associated D59.31
secondary D59.39
specified NEC D59.39
due to genetic disorder D59.32
familial D59.32
hereditary D59.32
infection-associated D59.31
secondary D59.39
Shiga toxin-producing E. coli [STEC] related
D59.31
specified NEC D59.39
typical D59.31
hemophagocytic, infection-associated D76.2
Henoch-Schönlein D69.0
hepatic flexure K59.89
hepatopulmonary K76.81

Syndrome (*Continued*)
hepatorenal K76.7
following delivery O90.41
postoperative or postprocedural K91.83
postpartum, puerperal O90.41
hepatourologic K76.7
hereditary alpha tryptasemia D89.44
Herter (-Gee) (nontropical sprue) K90.0
Heubner-Herter K90.0
Heyd's K76.7
Hilger's G90.09
histamine-like (fish poisoning) —*see* Poisoning,
fish
histiocytic D76.3
histiocytosis NEC D76.3
HIV infection, acute B20
Hoffmann-Werdnig G12.0
▌Hollander-Simons E88.19
Hoppe-Goldflam G70.00
with exacerbation (acute) G70.01
in crisis G70.01
Horner's G90.2
hungry bone E83.81
hunterian glossitis D51.0
Hunt's (herpetic geniculate ganglionitis)
(neuralgia) B02.21
dyssynergia cerebellaris myoclonica G11.19
Hutchinson's triad A50.53
hyperabduction G54.0
hyperammonemia-hyperornithinemia-
homocitrullinemia E72.4
hypereosinophilic (HES) D72.119
idiopathic (IHES) D72.110
lymphocytic variant (LHES) D72.111
myeloid D72.118
specified NEC D72.118
hyperimmunoglobulin D M04.1
hyperimmunoglobulin E (IgE) D82.4
hyperkalemic E87.5
hyperkinetic —*see* Hyperkinesia
hypermobility M35.7
hypernatremia E87.0
hyperosmolarity (*see also,* Diabetes, by type, with
hyperosmolarity) E87.0
hyperperfusion G97.82
hypersplenic D73.1
hypertransfusion, newborn P61.1
hyperventilation F45.8
hyperviscosity (of serum)
polycythemic D75.1
sclerothymic D58.8
hypoglycemic (familial) (neonatal) E16.2
hypokalemic E87.6
hyponatremic E87.1
hypopituitarism E23.0
hypoplastic left-heart Q23.4
hypopotassemia E87.6
hyposmolality E87.1
hypotension, maternal O26.5-•
hypothenar hammer I73.89
hypoventilation, obesity (OHS) E66.2
ICF (intravascular coagulation-fibrinolysis) D65
idiopathic
cardiorespiratory distress, newborn P22.0
nephrotic (infantile) N04.9
iliotibial band M76.3-•
immobility, immobilization (paraplegic) M62.3
immune effector cell-associated neurotoxicity
(ICANS) G92.00
grade
1 G92.01
2 G92.02
3 G92.03
4 G92.04
5 G92.05
unspecified G92.00
immune reconstitution D89.3
immune reconstitution inflammatory [IRIS] D89.3
immunity deficiency, combined D81.9
immunodeficiency
acquired —*see* Human, immunodeficiency
virus (HIV) disease
combined D81.9
impending coronary I20.0
impingement, shoulder M75.4-•
inappropriate secretion of antidiuretic hormone
E22.2
infant
gestational diabetes P70.0
of diabetic mother P70.1
infantilism (pituitary) E23.0
inferior vena cava I87.1

▶ New   ▌Revised   ~~deleted~~ Deleted   • Use Additional Character(s)

Syndrome *(Continued)*
  inspissated bile (newborn) P59.1
  institutional (childhood) F94.2
  insufficient sleep F51.12
  insulin resistance
    type A E88.811
    type B E88.818
  intermediate coronary (artery) I20.0
  interspinous ligament —*see* Spondylopathy,
      specified NEC
  intestinal
    carcinoid E34.09
    knot K56.2
  intravascular coagulation-fibrinolysis (ICF) D65
  iodine-deficiency, congenital E00.9
    type
      mixed E00.2
      myxedematous E00.1
      neurological E00.0
  IRDS (idiopathic respiratory distress, newborn)
      P22.0
  irritable
    bowel K58.9
      with
        constipation K58.1
        diarrhea K58.0
      mixed K58.2
      psychogenic F45.8
      specified NEC K58.8
    heart (psychogenic) F45.8
    weakness F48.8
  ischemic
    bowel (transient) K55.9
      chronic K55.1
      due to mesenteric artery insufficiency K55.1
    steal T82.898
  IVC (intravascular coagulopathy) D65
  Ivemark's Q89.01
  Jaccoud's —*see* Arthropathy, postrheumatic,
      chronic
  Jackson's G83.89
  Jakob-Creutzfeldt —*see* Creutzfeldt-Jakob
      disease or syndrome
  jaw-winking Q07.8
  Jervell-Lange-Nielsen I45.81
  jet lag G47.25
  Job's D71.8
  Joseph-Diamond-Blackfan D61.01
  jugular foramen G52.7
  Kabuki (type 1, due to KMT2D mutation) (type
      2, due to KDM6A mutation) Q89.81
  Kanner's (autism) F84.0
  Kartagener's Q89.3
  Kelly's D50.1
  Kimmelstiel-Wilson —*see* Diabetes, specified
      type, with Kimmelstiel-Wilson disease
  Kleefstra Q87.86
  Klein (e)-Levine G47.13
  Klippel-Feil (brevicollis) Q76.1
  Köhler-Pellegrini-Stieda —*see* Bursitis, tibial
      collateral
  König's K59.89
  Korsakoff (-Wernicke) (nonalcoholic) F04
    alcoholic F10.26
  Kostmann's D70.0
  Krabbe's congenital muscle hypoplasia Q79.8
  labyrinthine —*see* subcategory H83.2
  lacunar NEC G46.7
  Lambert-Eaton G70.80
    in
      neoplastic disease G73.1
      specified disease NEC G70.81
  Landau-Kleffner —*see* Epilepsy, specified NEC
  Larsen's Q74.8
  Lassueur Graham-Little Piccardi L66.19
  lateral
    cutaneous nerve of thigh G57.1-•
    medullary G46.4
  Launois' E22.0
  Laurence-Moon Q87.84
  Lawrence E88.12
  lazy
    leukocyte D70.8
    posture M62.3
  Lemierre I80.8
  Lennox-Gastaut G40.812
    intractable G40.814
      with status epilepticus G40.813
      without status epilepticus G40.814
    not intractable G40.812
      with status epilepticus G40.811
      without status epilepticus G40.812

Syndrome *(Continued)*
  lenticular, progressive E83.01
  Leopold-Levi's E05.90
  Lev's I44.2
  Li-Fraumeni Z15.01
  Lichtheim's D51.0
  Lightwood's N25.89
  Lignac (de Toni) (-Fanconi) (-Debré) E72.09
    with cystinosis E72.04
  Likoff's I20.89
  limbic epilepsy personality F07.0
  liver-kidney K76.7
  lobotomy F07.0
  Löffler's J82.89
  long arm 18 or 21 deletion Q93.89
  long QT I45.81
  Louis-Barré G11.3
  low
    atmospheric pressure T70.29
    back M54.50
    output (cardiac) I50.9
  lower radicular, newborn (birth injury) P14.8
  Luetscher's (dehydration) E86.0
  Lupus anticoagulant D68.62
  Lutembacher's Q21.19
  macrophage activation D76.1
    due to infection D76.2
  magnesium-deficiency R29.0
  Majeed M04.8
  Mal de Debarquement R42
  malabsorption K90.9
    postsurgical K91.2
  malformation, congenital, due to
    alcohol Q86.0
    exogenous cause NEC Q86.8
    hydantoin Q86.1
    warfarin Q86.2
  malignant
    carcinoid E34.00
    neuroleptic G21.0
  Mallory-Weiss K22.6
  mandibulofacial dysostosis Q75.4
  manic-depressive —*see* Disorder, bipolar
  maple-syrup-urine E71.0
  Marable's I77.4
  Marfan Q87.40
    with
      cardiovascular manifestations Q87.418
        aortic dilation Q87.410
      ocular manifestations Q87.42
      skeletal manifestations Q87.43
  Marie's (acromegaly) E22.0
  mast cell activation —*see* Activation, mast cell
  maternal hypotension —*see* Syndrome,
      hypotension, maternal
  May (-Hegglin) D72.0
  McArdle (-Schmidt) (-Pearson) E74.04
  McQuarrie's E16.2
  meconium plug (newborn) P76.0
  MED13L (mediator complex subunit 13L) Q87.85
  median arcuate ligament I77.4
  mediator complex subunit 13L (MED13L) Q87.85
  Meekeren-Ehlers-Danlos Q79.6
  megavitamin-B6 E67.2
  Meige G24.4
  MELAS E88.41
  Mendelson's O74.0
  MERRF (myoclonic epilepsy associated with
      ragged-red fibers) E88.42
  mesenteric
    artery (superior) K55.1
    vascular insufficiency K55.1
  metabolic E88.810
  metastatic carcinoid E34.00
  micrognathia-glossoptosis Q87.0
  midbrain NEC G93.89
  middle lobe (lung) J98.19
  middle radicular G54.0
  migraine —*see also* Migraine G43.909-•
  Mikulicz' K11.8
  milk-alkali E83.52
  Millard-Gubler G46.3
  Miller-Dieker Q93.88
  Miller-Fisher G61.0
  Minkowski-Chauffard D58.0
  Mirizzi's K83.1
  MNGIE (Mitochondrial Neurogastrointestinal
      Encephalopathy) E88.49
  Möbius, ophthalmoplegic migraine —*see*
      Migraine, ophthalmoplegic
  monofixation H50.42
  Morel-Moore M85.2

Syndrome *(Continued)*
  Morel-Morgagni M85.2
  Morgagni (-Morel) (-Stewart) M85.2
  Morgagni-Adams-Stokes I45.9
  Mounier-Kuhn Q32.4
    with bronchiectasis J47.9
      with
        exacerbation (acute) J47.1
        lower respiratory infection J47.0
    acquired J98.09
      with bronchiectasis J47.9
        with
          exacerbation (acute) J47.1
          lower respiratory infection J47.0
  Muckle-Wells M04.2
  mucocutaneous lymph node (acute febrile)
      (MCLS) M30.3
  multiple endocrine neoplasia (MEN) —*see*
      Neoplasia, endocrine, multiple (MEN}
  multiple operations —*see* Disorder, factitious
  multisystem inflammatory (in adults) (in
      children) M35.81
  myasthenic G70.9
    in
      diabetes mellitus —*see* Diabetes, amyotrophy
      endocrine disease NEC E34.9 [G73.3]
      neoplastic disease —*see also* Neoplasm
        D49.9 [G73.3]
      thyrotoxicosis (hyperthyroidism) E05.90
        [G73.3]
        with thyroid storm E05.91 [G73.3]
  myelodysplastic D46.9
    with
      5q deletion D46.C
      isolated del (5q) chromosomal abnormality
        D46.C
      multilineage dysplasia D46.A
        with ringed sideroblasts D46.B
    lesions, low grade D46.20
    specified NEC D46.Z
  myeloid hypereosinophilic D72.118
  myelopathic pain G89.0
  myeloproliferative (chronic) D47.1
  myofascial pain M79.18
  Naffziger's G54.0
  nail patella Q87.2
  NARP (Neuropathy, Ataxia and Retinitis
      pigmentosa) E88.49
  neonatal abstinence P96.1
  nephritic —*see also* Nephritis
    with edema —*see* Nephrosis
    acute N00.9
    chronic N03.9
    rapidly progressive N01.9
  nephrotic (congenital) —*see also* Nephrosis N04.9
    with
      C3
        glomerulonephritis N04.A
        glomerulopathy N04.A
          with dense deposit disease N04.6
      dense deposit disease N04.6
      diffuse
        crescentic glomerulonephritis N04.7
        endocapillary proliferative
          glomerulonephritis N04.4
        membranous glomerulonephritis N04.20
        mesangial proliferative
          glomerulonephritis N04.3
        mesangiocapillary glomerulonephritis
          N04.5
      focal and segmental glomerular lesions N04.1
      minor glomerular abnormality N04.0
      specified morphological changes NEC N04.8
    diabetic —*see* Diabetes, nephrosis
    specified type NEC with diffuse membranous
        glomerulonephritis N04.29
  neurologic neglect R41.4
  Nezelof's D81.4
  Niikawa-Kuroki Q89.81
  Nonne-Milroy-Meige Q82.0
  Nothnagel's vasomotor acroparesthesia I73.89
  obesity hypoventilation (OHS) E66.2
  obliterans
    bronchiolitis (see also Bronchiolitis,
      obliterative) J44.81
  oculomotor H51.9
  Ogilvie K59.81
  Oliver-McFarlane Q87.89
  ophthalmoplegia-cerebellar ataxia —*see*
      Strabismus, paralytic, third nerve
  oral allergy T78.19
  oral-facial-digital Q87.0

▶ New   ⇒ Revised   ~~deleted~~ Deleted   • Use Additional Character(s)

T

▶ New　　⇨ Revised　　~~deleted~~ Deleted　　● Use Additional Character(s)

▶ New   ⇒ Revised   ~~deleted~~ Deleted   ● Use Additional Character(s)

Tuberculosis, tubercular, tuberculous (Continued)
  sacrum A18.01
  salivary gland A18.83
  salpingitis (acute) (chronic) A18.17
  sandblaster's J65
  sclera A18.51
  scoliosis A18.01
  scrofulous A18.2
  scrotum A18.15
  seminal tract or vesicle A18.15
  senile A15.9
  septic —see Tuberculosis, miliary
  shoulder (joint) A18.02
    blade A18.03
  sigmoid A18.32
  sinus (any nasal) A15.8
    bone A18.03
    epididymis A18.15
  skeletal NEC A18.03
  skin (any site) (primary) A18.4
  small intestine A18.32
  soft palate A18.83
  spermatic cord A18.15
  spine, spinal (column) A18.01
    cord A17.81
    medulla A17.81
    membrane A17.0
    meninges A17.0
  spleen, splenitis A18.85
  spondylitis A18.01
  sternoclavicular joint A18.02
  stomach A18.83
  stonemason's J65
  subcutaneous tissue (cellular) (primary) A18.4
  subcutis (primary) A18.4
  subdeltoid bursa A18.83
  submaxillary (region) A18.83
  supraclavicular gland A18.2
  suprarenal (capsule) (gland) A18.7
  swelling, joint —see also category M01 (see also
      Tuberculosis, joint) A18.02
  symphysis pubis A18.02
  synovitis A18.09
    articular A18.02
    spine or vertebra A18.01
  systemic —see Tuberculosis, miliary
  tarsitis A18.4
  tendon (sheath) —see Tuberculosis, tenosynovitis
  tenosynovitis A18.09
    spine or vertebra A18.01
  testis A18.15
  throat A15.8
  thymus gland A18.82
  thyroid gland A18.81
  tongue A18.83
  tonsil, tonsillitis A15.8
  trachea, tracheal A15.5
    lymph gland or node A15.4
      primary (progressive) A15.7
  tracheobronchial A15.5
    lymph gland or node A15.4
      primary (progressive) A15.7
  tubal (acute) (chronic) A18.17
  tunica vaginalis A18.15
  ulcer (skin) (primary) A18.4
    bowel or intestine A18.32
    specified NEC - code under Tuberculosis, by
        site
  unspecified site A15.9
  ureter A18.11
  urethra, urethral (gland) A18.13
  urinary organ or tract A18.13
  uterus A18.17
  uveal tract A18.54
  uvula A18.83
  vagina A18.18
  vas deferens A18.15
  verruca, verrucosa (cutis) (primary) A18.4
  vertebra (column) A18.01
  vesiculitis A18.15
  vulva A18.18
  wrist (joint) A18.02
Tuberculum
  Carabelli —see Note at K00.2
  occlusal —see Note at K00.2
  paramolare K00.2
Tuberosity, entire maxillary M26.07
Tuberous sclerosis (brain) Q85.1
Tubo-ovarian —see condition
Tuboplasty, after previous sterilization Z31.0
  aftercare Z31.42

Tubotympanitis, catarrhal (chronic) —see Otitis,
    media, nonsuppurative, chronic, serous
Tularemia A21.9
  with
    conjunctivitis A21.1
    pneumonia A21.2
  abdominal A21.3
  bronchopneumonic A21.2
  conjunctivitis A21.1
  cryptogenic A21.3
  enteric A21.3
  gastrointestinal A21.3
  generalized A21.7
  ingestion A21.3
  intestinal A21.3
  oculoglandular A21.1
  ophthalmic A21.1
  pneumonia (any), pneumonic A21.2
  pulmonary A21.2
  sepsis A21.7
  specified NEC A21.8
  typhoidal A21.7
  ulceroglandular A21.0
Tularensis conjunctivitis A21.1
Tumefaction —see also Swelling
  liver —see Hypertrophy, liver
Tumor —see also Neoplasm, unspecified behavior,
    by site
  acinar cell —see Neoplasm, uncertain behavior,
      by site
  acinic cell —see Neoplasm, uncertain behavior,
      by site
  adenocarcinoid —see Neoplasm, malignant, by
      site
  adenomatoid —see also Neoplasm, benign, by
      site
    odontogenic —see Cyst, calcifying
        odontogenic
  adnexal (skin) —see Neoplasm, skin, benign,
      by site
  adrenal
    cortical (benign) D35.0-●
      malignant C74.0-●
    rest —see Neoplasm, benign, by site
  alpha-cell
    malignant
      pancreas C25.4
      specified site NEC —see Neoplasm,
          malignant, by site
      unspecified site C25.4
    pancreas D13.7
    specified site NEC —see Neoplasm, benign,
        by site
    unspecified site D13.7
  aneurysmal —see Aneurysm
  aortic body D44.7
    malignant C75.5
  Askin's —see Neoplasm, connective tissue,
      malignant
  basal cell —see also Neoplasm, skin, uncertain
      behavior D48.5
  Bednar —see Neoplasm, skin, malignant
  benign (unclassified) —see Neoplasm, benign,
      by site
  beta-cell
    malignant
      pancreas C25.4
      specified site NEC —see Neoplasm,
          malignant, by site
      unspecified site C25.4
    pancreas D13.7
    specified site NEC —see Neoplasm, benign,
        by site
    unspecified site D13.7
  Brenner D27.9
    borderline malignancy D39.1-●
    malignant C56-●
    proliferating D39.1
  bronchial alveolar, intravascular D38.1
  Brooke's —see Neoplasm, skin, benign
  brown fat —see Lipoma
  Burkitt —see Lymphoma, Burkitt
  calcifying epithelial odontogenic —see Cyst,
      calcifying odontogenic
  carcinoid D3A.00
    benign D3A.00
      appendix D3A.020
      ascending colon D3A.022
      bronchus (lung) D3A.090
      cecum D3A.021
      colon D3A.029

Tumor (Continued)
  carcinoid (Continued)
    benign (Continued)
      descending colon D3A.024
      duodenum D3A.010
      foregut NOS D3A.094
      hindgut NOS D3A.096
      ileum D3A.012
      jejunum D3A.011
      kidney D3A.093
      large intestine D3A.029
      lung (bronchus) D3A.090
      midgut NOS D3A.095
      rectum D3A.026
      sigmoid colon D3A.025
      small intestine D3A.019
      specified NEC D3A.098
      stomach D3A.092
      thymus D3A.091
      transverse colon D3A.023
    malignant C7A.00
      appendix C7A.020
      ascending colon C7A.022
      bronchus (lung) C7A.090
      cecum C7A.021
      colon C7A.029
      descending colon C7A.024
      duodenum C7A.010
      foregut NOS C7A.094
      hindgut NOS C7A.096
      ileum C7A.012
      jejunum C7A.011
      kidney C7A.093
      large intestine C7A.029
      lung (bronchus) C7A.090
      midgut NOS C7A.095
      rectum C7A.026
      sigmoid colon C7A.025
      small intestine C7A.019
      specified NEC C7A.098
      stomach C7A.092
      thymus C7A.091
      transverse colon C7A.023
    mesentery metastasis C7B.04
    secondary C7B.00
      bone C7B.03
      distant lymph nodes C7B.01
      liver C7B.02
      peritoneum C7B.04
      specified NEC C7B.09
  carotid body D44.6
    malignant C75.4
  cells —see also Neoplasm, unspecified behavior,
      by site
    benign —see Neoplasm, benign, by site
    malignant —see Neoplasm, malignant, by site
    uncertain whether benign or malignant —see
        Neoplasm, uncertain behavior, by site
  cervix, in pregnancy or childbirth —see
      Pregnancy, complicated by, tumor, cervix
  chondromatous giant cell —see Neoplasm, bone,
      benign
  chromaffin —see also Neoplasm, benign, by site
    malignant —see Neoplasm, malignant, by
        site
  Cock's peculiar L72.3
  Codman's —see Neoplasm, bone, benign
  dentigerous, mixed —see Cyst, calcifying
      odontogenic
  dermoid —see Neoplasm, benign, by site
    with malignant transformation C56-●
  desmoid (extra-abdominal) —see also Neoplasm,
      connective tissue, uncertain behavior
    abdominal —see Neoplasm, connective tissue,
        uncertain behavior
  embolus —see Neoplasm, secondary, by site
  embryonal (mixed) —see also Neoplasm,
      uncertain behavior, by site
    liver C22.7
  endodermal sinus
    specified site —see Neoplasm, malignant, by
        site
    unspecified site
      female C56.-●
      male C62.90
  epithelial
    benign —see Neoplasm, benign, by site
    malignant —see Neoplasm, malignant, by site
  Ewing's —see Neoplasm, bone, malignant, by site
  fatty —see Lipoma
  fibroid —see Leiomyoma

Tumor (Continued)
G cell
  malignant
    pancreas C25.4
    specified site NEC —see Neoplasm,
      malignant, by site
    unspecified site C25.4
  specified site —see Neoplasm, uncertain
    behavior, by site
  unspecified site D37.8
germ cell —see also Neoplasm, malignant, by site
  mixed —see Neoplasm, malignant,
    by site
ghost cell, odontogenic —see Cyst, calcifying
  odontogenic
giant cell —see also Neoplasm, uncertain
  behavior, by site
  bone D48.0
    malignant —see Neoplasm, bone, malignant
  chondromatous —see Neoplasm, bone, benign
  malignant —see Neoplasm, malignant,
    by site
  soft parts —see Neoplasm, connective tissue,
    uncertain behavior
    malignant —see Neoplasm, connective
      tissue, malignant
glomus D18.00
  intra-abdominal D18.03
  intracranial D18.02
  jugulare D44.7
    malignant C75.5
  skin D18.01
  specified site NEC D18.09
gonadal stromal —see Neoplasm, uncertain
  behavior, by site
granular cell —see also Neoplasm, connective
  tissue, benign
  malignant —see Neoplasm, connective tissue,
    malignant
granulosa cell D39.1-•
  juvenile D39.1-•
  malignant C56-•
granulosa cell-theca cell D39.1-•
  malignant C56-•
Grawitz's C64-•
hemorrhoidal —see Hemorrhoids
hilar cell D27-•
hilus cell D27-•
Hurthle cell (benign) D34
  malignant C73
hydatid —see Echinococcus
hypernephroid —see also Neoplasm, uncertain
  behavior, by site
interstitial cell —see also Neoplasm, uncertain
  behavior, by site
  benign —see Neoplasm, benign, by site
  malignant —see Neoplasm, malignant,
    by site
intravascular bronchial alveolar D38.1
islet cell —see Neoplasm, benign, by site
  malignant —see Neoplasm, malignant, by site
    pancreas C25.4
    specified site NEC —see Neoplasm,
      malignant, by site
    unspecified site C25.4
  pancreas D13.7
  specified site NEC —see Neoplasm, benign,
    by site
  unspecified site D13.7
juxtaglomerular D41.0-•
Klatskin's C24.0
Krukenberg's C79.6-•
Leydig cell —see Neoplasm, uncertain behavior,
  by site
  benign —see Neoplasm, benign, by site
    specified site —see Neoplasm, benign, by
      site
    unspecified site
      female D27.9
      male D29.20
  malignant —see Neoplasm, malignant, by site
    specified site —see Neoplasm, malignant,
      by site
    unspecified site
      female C56.9
      male C62.90
  specified site —see Neoplasm, uncertain
    behavior, by site
  unspecified site
    female D39.10
    male D40.10

Tumor (Continued)
lipid cell, ovary D27-•
lipoid cell, ovary D27-•
malignant —see also Neoplasm, malignant, by
  site C80.1
  fusiform cell (type) C80.1
  giant cell (type) C80.1
  localized, plasma cell —see Plasmacytoma,
    solitary
  mixed NEC C80.1
  small cell (type) C80.1
  spindle cell (type) C80.1
  unclassified C80.1
mast cell D47.09
melanotic, neuroectodermal —see Neoplasm,
  benign, by site
Merkel cell —see Carcinoma, Merkel cell
mesenchymal
  malignant —see Neoplasm, connective tissue,
    malignant
  mixed —see Neoplasm, connective tissue,
    uncertain behavior
mesodermal, mixed —see also Neoplasm,
  malignant, by site
  liver C22.4
mesonephric —see also Neoplasm, uncertain
  behavior, by site
  malignant —see Neoplasm, malignant, by site
metastatic
  from specified site —see Neoplasm, malignant,
    by site
  of specified site —see Neoplasm, malignant,
    by site
  to specified site —see Neoplasm, secondary,
    by site
mixed NEC —see also Neoplasm, benign, by site
  malignant —see Neoplasm, malignant, by site
mucinous of low malignant potential
  specified site —see Neoplasm, malignant, by
    site
  unspecified site C56.9
mucocarcinoid
  specified site —see Neoplasm, malignant, by
    site
  unspecified site C18.1
mucoepidermoid —see Neoplasm, uncertain
  behavior, by site
Müllerian, mixed
  specified site —see Neoplasm, malignant, by
    site
  unspecified site C54.9
myoepithelial —see Neoplasm, benign,
  by site
neuroectodermal (peripheral) —see Neoplasm,
  malignant, by site
  primitive
    specified site —see Neoplasm, malignant,
      by site
    unspecified site C71.9
neuroendocrine D3A.8
  malignant poorly differentiated C7A.1
  secondary NEC C7B.8
  specified NEC C7A.8
neurogenic olfactory C30.0
nonencapsulated sclerosing C73
odontogenic (adenomatoid) (benign) (calcifying
  epithelial) (keratocystic) (squamous) —see
  Cyst, calcifying odontogenic
  malignant C41.1
    upper jaw (bone) C41.0
ovarian stromal D39.1-•
ovary, in pregnancy —see Pregnancy,
  complicated by
pacinian —see Neoplasm, skin, benign
Pancoast's —see Pancoast's syndrome
papillary —see also Papilloma
  cystic D37.9
  mucinous of low malignant potential C56-•
    specified site —see Neoplasm, malignant,
      by site
    unspecified site C56.9
  serous of low malignant potential
    specified site —see Neoplasm, malignant,
      by site
    unspecified site C56.9
pelvic, in pregnancy or childbirth —see
  Pregnancy, complicated by
phantom F45.8
phyllodes D48.6-•
  benign D24-•
  malignant —see Neoplasm, breast, malignant

Tumor (Continued)
Pindborg —see Cyst, calcifying odontogenic
placental site trophoblastic D39.2
plasma cell (malignant) (localized) —see
  Plasmacytoma, solitary
polyvesicular vitelline
  specified site —see Neoplasm, malignant, by
    site
  unspecified site
    female C56.9
    male C62.90
Pott's puffy —see Osteomyelitis, specified NEC
Rathke's pouch D44.3
retinal anlage —see Neoplasm, benign, by site
salivary gland or duct type, mixed —see
  Neoplasm, salivary gland or duct, benign
  malignant —see Neoplasm, salivary gland or
    duct, malignant
Sampson's N80.10-•
Schmincke's —see Neoplasm, nasopharynx,
  malignant
sclerosing stromal D27-•
sebaceous —see Cyst, sebaceous
secondary —see Neoplasm, secondary, by
  site
  carcinoid C7B.00
    bone C7B.03
    distant lymph nodes C7B.01
    liver C7B.02
    peritoneum C7B.04
    specified NEC C7B.09
  neuroendocrine NEC C7B.8
serous of low malignant potential
  specified site —see Neoplasm, malignant, by
    site
  unspecified site C56.9
Sertoli cell —see Neoplasm, benign, by site
  with lipid storage
    specified site —see Neoplasm, benign, by
      site
    unspecified site
      female D27.9
      male D29.20
  specified site —see Neoplasm, benign, by site
  unspecified site
    female D27.9
    male D29.20
Sertoli-Leydig cell —see Neoplasm, benign, by
  site
  specified site —see Neoplasm, benign, by site
  unspecified site
    female D27.9
    male D29.20
sex cord(-stromal) —see Neoplasm, uncertain
  behavior, by site
  with annular tubules D39.1-•
skin appendage —see Neoplasm, skin,
  benign
smooth muscle —see Neoplasm, connective
  tissue, uncertain behavior
soft tissue
  benign —see Neoplasm, connective tissue,
    benign
  malignant —see Neoplasm, connective tissue,
    malignant
sternomastoid (congenital) Q68.0
stromal
  endometrial D39.0
  gastric D48.19
    benign D21.4
    malignant C49.A2
    uncertain behavior D48.19
  gastrointestinal C49.A-•
    benign D21.4
    esophagus C49.A1
    large intestine C49.A4
    malignant C49.A0
      colon C49.A4
      duodenum C49.A3
      esophagus C49.A1
      ileum C49.A3
      jejunum C49.A3
      Meckel diverticulum C49.A3
      large intestine C49.A4
      omentum C49.A9
      peritoneum C49.A9
      rectum C49.A5
      small intestine C49.A3
      specified site NEC C49.A9
      stomach C49.A2
    rectum C49.A5

▶ New   ⇒ Revised   ~~deleted~~ Deleted   • Use Additional Character(s)

▸ New   ➡ Revised   ~~deleted~~ Deleted   • Use Additional Character(s)

▶ New   ⇨ Revised   ~~deleted~~ Deleted   ● Use Additional Character(s)

Varix (*Continued*)
  gastric I86.4
  inflamed or infected I83.10
    ulcerated I83.209
  labia (majora) I86.3
  leg (asymptomatic) I83.9-●
    with
      edema I83.899
      inflammation I83.10
        with ulcer —*see* Varix, leg, with, ulcer,
          with inflammation by site
      pain I83.819
      specified complication NEC I83.899
      swelling I83.899
      ulcer I83.0-●
        with inflammation I83.2-●
        ankle I83.003
          with inflammation I83.203
        calf I83.002
          with inflammation I83.202
        foot NEC I83.005
          with inflammation I83.205
        heel I83.004
          with inflammation I83.204
        lower leg NEC I83.008
          with inflammation I83.208
        midfoot I83.004
          with inflammation I83.204
        thigh I83.001
          with inflammation I83.201
    bilateral (asymptomatic) I83.93
      with
        edema I83.893
        pain I83.813
        specified complication NEC I83.893
        swelling I83.893
        ulcer I83.0-●
          with inflammation I83.209
    left (asymptomatic) I83.92
      with
        edema I83.892
        inflammation I83.12
          with ulcer —*see* Varix, leg, with, ulcer,
            with inflammation by site
        pain I83.812
        specified complication NEC I83.892
        swelling I83.892
        ulcer I83.029
          with inflammation I83.229
          ankle I83.023
            with inflammation I83.223
          calf I83.022
            with inflammation I83.222
          foot NEC I83.025
            with inflammation I83.225
          heel I83.024
            with inflammation I83.224
          lower leg NEC I83.028
            with inflammation I83.228
          midfoot I83.024
            with inflammation I83.224
          thigh I83.021
            with inflammation I83.221
    right (asymptomatic) I83.91
      with
        edema I83.891
        inflammation I83.11
          with ulcer —*see* Varix, leg, with, ulcer,
            with inflammation by site
        pain I83.811
        specified complication NEC I83.891
        swelling I83.891
        ulcer I83.019
          with inflammation I83.219
          ankle I83.013
            with inflammation I83.213
          calf I83.012
            with inflammation I83.212
          foot NEC I83.015
            with inflammation I83.215
          heel I83.014
            with inflammation I83.214
          lower leg NEC I83.018
            with inflammation I83.218
          midfoot I83.014
            with inflammation I83.214
          thigh I83.011
            with inflammation I83.211
  nasal septum I86.8
  orbit I86.8
    congenital Q27.8
  ovary I86.2

Varix (*Continued*)
  papillary I78.1
  pelvis I86.2
  perineum I86.3
  pharynx I86.8
  placenta O43.89-●
  renal papilla I86.8
  retina H35.09
  scrotum (ulcerated) I86.1
  sigmoid colon I86.8
  specified site NEC I86.8
  spinal (cord) (vessels) I86.8
  spleen, splenic (vein) (with phlebolith) I86.8
  stomach I86.4
  sublingual I86.0
  ulcerated I83.009
    inflamed or infected I83.209
  uterine ligament I86.2
  vagina I86.8
  vocal cord I86.8
  vulva I86.3
Vas deferens —*see* condition
Vas deferentitis N49.1
Vasa previa O69.4
  hemorrhage from, affecting newborn P50.0
Vascular —*see also* condition
  loop on optic papilla Q14.2
  spasm I73.9
  spider I78.1
Vascularization, cornea —*see* Neovascularization,
  cornea
Vasculitis I77.6
  allergic D69.0
  ANCA (antineutrophilic cytoplasmic antibody)
    associated I77.82
  ANCA (antineutrophilic cytoplasmic antibody)
    positive I77.82
  antineutrophilic cytoplasmic antibody [ANCA]
    I77.82
  cryoglobulinemic D89.1
  disseminated I77.6
  hypocomplementemic M31.8
  kidney I77.89
  leukocytoclastic M31.0
  livedoid L95.0
  nodular L95.8
  retina H35.06-●
  rheumatic —*see* Fever, rheumatic
  rheumatoid —*see* Rheumatoid, vasculitis
  skin (limited to) L95.9
    specified NEC L95.8
  systemic M31.8
Vasculopathy, necrotizing M31.9
  cardiac allograft T86.290
  specified NEC M31.8
Vasitis (nodosa) N49.1
  tuberculous A18.15
Vasodilation I73.9
Vasomotor —*see* condition
Vasoplasty, after previous sterilization Z31.0
  aftercare Z31.42
Vasospasm (vasoconstriction) (*see also* Angiospasm)
  I73.9
  cerebral (cerebrovascular) (artery) I67.848
    reversible I67.841
  coronary I20.1
  nerve
    arm —*see* Mononeuropathy, upper limb
    brachial plexus G54.0
    cervical plexus G54.2
    leg —*see* Mononeuropathy, lower limb
    peripheral NOS I73.9
  retina (artery) —*see* Occlusion, artery, retina
Vasospastic —*see* condition
Vasovagal attack (paroxysmal) R55
  psychogenic F45.8
VATER syndrome Q87.2
Vater's ampulla —*see* condition
Vegetation, vegetative
  adenoid (nasal fossa) J35.8
  endocarditis (acute) (any valve) (subacute) I33.0
  heart (mycotic) (valve) I33.0
Veil
  Jackson's Q43.3
Vein, venous —*see* condition
Veldt sore —*see* Ulcer, skin
Velpeau's hernia —*see* Hernia, femoral
Venereal
  bubo A55
  disease A64
  granuloma inguinale A58
  lymphogranuloma (Durand-Nicolas-Favre) A55

Venofibrosis I87.8
Venom, venomous —*see* Table of Drugs and
  Chemicals, by animal or substance,
  poisoning
Venous —*see* condition
Ventilator lung, newborn P27.8
Ventral —*see* condition
Ventricle, ventricular —*see also* condition
  escape I49.3
  inversion Q20.5
Ventriculitis (cerebral) —*see also* Encephalitis
  G04.90
Ventriculostomy status Z98.2
Vernet's syndrome G52.7
Verneuil's disease (syphilitic bursitis) A52.78
Verruca (due to HPV) (filiformis) (simplex) (viral)
  (vulgaris) B07.9
  acuminata A63.0
  necrogenica (primary) (tuberculosa) A18.4
  plana B07.8
  plantaris B07.0
  seborrheica L82.1
    inflamed L82.0
  senile (seborrheic) L82.1
    inflamed L82.0
  tuberculosa (primary) A18.4
  venereal A63.0
Verrucosities —*see* Verruca
Verruga peruana, peruviana A44.1
Version
  cervix —*see* Malposition, uterus
  uterus (postinfectional) (postpartal, old) —*see*
    Malposition, uterus
Vertebra, vertebral —*see* condition
Vertical talus (congenital) Q66.80
  left foot Q66.82
  right foot Q66.81
Vertigo R42
  auditory —*see* Vertigo, aural
  aural H81.31-●
  benign paroxysmal (positional) H81.1-●
  central (origin) H81.4
  cerebral H81.4
  Dix and Hallpike (epidemic) —*see* Neuronitis,
    vestibular
  due to infrasound T75.23
  epidemic A88.1
    Dix and Hallpike —*see* Neuronitis,
      vestibular
    Pedersen's —*see* Neuronitis, vestibular
    vestibular neuronitis —*see* Neuronitis,
      vestibular
  hysterical F44.89
  infrasound T75.23
  labyrinthine —*see* subcategory H81.0
  laryngeal R05.4
  malignant positional H81.4
  Ménière's —*see* subcategory H81.40
  menopausal N95.11
  otogenic —*see* Vertigo, aural
  paroxysmal positional, benign —*see* Vertigo,
    benign paroxysmal
  Pedersen's (epidemic) —*see* Neuronitis,
    vestibular
  peripheral NEC H81.39-●
  positional
    benign paroxysmal —*see* Vertigo, benign
      paroxysmal
    malignant H81.4
Very-low-density-lipoprotein-type (VLDL)
  hyperlipoproteinemia E78.1
Vesania —*see* Psychosis
Vesical —*see* condition
Vesicle
  cutaneous R23.8
  seminal —*see* condition
  skin R23.8
Vesicocolic —*see* condition
Vesicoperineal —*see* condition
Vesicorectal —*see* condition
Vesicourethrorectal —*see* condition
Vesicovaginal —*see* condition
Vesicular —*see* condition
Vesiculitis (seminal) N49.0
  amebic A06.82
  gonorrheal (acute) (chronic) A54.23
  trichomonal A59.09
  tuberculous A18.15
Vestibulitis (ear) —*see also* subcategory H83.0
  nose (external) J34.89
  vulvar N94.810

▶ New   ➡ Revised   ~~deleted~~ Deleted   ● Use Additional Character(s)

▶ New   ⟹ Revised   ~~deleted~~ Deleted   ● Use Additional Character(s)

► New   ⇒ Revised   ~~deleted~~ Deleted   ● Use Additional Character(s)

ICD-10-CM
Table of Neoplasms

The list below gives the code numbers for neoplasms by anatomical site. For each site there are six possible code numbers according to whether the neoplasm in question is malignant, benign, in situ, of uncertain behavior, or of unspecified nature. The description of the neoplasm will often indicate which of the six columns is appropriate; e.g., malignant melanoma of skin, benign fibroadenoma of breast, carcinoma in situ of cervix uteri.

Where such descriptors are not present, the remainder of the Index should be consulted where guidance is given to the appropriate column for each morphological (histological) variety listed; e.g., Mesonephroma — *see Neoplasm, malignant;* Embryoma — *see also Neoplasm, uncertain behavior;* Disease, Bowen's — *see Neoplasm, skin, in situ.* However, the guidance in the Index can be overridden if one of the descriptors mentioned above is present; e.g., malignant adenoma of colon is coded to C18.9 and not to D12.6 as the adjective "Malignant" overrides the Index entry 'Adenoma — *see also Neoplasm, benign.*'

Codes listed with a dash -, following the code have a required additional character for laterality. The Tablular must be reviewed for the complete code.

	Malignant Primary	Malignant Secondary	Ca in situ	Benign	Uncertain Behavior	Unspecified Behavior
Neoplasm, neoplastic	C80.1	C79.9	D09.9	D36.9	D48.9	D49.9
abdomen, abdominal	C76.2	C79.8-●	D09.8	D36.7	D48.7	D49.89
cavity	C76.2	C79.8-●	D09.8	D36.7	D48.7	D49.89
organ	C76.2	C79.8-●	D09.8	D36.7	D48.7	D49.89
viscera	C76.2	C79.8-●	D09.8	D36.7	D48.7	D49.89
wall — *see also Neoplasm, abdomen, wall, skin*	C44.509	C79.2-●	D04.5	D23.5	D48.5	D49.2
connective tissue	C49.4	C79.8-●	—	D21.4	D48.1-●	D49.2
skin	C44.509					
basal cell carcinoma	C44.519	—	—	—	—	—
specified type NEC	C44.599	—	—	—	—	—
squamous cell carcinoma	C44.529	—	—	—	—	—
abdominopelvic	C76.8	C79.8-●	—	D36.7	D48.7	D49.89
accessory sinus — *see Neoplasm, sinus*						
acoustic nerve	C72.4-●	C79.49	—	D33.3	D43.3	D49.7
adenoid (pharynx) (tissue)	C11.1	C79.89	D00.08	D10.6	D37.05	D49.0
adipose tissue — *see also Neoplasm, connective tissue*	C49.4	C79.89	—	D21.9	D48.1-●	D49.2
adnexa (uterine)	C57.4	C79.89	D07.39	D28.7	D39.8	D49.59
adrenal	C74.9-●	C79.7-●	D09.3	D35.0-●	D44.1-●	D49.7
capsule	C74.9-●	C79.7-●	D09.3	D35.0-●	D44.1-●	D49.7
cortex	C74.0-●	C79.7-●	D09.3	D35.0-●	D44.1-●	D49.7
gland	C74.9-●	C79.7-●	D09.3	D35.0-●	D44.1-●	D49.7
medulla	C74.1-●	C79.7-●	D09.3	D35.0-●	D44.1-●	D49.7
ala nasi (external) — *see also Neoplasm, skin, nose*	C44.301	C79.2	D04.39	D23.39	D48.5	D49.2

	Malignant Primary	Malignant Secondary	Ca in situ	Benign	Uncertain Behavior	Unspecified Behavior
alimentary canal or tract NEC	C26.9	C78.80	D01.9	D13.99	D37.9	D49.0
alveolar	C03.9	C79.89	D00.03	D10.39	D37.09	D49.0
mucosa	C03.9	C79.89	D00.03	D10.39	D37.09	D49.0
lower	C03.1	C79.89	D00.03	D10.39	D37.09	D49.0
upper	C03.0	C79.89	D00.03	D10.39	D37.09	D49.0
ridge or process	C41.1	C79.51	—	D16.5-●	D48.0	D49.2
carcinoma	C03.9	C79.8-●	—	—	—	—
lower	C03.1	C79.8-●	—	—	—	—
upper	C03.0	C79.8-●	—	—	—	—
lower	C41.1	C79.51	—	D16.5-●	D48.0	D49.2
mucosa	C03.9	C79.89	D00.03	D10.39	D37.09	D49.0
lower	C03.1	C79.89	D00.03	D10.39	D37.09	D49.0
upper	C03.0	C79.89	D00.03	D10.39	D37.09	D49.0
upper	C41.0	C79.51	—	D16.4-●	D48.0	D49.2
sulcus	C06.1	C79.89	D00.02	D10.39	D37.09	D49.0
alveolus	C03.9	C79.89	D00.03	D10.39	D37.09	D49.0
lower	C03.1	C79.89	D00.03	D10.39	D37.09	D49.0
upper	C03.0	C79.89	D00.03	D10.39	D37.09	D49.0
ampulla of Vater	C24.1	C78.89	D01.5	D13.5	D37.6	D49.0
ankle NEC	C76.5-●	C79.89	D04.7-●	D36.7	D48.7	D49.89
anorectum, anorectal (junction)	C21.8	C78.5	D01.3	D12.9	D37.8	D49.0
antecubital fossa or space	C76.4-●	C79.89	D04.6-●	D36.7	D48.7	D49.89
antrum (Highmore) (maxillary)	C31.0	C78.39	D02.3	D14.0	D38.5	D49.1
pyloric	C16.3	C78.89	D00.2	D13.1	D37.1	D49.0
tympanicum	C30.1	C78.39	D02.3	D14.0	D38.5	D49.1
anus, anal	C21.0	C78.5	D01.3	D12.9	D37.8	D49.0
canal	C21.1	C78.5	D01.3	D12.9	D37.8	D49.0
cloacogenic zone	C21.2	C78.5	D01.3	D12.9	D37.8	D49.0
margin — *see also Neoplasm, anus, skin*	C44.500	C79.2	D04.5	D23.5	D48.5	D49.2
overlapping lesion with rectosigmoid junction or rectum	C21.8	—	—	—	—	—
skin	C44.500	C79.2	D04.5	D23.5	D48.5	D49.2
basal cell carcinoma	C44.510	—	—	—	—	—
specified type NEC	C44.590	—	—	—	—	—
squamous cell carcinoma	C44.520	—	—	—	—	—
sphincter	C21.1	C78.5	D01.3	D12.9	D37.8	D49.0
aorta (thoracic)	C49.3	C79.89	—	D21.3	D48.1-●	D49.2
abdominal	C49.4	C79.89	—	D21.4	D48.1-●	D49.2
aortic body	C75.5	C79.89	—	D35.6	D44.7	D49.7
aponeurosis	C49.9	C79.89	—	D21.9	D48.1-●	D49.2
palmar	C49.1-●	C79.89	—	D21.1-●	D48.1-●	D49.2
plantar	C49.2-●	C79.89	—	D21.2-●	D48.1-●	D49.2

	Malignant Primary	Malignant Secondary	Ca in situ	Benign	Uncertain Behavior	Unspecified Behavior
appendix	C18.1	C78.5	D01.0	D12.1	D37.3	D49.0
arachnoid	C70.9	C79.49	—	D32.9	D42.9	D49.7
cerebral	C70.0	C79.32	—	D32.0	D42.0	D49.7
spinal	C70.1	C79.49	—	D32.1	D42.1	D49.7
areola	C50.0-●	C79.81	D05.-	D24.-●	D48.6-●	D49.3
arm NEC	C76.4-●	C79.89	D04.6-●	D36.7	D48.7	D49.89
artery — *see Neoplasm, connective tissue*						
aryepiglottic fold	C13.1	C79.89	D00.08	D10.7	D37.05	D49.0
hypopharyngeal aspect	C13.1	C79.89	D00.08	D10.7	D37.05	D49.0
laryngeal aspect	C32.1	C78.39	D02.0	D14.1	D38.0	D49.1
marginal zone	C13.1	C79.89	D00.08	D10.7	D37.05	D49.0
arytenoid (cartilage)	C32.3	C78.39	D02.0	D14.1	D38.0	D49.1
fold — *see Neoplasm, aryepiglottic*						
associated with transplanted organ	C80.2	—	—	—	—	—
atlas	C41.2	C79.51	—	D16.6	D48.0	D49.2
atrium, cardiac	C38.0	C79.89	—	D15.1	D48.7	D49.89
auditory						
canal (external) (skin)	C44.20-●	C79.2	D04.2-●	D23.2-●	D48.5	D49.2
internal	C30.1	C78.39	D02.3	D14.0	D38.5	D49.1
nerve	C72.4-●	C79.49	—	D33.3	D43.3	D49.7
tube	C30.1	C78.39	D02.3	D14.0	D38.5	D49.1
opening	C11.2	C79.89	D00.08	D10.6	D37.05	D49.0
auricle, ear — *see also Neoplasm, skin, ear*	C44.20-●	C79.2	D04.2-●	D23.2-●	D48.5	D49.2
auricular canal (external) — *see also Neoplasm, skin, ear*	C44.20-●	C79.2	D04.2-●	D23.2-●	D48.5	D49.2
internal	C30.1	C78.39	D02.3	D14.0	D38.5	D49.2
autonomic nerve or nervous system NEC (*see Neoplasm, nerve, peripheral*)						
axilla, axillary	C76.1	C79.89	D09.8	D36.7	D48.7	D49.89
fold — *see also Neoplasm, skin, trunk*	C44.509	C79.2	D04.5	D23.5	D48.5	D49.2
back NEC	C76.8	C79.89	D04.5	D36.7	D48.7	D49.89
Bartholin's gland	C51.0	C79.82	D07.1	D28.0	D39.8	D49.59
basal ganglia	C71.0	C79.31	—	D33.0	D43.0	D49.6
basis pedunculi	C71.7	C79.31	—	D33.1	D43.1	D49.6
bile or biliary (tract)	C24.9	C78.89	D01.5	D13.5	D37.6	D49.0
canaliculi (biliferi) (intrahepatic)	C22.1	C78.7	D01.5	D13.4	D37.6	D49.0
canals, interlobular	C22.1	C78.89	D01.5	D13.4	D37.6	D49.0

	Malignant Primary	Malignant Secondary	Ca in situ	Benign	Uncertain Behavior	Unspecified Behavior
bile or biliary *(Continued)*						
duct or passage (common) (cystic) (extrahepatic)	C24.0	C78.89	D01.5	D13.5	D37.6	D49.0
interlobular	C22.1	C78.89	D01.5	D13.4	D37.6	D49.0
intrahepatic	C22.1	C78.7	D01.5	D13.4	D37.6	D49.0
and extrahepatic	C24.8	C78.89	D01.5	D13.5	D37.6	D49.0
bladder (urinary)	C67.9	C79.11	D09.0	D30.3	D41.4	D49.4
dome	C67.1	C79.11	D09.0	D30.3	D41.4	D49.4
neck	C67.5	C79.11	D09.0	D30.3	D41.4	D49.4
orifice	C67.9	C79.11	D09.0	D30.3	D41.4	D49.4
ureteric	C67.6	C79.11	D09.0	D30.3	D41.4	D49.4
urethral	C67.5	C79.11	D09.0	D30.3	D41.4	D49.4
overlapping lesion	C67.8	—	—	—	—	—
sphincter	C67.8	C79.11	D09.0	D30.3	D41.4	D49.4
trigone	C67.0	C79.11	D09.0	D30.3	D41.4	D49.4
urachus	C67.7	C79.11	D09.0	D30.3	D41.4	D49.4
wall	C67.9	C79.11	D09.0	D30.3	D41.4	D49.4
anterior	C67.3	C79.11	D09.0	D30.3	D41.4	D49.4
lateral	C67.2	C79.11	D09.0	D30.3	D41.4	D49.4
posterior	C67.4	C79.11	D09.0	D30.3	D41.4	D49.4
blood vessel — *see Neoplasm, connective tissue*						
bone (periosteum)	C41.9	C79.51	—	D16.9-●	D48.0	D49.2
acetabulum	C41.4	C79.51	—	D16.8-●	D48.0	D49.2
ankle	C40.3-●	C79.51	—	D16.3-●	—	—
arm NEC	C40.0-●	C79.51	—	D16.0-●	—	—
astragalus	C40.3-●	C79.51	—	D16.3-●	—	—
atlas	C41.2	C79.51	—	D16.6-●	D48.0	D49.2
axis	C41.2	C79.51	—	D16.6-●	D48.0	D49.2
back NEC	C41.2	C79.51	—	D16.6-●	D48.0	D49.2
calcaneus	C40.3-●	C79.51	—	D16.3-●	—	—
calvarium	C41.0	C79.51	—	D16.4-●	D48.0	D49.2
carpus (any)	C40.1-●	C79.51	—	D16.1-●	—	—
cartilage NEC	C41.9	C79.51	—	D16.9-●	D48.0	D49.2
clavicle	C41.3	C79.51	—	D16.7-●	D48.0	D49.2
clivus	C41.0	C79.51	—	D16.4-●	D48.0	D49.2
coccygeal vertebra	C41.4	C79.51	—	D16.8-●	D48.0	D49.2
coccyx	C41.4	C79.51	—	D16.8-●	D48.0	D49.2
costal cartilage	C41.3	C79.51	—	D16.7-●	D48.0	D49.2
costovertebral joint	C41.3	C79.51	—	D16.7-●	D48.0	D49.2
cranial	C41.0	C79.51	—	D16.4-●	D48.0	D49.2
cuboid	C40.3-●	C79.51	—	D16.3-●	—	—
cuneiform	C41.9	C79.51	—	D16.9-●	D48.0	D49.2
elbow	C40.0-●	C79.51	—	D16.0-●	—	—

◀ New　　▌ Revised　　~~deleted~~ Deleted　　● Use Additional Character(s)

	Malignant Primary	Malignant Secondary	Ca in situ	Benign	Uncertain Behavior	Unspecified Behavior
bone *(Continued)*						
ethmoid (labyrinth)	C41.0	C79.51	—	D16.4-•	D48.0	D49.2
face	C41.0	C79.51	—	D16.4-•	D48.0	D49.2
femur (any part)	C40.2-•	C79.51	—	D16.2-•	—	—
fibula (any part)	C40.2-•	C79.51	—	D16.2-•	—	—
finger (any)	C40.1-•	C79.51	—	D16.1-•	—	—
foot	C40.3-•	C79.51	—	D16.3-•	—	—
forearm	C40.0-•	C79.51	—	D16.0-•	—	—
frontal	C41.0	C79.51	—	D16.4-•	D48.0	D49.2
hand	C40.1-•	C79.51	—	D16.1-•	—	—
heel	C40.3-•	C79.51	—	D16.3-•	—	—
hip	C41.4	C79.51	—	D16.8-•	D48.0	D49.2
humerus (any part)	C40.0-•	C79.51	—	D16.0-•	—	—
hyoid	C41.0	C79.51	—	D16.4-•	D48.0	D49.2
ilium	C41.4	C79.51	—	D16.8-•	D48.0	D49.2
innominate	C41.4	C79.51	—	D16.8-•	D48.0	D49.2
intervertebral cartilage or disc	C41.2	C79.51	—	D16.6-•	D48.0	D49.2
ischium	C41.4	C79.51	—	D16.8-•	D48.0	D49.2
jaw (lower)	C41.1	C79.51	—	D16.5-•	D48.0	D49.2
knee	C40.2-•	C79.51	—	D16.2-•	—	—
leg NEC	C40.2-•	C79.51	—	D16.2-•	—	—
limb NEC	C40.9-•	C79.51	—	D16.9-•	—	—
lower (long bones)	C40.2-•	C79.51	—	D16.2-•	—	—
short bones	C40.3-•	C79.51	—	D16.3-•	—	—
upper (long bones)	C40.0-•	C79.51	—	D16.0-•	—	—
short bones	C40.1-•	C79.51	—	D16.1-•	—	—
malar	C41.0	C79.51	—	D16.4-•	D48.0	D49.2
mandible	C41.1	C79.51	—	D16.5-•	D48.0	D49.2
marrow NEC (any bone)	C96.9	C79.52	—	—	D47.9	D49.89
mastoid	C41.0	C79.51	—	D16.4-•	D48.0	D49.2
maxilla, maxillary (superior)	C41.0	C79.51	—	D16.4-•	D48.0	D49.2
inferior	C41.1	C79.51	—	D16.5-•	D48.0	D49.2
metacarpus (any)	C40.1-•	C79.51	—	D16.1-•	—	—
metatarsus (any)	C40.3-•	C79.51	—	D16.3-•	—	—
overlapping sites	C40.8-•	—	—	—	—	—
navicular						
ankle	C40.3-•	C79.51	—	—	—	—
hand	C40.1-•	C79.51	—	—	—	—
nose, nasal	C41.0	C79.51	—	D16.4-•	D48.0	D49.2
occipital	C41.0	C79.51	—	D16.4-•	D48.0	D49.2
orbit	C41.0	C79.51	—	D16.4-•	D48.0	D49.2
parietal	C41.0	C79.51	—	D16.4-•	D48.0	D49.2
patella	C40.2-•	C79.51	—	—	—	—
pelvic	C41.4	C79.51	—	D16.8	D48.0	D49.2

	Malignant Primary	Malignant Secondary	Ca in situ	Benign	Uncertain Behavior	Unspecified Behavior
bone *(Continued)*						
phalanges						
foot	C40.3-•	C79.51	—	—	—	—
hand	C40.1-•	C79.51	—	—	—	—
pubic	C41.4	C79.51	—	D16.8	D48.0	D49.2
radius (any part)	C40.0-•	C79.51	—	D16.0-•	—	—
rib	C41.3	C79.51	—	D16.7	D48.0	D49.2
sacral vertebra	C41.4	C79.51	—	D16.8	D48.0	D49.2
sacrum	C41.4	C79.51	—	D16.8	D48.0	D49.2
scaphoid	—	—	—	—	—	—
of ankle	C40.3-•	C79.51	—	—	—	—
of hand	C40.1-•	C79.51	—	—	—	—
scapula (any part)	C40.0-•	C79.51	—	D16.0-•	—	—
sella turcica	C41.0	C79.51	—	D16.4-•	D48.0	D49.2
shoulder	C40.0-•	C79.51	—	D16.0-•	—	—
skull	C41.0	C79.51	—	D16.4-•	D48.0	D49.2
sphenoid	C41.0	C79.51	—	D16.4-•	D48.0	D49.2
spine, spinal (column)	C41.2	C79.51	—	D16.6	D48.0	D49.2
coccyx	C41.4	C79.51	—	D16.8	D48.0	D49.2
sacrum	C41.4	C79.51	—	D16.8	D48.0	D49.2
sternum	C41.3	C79.51	—	D16.7	D48.0	D49.2
tarsus (any)	C40.3-•	C79.51	—	—	—	—
temporal	C41.0	C79.51	—	D16.4-•	D48.0	D49.2
thumb	C40.1-•	C79.51	—	—	—	—
tibia (any part)	C40.2-•	C79.51	—	—	—	—
toe (any)	C40.3-•	C79.51	—	—	—	—
trapezium	C40.1-•	C79.51	—	—	—	—
trapezoid	C40.1-•	C79.51	—	—	—	—
turbinate	C41.0	C79.51	—	D16.4-•	D48.0	D49.2
ulna (any part)	C40.0-•	C79.51	—	D16.0-•	—	—
unciform	C40.1-•	C79.51	—	—	—	—
vertebra (column)	C41.2	C79.51	—	D16.6	D48.0	D49.2
coccyx	C41.4	C79.51	—	D16.8	D48.0	D49.2
sacrum	C41.4	C79.51	—	D16.8	D48.0	D49.2
vomer	C41.0	C79.51	—	D16.4-•	D48.0	D49.2
wrist	C40.1-•	C79.51	—	—	—	—
xiphoid process	C41.3	C79.51	—	D16.7	D48.0	D49.2
zygomatic	C41.0	C79.51	—	D16.4-•	D48.0	D49.2
book-leaf (mouth)	C06.89	C79.89	D00.00	D10.39	D37.09	D49.0
bowel — *see Neoplasm, intestine*						
brachial plexus	C47.1-•	C79.89	—	D36.12	D48.2	D49.2
brain NEC	C71.9	C79.31	—	D33.2	D43.2	D49.6
basal ganglia	C71.0	C79.31	—	D33.0	D43.0	D49.6
cerebellopontine angle	C71.6	C79.31	—	D33.1	D43.1	D49.6

	Malignant Primary	Malignant Secondary	Ca in situ	Benign	Uncertain Behavior	Unspecified Behavior
brain NEC *(Continued)*						
cerebellum NOS	C71.6	C79.31	—	D33.1	D43.1	D49.6
cerebrum	C71.Ø	C79.31	—	D33.Ø	D43.Ø	D49.6
choroid plexus	C71.7	C79.31	—	D33.1	D43.1	D49.6
corpus callosum	C71.8	C79.31	—	D33.2	D43.2	D49.6
corpus striatum	C71.Ø	C79.31	—	D33.Ø	D43.Ø	D49.6
cortex (cerebral)	C71.Ø	C79.31	—	D33.Ø	D43.Ø	D49.6
frontal lobe	C71.1	C79.31	—	D33.Ø	D43.Ø	D49.6
globus pallidus	C71.Ø	C79.31	—	D33.Ø	D43.Ø	D49.6
hippocampus	C71.2	C79.31	—	D33.Ø	D43.Ø	D49.6
hypothalamus	C71.Ø	C79.31	—	D33.Ø	D43.Ø	D49.6
internal capsule	C71.Ø	C79.31	—	D33.Ø	D43.Ø	D49.6
medulla oblongata	C71.7	C79.31	—	D33.1	D43.1	D49.6
meninges	C70.Ø	C79.32	—	D32.Ø	D42.Ø	D49.7
midbrain	C71.7	C79.31	—	D33.1	D43.1	D49.6
occipital lobe	C71.4	C79.31	—	D33.Ø	D43.Ø	D49.6
overlapping lesion	C71.8	C79.31	—	—	—	—
parietal lobe	C71.3	C79.31	—	D33.Ø	D43.Ø	D49.6
peduncle	C71.7	C79.31	—	D33.1	D43.1	D49.6
pons	C71.7	C79.31	—	D33.1	D43.1	D49.6
stem	C71.7	C79.31	—	D33.1	D43.1	D49.6
tapetum	C71.8	C79.31	—	D33.2	D43.2	D49.6
temporal lobe	C71.2	C79.31	—	D33.Ø	D43.Ø	D49.6
thalamus	C71.Ø	C79.31	—	D33.Ø	D43.Ø	D49.6
uncus	C71.2	C79.31	—	D33.Ø	D43.Ø	D49.6
ventricle (floor)	C71.5	C79.31	—	D33.Ø	D43.Ø	D49.6
fourth	C71.7	C79.31	—	D33.1	D43.1	D49.6
branchial (cleft) (cyst) (vestiges)	C10.4	C79.89	D00.08	D10.5	D37.05	D49.Ø
breast (connective tissue) (glandular tissue) (soft parts)	C50.9-●	C79.81	D05.-●	D24.-●	D48.6-●	D49.3
areola	C50.Ø-●	C79.81	D05.-●	D24.-●	D48.6-●	D49.3
axillary tail	C50.6-●	C79.81	D05.-●	D24.-●	D48.6-●	D49.3
central portion	C50.1-●	C79.81	D05.-●	D24.-●	D48.6-●	D49.3
inflammatory	C50.A	—	—	—	—	—
inner	C50.8-●	C79.81	D05.-●	D24.-●	D48.6-●	D49.3
lower	C50.8-●	C79.81	D05.-●	D24.-●	D48.6-●	D49.3
lower-inner quadrant	C50.3-●	C79.81	D05.-●	D24.-●	D48.6-●	D49.3
lower-outer quadrant	C50.5-●	C79.81	D05.-●	D24.-●	D48.6-●	D49.3
mastectomy site (skin) — *see also Neoplasm, breast, skin*	C44.5Ø1	C79.2	—	—	—	—
specified as breast tissue	C50.8-●	C79.81	—	—	—	—
midline	C50.8-●	C79.81	D05.-●	D24.-●	D48.6-●	D49.3
nipple	C50.Ø-●	C79.81	D05.-●	D24.-●	D48.6-●	D49.3
outer	C50.8-●	C79.81	D05.-●	D24.-●	D48.6-●	D49.3

	Malignant Primary	Malignant Secondary	Ca in situ	Benign	Uncertain Behavior	Unspecified Behavior
overlapping lesion	C50.8-●	—	—	—	—	—
breast *(Continued)*						
skin	C44.5Ø1	C79.2	D04.5	D23.5	D48.5	D49.2
basal cell carcinoma	C44.511	—	—	—	—	—
specified type NEC	C44.591					
squamous cell carcinoma	C44.521	—	—	—	—	—
tail (axillary)	C50.6-●	C79.81	D05.-●	D24.-●	D48.6-●	D49.3
upper	C50.8-●	C79.81	D05.-●	D24.-●	D48.6-●	D49.3
upper-inner quadrant	C50.2-●	C79.81	D05.-●	D24.-●	D48.6-●	D49.3
upper-outer quadrant	C50.4-●	C79.81	D05.-●	D24.-●	D48.6-●	D49.3
broad ligament	C57.1	C79.82	D07.39	D28.2	D39.8	D49.59
bronchiogenic, bronchogenic (lung)	C34.9-●	C78.Ø-●	D02.2-●	D14.3-●	D38.1	D49.1
bronchiole	C34.9-●	C78.Ø-●	D02.2-●	D14.3-●	D38.1	D49.1
bronchus	C34.9-●	C78.Ø-●	D02.2-●	D14.3-●	D38.1	D49.1
carina	C34.Ø-●	C78.Ø-●	D02.2-●	D14.3-●	D38.1	D49.1
lower lobe of lung	C34.3-●	C78.Ø-●	D02.2-●	D14.3-●	D38.1	D49.1
main	C34.Ø-●	C78.Ø-●	D02.2-●	D14.3-●	D38.1	D49.1
middle lobe of lung	C34.2	C78.Ø-●	D02.21	D14.31	D38.1	D49.1
overlapping lesion	C34.8-●	—	—	—	—	—
upper lobe of lung	C34.1-●	C78.Ø-●	D02.2-●	D14.3-●	D38.1	D49.1
brow	C44.3Ø9	C79.2	D04.39	D23.39	D48.5	D49.2
basal cell carcinoma	C44.319					
specified type NEC	C44.399					
squamous cell carcinoma	C44.329					
buccal (cavity)	C06.9	C79.89	D00.00	D10.39	D37.09	D49.Ø
commissure	C06.Ø	C79.89	D00.02	D10.39	D37.09	D49.Ø
groove (lower) (upper)	C06.1	C79.89	D00.02	D10.39	D37.09	D49.Ø
mucosa	C06.Ø	C79.89	D00.02	D10.39	D37.09	D49.Ø
sulcus (lower) (upper)	C06.1	C79.89	D00.02	D10.39	D37.09	D49.Ø
bulbourethral gland	C68.Ø	C79.19	D09.19	D30.4	D41.3	D49.59
bursa — *see Neoplasm, connective tissue*						
buttock NEC	C76.3	C79.89	D04.5	D36.7	D48.7	D49.89
calf	C76.5-●	C79.89	D04.7-●	D36.7	D48.7	D49.89
calvarium	C41.Ø	C79.51	—	D16.4-●	D48.Ø	D49.2
calyx, renal	C65.-●	C79.Ø-●	D09.19	D30.1-●	D41.1-●	D49.51-●
canal						
anal	C21.1	C78.5	D01.3	D12.9	D37.8	D49.Ø
auditory (external) — *see also Neoplasm, skin, ear*	C44.20-●	C79.2	D04.2-●	D23.2-●	D48.5	D49.2
auricular (external) — *see also Neoplasm, skin, ear*	C44.20-●	C79.2	D04.2-●	D23.2-●	D48.5	D49.2
canaliculi, biliary (biliferi) (intrahepatic)	C22.1	C78.7	D01.5	D13.4	D37.6	D49.Ø

◀ New　　◀ Revised　　~~deleted~~ Deleted　　● Use Additional Character(s)

	Malignant Primary	Malignant Secondary	Ca in situ	Benign	Uncertain Behavior	Unspecified Behavior
canthus (eye) (inner) (outer)	C44.10-●	C79.2	D04.1-●	D23.1-●	D48.5	D49.2
basal cell carcinoma	C44.11-●	—	—	—	—	—
sebaceous cell	C44.13-●	—	—	—	—	—
specified type NEC	C44.19-●	—	—	—	—	—
squamous cell carcinoma	C44.12-●	—	—	—	—	—
capillary — *see Neoplasm, connective tissue*						
caput coli	C18.0	C78.5	D01.0	D12.0	D37.4	D49.0
carcinoid — *see Tumor, carcinoid*						
cardia (gastric)	C16.0	C78.89	D00.2	D13.1	D37.1	D49.0
cardiac orifice (stomach)	C16.0	C78.89	D00.2	D13.1	D37.1	D49.0
cardio-esophageal junction	C16.0	C78.89	D00.2	D13.1	D37.1	D49.0
cardio-esophagus	C16.0	C78.89	D00.2	D13.1	D37.1	D49.0
carina (bronchus)	C34.0-●	C78.0-●	D02.2-●	D14.3-●	D38.1	D49.1
carotid (artery)	C49.0	C79.89	—	D21.0	D48.1-●	D49.2
body	C75.4	C79.89	—	D35.5	D44.6	D49.7
carpus (any bone)	C40.1-●	C79.51	—	D16.1-●	—	—
cartilage (articular) (joint) NEC — *see also Neoplasm, bone*	C41.9	C79.51	—	D16.9-●	D48.0	D49.2
arytenoid	C32.3	C78.39	D02.0	D14.1	D38.0	D49.1
auricular	C49.0	C79.89	—	D21.0	D48.1-●	D49.2
bronchi	C34.0-●	C78.39	—	D14.3-●	D38.1	D49.1
costal	C41.3	C79.51	—	D16.7	D48.0	D49.2
cricoid	C32.3	C78.39	D02.0	D14.1	D38.0	D49.1
cuneiform	C32.3	C78.39	D02.0	D14.1	D38.0	D49.1
ear (external)	C49.0	C79.89	—	D21.0	D48.1-●	D49.2
ensiform	C41.3	C79.51	—	D16.7	D48.0	D49.2
epiglottis	C32.1	C78.39	D02.0	D14.1	D38.0	D49.1
anterior surface	C10.1	C79.89	D00.08	D10.5	D37.05	D49.0
eyelid	C49.0	C79.89	—	D21.0	D48.1-●	D49.2
intervertebral	C41.2	C79.51	—	D16.6	D48.0	D49.2
larynx, laryngeal	C32.3	C78.39	D02.0	D14.1	D38.0	D49.1
nose, nasal	C30.0	C78.39	D02.3	D14.0	D38.5	D49.1
pinna	C49.0	C79.89	—	D21.0	D48.1-●	D49.2
rib	C41.3	C79.51	—	D16.7	D48.0	D49.2
semilunar (knee)	C40.2-●	C79.51	—	D16.2-●	D48.0	D49.2
thyroid	C32.3	C78.39	D02.0	D14.1	D38.0	D49.1
trachea	C33	C78.39	D02.1	D14.2	D38.1	D49.1
cauda equina	C72.1	C79.49	—	D33.4	D43.4	D49.7
cavity						
buccal	C06.9	C79.89	D00.00	D10.30	D37.09	D49.0
nasal	C30.0	C78.39	D02.3	D14.0	D38.5	D49.1
oral	C06.9	C79.89	D00.00	D10.30	D37.09	D49.0

	Malignant Primary	Malignant Secondary	Ca in situ	Benign	Uncertain Behavior	Unspecified Behavior
cavity *(Continued)*						
peritoneal	C48.2	C78.6	—	D20.1	D48.4	D49.0
tympanic	C30.1	C78.39	D02.3	D14.0	D38.5	D49.1
cecum	C18.0	C78.5	D01.0	D12.0	D37.4	D49.0
central nervous system	C72.9	C79.40	—	—	—	—
cerebellopontine (angle)	C71.6	C79.31	—	D33.1	D43.1	D49.6
cerebellum, cerebellar	C71.6	C79.31	—	D33.1	D43.1	D49.6
~~cerebrum, cerebra (cortex) (hemisphere) (white matter)~~	~~C71.0~~	~~C79.31~~	—	~~D33.0~~	~~D43.0~~	~~D49.6~~
~~meninges~~	~~C70.0~~	~~C79.32~~	—	~~D32.0~~	~~D42.0~~	~~D49.7~~
~~peduncle~~	~~C71.7~~	~~C79.31~~	—	~~D33.1~~	~~D43.1~~	~~D49.6~~
~~ventricle~~	~~C71.5~~	~~C79.31~~	—	~~D33.0~~	~~D43.0~~	~~D49.6~~
~~fourth~~	~~C71.7~~	~~C79.31~~	—	~~D33.1~~	~~D43.1~~	~~D49.6~~
cerebrum, cerebral (cortex) (hemisphere) (white matter)	C71.0	C79.31	—	D33.0	D43.0	D49.6
meninges	C70.0	C79.32	—	D32.0	D42.0	D49.7
peduncle	C71.7	C79.31	—	D33.1	D43.1	D49.6
ventricle	C71.5	C79.31	—	D33.0	D43.0	D49.6
fourth	C71.7	C79.31	—	D33.1	D43.1	D49.6
cervical region	C76.0	C79.89	D09.8	D36.7	D48.7	D49.89
cervix (cervical) (uteri) (uterus)	C53.9	C79.82	D06.9	D26.0	D39.0	D49.59
canal	C53.0	C79.82	D06.0	D26.0	D39.0	D49.59
endocervix (canal) (gland)	C53.0	C79.82	D06.0	D26.0	D39.0	D49.59
exocervix	C53.1	C79.82	D06.1	D26.0	D39.0	D49.59
external os	C53.1	C79.82	D06.1	D26.0	D39.0	D49.59
internal os	C53.0	C79.82	D06.0	D26.0	D39.0	D49.59
nabothian gland	C53.0	C79.82	D06.0	D26.0	D39.0	D49.59
overlapping lesion	C53.8	—	—	—	—	—
squamocolumnar junction	C53.8	C79.82	D06.7	D26.0	D39.0	D49.59
stump	C53.8	C79.82	D06.7	D26.0	D39.0	D49.59
cheek	C76.0	C79.89	D09.8	D36.7	D48.7	D49.89
external	C44.309	C79.2	D04.39	D23.39	D48.5	D49.2
basal cell carcinoma	C44.319	—	—	—	—	—
specified type NEC	C44.399	—	—	—	—	—
squamous cell carcinoma	C44.329	—	—	—	—	—
inner aspect	C06.0	C79.89	D00.02	D10.39	D37.09	D49.0
internal	C06.0	C79.89	D00.02	D10.39	D37.09	D49.0
mucosa	C06.0	C79.89	D00.02	D10.39	D37.09	D49.0
chest (wall) NEC	C76.1	C79.89	D09.8	D36.7	D48.7	D49.89
chiasma opticum	C72.3-●	C79.49	—	D33.3	D43.3	D49.7
chin	C44.309	C79.2	D04.39	D23.39	D48.5	D49.2
basal cell carcinoma	C44.319	—	—	—	—	—
specified type NEC	C44.399	—	—	—	—	—
squamous cell carcinoma	C44.329	—	—	—	—	—

	Malignant Primary	Malignant Secondary	Ca in situ	Benign	Uncertain Behavior	Unspecified Behavior
choana	C11.3	C79.89	D00.08	D10.6	D37.05	D49.0
cholangiole	C22.1	C78.89	D01.5	D13.4	D37.6	D49.0
choledochal duct	C24.0	C78.89	D01.5	D13.5	D37.6	D49.0
choroid	C69.3-●	C79.49	D09.2-●	D31.3-●	D48.7	D49.81
plexus	C71.5	C79.31	—	D33.0	D43.0	D49.6
ciliary body	C69.4-●	C79.49	D09.2-●	D31.4-●	D48.7	D49.89
clavicle	C41.3	C79.51	—	D16.7	D48.0	D49.2
clitoris	C51.2	C79.82	D07.1	D28.0	D39.8	D49.59
clivus	C41.0	C79.51	—	D16.4-●	D48.0	D49.2
cloacogenic zone	C21.2	C78.5	D01.3	D12.9	D37.8	D49.0
coccygeal						
body or glomus	C49.5	C79.89	—	D21.5	D48.1-●	D49.2
vertebra	C41.4	C79.51	—	D16.8	D48.0	D49.2
coccyx	C41.4	C79.51	—	D16.8	D48.0	D49.2
colon — *see also Neoplasm, intestine, large*	C18.9	C78.5	—	—	—	—
with rectum	C19	C78.5	D01.1	D12.7	D37.5	D49.0
column, spinal — *see Neoplasm, spine*						
columnella — *see also Neoplasm, skin, face*	C44.390	C79.2	D04.39	D23.39	D48.5	D49.2
commissure						
labial, lip	C00.6	C79.89	D00.01	D10.39	D37.01	D49.0
laryngeal	C32.0	C78.39	D02.0	D14.1	D38.0	D49.1
common (bile) duct	C24.0	C78.89	D01.5	D13.5	D37.6	D49.0
concha — *see also Neoplasm, skin, ear*	C44.20-●	C79.2	D04.2-●	D23.2-●	D48.5	D49.2
nose	C30.0	C78.39	D02.3	D14.0	D38.5	D49.1
conjunctiva	C69.0-●	C79.49	D09.2-●	D31.0-●	D48.7	D49.89
connective tissue NEC	C49.9	C79.89	—	D21.9	D48.1-●	D49.2

Note: For neoplasms of connective tissue (blood vessel, bursa, fascia, ligament, muscle, peripheral nerves, sympathetic and parasympathetic nerves and ganglia, synovia, tendon, etc.) or of morphological types that indicate connective tissue, code according to the list under "Neoplasm, connective tissue." For sites that do not appear in this list, code to neoplasm of that site; e.g., fibrosarcoma, pancreas (C25.9)

Note: Morphological types that indicate connective tissue appear in their proper place in the alphabetic index with the instruction "*see Neoplasm, connective tissue ....*"

	Malignant Primary	Malignant Secondary	Ca in situ	Benign	Uncertain Behavior	Unspecified Behavior
abdomen	C49.4	C79.89	—	D21.4	D48.1-●	D49.2
abdominal wall	C49.4	C79.89	—	D21.4	D48.1-●	D49.2
ankle	C49.2-●	C79.89	—	D21.2-●	D48.1-●	D49.2
antecubital fossa or space	C49.1-●	C79.89	—	D21.1-●	D48.1-●	D49.2
arm	C49.1-●	C79.89	—	D21.1-●	D48.1-●	D49.2
auricle (ear)	C49.0	C79.89	—	D21.0	D48.1-●	D49.2

connective tissue NEC *(Continued)*	Malignant Primary	Malignant Secondary	Ca in situ	Benign	Uncertain Behavior	Unspecified Behavior
axilla	C49.3	C79.89	—	D21.3	D48.1-●	D49.2
back	C49.6	C79.89	—	D21.6	D48.1-●	D49.2
breast — *see Neoplasm, breast*						
buttock	C49.5	C79.89	—	D21.5	D48.1-●	D49.2
calf	C49.2-●	C79.89	—	D21.2-●	D48.1-●	D49.2
cervical region	C49.0	C79.89	—	D21.0	D48.1-●	D49.2
cheek	C49.0	C79.89	—	D21.0	D48.1-●	D49.2
chest (wall)	C49.3	C79.89	—	D21.3	D48.1-●	D49.2
chin	C49.0	C79.89	—	D21.0	D48.1-●	D49.2
diaphragm	C49.3	C79.89	—	D21.3	D48.1-●	D49.2
ear (external)	C49.0	C79.89	—	D21.0	D48.1-●	D49.2
elbow	C49.1-●	C79.89	—	D21.1-●	D48.1-●	D49.2
extrarectal	C49.5	C79.89	—	D21.5	D48.1-●	D49.2
extremity	C49.9	C79.89	—	D21.9	D48.1-●	D49.2
lower	C49.2-●	C79.89	—	D21.2-●	D48.1-●	D49.2
upper	C49.1-●	C79.89	—	D21.1-●	D48.1-●	D49.2
eyelid	C49.0	C79.89	—	D21.0	D48.1-●	D49.2
face	C49.0	C79.89	—	D21.0	D48.1-●	D49.2
finger	C49.1-●	C79.89	—	D21.1-●	D48.1-●	D49.2
flank	C49.6	C79.89	—	D21.6	D48.1-●	D49.2
foot	C49.2-●	C79.89	—	D21.2-●	D48.1-●	D49.2
forearm	C49.1-●	C79.89	—	D21.1-●	D48.1-●	D49.2
forehead	C49.0	C79.89	—	D21.0	D48.1-●	D49.2
gastric	C49.4	C79.89	—	D21.4	D48.1-●	D49.2
gastrointestinal	C49.4	C79.89	—	D21.4	D48.1-●	D49.2
gluteal region	C49.5	C79.89	—	D21.5	D48.1-●	D49.2
great vessels NEC	C49.3	C79.89	—	D21.3	D48.1-●	D49.2
groin	C49.5	C79.89	—	D21.5	D48.1-●	D49.2
hand	C49.1-●	C79.89	—	D21.1-●	D48.1-●	D49.2
head	C49.0	C79.89	—	D21.0	D48.1-●	D49.2
heel	C49.2-●	C79.89	—	D21.2-●	D48.1-●	D49.2
hip	C49.2-●	C79.89	—	D21.2-●	D48.1-●	D49.2
hypochondrium	C49.4	C79.89	—	D21.4	D48.1-●	D49.2
iliopsoas muscle	C49.5	C79.89	—	D21.5	D48.1-●	D49.2
infraclavicular region	C49.3	C79.89	—	D21.3	D48.1-●	D49.2
inguinal (canal) (region)	C49.5	C79.89	—	D21.5	D48.1-●	D49.2
intestinal	C49.4	C79.89	—	D21.4	D48.1-●	D49.2
intrathoracic	C49.3	C79.89	—	D21.3	D48.1-●	D49.2
ischiorectal fossa	C49.5	C79.89	—	D21.5	D48.1-●	D49.2
jaw	C03.9	C79.89	D00.03	D10.39	D48.1-●	D49.0
knee	C49.2-●	C79.89	—	D21.2-●	D48.1-●	D49.2
leg	C49.2-●	C79.89	—	D21.2-●	D48.1-●	D49.2

◀ New   ◀ Revised   ~~deleted~~ Deleted   ● Use Additional Character(s)

	Malignant Primary	Malignant Secondary	Ca in situ	Benign	Uncertain Behavior	Unspecified Behavior
connective tissue NEC *(Continued)*						
limb NEC	C49.9	C79.89	—	D21.9	D48.1-●	D49.2
lower	C49.2-●	C79.89	—	D21.2-●	D48.1-●	D49.2
upper	C49.1-●	C79.89	—	D21.1-●	D48.1-●	D49.2
nates	C49.5	C79.89	—	D21.5	D48.1-●	D49.2
neck	C49.0	C79.89	—	D21.0	D48.1-●	D49.2
orbit	C69.6-●	C79.49	D09.2-●	D31.6-●	D48.1-●	D49.89
overlapping lesion	C49.8	—		—	—	—
pararectal	C49.5	C79.89	—	D21.5	D48.1-●	D49.2
para-urethral	C49.5	C79.89	—	D21.5	D48.1-●	D49.2
paravaginal	C49.5	C79.89	—	D21.5	D48.1-●	D49.2
pelvis (floor)	C49.5	C79.89	—	D21.5	D48.1-●	D49.2
pelvo-abdominal	C49.8	C79.89	—	D21.6	D48.1-●	D49.2
perineum	C49.5	C79.89	—	D21.5	D48.1-●	D49.2
perirectal (tissue)	C49.5	C79.89	—	D21.5	D48.1-●	D49.2
periurethral (tissue)	C49.5	C79.89	—	D21.5	D48.1-●	D49.2
popliteal fossa or space	C49.2-●	C79.89	—	D21.2-●	D48.1-●	D49.2
presacral	C49.5	C79.89	—	D21.5	D48.1-●	D49.2
psoas muscle	C49.4	C79.89	—	D21.4	D48.1-●	D49.2
pterygoid fossa	C49.0	C79.89	—	D21.0	D48.1-●	D49.2
rectovaginal septum or wall	C49.5	C79.89	—	D21.5	D48.1-●	D49.2
rectovesical	C49.5	C79.89	—	D21.5	D48.1-●	D49.2
retroperitoneum	C48.0	C78.6	—	D20.0	D48.3	D49.0
sacrococcygeal region	C49.5	C79.89	—	D21.5	D48.1-●	D49.2
scalp	C49.0	C79.89	—	D21.0	D48.1-●	D49.2
scapular region	C49.3	C79.89	—	D21.3	D48.1-●	D49.2
shoulder	C49.1-●	C79.89	—	D21.1-●	D48.1-●	D49.2
skin (dermis) NEC — *see also Neoplasm, skin, by site*	C44.90	C79.2	D04.9	D23.9	D48.5	D49.2
stomach	C49.4	C79.89	—	D21.4	D48.1-●	D49.2
submental	C49.0	C79.89	—	D21.0	D48.1-●	D49.2
supraclavicular region	C49.0	C79.89	—	D21.0	D48.1-●	D49.2
temple	C49.0	C79.89	—	D21.0	D48.1-●	D49.2
temporal region	C49.0	C79.89	—	D21.0	D48.1-●	D49.2
thigh	C49.2-●	C79.89	—	D21.2-●	D48.1-●	D49.2
thoracic (duct) (wall)	C49.3	C79.89	—	D21.3	D48.1-●	D49.2
thorax	C49.3	C79.89	—	D21.3	D48.1-●	D49.2
thumb	C49.1-●	C79.89	—	D21.1-●	D48.1-●	D49.2
toe	C49.2-●	C79.89	—	D21.2-●	D48.1-●	D49.2
trunk	C49.6	C79.89	—	D21.6	D48.1-●	D49.2
umbilicus	C49.4	C79.89	—	D21.4	D48.1-●	D49.2
vesicorectal	C49.5	C79.89	—	D21.5	D48.1-●	D49.2
wrist	C49.1-●	C79.89	—	D21.1-●	D48.1-●	D49.2

	Malignant Primary	Malignant Secondary	Ca in situ	Benign	Uncertain Behavior	Unspecified Behavior
conus medullaris	C72.0	C79.49	—	D33.4	D43.4	D49.7
cord (true) (vocal)	C32.0	C78.39	D02.0	D14.1	D38.0	D49.1
false	C32.1	C78.39	D02.0	D14.1	D38.0	D49.1
spermatic	C63.1-●	C79.82	D07.69	D29.8	D40.8	D49.59
spinal (cervical) (lumbar) (thoracic)	C72.0	C79.49	—	D33.4	D43.4	D49.7
cornea (limbus)	C69.1-●	C79.49	D09.2-●	D31.1-●	D48.7	D49.89
corpus						
albicans	C56.-●	C79.6-●	D07.39	D27.-●	D39.1-●	D49.59
callosum, brain	C71.0	C79.31	—	D33.2	D43.2	D49.6
cavernosum	C60.2	C79.82	D07.4	D29.0	D40.8	D49.59
gastric	C16.2	C78.89	D00.2	D13.1	D37.1	D49.0
overlapping sites	C54.8	—		—	—	—
penis	C60.2	C79.82	D07.4	D29.0	D40.8	D49.59
striatum, cerebrum	C71.0	C79.31	—	D33.0	D43.0	D49.6
uteri	C54.9	C79.82	D07.0	D26.1	D39.0	D49.59
isthmus	C54.0	C79.82	D07.0	D26.1	D39.0	D49.59
cortex						
adrenal	C74.0-●	C79.7-●	D09.3	D35.0-●	D44.1-●	D49.7
cerebral	C71.0	C79.31	—	D33.0	D43.0	D49.6
costal cartilage	C41.3	C79.51	—	D16.7	D48.0	D49.2
costovertebral joint	C41.3	C79.51	—	D16.7	D48.0	D49.2
Cowper's gland	C68.0	C79.19	D09.19	D30.4	D41.3	D49.59
cranial (fossa, any)	C71.9	C79.31	—	D33.2	D43.2	D49.6
meninges	C70.0	C79.32	—	D32.0	D42.0	D49.7
nerve	C72.50	C79.49	—	D33.3	D43.3	D49.7
specified NEC	C72.59	C79.49	—	D33.3	D43.3	D49.7
craniobuccal pouch	C75.2	C79.89	D09.3	D35.2	D44.3	D49.7
craniopharyngeal (duct) (pouch)	C75.2	C79.89	D09.3	D35.3	D44.4	D49.7
cricoid	C13.0	C79.89	D00.08	D10.7	D37.05	D49.0
cartilage	C32.3	C78.39	D02.0	D14.1	D38.0	D49.1
cricopharynx	C13.0	C79.89	D00.08	D10.7	D37.05	D49.0
crypt of Morgagni	C21.8	C78.5	D01.3	D12.9	D37.8	D49.0
crystalline lens	C69.4-●	C79.49	D09.2-●	D31.4-●	D48.7	D49.89
cul-de-sac (Douglas')	C48.1	C78.6	—	D20.1	D48.4	D49.0
cuneiform cartilage	C32.3	C78.39	D02.0	D14.1	D38.0	D49.1
cutaneous — *see Neoplasm, skin*						
cutis — *see Neoplasm, skin*						
cystic (bile) duct (common)	C24.0	C78.89	D01.5	D13.5	D37.6	D49.0
dermis — *see Neoplasm, skin*						
diaphragm	C49.3	C79.89	—	D21.3	D48.1-●	D49.2
digestive organs, system, tube, or tract NEC	C26.9	C78.89	D01.9	D13.99	D37.9	D49.0

	Malignant Primary	Malignant Secondary	Ca in situ	Benign	Uncertain Behavior	Unspecified Behavior
disc, intervertebral	C41.2	C79.51	—	D16.6	D48.0	D49.2
disease, generalized	C80.0	—	—	—	—	—
disseminated	C80.0	—	—	—	—	—
Douglas' cul-de-sac or pouch	C48.1	C78.6	—	D20.1	D48.4	D49.0
duodenojejunal junction	C17.8	C78.4	D01.49	D13.39	D37.2	D49.0
duodenum	C17.0	C78.4	D01.49	D13.2	D37.2	D49.0
dura (cranial) (mater)	C70.9	C79.49	—	D32.9	D42.9	D49.7
cerebral	C70.0	C79.32	—	D32.0	D42.0	D49.7
spinal	C70.1	C79.49	—	D32.1	D42.1	D49.7
ear (external) — *see also Neoplasm, skin, ear*	C44.20-•	C79.2	D04.2-•	D23.2-•	D48.5	D49.2
auricle or auris — *see also Neoplasm, skin, ear*	C44.20-•	C79.2	D04.2-•	D23.2-•	D48.5	D49.2
canal, external — *see also Neoplasm, skin, ear*	C44.20-•	C79.2	D04.2-•	D23.2-•	D48.5	D49.2
cartilage	C49.0	C79.89	—	D21.0	D48.1-•	D49.2
external meatus — *see also Neoplasm, skin, ear*	C44.20-•	C79.2	D04.2-•	D23.2-•	D48.5	D49.2
inner	C30.1	C78.39	D02.3	D14.0	D38.5	D49.1
lobule — *see also Neoplasm, skin, ear*	C44.20-•	C79.2	D04.2-•	D23.2-•	D48.5	D49.2
middle	C30.1	C78.39	D02.3	D14.0	D38.5	D49.1
overlapping lesion with accessory sinuses	C31.8	—	—	—	—	—
skin	C44.20-•	C79.2	D04.2-•	D23.2-•	D48.5	D49.2
basal cell carcinoma	C44.21-•	—	—	—	—	—
specified type NEC	C44.29-•	—	—	—	—	—
squamous cell carcinoma	C44.22-•	—	—	—	—	—
earlobe	C44.20-•	C79.2	D04.2-•	D23.2-•	D48.5	D49.2
basal cell carcinoma	C44.21-•	—	—	—	—	—
specified type NEC	C44.29-•	—	—	—	—	—
squamous cell carcinoma	C44.22-•	—	—	—	—	—
ejaculatory duct	C63.7	C79.82	D07.69	D29.8	D40.8	D49.59
elbow NEC	C76.4-•	C79.89	D04.6-•	D36.7	D48.7	D49.89
endocardium	C38.0	C79.89	—	D15.1	D48.7	D49.89
endocervix (canal) (gland)	C53.0	C79.82	D06.0	D26.0	D39.0	D49.59
endocrine gland NEC	C75.9	C79.89	D09.3	D35.9	D44.9	D49.7
pluriglandular	C75.8	C79.89	D09.3	D35.7	D44.9	D49.7
endometrium (gland) (stroma)	C54.1	C79.82	D07.0	D26.1	D39.0	D49.59
ensiform cartilage	C41.3	C79.51	—	D16.7	D48.0	D49.2
enteric — *see Neoplasm, intestine*						
ependyma (brain)	C71.5	C79.31	—	D33.0	D43.0	D49.6
fourth ventricle	C71.7	C79.31	—	D33.1	D43.1	D49.6
epicardium	C38.0	C79.89	—	D15.1	D48.7	D49.89

	Malignant Primary	Malignant Secondary	Ca in situ	Benign	Uncertain Behavior	Unspecified Behavior
epididymis	C63.0-•	C79.82	D07.69	D29.3-•	D40.8	D49.59
epidural	C72.9	C79.49	—	D33.9	D43.9	D49.7
epiglottis	C32.1	C78.39	D02.0	D14.1	D38.0	D49.1
anterior aspect or surface	C10.1	C79.89	D00.08	D10.5	D37.05	D49.0
cartilage	C32.3	C78.39	D02.0	D14.1	D38.0	D49.1
free border (margin)	C10.1	C79.89	D00.08	D10.5	D37.05	D49.0
junctional region	C10.8	C79.89	D00.08	D10.5	D37.05	D49.0
posterior (laryngeal) surface	C32.1	C78.39	D02.0	D14.1	D38.0	D49.1
suprahyoid portion	C32.1	C78.39	D02.0	D14.1	D38.0	D49.1
esophagogastric junction	C16.0	C78.89	D00.2	D13.1	D37.1	D49.0
esophagus	C15.9	C78.89	D00.1	D13.0	D37.8	D49.0
abdominal	C15.5	C78.89	D00.1	D13.0	D37.8	D49.0
cervical	C15.3	C78.89	D00.1	D13.0	D37.8	D49.0
distal (third)	C15.5	C78.89	D00.1	D13.0	D37.8	D49.0
lower (third)	C15.5	C78.89	D00.1	D13.0	D37.8	D49.0
middle (third)	C15.4	C78.89	D00.1	D13.0	D37.8	D49.0
overlapping lesion	C15.8	—	—	—	—	—
proximal (third)	C15.3	C78.89	D00.1	D13.0	D37.8	D49.0
thoracic	C15.4	C78.89	D00.1	D13.0	D37.8	D49.0
upper (third)	C15.3	C78.89	D00.1	D13.0	D37.8	D49.0
ethmoid (sinus)	C31.1	C78.39	D02.3	D14.0	D38.5	D49.1
bone or labyrinth	C41.0	C79.51	—	D16.4-•	D48.0	D49.2
eustachian tube	C30.1	C78.39	D02.3	D14.0	D38.5	D49.1
exocervix	C53.1	C79.82	D06.1	D26.0	D39.0	D49.59
external						
meatus (ear) — *see also Neoplasm, skin, ear*	C44.20-•	C79.2	D04.2-•	D23.2-•	D48.5	D49.2
os, cervix uteri	C53.1	C79.82	D06.1	D26.0	D39.0	D49.59
extradural	C72.9	C79.49	—	D33.9	D43.9	D49.7
extrahepatic (bile) duct	C24.0	C78.89	D01.5	D13.5	D37.6	D49.0
overlapping lesion with gallbladder	C24.8	—	—	—	—	—
extraocular muscle	C69.6-•	C79.49	D09.2-•	D31.6-•	D48.7	D49.89
extrarectal	C76.3	C79.89	D09.8	D36.7	D48.7	D49.89
extremity	C76.8	C79.89	D04.8	D36.7	D48.7	D49.89
lower	C76.5-•	C79.89	D04.7-•	D36.7	D48.7	D49.89
upper	C76.4-•	C79.89	D04.6-•	D36.7	D48.7	D49.89
eye NEC	C69.9-•	C79.49	D09.2-•	D31.9-•	D48.7	D49.89
overlapping sites	C69.8-•	—	—	—	—	—
eyeball	C69.9-•	C79.49	D09.2-•	D31.9-•	D48.7	D49.89
eyebrow	C44.309	C79.2	D04.39	D23.39	D48.5	D49.2
basal cell carcinoma	C44.319	—	—	—	—	—
specified type NEC	C44.399	—	—	—	—	—
squamous cell carcinoma	C44.329	—	—	—	—	—

◄ New ◄ Revised ~~deleted~~ Deleted • Use Additional Character(s)

	Malignant Primary	Malignant Secondary	Ca in situ	Benign	Uncertain Behavior	Unspecified Behavior
eyelid (lower) (skin) (upper)	C44.10-●	—	—	—	—	—
basal cell carcinoma	C44.11-●	—	—	—	—	—
cartilage	C49.0	C79.89	—	D21.0	D48.1-●	D49.2
sebaceous cell	C44.13-●	—	—	—	—	—
specified type NEC	C44.19-●	—	—	—	—	—
squamous cell carcinoma	C44.12-●	—	—	—	—	—
face NEC	C76.0	C79.89	D04.39	D36.7	D48.7	D49.89
fallopian tube (accessory)	C57.0-●	C79.82	D07.39	D28.2	D39.8	D49.59
falx (cerebella) (cerebri)	C70.0	C79.32	—	D32.0	D42.0	D49.7
fascia — *see also Neoplasm, connective tissue*						
palmar	C49.1-●	C79.89	—	D21.1-●	D48.1-●	D49.2
plantar	C49.2-●	C79.89	—	D21.2-●	D48.1-●	D49.2
fatty tissue — *see Neoplasm, connective tissue*						
fauces, faucial NEC	C10.9	C79.89	D00.08	D10.5	D37.05	D49.0
pillars	C09.1	C79.89	D00.08	D10.5	D37.05	D49.0
tonsil	C09.9	C79.89	D00.08	D10.4	D37.05	D49.0
femur (any part)	C40.2-●	D48.1-●	—	D16.2-●	—	—
fetal membrane	C58	C79.82	D07.0	D26.7	D39.2	D49.59
fibrous tissue — *see Neoplasm, connective tissue*						
fibula (any part)	C40.2-●	C79.51	—	D16.2-●	—	—
filum terminale	C72.0	C79.49	—	D33.4	D43.4	D49.7
finger NEC	C76.4-●	C79.89	D04.6-●	D36.7	D48.7	D49.89
flank NEC	C76.8	C79.89	D04.5	D36.7	D48.7	D49.89
follicle, nabothian	C53.0	C79.82	D06.0	D26.0	D39.0	D49.59
foot NEC	C76.5-●	C79.89	D04.7-●	D36.7	D48.7	D49.89
forearm NEC	C76.4-●	C79.89	D04.6-●	D36.7	D48.7	D49.89
forehead (skin)	C44.309	C79.2	D04.39	D23.39	D48.5	D49.2
basal cell carcinoma	C44.319	—	—	—	—	—
specified type NEC	C44.399	—	—	—	—	—
squamous cell carcinoma	C44.329	—	—	—	—	—
foreskin	C60.0	C79.82	D07.4	D29.0	D40.8	D49.59
fornix						
pharyngeal	C11.3	C79.89	D00.08	D10.6	D37.05	D49.0
vagina	C52	C79.82	D07.2	D28.1	D39.8	D49.59
fossa (of)						
anterior (cranial)	C71.9	C79.31	—	D33.2	D43.2	D49.6
cranial	C71.9	C79.31	—	D33.2	D43.2	D49.6
ischiorectal	C76.3	C79.89	D09.8	D36.7	D48.7	D49.89
middle (cranial)	C71.9	C79.31	—	D33.2	D43.2	D49.6
piriform	C12	C79.89	D00.08	D10.7	D37.05	D49.0
pituitary	C75.1	C79.89	D09.3	D35.2	D44.3	D49.7
fossa (of) *(Continued)*						
posterior (cranial)	C71.9	C79.31	—	D33.2	D43.2	D49.6
pterygoid	C49.0	C79.89	—	D21.0	D48.1-●	D49.2
pyriform	C12	C79.89	D00.08	D10.7	D37.05	D49.0
Rosenmuller	C11.2	C79.89	D00.08	D10.6	D37.05	D49.0
tonsillar	C09.9	C79.89	D00.08	D10.5	D37.05	D49.0
fourchette	C51.9	C79.82	D07.1	D28.0	D39.8	D49.59
frenulum						
labii — *see Neoplasm, lip, internal*						
linguae	C02.2	C79.89	D00.07	D10.1	D37.02	D49.0
frontal						
bone	C41.0	C79.51	—	D16.4-●	D48.0	D49.2
lobe, brain	C71.1	C79.31	—	D33.0	D43.0	D49.6
pole	C71.1	C79.31	—	D33.0	D43.0	D49.6
sinus	C31.2	C78.39	D02.3	D14.0	D38.5	D49.1
fundus						
stomach	C16.1	C78.89	D00.2	D13.1	D37.1	D49.0
uterus	C54.3	C79.82	D07.0	D26.1	D39.0	D49.59
gall duct (extrahepatic)	C24.0	C78.89	D01.5	D13.5	D37.6	D49.0
intrahepatic	C22.1	C78.7	D01.5	D13.4	D37.6	D49.0
gallbladder	C23	C78.89	D01.5	D13.5	D37.6	D49.0
overlapping lesion with extrahepatic bile ducts	C24.8	—	—	—	—	—
ganglia — *see also Neoplasm, nerve, peripheral*	C47.9	C79.89	—	D36.10	D48.2	D49.2
basal	C71.0	C79.31	—	D33.0	D43.0	D49.6
cranial nerve	C72.50	C79.49	—	D33.3	D43.3	D49.7
Gartner's duct	C52	C79.82	D07.2	D28.1	D39.8	D49.59
gastric — *see Neoplasm, stomach*						
gastrocolic	C26.9	C78.89	D01.9	D13.99	D37.9	D49.0
gastroesophageal junction	C16.0	C78.89	D00.2	D13.1	D37.1	D49.0
gastrointestinal (tract) NEC	C26.9	C78.89	D01.9	D13.99	D37.9	D49.0
generalized	C80.0					
genital organ or tract						
female NEC	C57.9	C79.82	D07.30	D28.9	D39.9	D49.59
overlapping lesion	C57.8	—	—	—	—	—
specified site NEC	C57.7	C79.82	D07.39	D28.7	D39.8	D49.59
male NEC	C63.9	C79.82	D07.60	D29.9	D40.9	D49.59
overlapping lesion	C63.8	—	—	—	—	—
specified site NEC	C63.7	C79.82	D07.69	D29.8	D40.8	D49.59
genitourinary tract						
female	C57.9	C79.82	D07.30	D28.9	D39.9	D49.59
male	C63.9	C79.82	D07.60	D29.9	D40.9	D49.59

TABLE OF NEOPLASMS

	Malignant Primary	Malignant Secondary	Ca in situ	Benign	Uncertain Behavior	Unspecified Behavior
gingiva (alveolar) (marginal)	C03.9	C79.89	D00.03	D10.39	D37.09	D49.0
lower	C03.1	C79.89	D00.03	D10.39	D37.09	D49.0
mandibular	C03.1	C79.89	D00.03	D10.39	D37.09	D49.0
maxillary	C03.0	C79.89	D00.03	D10.39	D37.09	D49.0
upper	C03.0	C79.89	D00.03	D10.39	D37.09	D49.0
gland, glandular (lymphatic) (system) — *see also Neoplasm, lymph gland*						
endocrine NEC	C75.9	C79.89	D09.3	D35.9	D44.9	D49.7
salivary — *see Neoplasm, salivary gland*						
glans penis	C60.1	C79.82	D07.4	D29.0	D40.8	D49.59
globus pallidus	C71.0	C79.31	—	D33.0	D43.0	D49.6
glomus						
coccygeal	C49.5	C79.89	—	D21.5	D48.1-●	D49.2
jugularis	C75.5	C79.89	—	D35.6	D44.7	D49.7
glosso-epiglottic fold(s)	C10.1	C79.89	D00.08	D10.5	D37.05	D49.0
glossopalatine fold	C09.1	C79.89	D00.08	D10.5	D37.05	D49.0
glossopharyngeal sulcus	C09.0	C79.89	D00.08	D10.5	D37.05	D49.0
glottis	C32.0	C78.39	D02.0	D14.1	D38.0	D49.1
gluteal region	C76.3	C79.89	D04.5	D36.7	D48.7	D49.89
great vessels NEC	C49.3	C79.89	—	D21.3	D48.1-●	D49.2
groin NEC	C76.3	C79.89	D04.5	D36.7	D48.7	D49.89
gum	C03.9	C79.89	D00.03	D10.39	D37.09	D49.0
lower	C03.1	C79.89	D00.03	D10.39	D37.09	D49.0
upper	C03.0	C79.89	D00.03	D10.39	D37.09	D49.0
hand NEC	C76.4-●	C79.89	D04.6-●	D36.7	D48.7	D49.89
head NEC	C76.0	C79.89	D04.4	D36.7	D48.7	D49.89
heart	C38.0	C79.89	—	D15.1	D48.7	D49.89
heel NEC	C76.5-●	C79.89	D04.7-●	D36.7	D48.7	D49.89
helix — *see also Neoplasm, skin, ear*	C44.20-●	C79.2	D04.2-●	D23.2-●	D48.5	D49.2
hematopoietic, hemopoietic tissue NEC	C96.9	—	—	—	—	—
specified NEC	C96.Z	—	—	—	—	—
hemisphere, cerebral	C71.0	C79.31	—	D33.0	D43.0	D49.6
hemorrhoidal zone	C21.1	C78.5	D01.3	D12.9	D37.8	D49.0
hepatic — *see also Index to disease, by histology*	C22.9	C78.7	D01.5	D13.4	D37.6	D49.0
duct (bile)	C24.0	C78.89	D01.5	D13.5	D37.6	D49.0
flexure (colon)	C18.3	C78.5	D01.0	D12.3	D37.4	D49.0
primary	C22.8	C78.7	D01.5	D13.4	D37.6	D49.0
hepatobiliary	C24.9	C79.89	D01.5	D13.5	D37.6	D49.0
hepatoblastoma	C22.2	C78.7	D01.5	D13.4	D37.6	D49.0
hepatoma	C22.0	C78.7	D01.5	D13.4	D37.6	D49.0

	Malignant Primary	Malignant Secondary	Ca in situ	Benign	Uncertain Behavior	Unspecified Behavior
hilus of lung	C34.0-●	C78.0-●	D02.2-●	D14.3-●	D38.1	D49.1
hip NEC	C76.5-●	C79.89	D04.7-●	D36.7	D48.7	D49.89
hippocampus, brain	C71.2	C79.31	—	D33.0	D43.0	D49.6
humerus (any part)	C40.0-●	C79.51	—	D16.0-●	—	—
hymen	C52	C79.82	D07.2	D28.1	D39.8	D49.59
hypopharynx, hypopharyngeal NEC	C13.9	C79.89	D00.08	D10.7	D37.05	D49.0
overlapping lesion	C13.8	—	—	—	—	—
postcricoid region	C13.0	C79.89	D00.08	D10.7	D37.05	D49.0
posterior wall	C13.2	C79.89	D00.08	D10.7	D37.05	D49.0
pyriform fossa (sinus)	C12	C79.89	D00.08	D10.7	D37.05	D49.0
hypophysis	C75.1	C79.89	D09.3	D35.2	D44.3	D49.7
hypothalamus	C71.0	C79.31	—	D33.0	D43.0	D49.6
ileocecum, ileocecal (coil) (junction) (valve)	C18.0	C78.5	D01.0	D12.0	D37.4	D49.0
ileum	C17.2	C78.4	D01.49	D13.39	D37.2	D49.0
ilium	C41.4	C79.51	—	D16.8	D48.0	D49.2
immunoproliferative NEC	C88.9	—	—	—	—	—
infraclavicular (region)	C76.1	C79.89	D04.5	D36.7	D48.7	D49.89
inguinal (region)	C76.3	C79.89	D04.5	D36.7	D48.7	D49.89
insula	C71.0	C79.31	—	D33.0	D43.0	D49.6
insular tissue (pancreas)	C25.4	C78.89	D01.7	D13.7	D37.8	D49.0
brain	C71.0	C79.31	—	D33.0	D43.0	D49.6
interarytenoid fold	C13.1	C79.89	D00.08	D10.7	D37.05	D49.0
hypopharyngeal aspect	C13.1	C79.89	D00.08	D10.7	D37.05	D49.0
laryngeal aspect	C32.1	C78.39	D02.0	D14.1	D38.0	D49.1
marginal zone	C13.1	C79.89	D00.08	D10.7	D37.05	D49.0
interdental papillae	C03.9	C79.89	D00.03	D10.39	D37.09	D49.0
lower	C03.1	C79.89	D00.03	D10.39	D37.09	D49.0
upper	C03.0	C79.89	D00.03	D10.39	D37.09	D49.0
internal						
capsule	C71.0	C79.31	—	D33.0	D43.0	D49.6
os (cervix)	C53.0	C79.82	D06.0	D26.0	D39.0	D49.59
intervertebral cartilage or disc	C41.2	C79.51	—	D16.6	D48.0	D49.2
intestine, intestinal	C26.0	C78.80	D01.40	D13.99	D37.8	D49.0
large	C18.9	C78.5	D01.0	D12.6	D37.4	D49.0
appendix	C18.1	C78.5	D01.0	D12.1	D37.3	D49.0
caput coli	C18.0	C78.5	D01.0	D12.0	D37.4	D49.0
cecum	C18.0	C78.5	D01.0	D12.0	D37.4	D49.0
colon	C18.9	C78.5	D01.0	D12.6	D37.4	D49.0
and rectum	C19	C78.5	D01.1	D12.7	D37.5	D49.0
ascending	C18.2	C78.5	D01.0	D12.2	D37.4	D49.0
caput	C18.0	C78.5	D01.0	D12.0	D37.4	D49.0
descending	C18.6	C78.5	D01.0	D12.4	D37.4	D49.0

◄ New   ⬅ Revised   ~~deleted~~ Deleted   ● Use Additional Character(s)

	Malignant Primary	Malignant Secondary	Ca in situ	Benign	Uncertain Behavior	Unspecified Behavior
intestine, intestinal *(Continued)*						
large *(Continued)*						
colon *(Continued)*						
distal	C18.6	C78.5	D01.0	D12.4	D37.4	D49.0
left	C18.6	C78.5	D01.0	D12.4	D37.4	D49.0
overlapping lesion	C18.8	—	—	—	—	—
pelvic	C18.7	C78.5	D01.0	D12.5	D37.4	D49.0
right	C18.2	C78.5	D01.0	D12.2	D37.4	D49.0
sigmoid (flexure)	C18.7	C78.5	D01.0	D12.5	D37.4	D49.0
transverse	C18.4	C78.5	D01.0	D12.3	D37.4	D49.0
hepatic flexure	C18.3	C78.5	D01.0	D12.3	D37.4	D49.0
ileocecum, ileocecal (coil) (valve)	C18.0	C78.5	D01.0	D12.0	D37.4	D49.0
overlapping lesion	C18.8	—	—	—	—	—
sigmoid flexure (lower) (upper)	C18.7	C78.5	D01.0	D12.5	D37.4	D49.0
splenic flexure	C18.5	C78.5	D01.0	D12.3	D37.4	D49.0
small	C17.9	C78.4	D01.40	D13.30	D37.2	D49.0
duodenum	C17.0	C78.4	D01.49	D13.2	D37.2	D49.0
ileum	C17.2	C78.4	D01.49	D13.39	D37.2	D49.0
jejunum	C17.1	C78.4	D01.49	D13.39	D37.2	D49.0
overlapping lesion	C17.8	—	—	—	—	—
tract NEC	C26.0	C78.89	D01.40	D13.99	D37.8	D49.0
intra-abdominal	C76.2	C79.89	D09.8	D36.7	D48.7	D49.89
intracranial NEC	C71.9	C79.31	—	D33.2	D43.2	D49.6
intrahepatic (bile) duct	C22.1	C78.7	D01.5	D13.4	D37.6	D49.0
intraocular	C69.9-●	C79.49	D09.2-●	D31.9-●	D48.7	D49.89
intraorbital	C69.6-●	C79.49	D09.2-●	D31.6-●	D48.7	D49.89
intrasellar	C75.1	C79.89	D09.3	D35.2	D44.3	D49.7
intrathoracic (cavity) (organs)	C76.1	C79.89	D09.8	D15.9	D48.7	D49.89
specified NEC	C76.1	C79.89	D09.8	D15.7	—	—
iris	C69.4-●	C79.49	D09.2-●	D31.4-●	D48.7	D49.89
ischiorectal (fossa)	C76.3	C79.89	D09.8	D36.7	D48.7	D49.89
ischium	C41.4	C79.51	—	D16.8	D48.0	D49.2
island of Reil	C71.0	C79.31	—	D33.0	D43.0	D49.6
islands or islets of Langerhans	C25.4	C78.89	D01.7	D13.7	D37.8	D49.0
isthmus uteri	C54.0	C79.82	D07.0	D26.1	D39.0	D49.59
jaw	C76.0	C79.89	D09.8	D36.7	D48.7	D49.89
bone	C41.1	C79.51	—	D16.5-●	D48.0	D49.2
lower	C41.1	C79.51	—	D16.5-●		
upper	C41.0	C79.51	—	D16.4-●	—	—
carcinoma (any type) (lower) (upper)	C76.0	C79.89				
skin — *see also* Neoplasm, skin, face	C44.309	C79.2	D04.39	D23.39	D48.5	D49.2

	Malignant Primary	Malignant Secondary	Ca in situ	Benign	Uncertain Behavior	Unspecified Behavior
jaw *(Continued)*						
soft tissues	C03.9	C79.89	D00.03	D10.39	D37.09	D49.0
lower	C03.1	C79.89	D00.03	D10.39	D37.09	D49.0
upper	C03.0	C79.89	D00.03	D10.39	D37.09	D49.0
jejunum	C17.1	C78.4	D01.49	D13.39	D37.2	D49.0
joint NEC — *see also* Neoplasm, bone	C41.9	C79.51	—	D16.9-●	D48.0	D49.2
acromioclavicular	C40.0-●	C79.51	—	D16.0-●	—	—
bursa or synovial membrane — *see* Neoplasm, connective tissue						
costovertebral	C41.3	C79.51	—	D16.7	D48.0	D49.2
sternocostal	C41.3	C79.51	—	D16.7	D48.0	D49.2
temporomandibular	C41.1	C79.51	—	D16.5-●	D48.0	D49.2
junction						
anorectal	C21.8	C78.5	D01.3	D12.9	D37.8	D49.0
cardioesophageal	C16.0	C78.89	D00.2	D13.1	D37.1	D49.0
esophagogastric	C16.0	C78.89	D00.2	D13.1	D37.1	D49.0
gastroesophageal	C16.0	C78.89	D00.2	D13.1	D37.1	D49.0
hard and soft palate	C05.9	C79.89	D00.00	D10.39	D37.09	D49.0
ileocecal	C18.0	C78.5	D01.0	D12.0	D37.4	D49.0
pelvirectal	C19	C78.5	D01.1	D12.7	D37.5	D49.0
pelviureteric	C65.-●	C79.0-●	D09.19	D30.1-●	D41.1-●	D49.59
rectosigmoid	C19	C78.5	D01.1	D12.7	D37.5	D49.0
squamocolumnar, of cervix	C53.8	C79.82	D06.7	D26.0	D39.0	D49.59
Kaposi's sarcoma — *see* Kaposi's, sarcoma						
kidney (parenchymal)	C64.-●	C79.0-●	D09.19	D30.0-●	D41.0-●	D49.51-●
calyx	C65.-●	C79.0-●	D09.19	D30.1-●	D41.1-●	D49.51-●
hilus	C65.-●	C79.0-●	D09.19	D30.1-●	D41.1-●	D49.51-●
pelvis	C65.-●	C79.0-●	D09.19	D30.1-●	D41.1-●	D49.51-●
knee NEC	C76.5-●	C79.89	D04.7-●	D36.7	D48.7	D49.89
labia (skin)	C51.9	C79.82	D07.1	D28.0	D39.8	D49.59
majora	C51.0	C79.82	D07.1	D28.0	D39.8	D49.59
minora	C51.1	C79.82	D07.1	D28.0	D39.8	D49.59
labial — *see also* Neoplasm, lip	C00.9	C79.89	D00.01	D10.0	D37.01	D49.0
sulcus (lower) (upper)	C06.1	C79.89	D00.02	D10.39	D37.09	D49.0
labium (skin)	C51.9	C79.82	D07.1	D28.0	D39.8	D49.59
majus	C51.0	C79.82	D07.1	D28.0	D39.8	D49.59
minus	C51.1	C79.82	D07.1	D28.0	D39.8	D49.59
lacrimal						
canaliculi	C69.5-●	C79.49	D09.2-●	D31.5-●	D48.7	D49.89
duct (nasal)	C69.5-●	C79.49	D09.2-●	D31.5-●	D48.7	D49.89
gland	C69.5-●	C79.49	D09.2-●	D31.5-●	D48.7	D49.89

	Malignant Primary	Malignant Secondary	Ca in situ	Benign	Uncertain Behavior	Unspecified Behavior
lacrimal (*Continued*)						
punctum	C69.5-•	C79.49	D09.2-•	D31.5-•	D48.7	D49.89
sac	C69.5-•	C79.49	D09.2-•	D31.5-•	D48.7	D49.89
Langerhans, islands or islets	C25.4	C78.89	D01.7	D13.7	D37.8	D49.0
laryngopharynx	C13.9	C79.89	D00.08	D10.7	D37.05	D49.0
larynx, laryngeal NEC	C32.9	C78.39	D02.0	D14.1	D38.0	D49.1
aryepiglottic fold	C32.1	C78.39	D02.0	D14.1	D38.0	D49.1
cartilage (arytenoid) (cricoid) (cuneiform) (thyroid)	C32.3	C78.39	D02.0	D14.1	D38.0	D49.1
commissure (anterior) (posterior)	C32.0	C78.39	D02.0	D14.1	D38.0	D49.1
extrinsic NEC	C32.1	C78.39	D02.0	D14.1	D38.0	D49.1
meaning hypopharynx	C13.9	C79.89	D00.08	D10.7	D37.05	D49.0
interarytenoid fold	C32.1	C78.39	D02.0	D14.1	D38.0	D49.1
intrinsic	C32.0	C78.39	D02.0	D14.1	D38.0	D49.1
overlapping lesion	C32.8	—	—	—	—	—
ventricular band	C32.1	C78.39	D02.0	D14.1	D38.0	D49.1
leg NEC	C76.5-•	C79.89	D04.7-•	D36.7	D48.7	D49.89
lens, crystalline	C69.4-•	C79.49	D09.2-•	D31.4-•	D48.7	D49.89
lid (lower) (upper)	C44.10-•	C79.2	D04.1-•	D23.1-•	D48.5	D49.2
basal cell carcinoma	C44.11-•	—	—	—	—	—
sebaceous cell	C44.13-•	—	—	—	—	—
specified type NEC	C44.19-•	—	—	—	—	—
squamous cell carcinoma	C44.12-•	—	—	—	—	—
ligament — *see also Neoplasm, connective tissue*						
broad	C57.1-•	C79.82	D07.39	D28.2	D39.8	D49.59
Mackenrodt's	C57.7	C79.82	D07.39	D28.7	D39.8	D49.59
non-uterine — *see Neoplasm, connective tissue*						
round	C57.2	C79.82	—	D28.2	D39.8	D49.59
sacro-uterine	C57.3	C79.82	—	D28.2	D39.8	D49.59
uterine	C57.3	C79.82	—	D28.2	D39.8	D49.59
utero-ovarian	C57.7	C79.82	D07.39	D28.2	D39.8	D49.59
uterosacral	C57.3	C79.82	—	D28.2	D39.8	D49.59
limb	C76.8	C79.89	D04.8	D36.7	D48.7	D49.89
lower	C76.5-•	C79.89	D04.7-•	D36.7	D48.7	D49.89
upper	C76.4-•	C79.89	D04.6-•	D36.7	D48.7	D49.89
limbus of cornea	C69.1-•	C79.49	D09.2-•	D31.1-•	D48.7	D49.89
lingual NEC — *see also Neoplasm, tongue*	C02.9	C79.89	D00.07	D10.1	D37.02	D49.0
lingula, lung	C34.1-•	C78.0-•	D02.2-•	D14.3-•	D38.1	D49.1
lip	C00.9	C79.89	D00.01	D10.0	D37.01	D49.0
buccal aspect — *see Neoplasm, lip, internal*						
commissure	C00.6	C79.89	D00.01	D10.0	D37.01	D49.0

	Malignant Primary	Malignant Secondary	Ca in situ	Benign	Uncertain Behavior	Unspecified Behavior
lip (*Continued*)						
external	C00.2	C79.89	D00.01	D10.0	D37.01	D49.0
lower	C00.1	C79.89	D00.01	D10.0	D37.01	D49.0
upper	C00.0	C79.89	D00.01	D10.0	D37.01	D49.0
frenulum — *see Neoplasm, lip, internal*						
inner aspect — *see Neoplasm, lip, internal*						
internal	C00.5	C79.89	D00.01	D10.0	D37.01	D49.0
lower	C00.4	C79.89	D00.01	D10.0	D37.01	D49.0
upper	C00.3	C79.89	D00.01	D10.0	D37.01	D49.0
lipstick area	C00.2	C79.89	D00.01	D10.0	D37.01	D49.0
lower	C00.1	C79.89	D00.01	D10.0	D37.01	D49.0
upper	C00.0	C79.89	D00.01	D10.0	D37.01	D49.0
lower	C00.1	C79.89	D00.01	D10.0	D37.01	D49.0
internal	C00.4	C79.89	D00.01	D10.0	D37.01	D49.0
mucosa — *see Neoplasm, lip, internal*						
oral aspect — *see Neoplasm, lip, internal*						
overlapping lesion	C00.8	—	—	—	—	—
with oral cavity or pharynx	C14.8	—	—	—	—	—
skin (commissure) (lower) (upper)	C44.00	C79.2	D04.0	D23.0	D48.5	D49.2
basal cell carcinoma	C44.01	—	—	—	—	—
specified type NEC	C44.09	—	—	—	—	—
squamous cell carcinoma	C44.02	—	—	—	—	—
upper	C00.0	C79.89	D00.01	D10.0	D37.01	D49.0
internal	C00.3	C79.89	D00.01	D10.0	D37.01	D49.0
vermilion border	C00.2	C79.89	D00.01	D10.0	D37.01	D49.0
lower	C00.1	C79.89	D00.01	D10.0	D37.01	D49.0
upper	C00.0	C79.89	D00.01	D10.0	D37.01	D49.0
lipomatous — *see Lipoma, by site*						
liver — *see also Index to disease, by histology*	C22.9	C78.7	D01.5	D13.4	D37.6	D49.0
primary	C22.8	C78.7	D01.5	D13.4	D37.6	D49.0
lumbosacral plexus	C47.5	C79.89	—	D36.16	D48.2	D49.2
lung	C34.9-•	C78.0-•	D02.2-•	D14.3-•	D38.1	D49.1
azygos lobe	C34.1-•	C78.0-•	D02.2-•	D14.3-•	D38.1	D49.1
carina	C34.0-•	C78.0-•	D02.2-•	D14.3-•	D38.1	D49.1
hilus	C34.0-•	C78.0-•	D02.2-•	D14.3-•	D38.1	D49.1
lingula	C34.1-•	C78.0-•	D02.2-•	D14.3-•	D38.1	D49.1
lobe NEC	C34.9-•	C78.0-•	D02.2-•	D14.3-•	D38.1	D49.1
lower lobe	C34.3-•	C78.0-•	D02.2-•	D14.3-•	D38.1	D49.1
main bronchus	C34.0-•	C78.0-•	D02.2-•	D14.3-•	D38.1	D49.1

◄ New   ◄ Revised   ~~deleted~~ Deleted   • Use Additional Character(s)

	Malignant Primary	Malignant Secondary	Ca in situ	Benign	Uncertain Behavior	Unspecified Behavior
lung *(Continued)*						
mesothelioma — *see* Mesothelioma						
middle lobe	C34.2	C78.0-●	D02.21	D14.31	D38.1	D49.1
overlapping lesion	C34.8-●	—	—	—	—	—
upper lobe	C34.1-●	C78.0-●	D02.2-●	D14.3-●	D38.1	D49.1
lymph, lymphatic channel NEC	C49.9	C79.89	—	D21.9	D48.1-●	D49.2
gland (secondary)	—	C77.9	—	D36.0	D48.7	D49.89
abdominal	—	C77.2	—	D36.0	D48.7	D49.89
aortic	—	C77.2	—	D36.0	D48.7	D49.89
arm	—	C77.3	—	D36.0	D48.7	D49.89
auricular (anterior) (posterior)	—	C77.0	—	D36.0	D48.7	D49.89
axilla, axillary	—	C77.3	—	D36.0	D48.7	D49.89
brachial	—	C77.3	—	D36.0	D48.7	D49.89
bronchial	—	C77.1	—	D36.0	D48.7	D49.89
bronchopulmonary	—	C77.1	—	D36.0	D48.7	D49.89
celiac	—	C77.2	—	D36.0	D48.7	D49.89
cervical	—	C77.0	—	D36.0	D48.7	D49.89
cervicofacial	—	C77.0	—	D36.0	D48.7	D49.89
Cloquet	—	C77.4	—	D36.0	D48.7	D49.89
colic	—	C77.2	—	D36.0	D48.7	D49.89
common duct	—	C77.2	—	D36.0	D48.7	D49.89
cubital	—	C77.3	—	D36.0	D48.7	D49.89
diaphragmatic	—	C77.1	—	D36.0	D48.7	D49.89
epigastric, inferior	—	C77.1	—	D36.0	D48.7	D49.89
epitrochlear	—	C77.3	—	D36.0	D48.7	D49.89
esophageal	—	C77.1	—	D36.0	D48.7	D49.89
face	—	C77.0	—	D36.0	D48.7	D49.89
femoral	—	C77.4	—	D36.0	D48.7	D49.89
gastric	—	C77.2	—	D36.0	D48.7	D49.89
groin	—	C77.4	—	D36.0	D48.7	D49.89
head	—	C77.0	—	D36.0	D48.7	D49.89
hepatic	—	C77.2	—	D36.0	D48.7	D49.89
hilar (pulmonary)	—	C77.1	—	D36.0	D48.7	D49.89
splenic	—	C77.2	—	D36.0	D48.7	D49.89
hypogastric	—	C77.5	—	D36.0	D48.7	D49.89
ileocolic	—	C77.2	—	D36.0	D48.7	D49.89
iliac	—	C77.5	—	D36.0	D48.7	D49.89
infraclavicular	—	C77.3	—	D36.0	D48.7	D49.89
inguina, inguinal	—	C77.4	—	D36.0	D48.7	D49.89
innominate	—	C77.1	—	D36.0	D48.7	D49.89
intercostal	—	C77.1	—	D36.0	D48.7	D49.89
intestinal	—	C77.2	—	D36.0	D48.7	D49.89
intrabdominal	—	C77.2	—	D36.0	D48.7	D49.89
intrapelvic	—	C77.5	—	D36.0	D48.7	D49.89

	Malignant Primary	Malignant Secondary	Ca in situ	Benign	Uncertain Behavior	Unspecified Behavior
lymph, lymphatic channel NEC *(Continued)*						
gland *(Continued)*						
intrathoracic	—	C77.1	—	D36.0	D48.7	D49.89
jugular	—	C77.0	—	D36.0	D48.7	D49.89
leg	—	C77.4	—	D36.0	D48.7	D49.89
limb						
lower	—	C77.4	—	D36.0	D48.7	D49.89
upper	—	C77.3	—	D36.0	D48.7	D49.89
lower limb	—	C77.4	—	D36.0	D48.7	D49.89
lumbar	—	C77.2	—	D36.0	D48.7	D49.89
mandibular	—	C77.0	—	D36.0	D48.7	D49.89
mediastinal	—	C77.1	—	D36.0	D48.7	D49.89
mesenteric (inferior) (superior)	—	C77.2	—	D36.0	D48.7	D49.89
midcolic	—	C77.2	—	D36.0	D48.7	D49.89
multiple sites in categories C77.0 - C77.5	—	C77.8	—	D36.0	D48.7	D49.89
neck	—	C77.0	—	D36.0	D48.7	D49.89
obturator	—	C77.5	—	D36.0	D48.7	D49.89
occipital	—	C77.0	—	D36.0	D48.7	D49.89
pancreatic	—	C77.2	—	D36.0	D48.7	D49.89
para-aortic	—	C77.2	—	D36.0	D48.7	D49.89
paracervical	—	C77.5	—	D36.0	D48.7	D49.89
parametrial	—	C77.5	—	D36.0	D48.7	D49.89
parasternal	—	C77.1	—	D36.0	D48.7	D49.89
parotid	—	C77.0	—	D36.0	D48.7	D49.89
pectoral	—	C77.3	—	D36.0	D48.7	D49.89
pelvic	—	C77.5	—	D36.0	D48.7	D49.89
peri-aortic	—	C77.2	—	D36.0	D48.7	D49.89
peripancreatic	—	C77.2	—	D36.0	D48.7	D49.89
popliteal	—	C77.4	—	D36.0	D48.7	D49.89
porta hepatis	—	C77.2	—	D36.0	D48.7	D49.89
portal	—	C77.2	—	D36.0	D48.7	D49.89
preauricular	—	C77.0	—	D36.0	D48.7	D49.89
prelaryngeal	—	C77.0	—	D36.0	D48.7	D49.89
presymphysial	—	C77.5	—	D36.0	D48.7	D49.89
pretracheal	—	C77.0	—	D36.0	D48.7	D49.89
primary (any site) NEC	C96.9	—	—	—	—	—
pulmonary (hiler)	—	C77.1	—	D36.0	D48.7	D49.89
pyloric	—	C77.2	—	D36.0	D48.7	D49.89
retroperitoneal	—	C77.2	—	D36.0	D48.7	D49.89
retropharyngeal	—	C77.0	—	D36.0	D48.7	D49.89
Rosenmuller's	—	C77.4	—	D36.0	D48.7	D49.89
sacral	—	C77.5	—	D36.0	D48.7	D49.89

TABLE OF NEOPLASMS

	Malignant Primary	Malignant Secondary	Ca in situ	Benign	Uncertain Behavior	Unspecified Behavior
lymph, lymphatic channel NEC *(Continued)*						
gland *(Continued)*						
scalene	—	C77.0	—	D36.0	D48.7	D49.89
site NEC	—	C77.9	—	D36.0	D48.7	D49.89
splenic (hilar)	—	C77.2	—	D36.0	D48.7	D49.89
subclavicular	—	C77.3	—	D36.0	D48.7	D49.89
subinguinal	—	C77.4	—	D36.0	D48.7	D49.89
sublingual	—	C77.0	—	D36.0	D48.7	D49.89
submandibular	—	C77.0	—	D36.0	D48.7	D49.89
submaxillary	—	C77.0	—	D36.0	D48.7	D49.89
submental	—	C77.0	—	D36.0	D48.7	D49.89
subscapular	—	C77.3	—	D36.0	D48.7	D49.89
supraclavicular	—	C77.0	—	D36.0	D48.7	D49.89
thoracic	—	C77.1	—	D36.0	D48.7	D49.89
tibial	—	C77.4	—	D36.0	D48.7	D49.89
tracheal	—	C77.1	—	D36.0	D48.7	D49.89
tracheobronchial	—	C77.1	—	D36.0	D48.7	D49.89
upper limb	—	C77.3	—	D36.0	D48.7	D49.89
Virchow's	—	C77.0	—	D36.0	D48.7	D49.89
node — *see also Neoplasm, lymph gland*						
primary NEC	C96.9	—	—	—	—	—
vessel — *see also Neoplasm, connective tissue*	C49.9	C79.89	—	D21.9	D48.1-●	D49.2
Mackenrodt's ligament	C57.7	C79.82	D07.39	D28.7	D39.8	D49.59
malar	C41.0	C79.51	—	D16.4-●	D48.0	D49.2
region — *see Neoplasm, cheek*						
mammary gland — *see Neoplasm, breast*						
mandible	C41.1	C79.51	—	D16.5-●	D48.0	D49.2
alveolar						
mucosa (carcinoma)	C03.1	C79.89	D00.03	D10.39	D37.09	D49.0
ridge or process	C41.1	C79.51	—	D16.5-●	D48.0	D49.2
marrow (bone) NEC	C96.9	C79.52	—	—	D47.9	D49.89
mastectomy site (skin) — *see also Neoplasm, breast, skin*	C44.501	C79.2	—	—	—	—
specified as breast tissue	C50.8-●	C79.81	—	—	—	—
mastoid (air cells) (antrum) (cavity)	C30.1	C78.39	D02.3	D14.0	D38.5	D49.1
bone or process	C41.0	C79.51	—	D16.4-●	D48.0	D49.2
maxilla, maxillary (superior)	C41.0	C79.51	—	D16.4-●	D48.0	D49.2
alveolar						
mucosa	C03.0	C79.89	D00.03	D10.39	D37.09	D49.0
ridge or process (carcinoma)	C41.0	C79.51	—	D16.4-●	D48.0	D49.2
antrum	C31.0	C78.39	D02.3	D14.0	D38.5	D49.1

	Malignant Primary	Malignant Secondary	Ca in situ	Benign	Uncertain Behavior	Unspecified Behavior
maxilla, maxillary *(Continued)*						
carcinoma	C03.0	C79.51	—	—	—	—
inferior — *see Neoplasm, mandible*						
sinus	C31.0	C78.39	D02.3	D14.0	D38.5	D49.1
meatus external (ear) — *see also Neoplasm, skin, ear*	C44.20-●	C79.2	D04.2-●	D23.2-●	D48.5	D49.2
Meckel diverticulum, malignant	C17.3	C78.4	D01.49	D13.39	D37.2	D49.0
mediastinum, mediastinal	C38.3	C78.1	—	D15.2	D38.3	D49.89
anterior	C38.1	C78.1	—	D15.2	D38.3	D49.89
posterior	C38.2	C78.1	—	D15.2	D38.3	D49.89
medulla						
adrenal	C74.1-●	C79.7-●	D09.3	D35.0-●	D44.1-●	D49.7
oblongata	C71.7	C79.31	—	D33.1	D43.1	D49.6
meibomian gland	C44.10-●	C79.2	D04.1-●	D23.1-●	D48.5	D49.2
basal cell carcinoma	C44.11-●	—	—	—	—	—
sebaceous cell	C44.13-●	—	—	—	—	—
specified type NEC	C44.19-●	—	—	—	—	—
squamous cell carcinoma	C44.12-●	—	—	—	—	—
melanoma — *see Melanoma*						
meninges	C70.9	C79.49	—	D32.9	D42.9	D49.7
brain	C70.0	C79.32	—	D32.0	D42.0	D49.7
cerebral	C70.0	C79.32	—	D32.0	D42.0	D49.7
cranial	C70.0	C79.32	—	D32.0	D42.0	D49.7
intracranial	C70.0	C79.32	—	D32.0	D42.0	D49.7
spinal (cord)	C70.1	C79.49	—	D32.1	D42.1	D49.7
meniscus, knee joint (lateral) (medial)	C40.2-●	C79.51	—	D16.2-●	D48.0	D49.2
Merkel cell — *see Carcinoma, Merkel cell*						
mesentery, mesenteric	C48.1	C78.6	—	D20.1	D48.4	D49.0
mesoappendix	C48.1	C78.6	—	D20.1	D48.4	D49.0
mesocolon	C48.1	C78.6	—	D20.1	D48.4	D49.0
mesopharynx — *see Neoplasm, oropharynx*						
mesosalpinx	C57.1	C79.82	D07.39	D28.2	D39.8	D49.59
mesothelial tissue — *see Mesothelioma*						
mesothelioma — *see Mesothelioma*						
mesovarium	C57.1	C79.82	D07.39	D28.2	D39.8	D49.59
metacarpus (any bone)	C40.1-●	C79.51	—	D16.1-●	—	—
metastatic NEC — *see also Neoplasm, by site, secondary*	—	C79.9	—	—	—	—
metatarsus (any bone)	C40.3-●	C79.51	—	D16.3-●	—	—
midbrain	C71.7	C79.31	—	D33.1	D43.1	D49.6

◀ New　◀ Revised　~~deleted~~ Deleted　● Use Additional Character(s)

	Malignant Primary	Malignant Secondary	Ca in situ	Benign	Uncertain Behavior	Unspecified Behavior
milk duct — *see Neoplasm, breast*						
mons						
pubis	C51.9	C79.82	D07.1	D28.0	D39.8	D49.59
veneris	C51.9	C79.82	D07.1	D28.0	D39.8	D49.59
motor tract	C72.9	C79.49	—	D33.9	D43.9	D49.7
brain	C71.9	C79.31	—	D33.2	D43.2	D49.6
cauda equina	C72.1	C79.49	—	D33.4	D43.4	D49.7
spinal	C72.0	C79.49	—	D33.4	D43.4	D49.7
mouth	C06.9	C79.89	D00.00	D10.30	D37.09	D49.0
book-leaf	C06.89	C79.89	—	—	—	—
floor	C04.9	C79.89	D00.06	D10.2	D37.09	D49.0
anterior portion	C04.0	C79.89	D00.06	D10.2	D37.09	D49.0
lateral portion	C04.1	C79.89	D00.06	D10.2	D37.09	D49.0
overlapping lesion	C04.8	—	—	—	—	—
overlapping NEC	C06.80	—	—	—	—	—
roof	C05.9	C79.89	D00.00	D10.39	D37.09	D49.0
specified part NEC	C06.89	C79.89	D00.00	D10.39	D37.09	D49.0
vestibule	C06.1	C79.89	D00.00	D10.39	D37.09	D49.0
mucosa						
alveolar (ridge or process)	C03.9	C79.89	D00.03	D10.39	D37.09	D49.0
lower	C03.1	C79.89	D00.03	D10.39	D37.09	D49.0
upper	C03.0	C79.89	D00.03	D10.39	D37.09	D49.0
buccal	C06.0	C79.89	D00.02	D10.39	D37.09	D49.0
cheek	C06.0	C79.89	D00.02	D10.39	D37.09	D49.0
lip — *see Neoplasm, lip, internal*						
nasal	C30.0	C78.39	D02.3	D14.0	D38.5	D49.1
oral	C06.0	C79.89	D00.02	D10.39	D37.09	D49.0
Mullerian duct						
female	C57.7	C79.82	D07.39	D28.7	D39.8	D49.59
male	C63.7	C79.82	D07.69	D29.8	D40.8	D49.59
muscle — *see also Neoplasm, connective tissue*						
extraocular	C69.6-●	C79.49	D09.2-●	D31.6-●	D48.7	D49.89
myocardium	C38.0	C79.89	—	D15.1	D48.7	D49.89
myometrium	C54.2	C79.82	D07.0	D26.1	D39.0	D49.59
myopericardium	C38.0	C79.89	—	D15.1	D48.7	D49.89
nabothian gland (follicle)	C53.0	C79.82	D06.0	D26.0	D39.0	D49.59
nail — *see also Neoplasm, skin, limb*	C44.90	C79.2	D04.9	D23.9	D48.5	D49.2
finger — *see also Neoplasm, skin, limb, upper*	C44.60-●	C79.2	D04.6-●	D23.6-●	D48.5	D49.2
toe — *see also Neoplasm, skin, limb, lower*	C44.70-●	C79.2	D04.7-●	D23.7-●	D48.5	D49.2
nares, naris (anterior) (posterior)	C30.0	C78.39	D02.3	D14.0	D38.5	D49.1
nasal — *see Neoplasm, nose*						

	Malignant Primary	Malignant Secondary	Ca in situ	Benign	Uncertain Behavior	Unspecified Behavior
nasolabial groove — *see also Neoplasm, skin, face*	C44.309	C79.2	D04.39	D23.39	D48.5	D49.2
nasolacrimal duct	C69.5-●	C79.49	D09.2-●	D31.5-●	D48.7	D49.89
nasopharynx, nasopharyngeal	C11.9	C79.89	D00.08	D10.6	D37.05	D49.0
floor	C11.3	C79.89	D00.08	D10.6	D37.05	D49.0
overlapping lesion	C11.8	—	—	—	—	—
roof	C11.0	C79.89	D00.08	D10.6	D37.05	D49.0
wall	C11.9	C79.89	D00.08	D10.6	D37.05	D49.0
anterior	C11.3	C79.89	D00.08	D10.6	D37.05	D49.0
lateral	C11.2	C79.89	D00.08	D10.6	D37.05	D49.0
posterior	C11.1	C79.89	D00.08	D10.6	D37.05	D49.0
superior	C11.0	C79.89	D00.08	D10.6	D37.05	D49.0
nates — *see also Neoplasm, skin, trunk*	C44.509	C79.2	D04.5	D23.5	D48.5	D49.2
neck NEC	C76.0	C79.89	D09.8	D36.7	D48.7	D49.89
skin	C44.40	—	—	—	—	—
basal cell carcinoma	C44.41					
specified type NEC	C44.49	—	—	—	—	—
squamous cell carcinoma	C44.42					
nerve (ganglion)	C47.9	C79.89	—	D36.10	D48.2	D49.2
abducens	C72.59	C79.49	—	D33.3	D43.3	D49.7
accessory (spinal)	C72.59	C79.49	—	D33.3	D43.3	D49.7
acoustic	C72.4-●	C79.49	—	D33.3	D43.3	D49.7
auditory	C72.4-●	C79.49	—	D33.3	D43.3	D49.7
autonomic NEC — *see also Neoplasm, nerve, peripheral*	C47.9	C79.89	—	D36.10	D48.2	D49.2
brachial	C47.1-●	C79.89	—	D36.12	D48.2	D49.2
cranial	C72.50	C79.49	—	D33.3	D43.3	D49.7
specified NEC	C72.59	C79.49	—	D33.3	D43.3	D49.7
facial	C72.59	C79.49	—	D33.3	D43.3	D49.7
femoral	C47.2-●	C79.89	—	D36.13	D48.2	D49.2
ganglion NEC — *see also Neoplasm, nerve, peripheral*	C47.9	C79.89	—	D36.10	D48.2	D49.2
glossopharyngeal	C72.59	C79.49	—	D33.3	D43.3	D49.7
hypoglossal	C72.59	C79.49	—	D33.3	D43.3	D49.7
intercostal	C47.3	C79.89	—	D36.14	D48.2	D49.2
lumbar	C47.6	C79.89	—	D36.17	D48.2	D49.2
median	C47.1-●	C79.89	—	D36.12	D48.2	D49.2
obturator	C47.2-●	C79.89	—	D36.13	D48.2	D49.2
oculomotor	C72.59	C79.49	—	D33.3	D43.3	D49.7
olfactory	C47.2-●	C79.49	—	D33.3	D43.3	D49.7
optic	C72.3-●	C79.49	—	D33.3	D43.3	D49.7
parasympathetic NEC	C47.9	C79.89	—	D36.10	D48.2	D49.2

	Malignant Primary	Malignant Secondary	Ca in situ	Benign	Uncertain Behavior	Unspecified Behavior
nerve *(Continued)*						
peripheral NEC	C47.9	C79.89	—	D36.10	D48.2	D49.2
abdomen	C47.4	C79.89	—	D36.15	D48.2	D49.2
abdominal wall	C47.4	C79.89	—	D36.15	D48.2	D49.2
ankle	C47.2-●	C79.89	—	D36.13	D48.2	D49.2
antecubital fossa or space	C47.1-●	C79.89	—	D36.12	D48.2	D49.2
arm	C47.1-●	C79.89	—	D36.12	D48.2	D49.2
auricle (ear)	C47.0	C79.89	—	D36.11	D48.2	D49.2
axilla	C47.3	C79.89	—	D36.12	D48.2	D49.2
back	C47.6	C79.89	—	D36.17	D48.2	D49.2
buttock	C47.5	C79.89	—	D36.16	D48.2	D49.2
calf	C47.2-●	C79.89	—	D36.13	D48.2	D49.2
cervical region	C47.0	C79.89	—	D36.11	D48.2	D49.2
cheek	C47.0	C79.89	—	D36.11	D48.2	D49.2
chest (wall)	C47.3	C79.89	—	D36.14	D48.2	D49.2
chin	C47.0	C79.89	—	D36.11	D48.2	D49.2
ear (external)	C47.0	C79.89	—	D36.11	D48.2	D49.2
elbow	C47.1-●	C79.89	—	D36.12	D48.2	D49.2
extrarectal	C47.5	C79.89	—	D36.16	D48.2	D49.2
extremity	C47.9	C79.89	—	D36.10	D48.2	D49.2
lower	C47.2-●	C79.89	—	D36.13	D48.2	D49.2
upper	C47.1-●	C79.89	—	D36.12	D48.2	D49.2
eyelid	C47.0	C79.89	—	D36.11	D48.2	D49.2
face	C47.0	C79.89	—	D36.11	D48.2	D49.2
finger	C47.1-●	C79.89	—	D36.12	D48.2	D49.2
flank	C47.6	C79.89	—	D36.17	D48.2	D49.2
foot	C47.2-●	C79.89	—	D36.13	D48.2	D49.2
forearm	C47.1-●	C79.89	—	D36.12	D48.2	D49.2
forehead	C47.0	C79.89	—	D36.11	D48.2	D49.2
gluteal region	C47.5	C79.89	—	D36.16	D48.2	D49.2
groin	C47.5	C79.89	—	D36.16	D48.2	D49.2
hand	C47.1-●	C79.89	—	D36.12	D48.2	D49.2
head	C47.0	C79.89	—	D36.11	D48.2	D49.2
heel	C47.2-●	C79.89	—	D36.13	D48.2	D49.2
hip	C47.2-●	C79.89	—	D36.13	D48.2	D49.2
infraclavicular region	C47.3	C79.89	—	D36.14	D48.2	D49.2
inguinal (canal) (region)	C47.5	C79.89	—	D36.16	D48.2	D49.2
intrathoracic	C47.3	C79.89	—	D36.14	D48.2	D49.2
ischiorectal fossa	C47.5	C79.89	—	D36.16	D48.2	D49.2
knee	C47.2-●	C79.89	—	D36.13	D48.2	D49.2
leg	C47.2-●	C79.89	—	D36.13	D48.2	D49.2
limb NEC	C47.9	C79.89	—	D36.10	D48.2	D49.2
lower	C47.2-●	C79.89	—	D36.13	D48.2	D49.2
upper	C47.1-●	C79.89	—	D36.12	D48.2	D49.2
nerve *(Continued)*						
peripheral NEC *(Continued)*						
nates	C47.5	C79.89	—	D36.16	D48.2	D49.2
neck	C47.0	C79.89	—	D36.11	D48.2	D49.2
orbit	C69.6-●	C79.49	—	D31.6-●	D48.7	D49.2
pararectal	C47.5	C79.89	—	D36.16	D48.2	D49.2
paraurethral	C47.5	C79.89	—	D36.16	D48.2	D49.2
paravaginal	C47.5	C79.89	—	D36.16	D48.2	D49.2
pelvis (floor)	C47.5	C79.89	—	D36.16	D48.2	D49.2
pelvoabdominal	C47.8	C79.89	—	D36.17	D48.2	D49.2
perineum	C47.5	C79.89	—	D36.16	D48.2	D49.2
perirectal (tissue)	C47.5	C79.89	—	D36.16	D48.2	D49.2
periurethral (tissue)	C47.5	C79.89	—	D36.16	D48.2	D49.2
popliteal fossa or space	C47.2-●	C79.89	—	D36.13	D48.2	D49.2
presacral	C47.5	C79.89	—	D36.16	D48.2	D49.2
pterygoid fossa	C47.0	C79.89	—	D36.11	D48.2	D49.2
rectovaginal septum or wall	C47.5	C79.89	—	D36.16	D48.2	D49.2
rectovesical	C47.5	C79.89	—	D36.16	D48.2	D49.2
sacrococcygeal region	C47.5	C79.89	—	D36.16	D48.2	D49.2
scalp	C47.0	C79.89	—	D36.11	D48.2	D49.2
scapular region	C47.3	C79.89	—	D36.14	D48.2	D49.2
shoulder	C47.1-●	C79.89	—	D36.12	D48.2	D49.2
submental	C47.0	C79.89	—	D36.11	D48.2	D49.2
supraclavicular region	C47.0	C79.89	—	D36.11	D48.2	D49.2
temple	C47.0	C79.89	—	D36.11	D48.2	D49.2
temporal region	C47.0	C79.89	—	D36.11	D48.2	D49.2
thigh	C47.2-●	C79.89	—	D36.13	D48.2	D49.2
thoracic (duct) (wall)	C47.3	C79.89	—	D36.14	D48.2	D49.2
thorax	C47.3	C79.89	—	D36.14	D48.2	D49.2
thumb	C47.1-●	C79.89	—	D36.12	D48.2	D49.2
toe	C47.2-●	C79.89	—	D36.13	D48.2	D49.2
trunk	C47.6	C79.89	—	D36.17	D48.2	D49.2
umbilicus	C47.4	C79.89	—	D36.15	D48.2	D49.2
vesicorectal	C47.5	C79.89	—	D36.16	D48.2	D49.2
wrist	C47.1-●	C79.89	—	D36.12	D48.2	D49.2
radial	C47.1-●	C79.89	—	D36.12	D48.2	D49.2
sacral	C47.5	C79.89	—	D36.16	D48.2	D49.2
sciatic	C47.2-●	C79.89	—	D36.13	D48.2	D49.2
spinal NEC	C47.9	C79.89	—	D36.10	D48.2	D49.2
accessory	C72.59	C79.49	—	D33.3	D43.3	D49.7
sympathetic NEC — *see also Neoplasm, nerve, peripheral*	C47.9	C79.89	—	D36.10	D48.2	D49.2
trigeminal	C72.59	C79.49	—	D33.3	D43.3	D49.7

◀ New　◀ Revised　~~deleted~~ Deleted　● Use Additional Character(s)

TABLE OF NEOPLASMS

	Malignant Primary	Malignant Secondary	Ca in situ	Benign	Uncertain Behavior	Unspecified Behavior
nerve *(Continued)*						
trochlear	C72.59	C79.49	—	D33.3	D43.3	D49.7
ulnar	C47.1-●	C79.89	—	D36.12	D48.2	D49.2
vagus	C72.59	C79.49	—	D33.3	D43.3	D49.7
nervous system (central)	C72.9	C79.40	—	D33.9	D43.9	D49.7
autonomic — *see Neoplasm, nerve, peripheral*						
parasympathetic — *see Neoplasm, nerve, peripheral*						
specified site NEC	—	C79.49	—	D33.7	D43.8	—
sympathetic — *see Neoplasm, nerve, peripheral*						
nevus — *see Nevus*						
nipple	C50.0-●	C79.81	D05.-●	D24.-●	—	—
nose, nasal	C76.0	C79.89	D09.8	D36.7	D48.7	D49.89
ala (external) (nasi) — *see also Neoplasm, nose, skin*	C44.301	C79.2	D04.39	D23.39	D48.5	D49.2
bone	C41.0	C79.51	—	D16.4-●	D48.0	D49.2
cartilage	C30.0	C78.39	D02.3	D14.0	D38.5	D49.1
cavity	C30.0	C78.39	D02.3	D14.0	D38.5	D49.1
choana	C11.3	C79.89	D00.08	D10.6	D37.05	D49.0
external (skin) — *see also Neoplasm, nose, skin*	C44.301	C79.2	D04.39	D23.39	D48.5	D49.2
fossa	C30.0	C78.39	D02.3	D14.0	D38.5	D49.1
internal	C30.0	C78.39	D02.3	D14.0	D38.5	D49.1
mucosa	C30.0	C78.39	D02.3	D14.0	D38.5	D49.1
septum	C30.0	C78.39	D02.3	D14.0	D38.5	D49.1
posterior margin	C11.3	C79.89	D00.08	D10.6	D37.05	D49.0
sinus — *see Neoplasm, sinus*						
skin	C44.301	C79.2	D04.39	D23.39	D48.5	D49.2
basal cell carcinoma	C44.311	—	—	—	—	—
specified type NEC	C44.391	—	—	—	—	—
squamous cell carcinoma	C44.321	—	—	—	—	—
turbinate (mucosa)	C30.0	C78.39	D02.3	D14.0	D38.5	D49.1
bone	C41.0	C79.51	—	D16.4-●	D48.0	D49.2
vestibule	C30.0	C78.39	D02.3	D14.0	D38.5	D49.1
nostril	C30.0	C78.39	D02.3	D14.0	D38.5	D49.1
nucleus pulposus	C41.2	C79.51	—	D16.6	D48.0	D49.2
occipital						
bone	C41.0	C79.51	—	D16.4-●	D48.0	D49.2
lobe or pole, brain	C71.4	C79.31	—	D33.0	D43.0	D49.6
odontogenic — *see Neoplasm, jaw, bone*						

	Malignant Primary	Malignant Secondary	Ca in situ	Benign	Uncertain Behavior	Unspecified Behavior
olfactory nerve or bulb	C72.2-●	C79.49	—	D33.3	D43.3	D49.7
olive (brain)	C71.7	C79.31	—	D33.1	D43.1	D49.6
omentum	C48.1	C78.6	—	D20.1	D48.4	D49.0
operculum (brain)	C71.0	C79.31	—	D33.0	D43.0	D49.6
optic nerve, chiasm, or tract	C72.3-●	C79.49	—	D33.3	D43.3	D49.7
oral (cavity)	C06.9	C79.89	D00.00	D10.30	D37.09	D49.0
ill-defined	C14.8	C79.89	D00.00	D10.30	D37.09	D49.0
mucosa	C06.0	C79.89	D00.02	D10.39	D37.09	D49.0
orbit	C69.6-●	C79.49	D09.2-●	D31.6-●	D48.7	D49.89
autonomic nerve	C69.6-●	C79.49	—	D31.6-●	D48.7	D49.2
bone	C41.0	C79.51	—	D16.4-●	D48.0	D49.2
eye	C69.6-●	C79.49	D09.2-●	D31.6-●	D48.7	D49.89
peripheral nerves	C69.6-●	C79.49	—	D31.6-●	D48.7	D49.2
soft parts	C69.6-●	C79.49	D09.2-●	D31.6-●	D48.7	D49.89
organ of Zuckerkandl	C75.5	C79.89	—	D35.6	D44.7	D49.7
oropharynx	C10.9	C79.89	D00.08	D10.5	D37.05	D49.0
branchial cleft (vestige)	C10.4	C79.89	D00.08	D10.5	D37.05	D49.0
junctional region	C10.8	C79.89	D00.08	D10.5	D37.05	D49.0
lateral wall	C10.2	C79.89	D00.08	D10.5	D37.05	D49.0
overlapping lesion	C10.8	—	—	—	—	—
pillars or fauces	C09.1	C79.89	D00.08	D10.5	D37.05	D49.0
posterior wall	C10.3	C79.89	D00.08	D10.5	D37.05	D49.0
vallecula	C10.0	C79.89	D00.08	D10.5	D37.05	D49.0
os						
external	C53.1	C79.82	D06.1	D26.0	D39.0	D49.59
internal	C53.0	C79.82	D06.0	D26.0	D39.0	D49.59
ovary	C56.-●	C79.6-●	D07.39	D27.-●	D39.1-●	D49.59
oviduct	C57.0-●	C79.82	D07.39	D28.2	D39.8	D49.59
palate	C05.9	C79.89	D00.00	D10.39	D37.09	D49.0
hard	C05.0	C79.89	D00.05	D10.39	D37.09	D49.0
junction of hard and soft palate	C05.9	C79.89	D00.00	D10.39	D37.09	D49.0
overlapping lesions	C05.8	—	—	—	—	—
soft	C05.1	C79.89	D00.04	D10.39	D37.09	D49.0
nasopharyngeal surface	C11.3	C79.89	D00.08	D10.6	D37.05	D49.0
posterior surface	C11.3	C79.89	D00.08	D10.6	D37.05	D49.0
superior surface	C11.3	C79.89	D00.08	D10.6	D37.05	D49.0
palatoglossal arch	C09.1	C79.89	D00.00	D10.5	D37.09	D49.0
palatopharyngeal arch	C09.1	C79.89	D00.00	D10.5	D37.09	D49.0
pallium	C71.0	C79.31	—	D33.0	D43.0	D49.6
palpebra	C44.10-●	C79.2	D04.1-●	D23.1-●	D48.5	D49.2
basal cell carcinoma	C44.11-●	—	—	—	—	—
sebaceous cell	C44.13-●	—	—	—	—	—
specified type NEC	C44.19-●	—	—	—	—	—
squamous cell carcinoma	C44.12-●	—	—	—	—	—

	Malignant Primary	Malignant Secondary	Ca in situ	Benign	Uncertain Behavior	Unspecified Behavior
pancreas	C25.9	C78.89	D01.7	D13.6	D37.8	D49.0
body	C25.1	C78.89	D01.7	D13.6	D37.8	D49.0
duct (of Santorini) (of Wirsung)	C25.3	C78.89	D01.7	D13.6	D37.8	D49.0
ectopic tissue	C25.7	C78.89	—	D13.6	D37.8	D49.0
head	C25.0	C78.89	D01.7	D13.6	D37.8	D49.0
islet cells	C25.4	C78.89	D01.7	D13.7	D37.8	D49.0
neck	C25.7	C78.89	D01.7	D13.6	D37.8	D49.0
overlapping lesion	C25.8	—	—	—	—	—
tail	C25.2	C78.89	D01.7	D13.6	D37.8	D49.0
para-aortic body	C75.5	C79.89	—	D35.6	D44.7	D49.7
paraganglion NEC	C75.5	C79.89	—	D35.6	D44.7	D49.7
parametrium	C57.3	C79.82	—	D28.2	D39.8	D49.59
paranephric	C48.0	C78.6	—	D20.0	D48.3	D49.0
pararectal	C76.3	C79.89	—	D36.7	D48.7	D49.89
parasagittal (region)	C76.0	C79.89	D09.8	D36.7	D48.7	D49.89
parasellar	C72.9	C79.49	—	D33.9	D43.8	D49.7
parathyroid (gland)	C75.0	C79.89	D09.3	D35.1	D44.2	D49.7
paraurethral	C76.3	C79.89	—	D36.7	D48.7	D49.89
gland	C68.1	C79.19	D09.19	D30.8	D41.8	D49.59
paravaginal	C76.3	C79.89	—	D36.7	D48.7	D49.89
parenchyma, kidney	C64.-•	C79.0-•	D09.19	D30.0-•	D41.0-•	D49.51-•
parietal						
bone	C41.0	C79.51	—	D16.4-•	D48.0	D49.2
lobe, brain	C71.3	C79.31	—	D33.0	D43.0	D49.6
paroophoron	C57.1	C79.82	D07.39	D28.2	D39.8	D49.59
parotid (duct) (gland)	C07	C79.89	D00.00	D11.0	D37.030	D49.0
parovarium	C57.1	C79.82	D07.39	D28.2	D39.8	D49.59
patella	C40.2-•	C79.51	—	—	—	—
peduncle, cerebral	C71.7	C79.31	—	D33.1	D43.1	D49.6
pelvirectal junction	C19	C78.5	D01.1	D12.7	D37.5	D49.0
pelvis, pelvic	C76.3	C79.89	D09.8	D36.7	D48.7	D49.89
bone	C41.4	C79.51	—	D16.8	D48.0	D49.2
floor	C76.3	C79.89	D09.8	D36.7	D48.7	D49.89
renal	C65.-•	C79.0-•	D09.19	D30.1-•	D41.1-•	D49.51-•
viscera	C76.3	C79.89	D09.8	D36.7	D48.7	D49.89
wall	C76.3	C79.89	D09.8	D36.7	D48.7	D49.89
pelvo-abdominal	C76.8	C79.89	D09.8	D36.7	D48.7	D49.89
penis	C60.9	C79.82	D07.4	D29.0	D40.8	D49.59
body	C60.2	C79.82	D07.4	D29.0	D40.8	D49.59
corpus (cavernosum)	C60.2	C79.82	D07.4	D29.0	D40.8	D49.59
glans	C60.1	C79.82	D07.4	D29.0	D40.8	D49.59
overlapping sites	C60.8	—	—	—	—	—
skin NEC	C60.9	C79.82	D07.4	D29.0	D40.8	D49.59

	Malignant Primary	Malignant Secondary	Ca in situ	Benign	Uncertain Behavior	Unspecified Behavior
periadrenal (tissue)	C48.0	C78.6	—	D20.0	D48.3	D49.0
perianal (skin) — see also Neoplasm, anus, skin	C44.500	C79.2	D04.5	D23.5	D48.5	D49.2
pericardium	C38.0	C79.89	—	D15.1	D48.7	D49.89
perinephric	C48.0	C78.6	—	D20.0	D48.3	D49.0
perineum	C76.3	C79.89	D09.8	D36.7	D48.7	D49.89
periodontal tissue NEC	C03.9	C79.89	D00.03	D10.39	D37.09	D49.0
periosteum — see Neoplasm, bone						
peripancreatic	C48.0	C78.6	—	D20.0	D48.3	D49.0
peripheral nerve NEC	C47.9	C79.89	—	D36.10	D48.2	D49.2
perirectal (tissue)	C76.3	C79.89	—	D36.7	D48.7	D49.89
perirenal (tissue)	C48.0	C78.6	—	D20.0	D48.3	D49.0
peritoneum, peritoneal (cavity)	C48.2	C78.6	—	D20.1	D48.4	D49.0
benign mesothelial tissue — see Mesothelioma, benign						
overlapping lesion	C48.8	—	—	—	—	—
with digestive organs	C26.9	—	—	—	—	—
parietal	C48.1	C78.6	—	D20.1	D48.4	D49.0
pelvic	C48.1	C78.6	—	D20.1	D48.4	D49.0
specified part NEC	C48.1	C78.6	—	D20.1	D48.4	D49.0
peritonsillar (tissue)	C76.0	C79.89	D09.8	D36.7	D48.7	D49.89
periurethral tissue	C76.3	C79.89	—	D36.7	D48.7	D49.89
phalanges						
foot	C40.3-•	C79.51	—	D16.3-•	—	—
hand	C40.1-•	C79.51	—	D16.1-•	—	—
pharynx, pharyngeal	C14.0	C79.89	D00.08	D10.9	D37.05	D49.0
bursa	C11.1	C79.89	D00.08	D10.6	D37.05	D49.0
fornix	C11.3	C79.89	D00.08	D10.6	D37.05	D49.0
recess	C11.2	C79.89	D00.08	D10.6	D37.05	D49.0
region	C14.0	C79.89	D00.08	D10.9	D37.05	D49.0
tonsil	C11.1	C79.89	D00.08	D10.6	D37.05	D49.0
wall (lateral) (posterior)	C14.0	C79.89	D00.08	D10.9	D37.05	D49.0
pia mater	C70.9	C79.40	—	D32.9	D42.9	D49.7
cerebral	C70.0	C79.32	—	D32.0	D42.0	D49.7
cranial	C70.0	C79.32	—	D32.0	D42.0	D49.7
spinal	C70.1	C79.49	—	D32.1	D42.1	D49.7
pillars of fauces	C09.1	C79.89	D00.08	D10.5	D37.05	D49.0
pineal (body) (gland)	C75.3	C79.89	D09.3	D35.4	D44.5	D49.7
pinna (ear) NEC — see also Neoplasm, skin, ear	C44.20-•	C79.2	D04.2-•	D23.2-•	D48.5	D49.2
piriform fossa or sinus	C12	C79.89	D00.08	D10.7	D37.05	D49.0
pituitary (body) (fossa) (gland) (lobe)	C75.1	C79.89	D09.3	D35.2	D44.3	D49.7

◄ New   ◄ Revised   ~~deleted~~ Deleted   • Use Additional Character(s)

	Malignant Primary	Malignant Secondary	Ca in situ	Benign	Uncertain Behavior	Unspecified Behavior
placenta	C58	C79.82	D07.0	D26.7	D39.2	D49.59
pleura, pleural (cavity)	C38.4	C78.2	—	D19.0	D38.2	D49.1
overlapping lesion with heart or mediastinum	C38.8	—	—	—	—	—
parietal	C38.4	C78.2	—	D19.0	D38.2	D49.1
visceral	C38.4	C78.2	—	D19.0	D38.2	D49.1
plexus						
brachial	C47.1-●	C79.89	—	D36.12	D48.2	D49.2
cervical	C47.0	C79.89	—	D36.11	D48.2	D49.2
choroid	C71.5	C79.31	—	D33.0	D43.0	D49.6
lumbosacral	C47.5	C79.89	—	D36.16	D48.2	D49.2
sacral	C47.5	C79.89	—	D36.16	D48.2	D49.2
pluriendocrine	C75.8	C79.89	D09.3	D35.7	D44.9	D49.7
pole						
frontal	C71.1	C79.31	—	D33.0	D43.0	D49.6
occipital	C71.4	C79.31	—	D33.0	D43.0	D49.6
pons (varolii)	C71.7	C79.31	—	D33.1	D43.1	D49.6
popliteal fossa or space	C76.5-●	C79.89	D04.7-●	D36.7	D48.7	D49.89
postcricoid (region)	C13.0	C79.89	D00.08	D10.7	D37.05	D49.0
posterior fossa (cranial)	C71.9	C79.31	—	D33.2	D43.2	D49.6
postnasal space	C11.9	C79.89	D00.08	D10.6	D37.05	D49.0
prepuce	C60.0	C79.82	D07.4	D29.0	D40.8	D49.59
prepylorus	C16.4	C78.89	D00.2	D13.1	D37.1	D49.0
presacral (region)	C76.3	C79.89	—	D36.7	D48.7	D49.89
prostate (gland)	C61	C79.82	D07.5	D29.1	D40.0	D49.59
utricle	C68.0	C79.19	D09.19	D30.4	D41.3	D49.59
pterygoid fossa	C49.0	C79.89	—	D21.0	D48.1-●	D49.2
pubic bone	C41.4	C79.51	—	D16.8	D48.0	D49.2
pudenda, pudendum (femaie)	C51.9	C79.82	D07.1	D28.0	D39.8	D49.59
pulmonary — see also Neoplasm, lung	C34.9-●	C78.0-●	D02.2-●	D14.3-●	D38.1	D49.1
putamen	C71.0	C79.31	—	D33.0	D43.0	D49.6
pyloric						
antrum	C16.3	C78.89	D00.2	D13.1	D37.1	D49.0
canal	C16.4	C78.89	D00.2	D13.1	D37.1	D49.0
pylorus	C16.4	C78.89	D00.2	D13.1	D37.1	D49.0
pyramid (brain)	C71.7	C79.31	—	D33.1	D43.1	D49.6
pyriform fossa or sinus	C12	C79.89	D00.08	D10.7	D37.05	D49.0
radius (any part)	C40.0-●	C79.51	—	D16.0-●	—	—
Rathke's pouch	C75.1	C79.89	D09.3	D35.2	D44.3	D49.7
rectosigmoid (junction)	C19	C78.5	D01.1	D12.7	D37.5	D49.0
overlapping lesion with anus or rectum	C21.8	—	—	—	—	—
rectouterine pouch	C48.1	C78.6	—	D20.1	D48.4	D49.0
rectovaginal septum or wall	C76.3	C79.89	D09.8	D36.7	D48.7	D49.89
rectovesical septum	C76.3	C79.89	D09.8	D36.7	D48.7	D49.89
rectum (ampulla)	C20	C78.5	D01.2	D12.8	D37.5	D49.0
and colon	C19	C78.5	D01.1	D12.7	D37.5	D49.0
overlapping lesion with anus or rectosigmoid junction	C21.8	—	—	—	—	—
renal	C64.-●	C79.0-●	D09.19	D30.0-●	D41.0-●	D49.51-●
calyx	C65.-●	C79.0-●	D09.19	D30.1-●	D41.1-●	D49.51-●
hilus	C65.-●	C79.0-●	D09.19	D30.1-●	D41.1-●	D49.51-●
parenchyma	C64.-●	C79.0-●	D09.19	D30.0-●	D41.0-●	D49.51-●
pelvis	C65.-●	C79.0-●	D09.19	D30.1-●	D41.1-●	D49.51-●
respiratory						
organs or system NEC	C39.9	C78.30	D02.4	D14.4	D38.6	D49.1
tract NEC	C39.9	C78.30	D02.4	D14.4	D38.5	D49.1
upper	C39.0	C78.30	D02.4	D14.4	D38.5	D49.1
retina	C69.2-●	C79.49	D09.2-●	D31.2-●	D48.7	D49.81
retrobulbar	C69.6-●	C79.49	—	D31.6-●	D48.7	D49.89
retrocecal	C48.0	C78.6	—	D20.0	D48.3	D49.0
retromolar (area) (triangle) (trigone)	C06.2	C79.89	D00.00	D10.39	D37.09	D49.0
retro-orbital	C76.0	C79.89	D09.8	D36.7	D48.7	D49.89
retroperitoneal (space) (tissue)	C48.0	C78.6	—	D20.0	D48.3	D49.0
retroperitoneum	C48.0	C78.6	—	D20.0	D48.3	D49.0
retropharyngeal	C14.0	C79.89	D00.08	D10.9	D37.05	D49.0
retrovesical (septum)	C76.3	C79.89	D09.8	D36.7	D48.7	D49.89
rhinencephalon	C71.0	C79.31	—	D33.0	D43.0	D49.6
rib	C41.3	C79.51	—	D16.7	D48.0	D49.2
Rosenmuller's fossa	C11.2	C79.89	D00.08	D10.6	D37.05	D49.0
round ligament	C57.2	C79.82	—	D28.2	D39.8	D49.59
sacrococcyx, sacrococcygeal	C41.4	C79.51	—	D16.8	D48.0	D49.2
region	C76.3	C79.89	D09.8	D36.7	D48.7	D49.89
sacrouterine ligament	C57.3	C79.82	—	D28.2	D39.8	D49.59
sacrum, sacral (vertebra)	C41.4	C79.51	—	D16.8	D48.0	D49.2
salivary gland or duct (major)	C08.9	C79.89	D00.00	D11.9	D37.039	D49.0
minor NEC	C06.9	C79.89	D00.00	D10.39	D37.04	D49.0
overlapping lesion	C08.9	—	—	—	—	—
parotid	C07	C79.89	D00.00	D11.0	D37.030	D49.0
pluriglandular	C08.9	C79.89	D00.00	D11.9	D37.039	D49.0
sublingual	C08.1	C79.89	D00.00	D11.7	D37.031	D49.0
submandibular	C08.0	C79.89	D00.00	D11.7	D37.032	D49.0
submaxillary	C08.0	C79.89	D00.00	D11.7	D37.032	D49.0
salpinx (uterine)	C57.0-●	C79.82	D07.39	D28.2	D39.8	D49.59
Santorini's duct	C25.3	C78.89	D01.7	D13.6	D37.8	D49.0

◄ New   ◄ Revised   ~~deleted~~ Deleted   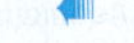 Use Additional Character(s)   **451**

TABLE OF NEOPLASMS

	Malignant Primary	Malignant Secondary	Ca in situ	Benign	Uncertain Behavior	Unspecified Behavior
scalp	C44.40	C79.2	D04.4	D23.4	D48.5	D49.2
basal cell carcinoma	C44.41	—	—	—	—	—
specified type NEC	C44.49	—	—	—	—	—
squamous cell carcinoma	C44.42	—	—	—	—	—
scapula (any part)	C40.0-•	C79.51	—	D16.0-•	—	—
scapular region	C76.1	C79.89	D09.8	D36.7	D48.7	D49.89
scar NEC — *see also Neoplasm, skin, by site*	C44.90	C79.2	D04.9	D23.9	D48.5	D49.2
sciatic nerve	C47.2-•	C79.89	—	D36.13	D48.2	D49.2
sclera	C69.4-•	C79.49	D09.2-•	D31.4-•	D48.7	D49.89
scrotum (skin)	C63.2	C79.82	D07.61	D29.4	D40.8	D49.59
sebaceous gland — *see Neoplasm, skin*						
sella turcica	C75.1	C79.89	D09.3	D35.2	D44.3	D49.7
bone	C41.0	C79.51	—	D16.4-•	D48.0	D49.2
semilunar cartilage (knee)	C40.2-•	C79.51	—	D16.2-•	D48.0	D49.2
seminal vesicle	C63.7	C79.82	D07.69	D29.8	D40.8	D49.59
septum						
nasal	C30.0	C78.39	D02.3	D14.0	D38.5	D49.1
posterior margin	C11.3	C79.89	D00.08	D10.6	D37.05	D49.0
rectovaginal	C76.3	C79.89	D09.8	D36.7	D48.7	D49.89
rectovesical	C76.3	C79.89	D09.8	D36.7	D48.7	D49.89
urethrovaginal	C57.9	C79.82	D07.30	D28.9	D39.9	D49.59
vesicovaginal	C57.9	C79.82	D07.30	D28.9	D39.9	D49.59
shoulder NEC	C76.4-•	C79.89	D04.6-•	D36.7	D48.7	D49.89
sigmoid flexure (lower) (upper)	C18.7	C78.5	D01.0	D12.5	D37.4	D49.0
sinus (accessory)	C31.9	C78.39	D02.3	D14.0	D38.5	D49.1
bone (any)	C41.0	C79.51	—	D16.4-•	D48.0	D49.2
ethmoidal	C31.1	C78.39	D02.3	D14.0	D38.5	D49.1
frontal	C31.2	C78.39	D02.3	D14.0	D38.5	D49.1
maxillary	C31.0	C78.39	D02.3	D14.0	D38.5	D49.1
nasal, paranasal NEC	C31.9	C78.39	D02.3	D14.0	D38.5	D49.1
overlapping lesion	C31.8	—	—	—	—	—
pyriform	C12	C79.89	D00.08	D10.7	D37.05	D49.0
sphenoid	C31.3	C78.39	D02.3	D14.0	D38.5	D49.1
skeleton, skeletal NEC	C41.9	C79.51	—	D16.9-•	D48.0	D49.2
Skene's gland	C68.1	C79.19	D09.19	D30.8	D41.8	D49.59
skin NOS	C44.90	C79.2	D04.9	D23.9	D48.5	D49.2
abdominal wall	C44.509	C79.2	D04.5	D23.5	D48.5	D49.2
basal cell carcinoma	C44.519	—	—	—	—	—
specified type NEC	C44.599	—	—	—	—	—
squamous cell carcinoma	C44.529	—	—	—	—	—

skin NOS *(Continued)*	Malignant Primary	Malignant Secondary	Ca in situ	Benign	Uncertain Behavior	Unspecified Behavior
ala nasi — *see also Neoplasm, nose, skin*	C44.301	C79.2	D04.39	D23.39	D48.5	D49.2
ankle — *see also Neoplasm, skin, limb, lower*	C44.70-•	C79.2	D04.7-•	D23.7-•	D48.5	D49.2
antecubital space — *see also Neoplasm, skin, limb, upper*	C44.60-•	C79.2	D04.6-•	D23.6-•	D48.5	D49.2
anus	C44.500	C79.2	D04.5	D23.5	D48.5	D49.2
basal cell carcinoma	C44.510	—	—	—	—	—
specified type NEC	C44.590	—	—	—	—	—
squamous cell carcinoma	C44.520	—	—	—	—	—
arm — *see also Neoplasm, skin, limb, upper*	C44.60-•	C79.2	D04.6-•	D23.6-•	D48.5	D49.2
auditory canal (external) — *see also Neoplasm, skin, ear*	C44.20-•	C79.2	D04.2-•	D23.2-•	D48.5	D49.2
auricle (ear) — *see also Neoplasm, skin, ear*	C44.20-•	C79.2	D04.2-•	D23.2-•	D48.5	D49.2
auricular canal (external) — *see also Neoplasm, skin, ear*	C44.20-•	C79.2	D04.2-•	D23.2-•	D48.5	D49.2
axilla, axillary fold — *see also Neoplasm, skin, trunk*	C44.509	C79.2	D04.5	D23.5	D48.5	D49.2
back — *see also Neoplasm, skin, trunk*	C44.509	C79.2	D04.5	D23.5	D48.5	D49.2
basal cell carcinoma	C44.91					
breast	C44.501	C79.2	D04.5	D23.5	D48.5	D49.2
basal cell carcinoma	C44.511	—	—	—	—	—
specified type NEC	C44.591	—	—	—	—	—
squamous cell carcinoma	C44.521	—	—	—	—	—
brow — *see also Neoplasm, skin, face*	C44.309	C79.2	D04.39	D23.39	D48.5	D49.2
buttock — *see also Neoplasm, skin, trunk*	C44.509	C79.2	D04.5	D23.5	D48.5	D49.2
calf — *see also Neoplasm, skin, limb, lower*	C44.70-•	C79.2	D04.7-•	D23.7-•	D48.5	D49.2
canthus (eye) (inner) (outer)	C44.10-•	C79.2	D04.1-•	D23.1-•	D48.5	D49.2
basal cell carcinoma	C44.11-•	—	—	—	—	—
sebaceous cell	C44.13-•	—	—	—	—	—
specified type NEC	C44.19-•	—	—	—	—	—
squamous cell carcinoma	C44.12-•	—	—	—	—	—
cervical region — *see also Neoplasm, skin, neck*	C44.40	C79.2	D04.4	D23.4	D48.5	D49.2
cheek (external) — *see also Neoplasm, skin, face*	C44.309	C79.2	D04.39	D23.39	D48.5	D49.2

◄ New   ◄ Revised   ~~deleted~~ Deleted   • Use Additional Character(s)

	Malignant Primary	Malignant Secondary	Ca in situ	Benign	Uncertain Behavior	Unspecified Behavior
skin NOS *(Continued)*						
chest (wall) — *see also Neoplasm, skin, trunk*	C44.509	C79.2	D04.5	D23.5	D48.5	D49.2
chin — *see also Neoplasm, skin, face*	C44.309	C79.2	D04.39	D23.39	D48.5	D49.2
clavicular area — *see also Neoplasm, skin, trunk*	C44.509	C79.2	D04.5	D23.5	D48.5	D49.2
clitoris	C51.2	C79.82	D07.1	D28.0	D39.8	D49.59
columnella — *see also Neoplasm, skin, face*	C44.309	C79.2	D04.39	D23.39	D48.5	D49.2
concha — *see also Neoplasm, skin, ear*	C44.20-●	C79.2	D04.2-●	D23.2-●	D48.5	D49.2
ear (external)	C44.20-●	C79.2	D04.2-●	D23.2-●	D48.5	D49.2
basal cell carcinoma	C44.21-●	—	—	—	—	—
specified type NEC	C44.29-●	—	—	—	—	—
squamous cell carcinoma	C44.22-●	—	—	—	—	—
elbow — *see also Neoplasm, skin, limb, upper*	C44.60-●	C79.2	D04.6-●	D23.6-●	D48.5	D49.2
eyebrow — *see also Neoplasm, skin, face*	C44.309	C79.2	D04.39	D23.39	D48.5	D49.2
eyelid	C44.10-●	C79.2	D04.1-●	D23.1-●	D48.5	D49.2
basal cell carcinoma	C44.11-●	—	—	—	—	—
sebaceous cell	C44.13-●	—	—	—	—	—
specified type NEC	C44.19-●	—	—	—	—	—
squamous cell carcinoma	C44.12-●	—	—	—	—	—
face NOS	C44.300	C79.2	D04.30	D23.30	D48.5	D49.2
basal cell carcinoma	C44.310	—	—	—	—	—
specified type NEC	C44.390	—	—	—	—	—
squamous cell carcinoma	C44.320	—	—	—	—	—
female genital organs (external)	C51.9	C79.82	D07.1	D28.0	D39.8	D49.59
clitoris	C51.2	C79.82	D07.1	D28.0	D39.8	D49.59
labium NEC	C51.9	C79.82	D07.1	D28.0	D39.8	D49.59
majus	C51.0	C79.82	D07.1	D28.0	D39.8	D49.59
minus	C51.1	C79.82	D07.1	D28.0	D39.8	D49.59
pudendum	C51.9	C79.82	D07.1	D28.0	D39.8	D49.59
vulva	C51.9	C79.82	D07.1	D28.0	D39.8	D49.59
finger — *see also Neoplasm, skin, limb, upper*	C44.60-●	C79.2	D04.6-●	D23.6-●	D48.5	D49.2
flank — *see also Neoplasm, skin, trunk*	C44.509	C79.2	D04.5	D23.5	D48.5	D49.2
foot — *see also Neoplasm, skin, limb, lower*	C44.70-●	C79.2	D04.7-●	D23.7-●	D48.5	D49.2
forearm — *see also Neoplasm, skin, limb, upper*	C44.60-●	C79.2	D04.6-●	D23.6-●	D48.5	D49.2
skin NOS *(Continued)*						
forehead — *see also Neoplasm, skin, face*	C44.309	C79.2	D04.39	D23.39	D48.5	D49.2
glabella — *see also Neoplasm, skin, face*	C44.309	C79.2	D04.39	D23.39	D48.5	D49.2
gluteal region — *see also Neoplasm, skin, trunk*	C44.509	C79.2	D04.5	D23.5	D48.5	D49.2
groin — *see also Neoplasm, skin, trunk*	C44.509	C79.2	D04.5	D23.5	D48.5	D49.2
hand — *see also Neoplasm, skin, limb, upper*	C44.60-●	C79.2	D04.6-●	D23.6-●	D48.5	D49.2
head NEC — *see also Neoplasm, skin, scalp*	C44.40	C79.2	D04.4	D23.4	D48.5	D49.2
heel — *see also Neoplasm, skin, limb, lower*	C44.70-●	C79.2	D04.7-●	D23.7-●	D48.5	D49.2
helix — *see also Neoplasm, skin, ear*	C44.20-●	C79.2	D04.2-●	D23.2-●	D48.5	D49.2
hip — *see also Neoplasm, skin, limb, lower*	C44.70-●	C79.2	D04.7-●	D23.7-●	D48.5	D49.2
infraclavicular region — *see also Neoplasm, skin, trunk*	C44.509	C79.2	D04.5	D23.5	D48.5	D49.2
inguinal region — *see also Neoplasm, skin, trunk*	C44.509	C79.2	D04.5	D23.5	D48.5	D49.2
jaw — *see also Neoplasm, skin, face*	C44.309	C79.2	D04.39	D23.39	D48.5	D49.2
Kaposi's sarcoma — *see Kaposi's, sarcoma, skin*						
knee — *see also Neoplasm, skin, limb, lower*	C44.70-●	C79.2	D04.7-●	D23.7-●	D48.5	D49.2
labia						
majora	C51.0	C79.82	D07.1	D28.0	D39.8	D49.59
minora	C51.1	C79.82	D07.1	D28.0	D39.8	D49.59
leg — *see also Neoplasm, skin, limb, lower*	C44.70-●	C79.2	D04.7-●	D23.7-●	D48.5	D49.2
lid (lower) (upper)	C44.10-●	C79.2	D04.1-●	D23.1-●	D48.5	D49.2
basal cell carcinoma	C44.11-●	—	—	—	—	—
sebaceous cell	C44.13-●	—	—	—	—	—
specified type NEC	C44.19-●	—	—	—	—	—
squamous cell carcinoma	C44.12-●	—	—	—	—	—
limb NEC	C44.90	C79.2	D04.9	D23.9	D48.5	D49.2
basal cell carcinoma	C44.91					
lower	C44.70-●	C79.2	D04.7-●	D23.7-●	D48.5	D49.2
basal cell carcinoma	C44.71-●	—	—	—	—	—
specified type NEC	C44.79-●	—	—	—	—	—
squamous cell carcinoma	C44.72-●	—	—	—	—	—

	Malignant Primary	Malignant Secondary	Ca in situ	Benign	Uncertain Behavior	Unspecified Behavior
skin NOS *(Continued)*						
limb NEC *(Continued)*						
upper	C44.60-●	C79.2	D04.6-●	D23.6-●	D48.5	D49.2
basal cell carcinoma	C44.61-●	—	—	—	—	—
specified type NEC	C44.69-●	—	—	—	—	—
squamous cell carcinoma	C44.62-●	—	—	—	—	—
lip (lower) (upper)	C44.00	C79.2	D04.0	D23.0	D48.5	D49.2
basal cell carcinoma	C44.01	—	—	—	—	—
specified type NEC	C44.09	—	—	—	—	—
squamous cell carcinoma	C44.02	—	—	—	—	—
male genital organs	C63.9	C79.82	D07.60	D29.9	D40.8	D49.59
penis	C60.9	C79.82	D07.4	D29.0	D40.8	D49.59
prepuce	C60.0	C79.82	D07.4	D29.0	D40.8	D49.59
scrotum	C63.2	C79.82	D07.61	D29.4	D40.8	D49.59
mastectomy site (skin) — *see also Neoplasm, skin, breast*	C44.501	C79.2	—	—	—	—
specified as breast tissue	C50.8-●	C79.81	—	—	—	—
meatus, acoustic (external) — *also Neoplasm, skin, ear*	C44.20-●	C79.2	D04.2-●	D23.2-●	D48.5	D49.2
melanotic — *see Melanoma*						
Merkel cell — *see Carcinoma, Merkel cell*						
nates — *see also Neoplasm, skin, trunk*	C44.509	C79.2	D04.5	D23.5	D48.5	D49.2
neck	C44.40	C79.2	D04.4	D23.4	D48.5	D49.2
basal cell carcinoma	C44.41	—	—	—	—	—
specified type NEC	C44.49	—	—	—	—	—
squamous cell carcinoma	C44.42	—	—	—	—	—
nevus — *see Nevus, skin*						
nose (external) — *see also Neoplasm, nose, skin*	C44.301	C79.2	D04.39	D23.39	D48.5	D49.2
overlapping lesion	C44.80					
basal cell carcinoma	C44.81	—	—	—	—	—
specified type NEC	C44.89	—	—	—	—	—
squamous cell carcinoma	C44.82	—	—	—	—	—
palm — *see also Neoplasm, skin, limb, upper*	C44.60-●	C79.2	D04.6-●	D23.6-●	D48.5	D49.2
palpebra	C44.10-●	C79.2	D04.1-●	D23.1-●	D48.5	D49.2
basal cell carcinoma	C44.11-●	—	—	—	—	—
sebaceous cell	C44.13-●	—	—	—	—	—
specified type NEC	C44.19-●	—	—	—	—	—
squamous cell carcinoma	C44.12-●	—	—	—	—	—
penis NEC	C60.9	C79.82	D07.4	D29.0	D40.8	D49.59
skin NOS *(Continued)*						
perianal — *see also Neoplasm, skin, anus*	C44.500	C79.2	D04.5	D23.5	D48.5	D49.2
perineum — *see also Neoplasm, skin, anus*	C44.500	C79.2	D04.5	D23.5	D48.5	D49.2
pinna — *see also Neoplasm, skin, ear*	C44.20-●	C79.2	D04.2-●	D23.2-●	D48.5	D49.2
plantar — *see also Neoplasm, skin, limb, lower*	C44.70-●	C79.2	D04.7-●	D23.7-●	D48.5	D49.2
popliteal fossa or space — *also Neoplasm, skin, limb, lower*	C44.70-●	C79.2	D04.7-●	D23.7-●	D48.5	D49.2
prepuce	C60.0	C79.82	D07.4	D29.0	D40.8	D49.59
pubes — *see also Neoplasm, skin, trunk*	C44.509	C79.2	D04.5	D23.5	D48.5	D49.2
sacrococcygeal region — *see also Neoplasm, skin, trunk*	C44.509	C79.2	D04.5	D23.5	D48.5	D49.2
scalp	C44.40	C79.2	D04.4	D23.4	D48.5	D49.2
basal cell carcinoma	C44.41	—	—	—	—	—
specified type NEC	C44.49	—	—	—	—	—
squamous cell carcinoma	C44.42	—	—	—	—	—
scapular region — *see also Neoplasm, skin, trunk*	C44.509	C79.2	D04.5	D23.5	D48.5	D49.2
scrotum	C63.2	C79.82	D07.61	D29.4	D40.8	D49.59
shoulder — *see also Neoplasm, skin, limb, upper*	C44.60-●	C79.2	D04.6-●	D23.6-●	D48.5	D49.2
sole (foot) — *see also Neoplasm, skin, limb, lower*	C44.70-●	C79.2	D04.7-●	D23.7-●	D48.5	D49.2
specified sites NEC	C44.80	C79.2	D04.8	D23.9	D48.5	D49.2
basal cell carcinoma	C44.81	—	—	—	—	—
specified type NEC	C44.89	—	—	—	—	—
squamous cell carcinoma	C44.82	—	—	—	—	—
specified type NEC	C44.99					
squamous cell carcinoma	C44.92					
submammary fold — *see also Neoplasm, skin, trunk*	C44.509	C79.2	D04.5	D23.5	D48.5	D49.2
supraclavicular region — *see also Neoplasm, skin, neck*	C44.40	C79.2	D04.4	D23.4	D48.5	D49.2
temple — *see also Neoplasm, skin, face*	C44.309	C79.2	D04.39	D23.39	D48.5	D49.2
thigh — *see also Neoplasm, skin, limb, lower*	C44.70-●	C79.2	D04.7-●	D23.7-●	D48.5	D49.2
thoracic wall — *see also Neoplasm, skin, trunk*	C44.509	C79.2	D04.5	D23.5	D48.5	D49.2

◄ New   ◄ Revised   ~~deleted~~ Deleted   ● Use Additional Character(s)

	Malignant Primary	Malignant Secondary	Ca in situ	Benign	Uncertain Behavior	Unspecified Behavior
skin NOS *(Continued)*						
thumb—*see also Neoplasm, skin, limb, upper*	C44.60-•	C79.2	D04.6-•	D23.6-•	D48.5	D49.2
toe—*see also Neoplasm, skin, limb, lower*	C44.70-•	C79.2	D04.7-•	D23.7-•	D48.5	D49.2
tragus—*see also Neoplasm, skin, ear*	C44.20-•	C79.2	D04.2-•	D23.2-•	D48.5	D49.2
trunk	C44.509	C79.2	D04.5	D23.5	D48.5	D49.2
basal cell carcinoma	C44.519	—	—	—	—	—
specified type NEC	C44.599	—	—	—	—	—
squamous cell carcinoma	C44.529	—	—	—	—	—
umbilicus—*see also Neoplasm, skin, trunk*	C44.509	C79.2	D04.5	D23.5	D48.5	D49.2
vulva	C51.9	C79.82	D07.1	D28.0	D39.8	D49.59
overlapping lesion	C51.8	—	—	—	—	—
wrist—*see also Neoplasm, skin, limb, upper*	C44.60-•	C79.2	D04.6-•	D23.6-•	D48.5	D49.2
skull	C41.0	C79.51	—	D16.4-•	D48.0	D49.2
soft parts or tissues—*see Neoplasm, connective tissue*						
specified site NEC	C76.8	C79.89	D09.8	D36.7	D48.7	D49.89
spermatic cord	C63.1-•	C79.82	D07.69	D29.8	D40.8	D49.59
sphenoid	C31.3	C78.39	D02.3	D14.0	D38.5	D49.1
bone	C41.0	C79.51	—	D16.4-•	D48.0	D49.2
sinus	C31.3	C78.39	D02.3	D14.0	D38.5	D49.1
sphincter						
anal	C21.1	C78.5	D01.3	D12.9	D37.8	D49.0
of Oddi	C24.0	C78.89	D01.5	D13.5	D37.6	D49.0
spine, spinal (column)	C41.2	C79.51	—	D16.6	D48.0	D49.2
bulb	C71.7	C79.31	—	D33.1	D43.1	D49.6
coccyx	C41.4	C79.51	—	D16.8	D48.0	D49.2
cord (cervical) (lumbar) (sacral) (thoracic)	C72.0	C79.49	—	D33.4	D43.4	D49.7
dura mater	C70.1	C79.49	—	D32.1	D42.1	D49.7
lumbosacral	C41.2	C79.51	—	D16.6	D48.0	D49.2
marrow NEC	C96.9	C79.52	—	—	D47.9	D49.89
membrane	C70.1	C79.49	—	D32.1	D42.1	D49.7
meninges	C70.1	C79.49	—	D32.1	D42.1	D49.7
nerve (root)	C47.9	C79.89	—	D36.10	D48.2	D49.2
pia mater	C70.1	C79.49	—	D32.1	D42.1	D49.7
root	C47.9	C79.89	—	D36.10	D48.2	D49.2
sacrum	C41.4	C79.51	—	D16.8	D48.0	D49.2
spleen, splenic NEC	C26.1	C78.89	D01.7	D13.99	D37.8	D49.0
flexure (colon)	C18.5	C78.5	D01.0	D12.3	D37.4	D49.0

	Malignant Primary	Malignant Secondary	Ca in situ	Benign	Uncertain Behavior	Unspecified Behavior
stem, brain	C71.7	C79.31	—	D33.1	D43.1	D49.6
Stensen's duct	C07	C79.89	D00.00	D11.0	D37.030	D49.0
sternum	C41.3	C79.51	—	D16.7	D48.0	D49.2
stomach	C16.9	C78.89	D00.2	D13.1	D37.1	D49.0
antrum (pyloric)	C16.3	C78.89	D00.2	D13.1	D37.1	D49.0
body	C16.2	C78.89	D00.2	D13.1	D37.1	D49.0
cardia	C16.0	C78.89	D00.2	D13.1	D37.1	D49.0
cardiac orifice	C16.0	C78.89	D00.2	D13.1	D37.1	D49.0
corpus	C16.2	C78.89	D00.2	D13.1	D37.1	D49.0
fundus	C16.1	C78.89	D00.2	D13.1	D37.1	D49.0
greater curvature NEC	C16.6	C78.89	D00.2	D13.1	D37.1	D49.0
lesser curvature NEC	C16.5	C78.89	D00.2	D13.1	D37.1	D49.0
overlapping lesion	C16.8	—	—	—	—	—
prepylorus	C16.4	C78.89	D00.2	D13.1	D37.1	D49.0
pylorus	C16.4	C78.89	D00.2	D13.1	D37.1	D49.0
wall NEC	C16.9	C78.89	D00.2	D13.1	D37.1	D49.0
anterior NEC	C16.8	C78.89	D00.2	D13.1	D37.1	D49.0
posterior NEC	C16.8	C78.89	D00.2	D13.1	D37.1	D49.0
stroma, endometrial	C54.1	C79.82	D07.0	D26.1	D39.0	D49.59
stump, cervical	C53.8	C79.82	D06.7	D26.0	D39.0	D49.59
subcutaneous (nodule) (tissue) NEC—*see Neoplasm, connective tissue*						
subdural	C70.9	C79.32	—	D32.9	D42.9	D49.7
subglottis, subglottic	C32.2	C78.39	D02.0	D14.1	D38.0	D49.1
sublingual	C04.9	C79.89	D00.06	D10.2	D37.09	D49.0
gland or duct	C08.1	C79.89	D00.00	D11.7	D37.031	D49.0
submandibular gland	C08.0	C79.89	D00.00	D11.7	D37.032	D49.0
submaxillary gland or duct	C08.0	C79.89	D00.00	D11.7	D37.032	D49.0
submental	C76.0	C79.89	D09.8	D36.7	D48.7	D49.89
subpleural	C34.9-•	C78.0-•	D02.2-•	D14.3-•	D38.1	D49.1
substernal	C38.1	C78.1	—	D15.2	D38.3	D49.89
sudoriferous, sudoriparous gland, site unspecified	C44.90	C79.2	D04.9	D23.9	D48.5	D49.2
specified site—*see Neoplasm, skin*						
supraclavicular region	C76.0	C79.89	D09.8	D36.7	D48.7	D49.89
supraglottis	C32.1	C78.39	D02.0	D14.1	D38.0	D49.1
suprarenal	C74.9-•	C79.7-•	D09.3	D35.0-•	D44.1-•	D49.7
capsule	C74.9-•	C79.7-•	D09.3	D35.0-•	D44.1-•	D49.7
cortex	C74.0-•	C79.7-•	D09.3	D35.0-•	D44.1-•	D49.7
gland	C74.9-•	C79.7-•	D09.3	D35.0-•	D44.1-•	D49.7
medulla	C74.1-•	C79.7-•	D09.3	D35.0-•	D44.1-•	D49.7

TABLE OF NEOPLASMS

◄ New   ◄ Revised   ~~deleted~~ Deleted   • Use Additional Character(s)

TABLE OF NEOPLASMS

	Malignant Primary	Malignant Secondary	Ca in situ	Benign	Uncertain Behavior	Unspecified Behavior
suprasellar (region)	C71.9	C79.31	—	D33.2	D43.2	D49.6
supratentorial (brain) NEC	C71.0	C79.31	—	D33.0	D43.0	D49.6
sweat gland (apocrine) (eccrine), site unspecified	C44.90	C79.2	D04.9	D23.9	D48.5	D49.2
specified site — *see Neoplasm, skin*						
sympathetic nerve or nervous system NEC	C47.9	C79.89	—	D36.10	D48.2	D49.2
symphysis pubis	C41.4	C79.51	—	D16.8	D48.0	D49.2
synovial membrane — *see Neoplasm, connective tissue*						
tapetum, brain	C71.8	C79.31	—	D33.2	D43.2	D49.6
tarsus (any bone)	C40.3-•	C79.51	—	D16.3-•	—	—
temple (skin) — *see also Neoplasm, skin, face*	C44.309	C79.2	D04.39	D23.39	D48.5	D49.2
temporal						
bone	C41.0	C79.51	—	D16.4-•	D48.0	D49.2
lobe or pole	C71.2	C79.31	—	D33.0	D43.0	D49.6
region	C76.0	C79.89	D09.8	D36.7	D48.7	D49.89
skin — *see also Neoplasm, skin, face*	C44.309	C79.2	D04.39	D23.39	D48.5	D49.2
tendon (sheath) — *see Neoplasm, connective tissue*						
tentorium (cerebelli)	C70.0	C79.32	—	D32.0	D42.0	D49.7
testis, testes	C62.9-•	C79.82	D07.69	D29.2-•	D40.1-•	D49.59
descended	C62.1-•	C79.82	D07.69	D29.2-•	D40.1-•	D49.59
ectopic	C62.0-•	C79.82	D07.69	D29.2-•	D40.1-•	D49.59
retained	C62.0-•	C79.82	D07.69	D29.2-•	D40.1-•	D49.59
scrotal	C62.1-•	C79.82	D07.69	D29.2-•	D40.1-•	D49.59
undescended	C62.0-•	C79.82	D07.69	D29.2-•	D40.1-•	D49.59
unspecified whether descended or undescended	C62.9-•	C79.82	D07.69	D29.2-•	D40.1-•	D49.59
thalamus	C71.0	C79.31	—	D33.0	D43.0	D49.6
thigh NEC	C76.5-•	C79.89	D04.7-•	D36.7	D48.7	D49.89
thorax, thoracic (cavity) (organs NEC)	C76.1	C79.89	D09.8	D36.7	D48.7	D49.89
duct	C49.3	C79.89	—	D21.3	D48.1-•	D49.2
wall NEC	C76.1	C79.89	D09.8	D36.7	D48.7	D49.89
throat	C14.0	C79.89	D00.08	D10.9	D37.05	D49.0
thumb NEC	C76.4-•	C79.89	D04.6-•	D36.7	D48.7	D49.89
thymus (gland)	C37	C79.89	D09.3	D15.0	D38.4	D49.89
thyroglossal duct	C73	C79.89	D09.3	D34	D44.0	D49.7
thyroid (gland)	C73	C79.89	D09.3	D34	D44.0	D49.7
cartilage	C32.3	C78.39	D02.0	D14.1	D38.0	D49.1

	Malignant Primary	Malignant Secondary	Ca in situ	Benign	Uncertain Behavior	Unspecified Behavior
tibia (any part)	C40.2-•	C79.51	—	D16.2-•	—	—
toe NEC	C76.5-•	C79.89	D04.7-•	D36.7	D48.7	D49.89
tongue	C02.9	C79.89	D00.07	D10.1	D37.02	D49.0
anterior (two-thirds) NEC	C02.3	C79.89	D00.07	D10.1	D37.02	D49.0
dorsal surface	C02.0	C79.89	D00.07	D10.1	D37.02	D49.0
ventral surface	C02.2	C79.89	D00.07	D10.1	D37.02	D49.0
base (dorsal surface)	C01	C79.89	D00.07	D10.1	D37.02	D49.0
border (lateral)	C02.1	C79.89	D00.07	D10.1	D37.02	D49.0
dorsal surface NEC	C02.0	C79.89	D00.07	D10.1	D37.02	D49.0
fixed part NEC	C01	C79.89	D00.07	D10.1	D37.02	D49.0
foreamen cecum	C02.0	C79.89	D00.07	D10.1	D37.02	D49.0
frenulum linguae	C02.2	C79.89	D00.07	D10.1	D37.02	D49.0
junctional zone	C02.8	C79.89	D00.07	D10.1	D37.02	D49.0
margin (lateral)	C02.1	C79.89	D00.07	D10.1	D37.02	D49.0
midline NEC	C02.0	C79.89	D00.07	D10.1	D37.02	D49.0
mobile part NEC	C02.3	C79.89	D00.07	D10.1	D37.02	D49.0
overlapping lesion	C02.8	—	—	—	—	—
posterior (third)	C01	C79.89	D00.07	D10.1	D37.02	D49.0
root	C01	C79.89	D00.07	D10.1	D37.02	D49.0
surface (dorsal)	C02.0	C79.89	D00.07	D10.1	D37.02	D49.0
base	C01	C79.89	D00.07	D10.1	D37.02	D49.0
ventral	C02.2	C79.89	D00.07	D10.1	D37.02	D49.0
tip	C02.1	C79.89	D00.07	D10.1	D37.02	D49.0
tonsil	C02.4	C79.89	D00.07	D10.1	D37.02	D49.0
tonsil	C09.9	C79.89	D00.08	D10.4	D37.05	D49.0
fauces, faucial	C09.9	C79.89	D00.08	D10.4	D37.05	D49.0
lingual	C02.4	C79.89	D00.07	D10.1	D37.02	D49.0
overlapping sites	C09.8	—	—	—	—	—
palatine	C09.9	C79.89	D00.08	D10.4	D37.05	D49.0
pharyngeal	C11.1	C79.89	D00.08	D10.6	D37.05	D49.0
pillar (anterior) (posterior)	C09.1	C79.89	D00.08	D10.5	D37.05	D49.0
tonsillar fossa	C09.0	C79.89	D00.08	D10.5	D37.05	D49.0
tooth socket NEC	C03.9	C79.89	D00.03	D10.39	D37.09	D49.0
trachea (cartilage) (mucosa)	C33	C78.39	D02.1	D14.2	D38.1	D49.1
overlapping lesion with bronchus or lung	C34.8-•	—	—	—	—	—
tracheobronchial	C34.8-•	C78.39	D02.1	D14.2	D38.1	D49.1
overlapping lesion with lung	C34.8-•	—	—	—	—	—
tragus — *see also Neoplasm, skin, ear*	C44.20-•	C79.2	D04.2-•	D23.2-•	D48.5	D49.2
trunk NEC	C76.8	C79.89	D04.5	D36.7	D48.7	D49.89
tubo-ovarian	C57.8	C79.82	D07.39	D28.7	D39.8	D49.59
tunica vaginalis	C63.7	C79.82	D07.69	D29.8	D40.8	D49.59

◄ New   ◄ Revised   ~~deleted~~ Deleted   • Use Additional Character(s)

	Malignant Primary	Malignant Secondary	Ca in situ	Benign	Uncertain Behavior	Unspecified Behavior
turbinate (bone)	C41.0	C79.51	—	D16.4-•	D48.0	D49.2
nasal	C30.0	C78.39	D02.3	D14.0	D38.5	D49.1
tympanic cavity	C30.1	C78.39	D02.3	D14.0	D38.5	D49.1
ulna (any part)	C40.0-•	C79.51		D16.0-•	—	—
umbilicus, umbilical — *see also Neoplasm, skin, trunk*	C44.509	C79.2	D04.5	D23.5	D48.5	D49.2
uncus, brain	C71.2	C79.31	—	D33.0	D43.0	D49.6
unknown site or unspecified	C80.1	C79.9	D09.9	D36.9	D48.9	D49.9
urachus	C67.7	C79.11	D09.0	D30.3	D41.4	D49.4
ureter, ureteral	C66.-•	C79.19	D09.19	D30.2-•	D41.2-•	D49.59
orifice (bladder)	C67.6	C79.11	D09.0	D30.3	D41.4	D49.4
ureter-bladder (junction)	C67.6	C79.11	D09.0	D30.3	D41.4	D49.4
urethra, urethral (gland)	C68.0	C79.19	D09.19	D30.4	D41.3	D49.59
orifice, internal	C67.5	C79.11	D09.0	D30.3	D41.4	D49.4
urethrovaginal (septum)	C57.9	C79.82	D07.30	D28.9	D39.8	D49.59
urinary organ or system	C68.9	C79.10	D09.10	D30.9	D41.9	D49.59
bladder — *see Neoplasm, bladder*						
overlapping lesion	C68.8	—	—	—	—	—
specified sites NEC	C68.8	C79.19	D09.19	D30.8	D41.8	D49.59
utero-ovarian	C57.8	C79.82	D07.39	D28.7	D39.8	D49.59
ligament	C57.1	C79.82	D07.39	D28.2	D39.8	D49.59
uterosacral ligament	C57.3	C79.82	—	D28.2	D39.8	D49.59
uterus, uteri, uterine	C55	C79.82	D07.0	D26.9	D39.0	D49.59
adnexa NEC	C57.4	C79.82	D07.39	D28.7	D39.8	D49.59
body	C54.9	C79.82	D07.0	D26.1	D39.0	D49.59
cervix	C53.9	C79.82	D06.9	D26.0	D39.0	D49.59
cornu	C54.9	C79.82	D07.0	D26.1	D39.0	D49.59
corpus	C54.9	C79.82	D07.0	D26.1	D39.0	D49.59
endocervix (canal) (gland)	C53.0	C79.82	D06.0	D26.0	D39.0	D49.59
endometrium	C54.1	C79.82	D07.0	D26.1	D39.0	D49.59
exocervix	C53.1	C79.82	D06.1	D26.0	D39.0	D49.59
external os	C53.1	C79.82	D06.1	D26.0	D39.0	D49.59
fundus	C54.3	C79.82	D07.0	D26.1	D39.0	D49.59
internal os	C53.0	C79.82	D06.0	D26.0	D39.0	D49.59
isthmus	C54.0	C79.82	D07.0	D26.1	D39.0	D49.59
ligament	C57.3	C79.82	—	D28.2	D39.8	D49.59
broad	C57.1	C79.82	D07.39	D28.2	D39.8	D49.59
round	C57.2	C79.82	—	D28.2	D39.8	D49.59
lower segment	C54.0	C79.82	D07.0	D26.1	D39.0	D49.59
myometrium	C54.2	C79.82	D07.0	D26.1	D39.0	D49.59
overlapping sites	C54.8	—	—	—	—	—
squamocolumnar junction	C53.8	C79.82	D06.7	D26.0	D39.0	D49.59
tube	C57.0-•	C79.82	D07.39	D28.2	D39.8	D49.59

	Malignant Primary	Malignant Secondary	Ca in situ	Benign	Uncertain Behavior	Unspecified Behavior
utricle, prostatic	C68.0	C79.19	D09.19	D30.4	D41.3	D49.59
uveal tract	C69.4-•	C79.49	D09.2-•	D31.4-•	D48.7	D49.89
uvula	C05.2	C79.89	D00.04	D10.39	D37.09	D49.0
vagina, vaginal (fornix) (vault) (wall)	C52	C79.82	D07.2	D28.1	D39.8	D49.59
vaginovesical	C57.9	C79.82	D07.30	D28.9	D39.9	D49.59
septum	C57.9	C79.82	D07.30	D28.9	D39.9	D49.59
vallecula (epiglottis)	C10.0	C79.89	D00.08	D10.5	D37.05	D49.0
vas deferens	C63.1-•	C79.82	D07.69	D29.8	D40.8	D49.59
vascular — *see Neoplasm, connective tissue*						
Vater's ampulla	C24.1	C78.89	D01.5	D13.5	D37.6	D49.0
vein, venous — *see Neoplasm, connective tissue*						
vena cava (abdominal) (inferior)	C49.4	C79.89	—	D21.4	D48.1-•	D49.2
superior	C49.3	C79.89	—	D21.3	D48.1-•	D49.2
ventricle (cerebral) (floor) (lateral) (third)	C71.5	C79.31	—	D33.0	D43.0	D49.6
cardiac (left) (right)	C38.0	C79.89		D15.1	D48.7	D49.89
fourth	C71.7	C79.31	—	D33.1	D43.1	D49.6
ventricular band of larynx	C32.1	C78.39	D02.0	D14.1	D38.0	D49.1
ventriculus — *see Neoplasm, stomach*						
vermillion border — *see Neoplasm, lip*						
vermis, cerebellum	C71.6	C79.31	—	D33.1	D43.1	D49.6
vertebra (column)	C41.2	C79.51	—	D16.6	D48.0	D49.2
coccyx	C41.4	C79.51	—	D16.8-•	D48.0	D49.2
marrow NEC	C96.9	C79.52	—	—	D47.9	D49.89
sacrum	C41.4	C79.51	—	D16.8-•	D48.0	D49.2
vesical — *see Neoplasm, bladder*						
vesicle, seminal	C63.7	C79.82	D07.69	D29.8	D40.8	D49.59
vesicocervical tissue	C57.9	C79.82	D07.30	D28.9	D39.9	D49.59
vesicorectal	C76.3	C79.82	D09.8	D36.7	D48.7	D49.89
vesicovaginal	C57.9	C79.82	D07.30	D28.9	D39.9	D49.59
septum	C57.9	C79.82	D07.30	D28.9	D39.8	D49.59
vessel (blood) — *see Neoplasm, connective tissue*						
vestibular gland, greater	C51.0	C79.82	D07.1	D28.0	D39.8	D49.59
vestibule						
mouth	C06.1	C79.89	D00.00	D10.39	D37.09	D49.0
nose	C30.0	C78.39	D02.3	D14.0	D38.5	D49.1
Virchow's gland	C77.0	C77.0	—	D36.0	D48.7	D49.89

	Malignant Primary	Malignant Secondary	Ca in situ	Benign	Uncertain Behavior	Unspecified Behavior
viscera NEC	C76.8	C79.89	D09.8	D36.7	D48.7	D49.89
vocal cords (true)	C32.0	C78.39	D02.0	D14.1	D38.0	D49.1
false	C32.1	C78.39	D02.0	D14.1	D38.0	D49.1
vomer	C41.0	C79.51	—	D16.4-●	D48.0	D49.2
vulva	C51.9	C79.82	D07.1	D28.0	D39.8	D49.59
vulvovaginal gland	C51.0	C79.82	D07.1	D28.0	D39.8	D49.59
Waldeyer's ring	C14.2	C79.89	D00.08	D10.9	D37.05	D49.0
Wharton's duct	C08.0	C79.89	D00.00	D11.7	D37.032	D49.0
white matter (central) (cerebral)	C71.0	C79.31	—	D33.0	D43.0	D49.6

	Malignant Primary	Malignant Secondary	Ca in situ	Benign	Uncertain Behavior	Unspecified Behavior
windpipe	C33	C78.39	D02.1	D14.2	D38.1	D49.1
Wirsung's duct	C25.3	C78.89	D01.7	D13.6	D37.8	D49.0
wolffian (body) (duct)						
female	C57.7	C79.82	D07.39	D28.7	D39.8	D49.59
male	C63.7	C79.82	D07.69	D29.8	D40.8	D49.59
womb — *see Neoplasm, uterus*						
wrist NEC	C76.4-●	C79.89	D04.6-●	D36.7	D48.7	D49.89
xiphoid process	C41.3	C79.51	—	D16.7	D48.0	D49.2
Zuckerkandl organ	C75.5	C79.89	—	D35.6	D44.7	D49.7

◄ New   ◀ Revised   ~~deleted~~ Deleted   ● Use Additional Character(s)

ICD-10-CM
Table of Drugs and Chemicals

Substance	Poisoning, Accidental (Unintentional)	Poisoning, Intentional Self-Harm	Poisoning, Assault	Poisoning, Undetermined	Adverse Effect	Underdosing
#						
1-propanol	T51.3X1	T51.3X2	T51.3X3	T51.3X4	—	—
2-propanol	T51.2X1	T51.2X2	T51.2X3	T51.2X4	—	—
2,4-D (dichlorophen-oxyacetic acid)	T60.3X1	T60.3X2	T60.3X3	T60.3X4	—	—
2,4-toluene diisocyanate	T65.0X1	T65.0X2	T65.0X3	T65.0X4	—	—
2,4,5-T (trichloro-phenoxyacetic acid)	T60.1X1	T60.1X2	T60.1X3	T60.1X4	—	—
3,4-methylenedioxy-methamphetamine	T43.641	T43.642	T43.643	T43.644	—	—
14-hydroxydihydro-morphinone	T40.2X1	T40.2X2	T40.2X3	T40.2X4	T40.2X5	T40.2X6
A						
ABOB	T37.5X1	T37.5X2	T37.5X3	T37.5X4	T37.5X5	T37.5X6
Abrine	T62.2X1	T62.2X2	T62.2X3	T62.2X4		
Abrus (seed)	T62.2X1	T62.2X2	T62.2X3	T62.2X4		
Absinthe	T51.0X1	T51.0X2	T51.0X3	T51.0X4	—	—
beverage	T51.0X1	T51.0X2	T51.0X3	T51.0X4		
Acaricide	T60.8X1	T60.8X2	T60.8X3	T60.8X4		
Acebutolol	T44.7X1	T44.7X2	T44.7X3	T44.7X4	T44.7X5	T44.7X6
Acecarbromal	T42.6X1	T42.6X2	T42.6X3	T42.6X4	T42.6X5	T42.6X6
Aceclidine	T44.1X1	T44.1X2	T44.1X3	T44.1X4	T44.1X5	T44.1X6
Acedapsone	T37.0X1	T37.0X2	T37.0X3	T37.0X4	T37.0X5	T37.0X6
Acefylline piperazine	T48.6X1	T48.6X2	T48.6X3	T48.6X4	T48.6X5	T48.6X6
Acemorphan	T40.2X1	T40.2X2	T40.2X3	T40.2X4	T40.2X5	T40.2X6
Acenocoumarin	T45.511	T45.512	T45.513	T45.514	T45.515	T45.516
Acenocoumarol	T45.511	T45.512	T45.513	T45.514	T45.515	T45.516
Acepifylline	T48.6X1	T48.6X2	T48.6X3	T48.6X4	T48.6X5	T48.6X6
Acepromazine	T43.3X1	T43.3X2	T43.3X3	T43.3X4	T43.3X5	T43.3X6
Acesulfamethoxypyridazine	T37.0X1	T37.0X2	T37.0X3	T37.0X4	T37.0X5	T37.0X6
Acetal	T52.8X1	T52.8X2	T52.8X3	T52.8X4		
Acetaldehyde (vapor)	T52.8X1	T52.8X2	T52.8X3	T52.8X4	—	—
liquid	T65.891	T65.892	T65.893	T65.894	—	—
P-Acetamidophenol	T39.1X1	T39.1X2	T39.1X3	T39.1X4	T39.1X5	T39.1X6
Acetaminophen	T39.1X1	T39.1X2	T39.1X3	T39.1X4	T39.1X5	T39.1X6
Acetaminosalol	T39.1X1	T39.1X2	T39.1X3	T39.1X4	T39.1X5	T39.1X6
Acetanilide	T39.1X1	T39.1X2	T39.1X3	T39.1X4	T39.1X5	T39.1X6
Acetarsol	T37.3X1	T37.3X2	T37.3X3	T37.3X4	T37.3X5	T37.3X6
Acetazolamide	T50.2X1	T50.2X2	T50.2X3	T50.2X4	T50.2X5	T50.2X6
Acetiamine	T45.2X1	T45.2X2	T45.2X3	T45.2X4	T45.2X5	T45.2X6
Acetic						
acid	T54.2X1	T54.2X2	T54.2X3	T54.2X4	—	—
with sodium acetate (ointment)	T49.3X1	T49.3X2	T49.3X3	T49.3X4	T49.3X5	T49.3X6

Substance	Poisoning, Accidental (Unintentional)	Poisoning, Intentional Self-Harm	Poisoning, Assault	Poisoning, Undetermined	Adverse Effect	Underdosing
Acetic (Continued)						
acid (Continued)						
ester (solvent) (vapor)	T52.8X1	T52.8X2	T52.8X3	T52.8X4	—	—
irrigating solution	T50.3X1	T50.3X2	T50.3X3	T50.3X4	T50.3X5	T50.3X6
medicinal (lotion)	T49.2X1	T49.2X2	T49.2X3	T49.2X4	T49.2X5	T49.2X6
anhydride	T65.891	T65.892	T65.893	T65.894	—	—
ether (vapor)	T52.8X1	T52.8X2	T52.8X3	T52.8X4	—	—
Acetohexamide	T38.3X1	T38.3X2	T38.3X3	T38.3X4	T38.3X5	T38.3X6
Acetohydroxamic acid	T50.991	T50.992	T50.993	T50.994	T50.995	T50.996
Acetomenaphthone	T45.7X1	T45.7X2	T45.7X3	T45.7X4	T45.7X5	T45.7X6
Acetomorphine	T40.1X1	T40.1X2	T40.1X3	T40.1X4	—	—
Acetone (oils)	T52.4X1	T52.4X2	T52.4X3	T52.4X4	—	—
chlorinated	T52.4X1	T52.4X2	T52.4X3	T52.4X4	—	—
vapor	T52.4X1	T52.4X2	T52.4X3	T52.4X4	—	—
Acetonitrile	T52.8X1	T52.8X2	T52.8X3	T52.8X4	—	—
Acetophenazine	T43.3X1	T43.3X2	T43.3X3	T43.3X4	T43.3X5	T43.3X6
Acetophenetedin	T39.1X1	T39.1X2	T39.1X3	T39.1X4	T39.1X5	T39.1X6
Acetophenone	T52.4X1	T52.4X2	T52.4X3	T52.4X4	—	—
Acetorphine	T40.2X1	T40.2X2	T40.2X3	T40.2X4	—	—
Acetosulfone (sodium)	T37.1X1	T37.1X2	T37.1X3	T37.1X4	T37.1X5	T37.1X6
Acetrizoate (sodium)	T50.8X1	T50.8X2	T50.8X3	T50.8X4	T50.8X5	T50.8X6
Acetylcarbromal	T42.6X1	T42.6X2	T42.6X3	T42.6X4	T42.6X5	T42.6X6
Acetrizoic acid	T50.8X1	T50.8X2	T50.8X3	T50.8X4	T50.8X5	T50.8X6
Acetyl						
bromide	T53.6X1	T53.6X2	T53.6X3	T53.6X4	—	—
chloride	T53.6X1	T53.6X2	T53.6X3	T53.6X4	—	—
Acetylcholine						
chloride	T44.1X1	T44.1X2	T44.1X3	T44.1X4	T44.1X5	T44.1X6
derivative	T44.1X1	T44.1X2	T44.1X3	T44.1X4	T44.1X5	T44.1X6
Acetylcysteine	T48.4X1	T48.4X2	T48.4X3	T48.4X4	T48.4X5	T48.4X6
Acetyldigitoxin	T46.0X1	T46.0X2	T46.0X3	T46.0X4	T46.0X5	T46.0X6
Acetyldigoxin	T46.0X1	T46.0X2	T46.0X3	T46.0X4	T46.0X5	T46.0X6
Acetyldihydrocodeine	T40.2X1	T40.2X2	T40.2X3	T40.2X4	—	—
Acetyldihydrocodeinone	T40.2X1	T40.2X2	T40.2X3	T40.2X4	—	—
Acetylene (gas)	T59.891	T59.892	T59.893	T59.894	—	—
dichloride	T53.6X1	T53.6X2	T53.6X3	T53.6X4	—	—
incomplete combustion of	T58.11	T58.12	T58.13	T58.14		
industrial	T59.891	T59.892	T59.893	T59.894	—	—
tetrachloride	T53.6X1	T53.6X2	T53.6X3	T53.6X4	—	—
vapor	T53.6X1	T53.6X2	T53.6X3	T53.6X4	—	—
Acetylphenylhydrazine	T39.8X1	T39.8X2	T39.8X3	T39.8X4	T39.8X5	T39.8X6
Acetylpheneturide	T42.6X1	T42.6X2	T42.6X3	T42.6X4	T42.6X5	T42.6X6

Substance	Poisoning, Accidental (Unintentional)	Poisoning, Intentional Self-Harm	Poisoning, Assault	Poisoning, Undetermined	Adverse Effect	Underdosing
Acetylsalicylic acid (salts)	T39.0X1	T39.0X2	T39.0X3	T39.0X4	T39.0X5	T39.0X6
enteric coated	T39.0X1	T39.0X2	T39.0X3	T39.0X4	T39.0X5	T39.0X6
Acetylsulfamethoxypyridazine	T37.0X1	T37.0X2	T37.0X3	T37.0X4	T37.0X5	T37.0X6
Achromycin	T36.4X1	T36.4X2	T36.4X3	T36.4X4	T36.4X5	T36.4X6
ophthalmic preparation	T49.5X1	T49.5X2	T49.5X3	T49.5X4	T49.5X5	T49.5X6
topical NEC	T49.0X1	T49.0X2	T49.0X3	T49.0X4	T49.0X5	T49.0X6
Aciclovir	T37.5X1	T37.5X2	T37.5X3	T37.5X4	T37.5X5	T37.5X6
Acid (corrosive) NEC	T54.2X1	T54.2X2	T54.2X3	T54.2X4	—	—
Acidifying agent NEC	T50.901	T50.902	T50.903	T50.904	T50.905	T50.906
Acipimox	T46.6X1	T46.6X2	T46.6X3	T46.6X4	T46.6X5	T46.6X6
Acitretin	T50.991	T50.992	T50.993	T50.994	T50.995	T50.996
Aclarubicin	T45.1X1	T45.1X2	T45.1X3	T45.1X4	T45.1X5	T45.1X6
Aclatonium napadisilate	T48.1X1	T48.1X2	T48.1X3	T48.1X4	T48.1X5	T48.1X6
Aconite (wild)	T46.991	T46.992	T46.993	T46.994	T46.995	T46.996
Aconitine	T46.991	T46.992	T46.993	T46.994	T46.995	T46.996
Aconitum ferox	T46.991	T46.992	T46.993	T46.994	T46.995	T46.996
Acridine	T65.6X1	T65.6X2	T65.6X3	T65.6X4	—	—
vapor	T59.891	T59.892	T59.893	T59.894	—	—
Acriflavine	T37.91	T37.92	T37.93	T37.94	T37.95	T37.96
Acriflavinium chloride	T49.0X1	T49.0X2	T49.0X3	T49.0X4	T49.0X5	T49.0X6
Acrinol	T49.0X1	T49.0X2	T49.0X3	T49.0X4	T49.0X5	T49.0X6
Acrisorcin	T49.0X1	T49.0X2	T49.0X3	T49.0X4	T49.0X5	T49.0X6
Acrivastine	T45.0X1	T45.0X2	T45.0X3	T45.0X4	T45.0X5	T45.0X6
Acrolein (gas)	T59.891	T59.892	T59.893	T59.894	—	—
liquid	T54.1X1	T54.1X2	T54.1X3	T54.1X4	—	—
Acrylamide	T65.891	T65.892	T65.893	T65.894	—	—
Acrylic resin	T49.3X1	T49.3X2	T49.3X3	T49.3X4	T49.3X5	T49.3X6
Acrylonitrile	T65.891	T65.892	T65.893	T65.894	—	—
Actaea spicata	T62.2X1	T62.2X2	T62.2X3	T62.2X4	—	—
berry	T62.1X1	T62.1X2	T62.1X3	T62.1X4	—	—
Acterol	T37.3X1	T37.3X2	T37.3X3	T37.3X4	T37.3X5	T37.3X6
ACTH	T38.811	T38.812	T38.813	T38.814	T38.815	T38.816
Actinomycin C	T45.1X1	T45.1X2	T45.1X3	T45.1X4	T45.1X5	T45.1X6
Actinomycin D	T45.1X1	T45.1X2	T45.1X3	T45.1X4	T45.1X5	T45.1X6
Activated charcoal — *see also Charcoal, medicinal*	T47.6X1	T47.6X2	T47.6X3	T47.6X4	T47.6X5	T47.6X6
Acyclovir	T37.5X1	T37.5X2	T37.5X3	T37.5X4	T37.5X5	T37.5X6
Adenine	T45.2X1	T45.2X2	T45.2X3	T45.2X4	T45.2X5	T45.2X6
arabinoside	T37.5X1	T37.5X2	T37.5X3	T37.5X4	T37.5X5	T37.5X6
Adenosine (phosphate)	T46.2X1	T46.2X2	T46.2X3	T46.2X4	T46.2X5	T46.2X6
ADH	T38.891	T38.892	T38.893	T38.894	T38.895	T38.896
Adhesive NEC	T65.891	T65.892	T65.893	T65.894	—	—

Substance	Poisoning, Accidental (Unintentional)	Poisoning, Intentional Self-Harm	Poisoning, Assault	Poisoning, Undetermined	Adverse Effect	Underdosing
Adicillin	T36.0X1	T36.0X2	T36.0X3	T36.0X4	T36.0X5	T36.0X6
Adiphenine	T44.3X1	T44.3X2	T44.3X3	T44.3X4	T44.3X5	T44.3X6
Adipiodone	T50.8X1	T50.8X2	T50.8X3	T50.8X4	T50.8X5	T50.8X6
Adjunct, pharmaceutical	T50.901	T50.902	T50.903	T50.904	T50.905	T50.906
Adrenal (extract, cortex or medulla) (glucocorticoids) (hormones) (mineralo corticoids)	T38.0X1	T38.0X2	T38.0X3	T38.0X4	T38.0X5	T38.0X6
ENT agent	T49.6X1	T49.6X2	T49.6X3	T49.6X4	T49.6X5	T49.6X6
ophthalmic preparation	T49.5X1	T49.5X2	T49.5X3	T49.5X4	T49.5X5	T49.5X6
topical NEC	T49.0X1	T49.0X2	T49.0X3	T49.0X4	T49.0X5	T49.0X6
Adrenaline	T44.5X1	T44.5X2	T44.5X3	T44.5X4	T44.5X5	T44.5X6
Adrenalin — *see Adrenaline*						
Adrenergic NEC	T44.901	T44.902	T44.903	T44.904	T44.905	T44.906
blocking agent NEC	T44.8X1	T44.8X2	T44.8X3	T44.8X4	T44.8X5	T44.8X6
beta, heart	T44.7X1	T44.7X2	T44.7X3	T44.7X4	T44.7X5	T44.7X6
specified NEC	T44.991	T44.992	T44.993	T44.994	T44.995	T44.996
Adrenochrome						
(mono) semicarbazone	T46.991	T46.992	T46.993	T46.994	T46.995	T46.996
derivative	T46.991	T46.992	T46.993	T46.994	T46.995	T46.996
Adrenocorticotrophic hormone	T38.811	T38.812	T38.813	T38.814	T38.815	T38.816
Adrenocorticotrophin	T38.811	T38.812	T38.813	T38.814	T38.815	T38.816
Adriamycin	T45.1X1	T45.1X2	T45.1X3	T45.1X4	T45.1X5	T45.1X6
Aerosol spray NEC	T65.91	T65.92	T65.93	T65.94	—	—
Aerosporin	T36.8X1	T36.8X2	T36.8X3	T36.8X4	T36.8X5	T36.8X6
ENT agent	T49.6X1	T49.6X2	T49.6X3	T49.6X4	T49.6X5	T49.6X6
ophthalmic preparation	T49.5X1	T49.5X2	T49.5X3	T49.5X4	T49.5X5	T49.5X6
topical NEC	T49.0X1	T49.0X2	T49.0X3	T49.0X4	T49.0X5	T49.0X6
Aethusa cynapium	T62.2X1	T62.2X2	T62.2X3	T62.2X4	—	—
Afghanistan black	T40.711	T40.712	T40.713	T40.714	T40.715	T40.716
Aflatoxin	T64.01	T64.02	T64.03	T64.04	—	—
Afloqualone	T42.8X1	T42.8X2	T42.8X3	T42.8X4	T42.8X5	T42.8X6
African boxwood	T62.2X1	T62.2X2	T62.2X3	T62.2X4	—	—
Agar	T47.4X1	T47.4X2	T47.4X3	T47.4X4	T47.4X5	T47.4X6
Agonist						
predominantly						
alpha-adrenoreceptor	T44.4X1	T44.4X2	T44.4X3	T44.4X4	T44.4X5	T44.4X6
beta-adrenoreceptor	T44.5X1	T44.5X2	T44.5X3	T44.5X4	T44.5X5	T44.5X6
Agricultural agent NEC	T65.91	T65.92	T65.93	T65.94	—	—
Agrypnal	T42.3X1	T42.3X2	T42.3X3	T42.3X4	T42.3X5	T42.3X6
AHLG	T50.Z11	T50.Z12	T50.Z13	T50.Z14	T50.Z15	T50.Z16
Air contaminant(s), source/type NOS	T65.91	T65.92	T65.93	T65.94	—	—

◄ New   ◄ Revised   ~~deleted~~ Deleted

Substance	External Cause (T-Code)					
	Poisoning, Accidental (Unintentional)	Poisoning, Intentional Self-Harm	Poisoning, Assault	Poisoning, Undetermined	Adverse Effect	Underdosing
Ajmaline	T46.2X1	T46.2X2	T46.2X3	T46.2X4	T46.2X5	T46.2X6
Akritoin	T37.8X1	T37.8X2	T37.8X3	T37.8X4	T37.8X5	T37.8X6
Akee	T62.1X1	T62.1X2	T62.1X3	T62.1X4	—	—
Akrinol	T49.0X1	T49.0X2	T49.0X3	T49.0X4	T49.0X5	T49.0X6
Alacepril	T46.4X1	T46.4X2	T46.4X3	T46.4X4	T46.4X5	T46.4X6
Alantolactone	T37.4X1	T37.4X2	T37.4X3	T37.4X4	T37.4X5	T37.4X6
Albamycin	T36.8X1	T36.8X2	T36.8X3	T36.8X4	T36.8X5	T36.8X6
Albendazole	T37.4X1	T37.4X2	T37.4X3	T37.4X4	T37.4X5	T37.4X6
Albumin						
bovine	T45.8X1	T45.8X2	T45.8X3	T45.8X4	T45.8X5	T45.8X6
human serum	T45.8X1	T45.8X2	T45.8X3	T45.8X4	T45.8X5	T45.8X6
salt-poor	T45.8X1	T45.8X2	T45.8X3	T45.8X4	T45.8X5	T45.8X6
normal human serum	T45.8X1	T45.8X2	T45.8X3	T45.8X4	T45.8X5	T45.8X6
Albuterol	T48.6X1	T48.6X2	T48.6X3	T48.6X4	T48.6X5	T48.6X6
Albutoin	T42.0X1	T42.0X2	T42.0X3	T42.0X4	T42.0X5	T42.0X6
Alclometasone	T49.0X1	T49.0X2	T49.0X3	T49.0X4	T49.0X5	T49.0X6
Alcohol	T51.91	T51.92	T51.93	T51.94	—	—
absolute	T51.0X1	T51.0X2	T51.0X3	T51.0X4	—	—
beverage	T51.0X1	T51.0X2	T51.0X3	T51.0X4	—	—
allyl	T51.8X1	T51.8X2	T51.8X3	T51.8X4	—	—
amyl	T51.3X1	T51.3X2	T51.3X3	T51.3X4	—	—
antifreeze	T51.1X1	T51.1X2	T51.1X3	T51.1X4	—	—
beverage	T51.0X1	T51.0X2	T51.0X3	T51.0X4	—	—
butyl	T51.3X1	T51.3X2	T51.3X3	T51.3X4	—	—
dehydrated	T51.0X1	T51.0X2	T51.0X3	T51.0X4	—	—
beverage	T51.0X1	T51.0X2	T51.0X3	T51.0X4	—	—
denatured	T51.0X1	T51.0X2	T51.0X3	T51.0X4	—	—
deterrent NEC	T50.6X1	T50.6X2	T50.6X3	T50.6X4	T50.6X5	T50.6X6
diagnostic (gastric function)	T50.8X1	T50.8X2	T50.8X3	T50.8X4	T50.8X5	T50.8X6
ethyl	T51.0X1	T51.0X2	T51.0X3	T51.0X4	—	—
beverage	T51.0X1	T51.0X2	T51.0X3	T51.0X4	—	—
grain	T51.0X1	T51.0X2	T51.0X3	T51.0X4	—	—
beverage	T51.0X1	T51.0X2	T51.0X3	T51.0X4	—	—
industrial	T51.0X1	T51.0X2	T51.0X3	T51.0X4	—	—
isopropyl	T51.2X1	T51.2X2	T51.2X3	T51.2X4	—	—
methyl	T51.1X1	T51.1X2	T51.1X3	T51.1X4	—	—
preparation for consumption	T51.0X1	T51.0X2	T51.0X3	T51.0X4	—	—
propyl	T51.3X1	T51.3X2	T51.3X3	T51.3X4	—	—
secondary	T51.2X1	T51.2X2	T51.2X3	T51.2X4	—	—
radiator	T51.1X1	T51.1X2	T51.1X3	T51.1X4	—	—
rubbing	T51.2X1	T51.2X2	T51.2X3	T51.2X4	—	—
specified type NEC	T51.8X1	T51.8X2	T51.8X3	T51.8X4	—	—

Substance	External Cause (T-Code)					
	Poisoning, Accidental (Unintentional)	Poisoning, Intentional Self-Harm	Poisoning, Assault	Poisoning, Undetermined	Adverse Effect	Underdosing
Alcohol *(Continued)*						
surgical	T51.0X1	T51.0X2	T51.0X3	T51.0X4	—	—
vapor (from any type of Alcohol)	T59.891	T59.892	T59.893	T59.894	—	—
wood	T51.1X1	T51.1X2	T51.1X3	T51.1X4	—	—
Alcuronium (chloride)	T48.1X1	T48.1X2	T48.1X3	T48.1X4	T48.1X5	T48.1X6
Aldactone	T50.0X1	T50.0X2	T50.0X3	T50.0X4	T50.0X5	T50.0X6
Aldesulfone sodium	T37.1X1	T37.1X2	T37.1X3	T37.1X4	T37.1X5	T37.1X6
Aldicarb	T60.0X1	T60.0X2	T60.0X3	T60.0X4	—	—
Aldomet	T46.5X1	T46.5X2	T46.5X3	T46.5X4	T46.5X5	T46.5X6
Aldosterone	T50.0X1	T50.0X2	T50.0X3	T50.0X4	T50.0X5	T50.0X6
Aldrin (dust)	T60.1X1	T60.1X2	T60.1X3	T60.1X4	—	—
Aleve — *see Naproxen*						
Alexitol sodium	T47.1X1	T47.1X2	T47.1X3	T47.1X4	T47.1X5	T47.1X6
Alfacalcidol	T45.2X1	T45.2X2	T45.2X3	T45.2X4	T45.2X5	T45.2X6
Alfadolone	T41.1X1	T41.1X2	T41.1X3	T41.1X4	T41.1X5	T41.1X6
Alfaxalone	T41.1X1	T41.1X2	T41.1X3	T41.1X4	T41.1X5	T41.1X6
Alfentanil	T40.411	T40.412	T40.413	T40.414	T40.415	T40.416
Alfuzosin (hydrochloride)	T44.8X1	T44.8X2	T44.8X3	T44.8X4	T44.8X5	T44.8X6
Algae (harmful) (toxin)	T65.821	T65.822	T65.823	T65.824	—	—
Algeldrate	T47.1X1	T47.1X2	T47.1X3	T47.1X4	T47.1X5	T47.1X6
Algin	T47.8X1	T47.8X2	T47.8X3	T47.8X4	T47.8X5	T47.8X6
Alglucerase	T45.3X1	T45.3X2	T45.3X3	T45.3X4	T45.3X5	T45.3X6
Alidase	T45.3X1	T45.3X2	T45.3X3	T45.3X4	T45.3X5	T45.3X6
Alimemazine	T43.3X1	T43.3X2	T43.3X3	T43.3X4	T43.3X5	T43.3X6
Aliphatic thiocyanates	T65.0X1	T65.0X2	T65.0X3	T65.0X4	—	—
Alizapride	T45.0X1	T45.0X2	T45.0X3	T45.0X4	T45.0X5	T45.0X6
Alkali (caustic)	T54.3X1	T54.3X2	T54.3X3	T54.3X4	—	—
Alkalizing agent NEC	T50.901	T50.902	T50.903	T50.904	T50.905	T50.906
Alkaline antiseptic solution (aromatic)	T49.6X1	T49.6X2	T49.6X3	T49.6X4	T49.6X5	T49.6X6
Alkalinizing agents (medicinal)	T50.901	T50.902	T50.903	T50.904	T50.905	T50.906
Alka-seltzer	T39.011	T39.012	T39.013	T39.014	T39.015	T39.016
Alkavervir	T46.5X1	T46.5X2	T46.5X3	T46.5X4	T46.5X5	T46.5X6
Alkonium (bromide)	T49.0X1	T49.0X2	T49.0X3	T49.0X4	T49.0X5	T49.0X6
Alkylating drug NEC	T45.1X1	T45.1X2	T45.1X3	T45.1X4	T45.1X5	T45.1X6
antimyeloproliferative	T45.1X1	T45.1X2	T45.1X3	T45.1X4	T45.1X5	T45.1X6
lymphatic	T45.1X1	T45.1X2	T45.1X3	T45.1X4	T45.1X5	T45.1X6
Alkylisocyanate	T65.0X1	T65.0X2	T65.0X3	T65.0X4	—	—
Allantoin	T49.411	T49.412	T49.413	T49.414	T49.415	T49.416
Allegron	T43.0X1	T43.0X2	T43.0X3	T43.0X4	T43.0X5	T43.0X6
Allethrin	T49.0X1	T49.0X2	T49.0X3	T49.0X4	T49.0X5	T49.0X6
Allobarbital	T42.3X1	T42.3X2	T42.3X3	T42.3X4	T42.3X5	T42.3X6

Substance	Poisoning, Accidental (Unintentional)	Poisoning, Intentional Self-Harm	Poisoning, Assault	Poisoning, Undetermined	Adverse Effect	Underdosing
Allopurinol	T50.4X1	T50.4X2	T50.4X3	T50.4X4	T50.4X5	T50.4X6
Allyl						
alcohol	T51.8X1	T51.8X2	T51.8X3	T51.8X4	—	—
disulfide	T46.6X1	T46.6X2	T46.6X3	T46.6X4	T46.6X5	T46.6X6
Allylestrenol	T38.5X1	T38.5X2	T38.5X3	T38.5X4	T38.5X5	T38.5X6
Allylisopropylacetylurea	T42.6X1	T42.6X2	T42.6X3	T42.6X4	T42.6X5	T42.6X6
Allylisopropylmalonylurea	T42.3X1	T42.3X2	T42.3X3	T42.3X4	T42.3X5	T42.3X6
Allylthiourea	T49.3X1	T49.3X2	T49.3X3	T49.3X4	T49.3X5	T49.3X6
Allyltribromide	T42.6X1	T42.6X2	T42.6X3	T42.6X4	T42.6X5	T42.6X6
Allypropymal	T42.3X1	T42.3X2	T42.3X3	T42.3X4	T42.3X5	T42.3X6
Almagate	T47.1X1	T47.1X2	T47.1X3	T47.1X4	T47.1X5	T47.1X6
Almasilate	T47.1X1	T47.1X2	T47.1X3	T47.1X4	T47.1X5	T47.1X6
Almitrine	T50.7X1	T50.7X2	T50.7X3	T50.7X4	T50.7X5	T50.7X6
Aloes	T47.2X1	T47.2X2	T47.2X3	T47.2X4	T47.2X5	T47.2X6
Aloglutamol	T47.1X1	T47.1X2	T47.1X3	T47.1X4	T47.1X5	T47.1X6
Aloin	T47.2X1	T47.2X2	T47.2X3	T47.2X4	T47.2X5	T47.2X6
Aloxidone	T42.2X1	T42.2X2	T42.2X3	T42.2X4	T42.2X5	T42.2X6
Alpha						
acetyldigoxin	T46.0X1	T46.0X2	T46.0X3	T46.0X4	T46.0X5	T46.0X6
adrenergic blocking drug	T44.6X1	T44.6X2	T44.6X3	T44.6X4	T44.6X5	T44.6X6
amylase	T45.3X1	T45.3X2	T45.3X3	T45.3X4	T45.3X5	T45.3X6
tocoferol (acetate)	T45.2X1	T45.2X2	T45.2X3	T45.2X4	T45.2X5	T45.2X6
tocopherol	T45.2X1	T45.2X2	T45.2X3	T45.2X4	T45.2X5	T45.2X6
Alphadolone	T41.1X1	T41.1X2	T41.1X3	T41.1X4	T41.1X5	T41.1X6
Alphaprodine	T40.491	T40.492	T40.493	T40.494	T40.495	T40.496
Alphaxalone	T41.1X1	T41.1X2	T41.1X3	T41.1X4	T41.1X5	T41.1X6
Alprazolam	T42.4X1	T42.4X2	T42.4X3	T42.4X4	T42.4X5	T42.4X6
Alprenolol	T44.7X1	T44.7X2	T44.7X3	T44.7X4	T44.7X5	T44.7X6
Alprostadil	T46.7X1	T46.7X2	T46.7X3	T46.7X4	T46.7X5	T46.7X6
Alsactide	T38.811	T38.812	T38.813	T38.814	T38.815	T38.816
Alseroxylon	T46.5X1	T46.5X2	T46.5X3	T46.5X4	T46.5X5	T46.5X6
Alteplase	T45.611	T45.612	T45.613	T45.614	T45.615	T45.616
Altizide	T50.2X1	T50.2X2	T50.2X3	T50.2X4	T50.2X5	T50.2X6
Altretamine	T45.1X1	T45.1X2	T45.1X3	T45.1X4	T45.1X5	T45.1X6
Alum (medicinal)	T49.4X1	T49.4X2	T49.4X3	T49.4X4	T49.4X5	T49.4X6
nonmedicinal (ammonium) (potassium)	T56.891	T56.892	T56.893	T56.894	—	—
Aluminium, aluminum						
acetate	T49.2X1	T49.2X2	T49.2X3	T49.2X4	T49.2X5	T49.2X6
solution	T49.0X1	T49.0X2	T49.0X3	T49.0X4	T49.0X5	T49.0X6
aspirin	T39.011	T39.012	T39.013	T39.014	T39.015	T39.016
bis (acetylsalicylate)	T39.011	T39.012	T39.013	T39.014	T39.015	T39.016

Substance	Poisoning, Accidental (Unintentional)	Poisoning, Intentional Self-Harm	Poisoning, Assault	Poisoning, Undetermined	Adverse Effect	Underdosing
Aluminium, aluminum (Continued)						
carbonate (gel, basic)	T47.1X1	T47.1X2	T47.1X3	T47.1X4	T47.1X5	T47.1X6
chlorhydroxide-complex	T47.1X1	T47.1X2	T47.1X3	T47.1X4	T47.1X5	T47.1X6
chloride	T49.2X1	T49.2X2	T49.2X3	T49.2X4	T49.2X5	T49.2X6
clofibrate	T46.6X1	T46.6X2	T46.6X3	T46.6X4	T46.6X5	T46.6X6
diacetate	T49.2X1	T49.2X2	T49.2X3	T49.2X4	T49.2X5	T49.2X6
glycinate	T47.1X1	T47.1X2	T47.1X3	T47.1X4	T47.1X5	T47.1X6
hydroxide (gel)	T47.1X1	T47.1X2	T47.1X3	T47.1X4	T47.1X5	T47.1X6
hydroxide-magnesium carb. gel	T47.1X1	T47.1X2	T47.1X3	T47.1X4	T47.1X5	T47.1X6
magnesium silicate	T47.1X1	T47.1X2	T47.1X3	T47.1X4	T47.1X5	T47.1X6
nicotinate	T46.7X1	T46.7X2	T46.7X3	T46.7X4	T46.7X5	T46.7X6
ointment (surgical) (topical)	T49.3X1	T49.3X2	T49.3X3	T49.3X4	T49.3X5	T49.3X6
phosphate	T47.1X1	T47.1X2	T47.1X3	T47.1X4	T47.1X5	T47.1X6
salicylate	T39.091	T39.092	T39.093	T39.094	T39.095	T39.096
silicate	T47.1X1	T47.1X2	T47.1X3	T47.1X4	T47.1X5	T47.1X6
sodium silicate	T47.1X1	T47.1X2	T47.1X3	T47.1X4	T47.1X5	T47.1X6
subacetate	T49.2X1	T49.2X2	T49.2X3	T49.2X4	T49.2X5	T49.2X6
sulfate	T49.0X1	T49.0X2	T49.0X3	T49.0X4	T49.0X5	T49.0X6
tannate	T47.6X1	T47.6X2	T47.6X3	T47.6X4	T47.6X5	T47.6X6
topical NEC	T49.3X1	T49.3X2	T49.3X3	T49.3X4	T49.3X5	T49.3X6
Alurate	T42.3X1	T42.3X2	T42.3X3	T42.3X4	T42.3X5	T42.3X6
Alverine	T44.3X1	T44.3X2	T44.3X3	T44.3X4	T44.3X5	T44.3X6
Alvodine	T40.2X1	T40.2X2	T40.2X3	T40.2X4	T40.2X5	T40.2X6
Amanita phalloides	T62.0X1	T62.0X2	T62.0X3	T62.0X4	—	—
Amanitine	T62.0X1	T62.0X2	T62.0X3	T62.0X4	—	—
Amantadine	T42.8X1	T42.8X2	T42.8X3	T42.8X4	T42.8X5	T42.8X6
Ambazone	T49.6X1	T49.6X2	T49.6X3	T49.6X4	T49.6X5	T49.6X6
Ambenonium (chloride)	T44.0X1	T44.0X2	T44.0X3	T44.0X4	T44.0X5	T44.0X6
Ambroxol	T48.4X1	T48.4X2	T48.4X3	T48.4X4	T48.4X5	T48.4X6
Ambuphylline	T48.6X1	T48.6X2	T48.6X3	T48.6X4	T48.6X5	T48.6X6
Ambutonium bromide	T44.3X1	T44.3X2	T44.3X3	T44.3X4	T44.3X5	T44.3X6
Amcinonide	T49.0X1	T49.0X2	T49.0X3	T49.0X4	T49.0X5	T49.0X6
Amdinocilline	T36.0X1	T36.0X2	T36.0X3	T36.0X4	T36.0X5	T36.0X6
Ametazole	T50.8X1	T50.8X2	T50.8X3	T50.8X4	T50.8X5	T50.8X6
Amethocaine	T41.3X1	T41.3X2	T41.3X3	T41.3X4	T41.3X5	T41.3X6
regional	T41.3X1	T41.3X2	T41.3X3	T41.3X4	T41.3X5	T41.3X6
spinal	T41.3X1	T41.3X2	T41.3X3	T41.3X4	T41.3X5	T41.3X6
Amethopterin	T45.1X1	T45.1X2	T45.1X3	T45.1X4	T45.1X5	T45.1X6
Amezinium metilsulfate	T44.991	T44.992	T44.993	T44.994	T44.995	T44.996
Amfebutamone	T43.291	T43.292	T43.293	T43.294	T43.295	T43.296
Amfepramone	T50.5X1	T50.5X2	T50.5X3	T50.5X4	T50.5X5	T50.5X6

Substance	Poisoning, Accidental (Unintentional)	Poisoning, Intentional Self-Harm	Poisoning, Assault	Poisoning, Undetermined	Adverse Effect	Underdosing
Amfetamine	T43.621	T43.622	T43.623	T43.624	T43.625	T43.626
Amfetaminil	T43.621	T43.622	T43.623	T43.624	T43.625	T43.626
Amfomycin	T36.8X1	T36.8X2	T36.8X3	T36.8X4	T36.8X5	T36.8X6
Amidefrine mesilate	T48.5X1	T48.5X2	T48.5X3	T48.5X4	T48.5X5	T48.5X6
Amidone	T40.3X1	T40.3X2	T40.3X3	T40.3X4	T40.3X5	T40.3X6
Amidopyrine	T39.2X1	T39.2X2	T39.2X3	T39.2X4	T39.2X5	T39.2X6
Amidotrizoate	T50.8X1	T50.8X2	T50.8X3	T50.8X4	T50.8X5	T50.8X6
Amiflamine	T43.1X1	T43.1X2	T43.1X3	T43.1X4	T43.1X5	T43.1X6
Amikacin	T36.5X1	T36.5X2	T36.5X3	T36.5X4	T36.5X5	T36.5X6
Amikhelline	T46.3X1	T46.3X2	T46.3X3	T46.3X4	T46.3X5	T46.3X6
Amiloride	T50.2X1	T50.2X2	T50.2X3	T50.2X4	T50.2X5	T50.2X6
Aminacrine	T49.0X1	T49.0X2	T49.0X3	T49.0X4	T49.0X5	T49.0X6
Amineptine	T43.011	T43.012	T43.013	T43.014	T43.015	T43.016
Aminitrozole	T37.3X1	T37.3X2	T37.3X3	T37.3X4	T37.3X5	T37.3X6
Aminoacetic acid (derivatives)	T50.3X1	T50.3X2	T50.3X3	T50.3X4	T50.3X5	T50.3X6
Amino acids	T50.3X1	T50.3X2	T50.3X3	T50.3X4	T50.3X5	T50.3X6
Aminoacridine	T49.0X1	T49.0X2	T49.0X3	T49.0X4	T49.0X5	T49.0X6
Aminobenzoic acid (-p)	T49.3X1	T49.3X2	T49.3X3	T49.3X4	T49.3X5	T49.3X6
4-Aminobutyric acid	T43.8X1	T43.8X2	T43.8X3	T43.8X4	T43.8X5	T43.8X6
Aminocaproic acid	T45.621	T45.622	T45.623	T45.624	T45.625	T45.626
Aminofenazone	T39.2X1	T39.2X2	T39.2X3	T39.2X4	T39.2X5	T39.2X6
Aminoethylisothiourium	T45.8X1	T45.8X2	T45.8X3	T45.8X4	T45.8X5	T45.8X6
Aminoglutethimide	T45.1X1	T45.1X2	T45.1X3	T45.1X4	T45.1X5	T45.1X6
Aminohippuric acid	T50.8X1	T50.8X2	T50.8X3	T50.8X4	T50.8X5	T50.8X6
Aminomethylbenzoic acid	T45.691	T45.692	T45.693	T45.694	T45.695	T45.696
Aminometradine	T50.2X1	T50.2X2	T50.2X3	T50.2X4	T50.2X5	T50.2X6
Aminopentamide	T44.3X1	T44.3X2	T44.3X3	T44.3X4	T44.3X5	T44.3X6
Aminophenazone	T39.2X1	T39.2X2	T39.2X3	T39.2X4	T39.2X5	T39.2X6
Aminophenol	T54.0X1	T54.0X2	T54.0X3	T54.0X4	—	—
4-Aminophenol derivatives	T39.1X1	T39.1X2	T39.1X3	T39.1X4	T39.1X5	T39.1X6
Aminophenylpyridone	T43.591	T43.592	T43.593	T43.594	T43.595	T43.596
Aminophylline	T48.6X1	T48.6X2	T48.6X3	T48.6X4	T48.6X5	T48.6X6
Aminopterin sodium	T45.1X1	T45.1X2	T45.1X3	T45.1X4	T45.1X5	T45.1X6
Aminopyrine	T39.2X1	T39.2X2	T39.2X3	T39.2X4	T39.2X5	T39.2X6
8-Aminoquinoline drugs	T37.2X1	T37.2X2	T37.2X3	T37.2X4	T37.2X5	T37.2X6
Aminorex	T50.5X1	T50.5X2	T50.5X3	T50.5X4	T50.5X5	T50.5X6
Aminosalicylic acid	T37.1X1	T37.1X2	T37.1X3	T37.1X4	T37.1X5	T37.1X6
Aminosalylum	T37.1X1	T37.1X2	T37.1X3	T37.1X4	T37.1X5	T37.1X6
Amiodarone	T46.2X1	T46.2X2	T46.2X3	T46.2X4	T46.2X5	T46.2X6
Amiphenazole	T50.7X1	T50.7X2	T50.7X3	T50.7X4	T50.7X5	T50.7X6
Amiquinsin	T46.5X1	T46.5X2	T46.5X3	T46.5X4	T46.5X5	T46.5X6
Amisometradine	T50.2X1	T50.2X2	T50.2X3	T50.2X4	T50.2X5	T50.2X6

Substance	Poisoning, Accidental (Unintentional)	Poisoning, Intentional Self-Harm	Poisoning, Assault	Poisoning, Undetermined	Adverse Effect	Underdosing
Amisulpride	T43.591	T43.592	T43.593	T43.594	T43.595	T43.596
Amitriptyline	T43.021	T43.022	T43.023	T43.024	T43.025	T43.026
Amitriptylinoxide	T43.021	T43.022	T43.023	T43.024	T43.025	T43.026
Amlexanox	T48.6X1	T48.6X2	T48.6X3	T48.6X4	T48.6X5	T48.6X6
Ammonia (fumes) (gas) (vapor)	T59.891	T59.892	T59.893	T59.894	—	—
aromatic spirit	T48.991	T48.992	T48.993	T48.994	T48.995	T48.996
liquid (household)	T54.3X1	T54.3X2	T54.3X3	T54.3X4	—	—
Ammoniated mercury	T49.0X1	T49.0X2	T49.0X3	T49.0X4	T49.0X5	T49.0X6
Ammonium						
acid tartrate	T49.5X1	T49.5X2	T49.5X3	T49.5X4	T49.5X5	T49.5X6
bromide	T42.6X1	T42.6X2	T42.6X3	T42.6X4	T42.6X5	T42.6X6
carbonate	T54.3X1	T54.3X2	T54.3X3	T54.3X4	—	—
chloride	T50.991	T50.992	T50.993	T50.994	T50.995	T50.996
expectorant	T48.4X1	T48.4X2	T48.4X3	T48.4X4	T48.4X5	T48.4X6
compounds (household) NEC	T54.3X1	T54.3X2	T54.3X3	T54.3X4	—	—
fumes (any usage)	T59.891	T59.892	T59.893	T59.894	—	—
industrial	T54.3X1	T54.3X2	T54.3X3	T54.3X4	—	—
ichthyosulronate	T49.4X1	T49.4X2	T49.4X3	T49.4X4	T49.4X5	T49.4X6
mandelate	T37.91	T37.92	T37.93	T37.94	T37.95	T37.96
sulfamate	T60.3X1	T60.3X2	T60.3X3	T60.3X4	—	—
sulfonate resin	T47.8X1	T47.8X2	T47.8X3	T47.8X4	T47.8X5	T47.8X6
Amobarbital (sodium)	T42.3X1	T42.3X2	T42.3X3	T42.3X4	T42.3X5	T42.3X6
Amodiaquine	T37.2X1	T37.2X2	T37.2X3	T37.2X4	T37.2X5	T37.2X6
Amopyroquin(e)	T37.2X1	T37.2X2	T37.2X3	T37.2X4	T37.2X5	T37.2X6
Amoxapine	T43.011	T43.012	T43.013	T43.014	T43.015	T43.016
Amoxicillin	T36.0X1	T36.0X2	T36.0X3	T36.0X4	T36.0X5	T36.0X6
Amperozide	T43.591	T43.592	T43.593	T43.594	T43.595	T43.596
Amphenidone	T43.591	T43.592	T43.593	T43.594	T43.595	T43.596
Amphetamine NEC	T43.621	T43.622	T43.623	T43.624	T43.625	T43.626
Amphomycin	T36.8X1	T36.8X2	T36.8X3	T36.8X4	T36.8X5	T36.8X6
Amphotalide	T37.4X1	T37.4X2	T37.4X3	T37.4X4	T37.4X5	T37.4X6
Amphotericin B	T36.7X1	T36.7X2	T36.7X3	T36.7X4	T36.7X5	T36.7X6
topical	T49.0X1	T49.0X2	T49.0X3	T49.0X4	T49.0X5	T49.0X6
Ampicillin	T36.0X1	T36.0X2	T36.0X3	T36.0X4	T36.0X5	T36.0X6
Amprotropine	T44.3X1	T44.3X2	T44.3X3	T44.3X4	T44.3X5	T44.3X6
Amsacrine	T45.1X1	T45.1X2	T45.1X3	T45.1X4	T45.1X5	T45.1X6
Amygdaline	T62.2X1	T62.2X2	T62.2X3	T62.2X4	—	—
Amyl						
acetate	T52.8X1	T52.8X2	T52.8X3	T52.8X4	—	—
vapor	T59.891	T59.892	T59.893	T59.894	—	—
alcohol	T51.3X1	T51.3X2	T51.3X3	T51.3X4	—	—
chloride	T53.6X1	T53.6X2	T53.6X3	T53.6X4	—	—

Substance	Poisoning, Accidental (Unintentional)	Poisoning, Intentional Self-Harm	Poisoning, Assault	Poisoning, Undetermined	Adverse Effect	Underdosing
Amyl *(Continued)*						
formate	T52.8X1	T52.8X2	T52.8X3	T52.8X4	—	—
nitrite	T46.3X1	T46.3X2	T46.3X3	T46.3X4	T46.3X5	T46.3X6
propionate	T65.891	T65.892	T65.893	T65.894	—	—
Amylase	T47.5X1	T47.5X2	T47.5X3	T47.5X4	T47.5X5	T47.5X6
Amyleine, regional	T41.3X1	T41.3X2	T41.3X3	T41.3X4	T41.3X5	T41.3X6
Amylene						
dichloride	T53.6X1	T53.6X2	T53.6X3	T53.6X4	—	—
hydrate	T51.3X1	T51.3X2	T51.3X3	T51.3X4	—	—
Amylmetacresol	T49.6X1	T49.6X2	T49.6X3	T49.6X4	T49.6X5	T49.6X6
Amylobarbitone	T42.3X1	T42.3X2	T42.3X3	T42.3X4	T42.3X5	T42.3X6
Amylocaine, regional	T41.3X1	T41.3X2	T41.3X3	T41.3X4	T41.3X5	T41.3X6
infiltration (subcutaneous)	T41.3X1	T41.3X2	T41.3X3	T41.3X4	T41.3X5	T41.3X6
nerve block (peripheral) (plexus)	T41.3X1	T41.3X2	T41.3X3	T41.3X4	T41.3X5	T41.3X6
spinal	T41.3X1	T41.3X2	T41.3X3	T41.3X4	T41.3X5	T41.3X6
topical (surface)	T41.3X1	T41.3X2	T41.3X3	T41.3X4	T41.3X5	T41.3X6
Amylopectin	T47.6X1	T47.6X2	T47.6X3	T47.6X4	T47.6X5	T47.6X6
Amytal (sodium)	T42.3X1	T42.3X2	T42.3X3	T42.3X4	T42.3X5	T42.3X6
Anabolic steroid	T38.7X1	T38.7X2	T38.7X3	T38.7X4	T38.7X5	T38.7X6
Analeptic NEC	T50.7X1	T50.7X2	T50.7X3	T50.7X4	T50.7X5	T50.7X6
Analgesic	T39.91	T39.92	T39.93	T39.94	T39.95	T39.96
anti-inflammatory NEC	T39.91	T39.92	T39.93	T39.94	T39.95	T39.96
propionic acid derivative	T39.311	T39.312	T39.313	T39.314	T39.315	T39.316
antirheumatic NEC	T39.4X1	T39.4X2	T39.4X3	T39.4X4	T39.4X5	T39.4X6
aromatic NEC	T39.1X1	T39.1X2	T39.1X3	T39.1X4	T39.1X5	T39.1X6
narcotic NEC	T40.601	T40.602	T40.603	T40.604	T40.605	T40.606
combination	T40.601	T40.602	T40.603	T40.604	T40.605	T40.606
obstetric	T40.601	T40.602	T40.603	T40.604	T40.605	T40.606
non-narcotic NEC	T39.91	T39.92	T39.93	T39.94	T39.95	T39.96
combination	T39.91	T39.92	T39.93	T39.94	T39.95	T39.96
pyrazole	T39.2X1	T39.2X2	T39.2X3	T39.2X4	T39.2X5	T39.2X6
specified NEC	T39.8X1	T39.8X2	T39.8X3	T39.8X4	T39.8X5	T39.8X6
Analgin	T39.2X1	T39.2X2	T39.2X3	T39.2X4	T39.2X5	T39.2X6
Anamirta cocculus	T62.1X1	T62.1X2	T62.1X3	T62.1X4	—	—
Ancillin	T36.0X1	T36.0X2	T36.0X3	T36.0X4	T36.0X5	T36.0X6
Ancrod	T45.691	T45.692	T45.693	T45.694	T45.695	T45.696
Androgen	T38.7X1	T38.7X2	T38.7X3	T38.7X4	T38.7X5	T38.7X6
Androgen-estrogen mixture	T38.7X1	T38.7X2	T38.7X3	T38.7X4	T38.7X5	T38.7X6
Androstalone	T38.7X1	T38.7X2	T38.7X3	T38.7X4	T38.7X5	T38.7X6
Androstanolone	T38.7X1	T38.7X2	T38.7X3	T38.7X4	T38.7X5	T38.7X6
Androsterone	T38.7X1	T38.7X2	T38.7X3	T38.7X4	T38.7X5	T38.7X6

Substance	Poisoning, Accidental (Unintentional)	Poisoning, Intentional Self-Harm	Poisoning, Assault	Poisoning, Undetermined	Adverse Effect	Underdosing
Anemone pulsatilla	T62.2X1	T62.2X2	T62.2X3	T62.2X4	—	—
Anesthesia						
caudal	T41.3X1	T41.3X2	T41.3X3	T41.3X4	T41.3X5	T41.3X6
endotracheal	T41.0X1	T41.0X2	T41.0X3	T41.0X4	T41.0X5	T41.0X6
epidural	T41.3X1	T41.3X2	T41.3X3	T41.3X4	T41.3X5	T41.3X6
inhalation	T41.0X1	T41.0X2	T41.0X3	T41.0X4	T41.0X5	T41.0X6
local	T41.3X1	T41.3X2	T41.3X3	T41.3X4	T41.3X5	T41.3X6
mucosal	T41.3X1	T41.3X2	T41.3X3	T41.3X4	T41.3X5	T41.3X6
muscle relaxation	T48.1X1	T48.1X2	T48.1X3	T48.1X4	T48.1X5	T48.1X6
nerve blocking	T41.3X1	T41.3X2	T41.3X3	T41.3X4	T41.3X5	T41.3X6
plexus blocking	T41.3X1	T41.3X2	T41.3X3	T41.3X4	T41.3X5	T41.3X6
potentiated	T41.201	T41.202	T41.203	T41.204	T41.205	T41.206
rectal	T41.201	T41.202	T41.203	T41.204	T41.205	T41.206
general	T41.201	T41.202	T41.203	T41.204	T41.205	T41.206
local	T41.3X1	T41.3X2	T41.3X3	T41.3X4	T41.3X5	T41.3X6
regional	T41.3X1	T41.3X2	T41.3X3	T41.3X4	T41.3X5	T41.3X6
surface	T41.3X1	T41.3X2	T41.3X3	T41.3X4	T41.3X5	T41.3X6
Anesthetic NEC — *see also Anesthesia*	T41.41	T41.42	T41.43	T41.44	T41.45	T41.46
with muscle relaxant	T41.201	T41.202	T41.203	T41.204	T41.205	T41.206
general	T41.201	T41.202	T41.203	T41.204	T41.205	T41.206
local	T41.3X1	T41.3X2	T41.3X3	T41.3X4	T41.3X5	T41.3X6
gaseous NEC	T41.0X1	T41.0X2	T41.0X3	T41.0X4	T41.0X5	T41.0X6
general NEC	T41.201	T41.202	T41.203	T41.204	T41.205	T41.206
halogenated hydrocarbon derivatives NEC	T41.0X1	T41.0X2	T41.0X3	T41.0X4	T41.0X5	T41.0X6
infiltration NEC	T41.3X1	T41.3X2	T41.3X3	T41.3X4	T41.3X5	T41.3X6
intravenous NEC	T41.1X1	T41.1X2	T41.1X3	T41.1X4	T41.1X5	T41.1X6
local NEC	T41.3X1	T41.3X2	T41.3X3	T41.3X4	T41.3X5	T41.3X6
rectal	T41.201	T41.202	T41.203	T41.204	T41.205	T41.206
general	T41.201	T41.202	T41.203	T41.204	T41.205	T41.206
local	T41.3X1	T41.3X2	T41.3X3	T41.3X4	T41.3X5	T41.3X6
regional NEC	T41.3X1	T41.3X2	T41.3X3	T41.3X4	T41.3X5	T41.3X6
spinal NEC	T41.3X1	T41.3X2	T41.3X3	T41.3X4	T41.3X5	T41.3X6
thiobarbiturate	T41.1X1	T41.1X2	T41.1X3	T41.1X4	T41.1X5	T41.1X6
topical	T41.3X1	T41.3X2	T41.3X3	T41.3X4	T41.3X5	T41.3X6
Aneurine	T45.2X1	T45.2X2	T45.2X3	T45.2X4	T45.2X5	T45.2X6
Angio-Conray	T50.8X1	T50.8X2	T50.8X3	T50.8X4	T50.8X5	T50.8X6
Angiotensin	T44.5X1	T44.5X2	T44.5X3	T44.5X4	T44.5X5	T44.5X6
Angiotensinamide	T44.991	T44.992	T44.993	T44.994	T44.995	T44.996
Anhydrohydroxy-progesterone	T38.5X1	T38.5X2	T38.5X3	T38.5X4	T38.5X5	T38.5X6
Anhydron	T50.2X1	T50.2X2	T50.2X3	T50.2X4	T50.2X5	T50.2X6
Anileridine	T40.491	T40.492	T40.493	T40.494	T40.495	T40.496

Substance	Poisoning, Accidental (Unintentional)	Poisoning, Intentional Self-Harm	Poisoning, Assault	Poisoning, Undetermined	Adverse Effect	Underdosing
Aniline (dye) (liquid)	T65.3X1	T65.3X2	T65.3X3	T65.3X4	—	—
analgesic	T39.1X1	T39.1X2	T39.1X3	T39.1X4	T39.1X5	T39.1X6
derivatives, therapeutic NEC	T39.1X1	T39.1X2	T39.1X3	T39.1X4	T39.1X5	T39.1X6
vapor	T65.3X1	T65.3X2	T65.3X3	T65.3X4		
Anise oil	T47.5X1	T47.5X2	T47.5X3	T47.5X4	T47.5X5	T47.5X6
Aniscoropine	T44.3X1	T44.3X2	T44.3X3	T44.3X4	T44.3X5	T44.3X6
Anisidine	T65.3X1	T65.3X2	T65.3X3	T65.3X4	—	—
Anisindione	T45.511	T45.512	T45.513	T45.514	T45.515	T45.516
Anisotropine methyl-bromide	T44.3X1	T44.3X2	T44.3X3	T44.3X4	T44.3X5	T44.3X6
Anistreplase	T45.611	T45.612	T45.613	T45.614	T45.615	T45.616
Anorexiant (central)	T50.5X1	T50.5X2	T50.5X3	T50.5X4	T50.5X5	T50.5X6
Anorexic agents	T50.5X1	T50.5X2	T50.5X3	T50.5X4	T50.5X5	T50.5X6
Ansamycin	T36.6X1	T36.6X2	T36.6X3	T36.6X4	T36.6X5	T36.6X6
Ant (bite) (sting)	T63.421	T63.422	T63.423	T63.424	—	—
Antabuse	T50.6X1	T50.6X2	T50.6X3	T50.6X4	T50.6X5	T50.6X6
Ant poison — see Insecticide						
Antacid NEC	T47.1X1	T47.1X2	T47.1X3	T47.1X4	T47.1X5	T47.1X6
Antagonist						
Aldosterone	T50.0X1	T50.0X2	T50.0X3	T50.0X4	T50.0X5	T50.0X6
alpha-adrenoreceptor	T44.6X1	T44.6X2	T44.6X3	T44.6X4	T44.6X5	T44.6X6
anticoagulant	T45.7X1	T45.7X2	T45.7X3	T45.7X4	T45.7X5	T45.7X6
beta-adrenoreceptor	T44.7X1	T44.7X2	T44.7X3	T44.7X4	T44.7X5	T44.7X6
extrapyramidal NEC	T44.3X1	T44.3X2	T44.3X3	T44.3X4	T44.3X5	T44.3X6
folic acid	T45.1X1	T45.1X2	T45.1X3	T45.1X4	T45.1X5	T45.1X6
H2 receptor	T47.0X1	T47.0X2	T47.0X3	T47.0X4	T47.0X5	T47.0X6
heavy metal	T45.8X1	T45.8X2	T45.8X3	T45.8X4	T45.8X5	T45.8X6
narcotic analgesic	T50.7X1	T50.7X2	T50.7X3	T50.7X4	T50.7X5	T50.7X6
opiate	T50.7X1	T50.7X2	T50.7X3	T50.7X4	T50.7X5	T50.7X6
pyrimidine	T45.1X1	T45.1X2	T45.1X3	T45.1X4	T45.1X5	T45.1X6
serotonin	T46.5X1	T46.5X2	T46.5X3	T46.5X4	T46.5X5	T46.5X6
Antazolin(e)	T45.0X1	T45.0X2	T45.0X3	T45.0X4	T45.0X5	T45.0X6
Anterior pituitary hormone NEC	T38.811	T38.812	T38.813	T38.814	T38.815	T38.816
Anthelmintic NEC	T37.4X1	T37.4X2	T37.4X3	T37.4X4	T37.4X5	T37.4X6
Anthiolimine	T37.4X1	T37.4X2	T37.4X3	T37.4X4	T37.4X5	T37.4X6
Anthralin	T49.4X1	T49.4X2	T49.4X3	T49.4X4	T49.4X5	T49.4X6
Anthramycin	T45.1X1	T45.1X2	T45.1X3	T45.1X4	T45.1X5	T45.1X6
Antiadrenergic NEC	T44.8X1	T44.8X2	T44.8X3	T44.8X4	T44.8X5	T44.8X6
Antiallergic NEC	T45.0X1	T45.0X2	T45.0X3	T45.0X4	T45.0X5	T45.0X6
Anti-anemic (drug) (preparation)	T45.8X1	T45.8X2	T45.8X3	T45.8X4	T45.8X5	T45.8X6
Antiandrogen NEC	T38.6X1	T38.6X2	T38.6X3	T38.6X4	T38.6X5	T38.6X6
Antianxiety drug NEC	T43.501	T43.502	T43.503	T43.504	T43.505	T43.506
Antiaris toxicaria	T65.891	T65.892	T65.893	T65.894	—	—

Substance	Poisoning, Accidental (Unintentional)	Poisoning, Intentional Self-Harm	Poisoning, Assault	Poisoning, Undetermined	Adverse Effect	Underdosing
Antiarteriosclerotic drug	T46.6X1	T46.6X2	T46.6X3	T46.6X4	T46.6X5	T46.6X6
Antiasthmatic drug NEC	T48.6X1	T48.6X2	T48.6X3	T48.6X4	T48.6X5	T48.6X6
Antibiotic NEC	T36.91	T36.92	T36.93	T36.94	T36.95	T36.96
aminoglycoside	T36.5X1	T36.5X2	T36.5X3	T36.5X3	T36.5X5	T36.5X6
anticancer	T45.1X1	T45.1X2	T45.1X3	T45.1X4	T45.1X5	T45.1X6
antifungal	T36.7X1	T36.7X2	T36.7X3	T36.7X4	T36.7X5	T36.7X6
antimycobacterial	T36.5X1	T36.5X2	T36.5X3	T36.5X4	T36.5X5	T36.5X6
antineoplastic	T45.1X1	T45.1X2	T45.1X3	T45.1X4	T45.1X5	T45.1X6
cephalosporin (group)	T36.1X1	T36.1X2	T36.1X3	T36.1X4	T36.1X5	T36.1X6
chloramphenicol (group)	T36.2X1	T36.2X2	T36.2X3	T36.2X4	T36.2X5	T36.2X6
ENT	T49.6X1	T49.6X2	T49.6X3	T49.6X4	T49.6X5	T49.6X6
eye	T49.5X1	T49.5X2	T49.5X3	T49.5X4	T49.5X5	T49.5X6
fungicidal (local)	T49.0X1	T49.0X2	T49.0X3	T49.0X4	T49.0X5	T49.0X6
intestinal	T36.8X1	T36.8X2	T36.8X3	T36.8X4	T36.8X5	T36.8X6
b-lactam NEC	T36.1X1	T36.1X2	T36.1X3	T36.1X4	T36.1X5	T36.1X6
local	T49.0X1	T49.0X2	T49.0X3	T49.0X4	T49.0X5	T49.0X6
macrolides	T36.3X1	T36.3X2	T36.3X3	T36.3X4	T36.3X5	T36.3X6
polypeptide	T36.8X1	T36.8X2	T36.8X3	T36.8X4	T36.8X5	T36.8X6
specified NEC	T36.8X1	T36.8X2	T36.8X3	T36.8X4	T36.8X5	T36.8X6
tetracycline (group)	T36.4X1	T36.4X2	T36.4X3	T36.4X4	T36.4X5	T36.4X6
throat	T49.6X1	T49.6X2	T49.6X3	T49.6X4	T49.6X5	T49.6X6
Anticancer agents NEC	T45.1X1	T45.1X2	T45.1X3	T45.1X4	T45.1X5	T45.1X6
Anticholesterolemic drug NEC	T46.6X1	T46.6X2	T46.6X3	T46.6X4	T46.6X5	T46.6X6
Anticholinergic NEC	T44.3X1	T44.3X2	T44.3X3	T44.3X4	T44.3X5	T44.3X6
Anticholinesterase	T44.0X1	T44.0X2	T44.0X3	T44.0X4	T44.0X5	T44.0X6
organophosphorus	T44.0X1	T44.0X2	T44.0X3	T44.0X4	T44.0X5	T44.0X6
insecticide	T60.0X1	T60.0X2	T60.0X3	T60.0X4	—	—
nerve gas	T59.891	T59.892	T59.893	T59.894	—	—
reversible	T44.0X1	T44.0X2	T44.0X3	T44.0X4	T44.0X5	T44.0X6
ophthalmological	T49.5X1	T49.5X2	T49.5X3	T49.5X4	T49.5X5	T49.5X6
Anticoagulant NEC	T45.511	T45.512	T45.513	T45.514	T45.515	T45.516
Antagonist	T45.7X1	T45.7X2	T45.7X4	T45.7X4	T45.7X5	T45.7X6
Anti-common-cold drug NEC	T48.5X1	T48.5X2	T48.5X3	T48.5X4	T48.5X5	T48.5X6
Anticonvulsant	T42.71	T42.72	T42.73	T42.74	T42.75	T42.76
barbiturate	T42.3X1	T42.3X2	T42.3X3	T42.3X4	T42.3X5	T42.3X6
combination (with barbiturate)	T42.3X1	T42.3X2	T42.3X3	T42.3X4	T42.3X5	T42.3X6
hydantoin	T42.0X1	T42.0X2	T42.0X3	T42.0X4	T42.0X5	T42.0X6
hypnotic NEC	T42.6X1	T42.6X2	T42.6X3	T42.6X4	T42.6X5	T42.6X6
oxazolidinedione	T42.2X1	T42.2X2	T42.2X3	T42.2X4	T42.2X5	T42.2X6
pyrimidinedione	T42.6X1	T42.6X2	T42.6X3	T42.6X4	T42.6X5	T42.6X6
specified NEC	T42.6X1	T42.6X2	T42.6X3	T42.6X4	T42.6X5	T42.6X6
succinimide	T42.2X1	T42.2X2	T42.2X3	T42.2X4	T42.2X5	T42.2X6

Substance	Poisoning, Accidental (Unintentional)	Poisoning, Intentional Self-Harm	Poisoning, Assault	Poisoning, Undetermined	Adverse Effect	Underdosing
Anti-D immunoglobulin (human)	T50.Z11	T50.Z12	T50.Z13	T50.Z14	T50.Z15	T50.Z16
Antidepressant NEC	T43.201	T43.202	T43.203	T43.204	T43.205	T43.206
monoamine oxidase inhibitor	T43.1X1	T43.1X2	T43.1X3	T43.1X4	T43.1X5	T43.1X6
selective serotonin norepinephrine reuptake inhibitor	T43.211	T43.212	T43.213	T43.214	T43.215	T43.216
selective serotonin reuptake inhibitor	T43.221	T43.222	T43.223	T43.224	T43.225	T43.226
specified NEC	T43.291	T43.292	T43.293	T43.294	T43.295	T43.296
tetracyclic	T43.021	T43.022	T43.023	T43.024	T43.025	T43.026
triazolopyridine	T43.221	T43.222	T43.223	T43.224	T43.225	T43.226
tricyclic	T43.011	T43.012	T43.013	T43.014	T43.015	T43.016
Antidiabetic NEC	T38.3X1	T38.3X2	T38.3X3	T38.3X4	T38.3X5	T38.3X6
biguanide	T38.3X1	T38.3X2	T38.3X3	T38.3X4	T38.3X5	T38.3X6
and sulfonyl combined	T38.3X1	T38.3X2	T38.3X3	T38.3X4	T38.3X5	T38.3X6
combined	T38.3X1	T38.3X2	T38.3X3	T38.3X4	T38.3X5	T38.3X6
sulfonylurea	T38.3X1	T38.3X2	T38.3X3	T38.3X4	T38.3X5	T38.3X6
Antidiarrheal drug NEC	T47.6X1	T47.6X2	T47.6X3	T47.6X4	T47.6X5	T47.6X6
absorbent	T47.6X1	T47.6X2	T47.6X3	T47.6X4	T47.6X5	T47.6X6
Antidiphtheria serum	T50.Z11	T50.Z12	T50.Z13	T50.Z14	T50.Z15	T50.Z16
Antidiuretic hormone	T38.891	T38.892	T38.893	T38.894	T38.895	T38.896
Antidote NEC	T50.6X1	T50.6X2	T50.6X3	T50.6X4	T50.6X5	T50.6X6
heavy metal	T45.8X1	T45.8X2	T45.8X3	T45.8X4	T45.8X5	T45.8X6
Antidysrhythmic NEC	T46.2X1	T46.2X2	T46.2X3	T46.2X4	T46.2X5	T46.2X6
Antiemetic drug	T45.0X1	T45.0X2	T45.0X3	T45.0X4	T45.0X5	T45.0X6
Antiepilepsy agent	T42.71	T42.72	T42.73	T42.74	T42.75	T42.76
combination	T42.5X1	T42.5X2	T42.5X3	T42.5X4	T42.5X5	T42.5X6
mixed	T42.5X1	T42.5X2	T42.5X3	T42.5X4	T42.5X5	T42.5X6
specified, NEC	T42.6X1	T42.6X2	T42.6X3	T42.6X4	T42.6X5	T42.6X6
Antiestrogen NEC	T38.6X1	T38.6X2	T38.6X3	T38.6X4	T38.6X5	T38.6X6
Antifertility pill	T38.4X1	T38.4X2	T38.4X3	T38.4X4	T38.4X5	T38.4X6
Antifibrinolytic drug	T45.621	T45.622	T45.623	T45.624	T45.625	T45.626
Antifilarial drug	T37.4X1	T37.4X2	T37.4X3	T37.4X4	T37.4X5	T37.4X6
Antiflatulent	T47.5X1	T47.5X2	T47.5X3	T47.5X4	T47.5X5	T47.5X6
Antifreeze	T65.91	T65.92	T65.93	T65.94	—	—
alcohol	T51.1X1	T51.1X2	T51.1X3	T51.1X4	—	—
ethylene glycol	T51.8X1	T51.8X2	T51.8X3	T51.8X4	—	—
Antifungal						
antibiotic (systemic)	T36.7X1	T36.7X2	T36.7X3	T36.7X4	T36.7X5	T36.7X6
anti-infective NEC	T37.91	T37.92	T37.93	T37.94	T37.95	T37.96
disinfectant, local	T49.0X1	T49.0X2	T49.0X3	T49.0X4	T49.0X5	T49.0X6
nonmedicinal (spray)	T60.3X1	T60.3X2	T60.3X3	T60.3X4	—	—
topical	T49.0X1	T49.0X2	T49.0X3	T49.0X4	T49.0X5	T49.0X6

Substance	Poisoning, Accidental (Unintentional)	Poisoning, Intentional Self-Harm	Poisoning, Assault	Poisoning, Undetermined	Adverse Effect	Underdosing
Anti-gastric-secretion drug NEC	T47.1X1	T47.1X2	T47.1X3	T47.1X4	T47.1X5	T47.1X6
Antigonadotrophin NEC	T38.6X1	T38.6X2	T38.6X3	T38.6X4	T38.6X5	T38.6X6
Antihallucinogen	T43.501	T43.502	T43.503	T43.504	T43.505	T43.506
Antihelmintics	T37.4X1	T37.4X2	T37.4X3	T37.4X4	T37.4X5	T37.4X6
Antihemophilic						
factor	T45.8X1	T45.8X2	T45.8X3	T45.8X4	T45.8X5	T45.8X6
fraction	T45.8X1	T45.8X2	T45.8X3	T45.8X4	T45.8X5	T45.8X6
globulin concentrate	T45.7X1	T45.7X2	T45.7X3	T45.7X4	T45.7X5	T45.7X6
human plasma	T45.8X1	T45.8X2	T45.8X3	T45.8X4	T45.8X5	T45.8X6
plasma, dried	T45.7X1	T45.7X2	T45.7X3	T45.7X4	T45.7X5	T45.7X6
Antihemorrhoidal preparation	T49.2X1	T49.2X2	T49.2X3	T49.2X4	T49.2X5	T49.2X6
Antiheparin drug	T45.7X1	T45.7X2	T45.7X3	T45.7X4	T45.7X5	T45.7X6
Antihistamine	T45.0X1	T45.0X2	T45.0X3	T45.0X4	T45.0X5	T45.0X6
Antihookworm drug	T37.4X1	T37.4X2	T37.4X3	T37.4X4	T37.4X5	T37.4X6
Anti-human lymphocytic globulin	T50.Z11	T50.Z12	T50.Z13	T50.Z14	T50.Z15	T50.Z16
Antihyperlipidemic drug	T46.6X1	T46.6X2	T46.6X3	T46.6X4	T46.6X5	T46.6X6
Antihypertensive drug NEC	T46.5X1	T46.5X2	T46.5X3	T46.5X4	T46.5X5	T46.5X6
Anti-infective NEC	T37.91	T37.92	T37.93	T37.94	T37.95	T37.96
anthelmintic	T37.4X1	T37.4X2	T37.4X3	T37.4X4	T37.4X5	T37.4X6
antibiotics	T36.91	T36.92	T36.93	T36.94	T36.95	T36.96
specified NEC	T36.8X1	T36.8X2	T36.8X3	T36.8X4	T36.8X5	T36.8X6
antimalarial	T37.2X1	T37.2X2	T37.2X3	T37.2X4	T37.2X5	T37.2X6
antimycobacterial NEC	T37.1X1	T37.1X2	T37.1X3	T37.1X4	T37.1X5	T37.1X6
antibiotics	T36.5X1	T36.5X2	T36.5X3	T36.5X4	T36.5X5	T36.5X6
antiprotozoal NEC	T37.3X1	T37.3X2	T37.3X3	T37.3X4	T37.3X5	T37.3X6
blood	T37.2X1	T37.2X2	T37.2X3	T37.2X4	T37.2X5	T37.2X6
antiviral	T37.5X1	T37.5X2	T37.5X3	T37.5X4	T37.5X5	T37.5X6
arsenical	T37.8X1	T37.8X2	T37.8X3	T37.8X4	T37.8X5	T37.8X6
bismuth, local	T49.0X1	T49.0X2	T49.0X3	T49.0X4	T49.0X5	T49.0X6
ENT	T49.6X1	T49.6X2	T49.6X3	T49.6X4	T49.6X5	T49.6X6
eye NEC	T49.5X1	T49.5X2	T49.5X3	T49.5X4	T49.5X5	T49.5X6
heavy metals NEC	T37.8X1	T37.8X2	T37.8X3	T37.8X4	T37.8X5	T37.8X6
local NEC	T49.0X1	T49.0X2	T49.0X3	T49.0X4	T49.0X5	T49.0X6
specified NEC	T49.0X1	T49.0X2	T49.0X3	T49.0X4	T49.0X5	T49.0X6
mixed	T37.91	T37.92	T37.93	T37.94	T37.95	T37.96
ophthalmic preparation	T49.5X1	T49.5X2	T49.5X3	T49.5X4	T49.5X5	T49.5X6
topical NEC	T49.0X1	T49.0X2	T49.0X3	T49.0X4	T49.0X5	T49.0X6
Anti-inflammatory drug NEC	T49.0X1	T49.0X2	T49.0X3	T49.0X4	T49.0X5	T49.0X6
local	T49.0X1	T49.0X2	T49.0X3	T49.0X4	T49.0X5	T49.0X6
nonsteroidal NEC	T39.391	T39.392	T39.393	T39.394	T39.395	T39.396
propionic acid derivative	T39.311	T39.312	T39.313	T39.314	T39.315	T39.316
specified NEC	T39.391	T39.392	T39.393	T39.394	T39.395	T39.396

◄ New　　◄ Revised　　~~deleted~~ Deleted

Substance	Poisoning, Accidental (Unintentional)	Poisoning, Intentional Self-Harm	Poisoning, Assault	Poisoning, Undetermined	Adverse Effect	Underdosing
Antikaluretic	T50.3X1	T50.3X2	T50.3X3	T50.3X4	T50.3X5	T50.3X6
Antiknock (tetraethyl lead)	T56.0X1	T56.0X2	T56.0X3	T56.0X4	—	—
Antilipemic drug NEC	T46.6X1	T46.6X2	T46.6X3	T46.6X4	T46.6X5	T46.6X6
Antimalarial	T37.2X1	T37.2X2	T37.2X3	T37.2X4	T37.2X5	T37.2X6
prophylactic NEC	T37.2X1	T37.2X2	T37.2X3	T37.2X4	T37.2X5	T37.2X6
pyrimidine derivative	T37.2X1	T37.2X2	T37.2X3	T37.2X4	T37.2X5	T37.2X6
Antimetabolite	T45.1X1	T45.1X2	T45.1X3	T45.1X4	T45.1X5	T45.1X6
Antimitotic agent	T45.1X1	T45.1X2	T45.1X3	T45.1X4	T45.1X5	T45.1X6
Antimony (compounds) (vapor) NEC	T56.891	T56.892	T56.893	T56.894	—	—
anti-infectives	T37.8X1	T37.8X2	T37.8X3	T37.8X4	T37.8X5	T37.8X6
dimercaptosuccinate	T37.3X1	T37.3X2	T37.3X3	T37.3X4	T37.3X5	T37.3X6
hydride	T56.891	T56.892	T56.893	T56.894	—	—
pesticide (vapor)	T60.8X1	T60.8X2	T60.8X3	T60.8X4	—	—
potassium (sodium) tartrate	T37.8X1	T37.8X2	T37.8X3	T37.8X4	T37.8X5	T37.8X6
sodium dimercaptosuccinate	T37.3X1	T37.3X2	T37.3X3	T37.3X4	T37.3X5	T37.3X6
tartrated	T37.8X1	T37.8X2	T37.8X3	T37.8X4	T37.8X5	T37.8X6
Antimuscarinic NEC	T44.3X1	T44.3X2	T44.3X3	T44.3X4	T44.3X5	T44.3X6
Antimycobacterial drug NEC	T37.1X1	T37.1X2	T37.1X3	T37.1X4	T37.1X5	T37.1X6
antibiotics	T36.5X1	T36.5X2	T36.5X3	T36.5X4	T36.5X5	T36.5X6
combination	T37.1X1	T37.1X2	T37.1X3	T37.1X4	T37.1X5	T37.1X6
Antinausea drug	T45.0X1	T45.0X2	T45.0X3	T45.0X4	T45.0X5	T45.0X6
Antinematode drug	T37.4X1	T37.4X2	T37.4X3	T37.4X4	T37.4X5	T37.4X6
Antineoplastic NEC	T45.1X1	T45.1X2	T45.1X3	T45.1X4	T45.1X5	T45.1X6
alkaloidal	T45.1X1	T45.1X2	T45.1X3	T45.1X4	T45.1X5	T45.1X6
antibiotics	T45.1X1	T45.1X2	T45.1X3	T45.1X4	T45.1X5	T45.1X6
combination	T45.1X1	T45.1X2	T45.1X3	T45.1X4	T45.1X5	T45.1X6
estrogen	T38.5X1	T38.5X2	T38.5X3	T38.5X4	T38.5X5	T38.5X6
steroid	T38.7X1	T38.7X2	T38.7X3	T38.7X4	T38.7X5	T38.7X6
Antiparasitic drug (systemic)	T37.91	T37.92	T37.93	T37.94	T37.95	T37.96
local	T49.0X1	T49.0X2	T49.0X3	T49.0X4	T49.0X5	T49.0X6
specified NEC	T37.8X1	T37.8X2	T37.8X3	T37.8X4	T37.8X5	T37.8X6
Antiparkinsonism drug NEC	T42.8X1	T42.8X2	T42.8X3	T42.8X4	T42.8X5	T42.8X6
Antiperspirant NEC	T49.2X1	T49.2X2	T49.2X3	T49.2X4	T49.2X5	T49.2X6
Antiphlogistic NEC	T39.4X1	T39.4X2	T39.4X3	T39.4X4	T39.4X5	T39.4X6
Antiplatyhelmintic drug	T37.4X1	T37.4X2	T37.4X3	T37.4X4	T37.4X5	T37.4X6
Antiprotozoal drug NEC	T37.3X1	T37.3X2	T37.3X3	T37.3X4	T37.3X5	T37.3X6
blood	T37.2X1	T37.2X2	T37.2X3	T37.2X4	T37.2X5	T37.2X6
local	T49.0X1	T49.0X2	T49.0X3	T49.0X4	T49.0X5	T49.0X6
Antipruritic drug NEC	T49.1X1	T49.1X2	T49.1X3	T49.1X4	T49.1X5	T49.1X6
Antipsychotic drug	T43.501	T43.502	T43.503	T43.504	T43.505	T43.506
specified NEC	T43.591	T43.592	T43.593	T43.594	T43.595	T43.596

Substance	Poisoning, Accidental (Unintentional)	Poisoning, Intentional Self-Harm	Poisoning, Assault	Poisoning, Undetermined	Adverse Effect	Underdosing
Antipyretic	T39.91	T39.92	T39.93	T39.94	T39.95	T39.96
specified NEC	T39.8X1	T39.8X2	T39.8X3	T39.8X4	T39.8X5	T39.8X6
Antipyrine	T39.2X1	T39.2X2	T39.2X3	T39.2X4	T39.2X5	T39.2X6
Antirabies hyperimmune serum	T50.Z11	T50.Z12	T50.Z13	T50.Z14	T50.Z15	T50.Z16
Antirheumatic NEC	T39.4X1	T39.4X2	T39.4X3	T39.4X4	T39.4X5	T39.4X6
Antirigidity drug NEC	T42.8X1	T42.8X2	T42.8X3	T42.8X4	T42.8X5	T42.8X6
Antischistosomal drug	T37.4X1	T37.4X2	T37.4X3	T37.4X4	T37.4X5	T37.4X6
Antiscorpion sera	T50.Z11	T50.Z12	T50.Z13	T50.Z14	T50.Z15	T50.Z16
Antiseborrheics	T49.4X1	T49.4X2	T49.4X3	T49.4X4	T49.4X5	T49.4X6
Antiseptics (external) (medicinal)	T49.0X1	T49.0X2	T49.0X3	T49.0X4	T49.0X5	T49.0X6
Antistine	T45.0X1	T45.0X2	T45.0X3	T45.0X4	T45.0X5	T45.0X6
Antitapeworm drug	T37.4X1	T37.4X2	T37.4X3	T37.4X4	T37.4X5	T37.4X6
Antitetanus immunoglobulin	T50.Z11	T50.Z12	T50.Z13	T50.Z14	T50.Z15	T50.Z16
Antithrombotic	T45.521	T45.522	T45.523	T45.524	T45.525	T45.526
Antithyroid drug NEC	T38.2X1	T38.2X2	T38.2X3	T38.2X4	T38.2X5	T38.2X6
Antitoxin	T50.Z11	T50.Z12	T50.Z13	T50.Z14	T50.Z15	T50.Z16
diphtheria	T50.Z11	T50.Z12	T50.Z13	T50.Z14	T50.Z15	T50.Z16
gas gangrene	T50.Z11	T50.Z12	T50.Z13	T50.Z14	T50.Z15	T50.Z16
tetanus	T50.Z11	T50.Z12	T50.Z13	T50.Z14	T50.Z15	T50.Z16
Antitoxin, any	T50.901	T50.902	T50.903	T50.904	T50.905	T50.906
Antitrichomonal drug	T37.3X1	T37.3X2	T37.3X3	T37.3X4	T37.3X5	T37.3X6
Antituberculars	T37.1X1	T37.1X2	T37.1X3	T37.1X4	T37.1X5	T37.1X6
antibiotics	T36.5X1	T36.5X2	T36.5X3	T36.5X4	T36.5X5	T36.5X6
Antitussive NEC	T48.3X1	T48.3X2	T48.3X3	T48.3X4	T48.3X5	T48.3X6
codeine mixture	T40.2X1	T40.2X2	T40.2X3	T40.2X4	T40.2X5	T40.2X6
opiate	T40.2X1	T40.2X2	T40.2X3	T40.2X4	T40.2X5	T40.2X6
Antivaricose drug	T46.8X1	T46.8X2	T46.8X3	T46.8X4	T46.8X5	T46.8X6
Antivenin, antivenom (sera)	T50.Z11	T50.Z12	T50.Z13	T50.Z14	T50.Z15	T50.Z16
crotaline	T50.Z11	T50.Z12	T50.Z13	T50.Z14	T50.Z15	T50.Z16
spider bite	T50.Z11	T50.Z12	T50.Z13	T50.Z14	T50.Z15	T50.Z16
Antivertigo drug	T45.0X1	T45.0X2	T45.0X3	T45.0X4	T45.0X5	T45.0X6
Antiviral drug NEC	T37.5X1	T37.5X2	T37.5X3	T37.5X4	T37.5X5	T37.5X6
eye	T49.5X1	T49.5X2	T49.5X3	T49.5X4	T49.5X5	T49.5X6
Antiwhipworm drug	T37.4X1	T37.4X2	T37.4X3	T37.4X4	T37.4X5	
Ant poisons — see Pesticides						
Antrol — see also by specific chemical substance	T60.91	T60.92	T60.93	T60.94	—	—
fungicide	T60.91	T60.92	T60.93	T60.94	—	—
ANTU (alpha naphthylthiourea)	T60.4X1	T60.4X2	T60.4X3	T60.4X4	—	—
Apalcillin	T36.0X1	T36.0X2	T36.0X3	T36.0X4	T36.0X5	T36.0X6
APC	T48.5X1	T48.5X2	T48.5X3	T48.5X4	T48.5X5	T48.5X6
Aplonidine	T44.4X1	T44.4X2	T44.4X3	T44.4X4	T44.4X5	T44.4X6
Apomorphine	T47.7X1	T47.7X2	T47.7X3	T47.7X4	T47.7X5	T47.7X6

TABLE OF DRUGS AND CHEMICALS

Substance	External Cause (T-Code)					
	Poisoning, Accidental (Unintentional)	Poisoning, Intentional Self-Harm	Poisoning, Assault	Poisoning, Undetermined	Adverse Effect	Underdosing
Appetite depressants, central	T50.5X1	T50.5X2	T50.5X3	T50.5X4	T50.5X5	T50.5X6
Apraclonidine (hydrochloride)	T44.4X1	T44.4X2	T44.4X3	T44.4X4	T44.4X5	T44.4X6
Apresoline	T46.5X1	T46.5X2	T46.5X3	T46.5X4	T46.5X5	T46.5X6
Aprindine	T46.2X1	T46.2X2	T46.2X3	T46.2X4	T46.2X5	T46.2X6
Aprobarbital	T42.3X1	T42.3X2	T42.3X3	T42.3X4	T42.3X5	T42.3X6
Apronalide	T42.6X1	T42.6X2	T42.6X3	T42.6X4	T42.6X5	T42.6X6
Aprotinin	T45.621	T45.622	T45.623	T45.624	T45.625	T45.626
Aptocaine	T41.3X1	T41.3X2	T41.3X3	T41.3X3	T41.3X5	T41.3X6
Aqua fortis	T54.2X1	T54.2X2	T54.2X3	T54.2X4	—	—
Ara-A	T37.5X1	T37.5X2	T37.5X3	T37.5X4	T37.5X5	T37.5X6
Ara-C	T45.1X1	T45.1X2	T45.1X3	T45.1X4	T45.1X5	T45.1X6
Arachis oil	T49.3X1	T49.3X2	T49.3X3	T49.3X4	T49.3X5	T49.3X6
cathartic	T47.4X1	T47.4X2	T47.4X3	T47.4X4	T47.4X5	T47.4X6
Aralen	T37.2X1	T37.2X2	T37.2X3	T37.2X4	T37.2X5	T37.2X6
Arecoline	T44.1X1	T44.1X2	T44.1X3	T44.1X4	T44.1X5	T44.1X6
Arginine	T50.991	T50.992	T50.993	T50.994	T50.995	T50.996
glutamate	T50.991	T50.992	T50.993	T50.994	T50.995	T50.996
Argyrol	T49.0X1	T49.0X2	T49.0X3	T49.0X4	T49.0X5	T49.0X6
ENT agent	T49.6X1	T49.6X2	T49.6X3	T49.6X4	T49.6X5	T49.6X6
ophthalmic preparation	T49.5X1	T49.5X2	T49.5X3	T49.5X4	T49.5X5	T49.5X6
Aristocort	T38.0X1	T38.0X2	T38.0X3	T38.0X4	T38.0X5	T38.0X6
ENT agent	T49.6X1	T49.6X2	T49.6X3	T49.6X4	T49.6X5	T49.6X6
ophthalmic preparation	T49.5X1	T49.5X2	T49.5X3	T49.5X4	T49.5X5	T49.5X6
topical NEC	T49.0X1	T49.0X2	T49.0X3	T49.0X4	T49.0X5	T49.0X6
Aromatics, corrosive	T54.1X1	T54.1X2	T54.1X3	T54.1X4	—	—
disinfectants	T54.1X1	T54.1X2	T54.1X3	T54.1X4	—	—
Arsenate of lead	T57.0X1	T57.0X2	T57.0X3	T57.0X4	—	—
herbicide	T57.0X1	T57.0X2	T57.0X3	T57.0X4	—	—
Arsenic, arsenicals (compounds) (dust) (vapor) NEC	T57.0X1	T57.0X2	T57.0X3	T57.0X4	—	—
anti-infectives	T37.8X1	T37.8X2	T37.8X3	T37.8X4	T37.8X5	T37.8X6
pesticide (dust) (fumes)	T57.0X1	T57.0X2	T57.0X3	T57.0X4	—	—
Arsine (gas)	T57.0X1	T57.0X2	T57.0X3	T57.0X4	—	—
Arsphenamine (silver)	T37.8X1	T37.8X2	T37.8X3	T37.8X4	T37.8X5	T37.8X6
Arsthinol	T37.3X1	T37.3X2	T37.3X3	T37.3X4	T37.3X5	T37.3X6
Artane	T44.3X1	T44.3X2	T44.3X3	T44.3X4	T44.3X5	T44.3X6
Arthropod (venomous) NEC	T63.481	T63.482	T63.483	T63.484	—	—
Articaine	T41.3X1	T41.3X2	T41.3X3	T41.3X4	T41.3X5	T41.3X6
Asbestos	T57.8X1	T57.8X2	T57.8X3	T57.8X4	—	—
Ascaridole	T37.4X1	T37.4X2	T37.4X3	T37.4X4	T37.4X5	T37.4X6
Ascorbic acid	T45.2X1	T45.2X2	T45.2X3	T45.2X4	T45.2X5	T45.2X6
Asiaticoside	T49.0X1	T49.0X2	T49.0X3	T49.0X4	T49.0X5	T49.0X6

Substance	External Cause (T-Code)					
	Poisoning, Accidental (Unintentional)	Poisoning, Intentional Self-Harm	Poisoning, Assault	Poisoning, Undetermined	Adverse Effect	Underdosing
Asparaginase	T45.1X1	T45.1X2	T45.1X3	T45.1X4	T45.1X5	T45.1X6
Aspidium (oleoresin)	T37.4X1	T37.4X2	T37.4X3	T37.4X4	T37.4X5	T37.4X6
Aspirin (aluminum) (soluble)	T39.011	T39.012	T39.013	T39.014	T39.015	T39.016
Aspoxicillin	T36.0X1	T36.0X2	T36.0X3	T36.0X4	T36.0X5	T36.0X6
Astemizole	T45.0X1	T45.0X2	T45.0X3	T45.0X4	T45.0X5	T45.0X6
Astringent (local)	T49.2X1	T49.2X2	T49.2X3	T49.2X4	T49.2X5	T49.2X6
specified NEC	T49.2X1	T49.2X2	T49.2X3	T49.2X4	T49.2X5	T49.2X6
Astromicin	T36.5X1	T36.5X2	T36.5X3	T36.5X4	T36.5X5	T36.5X6
Ataractic drug NEC	T43.501	T43.502	T43.503	T43.504	T43.505	T43.506
Atenolol	T44.7X1	T44.7X2	T44.7X3	T44.7X4	T44.7X5	T44.7X6
Atonia drug, intestinal	T47.4X1	T47.4X2	T47.4X3	T47.4X4	T47.4X5	T47.4X6
Atophan	T50.4X1	T50.4X2	T50.4X3	T50.4X4	T50.4X5	T50.4X6
Atracurium besilate	T48.1X1	T48.1X2	T48.1X3	T48.1X4	T48.1X5	T48.1X6
Atropine	T44.3X1	T44.3X2	T44.3X3	T44.3X4	T44.3X5	T44.3X6
derivative	T44.3X1	T44.3X2	T44.3X3	T44.3X4	T44.3X5	T44.3X6
methonitrate	T44.3X1	T44.3X2	T44.3X3	T44.3X4	T44.3X5	T44.3X6
Attapulgite	T47.6X1	T47.6X2	T47.6X3	T47.6X4	T47.6X5	T47.6X6
Attenuvax	T50.991	T50.992	T50.993	T50.994	T50.995	T50.996
Auramine	T65.891	T65.892	T65.893	T65.894	—	—
dye	T65.6X1	T65.6X2	T65.6X3	T65.6X4	—	—
fungicide	T60.3X1	T60.3X2	T60.3X3	T60.3X4	—	—
Auranofin	T39.4X1	T39.4X2	T39.4X3	T39.4X4	T39.4X5	T39.4X6
Aurantiin	T46.991	T46.992	T46.993	T46.994	T46.995	T46.996
Aureomycin	T36.4X1	T36.4X2	T36.4X3	T36.4X4	T36.4X5	T36.4X6
ophthalmic preparation	T49.5X1	T49.5X2	T49.5X3	T49.5X4	T49.5X5	T49.5X6
topical NEC	T49.0X1	T49.0X2	T49.0X3	T49.0X4	T49.0X5	T49.0X6
Aurothioglucose	T39.4X1	T39.4X2	T39.4X3	T39.4X4	T39.4X5	T39.4X6
Aurothioglycanide	T39.4X1	T39.4X2	T39.4X3	T39.4X4	T39.4X5	T39.4X6
Aurothiomalate sodium	T39.4X1	T39.4X2	T39.4X3	T39.4X4	T39.4X5	T39.4X6
Aurotioprol	T39.4X1	T39.4X2	T39.4X3	T39.4X4	T39.4X5	T39.4X6
Automobile fuel	T52.0X1	T52.0X2	T52.0X3	T52.0X4	—	—
Autonomic nervous system agent NEC	T44.901	T44.902	T44.903	T44.904	T44.905	T44.906
Avlosulfon	T37.1X1	T37.1X2	T37.1X3	T37.1X4	T37.1X5	T37.1X6
Avomine	T42.6X1	T42.6X2	T42.6X3	T42.6X4	T42.6X5	T42.6X6
Axerophthol	T45.2X1	T45.2X2	T45.2X3	T45.2X4	T45.2X5	T45.2X6
Azacitidine	T45.1X1	T45.1X2	T45.1X3	T45.1X4	T45.1X5	T45.1X6
Azacyclonol	T43.591	T43.592	T43.593	T43.594	T43.595	T43.596
Azadirachta	T60.2X1	T60.2X2	T60.2X3	T60.2X4	—	—
Azanidazole	T37.3X1	T37.3X2	T37.3X3	T37.3X4	T37.3X5	T37.3X6
Azapetine	T46.7X1	T46.7X2	T46.7X3	T46.7X4	T46.7X5	T46.7X6
Azapropazone	T39.2X1	T39.2X2	T39.2X3	T39.2X4	T39.2X5	T39.2X6

◄ New ◄ Revised ~~deleted~~ Deleted

Substance	Poisoning, Accidental (Unintentional)	Poisoning, Intentional Self-Harm	Poisoning, Assault	Poisoning, Undetermined	Adverse Effect	Underdosing
Azaribine	T45.1X1	T45.1X2	T45.1X3	T45.1X4	T45.1X5	T45.1X6
Azaserine	T45.1X1	T45.1X2	T45.1X3	T45.1X4	T45.1X5	T45.1X6
Azatadine	T45.0X1	T45.0X2	T45.0X3	T45.0X4	T45.0X5	T45.0X6
Azatepa	T45.1X1	T45.1X2	T45.1X3	T45.1X4	T45.1X5	T45.1X6
Azathioprine	T45.1X1	T45.1X2	T45.1X3	T45.1X4	T45.1X5	T45.1X6
Azelaic acid	T49.0X1	T49.0X2	T49.0X3	T49.0X4	T49.0X5	T49.0X6
Azelastine	T45.0X1	T45.0X2	T45.0X3	T45.0X4	T45.0X5	T45.0X6
Azidocillin	T36.0X1	T36.0X2	T36.0X3	T36.0X4	T36.0X5	T36.0X6
Azidothymidine	T37.5X1	T37.5X2	T37.5X3	T37.5X4	T37.5X5	T37.5X6
Azinphos (ethyl) (methyl)	T60.0X1	T60.0X2	T60.0X3	T60.0X4	—	—
Aziridine (chelating)	T54.1X1	T54.1X2	T54.1X3	T54.1X4	—	—
Azithromycin	T36.3X1	T36.3X2	T36.3X3	T36.3X4	T36.3X5	T36.3X6
Azlocillin	T36.01	T36.02	T36.03	T36.04	T36.05	T36.06
Azobenzene smoke	T65.3X1	T65.3X2	T65.3X3	T65.3X4	—	—
acaricide	T60.8X1	T60.8X2	T60.8X3	T60.8X4	—	—
Azosulfamide	T37.0X1	T37.0X2	T37.0X3	T37.0X4	T37.0X5	T37.0X6
AZT	T37.5X1	T37.5X2	T37.5X3	T37.5X4	T37.5X5	T37.5X6
Aztreonam	T36.1X1	T36.1X2	T36.1X3	T36.1X4	T36.1X5	T36.1X6
Azulfidine	T37.0X1	T37.0X2	T37.0X3	T37.0X4	T37.0X5	T37.0X6
Azuresin	T50.8X1	T50.8X2	T50.8X3	T50.8X4	T50.8X5	T50.8X6
B						
Bacampicillin	T36.0X1	T36.0X2	T36.0X3	T36.0X4	T36.0X5	T36.0X6
Bacillus						
lactobacillus	T47.8X1	T47.8X2	T47.8X3	T47.8X4	T47.8X5	T47.8X6
subtilis	T47.6X1	T47.6X2	T47.6X3	T47.6X4	T47.6X5	T47.6X6
Bacimycin	T49.0X1	T49.0X2	T49.0X3	T49.0X4	T49.0X5	T49.0X6
ophthalmic preparation	T49.5X1	T49.5X2	T49.5X3	T49.5X4	T49.5X5	T49.5X6
Bacitracin zinc	T49.0X1	T49.0X2	T49.0X3	T49.0X4	T49.0X5	T49.0X6
with neomycin	T49.0X1	T49.0X2	T49.0X3	T49.0X4	T49.0X5	T49.0X6
ENT agent	T49.6X1	T49.6X2	T49.6X3	T49.6X4	T49.6X5	T49.6X6
ophthalmic preparation	T49.5X1	T49.5X2	T49.5X3	T49.5X4	T49.5X5	T49.5X6
topical NEC	T49.0X1	T49.0X2	T49.0X3	T49.0X4	T49.0X5	T49.0X6
Baclofen	T42.8X1	T42.8X2	T42.8X3	T42.8X4	T42.8X5	T42.8X6
Baking soda	T50.991	T50.992	T50.993	T50.994	T50.995	T50.996
BAL	T45.8X1	T45.8X2	T45.8X3	T45.8X4	T45.8X5	T45.8X6
Bambuterol	T48.6X1	T48.6X2	T48.6X3	T48.6X4	T48.6X5	T48.6X6
Bamethan (sulfate)	T46.7X1	T46.7X2	T46.7X3	T46.7X4	T46.7X5	T46.7X6
Bamifylline	T48.6X1	T48.6X2	T48.6X3	T48.6X4	T48.6X5	T48.6X6
Bamipine	T45.0X1	T45.0X2	T45.0X3	T45.0X4	T45.0X5	T45.0X6
Baneberry — *see Actaea spicata*						
Banewort — *see Belladonna*						

Substance	Poisoning, Accidental (Unintentional)	Poisoning, Intentional Self-Harm	Poisoning, Assault	Poisoning, Undetermined	Adverse Effect	Underdosing
Barbenyl	T42.3X1	T42.3X2	T42.3X3	T42.3X4	T42.3X5	T42.3X6
Barbexaclone	T42.6X1	T42.6X2	T42.6X3	T42.6X4	T42.6X5	T42.6X6
Barbital	T42.3X1	T42.3X2	T42.3X3	T42.3X4	T42.3X5	T42.3X6
sodium	T42.3X1	T42.3X2	T42.3X3	T42.3X4	T42.3X5	T42.3X6
Barbitone	T42.3X1	T42.3X2	T42.3X3	T42.3X4	T42.3X5	T42.3X6
Barbiturate NEC	T42.3X1	T42.3X2	T42.3X3	T42.3X4	T42.3X5	T42.3X6
with tranquilizer	T42.3X1	T42.3X2	T42.3X3	T42.3X4	T42.3X5	T42.3X6
anesthetic (intravenous)	T41.1X1	T41.1X2	T41.1X3	T41.1X4	T41.1X5	T41.1X6
Barium (carbonate) (chloride) (sulfite)	T57.8X1	T57.8X2	T57.8X3	T57.8X4	—	—
diagnostic agent	T50.8X1	T50.8X2	T50.8X3	T50.8X4	T50.8X5	T50.8X6
pesticide	T60.4X1	T60.4X2	T60.4X3	T60.4X4	—	—
rodenticide	T60.4X1	T60.4X2	T60.4X3	T60.4X4	—	—
sulfate (medicinal)	T50.8X1	T50.8X2	T50.8X3	T50.8X4	T50.8X5	T50.8X6
Barrier cream	T49.3X1	T49.3X2	T49.3X3	T49.3X4	T49.3X5	T49.3X6
Basic fuchsin	T49.0X1	T49.0X2	T49.0X3	T49.0X4	T49.0X5	T49.0X6
Battery acid or fluid	T54.2X1	T54.2X2	T54.2X3	T54.2X4		
Bay rum	T51.8X1	T51.8X2	T51.8X3	T51.8X4	—	—
BCG (vaccine)	T50.A91	T50.A92	T50.A93	T50.A94	T50.A95	T50.A96
BCNU	T45.1X1	T45.1X2	T45.1X3	T45.1X4	T45.1X5	T45.1X6
Bearsfoot	T62.2X1	T62.2X2	T62.2X3	T62.2X4		
Beclamide	T42.6X1	T42.6X2	T42.6X3	T42.6X4	T42.6X5	T42.6X6
Beclomethasone	T44.5X1	T44.5X2	T44.5X3	T44.5X4	T44.5X5	T44.5X6
Bee (sting) (venom)	T63.441	T63.442	T63.443	T63.444	—	—
Befunolol	T49.5X1	T49.5X2	T49.5X3	T49.5X4	T49.5X5	T49.5X6
Bekanamycin	T36.5X1	T36.5X2	T36.5X3	T36.5X4	T36.5X5	T36.5X6
Belladonna — *see also Nightshade*						
alkaloids	T44.3X1	T44.3X2	T44.3X3	T44.3X4	T44.3X5	T44.3X6
extract	T44.3X1	T44.3X2	T44.3X3	T44.3X4	T44.3X5	T44.3X6
herb	T44.3X1	T44.3X2	T44.3X3	T44.3X4	T44.3X5	T44.3X6
Bemegride	T50.7X1	T50.7X2	T50.7X3	T50.7X4	T50.7X5	T50.7X6
Benactyzine	T44.3X1	T44.3X2	T44.3X3	T44.3X4	T44.3X5	T44.3X6
Benadryl	T45.0X1	T45.0X2	T45.0X3	T45.0X4	T45.0X5	T45.0X6
Benaprizine	T44.3X1	T44.3X2	T44.3X3	T44.3X4	T44.3X5	T44.3X6
Benazepril	T46.4X1	T46.4X2	T46.4X3	T46.4X4	T46.4X5	T46.4X6
Bencyclane	T46.7X1	T46.7X2	T46.7X3	T46.7X4	T46.7X5	T46.7X6
Bendazol	T46.3X1	T46.3X2	T46.3X3	T46.3X4	T46.3X5	T46.3X6
Bendrofluazide	T50.2X1	T50.2X2	T50.2X3	T50.2X4	T50.2X5	T50.2X6
Bendroflumethiazide	T50.2X1	T50.2X2	T50.2X3	T50.2X4	T50.2X5	T50.2X6
Benemid	T50.4X1	T50.4X2	T50.4X3	T50.4X4	T50.4X5	T50.4X6
Benethamine penicillin	T36.0X1	T36.0X2	T36.0X3	T36.0X4	T36.0X5	T36.0X6
Benisone	T49.0X1	T49.0X2	T49.0X3	T49.0X4	T49.0X5	T49.0X6

TABLE OF DRUGS AND CHEMICALS

Substance	External Cause (T-Code)					
	Poisoning, Accidental (Unintentional)	Poisoning, Intentional Self-Harm	Poisoning, Assault	Poisoning, Undetermined	Adverse Effect	Underdosing
Benexate	T47.1X1	T47.1X2	T47.1X3	T47.1X4	T47.1X5	T47.1X6
Benfluorex	T46.6X1	T46.6X2	T46.6X3	T46.6X4	T46.6X5	T46.6X6
Benfotiamine	T45.2X1	T45.2X2	T45.2X3	T45.2X4	T45.2X5	T45.2X6
Benomyl	T60.0X1	T60.0X2	T60.0X3	T60.0X4	—	—
Benoquin	T49.8X1	T49.8X2	T49.8X3	T49.8X4	T49.8X5	T49.8X6
Benoxinate	T41.3X1	T41.3X2	T41.3X3	T41.3X4	T41.3X5	T41.3X6
Benperidol	T43.4X1	T43.4X2	T43.4X3	T43.4X4	T43.4X5	T43.4X6
Benproperine	T48.3X1	T48.3X2	T48.3X3	T48.3X4	T48.3X5	T48.3X6
Benserazide	T42.8X1	T42.8X2	T42.8X3	T42.8X4	T42.8X5	T42.8X6
Bentazepam	T42.4X1	T42.4X2	T42.4X3	T42.4X4	T42.4X5	T42.4X6
Bentiromide	T50.8X1	T50.8X2	T50.8X3	T50.8X4	T50.8X5	T50.8X6
Bentonite	T49.3X1	T49.3X2	T49.3X3	T49.3X4	T49.3X5	T49.3X6
Benzalbutyramide	T46.6X1	T46.6X2	T46.6X3	T46.6X4	T46.6X5	T46.6X6
Benzalkonium (chloride)	T49.0X1	T49.0X2	T49.0X3	T49.0X4	T49.0X5	T49.0X6
ophthalmic preparation	T49.5X1	T49.5X2	T49.5X3	T49.5X4	T49.5X5	T49.5X6
Benzamine	T41.3X1	T41.3X2	T41.3X3	T41.3X4	T41.3X5	T41.3X6
lactate	T49.1X1	T49.1X2	T49.1X3	T49.1X4	T49.1X5	T49.1X6
Benzamidosalicylate (calcium)	T37.1X1	T37.1X2	T37.1X3	T37.1X4	T37.1X5	T37.1X6
Benzamphetamine	T50.5X1	T50.5X2	T50.5X3	T50.5X4	T50.5X5	T50.5X6
Benzapril hydrochloride	T46.5X1	T46.5X2	T46.5X3	T46.5X4	T46.5X5	T46.5X6
Benzathine benzylpenicillin	T36.0X1	T36.0X2	T36.0X3	T36.0X4	T36.0X5	T36.0X6
Benzathine penicillin	T36.0X1	T36.0X2	T36.0X3	T36.0X4	T36.0X5	T36.0X6
Benzatropine	T42.8X1	T42.8X2	T42.8X3	T42.8X4	T42.8X5	T42.8X6
Benzbromarone	T50.4X1	T50.4X2	T50.4X3	T50.4X4	T50.4X5	T50.4X6
Benzcarbimine	T45.1X1	T45.1X2	T45.1X3	T45.1X4	T45.1X5	T45.1X6
Benzedrex	T44.991	T44.992	T44.993	T44.994	T44.995	T44.996
Benzedrine (amphetamine)	T43.621	T43.622	T43.623	T43.624	T43.625	T43.626
Benzenamine	T65.3X1	T65.3X2	T65.3X3	T65.3X4	—	—
Benzene	T52.1X1	T52.1X2	T52.1X3	T52.1X4	—	—
homologues (acetyl) (dimethyl) (methyl) (solvent)	T52.2X1	T52.2X2	T52.2X3	T52.2X4	—	—
Benzethonium (chloride)	T49.0X1	T49.0X2	T49.0X3	T49.0X4	T49.0X5	T49.0X6
Benzfetamine	T50.5X1	T50.5X2	T50.5X3	T50.5X4	T50.5X5	T50.5X6
Benzhexol	T44.3X1	T44.3X2	T44.3X3	T44.3X4	T44.3X5	T44.3X6
Benzhydramine (chloride)	T45.0X1	T45.0X2	T45.0X3	T45.0X4	T45.0X5	T45.0X6
Benzidine	T65.891	T65.892	T65.893	T65.894	—	—
Benzilonium bromide	T44.3X1	T44.3X2	T44.3X3	T44.3X4	T44.3X5	T44.3X6
Benzimidazole	T60.3X1	T60.3X2	T60.3X3	T60.3X4	—	—
Benzin(e) — see Ligroin						
Benziodarone	T46.3X1	T46.3X2	T46.3X3	T46.3X4	T46.3X5	T46.3X6
Benznidazole	T37.3X1	T37.3X2	T37.3X3	T37.3X4	T37.3X5	T37.3X6
Benzocaine	T41.3X1	T41.3X2	T41.3X3	T41.3X4	T41.3X5	T41.3X6

Substance	External Cause (T-Code)					
	Poisoning, Accidental (Unintentional)	Poisoning, Intentional Self-Harm	Poisoning, Assault	Poisoning, Undetermined	Adverse Effect	Underdosing
Benzoctamine	T43.0X1	T43.0X2	T43.0X3	T43.0X4	T43.0X5	T43.0X6
Benzodiapin	T42.4X1	T42.4X2	T42.4X3	T42.4X4	T42.4X5	T42.4X6
Benzodiazepine NEC	T42.4X1	T42.4X2	T42.4X3	T42.4X4	T42.4X5	T42.4X6
Benzoic acid	T49.0X1	T49.0X2	T49.0X3	T49.0X4	T49.0X5	T49.0X6
with salicylic acid	T49.0X1	T49.0X2	T49.0X3	T49.0X4	T49.0X5	T49.0X6
Benzoin (tincture)	T48.5X1	T48.5X2	T48.5X3	T48.5X4	T48.5X5	T48.5X6
Benzol (benzene)	T52.1X1	T52.1X2	T52.1X3	T52.1X4	—	—
vapor	T52.0X1	T52.0X2	T52.0X3	T52.0X4	—	—
Benzomorphan	T40.2X1	T40.2X2	T40.2X3	T40.2X4	T40.2X5	T40.2X6
Benzonatate	T48.3X1	T48.3X2	T48.3X3	T48.3X4	T48.3X5	T48.3X6
Benzophenones	T49.3X1	T49.3X2	T49.3X3	T49.3X4	T49.3X5	T49.3X6
Benzopyrone	T46.991	T46.992	T46.993	T46.994	T46.995	T46.996
Benzothiadiazides	T50.2X1	T50.2X2	T50.2X3	T50.2X4	T50.2X5	T50.2X6
Benzoxonium chloride	T49.0X1	T49.0X2	T49.0X3	T49.0X4	T49.0X5	T49.0X6
Benzoyl peroxide	T49.0X1	T49.0X2	T49.0X3	T49.0X4	T49.0X5	T49.0X6
Benzoylpas calcium	T37.1X1	T37.1X2	T37.1X3	T37.1X4	T37.1X5	T37.1X6
Benzperidin	T43.591	T43.592	T43.593	T43.594	T43.595	T43.596
Benzperidol	T43.591	T43.592	T43.593	T43.594	T43.595	T43.596
Benzphetamine	T50.5X1	T50.5X2	T50.5X3	T50.5X4	T50.5X5	T50.5X6
Benzpyrinium bromide	T44.1X1	T44.1X2	T44.1X3	T44.1X4	T44.1X5	T44.1X6
Benzquinamide	T45.0X1	T45.0X2	T45.0X3	T45.0X4	T45.0X5	T45.0X6
Benzthiazide	T50.2X1	T50.2X2	T50.2X3	T50.2X4	T50.2X5	T50.2X6
Benztropine						
anticholinergic	T44.3X1	T44.3X2	T44.3X3	T44.3X4	T44.3X5	T44.3X6
antiparkinson	T42.8X1	T42.8X2	T42.8X3	T42.8X4	T42.8X5	T42.8X6
Benzydamine	T49.0X1	T49.0X2	T49.0X3	T49.0X4	T49.0X5	T49.0X6
Benzyl						
acetate	T52.8X1	T52.8X2	T52.8X3	T52.8X4	—	—
alcohol	T49.0X1	T49.0X2	T49.0X3	T49.0X4	T49.0X5	T49.0X6
benzoate	T49.0X1	T49.0X2	T49.0X3	T49.0X4	T49.0X5	T49.0X6
Benzoic acid	T49.0X1	T49.0X2	T49.0X3	T49.0X4	T49.0X5	T49.0X6
morphine	T40.2X1	T40.2X2	T40.2X3	T40.2X4		
nicotinate	T46.6X1	T46.6X2	T46.6X3	T46.6X4	T46.6X5	T46.6X6
penicillin	T36.0X1	T36.0X2	T36.0X3	T36.0X4	T36.0X5	T36.0X6
Benzylhydrochlorthiazide	T50.2X1	T50.2X2	T50.2X3	T50.2X4	T50.2X5	T50.2X6
Benzylpenicillin	T36.0X1	T36.0X2	T36.0X3	T36.0X4	T36.0X5	T36.0X6
Benzylthiouracil	T38.2X1	T38.2X2	T38.2X3	T38.2X4	T38.2X5	T38.2X6
Bephenium hydroxy-naphthoate	T37.4X1	T37.4X2	T37.4X3	T37.4X4	T37.4X5	T37.4X6
Bepridil	T46.1X1	T46.1X2	T46.1X3	T46.1X4	T46.1X5	T46.1X6
Bergamot oil	T65.891	T65.892	T65.893	T65.894	—	—
Bergapten	T50.991	T50.992	T50.993	T50.994	T50.995	T50.996
Berries, poisonous	T62.1X1	T62.1X2	T62.1X3	T62.1X4	—	—

◄ New   ◄ Revised   ~~deleted~~ Deleted

Substance	Poisoning, Accidental (Unintentional)	Poisoning, Intentional Self-Harm	Poisoning, Assault	Poisoning, Undetermined	Adverse Effect	Underdosing
Beryllium (compounds)	T56.7X1	T56.7X2	T56.7X3	T56.7X4	—	—
b-acetyldigoxin	T46.0X1	T46.0X2	T46.0X3	T46.0X4	T46.0X5	T46.0X6
beta adrenergic blocking agent, heart	T44.7X1	T44.7X2	T44.7X3	T44.7X4	T44.7X5	T44.7X6
b-benzalbutyramide	T46.6X1	T46.6X2	T46.6X3	T46.6X4	T46.6X5	T46.6X6
Betacarotene	T45.2X1	T45.2X2	T45.2X3	T45.2X4	T45.2X5	T45.2X6
b-eucaine	T49.1X1	T49.1X2	T49.1X3	T49.1X4	T49.1X5	T49.1X6
Beta-Chlor	T42.6X1	T42.6X2	T42.6X3	T42.6X4	T42.6X5	T42.6X6
b-galactosidase	T47.5X1	T47.5X2	T47.5X3	T47.5X4	T47.5X5	T47.5X6
Betahistine	T46.7X1	T46.7X2	T46.7X3	T46.7X4	T46.7X5	T46.7X6
Betaine	T47.5X1	T47.5X2	T47.5X3	T47.5X4	T47.5X5	T47.5X6
Betamethasone	T49.0X1	T49.0X2	T49.0X3	T49.0X4	T49.0X5	T49.0X6
topical	T49.0X1	T49.0X2	T49.0X3	T49.0X4	T49.0X5	T49.0X6
Betamicin	T36.8X1	T36.8X2	T36.8X3	T36.8X4	T36.8X5	T36.8X6
Betanidine	T46.5X1	T46.5X2	T46.5X3	T46.5X4	T46.5X5	T46.5X6
b-sitosterol(s)	T46.6X1	T46.6X2	T46.6X3	T46.6X4	T46.6X5	T46.6X6
Betaxolol	T44.7X1	T44.7X2	T44.7X3	T44.7X4	T44.7X5	T44.7X6
Betazole	T50.8X1	T50.8X2	T50.8X3	T50.8X4	T50.8X5	T50.8X6
Bethanechol	T44.1X1	T44.1X2	T44.1X3	T44.1X4	T44.1X5	T44.1X6
chloride	T44.1X1	T44.1X2	T44.1X3	T44.1X4	T44.1X5	T44.1X6
Bethanidine	T46.5X1	T46.5X2	T46.5X3	T46.5X4	T46.5X5	T46.5X6
Betoxycaine	T41.3X1	T41.3X2	T41.3X3	T41.3X4	T41.3X5	T41.3X6
Betula oil	T49.3X1	T49.3X2	T49.3X3	T49.3X4	T49.3X5	T49.3X6
Bevantolol	T44.7X1	T44.7X2	T44.7X3	T44.7X4	T44.7X5	T44.7X6
Bevonium metilsulfate	T44.3X1	T44.3X2	T44.3X3	T44.3X4	T44.3X5	T44.3X6
Bezafibrate	T46.6X1	T46.6X2	T46.6X3	T46.6X4	T46.6X5	T46.6X6
Bezitramide	T40.491	T40.492	T40.493	T40.494	T40.495	T40.496
BHA	T50.991	T50.992	T50.993	T50.994	T50.995	T50.996
Bhang	T40.711	T40.712	T40.713	T40.714	T40.715	T40.716
BHC (medicinal)	T49.0X1	T49.0X2	T49.0X3	T49.0X4	T49.0X5	T49.0X6
nonmedicinal (vapor)	T53.6X1	T53.6X2	T53.6X3	T53.6X4	—	—
Bialamicol	T37.3X1	T37.3X2	T37.3X3	T37.3X4	T37.3X5	T37.3X6
Bibenzonium bromide	T48.3X1	T48.3X2	T48.3X3	T48.3X4	T48.3X5	T48.3X6
Bibrocathol	T49.5X1	T49.5X2	T49.5X3	T49.5X4	T49.5X5	T49.5X6
Bichloride of mercury — see Mercury, chloride						
Bichromates (calcium) (potassium) (sodium) (crystals)	T57.8X1	T57.8X2	T57.8X3	T57.8X4	—	—
fumes	T56.2X1	T56.2X2	T56.2X3	T56.2X4	—	—
Biclotymol	T49.6X1	T49.6X2	T49.6X3	T49.6X4	T49.6X5	T49.6X6
Bicuculline	T50.7X1	T50.7X2	T50.7X3	T50.7X4	T50.7X5	T50.7X6
Bifemelane	T43.291	T43.292	T43.293	T43.294	T43.295	T43.296
Biguanide derivatives, oral	T38.3X1	T38.3X2	T38.3X3	T38.3X4	T38.3X5	T38.3X6

Substance	Poisoning, Accidental (Unintentional)	Poisoning, Intentional Self-Harm	Poisoning, Assault	Poisoning, Undetermined	Adverse Effect	Underdosing
Biligrafin	T50.8X1	T50.8X2	T50.8X3	T50.8X4	T50.8X5	T50.8X6
Bile salts	T47.5X1	T47.5X2	T47.5X3	T47.5X4	T47.5X5	T47.5X6
Bilopaque	T50.8X1	T50.8X2	T50.8X3	T50.8X4	T50.8X5	T50.8X6
Binifibrate	T46.6X1	T46.6X2	T46.6X3	T46.6X4	T46.6X5	T46.6X6
Binitrobenzol	T65.3X1	T65.3X2	T65.3X3	T65.3X4	—	—
Bioflavonoid(s)	T46.991	T46.992	T46.993	T46.994	T46.995	T46.996
Biological substance NEC	T50.901	T50.902	T50.903	T50.904	T50.905	T50.906
Biotin	T45.2X1	T45.2X2	T45.2X3	T45.2X4	T45.2X5	T45.2X6
Biperiden	T44.3X1	T44.3X2	T44.3X3	T44.3X4	T44.3X5	T44.3X6
Bisacodyl	T47.2X1	T47.2X2	T47.2X3	T47.2X4	T47.2X5	T47.2X6
Bisbentiamine	T45.2X1	T45.2X2	T45.2X3	T45.2X4	T45.2X5	T45.2X6
Bisbutiamine	T45.2X1	T45.2X2	T45.2X3	T45.2X4	T45.2X5	T45.2X6
Bisdequalinium (salts) (diacetate)	T49.6X1	T49.6X2	T49.6X3	T49.6X4	T49.6X5	T49.6X6
Bishydroxycoumarin	T45.511	T45.512	T45.513	T45.514	T45.515	T45.516
Bismarsen	T37.8X1	T37.8X2	T37.8X3	T37.8X4	T37.8X5	T37.8X6
Bismuth salts	T47.6X1	T47.6X2	T47.6X3	T47.6X4	T47.6X5	T47.6X6
aluminate	T47.1X1	T47.1X2	T47.1X3	T47.1X4	T47.1X5	T47.1X6
anti-infectives	T37.8X1	T37.8X2	T37.8X3	T37.8X4	T37.8X5	T37.8X6
formic iodide	T49.0X1	T49.0X2	T49.0X3	T49.0X4	T49.0X5	T49.0X6
glycolylarsenate	T49.0X1	T49.0X2	T49.0X3	T49.0X4	T49.0X5	T49.0X6
nonmedicinal (compounds) NEC	T65.91	T65.92	T65.93	T65.94	—	—
subcarbonate	T47.6X1	T47.6X2	T47.6X3	T47.6X4	T47.6X5	T47.6X6
subsalicylate	T37.8X1	T37.8X2	T37.8X3	T37.8X4	T37.8X5	T37.8X6
sulfarsphenamine	T37.8X1	T37.8X2	T37.8X3	T37.8X4	T37.8X5	T37.8X6
Bisoprolol	T44.7X1	T44.7X2	T44.7X3	T44.7X4	T44.7X5	T44.7X6
Bisoxatin	T47.2X1	T47.2X2	T47.2X3	T47.2X4	T47.2X5	T47.2X6
Bisulepin (hydrochloride)	T45.0X1	T45.0X2	T45.0X3	T45.0X4	T45.0X5	T45.0X6
Bithionol	T37.8X1	T37.8X2	T37.8X3	T37.8X4	T37.8X5	T37.8X6
anthelmintic	T37.4X1	T37.4X2	T37.4X3	T37.4X4	T37.4X5	T37.4X6
Bitolterol	T48.6X1	T48.6X2	T48.6X3	T48.6X4	T48.6X5	T48.6X6
Bitoscanate	T37.4X1	T37.4X2	T37.4X3	T37.4X4	T37.4X5	T37.4X6
Bitter almond oil	T62.8X1	T62.8X2	T62.8X3	T62.8X4	—	—
Bittersweet	T62.2X1	T62.2X2	T62.2X3	T62.2X4	—	—
Black						
flag	T60.91	T60.92	T60.93	T60.94	—	—
henbane	T62.2X1	T62.2X2	T62.2X3	T62.2X4	—	—
leaf (40)	T60.91	T60.92	T60.93	T60.94	—	—
widow spider (bite)	T63.311	T63.312	T63.313	T63.314	—	—
antivenin	T50.Z11	T50.Z12	T50.Z13	T50.Z14	T50.Z15	T50.Z16
Blast furnace gas (carbon monoxide from)	T58.8X1	T58.8X2	T58.8X3	T58.8X4	—	—
Bleach	T54.91	T54.92	T54.93	T54.94	—	—

TABLE OF DRUGS AND CHEMICALS

Substance	Poisoning, Accidental (Unintentional)	Poisoning, Intentional Self-Harm	Poisoning, Assault	Poisoning, Undetermined	Adverse Effect	Underdosing
Bleaching agent (medicinal)	T49.4X1	T49.4X2	T49.4X3	T49.4X4	T49.4X5	T49.4X6
Bleomycin	T45.1X1	T45.1X2	T45.1X3	T45.1X4	T45.1X5	T45.1X6
Blockain	T41.3X1	T41.3X2	T41.3X3	T41.3X4	T41.3X5	T41.3X6
infiltration (subcutaneous)	T41.3X1	T41.3X2	T41.3X3	T41.3X4	T41.3X5	T41.3X6
nerve block (peripheral) (plexus)	T41.3X1	T41.3X2	T41.3X3	T41.3X4	T41.3X5	T41.3X6
topical (surface)	T41.3X1	T41.3X2	T41.3X3	T41.3X4	T41.3X5	T41.3X6
Blockers, calcium channel	T46.1X1	T46.1X2	T46.1X3	T46.1X4	T46.1X5	T46.1X6
Blood (derivatives) (natural) (plasma) (whole)	T45.8X1	T45.8X2	T45.8X3	T45.8X4	T45.8X5	T45.8X6
dried	T45.8X1	T45.8X2	T45.8X3	T45.8X4	T45.8X5	T45.8X6
drug affecting NEC	T45.91	T45.92	T45.93	T45.94	T45.95	T45.96
expander NEC	T45.8X1	T45.8X2	T45.8X3	T45.8X4	T45.8X5	T45.8X6
fraction NEC	T45.8X1	T45.8X2	T45.8X3	T45.8X4	T45.8X5	T45.8X6
substitute (macromolecular)	T45.8X1	T45.8X2	T45.8X3	T45.8X4	T45.8X5	T45.8X6
Blue velvet	T40.2X1	T40.2X2	T40.2X3	T40.2X4	—	—
Bone meal	T62.8X1	T62.8X2	T62.8X3	T62.8X4	—	—
Bonine	T45.0X1	T45.0X2	T45.0X3	T45.0X4	T45.0X5	T45.0X6
Bopindolol	T44.7X1	T44.7X2	T44.7X3	T44.7X4	T44.7X5	T44.7X6
Boracic acid	T49.0X1	T49.0X2	T49.0X3	T49.0X4	T49.0X5	T49.0X6
ENT agent	T49.6X1	T49.6X2	T49.6X3	T49.6X4	T49.6X5	T49.6X6
ophthalmic preparation	T49.5X1	T49.5X2	T49.5X3	T49.5X4	T49.5X5	T49.5X6
Borane complex	T57.8X1	T57.8X2	T57.8X3	T57.8X4	—	—
Borate(s)	T57.8X1	T57.8X2	T57.8X3	T57.8X4	—	—
buffer	T50.991	T50.992	T50.993	T50.994	T50.995	T50.996
cleanser	T54.91	T54.92	T54.93	T54.94	—	—
sodium	T57.8X1	T57.8X2	T57.8X3	T57.8X4	—	—
Borax (cleanser)	T54.91	T54.92	T54.93	T54.94	—	—
Bordeaux mixture	T60.3X1	T60.3X2	T60.3X3	T60.3X4	—	—
Boric acid	T49.0X1	T49.0X2	T49.0X3	T49.0X4	T49.0X5	T49.0X6
ENT agent	T49.6X1	T49.6X2	T49.6X3	T49.6X4	T49.6X5	T49.6X6
ophthalmic preparation	T49.5X1	T49.5X2	T49.5X3	T49.5X4	T49.5X5	T49.5X6
Bornaprine	T44.3X1	T44.3X2	T44.3X3	T44.3X4	T44.3X5	T44.3X6
Boron	T57.8X1	T57.8X2	T57.8X3	T57.8X4	—	—
hydride NEC	T57.8X1	T57.8X2	T57.8X3	T57.8X4	—	—
fumes or gas	T57.8X1	T57.8X2	T57.8X3	T57.8X4	—	—
trifluoride	T59.891	T59.892	T59.893	T59.894	—	—
Botox	T48.291	T48.292	T48.293	T48.294	T48.295	T48.296
Botulinus anti-toxin (type A, B)	T50.Z11	T50.Z12	T50.Z13	T50.Z14	T50.Z15	T50.Z16
Brake fluid vapor	T59.891	T59.892	T59.893	T59.894	—	—
Brallobarbital	T42.3X1	T42.3X2	T42.3X3	T42.3X4	T42.3X5	T42.3X6
Bran (wheat)	T47.4X1	T47.4X2	T47.4X3	T47.4X4	T47.4X5	T47.4X6
Brass (fumes)	T56.891	T56.892	T56.893	T56.894	—	—

Substance	Poisoning, Accidental (Unintentional)	Poisoning, Intentional Self-Harm	Poisoning, Assault	Poisoning, Undetermined	Adverse Effect	Underdosing
Brasso	T52.0X1	T52.0X2	T52.0X3	T52.0X4	—	—
Bretylium tosilate	T46.2X1	T46.2X2	T46.2X3	T46.2X4	T46.2X5	T46.2X6
Brevital (sodium)	T41.1X1	T41.1X2	T41.1X3	T41.1X4	T41.1X5	T41.1X6
Brinase	T45.3X1	T45.3X2	T45.3X3	T45.3X4	T45.3X5	T45.3X6
British antilewisite	T45.8X1	T45.8X2	T45.8X3	T45.8X4	T45.8X5	T45.8X6
Brodifacoum	T60.4X1	T60.4X2	T60.4X3	T60.4X4	—	—
Bromal (hydrate)	T42.6X1	T42.6X2	T42.6X3	T42.6X4	T42.6X5	T42.6X6
Bromazepam	T42.4X1	T42.4X2	T42.4X3	T42.4X4	T42.4X5	T42.4X6
Bromazine	T45.0X1	T45.0X2	T45.0X3	T45.0X4	T45.0X5	T45.0X6
Brombenzylcyanide	T59.3X1	T59.3X2	T59.3X3	T59.3X4	—	—
Bromelains	T45.3X1	T45.3X2	T45.3X3	T45.3X4	T45.3X5	T45.3X6
Bromethalin	T60.4X1	T60.4X2	T60.4X3	T60.4X4	—	—
Bromhexine	T48.4X1	T48.4X2	T48.4X3	T48.4X4	T48.4X5	T48.4X6
Bromide salts	T42.6X1	T42.6X2	T42.6X3	T42.6X4	T42.6X5	T42.6X6
Bromindione	T45.511	T45.512	T45.513	T45.514	T45.515	T45.516
Bromine						
compounds (medicinal)	T42.6X1	T42.6X2	T42.6X3	T42.6X4	T42.6X5	T42.6X6
sedative	T42.6X1	T42.6X2	T42.6X3	T42.6X4	T42.6X5	T42.6X6
vapor	T59.891	T59.892	T59.893	T59.894	—	—
Bromisovalum	T42.6X1	T42.6X2	T42.6X3	T42.6X4	T42.6X5	T42.6X6
Bromisoval	T42.6X1	T42.6X2	T42.6X3	T42.6X4	T42.6X5	T42.6X6
Bromobenzylcyanide	T59.3X1	T59.3X2	T59.3X3	T59.3X4	—	—
Bromochlorosalicylanilide	T49.0X1	T49.0X2	T49.0X3	T49.0X4	T49.0X5	T49.0X6
Bromocriptine	T42.8X1	T42.8X2	T42.8X3	T42.8X4	T42.8X5	T42.8X6
Bromodiphenhydramine	T45.0X1	T45.0X2	T45.0X3	T45.0X4	T45.0X5	T45.0X6
Bromoform	T42.6X1	T42.6X2	T42.6X3	T42.6X4	T42.6X5	T42.6X6
Bromophenol blue reagent	T50.991	T50.992	T50.993	T50.994	T50.995	T50.996
Bromopride	T47.8X1	T47.8X2	T47.8X3	T47.8X4	T47.8X5	T47.8X6
Bromosalicylchloranitide	T49.0X1	T49.0X2	T49.0X3	T49.0X4	T49.0X5	T49.0X6
Bromosalicylhydroxamic acid	T37.1X1	T37.1X2	T37.1X3	T37.1X4	T37.1X5	T37.1X6
Bromo-seltzer	T39.1X1	T39.1X2	T39.1X3	T39.1X4	T39.1X5	T39.1X6
Bromoxynil	T60.3X1	T60.3X2	T60.3X3	T60.3X4	—	—
Bromperidol	T43.4X1	T43.4X2	T43.4X3	T43.4X4	T43.4X5	T43.4X6
Brompheniramine	T45.0X1	T45.0X2	T45.0X3	T45.0X4	T45.0X5	T45.0X6
Bromsulfophthalein	T50.8X1	T50.8X2	T50.8X3	T50.8X4	T50.8X5	T50.8X6
Bromural	T42.6X1	T42.6X2	T42.6X3	T42.6X4	T42.6X5	T42.6X6
Bromvaletone	T42.6X1	T42.6X2	T42.6X3	T42.6X4	T42.6X5	T42.6X6
Bronchodilator NEC	T48.6X1	T48.6X2	T48.6X3	T48.6X4	T48.6X5	T48.6X6
Brotizolam	T42.4X1	T42.4X2	T42.4X3	T42.4X4	T42.4X5	T42.4X6
Brovincamine	T46.7X1	T46.7X2	T46.7X3	T46.7X4	T46.7X5	T46.7X6
Brown spider (bite) (venom)	T63.391	T63.392	T63.393	T63.394	—	—

◄ New   ◄ Revised   ~~deleted~~ Deleted

Substance	Poisoning, Accidental (Unintentional)	Poisoning, Intentional Self-Harm	Poisoning, Assault	Poisoning, Undetermined	Adverse Effect	Underdosing
Brown recluse spider (bite) (venom)	T63.331	T63.332	T63.333	T63.334	—	—
Broxaterol	T48.6X1	T48.6X2	T48.6X3	T48.6X4	T48.6X5	T48.6X6
Broxuridine	T45.1X1	T45.1X2	T45.1X3	T45.1X4	T45.1X5	T45.1X6
Broxyquinoline	T37.8X1	T37.8X2	T37.8X3	T37.8X4	T37.8X5	T37.8X6
Bruceine	T48.291	T48.292	T48.293	T48.294	T48.295	T48.296
Brucia	T62.2X1	T62.2X2	T62.2X3	T62.2X4	—	—
Brucine	T65.1X1	T65.1X2	T65.1X3	T65.1X4	—	—
Brunswick green — see Copper						
Bruten — see Ibuprofen						
Bryonia	T47.2X1	T47.2X2	T47.2X3	T47.2X4	T47.2X5	T47.2X6
Buclizine	T45.0X1	T45.0X2	T45.0X3	T45.0X4	T45.0X5	T45.0X6
Buclosamide	T49.0X1	T49.0X2	T49.0X3	T49.0X4	T49.0X5	T49.0X6
Budesonide	T44.5X1	T44.5X2	T44.5X3	T44.5X4	T44.5X5	T44.5X6
Budralazine	T46.5X1	T46.5X2	T46.5X3	T46.5X4	T46.5X5	T46.5X6
Bufferin	T39.011	T39.012	T39.013	T39.014	T39.015	T39.016
Buflomedil	T46.7X1	T46.7X2	T46.7X3	T46.7X4	T46.7X5	T46.7X6
Buformin	T38.3X1	T38.3X2	T38.3X3	T38.3X4	T38.3X5	T38.3X6
Bufotenine	T40.991	T40.992	T40.993	T40.994	—	—
Bufrolin	T48.6X1	T48.6X2	T48.6X3	T48.6X4	T48.6X5	T48.6X6
Bufylline	T48.6X1	T48.6X2	T48.6X3	T48.6X4	T48.6X5	T48.6X6
Bulk filler	T50.5X1	T50.5X2	T50.5X3	T50.5X4	T50.5X5	T50.5X6
cathartic	T47.4X1	T47.4X2	T47.4X3	T47.4X4	T47.4X5	T47.4X6
Bumetanide	T50.1X1	T50.1X2	T50.1X3	T50.1X4	T50.1X5	T50.1X6
Bunaftine	T46.2X1	T46.2X2	T46.2X3	T46.2X4	T46.2X5	T46.2X6
Bunamiodyl	T50.8X1	T50.8X2	T50.8X3	T50.8X4	T50.8X5	T50.8X6
Bunazosin	T44.6X1	T44.6X2	T44.6X3	T44.6X4	T44.6X5	T44.6X6
Bunitrolol	T44.7X1	T44.7X2	T44.7X3	T44.7X4	T44.7X5	T44.7X6
Buphenine	T46.7X1	T46.7X2	T46.7X3	T46.7X4	T46.7X5	T46.7X6
Bupivacaine	T41.3X1	T41.3X2	T41.3X3	T41.3X4	T41.3X5	T41.3X6
infiltration (subcutaneous)	T41.3X1	T41.3X2	T41.3X3	T41.3X4	T41.3X5	T41.3X6
nerve block (peripheral) (plexus)	T41.3X1	T41.3X2	T41.3X3	T41.3X4	T41.3X5	T41.3X6
spinal	T41.3X1	T41.3X2	T41.3X3	T41.3X4	T41.3X5	T41.3X6
Bupranolol	T44.7X1	T44.7X2	T44.7X3	T44.7X4	T44.7X5	T44.7X6
Buprenorphine	T40.491	T40.492	T40.493	T40.494	T40.495	T40.496
Bupropion	T43.291	T43.292	T43.293	T43.294	T43.295	T43.296
Burimamide	T47.1X1	T47.1X2	T47.1X3	T47.1X4	T47.1X5	T47.1X6
Buserelin	T38.891	T38.892	T38.893	T38.894	T38.895	T38.896
Buspirone	T43.591	T43.592	T43.593	T43.594	T43.595	T43.596
Busulfan, busulphan	T45.1X1	T45.1X2	T45.1X3	T45.1X4	T45.1X5	T45.1X6
Butabarbital (sodium)	T42.3X1	T42.3X2	T42.3X3	T42.3X4	T42.3X5	T42.3X6
Butabarbitone	T42.3X1	T42.3X2	T42.3X3	T42.3X4	T42.3X5	T42.3X6

Substance	Poisoning, Accidental (Unintentional)	Poisoning, Intentional Self-Harm	Poisoning, Assault	Poisoning, Undetermined	Adverse Effect	Underdosing
Butabarpal	T42.3X1	T42.3X2	T42.3X3	T42.3X4	T42.3X5	T42.3X6
Butacaine	T41.3X1	T41.3X2	T41.3X3	T41.3X4	T41.3X5	T41.3X6
Butalamine	T46.7X1	T46.7X2	T46.7X3	T46.7X4	T46.7X5	T46.7X6
Butalbital	T42.3X1	T42.3X2	T42.3X3	T42.3X4	T42.3X5	T42.3X6
Butallylonal	T42.3X1	T42.3X2	T42.3X3	T42.3X4	T42.3X5	T42.3X6
Butamben	T41.3X1	T41.3X2	T41.3X3	T41.3X4	T41.3X5	T41.3X6
Butamirate	T48.3X1	T48.3X2	T48.3X3	T48.3X4	T48.3X5	T48.3X6
Butane (distributed in mobile container)	T59.891	T59.892	T59.893	T59.894	—	—
distributed through pipes	T59.891	T59.892	T59.893	T59.894	—	—
incomplete combustion	T58.11	T58.12	T58.13	T58.14	—	—
Butanilicaine	T41.3X1	T41.3X2	T41.3X3	T41.3X4	T41.3X5	T41.3X6
Butanol	T51.3X1	T51.3X2	T51.3X3	T51.3X4	—	—
Butanone, 2-butanone	T52.4X1	T52.4X2	T52.4X3	T52.4X4	—	—
Butantrone	T49.4X1	T49.4X2	T49.4X3	T49.4X4	T49.4X5	T49.4X6
Butaperazine	T43.3X1	T43.3X2	T43.3X3	T43.3X4	T43.3X5	T43.3X6
Butazolidin	T39.2X1	T39.2X2	T39.2X3	T39.2X4	T39.2X5	T39.2X6
Butetamate	T48.6X1	T48.6X2	T48.6X3	T48.6X4	T48.6X5	T48.6X6
Butethal	T42.3X1	T42.3X2	T42.3X3	T42.3X4	T42.3X5	T42.3X6
Butethamate	T44.3X1	T44.3X2	T44.3X3	T44.3X4	T44.3X5	T44.3X6
Buthalitone (sodium)	T41.1X1	T41.1X2	T41.1X3	T41.1X4	T41.1X5	T41.1X6
Butisol (sodium)	T42.3X1	T42.3X2	T42.3X3	T42.3X4	T42.3X5	T42.3X6
Butizide	T50.2X1	T50.2X2	T50.2X3	T50.2X4	T50.2X5	T50.2X6
Butobarbital	T42.3X1	T42.3X2	T42.3X3	T42.3X4	T42.3X5	T42.3X6
sodium	T42.3X1	T42.3X2	T42.3X3	T42.3X4	T42.3X5	T42.3X6
Butobarbitone	T42.3X1	T42.3X2	T42.3X3	T42.3X4	T42.3X5	T42.3X6
Butoconazole (nitrate)	T49.0X1	T49.0X2	T49.0X3	T49.0X4	T49.0X5	T49.0X6
Butorphanol	T40.491	T40.492	T40.493	T40.494	T40.495	T40.496
Butriptyline	T43.011	T43.012	T43.013	T43.014	T43.015	T43.016
Butropium bromide	T44.3X1	T44.3X2	T44.3X3	T44.3X4	T44.3X5	T44.3X6
Buttercups	T62.2X1	T62.2X2	T62.2X3	T62.2X4	—	—
Butter of antimony — see Antimony						
Butyl						
acetate (secondary)	T52.8X1	T52.8X2	T52.8X3	T52.8X4		
alcohol	T51.3X1	T51.3X2	T51.3X3	T51.3X4	—	—
aminobenzoate	T41.3X1	T41.3X2	T41.3X3	T41.3X4	T41.3X5	T41.3X6
butyrate	T52.8X1	T52.8X2	T52.8X3	T52.8X4		
carbinol	T51.3X1	T51.3X2	T51.3X3	T51.3X4		
carbitol	T52.3X1	T52.3X2	T52.3X3	T52.3X4		
cellosolve	T52.3X1	T52.3X2	T52.3X3	T52.3X4		—
chloral (hydrate)	T42.6X1	T42.6X2	T42.6X3	T42.6X4	T42.6X5	T42.6X6
formate	T52.8X1	T52.8X2	T52.8X3	T52.8X4	—	—

TABLE OF DRUGS AND CHEMICALS

Substance	Poisoning, Accidental (Unintentional)	Poisoning, Intentional Self-Harm	Poisoning, Assault	Poisoning, Undetermined	Adverse Effect	Underdosing
Butyl *(Continued)*						
lactate	T52.8X1	T52.8X2	T52.8X3	T52.8X4	—	—
propionate	T52.8X1	T52.8X2	T52.8X3	T52.8X4	—	—
scopolamine bromide	T44.3X1	T44.3X2	T44.3X3	T44.3X4	T44.3X5	T44.3X6
thiobarbital sodium	T41.1X1	T41.1X2	T41.1X3	T41.1X4	T41.1X5	T41.1X6
Butylated hydroxy-anisole	T50.991	T50.992	T50.993	T50.994	T50.995	T50.996
Butylchloral hydrate	T42.6X1	T42.6X2	T42.6X3	T42.6X4	T42.6X5	T42.6X6
Butyltoluene	T52.2X1	T52.2X2	T52.2X3	T52.2X4	—	—
Butyn	T41.3X1	T41.3X2	T41.3X3	T41.3X4	T41.3X5	T41.3X6
Butyrophenone (-based tranquilizers)	T43.4X1	T43.4X2	T43.4X3	T43.4X4	T43.4X5	T43.4X6
C						
Cabergoline	T42.8X1	T42.8X2	T42.8X3	T42.8X4	T42.8X5	T42.8X6
Cacodyl, cacodylic acid	T57.0X1	T57.0X2	T57.0X3	T57.0X4	—	—
Cactinomycin	T45.1X1	T45.1X2	T45.1X3	T45.1X4	T45.1X5	T45.1X6
Cade oil	T49.4X1	T49.4X2	T49.4X3	T49.4X4	T49.4X5	T49.4X6
Cadexomer iodine	T49.0X1	T49.0X2	T49.0X3	T49.0X4	T49.0X5	T49.0X6
Cadmium (chloride) (fumes) (oxide)	T56.3X1	T56.3X2	T56.3X3	T56.3X4	—	—
sulfide (medicinal) NEC	T49.4X1	T49.4X2	T49.4X3	T49.4X4	T49.4X5	T49.4X6
Cadralazine	T46.5X1	T46.5X2	T46.5X3	T46.5X4	T46.5X5	T46.5X6
Caffeine	T43.611	T43.612	T43.613	T43.614	T43.615	T43.616
Calabar bean	T62.2X1	T62.2X2	T62.2X3	T62.2X4	—	—
Caladium seguinum	T62.2X1	T62.2X2	T62.2X3	T62.2X4	—	—
Calamine (lotion)	T49.3X1	T49.3X2	T49.3X3	T49.3X4	T49.3X5	T49.3X6
Calcifediol	T45.2X1	T45.2X2	T45.2X3	T45.2X4	T45.2X5	T45.2X6
Calciferol	T45.2X1	T45.2X2	T45.2X3	T45.2X4	T45.2X5	T45.2X6
Calcitonin	T50.991	T50.992	T50.993	T50.994	T50.995	T50.996
Calcitriol	T45.2X1	T45.2X2	T45.2X3	T45.2X4	T45.2X5	T45.2X6
Calcium	T50.3X1	T50.3X2	T50.3X3	T50.3X4	T50.3X5	T50.3X6
actylsalicylate	T39.011	T39.012	T39.013	T39.014	T39.015	T39.016
benzamidosalicylate	T37.1X1	T37.1X2	T37.1X3	T37.1X4	T37.1X5	T37.1X6
bromide	T42.6X1	T42.6X2	T42.6X3	T42.6X4	T42.6X5	T42.6X6
bromolactobionate	T42.6X1	T42.6X2	T42.6X3	T42.6X4	T42.6X5	T42.6X6
carbaspirin	T39.011	T39.012	T39.013	T39.014	T39.015	T39.016
carbimide	T50.6X1	T50.6X2	T50.6X3	T50.6X4	T50.6X5	T50.6X6
carbonate	T47.1X1	T47.1X2	T47.1X3	T47.1X4	T47.1X5	T47.1X6
chloride	T50.991	T50.992	T50.993	T50.994	T50.995	T50.996
anhydrous	T50.991	T50.992	T50.993	T50.994	T50.995	T50.996
cyanide	T57.8X1	T57.8X2	T57.8X3	T57.8X4	—	—
dioctyl sulfosuccinate	T47.4X1	T47.4X2	T47.4X3	T47.4X4	T47.4X5	T47.4X6
disodium edathamil	T45.8X1	T45.8X2	T45.8X3	T45.8X4	T45.8X5	T45.8X6

Substance	Poisoning, Accidental (Unintentional)	Poisoning, Intentional Self-Harm	Poisoning, Assault	Poisoning, Undetermined	Adverse Effect	Underdosing
Calcium *(Continued)*						
disodium edetate	T45.8X1	T45.8X2	T45.8X3	T45.8X4	T45.8X5	T45.8X6
dobesilate	T46.991	T46.992	T46.993	T46.994	T46.995	T46.996
EDTA	T45.8X1	T45.8X2	T45.8X3	T45.8X4	T45.8X5	T45.8X6
ferrous citrate	T45.4X1	T45.4X2	T45.4X3	T45.4X4	T45.4X5	T45.4X6
folinate	T45.8X1	T45.8X2	T45.8X3	T45.8X4	T45.8X5	T45.8X6
glubionate	T50.3X1	T50.3X2	T50.3X3	T50.3X4	T50.3X5	T50.3X6
gluconate	T50.3X1	T50.3X2	T50.3X3	T50.3X4	T50.3X5	T50.3X6
gluconogalactogluconate	T50.3X1	T50.3X2	T50.3X3	T50.3X4	T50.3X5	T50.3X6
hydrate, hydroxide	T54.3X1	T54.3X2	T54.3X3	T54.3X4	—	—
hypochlorite	T54.3X1	T54.3X2	T54.3X3	T54.3X4	—	—
iodide	T48.4X1	T48.4X2	T48.4X3	T48.4X4	T48.4X5	T48.4X6
ipodate	T50.8X1	T50.8X2	T50.8X3	T50.8X4	T50.8X5	T50.8X6
lactate	T50.3X1	T50.3X2	T50.3X3	T50.3X4	T50.3X5	T50.3X6
leucovorin	T45.8X1	T45.8X2	T45.8X3	T45.8X4	T45.8X5	T45.8X6
mandelate	T37.91	T37.92	T37.93	T37.94	T37.95	T37.96
oxide	T54.3X1	T54.3X2	T54.3X3	T54.3X4	—	—
pantothenate	T45.2X1	T45.2X2	T45.2X3	T45.2X4	T45.2X5	T45.2X6
phosphate	T50.3X1	T50.3X2	T50.3X3	T50.3X4	T50.3X5	T50.3X6
salicylate	T39.091	T39.092	T39.093	T39.094	T39.095	T39.096
salts	T50.3X1	T50.3X2	T50.3X3	T50.3X4	T50.3X5	T50.3X6
Calculus-dissolving drug	T50.991	T50.992	T50.993	T50.994	T50.995	T50.996
Calomel	T49.0X1	T49.0X2	T49.0X3	T49.0X4	T49.0X5	T49.0X6
Caloric agent	T50.3X1	T50.3X2	T50.3X3	T50.3X4	T50.3X5	T50.3X6
Calusterone	T38.7X1	T38.7X2	T38.7X3	T38.7X4	T38.7X5	T38.7X6
Camazepam	T42.4X1	T42.4X2	T42.4X3	T42.4X4	T42.4X5	T42.4X6
Camomile	T49.0X1	T49.0X2	T49.0X3	T49.0X4	T49.0X5	T49.0X6
Camoquin	T37.2X1	T37.2X2	T37.2X3	T37.2X4	T37.2X5	T37.2X6
Camphor						
insecticide	T60.2X1	T60.2X2	T60.2X3	T60.2X4	—	—
medicinal	T49.8X1	T49.8X2	T49.8X3	T49.8X4	T49.8X5	T49.8X6
Camylofin	T44.3X1	T44.3X2	T44.3X3	T44.3X4	T44.3X5	T44.3X6
Cancer chemotherapy drug regimen	T45.1X1	T45.1X2	T45.1X3	T45.1X4	T45.1X5	T45.1X6
Candeptin	T49.0X1	T49.0X2	T49.0X3	T49.0X4	T49.0X5	T49.0X6
Candicidin	T49.0X1	T49.0X2	T49.0X3	T49.0X4	T49.0X5	T49.0X6
Cannabinoids, synthetic	T40.721	T40.722	T40.723	T40.724	T40.725	T40.726
Cannabinol	T40.711	T40.712	T40.713	T40.714	T40.715	T40.716
Cannabis (derivatives)	T40.711	T40.712	T40.713	T40.714	T40.715	T40.716
Canned heat	T51.1X1	T51.1X2	T51.1X3	T51.1X4	—	—
Canrenoic acid	T50.0X1	T50.0X2	T50.0X3	T50.0X4	T50.0X5	T50.0X6
Canrenone	T50.0X1	T50.0X2	T50.0X3	T50.0X4	T50.0X5	T50.0X6

◀ New   ◀ Revised   ~~deleted~~ Deleted

Substance	Poisoning, Accidental (Unintentional)	Poisoning, Intentional Self-Harm	Poisoning, Assault	Poisoning, Undetermined	Adverse Effect	Underdosing
Cantharides, cantharidin, cantharis	T49.8X1	T49.8X2	T49.8X3	T49.8X4	T49.8X5	T49.8X6
Canthaxanthin	T50.991	T50.992	T50.993	T50.994	T50.995	T50.996
Capillary-active drug NEC	T46.901	T46.902	T46.903	T46.904	T46.905	T46.906
Capreomycin	T36.8X1	T36.8X2	T36.8X3	T36.8X4	T36.8X5	T36.8X6
Capsicum	T49.4X1	T49.4X2	T49.4X3	T49.4X4	T49.4X5	T49.4X6
Captafol	T60.3X1	T60.3X2	T60.3X3	T60.3X4	—	—
Captan	T60.3X1	T60.3X2	T60.3X3	T60.3X4	—	—
Captodiame, captodiamine	T43.591	T43.592	T43.593	T43.594	T43.595	T43.596
Captopril	T46.4X1	T46.4X2	T46.4X3	T46.4X4	T46.4X5	T46.4X6
Caramiphen	T44.3X1	T44.3X2	T44.3X3	T44.3X4	T44.3X5	T44.3X6
Carazolol	T44.7X1	T44.7X2	T44.7X3	T44.7X4	T44.7X5	T44.7X6
Carbachol	T44.1X1	T44.1X2	T44.1X3	T44.1X4	T44.1X5	T44.1X6
Carbacrylamine (resin)	T50.3X1	T50.3X2	T50.3X3	T50.3X4	T50.3X5	T50.3X6
Carbamate (insecticide)	T60.0X1	T60.0X2	T60.0X3	T60.0X4	—	—
Carbamate (sedative)	T42.6X1	T42.6X2	T42.6X3	T42.6X4	T42.6X5	T42.6X6
herbicide	T60.0X1	T60.0X2	T60.0X3	T60.0X4	—	—
insecticide	T60.0X1	T60.0X2	T60.0X3	T60.0X4	—	—
Carbamazepine	T42.1X1	T42.1X2	T42.1X3	T42.1X4	T42.1X5	T42.1X6
Carbamide	T47.3X1	T47.3X2	T47.3X3	T47.3X4	T47.3X5	T47.3X6
peroxide	T49.0X1	T49.0X2	T49.0X3	T49.0X4	T49.0X5	T49.0X6
topical	T49.8X1	T49.8X2	T49.8X3	T49.8X4	T49.8X5	T49.8X6
Carbamylcholine chloride	T44.1X1	T44.1X2	T44.1X3	T44.1X4	T44.1X5	T44.1X6
Carbaril	T60.0X1	T60.0X2	T60.0X3	T60.0X4	—	—
Carbarsone	T37.3X1	T37.3X2	T37.3X3	T37.3X4	T37.3X5	T37.3X6
Carbaryl	T60.0X1	T60.0X2	T60.0X3	T60.0X4	—	—
Carbaspirin	T39.011	T39.012	T39.013	T39.014	T39.015	T39.016
Carbazochrome (salicylate) (sodium sulfonate)	T49.4X1	T49.4X2	T49.4X3	T49.4X4	T49.4X5	T49.4X6
Carbenicillin	T36.0X1	T36.0X2	T36.0X3	T36.0X4	T36.0X5	T36.0X6
Carbenoxolone	T47.1X1	T47.1X2	T47.1X3	T47.1X4	T47.1X5	T47.1X6
Carbetapentane	T48.3X1	T48.3X2	T48.3X3	T48.3X4	T48.3X5	T48.3X6
Carbethyl salicylate	T39.091	T39.092	T39.093	T39.094	T39.095	T39.096
Carbidopa (with levodopa)	T42.8X1	T42.8X2	T42.8X3	T42.8X4	T42.8X5	T42.8X6
Carbimazole	T38.2X1	T38.2X2	T38.2X3	T38.2X4	T38.2X5	T38.2X6
Carbinol	T51.1X1	T51.1X2	T51.1X3	T51.1X4	—	—
Carbinoxamine	T45.0X1	T45.0X2	T45.0X3	T45.0X4	T45.0X5	T45.0X6
Carbiphene	T39.8X1	T39.8X2	T39.8X3	T39.8X4	T39.8X5	T39.8X6
Carbitol	T52.3X1	T52.3X2	T52.3X3	T52.3X4	—	—
Carbocaine	T41.3X1	T41.3X2	T41.3X3	T41.3X4	T41.3X5	T41.3X6
infiltration (subcutaneous)	T41.3X1	T41.3X2	T41.3X3	T41.3X4	T41.3X5	T41.3X6
nerve block (peripheral) (plexus)	T41.3X1	T41.3X2	T41.3X3	T41.3X4	T41.3X5	T41.3X6
topical (surface)	T41.3X1	T41.3X2	T41.3X3	T41.3X4	T41.3X5	T41.3X6

Substance	Poisoning, Accidental (Unintentional)	Poisoning, Intentional Self-Harm	Poisoning, Assault	Poisoning, Undetermined	Adverse Effect	Underdosing
Carbo medicinalis	T47.6X1	T47.6X2	T47.6X3	T47.6X4	T47.6X5	T47.6X6
Carbomycin	T36.8X1	T36.8X2	T36.8X3	T36.8X4	T36.8X5	T36.8X6
Carbocisteine	T48.4X1	T48.4X2	T48.4X3	T48.4X4	T48.4X5	T48.4X6
Carbocromen	T46.3X1	T46.3X2	T46.3X3	T46.3X4	T46.3X5	T46.3X6
Carbol fuchsin	T49.0X1	T49.0X2	T49.0X3	T49.0X4	T49.0X5	T49.0X6
Carbolic acid — *see also* Phenol	T54.0X1	T54.0X2	T54.0X3	T54.0X4	—	—
Carbolonium (bromide)	T48.1X1	T48.1X2	T48.1X3	T48.1X4	T48.1X5	T48.1X6
Carbon						
bisulfide (liquid)	T65.4X1	T65.4X2	T65.4X3	T65.4X4	—	—
vapor	T65.4X1	T65.4X2	T65.4X3	T65.4X4	—	—
dioxide (gas)	T59.7X1	T59.7X2	T59.7X3	T59.7X4	—	—
medicinal	T41.5X1	T41.5X2	T41.5X3	T41.5X4	T41.5X5	T41.5X6
nonmedicinal	T59.7X1	T59.7X2	T59.7X3	T59.7X4	—	—
snow	T49.4X1	T49.4X2	T49.4X3	T49.4X4	T49.4X5	T49.4X6
disulfide (liquid)	T65.4X1	T65.4X2	T65.4X3	T65.4X4	—	—
vapor	T65.4X1	T65.4X2	T65.4X3	T65.4X4	—	—
monoxide (from incomplete combustion)	T58.91	T58.92	T58.93	T58.94	—	—
blast furnace gas	T58.8X1	T58.8X2	T58.8X3	T58.8X4	—	—
butane (distributed in mobile container)	T58.11	T58.12	T58.13	T58.14	—	—
distributed through pipes	T58.11	T58.12	T58.13	T58.14	—	—
charcoal fumes	T58.2X1	T58.2X2	T58.2X3	T58.2X4	—	—
coal	T58.2X1	T58.2X2	T58.2X3	T58.2X4	—	—
coke (in domestic stoves, fireplaces)	T58.2X1	T58.2X2	T58.2X3	T58.2X4	—	—
gas (piped)	T58.11	T58.12	T58.13	T58.14	—	—
solid (in domestic stoves, fireplaces)	T58.2X1	T58.2X2	T58.2X3	T58.2X4	—	—
exhaust gas (motor) not in transit	T58.01	T58.02	T58.03	T58.04	—	—
combustion engine, any not in watercraft	T58.01	T58.02	T58.03	T58.04	—	—
farm tractor, not in transit	T58.01	T58.02	T58.03	T58.04	—	—
gas engine	T58.01	T58.02	T58.03	T58.04	—	—
motor pump	T58.01	T58.02	T58.03	T58.04	—	—
motor vehicle, not in transit	T58.01	T58.02	T58.03	T58.04	—	—
fuel (in domestic use)	T58.2X1	T58.2X2	T58.2X3	T58.2X4	—	—
gas (piped)	T58.11	T58.12	T58.13	T58.14	—	—
in mobile container	T58.11	T58.12	T58.13	T58.14	—	—
utility	T58.11	T58.12	T58.13	T58.14	—	—
in mobile container	T58.11	T58.12	T58.13	T58.14	—	—
piped (natural)	T58.11	T58.12	T58.13	T58.14	—	—

TABLE OF DRUGS AND CHEMICALS

Substance	External Cause (T-Code)					
	Poisoning, Accidental (Unintentional)	Poisoning, Intentional Self-Harm	Poisoning, Assault	Poisoning, Undetermined	Adverse Effect	Underdosing
Carbon (Continued)						
monoxide (Continued)						
illuminating gas	T58.11	T58.12	T58.13	T58.14	—	—
industrial fuels or gases, any	T58.8X1	T58.8X2	T58.8X3	T58.8X4	—	—
kerosene (in domestic stoves, fireplaces)	T58.2X1	T58.2X2	T58.2X3	T58.2X4	—	—
kiln gas or vapor	T58.8X1	T58.8X2	T58.8X3	T58.8X4	—	—
motor exhaust gas, not in transit	T58.01	T58.02	T58.03	T58.04	—	—
piped gas (manufactured) (natural)	T58.11	T58.12	T58.13	T58.14	—	—
producer gas	T58.8X1	T58.8X2	T58.8X3	T58.8X4	—	—
propane (distributed in mobile container)	T58.11	T58.12	T58.13	T58.14	—	—
distributed through pipes	T58.11	T58.12	T58.13	T58.14	—	—
specified source NEC	T58.8X1	T58.8X2	T58.8X3	T58.8X4	—	—
stove gas	T58.11	T58.12	T58.13	T58.14	—	—
piped	T58.11	T58.12	T58.13	T58.14	—	—
utility gas	T58.11	T58.12	T58.13	T58.14	—	—
piped	T58.11	T58.12	T58.13	T58.14	—	—
water gas	T58.11	T58.12	T58.13	T58.14	—	—
wood (in domestic stoves, fireplaces)	T58.2X1	T58.2X2	T58.2X3	T58.2X4	—	—
tetrachloride (vapor) NEC	T53.0X1	T53.0X2	T53.0X3	T53.0X4	—	—
liquid (cleansing agent) NEC	T53.0X1	T53.0X2	T53.0X3	T53.0X4	—	—
solvent	T53.0X1	T53.0X2	T53.0X3	T53.0X4	—	—
Carbonic acid gas	T59.7X1	T59.7X2	T59.7X3	T59.7X4	—	—
anhydrase inhibitor NEC	T50.2X1	T50.2X2	T50.2X3	T50.2X4	T50.2X5	T50.2X6
Carbophenothion	T60.0X1	T60.0X2	T60.0X3	T60.0X4	—	—
Carboplatin	T45.1X1	T45.1X2	T45.1X3	T45.1X4	T45.1X5	T45.1X6
Carboprost	T48.0X1	T48.0X2	T48.0X3	T48.0X4	T48.0X5	T48.0X6
Carboquone	T45.1X1	T45.1X2	T45.1X3	T45.1X4	T45.1X5	T45.1X6
Carbowax	T49.3X1	T49.3X2	T49.3X3	T49.3X4	T49.3X5	T49.3X6
Carboxymethyl-cellulose	T47.4X1	T47.4X2	T47.4X3	T47.4X4	T47.4X5	T47.4X6
S-Carboxymethyl-cysteine	T48.4X1	T48.4X2	T48.4X3	T48.4X4	T48.4X5	T48.4X6
Carbrital	T42.3X1	T42.3X2	T42.3X3	T42.3X4	T42.3X5	T42.3X6
Carbromal	T42.6X1	T42.6X2	T42.6X3	T42.6X4	T42.6X5	T42.6X6
Carbutamide	T38.3X1	T38.3X2	T38.3X3	T38.3X4	T38.3X5	T38.3X6
Carbuterol	T48.6X1	T48.6X2	T48.6X3	T48.6X4	T48.6X5	T48.6X6
Cardiac						
depressants	T46.2X1	T46.2X2	T46.2X3	T46.2X4	T46.2X5	T46.2X6
rhythm regulator	T46.2X1	T46.2X2	T46.2X3	T46.2X4	T46.2X5	T46.2X6
specified NEC	T46.2X1	T46.2X2	T46.2X3	T46.2X4	T46.2X5	T46.2X6

Substance	External Cause (T-Code)					
	Poisoning, Accidental (Unintentional)	Poisoning, Intentional Self-Harm	Poisoning, Assault	Poisoning, Undetermined	Adverse Effect	Underdosing
Cardiografin	T50.8X1	T50.8X2	T50.8X3	T50.8X4	T50.8X5	T50.8X6
Cardio-green	T50.8X1	T50.8X2	T50.8X3	T50.8X4	T50.8X5	T50.8X6
Cardiotonic (glycoside) NEC	T46.0X1	T46.0X2	T46.0X3	T46.0X4	T46.0X5	T46.0X6
Cardiovascular drug NEC	T46.901	T46.902	T46.903	T46.904	T46.905	T46.906
Cardrase	T50.2X1	T50.2X2	T50.2X3	T50.2X4	T50.2X5	T50.2X6
Carfusin	T49.0X1	T49.0X2	T49.0X3	T49.0X4	T49.0X5	T49.0X6
Carfecillin	T36.0X1	T36.0X2	T36.0X3	T36.0X4	T36.0X5	T36.0X6
Carfenazine	T43.3X1	T43.3X2	T43.3X3	T43.3X4	T43.3X5	T43.3X6
Carindacillin	T36.0X1	T36.0X2	T36.0X3	T36.0X4	T36.0X5	T36.0X6
Carisoprodol	T42.8X1	T42.8X2	T42.8X3	T42.8X4	T42.8X5	T42.8X6
Carmellose	T47.4X1	T47.4X2	T47.4X3	T47.4X4	T47.4X5	T47.4X6
Carminative	T47.5X1	T47.5X2	T47.5X3	T47.5X4	T47.5X5	T47.5X6
Carmofur	T45.1X1	T45.1X2	T45.1X3	T45.1X4	T45.1X5	T45.1X6
Carmustine	T45.1X1	T45.1X2	T45.1X3	T45.1X4	T45.1X5	T45.1X6
Carotene	T45.2X1	T45.2X2	T45.2X3	T45.2X4	T45.2X5	T45.2X6
Carphenazine	T43.3X1	T43.3X2	T43.3X3	T43.3X4	T43.3X5	T43.3X6
Carpipramine	T42.4X1	T42.4X2	T42.4X3	T42.4X4	T42.4X5	T42.4X6
Carprofen	T39.311	T39.312	T39.313	T39.314	T39.315	T39.316
Carpronium chloride	T44.3X1	T44.3X2	T44.3X3	T44.3X4	T44.3X5	T44.3X6
Carrageenan	T47.8X1	T47.8X2	T47.8X3	T47.8X4	T47.8X5	T47.8X6
Carteolol	T44.7X1	T44.7X2	T44.7X3	T44.7X4	T44.7X5	T44.7X6
Carter's Little Pills	T47.2X1	T47.2X2	T47.2X3	T47.2X4	T47.2X5	T47.2X6
Cascara (sagrada)	T47.2X1	T47.2X2	T47.2X3	T47.2X4	T47.2X5	T47.2X6
Cassava	T62.2X1	T62.2X2	T62.2X3	T62.2X4	—	—
Castellani's paint	T49.0X1	T49.0X2	T49.0X3	T49.0X4	T49.0X5	T49.0X6
Castor						
bean	T62.2X1	T62.2X2	T62.2X3	T62.2X4	—	—
oil	T47.2X1	T47.2X2	T47.2X3	T47.2X4	T47.2X5	T47.2X6
Catalase	T45.3X1	T45.3X2	T45.3X3	T45.3X4	T45.3X5	T45.3X6
Caterpillar (sting)	T63.431	T63.432	T63.433	T63.434	—	—
Catha (edulis) (tea)	T43.691	T43.692	T43.693	T43.694	—	—
Cathartic NEC	T47.4X1	T47.4X2	T47.4X3	T47.4X4	T47.4X5	T47.4X6
anthracene derivative	T47.2X1	T47.2X2	T47.2X3	T47.2X4	T47.2X5	T47.2X6
bulk	T47.4X1	T47.4X2	T47.4X3	T47.4X4	T47.4X5	T47.4X6
contact	T47.2X1	T47.2X2	T47.2X3	T47.2X4	T47.2X5	T47.2X6
emollient NEC	T47.4X1	T47.4X2	T47.4X3	T47.4X4	T47.4X5	T47.4X6
irritant NEC	T47.2X1	T47.2X2	T47.2X3	T47.2X4	T47.2X5	T47.2X6
mucilage	T47.4X1	T47.4X2	T47.4X3	T47.4X4	T47.4X5	T47.4X6
saline	T47.3X1	T47.3X2	T47.3X3	T47.3X4	T47.3X5	T47.3X6
vegetable	T47.2X1	T47.2X2	T47.2X3	T47.2X4	T47.2X5	T47.2X6
Cathine	T50.5X1	T50.5X2	T50.5X3	T50.5X4	T50.5X5	T50.5X6
Cathomycin	T36.8X1	T36.8X2	T36.8X3	T36.8X4	T36.8X5	T36.8X6

◀ New ◀ Revised ~~deleted~~ Deleted

Substance	Poisoning, Accidental (Unintentional)	Poisoning, Intentional Self-Harm	Poisoning, Assault	Poisoning, Undetermined	Adverse Effect	Underdosing
Cation exchange resin	T5Ø.3X1	T5Ø.3X2	T5Ø.3X3	T5Ø.3X4	T5Ø.3X5	T5Ø.3X6
Caustic(s) NEC	T54.91	T54.92	T54.93	T54.94	—	—
alkali	T54.3X1	T54.3X2	T54.3X3	T54.3X4	—	—
hydroxide	T54.3X1	T54.3X2	T54.3X3	T54.3X4	—	—
potash	T54.3X1	T54.3X2	T54.3X3	T54.3X4	—	—
soda	T54.3X1	T54.3X2	T54.3X3	T54.3X4	—	—
specified NEC	T54.91	T54.92	T54.93	T54.94	—	—
Ceepryn	T49.ØX1	T49.ØX2	T49.ØX3	T49.ØX4	T49.ØX5	T49.ØX6
ENT agent	T49.6X1	T49.6X2	T49.6X3	T49.6X4	T49.6X5	T49.6X6
lozenges	T49.6X1	T49.6X2	T49.6X3	T49.6X4	T49.6X5	T49.6X6
Cefacetrile	T36.1X1	T36.1X2	T36.1X3	T36.1X4	T36.1X5	T36.1X6
Cefaclor	T36.1X1	T36.1X2	T36.1X3	T36.1X4	T36.1X5	T36.1X6
Cefadroxil	T36.1X1	T36.1X2	T36.1X3	T36.1X4	T36.1X5	T36.1X6
Cefalexin	T36.1X1	T36.1X2	T36.1X3	T36.1X4	T36.1X5	T36.1X6
Cefaloglycin	T36.1X1	T36.1X2	T36.1X3	T36.1X4	T36.1X5	T36.1X6
Cefaloridine	T36.1X1	T36.1X2	T36.1X3	T36.1X4	T36.1X5	T36.1X6
Cefalosporins	T36.1X1	T36.1X2	T36.1X3	T36.1X4	T36.1X5	T36.1X6
Cefalotin	T36.1X1	T36.1X2	T36.1X3	T36.1X4	T36.1X5	T36.1X6
Cefamandole	T36.1X1	T36.1X2	T36.1X3	T36.1X4	T36.1X5	T36.1X6
Cefamycin antibiotic	T36.1X1	T36.1X2	T36.1X3	T36.1X4	T36.1X5	T36.1X6
Cefapirin	T36.1X1	T36.1X2	T36.1X3	T36.1X4	T36.1X5	T36.1X6
Cefatrizine	T36.1X1	T36.1X2	T36.1X3	T36.1X4	T36.1X5	T36.1X6
Cefazedone	T36.1X1	T36.1X2	T36.1X3	T36.1X4	T36.1X5	T36.1X6
Cefazolin	T36.1X1	T36.1X2	T36.1X3	T36.1X4	T36.1X5	T36.1X6
Cefbuperazone	T36.1X1	T36.1X2	T36.1X3	T36.1X4	T36.1X5	T36.1X6
Cefetamet	T36.1X1	T36.1X2	T36.1X3	T36.1X4	T36.1X5	T36.1X6
Cefixime	T36.1X1	T36.1X2	T36.1X3	T36.1X4	T36.1X5	T36.1X6
Cefmenoxime	T36.1X1	T36.1X2	T36.1X3	T36.1X4	T36.1X5	T36.1X6
Cefmetazole	T36.1X1	T36.1X2	T36.1X3	T36.1X4	T36.1X5	T36.1X6
Cefminox	T36.1X1	T36.1X2	T36.1X3	T36.1X4	T36.1X5	T36.1X6
Cefonicid	T36.1X1	T36.1X2	T36.1X3	T36.1X4	T36.1X5	T36.1X6
Cefoperazone	T36.1X1	T36.1X2	T36.1X3	T36.1X4	T36.1X5	T36.1X6
Ceforanide	T36.1X1	T36.1X2	T36.1X3	T36.1X4	T36.1X5	T36.1X6
Cefotaxime	T36.1X1	T36.1X2	T36.1X3	T36.1X4	T36.1X5	T36.1X6
Cefotetan	T36.1X1	T36.1X2	T36.1X3	T36.1X4	T36.1X5	T36.1X6
Cefotiam	T36.1X1	T36.1X2	T36.1X3	T36.1X4	T36.1X5	T36.1X6
Cefoxitin	T36.1X1	T36.1X2	T36.1X3	T36.1X4	T36.1X5	T36.1X6
Cefpimizole	T36.1X1	T36.1X2	T36.1X3	T36.1X4	T36.1X5	T36.1X6
Cefpiramide	T36.1X1	T36.1X2	T36.1X3	T36.1X4	T36.1X5	T36.1X6
Cefradine	T36.1X1	T36.1X2	T36.1X3	T36.1X4	T36.1X5	T36.1X6
Cefroxadine	T36.1X1	T36.1X2	T36.1X3	T36.1X4	T36.1X5	T36.1X6
Cefsulodin	T36.1X1	T36.1X2	T36.1X3	T36.1X4	T36.1X5	T36.1X6

Substance	Poisoning, Accidental (Unintentional)	Poisoning, Intentional Self-Harm	Poisoning, Assault	Poisoning, Undetermined	Adverse Effect	Underdosing
Ceftazidime	T36.1X1	T36.1X2	T36.1X3	T36.1X4	T36.1X5	T36.1X6
Cefteram	T36.1X1	T36.1X2	T36.1X3	T36.1X4	T36.1X5	T36.1X6
Ceftezole	T36.1X1	T36.1X2	T36.1X3	T36.1X4	T36.1X5	T36.1X6
Ceftizoxime	T36.1X1	T36.1X2	T36.1X3	T36.1X4	T36.1X5	T36.1X6
Ceftriaxone	T36.1X1	T36.1X2	T36.1X3	T36.1X4	T36.1X5	T36.1X6
Cefuroxime	T36.1X1	T36.1X2	T36.1X3	T36.1X4	T36.1X5	T36.1X6
Cefuzonam	T36.1X1	T36.1X2	T36.1X3	T36.1X4	T36.1X5	T36.1X6
Celestone	T38.ØX1	T38.ØX2	T38.ØX3	T38.ØX4	T38.ØX5	T38.ØX6
topical	T49.ØX1	T49.ØX2	T49.ØX3	T49.ØX4	T49.ØX5	T49.ØX6
Celiprolol	T44.7X1	T44.7X2	T44.7X3	T44.7X4	T44.7X5	T44.7X6
Cellosolve	T52.91	T52.92	T52.93	T52.94	—	—
Cell stimulants and proliferants	T49.8X1	T49.8X2	T49.8X3	T49.8X4	T49.8X5	T49.8X6
Cellulose						
cathartic	T47.4X1	T47.4X2	T47.4X3	T47.4X4	T47.4X5	T47.4X6
hydroxyethyl	T47.4X1	T47.4X2	T47.4X3	T47.4X4	T47.4X5	T47.4X6
nitrates (topical)	T49.3X1	T49.3X2	T49.3X3	T49.3X4	T49.3X5	T49.3X6
oxidized	T49.4X1	T49.4X2	T49.4X3	T49.4X4	T49.4X5	T49.4X6
Centipede (bite)	T63.411	T63.412	T63.413	T63.414	—	—
Central nervous system						
depressants	T42.71	T42.72	T42.73	T42.74	T42.75	T42.76
anesthetic (general) NEC	T41.2Ø1	T41.2Ø2	T41.2Ø3	T41.2Ø4	T41.2Ø5	T41.2Ø6
gases NEC	T41.ØX1	T41.ØX2	T41.ØX3	T41.ØX4	T41.ØX5	T41.ØX6
intravenous	T41.1X1	T41.1X2	T41.1X3	T41.1X4	T41.1X5	T41.1X6
barbiturates	T42.3X1	T42.3X2	T42.3X3	T42.3X4	T42.3X5	T42.3X6
benzodiazepines	T42.4X1	T42.4X2	T42.4X3	T42.4X4	T42.4X5	T42.4X6
bromides	T42.6X1	T42.6X2	T42.6X3	T42.6X4	T42.6X5	T42.6X6
cannabis sativa	T4Ø.711	T4Ø.712	T4Ø.713	T4Ø.714	T4Ø.715	T4Ø.716
chloral hydrate	T42.6X1	T42.6X2	T42.6X3	T42.6X4	T42.6X5	T42.6X6
ethanol	T51.ØX1	T51.ØX2	T51.ØX3	T51.ØX4	—	—
hallucinogenics	T4Ø.9Ø1	T4Ø.9Ø2	T4Ø.9Ø3	T4Ø.9Ø4	T4Ø.9Ø5	T4Ø.9Ø6
hypnotics	T42.71	T42.72	T42.73	T42.74	T42.75	T42.76
specified NEC	T42.6X1	T42.6X2	T42.6X3	T42.6X4	T42.6X5	T42.6X6
muscle relaxants	T42.8X1	T42.8X2	T42.8X3	T42.8X4	T42.8X5	T42.8X6
paraldehyde	T42.6X1	T42.6X2	T42.6X3	T42.6X4	T42.6X5	T42.6X6
sedatives; sedative-hypnotics	T42.71	T42.72	T42.73	T42.74	T42.75	T42.76
mixed NEC	T42.6X1	T42.6X2	T42.6X3	T42.6X4	T42.6X5	T42.6X6
specified NEC	T42.6X1	T42.6X2	T42.6X3	T42.6X4	T42.6X5	T42.6X6
muscle-tone depressants	T42.8X1	T42.8X2	T42.8X3	T42.8X4	T42.8X5	T42.8X6
stimulants	T43.6Ø1	T43.6Ø2	T43.6Ø3	T43.6Ø4	T43.6Ø5	T43.6Ø6
amphetamines	T43.621	T43.622	T43.623	T43.624	T43.625	T43.626
analeptics	T5Ø.7X1	T5Ø.7X2	T5Ø.7X3	T5Ø.7X4	T5Ø.7X5	T5Ø.7X6

Substance	Poisoning, Accidental (Unintentional)	Poisoning, Intentional Self-Harm	Poisoning, Assault	Poisoning, Undetermined	Adverse Effect	Underdosing
Central nervous system (Continued)						
stimulants (Continued)						
antidepressants	T43.2Ø1	T43.2Ø2	T43.2Ø3	T43.2Ø4	T43.2Ø5	T43.2Ø6
opiate antagonists	T50.7X1	T50.7X2	T50.7X3	T50.7X4	T50.7X5	T50.7X6
specified NEC	T43.691	T43.692	T43.693	T43.694	T43.695	T43.696
Cephalexin	T36.1X1	T36.1X2	T36.1X3	T36.1X4	T36.1X5	T36.1X6
Cephaloglycin	T36.1X1	T36.1X2	T36.1X3	T36.1X4	T36.1X5	T36.1X6
Cephaloridine	T36.1X1	T36.1X2	T36.1X3	T36.1X4	T36.1X5	T36.1X6
Cephalosporins	T36.1X1	T36.1X2	T36.1X3	T36.1X4	T36.1X5	T36.1X6
N (adicillin)	T36.ØX1	T36.ØX2	T36.ØX3	T36.ØX4	T36.ØX5	T36.ØX6
Cephalothin	T36.1X1	T36.1X2	T36.1X3	T36.1X4	T36.1X5	T36.1X6
Cephalotin	T36.1X1	T36.1X2	T36.1X3	T36.1X4	T36.1X5	T36.1X6
Cephradine	T36.1X1	T36.1X2	T36.1X3	T36.1X4	T36.1X5	T36.1X6
Cerbera (odallam)	T62.2X1	T62.2X2	T62.2X3	T62.2X4	—	—
Cerberin	T46.ØX1	T46.ØX2	T46.ØX3	T46.ØX4	T46.ØX5	T46.ØX6
Cerebral stimulants	T43.6Ø1	T43.6Ø2	T43.6Ø3	T43.6Ø4	T43.6Ø5	T43.6Ø6
psychotherapeutic	T43.6Ø1	T43.6Ø2	T43.6Ø3	T43.6Ø4	T43.6Ø5	T43.6Ø6
specified NEC	T43.691	T43.692	T43.693	T43.694	T43.695	T43.696
Cerium oxalate	T45.ØX1	T45.ØX2	T45.ØX3	T45.ØX4	T45.ØX5	T45.ØX6
Cerous oxalate	T45.ØX1	T45.ØX2	T45.ØX3	T45.ØX4	T45.ØX5	T45.ØX6
Ceruletide	T50.8X1	T50.8X2	T50.8X3	T50.8X4	T50.8X5	T50.8X6
Cetalkonium (chloride)	T49.ØX1	T49.ØX2	T49.ØX3	T49.ØX4	T49.ØX5	T49.ØX6
Cethexonium chloride	T49.ØX1	T49.ØX2	T49.ØX3	T49.ØX4	T49.ØX5	T49.ØX6
Cetiedil	T46.7X1	T46.7X2	T46.7X3	T46.7X4	T46.7X5	T46.7X6
Cetirizine	T45.ØX1	T45.ØX2	T45.ØX3	T45.ØX4	T45.ØX5	T45.ØX6
Cetomacrogol	T50.991	T50.992	T50.993	T50.994	T50.995	T50.996
Cetotiamine	T45.2X1	T45.2X2	T45.2X3	T45.2X4	T45.2X5	T45.2X6
Cetoxime	T45.ØX1	T45.ØX2	T45.ØX3	T45.ØX4	T45.ØX5	T45.ØX6
Cetraxate	T47.1X1	T47.1X2	T47.1X3	T47.1X4	T47.1X5	T47.1X6
Cetrimide	T49.ØX1	T49.ØX2	T49.ØX3	T49.ØX4	T49.ØX5	T49.ØX6
Cetrimonium (bromide)	T49.ØX1	T49.ØX2	T49.ØX3	T49.ØX4	T49.ØX5	T49.ØX6
Cetylpyridinium chloride	T49.ØX1	T49.ØX2	T49.ØX3	T49.ØX4	T49.ØX5	T49.ØX6
ENT agent	T49.6X1	T49.6X2	T49.6X3	T49.6X4	T49.6X5	T49.6X6
lozenges	T49.6X1	T49.6X2	T49.6X3	T49.6X4	T49.6X5	T49.6X6
Cevadillasee Sabadilla						
Cevitamic acid	T45.2X1	T45.2X2	T45.2X3	T45.2X4	T45.2X5	T45.2X6
Chalk, precipitated	T47.1X1	T47.1X2	T47.1X3	T47.1X4	T47.1X5	T47.1X6
Chamomile	T49.ØX1	T49.ØX2	T49.ØX3	T49.ØX4	T49.ØX5	T49.ØX6
Ch'an su	T46.ØX1	T46.ØX2	T46.ØX3	T46.ØX4	T46.ØX5	T46.ØX6
Charcoal	T47.6X1	T47.6X2	T47.6X3	T47.6X4	T47.6X5	T47.6X6
activated — see also Charcoal, medicinal	T47.6X1	T47.6X2	T47.6X3	T47.6X4	T47.6X5	T47.6X6

Substance	Poisoning, Accidental (Unintentional)	Poisoning, Intentional Self-Harm	Poisoning, Assault	Poisoning, Undetermined	Adverse Effect	Underdosing
Charcoal (Continued)						
fumes (Carbon monoxide)	T58.2X1	T58.2X2	T58.2X3	T58.2X4	—	—
industrial	T58.8X1	T58.8X2	T58.8X3	T58.8X4	—	—
medicinal (activated)	T47.6X1	T47.6X2	T47.6X3	T47.6X4	T47.6X5	T47.6X6
antidiarrheal	T47.6X1	T47.6X2	T47.6X3	T47.6X4	T47.6X5	T47.6X6
poison control	T47.8X1	T47.8X2	T47.8X3	T47.8X4	T47.8X5	T47.8X6
specified use other than for diarrhea	T47.8X1	T47.8X2	T47.8X3	T47.8X4	T47.8X5	T47.8X6
topical	T49.8X1	T49.8X2	T49.8X3	T49.8X4	T49.8X5	T49.8X6
Chaulmosulfone	T37.1X1	T37.1X2	T37.1X3	T37.1X4	T37.1X5	T37.1X6
Chelating agent NEC	T50.6X1	T50.6X2	T50.6X3	T50.6X4	T50.6X5	T50.6X6
Chelidonium majus	T62.2X1	T62.2X2	T62.2X3	T62.2X4	—	—
Chemical substance NEC	T65.91	T65.92	T65.93	T65.94	—	—
Chenodeoxycholic acid	T47.5X1	T47.5X2	T47.5X3	T47.5X4	T47.5X5	T47.5X6
Chenodiol	T47.5X1	T47.5X2	T47.5X3	T47.5X4	T47.5X5	T47.5X6
Chenopodium	T37.4X1	T37.4X2	T37.4X3	T37.4X4	T37.4X5	T37.4X6
Cherry laurel	T62.2X1	T62.2X2	T62.2X3	T62.2X4	—	—
Chinidin(e)	T46.2X1	T46.2X2	T46.2X3	T46.2X4	T46.2X5	T46.2X6
Chiniofon	T37.8X1	T37.8X2	T37.8X3	T37.8X4	T37.8X5	T37.8X6
Chlophedianol	T48.3X1	T48.3X2	T48.3X3	T48.3X4	T48.3X5	T48.3X6
Chloral	T42.6X1	T42.6X2	T42.6X3	T42.6X4	T42.6X5	T42.6X6
derivative	T42.6X1	T42.6X2	T42.6X3	T42.6X4	T42.6X5	T42.6X6
hydrate	T42.6X1	T42.6X2	T42.6X3	T42.6X4	T42.6X5	T42.6X6
Chloralamide	T42.6X1	T42.6X2	T42.6X3	T42.6X4	T42.6X5	T42.6X6
Chloralodol	T42.6X1	T42.6X2	T42.6X3	T42.6X4	T42.6X5	T42.6X6
Chloralose	T60.4X1	T60.4X2	T60.4X3	T60.4X4	—	—
Chlorambucil	T45.1X1	T45.1X2	T45.1X3	T45.1X4	T45.1X5	T45.1X6
Chloramine	T57.8X1	T57.8X2	T57.8X3	T57.8X4	—	—
T	T49.ØX1	T49.ØX2	T49.ØX3	T49.ØX4	T49.ØX5	T49.ØX6
topical	T49.ØX1	T49.ØX2	T49.ØX3	T49.ØX4	T49.ØX5	T49.ØX6
Chloramphenicol	T36.2X1	T36.2X2	T36.2X3	T36.2X4	T36.2X5	T36.2X6
ENT agent	T49.6X1	T49.6X2	T49.6X3	T49.6X4	T49.6X5	T49.6X6
ophthalmic preparation	T49.5X1	T49.5X2	T49.5X3	T49.5X4	T49.5X5	T49.5X6
topical NEC	T49.ØX1	T49.ØX2	T49.ØX3	T49.ØX4	T49.ØX5	T49.ØX6
Chlorate (potassium) (sodium) NEC	T60.3X1	T60.3X2	T60.3X3	T60.3X4	—	—
herbicide	T60.3X1	T60.3X2	T60.3X3	T60.3X4	—	—
Chlorazanil	T50.2X1	T50.2X2	T50.2X3	T50.2X4	T50.2X5	T50.2X6
Chlorbenzene, chlorbenzol	T53.7X1	T53.7X2	T53.7X3	T53.7X4	—	—
Chlorbenzoxamine	T44.3X1	T44.3X2	T44.3X3	T44.3X4	T44.3X5	T44.3X6
Chlorbutol	T42.6X1	T42.6X2	T42.6X3	T42.6X4	T42.6X5	T42.6X6
Chlorcyclizine	T45.ØX1	T45.ØX2	T45.ØX3	T45.ØX4	T45.ØX5	T45.ØX6

◄ New   ◄ Revised   ~~deleted~~ Deleted

Substance	Poisoning, Accidental (Unintentional)	Poisoning, Intentional Self-Harm	Poisoning, Assault	Poisoning, Undetermined	Adverse Effect	Underdosing
Chlordan(e) (dust)	T60.1X1	T60.1X2	T60.1X3	T60.1X4	—	—
Chlordantoin	T49.0X1	T49.0X2	T49.0X3	T49.0X4	T49.0X5	T49.0X6
Chlordiazepoxide	T42.4X1	T42.4X2	T42.4X3	T42.4X4	T42.4X5	T42.4X6
Chlordiethyl benzamide	T49.3X1	T49.3X2	T49.3X3	T49.3X4	T49.3X5	T49.3X6
Chloresium	T49.8X1	T49.8X2	T49.8X3	T49.8X4	T49.8X5	T49.8X6
Chlorethiazol	T42.6X1	T42.6X2	T42.6X3	T42.6X4	T42.6X5	T42.6X6
Chlorethyl — see Ethyl, chloride						
Chloretone	T42.6X1	T42.6X2	T42.6X3	T42.6X4	T42.6X5	T42.6X6
Chlorex	T53.6X1	T53.6X2	T53.6X3	T53.6X4	—	—
insecticide	T60.1X1	T60.1X2	T60.1X3	T60.1X4	—	—
Chlorfenvinphos	T60.0X1	T60.0X2	T60.0X3	T60.0X4	—	—
Chlorhexadol	T42.6X1	T42.6X2	T42.6X3	T42.6X4	T42.6X5	T42.6X6
Chlorhexamide	T45.1X1	T45.1X2	T45.1X3	T45.1X4	T45.1X5	T45.1X6
Chlorhexidine	T49.0X1	T49.0X2	T49.0X3	T49.0X4	T49.0X5	T49.0X6
Chlorhydroxyquinolin	T49.0X1	T49.0X2	T49.0X3	T49.0X4	T49.0X5	T49.0X6
Chloride of lime (bleach)	T54.3X1	T54.3X2	T54.3X3	T54.3X4	—	—
Chlorimipramine	T43.011	T43.012	T43.013	T43.014	T43.015	T43.016
Chlorinated						
camphene	T53.6X1	T53.6X2	T53.6X3	T53.6X4	—	—
diphenyl	T53.7X1	T53.7X2	T53.7X3	T53.7X4	—	—
hydrocarbons NEC	T53.91	T53.92	T53.93	T53.94	—	—
solvents	T53.91	T53.92	T53.93	T53.94	—	—
lime (bleach)	T54.3X1	T54.3X2	T54.3X3	T54.3X4	—	—
and boric acid solution	T49.0X1	T49.0X2	T49.0X3	T49.0X4	T49.0X5	T49.0X6
naphthalene (insecticide)	T60.1X1	T60.1X2	T60.1X3	T60.1X4	—	—
industrial (non-pesticide)	T53.7X1	T53.7X2	T53.7X3	T53.7X4	—	—
pesticide NEC	T60.8X1	T60.8X2	T60.8X3	T60.8X4	—	—
soda — see also Sodium hypochlorite						
solution	T49.0X1	T49.0X2	T49.0X3	T49.0X4	T49.0X5	T49.0X6
Chlorine (fumes) (gas)	T59.4X1	T59.4X2	T59.4X3	T59.4X4	—	—
bleach	T54.3X1	T54.3X2	T54.3X3	T54.3X4	—	—
compound gas NEC	T59.4X1	T59.4X2	T59.4X3	T59.4X4	—	—
disinfectant	T59.4X1	T59.4X2	T59.4X3	T59.4X4	—	—
releasing agents NEC	T59.4X1	T59.4X2	T59.4X3	T59.4X4	—	—
Chlorisondamine chloride	T46.991	T46.992	T46.993	T46.994	T46.995	T46.996
Chlormadinone	T38.5X1	T38.5X2	T38.5X3	T38.5X4	T38.5X5	T38.5X6
Chlormephos	T60.0X1	T60.0X2	T60.0X3	T60.0X4	—	—
Chlormerodrin	T50.2X1	T50.2X2	T50.2X3	T50.2X4	T50.2X5	T50.2X6
Chlormethiazole	T42.6X1	T42.6X2	T42.6X3	T42.6X4	T42.6X5	T42.6X6
Chlormethine	T45.1X1	T45.1X2	T45.1X3	T45.1X4	T45.1X5	T45.1X6
Chlormethylenecycline	T36.4X1	T36.4X2	T36.4X3	T36.4X4	T36.4X5	T36.4X6

Substance	Poisoning, Accidental (Unintentional)	Poisoning, Intentional Self-Harm	Poisoning, Assault	Poisoning, Undetermined	Adverse Effect	Underdosing
Chlormezanone	T42.6X1	T42.6X2	T42.6X3	T42.6X4	T42.6X5	T42.6X6
Chloroacetic acid	T60.3X1	T60.3X2	T60.3X3	T60.3X4	—	—
Chloroacetone	T59.3X1	T59.3X2	T59.3X3	T59.3X4	—	—
Chloroacetophenone	T59.3X1	T59.3X2	T59.3X3	T59.3X4	—	—
Chloroaniline	T53.7X1	T53.7X2	T53.7X3	T53.7X4	—	—
Chlorobenzene, chlorobenzol	T53.7X1	T53.7X2	T53.7X3	T53.7X4	—	—
Chlorobromomethane (fire extinguisher)	T53.6X1	T53.6X2	T53.6X3	T53.6X4	—	—
Chlorobutanol	T49.0X1	T49.0X2	T49.0X3	T49.0X4	T49.0X5	T49.0X6
Chlorocresol	T49.0X1	T49.0X2	T49.0X3	T49.0X4	T49.0X5	T49.0X6
Chlorodehydro-methyltestosterone	T38.7X1	T38.7X2	T38.7X3	T38.7X4	T38.7X5	T38.7X6
Chlorodinitrobenzene	T53.7X1	T53.7X2	T53.7X3	T53.7X4	—	—
dust or vapor	T53.7X1	T53.7X2	T53.7X3	T53.7X4	—	—
Chlorodiphenyl	T53.7X1	T53.7X2	T53.7X3	T53.7X4	—	—
Chloroethane — see Ethyl, chloride						
Chloroethylene	T53.6X1	T53.6X2	T53.6X3	T53.6X4	—	—
Chlorofluorocarbons	T53.5X1	T53.5X2	T53.5X3	T53.5X4	—	—
Chloroform (fumes) (vapor)	T53.1X1	T53.1X2	T53.1X3	T53.1X4	—	—
anesthetic	T41.0X1	T41.0X2	T41.0X3	T41.0X4	T41.0X5	T41.0X6
solvent	T53.1X1	T53.1X2	T53.1X3	T53.1X4	—	—
water, concentrated	T41.0X1	T41.0X2	T41.0X3	T41.0X4	T41.0X5	T41.0X6
Chloroguanide	T37.2X1	T37.2X2	T37.2X3	T37.2X4	T37.2X5	T37.2X6
Chloromycetin	T36.2X1	T36.2X2	T36.2X3	T36.2X4	T36.2X5	T36.2X6
ENT agent	T49.6X1	T49.6X2	T49.6X3	T49.6X4	T49.6X5	T49.6X6
ophthalmic preparation	T49.5X1	T49.5X2	T49.5X3	T49.5X4	T49.5X5	T49.5X6
otic solution	T49.6X1	T49.6X2	T49.6X3	T49.6X4	T49.6X5	T49.6X6
topical NEC	T49.0X1	T49.0X2	T49.0X3	T49.0X4	T49.0X5	T49.0X6
Chloronitrobenzene	T53.7X1	T53.7X2	T53.7X3	T53.7X4	—	—
dust or vapor	T53.7X1	T53.7X2	T53.7X3	T53.7X4	—	—
Chlorophacinone	T60.4X1	T60.4X2	T60.4X3	T60.4X4	—	—
Chlorophenol	T53.7X1	T53.7X2	T53.7X3	T53.7X4	—	—
Chlorophenothane	T60.1X1	T60.1X2	T60.1X3	T60.1X4	—	—
Chlorophyll	T50.991	T50.992	T50.993	T50.994	T50.995	T50.996
Chloropicrin (fumes)	T53.6X1	T53.6X2	T53.6X3	T53.6X4	—	—
fumigant	T60.8X1	T60.8X2	T60.8X3	T60.8X4	—	—
fungicide	T60.3X1	T60.3X2	T60.3X3	T60.3X4	—	—
pesticide	T60.8X1	T60.8X2	T60.8X3	T60.8X4	—	—
Chloroprocaine	T41.3X1	T41.3X2	T41.3X3	T41.3X4	T41.3X5	T41.3X6
infiltration (subcutaneous)	T41.3X1	T41.3X2	T41.3X3	T41.3X4	T41.3X5	T41.3X6
nerve block (peripheral) (plexus)	T41.3X1	T41.3X2	T41.3X3	T41.3X4	T41.3X5	T41.3X6
spinal	T41.3X1	T41.3X2	T41.3X3	T41.3X4	T41.3X5	T41.3X6

◄ New   ◄ Revised   ~~deleted~~ Deleted

TABLE OF DRUGS AND CHEMICALS

Substance	External Cause (T-Code)					
	Poisoning, Accidental (Unintentional)	Poisoning, Intentional Self-Harm	Poisoning, Assault	Poisoning, Undetermined	Adverse Effect	Underdosing
Chloroptic	T49.5X1	T49.5X2	T49.5X3	T49.5X4	T49.5X5	T49.5X6
Chloropurine	T45.1X1	T45.1X2	T45.1X3	T45.1X4	T45.1X5	T45.1X6
Chloropyramine	T45.0X1	T45.0X2	T45.0X3	T45.0X4	T45.0X5	T45.0X6
Chloropyrifos	T60.0X1	T60.0X2	T60.0X3	T60.0X4	—	—
Chloropyrilene	T45.0X1	T45.0X2	T45.0X3	T45.0X4	T45.0X5	T45.0X6
Chloroquine	T37.2X1	T37.2X2	T37.2X3	T37.2X4	T37.2X5	T37.2X6
Chlorothalonil	T60.3X1	T60.3X2	T60.3X3	T60.3X4	—	—
Chlorothen	T45.0X1	T45.0X2	T45.0X3	T45.0X4	T45.0X5	T45.0X6
Chlorothiazide	T50.2X1	T50.2X2	T50.2X3	T50.2X4	T50.2X5	T50.2X6
Chlorothymol	T49.4X1	T49.4X2	T49.4X3	T49.4X4	T49.4X5	T49.4X6
Chlorotrianisene	T38.5X1	T38.5X2	T38.5X3	T38.5X4	T38.5X5	T38.5X6
Chlorovinyldichloro-arsine, not in war	T57.0X1	T57.0X2	T57.0X3	T57.0X4	—	—
Chloroxine	T49.4X1	T49.4X2	T49.4X3	T49.4X4	T49.4X5	T49.4X6
Chloroxylenol	T49.0X1	T49.0X2	T49.0X3	T49.0X4	T49.0X5	T49.0X6
Chlorphenamine	T45.0X1	T45.0X2	T45.0X3	T45.0X4	T45.0X5	T45.0X6
Chlorphenesin	T42.8X1	T42.8X2	T42.8X3	T42.8X4	T42.8X5	T42.8X6
topical (antifungal)	T49.0X1	T49.0X2	T49.0X3	T49.0X4	T49.0X5	T49.0X6
Chlorpheniramine	T45.0X1	T45.0X2	T45.0X3	T45.0X4	T45.0X5	T45.0X6
Chlorphenoxamine	T45.0X1	T45.0X2	T45.0X3	T45.0X4	T45.0X5	T45.0X6
Chlorphentermine	T50.5X1	T50.5X2	T50.5X3	T50.5X4	T50.5X5	T50.5X6
Chlorprocaine — see Chloroprocaine						
Chlorproguanil	T37.2X1	T37.2X2	T37.2X3	T37.2X4	T37.2X5	T37.2X6
Chlorpromazine	T43.3X1	T43.3X2	T43.3X3	T43.3X4	T43.3X5	T43.3X6
Chlorpropamide	T38.3X1	T38.3X2	T38.3X3	T38.3X4	T38.3X5	T38.3X6
Chlorprothixene	T43.4X1	T43.4X2	T43.4X3	T43.4X4	T43.4X5	T43.4X6
Chlorquinaldol	T49.0X1	T49.0X2	T49.0X3	T49.0X4	T49.0X5	T49.0X6
Chlorquinol	T49.0X1	T49.0X2	T49.0X3	T49.0X4	T49.0X5	T49.0X6
Chlortalidone	T50.2X1	T50.2X2	T50.2X3	T50.2X4	T50.2X5	T50.2X6
Chlortetracycline	T36.4X1	T36.4X2	T36.4X3	T36.4X4	T36.4X5	T36.4X6
Chlorthalidone	T50.2X1	T50.2X2	T50.2X3	T50.2X4	T50.2X5	T50.2X6
Chlorthiophos	T60.0X1	T60.0X2	T60.0X3	T60.0X4	—	—
Chlorotrianisene	T38.5X1	T38.5X2	T38.5X3	T38.5X4	T38.5X5	T38.5X6
Chlor-Trimeton	T45.0X1	T45.0X2	T45.0X3	T45.0X4	T45.0X5	T45.0X6
Chlorthion	T60.0X1	T60.0X2	T60.0X3	T60.0X4	—	—
Chlorzoxazone	T42.8X1	T42.8X2	T42.8X3	T42.8X4	T42.8X5	T42.8X6
Choke damp	T59.7X1	T59.7X2	T59.7X3	T59.7X4	—	—
Cholagogues	T47.5X1	T47.5X2	T47.5X3	T47.5X4	T47.5X5	T47.5X6
Cholebrine	T50.8X1	T50.8X2	T50.8X3	T50.8X4	T50.8X5	T50.8X6
Cholecalciferol	T45.2X1	T45.2X2	T45.2X3	T45.2X4	T45.2X5	T45.2X6
Cholecystokinin	T50.8X1	T50.8X2	T50.8X3	T50.8X4	T50.8X5	T50.8X6
Cholera vaccine	T50.A91	T50.A92	T50.A93	T50.A94	T50.A95	T50.A96

Substance	External Cause (T-Code)					
	Poisoning, Accidental (Unintentional)	Poisoning, Intentional Self-Harm	Poisoning, Assault	Poisoning, Undetermined	Adverse Effect	Underdosing
Choleretic	T47.5X1	T47.5X2	T47.5X3	T47.5X4	T47.5X5	T47.5X6
Cholesterol-lowering agents	T46.6X1	T46.6X2	T46.6X3	T46.6X4	T46.6X5	T46.6X6
Cholestyramine (resin)	T46.6X1	T46.6X2	T46.6X3	T46.6X4	T46.6X5	T46.6X6
Cholic acid	T47.5X1	T47.5X2	T47.5X3	T47.5X4	T47.5X5	T47.5X6
Choline	T48.6X1	T48.6X2	T48.6X3	T48.6X4	T48.6X5	T48.6X6
chloride	T50.991	T50.992	T50.993	T50.994	T50.995	T50.996
dihydrogen citrate	T50.991	T50.992	T50.993	T50.994	T50.995	T50.996
salicylate	T39.091	T39.092	T39.093	T39.094	T39.095	T39.096
theophyllinate	T48.6X1	T48.6X2	T48.6X3	T48.6X4	T48.6X5	T48.6X6
Cholinergic (drug) NEC	T44.1X1	T44.1X2	T44.1X3	T44.1X4	T44.1X5	T44.1X6
muscle tone enhancer	T44.1X1	T44.1X2	T44.1X3	T44.1X4	T44.1X5	T44.1X6
organophosphorus	T44.0X1	T44.0X2	T44.0X3	T44.0X4	T44.0X5	T44.0X6
insecticide	T60.0X1	T60.0X2	T60.0X3	T60.0X4	—	—
nerve gas	T59.891	T59.892	T59.893	T59.894		
trimethyl ammonium propanediol	T44.1X1	T44.1X2	T44.1X3	T44.1X4	T44.1X5	T44.1X6
Cholinesterase reactivator	T50.6X1	T50.6X2	T50.6X3	T50.6X4	T50.6X5	T50.6X6
Cholografin	T50.8X1	T50.8X2	T50.8X3	T50.8X4	T50.8X5	T50.8X6
Chorionic gonadotropin	T38.891	T38.892	T38.893	T38.894	T38.895	T38.896
Chromate	T56.2X1	T56.2X2	T56.2X3	T56.2X4	—	—
dust or mist	T56.2X1	T56.2X2	T56.2X3	T56.2X4	—	—
lead — see also Lead	T56.0X1	T56.0X2	T56.0X3	T56.0X4	—	—
paint	T56.0X1	T56.0X2	T56.0X3	T56.0X4	—	—
Chromic						
acid	T56.2X1	T56.2X2	T56.2X3	T56.2X4	—	—
dust or mist	T56.2X1	T56.2X2	T56.2X3	T56.2X4	—	—
phosphate 32P	T45.1X1	T45.1X2	T45.1X3	T45.1X4	T45.1X5	T45.1X6
Chromium	T56.2X1	T56.2X2	T56.2X3	T56.2X4	—	—
compounds — see Chromate						
sesquioxide	T50.8X1	T50.8X2	T50.8X3	T50.8X4	T50.8X5	T50.8X6
Chromomycin A3	T45.1X1	T45.1X2	T45.1X3	T45.1X4	T45.1X5	T45.1X6
Chromonar	T46.3X1	T46.3X2	T46.3X3	T46.3X4	T46.3X5	T46.3X6
Chromyl chloride	T56.2X1	T56.2X2	T56.2X3	T56.2X4	—	—
Chrysarobin	T49.4X1	T49.4X2	T49.4X3	T49.4X4	T49.4X5	T49.4X6
Chrysazin	T47.2X1	T47.2X2	T47.2X3	T47.2X4	T47.2X5	T47.2X6
Chymar	T45.3X1	T45.3X2	T45.3X3	T45.3X4	T45.3X5	T45.3X6
ophthalmic preparation	T49.5X1	T49.5X2	T49.5X3	T49.5X4	T49.5X5	T49.5X6
Chymopapain	T45.3X1	T45.3X2	T45.3X3	T45.3X4	T45.3X5	T45.3X6
Chymotrypsin	T45.3X1	T45.3X2	T45.3X3	T45.3X4	T45.3X5	T45.3X6
ophthalmic preparation	T49.5X1	T49.5X2	T49.5X3	T49.5X4	T49.5X5	T49.5X6
Cianidanol	T50.991	T50.992	T50.993	T50.994	T50.995	T50.996
Cianopramine	T43.011	T43.012	T43.013	T43.014	T43.015	T43.016
Cibenzoline	T46.2X1	T46.2X2	T46.2X3	T46.2X4	T46.2X5	T46.2X6

◄ New   ◄ Revised   ~~deleted~~ Deleted

Substance	Poisoning, Accidental (Unintentional)	Poisoning, Intentional Self-Harm	Poisoning, Assault	Poisoning, Undetermined	Adverse Effect	Underdosing
Ciclacillin	T36.0X1	T36.0X2	T36.0X3	T36.0X4	T36.0X5	T36.0X6
Ciclobarbital — *see Hexobarbital*						
Ciclonicate	T46.7X1	T46.7X2	T46.7X3	T46.7X4	T46.7X5	T46.7X6
Ciclopirox (olamine)	T49.0X1	T49.0X2	T49.0X3	T49.0X4	T49.0X5	T49.0X6
Ciclosporin	T45.1X1	T45.1X2	T45.1X3	T45.1X4	T45.1X5	T45.1X6
Cicuta maculata or virosa	T62.2X1	T62.2X2	T62.2X3	T62.2X4	—	—
Cicutoxin	T62.2X1	T62.2X2	T62.2X3	T62.2X4	—	—
Cigarette lighter fluid	T52.0X1	T52.0X2	T52.0X3	T52.0X4	—	—
Cigarettes (tobacco)	T65.221	T65.222	T65.223	T65.224		
Ciguatoxin	T61.01	T61.02	T61.03	T61.04	—	—
Cilazapril	T46.4X1	T46.4X2	T46.4X3	T46.4X4	T46.4X5	T46.4X6
Cimetidine	T47.0X1	T47.0X2	T47.0X3	T47.0X4	T47.0X5	T47.0X6
Cimetropium bromide	T44.3X1	T44.3X2	T44.3X3	T44.3X4	T44.3X5	T44.3X6
Cinchocaine	T41.3X1	T41.3X2	T41.3X3	T41.3X4	T41.3X5	T41.3X6
topical (surface)	T41.3X1	T41.3X2	T41.3X3	T41.3X4	T41.3X5	T41.3X6
Cinchona	T37.2X1	T37.2X2	T37.2X3	T37.2X4	T37.2X5	T37.2X6
Cinchonine alkaloids	T37.2X1	T37.2X2	T37.2X3	T37.2X4	T37.2X5	T37.2X6
Cinchophen	T50.4X1	T50.4X2	T50.4X3	T50.4X4	T50.4X5	T50.4X6
Cinepazide	T46.7X1	T46.7X2	T46.7X3	T46.7X4	T46.7X5	T46.7X6
Cinnamedrine	T48.5X1	T48.5X2	T48.5X3	T48.5X4	T48.5X5	T48.5X6
Cinnarizine	T45.0X1	T45.0X2	T45.0X3	T45.0X4	T45.0X5	T45.0X6
Cinoxacin	T37.8X1	T37.8X2	T37.8X3	T37.8X4	T37.8X5	T37.8X6
Ciprofibrate	T46.6X1	T46.6X2	T46.6X3	T46.6X4	T46.6X5	T46.6X6
Ciprofloxacin	T36.8X1	T36.8X2	T36.8X3	T36.8X4	T36.8X5	T36.8X6
Cisapride	T47.8X1	T47.8X2	T47.8X3	T47.8X4	T47.8X5	T47.8X6
Cisplatin	T45.1X1	T45.1X2	T45.1X3	T45.1X4	T45.1X5	T45.1X6
Citalopram	T43.221	T43.222	T43.223	T43.224	T43.225	T43.226
Citanest	T41.3X1	T41.3X2	T41.3X3	T41.3X4	T41.3X5	T41.3X6
infiltration (subcutaneous)	T41.3X1	T41.3X2	T41.3X3	T41.3X4	T41.3X5	T41.3X6
nerve block (peripheral) (plexus)	T41.3X1	T41.3X2	T41.3X3	T41.3X4	T41.3X5	T41.3X6
Citric acid	T47.5X1	T47.5X2	T47.5X3	T47.5X4	T47.5X5	T47.5X6
Citrovorum (factor)	T45.8X1	T45.8X2	T45.8X3	T45.8X4	T45.8X5	T45.8X6
Claviceps purpurea	T62.2X1	T62.2X2	T62.2X3	T62.2X4	—	—
Clavulanic acid	T36.1X1	T36.1X2	T36.1X3	T36.1X4	T36.1X5	T36.1X6
Cleaner, cleansing agent, type not specified	T65.891	T65.892	T65.893	T65.894	—	—
of paint or varnish	T52.91	T52.92	T52.93	T52.94	—	—
specified type NEC	T65.891	T65.892	T65.893	T65.894	—	—
Clebopride	T47.8X1	T47.8X2	T47.8X3	T47.8X4	T47.8X5	T47.8X6
Clefamide	T37.3X1	T37.3X2	T37.3X3	T37.3X4	T37.3X5	T37.3X6
Clemastine	T45.0X1	T45.0X2	T45.0X3	T45.0X4	T45.0X5	T45.0X6
Clematis vitalba	T62.2X1	T62.2X2	T62.2X3	T62.2X4	—	—

Substance	Poisoning, Accidental (Unintentional)	Poisoning, Intentional Self-Harm	Poisoning, Assault	Poisoning, Undetermined	Adverse Effect	Underdosing
Clemizole	T45.0X1	T45.0X2	T45.0X3	T45.0X4	T45.0X5	T45.0X6
penicillin	T36.0X1	T36.0X2	T36.0X3	T36.0X4	T36.0X5	T36.0X6
Clenbuterol	T48.6X1	T48.6X2	T48.6X3	T48.6X4	T48.6X5	T48.6X6
Clidinium bromide	T44.3X1	T44.3X2	T44.3X3	T44.3X4	T44.3X5	T44.3X6
Clindamycin	T36.8X1	T36.8X2	T36.8X3	T36.8X4	T36.8X5	T36.8X6
Clinofibrate	T46.6X1	T46.6X2	T46.6X3	T46.6X4	T46.6X5	T46.6X6
Clioquinol	T37.8X1	T37.8X2	T37.8X3	T37.8X4	T37.8X5	T37.8X6
Cliradon	T40.2X1	T40.2X2	T40.2X3	T40.2X4	—	—
Clobazam	T42.4X1	T42.4X2	T42.4X3	T42.4X4	T42.4X5	T42.4X6
Clobenzorex	T50.5X1	T50.5X2	T50.5X3	T50.5X4	T50.5X5	T50.5X6
Clobetasol	T49.0X1	T49.0X2	T49.0X3	T49.0X4	T49.0X5	T49.0X6
Clobetasone	T49.0X1	T49.0X2	T49.0X3	T49.0X4	T49.0X5	T49.0X6
Clobutinol	T48.3X1	T48.3X2	T48.3X3	T48.3X4	T48.3X5	T48.3X6
Clocapramine	T43.0X1	T43.0X2	T43.0X3	T43.0X4	T43.0X5	T43.0X6
Clocortolone	T38.0X1	T38.0X2	T38.0X3	T38.0X4	T38.0X5	T38.0X6
Clodantoin	T49.0X1	T49.0X2	T49.0X3	T49.0X4	T49.0X5	T49.0X6
Clodronic acid	T50.991	T50.992	T50.993	T50.994	T50.995	T50.996
Clofazimine	T37.1X1	T37.1X2	T37.1X3	T37.1X4	T37.1X5	T37.1X6
Clofedanol	T48.3X1	T48.3X2	T48.3X3	T48.3X4	T48.3X5	T48.3X6
Clofenamide	T50.2X1	T50.2X2	T50.2X3	T50.2X4	T50.2X5	T50.2X6
Clofenotane	T49.0X1	T49.0X2	T49.0X3	T49.0X4	T49.0X5	T49.0X6
Clofezone	T39.2X1	T39.2X2	T39.2X3	T39.2X4	T39.2X5	T39.2X6
Clofibrate	T46.6X1	T46.6X2	T46.6X3	T46.6X4	T46.6X5	T46.6X6
Clofibride	T46.6X1	T46.6X2	T46.6X3	T46.6X4	T46.6X5	T46.6X6
Cloforex	T50.5X1	T50.5X2	T50.5X3	T50.5X4	T50.5X5	T50.5X6
Clomacran	T43.0X1	T43.0X2	T43.0X3	T43.0X4	T43.0X5	T43.0X6
Clomethiazole	T42.6X1	T42.6X2	T42.6X3	T42.6X4	T42.6X5	T42.6X6
Clometocillin	T36.0X1	T36.0X2	T36.0X3	T36.0X4	T36.0X5	T36.0X6
Clomifene	T38.5X1	T38.5X2	T38.5X3	T38.5X4	T38.5X5	T38.5X6
Clomiphene	T38.5X1	T38.5X2	T38.5X3	T38.5X4	T38.5X5	T38.5X6
Clomipramine	T43.011	T43.012	T43.013	T43.014	T43.015	T43.016
Clomocycline	T36.4X1	T36.4X2	T36.4X3	T36.4X4	T36.4X5	T36.4X6
Clonazepam	T42.4X1	T42.4X2	T42.4X3	T42.4X4	T42.4X5	T42.4X6
Clonidine	T46.5X1	T46.5X2	T46.5X3	T46.5X4	T46.5X5	T46.5X6
Clonixin	T39.8X1	T39.8X2	T39.8X3	T39.8X4	T39.8X5	T39.8X6
Clopamide	T50.2X1	T50.2X2	T50.2X3	T50.2X4	T50.2X5	T50.2X6
Clopenthixol	T43.4X1	T43.4X2	T43.4X3	T43.4X4	T43.4X5	T43.4X6
Cloperastine	T48.3X1	T48.3X2	T48.3X3	T48.3X4	T48.3X5	T48.3X6
Clophedianol	T48.3X1	T48.3X2	T48.3X3	T48.3X4	T48.3X5	T48.3X6
Cloponone	T36.2X1	T36.2X2	T36.2X3	T36.2X4	T36.2X5	T36.2X6
Cloprednol	T38.0X1	T38.0X2	T38.0X3	T38.0X4	T38.0X5	T38.0X6
Cloral betaine	T42.6X1	T42.6X2	T42.6X3	T42.6X4	T42.6X5	T42.6X6

Substance	External Cause (T-Code)					
	Poisoning, Accidental (Unintentional)	Poisoning, Intentional Self-Harm	Poisoning, Assault	Poisoning, Undetermined	Adverse Effect	Underdosing
Cloramfenicol	T36.2X1	T36.2X2	T36.2X3	T36.2X4	T36.2X5	T36.2X6
Clorazepate (dipotassium)	T42.4X1	T42.4X2	T42.4X3	T42.4X4	T42.4X5	T42.4X6
Clorexolone	T50.2X1	T50.2X2	T50.2X3	T50.2X4	T50.2X5	T50.2X6
Clorox (bleach)	T54.91	T54.92	T54.93	T54.94	—	—
Clorfenamine	T45.0X1	T45.0X2	T45.0X3	T45.0X4	T45.0X5	T45.0X6
Clorgiline	T43.1X1	T43.1X2	T43.1X3	T43.1X4	T43.1X5	T43.1X6
Clorotepine	T44.3X1	T44.3X2	T44.3X3	T44.3X4	T44.3X5	T44.3X6
Clorprenaline	T48.6X1	T48.6X2	T48.6X3	T48.6X4	T48.6X5	T48.6X6
Clortermine	T50.5X1	T50.5X2	T50.5X3	T50.5X4	T50.5X5	T50.5X6
Clotiapine	T43.591	T43.592	T43.593	T43.594	T43.595	T43.596
Clotiazepam	T42.4X1	T42.4X2	T42.4X3	T42.4X4	T42.4X5	T42.4X6
Clotibric acid	T46.6X1	T46.6X2	T46.6X3	T46.6X4	T46.6X5	T46.6X6
Clotrimazole	T49.0X1	T49.0X2	T49.0X3	T49.0X4	T49.0X5	T49.0X6
Cloxacillin	T36.0X1	T36.0X2	T36.0X3	T36.0X4	T36.0X5	T36.0X6
Cloxazolam	T42.4X1	T42.4X2	T42.4X3	T42.4X4	T42.4X5	T42.4X6
Cloxiquine	T49.0X1	T49.0X2	T49.0X3	T49.0X4	T49.0X5	T49.0X6
Clozapine	T42.4X1	T42.4X2	T42.4X3	T42.4X4	T42.4X5	T42.4X6
Coagulant NEC	T45.7X1	T45.7X2	T45.7X3	T45.7X4	T45.7X5	T45.7X6
Coal (carbon monoxide from) — see also Carbon, monoxide, coal	T58.2X1	T58.2X2	T58.2X3	T58.2X4	—	—
oil — see Kerosene						
tar	T49.1X1	T49.1X2	T49.1X3	T49.1X4	T49.1X5	T49.1X6
fumes	T59.891	T59.892	T59.893	T59.894	—	—
medicinal (ointment)	T49.4X1	T49.4X2	T49.4X3	T49.4X4	T49.4X5	T49.4X6
analgesics NEC	T39.2X1	T39.2X2	T39.2X3	T39.2X4	T39.2X5	T39.2X6
naphtha (solvent)	T52.0X1	T52.0X2	T52.0X3	T52.0X4		
Cobalamine	T45.2X1	T45.2X2	T45.2X3	T45.2X4	T45.2X5	T45.2X6
Cobalt (nonmedicinal) (fumes) (industrial)	T56.891	T56.892	T56.893	T56.894		
medicinal (trace) (chloride)	T45.8X1	T45.8X2	T45.8X3	T45.8X4	T45.8X5	T45.8X6
Cobra (venom)	T63.041	T63.042	T63.043	T63.044		
Coca (leaf)	T40.5X1	T40.5X2	T40.5X3	T40.5X4	T40.5X5	T40.5X6
Cocaine	T40.5X1	T40.5X2	T40.5X3	T40.5X4	T40.5X5	T40.5X6
topical anesthetic	T41.3X1	T41.3X2	T41.3X3	T41.3X4	T41.3X5	T41.3X6
Cocarboxylase	T45.3X1	T45.3X2	T45.3X3	T45.3X4	T45.3X5	T45.3X6
Coccidioidin	T50.8X1	T50.8X2	T50.8X3	T50.8X4	T50.8X5	T50.8X6
Cocculus indicus	T62.1X1	T62.1X2	T62.1X3	T62.1X4		
Cochineal	T65.6X1	T65.6X2	T65.6X3	T65.6X4		
medicinal products	T50.991	T50.992	T50.993	T50.994	T50.995	T50.996
Codeine	T40.2X1	T40.2X2	T40.2X3	T40.2X4	T40.2X5	T40.2X6
Cod-liver oil	T45.2X1	T45.2X2	T45.2X3	T45.2X4	T45.2X5	T45.2X6

Substance	External Cause (T-Code)					
	Poisoning, Accidental (Unintentional)	Poisoning, Intentional Self-Harm	Poisoning, Assault	Poisoning, Undetermined	Adverse Effect	Underdosing
Coenzyme A	T50.991	T50.992	T50.993	T50.994	T50.995	T50.996
Coffee	T62.8X1	T62.8X2	T62.8X3	T62.8X4	—	—
Cogalactoisomerase	T50.991	T50.992	T50.993	T50.994	T50.995	T50.996
Cogentin	T44.3X1	T44.3X2	T44.3X3	T44.3X4	T44.3X5	T44.3X6
Coke fumes or gas (carbon monoxide)	T58.2X1	T58.2X2	T58.2X3	T58.2X4		
industrial use	T58.8X1	T58.8X2	T58.8X3	T58.8X4	—	—
Colace	T47.4X1	T47.4X2	T47.4X3	T47.4X4	T47.4X5	T47.4X6
Colaspase	T45.1X1	T45.1X2	T45.1X3	T45.1X4	T45.1X5	T45.1X6
Colchicine	T50.4X1	T50.4X2	T50.4X3	T50.4X4	T50.4X5	T50.4X6
Colchicum	T62.2X1	T62.2X2	T62.2X3	T62.2X4	—	—
Cold cream	T49.3X1	T49.3X2	T49.3X3	T49.3X4	T49.3X5	T49.3X6
Colecalciferol	T45.2X1	T45.2X2	T45.2X3	T45.2X4	T45.2X5	T45.2X6
Colestipol	T46.6X1	T46.6X2	T46.6X3	T46.6X4	T46.6X5	T46.6X6
Colestyramine	T46.6X1	T46.6X2	T46.6X3	T46.6X4	T46.6X5	T46.6X6
Colimycin	T36.8X1	T36.8X2	T36.8X3	T36.8X4	T36.8X5	T36.8X6
Colistimethate	T36.8X1	T36.8X2	T36.8X3	T36.8X4	T36.8X5	T36.8X6
Colistin	T36.8X1	T36.8X2	T36.8X3	T36.8X4	T36.8X5	T36.8X6
sulfate (eye preparation)	T49.5X1	T49.5X2	T49.5X3	T49.5X4	T49.5X5	T49.5X6
Collagen	T50.991	T50.992	T50.993	T50.994	T50.995	T50.996
Collagenase	T49.4X1	T49.4X2	T49.4X3	T49.4X4	T49.4X5	T49.4X6
Collodion	T49.3X1	T49.3X2	T49.3X3	T49.3X4	T49.3X5	T49.3X6
Colocynth	T47.2X1	T47.2X2	T47.2X3	T47.2X4	T47.2X5	T47.2X6
Colophony adhesive	T49.3X1	T49.3X2	T49.3X3	T49.3X4	T49.3X5	T49.3X6
Colorant — see also Dye	T50.991	T50.992	T50.993	T50.994	T50.995	T50.996
Coloring matter — see Dye(s)						
Combustion gas (after combustion) — see Carbon, monoxide						
prior to combustion	T59.891	T59.892	T59.893	T59.894	—	—
Compazine	T43.3X1	T43.3X2	T43.3X3	T43.3X4	T43.3X5	T43.3X6
Compound						
42 (warfarin)	T60.4X1	T60.4X2	T60.4X3	T60.4X4	—	—
269 (endrin)	T60.1X1	T60.1X2	T60.1X3	T60.1X4	—	—
497 (dieldrin)	T60.1X1	T60.1X2	T60.1X3	T60.1X4	—	—
1080 (sodium fluoroacetate)	T60.4X1	T60.4X2	T60.4X3	T60.4X4	—	—
3422 (parathion)	T60.0X1	T60.0X2	T60.0X3	T60.0X4	—	—
3911 (phorate)	T60.0X1	T60.0X2	T60.0X3	T60.0X4	—	—
3956 (toxaphene)	T60.1X1	T60.1X2	T60.1X3	T60.1X4	—	—
4049 (malathion)	T60.0X1	T60.0X2	T60.0X3	T60.0X4	—	—
4069 (malathion)	T60.0X1	T60.0X2	T60.0X3	T60.0X4	—	—
4124 (dicapthon)	T60.0X1	T60.0X2	T60.0X3	T60.0X4	—	—

◄ New   ◄ Revised   ~~deleted~~ Deleted

Substance	Poisoning, Accidental (Unintentional)	Poisoning, Intentional Self-Harm	Poisoning, Assault	Poisoning, Undetermined	Adverse Effect	Underdosing
Compound *(Continued)*						
E (cortisone)	T38.0X1	T38.0X2	T38.0X3	T38.0X4	T38.0X5	T38.0X6
F (hydrocortisone)	T38.0X1	T38.0X2	T38.0X3	T38.0X4	T38.0X5	T38.0X6
Congener, anabolic	T38.7X1	T38.7X2	T38.7X3	T38.7X4	T38.7X5	T38.7X6
Congo red	T50.8X1	T50.8X2	T50.8X3	T50.8X4	T50.8X5	T50.8X6
Coniine, conine	T62.2X1	T62.2X2	T62.2X3	T62.2X4	—	—
Conium (maculatum)	T62.2X1	T62.2X2	T62.2X3	T62.2X4	—	—
Conjugated estrogenic substances	T38.5X1	T38.5X2	T38.5X3	T38.5X4	T38.5X5	T38.5X6
Contac	T48.5X1	T48.5X2	T48.5X3	T48.5X4	T48.5X5	T48.5X6
Contact lens solution	T49.5X1	T49.5X2	T49.5X3	T49.5X4	T49.5X5	T49.5X6
Contraceptive (oral)	T38.4X1	T38.4X2	T38.4X3	T38.4X4	T38.4X5	T38.4X6
vaginal	T49.8X1	T49.8X2	T49.8X3	T49.8X4	T49.8X5	T49.8X6
Contrast medium, radiography	T50.8X1	T50.8X2	T50.8X3	T50.8X4	T50.8X5	T50.8X6
Convallaria glycosides	T46.0X1	T46.0X2	T46.0X3	T46.0X4	T46.0X5	T46.0X6
Convallaria majalis	T62.2X1	T62.2X2	T62.2X3	T62.2X4	—	—
berry	T62.1X1	T62.1X2	T62.1X3	T62.1X4	—	—
Copper (dust) (fumes) (nonmedicinal) NEC	T56.4X1	T56.4X2	T56.4X3	T56.4X4	—	—
arsenate, arsenite	T57.0X1	T57.0X2	T57.0X3	T57.0X4	—	—
insecticide	T60.2X1	T60.2X2	T60.2X3	T60.2X4	—	—
emetic	T47.7X1	T47.7X2	T47.7X3	T47.7X4	T47.7X5	T47.7X6
fungicide	T60.3X1	T60.3X2	T60.3X3	T60.3X4	—	—
gluconate	T49.0X1	T49.0X2	T49.0X3	T49.0X4	T49.0X5	T49.0X6
insecticide	T60.2X1	T60.2X2	T60.2X3	T60.2X4	—	—
medicinal (trace)	T45.8X1	T45.8X2	T45.8X3	T45.8X4	T45.8X5	T45.8X6
oleate	T49.0X1	T49.0X2	T49.0X3	T49.0X4	T49.0X5	T49.0X6
sulfate	T56.4X1	T56.4X2	T56.4X3	T56.4X4	—	—
cupric	T56.4X1	T56.4X2	T56.4X3	T56.4X4	—	—
fungicide	T60.3X1	T60.3X2	T60.3X3	T60.3X4	—	—
medicinal						
ear	T49.6X1	T49.6X2	T49.6X3	T49.6X4	T49.6X5	T49.6X6
emetic	T47.7X1	T47.7X2	T47.7X3	T47.7X4	T47.7X5	T47.7X6
eye	T49.5X1	T49.5X2	T49.5X3	T49.5X4	T49.5X5	T49.5X6
cuprous	T56.4X1	T56.4X2	T56.4X3	T56.4X4	—	—
fungicide	T60.3X1	T60.3X2	T60.3X3	T60.3X4	—	—
medicinal						
ear	T49.6X1	T49.6X2	T49.6X3	T49.6X4	T49.6X5	T49.6X6
emetic	T47.7X1	T47.7X2	T47.7X3	T47.7X4	T47.7X5	T47.7X6
eye	T49.5X1	T49.5X2	T49.5X3	T49.5X4	T49.5X5	T49.5X6
Copperhead snake (bite) (venom)	T63.061	T63.062	T63.063	T63.064	—	—
Coral (sting)	T63.691	T63.692	T63.693	T63.694	—	—
snake (bite) (venom)	T63.021	T63.022	T63.023	T63.024	—	—

Substance	Poisoning, Accidental (Unintentional)	Poisoning, Intentional Self-Harm	Poisoning, Assault	Poisoning, Undetermined	Adverse Effect	Underdosing
Corbadrine	T49.6X1	T49.6X2	T49.6X3	T49.6X4	T49.6X5	T49.6X6
Cordran	T49.0X1	T49.0X2	T49.0X3	T49.0X4	T49.0X5	T49.0X6
Cordite	T65.891	T65.892	T65.893	T65.894	—	—
vapor	T59.891	T59.892	T59.893	T59.894	—	—
Corn cures	T49.4X1	T49.4X2	T49.4X3	T49.4X4	T49.4X5	T49.4X6
Cornhusker's lotion	T49.3X1	T49.3X2	T49.3X3	T49.3X4	T49.3X5	T49.3X6
Corn starch	T49.3X1	T49.3X2	T49.3X3	T49.3X4	T49.3X5	T49.3X6
Coronary vasodilator NEC	T46.3X1	T46.3X2	T46.3X3	T46.3X4	T46.3X5	T46.3X6
Corrosive NEC	T54.91	T54.92	T54.93	T54.94	—	—
acid NEC	T54.2X1	T54.2X2	T54.2X3	T54.2X4	—	—
aromatics	T54.1X1	T54.1X2	T54.1X3	T54.1X4	—	—
disinfectant	T54.1X1	T54.1X2	T54.1X3	T54.1X4	—	—
fumes NEC	T54.91	T54.92	T54.93	T54.94	—	—
specified NEC	T54.91	T54.92	T54.93	T54.94	—	—
sublimate	T56.1X1	T56.1X2	T56.1X3	T56.1X4	—	—
Cortate	T38.0X1	T38.0X2	T38.0X3	T38.0X4	T38.0X5	T38.0X6
Cort-Dome	T38.0X1	T38.0X2	T38.0X3	T38.0X4	T38.0X5	T38.0X6
ENT agent	T49.6X1	T49.6X2	T49.6X3	T49.6X4	T49.6X5	T49.6X6
ophthalmic preparation	T49.5X1	T49.5X2	T49.5X3	T49.5X4	T49.5X5	T49.5X6
topical NEC	T49.0X1	T49.0X2	T49.0X3	T49.0X4	T49.0X5	T49.0X6
Cortef	T38.0X1	T38.0X2	T38.0X3	T38.0X4	T38.0X5	T38.0X6
ENT agent	T49.6X1	T49.6X2	T49.6X3	T49.6X4	T49.6X5	T49.6X6
ophthalmic preparation	T49.5X1	T49.5X2	T49.5X3	T49.5X4	T49.5X5	T49.5X6
topical NEC	T49.0X1	T49.0X2	T49.0X3	T49.0X4	T49.0X5	T49.0X6
Corticosteroid	T38.0X1	T38.0X2	T38.0X3	T38.0X4	T38.0X5	T38.0X6
ENT agent	T49.6X1	T49.6X2	T49.6X3	T49.6X4	T49.6X5	T49.6X6
mineral	T50.0X1	T50.0X2	T50.0X3	T50.0X4	T50.0X5	T50.0X6
ophthalmic	T49.5X1	T49.5X2	T49.5X3	T49.5X4	T49.5X5	T49.5X6
topical NEC	T49.0X1	T49.0X2	T49.0X3	T49.0X4	T49.0X5	T49.0X6
Corticotropin	T38.811	T38.812	T38.813	T38.814	T38.815	T38.816
Cortisol	T49.0X1	T49.0X2	T49.0X3	T49.0X4	T49.0X5	T49.0X6
ENT agent	T49.6X1	T49.6X2	T49.6X3	T49.6X4	T49.6X5	T49.6X6
ophthalmic preparation	T49.5X1	T49.5X2	T49.5X3	T49.5X4	T49.5X5	T49.5X6
topical NEC	T49.0X1	T49.0X2	T49.0X3	T49.0X4	T49.0X5	T49.0X6
Cortisone (acetate)	T38.0X1	T38.0X2	T38.0X3	T38.0X4	T38.0X5	T38.0X6
ENT agent	T49.6X1	T49.6X2	T49.6X3	T49.6X4	T49.6X5	T49.6X6
ophthalmic preparation	T49.5X1	T49.5X2	T49.5X3	T49.5X4	T49.5X5	T49.5X6
topical NEC	T49.0X1	T49.0X2	T49.0X3	T49.0X4	T49.0X5	T49.0X6
Cortivazol	T38.0X1	T38.0X2	T38.0X3	T38.0X4	T38.0X5	T38.0X6
Cortogen	T38.0X1	T38.0X2	T38.0X3	T38.0X4	T38.0X5	T38.0X6
ENT agent	T49.6X1	T49.6X2	T49.6X3	T49.6X4	T49.6X5	T49.6X6
ophthalmic preparation	T49.5X1	T49.5X2	T49.5X3	T49.5X4	T49.5X5	T49.5X6

Substance	External Cause (T-Code)					
	Poisoning, Accidental (Unintentional)	Poisoning, Intentional Self-Harm	Poisoning, Assault	Poisoning, Undetermined	Adverse Effect	Underdosing
Cortone	T38.0X1	T38.0X2	T38.0X3	T38.0X4	T38.0X5	T38.0X6
ENT agent	T49.6X1	T49.6X2	T49.6X3	T49.6X4	T49.6X5	T49.6X6
ophthalmic preparation	T49.5X1	T49.5X2	T49.5X3	T49.5X4	T49.5X5	T49.5X6
Cortril	T38.0X1	T38.0X2	T38.0X3	T38.0X4	T38.0X5	T38.0X6
ENT agent	T49.6X1	T49.6X2	T49.6X3	T49.6X4	T49.6X5	T49.6X6
ophthalmic preparation	T49.5X1	T49.5X2	T49.5X3	T49.5X4	T49.5X5	T49.5X6
topical NEC	T49.0X1	T49.0X2	T49.0X3	T49.0X4	T49.0X5	T49.0X6
Corynebacterium parvum	T45.1X1	T45.1X2	T45.1X3	T45.1X4	T45.1X5	T45.1X6
Cosmetic preparation	T49.8X1	T49.8X2	T49.8X3	T49.8X4	T49.8X5	T49.8X6
Cosmetics	T49.8X1	T49.8X2	T49.8X3	T49.8X4	T49.8X5	T49.8X6
Cosyntropin	T38.811	T38.812	T38.813	T38.814	T38.815	T38.816
Cotarnine	T45.7X1	T45.7X2	T45.7X3	T45.7X4	T45.7X5	T45.7X6
Co-trimoxazole	T36.8X1	T36.8X2	T36.8X3	T36.8X4	T36.8X5	T36.8X6
Cottonseed oil	T49.3X1	T49.3X2	T49.3X3	T49.3X4	T49.3X5	T49.3X6
Cough mixture (syrup)	T48.4X1	T48.4X2	T48.4X3	T48.4X4	T48.4X5	T48.4X6
containing opiates	T40.2X1	T40.2X2	T40.2X3	T40.2X4	T40.2X5	T40.2X6
expectorants	T48.4X1	T48.4X2	T48.4X3	T48.4X4	T48.4X5	T48.4X6
Coumadin	T45.511	T45.512	T45.513	T45.514	T45.515	T45.516
rodenticide	T60.4X1	T60.4X2	T60.4X3	T60.4X4	—	—
Coumaphos	T60.0X1	T60.0X2	T60.0X3	T60.0X4	—	—
Coumarin	T45.511	T45.512	T45.513	T45.514	T45.515	T45.516
Coumetarol	T45.511	T45.512	T45.513	T45.514	T45.515	T45.516
Cowbane	T62.2X1	T62.2X2	T62.2X3	T62.2X4	—	—
Cozyme	T45.2X1	T45.2X2	T45.2X3	T45.2X4	T45.2X5	T45.2X6
Crack	T40.5X1	T40.5X2	T40.5X3	T40.5X4	—	—
Crataegus extract	T46.0X1	T46.0X2	T46.0X3	T46.0X4	T46.0X5	T46.0X6
Creolin	T54.1X1	T54.1X2	T54.1X3	T54.1X4	—	—
disinfectant	T54.1X1	T54.1X2	T54.1X3	T54.1X4	—	—
Creosol (compound)	T49.0X1	T49.0X2	T49.0X3	T49.0X4	T49.0X5	T49.0X6
Creosote (coal tar) (beechwood)	T49.0X1	T49.0X2	T49.0X3	T49.0X4	T49.0X5	T49.0X6
medicinal (expectorant)	T48.4X1	T48.4X2	T48.4X3	T48.4X4	T48.4X5	T48.4X6
syrup	T48.4X1	T48.4X2	T48.4X3	T48.4X4	T48.4X5	T48.4X6
Cresol(s)	T49.0X1	T49.0X2	T49.0X3	T49.0X4	T49.0X5	T49.0X6
and soap solution	T49.0X1	T49.0X2	T49.0X3	T49.0X4	T49.0X5	T49.0X6
Cresyl acetate	T49.0X1	T49.0X2	T49.0X3	T49.0X4	T49.0X5	T49.0X6
Cresylic acid	T49.0X1	T49.0X2	T49.0X3	T49.0X4	T49.0X5	T49.0X6
Crimidine	T60.4X1	T60.4X2	T60.4X3	T60.4X4	—	—
Croconazole	T37.8X1	T37.8X2	T37.8X3	T37.8X4	T37.8X5	T37.8X6
Cromoglicic acid	T48.6X1	T48.6X2	T48.6X3	T48.6X4	T48.6X5	T48.6X6
Cromolyn	T48.6X1	T48.6X2	T48.6X3	T48.6X4	T48.6X5	T48.6X6
Cromonar	T46.3X1	T46.3X2	T46.3X3	T46.3X4	T46.3X5	T46.3X6

Substance	External Cause (T-Code)					
	Poisoning, Accidental (Unintentional)	Poisoning, Intentional Self-Harm	Poisoning, Assault	Poisoning, Undetermined	Adverse Effect	Underdosing
Cropropamide	T39.8X1	T39.8X2	T39.8X3	T39.8X4	T39.8X5	T39.8X6
with crotethamide	T50.7X1	T50.7X2	T50.7X3	T50.7X4	T50.7X5	T50.7X6
Crotamiton	T49.0X1	T49.0X2	T49.0X3	T49.0X4	T49.0X5	T49.0X6
Crotethamide	T39.8X1	T39.8X2	T39.8X3	T39.8X4	T39.8X5	T39.8X6
with cropropamide	T50.7X1	T50.7X2	T50.7X3	T50.7X4	T50.7X5	T50.7X6
Croton (oil)	T47.2X1	T47.2X2	T47.2X3	T47.2X4	T47.2X5	T47.2X6
chloral	T42.6X1	T42.6X2	T42.6X3	T42.6X4	T42.6X5	T42.6X6
Crude oil	T52.0X1	T52.0X2	T52.0X3	T52.0X4	—	—
Cryogenine	T39.8X1	T39.8X2	T39.8X3	T39.8X4	T39.8X5	T39.8X6
Cryolite (vapor)	T60.1X1	T60.1X2	T60.1X3	T60.1X4	—	—
insecticide	T60.1X1	T60.1X2	T60.1X3	T60.1X4	—	—
Cryptenamine (tannates)	T46.5X1	T46.5X2	T46.5X3	T46.5X4	T46.5X5	T46.5X6
Crystal violet	T49.0X1	T49.0X2	T49.0X3	T49.0X4	T49.0X5	T49.0X6
Cuckoopint	T62.2X1	T62.2X2	T62.2X3	T62.2X4	—	—
Cumetharol	T45.511	T45.512	T45.513	T45.514	T45.515	T45.516
Cupric						
acetate	T60.3X1	T60.3X2	T60.3X3	T60.3X4	—	—
acetoarsenite	T57.0X1	T57.0X2	T57.0X3	T57.0X4	—	—
arsenate	T57.0X1	T57.0X2	T57.0X3	T57.0X4	—	—
gluconate	T49.0X1	T49.0X2	T49.0X3	T49.0X4	T49.0X5	T49.0X6
oleate	T49.0X1	T49.0X2	T49.0X3	T49.0X4	T49.0X5	T49.0X6
sulfate	T56.4X1	T56.4X2	T56.4X3	T56.4X4	—	—
Cuprous sulfate — *see also* Copper, sulfate	T56.4X1	T56.4X2	T56.4X3	T56.4X4	—	—
Curare, curarine	T48.1X1	T48.1X2	T48.1X3	T48.1X4	T48.1X5	T48.1X6
Cyamemazine	T43.3X1	T43.3X2	T43.3X3	T43.3X4	T43.3X5	T43.3X6
Cyamopsis tetragonoloba	T46.6X1	T46.6X2	T46.6X3	T46.6X4	T46.6X5	T46.6X6
Cyanacetyl hydrazide	T37.1X1	T37.1X2	T37.1X3	T37.1X4	T37.1X5	T37.1X6
Cyanic acid (gas)	T59.891	T59.892	T59.893	T59.894		
Cyanide(s) (compounds) (potassium) (sodium) NEC	T65.0X1	T65.0X2	T65.0X3	T65.0X4		
dust or gas (inhalation) NEC	T57.3X1	T57.3X2	T57.3X3	T57.3X4		
fumigant	T65.0X1	T65.0X2	T65.0X3	T65.0X4		
hydrogen	T57.3X1	T57.3X2	T57.3X3	T57.3X4		
mercuric — *see Mercury*						
pesticide (dust) (fumes)	T65.0X1	T65.0X2	T65.0X3	T65.0X4	—	—
Cyanoacrylate adhesive	T49.3X1	T49.3X2	T49.3X3	T49.3X4	T49.3X5	T49.3X6
Cyanocobalamin	T45.8X1	T45.8X2	T45.8X3	T45.8X4	T45.8X5	T45.8X6
Cyanogen (chloride) (gas) NEC	T59.891	T59.892	T59.893	T59.894		
Cyclacillin	T36.0X1	T36.0X2	T36.0X3	T36.0X4	T36.0X5	T36.0X6
Cyclaine	T41.3X1	T41.3X2	T41.3X3	T41.3X4	T41.3X5	T41.3X6
Cyclamate	T50.991	T50.992	T50.993	T50.994	T50.995	T50.996

◀ New ◀ Revised ~~deleted~~ Deleted

Substance	External Cause (T-Code)					
	Poisoning, Accidental (Unintentional)	Poisoning, Intentional Self-Harm	Poisoning, Assault	Poisoning, Undetermined	Adverse Effect	Underdosing
Cyclamen europaeum	T62.2X1	T62.2X2	T62.2X3	T62.2X4	—	—
Cyclandelate	T46.7X1	T46.7X2	T46.7X3	T46.7X4	T46.7X5	T46.7X6
Cyclazocine	T50.7X1	T50.7X2	T50.7X3	T50.7X4	T50.7X5	T50.7X6
Cyclizine	T45.0X1	T45.0X2	T45.0X3	T45.0X4	T45.0X5	T45.0X6
Cyclobarbital	T42.3X1	T42.3X2	T42.3X3	T42.3X4	T42.3X5	T42.3X6
Cyclobarbitone	T42.3X1	T42.3X2	T42.3X3	T42.3X4	T42.3X5	T42.3X6
Cyclobenzaprine	T48.1X1	T48.1X2	T48.1X3	T48.1X4	T48.1X5	T48.1X6
Cyclodrine	T44.3X1	T44.3X2	T44.3X3	T44.3X4	T44.3X5	T44.3X6
Cycloguanil embonate	T37.2X1	T37.2X2	T37.2X3	T37.2X4	T37.2X5	T37.2X6
Cycloheptadiene	T43.291	T43.292	T43.293	T43.294	T43.295	T43.296
Cyclohexane	T52.8X1	T52.8X2	T52.8X3	T52.8X4	—	—
Cyclohexanol	T51.8X1	T51.8X2	T51.8X3	T51.8X4	—	—
Cyclohexanone	T52.4X1	T52.4X2	T52.4X3	T52.4X4	—	—
Cycloheximide	T60.3X1	T60.3X2	T60.3X3	T60.3X4	—	—
Cyclohexyl acetate	T52.8X1	T52.8X2	T52.8X3	T52.8X4	—	—
Cycloleucin	T45.1X1	T45.1X2	T45.1X3	T45.1X4	T45.1X5	T45.1X6
Cyclomethycaine	T41.3X1	T41.3X2	T41.3X3	T41.3X4	T41.3X5	T41.3X6
Cyclopentamine	T44.4X1	T44.4X2	T44.4X3	T44.4X4	T44.4X5	T44.4X6
Cyclopenthiazide	T50.2X1	T50.2X2	T50.2X3	T50.2X4	T50.2X5	T50.2X6
Cyclopentolate	T44.3X1	T44.3X2	T44.3X3	T44.3X4	T44.3X5	T44.3X6
Cyclophosphamide	T45.1X1	T45.1X2	T45.1X3	T45.1X4	T45.1X5	T45.1X6
Cycloplegic drug	T49.5X1	T49.5X2	T49.5X3	T49.5X4	T49.5X5	T49.5X6
Cyclopropane	T41.291	T41.292	T41.293	T41.294	T41.295	T41.296
Cyclopyrabital	T39.8X1	T39.8X2	T39.8X3	T39.8X4	T39.8X5	T39.8X6
Cycloserine	T37.1X1	T37.1X2	T37.1X3	T37.1X4	T37.1X5	T37.1X6
Cyclosporin	T45.1X1	T45.1X2	T45.1X3	T45.1X4	T45.1X5	T45.1X6
Cyclothiazide	T50.2X1	T50.2X2	T50.2X3	T50.2X4	T50.2X5	T50.2X6
Cycrimine	T44.3X1	T44.3X2	T44.3X3	T44.3X4	T44.3X5	T44.3X6
Cyhalothrin	T60.1X1	T60.1X2	T60.1X3	T60.1X4	—	—
Cymarin	T46.0X1	T46.0X2	T46.0X3	T46.0X4	T46.0X5	T46.0X6
Cypermethrin	T60.1X1	T60.1X2	T60.1X3	T60.1X4	—	—
Cyphenothrin	T60.2X1	T60.2X2	T60.2X3	T60.2X4	—	—
Cyproheptadine	T45.0X1	T45.0X2	T45.0X3	T45.0X4	T45.0X5	T45.0X6
Cyprolidol	T43.291	T43.292	T43.293	T43.294	T43.295	T43.296
Cyproterone	T38.6X1	T38.6X2	T38.6X3	T38.6X4	T38.6X5	T38.6X6
Cysteamine	T50.6X1	T50.6X2	T50.6X3	T50.6X4	T50.6X5	T50.6X6
Cytarabine	T45.1X1	T45.1X2	T45.1X3	T45.1X4	T45.1X5	T45.1X6
Cytisus						
laburnum	T62.2X1	T62.2X2	T62.2X3	T62.2X4	—	—
scoparius	T62.2X1	T62.2X2	T62.2X3	T62.2X4	—	—
Cytochrome C	T47.5X1	T47.5X2	T47.5X3	T47.5X4	T47.5X5	T47.5X6
Cytomel	T38.1X1	T38.1X2	T38.1X3	T38.1X4	T38.1X5	T38.1X6
Cytosine arabinoside	T45.1X1	T45.1X2	T45.1X3	T45.1X4	T45.1X5	T45.1X6
Cytoxan	T45.1X1	T45.1X2	T45.1X3	T45.1X4	T45.1X5	T45.1X6
Cytozyme	T45.7X1	T45.7X2	T45.7X3	T45.7X4	T45.7X5	T45.7X6
2,4-D	T60.3X1	T60.3X2	T60.3X3	T60.3X4	—	—
D						
Dacarbazine	T45.1X1	T45.1X2	T45.1X3	T45.1X4	T45.1X5	T45.1X6
Dactinomycin	T45.1X1	T45.1X2	T45.1X3	T45.1X4	T45.1X5	T45.1X6
DADPS	T37.1X1	T37.1X2	T37.1X3	T37.1X4	T37.1X5	T37.1X6
Dakin's solution	T49.0X1	T49.0X2	T49.0X3	T49.0X4	T49.0X5	T49.0X6
Dalapon (sodium)	T60.3X1	T60.3X2	T60.3X3	T60.3X4	—	—
Dalmane	T42.4X1	T42.4X2	T42.4X3	T42.4X4	T42.4X5	T42.4X6
Danazol	T38.6X1	T38.6X2	T38.6X3	T38.6X4	T38.6X5	T38.6X6
Danilone	T45.511	T45.512	T45.513	T45.514	T45.515	T45.516
Danthron	T47.2X1	T47.2X2	T47.2X3	T47.2X4	T47.2X5	T47.2X6
Dantrolene	T42.8X1	T42.8X2	T42.8X3	T42.8X4	T42.8X5	T42.8X6
Dantron	T47.2X1	T47.2X2	T47.2X3	T47.2X4	T47.2X5	T47.2X6
Daphne (gnidium) (mezereum)	T62.2X1	T62.2X2	T62.2X3	T62.2X4	—	—
berry	T62.1X1	T62.1X2	T62.1X3	T62.1X4	—	—
Dapsone	T37.1X1	T37.1X2	T37.1X3	T37.1X4	T37.1X5	T37.1X6
Daraprim	T37.2X1	T37.2X2	T37.2X3	T37.2X4	T37.2X5	T37.2X6
Darnel	T62.2X1	T62.2X2	T62.2X3	T62.2X4	—	—
Darvon	T39.8X1	T39.8X2	T39.8X3	T39.8X4	T39.8X5	T39.8X6
Daunomycin	T45.1X1	T45.1X2	T45.1X3	T45.1X4	T45.1X5	T45.1X6
Daunorubicin	T45.1X1	T45.1X2	T45.1X3	T45.1X4	T45.1X5	T45.1X6
DBI	T38.3X1	T38.3X2	T38.3X3	T38.3X4	T38.3X5	T38.3X6
D-Con	T60.91	T60.92	T60.93	T60.94	—	—
insecticide	T60.2X1	T60.2X2	T60.2X3	T60.2X4	—	—
rodenticide	T60.4X1	T60.4X2	T60.4X3	T60.4X4	—	—
DDAVP	T38.891	T38.892	T38.893	T38.894	T38.895	T38.896
DDE (bis(chlorophenyl)-dichloroethylene)	T60.2X1	T60.2X2	T60.2X3	T60.2X4	—	—
DDS	T37.1X1	T37.1X2	T37.1X3	T37.1X4	T37.1X5	T37.1X6
DDT (dust)	T60.1X1	T60.1X2	T60.1X3	T60.1X4	—	—
Deadly nightshade — see also Belladonna	T62.2X1	T62.2X2	T62.2X3	T62.2X4	—	—
berry	T62.1X1	T62.1X2	T62.1X3	T62.1X4	—	—
Deamino-D-arginine vasopressin	T38.891	T38.892	T38.893	T38.894	T38.895	T38.896
Deanol (aceglumate)	T50.991	T50.992	T50.993	T50.994	T50.995	T50.996
Debrisoquine	T46.5X1	T46.5X2	T46.5X3	T46.5X4	T46.5X5	T46.5X6
Decaborane	T57.8X1	T57.8X2	T57.8X3	T57.8X4	—	—
fumes	T59.891	T59.892	T59.893	T59.894	—	—

Substance	External Cause (T-Code) Poisoning, Accidental (Unintentional)	Poisoning, Intentional Self-Harm	Poisoning, Assault	Poisoning, Undetermined	Adverse Effect	Underdosing
Decadron	T38.0X1	T38.0X2	T38.0X3	T38.0X4	T38.0X5	T38.0X6
ENT agent	T49.6X1	T49.6X2	T49.6X3	T49.6X4	T49.6X5	T49.6X6
ophthalmic preparation	T49.5X1	T49.5X2	T49.5X3	T49.5X4	T49.5X5	T49.5X6
topical NEC	T49.0X1	T49.0X2	T49.0X3	T49.0X4	T49.0X5	T49.0X6
Decahydronaphthalene	T52.8X1	T52.8X2	T52.8X3	T52.8X4	—	—
Decalin	T52.8X1	T52.8X2	T52.8X3	T52.8X4	—	—
Decamethonium (bromide)	T48.1X1	T48.1X2	T48.1X3	T48.1X4	T48.1X5	T48.1X6
Decholin	T47.5X1	T47.5X2	T47.5X3	T47.5X4	T47.5X5	T47.5X6
Declomycin	T36.4X1	T36.4X2	T36.4X3	T36.4X4	T36.4X5	T36.4X6
Decongestant, nasal (mucosa)	T48.5X1	T48.5X2	T48.5X3	T48.5X4	T48.5X5	T48.5X6
combination	T48.5X1	T48.5X2	T48.5X3	T48.5X4	T48.5X5	T48.5X6
Deet	T60.8X1	T60.8X2	T60.8X3	T60.8X4	—	—
Deferoxamine	T45.8X1	T45.8X2	T45.8X3	T45.8X4	T45.8X5	T45.8X6
Deflazacort	T38.0X1	T38.0X2	T38.0X3	T38.0X4	T38.0X5	T38.0X6
Deglycyrrhizinized extract of licorice	T48.4X1	T48.4X2	T48.4X3	T48.4X4	T48.4X5	T48.4X6
Dehydrocholic acid	T47.5X1	T47.5X2	T47.5X3	T47.5X4	T47.5X5	T47.5X6
Dehydroemetine	T37.3X1	T37.3X2	T37.3X3	T37.3X4	T37.3X5	T37.3X6
Dekalin	T52.8X1	T52.8X2	T52.8X3	T52.8X4	—	—
Delalutin	T38.5X1	T38.5X2	T38.5X3	T38.5X4	T38.5X5	T38.5X6
Delphinium	T62.2X1	T62.2X2	T62.2X3	T62.2X4	—	—
Deltasone	T38.0X1	T38.0X2	T38.0X3	T38.0X4	T38.0X5	T38.0X6
Deltra	T38.0X1	T38.0X2	T38.0X3	T38.0X4	T38.0X5	T38.0X6
Delvinal	T42.3X1	T42.3X2	T42.3X3	T42.3X4	T42.3X5	T42.3X6
Delorazepam	T42.4X1	T42.4X2	T42.4X3	T42.4X4	T42.4X5	T42.4X6
Deltamethrin	T60.1X1	T60.1X2	T60.1X3	T60.1X4	—	—
Demecarium (bromide)	T49.5X1	T49.5X2	T49.5X3	T49.5X4	T49.5X5	T49.5X6
Demeclocycline	T36.4X1	T36.4X2	T36.4X3	T36.4X4	T36.4X5	T36.4X6
Demecolcine	T45.1X1	T45.1X2	T45.1X3	T45.1X4	T45.1X5	T45.1X6
Demegestone	T38.5X1	T38.5X2	T38.5X3	T38.5X4	T38.5X5	T38.5X6
Demelanizing agents	T49.8X1	T49.8X2	T49.8X3	T49.8X4	T49.8X5	T49.8X6
Demephion -O and -S	T60.0X1	T60.0X2	T60.0X3	T60.0X4	—	—
Demerol	T40.2X1	T40.2X2	T40.2X3	T40.2X4	T40.2X5	T40.2X6
Demethylchlortetracycline	T36.4X1	T36.4X2	T36.4X3	T36.4X4	T36.4X5	T36.4X6
Demethyltetracycline	T36.4X1	T36.4X2	T36.4X3	T36.4X4	T36.4X5	T36.4X6
Demeton -O and -S	T60.0X1	T60.0X2	T60.0X3	T60.0X4	—	—
Demulcent (external)	T49.3X1	T49.3X2	T49.3X3	T49.3X4	T49.3X5	T49.3X6
specified NEC	T49.3X1	T49.3X2	T49.3X3	T49.3X4	T49.3X5	T49.3X6
Demulen	T38.4X1	T38.4X2	T38.4X3	T38.4X4	T38.4X5	T38.4X6
Denatured alcohol	T51.0X1	T51.0X2	T51.0X3	T51.0X4	—	—
Dendrid	T49.5X1	T49.5X2	T49.5X3	T49.5X4	T49.5X5	T49.5X6
Dental drug, topical application NEC	T49.7X1	T49.7X2	T49.7X3	T49.7X4	T49.7X5	T49.7X6

Substance	External Cause (T-Code) Poisoning, Accidental (Unintentional)	Poisoning, Intentional Self-Harm	Poisoning, Assault	Poisoning, Undetermined	Adverse Effect	Underdosing
Dentifrice	T49.7X1	T49.7X2	T49.7X3	T49.7X4	T49.7X5	T49.7X6
Deodorant spray (feminine hygiene)	T49.8X1	T49.8X2	T49.8X3	T49.8X4	T49.8X5	T49.8X6
Deoxycortone	T50.0X1	T50.0X2	T50.0X3	T50.0X4	T50.0X5	T50.0X6
2-Deoxy-5-fluorouridine	T45.1X1	T45.1X2	T45.1X3	T45.1X4	T45.1X5	T45.1X6
5-Deoxy-5-fluorouridine	T45.1X1	T45.1X2	T45.1X3	T45.1X4	T45.1X5	T45.1X6
Deoxyribonuclease (pancreatic)	T45.3X1	T45.3X2	T45.3X3	T45.3X4	T45.3X5	T45.3X6
Depilatory	T49.4X1	T49.4X2	T49.4X3	T49.4X4	T49.4X5	T49.4X6
Deprenalin	T42.8X1	T42.8X2	T42.8X3	T42.8X4	T42.8X5	T42.8X6
Deprenyl	T42.8X1	T42.8X2	T42.8X3	T42.8X4	T42.8X5	T42.8X6
Depressant, appetite	T50.5X1	T50.5X2	T50.5X3	T50.5X4	T50.5X5	T50.5X6
Depressant						
appetite, central	T50.5X1	T50.5X2	T50.5X3	T50.5X4	T50.5X5	T50.5X6
cardiac	T46.2X1	T46.2X2	T46.2X3	T46.2X4	T46.2X5	T46.2X6
central nervous system (anesthetic) — *see also Central nervous system, depressants*	T42.71	T42.72	T42.73	T42.74	T42.75	T42.76
general anesthetic	T41.201	T41.202	T41.203	T41.204	T41.205	T41.206
muscle tone	T42.8X1	T42.8X2	T42.8X3	T42.8X4	T42.8X5	T42.8X6
muscle tone, central	T42.8X1	T42.8X2	T42.8X3	T42.8X4	T42.8X5	T42.8X6
psychotherapeutic	T43.501	T43.502	T43.503	T43.504	T43.505	T43.506
Deptropine	T45.0X1	T45.0X2	T45.0X3	T45.0X4	T45.0X5	T45.0X6
Dequalinium (chloride)	T49.0X1	T49.0X2	T49.0X3	T49.0X4	T49.0X5	T49.0X6
Derris root	T60.2X1	T60.2X2	T60.2X3	T60.2X4	—	—
Deserpidine	T43.011	T43.012	T43.013	T43.014	T43.015	T43.016
Desferrioxamine	T45.8X1	T45.8X2	T45.8X3	T45.8X4	T45.8X5	T45.8X6
Desipramine	T43.0X1	T43.0X2	T43.0X3	T43.0X4	T43.0X5	T43.0X6
Deslanoside	T46.0X1	T46.0X2	T46.0X3	T46.0X4	T46.0X5	T46.0X6
Desloughing agent	T49.4X1	T49.4X2	T49.4X3	T49.4X4	T49.4X5	T49.4X6
Desmethylimipramine	T43.011	T43.012	T43.013	T43.014	T43.015	T43.016
Desmopressin	T38.891	T38.892	T38.893	T38.894	T38.895	T38.896
Desocodeine	T40.2X1	T40.2X2	T40.2X3	T40.2X4	T40.2X5	T40.2X6
Desogestrel	T38.5X1	T38.5X2	T38.5X3	T38.5X4	T38.5X5	T38.5X6
Desomorphine	T40.2X1	T40.2X2	T40.2X3	T40.2X4	—	—
Desonide	T49.0X1	T49.0X2	T49.0X3	T49.0X4	T49.0X5	T49.0X6
Desoximetasone	T49.0X1	T49.0X2	T49.0X3	T49.0X4	T49.0X5	T49.0X6
Desoxycorticosteroid	T50.0X1	T50.0X2	T50.0X3	T50.0X4	T50.0X5	T50.0X6
Desoxycortone	T50.0X1	T50.0X2	T50.0X3	T50.0X4	T50.0X5	T50.0X6
Desoxyephedrine	T43.651	T43.652	T43.653	T43.654	T43.655	T43.656
Detaxtran	T46.6X1	T46.6X2	T46.6X3	T46.6X4	T46.6X5	T46.6X6
Detergent	T49.2X1	T49.2X2	T49.2X3	T49.2X4	T49.2X5	T49.2X6
external medication	T49.2X1	T49.2X2	T49.2X3	T49.2X4	T49.2X5	T49.2X6
local	T49.2X1	T49.2X2	T49.2X3	T49.2X4	T49.2X5	T49.2X6

◄ New   ◄ Revised   ~~deleted~~ Deleted

Substance	External Cause (T-Code)					
	Poisoning, Accidental (Unintentional)	Poisoning, Intentional Self-Harm	Poisoning, Assault	Poisoning, Undetermined	Adverse Effect	Underdosing
Detergent *(Continued)*						
medicinal	T49.2X1	T49.2X2	T49.2X3	T49.2X4	T49.2X5	T49.2X6
nonmedicinal	T55.1X1	T55.1X2	T55.1X3	T55.1X4	—	—
specified NEC	T55.1X1	T55.1X2	T55.1X3	T55.1X4	T55.1X5	T55.1X6
Deterrent, alcohol	T50.6X1	T50.6X2	T50.6X3	T50.6X4	T50.6X5	T50.6X6
Detoxifying agent	T50.6X1	T50.6X2	T50.6X3	T50.6X4	T50.6X5	T50.6X6
Detrothyronine	T38.1X1	T38.1X2	T38.1X3	T38.1X4	T38.1X5	T38.1X6
Dettol (external medication)	T49.0X1	T49.0X2	T49.0X3	T49.0X4	T49.0X5	T49.0X6
Dexamethasone	T38.0X1	T38.0X2	T38.0X3	T38.0X4	T38.0X5	T38.0X6
ENT agent	T49.6X1	T49.6X2	T49.6X3	T49.6X4	T49.6X5	T49.6X6
ophthalmic preparation	T49.5X1	T49.5X2	T49.5X3	T49.5X4	T49.5X5	T49.5X6
topical NEC	T49.0X1	T49.0X2	T49.0X3	T49.0X4	T49.0X5	T49.0X6
Dexamfetamine	T43.621	T43.622	T43.623	T43.624	T43.625	T43.626
Dexamphetamine	T43.621	T43.622	T43.623	T43.624	T43.625	T43.626
Dexbrompheniramine	T45.0X1	T45.0X2	T45.0X3	T45.0X4	T45.0X5	T45.0X6
Dexchlorpheniramine	T45.0X1	T45.0X2	T45.0X3	T45.0X4	T45.0X5	T45.0X6
Dexedrine	T43.621	T43.622	T43.623	T43.624	T43.625	T43.626
Dexetimide	T44.3X1	T44.3X2	T44.3X3	T44.3X4	T44.3X5	T44.3X6
Dexfenfluramine	T50.5X1	T50.5X2	T50.5X3	T50.5X4	T50.5X5	T50.5X6
Dexpanthenol	T45.2X1	T45.2X2	T45.2X3	T45.2X4	T45.2X5	T45.2X6
Dextran (40) (70) (150)	T45.8X1	T45.8X2	T45.8X3	T45.8X4	T45.8X5	T45.8X6
Dextriferron	T45.4X1	T45.4X2	T45.4X3	T45.4X4	T45.4X5	T45.4X6
Dextroamphetamine	T43.621	T43.622	T43.623	T43.624	T43.625	T43.626
Dextro calcium pantothenate	T45.2X1	T45.2X2	T45.2X3	T45.2X4	T45.2X5	T45.2X6
Dextromethorphan	T48.3X1	T48.3X2	T48.3X3	T48.3X4	T48.3X5	T48.3X6
Dextromoramide	T40.491	T40.492	T40.493	T40.494	—	—
topical	T49.8X1	T49.8X2	T49.8X3	T49.8X4	T49.8X5	T49.8X6
Dextro pantothenyl alcohol	T45.2X1	T45.2X2	T45.2X3	T45.2X4	T45.2X5	T45.2X6
Dextropropoxyphene	T40.491	T40.492	T40.493	T40.494	T40.495	T40.496
Dextrorphan	T40.2X1	T40.2X2	T40.2X3	T40.2X4	T40.2X5	T40.2X6
Dextrose	T50.3X1	T50.3X2	T50.3X3	T50.3X4	T50.3X5	T50.3X6
concentrated solution, intravenous	T46.8X1	T46.8X2	T46.8X3	T46.8X4	T46.8X5	T46.8X6
Dextrothyroxin	T38.1X1	T38.1X2	T38.1X3	T38.1X4	T38.1X5	T38.1X6
Dextrothyroxine sodium	T38.1X1	T38.1X2	T38.1X3	T38.1X4	T38.1X5	T38.1X6
DFP	T44.0X1	T44.0X2	T44.0X3	T44.0X4	T44.0X5	T44.0X6
DHE	T37.3X1	T37.3X2	T37.3X3	T37.3X4	T37.3X5	T37.3X6
45	T46.5X1	T46.5X2	T46.5X3	T46.5X4	T46.5X5	T46.5X6
Diabinese	T38.3X1	T38.3X2	T38.3X3	T38.3X4	T38.3X5	T38.3X6
Diacetone alcohol	T52.4X1	T52.4X2	T52.4X3	T52.4X4	—	—
Diacetyl monoxime	T50.991	T50.992	T50.993	T50.994	—	—
Diacetylmorphine	T40.1X1	T40.1X2	T40.1X3	T40.1X4		

Substance	External Cause (T-Code)					
	Poisoning, Accidental (Unintentional)	Poisoning, Intentional Self-Harm	Poisoning, Assault	Poisoning, Undetermined	Adverse Effect	Underdosing
Diachylon plaster	T49.4X1	T49.4X2	T49.4X3	T49.4X4	T49.4X5	T49.4X6
Diaethylstilboestrolum	T38.5X1	T38.5X2	T38.5X3	T38.5X4	T38.5X5	T38.5X6
Diagnostic agent NEC	T50.8X1	T50.8X2	T50.8X3	T50.8X4	T50.8X5	T50.8X6
Dial (soap)	T49.2X1	T49.2X2	T49.2X3	T49.2X4	T49.2X5	T49.2X6
sedative	T42.3X1	T42.3X2	T42.3X3	T42.3X4	T42.3X5	T42.3X6
Dialkyl carbonate	T52.91	T52.92	T52.93	T52.94	—	—
Diallylbarbituric acid	T42.3X1	T42.3X2	T42.3X3	T42.3X4	T42.3X5	T42.3X6
Diallymal	T42.3X1	T42.3X2	T42.3X3	T42.3X4	T42.3X5	T42.3X6
Dialysis solution (intraperitoneal)	T50.3X1	T50.3X2	T50.3X3	T50.3X4	T50.3X5	T50.3X6
Diaminodiphenylsulfone	T37.1X1	T37.1X2	T37.1X3	T37.1X4	T37.1X5	T37.1X6
Diamorphine	T40.1X1	T40.1X2	T40.1X3	T40.1X4	—	—
Diamox	T50.2X1	T50.2X2	T50.2X3	T50.2X4	T50.2X5	T50.2X6
Diamthazole	T49.0X1	T49.0X2	T49.0X3	T49.0X4	T49.0X5	T49.0X6
Dianthone	T47.2X1	T47.2X2	T47.2X3	T47.2X4	T47.2X5	T47.2X6
Diaphenylsulfone	T37.0X1	T37.0X2	T37.0X3	T37.0X4	T37.0X5	T37.0X6
Diasone (sodium)	T37.1X1	T37.1X2	T37.1X3	T37.1X4	T37.1X5	T37.1X6
Diastase	T47.5X1	T47.5X2	T47.5X3	T47.5X4	T47.5X5	T47.5X6
Diatrizoate	T50.8X1	T50.8X2	T50.8X3	T50.8X4	T50.8X5	T50.8X6
Diazepam	T42.4X1	T42.4X2	T42.4X3	T42.4X4	T42.4X5	T42.4X6
Diazinon	T60.0X1	T60.0X2	T60.0X3	T60.0X4	—	—
Diazomethane (gas)	T59.891	T59.892	T59.893	T59.894	—	—
Diazoxide	T46.5X1	T46.5X2	T46.5X3	T46.5X4	T46.5X5	T46.5X6
Dibekacin	T36.5X1	T36.5X2	T36.5X3	T36.5X4	T36.5X5	T36.5X6
Dibenamine	T44.6X1	T44.6X2	T44.6X3	T44.6X4	T44.6X5	T44.6X6
Dibenzepin	T43.011	T43.012	T43.013	T43.014	T43.015	T43.016
Dibenzheptropine	T45.0X1	T45.0X2	T45.0X3	T45.0X4	T45.0X5	T45.0X6
Dibenzyline	T44.6X1	T44.6X2	T44.6X3	T44.6X4	T44.6X5	T44.6X6
Diborane (gas)	T59.891	T59.892	T59.893	T59.894	—	—
Dibromochloropropane	T60.8X1	T60.8X2	T60.8X3	T60.8X4	—	—
Dibromodulcitol	T45.1X1	T45.1X2	T45.1X3	T45.1X4	T45.1X5	T45.1X6
Dibromoethane	T53.6X1	T53.6X2	T53.6X3	T53.6X4	—	—
Dibromomannitol	T45.1X1	T45.1X2	T45.1X3	T45.1X4	T45.1X5	T45.1X6
Dibromopropamidine isethionate	T49.0X1	T49.0X2	T49.0X3	T49.0X4	T49.0X5	T49.0X6
Dibrompropamidine	T49.0X1	T49.0X2	T49.0X3	T49.0X4	T49.0X5	T49.0X6
Dibucaine	T41.3X1	T41.3X2	T41.3X3	T41.3X4	T41.3X5	T41.3X6
topical (surface)	T41.3X1	T41.3X2	T41.3X3	T41.3X4	T41.3X5	T41.3X6
Dibunate sodium	T48.3X1	T48.3X2	T48.3X3	T48.3X4	T48.3X5	T48.3X6
Dibutoline sulfate	T44.3X1	T44.3X2	T44.3X3	T44.3X4	T44.3X5	T44.3X6
Dicamba	T60.3X1	T60.3X2	T60.3X3	T60.3X4	—	—
Dicapthon	T60.0X1	T60.0X2	T60.0X3	T60.0X4	—	—
Dichlobenil	T60.3X1	T60.3X2	T60.3X3	T60.3X4	—	—
Dichlone	T60.3X1	T60.3X2	T60.3X3	T60.3X4	—	—

Substance	Poisoning, Accidental (Unintentional)	Poisoning, Intentional Self-Harm	Poisoning, Assault	Poisoning, Undetermined	Adverse Effect	Underdosing
Dichloralphenozone	T42.6X1	T42.6X2	T42.6X3	T42.6X4	T42.6X5	T42.6X6
Dichlorbenzidine	T65.3X1	T65.3X2	T65.3X3	T65.3X4	—	—
Dichlorhydrin	T52.8X1	T52.8X2	T52.8X3	T52.8X4	—	—
Dichlorhydroxyquinoline	T37.8X1	T37.8X2	T37.8X3	T37.8X4	T37.8X5	T37.8X6
Dichlorobenzene	T53.7X1	T53.7X2	T53.7X3	T53.7X4	—	—
Dichlorobenzyl alcohol	T49.6X1	T49.6X2	T49.6X3	T49.6X4	T49.6X5	T49.6X6
Dichlorodifluoromethane	T53.5X1	T53.5X2	T53.5X3	T53.5X4	—	—
Dichloroethane	T52.8X1	T52.8X2	T52.8X3	T52.8X4	—	—
Sym-Dichloroethyl ether	T53.6X1	T53.6X2	T53.6X3	T53.6X4	—	—
Dichloroethyl sulfide, not in war	T59.891	T59.892	T59.893	T59.894		
Dichloroethylene	T53.6X1	T53.6X2	T53.6X3	T53.6X4	—	—
Dichloroformoxine, not in war	T59.891	T59.892	T59.893	T59.894		
Dichlorohydrin, alpha-dichlorohydrin	T52.8X1	T52.8X2	T52.8X3	T52.8X4	—	—
Dichloromethane (solvent)	T53.4X1	T53.4X2	T53.4X3	T53.4X4	—	—
vapor	T53.4X1	T53.4X2	T53.4X3	T53.4X4	—	—
Dichloronaphthoquinone	T60.3X1	T60.3X2	T60.3X3	T60.3X4	—	—
Dichlorophen	T37.4X1	T37.4X2	T37.4X3	T37.4X4	T37.4X5	T37.4X6
2,4-Dichlorophenoxy-acetic acid	T60.3X1	T60.3X2	T60.3X3	T60.3X4	—	—
Dichloropropene	T60.3X1	T60.3X2	T60.3X3	T60.3X4	—	—
Dichloropropionic acid	T60.3X1	T60.3X2	T60.3X3	T60.3X4	—	—
Dichlorphenamide	T50.2X1	T50.2X2	T50.2X3	T50.2X4	T50.2X5	T50.2X6
Dichlorvos	T60.0X1	T60.0X2	T60.0X3	T60.0X4	—	—
Diclofenac	T39.391	T39.392	T39.393	T39.394	T39.395	T39.396
Diclofenamide	T50.2X1	T50.2X2	T50.2X3	T50.2X4	T50.2X5	T50.2X6
Diclofensine	T43.291	T43.292	T43.293	T43.294	T43.295	T43.296
Diclonixine	T39.8X1	T39.8X2	T39.8X3	T39.8X4	T39.8X5	T39.8X6
Dicloxacillin	T36.0X1	T36.0X2	T36.0X3	T36.0X4	T36.0X5	T36.0X6
Dicophane	T49.0X1	T49.0X2	T49.0X3	T49.0X4	T49.0X5	T49.0X6
Dicoumarol, dicoumarin, dicumarol	T45.511	T45.512	T45.513	T45.514	T45.515	T45.516
Dicrotophos	T60.0X1	T60.0X2	T60.0X3	T60.0X4	—	—
Dicyanogen (gas)	T65.0X1	T65.0X2	T65.0X3	T65.0X4	—	—
Dicyclomine	T44.3X1	T44.3X2	T44.3X3	T44.3X4	T44.3X5	T44.3X6
Dicycloverine	T44.3X1	T44.3X2	T44.3X3	T44.3X4	T44.3X5	T44.3X6
Dideoxycytidine	T37.5X1	T37.5X2	T37.5X3	T37.5X4	T37.5X5	T37.5X6
Dideoxyinosine	T37.5X1	T37.5X2	T37.5X3	T37.5X4	T37.5X5	T37.5X6
Dieldrin (vapor)	T60.1X1	T60.1X2	T60.1X3	T60.1X4	—	—
Diemal	T42.3X1	T42.3X2	T42.3X3	T42.3X4	T42.3X5	T42.3X6
Dienestrol	T38.5X1	T38.5X2	T38.5X3	T38.5X4	T38.5X5	T38.5X6
Dienoestrol	T38.5X1	T38.5X2	T38.5X3	T38.5X4	T38.5X5	T38.5X6
Dietetic drug NEC	T50.901	T50.902	T50.903	T50.904	T50.905	T50.906
Diethazine	T42.8X1	T42.8X2	T42.8X3	T42.8X4	T42.8X5	T42.8X6

Substance	Poisoning, Accidental (Unintentional)	Poisoning, Intentional Self-Harm	Poisoning, Assault	Poisoning, Undetermined	Adverse Effect	Underdosing
Diethyl						
barbituric acid	T42.3X1	T42.3X2	T42.3X3	T42.3X4	T42.3X5	T42.3X6
carbamazine	T37.4X1	T37.4X2	T37.4X3	T37.4X4	T37.4X5	T37.4X6
carbinol	T51.3X1	T51.3X2	T51.3X3	T51.3X4	—	—
carbonate	T52.8X1	T52.8X2	T52.8X3	T52.8X4	—	—
ether (vapor) — see also Ether	T41.0X1	T41.0X2	T41.0X3	T41.0X4	T41.0X5	T41.0X6
oxide	T52.8X1	T52.8X2	T52.8X3	T52.8X4	—	—
propion	T50.5X1	T50.5X2	T50.5X3	T50.5X4	T50.5X5	T50.5X6
stilbestrol	T38.5X1	T38.5X2	T38.5X3	T38.5X4	T38.5X5	T38.5X6
toluamide (nonmedicinal)	T60.8X1	T60.8X2	T60.8X3	T60.8X4	—	—
medicinal	T49.3X1	T49.3X2	T49.3X3	T49.3X4	T49.3X5	T49.3X6
Diethylcarbamazine	T37.4X1	T37.4X2	T37.4X3	T37.4X4	T37.4X5	T37.4X6
Diethylene						
dioxide	T52.8X1	T52.8X2	T52.8X3	T52.8X4	—	—
glycol (monoacetate) (monobutyl ether) (monoethyl ether)	T52.3X1	T52.3X2	T52.3X3	T52.3X4	—	—
Diethylhexylphthalate	T65.891	T65.892	T65.893	T65.894	—	—
Diethylpropion	T50.5X1	T50.5X2	T50.5X3	T50.5X4	T50.5X5	T50.5X6
Diethylstilbestrol	T38.5X1	T38.5X2	T38.5X3	T38.5X4	T38.5X5	T38.5X6
Diethylstilboestrol	T38.5X1	T38.5X2	T38.5X3	T38.5X4	T38.5X5	T38.5X6
Diethylsulfone-diethylmethane	T42.6X1	T42.6X2	T42.6X3	T42.6X4	T42.6X5	T42.6X6
Diethyltoluamide	T49.0X1	T49.0X2	T49.0X3	T49.0X4	T49.0X5	T49.0X6
Diethyltryptamine (DET)	T40.991	T40.992	T40.993	T40.994	—	—
Difebarbamate	T42.3X1	T42.3X2	T42.3X3	T42.3X4	T42.3X5	T42.3X6
Difencloxazine	T40.2X1	T40.2X2	T40.2X3	T40.2X4	T40.2X5	T40.2X6
Difenidol	T45.0X1	T45.0X2	T45.0X3	T45.0X4	T45.0X5	T45.0X6
Difenoxin	T47.6X1	T47.6X2	T47.6X3	T47.6X4	T47.6X5	T47.6X6
Difetarsone	T37.3X1	T37.3X2	T37.3X3	T37.3X4	T37.3X5	T37.3X6
Diffusin	T45.3X1	T45.3X2	T45.3X3	T45.3X4	T45.3X5	T45.3X6
Diflorasone	T49.0X1	T49.0X2	T49.0X3	T49.0X4	T49.0X5	T49.0X6
Diflubenzuron	T60.1X1	T60.1X2	T60.1X3	T60.1X4	—	—
Diflos	T44.0X1	T44.0X2	T44.0X3	T44.0X4	T44.0X5	T44.0X6
Diflucortolone	T49.0X1	T49.0X2	T49.0X3	T49.0X4	T49.0X5	T49.0X6
Diflunisal	T39.091	T39.092	T39.093	T39.094	T39.095	T39.096
Difluoromethyldopa	T42.8X1	T42.8X2	T42.8X3	T42.8X4	T42.8X5	T42.8X6
Difluorophate	T44.0X1	T44.0X2	T44.0X3	T44.0X4	T44.0X5	T44.0X6
Digestant NEC	T47.5X1	T47.5X2	T47.5X3	T47.5X4	T47.5X5	T47.5X6
Digitalin(e)	T46.0X1	T46.0X2	T46.0X3	T46.0X4	T46.0X5	T46.0X6
Digitalis (leaf) (glycoside)	T46.0X1	T46.0X2	T46.0X3	T46.0X4	T46.0X5	T46.0X6
lanata	T46.0X1	T46.0X2	T46.0X3	T46.0X4	T46.0X5	T46.0X6
purpurea	T46.0X1	T46.0X2	T46.0X3	T46.0X4	T46.0X5	T46.0X6
Digitoxin	T46.0X1	T46.0X2	T46.0X3	T46.0X4	T46.0X5	T46.0X6

◀ New   ◀ Revised   ~~deleted~~ Deleted

Substance	Poisoning, Accidental (Unintentional)	Poisoning, Intentional Self-Harm	Poisoning, Assault	Poisoning, Undetermined	Adverse Effect	Underdosing
Digitoxose	T46.0X1	T46.0X2	T46.0X3	T46.0X4	T46.0X5	T46.0X6
Digoxin	T46.0X1	T46.0X2	T46.0X3	T46.0X4	T46.0X5	T46.0X6
Digoxine	T46.0X1	T46.0X2	T46.0X3	T46.0X4	T46.0X5	T46.0X6
Dihydralazine	T46.5X1	T46.5X2	T46.5X3	T46.5X4	T46.5X5	T46.5X6
Dihydrazine	T46.5X1	T46.5X2	T46.5X3	T46.5X4	T46.5X5	T46.5X6
Dihydrocodeinone	T40.2X1	T40.2X2	T40.2X3	T40.2X4	T40.2X5	T40.2X6
Dihydroergocornine	T46.7X1	T46.7X2	T46.7X3	T46.7X4	T46.7X5	T46.7X6
Dihydroergocristine (mesilate)	T46.7X1	T46.7X2	T46.7X3	T46.7X4	T46.7X5	T46.7X6
Dihydroergokryptine	T46.7X1	T46.7X2	T46.7X3	T46.7X4	T46.7X5	T46.7X6
Dihydroergotamine	T46.5X1	T46.5X2	T46.5X3	T46.5X4	T46.5X5	T46.5X6
Dihydroergotoxine	T46.7X1	T46.7X2	T46.7X3	T46.7X4	T46.7X5	T46.7X6
mesilate	T46.7X1	T46.7X2	T46.7X3	T46.7X4	T46.7X5	T46.7X6
Dihydrohydroxycodein-one	T40.2X1	T40.2X2	T40.2X3	T40.2X4	T40.2X5	T40.2X6
Dihydrohydroxymorphinone	T40.2X1	T40.2X2	T40.2X3	T40.2X4	T40.2X5	T40.2X6
Dihydroisocodeine	T40.2X1	T40.2X2	T40.2X3	T40.2X4	T40.2X5	T40.2X6
Dihydromorphine	T40.2X1	T40.2X2	T40.2X3	T40.2X4	—	—
Dihydromorphinone	T40.2X1	T40.2X2	T40.2X3	T40.2X4	T40.2X5	T40.2X6
Dihydrostreptomycin	T36.5X1	T36.5X2	T36.5X3	T36.5X4	T36.5X5	T36.5X6
Dihydrotachysterol	T45.2X1	T45.2X2	T45.2X3	T45.2X4	T45.2X5	T45.2X6
Dihydroxyaluminum aminoacetate	T47.1X1	T47.1X2	T47.1X3	T47.1X4	T47.1X5	T47.1X6
Dihydroxyaluminum sodium carbonate	T47.1X1	T47.1X2	T47.1X3	T47.1X4	T47.1X5	T47.1X6
Dihydroxyanthraquinone	T47.2X1	T47.2X2	T47.2X3	T47.2X4	T47.2X5	T47.2X6
Dihydroxycodeinone	T40.2X1	T40.2X2	T40.2X3	T40.2X4	T40.2X5	T40.2X6
Dihydroxypropyl theophylline	T50.2X1	T50.2X2	T50.2X3	T50.2X4	T50.2X5	T50.2X6
Diiodohydroxyquin	T37.8X1	T37.8X2	T37.8X3	T37.8X4	T37.8X5	T37.8X6
topical	T49.0X1	T49.0X2	T49.0X3	T49.0X4	T49.0X5	T49.0X6
Diiodohydroxyquinoline	T37.8X1	T37.8X2	T37.8X3	T37.8X4	T37.8X5	T37.8X6
Diiodotyrosine	T38.2X1	T38.2X2	T38.2X3	T38.2X4	T38.2X5	T38.2X6
Diisopromine	T44.3X1	T44.3X2	T44.3X3	T44.3X4	T44.3X5	T44.3X6
Diisopropylamine	T46.3X1	T46.3X2	T46.3X3	T46.3X4	T46.3X5	T46.3X6
Diisopropylfluorophosphate	T44.0X1	T44.0X2	T44.0X3	T44.0X4	T44.0X5	T44.0X6
Dilantin	T42.0X1	T42.0X2	T42.0X3	T42.0X4	T42.0X5	T42.0X6
Dilaudid	T40.2X1	T40.2X2	T40.2X3	T40.2X4	T40.2X5	T40.2X6
Dilazep	T46.3X1	T46.3X2	T46.3X3	T46.3X4	T46.3X5	T46.3X6
Dill	T47.5X1	T47.5X2	T47.5X3	T47.5X4	T47.5X5	T47.5X6
Diloxanide	T37.3X1	T37.3X2	T37.3X3	T37.3X4	T37.3X5	T37.3X6
Diltiazem	T46.1X1	T46.1X2	T46.1X3	T46.1X4	T46.1X5	T46.1X6
Dimazole	T49.0X1	T49.0X2	T49.0X3	T49.0X4	T49.0X5	T49.0X6
Dimefline	T50.7X1	T50.7X2	T50.7X3	T50.7X4	T50.7X5	T50.7X6
Dimefox	T60.0X1	T60.0X2	T60.0X3	T60.0X4	—	—

Substance	Poisoning, Accidental (Unintentional)	Poisoning, Intentional Self-Harm	Poisoning, Assault	Poisoning, Undetermined	Adverse Effect	Underdosing
Dimemorfan	T48.3X1	T48.3X2	T48.3X3	T48.3X4	T48.3X5	T48.3X6
Dimenhydrinate	T45.0X1	T45.0X2	T45.0X3	T45.0X4	T45.0X5	T45.0X6
Dimercaprol (British anti-lewisite)	T45.8X1	T45.8X2	T45.8X3	T45.8X4	T45.8X5	T45.8X6
Dimercaptopropanol	T45.8X1	T45.8X2	T45.8X3	T45.8X4	T45.8X5	T45.8X6
Dimestrol	T38.5X1	T38.5X2	T38.5X3	T38.5X4	T38.5X5	T38.5X6
Dimetane	T45.0X1	T45.0X2	T45.0X3	T45.0X4	T45.0X5	T45.0X6
Dimethicone	T47.1X1	T47.1X2	T47.1X3	T47.1X4	T47.1X5	T47.1X6
Dimethindene	T45.0X1	T45.0X2	T45.0X3	T45.0X4	T45.0X5	T45.0X6
Dimethisoquin	T49.1X1	T49.1X2	T49.1X3	T49.1X4	T49.1X5	T49.1X6
Dimethisterone	T38.5X1	T38.5X2	T38.5X3	T38.5X4	T38.5X5	T38.5X6
Dimethoate	T60.0X1	T60.0X2	T60.0X3	T60.0X4	—	—
Dimethocaine	T41.3X1	T41.3X2	T41.3X3	T41.3X4	T41.3X5	T41.3X6
Dimethoxanate	T48.3X1	T48.3X2	T48.3X3	T48.3X4	T48.3X5	T48.3X6
Dimethyl						
arsine, arsinic acid	T57.0X1	T57.0X2	T57.0X3	T57.0X4		
carbinol	T51.2X1	T51.2X2	T51.2X3	T51.2X4		
carbonate	T52.8X1	T52.8X2	T52.8X3	T52.8X4		
diguanide	T38.3X1	T38.3X2	T38.3X3	T38.3X4	T38.3X5	T38.3X6
ketone	T52.4X1	T52.4X2	T52.4X3	T52.4X4		
vapor	T52.4X1	T52.4X2	T52.4X3	T52.4X4		
meperidine	T40.2X1	T40.2X2	T40.2X3	T40.2X4	T40.2X5	T40.2X6
parathion	T60.0X1	T60.0X2	T60.0X3	T60.0X4	—	
phthlate	T49.3X1	T49.3X2	T49.3X3	T49.3X4	T49.3X5	T49.3X6
polysiloxane	T47.8X1	T47.8X2	T47.8X3	T47.8X4	T47.8X5	T47.8X6
sulfate (fumes)	T59.891	T59.892	T59.893	T59.894	—	—
liquid	T65.891	T65.892	T65.893	T65.894	—	—
sulfoxide (nonmedicinal)	T52.8X1	T52.8X2	T52.8X3	T52.8X4		
medicinal	T49.4X1	T49.4X2	T49.4X3	T49.4X4	T49.4X5	T49.4X6
tryptamine	T40.991	T40.992	T40.993	T40.994		—
tubocurarine	T48.1X1	T48.1X2	T48.1X3	T48.1X4	T48.1X5	T48.1X6
Dimethylamine sulfate	T49.4X1	T49.4X2	T49.4X3	T49.4X4	T49.4X5	T49.4X6
Dimethylformamide	T52.8X1	T52.8X2	T52.8X3	T52.8X4		
Dimethyltubocurarinium chloride	T48.1X1	T48.1X2	T48.1X3	T48.1X4	T48.1X5	T48.1X6
Dimeticone	T47.1X1	T47.1X2	T47.1X3	T47.1X4	T47.1X5	T47.1X6
Dimetilan	T60.0X1	T60.0X2	T60.0X3	T60.0X4		
Dimetindene	T45.0X1	T45.0X2	T45.0X3	T45.0X4	T45.0X5	T45.0X6
Dimetotiazine	T43.3X1	T43.3X2	T43.3X3	T43.3X4	T43.3X5	T43.3X6
Dimorpholamine	T50.7X1	T50.7X2	T50.7X3	T50.7X4	T50.7X5	T50.7X6
Dimoxyline	T46.3X1	T46.3X2	T46.3X3	T46.3X4	T46.3X5	T46.3X6
Dinitrobenzene	T65.3X1	T65.3X2	T65.3X3	T65.3X4		
vapor	T59.891	T59.892	T59.893	T59.894	—	—

Substance	External Cause (T-Code)					
	Poisoning, Accidental (Unintentional)	Poisoning, Intentional Self-Harm	Poisoning, Assault	Poisoning, Undetermined	Adverse Effect	Underdosing
Dinitrobenzol	T65.3X1	T65.3X2	T65.3X3	T65.3X4	—	—
vapor	T59.891	T59.892	T59.893	T59.894	—	—
Dinitrobutylphenol	T65.3X1	T65.3X2	T65.3X3	T65.3X4		
Dinitro (-ortho-)cresol (pesticide) (spray)	T65.3X1	T65.3X2	T65.3X3	T65.3X4		
Dinitrocyclohexylphenol	T65.3X1	T65.3X2	T65.3X3	T65.3X4	—	—
Dinitrophenol	T65.3X1	T65.3X2	T65.3X3	T65.3X4	—	—
Dinoprost	T48.0X1	T48.0X2	T48.0X3	T48.0X4	T48.0X5	T48.0X6
Dinoprostone	T48.0X1	T48.0X2	T48.0X3	T48.0X4	T48.0X5	T48.0X6
Dinoseb	T60.3X1	T60.3X2	T60.3X3	T60.3X4		
Dioctyl sulfosuccinate (calcium) (sodium)	T47.4X1	T47.4X2	T47.4X3	T47.4X4	T47.4X5	T47.4X6
Diodone	T50.8X1	T50.8X2	T50.8X3	T50.8X4	T50.8X5	T50.8X6
Diodoquin	T37.8X1	T37.8X2	T37.8X3	T37.8X4	T37.8X5	T37.8X6
Dionin	T40.2X1	T40.2X2	T40.2X3	T40.2X4	T40.2X5	T40.2X6
Diosmin	T46.991	T46.992	T46.993	T46.994	T46.995	T46.996
Dioxane	T52.8X1	T52.8X2	T52.8X3	T52.8X4	—	—
Dioxathion	T60.0X1	T60.0X2	T60.0X3	T60.0X4	—	—
Dioxin	T53.7X1	T53.7X2	T53.7X3	T53.7X4	—	—
Dioxopromethazine	T43.3X1	T43.3X2	T43.3X3	T43.3X4	T43.3X5	T43.3X6
Dioxyline	T46.3X1	T46.3X2	T46.3X3	T46.3X4	T46.3X5	T46.3X6
Dipentene	T52.8X1	T52.8X2	T52.8X3	T52.8X4		
Diperodon	T41.3X1	T41.3X2	T41.3X3	T41.3X4	T41.3X5	T41.3X6
Diphacinone	T60.4X1	T60.4X2	T60.4X3	T60.4X4		
Diphemanil	T44.3X1	T44.3X2	T44.3X3	T44.3X4	T44.3X5	T44.3X6
metilsulfate	T44.3X1	T44.3X2	T44.3X3	T44.3X4	T44.3X5	T44.3X6
Diphenadione	T45.511	T45.512	T45.513	T45.514	T45.515	T45.516
rodenticide	T60.4X1	T60.4X2	T60.4X3	T60.4X4	—	—
Diphenhydramine	T45.0X1	T45.0X2	T45.0X3	T45.0X4	T45.0X5	T45.0X6
Diphenidol	T45.0X1	T45.0X2	T45.0X3	T45.0X4	T45.0X5	T45.0X6
Diphenoxylate	T47.6X1	T47.6X2	T47.6X3	T47.6X4	T47.6X5	T47.6X6
Diphenylamine	T65.3X1	T65.3X2	T65.3X3	T65.3X4	—	—
Diphenylbutazone	T39.2X1	T39.2X2	T39.2X3	T39.2X4	T39.2X5	T39.2X6
Diphenylchloroarsine, not in war	T57.0X1	T57.0X2	T57.0X3	T57.0X4	—	—
Diphenylhydantoin	T42.0X1	T42.0X2	T42.0X3	T42.0X4	T42.0X5	T42.0X6
Diphenylmethane dye	T52.1X1	T52.1X2	T52.1X3	T52.1X4	—	—
Diphenylpyraline	T45.0X1	T45.0X2	T45.0X3	T45.0X4	T45.0X5	T45.0X6
Diphtheria						
antitoxin	T50.Z11	T50.Z12	T50.Z13	T50.Z14	T50.Z15	T50.Z16
toxoid	T50.A91	T50.A92	T50.A93	T50.A94	T50.A95	T50.A96
with tetanus toxoid	T50.A21	T50.A22	T50.A23	T50.A24	T50.A25	T50.A26
with pertussis component	T50.A11	T50.A12	T50.A13	T50.A14	T50.A15	T50.A16

Substance	External Cause (T-Code)					
	Poisoning, Accidental (Unintentional)	Poisoning, Intentional Self-Harm	Poisoning, Assault	Poisoning, Undetermined	Adverse Effect	Underdosing
Diphtheria *(Continued)*						
vaccine (combination)	T50.A91	T50.A92	T50.A93	T50.A94	T50.A95	T50.A96
combination						
including pertussis	T50.A11	T50.A12	T50.A13	T50.A14	T50.A15	T50.A16
without pertussis	T50.A21	T50.A22	T50.A23	T50.A24	T50.A25	T50.A26
Diphylline	T50.2X1	T50.2X2	T50.2X3	T50.2X4	T50.2X5	T50.2X6
Dipipanone	T40.491	T40.492	T40.493	T40.494	—	—
Dipivefrine	T49.5X1	T49.5X2	T49.5X3	T49.5X4	T49.5X5	T49.5X6
Diplovax	T50.B91	T50.B92	T50.B93	T50.B94	T50.B95	T50.B96
Diprophylline	T50.2X1	T50.2X2	T50.2X3	T50.2X4	T50.2X5	T50.2X6
Dipropyline	T48.291	T48.292	T48.293	T48.294	T48.295	T48.296
Dipyridamole	T46.3X1	T46.3X2	T46.3X3	T46.3X4	T46.3X5	T46.3X6
Dipyrone	T39.2X1	T39.2X2	T39.2X3	T39.2X4	T39.2X5	T39.2X6
Diquat (dibromide)	T60.3X1	T60.3X2	T60.3X3	T60.3X4	—	—
Disinfectant	T65.891	T65.892	T65.893	T65.894	—	—
alkaline	T54.3X1	T54.3X2	T54.3X3	T54.3X4	—	—
aromatic	T54.1X1	T54.1X2	T54.1X3	T54.1X4	—	—
intestinal	T37.8X1	T37.8X2	T37.8X3	T37.8X4	T37.8X5	T37.8X6
Disipal	T42.8X1	T42.8X2	T42.8X3	T42.8X4	T42.8X5	T42.8X6
Disodium edetate	T50.6X1	T50.6X2	T50.6X3	T50.6X4	T50.6X5	T50.6X6
Disoprofol	T41.291	T41.292	T41.293	T41.294	T41.295	T41.296
Disopyramide	T46.2X1	T46.2X2	T46.2X3	T46.2X4	T46.2X5	T46.2X6
Distigmine (bromide)	T44.0X1	T44.0X2	T44.0X3	T44.0X4	T44.0X5	T44.0X6
Disulfamide	T50.2X1	T50.2X2	T50.2X3	T50.2X4	T50.2X5	T50.2X6
Disulfanilamide	T37.0X1	T37.0X2	T37.0X3	T37.0X4	T37.0X5	T37.0X6
Disulfiram	T50.6X1	T50.6X2	T50.6X3	T50.6X4	T50.6X5	T50.6X6
Disulfoton	T60.0X1	T60.0X2	T60.0X3	T60.0X4	—	—
Dithiazanine iodide	T37.4X1	T37.4X2	T37.4X3	T37.4X4	T37.4X5	T37.4X6
Dithiocarbamate	T60.0X1	T60.0X2	T60.0X3	T60.0X4	—	—
Dithranol	T49.4X1	T49.4X2	T49.4X3	T49.4X4	T49.4X5	T49.4X6
Diucardin	T50.2X1	T50.2X2	T50.2X3	T50.2X4	T50.2X5	T50.2X6
Diupres	T50.2X1	T50.2X2	T50.2X3	T50.2X4	T50.2X5	T50.2X6
Diuretic NEC	T50.2X1	T50.2X2	T50.2X3	T50.2X4	T50.2X5	T50.2X6
benzothiadiazine	T50.2X1	T50.2X2	T50.2X3	T50.2X4	T50.2X5	T50.2X6
carbonic acid anhydrase inhibitors	T50.2X1	T50.2X2	T50.2X3	T50.2X4	T50.2X5	T50.2X6
furfuryl NEC	T50.2X1	T50.2X2	T50.2X3	T50.2X4	T50.2X5	T50.2X6
loop (high-ceiling)	T50.1X1	T50.1X2	T50.1X3	T50.1X4	T50.1X5	T50.1X6
mercurial NEC	T50.2X1	T50.2X2	T50.2X3	T50.2X4	T50.2X5	T50.2X6
osmotic	T50.2X1	T50.2X2	T50.2X3	T50.2X4	T50.2X5	T50.2X6
purine NEC	T50.2X1	T50.2X2	T50.2X3	T50.2X4	T50.2X5	T50.2X6
saluretic NEC	T50.2X1	T50.2X2	T50.2X3	T50.2X4	T50.2X5	T50.2X6

◀ New   ◀ Revised   ~~deleted~~ Deleted

Substance	External Cause (T-Code)					
	Poisoning, Accidental (Unintentional)	Poisoning, Intentional Self-Harm	Poisoning, Assault	Poisoning, Undetermined	Adverse Effect	Underdosing
Diuretic NEC *(Continued)*						
sulfonamide	T50.2X1	T50.2X2	T50.2X3	T50.2X4	T50.2X5	T50.2X6
thiazide NEC	T50.2X1	T50.2X2	T50.2X3	T50.2X4	T50.2X5	T50.2X6
xanthine	T50.2X1	T50.2X2	T50.2X3	T50.2X4	T50.2X5	T50.2X6
Diurgin	T50.2X1	T50.2X2	T50.2X3	T50.2X4	T50.2X5	T50.2X6
Diuril	T50.2X1	T50.2X2	T50.2X3	T50.2X4	T50.2X5	T50.2X6
Diuron	T60.3X1	T60.3X2	T60.3X3	T60.3X4	—	—
Divalproex	T42.6X1	T42.6X2	T42.6X3	T42.6X4	T42.6X5	T42.6X6
Divinyl ether	T41.0X1	T41.0X2	T41.0X3	T41.0X4	T41.0X5	T41.0X6
Dixanthogen	T49.0X1	T49.0X2	T49.0X3	T49.0X4	T49.0X5	T49.0X6
Dixyrazine	T43.3X1	T43.3X2	T43.3X3	T43.3X4	T43.3X5	T43.3X6
D-lysergic acid diethylamide	T40.8X1	T40.8X2	T40.8X3	T40.8X4	—	—
DMCT	T36.4X1	T36.4X2	T36.4X3	T36.4X4	T36.4X5	T36.4X6
DMSO — *see Dimethyl, sulfoxide*						
DNBP	T60.3X1	T60.3X2	T60.3X3	T60.3X4	—	—
DNOC	T65.3X1	T65.3X2	T65.3X3	T65.3X4	—	—
DOCA	T38.0X1	T38.0X2	T38.0X3	T38.0X4	T38.0X5	T38.0X6
Dobutamine	T44.5X1	T44.5X2	T44.5X3	T44.5X4	T44.5X5	T44.5X6
Docusate sodium	T47.4X1	T47.4X2	T47.4X3	T47.4X4	T47.4X5	T47.4X6
Dodicin	T49.0X1	T49.0X2	T49.0X3	T49.0X4	T49.0X5	T49.0X6
Dofamium chloride	T49.0X1	T49.0X2	T49.0X3	T49.0X4	T49.0X5	T49.0X6
Dolophine	T40.3X1	T40.3X2	T40.3X3	T40.3X4	T40.3X5	T40.3X6
Doloxene	T39.8X1	T39.8X2	T39.8X3	T39.8X4	T39.8X5	T39.8X6
Domestic gas (after combustion) — *see Gas, utility*						
prior to combustion	T59.891	T59.892	T59.893	T59.894	—	—
Domiodol	T48.4X1	T48.4X2	T48.4X3	T48.4X4	T48.4X5	T48.4X6
Domiphen (bromide)	T49.0X1	T49.0X2	T49.0X3	T49.0X4	T49.0X5	T49.0X6
Domperidone	T45.0X1	T45.0X2	T45.0X3	T45.0X4	T45.0X5	T45.0X6
Dopa	T42.8X1	T42.8X2	T42.8X3	T42.8X4	T42.8X5	T42.8X6
Dopamine	T44.991	T44.992	T44.993	T44.994	T44.995	T44.996
Doriden	T42.6X1	T42.6X2	T42.6X3	T42.6X4	T42.6X5	T42.6X6
Dormiral	T42.3X1	T42.3X2	T42.3X3	T42.3X4	T42.3X5	T42.3X6
Dormison	T42.6X1	T42.6X2	T42.6X3	T42.6X4	T42.6X5	T42.6X6
Dornase	T48.4X1	T48.4X2	T48.4X3	T48.4X4	T48.4X5	T48.4X6
Dorsacaine	T41.3X1	T41.3X2	T41.3X3	T41.3X4	T41.3X5	T41.3X6
Dosulepin	T43.011	T43.012	T43.013	T43.014	T43.015	T43.016
Dothiepin	T43.011	T43.012	T43.013	T43.014	T43.015	T43.016
Doxantrazole	T48.6X1	T48.6X2	T48.6X3	T48.6X4	T48.6X5	T48.6X6
Doxapram	T50.7X1	T50.7X2	T50.7X3	T50.7X4	T50.7X5	T50.7X6
Doxazosin	T44.6X1	T44.6X2	T44.6X3	T44.6X4	T44.6X5	T44.6X6
Doxepin	T43.011	T43.012	T43.013	T43.014	T43.015	T43.016

Substance	External Cause (T-Code)					
	Poisoning, Accidental (Unintentional)	Poisoning, Intentional Self-Harm	Poisoning, Assault	Poisoning, Undetermined	Adverse Effect	Underdosing
Doxifluridine	T45.1X1	T45.1X2	T45.1X3	T45.1X4	T45.1X5	T45.1X6
Doxorubicin	T45.1X1	T45.1X2	T45.1X3	T45.1X4	T45.1X5	T45.1X6
Doxycycline	T36.4X1	T36.4X2	T36.4X3	T36.4X4	T36.4X5	T36.4X6
Doxylamine	T45.0X1	T45.0X2	T45.0X3	T45.0X4	T45.0X5	T45.0X6
Dramamine	T45.0X1	T45.0X2	T45.0X3	T45.0X4	T45.0X5	T45.0X6
Drano (drain cleaner)	T54.3X1	T54.3X2	T54.3X3	T54.3X4	—	—
Dressing, live pulp	T49.7X1	T49.7X2	T49.7X3	T49.7X4	T49.7X5	T49.7X6
Drocode	T40.2X1	T40.2X2	T40.2X3	T40.2X4	T40.2X5	T40.2X6
Dromoran	T40.2X1	T40.2X2	T40.2X3	T40.2X4	T40.2X5	T40.2X6
Dromostanolone	T38.7X1	T38.7X2	T38.7X3	T38.7X4	T38.7X5	T38.7X6
Dronabinol	T40.711	T40.712	T40.713	T40.714	T40.715	T40.716
Droperidol	T43.591	T43.592	T43.593	T43.594	T43.595	T43.596
Dropropizine	T48.3X1	T48.3X2	T48.3X3	T48.3X4	T48.3X5	T48.3X6
Drostanolone	T38.7X1	T38.7X2	T38.7X3	T38.7X4	T38.7X5	T38.7X6
Drotaverine	T44.3X1	T44.3X2	T44.3X3	T44.3X4	T44.3X5	T44.3X6
Drotrecogin alfa	T45.511	T45.512	T45.513	T45.514	T45.515	T45.516
Drug NEC	T50.901	T50.902	T50.903	T50.904	T50.905	T50.906
specified NEC	T50.991	T50.992	T50.993	T50.994	T50.995	T50.996
DTIC	T45.1X1	T45.1X2	T45.1X3	T45.1X4	T45.1X5	T45.1X6
Duboisine	T44.3X1	T44.3X2	T44.3X3	T44.3X4	T44.3X5	T44.3X6
Dulcolax	T47.2X1	T47.2X2	T47.2X3	T47.2X4	T47.2X5	T47.2X6
Duponol (C) (EP)	T49.2X1	T49.2X2	T49.2X3	T49.2X4	T49.2X5	T49.2X6
Durabolin	T38.7X1	T38.7X2	T38.7X3	T38.7X4	T38.7X5	T38.7X6
Dyclone	T41.3X1	T41.3X2	T41.3X3	T41.3X4	T41.3X5	T41.3X6
Dyclonine	T41.3X1	T41.3X2	T41.3X3	T41.3X4	T41.3X5	T41.3X6
Dydrogesterone	T38.5X1	T38.5X2	T38.5X3	T38.5X4	T38.5X5	T38.5X6
Dye NEC	T65.6X1	T65.6X2	T65.6X3	T65.6X4	—	—
antiseptic	T49.0X1	T49.0X2	T49.0X3	T49.0X4	T49.0X5	T49.0X6
diagnostic agents	T50.8X1	T50.8X2	T50.8X3	T50.8X4	T50.8X5	T50.8X6
pharmaceutical NEC	T50.901	T50.902	T50.903	T50.904	T50.905	T50.906
Dyflos	T44.0X1	T44.0X2	T44.0X3	T44.0X4	T44.0X5	T44.0X6
Dymelor	T38.3X1	T38.3X2	T38.3X3	T38.3X4	T38.3X5	T38.3X6
Dynamite	T65.3X1	T65.3X2	T65.3X3	T65.3X4	—	—
fumes	T59.891	T59.892	T59.893	T59.894	—	—
Dyphylline	T44.3X1	T44.3X2	T44.3X3	T44.3X4	T44.3X5	T44.3X6
E						
Ear drug NEC	T49.6X1	T49.6X2	T49.6X3	T49.6X4	T49.6X5	T49.6X6
Ear preparations	T49.6X1	T49.6X2	T49.6X3	T49.6X4	T49.6X5	T49.6X6
Econazole	T49.0X1	T49.0X2	T49.0X3	T49.0X4	T49.0X5	T49.0X6
Ecothiopate iodide	T49.5X1	T49.5X2	T49.5X3	T49.5X4	T49.5X5	T49.5X6
Echothiophate, echothiopate, ecothiopate	T49.5X1	T49.5X2	T49.5X3	T49.5X4	T49.5X5	T49.5X6

TABLE OF DRUGS AND CHEMICALS

Substance	Poisoning, Accidental (Unintentional)	Poisoning, Intentional Self-Harm	Poisoning, Assault	Poisoning, Undetermined	Adverse Effect	Underdosing
Ecstasy	T43.641	T43.642	T43.643	T43.644	—	—
Ectylurea	T42.6X1	T42.6X2	T42.6X3	T42.6X4	T42.6X5	T42.6X6
Edathamil disodium	T45.8X1	T45.8X2	T45.8X3	T45.8X4	T45.8X5	T45.8X6
Edecrin	T50.1X1	T50.1X2	T50.1X3	T50.1X4	T50.1X5	T50.1X6
Edetate, disodium (calcium)	T45.8X1	T45.8X2	T45.8X3	T45.8X4	T45.8X5	T45.8X6
Edoxudine	T49.5X1	T49.5X2	T49.5X3	T49.5X4	T49.5X5	T49.5X6
Edrophonium	T44.0X1	T44.0X2	T44.0X3	T44.0X4	T44.0X5	T44.0X6
chloride	T44.0X1	T44.0X2	T44.0X3	T44.0X4	T44.0X5	T44.0X6
EDTA	T50.6X1	T50.6X2	T50.6X3	T50.6X4	T50.6X5	T50.6X6
Eflornithine	T37.2X1	T37.2X2	T37.2X3	T37.2X4	T37.2X5	T37.2X6
Efloxate	T46.3X1	T46.3X2	T46.3X3	T46.3X4	T46.3X5	T46.3X6
Elase	T49.8X1	T49.8X2	T49.8X3	T49.8X4	T49.8X5	T49.8X6
Elastase	T47.5X1	T47.5X2	T47.5X3	T47.5X4	T47.5X5	T47.5X6
Elaterium	T47.2X1	T47.2X2	T47.2X3	T47.2X4	T47.2X5	T47.2X6
Elcatonin	T50.991	T50.992	T50.993	T50.994	T50.995	T50.996
Elder	T62.2X1	T62.2X2	T62.2X3	T62.2X4	—	—
berry (unripe)	T62.1X1	T62.1X2	T62.1X3	T62.1X4	—	—
Electrolyte balance drug	T50.3X1	T50.3X2	T50.3X3	T50.3X4	T50.3X5	T50.3X6
Electrolytes NEC	T50.3X1	T50.3X2	T50.3X3	T50.3X4	T50.3X5	T50.3X6
Electrolytic agent NEC	T50.3X1	T50.3X2	T50.3X3	T50.3X4	T50.3X5	T50.3X6
Elemental diet	T50.901	T50.902	T50.903	T50.904	T50.905	T50.906
Elliptinium acetate	T45.1X1	T45.1X2	T45.1X3	T45.1X4	T45.1X5	T45.1X6
Embramine	T45.0X1	T45.0X2	T45.0X3	T45.0X4	T45.0X5	T45.0X6
Emepronium (salts)	T44.3X1	T44.3X2	T44.3X3	T44.3X4	T44.3X5	T44.3X6
bromide	T44.3X1	T44.3X2	T44.3X3	T44.3X4	T44.3X5	T44.3X6
Emetic NEC	T47.7X1	T47.7X2	T47.7X3	T47.7X4	T47.7X5	T47.7X6
Emetine	T37.3X1	T37.3X2	T37.3X3	T37.3X4	T37.3X5	T37.3X6
Emollient NEC	T49.3X1	T49.3X2	T49.3X3	T49.3X4	T49.3X5	T49.3X6
Emorfazone	T39.8X1	T39.8X2	T39.8X3	T39.8X4	T39.8X5	T39.8X6
Emylcamate	T43.591	T43.592	T43.593	T43.594	T43.595	T43.596
Enalapril	T46.4X1	T46.4X2	T46.4X3	T46.4X4	T46.4X5	T46.4X6
Enalaprilat	T46.4X1	T46.4X2	T46.4X3	T46.4X4	T46.4X5	T46.4X6
Encainide	T46.2X1	T46.2X2	T46.2X3	T46.2X4	T46.2X5	T46.2X6
Endocaine	T41.3X1	T41.3X2	T41.3X3	T41.3X4	T41.3X5	T41.3X6
Endosulfan	T60.2X1	T60.2X2	T60.2X3	T60.2X4	—	—
Endothall	T60.3X1	T60.3X2	T60.3X3	T60.3X4	—	—
Endralazine	T46.5X1	T46.5X2	T46.5X3	T46.5X4	T46.5X5	T46.5X6
Endrin	T60.1X1	T60.1X2	T60.1X3	T60.1X4	—	—
Enflurane	T41.0X1	T41.0X2	T41.0X3	T41.0X4	T41.0X5	T41.0X6
Enhexymal	T42.3X1	T42.3X2	T42.3X3	T42.3X4	T42.3X5	T42.3X6
Enocitabine	T45.1X1	T45.1X2	T45.1X3	T45.1X4	T45.1X5	T45.1X6
Enovid	T38.4X1	T38.4X2	T38.4X3	T38.4X4	T38.4X5	T38.4X6

Substance	Poisoning, Accidental (Unintentional)	Poisoning, Intentional Self-Harm	Poisoning, Assault	Poisoning, Undetermined	Adverse Effect	Underdosing
Enoxacin	T36.8X1	T36.8X2	T36.8X3	T36.8X4	T36.8X5	T36.8X6
Enoxaparin (sodium)	T45.511	T45.512	T45.513	T45.514	T45.515	T45.516
Enpiprazole	T43.591	T43.592	T43.593	T43.594	T43.595	T43.596
Enprofylline	T48.6X1	T48.6X2	T48.6X3	T48.6X4	T48.6X5	T48.6X6
Enprostil	T47.1X1	T47.1X2	T47.1X3	T47.1X4	T47.1X5	T47.1X6
ENT preparations (anti-infectives)	T49.6X1	T49.6X2	T49.6X3	T49.6X4	T49.6X5	T49.6X6
Enviomycin	T36.8X1	T36.8X2	T36.8X3	T36.8X4	T36.8X5	T36.8X6
Enzodase	T45.3X1	T45.3X2	T45.3X3	T45.3X4	T45.3X5	T45.3X6
Enzyme NEC	T45.3X1	T45.3X2	T45.3X3	T45.3X4	T45.3X5	T45.3X6
depolymerizing	T49.8X1	T49.8X2	T49.8X3	T49.8X4	T49.8X5	T49.8X6
fibrolytic	T45.3X1	T45.3X2	T45.3X3	T45.3X4	T45.3X5	T45.3X6
gastric	T47.5X1	T47.5X2	T47.5X3	T47.5X4	T47.5X5	T47.5X6
intestinal	T47.5X1	T47.5X2	T47.5X3	T47.5X4	T47.5X5	T47.5X6
local action	T49.4X1	T49.4X2	T49.4X3	T49.4X4	T49.4X5	T49.4X6
proteolytic	T49.4X1	T49.4X2	T49.4X3	T49.4X4	T49.4X5	T49.4X6
thrombolytic	T45.3X1	T45.3X2	T45.3X3	T45.3X4	T45.3X5	T45.3X6
EPAB	T41.3X1	T41.3X2	T41.3X3	T41.3X4	T41.3X5	T41.3X6
Epanutin	T42.0X1	T42.0X2	T42.0X3	T42.0X4	T42.0X5	T42.0X6
Ephedra	T44.991	T44.992	T44.993	T44.994	T44.995	T44.996
Ephedrine	T44.991	T44.992	T44.993	T44.994	T44.995	T44.996
Epichlorhydrin, epichlorohydrin	T52.8X1	T52.8X2	T52.8X3	T52.8X4	—	—
Epicillin	T36.0X1	T36.0X2	T36.0X3	T36.0X4	T36.0X5	T36.0X6
Epiestriol	T38.5X1	T38.5X2	T38.5X3	T38.5X4	T38.5X5	T38.5X6
Epilim — see Sodium, valproate						
Epimestrol	T38.5X1	T38.5X2	T38.5X3	T38.5X4	T38.5X5	T38.5X6
Epinephrine	T44.5X1	T44.5X2	T44.5X3	T44.5X4	T44.5X5	T44.5X6
Epirubicin	T45.1X1	T45.1X2	T45.1X3	T45.1X4	T45.1X5	T45.1X6
Epitiostanol	T38.7X1	T38.7X2	T38.7X3	T38.7X4	T38.7X5	T38.7X6
Epitizide	T50.2X1	T50.2X2	T50.2X3	T50.2X4	T50.2X5	T50.2X6
EPN	T60.0X1	T60.0X2	T60.0X3	T60.0X4	—	—
EPO	T45.8X1	T45.8X2	T45.8X3	T45.8X4	T45.8X5	T45.8X6
Epoetin alpha	T45.8X1	T45.8X2	T45.8X3	T45.8X4	T45.8X5	T45.8X6
Epomediol	T50.991	T50.992	T50.993	T50.994	T50.995	T50.996
Epoprostenol	T45.521	T45.522	T45.523	T45.524	T45.525	T45.526
Epoxy resin	T65.891	T65.892	T65.893	T65.894	—	—
Eprazinone	T48.4X1	T48.4X2	T48.4X3	T48.4X4	T48.4X5	T48.4X6
Epsilon amino-caproic acid	T45.621	T45.622	T45.623	T45.624	T45.625	T45.626
Epsom salt	T47.3X1	T47.3X2	T47.3X3	T47.3X4	T47.3X5	T47.3X6
Eptazocine	T40.491	T40.492	T40.493	T40.494	T40.495	T40.496
Equanil	T43.591	T43.592	T43.593	T43.594	T43.595	T43.596
Equisetum	T62.2X1	T62.2X2	T62.2X3	T62.2X4	—	—
diuretic	T50.2X1	T50.2X2	T50.2X3	T50.2X4	T50.2X5	T50.2X6

◀ New   ◀ Revised   ~~deleted~~ Deleted

Substance	Poisoning, Accidental (Unintentional)	Poisoning, Intentional Self-Harm	Poisoning, Assault	Poisoning, Undetermined	Adverse Effect	Underdosing
Ergobasine	T48.ØX1	T48.ØX2	T48.ØX3	T48.ØX4	T48.ØX5	T48.ØX6
Ergocalciferol	T45.2X1	T45.2X2	T45.2X3	T45.2X4	T45.2X5	T45.2X6
Ergoloid mesylates	T46.7X1	T46.7X2	T46.7X3	T46.7X4	T46.7X5	T46.7X6
Ergometrine	T48.ØX1	T48.ØX2	T48.ØX3	T48.ØX4	T48.ØX5	T48.ØX6
Ergonovine	T48.ØX1	T48.ØX2	T48.ØX3	T48.ØX4	T48.ØX5	T48.ØX6
Ergot NEC	T64.81	T64.82	T64.83	T64.84	—	—
derivative	T48.ØX1	T48.ØX2	T48.ØX3	T48.ØX4	T48.ØX5	T48.ØX6
medicinal (alkaloids)	T48.ØX1	T48.ØX2	T48.ØX3	T48.ØX4	T48.ØX5	T48.ØX6
prepared	T48.ØX1	T48.ØX2	T48.ØX3	T48.ØX4	T48.ØX5	T48.ØX6
Ergotamine	T46.5X1	T46.5X2	T46.5X3	T46.5X4	T46.5X5	T46.5X6
Ergotocine	T48.ØX1	T48.ØX2	T48.ØX3	T48.ØX4	T48.ØX5	T48.ØX6
Ergotrate	T48.ØX1	T48.ØX2	T48.ØX3	T48.ØX4	T48.ØX5	T48.ØX6
Eritrityl tetranitrate	T46.3X1	T46.3X2	T46.3X3	T46.3X4	T46.3X5	T46.3X6
Erythrityl tetranitrate	T46.3X1	T46.3X2	T46.3X3	T46.3X4	T46.3X5	T46.3X6
Erythrol tetranitrate	T46.3X1	T46.3X2	T46.3X3	T46.3X4	T46.3X5	T46.3X6
Erythromycin (salts)	T36.3X1	T36.3X2	T36.3X3	T36.3X4	T36.3X5	T36.3X6
ophthalmic preparation	T49.5X1	T49.5X2	T49.5X3	T49.5X4	T49.5X5	T49.5X6
topical NEC	T49.ØX1	T49.ØX2	T49.ØX3	T49.ØX4	T49.ØX5	T49.ØX6
Erythropoietin	T45.8X1	T45.8X2	T45.8X3	T45.8X4	T45.8X5	T45.8X6
human	T45.8X1	T45.8X2	T45.8X3	T45.8X4	T45.8X5	T45.8X6
Escin	T46.991	T46.992	T46.993	T46.994	T46.995	T46.996
Esculin	T45.2X1	T45.2X2	T45.2X3	T45.2X4	T45.2X5	T45.2X6
Esculoside	T45.2X1	T45.2X2	T45.2X3	T45.2X4	T45.2X5	T45.2X6
ESDT (ether-soluble tar distillate)	T49.1X1	T49.1X2	T49.1X3	T49.1X4	T49.1X5	T49.1X6
Eserine	T49.5X1	T49.5X2	T49.5X3	T49.5X4	T49.5X5	T49.5X6
Esflurbiprofen	T39.311	T39.312	T39.313	T39.314	T39.315	T39.316
Eskabarb	T42.3X1	T42.3X2	T42.3X3	T42.3X4	T42.3X5	T42.3X6
Eskalith	T43.8X1	T43.8X2	T43.8X3	T43.8X4	T43.8X5	T43.8X6
Esmolol	T44.7X1	T44.7X2	T44.7X3	T44.7X4	T44.7X5	T44.7X6
Estanozolol	T38.7X1	T38.7X2	T38.7X3	T38.7X4	T38.7X5	T38.7X6
Estazolam	T42.4X1	T42.4X2	T42.4X3	T42.4X4	T42.4X5	T42.4X6
Estradiol	T38.5X1	T38.5X2	T38.5X3	T38.5X4	T38.5X5	T38.5X6
with testosterone	T38.7X1	T38.7X2	T38.7X3	T38.7X4	T38.7X5	T38.7X6
benzoate	T38.5X1	T38.5X2	T38.5X3	T38.5X4	T38.5X5	T38.5X6
Estramustine	T45.1X1	T45.1X2	T45.1X3	T45.1X4	T45.1X5	T45.1X6
Estriol	T38.5X1	T38.5X2	T38.5X3	T38.5X4	T38.5X5	T38.5X6
Estrogen	T38.5X1	T38.5X2	T38.5X3	T38.5X4	T38.5X5	T38.5X6
with progesterone	T38.5X1	T38.5X2	T38.5X3	T38.5X4	T38.5X5	T38.5X6
conjugated	T38.5X1	T38.5X2	T38.5X3	T38.5X4	T38.5X5	T38.5X6
Estrone	T38.5X1	T38.5X2	T38.5X3	T38.5X4	T38.5X5	T38.5X6
Estropipate	T38.5X1	T38.5X2	T38.5X3	T38.5X4	T38.5X5	T38.5X6

Substance	Poisoning, Accidental (Unintentional)	Poisoning, Intentional Self-Harm	Poisoning, Assault	Poisoning, Undetermined	Adverse Effect	Underdosing
Etacrynate sodium	T50.1X1	T50.1X2	T50.1X3	T50.1X4	T50.1X5	T50.1X6
Etacrynic acid	T50.1X1	T50.1X2	T50.1X3	T50.1X4	T50.1X5	T50.1X6
Etafedrine	T48.6X1	T48.6X2	T48.6X3	T48.6X4	T48.6X5	T48.6X6
Etafenone	T46.3X1	T46.3X2	T46.3X3	T46.3X4	T46.3X5	T46.3X6
Etambutol	T37.1X1	T37.1X2	T37.1X3	T37.1X4	T37.1X5	T37.1X6
Etamiphyllin	T48.6X1	T48.6X2	T48.6X3	T48.6X4	T48.6X5	T48.6X6
Etamivan	T50.7X1	T50.7X2	T50.7X3	T50.7X4	T50.7X5	T50.7X6
Etamsylate	T45.7X1	T45.7X2	T45.7X3	T45.7X4	T45.7X5	T45.7X6
Etebenecid	T50.4X1	T50.4X2	T50.4X3	T50.4X4	T50.4X5	T50.4X6
Ethacridine	T49.ØX1	T49.ØX2	T49.ØX3	T49.ØX4	T49.ØX5	T49.ØX6
Ethacrynic acid	T50.1X1	T50.1X2	T50.1X3	T50.1X4	T50.1X5	T50.1X6
Ethadione	T42.2X1	T42.2X2	T42.2X3	T42.2X4	T42.2X5	T42.2X6
Ethambutol	T37.1X1	T37.1X2	T37.1X3	T37.1X4	T37.1X5	T37.1X6
Ethamide	T50.2X1	T50.2X2	T50.2X3	T50.2X4	T50.2X5	T50.2X6
Ethamivan	T50.7X1	T50.7X2	T50.7X3	T50.7X4	T50.7X5	T50.7X6
Ethamsylate	T45.7X1	T45.7X2	T45.7X3	T45.7X4	T45.7X5	T45.7X6
Ethanol	T51.ØX1	T51.ØX2	T51.ØX3	T51.ØX4	—	—
beverage	T51.ØX1	T51.ØX2	T51.ØX3	T51.ØX4	—	—
Ethanolamine oleate	T46.8X1	T46.8X2	T46.8X3	T46.8X4	T46.8X5	T46.8X6
Ethaverine	T44.3X1	T44.3X2	T44.3X3	T44.3X4	T44.3X5	T44.3X6
Ethchlorvynol	T42.6X1	T42.6X2	T42.6X3	T42.6X4	T42.6X5	T42.6X6
Ethebenecid	T50.4X1	T50.4X2	T50.4X3	T50.4X4	T50.4X5	T50.4X6
Ether (vapor)	T41.ØX1	T41.ØX2	T41.ØX3	T41.ØX4	T41.ØX5	T41.ØX6
anesthetic	T41.ØX1	T41.ØX2	T41.ØX3	T41.ØX4	T41.ØX5	T41.ØX6
divinyl	T41.ØX1	T41.ØX2	T41.ØX3	T41.ØX4	T41.ØX5	T41.ØX6
ethyl (medicinal)	T41.ØX1	T41.ØX2	T41.ØX3	T41.ØX4	T41.ØX5	T41.ØX6
nonmedicinal	T52.8X1	T52.8X2	T52.8X3	T52.8X4	—	—
petroleum — *see Ligroin*						
solvent	T52.8X1	T52.8X2	T52.8X3	T52.8X4		
Ethiazide	T50.2X1	T50.2X2	T50.2X3	T50.2X4	T50.2X5	T50.2X6
Ethidium chloride (vapor)	T59.891	T59.892	T59.893	T59.894	—	—
Ethinamate	T42.6X1	T42.6X2	T42.6X3	T42.6X4	T42.6X5	T42.6X6
Ethinylestradiol, ethinyloestradiol	T38.5X1	T38.5X2	T38.5X3	T38.5X4	T38.5X5	T38.5X6
with						
levonorgestrel	T38.4X1	T38.4X2	T38.4X3	T38.4X4	T38.4X5	T38.4X6
norethisterone	T38.4X1	T38.4X2	T38.4X3	T38.4X4	T38.4X5	T38.4X6
Ethiodized oil (131 I)	T50.8X1	T50.8X2	T50.8X3	T50.8X4	T50.8X5	T50.8X6
Ethion	T60.ØX1	T60.ØX2	T60.ØX3	T60.ØX4	—	—
Ethionamide	T37.1X1	T37.1X2	T37.1X3	T37.1X4	T37.1X5	T37.1X6
Ethioniamide	T37.1X1	T37.1X2	T37.1X3	T37.1X4	T37.1X5	T37.1X6
Ethisterone	T38.5X1	T38.5X2	T38.5X3	T38.5X4	T38.5X5	T38.5X6
Ethobral	T42.3X1	T42.3X2	T42.3X3	T42.3X4	T42.3X5	T42.3X6

TABLE OF DRUGS AND CHEMICALS

Substance	External Cause (T-Code)					
	Poisoning, Accidental (Unintentional)	Poisoning, Intentional Self-Harm	Poisoning, Assault	Poisoning, Undetermined	Adverse Effect	Underdosing
Ethocaine (infiltration) (topical)	T41.3X1	T41.3X2	T41.3X3	T41.3X4	T41.3X5	T41.3X6
nerve block (peripheral) (plexus)	T41.3X1	T41.3X2	T41.3X3	T41.3X4	T41.3X5	T41.3X6
spinal	T41.3X1	T41.3X2	T41.3X3	T41.3X4	T41.3X5	T41.3X6
Ethoheptazine	T40.491	T40.492	T40.493	T40.494	T40.495	T40.496
Ethopropazine	T44.3X1	T44.3X2	T44.3X3	T44.3X4	T44.3X5	T44.3X6
Ethosuximide	T42.2X1	T42.2X2	T42.2X3	T42.2X4	T42.2X5	T42.2X6
Ethotoin	T42.0X1	T42.0X2	T42.0X3	T42.0X4	T42.0X5	T42.0X6
Ethoxazene	T37.91	T37.92	T37.93	T37.94	T37.95	T37.96
Ethoxazorutoside	T46.991	T46.992	T46.993	T46.994	T46.995	T46.996
2-Ethoxyethanol	T52.3X1	T52.3X2	T52.3X3	T52.3X4	—	—
Ethoxzolamide	T50.2X1	T50.2X2	T50.2X3	T50.2X4	T50.2X5	T50.2X6
Ethyl						
acetate	T52.8X1	T52.8X2	T52.8X3	T52.8X4	—	—
alcohol	T51.0X1	T51.0X2	T51.0X3	T51.0X4	—	—
beverage	T51.0X1	T51.0X2	T51.0X3	T51.0X4	—	—
aldehyde (vapor)	T59.891	T59.892	T59.893	T59.894	—	—
liquid	T52.8X1	T52.8X2	T52.8X3	T52.8X4	—	—
aminobenzoate	T41.3X1	T41.3X2	T41.3X3	T41.3X4	T41.3X5	T41.3X6
aminophenothiazine	T43.3X1	T43.3X2	T43.3X3	T43.3X4	T43.3X5	T43.3X6
benzoate	T52.8X1	T52.8X2	T52.8X3	T52.8X4	—	—
biscoumacetate	T45.511	T45.512	T45.513	T45.514	T45.515	T45.516
bromide (anesthetic)	T41.0X1	T41.0X2	T41.0X3	T41.0X4	T41.0X5	T41.0X6
carbamate	T45.1X1	T45.1X2	T45.1X3	T45.1X4	T45.1X5	T45.1X6
carbinol	T51.3X1	T51.3X2	T51.3X3	T51.3X4	—	—
carbonate	T52.8X1	T52.8X2	T52.8X3	T52.8X4	—	—
chaulmoograte	T37.1X1	T37.1X2	T37.1X3	T37.1X4	T37.1X5	T37.1X6
chloride (anesthetic)	T41.0X1	T41.0X2	T41.0X3	T41.0X4	T41.0X5	T41.0X6
anesthetic (local)	T41.3X1	T41.3X2	T41.3X3	T41.3X4	T41.3X5	T41.3X6
inhaled	T41.0X1	T41.0X2	T41.0X3	T41.0X4	T41.0X5	T41.0X6
local	T49.4X1	T49.4X2	T49.4X3	T49.4X4	T49.4X5	T49.4X6
solvent	T53.6X1	T53.6X2	T53.6X3	T53.6X4	—	—
dibunate	T48.3X1	T48.3X2	T48.3X3	T48.3X4	T48.3X5	T48.3X6
dichloroarsine (vapor)	T57.0X1	T57.0X2	T57.0X3	T57.0X4	—	—
estranol	T38.7X1	T38.7X2	T38.7X3	T38.7X4	T38.7X5	T38.7X6
ether — *see also Ether*	T52.8X1	T52.8X2	T52.8X3	T52.8X4	—	—
formate NEC (solvent)	T52.0X1	T52.0X2	T52.0X3	T52.0X4	—	—
fumarate	T49.4X1	T49.4X2	T49.4X3	T49.4X4	T49.4X5	T49.4X6
hydroxyisobutyrate NEC (solvent)	T52.8X1	T52.8X2	T52.8X3	T52.8X4	—	—
iodoacetate	T59.3X1	T59.3X2	T59.3X3	T59.3X4	—	—
lactate NEC (solvent)	T52.8X1	T52.8X2	T52.8X3	T52.8X4	—	—
loflazepate	T42.4X1	T42.4X2	T42.4X3	T42.4X4	T42.4X5	T42.4X6

Substance	External Cause (T-Code)					
	Poisoning, Accidental (Unintentional)	Poisoning, Intentional Self-Harm	Poisoning, Assault	Poisoning, Undetermined	Adverse Effect	Underdosing
Ethyl *(Continued)*						
mercuric chloride	T56.1X1	T56.1X2	T56.1X3	T56.1X4	—	—
methylcarbinol	T51.8X1	T51.8X2	T51.8X3	T51.8X4	—	—
morphine	T40.2X1	T40.2X2	T40.2X3	T40.2X4	T40.2X5	T40.2X6
noradrenaline	T48.6X1	T48.6X2	T48.6X3	T48.6X4	T48.6X5	T48.6X6
oxybutyrate NEC (solvent)	T52.8X1	T52.8X2	T52.8X3	T52.8X4	—	—
Ethylene (gas)	T59.891	T59.892	T59.893	T59.894	—	—
anesthetic (general)	T41.0X1	T41.0X2	T41.0X3	T41.0X4	T41.0X5	T41.0X6
chlorohydrin	T52.8X1	T52.8X2	T52.8X3	T52.8X4	—	—
vapor	T53.6X1	T53.6X2	T53.6X3	T53.6X4	—	—
dichloride	T52.8X1	T52.8X2	T52.8X3	T52.8X4	—	—
vapor	T53.6X1	T53.6X2	T53.6X3	T53.6X4	—	—
dinitrate	T52.3X1	T52.3X2	T52.3X3	T52.3X4	—	—
glycol(s)	T52.8X1	T52.8X2	T52.8X3	T52.8X4	—	—
dinitrate	T52.3X1	T52.3X2	T52.3X3	T52.3X4	—	—
monobutyl ether	T52.3X1	T52.3X2	T52.3X3	T52.3X4	—	—
imine	T54.1X1	T54.1X2	T54.1X3	T54.1X4	—	—
oxide (fumigant) (nonmedicinal)	T59.891	T59.892	T59.893	T59.894	—	—
medicinal	T49.0X1	T49.0X2	T49.0X3	T49.0X4	T49.0X5	T49.0X6
Ethylenediamine theophylline	T48.6X1	T48.6X2	T48.6X3	T48.6X4	T48.6X5	T48.6X6
Ethylenediaminetetra-acetic acid	T50.6X1	T50.6X2	T50.6X3	T50.6X4	T50.6X5	T50.6X6
Ethylenedinitrilotetra-acetate	T50.6X1	T50.6X2	T50.6X3	T50.6X4	T50.6X5	T50.6X6
Ethylestrenol	T38.7X1	T38.7X2	T38.7X3	T38.7X4	T38.7X5	T38.7X6
Ethylhydroxycellulose	T47.4X1	T47.4X2	T47.4X3	T47.4X4	T47.4X5	T47.4X6
Ethylidene						
chloride NEC	T53.6X1	T53.6X2	T53.6X3	T53.6X4	—	—
diacetate	T60.3X1	T60.3X2	T60.3X3	T60.3X4	—	—
dicoumarin	T45.511	T45.512	T45.513	T45.514	T45.515	T45.516
dicoumarol	T45.511	T45.512	T45.513	T45.514	T45.515	T45.516
diethyl ether	T52.0X1	T52.0X2	T52.0X3	T52.0X4	—	—
Ethylmorphine	T40.2X1	T40.2X2	T40.2X3	T40.2X4	T40.2X5	T40.2X6
Ethylnorepinephrine	T48.6X1	T48.6X2	T48.6X3	T48.6X4	T48.6X5	T48.6X6
Ethylparachlorophen-oxyisobutyrate	T46.6X1	T46.6X2	T46.6X3	T46.6X4	T46.6X5	T46.6X6
Ethynodiol	T38.4X1	T38.4X2	T38.4X3	T38.4X4	T38.4X5	T38.4X6
with mestranol diacetate	T38.4X1	T38.4X2	T38.4X3	T38.4X4	T38.4X5	T38.4X6
Etidocaine	T41.3X1	T41.3X2	T41.3X3	T41.3X4	T41.3X5	T41.3X6
infiltration (subcutaneous)	T41.3X1	T41.3X2	T41.3X3	T41.3X4	T41.3X5	T41.3X6
nerve (peripheral) (plexus)	T41.3X1	T41.3X2	T41.3X3	T41.3X4	T41.3X5	T41.3X6
Etidronate	T50.991	T50.992	T50.993	T50.994	T50.995	T50.996
Etidronic acid (disodium salt)	T50.991	T50.992	T50.993	T50.994	T50.995	T50.996
Etifoxine	T42.6X1	T42.6X2	T42.6X3	T42.6X4	T42.6X5	T42.6X6

◄ New   ◄ Revised   ~~deleted~~ Deleted

Substance	Poisoning, Accidental (Unintentional)	Poisoning, Intentional Self-Harm	Poisoning, Assault	Poisoning, Undetermined	Adverse Effect	Underdosing
Etilefrine	T44.4X1	T44.4X2	T44.4X3	T44.4X4	T44.4X5	T44.4X6
Etilfen	T42.3X1	T42.3X2	T42.3X3	T42.3X4	T42.3X5	T42.3X6
Etinodiol	T38.4X1	T38.4X2	T38.4X3	T38.4X4	T38.4X5	T38.4X6
Etiroxate	T46.6X1	T46.6X2	T46.6X3	T46.6X4	T46.6X5	T46.6X6
Etizolam	T42.4X1	T42.4X2	T42.4X3	T42.4X4	T42.4X5	T42.4X6
Etodolac	T39.391	T39.392	T39.393	T39.394	T39.395	T39.396
Etofamide	T37.3X1	T37.3X2	T37.3X3	T37.3X4	T37.3X5	T37.3X6
Etofibrate	T46.6X1	T46.6X2	T46.6X3	T46.6X4	T46.6X5	T46.6X6
Etofylline	T46.7X1	T46.7X2	T46.7X3	T46.7X4	T46.7X5	T46.7X6
clofibrate	T46.6X1	T46.6X2	T46.6X3	T46.6X4	T46.6X5	T46.6X6
Etoglucid	T45.1X1	T45.1X2	T45.1X3	T45.1X4	T45.1X5	T45.1X6
Etomidate	T41.1X1	T41.1X2	T41.1X3	T41.1X4	T41.1X5	T41.1X6
Etomide	T39.8X1	T39.8X2	T39.8X3	T39.8X4	T39.8X5	T39.8X6
Etomidoline	T44.3X1	T44.3X2	T44.3X3	T44.3X4	T44.3X5	T44.3X6
Etoposide	T45.1X1	T45.1X2	T45.1X3	T45.1X4	T45.1X5	T45.1X6
Etorphine	T40.2X1	T40.2X2	T40.2X3	T40.2X4	T40.2X5	T40.2X6
Etoval	T42.3X1	T42.3X2	T42.3X3	T42.3X4	T42.3X5	T42.3X6
Etozolin	T50.1X1	T50.1X2	T50.1X3	T50.1X4	T50.1X5	T50.1X6
Etretinate	T50.991	T50.992	T50.993	T50.994	T50.995	T50.996
Etryptamine	T43.691	T43.692	T43.693	T43.694	T43.695	T43.696
Etybenzatropine	T44.3X1	T44.3X2	T44.3X3	T44.3X4	T44.3X5	T44.3X6
Etynodiol	T38.4X1	T38.4X2	T38.4X3	T38.4X4	T38.4X5	T38.4X6
Eucaine	T41.3X1	T41.3X2	T41.3X3	T41.3X4	T41.3X5	T41.3X6
Eucalyptus oil	T49.7X1	T49.7X2	T49.7X3	T49.7X4	T49.7X5	T49.7X6
Eucatropine	T49.5X1	T49.5X2	T49.5X3	T49.5X4	T49.5X5	T49.5X6
Eucodal	T40.2X1	T40.2X2	T40.2X3	T40.2X4	T40.2X5	T40.2X6
Euneryl	T42.3X1	T42.3X2	T42.3X3	T42.3X4	T42.3X5	T42.3X6
Euphthalmine	T44.3X1	T44.3X2	T44.3X3	T44.3X4	T44.3X5	T44.3X6
Eurax	T49.0X1	T49.0X2	T49.0X3	T49.0X4	T49.0X5	T49.0X6
Euresol	T49.4X1	T49.4X2	T49.4X3	T49.4X4	T49.4X5	T49.4X6
Euthroid	T38.1X1	T38.1X2	T38.1X3	T38.1X4	T38.1X5	T38.1X6
Evans blue	T50.8X1	T50.8X2	T50.8X3	T50.8X4	T50.8X5	T50.8X6
Evipal	T42.3X1	T42.3X2	T42.3X3	T42.3X4	T42.3X5	T42.3X6
sodium	T41.1X1	T41.1X2	T41.1X3	T41.1X4	T41.1X5	T41.1X6
Evipan	T42.3X1	T42.3X2	T42.3X3	T42.3X4	T42.3X5	T42.3X6
sodium	T41.1X1	T41.1X2	T41.1X3	T41.1X4	T41.1X5	T41.1X6
Exalamide	T49.0X1	T49.0X2	T49.0X3	T49.0X4	T49.0X5	T49.0X6
Exalgin	T39.1X1	T39.1X2	T39.1X3	T39.1X4	T39.1X5	T39.1X6
Excipients, pharmaceutical	T50.901	T50.902	T50.903	T50.904	T50.905	T50.906
Exhaust gas (engine) (motor vehicle)	T58.01	T58.02	T58.03	T58.04	—	—
Ex-Lax (phenolphthalein)	T47.2X1	T47.2X2	T47.2X3	T47.2X4	T47.2X5	T47.2X6
Expectorant NEC	T48.4X1	T48.4X2	T48.4X3	T48.4X4	T48.4X5	T48.4X6

Substance	Poisoning, Accidental (Unintentional)	Poisoning, Intentional Self-Harm	Poisoning, Assault	Poisoning, Undetermined	Adverse Effect	Underdosing
Extended insulin zinc suspension	T38.3X1	T38.3X2	T38.3X3	T38.3X4	T38.3X5	T38.3X6
External medications (skin) (mucous membrane)	T49.91	T49.92	T49.93	T49.94	T49.95	T49.96
dental agent	T49.7X1	T49.7X2	T49.7X3	T49.7X4	T49.7X5	T49.7X6
ENT agent	T49.6X1	T49.6X2	T49.6X3	T49.6X4	T49.6X5	T49.6X6
ophthalmic preparation	T49.5X1	T49.5X2	T49.5X3	T49.5X4	T49.5X5	T49.5X6
specified NEC	T49.8X1	T49.8X2	T49.8X3	T49.8X4	T49.8X5	T49.8X6
Extrapyramidal antagonist NEC	T44.3X1	T44.3X2	T44.3X3	T44.3X4	T44.3X5	T44.3X6
Eye agents (anti-infective)	T49.5X1	T49.5X2	T49.5X3	T49.5X4	T49.5X5	T49.5X6
Eye drug NEC	T49.5X1	T49.5X2	T49.5X3	T49.5X4	T49.5X5	T49.5X6

F

Substance	Poisoning, Accidental (Unintentional)	Poisoning, Intentional Self-Harm	Poisoning, Assault	Poisoning, Undetermined	Adverse Effect	Underdosing
FAC (fluorouracil + doxorubicin + cyclophosphamide)	T45.1X1	T45.1X2	T45.1X3	T45.1X4	T45.1X5	T45.1X6
Factor						
I (fibrinogen)	T45.8X1	T45.8X2	T45.8X3	T45.8X4	T45.8X5	T45.8X6
III (thromboplastin)	T45.8X1	T45.8X2	T45.8X3	T45.8X4	T45.8X5	T45.8X6
VIII (antihemophilic Factor) (Concentrate)	T45.8X1	T45.8X2	T45.8X3	T45.8X4	T45.8X5	T45.8X6
IX complex	T45.7X1	T45.7X2	T45.7X3	T45.7X4	T45.7X5	T45.7X6
human	T45.8X1	T45.8X2	T45.8X3	T45.8X4	T45.8X5	T45.8X6
Famotidine	T47.0X1	T47.0X2	T47.0X3	T47.0X4	T47.0X5	T47.0X6
Fat suspension, intravenous	T50.991	T50.992	T50.993	T50.994	T50.995	T50.996
Fazadinium bromide	T48.1X1	T48.1X2	T48.1X3	T48.1X4	T48.1X5	T48.1X6
Febarbamate	T42.3X1	T42.3X2	T42.3X3	T42.3X4	T42.3X5	T42.3X6
Fecal softener	T47.4X1	T47.4X2	T47.4X3	T47.4X4	T47.4X5	T47.4X6
Fedrilate	T48.3X1	T48.3X2	T48.3X3	T48.3X4	T48.3X5	T48.3X6
Felodipine	T46.1X1	T46.1X2	T46.1X3	T46.1X4	T46.1X5	T46.1X6
Felypressin	T38.891	T38.892	T38.893	T38.894	T38.895	T38.896
Femoxetine	T43.221	T43.222	T43.223	T43.224	T43.225	T43.226
Fenalcomine	T46.3X1	T46.3X2	T46.3X3	T46.3X4	T46.3X5	T46.3X6
Fenamisal	T37.1X1	T37.1X2	T37.1X3	T37.1X4	T37.1X5	T37.1X6
Fenazone	T39.2X1	T39.2X2	T39.2X3	T39.2X4	T39.2X5	T39.2X6
Fenbendazole	T37.4X1	T37.4X2	T37.4X3	T37.4X4	T37.4X5	T37.4X6
Fenbutrazate	T50.5X1	T50.5X2	T50.5X3	T50.5X4	T50.5X5	T50.5X6
Fencamfamine	T43.691	T43.692	T43.693	T43.694	T43.695	T43.696
Fendiline	T46.1X1	T46.1X2	T46.1X3	T46.1X4	T46.1X5	T46.1X6
Fenetylline	T43.691	T43.692	T43.693	T43.694	T43.695	T43.696
Fenflumizole	T39.391	T39.392	T39.393	T39.394	T39.395	T39.396
Fenfluramine	T50.5X1	T50.5X2	T50.5X3	T50.5X4	T50.5X5	T50.5X6
Fenobarbital	T42.3X1	T42.3X2	T42.3X3	T42.3X4	T42.3X5	T42.3X6
Fenofibrate	T46.6X1	T46.6X2	T46.6X3	T46.6X4	T46.6X5	T46.6X6
Fenoprofen	T39.311	T39.312	T39.313	T39.314	T39.315	T39.316
Fenoterol	T48.6X1	T48.6X2	T48.6X3	T48.6X4	T48.6X5	T48.6X6

Substance	Poisoning, Accidental (Unintentional)	Poisoning, Intentional Self-Harm	Poisoning, Assault	Poisoning, Undetermined	Adverse Effect	Underdosing
Fenoverine	T44.3X1	T44.3X2	T44.3X3	T44.3X4	T44.3X5	T44.3X6
Fenoxazoline	T48.5X1	T48.5X2	T48.5X3	T48.5X4	T48.5X5	T48.5X6
Fenproporex	T50.5X1	T50.5X2	T50.5X3	T50.5X4	T50.5X5	T50.5X6
Fenquizone	T50.2X1	T50.2X2	T50.2X3	T50.2X4	T50.2X5	T50.2X6
Fentanyl (analogs)	T40.411	T40.412	T40.413	T40.414	T40.415	T40.416
Fentazin	T43.3X1	T43.3X2	T43.3X3	T43.3X4	T43.3X5	T43.3X6
Fenthion	T60.0X1	T60.0X2	T60.0X3	T60.0X4	—	—
Fenticlor	T49.0X1	T49.0X2	T49.0X3	T49.0X4	T49.0X5	T49.0X6
Fenylbutazone	T39.2X1	T39.2X2	T39.2X3	T39.2X4	T39.2X5	T39.2X6
Feprazone	T39.2X1	T39.2X2	T39.2X3	T39.2X4	T39.2X5	T39.2X6
Fer de lance (bite) (venom)	T63.061	T63.062	T63.063	T63.064	—	—
Ferric — *see also Iron*						
chloride	T45.4X1	T45.4X2	T45.4X3	T45.4X4	T45.4X5	T45.4X6
citrate	T45.4X1	T45.4X2	T45.4X3	T45.4X4	T45.4X5	T45.4X6
hydroxide						
colloidal	T45.4X1	T45.4X2	T45.4X3	T45.4X4	T45.4X5	T45.4X6
polymaltose	T45.4X1	T45.4X2	T45.4X3	T45.4X4	T45.4X5	T45.4X6
pyrophosphate	T45.4X1	T45.4X2	T45.4X3	T45.4X4	T45.4X5	T45.4X6
Ferritin	T45.4X1	T45.4X2	T45.4X3	T45.4X4	T45.4X5	T45.4X6
Ferrocholinate	T45.4X1	T45.4X2	T45.4X3	T45.4X4	T45.4X5	T45.4X6
Ferrodextrane	T45.4X1	T45.4X2	T45.4X3	T45.4X4	T45.4X5	T45.4X6
Ferropolimaler	T45.4X1	T45.4X2	T45.4X3	T45.4X4	T45.4X5	T45.4X6
Ferrous — *see also Iron*						
phosphate	T45.4X1	T45.4X2	T45.4X3	T45.4X4	T45.4X5	T45.4X6
salt	T45.4X1	T45.4X2	T45.4X3	T45.4X4	T45.4X5	T45.4X6
with folic acid	T45.4X1	T45.4X2	T45.4X3	T45.4X4	T45.4X5	T45.4X6
Ferrous fumarate, gluconate, lactate, salt NEC, sulfate (medicinal)	T45.4X1	T45.4X2	T45.4X3	T45.4X4	T45.4X5	T45.4X6
Ferrovanadium (fumes)	T59.891	T59.892	T59.893	T59.894	—	—
Ferrum — *see Iron*						
Fertilizers NEC	T65.891	T65.892	T65.893	T65.894	—	—
with herbicide mixture	T60.3X1	T60.3X2	T60.3X3	T60.3X4	—	—
Fetoxilate	T47.6X1	T47.6X2	T47.6X3	T47.6X4	T47.6X5	T47.6X6
Fiber, dietary	T47.4X1	T47.4X2	T47.4X3	T47.4X4	T47.4X5	T47.4X6
Fibrinogen (human)	T45.8X1	T45.8X2	T45.8X3	T45.8X4	T45.8X5	T45.8X6
Fibrinolysin (human)	T45.691	T45.692	T45.693	T45.694	T45.695	T45.696
Fibrinolysis						
affecting drug	T45.601	T45.602	T45.603	T45.604	T45.605	T45.606
inhibitor NEC	T45.621	T45.622	T45.623	T45.624	T45.625	T45.626
Fibrinolytic drug	T45.611	T45.612	T45.613	T45.614	T45.615	T45.616
Filix mas	T37.4X1	T37.4X2	T37.4X3	T37.4X4	T37.4X5	T37.4X6
Filtering cream	T49.3X1	T49.3X2	T49.3X3	T49.3X4	T49.3X5	T49.3X6

Substance	Poisoning, Accidental (Unintentional)	Poisoning, Intentional Self-Harm	Poisoning, Assault	Poisoning, Undetermined	Adverse Effect	Underdosing
Fiorinal	T39.011	T39.012	T39.013	T39.014	T39.015	T39.016
Firedamp	T59.891	T59.892	T59.893	T59.894	—	—
Fish, noxious, nonbacterial	T61.91	T61.92	T61.93	T61.94	—	—
ciguatera	T61.01	T61.02	T61.03	T61.04	—	—
scombroid	T61.11	T61.12	T61.13	T61.14	—	—
shell	T61.781	T61.782	T61.783	T61.784	—	—
specified NEC	T61.771	T61.772	T61.773	T61.774	—	—
Flagyl	T37.3X1	T37.3X2	T37.3X3	T37.3X4	T37.3X5	T37.3X6
Flavine adenine dinucleotide	T45.2X1	T45.2X2	T45.2X3	T45.2X4	T45.2X5	T45.2X6
Flavodic acid	T46.991	T46.992	T46.993	T46.994	T46.995	T46.996
Flavoxate	T44.3X1	T44.3X2	T44.3X3	T44.3X4	T44.3X5	T44.3X6
Flaxedil	T48.1X1	T48.1X2	T48.1X3	T48.1X4	T48.1X5	T48.1X6
Flaxseed (medicinal)	T49.3X1	T49.3X2	T49.3X3	T49.3X4	T49.3X5	T49.3X6
Flecainide	T46.2X1	T46.2X2	T46.2X3	T46.2X4	T46.2X5	T46.2X6
Fleroxacin	T36.8X1	T36.8X2	T36.8X3	T36.8X4	T36.8X5	T36.8X6
Floctafenine	T39.8X1	T39.8X2	T39.8X3	T39.8X4	T39.8X5	T39.8X6
Flomax	T44.6X1	T44.6X2	T44.6X3	T44.6X4	T44.6X5	T44.6X6
Flomoxef	T36.1X1	T36.1X2	T36.1X3	T36.1X4	T36.1X5	T36.1X6
Flopropione	T44.3X1	T44.3X2	T44.3X3	T44.3X4	T44.3X5	T44.3X6
Florantyrone	T47.5X1	T47.5X2	T47.5X3	T47.5X4	T47.5X5	T47.5X6
Floraquin	T37.8X1	T37.8X2	T37.8X3	T37.8X4	T37.8X5	T37.8X6
Florinef	T38.0X1	T38.0X2	T38.0X3	T38.0X4	T38.0X5	T38.0X6
ENT agent	T49.6X1	T49.6X2	T49.6X3	T49.6X4	T49.6X5	T49.6X6
ophthalmic preparation	T49.5X1	T49.5X2	T49.5X3	T49.5X4	T49.5X5	T49.5X6
topical NEC	T49.0X1	T49.0X2	T49.0X3	T49.0X4	T49.0X5	T49.0X6
Flowers of sulfur	T49.4X1	T49.4X2	T49.4X3	T49.4X4	T49.4X5	T49.4X6
Floxuridine	T45.1X1	T45.1X2	T45.1X3	T45.1X4	T45.1X5	T45.1X6
Fluanisone	T43.4X1	T43.4X2	T43.4X3	T43.4X4	T43.4X5	T43.4X6
Flubendazole	T37.4X1	T37.4X2	T37.4X3	T37.4X4	T37.4X5	T37.4X6
Fluclorolone acetonide	T49.0X1	T49.0X2	T49.0X3	T49.0X4	T49.0X5	T49.0X6
Flucloxacillin	T36.0X1	T36.0X2	T36.0X3	T36.0X4	T36.0X5	T36.0X6
Fluconazole	T37.8X1	T37.8X2	T37.8X3	T37.8X4	T37.8X5	T37.8X6
Flucytosine	T37.8X1	T37.8X2	T37.8X3	T37.8X4	T37.8X5	T37.8X6
Fludeoxyglucose (18F)	T50.8X1	T50.8X2	T50.8X3	T50.8X4	T50.8X5	T50.8X6
Fludiazepam	T42.4X1	T42.4X2	T42.4X3	T42.4X4	T42.4X5	T42.4X6
Fludrocortisone	T50.0X1	T50.0X2	T50.0X3	T50.0X4	T50.0X5	T50.0X6
ENT agent	T49.6X1	T49.6X2	T49.6X3	T49.6X4	T49.6X5	T49.6X6
ophthalmic preparation	T49.5X1	T49.5X2	T49.5X3	T49.5X4	T49.5X5	T49.5X6
topical NEC	T49.0X1	T49.0X2	T49.0X3	T49.0X4	T49.0X5	T49.0X6
Fludroxycortide	T49.0X1	T49.0X2	T49.0X3	T49.0X4	T49.0X5	T49.0X6
Flufenamic acid	T39.391	T39.392	T39.393	T39.394	T39.395	T39.396
Fluindione	T45.511	T45.512	T45.513	T45.514	T45.515	T45.516

◀ New   ◀ Revised   ~~deleted~~ Deleted

Substance	External Cause (T-Code)					
	Poisoning, Accidental (Unintentional)	Poisoning, Intentional Self-Harm	Poisoning, Assault	Poisoning, Undetermined	Adverse Effect	Underdosing
Flumequine	T37.8X1	T37.8X2	T37.8X3	T37.8X4	T37.8X5	T37.8X6
Flumethasone	T49.0X1	T49.0X2	T49.0X3	T49.0X4	T49.0X5	T49.0X6
Flumethiazide	T50.2X1	T50.2X2	T50.2X3	T50.2X4	T50.2X5	T50.2X6
Flumidin	T37.5X1	T37.5X2	T37.5X3	T37.5X4	T37.5X5	T37.5X6
Flunarizine	T46.7X1	T46.7X2	T46.7X3	T46.7X4	T46.7X5	T46.7X6
Flunidazole	T37.8X1	T37.8X2	T37.8X3	T37.8X4	T37.8X5	T37.8X6
Flunisolide	T48.6X1	T48.6X2	T48.6X3	T48.6X4	T48.6X5	T48.6X6
Flunitrazepam	T42.4X1	T42.4X2	T42.4X3	T42.4X4	T42.4X5	T42.4X6
Fluocinolone (acetonide)	T49.0X1	T49.0X2	T49.0X3	T49.0X4	T49.0X5	T49.0X6
Fluocinonide	T49.0X1	T49.0X2	T49.0X3	T49.0X4	T49.0X5	T49.0X6
Fluocortin (butyl)	T49.0X1	T49.0X2	T49.0X3	T49.0X4	T49.0X5	T49.0X6
Fluocortolone	T49.0X1	T49.0X2	T49.0X3	T49.0X4	T49.0X5	T49.0X6
Fluohydrocortisone	T38.0X1	T38.0X2	T38.0X3	T38.0X4	T38.0X5	T38.0X6
ENT agent	T49.6X1	T49.6X2	T49.6X3	T49.6X4	T49.6X5	T49.6X6
ophthalmic preparation	T49.5X1	T49.5X2	T49.5X3	T49.5X4	T49.5X5	T49.5X6
topical NEC	T49.0X1	T49.0X2	T49.0X3	T49.0X4	T49.0X5	T49.0X6
Fluonid	T49.0X1	T49.0X2	T49.0X3	T49.0X4	T49.0X5	T49.0X6
Fluopromazine	T43.3X1	T43.3X2	T43.3X3	T43.3X4	T43.3X5	T43.3X6
Fluoroacetate	T60.8X1	T60.8X2	T60.8X3	T60.8X4	—	—
Fluorescein	T50.8X1	T50.8X2	T50.8X3	T50.8X4	T50.8X5	T50.8X6
Fluorhydrocortisone	T50.0X1	T50.0X2	T50.0X3	T50.0X4	T50.0X5	T50.0X6
Fluoride (nonmedicinal) (pesticide) (sodium) NEC	T60.8X1	T60.8X2	T60.8X3	T60.8X4	—	—
hydrogen — *see Hydrofluoric acid*						
medicinal NEC	T50.991	T50.992	T50.993	T50.994	T50.995	T50.996
dental use	T49.7X1	T49.7X2	T49.7X3	T49.7X4	T49.7X5	T49.7X6
not pesticide NEC	T54.91	T54.92	T54.93	T54.94	—	—
stannous	T49.7X1	T49.7X2	T49.7X3	T49.7X4	T49.7X5	T49.7X6
Fluorinated corticosteroids	T38.0X1	T38.0X2	T38.0X3	T38.0X4	T38.0X5	T38.0X6
Fluorine (gas)	T59.5X1	T59.5X2	T59.5X3	T59.5X4	—	—
salt — *see Fluoride(s)*						
Fluoristan	T49.7X1	T49.7X2	T49.7X3	T49.7X4	T49.7X5	T49.7X6
Fluormetholone	T49.0X1	T49.0X2	T49.0X3	T49.0X4	T49.0X5	T49.0X6
Fluoroacetate	T60.8X1	T60.8X2	T60.8X3	T60.8X4	—	—
Fluorocarbon monomer	T53.6X1	T53.6X2	T53.6X3	T53.6X4	—	—
Fluorocytosine	T37.8X1	T37.8X2	T37.8X3	T37.8X4	T37.8X5	T37.8X6
Fluorodeoxyuridine	T45.1X1	T45.1X2	T45.1X3	T45.1X4	T45.1X5	T45.1X6
Fluorometholone	T49.0X1	T49.0X2	T49.0X3	T49.0X4	T49.0X5	T49.0X6
ophthalmic preparation	T49.5X1	T49.5X2	T49.5X3	T49.5X4	T49.5X5	T49.5X6
Fluorophosphate insecticide	T60.0X1	T60.0X2	T60.0X3	T60.0X4	—	—
Fluoroquinolone antibiotics	T36.AX1	T36.AX2	T36.AX3	T36.AX4	T36.AX5	T36.AX6
Fluorosol	T46.3X1	T46.3X2	T46.3X3	T46.3X4	T46.3X5	T46.3X6

Substance	External Cause (T-Code)					
	Poisoning, Accidental (Unintentional)	Poisoning, Intentional Self-Harm	Poisoning, Assault	Poisoning, Undetermined	Adverse Effect	Underdosing
Fluorouracil	T45.1X1	T45.1X2	T45.1X3	T45.1X4	T45.1X5	T45.1X6
Fluorphenylalanine	T49.5X1	T49.5X2	T49.5X3	T49.5X4	T49.5X5	T49.5X6
Fluothane	T41.0X1	T41.0X2	T41.0X3	T41.0X4	T41.0X5	T41.0X6
Fluoxetine	T43.221	T43.222	T43.223	T43.224	T43.225	T43.226
Fluoxymesterone	T38.7X1	T38.7X2	T38.7X3	T38.7X4	T38.7X5	T38.7X6
Flupenthixol	T43.4X1	T43.4X2	T43.4X3	T43.4X4	T43.4X5	T43.4X6
Flupentixol	T43.4X1	T43.4X2	T43.4X3	T43.4X4	T43.4X5	T43.4X6
Fluphenazine	T43.3X1	T43.3X2	T43.3X3	T43.3X4	T43.3X5	T43.3X6
Fluprednidene	T49.0X1	T49.0X2	T49.0X3	T49.0X4	T49.0X5	T49.0X6
Fluprednisolone	T38.0X1	T38.0X2	T38.0X3	T38.0X4	T38.0X5	T38.0X6
Fluradoline	T39.8X1	T39.8X2	T39.8X3	T39.8X4	T39.8X5	T39.8X6
Flurandrenolide	T49.0X1	T49.0X2	T49.0X3	T49.0X4	T49.0X5	T49.0X6
Flurandrenolone	T49.0X1	T49.0X2	T49.0X3	T49.0X4	T49.0X5	T49.0X6
Flurazepam	T42.4X1	T42.4X2	T42.4X3	T42.4X4	T42.4X5	T42.4X6
Flurbiprofen	T39.311	T39.312	T39.313	T39.314	T39.315	T39.316
Flurobate	T49.0X1	T49.0X2	T49.0X3	T49.0X4	T49.0X5	T49.0X6
Flurotyl	T43.291	T43.292	T43.293	T43.294	T43.295	T43.296
Fluroxene	T41.0X1	T41.0X2	T41.0X3	T41.0X4	T41.0X5	T41.0X6
Fluspirilene	T43.591	T43.592	T43.593	T43.594	T43.595	T43.596
Flutamide	T38.6X1	T38.6X2	T38.6X3	T38.6X4	T38.6X5	T38.6X6
Flutazolam	T42.4X1	T42.4X2	T42.4X3	T42.4X4	T42.4X5	T42.4X6
Fluticasone propionate	T38.0X1	T38.0X2	T38.0X3	T38.0X4	T38.0X5	T38.0X6
Flutoprazepam	T42.4X1	T42.4X2	T42.4X3	T42.4X4	T42.4X5	T42.4X6
Flutropium bromide	T48.6X1	T48.6X2	T48.6X3	T48.6X4	T48.6X5	T48.6X6
Fluvoxamine	T43.221	T43.222	T43.223	T43.224	T43.225	T43.226
Folacin	T45.8X1	T45.8X2	T45.8X3	T45.8X4	T45.8X5	T45.8X6
Folic acid	T45.8X1	T45.8X2	T45.8X3	T45.8X4	T45.8X5	T45.8X6
with ferrous salt	T45.2X1	T45.2X2	T45.2X3	T45.2X4	T45.2X5	T45.2X6
antagonist	T45.1X1	T45.1X2	T45.1X3	T45.1X4	T45.1X5	T45.1X6
Folinic acid	T45.8X1	T45.8X2	T45.8X3	T45.8X4	T45.8X5	T45.8X6
Folium stramoniae	T48.6X1	T48.6X2	T48.6X3	T48.6X4	T48.6X5	T48.6X6
Follicle-stimulating hormone, human	T38.811	T38.812	T38.813	T38.814	T38.815	T38.816
Folpet	T60.3X1	T60.3X2	T60.3X3	T60.3X4	—	—
Fominoben	T48.3X1	T48.3X2	T48.3X3	T48.3X4	T48.3X5	T48.3X6
Food, foodstuffs, noxious, nonbacterial, NEC	T62.91	T62.92	T62.93	T62.94	—	—
berries	T62.1X1	T62.1X2	T62.1X3	T62.1X4	—	—
fish — *see also Fish*	T61.91	T61.92	T61.93	T61.94	—	—
mushrooms	T62.0X1	T62.0X2	T62.0X3	T62.0X4	—	—
plants	T62.2X1	T62.2X2	T62.2X3	T62.2X4	—	—
seafood	T61.91	T61.92	T61.93	T61.94	—	—
specified NEC	T61.8X1	T61.8X2	T61.8X3	T61.8X4	—	—

TABLE OF DRUGS AND CHEMICALS

Substance	Poisoning, Accidental (Unintentional)	Poisoning, Intentional Self-Harm	Poisoning, Assault	Poisoning, Undetermined	Adverse Effect	Underdosing
Food, foodstuffs, noxious, nonbacterial, NEC *(Continued)*						
seeds	T62.2X1	T62.2X2	T62.2X3	T62.2X4	—	—
shellfish	T61.781	T61.782	T61.783	T61.784	—	—
specified NEC	T62.8X1	T62.8X2	T62.8X3	T62.8X4	—	—
Fool's parsley	T62.2X1	T62.2X2	T62.2X3	T62.2X4		
Formaldehyde (solution), gas or vapor	T59.2X1	T59.2X2	T59.2X3	T59.2X4	—	—
fungicide	T60.3X1	T60.3X2	T60.3X3	T60.3X4	—	—
Formalin	T59.2X1	T59.2X2	T59.2X3	T59.2X4	—	—
fungicide	T60.3X1	T60.3X2	T60.3X3	T60.3X4	—	—
vapor	T59.2X1	T59.2X2	T59.2X3	T59.2X4	—	—
Formic acid	T54.2X1	T54.2X2	T54.2X3	T54.2X4	—	—
vapor	T59.891	T59.892	T59.893	T59.894	—	—
Foscarnet sodium	T37.5X1	T37.5X2	T37.5X3	T37.5X4	T37.5X5	T37.5X6
Fosfestrol	T38.5X1	T38.5X2	T38.5X3	T38.5X4	T38.5X5	T38.5X6
Fosfomycin	T36.8X1	T36.8X2	T36.8X3	T36.8X4	T36.8X5	T36.8X6
Fosfonet sodium	T37.5X1	T37.5X2	T37.5X3	T37.5X4	T37.5X5	T37.5X6
Fosinopril	T46.4X1	T46.4X2	T46.4X3	T46.4X4	T46.4X5	T46.4X6
sodium	T46.4X1	T46.4X2	T46.4X3	T46.4X4	T46.4X5	T46.4X6
Fowler's solution	T57.0X1	T57.0X2	T57.0X3	T57.0X4	—	—
Foxglove	T62.2X1	T62.2X2	T62.2X3	T62.2X4	—	—
Framycetin	T36.5X1	T36.5X2	T36.5X3	T36.5X4	T36.5X5	T36.5X6
Frangula	T47.2X1	T47.2X2	T47.2X3	T47.2X4	T47.2X5	T47.2X6
extract	T47.2X1	T47.2X2	T47.2X3	T47.2X4	T47.2X5	T47.2X6
Frei antigen	T50.8X1	T50.8X2	T50.8X3	T50.8X4	T50.8X5	T50.8X6
Freon	T53.5X1	T53.5X2	T53.5X3	T53.5X4	—	—
Fructose	T50.3X1	T50.3X2	T50.3X3	T50.3X4	T50.3X5	T50.3X6
Frusemide	T50.1X1	T50.1X2	T50.1X3	T50.1X4	T50.1X5	T50.1X6
FSH	T38.811	T38.812	T38.813	T38.814	T38.815	T38.816
Ftorafur	T45.1X1	T45.1X2	T45.1X3	T45.1X4	T45.1X5	T45.1X6
Fuel						
automobile	T52.0X1	T52.0X2	T52.0X3	T52.0X4	—	—
exhaust gas, not in transit	T58.01	T58.02	T58.03	T58.04	—	—
vapor NEC	T52.0X1	T52.0X2	T52.0X3	T52.0X4	—	—
gas (domestic use) — *see also Carbon, monoxide, fuel, utility*	T59.891	T59.892	T59.893	T59.894	—	—
utility	T59.891	T59.892	T59.893	T59.894	—	—
in mobile container	T59.891	T59.892	T59.893	T59.894	—	—
incomplete combustion of — *see Carbon, monoxide, fuel, utility*						
piped (natural)	T59.891	T59.892	T59.893	T59.894		

Substance	Poisoning, Accidental (Unintentional)	Poisoning, Intentional Self-Harm	Poisoning, Assault	Poisoning, Undetermined	Adverse Effect	Underdosing
Fuel *(Continued)*						
industrial, incomplete combustion	T58.8X1	T58.8X2	T58.8X3	T58.8X4	—	—
Fugillin	T36.8X1	T36.8X2	T36.8X3	T36.8X4	T36.8X5	T36.8X6
Fulminate of mercury	T56.1X1	T56.1X2	T56.1X3	T56.1X4		
Fulvicin	T36.7X1	T36.7X2	T36.7X3	T36.7X4	T36.7X5	T36.7X6
Fumadil	T36.8X1	T36.8X2	T36.8X3	T36.8X4	T36.8X5	T36.8X6
Fumagillin	T36.8X1	T36.8X2	T36.8X3	T36.8X4	T36.8X5	T36.8X6
Fumaric acid	T49.4X1	T49.4X2	T49.4X3	T49.4X4	T49.4X5	T49.4X6
Fumes (from)	T59.91	T59.92	T59.93	T59.94	—	—
carbon monoxide — *see Carbon, monoxide*						
charcoal (domestic use) — *see Charcoal, fumes*						
chloroform — *see Chloroform*						
coke (in domestic stoves, fireplaces) — *see Coke, fumes*						
corrosive NEC	T54.91	T54.92	T54.93	T54.94	—	—
ether — *see Ether*						
freons	T53.5X1	T53.5X2	T53.5X3	T53.5X4	—	—
hydrocarbons	T59.891	T59.892	T59.893	T59.894	—	—
petroleum (liquefied)	T59.891	T59.892	T59.893	T59.894	—	—
distributed through pipes (pure or mixed with air)	T59.891	T59.892	T59.893	T59.894	—	—
lead — *see Lead*						
metal — *see Metals, or the specified metal*						
nitrogen dioxide	T59.0X1	T59.0X2	T59.0X3	T59.0X4	—	—
pesticides — *see Pesticide*						
petroleum (liquefied)	T59.891	T59.892	T59.893	T59.894	—	—
distributed through pipes (pure or mixed with air)	T59.891	T59.892	T59.893	T59.894	—	—
polyester	T59.891	T59.892	T59.893	T59.894	—	—
specified source NEC — *see also substance specified*	T59.891	T59.892	T59.893	T59.894	—	—
sulfur dioxide	T59.1X1	T59.1X2	T59.1X3	T59.1X4	—	—
Fumigant NEC	T60.91	T60.92	T60.93	T60.94	—	—
Fungi, noxious, used as food	T62.0X1	T62.0X2	T62.0X3	T62.0X4	—	—
Fungicide NEC (nonmedicinal)	T60.3X1	T60.3X2	T60.3X3	T60.3X4	—	—
Fungizone	T36.7X1	T36.7X2	T36.7X3	T36.7X4	T36.7X5	T36.7X6
topical	T49.0X1	T49.0X2	T49.0X3	T49.0X4	T49.0X5	T49.0X6
Furacin	T49.0X1	T49.0X2	T49.0X3	T49.0X4	T49.0X5	T49.0X6
Furadantin	T37.91	T37.92	T37.93	T37.94	T37.95	T37.96

◄ New   ◄ Revised   ~~deleted~~ Deleted

Substance	Poisoning, Accidental (Unintentional)	Poisoning, Intentional Self-Harm	Poisoning, Assault	Poisoning, Undetermined	Adverse Effect	Underdosing
Furazolidone	T37.8X1	T37.8X2	T37.8X3	T37.8X4	T37.8X5	T37.8X6
Furazolium chloride	T49.0X1	T49.0X2	T49.0X3	T49.0X4	T49.0X5	T49.0X6
Furfural	T52.8X1	T52.8X2	T52.8X3	T52.8X4	—	—
Furnace (coal burning) (domestic), gas from industrial	T58.2X1	T58.2X2	T58.2X3	T58.2X4	—	—
industrial	T58.8X1	T58.8X2	T58.8X3	T58.8X4	—	—
Furniture polish	T65.891	T65.892	T65.893	T65.894	—	—
Furosemide	T50.1X1	T50.1X2	T50.1X3	T50.1X4	T50.1X5	T50.1X6
Furoxone	T37.91	T37.92	T37.93	T37.94	T37.95	T37.96
Fursultiamine	T45.2X1	T45.2X2	T45.2X3	T45.2X4	T45.2X5	T45.2X6
Fusafungine	T36.8X1	T36.8X2	T36.8X3	T36.8X4	T36.8X5	T36.8X6
Fusel oil (any) (amyl) (butyl) (propyl), vapor	T51.3X1	T51.3X2	T51.3X3	T51.3X4	—	—
Fusidate (ethanolamine) (sodium)	T36.8X1	T36.8X2	T36.8X3	T36.8X4	T36.8X5	T36.8X6
Fusidic acid	T36.8X1	T36.8X2	T36.8X3	T36.8X4	T36.8X5	T36.8X6
Fytic acid, nonasodium	T50.6X1	T50.6X2	T50.6X3	T50.6X4	T50.6X5	T50.6X6
G						
GABA	T43.8X1	T43.8X2	T43.8X3	T43.8X4	T43.8X5	T43.8X6
Gadolinium	T56.821	T56.822	T56.823	T56.824	T56.825	—
Gadopentetic acid	T50.8X1	T50.8X2	T50.8X3	T50.8X4	T50.8X5	T50.8X6
Galactose	T50.3X1	T50.3X2	T50.3X3	T50.3X4	T50.3X5	T50.3X6
b-Galactosidase	T47.5X1	T47.5X2	T47.5X3	T47.5X4	T47.5X5	T47.5X6
Galantamine	T44.0X1	T44.0X2	T44.0X3	T44.0X4	T44.0X5	T44.0X6
Gallamine (triethiodide)	T48.1X1	T48.1X2	T48.1X3	T48.1X4	T48.1X5	T48.1X6
Gallium citrate	T50.991	T50.992	T50.993	T50.994	T50.995	T50.996
Gallopamil	T46.1X1	T46.1X2	T46.1X3	T46.1X4	T46.1X5	T46.1X6
Gamboge	T47.2X1	T47.2X2	T47.2X3	T47.2X4	T47.2X5	T47.2X6
Gamimune	T50.Z11	T50.Z12	T50.Z13	T50.Z14	T50.Z15	T50.Z16
Gamma-aminobutyric acid	T43.8X1	T43.8X2	T43.8X3	T43.8X4	T43.8X5	T43.8X6
Gamma-benzene hexachloride (medicinal)	T49.0X1	T49.0X2	T49.0X3	T49.0X4	T49.0X5	T49.0X6
nonmedicinal, vapor	T53.6X1	T53.6X2	T53.6X3	T53.6X4	—	—
Gamma-BHC (medicinal) — *see also Gamma-benzene hexachloride*	T49.0X1	T49.0X2	T49.0X3	T49.0X4	T49.0X5	T49.0X6
Gamma globulin	T50.Z11	T50.Z12	T50.Z13	T50.Z14	T50.Z15	T50.Z16
Gamulin	T50.Z11	T50.Z12	T50.Z13	T50.Z14	T50.Z15	T50.Z16
Ganciclovir (sodium)	T37.5X1	T37.5X2	T37.5X3	T37.5X4	T37.5X5	T37.5X6
Ganglionic blocking drug NEC	T44.2X1	T44.2X2	T44.2X3	T44.2X4	T44.2X5	T44.2X6
specified NEC	T44.2X1	T44.2X2	T44.2X3	T44.2X4	T44.2X5	T44.2X6
Ganja	T40.711	T40.712	T40.713	T40.714	T40.715	T40.716
Garamycin	T36.5X1	T36.5X2	T36.5X3	T36.5X4	T36.5X5	T36.5X6
ophthalmic preparation	T49.5X1	T49.5X2	T49.5X3	T49.5X4	T49.5X5	T49.5X6
topical NEC	T49.0X1	T49.0X2	T49.0X3	T49.0X4	T49.0X5	T49.0X6

Substance	Poisoning, Accidental (Unintentional)	Poisoning, Intentional Self-Harm	Poisoning, Assault	Poisoning, Undetermined	Adverse Effect	Underdosing
Gardenal	T42.3X1	T42.3X2	T42.3X3	T42.3X4	T42.3X5	T42.3X6
Gardepanyl	T42.3X1	T42.3X2	T42.3X3	T42.3X4	T42.3X5	T42.3X6
Gas NEC	T59.91	T59.92	T59.93	T59.94	—	—
acetylene	T59.891	T59.892	T59.893	T59.894	—	—
incomplete combustion of	T58.11	T58.12	T58.13	T58.14	—	—
air contaminants, source or type not specified	T59.91	T59.92	T59.93	T59.94	—	—
anesthetic	T41.0X1	T41.0X2	T41.0X3	T41.0X4	T41.0X5	T41.0X6
blast furnace	T58.8X1	T58.8X2	T58.8X3	T58.8X4	—	—
butane — *see* Butane						
carbon monoxide — *see* Carbon, monoxide						
chlorine	T59.4X1	T59.4X2	T59.4X3	T59.4X4	—	—
coal	T58.2X1	T58.2X2	T58.2X3	T58.2X4	—	—
cyanide	T57.3X1	T57.3X2	T57.3X3	T57.3X4	—	—
dicyanogen	T65.0X1	T65.0X2	T65.0X3	T65.0X4	—	—
domestic — *see* Domestic gas	T57.91	T57.92	T57.93	T57.94	—	—
exhaust	T57.91	T57.92	T57.93	T57.94	—	—
from utility (for cooking, heating, or lighting) (after combustion) — *see* Carbon, monoxide, fuel, utility						
prior to combustion	T59.891	T59.892	T59.893	T59.894	—	—
from wood or coal-burning stove or fireplace	T57.91	T57.92	T57.93	T57.94	—	—
fuel (domestic use) (after combustion) — *see also* Carbon, monoxide, fuel	T57.91	T57.92	T57.93	T57.94	—	—
industrial use	T58.8X1	T58.8X2	T58.8X3	T58.8X4	—	—
prior to combustion	T59.891	T59.892	T59.893	T59.894	—	—
utility	T59.891	T59.892	T59.893	T59.894	—	—
in mobile container	T59.891	T59.892	T59.893	T59.894	—	—
incomplete combustion of — *see* Carbon, monoxide, fuel, utility						
piped (natural)	T59.891	T59.892	T59.893	T59.894	—	—
garage	T58.01	T58.02	T58.03	T58.04	—	—
hydrocarbon NEC	T59.891	T59.892	T59.893	T59.894	—	—
incomplete combustion of — *see* Carbon, monoxide, fuel, utility						
liquefied — *see* Butane						
piped	T59.891	T59.892	T59.893	T59.894	—	—
hydrocyanic acid	T65.0X1	T65.0X2	T65.0X3	T65.0X4	—	—

TABLE OF DRUGS AND CHEMICALS

Substance	External Cause (T-Code)					
	Poisoning, Accidental (Unintentional)	Poisoning, Intentional Self-Harm	Poisoning, Assault	Poisoning, Undetermined	Adverse Effect	Underdosing
Gas NEC *(Continued)*						
illuminating (after combustion)	T58.11	T58.12	T58.13	T58.14	—	—
prior to combustion	T59.891	T59.892	T59.893	T59.894	—	—
incomplete combustion, any — see Carbon, monoxide						
kiln	T58.8X1	T58.8X2	T58.8X3	T58.8X4	—	—
lacrimogenic	T59.3X1	T59.3X2	T59.3X3	T59.3X4	—	—
liquefied petroleum — see Butane						
marsh	T59.891	T59.892	T59.893	T59.894	—	—
motor exhaust, not in transit	T58.01	T58.02	T58.03	T58.04	—	—
mustard, not in war	T59.891	T59.892	T59.893	T59.894	—	—
natural	T59.891	T59.892	T59.893	T59.894	—	—
nerve, not in war	T59.91	T59.92	T59.93	T59.94	—	—
oil	T52.0X1	T52.0X2	T52.0X3	T52.0X4	—	—
petroleum (liquefied) (distributed in mobile containers)	T59.891	T59.892	T59.893	T59.894	—	—
piped (pure or mixed with air)	T59.891	T59.892	T59.893	T59.894	—	—
piped (manufactured) (natural) NEC	T59.891	T59.892	T59.893	T59.894	—	—
producer	T58.8X1	T58.8X2	T58.8X3	T58.8X4	—	—
propane — see Propane						
refrigerant (chlorofluoro-carbon)	T53.5X1	T53.5X2	T53.5X3	T53.5X4	—	—
not chlorofluoro-carbon	T59.891	T59.892	T59.893	T59.894	—	—
sewer	T59.91	T59.92	T59.93	T59.94	—	—
specified source NEC	T59.91	T59.92	T59.93	T59.94	—	—
stove (after combustion)	T58.11	T58.12	T58.13	T58.14	—	—
tear	T59.3X1	T59.3X2	T59.3X3	T59.3X4	—	—
therapeutic	T41.5X1	T41.5X2	T41.5X3	T41.5X4	T41.5X5	T41.5X6
utility (for cooking, heating, or lighting) (piped) NEC	T59.891	T59.892	T59.893	T59.894	—	—
in mobile container	T59.891	T59.892	T59.893	T59.894	—	—
incomplete combustion of — see Carbon, monoxide, fuel, utility						
piped (natural)	T59.891	T59.892	T59.893	T59.894	—	—
water	T58.11	T58.12	T58.13	T58.14	—	—
incomplete combustion of — see Carbon, monoxide, fuel, utility						

Substance	External Cause (T-Code)					
	Poisoning, Accidental (Unintentional)	Poisoning, Intentional Self-Harm	Poisoning, Assault	Poisoning, Undetermined	Adverse Effect	Underdosing
Gaseous substance — *see Gas*						
Gasoline	T52.0X1	T52.0X2	T52.0X3	T52.0X4	—	—
vapor	T52.0X1	T52.0X2	T52.0X3	T52.0X4	—	—
Gastric enzymes	T47.5X1	T47.5X2	T47.5X3	T47.5X4	T47.5X5	T47.5X6
Gastrografin	T50.8X1	T50.8X2	T50.8X3	T50.8X4	T50.8X5	T50.8X6
Gastrointestinal drug	T47.91	T47.92	T47.93	T47.94	T47.95	T47.96
biological	T47.8X1	T47.8X2	T47.8X3	T47.8X4	T47.8X5	T47.8X6
specified NEC	T47.8X1	T47.8X2	T47.8X3	T47.8X4	T47.8X5	T47.8X6
Gaultheria procumbens	T62.2X1	T62.2X2	T62.2X3	T62.2X4	—	—
Gelatin (intravenous)	T45.8X1	T45.8X2	T45.8X3	T45.8X4	T45.8X5	T45.8X6
absorbable (sponge)	T45.7X1	T45.7X2	T45.7X3	T45.7X4	T45.7X5	T45.7X6
Gefarnate	T44.3X1	T44.3X2	T44.3X3	T44.3X4	T44.3X5	T44.3X6
Gelfilm	T49.8X1	T49.8X2	T49.8X3	T49.8X4	T49.8X5	T49.8X6
Gelfoam	T45.7X1	T45.7X2	T45.7X3	T45.7X4	T45.7X5	T45.7X6
Gelsemine	T50.991	T50.992	T50.993	T50.994	T50.995	T50.996
Gelsemium (sempervirens)	T62.2X1	T62.2X2	T62.2X3	T62.2X4	—	—
Gemeprost	T48.0X1	T48.0X2	T48.0X3	T48.0X4	T48.0X5	T48.0X6
Gemfibrozil	T46.6X1	T46.6X2	T46.6X3	T46.6X4	T46.6X5	T46.6X6
Gemonil	T42.3X1	T42.3X2	T42.3X3	T42.3X4	T42.3X5	T42.3X6
Gentamicin	T36.5X1	T36.5X2	T36.5X3	T36.5X4	T36.5X5	T36.5X6
ophthalmic preparation	T49.5X1	T49.5X2	T49.5X3	T49.5X4	T49.5X5	T49.5X6
topical NEC	T49.0X1	T49.0X2	T49.0X3	T49.0X4	T49.0X5	T49.0X6
Gentian	T47.5X1	T47.5X2	T47.5X3	T47.5X4	T47.5X5	T47.5X6
violet	T49.0X1	T49.0X2	T49.0X3	T49.0X4	T49.0X5	T49.0X6
Gepefrine	T44.4X1	T44.4X2	T44.4X3	T44.4X4	T44.4X5	T44.4X6
Gestonorone caproate	T38.5X1	T38.5X2	T38.5X3	T38.5X4	T38.5X5	T38.5X6
Gexane	T49.0X1	T49.0X2	T49.0X3	T49.0X4	T49.0X5	T49.0X6
Gila monster (venom)	T63.111	T63.112	T63.113	T63.114	—	—
Ginger	T47.5X1	T47.5X2	T47.5X3	T47.5X4	T47.5X5	T47.5X6
Jamaica — *see Jamaica, ginger*						
Gitalin	T46.0X1	T46.0X2	T46.0X3	T46.0X4	T46.0X5	T46.0X6
amorphous	T46.0X1	T46.0X2	T46.0X3	T46.0X4	T46.0X5	T46.0X6
Gitaloxin	T46.0X1	T46.0X2	T46.0X3	T46.0X4	T46.0X5	T46.0X6
Gitoxin	T46.0X1	T46.0X2	T46.0X3	T46.0X4	T46.0X5	T46.0X6
Glafenine	T39.8X1	T39.8X2	T39.8X3	T39.8X4	T39.8X5	T39.8X6
Glandular extract (medicinal) NEC	T50.Z91	T50.Z92	T50.Z93	T50.Z94	T50.Z95	T50.Z96
Glaucarubin	T37.3X1	T37.3X2	T37.3X3	T37.3X4	T37.3X5	T37.3X6
Glibenclamide	T38.3X1	T38.3X2	T38.3X3	T38.3X4	T38.3X5	T38.3X6
Glibornuride	T38.3X1	T38.3X2	T38.3X3	T38.3X4	T38.3X5	T38.3X6
Gliclazide	T38.3X1	T38.3X2	T38.3X3	T38.3X4	T38.3X5	T38.3X6
Glimidine	T38.3X1	T38.3X2	T38.3X3	T38.3X4	T38.3X5	T38.3X6

Substance	Poisoning, Accidental (Unintentional)	Poisoning, Intentional Self-Harm	Poisoning, Assault	Poisoning, Undetermined	Adverse Effect	Underdosing
Glipizide	T38.3X1	T38.3X2	T38.3X3	T38.3X4	T38.3X5	T38.3X6
Gliquidone	T38.3X1	T38.3X2	T38.3X3	T38.3X4	T38.3X5	T38.3X6
Glisolamide	T38.3X1	T38.3X2	T38.3X3	T38.3X4	T38.3X5	T38.3X6
Glisoxepide	T38.3X1	T38.3X2	T38.3X3	T38.3X4	T38.3X5	T38.3X6
Globin zinc insulin	T38.3X1	T38.3X2	T38.3X3	T38.3X4	T38.3X5	T38.3X6
Globulin						
antilymphocytic	T50.Z11	T50.Z12	T50.Z13	T50.Z14	T50.Z15	T50.Z16
antirhesus	T50.Z11	T50.Z12	T50.Z13	T50.Z14	T50.Z15	T50.Z16
antivenin	T50.Z11	T50.Z12	T50.Z13	T50.Z14	T50.Z15	T50.Z16
antiviral	T50.Z11	T50.Z12	T50.Z13	T50.Z14	T50.Z15	T50.Z16
Glucagon	T38.3X1	T38.3X2	T38.3X3	T38.3X4	T38.3X5	T38.3X6
Glucocorticoids	T38.0X1	T38.0X2	T38.0X3	T38.0X4	T38.0X5	T38.0X6
Glucocorticosteroid	T38.0X1	T38.0X2	T38.0X3	T38.0X4	T38.0X5	T38.0X6
Gluconic acid	T50.991	T50.992	T50.993	T50.994	T50.995	T50.996
Glucosamine sulfate	T39.4X1	T39.4X2	T39.4X3	T39.4X4	T39.4X5	T39.4X6
Glucose	T50.3X1	T50.3X2	T50.3X3	T50.3X4	T50.3X5	T50.3X6
with sodium chloride	T50.3X1	T50.3X2	T50.3X3	T50.3X4	T50.3X5	T50.3X6
Glucosulfone sodium	T37.1X1	T37.1X2	T37.1X3	T37.1X4	T37.1X5	T37.1X6
Glucurolactone	T47.8X1	T47.8X2	T47.8X3	T47.8X4	T47.8X5	T47.8X6
Glue NEC	T52.8X1	T52.8X2	T52.8X3	T52.8X4	—	—
Glutamic acid	T47.5X1	T47.5X2	T47.5X3	T47.5X4	T47.5X5	T47.5X6
Glutaral (medicinal)	T49.0X1	T49.0X2	T49.0X3	T49.0X4	T49.0X5	T49.0X6
nonmedicinal	T65.891	T65.892	T65.893	T65.894	—	—
Glutaraldehyde (nonmedicinal)	T65.891	T65.892	T65.893	T65.894	—	—
medicinal	T49.0X1	T49.0X2	T49.0X3	T49.0X4	T49.0X5	T49.0X6
Glutathione	T50.6X1	T50.6X2	T50.6X3	T50.6X4	T50.6X5	T50.6X6
Glutethimide	T42.6X1	T42.6X2	T42.6X3	T42.6X4	T42.6X5	T42.6X6
Glyburide	T38.3X1	T38.3X2	T38.3X3	T38.3X4	T38.3X5	T38.3X6
Glycerin	T47.4X1	T47.4X2	T47.4X3	T47.4X4	T47.4X5	T47.4X6
Glycerol	T47.4X1	T47.4X2	T47.4X3	T47.4X4	T47.4X5	T47.4X6
borax	T49.6X1	T49.6X2	T49.6X3	T49.6X4	T49.6X5	T49.6X6
intravenous	T50.3X1	T50.3X2	T50.3X3	T50.3X4	T50.3X5	T50.3X6
iodinated	T48.4X1	T48.4X2	T48.4X3	T48.4X4	T48.4X5	T48.4X6
Glycerophosphate	T50.991	T50.992	T50.993	T50.994	T50.995	T50.996
Glyceryl						
gualacolate	T48.4X1	T48.4X2	T48.4X3	T48.4X4	T48.4X5	T48.4X6
nitrate	T46.3X1	T46.3X2	T46.3X3	T46.3X4	T46.3X5	T46.3X6
triacetate (topical)	T49.0X1	T49.0X2	T49.0X3	T49.0X4	T49.0X5	T49.0X6
trinitrate	T46.3X1	T46.3X2	T46.3X3	T46.3X4	T46.3X5	T46.3X6
Glycine	T50.3X1	T50.3X2	T50.3X3	T50.3X4	T50.3X5	T50.3X6
Glyclopyramide	T38.3X1	T38.3X2	T38.3X3	T38.3X4	T38.3X5	T38.3X6
Glycobiarsol	T37.3X1	T37.3X2	T37.3X3	T37.3X4	T37.3X5	T37.3X6

Substance	Poisoning, Accidental (Unintentional)	Poisoning, Intentional Self-Harm	Poisoning, Assault	Poisoning, Undetermined	Adverse Effect	Underdosing
Glycols (ether)	T52.3X1	T52.3X2	T52.3X3	T52.3X4	—	—
Glyconiazide	T37.1X1	T37.1X2	T37.1X3	T37.1X4	T37.1X5	T37.1X6
Glycopyrrolate	T44.3X1	T44.3X2	T44.3X3	T44.3X4	T44.3X5	T44.3X6
Glycopyrronium	T44.3X1	T44.3X2	T44.3X3	T44.3X4	T44.3X5	T44.3X6
bromide	T44.3X1	T44.3X2	T44.3X3	T44.3X4	T44.3X5	T44.3X6
Glycoside, cardiac (stimulant)	T46.0X1	T46.0X2	T46.0X3	T46.0X4	T46.0X5	T46.0X6
Glycyclamide	T38.3X1	T38.3X2	T38.3X3	T38.3X4	T38.3X5	T38.3X6
Glycyrrhiza extract	T48.4X1	T48.4X2	T48.4X3	T48.4X4	T48.4X5	T48.4X6
Glycyrrhizic acid	T48.4X1	T48.4X2	T48.4X3	T48.4X4	T48.4X5	T48.4X6
Glycyrrhizinate potassium	T48.4X1	T48.4X2	T48.4X3	T48.4X4	T48.4X5	T48.4X6
Glymidine sodium	T38.3X1	T38.3X2	T38.3X3	T38.3X4	T38.3X5	T38.3X6
Glyphosate	T60.3X1	T60.3X2	T60.3X3	T60.3X4	—	—
Glyphylline	T48.6X1	T48.6X2	T48.6X3	T48.6X4	T48.6X5	T48.6X6
Gold						
colloidal (l98Au)	T45.1X1	T45.1X2	T45.1X3	T45.1X4	T45.1X5	T45.1X6
salts	T39.4X1	T39.4X2	T39.4X3	T39.4X4	T39.4X5	T39.4X6
Golden sulfide of antimony	T56.891	T56.892	T56.893	T56.894	—	—
Goldylocks	T62.2X1	T62.2X2	T62.2X3	T62.2X4	—	—
Gonadal tissue extract	T38.901	T38.902	T38.903	T38.904	T38.905	T38.906
female	T38.5X1	T38.5X2	T38.5X3	T38.5X4	T38.5X5	T38.5X6
male	T38.7X1	T38.7X2	T38.7X3	T38.7X4	T38.7X5	T38.7X6
Gonadorelin	T38.891	T38.892	T38.893	T38.894	T38.895	T38.896
Gonadotropin	T38.891	T38.892	T38.893	T38.894	T38.895	T38.896
chorionic	T38.891	T38.892	T38.893	T38.894	T38.895	T38.896
pituitary	T38.811	T38.812	T38.813	T38.814	T38.815	T38.816
Goserelin	T45.1X1	T45.1X2	T45.1X3	T45.1X4	T45.1X5	T45.1X6
Grain alcohol	T51.0X1	T51.0X2	T51.0X3	T51.0X4	—	—
Gramicidin	T49.0X1	T49.0X2	T49.0X3	T49.0X4	T49.0X5	T49.0X6
Granisetron	T45.0X1	T45.0X2	T45.0X3	T45.0X4	T45.0X5	T45.0X6
Gratiola officinalis	T62.2X1	T62.2X2	T62.2X3	T62.2X4	—	—
Grease	T65.891	T65.892	T65.893	T65.894	—	—
Green hellebore	T62.2X1	T62.2X2	T62.2X3	T62.2X4		
Green soap	T49.2X1	T49.2X2	T49.2X3	T49.2X4	T49.2X5	T49.2X6
Grifulvin	T36.7X1	T36.7X2	T36.7X3	T36.7X4	T36.7X5	T36.7X6
Griseofulvin	T36.7X1	T36.7X2	T36.7X3	T36.7X4	T36.7X5	T36.7X6
Growth hormone	T38.811	T38.812	T38.813	T38.814	T38.815	T38.816
Guaiacol derivatives	T48.4X1	T48.4X2	T48.4X3	T48.4X4	T48.4X5	T48.4X6
Guaiac reagent	T50.991	T50.992	T50.993	T50.994	T50.995	T50.996
Guaifenesin	T48.4X1	T48.4X2	T48.4X3	T48.4X4	T48.4X5	T48.4X6
Guaimesal	T48.4X1	T48.4X2	T48.4X3	T48.4X4	T48.4X5	T48.4X6
Guaiphenesin	T48.4X1	T48.4X2	T48.4X3	T48.4X4	T48.4X5	T48.4X6
Guamecycline	T36.4X1	T36.4X2	T36.4X3	T36.4X4	T36.4X5	T36.4X6

Substance	External Cause (T-Code)					
	Poisoning, Accidental (Unintentional)	Poisoning, Intentional Self-Harm	Poisoning, Assault	Poisoning, Undetermined	Adverse Effect	Underdosing
Guanabenz	T46.5X1	T46.5X2	T46.5X3	T46.5X4	T46.5X5	T46.5X6
Guanacline	T46.5X1	T46.5X2	T46.5X3	T46.5X4	T46.5X5	T46.5X6
Guanadrel	T46.5X1	T46.5X2	T46.5X3	T46.5X4	T46.5X5	T46.5X6
Guanatol	T37.2X1	T37.2X2	T37.2X3	T37.2X4	T37.2X5	T37.2X6
Guanethidine	T46.5X1	T46.5X2	T46.5X3	T46.5X4	T46.5X5	T46.5X6
Guanfacine	T46.5X1	T46.5X2	T46.5X3	T46.5X4	T46.5X5	T46.5X6
Guano	T65.891	T65.892	T65.893	T65.894	—	—
Guanochlor	T46.5X1	T46.5X2	T46.5X3	T46.5X4	T46.5X5	T46.5X6
Guanoclor	T46.5X1	T46.5X2	T46.5X3	T46.5X4	T46.5X5	T46.5X6
Guanoctine	T46.5X1	T46.5X2	T46.5X3	T46.5X4	T46.5X5	T46.5X6
Guanoxabenz	T46.5X1	T46.5X2	T46.5X3	T46.5X4	T46.5X5	T46.5X6
Guanoxan	T46.5X1	T46.5X2	T46.5X3	T46.5X4	T46.5X5	T46.5X6
Guar gum (medicinal)	T46.6X1	T46.6X2	T46.6X3	T46.6X4	T46.6X5	T46.6X6

H

Substance	Poisoning, Accidental (Unintentional)	Poisoning, Intentional Self-Harm	Poisoning, Assault	Poisoning, Undetermined	Adverse Effect	Underdosing
Hachimycin	T36.7X1	T36.7X2	T36.7X3	T36.7X4	T36.7X5	T36.7X6
Hair						
dye	T49.4X1	T49.4X2	T49.4X3	T49.4X4	T49.4X5	T49.4X6
preparation NEC	T49.4X1	T49.4X2	T49.4X3	T49.4X4	T49.4X5	T49.4X6
Halazepam	T42.4X1	T42.4X2	T42.4X3	T42.4X4	T42.4X5	T42.4X6
Halcinolone	T49.0X1	T49.0X2	T49.0X3	T49.0X4	T49.0X5	T49.0X6
Halcinonide	T49.0X1	T49.0X2	T49.0X3	T49.0X4	T49.0X5	T49.0X6
Halethazole	T49.0X1	T49.0X2	T49.0X3	T49.0X4	T49.0X5	T49.0X6
Hallucinogen NOS	T40.901	T40.902	T40.903	T40.904	T40.905	T40.906
specified NEC	T40.991	T40.992	T40.993	T40.994	T40.995	T40.996
Halofantrine	T37.2X1	T37.2X2	T37.2X3	T37.2X4	T37.2X5	T37.2X6
Halofenate	T46.6X1	T46.6X2	T46.6X3	T46.6X4	T46.6X5	T46.6X6
Halometasone	T49.0X1	T49.0X2	T49.0X3	T49.0X4	T49.0X5	T49.0X6
Haloperidol	T43.4X1	T43.4X2	T43.4X3	T43.4X4	T43.4X5	T43.4X6
Haloprogin	T49.0X1	T49.0X2	T49.0X3	T49.0X4	T49.0X5	T49.0X6
Halotex	T49.0X1	T49.0X2	T49.0X3	T49.0X4	T49.0X5	T49.0X6
Halothane	T41.0X1	T41.0X2	T41.0X3	T41.0X4	T41.0X5	T41.0X6
Haloxazolam	T42.4X1	T42.4X2	T42.4X3	T42.4X4	T42.4X5	T42.4X6
Halquinols	T49.0X1	T49.0X2	T49.0X3	T49.0X4	T49.0X5	T49.0X6
Hamamelis	T49.2X1	T49.2X2	T49.2X3	T49.2X4	T49.2X5	T49.2X6
Haptendextran	T45.8X1	T45.8X2	T45.8X3	T45.8X4	T45.8X5	T45.8X6
Harmonyl	T46.5X1	T46.5X2	T46.5X3	T46.5X4	T46.5X5	T46.5X6
Hartmann's solution	T50.3X1	T50.3X2	T50.3X3	T50.3X4	T50.3X5	T50.3X6
Hashish	T40.711	T40.712	T40.713	T40.714	T40.715	T40.716
Hawaiian Woodrose seeds	T40.991	T40.992	T40.993	T40.994	—	—
HCB	T60.3X1	T60.3X2	T60.3X3	T60.3X4	—	—
HCH	T53.6X1	T53.6X2	T53.6X3	T53.6X4	—	—
medicinal	T49.0X1	T49.0X2	T49.0X3	T49.0X4	T49.0X5	T49.0X6

Substance	External Cause (T-Code)					
	Poisoning, Accidental (Unintentional)	Poisoning, Intentional Self-Harm	Poisoning, Assault	Poisoning, Undetermined	Adverse Effect	Underdosing
HCN	T57.3X1	T57.3X2	T57.3X3	T57.3X4	—	—
Headache cures, drugs, powders NEC	T50.901	T50.902	T50.903	T50.904	T50.905	T50.906
Heavenly Blue (morning glory)	T40.991	T40.992	T40.993	T40.994	—	—
Heavy metal antidote	T45.8X1	T45.8X2	T45.8X3	T45.8X4	T45.8X5	T45.8X6
Hedaquinium	T49.0X1	T49.0X2	T49.0X3	T49.0X4	T49.0X5	T49.0X6
Hedge hyssop	T62.2X1	T62.2X2	T62.2X3	T62.2X4	—	—
Heet	T49.8X1	T49.8X2	T49.8X3	T49.8X4	T49.8X5	T49.8X6
Helium	T48.991	T48.992	T48.993	T48.994	T48.995	T48.996
Helenin	T37.4X1	T37.4X2	T37.4X3	T37.4X4	T37.4X5	T37.4X6
Hellebore (black) (green) (white)	T62.2X1	T62.2X2	T62.2X3	T62.2X4	—	—
Helium (nonmedicinal) NEC	T59.891	T59.892	T59.893	T59.894	—	—
medicinal	T48.991	T48.992	T48.993	T48.994	T48.995	T48.996
Hematin	T45.8X1	T45.8X2	T45.8X3	T45.8X4	T45.8X5	T45.8X6
Hematinic preparation	T45.8X1	T45.8X2	T45.8X3	T45.8X4	T45.8X5	T45.8X6
Hemlock	T62.2X1	T62.2X2	T62.2X3	T62.2X4	—	—
Hemostatic	T45.621	T45.622	T45.623	T45.624	T45.625	T45.626
drug, systemic	T45.621	T45.622	T45.623	T45.624	T45.625	T45.626
Hemostyptic	T49.4X1	T49.4X2	T49.4X3	T49.4X4	T49.4X5	T49.4X6
Henbane	T62.2X1	T62.2X2	T62.2X3	T62.2X4	—	—
Heparin (sodium)	T45.511	T45.512	T45.513	T45.514	T45.515	T45.516
action reverser	T45.7X1	T45.7X2	T45.7X3	T45.7X4	T45.7X5	T45.7X6
Heparin-fraction	T45.511	T45.512	T45.513	T45.514	T45.515	T45.516
Heparinoid (systemic)	T45.511	T45.512	T45.513	T45.514	T45.515	T45.516
Hepatic secretion stimulant	T47.8X1	T47.8X2	T47.8X3	T47.8X4	T47.8X5	T47.8X6
Hepatitis B						
immune globulin	T50.Z11	T50.Z12	T50.Z13	T50.Z14	T50.Z15	T50.Z16
vaccine	T50.B91	T50.B92	T50.B93	T50.B94	T50.B95	T50.B96
Hepronicate	T46.7X1	T46.7X2	T46.7X3	T46.7X4	T46.7X5	T46.7X6
Heptabarb	T42.3X1	T42.3X2	T42.3X3	T42.3X4	T42.3X5	T42.3X6
Heptabarbitone	T42.3X1	T42.3X2	T42.3X3	T42.3X4	T42.3X5	T42.3X6
Heptabarbital	T42.3X1	T42.3X2	T42.3X3	T42.3X4	T42.3X5	T42.3X6
Heptachlor	T60.1X1	T60.1X2	T60.1X3	T60.1X4	—	—
Heptalgin	T40.2X1	T40.2X2	T40.2X3	T40.2X4	T40.2X5	T40.2X6
Heptaminol	T46.3X1	T46.3X2	T46.3X3	T46.3X4	T46.3X5	T46.3X6
Herbicide NEC	T60.3X1	T60.3X2	T60.3X3	T60.3X4	—	—
Heroin	T40.1X1	T40.1X2	T40.1X3	T40.1X4	—	—
Herplex	T49.5X1	T49.5X2	T49.5X3	T49.5X4	T49.5X5	T49.5X6
HES	T45.8X1	T45.8X2	T45.8X3	T45.8X4	T45.8X5	T45.8X6
Hesperidin	T46.991	T46.992	T46.993	T46.994	T46.995	T46.996
Hetacillin	T36.0X1	T36.0X2	T36.0X3	T36.0X4	T36.0X5	T36.0X6

◀ New   ◀ Revised   ~~deleted~~ Deleted

Substance	Poisoning, Accidental (Unintentional)	Poisoning, Intentional Self-Harm	Poisoning, Assault	Poisoning, Undetermined	Adverse Effect	Underdosing
Hetastarch	T45.8X1	T45.8X2	T45.8X3	T45.8X4	T45.8X5	T45.8X6
HETP	T60.0X1	T60.0X2	T60.0X3	T60.0X4	—	—
Hexachlorobenzene (vapor)	T60.3X1	T60.3X2	T60.3X3	T60.3X4	—	—
Hexachlorocyclohexane	T53.6X1	T53.6X2	T53.6X3	T53.6X4	—	—
Hexachlorophene	T49.0X1	T49.0X2	T49.0X3	T49.0X4	T49.0X5	T49.0X6
Hexadiline	T46.3X1	T46.3X2	T46.3X3	T46.3X4	T46.3X5	T46.3X6
Hexadimethrine (bromide)	T45.7X1	T45.7X2	T45.7X3	T45.7X4	T45.7X5	T45.7X6
Hexadylamine	T46.3X1	T46.3X2	T46.3X3	T46.3X4	T46.3X5	T46.3X6
Hexaethyl tetraphosphate	T60.0X1	T60.0X2	T60.0X3	T60.0X4	—	—
Hexafluorenium bromide	T48.1X1	T48.1X2	T48.1X3	T48.1X4	T48.1X5	T48.1X6
Hexafluorodiethyl ether	T43.291	T43.292	T43.293	T43.294	T43.295	T43.296
Hexafluronium (bromide)	T48.1X1	T48.1X2	T48.1X3	T48.1X4	T48.1X5	T48.1X6
Hexahydrobenzol	T52.8X1	T52.8X2	T52.8X3	T52.8X4	—	—
Hexahydrocresol(s)	T51.8X1	T51.8X2	T51.8X3	T51.8X4	—	—
arsenide	T57.0X1	T57.0X2	T57.0X3	T57.0X4	—	—
arseniurated	T57.0X1	T57.0X2	T57.0X3	T57.0X4	—	—
cyanide	T57.3X1	T57.3X2	T57.3X3	T57.3X4	—	—
gas	T59.891	T59.892	T59.893	T59.894	—	—
Fluoride (liquid)	T57.8X1	T57.8X2	T57.8X3	T57.8X4	—	—
vapor	T59.891	T59.892	T59.893	T59.894	—	—
phophorated	T60.0X1	T60.0X2	T60.0X3	T60.0X4	—	—
sulfate	T57.8X1	T57.8X2	T57.8X3	T57.8X4	—	—
sulfide (gas)	T59.6X1	T59.6X2	T59.6X3	T59.6X4	—	—
arseniurated	T57.0X1	T57.0X2	T57.0X3	T57.0X4	—	—
sulfurated	T57.8X1	T57.8X2	T57.8X3	T57.8X4	—	—
Hexahydrophenol	T51.8X1	T51.8X2	T51.8X3	T51.8X4	—	—
Hexa-germ	T49.2X1	T49.2X2	T49.2X3	T49.2X4	T49.2X5	T49.2X6
Hexalen	T51.8X1	T51.8X2	T51.8X3	T51.8X4	—	—
Hexamethonium bromide	T44.2X1	T44.2X2	T44.2X3	T44.2X4	T44.2X5	T44.2X6
Hexamethylene	T52.8X1	T52.8X2	T52.8X3	T52.8X4	—	—
Hexamethylmelamine	T45.1X1	T45.1X2	T45.1X3	T45.1X4	T45.1X5	T45.1X6
Hexamidine	T49.0X1	T49.0X2	T49.0X3	T49.0X4	T49.0X5	T49.0X6
Hexamine (mandelate)	T37.8X1	T37.8X2	T37.8X3	T37.8X4	T37.8X5	T37.8X6
Hexanone, 2-hexanone	T52.4X1	T52.4X2	T52.4X3	T52.4X4	—	—
Hexanuorenium	T48.1X1	T48.1X2	T48.1X3	T48.1X4	T48.1X5	T48.1X6
Hexapropymate	T42.6X1	T42.6X2	T42.6X3	T42.6X4	T42.6X5	T42.6X6
Hexasonium iodide	T44.3X1	T44.3X2	T44.3X3	T44.3X4	T44.3X5	T44.3X6
Hexcarbacholine bromide	T48.1X1	T48.1X2	T48.1X3	T48.1X4	T48.1X5	T48.1X6
Hexemal	T42.3X1	T42.3X2	T42.3X3	T42.3X4	T42.3X5	T42.3X6
Hexestrol	T38.5X1	T38.5X2	T38.5X3	T38.5X4	T38.5X5	T38.5X6
Hexethal (sodium)	T42.3X1	T42.3X2	T42.3X3	T42.3X4	T42.3X5	T42.3X6
Hexetidine	T37.8X1	T37.8X2	T37.8X3	T37.8X4	T37.8X5	T37.8X6

Substance	Poisoning, Accidental (Unintentional)	Poisoning, Intentional Self-Harm	Poisoning, Assault	Poisoning, Undetermined	Adverse Effect	Underdosing
Hexobarbital	T42.3X1	T42.3X2	T42.3X3	T42.3X4	T42.3X5	T42.3X6
rectal	T41.291	T41.292	T41.293	T41.294	T41.295	T41.296
sodium	T41.1X1	T41.1X2	T41.1X3	T41.1X4	T41.1X5	T41.1X6
Hexobendine	T46.3X1	T46.3X2	T46.3X3	T46.3X4	T46.3X5	T46.3X6
Hexocyclium	T44.3X1	T44.3X2	T44.3X3	T44.3X4	T44.3X5	T44.3X6
metilsulfate	T44.3X1	T44.3X2	T44.3X3	T44.3X4	T44.3X5	T44.3X6
Hexoestrol	T38.5X1	T38.5X2	T38.5X3	T38.5X4	T38.5X5	T38.5X6
Hexone	T52.4X1	T52.4X2	T52.4X3	T52.4X4	—	—
Hexoprenaline	T48.6X1	T48.6X2	T48.6X3	T48.6X4	T48.6X5	T48.6X6
Hexylcaine	T41.3X1	T41.3X2	T41.3X3	T41.3X4	T41.3X5	T41.3X6
Hexylresorcinol	T52.2X1	T52.2X2	T52.2X3	T52.2X4	—	—
HGH (human growth hormone)	T38.811	T38.812	T38.813	T38.814	T38.815	T38.816
Hinkle's pills	T47.2X1	T47.2X2	T47.2X3	T47.2X4	T47.2X5	T47.2X6
Histalog	T50.8X1	T50.8X2	T50.8X3	T50.8X4	T50.8X5	T50.8X6
Histamine (phosphate)	T50.8X1	T50.8X2	T50.8X3	T50.8X4	T50.8X5	T50.8X6
Histoplasmin	T50.8X1	T50.8X2	T50.8X3	T50.8X4	T50.8X5	T50.8X6
Holly berries	T62.2X1	T62.2X2	T62.2X3	T62.2X4	—	—
Homatropine	T44.3X1	T44.3X2	T44.3X3	T44.3X4	T44.3X5	T44.3X6
methylbromide	T44.3X1	T44.3X2	T44.3X3	T44.3X4	T44.3X5	T44.3X6
Homochlorcyclizine	T45.0X1	T45.0X2	T45.0X3	T45.0X4	T45.0X5	T45.0X6
Homosalate	T49.3X1	T49.3X2	T49.3X3	T49.3X4	T49.3X5	T49.3X6
Homo-tet	T50.Z11	T50.Z12	T50.Z13	T50.Z14	T50.Z15	T50.Z16
Hormone	T38.801	T38.802	T38.803	T38.804	T38.805	T38.806
adrenal cortical steroids	T38.0X1	T38.0X2	T38.0X3	T38.0X4	T38.0X5	T38.0X6
androgenic	T38.7X1	T38.7X2	T38.7X3	T38.7X4	T38.7X5	T38.7X6
anterior pituitary NEC	T38.811	T38.812	T38.813	T38.814	T38.815	T38.816
antidiabetic agents	T38.3X1	T38.3X2	T38.3X3	T38.3X4	T38.3X5	T38.3X6
antidiuretic	T38.891	T38.892	T38.893	T38.894	T38.895	T38.896
cancer therapy	T45.1X1	T45.1X2	T45.1X3	T45.1X4	T45.1X5	T45.1X6
follicle stimulating	T38.811	T38.812	T38.813	T38.814	T38.815	T38.816
gonadotropic	T38.891	T38.892	T38.893	T38.894	T38.895	T38.896
pituitary	T38.811	T38.812	T38.813	T38.814	T38.815	T38.816
growth	T38.811	T38.812	T38.813	T38.814	T38.815	T38.816
luteinizing	T38.811	T38.812	T38.813	T38.814	T38.815	T38.816
ovarian	T38.5X1	T38.5X2	T38.5X3	T38.5X4	T38.5X5	T38.5X6
oxytocic	T48.0X1	T48.0X2	T48.0X3	T48.0X4	T48.0X5	T48.0X6
parathyroid (derivatives)	T50.991	T50.992	T50.993	T50.994	T50.995	T50.996
pituitary (posterior) NEC	T38.891	T38.892	T38.893	T38.894	T38.895	T38.896
anterior	T38.811	T38.812	T38.813	T38.814	T38.815	T38.816
specified, NEC	T38.891	T38.892	T38.893	T38.894	T38.895	T38.896
thyroid	T38.1X1	T38.1X2	T38.1X3	T38.1X4	T38.1X5	T38.1X6
Hornet (sting)	T63.451	T63.452	T63.453	T63.454	—	—

Substance	Poisoning, Accidental (Unintentional)	Poisoning, Intentional Self-Harm	Poisoning, Assault	Poisoning, Undetermined	Adverse Effect	Underdosing
Horse anti-human lymphocytic serum	T50.Z11	T50.Z12	T50.Z13	T50.Z14	T50.Z15	T50.Z16
Horticulture agent NEC	T65.91	T65.92	T65.93	T65.94	—	—
with pesticide	T60.91	T60.92	T60.93	T60.94	—	—
Human						
albumin	T45.8X1	T45.8X2	T45.8X3	T45.8X4	T45.8X5	T45.8X6
growth hormone (HGH)	T38.811	T38.812	T38.813	T38.814	T38.815	T38.816
immune serum	T50.Z11	T50.Z12	T50.Z13	T50.Z14	T50.Z15	T50.Z16
Hyaluronidase	T45.3X1	T45.3X2	T45.3X3	T45.3X4	T45.3X5	T45.3X6
Hyazyme	T45.3X1	T45.3X2	T45.3X3	T45.3X4	T45.3X5	T45.3X6
Hycodan	T40.2X1	T40.2X2	T40.2X3	T40.2X4	T40.2X5	T40.2X6
Hydantoin derivative NEC	T42.0X1	T42.0X2	T42.0X3	T42.0X4	T42.0X5	T42.0X6
Hydeltra	T38.0X1	T38.0X2	T38.0X3	T38.0X4	T38.0X5	T38.0X6
Hydergine	T44.6X1	T44.6X2	T44.6X3	T44.6X4	T44.6X5	T44.6X6
Hydrabamine penicillin	T36.0X1	T36.0X2	T36.0X3	T36.0X4	T36.0X5	T36.0X6
Hydralazine	T46.5X1	T46.5X2	T46.5X3	T46.5X4	T46.5X5	T46.5X6
Hydrargaphen	T49.0X1	T49.0X2	T49.0X3	T49.0X4	T49.0X5	T49.0X6
Hydrargyri amino-chloridum	T49.0X1	T49.0X2	T49.0X3	T49.0X4	T49.0X5	T49.0X6
Hydrastine	T48.291	T48.292	T48.293	T48.294	T48.295	T48.296
Hydrazine	T54.1X1	T54.1X2	T54.1X3	T54.1X4	—	—
monoamine oxidase inhibitors	T43.1X1	T43.1X2	T43.1X3	T43.1X4	T43.1X5	T43.1X6
Hydrazoic acid, azides	T54.2X1	T54.2X2	T54.2X3	T54.2X4	—	—
Hydriodic acid	T48.4X1	T48.4X2	T48.4X3	T48.4X4	T48.4X5	T48.4X6
Hydrocarbon gas	T59.891	T59.892	T59.893	T59.894		
incomplete combustion of— *see Carbon, monoxide, fuel, utility*						
liquefied (mobile container)	T59.891	T59.892	T59.893	T59.894	—	—
piped (natural)	T59.891	T59.892	T59.893	T59.894	—	—
Hydrochloric acid (liquid)	T54.2X1	T54.2X2	T54.2X3	T54.2X4	—	—
medicinal (digestant)	T47.5X1	T47.5X2	T47.5X3	T47.5X4	T47.5X5	T47.5X6
vapor	T59.891	T59.892	T59.893	T59.894	—	—
Hydrochlorothiazide	T50.2X1	T50.2X2	T50.2X3	T50.2X4	T50.2X5	T50.2X6
Hydrocodone	T40.2X1	T40.2X2	T40.2X3	T40.2X4	T40.2X5	T40.2X6
Hydrocortisone (derivatives)	T38.0X1	T38.0X2	T38.0X3	T38.0X4	T38.0X5	T38.0X6
aceponate	T49.0X1	T49.0X2	T49.0X3	T49.0X4	T49.0X5	T49.0X6
ENT agent	T49.6X1	T49.6X2	T49.6X3	T49.6X4	T49.6X5	T49.6X6
ophthalmic preparation	T49.5X1	T49.5X2	T49.5X3	T49.5X4	T49.5X5	T49.5X6
topical NEC	T49.0X1	T49.0X2	T49.0X3	T49.0X4	T49.0X5	T49.0X6
Hydrocortone	T38.0X1	T38.0X2	T38.0X3	T38.0X4	T38.0X5	T38.0X6
ENT agent	T49.6X1	T49.6X2	T49.6X3	T49.6X4	T49.6X5	T49.6X6
ophthalmic preparation	T49.5X1	T49.5X2	T49.5X3	T49.5X4	T49.5X5	T49.5X6
topical NEC	T49.0X1	T49.0X2	T49.0X3	T49.0X4	T49.0X5	T49.0X6

Substance	Poisoning, Accidental (Unintentional)	Poisoning, Intentional Self-Harm	Poisoning, Assault	Poisoning, Undetermined	Adverse Effect	Underdosing
Hydrocyanic acid (liquid)	T57.3X1	T57.3X2	T57.3X3	T57.3X4	—	—
gas	T65.0X1	T65.0X2	T65.0X3	T65.0X4	—	—
Hydroflumethiazide	T50.2X1	T50.2X2	T50.2X3	T50.2X4	T50.2X5	T50.2X6
Hydrofluoric acid (liquid)	T54.2X1	T54.2X2	T54.2X3	T54.2X4	—	—
vapor	T59.891	T59.892	T59.893	T59.894	—	—
Hydrogen	T59.891	T59.892	T59.893	T59.894	—	—
arsenide	T57.0X1	T57.0X2	T57.0X3	T57.0X4	—	—
arseniureted	T57.0X1	T57.0X2	T57.0X3	T57.0X4	—	—
chloride	T57.8X1	T57.8X2	T57.8X3	T57.8X4	—	—
cyanide (salts)	T57.3X1	T57.3X2	T57.3X3	T57.3X4	—	—
gas	T57.3X1	T57.3X2	T57.3X3	T57.3X4	—	—
Fluoride	T59.5X1	T59.5X2	T59.5X3	T59.5X4	—	—
vapor	T59.5X1	T59.5X2	T59.5X3	T59.5X4	—	—
peroxide	T49.0X1	T49.0X2	T49.0X3	T49.0X4	T49.0X5	T49.0X6
phosphureted	T57.1X1	T57.1X2	T57.1X3	T57.1X4	—	—
sulfide	T59.6X1	T59.6X2	T59.6X3	T59.6X4	—	—
arseniureted	T57.0X1	T57.0X2	T57.0X3	T57.0X4	—	—
sulfureted	T59.6X1	T59.6X2	T59.6X3	T59.6X4	—	—
Hydromethylpyridine	T46.7X1	T46.7X2	T46.7X3	T46.7X4	T46.7X5	T46.7X6
Hydromorphinol	T40.2X1	T40.2X2	T40.2X3	T40.2X4	—	—
Hydromorphinone	T40.2X1	T40.2X2	T40.2X3	T40.2X4	T40.2X5	T40.2X6
Hydromorphone	T40.2X1	T40.2X2	T40.2X3	T40.2X4	T40.2X5	T40.2X6
Hydromox	T50.2X1	T50.2X2	T50.2X3	T50.2X4	T50.2X5	T50.2X6
Hydrophilic lotion	T49.3X1	T49.3X2	T49.3X3	T49.3X4	T49.3X5	T49.3X6
Hydroquinidine	T46.2X1	T46.2X2	T46.2X3	T46.2X4	T46.2X5	T46.2X6
Hydroquinone	T52.2X1	T52.2X2	T52.2X3	T52.2X4	—	—
vapor	T59.891	T59.892	T59.893	T59.894	—	—
Hydrosulfuric acid (gas)	T59.6X1	T59.6X2	T59.6X3	T59.6X4	—	—
Hydrotalcite	T47.1X1	T47.1X2	T47.1X3	T47.1X4	T47.1X5	T47.1X6
Hydrous wool fat	T49.3X1	T49.3X2	T49.3X3	T49.3X4	T49.3X5	T49.3X6
Hydroxide, caustic	T54.3X1	T54.3X2	T54.3X3	T54.3X4	—	—
Hydroxocobalamin	T45.8X1	T45.8X2	T45.8X3	T45.8X4	T45.8X5	T45.8X6
Hydroxyamphetamine	T49.5X1	T49.5X2	T49.5X3	T49.5X4	T49.5X5	T49.5X6
Hydroxycarbamide	T45.1X1	T45.1X2	T45.1X3	T45.1X4	T45.1X5	T45.1X6
Hydroxychloroquine	T37.8X1	T37.8X2	T37.8X3	T37.8X4	T37.8X5	T37.8X6
Hydroxydihydrocodeinone	T40.2X1	T40.2X2	T40.2X3	T40.2X4	T40.2X5	T40.2X6
Hydroxyestrone	T38.5X1	T38.5X2	T38.5X3	T38.5X4	T38.5X5	T38.5X6
Hydroxyethyl starch	T45.8X1	T45.8X2	T45.8X3	T45.8X4	T45.8X5	T45.8X6
Hydroxymethylpentanone	T52.4X1	T52.4X2	T52.4X3	T52.4X4	—	—
Hydroxyphenamate	T43.591	T43.592	T43.593	T43.594	T43.595	T43.596
Hydroxyphenylbutazone	T39.2X1	T39.2X2	T39.2X3	T39.2X4	T39.2X5	T39.2X6

◄ New   ◄ Revised   ~~deleted~~ Deleted

Substance	Poisoning, Accidental (Unintentional)	Poisoning, Intentional Self-Harm	Poisoning, Assault	Poisoning, Undetermined	Adverse Effect	Underdosing
Hydroxyprogesterone	T38.5X1	T38.5X2	T38.5X3	T38.5X4	T38.5X5	T38.5X6
caproate	T38.5X1	T38.5X2	T38.5X3	T38.5X4	T38.5X5	T38.5X6
Hydroxyquinoline (derivatives) NEC	T37.8X1	T37.8X2	T37.8X3	T37.8X4	T37.8X5	T37.8X6
Hydroxystilbamidine	T37.3X1	T37.3X2	T37.3X3	T37.3X4	T37.3X5	T37.3X6
Hydroxytoluene (nonmedicinal)	T54.0X1	T54.0X2	T54.0X3	T54.0X4	—	—
medicinal	T49.0X1	T49.0X2	T49.0X3	T49.0X4	T49.0X5	T49.0X6
Hydroxyurea	T45.1X1	T45.1X2	T45.1X3	T45.1X4	T45.1X5	T45.1X6
Hydroxyzine	T43.591	T43.592	T43.593	T43.594	T43.595	T43.596
antiallergic	T45.0X1	T45.0X2	T45.0X3	T45.0X4	T45.0X5	T45.0X6
Hyoscine	T44.3X1	T44.3X2	T44.3X3	T44.3X4	T44.3X5	T44.3X6
Hyoscyamine	T44.3X1	T44.3X2	T44.3X3	T44.3X4	T44.3X5	T44.3X6
Hyoscyamus	T44.3X1	T44.3X2	T44.3X3	T44.3X4	T44.3X5	T44.3X6
dry extract	T44.3X1	T44.3X2	T44.3X3	T44.3X4	T44.3X5	T44.3X6
Hypaque	T50.8X1	T50.8X2	T50.8X3	T50.8X4	T50.8X5	T50.8X6
Hypertussis	T50.Z11	T50.Z12	T50.Z13	T50.Z14	T50.Z15	T50.Z16
Hypnotic	T42.71	T42.72	T42.73	T42.74	T42.75	T42.76
anticonvulsant	T42.71	T42.72	T42.73	T42.74	T42.75	T42.76
specified NEC	T42.6X1	T42.6X2	T42.6X3	T42.6X4	T42.6X5	T42.6X6
Hypochlorite	T49.0X1	T49.0X2	T49.0X3	T49.0X4	T49.0X5	T49.0X6
Hypophysis, posterior	T38.891	T38.892	T38.893	T38.894	T38.895	T38.896
Hypotensive NEC	T46.5X1	T46.5X2	T46.5X3	T46.5X4	T46.5X5	T46.5X6
Hypromellose	T49.5X1	T49.5X2	T49.5X3	T49.5X4	T49.5X5	T49.5X6

I

Substance	Poisoning, Accidental (Unintentional)	Poisoning, Intentional Self-Harm	Poisoning, Assault	Poisoning, Undetermined	Adverse Effect	Underdosing
Ibacitabine	T37.5X1	T37.5X2	T37.5X3	T37.5X4	T37.5X5	T37.5X6
Ibopamine	T44.991	T44.992	T44.993	T44.994	T44.995	T44.996
Ibufenac	T39.311	T39.312	T39.313	T39.314	T39.315	T39.316
Ibuprofen	T39.311	T39.312	T39.313	T39.314	T39.315	T39.316
Ibuproxam	T39.311	T39.312	T39.313	T39.314	T39.315	T39.316
Ibuterol	T48.6X1	T48.6X2	T48.6X3	T48.6X4	T48.6X5	T48.6X6
Ichthammol	T49.0X1	T49.0X2	T49.0X3	T49.0X4	T49.0X5	T49.0X6
Ichthyol	T49.4X1	T49.4X2	T49.4X3	T49.4X4	T49.4X5	T49.4X6
Idarubicin	T45.1X1	T45.1X2	T45.1X3	T45.1X4	T45.1X5	T45.1X6
Idrocilamide	T42.8X1	T42.8X2	T42.8X3	T42.8X4	T42.8X5	T42.8X6
Ifenprodil	T46.7X1	T46.7X2	T46.7X3	T46.7X4	T46.7X5	T46.7X6
Ifosfamide	T45.1X1	T45.1X2	T45.1X3	T45.1X4	T45.1X5	T45.1X6
Iletin	T38.3X1	T38.3X2	T38.3X3	T38.3X4	T38.3X5	T38.3X6
Ilex	T62.2X1	T62.2X2	T62.2X3	T62.2X4	—	—
Illuminating gas (after combustion)	T58.11	T58.12	T58.13	T58.14	—	—
prior to combustion	T59.891	T59.892	T59.893	T59.894	—	—
Ilopan	T45.2X1	T45.2X2	T45.2X3	T45.2X4	T45.2X5	T45.2X6

Substance	Poisoning, Accidental (Unintentional)	Poisoning, Intentional Self-Harm	Poisoning, Assault	Poisoning, Undetermined	Adverse Effect	Underdosing
Iloprost	T46.7X1	T46.7X2	T46.7X3	T46.7X4	T46.7X5	T46.7X6
Ilotycin	T36.3X1	T36.3X2	T36.3X3	T36.3X4	T36.3X5	T36.3X6
ophthalmic preparation	T49.5X1	T49.5X2	T49.5X3	T49.5X4	T49.5X5	T49.5X6
topical NEC	T49.0X1	T49.0X2	T49.0X3	T49.0X4	T49.0X5	T49.0X6
Imidazole-4-carboxamide	T45.1X1	T45.1X2	T45.1X3	T45.1X4	T45.1X5	T45.1X6
Imipenem	T36.0X1	T36.0X2	T36.0X3	T36.0X4	T36.0X5	T36.0X6
Imipramine	T43.011	T43.012	T43.013	T43.014	T43.015	T43.016
Iminostilbene	T42.1X1	T42.1X2	T42.1X3	T42.1X4	T42.1X5	T42.1X6
Immu-G	T50.Z11	T50.Z12	T50.Z13	T50.Z14	T50.Z15	T50.Z16
Immuglobin	T50.Z11	T50.Z12	T50.Z13	T50.Z14	T50.Z15	T50.Z16
Immune						
checkpoint inhibitors	T45.AX1	T45.AX2	T45.AX3	T45.AX4	T45.AX5	T45.AX6
globulin	T50.Z11	T50.Z12	T50.Z13	T50.Z14	T50.Z15	T50.Z16
serum globulin	T50.Z11	T50.Z12	T50.Z13	T50.Z14	T50.Z15	T50.Z16
Immunoglobin human (intravenous) (normal)	T50.Z11	T50.Z12	T50.Z13	T50.Z14	T50.Z15	T50.Z16
unmodified	T50.Z11	T50.Z12	T50.Z13	T50.Z14	T50.Z15	T50.Z16
Immunostimulant drug	T45.AX1	T45.AX2	T45.AX3	T45.AX4	T45.AX5	T45.AX6
Immunosuppressive drug	T45.1X1	T45.1X2	T45.1X3	T45.1X4	T45.1X5	T45.1X6
Immu-tetanus	T50.Z11	T50.Z12	T50.Z13	T50.Z14	T50.Z15	T50.Z16
Indalpine	T43.221	T43.222	T43.223	T43.224	T43.225	T43.226
Indanazoline	T48.5X1	T48.5X2	T48.5X3	T48.5X4	T48.5X5	T48.5X6
Indandione (derivatives)	T45.511	T45.512	T45.513	T45.514	T45.515	T45.516
Indapamide	T46.5X1	T46.5X2	T46.5X3	T46.5X4	T46.5X5	T46.5X6
Indendione (derivatives)	T45.511	T45.512	T45.513	T45.514	T45.515	T45.516
Indenolol	T44.7X1	T44.7X2	T44.7X3	T44.7X4	T44.7X5	T44.7X6
Inderal	T44.7X1	T44.7X2	T44.7X3	T44.7X4	T44.7X5	T44.7X6
Indian						
hemp	T40.711	T40.712	T40.713	T40.714	T40.715	T40.716
tobacco	T62.2X1	T62.2X2	T62.2X3	T62.2X4	—	—
Indigo carmine	T50.8X1	T50.8X2	T50.8X3	T50.8X4	T50.8X5	T50.8X6
Indobufen	T45.521	T45.522	T45.523	T45.524	T45.525	T45.526
Indocin	T39.2X1	T39.2X2	T39.2X3	T39.2X4	T39.2X5	T39.2X6
Indocyanine green	T50.8X1	T50.8X2	T50.8X3	T50.8X4	T50.8X5	T50.8X6
Indometacin	T39.391	T39.392	T39.393	T39.394	T39.395	T39.396
Indomethacin	T39.391	T39.392	T39.393	T39.394	T39.395	T39.396
farnesil	T39.4X1	T39.4X2	T39.4X3	T39.4X4	T39.4X5	T39.4X6
Indoramin	T44.6X1	T44.6X2	T44.6X3	T44.6X4	T44.6X5	T44.6X6
Industrial						
alcohol	T51.0X1	T51.0X2	T51.0X3	T51.0X4	—	—
fumes	T59.891	T59.892	T59.893	T59.894	—	—
solvents (fumes) (vapors)	T52.91	T52.92	T52.93	T52.94	—	—
Influenza vaccine	T50.B91	T50.B92	T50.B93	T50.B94	T50.B95	T50.B96

TABLE OF DRUGS AND CHEMICALS

Substance	External Cause (T-Code) Poisoning, Accidental (Unintentional)	Poisoning, Intentional Self-Harm	Poisoning, Assault	Poisoning, Undetermined	Adverse Effect	Underdosing
Ingested substance NEC	T65.91	T65.92	T65.93	T65.94	—	—
INH	T37.1X1	T37.1X2	T37.1X3	T37.1X4	T37.1X5	T37.1X6
Inhalation, gas (noxious) — *see Gas*						
Inhibitor						
angiotensin-converting enzyme	T46.4X1	T46.4X2	T46.4X3	T46.4X4	T46.4X5	T46.4X6
carbonic anhydrase	T50.2X1	T50.2X2	T50.2X3	T50.2X4	T50.2X5	T50.2X6
fibrinolysis	T45.621	T45.622	T45.623	T45.624	T45.625	T45.626
monoamine oxidase NEC	T43.1X1	T43.1X2	T43.1X3	T43.1X4	T43.1X5	T43.1X6
hydrazine	T43.1X1	T43.1X2	T43.1X3	T43.1X4	T43.1X5	T43.1X6
postsynaptic	T43.8X1	T43.8X2	T43.8X3	T43.8X4	T43.8X5	T43.8X6
prothrombin synthesis	T45.511	T45.512	T45.513	T45.514	T45.515	T45.516
Ink	T65.891	T65.892	T65.893	T65.894	—	—
Inorganic substance NEC	T57.91	T57.92	T57.93	T57.94	—	—
Inosine pranobex	T37.5X1	T37.5X2	T37.5X3	T37.5X4	T37.5X5	T37.5X6
Inositol	T50.991	T50.992	T50.993	T50.994	T50.995	T50.996
nicotinate	T46.7X1	T46.7X2	T46.7X3	T46.7X4	T46.7X5	T46.7X6
Inproquone	T45.1X1	T45.1X2	T45.1X3	T45.1X4	T45.1X5	T45.1X6
Insect (sting), venomous	T63.481	T63.482	T63.483	T63.484	—	—
ant	T63.421	T63.422	T63.423	T63.424	—	—
bee	T63.441	T63.442	T63.443	T63.444	—	—
caterpillar	T63.431	T63.432	T63.433	T63.434	—	—
hornet	T63.451	T63.452	T63.453	T63.454	—	—
wasp	T63.461	T63.462	T63.463	T63.464	—	—
Insecticide NEC	T60.91	T60.92	T60.93	T60.94	—	—
carbamate	T60.0X1	T60.0X2	T60.0X3	T60.0X4	—	—
chlorinated	T60.1X1	T60.1X2	T60.1X3	T60.1X4	—	—
mixed	T60.91	T60.92	T60.93	T60.94	—	—
organochlorine	T60.1X1	T60.1X2	T60.1X3	T60.1X4	—	—
organophosphorus	T60.0X1	T60.0X2	T60.0X3	T60.0X4	—	—
Insular tissue extract	T38.3X1	T38.3X2	T38.3X3	T38.3X4	T38.3X5	T38.3X6
Insulin (amorphous) (globin) (isophane) (Lente) (NPH) (Semilente) (Ultralente)	T38.3X1	T38.3X2	T38.3X3	T38.3X4	T38.3X5	T38.3X6
defalan	T38.3X1	T38.3X2	T38.3X3	T38.3X4	T38.3X5	T38.3X6
human	T38.3X1	T38.3X2	T38.3X3	T38.3X4	T38.3X5	T38.3X6
injection, soluble	T38.3X1	T38.3X2	T38.3X3	T38.3X4	T38.3X5	T38.3X6
biphasic	T38.3X1	T38.3X2	T38.3X3	T38.3X4	T38.3X5	T38.3X6
intermediate acting	T38.3X1	T38.3X2	T38.3X3	T38.3X4	T38.3X5	T38.3X6
protamine zinc	T38.3X1	T38.3X2	T38.3X3	T38.3X4	T38.3X5	T38.3X6
slow acting	T38.3X1	T38.3X2	T38.3X3	T38.3X4	T38.3X5	T38.3X6

Substance	External Cause (T-Code) Poisoning, Accidental (Unintentional)	Poisoning, Intentional Self-Harm	Poisoning, Assault	Poisoning, Undetermined	Adverse Effect	Underdosing
zinc						
protamine injection	T38.3X1	T38.3X2	T38.3X3	T38.3X4	T38.3X5	T38.3X6
suspension (amorphous) (crystalline)	T38.3X1	T38.3X2	T38.3X3	T38.3X4	T38.3X5	T38.3X6
Interferon (alpha) (beta) (gamma)	T37.5X1	T37.5X2	T37.5X3	T37.5X4	T37.5X5	T37.5X6
Intestinal motility control drug	T47.6X1	T47.6X2	T47.6X3	T47.6X4	T47.6X5	T47.6X6
biological	T47.8X1	T47.8X2	T47.8X3	T47.8X4	T47.8X5	T47.8X6
Intranarcon	T41.1X1	T41.1X2	T41.1X3	T41.1X4	T41.1X5	T41.1X6
Intravenous						
amino acids	T50.991	T50.992	T50.993	T50.994	T50.995	T50.996
fat suspension	T50.991	T50.992	T50.993	T50.994	T50.995	T50.996
Inulin	T50.8X1	T50.8X2	T50.8X3	T50.8X4	T50.8X5	T50.8X6
Invert sugar	T50.3X1	T50.3X2	T50.3X3	T50.3X4	T50.3X5	T50.3X6
Inza — *see Naproxen*						
Iobenzamic acid	T50.8X1	T50.8X2	T50.8X3	T50.8X4	T50.8X5	T50.8X6
Iocarmic acid	T50.8X1	T50.8X2	T50.8X3	T50.8X4	T50.8X5	T50.8X6
Iocetamic acid	T50.8X1	T50.8X2	T50.8X3	T50.8X4	T50.8X5	T50.8X6
Iodamide	T50.8X1	T50.8X2	T50.8X3	T50.8X4	T50.8X5	T50.8X6
Iodide NEC — *see also Iodine*	T49.0X1	T49.0X2	T49.0X3	T49.0X4	T49.0X5	T49.0X6
mercury (ointment)	T49.0X1	T49.0X2	T49.0X3	T49.0X4	T49.0X5	T49.0X6
methylate	T49.0X1	T49.0X2	T49.0X3	T49.0X4	T49.0X5	T49.0X6
potassium (expectorant) NEC	T48.4X1	T48.4X2	T48.4X3	T48.4X4	T48.4X5	T48.4X6
Iodinated						
contrast medium	T50.8X1	T50.8X2	T50.8X3	T50.8X4	T50.8X5	T50.8X6
glycerol	T48.4X1	T48.4X2	T48.4X3	T48.4X4	T48.4X5	T48.4X6
human serum albumin (131I)	T50.8X1	T50.8X2	T50.8X3	T50.8X4	T50.8X5	T50.8X6
Iodine (antiseptic, external) (tincture) NEC	T49.0X1	T49.0X2	T49.0X3	T49.0X4	T49.0X5	T49.0X6
125 — *see also Radiation sickness, and Exposure to radioactive isotopes*						
therapeutic	T50.991	T50.992	T50.993	T50.994	T50.995	T50.996
131 — *see also Radiation sickness, and Exposure to radioactive isotopes*						
therapeutic	T38.2X1	T38.2X2	T38.2X3	T38.2X4	T38.2X5	T38.2X6
diagnostic	T50.8X1	T50.8X2	T50.8X3	T50.8X4	T50.8X5	T50.8X6
for thyroid conditions (antithyroid)	T38.2X1	T38.2X2	T38.2X3	T38.2X4	T38.2X5	T38.2X6
solution	T49.0X1	T49.0X2	T49.0X3	T49.0X4	T49.0X5	T49.0X6
vapor	T59.891	T59.892	T59.893	T59.894	—	—
Iodipamide	T50.8X1	T50.8X2	T50.8X3	T50.8X4	T50.8X5	T50.8X6
Iodized (poppy seed) oil	T50.8X1	T50.8X2	T50.8X3	T50.8X4	T50.8X5	T50.8X6
Iodobismitol	T37.8X1	T37.8X2	T37.8X3	T37.8X4	T37.8X5	T37.8X6

◀ New   ◀ Revised   ~~deleted~~ Deleted

Substance	Poisoning, Accidental (Unintentional)	Poisoning, Intentional Self-Harm	Poisoning, Assault	Poisoning, Undetermined	Adverse Effect	Underdosing
Iodochlorhydroxyquin	T37.8X1	T37.8X2	T37.8X3	T37.8X4	T37.8X5	T37.8X6
topical	T49.0X1	T49.0X2	T49.0X3	T49.0X4	T49.0X5	T49.0X6
Iodochlorhydroxyquino-line	T37.8X1	T37.8X2	T37.8X3	T37.8X4	T37.8X5	T37.8X6
Iodocholesterol (1311)	T50.8X1	T50.8X2	T50.8X3	T50.8X4	T50.8X5	T50.8X6
Iodoform	T49.0X1	T49.0X2	T49.0X3	T49.0X4	T49.0X5	T49.0X6
Iodohippuric acid	T50.8X1	T50.8X2	T50.8X3	T50.8X4	T50.8X5	T50.8X6
Iodopanoic acid	T50.8X1	T50.8X2	T50.8X3	T50.8X4	T50.8X5	T50.8X6
Iodophthalein (sodium)	T50.8X1	T50.8X2	T50.8X3	T50.8X4	T50.8X5	T50.8X6
Iodopyracet	T50.8X1	T50.8X2	T50.8X3	T50.8X4	T50.8X5	T50.8X6
Iodoquinol	T37.8X1	T37.8X2	T37.8X3	T37.8X4	T37.8X5	T37.8X6
Iodoxamic acid	T50.8X1	T50.8X2	T50.8X3	T50.8X4	T50.8X5	T50.8X6
Iofendylate	T50.8X1	T50.8X2	T50.8X3	T50.8X4	T50.8X5	T50.8X6
Ioglycamic acid	T50.8X1	T50.8X2	T50.8X3	T50.8X4	T50.8X5	T50.8X6
Iohexol	T50.8X1	T50.8X2	T50.8X3	T50.8X4	T50.8X5	T50.8X6
Ion exchange resin						
anion	T47.8X1	T47.8X2	T47.8X3	T47.8X4	T47.8X5	T47.8X6
cation	T50.3X1	T50.3X2	T50.3X3	T50.3X4	T50.3X5	T50.3X6
cholestyramine	T46.6X1	T46.6X2	T46.6X3	T46.6X4	T46.6X5	T46.6X6
intestinal	T47.8X1	T47.8X2	T47.8X3	T47.8X4	T47.8X5	T47.8X6
Iopamidol	T50.8X1	T50.8X2	T50.8X3	T50.8X4	T50.8X5	T50.8X6
Iopanoic acid	T50.8X1	T50.8X2	T50.8X3	T50.8X4	T50.8X5	T50.8X6
Iophenoic acid	T50.8X1	T50.8X2	T50.8X3	T50.8X4	T50.8X5	T50.8X6
Iopodate, sodium	T50.8X1	T50.8X2	T50.8X3	T50.8X4	T50.8X5	T50.8X6
Iopodic acid	T50.8X1	T50.8X2	T50.8X3	T50.8X4	T50.8X5	T50.8X6
Iopromide	T50.8X1	T50.8X2	T50.8X3	T50.8X4	T50.8X5	T50.8X6
Iopydol	T50.8X1	T50.8X2	T50.8X3	T50.8X4	T50.8X5	T50.8X6
Iotalamic acid	T50.8X1	T50.8X2	T50.8X3	T50.8X4	T50.8X5	T50.8X6
Iothalamate	T50.8X1	T50.8X2	T50.8X3	T50.8X4	T50.8X5	T50.8X6
Iothiouracil	T38.2X1	T38.2X2	T38.2X3	T38.2X4	T38.2X5	T38.2X6
Iotrol	T50.8X1	T50.8X2	T50.8X3	T50.8X4	T50.8X5	T50.8X6
Iotrolan	T50.8X1	T50.8X2	T50.8X3	T50.8X4	T50.8X5	T50.8X6
Iotroxate	T50.8X1	T50.8X2	T50.8X3	T50.8X4	T50.8X5	T50.8X6
Iotroxic acid	T50.8X1	T50.8X2	T50.8X3	T50.8X4	T50.8X5	T50.8X6
Ioversol	T50.8X1	T50.8X2	T50.8X3	T50.8X4	T50.8X5	T50.8X6
Ioxaglate	T50.8X1	T50.8X2	T50.8X3	T50.8X4	T50.8X5	T50.8X6
Ioxaglic acid	T50.8X1	T50.8X2	T50.8X3	T50.8X4	T50.8X5	T50.8X6
Ioxitalamic acid	T50.8X1	T50.8X2	T50.8X3	T50.8X4	T50.8X5	T50.8X6
Ipecac	T47.7X1	T47.7X2	T47.7X3	T47.7X4	T47.7X5	T47.7X6
Ipecacuanha	T48.4X1	T48.4X2	T48.4X3	T48.4X4	T48.4X5	T48.4X6
Ipodate, calcium	T50.8X1	T50.8X2	T50.8X3	T50.8X4	T50.8X5	T50.8X6
Ipral	T42.3X1	T42.3X2	T42.3X3	T42.3X4	T42.3X5	T42.3X6
Ipratropium (bromide)	T48.6X1	T48.6X2	T48.6X3	T48.6X4	T48.6X5	T48.6X6

Substance	Poisoning, Accidental (Unintentional)	Poisoning, Intentional Self-Harm	Poisoning, Assault	Poisoning, Undetermined	Adverse Effect	Underdosing
Ipriflavone	T46.3X1	T46.3X2	T46.3X3	T46.3X4	T46.3X5	T46.3X6
Iprindole	T43.011	T43.012	T43.013	T43.014	T43.015	T43.016
Iproclozide	T43.1X1	T43.1X2	T43.1X3	T43.1X4	T43.1X5	T43.1X6
Iprofenin	T50.8X1	T50.8X2	T50.8X3	T50.8X4	T50.8X5	T50.8X6
Iproheptine	T49.2X1	T49.2X2	T49.2X3	T49.2X4	T49.2X5	T49.2X6
Iproniazid	T43.1X1	T43.1X2	T43.1X3	T43.1X4	T43.1X5	T43.1X6
Iproplatin	T45.1X1	T45.1X2	T45.1X3	T45.1X4	T45.1X5	T45.1X6
Iproveratril	T46.1X1	T46.1X2	T46.1X3	T46.1X4	T46.1X5	T46.1X6
Iron (compounds) (medicinal) NEC	T45.4X1	T45.4X2	T45.4X3	T45.4X4	T45.4X5	T45.4X6
ammonium	T45.4X1	T45.4X2	T45.4X3	T45.4X4	T45.4X5	T45.4X6
dextran injection	T45.4X1	T45.4X2	T45.4X3	T45.4X4	T45.4X5	T45.4X6
nonmedicinal	T56.891	T56.892	T56.893	T56.894	—	—
salts	T45.4X1	T45.4X2	T45.4X3	T45.4X4	T45.4X5	T45.4X6
sorbitex	T45.4X1	T45.4X2	T45.4X3	T45.4X4	T45.4X5	T45.4X6
sorbitol citric acid complex	T45.4X1	T45.4X2	T45.4X3	T45.4X4	T45.4X5	T45.4X6
Irrigating fluid (vaginal)	T49.8X1	T49.8X2	T49.8X3	T49.8X4	T49.8X5	T49.8X6
eye	T49.5X1	T49.5X2	T49.5X3	T49.5X4	T49.5X5	T49.5X6
Isepamicin	T36.5X1	T36.5X2	T36.5X3	T36.5X4	T36.5X5	T36.5X6
Isoaminile (citrate)	T48.3X1	T48.3X2	T48.3X3	T48.3X4	T48.3X5	T48.3X6
Isoamyl nitrite	T46.3X1	T46.3X2	T46.3X3	T46.3X4	T46.3X5	T46.3X6
Isobenzan	T60.1X1	T60.1X2	T60.1X3	T60.1X4	—	—
Isobutyl acetate	T52.8X1	T52.8X2	T52.8X3	T52.8X4	—	—
Isocarboxazid	T43.1X1	T43.1X2	T43.1X3	T43.1X4	T43.1X5	T43.1X6
Isoconazole	T49.0X1	T49.0X2	T49.0X3	T49.0X4	T49.0X5	T49.0X6
Isocyanate	T65.0X1	T65.0X2	T65.0X3	T65.0X4	—	
Isoephedrine	T44.991	T44.992	T44.993	T44.994	T44.995	T44.996
Isoetarine	T48.6X1	T48.6X2	T48.6X3	T48.6X4	T48.6X5	T48.6X6
Isoethadione	T42.2X1	T42.2X2	T42.2X3	T42.2X4	T42.2X5	T42.2X6
Isoetharine	T44.5X1	T44.5X2	T44.5X3	T44.5X4	T44.5X5	T44.5X6
Isoflurane	T41.0X1	T41.0X2	T41.0X3	T41.0X4	T41.0X5	T41.0X6
Isoflurophate	T44.0X1	T44.0X2	T44.0X3	T44.0X4	T44.0X5	T44.0X6
Isomaltose, ferric complex	T45.4X1	T45.4X2	T45.4X3	T45.4X4	T45.4X5	T45.4X6
Isometheptene	T44.3X1	T44.3X2	T44.3X3	T44.3X4	T44.3X5	T44.3X6
Isoniazid	T37.1X1	T37.1X2	T37.1X3	T37.1X4	T37.1X5	T37.1X6
with						
rifampicin	T36.6X1	T36.6X2	T36.6X3	T36.6X4	T36.6X5	T36.6X6
thioacetazone	T37.1X1	T37.1X2	T37.1X3	T37.1X4	T37.1X5	T37.1X6
Isonicotinic acid hydrazide	T37.1X1	T37.1X2	T37.1X3	T37.1X4	T37.1X5	T37.1X6
Isonipecaine	T40.491	T40.492	T40.493	T40.494	T40.495	T40.496
Isopentaquine	T37.2X1	T37.2X2	T37.2X3	T37.2X4	T37.2X5	T37.2X6
Isophane insulin	T38.3X1	T38.3X2	T38.3X3	T38.3X4	T38.3X5	T38.3X6
Isophorone	T65.891	T65.892	T65.893	T65.894	—	—

Substance	Poisoning, Accidental (Unintentional)	Poisoning, Intentional Self-Harm	Poisoning, Assault	Poisoning, Undetermined	Adverse Effect	Underdosing
Isophosphamide	T45.1X1	T45.1X2	T45.1X3	T45.1X4	T45.1X5	T45.1X6
Isopregnenone	T38.5X1	T38.5X2	T38.5X3	T38.5X4	T38.5X5	T38.5X6
Isoprenaline	T48.6X1	T48.6X2	T48.6X3	T48.6X4	T48.6X5	T48.6X6
Isopromethazine	T43.3X1	T43.3X2	T43.3X3	T43.3X4	T43.3X5	T43.3X6
Isopropamide	T44.3X1	T44.3X2	T44.3X3	T44.3X4	T44.3X5	T44.3X6
iodide	T44.3X1	T44.3X2	T44.3X3	T44.3X4	T44.3X5	T44.3X6
Isopropanol	T51.2X1	T51.2X2	T51.2X3	T51.2X4	—	—
Isopropyl						
acetate	T52.8X1	T52.8X2	T52.8X3	T52.8X4	—	—
alcohol	T51.2X1	T51.2X2	T51.2X3	T51.2X4	—	—
medicinal	T49.4X1	T49.4X2	T49.4X3	T49.4X4	T49.4X5	T49.4X6
ether	T52.8X1	T52.8X2	T52.8X3	T52.8X4	—	—
Isopropylaminophena-zone	T39.2X1	T39.2X2	T39.2X3	T39.2X4	T39.2X5	T39.2X6
Isoproterenol	T48.6X1	T48.6X2	T48.6X3	T48.6X4	T48.6X5	T48.6X6
Isosorbide dinitrate	T46.3X1	T46.3X2	T46.3X3	T46.3X4	T46.3X5	T46.3X6
Isothipendyl	T45.0X1	T45.0X2	T45.0X3	T45.0X4	T45.0X5	T45.0X6
Isotretinoin	T50.991	T50.992	T50.993	T50.994	T50.995	T50.996
Isoxazolyl penicillin	T36.0X1	T36.0X2	T36.0X3	T36.0X4	T36.0X5	T36.0X6
Isoxicam	T39.391	T39.392	T39.393	T39.394	T39.395	T39.396
Isoxsuprine	T46.7X1	T46.7X2	T46.7X3	T46.7X4	T46.7X5	T46.7X6
Ispagula	T47.4X1	T47.4X2	T47.4X3	T47.4X4	T47.4X5	T47.4X6
husk	T47.4X1	T47.4X2	T47.4X3	T47.4X4	T47.4X5	T47.4X6
Isradipine	T46.1X1	T46.1X2	T46.1X3	T46.1X4	T46.1X5	T46.1X6
I-thyroxine sodium	T38.1X1	T38.1X2	T38.1X3	T38.1X4	T38.1X5	T38.1X6
Itraconazole	T37.8X1	T37.8X2	T37.8X3	T37.8X4	T37.8X5	T37.8X6
Itramin tosilate	T46.3X1	T46.3X2	T46.3X3	T46.3X4	T46.3X5	T46.3X6
Ivermectin	T37.4X1	T37.4X2	T37.4X3	T37.4X4	T37.4X5	T37.4X6
Izoniazid	T37.1X1	T37.1X2	T37.1X3	T37.1X4	T37.1X5	T37.1X6
with thioacetazone	T37.1X1	T37.1X2	T37.1X3	T37.1X4	T37.1X5	T37.1X6

J

Substance	Poisoning, Accidental (Unintentional)	Poisoning, Intentional Self-Harm	Poisoning, Assault	Poisoning, Undetermined	Adverse Effect	Underdosing
Jalap	T47.2X1	T47.2X2	T47.2X3	T47.2X4	T47.2X5	T47.2X6
Jamaica						
dogwood (bark)	T39.8X1	T39.8X2	T39.8X3	T39.8X4	T39.8X5	T39.8X6
ginger	T65.891	T65.892	T65.893	T65.894	—	—
root	T62.2X1	T62.2X2	T62.2X3	T62.2X4	—	—
Jatropha	T62.2X1	T62.2X2	T62.2X3	T62.2X4	—	—
curcas	T62.2X1	T62.2X2	T62.2X3	T62.2X4	—	—
Jectofer	T45.4X1	T45.4X2	T45.4X3	T45.4X4	T45.4X5	T45.4X6
Jellyfish (sting)	T63.621	T63.622	T63.623	T63.624	—	—
Jequirity (bean)	T62.2X1	T62.2X2	T62.2X3	T62.2X4	—	—
Jimson weed (stramonium)	T62.2X1	T62.2X2	T62.2X3	T62.2X4	—	—
seeds	T62.2X1	T62.2X2	T62.2X3	T62.2X4	—	—

Substance	Poisoning, Accidental (Unintentional)	Poisoning, Intentional Self-Harm	Poisoning, Assault	Poisoning, Undetermined	Adverse Effect	Underdosing
Josamycin	T36.3X1	T36.3X2	T36.3X3	T36.3X4	T36.3X5	T36.3X6
Juniper tar	T49.1X1	T49.1X2	T49.1X3	T49.1X4	T49.1X5	T49.1X6

K

Substance	Poisoning, Accidental (Unintentional)	Poisoning, Intentional Self-Harm	Poisoning, Assault	Poisoning, Undetermined	Adverse Effect	Underdosing
Kallidinogenase	T46.7X1	T46.7X2	T46.7X3	T46.7X4	T46.7X5	T46.7X6
Kallikrein	T46.7X1	T46.7X2	T46.7X3	T46.7X4	T46.7X5	T46.7X6
Kanamycin	T36.5X1	T36.5X2	T36.5X3	T36.5X4	T36.5X5	T36.5X6
Kantrex	T36.5X1	T36.5X2	T36.5X3	T36.5X4	T36.5X5	T36.5X6
Kaolin	T47.6X1	T47.6X2	T47.6X3	T47.6X4	T47.6X5	T47.6X6
light	T47.6X1	T47.6X2	T47.6X3	T47.6X4	T47.6X5	T47.6X6
Karaya (gum)	T47.4X1	T47.4X2	T47.4X3	T47.4X4	T47.4X5	T47.4X6
Kebuzone	T39.2X1	T39.2X2	T39.2X3	T39.2X4	T39.2X5	T39.2X6
Kelevan	T60.1X1	T60.1X2	T60.1X3	T60.1X4	—	—
Kemithal	T41.1X1	T41.1X2	T41.1X3	T41.1X4	T41.1X5	T41.1X6
Kenacort	T38.0X1	T38.0X2	T38.0X3	T38.0X4	T38.0X5	T38.0X6
Keratolytic drug NEC	T49.4X1	T49.4X2	T49.4X3	T49.4X4	T49.4X5	T49.4X6
anthracene	T49.4X1	T49.4X2	T49.4X3	T49.4X4	T49.4X5	T49.4X6
Keratoplastic NEC	T49.4X1	T49.4X2	T49.4X3	T49.4X4	T49.4X5	T49.4X6
Kerosene, kerosine (fuel) (solvent) NEC	T52.0X1	T52.0X2	T52.0X3	T52.0X4	—	—
insecticide	T52.0X1	T52.0X2	T52.0X3	T52.0X4	—	—
vapor	T52.0X1	T52.0X2	T52.0X3	T52.0X4	—	—
Ketamine	T41.291	T41.292	T41.293	T41.294	T41.295	T41.296
Ketazolam	T42.4X1	T42.4X2	T42.4X3	T42.4X4	T42.4X5	T42.4X6
Ketazon	T39.2X1	T39.2X2	T39.2X3	T39.2X4	T39.2X5	T39.2X6
Ketobemidone	T40.491	T40.492	T40.493	T40.494	—	—
Ketoconazole	T49.0X1	T49.0X2	T49.0X3	T49.0X4	T49.0X5	T49.0X6
Ketols	T52.4X1	T52.4X2	T52.4X3	T52.4X4	—	—
Ketone oils	T52.4X1	T52.4X2	T52.4X3	T52.4X4	—	—
Ketoprofen	T39.311	T39.312	T39.313	T39.314	T39.315	T39.316
Ketorolac	T39.8X1	T39.8X2	T39.8X3	T39.8X4	T39.8X5	T39.8X6
Ketotifen	T45.0X1	T45.0X2	T45.0X3	T45.0X4	T45.0X5	T45.0X6
Khat	T43.691	T43.692	T43.693	T43.694	—	—
Khellin	T46.3X1	T46.3X2	T46.3X3	T46.3X4	T46.3X5	T46.3X6
Khelloside	T46.3X1	T46.3X2	T46.3X3	T46.3X4	T46.3X5	T46.3X6
Kiln gas or vapor (carbon monoxide)	T58.8X1	T58.8X2	T58.8X3	T58.8X4	—	—
Kitasamycin	T36.3X1	T36.3X2	T36.3X3	T36.3X4	T36.3X5	T36.3X6
Konsyl	T47.4X1	T47.4X2	T47.4X3	T47.4X4	T47.4X5	T47.4X6
Kosam seed	T62.2X1	T62.2X2	T62.2X3	T62.2X4	—	—
Krait (venom)	T63.091	T63.092	T63.093	T63.094	—	—
Kwell (insecticide)	T60.1X1	T60.1X2	T60.1X3	T60.1X4	—	—
anti-infective (topical)	T49.0X1	T49.0X2	T49.0X3	T49.0X4	T49.0X5	T49.0X6

◀ New   ◀ Revised   ~~deleted~~ Deleted

Substance	External Cause (T-Code)					
	Poisoning, Accidental (Unintentional)	Poisoning, Intentional Self-Harm	Poisoning, Assault	Poisoning, Undetermined	Adverse Effect	Underdosing
L						
Labetalol	T44.8X1	T44.8X2	T44.8X3	T44.8X4	T44.8X5	T44.8X6
Laburnum (seeds)	T62.2X1	T62.2X2	T62.2X3	T62.2X4	—	—
leaves	T62.2X1	T62.2X2	T62.2X3	T62.2X4	—	—
Lachesine	T49.5X1	T49.5X2	T49.5X3	T49.5X4	T49.5X5	T49.5X6
Lacidipine	T46.5X1	T46.5X2	T46.5X3	T46.5X4	T46.5X5	T46.5X6
Lacquer	T65.6X1	T65.6X2	T65.6X3	T65.6X4		
Lacrimogenic gas	T59.3X1	T59.3X2	T59.3X3	T59.3X4		
Lactated potassic saline	T50.3X1	T50.3X2	T50.3X3	T50.3X4	T50.3X5	T50.3X6
Lactic acid	T49.8X1	T49.8X2	T49.8X3	T49.8X4	T49.8X5	T49.8X6
Lactobacillus						
acidophilus	T47.6X1	T47.6X2	T47.6X3	T47.6X4	T47.6X5	T47.6X6
compound	T47.6X1	T47.6X2	T47.6X3	T47.6X4	T47.6X5	T47.6X6
bifidus, lyophilized	T47.6X1	T47.6X2	T47.6X3	T47.6X4	T47.6X5	T47.6X6
bulgaricus	T47.6X1	T47.6X2	T47.6X3	T47.6X4	T47.6X5	T47.6X6
sporogenes	T47.6X1	T47.6X2	T47.6X3	T47.6X4	T47.6X5	T47.6X6
Lactoflavin	T45.2X1	T45.2X2	T45.2X3	T45.2X4	T45.2X5	T45.2X6
Lactose (as excipient)	T50.901	T50.902	T50.903	T50.904	T50.905	T50.906
Lactuca (virosa) (extract)	T42.6X1	T42.6X2	T42.6X3	T42.6X4	T42.6X5	T42.6X6
Lactucarium	T42.6X1	T42.6X2	T42.6X3	T42.6X4	T42.6X5	T42.6X6
Lactulose	T47.3X1	T47.3X2	T47.3X3	T47.3X4	T47.3X5	T47.3X6
Laevo — *see Levo-*						
Lanatosides	T46.0X1	T46.0X2	T46.0X3	T46.0X4	T46.0X5	T46.0X6
Lanolin	T49.3X1	T49.3X2	T49.3X3	T49.3X4	T49.3X5	T49.3X6
Largactil	T43.3X1	T43.3X2	T43.3X3	T43.3X4	T43.3X5	T43.3X6
Larkspur	T62.2X1	T62.2X2	T62.2X3	T62.2X4	—	—
Laroxyl	T43.011	T43.012	T43.013	T43.014	T43.015	T43.016
Lassar's paste	T49.4X1	T49.4X2	T49.4X3	T49.4X4	T49.4X5	T49.4X6
Lasix	T50.1X1	T50.1X2	T50.1X3	T50.1X4	T50.1X5	T50.1X6
Latamoxef	T36.1X1	T36.1X2	T36.1X3	T36.1X4	T36.1X5	T36.1X6
Latex	T65.811	T65.812	T65.813	T65.814		
Lathyrus (seed)	T62.2X1	T62.2X2	T62.2X3	T62.2X4	—	—
Laudanum	T40.0X1	T40.0X2	T40.0X3	T40.0X4	T40.0X5	T40.0X6
Laudexium	T48.1X1	T48.1X2	T48.1X3	T48.1X4	T48.1X5	T48.1X6
Laughing gas	T41.0X1	T41.0X2	T41.0X3	T41.0X4	T41.0X5	T41.0X6
Laurel, black or cherry	T62.2X1	T62.2X2	T62.2X3	T62.2X4	—	—
Laurolinium	T49.0X1	T49.0X2	T49.0X3	T49.0X4	T49.0X5	T49.0X6
Lauryl sulfoacetate	T49.2X1	T49.2X2	T49.2X3	T49.2X4	T49.2X5	T49.2X6

Substance	External Cause (T-Code)					
	Poisoning, Accidental (Unintentional)	Poisoning, Intentional Self-Harm	Poisoning, Assault	Poisoning, Undetermined	Adverse Effect	Underdosing
Laxative NEC	T47.4X1	T47.4X2	T47.4X3	T47.4X4	T47.4X5	T47.4X6
osmotic	T47.3X1	T47.3X2	T47.3X3	T47.3X4	T47.3X5	T47.3X6
saline	T47.3X1	T47.3X2	T47.3X3	T47.3X4	T47.3X5	T47.3X6
stimulant	T47.2X1	T47.2X2	T47.2X3	T47.2X4	T47.2X5	T47.2X6
L-dopa	T42.8X1	T42.8X2	T42.8X3	T42.8X4	T42.8X5	T42.8X6
Lead (dust) (fumes) (vapor) NEC	T56.0X1	T56.0X2	T56.0X3	T56.0X4	—	—
acetate	T49.2X1	T49.2X2	T49.2X3	T49.2X4	T49.2X5	T49.2X6
alkyl (fuel additive)	T56.0X1	T56.0X2	T56.0X3	T56.0X4	—	—
anti-infectives	T37.8X1	T37.8X2	T37.8X3	T37.8X4	T37.8X5	T37.8X6
antiknock compound (tetraethyl)	T56.0X1	T56.0X2	T56.0X3	T56.0X4	—	—
arsenate, arsenite (dust) (herbicide) (insecticide) (vapor)	T57.0X1	T57.0X2	T57.0X3	T57.0X4	—	—
carbonate	T56.0X1	T56.0X2	T56.0X3	T56.0X4	—	—
paint	T56.0X1	T56.0X2	T56.0X3	T56.0X4	—	—
chromate	T56.0X1	T56.0X2	T56.0X3	T56.0X4	—	—
paint	T56.0X1	T56.0X2	T56.0X3	T56.0X4	—	—
dioxide	T56.0X1	T56.0X2	T56.0X3	T56.0X4	—	—
inorganic	T56.0X1	T56.0X2	T56.0X3	T56.0X4	—	—
iodide	T56.0X1	T56.0X2	T56.0X3	T56.0X4	—	—
pigment (paint)	T56.0X1	T56.0X2	T56.0X3	T56.0X4	—	—
monoxide (dust)	T56.0X1	T56.0X2	T56.0X3	T56.0X4	—	—
paint	T56.0X1	T56.0X2	T56.0X3	T56.0X4	—	—
organic	T56.0X1	T56.0X2	T56.0X3	T56.0X4	—	—
oxide	T56.0X1	T56.0X2	T56.0X3	T56.0X4	—	—
paint	T56.0X1	T56.0X2	T56.0X3	T56.0X4	—	—
paint	T56.0X1	T56.0X2	T56.0X3	T56.0X4	—	—
salts	T56.0X1	T56.0X2	T56.0X3	T56.0X4	—	—
specified compound NEC	T56.0X1	T56.0X2	T56.0X3	T56.0X4	—	—
tetra-ethyl	T56.0X1	T56.0X2	T56.0X3	T56.0X4	—	—
Lebanese red	T40.711	T40.712	T40.713	T40.714	T40.715	T40.716
Lefetamine	T39.8X1	T39.8X2	T39.8X3	T39.8X4	T39.8X5	T39.8X6
Lenperone	T43.4X1	T43.4X2	T43.4X3	T43.4X4	T43.4X5	T43.4X6
Lente Iletin (insulin)	T38.3X1	T38.3X2	T38.3X3	T38.3X4	T38.3X5	T38.3X6
Leptazol	T50.7X1	T50.7X2	T50.7X3	T50.7X4	T50.7X5	T50.7X6
Leptophos	T60.0X1	T60.0X2	T60.0X3	T60.0X4	—	—
Leritine	T40.2X1	T40.2X2	T40.2X3	T40.2X4	T40.2X5	T40.2X6
Letosteine	T48.4X1	T48.4X2	T48.4X3	T48.4X4	T48.4X5	T48.4X6
Letter	T38.1X1	T38.1X2	T38.1X3	T38.1X4	T38.1X5	T38.1X6
Lettuce opium	T42.6X1	T42.6X2	T42.6X3	T42.6X4	T42.6X5	T42.6X6
Leucinocaine	T41.3X1	T41.3X2	T41.3X3	T41.3X4	T41.3X5	T41.3X6

TABLE OF DRUGS AND CHEMICALS

Substance	Poisoning, Accidental (Unintentional)	Poisoning, Intentional Self-Harm	Poisoning, Assault	Poisoning, Undetermined	Adverse Effect	Underdosing
Leucocianidol	T46.991	T46.992	T46.993	T46.994	T46.995	T46.996
Leucovorin (factor)	T45.8X1	T45.8X2	T45.8X3	T45.8X4	T45.8X5	T45.8X6
Leukeran	T45.1X1	T45.1X2	T45.1X3	T45.1X4	T45.1X5	T45.1X6
Leuprolide	T38.891	T38.892	T38.893	T38.894	T38.895	T38.896
Levalbuterol	T48.6X1	T48.6X2	T48.6X3	T48.6X4	T48.6X5	T48.6X6
Levallorphan	T50.7X1	T50.7X2	T50.7X3	T50.7X4	T50.7X5	T50.7X6
Levamisole	T37.4X1	T37.4X2	T37.4X3	T37.4X4	T37.4X5	T37.4X6
Levanil	T42.6X1	T42.6X2	T42.6X3	T42.6X4	T42.6X5	T42.6X6
Levarterenol	T44.4X1	T44.4X2	T44.4X3	T44.4X4	T44.4X5	T44.4X6
Levdropropizine	T48.3X1	T48.3X2	T48.3X3	T48.3X4	T48.3X5	T48.3X6
Levobunolol	T49.5X1	T49.5X2	T49.5X3	T49.5X4	T49.5X5	T49.5X6
Levocabastine (hydrochloride)	T45.0X1	T45.0X2	T45.0X3	T45.0X4	T45.0X5	T45.0X6
Levocarnitine	T50.991	T50.992	T50.993	T50.994	T50.995	T50.996
Levodopa	T42.8X1	T42.8X2	T42.8X3	T42.8X4	T42.8X5	T42.8X6
with carbidopa	T42.8X1	T42.8X2	T42.8X3	T42.8X4	T42.8X5	T42.8X6
Levo-dromoran	T40.2X1	T40.2X2	T40.2X3	T40.2X4	T40.2X5	T40.2X6
Levoglutamide	T50.991	T50.992	T50.993	T50.994	T50.995	T50.996
Levoid	T38.1X1	T38.1X2	T38.1X3	T38.1X4	T38.1X5	T38.1X6
Levo-iso-methadone	T40.3X1	T40.3X2	T40.3X3	T40.3X4	T40.3X5	T40.3X6
Levomepromazine	T43.3X1	T43.3X2	T43.3X3	T43.3X4	T43.3X5	T43.3X6
Levonordefrin	T49.6X1	T49.6X2	T49.6X3	T49.6X4	T49.6X5	T49.6X6
Levonorgestrel	T38.4X1	T38.4X2	T38.4X3	T38.4X4	T38.4X5	T38.4X6
with ethinylestradiol	T38.5X1	T38.5X2	T38.5X3	T38.5X4	T38.5X5	T38.5X6
Levopromazine	T43.3X1	T43.3X2	T43.3X3	T43.3X4	T43.3X5	T43.3X6
Levoprome	T42.6X1	T42.6X2	T42.6X3	T42.6X4	T42.6X5	T42.6X6
Levopropoxyphene	T40.491	T40.492	T40.493	T40.494	T40.495	T40.496
Levopropylhexedrine	T50.5X1	T50.5X2	T50.5X3	T50.5X4	T50.5X5	T50.5X6
Levoproxyphylline	T48.6X1	T48.6X2	T48.6X3	T48.6X4	T48.6X5	T48.6X6
Levorphanol	T40.491	T40.492	T40.493	T40.494	T40.495	T40.496
Levothyroxine	T38.1X1	T38.1X2	T38.1X3	T38.1X4	T38.1X5	T38.1X6
sodium	T38.1X1	T38.1X2	T38.1X3	T38.1X4	T38.1X5	T38.1X6
Levsin	T44.3X1	T44.3X2	T44.3X3	T44.3X4	T44.3X5	T44.3X6
Levulose	T50.3X1	T50.3X2	T50.3X3	T50.3X4	T50.3X5	T50.3X6
Lewisite (gas), not in war	T57.0X1	T57.0X2	T57.0X3	T57.0X4	—	—
Librium	T42.4X1	T42.4X2	T42.4X3	T42.4X4	T42.4X5	T42.4X6
Lidex	T49.0X1	T49.0X2	T49.0X3	T49.0X4	T49.0X5	T49.0X6
Lidocaine	T41.3X1	T41.3X2	T41.3X3	T41.3X4	T41.3X5	T41.3X6
regional	T41.3X1	T41.3X2	T41.3X3	T41.3X4	T41.3X5	T41.3X6
spinal	T41.3X1	T41.3X2	T41.3X3	T41.3X4	T41.3X5	T41.3X6
Lidofenin	T50.8X1	T50.8X2	T50.8X3	T50.8X4	T50.8X5	T50.8X6
Lidoflazine	T46.1X1	T46.1X2	T46.1X3	T46.1X4	T46.1X5	T46.1X6
Lighter fluid	T52.0X1	T52.0X2	T52.0X3	T52.0X4	—	—

Substance	Poisoning, Accidental (Unintentional)	Poisoning, Intentional Self-Harm	Poisoning, Assault	Poisoning, Undetermined	Adverse Effect	Underdosing
Lignin hemicellulose	T47.6X1	T47.6X2	T47.6X3	T47.6X4	T47.6X5	T47.6X6
Lignocaine	T41.3X1	T41.3X2	T41.3X3	T41.3X4	T41.3X5	T41.3X6
regional	T41.3X1	T41.3X2	T41.3X3	T41.3X4	T41.3X5	T41.3X6
spinal	T41.3X1	T41.3X2	T41.3X3	T41.3X4	T41.3X5	T41.3X6
Ligroin(e) (solvent)	T52.0X1	T52.0X2	T52.0X3	T52.0X4	—	—
vapor	T59.891	T59.892	T59.893	T59.894	—	—
Ligustrum vulgare	T62.2X1	T62.2X2	T62.2X3	T62.2X4	—	—
Lily of the valley	T62.2X1	T62.2X2	T62.2X3	T62.2X4	—	—
Lime (chloride)	T54.3X1	T54.3X2	T54.3X3	T54.3X4	—	—
Limonene	T52.8X1	T52.8X2	T52.8X3	T52.8X4	—	—
Lincomycin	T36.8X1	T36.8X2	T36.8X3	T36.8X4	T36.8X5	T36.8X6
Lindane (insecticide) (nonmedicinal) (vapor)	T53.6X1	T53.6X2	T53.6X3	T53.6X4	—	—
medicinal	T49.0X1	T49.0X2	T49.0X3	T49.0X4	T49.0X5	T49.0X6
Liniments NEC	T49.91	T49.92	T49.93	T49.94	T49.95	T49.96
Linoleic acid	T46.6X1	T46.6X2	T46.6X3	T46.6X4	T46.6X5	T46.6X6
Linolenic acid	T46.6X1	T46.6X2	T46.6X3	T46.6X4	T46.6X5	T46.6X6
Linseed	T47.4X1	T47.4X2	T47.4X3	T47.4X4	T47.4X5	T47.4X6
Liothyronine	T38.1X1	T38.1X2	T38.1X3	T38.1X4	T38.1X5	T38.1X6
Liotrix	T38.1X1	T38.1X2	T38.1X3	T38.1X4	T38.1X5	T38.1X6
Lipancreatin	T47.5X1	T47.5X2	T47.5X3	T47.5X4	T47.5X5	T47.5X6
Lipo-alprostadil	T46.7X1	T46.7X2	T46.7X3	T46.7X4	T46.7X5	T46.7X6
Lipo-Lutin	T38.5X1	T38.5X2	T38.5X3	T38.5X4	T38.5X5	T38.5X6
Lipotropic drug NEC	T50.901	T50.902	T50.903	T50.904	T50.905	T50.906
Liquefied petroleum gases	T59.891	T59.892	T59.893	T59.894	—	—
piped (pure or mixed with air)	T59.891	T59.892	T59.893	T59.894	—	—
Liquid						
paraffin	T47.4X1	T47.4X2	T47.4X3	T47.4X4	T47.4X5	T47.4X6
petrolatum	T47.4X1	T47.4X2	T47.4X3	T47.4X4	T47.4X5	T47.4X6
topical	T49.3X1	T49.3X2	T49.3X3	T49.3X4	T49.3X5	T49.3X6
specified NEC	T65.891	T65.892	T65.893	T65.894	—	—
substance	T65.91	T65.92	T65.93	T65.94	—	—
Liquor creosolis compositus	T65.891	T65.892	T65.893	T65.894	—	—
Liquorice	T48.4X1	T48.4X2	T48.4X3	T48.4X4	T48.4X5	T48.4X6
extract	T47.8X1	T47.8X2	T47.8X3	T47.8X4	T47.8X5	T47.8X6
Lirugen	T50.991	T50.992	T50.993	T50.994	T50.995	T50.996
Lisinopril	T46.4X1	T46.4X2	T46.4X3	T46.4X4	T46.4X5	T46.4X6
Lisuride	T42.8X1	T42.8X2	T42.8X3	T42.8X4	T42.8X5	T42.8X6
Lithane	T43.8X1	T43.8X2	T43.8X3	T43.8X4	T43.8X5	T43.8X6
Lithium	T56.891	T56.892	T56.893	T56.894	—	—
gluconate	T43.591	T43.592	T43.593	T43.594	T43.595	T43.596
salts (carbonate)	T43.591	T43.592	T43.593	T43.594	T43.595	T43.596

◀ New   ◀ Revised   ~~deleted~~ Deleted

Substance	Poisoning, Accidental (Unintentional)	Poisoning, Intentional Self-Harm	Poisoning, Assault	Poisoning, Undetermined	Adverse Effect	Underdosing
Lithonate	T43.8X1	T43.8X2	T43.8X3	T43.8X4	T43.8X5	T43.8X6
Liver						
extract	T45.8X1	T45.8X2	T45.8X3	T45.8X4	T45.8X5	T45.8X6
for parenteral use	T45.8X1	T45.8X2	T45.8X3	T45.8X4	T45.8X5	T45.8X6
fraction 1	T45.8X1	T45.8X2	T45.8X3	T45.8X4	T45.8X5	T45.8X6
hydrolysate	T45.8X1	T45.8X2	T45.8X3	T45.8X4	T45.8X5	T45.8X6
Lizard (bite) (venom)	T63.121	T63.122	T63.123	T63.124	—	—
LMD	T45.8X1	T45.8X2	T45.8X3	T45.8X4	T45.8X5	T45.8X6
Lobelia	T62.2X1	T62.2X2	T62.2X3	T62.2X4	—	—
Lobeline	T50.7X1	T50.7X2	T50.7X3	T50.7X4	T50.7X5	T50.7X6
Local action drug NEC	T49.8X1	T49.8X2	T49.8X3	T49.8X4	T49.8X5	T49.8X6
Locorten	T49.0X1	T49.0X2	T49.0X3	T49.0X4	T49.0X5	T49.0X6
Lofepramine	T43.011	T43.012	T43.013	T43.014	T43.015	T43.016
Lolium temulentum	T62.2X1	T62.2X2	T62.2X3	T62.2X4	—	—
Lomotil	T47.6X1	T47.6X2	T47.6X3	T47.6X4	T47.6X5	T47.6X6
Lomustine	T45.1X1	T45.1X2	T45.1X3	T45.1X4	T45.1X5	T45.1X6
Lonidamine	T45.1X1	T45.1X2	T45.1X3	T45.1X4	T45.1X5	T45.1X6
Loperamide	T47.6X1	T47.6X2	T47.6X3	T47.6X4	T47.6X5	T47.6X6
Loprazolam	T42.4X1	T42.4X2	T42.4X3	T42.4X4	T42.4X5	T42.4X6
Lorajmine	T46.2X1	T46.2X2	T46.2X3	T46.2X4	T46.2X5	T46.2X6
Loratidine	T45.0X1	T45.0X2	T45.0X3	T45.0X4	T45.0X5	T45.0X6
Lorazepam	T42.4X1	T42.4X2	T42.4X3	T42.4X4	T42.4X5	T42.4X6
Lorcainide	T46.2X1	T46.2X2	T46.2X3	T46.2X4	T46.2X5	T46.2X6
Lormetazepam	T42.4X1	T42.4X2	T42.4X3	T42.4X4	T42.4X5	T42.4X6
Lotions NEC	T49.91	T49.92	T49.93	T49.94	T49.95	T49.96
Lotusate	T42.3X1	T42.3X2	T42.3X3	T42.3X4	T42.3X5	T42.3X6
Lovastatin	T46.6X1	T46.6X2	T46.6X3	T46.6X4	T46.6X5	T46.6X6
Loxapine	T43.591	T43.592	T43.593	T43.594	T43.595	T43.596
Lowila	T49.2X1	T49.2X2	T49.2X3	T49.2X4	T49.2X5	T49.2X6
Lozenges (throat)	T49.6X1	T49.6X2	T49.6X3	T49.6X4	T49.6X5	T49.6X6
LSD	T40.8X1	T40.8X2	T40.8X3	T40.8X4	—	—
L-Tryptophan — see Amino acid						
Lubricant, eye	T49.5X1	T49.5X2	T49.5X3	T49.5X4	T49.5X5	T49.5X6
Lubricating oil NEC	T52.0X1	T52.0X2	T52.0X3	T52.0X4	—	—
Lucanthone	T37.4X1	T37.4X2	T37.4X3	T37.4X4	T37.4X5	T37.4X6
Luminal	T42.3X1	T42.3X2	T42.3X3	T42.3X4	T42.3X5	T42.3X6
Lung irritant (gas) NEC	T59.91	T59.92	T59.93	T59.94		
Luteinizing hormone	T38.811	T38.812	T38.813	T38.814	T38.815	T38.816
Lutocylol	T38.5X1	T38.5X2	T38.5X3	T38.5X4	T38.5X5	T38.5X6
Lutromone	T38.5X1	T38.5X2	T38.5X3	T38.5X4	T38.5X5	T38.5X6
Lututrin	T48.291	T48.292	T48.293	T48.294	T48.295	T48.296
Lye (Concentrated)	T54.3X1	T54.3X2	T54.3X3	T54.3X4	—	—

Substance	Poisoning, Accidental (Unintentional)	Poisoning, Intentional Self-Harm	Poisoning, Assault	Poisoning, Undetermined	Adverse Effect	Underdosing
Lygranum (skin test)	T50.8X1	T50.8X2	T50.8X3	T50.8X4	T50.8X5	T50.8X6
Lymecycline	T36.4X1	T36.4X2	T36.4X3	T36.4X4	T36.4X5	T36.4X6
Lymphogranuloma venereum antigen	T50.8X1	T50.8X2	T50.8X3	T50.8X4	T50.8X5	T50.8X6
Lynestrenol	T38.4X1	T38.4X2	T38.4X3	T38.4X4	T38.4X5	T38.4X6
Lypressin	T38.891	T38.892	T38.893	T38.894	T38.895	T38.896
Lyovac Sodium Edecrin	T50.1X1	T50.1X2	T50.1X3	T50.1X4	T50.1X5	T50.1X6
Lysergic acid diethylamide	T40.8X1	T40.8X2	T40.8X3	T40.8X4	—	—
Lysergide	T40.8X1	T40.8X2	T40.8X3	T40.8X4	—	—
Lysine vasopressin	T38.891	T38.892	T38.893	T38.894	T38.895	T38.896
Lysol	T54.1X1	T54.1X2	T54.1X3	T54.1X4	—	—
Lysozyme	T49.0X1	T49.0X2	T49.0X3	T49.0X4	T49.0X5	T49.0X6
Lytta (vitatta)	T49.8X1	T49.8X2	T49.8X3	T49.8X4	T49.8X5	T49.8X6

M

Substance	Poisoning, Accidental (Unintentional)	Poisoning, Intentional Self-Harm	Poisoning, Assault	Poisoning, Undetermined	Adverse Effect	Underdosing
Mace	T59.3X1	T59.3X2	T59.3X3	T59.3X4	—	—
Macrogol	T50.991	T50.992	T50.993	T50.994	T50.995	T50.996
Macrolide						
anabolic drug	T38.7X1	T38.7X2	T38.7X3	T38.7X4	T38.7X5	T38.7X6
antibiotic	T36.3X1	T36.3X2	T36.3X3	T36.3X4	T36.3X5	T36.3X6
Mafenide	T49.0X1	T49.0X2	T49.0X3	T49.0X4	T49.0X5	T49.0X6
Magaldrate	T47.1X1	T47.1X2	T47.1X3	T47.1X4	T47.1X5	T47.1X6
Magic mushroom	T40.991	T40.992	T40.993	T40.994	—	—
Magnamycin	T36.8X1	T36.8X2	T36.8X3	T36.8X4	T36.8X5	T36.8X6
Magnesia magma	T47.1X1	T47.1X2	T47.1X3	T47.1X4	T47.1X5	T47.1X6
Magnesium NEC	T56.891	T56.892	T56.893	T56.894	—	—
carbonate	T47.1X1	T47.1X2	T47.1X3	T47.1X4	T47.1X5	T47.1X6
citrate	T47.4X1	T47.4X2	T47.4X3	T47.4X4	T47.4X5	T47.4X6
hydroxide	T47.1X1	T47.1X2	T47.1X3	T47.1X4	T47.1X5	T47.1X6
oxide	T47.1X1	T47.1X2	T47.1X3	T47.1X4	T47.1X5	T47.1X6
peroxide	T49.0X1	T49.0X2	T49.0X3	T49.0X4	T49.0X5	T49.0X6
salicylate	T39.091	T39.092	T39.093	T39.094	T39.095	T39.096
silicofluoride	T50.3X1	T50.3X2	T50.3X3	T50.3X4	T50.3X5	T50.3X6
sulfate	T47.4X1	T47.4X2	T47.4X3	T47.4X4	T47.4X5	T47.4X6
thiosulfate	T45.0X1	T45.0X2	T45.0X3	T45.0X4	T45.0X5	T45.0X6
trisilicate	T47.1X1	T47.1X2	T47.1X3	T47.1X4	T47.1X5	T47.1X6
Malathion (medicinal)	T49.0X1	T49.0X2	T49.0X3	T49.0X4	T49.0X5	T49.0X6
insecticide	T60.0X1	T60.0X2	T60.0X3	T60.0X4	—	—
Male fern extract	T37.4X1	T37.4X2	T37.4X3	T37.4X4	T37.4X5	T37.4X6
M-AMSA	T45.1X1	T45.1X2	T45.1X3	T45.1X4	T45.1X5	T45.1X6
Mandelic acid	T37.8X1	T37.8X2	T37.8X3	T37.8X4	T37.8X5	T37.8X6
Manganese (dioxide) (salts)	T57.2X1	T57.2X2	T57.2X3	T57.2X4	—	—
medicinal	T50.991	T50.992	T50.993	T50.994	T50.995	T50.996

TABLE OF DRUGS AND CHEMICALS

Substance	External Cause (T-Code)					
	Poisoning, Accidental (Unintentional)	Poisoning, Intentional Self-Harm	Poisoning, Assault	Poisoning, Undetermined	Adverse Effect	Underdosing
Mannitol	T47.3X1	T47.3X2	T47.3X3	T47.3X4	T47.3X5	T47.3X6
hexanitrate	T46.3X1	T46.3X2	T46.3X3	T46.3X4	T46.3X5	T46.3X6
Mannomustine	T45.1X1	T45.1X2	T45.1X3	T45.1X4	T45.1X5	T45.1X6
MAO inhibitors	T43.1X1	T43.1X2	T43.1X3	T43.1X4	T43.1X5	T43.1X6
Mapharsen	T37.8X1	T37.8X2	T37.8X3	T37.8X4	T37.8X5	T37.8X6
Maphenide	T49.0X1	T49.0X2	T49.0X3	T49.0X4	T49.0X5	T49.0X6
Maprotiline	T43.021	T43.022	T43.023	T43.024	T43.025	T43.026
Marcaine	T41.3X1	T41.3X2	T41.3X3	T41.3X4	T41.3X5	T41.3X6
infiltration (subcutaneous)	T41.3X1	T41.3X2	T41.3X3	T41.3X4	T41.3X5	T41.3X6
nerve block (peripheral) (plexus)	T41.3X1	T41.3X2	T41.3X3	T41.3X4	T41.3X5	T41.3X6
Marezine	T45.0X1	T45.0X2	T45.0X3	T45.0X4	T45.0X5	T45.0X6
Marihuana	T40.711	T40.712	T40.713	T40.714	T40.715	T40.716
Marijuana	T40.711	T40.712	T40.713	T40.714	T40.715	T40.716
Marine (sting)	T63.691	T63.692	T63.693	T63.694	—	—
animals (sting)	T63.691	T63.692	T63.693	T63.694	—	—
plants (sting)	T63.711	T63.712	T63.713	T63.714	—	—
Marplan	T43.1X1	T43.1X2	T43.1X3	T43.1X4	T43.1X5	T43.1X6
Marsh gas	T59.891	T59.892	T59.893	T59.894	—	—
Marsilid	T43.1X1	T43.1X2	T43.1X3	T43.1X4	T43.1X5	T43.1X6
Matulane	T45.1X1	T45.1X2	T45.1X3	T45.1X4	T45.1X5	T45.1X6
Mazindol	T50.5X1	T50.5X2	T50.5X3	T50.5X4	T50.5X5	T50.5X6
MCPA	T60.3X1	T60.3X2	T60.3X3	T60.3X4	—	—
MDMA	T43.641	T43.642	T43.643	T43.644	—	—
Meadow saffron	T62.2X1	T62.2X2	T62.2X3	T62.2X4	—	—
Measles virus vaccine (attenuated)	T50.B91	T50.B92	T50.B93	T50.B94	T50.B95	T50.B96
Meat, noxious	T62.8X1	T62.8X2	T62.8X3	T62.8X4	—	—
Meballymal	T42.3X1	T42.3X2	T42.3X3	T42.3X4	T42.3X5	T42.3X6
Mebanazine	T43.1X1	T43.1X2	T43.1X3	T43.1X4	T43.1X5	T43.1X6
Mebaral	T42.3X1	T42.3X2	T42.3X3	T42.3X4	T42.3X5	T42.3X6
Mebendazole	T37.4X1	T37.4X2	T37.4X3	T37.4X4	T37.4X5	T37.4X6
Mebeverine	T44.3X1	T44.3X2	T44.3X3	T44.3X4	T44.3X5	T44.3X6
Mebhydrolin	T45.0X1	T45.0X2	T45.0X3	T45.0X4	T45.0X5	T45.0X6
Mebumal	T42.3X1	T42.3X2	T42.3X3	T42.3X4	T42.3X5	T42.3X6
Mebutamate	T43.591	T43.592	T43.593	T43.594	T43.595	T43.596
Mecamylamine	T44.2X1	T44.2X2	T44.2X3	T44.2X4	T44.2X5	T44.2X6
Mechlorethamine	T45.1X1	T45.1X2	T45.1X3	T45.1X4	T45.1X5	T45.1X6
Mecillinam	T36.0X1	T36.0X2	T36.0X3	T36.0X4	T36.0X5	T36.0X6
Meclizine (hydrochloride)	T45.0X1	T45.0X2	T45.0X3	T45.0X4	T45.0X5	T45.0X6
Meclocycline	T36.4X1	T36.4X2	T36.4X3	T36.4X4	T36.4X5	T36.4X6
Meclofenamate	T39.391	T39.392	T39.393	T39.394	T39.395	T39.396
Meclofenamic acid	T39.391	T39.392	T39.393	T39.394	T39.395	T39.396

Substance	External Cause (T-Code)					
	Poisoning, Accidental (Unintentional)	Poisoning, Intentional Self-Harm	Poisoning, Assault	Poisoning, Undetermined	Adverse Effect	Underdosing
Meclofenoxate	T43.691	T43.692	T43.693	T43.694	T43.695	T43.696
Meclozine	T45.0X1	T45.0X2	T45.0X3	T45.0X4	T45.0X5	T45.0X6
Mecobalamin	T45.8X1	T45.8X2	T45.8X3	T45.8X4	T45.8X5	T45.8X6
Mecoprop	T60.3X1	T60.3X2	T60.3X3	T60.3X4	—	—
Mecrilate	T49.3X1	T49.3X2	T49.3X3	T49.3X4	T49.3X5	T49.3X6
Mecysteine	T48.4X1	T48.4X2	T48.4X3	T48.4X4	T48.4X5	T48.4X6
Medazepam	T42.4X1	T42.4X2	T42.4X3	T42.4X4	T42.4X5	T42.4X6
Medicament NEC	T50.901	T50.902	T50.903	T50.904	T50.905	T50.906
Medinal	T42.3X1	T42.3X2	T42.3X3	T42.3X4	T42.3X5	T42.3X6
Medomin	T42.3X1	T42.3X2	T42.3X3	T42.3X4	T42.3X5	T42.3X6
Medrogestone	T38.5X1	T38.5X2	T38.5X3	T38.5X4	T38.5X5	T38.5X6
Medroxalol	T44.8X1	T44.8X2	T44.8X3	T44.8X4	T44.8X5	T44.8X6
Medroxyprogesterone acetate (depot)	T38.5X1	T38.5X2	T38.5X3	T38.5X4	T38.5X5	T38.5X6
Medrysone	T49.0X1	T49.0X2	T49.0X3	T49.0X4	T49.0X5	T49.0X6
Mefenamic acid	T39.391	T39.392	T39.393	T39.394	T39.395	T39.396
Mefenorex	T50.5X1	T50.5X2	T50.5X3	T50.5X4	T50.5X5	T50.5X6
Mefloquine	T37.2X1	T37.2X2	T37.2X3	T37.2X4	T37.2X5	T37.2X6
Mefruside	T50.2X1	T50.2X2	T50.2X3	T50.2X4	T50.2X5	T50.2X6
Megahallucinogen	T40.901	T40.902	T40.903	T40.904	T40.905	T40.906
Megestrol	T38.5X1	T38.5X2	T38.5X3	T38.5X4	T38.5X5	T38.5X6
Meglumine						
antimoniate	T37.8X1	T37.8X2	T37.8X3	T37.8X4	T37.8X5	T37.8X6
diatrizoate	T50.8X1	T50.8X2	T50.8X3	T50.8X4	T50.8X5	T50.8X6
iodipamide	T50.8X1	T50.8X2	T50.8X3	T50.8X4	T50.8X5	T50.8X6
iotroxate	T50.8X1	T50.8X2	T50.8X3	T50.8X4	T50.8X5	T50.8X6
MEK (methyl ethyl ketone)	T52.4X1	T52.4X2	T52.4X3	T52.4X4	—	—
Meladrazine	T44.3X1	T44.3X2	T44.3X3	T44.3X4	T44.3X5	T44.3X6
Meladinin	T49.3X1	T49.3X2	T49.3X3	T49.3X4	T49.3X5	T49.3X6
Melaleuca alternifolia oil	T49.0X1	T49.0X2	T49.0X3	T49.0X4	T49.0X5	T49.0X6
Melanizing agents	T49.3X1	T49.3X2	T49.3X3	T49.3X4	T49.3X5	T49.3X6
Melanocyte-stimulating hormone	T38.891	T38.892	T38.893	T38.894	T38.895	T38.896
Melarsonyl potassium	T37.3X1	T37.3X2	T37.3X3	T37.3X4	T37.3X5	T37.3X6
Melarsoprol	T37.3X1	T37.3X2	T37.3X3	T37.3X4	T37.3X5	T37.3X6
Melia azedarach	T62.2X1	T62.2X2	T62.2X3	T62.2X4	—	—
Melitracen	T43.011	T43.012	T43.013	T43.014	T43.015	T43.016
Mellaril	T43.3X1	T43.3X2	T43.3X3	T43.3X4	T43.3X5	T43.3X6
Meloxine	T49.3X1	T49.3X2	T49.3X3	T49.3X4	T49.3X5	T49.3X6
Melperone	T43.4X1	T43.4X2	T43.4X3	T43.4X4	T43.4X5	T43.4X6
Melphalan	T45.1X1	T45.1X2	T45.1X3	T45.1X4	T45.1X5	T45.1X6
Memantine	T43.8X1	T43.8X2	T43.8X3	T43.8X4	T43.8X5	T43.8X6

◀ New   ◀ Revised   ~~deleted~~ Deleted

Substance	Poisoning, Accidental (Unintentional)	Poisoning, Intentional Self-Harm	Poisoning, Assault	Poisoning, Undetermined	Adverse Effect	Underdosing
Menadiol	T45.7X1	T45.7X2	T45.7X3	T45.7X4	T45.7X5	T45.7X6
sodium sulfate	T45.7X1	T45.7X2	T45.7X3	T45.7X4	T45.7X5	T45.7X6
Menadione	T45.7X1	T45.7X2	T45.7X3	T45.7X4	T45.7X5	T45.7X6
sodium bisulfite	T45.7X1	T45.7X2	T45.7X3	T45.7X4	T45.7X5	T45.7X6
Menaphthone	T45.7X1	T45.7X2	T45.7X3	T45.7X4	T45.7X5	T45.7X6
Menaquinone	T45.7X1	T45.7X2	T45.7X3	T45.7X4	T45.7X5	T45.7X6
Menatetrenone	T45.7X1	T45.7X2	T45.7X3	T45.7X4	T45.7X5	T45.7X6
Meningococcal vaccine	T50.A91	T50.A92	T50.A93	T50.A94	T50.A95	T50.A96
Menningovax (-AC) (-C)	T50.A91	T50.A92	T50.A93	T50.A94	T50.A95	T50.A96
Menotropins	T38.811	T38.812	T38.813	T38.814	T38.815	T38.816
Menthol	T48.5X1	T48.5X2	T48.5X3	T48.5X4	T48.5X5	T48.5X6
Mepacrine	T37.2X1	T37.2X2	T37.2X3	T37.2X4	T37.2X5	T37.2X6
Meparfynol	T42.6X1	T42.6X2	T42.6X3	T42.6X4	T42.6X5	T42.6X6
Mepartricin	T36.7X1	T36.7X2	T36.7X3	T36.7X4	T36.7X5	T36.7X6
Mepazine	T43.3X1	T43.3X2	T43.3X3	T43.3X4	T43.3X5	T43.3X6
Mepenzolate	T44.3X1	T44.3X2	T44.3X3	T44.3X4	T44.3X5	T44.3X6
bromide	T44.3X1	T44.3X2	T44.3X3	T44.3X4	T44.3X5	T44.3X6
Meperidine	T40.491	T40.492	T40.493	T40.494	T40.495	T40.496
Mephebarbital	T42.3X1	T42.3X2	T42.3X3	T42.3X4	T42.3X5	T42.3X6
Mephenamin(e)	T42.8X1	T42.8X2	T42.8X3	T42.8X4	T42.8X5	T42.8X6
Mephenesin	T42.8X1	T42.8X2	T42.8X3	T42.8X4	T42.8X5	T42.8X6
Mephenhydramine	T45.0X1	T45.0X2	T45.0X3	T45.0X4	T45.0X5	T45.0X6
Mephenoxalone	T42.8X1	T42.8X2	T42.8X3	T42.8X4	T42.8X5	T42.8X6
Mephentermine	T44.991	T44.992	T44.993	T44.994	T44.995	T44.996
Mephenytoin	T42.0X1	T42.0X2	T42.0X3	T42.0X4	T42.0X5	T42.0X6
with phenobarbital	T42.3X1	T42.3X2	T42.3X3	T42.3X4	T42.3X5	T42.3X6
Mephobarbital	T42.3X1	T42.3X2	T42.3X3	T42.3X4	T42.3X5	T42.3X6
Mephosfolan	T60.0X1	T60.0X2	T60.0X3	T60.0X4	—	—
Mepindolol	T44.7X1	T44.7X2	T44.7X3	T44.7X4	T44.7X5	T44.7X6
Mepiperphenidol	T44.3X1	T44.3X2	T44.3X3	T44.3X4	T44.3X5	T44.3X6
Mepitiostane	T38.7X1	T38.7X2	T38.7X3	T38.7X4	T38.7X5	T38.7X6
Mepivacaine	T41.3X1	T41.3X2	T41.3X3	T41.3X4	T41.3X5	T41.3X6
epidural	T41.3X1	T41.3X2	T41.3X3	T41.3X4	T41.3X5	T41.3X6
Meprednisone	T38.0X1	T38.0X2	T38.0X3	T38.0X4	T38.0X5	T38.0X6
Meprobam	T43.591	T43.592	T43.593	T43.594	T43.595	T43.596
Meprobamate	T43.591	T43.592	T43.593	T43.594	T43.595	T43.596
Meproscillarin	T46.0X1	T46.0X2	T46.0X3	T46.0X4	T46.0X5	T46.0X6
Meprylcaine	T41.3X1	T41.3X2	T41.3X3	T41.3X4	T41.3X5	T41.3X6
Meptazinol	T39.8X1	T39.8X2	T39.8X3	T39.8X4	T39.8X5	T39.8X6
Mepyramine	T45.0X1	T45.0X2	T45.0X3	T45.0X4	T45.0X5	T45.0X6
Mequitazine	T43.3X1	T43.3X2	T43.3X3	T43.3X4	T43.3X5	T43.3X6
Meralluride	T50.2X1	T50.2X2	T50.2X3	T50.2X4	T50.2X5	T50.2X6

Substance	Poisoning, Accidental (Unintentional)	Poisoning, Intentional Self-Harm	Poisoning, Assault	Poisoning, Undetermined	Adverse Effect	Underdosing
Merbaphen	T50.2X1	T50.2X2	T50.2X3	T50.2X4	T50.2X5	T50.2X6
Merbromin	T49.0X1	T49.0X2	T49.0X3	T49.0X4	T49.0X5	T49.0X6
Mercaptobenzothiazole salts	T49.0X1	T49.0X2	T49.0X3	T49.0X4	T49.0X5	T49.0X6
Mercaptomerin	T50.2X1	T50.2X2	T50.2X3	T50.2X4	T50.2X5	T50.2X6
Mercaptopurine	T45.1X1	T45.1X2	T45.1X3	T45.1X4	T45.1X5	T45.1X6
Mercumatilin	T50.2X1	T50.2X2	T50.2X3	T50.2X4	T50.2X5	T50.2X6
Mercuramide	T50.2X1	T50.2X2	T50.2X3	T50.2X4	T50.2X5	T50.2X6
Mercurochrome	T49.0X1	T49.0X2	T49.0X3	T49.0X4	T49.0X5	T49.0X6
Mercurophylline	T50.2X1	T50.2X2	T50.2X3	T50.2X4	T50.2X5	T50.2X6
Mercury, mercurial, mercuric, mercurous (compounds) (cyanide) (fumes) (nonmedicinal) (vapor) NEC	T56.1X1	T56.1X2	T56.1X3	T56.1X4	—	—
ammoniated	T49.0X1	T49.0X2	T49.0X3	T49.0X4	T49.0X5	T49.0X6
anti-infective						
local	T49.0X1	T49.0X2	T49.0X3	T49.0X4	T49.0X5	T49.0X6
systemic	T37.8X1	T37.8X2	T37.8X3	T37.8X4	T37.8X5	T37.8X6
topical	T49.0X1	T49.0X2	T49.0X3	T49.0X4	T49.0X5	T49.0X6
chloride (ammoniated)	T49.0X1	T49.0X2	T49.0X3	T49.0X4	T49.0X5	T49.0X6
fungicide	T56.1X1	T56.1X2	T56.1X3	T56.1X4	—	—
diuretic NEC	T50.2X1	T50.2X2	T50.2X3	T50.2X4	T50.2X5	T50.2X6
fungicide	T56.1X1	T56.1X2	T56.1X3	T56.1X4	—	—
organic (fungicide)	T56.1X1	T56.1X2	T56.1X3	T56.1X4	—	—
oxide, yellow	T49.0X1	T49.0X2	T49.0X3	T49.0X4	T49.0X5	T49.0X6
Mersalyl	T50.2X1	T50.2X2	T50.2X3	T50.2X4	T50.2X5	T50.2X6
Merthiolate	T49.0X1	T49.0X2	T49.0X3	T49.0X4	T49.0X5	T49.0X6
ophthalmic preparation	T49.5X1	T49.5X2	T49.5X3	T49.5X4	T49.5X5	T49.5X6
Meruvax	T50.B91	T50.B92	T50.B93	T50.B94	T50.B95	T50.B96
Mesalazine	T47.8X1	T47.8X2	T47.8X3	T47.8X4	T47.8X5	T47.8X6
Mescal buttons	T40.991	T40.992	T40.993	T40.994	—	—
Mescaline	T40.991	T40.992	T40.993	T40.994	—	—
Mesna	T48.4X1	T48.4X2	T48.4X3	T48.4X4	T48.4X5	T48.4X6
Mesoglycan	T46.6X1	T46.6X2	T46.6X3	T46.6X4	T46.6X5	T46.6X6
Mesoridazine	T43.3X1	T43.3X2	T43.3X3	T43.3X4	T43.3X5	T43.3X6
Mestanolone	T38.7X1	T38.7X2	T38.7X3	T38.7X4	T38.7X5	T38.7X6
Mesterolone	T38.7X1	T38.7X2	T38.7X3	T38.7X4	T38.7X5	T38.7X6
Mestranol	T38.5X1	T38.5X2	T38.5X3	T38.5X4	T38.5X5	T38.5X6
Mesulergine	T42.8X1	T42.8X2	T42.8X3	T42.8X4	T42.8X5	T42.8X6
Mesulfen	T49.0X1	T49.0X2	T49.0X3	T49.0X4	T49.0X5	T49.0X6
Mesuximide	T42.2X1	T42.2X2	T42.2X3	T42.2X4	T42.2X5	T42.2X6
Metabutethamine	T41.3X1	T41.3X2	T41.3X3	T41.3X4	T41.3X5	T41.3X6
Metactesylacetate	T49.0X1	T49.0X2	T49.0X3	T49.0X4	T49.0X5	T49.0X6
Metacycline	T36.4X1	T36.4X2	T36.4X3	T36.4X4	T36.4X5	T36.4X6

◀ New   ◀ Revised   ~~deleted~~ Deleted

Substance	Poisoning, Accidental (Unintentional)	Poisoning, Intentional Self-Harm	Poisoning, Assault	Poisoning, Undetermined	Adverse Effect	Underdosing
Metaldehyde (snail killer) NEC	T60.8X1	T60.8X2	T60.8X3	T60.8X4	—	—
Metals (heavy) (nonmedicinal)	T56.91	T56.92	T56.93	T56.94	—	—
dust, fumes, or vapor NEC	T56.91	T56.92	T56.93	T56.94	—	—
gadolinium	T56.821	T56.822	T56.823	T56.824	T56.825	—
light NEC	T56.91	T56.92	T56.93	T56.94	—	—
dust, fumes, or vapor NEC	T56.91	T56.92	T56.93	T56.94	—	—
specified NEC	T56.891	T56.892	T56.893	T56.894	—	—
thallium	T56.811	T56.812	T56.813	T56.814	—	—
Metamfetamine	T43.651	T43.652	T43.652	T43.654	T43.655	T43.656
Metamizole sodium	T39.2X1	T39.2X2	T39.2X3	T39.2X4	T39.2X5	T39.2X6
Metampicillin	T36.0X1	T36.0X2	T36.0X3	T36.0X4	T36.0X5	T36.0X6
Metamucil	T47.4X1	T47.4X2	T47.4X3	T47.4X4	T47.4X5	T47.4X6
Metaphen	T49.0X1	T49.0X2	T49.0X3	T49.0X4	T49.0X5	T49.0X6
Metandienone	T38.7X1	T38.7X2	T38.7X3	T38.7X4	T38.7X5	T38.7X6
Metandrostenolone	T38.7X1	T38.7X2	T38.7X3	T38.7X4	T38.7X5	T38.7X6
Metaphos	T60.0X1	T60.0X2	T60.0X3	T60.0X4	—	—
Metapramine	T43.011	T43.012	T43.013	T43.014	T43.015	T43.016
Metaproterenol	T48.291	T48.292	T48.293	T48.294	T48.295	T48.296
Metaraminol	T44.4X1	T44.4X2	T44.4X3	T44.4X4	T44.4X5	T44.4X6
Metaxalone	T42.8X1	T42.8X2	T42.8X3	T42.8X4	T42.8X5	T42.8X6
Metenolone	T38.7X1	T38.7X2	T38.7X3	T38.7X4	T38.7X5	T38.7X6
Metergoline	T42.8X1	T42.8X2	T42.8X3	T42.8X4	T42.8X5	T42.8X6
Metescufylline	T46.991	T46.992	T46.993	T46.994	T46.995	T46.996
Metetoin	T42.0X1	T42.0X2	T42.0X3	T42.0X4	T42.0X5	T42.0X6
Metformin	T38.3X1	T38.3X2	T38.3X3	T38.3X4	T38.3X5	T38.3X6
Methacholine	T44.1X1	T44.1X2	T44.1X3	T44.1X4	T44.1X5	T44.1X6
Methacycline	T36.4X1	T36.4X2	T36.4X3	T36.4X4	T36.4X5	T36.4X6
Methadone	T40.3X1	T40.3X2	T40.3X3	T40.3X4	T40.3X5	T40.3X6
Methallenestril	T38.5X1	T38.5X2	T38.5X3	T38.5X4	T38.5X5	T38.5X6
Methallenoestril	T38.5X1	T38.5X2	T38.5X3	T38.5X4	T38.5X5	T38.5X6
Methamphetamine	T43.651	T43.652	T43.652	T43.654	T43.655	T43.656
Methampyrone	T39.2X1	T39.2X2	T39.2X3	T39.2X4	T39.2X5	T39.2X6
Methandienone	T38.7X1	T38.7X2	T38.7X3	T38.7X4	T38.7X5	T38.7X6
Methandriol	T38.7X1	T38.7X2	T38.7X3	T38.7X4	T38.7X5	T38.7X6
Methandrostenolone	T38.7X1	T38.7X2	T38.7X3	T38.7X4	T38.7X5	T38.7X6
Methane	T59.891	T59.892	T59.893	T59.894	—	—
Methanethiol	T59.891	T59.892	T59.893	T59.894	—	—
Methaniazide	T37.1X1	T37.1X2	T37.1X3	T37.1X4	T37.1X5	T37.1X6
Methanol (vapor)	T51.1X1	T51.1X2	T51.1X3	T51.1X4	—	—
Methantheline	T44.3X1	T44.3X2	T44.3X3	T44.3X4	T44.3X5	T44.3X6
Methanthelinium bromide	T44.3X1	T44.3X2	T44.3X3	T44.3X4	T44.3X5	T44.3X6
Methaphenilene	T45.0X1	T45.0X2	T45.0X3	T45.0X4	T45.0X5	T45.0X6

Substance	Poisoning, Accidental (Unintentional)	Poisoning, Intentional Self-Harm	Poisoning, Assault	Poisoning, Undetermined	Adverse Effect	Underdosing
Methapyrilene	T45.0X1	T45.0X2	T45.0X3	T45.0X4	T45.0X5	T45.0X6
Methaqualone (compound)	T42.6X1	T42.6X2	T42.6X3	T42.6X4	T42.6X5	T42.6X6
Metharbital	T42.3X1	T42.3X2	T42.3X3	T42.3X4	T42.3X5	T42.3X6
Methazolamide	T50.2X1	T50.2X2	T50.2X3	T50.2X4	T50.2X5	T50.2X6
Methdilazine	T43.3X1	T43.3X2	T43.3X3	T43.3X4	T43.3X5	T43.3X6
Methedrine	T43.651	T43.652	T43.652	T43.654	T43.655	T43.656
Methenamine (mandelate)	T37.8X1	T37.8X2	T37.8X3	T37.8X4	T37.8X5	T37.8X6
Methenolone	T38.7X1	T38.7X2	T38.7X3	T38.7X4	T38.7X5	T38.7X6
Methergine	T48.0X1	T48.0X2	T48.0X3	T48.0X4	T48.0X5	T48.0X6
Methetoin	T42.0X1	T42.0X2	T42.0X3	T42.0X4	T42.0X5	T42.0X6
Methiacil	T38.2X1	T38.2X2	T38.2X3	T38.2X4	T38.2X5	T38.2X6
Methicillin	T36.0X1	T36.0X2	T36.0X3	T36.0X4	T36.0X5	T36.0X6
Methimazole	T38.2X1	T38.2X2	T38.2X3	T38.2X4	T38.2X5	T38.2X6
Methiodal sodium	T50.8X1	T50.8X2	T50.8X3	T50.8X4	T50.8X5	T50.8X6
Methionine	T50.991	T50.992	T50.993	T50.994	T50.995	T50.996
Methisazone	T37.5X1	T37.5X2	T37.5X3	T37.5X4	T37.5X5	T37.5X6
Methisoprinol	T37.5X1	T37.5X2	T37.5X3	T37.5X4	T37.5X5	T37.5X6
Methitural	T42.3X1	T42.3X2	T42.3X3	T42.3X4	T42.3X5	T42.3X6
Methixene	T44.3X1	T44.3X2	T44.3X3	T44.3X4	T44.3X5	T44.3X6
Methobarbital, methobarbitone	T42.3X1	T42.3X2	T42.3X3	T42.3X4	T42.3X5	T42.3X6
Methocarbamol	T42.8X1	T42.8X2	T42.8X3	T42.8X4	T42.8X5	T42.8X6
skeletal muscle relaxant	T48.1X1	T48.1X2	T48.1X3	T48.1X4	T48.1X5	T48.1X6
Methohexital	T41.1X1	T41.1X2	T41.1X3	T41.1X4	T41.1X5	T41.1X6
Methohexitone	T41.1X1	T41.1X2	T41.1X3	T41.1X4	T41.1X5	T41.1X6
Methoin	T42.0X1	T42.0X2	T42.0X3	T42.0X4	T42.0X5	T42.0X6
Methopholine	T39.8X1	T39.8X2	T39.8X3	T39.8X4	T39.8X5	T39.8X6
Methopromazine	T43.3X1	T43.3X2	T43.3X3	T43.3X4	T43.3X5	T43.3X6
Methorate	T48.3X1	T48.3X2	T48.3X3	T48.3X4	T48.3X5	T48.3X6
Methoserpidine	T46.5X1	T46.5X2	T46.5X3	T46.5X4	T46.5X5	T46.5X6
Methotrexate	T45.1X1	T45.1X2	T45.1X3	T45.1X4	T45.1X5	T45.1X6
Methotrimeprazine	T43.3X1	T43.3X2	T43.3X3	T43.3X4	T43.3X5	T43.3X6
Methoxa-Dome	T49.3X1	T49.3X2	T49.3X3	T49.3X4	T49.3X5	T49.3X6
Methoxamine	T44.4X1	T44.4X2	T44.4X3	T44.4X4	T44.4X5	T44.4X6
Methoxsalen	T50.991	T50.992	T50.993	T50.994	T50.995	T50.996
Methoxyaniline	T65.3X1	T65.3X2	T65.3X3	T65.3X4	—	—
Methoxybenzyl penicillin	T36.0X1	T36.0X2	T36.0X3	T36.0X4	T36.0X5	T36.0X6
Methoxychlor	T53.7X1	T53.7X2	T53.7X3	T53.7X4		
Methoxy-DDT	T53.7X1	T53.7X2	T53.7X3	T53.7X4		
2-Methoxyethanol	T52.3X1	T52.3X2	T52.3X3	T52.3X4	—	—
Methoxyflurane	T41.0X1	T41.0X2	T41.0X3	T41.0X4	T41.0X5	T41.0X6
Methoxyphenamine	T48.6X1	T48.6X2	T48.6X3	T48.6X4	T48.6X5	T48.6X6
Methoxypromazine	T43.3X1	T43.3X2	T43.3X3	T43.3X4	T43.3X5	T43.3X6

◄ New ◄ Revised ~~deleted~~ Deleted

Substance	Poisoning, Accidental (Unintentional)	Poisoning, Intentional Self-Harm	Poisoning, Assault	Poisoning, Undetermined	Adverse Effect	Underdosing
5-Methoxypsoralen (5-MOP)	T50.991	T50.992	T50.993	T50.994	T50.995	T50.996
8-Methoxypsoralen (8-MOP)	T50.991	T50.992	T50.993	T50.994	T50.995	T50.996
Methscopolamine bromide	T44.3X1	T44.3X2	T44.3X3	T44.3X4	T44.3X5	T44.3X6
Methsuximide	T42.2X1	T42.2X2	T42.2X3	T42.2X4	T42.2X5	T42.2X6
Methyclothiazide	T50.2X1	T50.2X2	T50.2X3	T50.2X4	T50.2X5	T50.2X6
Methyl						
acetate	T52.4X1	T52.4X2	T52.4X3	T52.4X4	—	—
acetone	T52.4X1	T52.4X2	T52.4X3	T52.4X4	—	—
acrylate	T65.891	T65.892	T65.893	T65.894	—	—
alcohol	T51.1X1	T51.1X2	T51.1X3	T51.1X4	—	—
aminophenol	T65.3X1	T65.3X2	T65.3X3	T65.3X4	—	—
amphetamine	T43.651	T43.652	T43.652	T43.654	T43.655	T43.656
androstanolone	T38.7X1	T38.7X2	T38.7X3	T38.7X4	T38.7X5	T38.7X6
atropine	T44.3X1	T44.3X2	T44.3X3	T44.3X4	T44.3X5	T44.3X6
benzene	T52.2X1	T52.2X2	T52.2X3	T52.2X4	—	—
benzoate	T52.8X1	T52.8X2	T52.8X3	T52.8X4	—	—
benzol	T52.2X1	T52.2X2	T52.2X3	T52.2X4	—	—
bromide (gas)	T59.891	T59.892	T59.893	T59.894	—	—
fumigant	T60.8X1	T60.8X2	T60.8X3	T60.8X4	—	—
butanol	T51.3X1	T51.3X2	T51.3X3	T51.3X4	—	—
carbinol	T51.1X1	T51.1X2	T51.1X3	T51.1X4	—	—
carbonate	T52.8X1	T52.8X2	T52.8X3	T52.8X4	—	—
CCNU	T45.1X1	T45.1X2	T45.1X3	T45.1X4	T45.1X5	T45.1X6
cellosolve	T52.91	T52.92	T52.93	T52.94	—	—
cellulose	T47.4X1	T47.4X2	T47.4X3	T47.4X4	T47.4X5	T47.4X6
chloride (gas)	T59.891	T59.892	T59.893	T59.894	—	—
chloroformate	T59.3X1	T59.3X2	T59.3X3	T59.3X4	—	—
cyclohexane	T52.8X1	T52.8X2	T52.8X3	T52.8X4	—	—
cyclohexanol	T51.8X1	T51.8X2	T51.8X3	T51.8X4	—	—
cyclohexanone	T52.8X1	T52.8X2	T52.8X3	T52.8X4	—	—
cyclohexyl acetate	T52.8X1	T52.8X2	T52.8X3	T52.8X4	—	—
demeton	T60.0X1	T60.0X2	T60.0X3	T60.0X4	—	—
dihydromorphinone	T40.2X1	T40.2X2	T40.2X3	T40.2X4	T40.2X5	T40.2X6
ergometrine	T48.0X1	T48.0X2	T48.0X3	T48.0X4	T48.0X5	T48.0X6
ergonovine	T48.0X1	T48.0X2	T48.0X3	T48.0X4	T48.0X5	T48.0X6
ethyl ketone	T52.4X1	T52.4X2	T52.4X3	T52.4X4	—	—
glucamine antimonate	T37.8X1	T37.8X2	T37.8X3	T37.8X4	T37.8X5	T37.8X6
hydrazine	T65.891	T65.892	T65.893	T65.894	—	—
iodide	T65.891	T65.892	T65.893	T65.894	—	—
isobutyl ketone	T52.4X1	T52.4X2	T52.4X3	T52.4X4	—	—
isothiocyanate	T60.3X1	T60.3X2	T60.3X3	T60.3X4	—	—
mercaptan	T59.891	T59.892	T59.893	T59.894	—	—

Substance	Poisoning, Accidental (Unintentional)	Poisoning, Intentional Self-Harm	Poisoning, Assault	Poisoning, Undetermined	Adverse Effect	Underdosing
Methyl (Continued)						
morphine NEC	T40.2X1	T40.2X2	T40.2X3	T40.2X4	T40.2X5	T40.2X6
nicotinate	T49.4X1	T49.4X2	T49.4X3	T49.4X4	T49.4X5	T49.4X6
paraben	T49.0X1	T49.0X2	T49.0X3	T49.0X4	T49.0X5	T49.0X6
parafynol	T42.6X1	T42.6X2	T42.6X3	T42.6X4	T42.6X5	T42.6X6
parathion	T60.0X1	T60.0X2	T60.0X3	T60.0X4	—	—
peridol	T43.4X1	T43.4X2	T43.4X3	T43.4X4	T43.4X5	T43.4X6
phenidate	T43.631	T43.632	T43.633	T43.634	T43.635	T43.636
prednisolone	T38.0X1	T38.0X2	T38.0X3	T38.0X4	T38.0X5	T38.0X6
ENT agent	T49.6X1	T49.6X2	T49.6X3	T49.6X4	T49.6X5	T49.6X6
ophthalmic preparation	T49.5X1	T49.5X2	T49.5X3	T49.5X4	T49.5X5	T49.5X6
topical NEC	T49.0X1	T49.0X2	T49.0X3	T49.0X4	T49.0X5	T49.0X6
propylcarbinol	T51.3X1	T51.3X2	T51.3X3	T51.3X4	—	—
rosaniline NEC	T49.0X1	T49.0X2	T49.0X3	T49.0X4	T49.0X5	T49.0X6
salicylate	T49.2X1	T49.2X2	T49.2X3	T49.2X4	T49.2X5	T49.2X6
sulfate (fumes)	T59.891	T59.892	T59.893	T59.894	—	—
liquid	T52.8X1	T52.8X2	T52.8X3	T52.8X4	—	—
sulfonal	T42.6X1	T42.6X2	T42.6X3	T42.6X4	T42.6X5	T42.6X6
testosterone	T38.7X1	T38.7X2	T38.7X3	T38.7X4	T38.7X5	T38.7X6
thiouracil	T38.2X1	T38.2X2	T38.2X3	T38.2X4	T38.2X5	T38.2X6
Methylamphetamine	T43.651	T43.652	T43.652	T43.654	T43.655	T43.656
Methylated spirit	T51.1X1	T51.1X2	T51.1X3	T51.1X4	—	—
Methylatropine nitrate	T44.3X1	T44.3X2	T44.3X3	T44.3X4	T44.3X5	T44.3X6
Methylbenactyzium bromide	T44.3X1	T44.3X2	T44.3X3	T44.3X4	T44.3X5	T44.3X6
Methylbenzethonium chloride	T49.0X1	T49.0X2	T49.0X3	T49.0X4	T49.0X5	T49.0X6
Methylcellulose	T47.4X1	T47.4X2	T47.4X3	T47.4X4	T47.4X5	T47.4X6
laxative	T47.4X1	T47.4X2	T47.4X3	T47.4X4	T47.4X5	T47.4X6
Methylchlorophenoxy-acetic acid	T60.3X1	T60.3X2	T60.3X3	T60.3X4	—	—
Methyldopa	T46.5X1	T46.5X2	T46.5X3	T46.5X4	T46.5X5	T46.5X6
Methyldopate	T46.5X1	T46.5X2	T46.5X3	T46.5X4	T46.5X5	T46.5X6
Methylene						
blue	T50.6X1	T50.6X2	T50.6X3	T50.6X4	T50.6X5	T50.6X6
chloride or dichloride (solvent) NEC	T53.4X1	T53.4X2	T53.4X3	T53.4X4	—	—
Methylenedioxyamphet-amine	T43.621	T43.622	T43.623	T43.624	T43.625	T43.626
Methylenedioxymethamphetamine	T43.641	T43.642	T43.643	T43.644	—	—
Methylergometrine	T48.0X1	T48.0X2	T48.0X3	T48.0X4	T48.0X5	T48.0X6
Methylergonovine	T48.0X1	T48.0X2	T48.0X3	T48.0X4	T48.0X5	T48.0X6
Methylestrenolone	T38.5X1	T38.5X2	T38.5X3	T38.5X4	T38.5X5	T38.5X6
Methylethyl cellulose	T50.991	T50.992	T50.993	T50.994	T50.995	T50.996
Methylhexabital	T42.3X1	T42.3X2	T42.3X3	T42.3X4	T42.3X5	T42.3X6
Methylmorphine	T40.2X1	T40.2X2	T40.2X3	T40.2X4	T40.2X5	T40.2X6

Substance	Poisoning, Accidental (Unintentional)	Poisoning, Intentional Self-Harm	Poisoning, Assault	Poisoning, Undetermined	Adverse Effect	Underdosing
Methylparaben (ophthalmic)	T49.5X1	T49.5X2	T49.5X3	T49.5X4	T49.5X5	T49.5X6
Methylparafynol	T42.6X1	T42.6X2	T42.6X3	T42.6X4	T42.6X5	T42.6X6
Methylpentynol, methylpenthynol	T42.6X1	T42.6X2	T42.6X3	T42.6X4	T42.6X5	T42.6X6
Methylphenidate	T43.631	T43.632	T43.633	T43.634	T43.635	T43.636
Methylphenobarbital	T42.3X1	T42.3X2	T42.3X3	T42.3X4	T42.3X5	T42.3X6
Methylpolysiloxane	T47.1X1	T47.1X2	T47.1X3	T47.1X4	T47.1X5	T47.1X6
Methylprednisolone — see Methyl, prednisolone						
Methylrosaniline	T49.0X1	T49.0X2	T49.0X3	T49.0X4	T49.0X5	T49.0X6
Methylrosanilinium chloride	T49.0X1	T49.0X2	T49.0X3	T49.0X4	T49.0X5	T49.0X6
Methyltestosterone	T38.7X1	T38.7X2	T38.7X3	T38.7X4	T38.7X5	T38.7X6
Methylthionine chloride	T50.6X1	T50.6X2	T50.6X3	T50.6X4	T50.6X5	T50.6X6
Methylthioninium chloride	T50.6X1	T50.6X2	T50.6X3	T50.6X4	T50.6X5	T50.6X6
Methylthiouracil	T38.2X1	T38.2X2	T38.2X3	T38.2X4	T38.2X5	T38.2X6
Methyprylon	T42.6X1	T42.6X2	T42.6X3	T42.6X4	T42.6X5	T42.6X6
Methysergide	T46.5X1	T46.5X2	T46.5X3	T46.5X4	T46.5X5	T46.5X6
Metiamide	T47.1X1	T47.1X2	T47.1X3	T47.1X4	T47.1X5	T47.1X6
Meticillin	T36.0X1	T36.0X2	T36.0X3	T36.0X5		T36.0X6
Meticrane	T50.2X1	T50.2X2	T50.2X3	T50.2X4	T50.2X5	T50.2X6
Metildigoxin	T46.0X1	T46.0X2	T46.0X3	T46.0X4	T46.0X5	T46.0X6
Metipranolol	T49.5X1	T49.5X2	T49.5X3	T49.5X4	T49.5X5	T49.5X6
Metirosine	T46.5X1	T46.5X2	T46.5X3	T46.5X4	T46.5X5	T46.5X6
Metisazone	T37.5X1	T37.5X2	T37.5X3	T37.5X4	T37.5X5	T37.5X6
Metixene	T44.3X1	T44.3X2	T44.3X3	T44.3X4	T44.3X5	T44.3X6
Metizoline	T48.5X1	T48.5X2	T48.5X3	T48.5X4	T48.5X5	T48.5X6
Metoclopramide	T45.0X1	T45.0X2	T45.0X3	T45.0X4	T45.0X5	T45.0X6
Metofenazate	T43.3X1	T43.3X2	T43.3X3	T43.3X4	T43.3X5	T43.3X6
Metofoline	T39.8X1	T39.8X2	T39.8X3	T39.8X4	T39.8X5	T39.8X6
Metolazone	T50.2X1	T50.2X2	T50.2X3	T50.2X4	T50.2X5	T50.2X6
Metopon	T40.2X1	T40.2X2	T40.2X3	T40.2X4	T40.2X5	T40.2X6
Metoprine	T45.1X1	T45.1X2	T45.1X3	T45.1X4	T45.1X5	T45.1X6
Metoprolol	T44.7X1	T44.7X2	T44.7X3	T44.7X4	T44.7X5	T44.7X6
Metrifonate	T60.0X1	T60.0X2	T60.0X3	T60.0X4	—	—
Metrizamide	T50.8X1	T50.8X2	T50.8X3	T50.8X4	T50.8X5	T50.8X6
Metrizoic acid	T50.8X1	T50.8X2	T50.8X3	T50.8X4	T50.8X5	T50.8X6
Metronidazole	T37.8X1	T37.8X2	T37.8X3	T37.8X4	T37.8X5	T37.8X6
Metycaine	T41.3X1	T41.3X2	T41.3X3	T41.3X4	T41.3X5	T41.3X6
infiltration (subcutaneous)	T41.3X1	T41.3X2	T41.3X3	T41.3X4	T41.3X5	T41.3X6
nerve block (peripheral) (plexus)	T41.3X1	T41.3X2	T41.3X3	T41.3X4	T41.3X5	T41.3X6
topical (surface)	T41.3X1	T41.3X2	T41.3X3	T41.3X4	T41.3X5	T41.3X6
Metyrapone	T50.8X1	T50.8X2	T50.8X3	T50.8X4	T50.8X5	T50.8X6
Mevinphos	T60.0X1	T60.0X2	T60.0X3	T60.0X4	—	—

Substance	Poisoning, Accidental (Unintentional)	Poisoning, Intentional Self-Harm	Poisoning, Assault	Poisoning, Undetermined	Adverse Effect	Underdosing
Mexazolam	T42.4X1	T42.4X2	T42.4X3	T42.4X4	T42.4X5	T42.4X6
Mexenone	T49.3X1	T49.3X2	T49.3X3	T49.3X4	T49.3X5	T49.3X6
Mexiletine	T46.2X1	T46.2X2	T46.2X3	T46.2X4	T46.2X5	T46.2X6
Mezereon	T62.2X1	T62.2X2	T62.2X3	T62.2X4	—	—
berries	T62.1X1	T62.1X2	T62.1X3	T62.1X4	—	—
Mezlocillin	T36.0X1	T36.0X2	T36.0X3	T36.0X4	T36.0X5	T36.0X6
Mianserin	T43.021	T43.022	T43.023	T43.024	T43.025	T43.026
Micatin	T49.0X1	T49.0X2	T49.0X3	T49.0X4	T49.0X5	T49.0X6
Miconazole	T49.0X1	T49.0X2	T49.0X3	T49.0X4	T49.0X5	T49.0X6
Micronomicin	T36.5X1	T36.5X2	T36.5X3	T36.5X4	T36.5X5	T36.5X6
Midazolam	T42.4X1	T42.4X2	T42.4X3	T42.4X4	T42.4X5	T42.4X6
Midecamycin	T36.3X1	T36.3X2	T36.3X3	T36.3X4	T36.3X5	T36.3X6
Mifepristone	T38.6X1	T38.6X2	T38.6X3	T38.6X4	T38.6X5	T38.6X6
Milk of magnesia	T47.1X1	T47.1X2	T47.1X3	T47.1X4	T47.1X5	T47.1X6
Millipede (tropical) (venomous)	T63.411	T63.412	T63.413	T63.414	—	—
Miltown	T43.591	T43.592	T43.593	T43.594	T43.595	T43.596
Milverine	T44.3X1	T44.3X2	T44.3X3	T44.3X4	T44.3X5	T44.3X6
Minaprine	T43.291	T43.292	T43.293	T43.294	T43.295	T43.296
Minaxolone	T41.291	T41.292	T41.293	T41.294	T41.295	T41.296
Mineral						
acids	T54.2X1	T54.2X2	T54.2X3	T54.2X4	—	—
oil (laxative) (medicinal)	T47.4X1	T47.4X2	T47.4X3	T47.4X4	T47.4X5	T47.4X6
emulsion	T47.2X1	T47.2X2	T47.2X3	T47.2X4	T47.2X5	T47.2X6
nonmedicinal	T52.0X1	T52.0X2	T52.0X3	T52.0X4	—	—
topical	T49.3X1	T49.3X2	T49.3X3	T49.3X4	T49.3X5	T49.3X6
salt NEC	T50.3X1	T50.3X2	T50.3X3	T50.3X4	T50.3X5	T50.3X6
spirits	T52.0X1	T52.0X2	T52.0X3	T52.0X4	—	—
Mineralocorticosteroid	T50.0X1	T50.0X2	T50.0X3	T50.0X4	T50.0X5	T50.0X6
Minocycline	T36.4X1	T36.4X2	T36.4X3	T36.4X4	T36.4X5	T36.4X6
Minoxidil	T46.7X1	T46.7X2	T46.7X3	T46.7X4	T46.7X5	T46.7X6
Miokamycin	T36.3X1	T36.3X2	T36.3X3	T36.3X4	T36.3X5	T36.3X6
Miotic drug	T49.5X1	T49.5X2	T49.5X3	T49.5X4	T49.5X5	T49.5X6
Mipafox	T60.0X1	T60.0X2	T60.0X3	T60.0X4	—	—
Mirex	T60.1X1	T60.1X2	T60.1X3	T60.1X4	—	—
Mirtazapine	T43.021	T43.022	T43.023	T43.024	T43.025	T43.026
Misonidazole	T37.3X1	T37.3X2	T37.3X3	T37.3X4	T37.3X5	T37.3X6
Misoprostol	T47.1X1	T47.1X2	T47.1X3	T47.1X4	T47.1X5	T47.1X6
Mithramycin	T45.1X1	T45.1X2	T45.1X3	T45.1X4	T45.1X5	T45.1X6
Mitobronitol	T45.1X1	T45.1X2	T45.1X3	T45.1X4	T45.1X5	T45.1X6
Mitoguazone	T45.1X1	T45.1X2	T45.1X3	T45.1X4	T45.1X5	T45.1X6
Mitolactol	T45.1X1	T45.1X2	T45.1X3	T45.1X4	T45.1X5	T45.1X6
Mitomycin	T45.1X1	T45.1X2	T45.1X3	T45.1X4	T45.1X5	T45.1X6

◄ New   ◄ Revised   ~~deleted~~ Deleted

Substance	External Cause (T-Code) Poisoning, Accidental (Unintentional)	Poisoning, Intentional Self-Harm	Poisoning, Assault	Poisoning, Undetermined	Adverse Effect	Underdosing
Mitopodozide	T45.1X1	T45.1X2	T45.1X3	T45.1X4	T45.1X5	T45.1X6
Mitotane	T45.1X1	T45.1X2	T45.1X3	T45.1X4	T45.1X5	T45.1X6
Mitoxantrone	T45.1X1	T45.1X2	T45.1X3	T45.1X4	T45.1X5	T45.1X6
Mivacurium chloride	T48.1X1	T48.1X2	T48.1X3	T48.1X4	T48.1X5	T48.1X6
Miyari bacteria	T47.6X1	T47.6X2	T47.6X3	T47.6X4	T47.6X5	T47.6X6
Moclobemide	T43.1X1	T43.1X2	T43.1X3	T43.1X4	T43.1X5	T43.1X6
Moderil	T46.5X1	T46.5X2	T46.5X3	T46.5X4	T46.5X5	T46.5X6
Mofebutazone	T39.2X1	T39.2X2	T39.2X3	T39.2X4	T39.2X5	T39.2X6
Mogadon — *see Nitrazepam*						
Molindone	T43.591	T43.592	T43.593	T43.594	T43.595	T43.596
Molsidomine	T46.3X1	T46.3X2	T46.3X3	T46.3X4	T46.3X5	T46.3X6
Mometasone	T49.0X1	T49.0X2	T49.0X3	T49.0X4	T49.0X5	T49.0X6
Monistat	T49.0X1	T49.0X2	T49.0X3	T49.0X4	T49.0X5	T49.0X6
Monkshood	T62.2X1	T62.2X2	T62.2X3	T62.2X4	—	—
Monoamine oxidase inhibitor NEC	T43.1X1	T43.1X2	T43.1X3	T43.1X4	T43.1X5	T43.1X6
hydrazine	T43.1X1	T43.1X2	T43.1X3	T43.1X4	T43.1X5	T43.1X6
Monobenzone	T49.4X1	T49.4X2	T49.4X3	T49.4X4	T49.4X5	T49.4X6
Monochloroacetic acid	T60.3X1	T60.3X2	T60.3X3	T60.3X4	—	—
Monochlorobenzene	T53.7X1	T53.7X2	T53.7X3	T53.7X4	—	—
Monoethanolamine	T46.8X1	T46.8X2	T46.8X3	T46.8X4	T46.8X5	T46.8X6
oleate	T46.8X1	T46.8X2	T46.8X3	T46.8X4	T46.8X5	T46.8X6
Monooctanoin	T50.991	T50.992	T50.993	T50.994	T50.995	T50.996
Monophenylbutazone	T39.2X1	T39.2X2	T39.2X3	T39.2X4	T39.2X5	T39.2X6
Monosodium glutamate	T65.891	T65.892	T65.893	T65.894	—	—
Monosulfiram	T49.0X1	T49.0X2	T49.0X3	T49.0X4	T49.0X5	T49.0X6
Monoxide, carbon — *see Carbon, monoxide*	T57.91	T57.92	T57.93	T57.94	—	—
Monoxidine hydrochloride	T46.1X1	T46.1X2	T46.1X3	T46.1X4	T46.1X5	T46.1X6
Monuron	T60.3X1	T60.3X2	T60.3X3	T60.3X4	—	—
Moperone	T43.4X1	T43.4X2	T43.4X3	T43.4X4	T43.4X5	T43.4X6
Mopidamol	T45.1X1	T45.1X2	T45.1X3	T45.1X4	T45.1X5	T45.1X6
MOPP (mechlorethamine + vincristine + prednisone + procarbazine)	T45.1X1	T45.1X2	T45.1X3	T45.1X4	T45.1X5	T45.1X6
Morfin	T40.2X1	T40.2X2	T40.2X3	T40.2X4	T40.2X5	T40.2X6
Morinamide	T37.1X1	T37.1X2	T37.1X3	T37.1X4	T37.1X5	T37.1X6
Morning glory seeds	T40.991	T40.992	T40.993	T40.994	—	—
Moroxydine	T37.5X1	T37.5X2	T37.5X3	T37.5X4	T37.5X5	T37.5X6
Morphazinamide	T37.1X1	T37.1X2	T37.1X3	T37.1X4	T37.1X5	T37.1X6
Morphine	T40.2X1	T40.2X2	T40.2X3	T40.2X4	T40.2X5	T40.2X6
antagonist	T50.7X1	T50.7X2	T50.7X3	T50.7X4	T50.7X5	T50.7X6
Morpholinylethylmorphine	T40.2X1	T40.2X2	T40.2X3	T40.2X4	—	—
Morsuximide	T42.2X1	T42.2X2	T42.2X3	T42.2X4	T42.2X5	T42.2X6

Substance	External Cause (T-Code) Poisoning, Accidental (Unintentional)	Poisoning, Intentional Self-Harm	Poisoning, Assault	Poisoning, Undetermined	Adverse Effect	Underdosing
Mosapramine	T43.591	T43.592	T43.593	T43.594	T43.595	T43.596
Moth balls — *see also Pesticide*	T60.2X1	T60.2X2	T60.2X3	T60.2X4	—	—
naphthalene	T60.2X1	T60.2X2	T60.2X3	T60.2X4	—	—
paradichlorobenzene	T60.1X1	T60.1X2	T60.1X3	T60.1X4	—	—
Motor exhaust gas	T58.01	T58.02	T58.03	T58.04		
Mouthwash (antiseptic) (zinc chloride)	T49.6X1	T49.6X2	T49.6X3	T49.6X4	T49.6X5	T49.6X6
Moxastine	T45.0X1	T45.0X2	T45.0X3	T45.0X4	T45.0X5	T45.0X6
Moxaverine	T44.3X1	T44.3X2	T44.3X3	T44.3X4	T44.3X5	T44.3X6
Moxifensine	T43.291	T43.292	T43.293	T43.294	T43.295	T43.296
Moxisylyte	T46.7X1	T46.7X2	T46.7X3	T46.7X4	T46.7X5	T46.7X6
Mucilage, plant	T47.4X1	T47.4X2	T47.4X3	T47.4X4	T47.4X5	T47.4X6
Mucolytic drug	T48.4X1	T48.4X2	T48.4X3	T48.4X4	T48.4X5	T48.4X6
Mucomyst	T48.4X1	T48.4X2	T48.4X3	T48.4X4	T48.4X5	T48.4X6
Mucous membrane agents (external)	T49.91	T49.92	T49.93	T49.94	T49.95	T49.96
specified NEC	T49.8X1	T49.8X2	T49.8X3	T49.8X4	T49.8X5	T49.8X6
Multiple unspecified drugs, medicaments and biological substances	T50.911	T50.912	T50.913	T50.914	T50.915	T50.916
Mumps						
immune globulin (human)	T50.Z11	T50.Z12	T50.Z13	T50.Z14	T50.Z15	T50.Z16
skin test antigen	T50.8X1	T50.8X2	T50.8X3	T50.8X4	T50.8X5	T50.8X6
vaccine	T50.B91	T50.B92	T50.B93	T50.B94	T50.B95	T50.B96
Mumpsvax	T50.B91	T50.B92	T50.B93	T50.B94	T50.B95	T50.B96
Mupirocin	T49.0X1	T49.0X2	T49.0X3	T49.0X4	T49.0X5	T49.0X6
Muriatic acid — *see Hydrochloric acid*						
Muromonab-CD3	T45.1X1	T45.1X2	T45.1X3	T45.1X4	T45.1X5	T45.1X6
Muscle relaxant — *see Relaxant, muscle*						
Muscle-action drug NEC	T48.201	T48.202	T48.203	T48.204	T48.205	T48.206
Muscle affecting agents NEC	T48.201	T48.202	T48.203	T48.204	T48.205	T48.206
oxytocic	T48.0X1	T48.0X2	T48.0X3	T48.0X4	T48.0X5	T48.0X6
relaxants	T48.201	T48.202	T48.203	T48.204	T48.205	T48.206
central nervous system	T42.8X1	T42.8X2	T42.8X3	T42.8X4	T42.8X5	T42.8X6
skeletal	T48.1X1	T48.1X2	T48.1X3	T48.1X4	T48.1X5	T48.1X6
smooth	T44.3X1	T44.3X2	T44.3X3	T44.3X4	T44.3X5	T44.3X6
Muscle-tone depressant, central NEC	T42.8X1	T42.8X2	T42.8X3	T42.8X4	T42.8X5	T42.8X6
specified NEC	T42.8X1	T42.8X2	T42.8X3	T42.8X4	T42.8X5	T42.8X6
Mushroom, noxious	T62.0X1	T62.0X2	T62.0X3	T62.0X4	—	—
Mussel, noxious	T61.781	T61.782	T61.783	T61.784	—	—

TABLE OF DRUGS AND CHEMICALS

Substance	Poisoning, Accidental (Unintentional)	Poisoning, Intentional Self-Harm	Poisoning, Assault	Poisoning, Undetermined	Adverse Effect	Underdosing
Mustard (emetic)	T47.7X1	T47.7X2	T47.7X3	T47.7X4	T47.7X5	T47.7X6
black	T47.7X1	T47.7X2	T47.7X3	T47.7X4	T47.7X5	T47.7X6
gas, not in war	T59.91	T59.92	T59.93	T59.94	—	—
nitrogen	T45.1X1	T45.1X2	T45.1X3	T45.1X4	T45.1X5	T45.1X6
Mustine	T45.1X1	T45.1X2	T45.1X3	T45.1X4	T45.1X5	T45.1X6
M-vac	T45.1X1	T45.1X2	T45.1X3	T45.1X4	T45.1X5	T45.1X6
Mycifradin	T36.5X1	T36.5X2	T36.5X3	T36.5X4	T36.5X5	T36.5X6
topical	T49.0X1	T49.0X2	T49.0X3	T49.0X4	T49.0X5	T49.0X6
Mycitracin	T36.8X1	T36.8X2	T36.8X3	T36.8X4	T36.8X5	T36.8X6
ophthalmic preparation	T49.5X1	T49.5X2	T49.5X3	T49.5X4	T49.5X5	T49.5X6
Mycostatin	T36.7X1	T36.7X2	T36.7X3	T36.7X4	T36.7X5	T36.7X6
topical	T49.0X1	T49.0X2	T49.0X3	T49.0X4	T49.0X5	T49.0X6
Mycotoxins	T64.81	T64.82	T64.83	T64.84	—	—
aflatoxin	T64.01	T64.02	T64.03	T64.04	—	—
specified NEC	T64.81	T64.82	T64.83	T64.84	—	—
Mydriacyl	T44.3X1	T44.3X2	T44.3X3	T44.3X4	T44.3X5	T44.3X6
Mydriatic drug	T49.5X1	T49.5X2	T49.5X3	T49.5X4	T49.5X5	T49.5X6
Myelobromal	T45.1X1	T45.1X2	T45.1X3	T45.1X4	T45.1X5	T45.1X6
Myleran	T45.1X1	T45.1X2	T45.1X3	T45.1X4	T45.1X5	T45.1X6
Myochrysin(e)	T39.2X1	T39.2X2	T39.2X3	T39.2X4	T39.2X5	T39.2X6
Myoneural blocking agents	T48.1X1	T48.1X2	T48.1X3	T48.1X4	T48.1X5	T48.1X6
Myralact	T49.0X1	T49.0X2	T49.0X3	T49.0X4	T49.0X5	T49.0X6
Myristica fragrans	T62.2X1	T62.2X2	T62.2X3	T62.2X4	—	—
Myristicin	T65.891	T65.892	T65.893	T65.894		
Mysoline	T42.3X1	T42.3X2	T42.3X3	T42.3X4	T42.3X5	T42.3X6

N

Substance	Poisoning, Accidental (Unintentional)	Poisoning, Intentional Self-Harm	Poisoning, Assault	Poisoning, Undetermined	Adverse Effect	Underdosing
Nabilone	T40.711	T40.712	T40.713	T40.714	T40.715	T40.716
Nabumetone	T39.391	T39.392	T39.393	T39.394	T39.395	T39.396
Nadolol	T44.7X1	T44.7X2	T44.7X3	T44.7X4	T44.7X5	T44.7X6
Nafcillin	T36.0X1	T36.0X2	T36.0X3	T36.0X4	T36.0X5	T36.0X6
Nafoxidine	T38.6X1	T38.6X2	T38.6X3	T38.6X4	T38.6X5	T38.6X6
Naftazone	T46.991	T46.992	T46.993	T46.994	T46.995	T46.996
Naftidrofuryl (oxalate)	T46.7X1	T46.7X2	T46.7X3	T46.7X4	T46.7X5	T46.7X6
Naftifine	T49.0X1	T49.0X2	T49.0X3	T49.0X4	T49.0X5	T49.0X6
Nail polish remover	T52.91	T52.92	T52.93	T52.94	—	—
Nalbuphine	T40.491	T40.492	T40.493	T40.494	T40.495	T40.496
Naled	T60.0X1	T60.0X2	T60.0X3	T60.0X4	—	—
Nalidixic acid	T37.8X1	T37.8X2	T37.8X3	T37.8X4	T37.8X5	T37.8X6
Nalorphine	T50.7X1	T50.7X2	T50.7X3	T50.7X4	T50.7X5	T50.7X6
Naloxone	T50.7X1	T50.7X2	T50.7X3	T50.7X4	T50.7X5	T50.7X6
Naltrexone	T50.7X1	T50.7X2	T50.7X3	T50.7X4	T50.7X5	T50.7X6
Namenda	T43.8X1	T43.8X2	T43.8X3	T43.8X4	T43.8X5	T43.8X6

Substance	Poisoning, Accidental (Unintentional)	Poisoning, Intentional Self-Harm	Poisoning, Assault	Poisoning, Undetermined	Adverse Effect	Underdosing
Nandrolone	T38.7X1	T38.7X2	T38.7X3	T38.7X4	T38.7X5	T38.7X6
Naphazoline	T48.5X1	T48.5X2	T48.5X3	T48.5X4	T48.5X5	T48.5X6
Naphtha (painters') (petroleum)	T52.0X1	T52.0X2	T52.0X3	T52.0X4	—	—
solvent	T52.0X1	T52.0X2	T52.0X3	T52.0X4	—	—
vapor	T52.0X1	T52.0X2	T52.0X3	T52.0X4	—	—
Naphthalene (non-chlorinated)	T60.2X1	T60.2X2	T60.2X3	T60.2X4		
chlorinated	T60.1X1	T60.1X2	T60.1X3	T60.1X4		
vapor	T60.1X1	T60.1X2	T60.1X3	T60.1X4		
insecticide or moth repellent	T60.2X1	T60.2X2	T60.2X3	T60.2X4		
chlorinated	T60.1X1	T60.1X2	T60.1X3	T60.1X4		
vapor	T60.2X1	T60.2X2	T60.2X3	T60.2X4		
chlorinated	T60.1X1	T60.1X2	T60.1X3	T60.1X4		
Naphthol	T65.891	T65.892	T65.893	T65.894		
Naphthylamine	T65.891	T65.892	T65.893	T65.894		
Naphthylthiourea (ANTU)	T60.4X1	T60.4X2	T60.4X3	T60.4X4		
Naprosyn — see Naproxen						
Naproxen	T39.311	T39.312	T39.313	T39.314	T39.315	T39.316
Narcotic (drug)	T40.601	T40.602	T40.603	T40.604	T40.605	T40.606
analgesic NEC	T40.601	T40.602	T40.603	T40.604	T40.605	T40.606
antagonist	T50.7X1	T50.7X2	T50.7X3	T50.7X4	T50.7X5	T50.7X6
specified NEC	T40.691	T40.692	T40.693	T40.694	T40.695	T40.696
synthetic	T40.491	T40.492	T40.493	T40.494	T40.495	T40.496
Narcotine	T48.3X1	T48.3X2	T48.3X3	T48.3X4	T48.3X5	T48.3X6
Nardil	T43.1X1	T43.1X2	T43.1X3	T43.1X4	T43.1X5	T43.1X6
Nasal drug NEC	T49.6X1	T49.6X2	T49.6X3	T49.6X4	T49.6X5	T49.6X6
Natamycin	T49.0X1	T49.0X2	T49.0X3	T49.0X4	T49.0X5	T49.0X6
Natrium cyanide — see Cyanide(s)						
Natural gas	T59.891	T59.892	T59.893	T59.894	—	—
incomplete combustion	T57.91	T57.92	T57.93	T57.94		
Natural						
blood (product)	T45.8X1	T45.8X2	T45.8X3	T45.8X4	T45.8X5	T45.8X6
gas (piped)	T59.891	T59.892	T59.893	T59.894	—	—
incomplete combustion	T58.11	T58.12	T58.13	T58.14	—	—
Nealbarbital	T42.3X1	T42.3X2	T42.3X3	T42.3X4	T42.3X5	T42.3X6
Nectadon	T48.3X1	T48.3X2	T48.3X3	T48.3X4	T48.3X5	T48.3X6
Nedocromil	T48.6X1	T48.6X2	T48.6X3	T48.6X4	T48.6X5	T48.6X6
Nefopam	T39.8X1	T39.8X2	T39.8X3	T39.8X4	T39.8X5	T39.8X6
Nematocyst (sting)	T63.691	T63.692	T63.693	T63.694	—	—
Nembutal	T42.3X1	T42.3X2	T42.3X3	T42.3X4	T42.3X5	T42.3X6
Nemonapride	T43.591	T43.592	T43.593	T43.594	T43.595	T43.596
Neoarsphenamine	T37.8X1	T37.8X2	T37.8X3	T37.8X4	T37.8X5	T37.8X6

◄ New   ◄ Revised   ~~deleted~~ Deleted

Substance	Poisoning, Accidental (Unintentional)	Poisoning, Intentional Self-Harm	Poisoning, Assault	Poisoning, Undetermined	Adverse Effect	Underdosing
Neocinchophen	T50.4X1	T50.4X2	T50.4X3	T50.4X4	T50.4X5	T50.4X6
Neomycin (derivatives)	T36.5X1	T36.5X2	T36.5X3	T36.5X4	T36.5X5	T36.5X6
with						
bacitracin	T49.0X1	T49.0X2	T49.0X3	T49.0X4	T49.0X5	T49.0X6
neostigmine	T44.0X1	T44.0X2	T44.0X3	T44.0X4	T44.0X5	T44.0X6
ENT agent	T49.6X1	T49.6X2	T49.6X3	T49.6X4	T49.6X5	T49.6X6
ophthalmic preparation	T49.5X1	T49.5X2	T49.5X3	T49.5X4	T49.5X5	T49.5X6
topical NEC	T49.0X1	T49.0X2	T49.0X3	T49.0X4	T49.0X5	T49.0X6
Neonal	T42.3X1	T42.3X2	T42.3X3	T42.3X4	T42.3X5	T42.3X6
Neoprontosil	T37.0X1	T37.0X2	T37.0X3	T37.0X4	T37.0X5	T37.0X6
Neosalvarsan	T37.8X1	T37.8X2	T37.8X3	T37.8X4	T37.8X5	T37.8X6
Neosilversalvarsan	T37.8X1	T37.8X2	T37.8X3	T37.8X4	T37.8X5	T37.8X6
Neosporin	T36.8X1	T36.8X2	T36.8X3	T36.8X4	T36.8X5	T36.8X6
ENT agent	T49.6X1	T49.6X2	T49.6X3	T49.6X4	T49.6X5	T49.6X6
ophthalmic preparation	T49.5X1	T49.5X2	T49.5X3	T49.5X4	T49.5X5	T49.5X6
topical NEC	T49.0X1	T49.0X2	T49.0X3	T49.0X4	T49.0X5	T49.0X6
Neostigmine bromide	T44.0X1	T44.0X2	T44.0X3	T44.0X4	T44.0X5	T44.0X6
Neraval	T42.3X1	T42.3X2	T42.3X3	T42.3X4	T42.3X5	T42.3X6
Neravan	T42.3X1	T42.3X2	T42.3X3	T42.3X4	T42.3X5	T42.3X6
Nerium oleander	T62.2X1	T62.2X2	T62.2X3	T62.2X4	—	—
Nerve gas, not in war	T59.91	T59.92	T59.93	T59.94	—	—
Nesacaine	T41.3X1	T41.3X2	T41.3X3	T41.3X4	T41.3X5	T41.3X6
infiltration (subcutaneous)	T41.3X1	T41.3X2	T41.3X3	T41.3X4	T41.3X5	T41.3X6
nerve block (peripheral) (plexus)	T41.3X1	T41.3X2	T41.3X3	T41.3X4	T41.3X5	T41.3X6
Netilmicin	T36.5X1	T36.5X2	T36.5X3	T36.5X4	T36.5X5	T36.5X6
Neurobarb	T42.3X1	T42.3X2	T42.3X3	T42.3X4	T42.3X5	T42.3X6
Neuroleptic drug NEC	T43.501	T43.502	T43.503	T43.504	T43.505	T43.506
Neuromuscular blocking drug	T48.1X1	T48.1X2	T48.1X3	T48.1X4	T48.1X5	T48.1X6
Neutral insulin injection	T38.3X1	T38.3X2	T38.3X3	T38.3X4	T38.3X5	T38.3X6
Neutral spirits	T51.0X1	T51.0X2	T51.0X3	T51.0X4	—	—
beverage	T51.0X1	T51.0X2	T51.0X3	T51.0X4	—	—
Niacin	T46.7X1	T46.7X2	T46.7X3	T46.7X4	T46.7X5	T46.7X6
Niacinamide	T45.2X1	T45.2X2	T45.2X3	T45.2X4	T45.2X5	T45.2X6
Nialamide	T43.1X1	T43.1X2	T43.1X3	T43.1X4	T43.1X5	T43.1X6
Niaprazine	T42.6X1	T42.6X2	T42.6X3	T42.6X4	T42.6X5	T42.6X6
Nicametate	T46.7X1	T46.7X2	T46.7X3	T46.7X4	T46.7X5	T46.7X6
Nicardipine	T46.1X1	T46.1X2	T46.1X3	T46.1X4	T46.1X5	T46.1X6
Nicergoline	T46.7X1	T46.7X2	T46.7X3	T46.7X4	T46.7X5	T46.7X6
Nickel (carbonyl) (tetra-carbonyl) (fumes) (vapor)	T56.891	T56.892	T56.893	T56.894	—	—

Substance	Poisoning, Accidental (Unintentional)	Poisoning, Intentional Self-Harm	Poisoning, Assault	Poisoning, Undetermined	Adverse Effect	Underdosing
Nickelocene	T56.891	T56.892	T56.893	T56.894	—	—
Niclosamide	T37.4X1	T37.4X2	T37.4X3	T37.4X4	T37.4X5	T37.4X6
Nicofuranose	T46.7X1	T46.7X2	T46.7X3	T46.7X4	T46.7X5	T46.7X6
Nicomorphine	T40.2X1	T40.2X2	T40.2X3	T40.2X4	—	—
Nicorandil	T46.3X1	T46.3X2	T46.3X3	T46.3X4	T46.3X5	T46.3X6
Nicotiana (plant)	T62.2X1	T62.2X2	T62.2X3	T62.2X4	—	—
Nicotinamide	T45.2X1	T45.2X2	T45.2X3	T45.2X4	T45.2X5	T45.2X6
Nicotine (insecticide) (spray) (sulfate) NEC	T60.2X1	T60.2X2	T60.2X3	T60.2X4		
from tobacco	T65.291	T65.292	T65.293	T65.294		
cigarettes	T65.221	T65.222	T65.223	T65.224	—	—
not insecticide	T65.291	T65.292	T65.293	T65.294	—	—
Nicotinic acid	T46.7X1	T46.7X2	T46.7X3	T46.7X4	T46.7X5	T46.7X6
Nicotinyl alcohol	T46.7X1	T46.7X2	T46.7X3	T46.7X4	T46.7X5	T46.7X6
Nicoumalone	T45.511	T45.512	T45.513	T45.514	T45.515	T45.516
Nifedipine	T46.1X1	T46.1X2	T46.1X3	T46.1X4	T46.1X5	T46.1X6
Nifenazone	T39.2X1	T39.2X2	T39.2X3	T39.2X4	T39.2X5	T39.2X6
Nifuraldezone	T37.91	T37.92	T37.93	T37.94	T37.95	T37.96
Nifuratel	T37.8X1	T37.8X2	T37.8X3	T37.8X4	T37.8X5	T37.8X6
Nifurtimox	T37.3X1	T37.3X2	T37.3X3	T37.3X4	T37.3X5	T37.3X6
Nifurtoinol	T37.8X1	T37.8X2	T37.8X3	T37.8X4	T37.8X5	T37.8X6
Nightshade, deadly (solanum) — see also Belladonna	T62.2X1	T62.2X2	T62.2X3	T62.2X4	—	—
berry	T62.1X1	T62.1X2	T62.1X3	T62.1X4	—	—
Nikethamide	T50.7X1	T50.7X2	T50.7X3	T50.7X4	T50.7X5	T50.7X6
Nilstat	T36.7X1	T36.7X2	T36.7X3	T36.7X4	T36.7X5	T36.7X6
topical	T49.0X1	T49.0X2	T49.0X3	T49.0X4	T49.0X5	T49.0X6
Nilutamide	T38.6X1	T38.6X2	T38.6X3	T38.6X4	T38.6X5	T38.6X6
Nimesulide	T39.391	T39.392	T39.393	T39.394	T39.395	T39.396
Nimetazepam	T42.4X1	T42.4X2	T42.4X3	T42.4X4	T42.4X5	T42.4X6
Nimodipine	T46.1X1	T46.1X2	T46.1X3	T46.1X4	T46.1X5	T46.1X6
Nimorazole	T37.3X1	T37.3X2	T37.3X3	T37.3X4	T37.3X5	T37.3X6
Nimustine	T45.1X1	T45.1X2	T45.1X3	T45.1X4	T45.1X5	T45.1X6
Niridazole	T37.4X1	T37.4X2	T37.4X3	T37.4X4	T37.4X5	T37.4X6
Nisentil	T40.2X1	T40.2X2	T40.2X3	T40.2X4	T40.2X5	T40.2X6
Nisoldipine	T46.1X1	T46.1X2	T46.1X3	T46.1X4	T46.1X5	T46.1X6
Nitramine	T65.3X1	T65.3X2	T65.3X3	T65.3X4	—	—
Nitrate, organic	T46.3X1	T46.3X2	T46.3X3	T46.3X4	T46.3X5	T46.3X6
Nitrazepam	T42.4X1	T42.4X2	T42.4X3	T42.4X4	T42.4X5	T42.4X6
Nitrefazole	T50.6X1	T50.6X2	T50.6X3	T50.6X4	T50.6X5	T50.6X6
Nitrendipine	T46.1X1	T46.1X2	T46.1X3	T46.1X4	T46.1X5	T46.1X6

TABLE OF DRUGS AND CHEMICALS

Substance	External Cause (T-Code)					
	Poisoning, Accidental (Unintentional)	Poisoning, Intentional Self-Harm	Poisoning, Assault	Poisoning, Undetermined	Adverse Effect	Underdosing
Nitric						
acid (liquid)	T54.2X1	T54.2X2	T54.2X3	T54.2X4	—	—
vapor	T59.891	T59.892	T59.893	T59.894	—	—
oxide (gas)	T59.0X1	T59.0X2	T59.0X3	T59.0X4	—	—
Nitrimidazine	T37.3X1	T37.3X2	T37.3X3	T37.3X4	T37.3X5	T37.3X6
Nitrite, amyl (medicinal) (vapor)	T46.3X1	T46.3X2	T46.3X3	T46.3X4	T46.3X5	T46.3X6
Nitroaniline	T65.3X1	T65.3X2	T65.3X3	T65.3X4		
vapor	T59.891	T59.892	T59.893	T59.894		
Nitrobenzene, nitrobenzol	T65.3X1	T65.3X2	T65.3X3	T65.3X4		
vapor	T65.3X1	T65.3X2	T65.3X3	T65.3X4		
Nitrocellulose	T65.891	T65.892	T65.893	T65.894		
lacquer	T65.891	T65.892	T65.893	T65.894		
Nitrodiphenyl	T65.3X1	T65.3X2	T65.3X3	T65.3X4		
Nitrofural	T49.0X1	T49.0X2	T49.0X3	T49.0X4	T49.0X5	T49.0X6
Nitrofurantoin	T37.8X1	T37.8X2	T37.8X3	T37.8X4	T37.8X5	T37.8X6
Nitrofurazone	T49.0X1	T49.0X2	T49.0X3	T49.0X4	T49.0X5	T49.0X6
Nitrogen	T59.0X1	T59.0X2	T59.0X3	T59.0X4	—	—
mustard	T45.1X1	T45.1X2	T45.1X3	T45.1X4	T45.1X5	T45.1X6
Nitroglycerin, nitro-glycerol (medicinal)	T46.3X1	T46.3X2	T46.3X3	T46.3X4	T46.3X5	T46.3X6
nonmedicinal	T65.5X1	T65.5X2	T65.5X3	T65.5X4	—	—
fumes	T65.5X1	T65.5X2	T65.5X3	T65.5X4	—	—
Nitroglycol	T52.3X1	T52.3X2	T52.3X3	T52.3X4		
Nitrohydrochloric acid	T54.2X1	T54.2X2	T54.2X3	T54.2X4	—	—
Nitromersol	T49.0X1	T49.0X2	T49.0X3	T49.0X4	T49.0X5	T49.0X6
Nitronaphthalene	T65.891	T65.892	T65.893	T65.894		
Nitrophenol	T54.0X1	T54.0X2	T54.0X3	T54.0X4		
Nitropropane	T52.8X1	T52.8X2	T52.8X3	T52.8X4	—	—
Nitroprusside	T46.5X1	T46.5X2	T46.5X3	T46.5X4	T46.5X5	T46.5X6
Nitrosodimethylamine	T65.3X1	T65.3X2	T65.3X3	T65.3X4		
Nitrothiazol	T37.4X1	T37.4X2	T37.4X3	T37.4X4	T37.4X5	T37.4X6
Nitrotoluene, nitrotoluol	T65.3X1	T65.3X2	T65.3X3	T65.3X4		
vapor	T65.3X1	T65.3X2	T65.3X3	T65.3X4		
Nitrous						
acid (liquid)	T54.2X1	T54.2X2	T54.2X3	T54.2X4	—	—
fumes	T59.891	T59.892	T59.893	T59.894	—	—
ether spirit	T46.3X1	T46.3X2	T46.3X3	T46.3X4	T46.3X5	T46.3X6
oxide	T41.0X1	T41.0X2	T41.0X3	T41.0X4	T41.0X5	T41.0X6
Nitroxoline	T37.8X1	T37.8X2	T37.8X3	T37.8X4	T37.8X5	T37.8X6
Nitrozone	T49.0X1	T49.0X2	T49.0X3	T49.0X4	T49.0X5	T49.0X6
Nizatidine	T47.0X1	T47.0X2	T47.0X3	T47.0X4	T47.0X5	T47.0X6

Substance	External Cause (T-Code)					
	Poisoning, Accidental (Unintentional)	Poisoning, Intentional Self-Harm	Poisoning, Assault	Poisoning, Undetermined	Adverse Effect	Underdosing
Nizofenone	T43.8X1	T43.8X2	T43.8X3	T43.8X4	T43.8X5	T43.8X6
Noctec	T42.6X1	T42.6X2	T42.6X3	T42.6X4	T42.6X5	T42.6X6
Noludar	T42.6X1	T42.6X2	T42.6X3	T42.6X4	T42.6X5	T42.6X6
Noptil	T42.3X1	T42.3X2	T42.3X3	T42.3X4	T42.3X5	T42.3X6
Nomegestrol	T38.5X1	T38.5X2	T38.5X3	T38.5X4	T38.5X5	T38.5X6
Nomifensine	T43.291	T43.292	T43.293	T43.294	T43.295	T43.296
Nonoxinol	T49.8X1	T49.8X2	T49.8X3	T49.8X4	T49.8X5	T49.8X6
Nonylphenoxy (polyethoxy-ethanol)	T49.8X1	T49.8X2	T49.8X3	T49.8X4	T49.8X5	T49.8X6
Noptil	T42.3X1	T42.3X2	T42.3X3	T42.3X4	T42.3X5	T42.3X6
Noradrenaline	T44.4X1	T44.4X2	T44.4X3	T44.4X4	T44.4X5	T44.4X6
Noramidopyrine	T39.2X1	T39.2X2	T39.2X3	T39.2X4	T39.2X5	T39.2X6
methanesulfonate sodium	T39.2X1	T39.2X2	T39.2X3	T39.2X4	T39.2X5	T39.2X6
Norbormide	T60.4X1	T60.4X2	T60.4X3	T60.4X4	—	—
Nordazepam	T42.4X1	T42.4X2	T42.4X3	T42.4X4	T42.4X5	T42.4X6
Norepinephrine	T44.4X1	T44.4X2	T44.4X3	T44.4X4	T44.4X5	T44.4X6
Norethandrolone	T38.7X1	T38.7X2	T38.7X3	T38.7X4	T38.7X5	T38.7X6
Norethindrone	T38.4X1	T38.4X2	T38.4X3	T38.4X4	T38.4X5	T38.4X6
Norethisterone (acetate) (enantate)	T38.4X1	T38.4X2	T38.4X3	T38.4X4	T38.4X5	T38.4X6
with ethinylestradiol	T38.5X1	T38.5X2	T38.5X3	T38.5X4	T38.5X5	T38.5X6
Noretynodrel	T38.5X1	T38.5X2	T38.5X3	T38.5X4	T38.5X5	T38.5X6
Norfenefrine	T44.4X1	T44.4X2	T44.4X3	T44.4X4	T44.4X5	T44.4X6
Norfloxacin	T36.8X1	T36.8X2	T36.8X3	T36.8X4	T36.8X5	T36.8X6
Norgestrel	T38.4X1	T38.4X2	T38.4X3	T38.4X4	T38.4X5	T38.4X6
Norgestrienone	T38.4X1	T38.4X2	T38.4X3	T38.4X4	T38.4X5	T38.4X6
Norlestrin	T38.4X1	T38.4X2	T38.4X3	T38.4X4	T38.4X5	T38.4X6
Norlutin	T38.4X1	T38.4X2	T38.4X3	T38.4X4	T38.4X5	T38.4X6
Normal serum albumin (human), salt-poor	T45.8X1	T45.8X2	T45.8X3	T45.8X4	T45.8X5	T45.8X6
Normethandrone	T38.5X1	T38.5X2	T38.5X3	T38.5X4	T38.5X5	T38.5X6
Normison — see Benzodiazepines						
Normorphine	T40.2X1	T40.2X2	T40.2X3	T40.2X4	—	—
Norpseudoephedrine	T50.5X1	T50.5X2	T50.5X3	T50.5X4	T50.5X5	T50.5X6
Nortestosterone (furanpropionate)	T38.7X1	T38.7X2	T38.7X3	T38.7X4	T38.7X5	T38.7X6
Nortriptyline	T43.011	T43.012	T43.013	T43.014	T43.015	T43.016
Noscapine	T48.3X1	T48.3X2	T48.3X3	T48.3X4	T48.3X5	T48.3X6
Nose preparations	T49.6X1	T49.6X2	T49.6X3	T49.6X4	T49.6X5	T49.6X6
Novobiocin	T36.5X1	T36.5X2	T36.5X3	T36.5X4	T36.5X5	T36.5X6
Novocain (infiltration) (topical)	T41.3X1	T41.3X2	T41.3X3	T41.3X4	T41.3X5	T41.3X6
nerve block (peripheral) (plexus)	T41.3X1	T41.3X2	T41.3X3	T41.3X4	T41.3X5	T41.3X6
spinal	T41.3X1	T41.3X2	T41.3X3	T41.3X4	T41.3X5	T41.3X6

◀ New   ◀ Revised   ~~deleted~~ Deleted

TABLE OF DRUGS AND CHEMICALS

Substance	Poisoning, Accidental (Unintentional)	Poisoning, Intentional Self-Harm	Poisoning, Assault	Poisoning, Undetermined	Adverse Effect	Underdosing
Noxious foodstuff	T62.91	T62.92	T62.93	T62.94	—	—
specified NEC	T62.8X1	T62.8X2	T62.8X3	T62.8X4	—	—
Noxiptiline	T43.011	T43.012	T43.013	T43.014	T43.015	T43.016
Noxytiolin	T49.0X1	T49.0X2	T49.0X3	T49.0X4	T49.0X5	T49.0X6
NPH Iletin (insulin)	T38.3X1	T38.3X2	T38.3X3	T38.3X4	T38.3X5	T38.3X6
Numorphan	T40.2X1	T40.2X2	T40.2X3	T40.2X4	T40.2X5	T40.2X6
Nunol	T42.3X1	T42.3X2	T42.3X3	T42.3X4	T42.3X5	T42.3X6
Nupercaine (spinal anesthetic)	T41.3X1	T41.3X2	T41.3X3	T41.3X4	T41.3X5	T41.3X6
topical (surface)	T41.3X1	T41.3X2	T41.3X3	T41.3X4	T41.3X5	T41.3X6
Nutmeg oil (liniment)	T49.3X1	T49.3X2	T49.3X3	T49.3X4	T49.3X5	T49.3X6
Nutritional supplement	T50.901	T50.902	T50.903	T50.904	T50.905	T50.906
Nux vomica	T65.1X1	T65.1X2	T65.1X3	T65.1X4	—	—
Nydrazid	T37.1X1	T37.1X2	T37.1X3	T37.1X4	T37.1X5	T37.1X6
Nylidrin	T46.7X1	T46.7X2	T46.7X3	T46.7X4	T46.7X5	T46.7X6
Nystatin	T36.7X1	T36.7X2	T36.7X3	T36.7X4	T36.7X5	T36.7X6
topical	T49.0X1	T49.0X2	T49.0X3	T49.0X4	T49.0X5	T49.0X6
Nytol	T45.0X1	T45.0X2	T45.0X3	T45.0X4	T45.0X5	T45.0X6
O						
Obidoxime chloride	T50.6X1	T50.6X2	T50.6X3	T50.6X4	T50.6X5	T50.6X6
Octafonium (chloride)	T49.3X1	T49.3X2	T49.3X3	T49.3X4	T49.3X5	T49.3X6
Octamethyl pyrophosphoramide	T60.0X1	T60.0X2	T60.0X3	T60.0X4	—	—
Octanoin	T50.991	T50.992	T50.993	T50.994	T50.995	T50.996
Octatropine methylbromide	T44.3X1	T44.3X2	T44.3X3	T44.3X4	T44.3X5	T44.3X6
Octotiamine	T45.2X1	T45.2X2	T45.2X3	T45.2X4	T45.2X5	T45.2X6
Octoxinol (9)	T49.8X1	T49.8X2	T49.8X3	T49.8X4	T49.8X5	T49.8X6
Octreotide	T38.991	T38.992	T38.993	T38.994	T38.995	T38.996
Octyl nitrite	T46.3X1	T46.3X2	T46.3X3	T46.3X4	T46.3X5	T46.3X6
Oestradiol	T38.5X1	T38.5X2	T38.5X3	T38.5X4	T38.5X5	T38.5X6
Oestriol	T38.5X1	T38.5X2	T38.5X3	T38.5X4	T38.5X5	T38.5X6
Oestrogen	T38.5X1	T38.5X2	T38.5X3	T38.5X4	T38.5X5	T38.5X6
Oestrone	T38.5X1	T38.5X2	T38.5X3	T38.5X4	T38.5X5	T38.5X6
Ofloxacin	T36.8X1	T36.8X2	T36.8X3	T36.8X4	T36.8X5	T36.8X6
Oil (of)	T65.891	T65.892	T65.893	T65.894	—	—
bitter almond	T62.8X1	T62.8X2	T62.8X3	T62.8X4	—	—
cloves	T49.7X1	T49.7X2	T49.7X3	T49.7X4	T49.7X5	T49.7X6
colors	T65.6X1	T65.6X2	T65.6X3	T65.6X4	—	—
fumes	T59.891	T59.892	T59.893	T59.894	—	—
lubricating	T52.0X1	T52.0X2	T52.0X3	T52.0X4	—	—
Niobe	T52.8X1	T52.8X2	T52.8X3	T52.8X4	—	—
Oil (of) *(Continued)*						
vitriol (liquid)	T54.2X1	T54.2X2	T54.2X3	T54.2X4	—	—
fumes	T54.2X1	T54.2X2	T54.2X3	T54.2X4	—	—
wintergreen (bitter) NEC	T49.3X1	T49.3X2	T49.3X3	T49.3X4	T49.3X5	T49.3X6
Oily preparation (for skin)	T49.3X1	T49.3X2	T49.3X3	T49.3X4	T49.3X5	T49.3X6
Ointment NEC	T49.3X1	T49.3X2	T49.3X3	T49.3X4	T49.3X5	T49.3X6
Olanzapine	T43.591	T43.592	T43.593	T43.594	T43.595	T43.596
Oleander	T62.2X1	T62.2X2	T62.2X3	T62.2X4	—	—
Oleandomycin	T36.3X1	T36.3X2	T36.3X3	T36.3X4	T36.3X5	T36.3X6
Oleandrin	T46.0X1	T46.0X2	T46.0X3	T46.0X4	T46.0X5	T46.0X6
Oleic acid	T46.6X1	T46.6X2	T46.6X3	T46.6X4	T46.6X5	T46.6X6
Oleovitamin A	T45.2X1	T45.2X2	T45.2X3	T45.2X4	T45.2X5	T45.2X6
Oleum ricini	T47.2X1	T47.2X2	T47.2X3	T47.2X4	T47.2X5	T47.2X6
Olive oil (medicinal) NEC	T47.4X1	T47.4X2	T47.4X3	T47.4X4	T47.4X5	T47.4X6
Olivomycin	T45.1X1	T45.1X2	T45.1X3	T45.1X4	T45.1X5	T45.1X6
Olsalazine	T47.8X1	T47.8X2	T47.8X3	T47.8X4	T47.8X5	T47.8X6
Omeprazole	T47.1X1	T47.1X2	T47.1X3	T47.1X4	T47.1X5	T47.1X6
OMPA	T60.0X1	T60.0X2	T60.0X3	T60.0X4	—	—
Ondansetron	T45.0X1	T45.0X2	T45.0X3	T45.0X4	T45.0X5	T45.0X6
Oncovin	T45.1X1	T45.1X2	T45.1X3	T45.1X4	T45.1X5	T45.1X6
Ophthaine	T41.3X1	T41.3X2	T41.3X3	T41.3X4	T41.3X5	T41.3X6
Ophthetic	T41.3X1	T41.3X2	T41.3X3	T41.3X4	T41.3X5	T41.3X6
Opiate NEC	T40.601	T40.602	T40.603	T40.604	T40.605	T40.606
antagonists	T50.7X1	T50.7X2	T50.7X3	T50.7X4	T50.7X5	T50.7X6
Opioid NEC	T40.2X1	T40.2X2	T40.2X3	T40.2X4	T40.2X5	T40.2X6
Opipramol	T43.011	T43.012	T43.013	T43.014	T43.015	T43.016
Opium alkaloids (total)	T40.0X1	T40.0X2	T40.0X3	T40.0X4	T40.0X5	T40.0X6
standardized powdered	T40.0X1	T40.0X2	T40.0X3	T40.0X4	T40.0X5	T40.0X6
tincture (camphorated)	T40.0X1	T40.0X2	T40.0X3	T40.0X4	T40.0X5	T40.0X6
Oracon	T38.4X1	T38.4X2	T38.4X3	T38.4X4	T38.4X5	T38.4X6
Oragrafin	T50.8X1	T50.8X2	T50.8X3	T50.8X4	T50.8X5	T50.8X6
Oral contraceptives	T38.4X1	T38.4X2	T38.4X3	T38.4X4	T38.4X5	T38.4X6
Oral rehydration salts	T50.3X1	T50.3X2	T50.3X3	T50.3X4	T50.3X5	T50.3X6
Orazamide	T50.991	T50.992	T50.993	T50.994	T50.995	T50.996
Orciprenaline	T48.291	T48.292	T48.293	T48.294	T48.295	T48.296
Organidin	T48.4X1	T48.4X2	T48.4X3	T48.4X4	T48.4X5	T48.4X6
Organonitrate NEC	T46.3X1	T46.3X2	T46.3X3	T46.3X4	T46.3X5	T46.3X6
Organophosphates	T60.0X1	T60.0X2	T60.0X3	T60.0X4	—	—
Orimune	T50.B91	T50.B92	T50.B93	T50.B94	T50.B95	T50.B96
Orinase	T38.3X1	T38.3X2	T38.3X3	T38.3X4	T38.3X5	T38.3X6
Ormeloxifene	T38.6X1	T38.6X2	T38.6X3	T38.6X4	T38.6X5	T38.6X6

TABLE OF DRUGS AND CHEMICALS

Substance	Poisoning, Accidental (Unintentional)	Poisoning, Intentional Self-Harm	Poisoning, Assault	Poisoning, Undetermined	Adverse Effect	Underdosing
Ornidazole	T37.3X1	T37.3X2	T37.3X3	T37.3X4	T37.3X5	T37.3X6
Ornithine aspartate	T50.991	T50.992	T50.993	T50.994	T50.995	T50.996
Ornoprostil	T47.1X1	T47.1X2	T47.1X3	T47.1X4	T47.1X5	T47.1X6
Orphenadrine (hydrochloride)	T42.8X1	T42.8X2	T42.8X3	T42.8X4	T42.8X5	T42.8X6
Ortal (sodium)	T42.3X1	T42.3X2	T42.3X3	T42.3X4	T42.3X5	T42.3X6
Orthoboric acid	T49.0X1	T49.0X2	T49.0X3	T49.0X4	T49.0X5	T49.0X6
ENT agent	T49.6X1	T49.6X2	T49.6X3	T49.6X4	T49.6X5	T49.6X6
ophthalmic preparation	T49.5X1	T49.5X2	T49.5X3	T49.5X4	T49.5X5	T49.5X6
Orthocaine	T41.3X1	T41.3X2	T41.3X3	T41.3X4	T41.3X5	T41.3X6
Orthodichlorobenzene	T53.7X1	T53.7X2	T53.7X3	T53.7X4	—	—
Ortho-Novum	T38.4X1	T38.4X2	T38.4X3	T38.4X4	T38.4X5	T38.4X6
Orthotolidine (reagent)	T54.2X1	T54.2X2	T54.2X3	T54.2X4	—	—
Osmic acid (liquid)	T54.2X1	T54.2X2	T54.2X3	T54.2X4	—	—
fumes	T54.2X1	T54.2X2	T54.2X3	T54.2X4	—	—
Osmotic diuretics	T50.2X1	T50.2X2	T50.2X3	T50.2X4	T50.2X5	T50.2X6
Otilonium bromide	T44.3X1	T44.3X2	T44.3X3	T44.3X4	T44.3X5	T44.3X6
Otorhinolaryngological drug NEC	T49.6X1	T49.6X2	T49.6X3	T49.6X4	T49.6X5	T49.6X6
Ouabain(e)	T46.0X1	T46.0X2	T46.0X3	T46.0X4	T46.0X5	T46.0X6
Ovarian						
hormone	T38.5X1	T38.5X2	T38.5X3	T38.5X4	T38.5X5	T38.5X6
stimulant	T38.5X1	T38.5X2	T38.5X3	T38.5X4	T38.5X5	T38.5X6
Ovral	T38.4X1	T38.4X2	T38.4X3	T38.4X4	T38.4X5	T38.4X6
Ovulen	T38.4X1	T38.4X2	T38.4X3	T38.4X4	T38.4X5	T38.4X6
Oxacillin	T36.0X1	T36.0X2	T36.0X3	T36.0X4	T36.0X5	T36.0X6
Oxalic acid	T54.2X1	T54.2X2	T54.2X3	T54.2X4	—	—
ammonium salt	T50.991	T50.992	T50.993	T50.994	T50.995	T50.996
Oxamniquine	T37.4X1	T37.4X2	T37.4X3	T37.4X4	T37.4X5	T37.4X6
Oxanamide	T43.591	T43.592	T43.593	T43.594	T43.595	T43.596
Oxandrolone	T38.7X1	T38.7X2	T38.7X3	T38.7X4	T38.7X5	T38.7X6
Oxantel	T37.4X1	T37.4X2	T37.4X3	T37.4X4	T37.4X5	T37.4X6
Oxapium iodide	T44.3X1	T44.3X2	T44.3X3	T44.3X4	T44.3X5	T44.3X6
Oxaprotiline	T43.021	T43.022	T43.023	T43.024	T43.025	T43.026
Oxaprozin	T39.311	T39.312	T39.313	T39.314	T39.315	T39.316
Oxatomide	T45.0X1	T45.0X2	T45.0X3	T45.0X4	T45.0X5	T45.0X6
Oxazepam	T42.4X1	T42.4X2	T42.4X3	T42.4X4	T42.4X5	T42.4X6
Oxazimedrine	T50.5X1	T50.5X2	T50.5X3	T50.5X4	T50.5X5	T50.5X6
Oxazolam	T42.4X1	T42.4X2	T42.4X3	T42.4X4	T42.4X5	T42.4X6
Oxazolidine derivatives	T42.2X1	T42.2X2	T42.2X3	T42.2X4	T42.2X5	T42.2X6
Oxazolidinedione (derivative)	T42.2X1	T42.2X2	T42.2X3	T42.2X4	T42.2X5	T42.2X6
Ox bile extract	T47.5X1	T47.5X2	T47.5X3	T47.5X4	T47.5X5	T47.5X6
Oxcarbazepine	T42.1X1	T42.1X2	T42.1X3	T42.1X4	T42.1X5	T42.1X6
Oxedrine	T44.4X1	T44.4X2	T44.4X3	T44.4X4	T44.4X5	T44.4X6

Substance	Poisoning, Accidental (Unintentional)	Poisoning, Intentional Self-Harm	Poisoning, Assault	Poisoning, Undetermined	Adverse Effect	Underdosing
Oxeladin (citrate)	T48.3X1	T48.3X2	T48.3X3	T48.3X4	T48.3X5	T48.3X6
Oxendolone	T38.5X1	T38.5X2	T38.5X3	T38.5X4	T38.5X5	T38.5X6
Oxetacaine	T41.3X1	T41.3X2	T41.3X3	T41.3X4	T41.3X5	T41.3X6
Oxethazine	T41.3X1	T41.3X2	T41.3X3	T41.3X4	T41.3X5	T41.3X6
Oxetorone	T39.8X1	T39.8X2	T39.8X3	T39.8X4	T39.8X5	T39.8X6
Oxiconazole	T49.0X1	T49.0X2	T49.0X3	T49.0X4	T49.0X5	T49.0X6
Oxidizing agent NEC	T54.91	T54.92	T54.93	T54.94	—	—
Oxipurinol	T50.4X1	T50.4X2	T50.4X3	T50.4X4	T50.4X5	T50.4X6
Oxitriptan	T43.291	T43.292	T43.293	T43.294	T43.295	T43.296
Oxitropium bromide	T48.6X1	T48.6X2	T48.6X3	T48.6X4	T48.6X5	T48.6X6
Oxodipine	T46.1X1	T46.1X2	T46.1X3	T46.1X4	T46.1X5	T46.1X6
Oxolamine	T48.3X1	T48.3X2	T48.3X3	T48.3X4	T48.3X5	T48.3X6
Oxolinic acid	T37.8X1	T37.8X2	T37.8X3	T37.8X4	T37.8X5	T37.8X6
Oxomemazine	T43.3X1	T43.3X2	T43.3X3	T43.3X4	T43.3X5	T43.3X6
Oxophenarsine	T37.3X1	T37.3X2	T37.3X3	T37.3X4	T37.3X5	T37.3X6
Oxprenolol	T44.7X1	T44.7X2	T44.7X3	T44.7X4	T44.7X5	T44.7X6
Oxsoralen	T49.3X1	T49.3X2	T49.3X3	T49.3X4	T49.3X5	T49.3X6
Oxtriphylline	T48.6X1	T48.6X2	T48.6X3	T48.6X4	T48.6X5	T48.6X6
Oxybate sodium	T41.291	T41.292	T41.293	T41.294	T41.295	T41.296
Oxybuprocaine	T41.3X1	T41.3X2	T41.3X3	T41.3X4	T41.3X5	T41.3X6
Oxybutynin	T44.3X1	T44.3X2	T44.3X3	T44.3X4	T44.3X5	T44.3X6
Oxychlorosene	T49.0X1	T49.0X2	T49.0X3	T49.0X4	T49.0X5	T49.0X6
Oxycodone	T40.2X1	T40.2X2	T40.2X3	T40.2X4	T40.2X5	T40.2X6
Oxyfedrine	T46.3X1	T46.3X2	T46.3X3	T46.3X4	T46.3X5	T46.3X6
Oxygen	T41.5X1	T41.5X2	T41.5X3	T41.5X4	T41.5X5	T41.5X6
Oxylone	T49.0X1	T49.0X2	T49.0X3	T49.0X4	T49.0X5	T49.0X6
ophthalmic preparation	T49.5X1	T49.5X2	T49.5X3	T49.5X4	T49.5X5	T49.5X6
Oxymesterone	T38.7X1	T38.7X2	T38.7X3	T38.7X4	T38.7X5	T38.7X6
Oxymetazoline	T48.5X1	T48.5X2	T48.5X3	T48.5X4	T48.5X5	T48.5X6
Oxymetholone	T38.7X1	T38.7X2	T38.7X3	T38.7X4	T38.7X5	T38.7X6
Oxymorphone	T40.2X1	T40.2X2	T40.2X3	T40.2X4	T40.2X5	T40.2X6
Oxypertine	T43.591	T43.592	T43.593	T43.594	T43.595	T43.596
Oxyphenbutazone	T39.2X1	T39.2X2	T39.2X3	T39.2X4	T39.2X5	T39.2X6
Oxyphencyclimine	T44.3X1	T44.3X2	T44.3X3	T44.3X4	T44.3X5	T44.3X6
Oxyphenisatine	T47.2X1	T47.2X2	T47.2X3	T47.2X4	T47.2X5	T47.2X6
Oxyphenonium bromide	T44.3X1	T44.3X2	T44.3X3	T44.3X4	T44.3X5	T44.3X6
Oxypolygelatin	T45.8X1	T45.8X2	T45.8X3	T45.8X4	T45.8X5	T45.8X6
Oxyquinoline (derivatives)	T37.8X1	T37.8X2	T37.8X3	T37.8X4	T37.8X5	T37.8X6
Oxytetracycline	T36.4X1	T36.4X2	T36.4X3	T36.4X4	T36.4X5	T36.4X6
Oxytocic drug NEC	T48.0X1	T48.0X2	T48.0X3	T48.0X4	T48.0X5	T48.0X6
Oxytocin (synthetic)	T48.0X1	T48.0X2	T48.0X3	T48.0X4	T48.0X5	T48.0X6
Ozone	T59.891	T59.892	T59.893	T59.894	—	—

◄ New   ◄ Revised   ~~deleted~~ Deleted

Substance	External Cause (T-Code)					
	Poisoning, Accidental (Unintentional)	Poisoning, Intentional Self-Harm	Poisoning, Assault	Poisoning, Undetermined	Adverse Effect	Underdosing
P						
PABA	T49.3X1	T49.3X2	T49.3X3	T49.3X4	T49.3X5	T49.3X6
Packed red cells	T45.8X1	T45.8X2	T45.8X3	T45.8X4	T45.8X5	T45.8X6
Padimate	T49.3X1	T49.3X2	T49.3X3	T49.3X4	T49.3X5	T49.3X6
Paint NEC	T65.6X1	T65.6X2	T65.6X3	T65.6X4	—	—
cleaner	T52.91	T52.92	T52.93	T52.94	—	—
fumes NEC	T59.891	T59.892	T59.893	T59.894	—	—
lead (fumes)	T56.0X1	T56.0X2	T56.0X3	T56.0X4	—	—
solvent NEC	T52.8X1	T52.8X2	T52.8X3	T52.8X4	—	—
stripper	T52.8X1	T52.8X2	T52.8X3	T52.8X4	—	—
Palfium	T40.2X1	T40.2X2	T40.2X3	T40.2X4	—	—
Palm kernel oil	T50.991	T50.992	T50.993	T50.994	T50.995	T50.996
Paludrine	T37.2X1	T37.2X2	T37.2X2	T37.2X4	T37.2X5	T37.2X6
PAM (pralidoxime)	T50.6X1	T50.6X2	T50.6X3	T50.6X4	T50.6X5	T50.6X6
Pamaquine (naphthoute)	T37.2X1	T37.2X2	T37.2X3	T37.2X4	T37.2X5	T37.2X6
Panadol	T39.1X1	T39.1X2	T39.1X3	T39.1X4	T39.1X5	T39.1X6
Pancreatic						
digestive secretion stimulant	T47.8X1	T47.8X2	T47.8X3	T47.8X4	T47.8X5	T47.8X6
dornase	T45.3X1	T45.3X2	T45.3X3	T45.3X4	T45.3X5	T45.3X6
Pancreatin	T47.5X1	T47.5X2	T47.5X3	T47.5X4	T47.5X5	T47.5X6
Pancrelipase	T47.5X1	T47.5X2	T47.5X3	T47.5X4	T47.5X5	T47.5X6
Pancuronium (bromide)	T48.1X1	T48.1X2	T48.1X3	T48.1X4	T48.1X5	T48.1X6
Pangamic acid	T45.2X1	T45.2X2	T45.2X3	T45.2X4	T45.2X5	T45.2X6
Panthenol	T45.2X1	T45.2X2	T45.2X3	T45.2X4	T45.2X5	T45.2X6
topical	T49.8X1	T49.8X2	T49.8X3	T49.8X4	T49.8X5	T49.8X6
Pantopon	T40.0X1	T40.0X2	T40.0X3	T40.0X4	T40.0X5	T40.0X6
Pantothenic acid	T45.2X1	T45.2X2	T45.2X3	T45.2X4	T45.2X5	T45.2X6
Panwarfin	T45.511	T45.512	T45.513	T45.514	T45.515	T45.516
Papain	T47.5X1	T47.5X2	T47.5X3	T47.5X4	T47.5X5	T47.5X6
digestant	T47.5X1	T47.5X2	T47.5X3	T47.5X4	T47.5X5	T47.5X6
Papaveretum	T40.0X1	T40.0X2	T40.0X3	T40.0X4	T40.0X5	T40.0X6
Papaverine	T44.3X1	T44.3X2	T44.3X3	T44.3X4	T44.3X5	T44.3X6
Para-acetamidophenol	T39.1X1	T39.1X2	T39.1X3	T39.1X4	T39.1X5	T39.1X6
Para-aminobenzoic acid	T49.3X1	T49.3X2	T49.3X3	T49.3X4	T49.3X5	T49.3X6
Para-aminophenol derivatives	T39.1X1	T39.1X2	T39.1X3	T39.1X4	T39.1X5	T39.1X6
Para-aminosalicylic acid	T37.1X1	T37.1X2	T37.1X3	T37.1X4	T37.1X5	T37.1X6
Paracetaldehyde	T42.6X1	T42.6X2	T42.6X3	T42.6X4	T42.6X5	T42.6X6
Paracetamol	T39.1X1	T39.1X2	T39.1X3	T39.1X4	T39.1X5	T39.1X6
Parachlorophenol (camphorated)	T49.0X1	T49.0X2	T49.0X3	T49.0X4	T49.0X5	T49.0X6
Paracodin	T40.2X1	T40.2X2	T40.2X3	T40.2X4	T40.2X5	T40.2X6
Paradione	T42.2X1	T42.2X2	T42.2X3	T42.2X4	T42.2X5	T42.2X6

Substance	External Cause (T-Code)					
	Poisoning, Accidental (Unintentional)	Poisoning, Intentional Self-Harm	Poisoning, Assault	Poisoning, Undetermined	Adverse Effect	Underdosing
Paraffin(s) (wax)	T52.0X1	T52.0X2	T52.0X3	T52.0X4	—	—
liquid (medicinal)	T47.4X1	T47.4X2	T47.4X3	T47.4X4	T47.4X5	T47.4X6
nonmedicinal	T52.0X1	T52.0X2	T52.0X3	T52.0X4	—	—
Paraformaldehyde	T60.3X1	T60.3X2	T60.3X3	T60.3X4	—	—
Paraldehyde	T42.6X1	T42.6X2	T42.6X3	T42.6X4	T42.6X5	T42.6X6
Paramethadione	T42.2X1	T42.2X2	T42.2X3	T42.2X4	T42.2X5	T42.2X6
Paramethasone	T38.0X1	T38.0X2	T38.0X3	T38.0X4	T38.0X5	T38.0X6
acetate	T49.0X1	T49.0X2	T49.0X3	T49.0X4	T49.0X5	T49.0X6
Paraoxon	T60.0X1	T60.0X2	T60.0X3	T60.0X4	—	—
Paraquat	T60.3X1	T60.3X2	T60.3X3	T60.3X4	—	—
Parasympatholytic NEC	T44.3X1	T44.3X2	T44.3X3	T44.3X4	T44.3X5	T44.3X6
Parasympathomimetic drug NEC	T44.1X1	T44.1X2	T44.1X3	T44.1X4	T44.1X5	T44.1X6
Parathion	T60.0X1	T60.0X2	T60.0X3	T60.0X4	—	—
Parathormone	T50.991	T50.992	T50.993	T50.994	T50.995	T50.996
Parathyroid extract	T50.991	T50.992	T50.993	T50.994	T50.995	T50.996
Paratyphoid vaccine	T50.A91	T50.A92	T50.A93	T50.A94	T50.A95	T50.A96
Paredrine	T44.4X1	T44.4X2	T44.4X3	T44.4X4	T44.4X5	T44.4X6
Paregoric	T40.0X1	T40.0X2	T40.0X3	T40.0X4	T40.0X5	T40.0X6
Pargyline	T46.5X1	T46.5X2	T46.5X3	T46.5X4	T46.5X5	T46.5X6
Paris green	T57.0X1	T57.0X2	T57.0X3	T57.0X4	—	—
insecticide	T57.0X1	T57.0X2	T57.0X3	T57.0X4	—	—
Parnate	T43.1X1	T43.1X2	T43.1X3	T43.1X4	T43.1X5	T43.1X6
Paromomycin	T36.5X1	T36.5X2	T36.5X3	T36.5X4	T36.5X5	T36.5X6
Paroxypropione	T45.1X1	T45.1X2	T45.1X3	T45.1X4	T45.1X5	T45.1X6
Parzone	T40.2X1	T40.2X2	T40.2X3	T40.2X4	T40.2X5	T40.2X6
PAS	T37.1X1	T37.1X2	T37.1X3	T37.1X4	T37.1X5	T37.1X6
Pasiniazid	T37.1X1	T37.1X2	T37.1X3	T37.1X4	T37.1X5	T37.1X6
PBB (polybrominated biphenyls)	T65.891	T65.892	T65.893	T65.894	—	—
PCB	T65.891	T65.892	T65.893	T65.894	—	—
PCP						
meaning pentachlorophenol	T60.1X1	T60.1X2	T60.1X3	T60.1X4	—	—
fungicide	T60.3X1	T60.3X2	T60.3X3	T60.3X4	—	—
herbicide	T60.3X1	T60.3X2	T60.3X3	T60.3X4	—	—
insecticide	T60.1X1	T60.1X2	T60.1X3	T60.1X4	—	—
meaning phencyclidine	T40.991	T40.992	T40.993	T40.994	—	—
Peach kernel oil (emulsion)	T47.4X1	T47.4X2	T47.4X3	T47.4X4	T47.4X5	T47.4X6
Peanut oil (emulsion) NEC	T47.4X1	T47.4X2	T47.4X3	T47.4X4	T47.4X5	T47.4X6
topical	T49.3X1	T49.3X2	T49.3X3	T49.3X4	T49.3X5	T49.3X6
Pearly Gates (morning glory seeds)	T40.991	T40.992	T40.993	T40.994	—	—
Pecazine	T43.3X1	T43.3X2	T43.3X3	T43.3X4	T43.3X5	T43.3X6
Pectin	T47.6X1	T47.6X2	T47.6X3	T47.6X4	T47.6X5	T47.6X6

Substance	External Cause (T-Code)					
	Poisoning, Accidental (Unintentional)	Poisoning, Intentional Self-Harm	Poisoning, Assault	Poisoning, Undetermined	Adverse Effect	Underdosing
Pefloxacin	T37.8X1	T37.8X2	T37.8X3	T37.8X4	T37.8X5	T37.8X6
Pegademase, bovine	T50.Z91	T50.Z92	T50.Z93	T50.Z94	T50.Z95	T50.Z96
Pelletierine tannate	T37.4X1	T37.4X2	T37.4X3	T37.4X4	T37.4X5	T37.4X6
Pemirolast (potassium)	T48.6X1	T48.6X2	T48.6X3	T48.6X4	T48.6X5	T48.6X6
Pemoline	T50.7X1	T50.7X2	T50.7X3	T50.7X4	T50.7X5	T50.7X6
Pempidine	T44.2X1	T44.2X2	T44.2X3	T44.2X4	T44.2X5	T44.2X6
Penamecillin	T36.0X1	T36.0X2	T36.0X3	T36.0X4	T36.0X5	T36.0X6
Penbutolol	T44.7X1	T44.7X2	T44.7X3	T44.7X4	T44.7X5	T44.7X6
Penethamate	T36.0X1	T36.0X2	T36.0X3	T36.0X4	T36.0X5	T36.0X6
Penfluridol	T43.591	T43.592	T43.593	T43.594	T43.595	T43.596
Penflutizide	T50.2X1	T50.2X2	T50.2X3	T50.2X4	T50.2X5	T50.2X6
Pengitoxin	T46.0X1	T46.0X2	T46.0X3	T46.0X4	T46.0X5	T46.0X6
Penicillamine	T50.6X1	T50.6X2	T50.6X3	T50.6X4	T50.6X5	T50.6X6
Penicillin (any)	T36.0X1	T36.0X2	T36.0X3	T36.0X4	T36.0X5	T36.0X6
Penicillinase	T45.3X1	T45.3X2	T45.3X3	T45.3X4	T45.3X5	T45.3X6
Penicilloyl polylysine	T50.8X1	T50.8X2	T50.8X3	T50.8X4	T50.8X5	T50.8X6
Penimepicycline	T36.4X1	T36.4X2	T36.4X3	T36.4X4	T36.4X5	T36.4X6
Pentachloroethane	T53.6X1	T53.6X2	T53.6X3	T53.6X4	—	—
Pentachloronaphthalene	T53.7X1	T53.7X2	T53.7X3	T53.7X4	—	—
Pentachlorophenol (pesticide)	T60.1X1	T60.1X2	T60.1X3	T60.1X4	—	—
fungicide	T60.3X1	T60.3X2	T60.3X3	T60.3X4	—	—
herbicide	T60.3X1	T60.3X2	T60.3X3	T60.3X4	—	—
insecticide	T60.1X1	T60.1X2	T60.1X3	T60.1X4	—	—
Pentaerythritol tetranitrate	T46.3X1	T46.3X2	T46.3X3	T46.3X4	T46.3X5	T46.3X6
Pentaerythritol	T46.3X1	T46.3X2	T46.3X3	T46.3X4	T46.3X5	T46.3X6
chloral	T42.6X1	T42.6X2	T42.6X3	T42.6X4	T42.6X5	T42.6X6
tetranitrate NEC	T46.3X1	T46.3X2	T46.3X3	T46.3X4	T46.3X5	T46.3X6
Pentagastrin	T50.8X1	T50.8X2	T50.8X3	T50.8X4	T50.8X5	T50.8X6
Pentalin	T53.6X1	T53.6X2	T53.6X3	T53.6X4	—	—
Pentamethonium bromide	T44.2X1	T44.2X2	T44.2X3	T44.2X4	T44.2X5	T44.2X6
Pentamidine	T37.3X1	T37.3X2	T37.3X3	T37.3X4	T37.3X5	T37.3X6
Pentanol	T51.3X1	T51.3X2	T51.3X3	T51.3X4	—	—
Pentapyrrolinium (bitartrate)	T44.2X1	T44.2X2	T44.2X3	T44.2X4	T44.2X5	T44.2X6
Pentaquine	T37.2X1	T37.2X2	T37.2X3	T37.2X4	T37.2X5	T37.2X6
Pentazocine	T40.491	T40.492	T40.493	T40.494	T40.495	T40.496
Pentetrazole	T50.7X1	T50.7X2	T50.7X3	T50.7X4	T50.7X5	T50.7X6
Penthienate bromide	T44.3X1	T44.3X2	T44.3X3	T44.3X4	T44.3X5	T44.3X6
Pentifylline	T46.7X1	T46.7X2	T46.7X3	T46.7X4	T46.7X5	T46.7X6
Pentobarbital	T42.3X1	T42.3X2	T42.3X3	T42.3X4	T42.3X5	T42.3X6
sodium	T42.3X1	T42.3X2	T42.3X3	T42.3X4	T42.3X5	T42.3X6
Pentobarbitone	T42.3X1	T42.3X2	T42.3X3	T42.3X4	T42.3X5	T42.3X6
Pentolonium tartrate	T44.2X1	T44.2X2	T44.2X3	T44.2X4	T44.2X5	T44.2X6

Substance	External Cause (T-Code)					
	Poisoning, Accidental (Unintentional)	Poisoning, Intentional Self-Harm	Poisoning, Assault	Poisoning, Undetermined	Adverse Effect	Underdosing
Pentosan polysulfate (sodium)	T39.8X1	T39.8X2	T39.8X3	T39.8X4	T39.8X5	T39.8X6
Pentostatin	T45.1X1	T45.1X2	T45.1X3	T45.1X4	T45.1X5	T45.1X6
Pentothal	T41.1X1	T41.1X2	T41.1X3	T41.1X4	T41.1X5	T41.1X6
Pentoxifylline	T46.7X1	T46.7X2	T46.7X3	T46.7X4	T46.7X5	T46.7X6
Pentoxyverine	T48.3X1	T48.3X2	T48.3X3	T48.3X4	T48.3X5	T48.3X6
Pentrinat	T46.3X1	T46.3X2	T46.3X3	T46.3X4	T46.3X5	T46.3X6
Pentylenetetrazole	T50.7X1	T50.7X2	T50.7X3	T50.7X4	T50.7X5	T50.7X6
Pentylsalicylamide	T37.1X1	T37.1X2	T37.1X3	T37.1X4	T37.1X5	T37.1X6
Pentymal	T42.3X1	T42.3X2	T42.3X3	T42.3X4	T42.3X5	T42.3X6
Peplomycin	T45.1X1	T45.1X2	T45.1X3	T45.1X4	T45.1X5	T45.1X6
Peppermint (oil)	T47.5X1	T47.5X2	T47.5X3	T47.5X4	T47.5X5	T47.5X6
Pepsin	T47.5X1	T47.5X2	T47.5X3	T47.5X4	T47.5X5	T47.5X6
digestant	T47.5X1	T47.5X2	T47.5X3	T47.5X4	T47.5X5	T47.5X6
Pepstatin	T47.1X1	T47.1X2	T47.1X3	T47.1X4	T47.1X5	T47.1X6
Peptavlon	T50.8X1	T50.8X2	T50.8X3	T50.8X4	T50.8X5	T50.8X6
Perazine	T43.3X1	T43.3X2	T43.3X3	T43.3X4	T43.3X5	T43.3X6
Percaine (spinal)	T41.3X1	T41.3X2	T41.3X3	T41.3X4	T41.3X5	T41.3X6
topical (surface)	T41.3X1	T41.3X2	T41.3X3	T41.3X4	T41.3X5	T41.3X6
Perchloroethylene	T53.3X1	T53.3X2	T53.3X3	T53.3X4	—	—
medicinal	T37.4X1	T37.4X2	T37.4X3	T37.4X4	T37.4X5	T37.4X6
vapor	T53.3X1	T53.3X2	T53.3X3	T53.3X4	—	—
Percodan	T40.2X1	T40.2X2	T40.2X3	T40.2X4	T40.2X5	T40.2X6
Percogesic — see also Acetaminophen	T45.0X1	T45.0X2	T45.0X3	T45.0X4	T45.0X5	T45.0X6
Percorten	T38.0X1	T38.0X2	T38.0X3	T38.0X4	T38.0X5	T38.0X6
Pergolide	T42.8X1	T42.8X2	T42.8X3	T42.8X4	T42.8X5	T42.8X6
Pergonal	T38.811	T38.812	T38.813	T38.814	T38.815	T38.816
Perhexilene	T46.3X1	T46.3X2	T46.3X3	T46.3X4	T46.3X5	T46.3X6
Perhexiline (maleate)	T46.3X1	T46.3X2	T46.3X3	T46.3X4	T46.3X5	T46.3X6
Periactin	T45.0X1	T45.0X2	T45.0X3	T45.0X4	T45.0X5	T45.0X6
Periciazine	T43.3X1	T43.3X2	T43.3X3	T43.3X4	T43.3X5	T43.3X6
Periclor	T42.6X1	T42.6X2	T42.6X3	T42.6X4	T42.6X5	T42.6X6
Perindopril	T46.4X1	T46.4X2	T46.4X3	T46.4X4	T46.4X5	T46.4X6
Perisoxal	T39.8X1	T39.8X2	T39.8X3	T39.8X4	T39.8X5	T39.8X6
Peritrate	T46.3X1	T46.3X2	T46.3X3	T46.3X4	T46.3X5	T46.3X6
Peritoneal dialysis solution	T50.3X1	T50.3X2	T50.3X3	T50.3X4	T50.3X5	T50.3X6
Perlapine	T42.4X1	T42.4X2	T42.4X3	T42.4X4	T42.4X5	T42.4X6
Permanganate	T65.891	T65.892	T65.893	T65.894	—	—
Permethrin	T60.1X1	T60.1X2	T60.1X3	T60.1X4	—	—
Pernocton	T42.3X1	T42.3X2	T42.3X3	T42.3X4	T42.3X5	T42.3X6
Pernoston	T42.3X1	T42.3X2	T42.3X3	T42.3X4	T42.3X5	T42.3X6
Peronine	T40.2X1	T40.2X2	T40.2X3	T40.2X4	—	—
Perphenazine	T43.3X1	T43.3X2	T43.3X3	T43.3X4	T43.3X5	T43.3X6

◄ New   ◄ Revised   ~~deleted~~ Deleted

Substance	Poisoning, Accidental (Unintentional)	Poisoning, Intentional Self-Harm	Poisoning, Assault	Poisoning, Undetermined	Adverse Effect	Underdosing
Pertofrane	T43.011	T43.012	T43.013	T43.014	T43.015	T43.016
Pertussis						
immune serum (human)	T50.Z11	T50.Z12	T50.Z13	T50.Z14	T50.Z15	T50.Z16
vaccine (with diphtheria toxoid) (with tetanus toxoid)	T50.A11	T50.A12	T50.A13	T50.A14	T50.A15	T50.A16
Peruvian balsam	T49.0X1	T49.0X2	T49.0X3	T49.0X4	T49.0X5	T49.0X6
Peruvoside	T46.0X1	T46.0X2	T46.0X3	T46.0X4	T46.0X5	T46.0X6
Pesticide (dust) (fumes) (vapor) NEC	T60.91	T60.92	T60.93	T60.94	—	—
arsenic	T57.0X1	T57.0X2	T57.0X3	T57.0X4	—	—
chlorinated	T60.1X1	T60.1X2	T60.1X3	T60.1X4	—	—
cyanide	T65.0X1	T65.0X2	T65.0X3	T65.0X4	—	—
kerosene	T52.0X1	T52.0X2	T52.0X3	T52.0X4	—	—
mixture (of compounds)	T60.91	T60.92	T60.93	T60.94	—	—
naphthalene	T60.2X1	T60.2X2	T60.2X3	T60.2X4	—	—
organochlorine (compounds)	T60.1X1	T60.1X2	T60.1X3	T60.1X4	—	—
petroleum (distillate) (products) NEC	T60.8X1	T60.8X2	T60.8X3	T60.8X4	—	—
specified ingredient NEC	T60.8X1	T60.8X2	T60.8X3	T60.8X4	—	—
strychnine	T65.1X1	T65.1X2	T65.1X3	T65.1X4	—	—
thallium	T60.4X1	T60.4X2	T60.4X3	T60.4X4	—	—
Pethidine	T40.491	T40.492	T40.493	T40.494	T40.495	T40.496
Petrichloral	T42.6X1	T42.6X2	T42.6X3	T42.6X4	T42.6X5	T42.6X6
Petrol	T52.0X1	T52.0X2	T52.0X3	T52.0X4	—	—
vapor	T52.0X1	T52.0X2	T52.0X3	T52.0X4	—	—
Petrolatum	T49.3X1	T49.3X2	T49.3X3	T49.3X4	T49.3X5	T49.3X6
hydrophilic	T49.3X1	T49.3X2	T49.3X3	T49.3X4	T49.3X5	T49.3X6
liquid	T47.4X1	T47.4X2	T47.4X3	T47.4X4	T47.4X5	T47.4X6
topical	T49.3X1	T49.3X2	T49.3X3	T49.3X4	T49.3X5	T49.3X6
nonmedicinal	T52.0X1	T52.0X2	T52.0X3	T52.0X4	—	—
red veterinary	T49.3X1	T49.3X2	T49.3X3	T49.3X4	T49.3X5	T49.3X6
white	T49.3X1	T49.3X2	T49.3X3	T49.3X4	T49.3X5	T49.3X6
Petroleum (products) NEC	T52.0X1	T52.0X2	T52.0X3	T52.0X4	—	—
benzine(s) — see Ligroin						
ether — see Ligroin						
jelly — see Petrolatum						
naphtha — see Ligroin						
pesticide	T60.8X1	T60.8X2	T60.8X3	T60.8X4	—	—
solids	T52.0X1	T52.0X2	T52.0X3	T52.0X4	—	—
solvents	T52.0X1	T52.0X2	T52.0X3	T52.0X4	—	—
vapor	T52.0X1	T52.0X2	T52.0X3	T52.0X4	—	—
Peyote	T40.991	T40.992	T40.993	T40.994	—	—
Phanodorm, phanodorn	T42.3X1	T42.3X2	T42.3X3	T42.3X4	T42.3X5	T42.3X6

Substance	Poisoning, Accidental (Unintentional)	Poisoning, Intentional Self-Harm	Poisoning, Assault	Poisoning, Undetermined	Adverse Effect	Underdosing
Phanquinone	T37.3X1	T37.3X2	T37.3X3	T37.3X4	T37.3X5	T37.3X6
Phanquone	T37.3X1	T37.3X2	T37.3X3	T37.3X4	T37.3X5	T37.3X6
Pharmaceutical						
adjunct NEC	T50.901	T50.902	T50.903	T50.904	T50.905	T50.906
excipient NEC	T50.901	T50.902	T50.903	T50.904	T50.905	T50.906
sweetener	T50.901	T50.902	T50.903	T50.904	T50.905	T50.906
viscous agent	T50.901	T50.902	T50.903	T50.904	T50.905	T50.906
Phemitone	T42.3X1	T42.3X2	T42.3X3	T42.3X4	T42.3X5	T42.3X6
Phenacaine	T41.3X1	T41.3X2	T41.3X3	T41.3X4	T41.3X5	T41.3X6
Phenacemide	T42.6X1	T42.6X2	T42.6X3	T42.6X4	T42.6X5	T42.6X6
Phenacetin	T39.1X1	T39.1X2	T39.1X3	T39.1X4	T39.1X5	T39.1X6
Phenadoxone	T40.2X1	T40.2X2	T40.2X3	T40.2X4	—	—
Phenaglycodol	T43.591	T43.592	T43.593	T43.594	T43.595	T43.596
Phenantoin	T42.0X1	T42.0X2	T42.0X3	T42.0X4	T42.0X5	T42.0X6
Phenaphthazine reagent	T50.991	T50.992	T50.993	T50.994	T50.995	T50.996
Phenazocine	T40.491	T40.492	T40.493	T40.494	T40.495	T40.496
Phenazone	T39.2X1	T39.2X2	T39.2X3	T39.2X4	T39.2X5	T39.2X6
Phenazopyridine	T39.8X1	T39.8X2	T39.8X3	T39.8X4	T39.8X5	T39.8X6
Phenbenicillin	T36.0X1	T36.0X2	T36.0X3	T36.0X4	T36.0X5	T36.0X6
Phenbutrazate	T50.5X1	T50.5X2	T50.5X3	T50.5X4	T50.5X5	T50.5X6
Phencyclidine	T40.991	T40.992	T40.993	T40.994	T40.995	T40.996
Phendimetrazine	T50.5X1	T50.5X2	T50.5X3	T50.5X4	T50.5X5	T50.5X6
Phenelzine	T43.1X1	T43.1X2	T43.1X3	T43.1X4	T43.1X5	T43.1X6
Phenemal	T42.3X1	T42.3X2	T42.3X3	T42.3X4	T42.3X5	T42.3X6
Phenergan	T42.6X1	T42.6X2	T42.6X3	T42.6X4	T42.6X5	T42.6X6
Pheneticillin	T36.0X1	T36.0X2	T36.0X3	T36.0X4	T36.0X5	T36.0X6
Pheneturide	T42.6X1	T42.6X2	T42.6X3	T42.6X4	T42.6X5	T42.6X6
Phenformin	T38.3X1	T38.3X2	T38.3X3	T38.3X4	T38.3X5	T38.3X6
Phenglutarimide	T44.3X1	T44.3X2	T44.3X3	T44.3X4	T44.3X5	T44.3X6
Phenicarbazide	T39.8X1	T39.8X2	T39.8X3	T39.8X4	T39.8X5	T39.8X6
Phenindamine	T45.0X1	T45.0X2	T45.0X3	T45.0X4	T45.0X5	T45.0X6
Phenindione	T45.511	T45.512	T45.513	T45.514	T45.515	T45.516
Pheniprazine	T43.1X1	T43.1X2	T43.1X3	T43.1X4	T43.1X5	T43.1X6
Pheniramine	T45.0X1	T45.0X2	T45.0X3	T45.0X4	T45.0X5	T45.0X6
Phenisatin	T47.2X1	T47.2X2	T47.2X3	T47.2X4	T47.2X5	T47.2X6
Phenmetrazine	T50.5X1	T50.5X2	T50.5X3	T50.5X4	T50.5X5	T50.5X6
Phenobal	T42.3X1	T42.3X2	T42.3X3	T42.3X4	T42.3X5	T42.3X6
Phenobarbital	T42.3X1	T42.3X2	T42.3X3	T42.3X4	T42.3X5	T42.3X6
with						
mephenytoin	T42.3X1	T42.3X2	T42.3X3	T42.3X4	T42.3X5	T42.3X6
phenytoin	T42.3X1	T42.3X2	T42.3X3	T42.3X4	T42.3X5	T42.3X6
sodium	T42.3X1	T42.3X2	T42.3X3	T42.3X4	T42.3X5	T42.3X6

◀ New   ◀ Revised   ~~deleted~~ Deleted

Substance	Poisoning, Accidental (Unintentional)	Poisoning, Intentional Self-Harm	Poisoning, Assault	Poisoning, Undetermined	Adverse Effect	Underdosing
Phenobarbitone	T42.3X1	T42.3X2	T42.3X3	T42.3X4	T42.3X5	T42.3X6
Phenobutiodil	T50.8X1	T50.8X2	T50.8X3	T50.8X4	T50.8X5	T50.8X6
Phenoctide	T49.0X1	T49.0X2	T49.0X3	T49.0X4	T49.0X5	T49.0X6
Phenol	T49.0X1	T49.0X2	T49.0X3	T49.0X4	T49.0X5	T49.0X6
disinfectant	T54.0X1	T54.0X2	T54.0X3	T54.0X4	—	—
in oil injection	T46.8X1	T46.8X2	T46.8X3	T46.8X4	T46.8X5	T46.8X6
medicinal	T49.1X1	T49.1X2	T49.1X3	T49.1X4	T49.1X5	T49.1X6
nonmedicinal NEC	T54.0X1	T54.0X2	T54.0X3	T54.0X4	—	—
pesticide	T60.8X1	T60.8X2	T60.8X3	T60.8X4	—	—
red	T50.8X1	T50.8X2	T50.8X3	T50.8X4	T50.8X5	T50.8X6
Phenolic preparation	T49.1X1	T49.1X2	T49.1X3	T49.1X4	T49.1X5	T49.1X6
Phenolphthalein	T47.2X1	T47.2X2	T47.2X3	T47.2X4	T47.2X5	T47.2X6
Phenolsulfonphthalein	T50.8X1	T50.8X2	T50.8X3	T50.8X4	T50.8X5	T50.8X6
Phenomorphan	T40.2X1	T40.2X2	T40.2X3	T40.2X4	—	—
Phenonyl	T42.3X1	T42.3X2	T42.3X3	T42.3X4	T42.3X5	T42.3X6
Phenoperidine	T40.491	T40.492	T40.493	T40.494		
Phenopyrazone	T46.991	T46.992	T46.993	T46.994	T46.995	T46.996
Phenoquin	T50.4X1	T50.4X2	T50.4X3	T50.4X4	T50.4X5	T50.4X6
Phenothiazine (psychotropic) NEC	T43.3X1	T43.3X2	T43.3X3	T43.3X4	T43.3X5	T43.3X6
insecticide	T60.2X1	T60.2X2	T60.2X3	T60.2X4	—	—
Phenothrin	T49.0X1	T49.0X2	T49.0X3	T49.0X4	T49.0X5	T49.0X6
Phenoxybenzamine	T46.7X1	T46.7X2	T46.7X3	T46.7X4	T46.7X5	T46.7X6
Phenoxyethanol	T49.0X1	T49.0X2	T49.0X3	T49.0X4	T49.0X5	T49.0X6
Phenoxymethyl penicillin	T36.0X1	T36.0X2	T36.0X3	T36.0X4	T36.0X5	T36.0X6
Phenprobamate	T42.8X1	T42.8X2	T42.8X3	T42.8X4	T42.8X5	T42.8X6
Phenprocoumon	T45.511	T45.512	T45.513	T45.514	T45.515	T45.516
Phensuximide	T42.2X1	T42.2X2	T42.2X3	T42.2X4	T42.2X5	T42.2X6
Phentermine	T50.5X1	T50.5X2	T50.5X3	T50.5X4	T50.5X5	T50.5X6
Phenthicillin	T36.0X1	T36.0X2	T36.0X3	T36.0X4	T36.0X5	T36.0X6
Phentolamine	T46.7X1	T46.7X2	T46.7X3	T46.7X4	T46.7X5	T46.7X6
Phenyl						
butazone	T39.2X1	T39.2X2	T39.2X3	T39.2X4	T39.2X5	T39.2X6
enediamine	T65.3X1	T65.3X2	T65.3X3	T65.3X4	—	—
hydrazine	T65.3X1	T65.3X2	T65.3X3	T65.3X4	—	—
antineoplastic	T45.1X1	T45.1X2	T45.1X3	T45.1X4	T45.1X5	T45.1X6
mercuric compounds — *see* Mercury						
salicylate	T49.3X1	T49.3X2	T49.3X3	T49.3X4	T49.3X5	T49.3X6
Phenylalanine mustard	T45.1X1	T45.1X2	T45.1X3	T45.1X4	T45.1X5	T45.1X6
Phenylbutazone	T39.2X1	T39.2X2	T39.2X3	T39.2X4	T39.2X5	T39.2X6
Phenylenediamine	T65.3X1	T65.3X2	T65.3X3	T65.3X4	—	—
Phenylephrine	T44.4X1	T44.4X2	T44.4X3	T44.4X4	T44.4X5	T44.4X6
Phenylethylbiguanide	T38.3X1	T38.3X2	T38.3X3	T38.3X4	T38.3X5	T38.3X6
Phenylmercuric						
acetate	T49.0X1	T49.0X2	T49.0X3	T49.0X4	T49.0X5	T49.0X6
borate	T49.0X1	T49.0X2	T49.0X3	T49.0X4	T49.0X5	T49.0X6
nitrate	T49.0X1	T49.0X2	T49.0X3	T49.0X4	T49.0X5	T49.0X6
Phenylmethylbarbitone	T42.3X1	T42.3X2	T42.3X3	T42.3X4	T42.3X5	T42.3X6
Phenylpropanol	T47.5X1	T47.5X2	T47.5X3	T47.5X4	T47.5X5	T47.5X6
Phenylpropanolamine	T44.991	T44.992	T44.993	T44.994	T44.995	T44.996
Phenylsulfthion	T60.0X1	T60.0X2	T60.0X3	T60.0X4	—	—
Phenyltoloxamine	T45.0X1	T45.0X2	T45.0X3	T45.0X4	T45.0X5	T45.0X6
Phenyramidol, phenyramidon	T39.8X1	T39.8X2	T39.8X3	T39.8X4	T39.8X5	T39.8X6
Phenytoin	T42.0X1	T42.0X2	T42.0X3	T42.0X4	T42.0X5	T42.0X6
with Phenobarbital	T42.3X1	T42.3X2	T42.3X3	T42.3X4	T42.3X5	T42.3X6
pHisoHex	T49.2X1	T49.2X2	T49.2X3	T49.2X4	T49.2X5	T49.2X6
Pholcodine	T48.3X1	T48.3X2	T48.3X3	T48.3X4	T48.3X5	T48.3X6
Pholedrine	T46.991	T46.992	T46.993	T46.994	T46.995	T46.996
Phorate	T60.0X1	T60.0X2	T60.0X3	T60.0X4	—	—
Phosdrin	T60.0X1	T60.0X2	T60.0X3	T60.0X4	—	—
Phosfolan	T60.0X1	T60.0X2	T60.0X3	T60.0X4	—	—
Phosgene (gas)	T59.891	T59.892	T59.893	T59.894		
Phosphamidon	T60.0X1	T60.0X2	T60.0X3	T60.0X4	—	—
Phosphate	T65.891	T65.892	T65.893	T65.894		
laxative	T47.4X1	T47.4X2	T47.4X3	T47.4X4	T47.4X5	T47.4X6
organic	T60.0X1	T60.0X2	T60.0X3	T60.0X4	—	—
solvent	T52.91	T52.92	T52.93	T52.94		
tricresyl	T65.891	T65.892	T65.893	T65.894		
Phosphine	T57.1X1	T57.1X2	T57.1X3	T57.1X4		
fumigant	T57.1X1	T57.1X2	T57.1X3	T57.1X4		
Phospholine	T49.5X1	T49.5X2	T49.5X3	T49.5X4	T49.5X5	T49.5X6
Phosphoric acid	T54.2X1	T54.2X2	T54.2X3	T54.2X4		
Phosphorus (compound) NEC	T57.1X1	T57.1X2	T57.1X3	T57.1X4		
pesticide	T60.0X1	T60.0X2	T60.0X3	T60.0X4	—	—
Phthalates	T65.891	T65.892	T65.893	T65.894		
Phthalic anhydride	T65.891	T65.892	T65.893	T65.894		
Phthalimidoglutarimide	T42.6X1	T42.6X2	T42.6X3	T42.6X4	T42.6X5	T42.6X6
Phthalylsulfathiazole	T37.0X1	T37.0X2	T37.0X3	T37.0X4	T37.0X5	T37.0X6
Phylloquinone	T45.7X1	T45.7X2	T45.7X3	T45.7X4	T45.7X5	T45.7X6
Physeptone	T40.3X1	T40.3X2	T40.3X3	T40.3X4	T40.3X5	T40.3X6
Physostigma venenosum	T62.2X1	T62.2X2	T62.2X3	T62.2X4	—	—
Physostigmine	T49.5X1	T49.5X2	T49.5X3	T49.5X4	T49.5X5	T49.5X6
Phytolacca decandra	T62.2X1	T62.2X2	T62.2X3	T62.2X4	—	—
berries	T62.1X1	T62.1X2	T62.1X3	T62.1X4	—	—

◀ New   ◀ Revised   ~~deleted~~ Deleted

Substance	Poisoning, Accidental (Unintentional)	Poisoning, Intentional Self-Harm	Poisoning, Assault	Poisoning, Undetermined	Adverse Effect	Underdosing
Phytomenadione	T45.7X1	T45.7X2	T45.7X3	T45.7X4	T45.7X5	T45.7X6
Phytonadione	T45.7X1	T45.7X2	T45.7X3	T45.7X4	T45.7X5	T45.7X6
Picoperine	T48.3X1	T48.3X2	T48.3X3	T48.3X4	T48.3X5	T48.3X6
Picosulfate (sodium)	T47.2X1	T47.2X2	T47.2X3	T47.2X4	T47.2X5	T47.2X6
Picric (acid)	T54.2X1	T54.2X2	T54.2X3	T54.2X4	—	—
Picrotoxin	T50.7X1	T50.7X2	T50.7X3	T50.7X4	T50.7X5	T50.7X6
Piketoprofen	T49.0X1	T49.0X2	T49.0X3	T49.0X4	T49.0X5	T49.0X6
Pilocarpine	T44.1X1	T44.1X2	T44.1X3	T44.1X4	T44.1X5	T44.1X6
Pilocarpus (jaborandi) extract	T44.1X1	T44.1X2	T44.1X3	T44.1X4	T44.1X5	T44.1X6
Pilsicainide (hydrochloride)	T46.2X1	T46.2X2	T46.2X3	T46.2X4	T46.2X5	T46.2X6
Pimaricin	T36.7X1	T36.7X2	T36.7X3	T36.7X4	T36.7X5	T36.7X6
Pimeclone	T50.7X1	T50.7X2	T50.7X3	T50.7X4	T50.7X5	T50.7X6
Pimelic ketone	T52.8X1	T52.8X2	T52.8X3	T52.8X4	—	—
Pimethixene	T45.0X1	T45.0X2	T45.0X3	T45.0X4	T45.0X5	T45.0X6
Piminodine	T40.2X1	T40.2X2	T40.2X3	T40.2X4	T40.2X5	T40.2X6
Pimozide	T43.591	T43.592	T43.593	T43.594	T43.595	T43.596
Pinacidil	T46.5X1	T46.5X2	T46.5X3	T46.5X4	T46.5X5	T46.5X6
Pinaverium bromide	T44.3X1	T44.3X2	T44.3X3	T44.3X4	T44.3X5	T44.3X6
Pinazepam	T42.4X1	T42.4X2	T42.4X3	T42.4X4	T42.4X5	T42.4X6
Pindolol	T44.7X1	T44.7X2	T44.7X3	T44.7X4	T44.7X5	T44.7X6
Pindone	T60.4X1	T60.4X2	T60.4X3	T60.4X4	—	—
Pine oil (disinfectant)	T65.891	T65.892	T65.893	T65.894	—	—
Pinkroot	T37.4X1	T37.4X2	T37.4X3	T37.4X4	T37.4X5	T37.4X6
Pipadone	T40.2X1	T40.2X2	T40.2X3	T40.2X4	—	—
Pipamazine	T45.0X1	T45.0X2	T45.0X3	T45.0X4	T45.0X5	T45.0X6
Pipamperone	T43.4X1	T43.4X2	T43.4X3	T43.4X4	T43.4X5	T43.4X6
Pipazetate	T48.3X1	T48.3X2	T48.3X3	T48.3X4	T48.3X5	T48.3X6
Pipemidic acid	T37.8X1	T37.8X2	T37.8X3	T37.8X4	T37.8X5	T37.8X6
Pipenzolate bromide	T44.3X1	T44.3X2	T44.3X3	T44.3X4	T44.3X5	T44.3X6
Piperacetazine	T43.3X1	T43.3X2	T43.3X3	T43.3X4	T43.3X5	T43.3X6
Piperacillin	T36.0X1	T36.0X2	T36.0X3	T36.0X4	T36.0X5	T36.0X6
Piperazine	T37.4X1	T37.4X2	T37.4X3	T37.4X4	T37.4X5	T37.4X6
estrone sulfate	T38.5X1	T38.5X2	T38.5X3	T38.5X4	T38.5X5	T38.5X6
Piper cubeba	T62.2X1	T62.2X2	T62.2X3	T62.2X4	—	—
Piperidione	T48.3X1	T48.3X2	T48.3X3	T48.3X4	—	—
Piperidolate	T44.3X1	T44.3X2	T44.3X3	T44.3X4	T44.3X5	T44.3X6
Piperocaine	T41.3X1	T41.3X2	T41.3X3	T41.3X4	T41.3X5	T41.3X6
infiltration (subcutaneous)	T41.3X1	T41.3X2	T41.3X3	T41.3X4	T41.3X5	T41.3X6
nerve block (peripheral) (plexus)	T41.3X1	T41.3X2	T41.3X3	T41.3X4	T41.3X5	T41.3X6
topical (surface)	T41.3X1	T41.3X2	T41.3X3	T41.3X4	T41.3X5	T41.3X6
Piperonyl butoxide	T60.8X1	T60.8X2	T60.8X3	T60.8X4	—	—
Pipethanate	T44.3X1	T44.3X2	T44.3X3	T44.3X4	T44.3X5	T44.3X6

Substance	Poisoning, Accidental (Unintentional)	Poisoning, Intentional Self-Harm	Poisoning, Assault	Poisoning, Undetermined	Adverse Effect	Underdosing
Pipobroman	T45.1X1	T45.1X2	T45.1X3	T45.1X4	T45.1X5	T45.1X6
Pipofezine	T43.0X1	T43.0X2	T43.0X3	T43.0X4	T43.0X5	T43.0X6
Pipotiazine	T43.3X1	T43.3X2	T43.3X3	T43.3X4	T43.3X5	T43.3X6
Pipoxizine	T45.0X1	T45.0X2	T45.0X3	T45.0X4	T45.0X5	T45.0X6
Pipradrol	T43.691	T43.692	T43.693	T43.694	T43.695	T43.696
Piprinhydrinate	T45.0X1	T45.0X2	T45.0X3	T45.0X4	T45.0X5	T45.0X6
Pirarubicin	T45.1X1	T45.1X2	T45.1X3	T45.1X4	T45.1X5	T45.1X6
Pirazinamide	T37.1X1	T37.1X2	T37.1X3	T37.1X4	T37.1X5	T37.1X6
Pirbuterol	T48.6X1	T48.6X2	T48.6X3	T48.6X4	T48.6X5	T48.6X6
Pirenzepine	T47.1X1	T47.1X2	T47.1X3	T47.1X4	T47.1X5	T47.1X6
Piretanide	T50.1X1	T50.1X2	T50.1X3	T50.1X4	T50.1X5	T50.1X6
Piribedil	T42.8X1	T42.8X2	T42.8X3	T42.8X4	T42.8X5	T42.8X6
Piridoxilate	T46.3X1	T46.3X2	T46.3X3	T46.3X4	T46.3X5	T46.3X6
Piritramide	T40.491	T40.492	T40.493	T40.494	—	—
Pirlindole	T43.0X1	T43.0X2	T43.0X3	T43.0X4	T43.0X5	T43.0X6
Piromidic acid	T37.8X1	T37.8X2	T37.8X3	T37.8X4	T37.8X5	T37.8X6
Piroxicam	T39.391	T39.392	T39.393	T39.394	T39.395	T39.396
beta-cyclodextrin complex	T39.8X1	T39.8X2	T39.8X3	T39.8X4	T39.8X5	T39.8X6
Pirozadil	T46.6X1	T46.6X2	T46.6X3	T46.6X4	T46.6X5	T46.6X6
Piscidia (bark) (erythrina)	T39.8X1	T39.8X2	T39.8X3	T39.8X4	T39.8X5	T39.8X6
Pitch	T65.891	T65.892	T65.893	T65.894	—	—
Pitkin's solution	T41.3X1	T41.3X2	T41.3X3	T41.3X4	T41.3X5	T41.3X6
Pitocin	T48.0X1	T48.0X2	T48.0X3	T48.0X4	T48.0X5	T48.0X6
Pitressin (tannate)	T38.891	T38.892	T38.893	T38.894	T38.895	T38.896
Pituitary extracts (posterior)	T38.891	T38.892	T38.893	T38.894	T38.895	T38.896
anterior	T38.811	T38.812	T38.813	T38.814	T38.815	T38.816
Pituitrin	T38.891	T38.892	T38.893	T38.894	T38.895	T38.896
Pivampicillin	T36.0X1	T36.0X2	T36.0X3	T36.0X4	T36.0X5	T36.0X6
Pivmecillinam	T36.0X1	T36.0X2	T36.0X3	T36.0X4	T36.0X5	T36.0X6
Placental hormone	T38.891	T38.892	T38.893	T38.894	T38.895	T38.896
Placidyl	T42.6X1	T42.6X2	T42.6X3	T42.6X4	T42.6X5	T42.6X6
Plague vaccine	T50.A91	T50.A92	T50.A93	T50.A94	T50.A95	T50.A96
Plant						
food or fertilizer NEC	T65.891	T65.892	T65.893	T65.894	—	—
containing herbicide	T60.3X1	T60.3X2	T60.3X3	T60.3X4	—	—
noxious, used as food	T62.2X1	T62.2X2	T62.2X3	T62.2X4	—	—
berries	T62.1X1	T62.1X2	T62.1X3	T62.1X4	—	—
seeds	T62.2X1	T62.2X2	T62.2X3	T62.2X4	—	—
specified type NEC	T62.2X1	T62.2X2	T62.2X3	T62.2X4	—	—
Plasma	T45.8X1	T45.8X2	T45.8X3	T45.8X4	T45.8X5	T45.8X6
expander NEC	T45.8X1	T45.8X2	T45.8X3	T45.8X4	T45.8X5	T45.8X6
protein fraction (human)	T45.8X1	T45.8X2	T45.8X3	T45.8X4	T45.8X5	T45.8X6

◀ New   ◀ Revised   ~~deleted~~ Deleted

TABLE OF DRUGS AND CHEMICALS

Substance	Poisoning, Accidental (Unintentional)	Poisoning, Intentional Self-Harm	Poisoning, Assault	Poisoning, Undetermined	Adverse Effect	Underdosing
Plasmanate	T45.8X1	T45.8X2	T45.8X3	T45.8X4	T45.8X5	T45.8X6
Plasminogen (tissue) activator	T45.611	T45.612	T45.613	T45.614	T45.615	T45.616
Plaster dressing	T49.3X1	T49.3X2	T49.3X3	T49.3X4	T49.3X5	T49.3X6
Plastic dressing	T49.3X1	T49.3X2	T49.3X3	T49.3X4	T49.3X5	T49.3X6
Plegicil	T43.3X1	T43.3X2	T43.3X3	T43.3X4	T43.3X5	T43.3X6
Plicamycin	T45.1X1	T45.1X2	T45.1X3	T45.1X4	T45.1X5	T45.1X6
Podophyllotoxin	T49.8X1	T49.8X2	T49.8X3	T49.8X4	T49.8X5	T49.8X6
Podophyllum (resin)	T49.4X1	T49.4X2	T49.4X3	T49.4X4	T49.4X5	T49.4X6
Poison NEC	T65.91	T65.92	T65.93	T65.94	—	—
Poisonous berries	T62.1X1	T62.1X2	T62.1X3	T62.1X4	—	—
Pokeweed (any part)	T62.2X1	T62.2X2	T62.2X3	T62.2X4	—	—
Poldine metilsulfate	T44.3X1	T44.3X2	T44.3X3	T44.3X4	T44.3X5	T44.3X6
Polidexide (sulfate)	T46.6X1	T46.6X2	T46.6X3	T46.6X4	T46.6X5	T46.6X6
Polidocanol	T46.8X1	T46.8X2	T46.8X3	T46.8X4	T46.8X5	T46.8X6
Poliomyelitis vaccine	T50.B91	T50.B92	T50.B93	T50.B94	T50.B95	T50.B96
Polish (car) (floor) (furniture) (metal) (porcelain) (silver)	T65.891	T65.892	T65.893	T65.894	—	—
abrasive	T65.891	T65.892	T65.893	T65.894	—	—
porcelain	T65.891	T65.892	T65.893	T65.894	—	—
Poloxalkol	T47.4X1	T47.4X2	T47.4X3	T47.4X4	T47.4X5	T47.4X6
Poloxamer	T47.4X1	T47.4X2	T47.4X3	T47.4X4	T47.4X5	T47.4X6
Polyaminostyrene resins	T50.3X1	T50.3X2	T50.3X3	T50.3X4	T50.3X5	T50.3X6
Polycarbophil	T47.4X1	T47.4X2	T47.4X3	T47.4X4	T47.4X5	T47.4X6
Polychlorinated biphenyl	T65.891	T65.892	T65.893	T65.894	—	—
Polycycline	T36.4X1	T36.4X2	T36.4X3	T36.4X4	T36.4X5	T36.4X6
Polyester fumes	T59.891	T59.892	T59.893	T59.894	—	—
Polyester resin hardener	T52.91	T52.92	T52.93	T52.94	—	—
fumes	T59.891	T59.892	T59.893	T59.894	—	—
Polyestradiol phosphate	T38.5X1	T38.5X2	T38.5X3	T38.5X4	T38.5X5	T38.5X6
Polyethanolamine alkyl sulfate	T49.2X1	T49.2X2	T49.2X3	T49.2X4	T49.2X5	T49.2X6
Polyethylene adhesive	T49.3X1	T49.3X2	T49.3X3	T49.3X4	T49.3X5	T49.3X6
Polyferose	T45.4X1	T45.4X2	T45.4X3	T45.4X4	T45.4X5	T45.4X6
Polygeline	T45.8X1	T45.8X2	T45.8X3	T45.8X4	T45.8X5	T45.8X6
Polymyxin	T36.8X1	T36.8X2	T36.8X3	T36.8X4	T36.8X5	T36.8X6
B	T36.8X1	T36.8X2	T36.8X3	T36.8X4	T36.8X5	T36.8X6
ENT agent	T49.6X1	T49.6X2	T49.6X3	T49.6X4	T49.6X5	T49.6X6
ophthalmic preparation	T49.5X1	T49.5X2	T49.5X3	T49.5X4	T49.5X5	T49.5X6
topical NEC	T49.0X1	T49.0X2	T49.0X3	T49.0X4	T49.0X5	T49.0X6
E sulfate (eye preparation)	T49.5X1	T49.5X2	T49.5X3	T49.5X4	T49.5X5	T49.5X6
Polynoxylin	T49.0X1	T49.0X2	T49.0X3	T49.0X4	T49.0X5	T49.0X6
Polyoestradiol phosphate	T38.5X1	T38.5X2	T38.5X3	T38.5X4	T38.5X5	T38.5X6
Polyoxymethyleneurea	T49.0X1	T49.0X2	T49.0X3	T49.0X4	T49.0X5	T49.0X6

Substance	Poisoning, Accidental (Unintentional)	Poisoning, Intentional Self-Harm	Poisoning, Assault	Poisoning, Undetermined	Adverse Effect	Underdosing
Polysilane	T47.8X1	T47.8X2	T47.8X3	T47.8X4	T47.8X5	T47.8X6
Polytetrafluoroethylene (inhaled)	T59.891	T59.892	T59.893	T59.894	—	—
Polythiazide	T50.2X1	T50.2X2	T50.2X3	T50.2X4	T50.2X5	T50.2X6
Polyvidone	T45.8X1	T45.8X2	T45.8X3	T45.8X4	T45.8X5	T45.8X6
Polyvinylpyrrolidone	T45.8X1	T45.8X2	T45.8X3	T45.8X4	T45.8X5	T45.8X6
Pontocaine (hydrochloride) (infiltration) (topical)	T41.3X1	T41.3X2	T41.3X3	T41.3X4	T41.3X5	T41.3X6
nerve block (peripheral) (plexus)	T41.3X1	T41.3X2	T41.3X3	T41.3X4	T41.3X5	T41.3X6
spinal	T41.3X1	T41.3X2	T41.3X3	T41.3X4	T41.3X5	T41.3X6
Porfiromycin	T45.1X1	T45.1X2	T45.1X3	T45.1X4	T45.1X5	T45.1X6
Posterior pituitary hormone NEC	T38.891	T38.892	T38.893	T38.894	T38.895	T38.896
Pot	T40.711	T40.712	T40.713	T40.714	T40.715	T40.716
Potash (caustic)	T54.3X1	T54.3X2	T54.3X3	T54.3X4	—	—
Potassic saline injection (lactated)	T50.3X1	T50.3X2	T50.3X3	T50.3X4	T50.3X5	T50.3X6
Potassium (salts) NEC	T50.3X1	T50.3X2	T50.3X3	T50.3X4	T50.3X5	T50.3X6
aminobenzoate	T45.8X1	T45.8X2	T45.8X3	T45.8X4	T45.8X5	T45.8X6
aminosalicylate	T37.1X1	T37.1X2	T37.1X3	T37.1X4	T37.1X5	T37.1X6
antimony 'tartrate'	T37.8X1	T37.8X2	T37.8X3	T37.8X4	T37.8X5	T37.8X6
arsenite (solution)	T57.0X1	T57.0X2	T57.0X3	T57.0X4	—	—
bichromate	T56.2X1	T56.2X2	T56.2X3	T56.2X4	—	—
bisulfate	T47.3X1	T47.3X2	T47.3X3	T47.3X4	T47.3X5	T47.3X6
bromide	T42.6X1	T42.6X2	T42.6X3	T42.6X4	T42.6X5	T42.6X6
canrenoate	T50.0X1	T50.0X2	T50.0X3	T50.0X4	T50.0X5	T50.0X6
carbonate	T54.3X1	T54.3X2	T54.3X3	T54.3X4	—	—
chlorate NEC	T65.891	T65.892	T65.893	T65.894	—	—
chloride	T50.3X1	T50.3X2	T50.3X3	T50.3X4	T50.3X5	T50.3X6
citrate	T50.991	T50.992	T50.993	T50.994	T50.995	T50.996
cyanide	T65.0X1	T65.0X2	T65.0X3	T65.0X4	—	—
ferric hexacyanoferrate (medicinal)	T50.6X1	T50.6X2	T50.6X3	T50.6X4	T50.6X5	T50.6X6
nonmedicinal	T65.891	T65.892	T65.893	T65.894	—	—
Fluoride	T57.8X1	T57.8X2	T57.8X3	T57.8X4	—	—
glucaldrate	T47.1X1	T47.1X2	T47.1X3	T47.1X4	T47.1X5	T47.1X6
hydroxide	T54.3X1	T54.3X2	T54.3X3	T54.3X4	—	—
iodate	T49.0X1	T49.0X2	T49.0X3	T49.0X4	T49.0X5	T49.0X6
iodide	T48.4X1	T48.4X2	T48.4X3	T48.4X4	T48.4X5	T48.4X6
nitrate	T57.8X1	T57.8X2	T57.8X3	T57.8X4	—	—
oxalate	T65.891	T65.892	T65.893	T65.894	—	—
perchlorate (nonmedicinal) NEC	T65.891	T65.892	T65.893	T65.894	—	—
antithyroid	T38.2X1	T38.2X2	T38.2X3	T38.2X4	T38.2X5	T38.2X6
medicinal	T38.2X1	T38.2X2	T38.2X3	T38.2X4	T38.2X5	T38.2X6

Substance	Poisoning, Accidental (Unintentional)	Poisoning, Intentional Self-Harm	Poisoning, Assault	Poisoning, Undetermined	Adverse Effect	Underdosing
Permanganate (nonmedicinal)	T65.891	T65.892	T65.893	T65.894	—	—
medicinal	T49.0X1	T49.0X2	T49.0X3	T49.0X4	T49.0X5	T49.0X6
sulfate	T47.2X1	T47.2X2	T47.2X3	T47.2X4	T47.2X5	T47.2X6
Potassium-removing resin	T50.3X1	T50.3X2	T50.3X3	T50.3X4	T50.3X5	T50.3X6
Potassium-retaining drug	T50.3X1	T50.3X2	T50.3X3	T50.3X4	T50.3X5	T50.3X6
Povidone	T45.8X1	T45.8X2	T45.8X3	T45.8X4	T45.8X5	T45.8X6
iodine	T49.0X1	T49.0X2	T49.0X3	T49.0X4	T49.0X5	T49.0X6
Practolol	T44.7X1	T44.7X2	T44.7X3	T44.7X4	T44.7X5	T44.7X6
Prajmalium bitartrate	T46.2X1	T46.2X2	T46.2X3	T46.2X4	T46.2X5	T46.2X6
Pralidoxime (iodide)	T50.6X1	T50.6X2	T50.6X3	T50.6X4	T50.6X5	T50.6X6
chloride	T50.6X1	T50.6X2	T50.6X3	T50.6X4	T50.6X5	T50.6X6
Pramiverine	T44.3X1	T44.3X2	T44.3X3	T44.3X4	T44.3X5	T44.3X6
Pramocaine	T49.1X1	T49.1X2	T49.1X3	T49.1X4	T49.1X5	T49.1X6
Pramoxine	T49.1X1	T49.1X2	T49.1X3	T49.1X4	T49.1X5	T49.1X6
Prasterone	T38.7X1	T38.7X2	T38.7X3	T38.7X4	T38.7X5	T38.7X6
Pravastatin	T46.6X1	T46.6X2	T46.6X3	T46.6X4	T46.6X5	T46.6X6
Prazepam	T42.4X1	T42.4X2	T42.4X3	T42.4X4	T42.4X5	T42.4X6
Praziquantel	T37.4X1	T37.4X2	T37.4X3	T37.4X4	T37.4X5	T37.4X6
Prazitone	T43.291	T43.292	T43.293	T43.294	T43.295	T43.296
Prazosin	T44.6X1	T44.6X2	T44.6X3	T44.6X4	T44.6X5	T44.6X6
Prednicarbate	T49.0X1	T49.0X2	T49.0X3	T49.0X4	T49.0X5	T49.0X6
Prednimustine	T45.1X1	T45.1X2	T45.1X3	T45.1X4	T45.1X5	T45.1X6
Prednisolone	T38.0X1	T38.0X2	T38.0X3	T38.0X4	T38.0X5	T38.0X6
ENT agent	T49.6X1	T49.6X2	T49.6X3	T49.6X4	T49.6X5	T49.6X6
ophthalmic preparation	T49.5X1	T49.5X2	T49.5X3	T49.5X4	T49.5X5	T49.5X6
steaglate	T49.0X1	T49.0X2	T49.0X3	T49.0X4	T49.0X5	T49.0X6
topical NEC	T49.0X1	T49.0X2	T49.0X3	T49.0X4	T49.0X5	T49.0X6
Prednisone	T38.0X1	T38.0X2	T38.0X3	T38.0X4	T38.0X5	T38.0X6
Prednylidene	T38.0X1	T38.0X2	T38.0X3	T38.0X4	T38.0X5	T38.0X6
Pregnandiol	T38.5X1	T38.5X2	T38.5X3	T38.5X4	T38.5X5	T38.5X6
Pregneninolone	T38.5X1	T38.5X2	T38.5X3	T38.5X4	T38.5X5	T38.5X6
Preludin	T43.691	T43.692	T43.693	T43.694	T43.695	T43.696
Premarin	T38.5X1	T38.5X2	T38.5X3	T38.5X4	T38.5X5	T38.5X6
Premedication anesthetic	T41.201	T41.202	T41.203	T41.204	T41.205	T41.206
Prenalterol	T44.5X1	T44.5X2	T44.5X3	T44.5X4	T44.5X5	T44.5X6
Prenoxdiazine	T48.3X1	T48.3X2	T48.3X3	T48.3X4	T48.3X5	T48.3X6
Prenylamine	T46.3X1	T46.3X2	T46.3X3	T46.3X4	T46.3X5	T46.3X6
Preparation, local	T49.4X1	T49.4X2	T49.4X3	T49.4X4	T49.4X5	T49.4X6
Preparation H	T49.8X1	T49.8X2	T49.8X3	T49.8X4	T49.8X5	T49.8X6
Preservative (nonmedicinal)	T65.891	T65.892	T65.893	T65.894	—	—
medicinal	T50.901	T50.902	T50.903	T50.904	T50.905	T50.906
wood	T60.91	T60.92	T60.93	T60.94	—	—

Substance	Poisoning, Accidental (Unintentional)	Poisoning, Intentional Self-Harm	Poisoning, Assault	Poisoning, Undetermined	Adverse Effect	Underdosing
Prethcamide	T50.7X1	T50.7X2	T50.7X3	T50.7X4	T50.7X5	T50.7X6
Pride of China	T62.2X1	T62.2X2	T62.2X3	T62.2X4	—	—
Pridinol	T44.3X1	T44.3X2	T44.3X3	T44.3X4	T44.3X5	T44.3X6
Prifinium bromide	T44.3X1	T44.3X2	T44.3X3	T44.3X4	T44.3X5	T44.3X6
Prilocaine	T41.3X1	T41.3X2	T41.3X3	T41.3X4	T41.3X5	T41.3X6
infiltration (subcutaneous)	T41.3X1	T41.3X2	T41.3X3	T41.3X4	T41.3X5	T41.3X6
nerve block (peripheral) (plexus)	T41.3X1	T41.3X2	T41.3X3	T41.3X4	T41.3X5	T41.3X6
regional	T41.3X1	T41.3X2	T41.3X3	T41.3X4	T41.3X5	T41.3X6
Primaquine	T37.2X1	T37.2X2	T37.2X3	T37.2X4	T37.2X5	T37.2X6
Primidone	T42.6X1	T42.6X2	T42.6X3	T42.6X4	T42.6X5	T42.6X6
Primula (veris)	T62.2X1	T62.2X2	T62.2X3	T62.2X4	—	—
Prinadol	T40.2X1	T40.2X2	T40.2X3	T40.2X4	T40.2X5	T40.2X6
Priscol, Priscoline	T44.6X1	T44.6X2	T44.6X3	T44.6X4	T44.6X5	T44.6X6
Pristinamycin	T36.3X1	T36.3X2	T36.3X3	T36.3X4	T36.3X5	T36.3X6
Privet	T62.2X1	T62.2X2	T62.2X3	T62.2X4	—	—
berries	T62.1X1	T62.1X2	T62.1X3	T62.1X4	—	—
Privine	T44.4X1	T44.4X2	T44.4X3	T44.4X4	T44.4X5	T44.4X6
Pro-Banthine	T44.3X1	T44.3X2	T44.3X3	T44.3X4	T44.3X5	T44.3X6
Probarbital	T42.3X1	T42.3X2	T42.3X3	T42.3X4	T42.3X5	T42.3X6
Probenecid	T50.4X1	T50.4X2	T50.4X3	T50.4X4	T50.4X5	T50.4X6
Probucol	T46.6X1	T46.6X2	T46.6X3	T46.6X4	T46.6X5	T46.6X6
Procainamide	T46.2X1	T46.2X2	T46.2X3	T46.2X4	T46.2X5	T46.2X6
Procaine	T41.3X1	T41.3X2	T41.3X3	T41.3X4	T41.3X5	T41.3X6
benzylpenicillin	T36.0X1	T36.0X2	T36.0X3	T36.0X4	T36.0X5	T36.0X6
nerve block (periphreal) (plexus)	T41.3X1	T41.3X2	T41.3X3	T41.3X4	T41.3X5	T41.3X6
penicillin G	T36.0X1	T36.0X2	T36.0X3	T36.0X4	T36.0X5	T36.0X6
regional	T41.3X1	T41.3X2	T41.3X3	T41.3X4	T41.3X5	T41.3X6
spinal	T41.3X1	T41.3X2	T41.3X3	T41.3X4	T41.3X5	T41.3X6
Procalmidol	T43.591	T43.592	T43.593	T43.594	T43.595	T43.596
Procarbazine	T45.1X1	T45.1X2	T45.1X3	T45.1X4	T45.1X5	T45.1X6
Procaterol	T44.5X1	T44.5X2	T44.5X3	T44.5X4	T44.5X5	T44.5X6
Prochlorperazine	T43.3X1	T43.3X2	T43.3X3	T43.3X4	T43.3X5	T43.3X6
Procyclidine	T44.3X1	T44.3X2	T44.3X3	T44.3X4	T44.3X5	T44.3X6
Producer gas	T58.8X1	T58.8X2	T58.8X3	T58.8X4	—	—
Profadol	T40.491	T40.492	T40.493	T40.494	T40.495	T40.496
Profenamine	T44.3X1	T44.3X2	T44.3X3	T44.3X4	T44.3X5	T44.3X6
Profenil	T44.3X1	T44.3X2	T44.3X3	T44.3X4	T44.3X5	T44.3X6
Proflavine	T49.0X1	T49.0X2	T49.0X3	T49.0X4	T49.0X5	T49.0X6
Progabide	T42.6X1	T42.6X2	T42.6X3	T42.6X4	T42.6X5	T42.6X6
Progestin	T38.5X1	T38.5X2	T38.5X3	T38.5X4	T38.5X5	T38.5X6
oral contraceptive	T38.4X1	T38.4X2	T38.4X3	T38.4X4	T38.4X5	T38.4X6

Substance	External Cause (T-Code)					
	Poisoning, Accidental (Unintentional)	Poisoning, Intentional Self-Harm	Poisoning, Assault	Poisoning, Undetermined	Adverse Effect	Underdosing
Progesterone	T38.5X1	T38.5X2	T38.5X3	T38.5X4	T38.5X5	T38.5X6
Progestogen NEC	T38.5X1	T38.5X2	T38.5X3	T38.5X4	T38.5X5	T38.5X6
Progestone	T38.5X1	T38.5X2	T38.5X3	T38.5X4	T38.5X5	T38.5X6
Proglumide	T47.1X1	T47.1X2	T47.1X3	T47.1X4	T47.1X5	T47.1X6
Proguanil	T37.2X1	T37.2X2	T37.2X3	T37.2X4	T37.2X5	T37.2X6
Prolactin	T38.811	T38.812	T38.813	T38.814	T38.815	T38.816
Prolintane	T43.691	T43.692	T43.693	T43.694	T43.695	T43.696
Proloid	T38.1X1	T38.1X2	T38.1X3	T38.1X4	T38.1X5	T38.1X6
Proluton	T38.5X1	T38.5X2	T38.5X3	T38.5X4	T38.5X5	T38.5X6
Promacetin	T37.1X1	T37.1X2	T37.1X3	T37.1X4	T37.1X5	T37.1X6
Promazine	T43.3X1	T43.3X2	T43.3X3	T43.3X4	T43.3X5	T43.3X6
Promedol	T40.2X1	T40.2X2	T40.2X3	T40.2X4	—	—
Promegestone	T38.5X1	T38.5X2	T38.5X3	T38.5X4	T38.5X5	T38.5X6
Promethazine (teoclate)	T43.3X1	T43.3X2	T43.3X3	T43.3X4	T43.3X5	T43.3X6
Promin	T37.1X1	T37.1X2	T37.1X3	T37.1X4	T37.1X5	T37.1X6
Pronase	T45.3X1	T45.3X2	T45.3X3	T45.3X4	T45.3X5	T45.3X6
Pronestyl (hydrochloride)	T46.2X1	T46.2X2	T46.2X3	T46.2X4	T46.2X5	T46.2X6
Pronetalol	T44.7X1	T44.7X2	T44.7X3	T44.7X4	T44.7X5	T44.7X6
Prontosil	T37.0X1	T37.0X2	T37.0X3	T37.0X4	T37.0X5	T37.0X6
Propachlor	T60.3X1	T60.3X2	T60.3X3	T60.3X4	—	—
Propafenone	T46.2X1	T46.2X2	T46.2X3	T46.2X4	T46.2X5	T46.2X6
Propallylonal	T42.3X1	T42.3X2	T42.3X3	T42.3X4	T42.3X5	T42.3X6
Propamidine	T49.0X1	T49.0X2	T49.0X3	T49.0X4	T49.0X5	T49.0X6
Propane (distributed in mobile container)	T59.891	T59.892	T59.893	T59.894	—	—
distributed through pipes	T59.891	T59.892	T59.893	T59.894	—	—
incomplete combustion	T57.11	T57.12	T57.13	T57.14	—	—
Propanidid	T41.291	T41.292	T41.293	T41.294	T41.295	T41.296
Propanil	T60.3X1	T60.3X2	T60.3X3	T60.3X4	—	—
1-Propanol	T51.3X1	T51.3X2	T51.3X3	T51.3X4	—	—
2-Propanol	T51.2X1	T51.2X2	T51.2X3	T51.2X4	—	—
Propantheline	T44.3X1	T44.3X2	T44.3X3	T44.3X4	T44.3X5	T44.3X6
bromide	T44.3X1	T44.3X2	T44.3X3	T44.3X4	T44.3X5	T44.3X6
Proparacaine	T41.3X1	T41.3X2	T41.3X3	T41.3X4	T41.3X5	T41.3X6
Propatylnitrate	T46.3X1	T46.3X2	T46.3X3	T46.3X4	T46.3X5	T46.3X6
Propicillin	T36.0X1	T36.0X2	T36.0X3	T36.0X4	T36.0X5	T36.0X6
Propiolactone	T49.0X1	T49.0X2	T49.0X3	T49.0X4	T49.0X5	T49.0X6
Propiomazine	T45.0X1	T45.0X2	T45.0X3	T45.0X4	T45.0X5	T45.0X6
Propionaldehyde (medicinal)	T42.6X1	T42.6X2	T42.6X3	T42.6X4	T42.6X5	T42.6X6
Propionate (calcium) (sodium)	T49.0X1	T49.0X2	T49.0X3	T49.0X4	T49.0X5	T49.0X6
Propion gel	T49.0X1	T49.0X2	T49.0X3	T49.0X4	T49.0X5	T49.0X6

Substance	External Cause (T-Code)					
	Poisoning, Accidental (Unintentional)	Poisoning, Intentional Self-Harm	Poisoning, Assault	Poisoning, Undetermined	Adverse Effect	Underdosing
Propitocaine	T41.3X1	T41.3X2	T41.3X3	T41.3X4	T41.3X5	T41.3X6
infiltration (subcutaneous)	T41.3X1	T41.3X2	T41.3X3	T41.3X4	T41.3X5	T41.3X6
nerve block (peripheral) (plexus)	T41.3X1	T41.3X2	T41.3X3	T41.3X4	T41.3X5	T41.3X6
Propofol	T41.291	T41.292	T41.293	T41.294	T41.295	T41.296
Propoxur	T60.0X1	T60.0X2	T60.0X3	T60.0X4	—	—
Propoxycaine	T41.3X1	T41.3X2	T41.3X3	T41.3X4	T41.3X5	T41.3X6
infiltration (subcutaneous)	T41.3X1	T41.3X2	T41.3X3	T41.3X4	T41.3X5	T41.3X6
nerve block (peripheral) (plexus)	T41.3X1	T41.3X2	T41.3X3	T41.3X4	T41.3X5	T41.3X6
topical (surface)	T41.3X1	T41.3X2	T41.3X3	T41.3X4	T41.3X5	T41.3X6
Propoxyphene	T40.491	T40.492	T40.493	T40.494	T40.495	T40.496
Propranolol	T44.7X1	T44.7X2	T44.7X3	T44.7X4	T44.7X5	T44.7X6
Propyl						
alcohol	T51.3X1	T51.3X2	T51.3X3	T51.3X4	—	—
carbinol	T51.3X1	T51.3X2	T51.3X3	T51.3X4	—	—
hexadrine	T44.4X1	T44.4X2	T44.4X3	T44.4X4	T44.4X5	T44.4X6
iodone	T50.8X1	T50.8X2	T50.8X3	T50.8X4	T50.8X5	T50.8X6
thiouracil	T38.2X1	T38.2X2	T38.2X3	T38.2X4	T38.2X5	T38.2X6
Propylaminophenothiazine	T43.3X1	T43.3X2	T43.3X3	T43.3X4	T43.3X5	T43.3X6
Propylene	T59.891	T59.892	T59.893	T59.894	—	—
Propylhexedrine	T48.5X1	T48.5X2	T48.5X3	T48.5X4	T48.5X5	T48.5X6
Propyliodone	T50.8X1	T50.8X2	T50.8X3	T50.8X4	T50.8X5	T50.8X6
Propylthiouracil	T38.2X1	T38.2X2	T38.2X3	T38.2X4	T38.2X5	T38.2X6
Propylparaben (ophthalmic)	T49.5X1	T49.5X2	T49.5X3	T49.5X4	T49.5X5	T49.5X6
Propyphenazone	T39.2X1	T39.2X2	T39.2X3	T39.2X4	T39.2X5	T39.2X6
Proquazone	T39.391	T39.392	T39.393	T39.394	T39.395	T39.396
Proscillaridin	T46.0X1	T46.0X2	T46.0X3	T46.0X4	T46.0X5	T46.0X6
Prostacyclin	T45.521	T45.522	T45.523	T45.524	T45.525	T45.526
Prostaglandin (I2)	T45.521	T45.522	T45.523	T45.524	T45.525	T45.526
E1	T46.7X1	T46.7X2	T46.7X3	T46.7X4	T46.7X5	T46.7X6
E2	T48.0X1	T48.0X2	T48.0X3	T48.0X4	T48.0X5	T48.0X6
F2 alpha	T48.0X1	T48.0X2	T48.0X3	T48.0X4	T48.0X5	T48.0X6
Prostigmin	T44.0X1	T44.0X2	T44.0X3	T44.0X4	T44.0X5	T44.0X6
Prosultiamine	T45.2X1	T45.2X2	T45.2X3	T45.2X4	T45.2X5	T45.2X6
Protamine sulfate	T45.7X1	T45.7X2	T45.7X3	T45.7X4	T45.7X5	T45.7X6
zinc insulin	T38.3X1	T38.3X2	T38.3X3	T38.3X4	T38.3X5	T38.3X6
Protease	T47.5X1	T47.5X2	T47.5X3	T47.5X4	T47.5X5	T47.5X6
Protectant, skin NEC	T49.3X1	T49.3X2	T49.3X3	T49.3X4	T49.3X5	T49.3X6
Protein hydrolysate	T50.991	T50.992	T50.993	T50.994	T50.995	T50.996
Prothiaden — *see Dothiepin hydrochloride*						
Prothionamide	T37.1X1	T37.1X2	T37.1X3	T37.1X4	T37.1X5	T37.1X6

◀ New   ◀ Revised   ~~deleted~~ Deleted

Substance	Poisoning, Accidental (Unintentional)	Poisoning, Intentional Self-Harm	Poisoning, Assault	Poisoning, Undetermined	Adverse Effect	Underdosing
Prothipendyl	T43.591	T43.592	T43.593	T43.594	T43.595	T43.596
Prothoate	T60.0X1	T60.0X2	T60.0X3	T60.0X4	—	—
Prothrombin						
activator	T45.7X1	T45.7X2	T45.7X3	T45.7X4	T45.7X5	T45.7X6
synthesis inhibitor	T45.511	T45.512	T45.513	T45.514	T45.515	T45.516
Protionamide	T37.1X1	T37.1X2	T37.1X3	T37.1X4	T37.1X5	T37.1X6
Protirelin	T38.891	T38.892	T38.893	T38.894	T38.895	T38.896
Protokylol	T48.6X1	T48.6X2	T48.6X3	T48.6X4	T48.6X5	T48.6X6
Protopam	T50.6X1	T50.6X2	T50.6X3	T50.6X4	T50.6X5	T50.6X6
Protoveratrine(s) (A) (B)	T46.5X1	T46.5X2	T46.5X3	T46.5X4	T46.5X5	T46.5X6
Protriptyline	T43.011	T43.012	T43.013	T43.014	T43.015	T43.016
Provera	T38.5X1	T38.5X2	T38.5X3	T38.5X4	T38.5X5	T38.5X6
Provitamin A	T45.2X1	T45.2X2	T45.2X3	T45.2X4	T45.2X5	T45.2X6
Proxibarbal	T42.3X1	T42.3X2	T42.3X3	T42.3X4	T42.3X5	T42.3X6
Proxymetacaine	T41.3X1	T41.3X2	T41.3X3	T41.3X4	T41.3X5	T41.3X6
Proxyphylline	T48.6X1	T48.6X2	T48.6X3	T48.6X4	T48.6X5	T48.6X6
Prozac—*see* Fluoxetine hydrochloride						
Prunus						
laurocerasus	T62.2X1	T62.2X2	T62.2X3	T62.2X4	—	—
virginiana	T62.2X1	T62.2X2	T62.2X3	T62.2X4	—	—
Prussian blue						
commercial	T65.891	T65.892	T65.893	T65.894	—	—
therapeutic	T50.6X1	T50.6X2	T50.6X3	T50.6X4	T50.6X5	T50.6X6
Prussic acid	T65.0X1	T65.0X2	T65.0X3	T65.0X4	—	—
vapor	T57.3X1	T57.3X2	T57.3X3	T57.3X4	—	—
Pseudoephedrine	T44.991	T44.992	T44.993	T44.994	T44.995	T44.996
Psilocin	T40.991	T40.992	T40.993	T40.994	—	—
Psilocybin	T40.991	T40.992	T40.993	T40.994	—	—
Psilocybine	T40.991	T40.992	T40.993	T40.994	—	—
Psoralene (nonmedicinal)	T65.891	T65.892	T65.893	T65.894	—	—
Psoralens (medicinal)	T50.991	T50.992	T50.993	T50.994	T50.995	T50.996
PSP (phenolsulfonphthalein)	T50.8X1	T50.8X2	T50.8X3	T50.8X4	T50.8X5	T50.8X6
Psychodysleptic drug NOS	T40.901	T40.902	T40.903	T40.904	T40.905	T40.906
specified NEC	T40.991	T40.992	T40.993	T40.994	T40.995	T40.996
Psychostimulant	T43.601	T43.602	T43.603	T43.604	T43.605	T43.606
amphetamine	T43.621	T43.622	T43.623	T43.624	T43.625	T43.626
caffeine	T43.611	T43.612	T43.613	T43.614	T43.615	T43.616
methylphenidate	T43.631	T43.632	T43.633	T43.634	T43.635	T43.636
specified NEC	T43.691	T43.692	T43.693	T43.694	T43.695	T43.696
Psychotherapeutic drug NEC	T43.91	T43.92	T43.93	T43.94	T43.95	T43.96
antidepressants—*see also* Antidepressant	T43.201	T43.202	T43.203	T43.204	T43.205	T43.206

Substance	Poisoning, Accidental (Unintentional)	Poisoning, Intentional Self-Harm	Poisoning, Assault	Poisoning, Undetermined	Adverse Effect	Underdosing
Psychotherapeutic drug NEC *(Continued)*						
specified NEC	T43.8X1	T43.8X2	T43.8X3	T43.8X4	T43.8X5	T43.8X6
tranquilizers NEC	T43.501	T43.502	T43.503	T43.504	T43.505	T43.506
Psychotomimetic agents	T40.901	T40.902	T40.903	T40.904	T40.905	T40.906
Psychotropic drug NEC	T43.91	T43.92	T43.93	T43.94	T43.95	T43.96
specified NEC	T43.8X1	T43.8X2	T43.8X3	T43.8X4	T43.8X5	T43.8X6
Psyllium hydrophilic mucilloid	T47.4X1	T47.4X2	T47.4X3	T47.4X4	T47.4X5	T47.4X6
Pteroylglutamic acid	T45.8X1	T45.8X2	T45.8X3	T45.8X4	T45.8X5	T45.8X6
Pteroyltriglutamate	T45.1X1	T45.1X2	T45.1X3	T45.1X4	T45.1X5	T45.1X6
PTFE—*see* Polytetrafluoroethylene						
Pulp						
devitalizing paste	T49.7X1	T49.7X2	T49.7X3	T49.7X4	T49.7X5	T49.7X6
dressing	T49.7X1	T49.7X2	T49.7X3	T49.7X4	T49.7X5	T49.7X6
Pulsatilla	T62.2X1	T62.2X2	T62.2X3	T62.2X4	—	—
Pumpkin seed extract	T37.4X1	T37.4X2	T37.4X3	T37.4X4	T37.4X5	T37.4X6
Purex (bleach)	T54.91	T54.92	T54.93	T54.94	—	—
Purgative NEC—*see also* Cathartic	T47.4X1	T47.4X2	T47.4X3	T47.4X4	T47.4X5	T47.4X6
Purine analogue (antineoplastic)	T45.1X1	T45.1X2	T45.1X3	T45.1X4	T45.1X5	T45.1X6
Purine diuretics	T50.2X1	T50.2X2	T50.2X3	T50.2X4	T50.2X5	T50.2X6
Purinethol	T45.1X1	T45.1X2	T45.1X3	T45.1X4	T45.1X5	T45.1X6
PVP	T45.8X1	T45.8X2	T45.8X3	T45.8X4	T45.8X5	T45.8X6
Pyrabital	T39.8X1	T39.8X2	T39.8X3	T39.8X4	T39.8X5	T39.8X6
Pyramidon	T39.2X1	T39.2X2	T39.2X3	T39.2X4	T39.2X5	T39.2X6
Pyrantel	T37.4X1	T37.4X2	T37.4X3	T37.4X4	T37.4X5	T37.4X6
Pyrathiazine	T45.0X1	T45.0X2	T45.0X3	T45.0X4	T45.0X5	T45.0X6
Pyrazinamide	T37.1X1	T37.1X2	T37.1X3	T37.1X4	T37.1X5	T37.1X6
Pyrazinoic acid (amide)	T37.1X1	T37.1X2	T37.1X3	T37.1X4	T37.1X5	T37.1X6
Pyrazole (derivatives)	T39.2X1	T39.2X2	T39.2X3	T39.2X4	T39.2X5	T39.2X6
Pyrazolone analgesic NEC	T39.2X1	T39.2X2	T39.2X3	T39.2X4	T39.2X5	T39.2X6
Pyrethrin, pyrethrum (nonmedicinal)	T60.2X1	T60.2X2	T60.2X3	T60.2X4	—	—
Pyrethrum extract	T49.0X1	T49.0X2	T49.0X3	T49.0X4	T49.0X5	T49.0X6
Pyribenzamine	T45.0X1	T45.0X2	T45.0X3	T45.0X4	T45.0X5	T45.0X6
Pyridine	T52.8X1	T52.8X2	T52.8X3	T52.8X4	—	—
aldoxime methiodide	T50.6X1	T50.6X2	T50.6X3	T50.6X4	T50.6X5	T50.6X6
aldoxime methyl chloride	T50.6X1	T50.6X2	T50.6X3	T50.6X4	T50.6X5	T50.6X6
vapor	T59.891	T59.892	T59.893	T59.894	—	—
Pyridium	T39.8X1	T39.8X2	T39.8X3	T39.8X4	T39.8X5	T39.8X6
Pyridostigmine bromide	T44.0X1	T44.0X2	T44.0X3	T44.0X4	T44.0X5	T44.0X6
Pyridoxal phosphate	T45.2X1	T45.2X2	T45.2X3	T45.2X4	T45.2X5	T45.2X6

◄ New   ◄ Revised   ~~deleted~~ Deleted

Substance	External Cause (T-Code)					
	Poisoning, Accidental (Unintentional)	Poisoning, Intentional Self-Harm	Poisoning, Assault	Poisoning, Undetermined	Adverse Effect	Underdosing
Pyridoxine	T45.2X1	T45.2X2	T45.2X3	T45.2X4	T45.2X5	T45.2X6
Pyrilamine	T45.0X1	T45.0X2	T45.0X3	T45.0X4	T45.0X5	T45.0X6
Pyrimethamine	T37.2X1	T37.2X2	T37.2X3	T37.2X4	T37.2X5	T37.2X6
with sulfadoxine	T37.2X1	T37.2X2	T37.2X3	T37.2X4	T37.2X5	T37.2X6
Pyrimidine antagonist	T45.1X1	T45.1X2	T45.1X3	T45.1X4	T45.1X5	T45.1X6
Pyriminil	T60.4X1	T60.4X2	T60.4X3	T60.4X4	—	—
Pyrithione zinc	T49.4X1	T49.4X2	T49.4X3	T49.4X4	T49.4X5	T49.4X6
Pyrithyldione	T42.6X1	T42.6X2	T42.6X3	T42.6X4	T42.6X5	T42.6X6
Pyrogallic acid	T49.0X1	T49.0X2	T49.0X3	T49.0X4	T49.0X5	T49.0X6
Pyrogallol	T49.0X1	T49.0X2	T49.0X3	T49.0X4	T49.0X5	T49.0X6
Pyroxylin	T49.3X1	T49.3X2	T49.3X3	T49.3X4	T49.3X5	T49.3X6
Pyrrobutamine	T45.0X1	T45.0X2	T45.0X3	T45.0X4	T45.0X5	T45.0X6
Pyrrolizidine alkaloids	T62.8X1	T62.8X2	T62.8X3	T62.8X4	—	—
Pyrvinium chloride	T37.4X1	T37.4X2	T37.4X3	T37.4X4	T37.4X5	T37.4X6
PZI	T38.3X1	T38.3X2	T38.3X3	T38.3X4	T38.3X5	T38.3X6
Q						
Quaalude	T42.6X1	T42.6X2	T42.6X3	T42.6X4	T42.6X5	T42.6X6
Quarternary ammonium						
anti-infective	T49.0X1	T49.0X2	T49.0X3	T49.0X4	T49.0X5	T49.0X6
ganglion blocking	T44.2X1	T44.2X2	T44.2X3	T44.2X4	T44.2X5	T44.2X6
parasympatholytic	T44.3X1	T44.3X2	T44.3X3	T44.3X4	T44.3X5	T44.3X6
Quazepam	T42.4X1	T42.4X2	T42.4X3	T42.4X4	T42.4X5	T42.4X6
Quicklime	T54.3X1	T54.3X2	T54.3X3	T54.3X4	—	—
Quillaja extract	T48.4X1	T48.4X2	T48.4X3	T48.4X4	T48.4X5	T48.4X6
Quinacrine	T37.2X1	T37.2X2	T37.2X3	T37.2X4	T37.2X5	T37.2X6
Quinaglute	T46.2X1	T46.2X2	T46.2X3	T46.2X4	T46.2X5	T46.2X6
Quinalbarbital	T42.3X1	T42.3X2	T42.3X3	T42.3X4	T42.3X5	T42.3X6
Quinalbarbitone sodium	T42.3X1	T42.3X2	T42.3X3	T42.3X4	T42.3X5	T42.3X6
Quinalphos	T60.0X1	T60.0X2	T60.0X3	T60.0X4	—	—
Quinapril	T46.4X1	T46.4X2	T46.4X3	T46.4X4	T46.4X5	T46.4X6
Quinestradiol	T38.5X1	T38.5X2	T38.5X3	T38.5X4	T38.5X5	T38.5X6
Quinestradol	T38.5X1	T38.5X2	T38.5X3	T38.5X4	T38.5X5	T38.5X6
Quinestrol	T38.5X1	T38.5X2	T38.5X3	T38.5X4	T38.5X5	T38.5X6
Quinethazone	T50.2X1	T50.2X2	T50.2X3	T50.2X4	T50.2X5	T50.2X6
Quingestanol	T38.4X1	T38.4X2	T38.4X3	T38.4X4	T38.4X5	T38.4X6
Quinidine	T46.2X1	T46.2X2	T46.2X3	T46.2X4	T46.2X5	T46.2X6
Quinine	T37.2X1	T37.2X2	T37.2X3	T37.2X4	T37.2X5	T37.2X6
Quiniobine	T37.8X1	T37.8X2	T37.8X3	T37.8X4	T37.8X5	T37.8X6
Quinisocaine	T49.1X1	T49.1X2	T49.1X3	T49.1X4	T49.1X5	T49.1X6
Quinocide	T37.2X1	T37.2X2	T37.2X3	T37.2X4	T37.2X5	T37.2X6
Quinoline (derivatives) NEC	T37.8X1	T37.8X2	T37.8X3	T37.8X4	T37.8X5	T37.8X6

Substance	External Cause (T-Code)					
	Poisoning, Accidental (Unintentional)	Poisoning, Intentional Self-Harm	Poisoning, Assault	Poisoning, Undetermined	Adverse Effect	Underdosing
Quinupramine	T43.011	T43.012	T43.013	T43.014	T43.015	T43.016
Quotane	T41.3X1	T41.3X2	T41.3X3	T41.3X4	T41.3X5	T41.3X6
R						
Rabies						
immune globulin (human)	T50.Z11	T50.Z12	T50.Z13	T50.Z14	T50.Z15	T50.Z16
vaccine	T50.B91	T50.B92	T50.B93	T50.B94	T50.B95	T50.B96
Racemoramide	T40.2X1	T40.2X2	T40.2X3	T40.2X4	—	—
Racemorphan	T40.2X1	T40.2X2	T40.2X3	T40.2X4	T40.2X5	T40.2X6
Racepinefrin	T44.5X1	T44.5X2	T44.5X3	T44.5X4	T44.5X5	T44.5X6
Raclopride	T43.591	T43.592	T43.593	T43.594	T43.595	T43.596
Radiator alcohol	T51.1X1	T51.1X2	T51.1X3	T51.1X4	—	—
Radioactive drug NEC	T50.8X1	T50.8X2	T50.8X3	T50.8X4	T50.8X5	T50.8X6
Radio-opaque (drugs) (materials)	T50.8X1	T50.8X2	T50.8X3	T50.8X4	T50.8X5	T50.8X6
Ramifenazone	T39.2X1	T39.2X2	T39.2X3	T39.2X4	T39.2X5	T39.2X6
Ramipril	T46.4X1	T46.4X2	T46.4X3	T46.4X4	T46.4X5	T46.4X6
Ranitidine	T47.0X1	T47.0X2	T47.0X3	T47.0X4	T47.0X5	T47.0X6
Ranunculus	T62.2X1	T62.2X2	T62.2X3	T62.2X4	—	—
Rat poison NEC	T60.4X1	T60.4X2	T60.4X3	T60.4X4	—	—
Rattlesnake (venom)	T63.011	T63.012	T63.013	T63.014	—	—
Raubasine	T46.7X1	T46.7X2	T46.7X3	T46.7X4	T46.7X5	T46.7X6
Raudixin	T46.5X1	T46.5X2	T46.5X3	T46.5X4	T46.5X5	T46.5X6
Rautensin	T46.5X1	T46.5X2	T46.5X3	T46.5X4	T46.5X5	T46.5X6
Rautina	T46.5X1	T46.5X2	T46.5X3	T46.5X4	T46.5X5	T46.5X6
Rautotal	T46.5X1	T46.5X2	T46.5X3	T46.5X4	T46.5X5	T46.5X6
Rauwiloid	T46.5X1	T46.5X2	T46.5X3	T46.5X4	T46.5X5	T46.5X6
Rauwoldin	T46.5X1	T46.5X2	T46.5X3	T46.5X4	T46.5X5	T46.5X6
Rauwolfia (alkaloids)	T46.5X1	T46.5X2	T46.5X3	T46.5X4	T46.5X5	T46.5X6
Razoxane	T45.1X1	T45.1X2	T45.1X3	T45.1X4	T45.1X5	T45.1X6
Realgar	T57.0X1	T57.0X2	T57.0X3	T57.0X4	—	—
Recombinant (R) — see specific protein						
Red blood cells, packed	T45.8X1	T45.8X2	T45.8X3	T45.8X4	T45.8X5	T45.8X6
Red squill (scilliroside)	T60.4X1	T60.4X2	T60.4X3	T60.4X4	—	—
Reducing agent, industrial NEC	T65.891	T65.892	T65.893	T65.894		
Refrigerant gas (chlorofluoro-carbon)	T53.5X1	T53.5X2	T53.5X3	T53.5X4		
not chlorofluoro-carbon	T59.891	T59.892	T59.893	T59.894		
Regroton	T50.2X1	T50.2X2	T50.2X3	T50.2X4	T50.2X5	T50.2X6
Rehydration salts (oral)	T50.3X1	T50.3X2	T50.3X3	T50.3X4	T50.3X5	T50.3X6
Rela	T42.8X1	T42.8X2	T42.8X3	T42.8X4	T42.8X5	T42.8X6

Substance	Poisoning, Accidental (Unintentional)	Poisoning, Intentional Self-Harm	Poisoning, Assault	Poisoning, Undetermined	Adverse Effect	Underdosing
Relaxant, muscle						
anesthetic	T48.1X1	T48.1X2	T48.1X3	T48.1X4	T48.1X5	T43.1X6
central nervous system	T42.8X1	T42.8X2	T42.8X3	T42.8X4	T42.8X5	T42.8X6
skeletal NEC	T48.1X1	T48.1X2	T48.1X3	T48.1X4	T48.1X5	T48.1X6
smooth NEC	T44.3X1	T44.3X2	T44.3X3	T44.3X4	T44.3X5	T44.3X6
Remoxipride	T43.591	T43.592	T43.593	T43.594	T43.595	T43.596
Renese	T50.2X1	T50.2X2	T50.2X3	T50.2X4	T50.2X5	T50.2X6
Renografin	T50.8X1	T50.8X2	T50.8X3	T50.8X4	T50.8X5	T50.8X6
Replacement solution	T50.3X1	T50.3X2	T50.3X3	T50.3X4	T50.3X5	T50.3X6
Reproterol	T48.6X1	T48.6X2	T48.6X3	T48.6X4	T48.6X5	T48.6X6
Rescinnamine	T46.5X1	T46.5X2	T46.5X3	T46.5X4	T46.5X5	T46.5X6
Reserpin(e)	T46.5X1	T46.5X2	T46.5X3	T46.5X4	T46.5X5	T46.5X6
Resorcin, resorcinol (nonmedicinal)	T65.891	T65.892	T65.893	T65.894	—	—
medicinal	T49.4X1	T49.4X2	T49.4X3	T49.4X4	T49.4X5	T49.4X6
Respaire	T48.4X1	T48.4X2	T48.4X3	T48.4X4	T48.4X5	T48.4X6
Respiratory drug NEC	T48.901	T48.902	T48.903	T48.904	T48.905	T48.906
antiasthmatic NEC	T48.6X1	T48.6X2	T48.6X3	T48.6X4	T48.6X5	T48.6X6
anti-common-cold NEC	T48.5X1	T48.5X2	T48.5X3	T48.5X4	T48.5X5	T48.5X6
expectorant NEC	T48.4X1	T48.4X2	T48.4X3	T48.4X4	T48.4X5	T48.4X6
stimulant	T48.901	T48.902	T48.903	T48.904	T48.905	T48.906
Retinoic acid	T49.0X1	T49.0X2	T49.0X3	T49.0X4	T49.0X5	T49.0X6
Retinol	T45.2X1	T45.2X2	T45.2X3	T45.2X4	T45.2X5	T45.2X6
Rh (D) immune globulin (human)	T50.Z11	T50.Z12	T50.Z13	T50.Z14	T50.Z15	T50.Z16
Rhodine	T39.011	T39.012	T39.013	T39.014	T39.015	T39.016
RhoGAM	T50.Z11	T50.Z12	T50.Z13	T50.Z14	T50.Z15	T50.Z16
Rhubarb						
dry extract	T47.2X1	T47.2X2	T47.2X3	T47.2X4	T47.2X5	T47.2X6
tincture, compound	T47.2X1	T47.2X2	T47.2X3	T47.2X4	T47.2X5	T47.2X6
Ribavirin	T37.5X1	T37.5X2	T37.5X3	T37.5X4	T37.5X5	T37.5X6
Riboflavin	T45.2X1	T45.2X2	T45.2X3	T45.2X4	T45.2X5	T45.2X6
Ribostamycin	T36.5X1	T36.5X2	T36.5X3	T36.5X4	T36.5X5	T36.5X6
Ricin	T62.2X1	T62.2X2	T62.2X3	T62.2X4	—	—
Ricinus communis	T62.2X1	T62.2X2	T62.2X3	T62.2X4	—	—
Rickettsial vaccine NEC	T50.A91	T50.A92	T50.A93	T50.A94	T50.A95	T50.A96
Rifabutin	T36.6X1	T36.6X2	T36.6X3	T36.6X4	T36.6X5	T36.6X6
Rifamide	T36.6X1	T36.6X2	T36.6X3	T36.6X4	T36.6X5	T36.6X6
Rifampicin	T36.6X1	T36.6X2	T36.6X3	T36.6X4	T36.6X5	T36.6X6
with isoniazid	T37.1X1	T37.1X2	T37.1X3	T37.1X4	T37.1X5	T37.1X6
Rifampin	T36.6X1	T36.6X2	T36.6X3	T36.6X4	T36.6X5	T36.6X6
Rifamycin	T36.6X1	T36.6X2	T36.6X3	T36.6X4	T36.6X5	T36.6X6
Rifaximin	T36.6X1	T36.6X2	T36.6X3	T36.6X4	T36.6X5	T36.6X6
Rimantadine	T37.5X1	T37.5X2	T37.5X3	T37.5X4	T37.5X5	T37.5X6
Rimazolium metilsulfate	T39.8X1	T39.8X2	T39.8X3	T39.8X4	T39.8X5	T39.8X6
Rimifon	T37.1X1	T37.1X2	T37.1X3	T37.1X4	T37.1X5	T37.1X6
Rimiterol	T48.6X1	T48.6X2	T48.6X3	T48.6X4	T48.6X5	T48.6X6
Ringer (lactate) solution	T50.3X1	T50.3X2	T50.3X3	T50.3X4	T50.3X5	T50.3X6
Ristocetin	T36.8X1	T36.8X2	T36.8X3	T36.8X4	T36.8X5	T36.8X6
Ritalin	T43.631	T43.632	T43.633	T43.634	T43.635	T43.636
Ritodrine	T44.5X1	T44.5X2	T44.5X3	T44.5X4	T44.5X5	T44.5X6
Roach killer — *see Insecticide*						
Rociverine	T44.3X1	T44.3X2	T44.3X3	T44.3X4	T44.3X5	T44.3X6
Rocky Mountain spotted fever vaccine	T50.A91	T50.A92	T50.A93	T50.A94	T50.A95	T50.A96
Rodenticide NEC	T60.4X1	T60.4X2	T60.4X3	T60.4X4	—	—
Rohypnol	T42.4X1	T42.4X2	T42.4X3	T42.4X4	T42.4X5	T42.4X6
Rokitamycin	T36.3X1	T36.3X2	T36.3X3	T36.3X4	T36.3X5	T36.3X6
Rolaids	T47.1X1	T47.1X2	T47.1X3	T47.1X4	T47.1X5	T47.1X6
Rolitetracycline	T36.4X1	T36.4X2	T36.4X3	T36.4X4	T36.4X5	T36.4X6
Romilar	T48.3X1	T48.3X2	T48.3X3	T48.3X4	T48.3X5	T48.3X6
Ronifibrate	T46.6X1	T46.6X2	T46.6X3	T46.6X4	T46.6X5	T46.6X6
Rosaprostol	T47.1X1	T47.1X2	T47.1X3	T47.1X4	T47.1X5	T47.1X6
Rose bengal sodium (131I)	T50.8X1	T50.8X2	T50.8X3	T50.8X4	T50.8X5	T50.8X6
Rose water ointment	T49.3X1	T49.3X2	T49.3X3	T49.3X4	T49.3X5	T49.3X6
Rosoxacin	T37.8X1	T37.8X2	T37.8X3	T37.8X4	T37.8X5	T37.8X6
Rotenone	T60.2X1	T60.2X2	T60.2X3	T60.2X4	—	—
Rotoxamine	T45.0X1	T45.0X2	T45.0X3	T45.0X4	T45.0X5	T45.0X6
Rough-on-rats	T60.4X1	T60.4X2	T60.4X3	T60.4X4	—	—
Roxatidine	T47.0X1	T47.0X2	T47.0X3	T47.0X4	T47.0X5	T47.0X6
Roxithromycin	T36.3X1	T36.3X2	T36.3X3	T36.3X4	T36.3X5	T36.3X6
Rt-PA	T45.611	T45.612	T45.613	T45.614	T45.615	T45.616
Rubbing alcohol	T51.2X1	T51.2X2	T51.2X3	T51.2X4	—	—
Rubefacient	T49.4X1	T49.4X2	T49.4X3	T49.4X4	T49.4X5	T49.4X6
Rubella vaccine	T50.B91	T50.B92	T50.B93	T50.B94	T50.B95	T50.B96
Rubelogen	T50.B91	T50.B92	T50.B93	T50.B94	T50.B95	T50.B96
Rubeovax	T50.991	T50.992	T50.993	T50.994	T50.995	T50.996
Rubidium chloride Rb82	T50.8X1	T50.8X2	T50.8X3	T50.8X4	T50.8X5	T50.8X6
Rubidomycin	T45.1X1	T45.1X2	T45.1X3	T45.1X4	T45.1X5	T45.1X6
Rue	T62.2X1	T62.2X2	T62.2X3	T62.2X4	—	—
Rufocromomycin	T45.1X1	T45.1X2	T45.1X3	T45.1X4	T45.1X5	T45.1X6
Russel's viper venin	T45.7X1	T45.7X2	T45.7X3	T45.7X4	T45.7X5	T45.7X6
Ruta (graveolens)	T62.2X1	T62.2X2	T62.2X3	T62.2X4	—	—
Rutinum	T46.991	T46.992	T46.993	T46.994	T46.995	T46.996
Rutoside	T46.991	T46.992	T46.993	T46.994	T46.995	T46.996

Substance	Poisoning, Accidental (Unintentional)	Poisoning, Intentional Self-Harm	Poisoning, Assault	Poisoning, Undetermined	Adverse Effect	Underdosing
S						
Sabadilla (plant)	T62.2X1	T62.2X2	T62.2X3	T62.2X4	—	—
pesticide	T60.2X1	T60.2X2	T60.2X3	T60.2X4	—	—
Saccharated iron oxide	T45.8X1	T45.8X2	T45.8X3	T45.8X4	T45.8X5	T45.8X6
Saccharin	T50.901	T50.902	T50.903	T50.904	T50.905	T50.906
Saccharomyces boulardii	T47.6X1	T47.6X2	T47.6X3	T47.6X4	T47.6X5	T47.6X6
Safflower oil	T46.6X1	T46.6X2	T46.6X3	T46.6X4	T46.6X5	T46.6X6
Safrazine	T43.1X1	T43.1X2	T43.1X3	T43.1X4	T43.1X5	T43.1X6
Salazosulfapyridine	T37.0X1	T37.0X2	T37.0X3	T37.0X4	T37.0X5	T37.0X6
Salbutamol	T48.6X1	T48.6X2	T48.6X3	T48.6X4	T48.6X5	T48.6X6
Salicylamide	T39.091	T39.092	T39.093	T39.094	T39.095	T39.096
Salicylate NEC	T39.091	T39.092	T39.093	T39.094	T39.095	T39.096
methyl	T49.3X1	T49.3X2	T49.3X3	T49.3X4	T49.3X5	T49.3X6
theobromine calcium	T50.2X1	T50.2X2	T50.2X3	T50.2X4	T50.2X5	T50.2X6
Salicylazosulfapyridine	T37.0X1	T37.0X2	T37.0X3	T37.0X4	T37.0X5	T37.0X6
Salicylhydroxamic acid	T49.0X1	T49.0X2	T49.0X3	T49.0X4	T49.0X5	T49.0X6
Salicylic acid	T49.4X1	T49.4X2	T49.4X3	T49.4X4	T49.4X5	T49.4X6
with benzoic acid	T49.4X1	T49.4X2	T49.4X3	T49.4X4	T49.4X5	T49.4X6
congeners	T39.091	T39.092	T39.093	T39.094	T39.095	T39.096
derivative	T39.091	T39.092	T39.093	T39.094	T39.095	T39.096
salts	T39.091	T39.092	T39.093	T39.094	T39.095	T39.096
Salinazid	T37.1X1	T37.1X2	T37.1X3	T37.1X4	T37.1X5	T37.1X6
Salmeterol	T48.6X1	T48.6X2	T48.6X3	T48.6X4	T48.6X5	T48.6X6
Salol	T49.3X1	T49.3X2	T49.3X3	T49.3X4	T49.3X5	T49.3X6
Salsalate	T39.091	T39.092	T39.093	T39.094	T39.095	T39.096
Salt substitute	T50.901	T50.902	T50.903	T50.904	T50.905	T50.906
Salt-replacing drug	T50.901	T50.902	T50.903	T50.904	T50.905	T50.906
Salt-retaining mineralocorticoid	T50.0X1	T50.0X2	T50.0X3	T50.0X4	T50.0X5	T50.0X6
Saluretic NEC	T50.2X1	T50.2X2	T50.2X3	T50.2X4	T50.2X5	T50.2X6
Saluron	T50.2X1	T50.2X2	T50.2X3	T50.2X4	T50.2X5	T50.2X6
Salvarsan 606 (neosilver) (silver)	T37.8X1	T37.8X2	T37.8X3	T37.8X4	T37.8X5	T37.8X6
Sambucus canadensis	T62.2X1	T62.2X2	T62.2X3	T62.2X4	—	—
berry	T62.1X1	T62.1X2	T62.1X3	T62.1X4	—	—
Sandril	T46.5X1	T46.5X2	T46.5X3	T46.5X4	T46.5X5	T46.5X6
Sanguinaria canadensis	T62.2X1	T62.2X2	T62.2X3	T62.2X4	—	—
Saniflush (cleaner)	T54.2X1	T54.2X2	T54.2X3	T54.2X4	—	—
Santonin	T37.4X1	T37.4X2	T37.4X3	T37.4X4	T37.4X5	T37.4X6
Santyl	T49.8X1	T49.8X2	T49.8X3	T49.8X4	T49.8X5	T49.8X6
Saralasin	T46.5X1	T46.5X2	T46.5X3	T46.5X4	T46.5X5	T46.5X6
Sarcolysin	T45.1X1	T45.1X2	T45.1X3	T45.1X4	T45.1X5	T45.1X6
Sarkomycin	T45.1X1	T45.1X2	T45.1X3	T45.1X4	T45.1X5	T45.1X6
Saroten	T43.011	T43.012	T43.013	T43.014	T43.015	T43.016

Substance	Poisoning, Accidental (Unintentional)	Poisoning, Intentional Self-Harm	Poisoning, Assault	Poisoning, Undetermined	Adverse Effect	Underdosing
Saturnine — *see Lead*						
Savin (oil)	T49.4X1	T49.4X2	T49.4X3	T49.4X4	T49.4X5	T49.4X6
Scammony	T47.2X1	T47.2X2	T47.2X3	T47.2X4	T47.2X5	T47.2X6
Scarlet red	T49.8X1	T49.8X2	T49.8X3	T49.8X4	T49.8X5	T49.8X6
Scheele's green	T57.0X1	T57.0X2	T57.0X3	T57.0X4	—	—
insecticide	T57.0X1	T57.0X2	T57.0X3	T57.0X4	—	—
Schizontozide (blood) (tissue)	T37.2X1	T37.2X2	T37.2X3	T37.2X4	T37.2X5	T37.2X6
Schradan	T60.0X1	T60.0X2	T60.0X3	T60.0X4	—	—
Schweinfurth green	T57.0X1	T57.0X2	T57.0X3	T57.0X4	—	—
insecticide	T57.0X1	T57.0X2	T57.0X3	T57.0X4	—	—
Scilla, rat poison	T60.4X1	T60.4X2	T60.4X3	T60.4X4	—	—
Scillaren	T60.4X1	T60.4X2	T60.4X3	T60.4X4	—	—
Sclerosing agent	T46.8X1	T46.8X2	T46.8X3	T46.8X4	T46.8X5	T46.8X6
Scombrotoxin	T61.11	T61.12	T61.13	T61.14	—	—
Scopolamine	T44.3X1	T44.3X2	T44.3X3	T44.3X4	T44.3X5	T44.3X6
Scopolia extract	T44.3X1	T44.3X2	T44.3X3	T44.3X4	T44.3X5	T44.3X6
Scouring powder	T65.891	T65.892	T65.893	T65.894		
Sea						
anemone (sting)	T63.631	T63.632	T63.633	T63.634	—	—
cucumber (sting)	T63.691	T63.692	T63.693	T63.694	—	—
snake (bite) (venom)	T63.091	T63.092	T63.093	T63.094	—	—
urchin spine (puncture)	T63.691	T63.692	T63.693	T63.694	—	—
Seafood	T61.91	T61.92	T61.93	T61.94	—	—
specified NEC	T61.8X1	T61.8X2	T61.8X3	T61.8X4	—	—
Secbutabarbital	T42.3X1	T42.3X2	T42.3X3	T42.3X4	T42.3X5	T42.3X6
Secbutabarbitone	T42.3X1	T42.3X2	T42.3X3	T42.3X4	T42.3X5	T42.3X6
Secnidazole	T37.3X1	T37.3X2	T37.3X3	T37.3X4	T37.3X5	T37.3X6
Secobarbital	T42.3X1	T42.3X2	T42.3X3	T42.3X4	T42.3X5	T42.3X6
Seconal	T42.3X1	T42.3X2	T42.3X3	T42.3X4	T42.3X5	T42.3X6
Secretin	T50.8X1	T50.8X2	T50.8X3	T50.8X4	T50.8X5	T50.8X6
Sedative NEC	T42.71	T42.72	T42.73	T42.74	T42.75	T42.76
mixed NEC	T42.6X1	T42.6X2	T42.6X3	T42.6X4	T42.6X5	T42.6X6
Sedormid	T42.6X1	T42.6X2	T42.6X3	T42.6X4	T42.6X5	T42.6X6
Seed disinfectant or dressing	T60.8X1	T60.8X2	T60.8X3	T60.8X4	—	—
Seeds (poisonous)	T62.2X1	T62.2X2	T62.2X3	T62.2X4	—	—
Selegiline	T42.8X1	T42.8X2	T42.8X3	T42.8X4	T42.8X5	T42.8X6
Selenium NEC	T56.891	T56.892	T56.893	T56.894	—	—
disulfide or sulfide	T49.4X1	T49.4X2	T49.4X3	T49.4X4	T49.4X5	T49.4X6
fumes	T59.891	T59.892	T59.893	T59.894	—	—
sulfide	T49.4X1	T49.4X2	T49.4X3	T49.4X4	T49.4X5	T49.4X6
Selenomethionine (75Se)	T50.8X1	T50.8X2	T50.8X3	T50.8X4	T50.8X5	T50.8X6
Selsun	T49.4X1	T49.4X2	T49.4X3	T49.4X4	T49.4X5	T49.4X6

◀ New ◀ Revised ~~deleted~~ Deleted

Substance	Poisoning, Accidental (Unintentional)	Poisoning, Intentional Self-Harm	Poisoning, Assault	Poisoning, Undetermined	Adverse Effect	Underdosing
Semustine	T45.1X1	T45.1X2	T45.1X3	T45.1X4	T45.1X5	T45.1X6
Senega syrup	T48.4X1	T48.4X2	T48.4X3	T48.4X4	T48.4X5	T48.4X6
Senna	T47.2X1	T47.2X2	T47.2X3	T47.2X4	T47.2X5	T47.2X6
Sennoside A+B	T47.2X1	T47.2X2	T47.2X3	T47.2X4	T47.2X5	T47.2X6
Septisol	T49.2X1	T49.2X2	T49.2X3	T49.2X4	T49.2X5	T49.2X6
Seractide	T38.811	T38.812	T38.813	T38.814	T38.815	T38.816
Serax	T42.4X1	T42.4X2	T42.4X3	T42.4X4	T42.4X5	T42.4X6
Serenesil	T42.6X1	T42.6X2	T42.6X3	T42.6X4	T42.6X5	T42.6X6
Serenium (hydrochloride)	T37.91	T37.92	T37.93	T37.94	T37.95	T37.96
Serepax — see Oxazepam						
Sermorelin	T38.891	T38.892	T38.893	T38.894	T38.895	T38.896
Sernyl	T41.1X1	T41.1X2	T41.1X3	T41.1X4	T41.1X5	T41.1X6
Serotonin	T50.991	T50.992	T50.993	T50.994	T50.995	T50.996
Serpasil	T46.5X1	T46.5X2	T46.5X3	T46.5X4	T46.5X5	T46.5X6
Serrapeptase	T45.3X1	T45.3X2	T45.3X3	T45.3X4	T45.3X5	T45.3X6
Serum						
antibotulinus	T50.Z11	T50.Z12	T50.Z13	T50.Z14	T50.Z15	T50.Z16
anticytotoxic	T50.Z11	T50.Z12	T50.Z13	T50.Z14	T50.Z15	T50.Z16
antidiphtheria	T50.Z11	T50.Z12	T50.Z13	T50.Z14	T50.Z15	T50.Z16
antimeningococcus	T50.Z11	T50.Z12	T50.Z13	T50.Z14	T50.Z15	T50.Z16
anti-Rh	T50.Z11	T50.Z12	T50.Z13	T50.Z14	T50.Z15	T50.Z16
anti-snake-bite	T50.Z11	T50.Z12	T50.Z13	T50.Z14	T50.Z15	T50.Z16
antitetanic	T50.Z11	T50.Z12	T50.Z13	T50.Z14	T50.Z15	T50.Z16
antitoxic	T50.Z11	T50.Z12	T50.Z13	T50.Z14	T50.Z15	T50.Z16
complement (inhibitor)	T45.8X1	T45.8X2	T45.8X3	T45.8X4	T45.8X5	T45.8X6
convalescent	T50.Z11	T50.Z12	T50.Z13	T50.Z14	T50.Z15	T50.Z16
hemolytic complement	T45.8X1	T45.8X2	T45.8X3	T45.8X4	T45.8X5	T45.8X6
immune (human)	T50.Z11	T50.Z12	T50.Z13	T50.Z14	T50.Z15	T50.Z16
protective NEC	T50.Z11	T50.Z12	T50.Z13	T50.Z14	T50.Z15	T50.Z16
Setastine	T45.0X1	T45.0X2	T45.0X3	T45.0X4	T45.0X5	T45.0X6
Setoperone	T43.591	T43.592	T43.593	T43.594	T43.595	T43.596
Sewer gas	T59.91	T59.92	T59.93	T59.94	—	—
Shampoo	T55.0X1	T55.0X2	T55.0X3	T55.0X4	—	—
Shellfish, noxious, nonbacterial	T61.781	T61.782	T61.783	T61.784	—	—
Sildenafil	T46.7X1	T46.7X2	T46.7X3	T46.7X4	T46.7X5	T46.7X6
Silibinin	T50.991	T50.992	T50.993	T50.994	T50.995	T50.996
Silicone NEC	T65.891	T65.892	T65.893	T65.894	—	—
medicinal	T49.3X1	T49.3X2	T49.3X3	T49.3X4	T49.3X5	T49.3X6
Silvadene	T49.0X1	T49.0X2	T49.0X3	T49.0X4	T49.0X5	T49.0X6
Silver	T49.0X1	T49.0X2	T49.0X3	T49.0X4	T49.0X5	T49.0X6
anti-infectives	T49.0X1	T49.0X2	T49.0X3	T49.0X4	T49.0X5	T49.0X6
arsphenamine	T37.8X1	T37.8X2	T37.8X3	T37.8X4	T37.8X5	T37.8X6

Substance	Poisoning, Accidental (Unintentional)	Poisoning, Intentional Self-Harm	Poisoning, Assault	Poisoning, Undetermined	Adverse Effect	Underdosing
Silver (Continued)						
colloidal	T49.0X1	T49.0X2	T49.0X3	T49.0X4	T49.0X5	T49.0X6
nitrate	T49.0X1	T49.0X2	T49.0X3	T49.0X4	T49.0X5	T49.0X6
ophthalmic preparation	T49.5X1	T49.5X2	T49.5X3	T49.5X4	T49.5X5	T49.5X6
toughened (keratolytic)	T49.4X1	T49.4X2	T49.4X3	T49.4X4	T49.4X5	T49.4X6
nonmedicinal (dust)	T56.891	T56.892	T56.893	T56.894	—	—
protein	T49.5X1	T49.5X2	T49.5X3	T49.5X4	T49.5X5	T49.5X6
salvarsan	T37.8X1	T37.8X2	T37.8X3	T37.8X4	T37.8X5	T37.8X6
sulfadiazine	T49.4X1	T49.4X2	T49.4X3	T49.4X4	T49.4X5	T49.4X6
Silymarin	T50.991	T50.992	T50.993	T50.994	T50.995	T50.996
Simaldrate	T47.1X1	T47.1X2	T47.1X3	T47.1X4	T47.1X5	T47.1X6
Simazine	T60.3X1	T60.3X2	T60.3X3	T60.3X4	—	—
Simethicone	T47.1X1	T47.1X2	T47.1X3	T47.1X4	T47.1X5	T47.1X6
Simfibrate	T46.6X1	T46.6X2	T46.6X3	T46.6X4	T46.6X5	T46.6X6
Simvastatin	T46.6X1	T46.6X2	T46.6X3	T46.6X4	T46.6X5	T46.6X6
Sincalide	T50.8X1	T50.8X2	T50.8X3	T50.8X4	T50.8X5	T50.8X6
Sinequan	T43.011	T43.012	T43.013	T43.014	T43.015	T43.016
Singoserp	T46.5X1	T46.5X2	T46.5X3	T46.5X4	T46.5X5	T46.5X6
Sintrom	T45.511	T45.512	T45.513	T45.514	T45.515	T45.516
Sisomicin	T36.5X1	T36.5X2	T36.5X3	T36.5X4	T36.5X5	T36.5X6
Sitosterols	T46.6X1	T46.6X2	T46.6X3	T46.6X4	T46.6X5	T46.6X6
Skeletal muscle relaxants	T48.1X1	T48.1X2	T48.1X3	T48.1X4	T48.1X5	T48.1X6
Skin						
agents (external)	T49.91	T49.92	T49.93	T49.94	T49.95	T49.96
specified NEC	T49.8X1	T49.8X2	T49.8X3	T49.8X4	T49.8X5	T49.8X6
test antigen	T50.8X1	T50.8X2	T50.8X3	T50.8X4	T50.8X5	T50.8X6
Sleep-eze	T45.0X1	T45.0X2	T45.0X3	T45.0X4	T45.0X5	T45.0X6
Sleeping draught, pill	T42.71	T42.72	T42.73	T42.74	T42.75	T42.76
Smallpox vaccine	T50.B11	T50.B12	T50.B13	T50.B14	T50.B15	T50.B16
Smelter fumes NEC	T56.91	T56.92	T56.93	T56.94	—	—
Smog	T59.1X1	T59.1X2	T59.1X3	T59.1X4	—	—
Smoke NEC	T59.811	T59.812	T59.813	T59.814	—	—
Smooth muscle relaxant	T44.3X1	T44.3X2	T44.3X3	T44.3X4	T44.3X5	T44.3X6
Snail killer NEC	T60.8X1	T60.8X2	T60.8X3	T60.8X4	—	—
Snake venom or bite	T63.001	T63.002	T63.003	T63.004	—	—
hemocoagulase	T45.7X1	T45.7X2	T45.7X3	T45.7X4	T45.7X5	T45.7X6
Snuff	T65.211	T65.212	T65.213	T65.214	—	—
Soap (powder) (product)	T55.0X1	T55.0X2	T55.0X3	T55.0X4	—	—
enema	T47.4X1	T47.4X2	T47.4X3	T47.4X4	T47.4X5	T47.4X6
medicinal, soft	T49.2X1	T49.2X2	T49.2X3	T49.2X4	T49.2X5	T49.2X6
superfatted	T49.2X1	T49.2X2	T49.2X3	T49.2X4	T49.2X5	T49.2X6
Sobrerol	T48.4X1	T48.4X2	T48.4X3	T48.4X4	T48.4X5	T48.4X6

Substance	External Cause (T-Code)					
	Poisoning, Accidental (Unintentional)	Poisoning, Intentional Self-Harm	Poisoning, Assault	Poisoning, Undetermined	Adverse Effect	Underdosing
Soda (caustic)	T54.3X1	T54.3X2	T54.3X3	T54.3X4	—	—
bicarb	T47.1X1	T47.1X2	T47.1X3	T47.1X4	T47.1X5	T47.1X6
chlorinated — see Sodium, hypochlorite						
Sodium						
acetosulfone	T37.1X1	T37.1X2	T37.1X3	T37.1X4	T37.1X5	T37.1X6
acetrizoate	T50.8X1	T50.8X2	T50.8X3	T50.8X4	T50.8X5	T50.8X6
acid phosphate	T50.3X1	T50.3X2	T50.3X3	T50.3X4	T50.3X5	T50.3X6
alginate	T47.8X1	T47.8X2	T47.8X3	T47.8X4	T47.8X5	T47.8X6
amidotrizoate	T50.8X1	T50.8X2	T50.8X3	T50.8X4	T50.8X5	T50.8X6
aminopterin	T45.1X1	T45.1X2	T45.1X3	T45.1X4	T45.1X5	T45.1X6
amylosulfate	T47.8X1	T47.8X2	T47.8X3	T47.8X4	T47.8X5	T47.8X6
amytal	T42.3X1	T42.3X2	T42.3X3	T42.3X4	T42.3X5	T42.3X6
antimony gluconate	T37.3X1	T37.3X2	T37.3X3	T37.3X4	T37.3X5	T37.3X6
arsenate	T57.0X1	T57.0X2	T57.0X3	T57.0X4	—	—
aurothiomalate	T39.4X1	T39.4X2	T39.4X3	T39.4X4	T39.4X5	T39.4X6
aurothiosulfate	T39.4X1	T39.4X2	T39.4X3	T39.4X4	T39.4X5	T39.4X6
barbiturate	T42.3X1	T42.3X2	T42.3X3	T42.3X4	T42.3X5	T42.3X6
basic phosphate	T47.4X1	T47.4X2	T47.4X3	T47.4X4	T47.4X5	T47.4X6
bicarbonate	T47.1X1	T47.1X2	T47.1X3	T47.1X4	T47.1X5	T47.1X6
bichromate	T57.8X1	T57.8X2	T57.8X3	T57.8X4	—	—
biphosphate	T50.3X1	T50.3X2	T50.3X3	T50.3X4	T50.3X5	T50.3X6
bisulfate	T65.891	T65.892	T65.893	T65.894	—	—
borate						
cleanser	T57.8X1	T57.8X2	T57.8X3	T57.8X4	—	—
eye	T49.5X1	T49.5X2	T49.5X3	T49.5X4	T49.5X5	T49.5X6
therapeutic	T49.8X1	T49.8X2	T49.8X3	T49.8X4	T49.8X5	T49.8X6
bromide	T42.6X1	T42.6X2	T42.6X3	T42.6X4	T42.6X5	T42.6X6
cacodylate (nonmedicinal) NEC	T50.8X1	T50.8X2	T50.8X3	T50.8X4	T50.8X5	T50.8X6
anti-infective	T37.8X1	T37.8X2	T37.8X3	T37.8X4	T37.8X5	T37.8X6
herbicide	T60.3X1	T60.3X2	T60.3X3	T60.3X4	—	—
calcium edetate	T45.8X1	T45.8X2	T45.8X3	T45.8X4	T45.8X5	T45.8X6
carbonate NEC	T54.3X1	T54.3X2	T54.3X3	T54.3X4	—	—
chlorate NEC	T65.891	T65.892	T65.893	T65.894	—	—
herbicide	T54.91	T54.92	T54.93	T54.94	—	—
chloride	T50.3X1	T50.3X2	T50.3X3	T50.3X4	T50.3X5	T50.3X6
with glucose	T50.3X1	T50.3X2	T50.3X3	T50.3X4	T50.3X5	T50.3X6
chromate	T65.891	T65.892	T65.893	T65.894	—	—
citrate	T50.991	T50.992	T50.993	T50.994	T50.995	T50.996
cromoglicate	T48.6X1	T48.6X2	T48.6X3	T48.6X4	T48.6X5	T48.6X6
cyanide	T65.0X1	T65.0X2	T65.0X3	T65.0X4	—	—
cyclamate	T50.3X1	T50.3X2	T50.3X3	T50.3X4	T50.3X5	T50.3X6

Substance	External Cause (T-Code)					
	Poisoning, Accidental (Unintentional)	Poisoning, Intentional Self-Harm	Poisoning, Assault	Poisoning, Undetermined	Adverse Effect	Underdosing
Sodium (Continued)						
dehydrocholate	T45.8X1	T45.8X2	T45.8X3	T45.8X4	T45.8X5	T45.8X6
diatrizoate	T50.8X1	T50.8X2	T50.8X3	T50.8X4	T50.8X5	T50.8X6
dibunate	T48.4X1	T48.4X2	T48.4X3	T48.4X4	T48.4X5	T48.4X6
dioctyl sulfosuccinate	T47.4X1	T47.4X2	T47.4X3	T47.4X4	T47.4X5	T47.4X6
dipantoyl ferrate	T45.8X1	T45.8X2	T45.8X3	T45.8X4	T45.8X5	T45.8X6
edetate	T45.8X1	T45.8X2	T45.8X3	T45.8X4	T45.8X5	T45.8X6
ethacrynate	T50.1X1	T50.1X2	T50.1X3	T50.1X4	T50.1X5	T50.1X6
feredetate	T45.8X1	T45.8X2	T45.8X3	T45.8X4	T45.8X5	T45.8X6
Fluoride — see Fluoride						
fluoroacetate (dust) (pesticide)	T60.4X1	T60.4X2	T60.4X3	T60.4X4	—	—
free salt	T50.3X1	T50.3X2	T50.3X3	T50.3X4	T50.3X5	T50.3X6
fusidate	T36.8X1	T36.8X2	T36.8X3	T36.8X4	T36.8X5	T36.8X6
glucaldrate	T47.1X1	T47.1X2	T47.1X3	T47.1X4	T47.1X5	T47.1X6
glucosulfone	T37.1X1	T37.1X2	T37.1X3	T37.1X4	T37.1X5	T37.1X6
glutamate	T45.8X1	T45.8X2	T45.8X3	T45.8X4	T45.8X5	T45.8X6
hydrogen carbonate	T50.3X1	T50.3X2	T50.3X3	T50.3X4	T50.3X5	T50.3X6
hydroxide	T54.3X1	T54.3X2	T54.3X3	T54.3X4	—	—
hypochlorite (bleach) NEC	T54.3X1	T54.3X2	T54.3X3	T54.3X4	—	—
disinfectant	T54.3X1	T54.3X2	T54.3X3	T54.3X4	—	—
medicinal (anti-infective) (external)	T49.0X1	T49.0X2	T49.0X3	T49.0X4	T49.0X5	T49.0X6
vapor	T54.3X1	T54.3X2	T54.3X3	T54.3X4	—	—
hyposulfite	T49.0X1	T49.0X2	T49.0X3	T49.0X4	T49.0X5	T49.0X6
indigotin disulfonate	T50.8X1	T50.8X2	T50.8X3	T50.8X4	T50.8X5	T50.8X6
iodide	T50.991	T50.992	T50.993	T50.994	T50.995	T50.996
I-131	T50.8X1	T50.8X2	T50.8X3	T50.8X4	T50.8X5	T50.8X6
therapeutic	T38.2X1	T38.2X2	T38.2X3	T38.2X4	T38.2X5	T38.2X6
iodohippurate (131I)	T50.8X1	T50.8X2	T50.8X3	T50.8X4	T50.8X5	T50.8X6
iopodate	T50.8X1	T50.8X2	T50.8X3	T50.8X4	T50.8X5	T50.8X6
iothalamate	T50.8X1	T50.8X2	T50.8X3	T50.8X4	T50.8X5	T50.8X6
iron edetate	T45.4X1	T45.4X2	T45.4X3	T45.4X4	T45.4X5	T45.4X6
lactate (compound solution)	T45.8X1	T45.8X2	T45.8X3	T45.8X4	T45.8X5	T45.8X6
lauryl (sulfate)	T49.2X1	T49.2X2	T49.2X3	T49.2X4	T49.2X5	T49.2X6
(L)-triiodothyronine	T38.1X1	T38.1X2	T38.1X3	T38.1X4	T38.1X5	T38.1X6
magnesium citrate	T50.991	T50.992	T50.993	T50.994	T50.995	T50.996
mersalate	T50.2X1	T50.2X2	T50.2X3	T50.2X4	T50.2X5	T50.2X6
metasilicate	T65.891	T65.892	T65.893	T65.894	—	—
metrizoate	T50.8X1	T50.8X2	T50.8X3	T50.8X4	T50.8X5	T50.8X6
monofluoroacetate (pesticide)	T60.1X1	T60.1X2	T60.1X3	T60.1X4	—	—
morrhuate	T46.8X1	T46.8X2	T46.8X3	T46.8X4	T46.8X5	T46.8X6
nafcillin	T36.0X1	T36.0X2	T36.0X3	T36.0X4	T36.0X5	T36.0X6

◄ New ◄ Revised ~~deleted~~ Deleted

Substance	Poisoning, Accidental (Unintentional)	Poisoning, Intentional Self-Harm	Poisoning, Assault	Poisoning, Undetermined	Adverse Effect	Underdosing
Sodium *(Continued)*						
nitrate (oxidizing agent)	T65.891	T65.892	T65.893	T65.894	—	—
nitrite	T50.6X1	T50.6X2	T50.6X3	T50.6X4	T50.6X5	T50.6X6
nitroferricyanide	T46.5X1	T46.5X2	T46.5X3	T46.5X4	T46.5X5	T46.5X6
nitroprusside	T46.5X1	T46.5X2	T46.5X3	T46.5X4	T46.5X5	T46.5X6
oxalate	T65.891	T65.892	T65.893	T65.894	—	—
oxide/peroxide	T65.891	T65.892	T65.893	T65.894	—	—
oxybate	T41.291	T41.292	T41.293	T41.294	T41.295	T41.296
para-aminohippurate	T50.8X1	T50.8X2	T50.8X3	T50.8X4	T50.8X5	T50.8X6
perborate (nonmedicinal) NEC	T65.891	T65.892	T65.893	T65.894	—	—
medicinal	T49.0X1	T49.0X2	T49.0X3	T49.0X4	T49.0X5	T49.0X6
soap	T55.0X1	T55.0X2	T55.0X3	T55.0X4	—	—
percarbonate — *see Sodium, perborate*						
pertechnetate Tc99m	T50.8X1	T50.8X2	T50.8X3	T50.8X4	T50.8X5	T50.8X6
phosphate						
cellulose	T45.8X1	T45.8X2	T45.8X3	T45.8X4	T45.8X5	T45.8X6
dibasic	T47.2X1	T47.2X2	T47.2X3	T47.2X4	T47.2X5	T47.2X6
monobasic	T47.2X1	T47.2X2	T47.2X3	T47.2X4	T47.2X5	T47.2X6
phytate	T50.6X1	T50.6X2	T50.6X3	T50.6X4	T50.6X5	T50.6X6
picosulfate	T47.2X1	T47.2X2	T47.2X3	T47.2X4	T47.2X5	T47.2X6
polyhydroxyaluminium monocarbonate	T47.1X1	T47.1X2	T47.1X3	T47.1X4	T47.1X5	T47.1X6
polystyrene sulfonate	T50.3X1	T50.3X2	T50.3X3	T50.3X4	T50.3X5	T50.3X6
propionate	T49.0X1	T49.0X2	T49.0X3	T49.0X4	T49.0X5	T49.0X6
propyl hydroxybenzoate	T50.991	T50.992	T50.993	T50.994	T50.995	T50.996
psylliate	T46.8X1	T46.8X2	T46.8X3	T46.8X4	T46.8X5	T46.8X6
removing resins	T50.3X1	T50.3X2	T50.3X3	T50.3X4	T50.3X5	T50.3X6
salicylate	T39.091	T39.092	T39.093	T39.094	T39.095	T39.096
salt NEC	T50.3X1	T50.3X2	T50.3X3	T50.3X4	T50.3X5	T50.3X6
selenate	T60.2X1	T60.2X2	T60.2X3	T60.2X4	—	—
stibogluconate	T37.3X1	T37.3X2	T37.3X3	T37.3X4	T37.3X5	T37.3X6
sulfate	T47.4X1	T47.4X2	T47.4X3	T47.4X4	T47.4X5	T47.4X6
sulfoxone	T37.1X1	T37.1X2	T37.1X3	T37.1X4	T37.1X5	T37.1X6
tetradecyl sulfate	T46.8X1	T46.8X2	T46.8X3	T46.8X4	T46.8X5	T46.8X6
thiopental	T41.1X1	T41.1X2	T41.1X3	T41.1X4	T41.1X5	T41.1X6
thiosalicylate	T39.091	T39.092	T39.093	T39.094	T39.095	T39.096
thiosulfate	T50.6X1	T50.6X2	T50.6X3	T50.6X4	T50.6X5	T50.6X6
tolbutamide	T38.3X1	T38.3X2	T38.3X3	T38.3X4	T38.3X5	T38.3X6
l-triiodothyronine	T38.1X1	T38.1X2	T38.1X3	T38.1X4	T38.1X5	T38.1X6
tyropanoate	T50.8X1	T50.8X2	T50.8X3	T50.8X4	T50.8X5	T50.8X6
valproate	T42.6X1	T42.6X2	T42.6X3	T42.6X4	T42.6X5	T42.6X6
versenate	T50.6X1	T50.6X2	T50.6X3	T50.6X4	T50.6X5	T50.6X6

Substance	Poisoning, Accidental (Unintentional)	Poisoning, Intentional Self-Harm	Poisoning, Assault	Poisoning, Undetermined	Adverse Effect	Underdosing
Sodium-free salt	T50.901	T50.902	T50.903	T50.904	T50.905	T50.906
Sodium-removing resin	T50.3X1	T50.3X2	T50.3X3	T50.3X4	T50.3X5	T50.3X6
Soft soap	T55.0X1	T55.0X2	T55.0X3	T55.0X4	—	—
Solanine	T62.2X1	T62.2X2	T62.2X3	T62.2X4	—	—
berries	T62.1X1	T62.1X2	T62.1X3	T62.1X4	—	—
Solanum dulcamara	T62.2X1	T62.2X2	T62.2X3	T62.2X4	—	—
berries	T62.1X1	T62.1X2	T62.1X3	T62.1X4	—	—
Solapsone	T37.1X1	T37.1X2	T37.1X3	T37.1X4	T37.1X5	T37.1X6
Solar lotion	T49.3X1	T49.3X2	T49.3X3	T49.3X4	T49.3X5	T49.3X6
Solasulfone	T37.1X1	T37.1X2	T37.1X3	T37.1X4	T37.1X5	T37.1X6
Soldering fluid	T65.891	T65.892	T65.893	T65.894	—	—
Solid substance	T65.91	T65.92	T65.93	T65.94	—	—
specified NEC	T65.891	T65.892	T65.893	T65.894	—	—
Solvent, industrial NEC	T52.91	T52.92	T52.93	T52.94	—	—
naphtha	T52.0X1	T52.0X2	T52.0X3	T52.0X4	—	—
petroleum	T52.0X1	T52.0X2	T52.0X3	T52.0X4	—	—
specified NEC	T52.8X1	T52.8X2	T52.8X3	T52.8X4	—	—
Soma	T42.8X1	T42.8X2	T42.8X3	T42.8X4	T42.8X5	T42.8X6
Somatorelin	T38.891	T38.892	T38.893	T38.894	T38.895	T38.896
Somatostatin	T38.991	T38.992	T38.993	T38.994	T38.995	T38.996
Somatotropin	T38.811	T38.812	T38.813	T38.814	T38.815	T38.816
Somatrem	T38.811	T38.812	T38.813	T38.814	T38.815	T38.816
Somatropin	T38.811	T38.812	T38.813	T38.814	T38.815	T38.816
Sominex	T45.0X1	T45.0X2	T45.0X3	T45.0X4	T45.0X5	T45.0X6
Somnos	T42.6X1	T42.6X2	T42.6X3	T42.6X4	T42.6X5	T42.6X6
Somonal	T42.3X1	T42.3X2	T42.3X3	T42.3X4	T42.3X5	T42.3X6
Soneryl	T42.3X1	T42.3X2	T42.3X3	T42.3X4	T42.3X5	T42.3X6
Soothing syrup	T50.901	T50.902	T50.903	T50.904	T50.905	T50.906
Sopor	T42.6X1	T42.6X2	T42.6X3	T42.6X4	T42.6X5	T42.6X6
Soporific	T42.71	T42.72	T42.73	T42.74	T42.75	T42.76
Soporific drug	T42.71	T42.72	T42.73	T42.74	T42.75	T42.76
specified type NEC	T42.6X1	T42.6X2	T42.6X3	T42.6X4	T42.6X5	T42.6X6
Sorbide nitrate	T46.3X1	T46.3X2	T46.3X3	T46.3X4	T46.3X5	T46.3X6
Sorbitol	T47.4X1	T47.4X2	T47.4X3	T47.4X4	T47.4X5	T47.4X6
Sotalol	T44.7X1	T44.7X2	T44.7X3	T44.7X4	T44.7X5	T44.7X6
Sotradecol	T46.8X1	T46.8X2	T46.8X3	T46.8X4	T46.8X5	T46.8X6
Soysterol	T46.6X1	T46.6X2	T46.6X3	T46.6X4	T46.6X5	T46.6X6
Spacoline	T44.3X1	T44.3X2	T44.3X3	T44.3X4	T44.3X5	T44.3X6
Spanish fly	T49.8X1	T49.8X2	T49.8X3	T49.8X4	T49.8X5	T49.8X6
Sparine	T43.3X1	T43.3X2	T43.3X3	T43.3X4	T43.3X5	T43.3X6
Sparteine	T48.0X1	T48.0X2	T48.0X3	T48.0X4	T48.0X5	T48.0X6

TABLE OF DRUGS AND CHEMICALS

Substance	Poisoning, Accidental (Unintentional)	Poisoning, Intentional Self-Harm	Poisoning, Assault	Poisoning, Undetermined	Adverse Effect	Underdosing
Spasmolytic						
anticholinergics	T44.3X1	T44.3X2	T44.3X3	T44.3X4	T44.3X5	T44.3X6
autonomic	T44.3X1	T44.3X2	T44.3X3	T44.3X4	T44.3X5	T44.3X6
bronchial NEC	T48.6X1	T48.6X2	T48.6X3	T48.6X4	T48.6X5	T48.6X6
quaternary ammonium	T44.3X1	T44.3X2	T44.3X3	T44.3X4	T44.3X5	T44.3X6
skeletal muscle NEC	T48.1X1	T48.1X2	T48.1X3	T48.1X4	T48.1X5	T48.1X6
Spectinomycin	T36.5X1	T36.5X2	T36.5X3	T36.5X4	T36.5X5	T36.5X6
Speed	T43.651	T43.652	T43.652	T43.654	T43.655	T43.656
Spermicide	T49.8X1	T49.8X2	T49.8X3	T49.8X4	T49.8X5	T49.8X6
Spider (bite) (venom)	T63.391	T63.392	T63.393	T63.394	—	—
antivenin	T50.Z11	T50.Z12	T50.Z13	T50.Z14	T50.Z15	T50.Z16
Spigelia (root)	T37.4X1	T37.4X2	T37.4X3	T37.4X4	T37.4X5	T37.4X6
Spindle inactivator	T50.4X1	T50.4X2	T50.4X3	T50.4X4	T50.4X5	T50.4X6
Spiperone	T43.4X1	T43.4X2	T43.4X3	T43.4X4	T43.4X5	T43.4X6
Spiramycin	T36.3X1	T36.3X2	T36.3X3	T36.3X4	T36.3X5	T36.3X6
Spirapril	T46.4X1	T46.4X2	T46.4X3	T46.4X4	T46.4X5	T46.4X6
Spirilene	T43.591	T43.592	T43.593	T43.594	T43.595	T43.596
Spirit(s) (neutral) NEC	T51.0X1	T51.0X2	T51.0X3	T51.0X4	—	—
beverage	T51.0X1	T51.0X2	T51.0X3	T51.0X4	—	—
industrial	T51.0X1	T51.0X2	T51.0X3	T51.0X4	—	—
mineral	T52.0X1	T52.0X2	T52.0X3	T52.0X4	—	—
of salt — *see Hydrochloric acid*						
surgical	T51.0X1	T51.0X2	T51.0X3	T51.0X4	—	—
Spironolactone	T50.0X1	T50.0X2	T50.0X3	T50.0X4	T50.0X5	T50.0X6
Spiroperidol	T43.4X1	T43.4X2	T43.4X3	T43.4X4	T43.4X5	T43.4X6
Sponge, absorbable (gelatin)	T45.7X1	T45.7X2	T45.7X3	T45.7X4	T45.7X5	T45.7X6
Sporostacin	T49.0X1	T49.0X2	T49.0X3	T49.0X4	T49.0X5	T49.0X6
Spray (aerosol)	T65.91	T65.92	T65.93	T65.94	—	—
cosmetic	T65.891	T65.892	T65.893	T65.894	—	—
medicinal NEC	T50.901	T50.902	T50.903	T50.904	T50.905	T50.906
pesticides — *see Pesticide*						
specified content — *see specific substance*						
Spurge flax	T62.2X1	T62.2X2	T62.2X3	T62.2X4	—	—
Spurges	T62.2X1	T62.2X2	T62.2X3	T62.2X4	—	—
Sputum viscosity-lowering drug	T48.4X1	T48.4X2	T48.4X3	T48.4X4	T48.4X5	T48.4X6
Squill	T46.0X1	T46.0X2	T46.0X3	T46.0X4	T46.0X5	T46.0X6
rat poison	T60.4X1	T60.4X2	T60.4X3	T60.4X4	—	—
Squirting cucumber (cathartic)	T47.2X1	T47.2X2	T47.2X3	T47.2X4	T47.2X5	T47.2X6
Stains	T65.6X1	T65.6X2	T65.6X3	T65.6X4	—	—
Stannous fluoride	T49.7X1	T49.7X2	T49.7X3	T49.7X4	T49.7X5	T49.7X6
Stanolone	T38.7X1	T38.7X2	T38.7X3	T38.7X4	T38.7X5	T38.7X6

Substance	Poisoning, Accidental (Unintentional)	Poisoning, Intentional Self-Harm	Poisoning, Assault	Poisoning, Undetermined	Adverse Effect	Underdosing
Stanozolol	T38.7X1	T38.7X2	T38.7X3	T38.7X4	T38.7X5	T38.7X6
Staphisagria or stavesacre (pediculicide)	T49.0X1	T49.0X2	T49.0X3	T49.0X4	T49.0X5	T49.0X6
Starch	T50.901	T50.902	T50.903	T50.904	T50.905	T50.906
Stelazine	T43.3X1	T43.3X2	T43.3X3	T43.3X4	T43.3X5	T43.3X6
Stemetil	T43.3X1	T43.3X2	T43.3X3	T43.3X4	T43.3X5	T43.3X6
Stepronin	T48.4X1	T48.4X2	T48.4X3	T48.4X4	T48.4X5	T48.4X6
Sterculia	T47.4X1	T47.4X2	T47.4X3	T47.4X4	T47.4X5	T47.4X6
Sternutator gas	T59.891	T59.892	T59.893	T59.894	—	—
Steroid	T38.0X1	T38.0X2	T38.0X3	T38.0X4	T38.0X5	T38.0X6
anabolic	T38.7X1	T38.7X2	T38.7X3	T38.7X4	T38.7X5	T38.7X6
androgenic	T38.7X1	T38.7X2	T38.7X3	T38.7X4	T38.7X5	T38.7X6
antineoplastic, hormone	T38.7X1	T38.7X2	T38.7X3	T38.7X4	T38.7X5	T38.7X6
estrogen	T38.5X1	T38.5X2	T38.5X3	T38.5X4	T38.5X5	T38.5X6
ENT agent	T49.6X1	T49.6X2	T49.6X3	T49.6X4	T49.6X5	T49.6X6
ophthalmic preparation	T49.5X1	T49.5X2	T49.5X3	T49.5X4	T49.5X5	T49.5X6
topical NEC	T49.0X1	T49.0X2	T49.0X3	T49.0X4	T49.0X5	T49.0X6
Stibine	T56.891	T56.892	T56.893	T56.894	—	—
Stibogluconate	T37.3X1	T37.3X2	T37.3X3	T37.3X4	T37.3X5	T37.3X6
Stibophen	T37.4X1	T37.4X2	T37.4X3	T37.4X4	T37.4X5	T37.4X6
Stilbamidine (isetionate)	T37.3X1	T37.3X2	T37.3X3	T37.3X4	T37.3X5	T37.3X6
Stilbestrol	T38.5X1	T38.5X2	T38.5X3	T38.5X4	T38.5X5	T38.5X6
Stilboestrol	T38.5X1	T38.5X2	T38.5X3	T38.5X4	T38.5X5	T38.5X6
Stimulant						
central nervous system — *see also Psychostimulant*	T43.601	T43.602	T43.603	T43.604	T43.605	T43.606
analeptics	T50.7X1	T50.7X2	T50.7X3	T50.7X4	T50.7X5	T50.7X6
opiate antagonist	T50.7X1	T50.7X2	T50.7X3	T50.7X4	T50.7X5	T50.7X6
psychotherapeutic NEC — *see also Psychotherapeutic drug*	T43.601	T43.602	T43.603	T43.604	T43.605	T43.606
specified NEC	T43.691	T43.692	T43.693	T43.694	T43.695	T43.696
respiratory	T48.901	T48.902	T48.903	T48.904	T48.905	T48.906
Stone-dissolving drug	T50.901	T50.902	T50.903	T50.904	T50.905	T50.906
Storage battery (cells) (acid)	T54.2X1	T54.2X2	T54.2X3	T54.2X4	—	—
Stovaine	T41.3X1	T41.3X2	T41.3X3	T41.3X4	T41.3X5	T41.3X6
infiltration (subcutaneous)	T41.3X1	T41.3X2	T41.3X3	T41.3X4	T41.3X5	T41.3X6
nerve block (peripheral) (plexus)	T41.3X1	T41.3X2	T41.3X3	T41.3X4	T41.3X5	T41.3X6
spinal	T41.3X1	T41.3X2	T41.3X3	T41.3X4	T41.3X5	T41.3X6
topical (surface)	T41.3X1	T41.3X2	T41.3X3	T41.3X4	T41.3X5	T41.3X6
Stovarsal	T37.8X1	T37.8X2	T37.8X3	T37.8X4	T37.8X5	T37.8X6
Stove gas — *see Gas, stove*	T57.91	T57.92	T57.93	T57.94	—	—

◀ New   ◀ Revised   ~~deleted~~ Deleted

Substance	External Cause (T-Code)					
	Poisoning, Accidental (Unintentional)	Poisoning, Intentional Self-Harm	Poisoning, Assault	Poisoning, Undetermined	Adverse Effect	Underdosing
Stoxil	T49.5X1	T49.5X2	T49.5X3	T49.5X4	T49.5X5	T49.5X6
Stramonium	T48.6X1	T48.6X2	T48.6X3	T48.6X4	T48.6X5	T48.6X6
natural state	T62.2X1	T62.2X2	T62.2X3	T62.2X4	—	—
Streptodornase	T45.3X1	T45.3X2	T45.3X3	T45.3X4	T45.3X5	T45.3X6
Streptoduocin	T36.5X1	T36.5X2	T36.5X3	T36.5X4	T36.5X5	T36.5X6
Streptokinase	T45.611	T45.612	T45.613	T45.614	T45.615	T45.616
Streptomycin (derivative)	T36.5X1	T36.5X2	T36.5X3	T36.5X4	T36.5X5	T36.5X6
Streptonivicin	T36.5X1	T36.5X2	T36.5X3	T36.5X4	T36.5X5	T36.5X6
Streptovarycin	T36.5X1	T36.5X2	T36.5X3	T36.5X4	T36.5X5	T36.5X6
Streptozocin	T45.1X1	T45.1X2	T45.1X3	T45.1X4	T45.1X5	T45.1X6
Streptozotocin	T45.1X1	T45.1X2	T45.1X3	T45.1X4	T45.1X5	T45.1X6
Stripper (paint) (solvent)	T52.8X1	T52.8X2	T52.8X3	T52.8X4	—	—
Strobane	T60.1X1	T60.1X2	T60.1X3	T60.1X4	—	—
Strofantina	T46.0X1	T46.0X2	T46.0X3	T46.0X4	T46.0X5	T46.0X6
Strophanthin (g) (k)	T46.0X1	T46.0X2	T46.0X3	T46.0X4	T46.0X5	T46.0X6
Strophanthus	T46.0X1	T46.0X2	T46.0X3	T46.0X4	T46.0X5	T46.0X6
Strophantin	T46.0X1	T46.0X2	T46.0X3	T46.0X4	T46.0X5	T46.0X6
Strophantin-g	T46.0X1	T46.0X2	T46.0X3	T46.0X4	T46.0X5	T46.0X6
Strychnine (nonmedicinal) (pesticide) (salts)	T65.1X1	T65.1X2	T65.1X3	T65.1X4	—	—
medicinal	T48.291	T48.292	T48.293	T48.294	T48.295	T48.296
Strychnos (ignatii) — *see* Strychnine						
Styramate	T42.8X1	T42.8X2	T42.8X3	T42.8X4	T42.8X5	T42.8X6
Styrene	T65.891	T65.892	T65.893	T65.894	—	—
Succinimide, antiepileptic or anticonvulsant	T42.2X1	T42.2X2	T42.2X3	T42.2X4	T42.2X5	T42.2X6
mercuric — *see* Mercury						
Succinylcholine	T48.1X1	T48.1X2	T48.1X3	T48.1X4	T48.1X5	T48.1X6
Succinylsulfathiazole	T37.0X1	T37.0X2	T37.0X3	T37.0X4	T37.0X5	T37.0X6
Sucralfate	T47.1X1	T47.1X2	T47.1X3	T47.1X4	T47.1X5	T47.1X6
Sucrose	T50.3X1	T50.3X2	T50.3X3	T50.3X4	T50.3X5	T50.3X6
Sufentanil	T40.411	T40.412	T40.413	T40.414	T40.415	T40.416
Sulbactam	T36.0X1	T36.0X2	T36.0X3	T36.0X4	T36.0X5	T36.0X6
Sulbenicillin	T36.0X1	T36.0X2	T36.0X3	T36.0X4	T36.0X5	T36.0X6
Sulbentine	T49.0X1	T49.0X2	T49.0X3	T49.0X4	T49.0X5	T49.0X6
Sulfacetamide	T49.0X1	T49.0X2	T49.0X3	T49.0X4	T49.0X5	T49.0X6
ophthalmic preparation	T49.5X1	T49.5X2	T49.5X3	T49.5X4	T49.5X5	T49.5X6
Sulfachlorpyridazine	T37.0X1	T37.0X2	T37.0X3	T37.0X4	T37.0X5	T37.0X6
Sulfacitine	T37.0X1	T37.0X2	T37.0X3	T37.0X4	T37.0X5	T37.0X6
Sulfadiasulfone sodium	T37.0X1	T37.0X2	T37.0X3	T37.0X4	T37.0X5	T37.0X6
Sulfadiazine	T37.0X1	T37.0X2	T37.0X3	T37.0X4	T37.0X5	T37.0X6
silver (topical)	T49.0X1	T49.0X2	T49.0X3	T49.0X4	T49.0X5	T49.0X6

Substance	External Cause (T-Code)					
	Poisoning, Accidental (Unintentional)	Poisoning, Intentional Self-Harm	Poisoning, Assault	Poisoning, Undetermined	Adverse Effect	Underdosing
Sulfadimethoxine	T37.0X1	T37.0X2	T37.0X3	T37.0X4	T37.0X5	T37.0X6
Sulfadimidine	T37.0X1	T37.0X2	T37.0X3	T37.0X4	T37.0X5	T37.0X6
Sulfadoxine	T37.0X1	T37.0X2	T37.0X3	T37.0X4	T37.0X5	T37.0X6
with pyrimethamine	T37.2X1	T37.2X2	T37.2X3	T37.2X4	T37.2X5	T37.2X6
Sulfaethidole	T37.0X1	T37.0X2	T37.0X3	T37.0X4	T37.0X5	T37.0X6
Sulfafurazole	T37.0X1	T37.0X2	T37.0X3	T37.0X4	T37.0X5	T37.0X6
Sulfaguanidine	T37.0X1	T37.0X2	T37.0X3	T37.0X4	T37.0X5	T37.0X6
Sulfalene	T37.0X1	T37.0X2	T37.0X3	T37.0X4	T37.0X5	T37.0X6
Sulfaloxate	T37.0X1	T37.0X2	T37.0X3	T37.0X4	T37.0X5	T37.0X6
Sulfaloxic acid	T37.0X1	T37.0X2	T37.0X3	T37.0X4	T37.0X5	T37.0X6
Sulfamazone	T39.2X1	T39.2X2	T39.2X3	T39.2X4	T39.2X5	T39.2X6
Sulfamerazine	T37.0X1	T37.0X2	T37.0X3	T37.0X4	T37.0X5	T37.0X6
Sulfameter	T37.0X1	T37.0X2	T37.0X3	T37.0X4	T37.0X5	T37.0X6
Sulfamethazine	T37.0X1	T37.0X2	T37.0X3	T37.0X4	T37.0X5	T37.0X6
Sulfamethizole	T37.0X1	T37.0X2	T37.0X3	T37.0X4	T37.0X5	T37.0X6
Sulfamethoxazole	T37.0X1	T37.0X2	T37.0X3	T37.0X4	T37.0X5	T37.0X6
with trimethoprim	T36.8X1	T36.8X2	T36.8X3	T36.8X4	T36.8X5	T36.8X6
Sulfamethoxydiazine	T37.0X1	T37.0X2	T37.0X3	T37.0X4	T37.0X5	T37.0X6
Sulfamethoxypyridazine	T37.0X1	T37.0X2	T37.0X3	T37.0X4	T37.0X5	T37.0X6
Sulfamethylthiazole	T37.0X1	T37.0X2	T37.0X3	T37.0X4	T37.0X5	T37.0X6
Sulfametoxydiazine	T37.0X1	T37.0X2	T37.0X3	T37.0X4	T37.0X5	T37.0X6
Sulfamidopyrine	T39.2X1	T39.2X2	T39.2X3	T39.2X4	T39.2X5	T39.2X6
Sulfamonomethoxine	T37.0X1	T37.0X2	T37.0X3	T37.0X4	T37.0X5	T37.0X6
Sulfamoxole	T37.0X1	T37.0X2	T37.0X3	T37.0X4	T37.0X5	T37.0X6
Sulfamylon	T49.0X1	T49.0X2	T49.0X3	T49.0X4	T49.0X5	T49.0X6
Sulfan blue (diagnostic dye)	T50.8X1	T50.8X2	T50.8X3	T50.8X4	T50.8X5	T50.8X6
Sulfanilamide	T37.0X1	T37.0X2	T37.0X3	T37.0X4	T37.0X5	T37.0X6
Sulfanilylguanidine	T37.0X1	T37.0X2	T37.0X3	T37.0X4	T37.0X5	T37.0X6
Sulfaperin	T37.0X1	T37.0X2	T37.0X3	T37.0X4	T37.0X5	T37.0X6
Sulfaphenazole	T37.0X1	T37.0X2	T37.0X3	T37.0X4	T37.0X5	T37.0X6
Sulfaphenylthiazole	T37.0X1	T37.0X2	T37.0X3	T37.0X4	T37.0X5	T37.0X6
Sulfaproxyline	T37.0X1	T37.0X2	T37.0X3	T37.0X4	T37.0X5	T37.0X6
Sulfapyridine	T37.0X1	T37.0X2	T37.0X3	T37.0X4	T37.0X5	T37.0X6
Sulfapyrimidine	T37.0X1	T37.0X2	T37.0X3	T37.0X4	T37.0X5	T37.0X6
Sulfarsphenamine	T37.8X1	T37.8X2	T37.8X3	T37.8X4	T37.8X5	T37.8X6
Sulfasalazine	T37.0X1	T37.0X2	T37.0X3	T37.0X4	T37.0X5	T37.0X6
Sulfasuxidine	T37.0X1	T37.0X2	T37.0X3	T37.0X4	T37.0X5	T37.0X6
Sulfasymazine	T37.0X1	T37.0X2	T37.0X3	T37.0X4	T37.0X5	T37.0X6
Sulfated amylopectin	T47.8X1	T47.8X2	T47.8X3	T47.8X4	T47.8X5	T47.8X6
Sulfathiazole	T37.0X1	T37.0X2	T37.0X3	T37.0X4	T37.0X5	T37.0X6
Sulfatostearate	T49.2X1	T49.2X2	T49.2X3	T49.2X4	T49.2X5	T49.2X6
Sulfinpyrazone	T50.4X1	T50.4X2	T50.4X3	T50.4X4	T50.4X5	T50.4X6

Substance	Poisoning, Accidental (Unintentional)	Poisoning, Intentional Self-Harm	Poisoning, Assault	Poisoning, Undetermined	Adverse Effect	Underdosing
Sulfiram	T49.0X1	T49.0X2	T49.0X3	T49.0X4	T49.0X5	T49.0X6
Sulfisomidine	T37.0X1	T37.0X2	T37.0X3	T37.0X4	T37.0X5	T37.0X6
Sulfisoxazole	T37.0X1	T37.0X2	T37.0X3	T37.0X4	T37.0X5	T37.0X6
ophthalmic preparation	T49.5X1	T49.5X2	T49.5X3	T49.5X4	T49.5X5	T49.5X6
Sulfobromophthalein (sodium)	T50.8X1	T50.8X2	T50.8X3	T50.8X4	T50.8X5	T50.8X6
Sulfobromphthalein	T50.8X1	T50.8X2	T50.8X3	T50.8X4	T50.8X5	T50.8X6
Sulfogaiacol	T48.4X1	T48.4X2	T48.4X3	T48.4X4	T48.4X5	T48.4X6
Sulfomyxin	T36.8X1	T36.8X2	T36.8X3	T36.8X4	T36.8X5	T36.8X6
Sulfonal	T42.6X1	T42.6X2	T42.6X3	T42.6X4	T42.6X5	T42.6X6
Sulfonamide NEC	T37.0X1	T37.0X2	T37.0X3	T37.0X4	T37.0X5	T37.0X6
eye	T49.5X1	T49.5X2	T49.5X3	T49.5X4	T49.5X5	T49.5X6
Sulfonazide	T37.1X1	T37.1X2	T37.1X3	T37.1X4	T37.1X5	T37.1X6
Sulfones	T37.1X1	T37.1X2	T37.1X3	T37.1X4	T37.1X5	T37.1X6
Sulfonethylmethane	T42.6X1	T42.6X2	T42.6X3	T42.6X4	T42.6X5	T42.6X6
Sulfonmethane	T42.6X1	T42.6X2	T42.6X3	T42.6X4	T42.6X5	T42.6X6
Sulfonphthal, sulfonphthol	T50.8X1	T50.8X2	T50.8X3	T50.8X4	T50.8X5	T50.8X6
Sulfonylurea derivatives, oral	T38.3X1	T38.3X2	T38.3X3	T38.3X4	T38.3X5	T38.3X6
Sulforidazine	T43.3X1	T43.3X2	T43.3X3	T43.3X4	T43.3X5	T43.3X6
Sulfoxone	T37.1X1	T37.1X2	T37.1X3	T37.1X4	T37.1X5	T37.1X6
Sulfur, sulfurated, sulfuric, sulfurous, sulfuryl (compounds NEC) (medicinal)	T49.4X1	T49.4X2	T49.4X3	T49.4X4	T49.4X5	T49.4X6
acid	T54.2X1	T54.2X2	T54.2X3	T54.2X4	—	—
dioxide (gas)	T59.1X1	T59.1X2	T59.1X3	T59.1X4	—	—
ether — see Ether(s)						
hydrogen	T59.6X1	T59.6X2	T59.6X3	T59.6X4	—	—
medicinal (keratolytic) (ointment) NEC	T49.4X1	T49.4X2	T49.4X3	T49.4X4	T49.4X5	T49.4X6
ointment	T49.0X1	T49.0X2	T49.0X3	T49.0X4	T49.0X5	T49.0X6
pesticide (vapor)	T60.91	T60.92	T60.93	T60.94	—	—
vapor NEC	T59.891	T59.892	T59.893	T59.894	—	—
Sulfuric acid	T54.2X1	T54.2X2	T54.2X3	T54.2X4	—	—
Sulglicotide	T47.1X1	T47.1X2	T47.1X3	T47.1X4	T47.1X5	T47.1X6
Sulindac	T39.391	T39.392	T39.393	T39.394	T39.395	T39.396
Sulisatin	T47.2X1	T47.2X2	T47.2X3	T47.2X4	T47.2X5	T47.2X6
Sulisobenzone	T49.3X1	T49.3X2	T49.3X3	T49.3X4	T49.3X5	T49.3X6
Sulkowitch's reagent	T50.8X1	T50.8X2	T50.8X3	T50.8X4	T50.8X5	T50.8X6
Sulmetozine	T44.3X1	T44.3X2	T44.3X3	T44.3X4	T44.3X5	T44.3X6
Suloctidil	T46.7X1	T46.7X2	T46.7X3	T46.7X4	T46.7X5	T46.7X6
Sulph — see also Sulf-						
Sulphadiazine	T37.0X1	T37.0X2	T37.0X3	T37.0X4	T37.0X5	T37.0X6
Sulphadimethoxine	T37.0X1	T37.0X2	T37.0X3	T37.0X4	T37.0X5	T37.0X6
Sulphadimidine	T37.0X1	T37.0X2	T37.0X3	T37.0X4	T37.0X5	T37.0X6
Sulphadione	T37.1X1	T37.1X2	T37.1X3	T37.1X4	T37.1X5	T37.1X6
Sulphafurazole	T37.0X1	T37.0X2	T37.0X3	T37.0X4	T37.0X5	T37.0X6
Sulphamethizole	T37.0X1	T37.0X2	T37.0X3	T37.0X4	T37.0X5	T37.0X6
Sulphamethoxazole	T37.0X1	T37.0X2	T37.0X3	T37.0X4	T37.0X5	T37.0X6
Sulphan blue	T50.8X1	T50.8X2	T50.8X3	T50.8X4	T50.8X5	T50.8X6
Sulphaphenazole	T37.0X1	T37.0X2	T37.0X3	T37.0X4	T37.0X5	T37.0X6
Sulphapyridine	T37.0X1	T37.0X2	T37.0X3	T37.0X4	T37.0X5	T37.0X6
Sulphasalazine	T37.0X1	T37.0X2	T37.0X3	T37.0X4	T37.0X5	T37.0X6
Sulphinpyrazone	T50.4X1	T50.4X2	T50.4X3	T50.4X4	T50.4X5	T50.4X6
Sulpiride	T43.591	T43.592	T43.593	T43.594	T43.595	T43.596
Sulprostone	T48.0X1	T48.0X2	T48.0X3	T48.0X4	T48.0X5	T48.0X6
Sulpyrine	T39.2X1	T39.2X2	T39.2X3	T39.2X4	T39.2X5	T39.2X6
Sultamicillin	T36.0X1	T36.0X2	T36.0X3	T36.0X4	T36.0X5	T36.0X6
Sulthiame	T42.6X1	T42.6X2	T42.6X3	T42.6X4	T42.6X5	T42.6X6
Sultiame	T42.6X1	T42.6X2	T42.6X3	T42.6X4	T42.6X5	T42.6X6
Sultopride	T43.591	T43.592	T43.593	T43.594	T43.595	T43.596
Sumatriptan	T39.8X1	T39.8X2	T39.8X3	T39.8X4	T39.8X5	T39.8X6
Sunflower seed oil	T46.6X1	T46.6X2	T46.6X3	T46.6X4	T46.6X5	T46.6X6
Superinone	T48.4X1	T48.4X2	T48.4X3	T48.4X4	T48.4X5	T48.4X6
Suprofen	T39.311	T39.312	T39.313	T39.314	T39.315	T39.316
Suramin (sodium)	T37.4X1	T37.4X2	T37.4X3	T37.4X4	T37.4X5	T37.4X6
Surfacaine	T41.3X1	T41.3X2	T41.3X3	T41.3X4	T41.3X5	T41.3X6
Surital	T41.1X1	T41.1X2	T41.1X3	T41.1X4	T41.1X5	T41.1X6
Sutilains	T45.3X1	T45.3X2	T45.3X3	T45.3X4	T45.3X5	T45.3X6
Suxamethonium (chloride)	T48.1X1	T48.1X2	T48.1X3	T48.1X4	T48.1X5	T48.1X6
Suxethonium (chloride)	T48.1X1	T48.1X2	T48.1X3	T48.1X4	T48.1X5	T48.1X6
Suxibuzone	T39.2X1	T39.2X2	T39.2X3	T39.2X4	T39.2X5	T39.2X6
Sweet oil (birch)	T49.3X1	T49.3X2	T49.3X3	T49.3X4	T49.3X5	T49.3X6
Sweet niter spirit	T46.3X1	T46.3X2	T46.3X3	T46.3X4	T46.3X5	T46.3X6
Sweetener	T50.901	T50.902	T50.903	T50.904	T50.905	T50.906
Sym-dichloroethyl ether	T53.6X1	T53.6X2	T53.6X3	T53.6X4	—	—
Sympatholytic NEC	T44.8X1	T44.8X2	T44.8X3	T44.8X4	T44.8X5	T44.8X6
haloalkylamine	T44.8X1	T44.8X2	T44.8X3	T44.8X4	T44.8X5	T44.8X6
Sympathomimetic NEC	T44.901	T44.902	T44.903	T44.904	T44.905	T44.906
anti-common-cold	T48.5X1	T48.5X2	T48.5X3	T48.5X4	T48.5X5	T48.5X6
bronchodilator	T48.6X1	T48.6X2	T48.6X3	T48.6X4	T48.6X5	T48.6X6
specified NEC	T44.991	T44.992	T44.993	T44.994	T44.995	T44.996
Synagis	T50.B91	T50.B92	T50.B93	T50.B94	T50.B95	T50.B96
Synalar	T49.0X1	T49.0X2	T49.0X3	T49.0X4	T49.0X5	T49.0X6
Synthetic cannabinoids	T40.721	T40.722	T40.723	T40.724	T40.725	T40.726
Synthroid	T38.1X1	T38.1X2	T38.1X3	T38.1X4	T38.1X5	T38.1X6

◀ New   ◀ Revised   ~~deleted~~ Deleted

Substance	External Cause (T-Code)					
	Poisoning, Accidental (Unintentional)	Poisoning, Intentional Self-Harm	Poisoning, Assault	Poisoning, Undetermined	Adverse Effect	Underdosing
Syntocinon	T48.0X1	T48.0X2	T48.0X3	T48.0X4	T48.0X5	T48.0X6
Syrosingopine	T46.5X1	T46.5X2	T46.5X3	T46.5X4	T46.5X5	T46.5X6
Systemic drug	T45.91	T45.92	T45.93	T45.94	T45.95	T45.96
specified NEC	T45.8X1	T45.8X2	T45.8X3	T45.8X4	T45.8X5	T45.8X6
2,4,5-T	T60.3X1	T60.3X2	T60.3X3	T60.3X4	—	—
T						
Tablets — see also specified substance	T50.901	T50.902	T50.903	T50.904	T50.905	T50.906
Tace	T38.5X1	T38.5X2	T38.5X3	T38.5X4	T38.5X5	T38.5X6
Tacrine	T44.0X1	T44.0X2	T44.0X3	T44.0X4	T44.0X5	T44.0X6
Tadalafil	T46.7X1	T46.7X2	T46.7X3	T46.7X4	T46.7X5	T46.7X6
Talampicillin	T36.0X1	T36.0X2	T36.0X3	T36.0X4	T36.0X5	T36.0X6
Talbutal	T42.3X1	T42.3X2	T42.3X3	T42.3X4	T42.3X5	T42.3X6
Talc powder	T49.3X1	T49.3X2	T49.3X3	T49.3X4	T49.3X5	T49.3X6
Talcum	T49.3X1	T49.3X2	T49.3X3	T49.3X4	T49.3X5	T49.3X6
Taleranol	T38.6X1	T38.6X2	T38.6X3	T38.6X4	T38.6X5	T38.6X6
Tamoxifen	T38.6X1	T38.6X2	T38.6X3	T38.6X4	T38.6X5	T38.6X6
Tamsulosin	T44.6X1	T44.6X2	T44.6X3	T44.6X4	T44.6X5	T44.6X6
Tandearil, tanderil	T39.2X1	T39.2X2	T39.2X3	T39.2X4	T39.2X5	T39.2X6
Tannic acid	T49.2X1	T49.2X2	T49.2X3	T49.2X4	T49.2X5	T49.2X6
medicinal (astringent)	T49.2X1	T49.2X2	T49.2X3	T49.2X4	T49.2X5	T49.2X6
Tannin — see Tannic acid						
Tansy	T62.2X1	T62.2X2	T62.2X3	T62.2X4	—	—
TAO	T36.3X1	T36.3X2	T36.3X3	T36.3X4	T36.3X5	T36.3X6
Tapazole	T38.2X1	T38.2X2	T38.2X3	T38.2X4	T38.2X5	T38.2X6
Tar NEC	T52.0X1	T52.0X2	T52.0X3	T52.0X4	—	—
camphor	T60.1X1	T60.1X2	T60.1X3	T60.1X4	—	—
distillate	T49.1X1	T49.1X2	T49.1X3	T49.1X4	T49.1X5	T49.1X6
fumes	T59.891	T59.892	T59.893	T59.894	—	—
medicinal	T49.1X1	T49.1X2	T49.1X3	T49.1X4	T49.1X5	T49.1X6
ointment	T49.1X1	T49.1X2	T49.1X3	T49.1X4	T49.1X5	T49.1X6
Taractan	T43.591	T43.592	T43.593	T43.594	T43.595	T43.596
Tarantula (venomous)	T63.321	T63.322	T63.323	T63.324	—	—
Tartar emetic	T37.8X1	T37.8X2	T37.8X3	T37.8X4	T37.8X5	T37.8X6
Tartaric acid	T65.891	T65.892	T65.893	T65.894	—	—
Tartrated antimony (anti-infective)	T37.8X1	T37.8X2	T37.8X3	T37.8X4	T37.8X5	T37.8X6
Tartrate, laxative	T47.4X1	T47.4X2	T47.4X3	T47.4X4	T47.4X5	T47.4X6
Tauromustine	T45.1X1	T45.1X2	T45.1X3	T45.1X4	T45.1X5	T45.1X6
TCA — see Trichloroacetic acid						
TCDD	T53.7X1	T53.7X2	T53.7X3	T53.7X4	—	—
TDI (vapor)	T65.0X1	T65.0X2	T65.0X3	T65.0X4	—	—

Substance	External Cause (T-Code)					
	Poisoning, Accidental (Unintentional)	Poisoning, Intentional Self-Harm	Poisoning, Assault	Poisoning, Undetermined	Adverse Effect	Underdosing
Tear						
gas	T59.3X1	T59.3X2	T59.3X3	T59.3X4	—	—
solution	T49.5X1	T49.5X2	T49.5X3	T49.5X4	T49.5X5	T49.5X6
Teclothiazide	T50.2X1	T50.2X2	T50.2X3	T50.2X4	T50.2X5	T50.2X6
Teclozan	T37.3X1	T37.3X2	T37.3X3	T37.3X4	T37.3X5	T37.3X6
Tegafur	T45.1X1	T45.1X2	T45.1X3	T45.1X4	T45.1X5	T45.1X6
Tegretol	T42.1X1	T42.1X2	T42.1X3	T42.1X4	T42.1X5	T42.1X6
Teicoplanin	T36.8X1	T36.8X2	T36.8X3	T36.8X4	T36.8X5	T36.8X6
Telepaque	T50.8X1	T50.8X2	T50.8X3	T50.8X4	T50.8X5	T50.8X6
Tellurium	T56.891	T56.892	T56.893	T56.894	—	—
fumes	T56.891	T56.892	T56.893	T56.894	—	—
TEM	T45.1X1	T45.1X2	T45.1X3	T45.1X4	T45.1X5	T45.1X6
Temazepam	T42.4X1	T42.4X2	T42.4X3	T42.4X4	T42.4X5	T42.4X6
Temocillin	T36.0X1	T36.0X2	T36.0X3	T36.0X4	T36.0X5	T36.0X6
Tenamfetamine	T43.621	T43.622	T43.623	T43.624	T43.625	T43.626
Teniposide	T45.1X1	T45.1X2	T45.1X3	T45.1X4	T45.1X5	T45.1X6
Tenitramine	T46.3X1	T46.3X2	T46.3X3	T46.3X4	T46.3X5	T46.3X6
Tenoglicin	T48.4X1	T48.4X2	T48.4X3	T48.4X4	T48.4X5	T48.4X6
Tenonitrozole	T37.3X1	T37.3X2	T37.3X3	T37.3X4	T37.3X5	T37.3X6
Tenoxicam	T39.391	T39.392	T39.393	T39.394	T39.395	T39.396
TEPA	T45.1X1	T45.1X2	T45.1X3	T45.1X4	T45.1X5	T45.1X6
TEPP	T60.0X1	T60.0X2	T60.0X3	T60.0X4	—	—
Teprotide	T46.5X1	T46.5X2	T46.5X3	T46.5X4	T46.5X5	T46.5X6
Terazosin	T44.6X1	T44.6X2	T44.6X3	T44.6X4	T44.6X5	T44.6X6
Terbufos	T60.0X1	T60.0X2	T60.0X3	T60.0X4	—	—
Terbutaline	T48.6X1	T48.6X2	T48.6X3	T48.6X4	T48.6X5	T48.6X6
Terconazole	T49.0X1	T49.0X2	T49.0X3	T49.0X4	T49.0X5	T49.0X6
Terfenadine	T45.0X1	T45.0X2	T45.0X3	T45.0X4	T45.0X5	T45.0X6
Teriparatide (acetate)	T50.991	T50.992	T50.993	T50.994	T50.995	T50.996
Terizidone	T37.1X1	T37.1X2	T37.1X3	T37.1X4	T37.1X5	T37.1X6
Terlipressin	T38.891	T38.892	T38.893	T38.894	T38.895	T38.896
Terodiline	T46.3X1	T46.3X2	T46.3X3	T46.3X4	T46.3X5	T46.3X6
Teroxalene	T37.4X1	T37.4X2	T37.4X3	T37.4X4	T37.4X5	T37.4X6
Terpin(cis) hydrate	T48.4X1	T48.4X2	T48.4X3	T48.4X4	T48.4X5	T48.4X6
Terramycin	T36.4X1	T36.4X2	T36.4X3	T36.4X4	T36.4X5	T36.4X6
Tertatolol	T44.7X1	T44.7X2	T44.7X3	T44.7X4	T44.7X5	T44.7X6
Tessalon	T48.3X1	T48.3X2	T48.3X3	T48.3X4	T48.3X5	T48.3X6
Testolactone	T38.7X1	T38.7X2	T38.7X3	T38.7X4	T38.7X5	T38.7X6
Testosterone	T38.7X1	T38.7X2	T38.7X3	T38.7X4	T38.7X5	T38.7X6
Tetanus toxoid or vaccine	T50.A91	T50.A92	T50.A93	T50.A94	T50.A95	T50.A96
antitoxin	T50.Z11	T50.Z12	T50.Z13	T50.Z14	T50.Z15	T50.Z16
immune globulin (human)	T50.Z11	T50.Z12	T50.Z13	T50.Z14	T50.Z15	T50.Z16

◀ New   ◀ Revised   ~~deleted~~ Deleted

Substance	Poisoning, Accidental (Unintentional)	Poisoning, Intentional Self-Harm	Poisoning, Assault	Poisoning, Undetermined	Adverse Effect	Underdosing
Tetanus toxoid or vaccine (Continued)						
toxoid	T50.A91	T50.A92	T50.A93	T50.A94	T50.A95	T50.A96
with diphtheria toxoid	T50.A21	T50.A22	T50.A23	T50.A24	T50.A25	T50.A26
with pertussis	T50.A11	T50.A12	T50.A13	T50.A14	T50.A15	T50.A16
Tetrabenazine	T43.591	T43.592	T43.593	T43.594	T43.595	T43.596
Tetracaine	T41.3X1	T41.3X2	T41.3X3	T41.3X4	T41.3X5	T41.3X6
nerve block (peripheral) (plexus)	T41.3X1	T41.3X2	T41.3X3	T41.3X4	T41.3X5	T41.3X6
regional	T41.3X1	T41.3X2	T41.3X3	T41.3X4	T41.3X5	T41.3X6
spinal	T41.3X1	T41.3X2	T41.3X3	T41.3X4	T41.3X5	T41.3X6
Tetrachlorethylene — *see Tetrachloroethylene*						
Tetrachlormethiazide	T50.2X1	T50.2X2	T50.2X3	T50.2X4	T50.2X5	T50.2X6
2,3,7,8-Tetrachlorodibenzo-p-dioxin	T53.7X1	T53.7X2	T53.7X3	T53.7X4	—	—
Tetrachloroethane	T53.6X1	T53.6X2	T53.6X3	T53.6X4	—	—
vapor	T53.6X1	T53.6X2	T53.6X3	T53.6X4		
paint or varnish	T53.6X1	T53.6X2	T53.6X3	T53.6X4		
Tetrachloroethylene (liquid)	T53.3X1	T53.3X2	T53.3X3	T53.3X4		
medicinal	T37.4X1	T37.4X2	T37.4X3	T37.4X4	T37.4X5	T37.4X6
vapor	T53.3X1	T53.3X2	T53.3X3	T53.3X4		
Tetrachloromethane — *see Carbon tetrachloride*						
Tetracosactide	T38.811	T38.812	T38.813	T38.814	T38.815	T38.816
Tetracosactrin	T38.811	T38.812	T38.813	T38.814	T38.815	T38.816
Tetracycline	T36.4X1	T36.4X2	T36.4X3	T36.4X4	T36.4X5	T36.4X6
ophthalmic preparation	T49.5X1	T49.5X2	T49.5X3	T49.5X4	T49.5X5	T49.5X6
topical NEC	T49.0X1	T49.0X2	T49.0X3	T49.0X4	T49.0X5	T49.0X6
Tetradifon	T60.8X1	T60.8X2	T60.8X3	T60.8X4	—	—
Tetradotoxin	T61.771	T61.772	T61.773	T61.774		
Tetraethyl						
lead	T56.0X1	T56.0X2	T56.0X3	T56.0X4		
pyrophosphate	T60.0X1	T60.0X2	T60.0X3	T60.0X4	—	
Tetraethylammonium chloride	T44.2X1	T44.2X2	T44.2X3	T44.2X4	T44.2X5	T44.2X6
Tetraethylthiuram disulfide	T50.6X1	T50.6X2	T50.6X3	T50.6X4	T50.6X5	T50.6X6
Tetrahydroaminoacridine	T44.0X1	T44.0X2	T44.0X3	T44.0X4	T44.0X5	T44.0X6
Tetrahydrocannabinol	T40.711	T40.712	T40.713	T40.714	T40.715	T40.716
Tetrahydrofuran	T52.8X1	T52.8X2	T52.8X3	T52.8X4	—	—
Tetrahydronaphthalene	T52.8X1	T52.8X2	T52.8X3	T52.8X4	—	—
Tetrahydrozoline	T49.5X1	T49.5X2	T49.5X3	T49.5X4	T49.5X5	T49.5X6
Tetralin	T52.8X1	T52.8X2	T52.8X3	T52.8X4	—	—
Tetramethrin	T60.2X1	T60.2X2	T60.2X3	T60.2X4	—	—

Substance	Poisoning, Accidental (Unintentional)	Poisoning, Intentional Self-Harm	Poisoning, Assault	Poisoning, Undetermined	Adverse Effect	Underdosing
Tetramethylthiuram (disulfide) NEC	T60.3X1	T60.3X2	T60.3X3	T60.3X4	—	—
medicinal	T49.0X1	T49.0X2	T49.0X3	T49.0X4	T49.0X5	T49.0X6
Tetramisole	T37.4X1	T37.4X2	T37.4X3	T37.4X4	T37.4X5	T37.4X6
Tetranicotinoyl fructose	T46.7X1	T46.7X2	T46.7X3	T46.7X4	T46.7X5	T46.7X6
Tetronal	T42.6X1	T42.6X2	T42.6X3	T42.6X4	T42.6X5	T42.6X6
Tetrazepam	T42.4X1	T42.4X2	T42.4X3	T42.4X4	T42.4X5	T42.4X6
Tetryl	T65.3X1	T65.3X2	T65.3X3	T65.3X4	—	—
Tetrylammonium chloride	T44.2X1	T44.2X2	T44.2X3	T44.2X4	T44.2X5	T44.2X6
Tetryzoline	T49.5X1	T49.5X2	T49.5X3	T49.5X4	T49.5X5	T49.5X6
Thalidomide	T45.1X1	T45.1X2	T45.1X3	T45.1X4	T45.1X5	T45.1X6
Thallium (compounds) (dust) NEC	T56.811	T56.812	T56.813	T56.814	—	—
pesticide	T60.4X1	T60.4X2	T60.4X3	T60.4X4	—	—
THC	T40.711	T40.712	T40.713	T40.714	T40.715	T40.716
Thebacon	T48.3X1	T48.3X2	T48.3X3	T48.3X4	T48.3X5	T48.3X6
Thebaine	T40.2X1	T40.2X2	T40.2X3	T40.2X4	T40.2X5	T40.2X6
Thenoic acid	T49.6X1	T49.6X2	T49.6X3	T49.6X4	T49.6X5	T49.6X6
Thenyldiamine	T45.0X1	T45.0X2	T45.0X3	T45.0X4	T45.0X5	T45.0X6
Theobromine (calcium salicylate)	T48.6X1	T48.6X2	T48.6X3	T48.6X4	T48.6X5	T48.6X6
sodium salicylate	T48.6X1	T48.6X2	T48.6X3	T48.6X4	T48.6X5	T48.6X6
Theophyllamine	T48.6X1	T48.6X2	T48.6X3	T48.6X4	T48.6X5	T48.6X6
Theophylline	T48.6X1	T48.6X2	T48.6X3	T48.6X4	T48.6X5	T48.6X6
aminobenzoic acid	T48.6X1	T48.6X2	T48.6X3	T48.6X4	T48.6X5	T48.6X6
ethylenediamine	T48.6X1	T48.6X2	T48.6X3	T48.6X4	T48.6X5	T48.6X6
piperazine p-amino-benzoate	T48.6X1	T48.6X2	T48.6X3	T48.6X4	T48.6X5	T48.6X6
Thiabendazole	T37.4X1	T37.4X2	T37.4X3	T37.4X4	T37.4X5	T37.4X6
Thialbarbital	T41.1X1	T41.1X2	T41.1X3	T41.1X4	T41.1X5	T41.1X6
Thiamazole	T38.2X1	T38.2X2	T38.2X3	T38.2X4	T38.2X5	T38.2X6
Thiambutosine	T37.1X1	T37.1X2	T37.1X3	T37.1X4	T37.1X5	T37.1X6
Thiamine	T45.2X1	T45.2X2	T45.2X3	T45.2X4	T45.2X5	T45.2X6
Thiamphenicol	T36.2X1	T36.2X2	T36.2X3	T36.2X4	T36.2X5	T36.2X6
Thiamylal	T41.1X1	T41.1X2	T41.1X3	T41.1X4	T41.1X5	T41.1X6
sodium	T41.1X1	T41.1X2	T41.1X3	T41.1X4	T41.1X5	T41.1X6
Thiazesim	T43.291	T43.292	T43.293	T43.294	T43.295	T43.296
Thiazides (diuretics)	T50.2X1	T50.2X2	T50.2X3	T50.2X4	T50.2X5	T50.2X6
Thiazinamium metilsulfate	T43.3X1	T43.3X2	T43.3X3	T43.3X4	T43.3X5	T43.3X6
Thiethylperazine	T43.3X1	T43.3X2	T43.3X3	T43.3X4	T43.3X5	T43.3X6
Thimerosal	T49.0X1	T49.0X2	T49.0X3	T49.0X4	T49.0X5	T49.0X6
ophthalmic preparation	T49.5X1	T49.5X2	T49.5X3	T49.5X4	T49.5X5	T49.5X6
Thioacetazone	T37.1X1	T37.1X2	T37.1X3	T37.1X4	T37.1X5	T37.1X6
with isoniazid	T37.1X1	T37.1X2	T37.1X3	T37.1X4	T37.1X5	T37.1X6
Thiobarbital sodium	T41.1X1	T41.1X2	T41.1X3	T41.1X4	T41.1X5	T41.1X6

◀ New　　◀▶ Revised　　~~deleted~~ Deleted

Substance	Poisoning, Accidental (Unintentional)	Poisoning, Intentional Self-Harm	Poisoning, Assault	Poisoning, Undetermined	Adverse Effect	Underdosing
Thiobarbiturate anesthetic	T41.1X1	T41.1X2	T41.1X3	T41.1X4	T41.1X5	T41.1X6
Thiobismol	T37.8X1	T37.8X2	T37.8X3	T37.8X4	T37.8X5	T37.8X6
Thiobutabarbital sodium	T41.1X1	T41.1X2	T41.1X3	T41.1X4	T41.1X5	T41.1X6
Thiocarbamate (insecticide)	T60.0X1	T60.0X2	T60.0X3	T60.0X4	—	—
Thiocarbamide	T38.2X1	T38.2X2	T38.2X3	T38.2X4	T38.2X5	T38.2X6
Thiocarbarsone	T37.8X1	T37.8X2	T37.8X3	T37.8X4	T37.8X5	T37.8X6
Thiocarlide	T37.1X1	T37.1X2	T37.1X3	T37.1X4	T37.1X5	T37.1X6
Thioctamide	T50.991	T50.992	T50.993	T50.994	T50.995	T50.996
Thioctic acid	T50.991	T50.992	T50.993	T50.994	T50.995	T50.996
Thiofos	T60.0X1	T60.0X2	T60.0X3	T60.0X4	—	—
Thioglycolate	T49.4X1	T49.4X2	T49.4X3	T49.4X4	T49.4X5	T49.4X6
Thioglycolic acid	T65.891	T65.892	T65.893	T65.894	—	—
Thioguanine	T45.1X1	T45.1X2	T45.1X3	T45.1X4	T45.1X5	T45.1X6
Thiomercaptomerin	T50.2X1	T50.2X2	T50.2X3	T50.2X4	T50.2X5	T50.2X6
Thiomerin	T50.2X1	T50.2X2	T50.2X3	T50.2X4	T50.2X5	T50.2X6
Thiomersal	T49.0X1	T49.0X2	T49.0X3	T49.0X4	T49.0X5	T49.0X6
Thionazin	T60.0X1	T60.0X2	T60.0X3	T60.0X4	—	—
Thiopental (sodium)	T41.1X1	T41.1X2	T41.1X3	T41.1X4	T41.1X5	T41.1X6
Thiopentone (sodium)	T41.1X1	T41.1X2	T41.1X3	T41.1X4	T41.1X5	T41.1X6
Thiopropazate	T43.3X1	T43.3X2	T43.3X3	T43.3X4	T43.3X5	T43.3X6
Thioproperazine	T43.3X1	T43.3X2	T43.3X3	T43.3X4	T43.3X5	T43.3X6
Thioridazine	T43.3X1	T43.3X2	T43.3X3	T43.3X4	T43.3X5	T43.3X6
Thiosinamine	T49.3X1	T49.3X2	T49.3X3	T49.3X4	T49.3X5	T49.3X6
Thiotepa	T45.1X1	T45.1X2	T45.1X3	T45.1X4	T45.1X5	T45.1X6
Thiothixene	T43.4X1	T43.4X2	T43.4X3	T43.4X4	T43.4X5	T43.4X6
Thiouracil (benzyl) (methyl) (propyl)	T38.2X1	T38.2X2	T38.2X3	T38.2X4	T38.2X5	T38.2X6
Thiourea	T38.2X1	T38.2X2	T38.2X3	T38.2X4	T38.2X5	T38.2X6
Thiphenamil	T44.3X1	T44.3X2	T44.3X3	T44.3X4	T44.3X5	T44.3X6
Thiram	T60.3X1	T60.3X2	T60.3X3	T60.3X4	—	—
medicinal	T49.2X1	T49.2X2	T49.2X3	T49.2X4	T49.2X5	T49.2X6
Thonzylamine (systemic)	T45.0X1	T45.0X2	T45.0X3	T45.0X4	T45.0X5	T45.0X6
mucosal decongestant	T48.5X1	T48.5X2	T48.5X3	T48.5X4	T48.5X5	T48.5X6
Thorazine	T43.3X1	T43.3X2	T43.3X3	T43.3X4	T43.3X5	T43.3X6
Thorium dioxide suspension	T50.8X1	T50.8X2	T50.8X3	T50.8X4	T50.8X5	T50.8X6
Thornapple	T62.2X1	T62.2X2	T62.2X3	T62.2X4	—	—
Throat drug NEC	T49.6X1	T49.6X2	T49.6X3	T49.6X4	T49.6X5	T49.6X6
Thrombin	T45.7X1	T45.7X2	T45.7X3	T45.7X4	T45.7X5	T45.7X6
Thrombolysin	T45.611	T45.612	T45.613	T45.614	T45.615	T45.616
Thromboplastin	T45.7X1	T45.7X2	T45.7X3	T45.7X4	T45.7X5	T45.7X6
Thurfyl nicotinate	T46.7X1	T46.7X2	T46.7X3	T46.7X4	T46.7X5	T46.7X6
Thymol	T49.0X1	T49.0X2	T49.0X3	T49.0X4	T49.0X5	T49.0X6

Substance	Poisoning, Accidental (Unintentional)	Poisoning, Intentional Self-Harm	Poisoning, Assault	Poisoning, Undetermined	Adverse Effect	Underdosing
Thymopentin	T37.5X1	T37.5X2	T37.5X3	T37.5X4	T37.5X5	T37.5X6
Thymoxamine	T46.7X1	T46.7X2	T46.7X3	T46.7X4	T46.7X5	T46.7X6
Thymus extract	T38.891	T38.892	T38.893	T38.894	T38.895	T38.896
Thyreotrophic hormone	T38.811	T38.812	T38.813	T38.814	T38.815	T38.816
Thyroglobulin	T38.1X1	T38.1X2	T38.1X3	T38.1X4	T38.1X5	T38.1X6
Thyroid (hormone)	T38.1X1	T38.1X2	T38.1X3	T38.1X4	T38.1X5	T38.1X6
Thyrolar	T38.1X1	T38.1X2	T38.1X3	T38.1X4	T38.1X5	T38.1X6
Thyrotrophin	T38.811	T38.812	T38.813	T38.814	T38.815	T38.816
Thyrotropic hormone	T38.811	T38.812	T38.813	T38.814	T38.815	T38.816
Thyroxine	T38.1X1	T38.1X2	T38.1X3	T38.1X4	T38.1X5	T38.1X6
Tiabendazole	T37.4X1	T37.4X2	T37.4X3	T37.4X4	T37.4X5	T37.4X6
Tiamizide	T50.2X1	T50.2X2	T50.2X3	T50.2X4	T50.2X5	T50.2X6
Tianeptine	T43.291	T43.292	T43.293	T43.294	T43.295	T43.296
Tiapamil	T46.1X1	T46.1X2	T46.1X3	T46.1X4	T46.1X5	T46.1X6
Tiapride	T43.591	T43.592	T43.593	T43.594	T43.595	T43.596
Tiaprofenic acid	T39.311	T39.312	T39.313	T39.314	T39.315	T39.316
Tiaramide	T39.8X1	T39.8X2	T39.8X3	T39.8X4	T39.8X5	T39.8X6
Ticarcillin	T36.0X1	T36.0X2	T36.0X3	T36.0X4	T36.0X5	T36.0X6
Ticlatone	T49.0X1	T49.0X2	T49.0X3	T49.0X4	T49.0X5	T49.0X6
Ticlopidine	T45.521	T45.522	T45.523	T45.524	T45.525	T45.526
Ticrynafen	T50.1X1	T50.1X2	T50.1X3	T50.1X4	T50.1X5	T50.1X6
Tidiacic	T50.991	T50.992	T50.993	T50.994	T50.995	T50.996
Tiemonium	T44.3X1	T44.3X2	T44.3X3	T44.3X4	T44.3X5	T44.3X6
iodide	T44.3X1	T44.3X2	T44.3X3	T44.3X4	T44.3X5	T44.3X6
Tienilic acid	T50.1X1	T50.1X2	T50.1X3	T50.1X4	T50.1X5	T50.1X6
Tifenamil	T44.3X1	T44.3X2	T44.3X3	T44.3X4	T44.3X5	T44.3X6
Tigan	T45.0X1	T45.0X2	T45.0X3	T45.0X4	T45.0X5	T45.0X6
Tigloidine	T44.3X1	T44.3X2	T44.3X3	T44.3X4	T44.3X5	T44.3X6
Tilactase	T47.5X1	T47.5X2	T47.5X3	T47.5X4	T47.5X5	T47.5X6
Tiletamine	T41.291	T41.292	T41.293	T41.294	T41.295	T41.296
Tilidine	T40.441	T40.442	T40.443	T40.444	—	—
Timepidium bromide	T44.3X1	T44.3X2	T44.3X3	T44.3X4	T44.3X5	T44.3X6
Timiperone	T43.4X1	T43.4X2	T43.4X3	T43.4X4	T43.4X5	T43.4X6
Timolol	T44.7X1	T44.7X2	T44.7X3	T44.7X4	T44.7X5	T44.7X6
Tin (chloride) (dust) (oxide) NEC	T56.6X1	T56.6X2	T56.6X3	T56.6X4	—	—
anti-infectives	T37.8X1	T37.8X2	T37.8X3	T37.8X4	T37.8X5	T37.8X6
Tincture, iodine — see Iodine						
Tindal	T43.3X1	T43.3X2	T43.3X3	T43.3X4	T43.3X5	T43.3X6
Tinidazole	T37.3X1	T37.3X2	T37.3X3	T37.3X4	T37.3X5	T37.3X6
Tinoridine	T39.8X1	T39.8X2	T39.8X3	T39.8X4	T39.8X5	T39.8X6
Tiocarlide	T37.1X1	T37.1X2	T37.1X3	T37.1X4	T37.1X5	T37.1X6
Tioclomarol	T45.511	T45.512	T45.513	T45.514	T45.515	T45.516

Substance	External Cause (T-Code)					
	Poisoning, Accidental (Unintentional)	Poisoning, Intentional Self-Harm	Poisoning, Assault	Poisoning, Undetermined	Adverse Effect	Underdosing
Tioconazole	T49.0X1	T49.0X2	T49.0X3	T49.0X4	T49.0X5	T49.0X6
Tioguanine	T45.1X1	T45.1X2	T45.1X3	T45.1X4	T45.1X5	T45.1X6
Tiopronin	T50.991	T50.992	T50.993	T50.994	T50.995	T50.996
Tiotixene	T43.4X1	T43.4X2	T43.4X3	T43.4X4	T43.4X5	T43.4X6
Tioxolone	T49.4X1	T49.4X2	T49.4X3	T49.4X4	T49.4X5	T49.4X6
Tipepidine	T48.3X1	T48.3X2	T48.3X3	T48.3X4	T48.3X5	T48.3X6
Tiquizium bromide	T44.3X1	T44.3X2	T44.3X3	T44.3X4	T44.3X5	T44.3X6
Tiratricol	T38.1X1	T38.1X2	T38.1X3	T38.1X4	T38.1X5	T38.1X6
Tisopurine	T50.4X1	T50.4X2	T50.4X3	T50.4X4	T50.4X5	T50.4X6
Titanium (compounds) (vapor)	T56.891	T56.892	T56.893	T56.894	—	—
dioxide	T49.3X1	T49.3X2	T49.3X3	T49.3X4	T49.3X5	T49.3X6
ointment	T49.3X1	T49.3X2	T49.3X3	T49.3X4	T49.3X5	T49.3X6
oxide	T49.3X1	T49.3X2	T49.3X3	T49.3X4	T49.3X5	T49.3X6
tetrachloride	T56.891	T56.892	T56.893	T56.894	—	—
Titanocene	T56.891	T56.892	T56.893	T56.894	—	—
Titroid	T38.1X1	T38.1X2	T38.1X3	T38.1X4	T38.1X5	T38.1X6
Tizanidine	T42.8X1	T42.8X2	T42.8X3	T42.8X4	T42.8X5	T42.8X6
TMTD	T60.3X1	T60.3X2	T60.3X3	T60.3X4	—	—
TNT (fumes)	T65.3X1	T65.3X2	T65.3X3	T65.3X4	—	—
Toadstool	T62.0X1	T62.0X2	T62.0X3	T62.0X4	—	—
Tobacco NEC	T65.291	T65.292	T65.293	T65.294	—	—
cigarettes	T65.221	T65.222	T65.223	T65.224	—	—
Indian	T62.2X1	T62.2X2	T62.2X3	T62.2X4	—	—
smoke, second-hand	T65.221	T65.222	T65.223	T65.224	—	—
Tobramycin	T36.5X1	T36.5X2	T36.5X3	T36.5X4	T36.5X5	T36.5X6
Tocainide	T46.2X1	T46.2X2	T46.2X3	T46.2X4	T46.2X5	T46.2X6
Tocoferol	T45.2X1	T45.2X2	T45.2X3	T45.2X4	T45.2X5	T45.2X6
Tocopherol	T45.2X1	T45.2X2	T45.2X3	T45.2X4	T45.2X5	T45.2X6
acetate	T45.2X1	T45.2X2	T45.2X3	T45.2X4	T45.2X5	T45.2X6
Tocosamine	T48.0X1	T48.0X2	T48.0X3	T48.0X4	T48.0X5	T48.0X6
Todralazine	T46.5X1	T46.5X2	T46.5X3	T46.5X4	T46.5X5	T46.5X6
Tofisopam	T42.4X1	T42.4X2	T42.4X3	T42.4X4	T42.4X5	T42.4X6
Tofranil	T43.011	T43.012	T43.013	T43.014	T43.015	T43.016
Toilet deodorizer	T65.891	T65.892	T65.893	T65.894	—	—
Tolamolol	T44.7X1	T44.7X2	T44.7X3	T44.7X4	T44.7X5	T44.7X6
Tolazamide	T38.3X1	T38.3X2	T38.3X3	T38.3X4	T38.3X5	T38.3X6
Tolazoline	T46.7X1	T46.7X2	T46.7X3	T46.7X4	T46.7X5	T46.7X6
Tolbutamide (sodium)	T38.3X1	T38.3X2	T38.3X3	T38.3X4	T38.3X5	T38.3X6
Tolciclate	T49.0X1	T49.0X2	T49.0X3	T49.0X4	T49.0X5	T49.0X6
Tolmetin	T39.391	T39.392	T39.393	T39.394	T39.395	T39.396
Tolnaftate	T49.0X1	T49.0X2	T49.0X3	T49.0X4	T49.0X5	T49.0X6
Tolonidine	T46.5X1	T46.5X2	T46.5X3	T46.5X4	T46.5X5	T46.5X6

Substance	External Cause (T-Code)					
	Poisoning, Accidental (Unintentional)	Poisoning, Intentional Self-Harm	Poisoning, Assault	Poisoning, Undetermined	Adverse Effect	Underdosing
Toloxatone	T42.6X1	T42.6X2	T42.6X3	T42.6X4	T42.6X5	T42.6X6
Tolperisone	T44.3X1	T44.3X2	T44.3X3	T44.3X4	T44.3X5	T44.3X6
Tolserol	T42.8X1	T42.8X2	T42.8X3	T42.8X4	T42.8X5	T42.8X6
Toluene (liquid)	T52.2X1	T52.2X2	T52.2X3	T52.2X4	—	—
diisocyanate	T65.0X1	T65.0X2	T65.0X3	T65.0X4	—	—
Toluidine	T65.891	T65.892	T65.893	T65.894	—	—
vapor	T59.891	T59.892	T59.893	T59.894	—	—
Toluol (liquid)	T52.2X1	T52.2X2	T52.2X3	T52.2X4	—	—
vapor	T52.2X1	T52.2X2	T52.2X3	T52.2X4	—	—
Toluylenediamine	T65.3X1	T65.3X2	T65.3X3	T65.3X4	—	—
Tolylene-2,4-diisocyanate	T65.0X1	T65.0X2	T65.0X3	T65.0X4	—	—
Tonic NEC	T50.901	T50.902	T50.903	T50.904	T50.905	T50.906
Topical action drug NEC	T49.91	T49.92	T49.93	T49.94	T49.95	T49.96
ear, nose or throat	T49.6X1	T49.6X2	T49.6X3	T49.6X4	T49.6X5	T49.6X6
eye	T49.5X1	T49.5X2	T49.5X3	T49.5X4	T49.5X5	T49.5X6
skin	T49.91	T49.92	T49.93	T49.94	T49.95	T49.96
specified NEC	T49.8X1	T49.8X2	T49.8X3	T49.8X4	T49.8X5	T49.8X6
Toquizine	T44.3X1	T44.3X2	T44.3X3	T44.3X4	T44.3X5	T44.3X6
Toremifene	T38.6X1	T38.6X2	T38.6X3	T38.6X4	T38.6X5	T38.6X6
Tosylchloramide sodium	T49.8X1	T49.8X2	T49.8X3	T49.8X4	T49.8X5	T49.8X6
Toxaphene (dust) (spray)	T60.1X1	T60.1X2	T60.1X3	T60.1X4	—	—
Toxin, diphtheria (Schick Test)	T50.8X1	T50.8X2	T50.8X3	T50.8X4	T50.8X5	T50.8X6
Toxoid						
combined	T50.A21	T50.A22	T50.A23	T50.A24	T50.A25	T50.A26
diphtheria	T50.A91	T50.A92	T50.A93	T50.A94	T50.A95	T50.A96
tetanus	T50.A91	T50.A92	T50.A93	T50.A94	T50.A95	T50.A96
Trace element NEC	T45.8X1	T45.8X2	T45.8X3	T45.8X4	T45.8X5	T45.8X6
Tractor fuel NEC	T52.0X1	T52.0X2	T52.0X3	T52.0X4	—	—
Tragacanth	T50.991	T50.992	T50.993	T50.994	T50.995	T50.996
Tramadol	T40.421	T40.422	T40.423	T40.424	T40.425	T40.426
Tramazoline	T48.5X1	T48.5X2	T48.5X3	T48.5X4	T48.5X5	T48.5X6
Tranexamic acid	T45.621	T45.622	T45.623	T45.624	T45.625	T45.626
Tranilast	T45.0X1	T45.0X2	T45.0X3	T45.0X4	T45.0X5	T45.0X6
Tranquilizer NEC	T43.501	T43.502	T43.503	T43.504	T43.505	T43.506
with hypnotic or sedative	T42.6X1	T42.6X2	T42.6X3	T42.6X4	T42.6X5	T42.6X6
benzodiazepine NEC	T42.4X1	T42.4X2	T42.4X3	T42.4X4	T42.4X5	T42.4X6
butyrophenone NEC	T43.4X1	T43.4X2	T43.4X3	T43.4X4	T43.4X5	T43.4X6
carbamate	T43.591	T43.592	T43.593	T43.594	T43.595	T43.596
dimethylamine	T43.3X1	T43.3X2	T43.3X3	T43.3X4	T43.3X5	T43.3X6
ethylamine	T43.3X1	T43.3X2	T43.3X3	T43.3X4	T43.3X5	T43.3X6
hydroxyzine	T43.591	T43.592	T43.593	T43.594	T43.595	T43.596
major NEC	T43.501	T43.502	T43.503	T43.504	T43.505	T43.506

New ◀ Revised ◀ ~~deleted~~ Deleted

Substance	Poisoning, Accidental (Unintentional)	Poisoning, Intentional Self-Harm	Poisoning, Assault	Poisoning, Undetermined	Adverse Effect	Underdosing
Tranquilizer NEC *(Continued)*						
penothiazine NEC	T43.3X1	T43.3X2	T43.3X3	T43.3X4	T43.3X5	T43.3X6
phenothiazine-based	T43.3X1	T43.3X2	T43.3X3	T43.3X4	T43.3X5	T43.3X6
piperazine NEC	T43.3X1	T43.3X2	T43.3X3	T43.3X4	T43.3X5	T43.3X6
piperidine	T43.3X1	T43.3X2	T43.3X3	T43.3X4	T43.3X5	T43.3X6
propylamine	T43.3X1	T43.3X2	T43.3X3	T43.3X4	T43.3X5	T43.3X6
specified NEC	T43.591	T43.592	T43.593	T43.594	T43.595	T43.596
thioxanthene NEC	T43.591	T43.592	T43.593	T43.594	T43.595	T43.596
Tranxene	T42.4X1	T42.4X2	T42.4X3	T42.4X4	T42.4X5	T42.4X6
Tranylcypromine	T43.1X1	T43.1X2	T43.1X3	T43.1X4	T43.1X5	T43.1X6
Trapidil	T46.3X1	T46.3X2	T46.3X3	T46.3X4	T46.3X5	T46.3X6
Trasentine	T44.3X1	T44.3X2	T44.3X3	T44.3X4	T44.3X5	T44.3X6
Travert	T50.3X1	T50.3X2	T50.3X3	T50.3X4	T50.3X5	T50.3X6
Trazodone	T43.211	T43.212	T43.213	T43.214	T43.215	T43.216
Trecator	T37.1X1	T37.1X2	T37.1X3	T37.1X4	T37.1X5	T37.1X6
Treosulfan	T45.1X1	T45.1X2	T45.1X3	T45.1X4	T45.1X5	T45.1X6
Tretamine	T45.1X1	T45.1X2	T45.1X3	T45.1X4	T45.1X5	T45.1X6
Tretinoin	T49.0X1	T49.0X2	T49.0X3	T49.0X4	T49.0X5	T49.0X6
Tretoquinol	T48.6X1	T48.6X2	T48.6X3	T48.6X4	T48.6X5	T48.6X6
Triacetin	T49.0X1	T49.0X2	T49.0X3	T49.0X4	T49.0X5	T49.0X6
Triacetoxyanthracene	T49.4X1	T49.4X2	T49.4X3	T49.4X4	T49.4X5	T49.4X6
Triacetyloleandomycin	T36.3X1	T36.3X2	T36.3X3	T36.3X4	T36.3X5	T36.3X6
Triamcinolone	T38.0X1	T38.0X2	T38.0X3	T38.0X4	T38.0X5	T38.0X6
ENT agent	T49.6X1	T49.6X2	T49.6X3	T49.6X4	T49.6X5	T49.6X6
hexacetonide	T49.0X1	T49.0X2	T49.0X3	T49.0X4	T49.0X5	T49.0X6
ophthalmic preparation	T49.5X1	T49.5X2	T49.5X3	T49.5X4	T49.5X5	T49.5X6
topical NEC	T49.0X1	T49.0X2	T49.0X3	T49.0X4	T49.0X5	T49.0X6
Triampyzine	T44.3X1	T44.3X2	T44.3X3	T44.3X4	T44.3X5	T44.3X6
Triamterene	T50.2X1	T50.2X2	T50.2X3	T50.2X4	T50.2X5	T50.2X6
Triazine (herbicide)	T60.3X1	T60.3X2	T60.3X3	T60.3X4	—	—
Triaziquone	T45.1X1	T45.1X2	T45.1X3	T45.1X4	T45.1X5	T45.1X6
Triazolam	T42.4X1	T42.4X2	T42.4X3	T42.4X4	T42.4X5	T42.4X6
Triazole (herbicide)	T60.3X1	T60.3X2	T60.3X3	T60.3X4	—	—
Tribenoside	T46.991	T46.992	T46.993	T46.994	T46.995	T46.996
Tribromacetaldehyde	T42.6X1	T42.6X2	T42.6X3	T42.6X4	T42.6X5	T42.6X6
Tribromoethanol, rectal	T41.291	T41.292	T41.293	T41.294	T41.295	T41.296
Tribromomethane	T42.6X1	T42.6X2	T42.6X3	T42.6X4	T42.6X5	T42.6X6
Trichlorethane	T53.2X1	T53.2X2	T53.2X3	T53.2X4	—	—
Trichlorethylene	T53.2X1	T53.2X2	T53.2X3	T53.2X4	—	—
Trichlorfon	T60.0X1	T60.0X2	T60.0X3	T60.0X4	—	—
Trichlormethiazide	T50.2X1	T50.2X2	T50.2X3	T50.2X4	T50.2X5	T50.2X6
Trichlormethine	T45.1X1	T45.1X2	T45.1X3	T45.1X4	T45.1X5	T45.1X6

Substance	Poisoning, Accidental (Unintentional)	Poisoning, Intentional Self-Harm	Poisoning, Assault	Poisoning, Undetermined	Adverse Effect	Underdosing
Trichloroacetic acid, Trichloracetic acid	T54.2X1	T54.2X2	T54.2X3	T54.2X4	—	—
medicinal	T49.4X1	T49.4X2	T49.4X3	T49.4X4	T49.4X5	T49.4X6
Trichloroethane	T53.2X1	T53.2X2	T53.2X3	T53.2X4	—	—
Trichloroethanol	T42.6X1	T42.6X2	T42.6X3	T42.6X4	T42.6X5	T42.6X6
Trichloroethylene (liquid) (vapor)	T53.2X1	T53.2X2	T53.2X3	T53.2X4	—	—
anesthetic (gas)	T41.0X1	T41.0X2	T41.0X3	T41.0X4	T41.0X5	T41.0X6
vapor NEC	T53.2X1	T53.2X2	T53.2X3	T53.2X4	—	—
Trichloroethyl phosphate	T42.6X1	T42.6X2	T42.6X3	T42.6X4	T42.6X5	T42.6X6
Trichlorofluoromethane NEC	T53.5X1	T53.5X2	T53.5X3	T53.5X4	—	—
Trichloronate	T60.0X1	T60.0X2	T60.0X3	T60.0X4	—	—
2,4,5-Trichlorophen-oxyacetic acid	T60.3X1	T60.3X2	T60.3X3	T60.3X4	—	—
Trichloropropane	T53.6X1	T53.6X2	T53.6X3	T53.6X4	—	—
Trichlorotriethylamine	T45.1X1	T45.1X2	T45.1X3	T45.1X4	T45.1X5	T45.1X6
Trichomonacides NEC	T37.3X1	T37.3X2	T37.3X3	T37.3X4	T37.3X5	T37.3X6
Trichomycin	T36.7X1	T36.7X2	T36.7X3	T36.7X4	T36.7X5	T36.7X6
Triclobisonium chloride	T49.0X1	T49.0X2	T49.0X3	T49.0X4	T49.0X5	T49.0X6
Triclocarban	T49.0X1	T49.0X2	T49.0X3	T49.0X4	T49.0X5	T49.0X6
Triclofos	T42.6X1	T42.6X2	T42.6X3	T42.6X4	T42.6X5	T42.6X6
Triclosan	T49.0X1	T49.0X2	T49.0X3	T49.0X4	T49.0X5	T49.0X6
Tricresyl phosphate	T65.891	T65.892	T65.893	T65.894	—	—
solvent	T52.91	T52.92	T52.93	T52.94	—	—
Tricyclamol chloride	T44.3X1	T44.3X2	T44.3X3	T44.3X4	T44.3X5	T44.3X6
Tridesilon	T49.0X1	T49.0X2	T49.0X3	T49.0X4	T49.0X5	T49.0X6
Tridihexethyl iodide	T44.3X1	T44.3X2	T44.3X3	T44.3X4	T44.3X5	T44.3X6
Tridione	T42.2X1	T42.2X2	T42.2X3	T42.2X4	T42.2X5	T42.2X6
Trientine	T45.8X1	T45.8X2	T45.8X3	T45.8X4	T45.8X5	T45.8X6
Triethanolamine NEC	T54.3X1	T54.3X2	T54.3X3	T54.3X4	—	—
detergent	T54.3X1	T54.3X2	T54.3X3	T54.3X4	—	—
trinitrate (biphosphate)	T46.3X1	T46.3X2	T46.3X3	T46.3X4	T46.3X5	T46.3X6
Triethanomelamine	T45.1X1	T45.1X2	T45.1X3	T45.1X4	T45.1X5	T45.1X6
Triethylenemelamine	T45.1X1	T45.1X2	T45.1X3	T45.1X4	T45.1X5	T45.1X6
Triethylenephosphoramide	T45.1X1	T45.1X2	T45.1X3	T45.1X4	T45.1X5	T45.1X6
Triethylenethiophosphoramide	T45.1X1	T45.1X2	T45.1X3	T45.1X4	T45.1X5	T45.1X6
Trifluoperazine	T43.3X1	T43.3X2	T43.3X3	T43.3X4	T43.3X5	T43.3X6
Trifluoroethyl vinyl ether	T41.0X1	T41.0X2	T41.0X3	T41.0X4	T41.0X5	T41.0X6
Trifluperidol	T43.4X1	T43.4X2	T43.4X3	T43.4X4	T43.4X5	T43.4X6
Triflupromazine	T43.3X1	T43.3X2	T43.3X3	T43.3X4	T43.3X5	T43.3X6
Trifluridine	T37.5X1	T37.5X2	T37.5X3	T37.5X4	T37.5X5	T37.5X6
Triflusal	T45.521	T45.522	T45.523	T45.524	T45.525	T45.526
Trihexyphenidyl	T44.3X1	T44.3X2	T44.3X3	T44.3X4	T44.3X5	T44.3X6
Triiodothyronine	T38.1X1	T38.1X2	T38.1X3	T38.1X4	T38.1X5	T38.1X6

◄ New ◄ Revised ~~deleted~~ Deleted

TABLE OF DRUGS AND CHEMICALS

Substance	External Cause (T-Code)					
	Poisoning, Accidental (Unintentional)	Poisoning, Intentional Self-Harm	Poisoning, Assault	Poisoning, Undetermined	Adverse Effect	Underdosing
Trilene	T41.0X1	T41.0X2	T41.0X3	T41.0X4	T41.0X5	T41.0X6
Trilostane	T38.991	T38.992	T38.993	T38.994	T38.995	T38.996
Trimebutine	T44.3X1	T44.3X2	T44.3X3	T44.3X4	T44.3X5	T44.3X6
Trimecaine	T41.3X1	T41.3X2	T41.3X3	T41.3X4	T41.3X5	T41.3X6
Trimeprazine (tartrate)	T44.3X1	T44.3X2	T44.3X3	T44.3X4	T44.3X5	T44.3X6
Trimetaphan camsilate	T44.2X1	T44.2X2	T44.2X3	T44.2X4	T44.2X5	T44.2X6
Trimetazidine	T46.7X1	T46.7X2	T46.7X3	T46.7X4	T46.7X5	T46.7X6
Trimethadione	T42.2X1	T42.2X2	T42.2X3	T42.2X4	T42.2X5	T42.2X6
Trimethaphan	T44.2X1	T44.2X2	T44.2X3	T44.2X4	T44.2X5	T44.2X6
Trimethidinium	T44.2X1	T44.2X2	T44.2X3	T44.2X4	T44.2X5	T44.2X6
Trimethobenzamide	T45.0X1	T45.0X2	T45.0X3	T45.0X4	T45.0X5	T45.0X6
Trimethoprim	T37.8X1	T37.8X2	T37.8X3	T37.8X4	T37.8X5	T37.8X6
with sulfamethoxazole	T36.8X1	T36.8X2	T36.8X3	T36.8X4	T36.8X5	T36.8X6
Trimethylcarbinol	T51.3X1	T51.3X2	T51.3X3	T51.3X4	—	—
Trimethylpsoralen	T49.3X1	T49.3X2	T49.3X3	T49.3X4	T49.3X5	T49.3X6
Trimeton	T45.0X1	T45.0X2	T45.0X3	T45.0X4	T45.0X5	T45.0X6
Trimetrexate	T45.1X1	T45.1X2	T45.1X3	T45.1X4	T45.1X5	T45.1X6
Trimipramine	T43.011	T43.012	T43.013	T43.014	T43.015	T43.016
Trimustine	T45.1X1	T45.1X2	T45.1X3	T45.1X4	T45.1X5	T45.1X6
Trinitrine	T46.3X1	T46.3X2	T46.3X3	T46.3X4	T46.3X5	T46.3X6
Trinitrobenzol	T65.3X1	T65.3X2	T65.3X3	T65.3X4	—	—
Trinitrophenol	T65.3X1	T65.3X2	T65.3X3	T65.3X4	—	—
Trinitrotoluene (fumes)	T65.3X1	T65.3X2	T65.3X3	T65.3X4	—	—
Trional	T42.6X1	T42.6X2	T42.6X3	T42.6X4	T42.6X5	T42.6X6
Triorthocresyl phosphate	T65.891	T65.892	T65.893	T65.894	—	—
Trioxide of arsenic	T57.0X1	T57.0X2	T57.0X3	T57.0X4	—	—
Trioxysalen	T49.4X1	T49.4X2	T49.4X3	T49.4X4	T49.4X5	T49.4X6
Tripamide	T50.2X1	T50.2X2	T50.2X3	T50.2X4	T50.2X5	T50.2X6
Triparanol	T46.6X1	T46.6X2	T46.6X3	T46.6X4	T46.6X5	T46.6X6
Tripelennamine	T45.0X1	T45.0X2	T45.0X3	T45.0X4	T45.0X5	T45.0X6
Triperiden	T44.3X1	T44.3X2	T44.3X3	T44.3X4	T44.3X5	T44.3X6
Triperidol	T43.4X1	T43.4X2	T43.4X3	T43.4X4	T43.4X5	T43.4X6
Triphenylphosphate	T65.891	T65.892	T65.893	T65.894	—	—
Triple						
bromides	T42.6X1	T42.6X2	T42.6X3	T42.6X4	T42.6X5	T42.6X6
carbonate	T47.1X1	T47.1X2	T47.1X3	T47.1X4	T47.1X5	T47.1X6
vaccine						
DPT	T50.A11	T50.A12	T50.A13	T50.A14	T50.A15	T50.A16
including pertussis	T50.A11	T50.A12	T50.A13	T50.A14	T50.A15	T50.A16
MMR		T50.B91	T50.B92	—	—	—
Triprolidine	T45.0X1	T45.0X2	T45.0X3	T45.0X4	T45.0X5	T45.0X6
Trisodium hydrogen edetate	T50.6X1	T50.6X2	T50.6X3	T50.6X4	T50.6X5	T50.6X6

Substance	External Cause (T-Code)					
	Poisoning, Accidental (Unintentional)	Poisoning, Intentional Self-Harm	Poisoning, Assault	Poisoning, Undetermined	Adverse Effect	Underdosing
Trisoralen	T49.3X1	T49.3X2	T49.3X3	T49.3X4	T49.3X5	T49.3X6
Trisulfapyrimidines	T37.0X1	T37.0X2	T37.0X3	T37.0X4	T37.0X5	T37.0X6
Trithiozine	T44.3X1	T44.3X2	T44.3X3	T44.3X4	T44.3X5	T44.3X6
Tritiozine	T44.3X1	T44.3X2	T44.3X3	T44.3X4	T44.3X5	T44.3X6
Tritoqualine	T45.0X1	T45.0X2	T45.0X3	T45.0X4	T45.0X5	T45.0X6
Trofosfamide	T45.1X1	T45.1X2	T45.1X3	T45.1X4	T45.1X5	T45.1X6
Troleandomycin	T36.3X1	T36.3X2	T36.3X3	T36.3X4	T36.3X5	T36.3X6
Trolnitrate (phosphate)	T46.3X1	T46.3X2	T46.3X3	T46.3X4	T46.3X5	T46.3X6
Tromantadine	T37.5X1	T37.5X2	T37.5X3	T37.5X4	T37.5X5	T37.5X6
Trometamol	T50.2X1	T50.2X2	T50.2X3	T50.2X4	T50.2X5	T50.2X6
Tromethamine	T50.2X1	T50.2X2	T50.2X3	T50.2X4	T50.2X5	T50.2X6
Tronothane	T41.3X1	T41.3X2	T41.3X3	T41.3X4	T41.3X5	T41.3X6
Tropacine	T44.3X1	T44.3X2	T44.3X3	T44.3X4	T44.3X5	T44.3X6
Tropatepine	T44.3X1	T44.3X2	T44.3X3	T44.3X4	T44.3X5	T44.3X6
Tropicamide	T44.3X1	T44.3X2	T44.3X3	T44.3X4	T44.3X5	T44.3X6
Trospium chloride	T44.3X1	T44.3X2	T44.3X3	T44.3X4	T44.3X5	T44.3X6
Troxerutin	T46.991	T46.992	T46.993	T46.994	T46.995	T46.996
Troxidone	T42.2X1	T42.2X2	T42.2X3	T42.2X4	T42.2X5	T42.2X6
Tryparsamide	T37.3X1	T37.3X2	T37.3X3	T37.3X4	T37.3X5	T37.3X6
Trypsin	T45.3X1	T45.3X2	T45.3X3	T45.3X4	T45.3X5	T45.3X6
Tryptizol	T43.011	T43.012	T43.013	T43.014	T43.015	T43.016
TSH	T38.811	T38.812	T38.813	T38.814	T38.815	T38.816
Tuaminoheptane	T48.5X1	T48.5X2	T48.5X3	T48.5X4	T48.5X5	T48.5X6
Tuberculin, purified protein derivative (PPD)	T50.8X1	T50.8X2	T50.8X3	T50.8X4	T50.8X5	T50.8X6
Tubocurare	T48.1X1	T48.1X2	T48.1X3	T48.1X4	T48.1X5	T48.1X6
Tubocurarine (chloride)	T48.1X1	T48.1X2	T48.1X3	T48.1X4	T48.1X5	T48.1X6
Tulobuterol	T48.6X1	T48.6X2	T48.6X3	T48.6X4	T48.6X5	T48.6X6
Turpentine (spirits of)	T52.8X1	T52.8X2	T52.8X3	T52.8X4	—	—
vapor	T52.8X1	T52.8X2	T52.8X3	T52.8X4	—	—
Tybamate	T43.591	T43.592	T43.593	T43.594	T43.595	T43.596
Tyloxapol	T48.4X1	T48.4X2	T48.4X3	T48.4X4	T48.4X5	T48.4X6
Tymazoline	T48.5X1	T48.5X2	T48.5X3	T48.5X4	T48.5X5	T48.5X6
Typhoid-paratyphoid vaccine	T50.A91	T50.A92	T50.A93	T50.A94	T50.A95	T50.A96
Typhus vaccine	T50.A91	T50.A92	T50.A93	T50.A94	T50.A95	T50.A96
Tyropanoate	T50.8X1	T50.8X2	T50.8X3	T50.8X4	T50.8X5	T50.8X6
Tyrothricin	T49.6X1	T49.6X2	T49.6X3	T49.6X4	T49.6X5	T49.6X6
ENT agent	T49.6X1	T49.6X2	T49.6X3	T49.6X4	T49.6X5	T49.6X6
ophthalmic preparation	T49.5X1	T49.5X2	T49.5X3	T49.5X4	T49.5X5	T49.5X6
U						
Ufenamate	T39.391	T39.392	T39.393	T39.394	T39.395	T39.396
Ultraviolet light protectant	T49.3X1	T49.3X2	T49.3X3	T49.3X4	T49.3X5	T49.3X6

◀ New   ◀ Revised   ~~deleted~~ Deleted

Substance	Poisoning, Accidental (Unintentional)	Poisoning, Intentional Self-Harm	Poisoning, Assault	Poisoning, Undetermined	Adverse Effect	Underdosing
Undecenoic acid	T49.0X1	T49.0X2	T49.0X3	T49.0X4	T49.0X5	T49.0X6
Undecoylium	T49.0X1	T49.0X2	T49.0X3	T49.0X4	T49.0X5	T49.0X6
Undecylenic acid (derivatives)	T49.0X1	T49.0X2	T49.0X3	T49.0X4	T49.0X5	T49.0X6
Unna's boot	T49.3X1	T49.3X2	T49.3X3	T49.3X4	T49.3X5	T49.3X6
Unsaturated fatty acid	T46.6X1	T46.6X2	T46.6X3	T46.6X4	T46.6X5	T46.6X6
Uracil mustard	T45.1X1	T45.1X2	T45.1X3	T45.1X4	T45.1X5	T45.1X6
Uramustine	T45.1X1	T45.1X2	T45.1X3	T45.1X4	T45.1X5	T45.1X6
Urapidil	T46.5X1	T46.5X2	T46.5X3	T46.5X4	T46.5X5	T46.5X6
Urari	T48.1X1	T48.1X2	T48.1X3	T48.1X4	T48.1X5	T48.1X6
Urate oxidase	T50.4X1	T50.4X2	T50.4X3	T50.4X4	T50.4X5	T50.4X6
Urea	T47.3X1	T47.3X2	T47.3X3	T47.3X4	T47.3X5	T47.3X6
peroxide	T49.0X1	T49.0X2	T49.0X3	T49.0X4	T49.0X5	T49.0X6
stibamine	T37.4X1	T37.4X2	T37.4X3	T37.4X4	T37.4X5	T37.4X6
topical	T49.8X1	T49.8X2	T49.8X3	T49.8X4	T49.8X5	T49.8X6
Urethane	T45.1X1	T45.1X2	T45.1X3	T45.1X4	T45.1X5	T45.1X6
Urginea (maritima) (scilla) — *see Squill*						
Uric acid metabolism drug NEC	T50.4X1	T50.4X2	T50.4X3	T50.4X4	T50.4X5	T50.4X6
Uricosuric agent	T50.4X1	T50.4X2	T50.4X3	T50.4X4	T50.4X5	T50.4X6
Urinary anti-infective	T37.8X1	T37.8X2	T37.8X3	T37.8X4	T37.8X5	T37.8X6
Urofollitropin	T38.811	T38.812	T38.813	T38.814	T38.815	T38.816
Urokinase	T45.611	T45.612	T45.613	T45.614	T45.615	T45.616
Urokon	T50.8X1	T50.8X2	T50.8X3	T50.8X4	T50.8X5	T50.8X6
Ursodeoxycholic acid	T50.991	T50.992	T50.993	T50.994	T50.995	T50.996
Ursodiol	T50.991	T50.992	T50.993	T50.994	T50.995	T50.996
Urtica	T62.2X1	T62.2X2	T62.2X3	T62.2X4	—	—
Utility gas — *see Gas, utility*						

V

Substance	Poisoning, Accidental (Unintentional)	Poisoning, Intentional Self-Harm	Poisoning, Assault	Poisoning, Undetermined	Adverse Effect	Underdosing
Vaccine NEC	T50.Z91	T50.Z92	T50.Z93	T50.Z94	T50.Z95	T50.Z96
antineoplastic	T50.Z91	T50.Z92	T50.Z93	T50.Z94	T50.Z95	T50.Z96
bacterial NEC	T50.A91	T50.A92	T50.A93	T50.A94	T50.A95	T50.A96
with						
other bacterial component	T50.A91	T50.A92	T50.A93	T50.A94	T50.A95	T50.A96
pertussis component	T50.A91	T50.A92	T50.A93	T50.A94	T50.A95	T50.A96
viral-rickettsial component	T50.A91	T50.A92	T50.A93	T50.A94	T50.A95	T50.A96
mixed NEC	T50.A91	T50.A92	T50.A93	T50.A94	T50.A95	T50.A96
BCG	T50.A91	T50.A92	T50.A93	T50.A94	T50.A95	T50.A96
cholera	T50.A91	T50.A92	T50.A93	T50.A94	T50.A95	T50.A96
diphtheria	T50.A91	T50.A92	T50.A93	T50.A94	T50.A95	T50.A96
with tetanus	T50.A21	T50.A22	T50.A23	T50.A24	T50.A25	T50.A26
and pertussis	T50.A11	T50.A12	T50.A13	T50.A14	T50.A15	T50.A16

Substance	Poisoning, Accidental (Unintentional)	Poisoning, Intentional Self-Harm	Poisoning, Assault	Poisoning, Undetermined	Adverse Effect	Underdosing
Vaccine NEC *(Continued)*						
influenza	T50.B91	T50.B92	T50.B93	T50.B94	T50.B95	T50.B96
measles	T50.B91	T50.B92	T50.B93	T50.B94	T50.B95	T50.B96
with mumps and rubella	T50.B91	T50.B92	T50.B93	T50.B94	T50.B95	T50.B96
meningococcal	T50.A91	T50.A92	T50.A93	T50.A94	T50.A95	T50.A96
mumps	T50.B91	T50.B92	T50.B93	T50.B94	T50.B95	T50.B96
paratyphoid	T50.A91	T50.A92	T50.A93	T50.A94	T50.A95	T50.A96
pertussis	T50.A11	T50.A12	T50.A13	T50.A14	T50.A15	T50.A16
with diphtheria	T50.A11	T50.A12	T50.A13	T50.A14	T50.A15	T50.A16
and tetanus	T50.A11	T50.A12	T50.A13	T50.A14	T50.A15	T50.A16
plague	T50.A91	T50.A92	T50.A93	T50.A94	T50.A95	T50.A96
poliomyelitis	T50.B91	T50.B92	T50.B93	T50.B94	T50.B95	T50.B96
poliovirus	T50.B91	T50.B92	T50.B93	T50.B94	T50.B95	T50.B96
rabies	T50.B91	T50.B92	T50.B93	T50.B94	T50.B95	T50.B96
respiratory syncytial virus	T50.B91	T50.B92	T50.B93	T50.B94	T50.B95	T50.B96
rickettsial NEC	T50.A91	T50.A92	T50.A93	T50.A94	T50.A95	T50.A96
with						
bacterial component	T50.A21	T50.A22	T50.A23	T50.A24	T50.A25	T50.A26
Rocky Mountain spotted fever	T50.A91	T50.A92	T50.A93	T50.A94	T50.A95	T50.A96
rubella	T50.B91	T50.B92	T50.B93	T50.B94	T50.B95	T50.B96
sabin oral	T50.B91	T50.B92	T50.B93	T50.B94	T50.B95	T50.B96
smallpox	T50.B11	T50.B12	T50.B13	T50.B14	T50.B15	T50.B16
TAB	T50.A91	T50.A92	T50.A93	T50.A94	T50.A95	T50.A96
tetanus	T50.A91	T50.A92	T50.A93	T50.A94	T50.A95	T50.A96
typhoid	T50.A91	T50.A92	T50.A93	T50.A94	T50.A95	T50.A96
typhus	T50.A91	T50.A92	T50.A93	T50.A94	T50.A95	T50.A96
viral NEC	T50.B91	T50.B92	T50.B93	T50.B94	T50.B95	T50.B96
yellow fever	T50.B91	T50.B92	T50.B93	T50.B94	T50.B95	T50.B96
Vaccinia immune globulin	T50.Z11	T50.Z12	T50.Z13	T50.Z14	T50.Z15	T50.Z16
Vaginal contraceptives	T49.8X1	T49.8X2	T49.8X3	T49.8X4	T49.8X5	T49.8X6
Valerian						
root	T42.6X1	T42.6X2	T42.6X3	T42.6X4	T42.6X5	T42.6X6
tincture	T42.6X1	T42.6X2	T42.6X3	T42.6X4	T42.6X5	T42.6X6
Valethamate bromide	T44.3X1	T44.3X2	T44.3X3	T44.3X4	T44.3X5	T44.3X6
Valisone	T49.0X1	T49.0X2	T49.0X3	T49.0X4	T49.0X5	T49.0X6
Valium	T42.4X1	T42.4X2	T42.4X3	T42.4X4	T42.4X5	T42.4X6
Valmid	T42.6X1	T42.6X2	T42.6X3	T42.6X4	T42.6X5	T42.6X6
Valnoctamide	T42.6X1	T42.6X2	T42.6X3	T42.6X4	T42.6X5	T42.6X6
Valproate (sodium)	T42.6X1	T42.6X2	T42.6X3	T42.6X4	T42.6X5	T42.6X6
Valproic acid	T42.6X1	T42.6X2	T42.6X3	T42.6X4	T42.6X5	T42.6X6
Valpromide	T42.6X1	T42.6X2	T42.6X3	T42.6X4	T42.6X5	T42.6X6
Vanadium	T56.891	T56.892	T56.893	T56.894	—	—

TABLE OF DRUGS AND CHEMICALS

Substance	Poisoning, Accidental (Unintentional)	Poisoning, Intentional Self-Harm	Poisoning, Assault	Poisoning, Undetermined	Adverse Effect	Underdosing
Vancomycin	T36.8X1	T36.8X2	T36.8X3	T36.8X4	T36.8X5	T36.8X6
Vapor — *see also Gas*	T59.91	T59.92	T59.93	T59.94	—	—
kiln (carbon monoxide)	T58.8X1	T58.8X2	T58.8X3	T58.8X4	—	—
lead — *see Lead*						
specified source NEC	T59.891	T59.892	T59.893	T59.894	—	—
Vardenafil	T46.7X1	T46.7X2	T46.7X3	T46.7X4	T46.7X5	T46.7X6
Varicose reduction drug	T46.8X1	T46.8X2	T46.8X3	T46.8X4	T46.8X5	T46.8X6
Varnish	T65.4X1	T65.4X2	T65.4X3	T65.4X4	—	—
cleaner	T52.91	T52.92	T52.93	T52.94	—	—
Vaseline	T49.3X1	T49.3X2	T49.3X3	T49.3X4	T49.3X5	T49.3X6
Vasodilan	T46.7X1	T46.7X2	T46.7X3	T46.7X4	T46.7X5	T46.7X6
Vasodilator						
coronary NEC	T46.3X1	T46.3X2	T46.3X3	T46.3X4	T46.3X5	T46.3X6
peripheral NEC	T46.7X1	T46.7X2	T46.7X3	T46.7X4	T46.7X5	T46.7X6
Vasopressin	T38.891	T38.892	T38.893	T38.894	T38.895	T38.896
Vasopressor drugs	T38.891	T38.892	T38.893	T38.894	T38.895	T38.896
Vecuronium bromide	T48.1X1	T48.1X2	T48.1X3	T48.1X4	T48.1X5	T48.1X6
Vegetable extract, astringent	T49.2X1	T49.2X2	T49.2X3	T49.2X4	T49.2X5	T49.2X6
Venlafaxine	T43.211	T43.212	T43.213	T43.214	T43.215	T43.216
Venom, venomous (bite) (sting)	T63.91	T63.92	T63.93	T63.94	—	—
amphibian NEC	T63.831	T63.832	T63.833	T63.834	—	—
animal NEC	T63.891	T63.892	T63.893	T63.894	—	—
ant	T63.421	T63.422	T63.423	T63.424	—	—
arthropod NEC	T63.481	T63.482	T63.483	T63.484	—	—
bee	T63.441	T63.442	T63.443	T63.444	—	—
centipede	T63.411	T63.412	T63.413	T63.414	—	—
fish	T63.591	T63.592	T63.593	T63.594	—	—
frog	T63.811	T63.812	T63.813	T63.814	—	—
hornet	T63.451	T63.452	T63.453	T63.454	—	—
insect NEC	T63.481	T63.482	T63.483	T63.484	—	—
lizard	T63.121	T63.122	T63.123	T63.124	—	—
marine						
animals	T63.691	T63.692	T63.693	T63.694	—	—
bluebottle	T63.611	T63.612	T63.613	T63.614	—	—
jellyfish NEC	T63.621	T63.622	T63.623	T63.624	—	—
Portuguese Man-o-war	T63.611	T63.612	T63.613	T63.614	—	—
sea anemone	T63.631	T63.632	T63.633	T63.634	—	—
specified NEC	T63.691	T63.692	T63.693	T63.694	—	—
fish	T63.591	T63.592	T63.593	T63.594	—	—
plants	T63.711	T63.712	T63.713	T63.714	—	—
sting ray	T63.511	T63.512	T63.513	T63.514	—	—

Substance	Poisoning, Accidental (Unintentional)	Poisoning, Intentional Self-Harm	Poisoning, Assault	Poisoning, Undetermined	Adverse Effect	Underdosing
Venom, venomous *(Continued)*						
millipede (tropical)	T63.411	T63.412	T63.413	T63.414	—	—
plant NEC	T63.791	T63.792	T63.793	T63.794	—	—
marine	T63.711	T63.712	T63.713	T63.714	—	—
reptile	T63.191	T63.192	T63.193	T63.194	—	—
gila monster	T63.111	T63.112	T63.113	T63.114	—	—
lizard NEC	T63.121	T63.122	T63.123	T63.124	—	—
scorpion	T63.2X1	T63.2X2	T63.2X3	T63.2X4	—	—
snake	T63.001	T63.002	T63.003	T63.004	—	—
African NEC	T63.081	T63.082	T63.083	T63.084	—	—
American (North) (South) NEC	T63.061	T63.062	T63.063	T63.064	—	—
Asian	T63.081	T63.082	T63.083	T63.084	—	—
Australian	T63.071	T63.072	T63.073	T63.074	—	—
cobra	T63.041	T63.042	T63.043	T63.044	—	—
coral snake	T63.021	T63.022	T63.023	T63.024	—	—
rattlesnake	T63.011	T63.012	T63.013	T63.014	—	—
specified NEC	T63.091	T63.092	T63.093	T63.094	—	—
taipan	T63.031	T63.032	T63.033	T63.034	—	—
specified NEC	T63.891	T63.892	T63.893	T63.894	—	—
spider	T63.301	T63.302	T63.303	T63.304	—	—
black widow	T63.311	T63.312	T63.313	T63.314	—	—
brown recluse	T63.331	T63.332	T63.333	T63.334	—	—
specified NEC	T63.391	T63.392	T63.393	T63.394	—	—
tarantula	T63.321	T63.322	T63.323	T63.324	—	—
sting ray	T63.511	T63.512	T63.513	T63.514	—	—
toad	T63.821	T63.822	T63.823	T63.824	—	—
wasp	T63.461	T63.462	T63.463	T63.464	—	—
Venous sclerosing drug NEC	T46.8X1	T46.8X2	T46.8X3	T46.8X4	T46.8X5	T46.8X6
Ventolin — *see Albuterol*						
Verapamil	T46.1X1	T46.1X2	T46.1X3	T46.1X4	T46.1X5	T46.1X6
Veramon	T42.3X1	T42.3X2	T42.3X3	T42.3X4	T42.3X5	T42.3X6
Veratrine	T46.5X1	T46.5X2	T46.5X3	T46.5X4	T46.5X5	T46.5X6
Veratrum						
album	T62.2X1	T62.2X2	T62.2X3	T62.2X4	—	—
alkaloids	T46.5X1	T46.5X2	T46.5X3	T46.5X4	T46.5X5	T46.5X6
viride	T62.2X1	T62.2X2	T62.2X3	T62.2X4	—	—
Verdigris	T60.3X1	T60.3X2	T60.3X3	T60.3X4	—	—
Veronal	T42.3X1	T42.3X2	T42.3X3	T42.3X4	T42.3X5	T42.3X6
Veroxil	T37.4X1	T37.4X2	T37.4X3	T37.4X4	T37.4X5	T37.4X6
Versenate	T50.6X1	T50.6X2	T50.6X3	T50.6X4	T50.6X5	T50.6X6

◄ New   ◄ Revised   ~~deleted~~ Deleted

Substance	Poisoning, Accidental (Unintentional)	Poisoning, Intentional Self-Harm	Poisoning, Assault	Poisoning, Undetermined	Adverse Effect	Underdosing
Versidyne	T39.8X1	T39.8X2	T39.8X3	T39.8X4	T39.8X5	T39.8X6
Vetrabutine	T48.0X1	T48.0X2	T48.0X3	T48.0X4	T48.0X5	T48.0X6
Vidarabine	T37.5X1	T37.5X2	T37.5X3	T37.5X4	T37.5X5	T37.5X6
Vienna						
green	T57.0X1	T57.0X2	T57.0X3	T57.0X4	—	—
insecticide	T60.2X1	T60.2X2	T60.2X3	T60.2X4	—	—
red	T57.0X1	T57.0X2	T57.0X3	T57.0X4	—	—
pharmaceutical dye	T50.991	T50.992	T50.993	T50.994	T50.995	T50.996
Vigabatrin	T42.6X1	T42.6X2	T42.6X3	T42.6X4	T42.6X5	T42.6X6
Viloxazine	T43.291	T43.292	T43.293	T43.294	T43.295	T43.296
Viminol	T39.8X1	T39.8X2	T39.8X3	T39.8X4	T39.8X5	T39.8X6
Vinbarbital, vinbarbitone	T42.3X1	T42.3X2	T42.3X3	T42.3X4	T42.3X5	T42.3X6
Vinblastine	T45.1X1	T45.1X2	T45.1X3	T45.1X4	T45.1X5	T45.1X6
Vinburnine	T46.7X1	T46.7X2	T46.7X3	T46.7X4	T46.7X5	T46.7X6
Vincamine	T45.1X1	T45.1X2	T45.1X3	T45.1X4	T45.1X5	T45.1X6
Vincristine	T45.1X1	T45.1X2	T45.1X3	T45.1X4	T45.1X5	T45.1X6
Vindesine	T45.1X1	T45.1X2	T45.1X3	T45.1X4	T45.1X5	T45.1X6
Vinesthene, vinethene	T41.0X1	T41.0X2	T41.0X3	T41.0X4	T41.0X5	T41.0X6
Vinorelbine tartrate	T45.1X1	T45.1X2	T45.1X3	T45.1X4	T45.1X5	T45.1X6
Vinpocetine	T46.7X1	T46.7X2	T46.7X3	T46.7X4	T46.7X5	T46.7X6
Vinyl						
acetate	T65.891	T65.892	T65.893	T65.894	—	—
bital	T42.3X1	T42.3X2	T42.3X3	T42.3X4	T42.3X5	T42.3X6
bromide	T65.891	T65.892	T65.893	T65.894	—	—
chloride	T59.891	T59.892	T59.893	T59.894	—	—
ether	T41.0X1	T41.0X2	T41.0X3	T41.0X4	T41.0X5	T41.0X6
Vinylbital	T42.3X1	T42.3X2	T42.3X3	T42.3X4	T42.3X5	T42.3X6
Vinylidene chloride	T65.891	T65.892	T65.893	T65.894	—	—
Vioform	T37.8X1	T37.8X2	T37.8X3	T37.8X4	T37.8X5	T37.8X6
topical	T49.0X1	T49.0X2	T49.0X3	T49.0X4	T49.0X5	T49.0X6
Viomycin	T36.8X1	T36.8X2	T36.8X3	T36.8X4	T36.8X5	T36.8X6
Viosterol	T45.2X1	T45.2X2	T45.2X3	T45.2X4	T45.2X5	T45.2X6
Viper (venom)	T63.091	T63.092	T63.093	T63.094	—	—
Viprynium	T37.4X1	T37.4X2	T37.4X3	T37.4X4	T37.4X5	T37.4X6
Viquidil	T46.7X1	T46.7X2	T46.7X3	T46.7X4	T46.7X5	T46.7X6
Viral vaccine NEC	T50.B91	T50.B92	T50.B93	T50.B94	T50.B95	T50.B96
Virginiamycin	T36.8X1	T36.8X2	T36.8X3	T36.8X4	T36.8X5	T36.8X6
Virugon	T37.5X1	T37.5X2	T37.5X3	T37.5X4	T37.5X5	T37.5X6
Viscous agent	T50.901	T50.902	T50.903	T50.904	T50.905	T50.906
Visine	T49.5X1	T49.5X2	T49.5X3	T49.5X4	T49.5X5	T49.5X6
Visnadine	T46.3X1	T46.3X2	T46.3X3	T46.3X4	T46.3X5	T46.3X6

Substance	Poisoning, Accidental (Unintentional)	Poisoning, Intentional Self-Harm	Poisoning, Assault	Poisoning, Undetermined	Adverse Effect	Underdosing
Vitamin NEC	T45.2X1	T45.2X2	T45.2X3	T45.2X4	T45.2X5	T45.2X6
A	T45.2X1	T45.2X2	T45.2X3	T45.2X4	T45.2X5	T45.2X6
B NEC	T45.2X1	T45.2X2	T45.2X3	T45.2X4	T45.2X5	T45.2X6
nicotinic acid	T46.7X1	T46.7X2	T46.7X3	T46.7X4	T46.7X5	T46.7X6
B1	T45.2X1	T45.2X2	T45.2X3	T45.2X4	T45.2X5	T45.2X6
B2	T45.2X1	T45.2X2	T45.2X3	T45.2X4	T45.2X5	T45.2X6
B6	T45.2X1	T45.2X2	T45.2X3	T45.2X4	T45.2X5	T45.2X6
B12	T45.2X1	T45.2X2	T45.2X3	T45.2X4	T45.2X5	T45.2X6
B15	T45.2X1	T45.2X2	T45.2X3	T45.2X4	T45.2X5	T45.2X6
C	T45.2X1	T45.2X2	T45.2X3	T45.2X4	T45.2X5	T45.2X6
D	T45.2X1	T45.2X2	T45.2X3	T45.2X4	T45.2X5	T45.2X6
D2	T45.2X1	T45.2X2	T45.2X3	T45.2X4	T45.2X5	T45.2X6
D3	T45.2X1	T45.2X2	T45.2X3	T45.2X4	T45.2X5	T45.2X6
E	T45.2X1	T45.2X2	T45.2X3	T45.2X4	T45.2X5	T45.2X6
E acetate	T45.2X1	T45.2X2	T45.2X3	T45.2X4	T45.2X5	T45.2X6
hematopoietic	T45.8X1	T45.8X2	T45.8X3	T45.8X4	T45.8X5	T45.8X6
K NEC	T45.7X1	T45.7X2	T45.7X3	T45.7X4	T45.7X5	T45.7X6
K1	T45.7X1	T45.7X2	T45.7X3	T45.7X4	T45.7X5	T45.7X6
K2	T45.7X1	T45.7X2	T45.7X3	T45.7X4	T45.7X5	T45.7X6
PP	T45.2X1	T45.2X2	T45.2X3	T45.2X4	T45.2X5	T45.2X6
ulceroprotectant	T47.1X1	T47.1X2	T47.1X3	T47.1X4	T47.1X5	T47.1X6
Vleminckx's solution	T49.4X1	T49.4X2	T49.4X3	T49.4X4	T49.4X5	T49.4X6
Voltaren — see Diclofenac sodium						
W						
Warfarin	T45.511	T45.512	T45.513	T45.514	T45.515	T45.516
rodenticide	T60.4X1	T60.4X2	T60.4X3	T60.4X4	—	—
sodium	T45.511	T45.512	T45.513	T45.514	T45.515	T45.516
Wasp (sting)	T63.461	T63.462	T63.463	T63.464	—	—
Water						
balance drug	T50.3X1	T50.3X2	T50.3X3	T50.3X4	T50.3X5	T50.3X6
distilled	T50.3X1	T50.3X2	T50.3X3	T50.3X4	T50.3X5	T50.3X6
gas — see Gas, water						
incomplete combustion of — see Carbon, monoxide, fuel, utility						
hemlock	T62.2X1	T62.2X2	T62.2X3	T62.2X4	—	—
moccasin (venom)	T63.061	T63.062	T63.063	T63.064	—	—
purified	T50.3X1	T50.3X2	T50.3X3	T50.3X4	T50.3X5	T50.3X6
Wax (paraffin) (petroleum)	T52.0X1	T52.0X2	T52.0X3	T52.0X4	—	—
automobile	T65.891	T65.892	T65.893	T65.894	—	—
floor	T52.0X1	T52.0X2	T52.0X3	T52.0X4	—	—

TABLE OF DRUGS AND CHEMICALS

TABLE OF DRUGS AND CHEMICALS

Substance	Poisoning, Accidental (Unintentional)	Poisoning, Intentional Self-Harm	Poisoning, Assault	Poisoning, Undetermined	Adverse Effect	Underdosing
Weed killers NEC	T60.3X1	T60.3X2	T60.3X3	T60.3X4	—	—
Welldorm	T42.6X1	T42.6X2	T42.6X3	T42.6X4	T42.6X5	T42.6X6
White						
arsenic	T57.0X1	T57.0X2	T57.0X3	T57.0X4	—	—
hellebore	T62.2X1	T62.2X2	T62.2X3	T62.2X4	—	—
lotion (keratolytic)	T49.4X1	T49.4X2	T49.4X3	T49.4X4	T49.4X5	T49.4X6
spirit	T52.0X1	T52.0X2	T52.0X3	T52.0X4	—	—
Whitewash	T65.891	T65.892	T65.893	T65.894	—	—
Whole blood (human)	T45.8X1	T45.8X2	T45.8X3	T45.8X4	T45.8X5	T45.8X6
Wild						
black cherry	T62.2X1	T62.2X2	T62.2X3	T62.2X4	—	—
poisonous plants NEC	T62.2X1	T62.2X2	T62.2X3	T62.2X4	—	—
Window cleaning fluid	T65.891	T65.892	T65.893	T65.894	—	—
Wintergreen (oil)	T49.3X1	T49.3X2	T49.3X3	T49.3X4	T49.3X5	T49.3X6
Wisterine	T62.2X1	T62.2X2	T62.2X3	T62.2X4	—	—
Witch hazel	T49.2X1	T49.2X2	T49.2X3	T49.2X4	T49.2X5	T49.2X6
Wood alcohol or spirit	T51.1X1	T51.1X2	T51.1X3	T51.1X4	—	—
Wool fat (hydrous)	T49.3X1	T49.3X2	T49.3X3	T49.3X4	T49.3X5	T49.3X6
Woorali	T48.1X1	T48.1X2	T48.1X3	T48.1X4	T48.1X5	T48.1X6
Wormseed, American	T37.4X1	T37.4X2	T37.4X3	T37.4X4	T37.4X5	T37.4X6
X						
Xamoterol	T44.5X1	T44.5X2	T44.5X3	T44.5X4	T44.5X5	T44.5X6
Xanthine diuretics	T50.2X1	T50.2X2	T50.2X3	T50.2X4	T50.2X5	T50.2X6
Xanthinol nicotinate	T46.7X1	T46.7X2	T46.7X3	T46.7X4	T46.7X5	T46.7X6
Xanthotoxin	T49.3X1	T49.3X2	T49.3X3	T49.3X4	T49.3X5	T49.3X6
Xantinol nicotinate	T46.7X1	T46.7X2	T46.7X3	T46.7X4	T46.7X5	T46.7X6
Xantocillin	T36.0X1	T36.0X2	T36.0X3	T36.0X4	T36.0X5	T36.0X6
Xenon (127Xe) (133Xe)	T50.8X1	T50.8X2	T50.8X3	T50.8X4	T50.8X5	T50.8X6
Xenysalate	T49.4X1	T49.4X2	T49.4X3	T49.4X4	T49.4X5	T49.4X6
Xibornol	T37.8X1	T37.8X2	T37.8X3	T37.8X4	T37.8X5	T37.8X6
Xigris	T45.511	T45.512	T45.513	T45.514	T45.515	T45.516
Xipamide	T50.2X1	T50.2X2	T50.2X3	T50.2X4	T50.2X5	T50.2X6
Xylazine	T65.841	T65.842	T65.843	T65.844	—	—
Xylene (vapor)	T52.2X1	T52.2X2	T52.2X3	T52.2X4	—	—
Xylocaine (infiltration) (topical)	T41.3X1	T41.3X2	T41.3X3	T41.3X4	T41.3X5	T41.3X6
nerve block (peripheral) (plexus)	T41.3X1	T41.3X2	T41.3X3	T41.3X4	T41.3X5	T41.3X6
spinal	T41.3X1	T41.3X2	T41.3X3	T41.3X4	T41.3X5	T41.3X6
Xylol (vapor)	T52.2X1	T52.2X2	T52.2X3	T52.2X4	—	—
Xylometazoline	T48.5X1	T48.5X2	T48.5X3	T48.5X4	T48.5X5	T48.5X6

Substance	Poisoning, Accidental (Unintentional)	Poisoning, Intentional Self-Harm	Poisoning, Assault	Poisoning, Undetermined	Adverse Effect	Underdosing
Y						
Yeast	T45.2X1	T45.2X2	T45.2X3	T45.2X4	T45.2X5	T45.2X6
dried	T45.2X1	T45.2X2	T45.2X3	T45.2X4	T45.2X5	T45.2X6
Yellow						
fever vaccine	T50.B91	T50.B92	T50.B93	T50.B94	T50.B95	T50.B96
jasmine	T62.2X1	T62.2X2	T62.2X3	T62.2X4	—	—
phenolphthalein	T47.2X1	T47.2X2	T47.2X3	T47.2X4	T47.2X5	T47.2X6
Yew	T62.2X1	T62.2X2	T62.2X3	T62.2X4	—	—
Yohimbic acid	T40.991	T40.992	T40.993	T40.994	T40.995	T40.996
Z						
Zactane	T39.8X1	T39.8X2	T39.8X3	T39.8X4	T39.8X5	T39.8X6
Zalcitabine	T37.5X1	T37.5X2	T37.5X3	T37.5X4	T37.5X5	T37.5X6
Zaroxolyn	T50.2X1	T50.2X2	T50.2X3	T50.2X4	T50.2X5	T50.2X6
Zephiran (topical)	T49.0X1	T49.0X2	T49.0X3	T49.0X4	T49.0X5	T49.0X6
ophthalmic preparation	T49.5X1	T49.5X2	T49.5X3	T49.5X4	T49.5X5	T49.5X6
Zeranol	T38.7X1	T38.7X2	T38.7X3	T38.7X4	T38.7X5	T38.7X6
Zerone	T51.1X1	T51.1X2	T51.1X3	T51.1X4	—	—
Zidovudine	T37.5X1	T37.5X2	T37.5X3	T37.5X4	T37.5X5	T37.5X6
Zimeldine	T43.221	T43.222	T43.223	T43.224	T43.225	T43.226
Zinc (compounds) (fumes) (vapor) NEC	T56.5X1	T56.5X2	T56.5X3	T56.5X4	—	—
anti-infectives	T49.0X1	T49.0X2	T49.0X3	T49.0X4	T49.0X5	T49.0X6
antivaricose	T46.8X1	T46.8X2	T46.8X3	T46.8X4	T46.8X5	T46.8X6
bacitracin	T49.0X1	T49.0X2	T49.0X3	T49.0X4	T49.0X5	T49.0X6
chloride (mouthwash)	T49.6X1	T49.6X2	T49.6X3	T49.6X4	T49.6X5	T49.6X6
chromate	T56.5X1	T56.5X2	T56.5X3	T56.5X4	—	—
gelatin	T49.3X1	T49.3X2	T49.3X3	T49.3X4	T49.3X5	T49.3X6
oxide	T49.3X1	T49.3X2	T49.3X3	T49.3X4	T49.3X5	T49.3X6
plaster	T49.3X1	T49.3X2	T49.3X3	T49.3X4	T49.3X5	T49.3X6
peroxide	T49.0X1	T49.0X2	T49.0X3	T49.0X4	T49.0X5	T49.0X6
pesticides	T56.5X1	T56.5X2	T56.5X3	T56.5X4	—	—
phosphide	T60.4X1	T60.4X2	T60.4X3	T60.4X4	—	—
pyrithionate	T49.4X1	T49.4X2	T49.4X3	T49.4X4	T49.4X5	T49.4X6
stearate	T49.3X1	T49.3X2	T49.3X3	T49.3X4	T49.3X5	T49.3X6
sulfate	T49.5X1	T49.5X2	T49.5X3	T49.5X4	T49.5X5	T49.5X6
ENT agent	T49.6X1	T49.6X2	T49.6X3	T49.6X4	T49.6X5	T49.6X6
ophthalmic solution	T49.5X1	T49.5X2	T49.5X3	T49.5X4	T49.5X5	T49.5X6
topical NEC	T49.0X1	T49.0X2	T49.0X3	T49.0X4	T49.0X5	T49.0X6
undecylenate	T49.0X1	T49.0X2	T49.0X3	T49.0X4	T49.0X5	T49.0X6

◀ New   ◀ Revised   ~~deleted~~ Deleted

Substance	Poisoning, Accidental (Unintentional)	Poisoning, Intentional Self-Harm	Poisoning, Assault	Poisoning, Undetermined	Adverse Effect	Underdosing
Zineb	T60.0X1	T60.0X2	T60.0X3	T60.0X4	—	—
Zinostatin	T45.1X1	T45.1X2	T45.1X3	T45.1X4	T45.1X5	T45.1X6
Zipeprol	T48.3X1	T48.3X2	T48.3X3	T48.3X4	T48.3X5	T48.3X6
Zofenopril	T46.4X1	T46.4X2	T46.4X3	T46.4X4	T46.4X5	T46.4X6
Zolpidem	T42.6X1	T42.6X2	T42.6X3	T42.6X4	T42.6X5	T42.6X6
Zomepirac	T39.391	T39.392	T39.393	T39.394	T39.395	T39.396
Zopiclone	T42.6X1	T42.6X2	T42.6X3	T42.6X4	T42.6X5	T42.6X6

Substance	Poisoning, Accidental (Unintentional)	Poisoning, Intentional Self-Harm	Poisoning, Assault	Poisoning, Undetermined	Adverse Effect	Underdosing
Zorubicin	T45.1X1	T45.1X2	T45.1X3	T45.1X4	T45.1X5	T45.1X6
Zotepine	T43.591	T43.592	T43.593	T43.594	T43.595	T43.596
Zovant	T45.511	T45.512	T45.513	T45.514	T45.515	T45.516
Zoxazolamine	T42.8X1	T42.8X2	T42.8X3	T42.8X4	T42.8X5	T42.8X6
Zuclopenthixol	T43.4X1	T43.4X2	T43.4X3	T43.4X4	T43.4X5	T43.4X6
Zygadenus (venenosus)	T62.2X1	T62.2X2	T62.2X3	T62.2X4	—	—
Zyprexa	T43.591	T43.592	T43.593	T43.594	T43.595	T43.596

External Cause of Injuries Index

— A —

Abandonment (causing exposure to weather conditions) (with intent to injure or kill) NEC X58

Abuse (adult) (child) (mental) (physical) (sexual) X58

Accident (to) X58
  aircraft (in transit) (powered) —*see also* Accident, transport, aircraft
    due to, caused by cataclysm —*see* Forces of nature, by type
  animal-drawn vehicle —*see* Accident, transport, animal-drawn vehicle occupant
  animal-rider —*see* Accident, transport, animal-rider
  automobile —*see* Accident, transport, car occupant
  ~~bare foot water skiier V94.4~~
  ▶barefoot water skiier V94.4
  boat, boating —*see also* Accident, watercraft
    striking swimmer
      powered V94.11
      unpowered V94.12
  bus —*see* Accident, transport, bus occupant
  cable car, not on rails V98.0
    on rails —*see* Accident, transport, streetcar occupant
  car —*see* Accident, transport, car occupant
  caused by, due to
    animal NEC W64
    chain hoist W24.0
    cold (excessive) —*see* Exposure, cold
    corrosive liquid, substance —*see* Table of Drugs and Chemicals
    cutting or piercing instrument —*see* Contact, with, by type of instrument
    drive belt W24.0
    electric
      current —*see* Exposure, electric current
      motor —*see also* Contact, with, by type of machine W31.3
        current (of) W86.8
    environmental factor NEC X58
    explosive material —*see* Explosion
    fire, flames —*see* Exposure, fire
    firearm missile —*see* Discharge, firearm by type
    heat (excessive) —*see* Heat
    hot —*see* Contact, with, hot
    ignition —*see* Ignition
    lifting device W24.0
    lightning —*see* subcategory T75.0
      causing fire —*see* Exposure, fire
    machine, machinery —*see* Contact, with, by type of machine
    natural factor NEC X58
    pulley (block) W24.0
    radiation —*see* Radiation
    steam X13.1
      inhalation X13.0
      pipe X16
    thunderbolt —*see* subcategory T75.0
      causing fire —*see* Exposure, fire
    transmission device W24.1
  coach —*see* Accident, transport, bus occupant
  coal car —*see* Accident, transport, industrial vehicle occupant
  diving —*see also* Fall, into, water
    with
      drowning or submersion —*see* Drowning
  forklift —*see* Accident, transport, industrial vehicle occupant
  heavy transport vehicle NOS —*see* Accident, transport, truck occupant
  ice yacht V98.2
  in
    medical, surgical procedure
      as, or due to misadventure —*see* Misadventure
      causing an abnormal reaction or later complication without mention of misadventure —*see also* Complication of or following, by type of procedure Y84.9
  land yacht V98.1
  late effect of —*see* W00-X58 with 7th character S
  logging car —*see* Accident, transport, industrial vehicle occupant

Accident *(Continued)*
  machine, machinery —*see also* Contact, with, by type of machine
  on board watercraft V93.69
    explosion —*see* Explosion, in, watercraft
    fire —*see* Burn, on board watercraft
    powered craft V93.63
      ferry boat V93.61
      fishing boat V93.62
      jet ski V93.63
      liner V93.61
      merchant ship V93.60
      passenger ship V93.61
      sailboat V93.64
  mine tram —*see* Accident, transport, industrial vehicle occupant
  mobility scooter (motorized) —*see* Accident, transport, pedestrian, conveyance, specified type NEC
  motor scooter —*see* Accident, transport, motorcycle
  motor vehicle NOS (traffic) —*see also* Accident, transport V89.2
    nontraffic V89.0
    three-wheeled NOS —*see* Accident, transport, three-wheeled motor vehicle occupant
  motorcycle NOS —*see* Accident, transport, motorcycle
  nonmotor vehicle NOS (nontraffic) —*see also* Accident, transport V89.1
    traffic NOS V89.3
  nontraffic (victim's mode of transport NOS) V88.9
    collision (between) V88.7
      bus and truck V88.5
    ➡car and
      bus V88.3
      pickup V88.2
      three-wheeled motor vehicle V88.0
      train V88.6
      truck V88.4
      two-wheeled motor vehicle V88.0
      van V88.2
    ➡specified vehicle NEC and
      three-wheeled motor vehicle V88.1
      two-wheeled motor vehicle V88.1
    known mode of transport —*see* Accident, transport, by type of vehicle
    noncollision V88.8
  on board watercraft V93.89
    powered craft V93.83
      ferry boat V93.81
      fishing boat V93.82
      jet ski V93.83
      liner V93.81
      merchant ship V93.80
      passenger ship V93.81
    unpowered craft V93.88
      canoe V93.85
      inflatable V93.86
        in tow
          recreational V94.31
          specified NEC V94.32
      kayak V93.85
      sailboat V93.84
      surf-board V93.88
      water skis V93.87
      windsurfer V93.88
  parachutist V97.29
    entangled in object V97.21
    injured on landing V97.22
  pedal cycle —*see* Accident, transport, pedal cyclist
  pedestrian (on foot)
    with
      another pedestrian W51
        with fall W03
          due to ice or snow W00.0
        on pedestrian conveyance NEC V00.09
      rider of
        hoverboard V00.038
        Segway V00.038
        standing
          electric scooter V00.031
          micro-mobility pedestrian conveyance NEC V00.038
        roller skater (in-line) V00.01
        skate boarder V00.02
        transport vehicle —*see* Accident, transport
    on pedestrian conveyance —*see* Accident, transport, pedestrian, conveyance

Accident *(Continued)*
  pick-up truck or van —*see* Accident, transport, pickup truck occupant
  quarry truck —*see* Accident, transport, industrial vehicle occupant
  railway vehicle (any) (in motion) —*see* Accident, transport, railway vehicle occupant
    due to cataclysm —*see* Forces of nature, by type
  scooter (non-motorized) —*see* Accident, transport, pedestrian, conveyance, scooter
  sequelae of —*see* W00-X58 with 7th character S
  skateboard —*see* Accident, transport, pedestrian, conveyance, skateboard
  ski (ing) —*see* Accident, transport, pedestrian, conveyance
    lift V98.3
  specified cause NEC X58
  streetcar —*see* Accident, transport, streetcar occupant
  traffic (victim's mode of transport NOS) V87.9
    collision (between) V87.7
      bus and truck V87.5
    ➡car and
      bus V87.3
      pickup V87.2
      three-wheeled motor vehicle V87.0
      train V87.6
      truck V87.4
      two-wheeled motor vehicle V87.0
      van V87.2
    specified vehicle NEC V86.39
      and
        three-wheeled motor vehicle V87.1
        two-wheeled motor vehicle V87.1
      driver V86.09
      person on outside V86.29
      passenger V86.19
      while boarding or alighting V86.49
    known mode of transport —*see* Accident, transport, by type of vehicle
    noncollision V87.8
  transport (involving injury to) V99
    18 wheeler —*see* Accident, transport, truck occupant
    agricultural vehicle occupant (nontraffic) V84.9
      driver V84.5
      hanger-on V84.7
      passenger V84.6
      traffic V84.3
        driver V84.0
        hanger-on V84.2
        passenger V84.1
      while boarding or alighting V84.4
    aircraft NEC V97.89
      military NEC V97.818
        with civilian aircraft V97.810
        civilian injured by V97.811
      occupant injured (in)
        nonpowered craft accident V96.9
          balloon V96.00
            collision V96.03
            crash V96.01
            explosion V96.05
            fire V96.04
            forced landing V96.02
            specified type NEC V96.09
          glider V96.20
            collision V96.23
            crash V96.21
            explosion V96.25
            fire V96.24
            forced landing V96.22
            specified type NEC V96.29
          hang glider V96.10
            collision V96.13
            crash V96.11
            explosion V96.15
            fire V96.14
            forced landing V96.12
            specified type NEC V96.19
          specified craft NEC V96.8
        powered craft accident V95.9
          fixed wing NEC
            commercial V95.30
              collision V95.33
              crash V95.31

▶ New   ➡ Revised   ~~deleted~~ Deleted   ● Use Additional Character(s)

Accident (Continued)
  transport (Continued)
    aircraft (Continued)
      occupant injured (Continued)
        powered craft accident Continued)
          fixed wing (Continued)
            commercial I70.521 (Continued)
              explosion V95.35
              fire V95.34
              forced landing V95.32
              specified type NEC V95.39
            private V95.20
              collision V95.23
              crash V95.21
              explosion V95.25
              fire V95.24
              forced landing V95.22
              specified type NEC V95.29
          glider V95.10
            collision V95.13
            crash V95.11
            explosion V95.15
            fire V95.14
            forced landing V95.12
            specified type NEC V95.19
          helicopter V95.00
            collision V95.03
            crash V95.01
            explosion V95.05
            fire V95.04
            forced landing V95.02
            specified type NEC V95.09
          spacecraft V95.40
            collision V95.43
            crash V95.41
            explosion V95.45
            fire V95.44
            forced landing V95.42
            specified type NEC V95.49
          specified craft NEC V95.8
         ultralight V95.10
            collision V95.13
            crash V95.11
            explosion V95.15
            fire V95.14
            forced landing V95.12
            specified type NEC V95.19
        specified accident NEC V97.0
        while boarding or alighting
          V97.1
      person (injured by)
        falling from, in or on aircraft V97.0
        machinery on aircraft V97.89
        on ground with aircraft involvement
          V97.39
        rotating propeller V97.32
        struck by object falling from aircraft
          V97.31
        sucked into aircraft jet V97.33
        while boarding or alighting aircraft
          V97.1
    airport (battery-powered) passenger
      vehicle —see Accident, transport,
      industrial vehicle occupant
    all-terrain vehicle occupant (nontraffic)
      V86.95
      driver V86.55
      dune buggy —see Accident, transport, dune
        buggy occupant
      hanger-on V86.75
      passenger V86.65
      snowmobile —see Accident, transport,
        snowmobile occupant
      specified type NEC V86.99
        driver V86.59
        passenger V86.69
        person on outside V86.79
      traffic V86.35
        driver V86.05
        hanger-on V86.25
        passenger V86.15
      while boarding or alighting V86.45
    ambulance occupant (traffic) V86.31
      driver V86.01
      hanger-on V86.21
      nontraffic V86.91
        driver V86.51
        hanger-on V86.71
        passenger V86.61
      passenger V86.11
      while boarding or alighting V86.41

Accident (Continued)
  transport (Continued)
    animal-drawn vehicle occupant (in) V80.929
      collision (with)
        animal V80.12
          being ridden V80.711
        animal-drawn vehicle V80.721
        bus V80.42
        car V80.42
        fixed or stationary object V80.82
        military vehicle V80.920
        nonmotor vehicle V80.791
        pedal cycle V80.22
        pedestrian V80.12
        pickup V80.42
        railway train or vehicle V80.62
        specified motor vehicle NEC V80.52
        streetcar V80.731
        truck V80.42
        two-or three-wheeled motor vehicle
          V80.32
        van V80.42
      noncollision V80.02
      specified circumstance NEC V80. 928
    animal-rider V80.919
      collision (with)
        animal V80.11
          being ridden V80.710
        animal-drawn vehicle V80.720
        bus V80.41
        car V80.41
        fixed or stationary object V80.81
        military vehicle V80.910
        nonmotor vehicle V80.790
        pedal cycle V80.21
        pedestrian V80.11
        pickup V80.41
        railway train or vehicle V80.61
        specified motor vehicle NEC V80.51
        streetcar V80.730
        truck V80.41
        two- or three-wheeled motor vehicle
          V80.31
        van V80.41
      noncollision V80.018
        specified as horse rider V80.010
      specified circumstance NEC V80.918
    armored car —see Accident, transport, truck
      occupant
    battery-powered truck (baggage) (mail) —see
      Accident, transport, industrial vehicle
      occupant
    bus occupant V79.9
      collision (with)
        animal (traffic) V70.9
          being ridden (traffic) V76.9
            nontraffic V76.3
            while boarding or alighting V76.4
          nontraffic V70.3
          while boarding or alighting V70.4
        animal-drawn vehicle (traffic) V76.9
          nontraffic V76.3
          while boarding or alighting V76.4
        bus (traffic) V74.9
          nontraffic V74.3
          while boarding or alighting V74.4
        car (traffic) V73.9
          nontraffic V73.3
          while boarding or alighting V73.4
        motor vehicle NOS (traffic) V79.60
          nontraffic V79.20
          specified type NEC (traffic) V79.69
            nontraffic V79.29
        pedal cycle (traffic) V71.9
          nontraffic V71.3
          while boarding or alighting V71.4
        pickup truck (traffic) V73.9
          nontraffic V73.3
          while boarding or alighting V73.4
        railway vehicle (traffic) V75.9
          nontraffic V75.3
          while boarding or alighting V75.4
        specified vehicle NEC (traffic) V76.9
          nontraffic V76.3
          while boarding or alighting V76.4
        stationary object (traffic) V77.9
          nontraffic V77.3
          while boarding or alighting V77.4
        streetcar (traffic) V76.9
          nontraffic V76.3
          while boarding or alighting V76.4

Accident (Continued)
  transport (Continued)
    bus occupant (Continued)
      collision (Continued)
        three wheeled motor vehicle (traffic)
          V72.9
          nontraffic V72.3
          while boarding or alighting V72.4
        truck (traffic) V74.9
          nontraffic V74.3
          while boarding or alighting V74.4
        two wheeled motor vehicle (traffic) V72.9
          nontraffic V72.3
          while boarding or alighting V72.4
        van (traffic) V73.9
          nontraffic V73.3
          while boarding or alighting V73.4
      driver
        collision (with)
          animal (traffic) V70.5
            being ridden (traffic) V76.5
              nontraffic V76.0
            nontraffic V70.0
          animal-drawn vehicle (traffic)
            V76.5
            nontraffic V76.0
          bus (traffic) V74.5
            nontraffic V74.0
          car (traffic) V73.5
            nontraffic V73.0
          motor vehicle NOS (traffic) V79.40
            nontraffic V79.00
            specified type NEC (traffic) V79.49
              nontraffic V79.09
          pedal cycle (traffic) V71.5
            nontraffic V71.0
          pickup truck (traffic) V73.5
            nontraffic V73.0
          railway vehicle (traffic) V75.5
            nontraffic V75.0
          specified vehicle NEC (traffic)
            V76.5
            nontraffic V76.0
          stationary object (traffic) V77.5
            nontraffic V77.0
          streetcar (traffic) V76.5
            nontraffic V76.0
          three wheeled motor vehicle (traffic)
            V72.5
            nontraffic V72.0
          truck (traffic) V74.5
            nontraffic V74.0
          two wheeled motor vehicle (traffic)
            V72.5
            nontraffic V72.0
          van (traffic) V73.5
            nontraffic V73.0
        noncollision accident (traffic) V78.5
          nontraffic V78.0
      hanger-on
        collision (with)
          animal (traffic) V70.7
            being ridden (traffic) V76.7
              nontraffic V76.2
            nontraffic V70.2
          animal-drawn vehicle (traffic)
            V76.7
            nontraffic V76.2
          bus (traffic) V74.7
            nontraffic V74.2
          car (traffic) V73.7
            nontraffic V73.2
          pedal cycle (traffic) V71.7
            nontraffic V71.2
          pickup truck (traffic) V73.7
            nontraffic V73.2
          railway vehicle (traffic) V75.7
            nontraffic V75.2
          specified vehicle NEC (traffic)
            V76.7
            nontraffic V76.2
          stationary object (traffic) V77.7
            nontraffic V77.2
          streetcar (traffic) V76.7
            nontraffic V76.2
          three wheeled motor vehicle (traffic)
            V72.7
            nontraffic V72.2
          truck (traffic) V74.7
            nontraffic V74.2

A

Accident *(Continued)*
  transport *(Continued)*
    bus occupant *(Continued)*
      hanger-on *(Continued)*
        collision *(Continued)*
          two wheeled motor vehicle (traffic) V72.7
            nontraffic V72.2
          van (traffic) V73.7
            nontraffic V73.2
        noncollision accident (traffic) V78.7
          nontraffic V78.2
      noncollision accident (traffic) V78.9
        nontraffic V78.3
        while boarding or alighting V78.4
      nontraffic V79.3
      passenger
        collision (with)
          animal (traffic) V70.6
            being ridden (traffic) V76.6
              nontraffic V76.1
            nontraffic V70.1
          animal-drawn vehicle (traffic) V76.6
            nontraffic V76.1
          bus (traffic) V74.6
            nontraffic V74.1
          car (traffic) V73.6
            nontraffic V73.1
          motor vehicle NOS (traffic) V79.50
            nontraffic V79.10
            specified type NEC (traffic) V79.59
              nontraffic V79.19
          pedal cycle (traffic) V71.6
            nontraffic V71.1
          pickup truck (traffic) V73.6
            nontraffic V73.1
          railway vehicle (traffic) V75.6
            nontraffic V75.1
          specified vehicle NEC (traffic) V76.6
            nontraffic V76.1
          stationary object (traffic) V77.6
            nontraffic V77.1
          streetcar (traffic) V76.6
            nontraffic V76.1
          three wheeled motor vehicle (traffic) V72.6
            nontraffic V72.1
          truck (traffic) V74.6
            nontraffic V74.1
          two wheeled motor vehicle (traffic) V72.6
            nontraffic V72.1
          van (traffic) V73.6
            nontraffic V73.1
        noncollision accident (traffic) V78.6
          nontraffic V78.1
      specified type NEC V79.88
      military vehicle V79.81
    cable car, not on rails V98.0
      on rails —*see* Accident, transport, streetcar occupant
    car occupant V49.9
      ambulance occupant —*see* Accident, transport, ambulance occupant
      collision (with)
        animal (traffic) V40.9
          being ridden (traffic) V46.9
            nontraffic V46.3
            while boarding or alighting V46.4
          nontraffic V40.3
          while boarding or alighting V40.4
        animal-drawn vehicle (traffic) V46.9
          nontraffic V46.3
          while boarding or alighting V46.4
        bus (traffic) V44.9
          nontraffic V44.3
          while boarding or alighting V44.4
        car (traffic) V43.92
          nontraffic V43.32
          while boarding or alighting V43.42
        motor vehicle NOS (traffic) V49.60
          nontraffic V49.20
          specified type NEC (traffic) V49.69
            nontraffic V49.29
        pedal cycle (traffic) V41.9
          nontraffic V41.3
          while boarding or alighting V41.4
        pickup truck (traffic) V43.93
          nontraffic V43.33
          while boarding or alighting V43.43

Accident *(Continued)*
  transport *(Continued)*
    car occupant *(Continued)*
      collision *(Continued)*
        railway vehicle (traffic) V45.9
          nontraffic V45.3
          while boarding or alighting V45.4
        specified vehicle NEC (traffic) V46.9
          nontraffic V46.3
          while boarding or alighting V46.4
        sport utility vehicle (traffic) V43.91
          nontraffic V43.31
          while boarding or alighting V43.41
        stationary object (traffic) V47.9
          nontraffic V47.3
          while boarding or alighting V47.4
        streetcar (traffic) V46.9
          nontraffic V46.3
          while boarding or alighting V46.4
        three wheeled motor vehicle (traffic) V42.9
          nontraffic V42.3
          while boarding or alighting V42.4
        truck (traffic) V44.9
          nontraffic V44.3
          while boarding or alighting V44.4
        two wheeled motor vehicle (traffic) V42.9
          nontraffic V42.3
          while boarding or alighting V42.4
        van (traffic) V43.94
          nontraffic V43.34
          while boarding or alighting V43.44
      driver
        collision (with)
          animal (traffic) V40.5
            being ridden (traffic) V46.5
              nontraffic V46.0
            nontraffic V40.0
          animal-drawn vehicle (traffic) V46.5
            nontraffic V46.0
          bus (traffic) V44.5
            nontraffic V44.0
          car (traffic) V43.52
            nontraffic V43.02
          motor vehicle NOS (traffic) V49.40
            nontraffic V49.00
            specified type NEC (traffic) V49.49
              nontraffic V49.09
          pedal cycle (traffic) V41.5
            nontraffic V41.0
          pickup truck (traffic) V43.53
            nontraffic V43.03
          railway vehicle (traffic) V45.5
            nontraffic V45.0
          specified vehicle NEC (traffic) V46.5
            nontraffic V46.0
          sport utility vehicle (traffic) V43.51
            nontraffic V43.01
          stationary object (traffic) V47.5
            nontraffic V47.0
          streetcar (traffic) V46.5
            nontraffic V46.0
          three wheeled motor vehicle (traffic) V42.5
            nontraffic V42.0
          truck (traffic) V44.5
            nontraffic V44.0
          two wheeled motor vehicle (traffic) V42.5
            nontraffic V42.0
          van (traffic) V43.54
            nontraffic V43.04
        noncollision accident (traffic) V48.5
          nontraffic V48.0
      hanger-on
        collision (with)
          animal (traffic) V40.7
            being ridden (traffic) V46.7
              nontraffic V46.2
            nontraffic V40.2
          animal-drawn vehicle (traffic) V46.7
            nontraffic V46.2
          bus (traffic) V44.7
            nontraffic V44.2
          car (traffic) V43.72
            nontraffic V43.22
          pedal cycle (traffic) V41.7
            nontraffic V41.2
          pickup truck (traffic) V43.73
            nontraffic V43.23

Accident *(Continued)*
  transport *(Continued)*
    car occupant *(Continued)*
      hanger-on *(Continued)*
        collision *(Continued)*
          railway vehicle (traffic) V45.7
            nontraffic V45.2
          specified vehicle NEC (traffic) V46.7
            nontraffic V46.2
          sport utility vehicle (traffic) V43.71
            nontraffic V43.21
          stationary object (traffic) V47.7
            nontraffic V47.2
          streetcar (traffic) V46.7
            nontraffic V46.2
          three wheeled motor vehicle (traffic) V42.7
            nontraffic V42.2
          truck (traffic) V44.7
            nontraffic V44.2
          two wheeled motor vehicle (traffic) V42.7
            nontraffic V42.2
          van (traffic) V43.74
            nontraffic V43.24
        noncollision accident (traffic) V48.7
          nontraffic V48.2
      noncollision accident (traffic) V48.9
        nontraffic V48.3
        while boarding or alighting V48.4
      nontraffic V49.3
      passenger
        collision (with)
          animal (traffic) V40.6
            being ridden (traffic) V46.6
              nontraffic V46.1
            nontraffic V40.1
          animal-drawn vehicle (traffic) V46.6
            nontraffic V46.1
          bus (traffic) V44.6
            nontraffic V44.1
          car (traffic) V43.62
            nontraffic V43.12
          motor vehicle NOS (traffic) V49.50
            nontraffic V49.10
            specified type NEC (traffic) V49.59
              nontraffic V49.19
          pedal cycle (traffic) V41.6
            nontraffic V41.1
          pickup truck (traffic) V43.63
            nontraffic V43.13
          railway vehicle (traffic) V45.6
            nontraffic V45.1
          specified vehicle NEC (traffic) V46.6
            nontraffic V46.1
          sport utility vehicle (traffic) V43.61
            nontraffic V43.11
          stationary object (traffic) V47.6
            nontraffic V47.1
          streetcar (traffic) V46.6
            nontraffic V46.1
          three wheeled motor vehicle (traffic) V42.6
            nontraffic V42.1
          truck (traffic) V44.6
            nontraffic V44.1
          two wheeled motor vehicle (traffic) V42.6
            nontraffic V42.1
          van (traffic) V43.64
            nontraffic V43.14
        noncollision accident (traffic) V48.6
          nontraffic V48.1
      specified type NEC V49.88
      military vehicle V49.81
    coal car —*see* Accident, transport, industrial vehicle occupant
    construction vehicle occupant (nontraffic) V85.9
      driver V85.5
      hanger-on V85.7
      passenger V85.6
      traffic V85.3
        driver V85.0
        hanger-on V85.2
        passenger V85.1
      while boarding or alighting V85.4
    dirt bike rider (nontraffic) V86.96
      driver V86.56
      hanger-on V86.76
      passenger V86.66

Accident (Continued)
transport (Continued)
dirt bike rider (Continued)
traffic V86.36
driver V86.06
hanger-on V86.26
passenger V86.16
while boarding or alighting V86.46
due to cataclysm —see Forces of nature, by type
dune buggy occupant (nontraffic) V86.93
driver V86.53
hanger-on V86.73
passenger V86.63
traffic V86.33
driver V86.03
hanger-on V86.23
passenger V86.13
while boarding or alighting V86.43
e-bicycle —see Accident, transport, electric (assisted) bicyclist
e-bike —see Accident, transport, electric (assisted) bicyclist
electric (assisted) bicyclist V29.91
collision (with)
animal (traffic) V20.91
being ridden (traffic) V26.91
nontraffic V26.21
while boarding or alighting V26.31
nontraffic V20.21
while boarding or alighting V20.31
animal-drawn vehicle (traffic) V26.91
nontraffic V26.21
while boarding or alighting V26.31
bus (traffic) V24.91
nontraffic V24.21
while boarding or alighting V24.31
car (traffic) V23.91
nontraffic V23.21
while boarding or alighting V23.31
motor vehicle NOS (traffic) V29.601
nontraffic V29.201
specified type NEC (traffic) V29.691
nontraffic V29.291
pedal cycle (traffic) V21.91
nontraffic V21.21
while boarding or alighting V21.31
pedestrian V20.91
nontraffic V20.01
while boarding or alighting V20.31
pickup truck (traffic) V23.91
nontraffic V23.21
while boarding or alighting V23.31
railway vehicle (traffic) V25.91
nontraffic V25.21
while boarding or alighting V25.31
specified vehicle NEC (traffic) V26.91
nontraffic V26.21
while boarding or alighting V26.31
stationary object (traffic) V27.91
nontraffic V27.21
while boarding or alighting V27.31
streetcar (traffic) V26.91
nontraffic V26.21
while boarding or alighting V26.31
three wheeled motor vehicle (traffic) V22.91
nontraffic V22.21
while boarding or alighting V22.31
truck (traffic) V24.91
nontraffic V24.21
while boarding or alighting V24.31
two wheeled motor vehicle (traffic) V22.91
nontraffic V22.21
while boarding or alighting V22.31
van (traffic) V23.91
nontraffic V23.21
while boarding or alighting V23.31
driver
collision (with)
animal (traffic) V20.41
being ridden (traffic) V26.41
nontraffic V26.01
nontraffic V20.01
animal-drawn vehicle (traffic) V26.41
nontraffic V26.01
bus (traffic) V24.41
nontraffic V24.01

Accident (Continued)
transport (Continued)
bus occupant (Continued)
driver (Continued)
collision (Continued)
car (traffic) V23.41
nontraffic V23.01
motor vehicle NOS (traffic) V29.401
nontraffic V29.001
specified type NEC (traffic) V29.491
nontraffic V29.091
pedal cycle (traffic) V21.41
nontraffic V21.01
pedestrian
nontraffic V20.01
traffic V20.41
pickup truck (traffic) V23.41
nontraffic V23.01
railway vehicle (traffic) V25.41
nontraffic V25.01
specified vehicle NEC (traffic) V26.41
nontraffic V26.01
stationary object (traffic) V27.41
nontraffic V27.01
streetcar (traffic) V26.41
nontraffic V26.01
three wheeled motor vehicle (traffic) V22.41
nontraffic V22.01
truck (traffic) V24.41
nontraffic V24.01
two wheeled motor vehicle (traffic) V22.41
nontraffic V22.01
van (traffic) V23.41
nontraffic V23.01
noncollision accident (traffic) V28.41
nontraffic V28.01
noncollision accident (traffic) V28.91
nontraffic V28.21
while boarding or alighting V28.31
nontraffic V29.31
passenger
collision (with)
animal (traffic) V20.51
being ridden (traffic) V26.51
nontraffic V26.11
nontraffic V20.11
animal-drawn vehicle (traffic) V26.51
nontraffic V26.11
bus (traffic) V24.51
nontraffic V24.11
car (traffic) V23.51
nontraffic V23.11
motor vehicle NOS (traffic) V29.501
nontraffic V29.101
specified type NEC (traffic) V29.591
nontraffic V29.191
pedal cycle (traffic) V21.51
nontraffic V21.11
pedestrian
nontraffic V20.11
traffic V20.51
pickup truck (traffic) V23.51
nontraffic V23.11
railway vehicle (traffic) V25.51
nontraffic 25.11
specified vehicle NEC (traffic) V26.51
nontraffic V26.11
stationary object (traffic) V27.51
nontraffic V27.11
streetcar (traffic) V26.51
nontraffic V26.11
three wheeled motor vehicle (traffic) V22.51
nontraffic V22.11
truck (traffic) V24.51
nontraffic V24.11
two wheeled motor vehicle (traffic) V22.51
nontraffic V22.11
van (traffic) V23.51
nontraffic V23.11
noncollision accident (traffic) V28.51
nontraffic V28.11
specified type NEC V29.881
military vehicle V29.811
forklift —see Accident, transport, industrial vehicle occupant
go cart —see Accident, transport, all-terrain vehicle occupant

Accident (Continued)
transport (Continued)
golf cart —see Accident, transport, all-terrain vehicle occupant
heavy transport vehicle occupant —see Accident, transport, truck occupant
hoverboard V00.848
ice yacht V98.2
industrial vehicle occupant (nontraffic) V83.9
driver V83.5
hanger-on V83.7
passenger V83.6
traffic V83.3
driver V83.0
hanger-on V83.2
passenger V83.1
while boarding or alighting V83.4
interurban electric car —see Accident, transport, streetcar
land yacht V98.1
logging car —see Accident, transport, industrial vehicle occupant
military vehicle occupant (traffic) V86.34
driver V86.04
hanger-on V86.24
nontraffic V86.94
driver V86.54
hanger-on V86.74
passenger V86.64
passenger V86.14
while boarding or alighting V86.44
mine tram —see Accident, transport, industrial vehicle occupant
motor vehicle NEC occupant (traffic) V89.2
motorcoach —see Accident, transport, bus occupant
motor/cross bike rider —see also Accident, transport, dirt bike rider V86.96
motorcycle V29.99
collision (with)
animal (traffic) V20.99
being ridden (traffic) V26.99
nontraffic V26.29
while boarding or alighting V26.39
nontraffic V20.29
while boarding or alighting V20.39
animal-drawn vehicle (traffic) V26.99
nontraffic V26.29
while boarding or alighting V26.39
bus (traffic) V24.99
nontraffic V24.29
while boarding or alighting V24.39
car (traffic) V23.99
nontraffic V23.29
while boarding or alighting V23.39
motor vehicle NOS (traffic) V29.608
nontraffic V29.208
specified type NEC (traffic) V29.698
nontraffic V29.298
pedal cycle (traffic) V21.99
nontraffic V21.29
while boarding or alighting V21.39
pickup truck (traffic) V23.99
nontraffic V23.29
while boarding or alighting V23.39
railway vehicle (traffic) V25.99
nontraffic V25.29
while boarding or alighting V25.39
specified vehicle NEC (traffic) V26.99
nontraffic V26.29
while boarding or alighting V26.39
stationary object (traffic) V27.99
nontraffic V27.29
while boarding or alighting V27.39
streetcar (traffic) V26.99
nontraffic V26.29
while boarding or alighting V26.39
three wheeled motor vehicle (traffic) V22.99
nontraffic V22.29
while boarding or alighting V22.39
truck (traffic) V24.99
nontraffic V24.29
while boarding or alighting V24.39
two wheeled motor vehicle (traffic) V22.99
nontraffic V22.29
while boarding or alighting V22.39
van (traffic) V23.99
nontraffic V23.29
while boarding or alighting V23.39

▶ New   ⇒ Revised   ~~deleted~~ Deleted   ● Use Additional Character(s)

Accident *(Continued)*
transport *(Continued)*
pedal cyclist V19.9
collision (with)
animal (traffic) V10.9
being ridden (traffic) V16.9
nontraffic V16.2
while boarding or alighting
V16.3
nontraffic V10.2
while boarding or alighting V10.3
animal-drawn vehicle (traffic) V16.9
nontraffic V16.2
while boarding or alighting V16.3
bus (traffic) V14.9
nontraffic V14.2
while boarding or alighting V14.3
car (traffic) V13.9
nontraffic V13.2
while boarding or alighting V13.3
motor vehicle NOS (traffic) V19.60
nontraffic V19.20
specified type NEC (traffic) V19.69
nontraffic V19.29
pedal cycle (traffic) V11.9
nontraffic V11.2
while boarding or alighting V11.3
pickup truck (traffic) V13.9
nontraffic V13.2
while boarding or alighting V13.3
railway vehicle (traffic) V15.9
nontraffic V15.2
while boarding or alighting V15.3
specified vehicle NEC (traffic) V16.9
nontraffic V16.2
while boarding or alighting V16.3
stationary object (traffic) V17.9
nontraffic V17.2
while boarding or alighting V17.3
streetcar (traffic) V16.9
nontraffic V16.2
while boarding or alighting V16.3
three wheeled motor vehicle (traffic)
V12.9
nontraffic V12.2
while boarding or alighting V12.3
truck (traffic) V14.9
nontraffic V14.2
while boarding or alighting V14.3
two wheeled motor vehicle (traffic)
V12.9
nontraffic V12.2
while boarding or alighting V12.3
van (traffic) V13.9
nontraffic V13.2
while boarding or alighting V13.3
driver
collision (with)
animal (traffic) V10.4
being ridden (traffic) V16.4
nontraffic V16.0
nontraffic V10.0
animal-drawn vehicle (traffic) V16.4
nontraffic V16.0
bus (traffic) V14.4
nontraffic V14.0
car (traffic) V13.4
nontraffic V13.0
motor vehicle NOS (traffic) V19.40
nontraffic V19.00
specified type NEC (traffic)
V19.49
nontraffic V19.09
pedal cycle (traffic) V11.4
nontraffic V11.0
pickup truck (traffic) V13.4
nontraffic V13.0
railway vehicle (traffic) V15.4
nontraffic V15.0
specified vehicle NEC (traffic)
V16.4
nontraffic V16.0
stationary object (traffic) V17.4
nontraffic V17.0
streetcar (traffic) V16.4
nontraffic V16.0
three wheeled motor vehicle (traffic)
V12.4
nontraffic V12.0
truck (traffic) V14.4
nontraffic V14.0

Accident *(Continued)*
transport *(Continued)*
parachutist *(Continued)*
driver *(Continued)*
collision *(Continued)*
two wheeled motor vehicle (traffic)
V12.4
nontraffic V12.0
van (traffic) V13.4
nontraffic V13.0
noncollision accident (traffic) V18.4
nontraffic V18.0
noncollision accident (traffic) V18.9
nontraffic V18.2
while boarding or alighting V18.3
nontraffic V19.3
passenger
collision (with)
animal (traffic) V10.5
being ridden (traffic) V16.5
nontraffic V16.1
nontraffic V10.1
animal-drawn vehicle (traffic) V16.5
nontraffic V16.1
bus (traffic) V14.5
nontraffic V14.1
car (traffic) V13.5
nontraffic V13.1
motor vehicle NOS (traffic) V19.50
nontraffic V19.10
specified type NEC (traffic)
V19.59
nontraffic V19.19
pedal cycle (traffic) V11.5
nontraffic V11.1
pickup truck (traffic) V13.5
nontraffic V13.1
railway vehicle (traffic) V15.5
nontraffic V15.1
specified vehicle NEC (traffic) V16.5
nontraffic V16.1
stationary object (traffic) V17.5
nontraffic V17.1
streetcar (traffic) V16.5
nontraffic V16.1
three wheeled motor vehicle (traffic)
V12.5
nontraffic V12.1
truck (traffic) V14.5
nontraffic V14.1
two wheeled motor vehicle (traffic)
V12.5
nontraffic V12.1
van (traffic) V13.5
nontraffic V13.1
noncollision accident (traffic) V18.5
nontraffic V18.1
specified type NEC V19.88
military vehicle V19.81
pedestrian
conveyance (occupant) V09.9
baby stroller V00.828
collision (with) V09.9
animal being ridden or animal
drawn vehicle V06.99
nontraffic V06.09
traffic V06.19
bus or heavy transport V04.99
nontraffic V04.09
traffic V04.19
car V03.99
nontraffic V03.09
traffic V03.19
pedal cycle V01.99
nontraffic V01.09
traffic V01.19
pick-up truck or van V03.99
nontraffic V03.09
traffic V03.19
railway (train) (vehicle)
V05.99
nontraffic V05.09
traffic V05.19
stationary object V00.822
streetcar V06.99
nontraffic V06.09
traffic V06.19
two- or three-wheeled motor
vehicle V02.99
nontraffic V02.09
traffic V02.19

Accident *(Continued)*
transport *(Continued)*
pedestrian *(Continued)*
conveyance *(Continued)*
baby stroller *(Continued)*
collision *(Continued)*
vehicle V09.9
animal-drawn V06.99
nontraffic V06.09
traffic V06.19
motor
nontraffic V09.00
traffic V09.20
fall V00.821
nontraffic V09.1
involving motor vehicle NEC
V09.00
traffic V09.3
involving motor vehicle NEC
V09.20
flat-bottomed NEC V00.388
collision (with) V09.9
animal being ridden or animal
drawn vehicle V06.99
nontraffic V06.09
traffic V06.19
bus or heavy transport V04.99
nontraffic V04.09
traffic V04.19
car V03.99
nontraffic V03.09
traffic V03.19
pedal cycle V01.99
nontraffic V01.09
traffic V01.19
pick-up truck or van V03.99
nontraffic V03.09
traffic V03.19
railway (train) (vehicle) V05.99
nontraffic V05.09
traffic V05.19
stationary object V00.382
streetcar V06.99
nontraffic V06.09
traffic V06.19
two-or three-wheeled motor vehicle
V02.99
nontraffic V02.09
traffic V02.19
vehicle V09.9
animal-drawn V06.99
nontraffic V06.09
traffic V06.19
motor
nontraffic V09.00
traffic V09.20
fall V00.381
nontraffic V09.1
involving motor vehicle NEC V09.00
snow
board —*see* Accident, transport,
pedestrian, conveyance, snow
board
ski —*see* Accident, transport,
pedestrian, conveyance, skis
(snow)
traffic V09.3
involving motor vehicle NEC
V09.20
gliding type NEC V00.288
collision (with) V09.9
animal being ridden or animal
drawn vehicle V06.99
nontraffic V06.09
traffic V06.19
bus or heavy transport
V04.99
nontraffic V04.09
traffic V04.19
car V03.99
nontraffic V03.09
traffic V03.19
pedal cycle V01.99
nontraffic V01.09
traffic V01.19
pick-up truck or van V03.99
nontraffic V03.09
traffic V03.19
railway (train) (vehicle) V05.99
nontraffic V05.09
traffic V05.19

Accident (Continued)
  transport (Continued)
    pedestrian (Continued)
      conveyance (Continued)
        gliding type (Continued)
          collision (Continued)
            stationary object V00.282
            streetcar V06.99
              nontraffic V06.09
              traffic V06.19
            two- or three-wheeled motor
              vehicle V02.99
              nontraffic V02.09
              traffic V02.19
            vehicle V09.9
              animal-drawn V06.99
                nontraffic V06.09
                traffic V06.19
              motor
                nontraffic V09.00
                traffic V09.20
          fall V00.281
          heelies —see Accident, transport,
            pedestrian, conveyance,
            heelies
          hoverboard
            collision with
              animal being ridden or animal
                drawn vehicle V06.938
                nontraffic V06.038
                traffic V06.138
              bus or heavy transport
                V04.938
                nontraffic V04.038
                traffic V04.138
              car V03.938
                nontraffic V03.038
                traffic V03.138
              pedal cycle V01.938
                nontraffic V01.038
                traffic V01.138
              pick-up or van V03.938
                nontraffic V03.038
                traffic V03.138
              railway (train) (vehicle) V05.938
                nontraffic V05.038
                traffic V05.138
              streetcar V06.938
                nontraffic V06.038
                traffic V06.138
              three-wheeled motor vehicle
                V02.938
                nontraffic V02.038
                traffic V02.138
              two-wheeled motor vehicle
                V02.938
                nontraffic V02.038
                traffic V02.138
              vehicle, nonmotor, specified NEC
                V06.938
                nontraffic V06.038
                traffic V06.138
            fall V00.848
          ice skate —see Accident, transport,
            pedestrian, conveyance, ice skate
          nontraffic V09.1
            involving motor vehicle NEC
              V09.00
          Segway
            collision with
              animal being ridden or animal
                drawn vehicle V06.938
                nontraffic V06.038
                traffic V06.138
              bus or heavy transport V04.938
                nontraffic V04.038
                traffic V04.138
              car V03.938
                nontraffic V03.038
                traffic V03.138
              pedal cycle V01.938
                nontraffic V01.038
                traffic V01.138
              pick-up or van V03.038
                nontraffic V01.038
                traffic V03.138
              railway (train) (vehicle) V05.938
                nontraffic V05.038
                traffic V05.138
              streetcar V06.938
                nontraffic V06.038
                traffic V06.138

Accident (Continued)
  transport (Continued)
    pedestrian (Continued)
      conveyance (Continued)
        gliding type (Continued)
        Segway (Continued)
          collision with (Continued)
            three-wheeled motor vehicle
              V02.938
              nontraffic V02.038
               traffic V02.138
            two-wheeled motor vehicle
              V02.938
              nontraffic V02.038
               traffic V02.138
            vehicle, nonmotor, specified NEC
              V06.938
              nontraffic V06.038
              traffic V06.138
          fall V00.848
          sled —see Accident, transport,
            pedestrian, conveyance, sled
          standing
            electric scooter
              collision with
                 animal being ridden or animal
                  drawn vehicle
                  V06.931
                  nontraffic V06.031
                  traffic V06.131
                bus or heavy transport
                  V04.931
                  nontraffic V04.031
                  traffic V04.131
                car V03.931
                  nontraffic V03.031
                  traffic V03.131
                pedal cycle V01.931
                  nontraffic V01.031
                  traffic V01.131
                pick-up or van V03.931
                  nontraffic V03.031
                  traffic V03.131
                railway (train) (vehicle)
                  V05.931
                  nontraffic V05.031
                  traffic V05.131
                streetcar V06.931
                  nontraffic V06.031
                  traffic V06.131
                three-wheeled motor vehicle
                  V02.931
                  nontraffic V02.031
                  traffic V02.131
                two-wheeled motor vehicle
                  V02.931
                  nontraffic V02.031
                  traffic V02.131
                vehicle, nonmotor, specified
                  NEC V06.931
                  nontraffic V06.031
                  traffic V06.131
            fall V00.841
            micro-mobility pedestrian
              conveyance
              collision with
                 animal being ridden or animal
                  drawn vehicle
                  V06.938
                  nontraffic V06.038
                  traffic V06.138
                bus or heavy transport
                  V04.938
                  nontraffic V04.038
                  traffic V04.138
                car V03.938
                  nontraffic V03.038
                  traffic V03.138
                pedal cycle V01.938
                  nontraffic V01.038
                  traffic V01.138
                pick-up or van V03.938
                  nontraffic V03.038
                  traffic V03.138
                railway (train) (vehicle)
                  V05.938
                  nontraffic V05.038
                  traffic V05.138
                stationary object V00.842
                streetcar V06.938
                  nontraffic V06.038
                  traffic V06.138

Accident (Continued)
  transport (Continued)
    pedestrian (Continued)
      conveyance (Continued)
        gliding type (Continued)
        standing (Continued)
          micro-mobility pedestrian
            conveyance —(Continued)
            collision with (Continued)
              three-wheeled motor vehicle
              V02.938
              nontraffic V02.038
               traffic V02.138
              two-wheeled motor vehicle
              V02.938
               nontraffic V02.038
               traffic V02.138
              vehicle, nonmotor, specified
              NEC V06.938
              nontraffic V06.038
               traffic V06.138
            fall V00.848
            traffic V09.3
              involving motor vehicle NEC
                V09.20
            wheelies —see Accident, transport,
              pedestrian, conveyance,
               heelies
          heelies V00.158
            colliding with stationary object
              V00.152
            fall V00.151
          ice skates V00.218
            collision (with) V09.9
              animal being ridden or animal
                 drawn vehicle V06.99
                  nontraffic V06.09
                  traffic V06.19
              bus or heavy transport V04.99
                nontraffic V04.09
                traffic V04.19
              car V03.99
                nontraffic V03.09
                traffic V03.19
              pedal cycle V01.99
                nontraffic V01.09
                traffic V01.19
              pick-up truck or van V03.99
                nontraffic V03.09
                traffic V03.19
              railway (train) (vehicle) V05.99
                nontraffic V05.09
                traffic V05.19
              stationary object V00.212
              streetcar V06.99
                nontraffic V06.09
                traffic V06.19
              two- or three-wheeled motor
                vehicle V02.99
                nontraffic V02.09
                traffic V02.19
              vehicle V09.9
                animal-drawn V06.99
                  nontraffic V06.09
                  traffic V06.19
                motor
                  nontraffic V09.00
                  traffic V09.20
            fall V00.211
            nontraffic V09.1
              involving motor vehicle NEC
                V09.00
            traffic V09.3
               involving motor vehicle NEC
                V09.20
          motorized mobility scooter V00.838
            collision with stationary object
              V00.832
            fall from V00.831
          nontraffic V09.1
            involving motor vehicle V09.00
              military V09.01
              specified type NEC V09.09
          roller skates (non in-line) V00.128
            collision (with) V09.9
              animal being ridden or animal
                drawn vehicle V06.91
                nontraffic V06.01
                traffic V06.11
              bus or heavy transport V04.91
                nontraffic V04.01
                traffic V04.11

▶ New   ➡ Revised   ~~deleted~~ Deleted   ● Use Additional Character(s)

Accident *(Continued)*
  transport *(Continued)*
    pedestrian *(Continued)*
      conveyance *(Continued)*
        roller skates *(Continued)*
          collision *(Continued)*
            car V03.91
              nontraffic V03.01
              traffic V03.11
            pedal cycle V01.91
              nontraffic V01.01
              traffic V01.11
            pick-up truck or van V03.91
              nontraffic V03.01
              traffic V03.11
            railway (train) (vehicle) V05.91
              nontraffic V05.01
              traffic V05.11
            stationary object V00.122
            streetcar V06.91
              nontraffic V06.01
              traffic V06.11
            two- or three-wheeled motor vehicle V02.91
              nontraffic V02.01
              traffic V02.11
            vehicle V09.9
              animal-drawn V06.91
                nontraffic V06.01
                traffic V06.11
              motor
                nontraffic V09.00
                traffic V09.20
          fall V00.121
          in-line V00.118
            collision —*see also* Accident, transport, pedestrian, conveyance occupant, roller skates, collision
            with stationary object V00.112
            fall V00.111
            nontraffic V09.1
              involving motor vehicle NEC V09.00
            traffic V09.3
              involving motor vehicle NEC V09.20
        rolling shoes V00.158
         colliding with stationary object V00.152
         fall V00.151
        rolling type NEC V00.188
         collision (with) V09.9
          animal being ridden or animal drawn vehicle V06.99
           nontraffic V06.09
           traffic V06.19
          bus or heavy transport V04.99
           nontraffic V04.09
           traffic V04.19
          car V03.99
           nontraffic V03.09
           traffic V03.19
          pedal cycle V01.99
           nontraffic V01.09
           traffic V01.19
          pick-up truck or van V03.99
           nontraffic V03.09
           traffic V03.19
          railway (train) (vehicle) V05.99
           nontraffic V05.09
           traffic V05.19
          stationary object V00.182
          streetcar V06.99
           nontraffic V06.09
           traffic V06.19
          two- or three-wheeled motor vehicle V02.99
           nontraffic V02.09
           traffic V02.19
          vehicle V09.9
           animal-drawn V06.99
            nontraffic V06.09
            traffic V06.19
           motor
            nontraffic V09.00
            traffic V09.20

Accident *(Continued)*
  transport *(Continued)*
    pedestrian *(Continued)*
      conveyance *(Continued)*
        rolling type *(Continued)*
         fall V00.181
         in-line roller skate —*see* Accident, transport, pedestrian, conveyance, roller skate, in-line
         nontraffic V09.1
          involving motor vehicle NEC V09.00
         roller skate —*see* Accident, transport, pedestrian, conveyance, roller skate
         scooter (non-motorized) —*see* Accident, transport, pedestrian, conveyance, scooter
         skateboard —*see* Accident, transport, pedestrian, conveyance, skateboard
         traffic V09.3
          involving motor vehicle NEC V09.20
        scooter (non-motorized) V00.148
         collision (with) V09.9
          animal being ridden or animal drawn vehicle V06.99
           nontraffic V06.09
           traffic V06.19
          bus or heavy transport V04.99
           nontraffic V04.09
           traffic V04.19
          car V03.99
           nontraffic V03.09
           traffic V03.19
          pedal cycle V01.99
           nontraffic V01.09
           traffic V01.19
          pick-up truck or van V03.99
           nontraffic V03.09
           traffic V03.19
          railway (train) (vehicle) V05.99
           nontraffic V05.09
           traffic V05.19
          stationary object V00.142
          streetcar V06.99
           nontraffic V06.09
           traffic V06.19
          two- or three-wheeled motor vehicle V02.99
           nontraffic V02.09
           traffic V02.19
          vehicle V09.9
           animal-drawn V06.99
            nontraffic V06.09
            traffic V06.19
           motor
            nontraffic V09.00
            traffic V09.20
         fall V00.141
         nontraffic V09.1
          involving motor vehicle NEC V09.00
         traffic V09.3
          involving motor vehicle NEC V09.20
       skateboard V00.138
         collision (with) V09.9
          animal being ridden or animal drawn vehicle V06.92
           nontraffic V06.02
           traffic V06.12
          bus or heavy transport V04.92
           nontraffic V04.02
           traffic V04.12
          car V03.92
           nontraffic V03.02
           traffic V03.12
          pedal cycle V01.92
           nontraffic V01.02
           traffic V01.12
          pick-up truck or van V03.92
           nontraffic V03.02
           traffic V03.12
          railway (train) (vehicle) V05.92
           nontraffic V05.02
           traffic V05.12

Accident *(Continued)*
  transport *(Continued)*
    pedestrian *(Continued)*
      conveyance *(Continued)*
        skateboard *(Continued)*
         collision *(Continued)*
          stationary object V00.132
          streetcar V06.92
           nontraffic V06.02
           traffic V06.12
          two- or three-wheeled motor vehicle V02.92
           nontraffic V02.02
           traffic V02.12
          vehicle V09.9
           animal-drawn V06.92
            nontraffic V06.02
            traffic V06.12
           motor
            nontraffic V09.00
            traffic V09.20
         fall V00.131
         nontraffic V09.1
          involving motor vehicle NEC V09.00
         traffic V09.3
          involving motor vehicle NEC V09.20
       skis (snow) V00.328
         collision (with) V09.9
          animal being ridden or animal drawn vehicle V06.99
           nontraffic V06.09
           traffic V06.19
          bus or heavy transport V04.99
           nontraffic V04.09
           traffic V04.19
          car V03.99
           nontraffic V03.09
           traffic V03.19
          pedal cycle V01.99
           nontraffic V01.09
           traffic V01.19
          pick-up truck or van V03.99
           nontraffic V03.09
           traffic V03.19
          railway (train) (vehicle) V05.99
           nontraffic V05.09
           traffic V05.19
          stationary object V00.322
          streetcar V06.99
           nontraffic V06.09
           traffic V06.19
          two- or three-wheeled motor vehicle V02.99
           nontraffic V02.09
           traffic V02.19
          vehicle V09.9
           animal-drawn V06.99
            nontraffic V06.09
            traffic V06.19
           motor
            nontraffic V09.00
            traffic V09.20
         fall V00.321
         nontraffic V09.1
          involving motor vehicle NEC V09.00
         traffic V09.3
          involving motor vehicle NEC V09.20
       sled V00.228
         collision (with) V09.9
          animal being ridden or animal drawn vehicle V06.99
           nontraffic V06.09
           traffic V06.19
          bus or heavy transport V04.99
           nontraffic V04.09
           traffic V04.19
          car V03.99
           nontraffic V03.09
           traffic V03.19
          pedal cycle V01.99
           nontraffic V01.09
           traffic V01.19
          pick-up truck or van V03.99
           nontraffic V03.09
           traffic V03.19
          railway (train) (vehicle) V05.99
           nontraffic V05.09
           traffic V05.19

▶ New   ⟹ Revised   ~~deleted~~ Deleted   ● Use Additional Character(s)

Accident (*Continued*)
  transport (*Continued*)
    pedestrian (*Continued*)
      pickup truck occupant (*Continued*)
        specified vehicle NEC (traffic) V56.9
          nontraffic V56.3
          while boarding or alighting V56.4
        stationary object (traffic) V57.9
          nontraffic V57.3
          while boarding or alighting V57.4
        streetcar (traffic) V56.9
          nontraffic V56.3
          while boarding or alighting V56.4
        three wheeled motor vehicle (traffic)
          V52.9
          nontraffic V52.3
          while boarding or alighting V52.4
        truck (traffic) V54.9
          nontraffic V54.3
          while boarding or alighting V54.4
        two wheeled motor vehicle (traffic) V52.9
          nontraffic V52.3
          while boarding or alighting V52.4
        van (traffic) V53.9
          nontraffic V53.3
          while boarding or alighting V53.4
      driver
        collision (with)
          animal (traffic) V50.5
            being ridden (traffic) V56.5
              nontraffic V56.0
            nontraffic V50.0
          animal-drawn vehicle (traffic)
            V56.5
            nontraffic V56.0
          bus (traffic) V54.5
            nontraffic V54.0
          car (traffic) V53.5
            nontraffic V53.0
          motor vehicle NOS (traffic) V59.40
            nontraffic V59.00
            specified type NEC (traffic) V59.49
              nontraffic V59.09
          pedal cycle (traffic) V51.5
            nontraffic V51.0
          pickup truck (traffic) V53.5
            nontraffic V53.0
          railway vehicle (traffic) V55.5
            nontraffic V55.0
          specified vehicle NEC (traffic) V56.5
            nontraffic V56.0
          stationary object (traffic) V57.5
            nontraffic V57.0
          streetcar (traffic) V56.5
            nontraffic V56.0
          three wheeled motor vehicle (traffic)
            V52.5
            nontraffic V52.0
          truck (traffic) V54.5
            nontraffic V54.0
          two wheeled motor vehicle (traffic)
            V52.5
            nontraffic V52.0
          van (traffic) V53.5
            nontraffic V53.0
        noncollision accident (traffic) V58.5
          nontraffic V58.0
      hanger-on
        collision (with)
          animal (traffic) V50.7
            being ridden (traffic) V56.7
              nontraffic V56.2
            nontraffic V50.2
          animal-drawn vehicle (traffic) V56.7
            nontraffic V56.2
          bus (traffic) V54.7
            nontraffic V54.2
          car (traffic) V53.7
            nontraffic V53.2
          pedal cycle (traffic) V51.7
            nontraffic V51.2
          pickup truck (traffic) V53.7
            nontraffic V53.2
          railway vehicle (traffic) V55.7
            nontraffic V55.2
          specified vehicle NEC (traffic) V56.7
            nontraffic V56.2
          stationary object (traffic) V57.7
            nontraffic V57.2
          streetcar (traffic) V56.7
            nontraffic V56.2

Accident (*Continued*)
  transport (*Continued*)
    pedestrian (*Continued*)
      hanger-on (*Continued*)
        collision (*Continued*)
          three wheeled motor vehicle (traffic)
            V52.7
            nontraffic V52.2
          truck (traffic) V54.7
            nontraffic V54.2
          two wheeled motor vehicle (traffic)
            V52.7
            nontraffic V52.2
          van (traffic) V53.7
            nontraffic V53.2
        noncollision accident (traffic) V58.7
          nontraffic V58.2
      noncollision accident (traffic) V58.9
        nontraffic V58.3
        while boarding or alighting V58.4
      nontraffic V59.3
      passenger
        collision (with)
          animal (traffic) V50.6
            being ridden (traffic) V56.6
              nontraffic V56.1
            nontraffic V50.1
          animal-drawn vehicle (traffic) V56.6
            nontraffic V56.1
          bus (traffic) V54.6
            nontraffic V54.1
          car (traffic) V53.6
            nontraffic V53.1
          motor vehicle NOS (traffic) V59.50
            nontraffic V59.10
            specified type NEC (traffic) V59.59
              nontraffic V59.19
          pedal cycle (traffic) V51.6
            nontraffic V51.1
          pickup truck (traffic) V53.6
            nontraffic V53.1
          railway vehicle (traffic) V55.6
            nontraffic V55.1
          specified vehicle NEC (traffic) V56.6
            nontraffic V56.1
          stationary object (traffic) V57.6
            nontraffic V57.1
          streetcar (traffic) V56.6
            nontraffic V56.1
          three wheeled motor vehicle (traffic)
            V52.6
            nontraffic V52.1
          truck (traffic) V54.6
            nontraffic V54.1
          two wheeled motor vehicle (traffic)
            V52.6
            nontraffic V52.1
          van (traffic) V53.6
            nontraffic V53.1
        noncollision accident (traffic) V58.6
          nontraffic V58.1
        specified type NEC V59.88
        military vehicle V59.81
      quarry truck —*see* Accident, transport,
        industrial vehicle occupant
      race car —*see* Accident, transport, motor
        vehicle NEC occupant
      railway vehicle occupant V81.9
        collision (with) V81.3
          motor vehicle (non-military) (traffic)
            V81.1
            military V81.83
            nontraffic V81.0
          rolling stock V81.2
          specified object NEC V81.3
        during derailment V81.7
          with antecedent collision —*see* Accident,
            transport, railway vehicle occupant,
            collision
        explosion V81.81
        fall (in railway vehicle) V81.5
          during derailment V81.7
           with antecedent collision —*see*
            Accident, transport, railway
            vehicle occupant, collision
        from railway vehicle V81.6
          during derailment V81.7
           with antecedent collision —*see*
            Accident, transport, railway
            vehicle occupant, collision
        while boarding or alighting V81.4

Accident (*Continued*)
  transport (*Continued*)
    railway vehicle occupan (*Continued*)
      fire V81.81
      object falling onto train V81.82
      specified type NEC V81.89
      while boarding or alighting V81.4
    Segway V00.848
    ski lift V98.3
    snowmobile occupant (nontraffic) V86.92
      driver V86.52
      hanger-on V86.72
      passenger V86.62
      traffic V86.32
        driver V86.02
        hanger-on V86.22
        passenger V86.12
      while boarding or alighting V86.42
    specified NEC V98.8
    sport utility vehicle occupant —*see also*
      Accident, transport, pickup truck
      occupant
    streetcar occupant V82.9
      collision (with) V82.3
        motor vehicle (traffic) V82.1
          nontraffic V82.0
        rolling stock V82.2
      during derailment V82.7
        with antecedent collision —*see* Accident,
          transport, streetcar occupant,
          collision
      fall (in streetcar) V82.5
        during derailment V82.7
          with antecedent collision —*see*
           Accident, transport, streetcar
           occupant, collision
        from streetcar V82.6
          during derailment V82.7
           with antecedent collision —*see*
            Accident, transport, streetcar
            occupant, collision
          while boarding or alighting
           V82.4
      while boarding or alighting V82.4
      specified type NEC V82.8
      while boarding or alighting V82.4
    three-wheeled motor vehicle occupant V39.9
      collision (with)
        animal (traffic) V30.9
          being ridden (traffic) V36.9
           nontraffic V36.3
           while boarding or alighting V36.4
          nontraffic V30.3
          while boarding or alighting V30.4
        animal-drawn vehicle (traffic) V36.9
          nontraffic V36.3
          while boarding or alighting V36.4
        bus (traffic) V34.9
          nontraffic V34.3
          while boarding or alighting V34.4
        car (traffic) V33.9
          nontraffic V33.3
          while boarding or alighting V33.4
        motor vehicle NOS (traffic) V39.60
          nontraffic V39.20
          specified type NEC (traffic) V39.69
           nontraffic V39.29
        pedal cycle (traffic) V31.9
          nontraffic V31.3
          while boarding or alighting
           V31.4
        pickup truck (traffic) V33.9
          nontraffic V33.3
          while boarding or alighting
           V33.4
        railway vehicle (traffic) V35.9
          nontraffic V35.3
          while boarding or alighting V35.4
        specified vehicle NEC (traffic) V36.9
          nontraffic V36.3
          while boarding or alighting V36.4
        stationary object (traffic) V37.9
          nontraffic V37.3
          while boarding or alighting V37.4
        streetcar (traffic) V36.9
          nontraffic V36.3
          while boarding or alighting V36.4
        three wheeled motor vehicle (traffic)
          V32.9
          nontraffic V32.3
          while boarding or alighting V32.4

Accident (*Continued*)
  transport (*Continued*)
    three-wheeled motor vehicle
      occupant—(*Continued*)
      collision (*Continued*)
        truck (traffic) V34.9
          nontraffic V34.3
          while boarding or alighting V34.4
        two wheeled motor vehicle (traffic) V32.9
          nontraffic V32.3
          while boarding or alighting V32.4
        van (traffic) V33.9
          nontraffic V33.3
          while boarding or alighting V33.4
      driver
        collision (with)
          animal (traffic) V30.5
            being ridden (traffic) V36.5
              nontraffic V36.0
            nontraffic V30.0
          animal-drawn vehicle (traffic) V36.5
            nontraffic V36.0
          bus (traffic) V34.5
            nontraffic V34.0
          car (traffic) V33.5
            nontraffic V33.0
          motor vehicle NOS (traffic) V39.40
            nontraffic V39.00
            specified type NEC (traffic) V39.49
              nontraffic V39.09
          pedal cycle (traffic) V31.5
            nontraffic V31.0
          pickup truck (traffic) V33.5
            nontraffic V33.0
          railway vehicle (traffic) V35.5
            nontraffic V35.0
          specified vehicle NEC (traffic)
            V36.5
            nontraffic V36.0
          stationary object (traffic) V37.5
            nontraffic V37.0
          streetcar (traffic) V36.5
            nontraffic V36.0
          three wheeled motor vehicle (traffic)
            V32.5
            nontraffic V32.0
          truck (traffic) V34.5
            nontraffic V34.0
          two wheeled motor vehicle (traffic)
            V32.5
            nontraffic V32.0
          van (traffic) V33.5
            nontraffic V33.0
        noncollision accident (traffic) V38.5
          nontraffic V38.0
      hanger-on
        collision (with)
          animal (traffic) V30.7
            being ridden (traffic) V36.7
              nontraffic V36.2
            nontraffic V30.2
          animal-drawn vehicle (traffic) V36.7
            nontraffic V36.2
          bus (traffic) V34.7
            nontraffic V34.2
          car (traffic) V33.7
            nontraffic V33.2
          pedal cycle (traffic) V31.7
            nontraffic V31.2
          pickup truck (traffic) V33.7
            nontraffic V33.2
          railway vehicle (traffic) V35.7
            nontraffic V35.2
          specified vehicle NEC (traffic) V36.7
            nontraffic V36.2
          stationary object (traffic) V37.7
            nontraffic V37.2
          streetcar (traffic) V36.7
            nontraffic V36.2
          three wheeled motor vehicle (traffic)
            V32.7
            nontraffic V32.2
          truck (traffic) V34.7
            nontraffic V34.2
          two wheeled motor vehicle (traffic)
            V32.7
            nontraffic V32.2
          van (traffic) V33.7
            nontraffic V33.2
        noncollision accident (traffic) V38.7
          nontraffic V38.2

Accident (*Continued*)
  transport (*Continued*)
    three-wheeled motor vehicle
      occupant—(*Continued*)
      noncollision accident (traffic) V38.9
        nontraffic V38.3
        while boarding or alighting V38.4
      nontraffic V39.3
      passenger
        collision (with)
          animal (traffic) V30.6
            being ridden (traffic) V36.6
              nontraffic V36.1
            nontraffic V30.1
          animal-drawn vehicle (traffic) V36.6
            nontraffic V36.1
          bus (traffic) V34.6
            nontraffic V34.1
          car (traffic) V33.6
            nontraffic V33.1
          motor vehicle NOS (traffic) V39.50
            nontraffic V39.10
            specified type NEC (traffic) V39.59
              nontraffic V39.19
          pedal cycle (traffic) V31.6
            nontraffic V31.1
          pickup truck (traffic) V33.6
            nontraffic V33.1
          railway vehicle (traffic) V35.6
            nontraffic V35.1
          specified vehicle NEC (traffic) V36.6
            nontraffic V36.1
          stationary object (traffic) V37.6
            nontraffic V37.1
          streetcar (traffic) V36.6
            nontraffic V36.1
          three wheeled motor vehicle (traffic)
            V32.6
            nontraffic V32.1
          truck (traffic) V34.6
            nontraffic V34.1
          two wheeled motor vehicle (traffic)
            V32.6
            nontraffic V32.1
          van (traffic) V33.6
            nontraffic V33.1
        noncollision accident (traffic) V38.6
          nontraffic V38.1
      specified type NEC V39.89
        military vehicle V39.81
    tractor (farm) (and trailer) —*see* Accident,
      transport, agricultural vehicle occupant
    tram —*see* Accident, transport, streetcar
      in mine or quarry —*see* Accident, transport,
        industrial vehicle occupant
    trolley —*see* Accident, transport, streetcar
      in mine or quarry —*see* Accident, transport,
        industrial vehicle occupant
    truck (heavy) occupant V69.9
      collision (with)
        animal (traffic) V60.9
          being ridden (traffic) V66.9
            nontraffic V66.3
            while boarding or alighting V66.4
          nontraffic V60.3
          while boarding or alighting V60.4
        animal-drawn vehicle (traffic) V66.9
          nontraffic V66.3
          while boarding or alighting V66.4
        bus (traffic) V64.9
          nontraffic V64.3
          while boarding or alighting V64.4
        car (traffic) V63.9
          nontraffic V63.3
          while boarding or alighting V63.4
        motor vehicle NOS (traffic) V69.60
          nontraffic V69.20
          specified type NEC (traffic) V69.69
            nontraffic V69.29
        pedal cycle (traffic) V61.9
          nontraffic V61.3
          while boarding or alighting V61.4
        pickup truck (traffic) V63.9
          nontraffic V63.3
          while boarding or alighting V63.4
        railway vehicle (traffic) V65.9
          nontraffic V65.3
          while boarding or alighting V65.4
        specified vehicle NEC (traffic) V66.9
          nontraffic V66.3
          while boarding or alighting V66.4

Accident (*Continued*)
  transport (*Continued*)
    truck (heavy) occupant (*Continued*)
      collision (*Continued*)
        stationary object (traffic) V67.9
          nontraffic V67.3
          while boarding or alighting V67.4
        streetcar (traffic) V66.9
          nontraffic V66.3
          while boarding or alighting V66.4
        three wheeled motor vehicle (traffic)
          V62.9
          nontraffic V62.3
          while boarding or alighting V62.4
        truck (traffic) V64.9
          nontraffic V64.3
          while boarding or alighting V64.4
        two wheeled motor vehicle (traffic) V62.9
          nontraffic V62.3
          while boarding or alighting V62.4
        van (traffic) V63.9
          nontraffic V63.3
          while boarding or alighting V63.4
      driver
        collision (with)
          animal (traffic) V60.5
            being ridden (traffic) V66.5
              nontraffic V66.0
            nontraffic V60.0
          animal-drawn vehicle (traffic) V66.5
            nontraffic V66.0
          bus (traffic) V64.5
            nontraffic V64.0
          car (traffic) V63.5
            nontraffic V63.0
          motor vehicle NOS (traffic) V69.40
            nontraffic V69.00
            specified type NEC (traffic)
              V69.49
              nontraffic V69.09
          pedal cycle (traffic) V61.5
            nontraffic V61.0
          pickup truck (traffic) V63.5
            nontraffic V63.0
          railway vehicle (traffic) V65.5
            nontraffic V65.0
          specified vehicle NEC (traffic) V66.5
            nontraffic V66.0
          stationary object (traffic) V67.5
            nontraffic V67.0
          streetcar (traffic) V66.5
            nontraffic V66.0
          three wheeled motor vehicle (traffic)
            V62.5
            nontraffic V62.0
          truck (traffic) V64.5
            nontraffic V64.0
          two wheeled motor vehicle (traffic)
            V62.5
            nontraffic V62.0
          van (traffic) V63.5
            nontraffic V63.0
        noncollision accident (traffic) V68.5
          nontraffic V68.0
      dump —*see* Accident, transport,
        construction vehicle occupant
      hanger-on
        collision (with)
          animal (traffic) V60.7
            being ridden (traffic) V66.7
              nontraffic V66.2
            nontraffic V60.2
          animal-drawn vehicle (traffic)
            V66.7
            nontraffic V66.2
          bus (traffic) V64.7
            nontraffic V64.2
          car (traffic) V63.7
            nontraffic V63.2
          pedal cycle (traffic) V61.7
            nontraffic V61.2
          pickup truck (traffic) V63.7
            nontraffic V63.2
          railway vehicle (traffic) V65.7
            nontraffic V65.2
          specified vehicle NEC (traffic) V66.7
            nontraffic V66.2
          stationary object (traffic) V67.7
            nontraffic V67.2
          streetcar (traffic) V66.7
            nontraffic V66.2

▶ New   ⇒ Revised   ~~deleted~~ Deleted   ● Use Additional Character(s)

Accident *(Continued)*
  transport *(Continued)*
    truck (heavy) occupant *(Continued)*
      hanger-on *(Continued)*
        collision *(Continued)*
          three wheeled motor vehicle (traffic) V62.7
            nontraffic V62.2
          truck (traffic) V64.7
            nontraffic V64.2
          two wheeled motor vehicle (traffic) V62.7
            nontraffic V62.2
          van (traffic) V63.7
            nontraffic V63.2
        noncollision accident (traffic) V68.7
          nontraffic V68.2
      noncollision accident (traffic) V68.9
        nontraffic V68.3
        while boarding or alighting V68.4
      nontraffic V69.3
      passenger
        collision (with)
          animal (traffic) V60.6
            being ridden (traffic) V66.6
              nontraffic V66.1
            nontraffic V60.1
          animal-drawn vehicle (traffic) V66.6
            nontraffic V66.1
          bus (traffic) V64.6
            nontraffic V64.1
          car (traffic) V63.6
            nontraffic V63.1
          motor vehicle NOS (traffic) V69.50
            nontraffic V69.10
            specified type NEC (traffic) V69.59
              nontraffic V69.19
          pedal cycle (traffic) V61.6
            nontraffic V61.1
          pickup truck (traffic) V63.6
            nontraffic V63.1
          railway vehicle (traffic) V65.6
            nontraffic V65.1
          specified vehicle NEC (traffic) V66.6
            nontraffic V66.1
          stationary object (traffic) V67.6
            nontraffic V67.1
          streetcar (traffic) V66.6
            nontraffic V66.1
          three wheeled motor vehicle (traffic) V62.6
            nontraffic V62.1
          truck (traffic) V64.6
            nontraffic V64.1
          two wheeled motor vehicle (traffic) V62.6
            nontraffic V62.1
          van (traffic) V63.6
            nontraffic V63.1
        noncollision accident (traffic) V68.6
          nontraffic V68.1
    pickup —*see* Accident, transport, pickup truck occupant
    specified type NEC V69.88
      military vehicle V69.81
    van occupant V59.9
      collision (with)
        animal (traffic) V50.9
          being ridden (traffic) V56.9
            nontraffic V56.3
            while boarding or alighting V56.4
          nontraffic V50.3
          while boarding or alighting V50.4
        animal-drawn vehicle (traffic) V56.9
          nontraffic V56.3
          while boarding or alighting V56.4
        bus (traffic) V54.9
          nontraffic V54.3
          while boarding or alighting V54.4
        car (traffic) V53.9
          nontraffic V53.3
          while boarding or alighting V53.4
        motor vehicle NOS (traffic) V59.60
          nontraffic V59.20
          specified type NEC (traffic) V59.69
            nontraffic V59.29
        pedal cycle (traffic) V51.9
          nontraffic V51.3
          while boarding or alighting V51.4

Accident *(Continued)*
  transport *(Continued)*
    van occupant *(Continued)*
      collision *(Continued)*
        pickup truck (traffic) V53.9
          nontraffic V53.3
          while boarding or alighting V53.4
        railway vehicle (traffic) V55.9
          nontraffic V55.3
          while boarding or alighting V55.4
        specified vehicle NEC (traffic) V56.9
          nontraffic V56.3
          while boarding or alighting V56.4
        stationary object (traffic) V57.9
          nontraffic V57.3
          while boarding or alighting V57.4
        streetcar (traffic) V56.9
          nontraffic V56.3
          while boarding or alighting V56.4
        three wheeled motor vehicle (traffic) V52.9
          nontraffic V52.3
          while boarding or alighting V52.4
        truck (traffic) V54.9
          nontraffic V54.3
          while boarding or alighting V54.4
        two wheeled motor vehicle (traffic) V52.9
          nontraffic V52.3
          while boarding or alighting V52.4
        van (traffic) V53.9
          nontraffic V53.3
          while boarding or alighting V53.4
      driver
        collision (with)
          animal (traffic) V50.5
            being ridden (traffic) V56.5
              nontraffic V56.0
            nontraffic V50.0
          animal-drawn vehicle (traffic) V56.5
            nontraffic V56.0
          bus (traffic) V54.5
            nontraffic V54.0
          car (traffic) V53.5
            nontraffic V53.0
          motor vehicle NOS (traffic) V59.40
            nontraffic V59.00
            specified type NEC (traffic) V59.49
              nontraffic V59.09
          pedal cycle (traffic) V51.5
            nontraffic V51.0
          pickup truck (traffic) V53.5
            nontraffic V53.0
          railway vehicle (traffic) V55.5
            nontraffic V55.0
          specified vehicle NEC (traffic) V56.5
            nontraffic V56.0
          stationary object (traffic) V57.5
            nontraffic V57.0
          streetcar (traffic) V56.5
            nontraffic V56.0
          three wheeled motor vehicle (traffic) V52.5
            nontraffic V52.0
          truck (traffic) V54.5
            nontraffic V54.0
          two wheeled motor vehicle (traffic) V52.5
            nontraffic V52.0
          van (traffic) V53.5
            nontraffic V53.0
        noncollision accident (traffic) V58.5
          nontraffic V58.0
      hanger-on
        collision (with)
          animal (traffic) V50.7
            being ridden (traffic) V56.7
              nontraffic V56.2
            nontraffic V50.2
          animal-drawn vehicle (traffic) V56.7
            nontraffic V56.2
          bus (traffic) V54.7
            nontraffic V54.2
          car (traffic) V53.7
            nontraffic V53.2
          pedal cycle (traffic) V51.7
            nontraffic V51.2
          pickup truck (traffic) V53.7
            nontraffic V53.2
          railway vehicle (traffic) V55.7
            nontraffic V55.2

Accident *(Continued)*
  transport *(Continued)*
    van occupant *(Continued)*
      hanger-on *(Continued)*
        collision *(Continued)*
          specified vehicle NEC (traffic) V56.7
            nontraffic V56.2
          stationary object (traffic) V57.7
            nontraffic V57.2
          streetcar (traffic) V56.7
            nontraffic V56.2
          three wheeled motor vehicle (traffic) V52.7
            nontraffic V52.2
          truck (traffic) V54.7
            nontraffic V54.2
          two wheeled motor vehicle (traffic) V52.7
            nontraffic V52.2
          van (traffic) V53.7
            nontraffic V53.2
        noncollision accident (traffic) V58.7
          nontraffic V58.2
      noncollision accident (traffic) V58.9
        nontraffic V58.3
        while boarding or alighting V58.4
      nontraffic V59.3
      passenger
        collision (with)
          animal (traffic) V50.6
            being ridden (traffic) V56.6
              nontraffic V56.1
            nontraffic V50.1
          animal-drawn vehicle (traffic) V56.6
            nontraffic V56.1
          bus (traffic) V54.6
            nontraffic V54.1
          car (traffic) V53.6
            nontraffic V53.1
          motor vehicle NOS (traffic) V59.50
            nontraffic V59.10
            specified type NEC (traffic) V59.59
              nontraffic V59.19
          pedal cycle (traffic) V51.6
            nontraffic V51.1
          pickup truck (traffic) V53.6
            nontraffic V53.1
          railway vehicle (traffic) V55.6
            nontraffic V55.1
          specified vehicle NEC (traffic) V56.6
            nontraffic V56.1
          stationary object (traffic) V57.6
            nontraffic V57.1
          streetcar (traffic) V56.6
            nontraffic V56.1
          three wheeled motor vehicle (traffic) V52.6
            nontraffic V52.1
          truck (traffic) V54.6
            nontraffic V54.1
          two wheeled motor vehicle (traffic) V52.6
            nontraffic V52.1
          van (traffic) V53.6
            nontraffic V53.1
        noncollision accident (traffic) V58.6
          nontraffic V58.1
      specified type NEC V59.88
        military vehicle V59.81
    watercraft occupant —*see* Accident, watercraft
    vehicle NEC V89.9
      animal-drawn NEC —*see* Accident, transport, animal-drawn vehicle occupant
      special
        agricultural —*see* Accident, transport, agricultural vehicle occupant
        construction —*see* Accident, transport, construction vehicle occupant
        industrial —*see* Accident, transport, industrial vehicle occupant
        three-wheeled NEC (motorized) —*see* Accident, transport, three-wheeled motor vehicle occupant
    watercraft V94.9
      causing
        drowning —*see* Drowning, due to, accident to, watercraft
        injury NEC V91.89
          crushed between craft and object V91.19
            powered craft V91.13
              ferry boat V91.11
              fishing boat V91.12

Accident *(Continued)*
  watercraft *(Continued)*
    causing *(Continued)*
      injury *(Continued)*
        crushed between craft and
          object— *(Continued)*
          powered craft *(Continued)*
            jet ski V91.13
            liner V91.11
            merchant ship V91.10
            passenger ship V91.11
          unpowered craft V91.18
            canoe V91.15
            inflatable V91.16
            kayak V91.15
            sailboat V91.14
            surf-board V91.18
            windsurfer V91.18
        fall on board V91.29
          powered craft V91.23
            ferry boat V91.21
            fishing boat V91.22
            jet ski V91.23
            liner V91.21
            merchant ship V91.20
            passenger ship V91.21
          unpowered craft
            canoe V91.25
            inflatable V91.26
            kayak V91.25
            sailboat V91.24
        fire on board causing burn V91.09
          powered craft V91.03
            ferry boat V91.01
            fishing boat V91.02
            jet ski V91.03
            liner V91.01
            merchant ship V91.00
            passenger ship V91.01
          unpowered craft V91.08
            canoe V91.05
            inflatable V91.06
            kayak V91.05
            sailboat V91.04
            surf-board V91.08
            water skis V91.07
            windsurfer V91.08
        hit by falling object V91.39
          powered craft V91.33
            ferry boat V91.31
            fishing boat V91.32
            jet skis V91.33
            liner V91.31
            merchant ship V91.30
            passenger ship V91.31
          unpowered craft V91.38
            canoe V91.35
            inflatable V91.36
            kayak V91.35
            sailboat V91.34
            surf-board V91.38
            water skis V91.37
            windsurfer V91.38
        specified type NEC V91.89
          powered craft V91.83
            ferry boat V91.81
            fishing boat V91.82
            jet ski V91.83
            liner V91.81
            merchant ship V91.80
            passenger ship V91.81
          unpowered craft V91.88
            canoe V91.85
            inflatable V91.86
            kayak V91.85
            sailboat V91.84
            surf-board V91.88
            water skis V91.87
            windsurfer V91.88
    due to, caused by cataclysm —*see* Forces of
      nature, by type
    military NEC V94.818
      with civilian watercraft V94.810
      civilian in water injured by V94.811
    nonpowered, struck by
      nonpowered vessel V94.21
      powered vessel V94.22
    specified type NEC V94.89
    striking swimmer
      powered V94.11
      unpowered V94.12

Acid throwing (assault) Y08.89
Activity (involving) (of victim at time of event) Y93.9
  aerobic and step exercise (class) Y93.A3
  alpine skiing Y93.23
  animal care NEC Y93.K9
  arts and handcrafts NEC Y93.D9
  athletics NEC Y93.79
  athletics played as a team or group NEC Y93.69
  athletics played individually NEC Y93.59
  baking Y93.G3
  ▶ badminton Y93.73
  ballet Y93.41
  barbells Y93.B3
  BASE (Building, Antenna, Span, Earth) jumping
    Y93.33
  baseball Y93.64
  basketball Y93.67
  bathing (personal) Y93.E1
  beach volleyball Y93.68
  bike riding Y93.55
  blackout game Y93.85
  boogie boarding Y93.18
  bowling Y93.54
  boxing Y93.71
  brass instrument playing Y93.J4
  building construction Y93.H3
  bungee jumping Y93.34
  calisthenics Y93.A2
  canoeing (in calm and turbulent water) Y93.16
  capture the flag Y93.6A
  cardiorespiratory exercise NEC Y93.A9
  caregiving (providing) NEC Y93.F9
    bathing Y93.F1
    lifting Y93.F2
  cellular
    communication device Y93.C2
    telephone Y93.C2
  challenge course Y93.A5
  cheerleading Y93.45
  choking game Y93.85
  circuit training Y93.A4
  cleaning
    floor Y93.E5
  climbing NEC Y93.39
    mountain Y93.31
    rock Y93.31
    wall Y93.31
  clothing care and maintenance NEC Y93.E9
  combatives Y93.75
  computer
    keyboarding Y93.C1
    technology NEC Y93.C9
  confidence course Y93.A5
  construction (building) Y93.H3
  cooking and baking Y93.G3
  cool down exercises Y93.A2
  cricket Y93.69
  crocheting Y93.D1
  cross country skiing Y93.24
  dancing (all types) Y93.41
  digging
    dirt Y93.H1
  dirt digging Y93.H1
  dishwashing Y93.G1
  diving (platform) (springboard) Y93.12
    underwater Y93.15
  dodge ball Y93.6A
  downhill skiing Y93.23
  drum playing Y93.J2
  dumbbells Y93.B3
  electronic
    devices NEC Y93.C9
      hand held interactive Y93.C2
    game playing (using) (with)
      interactive device Y93.C2
      keyboard or other stationary device Y93.C1
  elliptical machine Y93.A1
  exercise(s)
    machines ((primarily) for)
      cardiorespiratory conditioning Y93.A1
      muscle strengthening Y93.B1
    muscle strengthening (non-machine) NEC
      Y93.B9
  external motion NEC Y93.I9
    rollercoaster Y93.I1
  fainting game Y93.85
  field hockey Y93.65
  figure skating (pairs) (singles) Y93.21
  flag football Y93.62
  floor mopping and cleaning Y93.E5
  food preparation and clean up Y93.G1

Activity *(Continued)*
  football (American) NOS Y93.61
    flag Y93.62
    tackle Y93.61
    touch Y93.62
  four square Y93.6A
  free weights Y93.B3
  frisbee (ultimate) Y93.74
  furniture
    building Y93.D3
    finishing Y93.D3
    repair Y93.D3
  game playing (electronic)
    using interactive device Y93.C2
    using keyboard or other stationary device
      Y93.C1
  gardening Y93.H2
  golf Y93.53
  grass drills Y93.A6
  grilling and smoking food Y93.G2
  grooming and shearing an animal Y93.K3
  guerilla drills Y93.A6
  gymnastics (rhythmic) Y93.43
  hand held interactive electronic device Y93.C2
  handball Y93.73
  handcrafts NEC Y93.D9
  hang gliding Y93.35
  hiking (on level or elevated terrain) Y93.01
  hockey (ice) Y93.22
    field Y93.65
  horseback riding Y93.52
  household (interior) maintenance NEC Y93.E9
  ice NEC Y93.29
    dancing Y93.21
    hockey Y93.22
    skating Y93.21
  inline roller skating Y93.51
  ironing Y93.E4
  judo Y93.75
  jumping (off) NEC Y93.39
    BASE (Building, Antenna, Span, Earth) Y93.33
    bungee Y93.34
    jacks Y93.A2
    rope Y93.56
  jumping jacks Y93.A2
  jumping rope Y93.56
  karate Y93.75
  kayaking (in calm and turbulent water) Y93.16
  keyboarding (computer) Y93.C1
  kickball Y93.6A
  knitting Y93.D1
  lacrosse Y93.65
  land maintenance NEC Y93.H9
  landscaping Y93.H2
  laundry Y93.E2
  machines (exercise)
    primarily for cardiorespiratory conditioning
      Y93.A1
    primarily for muscle strengthening Y93.B1
  maintenance
    exterior building NEC Y93.H9
    household (interior) NEC Y93.E9
    land Y93.H9
    property Y93.H9
  marching (on level or elevated terrain) Y93.01
  martial arts Y93.75
  microwave oven Y93.G3
  milking an animal Y93.K2
  mopping (floor) Y93.E5
  mountain climbing Y93.31
  muscle strengthening
    exercises (non-machine) NEC Y93.B9
    machines Y93.B1
  musical keyboard (electronic) playing Y93.J1
  nordic skiing Y93.24
  obstacle course Y93.A5
  ▶ outdoor, specified NEC Y93.L9
  oven (microwave) Y93.G3
  packing up and unpacking in moving to a new
    residence Y93.E6
  parasailing Y93.19
  pass out game Y93.85
  percussion instrument playing NEC Y93.J2
  personal
    bathing and showering Y93.E1
    hygiene NEC Y93.E8
    showering Y93.E1
  physical games generally associated with school
    recess, summer camp and children Y93.6A
  physical training NEC Y93.A9
  piano playing Y93.J1

Assault *(Continued)*
  steam X98.0
  striking against
    other person Y04.2
    sports equipment Y08.09
      baseball bat Y08.02
      hockey stick Y08.01
  struck by
    sports equipment Y08.09
      baseball bat Y08.02
      hockey stick Y08.01
  submersion —*see* Assault, drowning
  violence Y09
  weapon Y09
    blunt Y00
    cutting or piercing —*see* Assault, cutting or
      piercing instrument
    firearm —*see* Assault, firearm
  wound Y09
    cutting —*see* Assault, cutting or piercing
      instrument
    gunshot —*see* Assault, firearm
    knife X99.1
    piercing —*see* Assault, cutting or piercing
      instrument
    puncture —*see* Assault, cutting or piercing
      instrument
    stab —*see* Assault, cutting or piercing
      instrument
Attack by mammals NEC W55.89
Avalanche —*see* Landslide
Aviator's disease —*see* Air, pressure

B

Barotitis, barodontalgia, barosinusitis,
  barotrauma (otitic) (sinus) —*see* Air, pressure
Battered (baby) (child) (person) (syndrome)
  X58
Bayonet wound W26.1
  in
    legal intervention —*see* Legal, intervention,
      sharp object, bayonet
    war operations —*see* War operations,
      combat
  stated as undetermined whether accidental or
    intentional Y28.8
  suicide (attempt) X78.2
Bean in nose T17.1
Bed set on fire NEC —*see* Exposure, fire,
  uncontrolled, building, bed
Beheading (by guillotine)
  homicide X99.9
  legal execution —*see* Legal, intervention
Bending, injury in (prolonged) (static)
  X50.1
Bends —*see* Air, pressure, change
Bite, bitten by
  alligator W58.01
  arthropod (nonvenomous) NEC W57
  bull W55.21
  cat W55.01
  cow W55.21
  crocodile W58.11
  dog W54.0
  goat W55.31
  hoof stock NEC W55.31
  horse W55.11
  human being (accidentally) W50.3
    with intent to injure or kill Y04.1
    as, or caused by, a crowd or human stampede
      (with fall) W52
    assault Y04.1
    homicide (attempt) Y04.1
    in
      fight Y04.1
  insect (nonvenomous) W57
  lizard (nonvenomous) W59.01
  mammal NEC W55.81
    marine W56.31
  marine animal (nonvenomous) W56.81
  millipede W57
  moray eel W56.51
  mouse W53.01
  person(s) (accidentally) W50.3
    with intent to injure or kill Y04.1
    as, or caused by, a crowd or human stampede
      (with fall) W52
    assault Y04.1

Bite, bitten by *(Continued)*
  person(s) *(Continued)*
    homicide (attempt) Y04.1
    in
      fight Y04.1
  pig W55.41
  raccoon W55.51
  rat W53.11
  reptile W59.81
    lizard W59.01
    snake W59.11
    turtle W59.21
      terrestrial W59.81
  rodent W53.81
    mouse W53.01
    rat W53.11
    specified NEC W53.81
    squirrel W53.21
  shark W56.41
  sheep W55.31
  snake (nonvenomous) W59.11
  spider (nonvenomous) W57
  squirrel W53.21
Blast (air) **in war operations** —*see* War operations,
  blast
Blizzard X37.2
Blood alcohol level Y90.9
  20-39mg/100ml Y90.1
  40-59mg/100ml Y90.2
  60-79mg/100ml Y90.3
  80-99mg/100ml Y90.4
  100-119mg/100ml Y90.5
  120-199mg/100ml Y90.6
  200-239mg/100ml Y90.7
  less than 20mg/100ml Y90.0
  presence in blood, level not specified
    Y90.9
Blow X58
  by law-enforcing agent, police (on duty) —*see*
    Legal, intervention, manhandling
    blunt object —*see* Legal, intervention, blunt
      object
Blowing up —*see* Explosion
Brawl (hand) (fists) (foot) Y04.0
Breakage (accidental) (part of)
  ladder (causing fall) W11
  scaffolding (causing fall) W12
Broken
  glass, contact with —*see* Contact, with,
    glass
  power line (causing electric shock) W85
Bumping against, into (accidentally)
  object NEC W22.8
    with fall —*see* Fall, due to, bumping against,
      object
    caused by crowd or human stampede (with
      fall) W52
    sports equipment W21.9
  person(s) W51
    with fall W03
      due to ice or snow W00.0
    assault Y04.2
    caused by, a crowd or human stampede (with
      fall) W52
    homicide (attempt) Y04.2
  sports equipment W21.9
Burn, burned, burning (accidental) (by) (from)
  (on)
  acid NEC —*see* Table of Drugs and
    Chemicals
  bed linen —*see* Exposure, fire, uncontrolled, in
    building, bed
  blowtorch X08.8
    with ignition of clothing NEC X06.2
      nightwear X05
  bonfire, campfire (controlled) —*see also*
    Exposure, fire, controlled, not in
      building
    uncontrolled —*see* Exposure, fire,
      uncontrolled, not in building
  candle X08.8
    with ignition of clothing NEC X06.2
      nightwear X05
  caustic liquid, substance (external) (internal)
    NEC —*see* Table of Drugs and
      Chemicals
  chemical (external) (internal) —*see also* Table of
    Drugs and Chemicals
    in war operations —*see* War operations, fire
  cigar(s) or cigarette(s) X08.8
    with ignition of clothing NEC X06.2
      nightwear X05

Burn, burned, burning *(Continued)*
  clothes, clothing NEC (from controlled fire)
    X06.2
    with conflagration —*see* Exposure, fire,
      uncontrolled, building
      not in building or structure —*see* Exposure,
        fire, uncontrolled, not in building
  cooker (hot) X15.8
    stated as undetermined whether accidental or
      intentional Y27.3
    suicide (attempt) X77.3
  electric blanket X16
  engine (hot) X17
  fire, flames —*see* Exposure, fire
  flare, Very pistol —*see* Discharge, firearm NEC
  heat
    from appliance (electrical) (household) X15.8
      cooker X15.8
      hotplate X15.2
      kettle X15.8
      light bulb X15.8
      saucepan X15.3
      skillet X15.3
      stated as undetermined whether accidental
        or intentional Y27.3
      stove X15.0
      suicide (attempt) X77.3
      toaster X15.1
    in local application or packing during medical
      or surgical procedure
      Y63.5
  heating
    appliance, radiator or pipe X16
  homicide (attempt) —*see* Assault, burning
  hot
    air X14.1
    cooker X15.8
    drink X10.0
    engine X17
    fat X10.2
    fluid NEC X12
    food X10.1
    gases X14.1
    heating appliance X16
    household appliance NEC X15.8
    kettle X15.8
    liquid NEC X12
    machinery X17
    metal (molten) (liquid) NEC X18
    object (not producing fire or flames) NEC X19
    oil (cooking) X10.2
    pipe(s) X16
    radiator X16
    saucepan (glass) (metal) X15.3
    stove (kitchen) X15.0
    substance NEC X19
      caustic or corrosive NEC —*see* Table of
        Drugs and Chemicals
    toaster X15.1
    tool X17
    vapor X13.1
    water (tap) —*see* Contact, with, hot, tap water
  hotplate X15.2
    suicide (attempt) X77.3
  ignition —*see* Ignition
  in war operations —*see* War operations, fire
  inflicted by other person X97
    by hot objects, hot vapor, and steam —*see*
      Assault, burning, hot object
  internal, from swallowed caustic, corrosive
    liquid, substance —*see* Table of Drugs and
      Chemicals
  iron (hot) X15.8
    stated as undetermined whether accidental or
      intentional Y27.3
    suicide (attempt) X77.3
  kettle (hot) X15.8
    stated as undetermined whether accidental or
      intentional Y27.3
    suicide (attempt) X77.3
  lamp (flame) X08.8
    with ignition of clothing NEC X06.2
      nightwear X05
  lighter (cigar) (cigarette) X08.8
    with ignition of clothing NEC X06.2
      nightwear X05
  lightning —*see* subcategory T75.0
    causing fire —*see* Exposure, fire
  liquid (boiling) (hot) NEC X12
    stated as undetermined whether accidental or
      intentional Y27.2
    suicide (attempt) X77.2

  ▶ New   ⇨ Revised   ~~deleted~~ Deleted   ● Use Additional Character(s)

Burn, burned, burning (Continued)
local application of externally applied substance in medical or surgical care Y63.5
machinery (hot) X17
matches X08.8
with ignition of clothing NEC X06.2
nightwear X05
mattress —see Exposure, fire, uncontrolled, building, bed
medicament, externally applied Y63.5
metal (hot) (liquid) (molten) NEC X18
nightwear (nightclothes, nightdress, gown, pajamas, robe) X05
object (hot) NEC X19
on board watercraft
due to
accident to watercraft V91.09
powered craft V91.03
ferry boat V91.01
fishing boat V91.02
jet ski V91.03
liner V91.01
merchant ship V91.00
passenger ship V91.01
unpowered craft V91.08
canoe V91.05
inflatable V91.06
kayak V91.05
sailboat V91.04
surf-board V91.08
water skis V91.07
windsurfer V91.08
fire on board V93.09
ferry boat V93.01
fishing boat V93.02
jet ski V93.03
liner V93.01
merchant ship V93.00
passenger ship V93.01
powered craft NEC V93.03
sailboat V93.04
specified heat source NEC on board V93.19
ferry boat V93.11
fishing boat V93.12
jet ski V93.13
liner V93.11
merchant ship V93.10
passenger ship V93.11
powered craft NEC V93.13
sailboat V93.14
pipe (hot) X16
smoking X08.8
with ignition of clothing NEC X06.2
nightwear X05
powder —see Powder burn
radiator (hot) X16
saucepan (hot) (glass) (metal) X15.3
stated as undetermined whether accidental or intentional Y27.3
suicide (attempt) X77.3
self-inflicted X76
stated as undetermined whether accidental or intentional Y26
stated as undetermined whether accidental or intentional Y27.0
steam X13.1
pipe X16
stated as undetermined whether accidental or intentional Y27.8
stated as undetermined whether accidental or intentional Y27.0
suicide (attempt) X77.0
stove (hot) (kitchen) X15.0
stated as undetermined whether accidental or intentional Y27.3
suicide (attempt) X77.3
substance (hot) NEC X19
boiling X12
stated as undetermined whether accidental or intentional Y27.2
suicide (attempt) X77.2
molten (metal) X18
suicide (attempt) NEC X76
hot
household appliance X77.3
object X77.9
stated as undetermined whether accidental or intentional Y27.0
therapeutic misadventure
heat in local application or packing during medical or surgical procedure Y63.5
overdose of radiation Y63.2

Burn, burned, burning (Continued)
toaster (hot) X15.1
stated as undetermined whether accidental or intentional Y27.3
suicide (attempt) X77.3
tool (hot) X17
torch, welding X08.8
with ignition of clothing NEC X06.2
nightwear X05
trash fire (controlled) —see Exposure, fire, controlled, not in building
uncontrolled —see Exposure, fire, uncontrolled, not in building
vapor (hot) X13.1
stated as undetermined whether accidental or intentional Y27.0
suicide (attempt) X77.0
Very pistol —see Discharge, firearm NEC
Butted by animal W55.82
bull W55.22
cow W55.22
goat W55.32
horse W55.12
pig W55.42
sheep W55.32

— C —

Caisson disease —see Air, pressure, change
Campfire (exposure to) (controlled) —see also Exposure, fire, controlled, not in building
uncontrolled —see Exposure, fire, uncontrolled, not in building
Capital punishment (any means) —see Legal, intervention
Car sickness T75.3
Casualty (not due to war) NEC X58
war —see War operations
Cat
bite W55.01
scratch W55.03
Cataclysm, cataclysmic (any injury) NEC —see Forces of nature
Catching fire —see Exposure, fire
Caught
between
folding object W23.0
objects (moving) W23.0
and
machinery —see Contact, with, by type of machine
stationary W23.2
stationary W23.1
and moving W23.2
sliding door and door frame W23.0
by, in
machinery (moving parts of) —see Contact, with, by type of machine
washing-machine wringer W23.0
under packing crate (due to losing grip) W23.1
Cave-in caused by cataclysmic earth surface movement or eruption —see Landslide
Change(s) **in air pressure** —see Air, pressure, change
Choked, choking (on) (any object except food or vomitus)
food (bone) (seed) —see categories T17 and T18
vomitus T17.81-●
Civil insurrection —see War operations
Cloudburst (any injury) X37.8
Cold, exposure to (accidental) (excessive) (extreme) (natural) (place) **NEC** —see Exposure, cold
Collapse
building W20.1
burning (uncontrolled fire) X00.2
dam or man-made structure (causing earth movement) X36.0
machinery —see Contact, with, by type of machine
structure W20.1
burning (uncontrolled fire) X00.2
Collision (accidental) **NEC** —see also Accident, transport V89.9
pedestrian W51
with fall W03
due to ice or snow W00.0
involving pedestrian conveyance —see Accident, transport, pedestrian, conveyance

Collision (Continued)
with fall (Continued)
and
crowd or human stampede (with fall) W52
object W22.8
with fall —see Fall, due to, bumping against, object
person(s) —see Collision, pedestrian
transport vehicle NEC V89.9
and
avalanche, fallen or not moving —see Accident, transport
falling or moving —see Landslide
landslide, fallen or not moving —see Accident, transport
falling or moving —see Landslide
due to cataclysm —see Forces of nature, by type
intentional, purposeful suicide (attempt) —see Suicide, collision
Combustion, spontaneous —see Ignition
Complication (delayed) **of or following** (medical or surgical procedure) Y84.9
with misadventure —see Misadventure
amputation of limb(s) Y83.5
anastomosis (arteriovenous) (blood vessel) (gastrojejunal) (tendon) (natural or artificial material) Y83.2
aspiration (of fluid) Y84.4
tissue Y84.8
biopsy Y84.8
blood
sampling Y84.7
transfusion
procedure Y84.8
bypass Y83.2
catheterization (urinary) Y84.6
cardiac Y84.0
colostomy Y83.3
cystostomy Y83.3
dialysis (kidney) Y84.1
drug —see Table of Drugs and Chemicals
due to misadventure —see Misadventure
duodenostomy Y83.3
electroshock therapy Y84.3
external stoma, creation of Y83.3
formation of external stoma Y83.3
gastrostomy Y83.3
graft Y83.2
hypothermia (medically-induced) Y84.8
implant, implantation (of)
artificial
internal device (cardiac pacemaker) (electrodes in brain) (heart valve prosthesis) (orthopedic) Y83.1
material or tissue (for anastomosis or bypass) Y83.2
with creation of external stoma Y83.3
natural tissues (for anastomosis or bypass) Y83.2
with creation of external stoma Y83.3
infusion
procedure Y84.8
injection —see Table of Drugs and Chemicals
procedure Y84.8
insertion of gastric or duodenal sound Y84.5
insulin-shock therapy Y84.3
paracentesis (abdominal) (thoracic) (aspirative) Y84.4
procedures other than surgical operation —see Complication of or following, by type of procedure
radiological procedure or therapy Y84.2
removal of organ (partial) (total) NEC Y83.6
sampling
blood Y84.7
fluid NEC Y84.4
tissue Y84.8
shock therapy Y84.3
surgical operation NEC —see also Complication of or following, by type of operation Y83.9
reconstructive NEC Y83.4
with
anastomosis, bypass or graft Y83.2
formation of external stoma Y83.3
specified NEC Y83.8
transfusion —see also Table of Drugs and Chemicals
procedure Y84.8

B & C

Complication (Continued)
  transplant, transplantation (heart) (kidney)
    (liver) (whole organ, any) Y83.0
    partial organ Y83.4
  ureterostomy Y83.3
  vaccination —see also Table of Drugs and
    Chemicals
    procedure Y84.8
Compression
  divers' squeeze —see Air, pressure, change
  trachea by
    food (lodged in esophagus) —see categories
      T17 and T18
    vomitus (lodged in esophagus) T17.81-●
Conflagration —see Exposure, fire, uncontrolled
Constriction (external)
  hair W49.01
  jewelry W49.04
  ring W49.04
  rubber band W49.03
  specified item NEC W49.09
  string W49.02
  thread W49.02
Contact (accidental)
  with
    abrasive wheel (metalworking) W31.1
    alligator W58.09
      bite W58.01
      crushing W58.03
      strike W58.02
    amphibian W62.9
      frog W62.0
      toad W62.1
    animal (nonvenomous) NEC W64
      marine W56.89
        bite W56.81
        dolphin —see Contact, with, dolphin
        fish NEC —see Contact, with, fish
        mammal —see Contact, with, mammal,
          marine
        orca —see Contact, with, orca
        sea lion —see Contact, with, sea lion
        shark —see Contact, with, shark
        strike W56.82
    animate mechanical force NEC W64
    arrow W21.89
      not thrown, projected or falling W45.8
    arthropods (nonvenomous) W57
    axe W27.0
    band-saw (industrial) W31.2
    bayonet —see Bayonet wound
    bee(s) X58
    bench-saw (industrial) W31.2
    bird W61.99
      bite W61.91
      chicken —see Contact, with, chicken
      duck —see Contact, with, duck
      goose —see Contact, with, goose
      macaw —see Contact, with, macaw
      parrot —see Contact, with, parrot
      psittacine —see Contact, with, psittacine
      strike W61.92
      turkey —see Contact, with, turkey
    blender W29.0
    boiling water X12
      stated as undetermined whether accidental
        or intentional Y27.2
      suicide (attempt) X77.2
    bore, earth-drilling or mining (land) (seabed)
      W31.0
    buffalo —see Contact, with, hoof stock
      NEC
    bull W55.29
      bite W55.21
      gored W55.22
      strike W55.22
    bumper cars W31.81
    camel —see Contact, with, hoof stock NEC
    can
      lid W26.8
      opener W27.4
        powered W29.0
    cat W55.09
      bite W55.01
      scratch W55.03
    caterpillar (venomous) X58
    centipede (venomous) X58
    chain
      hoist W24.0
        agricultural operations Y30.89
      saw W29.3

Contact (Continued)
  with (Continued)
    chicken W61.39
      peck W61.33
      strike W61.32
    chisel W27.0
    circular saw W31.2
    cobra X58
    combine (harvester) W30.0
    conveyer belt W24.1
    cooker (hot) X15.8
      stated as undetermined whether accidental
        or intentional Y27.3
      suicide (attempt) X77.3
    coral X58
    cotton gin W31.82
    cow W55.29
      bite W55.21
      strike W55.22
    crane W24.0
      agricultural operations W30.89
    crocodile W58.19
      bite W58.11
      crushing W58.13
      strike W58.12
    dagger W26.1
      stated as undetermined whether accidental
        or intentional Y28.2
      suicide (attempt) X78.2
    dairy equipment W31.82
    dart W21.89
      not thrown, projected or falling W45.8
    deer —see Contact, with, hoof stock
      NEC
    derrick W24.0
      agricultural operations W30.89
        hay W30.2
    dog W54.8
      bite W54.0
      strike W54.1
    dolphin W56.09
      bite W56.01
      strike W56.02
    donkey —see Contact, with, hoof stock NEC
    drill (powered) W29.8
      earth (land) (seabed) W31.0
      nonpowered W27.8
    drive belt W24.0
      agricultural operations W30.89
    dry ice —see Exposure, cold, man-made
    dryer (clothes) (powered) (spin) W29.2
    duck W61.69
      bite W61.61
      strike W61.62
    earth(-)
      drilling machine (industrial) W31.0
      scraping machine in stationary use W31.83
    edge of stiff paper W26.2
    electric
      beater W29.0
      blanket X16
      fan W29.2
        commercial W31.82
      knife W29.1
      mixer W29.0
    elevator (building) W24.0
      agricultural operations W30.89
        grain W30.3
    engine(s), hot NEC X17
    excavating machine W31.0
    farm machine W30.9
    feces —see Contact, with, by type of animal
    fer de lance X58
    fish W56.59
      bite W56.51
      shark —see Contact, with, shark
      strike W56.52
    ▶ fishing hook W45.3
    flying horses W31.81
    forging (metalworking) machine W31.1
    fork W27.4
    forklift (truck) W24.0
      agricultural operations W30.89
    frog W62.0
    garden
      cultivator (powered) W29.3
        riding W30.89
      fork W27.1
    gas turbine W31.3
    Gila monster X58
    giraffe —see Contact, with, hoof stock NEC

Contact (Continued)
  with (Continued)
    glass (sharp) (broken) W25
      with subsequent fall W18.02
      assault X99.0
      due to fall —see Fall, by type
      stated as undetermined whether accidental
        or intentional Y28. 0
      suicide (attempt) X78.0
    goat W55.39
      bite W55.31
      strike W55.32
    goose W61.59
      bite W61.51
      strike W61.52
    hand
      saw W27.0
      tool (not powered) NEC W27.8
        powered W29.8
    harvester W30.0
    hay-derrick W30.2
    heat NEC X19
      from appliance (electrical) (household) —
        see Contact, with, hot, household
        appliance
      heating appliance X16
    heating
      appliance (hot) X16
      pad (electric) X16
    hedge-trimmer (powered) W29.3
    hoe W27.1
    hoist (chain) (shaft) NEC W24.0
      agricultural W30.89
    hoof stock NEC W55.39
      bite W55.31
      strike W55.32
    hornet(s) X58
    horse W55.19
      bite W55.11
      strike W55.12
    hot
      air X14.1
        inhalation X14.0
      cooker X15.8
      cooking
        pan X15.3
        pot X15.3
      drinks X10.0
      engine X17
      fats X10.2
      fluids NEC X12
        assault X98.2
        suicide (attempt) X77.2
        undetermined whether accidental or
          intentional Y27.2
      food X10.1
      gases X14.1
        inhalation X14.0
      heating appliance X16
      household appliance X15.8
        assault X98.3
        cooker X15.8
        hotplate X15.2
        kettle X15.8
        light bulb X15.8
        object NEC X19
          assault X98.8
          stated as undetermined whether
            accidental or intentional Y27.9
          suicide (attempt) X77.8
        saucepan X15.3
        skillet X15.3
        stated as undetermined whether
          accidental or intentional Y27.3
        stove X15.0
        suicide (attempt) X77.3
        toaster X15.1
      kettle X15.8
      light bulb X15.8
      liquid NEC —see also Burn X12
        drinks X10.0
        stated as undetermined whether
          accidental or intentional Y27.2
        suicide (attempt) X77.2
        tap water X11.8
          stated as undetermined whether
            accidental or intentional Y27.1
          suicide (attempt) X77.1
    machinery X17
    metal (molten) (liquid) NEC X18
    object (not producing fire or flames) NEC X19

   ➡ Revised   ~~deleted~~ Deleted   ● Use Additional Character(s)

C

C & D

Contact (Continued)
  with (Continued)
    sewing-machine (electric) (powered) W29.2
      not powered W27.8
    shaft (hoist) (lift) (transmission) NEC W24.0
      agricultural W30.89
    shark W56.49
      bite W56.41
      strike W56.42
    sharp object(s) W26.9
      specified NEC W26.8
    shears (hand) W27.2
      powered (industrial) W31.1
        domestic W29.2
    sheep W55.39
      bite W55.31
      strike W55.32
    shovel W27.8
      steam —see Accident, transport,
        construction vehicle
    snake (nonvenomous) W59.19
      bite W59.11
      crushing W59.13
      strike W59.12
    spade W27.1
    spider (venomous) X58
    spin-drier W29.2
    spinning machine W31.89
    splinter W45.8
    sports equipment W21.9
    staple gun (powered) W29.8
    steam X13.1
      engine W31.3
      inhalation X13.0
      pipe X16
      shovel W31.89
    stove (hot) (kitchen) X15.0
    substance, hot NEC X19
      molten (metal) X18
    sword W26.1
      assault X99.2
      stated as undetermined whether accidental
        or intentional
        Y28.2
      suicide (attempt) X78.2
    tarantula X58
    thresher W30.0
    tin can lid W26.8
    toad W62.1
    toaster (hot) X15.1
    tool W27.8
      hand (not powered) W27.8
        auger W27.0
        axe W27.0
        can opener W27.4
        chisel W27.0
        fork W27.4
        garden W27.1
        handsaw W27.0
        hoe W27.1
        ice-pick W27.4
        kitchen utensil W27.4
        manual
          lawn mower W27.1
          sewing machine W27.8
        meat grinder W27.4
        needle (sewing) W27.3
          hypodermic W46.0
            contaminated W46.1
        paper cutter W27.5
        pitchfork W27.1
        rake W27.1
        scissors W27.2
        screwdriver W27.0
        specified NEC W27.8
        workbench W27.0
      hot X17
      powered W29.8
        blender W29.0
          commercial W31.82
        can opener W29.0
          commercial W31.82
        chainsaw W29.3
        clothes dryer W29.2
          commercial W31.82
        dishwasher W29.2
          commercial W31.82
        edger W29.3
        electric fan W29.2
          commercial W31.82
        electric knife W29.1

Contact (Continued)
  with (Continued)
    tool (Continued)
      powered (Continued)
        food processor W29.0
          commercial W31.82
        garbage disposal W29.0
          commercial W31.82
        garden tool W29.3
        hedge trimmer W29.3
        ice maker W29.0
          commercial W31.82
        kitchen appliance W29.0
          commercial W31.82
        lawn mower W28
        meat grinder W29.0
          commercial W31.82
        mixer W29.0
          commercial W31.82
        rototiller W29.3
        sewing machine W29.2
          commercial W31.82
        washing machine W29.2
          commercial W31.82
    transmission device (belt, cable, chain, gear,
      pinion, shaft) W24.1
      agricultural operations W30.89
    turbine (gas) (water-driven) W31.3
    turkey W61.49
      peck W61.43
      strike W61.42
    turtle (nonvenomous) W59.29
      bite W59.21
      strike W59.22
      terrestrial W59.89
        bite W59.81
        crushing W59.83
        strike W59.82
    under-cutter W31.0
    urine —see Contact, with, by type of animal
    vehicle
      agricultural use (transport) —see Accident,
        transport, agricultural vehicle
        not on public highway W30.81
      industrial use (transport) —see
        Accident, transport, industrial vehicle
        not on public highway W31.83
      off-road use (transport) —see Accident,
        transport, all-terrain or off-road
        vehicle
        not on public highway W31.83
      special construction use (transport) —see
        Accident, transport, construction
        vehicle
        not on public highway W31.83
    venomous
      animal X58
      arthropods X58
      lizard X58
      marine animal NEC X58
      marine plant NEC X58
      millipedes (tropical) X58
      plant(s) X58
      snake X58
      spider X58
    viper X58
    washing-machine (powered) W29.2
    wasp X58
    weaving-machine W31.89
    winch W24.0
      agricultural operations W30.89
    wire NEC W24.0
      agricultural operations W30.89
    wood slivers W45.8
    yellow jacket X58
    zebra —see Contact, with, hoof stock NEC
  pressure W50.9
  stress W50.9
Coup de soleil X32
Crash
  aircraft (in transit) (powered) V95.9
    balloon V96.01
    fixed wing NEC (private) V95.21
      commercial V95.31
    glider V96.21
      hang V96.11
      powered V95.11
    helicopter V95.01
    in war operations —see War operations,
      destruction of aircraft
    microlight V95.11

Crash (Continued)
  aircraft (Continued)
    nonpowered V96.9
      specified NEC V96.8
    powered NEC V95.8
    stated as
      homicide (attempt) Y08.81
      suicide (attempt) X83.0
    ultralight V95.11
  spacecraft V95.41
  transport vehicle NEC —see also Accident,
    transport V89.9
    homicide (attempt) Y03.8
    motor NEC (traffic) V89.2
      homicide (attempt) Y03.8
      suicide (attempt) —see Suicide, collision
Cruelty (mental) (physical) (sexual) X58
Crushed (accidentally) X58
  between objects (moving) (stationary and
    moving) W23.0
    stationary W23.1
  by
    alligator W58.03
    avalanche NEC —see Landslide
    cave-in W20.0
      caused by cataclysmic earth surface
        movement —see Landslide
    crocodile W58.13
    crowd or human stampede W52
    falling
      aircraft W97.39
        in war operations —see War operations,
          destruction of aircraft
      earth, material W20.0
        caused by cataclysmic earth surface
          movement —see Landslide
      object NEC W20.8
    landslide NEC —see Landslide
    lizard (nonvenomous) W59.09
    machinery —see Contact, with, by type of
      machine
    reptile NEC W59.89
    snake (nonvenomous) W59.13
  in
    machinery —see Contact, with, by type of
      machine
Cut, cutting (any part of body) (accidental) —see
  also Contact, with, by object or machine
  during medical or surgical treatment as
    misadventure —see Index to Diseases and
    Injuries, Complications
  homicide (attempt) —see Assault, cutting or
    piercing instrument
  inflicted by other person —see Assault, cutting or
    piercing instrument
  legal
    execution —see Legal, intervention
    intervention —see Legal, intervention, sharp
      object
  machine NEC —see also Contact, with, by type of
    machine W31.9
  self-inflicted —see Suicide, cutting or piercing
    instrument
  suicide (attempt) —see Suicide, cutting or
    piercing instrument
Cyclone (any injury) X37.1

─────── **D** ───────

Decapitation (accidental circumstances) NEC X58
  homicide X99.9
  legal execution —see Legal, intervention
Dehydration from lack of water X58
Deprivation X58
Derailment (accidental)
  railway (rolling stock) (train) (vehicle) (without
    antecedent collision) V81.7
    with antecedent collision —see Accident,
      transport, railway vehicle occupant
  streetcar (without antecedent collision) V82.7
    with antecedent collision —see Accident,
      transport, streetcar occupant
Descent
  parachute (voluntary) (without accident to
    aircraft) V97.29
    due to accident to aircraft —see Accident,
      transport, aircraft
Desertion X58

▶ New   ⇨ Revised   ~~deleted~~ Deleted   ● Use Additional Character(s)

Destitution X58
Disability, late effect or sequela of injury —*see*
  Sequelae
Discharge (accidental)
  airgun W34.010
    assault X95.01
    homicide (attempt) X95.01
    stated as undetermined whether accidental or
      intentional Y24.0
    suicide (attempt) X74.01
  BB gun —*see* Discharge, airgun
  firearm (accidental) Y24.9
    accidental W34.00
    assault X95.9
    handgun (pistol) (revolver) Y22
      accidental W32.0
      assault X93
      homicide (attempt) X93
      legal intervention —*see* Legal, intervention,
        firearm, handgun
      stated as undetermined whether accidental
        or intentional Y22
      suicide (attempt) X72
    homicide (attempt) X95.9
    hunting rifle Y23.1
      accidental W33.02
      assault X94.1
      homicide (attempt) X94.1
      legal intervention
        injuring
          bystander Y35.032
          law enforcement personnel Y35.031
          suspect Y35.033
          unspecified person Y35.039
      stated as undetermined whether accidental
        or intentional Y23.1
      suicide (attempt) X73.1
    larger Y23.9
      accidental W33.00
      assault X94.9
      homicide (attempt) X94.9
      hunting rifle —*see* Discharge, firearm,
        hunting rifle
      legal intervention —*see* Legal, intervention,
        firearm by type of firearm
      machine gun —*see* Discharge, firearm,
        machine gun
      shotgun —*see* Discharge, firearm, shotgun
    specified NEC Y23.8
      accidental W33.09
      assault X94.8
      homicide (attempt) X94.8
      legal intervention
        injuring
          bystander Y35.092
          law enforcement personnel Y35.091
          suspect Y35.003
          unspecified person Y35.099
      stated as undetermined whether
        accidental or intentional Y23.8
      suicide (attempt) X73.8
    stated as undetermined whether accidental
      or intentional Y23.9
    suicide (attempt) X73.9
    legal intervention
      injuring
        bystander Y35.002
        law enforcement personnel Y35.001
        suspect Y35.003
        unspecified person Y35.009
      using rubber bullet
        injuring
          bystander Y35.042
          law enforcement personnel Y35.041
          suspect Y35.043
          unspecified person Y35.049
    machine gun Y23.3
      accidental W33.03
      assault X94.2
      homicide (attempt) X94.2
      legal intervention —*see* Legal, intervention,
        firearm, machine gun
      stated as undetermined whether accidental
        or intentional Y23.3
      suicide (attempt) X73.2
    pellet gun —*see* Discharge, airgun
    shotgun Y23.0
      accidental W33.01
      assault X94.0
      homicide (attempt) X94.0
      legal intervention —*see* Legal, intervention,
        firearm, specified NEC

Discharge (Continued)
  firearm (Continued)
    shotgun (Continued)
      stated as undetermined whether accidental
        or intentional Y23.0
      suicide (attempt) X73.0
    specified NEC W34.09
      assault X95.8
      homicide (attempt) X95.8
      legal intervention —*see* Legal, intervention,
        firearm, specified NEC
      stated as undetermined whether accidental
        or intentional Y24.8
      suicide (attempt) X74.8
    stated as undetermined whether accidental or
      intentional Y24.9
    suicide (attempt) X74.9
    Very pistol W34.09
      assault X95.8
      homicide (attempt) X95.8
      stated as undetermined whether accidental
        or intentional Y24.8
      suicide (attempt) X74.8
  firework(s) W39
    stated as undetermined whether accidental or
      intentional Y25
  gas-operated gun NEC W34.018
    airgun —*see* Discharge, airgun
    assault X95.09
    homicide (attempt) X95.09
    paintball gun —*see* Discharge, paintball gun
    stated as undetermined whether accidental or
      intentional Y24.8
    suicide (attempt) X74.09
  gun NEC —*see also* Discharge, firearm NEC
    air —*see* Discharge, airgun
    BB —*see* Discharge, airgun
    for single hand use —*see* Discharge, firearm,
      handgun
    hand —*see* Discharge, firearm, handgun
    machine —*see* Discharge, firearm, machine gun
    other specified —*see* Discharge, firearm NEC
    paintball —*see* Discharge, paintball gun
    pellet —*see* Discharge, airgun
  handgun —*see* Discharge, firearm, handgun
  machine gun —*see* Discharge, firearm, machine
    gun
  paintball gun W34.011
    assault X95.02
    homicide (attempt) X95.02
    stated as undetermined whether accidental or
      intentional Y24.8
    suicide (attempt) X74.02
  pistol —*see* Discharge, firearm, handgun
    flare —*see* Discharge, firearm, Very pistol
    pellet —*see* Discharge, airgun
    Very —*see* Discharge, firearm, Very pistol
  revolver —*see* Discharge, firearm, handgun
  rifle (hunting) —*see* Discharge, firearm, hunting
    rifle
  shotgun —*see* Discharge, firearm, shotgun
  spring-operated gun NEC W34.018
    assault X95.09
    homicide (attempt) X95.09
    stated as undetermined whether accidental or
      intentional Y24.8
    suicide (attempt) X74.09
Disease
  Andes W94.11
  aviator's —*see* Air, pressure
  range W94.11
Diver's disease, palsy, paralysis, squeeze —*see* Air,
  pressure
Diving (into water) —*see* Accident, diving
Dog bite W54.0
Dragged by transport vehicle NEC —*see also*
  Accident, transport V09.9
Drinking poison (accidental) —*see* Table of Drugs
  and Chemicals
Dropped (accidentally) **while being carried or
  supported by other person** W04
Drowning (accidental) W74
  assault X92.9
  due to
    accident (to)
      machinery —*see* Contact, with, by type of
        machine
      watercraft V90.89
        burning V90.29
          powered V90.23
            fishing boat V90.22
            jet ski V90.23

Drowning (Continued)
  due to (Continued)
    accident (Continued)
      watercraft (Continued)
        burning (Continued)
          powered (Continued)
            merchant ship V90.20
            passenger ship V90.21
          unpowered V90.28
            canoe V90.25
            inflatable V90.26
            kayak V90.25
            sailboat V90.24
            water skis V90.27
        crushed V90.39
          powered V90.33
            fishing boat V90.32
            jet ski V90.33
            merchant ship V90.30
            passenger ship V90.31
          unpowered V90.38
            canoe V90.35
            inflatable V90.36
            kayak V90.35
            sailboat V90.34
            water skis V90.37
        overturning V90.09
          powered V90.03
            fishing boat V90.02
            jet ski V90.03
            merchant ship V90.00
            passenger ship V90.01
          unpowered V90.08
            canoe V90.05
            inflatable V90.06
            kayak V90.05
            sailboat V90.04
        sinking V90.19
          powered V90.13
            fishing boat V90.12
            jet ski V90.13
            merchant ship V90.10
            passenger ship V90.11
          unpowered V90.18
            canoe V90.15
            inflatable V90.16
            kayak V90.15
            sailboat V90.14
        specified type NEC V90.89
          powered V90.83
            fishing boat V90.82
            jet ski V90.83
            merchant ship V90.80
            passenger ship V90.81
          unpowered V90.88
            canoe V90.85
            inflatable V90.86
            kayak V90.85
            sailboat V90.84
            water skis V90.87
    avalanche —*see* Landslide
    cataclysmic
      earth surface movement NEC —*see* Forces
        of nature, earth movement
      storm —*see* Forces of nature, cataclysmic
        storm
    cloudburst X37.8
    cyclone X37.1
    fall overboard (from) V92.09
      powered craft V92.03
        ferry boat V92.01
        fishing boat V92.02
        jet ski V92.03
        liner V92.01
        merchant ship V92.00
        passenger ship V92.01
      resulting from
        accident to watercraft —*see* Drowning,
          due to, accident to, watercraft
        being washed overboard (from) V92.29
          powered craft V92.23
            ferry boat V92.21
            fishing boat V92.22
            jet ski V92.23
            liner V92.21
            merchant ship V92.20
            passenger ship V92.21
          unpowered craft V92.28
            canoe V92.25
            inflatable V92.26
            kayak V92.25
            sailboat V92.24

Drowning *(Continued)*
  due to *(Continued)*
    fall overboard *(Continued)*
      resulting from *(Continued)*
        being washed overboard *(Continued)*
          unpowered craft *(Continued)*
            surf-board V92.28
            water skis V92.27
            windsurfer V92.28
        motion of watercraft V92.19
          powered craft V92.13
            ferry boat V92.11
            fishing boat V92.12
            jet ski V92.13
            liner V92.11
            merchant ship V92.10
            passenger ship V92.11
          unpowered craft
            canoe V92.15
            inflatable V92.16
             kayak V92.15
             sailboat V92.14
      unpowered craft V92.08
        canoe V92.05
        inflatable V92.06
        kayak V92.05
        sailboat V92.04
        surf-board V92.08
        water skis V92.07
        windsurfer V92.08
    hurricane X37.0
    jumping into water from watercraft (involved
      in accident) —*see also* Drowning, due to,
      accident to, watercraft
      without accident to or on watercraft W16.711
    tidal wave NEC —*see* Forces of nature, tidal
      wave
    torrential rain X37.8
  following
    fall
      into
        bathtub W16.211
        bucket W16.221
        fountain —*see* Drowning, following, fall,
          into, water, specified NEC
        quarry —*see* Drowning, following, fall,
          into, water, specified NEC
        reservoir —*see* Drowning, following, fall,
          into, water, specified NEC
        swimming-pool W16.011
          stated as undetermined whether
            accidental or intentional Y21.3
          striking
            bottom W16.021
            wall W16.031
          suicide (attempt) X71.2
        water NOS W16.41
          natural (lake) (open sea) (river)
            (stream) (pond) W16.111
            striking
              bottom W16.121
              side W16.131
          specified NEC W16.311
            striking
             bottom W16.321
             wall W16.331
      overboard NEC —*see* Drowning, due to, fall
        overboard
    jump or dive
      from boat W16.711
        striking bottom W16.721
      into
        fountain —*see* Drowning, following,
          jump or dive, into, water, specified
          NEC
        quarry —*see* Drowning, following, jump
          or dive, into, water, specified NEC
        reservoir —*see* Drowning, following,
          jump or dive, into, water, specified
          NEC
        swimming-pool W16.511
          striking
            bottom W16.521
            wall W16.531
          suicide (attempt) X71.2
        water NOS W16.91
          natural (lake) (open sea) (river)
            (stream) (pond) W16.611
          specified NEC W16.811
           striking
            bottom W16.821
            wall W16.831
          striking bottom W16.621

Drowning *(Continued)*
  homicide (attempt) X92.9
  in
    bathtub (accidental) W65
      assault X92.0
      following fall W16.211
        stated as undetermined whether
          accidental or intentional Y21.1
      stated as undetermined whether accidental
        or intentional Y21.0
      suicide (attempt) X71.0
    lake —*see* Drowning, in, natural water
    natural water (lake) (open sea) (river) (stream)
      (pond) W69
      assault X92.3
      following
        dive or jump W16.611
          striking bottom W16.621
        fall W16.111
          striking
            bottom W16.121
            side W16.131
      stated as undetermined whether accidental
        or intentional Y21.4
      suicide (attempt) X71.3
    quarry —*see* Drowning, in, specified place
      NEC
    quenching tank —*see* Drowning, in, specified
      place NEC
    reservoir —*see* Drowning, in, specified place
      NEC
    ▶resulting from accident to watercraft —*see*
      Drowning, due to, accident to, watercraft
    river —*see* Drowning, in, natural water
    sea —*see* Drowning, in, natural water
    specified place NEC W73
      assault X92.8
      following
        dive or jump W16.811
          striking
            bottom W16.821
            wall W16.831
        fall W16.311
          striking
            bottom W16.321
            wall W16.331
      stated as undetermined whether accidental
        or intentional Y21.8
      suicide (attempt) X71.8
    stream —*see* Drowning, in, natural water
    swimming-pool W67
      assault X92.1
        following fall X92.2
      following
        dive or jump W16.511
          striking
            bottom W16.521
            wall W16.531
        fall W16.011
          striking
            bottom W16.021
            wall W16.031
      stated as undetermined whether accidental
        or intentional Y21.2
        following fall Y21.3
      suicide (attempt) X71.1
        following fall X71.2
    war operations —*see* War operations,
      restriction of airway
  resulting from accident to watercraft —*see*
    Drowning, due to, accident, watercraft
  self-inflicted X71.9
  stated as undetermined whether accidental or
    intentional Y21.9
  suicide (attempt) X71.9

E

Earth (surface) movement NEC —*see* Forces of
  nature, earth movement
Earth falling (on) W20.0
  caused by cataclysmic earth surface movement or
    eruption —*see* Landslide
Earthquake (any injury) X34
Effect(s) (adverse) of
  air pressure (any) —*see* Air, pressure
  cold, excessive (exposure to) —*see* Exposure,
    cold
  heat (excessive) —*see* Heat
  hot place (weather) —*see* Heat

Effect *(Continued)*
  insolation X30
  late —*see* Sequelae
  motion —*see* Motion
  nuclear explosion or weapon in war operations —
    see War operations, nuclear weapon
  radiation —*see* Radiation
  travel —*see* Travel
Electric shock (accidental) (by) (in) —*see* Exposure,
  electric current
Electrocution (accidental) —*see* Exposure, electric
  current
**Endotracheal tube wrongly placed during
  anesthetic procedure** Y65.3
Entanglement
  in
    bed linen, causing suffocation —*see* category T71
    wheel of pedal cycle V19.88
Entry of foreign body or material —*see* Foreign
  body
~~Environmental pollution related condition —see Z57~~
▶**Environmental pollution related condition** —*see*
  category Z77
Execution, legal (any method) —*see* Legal,
  intervention
Exhaustion
  cold —*see* Exposure, cold
  due to excessive exertion —*see also* Overexertion
    X50.9
  heat —*see* Heat
Explosion (accidental) (of) (with secondary fire)
  W40.9
  acetylene W40.1
  aerosol can W36.1
  air tank (compressed) (in machinery) W36.2
  aircraft (in transit) (powered) NEC V95.9
    balloon V96.05
    fixed wing NEC (private) V95.25
      commercial V95.35
    glider V96.25
      hang V96.15
      powered V95.15
    helicopter V95.05
    in war operations —*see* War operations,
      destruction of aircraft
    microlight V95.15
    nonpowered V96.9
      specified NEC V96.8
    powered NEC V95.8
    stated as
      homicide (attempt) Y08.81
      suicide (attempt) X83.0
    ultralight V95.15
  anesthetic gas in operating room W40.1
  antipersonnel bomb W40.8
    assault X96.0
    homicide (attempt) X96.0
    suicide (attempt) X75
  assault X96.9
  bicycle tire W37.0
  blasting (cap) (materials) W40.0
  boiler (machinery), not on transport vehicle W35
    on watercraft —*see* Explosion, in, watercraft
  butane W40.1
  caused by other person X96.9
  coal gas W40.1
  detonator W40.0
  dump (munitions) W40.8
  dynamite W40.0
    in
      assault X96.8
      homicide (attempt) X96.8
      legal intervention
        injuring
          bystander Y35.112
          law enforcement personnel Y35.111
          suspect Y35.113
          unspecified person Y35.119
      suicide (attempt) X75
  explosive (material) W40.9
    gas W40.1
    in blasting operation W40.0
    specified NEC W40.8
      in
        assault X96.8
        homicide (attempt) X96.8
        legal intervention
          injuring
            bystander Y35.192
            law enforcement personnel Y35.191

Explosion *(Continued)*
explosive *(Continued)*
 specified *(Continued)*
  in *(Continued)*
   legal intervention *(Continued)*
    injuring *(Continued)*
     suspect Y35.193
     unspecified person Y35.199
    suicide (attempt) X75
factory (munitions) W40.8
fertilizer bomb W40.8
 assault X96.3
 homicide (attempt) X96.3
 suicide (attempt) X75
fire-damp W40.1
firearm (parts) NEC W34.19
 airgun W34.110
 BB gun W34.110
 gas, air or spring-operated gun NEC W34.118
 handgun W32.1
 hunting rifle W33.12
 larger firearm W33.10
  specified NEC W33.19
 machine gun W33.13
 paintball gun W34.111
 pellet gun W34.110
 shotgun W33.11
 Very pistol [flare] W34.19
fireworks W39
gas (coal) (explosive) W40.1
 cylinder W36.9
  aerosol can W36.1
  air tank W36.2
  pressurized W36.3
  specified NEC W36.8
gasoline (fumes) (tank) not in moving motor
  vehicle W40.1
 bomb W40.8
  assault X96.1
  homicide (attempt) X96.1
  suicide (attempt) X75
 in motor vehicle —*see* Accident, transport, by
  type of vehicle
grain store W40.8
grenade W40.8
 in
  assault X96.8
  homicide (attempt) X96.8
  legal intervention
   injuring
    bystander Y35.192
    law enforcement personnel Y35.191
    suspect Y35.193
    unspecified person Y35.199
  suicide (attempt) X75
handgun (parts) —*see* Explosion, firearm,
  handgun
homicide (attempt) X96.9
 antipersonnel bomb —*see* Explosion,
  antipersonnel bomb
 fertilizer bomb —*see* Explosion, fertilizer bomb
 gasoline bomb —*see* Explosion, gasoline bomb
 letter bomb —*see* Explosion, letter bomb
 pipe bomb —*see* Explosion, pipe bomb
 specified NEC X96.8
hose, pressurized W37.8
hot water heater, tank (in machinery) W35
 on watercraft —*see* Explosion, in, watercraft
in, on
 dump W40.8
 factory W40.8
 mine (of explosive gases) NEC W40.1
 watercraft V93.59
  powered craft V93.53
   ferry boat V93.51
   fishing boat V93.52
   jet ski V93.53
   liner V93.51
   merchant ship V93.50
   passenger ship V93.51
   sailboat V93.54
letter bomb W40.8
 assault X96.2
 homicide (attempt) X96.2
 suicide (attempt) X75
machinery —*see also* Contact, with, by type of
  machine
 on board watercraft —*see* Explosion, in,
  watercraft
 pressure vessel —*see* Explosion, by type of
  vessel

Explosion *(Continued)*
methane W40.1
mine W40.1
missile NEC W40.8
mortar bomb W40.8
 in
  assault X96.8
  homicide (attempt) X96.8
  legal intervention
   injuring
    bystander Y35.192
    law enforcement personnel Y35.191
    suspect Y35.193
    unspecified person Y35.199
  suicide (attempt) X75
munitions (dump) (factory) W40.8
pipe, pressurized W37.8
 bomb W40.8
  assault X96.4
  homicide (attempt) X96.4
  suicide (attempt) X75
pressure, pressurized
 cooker W38
 gas tank (in machinery) W36.3
 hose W37.8
 pipe W37.8
 specified device NEC W38
 tire W37.8
  bicycle W37.0
 vessel (in machinery) W38
propane W40.1
self-inflicted X75
shell (artillery) NEC W40.8
 during war operations —*see* War operations,
  explosion
 in
  legal intervention
   injuring
    bystander Y35.122
    law enforcement personnel Y35.121
    suspect Y35.123
    unspecified person Y35.129
  war —*see* War operations, explosion
spacecraft V95.45
stated as undetermined whether accidental or
  intentional Y25
steam or water lines (in machinery) W37.8
stove W40.9
suicide (attempt) X75
tire, pressurized W37.8
 bicycle W37.0
undetermined whether accidental or intentional
  Y25
vehicle tire NEC W37.8
 bicycle W37.0
war operations —*see* War operations, explosion
Exposure (to) X58
air pressure change —*see* Air, pressure
cold (accidental) (excessive) (extreme) (natural)
  (place) X31
 assault Y08.89
 due to
  man-made conditions W93.8
   dry ice (contact) W93.01
    inhalation W93.02
   liquid air (contact) (hydrogen) (nitrogen)
    W93.11
    inhalation W93.12
   refrigeration unit (deep freeze)
    W93.2
   suicide (attempt) X83.2
  weather (conditions) X31
 homicide (attempt) Y08.89
 self-inflicted X83.2
due to abandonment or neglect X58
electric current W86.8
 appliance (faulty) W86.8
  domestic W86.0
 caused by other person Y08.89
 conductor (faulty) W86.1
 control apparatus (faulty) W86.1
 electric power generating plant, distribution
  station W86.1
 electroshock gun —*see* Exposure, electric
  current, taser
 high-voltage cable W85
 homicide (attempt) Y08.89
 legal execution —*see* Legal, intervention,
  specified means NEC
 lightning —*see* subcategory T75.0
 live rail W86.8

Exposure *(Continued)*
electric current *(Continued)*
 misadventure in medical or surgical
  procedure in electroshock therapy Y63.4
 motor (electric) (faulty) W86.8
  domestic W86.0
 self-inflicted X83.1
 specified NEC W86.8
  domestic W86.0
 stun gun —*see* Exposure, electric current, taser
 suicide (attempt) X83.1
 taser W86.8
  assault Y08.89
  legal intervention —*see* category Y35
  self-harm (intentional) X83.8
  undetermined intent Y33
 third rail W86.8
 transformer (faulty) W86.1
 transmission lines W85
environmental tobacco smoke X58
excessive
 cold —*see* Exposure, cold
 heat (natural) NEC X30
  man-made W92
factor(s) NOS X58
 environmental NEC X58
  man-made NEC W99
  natural NEC —*see* Forces of nature
 specified NEC X58
fire, flames (accidental) X08.8
 assault X97
 campfire —*see* Exposure, fire, controlled, not
  in building
 controlled (in)
  with ignition (of) clothing —*see also*
   Ignition, clothes X06.2
   nightwear X05
  bonfire —*see* Exposure, fire, controlled, not
   in building
  brazier (in building or structure) —*see also*
   Exposure, fire, controlled, building
   not in building or structure —*see*
    Exposure, fire, controlled, not in
    building
  building or structure X02.0
   with
    fall from building X02.3
    from building X02.5
    injury due to building collapse X02.2
   ▶jump from building X02.5
    smoke inhalation X02.1
   hit by object from building X02.4
   specified mode of injury NEC X02.8
  fireplace, furnace or stove —*see* Exposure,
   fire, controlled, building
  not in building or structure X03.0
   with
    fall X03.3
    smoke inhalation X03.1
   hit by object X03.4
   specified mode of injury NEC X03.8
  trash —*see* Exposure, fire, controlled, not in
   building
 fireplace —*see* Exposure, fire, controlled,
  building
 fittings or furniture (in building or structure)
  (uncontrolled) —*see* Exposure, fire,
  uncontrolled, building
 forest (uncontrolled) —*see* Exposure, fire,
  uncontrolled, not in building
 grass (uncontrolled) —*see* Exposure, fire,
  uncontrolled, not in building
 hay (uncontrolled) —*see* Exposure, fire,
  uncontrolled, not in building
 homicide (attempt) X97
 ignition of highly flammable material X04
 in, of, on, starting in
  machinery —*see* Contact, with, by type of
   machine
  motor vehicle (in motion) —*see also*
   Accident, transport, occupant by type
   of vehicle V87.8
   with collision —*see* Collision
  railway rolling stock, train, vehicle V81.81
   with collision —*see* Accident, transport,
    railway vehicle occupant
  street car (in motion) V82.8
   with collision —*see* Accident, transport,
    streetcar occupant
  transport vehicle NEC —*see also* Accident,
   transport
   with collision —*see* Collision

E & F

Exposure (Continued)
  fire, flames (Continued)
    in, of, on, starting in (Continued)
      war operations —see also War operations,
        fire
        from nuclear explosion —see War
          operations, nuclear weapons
      watercraft (in transit) (not in transit) V91.09
        localized —see Burn, on board watercraft,
          due to, fire on board
        powered craft V91.03
          ferry boat V91.01
          fishing boat V91.02
          jet skis V91.03
          liner V91.01
          merchant ship V91.00
          passenger ship V91.01
        unpowered craft V91.08
          canoe V91.05
          inflatable V91.06
          kayak V91.05
          sailboat V91.04
          surf-board V91.08
          waterskis V91.07
          windsurfer V91.08
    lumber (uncontrolled) —see Exposure, fire,
      uncontrolled, not in building
    mine (uncontrolled) —see Exposure, fire,
      uncontrolled, not in building
    prairie (uncontrolled) —see Exposure, fire,
      uncontrolled, not in building
    resulting from
      explosion —see Explosion
      lightning X08.8
    self-inflicted X76
    specified NEC X08.8
    started by other person X97
    stated as undetermined whether accidental or
      intentional Y26
    stove —see Exposure, fire, controlled, building
    suicide (attempt) X76
    tunnel (uncontrolled) —see Exposure, fire,
      uncontrolled, not in building
    uncontrolled
      in building or structure X00.0
        with
          fall from building X00.3
          injury due to building collapse X00.2
          jump from building X00.5
          smoke inhalation X00.1
        bed X08.00
          due to
            cigarette X08.01
            specified material NEC X08.09
        furniture NEC X08.20
          due to
            cigarette X08.21
            specified material NEC X08.29
        hit by object from building X00.4
        sofa X08.10
          due to
            cigarette X08.11
            specified material NEC
              X08.19
        specified mode of injury NEC
          X00.8
      not in building or structure (any) X01.0
        with
          fall X01.3
          smoke inhalation X01.1
        hit by object X01.4
        specified mode of injury NEC X01.8
    undetermined whether accidental or
      intentional Y26
  forces of nature NEC —see Forces of nature
  G-forces (abnormal) W49.9
  gravitational forces (abnormal) W49.9
  heat (natural) NEC —see Heat
  high-pressure jet (hydraulic) (pneumatic) W49.9
  hydraulic jet W49.9
  inanimate mechanical force W49.9
  jet, high-pressure (hydraulic) (pneumatic) W49.9
  lightning —see subcategory T75.0
    causing fire —see Exposure, fire
  mechanical forces NEC W49.9
    animate NEC W64
    inanimate NEC W49.9
  noise W42.9
    supersonic W42.0
  noxious substance —see Table of Drugs and
    Chemicals
  pneumatic jet W49.9

Exposure (Continued)
  prolonged in deep-freeze unit or refrigerator
    W93.2
  radiation —see Radiation
  smoke —see also Exposure, fire
    tobacco, second hand Z77.22
  specified factors NEC X58
  sunlight X32
    man-made (sun lamp) W89.8
      tanning bed W89.1
  supersonic waves W42.0
  transmission line(s), electric W85
  vibration W49.9
  waves
    infrasound W49.9
    sound W42.9
    supersonic W42.0
  weather NEC —see Forces of nature

External cause status Y99.9
  child assisting in compensated work for family
    Y99.8
  civilian activity done for financial or other
    compensation Y99.0
  civilian activity done for income or pay
    Y99.0
  family member assisting in compensated work
    for other family member Y99.8
  hobby not done for income Y99.8
  leisure activity Y99.8
  military activity Y99.1
  off-duty activity of military personnel Y99.8
  recreation or sport not for income or while a
    student Y99.8
  specified NEC Y99.8
  student activity Y99.8
  volunteer activity Y99.2

——————— F ———————

Factors, supplemental
  alcohol
    blood level
      less than 20mg/100ml Y90.0
      presence in blood, level not specified Y90.9
      20-39mg/100ml Y90.1
      40-59mg/100ml Y90.2
      60-79mg/100ml Y90.3
      80-99mg/100ml Y90.4
      100-119mg/100ml Y90.5
      120-199mg/100ml Y90.6
      200-239mg/100ml Y90.7
      240mg/100ml or more Y90.8
      presence in blood, but level not specified
        Y90.9
  environmental-pollution-related condition —see
    Z57
  nosocomial condition Y95
  work-related condition Y99.0

Failure
  in suture or ligature during surgical procedure
    Y65.2
  mechanical, of instrument or apparatus (any)
    (during any medical or surgical procedure)
    Y65.8
  sterile precautions (during medical and surgical
    care) —see Misadventure, failure, sterile
    precautions, by type of procedure
  to
    introduce tube or instrument Y65.4
      endotracheal tube during anesthesia Y65.3
    make curve (transport vehicle) NEC —see
      Accident, transport
    remove tube or instrument Y65.4

Fall, falling (accidental) W19
  building W20.1
    burning (uncontrolled fire) X00.3
  down
    embankment W17.81
    escalator W10.0
    hill W17.81
    ladder W11
    ramp W10.2
    stairs, steps W10.9
  due to
    bumping against
      object W18.00
        sharp glass W18.02
        specified NEC W18.09
        sports equipment W18.01

Fall, falling (Continued)
  due to (Continued)
    bumping against (Continued)
      person W03
        due to ice or snow W00.0
        on pedestrian conveyance —see Accident,
          transport, pedestrian, conveyance
    collision with another person W03
      due to ice or snow W00.0
      involving pedestrian conveyance —see
        Accident, transport, pedestrian,
        conveyance
    grocery cart tipping over W17.82
    ice or snow W00.9
      from one level to another W00.2
      on stairs or steps W00.1
      involving pedestrian conveyance —see
        Accident, transport, pedestrian,
        conveyance
      on same level W00.0
    slipping (on moving sidewalk) W01.0
      with subsequent striking against object
        W01.10
        furniture W01.190
        sharp object W01.119
          glass W01.110
          power tool or machine W01.111
          specified NEC W01.118
        specified NEC W01.198
    striking against
      object W18.00
        sharp glass W18.02
        specified NEC W18.09
        sports equipment W18.01
      person W03
        due to ice or snow W00.0
        on pedestrian conveyance —see Accident,
          transport, pedestrian, conveyance
  earth (with asphyxia or suffocation (by
    pressure)) —see Earth, falling
  from, off, out of
    aircraft NEC (with accident to aircraft NEC)
      V97.0
      while boarding or alighting V97.1
    balcony W13.0
    bed W06
    boat, ship, watercraft NEC (with drowning or
      submersion) —see Drowning, due to, fall
      overboard
      with hitting bottom or object V94.0
    bridge W13.1
    building W13.9
      burning (uncontrolled fire) X00.3
    cavity W17.2
    chair W07
    cherry picker W17.89
    cliff W15
    dock W17.4
    embankment W17.81
    escalator W10.0
    flagpole W13.8
    furniture NEC W08
    grocery cart W17.82
    haystack W17.89
    high place NEC W17.89
      stated as undetermined whether accidental
        or intentional Y30
    hole W17.2
    incline W10.2
    ladder W11
    lifting device W17.89
    machine, machinery —see also Contact, with,
      by type of machine
      not in operation W17.89
    manhole W17.1
    mobile elevated work platform [MEWP] W17.89
    motorized mobility scooter W05.2
    one level to another NEC W17.89
      intentional, purposeful, suicide (attempt)
        X80
      stated as undetermined whether accidental
        or intentional Y30
    pit W17.2
    playground equipment W09.8
      jungle gym W09.2
      slide W09.0
      swing W09.1
    quarry W17.89
    railing W13.9
    ramp W10.2
    roof W13.2
    scaffolding W12

▶ New   ➡ Revised   ~~deleted~~ Deleted   ● Use Additional Character(s)

Incident, adverse
  device
    anesthesiology Y70.8
      accessory Y70.2
      diagnostic Y70.0
      miscellaneous Y70.8
      monitoring Y70.0
      prosthetic Y70.2
      rehabilitative Y70.1
      surgical Y70.3
      therapeutic Y70.1
    cardiovascular Y71.8
      accessory Y71.2
      diagnostic Y71.0
      miscellaneous Y71.8
      monitoring Y71.0
      prosthetic Y71.2
      rehabilitative Y71.1
      surgical Y71.3
      therapeutic Y71.1
    gastroenterology Y73.8
      accessory Y73.2
      diagnostic Y73.0
      miscellaneous Y73.8
      monitoring Y73.0
      prosthetic Y73.2
      rehabilitative Y73.1
      surgical Y73.3
      therapeutic Y73.1
    general
      hospital Y74.8
        accessory Y74.2
        diagnostic Y74.0
        miscellaneous Y74.8
        monitoring Y74.0
        prosthetic Y74.2
        rehabilitative Y74.1
        surgical Y74.3
        therapeutic Y74.1
      surgical Y81.8
        accessory Y81.2
        diagnostic Y81.0
        miscellaneous Y81.8
        monitoring Y81.0
        prosthetic Y81.2
        rehabilitative Y81.1
        surgical Y81.3
        therapeutic Y81.1
    gynecological Y76.8
      accessory Y76.2
      diagnostic Y76.0
      miscellaneous Y76.8
      monitoring Y76.0
      prosthetic Y76.2
      rehabilitative Y76.1
      surgical Y76.3
      therapeutic Y76.1
    medical Y82.9
      specified type NEC Y82.8
    neurological Y75.8
      accessory Y75.2
      diagnostic Y75.0
      miscellaneous Y75.8
      monitoring Y75.0
      prosthetic Y75.2
      rehabilitative Y75.1
      surgical Y75.3
      therapeutic Y75.1
    obstetrical Y76.8
      accessory Y76.2
      diagnostic Y76.0
      miscellaneous Y76.8
      monitoring Y76.0
      prosthetic Y76.2
      rehabilitative Y76.1
      surgical Y76.3
      therapeutic Y76.1
    ophthalmic Y77.8
      accessory Y77.2
      contact lens (rigid gas permeable)
        (soft) (hydrophilic)) Y77.11
      diagnostic Y77.0
      miscellaneous Y77.8
      monitoring Y77.0
      prosthetic Y77.2
      rehabilitative Y77.19
      surgical Y77.3
      therapeutic Y77.19
    orthopedic Y79.8
      accessory Y79.2
      diagnostic Y79.0
      miscellaneous Y79.8

Incident, adverse *(Continued)*
  device *(Continued)*
    orthopedic *(Continued)*
      monitoring Y79.0
      prosthetic Y79.2
      rehabilitative Y79.1
      surgical Y79.3
      therapeutic Y79.1
    otorhinolaryngological Y72.8
      accessory Y72.2
      diagnostic Y72.0
      miscellaneous Y72.8
      monitoring Y72.0
      prosthetic Y72.2
      rehabilitative Y72.1
      surgical Y72.3
      therapeutic Y72.1
    personal use Y74.8
      accessory Y74.2
      diagnostic Y74.0
      miscellaneous Y74.8
      monitoring Y74.0
      prosthetic Y74.2
      rehabilitative Y74.1
      surgical Y74.3
      therapeutic Y74.1
    physical medicine Y80.8
      accessory Y80.2
      diagnostic Y80.0
      miscellaneous Y80.8
      monitoring Y80.0
      prosthetic Y80.2
      rehabilitative Y80.1
      surgical Y80.3
      therapeutic Y80.1
    plastic surgical Y81.8
      accessory Y81.2
      diagnostic Y81.0
      miscellaneous Y81.8
      monitoring Y81.0
      prosthetic Y81.2
      rehabilitative Y81.1
      surgical Y81.3
      therapeutic Y81.1
    radiological Y78.8
      accessory Y78.2
      diagnostic Y78.0
      miscellaneous Y78.8
      monitoring Y78.0
      prosthetic Y78.2
      rehabilitative Y78.1
      surgical Y78.3
      therapeutic Y78.1
    urology Y73.8
      accessory Y73.2
      diagnostic Y73.0
      miscellaneous Y73.8
      monitoring Y73.0
      prosthetic Y73.2
      rehabilitative Y73.1
      surgical Y73.3
      therapeutic Y73.1

Incineration (accidental) —*see* Exposure, fire
Infanticide —*see* Assault
Infrasound waves (causing injury) W49.9
Ingestion
  foreign body (causing injury) (with
    obstruction) —*see* Foreign body, alimentary
    canal
  poisonous
    plant(s) X58
    substance NEC —*see* Table of Drugs and
      Chemicals
Inhalation
  excessively cold substance, man-made —*see*
    Exposure, cold, man-made
  food (any type) (into respiratory tract) (with
    asphyxia, obstruction respiratory tract,
    suffocation) —*see* categories T17
    and T18
  foreign body —*see* Foreign body, aspiration
  gastric contents (with asphyxia, obstruction
    respiratory passage, suffocation)
    T17.81-●
  hot air or gases X14.0
  liquid air, hydrogen, nitrogen W93.12
    suicide (attempt) X83.2
  steam X13.0
    assault X98.0
    stated as undetermined whether accidental or
      intentional Y27.0
    suicide (attempt) X77.0

Inhalation *(Continued)*
  toxic gas —*see* Table of Drugs and
    Chemicals
  vomitus (with asphyxia, obstruction respiratory
    passage, suffocation) T17.81-●
Injury, injured (accidental(ly)) **NOS** X58
  by, caused by, from
    assault —*see* Assault
    law-enforcing agent, police, in course of legal
      intervention —*see* Legal intervention
    suicide (attempt) X83.8
  due to, in
    civil insurrection —*see* War operations
    fight —*see also* Assault, fight Y04.0
    war operations —*see* War operations
  homicide —*see also* Assault Y09
  inflicted (by)
    in course of arrest (attempted), suppression
      of disturbance, maintenance of order,
      by law-enforcing agents —*see* Legal
      intervention
    other person
      stated as
        accidental X58
        intentional, homicide (attempt) —*see*
          Assault
        undetermined whether accidental or
          intentional Y33
  purposely (inflicted) by other person(s) —*see*
    Assault
  self-inflicted X83.8
    stated as accidental X58
  specified cause NEC X58
  undetermined whether accidental or intentional
    Y33
Insolation, effects X30
Insufficient nourishment X58
Interruption of respiration (by)
  food (lodged in esophagus) —*see* categories T17
    and T18
  vomitus (lodged in esophagus) T17.81-●
Intervention, legal —*see* Legal intervention
Intoxication
  drug —*see* Table of Drugs and Chemicals
  poison —*see* Table of Drugs and
    Chemicals

——————— **J** ———————

Jammed (accidentally)
  between objects (moving) (stationary and
    moving) W23.0
  stationary W23.1
Jumped, jumping
  before moving object NEC X81.8
    motor vehicle X81.0
    subway train X81.1
    train X81.1
    undetermined whether accidental or
      intentional Y31
  from
    boat (into water) voluntarily,
      without accident (to or on boat)
      W16.712
      with
        accident to or on boat —*see* Accident,
          watercraft
        drowning or submersion W16.711
          suicide (attempt) X71.3
        striking bottom W16.722
          causing drowning W16.721
    building —*see also* Jumped, from,
      high place W13.9
      burning (uncontrolled fire) X00.5
    high place NEC W17.89
      suicide (attempt) X80
      undetermined whether accidental or
        intentional Y30
    structure —*see also* Jumped, from, high place
      W13.9
      burning (uncontrolled fire) X00.5
  into water W16.92
    causing drowning W16.91
    from, off watercraft —*see* Jumped, from, boat
    in
      natural body W16.612
        causing drowning W16.611
        striking bottom W16.622
          causing drowning W16.621

Jumped, jumping (Continued)
  into water (Continued)
    in (Continued)
      specified place NEC W16.812
        causing drowning W16.811
        striking
          bottom W16.822
            causing drowning W16.821
          wall W16.832
            causing drowning W16.831
      swimming pool W16.512
        causing drowning W16.511
        striking
          bottom W16.522
            causing drowning W16.521
          wall W16.532
            causing drowning W16.531
  suicide (attempt) X71.3

K

Kicked by
animal NEC W55.82
person(s) (accidentally) W50.1
  with intent to injure or kill Y04.0
  as, or caused by, a crowd or human stampede
    (with fall) W52
  assault Y04.0
  homicide (attempt) Y04.0
  in
    fight Y04.0
    legal intervention
      injuring
        bystander Y35.812
        law enforcement personnel
          Y35.811
        suspect Y35.813
        unspecified person Y35.819

Kicking
against
  object W22.8
    sports equipment W21.9
    stationary W22.09
      sports equipment W21.89
  person —see Striking against, person
  sports equipment W21.9
carpet stretcher with knee X50.3
Killed, killing (accidentally) **NOS** —see also Injury
  X58
in
  action —see War operations
  brawl, fight (hand) (fists) (foot) Y04.0
    by weapon —see also Assault
      cutting, piercing —see Assault, cutting or
        piercing instrument
      firearm —see Discharge, firearm, by type,
        homicide
self
  stated as
    accident NOS X58
    suicide —see Suicide
    undetermined whether accidental or
      intentional Y33
Kneeling (prolonged) (static) X50.1
Knocked down (accidentally) (by) **NOS** X58
animal (not being ridden) NEC —see also Struck
  by, by type of animal
crowd or human stampede W52
person W51
  in brawl, fight Y04.0
transport vehicle NEC —see also Accident,
  transport V09.9

L

Laceration NEC —see Injury
Lack of
care (helpless person) (infant) (newborn) X58
food except as result of abandonment or neglect
  X58
  due to abandonment or neglect X58
water except as result of transport accident X58
  due to transport accident —see Accident,
    transport, by type
  helpless person, infant, newborn X58

Landslide (falling on transport vehicle) X36.1
  caused by collapse of man-made structure X36.0
Late effect —see Sequelae
Legal
execution (any method) —see Legal, intervention
intervention (by)
  baton —see Legal, intervention, blunt object,
    baton
  bayonet —see Legal, intervention, sharp
    object, bayonet
  blow —see Legal, intervention, manhandling
  blunt object
    baton
      injuring
        bystander Y35.312
        law enforcement personnel Y35.311
        suspect Y35.313
        unspecified person Y35.319
    injuring
      bystander Y35.302
      law enforcement personnel Y35.301
      suspect Y35.303
      unspecified person Y35.309
    specified NEC
      injuring
        bystander Y35.392
        law enforcement personnel Y35.391
        suspect Y35.393
        unspecified person Y35.399
    stave
      injuring
        bystander Y35.392
        law enforcement personnel Y35.391
        suspect Y35.393
        unspecified person Y35.399
  bomb —see Legal, intervention, explosive
  conducted energy device
    injuring
      bystander Y35.832
      law enforcement personnel Y35.831
      suspect Y35.833
      unspecified person Y35.839
  cutting or piercing instrument —see Legal,
    intervention, sharp object
  dynamite —see Legal, intervention, explosive,
    dynamite
  electroshock device (taser)
    injuring
      bystander Y35.832
      law enforcement personnel Y35.831
      suspect Y35.833
      unspecified person Y35.839
  explosive(s)
    dynamite
      injuring
        bystander Y35.112
        law enforcement personnel
          Y35.111
        suspect Y35.113
        unspecified person Y35.119
    grenade
      injuring
        bystander Y35.192
        law enforcement personnel Y35.191
        suspect Y35.193
        unspecified person Y35.199
    injuring
      bystander Y35.102
      law enforcement personnel Y35.101
      suspect Y35.103
      unspecified person Y35.109
    mortar bomb
      injuring
        bystander Y35.192
        law enforcement personnel
          Y35.191
        suspect Y35.193
        unspecified person Y35.199
    shell
      injuring
        bystander Y35.122
        law enforcement personnel
          Y35.121
        suspect Y35.123
        unspecified person Y35.129
    specified NEC
      injuring
        bystander Y35.192
        law enforcement personnel Y35.191
        suspect Y35.193
        unspecified person Y35.199

Legal (Continued)
intervention (by) (Continued)
  firearm(s) (discharge)
    handgun
      injuring
        bystander Y35.022
        law enforcement personnel Y35.021
        suspect Y35.023
        unspecified person Y35.029
    injuring
      bystander Y35.002
      law enforcement personnel Y35.001
      suspect Y35.003
      unspecified person Y35.009
    machine gun
      injuring
        bystander Y35.012
        law enforcement personnel Y35.011
        suspect Y35.013
        unspecified person Y35.019
    rifle pellet
      injuring
        bystander Y35.032
        law enforcement personnel Y35.031
        suspect Y35.033
        unspecified person Y35.039
    rubber bullet
      injuring
        bystander Y35.042
        law enforcement personnel Y35.041
        suspect Y35.043
        unspecified person Y35.049
    shotgun —see Legal, intervention, firearm,
      specified NEC
    specified NEC
      injuring
        bystander Y35.092
        law enforcement personnel Y35.091
        suspect Y35.093
        unspecified person Y35.099
  gas (asphyxiation) (poisoning)
    injuring
      bystander Y35.202
      law enforcement personnel Y35.201
      suspect Y35.203
      unspecified person Y35.209
    specified NEC
      injuring
        bystander Y35.292
        law enforcement personnel Y35.291
        suspect Y35.293
        unspecified person Y35.299
    tear gas
      injuring
        bystander Y35.212
        law enforcement personnel Y35.211
        suspect Y35.213
        unspecified person Y35.219
  grenade —see Legal, intervention, explosive,
    grenade
  injuring
    bystander Y35.92
    law enforcement personnel Y35.91
    suspect Y35.93
    unspecified person Y35.99
  late effect (of) —see with 7th character S
    Y35
  manhandling
    injuring
      bystander Y35.812
      law enforcement personnel Y35.811
      suspect Y35.813
      unspecified person Y35.819
  sequelae (of) —see with 7th character S Y35
  sharp objects
    bayonet
      injuring
        bystander Y35.412
        law enforcement personnel
          Y35.411
        suspect Y35.413
        unspecified person Y35.419
    injuring
      bystander Y35.402
      law enforcement personnel Y35.401
      suspect Y35.403
      unspecified person Y35.409
    specified NEC
      injuring
        bystander Y35.492
        law enforcement personnel Y35.491

M

L & M

▶ New   ➡ Revised   ~~deleted~~ Deleted   ● Use Additional Character(s)

M, N, O, & P

▶ New   ⇨ Revised   ~~deleted~~ Deleted   ● Use Additional Character(s)

Premature cessation (of) **surgical and medical care** Y66
Privation (food) (water) X58
Procedure (operation)
  correct, on wrong side or body part (wrong side) (wrong site) Y65.53
  intended for another patient done on wrong patient Y65.52
  performed on patient not scheduled for surgery Y65.52
  performed on wrong patient Y65.52
  wrong, performed on correct patient Y65.51
Prolonged
  sitting in transport vehicle —*see* Sitting
  stay in
    high altitude as cause of anoxia, barodontalgia, barotitis or hypoxia W94.11
    weightless environment X52
Pulling, excessive —*see also* Overexertion X50.9
Puncture, puncturing —*see also* Contact, with, by type of object or machine
  by
    plant thorns, spines, sharp leaves or other mechanisms NEC W60
  during medical or surgical treatment as misadventure —*see* Index to Diseases and Injuries, Complication(s)
Pushed, pushing (accidental) (injury in)
  by other person(s) (accidental) W51
    with fall W03
      due to ice or snow W00.0
    as, or caused by, a crowd or human stampede (with fall) W52
    before moving object NEC Y02.8
      motor vehicle Y02.0
      subway train Y02.1
      train Y02.1
    from
      high place NEC
        in accidental circumstances W17.89
        stated as
          intentional, homicide (attempt) Y01
          undetermined whether accidental or intentional Y30
      transport vehicle NEC —*see also* Accident, transport V89.9
        stated as
          intentional, homicide (attempt) Y08.89
    overexertion X50.9

R

Radiation (exposure to)
  arc lamps W89.0
  atomic power plant (malfunction) NEC W88.1
  complication of or abnormal reaction to medical radiotherapy Y84.2
  electromagnetic, ionizing W88.0
  gamma rays W88.1
  in
    war operations (from or following nuclear explosion) —*see also* War operations
  inadvertent exposure of patient (receiving test or therapy) Y63.3
  infrared (heaters and lamps) W90.1
    excessive heat from W92
  ionized, ionizing (particles, artificially accelerated)
    radioisotopes W88.1
    specified NEC W88.8
    x-rays W88.0
  isotopes, radioactive —*see* Radiation, radioactive isotopes
  laser(s) W90.2
    in war operations —*see* War operations
    misadventure in medical care Y63.2
  light sources (man-made visible and ultraviolet) W89.9
    natural X32
    specified NEC W89.8
    tanning bed W89.1
    welding light W89.0
  man-made visible light W89.9
    specified NEC W89.8
    tanning bed W89.1
    welding light W89.0

Radiation (*Continued*)
  microwave W90.8
  misadventure in medical or surgical procedure Y63.2
  natural NEC X39.08
    radon X39.01
  overdose (in medical or surgical procedure) Y63.2
  radar W90.0
  radioactive isotopes (any) W88.1
    atomic power plant malfunction W88.1
    misadventure in medical or surgical treatment Y63.2
  radiofrequency W90.0
  radium NEC W88.1
  sun X32
  ultraviolet (light) (man-made) W89.9
    natural X32
    specified NEC W89.8
    tanning bed W89.1
    welding light W89.0
  welding arc, torch, or light W89.0
    excessive heat from W92
  x-rays (hard) (soft) W88.0
Range disease W94.11
Rape (attempted) (confirmed) T74.2- ●
  suspected T76.2- ●
Rat bite W53.11
Reaching (prolonged) (static) X50.1
Reaction, abnormal to medical procedure —*see also* Complication of or following, by type of procedure Y84.9
  with misadventure —*see* Misadventure
  biologicals —*see* Table of Drugs and Chemicals
  drugs —*see* Table of Drugs and Chemicals
  vaccine —*see* Table of Drugs and Chemicals
Recoil
  airgun W34.110
  BB gun W34.110
  firearm NEC W34.19
  gas, air or spring-operated gun NEC W34.118
  handgun W32.1
  hunting rifle W33.12
  larger firearm W33.10
    specified NEC W33.19
  machine gun W33.13
  paintball gun W34.111
  pellet W34.110
  shotgun W33.11
  Very pistol [flare] W34.19
Reduction in
  atmospheric pressure —*see* Air, pressure, change
Rock falling on or hitting (accidentally) (person) W20.8
  in cave-in W20.0
Run over (accidentally) (by)
  animal (not being ridden) NEC W55.89
  machinery —*see* Contact, with, by specified type of machine
  transport vehicle NEC —*see also* Accident, transport V09.9
    intentional homicide (attempt) Y03.0
    motor NEC V09.20
      intentional homicide (attempt) Y03.0
Running
  before moving object X81.8
  motor vehicle X81.0
Running off, away
  animal (being ridden) —*see also* Accident, transport V80.918
    not being ridden W55.89
  animal-drawn vehicle NEC —*see also* Accident, transport V80.928
  highway, road(way), street
    transport vehicle NEC —*see also* Accident, transport V89.9
Rupture pressurized devices —*see* Explosion, by type of device

S

Saturnism —*see* Table of Drugs and Chemicals, lead
Scald, scalding (accidental) (by) (from) (in) X19
  air (hot) X14.1
  gases (hot) X14.1
  homicide (attempt) —*see* Assault, burning, hot object

Scald, scalding (*Continued*)
  inflicted by other person
    stated as intentional, homicide (attempt) —*see* Assault, burning, hot object
  liquid (boiling) (hot) NEC X12
    stated as undetermined whether accidental or intentional Y27.2
    suicide (attempt) X77.2
  local application of externally applied substance in medical or surgical care Y63.5
  metal (molten) (liquid) (hot) NEC X18
  self-inflicted X77.9
  stated as undetermined whether accidental or intentional Y27.8
  steam X13.1
    assault X98.0
    stated as undetermined whether accidental or intentional Y27.0
    suicide (attempt) X77.0
  suicide (attempt) X77.9
  vapor (hot) X13.1
    assault X98.0
    stated as undetermined whether accidental or intentional Y27.0
    suicide (attempt) X77.0
Scratched by
  cat W55.03
  person(s) (accidentally) W50.4
    with intent to injure or kill Y04.0
    as, or caused by, a crowd or human stampede (with fall) W52
    assault Y04.0
    homicide (attempt) Y04.0
    in
      fight Y04.0
      legal intervention
        injuring
          bystander Y35.892
          law enforcement personnel Y35.891
          suspect Y35.893
          unspecified person Y35.899
Seasickness T75.3
Self-harm NEC —*see also* External cause by type, undetermined whether accidental or intentional
  intentional —*see* Suicide
  poisoning NEC —*see* Table of drugs and biologicals, accident
Self-inflicted (injury) **NEC** —*see also* External cause by type, undetermined whether accidental or intentional
  intentional —*see* Suicide
  poisoning NEC —*see* Table of drugs and biologicals, accident
Sequelae (of)
  accident NEC —*see* W00-X58 with 7th character S
  assault (homicidal) (any means) —*see* X92-Y08 with 7th character S
  homicide, attempt (any means) —*see* X92-Y08 with 7th character S
  injury undetermined whether accidentally or purposely inflicted —*see* Y21-Y33 with 7th character S
  intentional self-harm (classifiable to X71-X83) —*see* X71-X83 with 7th character S
  legal intervention (*see* with 7th character S Y35)
  motor vehicle accident —*see* V00-V99 with 7th character S
  suicide, attempt (any means) —*see* X71-X83 with 7th character S
  transport accident —*see* V00-V99 with 7th character S
  war operations —*see* War operations
Shock
  electric —*see* Exposure, electric current
  from electric appliance (any) (faulty) W86.8
    domestic W86.0
    suicide (attempt) X83.1
Shooting, shot (accidental (ly)) —*see also* Discharge, firearm, by type
  herself or himself —*see* Discharge, firearm by type, self-inflicted
  homicide (attempt) —*see* Discharge, firearm by type, homicide
  in war operations —*see* War operations
  inflicted by other person —*see* Discharge, firearm by type, homicide
    accidental —*see* Discharge, firearm, by type of firearm

Shooting, shot *(Continued)*
legal
    execution —*see* Legal, intervention, firearm
    intervention —*see* Legal, intervention, firearm
  self-inflicted —*see* Discharge, firearm by type,
    suicide
    accidental —*see* Discharge, firearm, by type
      of firearm
  suicide (attempt) —*see* Discharge, firearm by
    type, suicide
Shoving (accidentally) **by other person** —*see*
  Pushed, by other person
Sickness
  alpine W94.11
  motion —*see* Motion
  mountain W94.11
Sinking (accidental)
  watercraft (causing drowning, submersion) —
    see also Drowning, due to, accident to,
    watercraft, sinking
    causing injury except drowning or
      submersion —*see* Accident, watercraft,
      causing, injury NEC
Siriasis X32
Sitting (prolonged) (static) X50.1
Slashed wrists —*see* Cut, self-inflicted
Slipping (accidental) (on same level) (with fall)
  W01.0
  without fall W18.40
    due to
      specified NEC W18.49
      stepping from one level to another W18.43
      stepping into hole or opening W18.42
      stepping on object W18.41
  on
    ice W00.0
      with skates —*see* Accident, transport,
        pedestrian, conveyance
    mud W01.0
    oil W01.0
    snow W00.0
      with skis —*see* Accident, transport,
        pedestrian, conveyance
    surface (slippery) (wet) NEC W01.0
Sliver, wood, contact with W45.8
Smoldering (due to fire) —*see* Exposure, fire
Sodomy (attempted) **by force** T74.2-●
Sound waves (causing injury) W42.9
  supersonic W42.0
Splinter, contact with W45.8
Stab, stabbing —*see* Cut
Standing (prolonged) (static) X50.1
Starvation X58
Status of external cause Y99.9
  child assisting in compensated work for family
    Y99.8
  civilian activity done for financial or other
    compensation Y99.0
  civilian activity done for income or pay Y99.0
  family member assisting in compensated work
    for other family member Y99.8
  hobby not done for income Y99.8
  leisure activity Y99.8
  military activity Y99.1
  off-duty activity of military personnel Y99.8
  recreation or sport not for income or while a
    student Y99.8
  specified NEC Y99.8
  student activity Y99.8
  volunteer activity Y99.2
Stepped on
  by
    animal (not being ridden) NEC W55.89
    crowd or human stampede W52
    person W50.0
Stepping on
  object W22.8
    with fall W18.31
    sports equipment W21.9
    stationary W22.09
      sports equipment W21.89
  person W51
    by crowd or human stampede W52
  sports equipment W21.9
Sting
  arthropod, nonvenomous W57
  insect, nonvenomous W57
Storm (cataclysmic) —*see* Forces of nature,
  cataclysmic storm

Straining, excessive —*see also* Overexertion X50.9
Strangling —*see* Strangulation
Strangulation (accidental) —*see* category T71
Strenuous movements —*see also* Overexertion X50.9
Striking against
  airbag (automobile) W22.10
    driver side W22.11
    front passenger side W22.12
    specified NEC W22.19
  bottom when
    diving or jumping into water (in)
      W16.822
      causing drowning W16.821
      from boat W16.722
        causing drowning W16.721
      natural body W16.622
        causing drowning W16.821
      swimming pool W16.522
        causing drowning W16.521
    falling into water (in) W16.322
      causing drowning W16.321
      fountain —*see* Striking against, bottom
        when, falling into water, specified
        NEC
      natural body W16.122
        causing drowning W16.121
      reservoir —*see* Striking against, bottom
        when, falling into water, specified
        NEC
      specified NEC W16.322
        causing drowning W16.321
      swimming pool W16.022
        causing drowning W16.021
  diving board (swimming-pool) W21.4
  object W22.8
    with
      drowning or submersion —*see* Drowning
      fall —*see* Fall, due to, bumping against,
        object
    caused by crowd or human stampede (with
      fall) W52
    furniture W22.03
    lamppost W22.02
    sports equipment W21.9
    stationary W22.09
      sports equipment W21.89
    wall W22.01
  person(s) W51
    with fall W03
      due to ice or snow W00.0
    as, or caused by, a crowd or human stampede
      (with fall) W52
    assault Y04.2
    homicide (attempt) Y04.2
  sports equipment W21.9
  wall (when) W22.01
    diving or jumping into water (in) W16.832
      causing drowning W16.831
      swimming pool W16.532
        causing drowning W16.531
    falling into water (in) W16.332
      causing drowning W16.331
      fountain —*see* Striking against, wall when,
        falling into water, specified NEC
      natural body W16.132
        causing drowning W16.131
      reservoir —*see* Striking against, wall when,
        falling into water, specified NEC
      specified NEC W16.332
        causing drowning W16.331
      swimming pool W16.032
        causing drowning W16.031
    swimming pool (when) W22.042
      causing drowning W22.041
      diving or jumping into water W16.532
        causing drowning W16.531
      falling into water W16.032
        causing drowning W16.031
Struck (accidentally) **by**
  airbag (automobile) W22.10
    driver side W22.11
    front passenger side W22.12
    specified NEC W22.19
  alligator W58.02
  animal (not being ridden) NEC W55.89
  avalanche —*see* Landslide
  ball (hit) (thrown) W21.00
    assault Y08.09
    baseball W21.03

Struck *(Continued)*
  ball *(Continued)*
    basketball W21.05
    football W21.01
    golf ball W21.04
    football W21.01
    soccer W21.02
    softball W21.07
    specified NEC W21.09
    volleyball W21.06
  bat or racquet
    baseball bat W21.11
      assault Y08.02
    golf club W21.13
      assault Y08.09
    specified NEC W21.19
      assault Y08.09
    tennis racquet W21.12
      assault Y08.09
  bullet —*see also* Discharge, firearm by type
    in war operations —*see* War operations
  crocodile W58.12
  dog W54.1
  flare, Very pistol —*see* Discharge, firearm NEC
  hailstones X39.8
  hockey (ice)
    field
      puck W21.221
      stick W21.211
    puck W21.220
    stick W21.210
      assault Y08.01
  landslide —*see* Landslide
  law-enforcement agent (on duty) —*see* Legal,
    intervention, manhandling
    with blunt object —*see* Legal, intervention,
      blunt object
  lightning —*see* subcategory T75.0
    causing fire —*see* Exposure, fire
  machine —*see* Contact, with, by type of machine
  mammal NEC W55.89
    marine W56.32
  marine animal W56.82
  missile
    firearm —*see* Discharge, firearm by type
    in war operations —*see* War operations,
      missile
  object W22.8
    blunt W22.8
      assault Y00
      suicide (attempt) X79
      undetermined whether accidental or
        intentional Y29
    falling W20.8
      from, in, on
        building W20.1
          burning (uncontrolled fire)
            X00.4
        cataclysmic
          earth surface movement NEC —*see*
            Landslide
          storm —*see* Forces of nature,
            cataclysmic storm
        cave-in W20.0
        earthquake X34
        machine (in operation) —*see* Contact,
          with, by type of machine
        structure W20.1
          burning X00.4
        transport vehicle (in motion) —*see*
          Accident, transport, by type of
          vehicle
  watercraft V93.49
    due to
      accident to craft V91.39
        powered craft V91.33
          ferry boat V91.31
          fishing boat V91.32
          jet ski V91.33
          liner V91.31
          merchant ship V91.30
          passenger ship V91.31
        unpowered craft V91.38
          canoe V91.35
          inflatable V91.36
          kayak V91.35
          sailboat V91.34
          surf-board V91.38
          windsurfer V91.38

 ▶ New   ➡ Revised   ~~deleted~~ Deleted   ● Use Additional Character(s)

Struck (Continued)
object (Continued)
  falling (Continued)
    from, in (Continued)
      watercraft (Continued)
        powered craft V93.43
          ferry boat V93.41
          fishing boat V93.42
          jet ski V93.43
          liner V93.41
          merchant ship V93.40
          passenger ship V93.41
        unpowered craft V93.48
          sailboat V93.44
          surf-board V93.48
          windsurfer V93.48
  moving NEC W20.8
  projected W20.8
    assault Y00
    in sports W21.9
      assault Y08.09
      ball W21.00
        baseball W21.03
        basketball W21.05
        football W21.01
        golf ball W21.04
        soccer W21.02
        softball W21.07
        specified NEC W21.09
        volleyball W21.06
      bat or racquet
        baseball bat W21.11
          assault Y08.02
        golf club W21.13
          assault Y08.09-●
        specified NEC W21.19
          assault Y08.09
        tennis racquet W21.12
          assault Y08.09
      hockey (ice)
        field
          puck W21.221
          stick W21.211
        puck W21.220
        stick W21.210
          assault Y08.01
      specified NEC W21.89
  set in motion by explosion —see Explosion
  thrown W20.8
    assault Y00
    in sports W21.9
      assault Y08.09
      ball W21.00
        baseball W21.03
        basketball W21.05
        football W21.01
        golf ball W21.04
        soccer W21.02
        soft ball W21.07
        specified NEC W21.09
        volleyball W21.06
      bat or racquet
        baseball bat W21.11
          assault Y08.02
        golf club W21.13
          assault Y08.09
        specified NEC W21.19
          assault Y08.09
        tennis racquet W21.12
          assault Y08.09
      hockey (ice)
        field
          puck W21.221
          stick W21.211
        puck W21.220
        stick W21.210
          assault Y08.01
      specified NEC W21.89
other person(s) W50.0
  with
    blunt object W22.8
      intentional, homicide (attempt) Y00
    sports equipment W21.9
    undetermined whether accidental or
      intentional Y29
  fall W03
    due to ice or snow W00.0
  as, or caused by, a crowd or human stampede
    (with fall) W52

Struck (Continued)
other person(s) (Continued)
  assault Y04.2
  homicide (attempt) Y04.2
  in legal intervention
    injuring
      bystander Y35.812
      law enforcement personnel
        Y35.811
      suspect Y35.813
      unspecified person Y35.819
  sports equipment W21.9
police (on duty) —see Legal, intervention,
  manhandling
  with blunt object —see Legal, intervention,
    blunt object
sports equipment W21.9
  assault Y08.09
  ball W21.00
    baseball W21.03
    basketball W21.05
    football W21.01
    golf ball W21.04
    soccer W21.02
    soft ball W21.07
    specified NEC W21.09
    volleyball W21.06
  bat or racquet
    baseball bat W21.11
      assault Y08.02
    golf club W21.13
      assault Y08.09
    specified NEC W21.19
    tennis racquet W21.12
      assault Y08.09
  cleats (shoe) W21.31
  foot wear NEC W21.39
  football helmet W21.81
  hockey (ice)
    field
      puck W21.221
      stick W21.211
    puck W21.220
    stick W21.210
      assault Y08.01
  skate blades W21.32
  specified NEC W21.89
    assault Y08.09
thunderbolt —see subcategory
  T75.0
  causing fire —see Exposure, fire
transport vehicle NEC —see also Accident,
  transport V09.9
  intentional, homicide (attempt) Y03.0
  motor NEC —see also Accident, transport
    V09.20
    homicide Y03.0
vehicle (transport) NEC —see Accident,
  transport, by type of vehicle
  stationary (falling from jack,
    hydraulic lift, ramp)
    W20.8

Stumbling
without fall W18.40
  due to
    specified NEC W18.49
    stepping from one level to another W18.43
    stepping into hole or opening W18.42
    stepping on object W18.41
  over
    animal NEC W01.0
      with fall W18.09
    carpet, rug or (small) object W22.8
      with fall W18.09
    person W51
      with fall W03
        due to ice or snow W00.0
Submersion (accidental) —see Drowning
Suffocation (accidental) (by external means)
  (by pressure) (mechanical) —see also category
  T71
due to, by
  avalanche —see Landslide
  explosion —see Explosion
  fire —see Exposure, fire
  food, any type (aspiration) (ingestion)
    (inhalation) —see categories T17 and T18
  ignition —see Ignition
  landslide —see Landslide

Suffocation (Continued)
due to, by (Continued)
  machine (ry) —see Contact, with, by type of
    machine
  vomitus (aspiration) (inhalation)
    T17.81-●
in
  burning building X00.8
Suicide, suicidal (attempted) (by) X83.8
blunt object X79
burning, burns X76
  hot object X77.9
    fluid NEC X77.2
    household appliance X77.3
    specified NEC X77.8
    steam X77.0
    tap water X77.1
    vapors X77.0
caustic substance —see Table of Drugs and
  Chemicals
cold, extreme X83.2
collision of motor vehicle with
  motor vehicle X82.0
  specified NEC X82.8
  train X82.1
  tree X82.2
crashing of aircraft X83.0
cut (any part of body) X78.9
cutting or piercing instrument X78.9
  dagger X78.2
  glass X78.0
  knife X78.1
  specified NEC X78.8
  sword X78.2
drowning (in) X71.9
  bathtub X71.0
  natural water X71.3
  specified NEC X71.8
  swimming pool X71.1
    following fall X71.2
electrocution X83.1
explosive(s) (material) X75
fire, flames X76
firearm X74.9
  airgun X74.01
  handgun X72
  hunting rifle X73.1
  larger X73.9
    specified NEC X73.8
  machine gun X73.2
  shotgun X73.0
  specified NEC X74.8
hanging X83.8
hot object —see Suicide, burning, hot object
jumping
  before moving object X81.8
    motor vehicle X81.0
    subway train X81.1
    train X81.1
  from high place X80
late effect of attempt —see X71-X83 with 7th
  character S
lying before moving object, train, vehicle
  X81.8
poisoning —see Table of Drugs and Chemicals
puncture (any part of body) —see Suicide,
  cutting or piercing instrument
scald —see Suicide, burning, hot object
sequelae of attempt —see X71-X83 with 7th
  character S
sharp object (any) —see Suicide, cutting or
  piercing instrument
shooting —see Suicide, firearm
specified means NEC X83.8
stab (any part of body) —see Suicide, cutting or
  piercing instrument
steam, hot vapors X77.0
strangulation X83.8
submersion —see Suicide, drowning
suffocation X83.8
wound NEC X83.8
Sunstroke X32
Supersonic waves (causing injury) W42.0
Surgical procedure, complication of (delayed or
  as an abnormal reaction without mention of
  misadventure) —see also Complication of or
  following, by type of procedure
due to or as a result of misadventure —see
  Misadventure

▶ New   ➡ Revised   ~~deleted~~ Deleted   ● Use Additional Character(s)

War operations *(Continued)*
  explosion *(Continued)*
    guided missile Y36.22-●
    improvised explosive device [IED]
      (person-borne) (roadside)
      (vehicle-borne) Y36.23-●
    land mine Y36.29-●
    marine mine (at sea) (in harbor) Y36.02-●
    marine weapon Y36.00-●
      specified NEC Y36.09-●
    own munitions or munitions launch
      device (accidental) Y36.24-●
    sea-based artillery shell Y36.03-●
    specified NEC Y36.29-●
    torpedo Y36.04-●
  fire Y36.30-●
    specified NEC Y36.39-●
  firearms
    discharge Y36.43-●
    pellets Y36.42-●
  flamethrower Y36.33-●
  fragments (from) (of)
    improvised explosive device [IED]
      (person-borne) (roadside)
      (vehicle-borne) Y36.26-●
    munitions Y36.25-●
    specified NEC Y36.29-●
    weapons Y36.27-●
  friendly fire Y36.92
  hand to hand (unarmed) combat Y36.44-●
  ▶HLB overpressure Y37.A2
  hot substances —*see* War operations, fire
  incendiary bullet Y36.32-●
  ▶LLB overpressure Y37.A1
  nuclear weapon (effects of) Y36.50-●
    acute radiation exposure Y36.54-●
    blast pressure Y36.51-●

War operations *(Continued)*
  nuclear weapon *(Continued)*
    direct blast Y36.51-●
    direct heat Y36.53-●
    fallout exposure Y36.54-●
    fireball Y36.53-●
    indirect blast (struck or crushed by blast
      debris) (being thrown by blast) Y36.52-●
    ionizing radiation (immediate exposure)
      Y36.54-●
    nuclear radiation Y36.54-●
    radiation
      ionizing (immediate exposure)
        Y36.54-●
      nuclear Y36.54-●
      thermal Y36.53-●
    secondary effects Y36.54-●
    specified NEC Y36.59-●
    thermal radiation Y36.53-●
  restriction of air (airway)
    intentional Y36.46-●
    unintentional Y36.47-●
  rubber bullets Y36.41-●
  shrapnel NOS Y36.29-●
  suffocation —*see* War operations, restriction of
    airways
  unconventional warfare NEC Y36.7X-●
  underwater blast NOS Y36.00-●
  warfare
    conventional NEC Y36.49-●
    unconventional NEC Y36.7X-●
  weapon of mass destruction [WMD] Y36.91
  weapons
    biological weapons Y36.6X-●
    chemical Y36.7X-●

War operations *(Continued)*
  weapons *(Continued)*
    nuclear (effects of) Y36.50-●
      acute radiation exposure Y36.54-●
      blast pressure Y36.51-●
      direct blast Y36.51-●
      direct heat Y36.53-●
      fallout exposure Y36.54-●
      fireball Y36.53-●
      radiation
        ionizing (immediate exposure) Y36.54-●
        nuclear Y36.54-●
        thermal Y36.53-●
      secondary effects Y36.54-●
      specified NEC Y36.59-●
    of mass destruction [WMD] Y36.91-●
Washed
  away by flood —*see* Flood
  off road by storm (transport vehicle) —*see* Forces
    of nature, cataclysmic storm
Weather exposure NEC —*see* Forces of nature
Weightlessness (causing injury) (effects of) (in
  spacecraft, real or simulated) X52
Work related condition Y99.0
Wound (accidental) **NEC** —*see also* Injury X58
  battle —*see also* War operations Y36.90
  gunshot —*see* Discharge, firearm by type
Wreck transport vehicle NEC —*see also* Accident,
  transport V89.9
Wrong
  device implanted into correct surgical site Y65.51
  fluid in infusion Y65.1
  patient, procedure performed on Y65.52
  procedure (operation) on correct patient Y65.51

ICD-10-CM Tabular List of Diseases and Injuries

CHAPTER 1

CERTAIN INFECTIOUS AND PARASITIC DISEASES (A00-B99)

OGCR Chapter-Specific Coding Guidelines

1. Chapter 1: Certain Infectious and Parasitic Diseases (A00-B99)

a. Human Immunodeficiency Virus (HIV) Infections

1) Code only confirmed cases

Code only confirmed cases of HIV infection/illness. This is an exception to the hospital inpatient guideline Section II, H.

In this context, "confirmation" does not require documentation of positive serology or culture for HIV; the provider's diagnostic statement that the patient is HIV positive, or has an HIV-related illness is sufficient.

2) Selection and sequencing of HIV codes

(a) Patient admitted for HIV-related condition

If a patient is admitted for an HIV-related condition, the principal diagnosis should be B20, Human immunodeficiency virus [HIV] disease followed by additional diagnosis codes for all reported HIV-related conditions.

(b) Patient with HIV disease admitted for unrelated condition

If a patient with HIV disease is admitted for an unrelated condition (such as a traumatic injury), the code for the unrelated condition (e.g., the nature of injury code) should be the principal diagnosis. Other diagnoses would be B20 followed by additional diagnosis codes for all reported HIV-related conditions.

(c) Whether the patient is newly diagnosed

Whether the patient is newly diagnosed or has had previous admissions/encounters for HIV conditions is irrelevant to the sequencing decision.

(d) Asymptomatic human immunodeficiency virus

Z21, Asymptomatic human immunodeficiency virus [HIV] infection status, is to be applied when the patient without any documentation of symptoms is listed as being "HIV positive," "known HIV," "HIV test positive," or similar terminology. Do not use this code if the term "AIDS" is used or if the patient is treated for any HIV-related illness or is described as having any condition(s) resulting from his/her HIV positive status; use B20 in these cases.

(e) Patients with inconclusive HIV serology

Patients with inconclusive HIV serology, but no definitive diagnosis or manifestations of the illness, may be assigned code R75, Inconclusive laboratory evidence of human immunodeficiency virus [HIV].

(f) Previously diagnosed HIV-related illness

Patients with any known prior diagnosis of an HIV-related illness should be coded to B20. Once a patient has developed an HIV-related illness, the patient should always be assigned code B20 on every subsequent admission/encounter. Patients previously diagnosed with any HIV illness (B20) should never be assigned to R75 or Z21, Asymptomatic human immunodeficiency virus [HIV] infection status.

(g) HIV Infection in Pregnancy, Childbirth and the Puerperium

During pregnancy, childbirth or the puerperium, a patient admitted (or presenting for a health care encounter) because of an HIV-related illness should receive a principal diagnosis code of O98.7-, Human immunodeficiency [HIV] disease complicating pregnancy, childbirth and the puerperium, followed by B20 and the code(s) for the HIV-related illness(es). Codes from Chapter 15 always take sequencing priority.

Patients with asymptomatic HIV infection status admitted (or presenting for a health care encounter) during pregnancy, childbirth, or the puerperium should receive codes of O98.7- and Z21.

(h) Encounters for testing for HIV

If a patient is being seen to determine his/her HIV status, use code Z11.4, Encounter for screening for human immunodeficiency virus [HIV]. Use additional codes for any associated high-risk behavior.

If a patient with signs or symptoms is being seen for HIV testing, code the signs and symptoms. An additional counseling code Z71.7, Human immunodeficiency virus [HIV] counseling, may be used if counseling is provided during the encounter for the test.

When a patient returns to be informed of his/her HIV test results and the test result is negative, use code Z71.7, Human immunodeficiency virus [HIV] counseling.

If the results are positive, see previous guidelines and assign codes as appropriate.

b. Infectious agents as the cause of diseases classified to other chapters

Certain infections are classified in chapters other than Chapter 1 and no organism is identified as part of the infection code. In these instances, it is necessary to use an additional code from Chapter 1 to identify the organism. A code from category B95, Streptococcus, Staphylococcus, and Enterococcus as the cause of diseases classified to other chapters, B96, Other bacterial agents as the cause of diseases classified to other chapters, or B97, Viral agents as the cause of diseases classified to other chapters, is to be used as an additional code to identify the organism. An instructional note will be found at the infection code advising that an additional organism code is required.

c. Infections resistant to antibiotics

Many bacterial infections are resistant to current antibiotics. It is necessary to identify all infections documented as antibiotic resistant. Assign a code from category Z16, Resistance to antimicrobial drugs, following the infection code only if the infection code does not identify drug resistance.

d. Sepsis, Severe Sepsis, and Septic Shock

1) Coding of Sepsis and Severe Sepsis

(a) Sepsis

For a diagnosis of sepsis, assign the appropriate code for the underlying systemic infection. If the type of infection or causal organism is not further specified, assign code A41.9, Sepsis, unspecified organism.

A code from subcategory R65.2, Severe sepsis, should not be assigned unless severe sepsis or an associated acute organ dysfunction is documented.

(i) Negative or inconclusive blood cultures and sepsis
Negative or inconclusive blood cultures do not preclude a diagnosis of sepsis in patients with clinical evidence of the condition, however, the provider should be queried.

(ii) Urosepsis
The term urosepsis is a nonspecific term. It is not to be considered synonymous with sepsis. It has no default code in the Alphabetic Index. Should a provider use this term, he/she must be queried for clarification.

(iii) Sepsis with organ dysfunction
If a patient has sepsis and associated acute organ dysfunction or multiple organ dysfunction (MOD), follow the instructions for coding severe sepsis.

(iv) Acute organ dysfunction that is not clearly associated with the sepsis
If a patient has sepsis and an acute organ dysfunction, but the medical record documentation indicates that the acute organ dysfunction is related to a medical condition other than the sepsis, do not assign a code from subcategory R65.2, Severe sepsis. An acute organ dysfunction must be associated with the sepsis in order to assign the severe sepsis code. If the documentation is not clear as to whether an acute organ dysfunction is related to the sepsis or another medical condition, query the provider.

(b) Severe sepsis

The coding of severe sepsis requires a minimum of 2 codes: first a code for the underlying systemic infection, followed by a code from subcategory R65.2, Severe sepsis. If the causal organism is not documented, assign code A41.9, Sepsis, unspecified organism, for the infection. Additional code(s) for the associated acute organ dysfunction are also required.

Due to the complex nature of severe sepsis, some cases may require querying the provider prior to assignment of the codes.

2) Septic shock

(a) Septic shock generally refers to circulatory failure associated with severe sepsis, and therefore, it represents a type of acute organ dysfunction.

For all cases of septic shock, the code for the systemic infection should be sequenced first, followed by code R65.21, Severe sepsis with septic shock or code T81.12, Postprocedural septic shock.

Any additional codes for the other acute organ dysfunctions should also be assigned. As noted in the sequencing instructions in the Tabular List, the code for septic shock cannot be assigned as a principal diagnosis.

3) Sequencing of severe sepsis

If severe sepsis is present on admission, and meets the definition of principal diagnosis, the underlying systemic infection should be assigned as principal diagnosis followed by the appropriate code from subcategory R65.2 as required by the sequencing rules in the Tabular List. A code from subcategory R65.2 can never be assigned as a principal diagnosis.

When severe sepsis develops during an encounter (it was not present on admission) the underlying systemic infection and the appropriate code from subcategory R65.2 should be assigned as secondary diagnoses.

Severe sepsis may be present on admission but the diagnosis may not be confirmed until sometime after admission. If the documentation is not clear whether severe sepsis was present on admission, the provider should be queried.

4) Sepsis and severe sepsis with a localized infection

If the reason for admission is both sepsis or severe sepsis and a localized infection, such as pneumonia or cellulitis, a code(s) for the underlying systemic infection should be assigned first and the code for the localized infection should be assigned as a secondary diagnosis. If the patient has severe sepsis, a code from subcategory R65.2 should also be assigned as a secondary diagnosis. If the patient is admitted with a localized infection, such as pneumonia, and sepsis/severe sepsis doesn't develop until after admission, the localized infection should be assigned first, followed by the appropriate sepsis/severe sepsis codes.

5) Sepsis due to a postprocedural infection

(a) Documentation of causal relationship

As with all postprocedural complications, code assignment is based on the provider's documentation of the relationship between the infection and the procedure.

(b) Sepsis due to a postprocedural infection

For infections following a procedure, a code from T81.40, to T81.43, Infection following a procedure, or O86.00 to O86.03, Infection of obstetric surgical wound, that identifies the site of the infection should be coded first, if known. Assign an additional code for sepsis following a procedure (T81.44) or sepsis following an obstetrical procedure (O86.04). Use an additional code to identify the infectious agent. If the patient has severe sepsis the appropriate code from subcategory R65.2 should also be assigned with the additional code(s) for any acute organ dysfunction.

For infections following infusion, transfusion, therapeutic injection, or immunization, a code from subcategory T80.2, Infections following infusion, transfusion, and therapeutic injection, or code T88.0-, Infection following immunization, should be coded first, followed by the code for the specific infection. If the patient has severe sepsis, the appropriate code from subcategory R65.2 should also be assigned, with the additional codes(s) for any acute organ dysfunction.

(c) Postprocedural infection and postprocedural septic shock

If a postprocedural infection has resulted in postprocedural septic shock, assign the codes indicated above for sepsis due to a postprocedural infection, followed by code T81.12-, Postprocedural septic shock. Do not assign code R65.21, Severe sepsis with septic shock. Additional code(s) should be assigned for any acute organ dysfunction.

6) Sepsis and severe sepsis associated with a noninfectious process (condition)

In some cases a noninfectious process (condition), such as trauma, may lead to an infection which can result in sepsis or severe sepsis. If sepsis or severe sepsis is documented as associated with a noninfectious condition, such as a burn or serious injury, and this condition meets the definition for principal diagnosis, the code for the noninfectious condition should be sequenced first, followed by the code for the resulting infection. If severe sepsis is present, a code from subcategory R65.2 should also be assigned with any associated organ dysfunction(s) codes. It is not necessary to assign a code from subcategory R65.1, Systemic inflammatory response syndrome (SIRS) of noninfectious origin, for these cases.

If the infection meets the definition of principal diagnosis it should be sequenced before the noninfectious condition. When both the associated noninfectious condition and the infection meet the definition of principal diagnosis either may be assigned as principal diagnosis.

Only one code from category R65, Symptoms and signs specifically associated with systemic inflammation and infection, should be assigned. Therefore, when a noninfectious condition leads to an infection resulting in severe sepsis, assign the appropriate code from subcategory R65.2, Severe sepsis. Do not additionally assign a code from subcategory R65.1, Systemic inflammatory response syndrome (SIRS) of noninfectious origin.
See Section I.C.18. SIRS due to non-infectious process

7) Sepsis and septic shock complicating abortion, pregnancy, childbirth, and the puerperium

See Section I.C.15. Sepsis and septic shock complicating abortion, pregnancy, childbirth and the puerperium

8) Newborn sepsis

See Section I.C.16. f. Bacterial sepsis of Newborn

e. Methicillin Resistant Staphylococcus aureus (MRSA) Conditions

1) Selection and sequencing of MRSA codes

(a) Combination codes for MRSA infection

When a patient is diagnosed with an infection that is due to methicillin resistant *Staphylococcus aureus* (MRSA), and that infection has a combination code that includes the causal organism (e.g., sepsis, pneumonia) assign the appropriate combination code for the condition (e.g., code A41.02, Sepsis due to Methicillin resistant Staphylococcus aureus or code J15.212, Pneumonia due to Methicillin resistant Staphylococcus aureus). Do not assign code B95.62, Methicillin resistant Staphylococcus aureus infection as the cause of diseases classified elsewhere, as an additional code because the combination code includes the type of infection and the MRSA organism. Do not assign a code from subcategory Z16.11, Resistance to penicillins, as an additional diagnosis.
See Section C.1. for instructions on coding and sequencing of sepsis and severe sepsis.

(b) Other codes for MRSA infection

When there is documentation of a current infection (e.g., wound infection, stitch abscess, urinary tract infection) due to MRSA, and that infection does not have a combination code that includes the causal organism, assign the appropriate code to identify the condition along with code B95.62, Methicillin resistant Staphylococcus aureus infection as the cause of diseases classified elsewhere for the MRSA infection. Do not assign a code from subcategory Z16.11, Resistance to penicillins.

(c) Methicillin susceptible Staphylococcus aureus (MSSA) and MRSA colonization

The condition or state of being colonized or carrying MSSA or MRSA is called colonization or carriage, while an individual person is described as being colonized or being a carrier. Colonization means that MSSA or MSRA is present on or in the body without necessarily causing illness. A positive MRSA colonization test might be documented by the provider as "MRSA screen positive" or "MRSA nasal swab positive".

Assign code Z22.322, Carrier or suspected carrier of Methicillin resistant Staphylococcus aureus, for patients documented as having MRSA colonization. Assign code Z22.321, Carrier or suspected carrier of Methicillin susceptible Staphylococcus aureus, for patient documented as having MSSA colonization. Colonization is not necessarily indicative of a disease process or as the cause of a specific condition the patient may have unless documented as such by the provider.

(d) MRSA colonization and infection

If a patient is documented as having both MRSA colonization and infection during a hospital admission, code Z22.322, Carrier or suspected carrier of Methicillin resistant Staphylococcus aureus, and a code for the MRSA infection may both be assigned.

f. Zika virus infections

1) Code only confirmed cases

Code only a confirmed diagnosis of Zika virus (A92.5, Zika virus disease) as documented by the provider. This is an exception to the hospital inpatient guideline Section II, H.

In this context, "confirmation" does not require documentation of the type of test performed; the physician's diagnostic statement that the condition is confirmed is sufficient. This code should be assigned regardless of the stated mode of transmission.

If the provider documents "suspected", "possible" or "probable" Zika, do not assign code A92.5. Assign a code(s) explaining the reason for encounter (such as fever, rash, or joint pain) or Z20.821, Contact with and (suspected) exposure to Zika virus.

CHAPTER 1

CERTAIN INFECTIOUS AND PARASITIC DISEASES (A00-B99)

Includes diseases generally recognized as communicable or transmissible

Use additional code to identify resistance to antimicrobial drugs (Z16.-)

Excludes1 certain localized infections - see body system-related chapters

Excludes2 carrier or suspected carrier of infectious disease (Z22.-)

infectious and parasitic diseases complicating pregnancy, childbirth and the puerperium (O98.-)

infectious and parasitic diseases specific to the perinatal period (P35-P39)

influenza and other acute respiratory infections (J00-J22)

This chapter contains the following blocks:

A00-A09	Intestinal infectious diseases
A15-A19	Tuberculosis
A20-A28	Certain zoonotic bacterial diseases
A30-A49	Other bacterial diseases
A50-A64	Infections with a predominantly sexual mode of transmission
A65-A69	Other spirochetal diseases
A70-A74	Other diseases caused by chlamydiae
A75-A79	Rickettsioses
A80-A89	Viral and prion infections of the central nervous system
A90-A99	Arthropod-borne viral fevers and viral hemorrhagic fevers
B00-B09	Viral infections characterized by skin and mucous membrane lesions
B10	Other human herpesviruses
B15-B19	Viral hepatitis
B20	Human immunodeficiency virus [HIV] disease
B25-B34	Other viral diseases
B35-B49	Mycoses
B50-B64	Protozoal diseases
B65-B83	Helminthiases
B85-B89	Pediculosis, acariasis and other infestations
B90-B94	Sequelae of infectious and parasitic diseases
B95-B97	Bacterial and viral infectious agents
B99	Other infectious diseases

INTESTINAL INFECTIOUS DISEASES (A00-A09)

● **A00** **Cholera**
A serious, often deadly, infectious disease of the small intestine

 A00.0 **Cholera due to Vibrio cholerae 01, biovar cholerae**
  Classical cholera

 A00.1 **Cholera due to Vibrio cholerae 01, biovar eltor**
  Cholera eltor

 A00.9 **Cholera, unspecified**

● **A01** **Typhoid and paratyphoid fevers**
Caused by Salmonella typhi and Salmonella paratyphi A, B, and C bacteria

 ● **A01.0** **Typhoid fever**
  Infection due to Salmonella typhi

  A01.00 **Typhoid fever, unspecified**

  A01.01 **Typhoid meningitis**

  A01.02 **Typhoid fever with heart involvement**
   Typhoid endocarditis
   Typhoid myocarditis

  A01.03 **Typhoid pneumonia** Ⓗ

  A01.04 **Typhoid arthritis** Ⓗ

  A01.05 **Typhoid osteomyelitis**

  A01.09 **Typhoid fever with other complications**

 A01.1 **Paratyphoid fever A**

 A01.2 **Paratyphoid fever B**

 A01.3 **Paratyphoid fever C**

 A01.4 **Paratyphoid fever, unspecified**
  Infection due to Salmonella paratyphi NOS

● **A02** **Other salmonella infections**
 Includes infection or foodborne intoxication due to any Salmonella species other than S. typhi and S. paratyphi

 A02.0 **Salmonella enteritis**
  Salmonellosis

 A02.1 **Salmonella sepsis** Ⓗ

 ● **A02.2** **Localized salmonella infections**

  A02.20 **Localized salmonella infection, unspecified**
   Specified in the documentation as localized, but unspecified as to type

  A02.21 **Salmonella meningitis**
   Specified as localized in the meninges

  A02.22 **Salmonella pneumonia** Ⓗ
   Specified as localized in the lungs

  A02.23 **Salmonella arthritis** Ⓗ
   Specified as localized in the joints

  A02.24 **Salmonella osteomyelitis** Ⓗ
   Specified as localized in bone

  A02.25 **Salmonella pyelonephritis**
   Salmonella tubulo-interstitial nephropathy

  A02.29 **Salmonella with other localized infection**
   Specified as localized (because it is still under localized heading) but does not assign into any of the above codes

 A02.8 **Other specified salmonella infections**
  Any specified salmonella infection which does NOT assign into any of the above codes (not specified as localized)

 A02.9 **Salmonella infection, unspecified**
  Unspecified in the documentation as to specific type of salmonella

● **A03** **Shigellosis**
An infectious disease caused by bacteria (Shigella)

 A03.0 **Shigellosis due to Shigella dysenteriae**
  Group A shigellosis [Shiga-Kruse dysentery]

 A03.1 **Shigellosis due to Shigella flexneri**
  Group B shigellosis

 A03.2 **Shigellosis due to Shigella boydii**
  Group C shigellosis

 A03.3 **Shigellosis due to Shigella sonnei**
  Group D shigellosis

 A03.8 **Other shigellosis**

 A03.9 **Shigellosis, unspecified**
  Bacillary dysentery NOS

● **A04** **Other bacterial intestinal infections**
 Excludes1 bacterial foodborne intoxications, NEC (A05.-)
  tuberculous enteritis (A18.32)

 A04.0 **Enteropathogenic Escherichia coli infection**
  Pertaining to or producing intestinal disease

 A04.1 **Enterotoxigenic Escherichia coli infection**
  Producing or containing intestinal toxin

Item 1–1 **Salmonella** is a bacterium that lives in the intestines of fowl and mammals and can spread to humans through improper food preparation and cooking. Salmonellosis is an infection with the bacterium. Symptoms include diarrhea, fever, and abdominal cramps 12 to 72 hours after infection. The illness usually lasts 4 to 7 days, and most persons recover without treatment. The diarrhea may be so severe that the patient needs to be hospitalized. Patients with immunocompromised systems in chronic, ill health are more likely to have the infection invade their bloodstream with life-threatening results. For example, patients with sickle cell disease are more prone to salmonella osteomyelitis than others.

▶ New ⇒ Revised ~~deleted~~ Deleted Excludes 1 Excludes 2 Includes Use additional Code first Code also Key words
OGCR Official Guidelines X Assign placeholder X ● Use Additional Character(s) ▶ Manifestation Code Ⓗ Hierarchical Condition Category **Coding Clinic**

A04.2 **Enteroinvasive** Escherichia coli infection
Capable of penetrating and spreading through intestinal mucosal epithelium

A04.3 **Enterohemorrhagic** Escherichia coli infection
Causing bloody diarrhea, resulting from microorganisms

A04.4 **Other** intestinal Escherichia coli infections
Escherichia coli enteritis NOS

A04.5 **Campylobacter** enteritis
Spiral shaped bacterium

A04.6 **Enteritis** due to Yersinia enterocolitica

    Excludes1   extraintestinal yersiniosis (A28.2)

Transmitted by infected food/water and person-to-person contact, affecting intestinal tract

● **A04.7** **Enterocolitis** due to Clostridium difficile
Clostridioides difficile colitis
Foodborne intoxication by Clostridium difficile
Pseudomembraneous colitis
Marked by fibrinous deposit (false membrane) with enmeshed necrotic cells

    A04.71   Enterocolitis due to Clostridium difficile, recurrent
       Coding Clinic: 2020, Q1, P18

    A04.72   Enterocolitis due to Clostridium difficile, **not** specified as recurrent

A04.8 **Other** specified bacterial intestinal infections

A04.9 **Bacterial** intestinal infection, **unspecified**
Bacterial enteritis NOS

● **A05** **Other** bacterial foodborne intoxications, not elsewhere classified

    Excludes1   Clostridium difficile foodborne intoxication and infection (A04.7-)
       Escherichia coli infection (A04.0-A04.4)
       listeriosis (A32.-)
       salmonella foodborne intoxication and infection (A02.-)
       toxic effect of noxious foodstuffs (T61-T62)

A05.0 **Foodborne** staphylococcal intoxication

A05.1 **Botulism** food poisoning
Botulism NOS
Classical foodborne intoxication due to Clostridium botulinum

    Excludes1   infant botulism (A48.51)
       wound botulism (A48.52)

A05.2 **Foodborne** Clostridium perfringens [Clostridium welchii] intoxication
Type A causes gas gangrene and necrotizing colitis; major cause of food poisoning in humans
Enteritis necroticans
Pig-bel

A05.3 **Foodborne** Vibrio parahaemolyticus intoxication
Organism that survives only in high salt environment (halophilic), major cause of gastroenteritis due to consumption of raw or improperly cooked fish/seafood

A05.4 **Foodborne** Bacillus cereus intoxication
Spore-forming species commonly found in soil, causes food poisoning from formation of intestinal toxins in contaminated foods

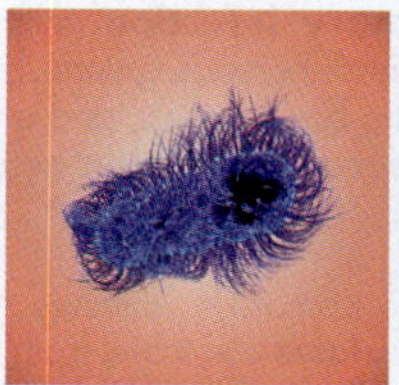

Figure 1-1 Electron micrograph of escherichia coli (E. coli) expressing P fimbriae. (Getty Image)

Item 1–2 *Escherichia coli [E. coli]* is a Gram-negative bacterium found in the intestinal tracts of humans and animals and is usually nonpathogenic. Pathogenic strains can cause diarrhea or pyogenic (pus-producing) infections. Can be a threat to food safety.

A05.5 **Foodborne** Vibrio vulnificus intoxication
Species that survives in high salt environment (halophilic) with infection by eating raw seafood causes septicemia and cellulitis

A05.8 **Other** specified bacterial foodborne intoxications

A05.9 **Bacterial** foodborne intoxication, **unspecified**

● **A06** **Amebiasis**
An intestinal illness caused by the microscopic parasite Entamoeba histolytica

    Includes   infection due to Entamoeba histolytica
    Excludes1   other protozoal intestinal diseases (A07.-)
    Excludes2   acanthamebiasis (B60.1-)
       Naegleriasis (B60.2)

A06.0 **Acute** amebic dysentery
Acute amebiasis
Intestinal amebiasis NOS

A06.1 **Chronic** intestinal amebiasis

A06.2 **Amebic** nondysenteric colitis
Pertaining to single cell microorganism

A06.3 **Ameboma** of intestine
Tumorlike mass produced by localized inflammation often in intestine
Ameboma NOS

A06.4 **Amebic** liver abscess
Hepatic amebiasis

A06.5 **Amebic** lung abscess
Amebic abscess of lung (and liver)

A06.6 **Amebic** brain abscess
Amebic abscess of brain (and liver) (and lung)

● **A06.7** **Cutaneous** amebiasis

● **A06.8** **Amebic** infection of other sites

    A06.81   Amebic cystitis

    A06.82   Other amebic genitourinary infections
       Amebic balanitis
       Amebic vesiculitis
       Amebic vulvovaginitis

    A06.89   Other amebic infections
       Amebic appendicitis
       Amebic splenic abscess

A06.9 **Amebiasis, unspecified**

● **A07** **Other** protozoal intestinal diseases

A07.0 **Balantidiasis**
Balantidial dysentery
Infection by protozoa that may cause diarrhea and dysentery, with ulceration of colonic mucous membranes

A07.1 **Giardiasis** [lambliasis]
Common infection in small intestine spread by contaminated food, water, or direct person-to-person contact

A07.2 **Cryptosporidiosis**
Human infection with protozoa usually seen as self-limited diarrhea in those who work with cattle

A07.3 **Isosporiasis**
Human intestinal disease caused by protozoa
Infection due to Isospora belli and Isospora hominis
Intestinal coccidiosis
Isosporosis

A07.4 **Cyclosporiasis**
Infection by protozoa with most common species infecting humans being C cayetanensis

A07.8 **Other** specified protozoal intestinal diseases
Intestinal microsporidiosis
Intestinal trichomoniasis
Sarcocystosis
Sarcosporidiosis

CHAPTER 1 (A00-B99)

CHAPTER 1 (A00–B99)

A07.9 **Protozoal intestinal disease, unspecified**
Flagellate diarrhea
Protozoal colitis
Protozoal diarrhea
Protozoal dysentery

● **A08** **Viral and other specified intestinal infections**
Excludes1 influenza with involvement of gastrointestinal
tract (J09.X3, J10.2, J11.2)

A08.0 **Rotaviral enteritis**
● **A08.1** **Acute gastroenteropathy due to Norwalk agent and
other small round viruses**
A08.11 **Acute gastroenteropathy due to Norwalk agent**
Acute gastroenteropathy due to Norovirus
Acute gastroenteropathy due to Norwalk-like
agent
A08.19 **Acute gastroenteropathy due to other small
round viruses**
Acute gastroenteropathy due to small round
virus [SRV] NOS

A08.2 **Adenoviral enteritis**
● **A08.3** **Other viral enteritis**
A08.31 **Calicivirus enteritis**
A08.32 **Astrovirus enteritis**
A08.39 **Other viral enteritis**
Coxsackie virus enteritis
Echovirus enteritis
Enterovirus enteritis NEC
Torovirus enteritis

A08.4 **Viral intestinal infection, unspecified**
Viral enteritis NOS
Viral gastroenteritis NOS
Viral gastroenteropathy NOS
Coding Clinic: 2016, Q3, P12

A08.8 **Other specified intestinal infections**

A09 **Infectious gastroenteritis and colitis, unspecified**
Infectious colitis NOS
Infectious enteritis NOS
Infectious gastroenteritis NOS
Excludes1 colitis NOS (K52.9)
diarrhea NOS (R19.7)
enteritis NOS (K52.9)
gastroenteritis NOS (K52.9)
noninfective gastroenteritis and colitis,
unspecified (K52.9)

TUBERCULOSIS (A15–A19)

Includes infections due to Mycobacterium tuberculosis
and Mycobacterium bovis
Excludes1 congenital tuberculosis (P37.0)
nonspecific reaction to test for tuberculosis
without active tuberculosis (R76.1-)
pneumoconiosis associated with tuberculosis, any
type in A15 (J65)
positive PPD (R76.11)
positive tuberculin skin test without active
tuberculosis (R76.11)
sequelae of tuberculosis (B90.-)
silicotuberculosis (J65)

● **A15** **Respiratory tuberculosis**
A15.0 **Tuberculosis of lung**
Tuberculous bronchiectasis
Chronic dilatation of bronchi
Tuberculous fibrosis of lung
Tuberculous pneumonia
Tuberculous pneumothorax
A15.4 **Tuberculosis of intrathoracic lymph nodes**
Tuberculosis of hilar lymph nodes
Tuberculosis of mediastinal lymph nodes
Tuberculosis of tracheobronchial lymph nodes
Excludes1 tuberculosis specified as primary (A15.7)

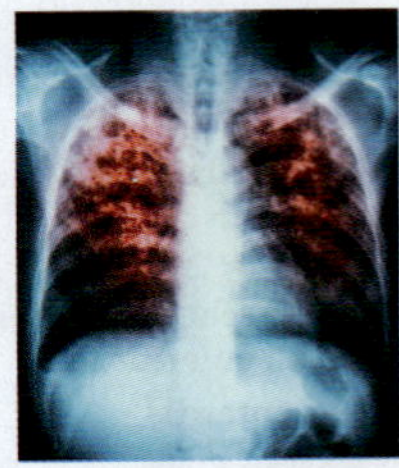

Figure 1-2 Far advanced bilateral pulmonary tuberculosis before and
after 8 months of treatment with streptomycin, PAS, and isoniazid. (Getty
Image)

A15.5 **Tuberculosis of larynx, trachea and
bronchus**
Tuberculosis of bronchus
Tuberculosis of glottis
Tuberculosis of larynx
Tuberculosis of trachea
A15.6 **Tuberculous pleurisy**
Tuberculosis of pleura
Tuberculous empyema
Excludes1 primary respiratory tuberculosis (A15.7)
A15.7 **Primary respiratory tuberculosis**
A15.8 **Other respiratory tuberculosis**
Mediastinal tuberculosis
Nasopharyngeal tuberculosis
Tuberculosis of nose
Tuberculosis of sinus [any nasal]
A15.9 **Respiratory tuberculosis unspecified**

● **A17** **Tuberculosis of nervous system**
A17.0 **Tuberculous meningitis**
Tuberculosis of meninges (cerebral) (spinal)
Tuberculous leptomeningitis
Excludes1 tuberculous meningoencephalitis
(A17.82)
A17.1 **Meningeal tuberculoma**
Tuberculoma of meninges (cerebral) (spinal)
Excludes2 tuberculoma of brain and spinal cord
(A17.81)
● **A17.8** **Other tuberculosis of nervous system**
A17.81 **Tuberculoma of brain and spinal
cord**
Tuberculous abscess of brain and spinal cord
A17.82 **Tuberculous meningoencephalitis**
*Inflammation of brain and meninges; AKA
cerebromeningitis and encephalomeningitis*
Tuberculous myelitis
A17.83 **Tuberculous neuritis**
Tuberculous mononeuropathy
A17.89 **Other tuberculosis of nervous
system**
Tuberculous polyneuropathy
A17.9 **Tuberculosis of nervous system, unspecified**

Item 1–3 Tuberculosis is a common and deadly infectious disease
caused by the *Mycobacterium tuberculosis* organism. The first tuberculosis
infection is called the **primary infection** and most commonly attacks the
lungs but can affect the central nervous system, lymphatic system, circulatory
system, genitourinary system, bones, joints, and even the skin. A **Ghon** lesion
is the **initial lesion.** A **secondary lesion** occurs when the tubercle bacilli
are carried to other areas.

Item 1–4 Although it primarily affects the lungs, the bacteria
Mycobacterium tuberculosis can travel from the pulmonary circulation to
virtually any organ in the body, much as a cancer metastasizes to a secondary
site. If the immune system becomes compromised by age or disease, what
would otherwise be a self-limiting primary tuberculosis in the lungs will develop
in other organs. These are known as extrapulmonary sites.

▶ New   ⇨ Revised   ~~deleted~~ Deleted   Excludes 1   Excludes 2   Includes   Use additional   Code first   Code also   Key words
OGCR Official Guidelines   X Assign placeholder X   ● Use Additional Character(s)   ▶ Manifestation Code   Hierarchical Condition Category   **Coding Clinic**

A18   Tuberculosis of other organs

A18.0   Tuberculosis of bones and joints

A18.01   Tuberculosis of spine
Pott's disease or curvature of spine
Tuberculous arthritis
Tuberculous osteomyelitis of spine
Tuberculous spondylitis

A18.02   Tuberculous arthritis of other joints
Tuberculosis of hip (joint)
Tuberculosis of knee (joint)

A18.03   Tuberculosis of other bones
Tuberculous mastoiditis
Tuberculous osteomyelitis

A18.09   Other musculoskeletal tuberculosis
Tuberculous myositis
Tuberculous synovitis
Tuberculous tenosynovitis

A18.1   Tuberculosis of genitourinary system

A18.10   Tuberculosis of genitourinary system, unspecified

A18.11   Tuberculosis of kidney and ureter

A18.12   Tuberculosis of bladder

A18.13   Tuberculosis of other urinary organs
Tuberculous urethritis

A18.14   Tuberculosis of prostate

A18.15   Tuberculosis of other male genital organs

A18.16   Tuberculosis of cervix

A18.17   Tuberculous female pelvic inflammatory disease
Tuberculous endometritis
Tuberculous oophoritis and salpingitis
Oophoritis = inflammation of ovary
Salpingitis = inflammation of fallopian tube

A18.18   Tuberculosis of other female genital organs
Tuberculous ulceration of vulva

A18.2   Tuberculous peripheral lymphadenopathy
Tuberculous adenitis

Excludes2   tuberculosis of bronchial and mediastinal lymph nodes (A15.4)
tuberculosis of mesenteric and retroperitoneal lymph nodes (A18.39)
tuberculous tracheobronchial adenopathy (A15.4)

A18.3   Tuberculosis of intestines, peritoneum and mesenteric glands

A18.31   Tuberculous peritonitis
Tuberculous ascites

A18.32   Tuberculous enteritis
Tuberculosis of anus and rectum
Tuberculosis of intestine (large) (small)

A18.39   Retroperitoneal tuberculosis
Tuberculosis of mesenteric glands
Tuberculosis of retroperitoneal (lymph glands)

A18.4   Tuberculosis of skin and subcutaneous tissue
Erythema induratum, tuberculous
Lupus exedens
Lupus vulgaris NOS
Lupus vulgaris of eyelid
Cutaneous tuberculosis characterized by reddish brown plaque on skin surrounded by papules and nodules
Scrofuloderma
Type of cutaneous tuberculosis, with direct extension of tuberculosis into skin from underlying structures; AKA tuberculosis colliquativa
Tuberculosis of external ear

Excludes2   lupus erythematosus (L93.-)
systemic lupus erythematosus (M32.-)

A18.5   Tuberculosis of eye

Excludes2   lupus vulgaris of eyelid (A18.4)

A18.50   Tuberculosis of eye, unspecified

A18.51   Tuberculous episcleritis
Inflammation of episclera and adjacent tissues

A18.52   Tuberculous keratitis
Tuberculous interstitial keratitis
Tuberculous keratoconjunctivitis (interstitial) (phlyctenular)
Inflammation of cornea and conjunctiva

A18.53   Tuberculous chorioretinitis
Inflammation of choroid and retina; retinochoroiditis

A18.54   Tuberculous iridocyclitis
Inflammation of iris and ciliary body

A18.59   Other tuberculosis of eye
Tuberculous conjunctivitis

A18.6   Tuberculosis of (inner) (middle) ear
Tuberculous otitis media

Excludes2   tuberculosis of external ear (A18.4)
tuberculous mastoiditis (A18.03)

A18.7   Tuberculosis of adrenal glands
Tuberculous Addison's disease

A18.8   Tuberculosis of other specified organs

A18.81   Tuberculosis of thyroid gland

A18.82   Tuberculosis of other endocrine glands
Tuberculosis of pituitary gland
Tuberculosis of thymus gland

A18.83   Tuberculosis of digestive tract organs, not elsewhere classified

Excludes1   tuberculosis of intestine (A18.32)

A18.84   Tuberculosis of heart
Tuberculous cardiomyopathy
Tuberculous endocarditis
Tuberculous myocarditis
Tuberculous pericarditis

A18.85   Tuberculosis of spleen

A18.89   Tuberculosis of other sites
Tuberculosis of muscle
Tuberculous cerebral arteritis

A19   Miliary tuberculosis

Includes   disseminated tuberculosis
generalized tuberculosis
tuberculous polyserositis

A19.0   Acute miliary tuberculosis of a single specified site

A19.1   Acute miliary tuberculosis of multiple sites

A19.2   Acute miliary tuberculosis, unspecified

A19.8   Other miliary tuberculosis

A19.9   Miliary tuberculosis, unspecified

Item 1–5   Miliary tuberculosis can be a life-threatening condition. If a tuberculous lesion enters a blood vessel, immense dissemination of tuberculous organisms can occur if the immune system is weak. High-risk populations—children under 4 years of age, the elderly, or the immunocompromised—are particularly prone to this type of infection. The lesions will have a millet seedlike appearance on chest x-ray. Bronchial washings and biopsy may aid in diagnosis.

CHAPTER 1 (A00-B99)

CERTAIN ZOONOTIC BACTERIAL DISEASES (A2Ø-A28)

● **A2Ø**   **Plague**
Infectious disease caused by a Yersinia pestis bacterium, transmitted by a rodent flea bite or handling of infected animal

    Includes   infection due to Yersinia pestis

A2Ø.Ø   **Bubonic plague**

A2Ø.1   **Cellulocutaneous plague**
Skin and subcutaneous tissue plague

A2Ø.2   **Pneumonic plague** Ⓗⓒⓒ

A2Ø.3   **Plague meningitis**

A2Ø.7   **Septicemic plague** Ⓗⓒⓒ

A2Ø.8   **Other forms of plague**
Abortive plague
Asymptomatic plague
Pestis minor
Systemic bacterial disease

A2Ø.9   **Plague, unspecified**

● **A21**   **Tularemia**
Caused by Francisella tularensis bacterium found in rodents, rabbits, and hares and transmitted to humans by contact with infected animal tissues or by ticks, biting flies, or mosquitoes

    Includes   deer-fly fever
infection due to Francisella tularensis
rabbit fever

Coding Clinic: 2Ø16, Q4, P25

A21.Ø   **Ulceroglandular tularemia**
Most common form of tularemia in humans is painful, swollen, erythematous papule at point of inoculation that ruptures to form shallow ulcer

A21.1   **Oculoglandular tularemia**
Primary site of entry is conjunctival sac, results in granulomatous corneal lesions
Ophthalmic tularemia

A21.2   **Pulmonary tularemia** Ⓗⓒⓒ

A21.3   **Gastrointestinal tularemia**
Abdominal tularemia

A21.7   **Generalized tularemia**

A21.8   **Other forms of tularemia**

A21.9   **Tularemia, unspecified**

● **A22**   **Anthrax**
An acute infectious disease caused by the spore-forming Bacillus anthracis; occurs in humans exposed to infected animals or tissue from infected animals

    Includes   infection due to Bacillus anthracis

A22.Ø   **Cutaneous anthrax**
Malignant carbuncle
Malignant pustule

A22.1   **Pulmonary anthrax** Ⓗⓒⓒ
Inhalation anthrax
Ragpicker's disease
Woolsorter's disease

A22.2   **Gastrointestinal anthrax**

A22.7   **Anthrax sepsis** Ⓗⓒⓒ
Infectious bacterial disease

A22.8   **Other forms of anthrax**
Anthrax meningitis

A22.9   **Anthrax, unspecified**

● **A23**   **Brucellosis**

    Includes   Malta fever
Mediterranean fever
undulant fever

A23.Ø   **Brucellosis due to Brucella melitensis**
Resulting in flu-like symptoms that may lead to chronic symptoms that include recurrent fevers, joint pain, and fatigue

A23.1   **Brucellosis due to Brucella abortus**
Most common cause of brucellosis in humans; AKA Bang bacillus

Item 1-6   Brucellosis: An infectious disease caused by the bacterium Brucella. Humans are infected by contact with contaminated animals or animal products. In humans brucellosis symptoms that are similar to the flu include fever, sweats, headaches, back pains, and physical weakness. Severe infections of the central nervous system or lining of the heart may occur. Brucellosis can also cause chronic symptoms that include recurrent fevers, joint pain, and fatigue.

A23.2   **Brucellosis due to Brucella suis**
Species found primarily in pigs, rabbits, and reindeer

A23.3   **Brucellosis due to Brucella canis**
Species that causes respiratory tract infection in humans

A23.8   **Other brucellosis**

A23.9   **Brucellosis, unspecified**

● **A24**   **Glanders and melioidosis**
Infection, usually of rodents, which spreads to other animals and humans, caused by Burkholderia pseudomallei through break in skin contaminated with infested soil or water

A24.Ø   **Glanders**
Infection due to Pseudomonas mallei
Malleus

A24.1   **Acute and fulminating melioidosis**
Melioidosis pneumonia
Melioidosis sepsis

A24.2   **Subacute and chronic melioidosis**

A24.3   **Other melioidosis**

A24.9   **Melioidosis, unspecified**
Infection due to Pseudomonas pseudomallei NOS
Whitmore's disease

● **A25**   **Rat-bite fevers**
RBF, infectious disease caused by Streptobacillus moniliformis or Spirillum minus.

A25.Ø   **Spirillosis**
Any disease condition caused by spirilla
Sodoku

A25.1   **Streptobacillosis**
Acute, febrile human illness caused by bacteria transmitted by rats in most cases, passed from rodent to human via rodent's urine or mucous secretions; AKA rat fever
Epidemic arthritic erythema
Haverhill fever
Streptobacillary rat-bite fever

A25.9   **Rat-bite fever, unspecified**

● **A26**   **Erysipeloid**
Infection with Erysipelothrix rhusiopathiae, occurring often as occupational disease resulting from handling infected fish, shellfish, meat, or poultry

A26.Ø   **Cutaneous erysipeloid**
Erythema migrans

A26.7   **Erysipelothrix sepsis** Ⓗⓒⓒ

A26.8   **Other forms of erysipeloid**

A26.9   **Erysipeloid, unspecified**

● **A27**   **Leptospirosis**
Occurs most commonly in the tropics

A27.Ø   **Leptospirosis icterohemorrhagica**
Leptospiral or spirochetal jaundice (hemorrhagic)
Weil's disease

● **A27.8**   **Other forms of leptospirosis**

    A27.81   **Aseptic meningitis in leptospirosis**

    A27.89   **Other forms of leptospirosis**

A27.9   **Leptospirosis, unspecified**

● **A28**   **Other zoonotic bacterial diseases, not elsewhere classified**

A28.Ø   **Pasteurellosis**
Infection of humans or other animals by species of Pasteurella

A28.1   **Cat-scratch disease**
Cat-scratch fever

A28.2 **Extraintestinal yersiniosis**
Infection from Yersinia enterocolitica; *AKA enteric yersiniosis, intestinal yersiniosis, Yersinia enteritis*
Excludes1 enteritis due to Yersinia enterocolitica (A04.6)
plague (A20.-)

A28.8 **Other specified zoonotic bacterial diseases, not elsewhere classified**

A28.9 **Zoonotic bacterial disease, unspecified**

OTHER BACTERIAL DISEASES (A30-A49)

● **A30** **Leprosy [Hansen's disease]**
Chronic infectious disease attacking the skin, peripheral nerves, and mucous membranes
Includes infection due to Mycobacterium leprae
Excludes1 sequelae of leprosy (B92)

A30.0 **Indeterminate leprosy**
I leprosy

A30.1 **Tuberculoid leprosy**
TT leprosy

A30.2 **Borderline tuberculoid leprosy**
BT leprosy

A30.3 **Borderline leprosy**
BB leprosy

A30.4 **Borderline lepromatous leprosy**
BL leprosy

A30.5 **Lepromatous leprosy**
LL leprosy

A30.8 **Other forms of leprosy**

A30.9 **Leprosy, unspecified**

● **A31** **Infection due to other mycobacteria**
Excludes2 leprosy (A30.-)
tuberculosis (A15-A19)

A31.0 **Pulmonary mycobacterial infection** 🅡🅒
Infection due to Mycobacterium avium
Infection due to Mycobacterium intracellulare [Battey bacillus]
Infection due to Mycobacterium kansasii

A31.1 **Cutaneous mycobacterial infection**
Buruli ulcer
Infection due to Mycobacterium marinum
Infection due to Mycobacterium ulcerans

A31.2 **Disseminated mycobacterium avium-intracellulare complex (DMAC)** 🅡🅒
MAC sepsis

A31.8 **Other mycobacterial infections**

A31.9 **Mycobacterial infection, unspecified**
Atypical mycobacterial infection NOS
Mycobacteriosis NOS

● **A32** **Listeriosis**
Infection caused by Listeria monocytogenes
Includes listerial foodborne infection
Excludes1 neonatal (disseminated) listeriosis (P37.2)

A32.0 **Cutaneous listeriosis**

● A32.1 **Listerial meningitis and meningoencephalitis**

A32.11 **Listerial meningitis**

A32.12 **Listerial meningoencephalitis**

A32.7 **Listerial sepsis** 🅡🅒

● A32.8 **Other forms of listeriosis**

A32.81 **Oculoglandular listeriosis**
Primary infection site is conjunctival sac, which if untreated may result in perforation of cornea and optic atrophy

A32.82 **Listerial endocarditis**
Exudative and proliferative inflammatory condition of endocardium caused by listeria bacteria

A32.89 **Other forms of listeriosis**
Listerial cerebral arteritis

A32.9 **Listeriosis, unspecified**

A33 **Tetanus neonatorum**   **N**
Neonate = newborn

A34 **Obstetrical tetanus**   **M**

A35 **Other tetanus**
Tetanus NOS
Excludes1 tetanus neonatorum (A33)
obstetrical tetanus (A34)

● A36 **Diphtheria**

A36.0 **Pharyngeal diphtheria**
Diphtheritic membranous angina
Tonsillar diphtheria

A36.1 **Nasopharyngeal diphtheria**

A36.2 **Laryngeal diphtheria**
Diphtheritic laryngotracheitis

A36.3 **Cutaneous diphtheria**
Excludes2 erythrasma (L08.1)

● A36.8 **Other diphtheria**

A36.81 **Diphtheritic cardiomyopathy** 🅡🅒
Diphtheritic myocarditis

A36.82 **Diphtheritic radiculomyelitis**

A36.83 **Diphtheritic polyneuritis**

A36.84 **Diphtheritic tubulo-interstitial nephropathy**

A36.85 **Diphtheritic cystitis**

A36.86 **Diphtheritic conjunctivitis**

A36.89 **Other diphtheritic complications**
Diphtheritic peritonitis

A36.9 **Diphtheria, unspecified**

● A37 **Whooping cough**
Pertussis is a highly contagious disease caused by the bacterium Bordetella pertussis and results in a whooping sounding cough.

● A37.0 **Whooping cough due to Bordetella pertussis**

A37.00 **Whooping cough due to Bordetella pertussis without pneumonia**
Paroxysmal cough due to Bordetella pertussis without pneumonia

A37.01 **Whooping cough due to Bordetella pertussis with pneumonia**
Paroxysmal cough due to Bordetella pertussis without pneumonia

● A37.1 **Whooping cough due to Bordetella parapertussis**

A37.10 **Whooping cough due to Bordetella parapertussis without pneumonia**

A37.11 **Whooping cough due to Bordetella parapertussis with pneumonia**

● A37.8 **Whooping cough due to other Bordetella species**

A37.80 **Whooping cough due to other Bordetella species without pneumonia**

A37.81 **Whooping cough due to other Bordetella species with pneumonia**

● A37.9 **Whooping cough, unspecified species**

A37.90 **Whooping cough, unspecified species without pneumonia**

A37.91 **Whooping cough, unspecified species with pneumonia**

Item 1-7 Diphtheria: A highly contagious bacterial disease that results in the formation of an adherent membrane in the throat that may lead to suffocation. In its most poisonous form, it attacks the heart and lungs. It is spread by direct physical contact or breathing the aerosolized secretions of infected individuals. The exact location is specified in the codes.

CHAPTER 1 (A00-B99)

CHAPTER 1 (A00–B99)

● A38　Scarlet fever
Most commonly caused by the bacteria Streptococcus pneumoniae and Neisseria meningitides

Includes　scarlatina

Excludes2　streptococcal sore throat (J02.0)

A38.0　Scarlet fever with **otitis media**

A38.1　Scarlet fever with **myocarditis**

A38.8　Scarlet fever with **other complications**

A38.9　Scarlet fever, **uncomplicated**
　　　　Scarlet fever, NOS

● A39　Meningococcal infection
Most commonly caused by the bacteria Streptococcus pneumoniae and Neisseria meningitides

A39.0　Meningococcal **meningitis**

A39.1　Waterhouse-Friderichsen syndrome 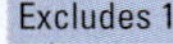
　　　Fulminating complication of meningococcemia
　　　Meningococcal hemorrhagic adrenalitis
　　　Meningococcic adrenal syndrome

A39.2　Acute meningococcemia

A39.3　Chronic meningococcemia

A39.4　Meningococcemia, **unspecified**

● A39.5　Meningococcal heart disease

A39.50　Meningococcal carditis, **unspecified**

A39.51　Meningococcal **endocarditis**

A39.52　Meningococcal **myocarditis**

A39.53　Meningococcal **pericarditis**

● A39.8　Other meningococcal infections

A39.81　Meningococcal **encephalitis**

A39.82　Meningococcal **retrobulbar neuritis**
　　　Optic neuritis in portion of optic nerve posterior to eyeball; AKA postocular optic neuritis

A39.83　Meningococcal **arthritis**

A39.84　**Postmeningococcal arthritis**

A39.89　Other meningococcal infections
　　　Meningococcal conjunctivitis

A39.9　Meningococcal infection, **unspecified**
　　　Meningococcal disease NOS

● A40　Streptococcal sepsis

Code first
, if applicable, postprocedural sepsis (T81.44-)
sepsis due to central venous catheter (T80.211-)
streptococcal sepsis during labor (O75.3)
streptococcal sepsis following abortion or ectopic or molar pregnancy (O03.37, O03.87, O04.87, O07.37, O08.82)
streptococcal sepsis following immunization (T88.0-)
streptococcal sepsis following infusion, transfusion or therapeutic injection (T80.22-, T80.29-)

Excludes1　neonatal (P36.0-P36.1)
　　　puerperal sepsis (O85)
　　　sepsis due to Streptococcus, group D (A41.81)

A40.0　Sepsis due to streptococcus, group **A**

A40.1　Sepsis due to streptococcus, group **B**
　　Coding Clinic: 2019, Q1, P14

A40.3　Sepsis due to **Streptococcus pneumoniae**
　　　Pneumococcal sepsis

A40.8　Other streptococcal sepsis

A40.9　Streptococcal sepsis, **unspecified**

● A41　Other sepsis

Code first
, if applicable, postprocedural sepsis (T81.44-)
sepsis due to central venous catheter (T80.211-)
sepsis during labor (O75.3)
sepsis following abortion, ectopic or molar pregnancy (O03.37, O03.87, O04.87, O07.37, O08.82)
sepsis following immunization (T88.0-)
sepsis following infusion, transfusion or therapeutic injection (T80.22-, T80.29-)

Excludes1　bacteremia NOS (R78.81)
　　　neonatal (P36.-)
　　　puerperal sepsis (O85)
　　　streptococcal sepsis (A40.-)

Excludes2　sepsis (due to) (in) actinomycotic (A42.7)
　　　sepsis (due to) (in) anthrax (A22.7)
　　　sepsis (due to) (in) candidal (B37.7)
　　　sepsis (due to) (in) Erysipelothrix (A26.7)
　　　sepsis (due to) (in) extraintestinal yersiniosis (A28.2)
　　　sepsis (due to) (in) gonococcal (A54.86)
　　　sepsis (due to) (in) herpesviral (B00.7)
　　　sepsis (due to) (in) listerial (A32.7)
　　　sepsis (due to) (in) melioidosis (A24.1)
　　　sepsis (due to) (in) meningococcal (A39.2-A39.4)
　　　sepsis (due to) (in) plague (A20.7)
　　　sepsis (due to) (in) tularemia (A21.7)
　　　toxic shock syndrome (A48.3)
　　Coding Clinic: 2022, Q1, P35; 2016, Q1, P39

● A41.0　Sepsis due to Staphylococcus aureus

A41.01　Sepsis due to Methicillin **susceptible** Staphylococcus aureus
　　　MSSA sepsis
　　　Staphylococcus aureus sepsis NOS

A41.02　Sepsis due to Methicillin **resistant** Staphylococcus aureus

A41.1　Sepsis due to **other specified staphylococcus**
　　　Coagulase negative staphylococcus sepsis
　　Coding Clinic: 2024, Q1, P19

A41.2　Sepsis due to **unspecified staphylococcus**

A41.3　Sepsis due to **Hemophilus influenzae**

A41.4　Sepsis due to **anaerobes**
　　Excludes1　gas gangrene (A48.0)

● A41.5　Sepsis due to other Gram-negative organisms

A41.50　**Gram-negative sepsis, unspecified**
　　　Gram-negative sepsis NOS

A41.51　Sepsis due to **Escherichia coli [E. coli]**
　　Coding Clinic: 2018, Q1, P16

A41.52　Sepsis due to **Pseudomonas**
　　　Pseudomonas aeruginosa

A41.53　Sepsis due to **Serratia**

A41.54　Sepsis due to Acinetobacter baumannii

A41.59　Other **Gram-negative sepsis**
　　Coding Clinic: 2019, Q1, P13

● A41.8　Other specified sepsis

A41.81　Sepsis due to **Enterococcus**

A41.89　Other specified sepsis
　　Coding Clinic: 2021, Q1, P33; 2016, Q3, P8-14

A41.9　Sepsis, **unspecified** organism
　　　Septicemia NOS
　　Coding Clinic: 2022, Q2, P5; Q1, P30; 2018, Q4, P18

● A42　Actinomycosis

Excludes1　actinomycetoma (B47.1)

A42.0　Pulmonary actinomycosis

A42.1　Abdominal actinomycosis

A42.2　Cervicofacial actinomycosis

A42.7　Actinomycotic sepsis

- **A42.8 Other forms of actinomycosis**
  - A42.81 Actinomycotic **meningitis**
  - A42.82 Actinomycotic **encephalitis**
  - A42.89 **Other** forms of actinomycosis
- A42.9 Actinomycosis, **unspecified**

- **A43 Nocardiosis**
  - A43.0 Pulmonary nocardiosis
  - A43.1 Cutaneous nocardiosis
  - A43.8 Other forms of nocardiosis
  - A43.9 Nocardiosis, **unspecified**

- **A44 Bartonellosis**
  - A44.0 **Systemic bartonellosis**
    Oroya fever
  - A44.1 Cutaneous and mucocutaneous bartonellosis
    Verruga peruana
  - A44.8 Other forms of bartonellosis
  - A44.9 Bartonellosis, **unspecified**

- A46 Erysipelas
  - **Excludes1** postpartum or puerperal erysipelas (O86.89)

- **A48 Other bacterial diseases, not elsewhere classified**
  - **Excludes1** actinomycetoma (B47.1)
  - A48.0 Gas gangrene
    Clostridial cellulitis
    Clostridial myonecrosis
    Coding Clinic: 2017, Q4, P102
  - A48.1 Legionnaires' disease
  - A48.2 Nonpneumonic Legionnaires' disease [Pontiac fever]
  - A48.3 Toxic shock syndrome
    Use additional code to identify the organism (B95, B96)
    - **Excludes1** endotoxic shock NOS (R57.8)
      sepsis NOS (A41.9)
    Coding Clinic: 2022, Q1, P35
  - A48.4 Brazilian purpuric fever
    Systemic Hemophilus aegyptius infection
  - **A48.5 Other specified botulism**
    Non-foodborne intoxication due to toxins of
    Clostridium botulinum [C. botulinum]
    - **Excludes1** food poisoning due to toxins of
      Clostridium botulinum (A05.1)
    - A48.51 **Infant botulism** P
    - A48.52 **Wound botulism**
      Non-foodborne botulism NOS
      Use additional code for associated wound
  - A48.8 Other specified bacterial diseases

- **A49 Bacterial infection of unspecified site**
  - **Excludes1** bacterial agents as the cause of diseases classified
    elsewhere (B95-B96)
    chlamydial infection NOS (A74.9)
    meningococcal infection NOS (A39.9)
    rickettsial infection NOS (A79.9)
    spirochetal infection NOS (A69.9)

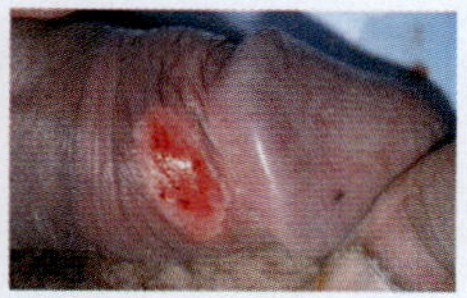

Figure 1-3 Chancre of primary syphilis. (From James WD, Berger TG, Elston DM: Andrews' Diseases of the Skin: Clinical Dermatology, Philadelphia, Saunders Elsevier, 2006)

Item 1-8 Gas gangrene is a necrotizing subcutaneous infection that will cause tissue death. Patients with poor circulation (e.g., diabetes, peripheral nephropathy) will have low oxygen content in their tissues (hypoxia), which allows the Clostridium bacteria to flourish. Gas gangrene often occurs at the site of a surgical wound or trauma. Onset is sudden and dramatic. Treatment can include debridement, amputation, and/or hyperbaric oxygen treatments.

Item 1-9 Syphilis, also known as lues, is the most serious of the venereal diseases caused by *Treponema pallidum*. The **primary** stage is characterized by an ulceration known as **chancre,** which usually appears on the genitals but can also develop on the anus, lips, tonsils, breasts, or fingers. Syphilis is easy to cure in its early stages. A single intramuscular injection of penicillin will usually cure a person who has had syphilis for less than a year.

The **secondary** stage is characterized by a rash that can affect any area of the body. **Latent** syphilis is divided into **early,** which is diagnosed within two years of infection, and **late,** which is diagnosed two years or more after infection. Additional doses of penicillin or another antibiotic are needed to treat someone who has had syphilis for longer than a year. For those allergic to penicillin, there are other antibiotic treatments. **Congenital** syphilis is also labeled **early** or **late** based on the time of diagnosis.

- **A49.0 Staphylococcal infection, unspecified site**
  - A49.01 **Methicillin susceptible Staphylococcus aureus**
    infection, unspecified site
    Methicillin susceptible Staphylococcus aureus
    (MSSA) infection
    Staphylococcus aureus infection NOS
  - A49.02 **Methicillin resistant Staphylococcus aureus**
    infection, unspecified site
    Methicillin resistant Staphylococcus aureus
    (MRSA) infection
  - A49.1 Streptococcal infection, **unspecified** site
  - A49.2 Hemophilus influenzae infection, **unspecified** site
    Any of seven bacterium of genus Haemophilus
  - A49.3 Mycoplasma infection, **unspecified** site
    *Bacterium of class Mollicutes, unusual group of bacteria
    distinguished by absence of cell wall*
  - A49.8 Other bacterial infections of **unspecified** site
  - A49.9 Bacterial infection, **unspecified**
    - **Excludes1** bacteremia NOS (R78.81)

INFECTIONS WITH A PREDOMINANTLY SEXUAL MODE OF TRANSMISSION (A50-A64)

- **Excludes1** nonspecific and nongonococcal urethritis (N34.1)
  Reiter's disease (M02.3-)
- **Excludes2** human immunodeficiency virus [HIV] disease
  (B20)

- **A50 Congenital syphilis**
  - **A50.0 Early congenital syphilis, symptomatic**
    Any congenital syphilitic condition specified as early or
    manifest less than two years after birth
    - A50.01 Early congenital syphilitic **oculopathy**
    - A50.02 Early congenital syphilitic **osteochondropathy**
    - A50.03 Early congenital syphilitic **pharyngitis**
      Early congenital syphilitic laryngitis
    - A50.04 Early congenital syphilitic **pneumonia**
    - A50.05 Early congenital syphilitic **rhinitis**
    - A50.06 Early **cutaneous** congenital syphilis
    - A50.07 Early **mucocutaneous** congenital syphilis
    - A50.08 Early **visceral** congenital syphilis
    - A50.09 Other early congenital syphilis, symptomatic
  - A50.1 Early congenital syphilis, **latent**
    Congenital syphilis without clinical manifestations,
    with positive serological reaction and negative
    spinal fluid test, less than two years after birth
  - A50.2 Early congenital syphilis, **unspecified**
    Congenital syphilis NOS less than two years after birth
  - **A50.3 Late congenital syphilitic oculopathy**
    - **Excludes1** Hutchinson's triad (A50.53)
    - A50.30 Late congenital syphilitic oculopathy,
      unspecified
    - A50.31 Late congenital syphilitic **interstitial keratitis**
    - A50.32 Late congenital syphilitic **chorioretinitis**
    - A50.39 **Other** late congenital syphilitic oculopathy

CHAPTER 1 (A00-B99)

● **A50.4 Late congenital neurosyphilis [juvenile neurosyphilis]**
Use additional code to identify any associated mental disorder

Excludes1 Hutchinson's triad (A50.53)

A50.40 Late congenital neurosyphilis, unspecified
Juvenile neurosyphilis NOS

A50.41 Late congenital syphilitic meningitis

A50.42 Late congenital syphilitic encephalitis

A50.43 Late congenital syphilitic polyneuropathy

A50.44 Late congenital syphilitic optic nerve atrophy

A50.45 Juvenile general paresis
Dementia paralytica juvenilis
Juvenile taboparetic neurosyphilis

A50.49 Other late congenital neurosyphilis
Juvenile tabes dorsalis

● **A50.5 Other late congenital syphilis, symptomatic**
Any congenital syphilitic condition specified as late or manifest two years or more after birth

A50.51 Clutton's joints

A50.52 Hutchinson's teeth

A50.53 Hutchinson's triad

A50.54 Late congenital cardiovascular syphilis

A50.55 Late congenital syphilitic arthropathy ℞

A50.56 Late congenital syphilitic osteochondropathy

A50.57 Syphilitic saddle nose

A50.59 Other late congenital syphilis, symptomatic

A50.6 Late congenital syphilis, latent
Congenital syphilis without clinical manifestations, with positive serological reaction and negative spinal fluid test, two years or more after birth.

A50.7 Late congenital syphilis, unspecified
Congenital syphilis NOS two years or more after birth.

A50.9 Congenital syphilis, unspecified

● **A51 Early syphilis**

A51.0 Primary genital syphilis
Syphilitic chancre NOS

A51.1 Primary anal syphilis

A51.2 Primary syphilis of other sites

● **A51.3 Secondary syphilis of skin and mucous membranes**

A51.31 Condyloma latum

A51.32 Syphilitic alopecia

A51.39 Other secondary syphilis of skin
Syphilitic leukoderma
Syphilitic mucous patch

Excludes1 late syphilitic leukoderma (A52.79)

● **A51.4 Other secondary syphilis**

A51.41 Secondary syphilitic meningitis

A51.42 Secondary syphilitic female pelvic disease

A51.43 Secondary syphilitic oculopathy
Secondary syphilitic chorioretinitis
Secondary syphilitic iridocyclitis, iritis
Secondary syphilitic uveitis

A51.44 Secondary syphilitic nephritis

A51.45 Secondary syphilitic hepatitis

A51.46 Secondary syphilitic osteopathy

A51.49 Other secondary syphilitic conditions
Secondary syphilitic lymphadenopathy
Secondary syphilitic myositis

A51.5 Early syphilis, latent
Syphilis (acquired) without clinical manifestations, with positive serological reaction and negative spinal fluid test, less than two years after infection.

A51.9 Early syphilis, unspecified

● **A52 Late syphilis**

● **A52.0 Cardiovascular and cerebrovascular syphilis**

A52.00 Cardiovascular syphilis, unspecified

A52.01 Syphilitic aneurysm of aorta

A52.02 Syphilitic aortitis

A52.03 Syphilitic endocarditis
Syphilitic aortic valve incompetence or stenosis
Syphilitic mitral valve stenosis
Syphilitic pulmonary valve regurgitation

A52.04 Syphilitic cerebral arteritis

A52.05 Other cerebrovascular syphilis
Syphilitic cerebral aneurysm (ruptured) (non-ruptured)
Syphilitic cerebral thrombosis

A52.06 Other syphilitic heart involvement
Syphilitic coronary artery disease
Syphilitic myocarditis
Syphilitic pericarditis

A52.09 Other cardiovascular syphilis

● **A52.1 Symptomatic neurosyphilis**

A52.10 Symptomatic neurosyphilis, unspecified

A52.11 Tabes dorsalis
Cognitive decline with progressive degeneration of posterior columns, roots, and ganglia of spinal cord, occur 15-20 years after initial infection of syphilis; AKA Duchenne disease
Locomotor ataxia (progressive)
Tabetic neurosyphilis

A52.12 Other cerebrospinal syphilis

A52.13 Late syphilitic meningitis

A52.14 Late syphilitic encephalitis

A52.15 Late syphilitic neuropathy
Late syphilitic acoustic neuritis
Late syphilitic optic (nerve) atrophy
Late syphilitic polyneuropathy
Late syphilitic retrobulbar neuritis

A52.16 Charcôt's arthropathy (tabetic)
Progressive musculoskeletal condition characterized by joint dislocation, fractures, and deformities, results in progressive destruction of bone and soft tissue of weight-bearing joints

A52.17 General paresis
Chronic meningoencephalitis results in loss of cortical function, or progressive dementia and generalized paralysis, occurring 10-20 years after initial infection of syphilis; AKA Bayle disease, dementia paralytica, paralytic dementiaparetic neurosyphilis, syphilitic meningoencephalitis
Dementia paralytica

A52.19 Other symptomatic neurosyphilis
Syphilitic parkinsonism

A52.2 Asymptomatic neurosyphilis

A52.3 Neurosyphilis, unspecified
Gumma (syphilitic)
Destructive lesions of syphilis
Syphilis (late)
Syphiloma
Coding Clinic: 2021, Q2, P6

● **A52.7 Other symptomatic late syphilis**

A52.71 Late syphilitic oculopathy
Late syphilitic chorioretinitis
Late syphilitic episcleritis

A52.72 Syphilis of lung and bronchus

A52.73 Symptomatic late syphilis of other respiratory organs

▶ New   ▶ Revised   ~~deleted~~ Deleted   Excludes 1   Excludes 2   Includes   Use additional   Code first   Code also   Key words
OGCR Official Guidelines   **X** Assign placeholder X   ● Use Additional Character(s)   ▶ Manifestation Code   ℞ Hierarchical Condition Category   **Coding Clinic**

A52.74   **Syphilis of liver and other viscera**
Late syphilitic peritonitis

A52.75   **Syphilis of kidney and ureter**
Syphilitic glomerular disease

A52.76   **Other genitourinary symptomatic late syphilis**
Late syphilitic female pelvic inflammatory disease

A52.77   **Syphilis of bone and joint**

A52.78   **Syphilis of other musculoskeletal tissue**
Late syphilitic bursitis
Syphilis [stage unspecified] of bursa
Syphilis [stage unspecified] of muscle
Syphilis [stage unspecified] of synovium
Syphilis [stage unspecified] of tendon

A52.79   **Other symptomatic late syphilis**
Late syphilitic leukoderma
Syphilis of adrenal gland
Syphilis of pituitary gland
Syphilis of thyroid gland
Syphilitic splenomegaly

> **Excludes1**   syphilitic leukoderma (secondary) (A51.39)

A52.8   **Late syphilis, latent**
Syphilis (acquired) without clinical manifestations, with positive serological reaction and negative spinal fluid test, two years or more after infection

A52.9   **Late syphilis, unspecified**

● **A53**   **Other and unspecified syphilis**

A53.0   **Latent syphilis, unspecified as early or late**
Latent syphilis NOS
Positive serological reaction for syphilis

A53.9   **Syphilis, unspecified**
Infection due to Treponema pallidum NOS
Syphilis (acquired) NOS

> **Excludes1**   syphilis NOS under two years of age (A50.2)

● **A54**   **Gonococcal infection**

● **A54.0**   **Gonococcal infection of lower genitourinary tract without periurethral or accessory gland abscess**

> **Excludes1**   gonococcal infection with genitourinary gland abscess (A54.1)
> gonococcal infection with periurethral abscess (A54.1)

A54.00   **Gonococcal infection of lower genitourinary tract, unspecified**

A54.01   **Gonococcal cystitis and urethritis, unspecified**

A54.02   **Gonococcal vulvovaginitis, unspecified**

A54.03   **Gonococcal cervicitis, unspecified**

A54.09   **Other gonococcal infection of lower genitourinary tract**

A54.1   **Gonococcal infection of lower genitourinary tract with periurethral and accessory gland abscess**
Gonococcal Bartholin's gland abscess

● **A54.2**   **Gonococcal pelviperitonitis and other gonococcal genitourinary infection**

A54.21   **Gonococcal infection of kidney and ureter**

A54.22   **Gonococcal prostatitis**

A54.23   **Gonococcal infection of other male genital organs**
Gonococcal epididymitis
Gonococcal orchitis

A54.24   **Gonococcal female pelvic inflammatory disease**
Gonococcal pelviperitonitis

> **Excludes1**   gonococcal peritonitis (A54.85)

A54.29   **Other gonococcal genitourinary infections**

Item 1-10 An STD (sexually transmitted disease) caused by **Neisseria gonorrhoeae** that flourishes in the warm, moist areas of the reproductive tract. Untreated gonorrhea spreads to other parts of the body, causing inflammation of the testes or prostate or pelvic inflammatory disease (PID).

● **A54.3**   **Gonococcal infection of eye**

A54.30   **Gonococcal infection of eye, unspecified**

A54.31   **Gonococcal conjunctivitis**
Form of bacterial conjunctivitis contracted by newborns during delivery; AKA neonatal conjunctivitis
Ophthalmia neonatorum due to gonococcus

A54.32   **Gonococcal iridocyclitis**
Inflammation of iris and of ciliary body due to gonococcal infection

A54.33   **Gonococcal keratitis**
Inflammation of cornea due to gonococcal infection; AKA keratoconjunctivitis, keratopathy

A54.39   **Other gonococcal eye infection**
Gonococcal endophthalmia

● **A54.4**   **Gonococcal infection of musculoskeletal system**

A54.40   **Gonococcal infection of musculoskeletal system, unspecified**

A54.41   **Gonococcal spondylopathy**
Disorder of vertebrae due to gonococcal infection; AKA rachiopathy

A54.42   **Gonococcal arthritis**

> **Excludes2**   gonococcal infection of spine (A54.41)

A54.43   **Gonococcal osteomyelitis**

> **Excludes2**   gonococcal infection of spine (A54.41)

A54.49   **Gonococcal infection of other musculoskeletal tissue**
Gonococcal bursitis
Gonococcal myositis
Gonococcal synovitis
Gonococcal tenosynovitis

A54.5   **Gonococcal pharyngitis**

A54.6   **Gonococcal infection of anus and rectum**

● **A54.8**   **Other gonococcal infections**

A54.81   **Gonococcal meningitis**

A54.82   **Gonococcal brain abscess**

A54.83   **Gonococcal heart infection**
Gonococcal endocarditis
Gonococcal myocarditis
Gonococcal pericarditis

A54.84   **Gonococcal pneumonia**

A54.85   **Gonococcal peritonitis**

> **Excludes1**   gonococcal pelviperitonitis (A54.24)

A54.86   **Gonococcal sepsis**

A54.89   **Other gonococcal infections**
Gonococcal keratoderma
Gonococcal lymphadenitis

A54.9   **Gonococcal infection, unspecified**

A55   **Chlamydial lymphogranuloma (venereum)**
Climatic or tropical bubo
Durand-Nicolas-Favre disease
Esthiomene
Lymphogranuloma inguinale

● **A56**   **Other sexually transmitted chlamydial diseases**

> **Includes**   sexually transmitted diseases due to Chlamydia trachomatis

> **Excludes1**   neonatal chlamydial conjunctivitis (P39.1)
> neonatal chlamydial pneumonia (P23.1)

> **Excludes2**   chlamydial lymphogranuloma (A55)
> conditions classified to A74.-

CHAPTER 1 (A00-B99)

● **A56.0 Chlamydial infection of lower genitourinary tract**
　　A56.00 Chlamydial infection of lower genitourinary tract, unspecified
　　A56.01 Chlamydial cystitis and urethritis
　　A56.02 Chlamydial vulvovaginitis
　　A56.09 Other chlamydial infection of lower genitourinary tract
　　　　Chlamydial cervicitis
● **A56.1 Chlamydial infection of pelviperitoneum and other genitourinary organs**
　　A56.11 Chlamydial female pelvic inflammatory disease
　　A56.19 Other chlamydial genitourinary infection
　　　　Chlamydial epididymitis
　　　　Chlamydial orchitis
　　A56.2 Chlamydial infection of genitourinary tract, unspecified
　　A56.3 Chlamydial infection of anus and rectum
　　A56.4 Chlamydial infection of pharynx
　　A56.8 Sexually transmitted chlamydial infection of other sites

A57 Chancroid
　　Ulcus molle
　　　Sexually transmitted infection caused by bacteria, Haemophilus ducreyi

A58 Granuloma inguinale
　　Chronic, progressive, ulcerative granulomatous disease
　　Donovanosis

● **A59 Trichomoniasis**
　　Excludes2　intestinal trichomoniasis (A07.8)
　　A common STD caused by a parasite, Trichomonas vaginalis
● **A59.0 Urogenital trichomoniasis**
　　A59.00 Urogenital trichomoniasis, unspecified
　　　　Fluor (vaginalis) due to Trichomonas
　　　　Leukorrhea (vaginalis) due to Trichomonas
　　A59.01 Trichomonal vulvovaginitis
　　A59.02 Trichomonal prostatitis
　　A59.03 Trichomonal cystitis and urethritis
　　A59.09 Other urogenital trichomoniasis
　　　　Common sexually transmitted disease (STD) caused by single-celled protozoan parasite; AKA trich
　　　　Trichomonas cervicitis
　　A59.8 Trichomoniasis of other sites
　　A59.9 Trichomoniasis, unspecified

● **A60 Anogenital herpesviral [herpes simplex] infections**
● **A60.0 Herpesviral infection of genitalia and urogenital tract**
　　A60.00 Herpesviral infection of urogenital system, unspecified
　　A60.01 Herpesviral infection of penis
　　A60.02 Herpesviral infection of other male genital organs
　　A60.03 Herpesviral cervicitis
　　A60.04 Herpesviral vulvovaginitis
　　　　Herpesviral [herpes simplex] ulceration
　　　　Herpesviral [herpes simplex] vaginitis
　　　　Herpesviral [herpes simplex] vulvitis
　　A60.09 Herpesviral infection of other urogenital tract
　　　　Coding Clinic: 2020, Q1, P20
　　A60.1 Herpesviral infection of perianal skin and rectum
　　A60.9 Anogenital herpesviral infection, unspecified

● **A63 Other predominantly sexually transmitted diseases, not elsewhere classified**
　　Excludes2　molluscum contagiosum (B08.1)
　　　　　　　papilloma of cervix (D26.0)
　　A63.0 Anogenital (venereal) warts
　　　　Anogenital warts due to (human) papillomavirus [HPV]
　　　　Condyloma acuminatum
　　A63.8 Other specified predominantly sexually transmitted diseases

A64 Unspecified sexually transmitted disease

OTHER SPIROCHETAL DISEASES (A65-A69)

　　Excludes2　leptospirosis (A27.-)
　　　　　　　syphilis (A50-A53)

A65 Nonvenereal syphilis
　　Bejel
　　Endemic syphilis
　　Njovera

● **A66 Yaws**
　　Endemic, infectious, tropical disease caused by spirochete, spread by direct contact; AKA frambesia, framboesia, frambesia tropica
　　Includes　bouba
　　　　　　frambesia (tropica)
　　　　　　pian
　　A66.0 Initial lesions of yaws
　　　　Chancre of yaws
　　　　Frambesia, initial or primary
　　　　Initial frambesial ulcer
　　　　Mother yaw
　　A66.1 Multiple papillomata and wet crab yaws
　　　　Frambesioma
　　　　Pianoma
　　　　Plantar or palmar papilloma of yaws
　　A66.2 Other early skin lesions of yaws
　　　　Cutaneous yaws, less than five years after infection
　　　　Early yaws (cutaneous)(macular)(maculopapular) (micropapular)(papular)
　　　　Frambeside of early yaws
　　A66.3 Hyperkeratosis of yaws
　　　　Hypertrophy of stratum corneum of skin in which there are small, hard, verrucous scales
　　　　Ghoul hand
　　　　Hyperkeratosis, palmar or plantar (early) (late) due to yaws
　　　　Worm-eaten soles
　　A66.4 Gummata and ulcers of yaws
　　　　Small, rubbery granuloma with necrotic center and inflamed characteristic of advanced stage of syphilis; AKA syphiloma
　　　　Gummatous frambeside
　　　　Nodular late yaws (ulcerated)
　　A66.5 Gangosa
　　　　Manifestation of yaws that develops in the soft palate and spreads eroding bone, cartilage, and soft tissue
　　　　Rhinopharyngitis mutilans
　　A66.6 Bone and joint lesions of yaws 🔮
　　　　Yaws ganglion
　　　　Yaws goundou
　　　　Yaws gumma, bone
　　　　Yaws gummatous osteitis or periostitis
　　　　Yaws hydrarthrosis
　　　　Yaws osteitis
　　　　Yaws periostitis (hypertrophic)
　　A66.7 Other manifestations of yaws
　　　　Juxta-articular nodules of yaws
　　　　Mucosal yaws
　　A66.8 Latent yaws
　　　　Yaws without clinical manifestations, with positive serology
　　A66.9 Yaws, unspecified

▶ New　　➡ Revised　　~~deleted~~ Deleted　　Excludes 1　　Excludes 2　　Includes　　Use additional　　Code first　　Code also　　Key words
OGCR Official Guidelines　　X Assign placeholder X　　● Use Additional Character(s)　　▶ Manifestation Code　　🔮 Hierarchical Condition Category　　**Coding Clinic**

Item 1–11 Cancrum oris, also known as **noma** or **gangrenous stomatitis,** begins as an ulcer of the gingiva and results in a progressive gangrenous process.

● **A67   Pinta [carate]**
Group of nonvenereal diseases caused by Treponema species

   A67.0   Primary lesions of pinta
     Chancre (primary) of pinta
     Papule (primary) of pinta

   A67.1   Intermediate lesions of pinta
     Erythematous plaques of pinta
     Hyperchromic lesions of pinta
     Hyperkeratosis of pinta
     Pintids

   A67.2   Late lesions of pinta
     Achromic skin lesions of pinta
     Cicatricial skin lesions of pinta
     Dyschromic skin lesions of pinta

   A67.3   Mixed lesions of pinta
     Achromic with hyperchromic skin lesions of pinta [carate]

   A67.9   Pinta, unspecified

● **A68   Relapsing fevers**
   Includes   recurrent fever
   Excludes2   Lyme disease (A69.2-)

   A68.0   Louse-borne relapsing fever
     Relapsing fever due to Borrelia recurrentis

   A68.1   Tick-borne relapsing fever
     Relapsing fever due to any Borrelia species other than Borrelia recurrentis

   A68.9   Relapsing fever, unspecified

● **A69   Other spirochetal infections**

   A69.0   Necrotizing ulcerative stomatitis
     Cancrum oris
     Fusospirochetal gangrene
     Noma
     Stomatitis gangrenosa

   A69.1   Other Vincent's infections
     Fusospirochetal pharyngitis
     Necrotizing ulcerative (acute) gingivitis
     Necrotizing ulcerative (acute) gingivostomatitis
     Spirochetal stomatitis
     Trench mouth
     Vincent's angina
     Vincent's gingivitis

   ● **A69.2   Lyme disease**
     Erythema chronicum migrans due to Borrelia burgdorferi

     A69.20   Lyme disease, unspecified
      Coding Clinic: 2021, Q4, P5

     A69.21   Meningitis due to Lyme disease

     A69.22   Other neurologic disorders in Lyme disease
      Cranial neuritis
      Meningoencephalitis
      Polyneuropathy

     A69.23   Arthritis due to Lyme disease

     A69.29   Other conditions associated with Lyme disease
      Myopericarditis due to Lyme disease
      Coding Clinic: 2016, Q3, P12

   A69.8   Other specified spirochetal infections

   A69.9   Spirochetal infection, unspecified

OTHER DISEASES CAUSED BY CHLAMYDIAE (A70–A74)

   Excludes1   sexually transmitted chlamydial diseases (A55-A56)

A70   Chlamydia psittaci infections
   Ornithosis
   Parrot fever
   Psittacosis

Item 1–12 Rickettsioses are diseases spread from ticks, lice, fleas, or mites to humans.
   Typhus is spread to humans chiefly by the fleas of rats.
   Endemic identifies a disease as being present in low numbers of humans at all times, whereas **epidemic** identifies a disease as being present in high numbers of humans at a specific time. Morbidity (death) is higher in epidemic diseases.
   Brill's disease, also known as **Brill-Zinsser disease,** is spread from human to human by body lice and also from the lice of flying squirrels. **Scrub typhus** is spread in the same ways as Brill's disease.
   Malaria is spread to humans by mosquitoes.

● **A71   Trachoma**
   Excludes1   sequelae of trachoma (B94.0)

   A71.0   Initial stage of trachoma
     Trachoma dubium

   A71.1   Active stage of trachoma
     Granular conjunctivitis (trachomatous)
     Trachomatous follicular conjunctivitis
     Trachomatous pannus

   A71.9   Trachoma, unspecified

● **A74   Other diseases caused by chlamydiae**
   Excludes1   neonatal chlamydial conjunctivitis (P39.1)
      neonatal chlamydial pneumonia (P23.1)
      Reiter's disease (M02.3-)
      sexually transmitted chlamydial diseases (A55-A56)
   Excludes2   chlamydial pneumonia (J16.0)

   A74.0   Chlamydial conjunctivitis
     Paratrachoma

   ● **A74.8   Other chlamydial diseases**

     A74.81   Chlamydial peritonitis

     A74.89   Other chlamydial diseases

   A74.9   Chlamydial infection, unspecified
     Chlamydiosis NOS

RICKETTSIOSES (A75-A79)

● **A75   Typhus fever**
   Excludes1   rickettsiosis due to Ehrlichia sennetsu (A79.81)

   A75.0   Epidemic louse-borne typhus fever due to Rickettsia prowazekii
     Organisms transmitted between humans via louse
     Classical typhus (fever)
     Epidemic (louse-borne) typhus

   A75.1   Recrudescent typhus [Brill's disease]
     Brill-Zinsser disease

   A75.2   Typhus fever due to Rickettsia typhi
     Murine (flea-borne) typhus

   A75.3   Typhus fever due to Rickettsia tsutsugamushi
     Scrub (mite-borne) typhus
     Tsutsugamushi fever
     Typhus fever due to Orientia Tsutsugamushi (scrub typhus)

   A75.9   Typhus fever, unspecified
     Typhus (fever) NOS

● **A77   Spotted fever [tick-borne rickettsioses]**

   A77.0   Spotted fever due to Rickettsia rickettsii
     Rocky Mountain spotted fever
     Sao Paulo fever

   A77.1   Spotted fever due to Rickettsia conorii
     African tick typhus
     Boutonneuse fever
     India tick typhus
     Kenya tick typhus
     Marseilles fever
     Mediterranean tick fever

   A77.2   Spotted fever due to Rickettsia siberica
     North Asian tick fever
     Siberian tick typhus

   A77.3   Spotted fever due to Rickettsia australis
     Queensland tick typhus

● **A77.4 Ehrlichiosis**
Type of tick-borne fever caused by bacteria infection

Excludes1   anaplasmosis [A. phagocytophilum]
(A79.82)
rickettsiosis due to Ehrlichia sennetsu (A79.81)
Coding Clinic: 2021, Q4, P5

A77.40 Ehrlichiosis, unspecified
Coding Clinic: 2021, Q4, P5

A77.41 Ehrlichiosis chaffeensis
[E. chaffeensis]

A77.49 Other ehrlichiosis
Ehrlichiosis due to E. ewingii
Ehrlichiosis due to E. muris euclairensis

A77.8 Other spotted fevers
Rickettsia 364D/R. philipii (Pacific Coast tick fever)
Spotted fever due to Rickettsia africae (African tick bite
fever)
Spotted fever due to Rickettsia parkeri]

A77.9 Spotted fever, unspecified
Tick-borne typhus NOS

A78 Q fever
Infection due to Coxiella burnetii
Nine Mile fever
Quadrilateral fever

● **A79 Other rickettsioses**
A79.0 Trench fever
Quintan fever
Wolhynian fever

A79.1 Rickettsialpox due to Rickettsia akari
Kew Garden fever
Vesicular rickettsiosis

● **A79.8 Other specified rickettsioses**
**A79.81 Rickettsiosis due to Ehrlichia
sennetsu**
Rickettsiosis due to Neorickettsia sennetsu

A79.82 Anaplasmosis [A. phagocytophilum]
Transfusion transmitted A. phagocytophilum
Coding Clinic: 2021, Q4, P5

A79.89 Other specified rickettsioses

A79.9 Rickettsiosis, unspecified
Rickettsial infection NOS

VIRAL AND PRION INFECTIONS OF THE CENTRAL NERVOUS SYSTEM (A80-A89)

Excludes1   postpolio syndrome (G14)
sequelae of poliomyelitis (B91)
sequelae of viral encephalitis (B94.1)

● **A80 Acute poliomyelitis**
Excludes1   acute flaccid myelitis (G04.82)

A80.0 Acute paralytic poliomyelitis, vaccine-associated

A80.1 Acute paralytic poliomyelitis, wild virus, imported

A80.2 Acute paralytic poliomyelitis, wild virus, indigenous

● **A80.3 Acute paralytic poliomyelitis, other and unspecified**

A80.30 Acute paralytic poliomyelitis, unspecified

A80.39 Other acute paralytic poliomyelitis

A80.4 Acute nonparalytic poliomyelitis

A80.9 Acute poliomyelitis, unspecified

● **A81 Atypical virus infections of central nervous system**
Includes   diseases of the central nervous system caused by
prions

Use additional, if applicable, code to identify:
dementia with anxiety (F02.84, F02.A4, F02.B4, F02.C4)
dementia with behavioral disturbance (F02.81-, F02.A1-, F02.
B1-, F02.C1-)
dementia with mood disturbance (F02.83, F02.A3, F02.B3,
F02.C3)
dementia with psychotic disturbance (F02.82, F02.A2, F02.
B2, F02.C2)
dementia without behavioral disturbance (F02.80, F02.A0,
F02.B0, F02.C0)
mild neurocognitive disorder due to known physiological
condition (F06.7-)

Item 1-13 Acute Poliomyelitis: Also called infantile paralysis and is
caused by the poliovirus, which enters the body orally and infects the intestinal
wall and then enters the blood stream and central nervous system, causing
muscle weakness and paralysis. This disease has been nearly eradicated with
the polio vaccine.

● **A81.0 Creutzfeldt-Jakob disease**
A81.00 Creutzfeldt-Jakob disease, unspecified
Jakob-Creutzfeldt disease, unspecified

A81.01 Variant Creutzfeldt-Jakob disease
vCJD

A81.09 Other Creutzfeldt-Jakob disease
CJD
Familial Creutzfeldt-Jakob disease
Iatrogenic Creutzfeldt-Jakob disease
Sporadic Creutzfeldt-Jakob disease
Subacute spongiform encephalopathy (with
dementia)

A81.1 Subacute sclerosing panencephalitis
*Type of viral encephalitis that causes parenchymatous lesions
in gray and white matter of brain*
Dawson's inclusion body encephalitis
Van Bogaert's sclerosing leukoencephalopathy

**A81.2 Progressive multifocal
leukoencephalopathy**
Group of diseases affecting white matter of brain
Multifocal leukoencephalopathy NOS

● **A81.8 Other atypical virus infections of central nervous
system**
A81.81 Kuru

**A81.82 Gerstmann-Sträussler-Scheinker
syndrome**
GSS syndrome

A81.83 Fatal familial insomnia
FFI

**A81.89 Other atypical virus infections of central
nervous system**

**A81.9 Atypical virus infection of central nervous system,
unspecified**
Prion diseases of the central nervous system NOS

● **A82 Rabies**
*Viral disease affecting the central nervous system and transmitted
from infected mammals to man*
A82.0 Sylvatic rabies
A82.1 Urban rabies
A82.9 Rabies, unspecified

● **A83 Mosquito-borne viral encephalitis**
*Inflammation of the brain caused most commonly by Herpes Simplex
virus*
Includes   mosquito-borne viral meningoencephalitis
Excludes2   Venezuelan equine encephalitis (A92.2)
West Nile fever (A92.3-)
West Nile virus (A92.3-)

A83.0 Japanese encephalitis
A83.1 Western equine encephalitis
A83.2 Eastern equine encephalitis
A83.3 St. Louis encephalitis
A83.4 Australian encephalitis
Kunjin virus disease
A83.5 California encephalitis
California meningoencephalitis
La Crosse encephalitis
A83.6 Rocio virus disease
Mosquito-borne virus
A83.8 Other mosquito-borne viral encephalitis
A83.9 Mosquito-borne viral encephalitis, unspecified

▶ New   ⇒ Revised   ~~deleted~~ Deleted   Excludes 1   Excludes 2   Includes   Use additional   Code first   Code also   Key words

    OGCR Official Guidelines   X Assign placeholder X   ● Use Additional Character(s)   ❱ Manifestation Code   Hierarchical Condition Category   **Coding Clinic**

Item 1-14 Encephalitis is an inflammation of the brain most often caused by a virus but may also be caused by a bacteria and most commonly transmitted by a mosquito. **Myelitis** is an inflammation of the spinal cord that may disrupt CNS function. Untreated myelitis may rapidly lead to permanent damage to the spinal cord. **Encephalomyelitis** is a general term for an inflammation of the brain and spinal cord.

A84 Tick-borne viral encephalitis

> **Includes** tick-borne viral meningoencephalitis

A84.0 Far Eastern tick-borne encephalitis [Russian spring-summer encephalitis]

A84.1 Central European tick-borne encephalitis

A84.8 Other tick-borne viral encephalitis

> **A84.81 Powassan virus disease**

> **A84.89 Other tick-borne viral encephalitis**
> Louping ill
> *Code first, if applicable, transfusion related infection (T80.22-)*

A84.9 Tick-borne viral encephalitis, unspecified

A85 Other viral encephalitis, not elsewhere classified

> **Includes** specified viral encephalomyelitis NEC
> specified viral meningoencephalitis NEC

> **Excludes1** encephalitis due to cytomegalovirus (B25.8)
> encephalitis due to herpesvirus NEC (B10.0-)
> encephalitis due to herpesvirus [herpes simplex] (B00.4)
> encephalitis due to measles virus (B05.0)
> encephalitis due to mumps virus (B26.2)
> encephalitis due to poliomyelitis virus (A80.-)
> encephalitis due to zoster (B02.0)
> lymphocytic choriomeningitis (A87.2)
> myalgic encephalomyelitis (G93.32)

A85.0 Enteroviral encephalitis
Enteroviral encephalomyelitis

A85.1 Adenoviral encephalitis
Adenoviral meningoencephalitis

A85.2 Arthropod-borne viral encephalitis, unspecified

> **Excludes1** West nile virus with encephalitis (A92.31)

A85.8 Other specified viral encephalitis
Encephalitis lethargica
Von Economo-Cruchet disease

A86 Unspecified viral encephalitis
Viral encephalomyelitis NOS
Viral meningoencephalitis NOS

A87 Viral meningitis

> **Excludes1** meningitis due to herpesvirus [herpes simplex] (B00.3)
> meningitis due to measles virus (B05.1)
> meningitis due to mumps virus (B26.1)
> meningitis due to poliomyelitis virus (A80.-)
> meningitis due to zoster (B02.1)

A87.0 Enteroviral meningitis
Group of common viruses responsible for the majority of viral meningitis
Coxsackievirus meningitis
Echovirus meningitis

A87.1 Adenoviral meningitis

A87.2 Lymphocytic choriomeningitis
Lymphocytic meningoencephalitis

A87.8 Other viral meningitis

A87.9 Viral meningitis, unspecified

A88 Other viral infections of central nervous system, not elsewhere classified

> **Excludes1** viral encephalitis NOS (A86)
> viral meningitis NOS (A87.9)

A88.0 Enteroviral exanthematous fever [Boston exanthem]
Infectious skin eruption

A88.1 Epidemic vertigo

A88.8 Other specified viral infections of central nervous system

A89 Unspecified viral infection of central nervous system

OGCR Section I. C.1.f.

Certain Infectious and Parasitic Diseases (A00-B99)

Zika virus infections

Code only confirmed cases

Code only a confirmed diagnosis of Zika virus (A92.5, Zika virus disease) as documented by the provider. This is an exception to the hospital inpatient guideline Section II, H.

In this context, "confirmation" does not require documentation of the type of test performed; the physician's diagnostic statement that the condition is confirmed is sufficient. This code should be assigned regardless of the stated mode of transmission.

If the provider documents "suspected", "possible" or "probable" Zika, do not assign code A92.5. Assign a code(s) explaining the reason for encounter (such as fever, rash, or joint pain) or Z20.828, Contact with and (suspected) exposure to other viral communicable diseases.

ARTHROPOD-BORNE VIRAL FEVERS AND VIRAL HEMORRHAGIC FEVERS (A90-A99)

A90 Dengue fever [classical dengue]
Acute, self-limited disease, characterized by fever, prostration, severe muscle pains, headache, rash, lymphadenopathy, and leukopenia, caused by dengue virus; AKA breakbone, dandy

> **Excludes1** dengue hemorrhagic fever (A91)

> **Coding Clinic: 2016, Q3, P13**

A91 Dengue hemorrhagic fever
Serious follow-up to regular dengue, with symptoms of hemorrhage

A92 Other mosquito-borne viral fevers

> **Excludes1** Ross River disease (B33.1)

A92.0 Chikungunya virus disease
Transmitted by mosquitoes
Chikungunya (hemorrhagic) fever

A92.1 O'nyong-nyong fever
Acute, nonfatal febrile disease transmitted by mosquitoes, which clinically resembles dengue and chikungunya

A92.2 Venezuelan equine fever
Venezuelan equine encephalitis
Venezuelan equine encephalomyelitis virus disease

A92.3 West Nile virus infection
West Nile fever

> **A92.30 West Nile virus infection, unspecified**
> West Nile fever NOS
> West Nile fever without complications
> West Nile virus NOS

> **A92.31 West Nile virus infection with encephalitis**
> West Nile encephalitis
> West Nile encephalomyelitis
> **Coding Clinic: 2016, Q3, P13**

> **A92.32 West Nile virus infection with other neurologic manifestation**
> *Use additional* code to specify the neurologic manifestation

> **A92.39 West Nile virus infection with other complications**
> *Use additional* code to specify the other conditions

A92.4 Rift Valley fever

CHAPTER 1 (A00-B99)

CHAPTER 1 (A00-B99)

A92.5   **Zika virus disease**
    Zika virus fever
    Zika virus infection
    Zika NOS
    Excludes1   congenital Zika virus disease (P35.4)
    Coding Clinic: 2016, Q4, P4-7, 121

A92.8   **Other specified mosquito-borne viral fevers**
A92.9   **Mosquito-borne viral fever, unspecified**

● **A93**   **Other arthropod-borne viral fevers, not elsewhere classified**

A93.0   **Oropouche virus disease**
    Tropical viral infection
    Oropouche fever

A93.1   **Sandfly fever**
    Pappataci fever
    Phlebotomus fever

A93.2   **Colorado tick fever**

A93.8   **Other specified arthropod-borne viral fevers**
    Piry virus disease
    Vesicular stomatitis virus disease [Indiana fever]

A94   **Unspecified arthropod-borne viral fever**
    Arboviral fever NOS
    Arbovirus infection NOS

● **A95**   **Yellow fever**
    Acute infectious disease transmitted by mosquitoes

A95.0   **Sylvatic yellow fever**
    Jungle yellow fever

A95.1   **Urban yellow fever**

A95.9   **Yellow fever, unspecified**

● **A96**   **Arenaviral hemorrhagic fever**
    Virus that causes various hemorrhagic fevers

A96.0   **Junin hemorrhagic fever**
    Argentinian hemorrhagic fever

A96.1   **Machupo hemorrhagic fever**
    Transmitted by contact with infected rodents
    Bolivian hemorrhagic fever

A96.2   **Lassa fever**
    Acute type of hemorrhagic fever caused by contact with
       disease carrying mouse or person

A96.8   **Other arenaviral hemorrhagic fevers**
A96.9   **Arenaviral hemorrhagic fever, unspecified**

● **A98**   **Other viral hemorrhagic fevers, not elsewhere classified**
    Excludes1   chikungunya hemorrhagic fever (A92.0)
              dengue hemorrhagic fever (A91)

A98.0   **Crimean-Congo hemorrhagic fever**
    Virus transmitted by ticks and contact with blood, secretions,
       or fluids from infected humans or animals
    Central Asian hemorrhagic fever

A98.1   **Omsk hemorrhagic fever**
    Transmitted to humans by bites of infected ticks or contact
       with infected muskrats

A98.2   **Kyasanur Forest disease**
    Transmitted via infected monkeys, voles, ticks

A98.3   **Marburg virus disease**
    Rare, acute, often fatal type of hemorrhagic fever

A98.4   **Ebola virus disease**

A98.5   **Hemorrhagic fever with renal syndrome**
    Epidemic hemorrhagic fever
    Korean hemorrhagic fever
    Russian hemorrhagic fever
    Hantaan virus disease
    Hantavirus disease with renal manifestations
    Nephropathia epidemica
    Songo fever
    Excludes1   hantavirus (cardio)-pulmonary syndrome
             (B33.4)

A98.8   **Other specified viral hemorrhagic fevers**

A99   **Unspecified viral hemorrhagic fever**

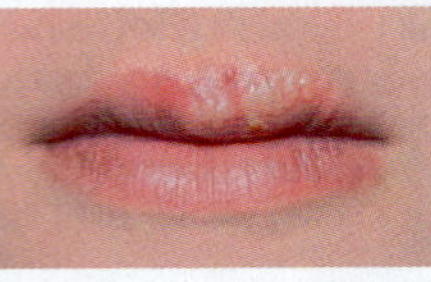

Figure 1-4 Primary herpes simplex in and around the mouth. The infection is usually acquired from siblings or parents and is readily transmitted to other direct contacts. (Getty Image)

Item 1–15   **Herpes** is a viral disease for which there is no cure. There are two types of the herpes simplex virus: **Type I** causes **cold sores** or **fever blisters,** and **Type II** causes **genital herpes.** The virus can be spread from a sore on the lips to the genitals or from the genitals to the lips.

VIRAL INFECTIONS CHARACTERIZED BY SKIN AND MUCOUS MEMBRANE LESIONS (B00-B09)

● **B00**   **Herpesviral [herpes simplex] infections**
    Excludes1   congenital herpesviral infections (P35.2)
    Excludes2   anogenital herpesviral infection (A60.-)
             gammaherpesviral mononucleosis (B27.0-)
             herpangina (B08.5)

B00.0   **Eczema herpeticum**
    Cutaneous eruption caused by herpes simplex virus (HSV)
       type 1, HSV-2, coxsackievirus A16, or vaccinia virus
    Kaposi's varicelliform eruption

B00.1   **Herpesviral vesicular dermatitis**
    Vesicle formation; characteristics include formation of blisters
       and scabs on feet and legs
    Herpes simplex facialis
    Herpes simplex labialis
    Herpes simplex otitis externa
    Vesicular dermatitis of ear
    Vesicular dermatitis of lip

B00.2   **Herpesviral gingivostomatitis and pharyngotonsillitis**
    Inflammation involving both gingivae and oral mucosa
    Herpesviral pharyngitis
    Inflammation of pharynx and tonsils; AKA
       tonsillopharyngitis

B00.3   **Herpesviral meningitis**

B00.4   **Herpesviral encephalitis**
    Herpesviral meningoencephalitis
    Simian B disease
    Excludes1   herpesviral encephalitis due to herpesvirus 6
             and 7 (B10.01, B10.09)
             non-simplex herpesviral encephalitis
             (B10.0-)

● **B00.5**   **Herpesviral ocular disease**

B00.50   **Herpesviral ocular disease, unspecified**

B00.51   **Herpesviral iridocyclitis**
    Herpesviral iritis
    Herpesviral uveitis, anterior

B00.52   **Herpesviral keratitis**
    Herpesviral keratoconjunctivitis

B00.53   **Herpesviral conjunctivitis**

B00.59   **Other herpesviral disease of eye**
    Herpesviral dermatitis of eyelid

B00.7   **Disseminated herpesviral disease** 🅗🅒🅒
    Herpesviral sepsis

● **B00.8**   **Other forms of herpesviral infections**

B00.81   **Herpesviral hepatitis**

B00.82   **Herpes simplex myelitis** 🅗🅒🅒

B00.89   **Other herpesviral infection**
    Herpesviral whitlow

B00.9   **Herpesviral infection, unspecified**
    Herpes simplex infection NOS

▶ New   ➡ Revised   ~~deleted~~ Deleted   Excludes 1   Excludes 2   Includes   Use additional   Code first   Code also   Key words

OGCR Official Guidelines   X Assign placeholder X   ● Use Additional Character(s)   ▶ Manifestation Code   🅗🅒🅒 Hierarchical Condition Category   Coding Clinic

● **B01**   **Varicella [chickenpox]**
Very contagious disease caused by the varicella zoster virus that results in an itchy outbreak of skin blisters (varicella). The same virus causes shingles (zoster).

   B01.0   Varicella meningitis

●   **B01.1**   Varicella encephalitis, myelitis and encephalomyelitis
     Postchickenpox encephalitis, myelitis and encephalomyelitis

     B01.11   Varicella encephalitis and encephalomyelitis
       Postchickenpox encephalitis and encephalomyelitis

     B01.12   Varicella myelitis
       Postchickenpox myelitis

   B01.2   Varicella pneumonia

●   **B01.8**   Varicella with other complications

     B01.81   Varicella keratitis

     B01.89   Other varicella complications

   B01.9   Varicella without complication
     Varicella NOS

● **B02**   **Zoster [herpes zoster]**

   Includes   shingles
     zona

   B02.0   Zoster encephalitis
     Zoster meningoencephalitis

   B02.1   Zoster meningitis

●   **B02.2**   Zoster with other nervous system involvement
     Coding Clinic: 2019, Q1, P18

     B02.21   Postherpetic geniculate ganglionitis

     B02.22   Postherpetic trigeminal neuralgia

     B02.23   Postherpetic polyneuropathy

     B02.24   Postherpetic myelitis
       Herpes zoster myelitis

     B02.29   Other postherpetic nervous system involvement
       Postherpetic radiculopathy

●   **B02.3**   Zoster ocular disease

     B02.30   Zoster ocular disease, unspecified

     B02.31   Zoster conjunctivitis

     B02.32   Zoster iridocyclitis

     B02.33   Zoster keratitis
       Herpes zoster keratoconjunctivitis

     B02.34   Zoster scleritis

     B02.39   Other herpes zoster eye disease
       Zoster blepharitis

   B02.7   Disseminated zoster

   B02.8   Zoster with other complications
     Herpes zoster otitis externa

   B02.9   Zoster without complications
     Zoster NOS

   B03   **Smallpox**
     Note: In 1980 the 33rd World Health Assembly declared that smallpox had been eradicated. The classification is maintained for surveillance purposes.

   B04   **Monkeypox**
     Mpox
     Disease occurring in captive monkeys and other mammals that may be transmitted to humans, clinically similar to smallpox
     Coding Clinic: 2022, Q3, P3

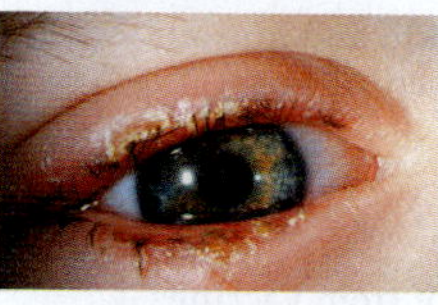

Figure 1-5   Photograph of eyelids with marginal blepharitis. (From Hoyt CS, Taylor D: Pediatric Ophthalmology and Strabismus, London, Elsevier Saunders, 2005)

Item 1–17 Blepharitis is a common condition in which the eyelid is swollen and yellow scaling and conjunctivitis develop. Usually the hair on the scalp and brow is involved.

● **B05**   **Measles**

   Includes   morbilli

   Excludes1   subacute sclerosing panencephalitis (A81.1)

   B05.0   Measles complicated by encephalitis
     Postmeasles encephalitis

   B05.1   Measles complicated by meningitis
     Postmeasles meningitis

   B05.2   Measles complicated by pneumonia
     Postmeasles pneumonia

   B05.3   Measles complicated by otitis media
     Postmeasles otitis media

   B05.4   Measles with intestinal complications

●   **B05.8**   Measles with other complications

     B05.81   Measles keratitis and keratoconjunctivitis

     B05.89   Other measles complications

   B05.9   Measles without complication
     Measles NOS

● **B06**   **Rubella [German measles]**

   Excludes1   congenital rubella (P35.0)

●   **B06.0**   Rubella with neurological complications

     B06.00   Rubella with neurological complication, unspecified

     B06.01   Rubella encephalitis
       Rubella meningoencephalitis

     B06.02   Rubella meningitis

     B06.09   Other neurological complications of rubella

●   **B06.8**   Rubella with other complications

     B06.81   Rubella pneumonia

     B06.82   Rubella arthritis

     B06.89   Other rubella complications

   B06.9   Rubella without complication
     Rubella NOS

● **B07**   **Viral warts**

   Includes   verruca simplex
     verruca vulgaris
     viral warts due to human papillomavirus

   Excludes2   anogenital (venereal) warts (A63.0)
     papilloma of bladder (D41.4)
     papilloma of cervix (D26.0)
     papilloma larynx (D14.1)

   B07.0   Plantar wart
     Verruca plantaris

   B07.8   Other viral warts
     Common wart
     Flat wart
     Verruca plana

   B07.9   Viral wart, unspecified

Item 1-16 Zoster: Also known as *shingles* and is caused by the same virus as chickenpox. After exposure, the virus lies dormant in nerve tissue and is activated by factors including aging, stress, suppression of the immune system, and certain medication. It begins as a unilateral rash that leads to blisters and sores on the skin. It may involve the nerve pathways of the eye, forehead, nose, and eyelids and may be very painful with long-term systemic effects.

CHAPTER 1 (A00-B99)

● **B08 Other viral infections characterized by skin and mucous membrane lesions, not elsewhere classified**
> **Excludes1**   vesicular stomatitis virus disease (A93.8)

● **B08.0 Other orthopoxvirus infections**
> **Excludes2**   monkeypox (B04)

● **B08.01 Cowpox and vaccinia not from vaccine**

B08.010 Cowpox

B08.011 Vaccinia not from vaccine
> **Excludes1**   vaccinia (from vaccination) (generalized) (T88.1)

B08.02 Orf virus disease
Contagious pustular dermatitis
Ecthyma contagiosum

B08.03 Pseudocowpox [milker's node]

B08.04 Paravaccinia, unspecified

B08.09 Other orthopoxvirus infections
Orthopoxvirus infection NOS

B08.1 Molluscum contagiosum
Various skin diseases characterized by soft, rounded, cutaneous lesions

● **B08.2 Exanthema subitum [sixth disease] Roseola infantum**
Acute, short-lived high fever in infants and young children followed by a rash mainly on the trunk, caused by human herpesvirus 6

B08.20 Exanthema subitum [sixth disease], unspecified
Roseola infantum, unspecified   P

B08.21 Exanthema subitum [sixth disease] due to human herpesvirus 6 Roseola infantum due to human herpesvirus 6   P
Virus results in sudden rash; infection results in lifelong persistence

B08.22 Exanthema subitum [sixth disease] due to human herpesvirus 7 Roseola infantum due to human herpesvirus 7   P

B08.3 Erythema infectiosum [fifth disease]
Moderately contagious, epidemic disease in children caused by B19 virus; onset of rash that begins as redness of cheeks, later there is rash on trunk and limbs; when this fades, there may be central clearing that leaves lacelike pattern

B08.4 Enteroviral vesicular stomatitis with exanthem
Hand, foot and mouth disease
Check your documentation—this code is HAND, foot, and mouth disease. Code B08.8 is foot and mouth disease.

B08.5 Enteroviral vesicular pharyngitis
Herpangina

● **B08.6 Parapoxvirus infections**

B08.60 Parapoxvirus infection, unspecified

B08.61 Bovine stomatitis

B08.62 Sealpox

B08.69 Other parapoxvirus infections

● **B08.7 Yatapoxvirus infections**

B08.70 Yatapoxvirus infection, unspecified

B08.71 Tanapox virus disease

B08.72 Yaba pox virus disease
Yaba monkey tumor disease

B08.79 Other yatapoxvirus infections

B08.8 Other specified viral infections characterized by skin and mucous membrane lesions
Enteroviral lymphonodular pharyngitis
Foot-and-mouth disease
Check your documentation. Code B08.4 is for HAND, foot, and mouth disease.
Poxvirus NEC

B09 Unspecified viral infection characterized by skin and mucous membrane lesions
Viral enanthema NOS
Viral exanthema NOS

OTHER HUMAN HERPESVIRUSES (B10)

● **B10 Other human herpesviruses**
> **Excludes2**   cytomegalovirus (B25.9)
> Epstein-Barr virus (B27.0-)
> herpes NOS (B00.9)
> herpes simplex (B00.-)
> herpes zoster (B02.-)
> human herpesvirus NOS (B00.-)
> human herpesvirus 1 and 2 (B00.-)
> human herpesvirus 3 (B01.-, B02.-)
> human herpesvirus 4 (B27.0-)
> human herpesvirus 5 (B25.-)
> varicella (B01.-)
> zoster (B02.-)

Coding Clinic: 2024, Q2, P21

● **B10.0 Other human herpesvirus encephalitis**
> **Excludes2**   herpes encephalitis NOS (B00.4)
> herpes simplex encephalitis (B00.4)
> human herpesvirus encephalitis (B00.4)
> simian B herpes virus encephalitis (B00.4)

B10.01 Human herpesvirus 6 encephalitis
Sudden rash or roseola

B10.09 Other human herpesvirus encephalitis
Human herpesvirus 7 encephalitis
Virus closely related to human herpesvirus 6, but not known to cause any disease

Coding Clinic: 2024, Q2, P21

● **B10.8 Other human herpesvirus infection**

B10.81 Human herpesvirus 6 infection
Causative agent of exanthema subitum that results in sudden rash

B10.82 Human herpesvirus 7 infection
Closely related to human herpesvirus 6, but not known cause any disease

B10.89 Other human herpesvirus infection
Human herpesvirus 8 infection
May be the cause of Kaposi sarcoma, a malignant tumor
Kaposi's sarcoma-associated herpesvirus infection

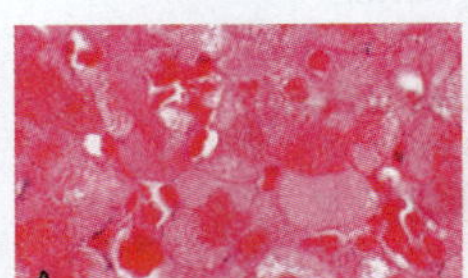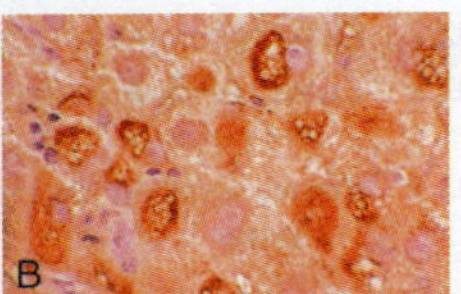

Figure 1-6   Hepatitis B viral infection. **A.** Liver parenchyma showing hepatocytes with diffuse granular cytoplasm, so-called ground glass hepatocytes (H&E). **B.** Immunoperoxidase stains from the same case, showing cytoplasmic inclusions of viral particles. (From Kumar: Robbins and Cotran: Pathologic Basis of Disease, ed 8, Saunders, An Imprint of Elsevier, 2009)

Item 1–18   Hepatitis A (HAV) was formerly called epidemic, infectious, short-incubation, or acute catarrhal jaundice hepatitis. The primary transmission mode is the oral–fecal route. **Hepatitis B (HBV)** was formerly called long-incubation period, serum, or homologous serum hepatitis. Transmission modes are through blood from infected persons and from body fluids of infected mother to neonate. **Hepatitis C (HCV),** caused by the hepatitis C virus, is primarily transfusion associated. **Hepatitis D (HDV),** also called delta hepatitis, is caused by the hepatitis D virus in patients formerly or currently infected with hepatitis B. **Hepatitis E (HEV)** is also called enterically transmitted non-A, non-B hepatitis. The primary transmission mode is the oral–fecal route, usually through contaminated water.

CHAPTER 1 (A00-B99)

▶ New   ⇨ Revised   ~~deleted~~ Deleted   Excludes 1   Excludes 2   Includes   Use additional   Code first   Code also   Key words
OGCR Official Guidelines   X Assign placeholder X   ● Use Additional Character(s)   ⬧ Manifestation Code   Ⓗ Hierarchical Condition Category   **Coding Clinic**

VIRAL HEPATITIS (B15-B19)

Excludes1 sequelae of viral hepatitis (B94.2)
Excludes2 cytomegaloviral hepatitis (B25.1)
     herpesviral [herpes simplex] hepatitis (B00.81)

● **B15 Acute hepatitis A**
   B15.0 Hepatitis A with hepatic coma
   B15.9 Hepatitis A without hepatic coma
     Hepatitis A (acute) (viral) NOS

● **B16 Acute hepatitis B**
   B16.0 Acute hepatitis B with delta-agent with hepatic coma
   B16.1 Acute hepatitis B with delta-agent without hepatic coma
   B16.2 Acute hepatitis B without delta-agent with hepatic coma
   B16.9 Acute hepatitis B without delta-agent and without hepatic coma
     Hepatitis B (acute) (viral) NOS
     Coding Clinic: 2016, Q3, P13

● **B17 Other acute viral hepatitis**
   B17.0 Acute delta-(super) infection of hepatitis B carrier
   ● **B17.1 Acute hepatitis C**
     B17.10 Acute hepatitis C without hepatic coma
       Acute hepatitis C NOS
     B17.11 Acute hepatitis C with hepatic coma
   B17.2 Acute hepatitis E
   B17.8 Other specified acute viral hepatitis
     Hepatitis non-A non-B (acute) (viral) NEC
   B17.9 Acute viral hepatitis, unspecified
     Acute hepatitis NOS
     Acute infectious hepatitis NOS

● **B18 Chronic viral hepatitis**
   Includes Carrier of viral hepatitis
   ▸ Use Additional code, if applicable, for ascites (R18.8)
   B18.0 Chronic viral hepatitis B with delta-agent
   B18.1 Chronic viral hepatitis B without delta-agent
     Carrier of viral hepatitis B
     Chronic (viral) hepatitis B
   B18.2 Chronic viral hepatitis C
     Carrier of viral hepatitis C
     Coding Clinic: 2018, Q1, P4; 2017, Q1, P41
   B18.8 Other chronic viral hepatitis
     Carrier of other viral hepatitis
   B18.9 Chronic viral hepatitis, unspecified
     Carrier of unspecified viral hepatitis

● **B19 Unspecified viral hepatitis**
   B19.0 Unspecified viral hepatitis with hepatic coma
   ● **B19.1 Unspecified viral hepatitis B**
     B19.10 Unspecified viral hepatitis B without hepatic coma
       Unspecified viral hepatitis B NOS
     B19.11 Unspecified viral hepatitis B with hepatic coma
   ● **B19.2 Unspecified viral hepatitis C**
     B19.20 Unspecified viral hepatitis C without hepatic coma
       Viral hepatitis C NOS
     B19.21 Unspecified viral hepatitis C with hepatic coma
   B19.9 Unspecified viral hepatitis without hepatic coma
     Viral hepatitis NOS

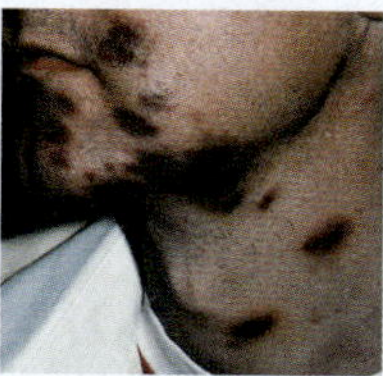

Figure 1-7 Kaposi's sarcoma. There are large confluent hyperpigmented patch-stage lesions with lymphedema. (From Kanski, JJ: Clinical Diagnosis in Ophthalmology, London, Elsevier Mosby, 2006)

Item 1–19 AIDS (acquired immune deficiency syndrome) is caused by **HIV** (human immunodeficiency virus). HIV affects certain white blood cells (T-4 lymphocytes) and destroys the ability of the cells to fight infections, making patients susceptible to a host of infectious diseases (e.g., *Pneumocystis carinii pneumonia [PCP], Kaposi's sarcoma,* and *lymphoma). AIDS-related complex (ARC)* is an early stage of AIDS in which tests for HIV are positive but the symptoms are mild.

OGCR Section I. C.1.a.

Certain Infectious and Parasitic Diseases (A00-B99)
a. Human Immunodeficiency Virus (HIV) Infections
   1) Code only confirmed cases
     Code only confirmed cases of HIV infection illness. This is an exception to the hospital inpatient guideline Section II, H.
     In this context, "confirmation" does not require documentation of positive serology or culture for HIV; the provider's diagnostic statement that the patient is HIV positive or has an HIV-related illness is sufficient.

HUMAN IMMUNODEFICIENCY VIRUS [HIV] DISEASE (B20)

B20 Human immunodeficiency virus [HIV] disease
   Includes acquired immune deficiency syndrome [AIDS]
     AIDS-related complex [ARC]
     HIV infection, symptomatic
   Code first Human immunodeficiency virus [HIV] disease complicating pregnancy, childbirth and the puerperium, if applicable (O98.7-)
   Use additional code(s) to identify all manifestations of HIV infection
   Excludes1 asymptomatic human immunodeficiency virus [HIV] infection status (Z21)
     exposure to HIV virus (Z20.6)
     inconclusive serologic evidence of HIV (R75)
   Coding Clinic: 2022, Q1, P36; 2021, Q2, P6; 2019, Q1, P9-11

OTHER VIRAL DISEASES (B25-B34)

● **B25 Cytomegaloviral disease**
   AKA: HCMV or Human Herpesvirus 5 (HHV-5)
   Excludes1 congenital cytomegalovirus infection (P35.1)
     cytomegaloviral mononucleosis (B27.1-)
   B25.0 Cytomegaloviral pneumonitis
   B25.1 Cytomegaloviral hepatitis
   B25.2 Cytomegaloviral pancreatitis
   B25.8 Other cytomegaloviral diseases
     Cytomegaloviral encephalitis
   B25.9 Cytomegaloviral disease, unspecified

● **B26 Mumps**
   Includes epidemic parotitis
     infectious parotitis
   Acute, contagious, viral disease
   B26.0 Mumps orchitis
   B26.1 Mumps meningitis
   B26.2 Mumps encephalitis
   B26.3 Mumps pancreatitis

CHAPTER 1 (A00-B99)

● **B26.8**   **Mumps with other complications**

    B26.81   **Mumps hepatitis**

    B26.82   **Mumps myocarditis**

    B26.83   **Mumps nephritis**

    B26.84   **Mumps polyneuropathy**

    B26.85   **Mumps arthritis**

    B26.89   **Other mumps complications**

   B26.9   **Mumps without complication**
Mumps NOS
Mumps parotitis NOS

● **B27**   **Infectious mononucleosis**

    Includes   glandular fever
monocytic angina
Pfeiffer's disease

● **B27.0**   **Gammaherpesviral mononucleosis**
AKA: Pfeiffer's disease, infective mononucleosis
Mononucleosis due to Epstein-Barr virus

    B27.00   **Gammaherpesviral mononucleosis without complication**
Infective mononucleosis

    B27.01   **Gammaherpesviral mononucleosis with polyneuropathy**

    B27.02   **Gammaherpesviral mononucleosis with meningitis**

    B27.09   **Gammaherpesviral mononucleosis with other complications**
Hepatomegaly in gammaherpesviral mononucleosis
Coding Clinic: 2025, Q2, P20; 2024, Q2, P21,22

● **B27.1**   **Cytomegaloviral mononucleosis**
Infectious disease resembling infectious mononucleosis

    B27.10   **Cytomegaloviral mononucleosis without complications**

    B27.11   **Cytomegaloviral mononucleosis with polyneuropathy**

    B27.12   **Cytomegaloviral mononucleosis with meningitis**

    B27.19   **Cytomegaloviral mononucleosis with other complication**
Hepatomegaly in cytomegaloviral mononucleosis

● **B27.8**   **Other infectious mononucleosis**

    B27.80   **Other infectious mononucleosis without complication**

    B27.81   **Other infectious mononucleosis with polyneuropathy**

    B27.82   **Other infectious mononucleosis with meningitis**

    B27.89   **Other infectious mononucleosis with other complication**
Hepatomegaly in other infectious mononucleosis

● **B27.9**   **Infectious mononucleosis, unspecified**

    B27.90   **Infectious mononucleosis, unspecified without complication**

    B27.91   **Infectious mononucleosis, unspecified with polyneuropathy**

    B27.92   **Infectious mononucleosis, unspecified with meningitis**

    B27.99   **Infectious mononucleosis, unspecified with other complication**
Hepatomegaly in unspecified infectious mononucleosis

● **B30**   **Viral conjunctivitis**

    Excludes1   herpesviral [herpes simplex] ocular disease (B00.5)
ocular zoster (B02.3)

   B30.0   **Keratoconjunctivitis due to adenovirus**
Epidemic keratoconjunctivitis
Shipyard eye

   B30.1   **Conjunctivitis due to adenovirus**
Acute adenoviral follicular conjunctivitis
Swimming-pool conjunctivitis

   B30.2   **Viral pharyngoconjunctivitis**

   B30.3   **Acute epidemic hemorrhagic conjunctivitis (enteroviral)**
Conjunctivitis due to coxsackievirus 24
Conjunctivitis due to enterovirus 70
Hemorrhagic conjunctivitis (acute)(epidemic)

   B30.8   **Other viral conjunctivitis**
Newcastle conjunctivitis

   B30.9   **Viral conjunctivitis, unspecified**

● **B33**   **Other viral diseases, not elsewhere classified**

   B33.0   **Epidemic myalgia**
Acute infectious disease, caused by group A coxsackie viruses or other enteroviruses with symptoms that include sudden pain in chest or upper abdomen with fever
Bornholm disease

   B33.1   **Ross River disease**
Epidemic polyarthritis and exanthema
Ross River fever

● **B33.2**   **Viral carditis**
Coxsackie (virus) carditis

    B33.20   **Viral carditis, unspecified**

    B33.21   **Viral endocarditis**

    B33.22   **Viral myocarditis**
Coding Clinic: 2025, Q1, P34

    B33.23   **Viral pericarditis**

    B33.24   **Viral cardiomyopathy**

   B33.3   **Retrovirus infections, not elsewhere classified**
Retrovirus infection NOS

   B33.4   **Hantavirus (cardio)-pulmonary syndrome [HPS] [HCPS]**
Hantavirus disease with pulmonary manifestations
Sin nombre virus disease

    Use additional code to identify any associated acute kidney failure (N17.9)

    Excludes1   hantavirus disease with renal manifestations (A98.5)
hemorrhagic fever with renal manifestations (A98.5)

   B33.8   **Other specified viral diseases**

    Excludes1   anogenital human papillomavirus infection (A63.0)
viral warts due to human papillomavirus infection (B07)

● **B34**   **Viral infection of unspecified site**

    Excludes1   anogenital human papillomavirus infection (A63.0)
cytomegaloviral disease NOS (B25.9)
herpesvirus [herpes simplex] infection NOS (B00.9)
retrovirus infection NOS (B33.3)
viral agents as the cause of diseases classified elsewhere (B97.-)
viral warts due to human papillomavirus infection (B07)

   B34.0   **Adenovirus infection, unspecified**

   B34.1   **Enterovirus infection, unspecified**
Intestinal tract infection
Coxsackievirus infection NOS
Echovirus infection NOS

B34.2 **Coronavirus infection, unspecified**
  Excludes1 COVID-19 (U07.1)
  pneumonia due to SARS-associated coronavirus (J12.81)

B34.3 **Parvovirus infection, unspecified**

B34.4 **Papovavirus infection, unspecified**

B34.8 **Other viral infections of unspecified site**

B34.9 **Viral infection, unspecified**
  Viremia NOS
  Coding Clinic: 2016, Q3, P10

MYCOSES (B35-B49)

Excludes2 hypersensitivity pneumonitis due to organic dust (J67.-)
  mycosis fungoides (C84.0-)

● **B35** **Dermatophytosis**
  AKA tinea or ringworm
  Includes favus
  infections due to species of Epidermophyton, Micro-sporum and Trichophyton
  tinea, any type except those in B36.-

B35.0 **Tinea barbae and tinea capitis**
  Beard ringworm
  Kerion
  Scalp ringworm
  Sycosis, mycotic

B35.1 **Tinea unguium**
  White patches or pits on surface or edges of nails, followed by infection under nail plate
  Dermatophytic onychia
  Dermatophytosis of nail
  Onychomycosis
  Ringworm of nails

B35.2 **Tinea manuum**
  Tinea of hands
  Dermatophytosis of hand
  Hand ringworm

B35.3 **Tinea pedis**
  Tinea affecting feet
  Athlete's foot
  Dermatophytosis of foot
  Foot ringworm

B35.4 **Tinea corporis**
  Infecting skin areas other than hands
  Ringworm of the body

B35.5 **Tinea imbricata**
  Chronic tropical tinea corporis; AKA Oriental ringworm, tinea inguinalis, tinea cruris
  Tokelau

B35.6 **Tinea cruris**
  In groin or perineal area, spreading to adjacent regions; AKA jock itch, eczema marginatum, ringworm of groin, or tinea inguinalis
  Dhobi itch
  Groin ringworm
  Jock itch

B35.8 **Other dermatophytoses**
  Disseminated dermatophytosis
  Granulomatous dermatophytosis

B35.9 **Dermatophytosis, unspecified**
  Ringworm NOS

● **B36** **Other superficial mycoses**

B36.0 **Pityriasis versicolor**
  Common, chronic, symptomless disorder that includes macular patches of various sizes and shapes; AKA liver spots
  Tinea flava
  Tinea versicolor

B36.1 **Tinea nigra**
  Minor fungal infection, with dark lesions, usually on skin of hands
  Keratomycosis nigricans palmaris
  Microsporosis nigra
  Pityriasis nigra

B36.2 **White piedra**
  White to light brown nodules on hair of beard, axilla, or groin; AKA trichosporosis
  Tinea blanca

B36.3 **Black piedra**
  Characterized by small black or brown nodules on shafts of scalp hair

B36.8 **Other specified superficial mycoses**

B36.9 **Superficial mycosis, unspecified**

● **B37** **Candidiasis**
  Includes candidosis
  moniliasis
  Excludes1 neonatal candidiasis (P37.5)

B37.0 **Candidal stomatitis**
  Oral thrush

B37.1 **Pulmonary candidiasis**
  Candidal bronchitis
  Candidal pneumonia

B37.2 **Candidiasis of skin and nail**
  Candidal onychia
  Candidal paronychia
  Excludes2 diaper dermatitis (L22)

B37.3 **Candidiasis of vulva and vagina**
  Candidal vulvovaginitis
  Monilial vulvovaginitis
  Vaginal thrush

  B37.31 **Acute candidiasis of vulva and vagina**
  Candidiasis of vulva and vagina NOS

  B37.32 **Chronic candidiasis of vulva and vagina**
  Recurrent candidiasis of vulva and vagina

● **B37.4** **Candidiasis of other urogenital sites**

  B37.41 **Candidal cystitis and urethritis**

  B37.42 **Candidal balanitis**
  Male condition only

  B37.49 **Other urogenital candidiasis**
  Candidal pyelonephritis

B37.5 **Candidal meningitis**

B37.6 **Candidal endocarditis**

B37.7 **Candidal sepsis**
  Disseminated candidiasis systemic candidiasis
  Coding Clinic: 2024, Q3, P13

● **B37.8** **Candidiasis of other sites**

  B37.81 **Candidal esophagitis**

  B37.82 **Candidal enteritis**
  Candidal proctitis

  B37.83 **Candidal cheilitis**
  Inflammation affecting lip

  B37.84 **Candidal otitis externa**
  Inflammation of external auditory canal

  B37.89 **Other sites of candidiasis**
  Infection manifested by invasive candidiasis
  Candidal osteomyelitis

B37.9 **Candidiasis, unspecified**
  Thrush NOS

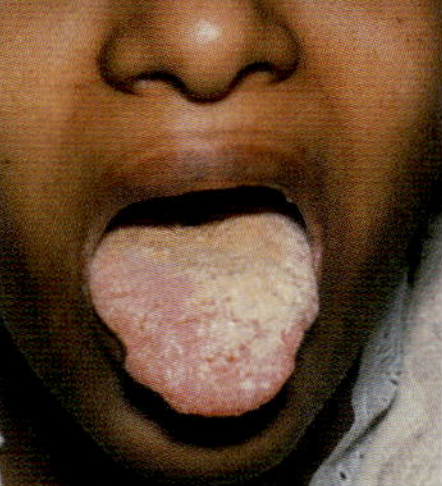

Figure 1-8 Oral candidiasis (thrush). (From James WD, Berger T, Elston D: Andrews' Diseases of the Skin: Clinical Dermatology, 11e, Saunders, 2011)

Item 1–20 Candidiasis, also called oidiomycosis or moniliasis, is a fungal infection. It most often appears on moist cutaneous areas of the body but can also be responsible for a variety of systemic infections such as endocarditis, meningitis, arthritis, and myositis. Antifungal medications cure most yeast infections.

CHAPTER 1 (A00-B99)

CHAPTER 1 (A00-B99)

Item 1-21　Bird and bat droppings that fall into the soil give rise to a fungus that can spread airborne spores. When inhaled into the lungs, these spores divide and multiply into lesions. Histoplasmosis capsulatum takes three forms: primary (lodged in the lungs only), chronic (resembles TB), and disseminated (infection has moved to other organs). This is an opportunistic infection in immunosuppressed patients.

● **B38**　**Coccidioidomycosis**
　　　Fungal disease; AKA coccidioidosis, coccidioidal granuloma, Posadas, or Posadas-Wernicke disease
　　B38.0　**Acute pulmonary** coccidioidomycosis
　　B38.1　**Chronic pulmonary** coccidioidomycosis
　　B38.2　**Pulmonary** coccidioidomycosis, **unspecified**
　　B38.3　**Cutaneous** coccidioidomycosis
　　B38.4　Coccidioidomycosis **meningitis**
　　B38.7　**Disseminated** coccidioidomycosis
　　　　　　Generalized coccidioidomycosis
　●　**B38.8**　**Other forms** of coccidioidomycosis
　　　　B38.81　**Prostatic** coccidioidomycosis
　　　　B38.89　**Other forms** of coccidioidomycosis
　　B38.9　Coccidioidomycosis, **unspecified**

● **B39**　**Histoplasmosis**
　　　Infection resulting from inhalation or ingestion of spores; AKA Darling disease

　　Code first *associated AIDS (B20)*
　　Use additional code for any associated manifestations, such as:
　　　　endocarditis (I39)
　　　　meningitis (G02)
　　　　pericarditis (I32)
　　　　retinitis (H32)
　　B39.0　**Acute pulmonary** histoplasmosis capsulati
　　B39.1　**Chronic pulmonary** histoplasmosis capsulati
　　B39.2　**Pulmonary** histoplasmosis capsulati, **unspecified**
　　B39.3　**Disseminated** histoplasmosis capsulati
　　　　　　Generalized histoplasmosis capsulati
　　B39.4　Histoplasmosis **capsulati, unspecified**
　　　　　　American histoplasmosis
　　B39.5　Histoplasmosis **duboisii**
　　　　　　African histoplasmosis
　　B39.9　Histoplasmosis, **unspecified**

● **B40**　**Blastomycosis**
　　　Rare and potentially fatal infection caused by inhaling fungus found in moist soil in temperate climates.

　　Excludes1　Brazilian blastomycosis (B41.-)
　　　　　　keloidal blastomycosis (B48.0)
　　B40.0　**Acute pulmonary** blastomycosis
　　B40.1　**Chronic pulmonary** blastomycosis
　　B40.2　**Pulmonary** blastomycosis, **unspecified**
　　B40.3　**Cutaneous** blastomycosis
　　B40.7　**Disseminated** blastomycosis
　　　　　　Generalized blastomycosis
　●　**B40.8**　Other forms of blastomycosis
　　　　B40.81　Blastomycotic **meningoencephalitis**
　　　　　　　　Meningomyelitis due to blastomycosis
　　　　B40.89　**Other forms** of blastomycosis
　　B40.9　Blastomycosis, **unspecified**

● **B41**　**Paracoccidioidomycosis**
　　　Fungal infection usually chronic that begins in lungs, spreads to mucocutaneous areas which may extend to skin, tonsils, gastrointestinal lymphatics, liver, and spleen; AKA Almeida or Lutz-Splendore-Almeida disease, Brazilian or South American blastomycosis, or paracoccidioidal granuloma

　　Includes　Brazilian blastomycosis
　　　　　　Lutz' disease
　　B41.0　**Pulmonary** paracoccidioidomycosis
　　B41.7　**Disseminated** paracoccidioidomycosis
　　　　　　Generalized paracoccidioidomycosis
　　B41.8　**Other forms** of paracoccidioidomycosis
　　B41.9　Paracoccidioidomycosis, **unspecified**

● **B42**　**Sporotrichosis**
　　　Chronic fungal infection with nodular lesions
　　B42.0　**Pulmonary** sporotrichosis
　　B42.1　**Lymphocutaneous** sporotrichosis
　　B42.7　**Disseminated** sporotrichosis
　　　　　　Generalized sporotrichosis
　●　**B42.8**　**Other forms** of sporotrichosis
　　　　B42.81　**Cerebral** sporotrichosis
　　　　　　　　Meningitis due to sporotrichosis
　　　　B42.82　**Sporotrichosis** arthritis
　　　　B42.89　**Other forms** of sporotrichosis
　　B42.9　Sporotrichosis, **unspecified**

● **B43**　**Chromomycosis and pheomycotic abscess**
　　　Chronic fungal infection of skin, initiated at site of puncture affecting lower limb or foot (mossy foot)
　　B43.0　**Cutaneous** chromomycosis
　　　　　　Dermatitis verrucosa
　　B43.1　**Pheomycotic brain abscess**
　　　　　　Cerebral chromomycosis
　　B43.2　**Subcutaneous** pheomycotic abscess and cyst
　　B43.8　**Other forms** of chromomycosis
　　B43.9　**Chromomycosis, unspecified**

● **B44**　**Aspergillosis**
　　　Infection marked by inflammatory lesions in skin, ear, orbit, nasal sinuses, lungs, and occasionally bones and meninges

　　Includes　aspergilloma
　　B44.0　**Invasive pulmonary** aspergillosis
　　B44.1　**Other pulmonary** aspergillosis
　　B44.2　**Tonsillar** aspergillosis
　　B44.7　**Disseminated** aspergillosis
　　　　　　Generalized aspergillosis
　●　**B44.8**　Other forms of aspergillosis
　　　　B44.81　**Allergic bronchopulmonary** aspergillosis
　　　　B44.89　**Other forms** of aspergillosis
　　B44.9　Aspergillosis, **unspecified**

● **B45**　**Cryptococcosis**
　　　Infection in the immunocompromised and fatal if left untreated; AKA torulosis, Buschke, or Busse-Buschke disease
　　B45.0　**Pulmonary** cryptococcosis
　　B45.1　**Cerebral** cryptococcosis
　　　　　　Cryptococcal meningitis
　　　　　　Cryptococcosis meningocerebralis
　　B45.2　**Cutaneous** cryptococcosis
　　B45.3　**Osseous** cryptococcosis
　　B45.7　**Disseminated** cryptococcosis
　　　　　　Generalized cryptococcosis
　　B45.8　**Other forms** of cryptococcosis
　　B45.9　**Cryptococcosis, unspecified**

▶ New　　⇨ Revised　　~~deleted~~ Deleted　　Excludes 1　　Excludes 2　　Includes　　Use additional　　Code first　　Code also　　Key words
OGCR Official Guidelines　　X Assign placeholder X　　● Use Additional Character(s)　　▌ Manifestation Code　　Ⓡⓒ Hierarchical Condition Category　　**Coding Clinic**

● B46   Zygomycosis
Fungal infections including subcutaneous lesions and infection of sinuses, brain, or lungs

     B46.0   Pulmonary mucormycosis HCC
         Fungal infection affecting lung

     B46.1   Rhinocerebral mucormycosis HCC

     B46.2   Gastrointestinal mucormycosis HCC

     B46.3   Cutaneous mucormycosis HCC
         Subcutaneous mucormycosis

     B46.4   Disseminated mucormycosis HCC
         Generalized mucormycosis

     B46.5   Mucormycosis, unspecified HCC

     B46.8   Other zygomycoses HCC
         Entomophthoromycosis

     B46.9   Zygomycosis, unspecified HCC
         Phycomycosis NOS

● B47   Mycetoma
Slow progressive, destructive fungal infection of cutaneous and subcutaneous tissues, fascia, and bone, primarily seen in foot (Madura foot) or leg

     B47.0   Eumycetoma
         Madura foot, mycotic Maduromycosis

     B47.1   Actinomycetoma

     B47.9   Mycetoma, unspecified
         Madura foot NOS

● B48   Other mycoses, not elsewhere classified

     B48.0   Lobomycosis
         Infection with symptoms of red, smooth, hard cutaneous nodules resembling keloids
         Keloidal blastomycosis
         Lobo's disease

     B48.1   Rhinosporidiosis
         Chronic, localized granulomatous fungal infection, affecting mucocutaneous tissues, usually of nose characterized by polyps, papillomas, and wartlike lesions

     B48.2   Allescheriasis
         Fungal infection
         Infection due to Pseudallescheria boydii
         Excludes1   eumycetoma (B47.0)

     B48.3   Geotrichosis
         Fungal infection usually of bronchi, lungs, mouth, or intestinal tract
         Geotrichum stomatitis

     B48.4   Penicillosis HCC
         Fungal infection
         Talaromycosis

     B48.8   Other specified mycoses HCC
         Adiaspiromycosis
         Infection of tissue and organs by Alternaria
         Infection of tissue and organs by Drechslera
         Infection of tissue and organs by Fusarium
         Infection of tissue and organs by saprophytic fungi NEC

B49   Unspecified mycosis
     Fungemia NOS

PROTOZOAL DISEASES (B50-B64)

     Excludes1   amebiasis (A06.-)
                other protozoal intestinal diseases (A07.-)

● B50   Plasmodium falciparum malaria
Severe form of malaria that can be fatal

     Includes   mixed infections of Plasmodium falciparum with any other Plasmodium species

     B50.0   Plasmodium falciparum malaria with cerebral complications
         Cerebral malaria NOS

     B50.8   Other severe and complicated Plasmodium falciparum malaria
         Severe or complicated Plasmodium falciparum malaria NOS

     B50.9   Plasmodium falciparum malaria, unspecified

● B51   Plasmodium vivax malaria

     Includes   mixed infections of Plasmodium vivax with other Plasmodium species, except Plasmodium falciparum

     Excludes1   plasmodium vivax with Plasmodium falciparum (B50.-)

     B51.0   Plasmodium vivax malaria with rupture of spleen

     B51.8   Plasmodium vivax malaria with other complications

     B51.9   Plasmodium vivax malaria without complication
         Plasmodium vivax malaria NOS

● B52   Plasmodium malariae malaria
Causes fever that recurs at approximately three-day intervals (quartan fever), longer than two-day (tertian) intervals of other malarial parasites

     Includes   mixed infections of Plasmodium malariae with other Plasmodium species, except Plasmodium falciparum and Plasmodium vivax

     Excludes1   plasmodium falciparum (B50.-)
                plasmodium vivax (B51.-)

     B52.0   Plasmodium malariae malaria with nephropathy

     B52.8   Plasmodium malariae malaria with other complications

     B52.9   Plasmodium malariae malaria without complication
         Plasmodium malariae malaria NOS

● B53   Other specified malaria

     B53.0   Plasmodium ovale malaria
         Least diagnosed type of malaria spread by female mosquitoes of rare species
         Excludes1   plasmodium ovale with Plasmodium falciparum (B50.-)
                plasmodium ovale with Plasmodium malariae (B52.-)
                plasmodium ovale with Plasmodium vivax (B51.-)

     B53.1   Malaria due to simian plasmodia
         Malaria-like disease (parasite infection)
         Excludes1   malaria due to simian plasmodia with Plasmodium falciparum (B50.-)
                malaria due to simian plasmodia with Plasmodium malariae (B52.-)
                malaria due to simian plasmodia with Plasmodium ovale (B53.0)
                malaria due to simian plasmodia with Plasmodium vivax (B51.-)

     B53.8   Other malaria, not elsewhere classified

● B54   Unspecified malaria

● B55   Leishmaniasis
Protozoal infection

     B55.0   Visceral leishmaniasis
         Kala-azar
         Post-kala-azar dermal leishmaniasis

     B55.1   Cutaneous leishmaniasis

     B55.2   Mucocutaneous leishmaniasis

     B55.9   Leishmaniasis, unspecified

CHAPTER 1 (A00-B99)

● **B56 African trypanosomiasis**
Human African trypanosomiasis (HAT) is transmitted by fly bites

B56.0 Gambiense trypanosomiasis
Infection due to Trypanosoma brucei gambiense
West African sleeping sickness

B56.1 Rhodesiense trypanosomiasis
East African sleeping sickness
Infection due to Trypanosoma brucei rhodesiense

B56.9 African trypanosomiasis, unspecified
Sleeping sickness NOS

● **B57 Chagas' disease**
Tropical parasitic disease

Includes   American trypanosomiasis
infection due to Trypanosoma cruzi

B57.0 Acute Chagas' disease with heart involvement
Acute Chagas' disease with myocarditis

B57.1 Acute Chagas' disease without heart involvement
Acute Chagas' disease NOS

B57.2 Chagas' disease (chronic) with heart involvement
American trypanosomiasis NOS
Chagas' disease (chronic) NOS
Chagas' disease (chronic) with myocarditis
Trypanosomiasis NOS

● **B57.3 Chagas' disease (chronic) with digestive system involvement**

B57.30 Chagas' disease with digestive system involvement, unspecified

B57.31 Megaesophagus in Chagas' disease

B57.32 Megacolon in Chagas' disease

B57.39 Other digestive system involvement in Chagas' disease

● **B57.4 Chagas' disease (chronic) with nervous system involvement**

B57.40 Chagas' disease with nervous system involvement, unspecified

B57.41 Meningitis in Chagas' disease

B57.42 Meningoencephalitis in Chagas' disease

B57.49 Other nervous system involvement in Chagas' disease

B57.5 Chagas' disease (chronic) with other organ involvement

● **B58 Toxoplasmosis**
Infection by protozoon transmitted in cysts in feces of cats

Includes   infection due to Toxoplasma gondii

Excludes1   congenital toxoplasmosis (P37.1)

● **B58.0 Toxoplasma oculopathy**

B58.00 Toxoplasma oculopathy, unspecified

B58.01 Toxoplasma chorioretinitis

B58.09 Other toxoplasma oculopathy
Toxoplasma uveitis

B58.1 Toxoplasma hepatitis

B58.2 Toxoplasma meningoencephalitis ℞

B58.3 Pulmonary toxoplasmosis ℞

● **B58.8 Toxoplasmosis with other organ involvement**

B58.81 Toxoplasma myocarditis

B58.82 Toxoplasma myositis

B58.83 Toxoplasma tubulo-interstitial nephropathy
Toxoplasma pyelonephritis

B58.89 Toxoplasmosis with other organ involvement

B58.9 Toxoplasmosis, unspecified

B59 Pneumocystosis ℞
Caused by fungus
Pneumonia due to Pneumocystis carinii
Pneumonia due to Pneumocystis jiroveci

● **B60 Other protozoal diseases, not elsewhere classified**

Excludes1   cryptosporidiosis (A07.2)
intestinal microsporidiosis (A07.8)
isosporiasis (A07.3)

B60.0 Babesiosis
Tickborne disease caused by microscopic organisms

B60.00 Babesiosis, unspecified
Babesiosis due to unspecified Babesia species
Piroplasmosis, unspecified

B60.01 Babesiosis due to Babesia microti
Infection due to B. microti

B60.02 Babesiosis due to Babesia duncani
Infection due to B. duncani and B. duncani-type species

B60.03 Babesiosis due to Babesia divergens
Babesiosis due to Babesia MO-1
Infection due to B. divergens and B. divergens-like strains

B60.09 Other babesiosis
Babesiosis due to Babesia KO-1
Babesiosis due to Babesia venatorum
Infection due to other Babesia species
Infection due to other protozoa of the order Piroplasmida
Other piroplasmosis

● **B60.1 Acanthamebiasis**

B60.10 Acanthamebiasis, unspecified

B60.11 Meningoencephalitis due to Acanthamoeba (culbertsoni)

B60.12 Conjunctivitis due to Acanthamoeba

B60.13 Keratoconjunctivitis due to Acanthamoeba

B60.19 Other acanthamebic disease

B60.2 Naegleriasis
Infection with microscopic organisms
Primary amebic meningoencephalitis

B60.8 Other specified protozoal diseases
Microsporidiosis

B64 Unspecified protozoal disease

HELMINTHIASES (B65-B83)

Diseases or infestations caused by parasitic worms

● **B65 Schistosomiasis [bilharziasis]**
Infection with flukes (flat parasitic worms)

Includes   snail fever

B65.0 Schistosomiasis due to Schistosoma haematobium [urinary schistosomiasis]

B65.1 Schistosomiasis due to Schistosoma mansoni [intestinal schistosomiasis]

B65.2 Schistosomiasis due to Schistosoma japonicum
Asiatic schistosomiasis

B65.3 Cercarial dermatitis
Swimmer's itch

B65.8 Other schistosomiasis
Infection due to Schistosoma intercalatum
Infection due to Schistosoma mattheei
Infection due to Schistosoma mekongi

Item 1–22 Toxoplasmosis is caused by the protozoa **Toxoplasma gondii,** of which the house cat can be a host. Human infection occurs when contact is made with materials containing the pathogen, such as feces, contaminated soil, or ingestion of infected lamb, goat, or pork. Of the infected, very few have symptoms because a healthy person's immune system keeps the parasite from causing illness. When the immune system is compromised, symptoms may occur. Clinical symptoms include flu-like symptoms, but the disease progresses to include the eyes and the brain in babies.

▶ New   ⇒ Revised   ~~deleted~~ Deleted   Excludes 1   Excludes 2   Includes   Use additional   Code first   Code also   Key words
OGCR Official Guidelines   X Assign placeholder X   ● Use Additional Character(s)   ❯ Manifestation Code   ℞ Hierarchical Condition Category   **Coding Clinic**

B65.9   Schistosomiasis, **unspecified**

● **B66**   **Other fluke infections**
Trematode (parasitic worms)

B66.0   **Opisthorchiasis**
Infection due to cat liver fluke
Infection due to Opisthorchis (felineus)(viverrini)

B66.1   **Clonorchiasis**
Chinese liver fluke disease
Infection due to Clonorchis sinensis
Oriental liver fluke disease

B66.2   **Dicroceliasis**
Liver fluke
Infection due to Dicrocoelium dendriticum
Lancet fluke infection

B66.3   **Fascioliasis**
Infection due to Fasciola gigantica
Infection due to Fasciola hepatica
Infection due to Fasciola indica
Sheep liver fluke disease

B66.4   **Paragonimiasis**
Infection due to Paragonimus species
Lung fluke disease
Pulmonary distomiasis

B66.5   **Fasciolopsiasis**
Largest intestinal fluke in humans
Infection due to Fasciolopsis buski
Intestinal distomiasis

B66.8   **Other specified fluke infections**
Echinostomiasis
Heterophyiasis
Metagonimiasis
Nanophyetiasis
Watsoniasis

B66.9   Fluke infection, **unspecified**

● **B67**   **Echinococcosis**
Larval forms of tapeworms usually of liver or lungs

   Includes   hydatidosis

B67.0   **Echinococcus granulosus infection of liver**

B67.1   **Echinococcus granulosus infection of lung**

B67.2   **Echinococcus granulosus infection of bone**

● B67.3   **Echinococcus granulosus infection, other and multiple sites**

    B67.31   **Echinococcus granulosus infection, thyroid gland**

    B67.32   **Echinococcus granulosus infection, multiple sites**

    B67.39   **Echinococcus granulosus infection, other sites**

B67.4   **Echinococcus granulosus infection, unspecified**
Dog tapeworm (infection)

B67.5   **Echinococcus multilocularis infection of liver**

● B67.6   **Echinococcus multilocularis infection, other and multiple sites**

    B67.61   **Echinococcus multilocularis infection, multiple sites**

    B67.69   **Echinococcus multilocularis infection, other sites**

B67.7   **Echinococcus multilocularis infection, unspecified**

B67.8   **Echinococcosis, unspecified, of liver**

● B67.9   **Echinococcosis, other and unspecified**

    B67.90   **Echinococcosis, unspecified**
Echinococcosis NOS

    B67.99   **Other echinococcosis**

Item 1-23 Echinococcosis: Also known as hydatid disease; is caused by Echinococcus granulosus, E. multilocularis, and E. vogeli tapeworms; and is contracted from infected food. Found in southern South America, the Mediterranean, the Middle East, central Asia, and Africa and uncommon in the United States but has been reported in California, New Mexico, Arizona and Utah. The disease is treated with medication over a long course, as it is resistive.

● **B68**   **Taeniasis**
Intestinal tapeworm (cestode) infection from raw or undercooked meat of infected animal

   Excludes1   cysticercosis (B69.-)

B68.0   **Taenia solium taeniasis**
Pork tapeworm (infection)

B68.1   **Taenia saginata taeniasis**
Beef tapeworm (infection)
Infection due to adult tapeworm Taenia saginata

B68.9   **Taeniasis, unspecified**

● **B69**   **Cysticercosis**
Systemic illness caused by the larvae of pork tapeworm

   Includes   cysticerciasis infection due to larval form of Taenia solium

B69.0   **Cysticercosis of central nervous system**

B69.1   **Cysticercosis of eye**

● B69.8   **Cysticercosis of other sites**

    B69.81   **Myositis in cysticercosis**

    B69.89   **Cysticercosis of other sites**

B69.9   **Cysticercosis, unspecified**

● **B70**   **Diphyllobothriasis and sparganosis**
Infection with tapeworms seen most often from inadequately cooked fish

B70.0   **Diphyllobothriasis**
Diphyllobothrium (adult) (latum) (pacificum) infection
Fish tapeworm (infection)

   Excludes2   larval diphyllobothriasis (B70.1)

B70.1   **Sparganosis**
Infection with migrating tapeworm larvae, which invade subcutaneous tissues, causing inflammation and fibrosis that resembles cellulitis
Infection due to Sparganum (mansoni) (proliferum)
Infection due to Spirometra larva
Larval diphyllobothriasis
Spirometrosis

● **B71**   **Other cestode infections**

B71.0   **Hymenolepiasis**
Intestinal infestation with tapeworms
Dwarf tapeworm infection
Rat tapeworm (infection)

B71.1   **Dipylidiasis**
Infection with tapeworm common to dogs and cats and seen in children having close contact with infected pets

B71.8   **Other specified cestode infections**
Infection by the larval stage of a tapeworm, usually through fruit or vegetables
Coenurosis

B71.9   **Cestode infection, unspecified**
Tapeworm (infection) NOS

B72   **Dracunculiasis**
Infection with roundworms

   Includes   guinea worm infection
infection due to Dracunculus medinensis

● **B73　Onchocerciasis**
Infection with parasitic worm
> **Includes**　onchocerca volvulus infection
> onchocercosis
> river blindness

● **B73.0　Onchocerciasis with eye disease**

B73.00　Onchocerciasis with eye involvement, unspecified

B73.01　Onchocerciasis with endophthalmitis

B73.02　Onchocerciasis with glaucoma

B73.09　Onchocerciasis with other eye involvement
Infestation of eyelid due to onchocerciasis

B73.1　Onchocerciasis without eye disease

● **B74　Filariasis**
Infestation with slender threadlike worms
> **Excludes2**　onchocerciasis (B73)
> tropical (pulmonary) eosinophilia NOS (J82.89)

B74.0　Filariasis due to Wuchereria bancrofti
Bancroftian elephantiasis
Bancroftian filariasis

B74.1　Filariasis due to Brugia malayi

B74.2　Filariasis due to Brugia timori

B74.3　Loiasis
Infection with round worms growing in subcutaneous connective tissue
Calabar swelling
Eyeworm disease of Africa
Loa loa infection

B74.4　Mansonelliasis
Infection with filarial parasite
Infection due to Mansonella ozzardi
Infection due to Mansonella perstans
Infection due to Mansonella streptocerca

B74.8　Other filariases
Dirofilariasis

B74.9　Filariasis, unspecified

B75　Trichinellosis
Infestation with parasitic roundworms ingested in undercooked contaminated meat
> **Includes**　infection due to Trichinella species trichiniasis

● **B76　Hookworm diseases**
Occurs in hot, humid parts of world where larvae are soil borne, enter digestive tract through skin of feet/legs or in contaminated food/water; AKA ground itch
> **Includes**　uncinariasis

B76.0　Ancylostomiasis
Infection due to Ancylostoma species

B76.1　Necatoriasis
Infection due to Necator americanus

B76.8　Other hookworm diseases

B76.9　Hookworm disease, unspecified
Cutaneous larva migrans NOS

● **B77　Ascariasis**
Infection by roundworm in small intestine
> **Includes**　ascaridiasis
> roundworm infection

B77.0　Ascariasis with intestinal complications

● **B77.8　Ascariasis with other complications**

B77.81　Ascariasis pneumonia

B77.89　Ascariasis with other complications

B77.9　Ascariasis, unspecified

● **B78　Strongyloidiasis**
Infection with adult female roundworms
> **Excludes1**　trichostrongyliasis (B81.2)

B78.0　Intestinal strongyloidiasis

B78.1　Cutaneous strongyloidiasis

B78.7　Disseminated strongyloidiasis

B78.9　Strongyloidiasis, unspecified

B79　Trichuriasis
Intestinal infection with roundworms
> **Includes**　trichocephaliasis
> whipworm (disease)(infection)

B80　Enterobiasis
Intestinal infection with pinworms
> **Includes**　oxyuriasis
> pinworm infection
> threadworm infection

● **B81　Other intestinal helminthiases, not elsewhere classified**
Diseases or infestations caused by parasitic worms
> **Excludes1**　angiostrongyliasis due to:
> Angiostrongylus cantonensis (B83.2)
> Parastrongylus cantonensis (B83.2)

B81.0　Anisakiasis
Roundworm infection via contaminated undercooked infected fish or marine mammals
Infection due to Anisakis larva

B81.1　Intestinal capillariasis
Infestation with of parasites (nematodes)
Capillariasis NOS
Infection due to Capillaria philippinensis
> **Excludes2**　hepatic capillariasis (B83.8)

B81.2　Trichostrongyliasis

B81.3　Intestinal angiostrongyliasis
Angiostrongyliasis due to:
Angiostrongylus costaricensis (B83.2)
Parastrongylus costaricensis (B83.2)

B81.4　Mixed intestinal helminthiases
Infection due to intestinal helminths classified to more than one of the categories B65.0-B81.3 and B81.8
Mixed helminthiasis NOS

B81.8　Other specified intestinal helminthiases
Infection due to Oesophagostomum species [esophagostomiasis]
Infection due to Ternidens diminutus [ternidensiasis]

● **B82　Unspecified intestinal parasitism**

B82.0　Intestinal helminthiasis, unspecified
Infected with worms

B82.9　Intestinal parasitism, unspecified

● **B83　Other helminthiases**
Caused by parasitic worms
> **Excludes1**　capillariasis NOS (B81.1)
> **Excludes2**　intestinal capillariasis (B81.1)

B83.0　Visceral larva migrans
Prolonged migration of nematode larvae
Toxocariasis

B83.1　Gnathostomiasis
Infection with nematode occurring from ingested undercooked fish contaminated with larvae; larvae migrate to subcutaneous tissue or deeper tissues, results are abscesses
Wandering swelling

B83.2　Angiostrongyliasis due to Parastrongylus cantonensis
Nematode infection caused by eating contaminated raw snails, slugs, or paratenic hosts such as prawns or crabs; larval worms migrate to central nervous system resulting in eosinophilic meningitis
Eosinophilic meningoencephalitis due to Parastrongylus cantonensis
> **Excludes2**　intestinal angiostrongyliasis (B81.3)

▶ New　　⇨ Revised　　~~deleted~~ Deleted　　Excludes 1　　Excludes 2　　Includes　　Use additional　　Code first　　Code also　　Key words
OGCR Official Guidelines　　X Assign placeholder X　　● Use Additional Character(s)　　▶ Manifestation Code　　Ⓡ Hierarchical Condition Category　　**Coding Clinic**

B83.3 Syngamiasis
Infestation with gapeworm from turkey, pheasant, guinea fowl, goose, and wild birds
Syngamosis

B83.4 Internal hirudiniasis
Infestation by leeches
> **Excludes2**   external hirudiniasis (B88.3)

B83.8 Other specified helminthiases
Parasitic worm infestation
Acanthocephaliasis
Gongylonemiasis
Hepatic capillariasis
Metastrongyliasis
Thelaziasis

B83.9 Helminthiasis, unspecified
Worms NOS
> **Excludes1**   intestinal helminthiasis NOS (B82.0)

PEDICULOSIS, ACARIASIS AND OTHER INFESTATIONS (B85-B89)

● **B85 Pediculosis and phthiriasis**
Infestation of lice

B85.0 Pediculosis due to Pediculus humanus capitis
Head-louse infestation

B85.1 Pediculosis due to Pediculus humanus corporis
Body-louse infestation

B85.2 Pediculosis, unspecified

B85.3 Phthiriasis
Crab or pubic lice
Infestation by crab-louse
Infestation by Phthirus pubis

B85.4 Mixed pediculosis and phthiriasis
Infestation classifiable to more than one of the categories B85.0-B85.3

B86 Scabies
Contagious dermatitis caused by mites
Sarcoptic itch

● **B87 Myiasis**
Infestation by fly maggots
> **Includes**   infestation by larva of flies

B87.0 Cutaneous myiasis
Creeping myiasis

B87.1 Wound myiasis
Traumatic myiasis

B87.2 Ocular myiasis

B87.3 Nasopharyngeal myiasis
Laryngeal myiasis

B87.4 Aural myiasis

● **B87.8 Myiasis of other sites**

B87.81 Genitourinary myiasis

B87.82 Intestinal myiasis

B87.89 Myiasis of other sites

B87.9 Myiasis, unspecified

● **B88 Other infestations**

B88.0 Other acariasis
~~Acarine dermatitis~~
~~Dermatitis due to Demodex species~~
~~Dermatitis due to Dermanyssus gallinae~~
~~Dermatitis due to Liponyssoides sanguineus~~
~~Trombiculosis~~
> **Excludes2**   scabies (B86)

▶ **B88.01 Infestation by Demodex mites**
▶ Demodex brevis infestation
▶ Demodex folliculorum infestation
▶ **Code also**, if applicable, eyelid inflammation (H01.8-)

▶ **B88.09 Other acariasis**
▶ Acarine dermatitis
▶ Dermatitis due to Dermanyssus gallinae
▶ Dermatitis due to Liponyssoides sanguineus
▶ Trombiculosis

B88.1 Tungiasis [sandflea infestation]
Inflammatory skin disease caused by infestation of fleas

B88.2 Other arthropod infestations
Scarabiasis

B88.3 External hirudiniasis
Leech infestation NOS
> **Excludes2**   internal hirudiniasis (B83.4)

B88.8 Other specified infestations
Infection of topical fresh water fish parasite
Ichthyoparasitism due to Vandellia cirrhosa
Linguatulosis
Porocephaliasis

B88.9 Infestation, unspecified
Infestation (skin) NOS
Infestation by mites NOS
Skin parasites NOS

B89 Unspecified parasitic disease

SEQUELAE OF INFECTIOUS AND PARASITIC DISEASES (B90-B94)

Note: Categories B90-B94 are to be used to indicate conditions in categories A00-B89 as the cause of sequelae, which are themselves classified elsewhere. The 'sequelae' include conditions specified as such; they also include residuals of diseases classifiable to the above categories if there is evidence that the disease itself is no longer present. Codes from these categories are not to be used for chronic infections. Code chronic current infections to active infectious disease as appropriate.

Code first condition resulting from (sequela) the infectious or parasitic disease

● **B90 Sequelae of tuberculosis**
Condition resulting from tuberculosis

B90.0 Sequelae of central nervous system tuberculosis

B90.1 Sequelae of genitourinary tuberculosis

B90.2 Sequelae of tuberculosis of bones and joints

B90.8 Sequelae of tuberculosis of other organs
> **Excludes2**   sequelae of respiratory tuberculosis (B90.9)

B90.9 Sequelae of respiratory and unspecified tuberculosis
Sequelae of tuberculosis NOS

B91 Sequelae of poliomyelitis
> **Excludes1**   postpolio syndrome (G14)

B92 Sequelae of leprosy

● **B94 Sequelae of other and unspecified infectious and parasitic diseases**

B94.0 Sequelae of trachoma

B94.1 Sequelae of viral encephalitis

B94.2 Sequelae of viral hepatitis

B94.8 Sequelae of other specified infectious and parasitic diseases
Coding Clinic: 2021, Q4, P102-106; 2021, Q1, P34,37,41,44,46,48

B94.9 Sequelae of unspecified infectious and parasitic disease
> **Excludes2**   post COVID-19 condition (U09.9)
Coding Clinic: 2017, Q4, P109

OGCR Section I.C.1.b.

Certain infectious and parasitic diseases

Infectious agents as the cause of diseases classified to other chapters

Certain infections are classified in chapters other than Chapter 1 and no organism is identified as part of the infection code. In these instances, it is necessary to use an additional code from Chapter 1 to identify the organism. A code from category B95, Streptococcus, Staphylococcus, and Enterococcus as the cause of diseases classified to other chapters, B96, Other bacterial agents as the cause of diseases classified to other chapters, or B97, Viral agents as the cause of diseases classified to other chapters, is to be used as an additional code to identify the organism. An instructional note will be found at the infection code advising that an additional organism code is required.

CHAPTER 1 (A00–B99)

BACTERIAL AND VIRAL INFECTIOUS AGENTS (B95-B97)

Note: These categories are provided for use as supplementary or additional codes to identify the infectious agent(s) in diseases classified elsewhere.

Code the disease first, then the bacterium. Do not report codes from B95-B97 for sepsis.

● **B95** **Streptococcus, Staphylococcus, and Enterococcus as the cause of diseases classified elsewhere**

  B95.0 **Streptococcus, group A, as the cause of diseases classified elsewhere**

  B95.1 **Streptococcus, group B, as the cause of diseases classified elsewhere**
     Coding Clinic: 2020, Q1, P10; 2019, Q2, P9-10; 2018, Q4, P23

  B95.2 **Enterococcus as the cause of diseases classified elsewhere**

  B95.3 **Streptococcus pneumoniae as the cause of diseases classified elsewhere**

  B95.4 **Other streptococcus as the cause of diseases classified elsewhere**
     Coding Clinic: 2025, Q1, P21

  B95.5 **Unspecified streptococcus as the cause of diseases classified elsewhere**

 ● **B95.6** **Staphylococcus aureus as the cause of diseases classified elsewhere**

    B95.61 **Methicillin susceptible Staphylococcus aureus infection as the cause of diseases classified elsewhere**
      Methicillin susceptible Staphylococcus aureus (MSSA) infection as the cause of diseases classified elsewhere
      Staphylococcus aureus infection NOS as the cause of diseases classified elsewhere

    B95.62 **Methicillin resistant Staphylococcus aureus infection as the cause of diseases classified elsewhere**
      Methicillin resistant staphylococcus aureus (MRSA) infection as the cause of diseases classified elsewhere
      Coding Clinic: 2016, Q1, P13

  B95.7 **Other staphylococcus as the cause of diseases classified elsewhere**

  B95.8 **Unspecified staphylococcus as the cause of diseases classified elsewhere**

● **B96** **Other bacterial agents as the cause of diseases classified elsewhere**

  B96.0 **Mycoplasma pneumoniae [M. pneumoniae] as the cause of diseases classified elsewhere**
     Pleuro-pneumonia-like-organism [PPLO]

  B96.1 **Klebsiella pneumoniae [K. pneumoniae] as the cause of diseases classified elsewhere**

 ● **B96.2** **Escherichia coli [E. coli] as the cause of diseases classified elsewhere**

    B96.20 **Unspecified Escherichia coli [E. coli] as the cause of diseases classified elsewhere**
      Escherichia coli [E. coli] NOS
      Coding Clinic: 2022, Q1, P31; 2018, Q4, P34; 2018, Q1, P16

    B96.21 **Shiga toxin-producing Escherichia coli [E. coli] [STEC] O157 as the cause of diseases classified elsewhere**
      E. coli O157:H- (nonmotile) with confirmation of Shiga toxin
      E. coli O157 with confirmation of Shiga toxin when H antigen is unknown, or is not H7
      O157:H7 Escherichia coli [E. coli] with or without confirmation of Shiga toxin-production
      Shiga toxin-producing Escherichia coli [E. coli] O157:H7 with or without confirmation of Shiga toxin-production
      STEC O157:H7 with or without confirmation of Shiga toxin-production

    B96.22 **Other specified Shiga toxin-producing Escherichia coli [E. coli] [STEC] as the cause of diseases classified elsewhere**
      Non-O157 Shiga toxin-producing Escherichia coli [E. coli]
      Non-O157 Shiga toxin-producing Escherichia coli [E. coli] with known O group

    B96.23 **Unspecified Shiga toxin-producing Escherichia coli [E. coli] [STEC] as the cause of diseases classified elsewhere**
      Shiga toxin-producing Escherichia coli [E. coli] with unspecified O group
      STEC NOS

    B96.29 **Other Escherichia coli [E. coli] as the cause of diseases classified elsewhere**
      Non-Shiga toxin-producing E. coli

  B96.3 **Hemophilus influenzae [H. influenzae] as the cause of diseases classified elsewhere**

  B96.4 **Proteus (mirabilis) (morganii) as the cause of diseases classified elsewhere**

  B96.5 **Pseudomonas (aeruginosa) (mallei) (pseudomallei) as the cause of diseases classified elsewhere**
     Coding Clinic: 2015, Q1, P18

  B96.6 **Bacteroides fragilis [B. fragilis] as the cause of diseases classified elsewhere**

  B96.7 **Clostridium perfringens [C. perfringens] as the cause of diseases classified elsewhere**

 ● **B96.8** **Other specified bacterial agents as the cause of diseases classified elsewhere**

    B96.81 **Helicobacter pylori [H. pylori] as the cause of diseases classified elsewhere**

    B96.82 **Vibrio vulnificus as the cause of diseases classified elsewhere**

    B96.83 **Acinetobacter baumannii as the cause of diseases classified elsewhere**

    B96.89 **Other specified bacterial agents as the cause of diseases classified elsewhere**

● **B97** **Viral agents as the cause of diseases classified elsewhere**

  B97.0 **Adenovirus as the cause of diseases classified elsewhere**

 ● **B97.1** **Enterovirus as the cause of diseases classified elsewhere**

    B97.10 **Unspecified enterovirus as the cause of diseases classified elsewhere**

    B97.11 **Coxsackievirus as the cause of diseases classified elsewhere**

    B97.12 **Echovirus as the cause of diseases classified elsewhere**

    B97.19 **Other enterovirus as the cause of diseases classified elsewhere**

 ● **B97.2** **Coronavirus as the cause of diseases classified elsewhere**

    B97.21 **SARS-associated coronavirus as the cause of diseases classified elsewhere**

      Excludes1 pneumonia due to SARS-associated coronavirus (J12.81)

    B97.29 **Other coronavirus as the cause of diseases classified elsewhere**

Item 1–24 **Retrovirus** develops by copying its RNA, genetic materials, into the DNA, which then produces new virus particles. It is from the Retroviridae virus family. **Human T-cell lymphotropic virus, Type I (HTLV-I),** is also called human T-cell leukemia virus, Type I, and is a retrovirus thought to cause T-cell leukemia/lymphoma. **Human T-cell lymphotropic virus, Type II (HTLV-II),** is also called human T-cell leukemia virus, Type II, and is a retrovirus associated with hematologic disorders.

    HIV-2 is one of the serotypes of HIV and is usually confined to West Africa, whereas **HIV-1** is found worldwide.

▶ New   ⇨ Revised   ~~deleted~~ Deleted   Excludes 1   Excludes 2   Includes   Use additional   Code first   Code also   Key words

OGCR Official Guidelines   X Assign placeholder X   ● Use Additional Character(s)   ▶ Manifestation Code   Hierarchical Condition Category   Coding Clinic

● **B97.3** **Retrovirus** as the cause of diseases classified elsewhere
    Excludes1   human immunodeficiency virus [HIV] disease (B20)

    B97.30   **Unspecified** retrovirus as the cause of diseases classified elsewhere

    B97.31   **Lentivirus** as the cause of diseases classified elsewhere

    B97.32   **Oncovirus** as the cause of diseases classified elsewhere

    B97.33   **Human T-cell lymphotrophic virus, type I [HTLV-I]** as the cause of diseases classified elsewhere

    B97.34   **Human T-cell lymphotrophic virus, type II [HTLV-II]** as the cause of diseases classified elsewhere

    B97.35   **Human immunodeficiency virus, type 2 [HIV 2]** as the cause of diseases classified elsewhere

    B97.39   **Other** retrovirus as the cause of diseases classified elsewhere

    B97.4   **Respiratory syncytial** virus as the cause of diseases classified elsewhere
       RSV as the cause of diseases classified elsewhere
       Code first related disorders, such as:
       otitis media (H65.-)
       upper respiratory infection (J06.9)
       Excludes1   acute bronchiolitis due to respiratory syncytial virus (RSV) (J21.0)
                acute bronchitis due to respiratory syncytial virus (RSV) (J20.5)
                respiratory syncytial virus (RSV) pneumonia (J12.1)

    B97.5   **Reovirus** as the cause of diseases classified elsewhere

    B97.6   **Parvovirus** as the cause of diseases classified elsewhere

    B97.7   **Papillomavirus** as the cause of diseases classified elsewhere

● **B97.8**   **Other viral agents** as the cause of diseases classified elsewhere

    B97.81   **Human metapneumovirus** as the cause of diseases classified elsewhere

    B97.89   **Other viral agents** as the cause of diseases classified elsewhere
       Coding Clinic: 2016, Q3, P8-10, 14

OTHER INFECTIOUS DISEASES (B99)

● **B99**   **Other and unspecified infectious diseases**

    B99.8   **Other** infectious disease

    B99.9   **Unspecified** infectious disease

CHAPTER 2

NEOPLASMS (C00-D49)

OGCR **Chapter-Specific Coding Guidelines**

2. Chapter 2: Neoplasms (C00-D49)
General guidelines
Chapter 2 of the ICD-10-CM contains the codes for most benign and all malignant neoplasms. Certain benign neoplasms, such as prostatic adenomas, may be found in the specific body system chapters. To properly code a neoplasm it is necessary to determine from the record if the neoplasm is benign, in-situ, malignant, or of uncertain histologic behavior. If malignant, any secondary (metastatic) sites should also be determined.

Primary malignant neoplasms overlapping site boundaries
A primary malignant neoplasm that overlaps two or more contiguous (next to each other) sites should be classified to the subcategory/code .8 ('overlapping lesion'), unless the combination is specifically indexed elsewhere. For multiple neoplasms of the same site that are not contiguous such as tumors in different quadrants of the same breast, codes for each site should be assigned.

Malignant neoplasm of ectopic tissue
Malignant neoplasms of ectopic tissue are to be coded to the site of origin mentioned, e.g., ectopic pancreatic malignant neoplasms involving the stomach are coded to malignant neoplasm of pancreas, unspecified (C25.9).
The neoplasm table in the Alphabetic Index should be referenced first. However, if the histological term is documented, that term should be referenced first, rather than going immediately to the Neoplasm Table, in order to determine which column in the Neoplasm Table is appropriate. For example, if the documentation indicates "adenoma," refer to the term in the Alphabetic Index to review the entries under this term and the instructional note to "see also neoplasm, by site, benign." The table provides the proper code based on the type of neoplasm and the site. It is important to select the proper column in the table that corresponds to the type of neoplasm. The Tabular List should then be referenced to verify that the correct code has been selected from the table and that a more specific site code does not exist.
See Section I.C.21. Factors influencing health status and contact with health services, Status, for information regarding Z15.0, codes for genetic susceptibility to cancer.

a. Treatment directed at the malignancy
If the treatment is directed at the malignancy, designate the malignancy as the principal diagnosis.
The only exception to this guideline is if a patient admission/encounter is solely for the administration of chemotherapy, immunotherapy or external beam radiation therapy, assign the appropriate Z51.— code as the first-listed or principal diagnosis, and the diagnosis or problem for which the service is being performed as a secondary diagnosis.

b. Treatment of secondary site
When a patient is admitted because of a primary neoplasm with metastasis and treatment is directed toward the secondary site only, the secondary neoplasm is designated as the principal diagnosis even though the primary malignancy is still present.

c. Coding and sequencing of complications
Coding and sequencing of complications associated with the malignancies or with the therapy thereof are subject to the following guidelines:

1) Anemia associated with malignancy
When admission/encounter is for management of an anemia associated with the malignancy, and the treatment is only for anemia, the appropriate code for the malignancy is sequenced as the principal or first-listed diagnosis followed by the appropriate code for the anemia (such as code D63.0, Anemia in neoplastic disease).

2) Anemia associated with chemotherapy, immunotherapy and radiation therapy
When the admission/encounter is for management of an anemia associated with an adverse effect of the administration of chemotherapy or immunotherapy and the only treatment is for the anemia, the anemia code is sequenced first followed by the appropriate codes for the neoplasm and the adverse effect (T45.1X5, Adverse effect of antineoplastic and immunosuppressive drugs).
When the admission/encounter is for management of an anemia associated with an adverse effect of radiotherapy, the anemia code should be sequenced first, followed by the appropriate neoplasm code and code Y84.2, Radiological procedure and radiotherapy as the cause of abnormal reaction of the patient, or of later complication, without mention of misadventure at the time of the procedure.

3) Management of dehydration due to the malignancy
When the admission/encounter is for management of dehydration due to the malignancy and only the dehydration is being treated (intravenous rehydration), the dehydration is sequenced first, followed by the code(s) for the malignancy.

4) Treatment of a complication resulting from a surgical procedure
When the admission/encounter is for treatment of a complication resulting from a surgical procedure, designate the complication as the principal or first-listed diagnosis if treatment is directed at resolving the complication.

d. Primary malignancy previously excised
When a primary malignancy has been previously excised or eradicated from its site and there is no further treatment directed to that site and there is no evidence of any existing primary malignancy at that site, a code from category Z85, Personal history of malignant neoplasm, should be used to indicate the former site of the malignancy. Any mention of extension, invasion, or metastasis to another site is coded as a secondary malignant neoplasm to that site. The secondary site may be the principal or first-listed with the Z85 code used as a secondary code.

e. Admissions/Encounters involving chemotherapy, immunotherapy and radiation therapy

1) Episode of care involves surgical removal of neoplasm
When an episode of care involves the surgical removal of a neoplasm, primary or secondary site, followed by adjunct chemotherapy or radiation treatment during the same episode of care, the code for the neoplasm should be assigned as principal or first-listed diagnosis.

2) Patient admission/encounter solely for administration of chemotherapy, immunotherapy and radiation therapy
If a patient admission/encounter is solely for the administration of chemotherapy, immunotherapy or external beam radiation therapy assign code Z51.0, Encounter for antineoplastic radiation therapy, or Z51.11, Encounter for antineoplastic chemotherapy, or Z51.12, Encounter for antineoplastic immunotherapy as the first-listed or principal diagnosis. If a patient receives more than one of these therapies during the same admission more than one of these codes may be assigned, in any sequence.
The malignancy for which the therapy is being administered should be assigned as a secondary diagnosis.
If a patient admission/encounter is for the insertion or implantation of radioactive elements (e.g., brachytherapy) the appropriate code for the malignancy is sequenced as the principal or first-listed diagnosis. Code Z51.0 should not be assigned.

3) Patient admitted for radiation therapy, chemotherapy or immunotherapy and develops complications
When a patient is admitted for the purpose of external beam radiotherapy, immunotherapy or chemotherapy and develops complications such as uncontrolled nausea and vomiting or dehydration, the principal or first-listed diagnosis is Z51.0, Encounter for antineoplastic radiation therapy, or Z51.11, Encounter for antineoplastic chemotherapy, or Z51.12, Encounter for antineoplastic immunotherapy followed by any codes for the complications.
When a patient is admitted for the purpose of insertion or implantation of radioactive elements (e.g., brachytherapy) and develops complications such as uncontrolled nausea and vomiting or dehydration, the principal or first-listed diagnosis is the appropriate code for the malignancy followed by any codes for the complications.

f. Admission/encounter to determine extent of malignancy
When the reason for admission/encounter is to determine the extent of the malignancy, or for a procedure such as paracentesis

or thoracentesis, the primary malignancy or appropriate metastatic site is designated as the principal or first-listed diagnosis, even though chemotherapy or radiotherapy is administered.

g. Symptoms, signs, and abnormal findings listed in Chapter 18 associated with neoplasms

Symptoms, signs, and ill-defined conditions listed in Chapter 18 characteristic of, or associated with, an existing primary or secondary site malignancy cannot be used to replace the malignancy as principal or first-listed diagnosis, regardless of the number of admissions or encounters for treatment and care of the neoplasm.

See Section I.C.21. Factors influencing health status and contact with health services, Encounter for prophylactic organ removal.

h. Admission/encounter for pain control/management

See Section I.C.6. for information on coding admission/encounter for pain control/management.

i. Malignancy in two or more noncontiguous sites

A patient may have more than one malignant tumor in the same organ. These tumors may represent different primaries or metastatic disease, depending on the site. Should the documentation be unclear, the provider should be queried as to the status of each tumor so that the correct codes can be assigned.

j. Disseminated malignant neoplasm, unspecified

Code C80.0, Disseminated malignant neoplasm, unspecified, is for use only in those cases where the patient has advanced metastatic disease and no known primary or secondary sites are specified. It should not be used in place of assigning codes for the primary site and all known secondary sites.

k. Malignant neoplasm without specification of site

Code C80.1, Malignant (primary) neoplasm, unspecified, equates to Cancer, unspecified. This code should only be used when no determination can be made as to the primary site of a malignancy. This code should rarely be used in the inpatient setting.

l. Sequencing of neoplasm codes

1) Encounter for treatment of primary malignancy

If the reason for the encounter is for treatment of a primary malignancy, assign the malignancy as the principal/first-listed diagnosis. The primary site is to be sequenced first, followed by any metastatic sites.

2) Encounter for treatment of secondary malignancy

When an encounter is for a primary malignancy with metastasis and treatment is directed toward the metastatic (secondary) site(s) only, the metastatic site(s) is designated as the principal/first-listed diagnosis. The primary malignancy is coded as an additional code.

3) Malignant neoplasm in a pregnant patient

When a pregnant woman has a malignant neoplasm, a code from subcategory O9A.1-, Malignant neoplasm complicating pregnancy, childbirth, and the puerperium, should be sequenced first, followed by the appropriate code from Chapter 2 to indicate the type of neoplasm.

4) Encounter for complication associated with a neoplasm

When an encounter is for management of a complication associated with a neoplasm, such as dehydration, and the treatment is only for the complication, the complication is coded first, followed by the appropriate code(s) for the neoplasm.

The exception to this guideline is anemia. When the admission/encounter is for management of an anemia associated with the malignancy, and the treatment is only for anemia, the appropriate code for the malignancy is sequenced as the principal or first-listed diagnosis followed by code D63.0, Anemia in neoplastic disease.

5) Complication from surgical procedure for treatment of a neoplasm

When an encounter is for treatment of a complication resulting from a surgical procedure performed for the treatment of the neoplasm, designate the complication as the principal/first-listed diagnosis. See guideline regarding the coding of a current malignancy versus personal history to determine if the code for the neoplasm should also be assigned.

6) Pathologic fracture due to a neoplasm

When an encounter is for a pathological fracture due to a neoplasm, and the focus of treatment is the fracture, a code from subcategory M84.5, Pathological fracture in neoplastic disease, should be sequenced first, followed by the code for the neoplasm.

If the focus of treatment is the neoplasm with an associated pathological fracture, the neoplasm code should be sequenced first, followed by a code from M84.5 for the pathological fracture.

m. Current malignancy versus personal history of malignancy

When a primary malignancy has been excised but further treatment, such as an additional surgery for the malignancy, radiation therapy or chemotherapy is directed to that site, the primary malignancy code should be used until treatment is completed.

When a primary malignancy has been previously excised or eradicated from its site, there is no further treatment (of the malignancy) directed to that site, and there is no evidence of any existing primary malignancy at that site, a code from category Z85, Personal history of malignant neoplasm, should be used to indicate the former site of the malignancy.

Subcategories Z85.0–Z85.7 should only be assigned for the former site of a primary malignancy, not the site of a secondary malignancy. Codes from subcategory Z85.8-, may be assigned for the former site(s) of either a primary or secondary malignancy included in this subcategory.

See Section I.C.21. Factors influencing health status and contact with health services, History (of)

n. Leukemia, Multiple Myeloma, and Malignant Plasma Cell Neoplasms in remission versus personal history

The categories for leukemia, and category C90, Multiple myeloma and malignant plasma cell neoplasms, have codes indicating whether or not the leukemia has achieved remission. There are also codes Z85.6, Personal history of leukemia, and Z85.79, Personal history of other malignant neoplasms of lymphoid, hematopoietic and related tissues. If the documentation is unclear, as to whether the leukemia has achieved remission, the provider should be queried.

See Section I.C.21. Factors influencing health status and contact with health services, History (of)

o. Aftercare following surgery for neoplasm

See Section I.C.21. Factors influencing health status and contact with health services, Aftercare

p. Follow-up care for completed treatment of a malignancy

See Section I.C.21. Factors influencing health status and contact with health services, Follow-up

q. Prophylactic organ removal for prevention of malignancy

See Section I.C. 21, Factors influencing health status and contact with health services, Prophylactic organ removal

r. Malignant neoplasm associated with transplanted organ

A malignant neoplasm of a transplanted organ should be coded as a transplant complication. Assign first the appropriate code from category T86.-, Complications of transplanted organs and tissue, followed by code C80.2, Malignant neoplasm associated with transplanted organ. Use an additional code for the specific malignancy.

Item 2–1 Neoplasm: Neo = new, plasm = growth, development, formation. This new growth (mass, tumor) can be malignant or benign, which is confirmed by the pathology report. Do not assign a code to a neoplasm until you review the pathology report. Certain CPT codes will specify benign or malignant lesion, so be certain the diagnosis code supports the procedure code.

CHAPTER 2

NEOPLASMS (C00-D49)

This chapter contains the following blocks:

C00-C14	Malignant neoplasms of lip, oral cavity and pharynx
C15-C26	Malignant neoplasms of digestive organs
C30-C39	Malignant neoplasms of respiratory and intrathoracic organs
C40-C41	Malignant neoplasms of bone and articular cartilage
C43-C44	Melanoma and other malignant neoplasms of skin
C45-C49	Malignant neoplasms of mesothelial and soft tissue
C50	Malignant neoplasms of breast
C51-C58	Malignant neoplasms of female genital organs
C60-C63	Malignant neoplasms of male genital organs
C64-C68	Malignant neoplasms of urinary tract
C69-C72	Malignant neoplasms of eye, brain and other parts of central nervous system
C73-C75	Malignant neoplasms of thyroid and other endocrine glands
C7A	Malignant neuroendocrine tumors
C7B	Secondary neuroendocrine tumors
C76-C80	Malignant neoplasms of ill-defined, other secondary and unspecified sites
C81-C96	Malignant neoplasms of lymphoid, hematopoietic and related tissue
D00-D09	In situ neoplasms
D10-D36	Benign neoplasms, except benign neuroendocrine tumors
D3A	Benign neuroendocrine tumors
D37-D48	Neoplasms of uncertain behavior, polycythemia vera and myelodysplastic syndromes
D49	Neoplasms of unspecified behavior

Notes: Functional activity

All neoplasms are classified in this chapter, whether they are functionally active or not. An additional code from Chapter 4 may be used, to identify functional activity associated with any neoplasm.

Morphology [Histology]

Chapter 2 classifies neoplasms primarily by site (topography), with broad groupings for behavior, malignant, in situ, benign, etc. The Table of Neoplasms should be used to identify the correct topography code. In a few cases, such as for malignant melanoma and certain neuroendocrine tumors, the morphology (histologic type) is included in the category and codes.

Primary malignant neoplasms overlapping site boundaries

A primary malignant neoplasm that overlaps two or more contiguous (next to each other) sites should be classified to the subcategory/code .8 ("overlapping lesion"), unless the combination is specifically indexed elsewhere. For multiple neoplasms of the same site that are not contiguous, such as tumors in different quadrants of the same breast, codes for each site should be assigned.

Malignant neoplasm of ectopic tissue

Malignant neoplasms of ectopic tissue are to be coded to the site mentioned, e.g., ectopic pancreatic malignant neoplasms are coded to pancreas, unspecified (C25.9).

MALIGNANT NEOPLASMS (C00-C96)

MALIGNANT NEOPLASMS, STATED OR PRESUMED TO BE PRIMARY (OF SPECIFIED SITES), AND CERTAIN SPECIFIED HISTOLOGIES, EXCEPT NEUROENDOCRINE, AND OF LYMPHOID, HEMATOPOIETIC AND RELATED TISSUE (C00-C75)

MALIGNANT NEOPLASMS OF LIP, ORAL CAVITY AND PHARYNX (C00-C14)

● **C00　Malignant neoplasm of lip**
　　Use additional code to identify:
　　　alcohol abuse and dependence (F10.-)
　　　history of tobacco dependence (Z87.891)
　　　tobacco dependence (F17.-)
　　　tobacco use (Z72.0)
　　Excludes1　malignant melanoma of lip (C43.0)
　　　　　　Merkel cell carcinoma of lip (C4A.0)
　　　　　　other and unspecified malignant neoplasm of skin of lip (C44.0-)

C00.0　Malignant neoplasm of external upper lip
　　Malignant neoplasm of lipstick area of upper lip
　　Malignant neoplasm of upper lip NOS
　　Malignant neoplasm of vermilion border of upper lip

C00.1　Malignant neoplasm of external lower lip
　　Malignant neoplasm of lower lip NOS
　　Malignant neoplasm of lipstick area of lower lip
　　Malignant neoplasm of vermilion border of lower lip

C00.2　Malignant neoplasm of external lip, unspecified
　　Malignant neoplasm of vermilion border of lip NOS

C00.3　Malignant neoplasm of upper lip, inner aspect
　　Malignant neoplasm of buccal aspect of upper lip
　　Malignant neoplasm of frenulum of upper lip
　　Malignant neoplasm of mucosa of upper lip
　　Malignant neoplasm of oral aspect of upper lip

C00.4　Malignant neoplasm of lower lip, inner aspect
　　Malignant neoplasm of buccal aspect of lower lip
　　Malignant neoplasm of frenulum of lower lip
　　Malignant neoplasm of mucosa of lower lip
　　Malignant neoplasm of oral aspect of lower lip

C00.5　Malignant neoplasm of lip, unspecified, inner aspect
　　Malignant neoplasm of buccal aspect of lip, unspecified
　　Malignant neoplasm of frenulum of lip, unspecified
　　Malignant neoplasm of mucosa of lip, unspecified
　　Malignant neoplasm of oral aspect of lip, unspecified

C00.6　Malignant neoplasm of commissure of lip, unspecified
　　Commissure: Site of union of corresponding parts

C00.8　Malignant neoplasm of overlapping sites of lip

C00.9　Malignant neoplasm of lip, unspecified

▶ New　➡ Revised　~~deleted~~ Deleted　Excludes 1　Excludes 2　Includes　Use additional　Code first　Code also　Key words
OGCR Official Guidelines　X Assign placeholder X　● Use Additional Character(s)　▶ Manifestation Code　🄷🄲 Hierarchical Condition Category　Coding Clinic

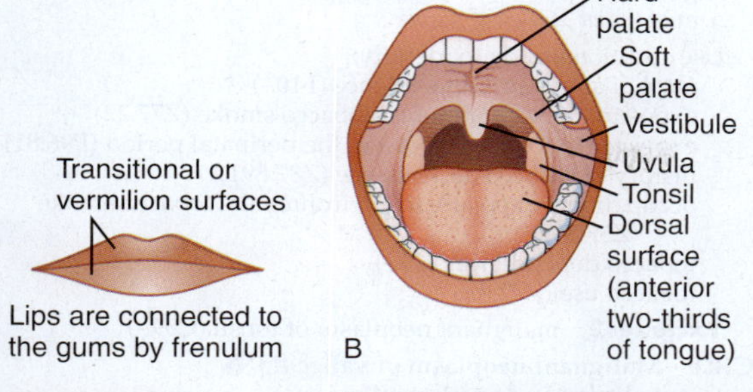

Figure 2-1 Anatomical structures of the mouth and lips. **A.** Transitional or vermilion borders. Lips are connected to the gums by frenulum. **B.** Dorsal surface. **C.** Ventral surface.

C01 Malignant neoplasm of base of tongue RCC
Malignant neoplasm of dorsal surface of base of tongue
Malignant neoplasm of fixed part of tongue NOS
Malignant neoplasm of posterior third of tongue

Use additional code to identify:
    alcohol abuse and dependence (F10.-)
    history of tobacco dependence (Z87.891)
    tobacco dependence (F17.-)
    tobacco use (Z72.0)

● **C02 Malignant neoplasm of other and unspecified parts of tongue**
Use additional code to identify:
    alcohol abuse and dependence (F10.-)
    history of tobacco dependence (Z87.891)
    tobacco dependence (F17.-)
    tobacco use (Z72.0)

C02.0 Malignant neoplasm of dorsal surface of tongue RCC
Malignant neoplasm of anterior two-thirds of tongue, dorsal surface

    Excludes2   malignant neoplasm of dorsal surface of base of tongue (C01)

C02.1 Malignant neoplasm of border of tongue RCC
Malignant neoplasm of tip of tongue

C02.2 Malignant neoplasm of ventral surface of tongue RCC
Malignant neoplasm of anterior two-thirds of tongue, ventral surface
Malignant neoplasm of frenulum linguae

C02.3 Malignant neoplasm of anterior two-thirds of tongue, part unspecified RCC
Malignant neoplasm of middle third of tongue NOS
Malignant neoplasm of mobile part of tongue NOS

C02.4 Malignant neoplasm of lingual tonsil RCC
Lingual tonsil: Aggregation of lymph follicles at root of tongue

    Excludes2   malignant neoplasm of tonsil NOS (C09.9)

C02.8 Malignant neoplasm of overlapping sites of tongue RCC
Malignant neoplasm of two or more contiguous sites of tongue

C02.9 Malignant neoplasm of tongue, unspecified RCC

● **C03 Malignant neoplasm of gum**
    Includes   malignant neoplasm of alveolar (ridge) mucosa
                     malignant neoplasm of gingiva

Use additional code to identify:
    alcohol abuse and dependence (F10.-)
    history of tobacco dependence (Z87.891)
    tobacco dependence (F17.-)
    tobacco use (Z72.0)

    Excludes2   malignant odontogenic neoplasms (C41.0-C41.1)

C03.0 Malignant neoplasm of upper gum RCC
C03.1 Malignant neoplasm of lower gum RCC
C03.9 Malignant neoplasm of gum, unspecified RCC

● **C04 Malignant neoplasm of floor of mouth**
Use additional code to identify:
    alcohol abuse and dependence (F10.-)
    history of tobacco dependence (Z87.891)
    tobacco dependence (F17.-)
    tobacco use (Z72.0)

C04.0 Malignant neoplasm of anterior floor of mouth RCC
Malignant neoplasm of anterior to the premolar-canine junction

C04.1 Malignant neoplasm of lateral floor of mouth RCC

C04.8 Malignant neoplasm of overlapping sites of floor of mouth RCC

C04.9 Malignant neoplasm of floor of mouth, unspecified RCC

● **C05 Malignant neoplasm of palate**
Use additional code to identify:
    alcohol abuse and dependence (F10.-)
    history of tobacco dependence (Z87.891)
    tobacco dependence (F17.-)
    tobacco use (Z72.0)

    Excludes1   Kaposi's sarcoma of palate (C46.2)

C05.0 Malignant neoplasm of hard palate RCC
C05.1 Malignant neoplasm of soft palate RCC

    Excludes2   malignant neoplasm of nasopharyngeal surface of soft palate (C11.3)

C05.2 Malignant neoplasm of uvula RCC
C05.8 Malignant neoplasm of overlapping sites of palate RCC
C05.9 Malignant neoplasm of palate, unspecified RCC
Malignant neoplasm of roof of mouth

● **C06 Malignant neoplasm of other and unspecified parts of mouth**
Use additional code to identify:
    alcohol abuse and dependence (F10.-)
    history of tobacco dependence (Z87.891)
    tobacco dependence (F17.-)
    tobacco use (Z72.0)

C06.0 Malignant neoplasm of cheek mucosa RCC
Malignant neoplasm of buccal mucosa NOS
Malignant neoplasm of internal cheek

C06.1 Malignant neoplasm of vestibule of mouth RCC
Malignant neoplasm of buccal sulcus (upper) (lower)
Malignant neoplasm of labial sulcus (upper) (lower)

C06.2 Malignant neoplasm of retromolar area RCC

● **C06.8 Malignant neoplasm of overlapping sites of other and unspecified parts of mouth**

    C06.80 Malignant neoplasm of overlapping sites of unspecified parts of mouth RCC

    C06.89 Malignant neoplasm of overlapping sites of other parts of mouth RCC
       'book leaf' neoplasm [ventral surface of tongue and floor of mouth]

C06.9 Malignant neoplasm of mouth, unspecified RCC
Malignant neoplasm of minor salivary gland, unspecified site
Malignant neoplasm of oral cavity NOS

CHAPTER 2 (C00-D49)

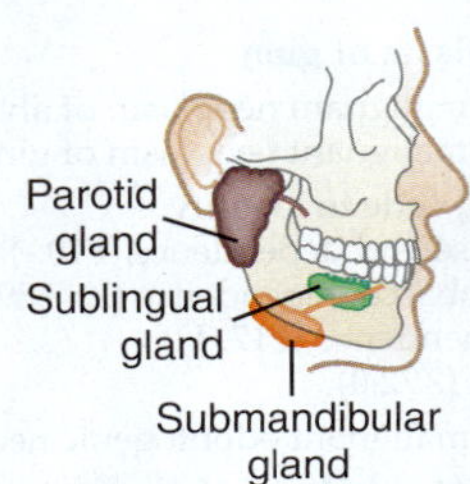

Figure 2-2 Major salivary glands.

C07 Malignant neoplasm of parotid gland Ⓗ

> **Use additional** code to identify:
> alcohol abuse and dependence (F10.-)
> exposure to environmental tobacco smoke (Z77.22)
> exposure to tobacco smoke in the perinatal period (P96.81)
> history of tobacco dependence (Z87.891)
> occupational exposure to environmental tobacco smoke (Z57.31)
> tobacco dependence (F17.-)
> tobacco use (Z72.0)

● **C08 Malignant neoplasm of other and unspecified major salivary glands**

> **Includes** malignant neoplasm of salivary ducts

> **Use additional** code to identify:
> alcohol abuse and dependence (F10.-)
> exposure to environmental tobacco smoke (Z77.22)
> exposure to tobacco smoke in the perinatal period (P96.81)
> history of tobacco dependence (Z87.891)
> occupational exposure to environmental tobacco smoke (Z57.31)
> tobacco dependence (F17.-)
> tobacco use (Z72.0)

> **Excludes1** malignant neoplasms of specified minor salivary glands which are classified according to their anatomical location

> **Excludes2** malignant neoplasms of minor salivary glands NOS (C06.9)
> malignant neoplasm of parotid gland (C07)

C08.0 **Malignant neoplasm of submandibular gland** Ⓗ
Malignant neoplasm of submaxillary gland

C08.1 **Malignant neoplasm of sublingual gland** Ⓗ

C08.9 **Malignant neoplasm of major salivary gland, unspecified** Ⓗ
Malignant neoplasm of salivary gland (major) NOS

★ **(See Plate 28 of the Anatomy Illustrations.)**

● **C09 Malignant neoplasm of tonsil**

> **Use additional** code to identify:
> alcohol abuse and dependence (F10.-)
> exposure to environmental tobacco smoke (Z77.22)
> exposure to tobacco smoke in the perinatal period (P96.81)
> history of tobacco dependence (Z87.891)
> occupational exposure to environmental tobacco smoke (Z57.31)
> tobacco dependence (F17.-)
> tobacco use (Z72.0)

> **Excludes2** malignant neoplasm of lingual tonsil (C02.4)
> malignant neoplasm of pharyngeal tonsil (C11.1)

C09.0 **Malignant neoplasm of tonsillar fossa** Ⓗ
Surface of palatine (two masses of lymphatic tissue on sides of throat) tonsils

C09.1 **Malignant neoplasm of tonsillar pillar (anterior) (posterior)** Ⓗ
Extension from palatine (two masses of lymphatic tissue on sides of throat) tonsils

C09.8 **Malignant neoplasm of overlapping sites of tonsil** Ⓗ

C09.9 **Malignant neoplasm of tonsil, unspecified** Ⓗ
Malignant neoplasm of tonsil NOS
Malignant neoplasm of faucial tonsils
Malignant neoplasm of palatine tonsils

● **C10 Malignant neoplasm of oropharynx**
Area of throat at back of mouth

> **Use additional** code to identify:
> alcohol abuse and dependence (F10.-)
> exposure to environmental tobacco smoke (Z77.22)
> exposure to tobacco smoke in the perinatal period (P96.81)
> history of tobacco dependence (Z87.891)
> occupational exposure to environmental tobacco smoke (Z57.31)
> tobacco dependence (F17.-)
> tobacco use (Z72.0)

> **Excludes2** malignant neoplasm of tonsil (C09.-)

C10.0 **Malignant neoplasm of vallecula** Ⓗ
Vallecula, depression or furrow

C10.1 **Malignant neoplasm of anterior surface of epiglottis** Ⓗ
Malignant neoplasm of epiglottis, free border [margin]
Malignant neoplasm of glossoepiglottic fold(s)

> **Excludes2** malignant neoplasm of epiglottis (suprahyoid portion) NOS (C32.1)

C10.2 **Malignant neoplasm of lateral wall of oropharynx** Ⓗ

C10.3 **Malignant neoplasm of posterior wall of oropharynx** Ⓗ

C10.4 **Malignant neoplasm of branchial cleft** Ⓗ
Congenital slitlike openings formed between branchial arches pharyngeal groove
Malignant neoplasm of branchial cyst [site of neoplasm]

C10.8 **Malignant neoplasm of overlapping sites of oropharynx** Ⓗ
Malignant neoplasm of junctional region of oropharynx

C10.9 **Malignant neoplasm of oropharynx, unspecified** Ⓗ

● **C11 Malignant neoplasm of nasopharynx**

> **Use additional** code to identify:
> exposure to environmental tobacco smoke (Z77.22)
> exposure to tobacco smoke in the perinatal period (P96.81)
> history of tobacco dependence (Z87.891)
> occupational exposure to environmental tobacco smoke (Z57.31)
> tobacco dependence (F17.-)
> tobacco use (Z72.0)

C11.0 **Malignant neoplasm of superior wall of nasopharynx** Ⓗ
Part of pharynx that lies above soft palate
Malignant neoplasm of roof of nasopharynx

C11.1 **Malignant neoplasm of posterior wall of nasopharynx** Ⓗ
Malignant neoplasm of adenoid
Malignant neoplasm of pharyngeal tonsil

C11.2 **Malignant neoplasm of lateral wall of nasopharynx** Ⓗ
Malignant neoplasm of fossa of Rosenmüller
Malignant neoplasm of opening of auditory tube
Malignant neoplasm of pharyngeal recess

C11.3 **Malignant neoplasm of anterior wall of nasopharynx** Ⓗ
Malignant neoplasm of floor of nasopharynx
Malignant neoplasm of nasopharyngeal (anterior) (posterior) surface of soft palate
Malignant neoplasm of posterior margin of nasal choana
Malignant neoplasm of posterior margin of nasal septum

C11.8 **Malignant neoplasm of overlapping sites of nasopharynx** Ⓗ

C11.9 **Malignant neoplasm of nasopharynx, unspecified** Ⓗ
Malignant neoplasm of nasopharyngeal wall NOS

C12 Malignant neoplasm of pyriform sinus Ⓗ
Malignant neoplasm of pyriform fossa

> **Use additional** code to identify:
> exposure to environmental tobacco smoke (Z77.22)
> exposure to tobacco smoke in the perinatal period (P96.81)
> history of tobacco dependence (Z87.891)
> occupational exposure to environmental tobacco smoke (Z57.31)
> tobacco dependence (F17.-)
> tobacco use (Z72.0)

▶ New   ⇨ Revised   ~~deleted~~ Deleted   Excludes 1   Excludes 2   Includes   Use additional   Code first   Code also   Key words

OGCR Official Guidelines   X Assign placeholder X   ● Use Additional Character(s)   ▌ Manifestation Code   Ⓗ Hierarchical Condition Category   **Coding Clinic**

● **C13**   Malignant neoplasm of **hypopharynx**

> Use additional code to identify:
> exposure to environmental tobacco smoke (Z77.22)
> exposure to tobacco smoke in the perinatal period (P96.81)
> history of tobacco dependence (Z87.891)
> occupational exposure to environmental tobacco smoke (Z57.31)
> tobacco dependence (F17.-)
> tobacco use (Z72.0)
>
> **Excludes2**   malignant neoplasm of pyriform sinus (C12)

C13.0   Malignant neoplasm of **postcricoid region** 🅗
> *Behind the cricoid cartilage of neck*

C13.1   Malignant neoplasm of **aryepiglottic fold, hypopharyngeal aspect** 🅗
> *Arytenoepiglottic fold, triangular opening between side of epiglottis and apex of arytenoid cartilage*
> Malignant neoplasm of aryepiglottic fold, marginal zone
> Malignant neoplasm of aryepiglottic fold NOS
> Malignant neoplasm of interarytenoid fold, marginal zone
> Malignant neoplasm of interarytenoid fold NOS
>
> **Excludes2**   malignant neoplasm of aryepiglottic fold or interarytenoid fold, laryngeal aspect (C32.1)

C13.2   Malignant neoplasm of **posterior wall of hypopharynx** 🅗

C13.8   Malignant neoplasm of **overlapping sites of hypopharynx** 🅗

C13.9   Malignant neoplasm of **hypopharynx, unspecified** 🅗
> Malignant neoplasm of hypopharyngeal wall NOS

● **C14**   Malignant neoplasm of **other and ill-defined sites in the lip, oral cavity and pharynx**

> Use additional code to identify:
> alcohol abuse and dependence (F10.-)
> exposure to environmental tobacco smoke (Z77.22)
> exposure to tobacco smoke in the perinatal period (P96.81)
> history of tobacco dependence (Z87.891)
> occupational exposure to environmental tobacco smoke (Z57.31)
> tobacco dependence (F17.-)
> tobacco use (Z72.0)
>
> **Excludes1**   malignant neoplasm of oral cavity NOS (C06.9)

C14.0   Malignant neoplasm of **pharynx, unspecified** 🅗

C14.2   Malignant neoplasm of **Waldeyer's ring** 🅗

C14.8   Malignant neoplasm of **overlapping sites of lip, oral cavity and pharynx** 🅗
> Primary malignant neoplasm of two or more contiguous sites of lip, oral cavity and pharynx
>
> **Excludes1**   'book leaf' neoplasm [ventral surface of tongue and floor of mouth] (C06.89)

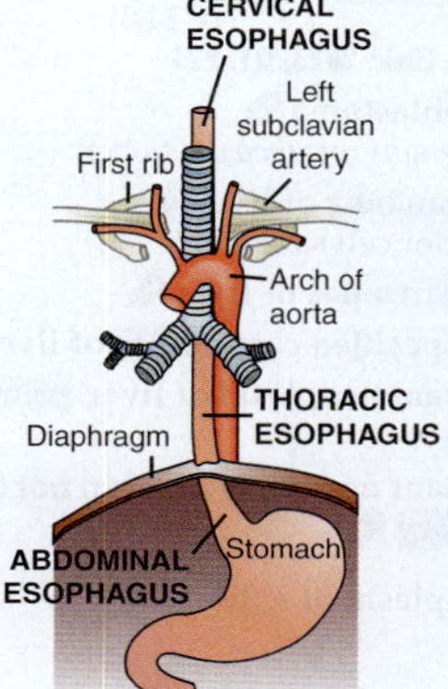

Figure 2-3   The esophagus is the muscular tube that connects the pharynx and the stomach. The 10 inch (25 cm) long esophagus is divided into three parts: **cervical, thoracic,** and **abdominal.**

MALIGNANT NEOPLASM OF DIGESTIVE ORGANS (C15-C26)

> **Excludes1**   Kaposi's sarcoma of gastrointestinal sites (C46.4)
>
> **Excludes2**   gastrointestinal stromal tumors (C49.A-)

● **C15**   Malignant neoplasms of **esophagus**

> Use additional code to identify:
> alcohol abuse and dependence (F10.-)

C15.3   Malignant neoplasm of **upper third of esophagus** 🅗

C15.4   Malignant neoplasm of **middle third of esophagus** 🅗

C15.5   Malignant neoplasm of **lower third of esophagus** 🅗
> **Excludes1**   malignant neoplasm of cardio-esophageal junction (C16.0)
>
> **Coding Clinic: 2022, Q3, P10**

C15.8   Malignant neoplasm of **overlapping sites of esophagus** 🅗

C15.9   Malignant neoplasm of **esophagus, unspecified** 🅗

● **C16**   Malignant neoplasm of **stomach**

> Use additional code to identify:
> alcohol abuse and dependence (F10.-)
>
> **Excludes2**   malignant carcinoid tumor of the stomach (C7A.092)

C16.0   Malignant neoplasm of **cardia** 🅗
> Malignant neoplasm of cardiac orifice
> Malignant neoplasm of cardio-esophageal junction
> Malignant neoplasm of esophagus and stomach
> Malignant neoplasm of gastro-esophageal junction

C16.1   Malignant neoplasm of **fundus of stomach** 🅗

C16.2   Malignant neoplasm of **body of stomach** 🅗

C16.3   Malignant neoplasm of **pyloric antrum** 🅗
> Malignant neoplasm of gastric antrum

C16.4   Malignant neoplasm of **pylorus** 🅗
> Malignant neoplasm of prepylorus
> Malignant neoplasm of pyloric canal

C16.5   Malignant neoplasm of **lesser curvature of stomach, unspecified** 🅗
> Malignant neoplasm of lesser curvature of stomach, not classifiable to C16.1-C16.4

C16.6   Malignant neoplasm of **greater curvature of stomach, unspecified** 🅗
> Malignant neoplasm of greater curvature of stomach, not classifiable to C16.0-C16.4

C16.8   Malignant neoplasm of **overlapping sites of stomach** 🅗

C16.9   Malignant neoplasm of **stomach, unspecified** 🅗
> Gastric cancer NOS

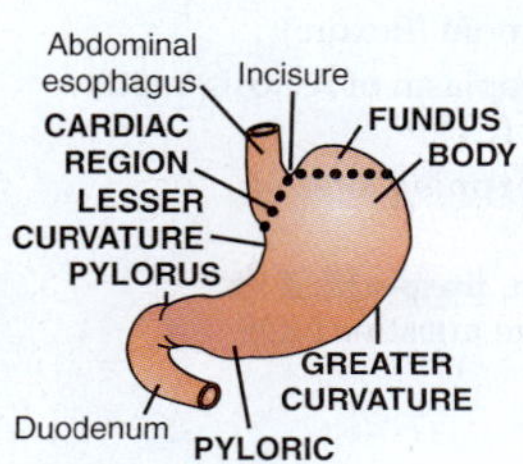

Figure 2-4   Parts of the stomach.

Item 2-2   The esophagus opens into the stomach through the **cardiac orifice,** also called the **cardioesophageal junction.** The **cardia** is adjacent to the cardiac orifice. The stomach widens into the **greater** and **lesser curvatures.** The **pyloric antrum** precedes the **pylorus,** which opens to the duodenum.

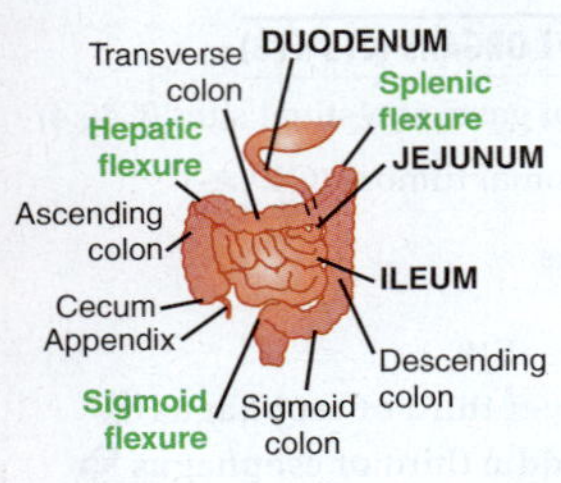

Figure 2-5 Small intestine and colon.

● **C17 Malignant neoplasm of small intestine**
   Excludes1 malignant carcinoid tumor of the small intestine (C7A.01)

   C17.0 Malignant neoplasm of duodenum 🅡
   First or proximal portion of small intestine, extending from pylorus to jejunum

   C17.1 Malignant neoplasm of jejunum 🅡
   Second section of small intestine, extending from duodenum to ileum

   C17.2 Malignant neoplasm of ileum 🅡
   Distal and longest portion of small intestine, extending from jejunum to cecum
      Excludes1 malignant neoplasm of ileocecal valve (C18.0)

   C17.3 Meckel's diverticulum, malignant 🅡
   Appendage of ileum
      Excludes1 Meckel's diverticulum, congenital (Q43.0)

   C17.8 Malignant neoplasm of overlapping sites of small intestine 🅡

   C17.9 Malignant neoplasm of small intestine, unspecified 🅡

● **C18 Malignant neoplasm of colon**
   Excludes1 malignant carcinoid tumors of the colon (C7A.02)

   C18.0 Malignant neoplasm of cecum 🅡
   First section of large intestine
   Malignant neoplasm of ileocecal valve

   C18.1 Malignant neoplasm of appendix 🅡
   Blind ended tube connected to the cecum; AKA vermiform appendix

   C18.2 Malignant neoplasm of ascending colon 🅡
   Ascending colon is between cecum and right colic flexure

   C18.3 Malignant neoplasm of hepatic flexure 🅡
   A flexure is a bending in a structure or organ. Note the three flexures illustrated in Figure 2–5.

   C18.4 Malignant neoplasm of transverse colon 🅡
   Portion of colon that runs transversely across upper part of abdomen, between right and left colic flexures

   C18.5 Malignant neoplasm of splenic flexure 🅡
   Bend at junction of transverse and descending colon

   C18.6 Malignant neoplasm of descending colon 🅡
   Portion between left colic flexure and sigmoid colon at pelvic brim; AKA iliac colon

   C18.7 Malignant neoplasm of sigmoid colon 🅡
   S-shaped part of colon extending from pelvic brim to third segment of sacrum
   Malignant neoplasm of sigmoid (flexure)
      Excludes1 malignant neoplasm of rectosigmoid junction (C19)

   C18.8 Malignant neoplasm of overlapping sites of colon 🅡

   C18.9 Malignant neoplasm of colon, unspecified 🅡
   Malignant neoplasm of large intestine NOS

● **C19 Malignant neoplasm of rectosigmoid junction** 🅡
   Malignant neoplasm of colon with rectum
   Malignant neoplasm of rectosigmoid (colon)
      Excludes1 malignant carcinoid tumors of the colon (C7A.02-)

● **C20 Malignant neoplasm of rectum** 🅡
   Malignant neoplasm of rectal ampulla
      Excludes1 malignant carcinoid tumor of the rectum (C7A.026)

● **C21 Malignant neoplasm of anus and anal canal**
      Excludes2 malignant carcinoid tumors of the colon (C7A.02-)
      malignant melanoma of anal margin (C43.51)
      malignant melanoma of anal skin (C43.51)
      malignant melanoma of perianal skin (C43.51)
      other and unspecified malignant neoplasm of anal margin (C44.500, C44.510, C44.520, C44.590)
      other and unspecified malignant neoplasm of anal skin (C44.500, C44.510, C44.520, C44.590)
      other and unspecified malignant neoplasm of perianal skin (C44.500, C44.510, C44.520, C44.590)

   C21.0 Malignant neoplasm of anus, unspecified 🅡
   C21.1 Malignant neoplasm of anal canal 🅡
   Terminal part of large intestine
   Malignant neoplasm of anal sphincter

   C21.2 Malignant neoplasm of cloacogenic zone 🅡

   C21.8 Malignant neoplasm of overlapping sites of rectum, anus and anal canal 🅡
   Malignant neoplasm of anorectal junction
   Malignant neoplasm of anorectum
   Primary malignant neoplasm of two or more contiguous sites of rectum, anus and anal canal

● **C22 Malignant neoplasm of liver and intrahepatic bile ducts**
   Intrahepatic: Within liver
   Use additional code to identify:
      alcohol abuse and dependence (F10.-)
      hepatitis B (B16.-, B18.0-B18.1) hepatitis C (B17.1-, B18.2)
      Excludes1 malignant neoplasm of biliary tract NOS (C24.9)
      secondary malignant neoplasm of liver and intrahepatic bile duct (C78.7)

   C22.0 Liver cell carcinoma 🅡
   Hepatocellular carcinoma
   Hepatoma

   C22.1 Intrahepatic bile duct carcinoma 🅡
   Cholangiocarcinoma
   Adenocarcinoma (cancer that originates in glandular tissue) arising from epithelium of intrahepatic bile ducts
      Excludes1 malignant neoplasm of hepatic duct (C24.0)
      Coding Clinic: 2023, Q1, P24

   C22.2 Hepatoblastoma 🅡
   Malignant intrahepatic tumor

   C22.3 Angiosarcoma of liver 🅡
   Kupffer cell sarcoma

   C22.4 Other sarcomas of liver 🅡
   C22.7 Other specified carcinomas of liver 🅡
   C22.8 Malignant neoplasm of liver, primary, unspecified as to type 🅡

   C22.9 Malignant neoplasm of liver, not specified as primary or secondary 🅡

   C23 Malignant neoplasm of gallbladder 🅡

▶ New   ⇨ Revised   ~~deleted~~ Deleted   Excludes 1   Excludes 2   Includes   Use additional   Code first   Code also   Key words
OGCR Official Guidelines   X Assign placeholder X   ● Use Additional Character(s)   ▸ Manifestation Code   🅡 Hierarchical Condition Category   **Coding Clinic**

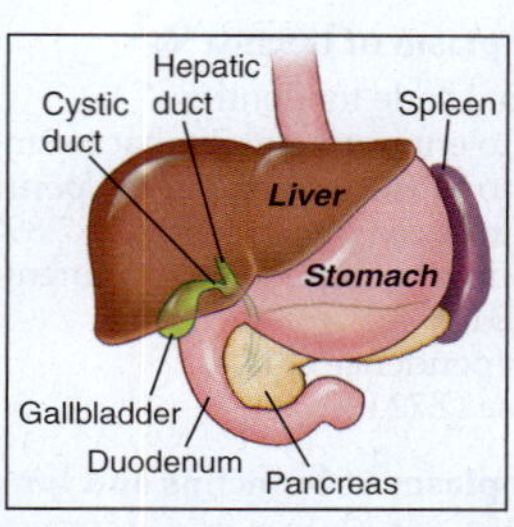

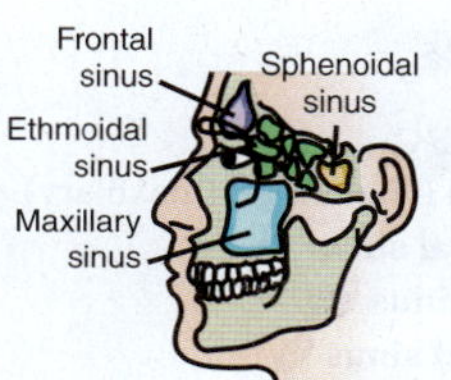

Figure 2-6 Diagram of liver, gallbladder, hepatic duct, pancreas, and spleen. (From Thibodeau and Patton: Anatomy and Physiology, ed 7, Mosby, 2010)

Figure 2-7 Paranasal sinuses. (From Buck CJ: Step-by-Step Medical Coding, ed 2016, St. Louis, Elsevier, 2016)

● **C24 Malignant neoplasm of other and unspecified parts of biliary tract**

> **Excludes1** malignant neoplasm of intrahepatic bile duct (C22.1)

C24.0 Malignant neoplasm of extrahepatic bile duct 🔁

Extrahepatic = outside the liver
Malignant neoplasm of biliary duct or passage NOS
Malignant neoplasm of common bile duct
Malignant neoplasm of cystic duct
Malignant neoplasm of hepatic duct

C24.1 Malignant neoplasm of ampulla of Vater 🔁
Union of pancreatic duct and common bile duct

C24.8 Malignant neoplasm of overlapping sites of biliary tract 🔁
Malignant neoplasm involving both intrahepatic and extrahepatic bile ducts
Primary malignant neoplasm of two or more contiguous sites of biliary tract

C24.9 Malignant neoplasm of biliary tract, unspecified 🔁

● **C25 Malignant neoplasm of pancreas**
Check documentation for specific site.

Code also if applicable exocrine pancreatic insufficiency (K86.81)

Use additional code to identify:
alcohol abuse and dependence (F10.-)

C25.0 Malignant neoplasm of head of pancreas 🔁

C25.1 Malignant neoplasm of body of pancreas 🔁
Coding Clinic: 2018, Q4, P40

C25.2 Malignant neoplasm of tail of pancreas 🔁

C25.3 Malignant neoplasm of pancreatic duct 🔁

C25.4 Malignant neoplasm of endocrine pancreas 🔁
Malignant neoplasm of islets of Langerhans
That part of the pancreas that acts as endocrine gland and consists of islets of Langerhans
Use additional code to identify any functional activity.

C25.7 Malignant neoplasm of other parts of pancreas 🔁
Malignant neoplasm of neck of pancreas

C25.8 Malignant neoplasm of overlapping sites of pancreas 🔁

C25.9 Malignant neoplasm of pancreas, unspecified 🔁

● **C26 Malignant neoplasm of other and ill-defined digestive organs**

> **Excludes1** malignant neoplasm of peritoneum and retroperitoneum (C48.-)

C26.0 Malignant neoplasm of intestinal tract, part unspecified 🔁
Malignant neoplasm of intestine NOS

C26.1 Malignant neoplasm of spleen 🔁

> **Excludes1** Hodgkin lymphoma (C81.-)
> non-Hodgkin lymphoma (C82-C85)

C26.9 Malignant neoplasm of ill-defined sites within the digestive system 🔁
Malignant neoplasm of alimentary canal or tract NOS
Malignant neoplasm of gastrointestinal tract NOS

> **Excludes1** malignant neoplasm of abdominal NOS (C76.2)
> malignant neoplasm of intra-abdominal NOS (C76.2)

MALIGNANT NEOPLASMS OF RESPIRATORY AND INTRATHORACIC ORGANS (C30-C39)

Includes malignant neoplasm of middle ear
Excludes1 mesothelioma (C45.-)

● **C30 Malignant neoplasm of nasal cavity and middle ear**

C30.0 Malignant neoplasm of nasal cavity 🔁
Malignant neoplasm of cartilage of nose
Malignant neoplasm of nasal concha
Malignant neoplasm of internal nose
Malignant neoplasm of septum of nose
Malignant neoplasm of vestibule of nose
Anterior part of nasal cavity

> **Excludes1** malignant neoplasm of nasal bone (C41.0)
> malignant neoplasm of nose NOS (C76.0)
> malignant neoplasm of olfactory bulb (C72.2-)
> malignant neoplasm of posterior margin of nasal septum and choana (C11.3)
> malignant melanoma of skin of nose (C43.31)
> malignant neoplasm of turbinates (C41.0)
> other and unspecified malignant neoplasm of skin of nose (C44.301, C44.311, C44.321, C44.391)

C30.1 Malignant neoplasm of middle ear 🔁
Malignant neoplasm of antrum tympanicum
Boney cavity or chamber
Malignant neoplasm of auditory tube
Malignant neoplasm of eustachian tube
Malignant neoplasm of inner ear
Malignant neoplasm of mastoid air cells
Malignant neoplasm of tympanic cavity

> **Excludes1** malignant neoplasm of auricular canal (external) (C43.2-, C44.2-)
> malignant neoplasm of bone of ear (meatus) (C41.0)
> malignant neoplasm of cartilage of ear (C49.0)
> malignant melanoma of skin of (external) ear (C43.2-)
> other and unspecified malignant neoplasm of skin of (external) ear (C44.2-)

Item 2–3 Islets of Langerhans (endocrine producing cells comprising 1% to 2% of the pancreatic mass) make and secrete hormones that regulate the body's production of insulin, glucagon, and stomach acid. Breakdown of the insulin-producing cells can cause diabetes mellitus. Islet cell tumors can be benign or malignant and include glucagonomas, insulinomas, gastrinomas, and neuroendocrine tumor. The neoplasm table must be consulted for the correct neoplasm code.

CHAPTER 2 (C00-D49)

● **C31 Malignant neoplasm of accessory sinuses**
    Paired sinuses in bones of face

   C31.0 Malignant neoplasm of maxillary sinus 🅡
        Malignant neoplasm of antrum (Highmore) (maxillary)

   C31.1 Malignant neoplasm of ethmoidal sinus 🅡

   C31.2 Malignant neoplasm of frontal sinus 🅡

   C31.3 Malignant neoplasm of sphenoid sinus 🅡

   C31.8 Malignant neoplasm of overlapping sites of accessory sinuses 🅡

   C31.9 Malignant neoplasm of accessory sinus, unspecified 🅡

● **C32 Malignant neoplasm of larynx**
    Use additional code to identify:
        alcohol abuse and dependence (F10.-)
        exposure to environmental tobacco smoke (Z77.22)
        exposure to tobacco smoke in the perinatal period (P96.81)
        history of tobacco dependence (Z87.891)
        occupational exposure to environmental tobacco smoke
            (Z57.31)
        tobacco dependence (F17.-)
        tobacco use (Z72.0)

   C32.0 Malignant neoplasm of glottis 🅡
        Vocal apparatus of larynx, consisting of true vocal cords (plicae vocales) and opening between them (rima glottidis)
        Malignant neoplasm of intrinsic larynx
        Malignant neoplasm of laryngeal commissure (anterior) (posterior)
        Malignant neoplasm of vocal cord (true) NOS
            True vocal cords ("lower vocal folds") produce vocalization when air from the lungs passes between them. Check your documentation. Code C32.1 is for malignant neoplasm of the false vocal cords.

   C32.1 Malignant neoplasm of supraglottis 🅡
        Area of pharynx above glottis
        Malignant neoplasm of aryepiglottic fold or interarytenoid fold, laryngeal aspect
        Malignant neoplasm of epiglottis (suprahyoid portion) NOS
        Malignant neoplasm of extrinsic larynx
        Malignant neoplasm of false vocal cord
            False vocal cords ("upper vocal folds") are not involved in vocalization. Check your documentation. Code C32.0 is for true vocal cords.
        Malignant neoplasm of posterior (laryngeal) surface of epiglottis
        Malignant neoplasm of ventricular bands

        Excludes2 malignant neoplasm of anterior surface of epiglottis (C10.1)
                    malignant neoplasm of aryepiglottic fold or interarytenoid fold, hypopharyngeal aspect (C13.1)
                    malignant neoplasm of aryepiglottic fold or interarytenoid fold, marginal zone (C13.1)
                    malignant neoplasm of aryepiglottic fold or interarytenoid fold NOS (C13.1)

   C32.2 Malignant neoplasm of subglottis 🅡
        Lowest part of larynx from just below vocal cords down to top of trachea

   C32.3 Malignant neoplasm of laryngeal cartilage 🅡
        Cartilages of larynx, including cricoid, thyroid, and epiglottic, and two each of arytenoid, corniculate, and cuneiform

   C32.8 Malignant neoplasm of overlapping sites of larynx 🅡

   C32.9 Malignant neoplasm of larynx, unspecified 🅡

● **C33 Malignant neoplasm of trachea** 🅡
    Use additional code to identify:
        exposure to environmental tobacco smoke (Z77.22)
        exposure to tobacco smoke in the perinatal period (P96.81)
        history of tobacco dependence (Z87.891)
        occupational exposure to environmental tobacco smoke
            (Z57.31)
        tobacco dependence (F17.-)
        tobacco use (Z72.0)

● **C34 Malignant neoplasm of bronchus and lung**
    Use additional code to identify:
        exposure to environmental tobacco smoke (Z77.22)
        exposure to tobacco smoke in the perinatal period (P96.81)
        history of tobacco dependence (Z87.891)
        occupational exposure to environmental tobacco smoke
            (Z57.31)
        tobacco dependence (F17.-)
        tobacco use (Z72.0)

        Excludes1 Kaposi's sarcoma of lung (C46.5-)
                    malignant carcinoid tumor of the bronchus and lung (C7A.090)
        Coding Clinic: 2023, Q1, P20

   ● **C34.0 Malignant neoplasm of main bronchus**
        Malignant neoplasm of carina
            Ridgelike structure
        Malignant neoplasm of hilus (of lung)
            Anatomic depression or pit

        C34.00 Malignant neoplasm of unspecified main bronchus 🅡

        C34.01 Malignant neoplasm of right main bronchus 🅡

        C34.02 Malignant neoplasm of left main bronchus 🅡

   ● **C34.1 Malignant neoplasm of upper lobe, bronchus or lung**

        C34.10 Malignant neoplasm of unspecified bronchus or lung 🅡

        C34.11 Malignant neoplasm of upper lobe, right bronchus or lung 🅡

        C34.12 Malignant neoplasm of upper lobe, left bronchus or lung 🅡

   C34.2 Malignant neoplasm of middle lobe, bronchus or lung 🅡

   ● **C34.3 Malignant neoplasm of lower lobe, bronchus or lung**

        C34.30 Malignant neoplasm of lower lobe, unspecified bronchus or lung 🅡

        C34.31 Malignant neoplasm of lower lobe, right bronchus or lung 🅡

        C34.32 Malignant neoplasm of lower lobe, left bronchus or lung 🅡

   ● **C34.8 Malignant neoplasm of overlapping sites of bronchus and lung**

        C34.80 Malignant neoplasm of overlapping sites of unspecified bronchus and lung 🅡

        C34.81 Malignant neoplasm of overlapping sites of right bronchus and lung 🅡

        C34.82 Malignant neoplasm of overlapping sites of left bronchus and lung 🅡

   ● **C34.9 Malignant neoplasm of unspecified part of bronchus or lung**

        C34.90 Malignant neoplasm of unspecified part of unspecified bronchus or lung 🅡
            Lung cancer NOS
            Coding Clinic: 2022, Q4, P23

        C34.91 Malignant neoplasm of unspecified part of right bronchus or lung 🅡

        C34.92 Malignant neoplasm of unspecified part of left bronchus or lung 🅡

   C37 Malignant neoplasm of thymus 🅡

        Excludes1 malignant carcinoid tumor of the thymus (C7A.091)

▶ New   ➡ Revised   ~~deleted~~ Deleted   Excludes 1   Excludes 2   Includes   Use additional   Code first   Code also   Key words

OGCR Official Guidelines   **X** Assign placeholder X   ● Use Additional Character(s)   🅛 Manifestation Code   🅡 Hierarchical Condition Category   **Coding Clinic**

● **C38 Malignant neoplasm of heart, mediastinum and pleura**

> **Excludes1** mesothelioma (C45.-)

C38.0 Malignant neoplasm of heart 🅡🅒🅒
Malignant neoplasm of pericardium

> **Excludes1** malignant neoplasm of great vessels (C49.3)

C38.1 Malignant neoplasm of anterior mediastinum 🅡🅒🅒

C38.2 Malignant neoplasm of posterior mediastinum 🅡🅒🅒

C38.3 Malignant neoplasm of mediastinum, part unspecified 🅡🅒🅒

C38.4 Malignant neoplasm of pleura 🅡🅒🅒

C38.8 Malignant neoplasm of overlapping sites of heart, mediastinum and pleura 🅡🅒🅒
Pleura are comprised of serous membrane that lines the thoracic cavity (parietal) and covers the lungs (visceral).

● **C39 Malignant neoplasm of other and ill-defined sites in the respiratory system and intrathoracic organs**
Intrathoracic: within thorax/chest

Use additional code to identify:
exposure to environmental tobacco smoke (Z77.22)
exposure to tobacco smoke in the perinatal period (P96.81)
history of tobacco dependence (Z87.891)
occupational exposure to environmental tobacco smoke (Z57.31)
tobacco dependence (F17.-)
tobacco use (Z72.0)

> **Excludes1** intrathoracic malignant neoplasm NOS (C76.1)
> thoracic malignant neoplasm NOS (C76.1)

C39.0 Malignant neoplasm of upper respiratory tract, part unspecified 🅡🅒🅒

C39.9 Malignant neoplasm of lower respiratory tract, part unspecified 🅡🅒🅒
Malignant neoplasm of respiratory tract NOS

MALIGNANT NEOPLASMS OF BONE AND ARTICULAR CARTILAGE (C40-C41)

> **Includes** malignant neoplasm of cartilage (articular) (joint)
> malignant neoplasm of periosteum
> **Excludes1** malignant neoplasm of bone marrow NOS (C96.9)
> malignant neoplasm of synovia (C49.-)

● **C40 Malignant neoplasm of bone and articular cartilage of limbs**
Use additional code to identify major osseous defect, if applicable (M89.7-)

● **C40.0 Malignant neoplasm of scapula and long bones of upper limb**

C40.00 Malignant neoplasm of scapula and long bones of unspecified upper limb 🅡🅒🅒

C40.01 Malignant neoplasm of scapula and long bones of right upper limb 🅡🅒🅒

C40.02 Malignant neoplasm of scapula and long bones of left upper limb 🅡🅒🅒

● **C40.1 Malignant neoplasm of short bones of upper limb**

C40.10 Malignant neoplasm of short bones of unspecified upper limb 🅡🅒🅒

C40.11 Malignant neoplasm of short bones of right upper limb 🅡🅒🅒

C40.12 Malignant neoplasm of short bones of left upper limb 🅡🅒🅒

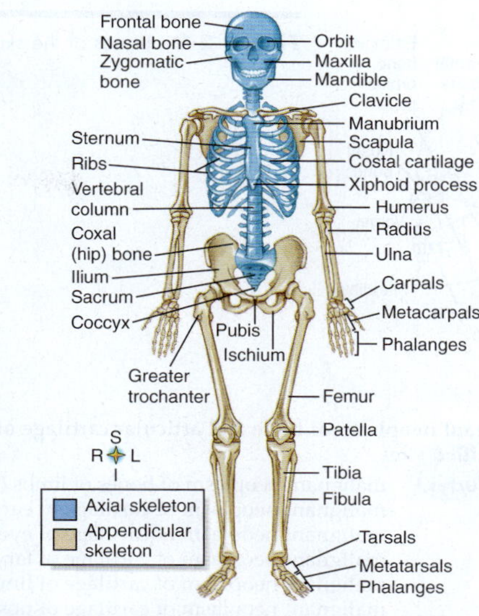

Figure 2-8 Diagram of skeleton of trunk and limbs with bones labeled. (From Thibodeau and Patton: Anatomy and Physiology, ed 7, Mosby, 2010)

● **C40.2 Malignant neoplasm of long bones of lower limb**

C40.20 Malignant neoplasm of long bones of unspecified lower limb 🅡🅒🅒

C40.21 Malignant neoplasm of long bones of right lower limb 🅡🅒🅒

C40.22 Malignant neoplasm of long bones of left lower limb 🅡🅒🅒

● **C40.3 Malignant neoplasm of short bones of lower limb**

C40.30 Malignant neoplasm of short bones of unspecified lower limb 🅡🅒🅒

C40.31 Malignant neoplasm of short bones of right lower limb 🅡🅒🅒

C40.32 Malignant neoplasm of short bones of left lower limb 🅡🅒🅒

● **C40.8 Malignant neoplasm of overlapping sites of bone and articular cartilage of limb**

C40.80 Malignant neoplasm of overlapping sites of bone and articular cartilage of unspecified limb 🅡🅒🅒

C40.81 Malignant neoplasm of overlapping sites of bone and articular cartilage of right limb 🅡🅒🅒

C40.82 Malignant neoplasm of overlapping sites of bone and articular cartilage of left limb 🅡🅒🅒

● **C40.9 Malignant neoplasm of unspecified bones and articular cartilage of limb**

C40.90 Malignant neoplasm of unspecified bones and articular cartilage of unspecified limb 🅡🅒🅒

C40.91 Malignant neoplasm of unspecified bones and articular cartilage of right limb 🅡🅒🅒

C40.92 Malignant neoplasm of unspecified bones and articular cartilage of left limb 🅡🅒🅒

N Newborn Age: 0   **P** Pediatric Age: 0–17   **M** Maternity DX: 9–64   **A** Adult Age: 15–124

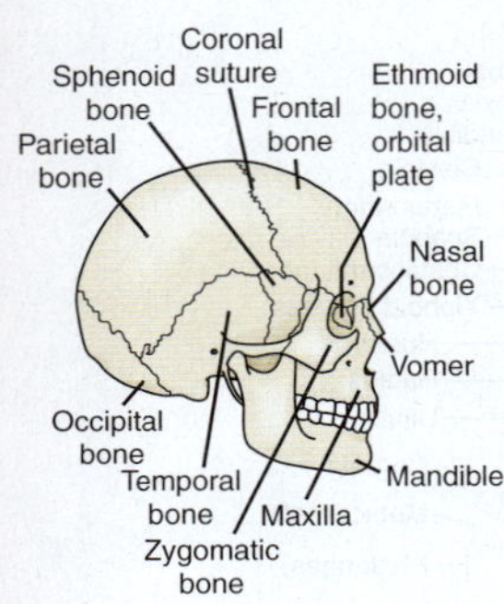

Figure 2-9   Bones of the skull.

● **C41 Malignant neoplasm of bone and articular cartilage of other and unspecified sites**

> **Excludes1**   malignant neoplasm of bones of limbs (C40.-)
> malignant neoplasm of cartilage of ear (C49.0)
> malignant neoplasm of cartilage of eyelid (C49.0)
> malignant neoplasm of cartilage of larynx (C32.3)
> malignant neoplasm of cartilage of limbs (C40.-)
> malignant neoplasm of cartilage of nose (C30.0)

C41.0 Malignant neoplasm of bones of skull and face 🅗
> Malignant neoplasm of maxilla (superior)
> Malignant neoplasm of orbital bone
>
> **Excludes2**   carcinoma, any type except intraosseous or odontogenic of:
> maxillary sinus (C31.0)
> upper jaw (C03.0)
> malignant neoplasm of jaw bone (lower) (C41.1)

C41.1 Malignant neoplasm of mandible 🅗
> Malignant neoplasm of inferior maxilla
> Malignant neoplasm of lower jaw bone
>
> **Excludes2**   carcinoma, any type except intraosseous or odontogenic of:
> jaw NOS (C03.9)
> lower (C03.1)
> malignant neoplasm of upper jaw bone (C41.0)

C41.2 Malignant neoplasm of vertebral column 🅗
> **Excludes1**   malignant neoplasm of sacrum and coccyx (C41.4)

C41.3 Malignant neoplasm of ribs, sternum and clavicle 🅗

C41.4 Malignant neoplasm of pelvic bones, sacrum and coccyx 🅗

C41.9 Malignant neoplasm of bone and articular cartilage, unspecified 🅗

MELANOMA AND OTHER MALIGNANT NEOPLASMS OF SKIN (C43-C44)

● **C43 Malignant melanoma of skin**

> **Excludes1**   melanoma in situ (D03.-)
> **Excludes2**   malignant melanoma of skin of genital organs (C51-C52, C60.-, C63.-)
> Merkel cell carcinoma (C4A.-)
> sites other than skin-code to malignant neoplasm of the site

C43.0 Malignant melanoma of lip 🅗
> **Excludes1**   malignant neoplasm of vermilion border of lip (C00.0-C00.2)

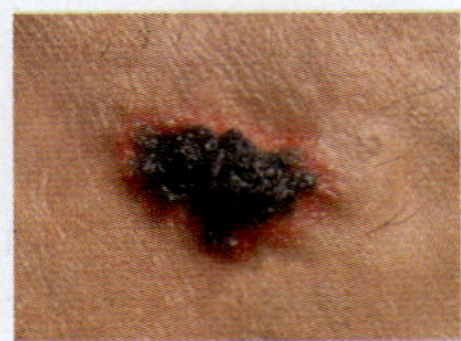

Figure 2-10   Malignant melanoma of skin. (Getty Image)

Item 2–4   Malignant melanoma is a serious form of skin cancer that affects the melanocytes (pigment-forming cells) and is caused by ultraviolet (UV) rays from the sun that damage skin. It is most commonly seen in the 40- to 60-year-olds with fair skin, blue or green eyes, and red or blond hair who sunburn easily.

Melanoma can spread very rapidly and is the most deadly form of skin cancer. It is less common than other types of skin cancer. The rate of melanoma is increasing and currently is the leading cause of death from skin disease.

● **C43.1 Malignant melanoma of eyelid, including canthus**
> *Canthus: Either corner of eye where upper and lower eyelids meet*

> **C43.10 Malignant melanoma of unspecified eyelid, including canthus** 🅗

● **C43.11 Malignant melanoma of right eyelid, including canthus** 🅗
> **C43.111 Malignant melanoma of right upper eyelid, including canthus** 🅗
> **C43.112 Malignant melanoma of right lower eyelid, including canthus** 🅗

● **C43.12 Malignant melanoma of left eyelid, including canthus** 🅗
> **C43.121 Malignant melanoma of left upper eyelid, including canthus** 🅗
> **C43.122 Malignant melanoma of left lower eyelid, including canthus** 🅗

● **C43.2 Malignant melanoma of ear and external auricular canal**
> **C43.20 Malignant melanoma of unspecified ear and external auricular canal** 🅗
> **C43.21 Malignant melanoma of right ear and external auricular canal** 🅗
> **C43.22 Malignant melanoma of left ear and external auricular canal** 🅗

● **C43.3 Malignant melanoma of other and unspecified parts of face**
> **C43.30 Malignant melanoma of unspecified part of face** 🅗
> **C43.31 Malignant melanoma of nose** 🅗
> **C43.39 Malignant melanoma of other parts of face** 🅗

C43.4 Malignant melanoma of scalp and neck 🅗

● **C43.5 Malignant melanoma of trunk**
> **Excludes2**   malignant neoplasm of anus NOS (C21.0)
> malignant neoplasm of scrotum (C63.2)

> **C43.51 Malignant melanoma of anal skin** 🅗
> Malignant melanoma of anal margin
> Malignant melanoma of perianal skin
> **C43.52 Malignant melanoma of skin of breast** 🅗
> **C43.59 Malignant melanoma of other part of trunk** 🅗

● **C43.6 Malignant melanoma of upper limb, including shoulder**
> **C43.60 Malignant melanoma of upper limb, including shoulder, unspecified side** 🅗
> **C43.61 Malignant melanoma of right upper limb, including shoulder** 🅗
> **C43.62 Malignant melanoma of left upper limb, including shoulder** 🅗

► New   ⇒ Revised   ~~deleted~~ Deleted   Excludes 1   Excludes 2   Includes   Use additional   Code first   Code also   Key words
OGCR Official Guidelines   **X** Assign placeholder X   ● Use Additional Character(s)   ▶ Manifestation Code   🅗 Hierarchical Condition Category   **Coding Clinic**

- **C43.7** Malignant melanoma of lower limb, including hip
  - **C43.70** Malignant melanoma of unspecified lower limb, including hip 🔲
  - **C43.71** Malignant melanoma of right lower limb, including hip 🔲
  - **C43.72** Malignant melanoma of left lower limb, including hip 🔲
- **C43.8** Malignant melanoma of overlapping sites of skin 🔲
- **C43.9** Malignant melanoma of skin, unspecified 🔲
  Malignant melanoma of unspecified site of skin
  Melanoma (malignant) NOS

- **C44** Other and unspecified malignant neoplasm of skin

  Includes   malignant neoplasm of sebaceous glands
  malignant neoplasm of sweat glands

  Excludes1   Kaposi's sarcoma of skin (C46.0)
  malignant melanoma of skin (C43.-)
  malignant neoplasm of skin of genital organs
      (C51-C52, C60.-, C63.2)
  Merkel cell carcinoma (C4A.-)

  - **C44.0** Other and unspecified malignant neoplasm of skin of lip

    Excludes1   malignant neoplasm of lip (C00.-)

    - **C44.00** Unspecified malignant neoplasm of skin of lip
    - **C44.01** Basal cell carcinoma of skin of lip
    - **C44.02** Squamous cell carcinoma of skin of lip
    - **C44.09** Other specified malignant neoplasm of skin of lip

  - **C44.1** Other and unspecified malignant neoplasm of skin of eyelid, including canthus

    Excludes1   connective tissue of eyelid (C49.0)

    - **C44.10** Unspecified malignant neoplasm of skin of eyelid, including canthus
      - **C44.101** Unspecified malignant neoplasm of skin of unspecified eyelid, including canthus
      - **C44.102** Unspecified malignant neoplasm of skin of right eyelid, including canthus
        - **C44.1021** Unspecified malignant neoplasm of skin of right upper eyelid, including canthus
        - **C44.1022** Unspecified malignant neoplasm of skin of right lower eyelid, including canthus
      - **C44.109** Unspecified malignant neoplasm of skin of left eyelid, including canthus
        - **C44.1091** Unspecified malignant neoplasm of skin of left upper eyelid, including canthus
        - **C44.1092** Unspecified malignant neoplasm of skin of left lower eyelid, including canthus
    - **C44.11** Basal cell carcinoma of skin of eyelid, including canthus
      - **C44.111** Basal cell carcinoma of skin of unspecified eyelid, including canthus
      - **C44.112** Basal cell carcinoma of skin of right eyelid, including canthus
        - **C44.1121** Basal cell carcinoma of skin of right upper eyelid, including canthus
        - **C44.1122** Basal cell carcinoma of skin of right lower eyelid, including canthus
      - **C44.119** Basal cell carcinoma of skin of left eyelid, including canthus
        - **C44.1191** Basal cell carcinoma of skin of left upper eyelid, including canthus
        - **C44.1192** Basal cell carcinoma of skin of left lower eyelid, including canthus
    - **C44.12** Squamous cell carcinoma of skin of eyelid, including canthus
      - **C44.121** Squamous cell carcinoma of skin of unspecified eyelid, including canthus
      - **C44.122** Squamous cell carcinoma of skin of right eyelid, including canthus
        - **C44.1221** Squamous cell carcinoma of skin of right upper eyelid, including canthus
        - **C44.1222** Squamous cell carcinoma of skin of right lower eyelid, including canthus
      - **C44.129** Squamous cell carcinoma of skin of left eyelid, including canthus
        - **C44.1291** Squamous cell carcinoma of skin of left upper eyelid, including canthus
        - **C44.1292** Squamous cell carcinoma of skin of left lower eyelid, including canthus
    - **C44.13** Sebaceous cell carcinoma of skin of eyelid, including canthus
      - **C44.131** Sebaceous cell carcinoma of skin of unspecified eyelid, including canthus
      - **C44.132** Sebaceous cell carcinoma of skin of right eyelid, including canthus
        - **C44.1321** Sebaceous cell carcinoma of skin of right upper eyelid, including canthus
        - **C44.1322** Sebaceous cell carcinoma of skin of right lower eyelid, including canthus
      - **C44.139** Sebaceous cell carcinoma of skin of left eyelid, including canthus
        - **C44.1391** Sebaceous cell carcinoma of skin of left upper eyelid, including canthus
        - **C44.1392** Sebaceous cell carcinoma of skin of left lower eyelid, including canthus
    - **C44.19** Other specified malignant neoplasm of skin of eyelid, including canthus
      - **C44.191** Other specified malignant neoplasm of skin of unspecified eyelid, including canthus
      - **C44.192** Other specified malignant neoplasm of skin of right eyelid, including canthus
        - **C44.1921** Other specified malignant neoplasm of skin of right upper eyelid, including canthus
        - **C44.1922** Other specified malignant neoplasm of skin of right lower eyelid, including canthus

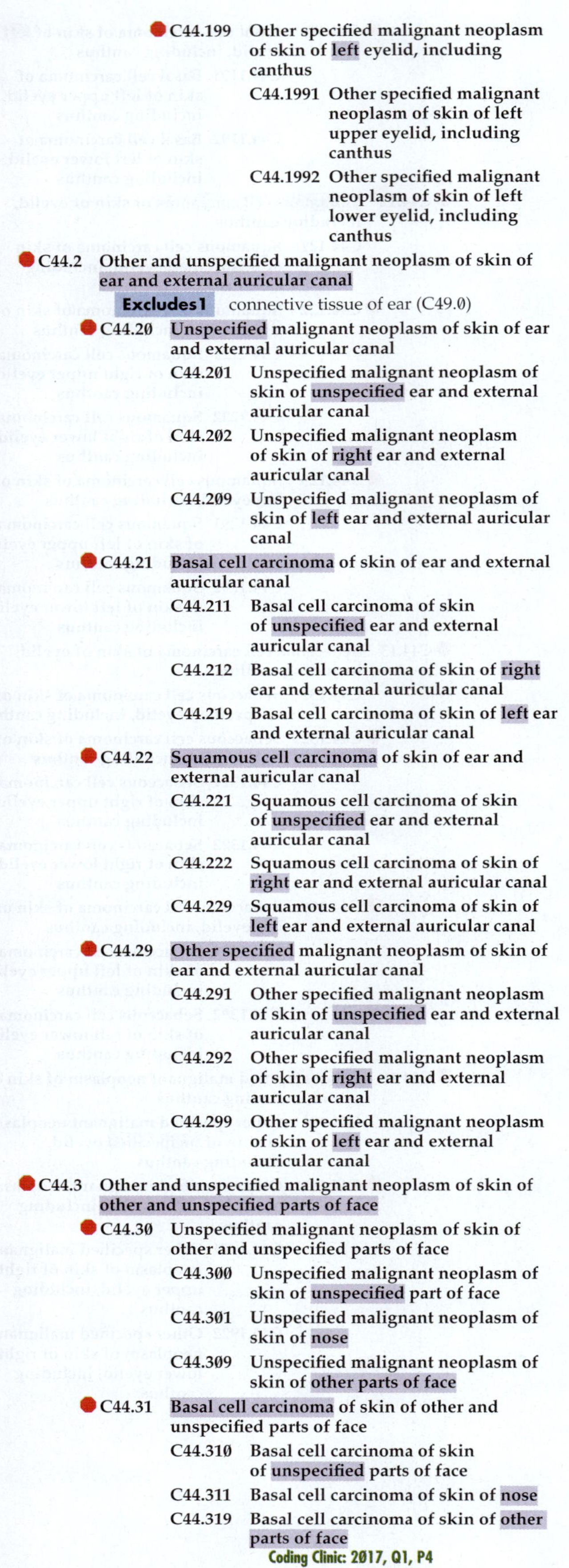

- **C44.199** Other specified malignant neoplasm of skin of left eyelid, including canthus
  - **C44.1991** Other specified malignant neoplasm of skin of left upper eyelid, including canthus
  - **C44.1992** Other specified malignant neoplasm of skin of left lower eyelid, including canthus
- **C44.2** Other and unspecified malignant neoplasm of skin of ear and external auricular canal

  Excludes1   connective tissue of ear (C49.0)
  - **C44.20** Unspecified malignant neoplasm of skin of ear and external auricular canal
    - **C44.201** Unspecified malignant neoplasm of skin of unspecified ear and external auricular canal
    - **C44.202** Unspecified malignant neoplasm of skin of right ear and external auricular canal
    - **C44.209** Unspecified malignant neoplasm of skin of left ear and external auricular canal
  - **C44.21** Basal cell carcinoma of skin of ear and external auricular canal
    - **C44.211** Basal cell carcinoma of skin of unspecified ear and external auricular canal
    - **C44.212** Basal cell carcinoma of skin of right ear and external auricular canal
    - **C44.219** Basal cell carcinoma of skin of left ear and external auricular canal
  - **C44.22** Squamous cell carcinoma of skin of ear and external auricular canal
    - **C44.221** Squamous cell carcinoma of skin of unspecified ear and external auricular canal
    - **C44.222** Squamous cell carcinoma of skin of right ear and external auricular canal
    - **C44.229** Squamous cell carcinoma of skin of left ear and external auricular canal
  - **C44.29** Other specified malignant neoplasm of skin of ear and external auricular canal
    - **C44.291** Other specified malignant neoplasm of skin of unspecified ear and external auricular canal
    - **C44.292** Other specified malignant neoplasm of skin of right ear and external auricular canal
    - **C44.299** Other specified malignant neoplasm of skin of left ear and external auricular canal
- **C44.3** Other and unspecified malignant neoplasm of skin of other and unspecified parts of face
  - **C44.30** Unspecified malignant neoplasm of skin of other and unspecified parts of face
    - **C44.300** Unspecified malignant neoplasm of skin of unspecified part of face
    - **C44.301** Unspecified malignant neoplasm of skin of nose
    - **C44.309** Unspecified malignant neoplasm of skin of other parts of face
  - **C44.31** Basal cell carcinoma of skin of other and unspecified parts of face
    - **C44.310** Basal cell carcinoma of skin of unspecified parts of face
    - **C44.311** Basal cell carcinoma of skin of nose
    - **C44.319** Basal cell carcinoma of skin of other parts of face
      Coding Clinic: 2017, Q1, P4

- **C44.32** Squamous cell carcinoma of skin of other and unspecified parts of face
  - **C44.320** Squamous cell carcinoma of skin of unspecified parts of face
  - **C44.321** Squamous cell carcinoma of skin of nose
  - **C44.329** Squamous cell carcinoma of skin of other parts of face
- **C44.39** Other specified malignant neoplasm of skin of other and unspecified parts of face
  - **C44.390** Other specified malignant neoplasm of skin of unspecified parts of face
  - **C44.391** Other specified malignant neoplasm of skin of nose
  - **C44.399** Other specified malignant neoplasm of skin of other parts of face
- **C44.4** Other and unspecified malignant neoplasm of skin of scalp and neck
  - **C44.40** Unspecified malignant neoplasm of skin of scalp and neck
  - **C44.41** Basal cell carcinoma of skin of scalp and neck
  - **C44.42** Squamous cell carcinoma of skin of scalp and neck
  - **C44.49** Other specified malignant neoplasm of skin of scalp and neck
- **C44.5** Other and unspecified malignant neoplasm of skin of trunk

  Excludes1   anus NOS (C21.0)
                 scrotum (C63.2)
  - **C44.50** Unspecified malignant neoplasm of skin of trunk
    - **C44.500** Unspecified malignant neoplasm of anal skin
Unspecified malignant neoplasm of anal margin
Unspecified malignant neoplasm of perianal skin
    - **C44.501** Unspecified malignant neoplasm of skin of breast
    - **C44.509** Unspecified malignant neoplasm of skin of other part of trunk
  - **C44.51** Basal cell carcinoma of skin of trunk
    - **C44.510** Basal cell carcinoma of anal skin
Basal cell carcinoma of anal margin
Basal cell carcinoma of perianal skin
    - **C44.511** Basal cell carcinoma of skin of breast
    - **C44.519** Basal cell carcinoma of skin of other part of trunk
  - **C44.52** Squamous cell carcinoma of skin of trunk
    - **C44.520** Squamous cell carcinoma of anal skin
Squamous cell carcinoma of anal margin
Squamous cell carcinoma of perianal skin
    - **C44.521** Squamous cell carcinoma of skin of breast
    - **C44.529** Squamous cell carcinoma of skin of other part of trunk
  - **C44.59** Other specified malignant neoplasm of skin of trunk
    - **C44.590** Other specified malignant neoplasm of anal skin
Other specified malignant neoplasm of anal margin
Other specified malignant neoplasm of perianal skin
    - **C44.591** Other specified malignant neoplasm of skin of breast
    - **C44.599** Other specified malignant neoplasm of skin of other part of trunk

▶ New   ⮕ Revised   ~~deleted~~ Deleted   Excludes 1   Excludes 2   Includes   Use additional   Code first   Code also   Key words

OGCR Official Guidelines   **X** Assign placeholder X   ● Use Additional Character(s)   ❱ Manifestation Code   Hierarchical Condition Category   **Coding Clinic**

● **C44.6**   **Other and unspecified malignant neoplasm of skin of upper limb, including shoulder**

  ● **C44.60**   **Unspecified** malignant neoplasm of skin of upper limb, including shoulder

     C44.601   Unspecified malignant neoplasm of skin of **unspecified** upper limb, including shoulder

     C44.602   Unspecified malignant neoplasm of skin of **right** upper limb, including shoulder

     C44.609   Unspecified malignant neoplasm of skin of **left** upper limb, including shoulder

  ● **C44.61**   **Basal cell carcinoma** of skin of upper limb, including shoulder

     C44.611   Basal cell carcinoma of skin of **unspecified** upper limb, including shoulder

     C44.612   Basal cell carcinoma of skin of **right** upper limb, including shoulder

     C44.619   Basal cell carcinoma of skin of **left** upper limb, including shoulder

  ● **C44.62**   **Squamous cell carcinoma** of skin of upper limb, including shoulder

     C44.621   Squamous cell carcinoma of skin of **unspecified** upper limb, including shoulder

     C44.622   Squamous cell carcinoma of skin of **right** upper limb, including shoulder

     C44.629   Squamous cell carcinoma of skin of **left** upper limb, including shoulder

  ● **C44.69**   **Other specified** malignant neoplasm of skin of upper limb, including shoulder

     C44.691   Other specified malignant neoplasm of skin of **unspecified** upper limb, including shoulder

     C44.692   Other specified malignant neoplasm of skin of **right** upper limb, including shoulder

     C44.699   Other specified malignant neoplasm of skin of **left** upper limb, including shoulder

● **C44.7**   **Other and unspecified malignant neoplasm of skin of lower limb, including hip**

  ● **C44.70**   **Unspecified** malignant neoplasm of skin of lower limb, including hip

     C44.701   Unspecified malignant neoplasm of skin of **unspecified** lower limb, including hip

     C44.702   Unspecified malignant neoplasm of skin of **right** lower limb, including hip

     C44.709   Unspecified malignant neoplasm of skin of **left** lower limb, including hip

  ● **C44.71**   **Basal cell carcinoma** of skin of lower limb, including hip

     C44.711   Basal cell carcinoma of skin of **unspecified** lower limb, including hip

     C44.712   Basal cell carcinoma of skin of **right** lower limb, including hip

     C44.719   Basal cell carcinoma of skin of **left** lower limb, including hip

  ● **C44.72**   **Squamous cell carcinoma** of skin of lower limb, including hip

     C44.721   Squamous cell carcinoma of skin of **unspecified** lower limb, including hip

     C44.722   Squamous cell carcinoma of skin of **right** lower limb, including hip

     C44.729   Squamous cell carcinoma of skin of **left** lower limb, including hip

  ● **C44.79**   **Other specified** malignant neoplasm of skin of lower limb, including hip

     C44.791   Other specified malignant neoplasm of skin of **unspecified** lower limb, including hip

     C44.792   Other specified malignant neoplasm of skin of **right** lower limb, including hip

     C44.799   Other specified malignant neoplasm of skin of **left** lower limb, including hip

● **C44.8**   **Other and unspecified malignant neoplasm of overlapping sites of skin**

     C44.80   **Unspecified** malignant neoplasm of overlapping sites of skin

     C44.81   **Basal cell carcinoma** of overlapping sites of skin

     C44.82   **Squamous cell carcinoma** of overlapping sites of skin

     C44.89   **Other** specified malignant neoplasm of overlapping sites of skin

● **C44.9**   **Other and unspecified malignant neoplasm of skin, unspecified**

     C44.90   **Unspecified** malignant neoplasm of skin, unspecified
        Malignant neoplasm of unspecified site of skin

     C44.91   **Basal cell carcinoma** of skin, unspecified

     C44.92   **Squamous cell carcinoma** of skin, unspecified

     C44.99   **Other** specified malignant neoplasm of skin, unspecified

MALIGNANT NEOPLASMS OF MESOTHELIAL AND SOFT TISSUE (C45-C49)

● **C45**   **Mesothelioma**
   Malignant cells develop in protective lining that covers internal organs (mesothelium) caused by exposure to asbestos

     C45.0   Mesothelioma of **pleura** 🔵
       Excludes1   other malignant neoplasm of pleura (C38.4)
       Coding Clinic: 2017, Q2, P11

     C45.1   Mesothelioma of **peritoneum** 🔵
       Mesothelioma of cul-de-sac
       Mesothelioma of mesentery
       Mesothelioma of mesocolon
       Mesothelioma of omentum
       Mesothelioma of peritoneum (parietal) (pelvic)
       Excludes1   other malignant neoplasm of soft tissue of peritoneum (C48.-)

     C45.2   Mesothelioma of **pericardium** 🔵
       Excludes1   other malignant neoplasm of pericardium (C38.0)

     C45.7   Mesothelioma of **other sites** 🔵

     C45.9   Mesothelioma, **unspecified** 🔵

● **C46**   **Kaposi's sarcoma**
   Code first any human immunodeficiency virus [HIV] disease (B20)

     C46.0   Kaposi's sarcoma of **skin** 🔵

     C46.1   Kaposi's sarcoma of **soft tissue** 🔵
       Kaposi's sarcoma of blood vessel
       Kaposi's sarcoma of connective tissue
       Kaposi's sarcoma of fascia
       Kaposi's sarcoma of ligament
       Kaposi's sarcoma of lymphatic(s) NEC
       Kaposi's sarcoma of muscle
       Excludes2   Kaposi's sarcoma of lymph glands and nodes (C46.3)

     C46.2   Kaposi's sarcoma of **palate** 🔵

     C46.3   Kaposi's sarcoma of **lymph nodes** 🔵

     C46.4   Kaposi's sarcoma of **gastrointestinal sites** 🔵

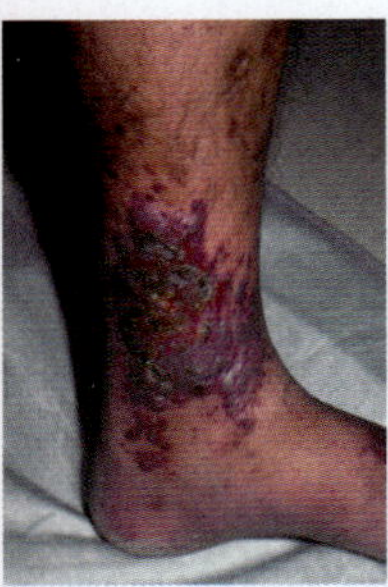

Figure 2-11 Kaposi's sarcoma. There are large confluent hyperpigmented patch-stage lesions with lymphedema. (From Goldman L, Ausiello D, Arend W, Armitage J, Clemmons D, Drazen J, Griggs R, et al: Cecil Medicine: Expert Consult, 23e, Saunders, 2007)

Item 2–5 Kaposi's sarcoma is a cancer that causes patches of abnormal tissue to grow under the skin; in the lining of the mouth, nose, and throat; or in other organs, often beginning and spreading to other organs. Patients who have had organ transplants or patients with AIDS are at high risk for this malignancy.

● **C46.5 Kaposi's sarcoma of lung**
    C46.50 Kaposi's sarcoma of unspecified lung
    C46.51 Kaposi's sarcoma of right lung
    C46.52 Kaposi's sarcoma of left lung
  C46.7 Kaposi's sarcoma of other sites
  C46.9 Kaposi's sarcoma, unspecified
    Kaposi's sarcoma of unspecified site

● **C47 Malignant neoplasm of peripheral nerves and autonomic nervous system**
  Includes malignant neoplasm of sympathetic and parasympathetic nerves and ganglia
  Excludes1 Kaposi's sarcoma of soft tissue (C46.1)

  C47.0 Malignant neoplasm of peripheral nerves of head, face and neck
    Excludes1 malignant neoplasm of peripheral nerves of orbit (C69.6-)

● **C47.1 Malignant neoplasm of peripheral nerves of upper limb, including shoulder**
    C47.10 Malignant neoplasm of peripheral nerves of unspecified upper limb, including shoulder
    C47.11 Malignant neoplasm of peripheral nerves of right upper limb, including shoulder
    C47.12 Malignant neoplasm of peripheral nerves of left upper limb, including shoulder

● **C47.2 Malignant neoplasm of peripheral nerves of lower limb, including hip**
    C47.20 Malignant neoplasm of peripheral nerves of unspecified lower limb, including hip
    C47.21 Malignant neoplasm of peripheral nerves of right lower limb, including hip
    C47.22 Malignant neoplasm of peripheral nerves of left lower limb, including hip

  C47.3 Malignant neoplasm of peripheral nerves of thorax
  C47.4 Malignant neoplasm of peripheral nerves of abdomen
  C47.5 Malignant neoplasm of peripheral nerves of pelvis
  C47.6 Malignant neoplasm of peripheral nerves of trunk, unspecified
    Malignant neoplasm of peripheral nerves of unspecified part of trunk
  C47.8 Malignant neoplasm of overlapping sites of peripheral nerves and autonomic nervous system
  C47.9 Malignant neoplasm of peripheral nerves and autonomic nervous system, unspecified
    Malignant neoplasm of unspecified site of peripheral nerves and autonomic nervous system

● **C48 Malignant neoplasm of retroperitoneum and peritoneum**
  Excludes1 Kaposi's sarcoma of connective tissue (C46.1)
    mesothelioma (C45.-)

  C48.0 Malignant neoplasm of retroperitoneum
    Behind/outside of peritoneum
  C48.1 Malignant neoplasm of specified parts of peritoneum
    Serous membrane lining abdominopelvic walls and covering viscera
    Malignant neoplasm of cul-de-sac
    Malignant neoplasm of mesentery
    Malignant neoplasm of mesocolon
    Malignant neoplasm of omentum
    Malignant neoplasm of parietal peritoneum
    Malignant neoplasm of pelvic peritoneum
  C48.2 Malignant neoplasm of peritoneum, unspecified
  C48.8 Malignant neoplasm of overlapping sites of retroperitoneum and peritoneum

● **C49 Malignant neoplasm of other connective and soft tissue**
  Includes malignant neoplasm of blood vessel
    malignant neoplasm of bursa
    malignant neoplasm of cartilage
    malignant neoplasm of fascia
    malignant neoplasm of fat
    malignant neoplasm of ligament, except uterine
    malignant neoplasm of lymphatic vessel
    malignant neoplasm of muscle
    malignant neoplasm of synovia
    malignant neoplasm of tendon (sheath)
  Excludes1 malignant neoplasm of cartilage (of):
    articular (C40-C41)
    larynx (C32.3)
    nose (C30.0)
    malignant neoplasm of connective tissue of breast (C50.-)
  Excludes2 Kaposi's sarcoma of soft tissue (C46.1)
    malignant neoplasm of heart (C38.0)
    malignant neoplasm of peripheral nerves and autonomic nervous system (C47.-)
    malignant neoplasm of peritoneum (C48.2)
    malignant neoplasm of retroperitoneum (C48.0)
    malignant neoplasm of uterine ligament (C57.3)
    mesothelioma (C45.-)

  C49.0 Malignant neoplasm of connective and soft tissue of head, face and neck
    Malignant neoplasm of connective tissue of ear
    Malignant neoplasm of connective tissue of eyelid
    Excludes1 connective tissue of orbit (C69.6-)

● **C49.1 Malignant neoplasm of connective and soft tissue of upper limb, including shoulder**
    C49.10 Malignant neoplasm of connective and soft tissue of unspecified upper limb, including shoulder
    C49.11 Malignant neoplasm of connective and soft tissue of right upper limb, including shoulder
    C49.12 Malignant neoplasm of connective and soft tissue of left upper limb, including shoulder

● **C49.2 Malignant neoplasm of connective and soft tissue of lower limb, including hip**
    C49.20 Malignant neoplasm of connective and soft tissue of unspecified lower limb, including hip
    C49.21 Malignant neoplasm of connective and soft tissue of right lower limb, including hip
    C49.22 Malignant neoplasm of connective and soft tissue of left lower limb, including hip

C49.3 Malignant neoplasm of connective and soft tissue of thorax 🔖
    Malignant neoplasm of axilla
    Malignant neoplasm of diaphragm
    Malignant neoplasm of great vessels
    Excludes1   malignant neoplasm of breast (C50.-)
                malignant neoplasm of heart (C38.0)
                malignant neoplasm of mediastinum
                    (C38.1-C38.3)
                malignant neoplasm of thymus (C37)
    Coding Clinic: 2015, Q3, P19

C49.4 Malignant neoplasm of connective and soft tissue of abdomen 🔖
    Malignant neoplasm of abdominal wall
    Malignant neoplasm of hypochondrium
    Coding Clinic: 2019, Q4, P44

C49.5 Malignant neoplasm of connective and soft tissue of pelvis 🔖
    Malignant neoplasm of buttock
    Malignant neoplasm of groin
    Malignant neoplasm of perineum

C49.6 Malignant neoplasm of connective and soft tissue of trunk, unspecified 🔖
    Malignant neoplasm of back NOS

C49.8 Malignant neoplasm of overlapping sites of connective and soft tissue 🔖
    Primary malignant neoplasm of two or more contiguous sites of connective and soft tissue

C49.9 Malignant neoplasm of connective and soft tissue, unspecified 🔖

● **C49.A Gastrointestinal stromal tumor**
    Coding Clinic: 2016, Q4, P8
    C49.A0 Gastrointestinal stromal tumor, unspecified site 🔖
    C49.A1 Gastrointestinal stromal tumor of esophagus 🔖
    C49.A2 Gastrointestinal stromal tumor of stomach 🔖
    C49.A3 Gastrointestinal stromal tumor of small intestine 🔖
    C49.A4 Gastrointestinal stromal tumor of large intestine 🔖
    C49.A5 Gastrointestinal stromal tumor of rectum 🔖
    C49.A9 Gastrointestinal stromal tumor of other sites 🔖

● **C4A Merkel cell carcinoma**
    C4A.0 Merkel cell carcinoma of lip 🔖
        Excludes1   malignant neoplasm of vermilion border of lip (C00.0-C00.2)

● **C4A.1 Merkel cell carcinoma of eyelid, including canthus**
    C4A.10 Merkel cell carcinoma of unspecified eyelid, including canthus 🔖
    ● **C4A.11 Merkel cell carcinoma of right eyelid, including canthus** 🔖
        C4A.111 Merkel cell carcinoma of right upper eyelid, including canthus 🔖
        C4A.112 Merkel cell carcinoma of right lower eyelid, including canthus 🔖
    ● **C4A.12 Merkel cell carcinoma of left eyelid, including canthus** 🔖
        C4A.121 Merkel cell carcinoma of left upper eyelid, including canthus 🔖
        C4A.122 Merkel cell carcinoma of left lower eyelid, including canthus 🔖

● **C4A.2 Merkel cell carcinoma of ear and external auricular canal**
    C4A.20 Merkel cell carcinoma of unspecified ear and external auricular canal 🔖
    C4A.21 Merkel cell carcinoma of right ear and external auricular canal 🔖
    C4A.22 Merkel cell carcinoma of left ear and external auricular canal 🔖

● **C4A.3 Merkel cell carcinoma of other and unspecified parts of face**
    C4A.30 Merkel cell carcinoma of unspecified part of face 🔖
    C4A.31 Merkel cell carcinoma of nose 🔖
    C4A.39 Merkel cell carcinoma of other parts of face 🔖

C4A.4 Merkel cell carcinoma of scalp and neck 🔖

● **C4A.5 Merkel cell carcinoma of trunk**
    Excludes2   malignant neoplasm of anus NOS (C21.0)
                malignant neoplasm of scrotum (C63.2)
    C4A.51 Merkel cell carcinoma of anal skin 🔖
        Merkel cell carcinoma of anal margin
        Merkel cell carcinoma of perianal skin
    C4A.52 Merkel cell carcinoma of skin of breast 🔖
    C4A.59 Merkel cell carcinoma of other part of trunk 🔖

● **C4A.6 Merkel cell carcinoma of upper limb, including shoulder**
    C4A.60 Merkel cell carcinoma of unspecified upper limb, including shoulder 🔖
    C4A.61 Merkel cell carcinoma of right upper limb, including shoulder 🔖
    C4A.62 Merkel cell carcinoma of left upper limb, including shoulder 🔖

● **C4A.7 Merkel cell carcinoma of lower limb, including hip**
    C4A.70 Merkel cell carcinoma of unspecified lower limb, including hip 🔖
    C4A.71 Merkel cell carcinoma of right lower limb, including hip 🔖
    C4A.72 Merkel cell carcinoma of left lower limb, including hip 🔖

C4A.8 Merkel cell carcinoma of overlapping sites 🔖

C4A.9 Merkel cell carcinoma, unspecified 🔖
    Merkel cell carcinoma of unspecified site
    Merkel cell carcinoma NOS

MALIGNANT NEOPLASMS OF BREAST (C50)

● **C50 Malignant neoplasm of breast**
    Includes   connective tissue of breast
             Paget's disease of breast
             Paget's disease of nipple
             Intraductal carcinoma of breast characterized by eczema-like inflammatory skin changes
    Use additional code to identify estrogen, and other hormones and factors receptor status (Z17.0, Z17.1)
    Excludes1   skin of breast (C44.501, C44.511, C44.521, C44.591)

● **C50.0 Malignant neoplasm of nipple and areola**
    ● **C50.01 Malignant neoplasm of nipple and areola, female**
        C50.011 Malignant neoplasm of nipple and areola, right female breast 🔖
        C50.012 Malignant neoplasm of nipple and areola, left female breast 🔖
        C50.019 Malignant neoplasm of nipple and areola, unspecified female breast 🔖

● **C50.02** Malignant neoplasm of nipple and areola, male
  C50.021 Malignant neoplasm of nipple and areola, right male breast ᴿᶜᶜ
  C50.022 Malignant neoplasm of nipple and areola, left male breast ᴿᶜᶜ
  C50.029 Malignant neoplasm of nipple and areola, unspecified male breast ᴿᶜᶜ

● **C50.1** Malignant neoplasm of central portion of breast
 ● **C50.11** Malignant neoplasm of central portion of breast, female
  C50.111 Malignant neoplasm of central portion of right female breast ᴿᶜᶜ
  C50.112 Malignant neoplasm of central portion of left female breast ᴿᶜᶜ
  C50.119 Malignant neoplasm of central portion of unspecified female breast ᴿᶜᶜ
 ● **C50.12** Malignant neoplasm of central portion of breast, male
  C50.121 Malignant neoplasm of central portion of right male breast ᴿᶜᶜ
  C50.122 Malignant neoplasm of central portion of left male breast ᴿᶜᶜ
  C50.129 Malignant neoplasm of central portion of unspecified male breast ᴿᶜᶜ

● **C50.2** Malignant neoplasm of upper-inner quadrant of breast
 ● **C50.21** Malignant neoplasm of upper-inner quadrant of breast, female
  C50.211 Malignant neoplasm of upper-inner quadrant of right female breast ᴿᶜᶜ
  C50.212 Malignant neoplasm of upper-inner quadrant of left female breast ᴿᶜᶜ
  C50.219 Malignant neoplasm of upper-inner quadrant of unspecified female breast ᴿᶜᶜ
 ● **C50.22** Malignant neoplasm of upper-inner quadrant of breast, male
  C50.221 Malignant neoplasm of upper-inner quadrant of right male breast ᴿᶜᶜ
  C50.222 Malignant neoplasm of upper-inner quadrant of left male breast ᴿᶜᶜ
  C50.229 Malignant neoplasm of upper-inner quadrant of unspecified male breast ᴿᶜᶜ

● **C50.3** Malignant neoplasm of lower-inner quadrant of breast
 ● **C50.31** Malignant neoplasm of lower-inner quadrant of breast, female
  C50.311 Malignant neoplasm of lower-inner quadrant of right female breast ᴿᶜᶜ
  C50.312 Malignant neoplasm of lower-inner quadrant of left female breast ᴿᶜᶜ
  C50.319 Malignant neoplasm of lower-inner quadrant of unspecified female breast ᴿᶜᶜ

● **C50.32** Malignant neoplasm of lower-inner quadrant of breast, male
  C50.321 Malignant neoplasm of lower-inner quadrant of right male breast ᴿᶜᶜ
  C50.322 Malignant neoplasm of lower-inner quadrant of left male breast ᴿᶜᶜ
  C50.329 Malignant neoplasm of lower-inner quadrant of unspecified male breast ᴿᶜᶜ

● **C50.4** Malignant neoplasm of upper-outer quadrant of breast
 ● **C50.41** Malignant neoplasm of upper-outer quadrant of breast, female
  C50.411 Malignant neoplasm of upper-outer quadrant of right female breast ᴿᶜᶜ
  C50.412 Malignant neoplasm of upper-outer quadrant of left female breast ᴿᶜᶜ
  C50.419 Malignant neoplasm of upper-outer quadrant of unspecified female breast ᴿᶜᶜ
 ● **C50.42** Malignant neoplasm of upper-outer quadrant of breast, male
  C50.421 Malignant neoplasm of upper-outer quadrant of right male breast ᴿᶜᶜ
  C50.422 Malignant neoplasm of upper-outer quadrant of left male breast ᴿᶜᶜ
  C50.429 Malignant neoplasm of upper-outer quadrant of unspecified male breast ᴿᶜᶜ

● **C50.5** Malignant neoplasm of lower-outer quadrant of breast
 ● **C50.51** Malignant neoplasm of lower-outer quadrant of breast, female
  C50.511 Malignant neoplasm of lower-outer quadrant of right female breast ᴿᶜᶜ
  C50.512 Malignant neoplasm of lower-outer quadrant of left female breast ᴿᶜᶜ
  C50.519 Malignant neoplasm of lower-outer quadrant of unspecified female breast ᴿᶜᶜ
 ● **C50.52** Malignant neoplasm of lower-outer quadrant of breast, male
  C50.521 Malignant neoplasm of lower-outer quadrant of right male breast ᴿᶜᶜ
  C50.522 Malignant neoplasm of lower-outer quadrant of left male breast ᴿᶜᶜ
  C50.529 Malignant neoplasm of lower-outer quadrant of unspecified male breast ᴿᶜᶜ

● **C50.6** Malignant neoplasm of axillary tail of breast
 ● **C50.61** Malignant neoplasm of axillary tail of breast, female
  C50.611 Malignant neoplasm of axillary tail of right female breast ᴿᶜᶜ
  C50.612 Malignant neoplasm of axillary tail of left female breast ᴿᶜᶜ
  C50.619 Malignant neoplasm of axillary tail of unspecified female breast ᴿᶜᶜ
 ● **C50.62** Malignant neoplasm of axillary tail of breast, male
  C50.621 Malignant neoplasm of axillary tail of right male breast ᴿᶜᶜ
  C50.622 Malignant neoplasm of axillary tail of left male breast ᴿᶜᶜ
  C50.629 Malignant neoplasm of axillary tail of unspecified male breast ᴿᶜᶜ

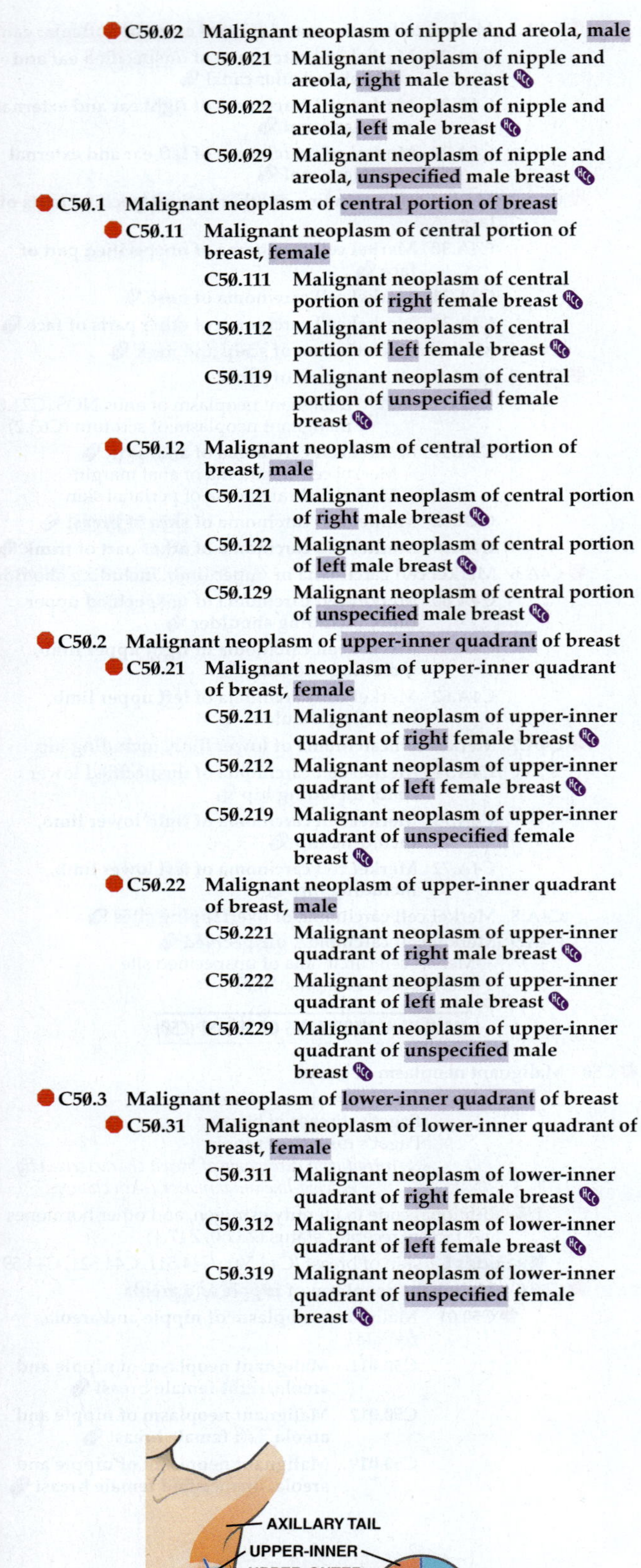

Figure 2-12 Female breast quadrants and axillary tail.

- **C50.8**   **Malignant neoplasm of overlapping sites of breast**
  - **C50.81**   **Malignant neoplasm of overlapping sites of breast, female**
    - **C50.811**   Malignant neoplasm of overlapping sites of right female breast
    - **C50.812**   Malignant neoplasm of overlapping sites of left female breast
    - **C50.819**   Malignant neoplasm of overlapping sites of unspecified female breast
  - **C50.82**   **Malignant neoplasm of overlapping sites of breast, male**
    - **C50.821**   Malignant neoplasm of overlapping sites of right male breast
    - **C50.822**   Malignant neoplasm of overlapping sites of left male breast
    - **C50.829**   Malignant neoplasm of overlapping sites of unspecified male breast
- **C50.9**   **Malignant neoplasm of breast of unspecified site**
  - **C50.91**   **Malignant neoplasm of breast of unspecified site, female**
    - **C50.911**   Malignant neoplasm of unspecified site of right female breast
    - **C50.912**   Malignant neoplasm of unspecified site of left female breast
      Coding Clinic: 2022, Q3, P11,15
    - **C50.919**   Malignant neoplasm of unspecified site of unspecified female breast
  - **C50.92**   **Malignant neoplasm of breast of unspecified site, male**
    - **C50.921**   Malignant neoplasm of unspecified site of right male breast
    - **C50.922**   Malignant neoplasm of unspecified site of left male breast
    - **C50.929**   Malignant neoplasm of unspecified site of unspecified male breast
- **C50.A**   **Malignant inflammatory neoplasm of breast**
  Inflammatory breast cancer (IBC)
  - **C50.A0**   **Malignant inflammatory neoplasm of unspecified breast**
  - **C50.A1**   **Malignant inflammatory neoplasm of right breast**
  - **C50.A2**   **Malignant inflammatory neoplasm of left breast**

MALIGNANT NEOPLASMS OF FEMALE GENITAL ORGANS (C51-C58)

> **Includes**   malignant neoplasm of skin of female genital organs

- **C51**   **Malignant neoplasm of vulva**
  > **Excludes1**   carcinoma in situ of vulva (D07.1)
  - **C51.0**   **Malignant neoplasm of labium majus**
    Outer folds of skin external female genitalia
    Malignant neoplasm of Bartholin's [greater vestibular] gland
  - **C51.1**   **Malignant neoplasm of labium minus**
    Two inner folds surrounding vulva in female genitalia
  - **C51.2**   **Malignant neoplasm of clitoris**
  - **C51.8**   **Malignant neoplasm of overlapping sites of vulva**
  - **C51.9**   **Malignant neoplasm of vulva, unspecified**
    Malignant neoplasm of external female genitalia NOS
    Malignant neoplasm of pudendum
- **C52**   **Malignant neoplasm of vagina**
  > **Excludes1**   carcinoma in situ of vagina (D07.2)
- **C53**   **Malignant neoplasm of cervix uteri**
  > **Excludes1**   carcinoma in situ of cervix uteri (D06.-)
  - **C53.0**   **Malignant neoplasm of endocervix**
    Inside the cervix
  - **C53.1**   **Malignant neoplasm of exocervix**
    Outside the cervix

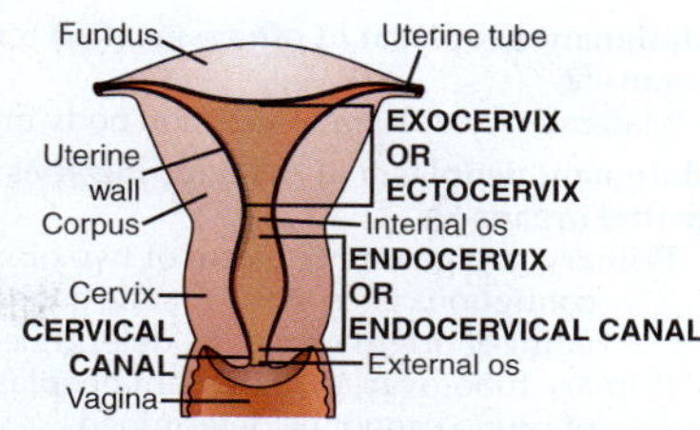

Figure 2-13   Cervix uteri.

- **C53.8**   **Malignant neoplasm of overlapping sites of cervix uteri**
- **C53.9**   **Malignant neoplasm of cervix uteri, unspecified**
  Coding Clinic: 2017, Q4, P103
- **C54**   **Malignant neoplasm of corpus uteri**
  - **C54.0**   **Malignant neoplasm of isthmus uteri**
    Constricted part of uterus between cervix and body
    Malignant neoplasm of lower uterine segment
  - **C54.1**   **Malignant neoplasm of endometrium**
    Lining of uterus
  - **C54.2**   **Malignant neoplasm of myometrium**
    Middle layer of uterine wall consisting of smooth muscle supporting stromal and vascular tissue
  - **C54.3**   **Malignant neoplasm of fundus uteri**
    Top rounded portion of uterus
  - **C54.8**   **Malignant neoplasm of overlapping sites of corpus uteri ♀**
    Main body of uterus
    Coding Clinic: 2023, Q3, P15
  - **C54.9**   **Malignant neoplasm of corpus uteri, unspecified**
- **C55**   **Malignant neoplasm of uterus, part unspecified**
- **C56**   **Malignant neoplasm of ovary**
  > **Use additional** code to identify any functional activity
  - **C56.1**   **Malignant neoplasm of right ovary**
    Coding Clinic: 2025, Q2, P16
  - **C56.2**   **Malignant neoplasm of left ovary**
  - **C56.3**   **Malignant neoplasm of bilateral ovaries**
  - **C56.9**   **Malignant neoplasm of unspecified ovary**
- **C57**   **Malignant neoplasm of other and unspecified female genital organs**
  - **C57.0**   **Malignant neoplasm of fallopian tube**
    Malignant neoplasm of oviduct
    Malignant neoplasm of uterine tube
    - **C57.00**   Malignant neoplasm of unspecified fallopian tube
    - **C57.01**   Malignant neoplasm of right fallopian tube
    - **C57.02**   Malignant neoplasm of left fallopian tube
  - **C57.1**   **Malignant neoplasm of broad ligament**
    - **C57.10**   Malignant neoplasm of unspecified broad ligament
    - **C57.11**   Malignant neoplasm of right broad ligament
    - **C57.12**   Malignant neoplasm of left broad ligament
  - **C57.2**   **Malignant neoplasm of round ligament**
    - **C57.20**   Malignant neoplasm of unspecified round ligament
    - **C57.21**   Malignant neoplasm of right round ligament
    - **C57.22**   Malignant neoplasm of left round ligament
  - **C57.3**   **Malignant neoplasm of parametrium**
    Malignant neoplasm of uterine ligament NOS
  - **C57.4**   **Malignant neoplasm of uterine adnexa, unspecified ♀**

C57.7 **Malignant neoplasm of other specified female genital organs** 🔴
Malignant neoplasm of wolffian body or duct

C57.8 **Malignant neoplasm of overlapping sites of female genital organs** 🔴
Primary malignant neoplasm of two or more contiguous sites of the female genital organs whose point of origin cannot be determined
Primary tubo-ovarian malignant neoplasm whose point of origin cannot be determined
Primary utero-ovarian malignant neoplasm whose point of origin cannot be determined

C57.9 **Malignant neoplasm of female genital organ, unspecified** 🔴
Malignant neoplasm of female genitourinary tract NOS

C58 **Malignant neoplasm of placenta** 🔴   **M**

Includes   choriocarcinoma NOS
chorionepithelioma NOS

Excludes1   chorioadenoma (destruens) (D39.2)
hydatidiform mole NOS (O01.9)
invasive hydatidiform mole (D39.2)
male choriocarcinoma NOS (C62.9-)
malignant hydatidiform mole (D39.2)

MALIGNANT NEOPLASMS OF MALE GENITAL ORGANS (C60-C63)

Includes   malignant neoplasm of skin of male genital organs

🔴 C60 **Malignant neoplasm of penis**

C60.0 **Malignant neoplasm of prepuce** 🔴
Malignant neoplasm of foreskin

C60.1 **Malignant neoplasm of glans penis** 🔴

C60.2 **Malignant neoplasm of body of penis** 🔴
Malignant neoplasm of corpus cavernosum

C60.8 **Malignant neoplasm of overlapping sites of penis** 🔴

C60.9 **Malignant neoplasm of penis, unspecified** 🔴
Malignant neoplasm of skin of penis NOS

C61 **Malignant neoplasm of prostate** 🔴
Use additional , if applicable, code to identify:
hormone sensitivity status (Z19.1-Z19.2)
rising PSA following treatment for malignant neoplasm of prostate (R97.21)

Excludes1   malignant neoplasm of seminal vesicle (C63.7)

🔴 C62 **Malignant neoplasm of testis**
Use additional code to identify any functional activity.

🔴 C62.0 **Malignant neoplasm of undescended testis**
Malignant neoplasm of ectopic testis
Malignant neoplasm of retained testis

C62.00 **Malignant neoplasm of unspecified undescended testis** 🔴

C62.01 **Malignant neoplasm of undescended right testis** 🔴

C62.02 **Malignant neoplasm of undescended left testis** 🔴

🔴 C62.1 **Malignant neoplasm of descended testis**
Malignant neoplasm of scrotal testis

C62.10 **Malignant neoplasm of unspecified descended testis, unspecified side** 🔴

C62.11 **Malignant neoplasm of descended right testis** 🔴

C62.12 **Malignant neoplasm of descended left testis** 🔴

🔴 C62.9 **Malignant neoplasm of testis, unspecified whether descended or undescended**

C62.90 **Malignant neoplasm of unspecified testis, unspecified whether descended or undescended** 🔴
Malignant neoplasm of testis NOS

C62.91 **Malignant neoplasm of right testis, unspecified whether descended or undescended** 🔴

C62.92 **Malignant neoplasm of left testis, unspecified whether descended or undescended** 🔴

🔴 C63 **Malignant neoplasm of other and unspecified male genital organs**

🔴 C63.0 **Malignant neoplasm of epididymis**

C63.00 **Malignant neoplasm of unspecified epididymis** 🔴

C63.01 **Malignant neoplasm of right epididymis** 🔴

C63.02 **Malignant neoplasm of left epididymis** 🔴

🔴 C63.1 **Malignant neoplasm of spermatic cord**

C63.10 **Malignant neoplasm of unspecified spermatic cord** 🔴

C63.11 **Malignant neoplasm of right spermatic cord** 🔴

C63.12 **Malignant neoplasm of left spermatic cord** 🔴

C63.2 **Malignant neoplasm of scrotum** 🔴
Malignant neoplasm of skin of scrotum

C63.7 **Malignant neoplasm of other specified male genital organs** 🔴
Malignant neoplasm of seminal vesicle
Malignant neoplasm of tunica vaginalis

C63.8 **Malignant neoplasm of overlapping sites of male genital organs** 🔴
Primary malignant neoplasm of two or more contiguous sites of male genital organs whose point of origin cannot be determined

C63.9 **Malignant neoplasm of male genital organ, unspecified** 🔴
Malignant neoplasm of male genitourinary tract NOS

MALIGNANT NEOPLASMS OF URINARY TRACT (C64-C68)

🔴 C64 **Malignant neoplasm of kidney, except renal pelvis**

Excludes1   malignant carcinoid tumor of the kidney (C7A.093)
malignant neoplasm of renal calyces (C65.-)
malignant neoplasm of renal pelvis (C65.-)

C64.1 **Malignant neoplasm of right kidney, except renal pelvis** 🔴
Coding Clinic: 2025, Q2, P12

C64.2 **Malignant neoplasm of left kidney, except renal pelvis** 🔴

C64.9 **Malignant neoplasm of unspecified kidney, except renal pelvis** 🔴

🔴 C65 **Malignant neoplasm of renal pelvis**

Includes   malignant neoplasm of pelviureteric junction
malignant neoplasm of renal calyces

C65.1 **Malignant neoplasm of right renal pelvis** 🔴

C65.2 **Malignant neoplasm of left renal pelvis** 🔴

C65.9 **Malignant neoplasm of unspecified renal pelvis** 🔴

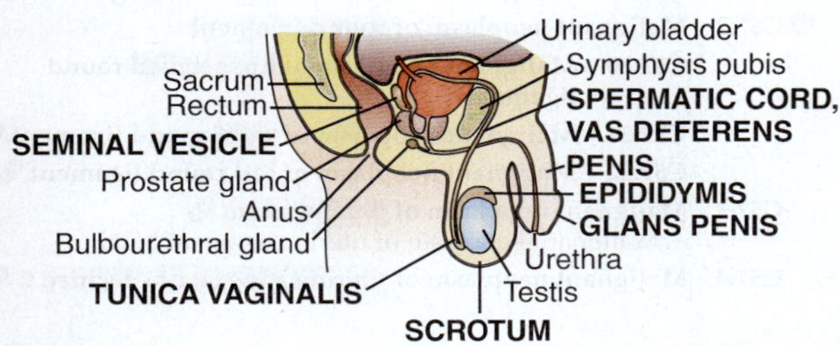

Figure 2-14 Penis and other male genital organs.

● **C66** **Malignant neoplasm of ureter**
  Excludes1 malignant neoplasm of ureteric orifice of bladder (C67.6)
  C66.1 Malignant neoplasm of right ureter
  C66.2 Malignant neoplasm of left ureter
  C66.9 Malignant neoplasm of unspecified ureter

● **C67** **Malignant neoplasm of bladder**
  C67.0 Malignant neoplasm of trigone of bladder
   Triangular area formed by three openings in the floor of urinary bladder
  C67.1 Malignant neoplasm of dome of bladder
   Vaulted roof
   Coding Clinic: 2023, Q3, P16
  C67.2 Malignant neoplasm of lateral wall of bladder
   Side walls
   Coding Clinic: 2023, Q3, P16
  C67.3 Malignant neoplasm of anterior wall of bladder
   Front wall
   Coding Clinic: 2023, Q3, P16
  C67.4 Malignant neoplasm of posterior wall of bladder
   Back wall
  C67.5 Malignant neoplasm of bladder neck
   Joining of bladder and urethra
   Malignant neoplasm of internal urethral orifice
   Coding Clinic: 2023, Q3, P16
  C67.6 Malignant neoplasm of ureteric orifice
   Opening from bladder to ureters
  C67.7 Malignant neoplasm of urachus
   Embryonic canal that connects the urinary bladder with the structure that forms the umbilical cord (allantois)
  C67.8 Malignant neoplasm of overlapping sites of bladder
  C67.9 Malignant neoplasm of bladder, unspecified
   Coding Clinic: 2017, Q1, P6; 2016, Q1, P19

● **C68** **Malignant neoplasm of other and unspecified urinary organs**
  Excludes1 malignant neoplasm of female genitourinary tract NOS (C57.9)
   malignant neoplasm of male genitourinary tract NOS (C63.9)
  C68.0 Malignant neoplasm of urethra
   Excludes1 malignant neoplasm of urethral orifice of bladder (C67.5)
  C68.1 Malignant neoplasm of paraurethral glands
   Group of glands of female urethra drained by paraurethral ducts; AKA Skene glands, female prostate
  C68.8 Malignant neoplasm of overlapping sites of urinary organs
   Primary malignant neoplasm of two or more contiguous sites of urinary organs whose point of origin cannot be determined
  C68.9 Malignant neoplasm of urinary organ, unspecified
   Malignant neoplasm of urinary system NOS

MALIGNANT NEOPLASMS OF EYE, BRAIN AND OTHER PARTS OF CENTRAL NERVOUS SYSTEM (C69-C72)

● **C69** **Malignant neoplasm of eye and adnexa**
  Excludes1 malignant neoplasm of connective tissue of eyelid (C49.0)
   malignant neoplasm of eyelid (skin) (C43.1-, C44.1-)
   malignant neoplasm of optic nerve (C72.3-)
● C69.0 Malignant neoplasm of conjunctiva
  C69.00 Malignant neoplasm of unspecified conjunctiva
  C69.01 Malignant neoplasm of right conjunctiva
  C69.02 Malignant neoplasm of left conjunctiva

● C69.1 Malignant neoplasm of cornea
  C69.10 Malignant neoplasm of unspecified cornea
  C69.11 Malignant neoplasm of right cornea
  C69.12 Malignant neoplasm of left cornea
● C69.2 Malignant neoplasm of retina
  Excludes1 dark area on retina (D49.81)
   neoplasm of unspecified behavior of retina and choroid (D49.81)
   retinal freckle (D49.81)
  C69.20 Malignant neoplasm of unspecified retina
  C69.21 Malignant neoplasm of right retina
  C69.22 Malignant neoplasm of left retina
● C69.3 Malignant neoplasm of choroid
  C69.30 Malignant neoplasm of unspecified choroid
  C69.31 Malignant neoplasm of right choroid
  C69.32 Malignant neoplasm of left choroid
● C69.4 Malignant neoplasm of ciliary body
  C69.40 Malignant neoplasm of unspecified ciliary body
  C69.41 Malignant neoplasm of right ciliary body
  C69.42 Malignant neoplasm of left ciliary body
● C69.5 Malignant neoplasm of lacrimal gland and duct
   Malignant neoplasm of lacrimal sac
   Malignant neoplasm of nasolacrimal duct
  C69.50 Malignant neoplasm of unspecified lacrimal gland and duct
  C69.51 Malignant neoplasm of right lacrimal gland and duct
  C69.52 Malignant neoplasm of left lacrimal gland and duct
● C69.6 Malignant neoplasm of orbit
   Malignant neoplasm of connective tissue of orbit
   Malignant neoplasm of extraocular muscle
   Malignant neoplasm of peripheral nerves of orbit
   Malignant neoplasm of retrobulbar tissue
   Malignant neoplasm of retro-ocular tissue
   Excludes1 malignant neoplasm of orbital bone (C41.0)
  C69.60 Malignant neoplasm of unspecified orbit
  C69.61 Malignant neoplasm of right orbit
  C69.62 Malignant neoplasm of left orbit
● C69.8 Malignant neoplasm of overlapping sites of eye and adnexa
  C69.80 Malignant neoplasm of overlapping sites of unspecified eye and adnexa
  C69.81 Malignant neoplasm of overlapping sites of right eye and adnexa
  C69.82 Malignant neoplasm of overlapping sites of left eye and adnexa
● C69.9 Malignant neoplasm of unspecified site of eye
   Malignant neoplasm of eyeball
  C69.90 Malignant neoplasm of unspecified site of unspecified eye
  C69.91 Malignant neoplasm of unspecified site of right eye
  C69.92 Malignant neoplasm of unspecified site of left eye

● **C70** **Malignant neoplasm of meninges**
  C70.0 Malignant neoplasm of cerebral meninges
  C70.1 Malignant neoplasm of spinal meninges
  C70.9 Malignant neoplasm of meninges, unspecified

CHAPTER 2 (C00-D49)

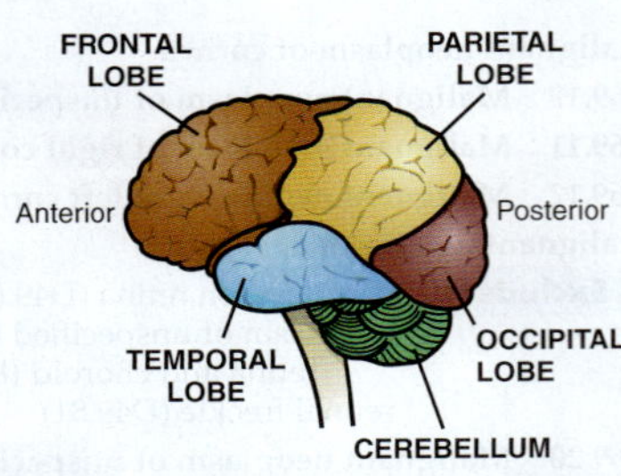

Figure 2-15 The brain.

- **C71**   **Malignant neoplasm of brain**
  - **Excludes1**   malignant neoplasm of cranial nerves (C72.2-C72.5)
    - retrobulbar malignant neoplasm (C69.6-)
  - **C71.0**   **Malignant neoplasm of cerebrum, except lobes and ventricles**
    - Malignant neoplasm of supratentorial NOS
  - **C71.1**   **Malignant neoplasm of frontal lobe**
  - **C71.2**   **Malignant neoplasm of temporal lobe**
  - **C71.3**   **Malignant neoplasm of parietal lobe**
  - **C71.4**   **Malignant neoplasm of occipital lobe**
  - **C71.5**   **Malignant neoplasm of cerebral ventricle**
    - **Excludes1**   malignant neoplasm of fourth cerebral ventricle (C71.7)
  - **C71.6**   **Malignant neoplasm of cerebellum**
  - **C71.7**   **Malignant neoplasm of brain stem**
    - Malignant neoplasm of fourth cerebral ventricle
    - Infratentorial malignant neoplasm NOS
  - **C71.8**   **Malignant neoplasm of overlapping sites of brain**
  - **C71.9**   **Malignant neoplasm of brain, unspecified**

- **C72**   **Malignant neoplasm of spinal cord, cranial nerves and other parts of central nervous system**
  - **Excludes1**   malignant neoplasm of meninges (C70.-)
    - malignant neoplasm of peripheral nerves and autonomic nervous system (C47.-)
  - **C72.0**   **Malignant neoplasm of spinal cord**
  - **C72.1**   **Malignant neoplasm of cauda equina**
    - *Lower end of spinal column*
  - **C72.2**   **Malignant neoplasm of olfactory nerve**
    - Malignant neoplasm of olfactory bulb
    - **C72.20**   **Malignant neoplasm of unspecified olfactory nerve**
    - **C72.21**   **Malignant neoplasm of right olfactory nerve**
    - **C72.22**   **Malignant neoplasm of left olfactory nerve**
  - **C72.3**   **Malignant neoplasm of optic nerve**
    - **C72.30**   **Malignant neoplasm of unspecified optic nerve**
    - **C72.31**   **Malignant neoplasm of right optic nerve**
    - **C72.32**   **Malignant neoplasm of left optic nerve**
  - **C72.4**   **Malignant neoplasm of acoustic nerve**
    - **C72.40**   **Malignant neoplasm of unspecified acoustic nerve**
    - **C72.41**   **Malignant neoplasm of right acoustic nerve**
    - **C72.42**   **Malignant neoplasm of left acoustic nerve**
  - **C72.5**   **Malignant neoplasm of other and unspecified cranial nerves**
    - **C72.50**   **Malignant neoplasm of unspecified cranial nerve**
      - Malignant neoplasm of cranial nerve NOS
    - **C72.59**   **Malignant neoplasm of other cranial nerves**
  - **C72.9**   **Malignant neoplasm of central nervous system, unspecified**
    - Malignant neoplasm of unspecified site of central nervous system
    - Malignant neoplasm of nervous system NOS

MALIGNANT NEOPLASMS OF THYROID AND OTHER ENDOCRINE GLANDS (C73-C75)

- **C73**   **Malignant neoplasm of thyroid gland**
  - Use additional code to identify any functional activity

- **C74**   **Malignant neoplasm of adrenal gland**
  - **C74.0**   **Malignant neoplasm of cortex of adrenal gland**
    - **C74.00**   **Malignant neoplasm of cortex of unspecified adrenal gland**
    - **C74.01**   **Malignant neoplasm of cortex of right adrenal gland**
    - **C74.02**   **Malignant neoplasm of cortex of left adrenal gland**
  - **C74.1**   **Malignant neoplasm of medulla of adrenal gland**
    - *Pair of glands situated on top of or above each kidney ("suprarenal")*
    - **C74.10**   **Malignant neoplasm of medulla of unspecified adrenal gland**
    - **C74.11**   **Malignant neoplasm of medulla of right adrenal gland**
    - **C74.12**   **Malignant neoplasm of medulla of left adrenal gland**
  - **C74.9**   **Malignant neoplasm of unspecified part of adrenal gland**
    - **C74.90**   **Malignant neoplasm of unspecified part of unspecified adrenal gland**
    - **C74.91**   **Malignant neoplasm of unspecified part of right adrenal gland**
    - **C74.92**   **Malignant neoplasm of unspecified part of left adrenal gland**

- **C75**   **Malignant neoplasm of other endocrine glands and related structures**
  - **Excludes1**   malignant carcinoid tumors (C7A.0-)
    - malignant neoplasm of adrenal gland (C74.-)
    - malignant neoplasm of endocrine pancreas (C25.4)
    - malignant neoplasm of islets of Langerhans (C25.4)
    - malignant neoplasm of ovary (C56.-)
    - malignant neoplasm of testis (C62.-)
    - malignant neoplasm of thymus (C37)
    - malignant neoplasm of thyroid gland (C73)
    - malignant neuroendocrine tumors (C7A.-)
  - **C75.0**   **Malignant neoplasm of parathyroid gland**
  - **C75.1**   **Malignant neoplasm of pituitary gland**
  - **C75.2**   **Malignant neoplasm of craniopharyngeal duct**
  - **C75.3**   **Malignant neoplasm of pineal gland**
  - **C75.4**   **Malignant neoplasm of carotid body**
  - **C75.5**   **Malignant neoplasm of aortic body and other paraganglia**
  - **C75.8**   **Malignant neoplasm with pluriglandular involvement, unspecified**
  - **C75.9**   **Malignant neoplasm of endocrine gland, unspecified**

MALIGNANT NEOPLASMS OF ILL-DEFINED, OTHER SECONDARY AND UNSPECIFIED SITES (C76-C80)

● **C76 Malignant neoplasm of other and ill-defined sites**

Excludes1   malignant neoplasm of female genitourinary tract NOS (C57.9)
malignant neoplasm of male genitourinary tract NOS (C63.9)
malignant neoplasm of lymphoid, hematopoietic and related tissue (C81-C96)
malignant neoplasm of skin (C44.-)
malignant neoplasm of unspecified site NOS (C80.1)

C76.0 Malignant neoplasm of head, face and neck
Malignant neoplasm of cheek NOS
Malignant neoplasm of nose NOS

C76.1 Malignant neoplasm of thorax
Intrathoracic malignant neoplasm NOS
Malignant neoplasm of axilla NOS
Thoracic malignant neoplasm NOS

C76.2 Malignant neoplasm of abdomen

C76.3 Malignant neoplasm of pelvis
Malignant neoplasm of groin NOS
Malignant neoplasm of sites overlapping systems within the pelvis
Rectovaginal (septum) malignant neoplasm
Between rectum and vagina
Rectovesical (septum) malignant neoplasm
Between rectum and urinary bladder; AKA vesicorectal

● **C76.4 Malignant neoplasm of upper limb**

C76.40   Malignant neoplasm of unspecified upper limb

C76.41   Malignant neoplasm of right upper limb

C76.42   Malignant neoplasm of left upper limb

● **C76.5 Malignant neoplasm of lower limb**

C76.50   Malignant neoplasm of unspecified lower limb

C76.51   Malignant neoplasm of right lower limb

C76.52   Malignant neoplasm of left lower limb

C76.8 Malignant neoplasm of other specified ill-defined sites
Malignant neoplasm of overlapping ill-defined sites

● **C77 Secondary and unspecified malignant neoplasm of lymph nodes**

Excludes1   malignant neoplasm of lymph nodes, specified as primary (C81-C86, C88, C96.-)
➡ mesentery metastasis of carcinoid tumor (C7B.04)
secondary carcinoid tumors of distant lymph nodes (C7B.01)

C77.0 Secondary and unspecified malignant neoplasm of lymph nodes of head, face and neck
Secondary and unspecified malignant neoplasm of supraclavicular lymph nodes
Coding Clinic: 2022, Q3, P15

C77.1 Secondary and unspecified malignant neoplasm of intrathoracic lymph nodes

C77.2 Secondary and unspecified malignant neoplasm of intra-abdominal lymph nodes

C77.3 Secondary and unspecified malignant neoplasm of axilla and upper limb lymph nodes
Secondary and unspecified malignant neoplasm of pectoral lymph nodes

C77.4 Secondary and unspecified malignant neoplasm of inguinal and lower limb lymph nodes

C77.5 Secondary and unspecified malignant neoplasm of intrapelvic lymph nodes

C77.8 Secondary and unspecified malignant neoplasm of lymph nodes of multiple regions

C77.9 Secondary and unspecified malignant neoplasm of lymph node, unspecified

Item 2–6 The adrenal glands are a pair of glands situated on top of or above each kidney ("suprarenal") and chiefly responsible for regulating the stress response through the synthesis of corticosteroids and catecholamines, including cortisol and adrenaline.

● **C78 Secondary malignant neoplasm of respiratory and digestive organs**

Excludes1   secondary carcinoid tumors of liver (C7B.02)
secondary carcinoid tumors of peritoneum (C7B.04)

Excludes2   lymph node metastases (C77.0)
Coding Clinic: 2023, Q1, P22

● **C78.0 Secondary malignant neoplasm of lung**

C78.00   Secondary malignant neoplasm of unspecified lung
Coding Clinic: 2022, Q3, P9

C78.01   Secondary malignant neoplasm of right lung
Coding Clinic: 2024, Q2, P11; 2023, Q3, P15

C78.02   Secondary malignant neoplasm of left lung
Coding Clinic: 2023, Q3, P15

C78.1 Secondary malignant neoplasm of mediastinum
Thoracic cavity between pleural cavities

C78.2 Secondary malignant neoplasm of pleura
Serous membrane covering lungs and lining thoracic cavity

● **C78.3 Secondary malignant neoplasm of other and unspecified respiratory organs**

C78.30   Secondary malignant neoplasm of unspecified respiratory organ

C78.39   Secondary malignant neoplasm of other respiratory organs

C78.4 Secondary malignant neoplasm of small intestine

C78.5 Secondary malignant neoplasm of large intestine and rectum

C78.6 Secondary malignant neoplasm of retroperitoneum and peritoneum
Coding Clinic: 2025, Q2, P16; 2017, Q2, P12

C78.7 Secondary malignant neoplasm of liver and intrahepatic bile duct
Coding Clinic: 2024, Q1, P25; 2022, Q3, P15

● **C78.8 Secondary malignant neoplasm of other and unspecified digestive organs**

C78.80   Secondary malignant neoplasm of unspecified digestive organ

C78.89   Secondary malignant neoplasm of other digestive organs
Code also exocrine pancreatic insufficiency (K86.81)

● **C79 Secondary malignant neoplasm of other and unspecified sites**

Excludes1   secondary carcinoid tumors (C7B.-)
secondary neuroendocrine tumors (C7B.-)
Coding Clinic: 2023, Q1, P22

● **C79.0 Secondary malignant neoplasm of kidney and renal pelvis**

C79.00   Secondary malignant neoplasm of unspecified kidney and renal pelvis

C79.01   Secondary malignant neoplasm of right kidney and renal pelvis

C79.02   Secondary malignant neoplasm of left kidney and renal pelvis

● **C79.1 Secondary malignant neoplasm of bladder and other and unspecified urinary organs**

C79.10   Secondary malignant neoplasm of unspecified urinary organs

C79.11   Secondary malignant neoplasm of bladder
Excludes2   lymph node metastases (C77.0)

C79.19   Secondary malignant neoplasm of other urinary organs

CHAPTER 2 (C00-D49)

CHAPTER 2 (C00-D49)

C79.2   Secondary malignant neoplasm of skin
         Excludes1   secondary Merkel cell carcinoma (C7B.1)

● C79.3 Secondary malignant neoplasm of brain and cerebral meninges
    C79.31   Secondary malignant neoplasm of brain
              Coding Clinic: 2022, Q3, P9,11
    C79.32   Secondary malignant neoplasm of cerebral meninges
              Coding Clinic: 2020, Q1, P13

● C79.4 Secondary malignant neoplasm of other and unspecified parts of nervous system
    C79.40   Secondary malignant neoplasm of unspecified part of nervous system
    C79.49   Secondary malignant neoplasm of other parts of nervous system

● C79.5 Secondary malignant neoplasm of bone and bone marrow
         Excludes1   secondary carcinoid tumors of bone (C7B.03)
    C79.51   Secondary malignant neoplasm of bone
              Coding Clinic: 2022, Q3, P15
    C79.52   Secondary malignant neoplasm of bone marrow

● C79.6 Secondary malignant neoplasm of ovary
    C79.60   Secondary malignant neoplasm of unspecified ovary
    C79.61   Secondary malignant neoplasm of right ovary
    C79.62   Secondary malignant neoplasm of left ovary
    C79.63   Secondary malignant neoplasm of bilateral ovaries

● C79.7 Secondary malignant neoplasm of adrenal gland
    C79.70   Secondary malignant neoplasm of unspecified adrenal gland
    C79.71   Secondary malignant neoplasm of right adrenal gland
    C79.72   Secondary malignant neoplasm of left adrenal gland

● C79.8 Secondary malignant neoplasm of other specified sites
    C79.81   Secondary malignant neoplasm of breast
    C79.82   Secondary malignant neoplasm of genital organs
              Coding Clinic: 2023, Q3, P15
    C79.89   Secondary malignant neoplasm of other specified sites
              Coding Clinic: 2017, Q2, P11

C79.9   Secondary malignant neoplasm of unspecified site
         Metastatic cancer NOS
         Metastatic disease NOS
         Excludes1   carcinomatosis NOS (C80.0)
                          generalized cancer NOS (C80.0)
                          malignant (primary) neoplasm of unspecified site (C80.1)
         Coding Clinic: 2023, Q2, P5

MALIGNANT NEUROENDOCRINE TUMORS (C7A)

● C7A Malignant neuroendocrine tumors
       Code also any associated multiple endocrine neoplasia [MEN] syndromes (E31.2-)
       Use additional code to identify any associated endocrine syndrome, such as:
            carcinoid syndrome (E34.00)
       Excludes2   malignant pancreatic islet cell tumors (C25.4)
                        Merkel cell carcinoma (C4A.-)

● C7A.0 Malignant carcinoid tumors
    C7A.00   Malignant carcinoid tumor of unspecified site
  ● C7A.01   Malignant carcinoid tumors of the small intestine
    C7A.010   Malignant carcinoid tumor of the duodenum
    C7A.011   Malignant carcinoid tumor of the jejunum
    C7A.012   Malignant carcinoid tumor of the ileum
    C7A.019   Malignant carcinoid tumor of the small intestine, unspecified portion
  ● C7A.02   Malignant carcinoid tumors of the appendix, large intestine, and rectum
    C7A.020   Malignant carcinoid tumor of the appendix
    C7A.021   Malignant carcinoid tumor of the cecum
    C7A.022   Malignant carcinoid tumor of the ascending colon
    C7A.023   Malignant carcinoid tumor of the transverse colon
    C7A.024   Malignant carcinoid tumor of the descending colon
    C7A.025   Malignant carcinoid tumor of the sigmoid colon
    C7A.026   Malignant carcinoid tumor of the rectum
    C7A.029   Malignant carcinoid tumor of the large intestine, unspecified portion
                  Malignant carcinoid tumor of the colon NOS
  ● C7A.09   Malignant carcinoid tumors of other sites
    C7A.090   Malignant carcinoid tumor of the bronchus and lung
    C7A.091   Malignant carcinoid tumor of the thymus
    C7A.092   Malignant carcinoid tumor of the stomach
    C7A.093   Malignant carcinoid tumor of the kidney
    C7A.094   Malignant carcinoid tumor of the foregut, unspecified
    C7A.095   Malignant carcinoid tumor of the midgut, unspecified
    C7A.096   Malignant carcinoid tumor of the hindgut, unspecified
    C7A.098   Malignant carcinoid tumors of other sites

C7A.1   Malignant poorly differentiated neuroendocrine tumors
         Malignant poorly differentiated neuroendocrine tumor NOS
         Malignant poorly differentiated neuroendocrine carcinoma, any site
         High grade neuroendocrine carcinoma, any site
         Coding Clinic: 2023, Q1, P21-22

C7A.8   Other malignant neuroendocrine tumors
         Secondary neuroendocrine tumors (C7B)
         Coding Clinic: 2019, Q3, P7

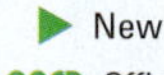 New   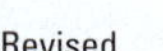 Revised   ~~deleted~~ Deleted   Excludes 1   Excludes 2   Includes   Use additional   Code first   Code also   Key words
OGCR Official Guidelines   X Assign placeholder X   ● Use Additional Character(s)   Manifestation Code   Hierarchical Condition Category   Coding Clinic

SECONDARY NEUROENDOCRINE TUMORS (C7B)

● **C7B   Secondary neuroendocrine tumors**
>> Use additional code to identify any functional activity

● **C7B.0   Secondary carcinoid tumors**

C7B.00   Secondary carcinoid tumors, unspecified site

C7B.01   Secondary carcinoid tumors of distant lymph nodes

C7B.02   Secondary carcinoid tumors of liver

C7B.03   Secondary carcinoid tumors of bone

C7B.04   Secondary carcinoid tumors of peritoneum
>> ➡ Mesentery metastasis of carcinoid tumor

C7B.09   Secondary carcinoid tumors of other sites

C7B.1   Secondary Merkel cell carcinoma
>> Merkel cell carcinoma nodal presentation
>> Merkel cell carcinoma visceral metastatic presentation

C7B.8   Other secondary neuroendocrine tumors
>> **Coding Clinic: 2024, Q2, P10; 2023, Q1, P21; 2019, Q3, P7**

OGCR   Section I.C.2.j and k

> Disseminated malignant neoplasm, unspecified
>
> j. Code C80.0, Disseminated malignant neoplasm, unspecified, is for use only in those cases where the patient has advanced metastatic disease and no known primary or secondary sites are specified. It should not be used in place of assigning codes for the primary site and all known secondary sites.
>
> Malignant neoplasm without specification of site
>
> k. Code C80.1, Malignant (primary) neoplasm, unspecified, equates to Cancer, unspecified. This code should only be used when no determination can be made as to the primary site of a malignancy. This code should rarely be used in the inpatient setting.

● **C80   Malignant neoplasm without specification of site**
>> **Excludes1**   malignant carcinoid tumor of unspecified site (C7A.00)
>> malignant neoplasm of specified multiple sites- code to each site

C80.0   **Disseminated malignant neoplasm, unspecified**
>> Carcinomatosis NOS
>> Generalized cancer, unspecified site (primary) (secondary)
>> Generalized malignancy, unspecified site (primary) (secondary)

C80.1   **Malignant (primary) neoplasm, unspecified**
>> Cancer NOS
>> Cancer unspecified site (primary)
>> Carcinoma unspecified site (primary)
>> Malignancy unspecified site (primary)
>> **Excludes1**   secondary malignant neoplasm of unspecified site (C79.9)

C80.2   **Malignant neoplasm associated with transplanted organ**
>> *Code first* complication of transplanted organ (T86.-)
>> Use additional code to identify the specific malignancy

★ **(See Plate 1 of the Anatomy Illustrations.)**

MALIGNANT NEOPLASMS OF LYMPHOID, HEMATOPOIETIC AND RELATED TISSUE (C81-C96)

>> **Excludes2**   Kaposi's sarcoma of lymph nodes (C46.3)
>> secondary and unspecified neoplasm of lymph nodes (C77.-)
>> secondary neoplasm of bone marrow (C79.52)
>> secondary neoplasm of spleen (C78.89)

● **C81   Hodgkin lymphoma**
>> *Form of malignant lymphoma with four types, nodular sclerosis, mixed cellularity, lymphocyte depleted, and lymphocyte predominant*
>> **Excludes1**   personal history of Hodgkin lymphoma (Z85.71)

● **C81.0   Nodular lymphocyte predominant Hodgkin lymphoma**
>> *Least aggressive, least common, typically no symptoms*
>> Lymphocytic-histiocytic predominance Hodgkin's disease

C81.00   Nodular lymphocyte predominant Hodgkin lymphoma, unspecified site

C81.01   Nodular lymphocyte predominant Hodgkin lymphoma, lymph nodes of head, face, and neck

C81.02   Nodular lymphocyte predominant Hodgkin lymphoma, intrathoracic lymph nodes

C81.03   Nodular lymphocyte predominant Hodgkin lymphoma, intra-abdominal lymph nodes

C81.04   Nodular lymphocyte predominant Hodgkin lymphoma, lymph nodes of axilla and upper limb

C81.05   Nodular lymphocyte predominant Hodgkin lymphoma, lymph nodes of inguinal region and lower limb

C81.06   Nodular lymphocyte predominant Hodgkin lymphoma, intrapelvic lymph nodes

C81.07   Nodular lymphocyte predominant Hodgkin lymphoma, spleen

C81.08   Nodular lymphocyte predominant Hodgkin lymphoma, lymph nodes of multiple sites

C81.09   Nodular lymphocyte predominant Hodgkin lymphoma, extranodal and solid organ sites

C81.0A   Nodular lymphocyte predominant Hodgkin lymphoma, in remission

● **C81.1   Nodular sclerosis Hodgkin lymphoma**
>> Nodular sclerosis classical Hodgkin lymphoma
>> *Moderately aggressive; most common in young adults*

C81.10   Nodular sclerosis Hodgkin lymphoma, unspecified site

C81.11   Nodular sclerosis Hodgkin lymphoma, lymph nodes of head, face, and neck

C81.12   Nodular sclerosis Hodgkin lymphoma, intrathoracic lymph nodes

C81.13   Nodular sclerosis Hodgkin lymphoma, intra-abdominal lymph nodes

C81.14   Nodular sclerosis Hodgkin lymphoma, lymph nodes of axilla and upper limb

C81.15   Nodular sclerosis Hodgkin lymphoma, lymph nodes of inguinal region and lower limb

C81.16   Nodular sclerosis Hodgkin lymphoma, intrapelvic lymph nodes

C81.17   Nodular sclerosis Hodgkin lymphoma, spleen

C81.18   Nodular sclerosis Hodgkin lymphoma, lymph nodes of multiple sites

C81.19   Nodular sclerosis Hodgkin lymphoma, extranodal and solid organ sites

C81.1A   Nodular sclerosis Hodgkin lymphoma, in remission

● **C81.2   Mixed cellularity Hodgkin lymphoma**
>> Mixed cellularity classical Hodgkin lymphoma
>> *A type of Hodgkin's that is moderately aggressive with mixed cell types*

C81.20   Mixed cellularity Hodgkin lymphoma, unspecified site

C81.21   Mixed cellularity Hodgkin lymphoma, lymph nodes of head, face, and neck

CHAPTER 2 (C00-D49)

C81.22   Mixed cellularity Hodgkin lymphoma, **intrathoracic** lymph nodes

C81.23   Mixed cellularity Hodgkin lymphoma, **intra-abdominal** lymph nodes

C81.24   Mixed cellularity Hodgkin lymphoma, lymph nodes of **axilla and upper limb**

C81.25   Mixed cellularity Hodgkin lymphoma, lymph nodes of **inguinal region and lower limb**

C81.26   Mixed cellularity Hodgkin lymphoma, **intrapelvic** lymph nodes

C81.27   Mixed cellularity Hodgkin lymphoma, **spleen**

C81.28   Mixed cellularity Hodgkin lymphoma, lymph nodes of **multiple sites**

C81.29   Mixed cellularity Hodgkin lymphoma, **extranodal and solid organ sites**

C81.2A   Mixed cellularity Hodgkin lymphoma, in remission

● **C81.3**   **Lymphocyte depleted** Hodgkin lymphoma
Lymphocyte depleted classical Hodgkin lymphoma
Most aggressive type with poor prognosis

C81.30   Lymphocyte depleted Hodgkin lymphoma, **unspecified site**

C81.31   Lymphocyte depleted Hodgkin lymphoma, lymph nodes of **head, face, and neck**

C81.32   Lymphocyte depleted Hodgkin lymphoma, **intrathoracic** lymph nodes

C81.33   Lymphocyte depleted Hodgkin lymphoma, **intra-abdominal** lymph nodes

C81.34   Lymphocyte depleted Hodgkin lymphoma, lymph nodes of **axilla and upper limb**

C81.35   Lymphocyte depleted Hodgkin lymphoma, lymph nodes of **inguinal region and lower limb**

C81.36   Lymphocyte depleted Hodgkin lymphoma, **intrapelvic** lymph nodes

C81.37   Lymphocyte depleted Hodgkin lymphoma, **spleen**

C81.38   Lymphocyte depleted Hodgkin lymphoma, lymph nodes of **multiple sites**

C81.39   Lymphocyte depleted Hodgkin lymphoma, **extranodal and solid organ sites**

C81.3A   Lymphocyte depleted Hodgkin lymphoma, in remission

● **C81.4**   **Lymphocyte-rich** Hodgkin lymphoma
Lymphocyte-rich classical Hodgkin lymphoma

   Excludes1   nodular lymphocyte predominant Hodgkin lymphoma (C81.0-)

C81.40   Lymphocyte-rich Hodgkin lymphoma, **unspecified site**

C81.41   Lymphocyte-rich Hodgkin lymphoma, lymph nodes of **head, face, and neck**

C81.42   Lymphocyte-rich Hodgkin lymphoma, **intrathoracic** lymph nodes

C81.43   Lymphocyte-rich Hodgkin lymphoma, **intra-abdominal** lymph nodes

C81.44   Lymphocyte-rich Hodgkin lymphoma, lymph nodes of **axilla and upper limb**

C81.45   Lymphocyte-rich Hodgkin lymphoma, lymph nodes of **inguinal region and lower limb**

C81.46   Lymphocyte-rich Hodgkin lymphoma, **intrapelvic** lymph nodes

C81.47   Lymphocyte-rich Hodgkin lymphoma, **spleen**

C81.48   Lymphocyte-rich Hodgkin lymphoma, lymph nodes of **multiple sites**

C81.49   Lymphocyte-rich Hodgkin lymphoma, **extranodal and solid organ sites**

C81.4A   Lymphocyte-rich Hodgkin lymphoma, in remission

● **C81.7**   **Other** Hodgkin lymphoma
Classical Hodgkin lymphoma NOS
Other classical Hodgkin lymphoma

C81.70   Other Hodgkin lymphoma, **unspecified site**

C81.71   Other Hodgkin lymphoma, lymph nodes of **head, face, and neck**

C81.72   Other Hodgkin lymphoma, **intrathoracic** lymph nodes

C81.73   Other Hodgkin lymphoma, **intra-abdominal** lymph nodes

C81.74   Other Hodgkin lymphoma, lymph nodes of **axilla and upper limb**

C81.75   Other Hodgkin lymphoma, lymph nodes of **inguinal region and lower limb**

C81.76   Other Hodgkin lymphoma, **intrapelvic** lymph nodes

C81.77   Other Hodgkin lymphoma, **spleen**

C81.78   Other Hodgkin lymphoma, lymph nodes of **multiple sites**

C81.79   Other Hodgkin lymphoma, **extranodal and solid organ sites**

C81.7A   Other Hodgkin lymphoma, in remission

● **C81.9**   Hodgkin lymphoma, **unspecified**

C81.90   Hodgkin lymphoma, unspecified, **unspecified site**

C81.91   Hodgkin lymphoma, unspecified, lymph nodes of **head, face, and neck**

C81.92   Hodgkin lymphoma, unspecified, **intrathoracic** lymph nodes

C81.93   Hodgkin lymphoma, unspecified, **intra-abdominal** lymph nodes

C81.94   Hodgkin lymphoma, unspecified, lymph nodes of **axilla and upper limb**

C81.95   Hodgkin lymphoma, unspecified, lymph nodes of **inguinal region and lower limb**

C81.96   Hodgkin lymphoma, unspecified, **intrapelvic** lymph nodes

C81.97   Hodgkin lymphoma, unspecified, **spleen**

C81.98   Hodgkin lymphoma, unspecified, lymph nodes of **multiple sites**

C81.99   Hodgkin lymphoma, unspecified, **extranodal and solid organ sites**

C81.9A   Hodgkin lymphoma, unspecified, in remission

● **C82**   **Follicular lymphoma**
Group of malignant lymphomas

   Includes   follicular lymphoma with or without diffuse areas

   Excludes1   mature T/NK-cell lymphomas (C84.-)
personal history of non-Hodgkin lymphoma (Z85.72)

● **C82.0**   Follicular lymphoma grade I

C82.00   Follicular lymphoma grade I, **unspecified site**

C82.01   Follicular lymphoma grade I, lymph nodes of **head, face, and neck**

C82.02   Follicular lymphoma grade I, **intrathoracic** lymph nodes

C82.03   Follicular lymphoma grade I, **intra-abdominal** lymph nodes

C82.04   Follicular lymphoma grade I, lymph nodes of **axilla and upper limb**

▶ New   ⇨ Revised   ~~deleted~~ Deleted   Excludes 1   Excludes 2   Includes   Use additional   Code first   Code also   Key words

OGCR Official Guidelines   X Assign placeholder X   ● Use Additional Character(s)   ▶ Manifestation Code   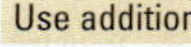 Hierarchical Condition Category   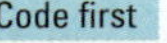 Coding Clinic

C82.05 Follicular lymphoma grade I, lymph nodes of inguinal region and lower limb ℞℞

C82.06 Follicular lymphoma grade I, **intrapelvic** lymph nodes ℞℞

C82.07 Follicular lymphoma grade I, **spleen** ℞℞

C82.08 Follicular lymphoma grade I, lymph nodes of **multiple sites** ℞℞

C82.09 Follicular lymphoma grade I, **extranodal and solid organ sites** ℞℞

C82.0A Follicular lymphoma grade I, in remission

● **C82.1 Follicular lymphoma grade II**

C82.10 Follicular lymphoma grade II, **unspecified site** ℞℞

C82.11 Follicular lymphoma grade II, lymph nodes of **head, face, and neck** ℞℞

C82.12 Follicular lymphoma grade II, **intrathoracic** lymph nodes ℞℞

C82.13 Follicular lymphoma grade II, **intra-abdominal** lymph nodes ℞℞

C82.14 Follicular lymphoma grade II, lymph nodes of **axilla and upper limb** ℞℞

C82.15 Follicular lymphoma grade II, lymph nodes of **inguinal region and lower limb** ℞℞

C82.16 Follicular lymphoma grade II, **intrapelvic** lymph nodes ℞℞

C82.17 Follicular lymphoma grade II, **spleen** ℞℞

C82.18 Follicular lymphoma grade II, lymph nodes of **multiple sites** ℞℞

C82.19 Follicular lymphoma grade II, **extranodal and solid organ sites** ℞℞

C82.1A Follicular lymphoma grade II, in remission

● **C82.2 Follicular lymphoma grade III, unspecified**

C82.20 Follicular lymphoma grade III, unspecified, **unspecified site** ℞℞

C82.21 Follicular lymphoma grade III, unspecified, lymph nodes of **head, face, and neck** ℞℞

C82.22 Follicular lymphoma grade III, unspecified, **intrathoracic lymph nodes** ℞℞

C82.23 Follicular lymphoma grade III, unspecified, **intra-abdominal** lymph nodes ℞℞

C82.24 Follicular lymphoma grade III, unspecified, lymph nodes of **axilla and upper limb** ℞℞

C82.25 Follicular lymphoma grade III, unspecified, lymph nodes of **inguinal region and lower limb** ℞℞

C82.26 Follicular lymphoma grade III, unspecified, **intrapelvic** lymph nodes ℞℞

C82.27 Follicular lymphoma grade III, unspecified, **spleen** ℞℞

C82.28 Follicular lymphoma grade III, unspecified, lymph nodes of **multiple sites** ℞℞

C82.29 Follicular lymphoma grade III, unspecified, **extranodal and solid organ sites** ℞℞

C82.2A Follicular lymphoma grade III, unspecified, in remission

● **C82.3 Follicular lymphoma grade IIIa**

C82.30 Follicular lymphoma grade IIIa, **unspecified site** ℞℞

C82.31 Follicular lymphoma grade IIIa, lymph nodes of **head, face, and neck** ℞℞

C82.32 Follicular lymphoma grade IIIa, **intrathoracic** lymph nodes ℞℞

C82.33 Follicular lymphoma grade IIIa, **intra-abdominal lymph nodes** ℞℞

C82.34 Follicular lymphoma grade IIIa, lymph nodes of **axilla and upper limb** ℞℞

C82.35 Follicular lymphoma grade IIIa, lymph nodes of **inguinal region and lower limb** ℞℞

C82.36 Follicular lymphoma grade IIIa, **intrapelvic** lymph nodes ℞℞

C82.37 Follicular lymphoma grade IIIa, **spleen** ℞℞

C82.38 Follicular lymphoma grade IIIa, lymph nodes of **multiple sites** ℞℞

C82.39 Follicular lymphoma grade IIIa, **extranodal and solid organ sites** ℞℞

C82.3A Follicular lymphoma grade IIIa, in remission

● **C82.4 Follicular lymphoma grade IIIb**

C82.40 Follicular lymphoma grade IIIb, **unspecified site** ℞℞

C82.41 Follicular lymphoma grade IIIb, lymph nodes of **head, face, and neck** ℞℞

C82.42 Follicular lymphoma grade IIIb, **intrathoracic** lymph nodes ℞℞

C82.43 Follicular lymphoma grade IIIb, **intra-abdominal** lymph nodes ℞℞

C82.44 Follicular lymphoma grade IIIb, lymph nodes of **axilla and upper limb** ℞℞

C82.45 Follicular lymphoma grade IIIb, lymph nodes of **inguinal region and lower limb** ℞℞

C82.46 Follicular lymphoma grade IIIb, **intrapelvic** lymph nodes ℞℞

C82.47 Follicular lymphoma grade IIIb, **spleen** ℞℞

C82.48 Follicular lymphoma grade IIIb, lymph nodes of **multiple sites** ℞℞

C82.49 Follicular lymphoma grade IIIb, **extranodal and solid organ sites** ℞℞

C82.4A Follicular lymphoma grade IIIb, in remission

● **C82.5 Diffuse follicle center lymphoma**

C82.50 Diffuse follicle center lymphoma, **unspecified site** ℞℞

C82.51 Diffuse follicle center lymphoma, lymph nodes of **head, face, and neck** ℞℞

C82.52 Diffuse follicle center lymphoma, **intrathoracic** lymph nodes ℞℞

C82.53 Diffuse follicle center lymphoma, **intra-abdominal** lymph nodes ℞℞

C82.54 Diffuse follicle center lymphoma, lymph nodes of **axilla and upper limb** ℞℞

C82.55 Diffuse follicle center lymphoma, lymph nodes of **inguinal region and lower limb** ℞℞

C82.56 Diffuse follicle center lymphoma, **intrapelvic** lymph nodes ℞℞

C82.57 Diffuse follicle center lymphoma, **spleen** ℞℞

C82.58 Diffuse follicle center lymphoma, lymph nodes of **multiple sites** ℞℞

C82.59 Diffuse follicle center lymphoma, **extranodal and solid organ sites** ℞℞

C82.5A Diffuse follicle center lymphoma, in remission

● **C82.6 Cutaneous follicle center lymphoma**

C82.60 Cutaneous follicle center lymphoma, **unspecified site** ℞℞

C82.61 Cutaneous follicle center lymphoma, lymph nodes of **head, face, and neck** ℞℞

C82.62 Cutaneous follicle center lymphoma, **intrathoracic** lymph nodes ℞℞

C82.63 Cutaneous follicle center lymphoma, intra-abdominal lymph nodes

C82.64 Cutaneous follicle center lymphoma, lymph nodes of axilla and upper limb

C82.65 Cutaneous follicle center lymphoma, lymph nodes of inguinal region and lower limb

C82.66 Cutaneous follicle center lymphoma, intrapelvic lymph nodes

C82.67 Cutaneous follicle center lymphoma, spleen

C82.68 Cutaneous follicle center lymphoma, lymph nodes of multiple sites

C82.69 Cutaneous follicle center lymphoma, extranodal and solid organ sites

C82.6A Cutaneous follicle center lymphoma, in remission

● **C82.8** **Other types of follicular lymphoma**

C82.80 Other types of follicular lymphoma, unspecified site

C82.81 Other types of follicular lymphoma, lymph nodes of head, face, and neck

C82.82 Other types of follicular lymphoma, intrathoracic lymph nodes

C82.83 Other types of follicular lymphoma, intra-abdominal lymph nodes

C82.84 Other types of follicular lymphoma, lymph nodes of axilla and upper limb

C82.85 Other types of follicular lymphoma, lymph nodes of inguinal region and lower limb

C82.86 Other types of follicular lymphoma, intra pelvic lymph nodes

C82.87 Other types of follicular lymphoma, spleen

C82.88 Other types of follicular lymphoma, lymph nodes of multiple sites

C82.89 Other types of follicular lymphoma, extranodal and solid organ sites

C82.8A Other types of follicular lymphoma, in remission

● **C82.9** **Follicular lymphoma, unspecified**

C82.90 Follicular lymphoma, unspecified, unspecified site

C82.91 Follicular lymphoma, unspecified, lymph nodes of head, face, and neck

C82.92 Follicular lymphoma, unspecified, intrathoracic lymph nodes

C82.93 Follicular lymphoma, unspecified, intra-abdominal lymph nodes

C82.94 Follicular lymphoma, unspecified, lymph nodes of axilla and upper limb

C82.95 Follicular lymphoma, unspecified, lymph nodes of inguinal region and lower limb

C82.96 Follicular lymphoma, unspecified, intra pelvic lymph nodes

C82.97 Follicular lymphoma, unspecified, spleen

C82.98 Follicular lymphoma, unspecified, lymph nodes of multiple sites

C82.99 Follicular lymphoma, unspecified, extranodal and solid organ sites

C82.9A Follicular lymphoma, unspecified, in remission

● **C83** **Non-follicular lymphoma**

> **Excludes1** personal history of non-Hodgkin lymphoma (Z85.72)

● **C83.0** **Small cell B-cell lymphoma**
Lymphoplasmacytic lymphoma
Nodal marginal zone lymphoma
Non-leukemic variant of B-CLL
Splenic marginal zone lymphoma

> **Excludes1** chronic lymphocytic leukemia (C91.1)
> mature T/NK-cell lymphomas (C84.-)
> Waldenström macroglobulinemia (C88.00)

Coding Clinic: 2023, Q1, P18-19

C83.00 Small cell B-cell lymphoma, unspecified site

C83.01 Small cell B-cell lymphoma, lymph nodes of head, face, and neck

C83.02 Small cell B-cell lymphoma, intrathoracic lymph nodes

C83.03 Small cell B-cell lymphoma, intra-abdominal lymph nodes

C83.04 Small cell B-cell lymphoma, lymph nodes of axilla and upper limb

C83.05 Small cell B-cell lymphoma, lymph nodes of inguinal region and lower limb

C83.06 Small cell B-cell lymphoma, intrapelvic lymph nodes

C83.07 Small cell B-cell lymphoma, spleen

C83.08 Small cell B-cell lymphoma, lymph nodes of multiple sites

C83.09 Small cell B-cell lymphoma, extranodal and solid organ sites

C83.0A Small cell B-cell lymphoma, in remission

● **C83.1** **Mantle cell lymphoma**
Centrocytic lymphoma
Malignant lymphomatous polyposis

C83.10 Mantle cell lymphoma, unspecified site

Coding Clinic: 2024, Q1, P24

C83.11 Mantle cell lymphoma, lymph nodes of head, face, and neck

C83.12 Mantle cell lymphoma, intrathoracic lymph nodes

C83.13 Mantle cell lymphoma, intra-abdominal lymph nodes

C83.14 Mantle cell lymphoma, lymph nodes of axilla and upper limb

C83.15 Mantle cell lymphoma, lymph nodes of inguinal region and lower limb

C83.16 Mantle cell lymphoma, intrapelvic lymph nodes

C83.17 Mantle cell lymphoma, spleen

C83.18 Mantle cell lymphoma, lymph nodes of multiple sites

C83.19 Mantle cell lymphoma, extranodal and solid organ sites

C83.1A Mantle cell lymphoma, in remission
Centrocytic lymphoma, in remission

● **C83.3** **Diffuse large B-cell lymphoma**
Anaplastic diffuse large B-cell lymphoma
CD30-positive diffuse large B-cell lymphoma
Centroblastic diffuse large B-cell lymphoma
Immunoblastic diffuse large B-cell lymphoma
Plasmablastic diffuse large B-cell lymphoma
Diffuse large B-cell lymphoma, subtype not specified
T-cell rich diffuse large B-cell lymphoma

> **Excludes1** mediastinal (thymic) large B-cell lymphoma (C85.2-)
> mature T/NK-cell lymphomas (C84.-)

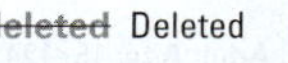 New   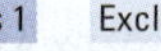 Revised   ~~deleted~~ Deleted   Excludes 1   Excludes 2   Includes   Use additional   Code first   Code also   Key words

OGCR Official Guidelines   **X** Assign placeholder X   ● Use Additional Character(s)   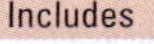 Manifestation Code   Hierarchical Condition Category   **Coding Clinic**

C83.30   **Diffuse large B-cell lymphoma, unspecified site** ᴿᶜ

C83.31   **Diffuse large B-cell lymphoma, lymph nodes of head, face, and neck** ᴿᶜ

C83.32   **Diffuse large B-cell lymphoma, intrathoracic lymph nodes** ᴿᶜ

C83.33   **Diffuse large B-cell lymphoma, intra-abdominal lymph nodes** ᴿᶜ

C83.34   **Diffuse large B-cell lymphoma, lymph nodes of axilla and upper limb** ᴿᶜ

C83.35   **Diffuse large B-cell lymphoma, lymph nodes of inguinal region and lower limb** ᴿᶜ

C83.36   **Diffuse large B-cell lymphoma, intrapelvic lymph nodes** ᴿᶜ

C83.37   **Diffuse large B-cell lymphoma, spleen** ᴿᶜ

C83.38   **Diffuse large B-cell lymphoma, lymph nodes of multiple sites** ᴿᶜ
    Coding Clinic: 2023, Q1, P22

C83.39   **Diffuse large B-cell lymphoma, extranodal and solid organ sites** ᴿᶜ
    Coding Clinic: 2023, Q1, P22

    C83.390   **Primary central nervous system lymphoma**
       PCNSL of brain
       PCNSL of meninges
       PCNSL of spinal cord
       PCNSL NOS

       Excludes1   Primary central nervous system lymphoma, Burkitt (C83.79)
            Primary central nervous system lymphoma, lymphoblastic (C83.59)
            Primary central nervous system lymphoma, other (C83.89)
            Primary central nervous system lymphoma, peripheral T-cell (C84.49)

       C83.398   **Diffuse large B-cell lymphoma of other extranodal and solid organ sites**

C83.3A   **Diffuse large B-cell lymphoma, in remission**

● C83.5   **Lymphoblastic (diffuse) lymphoma**
    Highly malignant type of non-Hodgkin lymphoma with diffuse infiltration
    B-precursor lymphoma
    Lymphoblastic B-cell lymphoma
    Lymphoblastic lymphoma NOS
    Lymphoblastic T-cell lymphoma
    T-precursor lymphoma

C83.50   **Lymphoblastic (diffuse) lymphoma, unspecified site** ᴿᶜ

C83.51   **Lymphoblastic (diffuse) lymphoma, lymph nodes of head, face, and neck** ᴿᶜ

C83.52   **Lymphoblastic (diffuse) lymphoma, intrathoracic lymph nodes** ᴿᶜ

C83.53   **Lymphoblastic (diffuse) lymphoma, intra-abdominal lymph nodes** ᴿᶜ

C83.54   **Lymphoblastic (diffuse) lymphoma, lymph nodes of axilla and upper limb** ᴿᶜ

C83.55   **Lymphoblastic (diffuse) lymphoma, lymph nodes of inguinal region and lower limb** ᴿᶜ

C83.56   **Lymphoblastic (diffuse) lymphoma, intrapelvic lymph nodes** ᴿᶜ

C83.57   **Lymphoblastic (diffuse) lymphoma, spleen** ᴿᶜ

C83.58   **Lymphoblastic (diffuse) lymphoma, lymph nodes of multiple sites** ᴿᶜ

C83.59   **Lymphoblastic (diffuse) lymphoma, extranodal and solid organ sites** ᴿᶜ

C83.5A   **Lymphoblastic (diffuse) lymphoma, in remission**

● C83.7   **Burkitt lymphoma**
    Form of small cell lymphoma
    Atypical Burkitt lymphoma
    Burkitt-like lymphoma

    Excludes1   mature B-cell leukemia Burkitt type (C91.A-)

C83.70   **Burkitt lymphoma, unspecified site** ᴿᶜ

C83.71   **Burkitt lymphoma, lymph nodes of head, face, and neck** ᴿᶜ

C83.72   **Burkitt lymphoma, intrathoracic lymph nodes** ᴿᶜ

C83.73   **Burkitt lymphoma, intra-abdominal lymph nodes** ᴿᶜ

C83.74   **Burkitt lymphoma, lymph nodes of axilla and upper limb** ᴿᶜ

C83.75   **Burkitt lymphoma, lymph nodes of inguinal region and lower limb** ᴿᶜ

C83.76   **Burkitt lymphoma, intrapelvic lymph nodes** ᴿᶜ

C83.77   **Burkitt lymphoma, spleen** ᴿᶜ

C83.78   **Burkitt lymphoma, lymph nodes of multiple sites** ᴿᶜ

C83.79   **Burkitt lymphoma, extranodal and solid organ sites** ᴿᶜ

C83.7A   **Burkitt lymphoma, in remission**

● C83.8   **Other non-follicular lymphoma**
    Intravascular large B-cell lymphoma
    Lymphoid granulomatosis
    Primary effusion B-cell lymphoma

    Excludes1   mediastinal (thymic) large B-cell lymphoma (C85.2-)
            T-cell rich B-cell lymphoma (C83.3-)

C83.80   **Other non-follicular lymphoma, unspecified site** ᴿᶜ

C83.81   **Other non-follicular lymphoma, lymph nodes of head, face, and neck** ᴿᶜ

C83.82   **Other non-follicular lymphoma, intrathoracic lymph nodes** ᴿᶜ

C83.83   **Other non-follicular lymphoma, intra-abdominal lymph nodes** ᴿᶜ

C83.84   **Other non-follicular lymphoma, lymph nodes of axilla and upper limb** ᴿᶜ

C83.85   **Other non-follicular lymphoma, lymph nodes of inguinal region and lower limb** ᴿᶜ

C83.86   **Other non-follicular lymphoma, intrapelvic lymph nodes** ᴿᶜ

C83.87   **Other non-follicular lymphoma, spleen** ᴿᶜ

C83.88   **Other non-follicular lymphoma, lymph nodes of multiple sites** ᴿᶜ

C83.89   **Other non-follicular lymphoma, extranodal and solid organ sites** ᴿᶜ

C83.8A   **Other non-follicular lymphoma, in remission**

● C83.9   **Non-follicular (diffuse) lymphoma, unspecified**

C83.90   **Non-follicular (diffuse) lymphoma, unspecified, unspecified site** ᴿᶜ

C83.91   **Non-follicular (diffuse) lymphoma, unspecified, lymph nodes of head, face, and neck** ᴿᶜ

C83.92   **Non-follicular (diffuse) lymphoma, unspecified, intrathoracic lymph nodes** ᴿᶜ

C83.93   **Non-follicular (diffuse) lymphoma, unspecified, intra-abdominal lymph nodes** ᴿᶜ

C83.94   Non-follicular (diffuse) lymphoma, unspecified, lymph nodes of axilla and upper limb 🅷🅲🅲

C83.95   Non-follicular (diffuse) lymphoma, unspecified, lymph nodes of inguinal region and lower limb 🅷🅲🅲

C83.96   Non-follicular (diffuse) lymphoma, unspecified, intrapelvic lymph nodes 🅷🅲🅲

C83.97   Non-follicular (diffuse) lymphoma, unspecified, spleen 🅷🅲🅲

C83.98   Non-follicular (diffuse) lymphoma, unspecified, lymph nodes of multiple sites 🅷🅲🅲

C83.99   Non-follicular (diffuse) lymphoma, unspecified, extranodal and solid organ sites 🅷🅲🅲

C83.9A   Non-follicular (diffuse) lymphoma, unspecified, in remission

● **C84**   **Mature T/NK-cell lymphomas**

> **Excludes1**   personal history of non-Hodgkin lymphoma (Z85.72)

● **C84.0**   **Mycosis fungoides**
Chronic or rapidly progressive form of cutaneous T-cell lymphoma; AKA granuloma fungoides

> **Excludes1**   peripheral T-cell lymphoma, not elsewhere classified (C84.4-)

C84.00   Mycosis fungoides, unspecified site 🅷🅲🅲

C84.01   Mycosis fungoides, lymph nodes of head, face, and neck 🅷🅲🅲

C84.02   Mycosis fungoides, intrathoracic lymph nodes 🅷🅲🅲

C84.03   Mycosis fungoides, intra-abdominal lymph nodes 🅷🅲🅲

C84.04   Mycosis fungoides, lymph nodes of axilla and upper limb 🅷🅲🅲

C84.05   Mycosis fungoides, lymph nodes of inguinal region and lower limb 🅷🅲🅲

C84.06   Mycosis fungoides, intrapelvic lymph nodes 🅷🅲🅲

C84.07   Mycosis fungoides, spleen 🅷🅲🅲

C84.08   Mycosis fungoides, lymph nodes of multiple sites 🅷🅲🅲

C84.09   Mycosis fungoides, extranodal and solid organ sites 🅷🅲🅲

C84.0A   Mycosis fungoides, in remission

● **C84.1**   **Sézary disease**
Type of cutaneous lymphoma affecting T-cells

C84.10   Sézary disease, unspecified site 🅷🅲🅲

C84.11   Sézary disease, lymph nodes of head, face, and neck 🅷🅲🅲

C84.12   Sézary disease, intrathoracic lymph nodes 🅷🅲🅲

C84.13   Sézary disease, intra-abdominal lymph nodes 🅷🅲🅲

C84.14   Sézary disease, lymph nodes of axilla and upper limb 🅷🅲🅲

C84.15   Sézary disease, lymph nodes of inguinal region and lower limb 🅷🅲🅲

C84.16   Sézary disease, intrapelvic lymph nodes 🅷🅲🅲

C84.17   Sézary disease, spleen 🅷🅲🅲

C84.18   Sézary disease, lymph nodes of multiple sites 🅷🅲🅲

C84.19   Sézary disease, extranodal and solid organ sites 🅷🅲🅲

C84.1A   Sézary disease, in remission

● **C84.4**   **Peripheral T-cell lymphoma, not elsewhere classified**
Diverse group of blood carcinomas originating from T-cells, requiring aggressive chemotherapy
Lennert's lymphoma
Lymphoepithelioid lymphoma
Mature T-cell lymphoma, not elsewhere classified

C84.40   Peripheral T-cell lymphoma, not elsewhere classified, unspecified site 🅷🅲🅲

C84.41   Peripheral T-cell lymphoma, not elsewhere classified, lymph nodes of head, face, and neck 🅷🅲🅲

C84.42   Peripheral T-cell lymphoma, not elsewhere classified, intrathoracic lymph nodes 🅷🅲🅲

C84.43   Peripheral T-cell lymphoma, not elsewhere classified, intra-abdominal lymph nodes 🅷🅲🅲

C84.44   Peripheral T-cell lymphoma, not elsewhere classified, lymph nodes of axilla and upper limb 🅷🅲🅲

C84.45   Peripheral T-cell lymphoma, not elsewhere classified, lymph nodes of inguinal region and lower limb 🅷🅲🅲

C84.46   Peripheral T-cell lymphoma, not elsewhere classified, intrapelvic lymph nodes 🅷🅲🅲

C84.47   Peripheral T-cell lymphoma, not elsewhere classified, spleen 🅷🅲🅲

C84.48   Peripheral T-cell lymphoma, not elsewhere classified, lymph nodes of multiple sites 🅷🅲🅲

C84.49   Peripheral T-cell lymphoma, not elsewhere classified, extranodal and solid organ sites 🅷🅲🅲

C84.4A   Peripheral T-cell lymphoma, not elsewhere classified, in remission

● **C84.6**   **Anaplastic large cell lymphoma, ALK-positive**
Anaplastic large cell lymphoma, CD30-positive

C84.60   Anaplastic large cell lymphoma, ALK-positive, unspecified site 🅷🅲🅲

C84.61   Anaplastic large cell lymphoma, ALK-positive, lymph nodes of head, face, and neck 🅷🅲🅲

C84.62   Anaplastic large cell lymphoma, ALK-positive, intrathoracic lymph nodes 🅷🅲🅲

C84.63   Anaplastic large cell lymphoma, ALK-positive, intra-abdominal lymph nodes 🅷🅲🅲

C84.64   Anaplastic large cell lymphoma, ALK-positive, lymph nodes of axilla and upper limb 🅷🅲🅲

C84.65   Anaplastic large cell lymphoma, ALK-positive, lymph nodes of inguinal region and lower limb 🅷🅲🅲

C84.66   Anaplastic large cell lymphoma, ALK-positive, intrapelvic lymph nodes 🅷🅲🅲

C84.67   Anaplastic large cell lymphoma, ALK-positive, spleen 🅷🅲🅲

C84.68   Anaplastic large cell lymphoma, ALK-positive, lymph nodes of multiple sites 🅷🅲🅲

C84.69   Anaplastic large cell lymphoma, ALK-positive, extranodal and solid organ sites 🅷🅲🅲

C84.6A   Anaplastic large cell lymphoma, ALK-positive, in remission

Item 2–7   Lymphosarcoma, also known as malignant lymphoma, is a cancer of the lymph system exhibiting abnormal cells encompassing an entire lymph node creating a diffuse pattern without any definite organization. Diffuse pattern lymphoma has a more unfavorable survival outlook than those with a follicular or nodular pattern. Reticulosarcoma is the most common aggressive form of non-Hodgkin lymphoma.

● **C84.7   Anaplastic large cell lymphoma, ALK-negative**

    Excludes1   primary cutaneous CD30-positive T-cell proliferations (C86.6-)

    C84.70   Anaplastic large cell lymphoma, ALK-negative, unspecified site

    C84.71   Anaplastic large cell lymphoma, ALK-negative, lymph nodes of head, face, and neck

    C84.72   Anaplastic large cell lymphoma, ALK-negative, intrathoracic lymph nodes

    C84.73   Anaplastic large cell lymphoma, ALK-negative, intra-abdominal lymph nodes

    C84.74   Anaplastic large cell lymphoma, ALK-negative, lymph nodes of axilla and upper limb

    C84.75   Anaplastic large cell lymphoma, ALK-negative, lymph nodes of inguinal region and lower limb

    C84.76   Anaplastic large cell lymphoma, ALK-negative, intrapelvic lymph nodes

    C84.77   Anaplastic large cell lymphoma, ALK-negative, spleen

    C84.78   Anaplastic large cell lymphoma, ALK-negative, lymph nodes of multiple sites

    C84.79   Anaplastic large cell lymphoma, ALK-negative, extranodal and solid organ sites

    C84.7A Anaplastic large cell lymphoma, ALK-negative, breast

       Breast implant associated anaplastic large cell lymphoma (BIA-ALCL)

       Use additional code to identify:

         breast implant status (Z98.82)

         personal history of breast implant removal (Z98.86)

    C84.7B   Anaplastic large cell lymphoma, ALK-negative, in remission

● **C84.9   Mature T/NK-cell lymphomas, unspecified**

    NK/T cell lymphoma NOS

    Excludes1   mature T-cell lymphoma, not elsewhere classified (C84.4-)

    C84.90   Mature T/NK-cell lymphomas, unspecified, unspecified site

    C84.91   Mature T/NK-cell lymphomas, unspecified, lymph nodes of head, face, and neck

    C84.92   Mature T/NK-cell lymphomas, unspecified, intrathoracic lymph nodes

    C84.93   Mature T/NK-cell lymphomas, unspecified, intra-abdominal lymph nodes

    C84.94   Mature T/NK-cell lymphomas, unspecified, lymph nodes of axilla and upper limb

    C84.95   Mature T/NK-cell lymphomas, unspecified, lymph nodes of inguinal region and lower limb

    C84.96   Mature T/NK-cell lymphomas, unspecified, intrapelvic lymph nodes

    C84.97   Mature T/NK-cell lymphomas, unspecified, spleen

    C84.98   Mature T/NK-cell lymphomas, unspecified, lymph nodes of multiple sites

    C84.99   Mature T/NK-cell lymphomas, unspecified, extranodal and solid organ sites

    C84.9A   Mature T/NK-cell lymphomas, unspecified, in remission

● **C84.A   Cutaneous T-cell lymphoma, unspecified**

    C84.A0   Cutaneous T-cell lymphoma, unspecified, unspecified site

    C84.A1   Cutaneous T-cell lymphoma, unspecified lymph nodes of head, face, and neck

    C84.A2   Cutaneous T-cell lymphoma, unspecified, intrathoracic lymph nodes

    C84.A3   Cutaneous T-cell lymphoma, unspecified, intra-abdominal lymph nodes

    C84.A4   Cutaneous T-cell lymphoma, unspecified, lymph nodes of axilla and upper limb

    C84.A5   Cutaneous T-cell lymphoma, unspecified, lymph nodes of inguinal region and lower limb

    C84.A6   Cutaneous T-cell lymphoma, unspecified, intrapelvic lymph nodes

    C84.A7   Cutaneous T-cell lymphoma, unspecified, spleen

       Coding Clinic: 2021, Q2, P7

    C84.A8   Cutaneous T-cell lymphoma, unspecified, lymph nodes of multiple sites

       Coding Clinic: 2021, Q2, P7

    C84.A9   Cutaneous T-cell lymphoma, unspecified, extranodal and solid organ sites

    C84.AA Cutaneous T-cell lymphoma, unspecified, in remission

● **C84.Z   Other mature T/NK-cell lymphomas**

    Note: If T-cell lineage or involvement is mentioned in conjunction with a specific lymphoma, code to the more specific description.

    Excludes1   angioimmunoblastic T-cell lymphoma (C86.50)

       blastic NK-cell lymphoma (C86.40)

       enteropathy-type T-cell lymphoma (C86.20)

       extranodal NK-cell lymphoma, nasal type (C86.00)

       hepatosplenic T-cell lymphoma (C86.10)

       primary cutaneous CD30-positive T-cell proliferations (C86.60)

       subcutaneous panniculitis-like T-cell lymphoma (C86.30)

       T-cell leukemia (C91.1-)

    C84.Z0   Other mature T/NK-cell lymphomas, unspecified site

    C84.Z1   Other mature T/NK-cell lymphomas, lymph nodes of head, face, and neck

    C84.Z2   Other mature T/NK-cell lymphomas, intrathoracic lymph nodes

    C84.Z3   Other mature T/NK-cell lymphomas, intra-abdominal lymph nodes

    C84.Z4   Other mature T/NK-cell lymphomas, lymph nodes of axilla and upper limb

    C84.Z5   Other mature T/NK-cell lymphomas, lymph nodes of inguinal region and lower limb

    C84.Z6   Other mature T/NK-cell lymphomas, intrapelvic lymph nodes

    C84.Z7   Other mature T/NK-cell lymphomas, spleen

    C84.Z8   Other mature T/NK-cell lymphomas, lymph nodes of multiple sites

    C84.Z9   Other mature T/NK-cell lymphomas, extranodal and solid organ sites

    C84.ZA   Other mature T/NK-cell lymphomas, in remission

● **C85   Other specified and unspecified types of non-Hodgkin lymphoma**

> **Excludes1**   other specified types of T/NK-cell lymphoma (C86.-)
> personal history of non-Hodgkin lymphoma (Z85.72)

- ● **C85.1   Unspecified B-cell lymphoma**

  Note: If B-cell lineage or involvement is mentioned in conjunction with a specific lymphoma, code to the more specific description.

  C85.10   Unspecified B-cell lymphoma, unspecified site

  C85.11   Unspecified B-cell lymphoma, lymph nodes of head, face, and neck

  C85.12   Unspecified B-cell lymphoma, intrathoracic lymph nodes

  C85.13   Unspecified B-cell lymphoma, intra-abdominal lymph nodes

  C85.14   Unspecified B-cell lymphoma, lymph nodes of axilla and upper limb

  C85.15   Unspecified B-cell lymphoma, lymph nodes of inguinal region and lower limb

  C85.16   Unspecified B-cell lymphoma, intrapelvic lymph nodes

  C85.17   Unspecified B-cell lymphoma, spleen

  C85.18   Unspecified B-cell lymphoma, lymph nodes of multiple sites

  C85.19   Unspecified B-cell lymphoma, extranodal and solid organ sites

  C85.1A   Unspecified B-cell lymphoma, in remission

- ● **C85.2   Mediastinal (thymic) large B-cell lymphoma**

  C85.20   Mediastinal (thymic) large B-cell lymphoma, unspecified site

  C85.21   Mediastinal (thymic) large B-cell lymphoma, lymph nodes of head, face, and neck

  C85.22   Mediastinal (thymic) large B-cell lymphoma, intrathoracic lymph nodes

  C85.23   Mediastinal (thymic) large B-cell lymphoma, intra-abdominal lymph nodes

  C85.24   Mediastinal (thymic) large B-cell lymphoma, lymph nodes of axilla and upper limb

  C85.25   Mediastinal (thymic) large B-cell lymphoma, lymph nodes of inguinal region and lower limb

  C85.26   Mediastinal (thymic) large B-cell lymphoma, intrapelvic lymph nodes

  C85.27   Mediastinal (thymic) large B-cell lymphoma, spleen

  C85.28   Mediastinal (thymic) large B-cell lymphoma, lymph nodes of multiple sites

  C85.29   Mediastinal (thymic) large B-cell lymphoma, extranodal and solid organ sites

  C85.2A   Mediastinal (thymic) large B-cell lymphoma, in remission

- ● **C85.8   Other specified types of non-Hodgkin lymphoma**

  C85.80   Other specified types of non-Hodgkin lymphoma, unspecified site

  C85.81   Other specified types of non-Hodgkin lymphoma, lymph nodes of head, face, and neck

  C85.82   Other specified types of non-Hodgkin lymphoma, intrathoracic lymph nodes

  C85.83   Other specified types of non-Hodgkin lymphoma, intra-abdominal lymph nodes

  C85.84   Other specified types of non-Hodgkin lymphoma, lymph nodes of axilla and upper limb

C85.85   Other specified types of non-Hodgkin lymphoma, lymph nodes of inguinal region and lower limb

C85.86   Other specified types of non-Hodgkin lymphoma, intrapelvic lymph nodes

C85.87   Other specified types of non-Hodgkin lymphoma, spleen

C85.88   Other specified types of non-Hodgkin lymphoma, lymph nodes of multiple sites

C85.89   Other specified types of non-Hodgkin lymphoma, extranodal and solid organ sites

C85.8A   Other specified types of non-Hodgkin lymphoma, in remission

● **C85.9   Non-Hodgkin lymphoma, unspecified**

Lymphoma NOS
Malignant lymphoma NOS
Non-Hodgkin lymphoma NOS

C85.90   Non-Hodgkin lymphoma, unspecified, unspecified site

C85.91   Non-Hodgkin lymphoma, unspecified, lymph nodes of head, face, and neck

C85.92   Non-Hodgkin lymphoma, unspecified, intrathoracic lymph nodes

C85.93   Non-Hodgkin lymphoma, unspecified, intra-abdominal lymph nodes

C85.94   Non-Hodgkin lymphoma, unspecified, lymph nodes of axilla and upper limb

C85.95   Non-Hodgkin lymphoma, unspecified, lymph nodes of inguinal region and lower limb

C85.96   Non-Hodgkin lymphoma, unspecified, intrapelvic lymph nodes

C85.97   Non-Hodgkin lymphoma, unspecified, spleen

C85.98   Non-Hodgkin lymphoma, unspecified, lymph nodes of multiple sites

C85.99   Non-Hodgkin lymphoma, unspecified, extranodal and solid organ sites

C85.9A   Non-Hodgkin lymphoma, unspecified, in remission

● **C86   Other specified types of T/NK-cell lymphoma**

> **Excludes1**   anaplastic large cell lymphoma, ALK negative (C84.7-)
> anaplastic large cell lymphoma, ALK positive (C84.6-)
> mature T/NK-cell lymphomas (C84.-)
> other specified types of non-Hodgkin lymphoma (C85.8-)

C86.0   Extranodal NK/T-cell lymphoma, nasal type

  C86.00   Extranodal NK/T-cell lymphoma, nasal type not having achieved remission

    Extranodal NK/T-cell lymphoma, nasal type NOS
    Extranodal NK/T-cell lymphoma, nasal type with failed remission

  C86.01   Extranodal NK/T-cell lymphoma, nasal type, in remission

C86.1   Hepatosplenic T-cell lymphoma

  Alpha-beta and gamma delta types

  C86.10   Hepatosplenic T-cell lymphoma not having achieved remission

    Hepatosplenic T-cell lymphoma NOS
    Hepatosplenic T-cell lymphoma with failed remission

  C86.11   Hepatosplenic T-cell lymphoma, in remission

C86.2   Enteropathy-type (intestinal) T-cell lymphoma

  Enteropathy associated T-cell lymphoma

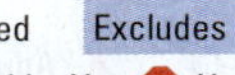

C86.20   Enteropathy-type (intestinal) T-cell lymphoma not having achieved remission
Enteropathy associated T-cell lymphoma NOS
Enteropathy associated T-cell lymphoma not having achieved remission
Enteropathy associated T-cell lymphoma with failed remission
Enteropathy-type (intestinal) T-cell lymphoma NOS
Enteropathy-type (intestinal) T-cell lymphoma with failed remission

C86.21   Enteropathy-type (intestinal) T-cell lymphoma, in remission
Enteropathy associated T-cell lymphoma, in remission

C86.3   Subcutaneous panniculitis-like T-cell lymphoma Ⓡ

C86.30   Subcutaneous panniculitis-like T-cell lymphoma not having achieved remission
Subcutaneous panniculitis-like T-cell lymphoma NOS
Subcutaneous panniculitis-like T-cell lymphoma with failed remission

C86.3   Subcutaneous panniculitis-like T-cell lymphoma, in remission

C86.4   Blastic NK-cell lymphoma Ⓡ
Blastic plasmacytoid dendritic cell neoplasm (BPDCN)

C86.40   Blastic NK-cell lymphoma not having achieved remission
Blastic NK-cell lymphoma NOS
Blastic NK-cell lymphoma with failed remission
Blastic plasmacytoid dendritic cell neoplasm (BPDCN) NOS
Blastic plasmacytoid dendritic cell neoplasm (BPDCN) not having achieved remission
Blastic plasmacytoid dendritic cell neoplasm (BPDCN) with failed remission

C86.41   Blastic NK-cell lymphoma, in remission
Blastic plasmacytoid dendritic cell neoplasm (BPDCN), in remission

C86.5   Angioimmunoblastic T-cell lymphoma Ⓡ
Angioimmunoblastic lymphadenopathy with dysproteinemia (AILD)

C86.50   Angioimmunoblastic T-cell lymphoma not having achieved remission
Angioimmunoblastic lymphadenopathy with dysproteinemia (AILD) NOS
Angioimmunoblastic lymphadenopathy with dysproteinemia (AILD) not having achieved remission
Angioimmunoblastic lymphadenopathy with dysproteinemia (AILD) with failed remission
Angioimmunoblastic T-cell lymphoma NOS
Angioimmunoblastic T-cell lymphoma with failed remission

C86.51   Angioimmunoblastic T-cell lymphoma, in remission
Angioimmunoblastic lymphadenopathy with dysproteinemia (AILD), in remission

C86.6   Primary cutaneous CD30-positive T-cell proliferations Ⓡ
Lymphomatoid papulosis
Primary cutaneous anaplastic large cell lymphoma
Primary cutaneous CD30-positive large T-cell lymphoma

C86.60   Primary cutaneous CD30-positive T-cell proliferations not having achieved remission
Lymphomatoid papulosis NOS
Lymphomatoid papulosis not having achieved remission
Lymphomatoid papulosis with failed remission
Primary cutaneous anaplastic large cell lymphoma NOS
Primary cutaneous anaplastic large cell lymphoma not having achieved remission
Primary cutaneous anaplastic large cell lymphoma with failed remission
Primary cutaneous CD30-positive large T-cell lymphoma NOS
Primary cutaneous CD30-positive large T-cell lymphoma not having achieved remission
Primary cutaneous CD30-positive large T-cell lymphoma with failed remission
Primary cutaneous CD30-positive T-cell proliferations NOS
Primary cutaneous CD30-positive T-cell proliferations with failed remission

C86.61   Primary cutaneous CD30-positive T-cell proliferations, in remission

🔴 **C88   Malignant immunoproliferative diseases and certain other B-cell lymphomas**
Diseases involving immune system

Excludes1 B-cell lymphoma, unspecified (C85.1-)
personal history of other malignant neoplasms of lymphoid, hematopoietic and related tissues (Z85.79)

C88.0   Waldenström's macroglobulinemia Ⓡ
Lymphoplasmacytic lymphoma with IgM-production
Macroglobulinemia (idiopathic) (primary)

Excludes1   small cell B-cell lymphoma (C83.0)

C88.00   Waldenström macroglobulinemia not having achieved remission
Lymphoplasmacytic lymphoma with IgM-production, NOS
Lymphoplasmacytic lymphoma with IgM-production not having achieved remission
Lymphoplasmacytic lymphoma with IgM-production with failed remission
Macroglobulinemia (idiopathic) (primary) NOS
Macroglobulinemia (idiopathic) (primary) not having achieved remission
Macroglobulinemia (idiopathic) (primary) with failed remission
Waldenström macroglobulinemia NOS
Waldenström macroglobulinemia with failed remission

C88.01   Waldenström macroglobulinemia, in remission

C88.2   Heavy chain disease Ⓡ
Franklin disease
Gamma heavy chain disease
Mu heavy chain disease

C88.20 **Heavy chain disease not having achieved remission**
Franklin disease NOS
Franklin disease not having achieved remission
Franklin disease with failed remission
Gamma heavy chain disease NOS
Gamma heavy chain disease not having achieved remission
Gamma heavy chain disease with failed remission
Heavy chain disease NOS
Heavy chain disease with failed remission
Mu heavy chain disease not having achieved remission
Mu heavy chain disease NOS
Mu heavy chain disease not having achieved remission
Mu heavy chain disease with failed remission

C88.21 **Heavy chain disease, in remission**

C88.3 **Immunoproliferative small intestinal disease** 🆁
Alpha heavy chain disease
Mediterranean lymphoma

C88.30 **Immunoproliferative small intestinal disease not having achieved remission**
Alpha heavy chain disease NOS
Alpha heavy chain disease not having achieved remission
Alpha heavy chain disease with failed remission
Immunoproliferative small intestinal disease NOS
Immunoproliferative small intestinal disease with failed remission
Mediterranean lymphoma NOS
Mediterranean lymphoma not having achieved remission
Mediterranean lymphoma with failed remission

C88.31 **Immunoproliferative small intestinal disease, in remission**

C88.4 **Extranodal marginal zone B-cell lymphoma of mucosa-associated lymphoid tissue [MALT-lymphoma]** 🆁
Lymphoma of skin-associated lymphoid tissue [SALT-lymphoma]
Lymphoma of bronchial-associated lymphoid tissue [BALT-lymphoma]

Excludes1 high malignant (diffuse large B-cell) lymphoma (C83.3-)

C88.40 **Extranodal marginal zone B-cell lymphoma of mucosa-associated lymphoid tissue [MALT-lymphoma] not having achieved remission**
Extranodal marginal zone B-cell lymphoma of mucosa-associated lymphoid tissue [MALT-lymphoma] NOS
Extranodal marginal zone B-cell lymphoma of mucosa-associated lymphoid tissue [MALT-lymphoma] with failed remission
Lymphoma of bronchial-associated lymphoid tissue [BALT-lymphoma] NOS
Lymphoma of bronchial-associated lymphoid tissue [BALT-lymphoma] not having achieved remission
Lymphoma of bronchial-associated lymphoid tissue [BALT-lymphoma] with failed remission
Lymphoma of skin-associated lymphoid tissue [SALT-lymphoma] NOS
Lymphoma of skin-associated lymphoid tissue [SALT-lymphoma] not having achieved remission
Lymphoma of skin-associated lymphoid tissue [SALT-lymphoma] with failed remission

C88.41 **Extranodal marginal zone B-cell**

Item 2–8 **Multiple myeloma** is a cancer of a plasma cell (a type of white blood cell) and is an incurable but treatable disease. Immunoproliferative neoplasm is a term for diseases (mostly cancers) in which the immune system cells proliferate.

C88.8 **Other malignant immunoproliferative diseases** 🆁

C88.80 **Other malignant immunoproliferative diseases not having achieved remission**
Other malignant immunoproliferative diseases NOS
Other malignant immunoproliferative diseases with failed remission

C88.81 **Other malignant immunoproliferative diseases, in remission**

C88.9 **Malignant immunoproliferative disease, unspecified** 🆁
Immunoproliferative disease NOS

C88.90 **Malignant immunoproliferative disease, unspecified not having achieved remission**
Immunoproliferative disease NOS
Immunoproliferative disease NOS not having achieved remission
Immunoproliferative disease NOS with failed remission
Malignant immunoproliferative disease, unspecified NOS
Malignant immunoproliferative disease, unspecified with failed remission

C88.91 **Malignant immunoproliferative disease, unspecified, in remission**

🔴 **C90** **Multiple myeloma and malignant plasma cell neoplasms**

Excludes1 personal history of other malignant neoplasms of lymphoid, hematopoietic and related tissues (Z85.79)

🔴 **C90.0** **Multiple myeloma**
Kahler's disease
Medullary plasmacytoma
Myelomatosis
Plasma cell myeloma

Excludes1 solitary myeloma (C90.3-)
solitary plasmacytoma (C90.3-)

C90.00 **Multiple myeloma not having achieved remission** 🆁
Multiple myeloma with failed remission
Multiple myeloma NOS

C90.01 **Multiple myeloma in remission** 🆁

C90.02 **Multiple myeloma in relapse** 🆁

🔴 **C90.1** **Plasma cell leukemia**
Rare type of acute leukemia
Plasmacytic leukemia
Coding Clinic: 2019, Q2, P30

C90.10 **Plasma cell leukemia not having achieved remission** 🆁
Plasma cell leukemia with failed remission
Plasma cell leukemia NOS
Coding Clinic: 2019, Q2, P30

C90.11 **Plasma cell leukemia in remission** 🆁

C90.12 **Plasma cell leukemia in relapse** 🆁

🔴 **C90.2** **Extramedullary plasmacytoma**
Malignant monoclonal plasma cell tumor growing in soft tissue; AKA plasma cell dyscrasias

C90.20 **Extramedullary plasmacytoma not having achieved remission** 🆁
Extramedullary plasmacytoma with failed remission
Extramedullary plasmacytoma NOS

C90.21 **Extramedullary plasmacytoma in remission** 🆁

C90.22 **Extramedullary plasmacytoma in relapse** 🆁

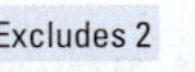
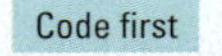

● **C90.3   Solitary plasmacytoma**
Localized malignant plasma cell tumor NOS
Plasmacytoma NOS
Solitary myeloma

    C90.30   Solitary plasmacytoma not having achieved remission 🔴
Solitary plasmacytoma with failed remission
Solitary plasmacytoma NOS

    C90.31   Solitary plasmacytoma in remission 🔴

    C90.32   Solitary plasmacytoma in relapse 🔴

● **C91   Lymphoid leukemia**
Type of leukemia affecting circulating cells of lymphoid origin

    Excludes1   personal history of leukemia (Z85.6)

● **C91.0   Acute lymphoblastic leukemia [ALL]**
Note: Codes in subcategory C91.0 should only be used for T-cell and B-cell precursor leukemia

    C91.00   Acute lymphoblastic leukemia not having achieved remission 🔴
Acute lymphoblastic leukemia with failed remission
Acute lymphoblastic leukemia NOS
Coding Clinic: 2022, Q1, P16

    C91.01   Acute lymphoblastic leukemia, in remission 🔴

    C91.02   Acute lymphoblastic leukemia, in relapse 🔴

● **C91.1   Chronic lymphocytic leukemia of B-cell type**
Lymphoplasmacytic leukemia
Richter syndrome

    Excludes1   lymphoplasmacytic lymphoma (C83.0-)
Coding Clinic: 2023, Q1, P18

    C91.10   Chronic lymphocytic leukemia of B-cell type not having achieved remission 🔴
Chronic lymphocytic leukemia of B-cell type with failed remission
Chronic lymphocytic leukemia of B-cell type NOS

    C91.11   Chronic lymphocytic leukemia of B-cell type in remission 🔴

    C91.12   Chronic lymphocytic leukemia of B-cell type in relapse 🔴

    Coding Clinic: 2023, Q1, P18

● **C91.3   Prolymphocytic leukemia of B-cell type**
Chronic leukemia with symptoms of large number of circulating lymphocytes

    C91.30   Prolymphocytic leukemia of B-cell type not having achieved remission 🔴
Prolymphocytic leukemia of B-cell type with failed remission
Prolymphocytic leukemia of B-cell type NOS

    C91.31   Prolymphocytic leukemia of B-cell type, in remission 🔴

    C91.32   Prolymphocytic leukemia of B-cell type, in relapse 🔴

● **C91.4   Hairy cell leukemia**
Chronic leukemia with splenomegaly and excessive number of abnormal large mononuclear cells covered by hairlike villi
Leukemic reticuloendotheliosis

    C91.40   Hairy cell leukemia not having achieved remission 🔴
Hairy cell leukemia with failed remission
Hairy cell leukemia NOS

    C91.41   Hairy cell leukemia, in remission 🔴

    C91.42   Hairy cell leukemia, in relapse 🔴

● **C91.5   Adult T-cell lymphoma/leukemia (HTLV-1-associated)**
Acute variant of adult T-cell lymphoma/leukemia (HTLV-1-associated)
Chronic variant of adult T-cell lymphoma/leukemia (HTLV-1-associated)
Lymphomatoid variant of adult T-cell lymphoma/leukemia (HTLV-1-associated)
Smouldering variant of adult T-cell lymphoma/leukemia (HTLV-1-associated)

    C91.50   Adult T-cell lymphoma/leukemia (HTLV-1-associated) not having achieved remission 🔴   **A**
Adult T-cell lymphoma/leukemia (HTLV-1-associated) with failed remission
Adult T-cell lymphoma/leukemia (HTLV-1-associated) NOS

    C91.51   Adult T-cell lymphoma/leukemia (HTLV-1-associated), in remission 🔴   **A**

    C91.52   Adult T-cell lymphoma/leukemia (HTLV-1-associated), in relapse 🔴   **A**

● **C91.6   Prolymphocytic leukemia of T-cell type**

    C91.60   Prolymphocytic leukemia of T-cell type not having achieved remission 🔴
Prolymphocytic leukemia of T-cell type with failed remission
Prolymphocytic leukemia of T-cell type NOS

    C91.61   Prolymphocytic leukemia of T-cell type, in remission 🔴

    C91.62   Prolymphocytic leukemia of T-cell type, in relapse 🔴

● **C91.9   Lymphoid leukemia, unspecified**

    C91.90   Lymphoid leukemia, unspecified not having achieved remission 🔴
Lymphoid leukemia with failed remission
Lymphoid leukemia NOS

    C91.91   Lymphoid leukemia, unspecified, in remission 🔴

    C91.92   Lymphoid leukemia, unspecified, in relapse 🔴

● **C91.A   Mature B-cell leukemia Burkitt-type**

    Excludes1   Burkitt lymphoma (C83.7-)

    C91.A0   Mature B-cell leukemia Burkitt-type not having achieved remission 🔴
Mature B-cell leukemia Burkitt-type with failed remission
Mature B-cell leukemia Burkitt-type NOS

    C91.A1   Mature B-cell leukemia Burkitt-type, in remission 🔴

    C91.A2   Mature B-cell leukemia Burkitt-type, in relapse 🔴

● **C91.Z   Other lymphoid leukemia**
T-cell large granular lymphocytic leukemia (associated with rheumatoid arthritis)

    C91.Z0   Other lymphoid leukemia not having achieved remission 🔴
Other lymphoid leukemia with failed remission
Other lymphoid leukemia NOS
Coding Clinic: 2019, Q2, P25

    C91.Z1   Other lymphoid leukemia, in remission 🔴

    C91.Z2   Other lymphoid leukemia, in relapse 🔴

Item 2–9   Leukemia is a cancer (acute or chronic) of the blood-forming tissues of the bone marrow. Blood cells all start out as stem cells. They mature and become red cells, white cells, or platelets. There are three main types of leukocytes (white cells that fight infection): monocytes, lymphocytes, and granulocytes. **Acute monocytic leukemia** (AML) affects monocytes. **Acute lymphoid leukemia** (ALL) affects lymphocytes, and **acute myeloid leukemia** (AML) affects cells that typically develop into white blood cells (not lymphocytes), though it may develop in other blood cells.

CHAPTER 2 (C00-D49)

CHAPTER 2 (C00–D49)

● **C92 Myeloid leukemia**

Code also, if applicable, pancytopenia (acquired) (D61.818)

Includes   granulocytic leukemia
myelogenous leukemia

Excludes1   personal history of leukemia (Z85.6)

Coding Clinic: 2019, Q1, P16

● **C92.0 Acute myeloblastic leukemia**

Acute myeloblastic leukemia, minimal differentiation
Acute myeloblastic leukemia (with maturation)
Acute myeloblastic leukemia 1/ETO
Acute myeloblastic leukemia M0
Acute myeloblastic leukemia M1
Acute myeloblastic leukemia M2
Acute myeloblastic leukemia with t(8;21)
Acute myeloblastic leukemia (without a FAB classification) NOS
Refractory anemia with excess blasts in transformation [RAEB T]

Excludes1   acute exacerbation of chronic myeloid leukemia (C92.10)
refractory anemia with excess of blasts not in transformation (D46.2-)

Coding Clinic: 2018, Q4, P87

C92.00 Acute myeloblastic leukemia, not having achieved remission Ⓡ

Acute myeloblastic leukemia with failed remission
Acute myeloblastic leukemia NOS

C92.01 Acute myeloblastic leukemia, in remission Ⓡ

Coding Clinic: 2021, Q3, P4

C92.02 Acute myeloblastic leukemia, in relapse Ⓡ

Coding Clinic: 2023, Q1, P23

● **C92.1 Chronic myeloid leukemia, BCR/ABL-positive**

Chronic myelogenous leukemia, Philadelphia chromosome (Ph1) positive
Chronic myelogenous leukemia, t(9;22) (q34;q11)
Chronic myelogenous leukemia with crisis of blast cells

Excludes1   atypical chronic myeloid leukemia BCR/ABL-negative (C92.2-)
chronic myelomonocytic leukemia (C93.1-)
chronic myeloproliferative disease (D47.1)

C92.10 Chronic myeloid leukemia, BCR/ABL-positive, not having achieved remission Ⓡ

Chronic myeloid leukemia, BCR/ABL-positive with failed remission
Chronic myeloid leukemia, BCR/ABL-positive NOS

Coding Clinic: 2017, Q1, P7

C92.11 Chronic myeloid leukemia, BCR/ABL-positive, in remission Ⓡ

C92.12 Chronic myeloid leukemia, BCR/ABL-positive, in relapse Ⓡ

● **C92.2 Atypical chronic myeloid leukemia, BCR/ABL-negative**

C92.20 Atypical chronic myeloid leukemia, BCR/ABL-negative, not having achieved remission Ⓡ

Atypical chronic myeloid leukemia, BCR/ABL-negative with failed remission
Atypical chronic myeloid leukemia, BCR/ABL-negative NOS

C92.21 Atypical chronic myeloid leukemia, BCR/ABL-negative, in remission Ⓡ

C92.22 Atypical chronic myeloid leukemia, BCR/ABL-negative, in relapse Ⓡ

● **C92.3 Myeloid sarcoma**

A malignant tumor of immature myeloid cells
Chloroma
Granulocytic sarcoma

C92.30 Myeloid sarcoma, not having achieved remission Ⓡ

Myeloid sarcoma with failed remission
Myeloid sarcoma NOS

C92.31 Myeloid sarcoma, in remission Ⓡ

C92.32 Myeloid sarcoma, in relapse Ⓡ

● **C92.4 Acute promyelocytic leukemia**

AML M3
AML Me with t(15;17) and variants

C92.40 Acute promyelocytic leukemia, not having achieved remission Ⓡ

Acute promyelocytic leukemia with failed remission
Acute promyelocytic leukemia NOS

C92.41 Acute promyelocytic leukemia, in remission Ⓡ

C92.42 Acute promyelocytic leukemia, in relapse Ⓡ

● **C92.5 Acute myelomonocytic leukemia**

AML M4
AML M4 Eo with inv(16) or t(16;16)

C92.50 Acute myelomonocytic leukemia, not having achieved remission Ⓡ

Acute myelomonocytic leukemia with failed remission
Acute myelomonocytic leukemia NOS

C92.51 Acute myelomonocytic leukemia, in remission Ⓡ

C92.52 Acute myelomonocytic leukemia, in relapse Ⓡ

● **C92.6 Acute myeloid leukemia with 11q23-abnormality**

Acute myeloid leukemia with variation of MLL-gene

C92.60 Acute myeloid leukemia with 11q23-abnormality not having achieved remission Ⓡ

Acute myeloid leukemia with 11q23-abnormality with failed remission
Acute myeloid leukemia with 11q23-abnormality NOS

C92.61 Acute myeloid leukemia with 11q23-abnormality in remission Ⓡ

C92.62 Acute myeloid leukemia with 11q23-abnormality in relapse Ⓡ

● **C92.9 Myeloid leukemia, unspecified**

C92.90 Myeloid leukemia, unspecified, not having achieved remission Ⓡ

Myeloid leukemia, unspecified with failed remission
Myeloid leukemia, unspecified NOS

C92.91 Myeloid leukemia, unspecified in remission Ⓡ

C92.92 Myeloid leukemia, unspecified in relapse Ⓡ

● **C92.A Acute myeloid leukemia with multilineage dysplasia**

Acute myeloid leukemia with dysplasia of remaining hematopoesis and/or myelodysplastic disease in its history

C92.A0 Acute myeloid leukemia with multilineage dysplasia, not having achieved remission Ⓡ

Acute myeloid leukemia with multilineage dysplasia with failed remission
Acute myeloid leukemia with multilineage dysplasia NOS

C92.A1 Acute myeloid leukemia with multilineage dysplasia, in remission Ⓡ

C92.A2 Acute myeloid leukemia with multilineage dysplasia, in relapse Ⓡ

▶ New   ➡ Revised   ~~deleted~~ Deleted   Excludes 1   Excludes 2   Includes   Use additional   Code first   Code also   Key words

OGCR Official Guidelines   **X** Assign placeholder X   ● Use Additional Character(s)   ▸ Manifestation Code   Ⓡ Hierarchical Condition Category   **Coding Clinic**

- **C92.Z   Other myeloid leukemia**
  - **C92.Z0   Other myeloid leukemia not having achieved remission**
    - Myeloid leukemia NEC with failed remission
    - Myeloid leukemia NEC
  - **C92.Z1   Other myeloid leukemia, in remission**
  - **C92.Z2   Other myeloid leukemia, in relapse**

- **C93   Monocytic leukemia**
  - **Includes**   monocytoid leukemia
  - **Excludes1**   personal history of leukemia (Z85.6)
  - **C93.0   Acute monoblastic/monocytic leukemia**
    - AML M5
    - AML M5a
    - AML M5b
    - **C93.00   Acute monoblastic/monocytic leukemia, not having achieved remission**
      - Acute monoblastic/monocytic leukemia with failed remission
      - Acute monoblastic/monocytic leukemia NOS
    - **C93.01   Acute monoblastic/monocytic leukemia, in remission**
    - **C93.02   Acute monoblastic/monocytic leukemia, in relapse**
  - **C93.1   Chronic myelomonocytic leukemia**
    - Chronic monocytic leukemia
    - CMML-1
    - CMML-2
    - CMML with eosinophilia
    - Code also, if applicable, eosinophilia (D72.18)
    - **C93.10   Chronic myelomonocytic leukemia not having achieved remission**
      - Chronic myelomonocytic leukemia with failed remission
      - Chronic myelomonocytic leukemia NOS
    - **C93.11   Chronic myelomonocytic leukemia, in remission**
    - **C93.12   Chronic myelomonocytic leukemia, in relapse**
  - **C93.3   Juvenile myelomonocytic leukemia**
    - **C93.30   Juvenile myelomonocytic leukemia, not having achieved remission**   **P**
      - Juvenile myelomonocytic leukemia with failed remission
      - Juvenile myelomonocytic leukemia NOS
    - **C93.31   Juvenile myelomonocytic leukemia, in remission**   **P**
    - **C93.32   Juvenile myelomonocytic leukemia, in relapse**   **P**
  - **C93.9   Monocytic leukemia, unspecified**
    - **C93.90   Monocytic leukemia, unspecified, not having achieved remission**
      - Monocytic leukemia, unspecified with failed remission
      - Monocytic leukemia, unspecified NOS
    - **C93.91   Monocytic leukemia, unspecified in remission**
    - **C93.92   Monocytic leukemia, unspecified in relapse**
  - **C93.Z   Other monocytic leukemia**
    - **C93.Z0   Other monocytic leukemia, not having achieved remission**
      - Other monocytic leukemia NOS
    - **C93.Z1   Other monocytic leukemia, in remission**
    - **C93.Z2   Other monocytic leukemia, in relapse**

- **C94   Other leukemias of specified cell type**
  - **Excludes1**   leukemic reticuloendotheliosis (C91.4-)
    - myelodysplastic syndromes (D46.-)
    - personal history of leukemia (Z85.6)
    - plasma cell leukemia (C90.1-)
  - **C94.0   Acute erythroid leukemia**
    - Acute myeloid leukemia M6(a)(b)
    - Erythroleukemia
    - **C94.00   Acute erythroid leukemia, not having achieved remission**
      - Acute erythroid leukemia with failed remission
      - Acute erythroid leukemia NOS
    - **C94.01   Acute erythroid leukemia, in remission**
    - **C94.02   Acute erythroid leukemia, in relapse**
  - **C94.2   Acute megakaryoblastic leukemia**
    - Acute myeloid leukemia M7
    - Acute megakaryocytic leukemia
    - **C94.20   Acute megakaryoblastic leukemia not having achieved remission**
      - Acute megakaryoblastic leukemia with failed remission
      - Acute megakaryoblastic leukemia NOS
    - **C94.21   Acute megakaryoblastic leukemia, in remission**
    - **C94.22   Acute megakaryoblastic leukemia, in relapse**
  - **C94.3   Mast cell leukemia**
    - **C94.30   Mast cell leukemia not having achieved remission**
      - Mast cell leukemia with failed remission
      - Mast cell leukemia NOS
    - **C94.31   Mast cell leukemia, in remission**
    - **C94.32   Mast cell leukemia, in relapse**
  - **C94.4   Acute panmyelosis with myelofibrosis**
    - Acute myelofibrosis
    - **Excludes1**   myelofibrosis NOS (D75.81)
      - secondary myelofibrosis NOS (D75.81)
    - **C94.40   Acute panmyelosis with myelofibrosis not having achieved remission**
      - Acute myelofibrosis NOS
      - Acute panmyelosis with myelofibrosis with failed remission
      - Acute panmyelosis NOS
    - **C94.41   Acute panmyelosis with myelofibrosis, in remission**
    - **C94.42   Acute panmyelosis with myelofibrosis, in relapse**
  - **C94.6   Myelodysplastic disease, not elsewhere classified**
    - Myelodysplastic/myeloproliferative neoplasm, unclassifiable
    - Myeloproliferative disease, not elsewhere classified
  - **C94.8   Other specified leukemias**
    - Aggressive NK-cell leukemia
    - Acute basophilic leukemia
    - Code also, if applicable, eosinophilia (D72.18)
    - **C94.80   Other specified leukemias not having achieved remission**
      - Other specified leukemia with failed remission
      - Other specified leukemias NOS
    - **C94.81   Other specified leukemias, in remission**
    - **C94.82   Other specified leukemias, in relapse**

● **C95   Leukemia of unspecified cell type**
     Excludes1   personal history of leukemia (Z85.6)

● **C95.0   Acute leukemia of unspecified cell type**
     Acute bilineal leukemia
     Acute mixed lineage leukemia
     Biphenotypic acute leukemia
     Stem cell leukemia of unclear lineage
       Excludes1   acute exacerbation of unspecified chronic leukemia (C95.10)

     C95.00   Acute leukemia of unspecified cell type not having achieved remission (RCC)
       Acute leukemia of unspecified cell type with failed remission
       Acute leukemia NOS

     C95.01   Acute leukemia of unspecified cell type, in remission (RCC)

     C95.02   Acute leukemia of unspecified cell type, in relapse (RCC)

● **C95.1   Chronic leukemia of unspecified cell type**
     C95.10   Chronic leukemia of unspecified cell type not having achieved remission (RCC)
       Chronic leukemia of unspecified cell type with failed remission
       Chronic leukemia NOS

     C95.11   Chronic leukemia of unspecified cell type, in remission (RCC)

     C95.12   Chronic leukemia of unspecified cell type, in relapse (RCC)

● **C95.9   Leukemia, unspecified**
     C95.90   Leukemia, unspecified not having achieved remission (RCC)
       Leukemia, unspecified with failed remission
       Leukemia NOS

     C95.91   Leukemia, unspecified, in remission (RCC)

     C95.92   Leukemia, unspecified, in relapse (RCC)

● **C96   Other and unspecified malignant neoplasms of lymphoid, hematopoietic and related tissue**
     Excludes1   personal history of other malignant neoplasms of lymphoid, hematopoietic and related tissues (Z85.79)

     C96.0   Multifocal and multisystemic (disseminated) Langerhans-cell histiocytosis (RCC)
       Histiocytosis X, multisystemic
       Letterer-Siwe disease
       Excludes1   adult pulmonary Langerhans cell histiocytosis (J84.82)
           multifocal and unisystemic Langerhans-cell histiocytosis (C96.5)
           unifocal Langerhans-cell histiocytosis (C96.6)

● **C96.2   Malignant mast cell neoplasm**
     Excludes1   indolent mastocytosis (D47.02)
           mast cell leukemia (C94.30)
           mastocytosis (congenital) (cutaneous) (Q82.2)

     C96.20   Malignant mast cell neoplasm, unspecified (RCC)

     C96.21   Aggressive systemic mastocytosis (RCC)

     C96.22   Mast cell sarcoma (RCC)

     C96.29   Other malignant mast cell neoplasm (RCC)

     C96.4   Sarcoma of dendritic cells (accessory cells) (RCC)
       Follicular dendritic cell sarcoma
       Interdigitating dendritic cell sarcoma
       Langerhans cell sarcoma

     C96.5   Multifocal and unisystemic Langerhans-cell histiocytosis (RCC)
       Hand-Schüller-Christian disease
       Histiocytosis X, multifocal
       Excludes1   multifocal and multisystemic (disseminated) Langerhans-cell histiocytosis (C96.0)
           unifocal Langerhans-cell histiocytosis (C96.6)

     C96.6   Unifocal Langerhans-cell histiocytosis (RCC)
       Eosinophilic granuloma
       Histiocytosis X, unifocal
       Histiocytosis X NOS
       Langerhans-cell histiocytosis NOS
       Excludes1   multifocal and multisysemic (disseminated) Langerhans-cell histiocytosis (C96.0)
           multifocal and unisystemic Langerhans-cell histiocytosis (C96.5)

     C96.9   Malignant neoplasm of lymphoid, hematopoietic and related tissue, unspecified (RCC)

     C96.A   Histiocytic sarcoma (RCC)
       Malignant histiocytosis

     C96.Z   Other specified malignant neoplasms of lymphoid, hematopoietic and related tissue (RCC)

IN SITU NEOPLASMS (D00-D09)

In situ is carcinoma involving cells in localized tissues that has not spread to nearby tissues

Includes   Bowen's disease
       erythroplasia
       grade III intraepithelial neoplasia
       Queyrat's erythroplasia

● **D00   Carcinoma in situ of oral cavity, esophagus and stomach**
     Excludes1   melanoma in situ (D03.-)

● **D00.0   Carcinoma in situ of lip, oral cavity and pharynx**
     Use additional code to identify:
     exposure to environmental tobacco smoke (Z77.22)
     exposure to tobacco smoke in the perinatal period (P96.81)
     history of tobacco dependence (Z87.891)
     occupational exposure to environmental tobacco smoke (Z57.31)
     tobacco dependence (F17.-)
     tobacco use (Z72.0)
       Excludes1   carcinoma in situ of aryepiglottic fold or interarytenoid fold, laryngeal aspect (D02.0)
           carcinoma in situ of epiglottis NOS (D02.0)
           carcinoma in situ of epiglottis suprahyoid portion (D02.0)
           carcinoma in situ of skin of lip (D03.0, D04.0)

     D00.00   Carcinoma in situ of oral cavity, unspecified site

     D00.01   Carcinoma in situ of labial mucosa and vermilion border

     D00.02   Carcinoma in situ of buccal mucosa

     D00.03   Carcinoma in situ of gingiva and edentulous alveolar ridge

     D00.04   Carcinoma in situ of soft palate

     D00.05   Carcinoma in situ of hard palate

     D00.06   Carcinoma in situ of floor of mouth

     D00.07   Carcinoma in situ of tongue

     D00.08   Carcinoma in situ of pharynx
       Carcinoma in situ of aryepiglottic fold NOS
       Carcinoma in situ of hypopharyngeal aspect of aryepiglottic fold
       Carcinoma in situ of marginal zone of aryepiglottic fold

     D00.1   Carcinoma in situ of esophagus

     D00.2   Carcinoma in situ of stomach

- **D01** Carcinoma in situ of **other and unspecified digestive organs**
    - **Excludes1**   melanoma in situ (D03.-)
  - **D01.0** Carcinoma in situ of **colon**
      - **Excludes1**   carcinoma in situ of rectosigmoid junction (D01.1)
  - **D01.1** Carcinoma in situ of **rectosigmoid junction**
  - **D01.2** Carcinoma in situ of **rectum**
  - **D01.3** Carcinoma in situ of **anus and anal canal**
      Anal intraepithelial neoplasia III [AIN III]
      Severe dysplasia of anus
      - **Excludes1**   anal intraepithelial neoplasia I and II [AIN I and AIN II] (K62.82)
          carcinoma in situ of anal margin (D04.5)
          carcinoma in situ of anal skin (D04.5)
          carcinoma in situ of perianal skin (D04.5)
  - **D01.4** Carcinoma in situ of **other and unspecified** parts of intestine
      - **Excludes1**   carcinoma in situ of ampulla of Vater (D01.5)
      - **D01.40** Carcinoma in situ of **unspecified** part of intestine
      - **D01.49** Carcinoma in situ of **other** parts of intestine
  - **D01.5** Carcinoma in situ of **liver, gallbladder and bile ducts**
      Carcinoma in situ of ampulla of Vater
  - **D01.7** Carcinoma in situ of **other specified digestive organs**
      Carcinoma in situ of pancreas
  - **D01.9** Carcinoma in situ of digestive organ, **unspecified**

- **D02** Carcinoma in situ of **middle ear and respiratory system**
    Use additional code to identify:
      exposure to environmental tobacco smoke (Z77.22)
      exposure to tobacco smoke in the perinatal period (P96.81)
      history of tobacco dependence (Z87.891)
      occupational exposure to environmental tobacco smoke (Z57.31)
      tobacco dependence (F17.-)
      tobacco use (Z72.0)
    - **Excludes1**   melanoma in situ (D03.-)
  - **D02.0** Carcinoma in situ of **larynx**
      Carcinoma in situ of aryepiglottic fold or interarytenoid fold, laryngeal aspect
      Carcinoma in situ of epiglottis (suprahyoid portion)
      - **Excludes1**   carcinoma in situ of aryepiglottic fold or interarytenoid fold NOS (D00.08)
          carcinoma in situ of hypopharyngeal aspect (D00.08)
          carcinoma in situ of marginal zone (D00.08)
  - **D02.1** Carcinoma in situ of **trachea**
  - **D02.2** Carcinoma in situ of **bronchus and lung**
      - **D02.20** Carcinoma in situ of **unspecified** bronchus and lung
      - **D02.21** Carcinoma in situ of **right** bronchus and lung
      - **D02.22** Carcinoma in situ of **left** bronchus and lung
  - **D02.3** Carcinoma in situ of **other parts of respiratory system**
      Carcinoma in situ of accessory sinuses
      Carcinoma in situ of middle ear
      Carcinoma in situ of nasal cavities
      - **Excludes1**   carcinoma in situ of ear (external) (skin) (D04.2-)
          carcinoma in situ of nose NOS (D09.8)
          carcinoma in situ of skin of nose (D04.3)
  - **D02.4** Carcinoma in situ of respiratory system, **unspecified**

- **D03** **Melanoma in situ**
  - **D03.0** Melanoma in situ of **lip**
  - **D03.1** Melanoma in situ of **eyelid, including canthus**
      - **D03.10** Melanoma in situ of **unspecified** eyelid, including canthus
      - **D03.11** Melanoma in situ of **right** eyelid, including canthus
        - **D03.111** Melanoma in situ of right upper eyelid, including canthus
        - **D03.112** Melanoma in situ of right lower eyelid, including canthus
      - **D03.12** Melanoma in situ of **left** eyelid, including canthus
        - **D03.121** Melanoma in situ of left upper eyelid, including canthus
        - **D03.122** Melanoma in situ of left lower eyelid, including canthus
  - **D03.2** Melanoma in situ of **ear and external auricular canal**
      - **D03.20** Melanoma in situ of **unspecified** ear and external auricular canal
      - **D03.21** Melanoma in situ of **right** ear and external auricular canal
      - **D03.22** Melanoma in situ of **left** ear and external auricular canal
  - **D03.3** Melanoma in situ of **other and unspecified parts of face**
      - **D03.30** Melanoma in situ of **unspecified** part of face
      - **D03.39** Melanoma in situ of **other** parts of face
  - **D03.4** Melanoma in situ of **scalp and neck**
  - **D03.5** Melanoma in situ of **trunk**
      - **D03.51** Melanoma in situ of **anal skin**
          Melanoma in situ of anal margin
          Melanoma in situ of perianal skin
      - **D03.52** Melanoma in situ of **breast (skin) (soft tissue)**
      - **D03.59** Melanoma in situ of **other** part of trunk
  - **D03.6** Melanoma in situ of **upper limb, including shoulder**
      - **D03.60** Melanoma in situ of **unspecified** upper limb, including shoulder
      - **D03.61** Melanoma in situ of **right** upper limb, including shoulder
      - **D03.62** Melanoma in situ of **left** upper limb, including shoulder
  - **D03.7** Melanoma in situ of **lower limb, including hip**
      - **D03.70** Melanoma in situ of **unspecified** lower limb, including hip
      - **D03.71** Melanoma in situ of **right** lower limb, including hip
      - **D03.72** Melanoma in situ of **left** lower limb, including hip
  - **D03.8** Melanoma in situ of **other sites**
      Melanoma in situ of scrotum
      - **Excludes1**   carcinoma in situ of scrotum (D07.61)
  - **D03.9** Melanoma in situ, **unspecified**

- **D04** Carcinoma in situ of **skin**
    - **Excludes1**   erythroplasia of Queyrat (penis) NOS (D07.4)
        melanoma in situ (D03.-)
  - **D04.0** Carcinoma in situ of **skin of lip**
      - **Excludes2**   carcinoma in situ of vermilion border of lip (D00.01)
  - **D04.1** Carcinoma in situ of skin of **eyelid, including canthus**
      - **D04.10** Carcinoma in situ of skin of **unspecified** eyelid, including canthus
      - **D04.11** Carcinoma in situ of skin of **right** eyelid, including canthus
        - **D04.111** Carcinoma in situ of skin of right upper eyelid, including canthus
        - **D04.112** Carcinoma in situ of skin of right lower eyelid, including canthus
      - **D04.12** Carcinoma in situ of skin of **left** eyelid, including canthus
        - **D04.121** Carcinoma in situ of skin of left upper eyelid, including canthus
        - **D04.122** Carcinoma in situ of skin of left lower eyelid, including canthus

CHAPTER 2 (C00-D49)

CHAPTER 2 (C00–D49)

● **D04.2** Carcinoma in situ of skin of ear and external auricular canal

    D04.20 Carcinoma in situ of skin of unspecified ear and external auricular canal

    D04.21 Carcinoma in situ of skin of right ear and external auricular canal

    D04.22 Carcinoma in situ of skin of left ear and external auricular canal

● **D04.3** Carcinoma in situ of skin of other and unspecified parts of face

    D04.30 Carcinoma in situ of skin of unspecified part of face

    D04.39 Carcinoma in situ of skin of other parts of face

D04.4 Carcinoma in situ of skin of scalp and neck

D04.5 Carcinoma in situ of skin of trunk
    Carcinoma in situ of anal margin
    Carcinoma in situ of anal skin
    Carcinoma in situ of perianal skin
    Carcinoma in situ of skin of breast

    Excludes 1   carcinoma in situ of anus NOS (D01.3)
         carcinoma in situ of scrotum (D07.61)
         carcinoma in situ of skin of genital organs (D07.-)

● **D04.6** Carcinoma in situ of skin of upper limb, including shoulder

    D04.60 Carcinoma in situ of skin of unspecified upper limb, including shoulder

    D04.61 Carcinoma in situ of skin of right upper limb, including shoulder

    D04.62 Carcinoma in situ of skin of left upper limb, including shoulder

● **D04.7** Carcinoma in situ of skin of lower limb, including hip

    D04.70 Carcinoma in situ of skin of unspecified lower limb, including hip

    D04.71 Carcinoma in situ of skin of right lower limb, including hip

    D04.72 Carcinoma in situ of skin of left lower limb, including hip

D04.8 Carcinoma in situ of skin of other sites

D04.9 Carcinoma in situ of skin, unspecified

● **D05** Carcinoma in situ of breast

    Excludes 1   carcinoma in situ of skin of breast (D04.5)
         melanoma in situ of breast (skin) (D03.5)
         Paget's disease of breast or nipple (C50.-)

    Excludes 2   malignant neoplasm of breast (C50.-)

● **D05.0** Lobular carcinoma in situ of breast

    D05.00 Lobular carcinoma in situ of unspecified breast

    D05.01 Lobular carcinoma in situ of right breast

    D05.02 Lobular carcinoma in situ of left breast

● **D05.1** Intraductal carcinoma in situ of breast

    D05.10 Intraductal carcinoma in situ of unspecified breast

    D05.11 Intraductal carcinoma in situ of right breast

    D05.12 Intraductal carcinoma in situ of left breast

● **D05.8** Other specified type of carcinoma in situ of breast

    D05.80 Other specified type of carcinoma in situ of unspecified breast

    D05.81 Other specified type of carcinoma in situ of right breast

    D05.82 Other specified type of carcinoma in situ of left breast

● **D05.9** Unspecified type of carcinoma in situ of breast

    D05.90 Unspecified type of carcinoma in situ of unspecified breast

    D05.91 Unspecified type of carcinoma in situ of right breast

    D05.92 Unspecified type of carcinoma in situ of left breast

● **D06** Carcinoma in situ of cervix uteri

    Includes   cervical adenocarcinoma in situ
         cervical intraepithelial glandular neoplasia
         cervical intraepithelial neoplasia III [CIN III]
         severe dysplasia of cervix uteri

    Excludes 1   cervical intraepithelial neoplasia II [CIN II] (N87.1)
         cytologic evidence of malignancy of cervix without histologic confirmation (R87.614)
         high grade squamous intraepithelial lesion (HGSIL) of cervix (R87.613)
         melanoma in situ of cervix (D03.5)
         moderate cervical dysplasia (N87.1)

D06.0 Carcinoma in situ of endocervix

D06.1 Carcinoma in situ of exocervix

D06.7 Carcinoma in situ of other parts of cervix

D06.9 Carcinoma in situ of cervix, unspecified

● **D07** Carcinoma in situ of other and unspecified genital organs

    Excludes 1   melanoma in situ of trunk (D03.5)

D07.0 Carcinoma in situ of endometrium

D07.1 Carcinoma in situ of vulva
    Severe dysplasia of vulva
    Vulvar intraepithelial neoplasia III [VIN III]

    Excludes 1   moderate dysplasia of vulva (N90.1)
         vulvar intraepithelial neoplasia II [VIN II] (N90.1)

D07.2 Carcinoma in situ of vagina
    Severe dysplasia of vagina
    Vaginal intraepithelial neoplasia III [VIN III]

    Excludes 1   moderate dysplasia of vagina (N89.1)
         vaginal intraepithelial neoplasia II [VIN II] (N89.1)

● **D07.3** Carcinoma in situ of other and unspecified female genital organs

    D07.30 Carcinoma in situ of unspecified female genital organs

    D07.39 Carcinoma in situ of other female genital organs

D07.4 Carcinoma in situ of penis
    Erythroplasia of Queyrat NOS

D07.5 Carcinoma in situ of prostate
    Prostatic intraepithelial neoplasia III (PIN III)
    Severe dysplasia of prostate

    Excludes 1   dysplasia (mild) (moderate) of prostate (N42.3-)
         prostatic intraepithelial neoplasia II [PIN II] (N42.3-)

● **D07.6** Carcinoma in situ of other and unspecified male genital organs

    D07.60 Carcinoma in situ of unspecified male genital organs

    D07.61 Carcinoma in situ of scrotum

    D07.69 Carcinoma in situ of other male genital organs

● **D09** Carcinoma in situ of other and unspecified sites

    Excludes 1   melanoma in situ (D03.-)

D09.0 Carcinoma in situ of bladder

● **D09.1** Carcinoma in situ of other and unspecified urinary organs

    D09.10 Carcinoma in situ of unspecified urinary organ

    D09.19 Carcinoma in situ of other urinary organs

● **D09.2** Carcinoma in situ of eye

    Excludes 1   carcinoma in situ of skin of eyelid (D04.1-)

    D09.20 Carcinoma in situ of unspecified eye

    D09.21 Carcinoma in situ of right eye

    D09.22 Carcinoma in situ of left eye

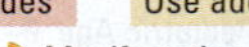

▶ New   ⇒ Revised   ~~deleted~~ Deleted   Excludes 1   Excludes 2   Includes   Use additional   Code first   Code also   Key words
OGCR Official Guidelines   X Assign placeholder X   ● Use Additional Character(s)   ▶ Manifestation Code   **HCC** Hierarchical Condition Category   **Coding Clinic**

D09.3   Carcinoma in situ of **thyroid and other endocrine glands**
> **Excludes1**   carcinoma in situ of endocrine pancreas (D01.7)
> carcinoma in situ of ovary (D07.39)
> carcinoma in situ of testis (D07.69)

D09.8   Carcinoma in situ of **other specified sites**

D09.9   Carcinoma in situ, **unspecified**

BENIGN NEOPLASMS, EXCEPT BENIGN NEUROENDOCRINE TUMORS (D10-D36)

● **D10**   Benign neoplasm of **mouth and pharynx**

D10.0   Benign neoplasm of **lip**
> Benign neoplasm of lip (frenulum) (inner aspect) (mucosa) (vermilion border)
> **Excludes1**   benign neoplasm of skin of lip (D22.0, D23.0)

D10.1   Benign neoplasm of **tongue**
> Benign neoplasm of lingual tonsil

D10.2   Benign neoplasm of **floor of mouth**

● D10.3   Benign neoplasm of **other and unspecified** parts of mouth

D10.30   Benign neoplasm of **unspecified** part of mouth

D10.39   Benign neoplasm of **other parts of mouth**
> Benign neoplasm of minor salivary gland NOS
> **Excludes1**   benign odontogenic neoplasms (D16.4-D16.5)
> benign neoplasm of mucosa of lip (D10.0)
> benign neoplasm of nasopharyngeal surface of soft palate (D10.6)

D10.4   Benign neoplasm of **tonsil**
> Benign neoplasm of tonsil (faucial) (palatine)
> **Excludes1**   benign neoplasm of lingual tonsil (D10.1)
> benign neoplasm of pharyngeal tonsil (D10.6)
> benign neoplasm of tonsillar fossa (D10.5)
> benign neoplasm of tonsillar pillars (D10.5)

D10.5   Benign neoplasm of **other parts of oropharynx**
> *Division of pharynx lying between soft palate and upper edge of epiglottis*
> Benign neoplasm of epiglottis, anterior aspect
> Benign neoplasm of tonsillar fossa
> Benign neoplasm of tonsillar pillars
> Benign neoplasm of vallecula
> **Excludes1**   benign neoplasm of epiglottis NOS (D14.1)
> benign neoplasm of epiglottis, suprahyoid portion (D14.1)

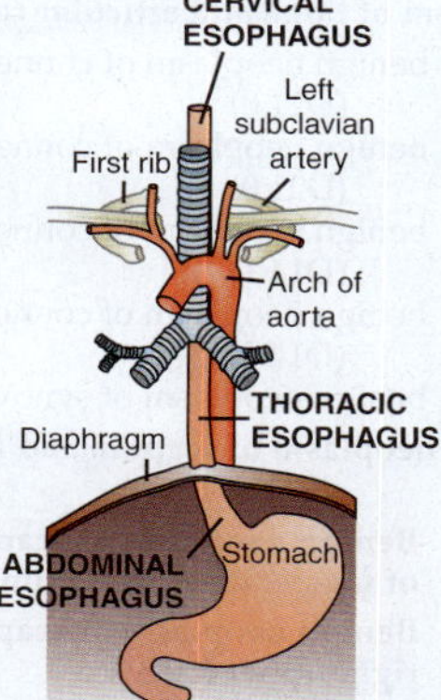

Figure 2-16   The esophagus is the muscular tube that connects the pharynx and the stomach. The 10 inch (25 cm) long esophagus is divided into three parts: **cervical, thoracic,** and **abdominal.**

D10.6   Benign neoplasm of **nasopharynx**
> *Segment of pharynx that lies above soft palate*
> Benign neoplasm of pharyngeal tonsil
> Benign neoplasm of posterior margin of septum and choanae

D10.7   Benign neoplasm of **hypopharynx**
> *Segment of pharynx that lies below upper edge of epiglottis and opens into larynx and esophagus*

D10.9   Benign neoplasm of **pharynx, unspecified**

● **D11**   Benign neoplasm of **major salivary glands**
> **Excludes1**   benign neoplasms of specified minor salivary glands which are classified according to their anatomical location
> benign neoplasms of minor salivary glands NOS (D10.39)

D11.0   Benign neoplasm of **parotid gland**

D11.7   Benign neoplasm of **other major salivary glands**
> Benign neoplasm of sublingual salivary gland
> Benign neoplasm of submandibular salivary gland

D11.9   Benign neoplasm of major salivary gland, **unspecified**

● **D12**   Benign neoplasm of **colon, rectum, anus and anal canal**
> **Excludes2**   benign carcinoid tumors of the large intestine and rectum (D3A.02-)
> polyp of colon NOS (K63.5)

> **Coding Clinic: 2017, Q1, P15; 2015, Q2, P14**

D12.0   Benign neoplasm of **cecum**
> Benign neoplasm of ileocecal valve

D12.1   Benign neoplasm of **appendix**
> **Excludes1**   benign carcinoid tumor of the appendix (D3A.020)

D12.2   Benign neoplasm of **ascending colon**
> **Coding Clinic: 2018, Q2, P14; 2017, Q1, P15**

D12.3   Benign neoplasm of **transverse colon**
> Benign neoplasm of hepatic flexure
> Benign neoplasm of splenic flexure
> *Flexure is a bending in a structure or organ. Note the three flexures illustrated in Figure 2–17. Hepatic = liver, sigmoid = colon, splenic = spleen.*
> **Coding Clinic: 2017, Q1, P16**

D12.4   Benign neoplasm of **descending colon**
> **Coding Clinic: 2015, Q2, P14**

D12.5   Benign neoplasm of **sigmoid colon**

D12.6   Benign neoplasm of **colon, unspecified**
> Adenomatosis of colon
> Benign neoplasm of large intestine NOS
> Polyposis (hereditary) of colon
> ~~**Excludes1**   inflammatory polyp of colon (K51.4-)~~
> ▶ **Excludes2**   inflammatory polyp of colon (K51.4-)
> **Coding Clinic: 2017, Q1, P8-9**

D12.7   Benign neoplasm of **rectosigmoid junction**
> *Angle where sigmoid colon becomes rectum*

D12.8   Benign neoplasm of **rectum**
> **Excludes1**   benign carcinoid tumor of the rectum (D3A.026)
> **Coding Clinic: 2018, Q1, P7**

D12.9   Benign neoplasm of **anus and anal canal**
> Benign neoplasm of anus NOS
> **Excludes1**   benign neoplasm of anal margin (D22.5, D23.5)
> benign neoplasm of anal skin (D22.5, D23.5)
> benign neoplasm of perianal skin (D22.5, D23.5)

CHAPTER 2 (C00-D49)

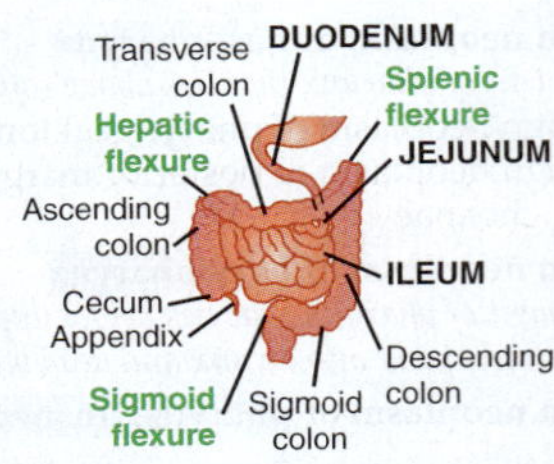

Figure 2-17 Small intestine and colon.

● **D13** Benign neoplasm of other and ill-defined parts of digestive system

    Excludes1   benign stromal tumors of digestive system (D21.4)

  D13.0 Benign neoplasm of esophagus

  D13.1 Benign neoplasm of stomach

    Excludes1   benign carcinoid tumor of the stomach (D3A.092)

  D13.2 Benign neoplasm of duodenum

    Excludes1   benign carcinoid tumor of the duodenum (D3A.010)

●   **D13.3** Benign neoplasm of other and unspecified parts of small intestine

    Excludes1   benign carcinoid tumors of the small intestine (D3A.01-)
        benign neoplasm of ileocecal valve (D12.0)

    D13.30 Benign neoplasm of unspecified part of small intestine

    D13.39 Benign neoplasm of other parts of small intestine

  D13.4 Benign neoplasm of liver
    Benign neoplasm of intrahepatic bile ducts

  D13.5 Benign neoplasm of extrahepatic bile ducts
    Extensions of common hepatic bile duct (tube that collects bile from liver)

  D13.6 Benign neoplasm of pancreas

    Excludes1   benign neoplasm of endocrine pancreas (D13.7)

  D13.7 Benign neoplasm of endocrine pancreas
    Pancreatic islets: Cells scattered throughout pancreas
    Islet cell tumor
    Benign neoplasm of islets of Langerhans
    Use additional code to identify any functional activity.

  D13.9 Benign neoplasm of ill-defined sites within the digestive system

  D13.91 Familial adenomatous polyposis
    Code also associated conditions, such as:
        benign neoplasm of colon (D12.6)
        malignant neoplasm of colon (C18.-)

  D13.99 Benign neoplasm of ill-defined sites within the digestive system
    Benign neoplasm of digestive system NOS
    Benign neoplasm of intestine NOS
    Benign neoplasm of spleen

● **D14** Benign neoplasm of middle ear and respiratory system

  D14.0 Benign neoplasm of middle ear, nasal cavity and accessory sinuses
    Benign neoplasm of cartilage of nose

    Excludes1   benign neoplasm of auricular canal (external) (D22.2-, D23.2-)
        benign neoplasm of bone of ear (D16.4)
        benign neoplasm of bone of nose (D16.4)
        benign neoplasm of cartilage of ear (D21.0)
        benign neoplasm of ear (external) (skin) (D22.2-, D23.2-)
        benign neoplasm of nose NOS (D36.7)
        benign neoplasm of skin of nose (D22.39, D23.39)
        benign neoplasm of olfactory bulb (D33.3)
        benign neoplasm of posterior margin of septum and choanae (D10.6)
        polyp of accessory sinus (J33.8)
        polyp of ear (middle) (H74.4)
        polyp of nasal (cavity) (J33.-)

  D14.1 Benign neoplasm of larynx
    Adenomatous polyp of larynx
    Benign neoplasm of epiglottis (suprahyoid portion)
    Horseshoe-shaped bone in anterior midline of neck between chin and thyroid cartilage

    Excludes1   benign neoplasm of epiglottis, anterior aspect (D10.5)
        polyp (nonadenomatous) of vocal cord or larynx (J38.1)

  D14.2 Benign neoplasm of trachea

●   **D14.3** Benign neoplasm of bronchus and lung

    Excludes1   benign carcinoid tumor of the bronchus and lung (D3A.090)

    D14.30 Benign neoplasm of unspecified bronchus and lung

    D14.31 Benign neoplasm of right bronchus and lung

    D14.32 Benign neoplasm of left bronchus and lung

  D14.4 Benign neoplasm of respiratory system, unspecified

● **D15** Benign neoplasm of other and unspecified intrathoracic organs

    Excludes1   benign neoplasm of mesothelial tissue (D19.-)

  D15.0 Benign neoplasm of thymus

    Excludes1   benign carcinoid tumor of the thymus (D3A.091)

  D15.1 Benign neoplasm of heart

    Excludes1   benign neoplasm of great vessels (D21.3)

  D15.2 Benign neoplasm of mediastinum
    Coding Clinic: 2024, Q3, P3

  D15.7 Benign neoplasm of other specified intrathoracic organs

  D15.9 Benign neoplasm of intrathoracic organ, unspecified

● **D16** Benign neoplasm of bone and articular cartilage

    Excludes1   benign neoplasm of connective tissue of ear (D21.0)
        benign neoplasm of connective tissue of eyelid (D21.0)
        benign neoplasm of connective tissue of larynx (D14.1)
        benign neoplasm of connective tissue of nose (D14.0)
        benign neoplasm of synovia (D21.-)

●   **D16.0** Benign neoplasm of scapula and long bones of upper limb

    D16.00 Benign neoplasm of scapula and long bones of unspecified upper limb

    D16.01 Benign neoplasm of scapula and long bones of right upper limb

    D16.02 Benign neoplasm of scapula and long bones of left upper limb

---

▶ New   ➡ Revised   ~~deleted~~ Deleted   Excludes 1   Excludes 2   Includes   Use additional   Code first   Code also   Key words

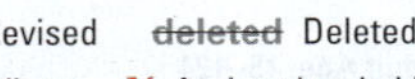 OGCR Official Guidelines   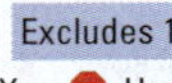 X Assign placeholder X   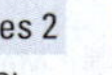 ● Use Additional Character(s)   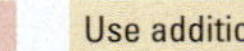 ▶ Manifestation Code   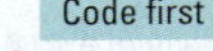 Hierarchical Condition Category   Coding Clinic

● **D16.1 Benign neoplasm of short bones of upper limb**

    D16.10 Benign neoplasm of short bones of unspecified upper limb

    D16.11 Benign neoplasm of short bones of right upper limb

    D16.12 Benign neoplasm of short bones of left upper limb

● **D16.2 Benign neoplasm of long bones of lower limb**

    D16.20 Benign neoplasm of long bones of unspecified lower limb

    D16.21 Benign neoplasm of long bones of right lower limb

    D16.22 Benign neoplasm of long bones of left lower limb

● **D16.3 Benign neoplasm of short bones of lower limb**

    D16.30 Benign neoplasm of short bones of unspecified lower limb

    D16.31 Benign neoplasm of short bones of right lower limb

    D16.32 Benign neoplasm of short bones of left lower limb

D16.4 Benign neoplasm of bones of skull and face
Benign neoplasm of maxilla (superior)
Benign neoplasm of orbital bone
Cavity or socket of skull in which eye and its appendages are located
Keratocyst of maxilla
Keratocystic odontogenic tumor of maxilla

    Excludes2 benign neoplasm of lower jaw bone (D16.5)

D16.5 Benign neoplasm of lower jaw bone
Keratocyst of mandible
Keratocystic odontogenic tumor of mandible

D16.6 Benign neoplasm of vertebral column

    Excludes1 benign neoplasm of sacrum and coccyx (D16.8)

D16.7 Benign neoplasm of ribs, sternum and clavicle

D16.8 Benign neoplasm of pelvic bones, sacrum and coccyx

D16.9 Benign neoplasm of bone and articular cartilage, unspecified

● **D17 Benign lipomatous neoplasm**
Slow-growing benign tumors (rubbery masses) of mature fat cells enclosed in a thin fibrous capsule

D17.0 Benign lipomatous neoplasm of skin and subcutaneous tissue of head, face and neck

D17.1 Benign lipomatous neoplasm of skin and subcutaneous tissue of trunk

● **D17.2 Benign lipomatous neoplasm of skin and subcutaneous tissue of limb**

    D17.20 Benign lipomatous neoplasm of skin and subcutaneous tissue of unspecified limb

    D17.21 Benign lipomatous neoplasm of skin and subcutaneous tissue of right arm

    D17.22 Benign lipomatous neoplasm of skin and subcutaneous tissue of left arm

    D17.23 Benign lipomatous neoplasm of skin and subcutaneous tissue of right leg

    D17.24 Benign lipomatous neoplasm of skin and subcutaneous tissue of left leg

● **D17.3 Benign lipomatous neoplasm of skin and subcutaneous tissue of other and unspecified sites**

    D17.30 Benign lipomatous neoplasm of skin and subcutaneous tissue of unspecified sites

    D17.39 Benign lipomatous neoplasm of skin and subcutaneous tissue of other sites

D17.4 Benign lipomatous neoplasm of intrathoracic organs

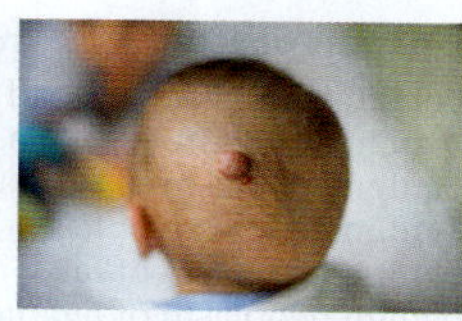

Figure 2-18 Hemangioma of skin and subcutaneous tissue. (Getty Image)

Item 2–10 Hemangiomas are abnormally dense collections of dilated capillaries that occur on the skin or in internal organs. Hemangiomas are both deep and superficial and undergo a rapid growth phase when the size increases rapidly, followed by a rest phase, in which the tumor changes very little, followed by an involutional phase in which the tumor begins to and can disappear altogether. **Lymphangiomas** or cystic hygroma are benign collections of overgrown lymph vessels and, although rare, may occur anywhere but most commonly on the head and neck of children and infants. Visceral organs, lungs, and gastrointestinal tract may also be involved.

D17.5 Benign lipomatous neoplasm of intra-abdominal organs

    Excludes1 benign lipomatous neoplasm of peritoneum and retroperitoneum (D17.79)

D17.6 Benign lipomatous neoplasm of spermatic cord

● **D17.7 Benign lipomatous neoplasm of other sites**

    D17.71 Benign lipomatous neoplasm of kidney

    D17.72 Benign lipomatous neoplasm of other genitourinary organ

    D17.79 Benign lipomatous neoplasm of other sites
Benign lipomatous neoplasm of peritoneum
Benign lipomatous neoplasm of retroperitoneum

D17.9 Benign lipomatous neoplasm, unspecified
Lipoma NOS

● **D18 Hemangioma and lymphangioma, any site**

    Excludes1 benign neoplasm of glomus jugulare (D35.6)
    blue or pigmented nevus (D22.-)
    nevus NOS (D22.-)
    vascular nevus (Q82.5)

● **D18.0 Hemangioma**
Common type of vascular malformation
Angioma NOS
Cavernous nevus

    D18.00 Hemangioma unspecified site

    D18.01 Hemangioma of skin and subcutaneous tissue

    D18.02 Hemangioma of intracranial structures

    D18.03 Hemangioma of intra-abdominal structures

    D18.09 Hemangioma of other sites

D18.1 Lymphangioma, any site
Coding Clinic: 2018, Q2, P13

● **D19 Benign neoplasm of mesothelial tissue**
Mesothelial tissue is the membrane lining several body cavities

    D19.0 Benign neoplasm of mesothelial tissue of pleura

    D19.1 Benign neoplasm of mesothelial tissue of peritoneum

    D19.7 Benign neoplasm of mesothelial tissue of other sites

    D19.9 Benign neoplasm of mesothelial tissue, unspecified
Benign mesothelioma NOS

● **D20 Benign neoplasm of soft tissue of retroperitoneum and peritoneum**

    Excludes1 benign lipomatous neoplasm of peritoneum and retroperitoneum (D17.79)
    benign neoplasm of mesothelial tissue (D19.-)

    D20.0 Benign neoplasm of soft tissue of retroperitoneum

    D20.1 Benign neoplasm of soft tissue of peritoneum

CHAPTER 2 (C00-D49)

CHAPTER 2 (C00-D49)

● **D21   Other benign neoplasms of connective and other soft tissue**

Includes   benign neoplasm of blood vessel
benign neoplasm of bursa
benign neoplasm of cartilage
benign neoplasm of fascia
benign neoplasm of fat
benign neoplasm of ligament, except uterine
benign neoplasm of lymphatic channel
benign neoplasm of muscle
benign neoplasm of synovia
benign neoplasm of tendon (sheath)
benign stromal tumors

Excludes1   benign neoplasm of articular cartilage (D16.-)
benign neoplasm of cartilage of larynx (D14.1)
benign neoplasm of cartilage of nose (D14.0)
benign neoplasm of connective tissue of breast (D24.-)
benign neoplasm of peripheral nerves and autonomic nervous system (D36.1-)
benign neoplasm of peritoneum (D20.1)
benign neoplasm of retroperitoneum (D20.0)
benign neoplasm of uterine ligament, any (D28.2)
benign neoplasm of vascular tissue (D18.-)
hemangioma (D18.0-)
lipomatous neoplasm (D17.-)
lymphangioma (D18.1)
uterine leiomyoma (D25.-)

D21.0   Benign neoplasm of connective and other soft tissue of head, face and neck
Benign neoplasm of connective tissue of ear
Benign neoplasm of connective tissue of eyelid

Excludes1   benign neoplasm of connective tissue of orbit (D31.6-)

● **D21.1   Benign neoplasm of connective and other soft tissue of upper limb, including shoulder**

D21.10   Benign neoplasm of connective and other soft tissue of unspecified upper limb, including shoulder

D21.11   Benign neoplasm of connective and other soft tissue of right upper limb, including shoulder

D21.12   Benign neoplasm of connective and other soft tissue of left upper limb, including shoulder

● **D21.2   Benign neoplasm of connective and other soft tissue of lower limb, including hip**

D21.20   Benign neoplasm of connective and other soft tissue of unspecified lower limb, including hip

D21.21   Benign neoplasm of connective and other soft tissue of right lower limb, including hip

D21.22   Benign neoplasm of connective and other soft tissue of left lower limb, including hip

D21.3   Benign neoplasm of connective and other soft tissue of thorax
Benign neoplasm of axilla
Benign neoplasm of diaphragm
Benign neoplasm of great vessels

Excludes1   benign neoplasm of heart (D15.1)
benign neoplasm of mediastinum (D15.2)
benign neoplasm of thymus (D15.0)

D21.4   Benign neoplasm of connective and other soft tissue of abdomen
Benign stromal tumors of abdomen

D21.5   Benign neoplasm of connective and other soft tissue of pelvis

Excludes1   benign neoplasm of any uterine ligament (D28.2)
uterine leiomyoma (D25.-)

D21.6   Benign neoplasm of connective and other soft tissue of trunk, unspecified
Benign neoplasm of connective and other soft tissue of back NOS

D21.9   Benign neoplasm of connective and other soft tissue, unspecified

● **D22   Melanocytic nevi**

Includes   atypical nevus
blue hairy pigmented nevus
nevus NOS

D22.0   Melanocytic nevi of lip
Skin lesions composed of nests of nevus cells with macules/papules

● **D22.1   Melanocytic nevi of eyelid, including canthus**

D22.10   Melanocytic nevi of unspecified eyelid, including canthus

● **D22.11   Melanocytic nevi of right eyelid, including canthus**

D22.111   Melanocytic nevi of right upper eyelid, including canthus

D22.112   Melanocytic nevi of right lower eyelid, including canthus

● **D22.12   Melanocytic nevi of left eyelid, including canthus**

D22.121   Melanocytic nevi of left upper eyelid, including canthus

D22.122   Melanocytic nevi of left lower eyelid, including canthus

● **D22.2   Melanocytic nevi of ear and external auricular canal**

D22.20   Melanocytic nevi of unspecified ear and external auricular canal

D22.21   Melanocytic nevi of right ear and external auricular canal

D22.22   Melanocytic nevi of left ear and external auricular canal

● **D22.3   Melanocytic nevi of other and unspecified parts of face**

D22.30   Melanocytic nevi of unspecified part of face

D22.39   Melanocytic nevi of other parts of face

D22.4   Melanocytic nevi of scalp and neck

D22.5   Melanocytic nevi of trunk
Melanocytic nevi of anal margin
Melanocytic nevi of anal skin
Melanocytic nevi of perianal skin
Melanocytic nevi of skin of breast

● **D22.6   Melanocytic nevi of upper limb, including shoulder**

D22.60   Melanocytic nevi of unspecified upper limb, including shoulder

D22.61   Melanocytic nevi of right upper limb, including shoulder

D22.62   Melanocytic nevi of left upper limb, including shoulder

● **D22.7   Melanocytic nevi of lower limb, including hip**

D22.70   Melanocytic nevi of unspecified lower limb, including hip

D22.71   Melanocytic nevi of right lower limb, including hip

D22.72   Melanocytic nevi of left lower limb, including hip

D22.9   Melanocytic nevi, unspecified

● **D23   Other benign neoplasms of skin**

Includes   benign neoplasm of hair follicles
benign neoplasm of sebaceous glands
benign neoplasm of sweat glands

Excludes1   benign lipomatous neoplasms of skin (D17.0-D17.3)

Excludes2   melanocytic nevi (D22.-)

D23.0   Other benign neoplasm of skin of lip

Excludes1   benign neoplasm of vermilion border of lip (D10.0)

● **D23.1   Other benign neoplasm of skin of eyelid, including canthus**

D23.10   Other benign neoplasm of skin unspecified of eyelid, including canthus

▶ New   ⇨ Revised   ~~deleted~~ Deleted   Excludes 1   Excludes 2   Includes   Use additional   Code first   Code also   Key words
OGCR Official Guidelines   X Assign placeholder X   ● Use Additional Character(s)   ▶ Manifestation Code   Hierarchical Condition Category   **Coding Clinic**

- **D23.11** Other benign neoplasm of skin of right eyelid, including canthus
    - D23.111 Other benign neoplasm of skin of right upper eyelid, including canthus
    - D23.112 Other benign neoplasm of skin of right lower eyelid, including canthus
    - **D23.12** Other benign neoplasm of skin of left eyelid, including canthus
        - D23.121 Other benign neoplasm of skin of left upper eyelid, including canthus
        - D23.122 Other benign neoplasm of skin of left lower eyelid, including canthus
- **D23.2** Other benign neoplasm of skin of ear and external auricular canal
    - D23.20 Other benign neoplasm of skin of unspecified ear and external auricular canal
    - D23.21 Other benign neoplasm of skin of right ear and external auricular canal
    - D23.22 Other benign neoplasm of skin of left ear and external auricular canal
- **D23.3** Other benign neoplasm of skin of other and unspecified parts of face
    - D23.30 Other benign neoplasm of skin of unspecified part of face
    - D23.39 Other benign neoplasm of skin of other parts of face
- D23.4 Other benign neoplasm of skin of scalp and neck
- D23.5 Other benign neoplasm of skin of trunk
    - Other benign neoplasm of anal margin
    - Other benign neoplasm of anal skin
    - Other benign neoplasm of perianal skin
    - Other benign neoplasm of skin of breast

    Excludes1   benign neoplasm of anus NOS (D12.9)
- **D23.6** Other benign neoplasm of skin of upper limb, including shoulder
    - D23.60 Other benign neoplasm of skin of unspecified upper limb, including shoulder
    - D23.61 Other benign neoplasm of skin of right upper limb, including shoulder
    - D23.62 Other benign neoplasm of skin of left upper limb, including shoulder
- **D23.7** Other benign neoplasm of skin of lower limb, including hip
    - D23.70 Other benign neoplasm of skin of unspecified lower limb, including hip
    - D23.71 Other benign neoplasm of skin of right lower limb, including hip
    - D23.72 Other benign neoplasm of skin of left lower limb, including hip
- D23.9 Other benign neoplasm of skin, unspecified
- **D24** Benign neoplasm of breast

    Includes   benign neoplasm of connective tissue of breast
    benign neoplasm of soft parts of breast
    fibroadenoma of breast

    Excludes2   adenofibrosis of breast (N60.2)
    benign cyst of breast (N60.-)
    benign mammary dysplasia (N60.-)
    benign neoplasm of skin of breast (D22.5, D23.5)
    fibrocystic disease of breast (N60.-)
    - D24.1 Benign neoplasm of right breast
        Coding Clinic: 2017, Q1, P5
    - D24.2 Benign neoplasm of left breast
    - D24.9 Benign neoplasm of unspecified breast

Item 2–11   Teratoma: terat = monster, oma = mass, tumor. Alternate terms: dermoid cyst of the ovary, ovarian teratoma. Teratomas are neoplasms and arise from germ cells (ovaries in female and testes in male) and can be benign or malignant. Teratomas have been known to contain hair, nails, and teeth, giving them a bizarre ("monster") appearance.

- **D25** Leiomyoma of uterus
    Benign tumors or nodules of the uterine wall

    Includes   uterine fibroid
    uterine fibromyoma
    uterine myoma
    - D25.0 Submucous leiomyoma of uterus
    - D25.1 Intramural leiomyoma of uterus
        Interstitial leiomyoma of uterus
    - D25.2 Subserosal leiomyoma of uterus
        Subperitoneal leiomyoma of uterus
    - D25.9 Leiomyoma of uterus, unspecified
- **D26** Other benign neoplasms of uterus
    - D26.0 Other benign neoplasm of cervix uteri
    - D26.1 Other benign neoplasm of corpus uteri
    - D26.7 Other benign neoplasm of other parts of uterus
    - D26.9 Other benign neoplasm of uterus, unspecified
- **D27** Benign neoplasm of ovary

    Use additional code to identify any functional activity.

    Excludes2   corpus albicans cyst (N83.2-)
    corpus luteum cyst (N83.1-)
    endometrial cyst (N80.1-)
    follicular (atretic) cyst (N83.0-)
    graafian follicle cyst (N83.0-)
    ovarian cyst NEC (N83.2-)
    ovarian retention cyst (N83.2-)
    - D27.0 Benign neoplasm of right ovary
    - D27.1 Benign neoplasm of left ovary
    - D27.9 Benign neoplasm of unspecified ovary
        Ovarian teratoma
- **D28** Benign neoplasm of other and unspecified female genital organs

    Includes   adenomatous polyp
    benign neoplasm of skin of female genital organs
    benign teratoma

    Excludes1   epoophoron cyst (Q50.5)
    fimbrial cyst (Q50.4)
    Gartner's duct cyst (Q52.4)
    parovarian cyst (Q50.5)
    - D28.0 Benign neoplasm of vulva
    - D28.1 Benign neoplasm of vagina
    - D28.2 Benign neoplasm of uterine tubes and ligaments
        Benign neoplasm of fallopian tube
        Benign neoplasm of uterine ligament (broad) (round)
    - D28.7 Benign neoplasm of other specified female genital organs
    - D28.9 Benign neoplasm of female genital organ, unspecified
- **D29** Benign neoplasm of male genital organs

    Includes   benign neoplasm of skin of male genital organs
    - D29.0 Benign neoplasm of penis
    - D29.1 Benign neoplasm of prostate

        Excludes1   enlarged prostate (N40.-)
    - **D29.2** Benign neoplasm of testis

        Use additional code to identify any functional activity.
        - D29.20 Benign neoplasm of unspecified testis
        - D29.21 Benign neoplasm of right testis
        - D29.22 Benign neoplasm of left testis
    - **D29.3** Benign neoplasm of epididymis
        - D29.30 Benign neoplasm of unspecified epididymis
        - D29.31 Benign neoplasm of right epididymis
        - D29.32 Benign neoplasm of left epididymis

CHAPTER 2 (C00-D49)

D29.4   Benign neoplasm of scrotum
    Benign neoplasm of skin of scrotum

D29.8   Benign neoplasm of other specified male genital organs
    Benign neoplasm of seminal vesicle
    Benign neoplasm of spermatic cord
    Benign neoplasm of tunica vaginalis

D29.9   Benign neoplasm of male genital organ, unspecified

● **D30   Benign neoplasm of urinary organs**

 ● **D30.0   Benign neoplasm of kidney**

    Excludes1   benign carcinoid tumor of the kidney (D3A.093)
        benign neoplasm of renal calyces (D30.1-)
        benign neoplasm of renal pelvis (D30.1-)

    D30.00   Benign neoplasm of unspecified kidney
    D30.01   Benign neoplasm of right kidney
    D30.02   Benign neoplasm of left kidney

 ● **D30.1   Benign neoplasm of renal pelvis**
    D30.10   Benign neoplasm of unspecified renal pelvis
    D30.11   Benign neoplasm of right renal pelvis
    D30.12   Benign neoplasm of left renal pelvis

 ● **D30.2   Benign neoplasm of ureter**

    Excludes1   benign neoplasm of ureteric orifice of bladder (D30.3)

    D30.20   Benign neoplasm of unspecified ureter
    D30.21   Benign neoplasm of right ureter
    D30.22   Benign neoplasm of left ureter

D30.3   Benign neoplasm of bladder
    Benign neoplasm of ureteric orifice of bladder
    Benign neoplasm of urethral orifice of bladder

D30.4   Benign neoplasm of urethra

    Excludes1   benign neoplasm of urethral orifice of bladder (D30.3)

D30.8   Benign neoplasm of other specified urinary organs
    Benign neoplasm of paraurethral glands

D30.9   Benign neoplasm of urinary organ, unspecified
    Benign neoplasm of urinary system NOS

● **D31   Benign neoplasm of eye and adnexa**

    Excludes1   benign neoplasm of connective tissue of eyelid (D21.0)
        benign neoplasm of optic nerve (D33.3)
        benign neoplasm of skin of eyelid (D22.1-, D23.1-)

 ● **D31.0   Benign neoplasm of conjunctiva**
    D31.00   Benign neoplasm of unspecified conjunctiva
    D31.01   Benign neoplasm of right conjunctiva
    D31.02   Benign neoplasm of left conjunctiva

 ● **D31.1   Benign neoplasm of cornea**
    D31.10   Benign neoplasm of unspecified cornea
    D31.11   Benign neoplasm of right cornea
    D31.12   Benign neoplasm of left cornea

 ● **D31.2   Benign neoplasm of retina**

    Excludes1   dark area on retina (D49.81)
        hemangioma of retina (D49.81)
        neoplasm of unspecified behavior of retina and choroid (D49.81)
        retinal freckle (D49.81)

    D31.20   Benign neoplasm of unspecified retina
    D31.21   Benign neoplasm of right retina
    D31.22   Benign neoplasm of left retina

 ● **D31.3   Benign neoplasm of choroid**
    D31.30   Benign neoplasm of unspecified choroid
    D31.31   Benign neoplasm of right choroid
    D31.32   Benign neoplasm of left choroid

 ● **D31.4   Benign neoplasm of ciliary body**
    D31.40   Benign neoplasm of unspecified ciliary body
    D31.41   Benign neoplasm of right ciliary body
    D31.42   Benign neoplasm of left ciliary body

 ● **D31.5   Benign neoplasm of lacrimal gland and duct**
    Benign neoplasm of lacrimal sac
    Benign neoplasm of nasolacrimal duct

    D31.50   Benign neoplasm of unspecified lacrimal gland and duct
    D31.51   Benign neoplasm of right lacrimal gland and duct
    D31.52   Benign neoplasm of left lacrimal gland and duct

 ● **D31.6   Benign neoplasm of unspecified site of orbit**
    Benign neoplasm of connective tissue of orbit
    Benign neoplasm of extraocular muscle
    Benign neoplasm of peripheral nerves of orbit
    Benign neoplasm of retrobulbar tissue
    Benign neoplasm of retro-ocular tissue

    Excludes1   benign neoplasm of orbital bone (D16.4)

    D31.60   Benign neoplasm of unspecified site of unspecified orbit
    D31.61   Benign neoplasm of unspecified site of right orbit
    D31.62   Benign neoplasm of unspecified site of left orbit

 ● **D31.9   Benign neoplasm of unspecified part of eye**
    Benign neoplasm of eyeball

    D31.90   Benign neoplasm of unspecified part of unspecified eye
    D31.91   Benign neoplasm of unspecified part of right eye
    D31.92   Benign neoplasm of unspecified part of left eye

● **D32   Benign neoplasm of meninges**

    D32.0   Benign neoplasm of cerebral meninges ⓗᶜᶜ
    D32.1   Benign neoplasm of spinal meninges ⓗᶜᶜ
    D32.9   Benign neoplasm of meninges, unspecified ⓗᶜᶜ
       Meningioma NOS

● **D33   Benign neoplasm of brain and other parts of central nervous system**

    Excludes1   angioma (D18.0-)
       benign neoplasm of meninges (D32.-)
       benign neoplasm of peripheral nerves and autonomic nervous system (D36.1-)
       hemangioma (D18.0-)
       neurofibromatosis (Q85.0-)
       retro-ocular benign neoplasm (D31.6-)

    D33.0   Benign neoplasm of brain, supratentorial ⓗᶜᶜ
    Benign neoplasm of cerebral ventricle
    Benign neoplasm of cerebrum
    Benign neoplasm of frontal lobe
    Benign neoplasm of occipital lobe
    Benign neoplasm of parietal lobe
    Benign neoplasm of temporal lobe

    Excludes1   benign neoplasm of fourth ventricle (D33.1)

    D33.1   Benign neoplasm of brain, infratentorial ⓗᶜᶜ
    Benign neoplasm of brain stem
    Benign neoplasm of cerebellum
    Benign neoplasm of fourth ventricle

    D33.2   Benign neoplasm of brain, unspecified ⓗᶜᶜ
    D33.3   Benign neoplasm of cranial nerves ⓗᶜᶜ
    Benign neoplasm of olfactory bulb

    D33.4   Benign neoplasm of spinal cord ⓗᶜᶜ
    D33.7   Benign neoplasm of other specified parts of central nervous system ⓗᶜᶜ
    D33.9   Benign neoplasm of central nervous system, unspecified ⓗᶜᶜ
    Benign neoplasm of nervous system (central) NOS

D34   Benign neoplasm of thyroid gland
    Use additional code to identify any functional activity.

● **D35**   Benign neoplasm of other and unspecified endocrine glands

Use additional code to identify any functional activity.

    Excludes1   benign neoplasm of endocrine pancreas (D13.7)
benign neoplasm of ovary (D27.-)
benign neoplasm of testis (D29.2.-)
benign neoplasm of thymus (D15.0)

   ● D35.0   Benign neoplasm of adrenal gland

     D35.00   Benign neoplasm of unspecified adrenal gland

     D35.01   Benign neoplasm of right adrenal gland

     D35.02   Benign neoplasm of left adrenal gland

   D35.1   Benign neoplasm of parathyroid gland

   D35.2   Benign neoplasm of pituitary gland

   D35.3   Benign neoplasm of craniopharyngeal duct

   D35.4   Benign neoplasm of pineal gland

   D35.5   Benign neoplasm of carotid body

   D35.6   Benign neoplasm of aortic body and other paraganglia
Benign tumor of glomus jugulare

   D35.7   Benign neoplasm of other specified endocrine glands

   D35.9   Benign neoplasm of endocrine gland, unspecified
Benign neoplasm of unspecified endocrine gland

● **D36**   Benign neoplasm of other and unspecified sites

   D36.0   Benign neoplasm of lymph nodes

     Excludes1   lymphangioma (D18.1)

   ● D36.1   Benign neoplasm of peripheral nerves and autonomic nervous system

     Excludes1   benign neoplasm of peripheral nerves of orbit (D31.6-)
neurofibromatosis (Q85.0-)

     D36.10   Benign neoplasm of peripheral nerves and autonomic nervous system, unspecified

     D36.11   Benign neoplasm of peripheral nerves and autonomic nervous system of face, head, and neck

     D36.12   Benign neoplasm of peripheral nerves and autonomic nervous system, upper limb, including shoulder

     D36.13   Benign neoplasm of peripheral nerves and autonomic nervous system of lower limb, including hip

     D36.14   Benign neoplasm of peripheral nerves and autonomic nervous system of thorax

     D36.15   Benign neoplasm of peripheral nerves and autonomic nervous system of abdomen

     D36.16   Benign neoplasm of peripheral nerves and autonomic nervous system of pelvis

     D36.17   Benign neoplasm of peripheral nerves and autonomic nervous system of trunk, unspecified

   D36.7   Benign neoplasm of other specified sites
Benign neoplasm of nose NOS
Benign neoplasm of back NOS

   D36.9   Benign neoplasm, unspecified site

NEOPLASMS OF UNCERTAIN BEHAVIOR, POLYCYTHEMIA VERA AND MYELODYSPLASTIC SYNDROMES (D37-D48)

Note: Categories D37-D44, and D48 classify by site neoplasms of uncertain behavior, i.e., histologic confirmation whether the neoplasm is malignant or benign cannot be made.

    Excludes1   neoplasms of unspecified behavior (D49.-)

● **D37**   Neoplasm of uncertain behavior of oral cavity and digestive organs

    Excludes1   stromal tumors of uncertain behavior of digestive system (D48.1-)

   ● D37.0   Neoplasm of uncertain behavior of lip, oral cavity and pharynx

     Excludes1   neoplasm of uncertain behavior of aryepiglottic fold or interarytenoid fold, laryngeal aspect (D38.0)
neoplasm of uncertain behavior of epiglottis NOS (D38.0)
neoplasm of uncertain behavior of skin of lip (D48.5)
neoplasm of uncertain behavior of suprahyoid portion of epiglottis (D38.0)

     D37.01   Neoplasm of uncertain behavior of lip
Neoplasm of uncertain behavior of vermilion border of lip

     D37.02   Neoplasm of uncertain behavior of tongue

   ● D37.03   Neoplasm of uncertain behavior of the major salivary glands

     D37.030   Neoplasm of uncertain behavior of the parotid salivary glands

     D37.031   Neoplasm of uncertain behavior of the sublingual salivary glands

     D37.032   Neoplasm of uncertain behavior of the submandibular salivary glands

     D37.039   Neoplasm of uncertain behavior of the major salivary glands, unspecified

     D37.04   Neoplasm of uncertain behavior of the minor salivary glands
Neoplasm of uncertain behavior of submucosal salivary glands of lip
Neoplasm of uncertain behavior of submucosal salivary glands of cheek
Neoplasm of uncertain behavior of submucosal salivary glands of hard palate
Neoplasm of uncertain behavior of submucosal salivary glands of soft palate

     D37.05   Neoplasm of uncertain behavior of pharynx
Neoplasm of uncertain behavior of aryepiglottic fold of pharynx NOS
Neoplasm of uncertain behavior of hypopharyngeal aspect of aryepiglottic fold of pharynx
Neoplasm of uncertain behavior of marginal zone of aryepiglottic fold of pharynx

     D37.09   Neoplasm of uncertain behavior of other specified sites of the oral cavity

   D37.1   Neoplasm of uncertain behavior of stomach

   D37.2   Neoplasm of uncertain behavior of small intestine

   D37.3   Neoplasm of uncertain behavior of appendix

   D37.4   Neoplasm of uncertain behavior of colon

   D37.5   Neoplasm of uncertain behavior of rectum
Neoplasm of uncertain behavior of rectosigmoid junction
Rectosigmoid junction: Angle where sigmoid colon becomes rectum

   D37.6   Neoplasm of uncertain behavior of liver, gallbladder and bile ducts
Neoplasm of uncertain behavior of ampulla of Vater
Ampulla of Vater: Enlarged segment of ducts from liver and pancreas at entry point to small intestine

CHAPTER 2 (C00-D49)

D37.8   Neoplasm of uncertain behavior of other specified digestive organs
Neoplasm of uncertain behavior of anal canal
Neoplasm of uncertain behavior of anal sphincter
Neoplasm of uncertain behavior of anus NOS
Neoplasm of uncertain behavior of esophagus
Neoplasm of uncertain behavior of intestine NOS
Neoplasm of uncertain behavior of pancreas

> **Excludes1**   neoplasm of uncertain behavior of anal margin (D48.5)
> neoplasm of uncertain behavior of anal skin (D48.5)
> neoplasm of uncertain behavior of perianal skin (D48.5)

D37.9   Neoplasm of uncertain behavior of digestive organ, unspecified

- **D38   Neoplasm of uncertain behavior of middle ear and respiratory and intrathoracic organs**

  > **Excludes1**   neoplasm of uncertain behavior of heart (D48.7)

  D38.0   Neoplasm of uncertain behavior of larynx
  Neoplasm of uncertain behavior of aryepiglottic fold or interarytenoid fold, laryngeal aspect
  Neoplasm of uncertain behavior of epiglottis (suprahyoid portion)

  > **Excludes1**   neoplasm of uncertain behavior of aryepiglottic fold or interarytenoid fold NOS (D37.05)
  > neoplasm of uncertain behavior of hypopharyngeal aspect of aryepiglottic fold (D37.05)
  > neoplasm of uncertain behavior of marginal zone of aryepiglottic fold (D37.05)

  D38.1   Neoplasm of uncertain behavior of trachea, bronchus and lung

  D38.2   Neoplasm of uncertain behavior of pleura

  D38.3   Neoplasm of uncertain behavior of mediastinum

  D38.4   Neoplasm of uncertain behavior of thymus

  D38.5   Neoplasm of uncertain behavior of other respiratory organs
  Neoplasm of uncertain behavior of accessory sinuses
  Neoplasm of uncertain behavior of cartilage of nose
  Neoplasm of uncertain behavior of middle ear
  Neoplasm of uncertain behavior of nasal cavities

  > **Excludes1**   neoplasm of uncertain behavior of ear (external) (skin) (D48.5)
  > neoplasm of uncertain behavior of nose NOS (D48.7)
  > neoplasm of uncertain behavior of skin of nose (D48.5)

  D38.6   Neoplasm of uncertain behavior of respiratory organ, unspecified

- **D39   Neoplasm of uncertain behavior of female genital organs**

  D39.0   Neoplasm of uncertain behavior of uterus

  - **D39.1   Neoplasm of uncertain behavior of ovary**

    Use additional code to identify any functional activity.

    D39.10   Neoplasm of uncertain behavior of unspecified ovary

    D39.11   Neoplasm of uncertain behavior of right ovary

    D39.12   Neoplasm of uncertain behavior of left ovary

  D39.2   Neoplasm of uncertain behavior of placentaM
  Chorioadenoma destruens
  Invasive hydatidiform mole
  Malignant hydatidiform mole

  > **Excludes1**   hydatidiform mole NOS (O01.9)

  Coding Clinic: 2023, Q3, P15

  D39.8   Neoplasm of uncertain behavior of other specified female genital organs
  Neoplasm of uncertain behavior of skin of female genital organs

  D39.9   Neoplasm of uncertain behavior of female genital organ, unspecified

BENIGN NEUROENDOCRINE TUMORS (D3A)

- **D3A   Benign neuroendocrine tumors**

  Code also any associated multiple endocrine neoplasia [MEN] syndromes (E31.2-)

  Use additional code to identify any associated endocrine syndrome, such as:
  carcinoid syndrome (E34.00)

  > **Excludes2**   benign pancreatic islet cell tumors (D13.7)

  - **D3A.0   Benign carcinoid tumors**

    D3A.00   Benign carcinoid tumor of unspecified site
    Carcinoid tumor NOS

    - **D3A.01   Benign carcinoid tumors of the small intestine**

      D3A.010   Benign carcinoid tumor of the duodenum

      D3A.011   Benign carcinoid tumor of the jejunum

      D3A.012   Benign carcinoid tumor of the ileum

      D3A.019   Benign carcinoid tumor of the small intestine, unspecified portion

    - **D3A.02   Benign carcinoid tumors of the appendix, large intestine, and rectum**

      D3A.020   Benign carcinoid tumor of the appendix

      D3A.021   Benign carcinoid tumor of the cecum

      D3A.022   Benign carcinoid tumor of the ascending colon

      D3A.023   Benign carcinoid tumor of the transverse colon

      D3A.024   Benign carcinoid tumor of the descending colon

      D3A.025   Benign carcinoid tumor of the sigmoid colon

      D3A.026   Benign carcinoid tumor of the rectum

      D3A.029   Benign carcinoid tumor of the large intestine, unspecified portion
      Benign carcinoid tumor of the colon NOS

    - **D3A.09   Benign carcinoid tumors of other sites**

      D3A.090   Benign carcinoid tumor of the bronchus and lung

      D3A.091   Benign carcinoid tumor of the thymus

      D3A.092   Benign carcinoid tumor of the stomach

      D3A.093   Benign carcinoid tumor of the kidney

      D3A.094   Benign carcinoid tumor of the foregut, unspecified

      D3A.095   Benign carcinoid tumor of the midgut, unspecified

      D3A.096   Benign carcinoid tumor of the hindgut, unspecified

      D3A.098   Benign carcinoid tumors of other sites

  D3A.8   Other benign neuroendocrine tumors
  Neuroendocrine tumor NOS

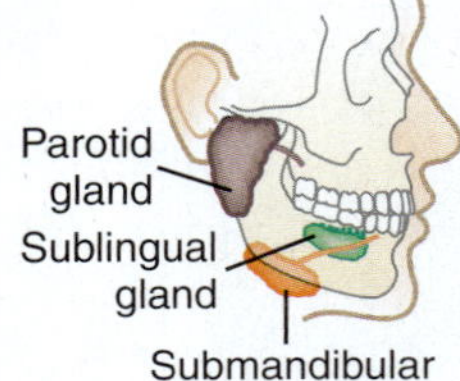

Figure 2-19   Major salivary glands.

> ▶ New   ➡ Revised   ~~deleted~~ Deleted   Excludes 1   Excludes 2   Includes   Use additional   Code first   Code also   Key words
> **OGCR** Official Guidelines   **X** Assign placeholder X   ● Use Additional Character(s)   ▸ Manifestation Code   🄷🄲 Hierarchical Condition Category   **Coding Clinic**

● D40 Neoplasm of uncertain behavior of male genital organs

    D40.0 Neoplasm of uncertain behavior of prostate

    ● D40.1 Neoplasm of uncertain behavior of testis

        D40.10 Neoplasm of uncertain behavior of unspecified testis

        D40.11 Neoplasm of uncertain behavior of right testis

        D40.12 Neoplasm of uncertain behavior of left testis

    D40.8 Neoplasm of uncertain behavior of other specified male genital organs

        Neoplasm of uncertain behavior of skin of male genital organs

    D40.9 Neoplasm of uncertain behavior of male genital organ, unspecified

● D41 Neoplasm of uncertain behavior of urinary organs

    ● D41.0 Neoplasm of uncertain behavior of kidney

        Excludes1 neoplasm of uncertain behavior of renal pelvis (D41.1-)

        D41.00 Neoplasm of uncertain behavior of unspecified kidney

        D41.01 Neoplasm of uncertain behavior of right kidney

        D41.02 Neoplasm of uncertain behavior of left kidney

    ● D41.1 Neoplasm of uncertain behavior of renal pelvis

        D41.10 Neoplasm of uncertain behavior of unspecified renal pelvis

        D41.11 Neoplasm of uncertain behavior of right renal pelvis

        D41.12 Neoplasm of uncertain behavior of left renal pelvis

    ● D41.2 Neoplasm of uncertain behavior of ureter

        D41.20 Neoplasm of uncertain behavior of unspecified ureter

        D41.21 Neoplasm of uncertain behavior of right ureter

        D41.22 Neoplasm of uncertain behavior of left ureter

    D41.3 Neoplasm of uncertain behavior of urethra

    D41.4 Neoplasm of uncertain behavior of bladder

    D41.8 Neoplasm of uncertain behavior of other specified urinary organs

    D41.9 Neoplasm of uncertain behavior of unspecified urinary organ

● D42 Neoplasm of uncertain behavior of meninges

    D42.0 Neoplasm of uncertain behavior of cerebral meninges

    D42.1 Neoplasm of uncertain behavior of spinal meninges

    D42.9 Neoplasm of uncertain behavior of meninges, unspecified

● D43 Neoplasm of uncertain behavior of brain and central nervous system

    Excludes1 neoplasm of uncertain behavior of peripheral nerves and autonomic nervous system (D48.2)

    D43.0 Neoplasm of uncertain behavior of brain, supratentorial

        Superior to tentorium of cerebellum

        Neoplasm of uncertain behavior of cerebral ventricle

        Neoplasm of uncertain behavior of cerebrum

        Neoplasm of uncertain behavior of frontal lobe

        Neoplasm of uncertain behavior of occipital lobe

        Neoplasm of uncertain behavior of parietal lobe

        Neoplasm of uncertain behavior of temporal lobe

        Excludes1 neoplasm of uncertain behavior of fourth ventricle (D43.1)

    D43.1 Neoplasm of uncertain behavior of brain, infratentorial

        Beneath the tentorium of cerebellum

        Neoplasm of uncertain behavior of brain stem

        Neoplasm of uncertain behavior of cerebellum

        Neoplasm of uncertain behavior of fourth ventricle

        Coding Clinic: 2023, Q2, P16

    D43.2 Neoplasm of uncertain behavior of brain, unspecified

    D43.3 Neoplasm of uncertain behavior of cranial nerves

    D43.4 Neoplasm of uncertain behavior of spinal cord

    D43.8 Neoplasm of uncertain behavior of other specified parts of central nervous system

    D43.9 Neoplasm of uncertain behavior of central nervous system, unspecified

        Neoplasm of uncertain behavior of nervous system (central) NOS

● D44 Neoplasm of uncertain behavior of endocrine glands

    Excludes1 multiple endocrine adenomatosis (E31.2-)
           multiple endocrine neoplasia (E31.2-)
           neoplasm of uncertain behavior of endocrine pancreas (D37.8)
           neoplasm of uncertain behavior of ovary (D39.1-)
           neoplasm of uncertain behavior of testis (D40.1-)
           neoplasm of uncertain behavior of thymus (D38.4)

    D44.0 Neoplasm of uncertain behavior of thyroid gland
        Coding Clinic: 2024, Q3, P3

    ● D44.1 Neoplasm of uncertain behavior of adrenal gland

        Use additional code to identify any functional activity.

        D44.10 Neoplasm of uncertain behavior of unspecified adrenal gland

        D44.11 Neoplasm of uncertain behavior of right adrenal gland

        D44.12 Neoplasm of uncertain behavior of left adrenal gland

    D44.2 Neoplasm of uncertain behavior of parathyroid gland

    D44.3 Neoplasm of uncertain behavior of pituitary gland

        Use additional code to identify any functional activity.

    D44.4 Neoplasm of uncertain behavior of craniopharyngeal duct

    D44.5 Neoplasm of uncertain behavior of pineal gland

    D44.6 Neoplasm of uncertain behavior of carotid body

    D44.7 Neoplasm of uncertain behavior of aortic body and other paraganglia
        Coding Clinic: 2016, Q4, P26

    D44.9 Neoplasm of uncertain behavior of unspecified endocrine gland

D45 Polycythemia vera

    Excludes1 familial polycythemia (D75.0)
           secondary polycythemia (D75.1)

    Primary polycythemia. Secondary polycythemia is D75.1. Check your documentation. Polycythemia is caused by too many red blood cells, which increase the thickness of blood (viscosity). This can cause engorgement of the spleen (splenomegaly) with extra RBCs and potential clot formation.

● D46 Myelodysplastic syndromes

    Use additional code for adverse effect, if applicable, to identify drug (T36-T50 with fifth or sixth character 5)

    Excludes2 drug-induced aplastic anemia (D61.1)

    D46.0 Refractory anemia without ring sideroblasts, so stated
        Refractory anemia without sideroblasts, without excess of blasts

    D46.1 Refractory anemia with ring sideroblasts RARS

    ● D46.2 Refractory anemia with excess of blasts [RAEB]
        Form of myelodysplasia with increased immature white blood cells (blasts) in bone marrow

        D46.20 Refractory anemia with excess of blasts, unspecified RAEB NOS

        D46.21 Refractory anemia with excess of blasts 1 RAEB 1
            Bone marrow disease which results in insufficient RBCs (anemia) in which level of blasts is less than 10%

        D46.22 Refractory anemia with excess of blasts 2 RAEB 2
            Bone marrow disease manifested by insufficient numbers of RBCs (anemia) with level of blasts 10-20%

D46.A   Refractory cytopenia with multilineage dysplasia

D46.B   Refractory cytopenia with multilineage dysplasia and ring sideroblasts
    RCMD RS

D46.C   Myelodysplastic syndrome with isolated del(5q) chromosomal abnormality
    Myelodysplastic syndrome with 5q deletion
    5q minus syndrome NOS

D46.4   Refractory anemia, unspecified

D46.Z   Other myelodysplastic syndromes
    Excludes1   chronic myelomonocytic leukemia (C93.1-)

D46.9   Myelodysplastic syndrome, unspecified
    Myelodysplasia NOS

● **D47**   **Other neoplasms of uncertain behavior of lymphoid, hematopoietic and related tissue**

    ● **D47.0**   **Mast cell neoplasms of uncertain behavior**
      Excludes1   congenital cutaneous mastocytosis (Q82.2)
        histiocytic neoplasms of uncertain behavior (D47.Z9)
        malignant mast cell neoplasm (C96.2-)

      D47.01   **Cutaneous mastocytosis**
        Diffuse cutaneous mastocytosis
        Maculopapular cutaneous mastocytosis
        Solitary mastocytoma
        Telangiectasia macularis eruptiva perstans
        Urticaria pigmentosa
        Excludes1   congenital (diffuse) (maculopapular) cutaneous mastocytosis (Q82.2)
          congenital urticaria pigmentosa (Q82.2)
          extracutaneous mastocytoma (D47.09)

      D47.02   **Systemic mastocytosis**
        Indolent systemic mastocytosis
        Isolated bone marrow mastocytosis
        Smoldering systemic mastocytosis
        Systemic mastocytosis, with an associated hematological non-mast cell lineage disease (SM-AHNMD)
        Code also if applicable, any associated hematological non-mast cell lineage disease, such as:
          acute myeloid leukemia (C92.6-, C92.A-)
          chronic myelomonocytic leukemia (C93.1-)
          essential thrombocytosis (D47.3)
          hypereosinophilic syndrome (D72.1)
          myelodysplastic syndrome (D46.9)
          myeloproliferative syndrome (D47.1)
          non-Hodgkin lymphoma (C82-C85)
          plasma cell myeloma (C90.0-)
          polycythemia vera (D45)
        Excludes1   aggressive systemic mastocytosis (C96.21)
          mast cell leukemia (C94.3-)

      D47.09   **Other mast cell neoplasms of uncertain behavior**
        Extracutaneous mastocytoma
        Mast cell tumor NOS
        Mastocytoma NOS
        Mastocytosis NOS

    D47.1   **Chronic myeloproliferative disease**
      Chronic neutrophilic leukemia
      Myeloproliferative disease, unspecified
      Excludes1   atypical chronic myeloid leukemia BCR/ABL-negative (C92.2-)
        chronic myeloid leukemia BCR/ABL-positive (C92.1-)
        myelofibrosis NOS (D75.81)
        myelophthisic anemia (D61.82)
        myelophthisis (D61.82)
        secondary myelofibrosis NOS (D75.81)

    D47.2   **Monoclonal gammopathy**
      Monoclonal gammopathy of undetermined significance [MGUS]
      Coding Clinic: 2021, Q3, P5

    D47.3   **Essential (hemorrhagic) thrombocythemia**
      Essential thrombocytosis
      Idiopathic hemorrhagic thrombocythemia
      Primary thrombocytosis
      Excludes2   reactive thrombocytosis (D75.838)
        secondary thrombocytosis (D75.838)
        thrombocythemia NOS (D75.839)
        thrombocytosis NOS (D75.839)

    D47.4   **Osteomyelofibrosis**
      Chronic idiopathic myelofibrosis
      Myelofibrosis (idiopathic) (with myeloid metaplasia)
      Myelosclerosis (megakaryocytic) with myeloid metaplasia
      Secondary myelofibrosis in myeloproliferative disease
      Excludes1   acute myelofibrosis (C94.4-)

    D47.9   **Neoplasm of uncertain behavior of lymphoid, hematopoietic and related tissue, unspecified**
      Lymphoproliferative disease NOS

    ● **D47.Z**   **Other specified neoplasms of uncertain behavior of lymphoid, hematopoietic and related tissue**

      D47.Z1   **Post-transplant lymphoproliferative disorder (PTLD)**
        Code first complications of transplanted organs and tissue (T86.-)

      D47.Z2   **Castleman disease**
        Code also if applicable, human herpesvirus 8 infection (B10.89)
        Excludes2   Kaposi's sarcoma (C46.-)
        Coding Clinic: 2016, Q4, P8

      D47.Z9   **Other specified neoplasms of uncertain behavior of lymphoid, hematopoietic and related tissue**
        Histiocytic tumors of uncertain behavior
        Coding Clinic: 2025, Q2, P19

● **D48**   **Neoplasm of uncertain behavior of other and unspecified sites**
    Excludes1   neurofibromatosis (nonmalignant) (Q85.0-)

    D48.0   **Neoplasm of uncertain behavior of bone and articular cartilage**
      Excludes1   neoplasm of uncertain behavior of cartilage of ear (D48.1-)
        neoplasm of uncertain behavior of cartilage of larynx (D38.0)
        neoplasm of uncertain behavior of cartilage of nose (D38.5)
        neoplasm of uncertain behavior of connective tissue of eyelid (D48.1-)
        neoplasm of uncertain behavior of synovia (D48.1-)

    ● **D48.1**   **Neoplasm of uncertain behavior of connective and other soft tissue**
      Neoplasm of uncertain behavior of connective tissue of ear
      Neoplasm of uncertain behavior of connective tissue of eyelid
      Stromal tumors of uncertain behavior of digestive system
      Excludes1   neoplasm of uncertain behavior of articular cartilage (D48.0)
        neoplasm of uncertain behavior of cartilage of larynx (D38.0)
        neoplasm of uncertain behavior of cartilage of nose (D38.5)
        neoplasm of uncertain behavior of connective tissue of breast (D48.6-)

      ● **D48.11**   **Desmoid tumor**
        ▶ Aggressive fibromatosis
        D48.110   Desmoid tumor of head and neck
        D48.111   Desmoid tumor of chest wall

▶ New   ⏩ Revised   ~~deleted~~ Deleted   Excludes 1   Excludes 2   Includes   Use additional   Code first   Code also   Key words
OGCR Official Guidelines   X Assign placeholder X   ● Use Additional Character(s)   ▶ Manifestation Code   Hierarchical Condition Category   **Coding Clinic**

D48.112 Desmoid tumor, intrathoracic

D48.113 Desmoid tumor of abdominal wall

D48.114 Desmoid tumor, intraabdomin
Desmoid tumor of pelvic cavity
Desmoid tumor, peritoneal, retroperitoneal

D48.115   Desmoid tumor of upper extremity and shoulder girdle

D48.116   Desmoid tumor of lower extremity and pelvic girdle
Desmoid tumor of buttock

D48.117   Desmoid tumor of back

D48.118   Desmoid tumor of other site

D48.119   Desmoid tumor of unspecified site

D48.19   Other specified neoplasm of uncertain behavior of connective and other soft tissue

D48.2   Neoplasm of uncertain behavior of peripheral nerves and autonomic nervous system

> **Excludes1**   neoplasm of uncertain behavior of peripheral nerves of orbit (D48.7)

D48.3   Neoplasm of uncertain behavior of retroperitoneum

D48.4   Neoplasm of uncertain behavior of peritoneum

D48.5   Neoplasm of uncertain behavior of skin
Neoplasm of uncertain behavior of anal margin
Neoplasm of uncertain behavior of anal skin
Neoplasm of uncertain behavior of perianal skin
Neoplasm of uncertain behavior of skin of breast

> **Excludes1**   neoplasm of uncertain behavior of anus NOS (D37.8)
> neoplasm of uncertain behavior of skin of genital organs (D39.8, D40.8)
> neoplasm of uncertain behavior of vermilion border of lip (D37.0)

● **D48.6   Neoplasm of uncertain behavior of breast**
Neoplasm of uncertain behavior of connective tissue of breast
Cystosarcoma phyllodes

> **Excludes1**   neoplasm of uncertain behavior of skin of breast (D48.5)

D48.60   Neoplasm of uncertain behavior of unspecified breast

D48.61   Neoplasm of uncertain behavior of right breast

D48.62   Neoplasm of uncertain behavior of left breast

D48.7   Neoplasm of uncertain behavior of other specified sites
Neoplasm of uncertain behavior of eye
Neoplasm of uncertain behavior of heart
Neoplasm of uncertain behavior of peripheral nerves of orbit

> **Excludes1**   neoplasm of uncertain behavior of connective tissue (D48.1-)
> neoplasm of uncertain behavior of skin of eyelid (D48.5)

D48.9   Neoplasm of uncertain behavior, unspecified

● **D49   Neoplasms of unspecified behavior**

Note: Category D49 classifies by site neoplasms of unspecified morphology and behavior. The term "mass," unless otherwise stated, is not to be regarded as a neoplastic growth.

> **Includes**   'growth' NOS
> neoplasm NOS
> new growth NOS
> tumor NOS

> **Excludes1**   neoplasms of uncertain behavior (D37-D44, D48)

D49.0   Neoplasm of unspecified behavior of digestive system

> **Excludes1**   neoplasm of unspecified behavior of margin of anus (D49.2)
> neoplasm of unspecified behavior of perianal skin (D49.2)
> neoplasm of unspecified behavior of skin of anus (D49.2)

D49.1   Neoplasm of unspecified behavior of respiratory system

D49.2   Neoplasm of unspecified behavior of bone, soft tissue, and skin

> **Excludes1**   neoplasm of unspecified behavior of anal canal (D49.0)
> neoplasm of unspecified behavior of anus NOS (D49.0)
> neoplasm of unspecified behavior of bone marrow (D49.89)
> neoplasm of unspecified behavior of cartilage of larynx (D49.1)
> neoplasm of unspecified behavior of cartilage of nose (D49.1)
> neoplasm of unspecified behavior of connective tissue of breast (D49.3)
> neoplasm of unspecified behavior of skin of genital organs (D49.59)
> neoplasm of unspecified behavior of vermilion border of lip (D49.0)

D49.3   Neoplasm of unspecified behavior of breast

> **Excludes1**   neoplasm of unspecified behavior of skin of breast (D49.2)

D49.4   Neoplasm of unspecified behavior of bladder

● **D49.5   Neoplasm of unspecified behavior of other genitourinary organs**

● **D49.51   Neoplasm of unspecified behavior of kidney**

D49.511   Neoplasm of unspecified behavior of right kidney
Coding Clinic: 2016, Q4, P9

D49.512   Neoplasm of unspecified behavior of left kidney
Coding Clinic: 2016, Q4, P9

D49.519   Neoplasm of unspecified behavior of unspecified kidney
Coding Clinic: 2016, Q4, P9

D49.59   Neoplasm of unspecified behavior of other genitourinary organ
Coding Clinic: 2016, Q4, P9

D49.6   Neoplasm of unspecified behavior of brain

> **Excludes1**   neoplasm of unspecified behavior of cerebral meninges (D49.7)
> neoplasm of unspecified behavior of cranial nerves (D49.7)

D49.7   Neoplasm of unspecified behavior of endocrine glands and other parts of nervous system

> **Excludes1**   neoplasm of unspecified behavior of peripheral, sympathetic, and parasympathetic nerves and ganglia (D49.2)

● **D49.8   Neoplasm of unspecified behavior of other specified sites**

> **Excludes1**   neoplasm of unspecified behavior of eyelid (skin) (D49.2)
> neoplasm of unspecified behavior of eyelid cartilage (D49.2)
> neoplasm of unspecified behavior of great vessels (D49.2)
> neoplasm of unspecified behavior of optic nerve (D49.7)

D49.81   Neoplasm of unspecified behavior of retina and choroid
Dark area on retina
Retinal freckle

D49.89   Neoplasm of unspecified behavior of other specified sites

D49.9   Neoplasm of unspecified behavior of unspecified site

OGCR **Chapter-Specific Coding Guidelines**

> 3. **Chapter 3: Disease of the blood and blood-forming organs and certain disorders involving the immune mechanism (D50-D89)**
> Reserved for future guideline expansion

CHAPTER 3

DISEASES OF THE BLOOD AND BLOOD-FORMING ORGANS AND CERTAIN DISORDERS INVOLVING THE IMMUNE MECHANISM (D50-D89)

Excludes2   autoimmune disease (systemic) NOS (M35.9)
certain conditions originating in the perinatal period (P00-P96)
complications of pregnancy, childbirth and the puerperium (O00-O9A)
congenital malformations, deformations and chromosomal abnormalities (Q00-Q99)
endocrine, nutritional and metabolic diseases (E00-E88)
human immunodeficiency virus [HIV] disease (B20)
injury, poisoning and certain other consequences of external causes (S00-T88)
neoplasms (C00-D49)
symptoms, signs and abnormal clinical and laboratory findings, not elsewhere classified (R00-R94)

This chapter contains the following blocks:

D50-D53	Nutritional anemias
D55-D59	Hemolytic anemias
D60-D64	Aplastic and other anemias and other bone marrow failure syndromes
D65-D69	Coagulation defects, purpura and other hemorrhagic conditions
D70-D77	Other disorders of blood and blood-forming organs
D78	Intraoperative and postprocedural complications of the spleen
D80-D89	Certain disorders involving the immune mechanism

NUTRITIONAL ANEMIAS (D50-D53)

● **D50   Iron deficiency anemia**
A disease characterized by a decrease in the number of red cells (hemoglobin) in the blood.

> **Includes**   asiderotic anemia
> hypochromic anemia

D50.0   Iron deficiency anemia secondary to blood loss (chronic)
Posthemorrhagic anemia (chronic)

> **Excludes1**   acute posthemorrhagic anemia (D62)
> congenital anemia from fetal blood loss (P61.3)

Coding Clinic: 2019, Q3, P17

D50.1   Sideropenic dysphagia
Weblike growth of membranes in throat that makes swallowing difficult
Kelly-Paterson syndrome
Plummer-Vinson syndrome

D50.8   Other iron deficiency anemias
Iron deficiency anemia due to inadequate dietary iron intake

D50.9   Iron deficiency anemia, unspecified

● **D51   Vitamin B12 deficiency anemia**

> **Excludes1**   vitamin B12 deficiency (E53.8)

D51.0   Vitamin B12 deficiency anemia due to intrinsic factor deficiency
Addison anemia
Biermer anemia
Pernicious (congenital) anemia
Congenital intrinsic factor deficiency

D51.1   Vitamin B12 deficiency anemia due to selective vitamin B12 malabsorption with proteinuria
Imerslund (Gräsbeck) syndrome
Megaloblastic hereditary anemia

D51.2   Transcobalamin II deficiency

D51.3   Other dietary vitamin B12 deficiency anemia
Vegan anemia

D51.8   Other vitamin B12 deficiency anemias

D51.9   Vitamin B12 deficiency anemia, unspecified

● **D52   Folate deficiency anemia**

> **Excludes1**   folate deficiency without anemia (E53.8)

D52.0   Dietary folate deficiency anemia
Nutritional megaloblastic anemia

D52.1   Drug-induced folate deficiency anemia

> **Use additional** code for adverse effect, if applicable, to identify drug (T36-T50 with fifth or sixth character 5)

D52.8   Other folate deficiency anemias

D52.9   Folate deficiency anemia, unspecified
Folic acid deficiency anemia NOS

● **D53   Other nutritional anemias**

> **Includes**   megaloblastic anemia unresponsive to vitamin B12 or folate therapy

D53.0   Protein deficiency anemia
Amino-acid deficiency anemia
Orotaciduric anemia

> **Excludes1**   Lesch-Nyhan syndrome (E79.1)

D53.1   Other megaloblastic anemias, not elsewhere classified
Megaloblastic anemia NOS

> **Excludes1**   Di Guglielmo's disease (C94.0)

D53.2   Scorbutic anemia
Anemia resulting from deficiency of ascorbic acid (vitamin C)

> **Excludes1**   scurvy (E54)

D53.8   Other specified nutritional anemias
Anemia associated with deficiency of copper
Anemia associated with deficiency of molybdenum
Anemia associated with deficiency of zinc

> ~~**Excludes1**   nutritional deficiencies without anemia, such as:~~
> ~~copper deficiency NOS (E61.0)~~
> ~~molybdenum deficiency NOS (E61.5)~~
> ~~zinc deficiency NOS (E60)~~

> ▶ **Excludes2**   nutritional deficiencies without anemia, such as:
> ▶ copper deficiency NOS (E61.0)
> ▶ molybdenum deficiency NOS (E61.5)
> ▶ zinc deficiency NOS (E60)

D53.9   Nutritional anemia, unspecified
Simple chronic anemia

> **Excludes1**   anemia NOS (D64.9)

Coding Clinic: 2018, Q4, P88

HEMOLYTIC ANEMIAS (D55-D59)

● **D55   Anemia due to enzyme disorders**

> **Excludes1**   drug-induced enzyme deficiency anemia (D59.2)

D55.0   Anemia due to glucose-6-phosphate dehydrogenase [G6PD] deficiency 🦠
Favism
G6PD deficiency anemia

> **Excludes1**   glucose-6-phosphate dehydrogenase (G6PD) deficiency without anemia (D75.A)

D55.1   Anemia due to other disorders of glutathione metabolism 🦠
Anemia (due to) enzyme deficiencies, except G6PD, related to the hexose monophosphate [HMP] shunt pathway
Anemia (due to) hemolytic nonspherocytic (hereditary), type I

● **D55.2 Anemia due to disorders of glycolytic enzymes** 🔍

    D55.21 Anemia due to pyruvate kinase deficiency
        PK deficiency anemia
        Pyruvate kinase deficiency anemia

    D55.29 Anemia due to other disorders of glycolytic enzymes
        Hexokinase deficiency anemia
        Triose-phosphate isomerase deficiency anemia

        Excludes1   disorders of glycolysis not associated with anemia (E74.81-)

D55.3 Anemia due to disorders of nucleotide metabolism 🔍

D55.8 Other anemias due to enzyme disorders 🔍

D55.9 Anemia due to enzyme disorder, unspecified 🔍

● **D56 Thalassemia**
    Hereditary disorders characterized by low production of hemoglobin or excessive destruction of red blood cells

    Excludes1   sickle-cell thalassemia (D57.4-)

    D56.0 Alpha thalassemia 🔍
        Alpha thalassemia major
        Hemoglobin H Constant Spring
        Hemoglobin H disease
        Hydrops fetalis due to alpha thalassemia
        Severe alpha thalassemia
        Triple gene defect alpha thalassemia

        Use additional code, if applicable, for hydrops fetalis due to alpha thalassemia (P56.99)

        Excludes1   alpha thalassemia trait or minor (D56.3)
                asymptomatic alpha thalassemia (D56.3)
                hydrops fetalis due to isoimmunization (P56.0)
                hydrops fetalis not due to immune hemolysis (P83.2)

    D56.1 Beta thalassemia 🔍
        Beta thalassemia major
        Cooley's anemia
        Homozygous beta thalassemia
        Severe beta thalassemia
        Thalassemia intermedia
        Thalassemia major

        Excludes1   beta thalassemia minor (D56.3)
                beta thalassemia trait (D56.3)
                delta-beta thalassemia (D56.2)
                hemoglobin E-beta thalassemia (D56.5)
                sickle-cell beta thalassemia (D57.4-)

    D56.2 Delta-beta thalassemia 🔍
        Homozygous delta-beta thalassemia

        Excludes1   delta-beta thalassemia minor (D56.3)
                delta-beta thalassemia trait (D56.3)

    D56.3 Thalassemia minor
    Genetic disorders that have in common defective production of hemoglobin
        Alpha thalassemia minor
        Alpha thalassemia silent carrier
        Alpha thalassemia trait
        Beta thalassemia minor
        Beta thalassemia trait
        Delta-beta thalassemia minor
        Delta-beta thalassemia trait
        Thalassemia trait NOS

        Excludes1   alpha thalassemia (D56.0)
                beta thalassemia (D56.1)
                delta-beta thalassemia (D56.2)
                hemoglobin E-beta thalassemia (D56.5)
                sickle-cell trait (D57.3)

    D56.4 Hereditary persistence of fetal hemoglobin [HPFH] 🔍
    Persistent production of hemoglobin

    D56.5 Hemoglobin E-beta thalassemia 🔍

        Excludes1   beta thalassemia (D56.1)
                beta thalassemia minor (D56.3)
                beta thalassemia trait (D56.3)
                delta-beta thalassemia (D56.2)
                delta-beta thalassemia trait (D56.3)
                hemoglobin E disease (D58.2)
                other hemoglobinopathies (D58.2)
                sickle-cell beta thalassemia (D57.4-)

    D56.8 Other thalassemias 🔍
        Dominant thalassemia
        Hemoglobin C thalassemia
        Mixed thalassemia
        Thalassemia with other hemoglobinopathy

        Excludes1   hemoglobin C disease (D58.2)
                hemoglobin E disease (D58.2)
                other hemoglobinopathies (D58.2)
                sickle cell anemia (D57.-)
                sickle-cell thalassemia (D57.4-)

    D56.9 Thalassemia, unspecified
        Mediterranean anemia (with other hemoglobinopathy)

● **D57 Sickle-cell disorders**
    Inherited disease in which red blood cells, normally disc-shaped, become crescent shaped

    Use additional code for any associated fever (R50.81)

    Excludes1   other hemoglobinopathies (D58.-)

    Coding Clinic: 2022, Q2, P29

● **D57.0 Hb-SS disease with crisis**
    Sickle-cell disease with crisis
    Hb-SS disease with (vaso-occlusive) pain

    D57.00 Hb-SS disease with crisis, unspecified 🔍
        Hb-SS disease with (painful) crisis NOS
        Hb-SS disease with (vaso-occlusive) pain NOS

    D57.01 Hb-SS disease with acute chest syndrome 🔍

    D57.02 Hb-SS disease with splenic sequestration 🔍
        Coding Clinic: 2025, Q1, P24

    D57.03 Hb-SS disease with cerebral vascular involvement
        Code also, if applicable, cerebral infarction (I63.-)

    D57.04 Hb-SS disease with dactylitis
        Coding Clinic: 2023, Q4, P7

    D57.09 Hb-SS disease with crisis with other specified complication
        Use additional code to identify complications, such as:
            cholelithiasis (K80.-)
            priapism (N48.32)

    D57.1 Sickle-cell disease without crisis Hb-SS disease without crisis 🔍
        Sickle-cell anemia NOS
        Sickle-cell disease NOS
        Sickle-cell disorder NOS

● **D57.2 Sickle-cell/Hb-C disease**
    Hb-SC disease
    Hb-S/Hb-C disease

    D57.20 Sickle-cell/Hb-C disease without crisis 🔍

● **D57.21 Sickle-cell/Hb-C disease with crisis**

    D57.211 Sickle-cell/Hb-C disease with acute chest syndrome 🔍

    D57.212 Sickle-cell/Hb-C disease with splenic sequestration 🔍

    D57.213 Sickle-cell/Hb-C disease with cerebral vascular involvement
        Code also, if applicable, cerebral infarction (I63.-)

    D57.214 Sickle-cell/Hb-C disease with dactylitis

    D57.218 Sickle-cell/Hb-C disease with crisis with other specified complication
        Use additional code to identify complications, such as:
            cholelithiasis (K80.-)
            priapism (N48.32)

CHAPTER 3 (D50-D89)

D57.219   **Sickle-cell/Hb-C disease with crisis, unspecified** 🅡🅒
    Sickle-cell/Hb-C disease with crisis NOS
    Sickle-cell/Hb-C disease with (vaso-occlusive) pain NOS

D57.3   **Sickle-cell trait** 🅡🅒
    Hb-S trait
    Heterozygous hemoglobin S

● **D57.4**   **Sickle-cell thalassemia**
    Sickle-cell beta thalassemia
    Thalassemia Hb-S disease

D57.40   **Sickle-cell thalassemia without crisis** 🅡🅒
    Microdrepanocytosis
    Sickle-cell thalassemia NOS

● **D57.41**   **Sickle-cell thalassemia, unspecified, with crisis**
    Sickle-cell "crisis" is precipitated when abnormally crescent-shaped red blood cells form clots and interrupt blood flow to major organs, causing severe pain and organ damage.
    Sickle-cell thalassemia with (painful) crisis NOS
    Sickle-cell thalassemia with (vaso-occlusive) pain NOS

D57.411   **Sickle-cell thalassemia, unspecified, with acute chest syndrome** 🅡🅒

D57.412   **Sickle-cell thalassemia with, unspecified, splenic sequestration** 🅡🅒

D57.413   **Sickle-cell thalassemia, unspecified, with cerebral vascular involvement**
    Code also, if applicable cerebral infarction (I63.-)

D57.414   **Sickle-cell thalassemia, unspecified, with dactylitis**

D57.418   **Sickle-cell thalassemia, unspecified, with crisis with other specified complication**
    Use additional code to identify complications, such as:
    cholelithiasis (K80.-)
    priapism (N48.32)

D57.419   **Sickle-cell thalassemia with, unspecified, crisis** 🅡🅒
    Sickle-cell thalassemia with (painful) crisis NOS
    Sickle-cell thalassemia with (vaso-occlusive) pain NOS

D57.42   **Sickle-cell thalassemia beta zero without crisis**
    HbS-beta zero without crisis
    Sickle-cell beta zero without crisis

● **D57.43**   **Sickle-cell thalassemia beta zero with crisis**
    HbS-beta zero with crisis
    Sickle-cell beta zero with crisis

D57.431   **Sickle-cell thalassemia beta zero with acute chest syndrome**
    HbS-beta zero with acute chest syndrome
    Sickle-cell beta zero with acute chest syndrome

D57.432   **Sickle-cell thalassemia beta zero with splenic sequestration**
    HbS-beta zero with splenic sequestration
    Sickle-cell beta zero with splenic sequestration

D57.433   **Sickle-cell thalassemia beta zero with cerebral vascular involvement**
    HbS-beta zero with cerebral vascular involvement
    Sickle-cell beta zero with cerebral vascular involvement
    Code also, if applicable cerebral infarction (I63.-)

D57.434   **Sickle-cell thalassemia beta zero with dactylitis**

D57.438   **Sickle-cell thalassemia beta zero with crisis with other specified complication**
    HbS-beta zero with other specified complication
    Sickle-cell beta zero with other specified complication
    Use additional code to identify complications, such as:
    cholelithiasis (K80.-)
    priapism (N48.32)

D57.439   **Sickle-cell thalassemia beta zero with crisis, unspecified**
    HbS-beta zero with other specified complication
    Sickle-cell beta zero with crisis unspecified
    Sickle-cell thalassemia beta zero with (painful) crisis NOS
    Sickle-cell thalassemia beta zero with (vaso-occlusive) pain NOS

D57.44   **Sickle-cell thalassemia beta plus without crisis**
    HbS-beta plus without crisis
    Sickle-cell beta plus without crisis

● **D57.45**   **Sickle-cell thalassemia beta plus with crisis**
    HbS-beta plus with crisis
    Sickle-cell beta plus with crisis

D57.451   **Sickle-cell thalassemia beta plus with acute chest syndrome**
    HbS-beta plus with acute chest syndrome
    Sickle-cell beta plus with acute chest syndrome

D57.452   **Sickle-cell thalassemia beta plus with splenic sequestration**
    HbS-beta plus with splenic sequestration
    Sickle-cell beta plus with splenic sequestration

D57.453   **Sickle-cell thalassemia beta plus with cerebral vascular involvement**
    HbS-beta plus with cerebral vascular involvement
    Sickle-cell beta plus with cerebral vascular involvement
    Code also, if applicable cerebral infarction (I63.-)

D57.454   **Sickle-cell thalassemia beta plus with dactylitis**

D57.458   **Sickle-cell thalassemia beta plus with crisis with other specified complication**
    HbS-beta plus with crisis with other specified complication
    Sickle-cell beta plus with crisis with other specified complication
    Use additional code to identify complications, such as:
    cholelithiasis (K80.-)
    priapism (N48.32)

D57.459 Sickle-cell thalassemia beta plus with crisis, unspecified
HbS-beta plus with crisis with unspecified complication
Sickle-cell beta plus with crisis with unspecified complication
Sickle-cell thalassemia beta plus with (painful) crisis NOS
Sickle-cell thalassemia beta plus with (vaso-occlusive) pain NOS

● **D57.8 Other sickle-cell disorders**
Hb-SD disease
Hb-SE disease

D57.80 Other sickle-cell disorders without crisis Ⓡ

● **D57.81 Other sickle-cell disorders with crisis**

D57.811 Other sickle-cell disorders with acute chest syndrome Ⓡ

D57.812 Other sickle-cell disorders with splenic sequestration Ⓡ

D57.813 Other sickle-cell disorders with cerebral vascular involvement
Code also, if applicable: cerebral infarction (I63.-)

D57.814 Other sickle-cell disorders with dactylitis

D57.818 Other sickle-cell disorders with crisis with other specified complication
Use additional code to identify complications, such as:
cholelithiasis (K80.-)
priapism (N48.32)

D57.819 Other sickle-cell disorders with crisis, unspecified Ⓡ
Other sickle-cell disorders with crisis NOS
Other sickle-cell disorders with (vaso-occlusive) pain NOS

● **D58 Other hereditary hemolytic anemias**
Genetic condition in which bone marrow is unable to compensate for premature destruction of red blood cells

Excludes1   hemolytic anemia of the newborn (P55.-)

D58.0 Hereditary spherocytosis Ⓡ
Presence of spherocytes (spherically shaped red blood cells)
Acholuric (familial) jaundice
Congenital (spherocytic) hemolytic icterus
Minkowski-Chauffard syndrome

D58.1 Hereditary elliptocytosis Ⓡ
Presence of large numbers of elliptocytes in blood
Elliptocytosis (congenital)
Ovalocytosis (congenital) (hereditary)

D58.2 Other hemoglobinopathies Ⓡ
Abnormal hemoglobin NOS
Congenital Heinz body anemia
Hb-C disease
Hb-D disease
Hb-E disease
Hemoglobinopathy NOS
Unstable hemoglobin hemolytic disease

Excludes1   familial polycythemia (D75.0)
Hb-M disease (D74.0)
hemoglobin E-beta thalassemia (D56.5)
hereditary persistence of fetal hemoglobin [HPFH] (D56.4)
high-altitude polycythemia (D75.1)
methemoglobinemia (D74.-)
other hemoglobinopathies with thalassemia (D56.8)

D58.8 Other specified hereditary hemolytic anemias Ⓡ
Stomatocytosis

D58.9 Hereditary hemolytic anemia, unspecified Ⓡ

● **D59 Acquired hemolytic anemia**

D59.0 Drug-induced autoimmune hemolytic anemia Ⓡ
Use additional code for adverse effect, if applicable, to identify drug (T36-T50 with fifth or sixth character 5)

D59.1 Other autoimmune hemolytic anemias Ⓡ
Excludes2   Evans syndrome (D69.41)
hemolytic disease of newborn (P55.-)
paroxysmal cold hemoglobinuria (D59.6)

D59.10 Autoimmune hemolytic anemia, unspecified

D59.11 Warm autoimmune hemolytic anemia
Warm type (primary) (secondary) (symptomatic) autoimmune hemolytic anemia
Warm type autoimmune hemolytic disease

D59.12 Cold autoimmune hemolytic anemia
Chronic cold hemagglutinin disease
Cold agglutinin disease
Cold agglutinin hemoglobinuria
Cold type (primary) (secondary) (symptomatic) autoimmune hemolytic anemia
Cold type autoimmune hemolytic disease

D59.13 Mixed type autoimmune hemolytic anemia
Mixed type autoimmune hemolytic disease
Mixed type, cold and warm, (primary) (secondary) (symptomatic) autoimmune hemolyticanemia

D59.19 Other autoimmune hemolytic anemia

D59.2 Drug-induced nonautoimmune hemolytic anemia Ⓡ
Drug-induced enzyme deficiency anemia
Use additional code for adverse effect, if applicable, to identify drug (T36-T50 with fifth or sixth character 5)

D59.3 Hemolytic-uremic syndrome Ⓡ
Code also, if applicable, any associated:
acute kidney failure (N17.-)
chronic kidney disease (N18.-)

D59.30 Hemolytic-uremic syndrome, unspecified
Hemolytic-uremic syndrome NOS

D59.31 Infection-associated hemolytic-uremic syndrome
Shiga toxin-producing E. coli [STEC] related hemolytic uremic syndrome
Typical hemolytic uremic syndrome
Use Additional code to identify associated infection, such as:
E. coli infection (B96.2-)
Human immunodeficiency virus [HIV] disease (B20)
Pneumococcal meningitis (G00.1)
Pneumococcal pneumonia (J13)
Sepsis due to Streptococcus pneumoniae (A40.3)
Shigella dysenteriae (A03.9)
Streptococcus pneumoniae as the cause of diseases classified elsewhere (B95.3)

D59.32 Hereditary hemolytic-uremic syndrome
Atypical hemolytic uremic syndrome with an identified genetic cause
Code also, if applicable:
defects in the complement system (D84.1)
methylmalonic acidemia (E71.120)

D59.39 Other hemolytic-uremic syndrome
Atypical (nongenetic) hemolytic uremic syndrome
Secondary hemolytic-uremic syndrome

Code first, if applicable, any associated:
COVID-19 (U07.1)
complications of kidney transplant (T86.1-)
complications of heart transplant (T86.2-)
complications of liver transplant (T86.4-)

Code also, if applicable, any associated condition, such as:
hypertensive emergency (I16.1)
malignant neoplasm (C00-C96)
systemic lupus erythematosus (M32.-)

Use Additional code, if applicable, for adverse effect to identify drug (T36-T50 with fifth or sixth character 5)

Coding Clinic: 2022, Q4, P6

D59.4 Other nonautoimmune hemolytic anemias
Mechanical hemolytic anemia
Microangiopathic hemolytic anemia
Toxic hemolytic anemia

D59.5 Paroxysmal nocturnal hemoglobinuria [Marchiafava-Micheli]
Excludes1   hemoglobinuria NOS (R82.3)

D59.6 Hemoglobinuria due to hemolysis from other external causes
Hemoglobinuria from exertion
March hemoglobinuria
Paroxysmal cold hemoglobinuria

Use additional code (Chapter 20) to identify external cause

Excludes1   hemoglobinuria NOS (R82.3)

D59.8 Other acquired hemolytic anemias

D59.9 Acquired hemolytic anemia, unspecified
Idiopathic hemolytic anemia, chronic

APLASTIC AND OTHER ANEMIAS AND OTHER BONE MARROW FAILURE SYNDROMES (D60-D64)

● **D60 Acquired pure red cell aplasia [erythroblastopenia]**
Deficiency of erythroblasts

Includes   red cell aplasia (acquired) (adult) (with thymoma)
Excludes1   congenital red cell aplasia (D61.01)

D60.0 Chronic acquired pure red cell aplasia
Lack of development of blood cell

D60.1 Transient acquired pure red cell aplasia

D60.8 Other acquired pure red cell aplasias

D60.9 Acquired pure red cell aplasia, unspecified

● **D61 Other aplastic anemias and other bone marrow failure syndromes**
Excludes2   neutropenia (D70.-)

● **D61.0 Constitutional aplastic anemia**
Condition where bone marrow is unable to produce blood cells

D61.01 Constitutional (pure) red blood cell aplasia
Blackfan-Diamond syndrome
Congenital (pure) red cell aplasia
Familial hypoplastic anemia
Primary (pure) red cell aplasia
Red cell (pure) aplasia of infants
Excludes1   acquired red cell aplasia (D60.9)

D61.02 Shwachman-Diamond syndrome
Code also, if applicable, associated conditions such as:
acute myeloblastic leukemia (C92.0-)
exocrine pancreatic insufficiency (K86.81)
myelodysplastic syndrome (D46.-)

Use additional code, if applicable, for genetic susceptibility to other malignant neoplasm(Z15.09)

D61.03 Fanconi anemia
Fanconi pancytopenia
Fanconi's anemia
Excludes1   Fanconi syndrome (E72.0-)

D61.09 Other constitutional aplastic anemia
Pancytopenia with malformations

D61.1 Drug-induced aplastic anemia
Use additional code for adverse effect, if applicable, to identify drug (T36-T50 with fifth or sixth character 5)

D61.2 Aplastic anemia due to other external agents
Code first, if applicable, toxic effects of substances chiefly nonmedicinal as to source (T51-T65)

D61.3 Idiopathic aplastic anemia

● **D61.8 Other specified aplastic anemias and other bone marrow failure syndromes**

● **D61.81 Pancytopenia**
Marked deficiency of all the blood elements: Red blood cells (erythrocytes), white blood cells (leukocytes), and platelets (thrombocytes). Check laboratory results.

Excludes1   pancytopenia (due to) (with) aplastic anemia (D61.9)
pancytopenia (due to) (with) bone marrow infiltration (D61.82)
pancytopenia (due to) (with) congenital (pure) red cell aplasia (D61.01)
pancytopenia (due to) (with) hairy cell leukemia (C91.4-)
pancytopenia (due to) (with) human immunodeficiency virus disease (B20.-)
pancytopenia (due to) (with) leukoerythroblastic anemia (D61.82)
pancytopenia (due to) (with) myeloproliferative disease (D47.1)

Excludes2   pancytopenia (due to) (with) myelodysplastic syndromes (D46.-)

D61.810 Antineoplastic chemotherapy induced pancytopenia
Excludes2   aplastic anemia due to antineoplastic chemotherapy (D61.1)

D61.811 Other drug-induced pancytopenia
Excludes2   aplastic anemia due to drugs (D61.1)

D61.818 Other pancytopenia
Coding Clinic: 2023, Q1, P23; 2019, Q1, P16

D61.82 Myelophthisis
Leukoerythroblastic anemia
Myelophthisic anemia
Panmyelophthisis
Code also the underlying disorder, such as:
malignant neoplasm of breast (C50.-)
tuberculosis (A15.-)

Excludes1   idiopathic myelofibrosis (D47.1)
myelofibrosis NOS (D75.81)
myelofibrosis with myeloid metaplasia (D47.4)
primary myelofibrosis (D47.1)
secondary myelofibrosis (D75.81)

D61.89 Other specified aplastic anemias and other bone marrow failure syndromes

D61.9   **Aplastic anemia, unspecified** 🔗
Hypoplastic anemia NOS
Medullary hypoplasia

D62   **Acute posthemorrhagic anemia**

> **Excludes1**   anemia due to chronic blood loss (D50.0)
> blood loss anemia NOS (D50.0)
> congenital anemia from fetal blood loss (P61.3)

Coding Clinic: 2019, Q3, P13,17

● **D63**   **Anemia in chronic diseases classified elsewhere**

▶ *D63.0*   *Anemia in neoplastic disease*

> *Code first neoplasm (C00-D49)*

> **Excludes1**   aplastic anemia due to antineoplastic
> chemotherapy (D61.1)

> **Excludes2**   anemia due to antineoplastic
> chemotherapy (D64.81)

OGCR   Section I.C.2.e.2.

2) Anemia associated with chemotherapy, immunotherapy and radiation therapy

When the admission/encounter is for management of an anemia associated with an adverse effect of the administration of chemotherapy or immunotherapy and the only treatment is for the anemia, the anemia code is sequenced first followed by the appropriate codes for the neoplasm and the adverse effect (T45.1X5, Adverse effect of antineoplastic and immunosuppressive drugs).

▶ *D63.1*   *Anemia in chronic kidney disease*
Erythropoietin resistant anemia (EPO resistant anemia)
Code first underlying chronic kidney disease (CKD) (N18.-)

▶ *D63.8*   *Anemia in other chronic diseases classified elsewhere*

> *Code first underlying disease, such as:*
> diphyllobothriasis (B70.0)
> hookworm disease (B76.0-B76.9)
> hypothyroidism (E00.0-E03.9)
> malaria (B50.0-B54)
> symptomatic late syphilis (A52.79)
> tuberculosis (A18.89)

● **D64**   **Other anemias**

> **Excludes1**   refractory anemia (D46.-)
> refractory anemia with excess blasts in
> transformation [RAEB T] (C92.0-)

D64.0   **Hereditary sideroblastic anemia** 🔗
Abnormal production RBCs (erythrocytes)
Sex-linked hypochromic sideroblastic anemia

▶ *D64.1*   *Secondary sideroblastic anemia due to disease* 🔗

> *Code first underlying disease*

D64.2   **Secondary sideroblastic anemia due to drugs and toxins** 🔗

> *Code first poisoning due to drug or toxin, if applicable
> (T36-T65 with fifth or sixth character 1-4)*

> Use additional code for adverse effect, if applicable, to
> identify drug (T36-T50 with fifth or sixth character 5)

D64.3   **Other sideroblastic anemias** 🔗
Sideroblastic anemia NOS
Pyridoxine-responsive sideroblastic anemia NEC

D64.4   **Congenital dyserythropoietic anemia**
Any of several rare hereditary anemias, mostly types of macrocytic anemia
Dyshematopoietic anemia (congenital)

> **Excludes1**   Blackfan-Diamond syndrome (D61.01)
> Di Guglielmo's disease (C94.0)

● **D64.8**   **Other specified anemias**

D64.81   **Anemia due to antineoplastic chemotherapy**
Antineoplastic chemotherapy induced anemia
aplastic anemia due to antineoplastic
chemotherapy (D61.1)

> **Excludes2**   anemia in neoplastic disease
> (D63.0)

Coding Clinic: 2023, Q3, P4; 2023, Q2, P18; 2021, Q3, P4

D64.89   **Other specified anemias**
Infantile pseudoleukemia

D64.9   **Anemia, unspecified**
Coding Clinic: 2018, Q4, P88; 2017, Q1, P7

COAGULATION DEFECTS, PURPURA AND OTHER HEMORRHAGIC CONDITIONS (D65-D69)

D65   **Disseminated intravascular coagulation [defibrination syndrome]** 🔗
Blood clots form and consume all coagulation proteins and platelets and disrupt normal coagulation, resulting in abnormal bleeding
Afibrinogenemia, acquired
Consumption coagulopathy
COVID-19 associated diffuse or disseminated intravascular coagulopathy
Diffuse or disseminated intravascular coagulation [DIC]
Fibrinolytic hemorrhage, acquired
Fibrinolytic purpura
Purpura fulminans

> Code also, if applicable, associated condition

> **Excludes1**   disseminated intravascular coagulation
> (complicating):
> abortion or ectopic or molar pregnancy
> (O00-O07, O08.1)
> in newborn (P60)
> pregnancy, childbirth and the puerperium
> (O45.0, O46.0, O67.0, O72.3)

Coding Clinic: 2022, Q4, P9; 2021, Q1, P39; 2019, Q2, P25

D66   **Hereditary factor VIII deficiency** 🔗
Inherited coagulation disorder carried by females but most often affecting males
Classical hemophilia
Deficiency factor VIII (with functional defect)
Hemophilia NOS
Hemophilia A

> **Excludes1**   factor VIII deficiency with vascular defect (D68.0-)

D67   **Hereditary factor IX deficiency** 🔗
Christmas disease
Factor IX deficiency (with functional defect)
Hemophilia B
Plasma thromboplastin component [PTC] deficiency

● **D68**   **Other coagulation defects**

> **Excludes1**   abnormal coagulation profile NOS (R79.1)

> **Excludes2**   coagulation defects complicating abortion or
> ectopic or molar pregnancy (O00-O07, O08.1)
> coagulation defects complicating pregnancy,
> childbirth and the puerperium (O45.0, O46.0,
> O67.0, O72.3)

Coding Clinic: 2016, Q1, P14

D68.0   **Von Willebrand disease** 🔗
Congenital bleeding disorder

> **Excludes1**   capillary fragility (hereditary) (D69.8)
> factor VIII deficiency NOS (D66)
> factor VIII deficiency with functional
> defect (D66)

D68.00   **Von Willebrand disease, unspecified**

D68.01   **Von Willebrand disease, type 1**
Partial quantitative deficiency of von
Willebrand factor
Type 1C von Willebrand disease
Coding Clinic: 2022, Q4, P9

● **D68.02**   **Von Willebrand disease, type 2**
Qualitative defects of von Willebrand factor

D68.020   **Von Willebrand disease, type 2A**
Qualitative defects of von
Willebrand factor with
decreased platelet adhesion and
selective deficiency of high-
molecular-weight multimers

D68.021   **Von Willebrand disease, type 2B**
Qualitative defects of von Willebrand factor with high-molecular-weight von Willebrand factor loss
Qualitative defects of von Willebrand factor with hyper-adhesive forms
Qualitative defects of von Willebrand factor with increased affinity for platelet glycoprotein lb

D68.022   **Von Willebrand disease, type 2M**
Qualitative defects of von Willebrand factor with defective platelet adhesion with anormal size distribution of von Willebrand factor multimers

D68.023   **Von Willebrand disease, type 2N**
Qualitative defects of von Willebrand factor with defective von Willebrand factor to factor VIII binding
Qualitative defects of von Willebrand factor with markedly decreased affinity for factor VIII

D68.029   **Von Willebrand disease, type 2, unspecified**
Qualitative defect in von Willebrand factor function, with no further subtyping

D68.03   **Von Willebrand disease, type 3**
(Near) complete absence of von Willebrand factor
Total quantitative deficiency of von Willebrand factor

D68.04   **Acquired von Willebrand disease**
Acquired von Willebrand syndrome

D68.09   **Other von Willebrand disease**
Platelet-type von Willebrand disease
Pseudo-von Willebrand disease
Code also, if applicable, qualitative platelet defects (D69.1)

D68.1   **Hereditary factor XI deficiency** 🅑
Deficiency of blood coagulation resulting in systemic blood-clotting defect
Hemophilia C
Plasma thromboplastin antecedent [PTA] deficiency
Rosenthal's disease

D68.2   **Hereditary deficiency of other clotting factors** 🅑
Blood clotting disorders caused by hereditary deficiencies of one or more clotting factors
AC globulin deficiency
Congenital afibrinogenemia
Deficiency of factor I [fibrinogen]
Deficiency of factor II [prothrombin]
Deficiency of factor V [labile]
Deficiency of factor VII [stable]
Deficiency of factor X [Stuart-Prower]
Deficiency of factor XII [Hageman]
Deficiency of factor XIII [fibrin stabilizing]
Dysfibrinogenemia (congenital)
Hypoproconvertinemia
Owren's disease
Proaccelerin deficiency
Coding Clinic: 2025, Q2, P3

● D68.3   **Hemorrhagic disorder due to circulating anticoagulants**
Blood clotting disorders caused by anticoagulants (warfarin and heparin)

● D68.31   **Hemorrhagic disorder due to intrinsic circulating anticoagulants, antibodies, or inhibitors**

D68.311   **Acquired hemophilia** 🅑
Autoimmune hemophilia
Autoimmune inhibitors to clotting factors
Secondary hemophilia

D68.312   **Antiphospholipid antibody with hemorrhagic disorder** 🅑
Lupus anticoagulant (LAC) with hemorrhagic disorder
Systemic lupus erythematosus [SLE] inhibitor with hemorrhagic disorder

Excludes1   ~~antiphospholipid antibody, finding without diagnosis (R76.0)~~
~~antiphospholipid antibody syndrome (D68.61)~~
~~antiphospholipid antibody with hypercoagulable state (D68.61)~~
~~lupus anticoagulant (LAC) finding without diagnosis (R76.0)~~
~~lupus anticoagulant (LAC) with hypercoagulable state (D68.62)~~
~~systemic lupus erythematosus [SLE] inhibitor finding without diagnosis (R76.0)~~
~~systemic lupus erythematosus [SLE] inhibitor with hypercoagulable state (D68.62)~~

▶ Excludes2   antiphospholipid antibody, finding without diagnosis (R76.0)
▶ antiphospholipid antibody syndrome (D68.61)
▶ antiphospholipid antibody with hypercoagulable state (D68.61)
▶ lupus anticoagulant (LAC) finding without diagnosis (R76.0)
▶ lupus anticoagulant (LAC) with hypercoagulable state (D68.62)
▶ systemic lupus erythematosus [SLE] inhibitor finding without diagnosis (R76.0)
▶ systemic lupus erythematosus [SLE] inhibitor with hypercoagulable state (D68.62)

▶ New   ➡ Revised   ~~deleted~~ Deleted   Excludes 1   Excludes 2   Includes   Use additional   Code first   Code also   Key words
OGCR Official Guidelines   X Assign placeholder X   ● Use Additional Character(s)   ▶ Manifestation Code   🅑 Hierarchical Condition Category   **Coding Clinic**

CHAPTER 3 (D50-D89)

D68.318 Other hemorrhagic disorder due to intrinsic circulating anticoagulants, antibodies, or inhibitors 🔍
    Antithromboplastinemia
    Antithromboplastinogenemia
    Hemorrhagic disorder due to intrinsic increase in antithrombin
    Hemorrhagic disorder due to intrinsic increase in anti-VIIIa
    Hemorrhagic disorder due to intrinsic increase in anti-IXa
    Hemorrhagic disorder due to intrinsic increase in anti-XIa

D68.32 Hemorrhagic disorder due to extrinsic circulating anticoagulants 🔍
    Drug-induced hemorrhagic disorder
    Hemorrhagic disorder due to increase in anti-IIa
    Hemorrhagic disorder due to increase in anti-Xa
    Hyperheparinemia
    Use additional code for adverse effect, if applicable, to identify drug (T45.515, T45.525)
    Coding Clinic: 2021, Q1, P5; 2016, Q1, P14-15

D68.4 Acquired coagulation factor deficiency 🔍
    Deficiency of coagulation factor due to liver disease
    Deficiency of coagulation factor due to vitamin K deficiency
    Excludes1 vitamin K deficiency of newborn (P53)

● **D68.5 Primary thrombophilia**
    AKA idiopathic thrombocytopenia, may be acquired or congenital and is a common cause of coagulation disorders.
    Primary hypercoagulable states
    Excludes1 antiphospholipid syndrome (D68.61)
        lupus anticoagulant (D68.62)
        secondary activated protein C resistance (D68.69)
        secondary antiphospholipid antibody syndrome (D68.69)
        secondary lupus anticoagulant with hypercoagulable state (D68.69)
        secondary systemic lupus erythematosus [SLE] inhibitor with hypercoagulable state (D68.69)
        systemic lupus erythematosus [SLE] inhibitor finding without diagnosis (R76.0)
        systemic lupus erythematosus [SLE] inhibitor with hemorrhagic disorder (D68.312)
        thrombotic thrombocytopenic purpura (M31.19)

D68.51 Activated protein C resistance 🔍
    Factor V Leiden mutation
    Coding Clinic: 2025, Q2, P3

D68.52 Prothrombin gene mutation 🔍

D68.59 Other primary thrombophilia 🔍
    Antithrombin III deficiency
    Hypercoagulable state NOS
    Primary hypercoagulable state NEC
    Primary thrombophilia NEC
    Protein C deficiency
    Protein S deficiency
    Thrombophilia NOS
    Coding Clinic: 2021, Q2, P8-9

● **D68.6 Other thrombophilia**
    Other hypercoagulable states
    Excludes1 diffuse or disseminated intravascular coagulation [DIC] (D65)
        heparin induced thrombocytopenia (HIT) (D75.82-)
        hyperhomocysteinemia (E72.11)

D68.61 Antiphospholipid syndrome 🔍
    Anticardiolipin syndrome
    Antiphospholipid antibody syndrome
    Excludes1 ~~anti-phospholipid antibody, finding without diagnosis (R76.0)~~
        ~~anti-phospholipid antibody with hemorrhagic disorder (D68.312)~~
        ~~lupus anticoagulant syndrome (D68.62)~~
    ▶ **Excludes2** anti-phospholipid antibody, finding without diagnosis (R76.0)
        ▶anti-phospholipid antibody with hemorrhagic disorder (D68.312)
        ▶lupus anticoagulant syndrome (D68.62)

D68.62 Lupus anticoagulant syndrome 🔍
    Lupus anticoagulant
    Presence of systemic lupus erythematosus [SLE] inhibitor
    Excludes1 ~~anticardiolipin syndrome (D68.61)~~
        ~~antiphospholipid syndrome (D68.61)~~
        ~~lupus anticoagulant (LAC) finding without diagnosis (R76.0)~~
        ~~lupus anticoagulant (LAC) with hemorrhagic disorder (D68.312)~~
    ▶ **Excludes2** anticardiolipin syndrome (D68.61)
        ▶antiphospholipid syndrome (D68.61)
        ▶lupus anticoagulant (LAC) finding without diagnosis (R76.0)
        ▶lupus anticoagulant (LAC) with hemorrhagic disorder (D68.312)

D68.69 Other thrombophilia 🔍
    COVID-19 associated hypercoagulability
    Hypercoagulable states NEC
    Secondary hypercoagulable state NOS
    Code also, if applicable, associated condition
    Coding Clinic: 2021, Q2, P8

D68.8 Other specified coagulation defects 🔍
    COVID-19 associated coagulopathy
    Code also, if applicable, associated condition
    Excludes1 hemorrhagic disease of newborn (P53)
    Coding Clinic: 2021, Q1, P39-40

D68.9 Coagulation defect, unspecified 🔍

● **D69 Purpura and other hemorrhagic conditions**
    Group of conditions characterized by small hemorrhages in skin, mucous membranes, or serosal surfaces
    Excludes1 benign hypergammaglobulinemic purpura (D89.0)
        cryoglobulinemic purpura (D89.1)
        essential (hemorrhagic) thrombocythemia (D47.3)
        hemorrhagic thrombocythemia (D47.3)
        purpura fulminans (D65)
        thrombotic thrombocytopenic purpura (M31.19)
        Waldenström hypergammaglobulinemic purpura (D89.0)

D69.0 Allergic purpura 🔍
    Allergic vasculitis
    Nonthrombocytopenic hemorrhagic purpura
    Nonthrombocytopenic idiopathic purpura
    Purpura anaphylactoid
    Purpura Henoch(-Schönlein)
    Purpura rheumatica
    Vascular purpura
    Excludes1 thrombocytopenic hemorrhagic purpura (D69.3)

CHAPTER 3 (D50–D89)

D69.1 Qualitative platelet defects 🅱
  Bernard-Soulier [giant platelet] syndrome
  Glanzmann's disease
  Grey platelet syndrome
  Thromboasthenia (hemorrhagic) (hereditary)
  Thrombocytopathy
  Excludes1 hemolytic-uremic syndrome (D59.3-)
  Excludes2 von Willebrand disease (D68.0-)

D69.2 Other nonthrombocytopenic purpura 🅱
  Purpura NOS
  Purpura simplex
  Senile purpura

D69.3 Immune thrombocytopenic purpura 🅱
  Hemorrhagic (thrombocytopenic) purpura
  Idiopathic thrombocytopenic purpura
  Tidal platelet dysgenesis

● **D69.4 Other primary thrombocytopenia**
  Excludes1 transient neonatal thrombocytopenia
                (P61.0)
                Wiskott-Aldrich syndrome (D82.0)

  D69.41 Evans syndrome 🅱
    Acquired hemolytic anemia and thrombocytopenia

  **D69.42 Congenital and hereditary thrombocytopenia
           purpura** 🅱
    Congenital thrombocytopenia
    Hereditary thrombocytopenia
    *Code first congenital or hereditary disorder,
       such as:*
        thrombocytopenia with absent radius (TAR
           syndrome) (Q87.2)

  D69.49 Other primary thrombocytopenia 🅱
    Megakaryocytic hypoplasia
    Primary thrombocytopenia NOS

● **D69.5 Secondary thrombocytopenia**
  *Acquired reduction of number of platelets required for blood
     clotting*
  Excludes1 heparin induced thrombocytopenia (HIT)
                (D75.82-)
                transient thrombocytopenia of newborn
                (P61.0)

  D69.51 Posttransfusion purpura
    Posttransfusion purpura from whole blood
       (fresh) or blood products PTP

  D69.59 Other secondary thrombocytopenia

D69.6 Thrombocytopenia, unspecified 🅱

D69.8 Other specified hemorrhagic conditions 🅱
  Capillary fragility (hereditary)
  Vascular pseudohemophilia

D69.9 Hemorrhagic condition, unspecified 🅱

OTHER DISORDERS OF BLOOD AND BLOOD-FORMING ORGANS (D70-D77)

● **D70 Neutropenia**
  Code also, if applicable, mucositis (J34.81, K12.3-, K92.81,
     N76.81)
  Decrease in number of neutrophils (type of white blood cell)
  Includes agranulocytosis
               decreased absolute neurophile count (ANC)
  Excludes1 neutropenic splenomegaly (D73.81)
                transient neonatal neutropenia (P61.5)

  D70.0 Congenital agranulocytosis 🅱
    Reduced numbers of neutrophils (type of white blood cell)
    Congenital neutropenia
    Infantile genetic agranulocytosis
    Kostmann's disease

  D70.1 Agranulocytosis secondary to cancer chemotherapy 🅱
    Decreased numbers of granulocytes (type of white blood cell)
    Code also underlying neoplasm
    Use additional code for adverse effect, if applicable, to
       identify drug (T45.1X5)

D70.2 Other drug-induced agranulocytosis 🅱
  Use additional code for adverse effect, if applicable,
     to identify drug (T36-T50 with fifth or sixth
     character 5)

D70.3 Neutropenia due to infection 🅱

D70.4 Cyclic neutropenia 🅱
  Chronic neutropenia (low number of type of white blood cell)
  Cyclic hematopoiesis
  Periodic neutropenia

D70.8 Other neutropenia 🅱

D70.9 Neutropenia, unspecified 🅱
  Coding Clinic: 2019, Q2, P25

● **D71 Functional disorders of polymorphonuclear neutrophils** 🅱
  Polymorphonuclear: varying shapes of nucleus; AKA PMNs
  ~~Cell membrane receptor complex [CR3] defect~~
  ~~Chronic (childhood) granulomatous disease~~
  ~~Congenital dysphagocytosis~~
  ~~Progressive septic granulomatosis~~

  ▶ **D71.1 Leukocyte adhesion deficiency**
    ▶ LAD-I
    ▶ LAD-II
    ▶ LAD-III
    ▶ Leukocyte adhesion deficiency type I
    ▶ Leukocyte adhesion deficiency type II
    ▶ Leukocyte adhesion deficiency type III

  ▶ **D71.8 Other functional disorders of polymorphonuclear
           neutrophils**
    ▶ Cell membrane receptor complex [CR3] defect
    ▶ Chronic (childhood) granulomatous disease
    ▶ Congenital dysphagocytosis
    ▶ Progressive septic granulomatosis

  ▶ **D71.9 Functional disorders of polymorphonuclear neutrophils,
           unspecified**

● **D72 Other disorders of white blood cells**
  Excludes1 basophilia (D72.824)
                immunity disorders (D80-D89)
                neutropenia (D70)
                preleukemia (syndrome) (D46.9)

  D72.0 Genetic anomalies of leukocytes
    Alder (granulation) (granulocyte) anomaly
    Alder syndrome
    Hereditary leukocytic hypersegmentation
    Hereditary leukocytic hyposegmentation
    Hereditary leukomelanopathy
    May-Hegglin (granulation) (granulocyte) anomaly
    May-Hegglin syndrome
    Pelger-Huët (granulation) (granulocyte) anomaly
    Pelger-Huët syndrome
    Excludes1 Chédiak (-Steinbrinck)-Higashi syndrome
                  (E70.330)

● **D72.1 Eosinophilia**
  *Formation and accumulation of high number of white cells in
     blood/tissue*
  Excludes2 Löffler's syndrome (J82.89)
                pulmonary eosinophilia (J82.-)

  D72.10 Eosinophilia, unspecified

● **D72.11 Hypereosinophilic syndrome [HES]**

    **D72.110 Idiopathic hypereosinophilic
             syndrome [IHES]**

    **D72.111 Lymphocytic Variant
             Hypereosinophilic Syndrome [LHES]**
      Lymphocyte variant
         hypereosinophilia
      Code also, if applicable, any
         associated lymphocytic
         neoplastic disorder

    D72.118 Other hypereosinophilic syndrome
      Episodic angioedema with
         eosinophilia
      Gleich's syndrome

    **D72.119 Hypereosinophilic syndrome [HES],
             unspecified**

D72.12   **Drug rash with eosinophilia and systemic symptoms syndrome**
DRESS syndrome
Use additional code for adverse effect, if applicable, to identify drug (T36-T50 with fifth or sixth character 5)

D72.18   *Eosinophilia in diseases classified elsewhere*
Code first underlying disease, such as:
chronic myelomonocytic leukemia (C93.1-)

D72.19   **Other eosinophilia**
Familial eosinophilia
Hereditary eosinophilia

● **D72.8**   **Other specified disorders of white blood cells**
Excludes1   leukemia (C91-C95)

● **D72.81**   **Decreased white blood cell count**
Excludes1   neutropenia (D70.-)

D72.810   **Lymphocytopenia**
Decreased lymphocytes
Reduction in number of lympho cytes in blood

D72.818   **Other decreased white blood cell count**
Basophilic leukopenia
Eosinophilic leukopenia
Monocytopenia
Other decreased leukocytes
Plasmacytopenia

D72.819   **Decreased white blood cell count, unspecified**
Decreased leukocytes, unspecified
Leukocytopenia, unspecified
Leukopenia
Excludes1   malignant leukopenia (D70.9)

● **D72.82**   **Elevated white blood cell count**
Excludes1   eosinophilia (D72.1)

D72.820   **Lymphocytosis (symptomatic)**
Elevated lymphocytes
Excess of normal lymphocytes

D72.821   **Monocytosis (symptomatic)**
Excludes1   infectious mononucleosis (B27.-)

D72.822   **Plasmacytosis**
Presence of excess plasma cells

D72.823   **Leukemoid reaction**
Basophilic leukemoid reaction
Leukemoid reaction NOS
Lymphocytic leukemoid reaction
Monocytic leukemoid reaction
Myelocytic leukemoid reaction
Neutrophilic leukemoid reaction

D72.824   **Basophilia**
Increase of basophils in blood

D72.825   **Bandemia**
Bandemia without diagnosis of specific infection
Excess number of band cells (immature white blood cells) released by bone marrow
Excludes1   confirmed infection -code to infection leukemia (C91.-, C92.-, C93.-, C94.-, C95.-)

D72.828   **Other elevated white blood cell count**

D72.829   **Elevated white blood cell count, unspecified**
Elevated leukocytes, unspecified
Leukocytosis, unspecified

D72.89   **Other specified disorders of white blood cells**
Abnormality of white blood cells NEC

D72.9   **Disorder of white blood cells, unspecified**
Abnormal leukocyte differential NOS

● **D73**   **Diseases of spleen**

D73.0   **Hyposplenism**
Diminished functioning of spleen
Atrophy of spleen
Excludes1   asplenia (congenital) (Q89.01)
postsurgical absence of spleen (Z90.81)
Coding Clinic: 2025, Q1, P24-25

D73.1   **Hypersplenism**
Accelerated function of spleen
Excludes1   neutropenic splenomegaly (D73.81)
primary splenic neutropenia (D73.81)
splenitis, splenomegaly in late syphilis (A52.79)
splenitis, splenomegaly in tuberculosis (A18.85)
splenomegaly NOS (R16.1)
splenomegaly congenital (Q89.0)

D73.2   **Chronic congestive splenomegaly**
Enlargement of spleen

D73.3   **Abscess of spleen**

D73.4   **Cyst of spleen**

D73.5   **Infarction of spleen**
Splenic rupture, nontraumatic
Torsion of spleen
Excludes1   rupture of spleen due to Plasmodium vivax malaria (B51.0)
traumatic rupture of spleen (S36.03-)

● **D73.8**   **Other diseases of spleen**

D73.81   **Neutropenic splenomegaly**
Werner-Schultz disease
Enlarged spleen responding to inadequate number of neutrophils

D73.89   **Other diseases of spleen**
Fibrosis of spleen NOS
Perisplenitis
Splenitis NOS

D73.9   **Disease of spleen, unspecified**

● **D74**   **Methemoglobinemia**
Excessive methemoglobin (form of hemoglobin)

D74.0   **Congenital methemoglobinemia**
Congenital NADH-methemoglobin reductase deficiency
Hemoglobin-M [Hb-M] disease
Methemoglobinemia, hereditary

D74.8   **Other methemoglobinemias**
Acquired methemoglobinemia (with sulfhemoglobinemia)
Toxic methemoglobinemia

D74.9   **Methemoglobinemia, unspecified**

● **D75**   **Other and unspecified diseases of blood and blood-forming organs**
Excludes2   acute lymphadenitis (L04.-)
chronic lymphadenitis (I88.1)
enlarged lymph nodes (R59.-)
hypergammaglobulinemia NOS (D89.2)
lymphadenitis NOS (I88.9)
mesenteric lymphadenitis (acute) (chronic) (I88.0)

D75.0   **Familial erythrocytosis**
Genetic mutation of gene that results in increased circulating RBCs
Benign polycythemia
Familial polycythemia
Excludes1   hereditary ovalocytosis (D58.1)

D75.1 Secondary polycythemia
Increase in total red cell mass
Acquired polycythemia
Emotional polycythemia
Erythrocytosis NOS
Hypoxemic polycythemia
Nephrogenous polycythemia
Polycythemia due to erythropoietin
Polycythemia due to fall in plasma volume
Polycythemia due to high altitude
Polycythemia due to stress
Polycythemia NOS
Relative polycythemia
> **Excludes1**   polycythemia neonatorum (P61.1)
> polycythemia vera (D45)

● **D75.8 Other specified diseases of blood and blood-forming organs**

▶ *D75.81 Myelofibrosis* 🝔
Replacing bone marrow by fibrous tissue
Myelofibrosis NOS
Secondary myelofibrosis NOS
> **Code first** the underlying disorder, such as:
> malignant neoplasm of breast (C50.-)
> **Use additional** code, if applicable,
> for associated therapy-related
> myelodysplastic syndrome (D46.-)
> **Use additional** code for adverse effect, if
> applicable, to identify drug (T45.1X5)
> **Excludes1**   acute myelofibrosis (C94.4-)
> idiopathic myelofibrosis (D47.1)
> leukoerythroblastic anemia
> (D61.82)
> myelofibrosis with myeloid
> metaplasia (D47.4)
> myelophthisic anemia (D61.82)
> myelophthisis (D61.82)
> primary myelofibrosis (D47.1)

D75.82 Heparin induced thrombocytopenia (HIT) 🝔
> **Use Additional** code, if applicable, for adverse
> effect of heparin (T45.515-)

D75.821 Non-immune heparin-induced thrombocytopenia
Non-immune HIT
Type 1 heparin-induced
thrombocytopenia

D75.822 Immune-mediated heparin-induced thrombocytopenia
Immune-mediated HIT
Type 2 heparin-induced
thrombocytopenia

D75.828 Other heparin-induced thrombocytopenia syndrome
Autoimmune heparin-induced
thrombocytopenia syndrome
Delayed-onset heparin-induced
thrombocytopenia
Persisting heparin-induced
thrombocytopenia

D75.829 Heparin-induced thrombocytopenia, unspecified

● **D75.83 Thrombocytosis**
> **Excludes2**   essential thrombocythemia (D47.3)

D75.838 Other thrombocytosis
Reactive thrombocytosis
Secondary thrombocytosis
> **Code also**, underlying condition, if
> known and applicable

D75.839 Thrombocytosis, unspecified
Thrombocythemia NOS
Thrombocytosis NOS

D75.84 Other platelet-activating anti-PF4 disorders
Spontaneous heparin-induced
thrombocytopenia syndrome (without
heparin exposure)
Thrombosis with thrombocytopenia syndrome
Vaccine-induced thrombotic thrombocytopenia
> **Use Additional** code, if applicable, for adverse
> effect of other viral vaccine (T50.B95-)

D75.89 Other specified diseases of blood and blood-forming organs

D75.9 Disease of blood and blood-forming organs, unspecified

D75.A Glucose-6-phosphate dehydrogenase (G6PD) deficiency without anemia
> **Excludes1**   glucose-6-phosphate dehydrogenase
> (G6PD) deficiency with anemia
> (D55.0)

● **D76 Other specified diseases with participation of lymphoreticular and reticulohistiocytic tissue**
> **Excludes1**   (Abt-) Letterer-Siwe disease (C96.0)
> eosinophilic granuloma (C96.6)
> Hand-Schüller-Christian disease (C96.5)
> histiocytic medullary reticulosis (C96.9)
> histiocytic sarcoma (C96.A)
> histiocytosis X, multifocal (C96.5)
> histiocytosis X, unifocal (C96.6)
> Langerhans-cell histiocytosis, multifocal (C96.5)
> Langerhans-cell histiocytosis NOS (C96.6)
> Langerhans-cell histiocytosis, unifocal (C96.6)
> leukemic reticuloendotheliosis (C91.4-)
> lipomelanotic reticulosis (I89.8)
> malignant histiocytosis (C96.A)
> malignant reticulosis (C86.0)
> nonlipid reticuloendotheliosis (C96.0)

D76.1 Hemophagocytic lymphohistiocytosis 🝔
Familial hemophagocytic reticulosis
Histiocytoses of mononuclear phagocytes

D76.2 Hemophagocytic syndrome, infection-associated 🝔
> **Use additional** code to identify infectious agent or
> disease.

D76.3 Other histiocytosis syndromes 🝔
Reticulohistiocytoma (giant-cell)
Sinus histiocytosis with massive lymphadenopathy
Xanthogranuloma

▶ *D77 Other disorders of blood and blood-forming organs in diseases classified elsewhere*
> **Code first** underlying disease, such as:
> amyloidosis (E85.-)
> congenital early syphilis (A50.0-)
> echinococcosis (B67.0-B67.9)
> malaria (B50.0-B54)
> schistosomiasis [bilharziasis] (B65.0-B65.9)
> vitamin C deficiency (E54)
> **Excludes1**   rupture of spleen due to Plasmodium vivax
> malaria (B51.0)
> splenitis, splenomegaly in late syphilis (A52.79)
> splenitis, splenomegaly in tuberculosis (A18.85)

INTRAOPERATIVE AND POSTPROCEDURAL COMPLICATIONS OF THE SPLEEN (D78)

● **D78 Intraoperative and postprocedural complications of the spleen**
Coding Clinic: 2016, Q4, P9

● **D78.0 Intraoperative hemorrhage and hematoma of the spleen complicating a procedure**
> **Excludes1**   intraoperative hemorrhage and
> hematoma of the spleen due to
> accidental puncture or laceration
> during a procedure (D78.1-)

D78.01 Intraoperative hemorrhage and hematoma of the spleen complicating a procedure on the spleen

D78.02 Intraoperative hemorrhage and hematoma of the spleen complicating other procedure

● **D78.1** **Accidental puncture and laceration of the spleen during a procedure**

    D78.11   Accidental puncture and laceration of the spleen during a procedure on the spleen

    D78.12   Accidental puncture and laceration of the spleen during other procedure
       Coding Clinic: 2022, Q1, P22-23

● **D78.2** **Postprocedural hemorrhage of the spleen following a procedure**

    D78.21   Postprocedural hemorrhage of the spleen following a procedure on the spleen

    D78.22   Postprocedural hemorrhage of the spleen following other procedure

● **D78.3** **Postprocedural hematoma and seroma of the spleen following a procedure**

    D78.31   Postprocedural hematoma of the spleen following a procedure on the spleen

    D78.32   Postprocedural hematoma of the spleen following other procedure

    D78.33   Postprocedural seroma of the spleen following a procedure on the spleen

    D78.34   Postprocedural seroma of the spleen following other procedure

● **D78.8** **Other intraoperative and postprocedural complications of the spleen**

    Use additional code, if applicable, to further specify disorder

    D78.81   Other intraoperative complications of the spleen

    D78.89   Other postprocedural complications of the spleen

CERTAIN DISORDERS INVOLVING THE IMMUNE MECHANISM (D80-D89)

    Includes   defects in the complement system
        immunodeficiency disorders, except human immunodeficiency virus [HIV] disease
        sarcoidosis

    Excludes1   autoimmune disease (systemic) NOS (M35.9)
        ➡ functional disorders of polymorphonuclear neutrophils (D71.-)
        human immunodeficiency virus [HIV] disease (B20)

● **D80** **Immunodeficiency with predominantly antibody defects**

    D80.0   **Hereditary hypogammaglobulinemia**
       Autosomal recessive agammaglobulinemia (Swiss type)
       X-linked agammaglobulinemia [Bruton] (with growth hormone deficiency)

    D80.1   **Nonfamilial hypogammaglobulinemia**
       Abnormally low levels of all classes of immunoglobulins
       Agammaglobulinemia with immunoglobulin-bearing B-lymphocytes
       Common variable agammaglobulinemia [CVAgamma]
       Hypogammaglobulinemia NOS

    D80.2   **Selective deficiency of immunoglobulin A [IgA]**

    D80.3   **Selective deficiency of immunoglobulin G [IgG] subclasses**

    D80.4   **Selective deficiency of immunoglobulin M [IgM]**

    D80.5   **Immunodeficiency with increased immunoglobulin M [IgM]**

    D80.6   **Antibody deficiency with near-normal immunoglobulins or with hyperimmunoglobulinemia**
       Abnormally high levels of immunoglobulins in serum

    D80.7   **Transient hypogammaglobulinemia of infancy**

    D80.8   **Other immunodeficiencies with predominantly antibody defects**
       Kappa light chain deficiency

    D80.9   **Immunodeficiency with predominantly antibody defects, unspecified**

● **D81** **Combined immunodeficiencies**

    Excludes1   autosomal recessive agammaglobulinemia (Swiss type) (D80.0)

    D81.0   **Severe combined immunodeficiency [SCID] with reticular dysgenesis**

    D81.1   **Severe combined immunodeficiency [SCID] with low T- and B-cell numbers**

    D81.2   **Severe combined immunodeficiency [SCID] with low or normal B-cell numbers**

●   D81.3   **Adenosine deaminase [ADA] deficiency**

    D81.30   **Adenosine deaminase deficiency, unspecified**
        ADA deficiency NOS

    D81.31   **Severe combined immunodeficiency due to adenosine deaminase deficiency**
        ADA deficiency with SCID
        Adenosine deaminase [ADA] deficiency with severe combined immunodeficiency

    D81.32   **Adenosine deaminase 2 deficiency**
        ADA2 deficiency
        Adenosine deaminase deficiency type 2
        Code also, if applicable, any associated manifestations, such as:
          polyarteritis nodosa (M30.0)
          stroke (I63.-)

    D81.39   **Other adenosine deaminase deficiency**
        Adenosine deaminase [ADA] deficiency type 1, NOS
        Adenosine deaminase [ADA] deficiency type 1, without SCID
        Adenosine deaminase [ADA] deficiency type 1, without severe combined immunodeficiency
        Partial ADA deficiency (type 1)
        Partial adenosine deaminase deficiency (type 1)

    D81.4   **Nezelof's syndrome**

    D81.5   **Purine nucleoside phosphorylase [PNP] deficiency**

    D81.6   **Major histocompatibility complex class I deficiency**
       Bare lymphocyte syndrome

    D81.7   **Major histocompatibility complex class II deficiency**

●   D81.8   **Other combined immunodeficiencies**

●   D81.81   **Biotin-dependent carboxylase deficiency**
       Multiple carboxylase deficiency

       Excludes1   biotin-dependent carboxylase deficiency due to dietary deficiency of biotin (E53.8)

    D81.810   **Biotinidase deficiency**

    D81.818   **Other biotin-dependent carboxylase deficiency**
        Holocarboxylase synthetase deficiency
        Other multiple carboxylase deficiency

    D81.819   **Biotin-dependent carboxylase deficiency, unspecified**
        Multiple carboxylase deficiency, unspecified

    D81.82   **Activated Phosphoinositide 3-kinase Delta Syndrome [APDS]**
       p110d-activating mutation causing senescent T cells, lymphadenopathy, and immunodeficiency [PASLI] disease
       Code also, if applicable, any associated manifestations, such as:
         bronchiectasis (J47.-)
         herpes virus infections (B00.-)
         other acute respiratory tract infections (J00-J06; J20-J22)
         other infections (A00-B99)
         pneumonia (J12-J18)

    D81.89   **Other combined immunodeficiencies**

CHAPTER 3 (D50-D89)

D81.9   Combined immunodeficiency, unspecified 🄷
     Severe combined immunodeficiency disorder [SCID] NOS

● **D82   Immunodeficiency associated with other major defects**

     Excludes1   ataxia telangiectasia [Louis-Bar] (G11.3)

D82.0   Wiskott-Aldrich syndrome 🄷
     X-linked immunodeficiency
     Immunodeficiency with thrombocytopenia and eczema

D82.1   Di George's syndrome 🄷
     Congenital disorder with defective development of third and fourth pharyngeal pouches
     Pharyngeal pouch syndrome
     Thymic alymphoplasia
     Thymic aplasia or hypoplasia with immunodeficiency
     Coding Clinic: 2019, Q3, P14

D82.2   Immunodeficiency with short-limbed stature 🄷

D82.3   Immunodeficiency following hereditary defective response to Epstein-Barr virus 🄷
     X-linked lymphoproliferative disease

D82.4   Hyperimmunoglobulin E [IgE] syndrome 🄷
     Suspected genetic defect that produces high levels of antibody immunoglobulin (IgE) that causes skin and lung infections and eczema

D82.8   Immunodeficiency associated with other specified major defects 🄷

D82.9   Immunodeficiency associated with major defect, unspecified 🄷

● **D83   Common variable immunodeficiency**

D83.0   Common variable immunodeficiency with predominant abnormalities of B-cell numbers and function 🄷

D83.1   Common variable immunodeficiency with predominant immunoregulatory T-cell disorders 🄷

D83.2   Common variable immunodeficiency with autoantibodies to B- or T-cells 🄷

D83.8   Other common variable immunodeficiencies 🄷

D83.9   Common variable immunodeficiency, unspecified 🄷

● **D84   Other immunodeficiencies**

D84.0   Lymphocyte function antigen-1 [LFA-1] defect 🄷

● **D84.1   Defects in the complement system** 🄷
     C1 esterase inhibitor [C1-INH] deficiency

D84.8   Other specified immunodeficiencies 🄷

     ▸ **D84.81   Immunodeficiency due to conditions classified elsewhere**
         Code first underlying condition, such as:
         chromosomal abnormalities (Q90-Q99)
         diabetes mellitus (E08-E13)
         malignant neoplasms (C00-C96)

         Excludes1   certain disorders involving the immune mechanism (D80-D83, D84.0, D84.1, D84.9)
                   human immunodeficiency virus [HIV] disease (B20)

● **D84.82   Immunodeficiency due to drugs and external causes**

     D84.821   Immunodeficiency due to drugs
         Immunodeficiency due to (current or past) medication
         Use additional code for adverse effect if applicable, to identify adverse effect of drug (T36-T50 with fifth or six character 5)
         Use additional code, if applicable, for associated long term (current) drug therapy drug or medication such as:
         long term (current) drug therapy systemic steroids (Z79.52)
         other long term (current) drug therapy (Z79.899)

     D84.822   Immunodeficiency due to external causes
         Code also, if applicable, radiological procedure and radiotherapy (Y84.2)
         Use additional code for external cause such as:
         exposure to ionizing radiation (W88)

     D84.89   Other immunodeficiencies

D84.9   Immunodeficiency, unspecified 🄷
     Immunocompromised NOS
     Immunodeficient NOS
     Immunosuppressed NOS

● **D86   Sarcoidosis**

D86.0   Sarcoidosis of lung 🄷

D86.1   Sarcoidosis of lymph nodes

D86.2   Sarcoidosis of lung with sarcoidosis of lymph nodes 🄷

D86.3   Sarcoidosis of skin

● **D86.8   Sarcoidosis of other sites**

     D86.81   Sarcoid meningitis

     D86.82   Multiple cranial nerve palsies in sarcoidosis 🄷

     D86.83   Sarcoid iridocyclitis
         Rare large tumor with irregular surface of iris

     D86.84   Sarcoid pyelonephritis
         Systemic disease of unknown etiology characterized by chronic granulomatous inflammation with tissue destruction of pelvis kidney
         Tubulo-interstitial nephropathy in sarcoidosis

     D86.85   Sarcoid myocarditis

     D86.86   Sarcoid arthropathy
         Polyarthritis in sarcoidosis

     D86.87   Sarcoid myositis
         Granumloma of muscle

     D86.89   Sarcoidosis of other sites
         Hepatic granuloma
         Uveoparotid fever [Heerfordt]

D86.9   Sarcoidosis, unspecified

● **D89   Other disorders involving the immune mechanism, not elsewhere classified**

     Excludes1   hyperglobulinemia NOS (R77.1)
                 monoclonal gammopathy (of undetermined significance) (D47.2)

     Excludes2   transplant failure and rejection (T86.-)

D89.0   Polyclonal hypergammaglobulinemia
     Benign hypergammaglobulinemic purpura
     Polyclonal gammopathy NOS

▶ New   ⇒ Revised   ~~deleted~~ Deleted   Excludes 1   Excludes 2   Includes   Use additional   Code first   Code also   Key words
OGCR Official Guidelines   X Assign placeholder X   ● Use Additional Character(s)   ▸ Manifestation Code   🄷 Hierarchical Condition Category   **Coding Clinic**

D89.1   Cryoglobulinemia 🔍
> *Cryoglobulin (proteins) in blood that precipitate temperatures below 98.6° F; usually symptomatic of underlying disease*

Cryoglobulinemic purpura
Cryoglobulinemic vasculitis
Essential cryoglobulinemia
Idiopathic cryoglobulinemia
Mixed cryoglobulinemia
Primary cryoglobulinemia
Secondary cryoglobulinemia

D89.2   Hypergammaglobulinemia, unspecified

D89.3   Immune reconstitution syndrome 🔍
Immune reconstitution inflammatory syndrome [IRIS]
Use additional code for adverse effect, if applicable, to identify drug (T36-T50 with fifth or sixth character 5)

Item 3-1 Sarcoidosis: A symptom of an inflammation producing tiny lumps of cells (granulomas) in various organs, most commonly the lungs and lymph nodes, that affect organ function. Cause is unknown occurring primarily in 20- to 40-year-olds, African-American, especially women, and those of Asian, German, Irish, Scandinavian, and Puerto Rican heritage.

● **D89.4   Mast cell activation syndrome and related disorders**
Excludes1   aggressive systemic mastocytosis (C96.21)
congenital cutaneous mastocytosis (Q82.2)
(non-congenital) cutaneous mastocytosis (D47.01)
(indolent) systemic mastocytosis (D47.02)
malignant mast cell neoplasm (C96.2-)
malignant mastocytoma (C96.29)
mast cell leukemia (C94.3-)
mast cell sarcoma (C96.22)
mastocytoma NOS (D47.09)
other mast cell neoplasms of uncertain behavior (D47.09)
systemic mastocytosis associated with a clonal hematologic non-mast cell lineage disease (SM-AHNMD) (D47.02)
Coding Clinic: 2016, Q4, P11

D89.40   Mast cell activation, unspecified 🔍
Mast cell activation disorder, unspecified
Mast cell activation syndrome, NOS

D89.41   Monoclonal mast cell activation syndrome 🔍
Coding Clinic: 2016, Q4, P11

D89.42   Idiopathic mast cell activation syndrome 🔍
Coding Clinic: 2016, Q4, P11

D89.44   Hereditary alpha tryptasemia
Use additional code, if applicable, for:
allergy status, other than to drugs and biological substances (Z91.0-)
personal history of anaphylaxis (Z87.892)

D89.43   Secondary mast cell activation 🔍
Secondary mast cell activation syndrome
Code also underlying etiology, if known
Coding Clinic: 2016, Q4, P11

D89.49   Other mast cell activation disorder 🔍
Other mast cell activation syndrome
Coding Clinic: 2016, Q4, P11

● **D89.8   Other specified disorders involving the immune mechanism, not elsewhere classified**

● **D89.81   Graft-versus-host disease**
Code first underlying cause, such as:
complications of transplanted organs and tissue (T86.-)
complications of blood transfusion (T80.89)
Use additional code to identify associated manifestations, such as:
desquamative dermatitis (L30.8)
diarrhea (R19.7)
elevated bilirubin (R17)
hair loss (L65.9)

D89.810   Acute graft-versus-host disease 🔍

D89.811   Chronic graft-versus-host disease 🔍
Coding Clinic: 2023, Q3, P20

D89.812   Acute on chronic graft-versus-host disease 🔍

D89.813   Graft-versus-host disease, unspecified 🔍

D89.82   Autoimmune lymphoproliferative syndrome [ALPS] 🔍

D89.84   IgG4-related disease
Immunoglobulin G4-related disease

● **D89.83   Cytokine release syndrome**
Code first underlying cause, such as:
complications following infusion, transfusion and therapeutic injection (T80.89-)
complications of transplanted organs and tissue (T86.-)
Use additional code to identify associated manifestations
code for adverse effect, if applicable, to identify immune checkpointinhibitors and immunostimulant drugs (T45.AX5)

D89.831   Cytokine release syndrome, grade 1

D89.832   Cytokine release syndrome, grade 2

D89.833   Cytokine release syndrome, grade 3

D89.834   Cytokine release syndrome, grade 4

D89.835   Cytokine release syndrome, grade 5

D89.839   Cytokine release syndrome, grade unspecified

D89.89   Other specified disorders involving the immune mechanism, not elsewhere classified 🔍
Excludes1   human immunodeficiency virus disease (B20)
Coding Clinic: 2017, Q4, P109

D89.9   Disorder involving the immune mechanism, unspecified 🔍
Immune disease NOS
Coding Clinic: 2015, Q3, P22

CHAPTER 3 (D50-D89)

CHAPTER 4

ENDOCRINE, NUTRITIONAL AND METABOLIC DISEASES (E00-E89)

OGCR Chapter-Specific Coding Guidelines

4. **Chapter 4: Endocrine, Nutritional, and Metabolic Diseases (E00-E89)**

   a. **Diabetes mellitus**

   The diabetes mellitus codes are combination codes that include the type of diabetes mellitus, the body system affected, and the complications affecting that body system. As many codes within a particular category as are necessary to describe all of the complications of the disease may be used. They should be sequenced based on the reason for a particular encounter. Assign as many codes from categories E08 – E13 as needed to identify all of the associated conditions that the patient has.

   1) **Type of diabetes**

   The age of a patient is not the sole determining factor, though most type 1 diabetics develop the condition before reaching puberty. For this reason type 1 diabetes mellitus is also referred to as juvenile diabetes.

   2) **Type of diabetes mellitus not documented**

   If the type of diabetes mellitus is not documented in the medical record the default is E11.-, Type 2 diabetes mellitus.

   3) **Diabetes mellitus and the use of insulin oral hypoglycemics**

   If the documentation in a medical record does not indicate the type of diabetes but does indicate that the patient uses insulin, code E11, Type 2 diabetes mellitus, should be assigned. An additional code should be assigned from category Z79 to identify the long-term (current) use of insulin or oral hypoglycemic drugs. If the patient is treated with both oral medications and insulin, only the code for long-term (current) use of insulin should be assigned. Code Z79.4 should not be assigned if insulin is given temporarily to bring a type 2 patient's blood sugar under control during an encounter.

   4) **Diabetes mellitus in pregnancy and gestational diabetes**

   See Section I.C.15. Diabetes mellitus in pregnancy.
   See Section I.C.15. Gestational (pregnancy induced) diabetes

   5) **Complications due to insulin pump malfunction**

   (a) **Underdose of insulin due to insulin pump failure**

   An underdose of insulin due to an insulin pump failure should be assigned to a code from subcategory T85.6, Mechanical complication of other specified internal and external prosthetic devices, implants and grafts, that specifies the type of pump malfunction, as the principal or first-listed code, followed by code T38.3X6-, Underdosing of insulin and oral hypoglycemic [antidiabetic] drugs. Additional codes for the type of diabetes mellitus and any associated complications due to the underdosing should also be assigned.

   (b) **Overdose of insulin due to insulin pump failure**

   The principal or first-listed code for an encounter due to an insulin pump malfunction resulting in an overdose of insulin, should also be T85.6-, Mechanical complication of other specified internal and external prosthetic devices, implants and grafts, followed by code T38.3X1-, Poisoning by insulin and oral hypoglycemic [antidiabetic] drugs, accidental (unintentional).

   6) **Secondary diabetes mellitus**

   Codes under categories E08, Diabetes mellitus due to underlying condition, E09, Drug or chemical induced diabetes mellitus and E13, Other specified diabetes mellitus, identify complications/manifestations associated with secondary diabetes mellitus. Secondary diabetes is always caused by another condition or event (e.g., cystic fibrosis, malignant neoplasm of pancreas, pancreatectomy, adverse effect of drug, or poisoning).

   (a) **Secondary diabetes mellitus and the use of insulin or hypoglycemic drugs**

   For patients with secondary diabetes mellitus who routinely use insulin or oral hypoglycemic drugs, an additional code from category Z79 should be assigned to identify the long-term (current) use of insulin or oral hypoglycemic drugs. If the patient is treated with both oral medications and insulin, only the code for long-term (current) use of insulin should be assigned. Code Z79.4 should not be assigned if insulin is given temporarily to bring a type 2 patient's blood sugar under control during an encounter.

   (b) **Assigning and sequencing secondary diabetes codes and its causes**

   The sequencing of the secondary diabetes codes in relationship to codes for the cause of the diabetes is based on the Tabular List instructions for categories E08, E09 and E13.

   (i) **Secondary diabetes mellitus due to pancreatectomy** For postpancreatectomy diabetes mellitus (lack of insulin due to the surgical removal of all or part of the pancreas), assign code E89.1, Postprocedural hypoinsulinemia. Assign a code from category E13 and a code from subcategory Z90.41-, Acquired absence of pancreas, as additional codes.

   (ii) **Secondary diabetes due to drugs** Secondary diabetes may be caused by an adverse effect of correctly administered medications, poisoning or sequela of poisoning.

   See Section I.C.19.e for coding of adverse effects and poisoning, and Section I.C.20 for external cause code reporting.

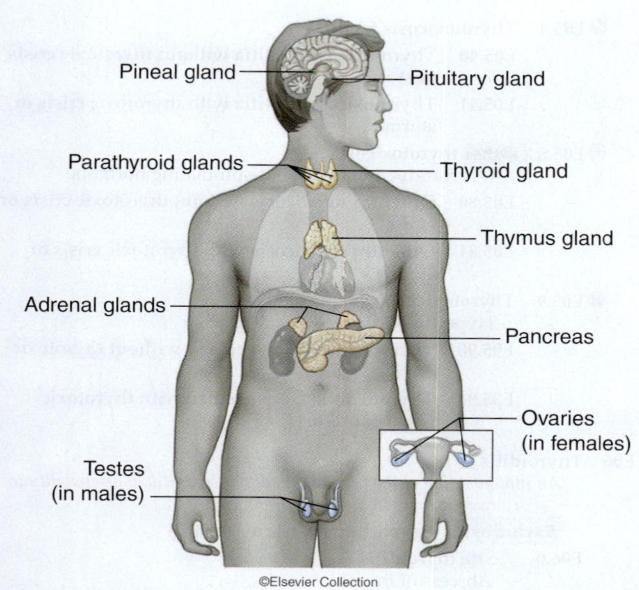

Figure 4-1   The endocrine system. ©Elsevier Collection.

CHAPTER 4

ENDOCRINE, NUTRITIONAL AND METABOLIC DISEASES (E00-E89)

All neoplasms, whether functionally active or not, are classified in Chapter 2. Appropriate codes in this chapter (i.e., E05.8, E07.0, E16-E31, E34.-) may be used as additional codes to indicate either functional activity by neoplasms and ectopic endocrine tissue or hyperfunction and hypofunction of endocrine glands associated with neoplasms and other conditions classified elsewhere.

Excludes1   transitory endocrine and metabolic disorders specific to newborn (P70-P74)

This chapter contains the following blocks:

E00-E07	Disorders of thyroid gland
E08-E13	Diabetes mellitus
E15-E16	Other disorders of glucose regulation and pancreatic internal secretion
E20-E35	Disorders of other endocrine glands
E36	Intraoperative complications of endocrine system
E40-E46	Malnutrition
E50-E64	Other nutritional deficiencies
E65-E68	Overweight, obesity and other hyperalimentation
E70-E88	Metabolic disorders
E89	Postprocedural endocrine and metabolic complications and disorders, not elsewhere classified

DISORDERS OF THYROID GLAND (E00-E07)

● **E00**   **Congenital iodine-deficiency syndrome**
    Use additional code (F70-F79) to identify associated intellectual disabilities.
    Excludes1   subclinical iodine-deficiency hypothyroidism (E02)

E00.0   **Congenital iodine-deficiency syndrome, neurological type**
    Endemic cretinism, neurological type

E00.1   **Congenital iodine-deficiency syndrome, myxedematous type**
    Dry, waxy type of swelling (nonpitting edema) with abnormal deposits of mucin in skin (mucinosis) and other tissues
    Endemic hypothyroid cretinism
    Endemic cretinism, myxedematous type

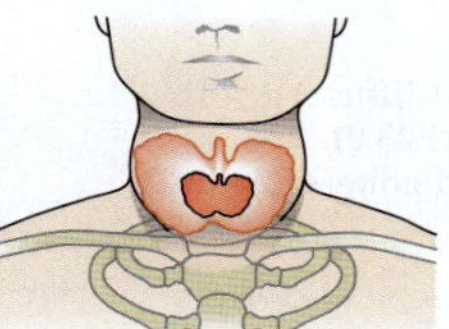

Figure 4-2   Goiter is an enlargement of the thyroid gland.

Item 4–1   Simple goiter indicates no nodules are present. The most common type of goiter is a **diffuse colloidal,** also called a **nontoxic** or **endemic** goiter.

E00.2   **Congenital iodine-deficiency syndrome, mixed type**
    Endemic cretinism, mixed type

E00.9   **Congenital iodine-deficiency syndrome, unspecified**
    Congenital iodine-deficiency hypothyroidism NOS
    Endemic cretinism NOS

● **E01**   **Iodine-deficiency related thyroid disorders and allied conditions**
    Excludes1   congenital iodine-deficiency syndrome (E00.-)
        subclinical iodine-deficiency hypothyroidism (E02)

E01.0   **Iodine-deficiency related diffuse (endemic) goiter**
    Thyroid gland is enlarged

E01.1   **Iodine-deficiency related multinodular (endemic) goiter**
    Iodine-deficiency related nodular goiter

E01.2   **Iodine-deficiency related (endemic) goiter, unspecified**
    Endemic goiter NOS

E01.8   **Other iodine-deficiency related thyroid disorders and allied conditions**
    Acquired iodine-deficiency hypothyroidism NOS

E02   **Subclinical iodine-deficiency hypothyroidism**
    Coding Clinic: 2021, Q1, P8-9

● **E03**   **Other hypothyroidism**
    Excludes1   iodine-deficiency related hypothyroidism (E00-E02)
        postprocedural hypothyroidism (E89.0)

E03.0   **Congenital hypothyroidism with diffuse goiter**
    Congenital parenchymatous goiter (nontoxic)
    Congenital goiter (nontoxic) NOS
    Excludes1   transitory congenital goiter with normal function (P72.0)

E03.1   **Congenital hypothyroidism without goiter**
    Aplasia of thyroid (with myxedema)
    Congenital atrophy of thyroid
    Congenital hypothyroidism NOS

E03.2   **Hypothyroidism due to medicaments and other exogenous substances**
    Code first poisoning due to drug or toxin, if applicable (T36-T65 with fifth or sixth character 1-4)
    Use additional code for adverse effect, if applicable, to identify drug (T36-T50 with fifth or sixth character 5)

E03.3   **Postinfectious hypothyroidism**

E03.4   **Atrophy of thyroid (acquired)**
    Excludes1   congenital atrophy of thyroid (E03.1)

E03.5   **Myxedema coma**
    Often fatal complication of long-term hypothyroidism

E03.8   **Other specified hypothyroidism**

E03.9   **Hypothyroidism, unspecified**
    Myxedema NOS
    Coding Clinic: 2021, Q1, P9

Item 4–2   Hypothyroidism is a condition in which there are insufficient levels of thyroxine. **Cretinism** is congenital hypothyroidism, which can result in mental and physical retardation.

CHAPTER 4 (E00-E89)

E04   Other nontoxic goiter
Excludes1   congenital goiter (NOS) (diffuse)
(parenchymatous) (E03.0)
iodine-deficiency related goiter (E00-E02)

E04.0   Nontoxic diffuse goiter
Thyroid gland is enlarged
Diffuse (colloid) nontoxic goiter
Simple nontoxic goiter

E04.1   Nontoxic single thyroid nodule
Colloid nodule (cystic) (thyroid)
Nontoxic uninodular goiter
Thyroid (cystic) nodule NOS

E04.2   Nontoxic multinodular goiter
Enlarged thyroid gland with multiple nodules
Cystic goiter NOS
Multinodular (cystic) goiter NOS

E04.8   Other specified nontoxic goiter

E04.9   Nontoxic goiter, unspecified
Goiter NOS
Nodular goiter (nontoxic) NOS

E05   Thyrotoxicosis [hyperthyroidism]
Enlarged thyroid gland with multiple nodules
Excludes1   chronic thyroiditis with transient thyrotoxicosis
(E06.2)
neonatal thyrotoxicosis (P72.1)

E05.0   Thyrotoxicosis with diffuse goiter
Exophthalmic or toxic goiter NOS
Graves' disease
Toxic diffuse goiter

E05.00   Thyrotoxicosis with diffuse goiter without thyrotoxic crisis or storm

E05.01   Thyrotoxicosis with diffuse goiter with thyrotoxic crisis or storm

E05.1   Thyrotoxicosis with toxic single thyroid nodule
Thyrotoxicosis with toxic uninodular goiter

E05.10   Thyrotoxicosis with toxic single thyroid nodule without thyrotoxic crisis or storm

E05.11   Thyrotoxicosis with toxic single thyroid nodule with thyrotoxic crisis or storm

E05.2   Thyrotoxicosis with toxic multinodular goiter
Toxic nodular goiter NOS

E05.20   Thyrotoxicosis with toxic multinodular goiter without thyrotoxic crisis or storm

E05.21   Thyrotoxicosis with toxic multinodular goiter with thyrotoxic crisis or storm

E05.3   Thyrotoxicosis from ectopic thyroid tissue

E05.30   Thyrotoxicosis from ectopic thyroid tissue without thyrotoxic crisis or storm

E05.31   Thyrotoxicosis from ectopic thyroid tissue with thyrotoxic crisis or storm

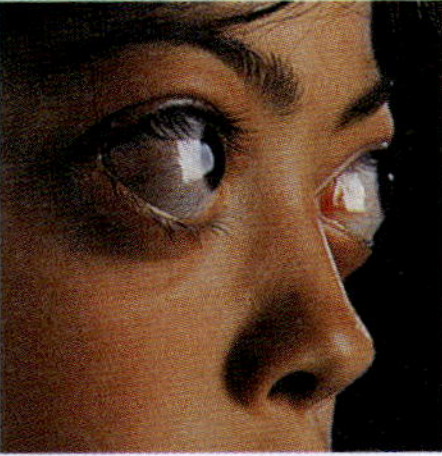

Figure 4-3   Graves' disease. In Graves' disease, exophthalmos often looks more pronounced than it actually is because of the extreme lid retraction that may occur. This patient, for instance, had minimal proptosis of the left eye but marked lid retraction. (From Lissauer T, Clayden G, and Craft A: Illustrated Textbook of Paediatrics, Edinburgh, Mosby, 2015)

Item 4–3   Thyrotoxicosis is a condition caused by excessive amounts of the thyroid hormone thyroxine production or hyperthyroidism. **Graves' disease is associated with hyperthyroidism** (known as **Basedow's disease** in Europe).

E05.4   Thyrotoxicosis factitia

E05.40   Thyrotoxicosis factitia without thyrotoxic crisis or storm

E05.41   Thyrotoxicosis factitia with thyrotoxic crisis or storm

E05.8   Other thyrotoxicosis
Overproduction of thyroid-stimulating hormone

E05.80   Other thyrotoxicosis without thyrotoxic crisis or storm

E05.81   Other thyrotoxicosis with thyrotoxic crisis or storm

E05.9   Thyrotoxicosis, unspecified
Hyperthyroidism NOS

E05.90   Thyrotoxicosis, unspecified without thyrotoxic crisis or storm

E05.91   Thyrotoxicosis, unspecified with thyrotoxic crisis or storm

E06   Thyroiditis
An inflammation of the thyroid gland which results in an inability to convert iodine into thyroid hormone
Excludes1   postpartum thyroiditis (O90.5)

E06.0   Acute thyroiditis
Abscess of thyroid
Pyogenic thyroiditis
Suppurative thyroiditis
Use additional code (B95-B97) to identify infectious agent.

E06.1   Subacute thyroiditis
Inflammation of thyroid gland following viral upper respiratory infection
de Quervain thyroiditis
Giant-cell thyroiditis
Granulomatous thyroiditis
Nonsuppurative thyroiditis
Viral thyroiditis
Excludes1   autoimmune thyroiditis (E06.3)

E06.2   Chronic thyroiditis with transient thyrotoxicosis
Chronic inflammation of thyroid gland with intermittent overproduction of thyroid hormone
Excludes1   autoimmune thyroiditis (E06.3)

E06.3   Autoimmune thyroiditis
Hashimoto's thyroiditis
Hashitoxicosis (transient)
Lymphadenoid goiter
Lymphocytic thyroiditis
Struma lymphomatosa
Coding Clinic: 2024, Q1, P14

E06.4   Drug-induced thyroiditis
Use additional code for adverse effect, if applicable, to identify drug (T36-T50 with fifth or sixth character 5)

E06.5   Other chronic thyroiditis
Chronic fibrous thyroiditis
Chronic thyroiditis NOS
Ligneous thyroiditis
Riedel thyroiditis

E06.9   Thyroiditis, unspecified

E07   Other disorders of thyroid

E07.0   Hypersecretion of calcitonin
C-cell hyperplasia of thyroid
Hypersecretion of thyrocalcitonin

E07.1   Dyshormogenetic goiter
Group of several types of goiter resulting from enzyme defects in hormone synthesis
Dyshormonogenetic goiter
Familial dyshormogenetic goiter
Pendred's syndrome
Excludes1   transitory congenital goiter with normal function (P72.0)

▶ New   ➡ Revised   ~~deleted~~ Deleted   Excludes 1   Excludes 2   Includes   Use additional   Code first   Code also   Key words
OGCR Official Guidelines   X Assign placeholder X   ● Use Additional Character(s)   ❙ Manifestation Code   Hierarchical Condition Category   **Coding Clinic**

● **E07.8**   **Other specified disorders of thyroid**

     E07.81   **Sick-euthyroid syndrome**
                Euthyroid sick-syndrome

     E07.89   **Other specified disorders of thyroid**
                Abnormality of thyroid-binding globulin
                Hemorrhage of thyroid
                Infarction of thyroid

   E07.9   **Disorder of thyroid, unspecified**

OGCR Section I.C.4.a.

Diabetes mellitus

The diabetes mellitus codes are combination codes that include the type of diabetes mellitus, body system affected, and the complications affecting that body system. As many codes within a particular category as are necessary to describe all of the complications of the disease may be used. They should be sequenced based on the reason for a particular visit. Assign as many codes from categories E08–E13 as needed to identify all of the associated conditions that the patient has.

DIABETES MELLITUS (E08-E13)

A metabolic disease that results in persistent hyperglycemia
Coding Clinic: 2016, Q4, P142

● **E08**   **Diabetes mellitus due to underlying condition**

     Code first the underlying condition, such as:
       congenital rubella (P35.0)
       Cushing's syndrome (E24.-)
       cystic fibrosis (E84.-)
       malignant neoplasm (C00-C96)
       malnutrition (E40-E46)
       pancreatitis and other diseases of the pancreas (K85-K86.-)

     Use additional code to identify control using:
       injectable non-insulin antidiabetic drugs (Z79.85)
       insulin (Z79.4)
       oral antidiabetic drugs (Z79.84)
       oral hypoglycemic drugs (Z79.84)

     Excludes1   drug or chemical induced diabetes mellitus (E09.-)
                   gestational diabetes (O24.4-)
                   neonatal diabetes mellitus (P70.2)
                   postpancreatectomy diabetes mellitus (E13.-)
                   postprocedural diabetes mellitus (E13.-)
                   secondary diabetes mellitus NEC (E13.-)
                   type 1 diabetes mellitus (E10.-)
                   type 2 diabetes mellitus (E11.-)

● **E08.0**   **Diabetes mellitus due to underlying condition with hyperosmolarity**

     E08.00   *Diabetes mellitus due to underlying condition with hyperosmolarity without nonketotic hyperglycemic-hyperosmolar coma (NKHHC)*

     E08.01   *Diabetes mellitus due to underlying condition with hyperosmolarity with coma*

● **E08.1**   **Diabetes mellitus due to underlying condition with ketoacidosis**

     E08.10   *Diabetes mellitus due to underlying condition with ketoacidosis without coma*

     E08.11   *Diabetes mellitus due to underlying condition with ketoacidosis with coma*

● **E08.2**   **Diabetes mellitus due to underlying condition with kidney complications**

     E08.21   *Diabetes mellitus due to underlying condition with diabetic nephropathy*
                Diabetes mellitus due to underlying condition with intercapillary glomerulosclerosis
                Diabetes mellitus due to underlying condition with intracapillary glomerulonephrosis
                Diabetes mellitus due to underlying condition with Kimmelstiel-Wilson disease

     E08.22   *Diabetes mellitus due to underlying condition with diabetic chronic kidney disease*
                Use additional code to identify stage of chronic kidney disease (N18.1-N18.6)

     E08.29   *Diabetes mellitus due to underlying condition with other diabetic kidney complication*
                Renal tubular degeneration in diabetes mellitus due to underlying condition

● **E08.3**   **Diabetes mellitus due to underlying condition with ophthalmic complications**
     Changes in blood vessels of retina in which blood vessels swell and leak fluid into retinal surface.
     Coding Clinic: 2016, Q4, P11

   ● **E08.31**   **Diabetes mellitus due to underlying condition with unspecified diabetic retinopathy**

     E08.311   *Diabetes mellitus due to underlying condition with unspecified diabetic retinopathy with macular edema*

     E08.319   *Diabetes mellitus due to underlying condition with unspecified diabetic retinopathy without macular edema*

   ● **E08.32**   **Diabetes mellitus due to underlying condition with mild nonproliferative diabetic retinopathy**
                Diabetes mellitus due to underlying condition with nonproliferative diabetic retinopathy NOS

                One of the following 7th characters is to be assigned to codes in subcategory E08.32 to designate laterality of the disease:

1	right eye
2	left eye
3	bilateral
9	unspecified eye

     E08.321   *Diabetes mellitus due to underlying condition with mild nonproliferative diabetic retinopathy with macular edema*

     E08.329   *Diabetes mellitus due to underlying condition with mild nonproliferative diabetic retinopathy without macular edema*

   ● **E08.33**   **Diabetes mellitus due to underlying condition with moderate nonproliferative diabetic retinopathy**

                One of the following 7th characters is to be assigned to codes in subcategory E08.33 to designate laterality of the disease:

1	right eye
2	left eye
3	bilateral
9	unspecified eye

     E08.331   *Diabetes mellitus due to underlying condition with moderate nonproliferative diabetic retinopathy with macular edema*

     E08.339   *Diabetes mellitus due to underlying condition with moderate nonproliferative diabetic retinopathy without macular edema*

CHAPTER 4 (E00-E89)

● **E08.34** **Diabetes mellitus due to underlying condition with severe nonproliferative diabetic retinopathy**

One of the following 7th characters is to be assigned to codes in subcategory E08.34 to designate laterality of the disease:

1	right eye
2	left eye
3	bilateral
9	unspecified eye

  ● ▌ *E08.341*   *Diabetes mellitus due to underlying condition with severe nonproliferative diabetic retinopathy with macular edema* ℞

  ● ▌ *E08.349*   *Diabetes mellitus due to underlying condition with severe nonproliferative diabetic retinopathy without macular edema* ℞

● **E08.35** **Diabetes mellitus due to underlying condition with proliferative diabetic retinopathy**

One of the following 7th characters is to be assigned to codes in subcategory E08.35 to designate laterality of the disease:

1	right eye
2	left eye
3	bilateral
9	unspecified eye

  ● ▌ *E08.351*   *Diabetes mellitus due to underlying condition with proliferative diabetic retinopathy with macular edema* ℞

  ● ▌ *E08.352*   *Diabetes mellitus due to underlying condition with proliferative diabetic retinopathy with traction retinal detachment involving the macula* ℞

  ● ▌ *E08.353*   *Diabetes mellitus due to underlying condition with proliferative diabetic retinopathy with traction retinal detachment not involving the macula* ℞

  ● ▌ *E08.354*   *Diabetes mellitus due to underlying condition with proliferative diabetic retinopathy with combined traction retinal detachment and rhegmatogenous retinal detachment* ℞

  ● ▌ *E08.355*   *Diabetes mellitus due to underlying condition with stable proliferative diabetic retinopathy* ℞

  ● ▌ *E08.359*   *Diabetes mellitus due to underlying condition with proliferative diabetic retinopathy without macular edema* ℞

 ▌ *E08.36*   *Diabetes mellitus due to underlying condition with diabetic cataract* ℞

X ● ▌ *E08.37*   *Diabetes mellitus due to underlying condition with diabetic macular edema, resolved following treatment* ℞

One of the following 7th characters is to be assigned to code E08.37 to designate laterality of the disease:

1	right eye
2	left eye
3	bilateral
9	unspecified eye

 ▌ *E08.39*   *Diabetes mellitus due to underlying condition with other diabetic ophthalmic complication* ℞

Use additional code to identify manifestation, such as:
diabetic glaucoma (H40-H42)

● **E08.4** **Diabetes mellitus due to underlying condition with neurological complications**

 ▌ *E08.40*   *Diabetes mellitus due to underlying condition with diabetic neuropathy, unspecified* ℞

 ▌ *E08.41*   *Diabetes mellitus due to underlying condition with diabetic mononeuropathy* ℞

 ▌ *E08.42*   *Diabetes mellitus due to underlying condition with diabetic polyneuropathy* ℞
Diabetes mellitus due to underlying condition with diabetic neuralgia

 ▌ *E08.43*   *Diabetes mellitus due to underlying condition with diabetic autonomic (poly)neuropathy* ℞
Diabetes mellitus due to underlying condition with diabetic gastroparesis

 ▌ *E08.44*   *Diabetes mellitus due to underlying condition with diabetic amyotrophy* ℞

 ▌ *E08.49*   *Diabetes mellitus due to underlying condition with other diabetic neurological complication* ℞

● **E08.5** **Diabetes mellitus due to underlying condition with circulatory complications**

 ▌ *E08.51*   *Diabetes mellitus due to underlying condition with diabetic peripheral angiopathy without gangrene* ℞

 ▌ *E08.52*   *Diabetes mellitus due to underlying condition with diabetic peripheral angiopathy with gangrene* ℞
Diabetes mellitus due to underlying condition with diabetic gangrene

 ▌ *E08.59*   *Diabetes mellitus due to underlying condition with other circulatory complications* ℞

● **E08.6** **Diabetes mellitus due to underlying condition with other specified complications**

● **E08.61** **Diabetes mellitus due to underlying condition with diabetic arthropathy**

 ▌ *E08.610*   *Diabetes mellitus due to underlying condition with diabetic neuropathic arthropathy* ℞
Diabetes mellitus due to underlying condition with Charcôt's joints

 ▌ *E08.618*   *Diabetes mellitus due to underlying condition with other diabetic arthropathy*

● **E08.62** **Diabetes mellitus due to underlying condition with skin complications**

 ▌ *E08.620*   *Diabetes mellitus due to underlying condition with diabetic dermatitis*
Diabetes mellitus due to underlying condition with diabetic necrobiosis lipoidica

 ▌ *E08.621*   *Diabetes mellitus due to underlying condition with foot ulcer* ℞
Use additional code to identify site of ulcer (L97.4-, L97.5-)

 ▌ *E08.622*   *Diabetes mellitus due to underlying condition with other skin ulcer* ℞
Use additional code to identify site of ulcer (L97.1-L97.9, L98.41-L98.49)

 ▌ *E08.628*   *Diabetes mellitus due to underlying condition with other skin complications* ℞

● **E08.63** **Diabetes mellitus due to underlying condition with oral complications**

 ▌ *E08.630*   *Diabetes mellitus due to underlying condition with periodontal disease* ℞

 ▌ *E08.638*   *Diabetes mellitus due to underlying condition with other oral complications* ℞

▶ New   ⟹ Revised   ~~deleted~~ Deleted   Excludes 1   Excludes 2   Includes   Use additional   Code first   Code also   Key words

OGCR Official Guidelines   X Assign placeholder X   ● Use Additional Character(s)   ▌ Manifestation Code   ℞ Hierarchical Condition Category   **Coding Clinic**

● **E08.64** **Diabetes mellitus due to underlying condition with hypoglycemia**
   Use additional code for hypoglycemia level, if applicable (E16.A-)

▶ *E08.641* *Diabetes mellitus due to underlying condition with hypoglycemia with coma* RCC

▶ *E08.649* *Diabetes mellitus due to underlying condition with hypoglycemia without coma* RCC

▶ *E08.65* *Diabetes mellitus due to underlying condition with hyperglycemia* RCC

▶ *E08.69* *Diabetes mellitus due to underlying condition with other specified complication* RCC
   Use additional code to identify complication

▶ *E08.8* *Diabetes mellitus due to underlying condition with unspecified complications* RCC

▶ *E08.9* *Diabetes mellitus due to underlying condition without complications* RCC

● **E09** **Drug or chemical induced diabetes mellitus**
   Code first poisoning due to drug or toxin, if applicable (T36-T65 with fifth or sixth character 1-4)
   Use additional code for adverse effect, if applicable, to identify drug (T36-T50 with fifth or sixth character 5)
   Use additional code to identify control using:
      injectable non-insulin antidiabetic drugs (Z79.85)
      insulin (Z79.4)
      oral antidiabetic drugs (Z79.84)
      oral hypoglycemic drugs (Z79.84)

   Excludes1   diabetes mellitus due to underlying condition (E08.-)
      gestational diabetes (O24.4-)
      neonatal diabetes mellitus (P70.2)
      postpancreatectomy diabetes mellitus (E13.-)
      postprocedural diabetes mellitus (E13.-)
      secondary diabetes mellitus NEC (E13.-)
      type 1 diabetes mellitus (E10.-)
      type 2 diabetes mellitus (E11.-)

● **E09.0** **Drug or chemical induced diabetes mellitus with hyperosmolarity**

   E09.00 **Drug or chemical induced diabetes mellitus with hyperosmolarity without nonketotic hyperglycemic-hyperosmolar coma (NKHHC)** RCC

   E09.01 **Drug or chemical induced diabetes mellitus with hyperosmolarity with coma** RCC

● **E09.1** **Drug or chemical induced diabetes mellitus with ketoacidosis**

   E09.10 **Drug or chemical induced diabetes mellitus with ketoacidosis without coma** RCC

   E09.11 **Drug or chemical induced diabetes mellitus with ketoacidosis with coma** RCC

● **E09.2** **Drug or chemical induced diabetes mellitus with kidney complications**

   E09.21 **Drug or chemical induced diabetes mellitus with diabetic nephropathy** RCC
      Drug or chemical induced diabetes mellitus with intercapillary glomerulosclerosis
      Drug or chemical induced diabetes mellitus with intracapillary glomerulonephrosis
      Drug or chemical induced diabetes mellitus with Kimmelstiel-Wilson disease

   E09.22 **Drug or chemical induced diabetes mellitus with diabetic chronic kidney disease** RCC
      Use additional code to identify stage of chronic kidney disease (N18.1-N18.6)

   E09.29 **Drug or chemical induced diabetes mellitus with other diabetic kidney complication** RCC
      Drug or chemical induced diabetes mellitus with renal tubular degeneration

● **E09.3** **Drug or chemical induced diabetes mellitus with ophthalmic complications**
      Coding Clinic: 2016, Q4, P11

● **E09.31** **Drug or chemical induced diabetes mellitus with unspecified diabetic retinopathy**

   E09.311 **Drug or chemical induced diabetes mellitus with unspecified diabetic retinopathy with macular edema** RCC

   E09.319 **Drug or chemical induced diabetes mellitus with unspecified diabetic retinopathy without macular edema** RCC

● **E09.32** **Drug or chemical induced diabetes mellitus with mild nonproliferative diabetic retinopathy**
      Drug or chemical induced diabetes mellitus with nonproliferative diabetic retinopathy NOS

      One of the following 7th characters is to be assigned to codes in subcategory E09.32 to designate laterality of the disease:

1	right eye
2	left eye
3	bilateral
9	unspecified eye

   ● **E09.321** **Drug or chemical induced diabetes mellitus with mild nonproliferative diabetic retinopathy with macular edema** RCC

   ● **E09.329** **Drug or chemical induced diabetes mellitus with mild nonproliferative diabetic retinopathy without macular edema** RCC

● **E09.33** **Drug or chemical induced diabetes mellitus with moderate nonproliferative diabetic retinopathy**

      One of the following 7th characters is to be assigned to codes in subcategory E09.33 to designate laterality of the disease:

1	right eye
2	left eye
3	bilateral
9	unspecified eye

   ● **E09.331** **Drug or chemical induced diabetes mellitus with moderate nonproliferative diabetic retinopathy with macular edema** RCC

   ● **E09.339** **Drug or chemical induced diabetes mellitus with moderate nonproliferative diabetic retinopathy without macular edema** RCC

● **E09.34** **Drug or chemical induced diabetes mellitus with severe nonproliferative diabetic retinopathy**

      One of the following 7th characters is to be assigned to codes in subcategory E09.34 to designate laterality of the disease:

1	right eye
2	left eye
3	bilateral
9	unspecified eye

   ● **E09.341** **Drug or chemical induced diabetes mellitus with severe nonproliferative diabetic retinopathy with macular edema** RCC

   ● **E09.349** **Drug or chemical induced diabetes mellitus with severe nonproliferative diabetic retinopathy without macular edema** RCC

CHAPTER 4 (E00-E89)

● **E09.35**   **Drug or chemical induced diabetes mellitus with proliferative diabetic retinopathy**

One of the following 7th characters is to be assigned to codes in subcategory E09.35 to designate laterality of the disease:

1	right eye
2	left eye
3	bilateral
9	unspecified eye

     ● **E09.351**   Drug or chemical induced diabetes mellitus with proliferative diabetic retinopathy with macular edema

     ● **E09.352**   Drug or chemical induced diabetes mellitus with proliferative diabetic retinopathy with traction retinal detachment involving the macula

     ● **E09.353**   Drug or chemical induced diabetes mellitus with proliferative diabetic retinopathy with traction retinal detachment not involving the macula

     ● **E09.354**   Drug or chemical induced diabetes mellitus with proliferative diabetic retinopathy with combined traction retinal detachment and rhegmatogenous retinal detachment

     ● **E09.355**   Drug or chemical induced diabetes mellitus with stable proliferative diabetic retinopathy

     ● **E09.359**   Drug or chemical induced diabetes mellitus with proliferative diabetic retinopathy without macular edema

   E09.36   Drug or chemical induced diabetes mellitus with diabetic cataract

X ● **E09.37**   **Drug or chemical induced diabetes mellitus with diabetic macular edema, resolved following treatment**

One of the following 7th characters is to be assigned to code E09.37 to designate laterality of the disease:

1	right eye
2	left eye
3	bilateral
9	unspecified eye

   E09.39   Drug or chemical induced diabetes mellitus with other diabetic ophthalmic complication

     Use additional code to identify manifestation, such as:
       diabetic glaucoma (H40-H42)

● **E09.4**   **Drug or chemical induced diabetes mellitus with neurological complications**

   E09.40   Drug or chemical induced diabetes mellitus with neurological complications with diabetic neuropathy, unspecified

   E09.41   Drug or chemical induced diabetes mellitus with neurological complications with diabetic mononeuropathy

   E09.42   Drug or chemical induced diabetes mellitus with neurological complications with diabetic polyneuropathy

     Drug or chemical induced diabetes mellitus with diabetic neuralgia

   E09.43   Drug or chemical induced diabetes mellitus with neurological complications with diabetic autonomic (poly)neuropathy

     Drug or chemical induced diabetes mellitus with diabetic gastroparesis

   E09.44   Drug or chemical induced diabetes mellitus with neurological complications with diabetic amyotrophy

   E09.49   Drug or chemical induced diabetes mellitus with neurological complications with other diabetic neurological complication

● **E09.5**   **Drug or chemical induced diabetes mellitus with circulatory complications**

   E09.51   Drug or chemical induced diabetes mellitus with diabetic peripheral angiopathy without gangrene

   E09.52   Drug or chemical induced diabetes mellitus with diabetic peripheral angiopathy with gangrene

     Drug or chemical induced diabetes mellitus with diabetic gangrene

   E09.59   Drug or chemical induced diabetes mellitus with other circulatory complications

● **E09.6**   **Drug or chemical induced diabetes mellitus with other specified complications**

   ● **E09.61**   Drug or chemical induced diabetes mellitus with diabetic arthropathy

     E09.610   Drug or chemical induced diabetes mellitus with diabetic neuropathic arthropathy

       Drug or chemical induced diabetes mellitus with Charcôt's joints

       Progressive degeneration of weight-bearing joint

     E09.618   Drug or chemical induced diabetes mellitus with other diabetic arthropathy

   ● **E09.62**   Drug or chemical induced diabetes mellitus with skin complications

     E09.620   Drug or chemical induced diabetes mellitus with diabetic dermatitis

       Drug or chemical induced diabetes mellitus with diabetic necrobiosis lipoidica

       Necrotizing skin condition

     E09.621   Drug or chemical induced diabetes mellitus with foot ulcer

       Use additional code to identify site of ulcer (L97.4-, L97.5-)

     E09.622   Drug or chemical induced diabetes mellitus with other skin ulcer

       Use additional code to identify site of ulcer (L97.1-L97.9, L98.41-L98.49)

     E09.628   Drug or chemical induced diabetes mellitus with other skin complications

   ● **E09.63**   Drug or chemical induced diabetes mellitus with oral complications

     E09.630   Drug or chemical induced diabetes mellitus with periodontal disease

     E09.638   Drug or chemical induced diabetes mellitus with other oral complications

   ● **E09.64**   Drug or chemical induced diabetes mellitus with hypoglycemia

     Use additional code for hypoglycemia level, if applicable (E16.A-)

     E09.641   Drug or chemical induced diabetes mellitus with hypoglycemia with coma

     E09.649   Drug or chemical induced diabetes mellitus with hypoglycemia without coma

     E09.65   Drug or chemical induced diabetes mellitus with hyperglycemia

     E09.69   Drug or chemical induced diabetes mellitus with other specified complication

       Use additional code to identify complication

   E09.8   Drug or chemical induced diabetes mellitus with unspecified complications

   E09.9   Drug or chemical induced diabetes mellitus without complications

---

▶ New   ⇨ Revised   ~~deleted~~ Deleted   Excludes 1   Excludes 2   Includes   Use additional   Code first   Code also   Key words

 OGCR Official Guidelines   **X** Assign placeholder X   ● Use Additional Character(s)   ▶ Manifestation Code   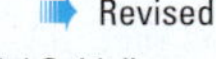 Hierarchical Condition Category   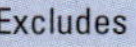 Coding Clinic

● **E10   Type 1 diabetes mellitus**

Includes   brittle diabetes (mellitus)
diabetes (mellitus) due to autoimmune process
diabetes (mellitus) due to immune mediated
pancreatic islet beta-cell destruction
idiopathic diabetes (mellitus)
juvenile onset diabetes (mellitus)
ketosis-prone diabetes (mellitus)

Excludes1   diabetes mellitus due to underlying condition
(E08.-)
drug or chemical induced diabetes mellitus
(E09.-)
gestational diabetes (O24.4-)
hyperglycemia NOS (R73.9)
neonatal diabetes mellitus (P70.2)
postpancreatectomy diabetes mellitus (E13.-)
postprocedural diabetes mellitus (E13.-)
secondary diabetes mellitus NEC (E13.-)
type 2 diabetes mellitus (E11.-)

● **E10.1   Type 1 diabetes mellitus with ketoacidosis**
*Acidosis accompanied by accumulation of ketone bodies
(ketosis) in body tissues and fluids*

**E10.10   Type 1 diabetes mellitus with ketoacidosis
without coma** _{RCC}
Coding Clinic: 2013, Q3, P20

**E10.11   Type 1 diabetes mellitus with ketoacidosis with
coma** _{RCC}

● **E10.2   Type 1 diabetes mellitus with kidney complications**

**E10.21   Type 1 diabetes mellitus with diabetic
nephropathy** _{RCC}
Type 1 diabetes mellitus with intercapillary
glomerulosclerosis
Type 1 diabetes mellitus with intracapillary
glomerulonephrosis
Type 1 diabetes mellitus with Kimmelstiel-
Wilson disease

**E10.22   Type 1 diabetes mellitus with diabetic chronic
kidney disease** _{RCC}
Use additional code to identify stage of chronic
kidney disease (N18.1-N18.6)

**E10.29   Type 1 diabetes mellitus with other diabetic
kidney complication** _{RCC}
Type 1 diabetes mellitus with renal tubular
degeneration
Coding Clinic: 2016, Q1, P13

● **E10.3   Type 1 diabetes mellitus with ophthalmic complications**
Coding Clinic: 2016, Q4, P11

● **E10.31   Type 1 diabetes mellitus with unspecified
diabetic retinopathy**

**E10.311   Type 1 diabetes mellitus
with unspecified diabetic retinopathy
with macular edema** _{RCC}

**E10.319   Type 1 diabetes mellitus
with unspecified diabetic retinopathy
without macular edema** _{RCC}

● **E10.32   Type 1 diabetes mellitus with mild
nonproliferative diabetic retinopathy**
Type 1 diabetes mellitus with nonproliferative
diabetic retinopathy NOS

One of the following 7th characters is to be
assigned to codes in subcategory E10.32 to
designate laterality of the disease:

1	right eye
2	left eye
3	bilateral
9	unspecified eye

● **E10.321   Type 1 diabetes mellitus with mild
nonproliferative diabetic retinopathy
with macular edema** _{RCC}

● **E10.329   Type 1 diabetes mellitus with mild
nonproliferative diabetic retinopathy
without macular edema** _{RCC}

● **E10.33   Type 1 diabetes mellitus with moderate
nonproliferative diabetic retinopathy**
One of the following 7th characters is to be
assigned to codes in subcategory E10.33 to
designate laterality of the disease:

1	right eye
2	left eye
3	bilateral
9	unspecified eye

● **E10.331   Type 1 diabetes mellitus with
moderate nonproliferative diabetic
retinopathy with macular edema** _{RCC}

● **E10.339   Type 1 diabetes mellitus with
moderate nonproliferative diabetic
retinopathy without macular
edema** _{RCC}

● **E10.34   Type 1 diabetes mellitus with severe
nonproliferative diabetic retinopathy**
One of the following 7th characters is to be
assigned to codes in subcategory E10.34 to
designate laterality of the disease:

1	right eye
2	left eye
3	bilateral
9	unspecified eye

● **E10.341   Type 1 diabetes mellitus with severe
nonproliferative diabetic retinopathy
with macular edema** _{RCC}

● **E10.349   Type 1 diabetes mellitus with severe
nonproliferative diabetic retinopathy
without macular edema** _{RCC}

● **E10.35   Type 1 diabetes mellitus with proliferative
diabetic retinopathy**
One of the following 7th characters is to be
assigned to codes in subcategory E10.35 to
designate laterality of the disease:

1	right eye
2	left eye
3	bilateral
9	unspecified eye

● **E10.351   Type 1 diabetes mellitus with
proliferative diabetic retinopathy
with macular edema** _{RCC}

● **E10.352   Type 1 diabetes mellitus with
proliferative diabetic retinopathy
with traction retinal detachment
involving the macula** _{RCC}

● **E10.353   Type 1 diabetes mellitus with
proliferative diabetic retinopathy
with traction retinal detachment not
involving the macula** _{RCC}

● **E10.354   Type 1 diabetes mellitus with
proliferative diabetic retinopathy
with combined traction retinal
detachment and rhegmatogenous
retinal detachment** _{RCC}

● **E10.355   Type 1 diabetes mellitus with stable
proliferative diabetic retinopathy** _{RCC}

● **E10.359   Type 1 diabetes mellitus with
proliferative diabetic retinopathy
without macular edema** _{RCC}

**E10.36   Type 1 diabetes mellitus with diabetic
cataract** _{RCC}

X ● E10.37   **Type 1 diabetes mellitus with diabetic macular edema, resolved following treatment** ℞

One of the following 7th characters is to be assigned to code E10.37 to designate laterality of the disease:

1	right eye
2	left eye
3	bilateral
9	unspecified eye

E10.39   **Type 1 diabetes mellitus with other diabetic ophthalmic complication** ℞

Use additional code to identify manifestation, such as:
diabetic glaucoma (H40-H42)

● E10.4   **Type 1 diabetes mellitus with neurological complications**

E10.40   **Type 1 diabetes mellitus with diabetic neuropathy, unspecified** ℞

E10.41   **Type 1 diabetes mellitus with diabetic mononeuropathy** ℞

E10.42   **Type 1 diabetes mellitus with diabetic polyneuropathy** ℞

Type 1 diabetes mellitus with diabetic neuralgia

E10.43   **Type 1 diabetes mellitus with diabetic autonomic (poly)neuropathy** ℞

Type 1 diabetes mellitus with diabetic gastroparesis

E10.44   **Type 1 diabetes mellitus with diabetic amyotrophy** ℞

E10.49   **Type 1 diabetes mellitus with other diabetic neurological complication** ℞

● E10.5   **Type 1 diabetes mellitus with circulatory complications**

E10.51   **Type 1 diabetes mellitus with diabetic peripheral angiopathy without gangrene** ℞

E10.52   **Type 1 diabetes mellitus with diabetic peripheral angiopathy with gangrene** ℞

Type 1 diabetes mellitus with diabetic gangrene

E10.59   **Type 1 diabetes mellitus with other circulatory complications** ℞

● E10.6   **Type 1 diabetes mellitus with other specified complications**

● E10.61   **Type 1 diabetes mellitus with diabetic arthropathy**

E10.610   **Type 1 diabetes mellitus with diabetic neuropathic arthropathy** ℞

Type 1 diabetes mellitus with Charcôt's joints

E10.618   **Type 1 diabetes mellitus with other diabetic arthropathy** ℞

● E10.62   **Type 1 diabetes mellitus with skin complications**

E10.620   **Type 1 diabetes mellitus with diabetic dermatitis** ℞

Type 1 diabetes mellitus with diabetic necrobiosis lipoidica

E10.621   **Type 1 diabetes mellitus with foot ulcer** ℞

Use additional code to identify site of ulcer (L97.4-, L97.5-)

E10.622   **Type 1 diabetes mellitus with other skin ulcer** ℞

Use additional code to identify site of ulcer (L97.1-L97.9, L98.41-L98.49)

E10.628   **Type 1 diabetes mellitus with other skin complications** ℞

● E10.63   **Type 1 diabetes mellitus with oral complications**

E10.630   **Type 1 diabetes mellitus with periodontal disease** ℞

E10.638   **Type 1 diabetes mellitus with other oral complications** ℞

● E10.64   **Type 1 diabetes mellitus with hypoglycemia**

Use additional code for hypoglycemia level, if applicable (E16.A-)

E10.641   **Type 1 diabetes mellitus with hypoglycemia with coma** ℞

E10.649   **Type 1 diabetes mellitus with hypoglycemia without coma** ℞
Coding Clinic: 2016, Q1, P13

E10.65   **Type 1 diabetes mellitus with hyperglycemia** ℞
Coding Clinic: 2022, Q1, P29; 2013, Q3, P20

E10.69   **Type 1 diabetes mellitus with other specified complication** ℞

Use additional code to identify complication
Coding Clinic: 2022, Q1, P29

E10.8   **Type 1 diabetes mellitus with unspecified complications** ℞

E10.9   **Type 1 diabetes mellitus without complications** ℞

E10.A   **Type 1 diabetes mellitus, presymptomatic**
Early-stage type 1 diabetes mellitus

E10.A0   **Type 1 diabetes mellitus, presymptomatic, unspecified**

E10.A1   **Type 1 diabetes mellitus, presymptomatic, Stage 1**
Multiple confirmed islet autoantibodies with normoglycemia

E10.A2   **Type 1 diabetes mellitus, presymptomatic, Stage 2**
Confirmed islet autoimmunity with dysglycemia
Coding Clinic: 2024, Q4, P6

● E11   **Type 2 diabetes mellitus**

Includes   diabetes (mellitus) due to insulin secretory defect
diabetes NOS
insulin resistant diabetes (mellitus)

Use additional code to identify control using:
injectable non-insulin antidiabetic drugs (Z79.85)
insulin (Z79.4)
oral antidiabetic drugs (Z79.84)
oral hypoglycemic drugs (Z79.84)

Excludes 1   diabetes mellitus due to underlying condition (E08.-)
drug or chemical induced diabetes mellitus (E09.-)
gestational diabetes (O24.4-)
neonatal diabetes mellitus (P70.2)
postpancreatectomy diabetes mellitus (E13.-)
postprocedural diabetes mellitus (E13.-)
secondary diabetes mellitus NEC (E13.-)
type 1 diabetes mellitus (E10.-)
Coding Clinic: 2023, Q2, P10; 2020, Q1, P12; 2016, Q4, P121, Q2, P10

● E11.0   **Type 2 diabetes mellitus with hyperosmolarity**

E11.00   **Type 2 diabetes mellitus with hyperosmolarity without nonketotic hyperglycemic-hyperosmolar coma (NKHHC)** ℞
Coding Clinic: 2022, Q1, P28

E11.01   **Type 2 diabetes mellitus with hyperosmolarity with coma** ℞

● E11.1   **Type 2 diabetes mellitus with ketoacidosis**

E11.10   **Type 2 diabetes mellitus with ketoacidosis without coma** ℞
Coding Clinic: 2017, Q4, P6

E11.11   **Type 2 diabetes mellitus with ketoacidosis with coma** ℞

▶ New   ➡ Revised   ~~deleted~~ Deleted   Excludes 1   Excludes 2   Includes   Use additional   Code first   Code also   Key words

OGCR Official Guidelines   X Assign placeholder X   ● Use Additional Character(s)   ▶ Manifestation Code   ℞ Hierarchical Condition Category   Coding Clinic

● **E11.2   Type 2 diabetes mellitus with kidney complications**

E11.21   Type 2 diabetes mellitus with diabetic nephropathy ℞
   Type 2 diabetes mellitus with intercapillary glomerulosclerosis
   Type 2 diabetes mellitus with intracapillary glomerulonephrosis
   Type 2 diabetes mellitus with Kimmelstiel-Wilson disease
   Coding Clinic: 2019, Q3, P3

E11.22   Type 2 diabetes mellitus with diabetic chronic kidney disease ℞
   Use additional code to identify stage of chronic kidney disease (N18.1-N18.6)
   Coding Clinic: 2022, Q3, P16; 2019, Q3, P3; 2018, Q4, P88; 2016, Q2, P36, Q1, P13

E11.29   Type 2 diabetes mellitus with other diabetic kidney complication ℞
   Type 2 diabetes mellitus with renal tubular degeneration

● **E11.3   Type 2 diabetes mellitus with ophthalmic complications**
   Coding Clinic: 2016, Q4, P11

● **E11.31   Type 2 diabetes mellitus with unspecified diabetic retinopathy**

E11.311   Type 2 diabetes mellitus with unspecified diabetic retinopathy with macular edema ℞

E11.319   Type 2 diabetes mellitus with unspecified diabetic retinopathy without macular edema ℞
   Coding Clinic: 2013, Q3, P20

● **E11.32   Type 2 diabetes mellitus with mild nonproliferative diabetic retinopathy**
   Type 2 diabetes mellitus with nonproliferative diabetic retinopathy NOS

   One of the following 7th characters is to be assigned to codes in subcategory E11.32 to designate laterality of the disease:

1	right eye
2	left eye
3	bilateral
9	unspecified eye

● **E11.321   Type 2 diabetes mellitus with mild nonproliferative diabetic retinopathy with macular edema** ℞

● **E11.329   Type 2 diabetes mellitus with mild nonproliferative diabetic retinopathy without macular edema** ℞

● **E11.33   Type 2 diabetes mellitus with moderate nonproliferative diabetic retinopathy**

   One of the following 7th characters is to be assigned to codes in subcategory E11.33 to designate laterality of the disease:

1	right eye
2	left eye
3	bilateral
9	unspecified eye

● **E11.331   Type 2 diabetes mellitus with moderate nonproliferative diabetic retinopathy with macular edema** ℞

● **E11.339   Type 2 diabetes mellitus with moderate nonproliferative diabetic retinopathy without macular edema** ℞

● **E11.34   Type 2 diabetes mellitus with severe nonproliferative diabetic retinopathy**

   One of the following 7th characters is to be assigned to codes in subcategory E11.34 to designate laterality of the disease:

1	right eye
2	left eye
3	bilateral
9	unspecified eye

● **E11.341   Type 2 diabetes mellitus with severe nonproliferative diabetic retinopathy with macular edema** ℞

● **E11.349   Type 2 diabetes mellitus with severe nonproliferative diabetic retinopathy without macular edema** ℞

● **E11.35   Type 2 diabetes mellitus with proliferative diabetic retinopathy**

   One of the following 7th characters is to be assigned to codes in subcategory E11.35 to designate laterality of the disease:

1	right eye
2	left eye
3	bilateral
9	unspecified eye

● **E11.351   Type 2 diabetes mellitus with proliferative diabetic retinopathy with macular edema** ℞

● **E11.352   Type 2 diabetes mellitus with proliferative diabetic retinopathy with traction retinal detachment involving the macula** ℞

● **E11.353   Type 2 diabetes mellitus with proliferative diabetic retinopathy with traction retinal detachment not involving the macula** ℞

● **E11.354   Type 2 diabetes mellitus with proliferative diabetic retinopathy with combined traction retinal detachment and rhegmatogenous retinal detachment** ℞

● **E11.355   Type 2 diabetes mellitus with stable proliferative diabetic retinopathy** ℞

● **E11.359   Type 2 diabetes mellitus with proliferative diabetic retinopathy without macular edema** ℞

E11.36   Type 2 diabetes mellitus with diabetic cataract ℞
   Coding Clinic: 2019, Q2, P30-31; 2016, Q2, P36

X ● **E11.37   Type 2 diabetes mellitus with diabetic macular edema, resolved following treatment** ℞

   One of the following 7th characters is to be assigned to code E11.37 to designate laterality of the disease:

1	right eye
2	left eye
3	bilateral
9	unspecified eye

E11.39   Type 2 diabetes mellitus with other diabetic ophthalmic complication ℞
   Use additional code to identify manifestation, such as:
   diabetic glaucoma (H40-H42)
   Coding Clinic: 2023, Q3, P19

CHAPTER 4 (E00-E89)

● **E11.4**   **Type 2 diabetes mellitus with neurological complications**
Coding Clinic: 2022, Q3, P16

    E11.40   **Type 2 diabetes mellitus with diabetic neuropathy, unspecified**

    E11.41   **Type 2 diabetes mellitus with diabetic mononeuropathy**

    E11.42   **Type 2 diabetes mellitus with diabetic polyneuropathy**
       Type 2 diabetes mellitus with diabetic neuralgia
       Coding Clinic: 2020, Q1, P12; 2016, Q1, P13

    E11.43   **Type 2 diabetes mellitus with diabetic autonomic (poly)neuropathy**
       Type 2 diabetes mellitus with diabetic gastroparesis
       Coding Clinic: 2023, Q2, P9; 2016, Q2, P36

    E11.44   **Type 2 diabetes mellitus with diabetic amyotrophy**
       Coding Clinic: 2022, Q3, P15; 2016, Q2, P36

    E11.49   **Type 2 diabetes mellitus with other diabetic neurological complication**

● **E11.5**   **Type 2 diabetes mellitus with circulatory complications**

    E11.51   **Type 2 diabetes mellitus with diabetic peripheral angiopathy without gangrene**

    E11.52   **Type 2 diabetes mellitus with diabetic peripheral angiopathy with gangrene**
       Type 2 diabetes mellitus with diabetic gangrene
       Coding Clinic: 2017, Q4, P102

    E11.59   **Type 2 diabetes mellitus with other circulatory complications**

● **E11.6**   **Type 2 diabetes mellitus with other specified complications**

   ● **E11.61**   **Type 2 diabetes mellitus with diabetic arthropathy**

      E11.610   **Type 2 diabetes mellitus with diabetic neuropathic arthropathy**
         Type 2 diabetes mellitus with Charcôt's joints
         Coding Clinic: 2016, Q2, P36

      E11.618   **Type 2 diabetes mellitus with other diabetic arthropathy**
         Coding Clinic: 2018, Q2, P7; 2016, Q2, P36

   ● **E11.62**   **Type 2 diabetes mellitus with skin complications**

      E11.620   **Type 2 diabetes mellitus with diabetic dermatitis**
         Type 2 diabetes mellitus with diabetic necrobiosis lipoidica

      E11.621   **Type 2 diabetes mellitus with foot ulcer**
         Use additional code to identify site of ulcer (L97.4-, L97.5-)
         Coding Clinic: 2020, Q1, P12; 2016, Q1, P12

      E11.622   **Type 2 diabetes mellitus with other skin ulcer**
         Use additional code to identify site of ulcer (L97.1-L97.9, L98.41-L98.49)
         Coding Clinic: 2021, Q1, P8; 2017, Q4, P17

      E11.628   **Type 2 diabetes mellitus with other skin complications**

   ● **E11.63**   **Type 2 diabetes mellitus with oral complications**

      E11.630   **Type 2 diabetes mellitus with periodontal disease**

      E11.638   **Type 2 diabetes mellitus with other oral complications**

    E11.64   **Type 2 diabetes mellitus with hypoglycemia**
       Use additional code for hypoglycemia level, if applicable (E16.A-)

      E11.641   **Type 2 diabetes mellitus with hypoglycemia with coma**

      E11.649   **Type 2 diabetes mellitus with hypoglycemia without coma**
         Coding Clinic: 2016, Q3, P42; 2015, Q3, P21

    E11.65   **Type 2 diabetes mellitus with hyperglycemia**
       Coding Clinic: 2023, Q2, P10; 2022, Q1, P28; 2013, Q3, P20

    E11.69   **Type 2 diabetes mellitus with other specified complication**
       Use additional code to identify complication
       Coding Clinic: 2020, Q1, P12; 2016, Q4, P142

● **E11.8**   **Type 2 diabetes mellitus with unspecified complications**

● **E11.9**   **Type 2 diabetes mellitus without complications**
   ▶ **Excludes1**   type 2 diabetes mellitus, without complications in remission (E11.A)
     Coding Clinic: 2025, Q1, P35; 2023, Q3, P19; 2016, Q4, P142, Q2, P36

▶ **E11.A**   **Type 2 diabetes mellitus without complications in remission**
   ▶ **Excludes1**   type 2 diabetes mellitus, with complications (E11.0-E11.8)
     ▶ type 2 diabetes mellitus, without complications not in remission (E11.9)

● **E13**   **Other specified diabetes mellitus**

   Includes   diabetes mellitus due to genetic defects of beta-cell function
      diabetes mellitus due to genetic defects in insulin action
      postpancreatectomy diabetes mellitus
      postprocedural diabetes mellitus
      secondary diabetes mellitus NEC

   Use additional code to identify control using:
     injectable non-insulin antidiabetic drugs (Z79.85)
     insulin (Z79.4)
     oral antidiabetic drugs (Z79.84)
     oral hypoglycemic drugs (Z79.84)

   Excludes1   diabetes (mellitus) due to autoimmune process (E10.-)
      diabetes (mellitus) due to immune mediated pancreatic islet beta-cell destruction (E10.-)
      diabetes mellitus due to underlying condition (E08.-)
      drug or chemical induced diabetes mellitus (E09.-)
      gestational diabetes (O24.4-)
      neonatal diabetes mellitus (P70.2)
      type 1 diabetes mellitus (E10.-)

● **E13.0**   **Other specified diabetes mellitus with hyperosmolarity**

    E13.00   **Other specified diabetes mellitus with hyperosmolarity without nonketotic hyperglycemic-hyperosmolar coma (NKHHC)**

    E13.01   **Other specified diabetes mellitus with hyperosmolarity with coma**

● **E13.1**   **Other specified diabetes mellitus with ketoacidosis**

    E13.10   **Other specified diabetes mellitus with ketoacidosis without coma**
       Coding Clinic: 2016, Q2, P10; 2013, Q1, P26

    E13.11   **Other specified diabetes mellitus with ketoacidosis with coma**

● **E13.2**   **Other specified diabetes mellitus with kidney complications**

E13.21   Other specified diabetes mellitus with diabetic nephropathy ℞
    Other specified diabetes mellitus with intercapillary glomerulosclerosis
    Other specified diabetes mellitus with intracapillary glomerulonephrosis
    Other specified diabetes mellitus with Kimmelstiel-Wilson disease

E13.22   Other specified diabetes mellitus with diabetic chronic kidney disease ℞
    Use additional code to identify stage of chronic kidney disease (N18.1-N18.6)

E13.29   Other specified diabetes mellitus with other diabetic kidney complication ℞
    Other specified diabetes mellitus with renal tubular degeneration

● **E13.3   Other specified diabetes mellitus with ophthalmic complications**
    Coding Clinic: 2016, Q4, P11

● **E13.31   Other specified diabetes mellitus with unspecified diabetic retinopathy**

E13.311   Other specified diabetes mellitus with unspecified diabetic retinopathy with macular edema ℞

E13.319   Other specified diabetes mellitus with unspecified diabetic retinopathy without macular edema ℞

● **E13.32   Other specified diabetes mellitus with mild nonproliferative diabetic retinopathy**
    Other specified diabetes mellitus with nonproliferative diabetic retinopathy NOS

    One of the following 7th characters is to be assigned to codes in subcategory E13.32 to designate laterality of the disease:

1	right eye
2	left eye
3	bilateral
9	unspecified eye

● **E13.321   Other specified diabetes mellitus with mild nonproliferative diabetic retinopathy with macular edema** ℞

● **E13.329   Other specified diabetes mellitus with mild nonproliferative diabetic retinopathy without macular edema** ℞

● **E13.33   Other specified diabetes mellitus with moderate nonproliferative diabetic retinopathy**

    One of the following 7th characters is to be assigned to codes in subcategory E13.33 to designate laterality of the disease:

1	right eye
2	left eye
3	bilateral
9	unspecified eye

● **E13.331   Other specified diabetes mellitus with moderate nonproliferative diabetic retinopathy with macular edema** ℞

● **E13.339   Other specified diabetes mellitus with moderate nonproliferative diabetic retinopathy without macular edema** ℞

● **E13.34   Other specified diabetes mellitus with severe nonproliferative diabetic retinopathy**

    One of the following 7th characters is to be assigned to codes in subcategory E13.34 to designate laterality of the disease:

1	right eye
2	left eye
3	bilateral
9	unspecified eye

● **E13.341   Other specified diabetes mellitus with severe nonproliferative diabetic retinopathy with macular edema** ℞

● **E13.349   Other specified diabetes mellitus with severe nonproliferative diabetic retinopathy without macular edema** ℞

● **E13.35   Other specified diabetes mellitus with proliferative diabetic retinopathy**

    One of the following 7th characters is to be assigned to codes in subcategory E13.35 to designate laterality of the disease:

1	right eye
2	left eye
3	bilateral
9	unspecified eye

● **E13.351   Other specified diabetes mellitus with proliferative diabetic retinopathy with macular edema** ℞

● **E13.352   Other specified diabetes mellitus with proliferative diabetic retinopathy with traction retinal detachment involving the macula** ℞

● **E13.353   Other specified diabetes mellitus with proliferative diabetic retinopathy with traction retinal detachment not involving the macula** ℞

● **E13.354   Other specified diabetes mellitus with proliferative diabetic retinopathy with combined traction retinal detachment and rhegmatogenous retinal detachment** ℞

● **E13.355   Other specified diabetes mellitus with stable proliferative diabetic retinopathy** ℞

● **E13.359   Other specified diabetes mellitus with proliferative diabetic retinopathy without macular edema** ℞

E13.36   Other specified diabetes mellitus with diabetic cataract ℞

X ● **E13.37   Other specified diabetes mellitus with diabetic macular edema, resolved following treatment** ℞

    One of the following 7th characters is to be assigned to code E13.37 to designate laterality of the disease:

1	right eye
2	left eye
3	bilateral
9	unspecified eye

E13.39   Other specified diabetes mellitus with other diabetic ophthalmic complication ℞
    Use additional code to identify manifestation, such as:
    diabetic glaucoma (H40-H42)

● **E13.4   Other specified diabetes mellitus with neurological complications**

E13.40   Other specified diabetes mellitus with diabetic neuropathy, unspecified ℞

E13.41   Other specified diabetes mellitus with diabetic mononeuropathy ℞

E13.42   Other specified diabetes mellitus with diabetic polyneuropathy ℞
    Other specified diabetes mellitus with diabetic neuralgia

E13.43   Other specified diabetes mellitus with diabetic autonomic (poly)neuropathy ℞
    Other specified diabetes mellitus with diabetic gastroparesis

E13.44   Other specified diabetes mellitus with diabetic amyotrophy ⓗ

E13.49   Other specified diabetes mellitus with other diabetic neurological complication ⓗ

● **E13.5**   Other specified diabetes mellitus with circulatory complications

E13.51   Other specified diabetes mellitus with diabetic peripheral angiopathy without gangrene ⓗ

E13.52   Other specified diabetes mellitus with diabetic peripheral angiopathy with gangrene ⓗ
> Other specified diabetes mellitus with diabetic gangrene

E13.59   Other specified diabetes mellitus with other circulatory complications ⓗ

● **E13.6**   Other specified diabetes mellitus with other specified complications

● **E13.61**   Other specified diabetes mellitus with diabetic arthropathy

E13.610   Other specified diabetes mellitus with diabetic neuropathic arthropathy ⓗ
> Other specified diabetes mellitus with Charcôt's joints

E13.618   Other specified diabetes mellitus with other diabetic arthropathy ⓗ

● **E13.62**   Other specified diabetes mellitus with skin complications

E13.620   Other specified diabetes mellitus with diabetic dermatitis ⓗ
> Other specified diabetes mellitus with diabetic necrobiosis lipoidica

E13.621   Other specified diabetes mellitus with foot ulcer ⓗ
> **Use additional** code to identify site of ulcer (L97.4-, L97.5-)

E13.622   Other specified diabetes mellitus with other skin ulcer ⓗ
> **Use additional** code to identify site of ulcer (L97.1-L97.9, L98.41-L98.49)

E13.628   Other specified diabetes mellitus with other skin complications ⓗ

● **E13.63**   Other specified diabetes mellitus with oral complications

E13.630   Other specified diabetes mellitus with periodontal disease ⓗ

E13.638   Other specified diabetes mellitus with other oral complications ⓗ

● **E13.64**   Other specified diabetes mellitus with hypoglycemia
> **Use additional** code for hypoglycemia level, if applicable (E16.A-)

E13.641   Other specified diabetes mellitus with hypoglycemia with coma ⓗ

E13.649   Other specified diabetes mellitus with hypoglycemia without coma ⓗ

E13.65   Other specified diabetes mellitus with hyperglycemia ⓗ

E13.69   Other specified diabetes mellitus with other specified complication ⓗ
> **Use additional** code to identify complication

E13.8   Other specified diabetes mellitus with unspecified complications ⓗ

E13.9   Other specified diabetes mellitus without complications ⓗ

OTHER DISORDERS OF GLUCOSE REGULATION AND PANCREATIC INTERNAL SECRETION (E15-E16)

E15   Nondiabetic hypoglycemic coma ⓗ
> **Includes**   drug-induced insulin coma in nondiabetic
> hyperinsulinism with hypoglycemic coma
> hypoglycemic coma NOS

● **E16**   Other disorders of pancreatic internal secretion

E16.0   Drug-induced hypoglycemia without coma
> **Excludes1**   diabetes with hypoglycemia without coma (E09.649)
>
> **Use additional** code for hypoglycemia level, if applicable (E16.A-)

E16.1   Other hypoglycemia
> Functional hyperinsulinism
> Functional nonhyperinsulinemic hypoglycemia
> Hyperinsulinism NOS
> Hyperplasia of pancreatic islet beta cells NOS
>
> **Excludes1**   diabetes with hypoglycemia (E08.649, E10.649, E11.649, E13.649)
> hypoglycemia in infant of diabetic mother (P70.1)
> neonatal hypoglycemia (P70.4)
>
> **Use additional** code for hypoglycemia level, if applicable (E16.A-)
> **Coding Clinic: 2024, Q2, P10**

E16.2   Hypoglycemia, unspecified
> **Excludes1**   diabetes with hypoglycemia (E08.649, E10.649, E11.649, E13.649)
>
> **Use additional** code for hypoglycemia level, if applicable (E16.A-)
> **Coding Clinic: 2024, Q4, P53; 2016, Q3, P42**

E16.3   Increased secretion of glucagon
> Hyperplasia of pancreatic endocrine cells with glucagon excess

E16.4   Increased secretion of gastrin
> Hypergastrinemia
> Hyperplasia of pancreatic endocrine cells with gastrin excess
> Zollinger-Ellison syndrome

E16.8   Other specified disorders of pancreatic internal secretion
> Increased secretion from endocrine pancreas of growth hormone-releasing hormone
> Increased secretion from endocrine pancreas of pancreatic polypeptide
> Increased secretion from endocrine pancreas of somatostatin
> Increased secretion from endocrine pancreas of vasoactive-intestinal polypeptide

E16.9   Disorder of pancreatic internal secretion, unspecified
> Islet-cell hyperplasia NOS
> Pancreatic endocrine cell hyperplasia NOS

E16.A   Hypoglycemia level

E16.A1   Hypoglycemia level 1
> Decreased blood glucose level 1

E16.A2   Hypoglycemia level 2
> Decreased blood glucose level 2
> **Coding Clinic: 2024, Q4, P53**

E16.A3   Hypoglycemia level 3
> Decreased blood glucose level 3

DISORDERS OF OTHER ENDOCRINE GLANDS (E20-E35)

Excludes1   galactorrhea (N64.3)
gynecomastia (N62)

● **E20   Hypoparathyroidism**
Greatly reduced function of parathyroid glands; AKA parathyroid insufficiency

Excludes1   Di George's syndrome (D82.1)
postprocedural hypoparathyroidism (E89.2)
tetany NOS (R29.0)
transitory neonatal hypoparathyroidism (P71.4)

E20.0   Idiopathic hypoparathyroidism
Rare condition, unknown cause; short dwarf-like with round face

E20.1   Pseudohypoparathyroidism
Hereditary condition resembling hypoparathyroidism, but caused by inability to respond to parathyroid hormone

● **E20.8   Other hypoparathyroidism**

● **E20.81   Hypoparathyroidism due to impaired parathyroid hormone secretion**

E20.810   Autosomal dominant hypocalcemia
Autosomal dominant hypocalcemia type 1 (ADH1)
Autosomal dominant hypocalcemia type 2 (ADH2)
Code also, if applicable, any associated conditions, such as:
calculus of kidney (N20.0)
chronic kidney disease (N18.-)
respiratory distress (J80, R06.-)
seizure disorder (G40.-, R56.9)

E20.811   Secondary hypoparathyroidism in diseases classified elsewhere
Code first *underlying condition, if known*

E20.812   Autoimmune hypoparathyroidism
Code first, *if applicable, underlying condition such as:*
autoimmune polyglandular failure (E31.0)
Schmidt's syndrome (E31.0)

E20.818   Other specified hypoparathyroidism due to impaired parathyroid hormonesecretion
Familial isolated hypoparathyroidism

E20.819   Hypoparathyroidism due to impaired parathyroid hormone secretion,unspecified

E20.89   Other specified hypoparathyroidism
Familial hypoparathyroidism

E20.9   Hypoparathyroidism, unspecified
Parathyroid tetany

● **E21   Hyperparathyroidism and other disorders of parathyroid gland**

Excludes1   adult osteomalacia (M83.-)
ectopic hyperparathyroidism (E34.2)
hungry bone syndrome (E83.81)
infantile and juvenile osteomalacia (E55.0)

Excludes2   familial hypocalciuric hypercalcemia (E83.52)

E21.0   Primary hyperparathyroidism
Hyperplasia of parathyroid
Osteitis fibrosa cystica generalisata [von Recklinghausen's disease of bone]

E21.1   Secondary hyperparathyroidism, not elsewhere classified
Excludes1   secondary hyperparathyroidism of renal origin (N25.81)

Item 4–4   Hyperparathyroidism is an overactive parathyroid gland that secretes excessive parathormone, causing increased levels of circulating calcium. This results in a loss of calcium in the bone (osteoporosis).
Hypoparathyroidism is an underactive parathyroid gland that results in decreased levels of circulating calcium. The primary manifestation is **tetany,** a continuous muscle spasm.

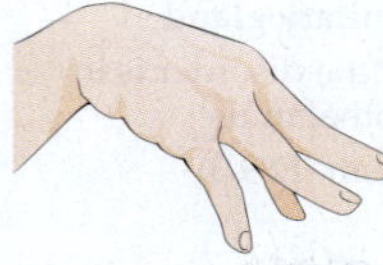

Figure 4-4   Tetany caused by hypoparathyroidism.

E21.2   Other hyperparathyroidism
Tertiary hyperparathyroidism
Excludes1   familial hypocalciuric hypercalcemia (E83.52)

E21.3   Hyperparathyroidism, unspecified

E21.4   Other specified disorders of parathyroid gland

E21.5   Disorder of parathyroid gland, unspecified

● **E22   Hyperfunction of pituitary gland**

Excludes1   Cushing's syndrome (E24.-)
Nelson's syndrome (E24.1)
overproduction of ACTH not associated with Cushing's disease (E27.0)
overproduction of pituitary ACTH (E24.0)
overproduction of thyroid-stimulating hormone (E05.8-)

E22.0   Acromegaly and pituitary gigantism
Chronic disease caused by hypersecretion of growth hormone
Overproduction of growth hormone
Excludes1   constitutional gigantism (E34.4)
constitutional tall stature (E34.4)
increased secretion from endocrine pancreas of growth hormone-releasing hormone (E16.8)

E22.1   Hyperprolactinemia
Increased levels of prolactin
Use additional code for adverse effect, if applicable, to identify drug (T36-T50 with fifth or sixth character 5)

E22.2   Syndrome of inappropriate secretion of antidiuretic hormone

E22.8   Other hyperfunction of pituitary gland
Central precocious puberty

E22.9   Hyperfunction of pituitary gland, unspecified

Item 4–5   Hyperadrenalism is overactivity of the adrenal cortex, which secretes corticosteroid hormones. Excessive glucocorticoid hormone results in hyperglycemia **(Cushing's syndrome),** and excessive aldosterone results in **Conn's syndrome. Adrenogenital syndrome** is the result of excessive secretion of androgens, male hormones, which stimulates premature sexual development. **Hypoadrenalism, Addison's disease,** is a condition in which the adrenal glands atrophy.

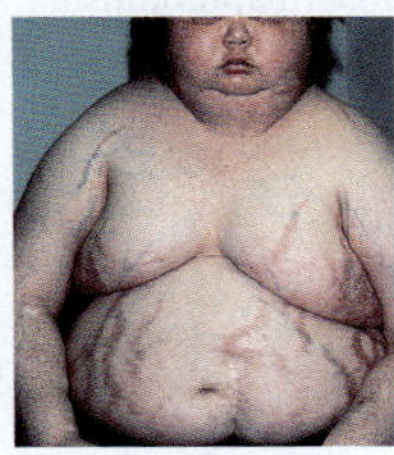

Figure 4-5   Centripetal and generalized obesity and dorsal kyphosis in a woman with Cushing's disease. (From Salvo SG: Mosby's Pathology for Massage Therapists, St. Louis, MO: Mosby/Elsevier, 2009)

CHAPTER 4 (E00–E89)

● **E23 Hypofunction and other disorders of the pituitary gland**

| **Includes** | the listed conditions whether the disorder is in the pituitary or the hypothalamus |

| **Excludes1** | postprocedural hypopituitarism (E89.3) |

E23.0 Hypopituitarism 🅗
- Fertile eunuch syndrome
- Hypogonadotropic hypogonadism
- Idiopathic growth hormone deficiency
- Isolated deficiency of gonadotropin
- Isolated deficiency of growth hormone
- Isolated deficiency of pituitary hormone
- Kallmann's syndrome
- Lorain-Levi short stature
- Necrosis of pituitary gland (postpartum)
- Panhypopituitarism
- Pituitary cachexia
- Pituitary insufficiency NOS
- Pituitary short stature
- Sheehan's syndrome
- Simmonds' disease

Coding Clinic: 2024, Q1, P15

E23.1 Drug-induced hypopituitarism 🅗

| **Use additional** | code for adverse effect, if applicable, to identify drug (T36-T50 with fifth or sixth character 5) |

E23.2 Diabetes insipidus 🅗

| **Excludes1** | nephrogenic diabetes insipidus (N25.1) |

E23.3 Hypothalamic dysfunction, not elsewhere classified 🅗

| **Excludes1** | Prader-Willi syndrome (Q87.11) Russell-Silver syndrome (Q87.19) |

Coding Clinic: 2024, Q1, P15

E23.6 Other disorders of pituitary gland 🅗
- Abscess of pituitary
- Adiposogenital dystrophy

E23.7 Disorder of pituitary gland, unspecified 🅗

● **E24 Cushing's syndrome**

| **Excludes1** | congenital adrenal hyperplasia (E25.0) |

E24.0 Pituitary-dependent Cushing's disease 🅗
- Overproduction of pituitary ACTH
- Pituitary-dependent hypercorticalism

E24.1 Nelson's syndrome 🅗

E24.2 Drug-induced Cushing's syndrome 🅗

| **Use additional** | code for adverse effect, if applicable, to identify drug (T36-T50 with fifth or sixth character 5) |

E24.3 Ectopic ACTH syndrome 🅗

E24.4 Alcohol-induced pseudo-Cushing's syndrome 🅗

E24.8 Other Cushing's syndrome 🅗

E24.9 Cushing's syndrome, unspecified 🅗

● **E25 Adrenogenital disorders**

Disorder of production of steroid hormone in adrenal gland

| **Includes** | adrenogenital syndromes, virilizing or feminizing, whether acquired or due to adrenal hyperplasia consequent on inborn enzyme defects in hormone synthesis female adrenal pseudohermaphroditism female heterosexual precocious pseudopuberty male isosexual precocious pseudopuberty male macrogenitosomia praecox male sexual precocity with adrenal hyperplasia male virilization (female) |

| **Excludes1** | indeterminate sex and pseudohermaphroditism (Q56) chromosomal abnormalities (Q90-Q99) |

E25.0 Congenital adrenogenital disorders associated with enzyme deficiency
- Congenital adrenal hyperplasia
- 21-Hydroxylase deficiency
- Salt-losing congenital adrenal hyperplasia

E25.8 Other adrenogenital disorders 🅗
- Idiopathic adrenogenital disorder

| **Use additional** | code for adverse effect, if applicable, to identify drug (T36-T50 with fifth or sixth character 5) |

E25.9 Adrenogenital disorder, unspecified 🅗
- Adrenogenital syndrome NOS

● **E26 Hyperaldosteronism**

Abnormality of electrolyte metabolism caused by excessive secretion of aldosterone

● **E26.0 Primary hyperaldosteronism**

E26.01 Conn's syndrome 🅗

| **Code also** | adrenal adenoma (D35.0-) |

E26.02 Glucocorticoid-remediable aldosteronism 🅗
- Familial aldosteronism type I

E26.09 Other primary hyperaldosteronism 🅗
- Primary aldosteronism due to adrenal hyperplasia (bilateral)

E26.1 Secondary hyperaldosteronism 🅗

● **E26.8 Other hyperaldosteronism**

E26.81 Bartter's syndrome 🅗

E26.89 Other hyperaldosteronism 🅗

E26.9 Hyperaldosteronism, unspecified 🅗
- Aldosteronism NOS
- Hyperaldosteronism NOS

● **E27 Other disorders of adrenal gland**

E27.0 Other adrenocortical overactivity 🅗
- Overproduction of ACTH, not associated with Cushing's disease
- Premature adrenarche

| **Excludes1** | Cushing's syndrome (E24.-) |

E27.1 Primary adrenocortical insufficiency 🅗
- Addison's disease
- Autoimmune adrenalitis

| **Excludes1** | Addison only phenotype adrenoleukodystrophy (E71.528) amyloidosis (E85.-) tuberculous Addison's disease (A18.7) Waterhouse-Friderichsen syndrome (A39.1) |

E27.2 Addisonian crisis 🅗

Acute onset of adrenocortical insufficiency
- Adrenal crisis
- Adrenocortical crisis

E27.3 Drug-induced adrenocortical insufficiency 🅗

| **Use additional** | code for adverse effect, if applicable, to identify drug (T36-T50 with fifth or sixth character 5) |

● **E27.4 Other and unspecified adrenocortical insufficiency**

| **Excludes1** | adrenoleukodystrophy [Addison-Schilder] (E71.528) Waterhouse-Friderichsen syndrome (A39.1) |

E27.40 Unspecified adrenocortical insufficiency 🅗
- Adrenocortical insufficiency NOS
- Hypoaldosteronism

Coding Clinic: 2024, Q1, P15

E27.49 Other adrenocortical insufficiency 🅗
- Adrenal hemorrhage
- Adrenal infarction

Coding Clinic: 2024, Q1, P15

E27.5 Adrenomedullary hyperfunction 🅗
- Adrenomedullary hyperplasia
- Catecholamine hypersecretion

▶ Code also, if applicable:
- ▶ malignant pheochromocytoma (C74.1-)
- ▶ pheochromocytoma (benign) (D35.0-)
- ▶ secondary hypertension (I15.2)

E27.8 Other specified disorders of adrenal gland 🅗
- Abnormality of cortisol-binding globulin

E27.9 Disorder of adrenal gland, unspecified 🅗

▶ New ➡ Revised ~~deleted~~ Deleted | Excludes 1 | | Excludes 2 | | Includes | | Use additional | | Code first | | Code also | | Key words |

OGCR Official Guidelines **X** Assign placeholder X ● Use Additional Character(s) ▸ Manifestation Code 🅗 Hierarchical Condition Category **Coding Clinic**

● **E28 Ovarian dysfunction**
   Excludes1   isolated gonadotropin deficiency (E23.0)
           postprocedural ovarian failure (E89.4-)

   E28.0 Estrogen excess
     Use additional code for adverse effect, if applicable, to identify drug (T36-T50 with fifth or sixth character 5)

   E28.1 Androgen excess
     Hypersecretion of ovarian androgens
     Use additional code for adverse effect, if applicable, to identify drug (T36-T50 with fifth or sixth character 5)

   E28.2 Polycystic ovarian syndrome
     Sclerocystic ovary syndrome
     Stein-Leventhal syndrome
     Coding Clinic: 2022, Q2, P16

   ● **E28.3 Primary ovarian failure**
     Excludes1   pure gonadal dysgenesis (Q99.1)
            Turner's syndrome (Q96.-)

     ● **E28.31 Premature menopause**
       E28.310 Symptomatic premature menopause A
         Symptoms such as flushing, sleeplessness, headache, lack of concentration, associated with premature menopause

       E28.319 Asymptomatic premature menopause A
         Premature menopause NOS

     E28.39 Other primary ovarian failure
       Decreased estrogen
       Resistant ovary syndrome

   E28.8 Other ovarian dysfunction
     Ovarian hyperfunction NOS
     Excludes1   postprocedural ovarian failure (E89.4-)

   E28.9 Ovarian dysfunction, unspecified

● **E29 Testicular dysfunction**
   Excludes1   androgen insensitivity syndrome (E34.5-)
           azoospermia or oligospermia NOS (N46.0-N46.1)
           isolated gonadotropin deficiency (E23.0)
           Klinefelter's syndrome (Q98.0-Q98.1, Q98.4)

   E29.0 Testicular hyperfunction
     Hypersecretion of testicular hormones

   E29.1 Testicular hypofunction
     Defective biosynthesis of testicular androgen NOS
     5-delta-Reductase deficiency (with male pseudohermaphroditism)
     Testicular hypogonadism NOS
     Use additional code for adverse effect, if applicable, to identify drug (T36-T50 with fifth or sixth character 5)
     Excludes1   postprocedural testicular hypofunction (E89.5)

   E29.8 Other testicular dysfunction

   E29.9 Testicular dysfunction, unspecified

● **E30 Disorders of puberty, not elsewhere classified**

   E30.0 Delayed puberty
     Constitutional delay of puberty
     Delayed sexual development

   E30.1 Precocious puberty P
     Sexual maturation at earlier age than normal, or before age 8 in girls and 9 in boys, usually hormonal; AKA sexual precocity or pubertas praecox
     Precocious menstruation
     Excludes1   Albright (-McCune) (-Sternberg) syndrome (Q78.1)
           central precocious puberty (E22.8)
           congenital adrenal hyperplasia (E25.0)
           female heterosexual precocious pseudopuberty (E25.-)
           male isosexual precocious pseudopuberty (E25.-)

   E30.8 Other disorders of puberty P
     Premature thelarche

   E30.9 Disorder of puberty, unspecified

● **E31 Polyglandular dysfunction**
   Excludes1   ataxia telangiectasia [Louis-Bar] (G11.3)
           dystrophia myotonica [Steinert] (G71.11)
           pseudohypoparathyroidism (E20.1)

   E31.0 Autoimmune polyglandular failure RCC
     Schmidt's syndrome

   E31.1 Polyglandular hyperfunction RCC
     Excludes1   multiple endocrine adenomatosis (E31.2-)
           multiple endocrine neoplasia (E31.2-)

   ● **E31.2 Multiple endocrine neoplasia [MEN] syndromes**
     Adenomatous hyperplasia and malignant tumors in endocrine glands
     Multiple endocrine adenomatosis
     Code also any associated malignancies and other conditions associated with the syndromes

     E31.20 Multiple endocrine neoplasia [MEN] syndrome, unspecified RCC
       Multiple endocrine adenomatosis NOS
       Multiple endocrine neoplasia [MEN] syndrome NOS

     E31.21 Multiple endocrine neoplasia [MEN] type I RCC
       Wermer's syndrome

     E31.22 Multiple endocrine neoplasia [MEN] type IIA RCC
       Sipple's syndrome

     E31.23 Multiple endocrine neoplasia [MEN] type IIB RCC

   E31.8 Other polyglandular dysfunction RCC

   E31.9 Polyglandular dysfunction, unspecified RCC

● **E32 Diseases of thymus**
   Excludes1   aplasia or hypoplasia of thymus with immunodeficiency (D82.1)
           myasthenia gravis (G70.0)

   E32.0 Persistent hyperplasia of thymus RCC
     Hypertrophy of thymus

   E32.1 Abscess of thymus RCC

   E32.8 Other diseases of thymus RCC
     Excludes1   aplasia or hypoplasia with immunodeficiency (D82.1)
           thymoma (D15.0)

   E32.9 Disease of thymus, unspecified RCC

● **E34 Other endocrine disorders**
   Excludes1   pseudohypoparathyroidism (E20.1)

   E34.0 Carcinoid syndrome RCC
     Code also the underlying disorder, such as:
     primary neuroendocrine tumors (C7A.-)
     secondary neuroendocrine tumors (C7B.-)

     E34.00 Carcinoid syndrome, unspecified
       Carcinoid disease, unspecified

     E34.01 Carcinoid heart syndrome
       Carcinoid heart disease
       Hedinger syndrome
       Coding Clinic: 2024, Q4, P8

     E34.09 Other carcinoid syndrome
       Carcinoid disease NEC
       Carcinoid syndrome NEC
       Other carcinoid disease

   E34.1 Other hypersecretion of intestinal hormones

   E34.2 Ectopic hormone secretion, not elsewhere classified
     Excludes1   ectopic ACTH syndrome (E24.3)

CHAPTER 4 (E00-E89)

E34.3   Short stature due to endocrine disorder

> **Excludes1**   achondroplastic short stature (Q77.4)
> hypochondroplastic short stature (Q77.4)
> nutritional short stature (E45)
> pituitary short stature (E23.0)
> progeria (E34.8)
> renal short stature (N25.0)
> Russell-Silver syndrome (Q87.19)
> short-limbed stature with immunodeficiency (D82.2)
> short stature due to endocrine disorder (E34.3-)
> short stature in specific dysmorphic syndromes - code to syndrome - see Alphabetical Index
> short stature NOS (R62.52)

E34.30   Short stature due to endocrine disorder, unspecified

E34.31   Constitutional short stature
Constitutional delay of growth, puberty, or maturation

● **E34.32   Genetic causes of short stature**

E34.321   Primary insulin-like growth factor-1 (IGF-1) deficiency
Acid-labile subunit gene (IGFALS) defect
Growth hormone gene 1 (GH1) defect with growth hormone neutralizing antibodies
Growth hormone insensitivity syndrome (GHIS)
Insulin-like growth factor 1 gene (IGF1) defect
Laron type short stature
Severe primary insulin-like growth factor-1 deficiency (SPIGFD)
Signal transducer and activator of transcription 5B gene (STAT5b) defect

E34.322   Insulin-like growth factor-1 (IGF-1) resistance
Genetic syndrome with resistance to insulin-like growth factor-1
Insulin-like growth factor-1 receptor (IGF-1R) defect
Post-insulin-like growth factor-1 receptor signaling defect

E34.328   Other genetic causes of short stature
Short stature due to ACAN gene variant
Short stature due to aggrecan deficiency
Short stature due to NPR-2 gene variant

E34.329   Unspecified genetic causes of short stature

● **E34.39   Other short stature due to endocrine disorder**

E34.4   Constitutional tall stature ᴴᶜᶜ
Constitutional gigantism

● **E34.5   Androgen insensitivity syndrome**

E34.50   Androgen insensitivity syndrome, unspecified
Androgen insensitivity NOS

E34.51   Complete androgen insensitivity syndrome
Complete androgen insensitivity
de Quervain syndrome
Goldberg-Maxwell syndrome

E34.52   Partial androgen insensitivity syndrome
Partial androgen insensitivity
Reifenstein syndrome

E34.8   Other specified endocrine disorders
Pineal gland dysfunction
Progeria

> **Excludes2**   pseudohypoparathyroidism (E20.1)

E34.9   Endocrine disorder, unspecified
Endocrine disturbance NOS
Hormone disturbance NOS

▶ **E35   Disorders of endocrine glands in diseases classified elsewhere**

Code first underlying disease, such as:
late congenital syphilis of thymus gland [Dubois disease] (A50.9)

Use additional code, if applicable, to identify:
sequelae of tuberculosis of other organs (B90.8)

> **Excludes1**   Echinococcus granulosus infection of thyroid gland (B67.3)
> meningococcal hemorrhagic adrenalitis (A39.1)
> syphilis of endocrine gland (A52.79)
> tuberculosis of adrenal gland, except calcification (A18.7)
> tuberculosis of endocrine gland NEC (A18.82)
> tuberculosis of thyroid gland (A18.81)
> Waterhouse-Friderichsen syndrome (A39.1)

INTRAOPERATIVE COMPLICATIONS OF ENDOCRINE SYSTEM (E36)

● **E36   Intraoperative complications of endocrine system**

> **Excludes2**   postprocedural endocrine and metabolic complications and disorders, not elsewhere classified (E89.-)

● **E36.0   Intraoperative hemorrhage and hematoma of an endocrine system organ or structure complicating a procedure**

> **Excludes1**   intraoperative hemorrhage and hematoma of an endocrine system organ or structure due to accidental puncture or laceration during a procedure (E36.1-)

E36.01   Intraoperative hemorrhage and hematoma of an endocrine system organ or structure complicating an endocrine system procedure
Coding Clinic: 2020, Q1, P19

E36.02   Intraoperative hemorrhage and hematoma of an endocrine system organ or structure complicating other procedure

● **E36.1   Accidental puncture and laceration of an endocrine system organ or structure during a procedure**

E36.11   Accidental puncture and laceration of an endocrine system organ or structure during an endocrine system procedure

E36.12   Accidental puncture and laceration of an endocrine system organ or structure during other procedure

E36.8   Other intraoperative complications of endocrine system
Use additional code, if applicable, to further specify disorder

MALNUTRITION (E40-E46)

> **Excludes1**   intestinal malabsorption (K90.-)
> sequelae of protein-calorie malnutrition (E64.0)

> **Excludes2**   nutritional anemias (D50-D53)
> starvation (T73.0)

E40   Kwashiorkor ᴴᶜᶜ
Malnutrition produced by severe protein deficiency
Severe malnutrition with nutritional edema with dyspigmentation of skin and hair

> **Excludes1**   marasmic kwashiorkor (E42)

Coding Clinic: 22017, Q3, P25

E41   Nutritional marasmus ᴴᶜᶜ
Severe malnutrition with marasmus

> **Excludes1**   marasmic kwashiorkor (E42)

Coding Clinic: 2017, Q3, P24-25

E42   Marasmic kwashiorkor ᴴᶜᶜ
Severe protein malnutrition
Intermediate form severe protein-calorie malnutrition
Severe protein-calorie malnutrition with signs of both kwashiorkor and marasmus
Coding Clinic: 2017, Q3, P25

▶ New   ⇛ Revised   ~~deleted~~ Deleted   Excludes 1   Excludes 2   Includes   Use additional   Code first   Code also   Key words
OGCR Official Guidelines   **X** Assign placeholder X   ● Use Additional Character(s)   ▶ Manifestation Code   ᴴᶜᶜ Hierarchical Condition Category   **Coding Clinic**

E43 Unspecified severe protein-calorie malnutrition 🟣
Starvation edema
Coding Clinic: 2023, Q4, P15; 2022, Q1, P13; 2020, Q1, P5-6; 2017, Q4, P108-109; 2017, Q3, P25

● **E44 Protein-calorie malnutrition of moderate and mild degree**
E44.0 Moderate protein-calorie malnutrition 🟣
E44.1 Mild protein-calorie malnutrition 🟣

E45 Retarded development following protein-calorie malnutrition 🟣
Nutritional short stature
Nutritional stunting
Physical retardation due to malnutrition

E46 Unspecified protein-calorie malnutrition 🟣
Malnutrition NOS
Protein-calorie imbalance NOS
Excludes1 nutritional deficiency NOS (E63.9)
Coding Clinic: 2017, Q3, P25

OTHER NUTRITIONAL DEFICIENCIES (E50-E64)

Excludes2 nutritional anemias (D50-D53)

● **E50 Vitamin A deficiency**
Excludes1 sequelae of vitamin A deficiency (E64.1)
E50.0 Vitamin A deficiency with conjunctival xerosis
E50.1 Vitamin A deficiency with Bitot's spot and conjunctival xerosis
Bitot's spot in the young child
E50.2 Vitamin A deficiency with corneal xerosis
E50.3 Vitamin A deficiency with corneal ulceration and xerosis
E50.4 Vitamin A deficiency with keratomalacia
Eye disorder that results in dry cornea caused by vitamin A deficiency
E50.5 Vitamin A deficiency with night blindness
E50.6 Vitamin A deficiency with xerophthalmic scars of cornea
Abnormal dryness and thickening of conjunctiva and cornea due to vitamin A deficiency
E50.7 Other ocular manifestations of vitamin A deficiency
Xerophthalmia NOS
E50.8 Other manifestations of vitamin A deficiency
Follicular keratosis
Xeroderma
E50.9 Vitamin A deficiency, unspecified
Hypovitaminosis A NOS

● **E51 Thiamine deficiency**
Excludes1 sequelae of thiamine deficiency (E64.8)
● **E51.1 Beriberi**
E51.11 Dry beriberi
Thiamine deficiency with nervous system manifestation most often caused by excessive alcohol consumption
Beriberi NOS
Beriberi with polyneuropathy
E51.12 Wet beriberi
Thiamine deficiency with cardiovascular manifestation most often caused by excessive alcohol consumption
Beriberi with cardiovascular manifestations
Cardiovascular beriberi
Shoshin disease
E51.2 Wernicke's encephalopathy
Acute disease of brain due to thiamine deficiency most often associated with excessive alcohol consumption
E51.8 Other manifestations of thiamine deficiency
E51.9 Thiamine deficiency, unspecified

E52 Niacin deficiency [pellagra]
Niacin (-tryptophan) deficiency
Nicotinamide deficiency
Pellagra (alcoholic)
Excludes1 sequelae of niacin deficiency (E64.8)

● **E53 Deficiency of other B group vitamins**
Excludes1 sequelae of vitamin B deficiency (E64.8)
E53.0 Riboflavin deficiency
Ariboflavinosis
Vitamin B2 deficiency
E53.1 Pyridoxine deficiency
Vitamin B6 deficiency
Excludes1 pyridoxine-responsive sideroblastic anemia (D64.3)
E53.8 Deficiency of other specified B group vitamins
Biotin deficiency
Cyanocobalamin deficiency
Folate deficiency
Folic acid deficiency
Pantothenic acid deficiency
Vitamin B12 deficiency
Excludes1 folate deficiency anemia (D52.-)
vitamin B12 deficiency anemia (D51.-)
E53.9 Vitamin B deficiency, unspecified

E54 Ascorbic acid deficiency
Deficiency of vitamin C
Scurvy
Excludes1 scorbutic anemia (D53.2)
sequelae of vitamin C deficiency (E64.2)

● **E55 Vitamin D deficiency**
Excludes1 adult osteomalacia (M83.-)
osteoporosis (M80.-)
sequelae of rickets (E64.3)
E55.0 Rickets, active
Infantile osteomalacia
Juvenile osteomalacia
Softening of bone
Excludes1 celiac rickets (K90.0)
Crohn's rickets (K50.-)
hereditary vitamin D-dependent rickets (E83.32)
inactive rickets (E64.3)
renal rickets (N25.0)
sequelae of rickets (E64.3)
vitamin D-resistant rickets (E83.31)
E55.9 Vitamin D deficiency, unspecified
Avitaminosis D

Item 4–6 Bitot's spots are the result of a buildup of keratin debris found on the superficial surface the conjunctiva; oval, triangular, or irregular in shape; and a sign of vitamin A deficiency and associated with night blindness. The disease may progress to **keratomalacia,** which can result in eventual prolapse of the iris and loss of the lens.

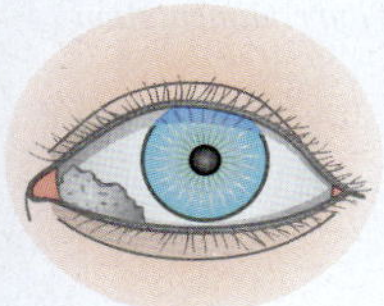

Figure 4-6 Bitot's spot on the conjunctiva.

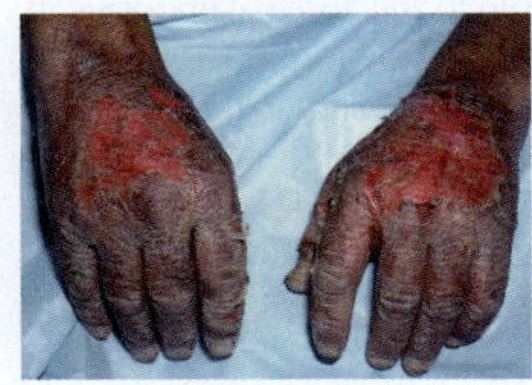

Figure 4-7 The sharply demarcated, characteristic scaling dermatitis of pellagra. (From James WD, Berger TG, Elston DM: Andrews' Diseases of the Skin: Clinical Dermatology, Philadelphia, Saunders Elsevier, 2006)

Item 4–7 Pellagra is associated with a deficiency of niacin and its precursor, **tryptophan.** Characteristics of the condition include diarrhea, dermatitis on exposed skin surfaces, dementia, and death. It is prevalent in developing countries where nutrition is inadequate. **Beriberi** is associated with thiamine deficiency.

● **E56**   **Other vitamin deficiencies**

     Excludes1   sequelae of other vitamin deficiencies (E64.8)

     E56.0   **Deficiency of vitamin E**

     E56.1   **Deficiency of vitamin K**

         Excludes1   deficiency of coagulation factor due to vitamin K deficiency (D68.4)

                 vitamin K deficiency of newborn (P53)

     E56.8   **Deficiency of other vitamins**

     E56.9   **Vitamin deficiency, unspecified**

E58   **Dietary calcium deficiency**

     Excludes1   disorders of calcium metabolism (E83.5-)

                sequelae of calcium deficiency (E64.8)

E59   **Dietary selenium deficiency**

     Keshan disease

     Excludes1   sequelae of selenium deficiency (E64.8)

E60   **Dietary zinc deficiency**

● **E61**   **Deficiency of other nutrient elements**

     Use additional code for adverse effect, if applicable, to identify drug (T36-T50 with fifth or sixth character 5)

     Excludes1   disorders of mineral metabolism (E83.-)

                iodine deficiency related thyroid disorders (E00-E02)

                sequelae of malnutrition and other nutritional deficiencies (E64.-)

     E61.0   **Copper deficiency**

     E61.1   **Iron deficiency**

         Excludes1   iron deficiency anemia (D50.-)

     E61.2   **Magnesium deficiency**

     E61.3   **Manganese deficiency**

     E61.4   **Chromium deficiency**

     E61.5   **Molybdenum deficiency**

     E61.6   **Vanadium deficiency**

     E61.7   **Deficiency of multiple nutrient elements**

     E61.8   **Deficiency of other specified nutrient elements**

     E61.9   **Deficiency of nutrient element, unspecified**

● **E63**   **Other nutritional deficiencies**

     Excludes2   dehydration (E86.0)

                failure to thrive, adult (R62.7)

                failure to thrive, child (R62.51)

                feeding problems in newborn (P92.-)

                sequelae of malnutrition and other nutritional deficiencies (E64.-)

     E63.0   **Essential fatty acid [EFA] deficiency**

     E63.1   **Imbalance of constituents of food intake**

     E63.8   **Other specified nutritional deficiencies**

     E63.9   **Nutritional deficiency, unspecified**

● **E64**   **Sequelae of malnutrition and other nutritional deficiencies**

     Pathological condition resulting from disease, injury, or other trauma

     Note: This category is to be used to indicate conditions in categories E43, E44, E46, E50-E63 as the cause of sequelae, which are themselves classified elsewhere. The "sequelae" include conditions specified as such; they also include the late effects of diseases classifiable to the above categories if the disease itself is no longer present

     Code first condition resulting from (sequela) of malnutrition and other nutritional deficiencies

     E64.0   **Sequelae of protein-calorie malnutrition** ⓗ

         Excludes2   retarded development following protein-calorie malnutrition (E45)

     E64.1   **Sequelae of vitamin A deficiency**

     E64.2   **Sequelae of vitamin C deficiency**

     E64.3   **Sequelae of rickets**

     E64.8   **Sequelae of other nutritional deficiencies**

     E64.9   **Sequelae of unspecified nutritional deficiency**

OVERWEIGHT, OBESITY AND OTHER HYPERALIMENTATION (E65-E68)

E65   **Localized adiposity**

     Fat pad

● **E66**   **Overweight and obesity**

     Code first obesity complicating pregnancy, childbirth and the puerperium, if applicable (O99.21-)

     Use additional code to identify body mass index (BMI), if known, for adults (Z68.1-Z68.45) or pediatrics (Z68.5-)

     Excludes2   adiposogenital dystrophy E23.6)

                lipomatosis NOS (E88.2)

                lipomatosis dolorosa [Dercum] (E88.2)

                Prader-Willi syndrome (Q87.11)

     Coding Clinic: 2022, Q3, P7; 2018, Q4, P80

● **E66.0**   **Obesity due to excess calories**

     E66.01   **Morbid (severe) obesity due to excess calories** ⓗ

         Excludes1   morbid (severe) obesity with alveolar hypoventilation (E66.2)

         Coding Clinic: 2025, Q1, P17; 2022, Q3, P6; 2022, Q2, P9; 2018, Q4, P79

     E66.09   **Other obesity due to excess calories**

     E66.1   **Drug-induced obesity**

         Use additional code for adverse effect, if applicable, to identify drug (T36-T50 with fifth or sixth character 5)

         Coding Clinic: 2022, Q3, P6

     E66.2   **Morbid (severe) obesity with alveolar hypoventilation** ⓗ

         Uncommon condition of unknown cause leading to inadequate ventilation in lungs, even though lungs and airways are normal

         Obesity hypoventilation syndrome (OHS)

         Pickwickian syndrome

     E66.3   **Overweight**

     E66.8   **Other obesity**

         E66.81   **Obesity class**

             E66.811   **Obesity, class 1**

             E66.812   **Obesity, class 2**

             Coding Clinic: 2024, Q4, P11

             E66.813   **Obesity, class 3**

             Coding Clinic: 2025, Q1, P17

         E66.89   **Other obesity not elsewhere classified**

     E66.9   **Obesity, unspecified**

         Obesity NOS

         Coding Clinic: 2021, Q2, P10-11

● **E67**   **Other hyperalimentation**

     Ingestion of more than optimal amount of nutrients

     Excludes1   hyperalimentation NOS (R63.2)

                sequelae of hyperalimentation (E68)

     E67.0   **Hypervitaminosis A**

     E67.1   **Hypercarotenemia**

     E67.2   **Megavitamin-B6 syndrome**

     E67.3   **Hypervitaminosis D**

     E67.8   **Other specified hyperalimentation**

E68   **Sequelae of hyperalimentation**

     Code first condition resulting from (sequela) of hyperalimentation

---

▶ New   ⟹ Revised   ~~deleted~~ Deleted   Excludes 1   Excludes 2   Includes   Use additional   Code first   Code also   Key words

OGCR Official Guidelines   X Assign placeholder X   ● Use Additional Character(s)   ▶ Manifestation Code   ⓗ Hierarchical Condition Category   **Coding Clinic**

METABOLIC DISORDERS (E70-E88)

Excludes1 androgen insensitivity syndrome (E34.5-)
congenital adrenal hyperplasia (E25.0)
hemolytic anemias attributable to enzyme
   disorders (D55.-)
Marfan syndrome (Q87.4-)
5-alpha-reductase deficiency (E29.1)

Excludes2 Ehlers-Danlos syndromes (Q79.6-)

E70 **Disorders of aromatic amino-acid metabolism**

E70.0 **Classical phenylketonuria**
Inherited disorder that increases to harmful levels amino acid phenylalanine

E70.1 **Other hyperphenylalaninemias**

E70.2 **Disorders of tyrosine metabolism**

Excludes1 transitory tyrosinemia of newborn (P74.5)

E70.20 **Disorder of tyrosine metabolism, unspecified**
Tyrosine: Nonessential amino acid occurring in most proteins

E70.21 **Tyrosinemia**
Congenital amino acid metabolism
Hypertyrosinemia

E70.29 **Other disorders of tyrosine metabolism**
Alkaptonuria
Ochronosis

E70.3 **Albinism**
Congenital condition of reduced or absent pigment in eyes, skin, and hair

E70.30 **Albinism, unspecified**

E70.31 **Ocular albinism**

E70.310 **X-linked ocular albinism**

E70.311 **Autosomal recessive ocular albinism**

E70.318 **Other ocular albinism**

E70.319 **Ocular albinism, unspecified**

E70.32 **Oculocutaneous albinism**
Partial or total lack of melanin pigment in eyes

Excludes1 Chediak-Higashi syndrome
   (E70.330)
Hermansky-Pudlak syndrome
   (E70.331)

E70.320 **Tyrosinase negative oculocutaneous albinism**
Albinism I
Oculocutaneous albinism ty-neg

E70.321 **Tyrosinase positive oculocutaneous albinism**
Albinism II
Oculocutaneous albinism ty-pos

E70.328 **Other oculocutaneous albinism**
Cross syndrome

E70.329 **Oculocutaneous albinism, unspecified**

E70.33 **Albinism with hematologic abnormality**

E70.330 **Chediak-Higashi syndrome**

E70.331 **Hermansky-Pudlak syndrome**

E70.338 **Other albinism with hematologic abnormality**

E70.339 **Albinism with hematologic abnormality, unspecified**

E70.39 **Other specified albinism**
Piebaldism

E70.4 **Disorders of histidine metabolism**

E70.40 **Disorders of histidine metabolism, unspecified**

E70.41 **Histidinemia**

E70.49 **Other disorders of histidine metabolism**

E70.5 **Disorders of tryptophan metabolism**

E70.8 **Other disorders of aromatic amino-acid metabolism**

E70.81 **Aromatic L-amino acid decarboxylase deficiency**
AADC deficiency

E70.89 **Other disorders of aromatic amino-acid metabolism**

E70.9 **Disorder of aromatic amino-acid metabolism, unspecified**

E71 **Disorders of branched-chain amino-acid metabolism and fatty-acid metabolism**

E71.0 **Maple-syrup-urine disease**
Due to defect in amino acid catabolism, causing severe ketoacidosis with smell of maple syrup in urine and on body

E71.1 **Other disorders of branched-chain amino-acid metabolism**

E71.11 **Branched-chain organic acidurias**

E71.110 **Isovaleric acidemia**

E71.111 **3-methylglutaconic aciduria**

E71.118 **Other branched-chain organic acidurias**

E71.12 **Disorders of propionate metabolism**

E71.120 **Methylmalonic acidemia**

E71.121 **Propionic acidemia**

E71.128 **Other disorders of propionate metabolism**

E71.19 **Other disorders of branched-chain amino-acid metabolism**
Hyperleucine-isoleucinemia
Hypervalinemia

E71.2 **Disorder of branched-chain amino-acid metabolism, unspecified**

E71.3 **Disorders of fatty-acid metabolism**

Excludes1 peroxisomal disorders (E71.5)
Refsum's disease (G60.1)
Schilder's disease (G37.0)

Excludes2 carnitine deficiency due to inborn error of
   metabolism (E71.42)

E71.30 **Disorder of fatty-acid metabolism, unspecified**

E71.31 **Disorders of fatty-acid oxidation**

E71.310 **Long chain/very long chain acyl CoA dehydrogenase deficiency**
LCAD deficiency
VLCAD deficiency

E71.311 **Medium chain acyl CoA dehydrogenase deficiency**
MCAD deficiency

E71.312 **Short chain acyl CoA dehydrogenase deficiency**
SCAD deficiency

E71.313 **Glutaric aciduria type II**
Glutaric aciduria type II A
Glutaric aciduria type II B
Glutaric aciduria type II C

Excludes1 glutaric aciduria (type
   1) NOS (E72.3)

E71.314   **Muscle carnitine palmitoyltransferase deficiency** 🅡🅒

E71.318   **Other disorders of fatty-acid oxidation** 🅡🅒

E71.32   **Disorders of ketone metabolism** 🅡🅒

E71.39   **Other disorders of fatty-acid metabolism** 🅡🅒

🔴 **E71.4**   **Disorders of carnitine metabolism**

> **Excludes1**   muscle carnitine palmitoyltransferase deficiency (E71.314)

E71.40   **Disorder of carnitine metabolism, unspecified** 🅡🅒

E71.41   **Primary carnitine deficiency** 🅡🅒

E71.42   **Carnitine deficiency due to inborn errors of metabolism** 🅡🅒

> **Code also** associated inborn error or metabolism

E71.43   **Iatrogenic carnitine deficiency** 🅡🅒
> *Iatrogenic: Outcomes from activity of physicians*
> Carnitine deficiency due to hemodialysis
> Carnitine deficiency due to Valproic acid therapy

🔴 **E71.44**   **Other secondary carnitine deficiency**

E71.440   **Ruvalcaba-Myhre-Smith syndrome** 🅡🅒

E71.448   **Other secondary carnitine deficiency** 🅡🅒

🔴 **E71.5**   **Peroxisomal disorders**
> *Class of conditions which lead to disorders of lipid metabolism*

> **Excludes1**   Schilder's disease (G37.0)

E71.50   **Peroxisomal disorder, unspecified** 🅡🅒

🔴 **E71.51**   **Disorders of peroxisome biogenesis**
> Group 1 peroxisomal disorders

> **Excludes1**   Refsum's disease (G60.1)

E71.510   **Zellweger syndrome** 🅡🅒

E71.511   **Neonatal adrenoleukodystrophy** 🅡🅒

> **Excludes1**   X-linked adrenoleuko-dystrophy (E71.42-)

E71.518   **Other disorders of peroxisome biogenesis** 🅡🅒

🔴 **E71.52**   **X-linked adrenoleukodystrophy**

E71.520   **Childhood cerebral X-linked adrenoleukodystrophy** 🅡🅒

E71.521   **Adolescent X-linked adrenoleukodystrophy** 🅡🅒

E71.522   **Adrenomyeloneuropathy** 🅡🅒

E71.528   **Other X-linked adrenoleukodystrophy** 🅡🅒

> Addison only phenotype adrenoleukodystrophy
> Addison-Schilder adrenoleukodystrophy

E71.529   **X-linked adrenoleukodystrophy, unspecified type** 🅡🅒

E71.53   **Other group 2 peroxisomal disorders** 🅡🅒

🔴 **E71.54**   **Other peroxisomal disorders**

E71.540   **Rhizomelic chondrodysplasia punctata** 🅡🅒
> *Rare, severe, inherited disorder with limb shortening, bone and cartilage abnormalities, abnormal facial appearance, severe mental retardation, psychomotor retardation, and cataracts*

> **Excludes1**   ~~chondrodysplasia punctata NOS (Q77.3)~~

E71.541   **Zellweger-like syndrome** 🅡🅒

E71.542   **Other group 3 peroxisomal disorders** 🅡🅒

E71.548   **Other peroxisomal disorders** 🅡🅒

🔴 **E72**   **Other disorders of amino-acid metabolism**

> **Excludes1**   disorders of:
> aromatic amino-acid metabolism (E70.-)
> branched-chain amino-acid metabolism (E71.0-E71.2)
> fatty-acid metabolism (E71.3)
> purine and pyrimidine metabolism (E79.-)
> gout (M1A.-, M10.-)

🔴 **E72.0**   **Disorders of amino-acid transport**

> **Excludes1**   disorders of tryptophan metabolism (E70.5)

E72.00   **Disorders of amino-acid transport, unspecified** 🅡🅒

E72.01   **Cystinuria** 🅡🅒
> *Hereditary aminoaciduria due to impairment of renal transport with predominant symptom of urinary cystine calculi*

E72.02   **Hartnup's disease** 🅡🅒
> *Inborn error of metabolism*

E72.03   **Lowe's syndrome** 🅡🅒
> *X-linked disorder with rickets, hydrophthalmia, congenital glaucoma, cataracts, mental retardation, and renal tubule dysfunction*

> **Use additional** code for associated glaucoma (H42)

E72.04   **Cystinosis** 🅡🅒
> *Genetic disease with excessive depostits of amino acid cystine in cells*
> Fanconi (-de Toni) (-Debré) syndrome with cystinosis

> **Excludes1**   Fanconi (-de Toni) (-Debré) syndrome without cystinosis (E72.09)

E72.09   **Other disorders of amino-acid transport** 🅡🅒
> Fanconi (-de Toni) (-Debré) syndrome, unspecified

🔴 **E72.1**   **Disorders of sulfur-bearing amino-acid metabolism**

> **Excludes1**   cystinosis (E72.04)
> cystinuria (E72.01)
> transcobalamin II deficiency (D51.2)

E72.10   **Disorders of sulfur-bearing amino-acid metabolism, unspecified** 🅡🅒

E72.11   **Homocystinuria** 🅡🅒
> Cystathionine synthase deficiency

E72.12   **Methylenetetrahydrofolate reductase deficiency** 🅡🅒

E72.19   **Other disorders of sulfur-bearing amino-acid metabolism** 🅡🅒
> Cystathioninuria
> Methioninemia
> Sulfite oxidase deficiency

Item 4–8 Leukodystrophy is characterized by degeneration and/or failure of the myelin formation of the central nervous system and sometimes of the peripheral nervous system. The disease is inherited and progressive.

▶ New   ⇒ Revised   ~~deleted~~ Deleted   Excludes 1   Excludes 2   Includes   Use additional   Code first   Code also   Key words

OGCR Official Guidelines   **X** Assign placeholder X   🔴 Use Additional Character(s)   ▶ Manifestation Code   🅡🅒 Hierarchical Condition Category   **Coding Clinic**

● **E72.2** **Disorders of urea cycle metabolism**
- **Excludes1**   disorders of ornithine metabolism (E72.4)

E72.20 **Disorder of urea cycle metabolism, unspecified** RCC
     Hyperammonemia
     Elevated levels of ammonia
- **Excludes1**   hyperammonemia-hyperornithinemia-homocitrullinemia syndrome E72.4
     transient hyperammonemia of newborn (P74.6)

E72.21 **Argininemia** RCC
     Disorder in which deficiency of enzyme arginase causes build-up of arginine and ammonia in blood

E72.22 **Arginosuccinic aciduria** RCC
     Gene disorder of urea cycle resulting accumulation of ammonia

E72.23 **Citrullinemia** RCC
     Urea cycle disorder that causes ammonia and other toxic substances to accumulate in blood

E72.29 **Other disorders of urea cycle metabolism** RCC

E72.3 **Disorders of lysine and hydroxylysine metabolism** RCC
     Glutaric aciduria NOS
     Glutaric aciduria (type I)
     Hydroxylysinemia
     Hyperlysinemia
- **Excludes1**   glutaric aciduria type II (E71.313)
     Refsum's disease (G60.1)
     Zellweger syndrome (E71.510)

E72.4 **Disorders of ornithine metabolism**
     Hyperammonemia-Hyperornithinemia-Homocitrullinemia syndrome
     Ornithinemia (types I, II)
     Ornithine transcarbamylase deficiency
- **Excludes1**   hereditary choroidal dystrophy (H31.2-)

● **E72.5** **Disorders of glycine metabolism**

E72.50 **Disorder of glycine metabolism, unspecified** RCC

E72.51 **Non-ketotic hyperglycinemia**

E72.52 **Trimethylaminuria**

● **E72.53** **Primary hyperoxaluria** RCC
     Oxalosis
     Oxaluria
- **Excludes1**   secondary hyperoxaluria (E72.54-)

▶ **E72.530** **Primary hyperoxaluria, type 1**

▶ **E72.538** **Other specified primary hyperoxaluria**
     ▶ Primary hyperoxaluria, type 2
     ▶ Primary hyperoxaluria, type 3

▶ **E72.539** **Primary hyperoxaluria, unspecified**

▶ **E72.54** **Secondary hyperoxaluria**
- **Excludes1**   primary hyperoxaluria (E72.53-)

▶ **E72.540** **Dietary hyperoxaluria**

▶ **E72.541** **Enteric hyperoxaluria**

▶ **E72.548** **Other secondary hyperoxaluria**

▶ **E72.549** **Secondary hyperoxaluria, unspecified**

E72.59 **Other disorders of glycine metabolism** RCC
     D-glycericacidemia
     Hyperhydroxyprolinemia
     Hyperprolinemia (types I, II)
     Sarcosinemia

● **E72.8** **Other specified disorders of amino-acid metabolism** RCC

E72.81 **Disorders of gamma aminobutyric acid metabolism** RCC
     4-hydroxybutyric aciduria
     Disorders of GABA metabolism
     GABA metabolic defect
     GABA transaminase deficiency
     GABA-T deficiency
     Gamma-hydroxybutyric aciduria
     SSADHD
     Succinic semialdehyde dehydrogenase deficiency

E72.89 **Other specified disorders of amino-acid metabolism** RCC
     Disorders of beta-amino-acid metabolism
     Disorders of gamma-glutamyl cycle

E72.9 **Disorder of amino-acid metabolism, unspecified** RCC

● **E73** **Lactose intolerance**
     Intolerance for lactose, due to inherited deficiency of lactase activity in intestinal mucosa

E73.0 **Congenital lactase deficiency**

E73.1 **Secondary lactase deficiency**

E73.8 **Other lactose intolerance**

E73.9 **Lactose intolerance, unspecified**

● **E74** **Other disorders of carbohydrate metabolism**
- **Excludes1**   diabetes mellitus (E08-E13)
     hypoglycemia NOS (E16.2)
     increased secretion of glucagon (E16.3)
     mucopolysaccharidosis (E76.0-E76.3)

● **E74.0** **Glycogen storage disease**

E74.00 **Glycogen storage disease, unspecified** RCC

E74.01 **von Gierke's disease** RCC
     Type I glycogen storage disease

E74.02 **Pompe disease** RCC
     Cardiac glycogenosis
     Type II glycogen storage disease

E74.03 **Cori disease** RCC
     Forbes' disease
     Type III glycogen storage disease

E74.04 **McArdle disease** RCC
     Type V glycogen storage disease

E74.05 **Lysosome-associated membrane protein 2 [LAMP2] deficiency**
     Danon disease
     Code also, if applicable, associated manifestations such as:
     dilated cardiomyopathy (I42.0)
     obstructive hypertrophic cardiomyopathy (I42.1)

E74.09 **Other glycogen storage disease** RCC
     Andersen disease
     Glycogen storage disease, types 0, IV, VI-XI
     Hers disease
     Liver phosphorylase deficiency
     Muscle phosphofructokinase deficiency
     Tauri disease

● **E74.1** **Disorders of fructose metabolism**
- **Excludes1**   muscle phosphofructokinase deficiency (E74.09)

E74.10 **Disorder of fructose metabolism, unspecified**

E74.11 **Essential fructosuria**
     Fructokinase deficiency

E74.12 **Hereditary fructose intolerance**
     Fructosemia

E74.19 **Other disorders of fructose metabolism**
     Fructose-1, 6-diphosphatase deficiency

● **E74.2** **Disorders of galactose metabolism**

E74.20 **Disorders of galactose metabolism, unspecified** RCC

CHAPTER 4 (E00-E89)

E74.21　**Galactosemia** 🔵
Genetic disorders resulting from defective simple sugar (galactose) metabolism

E74.29　**Other disorders of galactose metabolism** 🔵
Galactokinase deficiency

● E74.3　**Other disorders of intestinal carbohydrate absorption**
　　Excludes2　lactose intolerance (E73.-)

E74.31　**Sucrase-isomaltase deficiency**
Deficiency in metabolism in intestinal mucosa results in malabsorption of sucrose and starch

E74.39　**Other disorders of intestinal carbohydrate absorption**
Disorder of intestinal carbohydrate absorption NOS
Glucose-galactose malabsorption
Sucrase deficiency

E74.4　**Disorders of pyruvate metabolism and gluconeogenesis** 🔵
Deficiency of phosphoenolpyruvate carboxykinase
Deficiency of pyruvate carboxylase
Deficiency of pyruvate dehydrogenase
　　Excludes1　disorders of pyruvate metabolism and gluconeogenesis with anemia (D55.-)
Leigh's syndrome (G31.82)

● E74.8　**Other specified disorders of carbohydrate metabolism** 🔵

● E74.81　**Disorders of glucose transport, not elsewhere classified**

E74.810　**Glucose transporter protein type 1 deficiency**
De Vivo syndrome
Glucose transport defect, blood-brain barrier
GLUT1 deficiency
GLUT1 deficiency syndrome 1, infantile onset
GLUT1 deficiency syndrome 2, childhood onset

E74.818　**Other disorders of glucose transport**
(Familial) renal glycosuria

E74.819　**Disorders of glucose transport, unspecified**

E74.82　**Disorders of citrate metabolism**

E74.820　**SLC13A5 Citrate Transporter Disorder**

E74.829　**Other disorders of citrate metabolism**

E74.89　**Other specified disorders of carbohydrate metabolism**
Essential pentosuria
Coding Clinic: 2023, Q3, P3

E74.9　**Disorder of carbohydrate metabolism, unspecified** 🔵

● E75　**Disorders of sphingolipid metabolism and other lipid storage disorders**
　　Excludes1　mucolipidosis, types I-III (E77.0-E77.1)
Refsum's disease (G60.1)

● E75.0　**GM2 gangliosidosis**
Rare metabolic disorder that causes destruction of nerve cells of brain and spinal cord

E75.00　**GM2 gangliosidosis, unspecified**

E75.01　**Sandhoff disease**

E75.02　**Tay-Sachs disease**

E75.09　**Other GM2 gangliosidosis**
Adult GM2 gangliosidosis
Juvenile GM2 gangliosidosis

● E75.1　**Other and unspecified gangliosidosis**

E75.10　**Unspecified gangliosidosis**
Gangliosidosis NOS

E75.11　**Mucolipidosis IV**
Disorder with symptoms of psychomotor retardation and severe visual impairment

E75.19　**Other gangliosidosis**
GM1 gangliosidosis
GM3 gangliosidosis

● E75.2　**Other sphingolipidosis**
Lysosomal (a particle in a cytoplasm cell that contains digestive enzymes) storage diseases with symptoms of abnormal storage of amino acids
　　Excludes1　adrenoleukodystrophy [Addison-Schilder] (E71.528)

E75.21　**Fabry (-Anderson) disease** 🔵

E75.22　**Gaucher disease** 🔵

E75.23　**Krabbe disease**

● E75.24　**Niemann-Pick disease**
Acid sphingomyelinase deficiency (ASMD)

E75.240　**Niemann-Pick disease type A** 🔵
Acid sphingomyelinase deficiency type A (ASMD type A)
Infantile neurovisceral acid sphingomyelinase deficiency

E75.241　**Niemann-Pick disease type B** 🔵
Acid sphingomyelinase deficiency type B (ASMD type B)
Chronic visceral acid sphingomyelinase deficiency

E75.242　**Niemann-Pick disease type C** 🔵

E75.243　**Niemann-Pick disease type D** 🔵

E75.244　**Niemann-Pick disease type A/B**
Acid sphingomyelinase deficiency type A/B (ASMD type A/B)
Chronic neurovisceral acid sphingomyelinase deficiency

E75.248　**Other Niemann-Pick disease** 🔵

E75.249　**Niemann-Pick disease, unspecified** 🔵
Acid sphingomyelinase deficiency (ASMD) NOS

E75.25　**Metachromatic leukodystrophy**

E75.26　**Sulfatase deficiency**
Multiple sulfatase deficiency (MSD)

E75.27　**Pelizaeus-Merzbacher disease**

E75.28　**Canavan disease**

E75.29　**Other sphingolipidosis**
Farber's syndrome
Sulfatide lipidosis

E75.3　**Sphingolipidosis, unspecified** 🔵

E75.4　**Neuronal ceroid lipofuscinosis**
Batten disease
Bielschowsky-Jansky disease
Kufs disease
Spielmeyer-Vogt disease

E75.5　**Other lipid storage disorders**
Cerebrotendinous cholesterosis [van Bogaert-Scherer-Epstein]
Wolman's disease

E75.6　**Lipid storage disorder, unspecified**

● E76　**Disorders of glycosaminoglycan metabolism**

● E76.0　**Mucopolysaccharidosis, type I**
Inborn metabolic disorder of enzymes that break down carbohydrates

E76.01　**Hurler's syndrome** 🔵

E76.02　**Hurler-Scheie syndrome** 🔵

E76.03　**Scheie's syndrome** 🔵

E76.1　**Mucopolysaccharidosis, type II** 🔵
Inborn metabolic disorder of enzymes that break down carbohydrates occurs in 2-4 year old males
Hunter's syndrome

● **E76.2**   **Other mucopolysaccharidoses**
  ● **E76.21**   Morquio mucopolysaccharidoses
     E76.210   **Morquio A mucopolysaccharidoses** Ⓡⓒ
       Classic Morquio syndrome
       Morquio syndrome A
       Mucopolysaccharidosis, type IVA
     E76.211   **Morquio B mucopolysaccharidoses** Ⓡⓒ
       Morquio-like
         mucopolysaccharidoses
       Morquio-like syndrome
       Morquio syndrome B
       Mucopolysaccharidosis, type IVB
     E76.219   **Morquio mucopolysaccharidoses, unspecified** Ⓡⓒ
       Morquio syndrome
       Mucopolysaccharidosis, type IV
  ● **E76.22**   **Sanfilippo mucopolysaccharidoses** Ⓡⓒ
     Mucopolysaccharidosis, type III (A) (B) (C) (D)
     Sanfilippo A syndrome
     Sanfilippo B syndrome
     Sanfilippo C syndrome
     Sanfilippo D syndrome
     E76.29   **Other mucopolysaccharidoses** Ⓡⓒ
       beta-Glucuronidase deficiency
       Maroteaux-Lamy (mild) (severe) syndrome
       Mucopolysaccharidosis, types VI, VII
  E76.3   Mucopolysaccharidosis, **unspecified** Ⓡⓒ
  E76.8   Other disorders of glucosaminoglycan metabolism Ⓡⓒ
  E76.9   Glucosaminoglycan metabolism disorder, **unspecified** Ⓡⓒ

● **E77**   **Disorders of glycoprotein metabolism**
  E77.0   **Defects in post-translational modification of lysosomal enzymes** Ⓡⓒ
     Mucolipidosis II [I-cell disease]
     Mucolipidosis III [pseudo-Hurler polydystrophy]
  E77.1   **Defects in glycoprotein degradation** Ⓡⓒ
     Aspartylglucosaminuria
     Fucosidosis
     Mannosidosis
     Sialidosis [mucolipidosis I]
  E77.8   Other disorders of glycoprotein metabolism Ⓡⓒ
  E77.9   Disorder of glycoprotein metabolism, **unspecified** Ⓡⓒ

● **E78**   **Disorders of lipoprotein metabolism and other lipidemias**
   Excludes1   sphingolipidosis (E75.0-E75.3)
 ● **E78.0**   **Pure hypercholesterolemia**
     Coding Clinic: 2016, Q4, P13
     E78.00   **Pure hypercholesterolemia, unspecified**
       Fredrickson's hyperlipoproteinemia, type IIa
       Hyperbetalipoproteinemia
       Low-density-lipoprotein-type [LDL]
         hyperlipoproteinemia
       (Pure) hypercholesterolemia NOS
       Coding Clinic: 2023, Q2, P9; 2022, Q2, P6; 2016, Q4, P13
   ● **E78.01**   **Familial hypercholesterolemia**
       Coding Clinic: 2016, Q4, P13
     ▶ **E78.010**   **Homozygous familial hypercholesterolemia [HoFH]**
     ▶ **E78.011**   **Heterozygous familial hypercholesterolemia [HeFH]**
     ▶ **E78.019**   **Familial hypercholesterolemia, unspecified**
       ▶ Familial hypercholesterolemia NOS
  E78.1   **Pure hyperglyceridemia**
     Elevated fasting triglycerides
     Endogenous hyperglyceridemia
     Fredrickson's hyperlipoproteinemia, type IV
     Hyperlipidemia, group B
     Hyperprebetalipoproteinemia
     Very-low-density-lipoprotein-type [VLDL]
       hyperlipoproteinemia

  E78.2   **Mixed hyperlipidemia**
     Broad- or floating-betalipoproteinemia
     Combined hyperlipidemia NOS
     Elevated cholesterol with elevated triglycerides NEC
     Fredrickson's hyperlipoproteinemia, type IIb or III
     Hyperbetalipoproteinemia with prebetalipoproteinemia
     Hypercholesteremia with endogenous hyperglyceridemia
     Hyperlipidemia, group C
     Tubo-eruptive xanthoma
     Xanthoma tuberosum
     Excludes1   cerebrotendinous cholesterosis [van
         Bogaert-Scherer-Epstein] (E75.5)
         familial combined hyperlipidemia (E78.49)
     Coding Clinic: 2023, Q2, P9-10; 2022, Q2, P6-7
  E78.3   **Hyperchylomicronemia**
     Chylomicron retention disease
     Fredrickson's hyperlipoproteinemia, type I or V
     Hyperlipidemia, group D
     Mixed hyperglyceridemia
 ● **E78.4**   **Other hyperlipidemia**
     E78.41   **Elevated Lipoprotein(a)**
       Elevated Lp(a)
     E78.49   **Other hyperlipidemia**
       Familial combined hyperlipidemia
  E78.5   **Hyperlipidemia, unspecified**
     Coding Clinic: 2022, Q2, P6
  E78.6   **Lipoprotein deficiency**
     Abetalipoproteinemia
     Depressed HDL cholesterol
     High-density lipoprotein deficiency
     Hypoalphalipoproteinemia
     Hypobetalipoproteinemia (familial)
     Lecithin cholesterol acyltransferase deficiency
     Tangier disease
 ● **E78.7**   **Disorders of bile acid and cholesterol metabolism**
     Excludes1   Niemann-Pick disease type C (E75.242)
     E78.70   **Disorder of bile acid and cholesterol metabolism, unspecified**
     E78.71   **Barth syndrome**
     E78.72   **Smith-Lemli-Opitz syndrome**
     E78.79   **Other disorders of bile acid and cholesterol metabolism**
       Coding Clinic: 2023, Q1, P27
 ● **E78.8**   **Other disorders of lipoprotein metabolism**
     E78.81   **Lipoid dermatoarthritis**
     E78.89   **Other lipoprotein metabolism disorders**
  E78.9   **Disorder of lipoprotein metabolism, unspecified**

● **E79**   **Disorders of purine and pyrimidine metabolism**
   Purines, along with pyrimidines, signal RNA and DNA production
   Excludes1   Ataxia-telangiectasia (Q87.19)
       Bloom's syndrome (Q82.8)
       Cockayne's syndrome (Q87.19)
       calculus of kidney (N20.0)
       combined immunodeficiency disorders (D81.-)
       Fanconi's anemia (D61.09)
       gout (M1A.-, M10.-)
       orotaciduric anemia (D53.0)
       progeria (E34.8)
       Werner's syndrome (E34.8)
       xeroderma pigmentosum (Q82.1)
  E79.0   **Hyperuricemia without signs of inflammatory arthritis and tophaceous disease**
     Asymptomatic hyperuricemia
  E79.1   **Lesch-Nyhan syndrome** Ⓡⓒ
     HGPRT deficiency
  E79.2   **Myoadenylate deaminase deficiency** Ⓡⓒ
 ● **E79.8**   **Other disorders of purine and pyrimidine metabolism** Ⓡⓒ
     E79.81   **Aicardi-Goutières syndrome**
     E79.82   **Hereditary xanthinuria**
     E79.89   **Other specified disorders of purine and pyrimidine metabolism**
  E79.9   **Disorder of purine and pyrimidine metabolism, unspecified** Ⓡⓒ

● **E80 Disorders of porphyrin and bilirubin metabolism**
Group of chemical compounds in RBCs that combine with iron to form heme

> **Includes**   defects of catalase and peroxidase

E80.0 Hereditary erythropoietic porphyria 🔴
     Congenital erythropoietic porphyria
     Erythropoietic protoporphyria

E80.1 Porphyria cutanea tarda 🔴

● **E80.2 Other and unspecified porphyria**
     E80.20 Unspecified porphyria 🔴
         Porphyria NOS
     E80.21 Acute intermittent (hepatic) porphyria 🔴
     E80.29 Other porphyria 🔴
         Hereditary coproporphyria

E80.3 Defects of catalase and peroxidase 🔴
     Acatalasia [Takahara]

E80.4 Gilbert syndrome

E80.5 Crigler-Najjar syndrome

E80.6 Other disorders of bilirubin metabolism
     Dubin-Johnson syndrome
     Rotor's syndrome
     Coding Clinic: 2022, Q3, P7

E80.7 Disorder of bilirubin metabolism, unspecified

● **E83 Disorders of mineral metabolism**

> **Excludes1**   dietary mineral deficiency (E58-E61)
>   parathyroid disorders (E20-E21)
>   vitamin D deficiency (E55.-)

● **E83.0 Disorders of copper metabolism**
     E83.00 Disorder of copper metabolism, unspecified
     E83.01 Wilson's disease

> **Code also** associated Kayser Fleischer ring (H18.04-)

     E83.09 Other disorders of copper metabolism
         Menkes' (kinky hair) (steely hair) disease

● **E83.1 Disorders of iron metabolism**

> **Excludes1**   iron deficiency anemia (D50.-)
>   sideroblastic anemia (D64.0-D64.3)

     E83.10 Disorder of iron metabolism, unspecified
●   **E83.11 Hemochromatosis**

> **Excludes1**   GALD (P78.84)
>   Gestational alloimmune liver disease (P78.84)
>   Neonatal hemochromatosis (P78.84)

         E83.110 Hereditary hemochromatosis 🔴
             Bronzed diabetes
             Pigmentary cirrhosis (of liver)
             Primary (hereditary) hemochromatosis
         E83.111 Hemochromatosis due to repeated red blood cell transfusions
             Iron overload due to repeated red blood cell transfusions
             Transfusion (red blood cell) associated hemochromatosis
         E83.118 Other hemochromatosis
         E83.119 Hemochromatosis, unspecified
     E83.19 Other disorders of iron metabolism

> **Use additional** code, if applicable, for idiopathic pulmonary hemosiderosis (J84.03)

E83.2 Disorders of zinc metabolism
     Acrodermatitis enteropathica

● **E83.3 Disorders of phosphorus metabolism and phosphatases**

> **Excludes1**   adult osteomalacia (M83.-)
>   osteoporosis (M80.-)

> ▶ **Excludes2**   disorders of pyrophosphate metabolism (E83.82-)

     E83.30 Disorder of phosphorus metabolism, unspecified
     E83.31 Familial hypophosphatemia
         Vitamin D-resistant osteomalacia
         Vitamin D-resistant rickets

> **Excludes1**   vitamin D-deficiency rickets (E55.0)

     E83.32 Hereditary vitamin D-dependent rickets (type 1) (type 2)
         25-hydroxyvitamin D 1-alpha-hydroxylase deficiency
         Pseudovitamin D deficiency
         Vitamin D receptor defect
     E83.39 Other disorders of phosphorus metabolism
         Acid phosphatase deficiency
         Hypophosphatasia

● **E83.4 Disorders of magnesium metabolism**
     E83.40 Disorders of magnesium metabolism, unspecified
     E83.41 Hypermagnesemia
         Coding Clinic: 2016, Q4, P55
     E83.42 Hypomagnesemia
     E83.49 Other disorders of magnesium metabolism

● **E83.5 Disorders of calcium metabolism**
     autoimmune hypoparathyroidism (E20.812)
     autosomal dominant hypocalcemia (E20.810)

> **Excludes1**   chondrocalcinosis (M11.1-M11.2)
>   hungry bone syndrome (E83.81)
>   hyperparathyroidism (E21.0-E21.3)
>   secondary hypoparathyroidism in diseases classified elsewhere (E20.811)

     E83.50 Unspecified disorder of calcium metabolism
     E83.51 Hypocalcemia
     E83.52 Hypercalcemia
         Familial hypocalciuric hypercalcemia
     E83.59 Other disorders of calcium metabolism
         Idiopathic hypercalciuria

● **E83.8 Other disorders of mineral metabolism**
     E83.81 Hungry bone syndrome
▶ ●   **E83.82 Disorders of pyrophosphate metabolism**
     ▶ **E83.820 Generalized arterial calcification of infancy with unspecified genetic causality**

> ▶ **Code also**, if applicable, associated conditions such as:
> ▶ heart failure (I50.-)
> ▶ other secondary hypertension (I15.8)

     ▶ **E83.821 ENPP1 deficiency causing generalized arterial calcification of infancy**

> ▶ **Code also**, if applicable, associated conditions such as:
> ▶ heart failure (I50.-)
> ▶ other secondary hypertension (I15.8)

     ▶ **E83.822 ENPP1 deficiency causing autosomal recessive hypophosphatemic rickets type 2**

> ▶ New   ◀ Revised   ~~deleted~~ Deleted   Excludes 1   Excludes 2   Includes   Use additional   Code first   Code also   Key words
> OGCR Official Guidelines   X Assign placeholder X   ● Use Additional Character(s)   ▶ Manifestation Code   🔴 Hierarchical Condition Category   **Coding Clinic**

▶ **E83.823** **ABCC6 deficiency causing generalized arterial calcification of infancy**
▶ Code also, if applicable, associated conditions such as:
▶ heart failure (I50.-)
▶ other secondary hypertension (I15.8)

▶ **E83.824** **ABCC6 deficiency causing pseudoxanthoma elasticum**

▶ **E83.825** **CD73 deficiency causing arterial calcification**

E83.89 **Other disorders of mineral metabolism**

E83.9 **Disorder of mineral metabolism, unspecified**

● **E84** **Cystic fibrosis**

Includes mucoviscidosis

Code also exocrine pancreatic insufficiency (K86.81)

E84.0 **Cystic fibrosis with pulmonary manifestations**
Use additional code to identify any infectious organism present, such as:
Pseudomonas (B96.5)
Coding Clinic: 2021, Q1, P24

● **E84.1** **Cystic fibrosis with intestinal manifestations**

E84.11 **Meconium ileus in cystic fibrosis**   **N**
Excludes1 meconium ileus not due to cystic fibrosis (P76.0)

E84.19 **Cystic fibrosis with other intestinal manifestations**
Distal intestinal obstruction syndrome

E84.8 **Cystic fibrosis with other manifestations**

E84.9 **Cystic fibrosis, unspecified**

● **E85** **Amyloidosis**
A disorder resulting from the abnormal deposition of a particular protein (amyloid) into tissues of the body
Excludes2 Alzheimer's disease (G30.0-)

E85.0 **Non-neuropathic heredofamilial amyloidosis**
Hereditary amyloid nephropathy
Code also associated disorders, such as:
autoinflammatory syndromes (M04.-)
Excludes2 Transthyretin-related (ATTR) familial amyloid cardiomyopathy (E85.4)

E85.1 **Neuropathic heredofamilial amyloidosis**
Amyloid polyneuropathy (Portuguese)
Transthyretin-related (ATTR) familial amyloid polyneuropathy
Coding Clinic: 2012, Q4, P100

E85.2 **Heredofamilial amyloidosis, unspecified**

E85.3 **Secondary systemic amyloidosis**
Hemodialysis-associated amyloidosis

E85.4 **Organ-limited amyloidosis**
Localized amyloidosis
Transthyretin-related (ATTR) familial amyloid cardiomyopathy

● **E85.8** **Other amyloidosis**

E85.81 **Light chain (AL) amyloidosis**
Coding Clinic: 2024, Q2, P9

E85.82 **Wild-type transthyretin-related (ATTR) amyloidosis**
Senile systemic amyloidosis (SSA)

E85.89 **Other amyloidosis**

E85.9 **Amyloidosis, unspecified**

● **E86** **Volume depletion**
Excludes1 dehydration of newborn (P74.1)
postprocedural hypovolemic shock (T81.19)
traumatic hypovolemic shock (T79.4)
Excludes2 hypovolemic shock NOS (R57.1)
Use additional code(s) for any associated disorders of electrolyte and acid-base balance (E87.-)
Coding Clinic: 2019, Q2, P7

E86.0 **Dehydration**
Excessive loss of body water
Coding Clinic: 2019, Q2, P7-8

E86.1 **Hypovolemia**
Diminished volume of circulating blood
Depletion of volume of plasma

E86.9 **Volume depletion, unspecified**
Coding Clinic: 2019, Q2, P7-8

● **E87** **Other disorders of fluid, electrolyte and acid-base balance**
Excludes1 diabetes insipidus (E23.2)
electrolyte imbalance associated with hyperemesis gravidarum (O21.1)
electrolyte imbalance following ectopic or molar pregnancy (O08.5)
familial periodic paralysis (G72.3)
metabolic acidemia in newborn, unspecified (P19.9)

E87.0 **Hyperosmolality and hypernatremia**
Sodium [Na] excess
Sodium [Na] overload
Excludes2 diabetes with hyperosmolarity (E08, E09, E11, E13 with final characters .00 or .01)
Coding Clinic: 2022, Q1, P29; 2018, Q2, P6

E87.1 **Hypo-osmolality and hyponatremia**
Sodium [Na] deficiency
Excludes1 syndrome of inappropriate secretion of antidiuretic hormone (E22.2)
Coding Clinic: 2018, Q2, P6

● **E87.2** **Acidosis**
Excludes1 diabetic acidosis - see categories E08-E10, E11, E13 with ketoacidosis

E87.20 **Acidosis, unspecified**
Lactic acidosis NOS
Metabolic acidosis NOS
Code also, if applicable, respiratory failure with hypercapnia (J96. with 5th character 2)

E87.21 **Acute metabolic acidosis**
Acute lactic acidosis
Coding Clinic: 2024, Q4, P17

E87.22 **Chronic metabolic acidosis**
Chronic lactic acidosis
Code first underlying etiology, if applicable
Coding Clinic: 2022, Q4, P14

E87.29 **Other acidosis**
Respiratory acidosis NOS
Excludes2 acute respiratory acidosis (J96.02)
chronic respiratory acidosis (J96.12)

E87.3 **Alkalosis**
Alkalosis NOS
Metabolic alkalosis
Respiratory alkalosis

E87.4 **Mixed disorder of acid-base balance**

E87.5 **Hyperkalemia**
Potassium [K] excess
Potassium [K] overload

E87.6 **Hypokalemia**
Potassium [K] deficiency

Item 4–9 Circulating fluid volume is regulated by the amount of water and sodium ingested, excreted by the kidneys into the urine, and lost through the gastrointestinal tract, lungs, and skin. To maintain blood volume within a normal range, the kidneys regulate the amount of water and sodium lost into the urine. Too much (**fluid overload**) or too little fluid volume (**volume depletion**) will affect blood pressure. Severe cases of vomiting, diarrhea, bleeding, and burns (fluid loss through exposed burn surface area) can contribute to fluid loss. Internal body environment must maintain a precise balance (homeostasis) between too much fluid and too little fluid. This complex balancing mechanism is critical to good health.

● **E87.7**   **Fluid overload**

> **Excludes1**   edema NOS (R60.9)
> fluid retention (R60.9)

   E87.70   **Fluid overload, unspecified**
> **Coding Clinic: 2023, Q1, P19**

   E87.71   **Transfusion associated circulatory overload**
> Fluid overload due to transfusion (blood) (blood components) TACO

   E87.79   **Other fluid overload**

E87.8   **Other disorders of electrolyte and fluid balance, not elsewhere classified**
> Electrolyte imbalance NOS
> Hyperchloremia
> Hypochloremia

● **E88**   **Other and unspecified metabolic disorders**

> Use additional codes for associated conditions

> **Excludes1**   histiocytosis X (chronic) (C96.6)

● **E88.0**   **Disorders of plasma-protein metabolism, not elsewhere classified**

> **Excludes1**   monoclonal gammopathy (of undetermined significance) (D47.2)
> polyclonal hypergammaglobulinemia (D89.0)
> Waldenström macroglobulinemia (C88.00)

> **Excludes2**   disorder of lipoprotein metabolism (E78.-)

   E88.01   **Alpha-1-antitrypsin deficiency AAT deficiency** 🆁🅲

   E88.02   **Plasminogen deficiency**
> Dysplasminogenemia
> Hypoplasminogenemia
> Type 1 plasminogen deficiency
> Type 2 plasminogen deficiency

> → Code also, if applicable, ligneous conjunctivitis (H10.51-)

> Use additional code for associated findings, such as:
> hydrocephalus (G91.4)
> otitis media (H67.-)
> respiratory disorder related to plasminogen deficiency (J99)

   E88.09   **Other disorders of plasma-protein metabolism, not elsewhere classified**
> Bisalbuminemia

● **E88.1**   **Lipodystrophy, not elsewhere classified**
> *Defective fat metabolism resulting in absence of subcutaneous fat*
> ~~Lipodystrophy NOS~~

> **Excludes1**   Whipple's disease (K90.81)

 ▶ **E88.10**   **Lipodystrophy, unspecified**
> ▶ Lipodystrophy NOS

 ▶ **E88.11**   **Partial lipodystrophy**
> ▶ Acquired partial lipodystrophy (APL)
> ▶ Barraquer-Simons lipodystrophy
> ▶ Familial partial lipodystrophy (FPLD)

 ▶ **E88.12**   **Generalized lipodystrophy**
> ▶ Acquired generalized lipodystrophy (AGL)
> ▶ Berardinelli-Siep syndrome
> ▶ Congenital generalized lipodystrophy (CGL)
> ▶ Lawrence syndrome

 ▶ **E88.13**   **Localized lipodystrophy**
> ▶ Injection lipodystrophy
> ▶ Insulin lipodystrophy

 ▶ **E88.14**   **HIV-associated lipodystrophy**
> ▶ Code first any human immunodeficiency virus [HIV] disease (B20)

> ▶ Use Additional code for adverse effect, if applicable, to identify drug (T37.5X5-)

 ▶ **E88.19**   **Other lipodystrophy, not elsewhere classified**

E88.2   **Lipomatosis, not elsewhere classified**
> *Abnormal tumorlike accumulations of fat in tissue*
> Lipomatosis NOS
> Lipomatosis (Check) dolorosa [Dercum]
> **Coding Clinic: 2025, Q1, P26**

E88.3   **Tumor lysis syndrome**
> Tumor lysis syndrome (spontaneous)
> Tumor lysis syndrome following antineoplastic drug chemotherapy

> Use additional code for adverse effect, if applicable, to identify drug (T45.1X5)
> **Coding Clinic: 2019, Q2, P25**

● **E88.4**   **Mitochondrial metabolism disorders**
> *Congenital disorder of metabolism*

> **Excludes1**   disorders of pyruvate metabolism (E74.4)
> Kearns-Sayre syndrome (H49.81)
> Leber's disease (H47.22)
> Leigh's encephalopathy (G31.82)
> Mitochondrial myopathy, NEC (G71.3)
> Reye's syndrome (G93.7)

   E88.40   **Mitochondrial metabolism disorder, unspecified** 🆁🅲

   E88.41   **MELAS syndrome** 🆁🅲
> Mitochondrial myopathy, encephalopathy, lactic acidosis and stroke-like episodes

   E88.42   **MERRF syndrome** 🆁🅲
> Myoclonic epilepsy associated with ragged-red fibers

> Code also progressive myoclonic epilepsy (G40.3-)

   E88.43   **Disorders of mitochondrial tRNA synthetases**
> ▶ ARS2-related mitochondrial disorders
> ▶ LBSL
> ▶ Leukoencephalopathy with brainstem - spinal cord involvement - lactate elevation
> ▶ Leukoencephalopathy with thalamus - brainstem involvement - high lactate
> ▶ LTBL
> ▶ Mitochondrial aminoacyl-tRNA synthetase disorders

> Code also, if applicable, associated condition such as:
> ▶ leukoencephalopathy (G93.49)

   E88.49   **Other mitochondrial metabolism disorders** 🆁🅲

● **E88.8**   **Other specified metabolic disorders**

● **E88.81**   **Metabolic syndrome and other insulin resistance**

> Use additional codes for associated manifestations, such as:
> obesity (E66.-)
> **Coding Clinic: 2022, Q3, P6-7**

   E88.810   **Metabolic syndrome**
> Dysmetabolic syndrome

   E88.811   **Insulin resistance syndrome, Type A**
> **Coding Clinic: 2023, Q4, P14**

   E88.818   **Other insulin resistance**
> Insulin resistance syndrome, Type B

   E88.819   **Insulin resistance, unspecified**

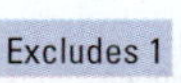

▶ New   ⇒ Revised   ~~deleted~~ Deleted   Excludes 1   Excludes 2   Includes   Use additional   Code first   Code also   Key words

OGCR Official Guidelines   **X** Assign placeholder X   ● Use Additional Character(s)   ▶ Manifestation Code   🆁🅲 Hierarchical Condition Category   **Coding Clinic**

E88.82   **Obesity due to disruption of MC4R pathway**
    Use additional code, if applicable, to identify associated manifestations, such as polyphagia (R63.2)
    Use additional code to identify body mass index (BMI), if known (Z68.-)
    Coding Clinic: 2024, Q4, P11

E88.89   **Other specified metabolic disorders**
    Launois-Bensaude adenolipomatosis
    Excludes1   adult pulmonary Langerhans cell histiocytosis (J84.82)

E88.9   **Metabolic disorder, unspecified**

E88.A   **Wasting disease (syndrome) due to underlying condition**
    Cachexia due to underlying condition
    Code first underlying condition
    Excludes1   cachexia NOS (R64)
              nutritional marasmus (E41)
    Excludes2   failure to thrive (R62.51, R62.7)
    Coding Clinic: 2023, Q4, P15

POSTPROCEDURAL ENDOCRINE AND METABOLIC COMPLICATIONS AND DISORDERS, NOT ELSEWHERE CLASSIFIED (E89)

● **E89   Postprocedural endocrine and metabolic complications and disorders, not elsewhere classified**
    Excludes2   intraoperative complications of endocrine system organ or structure (E36.0-, E36.1-, E36.8)

E89.0   **Postprocedural hypothyroidism**
    Postirradiation hypothyroidism
    Postsurgical hypothyroidism

E89.1   **Postprocedural hypoinsulinemia**
    Postpancreatectomy hyperglycemia
    Postsurgical hypoinsulinemia
    Code first, if applicable, diabetes mellitus (postpancreatectomy) (postprocedural) (E13.-)
    Use additional code, if applicable, to identify:
      acquired absence of pancreas (Z90.41-)
      insulin use (Z79.4)
    Excludes1   transient postprocedural hyperglycemia (R73.9)
              transient postprocedural hypoglycemia (E16.2)

E89.2   **Postprocedural hypoparathyroidism**
    Parathyroprival tetany
    Coding Clinic: 2023, Q3, P13

E89.3   **Postprocedural hypopituitarism**
    Postirradiation hypopituitarism

● E89.4   **Postprocedural ovarian failure**
    E89.40   **Asymptomatic postprocedural ovarian failure**
        Postprocedural ovarian failure NOS
    E89.41   **Symptomatic postprocedural ovarian failure**
        Symptoms such as flushing, sleeplessness, headache, lack of concentration, associated with postprocedural menopause

E89.5   **Postprocedural testicular hypofunction**

E89.6   **Postprocedural adrenocortical (-medullary) hypofunction**

● E89.8   **Other postprocedural endocrine and metabolic complications and disorders**
    Coding Clinic: 2016, Q4, P9
    ● E89.81   **Postprocedural hemorrhage of an endocrine system organ or structure following a procedure**
        E89.810   **Postprocedural hemorrhage of an endocrine system organ or structure following an endocrine system procedure**
        E89.811   **Postprocedural hemorrhage of an endocrine system organ or structure following other procedure**
    ● E89.82   **Postprocedural hematoma and seroma of an endocrine system organ or structure**
        E89.820   **Postprocedural hematoma of an endocrine system organ or structure following an endocrine system procedure**
        E89.821   **Postprocedural hematoma of an endocrine system organ or structure following other procedure**
        E89.822   **Postprocedural seroma of an endocrine system organ or structure following an endocrine system procedure**
        E89.823   **Postprocedural seroma of an endocrine system organ or structure following other procedure**

E89.89   **Other postprocedural endocrine and metabolic complications and disorders**
    Use additional code, if applicable, to further specify disorder

CHAPTER 4 (E00–E89)

CHAPTER 5

MENTAL, BEHAVIORAL AND NEURODEVELOPMENTAL DISORDERS (F01-F99)

OGCR Chapter-Specific Coding Guidelines

5. Chapter 5: Mental, Behavioral and Neurodevelopmental disorders (F01 – F99)

a. Pain disorders related to psychological factors

Assign code F45.41, for pain that is exclusively related to psychological disorders. As indicated by the Excludes 1 note under category G89, a code from category G89 should not be assigned with code F45.41

Code F45.42, Pain disorders with related psychological factors, should be used with a code from category G89, Pain, not elsewhere classified, if there is documentation of a psychological component for a patient with acute or chronic pain.

See Section I.C.6. Pain

b. Mental and behavioral disorders due to psychoactive substance use

1) In Remission

Selection of codes for "in remission" for categories F10-F19, Mental and behavioral disorders due to psychoactive substance use (categories F10-F19 with -11, -.21) requires the provider's clinical judgment. The appropriate codes for "in remission" are assigned only on the basis of provider documentation (as defined in the Official Guidelines for Coding and Reporting), unless otherwise instructed by the classification.

Mild substance use disorders in early or sustained remission are classified to the appropriate codes for substance abuse in remission, and moderate or severe substance use disorders in early or sustained remission are classified to the appropriate codes for substance dependence in remission.

2) Psychoactive Substance Use, Abuse and Dependence

When the provider documentation refers to use, abuse and dependence of the same substance (e.g., alcohol, opioid, cannabis, etc.), only one code should be assigned to identify the pattern of use based on the following hierarchy:

- If both use and abuse are documented, assign only the code for abuse
- If both abuse and dependence are documented, assign only the code for dependence
- If use, abuse and dependence are all documented, assign only the code for dependence
- If both use and dependence are documented, assign only the code for dependence

3) Psychoactive Substance Use, Unspecified

As with all other unspecified diagnoses, the codes for unspecified psychoactive substance use disorders (F10.9-, F11.9-, F12.9-, F13.9-, F14.9-, F15.9-, F16.9-, F19.9-, F19.9-) should only be assigned based on provider documentation and when they meet the definition of a reportable diagnosis (see Section III, Reporting Additional Diagnoses). These codes are to be used only when the psychoactive substance use is associated with a physical, mental or behavioral disorder, and such a relationship is documented by the provider.

c. Factitious Disorder

Factitious disorder imposed on self or Munchausen's syndrome is a disorder in which a person falsely reports or causes his or her own physical or psychological signs or symptoms. For patients with documented factitious disorder on self or Munchausen's syndrome, assign the appropriate code from subcategory F68.1-, Factitious disorder imposed on self.

Munchausen's syndrome by proxy (MSBP) is a disorder in which a caregiver (perpetrator) falsely reports or causes an illness or injury in another person (victim) under his or her care, such as a child, an elderly adult, or a person who has a disability. The condition is also referred to as "factitious disorder imposed on another" or "factitious disorder by proxy." The perpetrator, not the victim, receives this diagnosis. Assign code F68.A, Factitious disorder imposed on another, to the perpetrator's record. For the victim of a patient suffering from MSBP, assign the appropriate code from categories T74, Adult and child abuse, neglect and other maltreatment, confirmed, or T76, Adult and child abuse, neglect and other maltreatment, suspected.

See Section I.C.19.f. Adult and child abuse, neglect and other maltreatment

---

CHAPTER 5

MENTAL, BEHAVIORAL AND NEURODEVELOPMENTAL DISORDERS (F01-F99)

Includes disorders of psychological development

Excludes2 symptoms, signs and abnormal clinical laboratory findings, not elsewhere classified (R00-R99)

This chapter contains the following blocks:

F01-F09	Mental disorders due to known physiological conditions
F10-F19	Mental and behavioral disorders due to psychoactive substance use
F20-F29	Schizophrenia, schizotypal, delusional, and other non-mood psychotic disorders
F30-F39	Mood [affective] disorders
F40-F48	Anxiety, dissociative, stress-related, somatoform and other nonpsychotic mental disorders
F50-F59	Behavioral syndromes associated with physiological disturbances and physical factors
F60-F69	Disorders of adult personality and behavior
F70-F79	Intellectual disabilities
F80-F89	Pervasive and specific developmental disorders
F90-F98	Behavioral and emotional disorders with onset usually occurring in childhood and adolescence
F99	Unspecified mental disorder

MENTAL DISORDERS DUE TO KNOWN PHYSIOLOGICAL CONDITIONS (F01-F09)

This block comprises a range of mental disorders grouped together on the basis of their having in common a demonstrable etiology in cerebral disease, brain injury, or other insult leading to cerebral dysfunction. The dysfunction may be primary, as in diseases, injuries, and insults that affect the brain directly and selectively; or secondary, as in systemic diseases and disorders that attack the brain only as one of the multiple organs or systems of the body that are involved.

● **F01 Vascular dementia**

Vascular dementia as a result of infarction of the brain due to vascular disease, including hypertensive cerebrovascular disease.

Includes arteriosclerotic dementia

major neurocognitive disorder due to vascular disease
multi-infarct dementia

Code first, if applicable, any causal condition

● **F01.5 Vascular dementia, unspecified severity**

F01.50 Vascular dementia, unspecified severity, without behavioral disturbance, psychotic disturbance, mood disturbance, and anxiety   A

Major neurocognitive disorder due to vascular disease NOS

Vascular dementia NOS

Coding Clinic: 2021, Q2, P4

● **F01.51 Vascular dementia, unspecified severity, with behavioral disturbance**   A

▶ New   ➡ Revised   ~~deleted~~ Deleted   Excludes 1   Excludes 2   Includes   Use additional   Code first   Code also   Key words

OGCR Official Guidelines   **X** Assign placeholder X   ● Use Additional Character(s)   ▶ Manifestation Code   Hierarchical Condition Category   **Coding Clinic**

F01.511　Vascular dementia, unspecified severity, with agitation　A
　Major neurocognitive disorder due to vascular disease, unspecified severity, with aberrant motor behavior such as restlessness, rocking, pacing, or exit-seeking
　Major neurocognitive disorder due to vascular disease, unspecified severity, with verbal or physical behaviors such as profanity, shouting, threatening, anger, aggression, combativeness, or violence
　Vascular dementia, unspecified severity, with aberrant motor behavior such as restlessness, rocking, pacing, or exit-seeking
　Vascular dementia, unspecified severity, with verbal or physical behaviors such as profanity, shouting, threatening, anger, aggression, combativeness, or violence

F01.518　Vascular dementia, unspecified severity, with other behavioral disturbance　A
　Major neurocognitive disorder due to vascular disease, unspecified severity, with behavioral disturbances such as sleep disturbance, social disinhibition, or sexual disinhibition
　Vascular dementia, unspecified severity, with behavioral disturbances such as sleep disturbance, social disinhibition, or sexual disinhibition

Use Additional code, if applicable, to identify wandering in vascular dementia (Z91.83)

F01.52　Vascular dementia, unspecified severity, with psychotic disturbance　A
　Major neurocognitive disorder due to vascular disease, unspecified severity, with psychotic disturbance such as hallucinations, paranoia, suspiciousness, or delusional state
　Vascular dementia, unspecified severity, with psychotic disturbance such as hallucinations, paranoia, suspiciousness, or delusional state

F01.53　Vascular dementia, unspecified severity, with mood disturbance　A
　Major neurocognitive disorder due to vascular disease, unspecified severity, with mood disturbance such as depression, apathy, or anhedonia
　Vascular dementia, unspecified severity, with mood disturbance such as depression, apathy, or anhedonia

F01.54　Vascular dementia, unspecified severity, with anxiety　A
　Major neurocognitive disorder due to vascular disease, unspecified severity, with anxiety

● **F01.A　Vascular dementia, mild**
　　Excludes1　mild neurocognitive disorder due to known physiological condition with or without behavioral disturbance (F06.7-)

F01.A0　Vascular dementia, mild, without behavioral disturbance, psychotic disturbance, mood disturbance, and anxiety　A
　Major neurocognitive disorder due to vascular disease, mild, NOS
　Vascular dementia, mild, NOS

● **F01.A1　Vascular dementia, mild, with behavioral disturbance**

F01.A11　Vascular dementia, mild, with agitation　A
　Major neurocognitive disorder due to vascular disease, mild, with aberrant motor behavior such as restlessness, rocking, pacing, or exit-seeking
　Major neurocognitive disorder due to vascular disease, mild, with verbal or physical behaviors such as profanity, shouting, threatening, anger, aggression, combativeness, or violence
　Vascular dementia, mild, with aberrant motor behavior such as restlessness, rocking, pacing, or exit-seeking
　Vascular dementia, mild, with verbal or physical behaviors such as profanity, shouting, threatening, anger, aggression, combativeness, or violence

F01.A18　Vascular dementia, mild, with other behavioral disturbance　A
　Major neurocognitive disorder due to vascular disease, mild, with behavioral disturbances such as sleep disturbance, social disinhibition, or sexual disinhibition
　Vascular dementia, mild, with behavioral disturbances such as sleep disturbance, social disinhibition, or sexual disinhibition

Use Additional code, if applicable, to identify wandering in vascular dementia (Z91.83)

F01.A2　Vascular dementia, mild, with psychotic disturbance　A
　Major neurocognitive disorder due to vascular disease, mild, with psychotic disturbance such as hallucinations, paranoia, suspiciousness, or delusional state
　Vascular dementia, mild, with psychotic disturbance such as hallucinations, paranoia, suspiciousness, or delusional state

F01.A3　Vascular dementia, mild, with mood disturbance　A
　Major neurocognitive disorder due to vascular disease, mild, with mood disturbance such as depression, apathy, or anhedonia
　Vascular dementia, mild, with mood disturbance such as depression, apathy, or anhedonia

F01.A4　Vascular dementia, mild, with anxiety　A
　Major neurocognitive disorder due to vascular disease, mild, with anxiety

● **F01.B　Vascular dementia, moderate**

F01.B0　Vascular dementia, moderate, without behavioral disturbance, psychotic disturbance, mood disturbance, and anxiety　A
　Major neurocognitive disorder due to vascular disease, moderate, NOS
　Vascular dementia, moderate, NOS

● **F01.B1   Vascular dementia, moderate, with behavioral disturbance**

    F01.B11   Vascular dementia, moderate, with agitation A

        Major neurocognitive disorder due to vascular disease, moderate, with aberrant motor behavior such as restlessness, rocking, pacing, or exit-seeking

        Major neurocognitive disorder due to vascular disease, moderate, with verbal or physical behaviors such as profanity, shouting, threatening, anger, aggression, combativeness, or violence

        Vascular dementia, moderate, with aberrant motor behavior such as restlessness, rocking, pacing, or exit-seeking

        Vascular dementia, moderate, with verbal or physical behaviors such as profanity, shouting, threatening, anger, aggression, combativeness, or violence

    F01.B18   Vascular dementia, moderate, with other behavioral disturbance A

        Major neurocognitive disorder due to vascular disease, moderate, with behavioral disturbances such as sleep disturbance, social disinhibition, or sexual disinhibition

        Vascular dementia, moderate, with behavioral disturbances such as sleep disturbance, social disinhibition, or sexual disinhibition

        Use Additional code, if applicable, to identify wandering in vascular dementia (Z91.83)

    F01.B2   Vascular dementia, moderate, with psychotic disturbance A

        Major neurocognitive disorder due to vascular disease, moderate, with psychotic disturbance such as hallucinations, paranoia, suspiciousness, or delusional state

        Vascular dementia, moderate, with psychotic disturbance such as hallucinations, paranoia, suspiciousness, or delusional state

    F01.B3   Vascular dementia, moderate, with mood disturbance A

        Major neurocognitive disorder due to vascular disease, moderate, with mood disturbance such as depression, apathy, or anhedonia

        Vascular dementia, moderate, with mood disturbance such as depression, apathy, or anhedonia

    F01.B4   Vascular dementia, moderate, with anxiety A

        Major neurocognitive disorder due to vascular disease, moderate, with anxiety

● **F01.C   Vascular dementia, severe**

    F01.C0   Vascular dementia, severe, without behavioral disturbance, psychotic disturbance, mood disturbance, and anxiety A

        Major neurocognitive disorder due to vascular disease, severe, NOS

        Vascular dementia, severe, NOS

● **F01.C1   Vascular dementia, severe, with behavioral disturbance**

    F01.C11   Vascular dementia, severe, with agitation A

        Major neurocognitive disorder due to vascular disease, severe, with aberrant motor behavior such as restlessness, rocking, pacing, or exit-seeking

        Major neurocognitive disorder due to vascular disease, severe, with verbal or physical behaviors such as profanity, shouting, threatening, anger, aggression, combativeness, or violence

        Vascular dementia, severe, with aberrant motor behavior such as restlessness, rocking, pacing, or exit-seeking

        Vascular dementia, severe, with verbal or physical behaviors such as profanity, shouting, threatening, anger, aggression, combativeness, or violence

    F01.C18   Vascular dementia, severe, with other behavioral disturbance A

        Major neurocognitive disorder due to vascular disease, severe, with behavioral disturbances such as sleep disturbance, social disinhibition, or sexual disinhibition

        Vascular dementia, severe, with behavioral disturbances such as sleep disturbance, social disinhibition, or sexual disinhibition

        Use Additional code, if applicable, to identify wandering in vascular dementia (Z91.83)

    F01.C2   Vascular dementia, severe, with psychotic disturbance A

        Major neurocognitive disorder due to vascular disease, severe, with psychotic disturbance such as hallucinations, paranoia, suspiciousness, or delusional state

        Vascular dementia, severe, with psychotic disturbance such as hallucinations, paranoia, suspiciousness, or delusional state

    F01.C3   Vascular dementia, severe, with mood disturbance A

        Major neurocognitive disorder due to vascular disease, severe, with mood disturbance such as depression, apathy, or anhedonia

        Vascular dementia, severe, with mood disturbance such as depression, apathy, or anhedonia

    F01.C4   Vascular dementia, severe, with anxiety A

        Major neurocognitive disorder due to vascular disease, severe, with anxiety

● **F02   Dementia in other diseases classified elsewhere**
   Code first the underlying physiological condition, such as:
      Alzheimer's (G30.-)
      cerebral lipidosis (E75.4)
      Creutzfeldt-Jakob disease (A81.0-)
      epilepsy and recurrent seizures (G40.-)
      frontotemporal dementia (G31.09)
      hepatolenticular degeneration (E83.01)
      human immunodeficiency virus [HIV] disease (B20)
      Huntington's disease (G10)
      hypercalcemia (E83.52)
      hypothyroidism, acquired (E00-E03.-)
      intoxications (T36-T65)
      Jakob-Creutzfeldt disease (A81.0-)
      multiple sclerosis (G35.-)
      neurocognitive disorder with Lewy bodies (G31.83)
      neurosyphilis (A52.17)
      niacin deficiency [pellagra] (E52)
      other frontotemporal neurocognitive disorder (G31.90)
      Parkinson's disease (G20.-)
      Pick's disease (G31.01)
      polyarteritis nodosa (M30.0)
      prion disease (A81.9)
      systemic lupus erythematosus (M32.-)
      traumatic brain injury (S06.-)
      trypanosomiasis (B56.-, B57.-)
      vitamin B deficiency (E53.8)

   Includes   Major neurocognitive disorder in other diseases
                   classified elsewhere

   Excludes1   mild neurocognitive disorder due to known
                   physiological condition with or without
                   behavioral disturbance (F06.7-)

   Excludes2   dementia in alcohol and psychoactive substance
                   disorders (F10-F19, with .17, .27, .97)
                   vascular dementia (F01.5-, F01.A-, F01.B-, F01.C-)
   Coding Clinic: 2016, Q4, P141

● **F02.8   Dementia in other diseases classified elsewhere,
             unspecified severity**

   ▸ **F02.80   *Dementia in other diseases classified elsewhere,
                 unspecified severity, without behavioral
                 disturbance, psychotic disturbance, mood
                 disturbance, and anxiety***
                 Dementia in other diseases classified elsewhere
                 NOS
                 Major neurocognitive disorder in other
                 diseases classified elsewhere NOS
                 Coding Clinic: 2024, Q2, P9; 2017, Q1, P43; 2016, Q2, P6

● **F02.81   *Dementia in other diseases classified elsewhere,
             unspecified severity, with behavioral disturbance***
             Coding Clinic: 2017, Q2, P8, Q1, P43

   ▸ **F02.811   Dementia in other diseases classified
                  elsewhere, unspecified severity, with
                  agitation**
                  Dementia in other diseases classified
                     elsewhere, unspecified severity,
                     with aberrant motor behavior
                     such as restlessness, rocking,
                     pacing, or exit-seeking
                  Dementia in other diseases classified
                     elsewhere, unspecified severity,
                     with verbal or physical
                     behaviors such as profanity,
                     shouting, threatening, anger,
                     aggression, combativeness, or
                     violence
                  Major neurocognitive disorder
                     in other diseases classified
                     elsewhere, unspecified severity,
                     with aberrant motor behavior
                     such as restlessness, rocking,
                     pacing, or exit-seeking
                  Major neurocognitive disorder
                     in other diseases classified
                     elsewhere, unspecified severity,
                     with verbal or physical behaviors
                     such as profanity, shouting,
                     threatening, anger, aggression,
                     combativeness, or violence

   ▸ **F02.818   Dementia in other diseases
                  classified elsewhere, unspecified
                  severity, with other behavioral
                  disturbance**
                  Dementia in other diseases
                     classified elsewhere with
                     sleep disturbance, social
                     disinhibition, or sexual
                     disinhibition
                  Major neurocognitive disorder
                     in other diseases classified
                     elsewhere with sleep
                     disturbance, social
                     disinhibition, or sexual
                     disinhibition

      Use Additional code, if applicable, to identify
      wandering in dementia in conditions
      classified elsewhere (Z91.83)

   ▸ **F02.82   Dementia in other diseases classified
                 elsewhere, unspecified severity, with psychotic
                 disturbance**
                 Dementia in other diseases classified
                    elsewhere, unspecified severity,
                    with psychotic disturbance such as
                    hallucinations, paranoia, suspiciousness,
                    or delusional state
                 Major neurocognitive disorder in other
                    diseases classified elsewhere, unspecified,
                    with psychotic disturbance such as
                    hallucinations, paranoia, suspiciousness,
                    or delusional state

   ▸ **F02.83   Dementia in other diseases classified
                 elsewhere, unspecified severity, with mood
                 disturbance**
                 Dementia in other diseases classified
                    elsewhere, unspecified severity, with
                    mood disturbance such as depression,
                    apathy, or anhedonia
                 Major neurocognitive disorder in other
                    diseases classified elsewhere unspecified
                    severity, with mood disturbance such as
                    with depression, apathy, or anhedonia

CHAPTER 5 (F01-F99)

F02.84   **Dementia in other diseases classified elsewhere, unspecified severity, with anxiety**
Major neurocognitive disorder in other diseases classified elsewhere unspecified severity, with anxiety

● **F02.A**   **Dementia in other diseases classified elsewhere, mild**

     Excludes1   mild neurocognitive disorder due to known physiological condition with or without behavioral disturbance (F06.7-)

F02.A0   **Dementia in other diseases classified elsewhere, mild, without behavioral disturbance, psychotic disturbance, mood disturbance, and anxiety**
Dementia in other diseases classified elsewhere, mild, NOS
Major neurocognitive disorder in other diseases classified elsewhere, mild, NOS

● **F02.A1**   **Dementia in other diseases classified elsewhere, mild, with behavioral disturbance**

F02.A11   **Dementia in other diseases classified elsewhere, mild, with agitation**
Dementia in other diseases classified elsewhere, mild, with aberrant motor behavior such as restlessness, rocking, pacing, or exit-seeking
Dementia in other diseases classified elsewhere, mild, with verbal or physical behaviors such as profanity, shouting, threatening, anger, aggression, combativeness, or violence
Major neurocognitive disorder in other diseases classified elsewhere, mild, with aberrant motor behavior such as restlessness, rocking, pacing, or exit-seeking
Major neurocognitive disorder in other diseases classified elsewhere, mild, with verbal or physical behaviors such as profanity, shouting, threatening, anger, aggression, combativeness, or violence

F02.A18   **Dementia in other diseases classified elsewhere, mild, with other behavioral disturbance**
Dementia in other diseases classified elsewhere, mild, with behavioral disturbances such as sleep disturbance, social disinhibition, or sexual disinhibition
Major neurocognitive disorder in other diseases classified elsewhere, mild, with behavioral disturbances such as sleep disturbance, social disinhibition, or sexual disinhibition

Use Additional code, if applicable, to identify wandering in dementia in conditions classified elsewhere (Z91.83)

F02.A2   **Dementia in other diseases classified elsewhere, mild, with psychotic disturbance**
Dementia in other diseases classified elsewhere, mild, with psychotic disturbance such as hallucinations, paranoia, suspiciousness, or delusional state
Major neurocognitive disorder in other diseases classified elsewhere, mild, with psychotic disturbance such as hallucinations, paranoia, suspiciousness, or delusional state

F02.A3   **Dementia in other diseases classified elsewhere, mild, with mood disturbance**
Dementia in other diseases classified elsewhere, mild, with mood disturbance such as depression, apathy, or anhedonia
Major neurocognitive disorder in other diseases classified elsewhere, mild, with mood disturbance such as depression, apathy, or anhedonia

F02.A4   **Dementia in other diseases classified elsewhere, mild, with anxiety**
Major neurocognitive disorder in other diseases classified elsewhere, mild, with anxiety

● **F02.B**   **Dementia in other diseases classified elsewhere, moderate**

F02.B0   **Dementia in other diseases classified elsewhere, moderate, without behavioral disturbance, psychotic disturbance, mood disturbance, and anxiety**
Dementia in other diseases classified elsewhere, moderate, NOS
Major neurocognitive disorder in other diseases classified elsewhere, moderate, NOS

● **F02.B1**   **Dementia in other diseases classified elsewhere, moderate, with behavioral disturbance**

F02.B11   **Dementia in other diseases classified elsewhere, moderate, with agitation**
Dementia in other diseases classified elsewhere, moderate, with aberrant motor behavior such as restlessness, rocking, pacing, or exit-seeking
Dementia in other diseases classified elsewhere, moderate, with verbal or physical behaviors such as profanity, shouting, threatening, anger, aggression, combativeness, or violence
Major neurocognitive disorder in other diseases classified elsewhere, moderate, with aberrant motor behavior such as restlessness, rocking, pacing, or exit- seeking
Major neurocognitive disorder in other diseases classified elsewhere, moderate, with verbal or physical behaviors such as profanity, shouting, threatening, anger, aggression, combativeness, or violence

F02.B18   **Dementia in other diseases classified elsewhere, moderate, with other behavioral disturbance**
Dementia in other diseases classified elsewhere, moderate, with behavioral disturbances such as sleep disturbance, social disinhibition, or sexual disinhibition
Major neurocognitive disorder in other diseases classified elsewhere, moderate, with behavioral disturbance such as sleep disturbance, social disinhibition, or sexual disinhibition

Use Additional code, if applicable, to identify wandering in dementia in conditions classified elsewhere (Z91.83)

► New   ⇒ Revised   ~~deleted~~ Deleted   Excludes 1   Excludes 2   Includes   Use additional   Code first   Code also   Key words

OGCR Official Guidelines   X Assign placeholder X   ● Use Additional Character(s)   ► Manifestation Code   Hierarchical Condition Category   Coding Clinic

▶ **F02.B2   Dementia in other diseases classified elsewhere, moderate, with psychotic disturbance**

Dementia in other diseases classified elsewhere, moderate, with psychotic disturbance such as hallucinations, paranoia, suspiciousness, or delusional state

Major neurocognitive disorder in other diseases classified elsewhere, moderate, with psychotic disturbance such as hallucinations, paranoia, suspiciousness, or delusional state

▶ **F02.B3   Dementia in other diseases classified elsewhere, moderate, with mood disturbance**

Dementia in other diseases classified elsewhere, moderate, with mood disturbance such as depression, apathy, or anhedonia

Major neurocognitive disorder in other diseases classified elsewhere, moderate, with mood disturbance such as depression, apathy, or anhedonia

▶ **F02.B4   Dementia in other diseases classified elsewhere, moderate, with anxiety**

Major neurocognitive disorder in other diseases classified elsewhere, moderate, with anxiety

● **F02.C   Dementia in other diseases classified elsewhere, severe**

▶ **F02.C0   Dementia in other diseases classified elsewhere, severe, without behavioral disturbance, psychotic disturbance, mood disturbance, and anxiety**

Dementia in other diseases classified elsewhere, severe, NOS

Major neurocognitive disorder in other diseases classified elsewhere, severe, NOS

● **F02.C1   Dementia in other diseases classified elsewhere, severe, with behavioral disturbance**

▶ **F02.C11   Dementia in other diseases classified elsewhere, severe, with agitation**

Dementia in other diseases classified elsewhere, severe, with aberrant motor behavior such as restlessness, rocking, pacing, or exit-seeking

Dementia in other diseases classified elsewhere, severe, with verbal or physical behaviors such as profanity, shouting, threatening, anger, aggression, combativeness, or violence

Major neurocognitive disorder in other diseases classified elsewhere, severe, with aberrant motor behavior such as restlessness, rocking, pacing, or exit-seeking

Major neurocognitive disorder in other diseases classified elsewhere, severe, with verbal or physical behaviors such as profanity, shouting, threatening, anger, aggression, combativeness, or violence

Coding Clinic: 2022, Q4, P15

▶ **F02.C18   Dementia in other diseases classified elsewhere, severe, with other behavioral disturbance**

Dementia in other diseases classified elsewhere, severe, with behavioral disturbances such as sleep disturbance, social disinhibition, or sexual disinhibition

Major neurocognitive disorder in other diseases classified elsewhere, severe, with behavioral disturbances such as sleep disturbance, social disinhibition, or sexual disinhibition

Use Additional code, if applicable, to identify wandering in dementia in conditions classified elsewhere (Z91.83)

▶ **F02.C2   Dementia in other diseases classified elsewhere, severe, with psychotic disturbance**

Dementia in other diseases classified elsewhere, severe, with psychotic disturbance such as hallucinations, paranoia, suspiciousness, or delusional state

Major neurocognitive disorder in other diseases classified elsewhere, severe, with psychotic disturbance such as hallucinations, paranoia, suspiciousness, or delusional state

▶ **F02.C3   Dementia in other diseases classified elsewhere, severe, with mood disturbance**

Dementia in other diseases classified elsewhere, severe, with mood disturbance such as depression, apathy, or anhedonia

Major neurocognitive disorder in other diseases classified elsewhere, severe, with mood disturbance such as depression, apathy, or anhedonia

▶ **F02.C4   Dementia in other diseases classified elsewhere, severe, with anxiety**

Major neurocognitive disorder in other diseases classified elsewhere, severe, with anxiety

● **F03   Unspecified dementia**

Major neurocognitive disorder NOS
Presenile dementia NOS
Presenile psychosis NOS
Primary degenerative dementia NOS
Senile dementia NOS
Senile dementia depressed or paranoid type
Senile psychosis NOS

Excludes2   dementia with delirium or acute confusional state (F05)
mild memory disturbance due to known physiological condition (F06.8)

● **F03.9   Unspecified dementia, unspecified severity**

F03.90   Unspecified dementia, unspecified severity, without behavioral disturbance, psychotic disturbance, mood disturbance, and anxiety   A

Dementia NOS

Coding Clinic: 2024, Q2, P9; 2021, Q2, P4; 2012, Q4, P92

CHAPTER 5 (F01–F99)

Item 5-1 Psychosis was a term formerly applied to any mental disorder but is now restricted to disturbances of a great magnitude in which there is a personality disintegration and loss of contact with reality.

● **F03.91**   **Unspecified dementia with, unspecified severity, behavioral disturbance**

    F03.911   **Unspecified dementia, unspecified severity, with agitation**   A
      Unspecified dementia, unspecified severity, with aberrant motor behavior such as restlessness, rocking, pacing, or exit-seeking
      Unspecified dementia, unspecified severity, with verbal or physical behaviors such as profanity, shouting, threatening, anger, aggression, combativeness, or violence

    F03.918   **Unspecified dementia, unspecified severity, with other behavioral disturbance**   A
      Unspecified dementia, unspecified severity, with behavioral disturbances such as sleep disturbance, social disinhibition, or sexual disinhibition

      Use Additional code, if applicable, to identify wandering in unspecified dementia (Z91.83)

F03.92   **Unspecified dementia, unspecified severity, with psychotic disturbance**   A
   Unspecified dementia, unspecified severity, with psychotic disturbance such as hallucinations, paranoia, suspiciousness, or delusional state

F03.93   **Unspecified dementia, unspecified severity, with mood disturbance**   A
   Unspecified dementia, unspecified severity, with mood disturbance such as depression, apathy, or anhedonia

F03.94   **Unspecified dementia, unspecified severity, with anxiety**   A

● **F03.A**   **Unspecified dementia, mild**

   Excludes1   mild neurocognitive disorder due to known physiological condition with or without behavioral disturbance (F06.7-)

F03.A0   **Unspecified dementia, mild, without behavioral disturbance, psychotic disturbance, mood disturbance, and anxiety**   A
   Dementia, mild, NOS

● **F03.A1**   **Unspecified dementia, mild, with behavioral disturbance**

    F03.A11   **Unspecified dementia, mild, with agitation**   A
      Unspecified dementia, mild, with aberrant motor behavior such as restlessness, rocking, pacing, or exit-seeking
      Unspecified dementia, mild, with verbal or physical behaviors such as profanity, shouting, threatening, anger, aggression, combativeness, or violence

    F03.A18   **Unspecified dementia, mild, with other behavioral disturbance**   A
      Unspecified dementia, mild, with behavioral disturbances such as sleep disturbance, social disinhibition, or sexual disinhibition

      Use Additional code, if applicable, to identify wandering in unspecified dementia (Z91.83)

    F03.A2   **Unspecified dementia, mild, with psychotic disturbance**   A
      Unspecified dementia, mild, with psychotic disturbance such as hallucinations, paranoia, suspiciousness, or delusional state

    F03.A3   **Unspecified dementia, mild, with mood disturbance**   A
      Unspecified dementia, mild, with mood disturbance such as depression, apathy, or anhedonia

    F03.A4   **Unspecified dementia, mild, with anxiety**   A

● **F03.B**   **Unspecified dementia, moderate**

   F03.B0   **Unspecified dementia, moderate, without behavioral disturbance, psychotic disturbance, mood disturbance, and anxiety**   A
     Dementia, moderate, NOS

● **F03.B1**   **Unspecified dementia, moderate, with behavioral disturbance**

    F03.B11   **Unspecified dementia, moderate, with agitation**   A
      Unspecified dementia, moderate, with aberrant motor behavior such as restlessness, rocking, pacing, or exit-seeking
      Unspecified dementia, moderate, with verbal or physical behaviors such as profanity, shouting, threatening, anger, aggression, combativeness, or violence

    F03.B18   **Unspecified dementia, moderate, with other behavioral disturbance**   A
      Unspecified dementia, moderate, with behavioral disturbances such as sleep disturbance, social disinhibition, or sexual disinhibition

      Use Additional code, if applicable, to identify wandering in unspecified dementia (Z91.83)

    F03.B2   **Unspecified dementia, moderate, with psychotic disturbance**   A
      Unspecified dementia, moderate, with psychotic disturbance such as hallucinations, paranoia, suspiciousness, or delusional state

    F03.B3   **Unspecified dementia, moderate, with mood disturbance**   A
      Unspecified dementia, moderate, with mood disturbance such as depression, apathy, or anhedonia

    F03.B4   **Unspecified dementia, moderate, with anxiety**   A

● **F03.C**   **Unspecified dementia, severe**

   F03.C0   **Unspecified dementia, severe, without behavioral disturbance, psychotic disturbance, mood disturbance, and anxiety**   A
     Dementia, severe, NOS

▶ New   ⇒ Revised   ~~deleted~~ Deleted   Excludes 1   Excludes 2   Includes   Use additional   Code first   Code also   Key words

OGCR Official Guidelines   X Assign placeholder X   ● Use Additional Character(s)   ▸ Manifestation Code   Hierarchical Condition Category   Coding Clinic

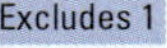

● **F03.C1　Unspecified dementia, severe, with behavioral disturbance**

　　F03.C11　Unspecified dementia, severe, with agitation　**A**

　　　　Unspecified dementia, severe, with aberrant motor behavior such as restlessness, rocking, pacing, or exit-seeking

　　　　Unspecified dementia, severe, with verbal or physical behaviors such as profanity, shouting, threatening, anger, aggression, combativeness, or violence

　　F03.C18　Unspecified dementia, severe, with other behavioral disturbance　**A**

　　　　Unspecified dementia, severe, with behavioral disturbances such as sleep disturbance, social disinhibition, or sexual disinhibition

　　　　Use Additional code, if applicable, to identify wandering in unspecified dementia (Z91.83)

F03.C2　Unspecified dementia, severe, with psychotic disturbance　**A**

　　Unspecified dementia, severe, with psychotic disturbance such as hallucinations, paranoia, suspiciousness, or delusional state

F03.C3　Unspecified dementia, severe, with mood disturbance　**A**

　　Unspecified dementia, severe, with mood disturbance such as depression, apathy, or anhedonia

　　Coding Clinic: 2023, Q4, P15

F03.C4　Unspecified dementia, severe, with anxiety　**A**

F04　Amnestic disorder due to known physiological condition

　Korsakov's psychosis or syndrome, nonalcoholic

　Code first the underlying physiological condition

　Excludes1　amnesia NOS (R41.3)
　　　　anterograde amnesia (R41.1)
　　　　dissociative amnesia (F44.0)
　　　　retrograde amnesia (R41.2)

　Excludes2　alcohol-induced or unspecified Korsakov's syndrome (F10.26, F10.96)
　　　　Korsakov's syndrome induced by other psychoactive substances (F13.26, F13.96, F19.16, F19.26, F19.96)

F05　Delirium due to known physiological condition

　Acute or subacute brain syndrome
　Acute or subacute confusional state (nonalcoholic)
　Acute or subacute infective psychosis
　Acute or subacute organic reaction
　Acute or subacute psycho-organic syndrome
　Delirium of mixed etiology
　Delirium superimposed on dementia
　Sundowning

　Code first the underlying physiological condition, such as:
　　dementia (F03.9-)

　Excludes1　delirium NOS (R41.0)

　Excludes2　delirium tremens alcohol-induced or unspecified (F10.231, F10.921)

　Coding Clinic: 2019, Q2, P34

● **F06　Other mental disorders due to known physiological condition**

　Includes　mental disorders due to endocrine disorder
　　　　mental disorders due to exogenous hormone
　　　　mental disorders due to exogenous toxic substance
　　　　mental disorders due to primary cerebral disease
　　　　mental disorders due to somatic illness
　　　　mental disorders due to systemic disease affecting the brain

　Code first the underlying physiological condition

　Excludes1　unspecified dementia (F03.0-)

　Excludes2　delirium due to known physiological condition (F05)
　　　　dementia as classified in F01-F02
　　　　other mental disorders associated with alcohol and other psychoactive substances (F10-F19)

F06.0　Psychotic disorder with hallucinations due to known physiological condition

　Organic hallucinatory state (nonalcoholic)

　Excludes2　hallucinations and perceptual disturbance induced by alcohol and other psychoactive substances (F10-F19 with .151, .251, .951)
　　　　schizophrenia (F20.-)

F06.1　Catatonic disorder due to known physiological condition

　Catatonia associated with another mental disorder
　Catatonia NOS

　Excludes1　catatonic stupor (R40.1)
　　　　stupor NOS (R40.1)

　Excludes2　catatonic schizophrenia (F20.2)
　　　　dissociative stupor (F44.2)

F06.2　Psychotic disorder with delusions due to known physiological condition

　Paranoid and paranoid-hallucinatory organic states
　Schizophrenia-like psychosis in epilepsy

　Excludes2　alcohol and drug-induced psychotic disorder (F10-F19 with .150, .250, .950)
　　　　brief psychotic disorder (F23)
　　　　delusional disorder (F22)
　　　　schizophrenia (F20.-)

● **F06.3　Mood disorder due to known physiological condition**

　Excludes2　mood disorders due to alcohol and other psychoactive substances (F10-F19 with .14, .24, .94)
　　　　mood disorders, not due to known physiological condition or unspecified (F30-F39)

　　F06.30　Mood disorder due to known physiological condition, unspecified

　　F06.31　Mood disorder due to known physiological condition with depressive features

　　　　Depressive disorder due to known physiological condition, with depressive features

　　F06.32　Mood disorder due to known physiological condition with major depressive-like episode

　　　　Depressive disorder due to known physiological condition, with major depressive-like episode

　　F06.33　Mood disorder due to known physiological condition with manic features

　　　　Bipolar and related disorder due to a known physiological condition, with manic features

　　　　Bipolar and related disorder due to known physiological condition, with manic- or hypomanic-like episodes

CHAPTER 5 (F01-F99)

F06.34 **Mood disorder due to known physiological condition with mixed features**
Bipolar and related disorder due to known physiological condition, with mixed features
Depressive disorder due to known physiological condition, with mixed features

F06.4 **Anxiety disorder due to known physiological condition**

> **Excludes2**   anxiety disorders due to alcohol and other psychoactive substances (F10-F19 with .180, .280, .980)
> anxiety disorders, not due to known physiological condition or unspecified (F40.-, F41.-)

● **F06.7** **Mild neurocognitive disorder due to known physiological condition**
Mild neurocognitive impairment due to a known physiological condition

> *Code first the underlying physiological condition, such as:*
> Alzheimer's disease (G30.-)
> human immunodeficiency virus [HIV] disease (B20)
> Huntington's disease (G10)
> Neurocognitive disorder with Lewy bodies (G31.83)
> other frontotemporal neurocognitive disorder (G31.09)
> Parkinson's disease (G20.-)
> systemic lupus erythematosus (M32.-)
> traumatic brain injury (S06.-)
> vitamin B deficiency (E53-)

> **Excludes1**   age related cognitive decline (R41.81)
> altered mental status (R41.82)
> cerebral degeneration (G31.9)
> change in mental status (R41.82)
> cognitive deficits following (sequelae of) cerebral hemorrhage or infarction (I69.01- I69.11-, I69.21-I69.31-, I69.81-I69.91-)
> dementia (F01.-, F02.-, F03.0-)
> mild cognitive impairment due to unknown or unspecified etiology (G31.84)
> neurologic neglect syndrome (R41.4)
> personality change, nonpsychotic (F68.8)

F06.70 **Mild neurocognitive disorder due to known physiological condition without behavioral disturbance**
Mild neurocognitive disorder due to known physiological condition, NOS

F06.71 **Mild neurocognitive disorder due to known physiological condition with behavioral disturbance**

F06.8 **Other specified mental disorders due to known physiological condition**
Epileptic psychosis NOS
Obsessive-compulsive and related disorder due to a known physiological condition
Organic dissociative disorder
Organic emotionally labile [asthenic] disorder

● **F07** **Personality and behavioral disorders due to known physiological condition**

> *Code first the underlying physiological condition*

F07.0 **Personality change due to known physiological condition**
Frontal lobe syndrome
Limbic epilepsy personality syndrome
Lobotomy syndrome
Organic personality disorder
Organic pseudopsychopathic personality
Organic pseudoretarded personality
Postleucotomy syndrome

> **Excludes1**   mild cognitive impairment (G31.84)
> postconcussional syndrome (F07.81)
> postencephalitic syndrome (F07.89)
> signs and symptoms involving emotional state (R45.-)

> **Excludes2**   specific personality disorder (F60.-)

● **F07.8** **Other personality and behavioral disorders due to known physiological condition**

F07.81 **Postconcussional syndrome**
Postcontusional syndrome (encephalopathy)
Post-traumatic brain syndrome, nonpsychotic
Use additional code to identify associated post-traumatic headache, if applicable (G44.3-)

> **Excludes1**   current concussion (brain) (S06.0-)
> postencephalitic syndrome (F07.89)

F07.89 **Other personality and behavioral disorders due to known physiological condition**
Postencephalitic syndrome
Damage to temporal brain lobes with memory loss and abnormal behavior
Right hemispheric organic affective disorder

F07.9 **Unspecified personality and behavioral disorder due to known physiological condition**
Organic psychosyndrome
Due to exposure to organic solvents

F09 **Unspecified mental disorder due to known physiological condition**
Mental disorder NOS due to known physiological condition
Organic brain syndrome NOS
Organic mental disorder NOS
Organic psychosis NOS
Symptomatic psychosis NOS

> *Code first the underlying physiological condition*

> **Excludes1**   mild neurocognitive disorder due to known physiological condition (F06.7-)
> psychosis NOS (F29)

MENTAL AND BEHAVIORAL DISORDERS DUE TO PSYCHOACTIVE SUBSTANCE USE (F10-F19)

● **F10** **Alcohol related disorders**
Use additional code for blood alcohol level, if applicable (Y90.-)
Coding Clinic: 2019, Q3, P8

● **F10.1** **Alcohol abuse**

> **Excludes1**   alcohol dependence (F10.2-)
> alcohol use, unspecified (F10.9-)

F10.10 **Alcohol abuse, uncomplicated**
Alcohol use disorder, mild

F10.11 **Alcohol abuse, in remission**
Alcohol use disorder, mild, in early remission
Alcohol use disorder, mild, in sustained remission
Coding Clinic: 2022, Q1, P25

● **F10.12** **Alcohol abuse with intoxication**

F10.120   **Alcohol abuse with intoxication, uncomplicated**

F10.121   **Alcohol abuse with intoxication, delirium**

F10.129   **Alcohol abuse with intoxication, unspecified**

● **F10.13** **Alcohol abuse, with withdrawal**

F10.130   **Alcohol abuse with withdrawal, uncomplicated**

F10.131   **Alcohol abuse with withdrawal delirium**

F10.132   **Alcohol abuse with withdrawal with perceptual disturbance**

F10.139   **Alcohol abuse with withdrawal, unspecified**

F10.14 **Alcohol abuse with alcohol-induced mood disorder**
Alcohol use disorder, mild, with alcohol-induced bipolar or related disorder
Alcohol use disorder, mild, with alcohol-induced depressive disorder

● **F10.15** **Alcohol abuse with alcohol-induced psychotic disorder**

F10.150   Alcohol abuse with alcohol-induced psychotic disorder with delusions

F10.151   Alcohol abuse with alcohol-induced psychotic disorder with hallucinations

F10.159   Alcohol abuse with alcohol-induced psychotic disorder, unspecified

● F10.18   Alcohol abuse with other alcohol-induced disorders
Coding Clinic: 2022, Q1, P33

F10.180   Alcohol abuse with alcohol-induced anxiety disorder
Coding Clinic: 2022, Q1, P33

F10.181   Alcohol abuse with alcohol-induced sexual dysfunction

F10.182   Alcohol abuse with alcohol-induced sleep disorder

F10.188   Alcohol abuse with other alcohol-induced disorder
Coding Clinic: 2022, Q1, P25

F10.19   Alcohol abuse with unspecified alcohol-induced disorder

● F10.2   Alcohol dependence

Excludes1   alcohol abuse (F10.1-)
alcohol use, unspecified (F10.9-)

Excludes2   toxic effect of alcohol (T51.0-)
Coding Clinic: 2019, Q3, P8

F10.20   Alcohol dependence, uncomplicated
Alcohol use disorder, moderate
Alcohol use disorder, severe
Coding Clinic: 2020, Q1, P9

F10.21   Alcohol dependence, in remission
Alcohol use disorder, moderate, in early remission
Alcohol use disorder, moderate, in sustained remission
Alcohol use disorder, severe, in early remission
Alcohol use disorder, severe, in sustained remission

● F10.22   Alcohol dependence with intoxication
Acute drunkenness (in alcoholism)

Excludes2   alcohol dependence with withdrawal (F10.23-)

F10.220   Alcohol dependence with intoxication, uncomplicated

F10.221   Alcohol dependence with intoxication delirium

F10.229   Alcohol dependence with intoxication, unspecified

● F10.23   Alcohol dependence with withdrawal

Excludes2   alcohol dependence with intoxication (F10.22-)

F10.230   Alcohol dependence with withdrawal, uncomplicated

F10.231   Alcohol dependence with withdrawal delirium

F10.232   Alcohol dependence with withdrawal with perceptual disturbance

F10.239   Alcohol dependence with withdrawal, unspecified
Coding Clinic: 2015, Q2, P15

F10.24   Alcohol dependence with alcohol-induced mood disorder
Alcohol use disorder, moderate, with alcohol-induced bipolar or related disorder
Alcohol use disorder, moderate, with alcohol-induced depressive disorder
Alcohol use disorder, severe, with alcohol-induced bipolar or related disorder
Alcohol use disorder, severe, with alcohol-induced depressive disorder

● F10.25   Alcohol dependence with alcohol-induced psychotic disorder

F10.250   Alcohol dependence with alcohol-induced psychotic disorder with delusions

F10.251   Alcohol dependence with alcohol-induced psychotic disorder with hallucinations

F10.259   Alcohol dependence with alcohol-induced psychotic disorder, unspecified

F10.26   Alcohol dependence with alcohol-induced persisting amnestic disorder
Alcohol use disorder, moderate, with alcohol-induced major neurocognitive disorder, amnestic-confabulatory type
Alcohol use disorder, severe, with alcohol-induced major neurocognitive disorder, amnestic-confabulatory type

F10.27   Alcohol dependence with alcohol-induced persisting dementia
Alcohol use disorder, moderate, with alcohol-induced major neurocognitive disorder, nonamnestic-confabulatory type
Alcohol use disorder, severe, with alcohol-induced major neurocognitive disorder, nonamnestic-confabulatory type

● F10.28   Alcohol dependence with other alcohol-induced disorders

F10.280   Alcohol dependence with alcohol-induced anxiety disorder

F10.281   Alcohol dependence with alcohol-induced sexual dysfunction

F10.282   Alcohol dependence with alcohol-induced sleep disorder

F10.288   Alcohol dependence with other alcohol-induced disorder
Alcohol use disorder, moderate, with alcohol-induced mild neurocognitive disorder
Alcohol use disorder, severe, with alcohol-induced mild neurocognitive disorder
Coding Clinic: 2020, Q1, P9

F10.29   Alcohol dependence with unspecified alcohol-induced disorder

● F10.9   Alcohol use, unspecified

Excludes1   alcohol abuse (F10.1-)
alcohol dependence (F10.2-)

F10.90   Alcohol use, unspecified, uncomplicated

F10.91   Alcohol use, unspecified, in remission

● F10.92   Alcohol use, unspecified with intoxication

F10.920   Alcohol use, unspecified with intoxication, uncomplicated

F10.921   Alcohol use, unspecified with intoxication delirium

F10.929   Alcohol use, unspecified with intoxication, unspecified

CHAPTER 5 (F01-F99)

● **F10.93** **Alcohol use, unspecified with withdrawal**
    F10.930 **Alcohol use, unspecified with withdrawal, uncomplicated**
    F10.931 **Alcohol use, unspecified with withdrawal delirium**
    F10.932 **Alcohol use, unspecified with withdrawal with perceptual disturbance**
    F10.939 **Alcohol use, unspecified with withdrawal, unspecified**
  F10.94 **Alcohol use, unspecified with alcohol-induced mood disorder** 🅡🅒
    Alcohol-induced bipolar or related disorder, without use disorder
    Alcohol-induced depressive disorder, without use disorder
● **F10.95** **Alcohol use, unspecified with alcohol-induced psychotic disorder**
    F10.950 **Alcohol use, unspecified with alcohol-induced psychotic disorder with delusions** 🅡🅒
    F10.951 **Alcohol use, unspecified with alcohol-induced psychotic disorder with hallucinations** 🅡🅒
    F10.959 **Alcohol use, unspecified with alcohol-induced psychotic disorder, unspecified** 🅡🅒
      Alcohol-induced psychotic disorder without use disorder
  F10.96 **Alcohol use, unspecified with alcohol-induced persisting amnestic disorder** 🅡🅒
    Alcohol-induced major neurocognitive disorder, amnestic-confabulatory type, without use disorder
  F10.97 **Alcohol use, unspecified with alcohol-induced persisting dementia** 🅡🅒
    Alcohol-induced major neurocognitive disorder, nonamnestic-confabulatory type, without use disorder
● **F10.98** **Alcohol use, unspecified with other alcohol-induced disorders**
    F10.980 **Alcohol use, unspecified with alcohol-induced anxiety disorder** 🅡🅒
      Alcohol-induced anxiety disorder, without use disorder
    F10.981 **Alcohol use, unspecified with alcohol-induced sexual dysfunction** 🅡🅒
      Alcohol-induced sexual dysfunction, without use disorder
    F10.982 **Alcohol use, unspecified with alcohol-induced sleep disorder** 🅡🅒
      Alcohol-induced sleep disorder, without use disorder
    F10.988 **Alcohol use, unspecified with other alcohol-induced disorder** 🅡🅒
      Alcohol-induced mild neurocognitive disorder, without use disorder
      Coding Clinic: 2019, Q3, P8
  F10.99 **Alcohol use, unspecified with unspecified alcohol-induced disorder** 🅡🅒

● **F11** **Opioid related disorders**
  ● **F11.1** **Opioid abuse**
    Excludes1   opioid dependence (F11.2-)
             opioid use, unspecified (F11.9-)
    F11.10 **Opioid abuse, uncomplicated**
      Opioid use disorder, mild
    F11.11 **Opioid abuse, in remission**
      Opioid use disorder, mild, in early remission
      Opioid use disorder, mild, in sustained remission
  ● **F11.12** **Opioid abuse with intoxication**
    F11.120 **Opioid abuse with intoxication, uncomplicated** 🅡🅒
    F11.121 **Opioid abuse with intoxication delirium** 🅡🅒
    F11.122 **Opioid abuse with intoxication with perceptual disturbance** 🅡🅒
    F11.129 **Opioid abuse with intoxication, unspecified** 🅡🅒
    F11.13 **Opioid abuse with withdrawal**
    F11.14 **Opioid abuse with opioid-induced mood disorder** 🅡🅒
      Opioid use disorder, mild, with opioid-induced depressive disorder
  ● **F11.15** **Opioid abuse with opioid-induced psychotic disorder**
    F11.150 **Opioid abuse with opioid-induced psychotic disorder with delusions** 🅡🅒
    F11.151 **Opioid abuse with opioid-induced psychotic disorder with hallucinations** 🅡🅒
    F11.159 **Opioid abuse with opioid-induced psychotic disorder, unspecified** 🅡🅒
  ● **F11.18** **Opioid abuse with other opioid-induced disorder**
    F11.181 **Opioid abuse with opioid-induced sexual dysfunction** 🅡🅒
    F11.182 **Opioid abuse with opioid-induced sleep disorder** 🅡🅒
    F11.188 **Opioid abuse with other opioid-induced disorder** 🅡🅒
      Opioid-associated amnestic syndrome with opioid abuse
    F11.19 **Opioid abuse with unspecified opioid-induced disorder** 🅡🅒
  ● **F11.2** **Opioid dependence**
    Excludes1   opioid abuse (F11.1-)
             opioid use, unspecified (F11.9-)
    Excludes2   opioid poisoning (T40.0—T40.2-)
    F11.20 **Opioid dependence, uncomplicated** 🅡🅒
      Opioid use disorder, moderate
      Opioid use disorder, severe
    F11.21 **Opioid dependence, in remission** 🅡🅒
      Opioid use disorder, moderate, in early remission
      Opioid use disorder, moderate, in sustained remission
      Opioid use disorder, severe, in early remission
      Opioid use disorder, severe, in sustained remission
  ● **F11.22** **Opioid dependence with intoxication**
    Excludes1   opioid dependence with withdrawal (F11.23)
    F11.220 **Opioid dependence with intoxication, uncomplicated** 🅡🅒
    F11.221 **Opioid dependence with intoxication delirium** 🅡🅒
    F11.222 **Opioid dependence with intoxication with perceptual disturbance** 🅡🅒
    F11.229 **Opioid dependence with intoxication, unspecified** 🅡🅒

▶ New   ➡ Revised   ~~deleted~~ Deleted   Excludes 1   Excludes 2   Includes   Use additional   Code first   Code also   Key words
OGCR Official Guidelines   **X** Assign placeholder X   ● Use Additional Character(s)   ▌ Manifestation Code   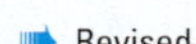 Hierarchical Condition Category   **Coding Clinic**

CHAPTER 5 (F01-F99)

F11.23   **Opioid dependence with withdrawal** 🔴
    Excludes1   opioid dependence with intoxication (F11.22-)

F11.24   **Opioid dependence with opioid-induced mood disorder** 🔴
    Opioid use disorder, moderate, with opioid-induced depressive disorder

● **F11.25**   **Opioid dependence with opioid-induced psychotic disorder**
    F11.250   **Opioid dependence with opioid-induced psychotic disorder with delusions**
    F11.251   **Opioid dependence with opioid-induced psychotic disorder with hallucinations** 🔴
    F11.259   **Opioid dependence with opioid-induced psychotic disorder, unspecified** 🔴

● **F11.28**   **Opioid dependence with other opioid-induced disorder**
    F11.281   **Opioid dependence with opioid-induced sexual dysfunction** 🔴
    F11.282   **Opioid dependence with opioid-induced sleep disorder** 🔴
    F11.288   **Opioid dependence with other opioid-induced disorder** 🔴
    F11.29   **Opioid dependence with unspecified opioid-induced disorder** 🔴

● **F11.9**   **Opioid use, unspecified**
    Excludes1   opioid abuse (F11.1-)
               opioid dependence (F11.2-)
    F11.90   **Opioid use, unspecified, uncomplicated**
    F11.91   **Opioid use, unspecified, in remission**
●   **F11.92**   **Opioid use, unspecified with intoxication**
    Excludes1   opioid use, unspecified with withdrawal (F11.93)
    F11.920   **Opioid use, unspecified with intoxication, uncomplicated** 🔴
    F11.921   **Opioid use, unspecified with intoxication delirium** 🔴
           Opioid-induced delirium
    F11.922   **Opioid use, unspecified with intoxication with perceptual disturbance** 🔴
    F11.929   **Opioid use, unspecified with intoxication, unspecified** 🔴

    F11.93   **Opioid use, unspecified with withdrawal** 🔴
    Excludes1   opioid use, unspecified with intoxication (F11.92-)
    F11.94   **Opioid use, unspecified with opioid-induced mood disorder** 🔴
          Opioid-induced depressive disorder, without use disorder

● **F11.95**   **Opioid use, unspecified with opioid-induced psychotic disorder**
    F11.950   **Opioid use, unspecified with opioid-induced psychotic disorder with delusions** 🔴
    F11.951   **Opioid use, unspecified with opioid-induced psychotic disorder with hallucinations** 🔴
    F11.959   **Opioid use, unspecified with opioid-induced psychotic disorder, unspecified** 🔴

● **F11.98**   **Opioid use, unspecified with other specified opioid-induced disorder**
    F11.981   **Opioid use, unspecified with opioid-induced sexual dysfunction** 🔴
          Opioid-induced sexual dysfunction, without use disorder
    F11.982   **Opioid use, unspecified with opioid-induced sleep disorder** 🔴
          Opioid-induced sleep disorder, without use disorder
    F11.988   **Opioid use, unspecified with other opioid-induced disorder** 🔴
          Opioid-associated amnestic syndrome with opioid abuse
          Opioid-induced anxiety disorder, without use disorder
    F11.99   **Opioid use, unspecified with unspecified opioid-induced disorder** 🔴

● **F12**   **Cannabis related disorders**
    Includes   marijuana
    Coding Clinic: 2020, Q1, P8
●   **F12.1**   **Cannabis abuse**
    Excludes1   cannabis dependence (F12.2-)
               cannabis use, unspecified (F12.9-)
    F12.10   **Cannabis abuse, uncomplicated**
          Cannabis use disorder, mild
    F12.11   **Cannabis abuse, in remission**
          Cannabis use disorder, mild, in early remission
          Cannabis use disorder, mild, in sustained remission
●   **F12.12**   **Cannabis abuse with intoxication**
    F12.120   **Cannabis abuse with intoxication, uncomplicated** 🔴
    F12.121   **Cannabis abuse with intoxication delirium** 🔴
    F12.122   **Cannabis abuse with intoxication with perceptual disturbance** 🔴
    F12.129   **Cannabis abuse with intoxication, unspecified** 🔴
    F12.13   **Cannabis abuse with withdrawal**
●   **F12.15**   **Cannabis abuse with psychotic disorder**
    F12.150   **Cannabis abuse with psychotic disorder with delusions** 🔴
    F12.151   **Cannabis abuse with psychotic disorder with hallucinations** 🔴
    F12.159   **Cannabis abuse with psychotic disorder, unspecified** 🔴
●   **F12.18**   **Cannabis abuse with other cannabis-induced disorder**
    F12.180   **Cannabis abuse with cannabis-induced anxiety disorder** 🔴
    F12.188   **Cannabis abuse with other cannabis-induced disorder** 🔴
          Cannabis use disorder, mild, with cannabis-induced sleep disorder
          Opioid-associated amnestic syndrome with opioid abuse
    F12.19   **Cannabis abuse with unspecified cannabis-induced disorder** 🔴
●   **F12.2**   **Cannabis dependence**
    Excludes1   cannabis abuse (F12.1-)
               cannabis use, unspecified (F12.9-)
    Excludes2   cannabis poisoning (T40.7-)
    F12.20   **Cannabis dependence, uncomplicated** 🔴
          Cannabis use disorder, moderate
          Cannabis use disorder, severe

CHAPTER 5 (F01-F99)

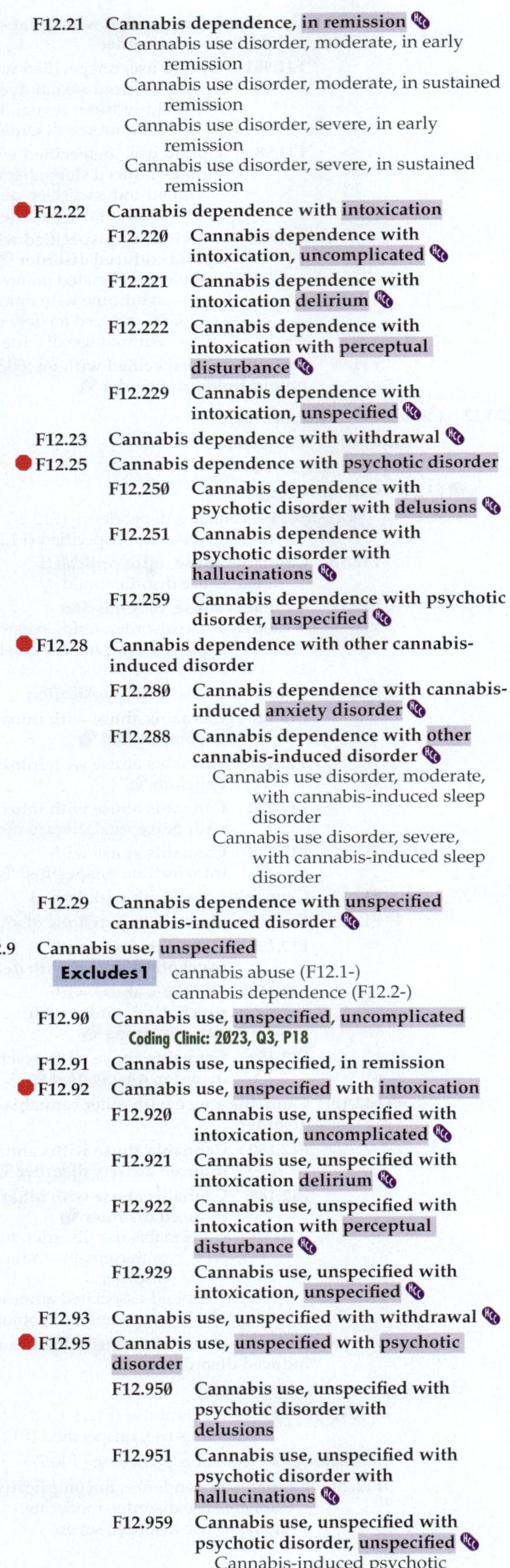

F12.21   Cannabis dependence, in remission
> Cannabis use disorder, moderate, in early remission
> Cannabis use disorder, moderate, in sustained remission
> Cannabis use disorder, severe, in early remission
> Cannabis use disorder, severe, in sustained remission

● **F12.22**   Cannabis dependence with intoxication

F12.220   Cannabis dependence with intoxication, uncomplicated

F12.221   Cannabis dependence with intoxication delirium

F12.222   Cannabis dependence with intoxication with perceptual disturbance

F12.229   Cannabis dependence with intoxication, unspecified

F12.23   Cannabis dependence with withdrawal

● **F12.25**   Cannabis dependence with psychotic disorder

F12.250   Cannabis dependence with psychotic disorder with delusions

F12.251   Cannabis dependence with psychotic disorder with hallucinations

F12.259   Cannabis dependence with psychotic disorder, unspecified

● **F12.28**   Cannabis dependence with other cannabis-induced disorder

F12.280   Cannabis dependence with cannabis-induced anxiety disorder

F12.288   Cannabis dependence with other cannabis-induced disorder
> Cannabis use disorder, moderate, with cannabis-induced sleep disorder
> Cannabis use disorder, severe, with cannabis-induced sleep disorder

F12.29   Cannabis dependence with unspecified cannabis-induced disorder

● **F12.9**   Cannabis use, unspecified

> **Excludes1**   cannabis abuse (F12.1-)
> cannabis dependence (F12.2-)

F12.90   Cannabis use, unspecified, uncomplicated
Coding Clinic: 2023, Q3, P18

F12.91   Cannabis use, unspecified, in remission

● **F12.92**   Cannabis use, unspecified with intoxication

F12.920   Cannabis use, unspecified with intoxication, uncomplicated

F12.921   Cannabis use, unspecified with intoxication delirium

F12.922   Cannabis use, unspecified with intoxication with perceptual disturbance

F12.929   Cannabis use, unspecified with intoxication, unspecified

F12.93   Cannabis use, unspecified with withdrawal

● **F12.95**   Cannabis use, unspecified with psychotic disorder

F12.950   Cannabis use, unspecified with psychotic disorder with delusions

F12.951   Cannabis use, unspecified with psychotic disorder with hallucinations

F12.959   Cannabis use, unspecified with psychotic disorder, unspecified
> Cannabis-induced psychotic disorder, without use disorder

● **F12.98**   Cannabis use, unspecified with other cannabis-induced disorder

F12.980   Cannabis use, unspecified with anxiety disorder
> Cannabis-induced anxiety disorder, without use disorder

F12.988   Cannabis use, unspecified with other cannabis-induced disorder
> Cannabis-induced sleep disorder, without use disorder

F12.99   Cannabis use, unspecified with unspecified cannabis-induced disorder

● **F13**   Sedative, hypnotic, or anxiolytic related disorders

● **F13.1**   Sedative, hypnotic or anxiolytic-related abuse

> **Excludes1**   sedative, hypnotic or anxiolytic-related dependence (F13.2-)
> sedative, hypnotic, or anxiolytic use, unspecified (F13.9-)

F13.10   Sedative, hypnotic or anxiolytic abuse, uncomplicated
> Sedative, hypnotic, or anxiolytic use disorder, mild

F13.11   Sedative, hypnotic or anxiolytic abuse, in remission
> Sedative, hypnotic or anxiolytic use disorder, mild, in early remission
> Sedative, hypnotic or anxiolytic use disorder, mild, in sustained remission

● **F13.12**   Sedative, hypnotic or anxiolytic abuse with intoxication

F13.120   Sedative, hypnotic or anxiolytic abuse with intoxication, uncomplicated

F13.121   Sedative, hypnotic or anxiolytic abuse with intoxication delirium

F13.129   Sedative, hypnotic or anxiolytic abuse with intoxication, unspecified

● **F13.13**   Sedative, hypnotic or anxiolytic abuse with withdrawal

F13.130   Sedative, hypnotic or anxiolytic abuse with withdrawal, uncomplicated

F13.131   Sedative, hypnotic or anxiolytic abuse with withdrawal delirium

F13.132   Sedative, hypnotic or anxiolytic abuse with withdrawal with perceptual disturbance

F13.139   Sedative, hypnotic or anxiolytic abuse with withdrawal, unspecified

F13.14   Sedative, hypnotic or anxiolytic abuse with sedative, hypnotic or anxiolytic-induced mood disorder
> Sedative, hypnotic, or anxiolytic use disorder, mild, with sedative, hypnotic, or anxiolytic-induced bipolar or related disorder
> Sedative, hypnotic, or anxiolytic use disorder, mild, with sedative, hypnotic, or anxiolytic-induced depressive disorder

● **F13.15**   Sedative, hypnotic or anxiolytic abuse with sedative, hypnotic or anxiolytic-induced psychotic disorder

F13.150   Sedative, hypnotic or anxiolytic abuse with sedative, hypnotic or anxiolytic-induced psychotic disorder with delusions

F13.151   Sedative, hypnotic or anxiolytic abuse with sedative, hypnotic or anxiolytic-induced psychotic disorder with hallucinations

F13.159 Sedative, hypnotic or anxiolytic abuse with sedative, hypnotic or anxiolytic-induced psychotic disorder, unspecified

● **F13.18** Sedative, hypnotic or anxiolytic abuse with other sedative, hypnotic or anxiolytic-induced disorders

F13.180 Sedative, hypnotic or anxiolytic abuse with sedative, hypnotic or anxiolytic-induced anxiety disorder

F13.181 Sedative, hypnotic or anxiolytic abuse with sedative, hypnotic or anxiolytic-induced sexual dysfunction

F13.182 Sedative, hypnotic or anxiolytic abuse with sedative, hypnotic or anxiolytic-induced sleep disorder

F13.188 Sedative, hypnotic or anxiolytic abuse with other sedative, hypnotic or anxiolytic-induced disorder

F13.19 Sedative, hypnotic or anxiolytic abuse with unspecified sedative, hypnotic or anxiolytic-induced disorder

● **F13.2** Sedative, hypnotic or anxiolytic-related dependence

> **Excludes1** sedative, hypnotic or anxiolytic-related abuse (F13.1-)
> sedative, hypnotic, or anxiolytic use, unspecified (F13.9-)

> **Excludes2** sedative, hypnotic, or anxiolytic poisoning (T42.-)

F13.20 Sedative, hypnotic or anxiolytic dependence, uncomplicated

F13.21 Sedative, hypnotic or anxiolytic dependence, in remission
> Sedative, hypnotic or anxiolytic use disorder, moderate, in early remission
> Sedative, hypnotic or anxiolytic use disorder, moderate, in sustained remission
> Sedative, hypnotic or anxiolytic use disorder, severe, in early remission
> Sedative, hypnotic or anxiolytic use disorder, severe, in sustained remission

● **F13.22** Sedative, hypnotic or anxiolytic dependence with intoxication

> **Excludes1** sedative, hypnotic or anxiolytic dependence with withdrawal (F13.23-)

F13.220 Sedative, hypnotic or anxiolytic dependence with intoxication, uncomplicated

F13.221 Sedative, hypnotic or anxiolytic dependence with intoxication delirium

F13.229 Sedative, hypnotic or anxiolytic dependence with intoxication, unspecified

● **F13.23** Sedative, hypnotic or anxiolytic dependence with withdrawal
> Sedative, hypnotic, or anxiolytic use disorder, moderate
> Sedative, hypnotic, or anxiolytic use disorder, severe

> **Excludes1** sedative, hypnotic or anxiolytic dependence with intoxication (F13.22-)

F13.230 Sedative, hypnotic or anxiolytic dependence with withdrawal, uncomplicated

F13.231 Sedative, hypnotic or anxiolytic dependence with withdrawal delirium

F13.232 Sedative, hypnotic or anxiolytic dependence with withdrawal with perceptual disturbance
> Sedative, hypnotic, or anxiolytic withdrawal with perceptual disturbances

F13.239 Sedative, hypnotic or anxiolytic dependence with withdrawal, unspecified
> Sedative, hypnotic, or anxiolytic withdrawal without perceptual disturbances

F13.24 Sedative, hypnotic or anxiolytic dependence with sedative, hypnotic or anxiolytic-induced mood disorder
> Sedative, hypnotic, or anxiolytic use disorder, moderate, with sedative, hypnotic, or anxiolytic-induced bipolar or related disorder
> Sedative, hypnotic, or anxiolytic use disorder, moderate, with sedative, hypnotic, or anxiolytic-induced depressive disorder
> Sedative, hypnotic, or anxiolytic use disorder, severe, with sedative, hypnotic, or anxiolytic-induced bipolar or related disorder
> Sedative, hypnotic, or anxiolytic use disorder, severe, with sedative, hypnotic, or anxiolytic-induced depressive disorder

● **F13.25** Sedative, hypnotic or anxiolytic dependence with sedative, hypnotic or anxiolytic-induced psychotic disorder

F13.250 Sedative, hypnotic or anxiolytic dependence with sedative, hypnotic or anxiolytic-induced psychotic disorder with delusions

F13.251 Sedative, hypnotic or anxiolytic dependence with sedative, hypnotic or anxiolytic-induced psychotic disorder with hallucinations

F13.259 Sedative, hypnotic or anxiolytic dependence with sedative, hypnotic or anxiolytic-induced psychotic disorder, unspecified

F13.26 Sedative, hypnotic or anxiolytic dependence with sedative, hypnotic or anxiolytic-induced persisting amnestic disorder

F13.27 Sedative, hypnotic or anxiolytic dependence with sedative, hypnotic or anxiolytic-induced persisting dementia
> Sedative, hypnotic, or anxiolytic use disorder, moderate, with sedative, hypnotic, or anxiolytic-induced major neurocognitive disorder
> Sedative, hypnotic, or anxiolytic use disorder, severe, with sedative, hypnotic, or anxiolytic-induced major neurocognitive disorder

● **F13.28** Sedative, hypnotic or anxiolytic dependence with other sedative, hypnotic or anxiolytic-induced disorders

F13.280 Sedative, hypnotic or anxiolytic dependence with sedative, hypnotic or anxiolytic-induced anxiety disorder

F13.281 Sedative, hypnotic or anxiolytic dependence with sedative, hypnotic or anxiolytic-induced sexual dysfunction

CHAPTER 5 (F01-F99)

F13.282 Sedative, hypnotic or anxiolytic dependence with sedative, hypnotic or anxiolytic-induced sleep disorder

F13.288 Sedative, hypnotic or anxiolytic dependence with other sedative, hypnotic or anxiolytic-induced disorder
> Sedative, hypnotic, or anxiolytic use disorder, moderate, with sedative, hypnotic, or anxiolytic-induced mild neurocognitive disorder
> Sedative, hypnotic, or anxiolytic use disorder, severe, with sedative, hypnotic, or anxiolytic-induced mild neurocognitive disorder

F13.29 Sedative, hypnotic or anxiolytic dependence with unspecified sedative, hypnotic or anxiolytic-induced disorder

● **F13.9** Sedative, hypnotic or anxiolytic-related use, unspecified
> **Excludes1**   sedative, hypnotic or anxiolytic-related abuse (F13.1-)
> sedative, hypnotic or anxiolytic-related dependence (F13.2-)

F13.90 Sedative, hypnotic, or anxiolytic use, unspecified, uncomplicated

F13.91 Sedative, hypnotic or anxiolytic use, unspecified, in remission

● **F13.92** Sedative, hypnotic or anxiolytic use, unspecified with intoxication
> **Excludes1**   sedative, hypnotic or anxiolytic use, unspecified with withdrawal (F13.93-)

F13.920 Sedative, hypnotic or anxiolytic use, unspecified with intoxication, uncomplicated

F13.921 Sedative, hypnotic or anxiolytic use, unspecified with intoxication delirium
> Sedative, hypnotic, or anxiolytic-induced delirium

F13.929 Sedative, hypnotic or anxiolytic use, unspecified with intoxication, unspecified

● **F13.93** Sedative, hypnotic or anxiolytic use, unspecified with withdrawal
> **Excludes1**   sedative, hypnotic or anxiolytic use, unspecified with intoxication (F13.92-)

F13.930 Sedative, hypnotic or anxiolytic use, unspecified with withdrawal, uncomplicated

F13.931 Sedative, hypnotic or anxiolytic use, unspecified with withdrawal delirium

F13.932 Sedative, hypnotic or anxiolytic use, unspecified with withdrawal with perceptual disturbances

F13.939 Sedative, hypnotic or anxiolytic use, unspecified with withdrawal, unspecified

F13.94 Sedative, hypnotic or anxiolytic use, unspecified with sedative, hypnotic or anxiolytic-induced mood disorder
> Sedative, hypnotic, or anxiolytic-induced bipolar or related disorder, without use disorder
> Sedative, hypnotic, or anxiolytic-induced depressive disorder, without use disorder

● **F13.95** Sedative, hypnotic or anxiolytic use, unspecified with sedative, hypnotic or anxiolytic-induced psychotic disorder

F13.950 Sedative, hypnotic or anxiolytic use, unspecified with sedative, hypnotic or anxiolytic-induced psychotic disorder with delusions

F13.951 Sedative, hypnotic or anxiolytic use, unspecified with sedative, hypnotic or anxiolytic-induced psychotic disorder with hallucinations

F13.959 Sedative, hypnotic or anxiolytic use, unspecified with sedative, hypnotic or anxiolytic-induced psychotic disorder, unspecified
> Sedative, hypnotic, or anxiolytic-induced psychotic disorder, without use disorder

F13.96 Sedative, hypnotic or anxiolytic use, unspecified with sedative, hypnotic or anxiolytic-induced persisting amnestic disorder

F13.97 Sedative, hypnotic or anxiolytic use, unspecified with sedative, hypnotic or anxiolytic-induced persisting dementia
> Sedative, hypnotic, or anxiolytic-induced major neurocognitive disorder, without use disorder

● **F13.98** Sedative, hypnotic or anxiolytic use, unspecified with other sedative, hypnotic or anxiolytic-induced disorders

F13.980 Sedative, hypnotic or anxiolytic use, unspecified with sedative, hypnotic or anxiolytic-induced anxiety disorder
> Sedative, hypnotic, or anxiolytic-induced anxiety disorder, without use disorder

F13.981 Sedative, hypnotic or anxiolytic use, unspecified with sedative, hypnotic or anxiolytic-induced sexual dysfunction
> Sedative, hypnotic, or anxiolytic-induced sexual dysfunction disorder, without use disorder

F13.982 Sedative, hypnotic or anxiolytic use, unspecified with sedative, hypnotic or anxiolytic-induced sleep disorder
> Sedative, hypnotic, or anxiolytic-induced sleep disorder, without use disorder

F13.988 Sedative, hypnotic or anxiolytic use, unspecified with other sedative, hypnotic or anxiolytic-induced disorder
> Sedative, hypnotic, or anxiolytic-induced mild neurocognitive disorder

F13.99 Sedative, hypnotic or anxiolytic use, unspecified with unspecified sedative, hypnotic or anxiolytic-induced disorder

● **F14 Cocaine related disorders**
    Excludes2 other stimulant-related disorders (F15.-)

  ● **F14.1 Cocaine abuse**
      Excludes1 cocaine dependence (F14.2-)
             cocaine use, unspecified (F14.9-)
    F14.10 **Cocaine abuse, uncomplicated**
        Cocaine use disorder, mild
    F14.11 **Cocaine abuse, in remission**
        Cocaine use disorder, mild, in early remission
        Cocaine use disorder, mild, in sustained remission
    ● **F14.12 Cocaine abuse with intoxication**
        F14.120 **Cocaine abuse with intoxication, uncomplicated** ℞
        F14.121 **Cocaine abuse with intoxication with delirium** ℞
        F14.122 **Cocaine abuse with intoxication with perceptual disturbance** ℞
        F14.129 **Cocaine abuse with intoxication, unspecified** ℞
    F14.13 **Cocaine abuse, unspecified with withdrawal**
    F14.14 **Cocaine abuse with cocaine-induced mood disorder** ℞
        Cocaine use disorder, mild, with cocaine-induced bipolar or related disorder
        Cocaine use disorder, mild, with cocaine-induced depressive disorder
    ● **F14.15 Cocaine abuse with cocaine-induced psychotic disorder**
        F14.150 **Cocaine abuse with cocaine-induced psychotic disorder with delusions** ℞
        F14.151 **Cocaine abuse with cocaine-induced psychotic disorder with hallucinations** ℞
        F14.159 **Cocaine abuse with cocaine-induced psychotic disorder, unspecified** ℞
    ● **F14.18 Cocaine abuse with other cocaine-induced disorder**
        F14.180 **Cocaine abuse with cocaine-induced anxiety disorder** ℞
        F14.181 **Cocaine abuse with cocaine-induced sexual dysfunction** ℞
        F14.182 **Cocaine abuse with cocaine-induced sleep disorder** ℞
        F14.188 **Cocaine abuse with other cocaine-induced disorder** ℞
            Cocaine use disorder, mild, with cocaine-induced obsessive-compulsive or related disorder
    F14.19 **Cocaine abuse with unspecified cocaine-induced disorder** ℞

  ● **F14.2 Cocaine dependence**
      Excludes1 cocaine abuse (F14.1-)
             cocaine use, unspecified (F14.9-)
      Excludes2 cocaine poisoning (T40.5-)
    F14.20 **Cocaine dependence, uncomplicated** ℞
        Cocaine use disorder, moderate
        Cocaine use disorder, severe
    F14.21 **Cocaine dependence, in remission** ℞
        Cocaine use disorder, moderate, in early remission
        Cocaine use disorder, moderate, in sustained remission
        Cocaine use disorder, severe, in early remission
        Cocaine use disorder, severe, in sustained remission
        Coding Clinic: 2017, Q2, P27

  ● **F14.22 Cocaine dependence with intoxication**
      Excludes1 cocaine dependence with withdrawal (F14.23)
        F14.220 **Cocaine dependence with intoxication, uncomplicated** ℞
        F14.221 **Cocaine dependence with intoxication delirium** ℞
        F14.222 **Cocaine dependence with intoxication with perceptual disturbance** ℞
        F14.229 **Cocaine dependence with intoxication, unspecified** ℞
    F14.23 **Cocaine dependence with withdrawal** ℞
      Excludes1 cocaine dependence with intoxication (F14.22-)
    F14.24 **Cocaine dependence with cocaine-induced mood disorder** ℞
        Cocaine use disorder, moderate, with cocaine-induced bipolar or related disorder
        Cocaine use disorder, moderate, with cocaine-induced depressive disorder
        Cocaine use disorder, severe, with cocaine-induced bipolar or related disorder
        Cocaine use disorder, severe, with cocaine-induced depressive disorder
    ● **F14.25 Cocaine dependence with cocaine-induced psychotic disorder**
        F14.250 **Cocaine dependence with cocaine-induced psychotic disorder with delusions** ℞
        F14.251 **Cocaine dependence with cocaine-induced psychotic disorder with hallucinations** ℞
        F14.259 **Cocaine dependence with cocaine-induced psychotic disorder, unspecified** ℞
    ● **F14.28 Cocaine dependence with other cocaine-induced disorder**
        F14.280 **Cocaine dependence with cocaine-induced anxiety disorder** ℞
        F14.281 **Cocaine dependence with cocaine-induced sexual dysfunction** ℞
        F14.282 **Cocaine dependence with cocaine-induced sleep disorder** ℞
        F14.288 **Cocaine dependence with other cocaine-induced disorder** ℞
            Cocaine use disorder, moderate, with cocaine-induced obsessive-compulsive or related disorder
            Cocaine use disorder, severe, with cocaine-induced obsessive-compulsive or related disorder
    F14.29 **Cocaine dependence with unspecified cocaine-induced disorder** ℞

  ● **F14.9 Cocaine use, unspecified**
      Excludes1 cocaine abuse (F14.1-)
             cocaine dependence (F14.2-)
    F14.90 **Cocaine use, unspecified, uncomplicated**
        Coding Clinic: 2018, Q2, P11
    F14.91 **Cocaine use, unspecified, in remission**
    ● **F14.92 Cocaine use, unspecified with intoxication**
        F14.920 **Cocaine use, unspecified with intoxication, uncomplicated** ℞
        F14.921 **Cocaine use, unspecified with intoxication delirium** ℞

F14.922 Cocaine use, unspecified with intoxication with perceptual disturbance `Rcc`

F14.929 Cocaine use, unspecified with intoxication, unspecified `Rcc`

F14.93 Cocaine use, unspecified with withdrawal

F14.94 Cocaine use, unspecified with cocaine-induced mood disorder `Rcc`
Cocaine-induced bipolar or related disorder, without use disorder
Cocaine-induced depressive disorder, without use disorder

● **F14.95 Cocaine use, unspecified with cocaine-induced psychotic disorder**

F14.950 Cocaine use, unspecified with cocaine-induced psychotic disorder with delusions `Rcc`

F14.951 Cocaine use, unspecified with cocaine-induced psychotic disorder with hallucinations `Rcc`

F14.959 Cocaine use, unspecified with cocaine-induced psychotic disorder, unspecified `Rcc`
Cocaine-induced psychotic disorder, without use disorder

● **F14.98 Cocaine use, unspecified with other specified cocaine-induced disorder**

F14.980 Cocaine use, unspecified with cocaine-induced anxiety disorder `Rcc`
Cocaine-induced anxiety disorder, without use disorder

F14.981 Cocaine use, unspecified with cocaine-induced sexual dysfunction `Rcc`
Cocaine-induced sexual dysfunction, without use disorder

F14.982 Cocaine use, unspecified with cocaine-induced sleep disorder `Rcc`
Cocaine-induced sleep disorder, without use disorder

F14.988 Cocaine use, unspecified with other cocaine-induced disorder `Rcc`
Cocaine-induced obsessive-compulsive or related disorder

F14.99 Cocaine use, unspecified with unspecified cocaine-induced disorder `Rcc`

● **F15 Other stimulant related disorders**

Includes	amphetamine-related disorders caffeine

Excludes2 cocaine-related disorders (F14.-)

● **F15.1 Other stimulant abuse**

Excludes1 other stimulant dependence (F15.2-)
other stimulant use, unspecified (F15.9-)

F15.10 Other stimulant abuse, uncomplicated
Amphetamine type substance use disorder, mild
Other or unspecified stimulant use disorder, mild

F15.11 Other stimulant abuse, in remission
Amphetamine type substance use disorder, mild, in early remission
Amphetamine type substance use disorder, mild, in sustained remission
Other or unspecified stimulant use disorder, mild, in early remission
Other or unspecified stimulant use disorder, mild, in sustained remission
Coding Clinic: 2021, Q3, P8

● **F15.12 Other stimulant abuse with intoxication**

F15.120 Other stimulant abuse with intoxication, uncomplicated `Rcc`

F15.121 Other stimulant abuse with intoxication delirium `Rcc`

F15.122 Other stimulant abuse with intoxication with perceptual disturbance `Rcc`
Amphetamine or other stimulant use disorder, mild, with amphetamine or other stimulant intoxication, with perceptual disturbances

F15.129 Other stimulant abuse with intoxication, unspecified `Rcc`
Amphetamine or other stimulant use disorder, mild, with amphetamine or other stimulant intoxication, without perceptual disturbances

F15.13 Other stimulant abuse with withdrawal

F15.14 Other stimulant abuse with stimulant-induced mood disorder `Rcc`
Amphetamine or other stimulant use disorder, mild, with amphetamine or other stimulant-induced bipolar or related disorder
Amphetamine or other stimulant use disorder, mild, with amphetamine or other stimulant-induced depressive disorder

● **F15.15 Other stimulant abuse with stimulant-induced psychotic disorder**

F15.150 Other stimulant abuse with stimulant-induced psychotic disorder with delusions `Rcc`

F15.151 Other stimulant abuse with stimulant-induced psychotic disorder with hallucinations `Rcc`

F15.159 Other stimulant abuse with stimulant-induced psychotic disorder, unspecified `Rcc`

● **F15.18 Other stimulant abuse with other stimulant-induced disorder**

F15.180 Other stimulant abuse with stimulant-induced anxiety disorder `Rcc`

F15.181 Other stimulant abuse with stimulant-induced sexual dysfunction `Rcc`

F15.182 Other stimulant abuse with stimulant-induced sleep disorder `Rcc`

F15.188 Other stimulant abuse with other stimulant-induced disorder `Rcc`
Amphetamine or other stimulant use disorder, mild, with amphetamine or other stimulant-induced obsessive-compulsive or related disorder

F15.19 Other stimulant abuse with unspecified stimulant-induced disorder `Rcc`

● **F15.2 Other stimulant dependence**

Excludes1 other stimulant abuse (F15.1-)
other stimulant use, unspecified (F15.9-)

F15.20 Other stimulant dependence, uncomplicated `Rcc`
Amphetamine type substance use disorder, moderate
Amphetamine type substance use disorder, severe
Other or unspecified stimulant use disorder, moderate
Other or unspecified stimulant use disorder, severe

F15.21   **Other stimulant dependence, in remission**
    Amphetamine type substance use disorder, moderate, in early remission
    Amphetamine type substance use disorder, moderate, in sustained remission
    Amphetamine type substance use disorder, severe, in early remission
    Amphetamine type substance use disorder, severe, in sustained remission
    Other or unspecified stimulant use disorder, moderate, in early remission
    Other or unspecified stimulant use disorder, moderate, in sustained remission
    Other or unspecified stimulant use disorder, severe, in early remission
    Other or unspecified stimulant use disorder, severe, in sustained remission

● **F15.22**   **Other stimulant dependence with intoxication**
    Excludes1   other stimulant dependence with withdrawal (F15.23)

F15.220   **Other stimulant dependence with intoxication, uncomplicated**

F15.221   **Other stimulant dependence with intoxication delirium**

F15.222   **Other stimulant dependence with intoxication with perceptual disturbance**
    Amphetamine or other stimulant use disorder, moderate, with amphetamine or other stimulant intoxication, with perceptual disturbances
    Amphetamine or other stimulant use disorder, severe, with amphetamine or other stimulant intoxication, with perceptual disturbances

F15.229   **Other stimulant dependence with intoxication, unspecified**
    Amphetamine or other stimulant use disorder, moderate, with amphetamine or other stimulant intoxication, without perceptual disturbances
    Amphetamine or other stimulant use disorder, severe, with amphetamine or other stimulant intoxication, without perceptual disturbances

F15.23   **Other stimulant dependence with withdrawal**
    Amphetamine or other stimulant withdrawal
    Excludes1   other stimulant dependence with intoxication (F15.22-)

F15.24   **Other stimulant dependence with stimulant-induced mood disorder**
    Amphetamine or other stimulant use disorder, moderate, with amphetamine or other stimulant-induced bipolar or related disorder
    Amphetamine or other stimulant use disorder, moderate, with amphetamine or other stimulant-induced depressive disorder
    Amphetamine or other stimulant use disorder, severe, with amphetamine or other stimulant-induced bipolar or related disorder
    Amphetamine or other stimulant use disorder, severe, with amphetamine or other stimulant-induced depressive disorder

● **F15.25**   **Other stimulant dependence with stimulant-induced psychotic disorder**

F15.250   **Other stimulant dependence with stimulant-induced psychotic disorder with delusions**

F15.251   **Other stimulant dependence with stimulant-induced psychotic disorder with hallucinations**

F15.259   **Other stimulant dependence with stimulant-induced psychotic disorder, unspecified**

● **F15.28**   **Other stimulant dependence with other stimulant-induced disorder**

F15.280   **Other stimulant dependence with stimulant-induced anxiety disorder**

F15.281   **Other stimulant dependence with stimulant-induced sexual dysfunction**

F15.282   **Other stimulant dependence with stimulant-induced sleep disorder**

F15.288   **Other stimulant dependence with other stimulant-induced disorder**
    Amphetamine or other stimulant use disorder, moderate, with amphetamine or other stimulant-induced obsessive-compulsive or related disorder
    Amphetamine or other stimulant use disorder, severe, with amphetamine or other stimulant-induced obsessive-compulsive or related disorder

F15.29   **Other stimulant dependence with unspecified stimulant-induced disorder**

● **F15.9**   **Other stimulant use, unspecified**
    Excludes1   other stimulant abuse (F15.1-)
        other stimulant dependence (F15.2-)

F15.90   **Other stimulant use, unspecified, uncomplicated**
    Coding Clinic: 2022, Q4, P46

F15.91   **Other stimulant use, unspecified, in remission**

● **F15.92**   **Other stimulant use, unspecified with intoxication**
    Excludes1   other stimulant use, unspecified with withdrawal (F15.93)

F15.920   **Other stimulant use, unspecified with intoxication, uncomplicated**

F15.921   **Other stimulant use, unspecified with intoxication delirium**
    Amphetamine or other stimulant-induced delirium

F15.922   **Other stimulant use, unspecified with intoxication with perceptual disturbance**

F15.929   **Other stimulant use, unspecified with intoxication, unspecified**
    Caffeine intoxication

F15.93   **Other stimulant use, unspecified with withdrawal**
    Caffeine withdrawal
    Excludes1   other stimulant use, unspecified with intoxication (F15.92-)

F15.94   **Other stimulant use, unspecified with stimulant-induced mood disorder**
    Amphetamine or other stimulant-induced bipolar or related disorder, without use disorder
    Amphetamine or other stimulant-induced depressive disorder, without use disorder

● **F15.95**   **Other stimulant use, unspecified with stimulant-induced psychotic disorder**

F15.950   **Other stimulant use, unspecified with stimulant-induced psychotic disorder with delusions**

F15.951   Other stimulant use, unspecified with stimulant-induced psychotic disorder with hallucinations ⬓

F15.959   Other stimulant use, unspecified with stimulant-induced psychotic disorder, unspecified ⬓
- Amphetamine or other stimulant-induced psychotic disorder, without use disorder

● **F15.98   Other stimulant use, unspecified with other stimulant-induced disorder**

F15.980   Other stimulant use, unspecified with stimulant-induced anxiety disorder ⬓
- Amphetamine or other stimulant-induced anxiety disorder, without use disorder
- Caffeine-induced anxiety disorder, without use disorder

F15.981   Other stimulant use, unspecified with stimulant-induced sexual dysfunction ⬓
- Amphetamine or other stimulant-induced sexual dysfunction, without use disorder

F15.982   Other stimulant use, unspecified with stimulant-induced sleep disorder ⬓
- Amphetamine or other stimulant-induced sleep disorder, without use disorder
- Caffeine-induced sleep disorder, without use disorder

F15.988   Other stimulant use, unspecified with other stimulant-induced disorder ⬓
- Amphetamine or other stimulant-induced obsessive-compulsive or related disorder, without use disorder

F15.99   Other stimulant use, unspecified with unspecified stimulant-induced disorder ⬓

● **F16   Hallucinogen related disorders**

    Includes   ecstasy
- PCP
- phencyclidine

● **F16.1   Hallucinogen abuse**

    Excludes 1   hallucinogen dependence (F16.2-)
- hallucinogen use, unspecified (F16.9-)

F16.10   Hallucinogen abuse, uncomplicated
- Other hallucinogen use disorder, mild
- Phencyclidine use disorder, mild
- **Coding Clinic: 2018, Q4, P31**

F16.11   Hallucinogen abuse, in remission
- Other hallucinogen use disorder, mild, in early remission
- Other hallucinogen use disorder, mild, in sustained remission
- Phencyclidine use disorder, mild, in early remission
- Phencyclidine use disorder, mild, in sustained remission

● F16.12   Hallucinogen abuse with intoxication

F16.120   Hallucinogen abuse with intoxication, uncomplicated ⬓

F16.121   Hallucinogen abuse with intoxication with delirium ⬓

F16.122   Hallucinogen abuse with intoxication with perceptual disturbance ⬓

F16.129   Hallucinogen abuse with intoxication, unspecified ⬓

F16.14   Hallucinogen abuse with hallucinogen-induced mood disorder ⬓
- Other hallucinogen use disorder, mild, with other hallucinogen-induced bipolar or related disorder
- Other hallucinogen use disorder, mild, with other hallucinogen-induced depressive disorder
- Phencyclidine use disorder, mild, with phencyclidine-induced bipolar or related disorder
- Phencyclidine use disorder, mild, with phencyclidine-induced depressive disorder

● F16.15   Hallucinogen abuse with hallucinogen-induced psychotic disorder

F16.150   Hallucinogen abuse with hallucinogen-induced psychotic disorder with delusions ⬓

F16.151   Hallucinogen abuse with hallucinogen-induced psychotic disorder with hallucinations ⬓

F16.159   Hallucinogen abuse with hallucinogen-induced psychotic disorder, unspecified ⬓

● F16.18   Hallucinogen abuse with other hallucinogen-induced disorder

F16.180   Hallucinogen abuse with hallucinogen-induced anxiety disorder ⬓

F16.183   Hallucinogen abuse with hallucinogen persisting perception disorder (flashbacks) ⬓

F16.188   Hallucinogen abuse with other hallucinogen-induced disorder ⬓

F16.19   Hallucinogen abuse with unspecified hallucinogen-induced disorder ⬓

● **F16.2   Hallucinogen dependence**

    Excludes 1   hallucinogen abuse (F16.1-)
- hallucinogen use, unspecified (F16.9-)

F16.20   Hallucinogen dependence, uncomplicated ⬓
- Other hallucinogen use disorder, moderate
- Other hallucinogen use disorder, severe
- Phencyclidine use disorder, moderate
- Phencyclidine use disorder, severe

F16.21   Hallucinogen dependence, in remission ⬓
- Other hallucinogen use disorder, moderate, in early remission
- Other hallucinogen use disorder, moderate, in sustained remission
- Other hallucinogen use disorder, severe, in early remission
- Other hallucinogen use disorder, severe, in sustained remission
- Phencyclidine use disorder, moderate, in early remission
- Phencyclidine use disorder, moderate, in sustained remission
- Phencyclidine use disorder, severe, in early remission
- Phencyclidine use disorder, severe, in sustained remission

● F16.22   Hallucinogen dependence with intoxication

F16.220   Hallucinogen dependence with intoxication, uncomplicated ⬓

F16.221   Hallucinogen dependence with intoxication with delirium ⬓

F16.229   Hallucinogen dependence with intoxication, unspecified ⬓

▶ New   ⇨ Revised   ~~deleted~~ Deleted   Excludes 1   Excludes 2   Includes   Use additional   Code first   Code also   Key words

OGCR Official Guidelines   X Assign placeholder X   ● Use Additional Character(s)   ⬧ Manifestation Code   ⬓ Hierarchical Condition Category   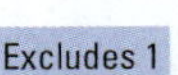 **Coding Clinic**

F16.24 **Hallucinogen dependence with hallucinogen-induced mood disorder** ℞

Other hallucinogen use disorder, moderate, with other hallucinogen-induced bipolar or related disorder

Other hallucinogen use disorder, moderate, with other hallucinogen-induced depressive disorder

Other hallucinogen use disorder, severe, with other hallucinogen-induced bipolar or related disorder

Other hallucinogen use disorder, severe, with other hallucinogen-induced depressive disorder

Phencyclidine use disorder, moderate, with phencyclidine-induced bipolar or related disorder

Phencyclidine use disorder, moderate, with phencyclidine-induced depressive disorder

Phencyclidine use disorder, severe, with phencyclidine-induced bipolar or related disorder

Phencyclidine use disorder, severe, with phencyclidine-induced depressive disorder

● **F16.25** **Hallucinogen dependence with hallucinogen-induced psychotic disorder**

F16.250 **Hallucinogen dependence with hallucinogen-induced psychotic disorder with delusions** ℞

F16.251 **Hallucinogen dependence with hallucinogen-induced psychotic disorder with hallucinations** ℞

F16.259 **Hallucinogen dependence with hallucinogen-induced psychotic disorder, unspecified** ℞

● **F16.28** **Hallucinogen dependence with other hallucinogen-induced disorder**

F16.280 **Hallucinogen dependence with hallucinogen-induced anxiety disorder** ℞

F16.283 **Hallucinogen dependence with hallucinogen persisting perception disorder (flashbacks)** ℞

F16.288 **Hallucinogen dependence with other hallucinogen-induced disorder** ℞

F16.29 **Hallucinogen dependence with unspecified hallucinogen-induced disorder** ℞

● **F16.9** **Hallucinogen use, unspecified**

Excludes1   hallucinogen abuse (F16.1-)
hallucinogen dependence (F16.2-)

F16.90 **Hallucinogen use, unspecified, uncomplicated**

F16.91 **Hallucinogen use, unspecified, in remission**

● **F16.92** **Hallucinogen use, unspecified with intoxication**

F16.920 **Hallucinogen use, unspecified with intoxication, uncomplicated** ℞

F16.921 **Hallucinogen use, unspecified with intoxication with delirium** ℞

Other hallucinogen intoxication delirium

F16.929 **Hallucinogen use, unspecified with intoxication, unspecified** ℞

F16.94 **Hallucinogen use, unspecified with hallucinogen-induced mood disorder** ℞

Other hallucinogen-induced bipolar or related disorder, without use disorder

Other hallucinogen-induced depressive disorder, without use disorder

Phencyclidine-induced bipolar or related disorder, without use disorder

Phencyclidine-induced depressive disorder, without use disorder

● **F16.95** **Hallucinogen use, unspecified with hallucinogen-induced psychotic disorder**

F16.950 **Hallucinogen use, unspecified with hallucinogen-induced psychotic disorder with delusions** ℞

F16.951 **Hallucinogen use, unspecified with hallucinogen-induced psychotic disorder with hallucinations** ℞

F16.959 **Hallucinogen use, unspecified with hallucinogen-induced psychotic disorder, unspecified**

Other hallucinogen-induced psychotic disorder, without use disorder

Phencyclidine-induced psychotic disorder, without use disorder

● **F16.98** **Hallucinogen use, unspecified with other specified hallucinogen-induced disorder**

F16.980 **Hallucinogen use, unspecified with hallucinogen-induced anxiety disorder** ℞

Other hallucinogen-induced anxiety disorder, without use disorder

Phencyclidine-induced anxiety disorder, without use disorder

F16.983 **Hallucinogen use, unspecified with hallucinogen persisting perception disorder (flashbacks)** ℞

F16.988 **Hallucinogen use, unspecified with other hallucinogen-induced disorder** ℞

F16.99 **Hallucinogen use, unspecified with unspecified hallucinogen-induced disorder** ℞

● **F17** **Nicotine dependence**

Excludes1   history of tobacco dependence (Z87.891)
tobacco use NOS (Z72.0)

Excludes2   tobacco use (smoking) during pregnancy, childbirth and the puerperium (O99.33-)
toxic effect of nicotine (T65.2-)

● **F17.2** **Nicotine dependence**

● **F17.20** **Nicotine dependence, unspecified**

F17.200 **Nicotine dependence, unspecified, uncomplicated**

Tobacco use disorder, mild
Tobacco use disorder, moderate
Tobacco use disorder, severe

Coding Clinic: 2016, Q1, P37

F17.201 **Nicotine dependence, unspecified, in remission**

Tobacco use disorder, mild, in early remission

Tobacco use disorder, mild, in sustained remission

Tobacco use disorder, moderate, in early remission

Tobacco use disorder, moderate, in sustained remission

Tobacco use disorder, severe, in early remission

Tobacco use disorder, severe, in sustained remission

F17.203   Nicotine dependence unspecified, with **withdrawal**
      Tobacco withdrawal

F17.208   Nicotine dependence, unspecified, with **other nicotine-induced disorders**

F17.209   Nicotine dependence, unspecified, with **unspecified** nicotine-induced disorders

● F17.21   Nicotine dependence, **cigarettes**

F17.210   Nicotine dependence, cigarettes, **uncomplicated**
      Coding Clinic: 2017, Q2, P28-29

F17.211   Nicotine dependence, cigarettes, **in remission**
      Tobacco use disorder, cigarettes, mild, in early remission
      Tobacco use disorder, cigarettes, mild, in sustained remission
      Tobacco use disorder, cigarettes, moderate, in early remission
      Tobacco use disorder, cigarettes, moderate, in sustained remission
      Tobacco use disorder, cigarettes, severe, in early remission
      Tobacco use disorder, cigarettes, severe, in sustained remission

F17.213   Nicotine dependence, cigarettes, with **withdrawal**

F17.218   Nicotine dependence, cigarettes, with other nicotine-induced disorders

F17.219   Nicotine dependence, cigarettes, with **unspecified** nicotine-induced disorders

● F17.22   Nicotine dependence, **chewing tobacco**

F17.220   Nicotine dependence, chewing tobacco, **uncomplicated**

F17.221   Nicotine dependence, chewing tobacco, **in remission**
      Tobacco use disorder, chewing tobacco, mild, in early remission
      Tobacco use disorder, chewing tobacco, mild, in sustained remission
      Tobacco use disorder, chewing tobacco, moderate, in early remission
      Tobacco use disorder, chewing tobacco, moderate, in sustained remission
      Tobacco use disorder, chewing tobacco, severe, in early remission
      Tobacco use disorder, chewing tobacco, severe, in sustained remission

F17.223   Nicotine dependence, chewing tobacco, with **withdrawal**

F17.228   Nicotine dependence, chewing tobacco, with **other nicotine-induced disorders**

F17.229   Nicotine dependence, chewing tobacco, with **unspecified** nicotine-induced disorders

● F17.29   Nicotine dependence, **other tobacco product**

F17.290   Nicotine dependence, other tobacco product, **uncomplicated**
      Coding Clinic: 2017, Q2, P28-29

F17.291   Nicotine dependence, other tobacco product, **in remission**
      Tobacco use disorder, other tobacco product, mild, in early remission
      Tobacco use disorder, other tobacco product, mild, in sustained remission
      Tobacco use disorder, other tobacco product, moderate, in early remission
      Tobacco use disorder, other tobacco product, moderate, in sustained remission
      Tobacco use disorder, other tobacco product, severe, in early remission
      Tobacco use disorder, other tobacco product, severe, in sustained remission

F17.293   Nicotine dependence, other tobacco product, with **withdrawal**

F17.298   Nicotine dependence, other tobacco product, with **other nicotine-induced disorders**

F17.299   Nicotine dependence, other tobacco product, with **unspecified** nicotine-induced disorders

● F18   Inhalant related disorders
    Includes   volatile solvents

● F18.1   Inhalant abuse
    Excludes1   inhalant dependence (F18.2-)
              inhalant use, unspecified (F18.9-)

F18.10   Inhalant abuse, **uncomplicated**
      Inhalant use disorder, mild

F18.11   Inhalant abuse, **in remission**
      Inhalant use disorder, mild, in early remission
      Inhalant use disorder, mild, in sustained remission

● F18.12   Inhalant abuse with **intoxication**

F18.120   Inhalant abuse with intoxication, **uncomplicated** 🅡🅒

F18.121   Inhalant abuse with intoxication **delirium** 🅡🅒

F18.129   Inhalant abuse with intoxication, **unspecified** 🅡🅒

F18.14   Inhalant abuse with inhalant-induced **mood disorder** 🅡🅒
      Inhalant use disorder, mild, with inhalant-induced depressive disorder

● F18.15   Inhalant abuse with inhalant-induced **psychotic disorder**

F18.150   Inhalant abuse with inhalant-induced psychotic disorder with **delusions** 🅡🅒

F18.151   Inhalant abuse with inhalant-induced psychotic disorder with **hallucinations** 🅡🅒

F18.159   Inhalant abuse with inhalant-induced psychotic disorder, **unspecified** 🅡🅒

F18.17   Inhalant abuse with inhalant-induced **dementia** 🅡🅒
      Inhalant use disorder, mild, with inhalant-induced major neurocognitive disorder

● F18.18   Inhalant abuse with other inhalant-induced disorders

F18.180   Inhalant abuse with inhalant-induced **anxiety disorder** 🅡🅒

F18.188   Inhalant abuse with **other inhalant-induced** disorder ℞
    Inhalant use disorder, mild, with inhalant-induced mild neurocognitive disorder

F18.19   Inhalant abuse with **unspecified inhalant-induced** disorder ℞

● **F18.2**   Inhalant **dependence**
    Excludes1   inhalant abuse (F18.1-)
           inhalant use, unspecified (F18.9-)

F18.20   Inhalant dependence, **uncomplicated** ℞
    Inhalant use disorder, moderate
    Inhalant use disorder, severe

F18.21   Inhalant dependence, in remission ℞
    Inhalant use disorder, moderate, in early remission
    Inhalant use disorder, moderate, in sustained remission
    Inhalant use disorder, severe, in early remission
    Inhalant use disorder, severe, in sustained remission

● **F18.22**   Inhalant dependence with **intoxication**

F18.220   Inhalant dependence with intoxication, **uncomplicated** ℞

F18.221   Inhalant dependence with intoxication delirium ℞

F18.229   Inhalant dependence with intoxication, **unspecified** ℞

F18.24   Inhalant dependence with inhalant-induced **mood disorder** ℞
    Inhalant use disorder, moderate, with inhalant-induced depressive disorder
    Inhalant use disorder, severe, with inhalant-induced depressive disorder

● **F18.25**   Inhalant dependence with inhalant-induced **psychotic disorder**

F18.250   Inhalant dependence with inhalant-induced psychotic disorder with **delusions** ℞

F18.251   Inhalant dependence with inhalant-induced psychotic disorder with **hallucinations** ℞

F18.259   Inhalant dependence with inhalant-induced psychotic disorder, **unspecified** ℞

F18.27   Inhalant dependence with inhalant-induced **dementia** ℞
    Inhalant use disorder, moderate, with inhalant-induced major neurocognitive disorder
    Inhalant use disorder, severe, with inhalant-induced major neurocognitive disorder

● **F18.28**   Inhalant dependence with other inhalant-induced disorders

F18.280   Inhalant dependence with inhalant-induced **anxiety disorder** ℞

F18.288   Inhalant dependence with **other inhalant-induced** disorder ℞
    Inhalant use disorder, moderate, with inhalant-induced mild neurocognitive disorder
    Inhalant use disorder, severe, with inhalant-induced mild neurocognitive disorder

F18.29   Inhalant dependence with **unspecified inhalant-induced** disorder ℞

● **F18.9**   Inhalant use, unspecified
    Excludes1   inhalant abuse (F18.1-)
           inhalant dependence (F18.2-)

F18.90   Inhalant use, **unspecified, uncomplicated**

F18.91   Inhalant use, unspecified, in remission

● **F18.92**   Inhalant use, **unspecified** with **intoxication**

F18.920   Inhalant use, unspecified with intoxication, **uncomplicated** ℞

F18.921   Inhalant use, unspecified with intoxication with **delirium** ℞

F18.929   Inhalant use, unspecified with intoxication, **unspecified** ℞

F18.94   Inhalant use, **unspecified** with inhalant-induced **mood disorder** ℞
    Inhalant-induced depressive disorder

● **F18.95**   Inhalant use, **unspecified** with inhalant-induced **psychotic disorder**

F18.950   Inhalant use, unspecified with inhalant-induced psychotic disorder with **delusions** ℞

F18.951   Inhalant use, unspecified with inhalant-induced psychotic disorder with **hallucinations** ℞

F18.959   Inhalant use, unspecified with inhalant-induced psychotic disorder, **unspecified** ℞

F18.97   Inhalant use, **unspecified** with inhalant-induced **persisting dementia** ℞
    Inhalant-induced major neurocognitive disorder

● **F18.98**   Inhalant use, **unspecified** with other inhalant-induced disorders

F18.980   Inhalant use, unspecified with inhalant-induced **anxiety disorder** ℞

F18.988   Inhalant use, unspecified with **other** inhalant-induced disorder ℞
    Inhalant-induced mild neurocognitive disorder

F18.99   Inhalant use, unspecified with **unspecified** inhalant-induced disorder ℞

● **F19**   Other psychoactive substance related disorders
    Includes   polysubstance drug use (indiscriminate drug use)

● **F19.1**   Other psychoactive substance **abuse**
    Excludes1   other psychoactive substance dependence (F19.2-)
           other psychoactive substance use, unspecified (F19.9-)

F19.10   Other psychoactive substance abuse, **uncomplicated**
    Other (or unknown) substance use disorder, mild

F19.11   Other psychoactive substance abuse, **in remission**
    Other (or unknown) substance use disorder, mild, in early remission
    Other (or unknown) substance use disorder, mild, in sustained remission

● **F19.12**   Other psychoactive substance abuse with **intoxication**

F19.120   Other psychoactive substance abuse with intoxication, **uncomplicated** ℞

F19.121   Other psychoactive substance abuse with intoxication delirium ℞

F19.122   Other psychoactive substance abuse with intoxication with **perceptual disturbances** ℞

F19.129   Other psychoactive substance abuse with intoxication, **unspecified** ℞

● **F19.13** **Other psychoactive substance abuse with withdrawal**

  F19.130 Other psychoactive substance abuse with withdrawal, uncomplicated

  F19.131 Other psychoactive substance abuse with withdrawal delirium

  F19.132 Other psychoactive substance abuse with withdrawal with perceptual disturbance

  F19.139 Other psychoactive substance abuse with withdrawal, unspecified
  Coding Clinic: 2023, Q3, P16

F19.14 **Other psychoactive substance abuse with psychoactive substance-induced mood disorder** 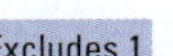
  Other (or unknown) substance use disorder, mild, with other (or unknown) substance-induced bipolar or related disorder
  Other (or unknown) substance use disorder, mild, with other (or unknown) substance-induced depressive disorder

● **F19.15** **Other psychoactive substance abuse with psychoactive substance-induced psychotic disorder**

  F19.150 Other psychoactive substance abuse with psychoactive substance-induced psychotic disorder with delusions

  F19.151 Other psychoactive substance abuse with psychoactive substance-induced psychotic disorder with hallucinations

  F19.159 Other psychoactive substance abuse with psychoactive substance-induced psychotic disorder, unspecified

F19.16 **Other psychoactive substance abuse with psychoactive substance-induced persisting amnestic disorder**

F19.17 **Other psychoactive substance abuse with psychoactive substance-induced persisting dementia**
  Other (or unknown) substance use disorder, mild, with other (or unknown) substance-induced major neurocognitive disorder

● **F19.18** **Other psychoactive substance abuse with other psychoactive substance-induced disorders**

  F19.180 Other psychoactive substance abuse with psychoactive substance-induced anxiety disorder

  F19.181 Other psychoactive substance abuse with psychoactive substance-induced sexual dysfunction

  F19.182 Other psychoactive substance abuse with psychoactive substance-induced sleep disorder

  F19.188 Other psychoactive substance abuse with other psychoactive substance-induced disorder
    Other (or unknown) substance use disorder, mild, with other (or unknown) substance-induced mild neurocognitive disorder
    Other (or unknown) substance use disorder, mild, with other (or unknown) substance-induced obsessive-compulsive or related disorder

F19.19 **Other psychoactive substance abuse with unspecified psychoactive substance-induced disorder**

● **F19.2** **Other psychoactive substance dependence**
  Excludes1 other psychoactive substance abuse (F19.1-)
    other psychoactive substance use, unspecified (F19.9-)

F19.20 **Other psychoactive substance dependence, uncomplicated**
    Other (or unknown) substance use disorder, moderate
    Other (or unknown) substance use disorder, severe

F19.21 **Other psychoactive substance dependence, in remission**
    Other (or unknown) substance use disorder, moderate, in early remission
    Other (or unknown) substance use disorder, moderate, in sustained remission
    Other (or unknown) substance use disorder, severe, in early remission
    Other (or unknown) substance use disorder, severe, in sustained remission

● **F19.22** **Other psychoactive substance dependence with intoxication**
  Excludes1 other psychoactive substance dependence with withdrawal (F19.23-)

  F19.220 Other psychoactive substance dependence with intoxication, uncomplicated

  F19.221 Other psychoactive substance dependence with intoxication delirium

  F19.222 Other psychoactive substance dependence with intoxication with perceptual disturbance

  F19.229 Other psychoactive substance dependence with intoxication, unspecified

● **F19.23** **Other psychoactive substance dependence with withdrawal**
  Excludes1 other psychoactive substance dependence with intoxication (F19.22-)

  F19.230 Other psychoactive substance dependence with withdrawal, uncomplicated

  F19.231 Other psychoactive substance dependence with withdrawal delirium

  F19.232 Other psychoactive substance dependence with withdrawal with perceptual disturbance

  F19.239 Other psychoactive substance dependence with withdrawal, unspecified

F19.24 **Other psychoactive substance dependence with psychoactive substance-induced mood disorder**
    Other (or unknown) substance use disorder, moderate, with other (or unknown) substance-induced bipolar or related disorder
    Other (or unknown) substance use disorder, moderate, with other (or unknown) substance-induced depressive disorder
    Other (or unknown) substance use disorder, severe, with other (or unknown) substance-induced bipolar or related disorder
    Other (or unknown) substance use disorder, severe, with other (or unknown) substance-induced depressive disorder

● **F19.25** **Other psychoactive substance dependence with psychoactive substance-induced psychotic disorder**

  F19.250 Other psychoactive substance dependence with psychoactive substance-induced psychotic disorder with delusions

  F19.251 Other psychoactive substance dependence with psychoactive substance-induced psychotic disorder with hallucinations

  F19.259 Other psychoactive substance dependence with psychoactive substance-induced psychotic disorder, unspecified

F19.26 **Other psychoactive substance dependence with psychoactive substance-induced persisting amnestic disorder**

F19.27 **Other psychoactive substance dependence with psychoactive substance-induced persisting dementia**

  Other (or unknown) substance use disorder, moderate, with other (or unknown) substance-induced major neurocognitive disorder

  Other (or unknown) substance use disorder, severe, with other (or unknown) substance-induced major neurocognitive disorder

● **F19.28** **Other psychoactive substance dependence with other psychoactive substance-induced disorders**

  F19.280 Other psychoactive substance dependence with psychoactive substance-induced anxiety disorder

  F19.281 Other psychoactive substance dependence with psychoactive substance-induced sexual dysfunction

  F19.282 Other psychoactive substance dependence with psychoactive substance-induced sleep disorder

  F19.288 Other psychoactive substance dependence with other psychoactive substance-induced disorder

    Other (or unknown) substance use disorder, moderate, with other (or unknown) substance-induced mild neurocognitive disorder

    Other (or unknown) substance use disorder, severe, with other (or unknown) substance-induced mild neurocognitive disorder

    Other (or unknown) substance use disorder, moderate, with other (or unknown) substance-induced obsessive-compulsive or related disorder

    Other (or unknown) substance use disorder, severe, with other (or unknown) substance-induced obsessive-compulsive or related disorder

F19.29 **Other psychoactive substance dependence with unspecified psychoactive substance-induced disorder**

● **F19.9** **Other psychoactive substance use, unspecified**

  Excludes1 other psychoactive substance abuse (F19.1-)
      other psychoactive substance dependence (F19.2-)

  F19.90 **Other psychoactive substance use, unspecified, uncomplicated**

F19.91 Other psychoactive substance use, unspecified, in remission

● **F19.92** Other psychoactive substance use, unspecified with intoxication

  Excludes1 other psychoactive substance use, unspecified with withdrawal (F19.93)

  F19.920 Other psychoactive substance use, unspecified with intoxication, uncomplicated

  F19.921 Other psychoactive substance use, unspecified with intoxication with delirium
    Other (or unknown) substance-induced delirium

  F19.922 Other psychoactive substance use, unspecified with intoxication with perceptual disturbance

  F19.929 Other psychoactive substance use, unspecified with intoxication, unspecified

● **F19.93** Other psychoactive substance use, unspecified with withdrawal

  Excludes1 other psychoactive substance use, unspecified with intoxication (F19.92-)

  F19.930 Other psychoactive substance use, unspecified with withdrawal, uncomplicated

  F19.931 Other psychoactive substance use, unspecified with withdrawal delirium

  F19.932 Other psychoactive substance use, unspecified with withdrawal with perceptual disturbance

  F19.939 Other psychoactive substance use, unspecified with withdrawal, unspecified

F19.94 Other psychoactive substance use, unspecified with psychoactive substance-induced mood disorder

  Other (or unknown) substance-induced bipolar or related disorder, without use disorder

  Other (or unknown) substance-induced depressive disorder, without use disorder

● **F19.95** Other psychoactive substance use, unspecified with psychoactive substance-induced psychotic disorder

  F19.950 Other psychoactive substance use, unspecified with psychoactive substance-induced psychotic disorder with delusions

  F19.951 Other psychoactive substance use, unspecified with psychoactive substance-induced psychotic disorder with hallucinations

  F19.959 Other psychoactive substance use, unspecified with psychoactive substance-induced psychotic disorder, unspecified
    Other or unknown substance-induced psychotic disorder, without use disorder

F19.96 Other psychoactive substance use, unspecified with psychoactive substance-induced persisting amnestic disorder

F19.97 Other psychoactive substance use, unspecified with psychoactive substance-induced persisting dementia
  Other (or unknown) substance-induced major neurocognitive disorder, without use disorder

● **F19.98** **Other psychoactive substance use, unspecified with other psychoactive substance-induced disorders**

    F19.980 **Other psychoactive substance use, unspecified with psychoactive substance-induced anxiety disorder** 🅡🅒
        Other (or unknown) substance-induced anxiety disorder, without use disorder

    F19.981 **Other psychoactive substance use, unspecified with psychoactive substance-induced sexual dysfunction** 🅡🅒
        Other (or unknown) substance-induced sexual dysfunction, without use disorder

    F19.982 **Other psychoactive substance use, unspecified with psychoactive substance-induced sleep disorder** 🅡🅒
        Other (or unknown) substance-induced sleep disorder, without use disorder

    F19.988 **Other psychoactive substance use, unspecified with other psychoactive substance-induced disorder** 🅡🅒
        Other (or unknown) substance-induced mild neurocognitive disorder, without use disorder
        Other (or unknown) substance-induced obsessive-compulsive or related disorder, without use disorder

  F19.99 **Other psychoactive substance use, unspecified with unspecified psychoactive substance-induced disorder** 🅡🅒

SCHIZOPHRENIA, SCHIZOTYPAL, DELUSIONAL, AND OTHER NON-MOOD PSYCHOTIC DISORDERS (F20-F29)

● **F20** **Schizophrenia**
Personality disorders characterized by multiple mental and behavioral irregularities (may exhibit disorganized thinking, delusions, and auditory hallucinations)

  Excludes1 brief psychotic disorder (F23)
            cyclic schizophrenia (F25.0)
            mood [affective] disorders with psychotic symptoms (F30.2, F31.2, F31.5, F31.64, F32.3, F33.3)
            schizoaffective disorder (F25.-)
            schizophrenic reaction NOS (F23)

  Excludes2 schizophrenic reaction in:
            alcoholism (F10.15-, F10.25-, F10.95-)
            brain disease (F06.2)
            epilepsy (F06.2)
            psychoactive drug use (F11-F19 with .15, .25, .95)
            schizotypal disorder (F21)

Use additional code, if applicable, to identify:
    other specified cognitive deficit (R41.84-)
Coding Clinic: 2019, Q2, P32

  F20.0 **Paranoid schizophrenia** 🅡🅒
    Paraphrenic schizophrenia
    Excludes1 involutional paranoid state (F22)
            paranoia (F22)

  F20.1 **Disorganized schizophrenia** 🅡🅒
    Hebephrenic schizophrenia
    Hebephrenia

  F20.2 **Catatonic schizophrenia** 🅡🅒
    Schizophrenic catalepsy
    Schizophrenic catatonia
    Schizophrenic flexibilitas cerea
    Excludes1 catatonic stupor (R40.1)

  F20.3 **Undifferentiated schizophrenia** 🅡🅒
    Atypical schizophrenia
    Excludes1 acute schizophrenia-like psychotic disorder (F23)
    Excludes2 post-schizophrenic depression (F32.89)

  F20.5 **Residual schizophrenia** 🅡🅒
    Restzustand (schizophrenic)
    Schizophrenic residual state

● **F20.8** **Other schizophrenia**
  F20.81 **Schizophreniform disorder** 🅡🅒
    Schizophreniform psychosis NOS
  F20.89 **Other schizophrenia** 🅡🅒
    Cenesthopathic schizophrenia
    Simple schizophrenia

  F20.9 **Schizophrenia, unspecified** 🅡🅒
Coding Clinic: 2019, Q2, P32

F21 **Schizotypal disorder**
Personality disorder characterized by need for social isolation, odd behavior and thinking, and often unconventional beliefs

  Borderline schizophrenia
  Latent schizophrenia
  Latent schizophrenic reaction
  Prepsychotic schizophrenia
  Prodromal schizophrenia
  Pseudoneurotic schizophrenia
  Pseudopsychopathic schizophrenia
  Schizotypal personality disorder
  Excludes2 Asperger's syndrome (F84.5)
            schizoid personality disorder (F60.1)

F22 **Delusional disorders** 🅡🅒
  Delusional dysmorphophobia
  Involutional paranoid state
  Paranoia
  Paranoia querulans
  Paranoid psychosis
  Paranoid state
  Paraphrenia (late)
  Sensitiver Beziehungswahn
  Excludes1 mood [affective] disorders with psychotic symptoms (F30.2, F31.2, F31.5, F31.64, F32.3, F33.3)
            paranoid schizophrenia (F20.0)
  Excludes2 paranoid personality disorder (F60.0)
            paranoid psychosis, psychogenic (F23)
            paranoid reaction (F23)

F23 **Brief psychotic disorder**
  Paranoid reaction
  Psychogenic paranoid psychosis
  Excludes2 mood [affective] disorders with psychotic symptoms (F30.2, F31.2, F31.5, F31.64, F32.3, F33.3)
Coding Clinic: 2019, Q2, P32

F24 **Shared psychotic disorder** 🅡🅒
  Folie à deux
  Induced paranoid disorder
  Induced psychotic disorder

● **F25** **Schizoaffective disorders**
Mental disorder exhibiting major depressive episode, manic episode, or mixed episode occurs with symptoms of schizophrenia, and mood disorder

  Excludes1 mood [affective] disorders with psychotic symptoms (F30.2, F31.2, F31.5, F31.64, F32.3, F33.3)
            schizophrenia (F20.-)

  F25.0 **Schizoaffective disorder, bipolar type** 🅡🅒
    Cyclic schizophrenia
    Schizoaffective disorder, manic type
    Schizoaffective disorder, mixed type
    Schizoaffective psychosis, bipolar type

  F25.1 **Schizoaffective disorder, depressive type** 🅡🅒
    Schizoaffective psychosis, depressive type

F25.8   Other schizoaffective disorders

F25.9   Schizoaffective disorder, unspecified
        Schizoaffective psychosis NOS

F28 **Other psychotic disorder not due to a substance or known physiological condition**
      Chronic hallucinatory psychosis
      Other specified schizophrenia spectrum and other psychotic disorder

F29 **Unspecified psychosis not due to a substance or known physiological condition**
      Psychosis NOS
      Unspecified schizophrenia spectrum and other psychotic disorder

      Excludes1 mental disorder NOS (F99)
                 unspecified mental disorder due to known physiological condition (F09)

MOOD [AFFECTIVE] DISORDERS (F30-F39)

● **F30** **Manic episode**
      Elevated, expansive, or irritable mood

      Includes bipolar disorder, single manic episode
                mixed affective episode

      Excludes1 bipolar disorder (F31.-)
                 major depressive disorder, single episode (F32.-)
                 major depressive disorder, recurrent (F33.-)

  ● **F30.1** **Manic episode without psychotic symptoms**

      F30.10 **Manic episode without psychotic symptoms, unspecified**

      F30.11 **Manic episode without psychotic symptoms, mild**

      F30.12 **Manic episode without psychotic symptoms, moderate**

      F30.13 **Manic episode, severe, without psychotic symptoms**

    F30.2 **Manic episode, severe with psychotic symptoms**
        Manic stupor
        Mania with mood-congruent psychotic symptoms
        Mania with mood-incongruent psychotic symptoms

    F30.3 **Manic episode in partial remission**

    F30.4 **Manic episode in full remission**

    F30.8 **Other manic episodes**
        Abnormality of mood resembling mania but less intense
        Hypomania

    F30.9 **Manic episode, unspecified**
        Mania NOS

● **F31** **Bipolar disorder**
      Mood disorders with history of manic, mixed, or hypomanic episodes

      Includes bipolar I disorder
                bipolar type I disorder
                manic-depressive illness
                manic-depressive psychosis
                manic-depressive reaction
                seasonal bipolar disorder

      Excludes1 bipolar disorder, single manic episode (F30.-)
                 major depressive disorder, single episode (F32.-)
                 major depressive disorder, recurrent (F33.-)

      Excludes2 cyclothymia (F34.0)

      Coding Clinic: 2020, Q1, P23

    F31.0 **Bipolar disorder, current episode hypomanic**

  ● **F31.1** **Bipolar disorder, current episode manic without psychotic features**

      F31.10 **Bipolar disorder, current episode manic without psychotic features, unspecified**

      F31.11 **Bipolar disorder, current episode manic without psychotic features, mild**

      F31.12 **Bipolar disorder, current episode manic without psychotic features, moderate**

      F31.13 **Bipolar disorder, current episode manic without psychotic features, severe**

    F31.2 **Bipolar disorder, current episode manic severe with psychotic features**
        Bipolar disorder, current episode manic with mood-congruent psychotic symptoms
        Bipolar disorder, current episode manic with mood-incongruent psychotic symptoms
        Bipolar I disorder, current or most recent episode manic with psychotic features

  ● **F31.3** **Bipolar disorder, current episode depressed, mild or moderate severity**

      F31.30 **Bipolar disorder, current episode depressed, mild or moderate severity, unspecified**

      F31.31 **Bipolar disorder, current episode depressed, mild**

      F31.32 **Bipolar disorder, current episode depressed, moderate**

    F31.4 **Bipolar disorder, current episode depressed, severe, without psychotic features**

    F31.5 **Bipolar disorder, current episode depressed, severe, with psychotic features**
        Bipolar disorder, current episode depressed with mood-incongruent psychotic symptoms
        Bipolar disorder, current episode depressed with mood-congruent psychotic symptoms
        Bipolar I disorder, current or most recent episode depressed, with psychotic features

  ● **F31.6** **Bipolar disorder, current episode mixed**

      F31.60 **Bipolar disorder, current episode mixed, unspecified**

      F31.61 **Bipolar disorder, current episode mixed, mild**

      F31.62 **Bipolar disorder, current episode mixed, moderate**

      F31.63 **Bipolar disorder, current episode mixed, severe, without psychotic features**

      F31.64 **Bipolar disorder, current episode mixed, severe, with psychotic features**
        Bipolar disorder, current episode mixed with mood-congruent psychotic symptoms
        Bipolar disorder, current episode mixed with mood-incongruent psychotic symptoms

  ● **F31.7** **Bipolar disorder, currently in remission**

      F31.70 **Bipolar disorder, currently in remission, most recent episode unspecified**

      F31.71 **Bipolar disorder, in partial remission, most recent episode hypomanic**

      F31.72 **Bipolar disorder, in full remission, most recent episode hypomanic**

      F31.73 **Bipolar disorder, in partial remission, most recent episode manic**

      F31.74 **Bipolar disorder, in full remission, most recent episode manic**

      F31.75 **Bipolar disorder, in partial remission, most recent episode depressed**

      F31.76 **Bipolar disorder, in full remission, most recent episode depressed**

      F31.77 **Bipolar disorder, in partial remission, most recent episode mixed**

      F31.78 **Bipolar disorder, in full remission, most recent episode mixed**

  ● **F31.8** **Other bipolar disorders**

      F31.81 **Bipolar II disorder**
          Bipolar disorder, type 2

      F31.89 **Other bipolar disorder**
          Recurrent manic episodes NOS

    F31.9 **Bipolar disorder, unspecified**
        Manic depression
      Coding Clinic: 2020, Q1, P23

CHAPTER 5 (F01-F99)

● F32   Depressive episode

Includes   single episode of agitated depression
single episode of depressive reaction
single episode of major depression
single episode of psychogenic depression
single episode of reactive depression
single episode of vital depression

Excludes1   bipolar disorder (F31.-)
manic episode (F30.-)
recurrent depressive disorder (F33.-)

Excludes2   adjustment disorder (F43.2)

F32.0   Major depressive disorder, single episode, mild ᴴᴄᴄ

F32.1   Major depressive disorder, single episode, moderate ᴴᴄᴄ

F32.2   Major depressive disorder, single episode, severe without psychotic features ᴴᴄᴄ
    Coding Clinic: 2024, Q4, P54

F32.3   Major depressive disorder, single episode, severe with psychotic features ᴴᴄᴄ
Single episode of major depression with mood-congruent psychotic symptoms
Single episode of major depression with mood-incongruent psychotic symptoms
Single episode of major depression with psychotic symptoms
Single episode of psychogenic depressive psychosis
Single episode of psychotic depression
Single episode of reactive depressive psychosis

F32.4   Major depressive disorder, single episode, in partial remission ᴴᴄᴄ

F32.5   Major depressive disorder, single episode, in full remission ᴴᴄᴄ

● F32.8   Other depressive episodes

F32.81   Premenstrual dysphoric disorder
    Excludes1   premenstrual tension syndrome (N94.3)
    Coding Clinic: 2016, Q4, P14

F32.89   Other specified depressive episodes
Atypical depression
Post-schizophrenic depression
Single episode of 'masked' depression NOS
    Coding Clinic: 2016, Q4, P14

F32.9   Major depressive disorder, single episode, unspecified
Major depression NOS
    Coding Clinic: 2021, Q1, P10

F32.A   Depression, unspecified
Depression NOS
Depressive disorder NOS
    Coding Clinic: 2023, Q4, P15; 2021, Q4, P10

● F33   Major depressive disorder, recurrent

Includes   recurrent episodes of depressive reaction
recurrent episodes of endogenous depression
recurrent episodes of major depression
recurrent episodes of psychogenic depression
recurrent episodes of reactive depression
recurrent episodes of seasonal affective disorder
recurrent episodes of seasonal depressive disorder
recurrent episodes of vital depression

Excludes1   bipolar disorder (F31.-)
manic episode (F30.-)
    Coding Clinic: 2020, Q1, P23

F33.0   Major depressive disorder, recurrent, mild ᴴᴄᴄ

F33.1   Major depressive disorder, recurrent, moderate ᴴᴄᴄ

F33.2   Major depressive disorder, recurrent severe without psychotic features ᴴᴄᴄ

F33.3   Major depressive disorder, recurrent, severe with psychotic symptoms ᴴᴄᴄ
Endogenous depression with psychotic symptoms
Major depressive disorder, recurrent, with psychotic features
Recurrent severe episodes of major depression with mood-congruent psychotic symptoms
Recurrent severe episodes of major depression with mood-incongruent psychotic symptoms
Recurrent severe episodes of major depression with psychotic symptoms
Recurrent severe episodes of psychogenic depressive psychosis
Recurrent severe episodes of psychotic depression
Recurrent severe episodes of reactive depressive psychosis

● F33.4   Major depressive disorder, recurrent, in remission

F33.40   Major depressive disorder, recurrent, in remission, unspecified ᴴᴄᴄ

F33.41   Major depressive disorder, recurrent, in partial remission ᴴᴄᴄ

F33.42   Major depressive disorder, recurrent, in full remission ᴴᴄᴄ

F33.8   Other recurrent depressive disorders ᴴᴄᴄ
Recurrent brief depressive episodes

F33.9   Major depressive disorder, recurrent, unspecified ᴴᴄᴄ
Monopolar depression NOS

● F34   Persistent mood [affective] disorders

F34.0   Cyclothymic disorder
Affective personality disorder
Cycloid personality
Cyclothymia
Cyclothymic personality

F34.1   Dysthymic disorder
Depressive neurosis
Depressive personality disorder
Dysthymia
Neurotic depression
Persistent anxiety depression
Persistent depressive disorder
    Excludes2   anxiety depression (mild or not persistent) (F41.8)

● F34.8   Other persistent mood [affective] disorders

F34.81   Disruptive mood dysregulation disorder ᴴᴄᴄ
    Coding Clinic: 2016, Q4, P14

F34.89   Other specified persistent mood disorders ᴴᴄᴄ
    Coding Clinic: 2016, Q4, P14

F34.9   Persistent mood [affective] disorder, unspecified ᴴᴄᴄ

● F39   Unspecified mood [affective] disorder ᴴᴄᴄ
Affective psychosis NOS

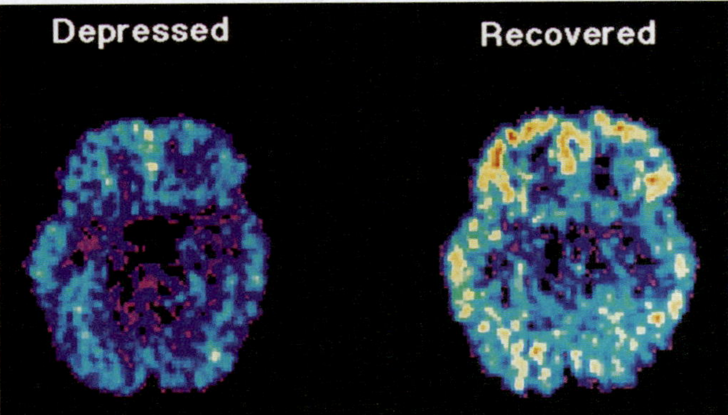

Figure 5-1   PET scan of depressed individual's brain before and after recovery. (From Fortinash KM: Psychiatric Mental Health Nursing, ed 4, St. Louis, Mosby, 2008)

▶ New   ⇒ Revised   ~~deleted~~ Deleted   Excludes 1   Excludes 2   Includes   Use additional   Code first   Code also   Key words
OGCR Official Guidelines   X Assign placeholder X   ● Use Additional Character(s)   ▶ Manifestation Code   ᴴᴄᴄ Hierarchical Condition Category   Coding Clinic

ANXIETY, DISSOCIATIVE, STRESS-RELATED, SOMATOFORM AND OTHER NONPSYCHOTIC MENTAL DISORDERS (F40-F48)

● **F40 Phobic anxiety disorders**
Irrational fear with avoidance of the feared subject, activity, or situation even though the individual knows that the reaction is excessive

● **F40.0 Agoraphobia**
Intense, irrational fear of open spaces

F40.00 Agoraphobia, unspecified

F40.01 Agoraphobia with panic disorder
Panic disorder with agoraphobia

Excludes1 panic disorder without agoraphobia (F41.0)

F40.02 Agoraphobia without panic disorder

● **F40.1 Social phobias**
Anthropophobia
Social anxiety disorder
Social anxiety disorder of childhood
Social neurosis

F40.10 Social phobia, unspecified

F40.11 Social phobia, generalized

● **F40.2 Specific (isolated) phobias**

Excludes2 dysmorphophobia (nondelusional) (F45.22)
nosophobia (F45.22)

● **F40.21 Animal type phobia**

F40.210 Arachnophobia
Fear of spiders

F40.218 Other animal type phobia

● **F40.22 Natural environment type phobia**

F40.220 Fear of thunderstorms

F40.228 Other natural environment type phobia

● **F40.23 Blood, injection, injury type phobia**

F40.230 Fear of blood

F40.231 Fear of injections and transfusions

F40.232 Fear of other medical care

F40.233 Fear of injury

● **F40.24 Situational type phobia**

F40.240 Claustrophobia
Fear of closed spaces

F40.241 Acrophobia
Fear of heights

F40.242 Fear of bridges

F40.243 Fear of flying

F40.248 Other situational type phobia

● **F40.29 Other specified phobia**

F40.290 Androphobia
Fear of men

F40.291 Gynephobia
Fear of women

F40.298 Other specified phobia

F40.8 Other phobic anxiety disorders
Phobic anxiety disorder of childhood

F40.9 Phobic anxiety disorder, unspecified
Phobia NOS
Phobic state NOS

● **F41 Other anxiety disorders**

Excludes2 anxiety in:
acute stress reaction (F43.0)
transient adjustment reaction (F43.2)
neurasthenia (F48.8)
psychophysiologic disorders (F45.-)
separation anxiety (F93.0)

F41.0 Panic disorder [episodic paroxysmal anxiety]
Panic attack
Panic state

Excludes1 panic disorder with agoraphobia (F40.01)

F41.1 Generalized anxiety disorder
Anxiety neurosis
Anxiety reaction
Anxiety state
Overanxious disorder

Excludes2 neurasthenia (F48.8)

F41.3 Other mixed anxiety disorders

F41.8 Other specified anxiety disorders
Anxiety depression (mild or not persistent)
Anxiety hysteria
Mixed anxiety and depressive disorder
Coding Clinic: 2021, Q1, P11

F41.9 Anxiety disorder, unspecified
Anxiety NOS
Coding Clinic: 2021, Q1, P11

● **F42 Obsessive-compulsive disorder**
Anxiety disorder with recurrent obsessions or compulsions

Excludes2 obsessive-compulsive personality (disorder) (F60.5)
➡ obsessive-compulsive symptoms occurring in depression (F32.-, F33.3)
obsessive-compulsive symptoms occurring in schizophrenia (F20.-)

F42.2 Mixed obsessional thoughts and acts
Coding Clinic: 2016, Q4, P15

F42.3 Hoarding disorder
Coding Clinic: 2016, Q4, P14-15

F42.4 Excoriation (skin-picking) disorder

Excludes1 factitial dermatitis (L98.1)
other specified behavioral and emotional disorders with onset usually occurring in early childhood and adolescence (F98.8)

Coding Clinic: 2016, Q4, P14-15

F42.8 Other obsessive-compulsive disorder
Anancastic neurosis
Obsessive-compulsive neurosis
Coding Clinic: 2016, Q4, P15

F42.9 Obsessive-compulsive disorder, unspecified
Coding Clinic: 2016, Q4, P15

● **F43 Reaction to severe stress and adjustment disorders**

F43.0 Acute stress reaction
Acute crisis reaction
Acute reaction to stress
Combat and operational stress reaction
Combat fatigue
Crisis state
Psychic shock

● **F43.1 Post-traumatic stress disorder (PTSD)**
Traumatic neurosis

F43.10 Post-traumatic stress disorder, unspecified

F43.11 Post-traumatic stress disorder, acute

F43.12 Post-traumatic stress disorder, chronic

● **F43.2 Adjustment disorders**
Culture shock
Grief reaction
Hospitalism in children

Excludes2 separation anxiety disorder of childhood (F93.0)

F43.20 Adjustment disorder, unspecified

F43.21 Adjustment disorder with depressed mood

F43.22 Adjustment disorder with anxiety

F43.23 Adjustment disorder with mixed anxiety and depressed mood

F43.24 Adjustment disorder with disturbance of conduct

F43.25 Adjustment disorder with mixed disturbance of emotions and conduct

F43.29 Adjustment disorder with other symptoms

● **F43.8   Other reactions to severe stress**
Other specified trauma and stressor-related disorder

   F43.81   Prolonged grief disorder
Complicated grief
Complicated grief disorder
Persistent complex bereavement disorder

   F43.89   Other reactions to severe stress

F43.9   Reaction to severe stress, unspecified
Trauma and stressor-related disorder, NOS

● **F44   Dissociative and conversion disorders**

   Includes   conversion hysteria
conversion reaction
hysteria
hysterical psychosis

   Excludes2   malingering [conscious simulation] (Z76.5)

F44.0   Dissociative amnesia
Sudden loss of memory for personal information

   Excludes1   amnesia NOS (R41.3)
anterograde amnesia (R41.1)
dissociative amnesia with dissociative
fugue (F44.1)
retrograde amnesia (R41.2)

   Excludes2   alcohol or other psychoactive substance-
induced amnestic disorder (F10, F13,
F19 with .26, .96)
amnestic disorder due to known
physiological condition (F04)
postictal amnesia in epilepsy (G40.-)

F44.1   Dissociative fugue
*Characterized by episode of sudden, unexpected travel with
amnesia for past and partial to total confusion about
identity or assumption of new identity*
Dissociative amnesia with dissociative fugue

   Excludes2   postictal fugue in epilepsy (G40.-)

F44.2   Dissociative stupor
*Profound diminution or absence of voluntary movement and
responsiveness to external stimuli*

   Excludes1   catatonic stupor (R40.1)
stupor NOS (R40.1)

   Excludes2   catatonic disorder due to known
physiological condition (F06.1)
depressive stupor (F32, F33)
manic stupor (F30, F31)

F44.4   Conversion disorder with motor symptom or deficit
Conversion disorder with abnormal movement
Conversion disorder with speech symptoms
Conversion disorder with swallowing symptoms
Conversion disorder with weakness/paralysis
Dissociative motor disorders
Psychogenic aphonia
Psychogenic dysphonia

F44.5   Conversion disorder with seizures or convulsions
Conversion disorder with attacks or seizures
Dissociative convulsions
Coding Clinic: 2019, Q1, P19

F44.6   Conversion disorder with sensory symptom or deficit
Conversion disorder with anesthesia or sensory loss
Conversion disorder with special sensory symptoms
Dissociative anesthesia and sensory loss
Psychogenic deafness

F44.7   Conversion disorder with mixed symptom presentation

● **F44.8   Other dissociative and conversion disorders**

   F44.81   Dissociative identity disorder
Multiple personality disorder

   F44.89   Other dissociative and conversion disorders
Ganser's syndrome
Psychogenic confusion
Psychogenic twilight state
Trance and possession disorders

F44.9   Dissociative and conversion disorder, unspecified
Dissociative disorder NOS

Pain disorders related to psychological factors
Assign code F45.41, for pain that is exclusively related to psychological
disorders. As indicated by the Excludes 1 note under category G89,
a code from category G89 should not be assigned with code F45.41
Code F45.42, Pain disorders with related psychological factors, should
be used with a code from category G89, Pain, not elsewhere classified,
if there is documentation of a psychological component for a patient
with acute or chronic pain.
See Section I.C.6. Pain

● **F45   Somatoform disorders**
*Mental disorders characterized by symptoms suggesting general
medical condition*

   Excludes2   dissociative and conversion disorders (F44.-)
factitious disorders (F68.1-, F68.A)
hair-plucking (F63.3)
lalling (F80.0)
lisping (F80.0)
malingering [conscious simulation] (Z76.5)
nail-biting (F98.8)
psychological or behavioral factors associated
with disorders or diseases classified
elsewhere (F54)
sexual dysfunction, not due to a substance or
known physiological condition (F52.-)
thumb-sucking (F98.8)
tic disorders (in childhood and adolescence) (F95.-)
Tourette's syndrome (F95.2)
trichotillomania (F63.3)

F45.0   Somatization disorder
Briquet's disorder
Multiple psychosomatic disorder

F45.1   Undifferentiated somatoform disorder
Somatic symptom disorder
Undifferentiated psychosomatic disorder

● **F45.2   Hypochondriacal disorders**
*Persistent, unrealistic preoccupation with possibility of
having serious disease*

   Excludes2   delusional dysmorphophobia (F22)
fixed delusions about bodily functions or
shape (F22)

   F45.20   Hypochondriacal disorder, unspecified

   F45.21   Hypochondriasis
Hypochondriacal neurosis
Illness anxiety disorder

   F45.22   Body dysmorphic disorder
Bigorexia
Dysmorphophobia (nondelusional)
Muscle dysmorphia
Nosophobia

   F45.29   Other hypochondriacal disorders

● **F45.4   Pain disorders related to psychological factors**

   Excludes1   pain NOS (R52)

   **F45.41   Pain disorder exclusively related to
psychological factors**
Somatoform pain disorder (persistent)

   F45.42   Pain disorder with related psychological factors
Code also associated acute or chronic pain
(G89.-)

F45.8   Other somatoform disorders
Psychogenic dysmenorrhea
Psychogenic dysphagia, including 'globus hystericus'
Psychogenic pruritus
Psychogenic torticollis
Somatoform autonomic dysfunction
Teeth grinding

   Excludes1   sleep related teeth grinding (G47.63)
Coding Clinic: 2016, Q4, P118

F45.9   Somatoform disorder, unspecified
Psychosomatic disorder NOS

● **F48　Other nonpsychotic mental disorders**
　F48.1　Depersonalization-derealization syndrome
　F48.2　Pseudobulbar affect
　　　Involuntary emotional expression disorder
　　　Code first underlying cause, if known, such as:
　　　　amyotrophic lateral sclerosis (G12.21)
　　　▶multiple sclerosis (G35.-)
　　　　sequelae of cerebrovascular disease (I69.-)
　　　　sequelae of traumatic intracranial injury (S06.-)
　F48.8　Other specified nonpsychotic mental disorders
　　　Dhat syndrome
　　　Neurasthenia
　　　Occupational neurosis, including writer's cramp
　　　Psychasthenia
　　　Psychasthenic neurosis
　　　Psychogenic syncope
　F48.9　Nonpsychotic mental disorder, unspecified
　　　Neurosis NOS

BEHAVIORAL SYNDROMES ASSOCIATED WITH PHYSIOLOGICAL DISTURBANCES AND PHYSICAL FACTORS (F50-F59)

● **F50　Eating disorders**
　Excludes1　anorexia NOS (R63.0)
　　　　　　feeding problems of newborn (P92.-)
　　　　　　polyphagia (R63.2)
　Excludes2　feeding difficulties (R63.3-)
　　　　　　feeding disorder in infancy or childhood (F98.2-)
　● **F50.0　Anorexia nervosa**
　　Excludes1　loss of appetite (R63.0)
　　　　　　　psychogenic loss of appetite (F50.89)
　　F50.00　Anorexia nervosa, unspecified
　　F50.01　Anorexia nervosa, restricting type
　　　F50.010　Anorexia nervosa, restricting type, mild
　　　　　Anorexia nervosa, restricting type, with a body mass index greater than or equal to 17 kg/m2
　　　F50.011　Anorexia nervosa, restricting type, moderate
　　　　　Anorexia nervosa, restricting type, with a body mass index of 16.0-16.99 kg/m2
　　　F50.012　Anorexia nervosa, restricting type, severe
　　　　　Anorexia nervosa, restricting type, with a body mass index of 15.0-15.99 kg/m2
　　　　　Coding Clinic: 2024, Q4, P13
　　　F50.013　Anorexia nervosa, restricting type, extreme
　　　　　Anorexia nervosa, restricting type, with a body mass index of less than 15.0 kg/m2
　　　F50.014　Anorexia nervosa, restricting type, in remission
　　　　　Anorexia nervosa, restricting type, in full remission
　　　　　Anorexia nervosa, restricting type, in partial remission
　　　F50.019　Anorexia nervosa, restricting type, unspecified
　　F50.02　Anorexia nervosa, binge eating/purging type
　　　Excludes1　bulimia nervosa (F50.02-)
　　　　　Coding Clinic: 2022, Q1, P13
　　　F50.020　Anorexia nervosa, binge eating/purging type, mild
　　　　　Anorexia nervosa, binge eating/purging type, with a body mass index greater thanor equal to 17 kg/m2

　　　F50.021　Anorexia nervosa, binge eating/purging type, moderate
　　　　　Anorexia nervosa, binge eating/purging type, with a body mass index of 16.0-16.99kg/m2
　　　F50.022　Anorexia nervosa, binge eating/purging type, severe
　　　　　Anorexia nervosa, binge eating/purging type, with a body mass index of 15.0-15.99kg/m2
　　　F50.023　Anorexia nervosa, binge eating/purging type, extreme
　　　　　Anorexia nervosa, binge eating/purging type, with a body mass index of less than 15.0 kg/m2
　　　　　Coding Clinic: 2024, Q4, P14
　　　F50.024　Anorexia nervosa, binge eating/purging type, in remission
　　　　　Anorexia nervosa, binge eating/purging type, in full remission
　　　　　Anorexia nervosa, binge eating/purging type, in partial remission
　　　F50.029　Anorexia nervosa, binge eating/purging type, unspecified
　● **F50.2　Bulimia nervosa**
　　　Bulimia NOS
　　　Hyperorexia nervosa
　　Excludes1　anorexia nervosa, binge eating/purging type (F50.02-)
　　F50.20　Bulimia nervosa, unspecified
　　F50.21　Bulimia nervosa, mild
　　　　Bulimia nervosa with 1-3 episodes of inappropriate compensatory behavior per week
　　F50.22　Bulimia nervosa, moderate
　　　　Bulimia nervosa with 4-7 episodes of inappropriate compensatory behavior per week
　　F50.23　Bulimia nervosa, severe
　　　　Bulimia nervosa with 8-13 episodes of inappropriate compensatory behavior per week
　　F50.24　Bulimia nervosa, extreme
　　　　Bulimia nervosa with 14 or more episodes of inappropriate compensatory behavior per week
　　F50.25　Bulimia nervosa, in remission
　　　　Bulimia nervosa, in full remission
　　　　Bulimia nervosa, in partial remission
　● **F50.8　Other eating disorders**
　　F50.81　Binge eating disorder
　　　　Coding Clinic: 2016, Q4, P15
　　　F50.810　Binge eating disorder, mild
　　　　　Binge eating disorder with 1-3 binge eating episodes per week
　　　F50.811　Binge eating disorder, moderate
　　　　　Binge eating disorder with 4-7 binge eating episodes per week
　　　F50.812　Binge eating disorder, severe
　　　　　Binge eating disorder with 8-13 binge eating episodes per week
　　　F50.813　Binge eating disorder, extreme
　　　　　Binge eating disorder with 14 or more eating episodes per week
　　　F50.814　Binge eating disorder, in remission
　　　　　Binge eating disorder, in full remission
　　　　　Binge eating disorder, in partial remission
　　　F50.819　Binge eating disorder, unspecified

CHAPTER 5 (F01-F99)

F50.82 **Avoidant/restrictive food intake disorder**
Avoidant/restrictive food intake disorder, in remission

F50.83 **Pica in adults** A
Pica in adults, in remission
> **Excludes1** pica in infancy and childhood (F98.3)
Coding Clinic: 2024, Q4, P54

F50.84 **Rumination disorder in adults** A
Rumination disorder in adults, in remission
> **Excludes1** rumination disorder in infancy and childhood (F98.21)

F50.89 **Other specified eating disorder**
Psychogenic loss of appetite
Coding Clinic: 2016, Q4, P16

F50.9 **Eating disorder, unspecified**
Atypical anorexia nervosa
Atypical bulimia nervosa
Feeding or eating disorder, unspecified
Other specified feeding disorder

● **F51** **Sleep disorders not due to a substance or known physiological condition**
> **Excludes2** organic sleep disorders (G47.-)

● **F51.0** **Insomnia not due to a substance or known physiological condition**
> **Excludes2** alcohol related insomnia (F10.182, F10.282, F10.982)
> drug-related insomnia (F11.182, F11.982, F13.182, F13.282, F13.982, F14.182, F14.282, F14.982, F15.182, F15.282, F15.982, F19.182, F19.282, F19.982)
> insomnia NOS (G47.0-)
> insomnia due to known physiological condition (G47.0-)
> organic insomnia (G47.0-)
> sleep deprivation (Z72.820)

F51.01 **Primary insomnia**
Idiopathic insomnia

F51.02 **Adjustment insomnia**

F51.03 **Paradoxical insomnia**

F51.04 **Psychophysiologic insomnia**

F51.05 **Insomnia due to other mental disorder**
Code also associated mental disorder

F51.09 **Other insomnia not due to a substance or known physiological condition**

● **F51.1** **Hypersomnia not due to a substance or known physiological condition**
Hypersomnia: Excessive sleeping/sleepiness
> **Excludes2** alcohol related hypersomnia (F10.182, F10.282, F10.982)
> drug-related hypersomnia (F11.182, F11.282, F11.982, F13.182, F13.282, F13.982, F14.182, F14.282, F14.982, F15.182, F15.282, F15.982, F19.182, F19.282, F19.982)
> hypersomnia NOS (G47.10)
> hypersomnia due to known physiological condition (G47.10)
> idiopathic hypersomnia (G47.11, G47.12)
> narcolepsy (G47.4-)

F51.11 **Primary hypersomnia**

F51.12 **Insufficient sleep syndrome**
> **Excludes1** sleep deprivation (Z72.820)

F51.13 **Hypersomnia due to other mental disorder**
Code also associated mental disorder

F51.19 **Other hypersomnia not due to a substance or known physiological condition**

F51.3 **Sleepwalking [somnambulism]**
Non-rapid eye movement sleep arousal disorders, sleepwalking type

F51.4 **Sleep terrors [night terrors]**
Non-rapid eye movement sleep arousal disorders, sleep terror type

F51.5 **Nightmare disorder**
Dream anxiety disorder

F51.8 **Other sleep disorders not due to a substance or known physiological condition**

F51.9 **Sleep disorder not due to a substance or known physiological condition, unspecified**
Emotional sleep disorder NOS

● **F52** **Sexual dysfunction not due to a substance or known physiological condition**
> **Excludes2** Dhat syndrome (F48.8)

F52.0 **Hypoactive sexual desire disorder**
Total loss of feeling of sexual pleasure
Lack or loss of sexual desire
Male hypoactive sexual desire disorder
Sexual anhedonia
> **Excludes1** decreased libido (R68.82)

F52.1 **Sexual aversion disorder**
Sexual aversion and lack of sexual enjoyment

● **F52.2** **Sexual arousal disorders**
Failure of genital response

F52.21 **Male erectile disorder**
Erectile disorder
Psychogenic impotence
> **Excludes1** impotence of organic origin (N52.-)
> impotence NOS (N52.-)

F52.22 **Female sexual arousal disorder**
Female sexual interest/arousal disorder

● **F52.3** **Orgasmic disorder**
Inhibited orgasm
Psychogenic anorgasmy

F52.31 **Female orgasmic disorder**

F52.32 **Male orgasmic disorder**
Delayed ejaculation

F52.4 **Premature ejaculation**

F52.5 **Vaginismus not due to a substance or known physiological condition**
Psychogenic vaginismus
> **Excludes2** vaginismus (due to a known physiological condition) (N94.2)

F52.6 **Dyspareunia not due to a substance or known physiological condition**
Dyspareunia: Difficult or painful sexual intercourse
Genito-pelvic pain penetration disorder
Psychogenic dyspareunia
> **Excludes2** dyspareunia (due to a known physiological condition) (N94.1-)

F52.8 **Other sexual dysfunction not due to a substance or known physiological condition**
Excessive sexual drive
Nymphomania
Satyriasis

F52.9 **Unspecified sexual dysfunction not due to a substance or known physiological condition**
Sexual dysfunction NOS

● **F53** **Mental and behavioral disorders associated with the puerperium, not elsewhere classified**
　　Acute mental illness with sudden onset following childbirth with symptoms of affective psychosis, disorientation, and confusion are prevalent
　　Excludes1　mood disorders with psychotic features (F30.2, F31.2, F31.5, F31.64, F32.3, F33.3)
　　　　　　postpartum dysphoria (O90.6)
　　　　　　psychosis in schizophrenia, schizotypal, delusional, and other psychotic disorders (F20-F29)

　F53.0 **Postpartum depression**　　　　　　　　　**M**
　　　Postnatal depression, NOS
　　　Postpartum depression, NOS
　　　Coding Clinic: 2018, Q4, P8

　F53.1 **Puerperal psychosis**　　　　　　　　　**M**
　　　Postpartum psychosis
　　　Puerperal psychosis, NOS
　　　Coding Clinic: 2018, Q4, P9

▶ *F54* *Psychological and behavioral factors associated with disorders or diseases classified elsewhere*
　　Psychological factors affecting physical conditions
　　Code first the associated physical disorder, such as:
　　　asthma (J45.-)
　　　dermatitis (L23-L25)
　　　gastric ulcer (K25.-)
　　　mucous colitis (K58.-)
　　　ulcerative colitis (K51.-)
　　　urticaria (L50.-)
　　Excludes2　tension-type headache (G44.2)

● **F55** **Abuse of non-psychoactive substances**
　　Excludes2　abuse of psychoactive substances (F10-F19)

　F55.0　**Abuse of antacids**
　F55.1　**Abuse of herbal or folk remedies**
　　　Coding Clinic: 2023, Q3, P16
　F55.2　**Abuse of laxatives**
　F55.3　**Abuse of steroids or hormones**
　F55.4　**Abuse of vitamins**
　F55.8　**Abuse of other non-psychoactive substances**

　F59　**Unspecified behavioral syndromes associated with physiological disturbances and physical factors**
　　　Psychogenic physiological dysfunction NOS

DISORDERS OF ADULT PERSONALITY AND BEHAVIOR (F60-F69)

● **F60**　**Specific personality disorders**
　　Long-term patterns of thoughts and behaviors causing serious problems with relationships and work

　F60.0　**Paranoid personality disorder**
　　　Hostile, devious, and combative response to disappointments
　　　Expansive paranoid personality (disorder)
　　　Fanatic personality (disorder)
　　　Querulant personality (disorder)
　　　Paranoid personality (disorder)
　　　Sensitive paranoid personality (disorder)
　　　Excludes2　paranoia (F22)
　　　　　　paranoia querulans (F22)
　　　　　　paranoid psychosis (F22)
　　　　　　paranoid schizophrenia (F20.0)
　　　　　　paranoid state (F22)

　F60.1　**Schizoid personality disorder**
　　　Detachment from social relationships with minimal emotional experiences and expressions
　　　Excludes2　Asperger's syndrome (F84.5)
　　　　　　delusional disorder (F22)
　　　　　　schizoid disorder of childhood (F84.5)
　　　　　　schizophrenia (F20.-)
　　　　　　schizotypal disorder (F21)

　F60.2　**Antisocial personality disorder**
　　　Continuous and chronic antisocial behavior
　　　Amoral personality (disorder)
　　　Asocial personality (disorder)
　　　Dissocial personality disorder
　　　Psychopathic personality (disorder)
　　　Sociopathic personality (disorder)
　　　Excludes1　conduct disorders (F91.-)
　　　Excludes2　borderline personality disorder (F60.3)

　F60.3　**Borderline personality disorder**
　　　Instability of mood, self-image or sense of self, and interpersonal relationships
　　　Aggressive personality (disorder)
　　　Emotionally unstable personality disorder
　　　Explosive personality (disorder)
　　　Excludes2　antisocial personality disorder (F60.2)

　F60.4　**Histrionic personality disorder**
　　　Personality disorder with excessive emotional and attention-seeking behavior
　　　Hysterical personality (disorder)
　　　Psychoinfantile personality (disorder)

　F60.5　**Obsessive-compulsive personality disorder**
　　　Anankastic personality (disorder)
　　　Compulsive personality (disorder)
　　　Obsessional personality (disorder)
　　　Excludes2　obsessive-compulsive disorder (F42.-)

　F60.6　**Avoidant personality disorder**
　　　Anxious personality disorder

　F60.7　**Dependent personality disorder**
　　　Asthenic personality (disorder)
　　　Inadequate personality (disorder)
　　　Passive personality (disorder)

● **F60.8**　**Other specific personality disorders**

　　F60.81　**Narcissistic personality disorder**
　　　　Vanity, conceit, egotism or indifference to plight of others

　　F60.89　**Other specific personality disorders**
　　　　Eccentric personality disorder
　　　　'Haltlose' type personality disorder
　　　　Immature personality disorder
　　　　Passive-aggressive personality disorder
　　　　Psychoneurotic personality disorder
　　　　Self-defeating personality disorder

　F60.9　**Personality disorder, unspecified**
　　　Character disorder NOS
　　　Character neurosis NOS
　　　Pathological personality NOS

● **F63**　**Impulse disorders**
　　Excludes2　habitual excessive use of alcohol or psychoactive substances (F10-F19)
　　　　　　impulse disorders involving sexual behavior (F65.-)

　F63.0　**Pathological gambling**
　　　Compulsive gambling
　　　Gambling disorder
　　　Excludes1　gambling and betting NOS (Z72.6)
　　　Excludes2　excessive gambling by manic patients (F30, F31)
　　　　　　gambling in antisocial personality disorder (F60.2)

　F63.1　**Pyromania**
　　　Pathological fire-setting
　　　Excludes2　fire-setting (by) (in):
　　　　　　adult with antisocial personality disorder (F60.2)
　　　　　　alcohol or psychoactive substance intoxication (F10-F19)
　　　　　　conduct disorders (F91.-)
　　　　　　mental disorders due to known physiological condition (F01-F09)
　　　　　　schizophrenia (F20.-)

CHAPTER 5 (F01-F99)

CHAPTER 5 (F01-F99)

F63.2   **Kleptomania**
Pathological stealing

Excludes1   shoplifting as the reason for observation for suspected mental disorder (Z03.8)

Excludes2   depressive disorder with stealing (F31.-, F32.-, F33.-)
stealing due to underlying mental condition-code to mental condition
stealing in mental disorders due to known physiological condition (F01-F09)

F63.3   **Trichotillomania**
Hair plucking

Excludes2   other stereotyped movement disorder (F98.4)

● F63.8   **Other impulse disorders**

F63.81   **Intermittent explosive disorder**

F63.89   **Other impulse disorders**

F63.9   **Impulse disorder, unspecified**
Impulse control disorder NOS

● **F64   Gender identity disorders**

F64.0   **Transsexualism**
Gender identity disorder in adolescence and adulthood
Gender incongruence in adolescents and adults
Gender identity in adolescents and adults
Transgender

Excludes1   gender identity disorder of childhood (F64.2)

Coding Clinic: 2016, Q4, P16

F64.1   **Dual role transvestism**
Use additional code to identify sex reassignment status (Z87.890)

Excludes1   gender identity disorder in childhood (F64.2)

Excludes2   fetishistic transvestism (F65.1)

Coding Clinic: 2016, Q4, P16

F64.2   **Gender identity disorder of childhood**   P
Gender dysphoria in children
Gender incongruence of childhood

Excludes1   gender identity disorder in adolescence and adulthood (F64.0)

Excludes2   sexual maturation disorder (F66)

F64.8   **Other gender identity disorders**
Other specified gender dysphoria

F64.9   **Gender identity disorder, unspecified**
Gender dysphoria, unspecified
Gender incongruence, unspecified
Gender-role disorder NOS

● **F65   Paraphilias**

F65.0   **Fetishism**
Intense sexual urges and arousing fantasies using inanimate objects
Fetishistic disorder

F65.1   **Transvestic fetishism**
Intense sexual urges, arousal, or orgasm associated with fantasized/actual cross-dressing
Fetishistic transvestism
Transvestic disorder

F65.2   **Exhibitionism**
Exhibitionistic disorder

F65.3   **Voyeurism**
Sexual urges or arousal involving real or fantasized observation of unsuspecting people who are naked, disrobing, or engaging in sexual activity
Voyeuristic disorder

F65.4   **Pedophilia**
Pedophilic disorder

● F65.5   **Sadomasochism**

F65.50   **Sadomasochism, unspecified**

F65.51   **Sexual masochism**
Sexual masochism disorder

F65.52   **Sexual sadism**
Sexual sadism disorder

● F65.8   **Other paraphilias**

F65.81   **Frotteurism**
Sexual arousal or orgasm is achieved by rubbing up against another person (or fantasies of), in crowded place with unsuspecting victim
Frotteuristic disorder

F65.89   **Other paraphilias**
Necrophilia
Other specified paraphilic disorder

F65.9   **Paraphilia, unspecified**
Paraphilic disorder, unspecified
Sexual deviation NOS

F66   Other sexual disorders
Sexual maturation disorder
Sexual relationship disorder

● **F68   Other disorders of adult personality and behavior**

● F68.1   **Factitious disorder imposed on self**
Compensation neurosis
Elaboration of physical symptoms for psychological reasons
Hospital hopper syndrome
Münchhausen's syndrome
Peregrinating patient

Excludes2   factitial dermatitis (L98.1)
person feigning illness (with obvious motivation) (Z76.5)

F68.10   **Factitious disorder imposed on self, unspecified**

F68.11   **Factitious disorder imposed on self with predominantly psychological signs and symptoms**

F68.12   **Factitious disorder imposed on self with predominantly physical signs and symptoms**

F68.13   **Factitious disorder imposed on self with combined psychological and physical signs and symptoms**

F68.8   **Other specified disorders of adult personality and behavior**

F68.A   **Factitious disorder imposed on another**
Factitious disorder by proxy
Münchhausen's by proxy

F69   Unspecified disorder of adult personality and behavior   A

INTELLECTUAL DISABILITIES (F70-F79)

Code first any associated physical or developmental disorders

Excludes1   borderline intellectual functioning, IQ above 70 to 84 (R41.83)

F70   Mild intellectual disabilities
IQ level 50-55 to approximately 70
Mild mental subnormality

F71   Moderate intellectual disabilities
IQ level 35-40 to 50-55
Moderate mental subnormality

F72   Severe intellectual disabilities
IQ 20-25 to 35-40
Severe mental subnormality

F73   Profound intellectual disabilities
IQ level below 20-25
Profound mental subnormality

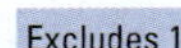

▶ New   ➡ Revised   ~~deleted~~ Deleted   Excludes 1   Excludes 2   Includes   Use additional   Code first   Code also   Key words

    OGCR Official Guidelines   X Assign placeholder X   ● Use Additional Character(s)   ▸ Manifestation Code   Ⓗⓒⓒ Hierarchical Condition Category   **Coding Clinic**

● **F78   Other intellectual disabilities**
  ● **F78.A   Other genetic related intellectual disabilities**
      F78.A1   SYNGAP1-related intellectual disability
          Code also, *if applicable, any associated:*
          autism spectrum disorder (F84.0)
          autistic disorder (F84.0)
          encephalopathy (G93.4-)
          epilepsy and recurrent seizures (G40.-)
          other pervasive developmental disorders
              (F84.8)
          pervasive developmental disorder, NOS (F84.9)

      F78.A9   Other genetic related intellectual disability
          Code also, *if applicable, any associated disorders*

  F79   Unspecified intellectual disabilities
          Mental deficiency NOS
          Mental subnormality NOS

PERVASIVE AND SPECIFIC DEVELOPMENTAL DISORDERS (F80-F89)

● **F80   Specific developmental disorders of speech and language**
  F80.0   Phonological disorder
          Communication disorder of unknown cause, characterized by
              failure to use age-appropriate sounds
          Dyslalia
          Functional speech articulation disorder
          Lalling
          Lisping
          Phonological developmental disorder
          Speech articulation developmental disorder
          Speech-sound disorder
          Excludes1   speech articulation impairment due to
                  aphasia NOS (R47.01)
                  speech articulation impairment due to
                      apraxia (R48.2)
          Excludes2   speech articulation impairment due to
                  hearing loss (F80.4)
                  speech articulation impairment due to
                      intellectual disabilities (F70-F79)
                  speech articulation impairment with
                      expressive language developmental
                      disorder (F80.1)
                  speech articulation impairment with
                      mixed receptive expressive language
                      developmental disorder (F80.2)

  F80.1   Expressive language disorder
          Developmental dysphasia or aphasia, expressive type
          Excludes1   mixed receptive-expressive language
                  disorder (F80.2)
                  dysphasia and aphasia NOS (R47.-)
          Excludes2   acquired aphasia with epilepsy [Landau-
                  Kleffner] (G40.80-)
                  intellectual disabilities (F70-F79)
                  pervasive developmental disorders
                      (F84.-)
                  selective mutism (F94.0)

  F80.2   Mixed receptive-expressive language disorder
          Developmental dysphasia or aphasia, receptive type
          Developmental Wernicke's aphasia
          Excludes1   central auditory processing disorder
                  (H93.25)
                  dysphasia or aphasia NOS (R47.-)
                  expressive language disorder (F80.1)
                  expressive type dysphasia or aphasia
                      (F80.1)
                  word deafness (H93.25)
          Excludes2   acquired aphasia with epilepsy [Landau-
                  Kleffner] (G40.80-)
                  intellectual disabilities (F70-F79)
                  pervasive developmental disorders (F84.-)
                  selective mutism (F94.0)

  F80.4   Speech and language development delay due to hearing loss
          Code also type of hearing loss (H90.-, H91.-)
  ● **F80.8   Other developmental disorders of speech or language**
      F80.81   Childhood onset fluency disorder
              Cluttering NOS
              Stuttering NOS
              Excludes1   adult onset fluency disorder
                      (F98.5)
                      fluency disorder in conditions
                          classified elsewhere (R47.82)
                      fluency disorder (stuttering)
                          following cerebrovascular
                          disease (I69. with final
                          characters -23)

      F80.82   Social pragmatic communication disorder
              Excludes1   Asperger's syndrome (F84.5)
                      autistic disorder (F84.0)
              Coding Clinic: 2016, Q4, P16

      F80.89   Other developmental disorders of speech and language
              Coding Clinic: 2017, Q1, P27

  F80.9   Developmental disorder of speech and language, unspecified
              Communication disorder NOS
              Language disorder NOS

● **F81   Specific developmental disorders of scholastic skills**
  F81.0   Specific reading disorder
          'Backward reading'
          Developmental dyslexia
          Specific learning disorder, with impairment in reading
          Specific reading retardation
          Excludes1   alexia NOS (R48.0)
                  dyslexia NOS (R48.0)

  F81.2   Mathematics disorder
          Developmental acalculia
          Developmental arithmetical disorder
          Developmental Gerstmann's syndrome
          Specific learning disorder, with impairment in
              mathematics
          Excludes1   acalculia NOS (R48.8)
          Excludes2   arithmetical difficulties associated with a
                  reading disorder (F81.0)
                  arithmetical difficulties associated with a
                      spelling disorder (F81.81)
                  arithmetical difficulties due to inadequate
                      teaching (Z55.8)

  ● **F81.8   Other developmental disorders of scholastic skills**
      F81.81   Disorder of written expression
              Specific learning disorder, with impairment in
                  written expression
              Specific spelling disorder

      F81.89   Other developmental disorders of scholastic skills

  F81.9   Developmental disorder of scholastic skills, unspecified
              Knowledge acquisition disability NOS
              Learning disability NOS
              Learning disorder NOS
              Coding Clinic: 2022, Q4, P41

  F82   Specific developmental disorder of motor function
          Clumsy child syndrome
          Developmental coordination disorder
          Developmental dyspraxia
          Excludes1   abnormalities of gait and mobility (R26.-)
                  lack of coordination (R27.-)
          Excludes2   lack of coordination secondary to intellectual
                  disabilities (F70-F79)

CHAPTER 5 (F01-F99)

● **F84 Pervasive developmental disorders**
  Code also any associated medical condition and intellectual disabilities

  F84.0 Autistic disorder
    Autism spectrum disorder
    Infantile autism
    Infantile psychosis
    Kanner's syndrome
    Excludes1 Asperger's syndrome (F84.5)
    Coding Clinic: 2022, Q4, P41; 2017, Q1, P27

  F84.2 Rett's syndrome
    Neurodevelopmental disorder
    Excludes1 Asperger's syndrome (F84.5)
                   Autistic disorder (F84.0)
                   other childhood disintegrative disorder
                   (F84.3)

  F84.3 Other childhood disintegrative disorder   P
    Dementia infantilis
    At least two years of normal development followed by significant loss of language abilities, social skills, bowel/bladder control, motor skills
    Disintegrative psychosis
    Heller's syndrome
    At least two years of normal development followed by significant loss of language abilities, social skills, bowel/bladder control, motor skills
    Symbiotic psychosis
    Abnormal relationship to mothering figure, characterized by intense separation anxiety, severe regression, giving up of useful speech, and autism
    Use additional code to identify any associated neurological condition.
    Excludes1 Asperger's syndrome (F84.5)
                   Autistic disorder (F84.0)
                   Rett's syndrome (F84.2)

  F84.5 Asperger's syndrome
    Developmental disorder
    Asperger's disorder
    Autistic psychopathy
    Schizoid disorder of childhood

  F84.8 Other pervasive developmental disorders
    Overactive disorder associated with intellectual disabilities and stereotyped movements

  F84.9 Pervasive developmental disorder, unspecified
    Atypical autism

F88 Other disorders of psychological development
    Developmental agnosia
    Global developmental delay
    Other specified neurodevelopmental disorder

F89 Unspecified disorder of psychological development
    Developmental disorder NOS
    Neurodevelopmental disorder NOS

BEHAVIORAL AND EMOTIONAL DISORDERS WITH ONSET USUALLY OCCURRING IN CHILDHOOD AND ADOLESCENCE (F90-F98)

Note: Codes within categories F90-F98 may be used regardless of the age of a patient. These disorders generally have onset within the childhood or adolescent years, but may continue throughout life or not be diagnosed until adulthood.

● **F90 Attention-deficit hyperactivity disorders**
    Attention deficit disorder with hyperactivity=ADHD
    Includes attention deficit disorder with hyperactivity
                  attention deficit syndrome with hyperactivity
    Excludes2 anxiety disorders (F40.-, F41.-)
                   mood [affective] disorders (F30-F39)
                   pervasive developmental disorders (F84.-)
                   schizophrenia (F20.-)

  F90.0 Attention-deficit hyperactivity disorder, predominantly inattentive type
    Attention-deficit/hyperactivity disorder, predominantly inattentive presentation

  F90.1 Attention-deficit hyperactivity disorder, predominantly hyperactive type
    Attention-deficit/hyperactivity disorder, predominantly hyperactive impulsive presentation

  F90.2 Attention-deficit hyperactivity disorder, combined type
    Attention-deficit/hyperactivity disorder, combined presentation

  F90.8 Attention-deficit hyperactivity disorder, other type

  F90.9 Attention-deficit hyperactivity disorder, unspecified type
    Attention-deficit hyperactivity disorder of childhood or adolescence NOS
    Attention-deficit hyperactivity disorder NOS

● **F91 Conduct disorders**
    Childhood/adolescence disruptive behavior disorder
    Excludes1 antisocial behavior (Z72.81-)
                   antisocial personality disorder (F60.2)
    Excludes2 conduct problems associated with attention-deficit hyperactivity disorder (F90.-)
                   mood [affective] disorders (F30-F39)
                   pervasive developmental disorders (F84.-)
                   schizophrenia (F20.-)

  F91.0 Conduct disorder confined to family context

  F91.1 Conduct disorder, childhood-onset type
    Unsocialized conduct disorder
    Conduct disorder, solitary aggressive type
    Unsocialized aggressive disorder

  F91.2 Conduct disorder, adolescent-onset type
    Socialized conduct disorder
    Conduct disorder, group type

  F91.3 Oppositional defiant disorder

  F91.8 Other conduct disorders
    Other specified conduct disorder
    Other specified disruptive disorder

  F91.9 Conduct disorder, unspecified
    Behavioral disorder NOS
    Conduct disorder NOS
    Disruptive behavior disorder NOS
    Disruptive disorder NOS

● **F93 Emotional disorders with onset specific to childhood**
  F93.0 Separation anxiety disorder of childhood
    Excludes2 mood [affective] disorders (F30-F39)
                   nonpsychotic mental disorders (F40-F48)
                   phobic anxiety disorder of childhood (F40.8)
                   social phobia (F40.1)

  F93.8 Other childhood emotional disorders
    Identity disorder
    Excludes2 gender identity disorder of childhood (F64.2)

  F93.9 Childhood emotional disorder, unspecified

● **F94 Disorders of social functioning with onset specific to childhood and adolescence**
  F94.0 Selective mutism
    Elective mutism
    Excludes2 pervasive developmental disorders (F84.-)
                   schizophrenia (F20.-)
                   specific developmental disorders of speech and language (F80.-)
                   transient mutism as part of separation anxiety in young children (F93.0)

Item 5–2 Enuresis: Bed wetting by children at night. Causes can be either psychological or medical (diabetes, urinary tract infections, or abnormalities). **Encopresis:** Overflow incontinence of bowels sometimes resulting from chronic constipation or fecal impaction. Check the documentation for additional diagnoses.

F94.1　Reactive attachment disorder of childhood
　　Use additional code to identify any associated failure to thrive or growth retardation

　　Excludes1　disinhibited attachment disorder of childhood (F94.2)
　　　　　normal variation in pattern of selective attachment

　　Excludes2　Asperger's syndrome (F84.5)
　　　　　maltreatment syndromes (T74.-)
　　　　　sexual or physical abuse in childhood, resulting in psychosocial problems (Z62.81-)

F94.2　Disinhibited attachment disorder of childhood
　　Affectionless psychopathy
　　Institutional syndrome

　　Excludes1　reactive attachment disorder of childhood (F94.1)

　　Excludes2　Asperger's syndrome (F84.5)
　　　　　attention-deficit hyperactivity disorders (F90.-)
　　　　　hospitalism in children (F43.2-)

F94.8　Other childhood disorders of social functioning

F94.9　Childhood disorder of social functioning, unspecified

● **F95　Tic disorder**
　　Involuntary twitch

F95.0　Transient tic disorder
　　Provisional tic disorder

F95.1　Chronic motor or vocal tic disorder

F95.2　Tourette's disorder
　　Combined vocal and multiple motor tic disorder [de la Tourette]
　　Tourette's syndrome

F95.8　Other tic disorders

F95.9　Tic disorder, unspecified
　　Tic NOS

● **F98　Other behavioral and emotional disorders with onset usually occurring in childhood and adolescence**

　　Excludes2　breath-holding spells (R06.89)
　　　　　gender identity disorder of childhood (F64.2)
　　　　　Kleine-Levin syndrome (G47.13)
　　　　　obsessive-compulsive disorder (F42.3-)
　　　　　sleep disorders not due to a substance or known physiological condition (F51.-)

F98.0　Enuresis not due to a substance or known physiological condition
　　Enuresis: Urinary incontinence
　　Enuresis (primary) (secondary) of nonorganic origin
　　Functional enuresis
　　Psychogenic enuresis
　　Urinary incontinence of nonorganic origin

　　Excludes1　enuresis NOS (R32)

F98.1　Encopresis not due to a substance or known physiological condition
　　Encopresis: Fecal incontinence
　　Functional encopresis
　　Incontinence of feces of nonorganic origin
　　Psychogenic encopresis

　　Use additional code to identify the cause of any coexisting constipation.

　　Excludes1　encopresis NOS (R15.-)

● **F98.2　Other feeding disorders of infancy and childhood**

　　Excludes2　anorexia nervosa and other eating disorders (F50.-)
　　　　　feeding difficulties (R63.3-)
　　　　　feeding problems of newborn (P92.-)
　　　　　pica of infancy or childhood (F98.3)

F98.21　Rumination disorder of infancy and childhood
　　Rumination disorder of infancy and childhood, in remission

　　Excludes1　rumination disorder in adults (F50.84)

F98.29　Other feeding disorders of infancy and early childhood

F98.3　Pica of infancy and childhood
　　Craving and eating substances such as paint, clay, or dirt to replace a nutritional deficit in the body.
　　Pica in infancy or childhood, in remission

　　Excludes1　pica in adults (F50.83)

F98.4　Stereotyped movement disorders
　　Stereotype/habit disorder

　　Excludes1　abnormal involuntary movements (R25.-)

　　Excludes2　compulsions in obsessive-compulsive disorder (F42.-)
　　　　　hair plucking (F63.3)
　　　　　movement disorders of organic origin (G20-G25)
　　　　　nail-biting (F98.8)
　　　　　nose-picking (F98.8)
　　　　　stereotypies that are part of a broader psychiatric condition (F01-F95)
　　　　　thumb-sucking (F98.8)
　　　　　tic disorders (F95.-)
　　　　　trichotillomania (F63.3)

F98.5　Adult onset fluency disorder

　　Excludes1　childhood onset fluency disorder (F80.81)
　　　　　dysphasia (R47.02)
　　　　　fluency disorder in conditions classified elsewhere (R47.82)
　　　　　fluency disorder (stuttering) following cerebrovascular disease (I69. with final characters -23)
　　　　　tic disorders (F95.-)

F98.8　Other specified behavioral and emotional disorders with onset usually occurring in childhood and adolescence
　　Excessive masturbation
　　Nail-biting
　　Nose-picking
　　Thumb-sucking

F98.9　Unspecified behavioral and emotional disorders with onset usually occurring in childhood and adolescence

---

UNSPECIFIED MENTAL DISORDER (F99)

F99　Mental disorder, not otherwise specified
　　Mental illness NOS

　　Excludes1　unspecified mental disorder due to known physiological condition (F09)

CHAPTER 5 (F01-F99)

CHAPTER 6

DISEASES OF THE NERVOUS SYSTEM (G00-G99)

OGCR Chapter-Specific Coding Guidelines

6. Chapter 6: Diseases of the Nervous System (G00-G99)

a. Dominant/nondominant side

Codes from category G81, Hemiplegia and hemiparesis, and subcategories, G83.1, Monoplegia of lower limb, G83.2, Monoplegia of upper limb, and G83.3, Monoplegia, unspecified, identify whether the dominant or nondominant side is affected. Should the affected side be documented, but not specified as dominant or nondominant, and the classification system does not indicate a default, code selection is as follows:

- For ambidextrous patients, the default should be dominant.
- If the left side is affected, the default is nondominant.
- If the right side is affected, the default is dominant.

b. Pain - Category G89

1) General coding information

Codes in category G89, Pain, not elsewhere classified, may be used in conjunction with codes from other categories and chapters to provide more detail about acute or chronic pain and neoplasm-related pain, unless otherwise indicated below.

If the pain is not specified as acute or chronic, post-thoracotomy, postprocedural, or neoplasm-related, do not assign codes from category G89.

A code from category G89 should not be assigned if the underlying (definitive) diagnosis is known, unless the reason for the encounter is pain control/management and not management of the underlying condition.

When an admission or encounter is for a procedure aimed at treating the underlying condition (e.g., spinal fusion, kyphoplasty), a code for the underlying condition (e.g., vertebral fracture, spinal stenosis) should be assigned as the principal diagnosis. No code from category G89 should be assigned.

(a) Category G89 Codes as Principal or First-Listed Diagnosis

Category G89 codes are acceptable as principal diagnosis or the first-listed code:

- When pain control or pain management is the reason for the admission/encounter (e.g., a patient with displaced intervertebral disc, nerve impingement and severe back pain presents for injection of steroid into the spinal canal). The underlying cause of the pain should be reported as an additional diagnosis, if known.
- When a patient is admitted for the insertion of a neurostimulator for pain control, assign the appropriate pain code as the principal or first-listed diagnosis. When an admission or encounter is for a procedure aimed at treating the underlying condition and a neurostimulator is inserted for pain control during the same admission/encounter, a code for the underlying condition should be assigned as the principal diagnosis and the appropriate pain code should be assigned as a secondary diagnosis.

(b) Use of Category G89 Codes in Conjunction with Site Specific Pain Codes

(i) Assigning Category G89 and Site-Specific Pain Codes

Codes from category G89 may be used in conjunction with codes that identify the site of pain (including codes from Chapter 18) if the category G89 code provides additional information. For example, if the code describes the site of the pain, but does not fully describe whether the pain is acute or chronic, then both codes should be assigned.

(ii) Sequencing of Category G89 Codes with Site-Specific Pain Codes

The sequencing of category G89 codes with site-specific pain codes (including Chapter 18 codes), is dependent on the circumstances of the encounter/admission as follows:

- If the encounter is for pain control or pain management, assign the code from category G89 followed by the code identifying the specific site of pain (e.g., encounter for pain management for acute neck pain from trauma is assigned code G89.11, Acute pain due to trauma, followed by code M54.2, Cervicalgia, to identify the site of pain).
- If the encounter is for any other reason except pain control or pain management, and a related definitive diagnosis has not been established (confirmed) by the provider, assign the code for the specific site of pain first, followed by the appropriate code from category G89.

2) Pain due to devices, implants and grafts

See Section I.C.19. Pain due to medical devices

3) Postoperative Pain

The provider's documentation should be used to guide the coding of postoperative pain, as well as *Section III. Reporting Additional Diagnoses* and *Section IV. Diagnostic Coding and Reporting in the Outpatient Setting*.

The default for post-thoracotomy and other postoperative pain not specified as acute or chronic is the code for the acute form.

Routine or expected postoperative pain immediately after surgery should not be coded.

(a) Postoperative pain not associated with specific postoperative complication

Postoperative pain not associated with a specific postoperative complication is assigned to the appropriate postoperative pain code in category G89.

(b) Postoperative pain associated with specific postoperative complication

Postoperative pain associated with a specific postoperative complication (such as painful wire sutures) is assigned to the appropriate code(s) found in Chapter 19, Injury, poisoning, and certain other consequences of external causes. If appropriate, use additional code(s) from category G89 to identify acute or chronic pain (G89.18 or G89.28).

4) Chronic pain

Chronic pain is classified to subcategory G89.2. There is no time frame defining when pain becomes chronic pain. The provider's documentation should be used to guide use of these codes.

5) Neoplasm Related Pain

Code G89.3 is assigned to pain documented as being related, associated or due to cancer, primary or secondary malignancy, or tumor. This code is assigned regardless of whether the pain is acute or chronic.

This code may be assigned as the principal or first-listed code when the stated reason for the admission/encounter is documented as pain control/pain management. The underlying neoplasm should be reported as an additional diagnosis.

When the reason for the admission/encounter is management of the neoplasm and the pain associated with the neoplasm is also documented, code G89.3 may be assigned as an additional diagnosis. It is not necessary to assign an additional code for the site of the pain.

See Section I.C.2 for instructions on the sequencing of neoplasms for all other stated reasons for the admission/encounter (except for pain control/pain management).

6) Chronic pain syndrome

Central pain syndrome (G89.0) and chronic pain syndrome (G89.4) are different than the term "chronic pain," and therefore codes should only be used when the provider has specifically documented this condition.

See Section I.C.5. Pain disorders related to psychological factors

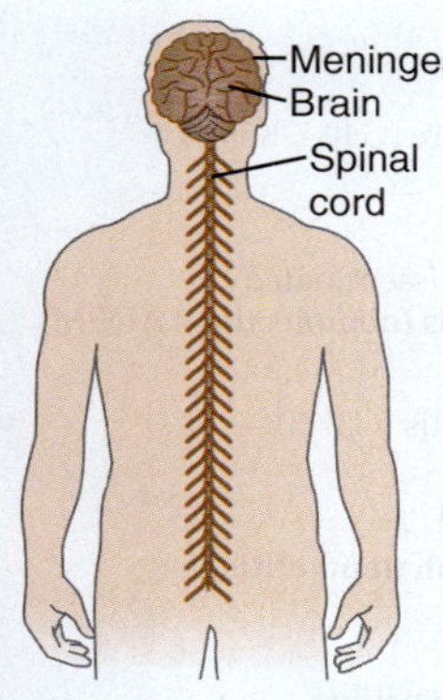

Figure 6-1 The brain and spinal cord make up the central nervous system.

Item 6–1 The two major classifications of the nervous system are the peripheral nervous system and the central nervous system (CNS). The central nervous system is composed of the brain and the spinal cord. The peripheral nervous system is composed of the parasympathetic and sympathetic systems. **Encephalitis** is the swelling of the brain. **Meningitis** is swelling of the covering of the brain, the meninges. Types and causes of brain infections are:

Type	Cause
purulent	bacterial
aseptic/abacterial	viral
chronic meningitis	mycobacterial and fungal

CHAPTER 6

DISEASES OF THE NERVOUS SYSTEM
(G00-G99)

Excludes2　certain conditions originating in the perinatal period (P04-P96)
certain infectious and parasitic diseases (A00-B99)
complications of pregnancy, childbirth and the puerperium (O00-O9A)
congenital malformations, deformations, and chromosomal abnormalities (Q00-Q99)
endocrine, nutritional and metabolic diseases (E00-E88)
injury, poisoning and certain other consequences of external causes (S00-T88)
neoplasms (C00-D49)
symptoms, signs and abnormal clinical and laboratory findings, not elsewhere classified (R00-R94)

This chapter contains the following blocks:

G00-G09	Inflammatory diseases of the central nervous system
G10-G14	Systemic atrophies primarily affecting the central nervous system
G20-G26	Extrapyramidal and movement disorders
G30-G32	Other degenerative diseases of the nervous system
G35-G37	Demyelinating diseases of the central nervous system
G40-G47	Episodic and paroxysmal disorders
G50-G59	Nerve, nerve root and plexus disorders
G60-G65	Polyneuropathies and other disorders of the peripheral nervous system
G70-G73	Diseases of myoneural junction and muscle
G80-G83	Cerebral palsy and other paralytic syndromes
G89-G99	Other disorders of the nervous system

INFLAMMATORY DISEASES OF THE CENTRAL NERVOUS SYSTEM (G00-G09)

● **G00　Bacterial meningitis, not elsewhere classified**
An infection of the cerebrospinal fluid surrounding the spinal cord and brain.

　　Includes　bacterial arachnoiditis
　　　　　bacterial leptomeningitis
　　　　　bacterial meningitis
　　　　　bacterial pachymeningitis

　　Excludes1　bacterial meningoencephalitis (G04.2)
　　　　　bacterial meningomyelitis (G04.2)

G00.0　Hemophilus meningitis
　　Meningitis due to Hemophilus influenzae

G00.1　Pneumococcal meningitis
　　Meningitis due to Streptococcal pneumoniae

G00.2　Streptococcal meningitis
　　Use additional code to further identify organism (B95.0-B95.5)

G00.3　Staphylococcal meningitis
　　Use additional code to further identify organism (B95.61-B95.8)

G00.8　Other bacterial meningitis
　　Meningitis due to Escherichia coli
　　Meningitis due to Friedländer bacillus
　　Meningitis due to Klebsiella
　　Use additional code to further identify organism (B96.-)

G00.9　Bacterial meningitis, unspecified
　　Meningitis due to gram-negative bacteria, unspecified
　　Purulent meningitis NOS
　　Pyogenic meningitis NOS
　　Suppurative meningitis NOS

▸ *G01　Meningitis in bacterial diseases classified elsewhere*

　　Code first underlying disease

　　Excludes1　meningitis (in):
　　　　gonococcal (A54.81)
　　　　leptospirosis (A27.81)
　　　　listeriosis (A32.11)
　　　　Lyme disease (A69.21)
　　　　meningococcal (A39.0)
　　　　neurosyphilis (A52.13)
　　　　tuberculosis (A17.0)
　　　　meningoencephalitis and meningomyelitis in bacterial diseases classified elsewhere (G05)

▸ *G02　Meningitis in other infectious and parasitic diseases classified elsewhere*

　　Code first underlying disease, such as:
　　African trypanosomiasis (B56.-)
　　poliovirus infection (A80.-)

　　Excludes1　candidal meningitis (B37.5)
　　　　coccidioidomycosis meningitis (B38.4)
　　　　cryptococcal meningitis (B45.1)
　　　　herpesviral [herpes simplex] meningitis (B00.3)
　　　　infectious mononucleosis complicated by meningitis (B27.- with fourth character 2)
　　　　measles complicated by meningitis (B05.1)
　　　　meningoencephalitis and meningomyelitis in other infectious and parasitic diseases classified elsewhere (G05)
　　　　mumps meningitis (B26.1)
　　　　rubella meningitis (B06.02)
　　　　varicella [chickenpox] meningitis (B01.0)
　　　　zoster meningitis (B02.1)

CHAPTER 6 (G00-G99)

CHAPTER 6 (G00–G99)

● **G03** **Meningitis due to other and unspecified causes**

Includes   arachnoiditis NOS
leptomeningitis NOS
meningitis NOS
pachymeningitis NOS

Excludes1   meningoencephalitis (G04.-)
meningomyelitis (G04.-)

G03.0 **Nonpyogenic meningitis**
Aseptic meningitis
Nonbacterial meningitis

G03.1 **Chronic meningitis**

G03.2 **Benign recurrent meningitis [Mollaret]**

G03.8 **Meningitis due to other specified causes**

G03.9 **Meningitis, unspecified**
Arachnoiditis (spinal) NOS

● **G04** **Encephalitis, myelitis and encephalomyelitis**

Includes   acute ascending myelitis
meningoencephalitis
meningomyelitis

Excludes1   encephalopathy NOS (G93.40)
other noninfectious acute disseminated
   encephalomyelitis (noninfectious ADEM)
   (G04.81)

Excludes2   acute transverse myelitis (G37.3)
alcoholic encephalopathy (G31.2)
multiple sclerosis (G35.-)
myalgic encephalomyelitis (G93.32)
subacute necrotizing myelitis (G37.4)
toxic encephalitis (G92.8)
toxic encephalopathy (G92.8)

● **G04.0** **Acute disseminated encephalitis and encephalomyelitis (ADEM)**

Excludes1   acute necrotizing hemorrhagic
   encephalopathy (G04.3-)

G04.00 **Acute disseminated encephalitis and encephalomyelitis, unspecified**

G04.01 *Postinfectious acute disseminated encephalitis and encephalomyelitis (postinfectious ADEM)*

Excludes1   post chickenpox encephalitis
   (B01.1)
post measles encephalitis (B05.0)
post measles myelitis (B05.1)

G04.02 **Postimmunization acute disseminated encephalitis, myelitis and encephalomyelitis**
Encephalitis, post immunization
Encephalomyelitis, post immunization

Use additional code to identify the vaccine
(T50.A-, T50.B-, T50.Z-)

G04.1 **Tropical spastic paraplegia** 🅡🅒

G04.2 **Bacterial meningoencephalitis and meningomyelitis, not elsewhere classified**

● **G04.3** **Acute necrotizing hemorrhagic encephalopathy**
Sudden and severe CNS disease with pathology of hemorrhages and necrosis of white matter

Excludes1   acute disseminated encephalitis and
   encephalomyelitis (G04.0-)

G04.30 **Acute necrotizing hemorrhagic encephalopathy, unspecified**

G04.31 **Postinfectious acute necrotizing hemorrhagic encephalopathy**

G04.32 **Postimmunization acute necrotizing hemorrhagic encephalopathy**

Use additional code to identify vaccine
(T50.A-, T50.B-, T50.Z-)

G04.39 **Other acute necrotizing hemorrhagic encephalopathy**

Code also underlying etiology, if applicable

● **G04.8** **Other encephalitis, myelitis and encephalomyelitis**

Code also any associated seizure (G40.-, R56.9)

G04.81 **Other encephalitis and encephalomyelitis**
Noninfectious acute disseminated
   encephalomyelitis (noninfectious ADEM)

G04.82 **Acute flaccid myelitis**

Excludes1   transverse myelitis (G37.3)

G04.89 **Other myelitis** 🅡🅒
Coding Clinic: 2020, Q1, P14

● **G04.9** **Encephalitis, myelitis and encephalomyelitis, unspecified**

G04.90 **Encephalitis and encephalomyelitis, unspecified**
Ventriculitis (cerebral) NOS

G04.91 **Myelitis, unspecified** 🅡🅒

● **G05** **Encephalitis, myelitis and encephalomyelitis in diseases classified elsewhere**

Code first *underlying disease, such as:*
congenital toxoplasmosis encephalitis, myelitis and
   encephalomyelitis (P37.1)
cytomegaloviral encephalitis, myelitis and encephalomyelitis
   (B25.8)
encephalitis, myelitis and encephalomyelitis (in) systemic
   lupus erythematosus (M32.19)
eosinophilic meningoencephalitis (B83.2)
human immunodeficiency virus [HIV] disease (B20)
poliovirus (A80.-)
suppurative otitis media (H66.01-H66.4)
systemic lupus erythematosus (M32.19)
trichinellosis (B75)

Excludes1   adenoviral encephalitis, myelitis and
   encephalomyelitis (A85.1)
encephalitis, myelitis and encephalomyelitis (in)
   measles (B05.0)
enteroviral encephalitis, myelitis and
   encephalomyelitis (A85.0)
herpesviral [herpes simplex] encephalitis,
   myelitis and encephalomyelitis (B00.4)
listerial encephalitis, myelitis and
   encephalomyelitis (A32.12)
meningococcal encephalitis, myelitis and
   encephalomyelitis (A39.81)
mumps encephalitis, myelitis and
   encephalomyelitis (B26.2)
postchickenpox encephalitis, myelitis and
   encephalomyelitis (B01.1-)
rubella encephalitis, myelitis and
   encephalomyelitis (B06.01)
toxoplasmosis encephalitis, myelitis and
   encephalomyelitis (B58.2)
zoster encephalitis, myelitis and
   encephalomyelitis (B02.0)

G05.3 *Encephalitis and encephalomyelitis in diseases classified elsewhere*
Meningoencephalitis in diseases classified elsewhere
Code first *underlying disease*

G05.4 *Myelitis in diseases classified elsewhere* 🅡🅒
Meningomyelitis in diseases classified elsewhere

● **G06** **Intracranial and intraspinal abscess and granuloma**
An accumulation of pus in either the brain or spinal cord

Use additional code (B95-B97) to identify infectious agent.

G06.0 **Intracranial abscess and granuloma**
Brain [any part] abscess (embolic)
Cerebellar abscess (embolic)
Cerebral abscess (embolic)
Intracranial epidural abscess or granuloma
Intracranial extradural abscess or granuloma
Intracranial subdural abscess or granuloma
Otogenic abscess (embolic)

Excludes1   tuberculous intracranial abscess and
   granuloma (A17.81)

▶ New   ▶ Revised   ~~deleted~~ Deleted   Excludes 1   Excludes 2   Includes   Use additional   Code first   Code also   Key words
OGCR Official Guidelines   **X** Assign placeholder X   ● Use Additional Character(s)   ▶ Manifestation Code   🅡🅒 Hierarchical Condition Category   **Coding Clinic**

Item 6–2 Huntington's chorea is an inherited degenerative disorder of the central nervous system and is characterized by ceaseless, jerky movements and progressive cognitive and behavioral deterioration.

G06.1   Intraspinal abscess and granuloma
     Abscess (embolic) of spinal cord [any part]
     Intraspinal epidural abscess or granuloma
     Intraspinal extradural abscess or granuloma
     Intraspinal subdural abscess or granuloma
     Excludes1   tuberculous intraspinal abscess and granuloma (A17.81)

G06.2   Extradural and subdural abscess, unspecified

G07   *Intracranial and intraspinal abscess and granuloma in diseases classified elsewhere*
     Code first underlying disease, such as:
       schistosomiasis granuloma of brain (B65.-)
     Excludes1   abscess of brain:
         amebic (A06.6)
         chromomycotic (B43.1)
         gonococcal (A54.82)
         tuberculous (A17.81)
         tuberculoma of meninges (A17.1)

G08   Intracranial and intraspinal phlebitis and thrombophlebitis
     Septic embolism of intracranial or intraspinal venous sinuses and veins
     Septic endophlebitis of intracranial or intraspinal venous sinuses and veins
     Septic phlebitis of intracranial or intraspinal venous sinuses and veins
     Septic thrombophlebitis of intracranial or intraspinal venous sinuses and veins
     Septic thrombosis of intracranial or intraspinal venous sinuses and veins
     Excludes1   intracranial phlebitis and thrombophlebitis complicating:
         abortion, ectopic or molar pregnancy (O00-O07, O08.7)
         pregnancy, childbirth and the puerperium (O22.5, O87.3)
         nonpyogenic intracranial phlebitis and thrombophlebitis (I67.6)
     Excludes2   intracranial phlebitis and thrombophlebitis complicating nonpyogenic intraspinal phlebitis and thrombophlebitis (G95.1)

G09   Sequelae of inflammatory diseases of central nervous system
     Note: Category G09 is to be used to indicate conditions whose primary classification is to G00-G08 as the cause of sequelae, themselves classifiable elsewhere. The 'sequelae' include conditions specified as residuals.
     Code first condition resulting from (sequela) of inflammatory diseases of central nervous system

SYSTEMIC ATROPHIES PRIMARILY AFFECTING THE CENTRAL NERVOUS SYSTEM (G10-G14)

G10   Huntington's disease 🟢
     Genetic disease with degeneration of cells of the nervous system, including brain
     Huntington's chorea
     Huntington's dementia
     Use Additional code, if applicable, to identify:
       dementia with anxiety (F02.84, F02.A4, F02.B4, F02.C4)
       dementia with behavioral disturbance (F02.81-, F02.A1-, F02.B1-, F02.C1-)
       dementia with mood disturbance (F02.83, F02.A3, F02.B3, F02.C3)
       dementia with psychotic disturbance (F02.82, F02.A2, F02.B2, F02.C2)
       dementia without behavioral disturbance (F02.80, F02.A0, F02.B0, F02.C0)
       mild neurocognitive disorder due to known physiological condition (F06.7-)

G11   Hereditary ataxia
     Genetic neurological disorder affecting coordination
     Excludes2   cerebral palsy (G80.-)
         hereditary and idiopathic neuropathy (G60.-)
         metabolic disorders (E70-E88)
     G11.0   Congenital nonprogressive ataxia 🟢

G11.1   Early-onset cerebellar ataxia 🟢
     G11.10   Early-onset cerebellar ataxia, unspecified
     G11.11   Friedreich ataxia
       Autosomal recessive Friedreich ataxia
       Friedreich ataxia with retained reflexes
     G11.19   Other early-onset cerebellar ataxia
       Early-onset cerebellar ataxia with essential tremor
       Early-onset cerebellar ataxia with myoclonus [Hunt's ataxia]
       Early-onset cerebellar ataxia with retained tendon reflexes
       X-linked recessive spinocerebellar ataxia

G11.2   Late-onset cerebellar ataxia 🟢   **A**

G11.3   Cerebellar ataxia with defective DNA repair 🟢
     Ataxia telangiectasia [Louis-Bar]
     Excludes2   Cockayne's syndrome (Q87.19)
         other disorders of purine and pyrimidine metabolism (E79.-)
         xeroderma pigmentosum (Q82.1)

G11.4   Hereditary spastic paraplegia 🟢

G11.5   Hypomyelination - hypogonadotropic hypogonadism - hypodontia
     4H syndrome
     Pol III-related leukodystrophy

G11.6   Leukodystrophy with vanishing white matter disease

G11.8   Other hereditary ataxias 🟢

G11.9   Hereditary ataxia, unspecified 🟢
     Hereditary cerebellar ataxia NOS
     Hereditary cerebellar degeneration
     Hereditary cerebellar disease
     Hereditary cerebellar syndrome

G12   Spinal muscular atrophy and related syndromes
     G12.0   Infantile spinal muscular atrophy, type I [Werdnig-Hoffman] 🟢

G12.1   Other inherited spinal muscular atrophy 🟢
     Adult form spinal muscular atrophy
     Childhood form, type II spinal muscular atrophy
     Distal spinal muscular atrophy
     Juvenile form, type III spinal muscular atrophy [Kugelberg-Welander]
     Progressive bulbar palsy of childhood [Fazio-Londe]
     Scapuloperoneal form spinal muscular atrophy

G12.2   Motor neuron disease
     Progressive disease of motor neurons that carry impluses to muscles to move
     G12.20   Motor neuron disease, unspecified 🟢
     G12.21   Amyotrophic lateral sclerosis 🟢   **A**
       Lou Gehrig's disease (ALS)
     G12.22   Progressive bulbar palsy 🟢
     G12.23   Primary lateral sclerosis 🟢
     G12.24   Familial motor neuron disease 🟢
     G12.25   Progressive spinal muscle atrophy 🟢
     G12.29   Other motor neuron disease 🟢

G12.8   Other spinal muscular atrophies and related syndromes 🟢

G12.9   Spinal muscular atrophy, unspecified 🟢

CHAPTER 6 (G00-G99)

● **G13** **Systemic atrophies primarily affecting central nervous system in diseases classified elsewhere**
▸ *G13.0* *Paraneoplastic neuromyopathy and neuropathy* 🅗🅒🅒
 Carcinomatous neuromyopathy
 Sensorial paraneoplastic neuropathy [Denny Brown]
 Code first underlying neoplasm (C00-D49)
▸ *G13.1* *Other systemic atrophy primarily affecting central nervous system in neoplastic disease* 🅗🅒🅒
 Paraneoplastic limbic encephalopathy
 Code first underlying neoplasm (C00-D49)
▸ *G13.2* *Systemic atrophy primarily affecting the central nervous system in myxedema*
 Code first underlying disease, such as:
  hypothyroidism (E03.-)
  myxedematous congenital iodine deficiency (E00.1)
▸ *G13.8* *Systemic atrophy primarily affecting central nervous system in other diseases classified elsewhere*
 Code first underlying disease

G14 **Postpolio syndrome**
 Includes Postpolio myelitic syndrome
 Excludes1 sequelae of poliomyelitis (B91)

EXTRAPYRAMIDAL AND MOVEMENT DISORDERS (G20-G26)

● **G20** **Parkinson's disease** 🅗🅒🅒
Progressive disease of the nervous system that affects muscle coordination
 Hemiparkinsonism
 Idiopathic Parkinsonism or Parkinson's disease
 Paralysis agitans
 Parkinsonism or Parkinson's disease NOS
 Primary Parkinsonism or Parkinson's disease
 Use additional code, if applicable, to identify:
  dementia with anxiety (F02.84, F02.A4, F02.B4, F02.C4)
  dementia with behavioral disturbance (F02.81-, F02.A1-, F02.B1-, F02.C1-)
  dementia with mood disturbance (F02.83, F02.A3, F02.B3, F02.C3)
  dementia with psychotic disturbance (F02.82, F02.A2, F02.B2, F02.C2)
  dementia without behavioral disturbance (F02.80, F02.A0, F02.B0, F02.C0)
  mild neurocognitive disorder due to known physiological condition (F06.7-)
 Coding Clinic: 2017, Q2, P7-8; 2016, Q2, P7
● **G20.A** **Parkinson's disease without dyskinesia**
 G20.A1 **Parkinson's disease without dyskinesia, without mention of fluctuations**
  Parkinson's disease NOS
  Parkinson's disease without dyskinesia, without mention of OFF episodes
 G20.A2 **Parkinson's disease without dyskinesia, with fluctuations**
  Parkinson's disease without dyskinesia, with OFF episodes
  Coding Clinic: 2023, Q4, P17
● **G20.B** **Parkinson's disease with dyskinesia**
 Excludes1 drug induced dystonia (G24.0-)
 G20.B1 **Parkinson's disease with dyskinesia, without mention of fluctuations**
  Parkinson's disease with dyskinesia, without mention of OFF episodes
  Coding Clinic: 2023, Q4, P16
 G20.B2 **Parkinson's disease with dyskinesia, with fluctuations**
  Parkinson's disease with dyskinesia, with OFF episodes
  Coding Clinic: 2023, Q4, P17
● **G20.C** **Parkinsonism, unspecified**
 Parkinsonism, NOS
 Excludes1 Parkinson's disease NOS (G20.A1)
  Parkinson's disease with dyskinesia (G20.B-)
  Parkinson's disease without dyskinesia (G20.A-)
  secondary parkinsonism (G20.-)

● **G21** **Secondary parkinsonism**
Symptoms of Parkinson's caused by medicines, illness, or other nervous system disorder
 Excludes1 Huntington's disease (G10)
  neurocognitive disorder with Lewy bodies (G31.83)
  Shy-Drager syndrome (G90.3)
  syphilitic Parkinsonism (A52.19)
 G21.0 **Malignant neuroleptic syndrome**
  Use additional code for adverse effect, if applicable, to identify drug (T43.3X5, T43.4X5, T43.505, T43.595)
  Excludes1 neuroleptic induced parkinsonism (G21.11)
● **G21.1** **Other drug-induced secondary parkinsonism**
 G21.11 **Neuroleptic induced parkinsonism** 🅗🅒🅒
  Use additional code for adverse effect, if applicable, to identify drug (T43.3X5, T43.4X5, T43.505, T43.595)
  Excludes1 malignant neuroleptic syndrome (G21.0)
 G21.19 **Other drug induced secondary parkinsonism** 🅗🅒🅒
  Other medication-induced parkinsonism
  Use additional code for adverse effect, if applicable, to identify drug (T36-T50 with fifth or sixth character 5)
 G21.2 **Secondary parkinsonism due to other external agents** 🅗🅒🅒
  Code first (T51-T65) to identify external agent
 G21.3 **Postencephalitic parkinsonism** 🅗🅒🅒
 G21.4 **Vascular parkinsonism** 🅗🅒🅒
 G21.8 **Other secondary parkinsonism** 🅗🅒🅒
 G21.9 **Secondary parkinsonism, unspecified** 🅗🅒🅒
● **G23** **Other degenerative diseases of basal ganglia**
 Excludes2 multi-system degeneration of the autonomic nervous system (G90.3)
 G23.0 **Hallervorden-Spatz disease** 🅗🅒🅒
  Pigmentary pallidal degeneration
 G23.1 **Progressive supranuclear ophthalmoplegia [Steele-Richardson-Olszewski]** 🅗🅒🅒
  Progressive supranuclear palsy
 G23.2 **Striatonigral degeneration** 🅗🅒🅒
 G23.3 **Hypomyelination with atrophy of the basal ganglia and cerebellum**
  H-ABC
  ▸ TUBB4A-related neurologic disorders
 G23.8 **Other specified degenerative diseases of basal ganglia** 🅗🅒🅒
  Calcification of basal ganglia
 G23.9 **Degenerative disease of basal ganglia, unspecified** 🅗🅒🅒
● **G24** **Dystonia**
Involuntary movements
 Includes dyskinesia
 Excludes2 athetoid cerebral palsy (G80.3)
● **G24.0** **Drug induced dystonia**
  Use additional code for adverse effect, if applicable, to identify drug (T36-T50 with fifth or sixth character 5)
 G24.01 **Drug induced subacute dyskinesia**
  Drug induced blepharospasm
  Drug induced orofacial dyskinesia
  Neuroleptic induced tardive dyskinesia
  Tardive dyskinesia
 G24.02 **Drug induced acute dystonia**
  Acute dystonic reaction to drugs
  Neuroleptic induced acute dystonia
 G24.09 **Other drug induced dystonia**

▸ New ➡ Revised ~~deleted~~ Deleted Excludes 1 Excludes 2 Includes Use additional Code first Code also Key words
OGCR Official Guidelines X Assign placeholder X ● Use Additional Character(s) ▸ Manifestation Code 🅗🅒🅒 Hierarchical Condition Category **Coding Clinic**

G24.1 Genetic torsion dystonia
Dystonia deformans progressiva
Dystonia musculorum deformans
Familial torsion dystonia
Idiopathic familial dystonia
Idiopathic (torsion) dystonia NOS
(Schwalbe-) Ziehen-Oppenheim disease

G24.2 Idiopathic nonfamilial dystonia

G24.3 Spasmodic torticollis
Head tilts toward one side and chin is elevated and turned toward opposite side (wry neck)

Excludes1 congenital torticollis (Q68.0)
hysterical torticollis (F44.4)
ocular torticollis (R29.891)
psychogenic torticollis (F45.8)
torticollis NOS (M43.6)
traumatic recurrent torticollis (S13.4)

G24.4 Idiopathic orofacial dystonia
Orofacial dyskinesia

Excludes1 drug induced orofacial dyskinesia (G24.01)

G24.5 Blepharospasm
Tonic spasm of orbicularis oculi muscle, producing closure of eyelids

Excludes1 drug induced blepharospasm (G24.01)

G24.8 Other dystonia
Acquired torsion dystonia NOS

G24.9 Dystonia, unspecified
Dyskinesia NOS

G25 Other extrapyramidal and movement disorders
Extrapyramidal: Other than pyramidal tracts

Excludes2 sleep related movement disorders (G47.6-)

G25.0 Essential tremor
Familial tremor

Excludes1 tremor NOS (R25.1)

G25.1 Drug-induced tremor
Use additional code for adverse effect, if applicable, to identify drug (T36-T50 with fifth or sixth character 5)

G25.2 Other specified forms of tremor
Intention tremor

G25.3 Myoclonus
Shocklike contractions muscle(s)
Drug-induced myoclonus
Palatal myoclonus
Use additional code for adverse effect, if applicable, to identify drug (T36-T50 with fifth or sixth character 5)

Excludes1 facial myokymia (G51.4)
myoclonic epilepsy (G40.-)

G25.4 Drug-induced chorea
Use additional code for adverse effect, if applicable, to identify drug (T36-T50 with fifth or sixth character 5)

G25.5 Other chorea
Continual, involuntary, jerky, movements
Chorea NOS

Excludes1 chorea NOS with heart involvement (I02.0)
Huntington's chorea (G10)
rheumatic chorea (I02.-)
Sydenham's chorea (I02.-)

G25.6 Drug induced tics and other tics of organic origin

G25.61 Drug induced tics
Use additional code for adverse effect, if applicable, to identify drug (T36-T50 with fifth or sixth character 5)

G25.69 Other tics of organic origin

Excludes1 habit spasm (F95.9)
tic NOS (F95.9)
Tourette's syndrome (F95.2)

G25.7 Other and unspecified drug induced movement disorders
Use additional code for adverse effect, if applicable, to identify drug (T36-T50 with fifth or sixth character 5)

G25.70 Drug induced movement disorder, unspecified

G25.71 Drug induced akathisia
Drug induced acathisia
Neuroleptic induced acute akathisia
Tardive akathisia

G25.79 Other drug induced movement disorders

G25.8 Other specified extrapyramidal and movement disorders

G25.81 Restless legs syndrome

G25.82 Stiff-man syndrome

G25.83 Benign shuddering attacks

G25.89 Other specified extrapyramidal and movement disorders

G25.9 Extrapyramidal and movement disorder, unspecified

G26 Extrapyramidal and movement disorders in diseases classified elsewhere
Code first underlying disease

OTHER DEGENERATIVE DISEASES OF THE NERVOUS SYSTEM (G30-G32)

G30 Alzheimer's disease
Progressive central neurodegenerative disorder

Includes Alzheimer's dementia senile and presenile forms

Use additional code, if applicable, to identify:
delirium, if applicable (F05)
dementia with anxiety (F02.84, F02.A4, F02.B4, F02.C4)
dementia with behavioral disturbance (F02.81-, F02.A1-, F02.B1-, F02.C1-)
dementia with mood disturbance (F02.83, F02.A3, F02.B3, F02.C3)
dementia with psychotic disturbance (F02.82, F02.A2, F02.B2, F02.C2)
dementia without behavioral disturbance (F02.80, F02.A0, F02.B0, F02.C0)
mild neurocognitive disorder due to known physiological condition (F06.7-)

Excludes1 senile degeneration of brain NEC (G31.1)
senile dementia NOS (F03.-)
senility NOS (R41.81)

G30.0 Alzheimer's disease with early onset

G30.1 Alzheimer's disease with late onset A
Coding Clinic: 2022, Q4, P15

G30.8 Other Alzheimer's disease

G30.9 Alzheimer's disease, unspecified
Coding Clinic: 2017, Q1, P43; 2016, Q2, P6; 2012, Q4, P95

G31 Other degenerative diseases of nervous system, not elsewhere classified
Use additional
code, if applicable, for codes G31.0-G31.83, G31.85-G31.9, to identify:
dementia with behavioral disturbance (F02.81-, F02.A1-, F02.B1-, F02.C1-)
dementia with mood disturbance (F02.83, F02.A3, F02.B3, F02.C3)
dementia with psychotic disturbance (F02.82, F02.A2, F02.B2, F02.C2)
dementia without behavioral disturbance (F02.80, F02.A0, F02.B0, F02.C0)
mild neurocognitive disorder due to known physiological condition (F06.7-)

Excludes2 Reye's syndrome (G93.7)

G31.0 Frontotemporal dementia

G31.01 Pick's disease
Primary progressive aphasia
Progressive isolated aphasia

CHAPTER 6 (G00-G99)

G31.09   Other frontotemporal neurocognitive disorder
Frontal dementia
Use Additional code, if applicable, to identify mild neurocognitive disorders due to known physiological condition (F06.7-)

G31.1   Senile degeneration of brain, not elsewhere classified
Excludes1   Alzheimer's disease (G30.-)
senility NOS (R41.81)

G31.2   Degeneration of nervous system due to alcohol
Alcoholic cerebellar ataxia
Alcoholic cerebellar degeneration
Alcoholic cerebral degeneration
Alcoholic encephalopathy
Dysfunction of the autonomic nervous system due to alcohol
Code also associated alcoholism (F10.-)

G31.8   Other specified degenerative diseases of nervous system

G31.80   Leukodystrophy, unspecified

G31.81   Alpers' disease
Rare neuronal degeneration of cerebral cortex disease of young children
Grey-matter degeneration
Coding Clinic: 2017, Q2, P7

G31.82   Leigh's disease
Rare neurometabolic disorder that affects central nervous system
Subacute necrotizing encephalopathy

G31.83   Neurocognitive disorder with Lewy bodies
Closely allied to Parkinson's Disease
Lewy body dementia
Lewy body disease
Use Additional code, if applicable, to identify mild neurocognitive disorders due to known physiological condition (F06.7-)
Coding Clinic: 2017, Q2, P7; 2016, Q4, P141

G31.84   Mild cognitive impairment of uncertain or unknown etiology
Mild cognitive disorder NOS
Mild neurocognitive disorder of uncertain or unknown etiology
Use Additional code to identify presence of:
alcohol abuse and dependence (F10.-)
exposure to environmental tobacco smoke (Z77.22)
history of tobacco dependence (Z87.891)
hypertension (I10-I1A)
occupational exposure to environmental tobacco smoke (Z57.31)
tobacco dependence (F17.-)
tobacco use (Z72.0)
Excludes1   age related cognitive decline (R41.81)
altered mental status (R41.82)
cerebral degeneration (G31.9)
cerebrovascular diseases (I60-I69)
change in mental status (R41.82)
cognitive deficits following (sequelae of) cerebral hemorrhage or infarction (I69.01-, I69.11-, I69.21-, I69.31-, I69.81-, I69.91-)
cognitive impairment due to intracranial or head injury (S06.-)
dementia (F01.-, F02.-, F03.-)
mild neurocognitive disorder due to a known physiological condition (F06.7-)
neurologic neglect syndrome (R41.4)
personality change, nonpsychotic (F68.8)
Coding Clinic: 2021, Q3, P3

G31.85   Corticobasal degeneration

G31.86   Alexander disease

G31.87   Primary progressive apraxia of speech

G31.89   Other specified degenerative diseases of nervous system

G31.9   Degenerative disease of nervous system, unspecified
Coding Clinic: 2021, Q3, P3

G32   Other degenerative disorders of nervous system in diseases classified elsewhere

G32.0   *Subacute combined degeneration of spinal cord in diseases classified elsewhere* HCC
Dana-Putnam syndrome
Sclerosis of spinal cord (combined) (dorsolateral) (posterolateral)
Code first underlying disease, such as:
other dietary vitamin B12 deficiency anemia
pernicious (D51.0)
vitamin B12 deficiency anemia, unspecified (D51.8)
Excludes1   syphilitic combined degeneration of spinal cord (A52.11)

G32.8   Other specified degenerative disorders of nervous system in diseases classified elsewhere
Code first underlying disease, such as:
amyloidosis cerebral degeneration (E85.-)
cerebral degeneration (due to) hypothyroidism (E00.0-E03.9)
cerebral degeneration (due to) neoplasm (C00-D49)
cerebral degeneration (due to) vitamin B deficiency, except thiamine (E52-E53.-)
Excludes1   superior hemorrhagic polioencephalitis [Wernicke's encephalopathy] (E51.2)

G32.81   *Cerebellar ataxia in diseases classified elsewhere* HCC
Code first underlying disease, such as:
celiac disease (with gluten ataxia) (K90.0)
cerebellar ataxia (in) neoplastic disease (paraneoplastic cerebellar degeneration) (C00-D49)
non-celiac gluten ataxia (M35.9)
Excludes1   systemic atrophy primarily affecting the central nervous system in alcoholic cerebellar ataxia (G31.2)
systemic atrophy primarily affecting the central nervous system in myxedema (G13.2)

G32.89   *Other specified degenerative disorders of nervous system in diseases classified elsewhere*
Degenerative encephalopathy in diseases classified elsewhere

DEMYELINATING DISEASES OF THE CENTRAL NERVOUS SYSTEM (G35-G37)

G35   Multiple sclerosis HCC
Destruction of central nervous system; four types: relapsing remitting, secondary progressive, primary progressive, and progressive relapsing
~~Disseminated multiple sclerosis~~
~~Generalized multiple sclerosis~~
~~Multiple sclerosis NOS~~
~~Multiple sclerosis of brain stem~~
~~Multiple sclerosis of cord~~
Coding Clinic: 2021, Q1, P7

G35.A   Relapsing-remitting multiple sclerosis
Excludes1   demyelinating disease of central nervous system, unspecified (G37.9)

G35.B   Primary progressive multiple sclerosis

G35.B0   Primary progressive multiple sclerosis, unspecified

G35.B1   Active primary progressive multiple sclerosis
Primary progressive multiple sclerosis with evidence of inflammatory disease activity

New   Revised   ~~deleted~~ Deleted   Excludes 1   Excludes 2   Includes   Use additional   Code first   Code also   Key words
OGCR Official Guidelines   X Assign placeholder X   Use Additional Character(s)   Manifestation Code   HCC Hierarchical Condition Category   Coding Clinic

Item 6–3   Multiple sclerosis (MS) is a nervous system disease affecting the brain and spinal cord by damaging the myelin sheath surrounding and protecting nerve cells. The damage slows down/blocks messages between the brain and body. Symptoms are visual disturbances, muscle weakness, coordination and balance issues, numbness, prickling, thinking and memory problems. The cause is unknown, though it is thought that it may be an autoimmune disease. It affects women more than men, between 20 and 40 years of age. MS can be mild, but it may cause the loss of ability to write, walk, and speak. There is no cure, but medication may slow or control symptoms.

▶ **G35.B2   Non-active primary progressive multiple sclerosis**
   ▶ Primary progressive multiple sclerosis without evidence of inflammatory disease activity

▶ ● **G35.C   Secondary progressive multiple sclerosis**
   ▶ **G35.CØ   Secondary progressive multiple sclerosis, unspecified**
   ▶ **G35.C1   Active secondary progressive multiple sclerosis**
      ▶ Secondary progressive multiple sclerosis with evidence of inflammatory disease activity
   ▶ **G35.C2   Non-active secondary progressive multiple sclerosis**
      ▶ Secondary progressive multiple sclerosis without evidence of inflammatory disease activity

▶ **G35.D   Multiple sclerosis, unspecified**
   ▶ Disseminated multiple sclerosis
   ▶ Generalized multiple sclerosis
   ▶ Multiple sclerosis NOS
   ▶ Multiple sclerosis of brain stem
   ▶ Multiple sclerosis of cord

● **G36   Other acute disseminated demyelination**
   Excludes1   postinfectious encephalitis and encephalomyelitis NOS (G04.01)

   G36.Ø   Neuromyelitis optica [Devic]
   Inflammatory disorder in which immune system attacks optic nerves and spinal cord producing inflammation of optic nerve (optic neuritis) and spinal cord (myelitis)
   Demyelination in optic neuritis
      Excludes1   optic neuritis NOS (H46)

   G36.1   Acute and subacute hemorrhagic leukoencephalitis [Hurst]
   G36.8   Other specified acute disseminated demyelination
   G36.9   Acute disseminated demyelination, unspecified

● **G37   Other demyelinating diseases of central nervous system**
   Destruction of central nervous system

   G37.Ø   Diffuse sclerosis of central nervous system
   Periaxial encephalitis
   Schilder's disease
      Excludes1   X linked adrenoleukodystrophy (E71.52-)

   G37.1   Central demyelination of corpus callosum
   G37.2   Central pontine myelinolysis
   Coding Clinic: 2022, Q2, P11
   G37.3   Acute transverse myelitis in demyelinating disease of central nervous system
   Acute transverse myelitis NOS
   Acute transverse myelopathy
      Excludes1   acute flaccid myelitis (G04.82)
      ▶ multiple sclerosis (G35.-)
         neuromyelitis optica [Devic] (G36.0)

   G37.4   Subacute necrotizing myelitis of central nervous system
   G37.5   Concentric sclerosis [Baló] of central nervous system

● **G37.8   Other specified demyelinating diseases of central nervous system**
   G37.81   Myelin oligodendrocyte glycoprotein antibody disease
   MOG antibody disease
      Code also associated manifestations, if known, such as:
      noninfectious acute disseminated encephalomyelitis (G04.81)
      neuromyelitis optica (G36.0)
   G37.89   Other specified demyelinating diseases of central nervous system

G37.9   Demyelinating disease of central nervous system, unspecified
   ▶ Clinically isolated syndromes

EPISODIC AND PAROXYSMAL DISORDERS (G4Ø-G47)

● **G4Ø   Epilepsy and recurrent seizures**
   Note: The following terms are to be considered equivalent to intractable: pharmacoresistant (pharmacologically resistant), treatment resistant, refractory (medically) and poorly controlled
      Excludes1   conversion disorder with seizures (F44.5)
      convulsions NOS (R56.9)
      post traumatic seizures (R56.1)
      seizure (convulsive) NOS (R56.9)
      seizure of newborn (P90)
      Excludes2   hippocampal sclerosis (G93.81)
      mesial temporal sclerosis (G93.81)
      temporal sclerosis (G93.81)
      Todd's paralysis (G83.84)

● **G4Ø.Ø   Localization-related (focal) (partial) idiopathic epilepsy and epileptic syndromes with seizures of localized onset**
   Benign childhood epilepsy with centrotemporal EEG spikes
   Childhood epilepsy with occipital EEG paroxysms
      Excludes1   adult onset localization-related epilepsy (G40.1-, G40.2-)

   ● **G4Ø.ØØ   Localization-related (focal) (partial) idiopathic epilepsy and epileptic syndromes with seizures of localized onset, not intractable**
   Localization-related (focal) (partial) idiopathic epilepsy and epileptic syndromes with seizures of localized onset without intractability

      G4Ø.ØØ1   Localization-related (focal) (partial) idiopathic epilepsy and epileptic syndromes with seizures of localized onset, not intractable, with status epilepticus

      G4Ø.ØØ9   Localization-related (focal) (partial) idiopathic epilepsy and epileptic syndromes with seizures of localized onset, not intractable, without status epilepticus
      Localization-related (focal) (partial) idiopathic epilepsy and epileptic syndromes with seizures of localized onset NOS

   ● **G4Ø.Ø1   Localization-related (focal) (partial) idiopathic epilepsy and epileptic syndromes with seizures of localized onset, intractable**

      G4Ø.Ø11   Localization-related (focal) (partial) idiopathic epilepsy and epileptic syndromes with seizures of localized onset, intractable, with status epilepticus

      G4Ø.Ø19   Localization-related (focal) (partial) idiopathic epilepsy and epileptic syndromes with seizures of localized onset, intractable, without status epilepticus

CHAPTER 6 (GØØ-G99)

CHAPTER 6 (G00-G99)

● **G40.1** **Localization-related (focal) (partial) symptomatic epilepsy and epileptic syndromes with simple partial seizures**
    Attacks without alteration of consciousness
    Epilepsia partialis continua [Kozhevnikof]
    Simple partial seizures developing into secondarily generalized seizures

● **G40.10** **Localization-related (focal) (partial) symptomatic epilepsy and epileptic syndromes with simple partial seizures, not intractable**
    Localization-related (focal) (partial) symptomatic epilepsy and epileptic syndromes with simple partial seizures without intractability

    G40.101 **Localization-related (focal) (partial) symptomatic epilepsy and epileptic syndromes with simple partial seizures, not intractable, with status epilepticus** 🝖

    G40.109 **Localization-related (focal) (partial) symptomatic epilepsy and epileptic syndromes with simple partial seizures, not intractable, without status epilepticus** 🝖
        Localization-related (focal) (partial) symptomatic epilepsy and epileptic syndromes with simple partial seizures NOS
        Coding Clinic: 2023, Q3, P4

● **G40.11** **Localization-related (focal) (partial) symptomatic epilepsy and epileptic syndromes with simple partial seizures, intractable**

    G40.111 **Localization-related (focal) (partial) symptomatic epilepsy and epileptic syndromes with simple partial seizures, intractable, with status epilepticus** 🝖

    G40.119 **Localization-related (focal) (partial) symptomatic epilepsy and epileptic syndromes with simple partial seizures, intractable, without status epilepticus** 🝖

● **G40.2** **Localization-related (focal) (partial) symptomatic epilepsy and epileptic syndromes with complex partial seizures**
    Attacks with alteration of consciousness, often with automatisms
    Complex partial seizures developing into secondarily generalized seizures

● **G40.20** **Localization-related (focal) (partial) symptomatic epilepsy and epileptic syndromes with complex partial seizures, not intractable**
    Localization-related (focal) (partial) symptomatic epilepsy and epileptic syndromes with complex partial seizures without intractability

    G40.201 **Localization-related (focal) (partial) symptomatic epilepsy and epileptic syndromes with complex partial seizures, not intractable, with status epilepticus** 🝖

    G40.209 **Localization-related (focal) (partial) symptomatic epilepsy and epileptic syndromes with complex partial seizures, not intractable, without status epilepticus** 🝖
        Localization-related (focal) (partial) symptomatic epilepsy and epileptic syndromes with complex partial seizures NOS

● **G40.21** **Localization-related (focal) (partial) symptomatic epilepsy and epileptic syndromes with complex partial seizures, intractable**

    G40.211 **Localization-related (focal) (partial) symptomatic epilepsy and epileptic syndromes with complex partial seizures, intractable, with status epilepticus** 🝖

    G40.219 **Localization-related (focal) (partial) symptomatic epilepsy and epileptic syndromes with complex partial seizures, intractable, without status epilepticus** 🝖

● **G40.3** **Generalized idiopathic epilepsy and epileptic syndromes**
    Code also MERRF syndrome, if applicable (E88.42)

● **G40.30** **Generalized idiopathic epilepsy and epileptic syndromes, not intractable**
    Generalized idiopathic epilepsy and epileptic syndromes without intractability

    G40.301 **Generalized idiopathic epilepsy and epileptic syndromes, not intractable, with status epilepticus** 🝖

    G40.309 **Generalized idiopathic epilepsy and epileptic syndromes, not intractable, without status epilepticus** 🝖
        Generalized idiopathic epilepsy and epileptic syndromes NOS

● **G40.31** **Generalized idiopathic epilepsy and epileptic syndromes, intractable**

    G40.311 **Generalized idiopathic epilepsy and epileptic syndromes, intractable, with status epilepticus** 🝖

    G40.319 **Generalized idiopathic epilepsy and epileptic syndromes, intractable, without status epilepticus** 🝖

● **G40.4** **Other generalized epilepsy and epileptic syndromes**
    Epilepsy with grand mal seizures on awakening
    Epilepsy with myoclonic absences
    Epilepsy with myoclonic-astatic seizures
    Grand mal seizure NOS
    Nonspecific atonic epileptic seizures
    Nonspecific clonic epileptic seizures
    Nonspecific myoclonic epileptic seizures
    Nonspecific tonic epileptic seizures
    Nonspecific tonic-clonic epileptic seizures
    Symptomatic early myoclonic encephalopathy

● **G40.40** **Other generalized epilepsy and epileptic syndromes, not intractable**
    Other generalized epilepsy and epileptic syndromes without intractability
    Other generalized epilepsy and epileptic syndromes NOS

    G40.401 **Other generalized epilepsy and epileptic syndromes, not intractable, with status epilepticus** 🝖

    G40.409 **Other generalized epilepsy and epileptic syndromes, not intractable, without status epilepticus** 🝖

● **G40.41** **Other generalized epilepsy and epileptic syndromes, intractable**

    G40.411 **Other generalized epilepsy and epileptic syndromes, intractable, with status epilepticus** 🝖

    G40.419 **Other generalized epilepsy and epileptic syndromes, intractable, without status epilepticus** 🝖

G40.42   **Cyclin-Dependent Kinase-Like 5 Deficiency Disorder**
CDKL5
Use additional code, if known, to identify associated manifestations, such as:
    cortical blindness (H47.61-)
    global developmental delay (F88)

● **G40.5**   **Epileptic seizures related to external causes**
Epileptic seizures related to alcohol
Epileptic seizures related to drugs
Epileptic seizures related to hormonal changes
Epileptic seizures related to sleep deprivation
Epileptic seizures related to stress
Code also, if applicable, associated epilepsy and recurrent seizures (G40.-)
Use additional code for adverse effect, if applicable, to identify drug (T36-T50 with fifth or sixth character 5)

   ● **G40.50**   **Epileptic seizures related to external causes, not intractable**

     G40.501   **Epileptic seizures related to external causes, not intractable, with status epilepticus**

     G40.509   **Epileptic seizures related to external causes, not intractable, without status epilepticus**
       Epileptic seizures related to external causes, NOS

● **G40.8**   **Other epilepsy and recurrent seizures**
Epilepsies and epileptic syndromes undetermined as to whether they are focal or generalized
Landau-Kleffner syndrome

   ● **G40.80**   **Other epilepsy**

     G40.801   **Other epilepsy, not intractable, with status epilepticus**
       Other epilepsy without intractability with status epilepticus

     G40.802   **Other epilepsy, not intractable, without status epilepticus**
       Other epilepsy NOS
       Other epilepsy without intractability without status epilepticus

     G40.803   **Other epilepsy, intractable, with status epilepticus**

     G40.804   **Other epilepsy, intractable, without status epilepticus**

   ● **G40.81**   **Lennox-Gastaut syndrome**

     G40.811   **Lennox-Gastaut syndrome, not intractable, with status epilepticus**

     G40.812   **Lennox-Gastaut syndrome, not intractable, without status epilepticus**

     G40.813   **Lennox-Gastaut syndrome, intractable, with status epilepticus**

     G40.814   **Lennox-Gastaut syndrome, intractable, without status epilepticus**

   ● **G40.82**   **Epileptic spasms**
     Infantile spasms
     Salaam attacks
     West's syndrome

     G40.821   **Epileptic spasms, not intractable, with status epilepticus**

     G40.822   **Epileptic spasms, not intractable, without status epilepticus**

     G40.823   **Epileptic spasms, intractable, with status epilepticus**

     G40.824   **Epileptic spasms, intractable, without status epilepticus**

● **G40.83**   **Dravet syndrome**
Polymorphic epilepsy in infancy (PMEI)
Severe myoclonic epilepsy in infancy (SMEI)

     G40.833   **Dravet syndrome, intractable, with status epilepticus**

     G40.834   **Dravet syndrome, intractable, without status epilepticus**
       Dravet syndrome NOS

● **G40.84**   **KCNQ2-related epilepsy**

     G40.841   **KCNQ2-related epilepsy, not intractable, with status epilepticus**

     G40.842   **KCNQ2-related epilepsy, not intractable, without status epilepticus**
       KCNQ2-related epilepsy NOS

     G40.843   **KCNQ2-related epilepsy, intractable, with status epilepticus**

     G40.844   **KCNQ2-related epilepsy, intractable, without status epilepticus**

   G40.89   **Other seizures**
     Excludes1   post traumatic seizures (R56.1)
       recurrent seizures NOS (G40.909)
       seizure NOS (R56.9)

● **G40.9**   **Epilepsy, unspecified**

   ● **G40.90**   **Epilepsy, unspecified, not intractable**
     Epilepsy, unspecified, without intractability

     G40.901   **Epilepsy, unspecified, not intractable, with status epilepticus**

     G40.909   **Epilepsy, unspecified, not intractable, without status epilepticus**
       Epilepsy NOS
       Epileptic convulsions NOS
       Epileptic fits NOS
       Epileptic seizures NOS
       Recurrent seizures NOS
       Seizure disorder NOS
       Coding Clinic: 2024, Q2, P9; 2021, Q2, P3

   ● **G40.91**   **Epilepsy, unspecified, intractable**
     Intractable seizure disorder NOS

     G40.911   **Epilepsy, unspecified, intractable, with status epilepticus**

     G40.919   **Epilepsy, unspecified, intractable, without status epilepticus**

● **G40.A**   **Absence epileptic syndrome**
Childhood absence epilepsy [pyknolepsy]
Juvenile absence epilepsy
Absence epileptic syndrome, NOS

● **G40.A0**   **Absence epileptic syndrome, not intractable**

     G40.A01   **Absence epileptic syndrome, not intractable, with status epilepticus**

     G40.A09   **Absence epileptic syndrome, not intractable, without status epilepticus**

● **G40.A1**   **Absence epileptic syndrome, intractable**

     G40.A11   **Absence epileptic syndrome, intractable, with status epilepticus**

     G40.A19   **Absence epileptic syndrome, intractable, without status epilepticus**

● **G40.B**   **Juvenile myoclonic epilepsy [impulsive petit mal]**

● **G40.B0**   **Juvenile myoclonic epilepsy, not intractable**

     G40.B01   **Juvenile myoclonic epilepsy, not intractable, with status epilepticus**

     G40.B09   **Juvenile myoclonic epilepsy, not intractable, without status epilepticus**

CHAPTER 6 (G00-G99)

● **G40.B1**   Juvenile myoclonic epilepsy, intractable

     G40.B11   Juvenile myoclonic epilepsy, intractable, with status epilepticus

     G40.B19   Juvenile myoclonic epilepsy, intractable, without status epilepticus

● **G40.C**   Lafora progressive myoclonus epilepsy

     Lafora body disease

     Code also, if applicable, associated conditions such as dementia (F02.8-)

● **G40.C0**   Lafora progressive myoclonus epilepsy, not intractable

     G40.C01   Lafora progressive myoclonus epilepsy, not intractable, with status epilepticus

     G40.C09   Lafora progressive myoclonus epilepsy, not intractable, without status epilepticus

       Lafora progressive myoclonus epilepsy NOS

● **G40.C1**   Lafora progressive myoclonus epilepsy, intractable

     G40.C11   Lafora progressive myoclonus epilepsy, intractable, with status epilepticus

     G40.C19   Lafora progressive myoclonus epilepsy, intractable, without status epilepticus

● **G43**   **Migraine**

     Note: The following terms are to be considered equivalent to intractable: pharmacoresistant (pharmacologically resistant), treatment resistant, refractory (medically) and poorly controlled

     Use additional code for adverse effect, if applicable, to identify drug (T36-T50 with fifth or sixth character 5)

     Excludes1   headache NOS (R51.9)
                 lower half migraine (G44.00)

     Excludes2   headache syndromes (G44.-)

● **G43.0**   Migraine without aura

     Neurological disorder, generally recurring headaches without early symptom (aura)

     Common migraine

     Excludes1   chronic migraine without aura (G43.7-)

● **G43.00**   Migraine without aura, not intractable

     Neurological disorder, generally recurring headaches without early symptom (aura); resistant to cure, relief, or control

     Migraine without aura without mention of refractory migraine

     G43.001   Migraine without aura, not intractable, with status migrainosus

     G43.009   Migraine without aura, not intractable, without status migrainosus

       Migraine without aura NOS

● **G43.01**   Migraine without aura, intractable

     Intractable migraine: Not easily cured or managed; relentless pain from a migraine

     Migraine without aura with refractory migraine

     G43.011   Migraine without aura, intractable, with status migrainosus

     G43.019   Migraine without aura, intractable, without status migrainosus

● **G43.1**   Migraine with aura

     Basilar migraine

     Classical migraine

     Migraine equivalents

     Migraine preceded or accompanied by transient focal neurological phenomena

     Migraine triggered seizures

     Migraine with acute-onset aura

     Migraine with aura without headache (migraine equivalents)

     Migraine with prolonged aura

     Migraine with typical aura

     Retinal migraine

     Code also any associated seizure (G40.-, R56.9)
       chronic migraine with aura (G43.E-)

     Excludes1   persistent migraine aura (G43.5-, G43.6-)

● **G43.10**   Migraine with aura, not intractable

     Migraine with aura without mention of refractory migraine

     G43.101   Migraine with aura, not intractable, with status migrainosus

     G43.109   Migraine with aura, not intractable, without status migrainosus

       Migraine with aura NOS

● **G43.11**   Migraine with aura, intractable

     Migraine with aura with refractory migraine

     G43.111   Migraine with aura, intractable, with status migrainosus

     G43.119   Migraine with aura, intractable, without status migrainosus

● **G43.4**   Hemiplegic migraine

     Inherited migraine disorder causing temporary paralysis of one side of body followed by severe headache and nausea

     Familial migraine

     Sporadic migraine

● **G43.40**   Hemiplegic migraine, not intractable

     Hemiplegic migraine without refractory migraine

     G43.401   Hemiplegic migraine, not intractable, with status migrainosus

     G43.409   Hemiplegic migraine, not intractable, without status migrainosus

       Hemiplegic migraine NOS

       Coding Clinic: 2025, Q2, P18-19

● **G43.41**   Hemiplegic migraine, intractable

     Hemiplegic migraine with refractory migraine

     G43.411   Hemiplegic migraine, intractable, with status migrainosus

     G43.419   Hemiplegic migraine, intractable, without status migrainosus

● **G43.5**   Persistent migraine aura without cerebral infarction

● **G43.50**   Persistent migraine aura without cerebral infarction, not intractable

     Persistent migraine aura without cerebral infarction, without refractory migraine

     G43.501   Persistent migraine aura without cerebral infarction, not intractable, with status migrainosus

     G43.509   Persistent migraine aura without cerebral infarction, not intractable, without status migrainosus

       Persistent migraine aura NOS

● **G43.51**   Persistent migraine aura without cerebral infarction, intractable

     Persistent migraine aura without cerebral infarction, with refractory migraine

     G43.511   Persistent migraine aura without cerebral infarction, intractable, with status migrainosus

     G43.519   Persistent migraine aura without cerebral infarction, intractable, without status migrainosus

---

Item 6–4   Migraine headache is described as an intense pulsing or throbbing pain in one area of the head. It can be accompanied by extreme sensitivity to light (photophobic) and sound and is three times more common in women than in men. Symptoms include nausea and vomiting. Research indicates migraine headaches are caused by inherited abnormalities in genes that control the activities of certain cell populations in the brain.

▶ New   ⇒ Revised   ~~deleted~~ Deleted   Excludes 1   Excludes 2   Includes   Use additional   Code first   Code also   Key words

OGCR Official Guidelines   X Assign placeholder X   ● Use Additional Character(s)   ▌ Manifestation Code   Hierarchical Condition Category   Coding Clinic

● **G43.6 Persistent migraine aura with cerebral infarction**
Visual, motor, or psychic disturbances, paresthesias, and related neurologic abnormalities accompanying migraine

Code also the type of cerebral infarction (I63.-)

● **G43.60 Persistent migraine aura with cerebral infarction, not intractable**
Persistent migraine aura with cerebral infarction, without refractory migraine

G43.601 Persistent migraine aura with cerebral infarction, not intractable, with status migrainosus

G43.609 Persistent migraine aura with cerebral infarction, not intractable, without status migrainosus

● **G43.61 Persistent migraine aura with cerebral infarction, intractable**
Persistent migraine aura with cerebral infarction, with refractory migraine

G43.611 Persistent migraine aura with cerebral infarction, intractable, with status migrainosus

G43.619 Persistent migraine aura with cerebral infarction, intractable, without status migrainosus

● **G43.7 Chronic migraine without aura**
Transformed migraine

Excludes1   migraine without aura (G43.0-)

● **G43.70 Chronic migraine without aura, not intractable**
Chronic migraine without aura, without refractory migraine

G43.701 Chronic migraine without aura, not intractable, with status migrainosus

G43.709 Chronic migraine without aura, not intractable, without status migrainosus
Chronic migraine without aura NOS

● **G43.71 Chronic migraine without aura, intractable**
Chronic migraine without aura, with refractory migraine

G43.711 Chronic migraine without aura, intractable, with status migrainosus

G43.719 Chronic migraine without aura, intractable, without status migrainosus

● **G43.8 Other migraine**

● **G43.80 Other migraine, not intractable**
Other migraine, without refractory migraine

G43.801 Other migraine, not intractable, with status migrainosus

G43.809 Other migraine, not intractable, without status migrainosus

● **G43.81 Other migraine, intractable**
Other migraine, with refractory migraine

G43.811 Other migraine, intractable, with status migrainosus

G43.819 Other migraine, intractable, without status migrainosus

● **G43.82 Menstrual migraine, not intractable**
Menstrual headache, not intractable
Menstrual migraine, without refractory migraine
Menstrually related migraine, not intractable
Pre-menstrual headache, not intractable
Pre-menstrual migraine, not intractable
Pure menstrual migraine, not intractable

Code also associated premenstrual tension syndrome (N94.3)

G43.821 Menstrual migraine, not intractable, with status migrainosus ♀

G43.829 Menstrual migraine, not intractable, without status migrainosus ♀
Menstrual migraine NOS

● **G43.83 Menstrual migraine, intractable**
Menstrual headache, intractable
Menstrual migraine, with refractory migraine
Menstrually related migraine, intractable
Pre-menstrual headache, intractable
Pre-menstrual migraine, intractable
Pure menstrual migraine, intractable

Code also associated premenstrual tension syndrome (N94.3)

G43.831 Menstrual migraine, intractable, with status migrainosus ♀

G43.839 Menstrual migraine, intractable, without status migrainosus ♀

● **G43.9 Migraine, unspecified**

● **G43.90 Migraine, unspecified, not intractable**
Migraine, unspecified, without refractory migraine

G43.901 Migraine, unspecified, not intractable, with status migrainosus
Status migrainosus NOS

G43.909 Migraine, unspecified, not intractable, without status migrainosus
Migraine NOS

● **G43.91 Migraine, unspecified, intractable**
Migraine, unspecified, with refractory migraine

G43.911 Migraine, unspecified, intractable, with status migrainosus

G43.919 Migraine, unspecified, intractable, without status migrainosus

● **G43.A Cyclical vomiting**

Excludes1   cyclical vomiting syndrome unrelated to migraine (R11.15)

G43.A0 Cyclical vomiting, in migraine, not intractable
Cyclical vomiting, without refractory migraine

G43.A1 Cyclical vomiting, in migraine, intractable
Cyclical vomiting, with refractory migraine

● **G43.B Ophthalmoplegic migraine**

G43.B0 Ophthalmoplegic migraine, not intractable
Ophthalmoplegic migraine, without refractory migraine

G43.B1 Ophthalmoplegic migraine, intractable
Ophthalmoplegic migraine, with refractory migraine

● **G43.C Periodic headache syndromes in child or adult**

G43.C0 Periodic headache syndromes in child or adult, not intractable
Periodic headache syndromes in child or adult, without refractory migraine

G43.C1 Periodic headache syndromes in child or adult, intractable
Periodic headache syndromes in child or adult, with refractory migraine

● **G43.D Abdominal migraine**

G43.D0 Abdominal migraine, not intractable
Abdominal migraine, without refractory migraine

G43.D1 Abdominal migraine, intractable
Abdominal migraine, with refractory migraine

● **G43.E Chronic migraine with aura**

Excludes1   migraine with aura (G43.1-)

● **G43.E0 Chronic migraine with aura, not intractable**
Chronic migraine with aura, without refractory migraine

G43.E01 Chronic migraine with aura, not intractable, with status migrainosus

G43.E09 Chronic migraine with aura, not intractable, without status migrainosus
Chronic migraine with aura NOS

● **G43.E1　Chronic migraine with aura, intractable**
Chronic migraine with aura, with refractory migraine

G43.E11　Chronic migraine with aura, intractable, with status migrainosus

G43.E19　Chronic migraine with aura, intractable, without status migrainosus

● **G44　Other headache syndromes**

Excludes1　headache NOS (R51.9)

Excludes2　atypical facial pain (G50.1)
headache due to lumbar puncture (G97.1)
migraines (G43.-)
trigeminal neuralgia (G50.0)

● **G44.0　Cluster headaches and other trigeminal autonomic cephalgias (TAC)**

● **G44.00　Cluster headache syndrome, unspecified**
Ciliary neuralgia
Cluster headache NOS
Histamine cephalgia
Lower half migraine
Migrainous neuralgia

G44.001　Cluster headache syndrome, unspecified, intractable

G44.009　Cluster headache syndrome, unspecified, not intractable
Cluster headache syndrome NOS

● **G44.01　Episodic cluster headache**

G44.011　Episodic cluster headache, intractable

G44.019　Episodic cluster headache, not intractable
Episodic cluster headache NOS

● **G44.02　Chronic cluster headache**

G44.021　Chronic cluster headache, intractable

G44.029　Chronic cluster headache, not intractable
Chronic cluster headache NOS

● **G44.03　Episodic paroxysmal hemicrania**
Paroxysmal hemicrania NOS

G44.031　Episodic paroxysmal hemicrania, intractable

G44.039　Episodic paroxysmal hemicrania, not intractable
Episodic paroxysmal hemicrania NOS

● **G44.04　Chronic paroxysmal hemicrania**
Unilateral headache

G44.041　Chronic paroxysmal hemicrania, intractable

G44.049　Chronic paroxysmal hemicrania, not intractable
Chronic paroxysmal hemicrania NOS

● **G44.05　Short lasting unilateral neuralgiform headache with conjunctival injection and tearing (SUNCT)**

G44.051　Short lasting unilateral neuralgiform headache with conjunctival injection and tearing (SUNCT), intractable

G44.059　Short lasting unilateral neuralgiform headache with conjunctival injection and tearing (SUNCT), not intractable
Short lasting unilateral neuralgiform headache with conjunctival injection and tearing (SUNCT) NOS

● **G44.09　Other trigeminal autonomic cephalgias (TAC)**
Cluster headaches

G44.091　Other trigeminal autonomic cephalgias (TAC), intractable

G44.099　Other trigeminal autonomic cephalgias (TAC), not intractable

G44.1　Vascular headache, not elsewhere classified

Excludes2　cluster headache (G44.0)
complicated headache syndromes (G44.5-)
drug-induced headache (G44.4-)
migraine (G43.-)
other specified headache syndromes (G44.8-)
post-traumatic headache (G44.3-)
tension-type headache (G44.2-)

● **G44.2　Tension-type headache**

● **G44.20　Tension-type headache, unspecified**

G44.201　Tension-type headache, unspecified, intractable

G44.209　Tension-type headache, unspecified, not intractable
Tension headache NOS

● **G44.21　Episodic tension-type headache**

G44.211　Episodic tension-type headache, intractable

G44.219　Episodic tension-type headache, not intractable
Episodic tension-type headache NOS

● **G44.22　Chronic tension-type headache**

G44.221　Chronic tension-type headache, intractable

G44.229　Chronic tension-type headache, not intractable
Chronic tension-type headache NOS

● **G44.3　Post-traumatic headache**

● **G44.30　Post-traumatic headache, unspecified**

G44.301　Post-traumatic headache, unspecified, intractable

G44.309　Post-traumatic headache, unspecified, not intractable
Post-traumatic headache NOS

● **G44.31　Acute post-traumatic headache**

G44.311　Acute post-traumatic headache, intractable

G44.319　Acute post-traumatic headache, not intractable
Acute post-traumatic headache NOS

● **G44.32　Chronic post-traumatic headache**

G44.321　Chronic post-traumatic headache, intractable

G44.329　Chronic post-traumatic headache, not intractable
Chronic post-traumatic headache NOS

● **G44.4　Drug-induced headache, not elsewhere classified**
Medication overuse headache
Use additional code for adverse effect, if applicable, to identify drug (T36-T50 with fifth or sixth character 5)

G44.40　Drug-induced headache, not elsewhere classified, not intractable

G44.41　Drug-induced headache, not elsewhere classified, intractable

● **G44.5　Complicated headache syndromes**

G44.51　Hemicrania continua
Persistent unilateral headache

G44.52　New daily persistent headache (NDPH)

G44.53   **Primary thunderclap headache**

G44.59   **Other complicated headache syndrome**

● G44.8   **Other specified headache syndromes**

    Excludes2   headache with orthostatic or positional component, not elsewhere classified (R51.0)

G44.81   **Hypnic headache**
Benign primary headaches

G44.82   **Headache associated with sexual activity**
Orgasmic headache
Preorgasmic headache

G44.83   **Primary cough headache**

G44.84   **Primary exertional headache**

G44.85   **Primary stabbing headache**

G44.86   **Cervicogenic headache**
Code also associated cervical spinal condition, if known
Coding Clinic: 2021, Q4, P12

G44.89   **Other headache syndrome**

● G45   **Transient cerebral ischemic attacks and related syndromes**

    Excludes1   neonatal cerebral ischemia (P91.0)
transient retinal artery occlusion (H34.0-)
Coding Clinic: 2023, Q1, P37; 2018, Q2, P9

G45.0   **Vertebro-basilar artery syndrome**

G45.1   **Carotid artery syndrome (hemispheric)**

G45.2   **Multiple and bilateral precerebral artery syndromes**

G45.3   **Amaurosis fugax**
Transient visual loss in one eye

G45.4   **Transient global amnesia**
Episode of short-term memory loss, nonrecurrent, lasting few hours

    Excludes1   amnesia NOS (R41.3)

G45.8   **Other transient cerebral ischemic attacks and related syndromes**

G45.9   **Transient cerebral ischemic attack, unspecified**
Spasm of cerebral artery
TIA
Transient cerebral ischemia NOS

● G46   **Vascular syndromes of brain in cerebrovascular diseases**
Code first underlying cerebrovascular disease (I60-I69)

G46.0   **Middle cerebral artery syndrome**

G46.1   **Anterior cerebral artery syndrome**

G46.2   **Posterior cerebral artery syndrome**

G46.3   **Brain stem stroke syndrome**
Benedikt syndrome
Claude syndrome
Foville syndrome
Millard-Gubler syndrome
Wallenberg syndrome
Weber syndrome

G46.4   **Cerebellar stroke syndrome**

G46.5   **Pure motor lacunar syndrome**
Occlusion of single deep penetrating artery

G46.6   **Pure sensory lacunar syndrome**

G46.7   **Other lacunar syndromes**

G46.8   **Other vascular syndromes of brain in cerebrovascular diseases**

● G47   **Sleep disorders**

    Excludes2   nightmares (F51.5)
nonorganic sleep disorders (F51.-)
sleep terrors (F51.4)
sleepwalking (F51.3)

● G47.0   **Insomnia**

    Excludes2   alcohol related insomnia (F10.182, F10.282, F10.982)
drug-related insomnia (F11.182, F11.282, F11.982, F13.182, F13.282, F13.982, F14.182, F14.282, F14.982, F15.182, F15.282, F15.982, F19.182, F19.282, F19.982)
idiopathic insomnia (F51.01)
insomnia due to a mental disorder (F51.05)
insomnia not due to a substance or known physiological condition (F51.0-)
nonorganic insomnia (F51.0-)
primary insomnia (F51.01)
sleep apnea (G47.3-)

G47.00   **Insomnia, unspecified**
Insomnia NOS

G47.01   **Insomnia due to medical condition**
Code also associated medical condition

G47.09   **Other insomnia**

● G47.1   **Hypersomnia**

    Excludes2   alcohol-related hypersomnia (F10.182, F10.282, F10.982)
drug-related hypersomnia (F11.182, F11.282, F11.982, F13.182, F13.282, F13.982, F14.182, F14.282, F14.982, F15.182, F15.282, F15.982, F19.182, F19.282, F19.982)
hypersomnia due to a mental disorder (F51.13)
hypersomnia not due to a substance or known physiological condition (F51.1-)
primary hypersomnia (F51.11)
sleep apnea (G47.3-)

G47.10   **Hypersomnia, unspecified**
Hypersomnia NOS

G47.11   **Idiopathic hypersomnia with long sleep time**
Idiopathic hypersomnia NOS

G47.12   **Idiopathic hypersomnia without long sleep time**

G47.13   **Recurrent hypersomnia**
Kleine-Levin syndrome
Menstrual related hypersomnia

G47.14   **Hypersomnia due to medical condition**
Code also associated medical condition

G47.19   **Other hypersomnia**

● G47.2   **Circadian rhythm sleep disorders**
Disorders of the sleep wake schedule
Inversion of nyctohemeral rhythm
Inversion of sleep rhythm

G47.20   **Circadian rhythm sleep disorder, unspecified type**
Sleep wake schedule disorder NOS

G47.21   **Circadian rhythm sleep disorder, delayed sleep phase type**
Delayed sleep phase syndrome

G47.22   **Circadian rhythm sleep disorder, advanced sleep phase type**

G47.23   **Circadian rhythm sleep disorder, irregular sleep wake type**
Irregular sleep-wake pattern

G47.24   **Circadian rhythm sleep disorder, free running type**
Circadian rhythm sleep disorder, non-24-hour sleep-wake type

G47.25   **Circadian rhythm sleep disorder, jet lag type**

G47.26   **Circadian rhythm sleep disorder, shift work type**

▸ G47.27   *Circadian rhythm sleep disorder in conditions classified elsewhere*
Code first underlying condition

G47.29   **Other circadian rhythm sleep disorder**

CHAPTER 6 (G00-G99)

- **G47.3 Sleep apnea**
  Characterized by episodes in which breathing stops during sleep
  Code also any associated underlying condition
  Excludes1   apnea NOS (R06.81)
  Cheyne-Stokes breathing (R06.3)
  pickwickian syndrome (E66.2)
  sleep apnea of newborn (P28.3-)
  - **G47.30 Sleep apnea, unspecified**
    Sleep apnea NOS
  - **G47.31 Primary central sleep apnea**
    Idiopathic central sleep apnea
  - **G47.32 High altitude periodic breathing**
  - **G47.33 Obstructive sleep apnea (adult) (pediatric)**
    Obstructive sleep apnea hypopnea
    Excludes1   obstructive sleep apnea of newborn (P28.3-)
  - **G47.34 Idiopathic sleep related nonobstructive alveolar hypoventilation**
    Sleep related hypoxia
  - **G47.35 Congenital central alveolar hypoventilation syndrome**
  - ▸ **G47.36 *Sleep related hypoventilation in conditions classified elsewhere***
    Sleep related hypoxemia in conditions classified elsewhere
    Code first *underlying condition*
  - ▸ **G47.37 *Central sleep apnea in conditions classified elsewhere***
    Code first *underlying condition*
  - **G47.39 Other sleep apnea**
- **G47.4 Narcolepsy and cataplexy**
  Cataplexy is a disorder evidenced by seizures including minor slacking of the facial muscles to complete collapse and often affects people who have narcolepsy, a disorder in which there is great difficulty remaining awake during the daytime.
  - ● **G47.41 Narcolepsy**
    - **G47.411 Narcolepsy with cataplexy**
    - **G47.419 Narcolepsy without cataplexy**
      Narcolepsy NOS
  - ● **G47.42 Narcolepsy in conditions classified elsewhere**
    Code first *underlying condition*
    - ▸ **G47.421 *Narcolepsy in conditions classified elsewhere with cataplexy***
    - ▸ **G47.429 *Narcolepsy in conditions classified elsewhere without cataplexy***
- ● **G47.5 Parasomnia**
  Excludes1   alcohol induced parasomnia (F10.182, F10.282, F10.982)
  drug induced parasomnia (F11.182, F11.282, F11.982, F13.182, F13.282, F13.982, F14.182, F14.282, F14.982, F15.182, F15.282, F15.982, F19.182, F19.282, F19.982)
  parasomnia not due to a substance or known physiological condition (F51.8)
  - **G47.50 Parasomnia, unspecified**
    Parasomnia NOS
  - **G47.51 Confusional arousals**
  - **G47.52 REM sleep behavior disorder**
  - **G47.53 Recurrent isolated sleep paralysis**
  - ▸ **G47.54 *Parasomnia in conditions classified elsewhere***
    Code first *underlying condition*
  - **G47.59 Other parasomnia**
- ● **G47.6 Sleep related movement disorders**
  Excludes2   restless legs syndrome (G25.81)
  - **G47.61 Periodic limb movement disorder**
  - **G47.62 Sleep related leg cramps**

  - **G47.63 Sleep related bruxism**
    Excludes1   psychogenic bruxism (F45.8)
    Coding Clinic: 2016, Q4, P118
  - **G47.69 Other sleep related movement disorders**
- **G47.8 Other sleep disorders**
  Other specified sleep-wake disorder
- **G47.9 Sleep disorder, unspecified**
  Sleep disorder NOS
  Unspecified sleep-wake disorder

★ **(See Plate 6 of the Anatomy Illustrations.)**

NERVE, NERVE ROOT AND PLEXUS DISORDERS (G50-G59)

Excludes1   current traumatic nerve, nerve root and plexus disorders - see Injury, nerve by body region
neuralgia NOS (M79.2)
neuritis NOS (M79.2)
peripheral neuritis in pregnancy (O26.82-)
radiculitis NOS (M54.1-)

- ● **G50 Disorders of trigeminal nerve**
  Includes   disorders of 5th cranial nerve
  - **G50.0 Trigeminal neuralgia**
    Syndrome of paroxysmal facial pain
    Tic douloureux
  - **G50.1 Atypical facial pain**
  - **G50.8 Other disorders of trigeminal nerve**
  - **G50.9 Disorder of trigeminal nerve, unspecified**
- ● **G51 Facial nerve disorders**
  Includes   disorders of 7th cranial nerve
  - **G51.0 Bell's palsy**
    Facial palsy
  - **G51.1 Geniculate ganglionitis**
    Rare disorder with symptoms of severe pain deep in ear, spreading to ear canal, outer ear, mastoid or eye regions
    Excludes1   postherpetic geniculate ganglionitis (B02.21)
  - **G51.2 Melkersson's syndrome**
    Melkersson-Rosenthal syndrome
  - ● **G51.3 Clonic hemifacial spasm**
    - **G51.31 Clonic hemifacial spasm, right**
    - **G51.32 Clonic hemifacial spasm, left**
      Coding Clinic: 2018, Q4, P10
    - **G51.33 Clonic hemifacial spasm, bilateral**
    - **G51.39 Clonic hemifacial spasm, unspecified**
  - **G51.4 Facial myokymia**
    Involuntary facial muscle movement
  - **G51.8 Other disorders of facial nerve**
  - **G51.9 Disorder of facial nerve, unspecified**
- ● **G52 Disorders of other cranial nerves**
  Excludes2   disorders of acoustic [8th] nerve (H93.3)
  disorders of optic [2nd] nerve (H46, H47.0)
  paralytic strabismus due to nerve palsy (H49.0-H49.2)
  - **G52.0 Disorders of olfactory nerve**
    Disorders of 1st cranial nerve

Item 6–5 Trigeminal neuralgia, tic douloureux, is a pain syndrome diagnosed from the patient's history alone. The condition is characterized by pain and a brief facial spasm or tic. Pain is unilateral and follows the sensory distribution of cranial nerve V, typically radiating to the maxillary (V2) or mandibular (V3) area.

Item 6–6   The most common facial nerve disorder is **Bell's Palsy,** which occurs suddenly and results in facial drooping unilaterally. This disorder is the result of a reaction to a virus that causes the facial nerve in the ear to swell, resulting in pressure in the bony canal.

G52.1 Disorders of glossopharyngeal nerve
Disorder of 9th cranial nerve
Glossopharyngeal neuralgia

G52.2 Disorders of vagus nerve
Disorders of pneumogastric [10th] nerve

G52.3 Disorders of hypoglossal nerve
Disorders of 12th cranial nerve

G52.7 Disorders of multiple cranial nerves
Polyneuritis cranialis

G52.8 Disorders of other specified cranial nerves

G52.9 Cranial nerve disorder, unspecified

G53 *Cranial nerve disorders in diseases classified elsewhere*
Code first underlying disease, such as:
neoplasm (C00-D49)

Excludes1   multiple cranial nerve palsy in sarcoidosis (D86.82)
multiple cranial nerve palsy in syphilis (A52.15)
postherpetic geniculate ganglionitis (B02.21)
postherpetic trigeminal neuralgia (B02.22)

G54 Nerve root and plexus disorders
Raiculopathy (nerve root disorder) caused by pressure on nerve root, most common cause is herniation of intervertebral disk. Plexus disorders (plexopathies) are due to compression or injury.

Excludes1   current traumatic nerve root and plexus disorders - see nerve injury by body region
intervertebral disc disorders (M50-M51)
neuralgia or neuritis NOS (M79.2)
neuritis or radiculitis brachial NOS (M54.13)
neuritis or radiculitis lumbar NOS (M54.16)
neuritis or radiculitis lumbosacral NOS (M54.17)
neuritis or radiculitis thoracic NOS (M54.14)
radiculitis NOS (M54.10)
radiculopathy NOS (M54.10)
spondylosis (M47.-)

G54.0 Brachial plexus disorders
Thoracic outlet syndrome
Coding Clinic: 2023, Q2, P8

G54.1 Lumbosacral plexus disorders

G54.2 Cervical root disorders, not elsewhere classified

G54.3 Thoracic root disorders, not elsewhere classified

G54.4 Lumbosacral root disorders, not elsewhere classified

G54.5 Neuralgic amyotrophy
Parsonage-Aldren-Turner syndrome
Shoulder-girdle neuritis

Excludes1   neuralgic amyotrophy in diabetes mellitus (E08-E13 with .44)

G54.6 Phantom limb syndrome with pain 🔁
Sensations (cramping, itching) in a limb that no longer exists

G54.7 Phantom limb syndrome without pain 🔁
Phantom limb syndrome NOS

G54.8 Other nerve root and plexus disorders

G54.9 Nerve root and plexus disorder, unspecified

G55 *Nerve root and plexus compressions in diseases classified elsewhere*
Code first underlying disease, such as:
neoplasm (C00-D49)

Excludes1   nerve root compression (due to) (in) ankylosing spondylitis (M45.-)
nerve root compression (due to) (in)dorsopathies (M53.-, M54.-)
nerve root compression (due to) (in)intervertebral disc disorders (M50.1.-, M51.1.-)
nerve root compression (due to) (in) spondylopathies (M46.-, M48.-)
nerve root compression (due to) (in) spondylosis (M47.0-, M47.2.-)

★ **(See Plates 472 and 473 on pages 56 and 57.)**

G56 Mononeuropathies of upper limb

Excludes1   current traumatic nerve disorder - see nerve injury by body region

G56.0 Carpal tunnel syndrome

    G56.00   Carpal tunnel syndrome, **unspecified** upper limb

    G56.01   Carpal tunnel syndrome, **right** upper limb

    G56.02   Carpal tunnel syndrome, **left** upper limb

    G56.03   Carpal tunnel syndrome, **bilateral** upper limbs
    Coding Clinic: 2016, Q4, P17

G56.1 Other lesions of median nerve

    G56.10   Other lesions of median nerve, **unspecified** side

    G56.11   Other lesions of median nerve, **right** upper limb

    G56.12   Other lesions of median nerve, **left** upper limb

    G56.13   Other lesions of median nerve, **bilateral** upper limbs
    Coding Clinic: 2016, Q4, P17

G56.2 Lesion of ulnar nerve
Tardy ulnar nerve palsy

    G56.20   Lesion of ulnar nerve, **unspecified** upper limb

    G56.21   Lesion of ulnar nerve, **right** upper limb

    G56.22   Lesion of ulnar nerve, **left** upper limb

    G56.23   Lesion of ulnar nerve, **bilateral** upper limbs
    Coding Clinic: 2016, Q4, P17

G56.3 Lesion of radial nerve

    G56.30   Lesion of radial nerve, **unspecified** upper limb

    G56.31   Lesion of radial nerve, **right** upper limb

    G56.32   Lesion of radial nerve, **left** upper limb

    G56.33   Lesion of radial nerve, **bilateral** upper limbs
    Coding Clinic: 2016, Q4, P17

G56.4 Causalgia of upper limb
Intense burning pain and sensitivity to slight touch
Complex regional pain syndrome II of upper limb

Excludes1   complex regional pain syndrome I of lower limb (G90.52-)
complex regional pain syndrome I of upper limb (G90.51-)
complex regional pain syndrome II of lower limb (G57.7-)
reflex sympathetic dystrophy of lower limb (G90.52-)
reflex sympathetic dystrophy (G90.51-)

    G56.40   Causalgia of **unspecified** upper limb

    G56.41   Causalgia of **right** upper limb

    G56.42   Causalgia of **left** upper limb

    G56.43   Causalgia of **bilateral** upper limbs
    Coding Clinic: 2016, Q4, P17

G56.8 Other specified mononeuropathies of upper limb
Disease of a single nerve
Interdigital neuroma of upper limb

    G56.80   Other specified mononeuropathies of **unspecified** upper limb

    G56.81   Other specified mononeuropathies of **right** upper limb

    G56.82   Other specified mononeuropathies of **left** upper limb

    G56.83   Other specified mononeuropathies of **bilateral** upper limbs
    Coding Clinic: 2016, Q4, P17

G56.9 Unspecified mononeuropathy of upper limb
Disease of a single nerve

    G56.90   Unspecified mononeuropathy of **unspecified** upper limb

    G56.91   Unspecified mononeuropathy of **right** upper limb

    G56.92   Unspecified mononeuropathy of **left** upper limb

CHAPTER 6 (G00-G99)

G56.93   **Unspecified** mononeuropathy of **bilateral upper** limbs
        Coding Clinic: 2016, Q4, P17

● **G57   Mononeuropathies of lower limb**
    Excludes1   current traumatic nerve disorder - see nerve injury by body region

★ **(See Plates 544 and 545 on pages 58 and 59.)**

● **G57.0   Lesion of sciatic nerve**
    Excludes1   sciatica NOS (M54.3-)
    Excludes2   sciatica attributed to intervertebral disc disorder (M51.1.-)

G57.00   Lesion of sciatic nerve, **unspecified** lower limb

G57.01   Lesion of sciatic nerve, **right** lower limb

G57.02   Lesion of sciatic nerve, **left** lower limb

G57.03   Lesion of sciatic nerve, **bilateral** lower limbs
    Coding Clinic: 2016, Q4, P1

● **G57.1   Meralgia paresthetica**
Numbness or pain in outer thigh caused by injury to nerve
Lateral cutaneous nerve of thigh syndrome

G57.10   Meralgia paresthetica, **unspecified** lower limb

G57.11   Meralgia paresthetica, **right** lower limb

G57.12   Meralgia paresthetica, **left** lower limb

G57.13   Meralgia paresthetica, **bilateral** lower limbs
    Coding Clinic: 2016, Q4, P1

● **G57.2   Lesion of femoral nerve**

G57.20   Lesion of femoral nerve, **unspecified** lower limb

G57.21   Lesion of femoral nerve, **right** lower limb

G57.22   Lesion of femoral nerve, **left** lower limb

G57.23   Lesion of femoral nerve, **bilateral** lower limbs
    Coding Clinic: 2016, Q4, P1

● **G57.3   Lesion of lateral popliteal nerve**
Peroneal nerve palsy

G57.30   Lesion of lateral popliteal nerve, **unspecified** lower limb

G57.31   Lesion of lateral popliteal nerve, **right** lower limb

G57.32   Lesion of lateral popliteal nerve, **left** lower limb

G57.33   Lesion of lateral popliteal nerve, **bilateral** lower limbs
    Coding Clinic: 2016, Q4, P1

● **G57.4   Lesion of medial popliteal nerve**

G57.40   Lesion of medial popliteal nerve, **unspecified** lower limb

G57.41   Lesion of medial popliteal nerve, **right** lower limb

G57.42   Lesion of medial popliteal nerve, **left** lower limb

G57.43   Lesion of medial popliteal nerve, **bilateral** lower limbs
    Coding Clinic: 2016, Q4, P1

● **G57.5   Tarsal tunnel syndrome**

G57.50   Tarsal tunnel syndrome, **unspecified** lower limb

G57.51   Tarsal tunnel syndrome, **right** lower limb

G57.52   Tarsal tunnel syndrome, **left** lower limb

G57.53   Tarsal tunnel syndrome, **bilateral** lower limbs
    Coding Clinic: 2016, Q4, P1

● **G57.6   Lesion of plantar nerve**
Morton's metatarsalgia

G57.60   Lesion of plantar nerve, **unspecified** lower limb

G57.61   Lesion of plantar nerve, **right** lower limb

G57.62   Lesion of plantar nerve, **left** lower limb

G57.63   Lesion of plantar nerve, **bilateral** lower limbs
    Coding Clinic: 2016, Q4, P1

● **G57.7   Causalgia of lower limb**
Complex regional pain syndrome II of lower limb

    Excludes1   complex regional pain syndrome I of lower limb (G90.52-)
    complex regional pain syndrome I of upper limb (G90.51-)
    complex regional pain syndrome II of upper limb (G56.4-)
    reflex sympathetic dystrophy of lower limb (G90.52-)
    reflex sympathetic dystrophy of upper limb (G90.51-)

G57.70   Causalgia of **unspecified** lower limb

G57.71   Causalgia of **right** lower limb

G57.72   Causalgia of **left** lower limb

G57.73   Causalgia of **bilateral** lower limbs
    Coding Clinic: 2016, Q4, P1

● **G57.8   Other specified mononeuropathies of lower limb**
Interdigital neuroma of lower limb

G57.80   Other specified mononeuropathies of **unspecified** lower limb

G57.81   Other specified mononeuropathies of **right** lower limb

G57.82   Other specified mononeuropathies of **left** lower limb

G57.83   Other specified mononeuropathies of **bilateral** lower limbs
    Coding Clinic: 2016, Q4, P17

● **G57.9   Unspecified mononeuropathy of lower limb**

G57.90   Unspecified mononeuropathy of **unspecified** lower limb

G57.91   Unspecified mononeuropathy of **right** lower limb

G57.92   Unspecified mononeuropathy of **left** lower limb

G57.93   Unspecified mononeuropathy of **bilateral** lower limbs
    Coding Clinic: 2016, Q4, P17

● **G58   Other mononeuropathies**

G58.0   Intercostal neuropathy

G58.7   Mononeuritis multiplex

G58.8   Other specified mononeuropathies

G58.9   Mononeuropathy, **unspecified**

▸ G59   *Mononeuropathy in diseases classified elsewhere*
    Code first underlying disease
    Excludes1   diabetic mononeuropathy (E08-E13 with .41)
    syphilitic nerve paralysis (A52.19)
    syphilitic neuritis (A52.15)
    tuberculous mononeuropathy (A17.83)

POLYNEUROPATHIES AND OTHER DISORDERS OF THE PERIPHERAL NERVOUS SYSTEM (G60-G65)

    Excludes1   neuralgia NOS (M79.2)
    neuritis NOS (M79.2)
    peripheral neuritis in pregnancy (O26.82-)
    radiculitis NOS (M54.10)

● **G60   Hereditary and idiopathic neuropathy**

G60.0   **Hereditary motor and sensory neuropathy**
Charcot-Marie-Tooth disease
Déjerine-Sottas disease
Hereditary motor and sensory neuropathy, types I-IV
Hypertrophic neuropathy of infancy
Peroneal muscular atrophy (axonal type) (hypertrophic type)
Roussy-Lévy syndrome

G60.1   **Refsum's disease**
Genetic disorder affecting fatty acid metabolism
Infantile Refsum disease

G60.2   Neuropathy in association **with hereditary ataxia**

Item 6–7 The **peripheral nervous system** consists of 31 pairs of spinal nerves, 12 pairs of cranial nerves, and the autonomic nerves, which are divided into the parasympathetic and sympathetic nerves. The cranial nerves are: olfactory (I), optic (II), oculomotor (III), trochlear (IV), trigeminal (V), abducens (VI), facial (VII), vestibulocochlear (VIII), glossopharyngeal (IX), vagus (X), accessory (XI), and hypoglossal (XII).

G60.3   **Idiopathic progressive neuropathy**

G60.8   **Other hereditary and idiopathic neuropathies**
   Dominantly inherited sensory neuropathy
   Morvan's disease
   Nelaton's syndrome
   Recessively inherited sensory neuropathy

G60.9   **Hereditary and idiopathic neuropathy, unspecified**

● **G61   Inflammatory polyneuropathy**

G61.0   **Guillain-Barré syndrome**
   Autoimmune disease affecting peripheral nervous system
   Acute (post-)infective polyneuritis
   Miller Fisher Syndrome

G61.1   **Serum neuropathy**
   Use additional code for adverse effect, if applicable, to identify serum (T50.-)

● G61.8   **Other inflammatory polyneuropathies**

G61.81   **Chronic inflammatory demyelinating polyneuritis**

G61.82   **Multifocal motor neuropathy**
   MMN

G61.89   **Other inflammatory polyneuropathies**

G61.9   **Inflammatory polyneuropathy, unspecified**

● **G62   Other and unspecified polyneuropathies**

G62.0   **Drug-induced polyneuropathy**
   Use additional code for adverse effect, if applicable, to identify drug (T36-T50 with fifth or sixth character 5)

G62.1   **Alcoholic polyneuropathy**
   Malfunction of many peripheral nerves throughout the body
   Coding Clinic: 2019, Q3, P8

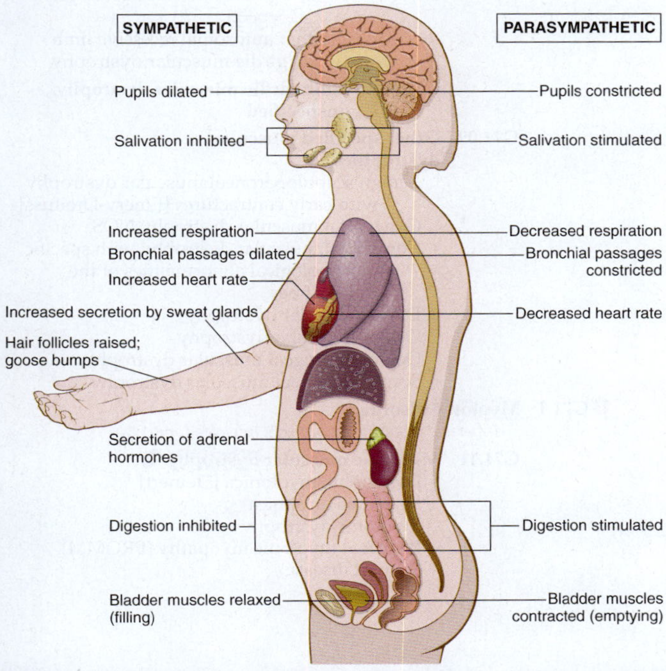

G62.2   **Polyneuropathy due to other toxic agents**
   Code first (T51-T65) *to identify toxic agent*

● G62.8   **Other specified polyneuropathies**

G62.81   **Critical illness polyneuropathy**
   Acute motor neuropathy

G62.82   **Radiation-induced polyneuropathy**
   Use additional external cause code (W88-W90, X39.0-) to identify cause
   Coding Clinic: 2016, Q4, P18

G62.89   **Other specified polyneuropathies**
   Coding Clinic: 2024, Q3, P11; 2016, Q2, P11

G62.9   **Polyneuropathy, unspecified**
   Neuropathy NOS

▶ *G63   Polyneuropathy in diseases classified elsewhere*
   Code first underlying disease, such as:
      amyloidosis (E85.-)
      endocrine disease, except diabetes (E00-E07, E15-E16, E20-E34)
      metabolic diseases (E70-E88)
      neoplasm (C00-D49)
      nutritional deficiency (E40-E64)

Excludes1   polyneuropathy (in):
      diabetes mellitus (E08-E13 with .42)
      diphtheria (A36.83)
      infectious mononucleosis complicated by polyneuropathy (B27.0-B27.9 with fifth character 1)
      Lyme disease (A69.22)
      mumps (B26.84)
      postherpetic (B02.23)
      rheumatoid arthritis (M05.5-)
      scleroderma (M34.83)
      systemic lupus erythematosus (M32.19)
   Coding Clinic: 2024, Q3, P11; 2023, Q3, P19-20; 2021, Q1, P7; 2012, Q4, P100

G64   **Other disorders of peripheral nervous system**
   Disorder of peripheral nervous system NOS

● G65   **Sequelae of inflammatory and toxic polyneuropathies**
   Code first condition resulting from (sequela) of inflammatory and toxic polyneuropathies

G65.0   **Sequelae of Guillain-Barré syndrome**

G65.1   **Sequelae of other inflammatory polyneuropathy**

G65.2   **Sequelae of toxic polyneuropathy**

DISEASES OF MYONEURAL JUNCTION AND MUSCLE (G70-G73)

● G70   **Myasthenia gravis and other myoneural disorders**
   Excludes1   botulism (A05.1, A48.51-A48.52)
      transient neonatal myasthenia gravis (P94.0)

● G70.0   **Myasthenia gravis**
   Acquired and results in fatigable muscle weakness exacerbated by activity and improved with rest

G70.00   **Myasthenia gravis without (acute) exacerbation**
   Myasthenia gravis NOS
   Coding Clinic: 2022, Q3, P16

G70.01   **Myasthenia gravis with (acute) exacerbation**
   Myasthenia gravis in crisis

G70.1   **Toxic myoneural disorders**
   Dysfunction at junction of muscle and motor nerve (myoneural junction)
   Code first (T51-T65) *to identify toxic agent*

G70.2   **Congenital and developmental myasthenia**

● G70.8   **Other specified myoneural disorders**

G70.80   **Lambert-Eaton syndrome, unspecified**
   Lambert-Eaton syndrome NOS

Figure 6-2   Actions of parasympathetic and sympathetic nerves. (From Chabner: The Language of Medicine, ed 9, St. Louis, Saunders, 2011)

CHAPTER 6 (G00-G99)

▶ **G70.81** *Lambert-Eaton syndrome in disease classified elsewhere* ᴴᶜᶜ

  Code first underlying disease

  Excludes1 Lambert-Eaton syndrome in neoplastic disease (G73.1)

  G70.89 **Other specified myoneural disorders** ᴴᶜᶜ

G70.9 **Myoneural disorder, unspecified** ᴴᶜᶜ

● **G71** **Primary disorders of muscles**

  Excludes2 arthrogryposis multiplex congenita (Q74.3)
  metabolic disorders (E70-E88)
  myositis (M60.-)

● **G71.0** **Muscular dystrophy** ᴴᶜᶜ

  G71.00 **Muscular dystrophy, unspecified** ᴴᶜᶜ

  G71.01 **Duchenne or Becker muscular dystrophy** ᴴᶜᶜ
  Autosomal recessive, childhood type, muscular dystrophy resembling Duchenne or Becker muscular dystrophy
  Benign [Becker] muscular dystrophy
  Severe [Duchenne] muscular dystrophy

  G71.02 **Facioscapulohumeral muscular dystrophy** ᴴᶜᶜ
  Scapulohumeral muscular dystrophy
  Coding Clinic: 2018, Q4, P12

  ● **G71.03** **Limb girdle muscular dystrophies**

  G71.031 **Autosomal dominant limb girdle muscular dystrophy**
  LGMD D4 calpain-3-related
  LGMD D5 collagen 6-related
  Limb girdle muscular dystrophy type 1

  G71.032 **Autosomal recessive limb girdle muscular dystrophy due to calpain-3 dysfunction**
  Limb girdle muscular dystrophy type 2A
  LGMD R1 calpain-3-related
  Primary calpainopathy

  G71.033 **Limb girdle muscular dystrophy due to dysferlin dysfunction**
  Dysferlinopathy
  LGMD R2 dysferlin-related
  Limb girdle muscular dystrophy type 2B
  Miyoshi Myopathy type 1

  ● **G71.034** **Limb girdle muscular dystrophy due to sarcoglycan dysfunction**

  G71.0340 **Limb girdle muscular dystrophy due to sarcoglycan dysfunction, unspecified**
  Sarcoglycanopathy, NOS

  G71.0341 **Limb girdle muscular dystrophy due to alpha sarcoglycan dysfunction**
  Alpha sarcoglycanopathy
  Limb-girdle muscular dystrophy due to alpha-sarcoglycan deficiency
  Limb girdle muscular dystrophy type 2D

  G71.0342 **Limb girdle muscular dystrophy due to beta sarcoglycan dysfunction**
  Beta sarcoglycanopathy
  Limb girdle muscular dystrophy due to beta-sarcoglycan deficiency
  Limb girdle muscular dystrophy type 2E

  G71.0349 **Limb girdle muscular dystrophy due to other sarcoglycan dysfunction**
  Delta sarcoglycanopathy
  Delta-sarcoglycan-related LGMD R6
  Gamma sarcoglycanopathy
  Gamma-sarcoglycan-related LGMD R5
  Limb girdle muscular dystrophy type 2C
  Limb girdle muscular dystrophy type 2F

  G71.035 **Limb girdle muscular dystrophy due to anoctamin-5 dysfunction**
  Anoctamin-5-related LGMD R12
  Anoctaminopathy
  Autosomal recessive limb girdle muscular dystrophy type 2L
  Miyoshi myopathy type 3

  ▶ **G71.036** **Limb girdle muscular dystrophy due to fukutin related protein dysfunction**
  ▶ LGMD R9 FKRP-related
  ▶ Limb girdle muscular dystrophy due to FKRP deficiency
  ▶ Limb girdle muscular dystrophy type 2I

  G71.038 **Other limb girdle muscular dystrophy**
  ~~LGMD R9 FKRP-related~~
  LGMD R22 collagen 6-related
  ~~Limb girdle muscular dystrophy due to fukutin related protein dysfunction~~
  ~~Limb girdle muscular dystrophy type 2I~~
  Other autosomal recessive limb girdle muscular dystrophy

  G71.039 **Limb girdle muscular dystrophy, unspecified**

  G71.09 **Other specified muscular dystrophies** ᴴᶜᶜ
  Benign scapuloperoneal muscular dystrophy with early contractures [Emery-Dreifuss]
  Congenital muscular dystrophy NOS
  Congenital muscular dystrophy with specific morphological abnormalities of the muscle fiber
  Distal muscular dystrophy
  Ocular muscular dystrophy
  Oculopharyngeal muscular dystrophy
  Scapuloperoneal muscular dystrophy

● **G71.1** **Myotonic disorders**
  Inherited disorder that affects muscles tone

  G71.11 **Myotonic muscular dystrophy** ᴴᶜᶜ
  Dystrophia myotonica [Steinert]
  Myotonia atrophica
  Myotonic dystrophy
  Proximal myotonic myopathy (PROMM)
  Steinert disease

Item 6–8 Muscular dystrophies (MD) are a group of rare inherited muscle diseases. Voluntary muscles become progressively weaker. In the late stages of MD, fat and connective tissue replace muscle fibers. In some types of muscular dystrophy, heart muscles, other involuntary muscles, and other organs are affected. **Myopathies** is a general term for neuromuscular diseases in which the muscle fibers dysfunction for any one of many reasons, resulting in muscular weakness.

G71.12 Myotonia congenita
Acetazolamide responsive myotonia congenita
Dominant myotonia congenita [Thomsen disease]
Myotonia levior
Recessive myotonia congenita [Becker disease]

G71.13 Myotonic chondrodystrophy
Chondrodystrophic myotonia
Congenital myotonic chondrodystrophy
Schwartz-Jampel disease

G71.14 Drug induced myotonia
Use additional code for adverse effect, if applicable, to identify drug (T36-T50 with fifth or sixth character 5)

G71.19 Other specified myotonic disorders
Myotonia fluctuans
Myotonia permanens
Neuromyotonia [Isaacs]
Paramyotonia congenita (of von Eulenburg)
Pseudomyotonia
Symptomatic myotonia

G71.2 Congenital myopathies
Excludes2 arthrogryposis multiplex congenita (Q74.3)

G71.20 Congenital myopathy, unspecified

G71.21 Nemaline myopathy

● **G71.22 Centronuclear myopathy**

G71.220 X-linked myotubular myopathy
Myotubular (centronuclear) myopathy

G71.228 Other centronuclear myopathy
Autosomal centronuclear myopathy
Autosomal dominant centronuclear myopathy
Autosomal recessive centronuclear myopathy
Centronuclear myopathy, NOS

G71.29 Other congenital myopathy
Central core disease
Minicore disease
Multicore disease
Multiminicore disease

G71.3 Mitochondrial myopathy, not elsewhere classified
Myopathies associated with increased number of enlarged, often abnormal, mitochondria in muscle fibers
Excludes1 Kearns-Sayre syndrome (H49.81)
Leber's disease (H47.21)
Leigh's encephalopathy (G31.82)
mitochondrial metabolism disorders (E88.4.-)
Reye's syndrome (G93.7)

G71.8 Other primary disorders of muscles

G71.9 Primary disorder of muscle, unspecified
Hereditary myopathy NOS

● **G72 Other and unspecified myopathies**
Excludes1 arthrogryposis multiplex congenita (Q74.3)
dermatopolymyositis (M33.-)
ischemic infarction of muscle (M62.2-)
myositis (M60.-)
polymyositis (M33.2.-)

G72.0 Drug-induced myopathy
Use additional code for adverse effect, if applicable, to identify drug (T36-T50 with fifth or sixth character 5)

G72.1 Alcoholic myopathy
Use additional code to identify alcoholism (F10.-)

G72.2 Myopathy due to other toxic agents
Code first (T51-T65) to identify toxic agent

G72.3 Periodic paralysis
Familial periodic paralysis
Hyperkalemic periodic paralysis (familial)
Hypokalemic periodic paralysis (familial)
Myotonic periodic paralysis (familial)
Normokalemic paralysis (familial)
Potassium sensitive periodic paralysis
Excludes1 paramyotonia congenita (of von Eulenburg) (G71.19)

● **G72.4 Inflammatory and immune myopathies, not elsewhere classified**

G72.41 Inclusion body myositis [IBM]

G72.49 Other inflammatory and immune myopathies, not elsewhere classified
Inflammatory myopathy NOS

● **G72.8 Other specified myopathies**

G72.81 Critical illness myopathy
Acute necrotizing myopathy
Acute quadriplegic myopathy
Intensive care (ICU) myopathy
Myopathy of critical illness

G72.89 Other specified myopathies

G72.9 Myopathy, unspecified

● **G73 Disorders of myoneural junction and muscle in diseases classified elsewhere**

▶ **G73.1 Lambert-Eaton syndrome in neoplastic disease**
Rare autoimmune disorder affecting calcium channels of nerve-muscle (neuromuscular) junction
Code first underlying neoplasm (C00-D49)
Excludes1 Lambert-Eaton syndrome not associated with neoplasm (G70.80-G70.81)

▶ **G73.3 Myasthenic syndromes in other diseases classified elsewhere**
Code first underlying disease, such as:
neoplasm (C00-D49)
thyrotoxicosis (E05.-)

▶ **G73.7 Myopathy in diseases classified elsewhere**
Code first underlying disease, such as:
glycogen storage disease (E74.0-)
hyperparathyroidism (E21.0, E21.3)
hypoparathyroidism (E20.-)
lipid storage disorders (E75.-)
Excludes1 myopathy in:
rheumatoid arthritis (M05.32)
sarcoidosis (D86.87)
scleroderma (M34.82)
Sjögren syndrome (M35.03)
systemic lupus erythematosus (M32.19)

CEREBRAL PALSY AND OTHER PARALYTIC SYNDROMES (G80-G83)

● **G80 Cerebral palsy**
Excludes1 hereditary spastic paraplegia (G11.4)

G80.0 Spastic quadriplegic cerebral palsy
Congenital spastic paralysis (cerebral)

G80.1 Spastic diplegic cerebral palsy
Spastic cerebral palsy NOS

G80.2 Spastic hemiplegic cerebral palsy

G80.3 Athetoid cerebral palsy
Result of damage to cerebellum or basal ganglia responsible for processing neuromuscular signals
Double athetosis (syndrome)
Dyskinetic cerebral palsy
Dystonic cerebral palsy
Vogt disease

G80.4 Ataxic cerebral palsy
Poor muscle tone and coordination

G80.8 Other cerebral palsy
Mixed cerebral palsy syndromes

G80.9 Cerebral palsy, unspecified
Cerebral palsy NOS

OGCR Section I.C.6.a.

Dominant/nondominant side

Codes from category G81, Hemiplegia and hemiparesis, and subcategories, G83.1, Monoplegia of lower limb, G83.2, Monoplegia of upper limb, and G83.3, Monoplegia, unspecified, identify whether the dominant and nondominant side is affected. Should the affected side be documented, but not specified as dominant or nondominant, and the classification system does not indicate a default, code selection is as follows:
- For ambidextrous patients, the default should be dominant.
- If the left side is affected, the default is nondominant.
- If the right side is affected, the default is dominant.

Item 6–9 Hemiplegia is complete paralysis of one side of the body—arm, leg, and trunk. **Hemiparesis** is a generalized weakness or incomplete paralysis of one side of the body. If most activities (eating, writing) are performed with the right hand, the right is the dominant side, and the left is the nondominant side. **Quadriplegia,** also called tetraplegia, is the complete paralysis of all four limbs. **Quadriparesis** is the incomplete paralysis of all four limbs. Nerve damage in C1–C4 is associated with lower limb paralysis, and C5–C7 damage is associated with upper limb paralysis. **Diplegia** is the paralysis of the upper limbs. **Monoplegia** is the complete paralysis of one limb.

● **G81   Hemiplegia and hemiparesis**
> **Note:** This category is to be used only when hemiplegia (complete)(incomplete) is reported without further specification, or is stated to be old or longstanding but of unspecified cause. The category is also for use in multiple coding to identify these types of hemiplegia resulting from any cause.

> **Excludes1**   congenital cerebral palsy (G80.-)
> hemiplegia and hemiparesis due to sequela of cerebrovascular disease (I69.05-, I69.15-, I69.25-, I69.35-, I69.85-, I69.95-)

> **Coding Clinic: 2012, Q4, P106**

● **G81.0   Flaccid hemiplegia**
> *Paralysis of half of body with loss of tone of muscles of paralyzed part and absence of tendon reflexes*

> G81.00   Flaccid hemiplegia affecting **unspecified side**
> G81.01   Flaccid hemiplegia affecting **right dominant side**
> G81.02   Flaccid hemiplegia affecting **left dominant side**
> G81.03   Flaccid hemiplegia affecting **right nondominant side**
> G81.04   Flaccid hemiplegia affecting **left nondominant side**

● **G81.1   Spastic hemiplegia**
> *Paralysis of half of body with spasticity of muscles of paralyzed part and increased tendon reflexes*

> G81.10   Spastic hemiplegia affecting **unspecified side**
> G81.11   Spastic hemiplegia affecting **right dominant side**
> G81.12   Spastic hemiplegia affecting **left dominant side**
> G81.13   Spastic hemiplegia affecting **right nondominant side**
> G81.14   Spastic hemiplegia affecting **left nondominant side**

● **G81.9   Hemiplegia, unspecified**
> G81.90   Hemiplegia, unspecified affecting **unspecified side**
> G81.91   Hemiplegia, unspecified affecting **right dominant side**
> G81.92   Hemiplegia, unspecified affecting **left dominant side**
> G81.93   Hemiplegia, unspecified affecting **right nondominant side**
> G81.94   Hemiplegia, unspecified affecting **left nondominant side**
> **Coding Clinic: 2015, Q1, P26**

● **G82   Paraplegia (paraparesis) and quadriplegia (quadriparesis)**
> **Note:** This category is to be used only when the listed conditions are reported without further specification, or are stated to be old or longstanding but of unspecified cause. The category is also for use in multiple coding to identify these conditions resulting from any cause.

> **Excludes1**   congenital cerebral palsy (G80.-)
> functional quadriplegia (R53.2)
> hysterical paralysis (F44.4)

● **G82.2   Paraplegia**
> Paralysis of both lower limbs NOS
> Paraparesis (lower) NOS
> Paraplegia (lower) NOS

> G82.20   Paraplegia, **unspecified**
> **Coding Clinic: 2017, Q3, P3**
> G82.21   Paraplegia, **complete**
> G82.22   Paraplegia, **incomplete**

● **G82.5   Quadriplegia**
> *Paralysis of all limbs; AKA tetraplegia*

> G82.50   Quadriplegia, **unspecified**
> G82.51   Quadriplegia, **C1-C4 complete**
> G82.52   Quadriplegia, **C1-C4 incomplete**
> **Coding Clinic: 2024, Q2, P23**
> G82.53   Quadriplegia, **C5-C7 complete**
> G82.54   Quadriplegia, **C5-C7 incomplete**

● **G83   Other paralytic syndromes**
> **Note:** This category is to be used only when the listed conditions are reported without further specification, or are stated to be old or longstanding but of unspecified cause. The category is also for use in multiple coding to identify these conditions resulting from any cause.

> **Includes**   paralysis (complete) (incomplete), except as in G80-G82

G83.0   Diplegia of upper limbs
> *Paralysis affecting limbs on both sides; AKA bilateral paralysis*
> Diplegia (upper)
> Paralysis of both upper limbs

● **G83.1   Monoplegia of lower limb**
> *Paralysis of limb on one side*
> Paralysis of lower limb

> **Excludes1**   monoplegia of lower limbs due to sequela of cerebrovascular disease (I69.04-, I69.14-, I69.24-, I69.34-, I69.84-, I69.94-)

> **Coding Clinic: 2012, Q4, P106**

> G83.10   Monoplegia of lower limb affecting **unspecified side**
> G83.11   Monoplegia of lower limb affecting **right dominant side**
> G83.12   Monoplegia of lower limb affecting **left dominant side**
> G83.13   Monoplegia of lower limb affecting **right nondominant side**
> G83.14   Monoplegia of lower limb affecting **left nondominant side**

● **G83.2   Monoplegia of upper limb**
> Paralysis of upper limb

> **Excludes1**   monoplegia of upper limbs due to sequela of cerebrovascular disease (I69.03-, I69.13-, I69.23-, I69.33-, I69.83-, I69.93-)

> **Coding Clinic: 2012, Q4, P106**

> G83.20   Monoplegia of upper limb affecting **unspecified side**
> G83.21   Monoplegia of upper limb affecting **right dominant side**
> G83.22   Monoplegia of upper limb affecting **left dominant side**

▶ New   ⇨ Revised   ~~deleted~~ Deleted   Excludes 1   Excludes 2   Includes   Use additional   Code first   Code also   Key words
OGCR Official Guidelines   **X** Assign placeholder X   ● Use Additional Character(s)   ▶ Manifestation Code   Hierarchical Condition Category   Coding Clinic

G83.23   **Monoplegia of upper limb affecting right nondominant side** RCC

G83.24   **Monoplegia of upper limb affecting left nondominant side** RCC

● G83.3   **Monoplegia, unspecified**
          Coding Clinic: 2012, Q4, P106

G83.30   **Monoplegia, unspecified affecting unspecified side** RCC

G83.31   **Monoplegia, unspecified affecting right dominant side** RCC

G83.32   **Monoplegia, unspecified affecting left dominant side** RCC

G83.33   **Monoplegia, unspecified affecting right nondominant side** RCC

G83.34   **Monoplegia, unspecified affecting left nondominant side** RCC

G83.4   **Cauda equina syndrome** RCC
         Aching pain due to compression of spinal nerve roots
         Neurogenic bladder due to cauda equina syndrome
         Excludes1   cord bladder NOS (G95.89)
                          neurogenic bladder NOS (N31.9)
         Coding Clinic: 2024, Q1, P18

G83.5   **Locked-in state** RCC
         Coding Clinic: 2022, Q2, P11

● G83.8   **Other specified paralytic syndromes**
         Excludes1   paralytic syndromes due to current spinal
                          cord injury-code to spinal cord
                          injury (S14, S24, S34)

G83.81   **Brown-Séquard syndrome** RCC
G83.82   **Anterior cord syndrome** RCC
G83.83   **Posterior cord syndrome** RCC
G83.84   **Todd's paralysis (postepileptic)** RCC
G83.89   **Other specified paralytic syndromes** RCC
G83.9   **Paralytic syndrome, unspecified** RCC

OTHER DISORDERS OF THE NERVOUS SYSTEM (G89-G99)

● G89   **Pain, not elsewhere classified**
        Code also related psychological factors associated with pain
        (F45.42)
        Excludes1   generalized pain NOS (R52)
                         pain disorders exclusively related to
                             psychological factors (F45.41)
                         pain NOS (R52)
        Excludes2   atypical face pain (G50.1)
                         headache syndromes (G44.-)
                         localized pain, unspecified type - code to pain by
                             site, such as:
                             abdomen pain (R10.-)
                             back pain (M54.9)
                             breast pain (N64.4)
                             chest pain (R07.1-R07.9)
                             ear pain (H92.0-)
                             eye pain (H57.1)
                             headache (R51.9)
                             joint pain (M25.5-)
                             limb pain (M79.6-)
                             lumbar region pain (M54.5-)
                             painful urination (R30.9)
                          ➡ pelvic and perineal pain (R10.2-)
                             shoulder pain (M25.51-)
                             spine pain (M54.-)
                             throat pain (R07.0)
                             tongue pain (K14.6)
                             tooth pain (K08.8)
                         renal colic (N23)
                         migraines (G43.-)
                         myalgia (M79.1-)
                         pain from prosthetic devices, implants, and grafts
                             (T82.84, T83.84, T84.84, T85.84-)
                         phantom limb syndrome with pain (G54.6)
                         vulvar vestibulitis (N94.810)
                         vulvodynia (N94.81-)

G89.0   **Central pain syndrome**
         *Neurological condition causing intractable pain resulting
             from damage to CNS*
         Déjérine-Roussy syndrome
         Myelopathic pain syndrome
         Thalamic pain syndrome (hyperesthetic)

● G89.1   **Acute pain, not elsewhere classified**
G89.11   **Acute pain due to trauma**
G89.12   **Acute post-thoracotomy pain**
          Post-thoracotomy pain NOS
G89.18   **Other acute postprocedural pain**
          Postoperative pain NOS
          Postprocedural pain NOS

● G89.2   **Chronic pain, not elsewhere classified**
         Excludes1   causalgia, lower limb (G57.7-)
                          causalgia, upper limb (G56.4-)
                          central pain syndrome (G89.0)
                          chronic pain syndrome (G89.4)
                          complex regional pain syndrome II, lower
                              limb (G57.7-)
                          complex regional pain syndrome II,
                              upper limb (G56.4-)
                          neoplasm related chronic pain (G89.3)
                          reflex sympathetic dystrophy (G90.5-)

G89.21   **Chronic pain due to trauma**
G89.22   **Chronic post-thoracotomy pain**
G89.28   **Other chronic postprocedural pain**
          Other chronic postoperative pain
G89.29   **Other chronic pain**
          Coding Clinic: 2023, Q3, P17

G89.3   **Neoplasm related pain (acute) (chronic)**
         Cancer associated pain
         Pain due to malignancy (primary) (secondary)
         Tumor associated pain

G89.4   **Chronic pain syndrome**
         Chronic pain associated with significant psychosocial
             dysfunction

● G90   **Disorders of autonomic nervous system**
        Excludes1   dysfunction of the autonomic nervous system
                         due to alcohol (G31.2)

● G90.0   **Idiopathic peripheral autonomic neuropathy**
G90.01   **Carotid sinus syncope**
          Carotid sinus syndrome
G90.09   **Other idiopathic peripheral autonomic
          neuropathy**
          Idiopathic peripheral autonomic neuropathy
          NOS

G90.1   **Familial dysautonomia [Riley-Day]** RCC
         Inherited disorder that affects nerve function

G90.2   **Horner's syndrome**
         Due to damage of the sympathetic nervous system
         Bernard(-Horner) syndrome
         Cervical sympathetic dystrophy or paralysis

G90.3   **Multi-system degeneration of the autonomic nervous
         system** RCC
         Neurogenic orthostatic hypotension [Shy-Drager]
         Excludes1   orthostatic hypotension NOS (I95.1)

G90.4   **Autonomic dysreflexia**
         Syndrome resulting from lesions of spinal cord
         Use additional code to identify the cause, such as:
             fecal impaction (K56.41)
             pressure ulcer (pressure area) (L89.-)
             urinary tract infection (N39.0)

● G90.5   **Complex regional pain syndrome I (CRPS I)**
         Reflex sympathetic dystrophy
         Excludes1   causalgia of lower limb (G57.7-)
                          causalgia of upper limb (G56.4-)
                          complex regional pain syndrome II of
                              lower limb (G57.7-)
                          complex regional pain syndrome II of
                              upper limb (G56.4-)

G90.50   **Complex regional pain syndrome I, unspecified**

CHAPTER 6 (G00-G99)

CHAPTER 6 (G00-G99)

● **G90.51** Complex regional pain syndrome I of upper limb

    G90.511 Complex regional pain syndrome I of right upper limb

    G90.512 Complex regional pain syndrome I of left upper limb

    G90.513 Complex regional pain syndrome I of upper limb, bilateral

    G90.519 Complex regional pain syndrome I of unspecified upper limb

● **G90.52** Complex regional pain syndrome I of lower limb

    G90.521 Complex regional pain syndrome I of right lower limb

    G90.522 Complex regional pain syndrome I of left lower limb

    G90.523 Complex regional pain syndrome I of lower limb, bilateral

    G90.529 Complex regional pain syndrome I of unspecified lower limb

    G90.59 Complex regional pain syndrome I of other specified site

G90.8 Other disorders of autonomic nervous system
Coding Clinic: 2023, Q2, P9

    G90.81 Serotonin syndrome
Serotonin toxicity

    Code first poisoning due to drug or toxin, such as:
linezolid (T36.8X- with sixth character 1-4)
monoamine oxidase inhibitors (T43.1X with sixth character 1-4)
selective serotonin and norepinephrine reuptake inhibitors [SSNRI] (T43.21 with sixth character 1-4)
selective serotonin reuptake inhibitors [SSRI] (T43.22 with sixth character 1-4)

    Use Additional code for adverse effect, if applicable, to identify drug, such as:
linezolid (T36.8X5)
monoamine oxidase inhibitors (T43.1X5)
selective serotonin and norepinephrine reuptake inhibitors [SSNRI](T43.215)
selective serotonin reuptake inhibitors [SSRI] (T43.225)

    Use Additional code, if applicable, to identify:
disseminated intravascular coagulation (D65)
hypertensive crisis (I16.-)
metabolic acidosis (E87.2-)
shock, not elsewhere classified (R57.-)
toxic encephalopathy (G92.-)
ventricular tachycardia (I47.2-)
Coding Clinic: 2024, Q4, P17

    G90.89 Other disorders of autonomic nervous system

G90.9 Disorder of the autonomic nervous system, unspecified

G90.A Postural orthostatic tachycardia syndrome [POTS]
Chronic orthostatic intolerance
Postural tachycardia syndrome
Coding Clinic: 2022, Q4, P20

G90.B LMNB1-related autosomal dominant leukodystrophy

● **G91** Hydrocephalus
Dilatation of cerebral ventricles, accompanied by accumulation of cerebrospinal fluid

    Includes acquired hydrocephalus
    Excludes1 Arnold-Chiari syndrome with hydrocephalus (Q07.-)
congenital hydrocephalus (Q03.-)
spina bifida with hydrocephalus (Q05.-)

G91.0 Communicating hydrocephalus
Secondary normal pressure hydrocephalus

G91.1 Obstructive hydrocephalus

G91.2 (Idiopathic) normal pressure hydrocephalus
Normal pressure hydrocephalus NOS

G91.3 Post-traumatic hydrocephalus, unspecified

▶ *G91.4* *Hydrocephalus in diseases classified elsewhere*
Code first underlying condition, such as:
congenital syphilis (A50.4-)
neoplasm (C00-D49)
plasminogen deficiency (E88.02)

    Excludes1 hydrocephalus due to congenital toxoplasmosis (P37.1)

G91.8 Other hydrocephalus

G91.9 Hydrocephalus, unspecified

G92 Toxic encephalopathy

● **G92.0** Immune effector cell-associated neurotoxicity syndrome
Code first underlying cause such as:
complications of immune effector cellular therapy (T80.82)

    Code also, if applicable, associated signs and symptoms, such as:
cerebral edema (G93.6)
unspecified convulsions (R56.9)

    G92.00 Immune effector cell-associated neurotoxicity syndrome, grade unspecified
ICANS, grade unspecified

    G92.01 Immune effector cell-associated neurotoxicity syndrome, grade 1
ICANS, grade 1

    G92.02 Immune effector cell-associated neurotoxicity syndrome, grade 2
ICANS, grade 2

    G92.03 Immune effector cell-associated neurotoxicity syndrome, grade 3
ICANS, grade 3

    G92.04 Immune effector cell-associated neurotoxicity syndrome, grade 4
ICANS, grade 4

    G92.05 Immune effector cell-associated neurotoxicity syndrome, grade 5
ICANS, grade 5

G92.8 Other toxic encephalopathy
Toxic encephalitis
Toxic metabolic encephalopathy

    Code first poisoning due to drug or toxin, if applicable, (T36-T65 with fifth or sixth character 1-4)

    Use Additional code for adverse effect, if applicable, to identify drug (T36-T50 with fifth or sixth character 5)
Coding Clinic: 2024, Q4, P17; 2024, Q2, P15; 2022, Q1, P53

G92.9 Unspecified toxic encephalopathy
Code first poisoning due to drug or toxin, if applicable, (T36-T65 with fifth or sixth character 1-4)

    Use Additional code for adverse effect, if applicable, to identify drug (T36-T50 with fifth or sixth character 5)

Disorder or disease of brain caused by chemicals
Coding Clinic: 2021, Q1, P13; 2017, Q1, P39-40

● **G93** Other disorders of brain

G93.0 Cerebral cysts
Arachnoid cyst
Porencephalic cyst, acquired

    Excludes1 acquired periventricular cysts of newborn (P91.1)
congenital cerebral cysts (Q04.6)

G93.1 Anoxic brain damage, not elsewhere classified 🅗🅒
Permanent brain damage by lack of oxygen perfusion through brain tissues.

    Excludes1 cerebral anoxia due to anesthesia during labor and delivery (O74.3)
cerebral anoxia due to anesthesia during the puerperium (O89.2)
neonatal anoxia (P84)

G93.2 Benign intracranial hypertension
Pseudotumor

> **Excludes1** hypertensive encephalopathy (I67.4)
> obstructive hydrocephalus (G91.1)

● G93.3 Postviral and related fatigue syndromes

> **Excludes1** chronic fatigue NOS (R53.82)

Use Additional code, if applicable, for post COVID-19 condition, unspecified (U09.9)

> **Excludes1** neurasthenia (F48.8)

G93.31 Postviral fatigue syndrome

G93.32 Myalgic encephalomyelitis/chronic fatigue syndrome
Chronic fatigue syndrome
ME/CFS
Myalgic encephalomyelitis

G93.39 Other post infection and related fatigue syndromes

● G93.4 Other and unspecified encephalopathy

> **Excludes2** alcoholic encephalopathy (G31.2)
> encephalopathy in diseases classified elsewhere (G94)
> hypertensive encephalopathy (I67.4)

Coding Clinic: 2024, Q2, P15; 2017, Q2, P9

G93.40 Encephalopathy, unspecified

G93.41 Metabolic encephalopathy
Septic encephalopathy
Coding Clinic: 2024, Q2, P15; 2017, Q2, P8; 2016, Q3, P42; 2015, Q3, P21

G93.42 Megalencephalic leukoencephalopathy with subcortical cysts

G93.43 Leukoencephalopathy with calcifications and cysts

G93.44 Adult-onset leukodystrophy with axonal spheroids
Adult-onset leukoencephalopathy with axonal spheroids and pigmented glia

G93.45 Developmental and epileptic encephalopathy
Early infantile epileptic encephalopathy
Code also if applicable, associated disorders such as:
developmental disorders of scholastic skills (F81.-)
developmental disorder of speech and language (F80.-)
epilepsy, by specific type (G40.-)
intellectual disabilities (F70-F79)
other neurodevelopmental disorder (F88)
pervasive developmental disorders (F84.-)

G93.49 Other encephalopathy
Encephalopathy NEC
Coding Clinic: 2021, Q2, P3; 2018, Q4, P16; 2018, Q2, P22; 2017, Q2, P9

G93.5 Compression of brain
Arnold-Chiari type 1 compression of brain
Compression of brain (stem)
Herniation of brain (stem)

> **Excludes1** traumatic compression of brain (S06.A-)

G93.6 Cerebral edema

> **Excludes1** cerebral edema due to birth injury (P11.0)
> traumatic cerebral edema (S06.1-)

Coding Clinic: 2022, Q3, P9,11

G93.7 Reye's syndrome   **P**
Life-threatening neurological condition, usually follows viral illness

Code first *(poisoning due to salicylates, if applicable (T39.0-, with sixth character 1-4)*

Use additional code for adverse effect due to salicylates, if applicable (T39.0-, with sixth character 5)

● G93.8 Other specified disorders of brain

G93.81 Temporal sclerosis
Hippocampal sclerosis
Mesial temporal sclerosis

G93.82 Brain death

G93.89 Other specified disorders of brain
Postradiation encephalopathy
Coding Clinic: 2024, Q2, P15,16; 2019, Q3, P9; 2016, Q4, P7

G93.9 Disorder of brain, unspecified

▶ G94 *Other disorders of brain in diseases classified elsewhere*
Code first *underlying disease*

> **Excludes1** encephalopathy in congenital syphilis (A50.49)
> encephalopathy in influenza (J09.X9, J10.81, J11.81)
> encephalopathy in syphilis (A52.19)
> hydrocephalus in diseases classified elsewhere (G91.4)

Coding Clinic: 2018, Q2, P22; 2017, Q2, P8

● G95 Other and unspecified diseases of spinal cord

> **Excludes2** myelitis (G04.-)

G95.0 Syringomyelia and syringobulbia

● G95.1 Vascular myelopathies

> **Excludes2** intraspinal phlebitis and thrombophlebitis, except non-pyogenic (G08)

G95.11 Acute infarction of spinal cord (embolic) (nonembolic)
Anoxia of spinal cord
Arterial thrombosis of spinal cord

G95.19 Other vascular myelopathies
Edema of spinal cord
Hematomyelia
Nonpyogenic intraspinal phlebitis and thrombophlebitis
Subacute necrotic myelopathy
Coding Clinic: 2024, Q3, P6; 2023, Q3, P21

● G95.2 Other and unspecified cord compression

G95.20 Unspecified cord compression

G95.29 Other cord compression

● G95.8 Other specified diseases of spinal cord

> **Excludes1** neurogenic bladder NOS (N31.9)
> neurogenic bladder due to cauda equina syndrome (G83.4)
> neuromuscular dysfunction of bladder without spinal cord lesion (N31.-)

G95.81 Conus medullaris syndrome
Damage to gray matter and/or nerve roots in lower end of spinal cord

G95.89 Other specified diseases of spinal cord
Cord bladder NOS
Drug-induced myelopathy
Radiation-induced myelopathy

> **Excludes1** myelopathy NOS (G95.9)

Coding Clinic: 2024, Q3, P6

G95.9 Disease of spinal cord, unspecified
Myelopathy NOS

● G96 Other disorders of central nervous system

● G96.0 Cerebrospinal fluid leak
Code also if applicable:
intracranial hypotension (G96.81-)

> **Excludes1** cerebrospinal fluid leak from spinal puncture (G97.0)

Coding Clinic: 2024, Q3, P7; 2018, Q2, P13

G96.00 Cerebrospinal fluid leak, unspecified
Code also if applicable:
head injury (S00-S09)

CHAPTER 6 (G00-G99)

G96.01   **Cranial cerebrospinal fluid leak, spontaneous**
Otorrhea due to spontaneous cerebrospinal fluid CSF leak
Rhinorrhea due to spontaneous cerebrospinal fluid CSF leak
Spontaneous cerebrospinal fluid leak from skull base

G96.02   **Spinal cerebrospinal fluid leak, spontaneous**
Spontaneous cerebrospinal fluid leak from spine

G96.08   **Other cranial cerebrospinal fluid leak**
Postoperative cranial cerebrospinal fluid leak
Traumatic cranial cerebrospinal fluid leak
Code also if applicable:
head injury (S00-S09)
Coding Clinic: 2024, Q3, P7

G96.09   **Other spinal cerebrospinal fluid leak**
Other spinal CSF leak
Postoperative spinal cerebrospinal fluid leak
Traumatic spinal cerebrospinal fluid leak
Code also if applicable:
head injury (S00-S09)
Coding Clinic: 2022, Q3, P24

● **G96.1**   **Disorders of meninges, not elsewhere classified**

G96.11   **Dural tear**
Code also intracranial hypotension, if applicable (G96.81-)
Excludes1   accidental puncture or laceration of dura during a procedure (G97.41)

G96.12   **Meningeal adhesions (cerebral) (spinal)**

● **G96.19**   **Other disorders of meninges, not elsewhere classified**

G96.191   **Perineural cyst**
Cervical nerve root cyst
Lumbar nerve root cyst
Sacral nerve root cyst
Tarlov cyst
Thoracic nerve root cyst

G96.198   **Other disorders of meninges, not elsewhere classified**

● **G96.8**   **Other specified disorders of central nervous system**

● **G96.81**   **Intracranial hypotension**
Code also any associated diagnoses, such as:
Brachial amyotrophy (G54.5)
Cerebrospinal fluid leak from spine (G96.02)
Cranial nerve disorders in diseases classified elsewhere (G53)
Nerve root and compressions in diseases classified elsewhere (G55)
Nonpyogenic thrombosis of intracranial venous system (I67.6)
Nontraumatic intracerebral hemorrhage (I61.-)
Nontraumatic subdural hemorrhage (I62.0-)
Other and unspecified cord compression (G95.2-)
Other secondary parkinsonism (G21.8)
Reversible cerebrovascular vasoconstriction syndrome (I67.841)
Spinal cord herniation (G95.89)
Stroke (I63.-)
Syringomyelia (G95.0)

G96.810   **Intracranial hypotension, unspecified**

G96.811   **Intracranial hypotension, spontaneous**
Coding Clinic: 2024, Q3, P7

G96.819   **Other intracranial hypotension**

G96.89   **Other specified disorders of central nervous system**

G96.9   **Disorder of central nervous system, unspecified**

● **G97**   **Intraoperative and postprocedural complications and disorders of nervous system, not elsewhere classified**
Excludes2   intraoperative and postprocedural cerebrovascular infarction (I97.81-, I97.82-)
Coding Clinic: 2016, Q4, P9

G97.0   **Cerebrospinal fluid leak from spinal puncture**
Code also any associated diagnoses or complications, such as:
intracranial hypotension following a procedure (G97.83-G97.84)

G97.1   **Other reaction to spinal and lumbar puncture**
Headache due to lumbar puncture
Other reaction to spinal dural puncture
Code also, if applicable, any associated headache with orthostatic component (R51.0)

G97.2   **Intracranial hypotension following ventricular shunting**
Code also any associated diagnoses or complications

● **G97.3**   **Intraoperative hemorrhage and hematoma of a nervous system organ or structure complicating a procedure**
Excludes1   intraoperative hemorrhage and hematoma of a nervous system organ or structure due to accidental puncture and laceration during a procedure (G97.4-)

G97.31   **Intraoperative hemorrhage and hematoma of a nervous system organ or structure complicating a nervous system procedure**

G97.32   **Intraoperative hemorrhage and hematoma of a nervous system organ or structure complicating other procedure**

● **G97.4**   **Accidental puncture and laceration of a nervous system organ or structure during a procedure**

G97.41   **Accidental puncture or laceration of dura during a procedure**
Incidental (inadvertent) durotomy
Code also any associated diagnoses or complications
Coding Clinic: 2024, Q1, P21

G97.48   **Accidental puncture and laceration of other nervous system organ or structure during a nervous system procedure**

G97.49   **Accidental puncture and laceration of other nervous system organ or structure during other procedure**

● **G97.5**   **Postprocedural hemorrhage of a nervous system organ or structure following a procedure**

G97.51   **Postprocedural hemorrhage of a nervous system organ or structure following a nervous system procedure**

G97.52   **Postprocedural hemorrhage of a nervous system organ or structure following other procedure**

● **G97.6**   **Postprocedural hematoma and seroma of a nervous system organ or structure following a procedure**

G97.61   **Postprocedural hematoma of a nervous system organ or structure following a nervous system procedure**

G97.62   **Postprocedural hematoma of a nervous system organ or structure following other procedure**
Coding Clinic: 2024, Q3, P5-6

G97.63   **Postprocedural seroma of a nervous system organ or structure following a nervous system procedure**

G97.64   **Postprocedural seroma of a nervous system organ or structure following other procedure**

▶ New   ➡ Revised   ~~deleted~~ Deleted   Excludes 1   Excludes 2   Includes   Use additional   Code first   Code also   Key words

OGCR Official Guidelines   X Assign placeholder X   ● Use Additional Character(s)   ▌ Manifestation Code   Hierarchical Condition Category   Coding Clinic

● **G97.8 Other intraoperative and postprocedural complications and disorders of nervous system**

Use additional code to further specify disorder

G97.81 Other intraoperative complications of nervous system

G97.82 Other postprocedural complications and disorders of nervous system
Coding Clinic: 2022, Q1, P35

G97.83 Intracranial hypotension following lumbar cerebrospinal fluid shunting

Code also any associated diagnoses or complications

G97.84 Intracranial hypotension following other procedure

Code also, if applicable:
accidental puncture or laceration of dura during a procedure (G97.41)
cerebrospinal fluid leak from spinal puncture (G97.0)

● **G98 Other disorders of nervous system not elsewhere classified**

Includes   nervous system disorder NOS

G98.0 Neurogenic arthritis, not elsewhere classified
Nonsyphilitic neurogenic arthropathy NEC
Nonsyphilitic neurogenic spondylopathy NEC

Excludes1   spondylopathy (in):
syringomyelia and syringobulbia (G95.0)
tabes dorsalis (A52.11)

G98.8 Other disorders of nervous system
Nervous system disorder NOS

● **G99 Other disorders of nervous system in diseases classified elsewhere**

▶ **G99.0 Autonomic neuropathy in diseases classified elsewhere**

Code first underlying disease, such as:
amyloidosis (E85.-)
gout (M1A.-, M10.-)
hyperthyroidism (E05.-)

Excludes1   diabetic autonomic neuropathy (E08-E13 with .43)

▶ **G99.2 Myelopathy in diseases classified elsewhere**

Code first underlying disease, such as:
neoplasm (C00-D49)

Excludes1   myelopathy in:
intervertebral disease (M50.0-, M51.0-)
spondylosis (M47.0-, M47.1-)

▶ **G99.8 Other specified disorders of nervous system in diseases classified elsewhere**

Code first underlying disorder, such as:
amyloidosis (E85.-)
avitaminosis (E56.-)

Excludes1   nervous system involvement in:
cysticercosis (B69.0)
rubella (B06.0-)
syphilis (A52.1-)

CHAPTER 7

DISEASES OF THE EYE AND ADNEXA
(H00-H59)

OGCR Chapter-Specific Coding Guidelines

7. Chapter 7: Diseases of the Eye and Adnexa (H00-H59)

a. Glaucoma

1) Assigning Glaucoma Codes

Assign as many codes from category H40, Glaucoma, as needed to identify the type of glaucoma, the affected eye, and the glaucoma stage.

2) Bilateral glaucoma with same type and stage

When a patient has bilateral glaucoma and both eyes are documented as being the same type and stage, and there is a code for bilateral glaucoma, report only the code for the type of glaucoma, bilateral, with the seventh character for the stage.

When a patient has bilateral glaucoma and both eyes are documented as being the same type and stage, and the classification does not provide a code for bilateral glaucoma (i.e., subcategories H40.10, H40.11, and H40.20) report only one code for the type of glaucoma with the appropriate seventh character for the stage.

3) Bilateral glaucoma stage with different types or stages

When a patient has bilateral glaucoma and each eye is documented as having a different type or stage, and the classification distinguishes laterality, assign the appropriate code for each eye rather than the code for bilateral glaucoma.

When a patient has bilateral glaucoma and each eye is documented as having a different type, and the classification does not distinguish laterality (i.e., subcategories H40.10, H40.11 and H40.20), assign one code for each type of glaucoma with the appropriate seventh character for the stage.

When a patient has bilateral glaucoma and each eye is documented as having the same type, but different stage, and the classification does not distinguish laterality (i.e., subcategories H40.10, H40.11, and H40.20), assign a code for the type of glaucoma for each eye with the seventh character for the specific glaucoma stage documented for each eye.

4) Patient admitted with glaucoma and stage evolves during the admission

If a patient is admitted with glaucoma and the stage progresses during the admission, assign the code for highest stage documented.

5) Indeterminate stage glaucoma

Assignment of the seventh character "4" for "indeterminate stage" should be based on the clinical documentation. The seventh character "4" is used for glaucomas whose stage cannot be clinically determined. This seventh character should not be confused with the seventh character "0", unspecified, which should be assigned when there is no documentation regarding the stage of the glaucoma.

b. Blindness

If "blindness" or "low vision" of both eyes is documented but the visual impairment category is not documented, assign code H54.3, Unqualified visual loss, both eyes. If "blindness" or "low vision" in one eye is documented but the visual impairment category is not documented, assign a code from H54.6-, Unqualified visual loss, one eye. If "blindness" or "visual loss" is documented without any information about whether one or both eyes are affected, assign code H54.7, Unspecified visual loss.

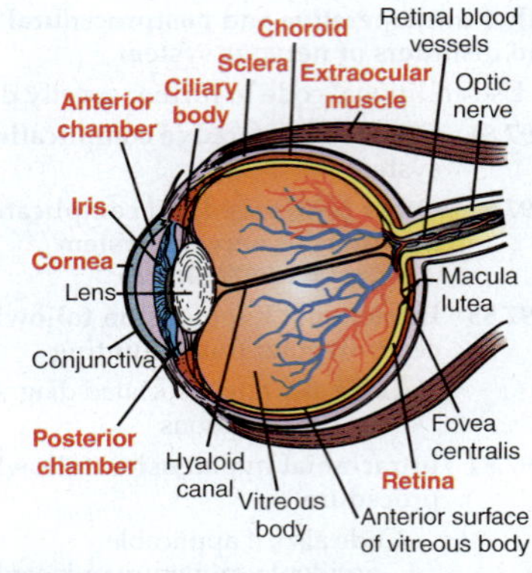

Figure 7-1 Eye and ocular adnexa. (From Buck CJ: Step-by-Step Medical Coding, ed 2016, St. Louis, Elsevier, 2016)

★ **(See Plate 15 of the Anatomy Illustrations.)**

CHAPTER 7

DISEASES OF THE EYE AND ADNEXA
(H00-H59)

Note: Use an external cause code following the code for the eye condition, if applicable, to identify the cause of the eye condition

Excludes2 certain conditions originating in the perinatal period (P04-P96)

certain infectious and parasitic diseases (A00-B99)

complications of pregnancy, childbirth and the puerperium (O00-O9A)

congenital malformations, deformations, and chromosomal abnormalities (Q00-Q99)

diabetes mellitus related eye conditions (E09.3-, E10.3-, E11.3-, E13.3-)

endocrine, nutritional and metabolic diseases (E00-E88)

injury (trauma) of eye and orbit (S05.-)

injury, poisoning and certain other consequences of external causes (S00-T88)

neoplasms (C00-D49)

symptoms, signs and abnormal clinical and laboratory findings, not elsewhere classified (R00-R94)

syphilis related eye disorders (A50.01, A50.3-, A51.43, A52.71)

This chapter contains the following blocks:

H00-H05	Disorders of eyelid, lacrimal system and orbit
H10-H11	Disorders of conjunctiva
H15-H22	Disorders of sclera, cornea, iris and ciliary body
H25-H28	Disorders of lens
H30-H36	Disorders of choroid and retina
H40-H42	Glaucoma
H43-H44	Disorders of vitreous body and globe
H46-H47	Disorders of optic nerve and visual pathways
H49-H52	Disorders of ocular muscles, binocular movement, accommodation and refraction
H53-H54	Visual disturbances and blindness
H55-H57	Other disorders of eye and adnexa
H59	Intraoperative and postprocedural complications and disorders of eye and adnexa, not elsewhere classified

DISORDERS OF EYELID, LACRIMAL SYSTEM AND ORBIT (H00-H05)

Excludes2   open wound of eyelid (S01.1-)
             superficial injury of eyelid (S00.1-, S00.2-)

● **H00** **Hordeolum and chalazion**
Hordeolum: inflammatory staphylococcal infection of sebaceous glands of eyelids; AKA stye. Chalazion: eyelid mass

● **H00.0** **Hordeolum (externum) (internum) of eyelid**
Bacterial infection (staphylococcus) of the sebaceous gland of the eyelid (stye)

● **H00.01** **Hordeolum externum**
Hordeolum NOS
Stye

H00.011 Hordeolum externum right upper eyelid

H00.012 Hordeolum externum right lower eyelid

H00.013 Hordeolum externum right eye, unspecified eyelid

H00.014 Hordeolum externum left upper eyelid

H00.015 Hordeolum externum left lower eyelid

H00.016 Hordeolum externum left eye, unspecified eyelid

H00.019 Hordeolum externum unspecified eye, unspecified eyelid

● **H00.02** **Hordeolum internum**
Infection of meibomian gland

H00.021 Hordeolum internum right upper eyelid

H00.022 Hordeolum internum right lower eyelid

H00.023 Hordeolum internum right eye, unspecified eyelid

H00.024 Hordeolum internum left upper eyelid

H00.025 Hordeolum internum left lower eyelid

H00.026 Hordeolum internum left eye, unspecified eyelid

H00.029 Hordeolum internum unspecified eye, unspecified eyelid

● **H00.03** **Abscess of eyelid**
Furuncle of eyelid

H00.031 Abscess of right upper eyelid

H00.032 Abscess of right lower eyelid

H00.033 Abscess of eyelid right eye, unspecified eyelid

H00.034 Abscess of left upper eyelid

H00.035 Abscess of left lower eyelid

H00.036 Abscess of eyelid left eye, unspecified eyelid

H00.039 Abscess of eyelid unspecified eye, unspecified eyelid

● **H00.1** **Chalazion**
Often caused by accumulation of meibomian gland secretions resulting from a blockage of duct.
Meibomian (gland) cyst

Excludes2   infected meibomian gland (H00.02-)

H00.11 Chalazion right upper eyelid

H00.12 Chalazion right lower eyelid

H00.13 Chalazion right eye, unspecified eyelid

H00.14 Chalazion left upper eyelid

H00.15 Chalazion left lower eyelid

H00.16 Chalazion left eye, unspecified eyelid

H00.19 Chalazion unspecified eye, unspecified eyelid

● **H01** **Other inflammation of eyelid**

● **H01.0** **Blepharitis**
Inflammation of eyelids

Excludes1   blepharoconjunctivitis (H10.5-)

● **H01.00** **Unspecified blepharitis**

H01.001 Unspecified blepharitis right upper eyelid

H01.002 Unspecified blepharitis right lower eyelid

H01.003 Unspecified blepharitis right eye, unspecified eyelid

H01.004 Unspecified blepharitis left upper eyelid

H01.005 Unspecified blepharitis left lower eyelid

H01.006 Unspecified blepharitis left eye, unspecified eyelid

H01.009 Unspecified blepharitis unspecified eye, unspecified eyelid

H01.00A Unspecified blepharitis right eye, upper and lower eyelids

H01.00B Unspecified blepharitis left eye, upper and lower eyelids

● **H01.01** **Ulcerative blepharitis**

H01.011 Ulcerative blepharitis right upper eyelid

H01.012 Ulcerative blepharitis right lower eyelid

H01.013 Ulcerative blepharitis right eye, unspecified eyelid

H01.014 Ulcerative blepharitis left upper eyelid

H01.015 Ulcerative blepharitis left lower eyelid

H01.016 Ulcerative blepharitis left eye, unspecified eyelid

H01.019 Ulcerative blepharitis unspecified eye, unspecified eyelid

H01.01A Ulcerative blepharitis right eye, upper and lower eyelids

H01.01B Ulcerative blepharitis left eye, upper and lower eyelids

● **H01.02** **Squamous blepharitis**

H01.021 Squamous blepharitis right upper eyelid

H01.022 Squamous blepharitis right lower eyelid

H01.023 Squamous blepharitis right eye, unspecified eyelid

H01.024 Squamous blepharitis left upper eyelid

H01.025 Squamous blepharitis left lower eyelid

H01.026 Squamous blepharitis left eye, unspecified eyelid

H01.029 Squamous blepharitis unspecified eye, unspecified eyelid

H01.02A Squamous blepharitis right eye, upper and lower eyelids

H01.02B Squamous blepharitis left eye, upper and lower eyelids

● **H01.1** **Noninfectious dermatoses of eyelid**

● **H01.11** **Allergic dermatitis of eyelid**
Contact dermatitis of eyelid

H01.111 Allergic dermatitis of right upper eyelid

H01.112 Allergic dermatitis of right lower eyelid

CHAPTER 7 (H00-H59)

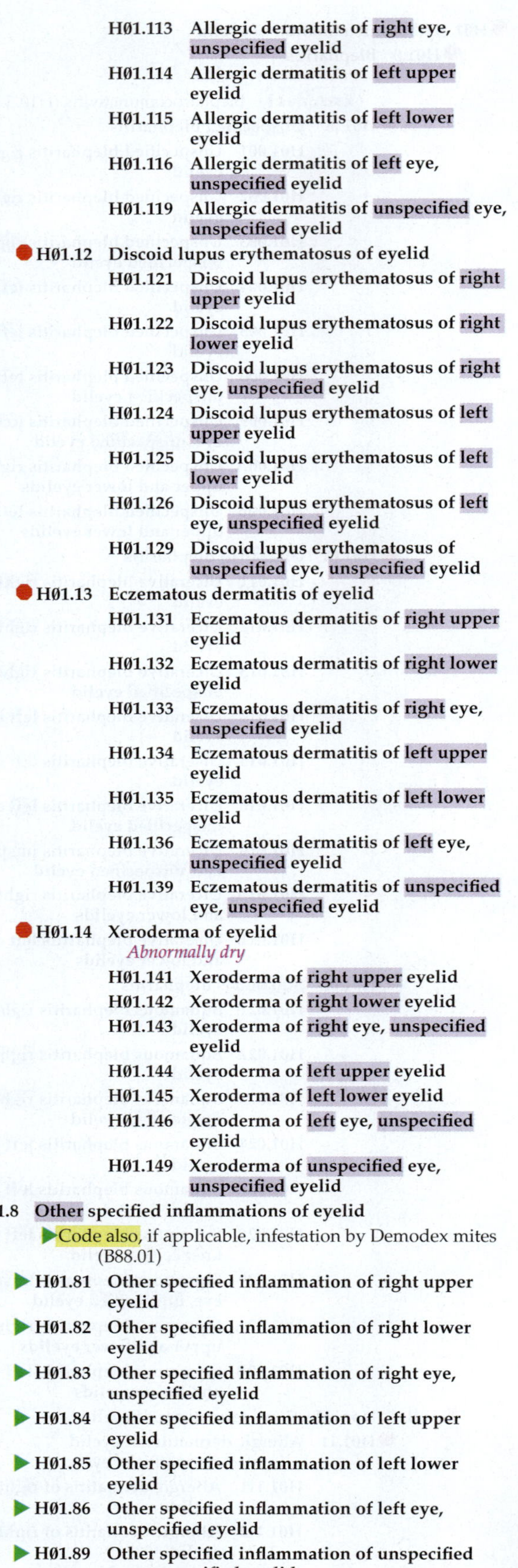

H01.113   Allergic dermatitis of right eye, unspecified eyelid

H01.114   Allergic dermatitis of left upper eyelid

H01.115   Allergic dermatitis of left lower eyelid

H01.116   Allergic dermatitis of left eye, unspecified eyelid

H01.119   Allergic dermatitis of unspecified eye, unspecified eyelid

● H01.12   **Discoid lupus erythematosus of eyelid**

H01.121   Discoid lupus erythematosus of right upper eyelid

H01.122   Discoid lupus erythematosus of right lower eyelid

H01.123   Discoid lupus erythematosus of right eye, unspecified eyelid

H01.124   Discoid lupus erythematosus of left upper eyelid

H01.125   Discoid lupus erythematosus of left lower eyelid

H01.126   Discoid lupus erythematosus of left eye, unspecified eyelid

H01.129   Discoid lupus erythematosus of unspecified eye, unspecified eyelid

● H01.13   **Eczematous dermatitis of eyelid**

H01.131   Eczematous dermatitis of right upper eyelid

H01.132   Eczematous dermatitis of right lower eyelid

H01.133   Eczematous dermatitis of right eye, unspecified eyelid

H01.134   Eczematous dermatitis of left upper eyelid

H01.135   Eczematous dermatitis of left lower eyelid

H01.136   Eczematous dermatitis of left eye, unspecified eyelid

H01.139   Eczematous dermatitis of unspecified eye, unspecified eyelid

● H01.14   **Xeroderma of eyelid**
Abnormally dry

H01.141   Xeroderma of right upper eyelid

H01.142   Xeroderma of right lower eyelid

H01.143   Xeroderma of right eye, unspecified eyelid

H01.144   Xeroderma of left upper eyelid

H01.145   Xeroderma of left lower eyelid

H01.146   Xeroderma of left eye, unspecified eyelid

H01.149   Xeroderma of unspecified eye, unspecified eyelid

● H01.8   **Other specified inflammations of eyelid**

▶ **Code also**, if applicable, infestation by Demodex mites (B88.01)

▶ H01.81   Other specified inflammation of right upper eyelid

▶ H01.82   Other specified inflammation of right lower eyelid

▶ H01.83   Other specified inflammation of right eye, unspecified eyelid

▶ H01.84   Other specified inflammation of left upper eyelid

▶ H01.85   Other specified inflammation of left lower eyelid

▶ H01.86   Other specified inflammation of left eye, unspecified eyelid

▶ H01.89   Other specified inflammation of unspecified eye, unspecified eyelid

▶ H01.8A   Other specified inflammation of right eye, upper and lower eyelids

▶ H01.8B   Other specified inflammation of left eye, upper and lower eyelids

H01.9   **Unspecified inflammation of eyelid**
Inflammation of eyelid NOS

● H02   **Other disorders of eyelid**
Turning inward (inversion) of eyelid margin and ingrowing eyelashes
Excludes1   congenital malformations of eyelid (Q10.0-Q10.3)

● H02.0   **Entropion and trichiasis of eyelid**

● H02.00   **Unspecified entropion of eyelid**

H02.001   Unspecified entropion of right upper eyelid

H02.002   Unspecified entropion of right lower eyelid

H02.003   Unspecified entropion of right eye, unspecified eyelid

H02.004   Unspecified entropion of left upper eyelid

H02.005   Unspecified entropion of left lower eyelid

H02.006   Unspecified entropion of left eye, unspecified eyelid

H02.009   Unspecified entropion of unspecified eye, unspecified eyelid

● H02.01   **Cicatricial entropion of eyelid**
Scar

H02.011   Cicatricial entropion of right upper eyelid

H02.012   Cicatricial entropion of right lower eyelid

H02.013   Cicatricial entropion of right eye, unspecified eyelid

H02.014   Cicatricial entropion of left upper eyelid

H02.015   Cicatricial entropion of left lower eyelid

H02.016   Cicatricial entropion of left eye, unspecified eyelid

H02.019   Cicatricial entropion of unspecified eye, unspecified eyelid

● H02.02   **Mechanical entropion of eyelid**
Turning inward (inversion) of eyelid margin due to lack of support

H02.021   Mechanical entropion of right upper eyelid

H02.022   Mechanical entropion of right lower eyelid

H02.023   Mechanical entropion of right eye, unspecified eyelid

H02.024   Mechanical entropion of left upper eyelid

H02.025   Mechanical entropion of left lower eyelid

H02.026   Mechanical entropion of left eye, unspecified eyelid

H02.029   Mechanical entropion of unspecified eye, unspecified eyelid

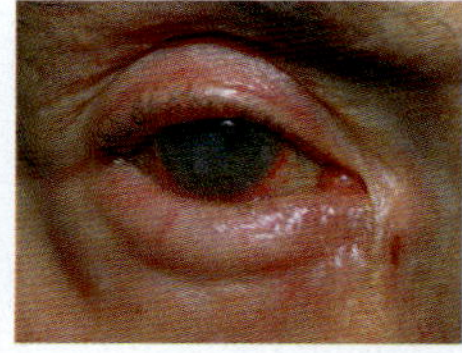

Figure 7-2   Right lower eyelid entropion. Note the inward rotation of the tarsal plate about the horizontal axis and the resultant contact between the mucocutaneous junction and ocular surface. (From Glynn M, Drake WM, Hutchison R: Hutchison's Clinical Methods: An Integrated Approach to Clinical Practice, Edinburgh, Saunders/Elsevier, 2012)

▶ New   ⇒ Revised   ~~deleted~~ Deleted   Excludes 1   Excludes 2   Includes   Use additional   Code first   Code also   Key words

OGCR Official Guidelines   X Assign placeholder X   ● Use Additional Character(s)   ▶ Manifestation Code   🔖 Hierarchical Condition Category   **Coding Clinic**

● **H02.03**   **Senile entropion of eyelid**
Turning inward (inversion) of eyelid margin due to aging

    H02.031   Senile entropion of right upper eyelid   **A**

    H02.032   Senile entropion of right lower eyelid   **A**

    H02.033   Senile entropion of right eye, unspecified eyelid   **A**

    H02.034   Senile entropion of left upper eyelid   **A**

    H02.035   Senile entropion of left lower eyelid   **A**

    H02.036   Senile entropion of left eye, unspecified eyelid   **A**

    H02.039   Senile entropion of unspecified eye, unspecified eyelid   **A**

● **H02.04**   **Spastic entropion of eyelid**
Turning inward (inversion) of eyelid margin caused by spasm of muscle

    H02.041   Spastic entropion of right upper eyelid

    H02.042   Spastic entropion of right lower eyelid

    H02.043   Spastic entropion of right eye, unspecified eyelid

    H02.044   Spastic entropion of left upper eyelid

    H02.045   Spastic entropion of left lower eyelid

    H02.046   Spastic entropion of left eye, unspecified eyelid

    H02.049   Spastic entropion of unspecified eye, unspecified eyelid

● **H02.05**   **Trichiasis without entropion**
Ingrowing hairs of eyelashes

    H02.051   Trichiasis without entropion right upper eyelid

    H02.052   Trichiasis without entropion right lower eyelid

    H02.053   Trichiasis without entropion right eye, unspecified eyelid

    H02.054   Trichiasis without entropion left upper eyelid

    H02.055   Trichiasis without entropion left lower eyelid

    H02.056   Trichiasis without entropion left eye, unspecified eyelid

    H02.059   Trichiasis without entropion unspecified eye, unspecified eyelid

● **H02.1**   **Ectropion of eyelid**
Eversion (pulling away) of eyelid

● **H02.10**   **Unspecified ectropion of eyelid**

    H02.101   Unspecified ectropion of right upper eyelid

    H02.102   Unspecified ectropion of right lower eyelid

    H02.103   Unspecified ectropion of right eye, unspecified eyelid

    H02.104   Unspecified ectropion of left upper eyelid

    H02.105   Unspecified ectropion of left lower eyelid

    H02.106   Unspecified ectropion of left eye, unspecified eyelid

    H02.109   Unspecified ectropion of unspecified eye, unspecified eyelid

● **H02.11**   **Cicatricial ectropion of eyelid**
Pulling of eyelid down and away from eye due to scar or tightening

    H02.111   Cicatricial ectropion of right upper eyelid

    H02.112   Cicatricial ectropion of right lower eyelid

    H02.113   Cicatricial ectropion of right eye, unspecified eyelid

    H02.114   Cicatricial ectropion of left upper eyelid

    H02.115   Cicatricial ectropion of left lower eyelid

    H02.116   Cicatricial ectropion of left eye, unspecified eyelid

    H02.119   Cicatricial ectropion of unspecified eye, unspecified eyelid

● **H02.12**   **Mechanical ectropion of eyelid**
Eversion (pulling away) of eyelid due to lack of support

    H02.121   Mechanical ectropion of right upper eyelid

    H02.122   Mechanical ectropion of right lower eyelid

    H02.123   Mechanical ectropion of right eye, unspecified eyelid

    H02.124   Mechanical ectropion of left upper eyelid

    H02.125   Mechanical ectropion of left lower eyelid

    H02.126   Mechanical ectropion of left eye, unspecified eyelid

    H02.129   Mechanical ectropion of unspecified eye, unspecified eyelid

● **H02.13**   **Senile ectropion of eyelid**
Eversion (pulling away) of eyelid due to age

    H02.131   Senile ectropion of right upper eyelid   **A**

    H02.132   Senile ectropion of right lower eyelid   **A**

    H02.133   Senile ectropion of right eye, unspecified eyelid   **A**

    H02.134   Senile ectropion of left upper eyelid   **A**

    H02.135   Senile ectropion of left lower eyelid   **A**

    H02.136   Senile ectropion of left eye, unspecified eyelid   **A**

    H02.139   Senile ectropion of unspecified eye, unspecified eyelid

● **H02.14**   **Spastic ectropion of eyelid**
Eversion (pulling away) of eyelid due to tonic muscle spasm

    H02.141   Spastic ectropion of right upper eyelid

    H02.142   Spastic ectropion of right lower eyelid

    H02.143   Spastic ectropion of right eye, unspecified eyelid

    H02.144   Spastic ectropion of left upper eyelid

    H02.145   Spastic ectropion of left lower eyelid

    H02.146   Spastic ectropion of left eye, unspecified eyelid

    H02.149   Spastic ectropion of unspecified eye, unspecified eyelid

● **H02.15**   **Paralytic ectropion of eyelid**

    H02.151   Paralytic ectropion of right upper eyelid

    H02.152   Paralytic ectropion of right lower eyelid

    H02.153   Paralytic ectropion of right eye, unspecified eyelid

    H02.154   Paralytic ectropion of left upper eyelid

    H02.155   Paralytic ectropion of left lower eyelid

    H02.156   Paralytic ectropion of left eye, unspecified eyelid

    H02.159   Paralytic ectropion of unspecified eye, unspecified eyelid

CHAPTER 7 (H00–H59)

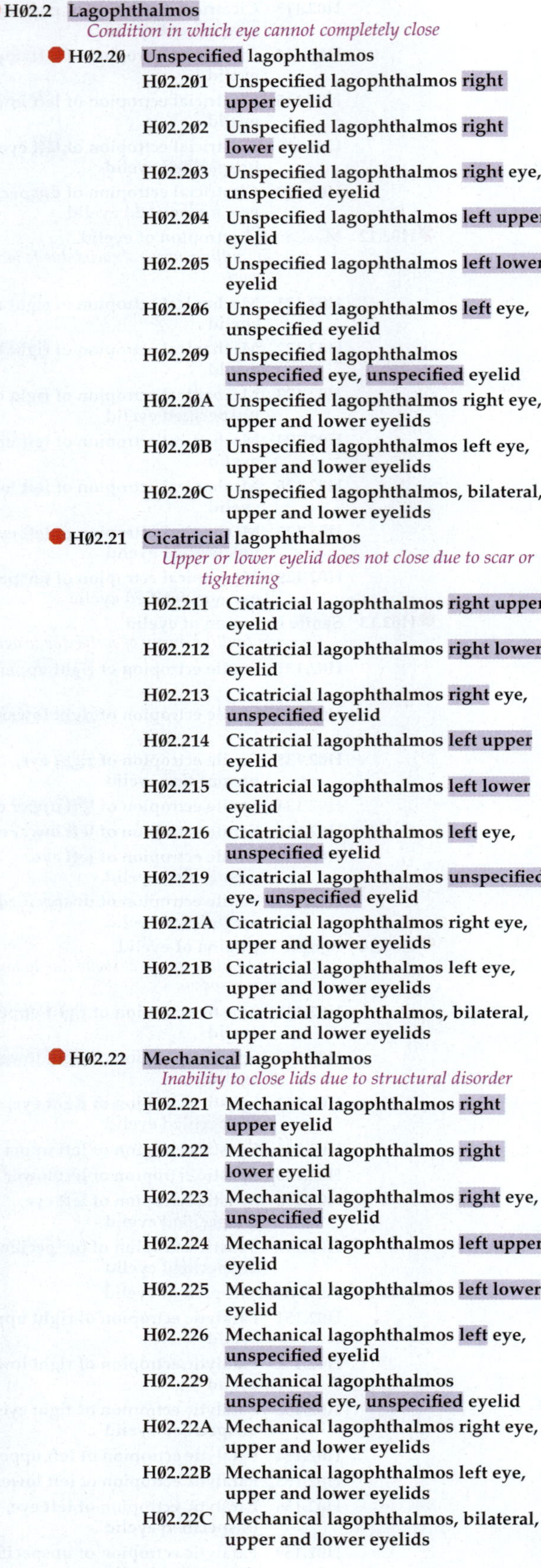

● **H02.2**   **Lagophthalmos**
Condition in which eye cannot completely close

  ● **H02.20**   **Unspecified** lagophthalmos

     H02.201   Unspecified lagophthalmos **right upper** eyelid

     H02.202   Unspecified lagophthalmos **right lower** eyelid

     H02.203   Unspecified lagophthalmos **right eye, unspecified** eyelid

     H02.204   Unspecified lagophthalmos **left upper** eyelid

     H02.205   Unspecified lagophthalmos **left lower** eyelid

     H02.206   Unspecified lagophthalmos **left eye, unspecified** eyelid

     H02.209   Unspecified lagophthalmos **unspecified eye, unspecified** eyelid

     H02.20A   Unspecified lagophthalmos right eye, upper and lower eyelids

     H02.20B   Unspecified lagophthalmos left eye, upper and lower eyelids

     H02.20C   Unspecified lagophthalmos, bilateral, upper and lower eyelids

  ● **H02.21**   **Cicatricial** lagophthalmos
Upper or lower eyelid does not close due to scar or tightening

     H02.211   Cicatricial lagophthalmos **right upper** eyelid

     H02.212   Cicatricial lagophthalmos **right lower** eyelid

     H02.213   Cicatricial lagophthalmos **right eye, unspecified** eyelid

     H02.214   Cicatricial lagophthalmos **left upper** eyelid

     H02.215   Cicatricial lagophthalmos **left lower** eyelid

     H02.216   Cicatricial lagophthalmos **left eye, unspecified** eyelid

     H02.219   Cicatricial lagophthalmos **unspecified eye, unspecified** eyelid

     H02.21A   Cicatricial lagophthalmos right eye, upper and lower eyelids

     H02.21B   Cicatricial lagophthalmos left eye, upper and lower eyelids

     H02.21C   Cicatricial lagophthalmos, bilateral, upper and lower eyelids

  ● **H02.22**   **Mechanical** lagophthalmos
Inability to close lids due to structural disorder

     H02.221   Mechanical lagophthalmos **right upper** eyelid

     H02.222   Mechanical lagophthalmos **right lower** eyelid

     H02.223   Mechanical lagophthalmos **right eye, unspecified** eyelid

     H02.224   Mechanical lagophthalmos **left upper** eyelid

     H02.225   Mechanical lagophthalmos **left lower** eyelid

     H02.226   Mechanical lagophthalmos **left eye, unspecified** eyelid

     H02.229   Mechanical lagophthalmos **unspecified eye, unspecified** eyelid

     H02.22A   Mechanical lagophthalmos right eye, upper and lower eyelids

     H02.22B   Mechanical lagophthalmos left eye, upper and lower eyelids

     H02.22C   Mechanical lagophthalmos, bilateral, upper and lower eyelids

  ● **H02.23**   **Paralytic** lagophthalmos
Eyelids do not close due to paralysis

     H02.231   Paralytic lagophthalmos **right upper** eyelid

     H02.232   Paralytic lagophthalmos **right lower** eyelid

     H02.233   Paralytic lagophthalmos **right eye, unspecified** eyelid

     H02.234   Paralytic lagophthalmos **left upper** eyelid

     H02.235   Paralytic lagophthalmos **left lower** eyelid

     H02.236   Paralytic lagophthalmos **left eye, unspecified** eyelid

     H02.239   Paralytic lagophthalmos **unspecified eye, unspecified** eyelid

     H02.23A   Paralytic lagophthalmos right eye, upper and lower eyelids

     H02.23B   Paralytic lagophthalmos left eye, upper and lower eyelids

     H02.23C   Paralytic lagophthalmos, bilateral, upper and lower eyelids

★ **(See Plate 17 of the Anatomy Illustrations.)**

● **H02.3**   **Blepharochalasis**
Relaxation of skin of eyelid, due to atrophy of intercellular tissue
Pseudoptosis

     H02.30   Blepharochalasis unspecified eye, **unspecified** eyelid

     H02.31   Blepharochalasis **right upper** eyelid

     H02.32   Blepharochalasis **right lower** eyelid

     H02.33   Blepharochalasis **right eye, unspecified** eyelid

     H02.34   Blepharochalasis **left upper** eyelid

     H02.35   Blepharochalasis **left lower** eyelid

     H02.36   Blepharochalasis **left eye, unspecified** eyelid

● **H02.4**   **Ptosis of eyelid**
Falling forward, drooping, sagging of eyelid

  ● **H02.40**   **Unspecified** ptosis of eyelid

     H02.401   Unspecified ptosis of **right** eyelid

     H02.402   Unspecified ptosis of **left** eyelid

     H02.403   Unspecified ptosis of **bilateral** eyelids

     H02.409   Unspecified ptosis of **unspecified** eyelid

  ● **H02.41**   **Mechanical** ptosis of eyelid

     H02.411   Mechanical ptosis of **right** eyelid

     H02.412   Mechanical ptosis of **left** eyelid

     H02.413   Mechanical ptosis of **bilateral** eyelids

     H02.419   Mechanical ptosis of **unspecified** eyelid

  ● **H02.42**   **Myogenic** ptosis of eyelid

     H02.421   Myogenic ptosis of **right** eyelid

     H02.422   Myogenic ptosis of **left** eyelid

     H02.423   Myogenic ptosis of **bilateral** eyelids

     H02.429   Myogenic ptosis of **unspecified** eyelid

  ● **H02.43**   **Paralytic** ptosis of eyelid
Neurogenic ptosis of eyelid

     H02.431   Paralytic ptosis of **right** eyelid

     H02.432   Paralytic ptosis of **left** eyelid

     H02.433   Paralytic ptosis of **bilateral** eyelids

     H02.439   Paralytic ptosis **unspecified** eyelid

Item 7–1   Ptosis of eyelid is drooping of the upper eyelid over the pupil when the eyes are fully opened resulting from nerve or muscle damage, which may require surgical correction.

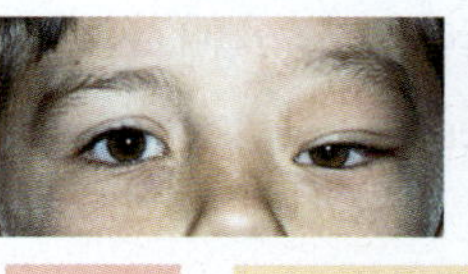

Figure 7-3   Ptosis of eyelid. (From Kanski JJ: Clinical Diagnosis in Ophthalmology, London, Elsevier Mosby, 2006)

● **H02.5 Other disorders affecting eyelid function**
  Excludes2 blepharospasm (G24.5)
      organic tic (G25.69)
      psychogenic tic (F95.-)
  ● **H02.51 Abnormal innervation syndrome**
    H02.511 Abnormal innervation syndrome right upper eyelid
    H02.512 Abnormal innervation syndrome right lower eyelid
    H02.513 Abnormal innervation syndrome right eye, unspecified eyelid
    H02.514 Abnormal innervation syndrome left upper eyelid
    H02.515 Abnormal innervation syndrome left lower eyelid
    H02.516 Abnormal innervation syndrome left eye, unspecified eyelid
    H02.519 Abnormal innervation syndrome unspecified eye, unspecified eyelid
  ● **H02.52 Blepharophimosis**
    Drooping of eyelid with reduced lid size
    Ankyloblepharon
    H02.521 Blepharophimosis right upper eyelid
    H02.522 Blepharophimosis right lower eyelid
    H02.523 Blepharophimosis right eye, unspecified eyelid
    H02.524 Blepharophimosis left upper eyelid
    H02.525 Blepharophimosis left lower eyelid
    H02.526 Blepharophimosis left eye, unspecified eyelid
    H02.529 Blepharophimosis unspecified eye, unspecified lid
  ● **H02.53 Eyelid retraction**
    Eyelid lag
    H02.531 Eyelid retraction right upper eyelid
    H02.532 Eyelid retraction right lower eyelid
    H02.533 Eyelid retraction right eye, unspecified eyelid
    H02.534 Eyelid retraction left upper eyelid
    H02.535 Eyelid retraction left lower eyelid
    H02.536 Eyelid retraction left eye, unspecified eyelid
    H02.539 Eyelid retraction unspecified eye, unspecified lid
    H02.59 Other disorders affecting eyelid function
    Deficient blink reflex
    Sensory disorders
● **H02.6 Xanthelasma of eyelid**
  Yellow-to-orange patches or pimples clustered together on eyelid
    H02.60 Xanthelasma of unspecified eye, unspecified eyelid
    H02.61 Xanthelasma of right upper eyelid
    H02.62 Xanthelasma of right lower eyelid
    H02.63 Xanthelasma of right eye, unspecified eyelid
    H02.64 Xanthelasma of left upper eyelid
    H02.65 Xanthelasma of left lower eyelid
    H02.66 Xanthelasma of left eye, unspecified eyelid
● **H02.7 Other and unspecified degenerative disorders of eyelid and periocular area**
    H02.70 Unspecified degenerative disorders of eyelid and periocular area
  ● **H02.71 Chloasma of eyelid and periocular area**
    Dyspigmentation of eyelid
    Hyperpigmentation of eyelid
    H02.711 Chloasma of right upper eyelid and periocular area
    H02.712 Chloasma of right lower eyelid and periocular area
    H02.713 Chloasma of right eye, unspecified eyelid and periocular area
    H02.714 Chloasma of left upper eyelid and periocular area
    H02.715 Chloasma of left lower eyelid and periocular area
    H02.716 Chloasma of left eye, unspecified eyelid and periocular area
    H02.719 Chloasma of unspecified eye, unspecified eyelid and periocular area
  ● **H02.72 Madarosis of eyelid and periocular area**
    Loss of eyelashes and/or eyebrows
    Hypotrichosis of eyelid
    H02.721 Madarosis of right upper eyelid and periocular area
    H02.722 Madarosis of right lower eyelid and periocular area
    H02.723 Madarosis of right eye, unspecified eyelid and periocular area
    H02.724 Madarosis of left upper eyelid and periocular area
    H02.725 Madarosis of left lower eyelid and periocular area
    H02.726 Madarosis of left eye, unspecified eyelid and periocular area
    H02.729 Madarosis of unspecified eye, unspecified eyelid and periocular area
  ● **H02.73 Vitiligo of eyelid and periocular area**
    Skin pigmentation disease characterized by white patches
    Hypopigmentation of eyelid
    H02.731 Vitiligo of right upper eyelid and periocular area
    H02.732 Vitiligo of right lower eyelid and periocular area
    H02.733 Vitiligo of right eye, unspecified eyelid and periocular area
    H02.734 Vitiligo of left upper eyelid and periocular area
    H02.735 Vitiligo of left lower eyelid and periocular area
    H02.736 Vitiligo of left eye, unspecified eyelid and periocular area
    H02.739 Vitiligo of unspecified eye, unspecified eyelid and periocular area
    H02.79 Other degenerative disorders of eyelid and periocular area
● **H02.8 Other specified disorders of eyelid**
  ● **H02.81 Retained foreign body in eyelid**
    Use additional code to identify the type of retained foreign body (Z18.-)
    Excludes1 laceration of eyelid with foreign body (S01.12-)
        retained intraocular foreign body (H44.6-, H44.7-)
        superficial foreign body of eyelid and periocular area (S00.25-)
    H02.811 Retained foreign body in right upper eyelid
    H02.812 Retained foreign body in right lower eyelid
    H02.813 Retained foreign body in right eye, unspecified eyelid
    H02.814 Retained foreign body in left upper eyelid
    H02.815 Retained foreign body in left lower eyelid
    H02.816 Retained foreign body in left eye, unspecified eyelid
    H02.819 Retained foreign body in unspecified eye, unspecified eyelid

● **H02.82** **Cysts of eyelid**
Sebaceous cyst of eyelid
    H02.821   Cysts of right upper eyelid
    H02.822   Cysts of right lower eyelid
    H02.823   Cysts of right eye, unspecified eyelid
    H02.824   Cysts of left upper eyelid
    H02.825   Cysts of left lower eyelid
    H02.826   Cysts of left eye, unspecified eyelid
    H02.829   Cysts of unspecified eye, unspecified eyelid

● **H02.83** **Dermatochalasis of eyelid**
Skin is inelastic and hangs loosely in folds
    H02.831   Dermatochalasis of right upper eyelid
    H02.832   Dermatochalasis of right lower eyelid
    H02.833   Dermatochalasis of right eye, unspecified eyelid
    H02.834   Dermatochalasis of left upper eyelid
    H02.835   Dermatochalasis of left lower eyelid
    H02.836   Dermatochalasis of left eye, unspecified eyelid
    H02.839   Dermatochalasis of unspecified eye, unspecified eyelid

● **H02.84** **Edema of eyelid**
Hyperemia of eyelid
    H02.841   Edema of right upper eyelid
    H02.842   Edema of right lower eyelid
    H02.843   Edema of right eye, unspecified eyelid
    H02.844   Edema of left upper eyelid
    H02.845   Edema of left lower eyelid
    H02.846   Edema of left eye, unspecified eyelid
    H02.849   Edema of unspecified eye, unspecified eyelid

● **H02.85** **Elephantiasis of eyelid**
Massive secondary lymphedema with hypertrophy of skin and subcutaneous tissues (pachyderma)
    H02.851   Elephantiasis of right upper eyelid
    H02.852   Elephantiasis of right lower eyelid
    H02.853   Elephantiasis of right eye, unspecified eyelid
    H02.854   Elephantiasis of left upper eyelid
    H02.855   Elephantiasis of left lower eyelid
    H02.856   Elephantiasis of left eye, unspecified eyelid
    H02.859   Elephantiasis of unspecified eye, unspecified eyelid

● **H02.86** **Hypertrichosis of eyelid**
Excessive growth of hair
    H02.861   Hypertrichosis of right upper eyelid
    H02.862   Hypertrichosis of right lower eyelid
    H02.863   Hypertrichosis of right eye, unspecified eyelid
    H02.864   Hypertrichosis of left upper eyelid
    H02.865   Hypertrichosis of left lower eyelid
    H02.866   Hypertrichosis of left eye, unspecified eyelid
    H02.869   Hypertrichosis of unspecified eye, unspecified eyelid

● **H02.87** **Vascular anomalies of eyelid**
    H02.871   Vascular anomalies of right upper eyelid
    H02.872   Vascular anomalies of right lower eyelid
    H02.873   Vascular anomalies of right eye, unspecified eyelid
    H02.874   Vascular anomalies of left upper eyelid
    H02.875   Vascular anomalies of left lower eyelid

    H02.876   Vascular anomalies of left eye, unspecified eyelid
    H02.879   Vascular anomalies of unspecified eye, unspecified eyelid

● **H02.88** **Meibomian gland dysfunction of eyelid**
    H02.881   Meibomian gland dysfunction right upper eyelid
    H02.882   Meibomian gland dysfunction right lower eyelid
    H02.883   Meibomian gland dysfunction of right eye, unspecified eyelid
    H02.884   Meibomian gland dysfunction left upper eyelid
    H02.885   Meibomian gland dysfunction left lower eyelid
    H02.886   Meibomian gland dysfunction of left eye, unspecified eyelid
    H02.889   Meibomian gland dysfunction of unspecified eye, unspecified eyelid
    H02.88A   Meibomian gland dysfunction right eye, upper and lower eyelids
    H02.88B   Meibomian gland dysfunction left eye, upper and lower eyelids

    H02.89   **Other specified disorders of eyelid**
          Hemorrhage of eyelid

    H02.9   **Unspecified disorder of eyelid**
          Disorder of eyelid NOS

● **H04** **Disorders of lacrimal system**
    Excludes1   congenital malformations of lacrimal system (Q10.4-Q10.6)

● **H04.0** **Dacryoadenitis**
Inflammation of lacrimal gland
● **H04.00** **Unspecified dacryoadenitis**
    H04.001   Unspecified dacryoadenitis, right lacrimal gland
    H04.002   Unspecified dacryoadenitis, left lacrimal gland
    H04.003   Unspecified dacryoadenitis, bilateral lacrimal glands
    H04.009   Unspecified dacryoadenitis, unspecified lacrimal gland

● **H04.01** **Acute dacryoadenitis**
    H04.011   Acute dacryoadenitis, right lacrimal gland
    H04.012   Acute dacryoadenitis, left lacrimal gland
    H04.013   Acute dacryoadenitis, bilateral lacrimal glands
    H04.019   Acute dacryoadenitis, unspecified lacrimal gland

★ **(See Plate 19 of the Anatomy Illustrations.)**

● **H04.02** **Chronic dacryoadenitis**
    H04.021   Chronic dacryoadenitis, right lacrimal gland
    H04.022   Chronic dacryoadenitis, left lacrimal gland
    H04.023   Chronic dacryoadenitis, bilateral lacrimal gland
    H04.029   Chronic dacryoadenitis, unspecified lacrimal gland

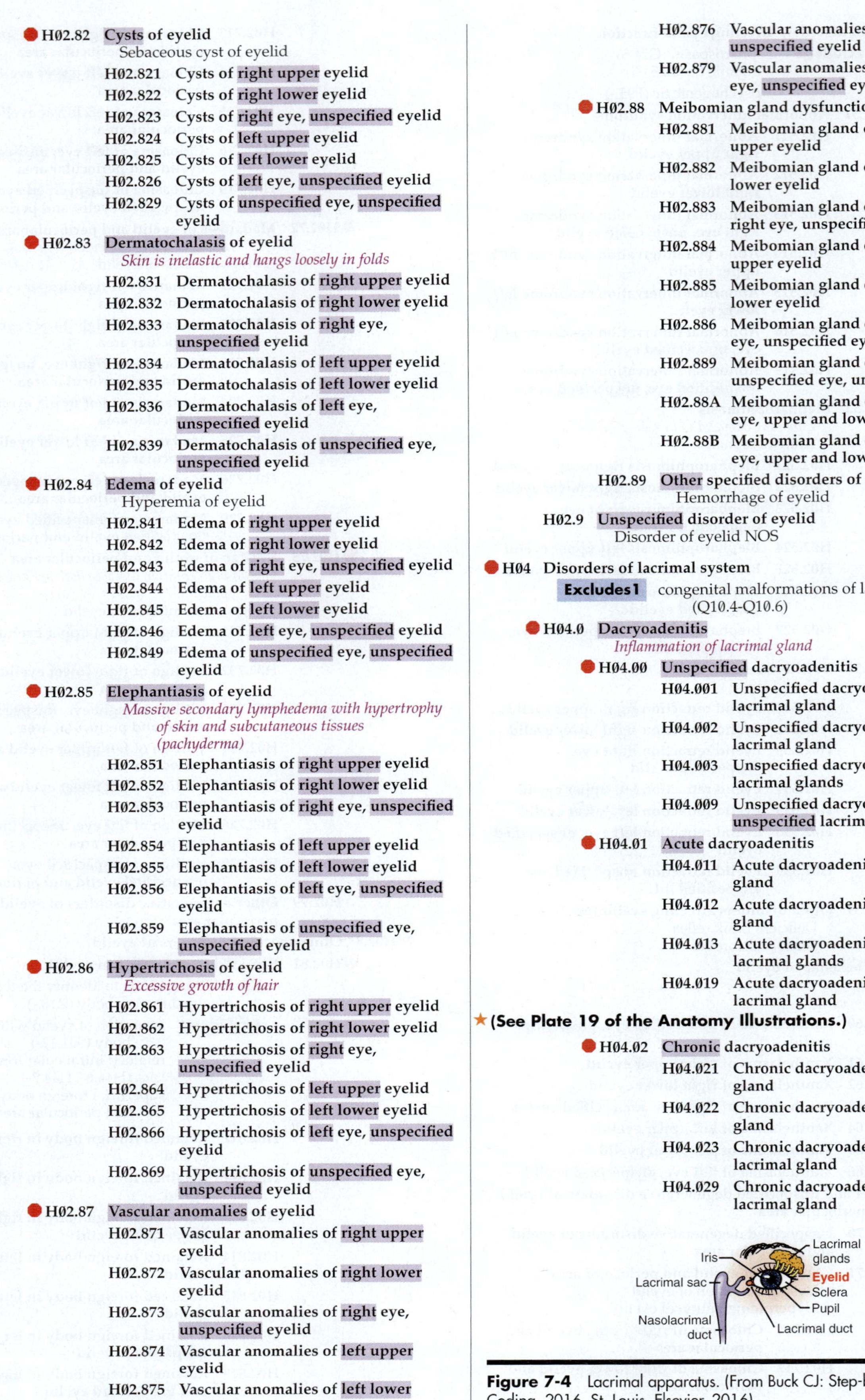

Figure 7-4 *Lacrimal apparatus. (From Buck CJ: Step-by-Step Medical Coding, 2016, St. Louis, Elsevier, 2016)*

● **H04.03**   **Chronic enlargement** of lacrimal gland
    H04.031   Chronic enlargement of **right** lacrimal gland
    H04.032   Chronic enlargement of **left** lacrimal gland
    H04.033   Chronic enlargement of **bilateral** lacrimal glands
    H04.039   Chronic enlargement of **unspecified** lacrimal gland

● **H04.1**   Other disorders of lacrimal gland
   ● **H04.11**   **Dacryops**
     Watery eye or distention of lacrimal duct due to fluid
     H04.111   Dacryops of **right** lacrimal gland
     H04.112   Dacryops of **left** lacrimal gland
     H04.113   Dacryops of **bilateral** lacrimal glands
     H04.119   Dacryops of **unspecified** lacrimal gland

   ● **H04.12**   **Dry eye syndrome**
     Tear film insufficiency, NOS
     H04.121   Dry eye syndrome of **right** lacrimal gland
     H04.122   Dry eye syndrome of **left** lacrimal gland
     H04.123   Dry eye syndrome of **bilateral** lacrimal glands
     H04.129   Dry eye syndrome of **unspecified** lacrimal gland

   ● **H04.13**   **Lacrimal cyst**
     Lacrimal cystic degeneration
     H04.131   Lacrimal cyst **right** lacrimal gland
     H04.132   Lacrimal cyst **left** lacrimal gland
     H04.133   Lacrimal cyst **bilateral** lacrimal glands
     H04.139   Lacrimal cyst **unspecified** lacrimal gland

   ● **H04.14**   **Primary** lacrimal gland atrophy
     H04.141   Primary lacrimal gland atrophy, **right** lacrimal gland
     H04.142   Primary lacrimal gland atrophy, **left** lacrimal gland
     H04.143   Primary lacrimal gland atrophy, **bilateral** lacrimal glands
     H04.149   Primary lacrimal gland atrophy, **unspecified** lacrimal gland

   ● **H04.15**   **Secondary** lacrimal gland atrophy
     H04.151   Secondary lacrimal gland atrophy, **right** lacrimal gland
     H04.152   Secondary lacrimal gland atrophy, **left** lacrimal gland
     H04.153   Secondary lacrimal gland atrophy, **bilateral** lacrimal glands
     H04.159   Secondary lacrimal gland atrophy, **unspecified** lacrimal gland

   ● **H04.16**   **Lacrimal gland dislocation**
     H04.161   Lacrimal gland dislocation, **right** lacrimal gland
     H04.162   Lacrimal gland dislocation, **left** lacrimal gland
     H04.163   Lacrimal gland dislocation, **bilateral** lacrimal glands
     H04.169   Lacrimal gland dislocation, **unspecified** lacrimal gland

     H04.19   Other specified disorders of lacrimal gland

● **H04.2**   **Epiphora**
     Overflow of tears due to stricture of lacrimal passages; AKA lacrimation
   ● **H04.20**   **Unspecified epiphora**
     H04.201   Unspecified epiphora, **right** side
     H04.202   Unspecified epiphora, **left** side
     H04.203   Unspecified epiphora, **bilateral**
     H04.209   Unspecified epiphora, **unspecified** side

● **H04.21**   Epiphora due to excess lacrimation
     H04.211   Epiphora due to excess lacrimation, **right** lacrimal gland
     H04.212   Epiphora due to excess lacrimation, **left** lacrimal gland
     H04.213   Epiphora due to excess lacrimation, **bilateral** lacrimal glands
     H04.219   Epiphora due to excess lacrimation, **unspecified** lacrimal gland

● **H04.22**   Epiphora due to insufficient drainage
     H04.221   Epiphora due to insufficient drainage, **right** side
     H04.222   Epiphora due to insufficient drainage, **left** side
     H04.223   Epiphora due to insufficient drainage, **bilateral**
     H04.229   Epiphora due to insufficient drainage, **unspecified** side

● **H04.3**   **Acute and unspecified inflammation of lacrimal passages**
     Excludes1   neonatal dacryocystitis (P39.1)
   ● **H04.30**   **Unspecified** dacryocystitis
     H04.301   Unspecified dacryocystitis of **right** lacrimal passage
     H04.302   Unspecified dacryocystitis of **left** lacrimal passage
     H04.303   Unspecified dacryocystitis of **bilateral** lacrimal passages
     H04.309   Unspecified dacryocystitis of **unspecified** lacrimal passage

   ● **H04.31**   **Phlegmonous** dacryocystitis
     Cellulitis of lacrimal sac
     H04.311   Phlegmonous dacryocystitis of **right** lacrimal passage
     H04.312   Phlegmonous dacryocystitis of **left** lacrimal passage
     H04.313   Phlegmonous dacryocystitis of **bilateral** lacrimal passages
     H04.319   Phlegmonous dacryocystitis of **unspecified** lacrimal passage

   ● **H04.32**   **Acute dacryocystitis**
     Acute dacryopericystitis
     H04.321   Acute dacryocystitis of **right** lacrimal passage
     H04.322   Acute dacryocystitis of **left** lacrimal passage
     H04.323   Acute dacryocystitis of **bilateral** lacrimal passages
     H04.329   Acute dacryocystitis of **unspecified** lacrimal passage

   ● **H04.33**   **Acute lacrimal canaliculitis**
     H04.331   Acute lacrimal canaliculitis of **right** lacrimal passage
     H04.332   Acute lacrimal canaliculitis of **left** lacrimal passage
     H04.333   Acute lacrimal canaliculitis of **bilateral** lacrimal passages
     H04.339   Acute lacrimal canaliculitis of **unspecified** lacrimal passage

● **H04.4**   **Chronic inflammation** of lacrimal passages
   ● **H04.41**   Chronic **dacryocystitis**
     Inflammation of lacrimal sac
     H04.411   Chronic dacryocystitis of **right** lacrimal passage
     H04.412   Chronic dacryocystitis of **left** lacrimal passage
     H04.413   Chronic dacryocystitis of **bilateral** lacrimal passages
     H04.419   Chronic dacryocystitis of **unspecified** lacrimal passage

CHAPTER 7 (H00–H59)

● **H04.42** Chronic lacrimal canaliculitis
  Inflammation of lacrimal ducts
  H04.421 Chronic lacrimal canaliculitis of right lacrimal passage
  H04.422 Chronic lacrimal canaliculitis of left lacrimal passage
  H04.423 Chronic lacrimal canaliculitis of bilateral lacrimal passages
  H04.429 Chronic lacrimal canaliculitis of unspecified lacrimal passage
● **H04.43** Chronic lacrimal mucocele
  Accumulation of mucous secretion
  H04.431 Chronic lacrimal mucocele of right lacrimal passage
  H04.432 Chronic lacrimal mucocele of left lacrimal passage
  H04.433 Chronic lacrimal mucocele of bilateral lacrimal passages
  H04.439 Chronic lacrimal mucocele of unspecified lacrimal passage
● **H04.5** Stenosis and insufficiency of lacrimal passages
 ● **H04.51** Dacryolith
  Concretion in lacrimal sac/duct; AKA lacrimal calculus
  H04.511 Dacryolith of right lacrimal passage
  H04.512 Dacryolith of left lacrimal passage
  H04.513 Dacryolith of bilateral lacrimal passages
  H04.519 Dacryolith of unspecified lacrimal passage
 ● **H04.52** Eversion of lacrimal punctum
  Turning out of lacrimal drainage opening
  H04.521 Eversion of right lacrimal punctum
  H04.522 Eversion of left lacrimal punctum
  H04.523 Eversion of bilateral lacrimal punctum
  H04.529 Eversion of unspecified lacrimal punctum
 ● **H04.53** Neonatal obstruction of nasolacrimal duct
  Excludes1 congenital stenosis and stricture of lacrimal duct (Q10.5)
  H04.531 Neonatal obstruction of right nasolacrimal duct **N**
  H04.532 Neonatal obstruction of left nasolacrimal duct **N**
  H04.533 Neonatal obstruction of bilateral nasolacrimal duct **N**
  H04.539 Neonatal obstruction of unspecified nasolacrimal duct **N**
 ● **H04.54** Stenosis of lacrimal canaliculi
  H04.541 Stenosis of right lacrimal canaliculi
  H04.542 Stenosis of left lacrimal canaliculi
  H04.543 Stenosis of bilateral lacrimal canaliculi
  H04.549 Stenosis of unspecified lacrimal canaliculi
 ● **H04.55** Acquired stenosis of nasolacrimal duct
  H04.551 Acquired stenosis of right nasolacrimal duct
  H04.552 Acquired stenosis of left nasolacrimal duct
  H04.553 Acquired stenosis of bilateral nasolacrimal duct
  H04.559 Acquired stenosis of unspecified nasolacrimal duct
 ● **H04.56** Stenosis of lacrimal punctum
  H04.561 Stenosis of right lacrimal punctum
  H04.562 Stenosis of left lacrimal punctum
  H04.563 Stenosis of bilateral lacrimal punctum
  H04.569 Stenosis of unspecified lacrimal punctum

 ● **H04.57** Stenosis of lacrimal sac
  H04.571 Stenosis of right lacrimal sac
  H04.572 Stenosis of left lacrimal sac
  H04.573 Stenosis of bilateral lacrimal sac
  H04.579 Stenosis of unspecified lacrimal sac
● **H04.6** Other changes of lacrimal passages
 ● **H04.61** Lacrimal fistula
  H04.611 Lacrimal fistula right lacrimal passage
  H04.612 Lacrimal fistula left lacrimal passage
  H04.613 Lacrimal fistula bilateral lacrimal passages
  H04.619 Lacrimal fistula unspecified lacrimal passage
 H04.69 Other changes of lacrimal passages
● **H04.8** Other disorders of lacrimal system
 ● **H04.81** Granuloma of lacrimal passages
  Inflammatory response due to infectious or noninfectious agents
  H04.811 Granuloma of right lacrimal passage
  H04.812 Granuloma of left lacrimal passage
  H04.813 Granuloma of bilateral lacrimal passages
  H04.819 Granuloma of unspecified lacrimal passage
 H04.89 Other disorders of lacrimal system
 H04.9 Disorder of lacrimal system, unspecified
● **H05** Disorders of orbit
  Excludes1 congenital malformation of orbit (Q10.7)
 ● **H05.0** Acute inflammation of orbit
  H05.00 Unspecified acute inflammation of orbit
  ● **H05.01** Cellulitis of orbit
   Infection of soft tissue of orbit
   Abscess of orbit
   H05.011 Cellulitis of right orbit
   H05.012 Cellulitis of left orbit
   H05.013 Cellulitis of bilateral orbits
   H05.019 Cellulitis of unspecified orbit
  ● **H05.02** Osteomyelitis of orbit
   Infection of boney orbit of eye
   H05.021 Osteomyelitis of right orbit
   H05.022 Osteomyelitis of left orbit
   H05.023 Osteomyelitis of bilateral orbits
   H05.029 Osteomyelitis of unspecified orbit
  ● **H05.03** Periostitis of orbit
   Inflammation of periosteum (membrane covering bone surface)
   H05.031 Periostitis of right orbit
   H05.032 Periostitis of left orbit
   H05.033 Periostitis of bilateral orbits
   H05.039 Periostitis of unspecified orbit
  ● **H05.04** Tenonitis of orbit
   Inflammation of tenon capsule (space enclosing fascia of Tenon between eyeball and fat of orbit)
   H05.041 Tenonitis of right orbit
   H05.042 Tenonitis of left orbit
   H05.043 Tenonitis of bilateral orbits
   H05.049 Tenonitis of unspecified orbit
 ● **H05.1** Chronic inflammatory disorders of orbit
  H05.10 Unspecified chronic inflammatory disorders of orbit
  ● **H05.11** Granuloma of orbit
   Pseudotumor (inflammatory) of orbit
   H05.111 Granuloma of right orbit
   H05.112 Granuloma of left orbit
   H05.113 Granuloma of bilateral orbits
   H05.119 Granuloma of unspecified orbit

- ● H05.12   Orbital myositis
  Inflammation of extraocular muscles of orbit
  - H05.121   Orbital myositis, right orbit
  - H05.122   Orbital myositis, left orbit
  - H05.123   Orbital myositis, bilateral
  - H05.129   Orbital myositis, unspecified orbit
- ● H05.2   Exophthalmic conditions
  Bulging eyes
  - H05.20   Unspecified exophthalmos
- ● H05.21   Displacement (lateral) of globe
  - H05.211   Displacement (lateral) of globe, right eye
  - H05.212   Displacement (lateral) of globe, left eye
  - H05.213   Displacement (lateral) of globe, bilateral
  - H05.219   Displacement (lateral) of globe, unspecified eye
- ● H05.22   Edema of orbit
  Orbital congestion
  - H05.221   Edema of right orbit
  - H05.222   Edema of left orbit
  - H05.223   Edema of bilateral orbit
  - H05.229   Edema of unspecified orbit
- ● H05.23   Hemorrhage of orbit
  - H05.231   Hemorrhage of right orbit
  - H05.232   Hemorrhage of left orbit
  - H05.233   Hemorrhage of bilateral orbit
  - H05.239   Hemorrhage of unspecified orbit
- ● H05.24   Constant exophthalmos
  Constant bulging eyes, often symptom of Graves disease
  - H05.241   Constant exophthalmos, right eye
  - H05.242   Constant exophthalmos, left eye
  - H05.243   Constant exophthalmos, bilateral
  - H05.249   Constant exophthalmos, unspecified eye
- ● H05.25   Intermittent exophthalmos
  Intermittent bulging eye occurring with bending forward or sharp turning of head
  - H05.251   Intermittent exophthalmos, right eye
  - H05.252   Intermittent exophthalmos, left eye
  - H05.253   Intermittent exophthalmos, bilateral
  - H05.259   Intermittent exophthalmos, unspecified eye
- ● H05.26   Pulsating exophthalmos
  Bulging eyes with pulsation and bruit, often due to aneurysm pushing eye forward
  - H05.261   Pulsating exophthalmos, right eye
  - H05.262   Pulsating exophthalmos, left eye
  - H05.263   Pulsating exophthalmos, bilateral
  - H05.269   Pulsating exophthalmos, unspecified eye
- ● H05.3   Deformity of orbit
  Excludes1   congenital deformity of orbit (Q10.7)
  hypertelorism (Q75.2)
  - H05.30   Unspecified deformity of orbit
- ● H05.31   Atrophy of orbit
  - H05.311   Atrophy of right orbit
  - H05.312   Atrophy of left orbit
  - H05.313   Atrophy of bilateral orbit
  - H05.319   Atrophy of unspecified orbit
- ● H05.32   Deformity of orbit due to bone disease
  Code also associated bone disease
  - H05.321   Deformity of right orbit due to bone disease
  - H05.322   Deformity of left orbit due to bone disease
  - H05.323   Deformity of bilateral orbits due to bone disease
  - H05.329   Deformity of unspecified orbit due to bone disease
- ● H05.33   Deformity of orbit due to trauma or surgery
  - H05.331   Deformity of right orbit due to trauma or surgery
  - H05.332   Deformity of left orbit due to trauma or surgery
  - H05.333   Deformity of bilateral orbits due to trauma or surgery
  - H05.339   Deformity of unspecified orbit due to trauma or surgery
- ● H05.34   Enlargement of orbit
  - H05.341   Enlargement of right orbit
  - H05.342   Enlargement of left orbit
  - H05.343   Enlargement of bilateral orbits
  - H05.349   Enlargement of unspecified orbit
- ● H05.35   Exostosis of orbit
  - H05.351   Exostosis of right orbit
  - H05.352   Exostosis of left orbit
  - H05.353   Exostosis of bilateral orbits
  - H05.359   Exostosis of unspecified orbit
- ● H05.4   Enophthalmos
  Recessed eyeball into orbit
  - H05.40   Unspecified enophthalmos
    - H05.401   Unspecified enophthalmos, right eye
    - H05.402   Unspecified enophthalmos, left eye
    - H05.403   Unspecified enophthalmos, bilateral
    - H05.409   Unspecified enophthalmos, unspecified eye
- ● H05.41   Enophthalmos due to atrophy of orbital tissue
  - H05.411   Enophthalmos due to atrophy of orbital tissue, right eye
  - H05.412   Enophthalmos due to atrophy of orbital tissue, left eye
  - H05.413   Enophthalmos due to atrophy of orbital tissue, bilateral
  - H05.419   Enophthalmos due to atrophy of orbital tissue, unspecified eye
- ● H05.42   Enophthalmos due to trauma or surgery
  - H05.421   Enophthalmos due to trauma or surgery, right eye
  - H05.422   Enophthalmos due to trauma or surgery, left eye
  - H05.423   Enophthalmos due to trauma or surgery, bilateral
  - H05.429   Enophthalmos due to trauma or surgery, unspecified eye

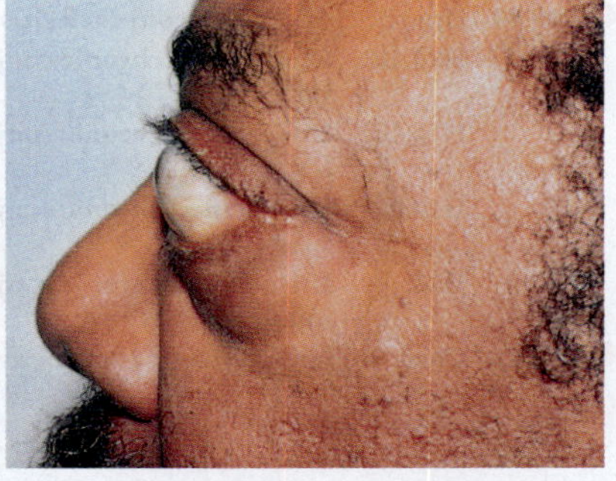

Figure 7-5   Exophthalmos. (From Black JM, Hokanson JH: Medical-Surgical Nursing: Clinical Management for Positive Outcomes, St. Louis, Saunders Elsevier, 2009)

CHAPTER 7 (H00-H59)

● **H05.5** **Retained (old) foreign body following penetrating wound of orbit**
Retrobulbar foreign body
Use additional code to identify the type of retained foreign body (Z18.-)

   Excludes1   current penetrating wound of orbit (S05.4-)

   Excludes2   retained foreign body of eyelid (H02.81-)
retained intraocular foreign body (H44.6-, H44.7-)

    H05.50   Retained (old) foreign body following penetrating wound of unspecified orbit

    H05.51   Retained (old) foreign body following penetrating wound of right orbit

    H05.52   Retained (old) foreign body following penetrating wound of left orbit

    H05.53   Retained (old) foreign body following penetrating wound of bilateral orbits

● **H05.8** **Other disorders of orbit**

  ● **H05.81**   **Cyst of orbit**
Encephalocele of orbit

     H05.811   Cyst of right orbit

     H05.812   Cyst of left orbit

     H05.813   Cyst of bilateral orbits

     H05.819   Cyst of unspecified orbit

  ● **H05.82**   **Myopathy of extraocular muscles**
Weakness of muscles of eye

     H05.821   Myopathy of extraocular muscles, right orbit

     H05.822   Myopathy of extraocular muscles, left orbit

     H05.823   Myopathy of extraocular muscles, bilateral

     H05.829   Myopathy of extraocular muscles, unspecified orbit

  ▶● **H05.83**   **Thyroid orbitopathy**
  ▶ Graves' ophthalmopathy
  ▶ Graves' orbitopathy
  ▶ Thyroid eye disease

    ▶ Code also, if applicable, any associated conditions such as:
    ▶ autoimmune thyroiditis (E06.3)
    ▶ thyrotoxicosis with diffuse goiter (E05.0-)

    ▶ **H05.831**   **Thyroid orbitopathy, right orbit**

    ▶ **H05.832**   **Thyroid orbitopathy, left orbit**

    ▶ **H05.833**   **Thyroid orbitopathy, bilateral**

    ▶ **H05.839**   **Thyroid orbitopathy, unspecified orbit**

     H05.89   Other disorders of orbit

   H05.9   Unspecified disorder of orbit

DISORDERS OF CONJUNCTIVA (H10-H11)

★ **(See Plate 18 of the Anatomy Illustrations.)**

● **H10** **Conjunctivitis**
Inflammation of membrane of the inside of the eyelid or on surface of eye (conjunctiva)

   Excludes1   keratoconjunctivitis (H16.2-)

  ● **H10.0** **Mucopurulent conjunctivitis**

    ● **H10.01**   **Acute follicular conjunctivitis**

      H10.011   Acute follicular conjunctivitis, right eye

      H10.012   Acute follicular conjunctivitis, left eye

      H10.013   Acute follicular conjunctivitis, bilateral

      H10.019   Acute follicular conjunctivitis, unspecified eye

    ● **H10.02**   **Other mucopurulent conjunctivitis**

      H10.021   Other mucopurulent conjunctivitis, right eye

      H10.022   Other mucopurulent conjunctivitis, left eye

      H10.023   Other mucopurulent conjunctivitis, bilateral

      H10.029   Other mucopurulent conjunctivitis, unspecified eye

  ● **H10.1** **Acute atopic conjunctivitis**
Acute papillary conjunctivitis

     H10.10   Acute atopic conjunctivitis, unspecified eye

     H10.11   Acute atopic conjunctivitis, right eye

     H10.12   Acute atopic conjunctivitis, left eye

     H10.13   Acute atopic conjunctivitis, bilateral

  ● **H10.2** **Other acute conjunctivitis**

    ● **H10.21**   **Acute toxic conjunctivitis**
Acute chemical conjunctivitis

      Code first (T51-T65) to identify chemical and intent

     Excludes1   burn and corrosion of eye and adnexa (T26.-)

      H10.211   Acute toxic conjunctivitis, right eye

      H10.212   Acute toxic conjunctivitis, left eye

      H10.213   Acute toxic conjunctivitis, bilateral

      H10.219   Acute toxic conjunctivitis, unspecified eye

    ● **H10.22**   **Pseudomembranous conjunctivitis**

      H10.221   Pseudomembranous conjunctivitis, right eye

      H10.222   Pseudomembranous conjunctivitis, left eye

      H10.223   Pseudomembranous conjunctivitis, bilateral

      H10.229   Pseudomembranous conjunctivitis, unspecified eye

    ● **H10.23**   **Serous conjunctivitis, except viral**

     Excludes1   viral conjunctivitis (B30.-)

      H10.231   Serous conjunctivitis, except viral, right eye

      H10.232   Serous conjunctivitis, except viral, left eye

      H10.233   Serous conjunctivitis, except viral, bilateral

      H10.239   Serous conjunctivitis, except viral, unspecified eye

  ● **H10.3** **Unspecified acute conjunctivitis**

    Excludes1   ophthalmia neonatorum NOS (P39.1)

     H10.30   Unspecified acute conjunctivitis, unspecified eye

     H10.31   Unspecified acute conjunctivitis, right eye

     H10.32   Unspecified acute conjunctivitis, left eye

     H10.33   Unspecified acute conjunctivitis, bilateral

  ● **H10.4** **Chronic conjunctivitis**

    ● **H10.40**   **Unspecified chronic conjunctivitis**

      H10.401   Unspecified chronic conjunctivitis, right eye

      H10.402   Unspecified chronic conjunctivitis, left eye

      H10.403   Unspecified chronic conjunctivitis, bilateral

      H10.409   Unspecified chronic conjunctivitis, unspecified eye

    ● **H10.41**   **Chronic giant papillary conjunctivitis**
Inflammation of membrane of the inside of the eyelid or on surface of eye often associated with contact lens wear

      H10.411   Chronic giant papillary conjunctivitis, right eye

      H10.412   Chronic giant papillary conjunctivitis, left eye

---

▶ New   ➡ Revised   ~~deleted~~ Deleted   Excludes 1   Excludes 2   Includes   Use additional   Code first   Code also   Key words

OGCR Official Guidelines   X Assign placeholder X   ● Use Additional Character(s)   ▶ Manifestation Code   Hierarchical Condition Category   Coding Clinic

H10.413   Chronic giant papillary conjunctivitis, **bilateral**

H10.419   Chronic giant papillary conjunctivitis, **unspecified eye**

● **H10.42**   Simple chronic conjunctivitis

H10.421   Simple chronic conjunctivitis, **right eye**

H10.422   Simple chronic conjunctivitis, **left eye**

H10.423   Simple chronic conjunctivitis, **bilateral**

H10.429   Simple chronic conjunctivitis, **unspecified eye**

● **H10.43**   Chronic follicular conjunctivitis

Inflammation of membrane of the inside of the eyelid or on surface of eye due to topical medications or infection

H10.431   Chronic follicular conjunctivitis, **right eye**

H10.432   Chronic follicular conjunctivitis, **left eye**

H10.433   Chronic follicular conjunctivitis, **bilateral**

H10.439   Chronic follicular conjunctivitis, **unspecified eye**

H10.44   Vernal conjunctivitis

Affecting children, especially boys in which there are flattened papules with thick, gelatinous exudate on conjunctivae on inside of upper lid

Excludes1   vernal keratoconjunctivitis with limbar and corneal involvement (H16.26-)

H10.45   Other chronic allergic conjunctivitis

● **H10.5**   Blepharoconjunctivitis

Inflammation of eyelids and conjunctiva

● **H10.50**   Unspecified blepharoconjunctivitis

H10.501   Unspecified blepharoconjunctivitis, **right eye**

H10.502   Unspecified blepharoconjunctivitis, **left eye**

H10.503   Unspecified blepharoconjunctivitis, **bilateral**

H10.509   Unspecified blepharoconjunctivitis, **unspecified eye**

● **H10.51**   Ligneous conjunctivitis

Code also underlying condition if known, such as:

plasminogen deficiency (E88.02)

H10.511   Ligneous conjunctivitis, **right eye**

H10.512   Ligneous conjunctivitis, **left eye**

H10.513   Ligneous conjunctivitis, **bilateral**

H10.519   Ligneous conjunctivitis, **unspecified eye**

● **H10.52**   Angular blepharoconjunctivitis

H10.521   Angular blepharoconjunctivitis, **right eye**

H10.522   Angular blepharoconjunctivitis, **left eye**

H10.523   Angular blepharoconjunctivitis, **bilateral**

H10.529   Angular blepharoconjunctivitis, **unspecified eye**

● **H10.53**   Contact blepharoconjunctivitis

H10.531   Contact blepharoconjunctivitis, **right eye**

H10.532   Contact blepharoconjunctivitis, **left eye**

H10.533   Contact blepharoconjunctivitis, **bilateral**

H10.539   Contact blepharoconjunctivitis, **unspecified eye**

● **H10.8**   Other conjunctivitis

● **H10.81**   Pingueculitis

Inflammation of a yellow, raised thickening on the white of the eye associated with chronic dry eyes

Excludes1   pinguecula (H11.15-)

H10.811   Pingueculitis, **right eye**

H10.812   Pingueculitis, **left eye**

H10.813   Pingueculitis, **bilateral**

H10.819   Pingueculitis, **unspecified eye**

● **H10.82**   Rosacea conjunctivitis

Code first underlying rosacea dermatitis (L71.-)

H10.821   Rosacea conjunctivitis, right eye

H10.822   Rosacea conjunctivitis, left eye

H10.823   Rosacea conjunctivitis, bilateral

Coding Clinic: 2018, Q4, P15

H10.829   Rosacea conjunctivitis, unspecified eye

H10.89   Other conjunctivitis

H10.9   Unspecified conjunctivitis

● **H11**   Other disorders of conjunctiva

Excludes1   keratoconjunctivitis (H16.2-)

● **H11.0**   Pterygium of eye

Excludes1   pseudopterygium (H11.81-)

● **H11.00**   Unspecified pterygium of eye

H11.001   Unspecified pterygium of **right eye**

H11.002   Unspecified pterygium of **left eye**

H11.003   Unspecified pterygium of eye, **bilateral**

H11.009   Unspecified pterygium of **unspecified eye**

● **H11.01**   Amyloid pterygium

H11.011   Amyloid pterygium of **right eye**

H11.012   Amyloid pterygium of **left eye**

H11.013   Amyloid pterygium of eye, **bilateral**

H11.019   Amyloid pterygium of **unspecified eye**

● **H11.02**   Central pterygium of eye

H11.021   Central pterygium of **right eye**

H11.022   Central pterygium of **left eye**

H11.023   Central pterygium of eye, **bilateral**

H11.029   Central pterygium of **unspecified eye**

● **H11.03**   Double pterygium of eye

H11.031   Double pterygium of **right eye**

H11.032   Double pterygium of **left eye**

H11.033   Double pterygium of eye, **bilateral**

H11.039   Double pterygium of **unspecified eye**

● **H11.04**   Peripheral pterygium of eye, **stationary**

H11.041   Peripheral pterygium, stationary, **right eye**

H11.042   Peripheral pterygium, stationary, **left eye**

H11.043   Peripheral pterygium, stationary, **bilateral**

H11.049   Peripheral pterygium, stationary, **unspecified eye**

● **H11.05**   Peripheral pterygium of eye, **progressive**

H11.051   Peripheral pterygium, progressive, **right eye**

H11.052   Peripheral pterygium, progressive, **left eye**

Item 7–2   **Pterygium** is Greek for batlike. The condition is characterized by a membrane that extends from the limbus to the center of the cornea and resembles a wing.

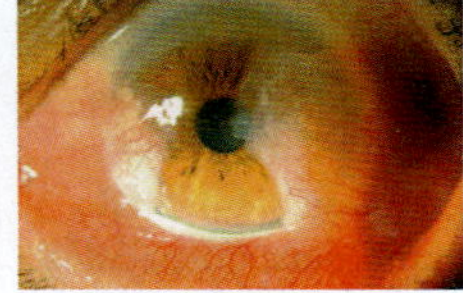

Figure 7-6   Double pterygium. Note both nasal and temporal pterygia in a 57-year-old farmer. (From Brightbill FS, McDonnell PJ: Corneal Surgery: Theory, Technique and Tissue, S.l., Mosby Elsevier, 2009)

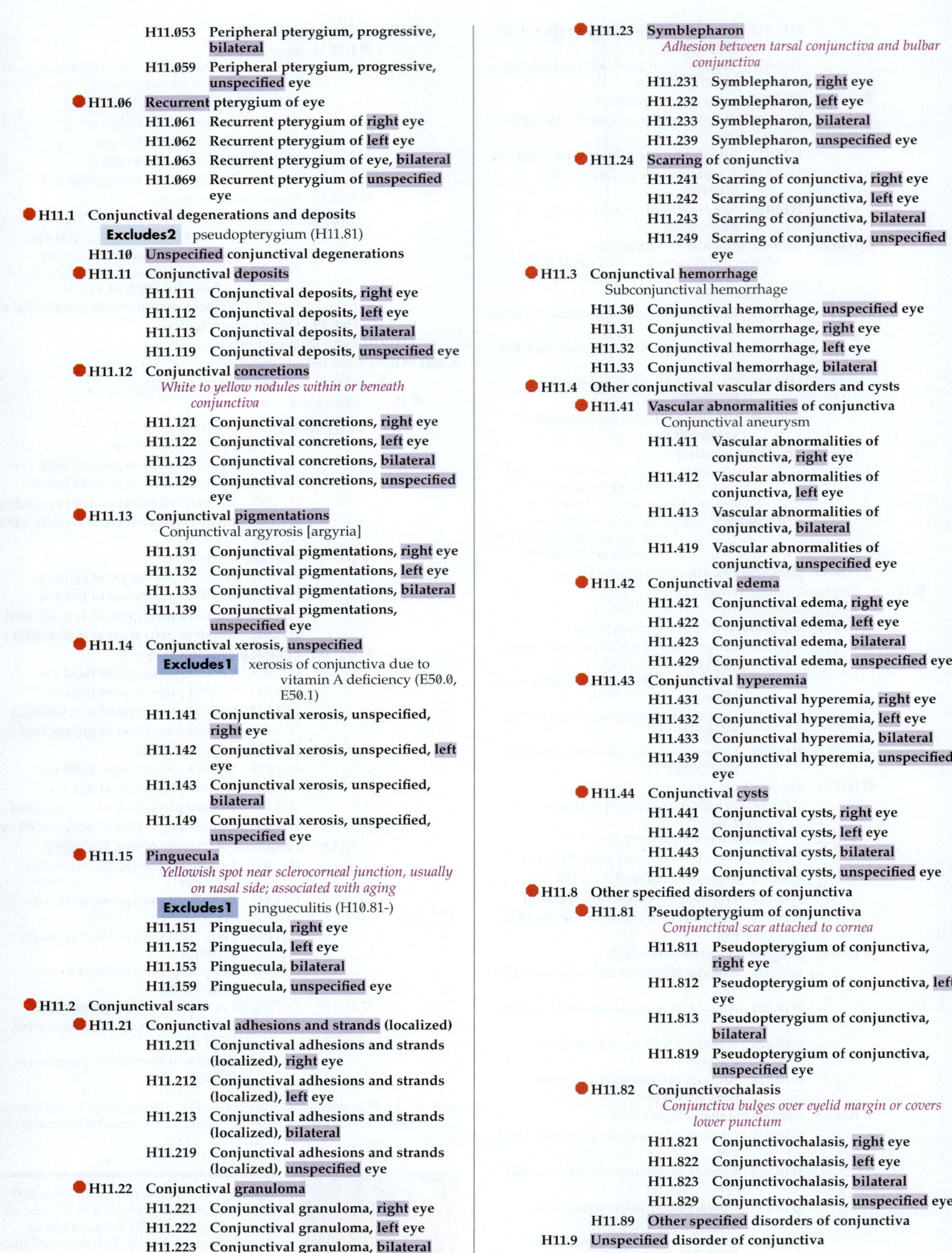

H11.053 Peripheral pterygium, progressive, bilateral

H11.059 Peripheral pterygium, progressive, unspecified eye

● **H11.06** Recurrent pterygium of eye

H11.061 Recurrent pterygium of right eye

H11.062 Recurrent pterygium of left eye

H11.063 Recurrent pterygium of eye, bilateral

H11.069 Recurrent pterygium of unspecified eye

● **H11.1** Conjunctival degenerations and deposits

Excludes2   pseudopterygium (H11.81)

H11.10 Unspecified conjunctival degenerations

● **H11.11** Conjunctival deposits

H11.111 Conjunctival deposits, right eye

H11.112 Conjunctival deposits, left eye

H11.113 Conjunctival deposits, bilateral

H11.119 Conjunctival deposits, unspecified eye

● **H11.12** Conjunctival concretions

White to yellow nodules within or beneath conjunctiva

H11.121 Conjunctival concretions, right eye

H11.122 Conjunctival concretions, left eye

H11.123 Conjunctival concretions, bilateral

H11.129 Conjunctival concretions, unspecified eye

● **H11.13** Conjunctival pigmentations

Conjunctival argyrosis [argyria]

H11.131 Conjunctival pigmentations, right eye

H11.132 Conjunctival pigmentations, left eye

H11.133 Conjunctival pigmentations, bilateral

H11.139 Conjunctival pigmentations, unspecified eye

● **H11.14** Conjunctival xerosis, unspecified

Excludes1   xerosis of conjunctiva due to vitamin A deficiency (E50.0, E50.1)

H11.141 Conjunctival xerosis, unspecified, right eye

H11.142 Conjunctival xerosis, unspecified, left eye

H11.143 Conjunctival xerosis, unspecified, bilateral

H11.149 Conjunctival xerosis, unspecified, unspecified eye

● **H11.15** Pinguecula

Yellowish spot near sclerocorneal junction, usually on nasal side; associated with aging

Excludes1   pingueculitis (H10.81-)

H11.151 Pinguecula, right eye

H11.152 Pinguecula, left eye

H11.153 Pinguecula, bilateral

H11.159 Pinguecula, unspecified eye

● **H11.2** Conjunctival scars

● **H11.21** Conjunctival adhesions and strands (localized)

H11.211 Conjunctival adhesions and strands (localized), right eye

H11.212 Conjunctival adhesions and strands (localized), left eye

H11.213 Conjunctival adhesions and strands (localized), bilateral

H11.219 Conjunctival adhesions and strands (localized), unspecified eye

● **H11.22** Conjunctival granuloma

H11.221 Conjunctival granuloma, right eye

H11.222 Conjunctival granuloma, left eye

H11.223 Conjunctival granuloma, bilateral

H11.229 Conjunctival granuloma, unspecified

● **H11.23** Symblepharon

Adhesion between tarsal conjunctiva and bulbar conjunctiva

H11.231 Symblepharon, right eye

H11.232 Symblepharon, left eye

H11.233 Symblepharon, bilateral

H11.239 Symblepharon, unspecified eye

● **H11.24** Scarring of conjunctiva

H11.241 Scarring of conjunctiva, right eye

H11.242 Scarring of conjunctiva, left eye

H11.243 Scarring of conjunctiva, bilateral

H11.249 Scarring of conjunctiva, unspecified eye

● **H11.3** Conjunctival hemorrhage

Subconjunctival hemorrhage

H11.30 Conjunctival hemorrhage, unspecified eye

H11.31 Conjunctival hemorrhage, right eye

H11.32 Conjunctival hemorrhage, left eye

H11.33 Conjunctival hemorrhage, bilateral

● **H11.4** Other conjunctival vascular disorders and cysts

● **H11.41** Vascular abnormalities of conjunctiva

Conjunctival aneurysm

H11.411 Vascular abnormalities of conjunctiva, right eye

H11.412 Vascular abnormalities of conjunctiva, left eye

H11.413 Vascular abnormalities of conjunctiva, bilateral

H11.419 Vascular abnormalities of conjunctiva, unspecified eye

● **H11.42** Conjunctival edema

H11.421 Conjunctival edema, right eye

H11.422 Conjunctival edema, left eye

H11.423 Conjunctival edema, bilateral

H11.429 Conjunctival edema, unspecified eye

● **H11.43** Conjunctival hyperemia

H11.431 Conjunctival hyperemia, right eye

H11.432 Conjunctival hyperemia, left eye

H11.433 Conjunctival hyperemia, bilateral

H11.439 Conjunctival hyperemia, unspecified eye

● **H11.44** Conjunctival cysts

H11.441 Conjunctival cysts, right eye

H11.442 Conjunctival cysts, left eye

H11.443 Conjunctival cysts, bilateral

H11.449 Conjunctival cysts, unspecified eye

● **H11.8** Other specified disorders of conjunctiva

● **H11.81** Pseudopterygium of conjunctiva

Conjunctival scar attached to cornea

H11.811 Pseudopterygium of conjunctiva, right eye

H11.812 Pseudopterygium of conjunctiva, left eye

H11.813 Pseudopterygium of conjunctiva, bilateral

H11.819 Pseudopterygium of conjunctiva, unspecified eye

● **H11.82** Conjunctivochalasis

Conjunctiva bulges over eyelid margin or covers lower punctum

H11.821 Conjunctivochalasis, right eye

H11.822 Conjunctivochalasis, left eye

H11.823 Conjunctivochalasis, bilateral

H11.829 Conjunctivochalasis, unspecified eye

H11.89 Other specified disorders of conjunctiva

H11.9 Unspecified disorder of conjunctiva

DISORDERS OF SCLERA, CORNEA, IRIS AND CILIARY BODY (H15-H22)

- ● **H15 Disorders of sclera**
  - ● **H15.Ø Scleritis**
    - *Inflammation of the white (sclera and episclera) of the eye.*
    - ● **H15.ØØ Unspecified scleritis**
      - H15.ØØ1 Unspecified scleritis, **right** eye
      - H15.ØØ2 Unspecified scleritis, **left** eye
      - H15.ØØ3 Unspecified scleritis, **bilateral**
      - H15.ØØ9 Unspecified scleritis, **unspecified** eye
    - ● **H15.Ø1 Anterior scleritis**
      - H15.Ø11 Anterior scleritis, **right** eye
      - H15.Ø12 Anterior scleritis, **left** eye
      - H15.Ø13 Anterior scleritis, **bilateral**
      - H15.Ø19 Anterior scleritis, **unspecified** eye
    - ● **H15.Ø2 Brawny scleritis**
      - *Swelling around the cornea that is gelantinous in appearance*
      - H15.Ø21 Brawny scleritis, **right** eye
      - H15.Ø22 Brawny scleritis, **left** eye
      - H15.Ø23 Brawny scleritis, **bilateral**
      - H15.Ø29 Brawny scleritis, **unspecified** eye
    - ● **H15.Ø3 Posterior scleritis**
      - Sclerotenonitis
      - H15.Ø31 Posterior scleritis, **right** eye
      - H15.Ø32 Posterior scleritis, **left** eye
      - H15.Ø33 Posterior scleritis, **bilateral**
      - H15.Ø39 Posterior scleritis, **unspecified** eye
    - ● **H15.Ø4 Scleritis with corneal involvement**
      - H15.Ø41 Scleritis with corneal involvement, **right** eye
      - H15.Ø42 Scleritis with corneal involvement, **left** eye
      - H15.Ø43 Scleritis with corneal involvement, **bilateral**
      - H15.Ø49 Scleritis with corneal involvement, **unspecified** eye
    - ● **H15.Ø5 Scleromalacia perforans**
      - *Necrotic without inflammation; usually associated with rheumatoid arthritis*
      - H15.Ø51 Scleromalacia perforans, **right** eye
      - H15.Ø52 Scleromalacia perforans, **left** eye
      - H15.Ø53 Scleromalacia perforans, **bilateral**
      - H15.Ø59 Scleromalacia perforans, **unspecified** eye
    - ● **H15.Ø9 Other scleritis**
      - Scleral abscess
      - H15.Ø91 Other scleritis, **right** eye
      - H15.Ø92 Other scleritis, **left** eye
      - H15.Ø93 Other scleritis, **bilateral**
      - H15.Ø99 Other scleritis, **unspecified** eye
  - ● **H15.1 Episcleritis**
    - *Inflammation of the white (sclera and episclera) of the eye.*
    - ● **H15.1Ø Unspecified episcleritis**
      - H15.1Ø1 Unspecified episcleritis, **right** eye
      - H15.1Ø2 Unspecified episcleritis, **left** eye
      - H15.1Ø3 Unspecified episcleritis, **bilateral**
      - H15.1Ø9 Unspecified episcleritis, **unspecified** eye
    - ● **H15.11 Episcleritis periodica fugax**
      - *Transient, recurrent inflammation of portion of episclera (connective tissue on the surface of the sclera)*
      - H15.111 Episcleritis periodica fugax, **right** eye
      - H15.112 Episcleritis periodica fugax, **left** eye
      - H15.113 Episcleritis periodica fugax, **bilateral**
      - H15.119 Episcleritis periodica fugax, **unspecified** eye
    - ● **H15.12 Nodular episcleritis**
      - *Characterized by tender, localized, moveable nodule within inflamed area*
      - H15.121 Nodular episcleritis, **right** eye
      - H15.122 Nodular episcleritis, **left** eye
      - H15.123 Nodular episcleritis, **bilateral**
      - H15.129 Nodular episcleritis, **unspecified** eye
  - ● **H15.8 Other disorders of sclera**
    - **Excludes2** blue sclera (Q13.5)
      - degenerative myopia (H44.2-)
    - ● **H15.81 Equatorial staphyloma**
      - H15.811 Equatorial staphyloma, **right** eye
      - H15.812 Equatorial staphyloma, **left** eye
      - H15.813 Equatorial staphyloma, **bilateral**
      - H15.819 Equatorial staphyloma, **unspecified** eye
    - ● **H15.82 Localized anterior staphyloma**
      - H15.821 Localized anterior staphyloma, **right** eye
      - H15.822 Localized anterior staphyloma, **left** eye
      - H15.823 Localized anterior staphyloma, **bilateral**
      - H15.829 Localized anterior staphyloma, **unspecified** eye
    - ● **H15.83 Staphyloma posticum**
      - H15.831 Staphyloma posticum, **right** eye
      - H15.832 Staphyloma posticum, **left** eye
      - H15.833 Staphyloma posticum, **bilateral**
      - H15.839 Staphyloma posticum, **unspecified** eye
    - ● **H15.84 Scleral ectasia**
      - H15.841 Scleral ectasia, **right** eye
      - H15.842 Scleral ectasia, **left** eye
      - H15.843 Scleral ectasia, **bilateral**
      - H15.849 Scleral ectasia, **unspecified** eye
    - ● **H15.85 Ring staphyloma**
      - H15.851 Ring staphyloma, **right** eye
      - H15.852 Ring staphyloma, **left** eye
      - H15.853 Ring staphyloma, **bilateral**
      - H15.859 Ring staphyloma, **unspecified** eye
    - **H15.89 Other disorders of sclera**
  - **H15.9 Unspecified disorder of sclera**
- ● **H16 Keratitis**
  - ● **H16.Ø Corneal ulcer**
    - ● **H16.ØØ Unspecified corneal ulcer**
      - H16.ØØ1 Unspecified corneal ulcer, **right** eye
      - H16.ØØ2 Unspecified corneal ulcer, **left** eye
      - H16.ØØ3 Unspecified corneal ulcer, **bilateral**
      - H16.ØØ9 Unspecified corneal ulcer, **unspecified** eye
    - ● **H16.Ø1 Central corneal ulcer**
      - H16.Ø11 Central corneal ulcer, **right** eye
      - H16.Ø12 Central corneal ulcer, **left** eye
      - H16.Ø13 Central corneal ulcer, **bilateral**
      - H16.Ø19 Central corneal ulcer, **unspecified** eye
    - ● **H16.Ø2 Ring corneal ulcer**
      - H16.Ø21 Ring corneal ulcer, **right** eye
      - H16.Ø22 Ring corneal ulcer, **left** eye
      - H16.Ø23 Ring corneal ulcer, **bilateral**
      - H16.Ø29 Ring corneal ulcer, **unspecified** eye
    - ● **H16.Ø3 Corneal ulcer with hypopyon**
      - H16.Ø31 Corneal ulcer with hypopyon, **right** eye
      - H16.Ø32 Corneal ulcer with hypopyon, **left** eye
      - H16.Ø33 Corneal ulcer with hypopyon, **bilateral**
      - H16.Ø39 Corneal ulcer with hypopyon, **unspecified** eye

CHAPTER 7 (HØØ-H59)

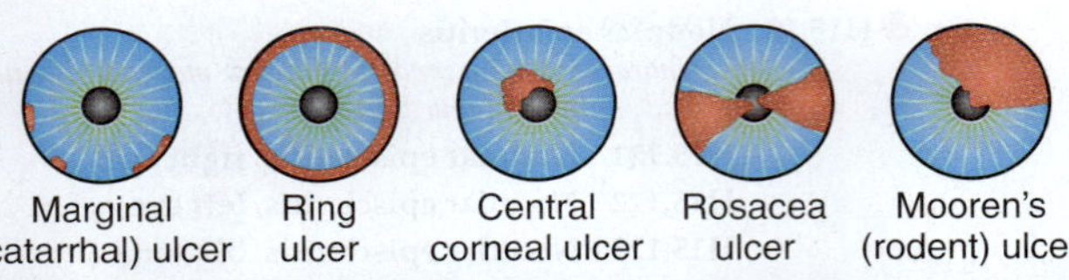

Figure 7-7 Corneal ulcers: marginal, ring, central corneal, rosacea, and Mooren's.

Item 7–3 An infected ulcer is usually called a **serpiginous** or **hypopyon** ulcer, which is a pus sac in the anterior chamber of the eye. **Marginal** ulcers are usually asymptomatic, not primary, and are often superficial and simple. More severe marginal ulcers spread to form a ring ulcer. **Ring** ulcers can extend around the entire corneal periphery. **Central corneal** ulcers develop when there is an abrasion to the epithelium and an infection develops in the eroded area. The **pyocyaneal** ulcer is the most serious corneal infection, which, if left untreated, can lead to loss of the eye.

- **H16.04   Marginal** corneal ulcer
  - H16.041   Marginal corneal ulcer, **right** eye
  - H16.042   Marginal corneal ulcer, **left** eye
  - H16.043   Marginal corneal ulcer, bilateral
  - H16.049   Marginal corneal ulcer, **unspecified** eye
- **H16.05   Mooren's** corneal ulcer
  - H16.051   Mooren's corneal ulcer, **right** eye
  - H16.052   Mooren's corneal ulcer, **left** eye
  - H16.053   Mooren's corneal ulcer, bilateral
  - H16.059   Mooren's corneal ulcer, **unspecified** eye
- **H16.06   Mycotic** corneal ulcer
  - H16.061   Mycotic corneal ulcer, **right** eye
  - H16.062   Mycotic corneal ulcer, **left** eye
  - H16.063   Mycotic corneal ulcer, bilateral
  - H16.069   Mycotic corneal ulcer, **unspecified** eye
- **H16.07   Perforated** corneal ulcer
  - H16.071   Perforated corneal ulcer, **right** eye
  - H16.072   Perforated corneal ulcer, **left** eye
  - H16.073   Perforated corneal ulcer, bilateral
  - H16.079   Perforated corneal ulcer, **unspecified** eye
- **H16.1   Other and unspecified superficial keratitis without conjunctivitis**
  - **H16.10   Unspecified** superficial keratitis
    - H16.101   Unspecified superficial keratitis, **right** eye
    - H16.102   Unspecified superficial keratitis, **left** eye
    - H16.103   Unspecified superficial keratitis, **bilateral**
    - H16.109   Unspecified superficial keratitis, **unspecified** eye
  - **H16.11   Macular** keratitis
    Areolar keratitis
    Nummular keratitis
    Stellate keratitis
    Striate keratitis
    - H16.111   Macular keratitis, **right** eye
    - H16.112   Macular keratitis, **left** eye
    - H16.113   Macular keratitis, **bilateral**
    - H16.119   Macular keratitis, **unspecified** eye
  - **H16.12   Filamentary** keratitis
    - H16.121   Filamentary keratitis, **right** eye
    - H16.122   Filamentary keratitis, **left** eye
    - H16.123   Filamentary keratitis, **bilateral**
    - H16.129   Filamentary keratitis, **unspecified** eye

- **H16.13   Photokeratitis**
  Snow blindness
  Welders' keratitis
  - H16.131   Photokeratitis, **right** eye
  - H16.132   Photokeratitis, **left** eye
  - H16.133   Photokeratitis, **bilateral**
  - H16.139   Photokeratitis, **unspecified** eye
- **H16.14   Punctate** keratitis
  - H16.141   Punctate keratitis, **right** eye
  - H16.142   Punctate keratitis, **left** eye
  - H16.143   Punctate keratitis, **bilateral**
  - H16.149   Punctate keratitis, **unspecified** eye
- **H16.2   Keratoconjunctivitis**
  - **H16.20   Unspecified** keratoconjunctivitis
    Superficial keratitis with conjunctivitis NOS
    - H16.201   Unspecified keratoconjunctivitis, **right** eye
    - H16.202   Unspecified keratoconjunctivitis, **left** eye
    - H16.203   Unspecified keratoconjunctivitis, **bilateral**
    - H16.209   Unspecified keratoconjunctivitis, **unspecified** eye
  - **H16.21   Exposure** keratoconjunctivitis
    - H16.211   Exposure keratoconjunctivitis, **right** eye
    - H16.212   Exposure keratoconjunctivitis, **left** eye
    - H16.213   Exposure keratoconjunctivitis, **bilateral**
    - H16.219   Exposure keratoconjunctivitis, **unspecified** eye
  - **H16.22   Keratoconjunctivitis sicca, not specified as Sjögren's**

    Excludes1   Sjögren's syndrome (M35.01)

    Coding Clinic: 2024, Q3, P16
    - H16.221   Keratoconjunctivitis sicca, not specified as Sjögren's, **right** eye
    - H16.222   Keratoconjunctivitis sicca, not specified as Sjögren's, **left** eye
    - H16.223   Keratoconjunctivitis sicca, not specified as Sjögren's, **bilateral**

      Coding Clinic: 2024, Q3, P16
    - H16.229   Keratoconjunctivitis sicca, not specified as Sjögren's, **unspecified** eye
  - **H16.23   Neurotrophic** keratoconjunctivitis
    - H16.231   Neurotrophic keratoconjunctivitis, **right** eye
    - H16.232   Neurotrophic keratoconjunctivitis, **left** eye
    - H16.233   Neurotrophic keratoconjunctivitis, **bilateral**
    - H16.239   Neurotrophic keratoconjunctivitis, **unspecified** eye
  - **H16.24   Ophthalmia nodosa**
    - H16.241   Ophthalmia nodosa, **right** eye
    - H16.242   Ophthalmia nodosa, **left** eye
    - H16.243   Ophthalmia nodosa, **bilateral**
    - H16.249   Ophthalmia nodosa, **unspecified** eye
  - **H16.25   Phlyctenular** keratoconjunctivitis
    - H16.251   Phlyctenular keratoconjunctivitis, **right** eye
    - H16.252   Phlyctenular keratoconjunctivitis, **left** eye
    - H16.253   Phlyctenular keratoconjunctivitis, **bilateral**
    - H16.259   Phlyctenular keratoconjunctivitis, **unspecified** eye

▶ New   ⇒ Revised   ~~deleted~~ Deleted   Excludes 1   Excludes 2   Includes   Use additional   Code first   Code also   Key words
OGCR Official Guidelines   X Assign placeholder X   ● Use Additional Character(s)   ▶ Manifestation Code   Hierarchical Condition Category   **Coding Clinic**

- **H16.26 Vernal keratoconjunctivitis, with limbar and corneal involvement**
  - **Excludes1** vernal conjunctivitis without limbar and corneal involvement (H10.44)
  - H16.261 Vernal keratoconjunctivitis, with limbar and corneal involvement, right eye
  - H16.262 Vernal keratoconjunctivitis, with limbar and corneal involvement, left eye
  - H16.263 Vernal keratoconjunctivitis, with limbar and corneal involvement, bilateral
  - H16.269 Vernal keratoconjunctivitis, with limbar and corneal involvement, unspecified eye
- **H16.29 Other keratoconjunctivitis**
  - H16.291 Other keratoconjunctivitis, right eye
  - H16.292 Other keratoconjunctivitis, left eye
  - H16.293 Other keratoconjunctivitis, bilateral
  - H16.299 Other keratoconjunctivitis, unspecified eye
- **H16.3 Interstitial and deep keratitis**
  - **H16.30 Unspecified interstitial keratitis**
    - H16.301 Unspecified interstitial keratitis, right eye
    - H16.302 Unspecified interstitial keratitis, left eye
    - H16.303 Unspecified interstitial keratitis, bilateral
    - H16.309 Unspecified interstitial keratitis, unspecified eye
  - **H16.31 Corneal abscess**
    - H16.311 Corneal abscess, right eye
    - H16.312 Corneal abscess, left eye
    - H16.313 Corneal abscess, bilateral
    - H16.319 Corneal abscess, unspecified eye
  - **H16.32 Diffuse interstitial keratitis**
    - Cogan's syndrome
    - H16.321 Diffuse interstitial keratitis, right eye
    - H16.322 Diffuse interstitial keratitis, left eye
    - H16.323 Diffuse interstitial keratitis, bilateral
    - H16.329 Diffuse interstitial keratitis, unspecified eye
  - **H16.33 Sclerosing keratitis**
    - H16.331 Sclerosing keratitis, right eye
    - H16.332 Sclerosing keratitis, left eye
    - H16.333 Sclerosing keratitis, bilateral
    - H16.339 Sclerosing keratitis, unspecified eye
  - **H16.39 Other interstitial and deep keratitis**
    - H16.391 Other interstitial and deep keratitis, right eye
    - H16.392 Other interstitial and deep keratitis, left eye
    - H16.393 Other interstitial and deep keratitis, bilateral
    - H16.399 Other interstitial and deep keratitis, unspecified eye
- **H16.4 Corneal neovascularization**
  - **H16.40 Unspecified corneal neovascularization**
    - H16.401 Unspecified corneal neovascularization, right eye
    - H16.402 Unspecified corneal neovascularization, left eye
    - H16.403 Unspecified corneal neovascularization, bilateral
    - H16.409 Unspecified corneal neovascularization, unspecified eye
  - **H16.41 Ghost vessels (corneal)**
    - H16.411 Ghost vessels (corneal), right eye
    - H16.412 Ghost vessels (corneal), left eye
    - H16.413 Ghost vessels (corneal), bilateral
    - H16.419 Ghost vessels (corneal), unspecified eye
  - **H16.42 Pannus (corneal)**
    - H16.421 Pannus (corneal), right eye
    - H16.422 Pannus (corneal), left eye
    - H16.423 Pannus (corneal), bilateral
    - H16.429 Pannus (corneal), unspecified eye
  - **H16.43 Localized vascularization of cornea**
    - H16.431 Localized vascularization of cornea, right eye
    - H16.432 Localized vascularization of cornea, left eye
    - H16.433 Localized vascularization of cornea, bilateral
    - H16.439 Localized vascularization of cornea, unspecified eye
  - **H16.44 Deep vascularization of cornea**
    - H16.441 Deep vascularization of cornea, right eye
    - H16.442 Deep vascularization of cornea, left eye
    - H16.443 Deep vascularization of cornea, bilateral
    - H16.449 Deep vascularization of cornea, unspecified eye
  - H16.8 Other keratitis
  - H16.9 Unspecified keratitis
- **H17 Corneal scars and opacities**
  - **H17.0 Adherent leukoma**
    - H17.00 Adherent leukoma, unspecified eye
    - H17.01 Adherent leukoma, right eye
    - H17.02 Adherent leukoma, left eye
    - H17.03 Adherent leukoma, bilateral
  - **H17.1 Central corneal opacity**
    - H17.10 Central corneal opacity, unspecified eye
    - H17.11 Central corneal opacity, right eye
    - H17.12 Central corneal opacity, left eye
    - H17.13 Central corneal opacity, bilateral
  - **H17.8 Other corneal scars and opacities**
    - **H17.81 Minor opacity of cornea**
      - Corneal nebula
      - H17.811 Minor opacity of cornea, right eye
      - H17.812 Minor opacity of cornea, left eye
      - H17.813 Minor opacity of cornea, bilateral
      - H17.819 Minor opacity of cornea, unspecified eye
    - **H17.82 Peripheral opacity of cornea**
      - H17.821 Peripheral opacity of cornea, right eye
      - H17.822 Peripheral opacity of cornea, left eye
      - H17.823 Peripheral opacity of cornea, bilateral
      - H17.829 Peripheral opacity of cornea, unspecified eye
    - H17.89 Other corneal scars and opacities
  - H17.9 Unspecified corneal scar and opacity
- **H18 Other disorders of cornea**
  - **H18.0 Corneal pigmentations and deposits**
    - **H18.00 Unspecified corneal deposit**
      - H18.001 Unspecified corneal deposit, right eye
      - H18.002 Unspecified corneal deposit, left eye
      - H18.003 Unspecified corneal deposit, bilateral
      - H18.009 Unspecified corneal deposit, unspecified eye

CHAPTER 7 (H00-H59)

● **H18.01** **Anterior** corneal pigmentations
      Staehli's line
   H18.011 Anterior corneal pigmentations, **right eye**
   H18.012 Anterior corneal pigmentations, **left eye**
   H18.013 Anterior corneal pigmentations, **bilateral**
   H18.019 Anterior corneal pigmentations, **unspecified eye**
● **H18.02** **Argentous** corneal deposits
   H18.021 Argentous corneal deposits, **right eye**
   H18.022 Argentous corneal deposits, **left eye**
   H18.023 Argentous corneal deposits, **bilateral**
   H18.029 Argentous corneal deposits, **unspecified eye**
● **H18.03** Corneal deposits in **metabolic disorders**
      Code also associated metabolic disorder
   H18.031 Corneal deposits in metabolic disorders, **right eye**
   H18.032 Corneal deposits in metabolic disorders, **left eye**
   H18.033 Corneal deposits in metabolic disorders, **bilateral**
   H18.039 Corneal deposits in metabolic disorders, **unspecified eye**
● **H18.04** **Kayser-Fleischer ring**
      Code also associated Wilson's disease (E83.01)
   H18.041 Kayser-Fleischer ring, **right eye**
   H18.042 Kayser-Fleischer ring, **left eye**
   H18.043 Kayser-Fleischer ring, **bilateral**
   H18.049 Kayser-Fleischer ring, **unspecified eye**
● **H18.05** **Posterior** corneal pigmentations
      Krukenberg's spindle
   H18.051 Posterior corneal pigmentations, **right eye**
   H18.052 Posterior corneal pigmentations, **left eye**
   H18.053 Posterior corneal pigmentations, **bilateral**
   H18.059 Posterior corneal pigmentations, **unspecified eye**
● **H18.06** **Stromal** corneal pigmentations
      Hematocornea
   H18.061 Stromal corneal pigmentations, **right eye**
   H18.062 Stromal corneal pigmentations, **left eye**
   H18.063 Stromal corneal pigmentations, **bilateral**
   H18.069 Stromal corneal pigmentations, **unspecified eye**
● **H18.1** Bullous keratopathy
   H18.10 Bullous keratopathy, **unspecified** eye
   H18.11 Bullous keratopathy, **right** eye
   H18.12 Bullous keratopathy, **left** eye
   H18.13 Bullous keratopathy, **bilateral**
● **H18.2** Other and unspecified corneal edema
   H18.20 **Unspecified** corneal edema
● **H18.21** Corneal edema **secondary to contact lens**
      Excludes2 other corneal disorders due to contact lens (H18.82-)
   H18.211 Corneal edema secondary to contact lens, **right eye**
   H18.212 Corneal edema secondary to contact lens, **left eye**
   H18.213 Corneal edema secondary to contact lens, **bilateral**
   H18.219 Corneal edema secondary to contact lens, **unspecified eye**

● **H18.22** Idiopathic corneal edema
   H18.221 Idiopathic corneal edema, **right eye**
   H18.222 Idiopathic corneal edema, **left eye**
   H18.223 Idiopathic corneal edema, **bilateral**
   H18.229 Idiopathic corneal edema, **unspecified eye**
● **H18.23** Secondary corneal edema
   H18.231 Secondary corneal edema, **right eye**
   H18.232 Secondary corneal edema, **left eye**
   H18.233 Secondary corneal edema, **bilateral**
   H18.239 Secondary corneal edema, **unspecified eye**
● **H18.3** Changes of corneal membranes
   H18.30 **Unspecified** corneal membrane change
● **H18.31** Folds and rupture in **Bowman's** membrane
   H18.311 Folds and rupture in Bowman's membrane, **right eye**
   H18.312 Folds and rupture in Bowman's membrane, **left eye**
   H18.313 Folds and rupture in Bowman's membrane, **bilateral**
   H18.319 Folds and rupture in Bowman's membrane, **unspecified eye**
● **H18.32** Folds in **Descemet's** membrane
   H18.321 Folds in Descemet's membrane, **right eye**
   H18.322 Folds in Descemet's membrane, **left eye**
   H18.323 Folds in Descemet's membrane, **bilateral**
   H18.329 Folds in Descemet's membrane, **unspecified eye**
● **H18.33** Rupture in **Descemet's** membrane
   H18.331 Rupture in Descemet's membrane, **right eye**
   H18.332 Rupture in Descemet's membrane, **left eye**
   H18.333 Rupture in Descemet's membrane, **bilateral**
   H18.339 Rupture in Descemet's membrane, **unspecified eye**
● **H18.4** Corneal degeneration
      Excludes1 Mooren's ulcer (H16.0-)
                     recurrent erosion of cornea (H18.83-)
   H18.40 **Unspecified** corneal degeneration
● **H18.41** **Arcus senilis**
      Senile corneal changes
   H18.411 Arcus senilis, **right eye**
   H18.412 Arcus senilis, **left eye**
   H18.413 Arcus senilis, **bilateral**
   H18.419 Arcus senilis, **unspecified** eye
● **H18.42** Band keratopathy
   H18.421 Band keratopathy, **right eye**
   H18.422 Band keratopathy, **left eye**
   H18.423 Band keratopathy, **bilateral**
   H18.429 Band keratopathy, **unspecified** eye
   H18.43 Other calcerous corneal degeneration
● **H18.44** Keratomalacia
      Excludes1 keratomalacia due to vitamin A deficiency (E50.4)
   H18.441 Keratomalacia, **right eye**
   H18.442 Keratomalacia, **left eye**
   H18.443 Keratomalacia, **bilateral**
   H18.449 Keratomalacia, **unspecified eye**

▶ New   ➡ Revised   ~~deleted~~ Deleted   Excludes 1   Excludes 2   Includes   Use additional   Code first   Code also   Key words
OGCR Official Guidelines   X Assign placeholder X   ● Use Additional Character(s)   ▶ Manifestation Code   Hierarchical Condition Category   **Coding Clinic**

● **H18.45 Nodular corneal degeneration**
  H18.451 Nodular corneal degeneration, right eye
  H18.452 Nodular corneal degeneration, left eye
  H18.453 Nodular corneal degeneration, bilateral
  H18.459 Nodular corneal degeneration, unspecified eye

● **H18.46 Peripheral corneal degeneration**
  H18.461 Peripheral corneal degeneration, right eye
  H18.462 Peripheral corneal degeneration, left eye
  H18.463 Peripheral corneal degeneration, bilateral
  H18.469 Peripheral corneal degeneration, unspecified eye

  H18.49 Other corneal degeneration

● H18.5 Hereditary corneal dystrophies

  ● H18.50 Unspecified hereditary corneal dystrophies
    H18.501 Unspecified hereditary corneal dystrophies, right eye
    H18.502 Unspecified hereditary corneal dystrophies, left eye
    H18.503 Unspecified hereditary corneal dystrophies, bilateral
    H18.509 Unspecified hereditary corneal dystrophies, unspecified eye

  ● H18.51 Endothelial corneal dystrophy
        Fuchs' dystrophy
    H18.511 Endothelial corneal dystrophy, right eye
    H18.512 Endothelial corneal dystrophy, left eye
    H18.513 Endothelial corneal dystrophy, bilateral
    H18.519 Endothelial corneal dystrophy, unspecified eye

  ● H18.52 Epithelial (juvenile) corneal dystrophy
    H18.521 Epithelial (juvenile) corneal dystrophy, right eye
    H18.522 Epithelial (juvenile) corneal dystrophy, left eye
    H18.523 Epithelial (juvenile) corneal dystrophy, bilateral
    H18.529 Epithelial (juvenile) corneal dystrophy, unspecified eye

  ● H18.53 Granular corneal dystrophy
    H18.531 Granular corneal dystrophy, right eye
    H18.532 Granular corneal dystrophy, left eye
    H18.533 Granular corneal dystrophy, bilateral
    H18.539 Granular corneal dystrophy, unspecified eye

  ● H18.54 Lattice corneal dystrophy
    H18.541 Lattice corneal dystrophy, right eye
    H18.542 Lattice corneal dystrophy, left eye
    H18.543 Lattice corneal dystrophy, bilateral
    H18.549 Lattice corneal dystrophy, unspecified eye

  ● H18.55 Macular corneal dystrophy
    H18.551 Macular corneal dystrophy, right eye
    H18.552 Macular corneal dystrophy, left eye
    H18.553 Macular corneal dystrophy, bilateral
    H18.559 Macular corneal dystrophy, unspecified eye

● **H18.59 Other hereditary corneal dystrophies**
  H18.591 Other hereditary corneal dystrophies, right eye
  H18.592 Other hereditary corneal dystrophies, left eye
  H18.593 Other hereditary corneal dystrophies, bilateral
  H18.599 Other hereditary corneal dystrophies, unspecified eye

● H18.6 Keratoconus

  ● H18.60 Keratoconus, unspecified
    H18.601 Keratoconus, unspecified, right eye
    H18.602 Keratoconus, unspecified, left eye
    H18.603 Keratoconus, unspecified, bilateral
    H18.609 Keratoconus, unspecified, unspecified eye

  ● H18.61 Keratoconus, stable
    H18.611 Keratoconus, stable, right eye
    H18.612 Keratoconus, stable, left eye
    H18.613 Keratoconus, stable, bilateral
    H18.619 Keratoconus, stable, unspecified eye

  ● H18.62 Keratoconus, unstable
        Acute hydrops
    H18.621 Keratoconus, unstable, right eye
    H18.622 Keratoconus, unstable, left eye
    H18.623 Keratoconus, unstable, bilateral
    H18.629 Keratoconus, unstable, unspecified eye

● H18.7 Other and unspecified corneal deformities
    Excludes1 congenital malformations of cornea (Q13.3-Q13.4)

  H18.70 Unspecified corneal deformity

  ● H18.71 Corneal ectasia
    H18.711 Corneal ectasia, right eye
    H18.712 Corneal ectasia, left eye
    H18.713 Corneal ectasia, bilateral
    H18.719 Corneal ectasia, unspecified eye

  ● H18.72 Corneal staphyloma
    H18.721 Corneal staphyloma, right eye
    H18.722 Corneal staphyloma, left eye
    H18.723 Corneal staphyloma, bilateral
    H18.729 Corneal staphyloma, unspecified eye

  ● H18.73 Descemetocele
    H18.731 Descemetocele, right eye
    H18.732 Descemetocele, left eye
    H18.733 Descemetocele, bilateral
    H18.739 Descemetocele, unspecified eye

  ● H18.79 Other corneal deformities
    H18.791 Other corneal deformities, right eye
    H18.792 Other corneal deformities, left eye
    H18.793 Other corneal deformities, bilateral
    H18.799 Other corneal deformities, unspecified eye

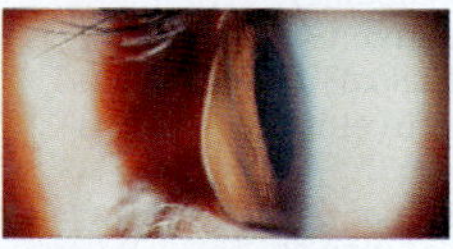

Figure 7-8 Lateral view of the displacement of the cone apex in keratoconus. (From Yanoff: Ophthalmology, ed 3, Mosby, Inc., 2008)

Item 7–4 Keratoconus results in corneal degeneration that begins in childhood, gradually changes the cornea from a round to cone shape, decreasing visual acuity. Treatment includes contact lenses. In severe cases the need for corneal transplant may be the treatment of choice; however, newer technologies may use high-frequency radio energy to shrink the edges of the cornea, pulling the central area back to a more normal shape. It can help delay or avoid the need for a corneal transplantation.

CHAPTER 7 (H00-H59)

CHAPTER 7 (H00-H59)

- ● H18.8   Other specified disorders of cornea
  - ● H18.81   **Anesthesia and hypoesthesia** of cornea
    - H18.811   Anesthesia and hypoesthesia of cornea, **right eye**
    - H18.812   Anesthesia and hypoesthesia of cornea, **left eye**
    - H18.813   Anesthesia and hypoesthesia of cornea, **bilateral**
    - H18.819   Anesthesia and hypoesthesia of cornea, **unspecified eye**
  - ● H18.82   Corneal disorder **due to contact lens**
    - **Excludes2**   corneal edema due to contact lens (H18.21-)
    - H18.821   **Corneal disorder due to contact lens, right eye**
    - H18.822   **Corneal disorder due to contact lens, left eye**
    - H18.823   **Corneal disorder due to contact lens, bilateral**
    - H18.829   **Corneal disorder due to contact lens, unspecified eye**
  - ● H18.83   **Recurrent erosion of cornea**
    - H18.831   **Recurrent erosion of cornea, right eye**
    - H18.832   **Recurrent erosion of cornea, left eye**
    - H18.833   **Recurrent erosion of cornea, bilateral**
    - H18.839   **Recurrent erosion of cornea, unspecified eye**
  - ● H18.89   **Other** specified disorders of cornea
    - H18.891   **Other specified disorders of cornea, right eye**
    - H18.892   **Other specified disorders of cornea, left eye**
    - H18.893   **Other specified disorders of cornea, bilateral**
    - H18.899   **Other specified disorders of cornea, unspecified eye**
  - H18.9   **Unspecified** disorder of cornea

- ● H20   Iridocyclitis
  - ● H20.0   **Acute and subacute** iridocyclitis
    - Acute anterior uveitis
    - Acute cyclitis
    - Acute iritis
    - Subacute anterior uveitis
    - Subacute cyclitis
    - Subacute iritis
    - **Excludes1**   iridocyclitis, iritis, uveitis (due to) (in) diabetes mellitus (E08-E13 with .39)
      iridocyclitis, iritis, uveitis (due to) (in) diphtheria (A36.89)
      iridocyclitis, iritis, uveitis (due to) (in) gonococcal (A54.32)
      iridocyclitis, iritis, uveitis (due to) (in) herpes (simplex) (B00.51)
      iridocyclitis, iritis, uveitis (due to) (in) herpes zoster (B02.32)
      iridocyclitis, iritis, uveitis (due to) (in) late congenital syphilis (A50.39)
      iridocyclitis, iritis, uveitis (due to) (in) late syphilis (A52.71)
      iridocyclitis, iritis, uveitis (due to) (in) sarcoidosis (D86.83)
      iridocyclitis, iritis, uveitis (due to) (in) syphilis (A51.43)
      iridocyclitis, iritis, uveitis (due to) (in) toxoplasmosis (B58.09)
      iridocyclitis, iritis, uveitis (due to) (in) tuberculosis (A18.54)
    - H20.00   **Unspecified acute and subacute iridocyclitis**

- ● H20.01   Primary iridocyclitis
  - H20.011   Primary iridocyclitis, **right** eye
  - H20.012   Primary iridocyclitis, **left** eye
  - H20.013   Primary iridocyclitis, **bilateral**
  - H20.019   Primary iridocyclitis, **unspecified** eye
- ● H20.02   **Recurrent** acute iridocyclitis
  - H20.021   Recurrent acute iridocyclitis, **right eye**
  - H20.022   Recurrent acute iridocyclitis, **left eye**
  - H20.023   Recurrent acute iridocyclitis, **bilateral**
  - H20.029   Recurrent acute iridocyclitis, **unspecified** eye
- ● H20.03   Secondary **infectious** iridocyclitis
  - H20.031   Secondary infectious iridocyclitis, **right eye**
  - H20.032   Secondary infectious iridocyclitis, **left eye**
  - H20.033   Secondary infectious iridocyclitis, **bilateral**
  - H20.039   Secondary infectious iridocyclitis, **unspecified** eye
- ● H20.04   Secondary **noninfectious** iridocyclitis
  - H20.041   Secondary noninfectious iridocyclitis, **right eye**
  - H20.042   Secondary noninfectious iridocyclitis, **left eye**
  - H20.043   Secondary noninfectious iridocyclitis, **bilateral**
  - H20.049   Secondary noninfectious iridocyclitis, **unspecified** eye
- ● H20.05   Hypopyon
  - H20.051   Hypopyon, **right eye**
  - H20.052   Hypopyon, **left eye**
  - H20.053   Hypopyon, **bilateral**
  - H20.059   Hypopyon, **unspecified** eye
- ● H20.1   Chronic iridocyclitis
  - **Use additional** code for any associated cataract (H26.21-)
  - **Excludes2**   posterior cyclitis (H30.2-)
  - H20.10   Chronic iridocyclitis, **unspecified** eye
  - H20.11   Chronic iridocyclitis, **right eye**
  - H20.12   Chronic iridocyclitis, **left eye**
  - H20.13   Chronic iridocyclitis, **bilateral**
- ● H20.2   **Lens-induced** iridocyclitis
  - H20.20   Lens-induced iridocyclitis, **unspecified** eye
  - H20.21   Lens-induced iridocyclitis, **right eye**
  - H20.22   Lens-induced iridocyclitis, **left eye**
  - H20.23   Lens-induced iridocyclitis, **bilateral**
- ● H20.8   Other iridocyclitis
  - **Excludes2**   glaucomatocyclitis crises (H40.4-)
    posterior cyclitis (H30.2-)
    sympathetic uveitis (H44.13-)
  - ● H20.81   **Fuchs' heterochromic** cyclitis
    - H20.811   Fuchs' heterochromic cyclitis, **right eye**
    - H20.812   Fuchs' heterochromic cyclitis, **left eye**
    - H20.813   Fuchs' heterochromic cyclitis, **bilateral**
    - H20.819   Fuchs' heterochromic cyclitis, **unspecified eye**

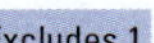

▶ New   ➡ Revised   ~~deleted~~ Deleted   Excludes 1   Excludes 2   Includes   Use additional   Code first   Code also   Key words

OGCR Official Guidelines   X Assign placeholder X   ● Use Additional Character(s)   ▶ Manifestation Code   Hierarchical Condition Category   **Coding Clinic**

● **H20.82**   Vogt-Koyanagi syndrome
    H20.821   Vogt-Koyanagi syndrome, **right** eye
    H20.822   Vogt-Koyanagi syndrome, **left** eye
    H20.823   Vogt-Koyanagi syndrome, **bilateral**
    H20.829   Vogt-Koyanagi syndrome, **unspecified** eye
H20.9   **Unspecified iridocyclitis**
    Uveitis NOS

● **H21**   Other disorders of iris and ciliary body
    Excludes2   sympathetic uveitis (H44.1-)
● **H21.0**   **Hyphema**
    Excludes1   traumatic hyphema (S05.1-)
    H21.00   Hyphema, **unspecified** eye
    H21.01   Hyphema, **right** eye
    H21.02   Hyphema, **left** eye
    H21.03   Hyphema, **bilateral**
● **H21.1**   **Other vascular disorders of iris and ciliary body**
    Neovascularization of iris or ciliary body
    Rubeosis iridis
    Rubeosis of iris
    ● **H21.1X**   Other vascular disorders of iris and ciliary body
      H21.1X1   Other vascular disorders of iris and ciliary body, **right** eye
      H21.1X2   Other vascular disorders of iris and ciliary body, **left** eye
      H21.1X3   Other vascular disorders of iris and ciliary body, **bilateral**
      H21.1X9   Other vascular disorders of iris and ciliary body, **unspecified** eye
● **H21.2**   **Degeneration of iris and ciliary body**
    ● **H21.21**   **Degeneration of chamber angle**
      H21.211   Degeneration of chamber angle, **right** eye
      H21.212   Degeneration of chamber angle, **left** eye
      H21.213   Degeneration of chamber angle, **bilateral**
      H21.219   Degeneration of chamber angle, **unspecified** eye
    ● **H21.22**   **Degeneration of ciliary body**
      H21.221   Degeneration of ciliary body, **right** eye
      H21.222   Degeneration of ciliary body, **left** eye
      H21.223   Degeneration of ciliary body, **bilateral**
      H21.229   Degeneration of ciliary body, **unspecified** eye
    ● **H21.23**   **Degeneration of iris (pigmentary)**
      Translucency of iris
      H21.231   Degeneration of iris (pigmentary), **right** eye
      H21.232   Degeneration of iris (pigmentary), **left** eye
      H21.233   Degeneration of iris (pigmentary), **bilateral**
      H21.239   Degeneration of iris (pigmentary), **unspecified** eye
    ● **H21.24**   **Degeneration of pupillary margin**
      H21.241   Degeneration of pupillary margin, **right** eye
      H21.242   Degeneration of pupillary margin, **left** eye
      H21.243   Degeneration of pupillary margin, **bilateral**
      H21.249   Degeneration of pupillary margin, **unspecified** eye

● **H21.25**   **Iridoschisis**
    H21.251   Iridoschisis, **right** eye
    H21.252   Iridoschisis, **left** eye
    H21.253   Iridoschisis, **bilateral**
    H21.259   Iridoschisis, **unspecified** eye
● **H21.26**   Iris **atrophy** (essential) (progressive)
    H21.261   Iris atrophy (essential) (progressive), **right** eye
    H21.262   Iris atrophy (essential) (progressive), **left** eye
    H21.263   Iris atrophy (essential) (progressive), **bilateral**
    H21.269   Iris atrophy (essential) (progressive), **unspecified** eye
● **H21.27**   **Miotic pupillary cyst**
    H21.271   Miotic pupillary cyst, **right** eye
    H21.272   Miotic pupillary cyst, **left** eye
    H21.273   Miotic pupillary cyst, **bilateral**
    H21.279   Miotic pupillary cyst, **unspecified** eye
    H21.29   **Other iris atrophy**
● **H21.3**   **Cyst of iris, ciliary body and anterior chamber**
    Excludes2   miotic pupillary cyst (H21.27-)
● **H21.30**   **Idiopathic** cysts of iris, ciliary body or anterior chamber
    Cyst of iris, ciliary body or anterior chamber NOS
    H21.301   Idiopathic cysts of iris, ciliary body or anterior chamber, **right** eye
    H21.302   Idiopathic cysts of iris, ciliary body or anterior chamber, **left** eye
    H21.303   Idiopathic cysts of iris, ciliary body or anterior chamber, **bilateral**
    H21.309   Idiopathic cysts of iris, ciliary body or anterior chamber, **unspecified** eye
● **H21.31**   **Exudative** cysts of iris or anterior chamber
    H21.311   Exudative cysts of iris or anterior chamber, **right** eye
    H21.312   Exudative cysts of iris or anterior chamber, **left** eye
    H21.313   Exudative cysts of iris or anterior chamber, **bilateral**
    H21.319   Exudative cysts of iris or anterior chamber, **unspecified** eye
● **H21.32**   **Implantation** cysts of iris, ciliary body or anterior chamber
    H21.321   Implantation cysts of iris, ciliary body or anterior chamber, **right** eye
    H21.322   Implantation cysts of iris, ciliary body or anterior chamber, **left** eye
    H21.323   Implantation cysts of iris, ciliary body or anterior chamber, **bilateral**
    H21.329   Implantation cysts of iris, ciliary body or anterior chamber, **unspecified** eye
● **H21.33**   **Parasitic** cyst of iris, ciliary body or anterior chamber
    H21.331   Parasitic cyst of iris, ciliary body or anterior chamber, **right** eye
    H21.332   Parasitic cyst of iris, ciliary body or anterior chamber, **left** eye
    H21.333   Parasitic cyst of iris, ciliary body or anterior chamber, **bilateral**
    H21.339   Parasitic cyst of iris, ciliary body or anterior chamber, **unspecified** eye

CHAPTER 7 (H00-H59)

● **H21.34**   Primary cyst of pars plana
    H21.341   Primary cyst of pars plana, **right eye**
    H21.342   Primary cyst of pars plana, **left eye**
    H21.343   Primary cyst of pars plana, **bilateral**
    H21.349   Primary cyst of pars plana, **unspecified eye**

● **H21.35**   Exudative cyst of pars plana
    H21.351   Exudative cyst of pars plana, **right eye**
    H21.352   Exudative cyst of pars plana, **left eye**
    H21.353   Exudative cyst of pars plana, **bilateral**
    H21.359   Exudative cyst of pars plana, **unspecified eye**

● **H21.4**   Pupillary membranes
    Iris bombé
    Pupillary occlusion
    Pupillary seclusion
    Excludes1   congenital pupillary membranes (Q13.8)
    H21.40   Pupillary membranes, **unspecified eye**
    H21.41   Pupillary membranes, **right eye**
    H21.42   Pupillary membranes, **left eye**
    H21.43   Pupillary membranes, **bilateral**

● **H21.5**   Other and unspecified adhesions and disruptions of iris and ciliary body
    Excludes1   corectopia (Q13.2)
●   **H21.50**   Unspecified adhesions of iris
    Synechia (iris) NOS
    H21.501   Unspecified adhesions of iris, **right eye**
    H21.502   Unspecified adhesions of iris, **left eye**
    H21.503   Unspecified adhesions of iris, **bilateral**
    H21.509   Unspecified adhesions of iris and ciliary body, **unspecified eye**

● **H21.51**   Anterior synechiae (iris)
    H21.511   Anterior synechiae (iris), **right eye**
    H21.512   Anterior synechiae (iris), **left eye**
    H21.513   Anterior synechiae (iris), **bilateral**
    H21.519   Anterior synechiae (iris), **unspecified eye**

● **H21.52**   Goniosynechiae
    H21.521   Goniosynechiae, **right eye**
    H21.522   Goniosynechiae, **left eye**
    H21.523   Goniosynechiae, **bilateral**
    H21.529   Goniosynechiae, **unspecified eye**

● **H21.53**   Iridodialysis
    H21.531   Iridodialysis, **right eye**
    H21.532   Iridodialysis, **left eye**
    H21.533   Iridodialysis, **bilateral**
    H21.539   Iridodialysis, **unspecified eye**

● **H21.54**   Posterior synechiae (iris)
    H21.541   Posterior synechiae (iris), **right eye**
    H21.542   Posterior synechiae (iris), **left eye**
    H21.543   Posterior synechiae (iris), **bilateral**
    H21.549   Posterior synechiae (iris), **unspecified eye**

● **H21.55**   Recession of chamber angle
    H21.551   Recession of chamber angle, **right eye**
    H21.552   Recession of chamber angle, **left eye**
    H21.553   Recession of chamber angle, **bilateral**
    H21.559   Recession of chamber angle, **unspecified eye**

● **H21.56**   Pupillary abnormalities
    Deformed pupil
    Ectopic pupil
    Rupture of sphincter, pupil
    Excludes1   congenital deformity of pupil (Q13.2-)
    H21.561   Pupillary abnormality, **right eye**
    H21.562   Pupillary abnormality, **left eye**
    H21.563   Pupillary abnormality, **bilateral**
    H21.569   Pupillary abnormality, **unspecified eye**

● **H21.8**   Other specified disorders of iris and ciliary body
    H21.81   Floppy iris syndrome
      Intraoperative floppy iris syndrome (IFIS)
      Use additional code for adverse effect, if applicable, to identify drug (T36-T50 with fifth or sixth character 5)
    H21.82   Plateau iris syndrome (post-iridectomy) (postprocedural)
    H21.89   Other specified disorders of iris and ciliary body
H21.9   Unspecified disorder of iris and ciliary body

▶ *H22*   *Disorders of iris and ciliary body in diseases classified elsewhere*
    Code first underlying disease, such as:
      gout (M1A.-, M10.-)
      leprosy (A30.-)
      parasitic disease (B89)

DISORDERS OF LENS (H25-H28)

● **H25**   Age-related cataract
    Senile cataract
    Excludes2   capsular glaucoma with pseudoexfoliation of lens (H40.1-)
●   **H25.0**   Age-related incipient cataract
●   **H25.01**   Cortical age-related cataract
    H25.011   Cortical age-related cataract, **right eye**   A
    H25.012   Cortical age-related cataract, **left eye**   A
    H25.013   Cortical age-related cataract, **bilateral**   A
    H25.019   Cortical age-related cataract, **unspecified eye**   A
●   **H25.03**   Anterior subcapsular polar age-related cataract
    H25.031   Anterior subcapsular polar age-related cataract, **right eye**   A
    H25.032   Anterior subcapsular polar age-related cataract, **left eye**   A
    H25.033   Anterior subcapsular polar age-related cataract, **bilateral**   A
    H25.039   Anterior subcapsular polar age-related cataract, **unspecified eye**   A

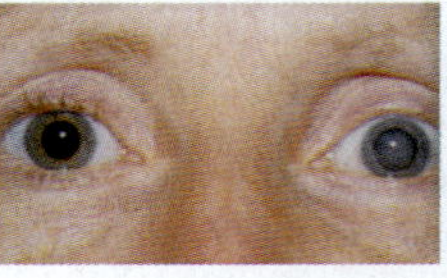

Figure 7-9   Age-related cataract. Nuclear sclerosis and cortical lens opacities are present. (From Ignatavicius DD, Workman ML: Medical-Surgical Nursing: Patient-Centered Collaborative Care, St. Louis, MO, Saunders/Elsevier, 2010)

Item 7–5   Senile cataracts are linked to the aging process. The most common area for the formation of a cataract is the cortical area of the lens. **Polar cataracts** can be either anterior or posterior. **Anterior polar cataracts** are more common and are small, white, capsular cataracts located on the anterior portion of the lens. **Total cataracts,** also called **complete** or **mature,** cause an opacity of all fibers of the lens. **Hypermature** describes a mature cataract with a swollen, milky cortex that covers the entire lens. **Immature**, also called **incipient,** cataracts have a clear cortex and are only slightly opaque. Treatment for all cataracts is the removal of the lens.

▶ New   ➡ Revised   ~~deleted~~ Deleted   Excludes 1   Excludes 2   Includes   Use additional   Code first   Code also   Key words
OGCR Official Guidelines   X Assign placeholder X   ● Use Additional Character(s)   ▶ Manifestation Code   Hierarchical Condition Category   **Coding Clinic**

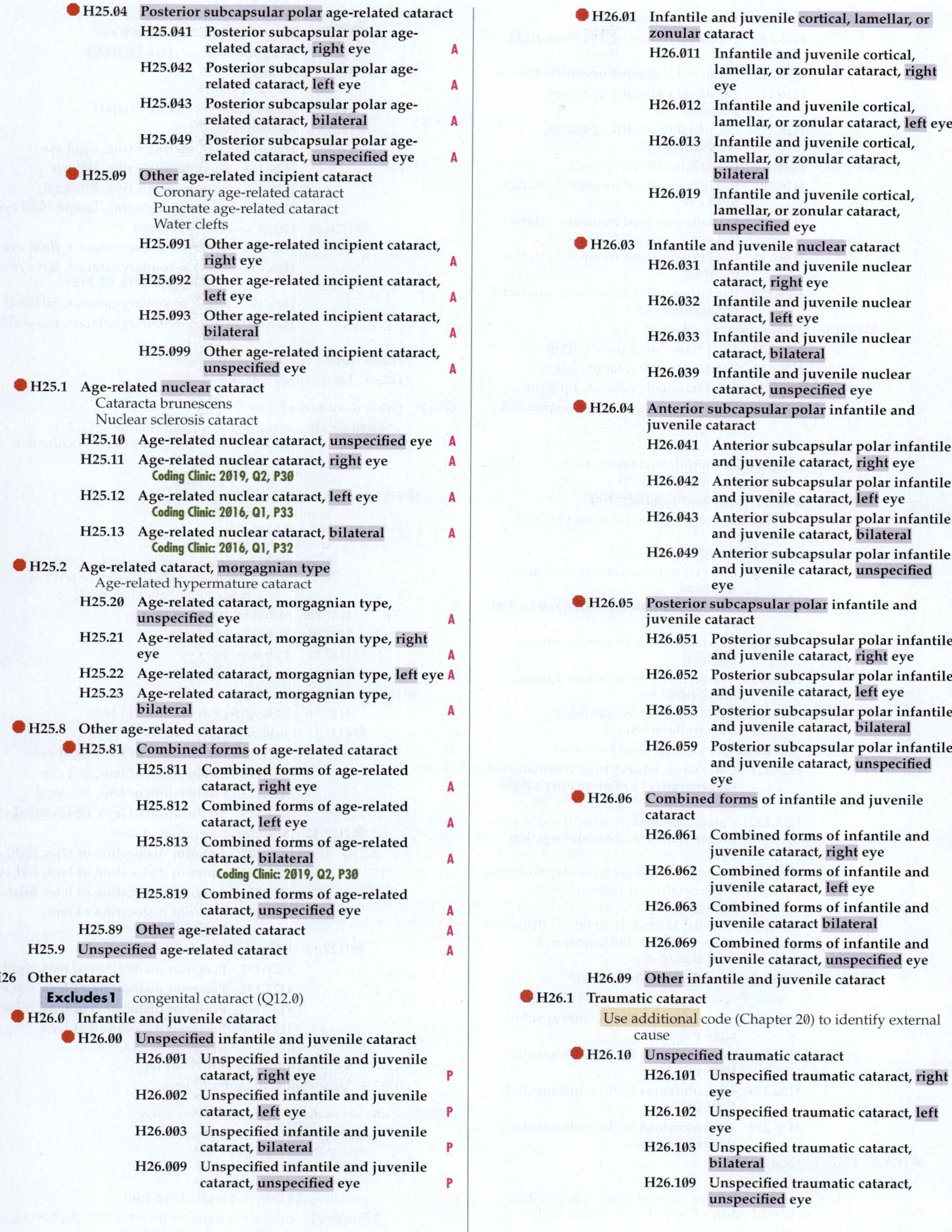

● **H25.04** **Posterior subcapsular polar age-related cataract**
  H25.041   Posterior subcapsular polar age-related cataract, right eye   A
  H25.042   Posterior subcapsular polar age-related cataract, left eye   A
  H25.043   Posterior subcapsular polar age-related cataract, bilateral   A
  H25.049   Posterior subcapsular polar age-related cataract, unspecified eye   A
● **H25.09** **Other age-related incipient cataract**
  Coronary age-related cataract
  Punctate age-related cataract
  Water clefts
  H25.091   Other age-related incipient cataract, right eye   A
  H25.092   Other age-related incipient cataract, left eye   A
  H25.093   Other age-related incipient cataract, bilateral   A
  H25.099   Other age-related incipient cataract, unspecified eye   A
● **H25.1** **Age-related nuclear cataract**
  Cataracta brunescens
  Nuclear sclerosis cataract
  H25.10   Age-related nuclear cataract, unspecified eye   A
  H25.11   Age-related nuclear cataract, right eye   A
      Coding Clinic: 2019, Q2, P30
  H25.12   Age-related nuclear cataract, left eye   A
      Coding Clinic: 2016, Q1, P33
  H25.13   Age-related nuclear cataract, bilateral   A
      Coding Clinic: 2016, Q1, P32
● **H25.2** **Age-related cataract, morgagnian type**
  Age-related hypermature cataract
  H25.20   Age-related cataract, morgagnian type, unspecified eye   A
  H25.21   Age-related cataract, morgagnian type, right eye   A
  H25.22   Age-related cataract, morgagnian type, left eye   A
  H25.23   Age-related cataract, morgagnian type, bilateral   A
● **H25.8** **Other age-related cataract**
  ● **H25.81** **Combined forms of age-related cataract**
      H25.811   Combined forms of age-related cataract, right eye   A
      H25.812   Combined forms of age-related cataract, left eye   A
      H25.813   Combined forms of age-related cataract, bilateral   A
          Coding Clinic: 2019, Q2, P30
      H25.819   Combined forms of age-related cataract, unspecified eye   A
  H25.89   Other age-related cataract   A
  H25.9   Unspecified age-related cataract   A
● **H26** **Other cataract**
  Excludes1   congenital cataract (Q12.0)
  ● **H26.0** **Infantile and juvenile cataract**
    ● **H26.00** **Unspecified infantile and juvenile cataract**
        H26.001   Unspecified infantile and juvenile cataract, right eye   P
        H26.002   Unspecified infantile and juvenile cataract, left eye   P
        H26.003   Unspecified infantile and juvenile cataract, bilateral   P
        H26.009   Unspecified infantile and juvenile cataract, unspecified eye   P

● **H26.01** **Infantile and juvenile cortical, lamellar, or zonular cataract**
    H26.011   Infantile and juvenile cortical, lamellar, or zonular cataract, right eye   P
    H26.012   Infantile and juvenile cortical, lamellar, or zonular cataract, left eye   P
    H26.013   Infantile and juvenile cortical, lamellar, or zonular cataract, bilateral   P
    H26.019   Infantile and juvenile cortical, lamellar, or zonular cataract, unspecified eye   P
● **H26.03** **Infantile and juvenile nuclear cataract**
    H26.031   Infantile and juvenile nuclear cataract, right eye   P
    H26.032   Infantile and juvenile nuclear cataract, left eye   P
    H26.033   Infantile and juvenile nuclear cataract, bilateral   P
    H26.039   Infantile and juvenile nuclear cataract, unspecified eye   P
● **H26.04** **Anterior subcapsular polar infantile and juvenile cataract**
    H26.041   Anterior subcapsular polar infantile and juvenile cataract, right eye   P
    H26.042   Anterior subcapsular polar infantile and juvenile cataract, left eye   P
    H26.043   Anterior subcapsular polar infantile and juvenile cataract, bilateral   P
    H26.049   Anterior subcapsular polar infantile and juvenile cataract, unspecified eye   P
● **H26.05** **Posterior subcapsular polar infantile and juvenile cataract**
    H26.051   Posterior subcapsular polar infantile and juvenile cataract, right eye   P
    H26.052   Posterior subcapsular polar infantile and juvenile cataract, left eye   P
    H26.053   Posterior subcapsular polar infantile and juvenile cataract, bilateral   P
    H26.059   Posterior subcapsular polar infantile and juvenile cataract, unspecified eye   P
● **H26.06** **Combined forms of infantile and juvenile cataract**
    H26.061   Combined forms of infantile and juvenile cataract, right eye   P
    H26.062   Combined forms of infantile and juvenile cataract, left eye   P
    H26.063   Combined forms of infantile and juvenile cataract bilateral   P
    H26.069   Combined forms of infantile and juvenile cataract, unspecified eye   P
  H26.09   Other infantile and juvenile cataract   P
● **H26.1** **Traumatic cataract**
  Use additional code (Chapter 20) to identify external cause
  ● **H26.10** **Unspecified traumatic cataract**
      H26.101   Unspecified traumatic cataract, right eye
      H26.102   Unspecified traumatic cataract, left eye
      H26.103   Unspecified traumatic cataract, bilateral
      H26.109   Unspecified traumatic cataract, unspecified eye

CHAPTER 7 (H00–H59)

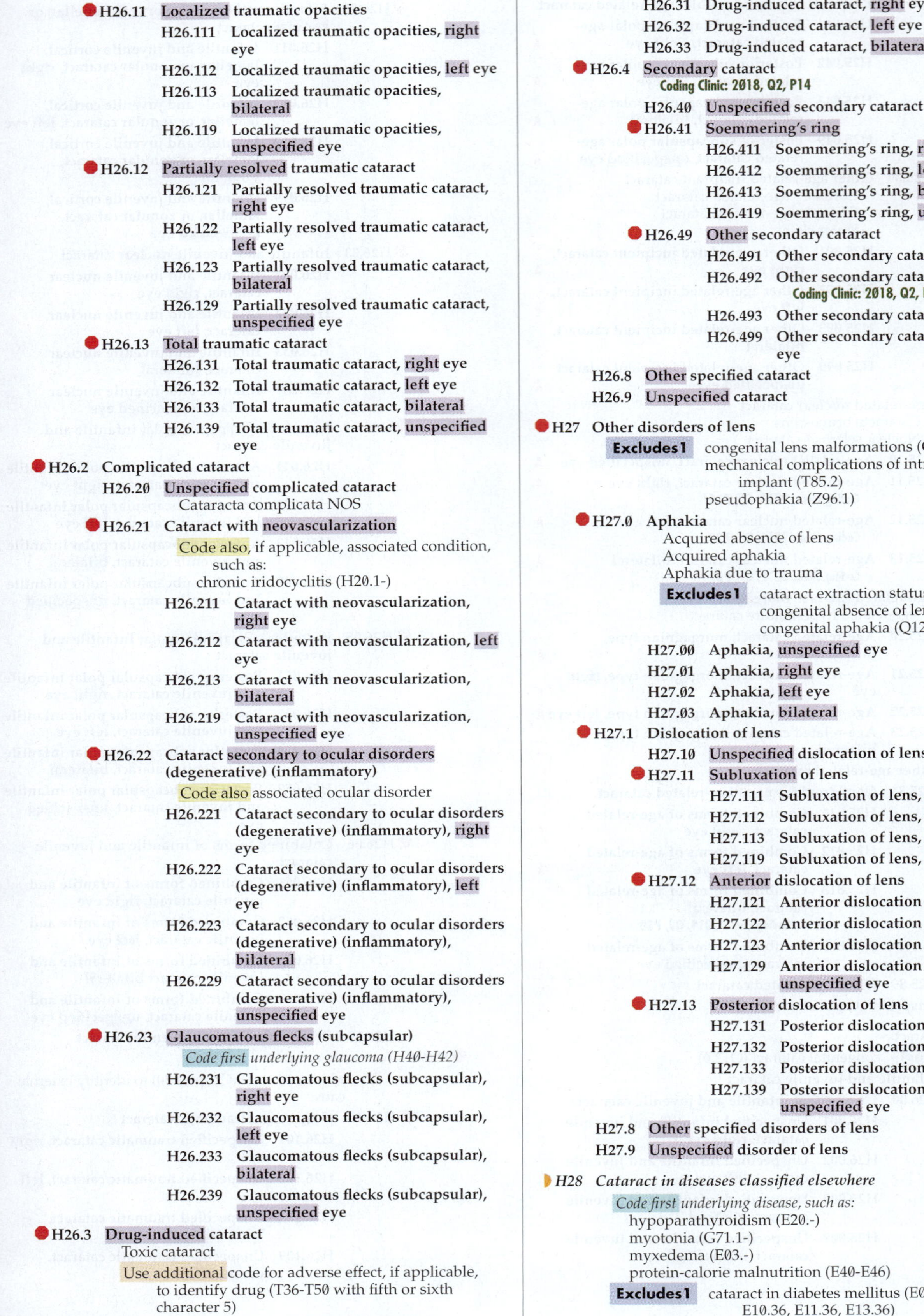

- **H26.11**   **Localized** traumatic opacities
  - H26.111   Localized traumatic opacities, **right eye**
  - H26.112   Localized traumatic opacities, **left eye**
  - H26.113   Localized traumatic opacities, **bilateral**
  - H26.119   Localized traumatic opacities, **unspecified eye**
- **H26.12**   **Partially resolved traumatic cataract**
  - H26.121   Partially resolved traumatic cataract, **right eye**
  - H26.122   Partially resolved traumatic cataract, **left eye**
  - H26.123   Partially resolved traumatic cataract, **bilateral**
  - H26.129   Partially resolved traumatic cataract, **unspecified eye**
- **H26.13**   **Total traumatic cataract**
  - H26.131   Total traumatic cataract, **right eye**
  - H26.132   Total traumatic cataract, **left eye**
  - H26.133   Total traumatic cataract, **bilateral**
  - H26.139   Total traumatic cataract, **unspecified eye**
- **H26.2**   **Complicated cataract**
  - **H26.20**   **Unspecified complicated cataract**
    Cataracta complicata NOS
  - **H26.21**   **Cataract with neovascularization**
    Code also, if applicable, associated condition, such as:
        chronic iridocyclitis (H20.1-)
    - H26.211   Cataract with neovascularization, **right eye**
    - H26.212   Cataract with neovascularization, **left eye**
    - H26.213   Cataract with neovascularization, **bilateral**
    - H26.219   Cataract with neovascularization, **unspecified eye**
  - **H26.22**   **Cataract secondary to ocular disorders (degenerative) (inflammatory)**
    Code also associated ocular disorder
    - H26.221   Cataract secondary to ocular disorders (degenerative) (inflammatory), **right eye**
    - H26.222   Cataract secondary to ocular disorders (degenerative) (inflammatory), **left eye**
    - H26.223   Cataract secondary to ocular disorders (degenerative) (inflammatory), **bilateral**
    - H26.229   Cataract secondary to ocular disorders (degenerative) (inflammatory), **unspecified eye**
  - **H26.23**   **Glaucomatous flecks (subcapsular)**
    Code first underlying glaucoma (H40-H42)
    - H26.231   Glaucomatous flecks (subcapsular), **right eye**
    - H26.232   Glaucomatous flecks (subcapsular), **left eye**
    - H26.233   Glaucomatous flecks (subcapsular), **bilateral**
    - H26.239   Glaucomatous flecks (subcapsular), **unspecified eye**
- **H26.3**   **Drug-induced cataract**
  Toxic cataract
  Use additional code for adverse effect, if applicable, to identify drug (T36-T50 with fifth or sixth character 5)
  - **H26.30**   **Drug-induced cataract, unspecified eye**
  - H26.31   Drug-induced cataract, **right eye**
  - H26.32   Drug-induced cataract, **left eye**
  - H26.33   Drug-induced cataract, **bilateral**
- **H26.4**   **Secondary cataract**
  Coding Clinic: 2018, Q2, P14
  - **H26.40**   **Unspecified secondary cataract**
  - **H26.41**   **Soemmering's ring**
    - H26.411   Soemmering's ring, **right eye**
    - H26.412   Soemmering's ring, **left eye**
    - H26.413   Soemmering's ring, **bilateral**
    - H26.419   Soemmering's ring, **unspecified eye**
  - **H26.49**   **Other secondary cataract**
    - H26.491   Other secondary cataract, **right eye**
    - H26.492   Other secondary cataract, **left eye**
      Coding Clinic: 2018, Q2, P13
    - H26.493   Other secondary cataract, **bilateral**
    - H26.499   Other secondary cataract, **unspecified eye**
- **H26.8**   Other specified cataract
- **H26.9**   Unspecified cataract
- **H27**   **Other disorders of lens**
  - **Excludes1**   congenital lens malformations (Q12.-)
    mechanical complications of intraocular lens implant (T85.2)
    pseudophakia (Z96.1)
  - **H27.0**   **Aphakia**
    Acquired absence of lens
    Acquired aphakia
    Aphakia due to trauma
    - **Excludes1**   cataract extraction status (Z98.4-)
      congenital absence of lens (Q12.3)
      congenital aphakia (Q12.3)
    - H27.00   Aphakia, **unspecified eye**
    - H27.01   Aphakia, **right eye**
    - H27.02   Aphakia, **left eye**
    - H27.03   Aphakia, **bilateral**
  - **H27.1**   **Dislocation of lens**
    - H27.10   Unspecified dislocation of lens
    - **H27.11**   **Subluxation of lens**
      - H27.111   Subluxation of lens, **right eye**
      - H27.112   Subluxation of lens, **left eye**
      - H27.113   Subluxation of lens, **bilateral**
      - H27.119   Subluxation of lens, **unspecified eye**
    - **H27.12**   **Anterior dislocation of lens**
      - H27.121   Anterior dislocation of lens, **right eye**
      - H27.122   Anterior dislocation of lens, **left eye**
      - H27.123   Anterior dislocation of lens, **bilateral**
      - H27.129   Anterior dislocation of lens, **unspecified eye**
    - **H27.13**   **Posterior dislocation of lens**
      - H27.131   Posterior dislocation of lens, **right eye**
      - H27.132   Posterior dislocation of lens, **left eye**
      - H27.133   Posterior dislocation of lens, **bilateral**
      - H27.139   Posterior dislocation of lens, **unspecified eye**
  - **H27.8**   Other specified disorders of lens
  - **H27.9**   Unspecified disorder of lens
- **H28**   *Cataract in diseases classified elsewhere*
  Code first underlying disease, such as:
      hypoparathyroidism (E20.-)
      myotonia (G71.1-)
      myxedema (E03.-)
      protein-calorie malnutrition (E40-E46)
  - **Excludes1**   cataract in diabetes mellitus (E08.36, E09.36, E10.36, E11.36, E13.36)

DISORDERS OF CHOROID AND RETINA (H30-H36)

★**(See Plate 16 of the Anatomy Illustrations.)**

● **H30** **Chorioretinal inflammation**
  ● **H30.0** **Focal chorioretinal inflammation**
    Focal chorioretinitis
    Focal choroiditis
    Focal retinitis
    Focal retinochoroiditis
    ● **H30.00** Unspecified focal chorioretinal inflammation
      Focal chorioretinitis NOS
      Focal choroiditis NOS
      Focal retinitis NOS
      Focal retinochoroiditis NOS
      H30.001   Unspecified focal chorioretinal inflammation, right eye
      H30.002   Unspecified focal chorioretinal inflammation, left eye
      H30.003   Unspecified focal chorioretinal inflammation, bilateral
      H30.009   Unspecified focal chorioretinal inflammation, unspecified eye
    ● **H30.01** Focal chorioretinal inflammation, juxtapapillary
      H30.011   Focal chorioretinal inflammation, juxtapapillary, right eye
      H30.012   Focal chorioretinal inflammation, juxtapapillary, left eye
      H30.013   Focal chorioretinal inflammation, juxtapapillary, bilateral
      H30.019   Focal chorioretinal inflammation, juxtapapillary, unspecified eye
    ● **H30.02** Focal chorioretinal inflammation of posterior pole
      H30.021   Focal chorioretinal inflammation of posterior pole, right eye
      H30.022   Focal chorioretinal inflammation of posterior pole, left eye
      H30.023   Focal chorioretinal inflammation of posterior pole, bilateral
      H30.029   Focal chorioretinal inflammation of posterior pole, unspecified eye
    ● **H30.03** Focal chorioretinal inflammation, peripheral
      H30.031   Focal chorioretinal inflammation, peripheral, right eye
      H30.032   Focal chorioretinal inflammation, peripheral, left eye
      H30.033   Focal chorioretinal inflammation, peripheral, bilateral
      H30.039   Focal chorioretinal inflammation, peripheral, unspecified eye
    ● **H30.04** Focal chorioretinal inflammation, macular or paramacular
      H30.041   Focal chorioretinal inflammation, macular or paramacular, right eye
      H30.042   Focal chorioretinal inflammation, macular or paramacular, left eye
      H30.043   Focal chorioretinal inflammation, macular or paramacular, bilateral
      H30.049   Focal chorioretinal inflammation, macular or paramacular, unspecified eye
  ● **H30.1** **Disseminated chorioretinal inflammation**
    Disseminated chorioretinitis
    Disseminated choroiditis
    Disseminated retinitis
    Disseminated retinochoroiditis
    Excludes2   exudative retinopathy (H35.02-)

  ● **H30.10** Unspecified disseminated chorioretinal inflammation
    Disseminated chorioretinitis NOS
    Disseminated choroiditis NOS
    Disseminated retinitis NOS
    Disseminated retinochoroiditis NOS
    H30.101   Unspecified disseminated chorioretinal inflammation, right eye
    H30.102   Unspecified disseminated chorioretinal inflammation, left eye
    H30.103   Unspecified disseminated chorioretinal inflammation, bilateral
    H30.109   Unspecified disseminated chorioretinal inflammation, unspecified eye
  ● **H30.11** Disseminated chorioretinal inflammation of posterior pole
    H30.111   Disseminated chorioretinal inflammation of posterior pole, right eye
    H30.112   Disseminated chorioretinal inflammation of posterior pole, left eye
    H30.113   Disseminated chorioretinal inflammation of posterior pole, bilateral
    H30.119   Disseminated chorioretinal inflammation of posterior pole, unspecified eye
  ● **H30.12** Disseminated chorioretinal inflammation, peripheral
    H30.121   Disseminated chorioretinal inflammation, peripheral right eye
    H30.122   Disseminated chorioretinal inflammation, peripheral, left eye
    H30.123   Disseminated chorioretinal inflammation, peripheral, bilateral
    H30.129   Disseminated chorioretinal inflammation, peripheral, unspecified eye
  ● **H30.13** Disseminated chorioretinal inflammation, generalized
    H30.131   Disseminated chorioretinal inflammation, generalized, right eye
    H30.132   Disseminated chorioretinal inflammation, generalized, left eye
    H30.133   Disseminated chorioretinal inflammation, generalized, bilateral
    H30.139   Disseminated chorioretinal inflammation, generalized, unspecified eye
  ● **H30.14** Acute posterior multifocal placoid pigment epitheliopathy
    H30.141   Acute posterior multifocal placoid pigment epitheliopathy, right eye
    H30.142   Acute posterior multifocal placoid pigment epitheliopathy, left eye
    H30.143   Acute posterior multifocal placoid pigment epitheliopathy, bilateral
    H30.149   Acute posterior multifocal placoid pigment epitheliopathy, unspecified eye
  ● **H30.2** **Posterior cyclitis**
    Pars planitis
    H30.20   Posterior cyclitis, unspecified eye
    H30.21   Posterior cyclitis, right eye
    H30.22   Posterior cyclitis, left eye
    H30.23   Posterior cyclitis, bilateral

CHAPTER 7 (H00-H59)

- **H30.8 Other chorioretinal inflammations**
  - **H30.81 Harada's disease**
    - H30.811 Harada's disease, right eye
    - H30.812 Harada's disease, left eye
    - H30.813 Harada's disease, bilateral
    - H30.819 Harada's disease, unspecified eye
  - **H30.89 Other chorioretinal inflammations**
    - H30.891 Other chorioretinal inflammations, right eye
    - H30.892 Other chorioretinal inflammations, left eye
    - H30.893 Other chorioretinal inflammations, bilateral
    - H30.899 Other chorioretinal inflammations, unspecified eye
- **H30.9 Unspecified chorioretinal inflammation**
  Chorioretinitis NOS
  Choroiditis NOS
  Neuroretinitis NOS
  Retinitis NOS
  Retinochoroiditis NOS
  - H30.90 Unspecified chorioretinal inflammation, unspecified eye
  - H30.91 Unspecified chorioretinal inflammation, right eye
  - H30.92 Unspecified chorioretinal inflammation, left eye
  - H30.93 Unspecified chorioretinal inflammation, bilateral

- **H31 Other disorders of choroid**
  - **H31.0 Chorioretinal scars**

    Excludes2 postsurgical chorioretinal scars (H59.81-)
    - **H31.00 Unspecified chorioretinal scars**
      - H31.001 Unspecified chorioretinal scars, right eye
      - H31.002 Unspecified chorioretinal scars, left eye
      - H31.003 Unspecified chorioretinal scars, bilateral
      - H31.009 Unspecified chorioretinal scars, unspecified eye
    - **H31.01 Macula scars of posterior pole (postinflammatory) (post-traumatic)**

      Excludes1 postprocedural chorioretinal scar (H59.81-)
      - H31.011 Macula scars of posterior pole (postinflammatory) (post-traumatic), right eye
      - H31.012 Macula scars of posterior pole (postinflammatory) (post-traumatic), left eye
      - H31.013 Macula scars of posterior pole (postinflammatory) (post-traumatic), bilateral
      - H31.019 Macula scars of posterior pole (postinflammatory) (post-traumatic), unspecified eye
    - **H31.02 Solar retinopathy**
      - H31.021 Solar retinopathy, right eye
      - H31.022 Solar retinopathy, left eye
      - H31.023 Solar retinopathy, bilateral
      - H31.029 Solar retinopathy, unspecified eye
  - **H31.09 Other chorioretinal scars**
    - H31.091 Other chorioretinal scars, right eye
    - H31.092 Other chorioretinal scars, left eye
    - H31.093 Other chorioretinal scars, bilateral
    - H31.099 Other chorioretinal scars, unspecified eye
  - **H31.1 Choroidal degeneration**

    Excludes2 angioid streaks of macula (H35.33)
    - **H31.10 Unspecified choroidal degeneration**
      Choroidal sclerosis NOS
      - H31.101 Choroidal degeneration, unspecified, right eye
      - H31.102 Choroidal degeneration, unspecified, left eye
      - H31.103 Choroidal degeneration, unspecified, bilateral
      - H31.109 Choroidal degeneration, unspecified eye
    - **H31.11 Age-related choroidal atrophy**
      - H31.111 Age-related choroidal atrophy, right eye A
      - H31.112 Age-related choroidal atrophy, left eye A
      - H31.113 Age-related choroidal atrophy, bilateral A
      - H31.119 Age-related choroidal atrophy, unspecified eye A
    - **H31.12 Diffuse secondary atrophy of choroid**
      - H31.121 Diffuse secondary atrophy of choroid, right eye
      - H31.122 Diffuse secondary atrophy of choroid, left eye
      - H31.123 Diffuse secondary atrophy of choroid, bilateral
      - H31.129 Diffuse secondary atrophy of choroid, unspecified eye
  - **H31.2 Hereditary choroidal dystrophy**

    Excludes2 hyperornithinemia (E72.4)
    ornithinemia (E72.4)
    - H31.20 Hereditary choroidal dystrophy, unspecified
    - H31.21 Choroideremia
    - H31.22 Choroidal dystrophy (central areolar) (generalized) (peripapillary)
    - H31.23 Gyrate atrophy, choroid
    - H31.29 Other hereditary choroidal dystrophy
  - **H31.3 Choroidal hemorrhage and rupture**
    - **H31.30 Unspecified choroidal hemorrhage**
      - H31.301 Unspecified choroidal hemorrhage, right eye
      - H31.302 Unspecified choroidal hemorrhage, left eye
      - H31.303 Unspecified choroidal hemorrhage, bilateral
      - H31.309 Unspecified choroidal hemorrhage, unspecified eye
    - **H31.31 Expulsive choroidal hemorrhage**
      - H31.311 Expulsive choroidal hemorrhage, right eye
      - H31.312 Expulsive choroidal hemorrhage, left eye
      - H31.313 Expulsive choroidal hemorrhage, bilateral
      - H31.319 Expulsive choroidal hemorrhage, unspecified eye

▶ New   ⇒ Revised   ~~deleted~~ Deleted   Excludes 1   Excludes 2   Includes   Use additional   Code first   Code also   Key words
OGCR Official Guidelines   X Assign placeholder X   ● Use Additional Character(s)   ▸ Manifestation Code   Hierarchical Condition Category   **Coding Clinic**

● H31.32   Choroidal rupture
    H31.321   Choroidal rupture, right eye
    H31.322   Choroidal rupture, left eye
    H31.323   Choroidal rupture, bilateral
    H31.329   Choroidal rupture, unspecified eye

● H31.4   Choroidal detachment
   ● H31.40   Unspecified choroidal detachment
    H31.401   Unspecified choroidal detachment, right eye
    H31.402   Unspecified choroidal detachment, left eye
    H31.403   Unspecified choroidal detachment, bilateral
    H31.409   Unspecified choroidal detachment, unspecified eye

   ● H31.41   Hemorrhagic choroidal detachment
    H31.411   Hemorrhagic choroidal detachment, right eye
    H31.412   Hemorrhagic choroidal detachment, left eye
    H31.413   Hemorrhagic choroidal detachment, bilateral
    H31.419   Hemorrhagic choroidal detachment, unspecified eye

   ● H31.42   Serous choroidal detachment
    H31.421   Serous choroidal detachment, right eye
    H31.422   Serous choroidal detachment, left eye
    H31.423   Serous choroidal detachment, bilateral
    H31.429   Serous choroidal detachment, unspecified eye

H31.8   Other specified disorders of choroid
H31.9   Unspecified disorder of choroid

▶ *H32*   *Chorioretinal disorders in diseases classified elsewhere*
   Code first underlying disease, such as:
    congenital toxoplasmosis (P37.1)
    histoplasmosis (B39.-)
    leprosy (A30.-)
   Excludes1   chorioretinitis (in):
     toxoplasmosis (acquired) (B58.01)
     tuberculosis (A18.53)

● H33   Retinal detachments and breaks
   Excludes1   detachment of retinal pigment epithelium (H35.72-, H35.73-)

   ● H33.0   Retinal detachment with retinal break
    Rhegmatogenous retinal detachment
    Excludes1   serous retinal detachment (without retinal break) (H33.2-)

    ● H33.00   Unspecified retinal detachment with retinal break
    H33.001   Unspecified retinal detachment with retinal break, right eye
    H33.002   Unspecified retinal detachment with retinal break, left eye
    H33.003   Unspecified retinal detachment with retinal break, bilateral
    H33.009   Unspecified retinal detachment with retinal break, unspecified eye

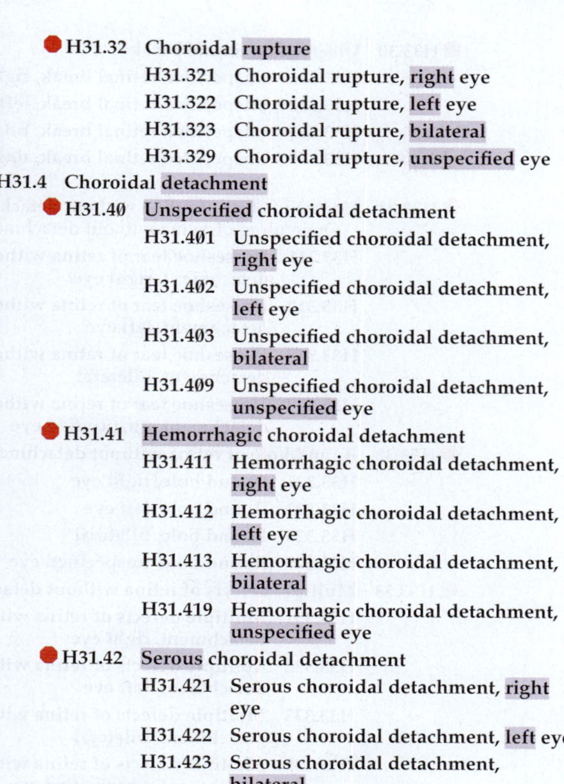
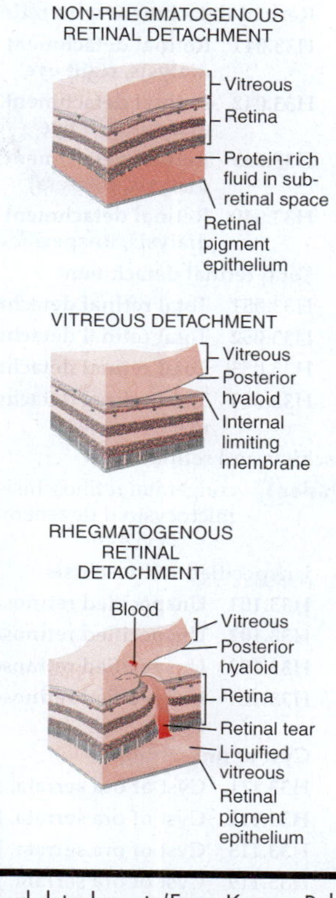

Figure 7-10   Retinal detachment. (From Kumar: Robbins and Cotran: Pathologic Basis of Disease, ed 7, Saunders, 2005)

Item 7–6   Retinal detachments and defects are conditions of the eye in which the retina separates from the underlying tissue. Initial detachment may be localized, requiring rapid treatment (medical emergency) to avoid the entire retina from detaching, which leads to vision loss and blindness.

   ● H33.01   Retinal detachment with single break
    H33.011   Retinal detachment with single break, right eye
    H33.012   Retinal detachment with single break, left eye
    H33.013   Retinal detachment with single break, bilateral
    H33.019   Retinal detachment with single break, unspecified eye

   ● H33.02   Retinal detachment with multiple breaks
    H33.021   Retinal detachment with multiple breaks, right eye
    H33.022   Retinal detachment with multiple breaks, left eye
    H33.023   Retinal detachment with multiple breaks, bilateral
    H33.029   Retinal detachment with multiple breaks, unspecified eye

   ● H33.03   Retinal detachment with giant retinal tear
    H33.031   Retinal detachment with giant retinal tear, right eye
    H33.032   Retinal detachment with giant retinal tear, left eye
    H33.033   Retinal detachment with giant retinal tear, bilateral
    H33.039   Retinal detachment with giant retinal tear, unspecified eye

CHAPTER 7 (H00-H59)

CHAPTER 7 (H00-H59)

● **H33.04 Retinal detachment with retinal dialysis**
  H33.041 Retinal detachment with retinal dialysis, **right eye**
  H33.042 Retinal detachment with retinal dialysis, **left eye**
  H33.043 Retinal detachment with retinal dialysis, **bilateral**
  H33.049 Retinal detachment with retinal dialysis, **unspecified eye**
● **H33.05 Total retinal detachment**
  H33.051 Total retinal detachment, **right eye**
  H33.052 Total retinal detachment, **left eye**
  H33.053 Total retinal detachment, **bilateral**
  H33.059 Total retinal detachment, **unspecified eye**
● **H33.1 Retinoschisis and retinal cysts**
  Excludes1 congenital retinoschisis (Q14.1)
    microcystoid degeneration of retina (H35.42-)
  ● **H33.10 Unspecified retinoschisis**
    H33.101 Unspecified retinoschisis, **right eye**
    H33.102 Unspecified retinoschisis, **left eye**
    H33.103 Unspecified retinoschisis, **bilateral**
    H33.109 Unspecified retinoschisis, **unspecified eye**
  ● **H33.11 Cyst of ora serrata**
    H33.111 Cyst of ora serrata, **right eye**
    H33.112 Cyst of ora serrata, **left eye**
    H33.113 Cyst of ora serrata, **bilateral**
    H33.119 Cyst of ora serrata, **unspecified eye**
  ● **H33.12 Parasitic cyst of retina**
    H33.121 Parasitic cyst of retina, **right eye**
    H33.122 Parasitic cyst of retina, **left eye**
    H33.123 Parasitic cyst of retina, **bilateral**
    H33.129 Parasitic cyst of retina, **unspecified eye**
  ● **H33.19 Other retinoschisis and retinal cysts**
    Pseudocyst of retina
    H33.191 Other retinoschisis and retinal cysts, **right eye**
    H33.192 Other retinoschisis and retinal cysts, **left eye**
    H33.193 Other retinoschisis and retinal cysts, **bilateral**
    H33.199 Other retinoschisis and retinal cysts, **unspecified eye**
● **H33.2 Serous retinal detachment**
  Retinal detachment NOS
  Retinal detachment without retinal break
  Excludes1 central serous chorioretinopathy (H35.71-)
  H33.20 Serous retinal detachment, **unspecified eye**
  H33.21 Serous retinal detachment, **right eye**
  H33.22 Serous retinal detachment, **left eye**
  H33.23 Serous retinal detachment, **bilateral**
● **H33.3 Retinal breaks without detachment**
  ~~**Excludes1**~~ ~~chorioretinal scars after surgery for detachment (H59.81-)~~
    ~~peripheral retinal degeneration without break (H35.4-)~~
  ▶ **Excludes2** chorioretinal scars after surgery for detachment (H59.81-)
    ▶peripheral retinal degeneration without break (H35.4-)

● **H33.30 Unspecified retinal break**
  H33.301 Unspecified retinal break, **right eye**
  H33.302 Unspecified retinal break, **left eye**
  H33.303 Unspecified retinal break, **bilateral**
  H33.309 Unspecified retinal break, **unspecified eye**
● **H33.31 Horseshoe tear of retina without detachment**
  Operculum of retina without detachment
  H33.311 Horseshoe tear of retina without detachment, **right eye**
  H33.312 Horseshoe tear of retina without detachment, **left eye**
  H33.313 Horseshoe tear of retina without detachment, **bilateral**
  H33.319 Horseshoe tear of retina without detachment, **unspecified eye**
● **H33.32 Round hole of retina without detachment**
  H33.321 Round hole, **right eye**
  H33.322 Round hole, **left eye**
  H33.323 Round hole, **bilateral**
  H33.329 Round hole, **unspecified eye**
● **H33.33 Multiple defects of retina without detachment**
  H33.331 Multiple defects of retina without detachment, **right eye**
  H33.332 Multiple defects of retina without detachment, **left eye**
  H33.333 Multiple defects of retina without detachment, **bilateral**
  H33.339 Multiple defects of retina without detachment, **unspecified eye**
● **H33.4 Traction detachment of retina**
  Proliferative vitreo-retinopathy with retinal detachment
  H33.40 Traction detachment of retina, **unspecified eye**
  H33.41 Traction detachment of retina, **right eye**
  H33.42 Traction detachment of retina, **left eye**
  H33.43 Traction detachment of retina, **bilateral**
H33.8 Other retinal detachments

● **H34 Retinal vascular occlusions**
  Blockage in vessel of the retina
  Excludes1 amaurosis fugax (G45.3)
● **H34.0 Transient retinal artery occlusion**
  H34.00 Transient retinal artery occlusion, **unspecified eye**
  H34.01 Transient retinal artery occlusion, **right eye**
  H34.02 Transient retinal artery occlusion, **left eye**
  H34.03 Transient retinal artery occlusion, **bilateral**
● **H34.1 Central retinal artery occlusion**
  H34.10 Central retinal artery occlusion, **unspecified** eye
  H34.11 Central retinal artery occlusion, **right eye**
  H34.12 Central retinal artery occlusion, **left eye**
  H34.13 Central retinal artery occlusion, **bilateral**
● **H34.2 Other retinal artery occlusions**
  ● **H34.21 Partial retinal artery occlusion**
    Hollenhorst's plaque
    Retinal microembolism
    H34.211 Partial retinal artery occlusion, **right eye**
    H34.212 Partial retinal artery occlusion, **left eye**
    H34.213 Partial retinal artery occlusion, **bilateral**
    H34.219 Partial retinal artery occlusion, **unspecified eye**

● H34.23   **Retinal artery branch occlusion**
    H34.231   Retinal artery branch occlusion, **right** eye
    H34.232   Retinal artery branch occlusion, **left** eye
    H34.233   Retinal artery branch occlusion, **bilateral**
    H34.239   Retinal artery branch occlusion, **unspecified eye**

● H34.8   **Other retinal vascular occlusions**
    Coding Clinic: 2016, Q4, P19

● H34.81   **Central retinal vein occlusion**

    One of the following 7th characters is to be assigned to codes in subcategory H34.81 to designate the severity of the occlusion:

> 0   with macular edema
> 1   with retinal neovascularization
> 2   stable
>   Old central retinal vein occlusion

  ● H34.811   **Central retinal vein occlusion, right** eye
  ● H34.812   **Central retinal vein occlusion, left** eye
  ● H34.813   **Central retinal vein occlusion, bilateral**
  ● H34.819   **Central retinal vein occlusion, unspecified eye**

● H34.82   **Venous engorgement**
    Incipient retinal vein occlusion
    Partial retinal vein occlusion
    H34.821   Venous engorgement, **right** eye
    H34.822   Venous engorgement, **left** eye
    H34.823   Venous engorgement, **bilateral**
    H34.829   Venous engorgement, **unspecified** eye

● H34.83   **Tributary (branch) retinal vein occlusion**

    One of the following 7th characters is to be assigned to codes in subcategory H34.83 to designate the severity of the occlusion:

> 0   with macular edema
> 1   with retinal neovascularization
> 2   stable
>   Old tributary (branch) retinal vein occlusion

  ● H34.831   **Tributary (branch) retinal vein occlusion, right** eye
  ● H34.832   **Tributary (branch) retinal vein occlusion, left** eye
  ● H34.833   **Tributary (branch) retinal vein occlusion, bilateral**
  ● H34.839   **Tributary (branch) retinal vein occlusion, unspecified** eye

    H34.9   **Unspecified retinal vascular occlusion**

● H35   **Other retinal disorders**

  Excludes2   diabetic retinal disorders (E08.311–E08.359, E09.311–E09.359, E10.311–E10.359, E11.311–E11.359, E13.311–E13.359)

● H35.0   **Background retinopathy and retinal vascular changes**
    Code also any associated hypertension (I10)
    OGCR Section I. C.9.a.5.

    Hypertensive Retinopathy
    Subcategory H35.0, Background retinopathy and retinal vascular changes, should be used with a code from category I10–I15, Hypertensive disease to include the systemic hypertension. The sequencing is based on the reason for the encounter.

● H35.00   **Unspecified background retinopathy**
● H35.01   **Changes in retinal vascular appearance**
    Retinal vascular sheathing
    H35.011   Changes in retinal vascular appearance, **right** eye
    H35.012   Changes in retinal vascular appearance, **left** eye
    H35.013   Changes in retinal vascular appearance, **bilateral**
    H35.019   Changes in retinal vascular appearance, **unspecified** eye

● H35.02   **Exudative retinopathy**
    Coats retinopathy
    H35.021   Exudative retinopathy, **right** eye
    H35.022   Exudative retinopathy, **left** eye
    H35.023   Exudative retinopathy, **bilateral**
    H35.029   Exudative retinopathy, **unspecified** eye

● H35.03   **Hypertensive retinopathy**
    H35.031   Hypertensive retinopathy, **right** eye
    H35.032   Hypertensive retinopathy, **left** eye
    H35.033   Hypertensive retinopathy, **bilateral**
    H35.039   Hypertensive retinopathy, **unspecified** eye

● H35.04   **Retinal micro-aneurysms, unspecified**
    H35.041   Retinal micro-aneurysms, unspecified, **right** eye
    H35.042   Retinal micro-aneurysms, unspecified, **left** eye
    H35.043   Retinal micro-aneurysms, unspecified, **bilateral**
    H35.049   Retinal micro-aneurysms, unspecified, **unspecified** eye

● H35.05   **Retinal neovascularization, unspecified**
    H35.051   Retinal neovascularization, unspecified, **right** eye
    H35.052   Retinal neovascularization, unspecified, **left** eye
    H35.053   Retinal neovascularization, unspecified, **bilateral**
    H35.059   Retinal neovascularization, unspecified, **unspecified** eye

● H35.06   **Retinal vasculitis**
    Eales disease
    Retinal perivasculitis
    H35.061   Retinal vasculitis, **right** eye
    H35.062   Retinal vasculitis, **left** eye
    H35.063   Retinal vasculitis, **bilateral**
    H35.069   Retinal vasculitis, **unspecified** eye

● H35.07   **Retinal telangiectasis**
    H35.071   Retinal telangiectasis, **right** eye
    H35.072   Retinal telangiectasis, **left** eye
    H35.073   Retinal telangiectasis, **bilateral**
    H35.079   Retinal telangiectasis, **unspecified** eye

    H35.09   **Other intraretinal microvascular abnormalities**
    Retinal varices

● H35.1   **Retinopathy of prematurity**
● H35.10   **Retinopathy of prematurity, unspecified**
    Retinopathy of prematurity NOS
    H35.101   Retinopathy of prematurity, unspecified, **right** eye
    H35.102   Retinopathy of prematurity, unspecified, **left** eye
    H35.103   Retinopathy of prematurity, unspecified, **bilateral**
    H35.109   Retinopathy of prematurity, unspecified, **unspecified** eye

CHAPTER 7 (H00-H59)

- **H35.11   Retinopathy of prematurity, stage 0**
  - H35.111   Retinopathy of prematurity, stage 0, right eye
  - H35.112   Retinopathy of prematurity, stage 0, left eye
  - H35.113   Retinopathy of prematurity, stage 0, bilateral
  - H35.119   Retinopathy of prematurity, stage 0, unspecified eye
- **H35.12   Retinopathy of prematurity, stage 1**
  - H35.121   Retinopathy of prematurity, stage 1, right eye
  - H35.122   Retinopathy of prematurity, stage 1, left eye
  - H35.123   Retinopathy of prematurity, stage 1, bilateral
  - H35.129   Retinopathy of prematurity, stage 1, unspecified eye
- **H35.13   Retinopathy of prematurity, stage 2**
  - H35.131   Retinopathy of prematurity, stage 2, right eye
  - H35.132   Retinopathy of prematurity, stage 2, left eye
  - H35.133   Retinopathy of prematurity, stage 2, bilateral
  - H35.139   Retinopathy of prematurity, stage 2, unspecified eye
- **H35.14   Retinopathy of prematurity, stage 3**
  - H35.141   Retinopathy of prematurity, stage 3, right eye
  - H35.142   Retinopathy of prematurity, stage 3, left eye
  - H35.143   Retinopathy of prematurity, stage 3, bilateral
  - H35.149   Retinopathy of prematurity, stage 3, unspecified eye
- **H35.15   Retinopathy of prematurity, stage 4**
  - H35.151   Retinopathy of prematurity, stage 4, right eye
  - H35.152   Retinopathy of prematurity, stage 4, left eye
  - H35.153   Retinopathy of prematurity, stage 4, bilateral
  - H35.159   Retinopathy of prematurity, stage 4, unspecified eye
- **H35.16   Retinopathy of prematurity, stage 5**
  - H35.161   Retinopathy of prematurity, stage 5, right eye
  - H35.162   Retinopathy of prematurity, stage 5, left eye
  - H35.163   Retinopathy of prematurity, stage 5, bilateral
  - H35.169   Retinopathy of prematurity, stage 5, unspecified eye
- **H35.17   Retrolental fibroplasia**
  - H35.171   Retrolental fibroplasia, right eye
  - H35.172   Retrolental fibroplasia, left eye
  - H35.173   Retrolental fibroplasia, bilateral
  - H35.179   Retrolental fibroplasia, unspecified eye
- **H35.2   Other non-diabetic proliferative retinopathy**

  Proliferative vitreo-retinopathy

Excludes1	proliferative vitreo-retinopathy with retinal detachment (H33.4-)

  Thaslassemia proliferative retinopathy

Excludes2	proliferative sickle-cell retinopathy (H36.82-)

  - **H35.20   Other non-diabetic proliferative retinopathy, unspecified eye**

- H35.21   Other non-diabetic proliferative retinopathy, right eye
- H35.22   Other non-diabetic proliferative retinopathy, left eye
- H35.23   Other non-diabetic proliferative retinopathy, bilateral
- **H35.3   Degeneration of macula and posterior pole**
  - **H35.30   Unspecified macular degeneration**   A

    Age-related macular degeneration
  - **H35.31   Nonexudative age-related macular degeneration**

    Atrophic age-related macular degeneration

    Dry age-related macular degeneration

    One of the following 7th characters is to be assigned to codes in subcategory H35.31 to designate the stage of the disease:

0	stage unspecified
1	early dry stage
2	intermediate dry stage
3	advanced atrophic without subfoveal involvement advanced dry stage
4	advanced atrophic with subfoveal involvement

    - **H35.311   Nonexudative age-related macular degeneration, right eye**   A

      Coding Clinic: 2016, Q4, P20-21
    - **H35.312   Nonexudative age-related macular degeneration, left eye**   A

      Coding Clinic: 2016, Q4, P20-21
    - **H35.313   Nonexudative age-related macular degeneration, bilateral**   A

      Coding Clinic: 2016, Q4, P20
    - **H35.319   Nonexudative age-related macular degeneration, unspecified eye**   A

      Coding Clinic: 2016, Q4, P20
  - **H35.32   Exudative age-related macular degeneration**

    Wet age-related macular degeneration

    One of the following 7th characters is to be assigned to codes in subcategory H35.32 to designate the stage of the disease:

0	stage unspecified
1	with active choroidal neovascularization
2	with inactive choroidal neovascularization with involuted or regressed neovascularization
3	with inactive scar

    Coding Clinic: 2016, Q4, P20
    - **H35.321   Exudative age-related macular degeneration, right eye**   A
    - **H35.322   Exudative age-related macular degeneration, left eye**   A
    - **H35.323   Exudative age-related macular degeneration, bilateral**   A
    - **H35.329   Exudative age-related macular degeneration, unspecified eye**   A
  - H35.33   **Angioid streaks** of macula
  - **H35.34   Macular cyst, hole, or pseudohole**
    - H35.341   Macular cyst, hole, or pseudohole, right eye
    - H35.342   Macular cyst, hole, or pseudohole, left eye
    - H35.343   Macular cyst, hole, or pseudohole, bilateral
    - H35.349   Macular cyst, hole, or pseudohole, unspecified eye

---

▶ New   ⇒ Revised   ~~deleted~~ Deleted   Excludes 1   Excludes 2   Includes   Use additional   Code first   Code also   Key words

OGCR Official Guidelines   **X** Assign placeholder X   ● Use Additional Character(s)   ▶ Manifestation Code   Hierarchical Condition Category   **Coding Clinic**

Item 7–7 Macular degeneration is typically age-related, chronic, and is evidenced by deterioration of the macula (the part of the retina that provides for central field vision), resulting in blurred vision or a blind spot in the center of visual field while not affecting peripheral vision.

- ● H35.35   Cystoid macular degeneration
  - **Excludes1**   cystoid macular edema following cataract surgery (H59.03-)
  - H35.351   Cystoid macular degeneration, right eye
  - H35.352   Cystoid macular degeneration, left eye
  - H35.353   Cystoid macular degeneration, bilateral
  - H35.359   Cystoid macular degeneration, unspecified eye
- ● H35.36   Drusen (degenerative) of macula
  - H35.361   Drusen (degenerative) of macula, right eye
    - **Coding Clinic: 2016, Q4, P21**
  - H35.362   Drusen (degenerative) of macula, left eye
    - **Coding Clinic: 2016, Q4, P21**
  - H35.363   Drusen (degenerative) of macula, bilateral
    - **Coding Clinic: 2017, Q1, P51**
  - H35.369   Drusen (degenerative) of macula, unspecified eye
- ● H35.37   Puckering of macula
  - H35.371   Puckering of macula, right eye
  - H35.372   Puckering of macula, left eye
  - H35.373   Puckering of macula, bilateral
  - H35.379   Puckering of macula, unspecified eye
- ● H35.38   Toxic maculopathy
  - *Code first* poisoning due to drug or toxin, if applicable (T36-T65 with fifth or sixth character 1-4)
  - **Use additional** code for adverse effect, if applicable, to identify drug (T36-T50 with fifth or sixth character 5)
  - H35.381   Toxic maculopathy, right eye
  - H35.382   Toxic maculopathy, left eye
  - H35.383   Toxic maculopathy, bilateral
  - H35.389   Toxic maculopathy, unspecified eye
- ● H35.4   Peripheral retinal degeneration
  - ~~**Excludes1** hereditary retinal degeneration (dystrophy) (H35.5-)~~
    ~~peripheral retinal degeneration with retinal break (H33.3-)~~
  - ▶ **Excludes2**   hereditary retinal degeneration (dystrophy) (H35.5-)
    - ▶ peripheral retinal degeneration with retinal break (H33.3-)
  - H35.40   Unspecified peripheral retinal degeneration
- ● H35.41   Lattice degeneration of retina
  - Palisade degeneration of retina
  - H35.411   Lattice degeneration of retina, right eye
  - H35.412   Lattice degeneration of retina, left eye
  - H35.413   Lattice degeneration of retina, bilateral
  - H35.419   Lattice degeneration of retina, unspecified eye
- ● H35.42   Microcystoid degeneration of retina
  - H35.421   Microcystoid degeneration of retina, right eye
  - H35.422   Microcystoid degeneration of retina, left eye
  - H35.423   Microcystoid degeneration of retina, bilateral
  - H35.429   Microcystoid degeneration of retina, unspecified eye
- ● H35.43   Paving stone degeneration of retina
  - H35.431   Paving stone degeneration of retina, right eye
  - H35.432   Paving stone degeneration of retina, left eye
  - H35.433   Paving stone degeneration of retina, bilateral
  - H35.439   Paving stone degeneration of retina, unspecified eye
- ● H35.44   Age-related reticular degeneration of retina
  - H35.441   Age-related reticular degeneration of retina, right eye   **A**
  - H35.442   Age-related reticular degeneration of retina, left eye   **A**
  - H35.443   Age-related reticular degeneration of retina, bilateral   **A**
  - H35.449   Age-related reticular degeneration of retina, unspecified eye   **A**
- ● H35.45   Secondary pigmentary degeneration
  - H35.451   Secondary pigmentary degeneration, right eye
  - H35.452   Secondary pigmentary degeneration, left eye
  - H35.453   Secondary pigmentary degeneration, bilateral
  - H35.459   Secondary pigmentary degeneration, unspecified eye
- ● H35.46   Secondary vitreoretinal degeneration
  - H35.461   Secondary vitreoretinal degeneration, right eye
  - H35.462   Secondary vitreoretinal degeneration, left eye
  - H35.463   Secondary vitreoretinal degeneration, bilateral
  - H35.469   Secondary vitreoretinal degeneration, unspecified eye
- ● H35.5   Hereditary retinal dystrophy
  - **Excludes1**   dystrophies primarily involving Bruch's membrane (H31.1-)
  - H35.50   Unspecified hereditary retinal dystrophy
  - H35.51   Vitreoretinal dystrophy
  - H35.52   Pigmentary retinal dystrophy
    - Albipunctate retinal dystrophy
    - Retinitis pigmentosa
    - Tapetoretinal dystrophy
  - H35.53   Other dystrophies primarily involving the sensory retina
    - Stargardt's disease
  - H35.54   Dystrophies primarily involving the retinal pigment epithelium
    - Vitelliform retinal dystrophy
- ● H35.6   Retinal hemorrhage
  - H35.60   Retinal hemorrhage, unspecified eye
  - H35.61   Retinal hemorrhage, right eye
  - H35.62   Retinal hemorrhage, left eye
  - H35.63   Retinal hemorrhage, bilateral
- ● H35.7   Separation of retinal layers
  - **Excludes1**   retinal detachment (serous) (H33.2-)
    - rhegmatogenous retinal detachment (H33.0-)
  - H35.70   Unspecified separation of retinal layers
- ● H35.71   Central serous chorioretinopathy
  - H35.711   Central serous chorioretinopathy, right eye
  - H35.712   Central serous chorioretinopathy, left eye

CHAPTER 7 (H00-H59)

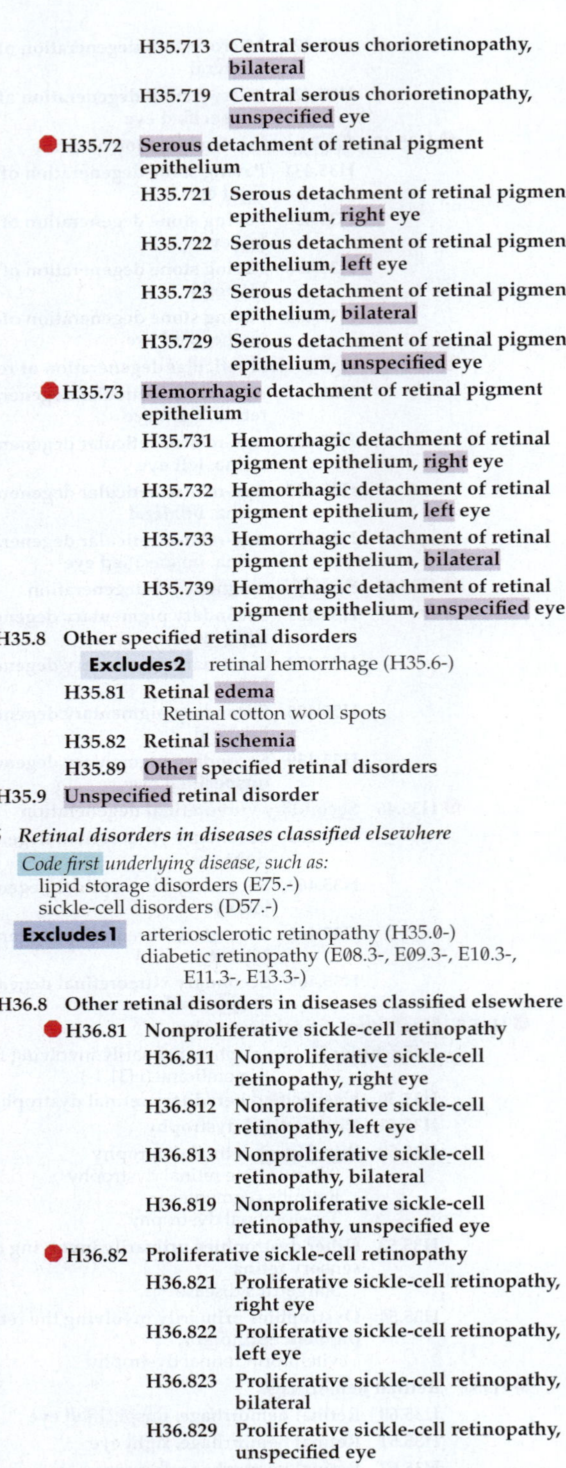

H35.713   Central serous chorioretinopathy, **bilateral**

H35.719   Central serous chorioretinopathy, **unspecified** eye

● **H35.72**   **Serous** detachment of retinal pigment epithelium

H35.721   Serous detachment of retinal pigment epithelium, **right eye**

H35.722   Serous detachment of retinal pigment epithelium, **left eye**

H35.723   Serous detachment of retinal pigment epithelium, **bilateral**

H35.729   Serous detachment of retinal pigment epithelium, **unspecified** eye

● **H35.73**   **Hemorrhagic** detachment of retinal pigment epithelium

H35.731   Hemorrhagic detachment of retinal pigment epithelium, **right eye**

H35.732   Hemorrhagic detachment of retinal pigment epithelium, **left eye**

H35.733   Hemorrhagic detachment of retinal pigment epithelium, **bilateral**

H35.739   Hemorrhagic detachment of retinal pigment epithelium, **unspecified** eye

● **H35.8**   **Other specified retinal disorders**

Excludes2   retinal hemorrhage (H35.6-)

H35.81   Retinal **edema**
Retinal cotton wool spots

H35.82   Retinal **ischemia**

H35.89   **Other** specified retinal disorders

H35.9   **Unspecified retinal disorder**

▶● **H36**   *Retinal disorders in diseases classified elsewhere*

Code first *underlying disease, such as:*
lipid storage disorders (E75.-)
sickle-cell disorders (D57.-)

Excludes1   arteriosclerotic retinopathy (H35.0-)
diabetic retinopathy (E08.3-, E09.3-, E10.3-, E11.3-, E13.3-)

● **H36.8**   **Other retinal disorders in diseases classified elsewhere**

● **H36.81**   **Nonproliferative sickle-cell retinopathy**

H36.811   Nonproliferative sickle-cell retinopathy, right eye

H36.812   Nonproliferative sickle-cell retinopathy, left eye

H36.813   Nonproliferative sickle-cell retinopathy, bilateral

H36.819   Nonproliferative sickle-cell retinopathy, unspecified eye

● **H36.82**   **Proliferative sickle-cell retinopathy**

H36.821   Proliferative sickle-cell retinopathy, right eye

H36.822   Proliferative sickle-cell retinopathy, left eye

H36.823   Proliferative sickle-cell retinopathy, bilateral

H36.829   Proliferative sickle-cell retinopathy, unspecified eye

● **H36.89**   **Other retinal disorders in diseases classified elsewhere**
Retinal dystrophy in lipid storage disorders

GLAUCOMA (H40-H42)

● **H40**   **Glaucoma**
Intraocular pressure (IOP) that is too high results from too much aqueous humor and because of excess production or inadequate drainage, optic nerve damage and vision loss may occur.

Excludes1   absolute glaucoma (H44.51-)
congenital glaucoma (Q15.0)
traumatic glaucoma due to birth injury (P15.3)

● **H40.0**   **Glaucoma suspect**

● **H40.00**   **Preglaucoma, unspecified**

H40.001   Preglaucoma, unspecified, **right** eye

H40.002   Preglaucoma, unspecified, **left** eye

H40.003   Preglaucoma, unspecified, **bilateral**

H40.009   Preglaucoma, unspecified, **unspecified** eye

● **H40.01**   **Open angle** with borderline findings, **low risk**
Open angle, low risk

H40.011   Open angle with borderline findings, low risk, **right eye**

H40.012   Open angle with borderline findings, low risk, **left eye**

H40.013   Open angle with borderline findings, low risk, **bilateral**

H40.019   Open angle with borderline findings, low risk, **unspecified eye**

● **H40.02**   **Open angle** with borderline findings, **high risk**
Open angle, high risk

H40.021   Open angle with borderline findings, high risk, **right eye**

H40.022   Open angle with borderline findings, high risk, **left eye**

H40.023   Open angle with borderline findings, high risk, **bilateral**

H40.029   Open angle with borderline findings, high risk, **unspecified eye**

● **H40.03**   **Anatomical narrow angle**
Primary angle closure suspect

H40.031   Anatomical narrow angle, **right eye**

H40.032   Anatomical narrow angle, **left eye**

H40.033   Anatomical narrow angle, **bilateral**

H40.039   Anatomical narrow angle, **unspecified** eye

● **H40.04**   **Steroid responder**

H40.041   Steroid responder, **right eye**

H40.042   Steroid responder, **left eye**

H40.043   Steroid responder, **bilateral**

H40.049   Steroid responder, **unspecified** eye

● **H40.05**   **Ocular hypertension**

H40.051   Ocular hypertension, **right eye**

H40.052   Ocular hypertension, **left eye**

H40.053   Ocular hypertension, **bilateral**

H40.059   Ocular hypertension, **unspecified** eye

● **H40.06**   **Primary angle closure without glaucoma damage**

H40.061   Primary angle closure without glaucoma damage, **right eye**

H40.062   Primary angle closure without glaucoma damage, **left eye**

H40.063   Primary angle closure without glaucoma damage, **bilateral**

H40.069   Primary angle closure without glaucoma damage, **unspecified** eye

● H40.1   **Open-angle glaucoma**
  X ● H40.10   **Unspecified open-angle glaucoma**
        One of the following 7th characters is to be
        assigned to code H40.10 to designate the
        stage of glaucoma

0	stage unspecified
1	mild stage
2	moderate stage
3	severe stage
4	indeterminate stage

  ● H40.11   **Primary open-angle glaucoma**
        Chronic simple glaucoma
        One of the following 7th characters is to be
        assigned to each code in subcategory
        H40.11 to designate the stage of
        glaucoma

0	stage unspecified
1	mild stage
2	moderate stage
3	severe stage
4	indeterminate stage

        Coding Clinic: 2016, Q4, P22
    ● H40.111   **Primary open-angle glaucoma, right
                eye**
                Coding Clinic: 2019, Q2, P31
    ● H40.112   **Primary open-angle glaucoma, left
                eye**
    ● H40.113   **Primary open-angle glaucoma,
                bilateral**
    ● H40.119   **Primary open-angle glaucoma,
                unspecified eye**
  ● H40.12   **Low-tension glaucoma**
        One of the following 7th characters is to be
        assigned to each code in subcategory
        H40.12 to designate the stage of
        glaucoma

0	stage unspecified
1	mild stage
2	moderate stage
3	severe stage
4	indeterminate stage

    ● H40.121   **Low-tension glaucoma, right eye**
    ● H40.122   **Low-tension glaucoma, left eye**
    ● H40.123   **Low-tension glaucoma, bilateral**
    ● H40.129   **Low-tension glaucoma, unspecified
                eye**
  ● H40.13   **Pigmentary glaucoma**
        One of the following 7th characters is to be
        assigned to each code in subcategory
        H40.13 to designate the stage of glaucoma

0	stage unspecified
1	mild stage
2	moderate stage
3	severe stage
4	indeterminate stage

    ● H40.131   **Pigmentary glaucoma, right eye**
    ● H40.132   **Pigmentary glaucoma, left eye**
    ● H40.133   **Pigmentary glaucoma, bilateral**
    ● H40.139   **Pigmentary glaucoma, unspecified
                eye**

● H40.14   **Capsular glaucoma with pseudoexfoliation of
            lens**
        One of the following 7th characters is to be
        assigned to each code in subcategory
        H40.14 to designate the stage of glaucoma

0	stage unspecified
1	mild stage
2	moderate stage
3	severe stage
4	indeterminate stage

    ● H40.141   **Capsular glaucoma with
                pseudoexfoliation of lens, right eye**
    ● H40.142   **Capsular glaucoma with
                pseudoexfoliation of lens, left eye**
    ● H40.143   **Capsular glaucoma with
                pseudoexfoliation of lens, bilateral**
    ● H40.149   **Capsular glaucoma with
                pseudoexfoliation of lens, unspecified
                eye**
  ● H40.15   **Residual stage of open-angle glaucoma**
    H40.151   **Residual stage of open-angle
                glaucoma, right eye**
    H40.152   **Residual stage of open-angle
                glaucoma, left eye**
    H40.153   **Residual stage of open-angle
                glaucoma, bilateral**
    H40.159   **Residual stage of open-angle
                glaucoma, unspecified eye**
● H40.2   **Primary angle-closure glaucoma**
      Excludes1   aqueous misdirection (H40.83-)
                      malignant glaucoma (H40.83-)
  X ● H40.20   **Unspecified primary angle-closure glaucoma**
        One of the following 7th characters is to be
        assigned to code H40.20 to designate the
        stage of glaucoma

0	stage unspecified
1	mild stage
2	moderate stage
3	severe stage
4	indeterminate stage

  ● H40.21   **Acute angle-closure glaucoma**
        Acute angle-closure glaucoma attack
        Acute angle-closure glaucoma crisis
    H40.211   **Acute angle-closure glaucoma, right
                eye**
    H40.212   **Acute angle-closure glaucoma, left
                eye**
    H40.213   **Acute angle-closure glaucoma,
                bilateral**
    H40.219   **Acute angle-closure glaucoma,
                unspecified eye**
  ● H40.22   **Chronic angle-closure glaucoma**
        Chronic primary angle closure glaucoma
        One of the following 7th characters is to be
        assigned to each code in subcategory
        H40.22 to designate the stage of
        glaucoma

0	stage unspecified
1	mild stage
2	moderate stage
3	severe stage
4	indeterminate stage

    ● H40.221   **Chronic angle-closure glaucoma, right
                eye**
    ● H40.222   **Chronic angle-closure glaucoma, left
                eye**

CHAPTER 7 (H00–H59)

● H40.223   Chronic angle-closure glaucoma, bilateral
● H40.229   Chronic angle-closure glaucoma, unspecified eye
● H40.23   Intermittent angle-closure glaucoma
    H40.231   Intermittent angle-closure glaucoma, right eye
    H40.232   Intermittent angle-closure glaucoma, left eye
    H40.233   Intermittent angle-closure glaucoma, bilateral
    H40.239   Intermittent angle-closure glaucoma, unspecified eye
● H40.24   Residual stage of angle-closure glaucoma
    H40.241   Residual stage of angle-closure glaucoma, right eye
    H40.242   Residual stage of angle-closure glaucoma, left eye
    H40.243   Residual stage of angle-closure glaucoma, bilateral
    H40.249   Residual stage of angle-closure glaucoma, unspecified eye

● H40.3   Glaucoma secondary to eye trauma
    Code also underlying condition
    One of the following 7th characters is to be assigned to each code in subcategory H40.3 to designate the stage of glaucoma

0	stage unspecified
1	mild stage
2	moderate stage
3	severe stage
4	indeterminate stage

    X ● H40.30   Glaucoma secondary to eye trauma, unspecified eye
    X ● H40.31   Glaucoma secondary to eye trauma, right eye
    X ● H40.32   Glaucoma secondary to eye trauma, left eye
    X ● H40.33   Glaucoma secondary to eye trauma, bilateral

● H40.4   Glaucoma secondary to eye inflammation
    Code also underlying condition
    One of the following 7th characters is to be assigned to each code in subcategory H40.4 to designate the stage of glaucoma

0	stage unspecified
1	mild stage
2	moderate stage
3	severe stage
4	indeterminate stage

    X ● H40.40   Glaucoma secondary to eye inflammation, unspecified eye
    X ● H40.41   Glaucoma secondary to eye inflammation, right eye
    X ● H40.42   Glaucoma secondary to eye inflammation, left eye
    X ● H40.43   Glaucoma secondary to eye inflammation, bilateral

● H40.5   Glaucoma secondary to other eye disorders
    Code also underlying eye disorder
    One of the following 7th characters is to be assigned to each code in subcategory H40.5 to designate the stage of glaucoma

0	stage unspecified
1	mild stage
2	moderate stage
3	severe stage
4	indeterminate stage

X ● H40.50   Glaucoma secondary to other eye disorders, unspecified eye
X ● H40.51   Glaucoma secondary to other eye disorders, right eye
X ● H40.52   Glaucoma secondary to other eye disorders, left eye
X ● H40.53   Glaucoma secondary to other eye disorders, bilateral

● H40.6   Glaucoma secondary to drugs
    Use additional code for adverse effect, if applicable, to identify drug (T36-T50 with fifth or sixth character 5)
    One of the following 7th characters is to be assigned to each code in subcategory H40.6 to designate the stage of glaucoma

0	stage unspecified
1	mild stage
2	moderate stage
3	severe stage
4	indeterminate stage

X ● H40.60   Glaucoma secondary to drugs, unspecified eye
X ● H40.61   Glaucoma secondary to drugs, right eye
X ● H40.62   Glaucoma secondary to drugs, left eye
X ● H40.63   Glaucoma secondary to drugs, bilateral

● H40.8   Other glaucoma
    ● H40.81   Glaucoma with increased episcleral venous pressure
        H40.811   Glaucoma with increased episcleral venous pressure, right eye
        H40.812   Glaucoma with increased episcleral venous pressure, left eye
        H40.813   Glaucoma with increased episcleral venous pressure, bilateral
        H40.819   Glaucoma with increased episcleral venous pressure, unspecified eye
    ● H40.82   Hypersecretion glaucoma
        H40.821   Hypersecretion glaucoma, right eye
        H40.822   Hypersecretion glaucoma, left eye
        H40.823   Hypersecretion glaucoma, bilateral
        H40.829   Hypersecretion glaucoma, unspecified eye
    ● H40.83   Aqueous misdirection
        Malignant glaucoma
        H40.831   Aqueous misdirection, right eye
        H40.832   Aqueous misdirection, left eye
        H40.833   Aqueous misdirection, bilateral
        H40.839   Aqueous misdirection, unspecified eye
    ▶ ● H40.84   Neovascular secondary angle closure glaucoma
        Code first the underlying condition such as:
        ▶ central retinal vein occlusion (H34.81)
        ▶ diabetes mellitus (E08.39, E09.39, E10.39, E11.39, E13.39)
        ▶ retinal ischemia (H35.82)
        ▶   H40.841 Neovascular secondary angle closure glaucoma, right eye
        ▶   H40.842 Neovascular secondary angle closure glaucoma, left eye
        ▶   H40.843 Neovascular secondary angle closure glaucoma, bilateral
        ▶   H40.849 Neovascular secondary angle closure glaucoma, unspecified eye
    H40.89   Other specified glaucoma
H40.9   Unspecified glaucoma

▶ New   ⇒ Revised   ~~deleted~~ Deleted   Excludes 1   Excludes 2   Includes   Use additional   Code first   Code also   Key words
OGCR Official Guidelines   X Assign placeholder X   ● Use Additional Character(s)   ▌ Manifestation Code   HCC Hierarchical Condition Category   Coding Clinic

H42 *Glaucoma in diseases classified elsewhere*

Code first underlying condition, such as:
amyloidosis (E85.-)
aniridia (Q13.1)
glaucoma (in) diabetes mellitus (E08.39, E09.39, E10.39, E11.39, E13.39)
Lowe's syndrome (E72.03)
Reiger anomaly (Q13.81)
specified metabolic disorder (E70-E88)

Excludes1 glaucoma (in) onchocerciasis (B73.02)
glaucoma (in) syphilis (A52.71)
glaucoma (in) tuberculous (A18.59)
▶neovascular secondary angle closure glaucoma (H40.84-)

DISORDERS OF VITREOUS BODY AND GLOBE (H43-H44)

● **H43** Disorders of vitreous body

● **H43.0** Vitreous prolapse

Excludes1 vitreous syndrome following cataract surgery (H59.0-)
traumatic vitreous prolapse (S05.2-)

    H43.00 Vitreous prolapse, unspecified eye
    H43.01 Vitreous prolapse, right eye
    H43.02 Vitreous prolapse, left eye
    H43.03 Vitreous prolapse, bilateral

● **H43.1** Vitreous hemorrhage
    H43.10 Vitreous hemorrhage, unspecified eye
    H43.11 Vitreous hemorrhage, right eye
    H43.12 Vitreous hemorrhage, left eye
    H43.13 Vitreous hemorrhage, bilateral

● **H43.2** Crystalline deposits in vitreous body
    H43.20 Crystalline deposits in vitreous body, unspecified eye
    H43.21 Crystalline deposits in vitreous body, right eye
    H43.22 Crystalline deposits in vitreous body, left eye
    H43.23 Crystalline deposits in vitreous body, bilateral

● **H43.3** Other vitreous opacities
●   **H43.31** Vitreous membranes and strands
    H43.311 Vitreous membranes and strands, right eye
    H43.312 Vitreous membranes and strands, left eye
    H43.313 Vitreous membranes and strands, bilateral
    H43.319 Vitreous membranes and strands, unspecified eye

●   **H43.39** Other vitreous opacities
Vitreous floaters
Small clumps of cells that float in the vitreous of the eye, appearing as black specks or dots in the field of vision and common in the aging eye.

    H43.391 Other vitreous opacities, right eye
    H43.392 Other vitreous opacities, left eye
    H43.393 Other vitreous opacities, bilateral
    H43.399 Other vitreous opacities, unspecified eye

● **H43.8** Other disorders of vitreous body

Excludes1 proliferative vitreo-retinopathy with retinal detachment (H33.4)

Excludes2 vitreous abscess (H44.02-)

●   **H43.81** Vitreous degeneration
Vitreous detachment
    H43.811 Vitreous degeneration, right eye
    H43.812 Vitreous degeneration, left eye
    H43.813 Vitreous degeneration, bilateral
    H43.819 Vitreous degeneration, unspecified eye

●   **H43.82** Vitreomacular adhesion
Vitreomacular traction
    H43.821 Vitreomacular adhesion, right eye A
    H43.822 Vitreomacular adhesion, left eye A
    H43.823 Vitreomacular adhesion, bilateral A
    H43.829 Vitreomacular adhesion, unspecified eye A

    H43.89 Other disorders of vitreous body
H43.9 Unspecified disorder of vitreous body

● **H44** Disorders of globe

Includes disorders affecting multiple structures of eye

● **H44.0** Purulent endophthalmitis

Use additional code to identify organism

Excludes1 bleb associated endophthalmitis (H59.4-)

●   **H44.00** Unspecified purulent endophthalmitis
    H44.001 Unspecified purulent endophthalmitis, right eye
    H44.002 Unspecified purulent endophthalmitis, left eye
    H44.003 Unspecified purulent endophthalmitis, bilateral
    H44.009 Unspecified purulent endophthalmitis, unspecified eye

●   **H44.01** Panophthalmitis (acute)
    H44.011 Panophthalmitis (acute), right eye
    H44.012 Panophthalmitis (acute), left eye
    H44.013 Panophthalmitis (acute), bilateral
    H44.019 Panophthalmitis (acute), unspecified eye

●   **H44.02** Vitreous abscess (chronic)
    H44.021 Vitreous abscess (chronic), right eye
    H44.022 Vitreous abscess (chronic), left eye
    H44.023 Vitreous abscess (chronic), bilateral
    H44.029 Vitreous abscess (chronic), unspecified eye

● **H44.1** Other endophthalmitis

Excludes1 bleb associated endophthalmitis (H59.4-)

Excludes2 ophthalmia nodosa (H16.2-)

●   **H44.11** Panuveitis
    H44.111 Panuveitis, right eye
    H44.112 Panuveitis, left eye
    H44.113 Panuveitis, bilateral
    H44.119 Panuveitis, unspecified eye

●   **H44.12** Parasitic endophthalmitis, unspecified
    H44.121 Parasitic endophthalmitis, unspecified, right eye
    H44.122 Parasitic endophthalmitis, unspecified, left eye
    H44.123 Parasitic endophthalmitis, unspecified, bilateral
    H44.129 Parasitic endophthalmitis, unspecified, unspecified eye

●   **H44.13** Sympathetic uveitis
    H44.131 Sympathetic uveitis, right eye
    H44.132 Sympathetic uveitis, left eye
    H44.133 Sympathetic uveitis, bilateral
    H44.139 Sympathetic uveitis, unspecified eye
    H44.19 Other endophthalmitis

CHAPTER 7 (H00-H59)

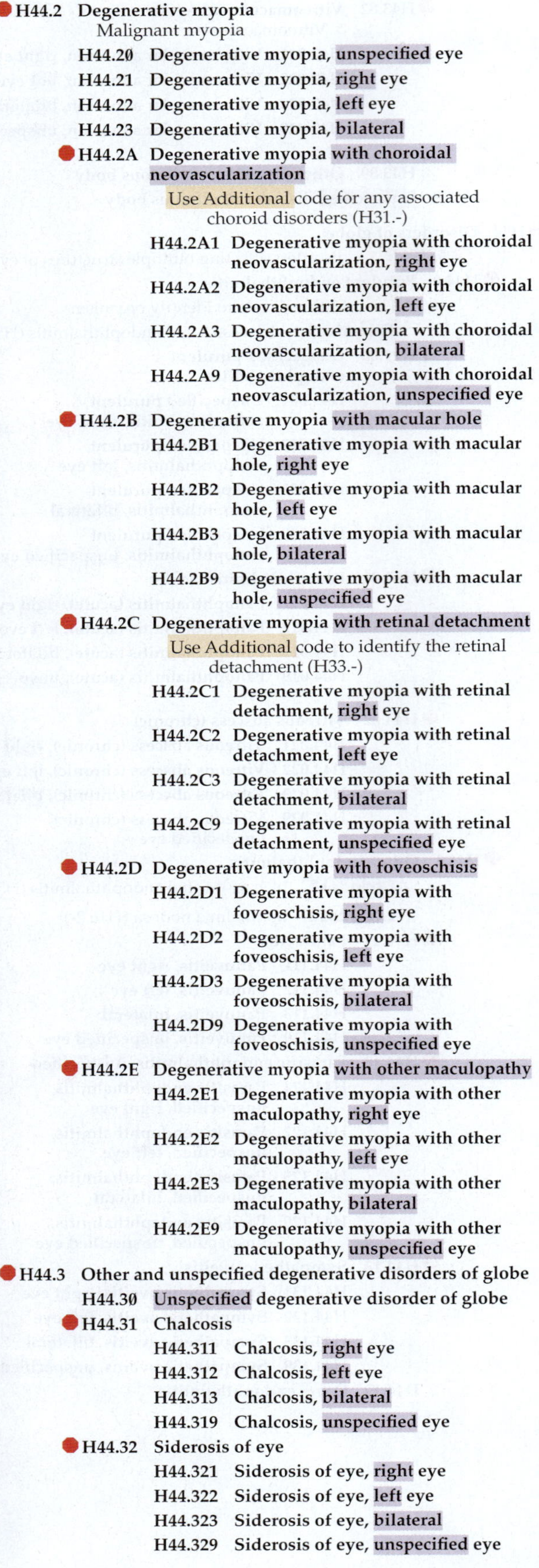

● **H44.2**   **Degenerative myopia**
    Malignant myopia

    H44.20   Degenerative myopia, unspecified eye

    H44.21   Degenerative myopia, right eye

    H44.22   Degenerative myopia, left eye

    H44.23   Degenerative myopia, bilateral

●   **H44.2A**   **Degenerative myopia with choroidal neovascularization**

      Use Additional code for any associated choroid disorders (H31.-)

    H44.2A1   Degenerative myopia with choroidal neovascularization, right eye

    H44.2A2   Degenerative myopia with choroidal neovascularization, left eye

    H44.2A3   Degenerative myopia with choroidal neovascularization, bilateral

    H44.2A9   Degenerative myopia with choroidal neovascularization, unspecified eye

●   **H44.2B**   **Degenerative myopia with macular hole**

    H44.2B1   Degenerative myopia with macular hole, right eye

    H44.2B2   Degenerative myopia with macular hole, left eye

    H44.2B3   Degenerative myopia with macular hole, bilateral

    H44.2B9   Degenerative myopia with macular hole, unspecified eye

●   **H44.2C**   **Degenerative myopia with retinal detachment**

      Use Additional code to identify the retinal detachment (H33.-)

    H44.2C1   Degenerative myopia with retinal detachment, right eye

    H44.2C2   Degenerative myopia with retinal detachment, left eye

    H44.2C3   Degenerative myopia with retinal detachment, bilateral

    H44.2C9   Degenerative myopia with retinal detachment, unspecified eye

●   **H44.2D**   **Degenerative myopia with foveoschisis**

    H44.2D1   Degenerative myopia with foveoschisis, right eye

    H44.2D2   Degenerative myopia with foveoschisis, left eye

    H44.2D3   Degenerative myopia with foveoschisis, bilateral

    H44.2D9   Degenerative myopia with foveoschisis, unspecified eye

●   **H44.2E**   **Degenerative myopia with other maculopathy**

    H44.2E1   Degenerative myopia with other maculopathy, right eye

    H44.2E2   Degenerative myopia with other maculopathy, left eye

    H44.2E3   Degenerative myopia with other maculopathy, bilateral

    H44.2E9   Degenerative myopia with other maculopathy, unspecified eye

● **H44.3**   **Other and unspecified degenerative disorders of globe**

    H44.30   Unspecified degenerative disorder of globe

●   **H44.31**   **Chalcosis**

    H44.311   Chalcosis, right eye

    H44.312   Chalcosis, left eye

    H44.313   Chalcosis, bilateral

    H44.319   Chalcosis, unspecified eye

●   **H44.32**   **Siderosis of eye**

    H44.321   Siderosis of eye, right eye

    H44.322   Siderosis of eye, left eye

    H44.323   Siderosis of eye, bilateral

    H44.329   Siderosis of eye, unspecified eye

●   **H44.39**   **Other degenerative disorders of globe**

    H44.391   Other degenerative disorders of globe, right eye

    H44.392   Other degenerative disorders of globe, left eye

    H44.393   Other degenerative disorders of globe, bilateral

    H44.399   Other degenerative disorders of globe, unspecified eye

● **H44.4**   **Hypotony of eye**

    H44.40   Unspecified hypotony of eye

●   **H44.41**   **Flat anterior chamber hypotony of eye**

    H44.411   Flat anterior chamber hypotony of right eye

    H44.412   Flat anterior chamber hypotony of left eye

    H44.413   Flat anterior chamber hypotony of eye, bilateral

    H44.419   Flat anterior chamber hypotony of unspecified eye

●   **H44.42**   **Hypotony of eye due to ocular fistula**

    H44.421   Hypotony of right eye due to ocular fistula

    H44.422   Hypotony of left eye due to ocular fistula

    H44.423   Hypotony of eye due to ocular fistula, bilateral

    H44.429   Hypotony of unspecified eye due to ocular fistula

●   **H44.43**   **Hypotony of eye due to other ocular disorders**

    H44.431   Hypotony of eye due to other ocular disorders, right eye

    H44.432   Hypotony of eye due to other ocular disorders, left eye

    H44.433   Hypotony of eye due to other ocular disorders, bilateral

    H44.439   Hypotony of eye due to other ocular disorders, unspecified eye

●   **H44.44**   **Primary hypotony of eye**

    H44.441   Primary hypotony of right eye

    H44.442   Primary hypotony of left eye

    H44.443   Primary hypotony of eye, bilateral

    H44.449   Primary hypotony of unspecified eye

● **H44.5**   **Degenerated conditions of globe**

    H44.50   Unspecified degenerated conditions of globe

●   **H44.51**   **Absolute glaucoma**

    H44.511   Absolute glaucoma, right eye

    H44.512   Absolute glaucoma, left eye

    H44.513   Absolute glaucoma, bilateral

    H44.519   Absolute glaucoma, unspecified eye

●   **H44.52**   **Atrophy of globe**
    Phthisis bulbi

    H44.521   Atrophy of globe, right eye

    H44.522   Atrophy of globe, left eye

    H44.523   Atrophy of globe, bilateral

    H44.529   Atrophy of globe, unspecified eye

●   **H44.53**   **Leucocoria**

    H44.531   Leucocoria, right eye

    H44.532   Leucocoria, left eye

    H44.533   Leucocoria, bilateral

    H44.539   Leucocoria, unspecified eye

● **H44.6**   **Retained (old) intraocular foreign body, magnetic**

> *Use additional* code to identify magnetic foreign body (Z18.11)
>
> **Excludes1**   current intraocular foreign body (S05.-)
>
> **Excludes2**   retained foreign body in eyelid (H02.81-)
> retained (old) foreign body following penetrating wound of orbit (H05.5-)
> retained (old) intraocular foreign body, nonmagnetic (H44.7-)

● **H44.60**   **Unspecified retained (old) intraocular foreign body, magnetic**

   H44.601   Unspecified retained (old) intraocular foreign body, magnetic, **right eye**

   H44.602   Unspecified retained (old) intraocular foreign body, magnetic, **left eye**

   H44.603   Unspecified retained (old) intraocular foreign body, magnetic, **bilateral**

   H44.609   Unspecified retained (old) intraocular foreign body, magnetic, **unspecified eye**

● **H44.61**   **Retained (old) magnetic foreign body in anterior chamber**

   H44.611   Retained (old) magnetic foreign body in anterior chamber, **right eye**

   H44.612   Retained (old) magnetic foreign body in anterior chamber, **left eye**

   H44.613   Retained (old) magnetic foreign body in anterior chamber, **bilateral**

   H44.619   Retained (old) magnetic foreign body in anterior chamber, **unspecified eye**

● **H44.62**   **Retained (old) magnetic foreign body in iris or ciliary body**

   H44.621   Retained (old) magnetic foreign body in iris or ciliary body, **right eye**

   H44.622   Retained (old) magnetic foreign body in iris or ciliary body, **left eye**

   H44.623   Retained (old) magnetic foreign body in iris or ciliary body, **bilateral**

   H44.629   Retained (old) magnetic foreign body in iris or ciliary body, **unspecified eye**

● **H44.63**   **Retained (old) magnetic foreign body in lens**

   H44.631   Retained (old) magnetic foreign body in lens, **right eye**

   H44.632   Retained (old) magnetic foreign body in lens, **left eye**

   H44.633   Retained (old) magnetic foreign body in lens, **bilateral**

   H44.639   Retained (old) magnetic foreign body in lens, **unspecified eye**

● **H44.64**   **Retained (old) magnetic foreign body in posterior wall of globe**

   H44.641   Retained (old) magnetic foreign body in posterior wall of globe, **right eye**

   H44.642   Retained (old) magnetic foreign body in posterior wall of globe, **left eye**

   H44.643   Retained (old) magnetic foreign body in posterior wall of globe, **bilateral**

   H44.649   Retained (old) magnetic foreign body in posterior wall of globe, **unspecified eye**

● **H44.65**   **Retained (old) magnetic foreign body in vitreous body**

   H44.651   Retained (old) magnetic foreign body in vitreous body, **right eye**

   H44.652   Retained (old) magnetic foreign body in vitreous body, **left eye**

   H44.653   Retained (old) magnetic foreign body in vitreous body, **bilateral**

   H44.659   Retained (old) magnetic foreign body in vitreous body, **unspecified eye**

● **H44.69**   **Retained (old) intraocular foreign body, magnetic, in other or multiple sites**

   H44.691   Retained (old) intraocular foreign body, magnetic, in other or multiple sites, **right eye**

   H44.692   Retained (old) intraocular foreign body, magnetic, in other or multiple sites, **left eye**

   H44.693   Retained (old) intraocular foreign body, magnetic, in other or multiple sites, **bilateral**

   H44.699   Retained (old) intraocular foreign body, magnetic, in other or multiple sites, **unspecified eye**

● **H44.7**   **Retained (old) intraocular foreign body, nonmagnetic**

> *Use additional* code to identify nonmagnetic foreign body (Z18.01-Z18.10, Z18.12, Z18.2-Z18.9)
>
> **Excludes1**   current intraocular foreign body (S05.-)
>
> **Excludes2**   retained foreign body in eyelid (H02.81-)
> retained (old) foreign body following penetrating wound of orbit (H05.5-)
> retained (old) intraocular foreign body, magnetic (H44.6-)

● **H44.70**   **Unspecified retained (old) intraocular foreign body, nonmagnetic**

   H44.701   Unspecified retained (old) intraocular foreign body, nonmagnetic, **right eye**

   H44.702   Unspecified retained (old) intraocular foreign body, nonmagnetic, **left eye**

   H44.703   Unspecified retained (old) intraocular foreign body, nonmagnetic, **bilateral**

   H44.709   Unspecified retained (old) intraocular foreign body, nonmagnetic, **unspecified eye**

> Retained (old) intraocular foreign body NOS

● **H44.71**   **Retained (nonmagnetic) (old) foreign body in anterior chamber**

   H44.711   Retained (nonmagnetic) (old) foreign body in anterior chamber, **right eye**

   H44.712   Retained (nonmagnetic) (old) foreign body in anterior chamber, **left eye**

   H44.713   Retained (nonmagnetic) (old) foreign body in anterior chamber, **bilateral**

   H44.719   Retained (nonmagnetic) (old) foreign body in anterior chamber, **unspecified eye**

● **H44.72**   **Retained (nonmagnetic) (old) foreign body in iris or ciliary body**

   H44.721   Retained (nonmagnetic) (old) foreign body in iris or ciliary body, **right eye**

   H44.722   Retained (nonmagnetic) (old) foreign body in iris or ciliary body, **left eye**

   H44.723   Retained (nonmagnetic) (old) foreign body in iris or ciliary body, **bilateral**

   H44.729   Retained (nonmagnetic) (old) foreign body in iris or ciliary body, **unspecified eye**

● **H44.73**   **Retained (nonmagnetic) (old) foreign body in lens**

   H44.731   Retained (nonmagnetic) (old) foreign body in lens, **right eye**

   H44.732   Retained (nonmagnetic) (old) foreign body in lens, **left eye**

   H44.733   Retained (nonmagnetic) (old) foreign body in lens, **bilateral**

   H44.739   Retained (nonmagnetic) (old) foreign body in lens, **unspecified eye**

CHAPTER 7 (H00-H59)

CHAPTER 7 (H00–H59)

● H44.74   Retained (nonmagnetic) (old) foreign body in posterior wall of globe
      H44.741   Retained (nonmagnetic) (old) foreign body in posterior wall of globe, right eye
      H44.742   Retained (nonmagnetic) (old) foreign body in posterior wall of globe, left eye
      H44.743   Retained (nonmagnetic) (old) foreign body in posterior wall of globe, bilateral
      H44.749   Retained (nonmagnetic) (old) foreign body in posterior wall of globe, unspecified eye

● H44.75   Retained (nonmagnetic) (old) foreign body in vitreous body
      H44.751   Retained (nonmagnetic) (old) foreign body in vitreous body, right eye
      H44.752   Retained (nonmagnetic) (old) foreign body in vitreous body, left eye
      H44.753   Retained (nonmagnetic) (old) foreign body in vitreous body, bilateral
      H44.759   Retained (nonmagnetic) (old) foreign body in vitreous body, unspecified eye

● H44.79   Retained (old) intraocular foreign body, nonmagnetic, in other or multiple sites
      H44.791   Retained (old) intraocular foreign body, nonmagnetic, in other or multiple sites, right eye
      H44.792   Retained (old) intraocular foreign body, nonmagnetic, in other or multiple sites, left eye
      H44.793   Retained (old) intraocular foreign body, nonmagnetic, in other or multiple sites, bilateral
      H44.799   Retained (old) intraocular foreign body, nonmagnetic, in other or multiple sites, unspecified eye

● H44.8   Other disorders of globe
  ● H44.81   Hemophthalmos
      H44.811   Hemophthalmos, right eye
      H44.812   Hemophthalmos, left eye
      H44.813   Hemophthalmos, bilateral
      H44.819   Hemophthalmos, unspecified eye
  ● H44.82   Luxation of globe
      H44.821   Luxation of globe, right eye
      H44.822   Luxation of globe, left eye
      H44.823   Luxation of globe, bilateral
      H44.829   Luxation of globe, unspecified eye
    H44.89   Other disorders of globe
H44.9   Unspecified disorder of globe

★ **(See Plate 7 of the Anatomy Illustrations.)**

DISORDERS OF OPTIC NERVE AND VISUAL PATHWAYS (H46-H47)

● H46   Optic neuritis
  Excludes2   ischemic optic neuropathy (H47.01-)
                neuromyelitis optica [Devic] (G36.0)
  ● H46.0   Optic papillitis
    H46.00   Optic papillitis, unspecified eye
    H46.01   Optic papillitis, right eye
    H46.02   Optic papillitis, left eye
    H46.03   Optic papillitis, bilateral

● H46.1   Retrobulbar neuritis
  Retrobulbar neuritis NOS
  Excludes1   syphilitic retrobulbar neuritis (A52.15)
    H46.10   Retrobulbar neuritis, unspecified eye
    H46.11   Retrobulbar neuritis, right eye
    H46.12   Retrobulbar neuritis, left eye
    H46.13   Retrobulbar neuritis, bilateral
H46.2   Nutritional optic neuropathy
H46.3   Toxic optic neuropathy
  Code first (T51-T65) to identify cause
H46.8   Other optic neuritis
H46.9   Unspecified optic neuritis
  Coding Clinic: 2023, Q3, P19

● H47   Other disorders of optic [2nd] nerve and visual pathways
  ● H47.0   Disorders of optic nerve, not elsewhere classified
    ● H47.01   Ischemic optic neuropathy
      H47.011   Ischemic optic neuropathy, right eye
      H47.012   Ischemic optic neuropathy, left eye
      H47.013   Ischemic optic neuropathy, bilateral
      H47.019   Ischemic optic neuropathy, unspecified eye
    ● H47.02   Hemorrhage in optic nerve sheath
      H47.021   Hemorrhage in optic nerve sheath, right eye
      H47.022   Hemorrhage in optic nerve sheath, left eye
      H47.023   Hemorrhage in optic nerve sheath, bilateral
      H47.029   Hemorrhage in optic nerve sheath, unspecified eye
    ● H47.03   Optic nerve hypoplasia
      H47.031   Optic nerve hypoplasia, right eye
      H47.032   Optic nerve hypoplasia, left eye
      H47.033   Optic nerve hypoplasia, bilateral
      H47.039   Optic nerve hypoplasia, unspecified eye
    ● H47.09   Other disorders of optic nerve, not elsewhere classified
      Compression of optic nerve
      H47.091   Other disorders of optic nerve, not elsewhere classified, right eye
      H47.092   Other disorders of optic nerve, not elsewhere classified, left eye
      H47.093   Other disorders of optic nerve, not elsewhere classified, bilateral
      H47.099   Other disorders of optic nerve, not elsewhere classified, unspecified eye
  ● H47.1   Papilledema
    H47.10   Unspecified papilledema
    H47.11   Papilledema associated with increased intracranial pressure
    H47.12   Papilledema associated with decreased ocular pressure
    H47.13   Papilledema associated with retinal disorder
  ● H47.14   Foster-Kennedy syndrome
      H47.141   Foster-Kennedy syndrome, right eye
      H47.142   Foster-Kennedy syndrome, left eye
      H47.143   Foster-Kennedy syndrome, bilateral
      H47.149   Foster-Kennedy syndrome, unspecified eye

▶ New   ▬▶ Revised   ~~deleted~~ Deleted   Excludes 1   Excludes 2   Includes   Use additional   Code first   Code also   Key words
OGCR Official Guidelines   X Assign placeholder X   ● Use Additional Character(s)   ▶ Manifestation Code   🞉 Hierarchical Condition Category   Coding Clinic

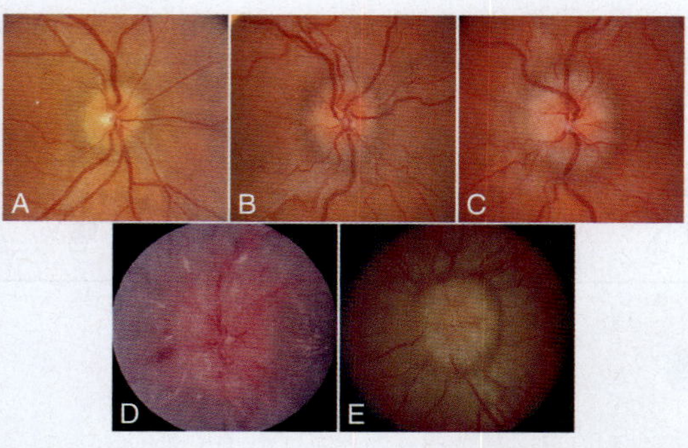

Figure 7-11 Stages of papilledema according to the Frisén grading scale. **A,** Very eary papilledema (Frisén stage 1). **B,** Early papilledema (Frisén stage 2). **C,** Moderate papilledema (Frisén stage 3). **D,** Marked papilledema (Frisén stage 4). **E,** Severe papilledema. (From Youmans JR, Winn HR: Youmans Neurological Surgery, Philadelphia, PA, Elsevier/Saunders, 2011)

Item 7–8 Papilledema is swelling of the optic disc caused by increased intracranial pressure. It is most often bilateral and occurs quickly (hours) or over weeks of time. It is a common symptom of a brain tumor. The term should not be used to describe optic disc swelling with underlying infectious, infiltrative, or inflammatory etiologies.

- ● H47.2 Optic atrophy
  - H47.20 Unspecified optic atrophy
  - ● H47.21 Primary optic atrophy
    - H47.211 Primary optic atrophy, right eye
    - H47.212 Primary optic atrophy, left eye
    - H47.213 Primary optic atrophy, bilateral
    - H47.219 Primary optic atrophy, unspecified eye
  - H47.22 Hereditary optic atrophy
    - Leber's optic atrophy
  - ● H47.23 Glaucomatous optic atrophy
    - H47.231 Glaucomatous optic atrophy, right eye
    - H47.232 Glaucomatous optic atrophy, left eye
    - H47.233 Glaucomatous optic atrophy, bilateral
    - H47.239 Glaucomatous optic atrophy, unspecified eye
  - ● H47.29 Other optic atrophy
    - Temporal pallor of optic disc
    - H47.291 Other optic atrophy, right eye
    - H47.292 Other optic atrophy, left eye
    - H47.293 Other optic atrophy, bilateral
    - H47.299 Other optic atrophy, unspecified eye
- ● H47.3 Other disorders of optic disc
  - ● H47.31 Coloboma of optic disc
    - H47.311 Coloboma of optic disc, right eye
    - H47.312 Coloboma of optic disc, left eye
    - H47.313 Coloboma of optic disc, bilateral
    - H47.319 Coloboma of optic disc, unspecified eye
  - ● H47.32 Drusen of optic disc
    - H47.321 Drusen of optic disc, right eye
    - H47.322 Drusen of optic disc, left eye
    - H47.323 Drusen of optic disc, bilateral
    - H47.329 Drusen of optic disc, unspecified eye
  - ● H47.33 Pseudopapilledema of optic disc
    - H47.331 Pseudopapilledema of optic disc, right eye
    - H47.332 Pseudopapilledema of optic disc, left eye
    - H47.333 Pseudopapilledema of optic disc, bilateral
    - H47.339 Pseudopapilledema of optic disc, unspecified eye
  - ● H47.39 Other disorders of optic disc
    - H47.391 Other disorders of optic disc, right eye
    - H47.392 Other disorders of optic disc, left eye
    - H47.393 Other disorders of optic disc, bilateral
    - H47.399 Other disorders of optic disc, unspecified eye
- ● H47.4 Disorders of optic chiasm
  - Code also underlying condition
  - H47.41 Disorders of optic chiasm in (due to) inflammatory disorders
  - H47.42 Disorders of optic chiasm in (due to) neoplasm
  - H47.43 Disorders of optic chiasm in (due to) vascular disorders
  - H47.49 Disorders of optic chiasm in (due to) other disorders
- ● H47.5 Disorders of other visual pathways
  - Disorders of optic tracts, geniculate nuclei and optic radiations
  - Code also underlying condition
  - ● H47.51 Disorders of visual pathways in (due to) inflammatory disorders
    - H47.511 Disorders of visual pathways in (due to) inflammatory disorders, right side
    - H47.512 Disorders of visual pathways in (due to) inflammatory disorders, left side
    - H47.519 Disorders of visual pathways in (due to) inflammatory disorders, unspecified side
  - ● H47.52 Disorders of visual pathways in (due to) neoplasm
    - H47.521 Disorders of visual pathways in (due to) neoplasm, right side
    - H47.522 Disorders of visual pathways in (due to) neoplasm, left side
    - H47.529 Disorders of visual pathways in (due to) neoplasm, unspecified side
  - ● H47.53 Disorders of visual pathways in (due to) vascular disorders
    - H47.531 Disorders of visual pathways in (due to) vascular disorders, right side
    - H47.532 Disorders of visual pathways in (due to) vascular disorders, left side
    - H47.539 Disorders of visual pathways in (due to) vascular disorders, unspecified side
- ● H47.6 Disorders of visual cortex
  - Code also underlying condition
  - Excludes1 injury to visual cortex S04.04-
  - ● H47.61 Cortical blindness
    - H47.611 Cortical blindness, right side of brain
    - H47.612 Cortical blindness, left side of brain
    - H47.619 Cortical blindness, unspecified side of brain

● **H47.62**   **Disorders of visual cortex in (due to) inflammatory disorders**
     H47.621   Disorders of visual cortex in (due to) inflammatory disorders, **right side of brain**
     H47.622   Disorders of visual cortex in (due to) inflammatory disorders, **left side of brain**
     H47.629   Disorders of visual cortex in (due to) inflammatory disorders, **unspecified** side of brain
● **H47.63**   Disorders of visual cortex in (due to) **neoplasm**
     H47.631   Disorders of visual cortex in (due to) neoplasm, **right side of brain**
     H47.632   Disorders of visual cortex in (due to) neoplasm, **left side of brain**
     H47.639   Disorders of visual cortex in (due to) neoplasm, **unspecified** side of brain
● **H47.64**   **Disorders of visual cortex in (due to) vascular disorders**
     H47.641   Disorders of visual cortex in (due to) vascular disorders, **right side of brain**
     H47.642   Disorders of visual cortex in (due to) vascular disorders, **left side of brain**
     H47.649   Disorders of visual cortex in (due to) vascular disorders, **unspecified** side of brain
H47.9   **Unspecified** disorder of visual pathways

DISORDERS OF OCULAR MUSCLES, BINOCULAR MOVEMENT, ACCOMMODATION AND REFRACTION (H49-H52)

Excludes2   nystagmus and other irregular eye movements (H55)

● **H49**   Paralytic strabismus
     Excludes2   internal ophthalmoplegia (H52.51-)
          internuclear ophthalmoplegia (H51.2-)
          progressive supranuclear ophthalmoplegia (G23.1)
● **H49.0**   Third [oculomotor] nerve palsy
     H49.00   Third [oculomotor] nerve palsy, **unspecified eye**
     H49.01   Third [oculomotor] nerve palsy, **right eye**
     H49.02   Third [oculomotor] nerve palsy, **left eye**
     H49.03   Third [oculomotor] nerve palsy, **bilateral**
● **H49.1**   Fourth [trochlear] nerve palsy
     H49.10   Fourth [trochlear] nerve palsy, **unspecified eye**
     H49.11   Fourth [trochlear] nerve palsy, **right eye**
     H49.12   Fourth [trochlear] nerve palsy, **left eye**
     H49.13   Fourth [trochlear] nerve palsy, **bilateral**
● **H49.2**   Sixth [abducent] nerve palsy
     H49.20   Sixth [abducent] nerve palsy, **unspecified eye**
     H49.21   Sixth [abducent] nerve palsy, **right eye**
     H49.22   Sixth [abducent] nerve palsy, **left eye**
     H49.23   Sixth [abducent] nerve palsy, **bilateral**
● **H49.3**   Total (external) ophthalmoplegia
     H49.30   Total (external) ophthalmoplegia, **unspecified eye**
     H49.31   Total (external) ophthalmoplegia, **right eye**
     H49.32   Total (external) ophthalmoplegia, **left eye**
     H49.33   Total (external) ophthalmoplegia, **bilateral**

Item 7-9   Strabismus or esotropia (crossed eyes) is a condition of the extraocular eye muscles, resulting in an inability of the eyes to focus and also affects depth perception.

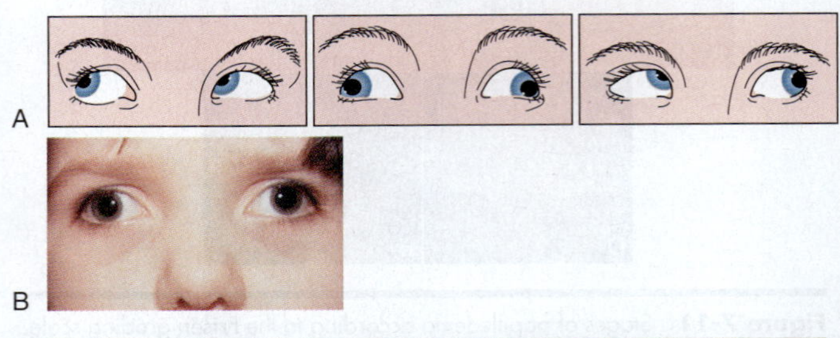

Figure 7-12   **A.** Image of strabismus. **B.** Exotropia. (**A** from Yanoff: Ophthalmology, ed 3, Mosby, Inc., 2008. **B** from Zitelli BJ, Davis HW, Pediatric Physical Diagnosis: Atlas of Pediatric Physical Diagnosis, Philadelphia, Elsevier Saunders, 2012)

● **H49.4**   Progressive external ophthalmoplegia
     Excludes1   Kearns-Sayre syndrome (H49.81-)
     H49.40   Progressive external ophthalmoplegia, **unspecified eye**
     H49.41   Progressive external ophthalmoplegia, **right eye**
     H49.42   Progressive external ophthalmoplegia, **left eye**
     H49.43   Progressive external ophthalmoplegia, **bilateral**
● **H49.8**   Other paralytic strabismus
●   **H49.81**   Kearns-Sayre syndrome
     Progressive external ophthalmoplegia with pigmentary retinopathy
     Code also, if applicable, other manifestations, such as:
         heart block (I45.9)
     H49.811   Kearns-Sayre syndrome, **right eye** ℍℂℂ
     H49.812   Kearns-Sayre syndrome, **left eye** ℍℂℂ
     H49.813   Kearns-Sayre syndrome, **bilateral** ℍℂℂ
     H49.819   Kearns-Sayre syndrome, **unspecified eye** ℍℂℂ
●   **H49.88**   Other paralytic strabismus
     External ophthalmoplegia NOS
     H49.881   Other paralytic strabismus, **right eye**
     H49.882   Other paralytic strabismus, **left eye**
     H49.883   Other paralytic strabismus, **bilateral**
     H49.889   Other paralytic strabismus, **unspecified** eye
H49.9   **Unspecified** paralytic strabismus

● **H50**   Other strabismus
●   **H50.0**   Esotropia
     Convergent concomitant strabismus
     Excludes1   intermittent esotropia (H50.31-, H50.32)
     H50.00   Unspecified esotropia
●   **H50.01**   Monocular esotropia
     H50.011   Monocular esotropia, **right eye**
     H50.012   Monocular esotropia, **left eye**
●   **H50.02**   Monocular esotropia with **A pattern**
     H50.021   Monocular esotropia with A pattern, **right eye**
     H50.022   Monocular esotropia with A pattern, **left eye**

▶ New   ⇨ Revised   ~~deleted~~ Deleted   Excludes 1   Excludes 2   Includes   Use additional   Code first   Code also   Key words
OGCR Official Guidelines   **X** Assign placeholder X   ● Use Additional Character(s)   ▶ Manifestation Code   ℍℂℂ Hierarchical Condition Category   **Coding Clinic**

- ● **H50.03**   Monocular esotropia with V pattern
  - **H50.031**   Monocular esotropia with V pattern, right eye
  - **H50.032**   Monocular esotropia with V pattern, left eye
- ● **H50.04**   Monocular esotropia with other noncomitancies
  - **H50.041**   Monocular esotropia with other noncomitancies, right eye
  - **H50.042**   Monocular esotropia with other noncomitancies, left eye
- **H50.05**   Alternating esotropia
- **H50.06**   Alternating esotropia with A pattern
- **H50.07**   Alternating esotropia with V pattern
- **H50.08**   Alternating esotropia with other noncomitancies
- ● **H50.1**   Exotropia

  Misalignment in which one eye deviates outward (away from nose) while the other fixates normally

  Divergent concomitant strabismus

  Excludes1   intermittent exotropia (H50.33-, H50.34)
  - **H50.10**   Unspecified exotropia
- ● **H50.11**   Monocular exotropia
  - **H50.111**   Monocular exotropia, right eye
  - **H50.112**   Monocular exotropia, left eye
- ● **H50.12**   Monocular exotropia with A pattern
  - **H50.121**   Monocular exotropia with A pattern, right eye
  - **H50.122**   Monocular exotropia with A pattern, left eye
- ● **H50.13**   Monocular exotropia with V pattern
  - **H50.131**   Monocular exotropia with V pattern, right eye
  - **H50.132**   Monocular exotropia with V pattern, left eye
- ● **H50.14**   Monocular exotropia with other noncomitancies
  - **H50.141**   Monocular exotropia with other noncomitancies, right eye
  - **H50.142**   Monocular exotropia with other noncomitancies, left eye
- **H50.15**   Alternating exotropia
- **H50.16**   Alternating exotropia with A pattern
- **H50.17**   Alternating exotropia with V pattern
- **H50.18**   Alternating exotropia with other noncomitancies
- ● **H50.2**   Vertical strabismus

  Hypertropia
  - **H50.21**   Vertical strabismus, right eye
  - **H50.22**   Vertical strabismus, left eye
- ● **H50.3**   Intermittent heterotropia

  Displacement of an organ or part of an organ from its normal position
  - **H50.30**   Unspecified intermittent heterotropia
- ● **H50.31**   Intermittent monocular esotropia
  - **H50.311**   Intermittent monocular esotropia, right eye
  - **H50.312**   Intermittent monocular esotropia, left eye
- **H50.32**   Intermittent alternating esotropia
- ● **H50.33**   Intermittent monocular exotropia
  - **H50.331**   Intermittent monocular exotropia, right eye
  - **H50.332**   Intermittent monocular exotropia, left eye
- **H50.34**   Intermittent alternating exotropia

- ● **H50.4**   Other and unspecified heterotropia
  - **H50.40**   Unspecified heterotropia
- ● **H50.41**   Cyclotropia
  - **H50.411**   Cyclotropia, right eye
  - **H50.412**   Cyclotropia, left eye
  - **H50.42**   Monofixation syndrome
  - **H50.43**   Accommodative component in esotropia
- ● **H50.5**   Heterophoria

  One or both eyes wander away from the position where both eyes are looking together in the same direction
  - **H50.50**   Unspecified heterophoria
  - **H50.51**   Esophoria

    Eye deviates inward (toward the nose)
  - **H50.52**   Exophoria

    Eye deviates outward (toward the ear)
  - **H50.53**   Vertical heterophoria
  - **H50.54**   Cyclophoria
  - **H50.55**   Alternating heterophoria
- ● **H50.6**   Mechanical strabismus
  - **H50.60**   Mechanical strabismus, unspecified
- ● **H50.61**   Brown's sheath syndrome
  - **H50.611**   Brown's sheath syndrome, right eye
  - **H50.612**   Brown's sheath syndrome, left eye
- ● **H50.62**   Inferior oblique muscle entrapment
  - **H50.621**   Inferior oblique muscle entrapment, right eye
  - **H50.622**   Inferior oblique muscle entrapment, left eye
  - **H50.629**   Inferior oblique muscle entrapment, unspecified eye
- ● **H50.63**   Inferior rectus muscle entrapment
  - **H50.631**   Inferior rectus muscle entrapment, right eye
  - **H50.632**   Inferior rectus muscle entrapment, left eye
  - **H50.639**   Inferior rectus muscle entrapment, unspecified eye
- ● **H50.64**   Lateral rectus muscle entrapment
  - **H50.641**   Lateral rectus muscle entrapment, right eye
  - **H50.642**   Lateral rectus muscle entrapment, left eye
  - **H50.649**   Lateral rectus muscle entrapment, unspecified eye
- ● **H50.65**   Medial rectus muscle entrapment
  - **H50.651**   Medial rectus muscle entrapment, right eye
  - **H50.652**   Medial rectus muscle entrapment, left eye
  - **H50.659**   Medial rectus muscle entrapment, unspecified eye
- ● **H50.66**   Superior oblique muscle entrapment
  - **H50.661**   Superior oblique muscle entrapment, right eye
  - **H50.662**   Superior oblique muscle entrapment, left eye
  - **H50.669**   Superior oblique muscle entrapment, unspecified eye
- ● **H50.67**   Superior rectus muscle entrapment
  - **H50.671**   Superior rectus muscle entrapment, right eye
  - **H50.672**   Superior rectus muscle entrapment, left eye
  - **H50.679**   Superior rectus muscle entrapment, unspecified eye

CHAPTER 7 (H00–H59)

● H50.68   Extraocular muscle entrapment, unspecified
     H50.681   Extraocular muscle entrapment, unspecified, **right eye**
     H50.682   Extraocular muscle entrapment, unspecified, **left eye**
     H50.689   Extraocular muscle entrapment, unspecified, **unspecified eye**
   H50.69   **Other mechanical strabismus**
     Strabismus due to adhesions
     Traumatic limitation of duction of eye muscle

● H50.8   Other specified strabismus
   ● H50.81   Duane's syndrome
     H50.811   Duane's syndrome, **right eye**
     H50.812   Duane's syndrome, **left eye**
   H50.89   Other specified strabismus
   H50.9   Unspecified strabismus

● **H51**   Other disorders of binocular movement
   H51.0   Palsy (spasm) of conjugate gaze
   ● H51.1   Convergence insufficiency and excess
     H51.11   Convergence **insufficiency**
     H51.12   Convergence **excess**
   ● H51.2   Internuclear ophthalmoplegia
     H51.20   Internuclear ophthalmoplegia, **unspecified eye**
     H51.21   Internuclear ophthalmoplegia, **right eye**
     H51.22   Internuclear ophthalmoplegia, **left eye**
     H51.23   Internuclear ophthalmoplegia, **bilateral**
   H51.8   Other specified disorders of binocular movement
   H51.9   Unspecified disorder of binocular movement

● **H52**   Disorders of refraction and accommodation
   ● H52.0   Hypermetropia
     H52.00   Hypermetropia, **unspecified** eye
     H52.01   Hypermetropia, **right eye**
     H52.02   Hypermetropia, **left eye**
     H52.03   Hypermetropia, **bilateral**
   ● H52.1   Myopia
     Excludes1   degenerative myopia (H44.2-)
     H52.10   Myopia, **unspecified** eye
     H52.11   Myopia, **right eye**
     H52.12   Myopia, **left eye**
     H52.13   Myopia, **bilateral**
   ● H52.2   Astigmatism
   ● H52.20   Unspecified astigmatism
     H52.201   Unspecified astigmatism, **right eye**
     H52.202   Unspecified astigmatism, **left eye**
     H52.203   Unspecified astigmatism, **bilateral**
     H52.209   Unspecified astigmatism, **unspecified** eye
   ● H52.21   Irregular astigmatism
     H52.211   Irregular astigmatism, **right eye**
     H52.212   Irregular astigmatism, **left eye**
     H52.213   Irregular astigmatism, **bilateral**
     H52.219   Irregular astigmatism, **unspecified eye**

● H52.22   Regular astigmatism
     H52.221   Regular astigmatism, **right eye**
     H52.222   Regular astigmatism, **left eye**
     H52.223   Regular astigmatism, **bilateral**
     H52.229   Regular astigmatism, **unspecified eye**
● H52.3   Anisometropia and aniseikonia
   H52.31   Anisometropia
   H52.32   Aniseikonia
   H52.4   Presbyopia
● H52.5   Disorders of accommodation
   ● H52.51   Internal ophthalmoplegia (complete) (total)
     H52.511   Internal ophthalmoplegia (complete) (total), **right eye**
     H52.512   Internal ophthalmoplegia (complete) (total), **left eye**
     H52.513   Internal ophthalmoplegia (complete) (total), **bilateral**
     H52.519   Internal ophthalmoplegia (complete) (total), **unspecified eye**
   ● H52.52   Paresis of accommodation
     H52.521   Paresis of accommodation, **right eye**
     H52.522   Paresis of accommodation, **left eye**
     H52.523   Paresis of accommodation, **bilateral**
     H52.529   Paresis of accommodation, **unspecified eye**
   ● H52.53   Spasm of accommodation
     H52.531   Spasm of accommodation, **right eye**
     H52.532   Spasm of accommodation, **left eye**
     H52.533   Spasm of accommodation, **bilateral**
     H52.539   Spasm of accommodation, **unspecified eye**
   H52.6   Other disorders of refraction
   H52.7   Unspecified disorder of refraction

VISUAL DISTURBANCES AND BLINDNESS (H53-H54)

● **H53**   Visual disturbances
   ● H53.0   Amblyopia ex anopsia
     ~~Excludes1~~   ~~amblyopia due to vitamin A deficiency (E50.5)~~
     ▶ **Excludes2**   strabismus (H50-)
   ● H53.00   Unspecified amblyopia
     H53.001   Unspecified amblyopia, **right eye**
     H53.002   Unspecified amblyopia, **left eye**
     H53.003   Unspecified amblyopia, **bilateral**
     H53.009   Unspecified amblyopia, **unspecified eye**
   ● H53.01   Deprivation amblyopia
     H53.011   Deprivation amblyopia, **right eye**
     H53.012   Deprivation amblyopia, **left eye**
     H53.013   Deprivation amblyopia, **bilateral**
     H53.019   Deprivation amblyopia, **unspecified eye**
   ● H53.02   Refractive amblyopia
     H53.021   Refractive amblyopia, **right eye**
     H53.022   Refractive amblyopia, **left eye**
     H53.023   Refractive amblyopia, **bilateral**
     H53.029   Refractive amblyopia, **unspecified eye**
   ● H53.03   Strabismic amblyopia
     Excludes1   strabismus (H50.-)
     H53.031   Strabismic amblyopia, **right eye**
     H53.032   Strabismic amblyopia, **left eye**
     H53.033   Strabismic amblyopia, **bilateral**
     H53.039   Strabismic amblyopia, **unspecified eye**

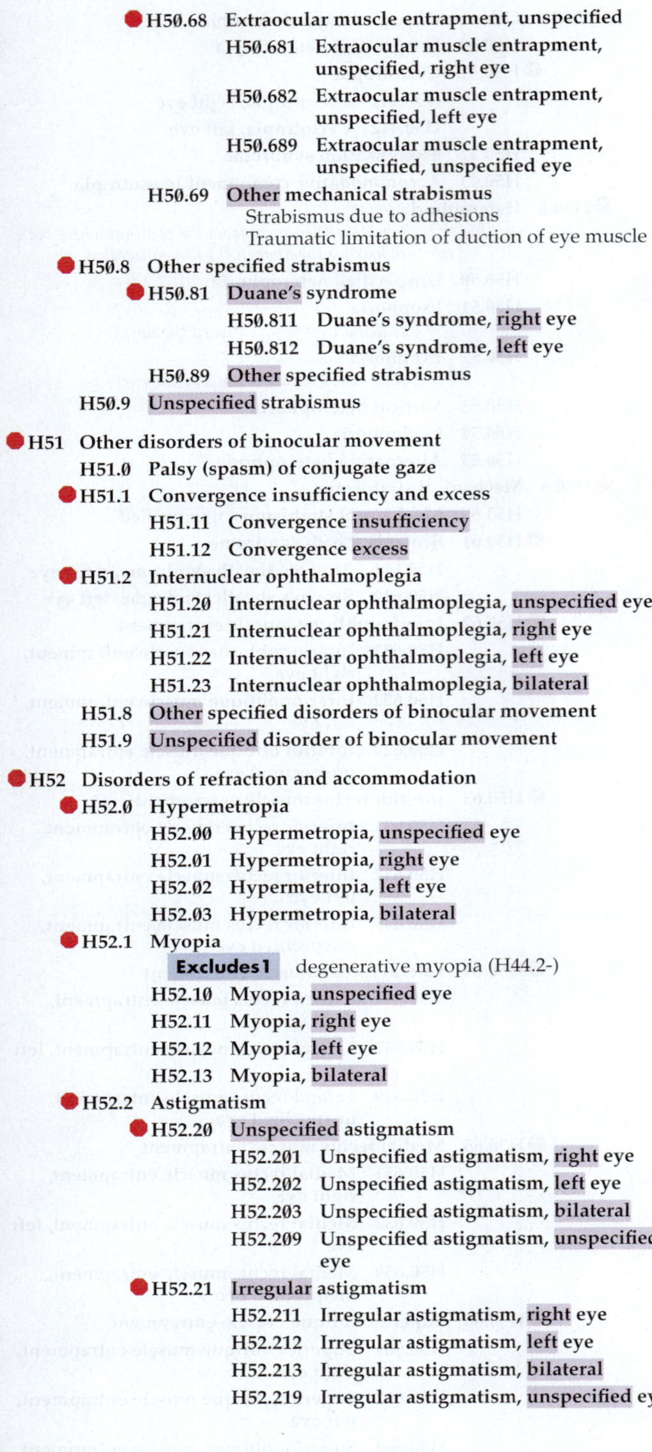

Item 7–10   Disorders of refraction: **Hypermetropia,** or farsightedness, means focus at a distance is adequate but not on close objects. **Myopia** is near-sightedness or short-sightedness and means the focus on nearby objects is clear but distant objects appear blurred. **Astigmatism** is warping of the curvature of the cornea so light rays entering do not meet a single focal point, resulting in a distorted image. **Anisometropia** is unequal refractive power in which one eye may be myopic (near-sighted) and the other hyperopic (far-sighted). **Presbyopia** is the loss of focus on near objects, which occurs with age because the lens loses elasticity.

▶ New   ⇨ Revised   ~~deleted~~ Deleted   Excludes 1   Excludes 2   Includes   Use additional   Code first   Code also   Key words
OGCR Official Guidelines   X Assign placeholder X   ● Use Additional Character(s)   ▸ Manifestation Code   Hierarchical Condition Category   Coding Clinic

● **H53.04　Amblyopia suspect**
　　Coding Clinic: 2016, Q4, P22

　　H53.041　Amblyopia suspect, right eye
　　H53.042　Amblyopia suspect, left eye
　　H53.043　Amblyopia suspect, bilateral
　　H53.049　Amblyopia suspect, unspecified eye

● **H53.1　Subjective visual disturbances**
　　Excludes1　subjective visual disturbances due to vitamin A deficiency (E50.5)
　　　　　　　　　visual hallucinations (R44.1)

　　H53.10　Unspecified subjective visual disturbances
　　H53.11　Day blindness
　　　　　　Hemeralopia
● 　H53.12　Transient visual loss
　　　　　　Scintillating scotoma
　　　　　　Excludes1　amaurosis fugax (G45.3-)
　　　　　　　　　　　　transient retinal artery occlusion (H34.0-)
　　　　　　Coding Clinic: 2022, Q1, P30

　　H53.121　Transient visual loss, right eye
　　H53.122　Transient visual loss, left eye
　　H53.123　Transient visual loss, bilateral
　　H53.129　Transient visual loss, unspecified eye
● 　H53.13　Sudden visual loss
　　H53.131　Sudden visual loss, right eye
　　H53.132　Sudden visual loss, left eye
　　H53.133　Sudden visual loss, bilateral
　　H53.139　Sudden visual loss, unspecified eye
● 　H53.14　Visual discomfort
　　　　　　Asthenopia
　　　　　　Photophobia
　　H53.141　Visual discomfort, right eye
　　H53.142　Visual discomfort, left eye
　　H53.143　Visual discomfort, bilateral
　　H53.149　Visual discomfort, unspecified
　　H53.15　Visual distortions of shape and size
　　　　　　Metamorphopsia
　　H53.16　Psychophysical visual disturbances
　　H53.19　Other subjective visual disturbances
　　　　　　Visual halos
　　　　　　Coding Clinic: 2022, Q1, P30

　H53.2　Diplopia
　　　　　Double vision
　　　　　Coding Clinic: 2022, Q3, P10
● H53.3　Other and unspecified disorders of binocular vision
　　H53.30　Unspecified disorder of binocular vision
　　H53.31　Abnormal retinal correspondence
　　H53.32　Fusion with defective stereopsis
　　H53.33　Simultaneous visual perception without fusion
　　H53.34　Suppression of binocular vision
● H53.4　Visual field defects
　　H53.40　Unspecified visual field defects
● 　H53.41　Scotoma involving central area
　　　　　　Central scotoma
　　H53.411　Scotoma involving central area, right eye
　　H53.412　Scotoma involving central area, left eye
　　H53.413　Scotoma involving central area, bilateral
　　H53.419　Scotoma involving central area, unspecified eye

● H53.42　Scotoma of blind spot area
　　　　　Enlarged blind spot
　　H53.421　Scotoma of blind spot area, right eye
　　H53.422　Scotoma of blind spot area, left eye
　　H53.423　Scotoma of blind spot area, bilateral
　　H53.429　Scotoma of blind spot area, unspecified eye
● H53.43　Sector or arcuate defects
　　　　　Arcuate scotoma
　　　　　Bjerrum scotoma
　　H53.431　Sector or arcuate defects, right eye
　　H53.432　Sector or arcuate defects, left eye
　　H53.433　Sector or arcuate defects, bilateral
　　H53.439　Sector or arcuate defects, unspecified eye
● H53.45　Other localized visual field defect
　　　　　Peripheral visual field defect
　　　　　Ring scotoma NOS
　　　　　Scotoma NOS
　　H53.451　Other localized visual field defect, right eye
　　H53.452　Other localized visual field defect, left eye
　　H53.453　Other localized visual field defect, bilateral
　　H53.459　Other localized visual field defect, unspecified eye
● H53.46　Homonymous bilateral field defects
　　　　　Homonymous hemianopia
　　　　　Homonymous hemianopsia
　　　　　Quadrant anopia
　　　　　Quadrant anopsia
　　H53.461　Homonymous bilateral field defects, right side
　　H53.462　Homonymous bilateral field defects, left side
　　H53.469　Homonymous bilateral field defects, unspecified side
　　　　　　Homonymous bilateral field defects NOS
　　H53.47　Heteronymous bilateral field defects
　　　　　　Heteronymous hemianop(s)ia
● H53.48　Generalized contraction of visual field
　　H53.481　Generalized contraction of visual field, right eye
　　H53.482　Generalized contraction of visual field, left eye
　　H53.483　Generalized contraction of visual field, bilateral
　　H53.489　Generalized contraction of visual field, unspecified eye
● H53.5　Color vision deficiencies
　　　　　Color blindness
　　　　　Excludes2　day blindness (H53.11)
　　H53.50　Unspecified color vision deficiencies
　　　　　　Color blindness NOS
　　H53.51　Achromatopsia
　　H53.52　Acquired color vision deficiency
　　H53.53　Deuteranomaly
　　　　　　Deuteranopia
　　H53.54　Protanomaly
　　　　　　Protanopia
　　H53.55　Tritanomaly
　　　　　　Tritanopia
　　H53.59　Other color vision deficiencies
● H53.6　Night blindness
　　　　　Excludes1　night blindness due to vitamin A deficiency (E50.5)
　　H53.60　Unspecified night blindness
　　H53.61　Abnormal dark adaptation curve

CHAPTER 7 (H00-H59)

H53.62   **Acquired night blindness**
H53.63   **Congenital night blindness**
H53.69   **Other night blindness**
● H53.7   **Vision sensitivity deficiencies**
    H53.71   **Glare sensitivity**
    H53.72   **Impaired contrast sensitivity**
H53.8   **Other visual disturbances**
H53.9   **Unspecified visual disturbance**

● H54   **Blindness and low vision**
    Note: For definition of visual impairment categories see table below.
    Code first any associated underlying cause of the blindness
    Excludes1   amaurosis fugax (G45.3)
● H54.0   **Blindness, both eyes**
    Visual impairment categories 3, 4, 5 in both eyes.
     ● H54.0X   **Blindness, both eyes, different category levels**
     H54.0X3   **Blindness right eye, category 3**
       H54.0X33   **Blindness right eye category 3, blindness left eye category 3**
       H54.0X34   **Blindness right eye category 3, blindness left eye category 4**
       H54.0X35   **Blindness right eye category 3, blindness left eye category 5**
     ● H54.0X4   **Blindness right eye, category 4**
       H54.0X43   **Blindness right eye category 4, blindness left eye category 3**
       H54.0X44   **Blindness right eye category 4, blindness left eye category 4**
       H54.0X45   **Blindness right eye category 4, blindness left eye category 5**
     ● H54.0X5   **Blindness right eye, category 5**
       H54.0X53   **Blindness right eye category 5, blindness left eye category 3**
       H54.0X54   **Blindness right eye category 5, blindness left eye category 4**
       H54.0X55   **Blindness right eye category 5, blindness left eye category 5**
● H54.1   **Blindness, one eye, low vision other eye**
    Visual impairment categories 3, 4, 5 in one eye, with categories 1 or 2 in the other eye.
    H54.10   **Blindness, one eye, low vision other eye, unspecified eyes**
     ● H54.11   **Blindness, right eye, low vision left eye**
       ● H54.113   **Blindness right eye category 3, low vision left eye**
       H54.1131   **Blindness right eye category 3, low vision left eye category 1**
       H54.1132   **Blindness right eye category 3, low vision left eye category 2**
       ● H54.114   **Blindness right eye category 4, low vision left eye**
       H54.1141   **Blindness right eye category 4, low vision left eye category 1**
       H54.1142   **Blindness right eye category 4, low vision left eye category 2**

● H54.115   **Blindness right eye category 5, low vision left eye**
     H54.1151   **Blindness right eye category 5, low vision left eye category 1**
     H54.1152   **Blindness right eye category 5, low vision left eye category 2**
● H54.12   **Blindness, left eye, low vision right eye**
    ● H54.121   **Low vision right eye category 1, blindness left eye**
     H54.1213   **Low vision right eye category 1, blindness left eye category 3**
     H54.1214   **Low vision right eye category 1, blindness left eye category 4**
     H54.1215   **Low vision right eye category 1, blindness left eye category 5**
    ● H54.122   **Low vision right eye category 2, blindness left eye**
     H54.1223   **Low vision right eye category 2, blindness left eye category 3**
     H54.1224   **Low vision right eye category 2, blindness left eye category 4**
     H54.1225   **Low vision right eye category 2, blindness left eye category 5**
● H54.2   **Low vision, both eyes**
    Visual impairment categories 1 or 2 in both eyes.
    ● H54.2X   **Low vision, both eyes, different category levels**
     ● H54.2X1   **Low vision, right eye, category 1**
     H54.2X11   **Low vision right eye category 1, low vision left eye category 1**
     H54.2X12   **Low vision right eye category 1, low vision left eye category 2**
     ● H54.2X2   **Low vision, right eye, category 2**
     H54.2X21   **Low vision right eye category 2, low vision left eye category 1**
     H54.2X22   **Low vision right eye category 2, low vision left eye category 2**
H54.3   **Unqualified visual loss, both eyes**
    Visual impairment category 9 in both eyes.
● H54.4   **Blindness, one eye**
    Visual impairment categories 3, 4, 5 in one eye [normal vision in other eye]
    H54.40   **Blindness, one eye, unspecified eye**
    ● H54.41   **Blindness, right eye, normal vision left eye**
     ● H54.413   **Blindness, right eye, category 3**
     H54.413A   **Blindness right eye category 3, normal vision left eye**
     ● H54.414   **Blindness, right eye, category 4**
     H54.414A   **Blindness right eye category 4, normal vision left eye**
     ● H54.415   **Blindness, right eye, category 5**
     H54.415A   **Blindness right eye category 5, normal vision left eye**

● **H54.42   Blindness, left eye, normal vision right eye**
　　● **H54.42A   Blindness, left eye, category 3-5**
　　　　H54.42A3   Blindness left eye category 3, normal vision right eye
　　　　H54.42A4   Blindness left eye category 4, normal vision right eye
　　　　H54.42A5   Blindness left eye category 5, normal vision right eye
● **H54.5   Low vision, one eye**
　　Visual impairment categories 1 or 2 in one eye [normal vision in other eye].
　　H54.50   Low vision, one eye, unspecified eye
　● **H54.51   Low vision, right eye, normal vision left eye**
　　● **H54.511   Low vision, right eye, category 1**
　　　　H54.511A   Low vision right eye category 1, normal vision left eye
　　● **H54.512   Low vision, right eye, category 2**
　　　　H54.512A   Low vision right eye category 2, normal vision left eye
　● **H54.52   Low vision, left eye, normal vision right eye**
　　● **H54.52A   Low vision, left eye, category 1-2**
　　　　H54.52A1   Low vision left eye category 1, normal vision right eye
　　　　H54.52A2   Low vision left eye category 2, normal vision right eye
● **H54.6   Unqualified visual loss, one eye**
　　Visual impairment category 9 in one eye [normal vision in other eye].
　　H54.60   Unqualified visual loss, one eye, unspecified
　　H54.61   Unqualified visual loss, right eye, normal vision left eye
　　H54.62   Unqualified visual loss, left eye, normal vision right eye

　　H54.7   Unspecified visual loss
　　　　Visual impairment category 9 NOS
　　H54.8   Legal blindness, as defined in USA
　　　　Blindness NOS according to USA definition
　　　　Excludes1   legal blindness with specification of impairment level (H54.0-H54.7)
　　　Note: The table below gives a classification of severity of visual impairment recommended by a WHO Study Group on the Prevention of Blindness, Geneva, 6-10 November 1972.

　　　The term "low vision" in category H54 comprises categories 1 and 2 of the table, the term "blindness" categories 3, 4, and 5, and the term "unqualified visual loss" category 9.

　　　If the extent of the visual field is taken into account, patients with a field no greater than 10 but greater than 5 around central fixation should be placed in category 3 and patients with a field no greater than 5 around central fixation should be placed in category 4, even if the central acuity is not impaired.

(Document 508 compliance requires all cells in the following table to be filled.)

	Visual acuity with best possible correction	
	Maximum less than:	**Minimum equal to or better than:**
—	6/18	6/60
3/10 (0.3)	1/10 (0.1)	—
20/70	20/200	—
—	6/60	3/60
1/10 (0.1)	1/20 (0.05)	—
20/200	20/400	—
—	3/60	1/60 (finger counting at one meter)
1/20 (0.05)	1/50 (0.02)	—
20/400	5/300 (20/1200)	—
—	1/60 (finger counting at one meter)	Light perception
1/50 (0.02)	—	—
5/300	—	—
—	No light perception	—
—	Undetermined or unspecified	—

OTHER DISORDERS OF EYE AND ADNEXA (H55-H57)

● **H55   Nystagmus and other irregular eye movements**
　● **H55.0   Nystagmus**
　　　Rapid, involuntary movements of the eyes in the horizontal or vertical direction
　　H55.00   Unspecified nystagmus
　　H55.01   Congenital nystagmus
　　H55.02   Latent nystagmus
　　H55.03   Visual deprivation nystagmus
　　H55.04   Dissociated nystagmus
　　H55.09   Other forms of nystagmus
　● **H55.8   Other irregular eye movements**
　　H55.81   Deficient saccadic eye movements
　　H55.82   Deficient smooth pursuit eye movements
　　H55.89   Other irregular eye movements

● **H57   Other disorders of eye and adnexa**
　● **H57.0   Anomalies of pupillary function**
　　H57.00   Unspecified anomaly of pupillary function
　　H57.01   Argyll Robertson pupil, atypical
　　　　Excludes1   syphilitic Argyll Robertson pupil (A52.19)
　　H57.02   Anisocoria
　　H57.03   Miosis
　　H57.04   Mydriasis
　● **H57.05   Tonic pupil**
　　　　H57.051   Tonic pupil, right eye
　　　　H57.052   Tonic pupil, left eye
　　　　H57.053   Tonic pupil, bilateral
　　　　H57.059   Tonic pupil, unspecified eye
　　H57.09   Other anomalies of pupillary function
　● **H57.1   Ocular pain**
　　H57.10   Ocular pain, unspecified eye
　　H57.11   Ocular pain, right eye
　　H57.12   Ocular pain, left eye
　　H57.13   Ocular pain, bilateral

CHAPTER 7 (H00–H59)

● **H57.8** **Other** specified disorders of eye and adnexa
  ● **H57.81** Brow ptosis
    H57.811 Brow ptosis, right
    H57.812 Brow ptosis, left
    H57.813 Brow ptosis, bilateral
    H57.819 Brow ptosis, unspecified
    H57.89 Other specified disorders of eye and adnexa
  ● **H57.8A** Foreign body sensation eye (ocular)
    H57.8A1 Foreign body sensation, right eye
    H57.8A2 Foreign body sensation, left eye
    H57.8A3 Foreign body sensation, bilateral eyes
    H57.8A9 Foreign body sensation, unspecified eye
  H57.9 **Unspecified** disorder of eye and adnexa

INTRAOPERATIVE AND POSTPROCEDURAL COMPLICATIONS AND DISORDERS OF EYE AND ADNEXA, NOT ELSEWHERE CLASSIFIED (H59)

● **H59** Intraoperative and postprocedural complications and disorders of eye and adnexa, not elsewhere classified
  Excludes1 mechanical complication of intraocular lens (T85.2)
        mechanical complication of other ocular prosthetic devices, implants and grafts (T85.3)
        pseudophakia (Z96.1)
        secondary cataracts (H26.4-)

● **H59.0** Disorders of the eye **following cataract surgery**
  ● **H59.01** **Keratopathy** (bullous aphakic) following cataract surgery
    Vitreal corneal syndrome
    Vitreous (touch) syndrome
    H59.011 Keratopathy (bullous aphakic) following cataract surgery, right eye
    H59.012 Keratopathy (bullous aphakic) following cataract surgery, left eye
    H59.013 Keratopathy (bullous aphakic) following cataract surgery, bilateral
    H59.019 Keratopathy (bullous aphakic) following cataract surgery, unspecified eye
  ● **H59.02** **Cataract** (lens) fragments in eye following cataract surgery
    H59.021 Cataract (lens) fragments in eye following cataract surgery, right eye
    H59.022 Cataract (lens) fragments in eye following cataract surgery, left eye
    H59.023 Cataract (lens) fragments in eye following cataract surgery, bilateral
    H59.029 Cataract (lens) fragments in eye following cataract surgery, unspecified eye
  ● **H59.03** **Cystoid macular edema** following cataract surgery
    H59.031 Cystoid macular edema following cataract surgery, right eye
    H59.032 Cystoid macular edema following cataract surgery, left eye
    H59.033 Cystoid macular edema following cataract surgery, bilateral
    H59.039 Cystoid macular edema following cataract surgery, unspecified eye
  ● **H59.09** **Other** disorders of the eye following cataract surgery
    H59.091 Other disorders of the right eye following cataract surgery
    H59.092 Other disorders of the left eye following cataract surgery
    H59.093 Other disorders of the eye following cataract surgery, bilateral
    H59.099 Other disorders of unspecified eye following cataract surgery

● **H59.1** Intraoperative **hemorrhage and hematoma** of eye and adnexa complicating a procedure
  Excludes1 intraoperative hemorrhage and hematoma of eye and adnexa due to accidental puncture or laceration during a procedure (H59.2-)
  ● **H59.11** Intraoperative hemorrhage and hematoma of eye and adnexa complicating an **ophthalmic procedure**
    H59.111 Intraoperative hemorrhage and hematoma of **right** eye and adnexa complicating an ophthalmic procedure
    H59.112 Intraoperative hemorrhage and hematoma of **left** eye and adnexa complicating an ophthalmic procedure
    H59.113 Intraoperative hemorrhage and hematoma of eye and adnexa complicating an ophthalmic procedure, **bilateral**
    H59.119 Intraoperative hemorrhage and hematoma of **unspecified** eye and adnexa complicating an ophthalmic procedure
  ● **H59.12** Intraoperative hemorrhage and hematoma of eye and adnexa complicating **other procedure**
    H59.121 Intraoperative hemorrhage and hematoma of **right** eye and adnexa complicating other procedure
    H59.122 Intraoperative hemorrhage and hematoma of **left** eye and adnexa complicating other procedure
    H59.123 Intraoperative hemorrhage and hematoma of eye and adnexa complicating other procedure, **bilateral**
    H59.129 Intraoperative hemorrhage and hematoma of **unspecified** eye and adnexa complicating other procedure

● **H59.2** Accidental **puncture and laceration** of eye and adnexa during a procedure
  ● **H59.21** Accidental puncture and laceration of eye and adnexa during an **ophthalmic procedure**
    H59.211 Accidental puncture and laceration of **right** eye and adnexa during an ophthalmic procedure
    H59.212 Accidental puncture and laceration of **left** eye and adnexa during an ophthalmic procedure
    H59.213 Accidental puncture and laceration of eye and adnexa during an ophthalmic procedure, **bilateral**
    H59.219 Accidental puncture and laceration of **unspecified** eye and adnexa during an ophthalmic procedure
  ● **H59.22** Accidental puncture and laceration of eye and adnexa during **other procedure**
    H59.221 Accidental puncture and laceration of **right** eye and adnexa during other procedure
    H59.222 Accidental puncture and laceration of **left** eye and adnexa during other procedure

        H59.223 Accidental puncture and laceration of eye and adnexa during other procedure, bilateral

        H59.229 Accidental puncture and laceration of unspecified eye and adnexa during other procedure

● H59.3 Postprocedural hemorrhage, hematoma, and seroma of eye and adnexa following other procedure
     Coding Clinic: 2016, Q4, P10

  ● H59.31 Postprocedural hemorrhage of eye and adnexa following an ophthalmic procedure

        H59.311 Postprocedural hemorrhage of right eye and adnexa following an ophthalmic procedure

        H59.312 Postprocedural hemorrhage of left eye and adnexa following an ophthalmic procedure

        H59.313 Postprocedural hemorrhage of eye and adnexa following an ophthalmic procedure, bilateral

        H59.319 Postprocedural hemorrhage of unspecified eye and adnexa following an ophthalmic procedure

  ● H59.32 Postprocedural hemorrhage of eye and adnexa following other procedure

        H59.321 Postprocedural hemorrhage of right eye and adnexa following other procedure

        H59.322 Postprocedural hemorrhage of left eye and adnexa following other procedure

        H59.323 Postprocedural hemorrhage of eye and adnexa following other procedure, bilateral

        H59.329 Postprocedural hemorrhage of unspecified eye and adnexa following other procedure

  ● H59.33 Postprocedural hematoma of eye and adnexa following an ophthalmic procedure

        H59.331 Postprocedural hematoma of right eye and adnexa following an ophthalmic procedure

        H59.332 Postprocedural hematoma of left eye and adnexa following an ophthalmic procedure

        H59.333 Postprocedural hematoma of eye and adnexa following an ophthalmic procedure, bilateral

        H59.339 Postprocedural hematoma of unspecified eye and adnexa following an ophthalmic procedure

  ● H59.34 Postprocedural hematoma of eye and adnexa following other procedure

        H59.341 Postprocedural hematoma of right eye and adnexa following other procedure

        H59.342 Postprocedural hematoma of left eye and adnexa following other procedure

        H59.343 Postprocedural hematoma of eye and adnexa following other procedure, bilateral

        H59.349 Postprocedural hematoma of unspecified eye and adnexa following other procedure

  ● H59.35 Postprocedural seroma of eye and adnexa following an ophthalmic procedure

        H59.351 Postprocedural seroma of right eye and adnexa following an ophthalmic procedure

        H59.352 Postprocedural seroma of left eye and adnexa following an ophthalmic procedure

        H59.353 Postprocedural seroma of eye and adnexa following an ophthalmic procedure, bilateral

        H59.359 Postprocedural seroma of unspecified eye and adnexa following an ophthalmic procedure

  ● H59.36 Postprocedural seroma of eye and adnexa following other procedure

        H59.361 Postprocedural seroma of right eye and adnexa following other procedure

        H59.362 Postprocedural seroma of left eye and adnexa following other procedure

        H59.363 Postprocedural seroma of eye and adnexa following other procedure, bilateral

        H59.369 Postprocedural seroma of unspecified eye and adnexa following other procedure

● H59.4 Inflammation (infection) of postprocedural bleb
     Postprocedural blebitis

     Excludes1 filtering (vitreous) bleb after glaucoma surgery status (Z98.83)

     H59.40 Inflammation (infection) of postprocedural bleb, unspecified

     H59.41 Inflammation (infection) of postprocedural bleb, stage 1

     H59.42 Inflammation (infection) of postprocedural bleb, stage 2

     H59.43 Inflammation (infection) of postprocedural bleb, stage 3
        Bleb endophthalmitis

● H59.8 Other intraoperative and postprocedural complications and disorders of eye and adnexa, not elsewhere classified

  ● H59.81 Chorioretinal scars after surgery for detachment

        H59.811 Chorioretinal scars after surgery for detachment, right eye

        H59.812 Chorioretinal scars after surgery for detachment, left eye

        H59.813 Chorioretinal scars after surgery for detachment, bilateral

        H59.819 Chorioretinal scars after surgery for detachment, unspecified eye

     H59.88 Other intraoperative complications of eye and adnexa, not elsewhere classified

     H59.89 Other postprocedural complications and disorders of eye and adnexa, not elsewhere classified

CHAPTER 7 (H00–H59)

CHAPTER 8

DISEASES OF THE EAR AND MASTOID PROCESS (H60-H95)

OGCR Chapter-Specific Coding Guidelines

 8. Chapter 8: Diseases of the Ear and Mastoid Process (H60-H95)
  Reserved for future guideline expansion

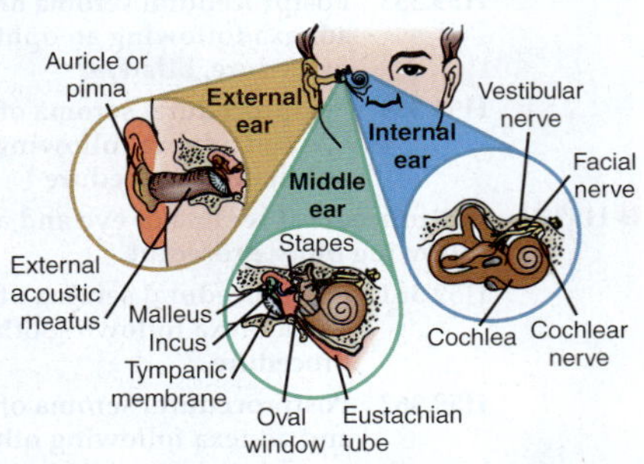

Figure 8-1 Auditory system. (From Buck CJ: Step-by-Step Medical Coding, ed 2016, St. Louis, Elsevier, 2016)

★ **(See Plate 20 of the Anatomy Illustrations.)**

CHAPTER 8

DISEASES OF THE EAR AND MASTOID PROCESS (H60-H95)

Note: Use an external cause code following the code for the ear condition, if applicable, to identify the cause of the ear condition

 Excludes2 certain conditions originating in the perinatal period (P04-P96)
  certain infectious and parasitic diseases (A00-B99)
  complications of pregnancy, childbirth and the puerperium (O00-O9A)
  congenital malformations, deformations and chromosomal abnormalities (Q00-Q99)
  endocrine, nutritional and metabolic diseases (E00-E88)
  injury, poisoning and certain other consequences of external causes (S00-T88)
  neoplasms (C00-D49)
  symptoms, signs and abnormal clinical and laboratory findings, not elsewhere classified (R00-R94)

This chapter contains the following blocks:

H60-H62	Diseases of external ear
H65-H75	Diseases of middle ear and mastoid
H80-H83	Diseases of inner ear
H90-H94	Other disorders of ear
H95	Intraoperative and postprocedural complications and disorders of ear and mastoid process, not elsewhere classified

DISEASES OF EXTERNAL EAR (H60-H62)

● **H60** **Otitis externa**
 ● **H60.0** **Abscess of external ear**
  Boil of external ear
  Carbuncle of auricle or external auditory canal
  Furuncle of external ear
  H60.00 Abscess of external ear, **unspecified** ear
  H60.01 Abscess of **right** external ear
  H60.02 Abscess of **left** external ear
  H60.03 Abscess of external ear, **bilateral**

● **H60.1** **Cellulitis of external ear**
 Cellulitis of auricle
 Cellulitis of external auditory canal
 H60.10 Cellulitis of external ear, **unspecified** ear
 H60.11 Cellulitis of **right** external ear
 H60.12 Cellulitis of **left** external ear
 H60.13 Cellulitis of external ear, **bilateral**

● **H60.2** **Malignant otitis externa**
 H60.20 Malignant otitis externa, **unspecified** ear
 H60.21 Malignant otitis externa, **right** ear
 H60.22 Malignant otitis externa, **left** ear
 H60.23 Malignant otitis externa, **bilateral**

● **H60.3** **Other infective otitis externa**
 ● **H60.31** **Diffuse otitis externa**
  H60.311 Diffuse otitis externa, **right** ear
  H60.312 Diffuse otitis externa, **left** ear
  H60.313 Diffuse otitis externa, **bilateral**
  H60.319 Diffuse otitis externa, **unspecified** ear
 ● **H60.32** **Hemorrhagic otitis externa**
  H60.321 Hemorrhagic otitis externa, **right** ear
  H60.322 Hemorrhagic otitis externa, **left** ear
  H60.323 Hemorrhagic otitis externa, **bilateral**
  H60.329 Hemorrhagic otitis externa, **unspecified** ear
 ● **H60.33** **Swimmer's ear**
  H60.331 Swimmer's ear, **right** ear
  H60.332 Swimmer's ear, **left** ear
  H60.333 Swimmer's ear, **bilateral**
  H60.339 Swimmer's ear, **unspecified** ear
 ● **H60.39** **Other infective otitis externa**
  H60.391 Other infective otitis externa, **right** ear
  H60.392 Other infective otitis externa, **left** ear
  H60.393 Other infective otitis externa, **bilateral**
  H60.399 Other infective otitis externa, **unspecified** ear

● **H60.4** **Cholesteatoma of external ear**
 Keratosis obturans of external ear (canal)
 Excludes2 cholesteatoma of middle ear (H71.-)
  recurrent cholesteatoma of postmastoidectomy cavity (H95.0-)
 H60.40 Cholesteatoma of external ear, **unspecified** ear
 H60.41 Cholesteatoma of **right** external ear
 H60.42 Cholesteatoma of **left** external ear
 H60.43 Cholesteatoma of external ear, **bilateral**

● **H60.5** **Acute noninfective otitis externa**
 ● **H60.50** **Unspecified** acute noninfective otitis externa
  Acute otitis externa NOS
  H60.501 Unspecified acute noninfective otitis externa, **right** ear
  H60.502 Unspecified acute noninfective otitis externa, **left** ear
  H60.503 Unspecified acute noninfective otitis externa, **bilateral**
  H60.509 Unspecified acute noninfective otitis externa, **unspecified** ear
 ● **H60.51** **Acute actinic otitis externa**
  H60.511 Acute actinic otitis externa, **right** ear
  H60.512 Acute actinic otitis externa, **left** ear
  H60.513 Acute actinic otitis externa, **bilateral**
  H60.519 Acute actinic otitis externa, **unspecified** ear

● **H60.52** Acute chemical otitis externa
    H60.521   Acute chemical otitis externa, right ear
    H60.522   Acute chemical otitis externa, left ear
    H60.523   Acute chemical otitis externa, bilateral
    H60.529   Acute chemical otitis externa, unspecified ear

● **H60.53** Acute contact otitis externa
    H60.531   Acute contact otitis externa, right ear
    H60.532   Acute contact otitis externa, left ear
    H60.533   Acute contact otitis externa, bilateral
    H60.539   Acute contact otitis externa, unspecified ear

● **H60.54** Acute eczematoid otitis externa
    H60.541   Acute eczematoid otitis externa, right ear
    H60.542   Acute eczematoid otitis externa, left ear
    H60.543   Acute eczematoid otitis externa, bilateral
    H60.549   Acute eczematoid otitis externa, unspecified ear

● **H60.55** Acute reactive otitis externa
    H60.551   Acute reactive otitis externa, right ear
    H60.552   Acute reactive otitis externa, left ear
    H60.553   Acute reactive otitis externa, bilateral
    H60.559   Acute reactive otitis externa, unspecified ear

● **H60.59** Other noninfective acute otitis externa
    H60.591   Other noninfective acute otitis externa, right ear
    H60.592   Other noninfective acute otitis externa, left ear
    H60.593   Other noninfective acute otitis externa, bilateral
    H60.599   Other noninfective acute otitis externa, unspecified ear

● **H60.6** Unspecified chronic otitis externa
    H60.60   Unspecified chronic otitis externa, unspecified ear
    H60.61   Unspecified chronic otitis externa, right ear
    H60.62   Unspecified chronic otitis externa, left ear
    H60.63   Unspecified chronic otitis externa, bilateral

● **H60.8** Other otitis externa
    ● **H60.8X** Other otitis externa
      H60.8X1   Other otitis externa, right ear
      H60.8X2   Other otitis externa, left ear
      H60.8X3   Other otitis externa, bilateral
      H60.8X9   Other otitis externa, unspecified ear

● **H60.9** Unspecified otitis externa
    H60.90   Unspecified otitis externa, unspecified ear
    H60.91   Unspecified otitis externa, right ear
    H60.92   Unspecified otitis externa, left ear
    H60.93   Unspecified otitis externa, bilateral

● **H61** Other disorders of external ear
   ● **H61.0** Chondritis and perichondritis of external ear
     Chondrodermatitis nodularis chronica helicis
     Perichondritis of auricle
     Perichondritis of pinna
    ● **H61.00** Unspecified perichondritis of external ear
      H61.001   Unspecified perichondritis of right external ear
      H61.002   Unspecified perichondritis of left external ear
      H61.003   Unspecified perichondritis of external ear, bilateral
      H61.009   Unspecified perichondritis of external ear, unspecified ear

● **H61.01** Acute perichondritis of external ear
    H61.011   Acute perichondritis of right external ear
    H61.012   Acute perichondritis of left external ear
    H61.013   Acute perichondritis of external ear, bilateral
    H61.019   Acute perichondritis of external ear, unspecified ear

● **H61.02** Chronic perichondritis of external ear
    H61.021   Chronic perichondritis of right external ear
    H61.022   Chronic perichondritis of left external ear
    H61.023   Chronic perichondritis of external ear, bilateral
    H61.029   Chronic perichondritis of external ear, unspecified ear

● **H61.03** Chondritis of external ear
    Chondritis of auricle
    Chondritis of pinna
    H61.031   Chondritis of right external ear
    H61.032   Chondritis of left external ear
      Coding Clinic: 2015, Q1, P18
    H61.033   Chondritis of external ear, bilateral
    H61.039   Chondritis of external ear, unspecified ear

● **H61.1** Noninfective disorders of pinna
    Excludes2   cauliflower ear (M95.1-)
              gouty tophi of ear (M1A.-)
   ● **H61.10** Unspecified noninfective disorders of pinna
     Disorder of pinna NOS
    H61.101   Unspecified noninfective disorders of pinna, right ear
    H61.102   Unspecified noninfective disorders of pinna, left ear
    H61.103   Unspecified noninfective disorders of pinna, bilateral
    H61.109   Unspecified noninfective disorders of pinna, unspecified ear

   ● **H61.11** Acquired deformity of pinna
     Acquired deformity of auricle
     Excludes2   cauliflower ear (M95.1-)
    H61.111   Acquired deformity of pinna, right ear
    H61.112   Acquired deformity of pinna, left ear
    H61.113   Acquired deformity of pinna, bilateral
    H61.119   Acquired deformity of pinna, unspecified ear

   ● **H61.12** Hematoma of pinna
     Hematoma of auricle
    H61.121   Hematoma of pinna, right ear
    H61.122   Hematoma of pinna, left ear
    H61.123   Hematoma of pinna, bilateral
    H61.129   Hematoma of pinna, unspecified ear

   ● **H61.19** Other noninfective disorders of pinna
    H61.191   Noninfective disorders of pinna, right ear
    H61.192   Noninfective disorders of pinna, left ear
    H61.193   Noninfective disorders of pinna, bilateral
    H61.199   Noninfective disorders of pinna, unspecified ear

CHAPTER 8 (H60–H95)

- **H61.2 Impacted cerumen**
  Wax in ear
  - H61.20   Impacted cerumen, **unspecified** ear
  - H61.21   Impacted cerumen, **right** ear
  - H61.22   Impacted cerumen, **left** ear
  - H61.23   Impacted cerumen, **bilateral**
- **H61.3 Acquired stenosis of external ear canal**
  Collapse of external ear canal
  > **Excludes1**   postprocedural stenosis of external ear canal (H95.81-)
  - **H61.30 Acquired stenosis of external ear canal, unspecified**
    - H61.301   Acquired stenosis of **right** external ear canal, unspecified
    - H61.302   Acquired stenosis of **left** external ear canal, unspecified
    - H61.303   Acquired stenosis of external ear canal, unspecified, **bilateral**
    - H61.309   Acquired stenosis of external ear canal, unspecified, **unspecified** ear
  - **H61.31 Acquired stenosis of external ear canal secondary to trauma**
    - H61.311   Acquired stenosis of **right** external ear canal secondary to trauma
    - H61.312   Acquired stenosis of **left** external ear canal secondary to trauma
    - H61.313   Acquired stenosis of external ear canal secondary to trauma, **bilateral**
    - H61.319   Acquired stenosis of external ear canal secondary to trauma, **unspecified** ear
  - **H61.32 Acquired stenosis of external ear canal secondary to inflammation and infection**
    - H61.321   Acquired stenosis of **right** external ear canal secondary to inflammation and infection
    - H61.322   Acquired stenosis of **left** external ear canal secondary to inflammation and infection
    - H61.323   Acquired stenosis of external ear canal secondary to inflammation and infection, **bilateral**
    - H61.329   Acquired stenosis of external ear canal secondary to inflammation and infection, **unspecified** ear
  - **H61.39 Other** acquired stenosis of external ear canal
    - H61.391   Other acquired stenosis of **right** external ear canal
    - H61.392   Other acquired stenosis of **left** external ear canal
    - H61.393   Other acquired stenosis of external ear canal, **bilateral**
    - H61.399   Other acquired stenosis of external ear canal, **unspecified** ear
- **H61.8 Other specified disorders of external ear**
  - **H61.81 Exostosis of external canal**
    - H61.811   Exostosis of **right** external canal
    - H61.812   Exostosis of **left** external canal
    - H61.813   Exostosis of external canal, **bilateral**
    - H61.819   Exostosis of external canal, **unspecified** ear
  - **H61.89 Other specified disorders of external ear**
    - H61.891   Other specified disorders of **right** external ear
    - H61.892   Other specified disorders of **left** external ear
    - H61.893   Other specified disorders of external ear, **bilateral**
    - H61.899   Other specified disorders of external ear, **unspecified** ear

- **H61.9 Disorder of external ear, unspecified**
  - H61.90   Disorder of external ear, unspecified, **unspecified** ear
  - H61.91   Disorder of **right** external ear, unspecified
  - H61.92   Disorder of **left** external ear, unspecified
  - H61.93   Disorder of external ear, unspecified, **bilateral**
- **H62 Disorders of external ear in diseases classified elsewhere**
  - **H62.4 Otitis externa in other diseases classified elsewhere**
    Code first underlying disease, such as:
      erysipelas (A46)
      impetigo (L01.0-)
    > **Excludes1**   otitis externa (in):
    >   candidiasis (B37.84)
    >   herpes viral [herpes simplex] (B00.1)
    >   herpes zoster (B02.8)
    - ▶ *H62.40*   *Otitis externa in other diseases classified elsewhere, unspecified ear*
    - ▶ *H62.41*   *Otitis externa in other diseases classified elsewhere, right ear*
    - ▶ *H62.42*   *Otitis externa in other diseases classified elsewhere, left ear*
    - ▶ *H62.43*   *Otitis externa in other diseases classified elsewhere, bilateral*
  - **H62.8 Other disorders of external ear in diseases classified elsewhere**
    Code first underlying disease, such as:
      gout (M1A.-, M10.-)
    - **H62.8X Other disorders of external ear in diseases classified elsewhere**
      - ▶ *H62.8X1*   *Other disorders of right external ear in diseases classified elsewhere*
      - ▶ *H62.8X2*   *Other disorders of left external ear in diseases classified elsewhere*
      - ▶ *H62.8X3*   *Other disorders of external ear in diseases classified elsewhere, bilateral*
      - ▶ *H62.8X9*   *Other disorders of external ear in diseases classified elsewhere, unspecified ear*

DISEASES OF MIDDLE EAR AND MASTOID (H65-H75)

★ **(See Plate 21 of the Anatomy Illustrations.)**

- **H65 Nonsuppurative otitis media**
  Bacterial or viral infection or inflammation of the middle ear; may result in fluid accumulation with pain and temporary hearing loss.
  > **Includes**   nonsuppurative otitis media with myringitis

  Use additional code for any associated perforated tympanic membrane (H72.-)

  Use additional code to identify:
    exposure to environmental tobacco smoke (Z77.22)
    exposure to tobacco smoke in the perinatal period (P96.81)
    history of tobacco dependence (Z87.891)
    infectious agent (B95-B97)
    occupational exposure to environmental tobacco smoke (Z57.31)
    tobacco dependence (F17.-)
    tobacco use (Z72.0)
  - **H65.0 Acute serous otitis media**
    Acute and subacute secretory otitis
    - H65.00   Acute serous otitis media, **unspecified** ear
    - H65.01   Acute serous otitis media, **right** ear
    - H65.02   Acute serous otitis media, **left** ear
    - H65.03   Acute serous otitis media, **bilateral**
    - H65.04   Acute serous otitis media, **recurrent, right ear**
    - H65.05   Acute serous otitis media, **recurrent, left ear**
    - H65.06   Acute serous otitis media, **recurrent, bilateral**
    - H65.07   Acute serous otitis media, **recurrent, unspecified ear**

● **H65.1** **Other acute nonsuppurative otitis media**

Excludes1 otitic barotrauma (T70.0)
otitis media (acute) NOS (H66.9)

● **H65.11** **Acute and subacute allergic otitis media (mucoid) (sanguinous) (serous)**

H65.111 **Acute and subacute allergic otitis media (mucoid) (sanguinous) (serous), right ear**

H65.112 **Acute and subacute allergic otitis media (mucoid) (sanguinous) (serous), left ear**

H65.113 **Acute and subacute allergic otitis media (mucoid) (sanguinous) (serous), bilateral**

H65.114 **Acute and subacute allergic otitis media (mucoid) (sanguinous) (serous), recurrent, right ear**

H65.115 **Acute and subacute allergic otitis media (mucoid) (sanguinous) (serous), recurrent, left ear**

H65.116 **Acute and subacute allergic otitis media (mucoid) (sanguinous) (serous), recurrent, bilateral**

H65.117 **Acute and subacute allergic otitis media (mucoid) (sanguinous) (serous), recurrent, unspecified ear**

H65.119 **Acute and subacute allergic otitis media (mucoid) (sanguinous) (serous), unspecified ear**

● **H65.19** **Other acute nonsuppurative otitis media**
Acute and subacute mucoid otitis media
Acute and subacute nonsuppurative otitis media NOS
Acute and subacute sanguinous otitis media
Acute and subacute seromucinous otitis media

H65.191 **Other acute nonsuppurative otitis media, right ear**

H65.192 **Other acute nonsuppurative otitis media, left ear**

H65.193 **Other acute nonsuppurative otitis media, bilateral**

H65.194 **Other acute nonsuppurative otitis media, recurrent, right ear**

H65.195 **Other acute nonsuppurative otitis media, recurrent, left ear**

H65.196 **Other acute nonsuppurative otitis media, recurrent, bilateral**

H65.197 **Other acute nonsuppurative otitis media recurrent, unspecified ear**

H65.199 **Other acute nonsuppurative otitis media, unspecified ear**

● **H65.2** **Chronic serous otitis media**
Chronic tubotympanal catarrh

H65.20 **Chronic serous otitis media, unspecified ear**

H65.21 **Chronic serous otitis media, right ear**

H65.22 **Chronic serous otitis media, left ear**

H65.23 **Chronic serous otitis media, bilateral**

● **H65.3** **Chronic mucoid otitis media**
Chronic mucinous otitis media
Chronic secretory otitis media
Chronic transudative otitis media
Glue ear

Excludes1 adhesive middle ear disease (H74.1)

H65.30 **Chronic mucoid otitis media, unspecified ear**

H65.31 **Chronic mucoid otitis media, right ear**

H65.32 **Chronic mucoid otitis media, left ear**

H65.33 **Chronic mucoid otitis media, bilateral**

● **H65.4** **Other chronic nonsuppurative otitis media**

● **H65.41** **Chronic allergic otitis media**

H65.411 **Chronic allergic otitis media, right ear**

H65.412 **Chronic allergic otitis media, left ear**

H65.413 **Chronic allergic otitis media, bilateral**

H65.419 **Chronic allergic otitis media, unspecified ear**

● **H65.49** **Other chronic nonsuppurative otitis media**
Chronic exudative otitis media
Chronic nonsuppurative otitis media NOS
Chronic otitis media with effusion (nonpurulent)
Chronic seromucinous otitis media

H65.491 **Other chronic nonsuppurative otitis media, right ear**

H65.492 **Other chronic nonsuppurative otitis media, left ear**

H65.493 **Other chronic nonsuppurative otitis media, bilateral**

H65.499 **Other chronic nonsuppurative otitis media, unspecified ear**

● **H65.9** **Unspecified nonsuppurative otitis media**
Allergic otitis media NOS
Catarrhal otitis media NOS
Exudative otitis media NOS
Mucoid otitis media NOS
Otitis media with effusion (nonpurulent) NOS
Secretory otitis media NOS
Seromucinous otitis media NOS
Serous otitis media NOS
Transudative otitis media NOS

H65.90 **Unspecified nonsuppurative otitis media, unspecified ear**

H65.91 **Unspecified nonsuppurative otitis media, right ear**

H65.92 **Unspecified nonsuppurative otitis media, left ear**

H65.93 **Unspecified nonsuppurative otitis media, bilateral**

● **H66** **Suppurative and unspecified otitis media**
Suppurative: Discharging pus

Includes suppurative and unspecified otitis media with myringitis

Use additional code to identify:
exposure to environmental tobacco smoke (Z77.22)
exposure to tobacco smoke in the perinatal period (P96.81)
history of tobacco dependence (Z87.891)
occupational exposure to environmental tobacco smoke (Z57.31)
tobacco dependence (F17.-)
tobacco use (Z72.0)

● **H66.0** **Acute suppurative otitis media**

● **H66.00** **Acute suppurative otitis media without spontaneous rupture of ear drum**

H66.001 **Acute suppurative otitis media without spontaneous rupture of ear drum, right ear**
Coding Clinic: 2016, Q1, P34

H66.002 **Acute suppurative otitis media without spontaneous rupture of ear drum, left ear**

H66.003 **Acute suppurative otitis media without spontaneous rupture of ear drum, bilateral**

H66.004 **Acute suppurative otitis media without spontaneous rupture of ear drum, recurrent, right ear**

H66.005 **Acute suppurative otitis media without spontaneous rupture of ear drum, recurrent, left ear**

H66.006 **Acute suppurative otitis media without spontaneous rupture of ear drum, recurrent, bilateral**

H66.007 **Acute suppurative otitis media without spontaneous rupture of ear drum, recurrent, unspecified ear**

H66.009 **Acute suppurative otitis media without spontaneous rupture of ear drum, unspecified ear**

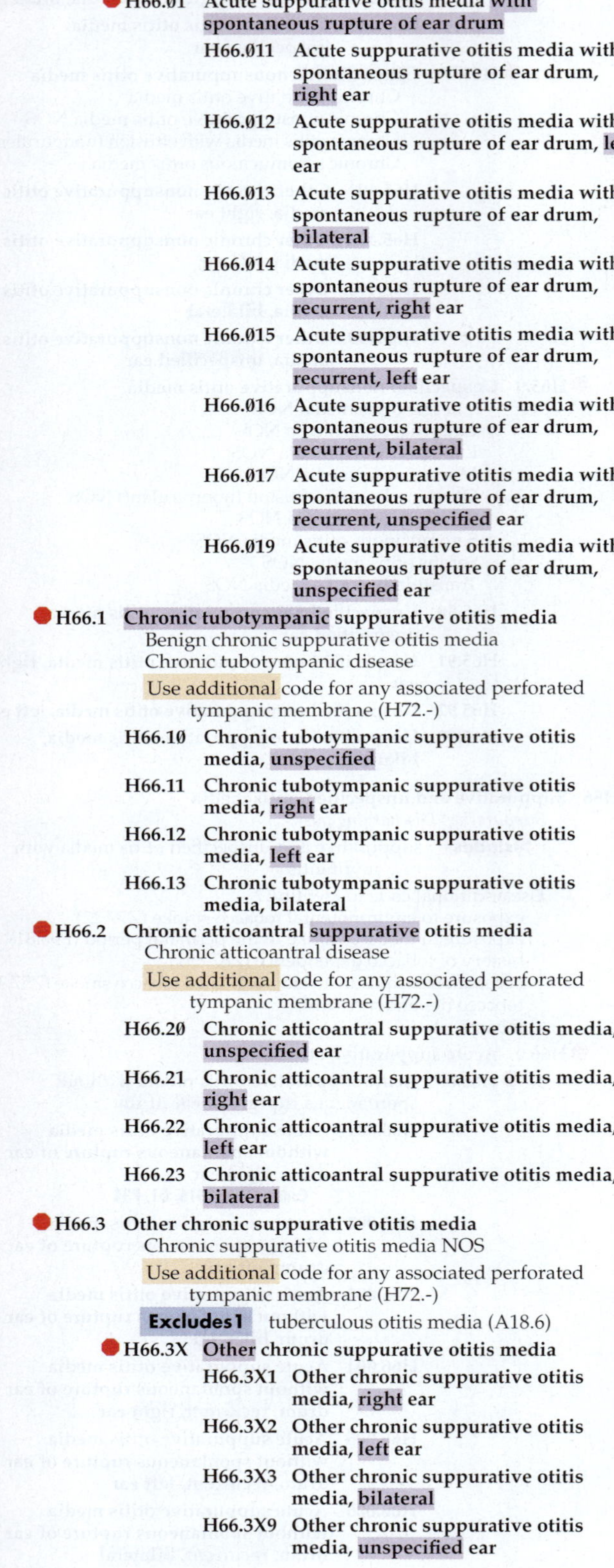

● **H66.01** Acute suppurative otitis media with spontaneous rupture of ear drum

　　H66.011 Acute suppurative otitis media with spontaneous rupture of ear drum, right ear

　　H66.012 Acute suppurative otitis media with spontaneous rupture of ear drum, left ear

　　H66.013 Acute suppurative otitis media with spontaneous rupture of ear drum, bilateral

　　H66.014 Acute suppurative otitis media with spontaneous rupture of ear drum, recurrent, right ear

　　H66.015 Acute suppurative otitis media with spontaneous rupture of ear drum, recurrent, left ear

　　H66.016 Acute suppurative otitis media with spontaneous rupture of ear drum, recurrent, bilateral

　　H66.017 Acute suppurative otitis media with spontaneous rupture of ear drum, recurrent, unspecified ear

　　H66.019 Acute suppurative otitis media with spontaneous rupture of ear drum, unspecified ear

● **H66.1** Chronic tubotympanic suppurative otitis media
　Benign chronic suppurative otitis media
　Chronic tubotympanic disease

　Use additional code for any associated perforated tympanic membrane (H72.-)

　　H66.10 Chronic tubotympanic suppurative otitis media, unspecified

　　H66.11 Chronic tubotympanic suppurative otitis media, right ear

　　H66.12 Chronic tubotympanic suppurative otitis media, left ear

　　H66.13 Chronic tubotympanic suppurative otitis media, bilateral

● **H66.2** Chronic atticoantral suppurative otitis media
　Chronic atticoantral disease

　Use additional code for any associated perforated tympanic membrane (H72.-)

　　H66.20 Chronic atticoantral suppurative otitis media, unspecified ear

　　H66.21 Chronic atticoantral suppurative otitis media, right ear

　　H66.22 Chronic atticoantral suppurative otitis media, left ear

　　H66.23 Chronic atticoantral suppurative otitis media, bilateral

● **H66.3** Other chronic suppurative otitis media
　Chronic suppurative otitis media NOS

　Use additional code for any associated perforated tympanic membrane (H72.-)

　Excludes1 tuberculous otitis media (A18.6)

● **H66.3X** Other chronic suppurative otitis media

　　H66.3X1 Other chronic suppurative otitis media, right ear

　　H66.3X2 Other chronic suppurative otitis media, left ear

　　H66.3X3 Other chronic suppurative otitis media, bilateral

　　H66.3X9 Other chronic suppurative otitis media, unspecified ear

● **H66.4** Suppurative otitis media, unspecified
　Purulent otitis media NOS

　Use additional code for any associated perforated tympanic membrane (H72.-)

　　H66.40 Suppurative otitis media, unspecified, unspecified ear

　　H66.41 Suppurative otitis media, unspecified, right ear

　　H66.42 Suppurative otitis media, unspecified, left ear

　　H66.43 Suppurative otitis media, unspecified, bilateral

● **H66.9** Otitis media, unspecified
　Otitis media NOS
　Acute otitis media NOS
　Chronic otitis media NOS

　Use additional code for any associated perforated tympanic membrane (H72.-)

　　H66.90 Otitis media, unspecified, unspecified ear

　　H66.91 Otitis media, unspecified, right ear

　　H66.92 Otitis media, unspecified, left ear

　　H66.93 Otitis media, unspecified, bilateral

● **H67** Otitis media in diseases classified elsewhere

　Code first underlying disease, such as:
　　plasminogen deficiency (E88.02)
　　viral disease NEC (B00-B34)

　Use additional code for any associated perforated tympanic membrane (H72.-)

　Excludes1 otitis media in:
　　　influenza (J09.X9, J10.83, J11.83)
　　　measles (B05.3)
　　　scarlet fever (A38.0)
　　　tuberculosis (A18.6)

▶ *H67.1 Otitis media in diseases classified elsewhere, right ear*

▶ *H67.2 Otitis media in diseases classified elsewhere, left ear*

▶ *H67.3 Otitis media in diseases classified elsewhere, bilateral*

▶ *H67.9 Otitis media in diseases classified elsewhere, unspecified ear*

● **H68** Eustachian salpingitis and obstruction

● **H68.0** Eustachian salpingitis

　● **H68.00** Unspecified Eustachian salpingitis

　　H68.001 Unspecified Eustachian salpingitis, right ear

　　H68.002 Unspecified Eustachian salpingitis, left ear

　　H68.003 Unspecified Eustachian salpingitis, bilateral

　　H68.009 Unspecified Eustachian salpingitis, unspecified ear

　● **H68.01** Acute Eustachian salpingitis

　　H68.011 Acute Eustachian salpingitis, right ear

　　H68.012 Acute Eustachian salpingitis, left ear

　　H68.013 Acute Eustachian salpingitis, bilateral

　　H68.019 Acute Eustachian salpingitis, unspecified ear

　● **H68.02** Chronic Eustachian salpingitis

　　H68.021 Chronic Eustachian salpingitis, right ear

　　H68.022 Chronic Eustachian salpingitis, left ear

　　H68.023 Chronic Eustachian salpingitis, bilateral

　　H68.029 Chronic Eustachian salpingitis, unspecified ear

● **H68.1**   **Obstruction of Eustachian tube**
     Stenosis of Eustachian tube
     Stricture of Eustachian tube
   ● **H68.10**   **Unspecified obstruction of Eustachian tube**
      H68.101   Unspecified obstruction of Eustachian tube, **right ear**
      H68.102   Unspecified obstruction of Eustachian tube, **left ear**
      H68.103   Unspecified obstruction of Eustachian tube, **bilateral**
      H68.109   Unspecified obstruction of Eustachian tube, **unspecified ear**
   ● **H68.11**   **Osseous obstruction of Eustachian tube**
      H68.111   Osseous obstruction of Eustachian tube, **right ear**
      H68.112   Osseous obstruction of Eustachian tube, **left ear**
      H68.113   Osseous obstruction of Eustachian tube, **bilateral**
      H68.119   Osseous obstruction of Eustachian tube, **unspecified ear**
   ● **H68.12**   **Intrinsic cartilagenous obstruction of Eustachian tube**
      H68.121   Intrinsic cartilagenous obstruction of Eustachian tube, **right ear**
      H68.122   Intrinsic cartilagenous obstruction of Eustachian tube, **left ear**
      H68.123   Intrinsic cartilagenous obstruction of Eustachian tube, **bilateral**
      H68.129   Intrinsic cartilagenous obstruction of Eustachian tube, **unspecified ear**
   ● **H68.13**   **Extrinsic cartilagenous obstruction of Eustachian tube**
     Compression of Eustachian tube
      H68.131   Extrinsic cartilagenous obstruction of Eustachian tube, **right ear**
      H68.132   Extrinsic cartilagenous obstruction of Eustachian tube, **left ear**
      H68.133   Extrinsic cartilagenous obstruction of Eustachian tube, **bilateral**
      H68.139   Extrinsic cartilagenous obstruction of Eustachian tube, **unspecified ear**

● **H69**   **Other and unspecified disorders of Eustachian tube**
   ● **H69.0**   **Patulous Eustachian tube**
      H69.00   Patulous Eustachian tube, **unspecified ear**
      H69.01   Patulous Eustachian tube, **right ear**
      H69.02   Patulous Eustachian tube, **left ear**
      H69.03   Patulous Eustachian tube, **bilateral**
   ● **H69.8**   **Other specified disorders of Eustachian tube**
      H69.80   Other specified disorders of Eustachian tube, **unspecified ear**
      H69.81   Other specified disorders of Eustachian tube, **right ear**
      H69.82   Other specified disorders of Eustachian tube, **left ear**
      H69.83   Other specified disorders of Eustachian tube, **bilateral**
   ● **H69.9**   **Unspecified Eustachian tube disorder**
      H69.90   Unspecified Eustachian tube disorder, **unspecified ear**
      H69.91   Unspecified Eustachian tube disorder, **right ear**
      H69.92   Unspecified Eustachian tube disorder, **left ear**
      H69.93   Unspecified Eustachian tube disorder, **bilateral**

● **H70**   **Mastoiditis and related conditions**
   ● **H70.0**   **Acute mastoiditis**
     Abscess of mastoid
     Empyema of mastoid
   ● **H70.00**   **Acute mastoiditis without complications**
      H70.001   Acute mastoiditis without complications, **right ear**
      H70.002   Acute mastoiditis without complications, **left ear**
      H70.003   Acute mastoiditis without complications, **bilateral**
      H70.009   Acute mastoiditis without complications, **unspecified ear**
   ● **H70.01**   **Subperiosteal abscess of mastoid**
      H70.011   Subperiosteal abscess of mastoid, **right ear**
      H70.012   Subperiosteal abscess of mastoid, **left ear**
      H70.013   Subperiosteal abscess of mastoid, **bilateral**
      H70.019   Subperiosteal abscess of mastoid, **unspecified ear**
   ● **H70.09**   **Acute mastoiditis with other complications**
      H70.091   Acute mastoiditis with other complications, **right ear**
      H70.092   Acute mastoiditis with other complications, **left ear**
      H70.093   Acute mastoiditis with other complications, **bilateral**
      H70.099   Acute mastoiditis with other complications, **unspecified ear**
   ● **H70.1**   **Chronic mastoiditis**
     Caries of mastoid
     Fistula of mastoid
     Excludes1   tuberculous mastoiditis (A18.03)
      H70.10   Chronic mastoiditis, **unspecified** ear
      H70.11   Chronic mastoiditis, **right ear**
      H70.12   Chronic mastoiditis, **left ear**
      H70.13   Chronic mastoiditis, **bilateral**
   ● **H70.2**   **Petrositis**
     Inflammation of petrous bone
   ● **H70.20**   **Unspecified petrositis**
      H70.201   Unspecified petrositis, **right ear**
      H70.202   Unspecified petrositis, **left ear**
      H70.203   Unspecified petrositis, **bilateral**
      H70.209   Unspecified petrositis, **unspecified ear**
   ● **H70.21**   **Acute petrositis**
      H70.211   Acute petrositis, **right ear**
      H70.212   Acute petrositis, **left ear**
      H70.213   Acute petrositis, **bilateral**
      H70.219   Acute petrositis, **unspecified ear**
   ● **H70.22**   **Chronic petrositis**
      H70.221   Chronic petrositis, **right ear**
      H70.222   Chronic petrositis, **left ear**
      H70.223   Chronic petrositis, **bilateral**
      H70.229   Chronic petrositis, **unspecified ear**

Item 8–1   **Mastoiditis** is an infection of the portion of the temporal bone of the skull that is behind the ear (mastoid process) caused by an untreated otitis media, leading to an infection of the surrounding structures which may include the brain.

CHAPTER 8 (H60–H95)

CHAPTER 8 (H60–H95)

● **H70.8 Other mastoiditis and related conditions**

  Excludes1   preauricular sinus and cyst (Q18.1)
             sinus, fistula, and cyst of branchial cleft (Q18.0)

  ● **H70.81 Postauricular fistula**
     H70.811   Postauricular fistula, right ear
     H70.812   Postauricular fistula, left ear
     H70.813   Postauricular fistula, bilateral
     H70.819   Postauricular fistula, unspecified ear

  ● **H70.89 Other mastoiditis and related conditions**
     H70.891   Other mastoiditis and related conditions, right ear
     H70.892   Other mastoiditis and related conditions, left ear
     H70.893   Other mastoiditis and related conditions, bilateral
     H70.899   Other mastoiditis and related conditions, unspecified ear

● **H70.9 Unspecified mastoiditis**
   H70.90   Unspecified mastoiditis, unspecified ear
   H70.91   Unspecified mastoiditis, right ear
   H70.92   Unspecified mastoiditis, left ear
   H70.93   Unspecified mastoiditis, bilateral

● **H71 Cholesteatoma of middle ear**

  Excludes2   cholesteatoma of external ear (H60.4-)
             recurrent cholesteatoma of postmastoidectomy cavity (H95.0-)

● **H71.0 Cholesteatoma of attic**
   H71.00   Cholesteatoma of attic, unspecified ear
   H71.01   Cholesteatoma of attic, right ear
   H71.02   Cholesteatoma of attic, left ear
     Coding Clinic: 2021, Q3, P9
   H71.03   Cholesteatoma of attic, bilateral

● **H71.1 Cholesteatoma of tympanum**
   H71.10   Cholesteatoma of tympanum, unspecified ear
   H71.11   Cholesteatoma of tympanum, right ear
   H71.12   Cholesteatoma of tympanum, left ear
   H71.13   Cholesteatoma of tympanum, bilateral

● **H71.2 Cholesteatoma of mastoid**
   H71.20   Cholesteatoma of mastoid, unspecified ear
   H71.21   Cholesteatoma of mastoid, right ear
   H71.22   Cholesteatoma of mastoid, left ear
     Coding Clinic: 2021, Q3, P9
   H71.23   Cholesteatoma of mastoid, bilateral

● **H71.3 Diffuse cholesteatosis**
     Coding Clinic: 2021, Q3, P9
   H71.30   Diffuse cholesteatosis, unspecified ear
   H71.31   Diffuse cholesteatosis, right ear
   H71.32   Diffuse cholesteatosis, left ear
   H71.33   Diffuse cholesteatosis, bilateral

● **H71.9 Unspecified cholesteatoma**
   H71.90   Unspecified cholesteatoma, unspecified ear
   H71.91   Unspecified cholesteatoma, right ear
   H71.92   Unspecified cholesteatoma, left ear
   H71.93   Unspecified cholesteatoma, bilateral

★ **(See Plate 22 of the Anatomy Illustrations.)**

● **H72 Perforation of tympanic membrane**
   Hole or rupture in ear drum

  Includes   persistent post-traumatic perforation of ear drum
           postinflammatory perforation of ear drum

  Code first any associated otitis media (H65.-, H66.1-, H66.2-, H66.3-, H66.4-, H66.9-, H67.-)

  Excludes1   acute suppurative otitis media with rupture of the tympanic membrane (H66.01-)
             traumatic rupture of ear drum (S09.2-)

● **H72.0 Central perforation of tympanic membrane**
   H72.00   Central perforation of tympanic membrane, unspecified ear
   H72.01   Central perforation of tympanic membrane, right ear
   H72.02   Central perforation of tympanic membrane, left ear
   H72.03   Central perforation of tympanic membrane, bilateral

● **H72.1 Attic perforation of tympanic membrane**
   Perforation of pars flaccida
   H72.10   Attic perforation of tympanic membrane, unspecified ear
   H72.11   Attic perforation of tympanic membrane, right ear
   H72.12   Attic perforation of tympanic membrane, left ear
   H72.13   Attic perforation of tympanic membrane, bilateral

● **H72.2 Other marginal perforations of tympanic membrane**
  ● **H72.2X Other marginal perforations of tympanic membrane**
     H72.2X1   Other marginal perforations of tympanic membrane, right ear
     H72.2X2   Other marginal perforations of tympanic membrane, left ear
     H72.2X3   Other marginal perforations of tympanic membrane, bilateral
     H72.2X9   Other marginal perforations of tympanic membrane, unspecified ear

● **H72.8 Other perforations of tympanic membrane**
  ● **H72.81 Multiple perforations of tympanic membrane**
     H72.811   Multiple perforations of tympanic membrane, right ear
     H72.812   Multiple perforations of tympanic membrane, left ear
     H72.813   Multiple perforations of tympanic membrane, bilateral
     H72.819   Multiple perforations of tympanic membrane, unspecified ear

  ● **H72.82 Total perforations of tympanic membrane**
     H72.821   Total perforations of tympanic membrane, right ear
     H72.822   Total perforations of tympanic membrane, left ear
     H72.823   Total perforations of tympanic membrane, bilateral
     H72.829   Total perforations of tympanic membrane, unspecified ear

● **H72.9 Unspecified perforation of tympanic membrane**
   H72.90   Unspecified perforation of tympanic membrane, unspecified ear
   H72.91   Unspecified perforation of tympanic membrane, right ear
   H72.92   Unspecified perforation of tympanic membrane, left ear
   H72.93   Unspecified perforation of tympanic membrane, bilateral

---

▶ New   ⇒ Revised   ~~deleted~~ Deleted   Excludes 1   Excludes 2   Includes   Use additional   Code first   Code also   Key words
OGCR Official Guidelines   **X** Assign placeholder X   ● Use Additional Character(s)   ▶ Manifestation Code   Hierarchical Condition Category   **Coding Clinic**

● **H73   Other disorders of tympanic membrane**
  ● **H73.0   Acute myringitis**
      Excludes1   acute myringitis with otitis media (H65, H66)
    ● **H73.00   Unspecified acute myringitis**
       Acute tympanitis NOS
       H73.001   Acute myringitis, **right** ear
       H73.002   Acute myringitis, **left** ear
       H73.003   Acute myringitis, **bilateral**
       H73.009   Acute myringitis, **unspecified** ear
    ● **H73.01   Bullous myringitis**
       H73.011   Bullous myringitis, **right** ear
       H73.012   Bullous myringitis, **left** ear
       H73.013   Bullous myringitis, **bilateral**
       H73.019   Bullous myringitis, **unspecified** ear
    ● **H73.09   Other acute myringitis**
       H73.091   Other acute myringitis, **right** ear
       H73.092   Other acute myringitis, **left** ear
       H73.093   Other acute myringitis, **bilateral**
       H73.099   Other acute myringitis, **unspecified** ear
  ● **H73.1   Chronic myringitis**
      Chronic tympanitis
      Excludes1   chronic myringitis with otitis media (H65, H66)
     H73.10   Chronic myringitis, **unspecified** ear
     H73.11   Chronic myringitis, **right** ear
     H73.12   Chronic myringitis, **left** ear
     H73.13   Chronic myringitis, **bilateral**
  ● **H73.2   Unspecified myringitis**
     H73.20   Unspecified myringitis, **unspecified** ear
     H73.21   Unspecified myringitis, **right** ear
     H73.22   Unspecified myringitis, **left** ear
     H73.23   Unspecified myringitis, **bilateral**
  ● **H73.8   Other specified disorders of tympanic membrane**
    ● **H73.81   Atrophic flaccid tympanic membrane**
       H73.811   Atrophic flaccid tympanic membrane, **right** ear
       H73.812   Atrophic flaccid tympanic membrane, **left** ear
       H73.813   Atrophic flaccid tympanic membrane, **bilateral**
       H73.819   Atrophic flaccid tympanic membrane, **unspecified** ear
    ● **H73.82   Atrophic nonflaccid tympanic membrane**
       H73.821   Atrophic nonflaccid tympanic membrane, **right** ear
       H73.822   Atrophic nonflaccid tympanic membrane, **left** ear
       H73.823   Atrophic nonflaccid tympanic membrane, **bilateral**
       H73.829   Atrophic nonflaccid tympanic membrane, **unspecified** ear
    ● **H73.89   Other specified disorders of tympanic membrane**
       H73.891   Other specified disorders of tympanic membrane, **right** ear
       H73.892   Other specified disorders of tympanic membrane, **left** ear
       H73.893   Other specified disorders of tympanic membrane, **bilateral**
       H73.899   Other specified disorders of tympanic membrane, **unspecified** ear

● **H73.9   Unspecified disorder of tympanic membrane**
     H73.90   Unspecified disorder of tympanic membrane, **unspecified** ear
     H73.91   Unspecified disorder of tympanic membrane, **right** ear
     H73.92   Unspecified disorder of tympanic membrane, **left** ear
     H73.93   Unspecified disorder of tympanic membrane, **bilateral**

● **H74   Other disorders of middle ear mastoid**
     Excludes2   mastoiditis (H70.-)
  ● **H74.0   Tympanosclerosis**
     H74.01   Tympanosclerosis, **right** ear
     H74.02   Tympanosclerosis, **left** ear
     H74.03   Tympanosclerosis, **bilateral**
     H74.09   Tympanosclerosis, **unspecified** ear
  ● **H74.1   Adhesive middle ear disease**
      Adhesive otitis
      Excludes1   glue ear (H65.3-)
     H74.11   Adhesive **right** middle ear disease
     H74.12   Adhesive **left** middle ear disease
     H74.13   Adhesive middle ear disease, **bilateral**
     H74.19   Adhesive middle ear disease, **unspecified** ear
  ● **H74.2   Discontinuity and dislocation of ear ossicles**
     H74.20   Discontinuity and dislocation of ear ossicles, **unspecified** ear
     H74.21   Discontinuity and dislocation of **right** ear ossicles
     H74.22   Discontinuity and dislocation of **left** ear ossicles
     H74.23   Discontinuity and dislocation of ear ossicles, **bilateral**
  ● **H74.3   Other acquired abnormalities of ear ossicles**
    ● **H74.31   Ankylosis of ear ossicles**
       H74.311   Ankylosis of ear ossicles, **right** ear
       H74.312   Ankylosis of ear ossicles, **left** ear
       H74.313   Ankylosis of ear ossicles, **bilateral**
       H74.319   Ankylosis of ear ossicles, **unspecified** ear
    ● **H74.32   Partial loss of ear ossicles**
       H74.321   Partial loss of ear ossicles, **right** ear
       H74.322   Partial loss of ear ossicles, **left** ear
       H74.323   Partial loss of ear ossicles, **bilateral**
       H74.329   Partial loss of ear ossicles, **unspecified** ear
    ● **H74.39   Other acquired abnormalities of ear ossicles**
       H74.391   Other acquired abnormalities of **right** ear ossicles
       H74.392   Other acquired abnormalities of **left** ear ossicles
       H74.393   Other acquired abnormalities of ear ossicles, **bilateral**
       H74.399   Other acquired abnormalities of ear ossicles, **unspecified** ear
  ● **H74.4   Polyp of middle ear**
     H74.40   Polyp of middle ear, **unspecified** ear
     H74.41   Polyp of **right** middle ear
     H74.42   Polyp of **left** middle ear
     H74.43   Polyp of middle ear, **bilateral**

CHAPTER 8 (H60–H95)

● **H74.8**   Other specified disorders of middle ear and mastoid

   ● **H74.8X**   Other specified disorders of middle ear and mastoid

     H74.8X1   Other specified disorders of right middle ear and mastoid

     H74.8X2   Other specified disorders of left middle ear and mastoid

     H74.8X3   Other specified disorders of middle ear and mastoid, bilateral

     H74.8X9   Other specified disorders of middle ear and mastoid, unspecified ear

● **H74.9**   Unspecified disorder of middle ear and mastoid

     H74.90   Unspecified disorder of middle ear and mastoid, unspecified ear

     H74.91   Unspecified disorder of right middle ear and mastoid

     H74.92   Unspecified disorder of left middle ear and mastoid

     H74.93   Unspecified disorder of middle ear and mastoid, bilateral

● **H75**   Other disorders of middle ear and mastoid in diseases classified elsewhere

    Code first underlying disease

   ● **H75.0**   Mastoiditis in infectious and parasitic diseases classified elsewhere

     Excludes1   mastoiditis (in):
       syphilis (A52.77)
       tuberculosis (A18.03)

     ▸ *H75.00*   *Mastoiditis in infectious and parasitic diseases classified elsewhere, unspecified ear*

     ▸ *H75.01*   *Mastoiditis in infectious and parasitic diseases classified elsewhere, right ear*

     ▸ *H75.02*   *Mastoiditis in infectious and parasitic diseases classified elsewhere, left ear*

     ▸ *H75.03*   *Mastoiditis in infectious and parasitic diseases classified elsewhere, bilateral*

   ● **H75.8**   Other specified disorders of middle ear and mastoid in diseases classified elsewhere

     ▸ *H75.80*   *Other specified disorders of middle ear and mastoid in diseases classified elsewhere, unspecified ear*

     ▸ *H75.81*   *Other specified disorders of right middle ear and mastoid in diseases classified elsewhere*

     ▸ *H75.82*   *Other specified disorders of left middle ear and mastoid in diseases classified elsewhere*

     ▸ *H75.83*   *Other specified disorders of middle ear and mastoid in diseases classified elsewhere, bilateral*

DISEASES OF INNER EAR (H80–H83)

★ **(See Plate 23 of the Anatomy Illustrations.)**

● **H80**   Otosclerosis

    Inherited middle ear spongelike bone growth causing hearing loss

     Includes   Otospongiosis

   ● **H80.0**   Otosclerosis involving oval window, nonobliterative

     H80.00   Otosclerosis involving oval window, nonobliterative, unspecified ear

     H80.01   Otosclerosis involving oval window, nonobliterative, right ear

     H80.02   Otosclerosis involving oval window, nonobliterative, left ear

     H80.03   Otosclerosis involving oval window, nonobliterative, bilateral

   ● **H80.1**   Otosclerosis involving oval window, obliterative

     H80.10   Otosclerosis involving oval window, obliterative, unspecified ear

     H80.11   Otosclerosis involving oval window, obliterative, right ear

     H80.12   Otosclerosis involving oval window, obliterative, left ear

     H80.13   Otosclerosis involving oval window, obliterative, bilateral

   ● **H80.2**   Cochlear otosclerosis

     Otosclerosis involving otic capsule
     Otosclerosis involving round window

     H80.20   Cochlear otosclerosis, unspecified ear

     H80.21   Cochlear otosclerosis, right ear

     H80.22   Cochlear otosclerosis, left ear

     H80.23   Cochlear otosclerosis, bilateral

   ● **H80.8**   Other otosclerosis

     H80.80   Other otosclerosis, unspecified ear

     H80.81   Other otosclerosis, right ear

     H80.82   Other otosclerosis, left ear

     H80.83   Other otosclerosis, bilateral

   ● **H80.9**   Unspecified otosclerosis

     H80.90   Unspecified otosclerosis, unspecified ear

     H80.91   Unspecified otosclerosis, right ear

     H80.92   Unspecified otosclerosis, left ear

     H80.93   Unspecified otosclerosis, bilateral

● **H81**   Disorders of vestibular function

     Excludes1   epidemic vertigo (A88.1)
       vertigo NOS (R42)

   ● **H81.0**   Ménière's disease

     Vestibular disorder that produces recurring symptoms including severe and intermittent hearing loss including the feeling of ear pressure or pain
     Labyrinthine hydrops
     Ménière's syndrome or vertigo

     H81.01   Ménière's disease, right ear

     H81.02   Ménière's disease, left ear

     H81.03   Ménière's disease, bilateral

     H81.09   Ménière's disease, unspecified ear

   ● **H81.1**   Benign paroxysmal vertigo

     H81.10   Benign paroxysmal vertigo, unspecified ear

     H81.11   Benign paroxysmal vertigo, right ear

     H81.12   Benign paroxysmal vertigo, left ear

     H81.13   Benign paroxysmal vertigo, bilateral

   ● **H81.2**   Vestibular neuronitis

     H81.20   Vestibular neuronitis, unspecified ear

     H81.21   Vestibular neuronitis, right ear

     H81.22   Vestibular neuronitis, left ear

     H81.23   Vestibular neuronitis, bilateral

   ● **H81.3**   Other peripheral vertigo

    ● **H81.31**   Aural vertigo

      H81.311   Aural vertigo, right ear

      H81.312   Aural vertigo, left ear

      H81.313   Aural vertigo, bilateral

      H81.319   Aural vertigo, unspecified ear

    ● **H81.39**   Other peripheral vertigo

     Lermoyez´ syndrome
     Otogenic vertigo
     Peripheral vertigo NOS

      H81.391   Other peripheral vertigo, right ear

      H81.392   Other peripheral vertigo, left ear

      H81.393   Other peripheral vertigo, bilateral

      H81.399   Other peripheral vertigo, unspecified ear

   H81.4   Vertigo of central origin
     Central positional nystagmus

- **H81.8   Other disorders of vestibular function**
  - **H81.8X   Other disorders of vestibular function**
    - H81.8X1   Other disorders of vestibular function, **right** ear
    - H81.8X2   Other disorders of vestibular function, **left** ear
    - H81.8X3   Other disorders of vestibular function, **bilateral**
    - H81.8X9   Other disorders of vestibular function, **unspecified** ear
      - **Coding Clinic: 2022, Q2, P12**
- **H81.9   Unspecified disorder of vestibular function**
  - Vertiginous syndrome NOS
  - H81.90   Unspecified disorder of vestibular function, **unspecified** ear
  - H81.91   Unspecified disorder of vestibular function, **right** ear
  - H81.92   Unspecified disorder of vestibular function, **left** ear
  - H81.93   Unspecified disorder of vestibular function, **bilateral**
- **H82   Vertiginous syndromes in diseases classified elsewhere**
  - *Code first* underlying disease
  - **Excludes1**   epidemic vertigo (A88.1)
  - *H82.1   Vertiginous syndromes in diseases classified elsewhere, right ear*
  - *H82.2   Vertiginous syndromes in diseases classified elsewhere, left ear*
  - *H82.3   Vertiginous syndromes in diseases classified elsewhere, bilateral*
  - *H82.9   Vertiginous syndromes in diseases classified elsewhere, unspecified ear*
- **H83   Other diseases of inner ear**
  - **H83.0   Labyrinthitis**
    - *Balance disorder that follows URI or head injury*
    - H83.01   Labyrinthitis, **right** ear
    - H83.02   Labyrinthitis, **left** ear
    - H83.03   Labyrinthitis, **bilateral**
    - H83.09   Labyrinthitis, **unspecified** ear
  - **H83.1   Labyrinthine fistula**
    - H83.11   Labyrinthine fistula, **right** ear
    - H83.12   Labyrinthine fistula, **left** ear
    - H83.13   Labyrinthine fistula, **bilateral**
    - H83.19   Labyrinthine fistula, **unspecified** ear
  - **H83.2   Labyrinthine dysfunction**
    - Labyrinthine hypersensitivity
    - Labyrinthine hypofunction
    - Labyrinthine loss of function
    - **H83.2X   Labyrinthine dysfunction**
      - H83.2X1   Labyrinthine dysfunction, **right** ear
      - H83.2X2   Labyrinthine dysfunction, **left** ear
      - H83.2X3   Labyrinthine dysfunction, **bilateral**
      - H83.2X9   Labyrinthine dysfunction, **unspecified** ear
  - **H83.3   Noise effects on inner ear**
    - Acoustic trauma of inner ear
    - Noise-induced hearing loss of inner ear
    - **H83.3X   Noise effects on inner ear**
      - H83.3X1   Noise effects on **right** inner ear
      - H83.3X2   Noise effects on **left** inner ear
      - H83.3X3   Noise effects on inner ear, **bilateral**
      - H83.3X9   Noise effects on inner ear, **unspecified** ear

- **H83.8   Other specified diseases of inner ear**
  - **H83.8X   Other specified diseases of inner ear**
    - H83.8X1   Other specified diseases of **right** inner ear
    - H83.8X2   Other specified diseases of **left** inner ear
    - H83.8X3   Other specified diseases of inner ear, **bilateral**
    - H83.8X9   Other specified diseases of inner ear, **unspecified** ear
- **H83.9   Unspecified disease of inner ear**
  - H83.90   Unspecified disease of inner ear, **unspecified** ear
  - H83.91   Unspecified disease of **right** inner ear
  - H83.92   Unspecified disease of **left** inner ear
  - H83.93   Unspecified disease of inner ear, **bilateral**

OTHER DISORDERS OF EAR (H90-H94)

- **H90   Conductive and sensorineural hearing loss**
  - **Excludes1**   deaf nonspeaking NEC (H91.3)
    - deafness NOS (H91.9-)
    - hearing loss NOS (H91.9-)
    - noise-induced hearing loss (H83.3-)
    - ototoxic hearing loss (H91.0-)
    - sudden (idiopathic) hearing loss (H91.2-)
  - H90.0   **Conductive** hearing loss, **bilateral**
  - **H90.1   Conductive hearing loss, unilateral with unrestricted hearing on the contralateral side**
    - H90.11   Conductive hearing loss, unilateral, **right** ear, with unrestricted hearing on the contralateral side
    - H90.12   Conductive hearing loss, unilateral, **left** ear, with unrestricted hearing on the contralateral side
  - H90.2   **Conductive** hearing loss, **unspecified**
    - Conductive deafness NOS
  - H90.3   **Sensorineural** hearing loss, **bilateral**
  - **H90.4   Sensorineural hearing loss, unilateral with unrestricted hearing on the contralateral side**
    - H90.41   Sensorineural hearing loss, unilateral, **right** ear, with unrestricted hearing on the contralateral side
    - H90.42   Sensorineural hearing loss, unilateral, **left** ear, with unrestricted hearing on the contralateral side
  - H90.5   **Unspecified sensorineural** hearing loss
    - Central hearing loss NOS
    - Congenital deafness NOS
    - Neural hearing loss NOS
    - Perceptive hearing loss NOS
    - Sensorineural deafness NOS
    - Sensory hearing loss NOS
    - **Excludes1**   abnormal auditory perception (H93.2-)
      - psychogenic deafness (F44.6)
  - H90.6   **Mixed** conductive and sensorineural hearing loss, **bilateral**
    - **Coding Clinic: 2015, Q2, P7**
  - **H90.7   Mixed conductive and sensorineural hearing loss, unilateral with unrestricted hearing on the contralateral side**
    - H90.71   Mixed conductive and sensorineural hearing loss, unilateral, **right** ear, with unrestricted hearing on the contralateral side
    - H90.72   Mixed conductive and sensorineural hearing loss, unilateral, **left** ear, with unrestricted hearing on the contralateral side
  - H90.8   **Mixed** conductive and sensorineural hearing loss, **unspecified**

CHAPTER 8 (H60-H95)

● **H90.A** Conductive and sensorineural hearing loss with restricted hearing on the contralateral side
  Coding Clinic: 2016, Q4, P23-24
- ● **H90.A1** Conductive hearing loss, unilateral, with restricted hearing on the contralateral side
  - **H90.A11** Conductive hearing loss, unilateral, right ear with restricted hearing on the contralateral side
  - **H90.A12** Conductive hearing loss, unilateral, left ear with restricted hearing on the contralateral side
    Coding Clinic: 2016, Q4, P25
- ● **H90.A2** Sensorineural hearing loss, unilateral, with restricted hearing on the contralateral side
  - **H90.A21** Sensorineural hearing loss, unilateral, right ear, with restricted hearing on the contralateral side
  - **H90.A22** Sensorineural hearing loss, unilateral, left ear, with restricted hearing on the contralateral side
- ● **H90.A3** Mixed conductive and sensorineural hearing loss, unilateral with restricted hearing on the contralateral side
  - **H90.A31** Mixed conductive and sensorineural hearing loss, unilateral, right ear with restricted hearing on the contralateral side
  - **H90.A32** Mixed conductive and sensorineural hearing loss, unilateral, left ear with restricted hearing on the contralateral side

● **H91** Other and unspecified hearing loss
  | **Excludes1** | abnormal auditory perception (H93.2-) |
  hearing loss as classified in H90.-
  impacted cerumen (H61.2-)
  noise-induced hearing loss (H83.3-)
  psychogenic deafness (F44.6)
  transient ischemic deafness (H93.01-)
- ● **H91.0** Ototoxic hearing loss
  Code first poisoning due to drug or toxin, if applicable (T36-T65 with fifth or sixth character 1-4)
  Use additional code for adverse effect, if applicable, to identify drug (T36-T50 with fifth or sixth character 5)
  - **H91.01** Ototoxic hearing loss, right ear
  - **H91.02** Ototoxic hearing loss, left ear
  - **H91.03** Ototoxic hearing loss, bilateral
  - **H91.09** Ototoxic hearing loss, unspecified ear
- ● **H91.1** Presbycusis
  Presbyacusia
  - **H91.10** Presbycusis, unspecified ear
  - **H91.11** Presbycusis, right ear
  - **H91.12** Presbycusis, left ear
  - **H91.13** Presbycusis, bilateral
- ● **H91.2** Sudden idiopathic hearing loss
  Sudden hearing loss NOS
  - **H91.20** Sudden idiopathic hearing loss, unspecified ear
  - **H91.21** Sudden idiopathic hearing loss, right ear
  - **H91.22** Sudden idiopathic hearing loss, left ear
  - **H91.23** Sudden idiopathic hearing loss, bilateral
  - **H91.3** Deaf nonspeaking, not elsewhere classified
- ● **H91.8** Other specified hearing loss
  - ● **H91.8X** Other specified hearing loss
    - **H91.8X1** Other specified hearing loss, right ear
    - **H91.8X2** Other specified hearing loss, left ear
    - **H91.8X3** Other specified hearing loss, bilateral
    - **H91.8X9** Other specified hearing loss, unspecified ear

- ● **H91.9** Unspecified hearing loss
  Deafness NOS
  High frequency deafness
  Low frequency deafness
  - **H91.90** Unspecified hearing loss, unspecified ear
  - **H91.91** Unspecified hearing loss, right ear
  - **H91.92** Unspecified hearing loss, left ear
  - **H91.93** Unspecified hearing loss, bilateral

● **H92** Otalgia and effusion of ear
- ● **H92.0** Otalgia
  - **H92.01** Otalgia, right ear
  - **H92.02** Otalgia, left ear
  - **H92.03** Otalgia, bilateral
  - **H92.09** Otalgia, unspecified ear
- ● **H92.1** Otorrhea
  | **Excludes1** | leakage of cerebrospinal fluid through ear (G96.0) |
  - **H92.10** Otorrhea, unspecified ear
  - **H92.11** Otorrhea, right ear
  - **H92.12** Otorrhea, left ear
  - **H92.13** Otorrhea, bilateral
- ● **H92.2** Otorrhagia
  | **Excludes1** | traumatic otorrhagia - code to injury |
  - **H92.20** Otorrhagia, unspecified ear
  - **H92.21** Otorrhagia, right ear
  - **H92.22** Otorrhagia, left ear
  - **H92.23** Otorrhagia, bilateral

● **H93** Other disorders of ear, not elsewhere classified
- ● **H93.0** Degenerative and vascular disorders of ear
  | **Excludes1** | presbycusis (H91.1) |
  - ● **H93.01** Transient ischemic deafness
    - **H93.011** Transient ischemic deafness, right ear
    - **H93.012** Transient ischemic deafness, left ear
    - **H93.013** Transient ischemic deafness, bilateral
    - **H93.019** Transient ischemic deafness, unspecified ear
  - ● **H93.09** Unspecified degenerative and vascular disorders of ear
    - **H93.091** Unspecified degenerative and vascular disorders of right ear
    - **H93.092** Unspecified degenerative and vascular disorders of left ear
    - **H93.093** Unspecified degenerative and vascular disorders of ear, bilateral
    - **H93.099** Unspecified degenerative and vascular disorders of unspecified ear
- ● **H93.1** Tinnitus
  Perception of sound (ringing, buzzing, humming, whistling tunes, or singing)
  - **H93.11** Tinnitus, right ear
  - **H93.12** Tinnitus, left ear
  - **H93.13** Tinnitus, bilateral
  - **H93.19** Tinnitus, unspecified ear
- ● **H93.A** Pulsatile tinnitus
  Coding Clinic: 2016, Q4, P25
  - **H93.A1** Pulsatile tinnitus, right ear
    Coding Clinic: 2023, Q2, P19; 2016, Q4, P26
  - **H93.A2** Pulsatile tinnitus, left ear
  - **H93.A3** Pulsatile tinnitus, bilateral
  - **H93.A9** Pulsatile tinnitus, unspecified ear

▶ New   ⇨ Revised   ~~deleted~~ Deleted   Excludes 1   Excludes 2   Includes   Use additional   Code first   Code also   Key words
OGCR Official Guidelines   **X** Assign placeholder X   ● Use Additional Character(s)   ⟩ Manifestation Code   ℞ Hierarchical Condition Category   **Coding Clinic**

● **H93.2 Other abnormal auditory perceptions**
Excludes2 auditory hallucinations (R44.0)
● **H93.21 Auditory recruitment**
H93.211 Auditory recruitment, right ear
H93.212 Auditory recruitment, left ear
H93.213 Auditory recruitment, bilateral
H93.219 Auditory recruitment, unspecified ear
● **H93.22 Diplacusis**
H93.221 Diplacusis, right ear
H93.222 Diplacusis, left ear
H93.223 Diplacusis, bilateral
H93.229 Diplacusis, unspecified ear
● **H93.23 Hyperacusis**
H93.231 Hyperacusis, right ear
H93.232 Hyperacusis, left ear
H93.233 Hyperacusis, bilateral
H93.239 Hyperacusis, unspecified ear
● **H93.24 Temporary auditory threshold shift**
H93.241 Temporary auditory threshold shift, right ear
H93.242 Temporary auditory threshold shift, left ear
H93.243 Temporary auditory threshold shift, bilateral
H93.249 Temporary auditory threshold shift, unspecified ear
H93.25 Central auditory processing disorder
Congenital auditory imperception
Word deafness
Excludes1 mixed receptive-expressive language disorder (F80.2)
● **H93.29 Other abnormal auditory perceptions**
H93.291 Other abnormal auditory perceptions, right ear
H93.292 Other abnormal auditory perceptions, left ear
H93.293 Other abnormal auditory perceptions, bilateral
H93.299 Other abnormal auditory perceptions, unspecified ear
● **H93.3 Disorders of acoustic nerve**
Disorder of 8th cranial nerve
Excludes1 acoustic neuroma (D33.3)
syphilitic acoustic neuritis (A52.15)
● **H93.3X Disorders of acoustic nerve**
H93.3X1 Disorders of right acoustic nerve
H93.3X2 Disorders of left acoustic nerve
H93.3X3 Disorders of bilateral acoustic nerves
H93.3X9 Disorders of unspecified acoustic nerve
● **H93.8 Other specified disorders of ear**
● **H93.8X Other specified disorders of ear**
H93.8X1 Other specified disorders of right ear
H93.8X2 Other specified disorders of left ear
H93.8X3 Other specified disorders of ear, bilateral
H93.8X9 Other specified disorders of ear, unspecified ear
● **H93.9 Unspecified disorder of ear**
H93.90 Unspecified disorder of ear, unspecified ear
H93.91 Unspecified disorder of right ear
H93.92 Unspecified disorder of left ear
H93.93 Unspecified disorder of ear, bilateral

● **H94 Other disorders of ear in diseases classified elsewhere**
● **H94.0 Acoustic neuritis in infectious and parasitic diseases classified elsewhere**
Code first underlying disease, such as:
parasitic disease (B65-B89)
Excludes1 acoustic neuritis (in):
herpes zoster (B02.29)
syphilis (A52.15)
H94.00 Acoustic neuritis in infectious and parasitic diseases classified elsewhere, unspecified ear
H94.01 Acoustic neuritis in infectious and parasitic diseases classified elsewhere, right ear
H94.02 Acoustic neuritis in infectious and parasitic diseases classified elsewhere, left ear
H94.03 Acoustic neuritis in infectious and parasitic diseases classified elsewhere, bilateral
● **H94.8 Other specified disorders of ear in diseases classified elsewhere**
Code first underlying disease, such as:
congenital syphilis (A50.0)
Excludes1 aural myiasis (B87.4)
syphilitic labyrinthitis (A52.79)
H94.80 Other specified disorders of ear in diseases classified elsewhere, unspecified ear
H94.81 Other specified disorders of right ear in diseases classified elsewhere
H94.82 Other specified disorders of left ear in diseases classified elsewhere
H94.83 Other specified disorders of ear in diseases classified elsewhere, bilateral

INTRAOPERATIVE AND POSTPROCEDURAL COMPLICATIONS AND DISORDERS OF EAR AND MASTOID PROCESS, NOT ELSEWHERE CLASSIFIED (H95)

● **H95 Intraoperative and postprocedural complications and disorders of ear and mastoid process, not elsewhere classified**
Coding Clinic: 2016, Q4, P10
● **H95.0 Recurrent cholesteatoma of postmastoidectomy cavity**
H95.00 Recurrent cholesteatoma of postmastoidectomy cavity, unspecified ear
H95.01 Recurrent cholesteatoma of postmastoidectomy cavity, right ear
H95.02 Recurrent cholesteatoma of postmastoidectomy cavity, left ear
H95.03 Recurrent cholesteatoma of postmastoidectomy cavity, bilateral ears
● **H95.1 Other disorders of ear and mastoid process following mastoidectomy**
● **H95.11 Chronic inflammation of postmastoidectomy cavity**
H95.111 Chronic inflammation of postmastoidectomy cavity, right ear
H95.112 Chronic inflammation of postmastoidectomy cavity, left ear
H95.113 Chronic inflammation of postmastoidectomy cavity, bilateral ears
H95.119 Chronic inflammation of postmastoidectomy cavity, unspecified ear
● **H95.12 Granulation of postmastoidectomy cavity**
H95.121 Granulation of postmastoidectomy cavity, right ear
H95.122 Granulation of postmastoidectomy cavity, left ear
H95.123 Granulation of postmastoidectomy cavity, bilateral ears
H95.129 Granulation of postmastoidectomy cavity, unspecified ear

CHAPTER 8 (H60-H95)

● H95.13　Mucosal cyst of postmastoidectomy cavity
　　　H95.131　Mucosal cyst of postmastoidectomy cavity, **right ear**
　　　H95.132　Mucosal cyst of postmastoidectomy cavity, **left ear**
　　　H95.133　Mucosal cyst of postmastoidectomy cavity, **bilateral ears**
　　　H95.139　Mucosal cyst of postmastoidectomy cavity, **unspecified ear**
● H95.19　Other disorders following mastoidectomy
　　　H95.191　Other disorders following mastoidectomy, **right ear**
　　　H95.192　Other disorders following mastoidectomy, **left ear**
　　　H95.193　Other disorders following mastoidectomy, **bilateral ears**
　　　H95.199　Other disorders following mastoidectomy, **unspecified ear**
● H95.2　Intraoperative hemorrhage and hematoma of ear and mastoid process complicating a procedure
　　　Excludes1　intraoperative hemorrhage and hematoma of ear and mastoid process due to accidental puncture or laceration during a procedure (H95.3-)
　　　H95.21　Intraoperative hemorrhage and hematoma of ear and mastoid process complicating a procedure on the **ear and mastoid process**
　　　H95.22　Intraoperative hemorrhage and hematoma of ear and mastoid process complicating **other procedure**
● H95.3　Accidental puncture and laceration of ear and mastoid process during a procedure
　　　H95.31　Accidental puncture and laceration of the ear and mastoid process during a procedure on the **ear and mastoid process**
　　　H95.32　Accidental puncture and laceration of the ear and mastoid process during **other procedure**
● H95.4　Postprocedural hemorrhage of ear and mastoid process following a procedure
　　　H95.41　Postprocedural hemorrhage of ear and mastoid process following a procedure on the **ear and mastoid process**
　　　H95.42　Postprocedural hemorrhage of ear and mastoid process following **other procedure**

● H95.5　Postprocedural hematoma and seroma of ear and mastoid process following a procedure
　　　H95.51　Postprocedural **hematoma** of ear and mastoid process following a procedure on the **ear and mastoid process**
　　　H95.52　Postprocedural **hematoma** of ear and mastoid process following **other procedure**
　　　H95.53　Postprocedural **seroma** of ear and mastoid process following a procedure on the **ear and mastoid process**
　　　H95.54　Postprocedural **seroma** of ear and mastoid process following **other procedure**
● H95.8　Other intraoperative and postprocedural complications and disorders of the ear and mastoid process, not elsewhere classified
　　　Excludes2　postprocedural complications and disorders following mastoidectomy (H95.0-, H95.1-)
● H95.81　Postprocedural stenosis of external ear canal
　　　H95.811　Postprocedural stenosis of **right** external ear canal
　　　H95.812　Postprocedural stenosis of **left** external ear canal
　　　H95.813　Postprocedural stenosis of external ear canal, **bilateral**
　　　H95.819　Postprocedural stenosis of **unspecified** external ear canal
　　　H95.88　Other intraoperative complications and disorders of the ear and mastoid process, not elsewhere classified
　　　　　　Use additional code, if applicable, to further specify disorder
　　　H95.89　Other postprocedural complications and disorders of the ear and mastoid process, not elsewhere classified
　　　　　　Use additional code, if applicable, to further specify disorder

CHAPTER 9

DISEASES OF THE CIRCULATORY SYSTEM (I00-I99)

OGCR Chapter-Specific Coding Guidelines

9. Chapter 9: Diseases of the Circulatory System (I00-I99)

a. Hypertension

The classification presumes a causal relationship between hypertension and heart involvement and between hypertension and kidney involvement, as the two conditions are linked by the term "with" in the Alphabetic Index. These conditions should be coded as related even in the absence of provider documentation explicitly linking them, unless the documentation clearly states the conditions are unrelated.

For hypertension and conditions not specifically linked by relational terms such as "with," "associated with" or "due to" in the classification, provider documentation must link the conditions in order to code them as related.

1) Hypertension with Heart Disease

Hypertension with heart conditions classified to I50.- or I51.4-I51.7, I51.89, I51.9, are assigned to, a code from category I11, Hypertensive heart disease. Use additional code(s) from category I50, Heart failure, to identify the type(s) of heart failure in those patients with heart failure.

The same heart conditions (I50.-, I51.4-I51.7, I51.89, I51.9) with hypertension, are coded separately if the provider has documented they are unrelated to the hypertension. Sequence according to the circumstances of the admission/encounter.

2) Hypertensive Chronic Kidney Disease

Assign codes from category I12, Hypertensive chronic kidney disease, when both hypertension and a condition classifiable to category N18, Chronic kidney disease (CKD), are present. CKD should not be coded as hypertensive if the provider indicates the CKD is not related to the hypertension.

The appropriate code from category N18 should be used as a secondary code with a code from category I12 to identify the stage of chronic kidney disease.

See Section I.C.14. Chronic kidney disease.

If a patient has hypertensive chronic kidney disease and acute renal failure, an additional code for the acute renal failure is required.

3) Hypertensive Heart and Chronic Kidney Disease

Assign codes from combination category I13, Hypertensive heart and chronic kidney disease, when there is hypertension with both heart and kidney involvement. If heart failure is present, assign an additional code from category I50 to identify the type of heart failure.

The appropriate code from category N18, Chronic kidney disease, should be used as a secondary code with a code from category I13 to identify the stage of chronic kidney disease.

See Section I.C.14. Chronic kidney disease.

The codes in category I13, Hypertensive heart and chronic kidney disease, are combination codes that include hypertension, heart disease and chronic kidney disease. The Includes note at I13 specifies that the conditions included at I11 and I12 are included together in I13. If a patient has hypertension, heart disease and chronic kidney disease then a code from I13 should be used, not individual codes for hypertension, heart disease and chronic kidney disease, or codes from I11 or I12.

For patients with both acute renal failure and chronic kidney disease an additional code for acute renal failure is required.

4) Hypertensive Cerebrovascular Disease

For hypertensive cerebrovascular disease, first assign the appropriate code from categories I60-I69, followed by the appropriate hypertension code.

5) Hypertensive Retinopathy

Subcategory H35.0, Background retinopathy and retinal vascular changes, should be used with a code from category I10 – I15, Hypertensive disease to include the systemic hypertension. The sequencing is based on the reason for the encounter.

6) Hypertension, Secondary

Secondary hypertension is due to an underlying condition. Two codes are required: one to identify the underlying etiology and one from category I15 to identify the hypertension. Sequencing of codes is determined by the reason for admission/encounter.

7) Hypertension, Transient

Assign code R03.0, Elevated blood pressure reading without diagnosis of hypertension, unless patient has an established diagnosis of hypertension. Assign code O13.-, Gestational [pregnancy-induced] hypertension without significant proteinuria, or O14.-, Pre-eclampsia, for transient hypertension of pregnancy.

8) Hypertension, Controlled

This diagnostic statement usually refers to an existing state of hypertension under control by therapy. Assign the appropriate code from categories I10-I15, Hypertensive diseases.

9) Hypertension, Uncontrolled

Uncontrolled hypertension may refer to untreated hypertension or hypertension not responding to current therapeutic regimen. In either case, assign the appropriate code from categories I10-I15, Hypertensive diseases.

10) Hypertensive Crisis

Assign a code from category I16, Hypertensive crisis, for documented hypertensive urgency, hypertensive emergency or unspecified hypertensive crisis. Code also any identified hypertensive disease (I10-I15). The sequencing is based on the reason for the encounter.

11) Pulmonary Hypertension

Pulmonary hypertension is classified to category I27, Other pulmonary heart diseases. For secondary pulmonary hypertension (I27.1, I27.2-), code also any associated conditions or adverse effects of drugs or toxins. The sequencing is based on the reason for the encounter, except for adverse effects of drugs.

See Section I.C.19.e Adverse Effects, Poisoning, Underdosing and Toxic Effects.

b. Atherosclerotic Coronary Artery Disease and Angina

ICD-10-CM has combination codes for atherosclerotic heart disease with angina pectoris. The subcategories for these codes are I25.11, Atherosclerotic heart disease of native coronary artery with angina pectoris and I25.7, Atherosclerosis of coronary artery bypass graft(s) and coronary artery of transplanted heart with angina pectoris.

When using one of these combination codes it is not necessary to use an additional code for angina pectoris. A causal relationship can be assumed in a patient with both atherosclerosis and angina pectoris, unless the documentation indicates the angina is due to something other than the atherosclerosis.

If a patient with coronary artery disease is admitted due to an acute myocardial infarction (AMI), the AMI should be sequenced before the coronary artery disease.

See Section I.C.9. Acute myocardial infarction (AMI).

c. Intraoperative and Postprocedural Cerebrovascular Accident

Medical record documentation should clearly specify the cause-and-effect relationship between the medical intervention and the cerebrovascular accident in order to assign a code for intraoperative or postprocedural cerebrovascular accident.

Proper code assignment depends on whether it was an infarction or hemorrhage and whether it occurred intraoperatively or postoperatively. If it was a cerebral hemorrhage, code assignment depends on the type of procedure performed.

d. Sequelae of Cerebrovascular Disease

1) Category I69, Sequelae of Cerebrovascular disease

Category I69 is used to indicate conditions classifiable to categories I60-I67 as the causes of sequela (neurologic deficits), themselves classified elsewhere. These "late effects" include neurologic deficits that persist after initial onset of conditions classifiable to categories I60-I67. The neurologic deficits caused by cerebrovascular disease may be present from the onset or may arise at any time after the onset of the condition classifiable to categories I60-I67.

Codes from category I69, Sequelae of cerebrovascular disease, that specify hemiplegia, hemiparesis and monoplegia identify whether the dominant or nondominant side is affected. Should the affected side be documented, but not specified as dominant or nondominant, and the classification system does not indicate a default, code selection is as follows:

- For ambidextrous patients, the default should be dominant.
- If the left side is affected, the default is nondominant.
- If the right side is affected, the default is dominant.

2) Codes from category I69 with codes from I60-I67

Codes from category I69 may assigned on a health care record with codes from I60-I67, if the patient has a current cerebrovascular disease and deficits from an old cerebrovascular disease.

3) Codes from category I69 and Personal history of transient ischemic attack (TIA) and cerebral infarction (Z86.73)

Codes from category I69 should not be assigned if the patient does not have neurologic deficits.

See Section I.C.21. 4. History (of) for use of personal history codes.

e. Acute myocardial infarction (AMI)

1) Type 1 ST elevation myocardial infarction (STEMI) and non-ST elevation myocardial infarction (NSTEMI)

The ICD-10-CM codes for acute type 1 myocardial infarction (AMI) identify the site, such as anterolateral wall or true posterior wall. Subcategories I21.0-I21.2 and code I21.3 are used for type 1 ST elevation myocardial infarction (STEMI). Code I21.4, non-ST elevation (NSTEMI) myocardial infarction, is used for type 1 non-ST elevation myocardial infarction (NSTEMI) and nontransmural MIs.

If a type 1 NSTEMI evolves to STEMI, assign the STEMI code. If a type 1 STEMI converts to NSTEMI due to thrombolytic therapy, it is still coded as STEMI.

For encounters occurring while the myocardial infarction is equal to, or less than, four weeks old, including transfers to another acute setting or a postacute setting, and the myocardial infarction meets the definition for "other diagnoses" (see Section III, Reporting Additional Diagnoses), codes from category I21 may continue to be reported. For encounters after the 4-week time frame and the patient is still receiving care related to the myocardial infarction, the appropriate aftercare code should be assigned, rather than a code from category I21. For old or healed myocardial infarctions not requiring further care, code I25.2, Old myocardial infarction, may be assigned.

2) Acute myocardial infarction, unspecified

Code I21.9, Acute myocardial infarction, unspecified, is the default for unspecified acute myocardial infarction or unspecified type. If only type 1 STEMI or transmural MI without the site is documented, assign code I21.3, ST elevation (STEMI) myocardial infarction of unspecified site.

3) AMI documented as nontransmural or subendocardial but site provided

If an AMI is documented as nontransmural or subendocardial, but the site is provided, it is still coded as a subendocardial AMI.

See Section I.C.21.3 for information on coding status post administration of tPA in a different facility within the last 24 hours.

4) Subsequent acute myocardial infarction

A code from category I22, Subsequent ST elevation (STEMI) and non-ST elevation (NSTEMI) myocardial infarction, is to be used when a patient who has suffered a type 1 or unspecified AMI has a new AMI within the 4-week time frame of the initial AMI. A code from category I22 must be used in conjunction with a code from category I21. The sequencing of the I22 and I21 codes depends on the circumstances of the encounter.

Do not assign code I22 for subsequent myocardial infarctions other than type 1 or unspecified. For subsequent type 2 AMI assign only code I21.A1. For subsequent type 4 or type 5 AMI, assign only code I21.A9.

If a subsequent myocardial infarction of one type occurs within 4 weeks of a myocardial infarction of a different type, assign the appropriate codes from category I21 to identify each type. Do not assign a code from I22. Codes from category I22 should only be assigned if both the initial and subsequent myocardial infarctions are type 1 or unspecified.

5) Other Types of Myocardial Infarction

The ICD-10-CM provides codes for different types of myocardial infarction. Type 1 myocardial infarctions are assigned to codes I21.0-I21.4 and I21.9.

Type 2 myocardial infarction, and myocardial infarction due to demand ischemia or secondary to ischemic balance, is assigned to code I21.A1, Myocardial infarction type 2 with a code for the underlying cause. Do not assign code I24.8, Other forms of acute ischemic heart disease for the demand ischemia. Sequencing of type 2 AMI or the underlying cause is dependent on the circumstances of admission. When a type 2 AMI code is described as NSTEMI or STEMI, only assign code I21.A1. Codes I21.01-I21.4 should only be assigned for type 1 AMIs.

Acute myocardial infarctions type 3, 4a, 4b, 4c, and 5 are assigned to code I21.A9, Other myocardial infarction type.

The "Code also" and "Code first" notes should be followed related to complications, and for coding of postprocedural myocardial infarctions during or following cardiac surgery.

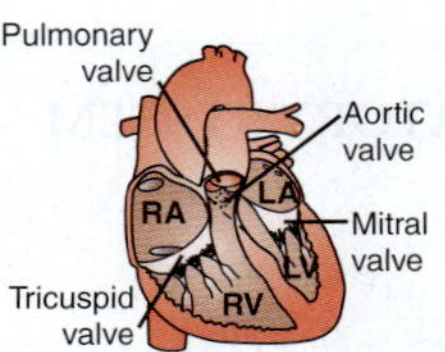

Figure 9-1 Cardiovascular valves.

Item 9–1 Rheumatic fever is the inflammation of the valve(s) of the heart, usually the mitral or aortic, which leads to valve damage. Rheumatic heart inflammations are usually **pericarditis** (sac surrounding heart), **endocarditis** (heart cavity), or **myocarditis** (heart muscle).

CHAPTER 9

DISEASES OF THE CIRCULATORY SYSTEM (IØØ-I99)

Excludes2   certain conditions originating in the perinatal period (P04-P96)
certain infectious and parasitic diseases (A00-B99)
complications of pregnancy, childbirth and the puerperium (O00-O9A)
congenital malformations, deformations, and chromosomal abnormalities (Q00-Q99)
endocrine, nutritional and metabolic diseases (E00-E88)
injury, poisoning and certain other consequences of external causes (S00-T88)
neoplasms (C00-D49)
symptoms, signs and abnormal clinical and laboratory findings, not elsewhere classified (R00-R94)
systemic connective tissue disorders (M30-M36)
transient cerebral ischemic attacks and related syndromes (G45.-)

This chapter contains the following blocks:

IØØ-IØ2	Acute rheumatic fever
IØ5-IØ9	Chronic rheumatic heart diseases
I10-I1A	Hypertensive diseases
I20-I25	Ischemic heart diseases
I26-I28	Pulmonary heart disease and diseases of pulmonary circulation
I30-I5A	Other forms of heart disease
I60-I69	Cerebrovascular diseases
I70-I79	Diseases of arteries, arterioles and capillaries
I80-I89	Diseases of veins, lymphatic vessels and lymph nodes, not elsewhere classified
I95-I99	Other and unspecified disorders of the circulatory system

ACUTE RHEUMATIC FEVER (IØØ-IØ2)

IØØ   **Rheumatic fever without heart involvement**

     Includes   arthritis, rheumatic, acute or subacute

     Excludes1   rheumatic fever with heart involvement (IØ1.0-IØ1.9)

● **IØ1**   **Rheumatic fever with heart involvement**

     Excludes1   chronic diseases of rheumatic origin (IØ5-IØ9) unless rheumatic fever is also present or there is evidence of reactivation or activity of the rheumatic process.

   IØ1.0   **Acute rheumatic pericarditis**
      Any condition in IØØ with pericarditis
      Rheumatic pericarditis (acute)

     Excludes1   acute pericarditis not specified as rheumatic (I30.-)

   IØ1.1   **Acute rheumatic endocarditis**
      Any condition in IØØ with endocarditis or valvulitis
      Acute rheumatic valvulitis

▶ New   ⇒ Revised   ~~deleted~~ Deleted   Excludes 1   Excludes 2   Includes   Use additional   Code first   Code also   Key words

OGCR Official Guidelines   ✗ Assign placeholder X   ● Use Additional Character(s)   ▶ Manifestation Code   🅗 Hierarchical Condition Category   **Coding Clinic**

Item 9–2 Rheumatic chorea, also called Sydenham's, juvenile, minor, simple, or St. Vitus' dance, is a major symptom of rheumatic fever and is characterized by ceaseless, involuntary, jerky, purposeless movements.

I01.2   **Acute rheumatic myocarditis**
      Any condition in I00 with myocarditis

I01.8   **Other acute rheumatic heart disease**
      Any condition in I00 with other or multiple types of heart involvement
      Acute rheumatic pancarditis

I01.9   **Acute rheumatic heart disease, unspecified**
      Any condition in I00 with unspecified type of heart involvement
      Rheumatic carditis, acute
      Rheumatic heart disease, active or acute

● **I02**   **Rheumatic chorea**
     Includes   Sydenham's chorea
     Excludes1   chorea NOS (G25.5)
        Huntington's chorea (G10)

I02.0   **Rheumatic chorea with heart involvement**
      Chorea NOS with heart involvement
      Rheumatic chorea with heart involvement of any type classifiable under I01.-

I02.9   **Rheumatic chorea without heart involvement**
      Rheumatic chorea NOS

CHRONIC RHEUMATIC HEART DISEASES (I05-I09)

● **I05**   **Rheumatic mitral valve diseases**
     Includes   conditions classifiable to both I05.0 and I05.2-I05.9, whether specified as rheumatic or not
     Excludes1   mitral valve disease specified as nonrheumatic (I34.-)
        mitral valve disease with aortic and/or tricuspid valve involvement (I08.-)

I05.0   **Rheumatic mitral stenosis**
      Mitral (valve) obstruction (rheumatic)

I05.1   **Rheumatic mitral insufficiency**
      Rheumatic mitral incompetence
      Rheumatic mitral regurgitation
      Excludes1   mitral insufficiency not specified as rheumatic (I34.0)

I05.2   **Rheumatic mitral stenosis with insufficiency**
      Rheumatic mitral stenosis with incompetence or regurgitation

I05.8   **Other rheumatic mitral valve diseases**
      Rheumatic mitral (valve) failure

I05.9   **Rheumatic mitral valve disease, unspecified**
      Rheumatic mitral (valve) disorder (chronic) NOS

● **I06**   **Rheumatic aortic valve diseases**
     Excludes1   aortic valve disease not specified as rheumatic (I35.-)
        aortic valve disease with mitral and/or tricuspid valve involvement (I08.-)

I06.0   **Rheumatic aortic stenosis**
      Rheumatic aortic (valve) obstruction

I06.1   **Rheumatic aortic insufficiency**
      Rheumatic aortic incompetence
      Rheumatic aortic regurgitation

I06.2   **Rheumatic aortic stenosis with insufficiency**
      Rheumatic aortic stenosis with incompetence or regurgitation

★**(See Plate 33 of the Anatomy Illustrations.)**

Item 9–4 Aortic stenosis is the narrowing of the aortic valve located between the left ventricle and the aorta. **Aortic insufficiency** is the improper closure of the aortic valve, which may lead to enlargement (hypertrophy) of the left ventricle.

I06.8   **Other rheumatic aortic valve diseases**

I06.9   **Rheumatic aortic valve disease, unspecified**
      Rheumatic aortic (valve) disease NOS

● **I07**   **Rheumatic tricuspid valve diseases**
     Includes   rheumatic tricuspid valve diseases specified as rheumatic or unspecified
     Excludes1   tricuspid valve disease specified as nonrheumatic (I36.-)
        tricuspid valve disease with aortic and/or mitral valve involvement (I08.-)
     Excludes2   tricuspid valve disease specified as nonrheumatic (I36.-)
        tricuspid valve disease with aortic and/or mitral valve involvement (I08.-)

I07.0   **Rheumatic tricuspid stenosis**
      Tricuspid (valve) stenosis (rheumatic)

I07.1   **Rheumatic tricuspid insufficiency**
      Tricuspid (valve) insufficiency (rheumatic)

I07.2   **Rheumatic tricuspid stenosis and insufficiency**

I07.8   **Other rheumatic tricuspid valve diseases**

I07.9   **Rheumatic tricuspid valve disease, unspecified**
      Rheumatic tricuspid valve disorder NOS

● **I08**   **Multiple valve diseases**
     Includes   multiple valve diseases specified as rheumatic or unspecified
     Excludes1   endocarditis, valve unspecified (I38)
        multiple valve disease specified a nonrheumatic (I34.-, I35.-, I36.-, I37.-, I38.-, Q22.-, Q23.-, Q24.8-)
        rheumatic valve disease NOS (I09.1)
     Coding Clinic: 2025, Q1, P19; 2019, Q2, P5

I08.0   **Rheumatic disorders of both mitral and aortic valves**
      Involvement of both mitral and aortic valves specified as rheumatic or unspecified
      Coding Clinic: 2025, Q1, P19; 2019, Q2, P5

I08.1   **Rheumatic disorders of both mitral and tricuspid valves**

I08.2   **Rheumatic disorders of both aortic and tricuspid valves**

I08.3   **Combined rheumatic disorders of mitral, aortic and tricuspid valves**

I08.8   **Other rheumatic multiple valve diseases**

I08.9   **Rheumatic multiple valve disease, unspecified**

● **I09**   **Other rheumatic heart diseases**

I09.0   **Rheumatic myocarditis**
      Excludes1   myocarditis not specified as rheumatic (I51.4)

I09.1   **Rheumatic diseases of endocardium, valve unspecified**
      Rheumatic endocarditis (chronic)
      Rheumatic valvulitis (chronic)
      Excludes1   endocarditis, valve unspecified (I38)

I09.2   **Chronic rheumatic pericarditis**
      Adherent pericardium, rheumatic
      Chronic rheumatic mediastinopericarditis
      Chronic rheumatic myopericarditis
      Excludes1   chronic pericarditis not specified as rheumatic (I31.-)

● **I09.8**   **Other specified rheumatic heart diseases**

I09.81   **Rheumatic heart failure**
      Use additional code to identify type of heart failure (I50.-)

I09.89   **Other specified rheumatic heart diseases**
      Rheumatic disease of pulmonary valve

I09.9   **Rheumatic heart disease, unspecified**
      Rheumatic carditis
      Excludes1   rheumatoid carditis (M05.31)

Item 9–3 Mitral stenosis is the narrowing of the mitral valve separating the left atrium from the left ventricle. **Mitral insufficiency** is the improper closure of the mitral valve, which may lead to enlargement (hypertrophy) of the left atrium.

CHAPTER 9 (I00-I99)

Item 9–5 Hypertension is caused by high arterial blood pressure in the arteries. **Essential, primary,** or **idiopathic** hypertension occurs without identifiable organic cause. **Secondary** hypertension is that which has an organic cause. **Malignant** hypertension is severely elevated blood pressure. **Benign** hypertension is mildly elevated blood pressure.

HYPERTENSIVE DISEASES (I10-I16)

Use additional code to identify:
exposure to environmental tobacco smoke (Z77.22)
history of tobacco dependence (Z87.891)
occupational exposure to environmental tobacco smoke (Z57.31)
tobacco dependence (F17.-)
tobacco use (Z72.0)

| **Excludes1** | neonatal hypertension (P29.2)
primary pulmonary hypertension (I27.0) |
| **Excludes2** | hypertensive disease complicating pregnancy, childbirth and the puerperium (O10-O11, O13-O16) |

I10   Essential (primary) hypertension

Includes	high blood pressure hypertension (arterial) (benign) (essential) (malignant) (primary) (systemic)
Excludes1	hypertensive disease complicating pregnancy, childbirth and the puerperium (O10-O11, O13-O16)
Excludes2	essential (primary) hypertension involving vessels of brain (I60-I69) essential (primary) hypertension involving vessels of eye (H35.0-)

Coding Clinic: 2023, Q4, P24-25,42

● **I11   Hypertensive heart disease**

| **Includes** | any condition in I50.- or I51.4-I51.7, I51.89, I51.9 due to hypertension |

I11.0   Hypertensive heart disease with heart failure Ⓗⓒ
Hypertensive heart failure
Use additional code to identify type of heart failure (I50.-)
Coding Clinic: 2017, Q1, P47

I11.9   Hypertensive heart disease without heart failure
Hypertensive heart disease NOS

OGCR Section I.C.9.a.2.

Hypertensive Chronic Kidney Disease
Assign codes from category I12, Hypertensive chronic kidney disease, when both hypertension and a condition classifiable to category N18, Chronic kidney disease (CKD), are present. CKD should not be coded as hypertensive if the physician has specifically documented a different cause.

The appropriate code from category N18 should be used as a secondary code with a code from category I12 to identify the stage of chronic kidney disease.
See Section I.C.14. Chronic kidney disease.

If a patient has hypertensive chronic kidney disease and acute renal failure, an additional code for the acute renal failure is required.

● **I12   Hypertensive chronic kidney disease**

Includes	any condition in N18 and N26 - due to hypertension arteriosclerosis of kidney arteriosclerotic nephritis (chronic) (interstitial) hypertensive nephropathy nephrosclerosis
Excludes1	hypertension due to kidney disease (I15.0, I15.1) renovascular hypertension (I15.0) secondary hypertension (I15.-)
Excludes2	acute kidney failure (N17.-)

Coding Clinic: 2018, Q4, P89; 2016, Q4, P123

I12.0   Hypertensive chronic kidney disease with stage 5 chronic kidney disease or end stage renal disease Ⓗⓒ
Use additional code to identify the stage of chronic kidney disease (N18.5, N18.6)
Coding Clinic: 2016, Q3, P23

I12.9   Hypertensive chronic kidney disease with stage 1 through stage 4 chronic kidney disease, or unspecified chronic kidney disease
Hypertensive chronic kidney disease NOS
Hypertensive renal disease NOS
Use additional code to identify the stage of chronic kidney disease (N18.1-N18.4, N18.9)
Coding Clinic: 2022, Q4, P6; 2018, Q4, P88

OGCR Section I.c.9.a.3.

Hypertensive Heart and Chronic Kidney Disease
Assign codes from combination category I13, Hypertensive heart and chronic kidney disease, when **there is hypertension with both heart and kidney involvement.** If heart failure is present, assign an additional code from category I50 to identify the type of heart failure.

The appropriate code from category N18, Chronic kidney disease, should be used as a secondary code with a code from category I13 to identify the stage of chronic kidney disease.
See Section I.C.14. Chronic kidney disease.

The codes in category I13, Hypertensive heart and chronic kidney disease, are combination codes that include hypertension, heart disease and chronic kidney disease. The Includes note at I13 specifies that the conditions included at I11 and I12 are included together in I13. If a patient has hypertension, heart disease and chronic kidney disease then a code from I13 should be used, not individual codes for hypertension, heart disease and chronic kidney disease, or codes from I11 or I12.

For patients with both acute renal failure and chronic kidney disease an additional code for acute renal failure is required.

● **I13   Hypertensive heart and chronic kidney disease**

| **Includes** | any condition in I11.- with any condition in I12.-
cardiorenal disease
cardiovascular renal disease |

Coding Clinic: 2022, Q4, P6

I13.0   Hypertensive heart and chronic kidney disease with heart failure and stage 1 through stage 4 chronic kidney disease, or unspecified chronic kidney disease Ⓗⓒ
Use additional code to identify type of heart failure (I50.-)
Use additional code to identify stage of chronic kidney disease (N18.1-N18.4, N18.9)

● **I13.1   Hypertensive heart and chronic kidney disease without heart failure**

I13.10   Hypertensive heart and chronic kidney disease without heart failure, with stage 1 through stage 4 chronic kidney disease, or unspecified chronic kidney disease
Hypertensive heart disease and hypertensive chronic kidney disease NOS
Use additional code to identify the stage of chronic kidney disease (N18.1-N18.4, N18.9)

I13.11   Hypertensive heart and chronic kidney disease without heart failure, with stage 5 chronic kidney disease, or end stage renal disease Ⓗⓒ
Use additional code to identify the stage of chronic kidney disease (N18.5, N18.6)

I13.2   Hypertensive heart and chronic kidney disease with heart failure and with stage 5 chronic kidney disease, or end stage renal disease Ⓗⓒ
Use additional code to identify type of heart failure (I50.-)
Use additional code to identify the stage of chronic kidney disease (N18.5, N18.6)

OGCR Section I.9.a.6.

Hypertension, Secondary
Secondary hypertension is due to an underlying condition. Two codes are required: one to identify the underlying etiology and one from category I15 to identify the hypertension. Sequencing of codes is determined by the reason for admission/encounter.

● **I15** **Secondary hypertension**
    Code also underlying condition
    Excludes1 postprocedural hypertension (I97.3)
    Excludes2 secondary hypertension involving vessels of
                 brain (I60-I69)
               secondary hypertension involving vessels of eye
                 (H35.0-)
   I15.0 **Renovascular hypertension**
   I15.1 **Hypertension secondary to other renal disorders**
        Coding Clinic: 2016, Q3, P23
   I15.2 **Hypertension secondary to endocrine disorders**
        Coding Clinic: 2023, Q2, P16-17
   I15.8 **Other secondary hypertension**
   I15.9 **Secondary hypertension, unspecified**

● **I16** **Hypertensive crisis**
    Code also any identified hypertensive disease (I10-I15, I1A)
    Coding Clinic: 2016, Q4, P26-27, 123
   I16.0 **Hypertensive urgency**
   I16.1 **Hypertensive emergency**
        Coding Clinic: 2023, Q4, P25
    Use Additional code, if applicable, to identify specific organ
        dysfunction, such as:
        acute kidney injury (N17.-)
        acute myocardial infarction (I21.-)
        acute pulmonary edema (left and/or right ventricular
            failure) (J81.0, I50.-)
        aortic dissection (I71.0-)
        cerebral hemorrhage (I60.-. I61.-, I62.-)
        cerebral infarction (I63.-)
        eclampsia (O15.-)
        hypertensive encephalopathy (I67.4)
        seizure (R56.9)
   I16.9 **Hypertensive crisis, unspecified**

● **I1A** **Other hypertension**
   I1A.0 **Resistant hypertension**
        Apparent treatment resistant hypertension
        Treatment resistant hypertension
        True resistant hypertension
        Code first specific type of existing hypertension, if known,
          such as:
            essential hypertension (I10)
            secondary hypertension (I15.-)
            Coding Clinic: 2023, Q4, P24-25

ISCHEMIC HEART DISEASES (I20-I25)

Code also the presence of hypertension (I10-I1A)

● **I20** **Angina pectoris**
    Chest pain/discomfort due to lack of oxygen to the heart muscle.
    Principal symptom of myocardial infarction.
    Use additional code to identify:
        exposure to environmental tobacco smoke (Z77.22)
        history of tobacco dependence (Z87.891)
        occupational exposure to environmental tobacco smoke (Z57.31)
        tobacco dependence (F17.-)
        tobacco use (Z72.0)
    Excludes1 angina pectoris with atherosclerotic heart disease
               of native coronary arteries (I25.1-)
               atherosclerosis of coronary artery bypass graft(s)
                 and coronary artery of transplanted heart
                 with angina pectoris (I25.7-)
               postinfarction angina (I23.7)
   I20.0 **Unstable angina** ℞
        Accelerated angina
        Crescendo angina
        De novo effort angina
        Intermediate coronary syndrome
        Preinfarction syndrome
        Worsening effort angina
   I20.1 **Angina pectoris with documented spasm** ℞
        Angiospastic angina
        Prinzmetal angina
        Spasm-induced angina
        Variant angina

   I20.2 **Refractory angina pectoris**
● **I20.8** **Other forms of angina pectoris** ℞
    Use additional code(s) for symptoms associated with
        angina equivalent
    I20.81 **Angina pectoris with coronary microvascular dysfunction**
        Angina pectoris with coronary microvascular
          disease
    I20.89 **Other forms of angina pectoris**
        Angina equivalent
        Angina of effort
        Coronary slow flow syndrome
        Stable angina
        Stenocardia
   I20.9 **Angina pectoris, unspecified** ℞
        Angina NOS
        Anginal syndrome
        Cardiac angina
        Ischemic chest pain

● **I21** **Acute myocardial infarction**
    Includes cardiac infarction
             coronary (artery) embolism
             coronary (artery) occlusion
             coronary (artery) rupture
             coronary (artery) thrombosis
             infarction of heart, myocardium, or ventricle
             myocardial infarction specified as acute or with a
                 stated duration of 4 weeks (28 days) or less
                 from onset
    Use additional code, if applicable, to identify:
        exposure to environmental tobacco smoke (Z77.22)
        history of tobacco dependence (Z87.891)
        occupational exposure to environmental tobacco smoke (Z57.31)
        status post administration of tPA (rtPA) in a different facility
          within the last 24 hours prior to admission to current
          facility (Z92.82)
        tobacco dependence (F17.-)
        tobacco use (Z72.0)
    Excludes2 old myocardial infarction (I25.2)
               postmyocardial infarction syndrome (I24.1)
               subsequent type 1 myocardial infarction (I22.-)
    Coding Clinic: 2016, Q4, P140; 2013, Q1, P25-26; 2012, Q4, P103
● **I21.0** **ST elevation (STEMI) myocardial infarction of anterior wall**
        Type 1 ST elevation myocardial infarction of anterior wall
        Coding Clinic: 2013, Q1, P26
    I21.01 **ST elevation (STEMI) myocardial infarction involving left main coronary artery** ℞
    I21.02 **ST elevation (STEMI) myocardial infarction involving left anterior descending coronary artery** ℞
        ST elevation (STEMI) myocardial infarction
          involving diagonal coronary artery
        Coding Clinic: 2013, Q1, P26
    I21.09 **ST elevation (STEMI) myocardial infarction involving other coronary artery of anterior wall** ℞
        Acute transmural myocardial infarction of
          anterior wall
        Anteroapical transmural (Q wave) infarction
          (acute)
        Anterolateral transmural (Q wave) infarction
          (acute)
        Anteroseptal transmural (Q wave) infarction
          (acute)
        Transmural (Q wave) infarction (acute) (of)
          anterior (wall) NOS
        Coding Clinic: 2012, Q4, P102, 104
● **I21.1** **ST elevation (STEMI) myocardial infarction of inferior wall**
        Type 1 ST elevation myocardial infarction of inferior wall
        Coding Clinic: 2013, Q1, P26

CHAPTER 9 (I00-I99)

CHAPTER 9 (I00-I99)

I21.11 **ST elevation (STEMI) myocardial infarction involving right coronary artery** 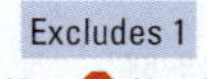
Inferoposterior transmural (Q wave) infarction (acute)

I21.19 **ST elevation (STEMI) myocardial infarction involving other coronary artery of inferior wall**
Acute transmural myocardial infarction of inferior wall
Inferolateral transmural (Q wave) infarction (acute)
Transmural (Q wave) infarction (acute) (of) diaphragmatic wall
Transmural (Q wave) infarction (acute) (of) inferior (wall) NOS

> **Excludes2** ST elevation (STEMI) myocardial infarction involving left circumflex coronary artery (I21.21)

Coding Clinic: 2012, Q4, P97

● **I21.2** **ST elevation (STEMI) myocardial infarction of other sites**
Type 1 ST elevation myocardial infarction of other sites
Coding Clinic: 2013, Q1, P26

I21.21 **ST elevation (STEMI) myocardial infarction involving left circumflex coronary artery**
ST elevation (STEMI) myocardial infarction involving oblique marginal coronary artery

I21.29 **ST elevation (STEMI) myocardial infarction involving other sites**
Acute transmural myocardial infarction of other sites
Apical-lateral transmural (Q wave) infarction (acute)
Basal-lateral transmural (Q wave) infarction (acute)
High lateral transmural (Q wave) infarction (acute)
Lateral (wall) NOS transmural (Q wave) infarction (acute)
Posterior (true) transmural (Q wave) infarction (acute)
Posterobasal transmural (Q wave) infarction (acute)
Posterolateral transmural (Q wave) infarction (acute)
Posteroseptal transmural (Q wave) infarction (acute)
Septal transmural (Q wave) infarction (acute) NOS

OGCR Section I.c.9.e.2.

Acute myocardial infarction, unspecified

Code I21.9, Acute myocardial infarction, unspecified, is the default for unspecified acute myocardial infarction or unspecified type. If only type 1 STEMI or transmural MI without the site is documented, assign I21.3, ST elevation (STEMI) myocardial infarction of unspecified site.

I21.3 **ST elevation (STEMI) myocardial infarction of unspecified site**
Acute transmural myocardial infarction of unspecified site
Transmural (Q wave) myocardial infarction NOS
Type 1 ST elevation myocardial infarction of unspecified site
Coding Clinic: 2013, Q1, P26

I21.4 **Non-ST elevation (NSTEMI) myocardial infarction**
Acute subendocardial myocardial infarction
Non-Q wave myocardial infarction NOS
Nontransmural myocardial infarction NOS
Type 1 non-ST elevation myocardial infarction
Coding Clinic: 2025, Q1, P20; 2024, Q1, P28; 2023, Q2, P29; 2021, Q3, P7; 2017, Q1, P44; 2015, Q2, P16; 2013, Q1, P26

I21.9 **Acute myocardial infarction, unspecified**
Myocardial infarction (acute) NOS

● **I21.A** **Other type of myocardial infarction**

I21.A1 **Myocardial infarction type 2**
Myocardial infarction due to demand ischemia
Myocardial infarction secondary to ischemic imbalance

> *Code first*, *if applicable, the underlying cause, such as:*
> anemia (D50.0-D64.9)
> chronic obstructive pulmonary disease (J44.-)
> paroxysmal tachycardia (I47.0-I47.9)
> shock (R57.0-R57.9)

Coding Clinic: 2017, Q4, P13-14

I21.A9 **Other myocardial infarction type**
Myocardial infarction associated with revascularization procedure
Myocardial infarction type 3
Myocardial infarction type 4a
Myocardial infarction type 4b
Myocardial infarction type 4c
Myocardial infarction type 5

> *Code first*, *if applicable, postprocedural myocardial infarction following cardiac surgery (I97.190), or postprocedural myocardial infarction during cardiac surgery (I97.790)*

> Code also complication, if known and applicable, such as:
> (acute) stent occlusion (T82.897-)
> (acute) stent stenosis (T82.857-)
> (acute) stent thrombosis (T82.865-)
> cardiac arrest due to underlying cardiac condition (I46.2)
> complication of percutaneous coronary intervention (PCI) (I97.89)
> occlusion of coronary artery bypass graft (T82.218-)

Coding Clinic: 2021, Q3, P6-7; 2019, Q2, P32-33

I21.B **Myocardial infarction with coronary microvascular dysfunction**
Myocardial infarction with coronary microvascular disease
Myocardial infarction with nonobstructive coronary arteries
[MINOCA] with microvascular disease

● **I22** **Subsequent ST elevation (STEMI) and non-ST elevation (NSTEMI) myocardial infarction**

> **Includes** acute myocardial infarction occurring within four weeks (28 days) of a previous acute myocardial infarction, regardless of site
> cardiac infarction
> coronary (artery) embolism
> coronary (artery) occlusion
> coronary (artery) rupture
> coronary (artery) thrombosis
> infarction of heart, myocardium, or ventricle
> recurrent myocardial infarction
> reinfarction of myocardium
> rupture of heart, myocardium, or ventricle
> subsequent type 1 myocardial infarction

> **Excludes1** subsequent myocardial infarction, type 2 (I21.A1)
> subsequent myocardial infarction of other type (type 3) (type 4) (type 5) (I21.A9)

Use additional code, if applicable, to identify:
exposure to environmental tobacco smoke (Z77.22)
history of tobacco dependence (Z87.891)
occupational exposure to environmental tobacco smoke (Z57.31)
status post administration of tPA (rtPA) in a different facility within the last 24 hours prior to admission to current facility (Z92.82)
tobacco dependence (F17.-)
tobacco use (Z72.0)
Coding Clinic: 2017, Q4, P14; 2013, Q1, P25; 2012, Q4, P103

▶ New   ⇨ Revised   ~~deleted~~ Deleted   Excludes 1   Excludes 2   Includes   Use additional   Code first   Code also   Key words
OGCR Official Guidelines   X Assign placeholder X   ● Use Additional Character(s)   ▸ Manifestation Code   Hierarchical Condition Category   **Coding Clinic**

I22.0   **Subsequent ST elevation (STEMI) myocardial infarction of anterior wall** 🗝
 Subsequent acute transmural myocardial infarction of anterior wall
 Subsequent transmural (Q wave) infarction (acute)(of) anterior (wall) NOS
 Subsequent anteroapical transmural (Q wave) infarction (acute)
 Subsequent anterolateral transmural (Q wave) infarction (acute)
 Subsequent anteroseptal transmural (Q wave) infarction (acute)

I22.1   **Subsequent ST elevation (STEMI) myocardial infarction of inferior wall** 🗝
 Subsequent acute transmural myocardial infarction of inferior wall
 Subsequent transmural (Q wave) infarction (acute)(of) diaphragmatic wall
 Subsequent transmural (Q wave) infarction (acute)(of) inferior (wall) NOS
 Subsequent inferolateral transmural (Q wave) infarction (acute)
 Subsequent inferoposterior transmural (Q wave) infarction (acute)
 Coding Clinic: 2012, Q4, P97, 102, 104

I22.2   **Subsequent non-ST elevation (NSTEMI) myocardial infarction** 🗝
 Subsequent acute subendocardial myocardial infarction
 Subsequent non-Q wave myocardial infarction NOS
 Subsequent nontransmural myocardial infarction NOS

I22.8   **Subsequent ST elevation (STEMI) myocardial infarction of other sites** 🗝
 Subsequent acute transmural myocardial infarction of other sites
 Subsequent apical-lateral transmural (Q wave) myocardial infarction (acute)
 Subsequent basal-lateral transmural (Q wave) myocardial infarction (acute)
 Subsequent high lateral transmural (Q wave) myocardial infarction (acute)
 Subsequent transmural (Q wave) myocardial infarction (acute)(of) lateral (wall) NOS
 Subsequent posterior (true) transmural (Q wave) myocardial infarction (acute)
 Subsequent posterobasal transmural (Q wave) myocardial infarction (acute)
 Subsequent posterolateral transmural (Q wave) myocardial infarction (acute)
 Subsequent posteroseptal transmural (Q wave) myocardial infarction (acute)
 Subsequent septal NOS transmural (Q wave) myocardial infarction (acute)

I22.9   **Subsequent ST elevation (STEMI) myocardial infarction of unspecified site** 🗝
 Subsequent acute myocardial infarction of unspecified site
 Subsequent myocardial infarction (acute) NOS

● **I23**   **Certain current complications following ST elevation (STEMI) and non-ST elevation (NSTEMI) myocardial infarction (within the 28 day period)**
 Coding Clinic: 2017, Q2, P11

I23.0   **Hemopericardium as current complication following acute myocardial infarction** 🗝   A
 Excludes1   hemopericardium not specified as current complication following acute myocardial infarction (I31.2)

I23.1   **Atrial septal defect as current complication following acute myocardial infarction** 🗝   A
 Excludes1   acquired atrial septal defect not specified as current complication following acute myocardial infarction (I51.0)

Item 9–6   Classification is based on the location of the atherosclerosis. **"Of native coronary artery"** indicates the atherosclerosis is within an original heart artery. **"Of autologous vein bypass graft"** indicates that the atherosclerosis is within a vein graft that was taken from within the patient. **"Of nonautologous biological bypass graft"** indicates the atherosclerosis is within a vessel grafted from other than the patient. **"Of artery bypass graft"** indicates the atherosclerosis is within an artery that was grafted from within the patient.

I23.2   **Ventricular septal defect as current complication following acute myocardial infarction** 🗝   A
 Excludes1   acquired ventricular septal defect not specified as current complication following acute myocardial infarction (I51.0)

I23.3   **Rupture of cardiac wall without hemopericardium as current complication following acute myocardial infarction** 🗝   A
 Coding Clinic: 2017, Q2, P11

I23.4   **Rupture of chordae tendineae as current complication following acute myocardial infarction** 🗝
 Excludes1   rupture of chordae tendineae not specified as current complication following acute myocardial infarction (I51.1)

I23.5   **Rupture of papillary muscle as current complication following acute myocardial infarction** 🗝
 Excludes1   rupture of papillary muscle not specified as current complication following acute myocardial infarction (I51.2)

I23.6   **Thrombosis of atrium, auricular appendage, and ventricle as current complications following acute myocardial infarction** 🗝   A
 Excludes1   thrombosis of atrium, auricular appendage, and ventricle not specified as current complication following acute myocardial infarction (I51.3)

I23.7   **Postinfarction angina** 🗝   A
 Coding Clinic: 2015, Q2, P16-17

I23.8   **Other current complications following acute myocardial infarction** 🗝   A

● **I24**   **Other acute ischemic heart diseases**
 Excludes1   angina pectoris (I20.-)
  transient myocardial ischemia in newborn (P29.4)
 Excludes2   non-ischemic myocardial injury (I5A)

I24.0   **Acute coronary thrombosis not resulting in myocardial infarction** 🗝
 Acute coronary (artery) (vein) embolism not resulting in myocardial infarction
 Acute coronary (artery) (vein) occlusion not resulting in myocardial infarction
 Acute coronary (artery) (vein) thromboembolism not resulting in myocardial infarction
 Excludes1   atherosclerotic heart disease (I25.1-)
 Coding Clinic: 2013, Q1, P24

I24.1   **Dressler's syndrome** 🗝
 Postmyocardial infarction syndrome
 Excludes1   postinfarction angina (I23.7)

● **I24.8**   **Other forms of acute ischemic heart disease** 🗝
 Excludes1   myocardial infarction due to demand ischemia (I21.A1)

 Coding Clinic: 2017, Q4, P13

I24.81   **Acute coronary microvascular dysfunction**
 Acute (presentation of) coronary microvascular disease

I24.89   **Other forms of acute ischemic heart disease**

CHAPTER 9 (I00-I99)

I24.9   **Acute ischemic heart disease, unspecified**

     Excludes1   ischemic heart disease (chronic) NOS (I25.9)

● **I25**   **Chronic ischemic heart disease**

     Excludes2   non-ischemic myocardial injury (I5A)

     Use additional code to identify:
       chronic total occlusion of coronary artery (I25.82)
       exposure to environmental tobacco smoke (Z77.22)
       history of tobacco dependence (Z87.891)
       occupational exposure to environmental tobacco smoke (Z57.31)
       tobacco dependence (F17.-)
       tobacco use (Z72.0)
       Coding Clinic: 2025, Q1, P20

★ **(See Plates 218 and 219 on pages 74 and 75.)**

   ● **I25.1**   **Atherosclerotic heart disease of native coronary artery**
       Disease in which fatty deposits form on the walls of arteries
       Atherosclerotic cardiovascular disease
       Coronary (artery) atheroma
       Coronary (artery) atherosclerosis
       Coronary (artery) disease
       Coronary (artery) sclerosis

       Use additional code, if applicable, to identify:
         coronary atherosclerosis due to calcified coronary lesion (I25.84)
         coronary atherosclerosis due to lipid rich plaque (I25.83)

       Excludes2   atheroembolism (I75.-)
           atherosclerosis of coronary artery bypass graft(s) and transplanted heart (I25.7-)

     I25.10   **Atherosclerotic heart disease of native coronary artery without angina pectoris**   A
       Atherosclerotic heart disease NOS
       Coding Clinic: 2024, Q1, P28; 2021, Q3, P6-7; 2015, Q2, P17; 2012, Q4, P92

OGCR   See Section I.9.b.

> **Atherosclerotic Coronary Artery Disease and Angina**
>
> ICD-10-CM has combination codes for atherosclerotic heart disease with angina pectoris. The subcategories for these codes are I25.11, Atherosclerotic heart disease of native coronary artery with angina pectoris and I25.7, Atherosclerosis of coronary artery bypass graft(s) and coronary artery of transplanted heart with angina pectoris.
>
> When using one of these combination codes it is not necessary to use an additional code for angina pectoris. A causal relationship can be assumed in a patient with both atherosclerosis and angina pectoris, unless the documentation indicates the angina is due to something other than the atherosclerosis.
>
> If a patient with coronary artery disease is admitted due to an acute myocardial infarction (AMI), the AMI should be sequenced before the coronary artery disease.
>
> *See Section I.C.9. Acute myocardial infarction (AMI).*

   ● **I25.11**   **Atherosclerotic heart disease of native coronary artery with angina pectoris**

     I25.110   **Atherosclerotic heart disease of native coronary artery with unstable angina pectoris** 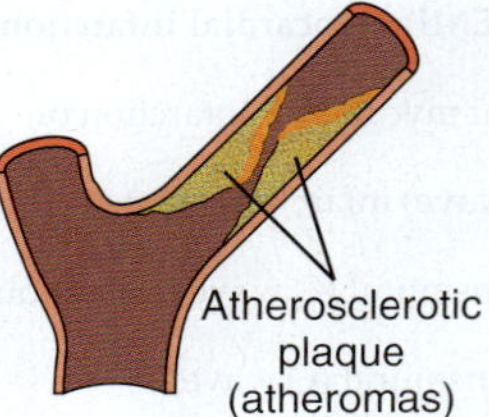   A

       Excludes1   unstable angina without atherosclerotic heart disease (I20.0)

     I25.111   **Atherosclerotic heart disease of native coronary artery with angina pectoris with documented spasm**   A

       Excludes1   angina pectoris with documented spasm without atherosclerotic heart disease (I20.1)

     I25.112   **Atherosclerotic heart disease of native coronary artery with refractory angina pectoris**   A

     I25.118   **Atherosclerotic heart disease of native coronary artery with other forms of angina pectoris**   A

       Excludes1   other forms of angina pectoris without atherosclerotic heart disease (I20.8-)
       Coding Clinic: 2015, Q2, P16-17

     I25.119   **Atherosclerotic heart disease of native coronary artery with unspecified angina pectoris**   A
       Atherosclerotic heart disease with angina NOS
       Atherosclerotic heart disease with ischemic chest pain

       Excludes1   unspecified angina pectoris without atherosclerotic heart disease (I20.9)

   I25.2   **Old myocardial infarction**
       Healed myocardial infarction
       Past myocardial infarction diagnosed by ECG or other investigation, but currently presenting no symptoms

   I25.3   **Aneurysm of heart**
       Mural aneurysm
       Ventricular aneurysm

   ● **I25.4**   **Coronary artery aneurysm and dissection**

     I25.41   **Coronary artery aneurysm**
       Coronary arteriovenous fistula, acquired

       Excludes1   congenital coronary (artery) aneurysm (Q24.5)

     I25.42   **Coronary artery dissection**

   I25.5   **Ischemic cardiomyopathy**

     Excludes2   coronary atherosclerosis (I25.1-, I25.7-)
     Coding Clinic: 2022, Q3, P18

   I25.6   **Silent myocardial ischemia**

   ● **I25.7**   **Atherosclerosis of coronary artery bypass graft(s) and coronary artery of transplanted heart with angina pectoris**

     Use additional code, if applicable, to identify:
       coronary atherosclerosis due to calcified coronary lesion (I25.84)
       coronary atherosclerosis due to lipid rich plaque (I25.83)

     Excludes1   atherosclerosis of bypass graft(s) of transplanted heart without angina pectoris (I25.812)
         atherosclerosis of coronary artery bypass graft(s) without angina pectoris (I25.810)
         atherosclerosis of native coronary artery of transplanted heart without angina pectoris (I25.811)

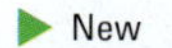

Figure 9-2   Atherosclerotic plaque.

▶ New   ➡ Revised   ~~deleted~~ Deleted   Excludes 1   Excludes 2   Includes   Use additional   Code first   Code also   Key words
OGCR Official Guidelines   X Assign placeholder X   ● Use Additional Character(s)   ▶ Manifestation Code   Hierarchical Condition Category   **Coding Clinic**

CHAPTER 9 (I00-I99)

● **I25.70** **Atherosclerosis of coronary artery bypass graft(s), unspecified, with angina pectoris**

I25.700 **Atherosclerosis of coronary artery bypass graft(s), unspecified, with unstable angina pectoris** 🔵   A

> **Excludes1**   unstable angina pectoris without atherosclerosis of coronary artery bypass graft (I20.0)

I25.701 **Atherosclerosis of coronary artery bypass graft(s), unspecified, with angina pectoris with documented spasm** 🔵   A

> **Excludes1**   angina pectoris with documented spasm without atherosclerosis of coronary artery bypass graft (I20.1)

I25.702 **Atherosclerosis of coronary artery bypass graft(s), unspecified, with refractory angina pectoris**   A

Coding Clinic: 2022, Q4, P22

I25.708 **Atherosclerosis of coronary artery bypass graft(s), unspecified, with other forms of angina pectoris** 🔵   A

> **Excludes1**   other forms of angina pectoris without atherosclerosis of coronary artery bypass graft (I20.8-)

I25.709 **Atherosclerosis of coronary artery bypass graft(s), unspecified, with unspecified angina pectoris** 🔵   A

> **Excludes1**   unspecified angina pectoris without atherosclerosis of coronary artery bypass graft (I20.9)

● **I25.71** **Atherosclerosis of autologous vein coronary artery bypass graft(s) with angina pectoris**

I25.710 **Atherosclerosis of autologous vein coronary artery bypass graft(s) with unstable angina pectoris** 🔵   A

> **Excludes1**   unstable angina without atherosclerosis of autologous vein coronary artery bypass graft(s) (I20.0)
>
> **Excludes2**   embolism or thrombus of coronary artery bypass graft(s) (T82.8-)

I25.711 **Atherosclerosis of autologous vein coronary artery bypass graft(s) with angina pectoris with documented spasm** 🔵   A

> **Excludes1**   angina pectoris with documented spasm without atherosclerosis of autologous vein coronary artery bypass graft(s) (I20.1)

I25.712 **Atherosclerosis of autologous vein coronary artery bypass graft(s) with refractory angina pectoris**   A

I25.718 **Atherosclerosis of autologous vein coronary artery bypass graft(s) with other forms of angina pectoris** 🔵   A

> **Excludes1**   other forms of angina pectoris without atherosclerosis of autologous vein coronary artery bypass graft(s) (I20.8-)

I25.719 **Atherosclerosis of autologous vein coronary artery bypass graft(s) with unspecified angina pectoris** 🔵   A

> **Excludes1**   unspecified angina pectoris without atherosclerosis of autologous vein coronary artery bypass graft(s) (I20.9)

● **I25.72** **Atherosclerosis of autologous artery coronary artery bypass graft(s) with angina pectoris**

Atherosclerosis of internal mammary artery graft with angina pectoris

I25.720 **Atherosclerosis of autologous artery coronary artery bypass graft(s) with unstable angina pectoris** 🔵   A

> **Excludes1**   unstable angina without atherosclerosis of autologous artery coronary artery bypass graft(s) (I20.0)

I25.721 **Atherosclerosis of autologous artery coronary artery bypass graft(s) with angina pectoris with documented spasm** 🔵   A

> **Excludes1**   angina pectoris with documented spasm without atherosclerosis of autologous artery coronary artery bypass graft(s) (I20.1)

I25.722 **Atherosclerosis of autologous artery coronary artery bypass graft(s) with refractory angina pectoris**   A

I25.728   Atherosclerosis of autologous artery coronary artery bypass graft(s) with other forms of angina pectoris 🅡   A

     Excludes 1   other forms of angina pectoris without atherosclerosis of autologous artery coronary artery bypass graft(s) (I20.8-)

I25.729   Atherosclerosis of autologous artery coronary artery bypass graft(s) with unspecified angina pectoris 🅡   A

     Excludes 1   unspecified angina pectoris without atherosclerosis of autologous artery coronary artery bypass graft(s) (I20.9)

● **I25.73**   Atherosclerosis of nonautologous biological coronary artery bypass graft(s) with angina pectoris

I25.730   Atherosclerosis of nonautologous biological coronary artery bypass graft(s) with unstable angina pectoris 🅡   A

     Excludes 1   unstable angina without atherosclerosis of nonautologous biological coronary artery bypass graft(s) (I20.0)

I25.731   Atherosclerosis of nonautologous biological coronary artery bypass graft(s) with angina pectoris with documented spasm 🅡   A

     Excludes 1   angina pectoris with documented spasm without atherosclerosis of nonautologous biological coronary artery bypass graft(s) (I20.1)

I25.732   Atherosclerosis of nonautologous biological coronary artery bypass graft(s) with refractory angina pectoris   A

I25.738   Atherosclerosis of nonautologous biological coronary artery bypass graft(s) with other forms of angina pectoris 🅡   A

     Excludes 1   other forms of angina pectoris without atherosclerosis of nonautologous biological coronary artery bypass graft(s) (I20.8-)

I25.739   Atherosclerosis of nonautologous biological coronary artery bypass graft(s) with unspecified angina pectoris 🅡   A

     Excludes 1   unspecified angina pectoris without atherosclerosis of nonautologous biological coronary artery bypass graft(s) (I20.9)

● **I25.75**   Atherosclerosis of native coronary artery of transplanted heart with angina pectoris

     Excludes 1   atherosclerosis of native coronary artery of transplanted heart without angina pectoris (I25.811)

I25.750   Atherosclerosis of native coronary artery of transplanted heart with unstable angina 🅡

I25.751   Atherosclerosis of native coronary artery of transplanted heart with angina pectoris with documented spasm 🅡

I25.752   Atherosclerosis of native coronary artery of transplanted heart with refractory angina pectoris   A

I25.758   Atherosclerosis of native coronary artery of transplanted heart with other forms of angina pectoris 🅡

I25.759   Atherosclerosis of native coronary artery of transplanted heart with unspecified angina pectoris 🅡

● **I25.76**   Atherosclerosis of bypass graft of coronary artery of transplanted heart with angina pectoris

     Excludes 1   atherosclerosis of bypass graft of coronary artery of transplanted heart without angina pectoris (I25.812)

I25.760   Atherosclerosis of bypass graft of coronary artery of transplanted heart with unstable angina 🅡   A

I25.761   Atherosclerosis of bypass graft of coronary artery of transplanted heart with angina pectoris with documented spasm 🅡   A

I25.762   Atherosclerosis of bypass graft of coronary artery of transplanted heart with refractory angina pectoris   A

I25.768   Atherosclerosis of bypass graft of coronary artery of transplanted heart with other forms of angina pectoris 🅡   A

I25.769   Atherosclerosis of bypass graft of coronary artery of transplanted heart with unspecified angina pectoris 🅡   A

● **I25.79** **Atherosclerosis of other coronary artery bypass graft(s) with angina pectoris**   **A**

I25.790 **Atherosclerosis of other coronary artery bypass graft(s) with unstable angina pectoris**

> **Excludes1**   unstable angina without atherosclerosis of other coronary artery bypass graft(s) (I20.0)

I25.791 **Atherosclerosis of other coronary artery bypass graft(s) with angina pectoris with documented spasm**   **A**

> **Excludes1**   angina pectoris with documented spasm without atherosclerosis of other coronary artery bypass graft(s) (I20.1)

I25.792 **Atherosclerosis of other coronary artery bypass graft(s) with refractory angina pectoris**   **A**

I25.798 **Atherosclerosis of other coronary artery bypass graft(s) with other forms of angina pectoris**   **A**

> **Excludes1**   other forms of angina pectoris without atherosclerosis of other coronary artery bypass graft(s) (I20.8-)

I25.799 **Atherosclerosis of other coronary artery bypass graft(s) with unspecified angina pectoris**   **A**

> **Excludes1**   unspecified angina pectoris without atherosclerosis of other coronary artery bypass graft(s) (I20.9)

● **I25.8** **Other forms of chronic ischemic heart disease**

● **I25.81** **Atherosclerosis of other coronary vessels without angina pectoris**

> Use additional code, if applicable, to identify:
> coronary atherosclerosis due to calcified coronary lesion (I25.84)
> coronary atherosclerosis due to lipid rich plaque (I25.83)

> **Excludes2**   atherosclerotic heart disease of native coronary artery without angina pectoris (I25.10)

I25.810 **Atherosclerosis of coronary artery bypass graft(s) without angina pectoris**   **A**

> Atherosclerosis of coronary artery bypass graft NOS

> **Excludes1**   atherosclerosis of coronary bypass graft(s) with angina pectoris (I25.70- -I25.73-, I25.79-)

> **Coding Clinic: 2016, Q4, P86**

I25.811 **Atherosclerosis of native coronary artery of transplanted heart without angina pectoris**

> Atherosclerosis of native coronary artery of transplanted heart NOS

> **Excludes1**   atherosclerosis of native coronary artery of transplanted heart with angina pectoris (I25.75-)

I25.812 **Atherosclerosis of bypass graft of coronary artery of transplanted heart without angina pectoris**   **A**

> Atherosclerosis of bypass graft of transplanted heart NOS

> **Excludes1**   atherosclerosis of bypass graft of transplanted heart with angina pectoris (I25.76)

I25.82 **Chronic total occlusion of coronary artery**

> Complete occlusion of coronary artery
> Total occlusion of coronary artery
> *Code first* coronary atherosclerosis (I25.1-, I25.7-, I25.81-)

> **Excludes1**   acute coronary occlusion with myocardial infarction (I21.0-I21.B, I22.-)
> acute coronary occlusion without myocardial infarction (I24.0)

I25.83 **Coronary atherosclerosis due to lipid rich plaque**   **A**

> *Code first* coronary atherosclerosis (I25.1-, I25.7-, I25.81-)

I25.84 **Coronary atherosclerosis due to calcified coronary lesion**

> Coronary atherosclerosis due to severely calcified coronary lesion
> *Code first* coronary atherosclerosis (I25.1-, I25.7-, I25.81-)

I25.85 **Chronic coronary microvascular dysfunction**

> Chronic (presentation of) coronary microvascular disease
> Coronary microvascular dysfunction NOS

I25.89 **Other forms of chronic ischemic heart disease**

I25.9 **Chronic ischemic heart disease, unspecified**

> Ischemic heart disease (chronic) NOS

PULMONARY HEART DISEASE AND DISEASES OF PULMONARY CIRCULATION (I26-I28)

● **I26** **Pulmonary embolism**

> **Includes**   cor pulmonale without embolism (I27.81)
> pulmonary (acute)(artery)(vein) infarction
> pulmonary (acute)(artery)(vein) thromboembolism
> pulmonary (acute)(artery)(vein) thrombosis

> **Excludes2**   chronic pulmonary embolism (I27.82)
> personal history of pulmonary embolism (Z86.711)
> pulmonary embolism due to trauma (T79.0, T79.1)
> pulmonary embolism due to complications of surgical and medical care (T80.0, T81.7-, T82.8-)
> pulmonary embolism complicating abortion, ectopic or molar pregnancy (O00-O07, O08.2)
> pulmonary embolism complicating pregnancy, childbirth and the puerperium (O88.-)
> septic (non-pulmonary) arterial embolism (I76)

> **Coding Clinic: 2021, Q2, P10**

Item 9–7 Pulmonary heart disease or **cor pulmonale** is right ventricle hypertrophy or RVH as a result of a respiratory disorder increasing back flow pressure to the right ventricle. Left untreated, cor pulmonale leads to right-heart failure and death.

CHAPTER 9 (I00-I99)

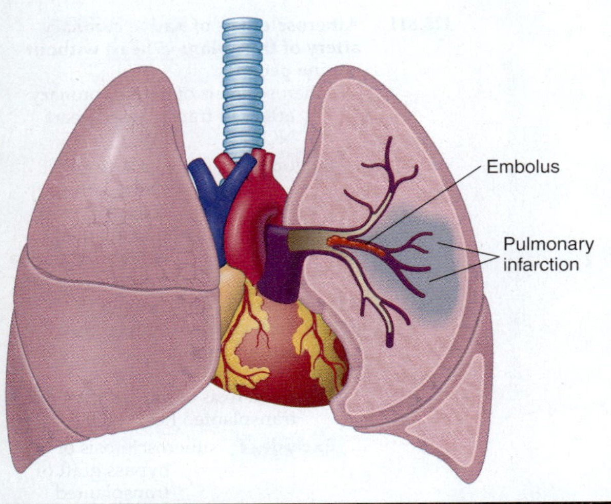

Figure 9-3   Pulmonary embolism. (From Chabner: The Language of Medicine, ed 8, St. Louis, Saunders, 2007)

● **I26.0**   **Pulmonary embolism with acute cor pulmonale**

    I26.01   **Septic pulmonary embolism with acute cor pulmonale** 🄷🄲🄲
       Code first underlying infection

    I26.02   **Saddle embolus of pulmonary artery with acute cor pulmonale** 🄷🄲🄲

    I26.03   **Cement embolism of pulmonary artery with acute cor pulmonale** 🄷🄲🄲
       Code first complication of other artery following a procedure (T81.718)

    I26.04   **Fat embolism of pulmonary artery with acute cor pulmonale** 🄷🄲🄲
       Code first, if applicable:
         complication of other artery following a procedure (T81.718)
         traumatic fat embolism (T79.1)

    I26.09   **Other pulmonary embolism with acute cor pulmonale** 🄷🄲🄲
       Acute cor pulmonale NOS
       Other thrombotic pulmonary embolism with acute cor pulmonale

● **I26.9**   **Pulmonary embolism without acute cor pulmonale**

    I26.90   **Septic pulmonary embolism without acute cor pulmonale** 🄷🄲🄲
       Code first underlying infection

    I26.92   **Saddle embolus of pulmonary artery without acute cor pulmonale** 🄷🄲🄲

    I26.93   **Single subsegmental thrombotic pulmonary embolism without acute cor pulmonale** 🄷🄲🄲
       Subsegmental pulmonary embolism NOS

    I26.94   **Multiple subsegmental thrombotic pulmonary emboli without acute cor pulmonale** 🄷🄲🄲
       Coding Clinic: 2022, Q2, P13; 2021, Q2, P10

    I26.95   **Cement embolism of pulmonary artery without acute cor pulmonale** 🄷🄲🄲
       Code first complication of other artery following a procedure (T81.718)
       Coding Clinic: 2024, Q4, P19

    I26.96   **Fat embolism of pulmonary artery without acute cor pulmonale** 🄷🄲🄲
       Code first, if applicable:
         complication of other artery following a procedure (T81.718)
         traumatic fat embolism (T79.1)
       Coding Clinic: 2024, Q4, P19

    I26.99   **Other pulmonary embolism without acute cor pulmonale** 🄷🄲🄲
       Acute pulmonary embolism NOS
       Other thrombotic pulmonary embolism with acute cor pulmonale
       Pulmonary embolism NOS
       Coding Clinic: 2022, Q2, P13; 2019, Q2, P22-23

● **I27**   **Other pulmonary heart diseases**

    I27.0   **Primary pulmonary hypertension** 🄷🄲🄲
       Heritable pulmonary arterial hypertension
       Idiopathic pulmonary arterial hypertension
       Primary group 1 pulmonary hypertension
       Primary pulmonary arterial hypertension

       Excludes1   persistent pulmonary hypertension of newborn (P29.30)
           pulmonary hypertension NOS (I27.20)
           secondary pulmonary arterial hypertension (I27.21)
           secondary pulmonary hypertension (I27.29)

    I27.1   **Kyphoscoliotic heart disease** 🄷🄲🄲

● **I27.2**   **Other secondary pulmonary hypertension**
       Code also associated underlying condition

       Excludes1   Eisenmenger's syndrome (I27.83)
       Coding Clinic: 2016, Q2, P8

    I27.20   **Pulmonary hypertension, unspecified** 🄷🄲🄲
       Pulmonary hypertension NOS

    I27.21   **Secondary pulmonary arterial hypertension** 🄷🄲🄲
       (Associated) (drug-induced) (toxin-induced) pulmonary arterial hypertension NOS
       (Associated) (drug-induced) (toxin-induced) (secondary) group 1 pulmonary hypertension
       Code also associated conditions if applicable, or adverse effects of drugs or toxins, such as:
       adverse effect of appetite depressants (T50.5X5)
       congenital heart disease (Q20-Q28)
       human immunodeficiency virus [HIV] disease (B20)
       polymyositis (M33.2-)
       portal hypertension (K76.6)
       rheumatoid arthritis (M05.-)
       schistosomiasis (B65.-)
       Sjögren syndrome (M35.0-)
       systemic sclerosis (M34.-)

    I27.22   **Pulmonary hypertension due to left heart disease** 🄷🄲🄲
       Group 2 pulmonary hypertension
       Code also associated left heart disease, if known, such as:
       multiple valve disease (I08.-)
       rheumatic mitral valve diseases (I05.-)
       rheumatic aortic valve diseases (I06.-)

    I27.23   **Pulmonary hypertension due to lung diseases and hypoxia** 🄷🄲🄲
       Group 3 pulmonary hypertension
       Code also associated lung disease, if known, such as:
       bronchiectasis (J47.-)
       cystic fibrosis with pulmonary manifestations (E84.0)
       interstitial lung disease (J84.-)
       pleural effusion (J90)
       sleep apnea (G47.3-)

    I27.24   **Chronic thromboembolic pulmonary hypertension** 🄷🄲🄲
       Group 4 pulmonary hypertension
       Code also associated pulmonary embolism, if applicable (I26.-, I27.82)

► New   ⇒ Revised   ~~deleted~~ Deleted   Excludes 1   Excludes 2   Includes   Use additional   Code first   Code also   Key words

OGCR Official Guidelines   X Assign placeholder X   ● Use Additional Character(s)   ▶ Manifestation Code   🄷🄲🄲 Hierarchical Condition Category   **Coding Clinic**

I27.29　**Other secondary pulmonary hypertension** 🄡🄒
　Group 5 pulmonary hypertension
　Pulmonary hypertension with unclear
　　multifactorial mechanisms
　Pulmonary hypertension due to hematologic
　　disorders
　Pulmonary hypertension due to metabolic
　　disorders
　Pulmonary hypertension due to other systemic
　　disorders
　Code also other associated disorders, if known,
　　such as:
　　chronic myeloid leukemia (C92.10-C92.22)
　　essential thrombocythemia (D47.3)
　　Gaucher disease (E75.22)
　　hypertensive chronic kidney disease with end
　　　stage renal disease (I12.0, I13.11,I13.2)
　　hyperthyroidism (E05.-)
　　hypothyroidism (E00-E03)
　　polycythemia vera (D45)
　　sarcoidosis (D86.-)

● I27.8　**Other specified pulmonary heart diseases**
　I27.81　**Cor pulmonale (chronic)** 🄡🄒
　　Cor pulmonale NOS
　　Code also, if applicable, right heart failure
　　　(I50.81-)
　　　Excludes 1　acute cor pulmonale (I26.0-)

　I27.82　**Chronic pulmonary embolism** 🄡🄒
　　Use additional code, if applicable, for
　　　associated long-term (current) use of
　　　anticoagulants (Z79.01)
　　　Excludes 1　personal history of pulmonary
　　　　　embolism (Z86.711)
　　Coding Clinic: 2021, Q2, P10

　I27.83　**Eisenmenger's syndrome** 🄡🄒
　　Eisenmenger's complex
　　(Irreversible) Eisenmenger's disease
　　Pulmonary hypertension with right to left
　　　shunt related to congenital heart disease
　　Code also underlying heart defect, if known,
　　　such as:
　　　atrial septal defect (Q21.1-)
　　　Eisenmenger's defect (Q21.8)
　　　patent ductus arteriosus (Q25.0)
　　　ventricular septal defect (Q21.0)

▶ ● I27.84　**Fontan related circulation**
　▶ I27.840　**Fontan-associated liver disease [FALD]**
　▶ I27.841　**Fontan-associated lymphatic**
　　　dysfunction
　　　▶ **Code also** associated conditions such
　　　　as:
　　　　▶chylothorax (J94.0)
　　　　▶Fontan associated protein-losing
　　　　　enteropathy (K90.89)
　　　　▶plastic (obstructive) bronchitis
　　　　　(J44.89)

　▶ I27.848　**Other Fontan-associated condition**
　　　▶ **Use Additional** code to specify the
　　　　Fontan associated condition

　▶ I27.849　**Fontan related circulation,**
　　　unspecified

　I27.89　**Other specified pulmonary heart diseases** 🄡🄒
　I27.9　**Pulmonary heart disease, unspecified** 🄡🄒
　　Chronic cardiopulmonary disease

● I28　**Other diseases of pulmonary vessels**
　I28.0　**Arteriovenous fistula of pulmonary vessels** 🄡🄒
　　　Excludes 1　congenital arteriovenous fistula (Q25.72)

　I28.1　**Aneurysm of pulmonary artery** 🄡🄒
　　　Excludes 1　congenital aneurysm (Q25.79)
　　　　　congenital arteriovenous aneurysm
　　　　　　(Q25.72)

I28.8　**Other diseases of pulmonary vessels** 🄡🄒
　Pulmonary arteritis
　Pulmonary endarteritis
　Rupture of pulmonary vessels
　Stenosis of pulmonary vessels
　Stricture of pulmonary vessels

I28.9　**Disease of pulmonary vessels, unspecified** 🄡🄒

OTHER FORMS OF HEART DISEASE (I30-I5A)

● I30　**Acute pericarditis**
　*Inflammation of pericardium (sac surrounding the heart) caused by
　an infection*
　　Includes　　acute mediastinopericarditis
　　　　acute myopericarditis
　　　　acute pericardial effusion
　　　　acute pleuropericarditis
　　　　acute pneumopericarditis

　　Excludes 1　Dressler's syndrome (I24.1)
　　　　rheumatic pericarditis (acute) (I01.0)
　　　　viral pericarditis due to Coxsackie virus (B33.23)

I30.0　**Acute nonspecific idiopathic pericarditis**
I30.1　**Infective pericarditis**
　Pneumococcal pericarditis
　Pneumopyopericardium
　Purulent pericarditis
　Pyopericarditis
　Pyopericardium
　Pyopneumopericardium
　Staphylococcal pericarditis
　Streptococcal pericarditis
　Suppurative pericarditis
　Viral pericarditis
　Use additional code (B95-B97) to identify infectious
　　agent
I30.8　**Other forms of acute pericarditis**
I30.9　**Acute pericarditis, unspecified**

● I31　**Other diseases of pericardium**
　　Excludes 1　diseases of pericardium specified as rheumatic
　　　　(I09.2)
　　　　postcardiotomy syndrome (I97.0)
　　　　traumatic injury to pericardium (S26.-)

I31.0　**Chronic adhesive pericarditis**
　Accretio cordis
　Adherent pericardium
　Adhesive mediastinopericarditis
I31.1　**Chronic constrictive pericarditis**
　Concretio cordis
　Pericardial calcification
I31.2　**Hemopericardium, not elsewhere classified**
　　Excludes 1　hemopericardium as current complication
　　　　following acute myocardial
　　　　infarction (I23.0)

● I31.3　**Pericardial effusion (noninflammatory)**
　　Excludes 1　acute pericardial effusion (I30.9)
　　Coding Clinic: 2019, Q1, P16
　▸ I31.31　**Malignant pericardial effusion in diseases**
　　　classified elsewhere
　　　Code first underlying neoplasm (C00-D49)
　　　Coding Clinic: 2022, Q4, P24
　I31.39　**Other pericardial effusion (noninflammatory)**
　　Chylopericardium
I31.4　**Cardiac tamponade**
　Code first underlying cause
I31.8　**Other specified diseases of pericardium**
　Epicardial plaques
　Focal pericardial adhesions
I31.9　**Disease of pericardium, unspecified**
　Pericarditis (chronic) NOS

CHAPTER 9 (I00-I99)

CHAPTER 9 (I00–I99)

▶ **I32** *Pericarditis in diseases classified elsewhere*
Code first underlying disease
　Excludes1　pericarditis (in):
　　　coxsackie (virus) (B33.23)
　　　gonococcal (A54.83)
　　　meningococcal (A39.53)
　　　rheumatoid (arthritis) (M05.31)
　　　syphilitic (A52.06)
　　　systemic lupus erythematosus (M32.12)
　　　tuberculosis (A18.84)

● **I33** **Acute and subacute endocarditis**
Inflammation/infection of lining of heart, affecting heart valves including replacement valves and is usually caused by a bacterial infection
　Excludes1　acute rheumatic endocarditis (I01.1)
　　　endocarditis NOS (I38)

　I33.0　**Acute and subacute infective endocarditis**
　　Bacterial endocarditis (acute) (subacute)
　　Infective endocarditis (acute) (subacute) NOS
　　Endocarditis lenta (acute) (subacute)
　　Malignant endocarditis (acute) (subacute)
　　Purulent endocarditis (acute) (subacute)
　　Septic endocarditis (acute) (subacute)
　　Ulcerative endocarditis (acute) (subacute)
　　Vegetative endocarditis (acute) (subacute)
　　Use additional code (B95-B97) to identify infectious agent
　　Coding Clinic: 2025, Q1, P19-20

　I33.9　**Acute and subacute endocarditis, unspecified**
　　Acute endocarditis NOS
　　Acute myoendocarditis NOS
　　Acute periendocarditis NOS
　　Subacute endocarditis NOS
　　Subacute myoendocarditis NOS
　　Subacute periendocarditis NOS

● **I34** **Nonrheumatic mitral valve disorders**
　Code also, if applicable:
　　nonrheumatic mitral (valve) annulus calcification (I34.81)
　Excludes1　mitral valve disease (I05.9)
　　　mitral valve failure (I05.8)
　　　mitral valve stenosis (I05.0)
　　　mitral valve disorder of unspecified cause with diseases of aortic and/or tricuspid valve(s) (I08.-)
　　　mitral valve disorder of unspecified cause with mitral stenosis or obstruction (I05.0)
　　　mitral valve disorder specified as congenital (Q23.2, Q23.9)
　　　mitral valve disorder specified as rheumatic (I05.-)

　I34.0　**Nonrheumatic mitral (valve) insufficiency**
　　Nonrheumatic mitral (valve) incompetence NOS
　　Nonrheumatic mitral (valve) regurgitation NOS
　　Coding Clinic: 2025, Q1, P19

　I34.1　**Nonrheumatic mitral (valve) prolapse**
　　Floppy nonrheumatic mitral valve syndrome
　　Excludes1　Marfan's syndrome (Q87.4-)

　I34.2　**Nonrheumatic mitral (valve) stenosis**
　　Code also, if applicable:
　　　nonrheumatic mitral (valve) annulus calcification (I34.81)

● **I34.8**　**Other nonrheumatic mitral valve disorders**

　　I34.81　**Nonrheumatic mitral (valve) annulus calcification**
　　　Nonrheumatic mitral (valve) annular calcification
　　　Mitral (valve) annulus calcification NOS
　　　Code also, if applicable:
　　　　nonrheumatic mitral (valve) insufficiency (I34.0)
　　　　nonrheumatic mitral (valve) stenosis (I34.2)

　　I34.89　**Other nonrheumatic mitral valve disorders**

　I34.9　**Nonrheumatic mitral valve disorder, unspecified**

● **I35** **Nonrheumatic aortic valve disorders**
　Code also, if applicable, bicuspid aortic valve (Q23.81)
　Excludes2　aortic valve disorder of unspecified cause but with diseases of mitral and/or tricuspid valve(s) (I08.-)
　　　aortic valve disorder specified as congenital (Q23.0, Q23.1)
　　　aortic valve disorder specified as rheumatic (I06.-)
　　　hypertrophic subaortic stenosis (I42.1)

　I35.0　**Nonrheumatic aortic (valve) stenosis**
　　Coding Clinic: 2024, Q4, P26

　I35.1　**Nonrheumatic aortic (valve) insufficiency**
　　Nonrheumatic aortic (valve) incompetence NOS
　　Nonrheumatic aortic (valve) regurgitation NOS

　I35.2　**Nonrheumatic aortic (valve) stenosis with insufficiency**

　I35.8　**Other nonrheumatic aortic valve disorders**

　I35.9　**Nonrheumatic aortic valve disorder, unspecified**

● **I36** **Nonrheumatic tricuspid valve disorders**
　Excludes1　tricuspid valve disorders of unspecified cause (I07.-)
　　　tricuspid valve disorders specified as congenital (Q22.4, Q22.8, Q22.9)
　　　tricuspid valve disorders specified as rheumatic (I07.-)
　　　tricuspid valve disorders with aortic and/or mitral valve involvement (I08.-)

　I36.0　**Nonrheumatic tricuspid (valve) stenosis**

　I36.1　**Nonrheumatic tricuspid (valve) insufficiency**
　　Nonrheumatic tricuspid (valve) incompetence
　　Nonrheumatic tricuspid (valve) regurgitation

　I36.2　**Nonrheumatic tricuspid (valve) stenosis with insufficiency**

　I36.8　**Other nonrheumatic tricuspid valve disorders**

　I36.9　**Nonrheumatic tricuspid valve disorder, unspecified**

● **I37** **Nonrheumatic pulmonary valve disorders**
　Excludes1　pulmonary valve disorder specified as congenital (Q22.1, Q22.2, Q22.3)
　　　pulmonary valve disorder specified as rheumatic (I09.89)

　I37.0　**Nonrheumatic pulmonary valve stenosis**

　I37.1　**Nonrheumatic pulmonary valve insufficiency**
　　Nonrheumatic pulmonary valve incompetence
　　Nonrheumatic pulmonary valve regurgitation

　I37.2　**Nonrheumatic pulmonary valve stenosis with insufficiency**

　I37.8　**Other nonrheumatic pulmonary valve disorders**

　I37.9　**Nonrheumatic pulmonary valve disorder, unspecified**

　I38　**Endocarditis, valve unspecified**
　　Includes　endocarditis (chronic) NOS
　　　valvular incompetence NOS
　　　valvular insufficiency NOS
　　　valvular regurgitation NOS
　　　valvular stenosis NOS
　　　valvulitis (chronic) NOS
　　Excludes1　congenital insufficiency of cardiac valve NOS (Q24.8)
　　　congenital stenosis of cardiac valve NOS (Q24.8)
　　　endocardial fibroelastosis (I42.4)
　　　endocarditis specified as rheumatic (I09.1)

▶ **I39** *Endocarditis and heart valve disorders in diseases classified elsewhere*
　Code first underlying disease, such as:
　　Q fever (A78)
　Excludes1　endocardial involvement in:
　　　candidiasis (B37.6)
　　　gonococcal infection (A54.83)
　　　Libman-Sacks disease (M32.11)
　　　listerosis (A32.82)
　　　meningococcal infection (A39.51)
　　　rheumatoid arthritis (M05.31)
　　　syphilis (A52.03)
　　　tuberculosis (A18.84)
　　　typhoid fever (A01.02)

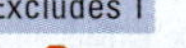

▶ New　⇒ Revised　~~deleted~~ Deleted　Excludes 1　Excludes 2　Includes　Use additional　Code first　Code also　Key words
OGCR Official Guidelines　X Assign placeholder X　● Use Additional Character(s)　▶ Manifestation Code　🅗 Hierarchical Condition Category　**Coding Clinic**

● **I40**   **Acute myocarditis**
Inflammation of heart muscle due to infection (viral/bacterial)

   Includes   subacute myocarditis

   Excludes1   acute rheumatic myocarditis (I01.2)

   I40.0   **Infective myocarditis**
      Septic myocarditis

      Use additional code (B95-B97) to identify infectious agent
      Coding Clinic: 2025, Q1, P34

   I40.1   **Isolated myocarditis**
      Fiedler's myocarditis
      Giant cell myocarditis
      Idiopathic myocarditis

   I40.8   **Other acute myocarditis**

   I40.9   **Acute myocarditis, unspecified**

▶ **I41**   *Myocarditis in diseases classified elsewhere*

   Code first underlying disease, such as:
      typhus (A75.0-A75.9)

   Excludes1   myocarditis (in):
        Chagas' disease (chronic) (B57.2)
        acute (B57.0)
        coxsackie (virus) infection (B33.22)
        diphtheritic (A36.81)
        gonococcal (A54.83)
        influenzal (J09.X9, J10.82, J11.82)
        meningococcal (A39.52)
        mumps (B26.82)
        rheumatoid arthritis (M05.31)
        sarcoid (D86.85)
        syphilis (A52.06)
        toxoplasmosis (B58.81)
        tuberculous (A18.84)

   Coding Clinic: 2025, Q1, P34

● **I42**   **Cardiomyopathy**
Disease of the heart muscle resulting in an abnormally enlarged, weakened, thickened, and/or stiffened muscles

   Includes   myocardiopathy

   Code first pre-existing cardiomyopathy complicating pregnancy and puerperium (O99.4)

   Excludes2   ischemic cardiomyopathy (I25.5)
      peripartum cardiomyopathy (O90.3)
      ventricular hypertrophy (I51.7)

   I42.0   **Dilated cardiomyopathy**
      Congestive cardiomyopathy

   I42.1   **Obstructive hypertrophic cardiomyopathy**
      Hypertrophic subaortic stenosis (idiopathic)

   I42.2   **Other hypertrophic cardiomyopathy**
      Nonobstructive hypertrophic cardiomyopathy

   I42.3   **Endomyocardial (eosinophilic) disease**
      Endomyocardial (tropical) fibrosis
      Löffler's endocarditis

   I42.4   **Endocardial fibroelastosis**
      Congenital cardiomyopathy
      Elastomyofibrosis

   I42.5   **Other restrictive cardiomyopathy**
      Constrictive cardiomyopathy NOS

   I42.6   **Alcoholic cardiomyopathy**
      Code also presence of alcoholism (F10.-)

   I42.7   **Cardiomyopathy due to drug and external agent**

      Code first poisoning due to drug or toxin, if applicable (T36-T65 with fifth or sixth character 1-4)

      Use additional code for adverse effect, if applicable, to identify drug (T36-T50 with fifth or sixth character 5)
      Coding Clinic: 2021, Q3, P8

   I42.8   **Other cardiomyopathies**

   I42.9   **Cardiomyopathy, unspecified**
      Cardiomyopathy (primary) (secondary) NOS

▶ **I43**   *Cardiomyopathy in diseases classified elsewhere*

   Code first underlying disease, such as:
      amyloidosis (E85.-)
      glycogen storage disease (E74.0-)
      gout (M10.0-)
      thyrotoxicosis (E05.0-E05.9-)

   Excludes1   cardiomyopathy (in):
        coxsackie (virus) (B33.24)
        diphtheria (A36.81)
        sarcoidosis (D86.85)
        tuberculosis (A18.84)

   Coding Clinic: 2024, Q2, P9

● **I44**   **Atrioventricular and left bundle-branch block**
Conduction problem resulting in arrhythmias/dysrhythmias due to a lack of electrical impulses being transmitted normally through the heart

   I44.0   **Atrioventricular block, first degree**

   I44.1   **Atrioventricular block, second degree**
      Atrioventricular block, type I and II
      Möbitz block, type I and II
      Second degree block, type I and II
      Wenckebach's block

   I44.2   **Atrioventricular block, complete**
      Complete heart block NOS
      Third degree block
      Coding Clinic: 2025, Q2, P4; 2019, Q2, P4

● **I44.3**   **Other and unspecified atrioventricular block**
      Atrioventricular block NOS

      I44.30   **Unspecified atrioventricular block**

      I44.39   **Other atrioventricular block**

   I44.4   **Left anterior fascicular block**

   I44.5   **Left posterior fascicular block**

● **I44.6**   **Other and unspecified fascicular block**

      I44.60   **Unspecified fascicular block**
         Left bundle-branch hemiblock NOS

      I44.69   **Other fascicular block**

   I44.7   **Left bundle-branch block, unspecified**

● **I45**   **Other conduction disorders**

   I45.0   **Right fascicular block**

● **I45.1**   **Other and unspecified right bundle-branch block**

      I45.10   **Unspecified right bundle-branch block**
         Right bundle-branch block NOS

      I45.19   **Other right bundle-branch block**

   I45.2   **Bifascicular block**

   I45.3   **Trifascicular block**

   I45.4   **Nonspecific intraventricular block**
      Bundle-branch block NOS

   I45.5   **Other specified heart block**
      Sinoatrial block
      Sinoauricular block

      Excludes1   heart block NOS (I45.9)

   I45.6   **Pre-excitation syndrome**
      Accelerated atrioventricular conduction
      Accessory atrioventricular conduction
      Anomalous atrioventricular excitation
      Lown-Ganong-Levine syndrome
      Pre-excitation atrioventricular conduction
      Wolff-Parkinson-White syndrome

● **I45.8**   **Other specified conduction disorders**

      I45.81   **Long QT syndrome**

      I45.89   **Other specified conduction disorders**
         Atrioventricular [AV] dissociation
         Interference dissociation
         Isorhythmic dissociation
         Nonparoxysmal AV nodal tachycardia
         Coding Clinic: 2013, Q2, P32

   I45.9   **Conduction disorder, unspecified**
      Heart block NOS
      Stokes-Adams syndrome

CHAPTER 9 (I00-I99)

● **I46   Cardiac arrest**
> **Excludes2**   cardiogenic shock (R57.0)

    I46.2   Cardiac arrest due to underlying cardiac condition ℞
> *Code first* underlying cardiac condition
> **Coding Clinic: 2024, Q1, P27**

    I46.8   Cardiac arrest due to other underlying condition ℞
> *Code first* underlying condition

    I46.9   Cardiac arrest, cause unspecified ℞

● **I47   Paroxysmal tachycardia**
> *Code first* tachycardia complicating:
> abortion or ectopic or molar pregnancy (O00–O07, O08.8)
> obstetric surgery and procedures (O75.4)
>
> **Excludes1**   tachycardia NOS (R00.0)
> sinoauricular tachycardia NOS (R00.0)
> sinus [sinusal] tachycardia NOS (R00.0)

    I47.0   Re-entry ventricular arrhythmia ℞

●   **I47.1   Supraventricular tachycardia** ℞

    I47.10   Supraventricular tachycardia, unspecified

    I47.11   Inappropriate sinus tachycardia, so stated
> IST

    I47.19   Other supraventricular tachycardia
> Atrial (paroxysmal) tachycardia
> Atrioventricular [AV] (paroxysmal) tachycardia
> Atrioventricular re-entrant (nodal) tachycardia [AVNRT] [AVRT]
> Junctional (paroxysmal) tachycardia
> Nodal (paroxysmal) tachycardia

●   **I47.2   Ventricular tachycardia** ℞

    I47.20   Ventricular tachycardia, unspecified

    I47.21   Torsades de pointes
> **Code also**, if applicable, long QT syndrome (I45.81)
> **Use Additional** code for adverse effect, if applicable, to identify drug (T36–T50 with fifth or sixth character 5)
> **Coding Clinic: 2022, Q4, P24**

    I47.29   Other ventricular tachycardia
> **Coding Clinic: 2021, Q3, P12; 2013, Q3, P23**

    I47.9   Paroxysmal tachycardia, unspecified ℞
> Bouveret (-Hoffman) syndrome

● **I48   Atrial fibrillation and flutter**
> *Most common abnormal heart rhythm (arrhythmia) presenting as irregular, rapid beating (tachycardia) of the heart's upper chamber.*

    I48.0   Paroxysmal atrial fibrillation ℞

●   **I48.1   Persistent atrial fibrillation** ℞
> *Rapid contractions of the upper heart chamber*
>
> **Excludes1**   Permanent atrial fibrillation (I48.21)
>
> **Coding Clinic: 2019, Q2, P3-4**

    I48.11   Longstanding persistent atrial fibrillation

    I48.19   Other persistent atrial fibrillation
> Chronic persistent atrial fibrillation
> Persistent atrial fibrillation, NOS

●   **I48.2   Chronic atrial fibrillation** ℞
> **Coding Clinic: 2019, Q2, P3**

    I48.20   Chronic atrial fibrillation, unspecified
> **Excludes1**   Chronic persistent atrial fibrillation (I48.19)

    I48.21   Permanent atrial fibrillation

    I48.3   Typical atrial flutter ℞
> Type I atrial flutter

    I48.4   Atypical atrial flutter ℞
> Type II atrial flutter

●   **I48.9   Unspecified atrial fibrillation and atrial flutter**

    I48.91   Unspecified atrial fibrillation ℞

    I48.92   Unspecified atrial flutter ℞

● **I49   Other cardiac arrhythmias**
> *Code first* cardiac arrhythmia complicating:
> abortion or ectopic or molar pregnancy (O00–O07, O08.8)
> obstetric surgery and procedures (O75.4)
>
> **Excludes2**   bradycardia NOS (R00.1)
> neonatal dysrhythmia (P29.1-)
> sinoatrial bradycardia (R00.1)
> sinus bradycardia (R00.1)
> vagal bradycardia (R00.1)

●   **I49.0   Ventricular fibrillation and flutter**

    I49.01   Ventricular fibrillation ℞

    I49.02   Ventricular flutter ℞

    I49.1   Atrial premature depolarization
> Atrial premature beats

    I49.2   Junctional premature depolarization ℞

    I49.3   Ventricular premature depolarization

●   **I49.4   Other and unspecified premature depolarization**

    I49.40   Unspecified premature depolarization
> Premature beats NOS

    I49.49   Other premature depolarization
> Ectopic beats
> Extrasystoles
> Extrasystolic arrhythmias
> Premature contractions

    I49.5   Sick sinus syndrome ℞
> Tachycardia-bradycardia syndrome
> **Coding Clinic: 2019, Q1, P33**

    I49.8   Other specified cardiac arrhythmias
> Brugada syndrome
> Coronary sinus rhythm disorder
> Ectopic rhythm disorder
> Nodal rhythm disorder
> **Coding Clinic: 2025, Q2, P4**

    I49.9   Cardiac arrhythmia, unspecified
> Arrhythmia (cardiac) NOS

● **I50   Heart failure**
> *Code first* heart failure complicating abortion or ectopic or molar pregnancy (O00–O07, O08.8)
> heart failure due to hypertension (I11.0)
> heart failure due to hypertension with chronic kidney disease (I13.-)
> heart failure following surgery (I97.13-)
> obstetric surgery and procedures (O75.4)
> rheumatic heart failure (I09.81)
>
> **Excludes2**   cardiac arrest (I46.-)
> neonatal cardiac failure (P20.0)
> **Coding Clinic: 2017, Q1, P47; 2016, Q4, P122-123, Q1, P38; 2015, Q2, P15**

Item 9–8 Congestive heart failure (CHF) is a condition in which the left ventricle of the heart cannot pump enough blood to the body. The blood flow from the heart slows or returns to the heart from the venous system (back flow) resulting in congestion (fluid accumulation) particularly in the abdomen. Most commonly, fluid collects in the lungs and results in shortness of breath, especially when in a reclining position.

I50.1 **Left ventricular failure, unspecified** 🚫
Cardiac asthma
Edema of lung with heart disease NOS
Edema of lung with heart failure
Left heart failure
Pulmonary edema with heart disease NOS
Pulmonary edema with heart failure
Excludes1 edema of lung without heart disease or heart failure (J81.-)
pulmonary edema without heart disease or failure (J81.-)

🔴 **I50.2** **Systolic (congestive) heart failure**
Heart failure with reduced ejection fraction [HFrEF]
Systolic left ventricular heart failure
Code also end stage heart failure, if applicable (I50.84)
Excludes1 combined systolic (congestive) and diastolic (congestive) heart failure (I50.4-)

I50.20 **Unspecified systolic (congestive) heart failure** 🚫

I50.21 **Acute systolic (congestive) heart failure** 🚫
Presenting a short and relatively severe episode

I50.22 **Chronic systolic (congestive) heart failure** 🚫
Long-lasting, presenting over time

I50.23 **Acute on chronic systolic (congestive) heart failure** 🚫
Combination code. What was a chronic condition now has an acute exacerbation (to make more severe).
Coding Clinic: 2013, Q2, P33

🔴 **I50.3** **Diastolic (congestive) heart failure**
Diastolic left ventricular heart failure
Heart failure with normal ejection fraction
Heart failure with preserved ejection fraction [HFpEF]
Code also end stage heart failure, if applicable (I50.84)
Excludes1 combined systolic (congestive) and diastolic (congestive) heart failure (I50.4-)

I50.30 **Unspecified diastolic (congestive) heart failure** 🚫

I50.31 **Acute diastolic (congestive) heart failure** 🚫
Coding Clinic: 2025, Q2, P5; 2017, Q1, P46

I50.32 **Chronic diastolic (congestive) heart failure** 🚫
Coding Clinic: 2023, Q3, P14

I50.33 **Acute on chronic diastolic (congestive) heart failure** 🚫
Coding Clinic: 2024, Q2, P10

🔴 **I50.4** **Combined systolic (congestive) and diastolic (congestive) heart failure**
Combined systolic and diastolic left ventricular heart failure
Heart failure with reduced ejection fraction and diastolic dysfunction
Code also end stage heart failure, if applicable (I50.84)

I50.40 **Unspecified combined systolic (congestive) and diastolic (congestive) heart failure** 🚫

I50.41 **Acute combined systolic (congestive) and diastolic (congestive) heart failure** 🚫

I50.42 **Chronic combined systolic (congestive) and diastolic (congestive) heart failure** 🚫

I50.43 **Acute on chronic combined systolic (congestive) and diastolic (congestive) heart failure** 🚫

🔴 **I50.8** **Other heart failure**
🔴 **I50.81** **Right heart failure**
Right ventricular failure

I50.810 **Right heart failure, unspecified** 🚫
Right heart failure without mention of left heart failure
Right ventricular failure NOS

I50.811 **Acute right heart failure** 🚫
Acute isolated right heart failure
Acute (isolated) right ventricular failure

I50.812 **Chronic right heart failure** 🚫
Chronic isolated right heart failure
Chronic (isolated) right ventricular failure

I50.813 **Acute on chronic right heart failure** 🚫
Acute on chronic isolated right heart failure
Acute on chronic (isolated) right ventricular failure
Acute decompensation of chronic (isolated) right ventricular failure
Acute exacerbation of chronic (isolated) right ventricular failure
Coding Clinic: 2023, Q3, P14

I50.814 **Right heart failure due to left heart failure** 🚫
Right ventricular failure secondary to left ventricular failure
Code also the type of left ventricular failure, if known (I50.2-I50.43)
Excludes1 Right heart failure with but not due to left heart failure (I50.82)

I50.82 **Biventricular heart failure** 🚫
Code also the type of left ventricular failure as systolic, diastolic, or combined, if known (I50.2-I50.43)

I50.83 **High output heart failure** 🚫

I50.84 **End stage heart failure** 🚫
Stage D heart failure
Code also the type of heart failure as systolic, diastolic, or combined, if known (I50.2-I50.43)
Coding Clinic: 2022, Q3, P17

I50.89 **Other heart failure** 🚫

I50.9 **Heart failure, unspecified** 🚫
Cardiac, heart or myocardial failure NOS
Congestive heart disease
Congestive heart failure NOS
Excludes2 fluid overload unrelated to congestive heart failure (E87.70)
Coding Clinic: 2017, Q1, P45-46; 2015, Q2, P15; 2012, Q4, P92

🔴 **I51** **Complications and ill-defined descriptions of heart disease**
~~**Excludes1** any condition in I51.4-I51.9 due to hypertension (I11.-)~~
~~any condition in I51.4-I51.9 due to hypertension and chronic kidney disease (I13.-)~~
~~heart disease specified as rheumatic (I00-I09)~~

▶ **Excludes2** heart disease specified as rheumatic (I00-I09)

I51.0 **Cardiac septal defect, acquired**   **A**
Acquired septal atrial defect (old)
Acquired septal auricular defect (old)
Acquired septal ventricular defect (old)
Excludes1 cardiac septal defect as current complication following acute myocardial infarction (I23.1, I23.2)

CHAPTER 9 (I00-I99)

I51.1 **Rupture of chordae tendineae, not elsewhere classified** Ⓡ

> **Excludes1** rupture of chordae tendineae as current complication following acute myocardial infarction (I23.4)

I51.2 **Rupture of papillary muscle, not elsewhere classified** Ⓡ

> **Excludes1** rupture of papillary muscle as current complication following acute myocardial infarction (I23.5)

I51.3 **Intracardiac thrombosis, not elsewhere classified**
Apical thrombosis (old)
Atrial thrombosis (old)
Auricular thrombosis (old)
Mural thrombosis (old)
Ventricular thrombosis (old)

> **Excludes1** intracardiac thrombosis as current complication following acute myocardial infarction (I23.6)

Coding Clinic: 2013, Q1, P24

I51.4 **Myocarditis, unspecified** Ⓡ
Chronic (interstitial) myocarditis
Myocardial fibrosis
Myocarditis NOS

> **Excludes1** acute or subacute myocarditis (I40.-)

Coding Clinic: 2016, Q4, P122

I51.5 **Myocardial degeneration** Ⓡ

> ▶ **Excludes1** myocardial degeneration due to hypertension (I11.-)
> ▶ myocardial degeneration due to hypertension and chronic kidney disease (I13.-)

Fatty degeneration of heart or myocardium
Myocardial disease
Senile degeneration of heart or myocardium

Coding Clinic: 2016, Q4, P122

I51.7 **Cardiomegaly**

> ▶ **Excludes1** cardiomegaly due to hypertension (I11.-)
> ▶ cardiomegaly due to hypertension and chronic kidney disease (I13.-)

Cardiac dilatation
Cardiac hypertrophy
Ventricular dilatation

Coding Clinic: 2016, Q4, P122

● **I51.8** **Other ill-defined heart diseases**
Coding Clinic: 2016, Q4, P122

I51.81 **Takotsubo syndrome**
Reversible left ventricular dysfunction following sudden emotional stress
Stress induced cardiomyopathy
Takotsubo cardiomyopathy
Transient left ventricular apical ballooning syndrome

I51.89 **Other ill-defined heart diseases**
Carditis (acute)(chronic)
Pancarditis (acute)(chronic)

Coding Clinic: 2019, Q2, P6

I51.9 **Heart disease, unspecified**
Coding Clinic: 2016, Q4, P122

▶ *I52* *Other heart disorders in diseases classified elsewhere*
Code first underlying disease, such as:
congenital syphilis (A50.5)
mucopolysaccharidosis (E76.3)
schistosomiasis (B65.0-B65.9)

> **Excludes1** heart disease (in):
> gonococcal infection (A54.83)
> meningococcal infection (A39.50)
> rheumatoid arthritis (M05.31)
> syphilis (A52.06)

CEREBROVASCULAR DISEASES (I60-I69)

Use additional code to identify presence of:
alcohol abuse and dependence (F10.-)
exposure to environmental tobacco smoke (Z77.22)
history of tobacco dependence (Z87.891)
hypertension (I10-I1A)
occupational exposure to environmental tobacco smoke (Z57.31)
tobacco dependence (F17.-)
tobacco use (Z72.0)

> **Excludes1** traumatic intracranial hemorrhage (S06.-)

Coding Clinic: 2015, Q4, P40

I5A **Non-ischemic myocardial injury (non-traumatic)**
Acute (non-ischemic) myocardial injury
Chronic (non-ischemic) myocardial injury
Unspecified (non-ischemic) myocardial injury

Code first the underlying cause, if known and applicable, such as:
acute kidney failure (N17.-)
acute myocarditis (I40.-)
cardiomyopathy (I42.-)
chronic kidney disease (CKD) (N18.-)
heart failure (I50.-)
hypertensive urgency (I16.0)
nonrheumatic aortic valve disorders (I35.-)
paroxysmal tachycardia (I47.-)
pulmonary embolism (I26.-)
pulmonary hypertension (I27.0, I27.2-)
sepsis (A41.-)
takotsubo syndrome (I51.81)

Use additional code, if known, to indicate National Institutes of Health Stroke Scale (NIHSS) score (R29.7-)

> **Excludes1** acute myocardial infarction (I21.-)
> injury of heart (S26.-)

> **Excludes2** other acute ischemic heart diseases (I24.-)

Coding Clinic: 2021, Q4, P15

● **I60** **Nontraumatic subarachnoid hemorrhage**

> **Excludes1** syphilitic ruptured cerebral aneurysm (A52.05)

> **Excludes2** sequelae of subarachnoid hemorrhage (I69.0-)

● **I60.0** **Nontraumatic subarachnoid hemorrhage from carotid siphon and bifurcation**

I60.00 **Nontraumatic subarachnoid hemorrhage from unspecified carotid siphon and bifurcation** Ⓡ

I60.01 **Nontraumatic subarachnoid hemorrhage from right carotid siphon and bifurcation**

I60.02 **Nontraumatic subarachnoid hemorrhage from left carotid siphon and bifurcation** Ⓡ

● **I60.1** **Nontraumatic subarachnoid hemorrhage from middle cerebral artery**

I60.10 **Nontraumatic subarachnoid hemorrhage from unspecified middle cerebral artery** Ⓡ

I60.11 **Nontraumatic subarachnoid hemorrhage from right middle cerebral artery** Ⓡ

I60.12 **Nontraumatic subarachnoid hemorrhage from left middle cerebral artery** Ⓡ

I60.2 **Nontraumatic subarachnoid hemorrhage from anterior communicating artery** Ⓡ

● **I60.3** **Nontraumatic subarachnoid hemorrhage from posterior communicating artery**

I60.30 **Nontraumatic subarachnoid hemorrhage from unspecified posterior communicating artery** Ⓡ

I60.31 **Nontraumatic subarachnoid hemorrhage from right posterior communicating artery** Ⓡ

I60.32 **Nontraumatic subarachnoid hemorrhage from left posterior communicating artery** Ⓡ

I60.4 **Nontraumatic subarachnoid hemorrhage from basilar artery** Ⓡ

▶ New   ➡ Revised   ~~deleted~~ Deleted   Excludes 1   Excludes 2   Includes   Use additional   Code first   Code also   Key words
OGCR Official Guidelines   X Assign placeholder X   ● Use Additional Character(s)   ▶ Manifestation Code   Ⓡ Hierarchical Condition Category   **Coding Clinic**

● **I60.5**   **Nontraumatic subarachnoid hemorrhage from vertebral artery**
    I60.50   Nontraumatic subarachnoid hemorrhage from **unspecified vertebral artery** ℞
    I60.51   Nontraumatic subarachnoid hemorrhage from **right vertebral artery** ℞
    I60.52   Nontraumatic subarachnoid hemorrhage from **left vertebral artery** ℞

I60.6   **Nontraumatic subarachnoid hemorrhage from other intracranial arteries** ℞

I60.7   **Nontraumatic subarachnoid hemorrhage from unspecified intracranial artery** ℞
    Ruptured (congenital) berry aneurysm
    Ruptured (congenital) cerebral aneurysm
    Subarachnoid hemorrhage (nontraumatic) from cerebral artery NOS
    Subarachnoid hemorrhage (nontraumatic) from communicating artery NOS
    Excludes1   berry aneurysm, nonruptured (I67.1)

I60.8   **Other nontraumatic subarachnoid hemorrhage** ℞
    Meningeal hemorrhage
    Rupture of cerebral arteriovenous malformation

I60.9   **Nontraumatic subarachnoid hemorrhage, unspecified** ℞

● **I61**   **Nontraumatic intracerebral hemorrhage**
    Use Additional code, if known, to indicate National Institutes of Health Stroke Scale (NIHSS) score (R29.7-)
    Excludes2   sequelae of intracerebral hemorrhage (I69.1-)
    Coding Clinic: 2017, Q2, P10

I61.0   **Nontraumatic intracerebral hemorrhage in hemisphere, subcortical** ℞
    Deep intracerebral hemorrhage (nontraumatic)
    Coding Clinic: 2016, Q4, P27

I61.1   **Nontraumatic intracerebral hemorrhage in hemisphere, cortical** ℞
    Cerebral lobe hemorrhage (nontraumatic)
    Superficial intracerebral hemorrhage (nontraumatic)
    Coding Clinic: 2016, Q4, P28

I61.2   **Nontraumatic intracerebral hemorrhage in hemisphere, unspecified** ℞

I61.3   **Nontraumatic intracerebral hemorrhage in brain stem** ℞
    Coding Clinic: 2023, Q4, P42

I61.4   **Nontraumatic intracerebral hemorrhage in cerebellum** ℞

I61.5   **Nontraumatic intracerebral hemorrhage, intraventricular** ℞

I61.6   **Nontraumatic intracerebral hemorrhage, multiple localized** ℞

I61.8   **Other nontraumatic intracerebral hemorrhage** ℞
    Coding Clinic: 2024, Q2, P25

I61.9   **Nontraumatic intracerebral hemorrhage, unspecified** ℞
    Coding Clinic: 2022, Q3, P9-10

● **I62**   **Other and unspecified nontraumatic intracranial hemorrhage**
    Use Additional code, if known, to indicate National Institutes of Health Stroke Scale (NIHSS) score (R29.7-)
    Excludes2   sequelae of intracranial hemorrhage (I69.2)

● **I62.0**   **Nontraumatic subdural hemorrhage**
    I62.00   Nontraumatic subdural hemorrhage, **unspecified** ℞
    I62.01   Nontraumatic **acute subdural hemorrhage** ℞
    I62.02   Nontraumatic **subacute subdural hemorrhage** ℞
    I62.03   Nontraumatic **chronic subdural hemorrhage** ℞

I62.1   **Nontraumatic extradural hemorrhage** ℞
    Nontraumatic epidural hemorrhage
    Coding Clinic: 2023, Q3, P22

I62.9   **Nontraumatic intracranial hemorrhage, unspecified** ℞

★ **(See Plate 31 of the Anatomy Illustrations.)**

● **I63**   **Cerebral infarction**
    Excludes1   neonatal cerebral infarction (P91.82-)
    Excludes2   chronic, without residual deficits (sequelae) (Z86.73)
    Includes   occlusion and stenosis of cerebral and precerebral arteries, resulting in cerebral infarction
    Use additional code, if applicable, to identify status post administration of tPA (rtPA) in a different facility within the last 24 hours prior to admission to current facility (Z92.82)
    Use additional code, if known, to indicate National Institutes of Health Stroke Scale (NIHSS) score (R29.7-)
    Excludes2   sequelae of cerebral infarction (I69.3-)
    Coding Clinic: 2016, Q4, P28, 61, 127

● **I63.0**   **Cerebral infarction due to thrombosis of precerebral arteries**
    I63.00   Cerebral infarction due to thrombosis of **unspecified precerebral artery** ℞

● **I63.01**   Cerebral infarction due to thrombosis of **vertebral** artery
      I63.011   Cerebral infarction due to thrombosis of **right vertebral artery** ℞
      I63.012   Cerebral infarction due to thrombosis of **left vertebral artery** ℞
      I63.013   Cerebral infarction due to thrombosis of **bilateral vertebral arteries** ℞
      I63.019   Cerebral infarction due to thrombosis of **unspecified vertebral artery** ℞

    I63.02   Cerebral infarction due to thrombosis of **basilar artery** ℞

● **I63.03**   Cerebral infarction due to thrombosis of **carotid artery**
      I63.031   Cerebral infarction due to thrombosis of **right carotid artery** ℞
      I63.032   Cerebral infarction due to thrombosis of **left carotid artery** ℞
      I63.033   Cerebral infarction due to thrombosis of **bilateral carotid arteries** ℞
      I63.039   Cerebral infarction due to thrombosis of **unspecified carotid artery** ℞

    I63.09   Cerebral infarction due to thrombosis of **other precerebral artery** ℞

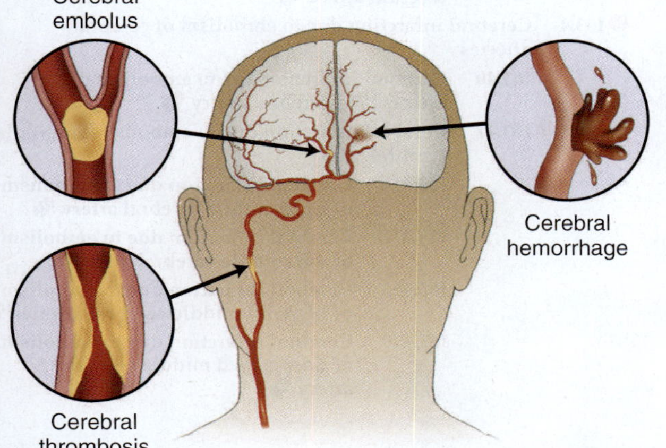

Figure 9-4   Events causing a stroke. (From Shiland: Mastering Healthcare Terminology, ed 1, St. Louis, Mosby, 2003)

● **I63.1**   Cerebral infarction due to embolism of precerebral arteries
  - **I63.10**   Cerebral infarction due to embolism of unspecified precerebral artery 🔴
  - ● **I63.11**   Cerebral infarction due to embolism of vertebral artery
    - **I63.111**   Cerebral infarction due to embolism of right vertebral artery 🔴
    - **I63.112**   Cerebral infarction due to embolism of left vertebral artery 🔴
    - **I63.113**   Cerebral infarction due to embolism of bilateral vertebral arteries 🔴
    - **I63.119**   Cerebral infarction due to embolism of unspecified vertebral artery 🔴
  - **I63.12**   Cerebral infarction due to embolism of basilar artery 🔴
  - ● **I63.13**   Cerebral infarction due to embolism of carotid artery
    - **I63.131**   Cerebral infarction due to embolism of right carotid artery 🔴
    - **I63.132**   Cerebral infarction due to embolism of left carotid artery 🔴
    - **I63.133**   Cerebral infarction due to embolism of bilateral carotid arteries 🔴
    - **I63.139**   Cerebral infarction due to embolism of unspecified carotid artery 🔴
  - **I63.19**   Cerebral infarction due to embolism of other precerebral artery 🔴

● **I63.2**   Cerebral infarction due to unspecified occlusion or stenosis of precerebral arteries
  - **I63.20**   Cerebral infarction due to unspecified occlusion or stenosis of unspecified precerebral arteries 🔴
  - ● **I63.21**   Cerebral infarction due to unspecified occlusion or stenosis of vertebral arteries
    - **I63.211**   Cerebral infarction due to unspecified occlusion or stenosis of right vertebral artery 🔴
    - **I63.212**   Cerebral infarction due to unspecified occlusion or stenosis of left vertebral artery 🔴
    - **I63.213**   Cerebral infarction due to unspecified occlusion or stenosis of bilateral vertebral arteries 🔴
    - **I63.219**   Cerebral infarction due to unspecified occlusion or stenosis of unspecified vertebral artery 🔴
  - **I63.22**   Cerebral infarction due to unspecified occlusion or stenosis of basilar artery 🔴
  - ● **I63.23**   Cerebral infarction due to unspecified occlusion or stenosis of carotid arteries
    - **I63.231**   Cerebral infarction due to unspecified occlusion or stenosis of right carotid arteries 🔴
    - **I63.232**   Cerebral infarction due to unspecified occlusion or stenosis of left carotid arteries 🔴
    - **I63.233**   Cerebral infarction due to unspecified occlusion or stenosis of bilateral carotid arteries 🔴
    - **I63.239**   Cerebral infarction due to unspecified occlusion or stenosis of unspecified carotid artery 🔴
  - **I63.29**   Cerebral infarction due to unspecified occlusion or stenosis of other precerebral arteries 🔴

● **I63.3**   Cerebral infarction due to thrombosis of cerebral arteries
  - **I63.30**   Cerebral infarction due to thrombosis of unspecified cerebral artery 🔴
  - ● **I63.31**   Cerebral infarction due to thrombosis of middle cerebral artery
    - **I63.311**   Cerebral infarction due to thrombosis of right middle cerebral artery 🔴
    - **I63.312**   Cerebral infarction due to thrombosis of left middle cerebral artery 🔴
    - **I63.313**   Cerebral infarction due to thrombosis of bilateral middle cerebral arteries 🔴
    - **I63.319**   Cerebral infarction due to thrombosis of unspecified middle cerebral artery 🔴
  - ● **I63.32**   Cerebral infarction due to thrombosis of anterior cerebral artery
    - **I63.321**   Cerebral infarction due to thrombosis of right anterior cerebral artery 🔴
    - **I63.322**   Cerebral infarction due to thrombosis of left anterior cerebral artery 🔴
    - **I63.323**   Cerebral infarction due to thrombosis of bilateral anterior cerebral arteries 🔴
    - **I63.329**   Cerebral infarction due to thrombosis of unspecified anterior cerebral artery 🔴
  - ● **I63.33**   Cerebral infarction due to thrombosis of posterior cerebral artery
    - **I63.331**   Cerebral infarction due to thrombosis of right posterior cerebral artery 🔴
    - **I63.332**   Cerebral infarction due to thrombosis of left posterior cerebral artery 🔴
    - **I63.333**   Cerebral infarction due to thrombosis of bilateral posterior cerebral arteries 🔴
    - **I63.339**   Cerebral infarction due to thrombosis of unspecified posterior cerebral artery 🔴
  - ● **I63.34**   Cerebral infarction due to thrombosis of cerebellar artery
    - **I63.341**   Cerebral infarction due to thrombosis of right cerebellar artery 🔴
    - **I63.342**   Cerebral infarction due to thrombosis of left cerebellar artery 🔴
    - **I63.343**   Cerebral infarction due to thrombosis of bilateral cerebellar arteries 🔴
    - **I63.349**   Cerebral infarction due to thrombosis of unspecified cerebellar artery 🔴
  - **I63.39**   Cerebral infarction due to thrombosis of other cerebral artery 🔴

● **I63.4**   Cerebral infarction due to embolism of cerebral arteries
  - **I63.40**   Cerebral infarction due to embolism of unspecified cerebral artery 🔴
  - ● **I63.41**   Cerebral infarction due to embolism of middle cerebral artery
    - **I63.411**   Cerebral infarction due to embolism of right middle cerebral artery 🔴
    - **I63.412**   Cerebral infarction due to embolism of left middle cerebral artery 🔴
    - **I63.413**   Cerebral infarction due to embolism of bilateral middle cerebral arteries 🔴
    - **I63.419**   Cerebral infarction due to embolism of unspecified middle cerebral artery 🔴

▶ New   ⇨ Revised   ~~deleted~~ Deleted   Excludes 1   Excludes 2   Includes   Use additional   Code first   Code also   Key words
OGCR Official Guidelines   X Assign placeholder X   ● Use Additional Character(s)   ▶ Manifestation Code   🔴 Hierarchical Condition Category   **Coding Clinic**

● **I63.42** Cerebral infarction due to embolism of anterior cerebral artery

    I63.421 Cerebral infarction due to embolism of right anterior cerebral artery 🆁

    I63.422 Cerebral infarction due to embolism of left anterior cerebral artery 🆁

    I63.423 Cerebral infarction due to embolism of bilateral anterior cerebral arteries 🆁

    I63.429 Cerebral infarction due to embolism of unspecified anterior cerebral artery 🆁

● **I63.43** Cerebral infarction due to embolism of posterior cerebral artery

    I63.431 Cerebral infarction due to embolism of right posterior cerebral artery 🆁

    I63.432 Cerebral infarction due to embolism of left posterior cerebral artery 🆁

    I63.433 Cerebral infarction due to embolism of bilateral posterior cerebral arteries 🆁

    I63.439 Cerebral infarction due to embolism of unspecified posterior cerebral artery 🆁

● **I63.44** Cerebral infarction due to embolism of cerebellar artery

    I63.441 Cerebral infarction due to embolism of right cerebellar artery 🆁

    I63.442 Cerebral infarction due to embolism of left cerebellar artery 🆁

    I63.443 Cerebral infarction due to embolism of bilateral cerebellar arteries 🆁

    I63.449 Cerebral infarction due to embolism of unspecified cerebellar artery 🆁

    I63.49 Cerebral infarction due to embolism of other cerebral artery 🆁

● **I63.5** Cerebral infarction due to unspecified occlusion or stenosis of cerebral arteries

    I63.50 Cerebral infarction due to unspecified occlusion or stenosis of unspecified cerebral artery 🆁

●   **I63.51** Cerebral infarction due to unspecified occlusion or stenosis of middle cerebral artery

    I63.511 Cerebral infarction due to unspecified occlusion or stenosis of right middle cerebral artery 🆁

    I63.512 Cerebral infarction due to unspecified occlusion or stenosis of left middle cerebral artery 🆁

    I63.513 Cerebral infarction due to unspecified occlusion or stenosis of bilateral middle cerebral arteries 🆁

    I63.519 Cerebral infarction due to unspecified occlusion or stenosis of unspecified middle cerebral artery 🆁

● **I63.52** Cerebral infarction due to unspecified occlusion or stenosis of anterior cerebral artery

    I63.521 Cerebral infarction due to unspecified occlusion or stenosis of right anterior cerebral artery 🆁

    I63.522 Cerebral infarction due to unspecified occlusion or stenosis of left anterior cerebral artery 🆁

    I63.523 Cerebral infarction due to unspecified occlusion or stenosis of bilateral anterior cerebral arteries 🆁

    I63.529 Cerebral infarction due to unspecified occlusion or stenosis of unspecified anterior cerebral artery 🆁

● **I63.53** Cerebral infarction due to unspecified occlusion or stenosis of posterior cerebral artery

    I63.531 Cerebral infarction due to unspecified occlusion or stenosis of right posterior cerebral artery 🆁

    I63.532 Cerebral infarction due to unspecified occlusion or stenosis of left posterior cerebral artery 🆁
        Coding Clinic: 2024, Q1, P32; 2017, Q2, P10

    I63.533 Cerebral infarction due to unspecified occlusion or stenosis of bilateral posterior cerebral arteries 🆁

    I63.539 Cerebral infarction due to unspecified occlusion or stenosis of unspecified posterior cerebral artery 🆁

● **I63.54** Cerebral infarction due to unspecified occlusion or stenosis of cerebellar artery

    I63.541 Cerebral infarction due to unspecified occlusion or stenosis of right cerebellar artery 🆁

    I63.542 Cerebral infarction due to unspecified occlusion or stenosis of left cerebellar artery 🆁

    I63.543 Cerebral infarction due to unspecified occlusion or stenosis of bilateral cerebellar arteries 🆁

    I63.549 Cerebral infarction due to unspecified occlusion or stenosis of unspecified cerebellar artery 🆁

    I63.59 Cerebral infarction due to unspecified occlusion or stenosis of other cerebral artery 🆁

  I63.6 Cerebral infarction due to cerebral venous thrombosis, nonpyogenic 🆁

● **I63.8** Other cerebral infarction 🆁

    I63.81 Other cerebral infarction due to occlusion or stenosis of small artery 🆁
        Lacunar infarction
        Coding Clinic: 2018, Q4, P16

    I63.89 Other cerebral infarction 🆁
        Coding Clinic: 2024, Q1, P26, 32; 2022, Q1, P25; 2017, Q2, P9

  I63.9 Cerebral infarction, unspecified 🆁
    Stroke NOS

    Excludes2 transient cerebral ischemic attacks and related syndromes (G45.-)
    Coding Clinic: 2016, Q4, P62; 2015, Q1, P26

● **I65** Occlusion and stenosis of precerebral arteries, not resulting in cerebral infarction

    Includes embolism of precerebral artery
        narrowing of precerebral artery
        obstruction (complete) (partial) of precerebral artery
        thrombosis of precerebral artery

    Excludes1 insufficiency, NOS, of precerebral artery (G45.-)
        insufficiency of precerebral arteries causing cerebral infarction (I63.0-I63.2)

● **I65.0** Occlusion and stenosis of vertebral artery

    I65.01 Occlusion and stenosis of right vertebral artery

    I65.02 Occlusion and stenosis of left vertebral artery

    I65.03 Occlusion and stenosis of bilateral vertebral arteries

    I65.09 Occlusion and stenosis of unspecified vertebral artery

  I65.1 Occlusion and stenosis of basilar artery

● **I65.2** Occlusion and stenosis of carotid artery

    I65.21 Occlusion and stenosis of right carotid artery

    I65.22 Occlusion and stenosis of left carotid artery

    I65.23 Occlusion and stenosis of bilateral carotid arteries
        Coding Clinic: 2021, Q1, P4

    I65.29 Occlusion and stenosis of unspecified carotid artery

CHAPTER 9 (I00-I99)

I65.8   Occlusion and stenosis of other precerebral arteries

I65.9   Occlusion and stenosis of unspecified precerebral artery
    Occlusion and stenosis of precerebral artery NOS

● I66   **Occlusion and stenosis of cerebral arteries, not resulting in cerebral infarction**

    Includes   embolism of cerebral artery
        narrowing of cerebral artery
        obstruction (complete) (partial) of cerebral artery
        thrombosis of cerebral artery

    Excludes1   occlusion and stenosis of cerebral artery causing cerebral infarction (I63.3-I63.5)

  ● I66.0   Occlusion and stenosis of middle cerebral artery

    I66.01   Occlusion and stenosis of right middle cerebral artery

    I66.02   Occlusion and stenosis of left middle cerebral artery

    I66.03   Occlusion and stenosis of bilateral middle cerebral arteries

    I66.09   Occlusion and stenosis of unspecified middle cerebral artery

  ● I66.1   Occlusion and stenosis of anterior cerebral artery

    I66.11   Occlusion and stenosis of right anterior cerebral artery

    I66.12   Occlusion and stenosis of left anterior cerebral artery

    I66.13   Occlusion and stenosis of bilateral anterior cerebral arteries

    I66.19   Occlusion and stenosis of unspecified anterior cerebral artery

  ● I66.2   Occlusion and stenosis of posterior cerebral artery

    I66.21   Occlusion and stenosis of right posterior cerebral artery

    I66.22   Occlusion and stenosis of left posterior cerebral artery

    I66.23   Occlusion and stenosis of bilateral posterior cerebral arteries

    I66.29   Occlusion and stenosis of unspecified posterior cerebral artery

  I66.3   Occlusion and stenosis of cerebellar arteries

  I66.8   Occlusion and stenosis of other cerebral arteries
    Occlusion and stenosis of perforating arteries

  I66.9   Occlusion and stenosis of unspecified cerebral artery

● I67   Other cerebrovascular diseases

    Excludes1   Occlusion and stenosis of cerebral artery causing cerebral infarction (I63.3-I63.5-)
        Occlusion and stenosis of precerebral artery causing cerebral infarction (I63.2-)

    Excludes2   sequelae of the listed conditions (I69.8)

  I67.0   Dissection of cerebral arteries, nonruptured 🅗

    Excludes1   ruptured cerebral arteries (I60.7)

    Coding Clinic: 2021, Q3, P5

  I67.1   Cerebral aneurysm, nonruptured
    Cerebral aneurysm NOS
    Cerebral arteriovenous fistula, acquired
    Internal carotid artery aneurysm, intracranial portion
    Internal carotid artery aneurysm, NOS

    Excludes1   congenital cerebral aneurysm, nonruptured (Q28.-)
        ruptured cerebral aneurysm (I60.7)

  I67.2   Cerebral atherosclerosis
    Atheroma of cerebral and precerebral arteries

  I67.3   Progressive vascular leukoencephalopathy
    Binswanger's disease

I67.4   Hypertensive encephalopathy
    Code also, if applicable, associated hypertensive conditions such as:
        essential (primary) hypertension (I10)
        hypertensive chronic kidney disease (I12.-)
        hypertensive heart and chronic kidney disease (I13.-)
        hypertensive heart disease (I11.-)

    Excludes2   insufficiency, NOS, of precerebral arteries (G45.2)

    Coding Clinic: 2023, Q4, P25

I67.5   Moyamoya disease

I67.6   Nonpyogenic thrombosis of intracranial venous system
    Nonpyogenic thrombosis of cerebral vein
    Nonpyogenic thrombosis of intracranial venous sinus

    Excludes1   nonpyogenic thrombosis of intracranial venous system causing infarction (I63.6)

I67.7   Cerebral arteritis, not elsewhere classified
    Granulomatous angiitis of the nervous system

    Excludes1   allergic granulomatous angiitis (M30.1)

● I67.8   Other specified cerebrovascular diseases

  I67.81   Acute cerebrovascular insufficiency
    Acute cerebrovascular insufficiency unspecified as to location or reversibility

  I67.82   Cerebral ischemia
    Chronic cerebral ischemia

  I67.83   Posterior reversible encephalopathy syndrome
    PRES

  ● I67.84   Cerebral vasospasm and vasoconstriction

    I67.841   Reversible cerebrovascular vasoconstriction syndrome
        Call-Fleming syndrome
        Code first underlying condition, if applicable, such as eclampsia (O15.00-O15.9)

    I67.848   Other cerebrovascular vasospasm and vasoconstriction

  ● I67.85   Hereditary cerebrovascular diseases

    I67.850   Cerebral autosomal dominant arteriopathy with subcortical infarcts and leukoencephalopathy
        CADASIL
        Code also any associated diagnoses, such as:
          epilepsy (G40.-), stroke (I63.-)
          vascular dementia (F01.-)

    I67.858   Other hereditary cerebrovascular disease

  I67.89   Other cerebrovascular disease
    Coding Clinic: 2023, Q2, P19

I67.9   Cerebrovascular disease, unspecified

● I68   Cerebrovascular disorders in diseases classified elsewhere

  ▶ I68.0   *Cerebral amyloid angiopathy*
    Code first underlying amyloidosis (E85.-)

  ▶ I68.2   *Cerebral arteritis in other diseases classified elsewhere*
    Code first underlying disease

    Excludes1   cerebral arteritis (in):
        listerosis (A32.89)
        systemic lupus erythematosus (M32.19)
        syphilis (A52.04)
        tuberculosis (A18.89)

A

▶ New   ⇒ Revised   ~~deleted~~ Deleted   Excludes 1   Excludes 2   Includes   Use additional   Code first   Code also   Key words
OGCR Official Guidelines   X Assign placeholder X   ● Use Additional Character(s)   ▶ Manifestation Code   🅗 Hierarchical Condition Category   **Coding Clinic**

I68.8 *Other cerebrovascular disorders in diseases classified elsewhere*

  Code first underlying disease

  Excludes1 syphilitic cerebral aneurysm (A52.05)

  OGCR Section I.c.9.d.

  Sequelae of Cerebrovascular Disease

  1) Category I69, Sequelae of Cerebrovascular disease

  Category I69 is used to indicate conditions classifiable to categories I60-I67 as the causes of sequela (neurologic deficits), themselves classified elsewhere. These "late effects" include neurologic deficits that persist after initial onset of conditions classifiable to categories I60-I67. The neurologic deficits caused by cerebrovascular disease may be present from the onset of may arise at any time after the onset of the condition classifiable to categories I60-I67.

  Codes from category I69, Sequelae of cerebrovascular disease, that specify hemiplegia, hemiparesis and monoplegia identify whether the dominant or nondominant side is affected. Should the affected side be documented, but not specified as dominant or nondominant, and the classification system does not indicate a default, code selection is as follows:

  For ambidextrous patients, the default should be dominant.

  If the left side is affected, the default is nondominant.

  If the right side is affected, the default is dominant.

  2) Codes from category I69 with codes from I60-I67

  Codes from category I69 may be assigned on a health care record with codes from I60-I67, if the patient has a current cerebrovascular disease and deficits from an old cerebrovascular disease.

● **I69** **Sequelae of cerebrovascular disease**

  Note: Category I69 is to be used to indicate conditions in I60-I67 as the cause of sequelae. The 'sequelae' include conditions specified as such or as residuals which may occur at any time after the onset of the causal condition.

  Excludes1 personal history of cerebral infarction without residual deficit (Z86.73)
    personal history of prolonged reversible ischemic neurologic deficit (PRIND) (Z86.73)
    personal history of reversible ischemic neurologcial deficit (RIND) (Z86.73)
    sequelae of traumatic intracranial injury (S06.-)

  Coding Clinic: 2016, Q4, P28; 2015, Q4, P40; 2012, Q4, P107

● **I69.0** **Sequelae of nontraumatic subarachnoid hemorrhage**

  I69.00 **Unspecified** sequelae of nontraumatic subarachnoid hemorrhage

 ● **I69.01** **Cognitive deficits** following nontraumatic subarachnoid hemorrhage

   I69.010 **Attention and concentration** deficit following nontraumatic subarachnoid hemorrhage

   I69.011 **Memory** deficit following nontraumatic subarachnoid hemorrhage

   I69.012 **Visuospatial** deficit and spatial neglect following nontraumatic subarachnoid hemorrhage

   I69.013 **Psychomotor** deficit following nontraumatic subarachnoid hemorrhage

   I69.014 **Frontal lobe and executive function** deficit following nontraumatic subarachnoid hemorrhage

   I69.015 **Cognitive social or emotional** deficit following nontraumatic subarachnoid hemorrhage

   I69.018 **Other symptoms and signs** involving cognitive functions following nontraumatic subarachnoid hemorrhage

   I69.019 **Unspecified** symptoms and signs involving cognitive functions following nontraumatic subarachnoid hemorrhage

 ● **I69.02** **Speech and language deficits** following nontraumatic subarachnoid hemorrhage

   I69.020 **Aphasia** following nontraumatic subarachnoid hemorrhage

   I69.021 **Dysphasia** following nontraumatic subarachnoid hemorrhage

   I69.022 **Dysarthria** following nontraumatic subarachnoid hemorrhage

   I69.023 **Fluency disorder** following nontraumatic subarachnoid hemorrhage
     Stuttering following nontraumatic subarachnoid hemorrhage

   I69.028 **Other speech and language deficits** following nontraumatic subarachnoid hemorrhage

 ● **I69.03** **Monoplegia of upper limb** following nontraumatic subarachnoid hemorrhage

   I69.031 Monoplegia of upper limb following nontraumatic subarachnoid hemorrhage affecting **right dominant side** ℞

   I69.032 Monoplegia of upper limb following nontraumatic subarachnoid hemorrhage affecting **left dominant side** ℞

   I69.033 Monoplegia of upper limb following nontraumatic subarachnoid hemorrhage affecting **right non-dominant side** ℞

   I69.034 Monoplegia of upper limb following nontraumatic subarachnoid hemorrhage affecting **left non-dominant side** ℞

   I69.039 Monoplegia of upper limb following nontraumatic subarachnoid hemorrhage affecting **unspecified side** ℞

 ● **I69.04** **Monoplegia of lower limb** following nontraumatic subarachnoid hemorrhage

   I69.041 Monoplegia of lower limb following nontraumatic subarachnoid hemorrhage affecting **right dominant side** ℞

   I69.042 Monoplegia of lower limb following nontraumatic subarachnoid hemorrhage affecting **left dominant side** ℞

   I69.043 Monoplegia of lower limb following nontraumatic subarachnoid hemorrhage affecting **right non-dominant side** ℞

   I69.044 Monoplegia of lower limb following nontraumatic subarachnoid hemorrhage affecting **left non-dominant side** ℞

   I69.049 Monoplegia of lower limb following nontraumatic subarachnoid hemorrhage affecting **unspecified side** ℞

 ● **I69.05** **Hemiplegia and hemiparesis** following nontraumatic subarachnoid hemorrhage

   I69.051 Hemiplegia and hemiparesis following nontraumatic subarachnoid hemorrhage affecting **right dominant side** ℞

   I69.052 Hemiplegia and hemiparesis following nontraumatic subarachnoid hemorrhage affecting **left dominant side** ℞

I69.Ø53 Hemiplegia and hemiparesis following nontraumatic subarachnoid hemorrhage affecting **right non-dominant side** ℞꜀

I69.Ø54 Hemiplegia and hemiparesis following nontraumatic subarachnoid hemorrhage affecting **left non-dominant side** ℞꜀

I69.Ø59 Hemiplegia and hemiparesis following nontraumatic subarachnoid hemorrhage affecting **unspecified side** ℞꜀

● **I69.Ø6** **Other paralytic syndrome** following nontraumatic subarachnoid hemorrhage

Use additional code to identify type of paralytic syndrome, such as:
locked-in state (G83.5)
quadriplegia (G82.5-)

Excludes1 hemiplegia/hemiparesis following nontraumatic subarachnoid hemorrhage (I69.Ø5-)
monoplegia of lower limb following nontraumatic subarachnoid hemorrhage (I69.Ø4-)
monoplegia of upper limb following nontraumatic subarachnoid hemorrhage (I69.Ø3-)

I69.Ø61 Other paralytic syndrome following nontraumatic subarachnoid hemorrhage affecting **right dominant side** ℞꜀

I69.Ø62 Other paralytic syndrome following nontraumatic subarachnoid hemorrhage affecting **left dominant side** ℞꜀

I69.Ø63 Other paralytic syndrome following nontraumatic subarachnoid hemorrhage affecting **right non-dominant side** ℞꜀

I69.Ø64 Other paralytic syndrome following nontraumatic subarachnoid hemorrhage affecting **left non-dominant side** ℞꜀

I69.Ø65 Other paralytic syndrome following nontraumatic subarachnoid hemorrhage, **bilateral** ℞꜀

I69.Ø69 Other paralytic syndrome following nontraumatic subarachnoid hemorrhage affecting **unspecified side** ℞꜀

● **I69.Ø9** **Other sequelae** of nontraumatic subarachnoid hemorrhage

I69.Ø90 **Apraxia** following nontraumatic subarachnoid hemorrhage

I69.Ø91 **Dysphagia** following nontraumatic subarachnoid hemorrhage

Use additional code to identify the type of dysphagia, if known (R13.11-R13.19)

I69.Ø92 **Facial weakness** following nontraumatic subarachnoid hemorrhage
Facial droop following nontraumatic subarachnoid hemorrhage

I69.Ø93 **Ataxia** following nontraumatic subarachnoid hemorrhage

I69.Ø98 **Other sequelae** following nontraumatic subarachnoid hemorrhage
Alterations of sensation following nontraumatic subarachnoid hemorrhage
Disturbance of vision following nontraumatic subarachnoid hemorrhage

Use additional code to identify the sequelae

● **I69.1** Sequelae of nontraumatic **intracerebral** hemorrhage

I69.1Ø **Unspecified** sequelae of nontraumatic intracerebral hemorrhage

● **I69.11** **Cognitive deficits** following nontraumatic intracerebral hemorrhage

I69.11Ø **Attention and concentration** deficit following nontraumatic intracerebral hemorrhage

I69.111 **Memory** deficit following nontraumatic intracerebral hemorrhage

I69.112 **Visuospatial** deficit and spatial neglect following nontraumatic intracerebral hemorrhage

I69.113 **Psychomotor** deficit following nontraumatic intracerebral hemorrhage

I69.114 **Frontal lobe and executive function** deficit following nontraumatic intracerebral hemorrhage

I69.115 **Cognitive social or emotional** deficit following nontraumatic intracerebral hemorrhage

I69.118 **Other symptoms and signs** involving cognitive functions following nontraumatic intracerebral hemorrhage

I69.119 **Unspecified** symptoms and signs involving cognitive functions following nontraumatic intracerebral hemorrhage

● **I69.12** **Speech and language deficits** following nontraumatic intracerebral hemorrhage

I69.12Ø **Aphasia** following nontraumatic intracerebral hemorrhage

I69.121 **Dysphasia** following nontraumatic intracerebral hemorrhage

I69.122 **Dysarthria** following nontraumatic intracerebral hemorrhage

I69.123 **Fluency disorder** following nontraumatic intracerebral hemorrhage
Stuttering following nontraumatic intracerebral hemorrhage

I69.128 **Other speech and language deficits** following nontraumatic intracerebral hemorrhage

● **I69.13** **Monoplegia of upper limb** following nontraumatic intracerebral hemorrhage

I69.131 Monoplegia of upper limb following nontraumatic intracerebral hemorrhage affecting **right dominant side** ℞꜀

I69.132 Monoplegia of upper limb following nontraumatic intracerebral hemorrhage affecting **left dominant side** ℞꜀

I69.133 Monoplegia of upper limb following nontraumatic intracerebral hemorrhage affecting **right non-dominant side** ℞꜀

I69.134   Monoplegia of upper limb following nontraumatic intracerebral hemorrhage affecting left non-dominant side ▨

I69.139   Monoplegia of upper limb following nontraumatic intracerebral hemorrhage affecting unspecified side ▨

● I69.14   **Monoplegia of lower limb following nontraumatic intracerebral hemorrhage**

I69.141   Monoplegia of lower limb following nontraumatic intracerebral hemorrhage affecting right dominant side ▨

I69.142   Monoplegia of lower limb following nontraumatic intracerebral hemorrhage affecting left dominant side ▨

I69.143   Monoplegia of lower limb following nontraumatic intracerebral hemorrhage affecting right non-dominant side ▨

I69.144   Monoplegia of lower limb following nontraumatic intracerebral hemorrhage affecting left non-dominant side ▨

I69.149   Monoplegia of lower limb following nontraumatic intracerebral hemorrhage affecting unspecified side ▨

● I69.15   **Hemiplegia and hemiparesis following nontraumatic intracerebral hemorrhage**

I69.151   Hemiplegia and hemiparesis following nontraumatic intracerebral hemorrhage affecting right dominant side ▨

I69.152   Hemiplegia and hemiparesis following nontraumatic intracerebral hemorrhage affecting left dominant side ▨

I69.153   Hemiplegia and hemiparesis following nontraumatic intracerebral hemorrhage affecting right non-dominant side ▨

I69.154   Hemiplegia and hemiparesis following nontraumatic intracerebral hemorrhage affecting left non-dominant side ▨

I69.159   Hemiplegia and hemiparesis following nontraumatic intracerebral hemorrhage affecting unspecified side ▨

● I69.16   **Other paralytic syndrome following nontraumatic intracerebral hemorrhage**

Use additional code to identify type of paralytic syndrome, such as:
locked-in state (G83.5)
quadriplegia (G82.5-)

Excludes1   hemiplegia/hemiparesis following nontraumatic intracerebral hemorrhage (I69.15-)
monoplegia of lower limb following nontraumatic intracerebral hemorrhage (I69.14-)
monoplegia of upper limb following nontraumatic intracerebral hemorrhage (I69.13-)

I69.161   Other paralytic syndrome following nontraumatic intracerebral hemorrhage affecting right dominant side ▨

I69.162   Other paralytic syndrome following nontraumatic intracerebral hemorrhage affecting left dominant side ▨

I69.163   Other paralytic syndrome following nontraumatic intracerebral hemorrhage affecting right non-dominant side ▨

I69.164   Other paralytic syndrome following nontraumatic intracerebral hemorrhage affecting left non-dominant side ▨

I69.165   Other paralytic syndrome following nontraumatic intracerebral hemorrhage, bilateral ▨

I69.169   Other paralytic syndrome following nontraumatic intracerebral hemorrhage affecting unspecified side ▨

● I69.19   **Other sequelae of nontraumatic intracerebral hemorrhage**

I69.190   **Apraxia following nontraumatic intracerebral hemorrhage**

I69.191   **Dysphagia following nontraumatic intracerebral hemorrhage**

Use additional code to identify the type of dysphagia, if known (R13.11-R13.19)

I69.192   **Facial weakness following nontraumatic intracerebral hemorrhage**
Facial droop following nontraumatic intracerebral hemorrhage

I69.193   **Ataxia following nontraumatic intracerebral hemorrhage**

I69.198   **Other sequelae of nontraumatic intracerebral hemorrhage**
Alteration of sensations following nontraumatic intracerebral hemorrhage
Disturbance of vision following nontraumatic intracerebral hemorrhage

Use additional code to identify the sequelae

● I69.2   **Sequelae of other nontraumatic intracranial hemorrhage**

I69.20   **Unspecified sequelae of other nontraumatic intracranial hemorrhage**

● I69.21   **Cognitive deficits following other nontraumatic intracranial hemorrhage**

I69.210   **Attention and concentration deficit following other nontraumatic intracranial hemorrhage**

I69.211   **Memory deficit following other nontraumatic intracranial hemorrhage**

I69.212   **Visuospatial deficit and spatial neglect following other nontraumatic intracranial hemorrhage**

I69.213   **Psychomotor deficit following other nontraumatic intracranial hemorrhage**

I69.214   **Frontal lobe and executive function deficit following other nontraumatic intracranial hemorrhage**

I69.215   **Cognitive social or emotional deficit following other nontraumatic intracranial hemorrhage**

I69.218   **Other symptoms and signs involving cognitive functions following other nontraumatic intracranial hemorrhage**

I69.219   **Unspecified symptoms and signs involving cognitive functions following other nontraumatic intracranial hemorrhage**

● **I69.22** **Speech and language deficits** following other nontraumatic intracranial hemorrhage

    I69.220 **Aphasia** following other nontraumatic intracranial hemorrhage

    I69.221 **Dysphasia** following other nontraumatic intracranial hemorrhage

    I69.222 **Dysarthria** following other nontraumatic intracranial hemorrhage

    I69.223 **Fluency disorder** following other nontraumatic intracranial hemorrhage
        Stuttering following other nontraumatic intracranial hemorrhage

    I69.228 **Other speech and language deficits** following other nontraumatic intracranial hemorrhage

● **I69.23** **Monoplegia of upper limb** following other nontraumatic intracranial hemorrhage

    I69.231 **Monoplegia of upper limb** following other nontraumatic intracranial hemorrhage affecting **right dominant side** ℞

    I69.232 **Monoplegia of upper limb** following other nontraumatic intracranial hemorrhage affecting **left dominant side** ℞

    I69.233 **Monoplegia of upper limb** following other nontraumatic intracranial hemorrhage affecting **right non-dominant side** ℞

    I69.234 **Monoplegia of upper limb** following other nontraumatic intracranial hemorrhage affecting **left non-dominant side** ℞

    I69.239 **Monoplegia of upper limb** following other nontraumatic intracranial hemorrhage affecting **unspecified side** ℞

● **I69.24** **Monoplegia of lower limb** following other nontraumatic intracranial hemorrhage

    I69.241 **Monoplegia of lower limb** following other nontraumatic intracranial hemorrhage affecting **right dominant side** ℞

    I69.242 **Monoplegia of lower limb** following other nontraumatic intracranial hemorrhage affecting **left dominant side** ℞

    I69.243 **Monoplegia of lower limb** following other nontraumatic intracranial hemorrhage affecting **right non-dominant side** ℞

    I69.244 **Monoplegia of lower limb** following other nontraumatic intracranial hemorrhage affecting **left non-dominant side** ℞

    I69.249 **Monoplegia of lower limb** following other nontraumatic intracranial hemorrhage affecting **unspecified side** ℞

● **I69.25** **Hemiplegia and hemiparesis** following other nontraumatic intracranial hemorrhage

    I69.251 **Hemiplegia and hemiparesis** following other nontraumatic intracranial hemorrhage affecting **right dominant side** ℞

    I69.252 **Hemiplegia and hemiparesis** following other nontraumatic intracranial hemorrhage affecting **left dominant side** ℞

    I69.253 **Hemiplegia and hemiparesis** following other nontraumatic intracranial hemorrhage affecting **right non-dominant side** ℞

    I69.254 **Hemiplegia and hemiparesis** following other nontraumatic intracranial hemorrhage affecting **left non-dominant side** ℞

    I69.259 **Hemiplegia and hemiparesis** following other nontraumatic intracranial hemorrhage affecting **unspecified side** ℞

● **I69.26** **Other paralytic syndrome** following other nontraumatic intracranial hemorrhage

    Use additional code to identify type of paralytic syndrome, such as:
      locked-in state (G83.5)
      quadriplegia (G82.5-)

    Excludes1 hemiplegia/hemiparesis following other nontraumatic intracranial hemorrhage (I69.25-)
        monoplegia of lower limb following other nontraumatic intracranial hemorrhage (I69.24-)
        monoplegia of upper limb following other nontraumatic intracranial hemorrhage (I69.23-)

    I69.261 **Other paralytic syndrome** following other nontraumatic intracranial hemorrhage affecting **right dominant side** ℞

    I69.262 **Other paralytic syndrome** following other nontraumatic intracranial hemorrhage affecting **left dominant side** ℞

    I69.263 **Other paralytic syndrome** following other nontraumatic intracranial hemorrhage affecting **right non-dominant side** ℞

    I69.264 **Other paralytic syndrome** following other nontraumatic intracranial hemorrhage affecting **left non-dominant side** ℞

    I69.265 **Other paralytic syndrome** following other nontraumatic intracranial hemorrhage, **bilateral** ℞

    I69.269 **Other paralytic syndrome** following other nontraumatic intracranial hemorrhage affecting **unspecified side** ℞

● **I69.29** **Other sequelae** of other nontraumatic intracranial hemorrhage

    I69.290 **Apraxia** following other nontraumatic intracranial hemorrhage

    I69.291 **Dysphagia** following other nontraumatic intracranial hemorrhage
      Use additional code to identify the type of dysphagia, if known (R13.11-R13.19)

    I69.292 **Facial weakness** following other nontraumatic intracranial hemorrhage
      Facial droop following other nontraumatic intracranial hemorrhage

    I69.293 **Ataxia** following other nontraumatic intracranial hemorrhage

▶ New ⇒ Revised ~~deleted~~ Deleted | Excludes 1 | Excludes 2 | Includes | Use additional | Code first | Code also | Key words
OGCR Official Guidelines   **X** Assign placeholder X   ● Use Additional Character(s)   ▶ Manifestation Code   ℞ Hierarchical Condition Category   **Coding Clinic**

I69.298 **Other sequelae of other nontraumatic intracranial hemorrhage**
Alteration of sensation following other nontraumatic intracranial hemorrhage
Disturbance of vision following other nontraumatic intracranial hemorrhage
Use additional code to identify the sequelae

● **I69.3** **Sequelae of cerebral infarction**
Sequelae of stroke NOS
Coding Clinic: 2012, Q4, P92, 95

I69.30 **Unspecified sequelae of cerebral infarction**

● **I69.31** **Cognitive deficits following cerebral infarction**

I69.310 **Attention and concentration deficit following cerebral infarction**

I69.311 **Memory deficit following cerebral infarction**

I69.312 **Visuospatial deficit and spatial neglect following cerebral infarction**

I69.313 **Psychomotor deficit following cerebral infarction**

I69.314 **Frontal lobe and executive function deficit following cerebral infarction**

I69.315 **Cognitive social or emotional deficit following cerebral infarction**

I69.318 **Other symptoms and signs involving cognitive functions following cerebral infarction**

I69.319 **Unspecified symptoms and signs involving cognitive functions following cerebral infarction**

● **I69.32** **Speech and language deficits following cerebral infarction**

I69.320 **Aphasia following cerebral infarction**

I69.321 **Dysphasia following cerebral infarction**
Coding Clinic: 2012, Q4, P91

I69.322 **Dysarthria following cerebral infarction**
Excludes2 transient ischemic attack (TIA) (G45.9)

I69.323 **Fluency disorder following cerebral infarction**
Stuttering following cerebral infarction

I69.328 **Other speech and language deficits following cerebral infarction**

● **I69.33** **Monoplegia of upper limb following cerebral infarction**
Coding Clinic: 2017, Q1, P47

I69.331 **Monoplegia of upper limb following cerebral infarction affecting right dominant side** ℞

I69.332 **Monoplegia of upper limb following cerebral infarction affecting left dominant side** ℞

I69.333 **Monoplegia of upper limb following cerebral infarction affecting right non-dominant side** ℞

I69.334 **Monoplegia of upper limb following cerebral infarction affecting left non-dominant side** ℞

I69.339 **Monoplegia of upper limb following cerebral infarction affecting unspecified side** ℞

● **I69.34** **Monoplegia of lower limb following cerebral infarction**
Coding Clinic: 2017, Q1, P47

I69.341 **Monoplegia of lower limb following cerebral infarction affecting right dominant side** ℞

I69.342 **Monoplegia of lower limb following cerebral infarction affecting left dominant side** ℞

I69.343 **Monoplegia of lower limb following cerebral infarction affecting right non-dominant side** ℞

I69.344 **Monoplegia of lower limb following cerebral infarction affecting left non-dominant side** ℞

I69.349 **Monoplegia of lower limb following cerebral infarction affecting unspecified side** ℞

● **I69.35** **Hemiplegia and hemiparesis following cerebral infarction**

I69.351 **Hemiplegia and hemiparesis following cerebral infarction affecting right dominant side** ℞
Excludes2 transient ischemic attack (TIA) (G45.9)
Coding Clinic: 2015, Q1, P25

I69.352 **Hemiplegia and hemiparesis following cerebral infarction affecting left dominant side** ℞

I69.353 **Hemiplegia and hemiparesis following cerebral infarction affecting right non-dominant side** ℞

I69.354 **Hemiplegia and hemiparesis following cerebral infarction affecting left non-dominant side** ℞
Coding Clinic: 2012, Q4, P91

I69.359 **Hemiplegia and hemiparesis following cerebral infarction affecting unspecified side** ℞

● **I69.36** **Other paralytic syndrome following cerebral infarction**
Use additional code to identify type of paralytic syndrome, such as:
locked-in state (G83.5)
quadriplegia (G82.5-)
Excludes1 hemiplegia/hemiparesis following cerebral infarction (I69.35-)
monoplegia of lower limb following cerebral infarction (I69.34-)
monoplegia of upper limb following cerebral infarction (I69.33-)

I69.361 **Other paralytic syndrome following cerebral infarction affecting right dominant side** ℞

I69.362 **Other paralytic syndrome following cerebral infarction affecting left dominant side** ℞

I69.363 **Other paralytic syndrome following cerebral infarction affecting right non-dominant side** ℞

I69.364 **Other paralytic syndrome following cerebral infarction affecting left non-dominant side** ℞

I69.365 **Other paralytic syndrome following cerebral infarction, bilateral** ℞

I69.369 **Other paralytic syndrome following cerebral infarction affecting unspecified side** ℞

CHAPTER 9 (I00-I99)

● **I69.39**   **Other sequelae of cerebral infarction**

    I69.390   **Apraxia following cerebral infarction**

    I69.391   **Dysphagia following cerebral infarction**

        Use additional code to identify the type of dysphagia, if known (R13.11-R13.19)

    I69.392   **Facial weakness following cerebral infarction**

        Facial droop following cerebral infarction

        Coding Clinic: 2024, Q2, P13

    I69.393   **Ataxia following cerebral infarction**

    I69.398   **Other sequelae of cerebral infarction**

        Alteration of sensation following cerebral infarction

        Disturbance of vision following cerebral infarction

        Use additional code to identify the sequelae

        Coding Clinic: 2024, Q2, P13

● **I69.8**   **Sequelae of other cerebrovascular diseases**

    Excludes1   sequelae of traumatic intracranial injury (S06.-)

    I69.80   **Unspecified sequelae of other cerebrovascular disease**

● **I69.81**   **Cognitive deficits following other cerebrovascular disease**

    I69.810   **Attention and concentration deficit following other cerebrovascular disease**

    I69.811   **Memory deficit following other cerebrovascular disease**

    I69.812   **Visuospatial deficit and spatial neglect following other cerebrovascular disease**

    I69.813   **Psychomotor deficit following other cerebrovascular disease**

    I69.814   **Frontal lobe and executive function deficit following other cerebrovascular disease**

    I69.815   **Cognitive social or emotional deficit following other cerebrovascular disease**

    I69.818   **Other symptoms and signs involving cognitive functions following other cerebrovascular disease**

    I69.819   **Unspecified symptoms and signs involving cognitive functions following other cerebrovascular disease**

● **I69.82**   **Speech and language deficits following other cerebrovascular disease**

    I69.820   **Aphasia following other cerebrovascular disease**

    I69.821   **Dysphasia following other cerebrovascular disease**

    I69.822   **Dysarthria following other cerebrovascular disease**

    I69.823   **Fluency disorder following other cerebrovascular disease**

        Stuttering following other cerebrovascular disease

    I69.828   **Other speech and language deficits following other cerebrovascular disease**

        Coding Clinic: 2019, Q3, P9

● **I69.83**   **Monoplegia of upper limb following other cerebrovascular disease**

    I69.831   **Monoplegia of upper limb following other cerebrovascular disease affecting right dominant side** 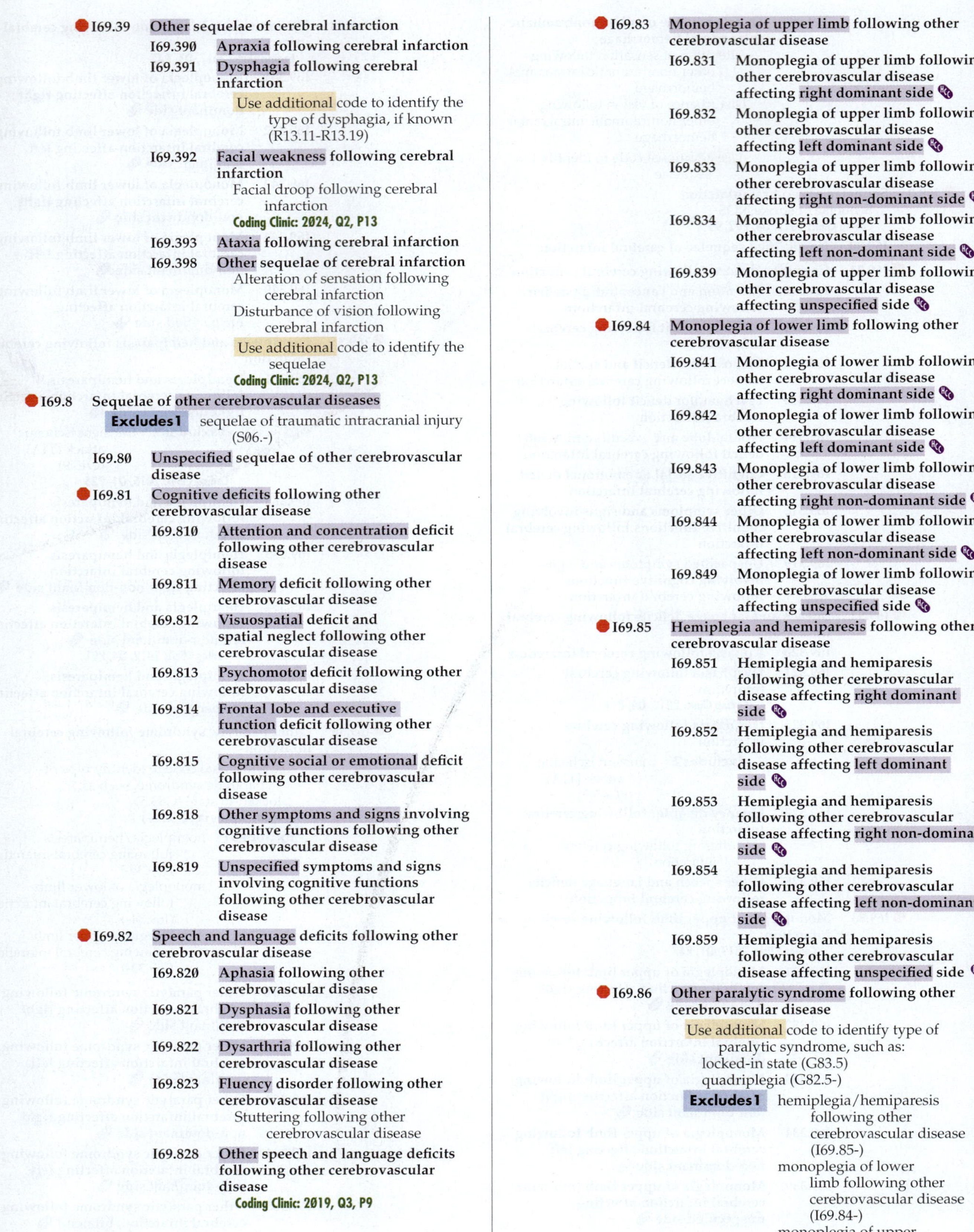

    I69.832   **Monoplegia of upper limb following other cerebrovascular disease affecting left dominant side**

    I69.833   **Monoplegia of upper limb following other cerebrovascular disease affecting right non-dominant side**

    I69.834   **Monoplegia of upper limb following other cerebrovascular disease affecting left non-dominant side**

    I69.839   **Monoplegia of upper limb following other cerebrovascular disease affecting unspecified side**

● **I69.84**   **Monoplegia of lower limb following other cerebrovascular disease**

    I69.841   **Monoplegia of lower limb following other cerebrovascular disease affecting right dominant side**

    I69.842   **Monoplegia of lower limb following other cerebrovascular disease affecting left dominant side**

    I69.843   **Monoplegia of lower limb following other cerebrovascular disease affecting right non-dominant side**

    I69.844   **Monoplegia of lower limb following other cerebrovascular disease affecting left non-dominant side**

    I69.849   **Monoplegia of lower limb following other cerebrovascular disease affecting unspecified side**

● **I69.85**   **Hemiplegia and hemiparesis following other cerebrovascular disease**

    I69.851   **Hemiplegia and hemiparesis following other cerebrovascular disease affecting right dominant side**

    I69.852   **Hemiplegia and hemiparesis following other cerebrovascular disease affecting left dominant side**

    I69.853   **Hemiplegia and hemiparesis following other cerebrovascular disease affecting right non-dominant side**

    I69.854   **Hemiplegia and hemiparesis following other cerebrovascular disease affecting left non-dominant side**

    I69.859   **Hemiplegia and hemiparesis following other cerebrovascular disease affecting unspecified side**

● **I69.86**   **Other paralytic syndrome following other cerebrovascular disease**

    Use additional code to identify type of paralytic syndrome, such as:
    locked-in state (G83.5)
    quadriplegia (G82.5-)

    Excludes1   hemiplegia/hemiparesis following other cerebrovascular disease (I69.85-)
        monoplegia of lower limb following other cerebrovascular disease (I69.84-)
        monoplegia of upper limb following other cerebrovascular disease (I69.83-)

I69.861   **Other paralytic syndrome following other cerebrovascular disease affecting right dominant side**

I69.862   **Other paralytic syndrome following other cerebrovascular disease affecting left dominant side**

I69.863   **Other paralytic syndrome following other cerebrovascular disease affecting right non-dominant side**

I69.864   **Other paralytic syndrome following other cerebrovascular disease affecting left non-dominant side**

I69.865   **Other paralytic syndrome following other cerebrovascular disease, bilateral**

I69.869   **Other paralytic syndrome following other cerebrovascular disease affecting unspecified side**

● **I69.89**   **Other sequelae of other cerebrovascular disease**

I69.890   **Apraxia following other cerebrovascular disease**

I69.891   **Dysphagia following other cerebrovascular disease**
> Use additional code to identify the type of dysphagia, if known (R13.11-R13.19)

I69.892   **Facial weakness following other cerebrovascular disease**
> Facial droop following other cerebrovascular disease

I69.893   **Ataxia following other cerebrovascular disease**

I69.898   **Other sequelae of other cerebrovascular disease**
> Alteration of sensation following other cerebrovascular disease
> Disturbance of vision following other cerebrovascular disease
> Use additional code to identify the sequelae

● **I69.9**   **Sequelae of unspecified cerebrovascular diseases**

> **Excludes1**   sequelae of stroke (I69.3)
> sequelae of traumatic intracranial injury (S06.-)

I69.90   **Unspecified sequelae of unspecified cerebrovascular disease**

● **I69.91**   **Cognitive deficits following unspecified cerebrovascular disease**

I69.910   **Attention and concentration deficit following unspecified cerebrovascular disease**

I69.911   **Memory deficit following unspecified cerebrovascular disease**

I69.912   **Visuospatial deficit and spatial neglect following unspecified cerebrovascular disease**

I69.913   **Psychomotor deficit following unspecified cerebrovascular disease**

I69.914   **Frontal lobe and executive function deficit following unspecified cerebrovascular disease**

I69.915   **Cognitive social or emotional deficit following unspecified cerebrovascular disease**

I69.918   **Other symptoms and signs involving cognitive functions following unspecified cerebrovascular disease**

I69.919   **Unspecified symptoms and signs involving cognitive functions following unspecified cerebrovascular disease**

● **I69.92**   **Speech and language deficits following unspecified cerebrovascular disease**

I69.920   **Aphasia following unspecified cerebrovascular disease**

I69.921   **Dysphasia following unspecified cerebrovascular disease**

I69.922   **Dysarthria following unspecified cerebrovascular disease**

I69.923   **Fluency disorder following unspecified cerebrovascular disease**
> Stuttering following unspecified cerebrovascular disease

I69.928   **Other speech and language deficits following unspecified cerebrovascular disease**

● **I69.93**   **Monoplegia of upper limb following unspecified cerebrovascular disease**

I69.931   **Monoplegia of upper limb following unspecified cerebrovascular disease affecting right dominant side**

I69.932   **Monoplegia of upper limb following unspecified cerebrovascular disease affecting left dominant side**

I69.933   **Monoplegia of upper limb following unspecified cerebrovascular disease affecting right non-dominant side**

I69.934   **Monoplegia of upper limb following unspecified cerebrovascular disease affecting left non-dominant side**

I69.939   **Monoplegia of upper limb following unspecified cerebrovascular disease affecting unspecified side**

● **I69.94**   **Monoplegia of lower limb following unspecified cerebrovascular disease**

I69.941   **Monoplegia of lower limb following unspecified cerebrovascular disease affecting right dominant side**

I69.942   **Monoplegia of lower limb following unspecified cerebrovascular disease affecting left dominant side**

I69.943   **Monoplegia of lower limb following unspecified cerebrovascular disease affecting right non-dominant side**

I69.944   **Monoplegia of lower limb following unspecified cerebrovascular disease affecting left non-dominant side**

I69.949   **Monoplegia of lower limb following unspecified cerebrovascular disease affecting unspecified side**

● **I69.95**   **Hemiplegia and hemiparesis following unspecified cerebrovascular disease**

I69.951   **Hemiplegia and hemiparesis following unspecified cerebrovascular disease affecting right dominant side**

I69.952   **Hemiplegia and hemiparesis following unspecified cerebrovascular disease affecting left dominant side**

I69.953   **Hemiplegia and hemiparesis following unspecified cerebrovascular disease affecting right non-dominant side**

CHAPTER 9 (I00-I99)

I69.954 Hemiplegia and hemiparesis following unspecified cerebrovascular disease affecting left non-dominant side

I69.959 Hemiplegia and hemiparesis following unspecified cerebrovascular disease affecting unspecified side

● **I69.96** Other paralytic syndrome following unspecified cerebrovascular disease

Use additional code to identify type of paralytic syndrome, such as:
locked-in state (G83.5)
quadriplegia (G82.5-)

Excludes1 hemiplegia/hemiparesis following unspecified cerebrovascular disease (I69.95-)
monoplegia of lower limb following unspecified cerebrovascular disease (I69.94-)
monoplegia of upper limb following unspecified cerebrovascular disease (I69.93-)

I69.961 Other paralytic syndrome following unspecified cerebrovascular disease affecting right dominant side

I69.962 Other paralytic syndrome following unspecified cerebrovascular disease affecting left dominant side

I69.963 Other paralytic syndrome following unspecified cerebrovascular disease affecting right non-dominant side

I69.964 Other paralytic syndrome following unspecified cerebrovascular disease affecting left non-dominant side

I69.965 Other paralytic syndrome following unspecified cerebrovascular disease, bilateral

I69.969 Other paralytic syndrome following unspecified cerebrovascular disease affecting unspecified side

● **I69.99** Other sequelae of unspecified cerebrovascular disease

I69.990 Apraxia following unspecified cerebrovascular disease

I69.991 Dysphagia following unspecified cerebrovascular disease

Use additional code to identify the type of dysphagia, if known (R13.11-R13.19)

I69.992 Facial weakness following unspecified cerebrovascular disease
Facial droop following unspecified cerebrovascular disease

I69.993 Ataxia following unspecified cerebrovascular disease

I69.998 Other sequelae following unspecified cerebrovascular disease
Alteration in sensation following unspecified cerebrovascular disease
Disturbance of vision following unspecified cerebrovascular disease

Use additional code to identify the sequelae

DISEASES OF ARTERIES, ARTERIOLES AND CAPILLARIES (I70-I79)

● **I70** Atherosclerosis

Includes arteriolosclerosis
arterial degeneration
arteriosclerosis
arteriosclerotic vascular disease
arteriovascular degeneration
atheroma
endarteritis deformans or obliterans
senile arteritis
senile endarteritis
vascular degeneration

Use additional code to identify:
exposure to environmental tobacco smoke (Z77.22)
history of tobacco dependence (Z87.891)
occupational exposure to environmental tobacco smoke (Z57.31)
tobacco dependence (F17.-)
tobacco use (Z72.0)

Excludes2 arteriosclerotic cardiovascular disease (I25.1-)
arteriosclerotic heart disease (I25.1-)
atheroembolism (I75.-)
cerebral atherosclerosis (I67.2)
coronary atherosclerosis (I25.1-)
mesenteric atherosclerosis (K55.1)
precerebral atherosclerosis (I67.2)
primary pulmonary atherosclerosis (I27.0)

I70.0 Atherosclerosis of aorta　A

I70.1 Atherosclerosis of renal artery　A
Goldblatt's kidney

Excludes2 atherosclerosis of renal arterioles (I12.-)

★ (See Plates 500, 501, and 502 on pages 60 – 62.)

● **I70.2** Atherosclerosis of native arteries of the extremities
Mönckeberg's (medial) sclerosis

Use additional code, if applicable, to identify chronic total occlusion of artery of extremity (I70.92)

Excludes2 atherosclerosis of bypass graft of extremities (I70.30-I70.79)

● **I70.20** Unspecified atherosclerosis of native arteries of extremities

I70.201 Unspecified atherosclerosis of native arteries of extremities, right leg　A

I70.202 Unspecified atherosclerosis of native arteries of extremities, left leg　A

I70.203 Unspecified atherosclerosis of native arteries of extremities, bilateral legs　A

I70.208 Unspecified atherosclerosis of native arteries of extremities, other extremity　A

I70.209 Unspecified atherosclerosis of native arteries of extremities, unspecified extremity　A

● **I70.21** Atherosclerosis of native arteries of extremities with intermittent claudication

I70.211 Atherosclerosis of native arteries of extremities with intermittent claudication, right leg　A

I70.212 Atherosclerosis of native arteries of extremities with intermittent claudication, left leg　A

I70.213 Atherosclerosis of native arteries of extremities with intermittent claudication, bilateral legs　A

I70.218 Atherosclerosis of native arteries of extremities with intermittent claudication, other extremity　A

I70.219 Atherosclerosis of native arteries of extremities with intermittent claudication, unspecified extremity　A

▶ New　➡ Revised　~~deleted~~ Deleted　Excludes 1　Excludes 2　Includes　Use additional　Code first　Code also　Key words
OGCR Official Guidelines　X Assign placeholder X　● Use Additional Character(s)　◗ Manifestation Code　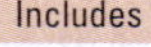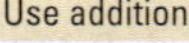 Hierarchical Condition Category　**Coding Clinic**

● **I70.22**   **Atherosclerosis of native arteries of extremities with rest pain**

   Includes   any condition classifiable to I70.21-
     chronic limb-threatening ischemia NOS of native arteries of extremities
     chronic limb-threatening ischemia of native arteries of extremities with rest pain
     critical limb ischemia NOS of native arteries of extremities
     critical limb ischemia of native arteries of extremities with rest pain

   I70.221   **Atherosclerosis of native arteries of extremities with rest pain, right leg** A

   I70.222   **Atherosclerosis of native arteries of extremities with rest pain, left leg** A

   I70.223   **Atherosclerosis of native arteries of extremities with rest pain, bilateral legs** A

   I70.228   **Atherosclerosis of native arteries of extremities with rest pain, other extremity** A

   I70.229   **Atherosclerosis of native arteries of extremities with rest pain, unspecified extremity** A

● **I70.23**   **Atherosclerosis of native arteries of right leg with ulceration**

   Includes   any condition classifiable to I70.211 and I70.221
     chronic limb-threatening ischemia of native arteries of right leg with ulceration
     critical limb ischemia of native arteries of right leg with ulceration

   Use additional code to identify severity of ulcer (L97.-)

   I70.231   **Atherosclerosis of native arteries of right leg with ulceration of thigh** A

   I70.232   **Atherosclerosis of native arteries of right leg with ulceration of calf** A

   I70.233   **Atherosclerosis of native arteries of right leg with ulceration of ankle** A

   I70.234   **Atherosclerosis of native arteries of right leg with ulceration of heel and midfoot** A
     Atherosclerosis of native arteries of right leg with ulceration of plantar surface of midfoot

   I70.235   **Atherosclerosis of native arteries of right leg with ulceration of other part of foot** A
     Atherosclerosis of native arteries of right leg extremities with ulceration of toe

   I70.238   **Atherosclerosis of native arteries of right leg with ulceration of other part of lower leg** A

   I70.239   **Atherosclerosis of native arteries of right leg with ulceration of unspecified site** A

● **I70.24**   **Atherosclerosis of native arteries of left leg with ulceration**

   Includes   any condition classifiable to I70.212 and I70.222
     chronic limb-threatening ischemia of native arteries of left leg with ulceration
     critical limb ischemia of native arteries of left leg with ulceration

   Use additional code to identify severity of ulcer (L97.-)

   I70.241   **Atherosclerosis of native arteries of left leg with ulceration of thigh** A

   I70.242   **Atherosclerosis of native arteries of left leg with ulceration of calf** A

   I70.243   **Atherosclerosis of native arteries of left leg with ulceration of ankle** A

   I70.244   **Atherosclerosis of native arteries of left leg with ulceration of heel and midfoot** A
     Atherosclerosis of native arteries of left leg with ulceration of plantar surface of midfoot

   I70.245   **Atherosclerosis of native arteries of left leg with ulceration of other part of foot** A
     Atherosclerosis of native arteries of left leg extremities with ulceration of toe

   I70.248   **Atherosclerosis of native arteries of left leg with ulceration of other part of lower leg** A

   I70.249   **Atherosclerosis of native arteries of left leg with ulceration of unspecified site** A

  I70.25   **Atherosclerosis of native arteries of other extremities with ulceration** A

   Includes   any condition classifiable to I70.218 and I70.228

   Use additional code to identify the severity of the ulcer (L98.49-)

● **I70.26**   **Atherosclerosis of native arteries of extremities with gangrene**

   Includes   any condition classifiable to I70.21-, I70.22-, I70.23-, I70.24-, and I70.25-
     chronic limb-threatening ischemia of native arteries of extremities with gangrene
     critical limb ischemia of native arteries of extremities with gangrene

   Use additional code to identify the severity of any ulcer (L97.-, L98.49-), if applicable

   I70.261   **Atherosclerosis of native arteries of extremities with gangrene, right leg** A

   I70.262   **Atherosclerosis of native arteries of extremities with gangrene, left leg** A

   I70.263   **Atherosclerosis of native arteries of extremities with gangrene, bilateral legs** A

CHAPTER 9 (I00-I99)

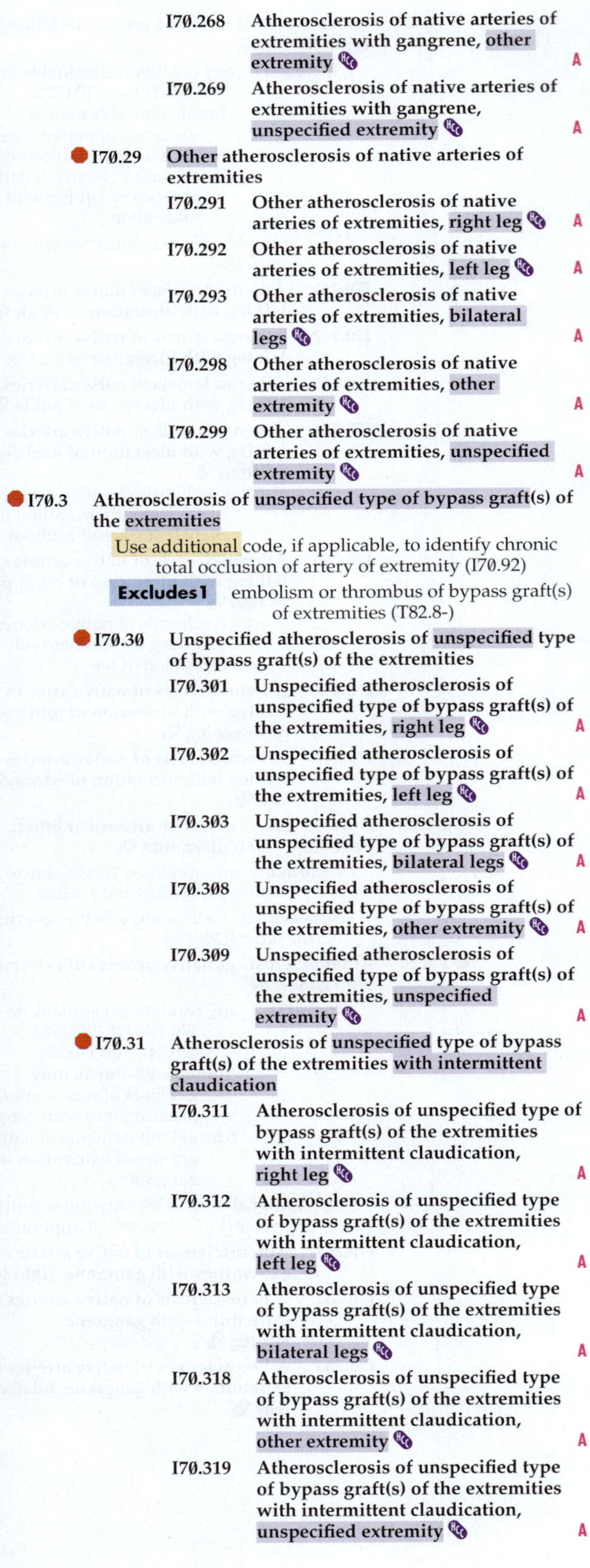

I70.268   Atherosclerosis of native arteries of extremities with gangrene, **other** extremity **Ⓗ**   A

I70.269   Atherosclerosis of native arteries of extremities with gangrene, **unspecified extremity** **Ⓗ**   A

● **I70.29**   Other atherosclerosis of native arteries of extremities

I70.291   Other atherosclerosis of native arteries of extremities, **right leg** **Ⓗ**   A

I70.292   Other atherosclerosis of native arteries of extremities, **left leg** **Ⓗ**   A

I70.293   Other atherosclerosis of native arteries of extremities, **bilateral legs** **Ⓗ**   A

I70.298   Other atherosclerosis of native arteries of extremities, **other** extremity **Ⓗ**   A

I70.299   Other atherosclerosis of native arteries of extremities, **unspecified extremity** **Ⓗ**   A

● **I70.3**   Atherosclerosis of **unspecified type of bypass graft(s) of the extremities**

Use additional code, if applicable, to identify chronic total occlusion of artery of extremity (I70.92)

Excludes1   embolism or thrombus of bypass graft(s) of extremities (T82.8-)

● **I70.30**   Unspecified atherosclerosis of **unspecified** type of bypass graft(s) of the extremities

I70.301   Unspecified atherosclerosis of unspecified type of bypass graft(s) of the extremities, **right leg** **Ⓗ**   A

I70.302   Unspecified atherosclerosis of unspecified type of bypass graft(s) of the extremities, **left leg** **Ⓗ**   A

I70.303   Unspecified atherosclerosis of unspecified type of bypass graft(s) of the extremities, **bilateral legs** **Ⓗ**   A

I70.308   Unspecified atherosclerosis of unspecified type of bypass graft(s) of the extremities, **other extremity** **Ⓗ**   A

I70.309   Unspecified atherosclerosis of unspecified type of bypass graft(s) of the extremities, **unspecified extremity** **Ⓗ**   A

● **I70.31**   Atherosclerosis of **unspecified type of bypass graft(s) of the extremities with intermittent claudication**

I70.311   Atherosclerosis of unspecified type of bypass graft(s) of the extremities with intermittent claudication, **right leg** **Ⓗ**   A

I70.312   Atherosclerosis of unspecified type of bypass graft(s) of the extremities with intermittent claudication, **left leg** **Ⓗ**   A

I70.313   Atherosclerosis of unspecified type of bypass graft(s) of the extremities with intermittent claudication, **bilateral legs** **Ⓗ**   A

I70.318   Atherosclerosis of unspecified type of bypass graft(s) of the extremities with intermittent claudication, **other extremity** **Ⓗ**   A

I70.319   Atherosclerosis of unspecified type of bypass graft(s) of the extremities with intermittent claudication, **unspecified extremity** **Ⓗ**   A

● **I70.32**   Atherosclerosis of **unspecified type of bypass graft(s) of the extremities with rest pain**

Includes   any condition classifiable to I70.31-
chronic limb-threatening ischemia NOS of unspecified type of bypass graft(s) of the extremities
chronic limb-threatening ischemia of unspecified type of bypass graft(s) of the extremities with rest pain, right leg
critical limb ischemia NOS of unspecified type of bypass graft(s) of the extremities
critical limb ischemia of unspecified type of bypass graft(s) of the extremities with rest pain

I70.321   Atherosclerosis of unspecified type of bypass graft(s) of the extremities with rest pain, **right leg** **Ⓗ**   A

I70.322   Atherosclerosis of unspecified type of bypass graft(s) of the extremities with rest pain, **left leg** **Ⓗ**   A

I70.323   Atherosclerosis of unspecified type of bypass graft(s) of the extremities with rest pain, **bilateral legs** **Ⓗ**   A

I70.328   Atherosclerosis of unspecified type of bypass graft(s) of the extremities with rest pain, **other extremity** **Ⓗ**   A

I70.329   Atherosclerosis of unspecified type of bypass graft(s) of the extremities with rest pain, **unspecified extremity** **Ⓗ**   A

● **I70.33**   Atherosclerosis of **unspecified type of bypass graft(s) of the right leg with ulceration**

Includes   any condition classifiable to I70.311 and I70.321
chronic limb-threatening ischemia of unspecified type of bypass graft(s) of the right leg with ulceration
critical limb ischemia of unspecified type of bypass graft(s) of the right leg with ulceration

Use additional code to identify severity of ulcer (L97.-)

I70.331   Atherosclerosis of unspecified type of bypass graft(s) of the right leg with ulceration of **thigh** **Ⓗ**   A

I70.332   Atherosclerosis of unspecified type of bypass graft(s) of the right leg with ulceration of **calf** **Ⓗ**   A

I70.333   Atherosclerosis of unspecified type of bypass graft(s) of the right leg with ulceration of **ankle** **Ⓗ**   A

I70.334   Atherosclerosis of unspecified **type of bypass graft(s) of the right leg with ulceration of heel and midfoot** **Ⓗ**   A

Atherosclerosis of unspecified type of bypass graft(s) of right leg with ulceration of plantar surface of midfoot

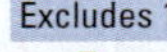

▶ New   ➡ Revised   ~~deleted~~ Deleted   Excludes 1   Excludes 2   Includes   Use additional   Code first   Code also   Key words

OGCR Official Guidelines   X Assign placeholder X   ● Use Additional Character(s)   ▶ Manifestation Code   Ⓗ Hierarchical Condition Category   **Coding Clinic**

I70.335   Atherosclerosis of unspecified type of bypass graft(s) of the right leg with ulceration of **other part of foot**   A
Atherosclerosis of unspecified type of bypass graft(s) of the right leg with ulceration of toe

I70.338   Atherosclerosis of unspecified type of bypass graft(s) of the right leg with ulceration of **other part of lower leg**   A

I70.339   Atherosclerosis of unspecified type of bypass graft(s) of the right leg with ulceration of **unspecified site**   A

● **I70.34**   Atherosclerosis of **unspecified type of bypass graft(s) of the left leg with ulceration**

   Includes   any condition classifiable to I70.312 and I70.322
chronic limb-threatening ischemia of unspecified type of bypass graft(s) of the left leg with ulceration
critical limb ischemia of unspecified type of bypass graft(s) of the left leg with ulceration

   Use additional code to identify severity of ulcer (L97.-)

I70.341   Atherosclerosis of unspecified type of bypass graft(s) of the left leg with ulceration of **thigh**   A

I70.342   Atherosclerosis of unspecified type of bypass graft(s) of the left leg with ulceration of **calf**   A

I70.343   Atherosclerosis of unspecified type of bypass graft(s) of the left leg with ulceration of **ankle**   A

I70.344   Atherosclerosis of unspecified type of bypass graft(s) of the left leg with ulceration of **heel and midfoot**   A
Atherosclerosis of unspecified type of bypass graft(s) of left leg with ulceration of plantar surface of midfoot

I70.345   Atherosclerosis of unspecified type of bypass graft(s) of the left leg with ulceration of **other part of foot**   A
Atherosclerosis of unspecified type of bypass graft(s) of the left leg with ulceration of toe

I70.348   Atherosclerosis of unspecified type of bypass graft(s) of the left leg with ulceration of **other part of lower leg**   A

I70.349   Atherosclerosis of unspecified type of bypass graft(s) of the left leg with ulceration of **unspecified site**   A

I70.35   Atherosclerosis of **unspecified type of bypass graft(s) of other extremity with ulceration**   A

   Includes   any condition classifiable to I70.318 and I70.328

   Use additional code to identify severity of ulcer (L98.49-)

● **I70.36**   Atherosclerosis of **unspecified type of bypass graft(s) of the extremities with gangrene**

   Includes   any condition classifiable to I70.31-, I70.32-, I70.33-, I70.34-, I70.35
chronic limb-threatening ischemia of unspecified type of bypass graft(s) of the extremities with gangrene
critical limb ischemia of unspecified type of bypass graft(s) of the extremities with gangrene

   Use additional code to identify the severity of any ulcer (L97.-, L98.49-), if applicable

I70.361   Atherosclerosis of unspecified type of bypass graft(s) of the extremities with gangrene, **right leg**   A

I70.362   Atherosclerosis of unspecified type of bypass graft(s) of the extremities with gangrene, **left leg**   A

I70.363   Atherosclerosis of unspecified type of bypass graft(s) of the extremities with gangrene, **bilateral legs**   A

I70.368   Atherosclerosis of unspecified type of bypass graft(s) of the extremities with gangrene, **other extremity**   A

I70.369   Atherosclerosis of unspecified type of bypass graft(s) of the extremities with gangrene, **unspecified extremity**   A

● **I70.39**   Other atherosclerosis of **unspecified type** of bypass graft(s) of the extremities

I70.391   Other atherosclerosis of unspecified type of bypass graft(s) of the extremities, **right leg**   A

I70.392   Other atherosclerosis of unspecified type of bypass graft(s) of the extremities, **left leg**   A

I70.393   Other atherosclerosis of unspecified type of bypass graft(s) of the extremities, **bilateral legs**   A

I70.398   Other atherosclerosis of unspecified type of bypass graft(s) of the extremities, **other extremity**   A

I70.399   Other atherosclerosis of unspecified type of bypass graft(s) of the extremities, **unspecified extremity**   A

● **I70.4**   Atherosclerosis of **autologous vein bypass graft(s) of the extremities**

   Use additional code, if applicable, to identify chronic total occlusion of artery of extremity (I70.92)

● **I70.40**   **Unspecified atherosclerosis of autologous vein bypass graft(s) of the extremities**

I70.401   Unspecified atherosclerosis of autologous vein bypass graft(s) of the extremities, **right leg**   A

I70.402   Unspecified atherosclerosis of autologous vein bypass graft(s) of the extremities, **left leg**   A

I70.403   Unspecified atherosclerosis of autologous vein bypass graft(s) of the extremities, **bilateral legs**   A

I70.408   Unspecified atherosclerosis of autologous vein bypass graft(s) of the extremities, **other extremity**   A

I70.409   Unspecified atherosclerosis of autologous vein bypass graft(s) of the extremities, **unspecified extremity**   A

● **I70.41** **Atherosclerosis of autologous vein bypass graft(s) of the extremities with intermittent claudication**

     I70.411 Atherosclerosis of autologous vein bypass graft(s) of the extremities with intermittent claudication, right leg 🅱   A

     I70.412 Atherosclerosis of autologous vein bypass graft(s) of the extremities with intermittent claudication, left leg 🅱   A

     I70.413 Atherosclerosis of autologous vein bypass graft(s) of the extremities with intermittent claudication, bilateral legs 🅱   A

     I70.418 Atherosclerosis of autologous vein bypass graft(s) of the extremities with intermittent claudication, other extremity 🅱   A

     I70.419 Atherosclerosis of autologous vein bypass graft(s) of the extremities with intermittent claudication, unspecified extremity 🅱   A

● **I70.42** **Atherosclerosis of autologous vein bypass graft(s) of the extremities with rest pain**

     Includes   any condition classifiable to I70.41-
           chronic limb-threatening ischemia NOS of autologous vein bypass graft(s) of the extremities
           chronic limb-threatening ischemia of autologous vein bypass graft(s) of the extremities with rest pain
           critical limb ischemia NOS of autologous vein bypass graft(s) of the extremities
           critical limb ischemia of autologous vein bypass graft(s) of the extremities with rest pain

     I70.421 Atherosclerosis of autologous vein bypass graft(s) of the extremities with rest pain, right leg 🅱   A

     I70.422 Atherosclerosis of autologous vein bypass graft(s) of the extremities with rest pain, left leg 🅱   A

     I70.423 Atherosclerosis of autologous vein bypass graft(s) of the extremities with rest pain, bilateral legs 🅱   A

     I70.428 Atherosclerosis of autologous vein bypass graft(s) of the extremities with rest pain, other extremity 🅱   A

     I70.429 Atherosclerosis of autologous vein bypass graft(s) of the extremities with rest pain, unspecified extremity 🅱   A

● **I70.43** **Atherosclerosis of autologous vein bypass graft(s) of the right leg with ulceration**

     Includes   any condition classifiable to I70.411 and I70.421
           chronic limb-threatening ischemia of autologous vein bypass graft(s) of the right leg with ulceration
           critical limb ischemia of autologous vein bypass graft(s) of the right leg with ulceration

     Use additional code to identify severity of ulcer (L97.-)

     I70.431 Atherosclerosis of autologous vein bypass graft(s) of the right leg with ulceration of thigh 🅱   A

     I70.432 Atherosclerosis of autologous vein bypass graft(s) of the right leg with ulceration of calf 🅱   A

     I70.433 Atherosclerosis of autologous vein bypass graft(s) of the right leg with ulceration of ankle 🅱   A

     I70.434 Atherosclerosis of autologous vein bypass graft(s) of the right leg with ulceration of heel and midfoot 🅱   A
           Atherosclerosis of autologous vein bypass graft(s) of right leg with ulceration of plantar surface of midfoot

     I70.435 Atherosclerosis of autologous vein bypass graft(s) of the right leg with ulceration of other part of foot 🅱   A
           Atherosclerosis of autologous vein bypass graft(s) of right leg with ulceration of toe

     I70.438 Atherosclerosis of autologous vein bypass graft(s) of the right leg with ulceration of other part of lower leg 🅱   A

     I70.439 Atherosclerosis of autologous vein bypass graft(s) of the right leg with ulceration of unspecified site 🅱   A

● **I70.44** **Atherosclerosis of autologous vein bypass graft(s) of the left leg with ulceration**

     Includes   any condition classifiable to I70.412 and I70.422
           chronic limb-threatening ischemia of autologous vein bypass graft(s) of the left leg with ulceration
           critical limb ischemia of autologous vein bypass graft(s) of the left leg with ulceration

     Use additional code to identify severity of ulcer (L97.-)

     I70.441 Atherosclerosis of autologous vein bypass graft(s) of the left leg with ulceration of thigh 🅱   A

     I70.442 Atherosclerosis of autologous vein bypass graft(s) of the left leg with ulceration of calf 🅱   A

     I70.443 Atherosclerosis of autologous vein bypass graft(s) of the left leg with ulceration of ankle 🅱   A

     I70.444 Atherosclerosis of autologous vein bypass graft(s) of the left leg with ulceration of heel and midfoot 🅱   A
           Atherosclerosis of autologous vein bypass graft(s) of left leg with ulceration of plantar surface of midfoot

     I70.445 Atherosclerosis of autologous vein bypass graft(s) of the left leg with ulceration of other part of foot 🅱   A
           Atherosclerosis of autologous vein bypass graft(s) of left leg with ulceration of toe

     I70.448 Atherosclerosis of autologous vein bypass graft(s) of the left leg with ulceration of other part of lower leg 🅱   A

     I70.449 Atherosclerosis of autologous vein bypass graft(s) of the left leg with ulceration of unspecified site 🅱   A

▶ New   ➡ Revised   ~~deleted~~ Deleted   Excludes 1   Excludes 2   Includes   Use additional   Code first   Code also   Key words
OGCR Official Guidelines   **X** Assign placeholder X   ● Use Additional Character(s)   ▶ Manifestation Code   🅱 Hierarchical Condition Category   **Coding Clinic**

I70.45 **Atherosclerosis of autologous vein bypass graft(s) of other extremity with ulceration** A

> **Includes** any condition classifiable to I70.418, I70.428, and I70.438

> **Use additional** code to identify severity of ulcer (L98.49-)

● **I70.46** **Atherosclerosis of autologous vein bypass graft(s) of the extremities with gangrene**

> **Includes** any condition classifiable to I70.41-, I70.42-, and I70.43-, I70.44-, I70.45
> chronic limb-threatening ischemia of autologous vein bypass graft(s) of the extremities with gangrene
> critical limb ischemia of autologous vein bypass graft(s) of the extremities with gangrene

> **Use additional** code to identify the severity of any ulcer (L97.-, L98.49-), if applicable

 I70.461 Atherosclerosis of autologous vein bypass graft(s) of the extremities with gangrene, **right leg** A

 I70.462 Atherosclerosis of autologous vein bypass graft(s) of the extremities with gangrene, **left leg** A

 I70.463 Atherosclerosis of autologous vein bypass graft(s) of the extremities with gangrene, **bilateral legs** A

 I70.468 Atherosclerosis of autologous vein bypass graft(s) of the extremities with gangrene, **other extremity** A

 I70.469 Atherosclerosis of autologous vein bypass graft(s) of the extremities with gangrene, **unspecified extremity** A

● **I70.49** **Other atherosclerosis of autologous vein bypass graft(s) of the extremities**

 I70.491 Other atherosclerosis of autologous vein bypass graft(s) of the extremities, **right leg** A

 I70.492 Other atherosclerosis of autologous vein bypass graft(s) of the extremities, **left leg** A

 I70.493 Other atherosclerosis of autologous vein bypass graft(s) of the extremities, **bilateral legs** A

 I70.498 Other atherosclerosis of autologous vein bypass graft(s) of the extremities, **other extremity** A

 I70.499 Other atherosclerosis of autologous vein bypass graft(s) of the extremities, **unspecified extremity** A

● **I70.5** **Atherosclerosis of nonautologous biological bypass graft(s) of the extremities**

> **Use additional** code, if applicable, to identify chronic total occlusion of artery of extremity (I70.92)

● **I70.50** **Unspecified atherosclerosis of nonautologous biological bypass graft(s) of the extremities**

 I70.501 Unspecified atherosclerosis of nonautologous biological bypass graft(s) of the extremities, **right leg** A

 I70.502 Unspecified atherosclerosis of nonautologous biological bypass graft(s) of the extremities, **left leg** A

I70.503 Unspecified atherosclerosis of nonautologous biological bypass graft(s) of the extremities, **bilateral legs** A

I70.508 Unspecified atherosclerosis of nonautologous biological bypass graft(s) of the extremities, **other extremity** A

I70.509 Unspecified atherosclerosis of nonautologous biological bypass graft(s) of the extremities, **unspecified extremity** A

● **I70.51** **Atherosclerosis of nonautologous biological bypass graft(s) of the extremities intermittent claudication**

 I70.511 Atherosclerosis of nonautologous biological bypass graft(s) of the extremities with intermittent claudication, **right leg** A

 I70.512 Atherosclerosis of nonautologous biological bypass graft(s) of the extremities with intermittent claudication, **left leg** A

 I70.513 Atherosclerosis of nonautologous biological bypass graft(s) of the extremities with intermittent claudication, **bilateral legs** A

 I70.518 Atherosclerosis of nonautologous biological bypass graft(s) of the extremities with intermittent claudication, **other extremity** A

 I70.519 Atherosclerosis of nonautologous biological bypass graft(s) of the extremities with intermittent claudication, **unspecified extremity** A

● **I70.52** **Atherosclerosis of nonautologous biological bypass graft(s) of the extremities with rest pain**

> **Includes** any condition classifiable to I70.51-
> chronic limb-threatening ischemia NOS of nonautologous biological bypass graft(s) of the extremities
> chronic limb-threatening ischemia of nonautologous biological bypass graft(s) of the extremities with rest pain
> critical limb ischemia NOS of nonautologous biological bypass graft(s) of the extremities
> critical limb ischemia of nonautologous biological bypass graft(s) of the extremities with rest pain

 I70.521 Atherosclerosis of nonautologous biological bypass graft(s) of the extremities with rest pain, **right leg** A

 I70.522 Atherosclerosis of nonautologous biological bypass graft(s) of the extremities with rest pain, **left leg** A

 I70.523 Atherosclerosis of nonautologous biological bypass graft(s) of the extremities with rest pain, **bilateral legs** A

CHAPTER 9 (I00-I99)

I70.528   Atherosclerosis of nonautologous biological bypass graft(s) of the extremities with rest pain, other extremity 🅡 A

I70.529   Atherosclerosis of nonautologous biological bypass graft(s) of the extremities with rest pain, unspecified extremity 🅡 A

● **I70.53**   Atherosclerosis of nonautologous biological bypass graft(s) of the right leg with ulceration

Includes   any condition classifiable to I70.511 and I70.521
chronic limb-threatening ischemia of nonautologous biological bypass graft(s) of the right leg with ulceration
critical limb ischemia of nonautologous biological bypass graft(s) of the right leg with ulceration

Use additional code to identify severity of ulcer (L97.-)

I70.531   Atherosclerosis of nonautologous biological bypass graft(s) of the right leg with ulceration of thigh 🅡 A

I70.532   Atherosclerosis of nonautologous biological bypass graft(s) of the right leg with ulceration of calf 🅡 A

I70.533   Atherosclerosis of nonautologous biological bypass graft(s) of the right leg with ulceration of ankle 🅡 A

I70.534   Atherosclerosis of nonautologous biological bypass graft(s) of the right leg with ulceration of heel and midfoot 🅡 A
Atherosclerosis of nonautologous biological bypass graft(s) of right leg with ulceration of plantar surface of midfoot

I70.535   Atherosclerosis of nonautologous biological bypass graft(s) of the right leg with ulceration of other part of foot 🅡 A
Atherosclerosis of nonautologous biological bypass graft(s) of the right leg with ulceration of toe

I70.538   Atherosclerosis of nonautologous biological bypass graft(s) of the right leg with ulceration of other part of lower leg 🅡 A

I70.539   Atherosclerosis of nonautologous biological bypass graft(s) of the right leg with ulceration of unspecified site 🅡 A

● **I70.54**   Atherosclerosis of nonautologous biological bypass graft(s) of the left leg with ulceration

Includes   any condition classifiable to I70.512 and I70.522
chronic limb-threatening ischemia of nonautologous biological bypass graft(s) of the left leg with ulceration
critical limb ischemia of nonautologous biological bypass graft(s) of the left leg with ulceration

Use additional code to identify severity of ulcer (L97.-)

I70.541   Atherosclerosis of nonautologous biological bypass graft(s) of the left leg with ulceration of thigh 🅡 A

I70.542   Atherosclerosis of nonautologous biological bypass graft(s) of the left leg with ulceration of calf 🅡 A

I70.543   Atherosclerosis of nonautologous biological bypass graft(s) of the left leg with ulceration of ankle 🅡 A

I70.544   Atherosclerosis of nonautologous biological bypass graft(s) of the left leg with ulceration of heel and midfoot 🅡 A
Atherosclerosis of nonautologous biological bypass graft(s) of left leg with ulceration of plantar surface of midfoot

I70.545   Atherosclerosis of nonautologous biological bypass graft(s) of the left leg with ulceration of other part of foot 🅡 A
Atherosclerosis of nonautologous biological bypass graft(s) of the left leg with ulceration of toe

I70.548   Atherosclerosis of nonautologous biological bypass graft(s) of the left leg with ulceration of other part of lower leg 🅡 A

I70.549   Atherosclerosis of nonautologous biological bypass graft(s) of the left leg with ulceration of unspecified site 🅡 A

I70.55   Atherosclerosis of nonautologous biological bypass graft(s) of other extremity with ulceration 🅡 A

Includes   any condition classifiable to I70.518, I70.528, and I70.538

Use additional code to identify severity of ulcer (L98.49)

● **I70.56**   Atherosclerosis of nonautologous biological bypass graft(s) of the extremities with gangrene

Includes   any condition classifiable to I70.51-, I70.52-, and I70.53-, I70.54-, I70.55
chronic limb-threatening ischemia of nonautologous biological bypass graft(s) of the extremities with gangrene
critical limb ischemia of nonautologous biological bypass graft(s) of the extremities with gangrene

Use additional code to identify the severity of any ulcer (L97.-, L98.49-), if applicable

I70.561   Atherosclerosis of nonautologous biological bypass graft(s) of the extremities with gangrene, right leg 🅡 A

I70.562   Atherosclerosis of nonautologous biological bypass graft(s) of the extremities with gangrene, left leg 🅡 A

I70.563   Atherosclerosis of nonautologous biological bypass graft(s) of the extremities with gangrene, bilateral legs 🅡 A

I70.568   Atherosclerosis of nonautologous biological bypass graft(s) of the extremities with gangrene, other extremity 🔒   **A**

I70.569   Atherosclerosis of nonautologous biological bypass graft(s) of the extremities with gangrene, unspecified extremity 🔒   **A**

● **I70.59   Other atherosclerosis of nonautologous biological bypass graft(s) of the extremities**

I70.591   Other atherosclerosis of nonautologous biological bypass graft(s) of the extremities, right leg 🔒   **A**

I70.592   Other atherosclerosis of nonautologous biological bypass graft(s) of the extremities, left leg 🔒   **A**

I70.593   Other atherosclerosis of nonautologous biological bypass graft(s) of the extremities, bilateral legs 🔒   **A**

I70.598   Other atherosclerosis of nonautologous biological bypass graft(s) of the extremities, other extremity 🔒   **A**

I70.599   Other atherosclerosis of nonautologous biological bypass graft(s) of the extremities, unspecified extremity 🔒   **A**

● **I70.6   Atherosclerosis of nonbiological bypass graft(s) of the extremities**

> Use additional code, if applicable, to identify chronic total occlusion of artery of extremity (I70.92)

● **I70.60   Unspecified atherosclerosis of nonbiological bypass graft(s) of the extremities**

I70.601   Unspecified atherosclerosis of nonbiological bypass graft(s) of the extremities, right leg 🔒   **A**

I70.602   Unspecified atherosclerosis of nonbiological bypass graft(s) of the extremities, left leg 🔒   **A**

I70.603   Unspecified atherosclerosis of nonbiological bypass graft(s) of the extremities, bilateral legs 🔒   **A**

I70.608   Unspecified atherosclerosis of nonbiological bypass graft(s) of the extremities, other extremity 🔒   **A**

I70.609   Unspecified atherosclerosis of nonbiological bypass graft(s) of the extremities, unspecified extremity 🔒   **A**

● **I70.61   Atherosclerosis of nonbiological bypass graft(s) of the extremities with intermittent claudication**

I70.611   Atherosclerosis of nonbiological bypass graft(s) of the extremities with intermittent claudication, right leg 🔒   **A**

I70.612   Atherosclerosis of nonbiological bypass graft(s) of the extremities with intermittent claudication, left leg 🔒   **A**

I70.613   Atherosclerosis of nonbiological bypass graft(s) of the extremities with intermittent claudication, bilateral legs 🔒   **A**

I70.618   Atherosclerosis of nonbiological bypass graft(s) of the extremities with intermittent claudication, other extremity 🔒   **A**

I70.619   Atherosclerosis of nonbiological bypass graft(s) of the extremities with intermittent claudication, unspecified extremity 🔒   **A**

● **I70.62   Atherosclerosis of nonbiological bypass graft(s) of the extremities with rest pain**

> **Includes**   any condition classifiable to I70.61-
> chronic limb-threatening ischemia NOS of nonbiological bypass graft(s) of the extremities
> chronic limb-threatening ischemia of nonbiological bypass graft(s) of the extremities with rest pain
> critical limb ischemia NOS of nonbiological bypass graft(s) of the extremities
> critical limb ischemia of nonbiological bypass graft(s) of the extremities with rest pain

I70.621   Atherosclerosis of nonbiological bypass graft(s) of the extremities with rest pain, right leg 🔒   **A**

I70.622   Atherosclerosis of nonbiological bypass graft(s) of the extremities with rest pain, left leg 🔒   **A**

I70.623   Atherosclerosis of nonbiological bypass graft(s) of the extremities with rest pain, bilateral legs 🔒   **A**

I70.628   Atherosclerosis of nonbiological bypass graft(s) of the extremities with rest pain, other extremity 🔒   **A**

I70.629   Atherosclerosis of nonbiological bypass graft(s) of the extremities with rest pain, unspecified extremity 🔒   **A**

● **I70.63   Atherosclerosis of nonbiological bypass graft(s) of the right leg with ulceration**

> **Includes**   any condition classifiable to I70.611 and I70.621
> chronic limb-threatening ischemia of nonbiological bypass graft(s) of the right leg with ulceration
> critical limb ischemia of nonbiological bypass graft(s) of the right leg with ulceration

> Use additional code to identify severity of ulcer (L97.-)

I70.631   Atherosclerosis of nonbiological bypass graft(s) of the right leg with ulceration of thigh 🔒   **A**

I70.632   Atherosclerosis of nonbiological bypass graft(s) of the right leg with ulceration of calf 🔒   **A**

I70.633   Atherosclerosis of nonbiological bypass graft(s) of the right leg with ulceration of ankle 🔒   **A**

I70.634   Atherosclerosis of nonbiological bypass graft(s) of the right leg with ulceration of heel and midfoot 🔒   **A**

> Atherosclerosis of nonbiological bypass graft(s) of right leg with ulceration of plantar surface of midfoot

I70.635   Atherosclerosis of nonbiological bypass graft(s) of the right leg with ulceration of other part of foot 🔒   **A**

> Atherosclerosis of nonbiological bypass graft(s) of the right leg with ulceration of toe

I70.638   Atherosclerosis of nonbiological bypass graft(s) of the right leg with ulceration of other part of lower leg ⓡ A

I70.639   Atherosclerosis of nonbiological bypass graft(s) of the right leg with ulceration of unspecified site ⓡ A

● **I70.64**   Atherosclerosis of nonbiological bypass graft(s) of the left leg with ulceration

> **Includes**   any condition classifiable to I70.612 and I70.622
>
> chronic limb-threatening ischemia of nonbiological bypass graft(s) of the left leg with ulceration
>
> critical limb ischemia of nonbiological bypass graft(s) of the left leg with ulceration

> Use additional code to identify severity of ulcer (L97.-)

I70.641   Atherosclerosis of nonbiological bypass graft(s) of the left leg with ulceration of thigh ⓡ A

I70.642   Atherosclerosis of nonbiological bypass graft(s) of the left leg with ulceration of calf ⓡ A

I70.643   Atherosclerosis of nonbiological bypass graft(s) of the left leg with ulceration of ankle ⓡ A

I70.644   Atherosclerosis of nonbiological bypass graft(s) of the left leg with ulceration of heel and midfoot ⓡ A

> Atherosclerosis of nonbiological bypass graft(s) of left leg with ulceration of plantar surface of midfoot

I70.645   Atherosclerosis of nonbiological bypass graft(s) of the left leg with ulceration of other part of foot ⓡ A

> Atherosclerosis of nonbiological bypass graft(s) of the left leg with ulceration of toe

I70.648   Atherosclerosis of nonbiological bypass graft(s) of the left leg with ulceration of other part of lower leg ⓡ A

I70.649   Atherosclerosis of nonbiological bypass graft(s) of the left leg with ulceration of unspecified site ⓡ A

I70.65   Atherosclerosis of nonbiological bypass graft(s) of other extremity with ulceration ⓡ A

> **Includes**   any condition classifiable to I70.618 and I70.628

> Use additional code to identify severity of ulcer (L98.49-)

● **I70.66**   Atherosclerosis of nonbiological bypass graft(s) of the extremities with gangrene

> **Includes**   any condition classifiable to I70.61-, I70.62-, I70.63-, I70.64-, I70.65
>
> chronic limb-threatening ischemia of nonbiological bypass graft(s) of the extremities with gangrene
>
> critical limb ischemia of nonbiological bypass graft(s) of the extremities with gangrene

> Use additional code to identify the severity of any ulcer (L97.-, L98.49-), if applicable

I70.661   Atherosclerosis of nonbiological bypass graft(s) of the extremities with gangrene, right leg ⓡ A

I70.662   Atherosclerosis of nonbiological bypass graft(s) of the extremities with gangrene, left leg ⓡ A

I70.663   Atherosclerosis of nonbiological bypass graft(s) of the extremities with gangrene, bilateral legs ⓡ A

I70.668   Atherosclerosis of nonbiological bypass graft(s) of the extremities with gangrene, other extremity ⓡ A

I70.669   Atherosclerosis of nonbiological bypass graft(s) of the extremities with gangrene, unspecified extremity ⓡ A

● **I70.69**   Other atherosclerosis of nonbiological bypass graft(s) of the extremities

I70.691   Other atherosclerosis of nonbiological bypass graft(s) of the extremities, right leg ⓡ A

I70.692   Other atherosclerosis of nonbiological bypass graft(s) of the extremities, left leg ⓡ A

I70.693   Other atherosclerosis of nonbiological bypass graft(s) of the extremities, bilateral legs ⓡ A

I70.698   Other atherosclerosis of nonbiological bypass graft(s) of the extremities, other extremity ⓡ A

I70.699   Other atherosclerosis of nonbiological bypass graft(s) of the extremities, unspecified extremity ⓡ A

● **I70.7**   Atherosclerosis of other type of bypass graft(s) of the extremities

> Use additional code, if applicable, to identify chronic total occlusion of artery of extremity (I70.92)

● **I70.70**   Unspecified atherosclerosis of other type of bypass graft(s) of the extremities

I70.701   Unspecified atherosclerosis of other type of bypass graft(s) of the extremities, right leg ⓡ A

I70.702   Unspecified atherosclerosis of other type of bypass graft(s) of the extremities, left leg ⓡ A

I70.703   Unspecified atherosclerosis of other type of bypass graft(s) of the extremities, bilateral legs ⓡ A

I70.708   Unspecified atherosclerosis of other type of bypass graft(s) of the extremities, other extremity ⓡ A

I70.709   Unspecified atherosclerosis of other type of bypass graft(s) of the extremities, unspecified extremity ⓡ A

● **I70.71**   Atherosclerosis of other type of bypass graft(s) of the extremities with intermittent claudication

I70.711   Atherosclerosis of other type of bypass graft(s) of the extremities with intermittent claudication, right leg ⓡ A

I70.712   Atherosclerosis of other type of bypass graft(s) of the extremities with intermittent claudication, left leg ⓡ A

I70.713   Atherosclerosis of other type of bypass graft(s) of the extremities with intermittent claudication, bilateral legs ⓡ A

I70.718   **Atherosclerosis of other type of bypass graft(s) of the extremities with intermittent claudication, other extremity** Rx   A

I70.719   **Atherosclerosis of other type of bypass graft(s) of the extremities with intermittent claudication, unspecified extremity** Rx   A

● **I70.72   Atherosclerosis of other type of bypass graft(s) of the extremities with rest pain**

  Includes   any condition classifiable to I70.71-
  chronic limb-threatening ischemia NOS of other type of bypass graft(s) of the extremities
  chronic limb-threatening ischemia of other type of bypass graft(s) of the extremities with rest pain
  critical limb ischemia NOS of other type of bypass graft(s) of the extremities
  critical limb ischemia of other type of bypass graft(s) of the extremities with rest pain

I70.721   **Atherosclerosis of other type of bypass graft(s) of the extremities with rest pain, right leg** Rx   A

I70.722   **Atherosclerosis of other type of bypass graft(s) of the extremities with rest pain, left leg** Rx   A

I70.723   **Atherosclerosis of other type of bypass graft(s) of the extremities with rest pain, bilateral legs** Rx   A

I70.728   **Atherosclerosis of other type of bypass graft(s) of the extremities with rest pain, other extremity** Rx   A

I70.729   **Atherosclerosis of other type of bypass graft(s) of the extremities with rest pain, unspecified extremity** Rx   A

● **I70.73   Atherosclerosis of other type of bypass graft(s) of the right leg with ulceration**

  Includes   any condition classifiable to I70.711 and I70.721
  chronic limb-threatening ischemia of other type of bypass graft(s) of the right leg with ulceration
  critical limb ischemia of other type of bypass graft(s) of the right leg with ulceration

  Use additional code to identify severity of ulcer (L97.-)

I70.731   **Atherosclerosis of other type of bypass graft(s) of the right leg with ulceration of thigh** Rx   A

I70.732   **Atherosclerosis of other type of bypass graft(s) of the right leg with ulceration of calf** Rx   A

I70.733   **Atherosclerosis of other type of bypass graft(s) of the right leg with ulceration of ankle** Rx   A

I70.734   **Atherosclerosis of other type of bypass graft(s) of the right leg with ulceration of heel and midfoot** Rx   A
  Atherosclerosis of other type of bypass graft(s) of right leg with ulceration of plantar surface of midfoot

I70.735   **Atherosclerosis of other type of bypass graft(s) of the right leg with ulceration of other part of foot** Rx   A
  Atherosclerosis of other type of bypass graft(s) of right leg with ulceration of toe

I70.738   **Atherosclerosis of other type of bypass graft(s) of the right leg with ulceration of other part of lower leg** Rx   A

I70.739   **Atherosclerosis of other type of bypass graft(s) of the right leg with ulceration of unspecified site** Rx   A

● **I70.74   Atherosclerosis of other type of bypass graft(s) of the left leg with ulceration**

  Includes   any condition classifiable to I70.712 and I70.722
  chronic limb-threatening ischemia of other type of bypass graft(s) of the left leg with ulceration
  critical limb ischemia of other type of bypass graft(s) of the left leg with ulceration

  Use additional code to identify severity of ulcer (L97.-)

I70.741   **Atherosclerosis of other type of bypass graft(s) of the left leg with ulceration of thigh** Rx   A

I70.742   **Atherosclerosis of other type of bypass graft(s) of the left leg with ulceration of calf** Rx   A

I70.743   **Atherosclerosis of other type of bypass graft(s) of the left leg with ulceration of ankle** Rx   A

I70.744   **Atherosclerosis of other type of bypass graft(s) of the left leg with ulceration of heel and midfoot** Rx   A
  Atherosclerosis of other type of bypass graft(s) of left leg with ulceration of plantar surface of midfoot

I70.745   **Atherosclerosis of other type of bypass graft(s) of the left leg with ulceration of other part of foot** Rx   A
  Atherosclerosis of other type of bypass graft(s) of left leg with ulceration of toe

I70.748   **Atherosclerosis of other type of bypass graft(s) of the left leg with ulceration of other part of lower leg** Rx   A

I70.749   **Atherosclerosis of other type of bypass graft(s) of the left leg with ulceration of unspecified site** Rx   A

I70.75   **Atherosclerosis of other type of bypass graft(s) of other extremity with ulceration** Rx   A

  Includes   any condition classifiable to I70.718 and I70.728

  Use additional code to identify severity of ulcer (L98.49)

CHAPTER 9 (IØØ-I99)

● **I70.76 Atherosclerosis of other type of bypass graft(s) of the extremities with gangrene**

> **Includes**   any condition classifiable to I70.71-, I70.72-, I70.73-, I70.74-, I70.75
> chronic limb-threatening ischemia of other type of bypass graft(s) of the extremities with gangrene
> critical limb ischemia of other type of bypass graft(s) of the extremities with gangrene

Use additional code to identify the severity of any ulcer (L97.-, L98.49-), if applicable

I70.761 **Atherosclerosis of other type of bypass graft(s) of the extremities with gangrene, right leg** 🜊   A

I70.762 **Atherosclerosis of other type of bypass graft(s) of the extremities with gangrene, left leg** 🜊   A

I70.763 **Atherosclerosis of other type of bypass graft(s) of the extremities with gangrene, bilateral legs** 🜊   A

I70.768 **Atherosclerosis of other type of bypass graft(s) of the extremities with gangrene, other extremity** 🜊   A

I70.769 **Atherosclerosis of other type of bypass graft(s) of the extremities with gangrene, unspecified extremity** 🜊   A

● **I70.79 Other atherosclerosis of other type of bypass graft(s) of the extremities**

I70.791 **Other atherosclerosis of other type of bypass graft(s) of the extremities, right leg** 🜊   A

I70.792 **Other atherosclerosis of other type of bypass graft(s) of the extremities, left leg** 🜊   A

I70.793 **Other atherosclerosis of other type of bypass graft(s) of the extremities, bilateral legs** 🜊   A

I70.798 **Other atherosclerosis of other type of bypass graft(s) of the extremities, other extremity** 🜊   A

I70.799 **Other atherosclerosis of other type of bypass graft(s) of the extremities, unspecified extremity** 🜊   A

I70.8 Atherosclerosis of **other arteries**   A

● I70.9 Other and unspecified atherosclerosis

> ▶ **Excludes2**   disorders of pyrophosphate metabolism (E83.82-)

I70.90 **Unspecified atherosclerosis**   A

I70.91 **Generalized atherosclerosis**   A

I70.92 **Chronic total occlusion of artery of the extremities** 🜊   A
Complete occlusion of artery of the extremities
Total occlusion of artery of the extremities
Code first atherosclerosis of arteries of the extremities (I70.2-, I70.3-, I70.4-, I70.5-, I70.6-, I70.7-)

● **I71   Aortic aneurysm and dissection**
Code first, if applicable:
syphilitic aortic aneurysm (A52.01)
traumatic aortic aneurysm (S25.09, S35.09)

● **I71.0   Dissection of aorta**

I71.00 **Dissection of unspecified site of aorta** 🜊

● I71.01 Dissection of **thoracic** aorta 🜊

I71.010 **Dissection of ascending aorta**
Coding Clinic: 2024, Q2, P17

I71.011 **Dissection of aortic arch**
Coding Clinic: 2024, Q2, P17

I71.012 **Dissection of descending thoracic aorta**
Coding Clinic: 2024, Q2, P17

I71.019 **Dissection of thoracic aorta, unspecified**

I71.02 Dissection of **abdominal aorta** 🜊

I71.03 Dissection of **thoracoabdominal aorta** 🜊

● I71.1   **Thoracic** aortic aneurysm, **ruptured** 🜊

I71.10 Thoracic aortic aneurysm, ruptured, unspecified

I71.11 Aneurysm of the ascending aorta, ruptured

I71.12 Aneurysm of the aortic arch, ruptured

I71.13 Aneurysm of the descending thoracic aorta, ruptured

● I71.2   Thoracic aortic aneurysm, **without rupture** 🜊

I71.20 Thoracic aortic aneurysm, without rupture, unspecified

I71.21 Aneurysm of the ascending aorta, without rupture

I71.22 Aneurysm of the aortic arch, without rupture

I71.23 Aneurysm of the descending thoracic aorta, without rupture

● I71.3   **Abdominal** aortic aneurysm, **ruptured** 🜊

I71.30 Abdominal aortic aneurysm, ruptured, unspecified

I71.31 Pararenal abdominal aortic aneurysm, ruptured

I71.32 Juxtarenal abdominal aortic aneurysm, ruptured

I71.33 Infrarenal abdominal aortic aneurysm, ruptured

● I71.4   **Abdominal** aortic aneurysm, **without rupture** 🜊

I71.40 Abdominal aortic aneurysm, without rupture, unspecified

I71.41 Pararenal abdominal aortic aneurysm, without rupture
Coding Clinic: 2024, Q2, P16

I71.42 Juxtarenal abdominal aortic aneurysm, without rupture

I71.43 Infrarenal abdominal aortic aneurysm, without rupture

● I71.5   **Thoracoabdominal** aortic aneurysm, **ruptured** 🜊

I71.50 Thoracoabdominal aortic aneurysm, ruptured, unspecified

I71.51 Supraceliac aneurysm of the thoracoabdominal aorta, ruptured

I71.52 Paravisceral aneurysm of the thoracoabdominal aorta, ruptured

● I71.6   **Thoracoabdominal** aortic aneurysm, **without rupture** 🜊

I71.60 Thoracoabdominal aortic aneurysm, without rupture, unspecified

I71.61 Supraceliac aneurysm of the thoracoabdominal aorta, without rupture

I71.62 Paravisceral aneurysm of the thoracoabdominal aorta, without rupture

I71.8 Aortic aneurysm of **unspecified** site, **ruptured** 🜊
Rupture of aorta NOS

I71.9 Aortic aneurysm of **unspecified** site, **without rupture** 🜊
Aneurysm of aorta
Dilatation of aorta
Hyaline necrosis of aorta

CHAPTER 9 (I00-I99)

▶ New   🔁 Revised   ~~deleted~~ Deleted   Excludes 1   Excludes 2   Includes   Use additional   Code first   Code also   Key words
OGCR Official Guidelines   X Assign placeholder X   ● Use Additional Character(s)   ▸ Manifestation Code   🜊 Hierarchical Condition Category   **Coding Clinic**

● **I72 Other aneurysm**

Includes aneurysm (cirsoid) (false) (ruptured)

Excludes2 acquired aneurysm (I77.0)
aneurysm (of) aorta (I71.-)
aneurysm (of) arteriovenous NOS (Q27.3-)
carotid artery dissection (I77.71)
cerebral (nonruptured) aneurysm (I67.1)
coronary aneurysm (I25.4)
coronary artery dissection (I25.42)
dissection of artery NEC (I77.79)
dissection of precerebral artery, congenital (nonruptured) (Q28.1)
heart aneurysm (I25.3)
iliac artery dissection (I77.72)
precerebral artery, congenital (nonruptured) (Q28.1)
pulmonary artery aneurysm (I28.1)
renal artery dissection (I77.73)
retinal aneurysm (H35.0)
ruptured cerebral aneurysm (I60.7)
varicose aneurysm (I77.0)
vertebral artery dissection (I77.74)

I72.0 Aneurysm of carotid artery
Aneurysm of common carotid artery
Aneurysm of external carotid artery
Aneurysm of internal carotid artery, extracranial portion

     Excludes1 aneurysm of internal carotid artery, intracranial portion (I67.1)
aneurysm of internal carotid artery NOS (I67.1)

I72.1 Aneurysm of artery of upper extremity

I72.2 Aneurysm of renal artery

I72.3 Aneurysm of iliac artery

I72.4 Aneurysm of artery of lower extremity
Coding Clinic: 2019, Q2, P22

I72.5 Aneurysm of other precerebral arteries
Aneurysm of basilar artery (trunk)

     Excludes2 aneurysm of carotid artery (I72.0)
aneurysm of vertebral artery (I72.6)
dissection of carotid artery (I77.71)
dissection of other precerebral arteries (I77.75)
dissection of vertebral artery (I77.74)
Coding Clinic 2016, Q4, P28

I72.6 Aneurysm of vertebral artery

     Excludes2 dissection of vertebral artery (I77.74)
Coding Clinic 2016, Q4, P28

I72.8 Aneurysm of other specified arteries

I72.9 Aneurysm of unspecified site

● **I73 Other peripheral vascular diseases**

Excludes2 chilblains (T69.1)
frostbite (T33-T34)
immersion hand or foot (T69.0-)
spasm of cerebral artery (G45.9)
Coding Clinic: 2018, Q4, P87-88

● **I73.0 Raynaud's syndrome**
Diminishing oxygen supply to fingers, toes, nose, and ears when exposed to temperature changes or stress
Raynaud's disease
Raynaud's phenomenon (secondary)

I73.00 Raynaud's syndrome without gangrene

I73.01 Raynaud's syndrome with gangrene

I73.1 Thromboangiitis obliterans [Buerger's disease]
Inflammatory occlusive disease resulting in poor circulation to the legs, feet, and sometimes the hands due to progressive inflammatory narrowing and eventually obliteration of the small arteries

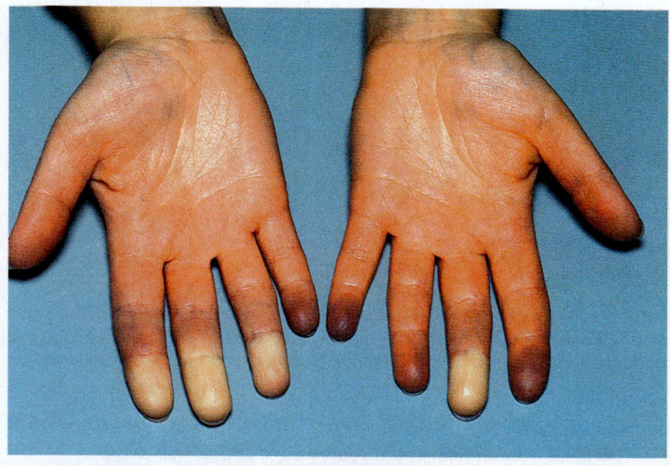

Figure 9-5 Raynaud's syndrome. (From Hallett: Comprehensive Vascular and Endovascular Surgery, ed 2, Philadelphia, Mosby Ltd., 2010)

● **I73.8 Other specified peripheral vascular diseases**

     Excludes1 diabetic (peripheral) angiopathy (E08-E13 with .51-.52)

I73.81 Erythromelalgia

I73.89 Other specified peripheral vascular diseases
Acrocyanosis
Erythrocyanosis
Simple acroparesthesia [Schultze's type]
Vasomotor acroparesthesia [Nothnagel's type]

I73.9 Peripheral vascular disease, unspecified
Intermittent claudication
Peripheral angiopathy NOS
Spasm of artery

     Excludes1 atherosclerosis of the extremities (I70.2—I70.7-)
Coding Clinic: 2018, Q4, P87

● **I74 Arterial embolism and thrombosis**

Includes embolic infarction
embolic occlusion
thrombotic infarction
thrombotic occlusion

Code first embolism and thrombosis complicating abortion or ectopic or molar pregnancy (O00-O07, O08.2)
embolism and thrombosis complicating pregnancy, childbirth and the puerperium (O88.-)

Excludes2 atheroembolism (I75.-)
basilar embolism and thrombosis (I63.0-I63.2, I65.1)
carotid embolism and thrombosis (I63.0-I63.2, I65.2)
cerebral embolism and thrombosis (I63.3-I63.5, I66.-)
coronary embolism and thrombosis (I21-I25)
mesenteric embolism and thrombosis (K55.0-)
ophthalmic embolism and thrombosis (H34.-)
precerebral embolism and thrombosis NOS (I63.0-I63.2, I65.9)
pulmonary embolism and thrombosis (I26.-)
renal embolism and thrombosis (N28.0)
retinal embolism and thrombosis (H34.-)
septic embolism and thrombosis (I76)
vertebral embolism and thrombosis (I63.0-I63.2, I65.0)
Coding Clinic: 2023, Q2, P7

CHAPTER 9 (I00-I99)

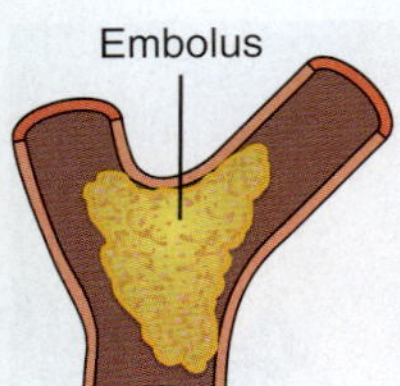

Figure 9-6 An arterial embolus.

Item 9–9 An **embolus** is a mass of undissolved matter present in the blood that is transported by the blood current. A **thrombus** is a blood clot that occludes or shuts off a vessel. When a thrombus is dislodged, it becomes an embolus.

● **I74.0 Embolism and thrombosis of abdominal aorta**
    I74.01 Saddle embolus of abdominal aorta 🇭🇨
    I74.09 Other arterial embolism and thrombosis of abdominal aorta 🇭🇨
       Aortic bifurcation syndrome
       Aortoiliac obstruction
       Leriche's syndrome

● **I74.1 Embolism and thrombosis of other and unspecified parts of aorta**
    I74.10 Embolism and thrombosis of unspecified parts of aorta 🇭🇨
    I74.11 Embolism and thrombosis of thoracic aorta 🇭🇨
    I74.19 Embolism and thrombosis of other parts of aorta 🇭🇨

   I74.2 Embolism and thrombosis of arteries of the upper extremities 🇭🇨

   I74.3 Embolism and thrombosis of arteries of the lower extremities 🇭🇨

   I74.4 Embolism and thrombosis of arteries of extremities, unspecified 🇭🇨
       Peripheral arterial embolism NOS

   I74.5 Embolism and thrombosis of iliac artery 🇭🇨
       Coding Clinic: 2023, Q2, P7

   I74.8 Embolism and thrombosis of other arteries 🇭🇨

   I74.9 Embolism and thrombosis of unspecified artery 🇭🇨

● **I75 Atheroembolism** 🇭🇨
   Includes   atherothrombotic microembolism
              cholesterol embolism

● **I75.0 Atheroembolism of extremities**
   ● **I75.01 Atheroembolism of upper extremity**
      I75.011 Atheroembolism of right upper extremity 🇭🇨
      I75.012 Atheroembolism of left upper extremity 🇭🇨
      I75.013 Atheroembolism of bilateral upper extremities 🇭🇨
      I75.019 Atheroembolism of unspecified upper extremity 🇭🇨
   ● **I75.02 Atheroembolism of lower extremity**
      I75.021 Atheroembolism of right lower extremity 🇭🇨
      I75.022 Atheroembolism of left lower extremity 🇭🇨
      I75.023 Atheroembolism of bilateral lower extremities 🇭🇨
      I75.029 Atheroembolism of unspecified lower extremity 🇭🇨

● **I75.8 Atheroembolism of other sites**
    I75.81 Atheroembolism of kidney 🇭🇨
       Use additional code for any associated acute kidney failure and chronic kidney disease (N17.-, N18.-)
    I75.89 Atheroembolism of other site 🇭🇨

   I76 Septic arterial embolism 🇭🇨
      Code first underlying infection, such as:
       infective endocarditis (I33.0)
       lung abscess (J85.-)
      Use additional code to identify the site of the embolism (I74.-)
      Excludes2   septic pulmonary embolism (I26.01, I26.90)

● **I77 Other disorders of arteries and arterioles**
      Excludes2   collagen (vascular) diseases (M30-M36)
                 hypersensitivity angiitis (M31.0)
                 pulmonary artery (I28.-)

   I77.0 Arteriovenous fistula, acquired 🇭🇨
       Aneurysmal varix
       Arteriovenous aneurysm, acquired
      Excludes1   arteriovenous aneurysm NOS (Q27.3-)
               presence of arteriovenous shunt (fistula) for dialysis (Z99.2)
               traumatic - see injury of blood vessel by body region
      Excludes2   cerebral (I67.1)
               coronary (I25.4)

   I77.1 Stricture of artery 🇭🇨
       Narrowing of artery
       Coding Clinic: 2021, Q3, P13

   I77.2 Rupture of artery 🇭🇨
       Erosion of artery
       Fistula of artery
       Ulcer of artery
      Excludes1   traumatic rupture of artery - see injury of blood vessel by body region

   I77.3 Arterial fibromuscular dysplasia 🇭🇨
       Fibromuscular hyperplasia (of) carotid artery
       Fibromuscular hyperplasia (of) renal artery

   I77.4 Celiac artery compression syndrome 🇭🇨
       Coding Clinic: 2021, Q3, P12-13

   I77.5 Necrosis of artery 🇭🇨

   I77.6 Arteritis, unspecified 🇭🇨
       Aortitis NOS
       Endarteritis NOS
      Excludes1   arteritis or endarteritis:
               aortic arch (M31.4)
               cerebral NEC (I67.7)
               coronary (I25.89)
               deformans (I70.-)
               giant cell (M31.5, M31.6)
               obliterans (I70.-)
               senile (I70.-)

● **I77.7 Other arterial dissection**
      Excludes2   dissection of aorta (I71.0-)
               dissection of coronary artery (I25.42)
    I77.70 Dissection of unspecified artery 🇭🇨
       Coding Clinic 2016, Q4, P28
    I77.71 Dissection of carotid artery 🇭🇨
    I77.72 Dissection of iliac artery 🇭🇨
    I77.73 Dissection of renal artery 🇭🇨
    I77.74 Dissection of vertebral artery 🇭🇨
      Excludes2   aneurysm of vertebral artery (I72.6)
       Coding Clinic 2024, Q1, P26

CHAPTER 9 (I00-I99)

I77.75　Dissection of other precerebral arteries ℞
Dissection of basilar artery (trunk)
> **Excludes2**　aneurysm of carotid artery (I72.0)
> aneurysm of other precerebral arteries (I72.5)
> aneurysm of vertebral artery (I72.6)
> dissection of carotid artery (I77.71)
> dissection of vertebral artery (I77.74)
> **Coding Clinic 2016, Q4, P28**

I77.76　Dissection of artery of upper extremity ℞
> **Coding Clinic 2016, Q4, P28**

I77.77　Dissection of artery of lower extremity ℞
> **Coding Clinic 2016, Q4, P28**

I77.79　Dissection of other specified artery ℞
> **Coding Clinic 2016, Q4, P28**

● **I77.8　Other specified disorders of arteries and arterioles**

I77.81　Aortic ectasia
Ectasis aorta
> **Excludes1**　aortic aneurysm and dissection (I71.-)

I77.810　Thoracic aortic ectasia ℞
I77.811　Abdominal aortic ectasia ℞
I77.812　Thoracoabdominal aortic ectasia ℞
I77.819　Aortic ectasia, unspecified site ℞

I77.82　Antineutrophilic cytoplasmic antibody [ANCA] vasculitis
ANCA associated vasculitis
ANCA positive vasculitis
> **Excludes2**　eosinophilic granulomatosis with polyangiitis (M30.1)
> granulomatosis with polyangiitis (M31.3-)
> microscopic polyangiitis (M31.7

I77.89　Other specified disorders of arteries and arterioles ℞
> **Coding Clinic 2021, Q1, P23**

I77.9　Disorder of arteries and arterioles, unspecified ℞
> **Coding Clinic 2021, Q1, P4**

● **I78　Diseases of capillaries**

I78.0　Hereditary hemorrhagic telangiectasia ℞
Rendu-Osler-Weber disease

I78.1　Nevus, non-neoplastic
Araneus nevus　　　　Spider nevus
Senile nevus　　　　　Stellar nevus
> **Excludes1**　nevus NOS (D22.-)
> vascular NOS (Q82.5)
>
> **Excludes2**　blue nevus (D22.-)
> flammeus nevus (Q82.5)
> hairy nevus (D22.-)
> melanocytic nevus (D22.-)
> pigmented nevus (D22.-)
> portwine nevus (Q82.5)
> sanguineous nevus (Q82.5)
> strawberry nevus (Q82.5)
> verrucous nevus (Q82.5)
> **Coding Clinic: 2019, Q1, P21**

I78.8　Other diseases of capillaries

I78.9　Disease of capillaries, unspecified

● **I79　Disorders of arteries, arterioles and capillaries in diseases classified elsewhere**

▶ **I79.0　Aneurysm of aorta in diseases classified elsewhere** ℞
Code first underlying disease
> **Excludes1**　syphilitic aneurysm (A52.01)

▶ **I79.1　Aortitis in diseases classified elsewhere** ℞
Code first underlying disease
> **Excludes1**　syphilitic aortitis (A52.02)

▶ **I79.8　Other disorders of arteries, arterioles and capillaries in diseases classified elsewhere** ℞
Code first underlying disease, such as:
amyloidosis (E85.-)
> **Excludes1**　diabetic (peripheral) angiopathy (E08-E13 with .51-.52)
> syphilitic endarteritis (A52.09)
> tuberculous endarteritis (A18.89)

DISEASES OF VEINS, LYMPHATIC VESSELS AND LYMPH NODES, NOT ELSEWHERE CLASSIFIED (I80-I89)

● **I80　Phlebitis and thrombophlebitis**
Inflammation of a vein with infiltration of walls (phlebitis)
> **Includes**　endophlebitis
> inflammation, vein
> periphlebitis
> suppurative phlebitis

➡ *Code first*, if applicable: phlebitis and thrombophlebitis complicating abortion, ectopic or molar pregnancy (O00-O07, O08.7)
phlebitis and thrombophlebitis complicating pregnancy, childbirth and the puerperium (O22.-, O87.-)
> **Excludes1**　venous embolism and thrombosis of lower extremities (I82.4-, I82.5-, I82.81-)

● **I80.0　Phlebitis and thrombophlebitis of superficial vessels of lower extremities**
Phlebitis and thrombophlebitis of femoropopliteal vein

I80.00　Phlebitis and thrombophlebitis of superficial vessels of unspecified lower extremity

I80.01　Phlebitis and thrombophlebitis of superficial vessels of right lower extremity

I80.02　Phlebitis and thrombophlebitis of superficial vessels of left lower extremity

I80.03　Phlebitis and thrombophlebitis of superficial vessels of lower extremities, bilateral

● **I80.1　Phlebitis and thrombophlebitis of femoral vein**
Phlebitis and thrombophlebitis of common femoral vein
Phlebitis and thrombophlebitis of deep femoral vein

I80.10　Phlebitis and thrombophlebitis of unspecified femoral vein ℞

I80.11　Phlebitis and thrombophlebitis of right femoral vein ℞

I80.12　Phlebitis and thrombophlebitis of left femoral vein ℞

I80.13　Phlebitis and thrombophlebitis of femoral vein, bilateral ℞

● **I80.2　Phlebitis and thrombophlebitis of other and unspecified deep vessels of lower extremities**

● **I80.20　Phlebitis and thrombophlebitis of unspecified deep vessels of lower extremities**

I80.201　Phlebitis and thrombophlebitis of unspecified deep vessels of right lower extremity ℞

I80.202　Phlebitis and thrombophlebitis of unspecified deep vessels of left lower extremity ℞

CHAPTER 9 (I00-I99)

CHAPTER 9 (I00–I99)

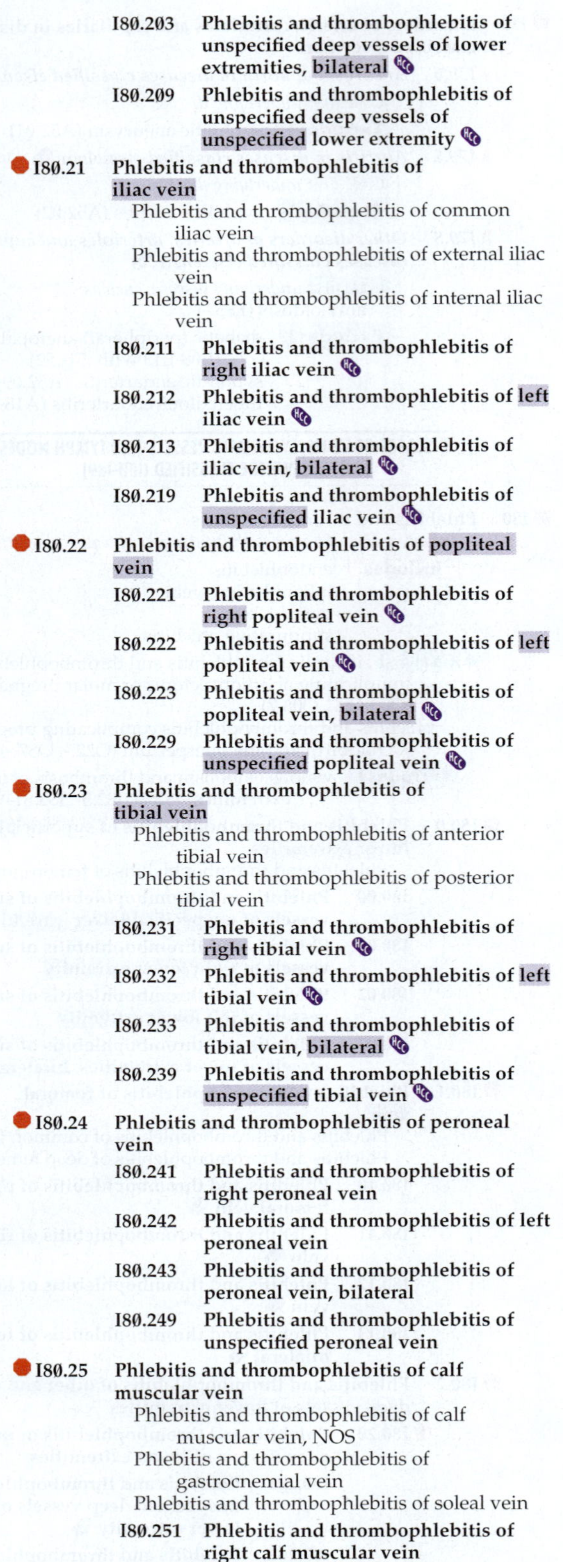

I80.203   Phlebitis and thrombophlebitis of unspecified deep vessels of lower extremities, bilateral Ⓗ

I80.209   Phlebitis and thrombophlebitis of unspecified deep vessels of unspecified lower extremity Ⓗ

● I80.21   Phlebitis and thrombophlebitis of iliac vein

Phlebitis and thrombophlebitis of common iliac vein

Phlebitis and thrombophlebitis of external iliac vein

Phlebitis and thrombophlebitis of internal iliac vein

    I80.211   Phlebitis and thrombophlebitis of right iliac vein Ⓗ

    I80.212   Phlebitis and thrombophlebitis of left iliac vein Ⓗ

    I80.213   Phlebitis and thrombophlebitis of iliac vein, bilateral Ⓗ

    I80.219   Phlebitis and thrombophlebitis of unspecified iliac vein Ⓗ

● I80.22   Phlebitis and thrombophlebitis of popliteal vein

    I80.221   Phlebitis and thrombophlebitis of right popliteal vein Ⓗ

    I80.222   Phlebitis and thrombophlebitis of left popliteal vein Ⓗ

    I80.223   Phlebitis and thrombophlebitis of popliteal vein, bilateral Ⓗ

    I80.229   Phlebitis and thrombophlebitis of unspecified popliteal vein Ⓗ

● I80.23   Phlebitis and thrombophlebitis of tibial vein

Phlebitis and thrombophlebitis of anterior tibial vein

Phlebitis and thrombophlebitis of posterior tibial vein

    I80.231   Phlebitis and thrombophlebitis of right tibial vein Ⓗ

    I80.232   Phlebitis and thrombophlebitis of left tibial vein Ⓗ

    I80.233   Phlebitis and thrombophlebitis of tibial vein, bilateral Ⓗ

    I80.239   Phlebitis and thrombophlebitis of unspecified tibial vein Ⓗ

● I80.24   Phlebitis and thrombophlebitis of peroneal vein

    I80.241   Phlebitis and thrombophlebitis of right peroneal vein

    I80.242   Phlebitis and thrombophlebitis of left peroneal vein

    I80.243   Phlebitis and thrombophlebitis of peroneal vein, bilateral

    I80.249   Phlebitis and thrombophlebitis of unspecified peroneal vein

● I80.25   Phlebitis and thrombophlebitis of calf muscular vein

Phlebitis and thrombophlebitis of calf muscular vein, NOS

Phlebitis and thrombophlebitis of gastrocnemial vein

Phlebitis and thrombophlebitis of soleal vein

    I80.251   Phlebitis and thrombophlebitis of right calf muscular vein

    I80.252   Phlebitis and thrombophlebitis of left calf muscular vein

    I80.253   Phlebitis and thrombophlebitis of calf muscular vein, bilateral

    I80.259   Phlebitis and thrombophlebitis of unspecified calf muscular vein

● I80.29   Phlebitis and thrombophlebitis of other deep vessels of lower extremities

    I80.291   Phlebitis and thrombophlebitis of other deep vessels of right lower extremity Ⓗ

    I80.292   Phlebitis and thrombophlebitis of other deep vessels of left lower extremity Ⓗ

    I80.293   Phlebitis and thrombophlebitis of other deep vessels of lower extremity, bilateral Ⓗ

    I80.299   Phlebitis and thrombophlebitis of other deep vessels of unspecified lower extremity Ⓗ

I80.3   Phlebitis and thrombophlebitis of lower extremities, unspecified

I80.8   Phlebitis and thrombophlebitis of other sites

I80.9   Phlebitis and thrombophlebitis of unspecified site

I81   **Portal vein thrombosis**

Portal (vein) obstruction

> **Excludes2**   hepatic vein thrombosis (I82.0)
> phlebitis of portal vein (K75.1)

Coding Clinic: 2019, Q4, P68

● I82   **Other venous embolism and thrombosis**

Code first venous embolism and thrombosis complicating:

abortion, ectopic or molar pregnancy (O00-O07, O08.7)

pregnancy, childbirth and the puerperium (O22.-, O87.-)

> **Excludes2**   venous embolism and thrombosis (of):
> cerebral (I63.6, I67.6)
> coronary (I21-I25)
> intracranial and intraspinal, septic or NOS (G08)
> intracranial, nonpyogenic (I67.6)
> intraspinal, nonpyogenic (G95.1)
> mesenteric (K55.0-)
> portal (I81)
> pulmonary (I26.-)

I82.0   **Budd-Chiari syndrome** Ⓗ

Hepatic vein thrombosis

I82.1   **Thrombophlebitis migrans**

"White leg" is the other term to describe a migrating thrombus.

● I82.2   **Embolism and thrombosis of vena cava and other thoracic veins**

  ● I82.21   Embolism and thrombosis of superior vena cava

    I82.210   **Acute embolism and thrombosis of superior vena cava** Ⓗ

Embolism and thrombosis of superior vena cava NOS

    I82.211   **Chronic embolism and thrombosis of superior vena cava** Ⓗ

  ● I82.22   Embolism and thrombosis of inferior vena cava

    I82.220   **Acute embolism and thrombosis of inferior vena cava** Ⓗ

Embolism and thrombosis of inferior vena cava NOS

    I82.221   **Chronic embolism and thrombosis of inferior vena cava** Ⓗ

▶ New   ⇨ Revised   ~~deleted~~ Deleted   Excludes 1   Excludes 2   Includes   Use additional   Code first   Code also   Key words

OGCR Official Guidelines   X Assign placeholder X   ● Use Additional Character(s)   ▶ Manifestation Code   Ⓗ Hierarchical Condition Category   **Coding Clinic** 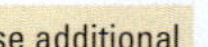

● **I82.29** **Embolism and thrombosis of other thoracic veins**
Embolism and thrombosis of brachiocephalic (innominate) vein

    I82.290 **Acute embolism and thrombosis of other thoracic veins** _{RCC}

    I82.291 **Chronic embolism and thrombosis of other thoracic veins** _{RCC}

I82.3 **Embolism and thrombosis of renal vein** _{RCC}

● **I82.4** **Acute embolism and thrombosis of deep veins of lower extremity**

    I82.40 **Acute embolism and thrombosis of unspecified deep veins of lower extremity**
Deep vein thrombosis NOS
DVT NOS

        Excludes1   acute embolism and thrombosis of unspecified deep veins of distal lower extremity (I82.4Z-)
acute embolism and thrombosis of unspecified deep veins of proximal lower extremity (I82.4Y-)

        I82.401 **Acute embolism and thrombosis of unspecified deep veins of right lower extremity** _{RCC}

        I82.402 **Acute embolism and thrombosis of unspecified deep veins of left lower extremity** _{RCC}

        I82.403 **Acute embolism and thrombosis of unspecified deep veins of lower extremity, bilateral** _{RCC}

        I82.409 **Acute embolism and thrombosis of unspecified deep veins of unspecified lower extremity** _{RCC}

● **I82.41** **Acute embolism and thrombosis of femoral vein**
Acute embolism and thrombosis of common femoral vein
Acute embolism and thrombosis of deep femoral vein

        I82.411 **Acute embolism and thrombosis of right femoral vein** _{RCC}

        I82.412 **Acute embolism and thrombosis of left femoral vein** _{RCC}
           Coding Clinic: 2023, Q3, P12

        I82.413 **Acute embolism and thrombosis of femoral vein, bilateral** _{RCC}

        I82.419 **Acute embolism and thrombosis of unspecified femoral vein** _{RCC}

● **I82.42** **Acute embolism and thrombosis of iliac vein**
Acute embolism and thrombosis of common iliac vein
Acute embolism and thrombosis of external iliac vein
Acute embolism and thrombosis of internal iliac vein

        I82.421 **Acute embolism and thrombosis of right iliac vein** _{RCC}

        I82.422 **Acute embolism and thrombosis of left iliac vein** _{RCC}

        I82.423 **Acute embolism and thrombosis of iliac vein, bilateral** _{RCC}

        I82.429 **Acute embolism and thrombosis of unspecified iliac vein** _{RCC}

● **I82.43** **Acute embolism and thrombosis of popliteal vein**

        I82.431 **Acute embolism and thrombosis of right popliteal vein** _{RCC}

        I82.432 **Acute embolism and thrombosis of left popliteal vein** _{RCC}

        I82.433 **Acute embolism and thrombosis of popliteal vein, bilateral** _{RCC}

        I82.439 **Acute embolism and thrombosis of unspecified popliteal vein** _{RCC}

● **I82.44** **Acute embolism and thrombosis of tibial vein**
Acute embolism and thrombosis of anterior tibial vein
Acute embolism and thrombosis of posterior tibial vein

        I82.441 **Acute embolism and thrombosis of right tibial vein** _{RCC}

        I82.442 **Acute embolism and thrombosis of left tibial vein** _{RCC}

        I82.443 **Acute embolism and thrombosis of tibial vein, bilateral** _{RCC}

        I82.449 **Acute embolism and thrombosis of unspecified tibial vein** _{RCC}

● **I82.45** **Acute embolism and thrombosis of peroneal vein**

        I82.451 **Acute embolism and thrombosis of right peroneal vein**

        I82.452 **Acute embolism and thrombosis of left peroneal vein**

        I82.453 **Acute embolism and thrombosis of peroneal vein, bilateral**

        I82.459 **Acute embolism and thrombosis of unspecified peroneal vein**

● **I82.46** **Acute embolism and thrombosis of calf muscular vein**
Acute embolism and thrombosis of calf muscular vein, NOS
Acute embolism and thrombosis of gastrocnemial vein
Acute embolism and thrombosis of soleal vein

        I82.461 **Acute embolism and thrombosis of right calf muscular vein**

        I82.462 **Acute embolism and thrombosis of left calf muscular vein**

        I82.463 **Acute embolism and thrombosis of calf muscular vein, bilateral**

        I82.469 **Acute embolism and thrombosis of unspecified calf muscular vein**

● **I82.49** **Acute embolism and thrombosis of other specified deep vein of lower extremity**

        I82.491 **Acute embolism and thrombosis of other specified deep vein of right lower extremity** _{RCC}

        I82.492 **Acute embolism and thrombosis of other specified deep vein of left lower extremity** _{RCC}

        I82.493 **Acute embolism and thrombosis of other specified deep vein of lower extremity, bilateral** _{RCC}

        I82.499 **Acute embolism and thrombosis of other specified deep vein of unspecified lower extremity** _{RCC}

● **I82.4Y** **Acute embolism and thrombosis of unspecified deep veins of proximal lower extremity**
Acute embolism and thrombosis of deep vein of thigh NOS
Acute embolism and thrombosis of deep vein of upper leg NOS

        I82.4Y1 **Acute embolism and thrombosis of unspecified deep veins of right proximal lower extremity** _{RCC}

CHAPTER 9 (I00-I99)

I82.4Y2   Acute embolism and thrombosis of unspecified deep veins of **left** proximal lower extremity

I82.4Y3   Acute embolism and thrombosis of unspecified deep veins of proximal lower extremity, **bilateral**

I82.4Y9   Acute embolism and thrombosis of unspecified deep veins of **unspecified** proximal lower extremity

● I82.4Z   Acute embolism and thrombosis of **unspecified deep veins of distal lower extremity**

     Acute embolism and thrombosis of deep vein of calf NOS

     Acute embolism and thrombosis of deep vein of lower leg NOS

I82.4Z1   Acute embolism and thrombosis of unspecified deep veins of **right** distal lower extremity

I82.4Z2   Acute embolism and thrombosis of unspecified deep veins of **left** distal lower extremity

I82.4Z3   Acute embolism and thrombosis of unspecified deep veins of distal lower extremity, **bilateral**

I82.4Z9   Acute embolism and thrombosis of unspecified deep veins of **unspecified** distal lower extremity

● I82.5   Chronic embolism and thrombosis of **deep veins of lower extremity**

     Use additional code, if applicable, for associated long-term (current) use of anticoagulants (Z79.01)

     Excludes1   personal history of venous embolism and thrombosis (Z86.718)

● I82.50   Chronic embolism and thrombosis of **unspecified** deep veins of lower extremity

     Excludes1   chronic embolism and thrombosis of unspecified deep veins of distal lower extremity (I82.5Z-)

         chronic embolism and thrombosis of unspecified deep veins of proximal lower extremity (I82.5Y-)

I82.501   Chronic embolism and thrombosis of unspecified deep veins of **right** lower extremity

I82.502   Chronic embolism and thrombosis of unspecified deep veins of **left** lower extremity

I82.503   Chronic embolism and thrombosis of unspecified deep veins of lower extremity, **bilateral**

I82.509   Chronic embolism and thrombosis of unspecified deep veins of **unspecified** lower extremity

● I82.51   Chronic embolism and thrombosis of **femoral vein**

     Chronic embolism and thrombosis of common femoral vein

     Chronic embolism and thrombosis of deep femoral vein

I82.511   Chronic embolism and thrombosis of **right** femoral vein

I82.512   Chronic embolism and thrombosis of **left** femoral vein

I82.513   Chronic embolism and thrombosis of femoral vein, **bilateral**

I82.519   Chronic embolism and thrombosis of **unspecified** femoral vein

Item 9–10   Varicose/Varicosities (varix = singular, varices = plural): Enlarged, engorged, tortuous, twisted vascular vessels (veins, arteries, lymphatics). As such, the condition can present in various parts of the body, although the most familiar locations are the lower extremities. A common complication of varices is thrombophlebitis. Varicosities of the anus and rectum are called hemorrhoids.

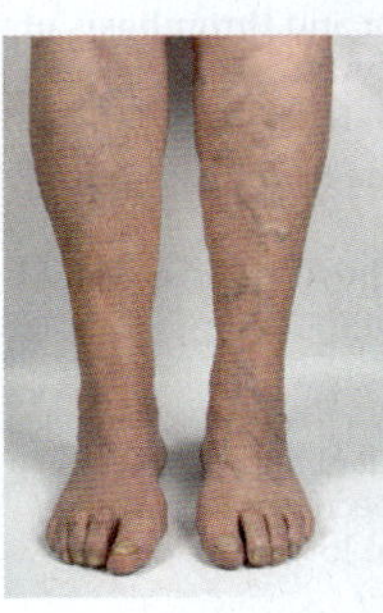

Figure 9-7   Varicose veins of the legs. (Getty Image)

● I82.52   Chronic embolism and thrombosis of **iliac vein**

     Chronic embolism and thrombosis of common iliac vein

     Chronic embolism and thrombosis of external iliac vein

     Chronic embolism and thrombosis of internal iliac vein

I82.521   Chronic embolism and thrombosis of **right iliac vein**

I82.522   Chronic embolism and thrombosis of **left iliac vein**

I82.523   Chronic embolism and thrombosis of iliac vein, **bilateral**

I82.529   Chronic embolism and thrombosis of **unspecified** iliac vein

● I82.53   Chronic embolism and thrombosis of **popliteal vein**

I82.531   Chronic embolism and thrombosis of **right** popliteal vein

I82.532   Chronic embolism and thrombosis of **left** popliteal vein

I82.533   Chronic embolism and thrombosis of popliteal vein, **bilateral**

I82.539   Chronic embolism and thrombosis of **unspecified** popliteal vein

● I82.54   Chronic embolism and thrombosis of **tibial vein**

     Chronic embolism and thrombosis of anterior tibial vein

     Chronic embolism and thrombosis of posterior tibial vein

I82.541   Chronic embolism and thrombosis of **right** tibial vein

I82.542   Chronic embolism and thrombosis of **left** tibial vein

I82.543   Chronic embolism and thrombosis of tibial vein, **bilateral**

I82.549   Chronic embolism and thrombosis of **unspecified** tibial vein

● I82.55   Chronic embolism and thrombosis of peroneal vein

I82.551   Chronic embolism and thrombosis of right peroneal vein

I82.552   Chronic embolism and thrombosis of left peroneal vein

I82.553   Chronic embolism and thrombosis of peroneal vein, bilateral

I82.559   Chronic embolism and thrombosis of unspecified peroneal vein

▶ New   ⇨ Revised   ~~deleted~~ Deleted   Excludes 1   Excludes 2   Includes   Use additional   Code first   Code also   Key words
OGCR Official Guidelines   **X** Assign placeholder X   ● Use Additional Character(s)   ▶ Manifestation Code   Hierarchical Condition Category   **Coding Clinic**

● **I82.56 Chronic embolism and thrombosis of calf muscular vein**
  Chronic embolism and thrombosis of calf muscular vein NOS
  Chronic embolism and thrombosis of gastrocnemial vein
  Chronic embolism and thrombosis of soleal vein

 I82.561 Chronic embolism and thrombosis of right calf muscular vein

 I82.562 Chronic embolism and thrombosis of left calf muscular vein

 I82.563 Chronic embolism and thrombosis of calf muscular vein, bilateral

 I82.569 Chronic embolism and thrombosis of unspecified calf muscular vein

● **I82.59 Chronic embolism and thrombosis of other specified deep vein of lower extremity**

 I82.591 Chronic embolism and thrombosis of other specified deep vein of right lower extremity HCC

 I82.592 Chronic embolism and thrombosis of other specified deep vein of left lower extremity HCC

 I82.593 Chronic embolism and thrombosis of other specified deep vein of lower extremity, bilateral HCC

 I82.599 Chronic embolism and thrombosis of other specified deep vein of unspecified lower extremity HCC

● **I82.5Y Chronic embolism and thrombosis of unspecified deep veins of proximal lower extremity**
  Chronic embolism and thrombosis of deep veins of thigh NOS
  Chronic embolism and thrombosis of deep veins of upper leg NOS

 I82.5Y1 Chronic embolism and thrombosis of unspecified deep veins of right proximal lower extremity HCC

 I82.5Y2 Chronic embolism and thrombosis of unspecified deep veins of left proximal lower extremity HCC

 I82.5Y3 Chronic embolism and thrombosis of unspecified deep veins of proximal lower extremity, bilateral HCC

 I82.5Y9 Chronic embolism and thrombosis of unspecified deep veins of unspecified proximal lower extremity HCC

● **I82.5Z Chronic embolism and thrombosis of unspecified deep veins of distal lower extremity**
  Chronic embolism and thrombosis of deep veins of calf NOS
  Chronic embolism and thrombosis of deep veins of lower leg NOS

 I82.5Z1 Chronic embolism and thrombosis of unspecified deep veins of right distal lower extremity HCC

 I82.5Z2 Chronic embolism and thrombosis of unspecified deep veins of left distal lower extremity HCC

 I82.5Z3 Chronic embolism and thrombosis of unspecified deep veins of distal lower extremity, bilateral HCC

 I82.5Z9 Chronic embolism and thrombosis of unspecified deep veins of unspecified distal lower extremity HCC

● **I82.6 Acute embolism and thrombosis of veins of upper extremity**

 ● **I82.60 Acute embolism and thrombosis of unspecified veins of upper extremity**

  I82.601 Acute embolism and thrombosis of unspecified veins of right upper extremity

  I82.602 Acute embolism and thrombosis of unspecified veins of left upper extremity

  I82.603 Acute embolism and thrombosis of unspecified veins of upper extremity, bilateral

  I82.609 Acute embolism and thrombosis of unspecified veins of unspecified upper extremity

 ● **I82.61 Acute embolism and thrombosis of superficial veins of upper extremity**
  Acute embolism and thrombosis of antecubital vein
  Acute embolism and thrombosis of basilic vein
  Acute embolism and thrombosis of cephalic vein

  I82.611 Acute embolism and thrombosis of superficial veins of right upper extremity

  I82.612 Acute embolism and thrombosis of superficial veins of left upper extremity

  I82.613 Acute embolism and thrombosis of superficial veins of upper extremity, bilateral

  I82.619 Acute embolism and thrombosis of superficial veins of unspecified upper extremity

 ● **I82.62 Acute embolism and thrombosis of deep veins of upper extremity**
  Acute embolism and thrombosis of brachal vein
  Acute embolism and thrombosis of radial vein
  Acute embolism and thrombosis of ulnar vein

  I82.621 Acute embolism and thrombosis of deep veins of right upper extremity HCC

  I82.622 Acute embolism and thrombosis of deep veins of left upper extremity HCC

  I82.623 Acute embolism and thrombosis of deep veins of upper extremity, bilateral HCC

  I82.629 Acute embolism and thrombosis of deep veins of unspecified upper extremity HCC

● **I82.7 Chronic embolism and thrombosis of veins of upper extremity**
  Use additional code, if applicable, for associated long-term (current) use of anticoagulants (Z79.01)
  Excludes1 personal history of venous embolism and thrombosis (Z86.718)

 ● **I82.70 Chronic embolism and thrombosis of unspecified veins of upper extremity**

  I82.701 Chronic embolism and thrombosis of unspecified veins of right upper extremity

  I82.702 Chronic embolism and thrombosis of unspecified veins of left upper extremity

  I82.703 Chronic embolism and thrombosis of unspecified veins of upper extremity, bilateral

  I82.709 Chronic embolism and thrombosis of unspecified veins of unspecified upper extremity

 ● **I82.71 Chronic embolism and thrombosis of superficial veins of upper extremity**
  Chronic embolism and thrombosis of antecubital vein
  Chronic embolism and thrombosis of basilic vein
  Chronic embolism and thrombosis of cephalic vein

  I82.711 Chronic embolism and thrombosis of superficial veins of right upper extremity

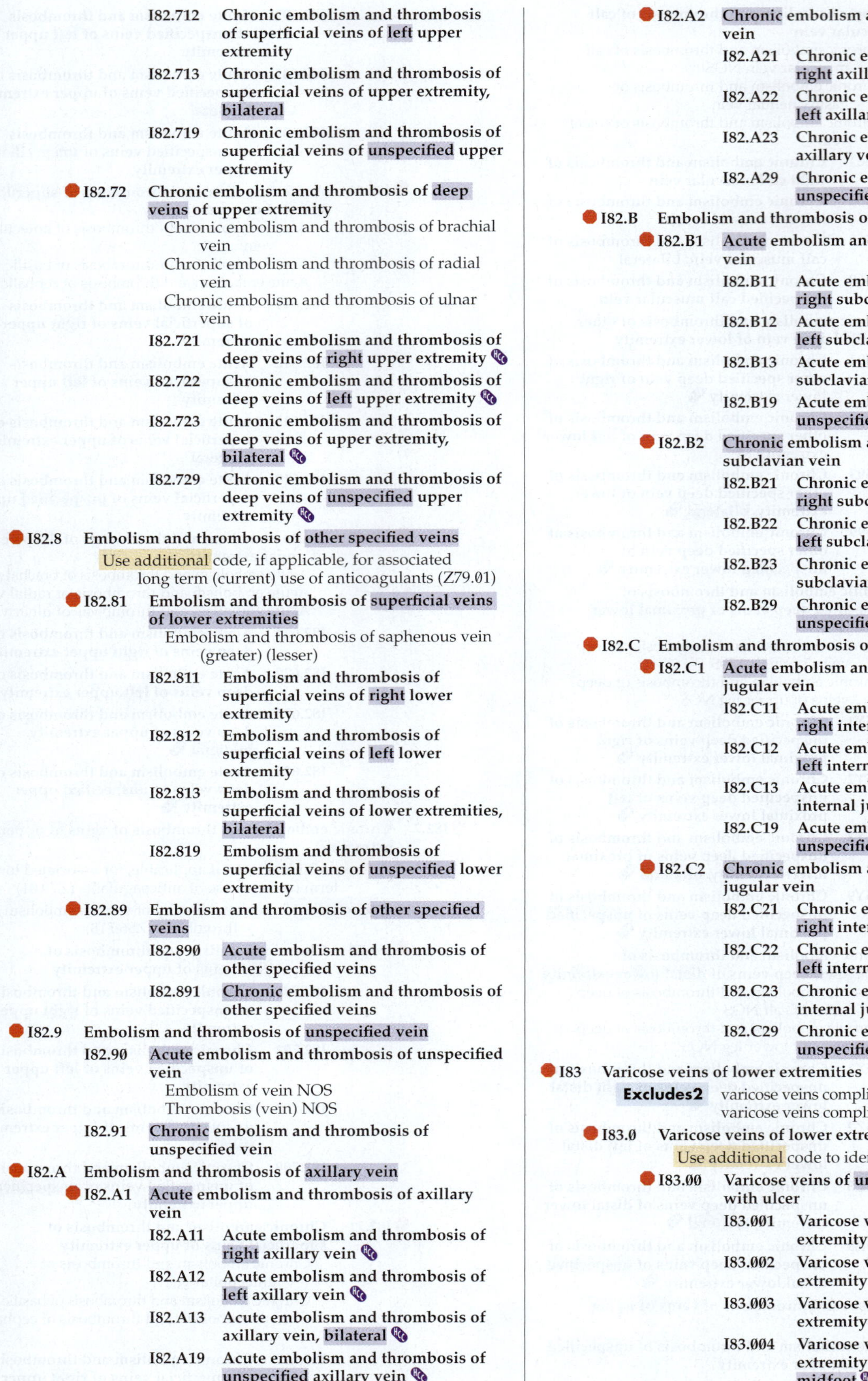

I82.712 Chronic embolism and thrombosis of superficial veins of **left** upper extremity

I82.713 Chronic embolism and thrombosis of superficial veins of upper extremity, **bilateral**

I82.719 Chronic embolism and thrombosis of superficial veins of **unspecified** upper extremity

● **I82.72** Chronic embolism and thrombosis of **deep veins** of upper extremity

Chronic embolism and thrombosis of brachial vein

Chronic embolism and thrombosis of radial vein

Chronic embolism and thrombosis of ulnar vein

I82.721 Chronic embolism and thrombosis of deep veins of **right** upper extremity ✚

I82.722 Chronic embolism and thrombosis of deep veins of **left** upper extremity ✚

I82.723 Chronic embolism and thrombosis of deep veins of upper extremity, **bilateral** ✚

I82.729 Chronic embolism and thrombosis of deep veins of **unspecified** upper extremity ✚

● **I82.8** Embolism and thrombosis of **other specified veins**

Use additional code, if applicable, for associated long term (current) use of anticoagulants (Z79.01)

● **I82.81** Embolism and thrombosis of **superficial veins of lower extremities**

Embolism and thrombosis of saphenous vein (greater) (lesser)

I82.811 Embolism and thrombosis of superficial veins of **right** lower extremity

I82.812 Embolism and thrombosis of superficial veins of **left** lower extremity

I82.813 Embolism and thrombosis of superficial veins of lower extremities, **bilateral**

I82.819 Embolism and thrombosis of superficial veins of **unspecified** lower extremity

● **I82.89** Embolism and thrombosis of **other specified veins**

I82.890 Acute embolism and thrombosis of other specified veins

I82.891 Chronic embolism and thrombosis of other specified veins

● **I82.9** Embolism and thrombosis of **unspecified vein**

I82.90 Acute embolism and thrombosis of unspecified vein

Embolism of vein NOS

Thrombosis (vein) NOS

I82.91 Chronic embolism and thrombosis of unspecified vein

● **I82.A** Embolism and thrombosis of **axillary vein**

● **I82.A1** Acute embolism and thrombosis of axillary vein

I82.A11 Acute embolism and thrombosis of **right** axillary vein

I82.A12 Acute embolism and thrombosis of **left** axillary vein

I82.A13 Acute embolism and thrombosis of axillary vein, **bilateral** ✚

I82.A19 Acute embolism and thrombosis of **unspecified** axillary vein ✚

● **I82.A2** Chronic embolism and thrombosis of axillary vein

I82.A21 Chronic embolism and thrombosis of **right** axillary vein ✚

I82.A22 Chronic embolism and thrombosis of **left** axillary vein ✚

I82.A23 Chronic embolism and thrombosis of axillary vein, **bilateral** ✚

I82.A29 Chronic embolism and thrombosis of **unspecified** axillary vein ✚

● **I82.B** Embolism and thrombosis of **subclavian vein**

● **I82.B1** **Acute** embolism and thrombosis of subclavian vein

I82.B11 Acute embolism and thrombosis of **right** subclavian vein ✚

I82.B12 Acute embolism and thrombosis of **left** subclavian vein ✚

I82.B13 Acute embolism and thrombosis of subclavian vein, **bilateral** ✚

I82.B19 Acute embolism and thrombosis of **unspecified** subclavian vein ✚

● **I82.B2** Chronic embolism and thrombosis of subclavian vein

I82.B21 Chronic embolism and thrombosis of **right** subclavian vein ✚

I82.B22 Chronic embolism and thrombosis of **left** subclavian vein ✚

I82.B23 Chronic embolism and thrombosis of subclavian vein, **bilateral** ✚

I82.B29 Chronic embolism and thrombosis of **unspecified** subclavian vein ✚

● **I82.C** Embolism and thrombosis of **internal jugular vein**

● **I82.C1** **Acute** embolism and thrombosis of internal jugular vein

I82.C11 Acute embolism and thrombosis of **right** internal jugular vein ✚

I82.C12 Acute embolism and thrombosis of **left** internal jugular vein ✚

I82.C13 Acute embolism and thrombosis of internal jugular vein, **bilateral** ✚

I82.C19 Acute embolism and thrombosis of **unspecified** internal jugular vein ✚

● **I82.C2** Chronic embolism and thrombosis of internal jugular vein

I82.C21 Chronic embolism and thrombosis of **right** internal jugular vein ✚

I82.C22 Chronic embolism and thrombosis of **left** internal jugular vein ✚

I82.C23 Chronic embolism and thrombosis of internal jugular vein, **bilateral** ✚

I82.C29 Chronic embolism and thrombosis of **unspecified** internal jugular vein ✚

● **I83** Varicose veins of lower extremities

Excludes2 varicose veins complicating pregnancy (O22.0-)
varicose veins complicating the puerperium (O87.4)

● **I83.0** Varicose veins of lower extremities with **ulcer**

Use additional code to identify severity of ulcer (L97.-)

● **I83.00** Varicose veins of **unspecified** lower extremity with ulcer

I83.001 Varicose veins of unspecified lower extremity with ulcer of **thigh** ✚   A

I83.002 Varicose veins of unspecified lower extremity with ulcer of **calf** ✚   A

I83.003 Varicose veins of unspecified lower extremity with ulcer of **ankle** ✚   A

I83.004 Varicose veins of unspecified lower extremity with ulcer of **heel and midfoot** ✚   A

Varicose veins of unspecified lower extremity with ulcer of plantar surface of midfoot

I83.005   Varicose veins of unspecified lower extremity with ulcer **other part of foot** 🆁🅲   A
　　　　Varicose veins of unspecified lower extremity with ulcer of toe

I83.008   Varicose veins of unspecified lower extremity with ulcer **other part of lower leg** 🆁🅲   A

I83.009   Varicose veins of unspecified lower extremity with ulcer of **unspecified site** 🆁🅲   A

● **I83.01   Varicose veins of right lower extremity with ulcer**

I83.011   Varicose veins of right lower extremity with ulcer of **thigh** 🆁🅲   A

I83.012   Varicose veins of right lower extremity with ulcer of **calf** 🆁🅲   A

I83.013   Varicose veins of right lower extremity with ulcer of **ankle** 🆁🅲   A

I83.014   Varicose veins of right lower extremity with ulcer of **heel and midfoot** 🆁🅲   A
　　　　Varicose veins of right lower extremity with ulcer of plantar surface of midfoot

I83.015   Varicose veins of right lower extremity with ulcer **other part of foot** 🆁🅲   A
　　　　Varicose veins of right lower extremity with ulcer of toe

I83.018   Varicose veins of right lower extremity with ulcer **other part of lower leg** 🆁🅲   A

I83.019   Varicose veins of right lower extremity with ulcer of **unspecified site** 🆁🅲   A

● **I83.02   Varicose veins of left lower extremity with ulcer**

I83.021   Varicose veins of left lower extremity with ulcer of **thigh** 🆁🅲   A

I83.022   Varicose veins of left lower extremity with ulcer of **calf** 🆁🅲   A

I83.023   Varicose veins of left lower extremity with ulcer of **ankle** 🆁🅲   A

I83.024   Varicose veins of left lower extremity with ulcer of **heel and midfoot** 🆁🅲   A
　　　　Varicose veins of left lower extremity with ulcer of plantar surface of midfoot

I83.025   Varicose veins of left lower extremity with ulcer **other part of foot** 🆁🅲   A
　　　　Varicose veins of left lower extremity with ulcer of toe

I83.028   Varicose veins of left lower extremity with ulcer **other part of lower leg** 🆁🅲   A

I83.029   Varicose veins of left lower extremity with ulcer of **unspecified site** 🆁🅲   A

● **I83.1   Varicose veins of lower extremities with inflammation**

I83.10   Varicose veins of **unspecified** lower extremity with inflammation   A

I83.11   Varicose veins of **right** lower extremity with inflammation   A

I83.12   Varicose veins of **left** lower extremity with inflammation   A

● **I83.2   Varicose veins of lower extremities with both ulcer and inflammation**

Use additional code to identify severity of ulcer (L97.-)

● **I83.20   Varicose veins of unspecified lower extremity with both ulcer and inflammation**

I83.201   Varicose veins of unspecified lower extremity with both ulcer of **thigh and inflammation** 🆁🅲   A

I83.202   Varicose veins of unspecified lower extremity with both ulcer of **calf and inflammation** 🆁🅲   A

I83.203   Varicose veins of unspecified lower extremity with both ulcer of **ankle and inflammation** 🆁🅲   A

I83.204   Varicose veins of unspecified lower extremity with both ulcer of **heel and midfoot and inflammation** 🆁🅲   A
　　　　Varicose veins of unspecified lower extremity with both ulcer of plantar surface of midfoot and inflammation

I83.205   Varicose veins of unspecified lower extremity with both ulcer **other part of foot and inflammation** 🆁🅲   A
　　　　Varicose veins of unspecified lower extremity with both ulcer of toe and inflammation

I83.208   Varicose veins of unspecified lower extremity with both ulcer of **other part of lower extremity and inflammation** 🆁🅲   A

I83.209   Varicose veins of unspecified lower extremity with both ulcer of **unspecified site and inflammation** 🆁🅲   A

● **I83.21   Varicose veins of right lower extremity with both ulcer and inflammation**

I83.211   Varicose veins of right lower extremity with both ulcer of **thigh and inflammation** 🆁🅲   A

I83.212   Varicose veins of right lower extremity with both ulcer of **calf and inflammation** 🆁🅲   A

I83.213   Varicose veins of right lower extremity with both ulcer of **ankle and inflammation** 🆁🅲   A

I83.214   Varicose veins of right lower extremity with both ulcer of **heel and midfoot and inflammation** 🆁🅲   A
　　　　Varicose veins of right lower extremity with both ulcer of plantar surface of midfoot and inflammation

I83.215   Varicose veins of right lower extremity with both ulcer **other part of foot and inflammation** 🆁🅲   A
　　　　Varicose veins of right lower extremity with both ulcer of toe and inflammation

I83.218   Varicose veins of right lower extremity with both ulcer of **other part of lower extremity and inflammation** 🆁🅲   A

I83.219   Varicose veins of right lower extremity with both ulcer of **unspecified site and inflammation** 🆁🅲   A

● **I83.22   Varicose veins of left lower extremity with both ulcer and inflammation**

I83.221   Varicose veins of left lower extremity with both ulcer of **thigh and inflammation** 🆁🅲   A

I83.222   Varicose veins of left lower extremity with both ulcer of **calf and inflammation** 🆁🅲   A

I83.223   Varicose veins of left lower extremity with both ulcer of **ankle and inflammation** 🆁🅲   A

I83.224   Varicose veins of left lower extremity with both ulcer of **heel and midfoot and inflammation** 🆁🅲   A
　　　　Varicose veins of left lower extremity with both ulcer of plantar surface of midfoot and inflammation

I83.225 Varicose veins of left lower extremity with both ulcer other part of foot and inflammation 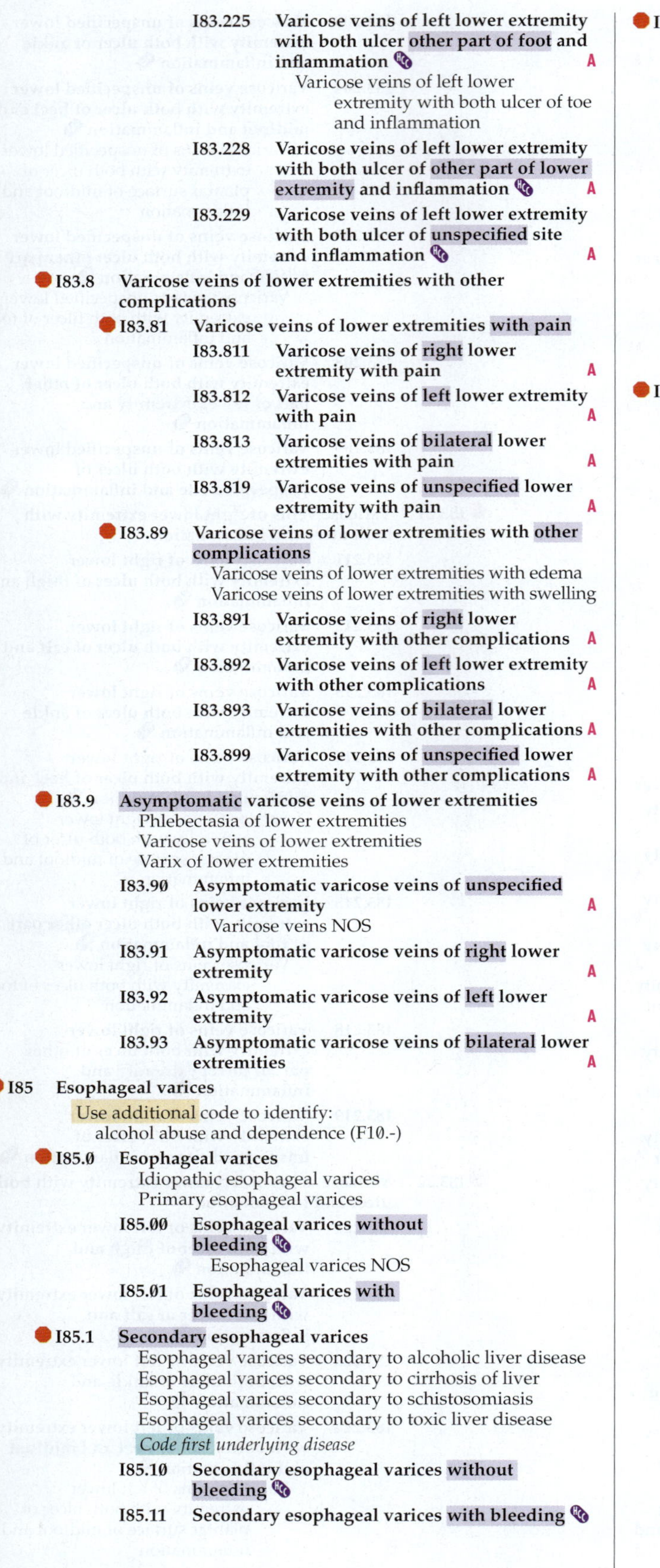   A

> Varicose veins of left lower extremity with both ulcer of toe and inflammation

I83.228 Varicose veins of left lower extremity with both ulcer of other part of lower extremity and inflammation   A

I83.229 Varicose veins of left lower extremity with both ulcer of unspecified site and inflammation   A

● **I83.8** Varicose veins of lower extremities with other complications

   ● **I83.81** Varicose veins of lower extremities with pain

     I83.811 Varicose veins of right lower extremity with pain   A

     I83.812 Varicose veins of left lower extremity with pain   A

     I83.813 Varicose veins of bilateral lower extremities with pain   A

     I83.819 Varicose veins of unspecified lower extremity with pain   A

   ● **I83.89** Varicose veins of lower extremities with other complications

> Varicose veins of lower extremities with edema
> Varicose veins of lower extremities with swelling

     I83.891 Varicose veins of right lower extremity with other complications   A

     I83.892 Varicose veins of left lower extremity with other complications   A

     I83.893 Varicose veins of bilateral lower extremities with other complications   A

     I83.899 Varicose veins of unspecified lower extremity with other complications   A

● **I83.9** Asymptomatic varicose veins of lower extremities

> Phlebectasia of lower extremities
> Varicose veins of lower extremities
> Varix of lower extremities

   I83.90 Asymptomatic varicose veins of unspecified lower extremity   A

> Varicose veins NOS

   I83.91 Asymptomatic varicose veins of right lower extremity   A

   I83.92 Asymptomatic varicose veins of left lower extremity   A

   I83.93 Asymptomatic varicose veins of bilateral lower extremities   A

● **I85** Esophageal varices

Use additional code to identify:
alcohol abuse and dependence (F10.-)

   ● **I85.0** Esophageal varices

> Idiopathic esophageal varices
> Primary esophageal varices

     I85.00 Esophageal varices without bleeding

> Esophageal varices NOS

     I85.01 Esophageal varices with bleeding

   ● **I85.1** Secondary esophageal varices

> Esophageal varices secondary to alcoholic liver disease
> Esophageal varices secondary to cirrhosis of liver
> Esophageal varices secondary to schistosomiasis
> Esophageal varices secondary to toxic liver disease

Code first *underlying disease*

     I85.10 Secondary esophageal varices without bleeding

     I85.11 Secondary esophageal varices with bleeding

● **I86** Varicose veins of other sites

> **Excludes1** varicose veins of unspecified site (I83.9-)
>
> **Excludes2** retinal varices (H35.0-)

   I86.0 Sublingual varices

   I86.1 Scrotal varices

> Varicocele

   I86.2 Pelvic varices

   I86.3 Vulval varices

> **Excludes1** vulval varices complicating childbirth and the puerperium (O87.8)
> vulval varices complicating pregnancy (O22.1-)

   I86.4 Gastric varices

   I86.8 Varicose veins of other specified sites   A

> Varicose ulcer of nasal septum

● **I87** Other disorders of veins

   ● **I87.0** Postthrombotic syndrome

> Chronic venous hypertension due to deep vein thrombosis
> Postphlebitic syndrome

> **Excludes1** chronic venous hypertension without deep vein thrombosis (I87.3-)

     ● **I87.00** Postthrombotic syndrome without complications

> Asymptomatic Postthrombotic syndrome

       I87.001 Postthrombotic syndrome without complications of right lower extremity

       I87.002 Postthrombotic syndrome without complications of left lower extremity

       I87.003 Postthrombotic syndrome without complications of bilateral lower extremity

       I87.009 Postthrombotic syndrome without complications of unspecified extremity

> Postthrombotic syndrome NOS

     ● **I87.01** Postthrombotic syndrome with ulcer

> **Use additional** code to specify site and severity of ulcer (L97.-)

       I87.011 Postthrombotic syndrome with ulcer of right lower extremity

       I87.012 Postthrombotic syndrome with ulcer of left lower extremity

       I87.013 Postthrombotic syndrome with ulcer of bilateral lower extremity

       I87.019 Postthrombotic syndrome with ulcer of unspecified lower extremity

     ● **I87.02** Postthrombotic syndrome with inflammation

       I87.021 Postthrombotic syndrome with inflammation of right lower extremity

       I87.022 Postthrombotic syndrome with inflammation of left lower extremity

       I87.023 Postthrombotic syndrome with inflammation of bilateral lower extremity

       I87.029 Postthrombotic syndrome with inflammation of unspecified lower extremity

     ● **I87.03** Postthrombotic syndrome with ulcer and inflammation

> **Use additional** code to specify site and severity of ulcer (L97.-)

       I87.031 Postthrombotic syndrome with ulcer and inflammation of right lower extremity

I87.032   Postthrombotic syndrome with ulcer and inflammation of left lower extremity ℞

I87.033   Postthrombotic syndrome with ulcer and inflammation of bilateral lower extremity ℞

I87.039   Postthrombotic syndrome with ulcer and inflammation of unspecified lower extremity ℞

● **I87.09   Postthrombotic syndrome with other complications**

I87.091   Postthrombotic syndrome with other complications of right lower extremity

I87.092   Postthrombotic syndrome with other complications of left lower extremity

I87.093   Postthrombotic syndrome with other complications of bilateral lower extremity

I87.099   Postthrombotic syndrome with other complications of unspecified lower extremity

I87.1   Compression of vein
Stricture of vein
Vena cava syndrome (inferior) (superior)

Excludes2   compression of pulmonary vein (I28.8)

Coding Clinic: 2023, Q2, P8

I87.2   Venous insufficiency (chronic) (peripheral)
Stasis dermatitis

Code also, if applicable, associated hypertensive conditions such as:
essential (primary) hypertension (I10)
hypertensive chronic kidney disease (I12.-)
hypertensive heart and chronic kidney disease (I13.-)
hypertensive heart disease (I11.-)

Use Additional code, if applicable, to specify site and severity of ulcer (L97.-)

Excludes1   stasis dermatitis with varicose veins of lower extremities (I83.1-, I83.2-)

Coding Clinic: 2 2025, Q1, P35; 024, Q1, P16

● **I87.3   Chronic venous hypertension (idiopathic)**
Stasis edema

Excludes1   chronic venous hypertension due to deep vein thrombosis (I87.0-)
varicose veins of lower extremities (I83.-)

● **I87.30   Chronic venous hypertension (idiopathic) without complications**
Asymptomatic chronic venous hypertension (idiopathic)

I87.301   Chronic venous hypertension (idiopathic) without complications of right lower extremity

I87.302   Chronic venous hypertension (idiopathic) without complications of left lower extremity

I87.303   Chronic venous hypertension (idiopathic) without complications of bilateral lower extremity

I87.309   Chronic venous hypertension (idiopathic) without complications of unspecified lower extremity
Chronic venous hypertension NOS

● **I87.31   Chronic venous hypertension (idiopathic) with ulcer**

Use additional code to specify site and severity of ulcer (L97.-)

I87.311   Chronic venous hypertension (idiopathic) with ulcer of right lower extremity ℞

I87.312   Chronic venous hypertension (idiopathic) with ulcer of left lower extremity ℞

I87.313   Chronic venous hypertension (idiopathic) with ulcer of bilateral lower extremity ℞

I87.319   Chronic venous hypertension (idiopathic) with ulcer of unspecified lower extremity ℞

● **I87.32   Chronic venous hypertension (idiopathic) with inflammation**

I87.321   Chronic venous hypertension (idiopathic) with inflammation of right lower extremity

I87.322   Chronic venous hypertension (idiopathic) with inflammation of left lower extremity

I87.323   Chronic venous hypertension (idiopathic) with inflammation of bilateral lower extremity

I87.329   Chronic venous hypertension (idiopathic) with inflammation of unspecified lower extremity

● **I87.33   Chronic venous hypertension (idiopathic) with ulcer and inflammation**

Use additional code to specify site and severity of ulcer (L97.-)

I87.331   Chronic venous hypertension (idiopathic) with ulcer and inflammation of right lower extremity ℞

I87.332   Chronic venous hypertension (idiopathic) with ulcer and inflammation of left lower extremity ℞

I87.333   Chronic venous hypertension (idiopathic) with ulcer and inflammation of bilateral lower extremity ℞

I87.339   Chronic venous hypertension (idiopathic) with ulcer and inflammation of unspecified lower extremity ℞

● **I87.39   Chronic venous hypertension (idiopathic) with other complications**

I87.391   Chronic venous hypertension (idiopathic) with other complications of right lower extremity

I87.392   Chronic venous hypertension (idiopathic) with other complications of left lower extremity

I87.393   Chronic venous hypertension (idiopathic) with other complications of bilateral lower extremity

I87.399   Chronic venous hypertension (idiopathic) with other complications of unspecified lower extremity

I87.8   Other specified disorders of veins
Phlebosclerosis
Venofibrosis

I87.9   Disorder of vein, unspecified

● **I88   Nonspecific lymphadenitis**

Excludes1   acute lymphadenitis, except mesenteric (L04.-)
enlarged lymph nodes NOS (R59.-)
human immunodeficiency virus [HIV] disease resulting in generalized lymphadenopathy (B20)

I88.0   Nonspecific mesenteric lymphadenitis
Mesenteric lymphadenitis (acute)(chronic)

I88.1   Chronic lymphadenitis, except mesenteric
Adenitis
Lymphadenitis

I88.8   Other nonspecific lymphadenitis

I88.9   Nonspecific lymphadenitis, unspecified
Lymphadenitis NOS

● **I89 Other noninfective disorders of lymphatic vessels and lymph nodes**

  Excludes1 chylocele, tunica vaginalis (nonfilarial) NOS (N50.89)
     enlarged lymph nodes NOS (R59.-)
     filarial chylocele (B74.-)
     hereditary lymphedema (Q82.0)

 I89.0 Lymphedema, not elsewhere classified
   Elephantiasis (nonfilarial) NOS
   Lymphangiectasis
   Obliteration, lymphatic vessel
   Praecox lymphedema
   Secondary lymphedema

   Excludes1 postmastectomy lymphedema (I97.2)
   Coding Clinic: 2024, Q1, P17

 I89.1 Lymphangitis
   Chronic lymphangitis
   Lymphangitis NOS
   Subacute lymphangitis

   Excludes1 acute lymphangitis (L03.-)

 I89.8 Other specified noninfective disorders of lymphatic vessels and lymph nodes
   Chylocele (nonfilarial)
   Chylous ascites
   Chylous cyst
   Lipomelanotic reticulosis
   Lymph node or vessel fistula
   Lymph node or vessel infarction
   Lymph node or vessel rupture

 I89.9 Noninfective disorder of lymphatic vessels and lymph nodes, unspecified
   Disease of lymphatic vessels NOS

OTHER AND UNSPECIFIED DISORDERS OF THE CIRCULATORY SYSTEM (I95-I99)

● **I95 Hypotension**
 Subnormal arterial blood pressure

  Excludes1 cardiovascular collapse (R57.9)
     maternal hypotension syndrome (O26.5-)
     nonspecific low blood pressure reading NOS (R03.1)

 I95.0 Idiopathic hypotension
 I95.1 Orthostatic hypotension
   Hypotension, postural
   Moving from a sitting or reclining position to a standing position precipitates a sudden drop in blood pressure (hypotension).

   Excludes1 neurogenic orthostatic hypotension [Shy-Drager] (G90.3)
     orthostatic hypotension due to drugs (I95.2)
   Coding Clinic: 2023, Q2, P9

 I95.2 Hypotension due to drugs
   Orthostatic hypotension due to drugs

   Use additional code for adverse effect, if applicable, to identify drug (T36-T50 with fifth or sixth character 5)

 I95.3 Hypotension of hemodialysis
   Intra-dialytic hypotension

 ● **I95.8 Other hypotension**
  I95.81 Postprocedural hypotension
  I95.89 Other hypotension
    Chronic hypotension

 I95.9 Hypotension, unspecified

I96 Gangrene, not elsewhere classified
 Gangrenous cellulitis

  Excludes1 gangrene in atherosclerosis of native arteries of the extremities (I70.26)
     gangrene of certain specified sites - *see* Alphabetical Index
     gangrene in hernia (K40.1, K40.4, K41.1, K41.4, K42.1, K43.1-, K44.1, K45.1, K46.1)
     gangrene in other peripheral vascular diseases (I73.-)
     gas gangrene (A48.0)
     pyoderma gangrenosum (L88)

  Excludes2 gangrene in diabetes mellitus (E08-E13 with .52)
  Coding Clinic: 2018, Q4, P87; 2017, Q3, P6; 2013, Q2, P35

● **I97 Intraoperative and postprocedural complications and disorders of circulatory system, not elsewhere classified**

  Excludes2 postprocedural shock (T81.1-)
  Coding Clinic: 2019, Q2, P22

 I97.0 Postcardiotomy syndrome
 ● **I97.1 Other postprocedural cardiac functional disturbances**

   Excludes2 acute pulmonary insufficiency following thoracic surgery (J95.1)
     intraoperative cardiac functional disturbances (I97.7-)

  ● **I97.11 Postprocedural cardiac insufficiency**
   I97.110 Postprocedural cardiac insufficiency following cardiac surgery
   I97.111 Postprocedural cardiac insufficiency following other surgery

  ● **I97.12 Postprocedural cardiac arrest**
   I97.120 Postprocedural cardiac arrest following cardiac surgery
   I97.121 Postprocedural cardiac arrest following other surgery

  ● **I97.13 Postprocedural heart failure**
   Use additional code to identify the heart failure (I50.-)

   I97.130 Postprocedural heart failure following cardiac surgery
   I97.131 Postprocedural heart failure following other surgery

  ● **I97.19 Other postprocedural cardiac functional disturbances**
   Use additional code, if applicable, to further specify disorder

   I97.190 Other postprocedural cardiac functional disturbances following cardiac surgery
    Use Additional code, if applicable, for type 4 or type 5 myocardial infarction, to further specify disorder
    Coding Clinic: 2019, Q2, P32-33

   I97.191 Other postprocedural cardiac functional disturbances following other surgery

 I97.2 Postmastectomy lymphedema syndrome A
   Elephantiasis due to mastectomy
   Obliteration of lymphatic vessels

 I97.3 Postprocedural hypertension
 ● **I97.4 Intraoperative hemorrhage and hematoma of a circulatory system organ or structure complicating a procedure**

   Excludes1 intraoperative hemorrhage and hematoma of a circulatory system organ or structure due to accidental puncture and laceration during a procedure (I97.5-)

   Excludes2 intraoperative cerebrovascular hemorrhage complicating a procedure (G97.3-)

  ● **I97.41 Intraoperative hemorrhage and hematoma of a circulatory system organ or structure complicating a circulatory system procedure**

   I97.410 Intraoperative hemorrhage and hematoma of a circulatory system organ or structure complicating a cardiac catheterization

   I97.411 Intraoperative hemorrhage and hematoma of a circulatory system organ or structure complicating a cardiac bypass

I97.418   Intraoperative hemorrhage and hematoma of a circulatory system organ or structure complicating other circulatory system procedure

I97.42   Intraoperative hemorrhage and hematoma of a circulatory system organ or structure complicating other procedure
> Coding Clinic: 2020, Q1, P20; 2016, Q4, P100

● **I97.5**   Accidental puncture and laceration of a circulatory system organ or structure during a procedure

> **Excludes2**   accidental puncture and laceration of brain during a procedure (G97.4-)

I97.51   Accidental puncture and laceration of a circulatory system organ or structure during a circulatory system procedure
> Coding Clinic: 2019, Q2, P24

I97.52   Accidental puncture and laceration of a circulatory system organ or structure during other procedure

● **I97.6**   Postprocedural hemorrhage, hematoma and seroma of a circulatory system organ or structure following a procedure

> **Excludes2**   postprocedural cerebrovascular hemorrhage complicating a procedure (G97.5-)

> Coding Clinic: 2016, Q4, P10

● **I97.61**   Postprocedural hemorrhage of a circulatory system organ or structure following a circulatory system procedure

I97.610   Postprocedural hemorrhage of a circulatory system organ or structure following a cardiac catheterization

I97.611   Postprocedural hemorrhage of a circulatory system organ or structure following cardiac bypass

I97.618   Postprocedural hemorrhage of a circulatory system organ or structure following other circulatory system procedure

● **I97.62**   Postprocedural hemorrhage, hematoma and seroma of a circulatory system organ or structure following other procedure

I97.620   Postprocedural hemorrhage of a circulatory system organ or structure following other procedure

I97.621   Postprocedural hematoma of a circulatory system organ or structure following other procedure

I97.622   Postprocedural seroma of a circulatory system organ or structure following other procedure

● **I97.63**   Postprocedural hematoma of a circulatory system organ or structure following a circulatory system procedure

I97.630   Postprocedural hematoma of a circulatory system organ or structure following a cardiac catheterization

I97.631   Postprocedural hematoma of a circulatory system organ or structure following cardiac bypass

I97.638   Postprocedural hematoma of a circulatory system organ or structure following other circulatory system procedure

● **I97.64**   Postprocedural seroma of a circulatory system organ or structure following a circulatory system procedure

I97.640   Postprocedural seroma of a circulatory system organ or structure following a cardiac catheterization

I97.641   Postprocedural seroma of a circulatory system organ or structure following cardiac bypass

I97.648   Postprocedural seroma of a circulatory system organ or structure following other circulatory system procedure

● **I97.7**   Intraoperative cardiac functional disturbances

> **Excludes2**   acute pulmonary insufficiency following thoracic surgery (J95.1)
> postprocedural cardiac functional disturbances (I97.1-)

● **I97.71**   Intraoperative cardiac arrest

I97.710   Intraoperative cardiac arrest during cardiac surgery

I97.711   Intraoperative cardiac arrest during other surgery

● **I97.79**   Other intraoperative cardiac functional disturbances
> Use additional code, if applicable, to further specify disorder

I97.790   Other intraoperative cardiac functional disturbances during cardiac surgery

I97.791   Other intraoperative cardiac functional disturbances during other surgery

● **I97.8**   Other intraoperative and postprocedural complications and disorders of the circulatory system, not elsewhere classified
> Use additional code, if applicable, to further specify disorder

● **I97.81**   Intraoperative cerebrovascular infarction

I97.810   Intraoperative cerebrovascular infarction during cardiac surgery

I97.811   Intraoperative cerebrovascular infarction during other surgery

● **I97.82**   Postprocedural cerebrovascular infarction

I97.820   Postprocedural cerebrovascular infarction following cardiac surgery

I97.821   Postprocedural cerebrovascular infarction following other surgery

I97.88   Other intraoperative complications of the circulatory system, not elsewhere classified

I97.89   Other postprocedural complications and disorders of the circulatory system, not elsewhere classified
> Coding Clinic: 2025, Q2, P5-6; 2024, Q1, P26; 2019, Q2, P32-33

● **I99**   Other and unspecified disorders of circulatory system

I99.8   Other disorder of circulatory system

I99.9   Unspecified disorder of circulatory system

CHAPTER 10

DISEASES OF THE RESPIRATORY SYSTEM (J00-J99)

OGCR Chapter-Specific Coding Guidelines

10. **Chapter 10: Diseases of the Respiratory System (J00-J99)**

a. **Chronic Obstructive Pulmonary Disease [COPD] and Asthma**

1) **Acute exacerbation of chronic obstructive bronchitis and asthma**

The codes in categories J44 and J45 distinguish between uncomplicated cases and those in acute exacerbation. An acute exacerbation is a worsening or a decompensation of a chronic condition. An acute exacerbation is not equivalent to an infection superimposed on a chronic condition, though an exacerbation may be triggered by an infection.

b. **Acute Respiratory Failure**

1) **Acute respiratory failure as principal diagnosis**

A code from subcategory J96.0, Acute respiratory failure, or subcategory J96.2, Acute and chronic respiratory failure, may be assigned as a principal diagnosis when it is the condition established after study to be chiefly responsible for occasioning the admission to the hospital, and the selection is supported by the Alphabetic Index and Tabular List. However, chapter-specific coding guidelines (such as obstetrics, poisoning, HIV, newborn) that provide sequencing direction take precedence.

2) **Acute respiratory failure as secondary diagnosis**

Respiratory failure may be listed as a secondary diagnosis if it occurs after admission, or if it is present on admission, but does not meet the definition of principal diagnosis.

3) **Sequencing of acute respiratory failure and another acute condition**

When a patient is admitted with respiratory failure and another acute condition (e.g., myocardial infarction, cerebrovascular accident, aspiration pneumonia), the principal diagnosis will not be the same in every situation. This applies whether the other acute condition is a respiratory or nonrespiratory condition. Selection of the principal diagnosis will be dependent on the circumstances of admission. If both the respiratory failure and the other acute condition are equally responsible for occasioning the admission to the hospital, and there are no chapter-specific sequencing rules, the guideline regarding two or more diagnoses that equally meet the definition for principal diagnosis (*Section II, C.*) may be applied in these situations.

If the documentation is not clear as to whether acute respiratory failure and another condition are equally responsible for occasioning the admission, query the provider for clarification.

c. **Influenza due to certain identified influenza viruses**

Code only confirmed cases of influenza due to certain identified influenza viruses (category J09), and due to other identified influenza virus (category J10). This is an exception to the hospital inpatient guideline Section II, H. (Uncertain Diagnosis).

In this context, "confirmation" does not require documentation of positive laboratory testing specific for avian or other novel influenza A or other identified influenza virus. However, coding should be based on the provider's diagnostic statement that the patient has avian influenza, or other novel influenza A, for category J09, or has another particular identified strain of influenza, such as H1N1 or H3N2, but not identified as novel or variant, for category J10.

If the provider records "suspected" or "possible" or "probable" avian influenza, or novel influenza, or other identified influenza, then the appropriate influenza code from category J11, Influenza due to unidentified influenza virus, should be assigned. A code from category J09, Influenza due to certain identified influenza viruses, should not be assigned nor should a code from category J10, Influenza due to other identified influenza virus.

d. **Ventilator associated Pneumonia**

1) **Documentation of Ventilator associated Pneumonia**

As with all procedural or postprocedural complications, code assignment is based on the provider's documentation of the relationship between the condition and the procedure.

Code J95.851, Ventilator associated pneumonia, should be assigned only when the provider has documented ventilator associated pneumonia (VAP). An additional code to identify the organism (e.g., Pseudomonas aeruginosa, code B96.5) should also be assigned. Do not assign an additional code from categories J12-J18 to identify the type of pneumonia.

Code J95.851 should not be assigned for cases where the patient has pneumonia and is on a mechanical ventilator and the provider has not specifically stated that the pneumonia is ventilator associated pneumonia. If the documentation is unclear as to whether the patient has a pneumonia that is a complication attributable to the mechanical ventilator, query the provider.

2) **Ventilator associated Pneumonia Develops after Admission**

A patient may be admitted with one type of pneumonia (e.g., code J13, Pneumonia due to Streptococcus pneumonia) and subsequently develop VAP. In this instance, the principal diagnosis would be the appropriate code from categories J12-J18 for the pneumonia diagnosed at the time of admission. Code J95.851, Ventilator associated pneumonia, would be assigned as an additional diagnosis when the provider has also documented the presence of ventilator associated pneumonia.

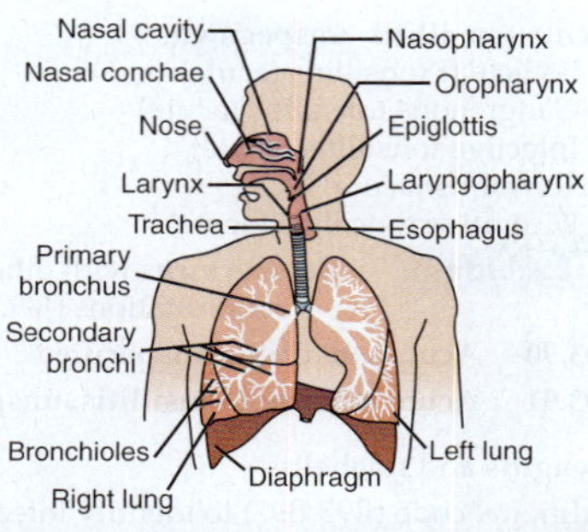

Figure 10-1 Respiratory system. (From Buck CJ: Step-by-Step Medical Coding, ed 2016, St. Louis, Elsevier, 2016)

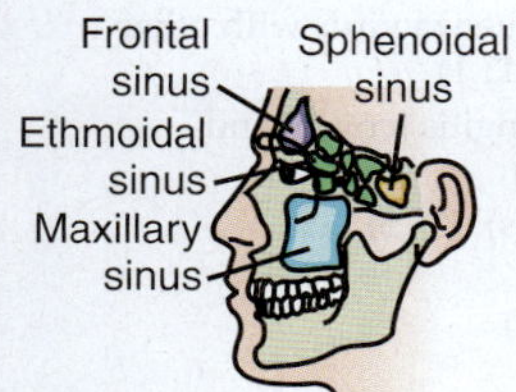

Figure 10-2 Paranasal sinuses. (From Buck CJ: Step-by-Step Medical Coding, ed 2016, St. Louis, Elsevier, 2016)

Item 10–1 Pharyngitis is painful inflammation of the pharynx (sore throat). Ninety percent of the infections are caused by a virus with the remaining being bacterial and rarely a fungus (candidiasis). Other irritants such as pollutants, chemicals, or smoke may cause similar symptoms.

CHAPTER 10

DISEASES OF THE RESPIRATORY SYSTEM (J00-J99)

Note: When a respiratory condition is described as occurring in more than one site and is not specifically indexed, it should be classified to the lower anatomic site (e.g., tracheobronchitis to bronchitis in J40).

Use additional code, where applicable, to identify:
exposure to environmental tobacco smoke (Z77.22)
exposure to tobacco smoke in the perinatal period (P96.81)
history of tobacco dependence (Z87.891)
occupational exposure to environmental tobacco smoke (Z57.31)
tobacco dependence (F17.-)
tobacco use (Z72.0)

Excludes2 certain conditions originating in the perinatal period (P04-P96)
certain infectious and parasitic diseases (A00-B99)
complications of pregnancy, childbirth and the puerperium (O00-O99A)
congenital malformations, deformations and chromosomal abnormalities (Q00-Q99)
endocrine, nutritional and metabolic diseases (E00-E88)
injury, poisoning and certain other consequences of external causes (S00-T88)
neoplasms (C00-D49)
smoke inhalation (T59.81-)
symptoms, signs and abnormal clinical and laboratory findings, not elsewhere classified (R00-R94)

This chapter contains the following blocks:

J00-J06	Acute upper respiratory infections
J09-J18	Influenza and pneumonia
J20-J22	Other acute lower respiratory infections
J30-J39	Other diseases of upper respiratory tract
J40-J4A	Chronic lower respiratory diseases
J60-J70	Lung diseases due to external agents
J80-J84	Other respiratory diseases principally affecting the interstitium
J85-J86	Suppurative and necrotic conditions of the lower respiratory tract
J90-J94	Other diseases of the pleura
J95	Intraoperative and postprocedural complications and disorders of respiratory system, not elsewhere classified
J96-J99	Other diseases of the respiratory system

ACUTE UPPER RESPIRATORY INFECTIONS (J00-J06)

Use Additional code, if applicable, to identify resistance to antimicrobial drugs (Z16.-)

Excludes1 chronic obstructive pulmonary disease with acute lower respiratory infection (J44.0)

J00 Acute nasopharyngitis [common cold]
Acute rhinitis
Coryza (acute)
Infective nasopharyngitis NOS
Infective rhinitis
Nasal catarrh, acute
Nasopharyngitis NOS

Excludes1 acute pharyngitis (J02.-)
acute sore throat NOS (J02.9)
influenza virus with other respiratory manifestations (J09.X2, J10.1, J11.1)
pharyngitis NOS (J02.9)
rhinitis NOS (J31.0)
sore throat NOS (J02.9)

Excludes2 allergic rhinitis (J30.1-J30.9)
chronic pharyngitis (J31.2)
chronic rhinitis (J31.0)
chronic sore throat (J31.2)
nasopharyngitis, chronic (J31.1)
vasomotor rhinitis (J30.0)

★ **(See Plate 27 of the Anatomy Illustrations.)**

● **J01 Acute sinusitis**
Includes acute abscess of sinus
acute empyema of sinus
acute infection of sinus
acute inflammation of sinus
acute suppuration of sinus

Use additional code (B95-B97) to identify infectious agent.

Excludes1 sinusitis NOS (J32.9)
Excludes2 chronic sinusitis (J32.0-J32.8)

● **J01.0 Acute maxillary sinusitis**
Acute antritis

   J01.00 Acute maxillary sinusitis, unspecified
   J01.01 Acute recurrent maxillary sinusitis

● **J01.1 Acute frontal sinusitis**
   J01.10 Acute frontal sinusitis, unspecified
   J01.11 Acute recurrent frontal sinusitis

● **J01.2 Acute ethmoidal sinusitis**
   J01.20 Acute ethmoidal sinusitis, unspecified
   J01.21 Acute recurrent ethmoidal sinusitis

● **J01.3 Acute sphenoidal sinusitis**
   J01.30 Acute sphenoidal sinusitis, unspecified
   J01.31 Acute recurrent sphenoidal sinusitis

● **J01.4 Acute pansinusitis**
   J01.40 Acute pansinusitis, unspecified
   J01.41 Acute recurrent pansinusitis

● **J01.8**   **Other acute sinusitis**
    J01.80   **Other acute sinusitis**
        Acute sinusitis involving more than one sinus but not pansinusitis
    J01.81   **Other acute recurrent sinusitis**
        Acute recurrent sinusitis involving more than one sinus but not pansinusitis
● **J01.9**   **Acute sinusitis, unspecified**
    J01.90   **Acute sinusitis, unspecified**
    J01.91   **Acute recurrent sinusitis, unspecified**

● **J02**   **Acute pharyngitis**
    Includes   acute sore throat
    Excludes1   acute laryngopharyngitis (J06.0)
        peritonsillar abscess (J36)
        pharyngeal abscess (J39.1)
        retropharyngeal abscess (J39.0)
    Excludes2   chronic pharyngitis (J31.2)
    J02.0   **Streptococcal pharyngitis**
        Septic pharyngitis
        Streptococcal sore throat
        Excludes2   scarlet fever (A38.-)
    J02.8   **Acute pharyngitis due to other specified organisms**
        Use additional code (B95-B97) to identify infectious agent
        Excludes1   pharyngitis due to coxsackie virus (B08.5)
            pharyngitis due to gonococcus (A54.5)
            acute pharyngitis due to herpes [simplex] virus (B00.2)
            acute pharyngitis due to infectious mononucleosis (B27.-)
            enteroviral vesicular pharyngitis (B08.5)
    J02.9   **Acute pharyngitis, unspecified**
        Gangrenous pharyngitis (acute)
        Infective pharyngitis (acute) NOS
        Pharyngitis (acute) NOS
        Sore throat (acute) NOS
        Suppurative pharyngitis (acute)
        Ulcerative pharyngitis (acute)
        Excludes1   influenza virus with other respiratory manifestations (J09.X2, J10.1, J11.1)

● **J03**   **Acute tonsillitis**
    Inflammation of pharyngeal tonsils caused by virus or bacteria
    Excludes1   acute sore throat (J02.-)
        hypertrophy of tonsils (J35.1)
        peritonsillar abscess (J36)
        sore throat NOS (J02.9)
        streptococcal sore throat (J02.0)
    Excludes2   chronic tonsillitis (J35.0)
    J03.0   **Streptococcal tonsillitis**
        J03.00   **Acute streptococcal tonsillitis, unspecified**
        J03.01   **Acute recurrent streptococcal tonsillitis**
    J03.8   **Acute tonsillitis due to other specified organisms**
        Use additional code (B95-B97) to identify infectious agent.
        Excludes1   diphtheritic tonsillitis (A36.0)
            herpesviral pharyngotonsillitis (B00.2)
            streptococcal tonsillitis (J03.0)
            tuberculous tonsillitis (A15.8)
            Vincent's tonsillitis (A69.1)
        J03.80   **Acute tonsillitis due to other specified organisms**
        J03.81   **Acute recurrent tonsillitis due to other specified organisms**

● **J03.9**   **Acute tonsillitis, unspecified**
    Follicular tonsillitis (acute)
    Gangrenous tonsillitis (acute)
    Infective tonsillitis (acute)
    Tonsillitis (acute) NOS
    Ulcerative tonsillitis (acute)
    Excludes1   influenza virus with other respiratory manifestations (J09.X2, J10.1, J11.1)
    J03.90   **Acute tonsillitis, unspecified**
    J03.91   **Acute recurrent tonsillitis, unspecified**

● **J04**   **Acute laryngitis and tracheitis**
    Use additional code (B95-B97) to identify infectious agent.
    Code also influenza, if present, such as:
        influenza due to identified novel influenza A virus with other respiratory manifestations (J09.X2)
        influenza due to other identified influenza virus with other respiratory manifestations (J10.1)
        influenza due to unidentified influenza virus with other respiratory manifestations (J11.1)
    Excludes1   acute obstructive laryngitis [croup] and epiglottitis (J05.-)
    Excludes2   laryngismus (stridulus) (J38.5)
    J04.0   **Acute laryngitis**
        Edematous laryngitis (acute)
        Laryngitis (acute) NOS
        Subglottic laryngitis (acute)
        Suppurative laryngitis (acute)
        Ulcerative laryngitis (acute)
        Excludes1   acute obstructive laryngitis (J05.0)
        Excludes2   chronic laryngitis (J37.0)
●   **J04.1**   **Acute tracheitis**
        Acute viral tracheitis
        Catarrhal tracheitis (acute)
        Tracheitis (acute) NOS
        Excludes2   chronic tracheitis (J42)
        J04.10   **Acute tracheitis without obstruction**
        J04.11   **Acute tracheitis with obstruction**
    J04.2   **Acute laryngotracheitis**
        Laryngotracheitis NOS
        Tracheitis (acute) with laryngitis (acute)
        Excludes1   acute obstructive laryngotracheitis (J05.0)
        Excludes2   chronic laryngotracheitis (J37.1)
●   **J04.3**   **Supraglottitis, unspecified**
        J04.30   **Supraglottitis, unspecified, without obstruction**
        J04.31   **Supraglottitis, unspecified, with obstruction**

● **J05**   **Acute obstructive laryngitis [croup] and epiglottitis**
    Use additional code (B95-B97) to identify infectious agent.
    Code also influenza, if present, such as:
        influenza due to identified novel influenza A virus with other respiratory manifestations (J09.X2)
        influenza due to other identified influenza virus with other respiratory manifestations (J10.1)
        influenza due to unidentified influenza virus with other respiratory manifestations (J11.1)
    J05.0   **Acute obstructive laryngitis [croup]**
        Obstructive laryngitis (acute) NOS
        Obstructive laryngotracheitis NOS
●   **J05.1**   **Acute epiglottitis**
        Excludes2   epiglottitis, chronic (J37.0)
        J05.10   **Acute epiglottitis without obstruction**
            Epiglottitis NOS
        J05.11   **Acute epiglottitis with obstruction**

Item 10–2   **Laryngitis** is an inflammation of the larynx (voice box) resulting in hoarse voice or the complete loss of the voice. **Tracheitis** is an inflammation of the trachea (often following a URI) commonly caused by *staphylococcus aureus* resulting in inspiratory stridor (crowing sound on inspiration) and a crouplike cough.

● **J06**   **Acute upper respiratory infections of multiple and unspecified sites**

    Excludes1   acute respiratory infection NOS (J22)
         influenza virus with other respiratory
           manifestations (J09.X2, J10.1, J11.1)
         streptococcal pharyngitis (J02.0)

    Coding Clinic: 2020, Q1, P22

  J06.0   **Acute laryngopharyngitis**

  J06.9   **Acute upper respiratory infection, unspecified**
      Upper respiratory disease, acute
      Upper respiratory infection NOS

      Use additional code (B95-B97) to identify infectious
        agent, if known, such as:
        respiratory syncytial virus (RSV) (B97.4)

INFLUENZA AND PNEUMONIA (J09-J18)

    Excludes2   allergic or eosinophilic pneumonia (J82)
         aspiration pneumonia NOS (J69.0)
         meconium pneumonia (P24.01)
         neonatal aspiration pneumonia (P24.-)
         pneumonia due to solids and liquids (J69.-)
         congenital pneumonia (P23.9)
         lipid pneumonia (J69.1)
         rheumatic pneumonia (I00)
         ventilator associated pneumonia (J95.851)

    Coding Clinic: 2020, Q1, P22

● **J09**   **Influenza due to certain identified influenza viruses**

    Excludes1   influenza A/H1N1 (J10.-)
         influenza due to other influenza viruses (J10.-)
         influenza due to unidentified influenza virus
           (J11.-)
         seasonal influenza due to other identified
           influenza virus (J10.-)
         seasonal influenza due to unidentified influenza
           virus (J11.-)

● **J09.X**   **Influenza due to identified novel influenza A virus**
      Avian influenza
      Bird influenza
      Influenza A/H5N1
      Influenza of other animal origin, not bird or swine
      Swine influenza virus (viruses that normally cause
        infections in pigs)

    Coding Clinic: 2016, Q3, P11

  J09.X1   **Influenza due to identified novel influenza A virus with pneumonia**

      Code also , if applicable, associated:
        lung abscess (J85.1)
        other specified type of pneumonia

  J09.X2   **Influenza due to identified novel influenza A virus with other respiratory manifestations**
      Influenza due to identified novel influenza A
        virus NOS
      Influenza due to identified novel influenza A
        virus with laryngitis
      Influenza due to identified novel influenza A
        virus with pharyngitis
      Influenza due to identified novel influenza A
        virus with upper respiratory symptoms

      Use additional code, if applicable, for
        associated:
        pleural effusion (J91.8)
        sinusitis (J01.-)

  J09.X3   **Influenza due to identified novel influenza A virus with gastrointestinal manifestations**
      Influenza due to identified novel influenza A
        virus gastroenteritis

      Excludes1   'intestinal flu' [viral
          gastroenteritis] (A08.-)

  J09.X9   **Influenza due to identified novel influenza A virus with other manifestations**
      Influenza due to identified novel influenza A
        virus with encephalopathy
      Influenza due to identified novel influenza A
        virus with myocarditis
      Influenza due to identified novel influenza A
        virus with otitis media

      Use additional code to identify manifestation

● **J10**   **Influenza due to other identified influenza virus**

    Includes   influenza A (non-novel)
         influenza B
         influenza C

    Excludes1   influenza due to avian influenza virus (J09.X-)
         influenza due to swine flu (J09.X-)
         influenza due to unidentified influenza virus
           (J11.-)

● **J10.0**   **Influenza due to other identified influenza virus with pneumonia**

      Code also associated lung abscess, if applicable (J85.1)

  J10.00   **Influenza due to other identified influenza virus with unspecified type of pneumonia**

  J10.01   **Influenza due to other identified influenza virus with the same other identified influenza virus pneumonia**

  J10.08   **Influenza due to other identified influenza virus with other specified pneumonia**

      Code also other specified type of pneumonia
      Coding Clinic: 2017, Q4, P96

  J10.1   **Influenza due to other identified influenza virus with other respiratory manifestations**
      Influenza due to other identified influenza virus NOS
      Influenza due to other identified influenza virus with
        laryngitis
      Influenza due to other identified influenza virus with
        pharyngitis
      Influenza due to other identified influenza virus with
        upper respiratory symptoms

      Use additional code for associated pleural effusion, if
        applicable (J91.8)
      Use additional code for associated sinusitis, if
        applicable (J01.-)
      Coding Clinic: 2016, Q3, P11

  J10.2   **Influenza due to other identified influenza virus with gastrointestinal manifestations**
      Influenza due to other identified influenza virus
        gastroenteritis

      Excludes1   'intestinal flu' [viral gastroenteritis]
         (A08.-)

● **J10.8**   **Influenza due to other identified influenza virus with other manifestations**

  J10.81   **Influenza due to other identified influenza virus with encephalopathy**

  J10.82   **Influenza due to other identified influenza virus with myocarditis**

  J10.83   **Influenza due to other identified influenza virus with otitis media**

      Use additional code for any associated
        perforated tympanic membrane (H72.-)

  J10.89   **Influenza due to other identified influenza virus with other manifestations**

      Use additional codes to identify the
        manifestations

● **J11**   **Influenza due to unidentified influenza virus**

● **J11.0**   **Influenza due to unidentified influenza virus with pneumonia**

      Code also associated lung abscess, if applicable (J85.1)

CHAPTER 10 (J00-J99)

J11.00 **Influenza due to unidentified influenza virus with unspecified type of pneumonia**
Influenza with pneumonia NOS
Coding Clinic: 2016, Q3, P12

J11.08 **Influenza due to unidentified influenza virus with specified pneumonia**
Code also other specified type of pneumonia

J11.1 **Influenza due to unidentified influenza virus with other respiratory manifestations**
Influenza NOS
Influenzal laryngitis NOS
Influenzal pharyngitis NOS
Influenza with upper respiratory symptoms NOS
Use additional code for associated pleural effusion, if applicable (J91.8)
Use additional code for associated sinusitis, if applicable (J01.-)

J11.2 **Influenza due to unidentified influenza virus with gastrointestinal manifestations**
Influenza gastroenteritis NOS
Excludes1 'intestinal flu' [viral gastroenteritis] (A08.-)

● **J11.8** **Influenza due to unidentified influenza virus with other manifestations**

J11.81 **Influenza due to unidentified influenza virus with encephalopathy**
Influenzal encephalopathy NOS

J11.82 **Influenza due to unidentified influenza virus with myocarditis**
Influenzal myocarditis NOS

J11.83 **Influenza due to unidentified influenza virus with otitis media**
Influenzal otitis media NOS
Use additional code for any associated perforated tympanic membrane (H72.-)

J11.89 **Influenza due to unidentified influenza virus with other manifestations**
Use additional codes to identify the manifestations

● **J12** **Viral pneumonia, not elsewhere classified**
Includes bronchopneumonia due to viruses other than influenza viruses
Code first associated influenza, if applicable (J09.X1, J10.0-, J11.0-)
Code also associated abscess, if applicable (J85.1)
Excludes2 aspiration pneumonia due to anesthesia during labor and delivery (O74.0)
aspiration pneumonia due to anesthesia during pregnancy (O29)
aspiration pneumonia due to anesthesia during puerperium (O89.0)
aspiration pneumonia due to solids and liquids (J69.-)
aspiration pneumonia NOS (J69.0)
congenital pneumonia (P23.0)
congenital rubella pneumonitis (P35.0)
interstitial pneumonia NOS (J84.9)
lipid pneumonia (J69.1)
neonatal aspiration pneumonia (P24.-)
Coding Clinic: 2021, Q1, P34

J12.0 **Adenoviral pneumonia**
J12.1 **Respiratory syncytial virus pneumonia**
RSV pneumonia
J12.2 **Parainfluenza virus pneumonia**
J12.3 **Human metapneumovirus pneumonia**
● **J12.8** **Other viral pneumonia**

J12.81 **Pneumonia due to SARS-associated coronavirus**
Severe acute respiratory syndrome NOS

J12.82 **Pneumonia due to coronavirus disease 2019**
Pneumonia due to 2019 novel coronavirus (SARS-CoV-2)
Pneumonia due to COVID-19
Code first COVID-19 (U07.1)
Coding Clinic: 2021, Q1, P33-34, 42, 47, 49

J12.89 **Other viral pneumonia**
Coding Clinic: 2021, Q1, P33-34

J12.9 **Viral pneumonia, unspecified**
J13 **Pneumonia due to Streptococcus pneumoniae** 🅰
Bronchopneumonia due to S. pneumoniae
Code first, if applicable, associated influenza, if applicable (J09.X1, J10.0-, J11.0-)
Code also, if applicable, any associated condition such as: abscess (J85.1)
aspiration pneumonia (J69.-)
Excludes1 congenital pneumonia due to S. pneumoniae (P23.6)
lobar pneumonia, unspecified organism (J18.1)
pneumonia due to other streptococci (J15.3-J15.4)

J14 **Pneumonia due to Hemophilus influenzae** 🅰
Bronchopneumonia due to H. influenzae
Code first, if applicable, associated influenza, if applicable (J09.X1, J10.0-, J11.0-)
Code also, if applicable, any associated condition such as: abscess (J85.1)
aspiration pneumonia (J69.-)
Excludes1 congenital pneumonia due to H. influenzae (P23.6)

● **J15** **Bacterial pneumonia, not elsewhere classified**
Includes bronchopneumonia due to bacteria other than S. pneumoniae and H. influenzae
Code first, if applicable, associated influenza, if applicable (J09.X1, J10.0-, J11.0-)
Code also, if applicable, any associated condition such as: abscess (J85.1)
aspiration pneumonia (J69.-)
Excludes1 chlamydial pneumonia (J16.0)
congenital pneumonia (P23.-)
Legionnaires' disease (A48.1)
spirochetal pneumonia (A69.8)

J15.0 **Pneumonia due to Klebsiella pneumoniae** 🅰
J15.1 **Pneumonia due to Pseudomonas** 🅰
● **J15.2** **Pneumonia due to staphylococcus**

J15.20 **Pneumonia due to staphylococcus, unspecified** 🅰

● **J15.21** **Pneumonia due to staphylococcus aureus**

J15.211 **Pneumonia due to Methicillin susceptible Staphylococcus aureus** 🅰
MSSA pneumonia
Pneumonia due to Staphylococcus aureus NOS

J15.212 **Pneumonia due to Methicillin resistant Staphylococcus aureus** 🅰

J15.29 **Pneumonia due to other staphylococcus** 🅰

Item 10–3 Pneumonia is an infection of the lungs, caused by a variety of microorganisms, including viruses, most commonly the Streptococcus pneumoniae (pneumococcus) bacteria, fungi, and parasites. Pneumonia occurs when the immune system is weakened, often by a URI or influenza.

▶ New   ⇒ Revised   ~~deleted~~ Deleted   Excludes 1   Excludes 2   Includes   Use additional   Code first   Code also   Key words
OGCR Official Guidelines   **X** Assign placeholder X   ● Use Additional Character(s)   ▸ Manifestation Code   🅰 Hierarchical Condition Category   **Coding Clinic**

J15.3   Pneumonia due to **streptococcus, group B** 🦠

J15.4   Pneumonia due to **other streptococci** 🦠

> **Excludes1**   pneumonia due to streptococcus, group B (J15.3)
> pneumonia due to Streptococcus pneumoniae (J13)

J15.5   Pneumonia due to **Escherichia coli** 🦠

● **J15.6**   Pneumonia due to **other Gram-negative bacteria** 🦠

J15.61   Pneumonia due to Acinetobacter baumannii

J15.69   Pneumonia due to other Gram-negative bacteria
> Pneumonia due to other aerobic Gram-negative bacteria
> Pneumonia due to Serratia marcescens

J15.7   Pneumonia due to **Mycoplasma pneumoniae**

J15.8   Pneumonia due to **other specified bacteria** 🦠

J15.9   **Unspecified bacterial pneumonia**
> Pneumonia due to gram-positive bacteria
> **Coding Clinic: 2017, Q4, P96**

● **J16**   **Pneumonia due to other infectious organisms, not elsewhere classified**

> *Code first*, if applicable, associated influenza, if applicable (J09.X1, J10.0-, J11.0-)

> Code also, if applicable, any associated condition such as:
> abscess (J85.1)
> aspiration pneumonia (J69.-)

> **Excludes1**   congenital pneumonia (P23.-)
> ornithosis (A70)
> pneumocystosis (B59)
> pneumonia NOS (J18.9)

J16.0   **Chlamydial pneumonia**

J16.8   Pneumonia due to **other specified infectious organisms**

▷ *J17*   *Pneumonia in diseases classified elsewhere*

> *Code first underlying disease, such as:*
> Q fever (A78)
> rheumatic fever (I00)
> schistosomiasis (B65.0-B65.9)

> Code also, if applicable, any associated condition such as:
> abscess (J85.1)
> aspiration pneumonia (J69.-)

> **Excludes1**   candidial pneumonia (B37.1)
> chlamydial pneumonia (J16.0)
> gonorrheal pneumonia (A54.84)
> histoplasmosis pneumonia (B39.0-B39.2)
> measles pneumonia (B05.2)
> nocardiosis pneumonia (A43.0)
> pneumocystosis (B59)
> pneumonia due to Pneumocystis carinii (B59)
> pneumonia due to Pneumocystis jiroveci (B59)
> pneumonia in actinomycosis (A42.0)
> pneumonia in anthrax (A22.1)
> pneumonia in ascariasis (B77.81)
> pneumonia in aspergillosis (B44.0-B44.1)
> pneumonia in coccidioidomycosis (B38.0-B38.2)
> pneumonia in cytomegalovirus disease (B25.0)
> pneumonia in toxoplasmosis (B58.3)
> rubella pneumonia (B06.81)
> salmonella pneumonia (A02.22)
> spirochetal infection NEC with pneumonia (A69.8)
> tularemia pneumonia (A21.2)
> typhoid fever with pneumonia (A01.03)
> varicella pneumonia (B01.2)
> whooping cough with pneumonia (A37 with fifth-character 1)

● **J18**   **Pneumonia, unspecified organism**

> *Code first, if applicable, associated influenza, if applicable (J09.X1, J10.0-, J11.0-)*

> Code also, if applicable, any associated condition such as:
> aspiration pneumonia (J69.-)

> **Excludes1**   congenital pneumonia (P23.0)
> drug-induced interstitial lung disorder (J70.2-J70.4)
> interstitial pneumonia NOS (J84.9)
> neonatal aspiration pneumonia (P24.-)
> pneumonitis due to fumes and vapors (J68.0)
> usual interstitial pneumonia (J84.178)

> **Excludes2**   abscess of lung with pneumonia (J85.1)
> aspiration pneumonia due to anesthesia during labor and delivery (O74.0)
> aspiration pneumonia due to anesthesia during pregnancy (O29)
> aspiration pneumonia due to anesthesia during puerperium (O89.0)
> aspiration pneumonia due to solids and liquids (J69.-)
> aspiration pneumonia NOS (J69.0)
> lipid pneumonia (J69.1)
> pneumonitis due to external agents (J67-J70)

J18.0   **Bronchopneumonia, unspecified organism**

> **Excludes1**   hypostatic bronchopneumonia (J18.2)
> lipid pneumonia (J69.1)

> **Excludes2**   acute bronchiolitis (J21.-)
> chronic bronchiolitis (J44.89)
> other specified chronic obstructive pulmonary disease (J44.89)

J18.1   **Lobar pneumonia, unspecified organism** 🦠
> **Coding Clinic: 2016, Q3, P15**

J18.2   **Hypostatic pneumonia, unspecified organism**
> Hypostatic bronchopneumonia
> Passive pneumonia

J18.8   **Other pneumonia, unspecified organism**

J18.9   **Pneumonia, unspecified organism**
> **Coding Clinic: Q3, P15; 2019, Q2, P28; Q1, P36; 2016, Q3, P15; 2012, Q4, P94**

OTHER ACUTE LOWER RESPIRATORY INFECTIONS (J20-J22)

> **Excludes2**   chronic obstructive pulmonary disease with acute lower respiratory infection (J44.0)

● **J20**   **Acute bronchitis**
> *Inflammation/irritation of the bronchial tubes lasting 2-3 weeks, most commonly caused by a virus*

> **Includes**   acute and subacute bronchitis (with) bronchospasm
> acute and subacute bronchitis (with) tracheitis
> acute and subacute bronchitis (with) tracheobronchitis, acute
> acute and subacute fibrinous bronchitis
> acute and subacute membranous bronchitis
> acute and subacute purulent bronchitis
> acute and subacute septic bronchitis

> **Excludes1**   bronchitis NOS (J40)
> tracheobronchitis NOS (J40)

> **Excludes2**   acute bronchitis with bronchiectasis (J47.0)
> acute bronchitis with chronic obstructive asthma (J44.0)
> acute bronchitis with chronic obstructive pulmonary disease (J44.0)
> allergic bronchitis NOS (J45.909)
> bronchitis due to chemicals, fumes and vapors (J68.0)
> chronic bronchitis NOS (J42)
> chronic mucopurulent bronchitis (J41.1)
> chronic obstructive bronchitis (J44.-)
> chronic obstructive tracheobronchitis (J44.-)
> chronic simple bronchitis (J41.0)
> chronic tracheobronchitis (J42)

J20.0   **Acute bronchitis due to Mycoplasma pneumoniae**

J20.1   **Acute bronchitis due to Hemophilus influenzae**

J20.2   **Acute bronchitis due to streptococcus**

CHAPTER 10 (J00–J99)

J20.3	**Acute bronchitis due to coxsackievirus**
J20.4	**Acute bronchitis due to parainfluenza virus**
J20.5	**Acute bronchitis due to respiratory syncytial virus**
	Acute bronchitis due to RSV
J20.6	**Acute bronchitis due to rhinovirus**
	Coding Clinic: 2016, Q3, P10
J20.7	**Acute bronchitis due to echovirus**
J20.8	**Acute bronchitis due to other specified organisms**
	Coding Clinic: 2016, Q3, P11
J20.9	**Acute bronchitis, unspecified**
	Coding Clinic: 2019, Q1, P35; 2016, Q3, P16

● **J21**   **Acute bronchiolitis**

Bronchiolitis obliterans with organizing pneumonia (BOOP) inflammation of bronchioles and surrounding tissue in lung

Includes   acute bronchiolitis with bronchospasm

Excludes2   respiratory bronchiolitis interstitial lung disease (J84.115)

J21.0	**Acute bronchiolitis due to respiratory syncytial virus**
	Acute bronchitis due to RSV
J21.1	**Acute bronchiolitis due to human metapneumovirus**
J21.8	**Acute bronchiolitis due to other specified organisms**
J21.9	**Acute bronchiolitis, unspecified**
	Bronchiolitis (acute)

Excludes1   chronic bronchiolitis (J44.89)

J22   **Unspecified acute lower respiratory infection**

Acute (lower) respiratory (tract) infection NOS

Excludes1   upper respiratory infection (acute) (J06.9)

Coding Clinic: 2020, Q1, P22-23

OTHER DISEASES OF UPPER RESPIRATORY TRACT (J30-J39)

● **J30**   **Vasomotor and allergic rhinitis**

Includes   spasmodic rhinorrhea

Excludes1   allergic rhinitis with asthma (bronchial) (J45.909)
rhinitis NOS (J31.0)

J30.0	**Vasomotor rhinitis**
J30.1	**Allergic rhinitis due to pollen**
	Allergy NOS due to pollen
	Hay fever
	Pollinosis
J30.2	**Other seasonal allergic rhinitis**
J30.5	**Allergic rhinitis due to food**
● **J30.8**	**Other allergic rhinitis**
J30.81	**Allergic rhinitis due to animal (cat) (dog) hair and dander**
J30.89	**Other allergic rhinitis**
	Perennial allergic rhinitis
J30.9	**Allergic rhinitis, unspecified**

● **J31**   **Chronic rhinitis, nasopharyngitis and pharyngitis**

J31.0   **Chronic rhinitis**

Atrophic rhinitis (chronic)
Granulomatous rhinitis (chronic)
Hypertrophic rhinitis (chronic)
Obstructive rhinitis (chronic)
Ozena
Purulent rhinitis (chronic)
Rhinitis (chronic) NOS
Ulcerative rhinitis (chronic)

Excludes1   allergic rhinitis (J30.1-J30.9)
vasomotor rhinitis (J30.0)

J31.1   **Chronic nasopharyngitis**

Excludes2   acute nasopharyngitis (J00)

J31.2   **Chronic pharyngitis**

Chronic sore throat
Atrophic pharyngitis (chronic)
Granular pharyngitis (chronic)
Hypertrophic pharyngitis (chronic)

Excludes2   acute pharyngitis (J02.9)

● **J32**   **Chronic sinusitis**

Includes   sinus abscess
sinus empyema
sinus infection
sinus suppuration

Excludes2   acute sinusitis (J01.-)

J32.0	**Chronic maxillary sinusitis**
	Antritis (chronic)
	Maxillary sinusitis NOS
J32.1	**Chronic frontal sinusitis**
	Frontal sinusitis NOS
J32.2	**Chronic ethmoidal sinusitis**
	Ethmoidal sinusitis NOS

Excludes1   Woakes' ethmoiditis (J33.1)

J32.3	**Chronic sphenoidal sinusitis**
	Sphenoidal sinusitis NOS
J32.4	**Chronic pansinusitis**
	Pansinusitis NOS
J32.8	**Other chronic sinusitis**
	Sinusitis (chronic) involving more than one sinus but not pansinusitis
J32.9	**Chronic sinusitis, unspecified**
	Sinusitis (chronic) NOS

● **J33**   **Nasal polyp**

Excludes1   adenomatous polyps (D14.0)

J33.0	**Polyp of nasal cavity**
	Choanal polyp
	Nasopharyngeal polyp
J33.1	**Polypoid sinus degeneration**
	Woakes' syndrome or ethmoiditis
J33.8	**Other polyp of sinus**
	Accessory polyp of sinus
	Ethmoidal polyp of sinus
	Maxillary polyp of sinus
	Sphenoidal polyp of sinus
J33.9	**Nasal polyp, unspecified**

● **J34**   **Other and unspecified disorders of nose and nasal sinuses**

Excludes2   varicose ulcer of nasal septum (I86.8)

J34.0	**Abscess, furuncle and carbuncle of nose**
	Cellulitis of nose
	Necrosis of nose
	Ulceration of nose
J34.1	**Cyst and mucocele of nose and nasal sinus**
J34.2	**Deviated nasal septum**
	Deflection or deviation of septum (nasal) (acquired)

Excludes1   congenital deviated nasal septum (Q67.4)

J34.3   **Hypertrophy of nasal turbinates**

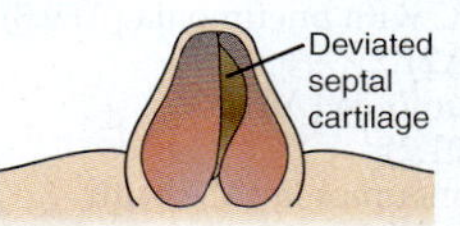

Figure 10-3   Deviated nasal septum.

Item 10–4   **Nasal polyps** are an abnormal growth of tissue (tumor) projecting from a mucous membrane and attached to the surface by a narrow elongated stalk (pedunculated). Nasal polyps usually originate in the ethmoid sinus but also may occur in the maxillary sinus. Symptoms are nasal block, sinusitis, anosmia, and secondary infections.

Item 10–5   A **deviated nasal septum** is the displacement of the septal cartilage that separates the nares. This displacement causes obstructed air flow through the nasal passages. A child can be born with this displacement (congenital), or the condition may be acquired through trauma, such as a sports injury. Symptoms include nasal block, sinusitis, and related secondary infections. Septoplasty is surgical repair of this condition.

▶ New   ⮕ Revised   ~~deleted~~ Deleted   Excludes 1   Excludes 2   Includes   Use additional   Code first   Code also   Key words

OGCR Official Guidelines   **X** Assign placeholder X   ● Use Additional Character(s)   ▸ Manifestation Code   Hierarchical Condition Category   **Coding Clinic**

● **J34.8 Other specified disorders of nose and nasal sinuses**

    J34.81 Nasal mucositis (ulcerative)

        Code also type of associated therapy, such as:
           antineoplastic and immunosuppressive drugs (T45.1X-)
           radiological procedure and radiotherapy (Y84.2)

        Excludes2 gastrointestinal mucositis (ulcerative) (K92.81)
              mucositis (ulcerative) of vagina and vulva (N76.81)
              oral mucositis (ulcerative) (K12.3-)

    ● **J34.82 Nasal valve collapse**
        Nasal valve compromise
        Nasal valve stenosis

        Code first underlying cause, such as:
          deviated nasal septum (J34.2)

        ● **J34.820 Internal nasal valve collapse**

            J34.8200 Internal nasal valve collapse, unspecified

            J34.8201 Internal nasal valve collapse, static
              Narrowing of the septum, head of the inferior turbinate and the upper lateral cartilage

            J34.8202 Internal nasal valve collapse, dynamic
              Collapse or falling of the upper, middle sidewall of the nose on inspiration

        ● **J34.821 External nasal valve collapse**

            J34.8210 External nasal valve collapse, unspecified

            J34.8211 External nasal valve collapse, static
              Fixed narrowing of the caudal septum, lower lateral cartilage, alar rim and nasal sill

            J34.8212 External nasal valve collapse, dynamic
              Collapse or falling of the lower sidewall or nostril of the nose on inspiration

        J34.829 Nasal valve collapse, unspecified
          Nasal valve collapse, NOS

    J34.89 Other specified disorders of nose and nasal sinuses
        Perforation of nasal septum NOS
        Rhinolith

    J34.9 Unspecified disorder of nose and nasal sinuses

● **J35 Chronic diseases of tonsils and adenoids**

    ● **J35.0 Chronic tonsillitis and adenoiditis**

        Excludes2 acute tonsillitis (J03.-)

        J35.01 Chronic tonsillitis

        J35.02 Chronic adenoiditis

        J35.03 Chronic tonsillitis and adenoiditis

    J35.1 Hypertrophy of tonsils
        Enlargement of tonsils

        Excludes1 hypertrophy of tonsils with tonsillitis (J35.0-)

    J35.2 Hypertrophy of adenoids
        Enlargement of adenoids

        Excludes1 hypertrophy of adenoids with adenoiditis (J35.0-)

    J35.3 Hypertrophy of tonsils with hypertrophy of adenoids

        Excludes1 hypertrophy of tonsils and adenoids with tonsillitis and adenoiditis (J35.03)

    J35.8 Other chronic diseases of tonsils and adenoids
        Adenoid vegetations
        Amygdalolith
        Calculus, tonsil
        Cicatrix of tonsil (and adenoid)
        Tonsillar tag
        Ulcer of tonsil

    J35.9 Chronic disease of tonsils and adenoids, unspecified
        Disease (chronic) of tonsils and adenoids NOS

J36 Peritonsillar abscess

    Includes abscess of tonsil
            peritonsillar cellulitis
            quinsy

    Use additional code (B95-B97) to identify infectious agent.

    Excludes1 acute tonsillitis (J03.-)
           chronic tonsillitis (J35.0)
           retropharyngeal abscess (J39.0)
           tonsillitis NOS (J03.9-)

● **J37 Chronic laryngitis and laryngotracheitis**

    Use additional code to identify:
        exposure to environmental tobacco smoke (Z77.22)
        exposure to tobacco smoke in the perinatal period (P96.81)
        history of tobacco dependence (Z87.891)
        infectious agent (B95-B97)
        occupational exposure to environmental tobacco smoke (Z57.31)
        tobacco dependence (F17.-)
        tobacco use (Z72.0)

    J37.0 Chronic laryngitis
        Catarrhal laryngitis
        Hypertrophic laryngitis
        Sicca laryngitis

        Excludes2 acute laryngitis (J04.0)
           obstructive (acute) laryngitis (J05.0)

    J37.1 Chronic laryngotracheitis
        Laryngitis, chronic, with tracheitis (chronic)
        Tracheitis, chronic, with laryngitis

        Excludes1 chronic tracheitis (J42)

        Excludes2 acute laryngotracheitis (J04.2)
           acute tracheitis (J04.1)

● **J38 Diseases of vocal cords and larynx, not elsewhere classified**

    Excludes1 congenital laryngeal stridor (P28.89)
           obstructive laryngitis (acute) (J05.0)
           postprocedural subglottic stenosis (J95.5)
           stridor (R06.1)
           ulcerative laryngitis (J04.0)

    ● **J38.0 Paralysis of vocal cords and larynx**
        Laryngoplegia
        Paralysis of glottis

        J38.00 Paralysis of vocal cords and larynx, unspecified

        J38.01 Paralysis of vocal cords and larynx, unilateral
           Coding Clinic: 2025, Q1, P27

        J38.02 Paralysis of vocal cords and larynx, bilateral

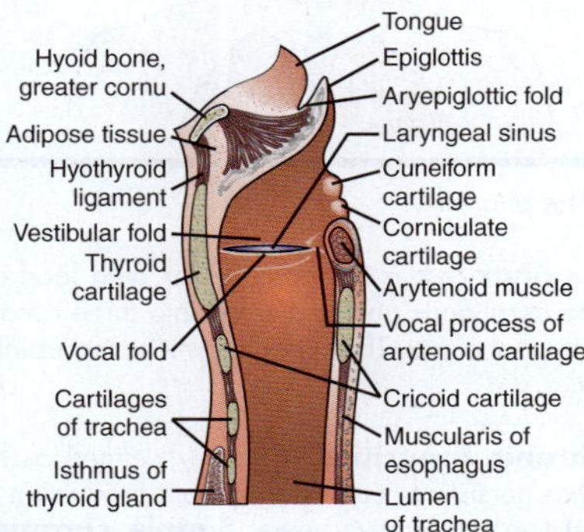

Figure 10-4 Coronal section of the larynx.

Item 10-6 The **larynx** extends from the tongue to the trachea and is divided into an upper and lower portion separated by folds. The framework of the larynx is cartilage composed of the single cricoid, thyroid, and epiglottic cartilages, and the paired arytenoid, cuneiform, and corniculate cartilages.

CHAPTER 10 (J00-J99)

J38.1 **Polyp of vocal cord and larynx**
    Excludes1 adenomatous polyps (D14.1)

J38.2 **Nodules of vocal cords**
    Chorditis (fibrinous)(nodosa)(tuberosa)
    Singer's nodes
    Teacher's nodes

J38.3 **Other diseases of vocal cords**
    Abscess of vocal cords
    Cellulitis of vocal cords
    Granuloma of vocal cords
    Leukokeratosis of vocal cords
    Leukoplakia of vocal cords

J38.4 **Edema of larynx**
    Edema (of) glottis
    Subglottic edema
    Supraglottic edema
    Excludes1 acute obstructive laryngitis [croup] (J05.0)
        edematous laryngitis (J04.0)

J38.5 **Laryngeal spasm**
    Laryngismus (stridulus)

J38.6 **Stenosis of larynx**

J38.7 **Other diseases of larynx**
    Abscess of larynx
    Cellulitis of larynx
    Disease of larynx NOS
    Necrosis of larynx
    Pachyderma of larynx
    Perichondritis of larynx
    Ulcer of larynx

● **J39** **Other diseases of upper respiratory tract**
    Excludes1 acute respiratory infection NOS (J22)
        acute upper respiratory infection (J06.9)
        upper respiratory inflammation due to chemicals, gases, fumes or vapors (J68.2)

J39.0 **Retropharyngeal and parapharyngeal abscess**
    Peripharyngeal abscess
    Excludes1 peritonsillar abscess (J36)

J39.1 **Other abscess of pharynx**
    Cellulitis of pharynx
    Nasopharyngeal abscess

J39.2 **Other diseases of pharynx**
    Cyst of pharynx
    Edema of pharynx
    Excludes2 chronic pharyngitis (J31.2)
        ulcerative pharyngitis (J02.9)

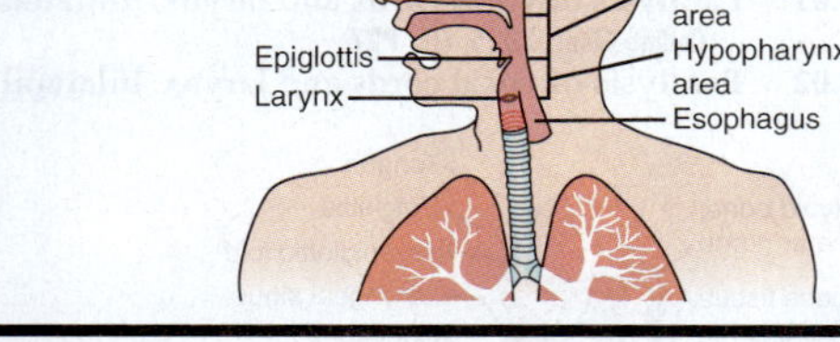

Figure 10-5 The pharynx.

Item 10–7 The **pharynx** is the passage for both food and air between the mouth and the esophagus and is divided into three areas: nasopharynx, oropharynx, and hypopharynx. The hypopharynx branches into the esophagus and the voice box.

Item 10–8 **Chronic bronchitis** is usually defined as being present in any patient who has persistent cough with sputum production for at least three months in at least two consecutive years. **Simple chronic bronchitis** is marked by a productive cough but no pathological airflow obstruction. **Chronic obstructive pulmonary disease (COPD)** is a group of conditions—bronchitis, emphysema, asthma, bronchiectasis, allergic alveolitis—marked by dyspnea. **Catarrhal** bronchitis is an acute form of bronchitis marked by profuse mucus and pus production (**mucopurulent** discharge). **Croupous** bronchitis, also known as pseudomembranous, fibrinous, plastic, exudative, or membranous, is marked by a violent cough and dyspnea.

J39.3 **Upper respiratory tract hypersensitivity reaction, site unspecified**
    Excludes1 hypersensitivity reaction of upper respiratory tract, such as:
        extrinsic allergic alveolitis (J67.9)
        pneumoconiosis (J60-J67.9)

J39.8 **Other specified diseases of upper respiratory tract**
    Coding Clinic: 2023, Q1, P30

J39.9 **Disease of upper respiratory tract, unspecified**

CHRONIC LOWER RESPIRATORY DISEASES (J40-J4A)

    Excludes1 bronchitis due to chemicals, gases, fumes and vapors (J68.0)
    Excludes2 cystic fibrosis (E84.-)

J40 **Bronchitis, not specified as acute or chronic**
    Bronchitis NOS
    Catarrhal bronchitis
    Bronchitis with tracheitis NOS
    Tracheobronchitis NOS
    Use additional code to identify:
        exposure to environmental tobacco smoke (Z77.22)
        exposure to tobacco smoke in the perinatal period (P96.81)
        history of tobacco dependence (Z87.891)
        occupational exposure to environmental tobacco smoke (Z57.31)
        tobacco dependence (F17.-)
        tobacco use (Z72.0)
    Excludes1 acute bronchitis (J20.-)
        allergic bronchitis NOS (J45.909)
        asthmatic bronchitis NOS (J45.9-)
        bronchitis due to chemicals, fumes and vapors (J68.0)

● **J41** **Simple and mucopurulent chronic bronchitis**
    Use additional code to identify:
        exposure to environmental tobacco smoke (Z77.22)
        exposure to tobacco smoke in the perinatal period (P96.81)
        history of tobacco dependence (Z87.891)
        occupational exposure to environmental tobacco smoke (Z57.31)
        tobacco dependence (F17.-)
        tobacco use (Z72.0)
    Excludes2 chronic bronchitis NOS (J42)
        chronic obstructive bronchitis (J44.-)

J41.0 **Simple chronic bronchitis** ℞℞

J41.1 **Mucopurulent chronic bronchitis** ℞℞

J41.8 **Mixed simple and mucopurulent chronic bronchitis** ℞℞

J42 **Unspecified chronic bronchitis** ℞℞
    Chronic bronchitis NOS
    Chronic tracheitis
    Chronic tracheobronchitis
    Use additional code to identify:
        exposure to environmental tobacco smoke (Z77.22)
        exposure to tobacco smoke in the perinatal period (P96.81)
        history of tobacco dependence (Z87.891)
        occupational exposure to environmental tobacco smoke (Z57.31)
        tobacco dependence (F17.-)
        tobacco use (Z72.0)
    Excludes1 bronchiolitis obliterans and bronchiolitis obliterans syndrome (J44.81)
        chronic asthmatic bronchitis (J44.-)
        chronic bronchitis with airways obstruction (J44.-)
        chronic emphysematous bronchitis (J44.-)
        chronic obstructive pulmonary disease NOS (J44.9)
        simple and mucopurulent chronic bronchitis (J41.-)

● **J43** **Emphysema**
    Excludes1 compensatory emphysema (J98.3)
        ~~emphysema due to inhalation of chemicals, gases, fumes or vapors (J68.4)~~
        interstitial emphysema (J98.2)
        mediastinal emphysema (J98.2)
        neonatal interstitial emphysema (P25.0)
        surgical (subcutaneous) emphysema (T81.82)
    Excludes2 emphysema with chronic (obstructive) bronchitis (J44.-)
        ▶emphysema due to inhalation of chemicals, gases, fumes or vapors (J68.4)
        emphysematous (obstructive) bronchitis (J44.-)
        traumatic subcutaneous emphysema (T79.7)
    Coding Clinic: 2024, Q2, P4

▶ New   ◀ Revised   ~~deleted~~ Deleted   Excludes 1   Excludes 2   Includes   Use additional   Code first   Code also   Key words

OGCR Official Guidelines   X Assign placeholder X   ● Use Additional Character(s)   ▶ Manifestation Code   ℞℞ Hierarchical Condition Category   Coding Clinic

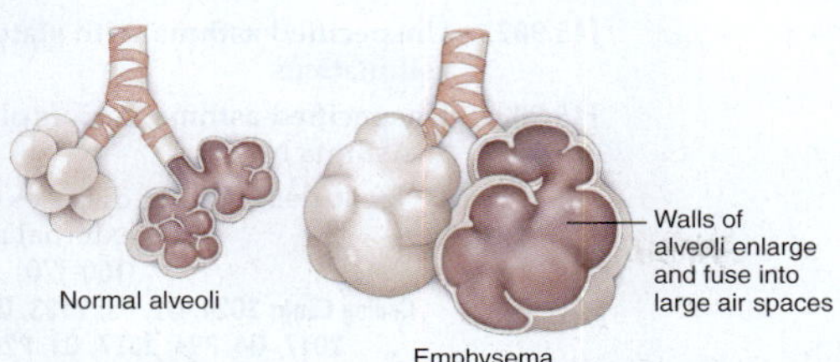

Figure 10-6   Emphysema. (From Shiland, BJ: Medical Terminology & Anatomy for ICD-10 Coding, ed 2, Mosby, 2015)

J43.0   **Unilateral pulmonary emphysema [MacLeod's syndrome]** 🏷
Swyer-James syndrome
Unilateral emphysema
Unilateral hyperlucent lung
Unilateral pulmonary artery functional hypoplasia
Unilateral transparency of lung

J43.1   **Panlobular emphysema** 🏷
Panacinar emphysema

J43.2   **Centrilobular emphysema** 🏷

J43.8   **Other emphysema** 🏷

J43.9   **Emphysema, unspecified** 🏷
Bullous emphysema (lung)(pulmonary)
Emphysema (lung)(pulmonary) NOS
Emphysematous bleb
Vesicular emphysema (lung)(pulmonary)
Coding Clinic: 2024, Q2, P4, 5; 2019, Q1, P35-37; 2017, Q4, P97-98

● **J44**   **Other chronic obstructive pulmonary disease**
Includes   asthma with chronic obstructive pulmonary disease
chronic asthmatic (obstructive) bronchitis
chronic bronchitis with airway obstruction
chronic bronchitis with emphysema
chronic emphysematous bronchitis
chronic obstructive asthma
chronic obstructive bronchitis
chronic obstructive tracheobronchitis
Code also type of asthma, if applicable (J45.-)
~~**Excludes1**~~   ~~chronic bronchitis NOS (J42)~~
~~chronic simple and mucopurulent bronchitis (J41.-)~~
~~chronic tracheitis (J42)~~
~~chronic tracheobronchitis (J42)~~

Excludes2   bronchiectasis (J47.-)
▶chronic bronchitis NOS (J42)
▶chronic simple and mucopurulent bronchitis (J41.-)
▶chronic tracheitis (J42)
▶chronic tracheobronchitis (J42)
emphysema without chronic bronchitis (J43.-)
Coding Clinic: 2024, Q2, P3-6; 2019, Q1, P34-36; 2017, Q4, P97; 2017, Q1, P25; 2016, Q3, P16

J44.0   **Chronic obstructive pulmonary disease with (acute) lower respiratory infection** 🏷
Code also to identify the infection
Coding Clinic: 2024, Q2, P6; 2019, Q1, P35-36; 2017, Q4, P96; 2017, Q2, P30, Q1, P24-25; 2016, Q3, P15-16

J44.1   **Chronic obstructive pulmonary disease with (acute) exacerbation** 🏷
Decompensated COPD
Decompensated COPD with (acute) exacerbation
Excludes2   chronic obstructive pulmonary disease [COPD] with acute bronchitis (J44.0)
lung diseases due to external agents (J60-J70)
Coding Clinic: 2024, Q2, P6; 2019, Q1, P34-35; 2017, Q4, P96; 2017, Q1, P26; 2016, Q3, P15-16, Q1, P36

● **J44.8**   **Other specified chronic obstructive pulmonary disease**
J44.81   **Bronchiolitis obliterans and bronchiolitis obliterans syndrome**
Obliterative bronchiolitis
Code first, if applicable:
complication of bone marrow transplant (T86.09)
complication of stem cell transplant (T86.5)
heart-lung transplant rejection (T86.31)
lung transplant rejection (T86.810)
other complications of heart-lung transplant (T86.39)
other complications of lung transplant (T86.818)
Code also, if applicable, associated conditions, such as:
chronic graft-versus-host disease (D89.811)
chronic lung allograft dysfunction (J4A.-)
chronic respiratory conditions due to chemicals, gases, fumes and vapors (J68.4)

J44.89   **Other specified chronic obstructive pulmonary disease**
Chronic asthmatic (obstructive) bronchitis
Chronic emphysematous bronchitis
Coding Clinic: 2024, Q2, P3

J44.9   **Chronic obstructive pulmonary disease, unspecified** 🏷
Chronic obstructive airway disease NOS
Chronic obstructive lung disease NOS
Excludes2   lung diseases due to external agents (J60-J70)
Coding Clinic: 2024, Q2, P3, 4, 6; 2019, Q1, P36; 2017, Q4, P96-97; 2017, Q1, P24-25; 2016, Q1, P37

● **J45**   **Asthma**
Allergic (predominantly) asthma
Allergic bronchitis NOS
Allergic rhinitis with asthma
Atopic asthma
Extrinsic allergic asthma
Hay fever with asthma
Idiosyncratic asthma
Intrinsic nonallergic asthma
Nonallergic asthma
Use additional code to identify:
eosinophilic asthma (J82.83)
exposure to environmental tobacco smoke (Z77.22)
exposure to tobacco smoke in the perinatal period (P96.81)
history of tobacco dependence (Z87.891)
occupational exposure to environmental tobacco smoke (Z57.31)
tobacco dependence (F17.-)
tobacco use (Z72.0)
Excludes1   detergent asthma (J69.8)
miner's asthma (J60)
wheezing NOS (R06.2)
wood asthma (J67.8)
Excludes2   asthma with chronic obstructive pulmonary disease (J44.89)
chronic asthmatic (obstructive) bronchitis (J44.89)
chronic obstructive asthma (J44.89)
other specified chronic obstructive pulmonary disease (J44.89)
Coding Clinic: 2024, Q2, P3; 2019, Q1, P37; 2017, Q1, P25

● **J45.2**   **Mild intermittent asthma**
J45.20   **Mild intermittent asthma, uncomplicated**
Mild intermittent asthma NOS
J45.21   **Mild intermittent asthma with (acute) exacerbation**
J45.22   **Mild intermittent asthma with status asthmaticus**

CHAPTER 10 (J00-J99)

Item 10–9   **Asthma** is a bronchial condition marked by airway obstruction, hyper-responsiveness, and inflammation. **Extrinsic** asthma, also known as allergic asthma, is characterized by the same symptoms that occur with exposure to allergens and is divided into the following types: **atopic, occupational, and allergic bronchopulmonary aspergillosis. Intrinsic** asthma occurs in patients who have no history of allergy or sensitivities to allergens and is divided into the following types: **nonreaginic** and **pharmacologic. Status asthmaticus** is the most severe form of asthma attack and can last for days or weeks.

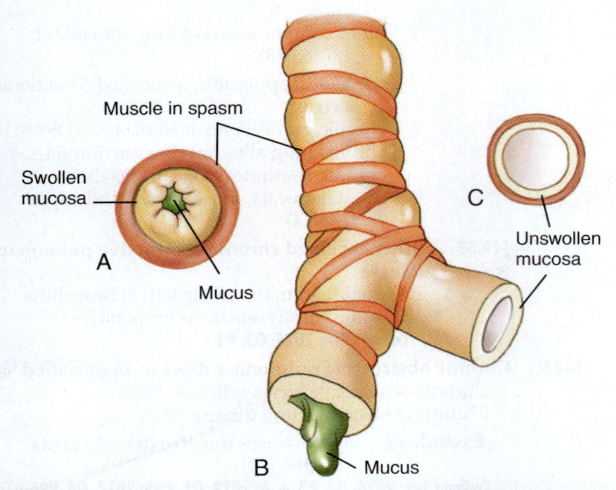

Figure 10-7   Factors causing expiratory obstruction in asthma. **A.** Cross section of a bronchiole occluded by muscle spasm, swollen mucosa, and mucus. **B.** Longitudinal section of an obstructed bronchiole. **C.** Cross section of a clear bronchiole. (From Shiland: Mastering Healthcare Terminology, ed 1, St. Louis, Mosby, 2003)

● **J45.3**   **Mild persistent** asthma

    J45.30   **Mild persistent asthma, uncomplicated**
       Mild persistent asthma NOS

    J45.31   **Mild persistent asthma with (acute) exacerbation**
       Coding Clinic: 2016, Q1, P35

    J45.32   **Mild persistent asthma with status asthmaticus**

● **J45.4**   **Moderate persistent** asthma

    J45.40   **Moderate persistent asthma, uncomplicated**
       Moderate persistent asthma NOS

    J45.41   **Moderate persistent asthma with (acute) exacerbation**
       Coding Clinic: 2017, Q1, P26

    J45.42   **Moderate persistent asthma with status asthmaticus**

● **J45.5**   **Severe persistent** asthma

    J45.50   **Severe persistent asthma, uncomplicated**
       Severe persistent asthma NOS

    J45.51   **Severe persistent asthma with (acute) exacerbation**

    J45.52   **Severe persistent asthma with status asthmaticus**

● **J45.9**   **Other and unspecified asthma**

   ● **J45.90**   **Unspecified asthma**
       Asthmatic bronchitis NOS
       Childhood asthma NOS
       Late onset asthma

      J45.901   **Unspecified asthma with (acute) exacerbation**
        Coding Clinic: 2017, Q4, P96

      J45.902   **Unspecified asthma with status asthmaticus**

      J45.909   **Unspecified asthma, uncomplicated**
        Asthma NOS

        Excludes2   lung diseases due to external agents (J60-J70)
         Coding Clinic: 2024, Q2, P3; 2023, Q1, P17; 2017, Q4, P96; 2017, Q1, P25

   ● **J45.99**   **Other asthma**

      J45.990   **Exercise induced bronchospasm**

      J45.991   **Cough variant asthma**

      J45.998   **Other asthma**

● **J47**   **Bronchiectasis**

    Includes   bronchiolectasis

    Use additional code to identify:
      exposure to environmental tobacco smoke (Z77.22)
      exposure to tobacco smoke in the perinatal period (P96.81)
      history of tobacco dependence (Z87.891)
      occupational exposure to environmental tobacco smoke (Z57.31)
      tobacco dependence (F17.-)
      tobacco use (Z72.0)

    Excludes1   congenital bronchiectasis (Q33.4)
      tuberculous bronchiectasis (current disease) (A15.0)
    Coding Clinic: 2024, Q2, P5,6

    J47.0   **Bronchiectasis with acute lower respiratory infection** Ⓗ
      Bronchiectasis with acute bronchitis
      Code also to identify infection, if applicable

    J47.1   **Bronchiectasis with (acute) exacerbation** Ⓗ
      Coding Clinic: 2021, Q1, P24

    J47.9   **Bronchiectasis, uncomplicated** Ⓗ
      Bronchiectasis NOS
      Coding Clinic: 2024, Q2, P5,6

LUNG DISEASES DUE TO EXTERNAL AGENTS (J60-J70)

    Excludes2   asthma (J45.-)
      malignant neoplasm of bronchus and lung (C34.-)

● **J4A**   **Chronic lung allograft dysfunction**

    Code first, if applicable:
      heart-lung transplant rejection (T86.31)
      lung transplant rejection (T86.810)
      other complications of heart-lung transplant (T86.39)
      other complications of lung transplant (T86.818)

    Code also, if applicable, bronchiolitis obliterans syndrome (J44.81)

    J4A.0   **Restrictive allograft syndrome**
      Code also, if applicable, for mixed chronic lung allograft dysfunction, bronchiolitis obliterans syndrome (J44.81)

    J4A.8   **Other chronic lung allograft dysfunction**

    J4A.9   **Chronic lung allograft dysfunction, unspecified**

J60   **Coalworker's pneumoconiosis** Ⓗ   A
    Anthracosilicosis
    Anthracosis
    Black lung disease
    Coalworker's lung

    Excludes1   coalworker pneumoconiosis with tuberculosis, any type in A15 (J65)

J61   **Pneumoconiosis due to asbestos and other mineral fibers** Ⓗ   A
    Asbestosis

    Excludes1   pleural plaque with asbestosis (J92.0)
      pneumoconiosis with tuberculosis, any type in A15 (J65)

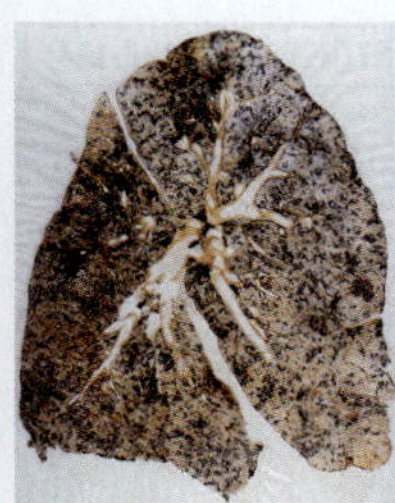

Figure 10-8 Progressive massive fibrosis superimposed on coal workers' pneumoconiosis. The large, blackened scars are located principally in the upper lobe. (From Frazier MS, Drzymkowski JW: Essentials of Human Diseases and Conditions, St. Louis, MO, Saunders, 2004)

Item 10–10 Pneumoconiosis refers to a lung condition resulting from exposure to inorganic or organic airborne particles, such as coal dust or moldy hay, as well as chemical fumes and vapors, such as insecticides. In this condition, the lungs retain the airborne particles.

● **J62 Pneumoconiosis due to dust containing silica**
    Includes   silicotic fibrosis (massive) of lung
    Excludes1   pneumoconiosis with tuberculosis, any type in A15 (J65)

   J62.0   **Pneumoconiosis due to talc dust**

   J62.8   **Pneumoconiosis due to other dust containing silica**
         Silicosis NOS

● **J63 Pneumoconiosis due to other inorganic dusts**
    Excludes1   pneumoconiosis with tuberculosis, any type in A15 (J65)
     Coding Clinic: 2019, Q3, P8

   J63.0   **Aluminosis (of lung)**

   J63.1   **Bauxite fibrosis (of lung)**

   J63.2   **Berylliosis**

   J63.3   **Graphite fibrosis (of lung)**

   J63.4   **Siderosis**
     Coding Clinic: 2019, Q3, P8

   J63.5   **Stannosis**

   J63.6   **Pneumoconiosis due to other specified inorganic dusts**

   J64 Unspecified pneumoconiosis
    Excludes1   pneumonoconiosis with tuberculosis, any type in A15 (J65)

   J65 Pneumoconiosis associated with tuberculosis
     Any condition in J60-J64 with tuberculosis, any type in A15
     Silicotuberculosis

● **J66 Airway disease due to specific organic dust**
    Excludes2   allergic alveolitis (J67.-)
         asbestosis (J61)
         bagassosis (J67.1)
         farmer's lung (J67.0)
         hypersensitivity pneumonitis due to organic dust (J67.-)
         reactive airways dysfunction syndrome (J68.3)

   J66.0   **Byssinosis**
         Airway disease due to cotton dust

   J66.1   **Flax-dressers' disease**

   J66.2   **Cannabinosis**

   J66.8   **Airway disease due to other specific organic dusts**

● **J67 Hypersensitivity pneumonitis due to organic dust**
    Includes   allergic alveolitis and pneumonitis due to inhaled organic dust and particles of fungal, actinomycetic or other origin
    Excludes1   pneumonitis due to inhalation of chemicals, gases, fumes or vapors (J68.0)

   J67.0   **Farmer's lung**
         Harvester's lung
         Haymaker's lung
         Moldy hay disease

   J67.1   **Bagassosis**
         Bagasse disease
         Bagasse pneumonitis

   J67.2   **Bird fancier's lung**
         Budgerigar fancier's disease or lung
         Pigeon fancier's disease or lung

   J67.3   **Suberosis**
         Corkhandler's disease or lung
         Corkworker's disease or lung

   J67.4   **Maltworker's lung**
         Alveolitis due to Aspergillus clavatus

   J67.5   **Mushroom-worker's lung**

   J67.6   **Maple-bark-stripper's lung**
         Alveolitis due to Cryptostroma corticale
         Cryptostromosis

   J67.7   **Air conditioner and humidifier lung**
         Allergic alveolitis due to fungal, thermophilic actinomycetes and other organisms growing in ventilation [air conditioning] systems

   J67.8   **Hypersensitivity pneumonitis due to other organic dusts**
         Cheese-washer's lung
         Coffee-worker's lung
         Fish-meal worker's lung
         Furrier's lung
         Sequoiosis

   J67.9   **Hypersensitivity pneumonitis due to unspecified organic dust**
         Allergic alveolitis (extrinsic) NOS
         Hypersensitivity pneumonitis NOS

● **J68 Respiratory conditions due to inhalation of chemicals, gases, fumes and vapors**
    Code first (T51-T65) *to identify cause*
    Use additional code to identify associated respiratory conditions, such as:
     acute respiratory failure (J96.0-)

   J68.0   **Bronchitis and pneumonitis due to chemicals, gases, fumes and vapors**
         Chemical bronchitis (acute)
     Coding Clinic: 2019, Q2, P31-32

   J68.1   **Pulmonary edema due to chemicals, gases, fumes and vapors**
         Chemical pulmonary edema (acute) (chronic)
      Excludes1   pulmonary edema (acute) (chronic) NOS (J81.-)

   J68.2   **Upper respiratory inflammation due to chemicals, gases, fumes and vapors, not elsewhere classified**

   J68.3   **Other acute and subacute respiratory conditions due to chemicals, gases, fumes and vapors**
         Reactive airways dysfunction syndrome

   J68.4   **Chronic respiratory conditions due to chemicals, gases, fumes and vapors**
     Code also, if applicable, chronic conditions, such as:
       emphysema (J43.-)
       obliterative bronchiolitis (J44.81)
       pulmonary fibrosis (J84.10)
      Excludes1   chronic pulmonary edema due to chemicals, gases, fumes and vapors (J68.1)

   J68.8   **Other respiratory conditions due to chemicals, gases, fumes and vapors**

   J68.9   **Unspecified respiratory condition due to chemicals, gases, fumes and vapors**

CHAPTER 10 (J00-J99)

● **J69 Pneumonitis due to solids and liquids**

Code also, if applicable, other types of pneumonias

Excludes1   neonatal aspiration syndromes (P24.-)
postprocedural pneumonitis (J95.4)

J69.0 Pneumonitis due to inhalation of food and vomit Ⓗ

Aspiration pneumonia NOS
Aspiration pneumonia (due to) food (regurgitated)
Aspiration pneumonia (due to) gastric secretions
Aspiration pneumonia (due to) milk
Aspiration pneumonia (due to) vomit

Code also any associated foreign body in respiratory tract (T17.-)

Excludes1   chemical pneumonitis due to anesthesia (J95.4)
obstetric aspiration pneumonitis (O74.0)

Coding Clinic: 2021, Q1, P34; 2019, Q2, P7, 31-32; 2017, Q1, P24

J69.1 Pneumonitis due to inhalation of oils and essences Ⓗ

Exogenous lipoid pneumonia
Lipid pneumonia NOS

Code first (T51-T65) to identify substance

Excludes1   endogenous lipoid pneumonia (J84.89)

J69.8 Pneumonitis due to inhalation of other solids and liquids Ⓗ

Pneumonitis due to aspiration of blood
Pneumonitis due to aspiration of detergent

Code first (T51-T65) to identify substance

● **J70 Respiratory conditions due to other external agents**

J70.0 Acute pulmonary manifestations due to radiation Ⓗ

Radiation pneumonitis

Use additional code (W88-W90, X39.0-) to identify the external cause

J70.1 Chronic and other pulmonary manifestations due to radiation Ⓗ

Fibrosis of lung following radiation

Use additional code (W88-W90, X39.0-) to identify the external cause

J70.2 Acute drug-induced interstitial lung disorders Ⓗ

Use additional code for adverse effect, if applicable, to identify drug (T36-T50 with fifth or sixth character 5)

Excludes1   interstitial pneumonia NOS (J84.9)
lymphoid interstitial pneumonia (J84.2)

Coding Clinic: 2019, Q2, P28

J70.3 Chronic drug-induced interstitial lung disorders Ⓗ

Use additional code for adverse effect, if applicable, to identify drug (T36-T50 with fifth or sixth character 5)

Excludes1   interstitial pneumonia NOS (J84.9)
lymphoid interstitial pneumonia (J84.2)

J70.4 Drug-induced interstitial lung disorders, unspecified Ⓗ

Use additional code for adverse effect, if applicable, to identify drug (T36-T50 with fifth or sixth character 5)

Excludes1   interstitial pneumonia NOS (J84.9)
lymphoid interstitial pneumonia (J84.2)

Coding Clinic: 2019, Q2, P28

J70.5 Respiratory conditions due to smoke inhalation Ⓗ

Code first smoke inhalation (T59.81-)

Excludes2   smoke inhalation due to chemicals, gases, fumes and vapors (J68.9)

J70.8 Respiratory conditions due to other specified external agents Ⓗ

Code first (T51-T65) to identify the external agent

J70.9 Respiratory conditions due to unspecified external agent Ⓗ

Code first (T51-T65) to identify the external agent

OTHER RESPIRATORY DISEASES PRINCIPALLY AFFECTING THE INTERSTITIUM (J80-J84)

J80 Acute respiratory distress syndrome Ⓗ

Acute respiratory distress syndrome in adult or child
Adult hyaline membrane disease

Excludes1   respiratory distress syndrome in newborn (perinatal) (P22.0)

Coding Clinic: 2017, Q1, P26-27

● **J81 Pulmonary edema**

Use additional code to identify:
exposure to environmental tobacco smoke (Z77.22)
history of tobacco dependence (Z87.891)
occupational exposure to environmental tobacco smoke (Z57.31)
tobacco dependence (F17.-)
tobacco use (Z72.0)

Excludes1   chemical (acute) pulmonary edema (J68.1)
hypostatic pneumonia (J18.2)
passive pneumonia (J18.2)
pulmonary edema due to external agents (J60-J70)
pulmonary edema with heart disease NOS (I50.1)
pulmonary edema with heart failure (I50.1)

J81.0 Acute pulmonary edema Ⓗ

Acute edema of lung

Coding Clinic: 2023, Q1, P25; 2017, Q1, P26

J81.1 Chronic pulmonary edema

Pulmonary congestion (chronic) (passive)
Pulmonary edema NOS

J82 Pulmonary eosinophilia, not elsewhere classified Ⓗ

Excludes2   pulmonary eosinophilia due to aspergillosis (B44.-)
pulmonary eosinophilia due to drugs (J70.2-J70.4)
pulmonary eosinophilia due to specified parasitic infection (B50-B83)
pulmonary eosinophilia due to systemic connective tissue disorders (M30-M36)
pulmonary infiltrate NOS (R91.8)

● **J82.8 Pulmonary eosinophilia, not elsewhere classified**

J82.81 Chronic eosinophilic pneumonia

Eosinophilic pneumonia, NOS

J82.82 Acute eosinophilic pneumonia

J82.83 Eosinophilic asthma

Code first asthma, by type, such as:
mild intermittent asthma (J45.2-)
mild persistent asthma (J45.3-)
moderate persistent asthma (J45.4-)
severe persistent asthma (J45.5-)

J82.89 Other pulmonary eosinophilia, not elsewhere classified

Allergic pneumonia
Löffler's pneumonia
Tropical (pulmonary) eosinophilia NOS

● **J84 Other interstitial pulmonary diseases**

Excludes1   drug-induced interstitial lung disorders (J70.2-J70.4)
interstitial emphysema (J98.2)

Excludes2   lung diseases due to external agents (J60-J70)

Coding Clinic: 2019, Q2, P28

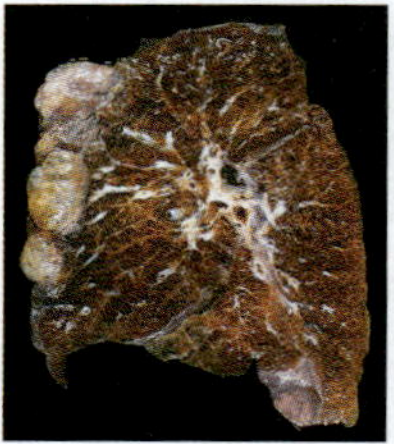

Figure 10-9 Bullous emphysema with large subpleural bullae *(upper left)*. (From Kumar: Robbins and Cotran: Pathologic Basis of Disease, ed 8, Saunders, An Imprint of Elsevier, 2009)

● **J84.0**   **Alveolar and parieto-alveolar conditions**

    J84.01   **Alveolar proteinosis** RCC

    J84.02   **Pulmonary alveolar microlithiasis** RCC

    J84.03   *Idiopathic pulmonary hemosiderosis* RCC
         Essential brown induration of lung
         Code first underlying disease, such as:
         disorders of iron metabolism (E83.1-)
         Code also, if applicable, associated condition
         Excludes1   acute idiopathic pulmonary hemorrhage in infants [AIPHI] (R04.81)

    J84.09   **Other alveolar and parieto-alveolar conditions** RCC

● **J84.1**   **Other interstitial pulmonary diseases with fibrosis**
    ▶ Code also, if applicable, pulmonary fibrosis (chronic) due to inhalation of chemicals, gases, fumes or vapors (J68.4)
    Excludes1   ~~pulmonary fibrosis (chronic) due to inhalation of chemicals, gases, fumes or vapors (J68.4)~~
                pulmonary fibrosis (chronic) following radiation (J70.1)

    J84.10   **Pulmonary fibrosis, unspecified** RCC
         Capillary fibrosis of lung
         Cirrhosis of lung (chronic) NOS
         Fibrosis of lung (atrophic) (chronic) (confluent) (massive) (perialveolar) (peribronchial) NOS
         Induration of lung (chronic) NOS
         Postinflammatory pulmonary fibrosis
         Coding Clinic: 2024, Q2, P20

● **J84.11**   **Idiopathic interstitial pneumonia**
         Excludes1   lymphoid interstitial pneumonia (J84.2)
                pneumocystis pneumonia (B59)

    J84.111   **Idiopathic interstitial pneumonia, not otherwise specified** RCC

    J84.112   **Idiopathic pulmonary fibrosis** RCC
         Cryptogenic fibrosing alveolitis
         Idiopathic fibrosing alveolitis

    J84.113   **Idiopathic non-specific interstitial pneumonitis** RCC
         Excludes1   non-specific interstitial pneumonia NOS, or due to known underlying cause (J84.89)

    J84.114   **Acute interstitial pneumonitis** RCC
         Hamman-Rich syndrome
         Excludes1   pneumocystis pneumonia (B59)

    J84.115   **Respiratory bronchiolitis interstitial lung disease** RCC

    J84.116   **Cryptogenic organizing pneumonia** RCC
         Excludes1   organizing pneumonia NOS, or due to known underlying cause (J84.89)

    J84.117   **Desquamative interstitial pneumonia** RCC

● **J84.17**   *Other interstitial pulmonary diseases with fibrosis in diseases classified elsewhere* RCC

    J84.170   *Interstitial lung disease with progressive fibrotic phenotype in diseases classified elsewhere*
         Progressive fibrotic interstitial lung disease
         Code first underlying disease, such as:
         lung diseases due to external agents (J60-J70)
         rheumatoid arthritis (M05.00-M06.9)
         sarcoidosis (D86.-)
         systemic connective tissue disorders (M30-M36)

    J84.178   *Other interstitial pulmonary diseases with fibrosis in diseases classified elsewhere*
         Interstitial pneumonia (nonspecific) (usual) due to collagen vascular disease
         Interstitial pneumonia (nonspecific) (usual) in diseases classified elsewhere
         Organizing pneumonia due to collagen vascular disease
         Organizing pneumonia in diseases classified elsewhere
         Code first underlying disease, such as:
         progressive systemic sclerosis (M34.0)
         rheumatoid arthritis (M05.00-M06.9)
         systemic lupus erythematosis (M32.0-M32.9)

J84.2   **Lymphoid interstitial pneumonia** RCC
    Lymphoid interstitial pneumonitis

● **J84.8**   **Other specified interstitial pulmonary diseases**
    Excludes1   exogenous lipoid pneumonia (J69.1)
                unspecified lipoid pneumonia (J69.1)

    J84.81   **Lymphangioleiomyomatosis** RCC
         Lymphangiomyomatosis

    J84.82   **Adult pulmonary Langerhans cell histiocytosis** RCC   **A**
         Adult PLCH

    J84.83   **Surfactant mutations of the lung** RCC

● **J84.84**   **Other interstitial lung diseases of childhood**

    J84.841   **Neuroendocrine cell hyperplasia of infancy** RCC

    J84.842   **Pulmonary interstitial glycogenosis** RCC

    J84.843   **Alveolar capillary dysplasia with vein misalignment** RCC

    J84.848   **Other interstitial lung diseases of childhood** RCC

CHAPTER 10 (J00-J99)

J84.89   **Other specified interstitial pulmonary diseases** 🅷
Endogenous lipoid pneumonia
Interstitial pneumonitis
Non-specific interstitial pneumonitis NOS
Organizing pneumonia NOS
> *Code first*, *if applicable*:
> poisoning due to drug or toxin (T51-T65 with fifth or sixth character to indicate intent), for toxic pneumonopathy
> underlying cause of pneumonopathy, if known
> *Use additional* code, for adverse effect, to identify drug (T36-T50 with fifth or sixth character 5), if drug-induced
> **Excludes1**   cryptogenic organizing pneumonia (J84.116)
> idiopathic non-specific interstitial pneumonitis (J84.113)
> lipoid pneumonia, exogenous or unspecified (J69.1)
> lymphoid interstitial pneumonia (J84.2)
> **Coding Clinic: 2021, Q4, P106-107; 2021, Q1, P48; 2019, Q2, P28**

J84.9   **Interstitial pulmonary disease, unspecified** 🅷
Interstitial pneumonia NOS

SUPPURATIVE AND NECROTIC CONDITIONS OF THE LOWER RESPIRATORY TRACT (J85-J86)

● **J85**   **Abscess of lung and mediastinum**
Use additional code (B95-B97) to identify infectious agent.

J85.0   **Gangrene and necrosis of lung** 🅷

J85.1   **Abscess of lung with pneumonia** 🅷
Code also the type of pneumonia

J85.2   **Abscess of lung without pneumonia** 🅷
Abscess of lung NOS

J85.3   **Abscess of mediastinum** 🅷

● **J86**   **Pyothorax**
Code also, if applicable, disruption of internal operation (surgical) wound (T81.32-)
Use additional code (B95-B97) to identify infectious agent.
Excludes1   abscess of lung (J85.-)
pyothorax due to tuberculosis (A15.6)

J86.0   **Pyothorax with fistula** 🅷
Bronchocutaneous fistula
Bronchopleural fistula
Hepatopleural fistula
Mediastinal fistula
Pleural fistula
Thoracic fistula
Any condition classifiable to J86.9 with fistula
Coding Clinic: 2024, Q3, P4

J86.9   **Pyothorax without fistula** 🅷
Abscess of pleura
Abscess of thorax
Empyema (chest) (lung) (pleura)
Fibrinopurulent pleurisy
Purulent pleurisy
Pyopneumothorax
Septic pleurisy
Seropurulent pleurisy
Suppurative pleurisy

OTHER DISEASES OF THE PLEURA (J90-J94)

J90   **Pleural effusion, not elsewhere classified**
Encysted pleurisy
Pleural effusion NOS
Pleurisy with effusion (exudative) (serous)
Excludes1   chylous (pleural) effusion (J94.0)
malignant pleural effusion (J91.0))
pleurisy NOS (R09.1)
tuberculous pleural effusion (A15.6)
Coding Clinic: 2015, Q2, P16

● **J91**   **Pleural effusion in conditions classified elsewhere**
Excludes2   pleural effusion in heart failure (I50.-)
pleural effusion in systemic lupus erythematosus (M32.13)

▶ **J91.0**   *Malignant pleural effusion*
Code first underlying neoplasm (C00-D49)
Coding Clinic: 2024, Q2, P11,12; 2022, Q3, P14-15

▶ **J91.8**   *Pleural effusion in other conditions classified elsewhere*
Code first underlying disease, such as:
filariasis (B74.0-B74.9)
influenza (J09.X2, J10.1, J11.1)
Coding Clinic: 2024, Q3, P4; 2015, Q2, P16

● **J92**   **Pleural plaque**
Includes   pleural thickening

J92.0   **Pleural plaque with presence of asbestos**

J92.9   **Pleural plaque without asbestos**
Pleural plaque NOS

● **J93**   **Pneumothorax and air leak**
Collapsed lung
Excludes1   congenital or perinatal pneumothorax (P25.1)
postprocedural air leak (J95.812)
postprocedural pneumothorax (J95.811)
traumatic pneumothorax (S27.0)
tuberculous (current disease) pneumothorax (A15.-)
pyopneumothorax (J86.-)

J93.0   **Spontaneous tension pneumothorax**
Tension pneumothorax (most serious type) occurs when air (positive pressure) collects in the pleural space

● **J93.1**   **Other spontaneous pneumothorax**

J93.11   **Primary spontaneous pneumothorax**

J93.12   **Secondary spontaneous pneumothorax**
Code first underlying condition, such as:
catamenial pneumothorax due to endometriosis (N80.B-)
cystic fibrosis (E84.-)
eosinophilic pneumonia (J82)
lymphangioleiomyomatosis (J84.81)
malignant neoplasm of bronchus and lung (C34.-)
Marfan syndrome (Q87.4-)
pneumonia due to Pneumocystis carinii (B59)
secondary malignant neoplasm of lung (C78.0-)
spontaneous rupture of the esophagus (K22.3)

● **J93.8**   **Other pneumothorax and air leak**

J93.81   **Chronic pneumothorax**

J93.82   **Other air leak**
Persistent air leak

J93.83   **Other pneumothorax**
Acute pneumothorax
Spontaneous pneumothorax NOS

J93.9   **Pneumothorax, unspecified**
Pneumothorax NOS

Item 10–11   **Empyema** is a condition in which pus accumulates in a body cavity. Empyema **with fistula** occurs when the pus passes from one cavity to another organ or structure.

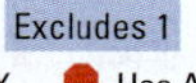

● **J94**   **Other pleural conditions**

    Excludes1   pleurisy NOS (R09.1)
        traumatic hemopneumothorax (S27.2)
        traumatic hemothorax (S27.1)
        tuberculous pleural conditions (current disease)
        (A15.-)

  J94.0   **Chylous effusion**
      Chyliform effusion

  J94.1   **Fibrothorax**

  J94.2   **Hemothorax**
      Hemopneumothorax

  J94.8   **Other specified pleural conditions**
      Hydropneumothorax
      Hydrothorax
      Coding Clinic: 2024, Q3, P4; 2021, Q1, P49

  J94.9   **Pleural condition, unspecified**

INTRAOPERATIVE AND POSTPROCEDURAL COMPLICATIONS AND DISORDERS OF RESPIRATORY SYSTEM, NOT ELSEWHERE CLASSIFIED (J95)

● **J95**   **Intraoperative and postprocedural complications and disorders of respiratory system, not elsewhere classified**

    Excludes2   aspiration pneumonia (J69.-)
        emphysema (subcutaneous) resulting from a
        procedure (T81.82)
        hypostatic pneumonia (J18.2)
        pulmonary manifestations due to radiation
        (J70.0- J70.1)

 ● **J95.0**   **Tracheostomy complications**

    J95.00   **Unspecified tracheostomy complication** Ⓡ

    J95.01   **Hemorrhage from tracheostomy stoma** Ⓡ

    J95.02   **Infection of tracheostomy stoma** Ⓡ

      Use additional code to identify type of
        infection, such as:
        cellulitis of neck (L03.221)
        sepsis (A40, A41.-)

    J95.03   **Malfunction of tracheostomy stoma** Ⓡ
      Mechanical complication of tracheostomy
        stoma
      Obstruction of tracheostomy airway
      Tracheal stenosis due to tracheostomy

    J95.04   **Tracheo-esophageal fistula following tracheostomy** Ⓡ

    J95.09   **Other tracheostomy complication** Ⓡ

  J95.1   **Acute pulmonary insufficiency following thoracic surgery** Ⓡ

    Excludes2   functional disturbances following cardiac
        surgery (I97.0, I97.1-)

  J95.2   **Acute pulmonary insufficiency following nonthoracic surgery** Ⓡ

    Excludes2   functional disturbances following cardiac
        surgery (I97.0, I97.1-)

  J95.3   **Chronic pulmonary insufficiency following surgery** Ⓡ

    Excludes2   functional disturbances following cardiac
        surgery (I97.0, I97.1-)

  J95.4   **Chemical pneumonitis due to anesthesia**
      Mendelson's syndrome
      Postprocedural aspiration pneumonia
      Use additional code for adverse effect, if applicable, to
        identify drug (T41.- with fifth or sixth character 5)

    Excludes1   aspiration pneumonitis due to anesthesia
        complicating labor and delivery
        (O74.0)
        aspiration pneumonitis due to anesthesia
        complicating pregnancy (O29)
        aspiration pneumonitis due to anesthesia
        complicating the puerperium
        (O89.01)

  J95.5   **Postprocedural subglottic stenosis**

● **J95.6**   **Intraoperative hemorrhage and hematoma of a respiratory system organ or structure complicating a procedure**

    Excludes1   intraoperative hemorrhage and
        hematoma of a respiratory system
        organ or structure due to accidental
        puncture and laceration during
        procedure (J95.7-)

    J95.61   **Intraoperative hemorrhage and hematoma of a respiratory system organ or structure complicating a respiratory system procedure**

    J95.62   **Intraoperative hemorrhage and hematoma of a respiratory system organ or structure complicating other procedure**

● **J95.7**   **Accidental puncture and laceration of a respiratory system organ or structure during a procedure**

    Excludes2   postprocedural pneumothorax (J95.811)

    J95.71   **Accidental puncture and laceration of a respiratory system organ or structure during a respiratory system procedure**

    J95.72   **Accidental puncture and laceration of a respiratory system organ or structure during other procedure**

● **J95.8**   **Other intraoperative and postprocedural complications and disorders of respiratory system, not elsewhere classified**
      Coding Clinic: 2016, Q4, P10

 ● **J95.81**   **Postprocedural pneumothorax and air leak**

      J95.811   **Postprocedural pneumothorax**
        Coding Clinic: 2021, Q1, P49

      J95.812   **Postprocedural air leak**

 ● **J95.82**   **Postprocedural respiratory failure**

      Excludes1   Respiratory failure in other
        conditions (J96.-)

      J95.821   **Acute postprocedural respiratory failure** Ⓡ
        Postprocedural respiratory failure
        NOS
        Coding Clinic: 2024, Q4, P19

      J95.822   **Acute and chronic postprocedural respiratory failure** Ⓡ

 ● **J95.83**   **Postprocedural hemorrhage of a respiratory system organ or structure following a procedure**

      J95.830   **Postprocedural hemorrhage of a respiratory system organ or structure following a respiratory system procedure**

      J95.831   **Postprocedural hemorrhage of a respiratory system organ or structure following other procedure**
        Coding Clinic: 2023, Q2, P28

    J95.84   **Transfusion-related acute lung injury (TRALI)**

 ● **J95.85**   **Complication of respirator [ventilator]**

      J95.850   **Mechanical complication of respirator** Ⓡ

        Excludes1   encounter for
          respirator
          [ventilator]
          dependence
          during power
          failure (Z99.12)

CHAPTER 10 (J00-J99)

J95.851   **Ventilator associated pneumonia** 🅷
Ventilator associated pneumonitis
   Use additional code to identify the organism, if known (B95.-, B96.-, B97.-)
     Excludes1   ventilator lung in newborn (P27.8)
     Coding Clinic: 2017, Q1, P25

J95.859   **Other complication of respirator [ventilator]** 🅷
     Coding Clinic: 2021, Q1, P49

● **J95.86**   **Postprocedural hematoma and seroma of a respiratory system organ or structure following a procedure**

J95.860   **Postprocedural hematoma of a respiratory system organ or structure following a respiratory system procedure**

J95.861   **Postprocedural hematoma of a respiratory system organ or structure following other procedure**

J95.862   **Postprocedural seroma of a respiratory system organ or structure following a respiratory system procedure**

J95.863   **Postprocedural seroma of a respiratory system organ or structure following other procedure**

J95.87   **Transfusion-associated dyspnea (TAD)**
     Excludes1   transfusion associated circulatory overload (TACO) (E87.71)
             transfusion-related acute lung injury (TRALI) (J95.84)

J95.88   **Other intraoperative complications of respiratory system, not elsewhere classified**

J95.89   **Other postprocedural complications and disorders of respiratory system, not elsewhere classified**
   Use additional code to identify disorder, such as:
     aspiration pneumonia (J69.-)
     bacterial or viral pneumonia (J12-J18)
     Excludes2   acute pulmonary insufficiency following thoracic surgery (J95.1)
             postprocedural subglottic stenosis (J95.5)

OTHER DISEASES OF THE RESPIRATORY SYSTEM (J96-J99)

● **J96**   **Respiratory failure, not elsewhere classified**
     Excludes1   acute respiratory distress syndrome (J80)
             cardiorespiratory failure (R09.2)
             newborn respiratory distress syndrome (P22.0)
             postprocedural respiratory failure (J95.82-)
             respiratory arrest (R09.2)
             respiratory arrest of newborn (P28.81)
             respiratory failure of newborn (P28.5)

● **J96.0**   **Acute respiratory failure**

J96.00   **Acute respiratory failure, unspecified whether with hypoxia or hypercapnia** 🅷
     Coding Clinic: 2016, Q3, P14

J96.01   **Acute respiratory failure with hypoxia** 🅷
     Coding Clinic: 2024, Q2, P11

J96.02   **Acute respiratory failure with hypercapnia** 🅷
   Acute respiratory acidosis

● **J96.1**   **Chronic respiratory failure**

J96.10   **Chronic respiratory failure, unspecified whether with hypoxia or hypercapnia** 🅷
     Coding Clinic: 2021, Q4, P105-106; 2021, Q1, P46; 2016, Q1, P38; 2015, Q1, P21

J96.11   **Chronic respiratory failure with hypoxia** 🅷

J96.12   **Chronic respiratory failure with hypercapnia** 🅷
   Chronic respiratory acidosis

● **J96.2**   **Acute and chronic respiratory failure**
   Acute on chronic respiratory failure

J96.20   **Acute and chronic respiratory failure, unspecified whether with hypoxia or hypercapnia** 🅷

J96.21   **Acute and chronic respiratory failure with hypoxia** 🅷

J96.22   **Acute and chronic respiratory failure with hypercapnia** 🅷

● **J96.9**   **Respiratory failure, unspecified**

J96.90   **Respiratory failure, unspecified, unspecified whether with hypoxia or hypercapnia** 🅷
     Coding Clinic: 2021, Q1, P44

J96.91   **Respiratory failure, unspecified with hypoxia** 🅷

J96.92   **Respiratory failure, unspecified with hypercapnia** 🅷

● **J98**   **Other respiratory disorders**
   Use additional code to identify:
     exposure to environmental tobacco smoke (Z77.22)
     exposure to tobacco smoke in the perinatal period (P96.81)
     history of tobacco dependence (Z87.891)
     occupational exposure to environmental tobacco smoke (Z57.31)
     tobacco dependence (F17.-)
     tobacco use (Z72.0)
     Excludes1   newborn apnea (P28.4-)
             newborn sleep apnea (P28.3-)
     Excludes2   apnea NOS (R06.81)
             sleep apnea (G47.3-)

● **J98.0**   **Diseases of bronchus, not elsewhere classified**

J98.01   **Acute bronchospasm**
     Excludes1   acute bronchiolitis with bronchospasm (J21.-)
             acute bronchitis with bronchospasm (J20.-)
             asthma (J45.-)
             exercise induced bronchospasm (J45.990)

J98.09   **Other diseases of bronchus, not elsewhere classified**
   Broncholithiasis
   Calcification of bronchus
   Stenosis of bronchus
   Tracheobronchial collapse
   Tracheobronchial dyskinesia
   Ulcer of bronchus
   Coding Clinic: 2022, Q3, P8

● **J98.1**   **Pulmonary collapse**
     Excludes1   therapeutic collapse of lung status (Z98.3)

J98.11   **Atelectasis**
     Excludes1   newborn atelectasis
             tuberculous atelectasis (current disease) (A15)

J98.19   **Other pulmonary collapse**

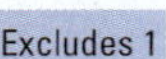

J98.2   **Interstitial emphysema** 🅡🅒
Mediastinal emphysema
Excludes1   emphysema NOS (J43.9)
emphysema in newborn (P25.0)
surgical emphysema (subcutaneous)
(T81.82)
traumatic subcutaneous emphysema
(T79.7)

J98.3   **Compensatory emphysema** 🅡🅒

J98.4   **Other disorders of lung**
Calcification of lung
Cystic lung disease (acquired)
Lung disease NOS
Pulmolithiasis
Excludes1   acute interstitial pneumonitis (J84.114)
pulmonary insufficiency following
surgery (J95.1-J95.2)
Coding Clinic: 2024, Q2, P20, 21

● **J98.5**   **Diseases of mediastinum, not elsewhere classified**
Excludes2   abscess of mediastinum (J85.3)
Coding Clinic: 2016, Q4, P29

J98.51   **Mediastinitis**
Code first underlying condition, if applicable, such
as postoperative mediastinitis (T81.-)

J98.59   **Other diseases of mediastinum, not elsewhere
classified**
Fibrosis of mediastinum
Hernia of mediastinum
Retraction of mediastinum

J98.6   **Disorders of diaphragm**
Diaphragmatitis
Paralysis of diaphragm
Relaxation of diaphragm
Excludes1   congenital malformation of diaphragm
NEC (Q79.1)
congenital diaphragmatic hernia (Q79.0)
Excludes2   diaphragmatic hernia (K44.-)

J98.8   **Other specified respiratory disorders**
Coding Clinic: 2025, Q2, P8

J98.9   **Respiratory disorder, unspecified**
Respiratory disease (chronic) NOS

▶ **J99**   ***Respiratory disorders in diseases classified elsewhere*** 🅡🅒
Code first underlying disease, such as:
amyloidosis (E85.-)
ankylosing spondylitis (M45.-)
congenital syphilis (A50.-)
cryoglobulinemia (D89.1)
early congenital syphilis (A50.-)
plasminogen deficiency (E88.02)
schistosomiasis (B65.0-B65.9)
Excludes1   respiratory disorders in:
amebiasis (A06.5)
blastomycosis (B40.0-B40.2)
candidiasis (B37.1)
coccidioidomycosis (B38.0-B38.2)
cystic fibrosis with pulmonary manifestations
(E84.0)
dermatomyositis (M33.01, M33.11)
histoplasmosis (B39.0-B39.2)
late syphilis (A52.72, A52.73)
polymyositis (M33.21)
Sjögren syndrome (M35.02)
systemic lupus erythematosus (M32.13)
systemic sclerosis (M34.81)
Wegener's granulomatosis (M31.30-M31.31)

CHAPTER 10 (J00-J99)

CHAPTER 11

DISEASES OF THE DIGESTIVE SYSTEM (K00-K95)

OGCR Chapter-Specific Coding Guidelines

11. **Chapter 11: Diseases of the Digestive System (K00-K95)**
Reserved for future guideline expansion

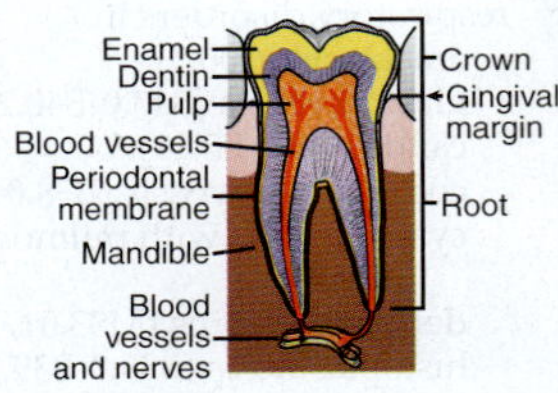

Figure 11-1 Anatomy of a tooth.

Item 11-1 **Anodontia** is the congenital absence of teeth. **Hypodontia** is partial anodontia. **Oligodontia** is the congenital absence of some teeth, whereas **supernumerary** is having more teeth than the normal number. **Mesiodens** are small extra teeth that often appear in pairs, although single small teeth are not uncommon.

CHAPTER 11

DISEASES OF THE DIGESTIVE SYSTEM (K00-K95)

Excludes2   certain conditions originating in the perinatal period (P04-P96)
certain infectious and parasitic diseases (A00-B99)
complications of pregnancy, childbirth and the puerperium (O00-O9A)
congenital malformations, deformations and chromosomal abnormalities (Q00-Q99)
endocrine, nutritional and metabolic diseases (E00-E88)
injury, poisoning and certain other consequences of external causes (S00-T88)
neoplasms (C00-D49)
symptoms, signs and abnormal clinical and laboratory findings, not elsewhere classified (R00-R94)

This chapter contains the following blocks:

K00-K14	Diseases of oral cavity and salivary glands
K20-K31	Diseases of esophagus, stomach and duodenum
K35-K38	Diseases of appendix
K40-K46	Hernia
K50-K52	Noninfective enteritis and colitis
K55-K64	Other diseases of intestines
K65-K68	Diseases of peritoneum and retroperitoneum
K70-K77	Diseases of liver
K80-K87	Disorders of gallbladder, biliary tract and pancreas
K90-K95	Other diseases of the digestive system

DISEASES OF ORAL CAVITY AND SALIVARY GLANDS (K00-K14)

● **K00**   **Disorders of tooth development and eruption**
   Excludes2   embedded and impacted teeth (K01.-)

K00.0   **Anodontia**
Hypodontia
Oligodontia
   Excludes1   acquired absence of teeth (K08.1-)

K00.1   **Supernumerary teeth**
Distomolar
Fourth molar
Mesiodens
Paramolar
Supplementary teeth
   Excludes2   supernumerary roots (K00.2)

K00.2   **Abnormalities of size and form of teeth**
Concrescence of teeth
Fusion of teeth
Gemination of teeth
Dens evaginatus
Dens in dente
Dens invaginatus
Enamel pearls
Macrodontia
Microdontia
Peg-shaped [conical] teeth
Supernumerary roots
Taurodontism
Tuberculum paramolare
   Excludes1   abnormalities of teeth due to congenital syphilis (A50.5)
tuberculum Carabelli, which is regarded as a normal variation and should not be coded

K00.3   **Mottled teeth**
Dental fluorosis
Mottling of enamel
Nonfluoride enamel opacities
   Excludes2   deposits [accretions] on teeth (K03.6)

K00.4   **Disturbances in tooth formation**
Aplasia and hypoplasia of cementum
Dilaceration of tooth
Enamel hypoplasia (neonatal) (postnatal) (prenatal)
Regional odontodysplasia
Turner's tooth
   Excludes1   Hutchinson's teeth and mulberry molars in congenital syphilis (A50.5)
   Excludes2   mottled teeth (K00.3)

K00.5   **Hereditary disturbances in tooth structure, not elsewhere classified**
Amelogenesis imperfecta
Dentinogenesis imperfecta
Odontogenesis imperfecta
Dentinal dysplasia
Shell teeth

K00.6   **Disturbances in tooth eruption**
Dentia praecox
Natal tooth
Neonatal tooth
Premature eruption of tooth
Premature shedding of primary [deciduous] tooth
Prenatal teeth
Retained [persistent] primary tooth
   Excludes2   embedded and impacted teeth (K01.-)

K00.7   **Teething syndrome**

K00.8   **Other disorders of tooth development**
Color changes during tooth formation
Intrinsic staining of teeth NOS
   Excludes2   posteruptive color changes (K03.7)

K00.9   **Disorder of tooth development, unspecified**
Disorder of odontogenesis NOS

● **K01**   **Embedded and impacted teeth**
   Excludes1   abnormal position of fully erupted teeth (M26.3-)

K01.0   **Embedded teeth**

K01.1   **Impacted teeth**

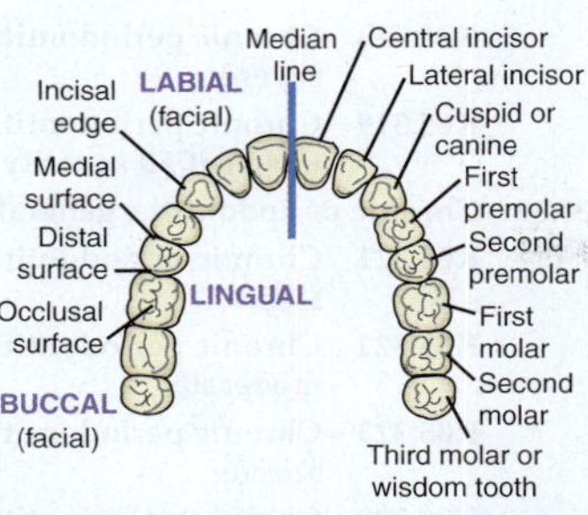

Figure 11-2 The permanent teeth within the dental arch.

Item 11–2 Each dental arch (jaw) normally contains 16 teeth. Tooth decay or **dental caries** is a disease of the enamel, dentin, and cementum of the tooth and can result in a cavity.

● **K02   Dental caries**
    Includes   caries of dentine
                    dental cavities
                    early childhood caries
                    pre-eruptive caries
                    recurrent caries (dentino enamel junction)
                        (enamel) (to the pulp)
                    tooth decay

    K02.3   **Arrested dental caries**
           Arrested coronal and root caries

●   K02.5   **Dental caries on pit and fissure surface**
           Dental caries on chewing surface of tooth

        K02.51   **Dental caries on pit and fissure surface limited to enamel**
              White spot lesions [initial caries] on pit and fissure surface of tooth

        K02.52   **Dental caries on pit and fissure surface penetrating into dentin**
              Primary dental caries, cervical origin

        K02.53   **Dental caries on pit and fissure surface penetrating into pulp**

●   K02.6   **Dental caries on smooth surface**

        K02.61   **Dental caries on smooth surface limited to enamel**
              White spot lesions [initial caries] on smooth surface of tooth

        K02.62   **Dental caries on smooth surface penetrating into dentin**

        K02.63   **Dental caries on smooth surface penetrating into pulp**

    K02.7   **Dental root caries**
    K02.9   **Dental caries, unspecified**

● **K03   Other diseases of hard tissues of teeth**
    Excludes2   bruxism (F45.8)
                      dental caries (K02.-)
                      teeth-grinding NOS (F45.8)

    K03.0   **Excessive attrition of teeth**
           Approximal wear of teeth
           Occlusal wear of teeth

    K03.1   **Abrasion of teeth**
           Dentifrice abrasion of teeth
           Habitual abrasion of teeth
           Occupational abrasion of teeth
           Ritual abrasion of teeth
           Traditional abrasion of teeth
           Wedge defect NOS

    K03.2   **Erosion of teeth**
           Erosion of teeth due to diet
           Erosion of teeth due to drugs and medicaments
           Erosion of teeth due to persistent vomiting
           Erosion of teeth NOS
           Idiopathic erosion of teeth
           Occupational erosion of teeth

    K03.3   **Pathological resorption of teeth**
           Internal granuloma of pulp
           Resorption of teeth (external)

    K03.4   **Hypercementosis**
           Cementation hyperplasia

    K03.5   **Ankylosis of teeth**

    K03.6   **Deposits [accretions] on teeth**
           Betel deposits [accretions] on teeth
           Black deposits [accretions] on teeth
           Extrinsic staining of teeth NOS
           Green deposits [accretions] on teeth
           Materia alba deposits [accretions] on teeth
           Orange deposits [accretions] on teeth
           Staining of teeth NOS
           Subgingival dental calculus
           Supragingival dental calculus
           Tobacco deposits [accretions] on teeth

    K03.7   **Posteruptive color changes of dental hard tissues**
        Excludes2   deposits [accretions] on teeth (K03.6)

●   K03.8   **Other specified diseases of hard tissues of teeth**
        K03.81   **Cracked tooth**
              Excludes1   asymptomatic craze lines in enamel - omit code
                                      broken or fractured tooth due to trauma (S02.5)

        K03.89   Other specified diseases of hard tissues of teeth
    K03.9   **Disease of hard tissues of teeth, unspecified**

● **K04   Diseases of pulp and periapical tissues**
    Coding Clinic: 2016, Q4, P29

●   K04.0   **Pulpitis**
           Acute pulpitis
           Chronic (hyperplastic) (ulcerative) pulpitis

        K04.01   **Reversible pulpitis**
        K04.02   **Irreversible pulpitis**

    K04.1   **Necrosis of pulp**
           Pulpal gangrene

    K04.2   **Pulp degeneration**
           Denticles
           Pulpal calcifications
           Pulpal stones

    K04.3   **Abnormal hard tissue formation in pulp**
           Secondary or irregular dentine

    K04.4   **Acute apical periodontitis of pulpal origin**
           Acute apical periodontitis NOS
         Excludes1   acute periodontitis (K05.2-)

    K04.5   **Chronic apical periodontitis**
           Apical or periapical granuloma
           Apical periodontitis NOS
         Excludes1   chronic periodontitis (K05.3-)

    K04.6   **Periapical abscess with sinus**
           Dental abscess with sinus
           Dentoalveolar abscess with sinus

    K04.7   **Periapical abscess without sinus**
           Dental abscess without sinus
           Dentoalveolar abscess without sinus

    K04.8   **Radicular cyst**
           Apical (periodontal) cyst
           Periapical cyst
           Residual radicular cyst
         Excludes2   lateral periodontal cyst (K09.0)

●   K04.9   **Other and unspecified diseases of pulp and periapical tissues**
        K04.90   **Unspecified diseases of pulp and periapical tissues**
        K04.99   **Other diseases of pulp and periapical tissues**

Item 11–3   Acute gingivitis, also known as orilitis or ulitis, is the short-term, severe inflammation of the gums (gingiva) caused by bacteria. **Chronic gingivitis** is persistent inflammation of the gums. When the gingivitis moves into the periodontium it is called periodontitis, also known as paradentitis.

● **K05   Gingivitis and periodontal diseases**

Use additional code to identify:
    alcohol abuse and dependence (F10.-)
    exposure to environmental tobacco smoke (Z77.22)
    exposure to tobacco smoke in the perinatal period (P96.81)
    history of tobacco dependence (Z87.891)
    occupational exposure to environmental tobacco smoke
      (Z57.31)
    tobacco dependence (F17.-)
    tobacco use (Z72.0)
Coding Clinic: 2016, Q4, P29

● **K05.0   Acute gingivitis**

    Excludes1   acute necrotizing ulcerative gingivitis
         (A69.1)
         herpesviral [herpes simplex]
           gingivostomatitis (B00.2)

    K05.00   Acute gingivitis, plaque induced
       Acute gingivitis NOS
       Plaque induced gingival disease

    K05.01   Acute gingivitis, non-plaque induced

● **K05.1   Chronic gingivitis**
    Desquamative gingivitis (chronic)
    Gingivitis (chronic) NOS
    Hyperplastic gingivitis (chronic)
    Pregnancy associated gingivitis
    Simple marginal gingivitis (chronic)
    Ulcerative gingivitis (chronic)

    Code first, if applicable, diseases of the digestive system
    complicating pregnancy (O99.61-)

    K05.10   Chronic gingivitis, plaque induced
       Chronic gingivitis NOS
       Gingivitis NOS

    K05.11   Chronic gingivitis, non-plaque induced

● **K05.2   Aggressive periodontitis**
    Acute pericoronitis

    Excludes1   acute apical periodontitis (K04.4)
         periapical abscess (K04.7)
         periapical abscess with sinus (K04.6)

    K05.20   Aggressive periodontitis, unspecified

●   **K05.21   Aggressive periodontitis, localized**
       Periodontal abscess

      K05.211   Aggressive periodontitis, localized, slight

      K05.212   Aggressive periodontitis, localized, moderate

      K05.213   Aggressive periodontitis, localized, severe

      K05.219   Aggressive periodontitis, localized, unspecified severity

●   **K05.22   Aggressive periodontitis, generalized**

      K05.221   Aggressive periodontitis, generalized, slight

      K05.222   Aggressive periodontitis, generalized, moderate

      K05.223   Aggressive periodontitis, generalized, severe

      K05.229   Aggressive periodontitis, generalized, unspecified severity

● **K05.3   Chronic periodontitis**
    Chronic pericoronitis
    Complex periodontitis
    Periodontitis NOS
    Simplex periodontitis

    Excludes1   chronic apical periodontitis (K04.5)

    K05.30   Chronic periodontitis, unspecified

●   **K05.31   Chronic periodontitis, localized**

      K05.311   Chronic periodontitis, localized, slight

      K05.312   Chronic periodontitis, localized, moderate

      K05.313   Chronic periodontitis, localized, severe

      K05.319   Chronic periodontitis, localized, unspecified severity

●   **K05.32   Chronic periodontitis, generalized**

      K05.321   Chronic periodontitis, generalized, slight

      K05.322   Chronic periodontitis, generalized, moderate

      K05.323   Chronic periodontitis, generalized, severe

      K05.329   Chronic periodontitis, generalized, unspecified severity

K05.4   Periodontosis
    Juvenile periodontosis

K05.5   Other periodontal diseases
    Combined periodontic-endodontic lesion
    Narrow gingival width (of periodontal soft tissue)

    Excludes2   leukoplakia of gingiva (K13.21)

K05.6   Periodontal disease, unspecified

● **K06   Other disorders of gingiva and edentulous alveolar ridge**

    Excludes2   acute gingivitis (K05.0)
         atrophy of edentulous alveolar ridge (K08.2)
         chronic gingivitis (K05.1)
         gingivitis NOS (K05.1)

Coding Clinic: 2016, Q4, P29

● **K06.0   Gingival recession**
    Gingival recession (postinfective) (postprocedural)

●   **K06.01   Gingival recession, localized**

      K06.010   Localized gingival recession, unspecified
         Localized gingival recession, NOS

      K06.011   Localized gingival recession, minimal

      K06.012   Localized gingival recession, moderate

      K06.013   Localized gingival recession, severe

●   **K06.02   Gingival recession, generalized**

      K06.020   Generalized gingival recession, unspecified
         Generalized gingival recession, NOS

      K06.021   Generalized gingival recession, minimal

      K06.022   Generalized gingival recession, moderate

      K06.023   Generalized gingival recession, severe

K06.1   Gingival enlargement
    Gingival fibromatosis

K06.2   Gingival and edentulous alveolar ridge lesions associated with trauma
    Irritative hyperplasia of edentulous ridge [denture hyperplasia]

    Use additional code (Chapter 20) to identify external
    cause or denture status (Z97.2)

K06.3   Horizontal alveolar bone loss

K06.8   Other specified disorders of gingiva and edentulous alveolar ridge
    Fibrous epulis
    Flabby alveolar ridge
    Giant cell epulis
    Peripheral giant cell granuloma of gingiva
    Pyogenic granuloma of gingiva
    Vertical ridge deficiency

    Excludes2   gingival cyst (K09.0)

K06.9   Disorder of gingiva and edentulous alveolar ridge, unspecified

K08 Other disorders of teeth and supporting structures
> **Excludes2** dentofacial anomalies [including malocclusion] (M26.-)
> disorders of jaw (M27.-)
>
> Coding Clinic: 2016, Q4, P29

K08.0 Exfoliation of teeth due to systemic causes
> Code also underlying systemic condition

K08.1 Complete loss of teeth
> Acquired loss of teeth, complete
>
> **Excludes1** congenital absence of teeth (K00.0)
> exfoliation of teeth due to systemic causes (K08.0)
> partial loss of teeth (K08.4-)

K08.10 Complete loss of teeth, unspecified cause
- K08.101 Complete loss of teeth, unspecified cause, class I
- K08.102 Complete loss of teeth, unspecified cause, class II
- K08.103 Complete loss of teeth, unspecified cause, class III
- K08.104 Complete loss of teeth, unspecified cause, class IV
- K08.109 Complete loss of teeth, unspecified cause, unspecified class
  - Edentulism NOS

K08.11 Complete loss of teeth due to trauma
- K08.111 Complete loss of teeth due to trauma, class I
- K08.112 Complete loss of teeth due to trauma, class II
- K08.113 Complete loss of teeth due to trauma, class III
- K08.114 Complete loss of teeth due to trauma, class IV
- K08.119 Complete loss of teeth due to trauma, unspecified class

K08.12 Complete loss of teeth due to periodontal diseases
- K08.121 Complete loss of teeth due to periodontal diseases, class I
- K08.122 Complete loss of teeth due to periodontal diseases, class II
- K08.123 Complete loss of teeth due to periodontal diseases, class III
- K08.124 Complete loss of teeth due to periodontal diseases, class IV
- K08.129 Complete loss of teeth due to periodontal diseases, unspecified class

K08.13 Complete loss of teeth due to caries
- K08.131 Complete loss of teeth due to caries, class I
- K08.132 Complete loss of teeth due to caries, class II
- K08.133 Complete loss of teeth due to caries, class III
- K08.134 Complete loss of teeth due to caries, class IV
- K08.139 Complete loss of teeth due to caries, unspecified class

K08.19 Complete loss of teeth due to other specified cause
- K08.191 Complete loss of teeth due to other specified cause, class I
- K08.192 Complete loss of teeth due to other specified cause, class II
- K08.193 Complete loss of teeth due to other specified cause, class III
- K08.194 Complete loss of teeth due to other specified cause, class IV
- K08.199 Complete loss of teeth due to other specified cause, unspecified class

K08.2 Atrophy of edentulous alveolar ridge
K08.20 Unspecified atrophy of edentulous alveolar ridge
> Atrophy of the mandible NOS
> Atrophy of the maxilla NOS

K08.21 Minimal atrophy of the mandible
> Minimal atrophy of the edentulous mandible

K08.22 Moderate atrophy of the mandible
> Moderate atrophy of the edentulous mandible

K08.23 Severe atrophy of the mandible
> Severe atrophy of the edentulous mandible

K08.24 Minimal atrophy of maxilla
> Minimal atrophy of the edentulous maxilla

K08.25 Moderate atrophy of the maxilla
> Moderate atrophy of the edentulous maxilla

K08.26 Severe atrophy of the maxilla
> Severe atrophy of the edentulous maxilla

K08.3 Retained dental root

K08.4 Partial loss of teeth
> Acquired loss of teeth, partial
>
> **Excludes1** complete loss of teeth (K08.1-)
> congenital absence of teeth (K00.0)
>
> **Excludes2** exfoliation of teeth due to systemic causes (K08.0)

K08.40 Partial loss of teeth, unspecified cause
- K08.401 Partial loss of teeth, unspecified cause, class I
- K08.402 Partial loss of teeth, unspecified cause, class II
- K08.403 Partial loss of teeth, unspecified cause, class III
- K08.404 Partial loss of teeth, unspecified cause, class IV
- K08.409 Partial loss of teeth, unspecified cause, unspecified class
  - Tooth extraction status NOS

K08.41 Partial loss of teeth due to trauma
- K08.411 Partial loss of teeth due to trauma, class I
- K08.412 Partial loss of teeth due to trauma, class II
- K08.413 Partial loss of teeth due to trauma, class III
- K08.414 Partial loss of teeth due to trauma, class IV
- K08.419 Partial loss of teeth due to trauma, unspecified class

K08.42 Partial loss of teeth due to periodontal diseases
- K08.421 Partial loss of teeth due to periodontal diseases, class I
- K08.422 Partial loss of teeth due to periodontal diseases, class II
- K08.423 Partial loss of teeth due to periodontal diseases, class III
- K08.424 Partial loss of teeth due to periodontal diseases, class IV
- K08.429 Partial loss of teeth due to periodontal diseases, unspecified class

K08.43 Partial loss of teeth due to caries
- K08.431 Partial loss of teeth due to caries, class I
- K08.432 Partial loss of teeth due to caries, class II
- K08.433 Partial loss of teeth due to caries, class III

CHAPTER 11 (K00-K95)

CHAPTER 11 (K00-K95)

K08.434 Partial loss of teeth due to caries, class IV

K08.439 Partial loss of teeth due to caries, unspecified class

● **K08.49** Partial loss of teeth due to other specified cause

K08.491 Partial loss of teeth due to other specified cause, class I

K08.492 Partial loss of teeth due to other specified cause, class II

K08.493 Partial loss of teeth due to other specified cause, class III

K08.494 Partial loss of teeth due to other specified cause, class IV

K08.499 Partial loss of teeth due to other specified cause, unspecified class

● **K08.5** Unsatisfactory restoration of tooth
Defective bridge, crown, filling
Defective dental restoration

 Excludes1 dental restoration status (Z98.811)

 Excludes2 endosseous dental implant failure (M27.6-)
     unsatisfactory endodontic treatment (M27.5-)

K08.50 Unsatisfactory restoration of tooth, unspecified
Defective dental restoration NOS

K08.51 Open restoration margins of tooth
Dental restoration failure of marginal integrity
Open margin on tooth restoration
Poor gingival margin to tooth restoration

K08.52 Unrepairable overhanging of dental restorative materials
Overhanging of tooth restoration

● **K08.53** Fractured dental restorative material

 Excludes1 cracked tooth (K03.81)
     traumatic fracture of tooth (S02.5)

K08.530 Fractured dental restorative material without loss of material

K08.531 Fractured dental restorative material with loss of material

K08.539 Fractured dental restorative material, unspecified

K08.54 Contour of existing restoration of tooth biologically incompatible with oral health
Dental restoration failure of periodontal anatomical integrity
Unacceptable contours of existing restoration of tooth
Unacceptable morphology of existing restoration of tooth

K08.55 Allergy to existing dental restorative material

 Use additional code to identify the specific type of allergy

K08.56 Poor aesthetic of existing restoration of tooth
Dental restoration aesthetically inadequate or displeasing

K08.59 Other unsatisfactory restoration of tooth
Other defective dental restoration

● **K08.8** Other specified disorders of teeth and supporting structures

K08.81 Primary occlusal trauma

K08.82 Secondary occlusal trauma

K08.89 Other specified disorders of teeth and supporting structures
Enlargement of alveolar ridge NOS
Insufficient anatomic crown height
Insufficient clinical crown length
Irregular alveolar process
Toothache NOS

K08.9 Disorder of teeth and supporting structures, unspecified

---

Item 11–4 **Atrophy** is wasting away of a tissue or organ, whereas **hypertrophy** is overdevelopment or enlargement of a tissue or organ. **Sialoadenitis** is salivary gland inflammation. **Parotitis** is the inflammation of the parotid gland. In the epidemic form, parotitis is also known as mumps. **Sialolithiasis** is the formation of calculus within a salivary gland. **Mucocele** is a polyp composed of mucus.

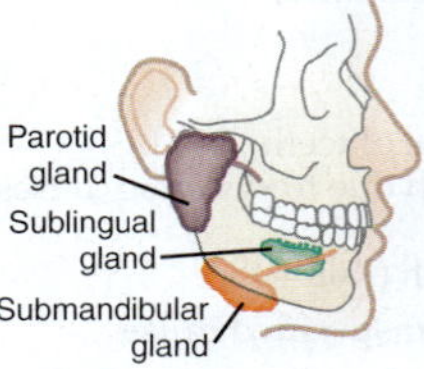

Figure 11-3 Major salivary glands.

● **K09** Cysts of oral region, not elsewhere classified

 Includes lesions showing histological features both of aneurysmal cyst and of another fibro-osseous lesion

 Excludes2 cysts of jaw (M27.0-, M27.4-)
     radicular cyst (K04.8)

K09.0 Developmental odontogenic cysts
Dentigerous cyst
Eruption cyst
Follicular cyst
Gingival cyst
Lateral periodontal cyst
Primordial cyst

 Excludes2 keratocysts (D16.4, D16.5)
     odontogenic keratocystic tumors (D16.4, D16.5)

K09.1 Developmental (nonodontogenic) cysts of oral region
Cyst (of) incisive canal
Cyst (of) palatine of papilla
Globulomaxillary cyst
Median palatal cyst
Nasoalveolar cyst
Nasolabial cyst
Nasopalatine duct cyst

K09.8 Other cysts of oral region, not elsewhere classified
Dermoid cyst
Epidermoid cyst
Lymphoepithelial cyst
Epstein's pearl

K09.9 Cyst of oral region, unspecified

★ **(See Plate 28 of the Anatomy Illustrations.)**

● **K11** Diseases of salivary glands

 Use additional code to identify:
 alcohol abuse and dependence (F10.-)
 exposure to environmental tobacco smoke (Z77.22)
 exposure to tobacco smoke in the perinatal period (P96.81)
 history of tobacco dependence (Z87.891)
 occupational exposure to environmental tobacco smoke (Z57.31)
 tobacco dependence (F17.-)
 tobacco use (Z72.0)

K11.0 Atrophy of salivary gland

K11.1 Hypertrophy of salivary gland

● **K11.2** Sialoadenitis
Parotitis

 Excludes1 epidemic parotitis (B26.-)
     mumps (B26.-)
     uveoparotid fever [Heerfordt] (D86.89)

K11.20 Sialoadenitis, unspecified

K11.21 Acute sialoadenitis

 Excludes1 acute recurrent sialoadenitis (K11.22)

K11.22 Acute recurrent sialoadenitis

K11.23 Chronic sialoadenitis

▶ New ⇨ Revised ~~deleted~~ Deleted Excludes 1 Excludes 2 Includes Use additional Code first Code also Key words

OGCR Official Guidelines X Assign placeholder X ● Use Additional Character(s) ▶ Manifestation Code Ⓗ Hierarchical Condition Category **Coding Clinic**

K11.3   **Abscess of salivary gland**

K11.4   **Fistula of salivary gland**

> **Excludes1**   congenital fistula of salivary gland (Q38.4)

K11.5   **Sialolithiasis**
Calculus of salivary gland or duct
Stone of salivary gland or duct

K11.6   **Mucocele of salivary gland**
Mucous extravasation cyst of salivary gland
Mucous retention cyst of salivary gland
Ranula

K11.7   **Disturbances of salivary secretion**
Hypoptyalism
Ptyalism
Xerostomia

> **Excludes2**   dry mouth NOS (R68.2)

K11.8   **Other diseases of salivary glands**
Benign lymphoepithelial lesion of salivary gland
Mikulicz' disease
Necrotizing sialometaplasia
Sialectasia
Stenosis of salivary duct
Stricture of salivary duct

> **Excludes1**   Sjögren syndrome (M35.0-)

K11.9   **Disease of salivary gland, unspecified**
Sialoadenopathy NOS

● **K12**   **Stomatitis and related lesions**
Use additional code to identify:
alcohol abuse and dependence (F10.-)
exposure to environmental tobacco smoke (Z77.22)
exposure to tobacco smoke in the perinatal period (P96.81)
history of tobacco dependence (Z87.891)
occupational exposure to environmental tobacco smoke (Z57.31)
tobacco dependence (F17.-)
tobacco use (Z72.0)

> **Excludes1**   cancrum oris (A69.0)
> cheilitis (K13.0)
> gangrenous stomatitis (A69.0)
> herpesviral [herpes simplex] gingivostomatitis (B00.2)
> noma (A69.0)

K12.0   **Recurrent oral aphthae**
Aphthous stomatitis (major) (minor)
Bednar's aphthae
Periadenitis mucosa necrotica recurrens
Recurrent aphthous ulcer
Stomatitis herpetiformis

K12.1   **Other forms of stomatitis**
Stomatitis NOS
Denture stomatitis
Ulcerative stomatitis
Vesicular stomatitis

> **Excludes1**   acute necrotizing ulcerative stomatitis (A69.1)
> Vincent's stomatitis (A69.1)

K12.2   **Cellulitis and abscess of mouth**
Cellulitis of mouth (floor)
Submandibular abscess

> **Excludes2**   abscess of salivary gland (K11.3)
> abscess of tongue (K14.0)
> periapical abscess (K04.6-K04.7)
> periodontal abscess (K05.21)
> peritonsillar abscess (J36)

● **K12.3**   **Oral mucositis (ulcerative)**
Mucositis (oral) (oropharyneal)

> **Excludes2**   gastrointestinal mucositis (ulcerative) (K92.81)
> mucositis (ulcerative) of vagina and vulva (N76.81)
> nasal mucositis (ulcerative) (J34.81)

K12.30   **Oral mucositis (ulcerative), unspecified**

K12.31   **Oral mucositis (ulcerative) due to antineoplastic therapy**
Use additional code for adverse effect, if applicable, to identify antineoplastic and immunosuppressive drugs (T45.1X5)
Use additional code for other antineoplastic therapy, such as:
radiological procedure and radiotherapy (Y84.2)

K12.32   **Oral mucositis (ulcerative) due to other drugs**
Use additional code for adverse effect, if applicable, to identify drug (T36-T50 with fifth or sixth character 5)

K12.33   **Oral mucositis (ulcerative) due to radiation**
Use additional external cause code (W88-W90, X39.0-) to identify cause

K12.39   **Other oral mucositis (ulcerative)**
Viral oral mucositis (ulcerative)

● **K13**   **Other diseases of lip and oral mucosa**

> **Includes**   epithelial disturbances of tongue

Use additional code to identify:
alcohol abuse and dependence (F10.-)
exposure to environmental tobacco smoke (Z77.22)
exposure to tobacco smoke in the perinatal period (P96.81)
history of tobacco dependence (Z87.891)
occupational exposure to environmental tobacco smoke (Z57.31)
tobacco dependence (F17.-)
tobacco use (Z72.0)

> **Excludes2**   certain disorders of gingiva and edentulous alveolar ridge (K05-K06)
> cysts of oral region (K09.-)
> diseases of tongue (K14.-)
> stomatitis and related lesions (K12.-)

K13.0   **Diseases of lips**
Abscess of lips
Angular cheilitis
Cellulitis of lips
Cheilitis NOS
Cheilodynia
Cheilosis
Exfoliative cheilitis
Fistula of lips
Glandular cheilitis
Hypertrophy of lips
Perlèche NEC

> **Excludes1**   ariboflavinosis (E53.0)
> cheilitis due to radiation-related disorders (L55-L59)
> congenital fistula of lips (Q38.0)
> congenital hypertrophy of lips (Q18.6)
> Perlèche due to candidiasis (B37.83)
> Perlèche due to riboflavin deficiency (E53.0)

K13.1   **Cheek and lip biting**

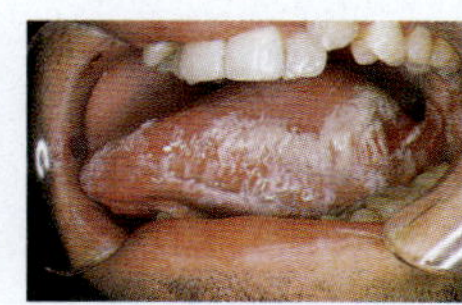

Figure 11-4   Oral leukoplakia and associated. (From Swartz MH: Textbook of Physical Diagnosis: History and Examination, Philadelphia, PA, Saunders/Elsevier, 2010)

Item 11–5   **Stomatitis** is the inflammation of the oral mucosa. **Mucositis** is the inflammation of the mucous membranes lining the digestive tract from the mouth to the anus. It is a common side effect of chemotherapy and of radiotherapy that involves any part of the digestive tract.

CHAPTER 11 (K00-K95)

● **K13.2 Leukoplakia and other disturbances of oral epithelium, including tongue**

> **Excludes1**   carcinoma in situ of oral epithelium (D00.0-)
> hairy leukoplakia (K13.3)

    K13.21 Leukoplakia of oral mucosa, including tongue
Considered precancerous and evidenced by thickened white patches of epithelium on mucous membranes
Leukokeratosis of oral mucosa
Leukoplakia of gingiva, lips, tongue

> **Excludes1**   hairy leukoplakia (K13.3)
> leukokeratosis nicotina palati (K13.24)

    K13.22 Minimal keratinized residual ridge mucosa
Minimal keratinization of alveolar ridge mucosa

    K13.23 Excessive keratinized residual ridge mucosa
Excessive keratinization of alveolar ridge mucosa

    K13.24 Leukokeratosis nicotina palati
Smoker's palate

    K13.29 Other disturbances of oral epithelium, including tongue
Erythroplakia of mouth or tongue
Focal epithelial hyperplasia of mouth or tongue
Leukoedema of mouth or tongue
Other oral epithelium disturbances

K13.3 Hairy leukoplakia

K13.4 Granuloma and granuloma-like lesions of oral mucosa
Eosinophilic granuloma
Granuloma pyogenicum
Verrucous xanthoma

K13.5 Oral submucous fibrosis
Submucous fibrosis of tongue

K13.6 Irritative hyperplasia of oral mucosa

> **Excludes2**   irritative hyperplasia of edentulous ridge [denture hyperplasia] (K06.2)

● **K13.7 Other and unspecified lesions of oral mucosa**

    K13.70 Unspecified lesions of oral mucosa

    K13.79 Other lesions of oral mucosa
Focal oral mucinosis
Coding Clinic: 2022, Q2, P8

★ **(See Plate 26 of the Anatomy Illustrations.)**

● **K14 Diseases of tongue**

Use additional code to identify:
alcohol abuse and dependence (F10.-)
exposure to environmental tobacco smoke (Z77.22)
history of tobacco dependence (Z87.891)
occupational exposure to environmental tobacco smoke (Z57.31)
tobacco dependence (F17.-)
tobacco use (Z72.0)

> **Excludes2**   erythroplakia (K13.29)
> focal epithelial hyperplasia (K13.29)
> leukoedema of tongue (K13.29)
> leukoplakia of tongue (K13.21)
> hairy leukoplakia (K13.3)
> macroglossia (congenital) (Q38.2)
> submucous fibrosis of tongue (K13.5)

K14.0 Glossitis
Abscess of tongue
Ulceration (traumatic) of tongue

> **Excludes1**   atrophic glossitis (K14.4)

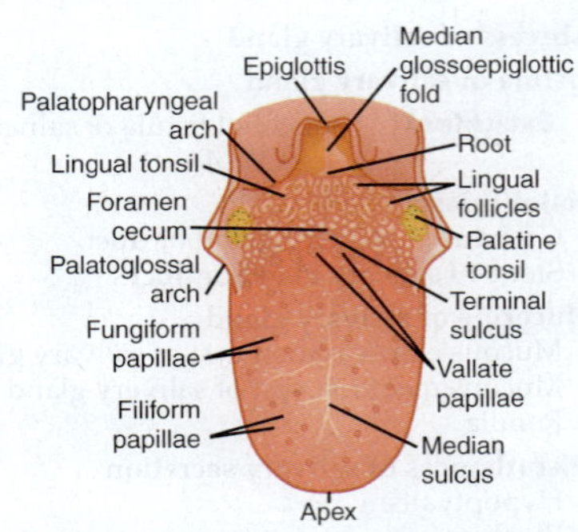

Figure 11-5   Structure of the tongue.

K14.1 Geographic tongue
Benign migratory glossitis
Glossitis areata exfoliativa

K14.2 Median rhomboid glossitis

K14.3 Hypertrophy of tongue papillae
Black hairy tongue
Coated tongue
Hypertrophy of foliate papillae
Lingua villosa nigra

K14.4 Atrophy of tongue papillae
Atrophic glossitis

K14.5 Plicated tongue
Fissured tongue   Scrotal tongue
Furrowed tongue

> **Excludes1**   fissured tongue, congenital (Q38.3)

K14.6 Glossodynia
Glossopyrosis   Painful tongue

K14.8 Other diseases of tongue
Atrophy of tongue   Glossocele
Crenated tongue   Glossoptosis
Enlargement of tongue   Hypertrophy of tongue

K14.9 Disease of tongue, unspecified
Glossopathy NOS

DISEASES OF ESOPHAGUS, STOMACH AND DUODENUM (K20-K31)

> **Excludes2**   hiatus hernia (K44.-)

● **K20 Esophagitis**

Use additional code to identify:
alcohol abuse and dependence (F10.-)

> **Excludes1**   erosion of esophagus (K22.1-)
> esophagitis with gastro-esophageal reflux disease (K21.0-)
> reflux esophagitis (K21.0-)
> ulcerative esophagitis (K22.1-)

> **Excludes2**   eosinophilic gastritis or gastroenteritis (K52.81)
> *Coding Clinic: 2023, Q1, P20*

K20.0 Eosinophilic esophagitis

● **K20.8 Other esophagitis**

    K20.80 Other esophagitis without bleeding
Abscess of esophagus
Other esophagitis NOS

    K20.81 Other esophagitis with bleeding

● **K20.9 Esophagitis, unspecified**

    K20.90 Esophagitis, unspecified without bleeding
Esophagitis NOS

    K20.91 Esophagitis, unspecified with bleeding

● **K21** Gastro-esophageal reflux disease

    Excludes1 newborn esophageal reflux (P78.83)

  ● **K21.0** Gastro-esophageal reflux disease with esophagitis

    K21.00 Gastro-esophageal reflux disease with esophagitis, without bleeding
        Reflux esophagitis

    K21.01 Gastro-esophageal reflux disease with esophagitis, with bleeding

  K21.9 Gastro-esophageal reflux disease without esophagitis
    Esophageal reflux NOS
    Coding Clinic: 2016, Q1, P18

● **K22** Other diseases of esophagus

    Excludes2 esophageal varices (I85.-)

  K22.0 **Achalasia of cardia**
    Achalasia NOS
    Cardiospasm

    Excludes1 congenital cardiospasm (Q39.5)

  ● **K22.1** **Ulcer of esophagus**
    Barrett's ulcer
    Erosion of esophagus
    Fungal ulcer of esophagus
    Peptic ulcer of esophagus
    Ulcer of esophagus due to ingestion of chemicals
    Ulcer of esophagus due to ingestion of drugs and medicaments
    Ulcerative esophagitis

    Code first poisoning due to drug or toxin, if applicable (T36-T65 with fifth or sixth character 1-4)

    Use additional code for adverse effect, if applicable, to identify drug (T36-T50 with fifth or sixth character 5)

    Excludes1 Barrett's esophagus (K22.87-)

    K22.10 Ulcer of esophagus without bleeding
        Ulcer of esophagus NOS

    K22.11 Ulcer of esophagus with bleeding

      Excludes2 bleeding esophageal varices (I85.01, I85.11)
      Coding Clinic: 2023, Q1, P20

  K22.2 **Esophageal obstruction**
    Compression of esophagus
    Constriction of esophagus
    Stenosis of esophagus
    Stricture of esophagus

    Excludes1 congenital stenosis or stricture of esophagus (Q39.3)
    Coding Clinic: 2024, Q2, P26

  K22.3 **Perforation of esophagus**
    Rupture of esophagus

    Excludes1 traumatic perforation of (thoracic) esophagus (S27.8-)

  K22.4 **Dyskinesia of esophagus**
    Difficulty in moving
    Corkscrew esophagus
    Diffuse esophageal spasm
    Spasm of esophagus

    Excludes1 cardiospasm (K22.0)
    Coding Clinic: 2025, Q2, P17

  K22.5 **Diverticulum of esophagus, acquired**
    Esophageal pouch, acquired

    Excludes1 diverticulum of esophagus (congenital) (Q39.6)

  K22.6 **Gastro-esophageal laceration-hemorrhage syndrome**
    Mallory-Weiss syndrome

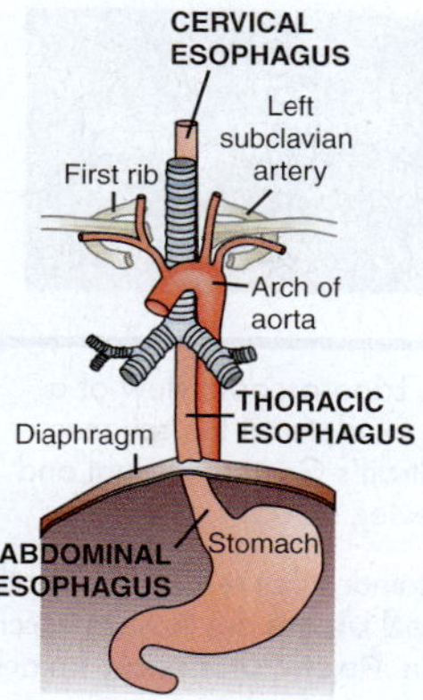

Figure 11-6 The esophagus is the muscular tube that connects the pharynx and the stomach. The 10-inch (25 cm) long esophagus is divided into three parts: **cervical, thoracic,** and **abdominal.**

Item 11–7 Achalasia is a condition in which the smooth muscle fibers of the esophagus do not relax. Most frequently, this condition occurs at the esophagogastric sphincter. **Cardiospasm,** also known as **megaesophagus,** is achalasia of the thoracic esophagus.

  ● **K22.7** **Barrett's esophagus**
    Barrett's disease
    Barrett's syndrome

    Excludes1 Barrett's ulcer (K22.1)
        malignant neoplasm of esophagus (C15.-)

    K22.70 Barrett's esophagus without dysplasia
        Barrett's esophagus NOS

   ● **K22.71** Barrett's esophagus with dysplasia

      K22.710 Barrett's esophagus with low grade dysplasia

      K22.711 Barrett's esophagus with high grade dysplasia

      K22.719 Barrett's esophagus with dysplasia, unspecified

  ● **K22.8** **Other specified diseases of esophagus**

    K22.81 **Esophageal polyp**

      Excludes1 benign neoplasm of esophagus (D13.0)

    K22.82 Esophagogastric junction polyp

      Excludes1 benign neoplasm of stomach (D13.1)

    K22.89 **Other specified disease of esophagus**
      Hemorrhage of esophagus NOS

      Excludes2 esophageal varices (I85.-)
        Paterson-Kelly syndrome (D50.1)
      Coding Clinic: 2024, Q2, P26; 2020, Q1, P16

  K22.9 Disease of esophagus, unspecified

▶ *K23* *Disorders of esophagus in diseases classified elsewhere*
    Code first underlying disease, such as:
    congenital syphilis (A50.5)

    Excludes1 late syphilis (A52.79)
        megaesophagus due to Chagas' disease (B57.31)
        tuberculosis (A18.83)

● **K25** **Gastric ulcer**

    Includes erosion (acute) of stomach
        pylorus ulcer (peptic)
        stomach ulcer (peptic)

    Use additional code to identify:
    alcohol abuse and dependence (F10.-)

    Excludes1 acute gastritis (K29.0-)
        peptic ulcer NOS (K27.-)

  K25.0 **Acute gastric ulcer with hemorrhage**
    Coding Clinic: 2023, Q1, P16

  K25.1 **Acute gastric ulcer with perforation**

  K25.2 **Acute gastric ulcer with both hemorrhage and perforation**

  K25.3 **Acute gastric ulcer without hemorrhage or perforation**

  K25.4 **Chronic or unspecified gastric ulcer with hemorrhage**
    Coding Clinic: 2017, Q3, P27

Item 11–6 Esophageal reflux is the return flow of the contents of the stomach to the esophagus and is referred to as GERD and/or "heartburn." **Gastroesophageal reflux** is the return flow of the contents of the stomach and duodenum to the esophagus. **Esophageal leukoplakia** are white areas on the mucous membrane of the esophagus for which no specific cause can be identified.

CHAPTER 11 (K00–K95)

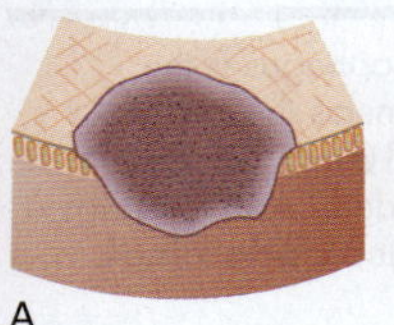 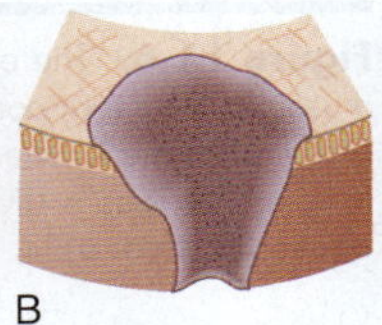 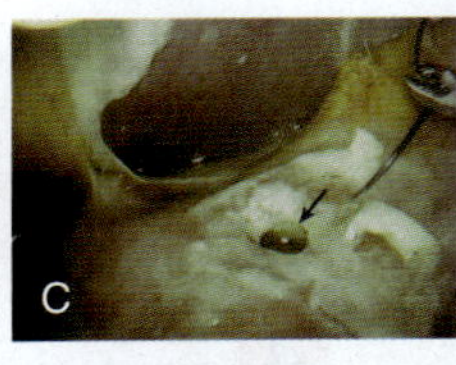

A   B   C

Figure 11-7 **A.** Ulcer. **B.** Perforated ulcer. **C.** Laparoscopic view of a perforated duodenal ulcer *(arrow)* with fibrinous exudate on the adjacent peritoneum. (**C** from Feldman: Sleisenger & Fordtran's Gastrointestinal and Liver Disease, ed 8, Saunders, An Imprint of Elsevier, 2006)

Item 11–8 **Gastric ulcers** are lesions of the stomach that result in the death of the tissue and a defect of the surface. **Perforated ulcers** are those in which the lesion penetrates the gastric wall, leaving a hole. **Peptic ulcers** are lesions of the stomach or the duodenum. **Peptic** refers to the gastric juice, pepsin.

K25.5   Chronic or unspecified gastric ulcer with perforation ᴴᶜᶜ

K25.6   Chronic or unspecified gastric ulcer with both hemorrhage and perforation ᴴᶜᶜ

K25.7   Chronic gastric ulcer without hemorrhage or perforation

K25.9   Gastric ulcer, unspecified as acute or chronic, without hemorrhage or perforation
    Coding Clinic: 2021, Q1, P12

● **K26   Duodenal ulcer**

   Includes   erosion (acute) of duodenum
               duodenum ulcer (peptic)
               postpyloric ulcer (peptic)

   Use additional code to identify:
     alcohol abuse and dependence (F10.-)

   Excludes1   peptic ulcer NOS (K27.-)

K26.0   **Acute duodenal ulcer with hemorrhage**

K26.1   **Acute duodenal ulcer with perforation** ᴴᶜᶜ

K26.2   **Acute duodenal ulcer with both hemorrhage and perforation** ᴴᶜᶜ

K26.3   **Acute duodenal ulcer without hemorrhage or perforation**

K26.4   **Chronic or unspecified duodenal ulcer with hemorrhage**
    Coding Clinic: 2016, Q1, P14

K26.5   **Chronic or unspecified duodenal ulcer with perforation** ᴴᶜᶜ

K26.6   **Chronic or unspecified duodenal ulcer with both hemorrhage and perforation** ᴴᶜᶜ

K26.7   **Chronic duodenal ulcer without hemorrhage or perforation**
    Coding Clinic: 2023, Q2, P11

K26.9   **Duodenal ulcer, unspecified as acute or chronic, without hemorrhage or perforation**

● **K27   Peptic ulcer, site unspecified**

   Includes   gastroduodenal ulcer NOS
               peptic ulcer NOS

   Use additional code to identify:
     alcohol abuse and dependence (F10.-)

   Excludes1   peptic ulcer of newborn (P78.82)

K27.0   **Acute peptic ulcer, site unspecified, with hemorrhage**

K27.1   **Acute peptic ulcer, site unspecified, with perforation** ᴴᶜᶜ

K27.2   **Acute peptic ulcer, site unspecified, with both hemorrhage and perforation** ᴴᶜᶜ

K27.3   **Acute peptic ulcer, site unspecified, without hemorrhage or perforation**

K27.4   **Chronic or unspecified peptic ulcer, site unspecified, with hemorrhage**

K27.5   **Chronic or unspecified peptic ulcer, site unspecified, with perforation** ᴴᶜᶜ

K27.6   **Chronic or unspecified peptic ulcer, site unspecified, with both hemorrhage and perforation** ᴴᶜᶜ

K27.7   **Chronic peptic ulcer, site unspecified, without hemorrhage or perforation**

K27.9   **Peptic ulcer, site unspecified, unspecified as acute or chronic, without hemorrhage or perforation**

● **K28   Gastrojejunal ulcer**

   Includes   anastomotic ulcer (peptic) or erosion
               gastrocolic ulcer (peptic) or erosion
               gastrointestinal ulcer (peptic) or erosion
               gastrojejunal ulcer (peptic) or erosion
               jejunal ulcer (peptic) or erosion
               marginal ulcer (peptic) or erosion
               stomal ulcer (peptic) or erosion

   Use additional code to identify:
     alcohol abuse and dependence (F10.-)

   Excludes1   primary ulcer of small intestine (K63.3)

K28.0   **Acute gastrojejunal ulcer with hemorrhage**

K28.1   **Acute gastrojejunal ulcer with perforation** ᴴᶜᶜ

K28.2   **Acute gastrojejunal ulcer with both hemorrhage and perforation** ᴴᶜᶜ

K28.3   **Acute gastrojejunal ulcer without hemorrhage or perforation**

K28.4   **Chronic or unspecified gastrojejunal ulcer with hemorrhage**
    Coding Clinic: 2023, Q3, P10

K28.5   **Chronic or unspecified gastrojejunal ulcer with perforation** ᴴᶜᶜ

K28.6   **Chronic or unspecified gastrojejunal ulcer with both hemorrhage and perforation** ᴴᶜᶜ

K28.7   **Chronic gastrojejunal ulcer without hemorrhage or perforation**

K28.9   **Gastrojejunal ulcer, unspecified as acute or chronic, without hemorrhage or perforation**

● **K29   Gastritis and duodenitis**

   Excludes1   eosinophilic gastritis or gastroenteritis (K52.81)
               Zollinger-Ellison syndrome (E16.4)

● **K29.0   Acute gastritis**

   Use additional code to identify:
     alcohol abuse and dependence (F10.-)

   Excludes1   erosion (acute) of stomach (K25.-)

K29.00   **Acute gastritis without bleeding**

K29.01   **Acute gastritis with bleeding**

● **K29.2   Alcoholic gastritis**

   Use additional code to identify:
     alcohol abuse and dependence (F10.-)

K29.20   **Alcoholic gastritis without bleeding**

K29.21   **Alcoholic gastritis with bleeding**

● **K29.3   Chronic superficial gastritis**

K29.30   **Chronic superficial gastritis without bleeding**

K29.31   **Chronic superficial gastritis with bleeding**

● **K29.4   Chronic atrophic gastritis**
    Gastric atrophy

K29.40   **Chronic atrophic gastritis without bleeding**

K29.41   **Chronic atrophic gastritis with bleeding**

● **K29.5   Unspecified chronic gastritis**
    Chronic antral gastritis
    Chronic fundal gastritis

K29.50   **Unspecified chronic gastritis without bleeding**

K29.51   **Unspecified chronic gastritis with bleeding**

● **K29.6   Other gastritis**
    Giant hypertrophic gastritis
    Granulomatous gastritis
    Ménétrier's disease

K29.60   **Other gastritis without bleeding**

K29.61   **Other gastritis with bleeding**

● **K29.7   Gastritis, unspecified**

K29.70   **Gastritis, unspecified, without bleeding**

K29.71   **Gastritis, unspecified, with bleeding**

▶ New   ➡ Revised   ~~deleted~~ Deleted   Excludes 1   Excludes 2   Includes   Use additional   Code first   Code also   Key words
OGCR Official Guidelines   X Assign placeholder X   ● Use Additional Character(s)   ▶ Manifestation Code   ᴴᶜᶜ Hierarchical Condition Category   **Coding Clinic**

CHAPTER 11 (K00-K95)

Item 11–9   **Gastritis** is a severe inflammation of the stomach. **Atrophic gastritis** is a chronic inflammation of the stomach that results in destruction of the cells of the mucosa of the stomach. Duodenitis is an inflammation of the duodenum, the first section of the small intestine.

● **K29.8   Duodenitis**
     K29.8Ø   Duodenitis without bleeding
        Coding Clinic: 2Ø25, Q2, P5
     K29.81   Duodenitis with bleeding
● **K29.9   Gastroduodenitis, unspecified**
     K29.9Ø   Gastroduodenitis, unspecified, without bleeding
     K29.91   Gastroduodenitis, unspecified, with bleeding

K3Ø   Functional dyspepsia
     Indigestion
     Excludes1   dyspepsia NOS (R10.13)
                 heartburn (R12)
                 nervous dyspepsia (F45.8)
                 neurotic dyspepsia (F45.8)
                 psychogenic dyspepsia (F45.8)

● **K31   Other diseases of stomach and duodenum**
     Includes   functional disorders of stomach
     Excludes2   diabetic gastroparesis (E08.43, E09.43, E10.43, E11.43, E13.43)
                 diverticulum of duodenum (K57.00-K57.13)

     K31.Ø   Acute dilatation of stomach
        Acute distention of stomach
     K31.1   Adult hypertrophic pyloric stenosis   A
        Pyloric stenosis NOS
        Excludes1   congenital or infantile pyloric stenosis (Q40.0)
        Coding Clinic: 2Ø23, Q3, P12
     K31.2   Hourglass stricture and stenosis of stomach
        Excludes1   congenital hourglass stomach (Q40.2)
                 hourglass contraction of stomach (K31.89)
     K31.3   Pylorospasm, not elsewhere classified
        Excludes1   congenital or infantile pylorospasm (Q40.0)
                 neurotic pylorospasm (F45.8)
                 psychogenic pylorospasm (F45.8)
     K31.4   Gastric diverticulum
        Excludes1   congenital diverticulum of stomach (Q40.2)
     K31.5   Obstruction of duodenum
        Constriction of duodenum
        Duodenal ileus (chronic)
        Stenosis of duodenum
           Narrowing
        Stricture of duodenum
           Narrowing
        Volvulus of duodenum
           Twisting/knotting
        Excludes1   congenital stenosis of duodenum (Q41.0)
     K31.6   Fistula of stomach and duodenum
        Gastrocolic fistula
        Gastrojejunocolic fistula
        Code also, if applicable, disruption of internal operation (surgical) wound (T81.32-)
     K31.7   Polyp of stomach and duodenum
        Excludes1   adenomatous polyp of stomach (D13.1)
        Coding Clinic: 2Ø2Ø, Q1, P16
●   **K31.8   Other specified diseases of stomach and duodenum**
     ● **K31.81   Angiodysplasia of stomach and duodenum**
        K31.811   Angiodysplasia of stomach and duodenum with bleeding
            Coding Clinic: 2Ø23, Q1, P16
        K31.819   Angiodysplasia of stomach and duodenum without bleeding
            Angiodysplasia of stomach and duodenum NOS
       K31.82   Dieulafoy lesion (hemorrhagic) of stomach and duodenum
          Excludes2   Dieulafoy lesion of intestine (K63.81)

Item 11–10   **Achlorhydria,** also known as gastric anacidity, is the absence of gastric acid.

     K31.83   Achlorhydria
     K31.84   Gastroparesis
        Gastroparalysis
        Code first underlying disease, if known, such as:
          anorexia nervosa (F50.0-)
          diabetes mellitus (E08.43, E09.43, E10.43, E11.43, E13.43)
          scleroderma (M34.-)
     K31.89   Other diseases of stomach and duodenum
        Coding Clinic: 2Ø24, Q2, P26; 2Ø2Ø, Q1, P16; 2Ø17, Q1, P28
     K31.9   Disease of stomach and duodenum, unspecified
●   **K31.A   Gastric intestinal metaplasia**
     K31.AØ   Gastric intestinal metaplasia, unspecified
        Gastric intestinal metaplasia indefinite for dysplasia
        Gastric intestinal metaplasia NOS
     ● **K31.A1   Gastric intestinal metaplasia without dysplasia**
        K31.A11   Gastric intestinal metaplasia without dysplasia, involving the antrum
        K31.A12   Gastric intestinal metaplasia without dysplasia, involving the body(corpus)
        K31.A13   Gastric intestinal metaplasia without dysplasia, involving the fundus involving the cardia
        K31.A14   Gastric intestinal metaplasia without dysplasia, involving the cardia
        K31.A15   Gastric intestinal metaplasia without dysplasia, involving multiple sites
        K31.A19   Gastric intestinal metaplasia without dysplasia, unspecified site
     ● **K31.A2   Gastric intestinal metaplasia with dysplasia**
        K31.A21   Gastric intestinal metaplasia with low grade dysplasia
        K31.A22   Gastric intestinal metaplasia with high grade dysplasia
        K31.A29   Gastric intestinal metaplasia with dysplasia, unspecified

DISEASES OF APPENDIX (K35-K38)

● **K35   Acute appendicitis**
●   **K35.2   Acute appendicitis with generalized peritonitis**
     ● **K35.2Ø   Acute appendicitis with generalized peritonitis, without abscess (Acute) appendicitis with generalized peritonitis NOS**
        Coding Clinic: 2Ø18, Q4, P18
        K35.2ØØ   Acute appendicitis with generalized peritonitis, without perforation or abscess
           (Acute) appendicitis with generalized peritonitis without rupture or perforation of appendix NOS
        K35.2Ø1   Acute appendicitis with generalized peritonitis, with perforation, without abscess
           Appendicitis (acute) with generalized (diffuse) peritonitis following rupture or perforation of appendix NOS
        K35.2Ø9   Acute appendicitis with generalized peritonitis, without abscess, unspecified as to perforation
           (Acute) appendicitis with generalized peritonitis NOS

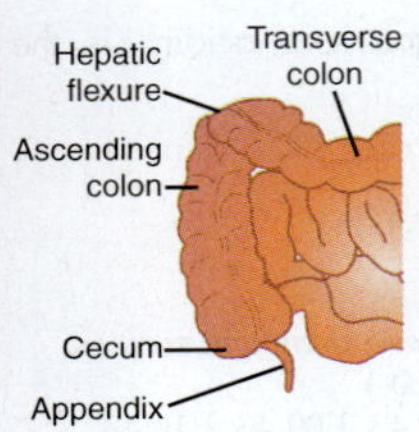

Figure 11-8 Acute appendicitis is the inflammation of the appendix, usually associated with obstruction. Most often this is a disease of adolescents and young adults.

● **K35.21 Acute appendicitis with generalized peritonitis, with abscess**

K35.210 Acute appendicitis with generalized peritonitis, without perforation, with abscess
(Acute) appendicitis with generalized peritonitis without rupture or perforation of appendix, with abscess

K35.211 Acute appendicitis with generalized peritonitis, with perforation and abscess
Appendicitis (acute) with generalized (diffuse) peritonitis following rupture or perforation of appendix, with abscess

K35.219 Acute appendicitis with generalized peritonitis, with abscess, unspecified as to perforation
(Acute) appendicitis with generalized peritonitis and abscess NOS

● **K35.3 Acute appendicitis with localized peritonitis**

K35.30 Acute appendicitis with localized peritonitis, without perforation or gangrene
Acute appendicitis with localized peritonitis NOS

K35.31 Acute appendicitis with localized peritonitis and gangrene, without perforation

K35.32 Acute appendicitis with perforation, localized peritonitis, and gangrene, without abscess
(Acute) appendicitis with perforation NOS
Perforated appendix NOS
Ruptured appendix (with localized peritonitis) NOS
Coding Clinic: 2020, Q1, P16; 2018, Q4, P18

K35.33 Acute appendicitis with perforation, localized peritonitis, and gangrene, with abscess
(Acute) appendicitis with (peritoneal) abscess NOS
Ruptured appendix with localized peritonitis and abscess

● **K35.8 Other and unspecified acute appendicitis**

K35.80 Unspecified acute appendicitis
Acute appendicitis NOS
Acute appendicitis without (localized) (generalized) peritonitis

● **K35.89 Other acute appendicitis**

K35.890 Other acute appendicitis without perforation or gangrene

K35.891 Other acute appendicitis without perforation, with gangrene
(Acute) appendicitis with gangrene NOS

K36 Other appendicitis
Chronic appendicitis
Recurrent appendicitis

K37 Unspecified appendicitis

Excludes1 unspecified appendicitis with peritonitis (K35.2-, K35.3)

● **K38 Other diseases of appendix**

K38.0 Hyperplasia of appendix

K38.1 Appendicular concretions
Fecalith of appendix
Stercolith of appendix

K38.2 Diverticulum of appendix

K38.3 Fistula of appendix

K38.8 Other specified diseases of appendix
Intussusception of appendix

K38.9 Disease of appendix, unspecified

HERNIA (K40-K46)

Note: Hernia with both gangrene and obstruction is classified to hernia with gangrene.

Includes acquired hernia
congenital [except diaphragmatic or hiatus] hernia
recurrent hernia

● **K40 Inguinal hernia**

Includes bubonocele
direct inguinal hernia
double inguinal hernia
indirect inguinal hernia
inguinal hernia NOS
oblique inguinal hernia
scrotal hernia

● **K40.0 Bilateral inguinal hernia, with obstruction, without gangrene**
Inguinal hernia (bilateral) causing obstruction without gangrene
Incarcerated inguinal hernia (bilateral) without gangrene
Irreducible inguinal hernia (bilateral) without gangrene
Strangulated inguinal hernia (bilateral) without gangrene

K40.00 Bilateral inguinal hernia, with obstruction, without gangrene, not specified as recurrent
Bilateral inguinal hernia, with obstruction, without gangrene NOS

K40.01 Bilateral inguinal hernia, with obstruction, without gangrene, recurrent

Item 11–11 Hernias of the groin are the most common type, accounting for 80 percent of all hernias. There are two major types of inguinal hernias: indirect (oblique) affecting men only and direct. **Indirect inguinal hernias** result when the intestines emerge through the abdominal wall in an indirect fashion through the inguinal canal. **Direct inguinal hernias** penetrate through the abdominal wall in a direct fashion. **Femoral hernias** occur at the femoral ring where the femoral vessels enter the thigh and is most common in women. An abdominal wall hernia is also called a ventral or epigastric hernia and occurs in both sexes. Classification is based on location of the hernia and whether there is obstruction or gangrene.

Ventral, epigastric, or incisional hernia occurs on the abdominal surface caused by musculature weakness or a tear at a previous surgical site and is evidenced by a bulge that changes in size, becoming larger with exertion. An **incarcerated** hernia is one in which the intestines become trapped in the hernia. A **strangulated** hernia is one in which the blood supply to the intestines is lost. **Hiatal hernia** occurs when a loop of the stomach protrudes upward through the small opening in the diaphragm through which the esophagus passes, leaving the abdominal cavity and entering the chest. It occurs in both sexes.

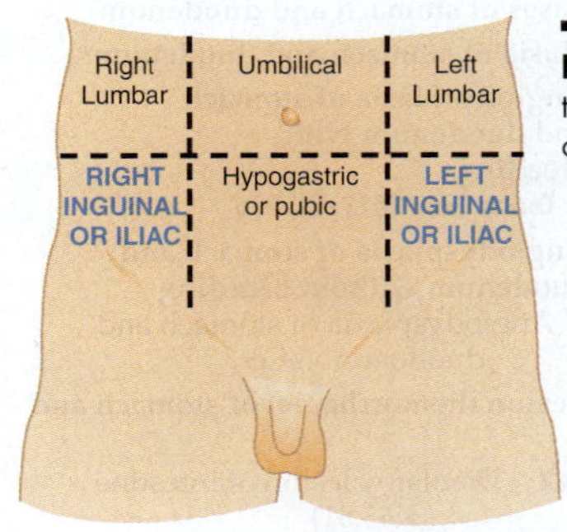

Figure 11-9 Inguinal hernias are those that are located in the inguinal or iliac areas of the abdomen.

▶ New ➡ Revised ~~deleted~~ Deleted Excludes 1 Excludes 2 Includes Use additional Code first Code also Key words
OGCR Official Guidelines **X** Assign placeholder X ● Use Additional Character(s) ▶ Manifestation Code Ⓡ Hierarchical Condition Category **Coding Clinic**

● **K40.1** **Bilateral inguinal hernia, with gangrene**

     K40.10 Bilateral inguinal hernia, with gangrene, **not specified as recurrent**
         Bilateral inguinal hernia, with gangrene NOS

     K40.11 Bilateral inguinal hernia, with gangrene, **recurrent**

● **K40.2** **Bilateral inguinal hernia, without obstruction or gangrene**

     K40.20 Bilateral inguinal hernia, without obstruction or gangrene, **not specified as recurrent**
         Bilateral inguinal hernia NOS

     K40.21 Bilateral inguinal hernia, without obstruction or gangrene, **recurrent**

● **K40.3** **Unilateral inguinal hernia, with obstruction, without gangrene**

     Inguinal hernia (unilateral) causing obstruction without gangrene

     Incarcerated inguinal hernia (unilateral) without gangrene

     Irreducible inguinal hernia (unilateral) without gangrene

     Strangulated inguinal hernia (unilateral) without gangrene

     K40.30 Unilateral inguinal hernia, with obstruction, without gangrene, **not specified as recurrent**
         Inguinal hernia, with obstruction NOS
         Unilateral inguinal hernia, with obstruction, without gangrene NOS

     K40.31 Unilateral inguinal hernia, with obstruction, without gangrene, **recurrent**

● **K40.4** **Unilateral inguinal hernia, with gangrene**

     K40.40 Unilateral inguinal hernia, with gangrene, **not specified as recurrent**
         Inguinal hernia with gangrene NOS
         Unilateral inguinal hernia with gangrene NOS

     K40.41 Unilateral inguinal hernia, with gangrene, **recurrent**

● **K40.9** **Unilateral inguinal hernia, without obstruction or gangrene**

     K40.90 Unilateral inguinal hernia, without obstruction or gangrene, **not specified as recurrent**
         Inguinal hernia NOS
         Unilateral inguinal hernia NOS
         Coding Clinic: 2021, Q3, P31

     K40.91 Unilateral inguinal hernia, without obstruction or gangrene, **recurrent**
         Coding Clinic: 2021, Q3, P31

● **K41** **Femoral hernia**

  ● **K41.0** **Bilateral femoral hernia, with obstruction, without gangrene**

     Femoral hernia (bilateral) causing obstruction, without gangrene

     Incarcerated femoral hernia (bilateral), without gangrene

     Irreducible femoral hernia (bilateral), without gangrene

     Strangulated femoral hernia (bilateral), without gangrene

     K41.00 Bilateral femoral hernia, with obstruction, without gangrene, **not specified as recurrent**
         Bilateral femoral hernia, with obstruction, without gangrene NOS

     K41.01 Bilateral femoral hernia, with obstruction, without gangrene, **recurrent**

  ● **K41.1** **Bilateral femoral hernia, with gangrene**

     K41.10 Bilateral femoral hernia, with gangrene, **not specified as recurrent**
         Bilateral femoral hernia, with gangrene NOS

     K41.11 Bilateral femoral hernia, with gangrene, **recurrent**

  ● **K41.2** **Bilateral femoral hernia, without obstruction or gangrene**

     K41.20 Bilateral femoral hernia, without obstruction or gangrene, **not specified as recurrent**
         Bilateral femoral hernia NOS

     K41.21 Bilateral femoral hernia, without obstruction or gangrene, **recurrent**

● **K41.3** **Unilateral femoral hernia, with obstruction, without gangrene**

     Femoral hernia (unilateral) causing obstruction, without gangrene

     Incarcerated femoral hernia (unilateral), without gangrene

     Irreducible femoral hernia (unilateral), without gangrene

     Strangulated femoral hernia (unilateral), without gangrene

     K41.30 Unilateral femoral hernia, with obstruction, without gangrene, **not specified as recurrent**
         Femoral hernia, with obstruction NOS
         Unilateral femoral hernia, with obstruction NOS

     K41.31 Unilateral femoral hernia, with obstruction, without gangrene, **recurrent**
         Coding Clinic: 2021, Q3, P30

● **K41.4** **Unilateral femoral hernia, with gangrene**

     K41.40 Unilateral femoral hernia, with gangrene, **not specified as recurrent**
         Femoral hernia, with gangrene NOS
         Unilateral femoral hernia, with gangrene NOS

     K41.41 Unilateral femoral hernia, with gangrene, **recurrent**

● **K41.9** **Unilateral femoral hernia, without obstruction or gangrene**

     K41.90 Unilateral femoral hernia, without obstruction or gangrene, **not specified as recurrent**
         Femoral hernia NOS
         Unilateral femoral hernia NOS
         Coding Clinic: 2021, Q3, P30-31

     K41.91 Unilateral femoral hernia, without obstruction or gangrene, **recurrent**

● **K42** **Umbilical hernia**

     Includes   paraumbilical hernia

     Excludes1   omphalocele (Q79.2)

     K42.0 **Umbilical hernia with obstruction, without gangrene**
         Umbilical hernia causing obstruction, without gangrene
         Incarcerated umbilical hernia, without gangrene
         Irreducible umbilical hernia, without gangrene
         Strangulated umbilical hernia, without gangrene

     K42.1 **Umbilical hernia with gangrene**
         Gangrenous umbilical hernia

     K42.9 **Umbilical hernia without obstruction or gangrene**
         Umbilical hernia NOS

● **K43** **Ventral hernia**

     K43.0 **Incisional hernia with obstruction, without gangrene**
         Incisional hernia causing obstruction, without gangrene
         Incarcerated incisional hernia, without gangrene
         Irreducible incisional hernia, without gangrene
         Strangulated incisional hernia, without gangrene

     K43.1 **Incisional hernia with gangrene**
         Gangrenous incisional hernia

     K43.2 **Incisional hernia without obstruction or gangrene**
         Incisional hernia NOS

     K43.3 **Parastomal hernia with obstruction, without gangrene**
         Incarcerated parastomal hernia, without gangrene
         Irreducible parastomal hernia, without gangrene
         Parastomal hernia causing obstruction, without gangrene
         Strangulated parastomal hernia, without gangrene

     K43.4 **Parastomal hernia with gangrene**
         Gangrenous parastomal hernia

     K43.5 **Parastomal hernia without obstruction or gangrene**
         Parastomal hernia NOS

CHAPTER 11 (K00–K95)

K43.6   **Other and unspecified ventral hernia with obstruction, without gangrene**
    Epigastric hernia causing obstruction, without gangrene
    Hypogastric hernia causing obstruction, without gangrene
    Incarcerated epigastric hernia without gangrene
    Incarcerated hypogastric hernia without gangrene
    Incarcerated midline hernia without gangrene
    Incarcerated spigelian hernia without gangrene
    Incarcerated subxiphoid hernia without gangrene
    Irreducible epigastric hernia without gangrene
    Irreducible hypogastric hernia without gangrene
    Irreducible midline hernia without gangrene
    Irreducible spigelian hernia without gangrene
    Irreducible subxiphoid hernia without gangrene
    Midline hernia causing obstruction, without gangrene
    Spigelian hernia causing obstruction, without gangrene
    Strangulated epigastric hernia without gangrene
    Strangulated hypogastric hernia without gangrene
    Strangulated midline hernia without gangrene
    Strangulated spigelian hernia without gangrene
    Strangulated subxiphoid hernia without gangrene
    Subxiphoid hernia causing obstruction, without gangrene

K43.7   **Other and unspecified ventral hernia with gangrene**
    Any condition listed under K43.6 specified as gangrenous

K43.9   **Ventral hernia without obstruction or gangrene**
    Epigastric hernia
    Ventral hernia NOS

● **K44**   **Diaphragmatic hernia**
    Includes   hiatus hernia (esophageal) (sliding)
         paraesophageal hernia

    Excludes1   congenital diaphragmatic hernia (Q79.0)
         congenital hiatus hernia (Q40.1)

K44.0   **Diaphragmatic hernia with obstruction, without gangrene**
    Diaphragmatic hernia causing obstruction
    Incarcerated diaphragmatic hernia
    Irreducible diaphragmatic hernia
    Strangulated diaphragmatic hernia
    Coding Clinic: 2022, Q2, P14

K44.1   **Diaphragmatic hernia with gangrene**
    Gangrenous diaphragmatic hernia

K44.9   **Diaphragmatic hernia without obstruction or gangrene**
    Diaphragmatic hernia NOS
    Coding Clinic: 2017, Q1, P7

● **K45**   **Other abdominal hernia**
    Includes   abdominal hernia, specified site NEC
         lumbar hernia
         obturator hernia
         pudendal hernia
         retroperitoneal hernia
         sciatic hernia

K45.0   **Other specified abdominal hernia with obstruction, without gangrene**
    Other specified abdominal hernia causing obstruction
    Other specified incarcerated abdominal hernia
    Other specified irreducible abdominal hernia
    Other specified strangulated abdominal hernia

K45.1   **Other specified abdominal hernia with gangrene**
    Any condition listed under K45 specified as gangrenous
    Coding Clinic: 2024, Q2, P22, 23

K45.8   **Other specified abdominal hernia without obstruction or gangrene**

● **K46**   **Unspecified abdominal hernia**
    Includes   enterocele
         epiplocele
         hernia NOS
         interstitial hernia
         intestinal hernia
         intra-abdominal hernia

    Excludes1   vaginal enterocele (N81.5)

Item 11–12 Crohn's disease, also known as **regional enteritis,** is a chronic inflammatory disease of the intestines. Classification is based on location in the small (duodenum, ileum, jejunum) or large (cecum, colon, rectum, anal canal) intestine.

K46.0   **Unspecified abdominal hernia with obstruction, without gangrene**
    Unspecified abdominal hernia causing obstruction
    Unspecified incarcerated abdominal hernia
    Unspecified irreducible abdominal hernia
    Unspecified strangulated abdominal hernia

K46.1   **Unspecified abdominal hernia with gangrene**
    Any condition listed under K46 specified as gangrenous

K46.9   **Unspecified abdominal hernia without obstruction or gangrene**
    Abdominal hernia NOS

★ **(See Plate 32 of the Anatomy Illustrations.)**

NONINFECTIVE ENTERITIS AND COLITIS (K50-K52)

    Includes   noninfective inflammatory bowel disease
    Excludes1   irritable bowel syndrome (K58.-)
         megacolon (K59.3-)

● **K50**   **Crohn's disease [regional enteritis]**
    Includes   granulomatous enteritis
    Use additional code to identify manifestations, such as:
         pyoderma gangrenosum (L88)
    Use Additional code to identify any associated fistulas, if applicable:
         anal fistula (K60.3-)
         anorectal fistula (K60.5-)
         rectal fistula (K60.4-)
    Excludes1   ulcerative colitis (K51.-)

● **K50.0**   **Crohn's disease of small intestine**
    Crohn's disease [regional enteritis] of duodenum
    Crohn's disease [regional enteritis] of ileum
    Crohn's disease [regional enteritis] of jejunum
    Regional ileitis
    Terminal ileitis
    Excludes1   Crohn's disease of both small and large intestine (K50.8-)

    K50.00   Crohn's disease of small intestine without complications 🅷🅲🅲

●   **K50.01**   Crohn's disease of small intestine with complications

      K50.011   Crohn's disease of small intestine with **rectal bleeding** 🅷🅲🅲

      K50.012   Crohn's disease of small intestine with **intestinal obstruction** 🅷🅲🅲

      K50.013   Crohn's disease of small intestine with **fistula** 🅷🅲🅲

      K50.014   Crohn's disease of small intestine with **abscess** 🅷🅲🅲
         Coding Clinic: 2012, Q4, P104

      K50.018   Crohn's disease of small intestine with **other complication** 🅷🅲🅲

      K50.019   Crohn's disease of small intestine with **unspecified complications** 🅷🅲🅲

● **K50.1**   **Crohn's disease of large intestine**
    Crohn's disease [regional enteritis] of colon
    Crohn's disease [regional enteritis] of large bowel
    Crohn's disease [regional enteritis] of rectum
    Granulomatous colitis
    Regional colitis
    Excludes1   Crohn's disease of both small and large intestine (K50.8)

    K50.10   Crohn's disease of large intestine without complications 🅷🅲🅲

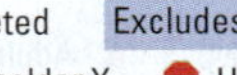

CHAPTER 11 (K00-K95)

▶ New   ⮕ Revised   ~~deleted~~ Deleted   Excludes 1   Excludes 2   Includes   Use additional   Code first   Code also   Key words

OGCR Official Guidelines   **X** Assign placeholder X   ● Use Additional Character(s)   ▶ Manifestation Code   🅷🅲🅲 Hierarchical Condition Category   **Coding Clinic**

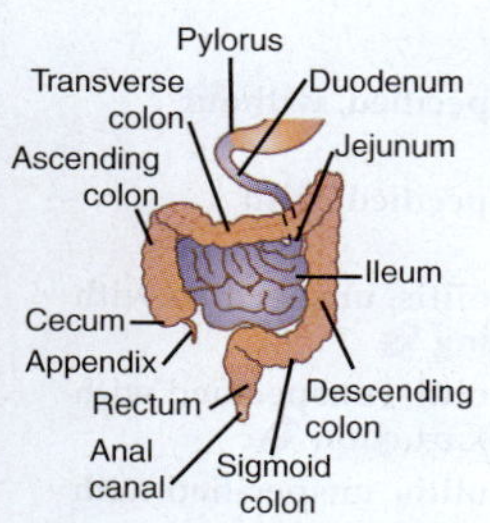

Figure 11-10   Small and large intestines.

Item 11–13 Ulcerative colitis attacks the colonic mucosa and forms abscesses. The disease involves the intestines. Classification is based on the location:
- Enterocolitis: large and small intestine
- Ileocolitis: ileum and colon
- Proctitis: rectum
- Proctosigmoiditis: sigmoid colon and rectum

● **K50.11**   **Crohn's disease of large intestine with complications**
  - **K50.111**   Crohn's disease of large intestine with **rectal bleeding** ℞
  - **K50.112**   Crohn's disease of large intestine with **intestinal obstruction** ℞
  - **K50.113**   Crohn's disease of large intestine with **fistula** ℞
  - **K50.114**   Crohn's disease of large intestine with **abscess** ℞
    Coding Clinic: 2012, Q4, P104
  - **K50.118**   Crohn's disease of large intestine with **other complication** ℞
  - **K50.119**   Crohn's disease of large intestine with **unspecified complications** ℞

● **K50.8**   Crohn's disease of **both small and large intestine**
  - **K50.80**   Crohn's disease of both small and large intestine **without complications** ℞
● **K50.81**   Crohn's disease of both small and large intestine with complications
  - **K50.811**   Crohn's disease of both small and large intestine with **rectal bleeding** ℞
  - **K50.812**   Crohn's disease of both small and large intestine with **intestinal obstruction** ℞
  - **K50.813**   Crohn's disease of both small and large intestine with **fistula** ℞
  - **K50.814**   Crohn's disease of both small and large intestine with **abscess** ℞
    Coding Clinic: 2012, Q4, P104
  - **K50.818**   Crohn's disease of both small and large intestine with **other complication** ℞
  - **K50.819**   Crohn's disease of both small and large intestine with **unspecified complications** ℞

● **K50.9**   Crohn's disease, unspecified
  - **K50.90**   Crohn's disease, unspecified, **without complications** ℞
    Crohn's disease NOS
    Regional enteritis NOS
● **K50.91**   Crohn's disease, unspecified, with complications
  - **K50.911**   Crohn's disease, unspecified, with **rectal bleeding** ℞
  - **K50.912**   Crohn's disease, unspecified, with **intestinal obstruction** ℞
  - **K50.913**   Crohn's disease, unspecified, with **fistula** ℞
  - **K50.914**   Crohn's disease, unspecified, with **abscess** ℞
    Coding Clinic: 2012, Q4, P104

  - **K50.918**   Crohn's disease, unspecified, with **other complication** ℞
  - **K50.919**   Crohn's disease, unspecified, with **unspecified complications** ℞

● **K51**   **Ulcerative colitis**
  Use additional code to identify manifestations, such as: pyoderma gangrenosum (L88)
  Use Additional code to identify any associated fistulas, if applicable:
    anal fistula (K60.3-)
    anorectal fistula (K60.5-)
    rectal fistula (K60.4-)
  Excludes1   Crohn's disease [regional enteritis] (K50.-)

● **K51.0**   **Ulcerative (chronic) pancolitis**
    Backwash ileitis
  - **K51.00**   **Ulcerative (chronic) pancolitis without complications** ℞
      Ulcerative (chronic) pancolitis NOS
● **K51.01**   **Ulcerative (chronic) pancolitis with complications**
  - **K51.011**   Ulcerative (chronic) pancolitis with **rectal bleeding** ℞
  - **K51.012**   Ulcerative (chronic) pancolitis with **intestinal obstruction** ℞
  - **K51.013**   Ulcerative (chronic) pancolitis with **fistula** ℞
  - **K51.014**   Ulcerative (chronic) pancolitis with **abscess** ℞
  - **K51.018**   Ulcerative (chronic) pancolitis with **other complication** ℞
  - **K51.019**   Ulcerative (chronic) pancolitis with **unspecified complications** ℞

● **K51.2**   Ulcerative (chronic) proctitis
  - **K51.20**   Ulcerative (chronic) proctitis **without complications** ℞
      Ulcerative (chronic) proctitis NOS
● **K51.21**   Ulcerative (chronic) proctitis with complications
  - **K51.211**   Ulcerative (chronic) proctitis with **rectal bleeding** ℞
  - **K51.212**   Ulcerative (chronic) proctitis with **intestinal obstruction** ℞
  - **K51.213**   Ulcerative (chronic) proctitis with **fistula** ℞
  - **K51.214**   Ulcerative (chronic) proctitis with **abscess** ℞
  - **K51.218**   Ulcerative (chronic) proctitis with **other complication** ℞
  - **K51.219**   Ulcerative (chronic) proctitis with **unspecified complications** ℞

● **K51.3**   Ulcerative (chronic) rectosigmoiditis
  - **K51.30**   Ulcerative (chronic) rectosigmoiditis **without complications** ℞
      Ulcerative (chronic) rectosigmoiditis NOS

● **K51.31**   Ulcerative (chronic) rectosigmoiditis with complications

    K51.311   Ulcerative (chronic) rectosigmoiditis with rectal bleeding 🅗

    K51.312   Ulcerative (chronic) rectosigmoiditis with intestinal obstruction 🅗

    K51.313   Ulcerative (chronic) rectosigmoiditis with fistula 🅗

    K51.314   Ulcerative (chronic) rectosigmoiditis with abscess 🅗

    K51.318   Ulcerative (chronic) rectosigmoiditis with other complication 🅗

    K51.319   Ulcerative (chronic) rectosigmoiditis with unspecified complications 🅗

● **K51.4**   Inflammatory polyps of colon

    Excludes2   adenomatous polyp of colon (D12.6)
      polyposis of colon (D12.6)
      polyps of colon NOS (K63.5)

    K51.40   Inflammatory polyps of colon without complications 🅗
      Inflammatory polyps of colon NOS

●   **K51.41**   Inflammatory polyps of colon with complications

    K51.411   Inflammatory polyps of colon with rectal bleeding 🅗

    K51.412   Inflammatory polyps of colon with intestinal obstruction 🅗

    K51.413   Inflammatory polyps of colon with fistula 🅗

    K51.414   Inflammatory polyps of colon with abscess 🅗

    K51.418   Inflammatory polyps of colon with other complication 🅗

    K51.419   Inflammatory polyps of colon with unspecified complications 🅗

● **K51.5**   Left sided colitis
    Left hemicolitis

    K51.50   Left sided colitis without complications 🅗
      Left sided colitis NOS

●   **K51.51**   Left sided colitis with complications

    K51.511   Left sided colitis with rectal bleeding 🅗

    K51.512   Left sided colitis with intestinal obstruction 🅗

    K51.513   Left sided colitis with fistula 🅗

    K51.514   Left sided colitis with abscess 🅗

    K51.518   Left sided colitis with other complication 🅗

    K51.519   Left sided colitis with unspecified complications 🅗

● **K51.8**   Other ulcerative colitis

    K51.80   Other ulcerative colitis without complications 🅗

●   **K51.81**   Other ulcerative colitis with complications

    K51.811   Other ulcerative colitis with rectal bleeding 🅗

    K51.812   Other ulcerative colitis with intestinal obstruction 🅗

    K51.813   Other ulcerative colitis with fistula 🅗

    K51.814   Other ulcerative colitis with abscess 🅗

    K51.818   Other ulcerative colitis with other complication 🅗

    K51.819   Other ulcerative colitis with unspecified complications 🅗

● **K51.9**   Ulcerative colitis, unspecified

    K51.90   Ulcerative colitis, unspecified, without complications 🅗

●   **K51.91**   Ulcerative colitis, unspecified, with complications

    K51.911   Ulcerative colitis, unspecified with rectal bleeding 🅗

    K51.912   Ulcerative colitis, unspecified with intestinal obstruction 🅗

    K51.913   Ulcerative colitis, unspecified with fistula 🅗

    K51.914   Ulcerative colitis, unspecified with abscess 🅗

    K51.918   Ulcerative colitis, unspecified with other complication 🅗

    K51.919   Ulcerative colitis, unspecified with unspecified complications 🅗

● **K52**   Other and unspecified noninfective gastroenteritis and colitis

    K52.0   Gastroenteritis and colitis due to radiation

    K52.1   Toxic gastroenteritis and colitis
      Drug-induced gastroenteritis and colitis

      Code first (T51-T65) to identify toxic agent

      Use additional code for adverse effect, if applicable, to identify drug (T36-T50 with fifth or sixth character 5)
      Coding Clinic: 2019, Q1, P17

●   **K52.2**   Allergic and dietetic gastroenteritis and colitis
      Food hypersensitivity gastroenteritis or colitis

      Use additional code to identify type of food allergy (Z91.01-, Z91.02-)

    Excludes2   allergic eosinophilic colitis (K52.82)
      allergic eosinophilic esophagitis (K20.0)
      allergic eosinophilic gastritis (K52.81)
      allergic eosinophilic gastroenteritis (K52.81)
      Coding Clinic: 2016, Q4, P30-31

    K52.21   Food protein-induced enterocolitis syndrome
      FPIES

      Use additional code for hypovolemic shock, if present (R57.1)

    K52.22   Food protein-induced enteropathy

    K52.29   Other allergic and dietetic gastroenteritis and colitis
      Allergic proctocolitis
      Food hypersensitivity gastroenteritis or colitis
      Food-induced eosinophilic proctocolitis
      Food protein-induced proctocolitis
      Immediate gastrointestinal hypersensitivity
      Milk protein-induced proctocolitis

    K52.3   Indeterminate colitis
      Colonic inflammatory bowel disease unclassified (IBDU)

    Excludes1   unspecified colitis (K52.9)

●   **K52.8**   Other specified noninfective gastroenteritis and colitis

    K52.81   Eosinophilic gastritis or gastroenteritis
      Eosinophilic enteritis

      Excludes2   eosinophilic esophagitis (K20.0)

    K52.82   Eosinophilic colitis

      Excludes2   allergic proctocolitis (K52.29)
      food-induced eosinophilic proctocolitis (K52.29)
      food protein-induced enterocolitis syndrome (FPIES) (K52.21)
      food protein-induced proctocolitis (K52.29)
      milk protein-induced proctocolitis (K52.29)

●   **K52.83**   Microscopic colitis
      Coding Clinic: 2016, Q4, P30-31

    K52.831   Collagenous colitis

    K52.832   Lymphocytic colitis

    K52.838   Other microscopic colitis

    K52.839   Microscopic colitis, unspecified

K52.89   **Other specified noninfective gastroenteritis and colitis**
Coding Clinic: 2019, Q1, P21

K52.9   **Noninfective gastroenteritis and colitis, unspecified**
Colitis NOS   Ileitis NOS
Enteritis NOS   Jejunitis NOS
Gastroenteritis NOS   Sigmoiditis NOS

Excludes1   diarrhea NOS (R19.7)
functional diarrhea (K59.1)
infectious gastroenteritis and colitis NOS (A09)
neonatal diarrhea (noninfective) (P78.3)
psychogenic diarrhea (F45.8)
Coding Clinic: 2021, Q3, P3-4

OTHER DISEASES OF INTESTINES (K55-K64)

● K55   Vascular disorders of intestine
Excludes1   necrotizing enterocolitis of newborn (P77.-)
Excludes2   angioectasia (angiodysplasia) duodenum (K31.81)

● K55.0   **Acute vascular disorders of intestine**
Infarction of appendices epiploicae
Mesenteric (artery) (vein) embolism
Mesenteric (artery) (vein) infarction
Mesenteric (artery) (vein) thrombosis
Coding Clinic: 2019, Q4, P68

● K55.01   **Acute (reversible) ischemia of small intestine**
Coding Clinic: 2016, Q4, P32

K55.011   **Focal (segmental) acute (reversible) ischemia of small intestine**

K55.012   **Diffuse acute (reversible) ischemia of small intestine**

K55.019   **Acute (reversible) ischemia of small intestine, extent unspecified**

● K55.02   **Acute infarction of small intestine**
Gangrene of small intestine
Necrosis of small intestine
Coding Clinic: 2016, Q4, P32

K55.021   **Focal (segmental) acute infarction of small intestine**

K55.022   **Diffuse acute infarction of small intestine**

K55.029   **Acute infarction of small intestine, extent unspecified**

● K55.03   **Acute (reversible) ischemia of large intestine**
Acute fulminant ischemic colitis
Subacute ischemic colitis
Coding Clinic: 2016, Q4, P32

K55.031   **Focal (segmental) acute (reversible) ischemia of large intestine**

K55.032   **Diffuse acute (reversible) ischemia of large intestine**

K55.039   **Acute (reversible) ischemia of large intestine, extent unspecified**
Coding Clinic: 2019, Q4, P68

● K55.04   **Acute infarction of large intestine**
Gangrene of large intestine
Necrosis of large intestine
Coding Clinic: 2016, Q4, P32

K55.041   **Focal (segmental) acute infarction of large intestine**

K55.042   **Diffuse acute infarction of large intestine**

K55.049   **Acute infarction of large intestine, extent unspecified**

● K55.05   **Acute (reversible) ischemia of intestine, part unspecified**

K55.051   **Focal (segmental) acute (reversible) ischemia of intestine, part unspecified**

K55.052   **Diffuse acute (reversible) ischemia of intestine, part unspecified**

K55.059   **Acute (reversible) ischemia of intestine, part and extent unspecified**

● K55.06   **Acute infarction of intestine, part unspecified**
Acute intestinal infarction
Gangrene of intestine
Necrosis of intestine

K55.061   **Focal (segmental) acute infarction of intestine, part unspecified**

K55.062   **Diffuse acute infarction of intestine, part unspecified**

K55.069   **Acute infarction of intestine, part and extent unspecified**

K55.1   **Chronic vascular disorders of intestine**
Chronic ischemic colitis
Chronic ischemic enteritis
Chronic ischemic enterocolitis
Ischemic stricture of intestine
Mesenteric atherosclerosis
Mesenteric vascular insufficiency

● K55.2   **Angiodysplasia of colon**
K55.20   **Angiodysplasia of colon without hemorrhage**
K55.21   **Angiodysplasia of colon with hemorrhage**

● K55.3   **Necrotizing enterocolitis**
Excludes1   necrotizing enterocolitis of newborn (P77.-)
Excludes2   necrotizing enterocolitis due to Clostridium difficile (A04.7-)

K55.30   **Necrotizing enterocolitis, unspecified**
Necrotizing enterocolitis, NOS

K55.31   **Stage 1 necrotizing enterocolitis**
Necrotizing enterocolitis without pneumatosis, without perforation
Coding Clinic: 2016, Q4, P32

K55.32   **Stage 2 necrotizing enterocolitis**
Necrotizing enterocolitis with pneumatosis, without perforation
Coding Clinic: 2016, Q4, P32

K55.33   **Stage 3 necrotizing enterocolitis**
Necrotizing enterocolitis with perforation
Necrotizing enterocolitis with pneumatosis and perforation
Coding Clinic: 2016, Q4, P32

K55.8   **Other vascular disorders of intestine**

K55.9   **Vascular disorder of intestine, unspecified**
Ischemic colitis
Ischemic enteritis
Ischemic enterocolitis

● K56   **Paralytic ileus and intestinal obstruction without hernia**
Excludes1   congenital stricture or stenosis of intestine (Q41-Q42)
cystic fibrosis with meconium ileus (E84.11)
ischemic stricture of intestine (K55.1)
meconium ileus NOS (P76.0)
neonatal intestinal obstructions classifiable to P76.-
obstruction of duodenum (K31.5)
postprocedural intestinal obstruction (K91.3-)
Excludes2   stenosis of anus or rectum (K62.4)

K56.0   **Paralytic ileus**
Paralysis of bowel
Paralysis of colon
Paralysis of intestine
Excludes1   gallstone ileus (K56.3)
ileus NOS (K56.7)
obstructive ileus NOS (K56.69-)

CHAPTER 11 (K00-K95)

K56.1   Intussusception 🅷🅲🅲
     Intussusception or invagination of bowel
     Intussusception or invagination of colon
     Intussusception or invagination of intestine
     Intussusception or invagination of rectum
     Excludes2   intussusception of appendix (K38.8)
     Coding Clinic: 2023, Q3, P12

K56.2   Volvulus 🅷🅲🅲
     Strangulation of colon or intestine
     Torsion of colon or intestine
     Twist of colon or intestine
     Excludes2   volvulus of duodenum (K31.5)
     Coding Clinic: 2024, Q2, P22

K56.3   Gallstone ileus 🅷🅲🅲
     Obstruction of intestine by gallstone

⬤ **K56.4   Other impaction of intestine**
     K56.41   Fecal impaction 🅷🅲🅲
         Excludes2   incomplete defecation (R15.0)
         Coding Clinic: 2024, Q2, P6
     K56.49   Other impaction of intestine 🅷🅲🅲

⬤ **K56.5   Intestinal adhesions [bands] with obstruction (postinfection)**
     Abdominal hernia due to adhesions with obstruction
     Peritoneal adhesions [bands] with intestinal obstruction (postinfection)
     K56.50   Intestinal adhesions [bands], unspecified as to partial versus complete obstruction 🅷🅲🅲
         Intestinal adhesions with obstruction NOS
     K56.51   Intestinal adhesions [bands], with partial obstruction 🅷🅲🅲
         Intestinal adhesions with incomplete obstruction
     K56.52   Intestinal adhesions [bands] with complete obstruction 🅷🅲🅲

⬤ **K56.6   Other and unspecified intestinal obstruction**
     ⬤ **K56.60   Unspecified intestinal obstruction**
         Coding Clinic: 2017, Q2, P12
         K56.600   Partial intestinal obstruction, unspecified as to cause 🅷🅲🅲
             Incomplete intestinal obstruction, NOS

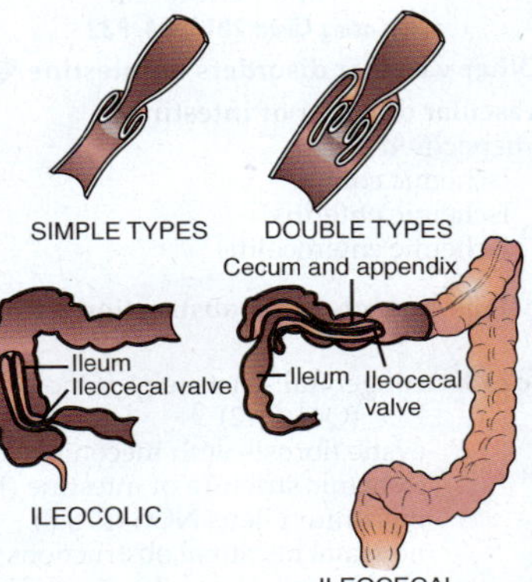

Figure 11-11   Types of intussusception.

Item 11–14   Intussusception is the prolapse (telescoping) of a part of the intestine into another adjacent part of the intestine. Intussusception may be enteric (ileoileal, jejunoileal, jejunojejunal), colic (colocolic), or intracolic (ileocecal, ileocolic).

Item 11–15   Volvulus is the twisting of a segment of the intestine, resulting in obstruction. Paralytic ileus is paralysis of the intestine. It need not be a complete paralysis, but it must prohibit the passage of food through the intestine and lead to intestinal blockage. It is a common aftermath of some types of surgery.

     K56.601   Complete intestinal obstruction, unspecified as to cause 🅷🅲🅲
     K56.609   Unspecified intestinal obstruction, unspecified as to partial versus complete obstruction 🅷🅲🅲
         Intestinal obstruction NOS

     ⬤ **K56.69   Other intestinal obstruction**
         Enterostenosis NOS
         Obstructive ileus NOS
         Occlusion of colon or intestine NOS
         Stenosis of colon or intestine NOS
         Stricture of colon or intestine NOS
         Coding Clinic: 2017, Q2, P12
         K56.690   Other partial intestinal obstruction 🅷🅲🅲
             Other incomplete intestinal obstruction
         K56.691   Other complete intestinal obstruction 🅷🅲🅲
         K56.699   Other intestinal obstruction unspecified as to partial versus complete obstruction 🅷🅲🅲
             Other intestinal obstruction, NEC
             Coding Clinic: 2023, Q3, P11

K56.7   Ileus, unspecified 🅷🅲🅲
     Excludes1   obstructive ileus (K56.69-)
     Excludes2   intestinal obstruction with hernia (K40-K46)
     Coding Clinic: 2017, Q1, P41

⬤ **K57   Diverticular disease of intestine**
     Code also if applicable peritonitis K65.-
     Excludes1   congenital diverticulum of intestine (Q43.8)
                 Meckel's diverticulum (Q43.0)
     Excludes2   diverticulum of appendix (K38.2)
     Coding Clinic: 2022, Q1, P26

⬤ **K57.0   Diverticulitis of small intestine with perforation and abscess**
     Excludes1   diverticulitis of both small and large intestine with perforation and abscess (K57.4-)
     K57.00   Diverticulitis of small intestine with perforation and abscess without bleeding
     K57.01   Diverticulitis of small intestine with perforation and abscess with bleeding

⬤ **K57.1   Diverticular disease of small intestine without perforation or abscess**
     Excludes1   diverticular disease of both small and large intestine without perforation or abscess (K57.5-)
     K57.10   Diverticulosis of small intestine without perforation or abscess without bleeding
         Diverticular disease of small intestine NOS
     K57.11   Diverticulosis of small intestine without perforation or abscess with bleeding
     K57.12   Diverticulitis of small intestine without perforation or abscess without bleeding
     K57.13   Diverticulitis of small intestine without perforation or abscess with bleeding

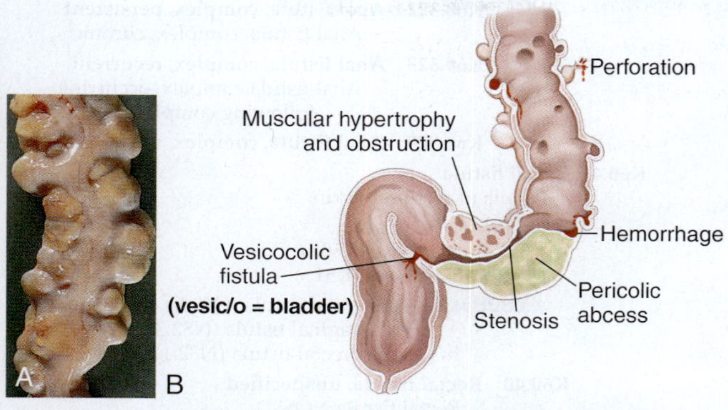

Figure 11-12 Diverticulosis. (From Shiland: Mastering Healthcare Terminology, ed 4, St. Louis, Mosby, 2012)

Item 11–16 **Diverticula** of the intestines are acquired herniations of the mucosa. Diverticulum (singular): Pocket or pouch that bulges outward through a weak spot (herniation) in the colon. Diverticula (plural). **Diverticulosis** is the condition of having diverticula. **Diverticulitis** is inflammation of these pouches or herniations. Classification is based on location (small intestine or colon) and whether it occurs with or without hemorrhage.

● **K57.2** **Diverticulitis of large intestine with perforation and abscess**

> **Excludes1**   diverticulitis of both small and large intestine with perforation and abscess (K57.4-)

> *Coding Clinic: 2022, Q1, P27*

K57.20 **Diverticulitis of large intestine with perforation and abscess without bleeding**
> *Coding Clinic: 2025, Q2, P6; 2022, Q1, P26*

K57.21 **Diverticulitis of large intestine with perforation and abscess with bleeding**

● **K57.3** **Diverticular disease of large intestine without perforation or abscess**

> **Excludes1**   diverticular disease of both small and large intestine without perforation or abscess (K57.5-)

K57.30 **Diverticulosis of large intestine without perforation or abscess without bleeding**
Diverticular disease of colon NOS

K57.31 **Diverticulosis of large intestine without perforation or abscess with bleeding**

K57.32 **Diverticulitis of large intestine without perforation or abscess without bleeding**

K57.33 **Diverticulitis of large intestine without perforation or abscess with bleeding**

● **K57.4** **Diverticulitis of both small and large intestine with perforation and abscess**

K57.40 **Diverticulitis of both small and large intestine with perforation and abscess without bleeding**

K57.41 **Diverticulitis of both small and large intestine with perforation and abscess with bleeding**

● **K57.5** **Diverticular disease of both small and large intestine without perforation or abscess**

K57.50 **Diverticulosis of both small and large intestine without perforation or abscess without bleeding**
Diverticular disease of both small and large intestine NOS

K57.51 **Diverticulosis of both small and large intestine without perforation or abscess with bleeding**

K57.52 **Diverticulitis of both small and large intestine without perforation or abscess without bleeding**

K57.53 **Diverticulitis of both small and large intestine without perforation or abscess with bleeding**

● **K57.8** **Diverticulitis of intestine, part unspecified, with perforation and abscess**

K57.80 **Diverticulitis of intestine, part unspecified, with perforation and abscess without bleeding**

K57.81 **Diverticulitis of intestine, part unspecified, with perforation and abscess with bleeding**

● **K57.9** **Diverticular disease of intestine, part unspecified, without perforation or abscess**

K57.90 **Diverticulosis of intestine, part unspecified, without perforation or abscess without bleeding**
Diverticular disease of intestine NOS
> *Coding Clinic: 2021, Q1, P12*

K57.91 **Diverticulosis of intestine, part unspecified, without perforation or abscess with bleeding**

K57.92 **Diverticulitis of intestine, part unspecified, without perforation or abscess without bleeding**

K57.93 **Diverticulitis of intestine, part unspecified, without perforation or abscess with bleeding**

● **K58** **Irritable bowel syndrome**

> **Includes**   irritable colon
> spastic colon

K58.0 **Irritable bowel syndrome with diarrhea**

K58.1 **Irritable bowel syndrome with constipation**
> *Coding Clinic: 2016, Q4, P32*

K58.2 **Mixed irritable bowel syndrome**
> *Coding Clinic: 2016, Q4, P32*

K58.8 **Other irritable bowel syndrome**
> *Coding Clinic: 2016, Q4, P32*

K58.9 **Irritable bowel syndrome without diarrhea**
Irritable bowel syndrome, unspecified

● **K59** **Other functional intestinal disorders**

> **Excludes1**   change in bowel habit NOS (R19.4)
> intestinal malabsorption (K90.-)
> psychogenic intestinal disorders (F45.8)

> **Excludes2**   functional disorders of stomach (K31.-)

● **K59.0** **Constipation**

> **Excludes2**   incomplete defecation (R15.0)
> *Coding Clinic: 2024, Q2, P6*

K59.00 **Constipation, unspecified**

K59.01 **Slow transit constipation**

K59.02 **Outlet dysfunction constipation**
> *Coding Clinic: 2023, Q1, P24*

K59.03 **Drug induced constipation**
> **Use additional** code for adverse effect, if applicable, to identify drug (T36-T50 with fifth or sixth character 5)
> *Coding Clinic: 2016, Q4, P33*

K59.04 **Chronic idiopathic constipation**
Functional constipation
> *Coding Clinic: 2016, Q4, P33*

K59.09 **Other constipation**
Chronic constipation

K59.1 Functional diarrhea

Excludes1   diarrhea NOS (R19.7)
irritable bowel syndrome with diarrhea (K58.0)

K59.2 Neurogenic bowel, not elsewhere classified

● **K59.3 Megacolon, not elsewhere classified**
Dilatation of colon
Code first, if applicable (T51-T65) to identify toxic agent
Excludes1   congenital megacolon (aganglionic) (Q43.1)
megacolon (due to) (in) Chagas' disease (B57.32)
megacolon (due to) (in) Clostridium difficile (A04.7-)
megacolon (due to) (in) Hirschsprung's disease (Q43.1)
Coding Clinic: 2016, Q4, P33

K59.31 Toxic megacolon (HCC)

K59.39 Other megacolon
Megacolon NOS

K59.4 Anal spasm
Proctalgia fugax

● **K59.8 Other specified functional intestinal disorders**

K59.81 Ogilvie syndrome
Acute colonic pseudo-obstruction (ACPO)

K59.89 Other specified functional intestinal disorders
Atony of colon
Pseudo-obstruction (acute) (chronic) of intestine

K59.9 Functional intestinal disorder, unspecified

● **K60 Fissure and fistula of anal and rectal regions**
Excludes1   fissure and fistula of anal and rectal regions with abscess or cellulitis (K61.-)
abscess or cellulitis off anal and rectal regions (K61.-)

Excludes2   anal sphincter tear (healed) (nontraumatic) (old) (K62.81)

K60.0 Acute anal fissure

K60.1 Chronic anal fissure

K60.2 Anal fissure, unspecified

K60.3 Anal fistula
Code first, if applicable:
Crohn's disease (K50.-)
ulcerative colitis (K51.-)
Excludes1   congenital fistula (Q43.6)

K60.30 Anal fistula, unspecified
Anal fistula NOS

● **K60.31 Anal fistula, simple**
Low intersphincteric anal fistula
Superficial anal fistula

K60.311 Anal fistula, simple, initial
Anal fistula, simple, new

K60.312 Anal fistula, simple, persistent
Anal fistula, simple, chronic

K60.313 Anal fistula, simple, recurrent
Anal fistula simple, occurring following complete healing

K60.319 Anal fistula, simple, unspecified

● **K60.32 Anal fistula, complex**
Extrasphincteric anal fistula
High intersphincteric anal fistula
Suprasphincteric anal fistula
Transsphincteric anal fistula
Code also, if applicable:
perianal abscess (K61.0)
rectovaginal fistula (N82.3)
stenosis of anus and rectum (K62.4)

K60.321 Anal fistula, complex, initial
Anal fistula, complex, new

K60.322 Anal fistula, complex, persistent
Anal fistula, complex, chronic

K60.323 Anal fistula, complex, recurrent
Anal fistula complex, occurring following complete healing

K60.329 Anal fistula, complex, unspecified

K60.4 Rectal fistula
Fistula of rectum to skin
Code first, if applicable:
Crohn's disease (K50.-)
ulcerative colitis (K51.-)
Excludes1   congenital fistula (Q43.6)
rectovaginal fistula (N82.3)
vesicorectal fistula (N32.1)

K60.40 Rectal fistula, unspecified
Rectal fistula NOS

● **K60.41 Rectal fistula, simple**
Low intersphincteric rectal fistula
Superficial rectal fistula

K60.411 Rectal fistula, simple, initial
Rectal, fistula, simple, new

K60.412 Rectal fistula, simple, persistent
Rectal fistula, simple, chronic

K60.413 Rectal fistula, simple, recurrent
Rectal fistula simple, occurring following complete healing

K60.419 Rectal fistula, simple, unspecified

● **K60.42 Rectal fistula, complex**
Extrasphincteric rectal fistula
High intersphincteric rectal fistula
Suprasphincteric rectal fistula
Transsphincteric rectal fistula
Code also, if applicable:
perianal abscess (K61.0)
rectovaginal fistula (N82.3)
stenosis of anus and rectum (K62.4)

K60.421 Rectal fistula, complex, initial
Rectal fistula, complex, new

K60.422 Rectal fistula, complex, persistent
Rectal fistula, complex, chronic

K60.423 Rectal fistula, complex, recurrent
Rectal fistula complex occurring following complete healing

K60.429 Rectal fistula, complex, unspecified

K60.5 Anorectal fistula
Code first, if applicable:
Crohn's disease (K50.-)
ulcerative colitis (K51.-)
Excludes1   congenital fistula (Q43.6)

K60.50 Anorectal fistula, unspecified
Anorectal fistula NOS

K60.51 Anorectal fistula, simple
Low intersphincteric anorectal fistula
Superficial anorectal fistula

K60.511 Anorectal fistula, simple, initial
Anorectal fistula, simple, new

K60.512 Anorectal fistula, simple, persistent
Anorectal fistula, simple, chronic

K60.513 Anorectal fistula, simple, recurrent
Anorectal fistula simple, occurring following complete healing

K60.519 Anorectal fistula, simple, unspecified

K60.52 Anorectal fistula, complex
Extrasphincteric anorectal fistula
High intersphincteric anorectal fistula
Suprasphincteric anorectal fistula
Transsphincteric anorectal fistula
Code also, if applicable:
perianal abscess (K61.0)
rectovaginal fistula (N82.3)
stenosis of anus and rectum (K62.4)

▶ New   ⇨ Revised   ~~deleted~~ Deleted   Excludes 1   Excludes 2   Includes   Use additional   Code first   Code also   Key words
OGCR Official Guidelines   X Assign placeholder X   ● Use Additional Character(s)   ▶ Manifestation Code   (HCC) Hierarchical Condition Category   Coding Clinic

K60.521   Anorectal fistula, complex, initial
     Anorectal fistula, complex, new

K60.522   Anorectal fistula, complex, persistent
     Anorectal fistula, complex, chronic

K60.523   Anorectal fistula, complex, recurrent
     Anorectal fistula complex, occurring
       following complete healing

K60.529   Anorectal fistula, complex, unspecified

● K61   Abscess of anal and rectal regions

Includes   abscess of anal and rectal regions
     cellulitis of anal and rectal regions

K61.0   Anal abscess
     Perianal abscess

     Excludes2   intrasphincteric abscess (K61.4)

K61.1   Rectal abscess
     Perirectal abscess

     Excludes1   ischiorectal abscess (K61.39)

     Coding Clinic: 2012, Q4, P104

K61.2   Anorectal abscess

K61.3   Ischiorectal abscess

     K61.31   Horseshoe abscess

     K61.39   Other ischiorectal abscess
       Abscess of ischiorectal fossa
       Ischiorectal abscess, NOS

K61.4   Intrasphincteric abscess
     Intersphincteric abscess

K61.5   Supralevator abscess

● K62   Other diseases of anus and rectum

Includes   anal canal

Excludes2   colostomy and enterostomy malfunction (K94.0-, K91.4-)
     fecal incontinence (R15.-)
     hemorrhoids (K64.-)

K62.0   Anal polyp
     Coding Clinic: 2018, Q1, P7

K62.1   Rectal polyp

     Excludes1   adenomatous polyp (D12.8)

     Coding Clinic: 2018, Q1, P7

K62.2   Anal prolapse
     Prolapse of anal canal

K62.3   Rectal prolapse
     Prolapse of rectal mucosa

K62.4   Stenosis of anus and rectum
     Stricture of anus (sphincter)

     Coding Clinic: 2019, Q2, P13

K62.5   Hemorrhage of anus and rectum

     Excludes1   gastrointestinal bleeding NOS (K92.2)
       melena (K92.1)
       neonatal rectal hemorrhage (P54.2)

K62.6   Ulcer of anus and rectum
     Solitary ulcer of anus and rectum
     Stercoral ulcer of anus and rectum

     Excludes1   fissure and fistula of anus and rectum (K60.-)
       ulcerative colitis (K51.-)

K62.7   Radiation proctitis
     Use additional code to identify the type of radiation
       (W88.-) or radiation therapy (Y84.2)
     Coding Clinic: 2019, Q1, P21

● K62.8   Other specified diseases of anus and rectum

     Excludes2   ulcerative proctitis (K51.2)

     K62.81   Anal sphincter tear (healed) (nontraumatic) (old)
       Tear of anus, nontraumatic

       Use additional code for any associated fecal
         incontinence (R15.-)

       Excludes2   anal fissure (K60.-)
         anal sphincter tear (healed)
           (old) complicating delivery
           (O34.7-)
         traumatic tear of anal sphincter
           (S31.831)

     K62.82   Dysplasia of anus
       Anal intraepithelial neoplasia I and II (AIN I
         and II) (histologically confirmed)
       Dysplasia of anus NOS
       Mild and moderate dysplasia of anus
         (histologically confirmed)

       Excludes1   abnormal results from anal
           cytologic examination
           without histologic
           confirmation (R85.61-)
         anal intraepithelial neoplasia III
           (D01.3)
         carcinoma in situ of anus (D01.3)
         HGSIL of anus (R85.613)
         severe dysplasia of anus (D01.3)

     K62.89   Other specified diseases of anus and rectum
       Proctitis NOS

       Use additional code for any associated fecal
         incontinence (R15.-)

K62.9   Disease of anus and rectum, unspecified

● K63   Other diseases of intestine

K63.0   Abscess of intestine

     Excludes1   abscess of intestine with Crohn's disease
       (K50.014, K50.114, K50.814, K50.914)
       abscess of intestine with diverticular
         disease (K57.0, K57.2, K57.4, K57.8)
       abscess of intestine with ulcerative colitis
         (K51.014, K51.214, K51.314, K51.414,
         K51.514, K51.814, K51.914)

     Excludes2   abscess of anal and rectal regions (K61.-)
       abscess of appendix (K35.3-)

K63.1   Perforation of intestine (nontraumatic)
     Perforation (nontraumatic) of rectum

     Excludes1   perforation (nontraumatic) of duodenum
         (K26.-)
       perforation (nontraumatic) of intestine
         with diverticular disease (K57.0,
         K57.2, K57.4, K57.8)

     Excludes2   perforation (nontraumatic) of appendix
         (K35.2-, K35.3)

     Coding Clinic: 2025, Q2, P9

K63.2   Fistula of intestine
     Code also, if applicable, disruption of internal
       operation (surgical) wound (T81.32-)

     Excludes1   fistula of duodenum (K31.6)
       fistula of intestine with Crohn's disease
         (K50.013, K50.113, K50.813, K50.913)
       fistula of intestine with ulcerative colitis
         (K51.013, K51.213, K51.313, K51.413,
         K51.513, K51.813, K51.913)

     Excludes2   fistula of anal and rectal regions (K60.-)
       fistula of appendix (K38.3)
       intestinal-genital fistula, female
         (N82.2-N82.4)
       vesicointestinal fistula (N32.1)

     Coding Clinic: 2017, Q3, P4

Item 11–17   A **fissure** is a groove in the surface, whereas a **fistula** is an abnormal passage. An **abscess** is an accumulation of pus in a tissue cavity resulting from a bacterial or parasitic infection.

CHAPTER 11 (K00-K95)

K63.3 **Ulcer of intestine**
       Primary ulcer of small intestine
       Excludes1   duodenal ulcer (K26.-)
                       gastrointestinal ulcer (K28.-)
                       gastrojejunal ulcer (K28.-)
                       jejunal ulcer (K28.-)
                       peptic ulcer, site unspecified (K27.-)
                       ulcer of intestine with perforation (K63.1)
                       ulcer of anus or rectum (K62.6)
                       ulcerative colitis (K51.-)

K63.4 **Enteroptosis**
K63.5 **Polyp of colon**
       Excludes2   adenomatous polyp of colon (D12.-)
                       inflammatory polyp of colon (K51.4-)
                       polyposis of colon (D12.6)
       Coding Clinic: 2019, Q1, P33; 2017, Q1, P15-16; 2015, Q2, P14

● K63.8 **Other specified diseases of intestine**
       K63.81   **Dieulafoy lesion of intestine**
                Excludes2   Dieulafoy lesion of stomach and
                                duodenum (K31.82)
       ● K63.82   **Intestinal microbial overgrowth**
             ● K63.821   **Small intestinal bacterial overgrowth**
                       K63.8211   **Small intestinal bacterial
                                   overgrowth, hydrogen-
                                   subtype**
                       K63.8212   **Small intestinal bacterial
                                   overgrowth, hydrogen
                                   sulfide-subtype**
                       K63.8219   **Small intestinal bacterial
                                   overgrowth, unspecified**
                 K63.822   **Small intestinal fungal overgrowth**
                 K63.829   **Intestinal methanogen overgrowth,
                            unspecified**
       K63.89   **Other specified diseases of intestine**
                Coding Clinic: 2013, Q2, P31
K63.9 **Disease of intestine, unspecified**

● K64 **Hemorrhoids and perianal venous thrombosis**
       Includes   piles
       Excludes1   hemorrhoids complicating childbirth and the
                       puerperium (O87.2)
                       hemorrhoids complicating pregnancy (O22.4)

K64.0 **First degree hemorrhoids**
       Grade/stage I hemorrhoids
       Hemorrhoids (bleeding) without prolapse outside of
       anal canal

K64.1 **Second degree hemorrhoids**
       Grade/stage II hemorrhoids
       Hemorrhoids (bleeding) that prolapse with straining,
       but retract spontaneously

K64.2 **Third degree hemorrhoids**
       Grade/stage III hemorrhoids
       Hemorrhoids (bleeding) that prolapse with straining
       and require manual replacement back inside anal
       canal

K64.3 **Fourth degree hemorrhoids**
       Grade/stage IV hemorrhoids
       Hemorrhoids (bleeding) with prolapsed tissue that
       cannot be manually replaced

K64.4 **Residual hemorrhoidal skin tags**
       External hemorrhoids, NOS
       Skin tags of anus

K64.5 **Perianal venous thrombosis**
       External hemorrhoids with thrombosis
       Perianal hematoma
       Thrombosed hemorrhoids NOS

K64.8 **Other hemorrhoids**
       Internal hemorrhoids, without mention of degree
       Prolapsed hemorrhoids, degree not specified

K64.9 **Unspecified hemorrhoids**
       Hemorrhoids (bleeding) NOS
       Hemorrhoids (bleeding) without mention of degree

DISEASES OF PERITONEUM AND RETROPERITONEUM (K65-K68)

● K65 **Peritonitis**
       Use additional code (B95-B97), to identify infectious agent, if
       known
       Code also if applicable diverticular disease of intestine (K57.-)
       Excludes1   acute appendicitis with generalized peritonitis
                       (K35.2-)
                       aseptic peritonitis (T81.6)
                       benign paroxysmal peritonitis (E85.0)
                       chemical peritonitis (T81.6)
                       gonococcal peritonitis (A54.85)
                       neonatal peritonitis (P78.0-P78.1)
                       pelvic peritonitis, female (N73.3-N73.5)
                       periodic familial peritonitis (E85.0)
                       peritonitis due to talc or other foreign substance
                       (T81.6)
                       peritonitis in chlamydia (A74.81)
                       peritonitis in diphtheria (A36.89)
                       peritonitis in syphilis (late) (A52.74)
                       peritonitis in tuberculosis (A18.31)
                       peritonitis with or following abortion or ectopic
                       or molar pregnancy (O00-O07, O08.0)
                       peritonitis with or following appendicitis (K35.-)
                       puerperal peritonitis (O85)
                       retroperitoneal infections (K68.-)
       Coding Clinic: 2022, Q1, P26

K65.0 **Generalized (acute) peritonitis** 🅷🅲🅲
       Pelvic peritonitis (acute), male
       Subphrenic peritonitis (acute)
       Suppurative peritonitis (acute)

K65.1 **Peritoneal abscess** 🅷🅲🅲
       Abdominopelvic abscess
       Abscess (of) omentum
       Abscess (of) peritoneum
       Mesenteric abscess
       Retrocecal abscess
       Subdiaphragmatic abscess
       Subhepatic abscess
       Subphrenic abscess
       Coding Clinic: 2024, Q1, P20; 2022, Q1, P26; 2019, Q1, P15

K65.2 **Spontaneous bacterial peritonitis** 🅷🅲🅲
       Excludes1   bacterial peritonitis NOS (K65.9)

K65.3 **Choleperitonitis** 🅷🅲🅲
       Peritonitis due to bile

K65.4 **Sclerosing mesenteritis** 🅷🅲🅲
       Fat necrosis of peritoneum
       (Idiopathic) sclerosing mesenteric fibrosis
       Mesenteric lipodystrophy
       Mesenteric panniculitis
       Retractile mesenteritis

K65.8 **Other peritonitis** 🅷🅲🅲
       Chronic proliferative peritonitis
       Peritonitis due to urine

K65.9 **Peritonitis, unspecified** 🅷🅲🅲
       Bacterial peritonitis NOS
       Coding Clinic: 2013, Q2, P31

● K66 **Other disorders of peritoneum**
       Excludes2   ascites (R18.-)
                       peritoneal effusion (chronic) (R18.8)

K66.0 **Peritoneal adhesions (postprocedural) (postinfection)**
       Adhesions (of) abdominal (wall)
       Adhesions (of) diaphragm
       Adhesions (of) intestine
       Adhesions (of) male pelvis
       Adhesions (of) omentum
       Adhesions (of) stomach
       Adhesive bands
       Mesenteric adhesions
       Excludes2   female pelvic adhesions [bands] (N73.6)
                       female pelvic postprocedural adhesions
                       (N99.4)

CHAPTER 11 (K00-K95)

Item 11–18 **Peritonitis** is an inflammation of the lining (peritoneum) of the abdominal cavity and surface of the intestines.

Item 11–19 **Retroperitoneal infections** occur between the posterior parietal peritoneum and posterior abdominal wall where the kidneys, adrenal glands, ureters, duodenum, ascending colon, descending colon, pancreas, and the large vessels and nerves are located.

K66.1 **Hemoperitoneum**
  Peritoneal hematoma
  Peritoneal hemorrhage
  Excludes1 traumatic hemoperitoneum (S36.8-)
  Excludes2 retroperitoneal hematoma (K68.3)
      retroperitoneal hemorrhage (K68.3)
  Coding Clinic: 2022, Q1, P22-23

K66.8 **Other specified disorders of peritoneum**
K66.9 **Disorder of peritoneum, unspecified**

K67 *Disorders of peritoneum in infectious diseases classified elsewhere* HCC
  Code first underlying disease, such as:
    congenital syphilis (A50.0)
    helminthiasis (B65.0-B83.9)
  Excludes1 peritonitis in chlamydia (A74.81)
      peritonitis in diphtheria (A36.89)
      peritonitis in gonococcal (A54.85)
      peritonitis in syphilis (late) (A52.74)
      peritonitis in tuberculosis (A18.31)

K68 **Disorders of retroperitoneum**
  K68.1 **Retroperitoneal abscess**
    K68.11 **Postprocedural retroperitoneal abscess**
        Excludes2 infection following procedure (T81.44)
    K68.12 **Psoas muscle abscess** HCC
    K68.19 **Other retroperitoneal abscess** HCC
        Coding Clinic: 2025, Q2, P6; 2019, Q1, P15
  K68.2 **Retroperitoneal fibrosis**
    Code also, if applicable, associated obstruction of ureter (N13.5)
  K68.3 **Retroperitoneal hematoma**
    Retroperitoneal hemorrhage
  K68.9 **Other disorders of retroperitoneum**

DISEASES OF LIVER (K70-K77)

  Excludes1 jaundice NOS (R17)
  Excludes2 hemochromatosis (E83.11-)
      Reye's syndrome (G93.7)
      viral hepatitis (B15-B19)
      Wilson's disease (E83.01)

K70 **Alcoholic liver disease**
  Use additional code to identify:
    alcohol abuse and dependence (F10.-)
  K70.0 **Alcoholic fatty liver**   A
  K70.1 **Alcoholic hepatitis**
    K70.10 **Alcoholic hepatitis without ascites**   A
    K70.11 **Alcoholic hepatitis with ascites**   A
  K70.2 **Alcoholic fibrosis and sclerosis of liver**   A
  K70.3 **Alcoholic cirrhosis of liver**
    Alcoholic cirrhosis NOS
    K70.30 **Alcoholic cirrhosis of liver without ascites** HCC   A
    K70.31 **Alcoholic cirrhosis of liver with ascites** HCC   A
        Coding Clinic: 2018, Q1, P5
  K70.4 **Alcoholic hepatic failure**
    Acute alcoholic hepatic failure
    Alcoholic hepatic failure NOS
    Chronic alcoholic hepatic failure
    Subacute alcoholic hepatic failure

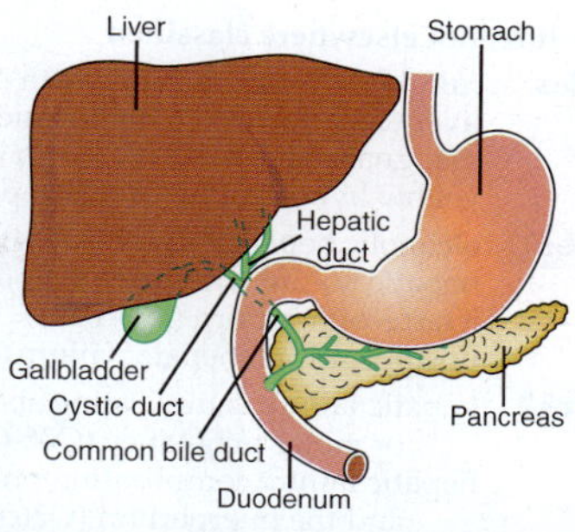

Figure 11-13 Liver and bile ducts.

Item 11–20 **Cirrhosis** is the progressive fibrosis of the liver resulting in loss of liver function. The main causes of cirrhosis of the liver are alcohol abuse, chronic hepatitis (inflammation of the liver), biliary disease, and excessive amounts of iron. **Alcoholic cirrhosis of the liver** is also called portal, Laënnec's, or fatty nutritional cirrhosis.

    K70.40 **Alcoholic hepatic failure without coma** HCC   A
    K70.41 **Alcoholic hepatic failure with coma** HCC   A
  K70.9 **Alcoholic liver disease, unspecified** HCC   A

K71 **Toxic liver disease**
  Includes drug-induced idiosyncratic (unpredictable) liver disease
      drug-induced toxic (predictable) liver disease
  Code first poisoning due to drug or toxin, if applicable (T36-T65 with fifth or sixth character 1-4)
  Use additional code for adverse effect, if applicable, to identify drug (T36-T50 with fifth or sixth character 5)
  Excludes2 alcoholic liver disease (K70.-)
      Budd-Chiari syndrome (I82.0)
  K71.0 **Toxic liver disease with cholestasis**
    Cholestasis with hepatocyte injury
    'Pure' cholestasis
  K71.1 **Toxic liver disease with hepatic necrosis**
    Hepatic failure (acute) (chronic) due to drugs
    K71.10 **Toxic liver disease with hepatic necrosis, without coma**
    K71.11 **Toxic liver disease with hepatic necrosis, with coma** HCC
  K71.2 **Toxic liver disease with acute hepatitis**
  K71.3 **Toxic liver disease with chronic persistent hepatitis**
  K71.4 **Toxic liver disease with chronic lobular hepatitis**
  K71.5 **Toxic liver disease with chronic active hepatitis**
    Toxic liver disease with lupoid hepatitis
    K71.50 **Toxic liver disease with chronic active hepatitis without ascites**
    K71.51 **Toxic liver disease with chronic active hepatitis with ascites**
        Coding Clinic: 2018, Q1, P4
  K71.6 **Toxic liver disease with hepatitis, not elsewhere classified**
  K71.7 **Toxic liver disease with fibrosis and cirrhosis of liver**
  K71.8 **Toxic liver disease with other disorders of liver**
    Toxic liver disease with focal nodular hyperplasia
    Toxic liver disease with hepatic granulomas
    Toxic liver disease with peliosis hepatis
    Toxic liver disease with veno-occlusive disease of liver
    Coding Clinic: 2024, Q1, P25
  K71.9 **Toxic liver disease, unspecified**

CHAPTER 11 (K00-K95)

● **K72**   **Hepatic failure, not elsewhere classified**

> **Includes**   fulminant hepatitis NEC, with hepatic failure
> liver (cell) necrosis with hepatic failure
> malignant hepatitis NEC, with hepatic failure
> yellow liver atrophy or dystrophy

> **Excludes1**   alcoholic hepatic failure (K70.4)
> hepatic failure with toxic liver disease (K71.1-)
> icterus of newborn (P55-P59)
> postprocedural hepatic failure (K91.82)

> **Excludes2**   hepatic failure complicating abortion or ectopic
> or molar pregnancy (O00-O07, O08.8)
> hepatic failure complicating pregnancy, childbirth
> and the puerperium (O26.6-)
> viral hepatitis with hepatic coma (B15-B19)

   ● **K72.0**   **Acute and subacute hepatic failure**
> Acute non-viral hepatitis NOS
> **Coding Clinic: 2015, Q2, P17**

     K72.00   **Acute and subacute hepatic failure without coma**
> **Coding Clinic: 2021, Q1, P13; 2015, Q2, P17**

     K72.01   **Acute and subacute hepatic failure with coma** Ⓗ

   ● **K72.1**   **Chronic hepatic failure**
> End stage liver disease

     K72.10   **Chronic hepatic failure without coma** Ⓗ
> **Coding Clinic: 2021, Q1, P13; 2017, Q1, P41**

     K72.11   **Chronic hepatic failure with coma** Ⓗ
> **Coding Clinic: 2020, Q1, P15**

   ● **K72.9**   **Hepatic failure, unspecified**

     K72.90   **Hepatic failure, unspecified without coma** Ⓗ
> **Coding Clinic: 2022, Q1, P53; 2018, Q4, P21**

     K72.91   **Hepatic failure, unspecified with coma** Ⓗ
> Hepatic coma NOS
> **Coding Clinic: 2016, Q2, P35**

● **K73**   **Chronic hepatitis, not elsewhere classified**

> **Excludes1**   alcoholic hepatitis (chronic) (K70.1-)
> drug-induced hepatitis (chronic) (K71.-)
> granulomatous hepatitis (chronic) NEC (K75.3)
> reactive, nonspecific hepatitis (chronic) (K75.2)
> viral hepatitis (chronic) (B15-B19)

   K73.0   **Chronic persistent hepatitis, not elsewhere classified** Ⓗ

   K73.1   **Chronic lobular hepatitis, not elsewhere classified** Ⓗ

   K73.2   **Chronic active hepatitis, not elsewhere classified** Ⓗ

   K73.8   **Other chronic hepatitis, not elsewhere classified** Ⓗ

   K73.9   **Chronic hepatitis, unspecified** Ⓗ

● **K74**   **Fibrosis and cirrhosis of liver**

> **Code also**, if applicable, viral hepatitis (acute) (chronic)
> (B15-B19)

> **Excludes1**   alcoholic cirrhosis (of liver) (K70.3)
> alcoholic fibrosis of liver (K70.2)
> cardiac sclerosis of liver (K76.1)
> cirrhosis (of liver) with toxic liver disease (K71.7)
> congenital cirrhosis (of liver) (P78.81)
> pigmentary cirrhosis (of liver) (E83.110)

   ● **K74.0**   **Hepatic fibrosis**
> **Code first** underlying liver disease, such as:
> nonalcoholic steatohepatitis (NASH) (K75.81)

     K74.00   **Hepatic fibrosis, unspecified**

     K74.01   **Hepatic fibrosis, early fibrosis**
> Hepatic fibrosis, stage F1 or stage F2

     K74.02   **Hepatic fibrosis, advanced fibrosis**
> Hepatic fibrosis, stage F3

> **Excludes1**   cirrhosis of liver (K74.6-)
> hepatic fibrosis, stage F4 (K74.6-)

   K74.1   **Hepatic sclerosis**

   K74.2   **Hepatic fibrosis with hepatic sclerosis**

   K74.3   **Primary biliary cirrhosis** Ⓗ
> Chronic nonsuppurative destructive cholangitis
> Primary biliary cholangitis

> **Excludes2**   primary sclerosing cholangitis (K83.01)

   K74.4   **Secondary biliary cirrhosis** Ⓗ

   K74.5   **Biliary cirrhosis, unspecified** Ⓗ

   ● **K74.6**   **Other and unspecified cirrhosis of liver**

     K74.60   **Unspecified cirrhosis of liver** Ⓗ
> Cirrhosis (of liver) NOS
> **Coding Clinic: 2018, Q1, P4**

     K74.69   **Other cirrhosis of liver** Ⓗ
> Cryptogenic cirrhosis (of liver)
> Macronodular cirrhosis (of liver)
> Micronodular cirrhosis (of liver)
> Mixed type cirrhosis (of liver)
> Portal cirrhosis (of liver)
> Postnecrotic cirrhosis (of liver)

● **K75**   **Other inflammatory liver diseases**

> **Excludes2**   toxic liver disease (K71.-)

   K75.0   **Abscess of liver**
> Cholangitic hepatic abscess
> Hematogenic hepatic abscess
> Hepatic abscess NOS
> Lymphogenic hepatic abscess
> Pylephlebitic hepatic abscess

> **Excludes1**   amebic liver abscess (A06.4)
> cholangitis without liver abscess (K83.09)
> pylephlebitis without liver abscess (K75.1)

> **Excludes2**   acute or subacute hepatitis NOS (B17.9)
> acute or subacute non-viral hepatitis (K72.0)
> chronic hepatitis NEC (K73.8)

   K75.1   **Phlebitis of portal vein**
> Pylephlebitis

> **Excludes1**   pylephlebitic liver abscess (K75.0)

   K75.2   **Nonspecific reactive hepatitis**

> **Excludes1**   acute or subacute hepatitis (K72.0-)
> chronic hepatitis NEC (K73.-)
> viral hepatitis (B15-B19)

   K75.3   **Granulomatous hepatitis, not elsewhere classified**

> **Excludes1**   acute or subacute hepatitis (K72.0-)
> chronic hepatitis NEC (K73.-)
> viral hepatitis (B15-B19)

   K75.4   **Autoimmune hepatitis** Ⓗ
> Lupoid hepatitis NEC

   ● **K75.8**   **Other specified inflammatory liver diseases**

     K75.81   **Nonalcoholic steatohepatitis (NASH)**
> ▶ Metabolic dysfunction-associated
> steatohepatitis (MASH)

> **Use additional** code, if applicable, hepatic
> fibrosis (K74.0-)

     K75.89   **Other specified inflammatory liver diseases**

   K75.9   **Inflammatory liver disease, unspecified**
> Hepatitis NOS

> **Excludes1**   acute or subacute hepatitis (K72.0-)
> chronic hepatitis NEC (K73.-)
> viral hepatitis (B15-B19)

> **Coding Clinic: 2015, Q2, P17**

● **K76**   **Other diseases of liver**
> ▶ Metabolic dysfunction-associated steatotic liver disease
> (MASLD)

> **Excludes2**   alcoholic liver disease (K70.-)
> amyloid degeneration of liver (E85.-)
> cystic disease of liver (congenital) (Q44.6)
> hepatic vein thrombosis (I82.0)
> hepatomegaly NOS (R16.0)
> pigmentary cirrhosis (of liver) (E83.110)
> portal vein thrombosis (I81)
> toxic liver disease (K71.-)

   K76.0   **Fatty (change of) liver, not elsewhere classified**
> Nonalcoholic fatty liver disease (NAFLD)

> **Excludes1**   nonalcoholic steatohepatitis (NASH)
> (K75.81)

● **New**   ➡ **Revised**   ~~deleted~~ **Deleted**   **Excludes 1**   **Excludes 2**   **Includes**   **Use additional**   **Code first**   **Code also**   **Key words**
OGCR Official Guidelines   **X** Assign placeholder X   ● Use Additional Character(s)   ❚ Manifestation Code   Ⓗ Hierarchical Condition Category   **Coding Clinic**

K76.1   **Chronic passive congestion of liver**
Cardiac cirrhosis
Cardiac sclerosis

K76.2   **Central hemorrhagic necrosis of liver**
Excludes1   liver necrosis with hepatic failure (K72.-)

K76.3   **Infarction of liver**

K76.4   **Peliosis hepatis**
Hepatic angiomatosis

K76.5   **Hepatic veno-occlusive disease**
Excludes1   Budd-Chiari syndrome (I82.0)

K76.6   **Portal hypertension** 🗝
Use additional code for any associated complications,
such as:
portal hypertensive gastropathy (K31.89)
Coding Clinic: 2020, Q1, P15

K76.7   **Hepatorenal syndrome** 🗝
Excludes1   hepatorenal syndrome following labor
and delivery (O90.41)
postprocedural hepatorenal syndrome
(K91.83)
Coding Clinic: 2025, Q1, P26

● **K76.8**   **Other specified diseases of liver**

K76.81   **Hepatopulmonary syndrome** 🗝
Code first underlying liver disease, such as:
alcoholic cirrhosis of liver (K70.3-)
cirrhosis of liver without mention of alcohol
(K74.6-)

K76.82   **Hepatic encephalopathy**
Hepatic encephalopathy, NOS
Hepatic encephalopathy without coma
Hepatocerebral intoxication
Portal-systemic encephalopathy
Code also underlying liver disease, such as:
acute and subacute hepatic failure without
coma (K72.00)
alcoholic hepatic failure without coma
(K70.40)
chronic hepatic failure without coma (K72.10)
hepatic failure with toxic liver disease
without coma (K71.10)
hepatic failure without coma (K72.90)
icterus of newborn (P55-P59)
postprocedural hepatic failure (K91.82)
viral hepatitis without hepatic coma (B15.9,
B16.1, B16.9, B17.10, B19.10, B19.20,
B19.9)
Excludes1   acute and subacute hepatic
failure with coma (K72.01)
alcoholic hepatic failure with coma (K70.41)
chronic hepatic failure with coma (K72.11)
hepatic failure with coma (K72.91)

K76.89   **Other specified diseases of liver**
Cyst (simple) of liver
Focal nodular hyperplasia of liver
Hepatoptosis

K76.9   **Liver disease, unspecified**

▶ **K77**   *Liver disorders in diseases classified elsewhere*
Code first underlying disease, such as:
amyloidosis (E85.-)
congenital syphilis (A50.0, A50.5)
congenital toxoplasmosis (P37.1)
infectious mononucleosis with liver disease (B27.0-B27.9
with fifth character 9)
schistosomiasis (B65.0-B65.9)
Excludes1   alcoholic hepatitis (K70.1-)
alcoholic liver disease (K70.-)
cytomegaloviral hepatitis (B25.1)
herpesviral [herpes simplex] hepatitis (B00.81)
mumps hepatitis (B26.81)
sarcoidosis with liver disease (D86.89)
secondary syphilis with liver disease (A51.45)
syphilis (late) with liver disease (A52.74)
toxoplasmosis (acquired) hepatitis (B58.1)
tuberculosis with liver disease (A18.83)

DISORDERS OF GALLBLADDER, BILIARY TRACT AND PANCREAS (K80–K87)

● **K80**   **Cholelithiasis**
Presence or formation of gallstones
Excludes1   retained cholelithiasis following cholecystectomy
(K91.86)

● **K80.0**   **Calculus of gallbladder with acute cholecystitis**
Any condition listed in K80.2 with acute cholecystitis
Use additional code if applicable for associated
gangrene of gallbladder (K82.A1), or perforation of
gallbladder (K82.A2)
*Check documentation for acute/chronic gallbladder/common
bile duct either with or without obstruction.*

K80.00   **Calculus of gallbladder with acute cholecystitis
without obstruction**
Coding Clinic: 2023, Q2, P12; 2018, Q4, P20

K80.01   **Calculus of gallbladder with acute cholecystitis
with obstruction**

● **K80.1**   **Calculus of gallbladder with other
cholecystitis**
Use additional code if applicable for associated
gangrene of gallbladder (K82.A1), or perforation of
gallbladder (K82.A2)

K80.10   **Calculus of gallbladder with chronic
cholecystitis without obstruction**
Cholelithiasis with cholecystitis NOS

K80.11   **Calculus of gallbladder with chronic
cholecystitis with obstruction**

K80.12   **Calculus of gallbladder with acute and chronic
cholecystitis without obstruction**

K80.13   **Calculus of gallbladder with acute and chronic
cholecystitis with obstruction**

K80.18   **Calculus of gallbladder with other cholecystitis
without obstruction**

K80.19   **Calculus of gallbladder with other cholecystitis
with obstruction**

● **K80.2**   **Calculus of gallbladder without cholecystitis**
Cholecystolithiasis without cholecystitis
Cholelithiasis (without cholecystitis)
Colic (recurrent) of gallbladder (without cholecystitis)
Gallstone (impacted) of cystic duct (without
cholecystitis)
Gallstone (impacted) of gallbladder (without
cholecystitis)

K80.20   **Calculus of gallbladder without cholecystitis
without obstruction**

K80.21   **Calculus of gallbladder without cholecystitis
with obstruction**

● **K80.3**   **Calculus of bile duct with cholangitis**
Any condition listed in K80.5 with cholangitis

K80.30   **Calculus of bile duct with cholangitis,
unspecified, without obstruction**

K80.31   **Calculus of bile duct with cholangitis,
unspecified, with obstruction**

K80.32   **Calculus of bile duct with acute cholangitis
without obstruction**

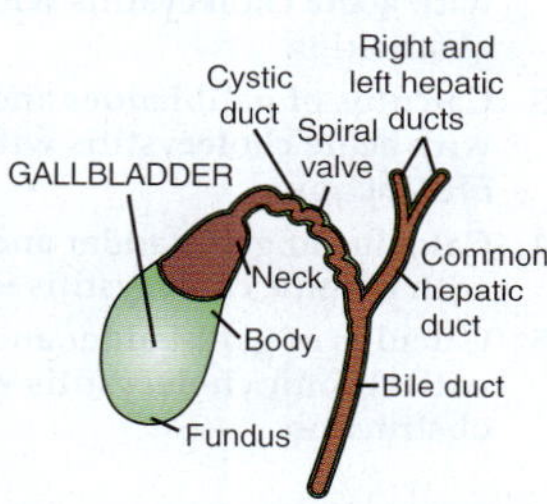

Figure 11-14   Gallbladder and bile ducts.

K80.33 **Calculus of bile duct with acute cholangitis with obstruction**

K80.34 **Calculus of bile duct with chronic cholangitis without obstruction**

K80.35 **Calculus of bile duct with chronic cholangitis with obstruction**

K80.36 **Calculus of bile duct with acute and chronic cholangitis without obstruction**

K80.37 **Calculus of bile duct with acute and chronic cholangitis with obstruction**

● K80.4 **Calculus of bile duct with cholecystitis**
Any condition listed in K80.5 with cholecystitis (with cholangitis)
Code also, if applicable, fistula of bile duct (K83.3)
Use additional code if applicable for associated gangrene of gallbladder (K82.A1), or perforation of gallbladder (K82.A2)

K80.40 **Calculus of bile duct with cholecystitis, unspecified, without obstruction**

K80.41 **Calculus of bile duct with cholecystitis, unspecified, with obstruction**
Coding Clinic: 2019, Q1, P18

K80.42 **Calculus of bile duct with acute cholecystitis without obstruction**

K80.43 **Calculus of bile duct with acute cholecystitis with obstruction**

K80.44 **Calculus of bile duct with chronic cholecystitis without obstruction**

K80.45 **Calculus of bile duct with chronic cholecystitis with obstruction**

K80.46 **Calculus of bile duct with acute and chronic cholecystitis without obstruction**

K80.47 **Calculus of bile duct with acute and chronic cholecystitis with obstruction**

● K80.5 **Calculus of bile duct without cholangitis or cholecystitis**
Choledocholithiasis (without cholangitis or cholecystitis)
Gallstone (impacted) of bile duct NOS (without cholangitis or cholecystitis)
Gallstone (impacted) of common duct (without cholangitis or cholecystitis)
Gallstone (impacted) of hepatic duct (without cholangitis or cholecystitis)
Hepatic cholelithiasis (without cholangitis or cholecystitis)
Hepatic colic (recurrent) (without cholangitis or cholecystitis)

K80.50 **Calculus of bile duct without cholangitis or cholecystitis without obstruction**

K80.51 **Calculus of bile duct without cholangitis or cholecystitis with obstruction**

● K80.6 **Calculus of gallbladder and bile duct with cholecystitis**
Use additional code if applicable for associated gangrene of gallbladder (K82.A1), or perforation of gallbladder (K82.A2)

K80.60 **Calculus of gallbladder and bile duct with cholecystitis, unspecified, without obstruction**

K80.61 **Calculus of gallbladder and bile duct with cholecystitis, unspecified, with obstruction**

K80.62 **Calculus of gallbladder and bile duct with acute cholecystitis without obstruction**

K80.63 **Calculus of gallbladder and bile duct with acute cholecystitis with obstruction**

K80.64 **Calculus of gallbladder and bile duct with chronic cholecystitis without obstruction**

K80.65 **Calculus of gallbladder and bile duct with chronic cholecystitis with obstruction**

K80.66 **Calculus of gallbladder and bile duct with acute and chronic cholecystitis without obstruction**

K80.67 **Calculus of gallbladder and bile duct with acute and chronic cholecystitis with obstruction**

● K80.7 **Calculus of gallbladder and bile duct without cholecystitis**

K80.70 **Calculus of gallbladder and bile duct without cholecystitis without obstruction**

K80.71 **Calculus of gallbladder and bile duct without cholecystitis with obstruction**

● K80.8 **Other cholelithiasis**

K80.80 **Other cholelithiasis without obstruction**

K80.81 **Other cholelithiasis with obstruction**

● K81 **Cholecystitis**
Chronic or acute inflammation of the gallbladder
Use additional code if applicable for associated gangrene of gallbladder (K82.A1), or perforation of gallbladder (K82.A2)
Excludes1 cholecystitis with cholelithiasis (K80.-)

K81.0 **Acute cholecystitis**
Abscess of gallbladder
Angiocholecystitis
Emphysematous (acute) cholecystitis
Empyema of gallbladder
Gangrene of gallbladder
Gangrenous cholecystitis
Suppurative cholecystitis

K81.1 **Chronic cholecystitis**

K81.2 **Acute cholecystitis with chronic cholecystitis**

K81.9 **Cholecystitis, unspecified**

● K82 **Other diseases of gallbladder**
Excludes1 nonvisualization of gallbladder (R93.2)
postcholecystectomy syndrome (K91.5)

K82.0 **Obstruction of gallbladder**
Occlusion of cystic duct or gallbladder without cholelithiasis
Stenosis of cystic duct or gallbladder without cholelithiasis
Stricture of cystic duct or gallbladder without cholelithiasis
Excludes1 obstruction of gallbladder with cholelithiasis (K80.-)

K82.1 **Hydrops of gallbladder**
Mucocele of gallbladder

K82.2 **Perforation of gallbladder**
Rupture of cystic duct or gallbladder
Excludes1 Perforation of gallbladder in cholecystitis (K82.A2)

K82.3 **Fistula of gallbladder**
Cholecystocolic fistula
Cholecystoduodenal fistula
Coding Clinic: 2019, Q1, P18

K82.4 **Cholesterolosis of gallbladder**
Strawberry gallbladder
Excludes1 cholesterolosis of gallbladder with cholecystitis (K81.-)
cholesterolosis of gallbladder with cholelithiasis (K80.-)

K82.8 **Other specified diseases of gallbladder**
Adhesions of cystic duct or gallbladder
Atrophy of cystic duct or gallbladder
Cyst of cystic duct or gallbladder
Dyskinesia of cystic duct or gallbladder
Hypertrophy of cystic duct or gallbladder
Nonfunctioning of cystic duct or gallbladder
Ulcer of cystic duct or gallbladder

K82.9　Disease of gallbladder, unspecified

● **K82.A　Disorders of gallbladder in diseases classified elsewhere**

　　Code first the type of cholecystitis (K81.-), or cholelithiasis with cholecystitis (K80.00-K80.19, K80.40-K80.47, K80.60-K80.67)

　　▶ **K82.A1　Gangrene of gallbladder in cholecystitis**
　　　　Coding Clinic: 2018, Q4, P20

　　● **K82.A2　Perforation of gallbladder in cholecystitis**
　　　　Coding Clinic: 2018, Q4, P20

● **K83　Other diseases of biliary tract**

　　Excludes1　postcholecystectomy syndrome (K91.5)
　　Excludes2　conditions involving the gallbladder (K81-K82)
　　　　　　　conditions involving the cystic duct (K81-K82)

● **K83.0　Cholangitis**

　　Excludes1　cholangitic liver abscess (K75.0)
　　　　　　　cholangitis with choledocholithiasis (K80.3-, K80.4-)

　　Excludes2　chronic nonsuppurative destructive cholangitis (K74.3)
　　　　　　　primary biliary cholangitis (K74.3)
　　　　　　　primary biliary cirrhosis (K74.3)

　　K83.01　Primary sclerosing cholangitis
　　　　Coding Clinic: 2018, Q4, P21

　　K83.09　Other cholangitis
　　　　Ascending cholangitis
　　　　Cholangitis NOS
　　　　Primary cholangitis
　　　　Recurrent cholangitis
　　　　Sclerosing cholangitis
　　　　Secondary cholangitis
　　　　Stenosing cholangitis
　　　　Suppurative cholangitis

K83.1　Obstruction of bile duct
　　Occlusion of bile duct without cholelithiasis
　　Stenosis of bile duct without cholelithiasis
　　Stricture of bile duct without cholelithiasis

　　Excludes1　congenital obstruction of bile duct (Q44.3)
　　　　　　　obstruction of bile duct with cholelithiasis (K80.-)

　　Coding Clinic: 2023, Q1, P27; 2016, Q1, P18

K83.2　Perforation of bile duct
　　Rupture of bile duct

K83.3　Fistula of bile duct
　　Choledochoduodenal fistula

K83.4　Spasm of sphincter of Oddi

K83.5　Biliary cyst

K83.8　Other specified diseases of biliary tract
　　Adhesions of biliary tract
　　Atrophy of biliary tract
　　Hypertrophy of biliary tract
　　Ulcer of biliary tract

K83.9　Disease of biliary tract, unspecified

● **K85　Acute pancreatitis**

　　Inflammatory process in which pancreatic enzymes autodigest the gland

　　Includes　acute (recurrent) pancreatitis
　　　　　　subacute pancreatitis

　　Coding Clinic: 2016, Q4, P34

● **K85.0　Idiopathic acute pancreatitis**

　　K85.00　Idiopathic acute pancreatitis without necrosis or infection

　　K85.01　Idiopathic acute pancreatitis with uninfected necrosis

　　K85.02　Idiopathic acute pancreatitis with infected necrosis

● **K85.1　Biliary acute pancreatitis**
　　Gallstone pancreatitis

　　K85.10　Biliary acute pancreatitis without necrosis or infection
　　　　Coding Clinic: 2023, Q2, P12

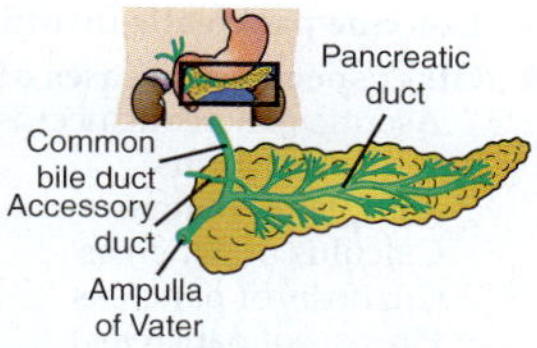

Figure 11-15　Pancreatic ductal system.

　　K85.11　Biliary acute pancreatitis with uninfected necrosis

　　K85.12　Biliary acute pancreatitis with infected necrosis

● **K85.2　Alcohol induced acute pancreatitis**

　　Excludes2　alcohol induced chronic pancreatitis (K86.0)

　　K85.20　Alcohol induced acute pancreatitis without necrosis or infection
　　　　Coding Clinic: 2020, Q1, P9

　　K85.21　Alcohol induced acute pancreatitis with uninfected necrosis

　　K85.22　Alcohol induced acute pancreatitis with infected necrosis

● **K85.3　Drug induced acute pancreatitis**

　　Use additional code for adverse effect, if applicable, to identify drug (T36-T50 with fifth or sixth character 5)

　　Use additional code to identify drug abuse and dependence (F11.-F17.-)

　　K85.30　Drug induced acute pancreatitis without necrosis or infection

　　K85.31　Drug induced acute pancreatitis with uninfected necrosis

　　K85.32　Drug induced acute pancreatitis with infected necrosis

● **K85.8　Other acute pancreatitis**

　　K85.80　Other acute pancreatitis without necrosis or infection

　　K85.81　Other acute pancreatitis with uninfected necrosis

　　K85.82　Other acute pancreatitis with infected necrosis

● **K85.9　Acute pancreatitis, unspecified**
　　Pancreatitis NOS

　　K85.90　Acute pancreatitis without necrosis or infection, unspecified

　　K85.91　Acute pancreatitis with uninfected necrosis, unspecified

　　K85.92　Acute pancreatitis with infected necrosis, unspecified

● **K86　Other diseases of pancreas**

　　Excludes2　fibrocystic disease of pancreas (E84.-)
　　　　　　　islet cell tumor (of pancreas) (D13.7)
　　　　　　　pancreatic steatorrhea (K90.3)

K86.0　Alcohol-induced chronic pancreatitis

　　Use additional code to identify:
　　　　alcohol abuse and dependence (F10.-)
　　Code also exocrine pancreatic insufficiency (K86.81)
　　Excludes2　alcohol induced acute pancreatitis (K85.2-)

K86.1　Other chronic pancreatitis
　　Chronic pancreatitis NOS
　　Infectious chronic pancreatitis
　　Recurrent chronic pancreatitis
　　Relapsing chronic pancreatitis
　　Code also exocrine pancreatic insufficiency (K86.81)

K86.2　Cyst of pancreas

K86.3　Pseudocyst of pancreas

● **K86.8　Other specified diseases of pancreas**
　　Coding Clinic: 2016, Q4, P34

CHAPTER 11 (K00-K95)

K86.81 **Exocrine pancreatic insufficiency**

K86.89 **Other specified diseases of pancreas**
　Aseptic pancreatic necrosis, unrelated to acute pancreatitis
　Atrophy of pancreas
　Calculus of pancreas
　Cirrhosis of pancreas
　Fibrosis of pancreas
　Pancreatic fat necrosis, unrelated to acute pancreatitis
　Pancreatic infantilism
　Pancreatic necrosis NOS, unrelated to acute pancreatitis
　Coding Clinic: 2024, Q3, P4

K86.9 **Disease of pancreas, unspecified**

▶ **K87** *Disorders of gallbladder, biliary tract and pancreas in diseases classified elsewhere*
　Code first underlying disease
　Excludes1　cytomegaloviral pancreatitis (B25.2)
　　mumps pancreatitis (B26.3)
　　syphilitic gallbladder (A52.74)
　　syphilitic pancreas (A52.74)
　　tuberculosis of gallbladder (A18.83)
　　tuberculosis of pancreas (A18.83)

OTHER DISEASES OF THE DIGESTIVE SYSTEM (K90-K95)

● **K90** **Intestinal malabsorption**
　Excludes1　intestinal malabsorption following gastrointestinal surgery (K91.2)

K90.0 **Celiac disease**
　Celiac disease with steatorrhea
　Celiac gluten-sensitive enteropathy
　Nontropical sprue
　Use additional code for associated disorders including:
　　dermatitis herpetiformis (L13.0)
　　gluten ataxia (G32.81)
　Code also exocrine pancreatic insufficiency (K86.81)

K90.1 **Tropical sprue**
　Sprue NOS
　Tropical steatorrhea

K90.2 **Blind loop syndrome, not elsewhere classified**
　Blind loop syndrome NOS
　Excludes1　congenital blind loop syndrome (Q43.8)
　　postsurgical blind loop syndrome (K91.2)

K90.3 **Pancreatic steatorrhea**

● **K90.4** **Other malabsorption due to intolerance**
　Excludes2　celiac gluten-sensitive enteropathy (K90.0)
　　lactose intolerance (E73.-)
　Coding Clinic: 2016, Q4, P35-36

K90.41 **Non-celiac gluten sensitivity**
　Gluten sensitivity NOS
　Non-celiac gluten sensitive enteropathy

K90.49 **Malabsorption due to intolerance, not elsewhere classified**
　Malabsorption due to intolerance to carbohydrate
　Malabsorption due to intolerance to fat
　Malabsorption due to intolerance to protein
　Malabsorption due to intolerance to starch

● **K90.8** **Other intestinal malabsorption**
K90.81 **Whipple's disease**
● **K90.82** **Short bowel syndrome**
　Short gut syndrome

K90.821 **Short bowel syndrome with colon in continuity**
　Short bowel syndrome with colonic continuity
　Coding Clinic: 2023, Q4, P32

K90.822 **Short bowel syndrome without colon in continuity**
　Short bowel syndrome without colonic continuity
　Coding Clinic: 2023, Q4, P33

K90.829 **Short bowel syndrome, unspecified**

K90.83 **Intestinal failure**
K90.89 **Other intestinal malabsorption**
K90.9 **Intestinal malabsorption, unspecified**
　Coding Clinic: 2017, Q4, P108-109

● **K91** **Intraoperative and postprocedural complications and disorders of digestive system, not elsewhere classified**
　Excludes2　complications of artificial opening of digestive system (K94.-)
　　complications of bariatric procedures (K95.-)
　　gastrojejunal ulcer (K28.-)
　　postprocedural (radiation) retroperitoneal abscess (K68.11)
　　radiation colitis (K52.0)
　　radiation gastroenteritis (K52.0)
　　radiation proctitis (K62.7)
　Coding Clinic: 2016, Q4, P10

K91.0 **Vomiting following gastrointestinal surgery**

K91.1 **Postgastric surgery syndromes**
　Dumping syndrome
　Postgastrectomy syndrome
　Postvagotomy syndrome

K91.2 **Postsurgical malabsorption, not elsewhere classified**
　Postsurgical blind loop syndrome
　Excludes1　malabsorption osteomalacia in adults (M83.2)
　　malabsorption osteoporosis, postsurgical (M80.8-, M81.8)

● **K91.3** **Postprocedural intestinal obstruction**
　Coding Clinic: 2017, Q1, P40-41

K91.30 **Postprocedural intestinal obstruction, unspecified as to partial versus complete**
　Postprocedural intestinal obstruction NOS

K91.31 **Postprocedural partial intestinal obstruction**
　Postprocedural incomplete intestinal obstruction

K91.32 **Postprocedural complete intestinal obstruction**

K91.5 **Postcholecystectomy syndrome**

● **K91.6** **Intraoperative hemorrhage and hematoma of a digestive system organ or structure complicating a procedure**
　Excludes1　intraoperative hemorrhage and hematoma of a digestive system organ or structure due to accidental puncture and laceration during a procedure (K91.7-)

K91.61 **Intraoperative hemorrhage and hematoma of a digestive system organ or structure complicating a digestive system procedure**
　Coding Clinic: 2020, Q1, P20

K91.62 **Intraoperative hemorrhage and hematoma of a digestive system organ or structure complicating other procedure**

● **K91.7** **Accidental puncture and laceration of a digestive system organ or structure during a procedure**

K91.71 **Accidental puncture and laceration of a digestive system organ or structure during a digestive system procedure**
　Coding Clinic: 2022, Q1, P51-52; 2021, Q2, P12

K91.72 **Accidental puncture and laceration of a digestive system organ or structure during other procedure**
　Coding Clinic: 2022, Q1, P51; 2019, Q2, P24

● **K91.8** **Other intraoperative and postprocedural complications and disorders of digestive system**

K91.81 **Other intraoperative complications of digestive system**

K91.82 **Postprocedural hepatic failure**

K91.83 **Postprocedural hepatorenal syndrome**

● **K91.84** **Postprocedural hemorrhage of a digestive system organ or structure following a procedure**

K91.840 **Postprocedural hemorrhage of a digestive system organ or structure following a digestive system procedure**
　Coding Clinic: 2016, Q1, P15

K91.841 **Postprocedural hemorrhage of a digestive system organ or structure following other procedure**

▶ New　　⇒ Revised　　~~deleted~~ Deleted　　Excludes 1　　Excludes 2　　Includes　　Use additional　　Code first　　Code also　　Key words
OGCR Official Guidelines　　X Assign placeholder X　　● Use Additional Character(s)　　▶ Manifestation Code　　Hierarchical Condition Category　　Coding Clinic

● **K91.85 Complications of intestinal pouch**

     K91.850 Pouchitis 🔗
          Inflammation of internal ileoanal pouch

     K91.858 Other complications of intestinal pouch 🔗
          Coding Clinic: 2019, Q2, P13

    K91.86 Retained cholelithiasis following cholecystectomy

● **K91.87 Postprocedural hematoma and seroma of a digestive system organ or structure following a procedure**

     K91.870 Postprocedural hematoma of a digestive system organ or structure following a digestive system procedure
          Coding Clinic: 2022, Q1, P24

     K91.871 Postprocedural hematoma of a digestive system organ or structure following other procedure

     K91.872 Postprocedural seroma of a digestive system organ or structure following a digestive system procedure

     K91.873 Postprocedural seroma of a digestive system organ or structure following other procedure

    K91.89 Other postprocedural complications and disorders of digestive system
      Use additional code, if applicable, to further specify disorder
      Excludes2   postprocedural retroperitoneal abscess (K68.11)
      Coding Clinic: 2017, Q1, P41

● **K92 Other diseases of digestive system**
    Excludes1   neonatal gastrointestinal hemorrhage (P54.0-P54.3)

   K92.0 Hematemesis

   K92.1 Melena
     Excludes1   occult blood in feces (R19.5)

   K92.2 Gastrointestinal hemorrhage, unspecified
     Gastric hemorrhage NOS
     Intestinal hemorrhage NOS
     Excludes1   acute hemorrhagic gastritis (K29.01)
         hemorrhage of anus and rectum (K62.5)
         angiodysplasia of stomach with hemorrhage (K31.811)
         diverticular disease with hemorrhage (K57.-)
         gastritis and duodenitis with hemorrhage (K29.-)
         peptic ulcer with hemorrhage (K25-K28)
     Coding Clinic: 2021, Q1, P12

● **K92.8 Other specified diseases of the digestive system**

     K92.81 Gastrointestinal mucositis (ulcerative)
       Code also type of associated therapy, such as:
         antineoplastic and immunosuppressive drugs (T45.1X-)
         radiological procedure and radiotherapy (Y84.2)
       Excludes2   mucositis (ulcerative) of vagina and vulva (N76.81)
          nasal mucositis (ulcerative) (J34.81)
          oral mucositis (ulcerative) (K12.3-)

     K92.89 Other specified diseases of the digestive system

   K92.9 Disease of digestive system, unspecified

● **K94 Complications of artificial openings of the digestive system**

● **K94.0 Colostomy complications**

     K94.00 Colostomy complication, unspecified 🔗
     K94.01 Colostomy hemorrhage 🔗
     K94.02 Colostomy infection 🔗
       Use additional code to specify type of infection, such as:
         cellulitis of abdominal wall (L03.311)
         sepsis (A40.-, A41.-)
     K94.03 Colostomy malfunction 🔗
       Mechanical complication of colostomy
     K94.09 Other complications of colostomy 🔗

● **K94.1 Enterostomy complications**

     K94.10 Enterostomy complication, unspecified 🔗
     K94.11 Enterostomy hemorrhage 🔗
     K94.12 Enterostomy infection 🔗
       Use additional code to specify type of infection, such as:
         cellulitis of abdominal wall (L03.311)
         sepsis (A40.-, A41.-)
     K94.13 Enterostomy malfunction 🔗
       Mechanical complication of enterostomy
       Coding Clinic: 2021, Q4, P18
     K94.19 Other complications of enterostomy 🔗

● **K94.2 Gastrostomy complications**

     K94.20 Gastrostomy complication, unspecified 🔗
     K94.21 Gastrostomy hemorrhage 🔗
     K94.22 Gastrostomy infection 🔗
       Use additional code to specify type of infection, such as:
         cellulitis of abdominal wall (L03.311)
         sepsis (A40.-, A41.-)
     K94.23 Gastrostomy malfunction 🔗
       Mechanical complication of gastrostomy
     K94.29 Other complications of gastrostomy 🔗

● **K94.3 Esophagostomy complications**

     K94.30 Esophagostomy complications, unspecified 🔗
     K94.31 Esophagostomy hemorrhage 🔗
     K94.32 Esophagostomy infection 🔗
       Use additional code to identify the infection
     K94.33 Esophagostomy malfunction 🔗
       Mechanical complication of esophagostomy
     K94.39 Other complications of esophagostomy 🔗

● **K95 Complications of bariatric procedures**

● **K95.0 Complications of gastric band procedure**

     K95.01 Infection due to gastric band procedure
       Use additional code to specify type of infection or organism, such as:
         bacterial and viral infectious agents (B95.-, B96.-)
         cellulitis of abdominal wall (L03.311)
         sepsis (A40.-, A41.-)
     K95.09 Other complications of gastric band procedure
       Use additional code, if applicable, to further specify complication

● **K95.8 Complications of other bariatric procedure**
     Excludes1   complications of gastric band surgery (K95.0-)

     K95.81 Infection due to other bariatric procedure
       Use additional code to specify type of infection or organism, such as:
         bacterial and viral infectious agents (B95.-, B96.-)
         cellulitis of abdominal wall (L03.311)
         sepsis (A40.-, A41.-)
     K95.89 Other complications of other bariatric procedure 🔗
       Use additional code, if applicable, to further specify complication

CHAPTER 11 (K00–K95)

CHAPTER 12

DISEASES OF THE SKIN AND SUBCUTANEOUS TISSUE (L00-L99)

OGCR Chapter-Specific Coding Guidelines

12.   Chapter 12: Diseases of the Skin and Subcutaneous Tissue (L00-L99)

a. Pressure ulcer stage codes

1) Pressure ulcer stages

Codes from category L89, Pressure ulcer, identify the site of the pressure ulcer as well as the stage of the ulcer.

The ICD-10-CM classifies pressure ulcer stages based on severity, which is designated by stages 1-4, unspecified stage and unstageable.

Assign as many codes from category L89 as needed to identify all the pressure ulcers the patient has, if applicable.

See Section I.B.14 for pressure ulcer stage documentation by clinicians other than patient's provider.

2) Unstageable pressure ulcers

Assignment of the code for unstageable pressure ulcer (L89.--0) should be based on the clinical documentation. These codes are used for pressure ulcers whose stage cannot be clinically determined (e.g., the ulcer is covered by eschar or has been treated with a skin or muscle graft) and pressure ulcers that are documented as deep tissue injury but not documented as due to trauma. This code should not be confused with the codes for unspecified stage (L89.--9). When there is no documentation regarding the stage of the pressure ulcer, assign the appropriate code for unspecified stage (L89.--9).

3) Documented pressure ulcer stage

Assignment of the pressure ulcer stage code should be guided by clinical documentation of the stage or documentation of the terms found in the Alphabetic Index. For clinical terms describing the stage that are not found in the Alphabetic Index, and there is no documentation of the stage, the provider should be queried.

4) Patients admitted with pressure ulcers documented as healed

No code is assigned if the documentation states that the pressure ulcer is completely healed.

5) Patients admitted with pressure ulcers documented as healing

Pressure ulcers described as healing should be assigned the appropriate pressure ulcer stage code based on the documentation in the medical record. If the documentation does not provide information about the stage of the healing pressure ulcer, assign the appropriate code for unspecified stage.

If the documentation is unclear as to whether the patient has a current (new) pressure ulcer or if the patient is being treated for a healing pressure ulcer, query the provider.

For ulcers that were present on admission but healed at the time of discharge, assign the code for the site and stage of the pressure ulcer at the time of admission.

6) Patient admitted with pressure ulcer evolving into another stage during the admission

If a patient is admitted to an inpatient hospital with a pressure ulcer at one stage and it progresses to a higher stage, two separate codes should be assigned: one code for the site and stage of the ulcer on admission and a second code for the same ulcer site and the highest stage reported during the stay.

b. Non-Pressure Chronic Ulcers

1) Patients admitted with non-pressure ulcers documented as healed

No code is assigned if the documentation states that the non-pressure ulcer is completely healed.

2) Patients admitted with non-pressure ulcers documented as healing

Non-pressure ulcers described as healing should be assigned the appropriate non-pressure ulcer code based on the documentation in the medical record. If the documentation does not provide information about the severity of the healing non-pressure ulcer, assign the appropriate code for unspecified severity.

If the documentation is unclear as to whether the patient has a current (new) non-pressure ulcer or if the patient is being treated for a healing non-pressure ulcer, query the provider.

For ulcers that were present on admission but healed at the time of discharge, assign the code for the site and severity of the non-pressure ulcer at the time of admission.

3) Patient admitted with non-pressure ulcer that progresses to another severity level during the admission

If a patient is admitted to an inpatient hospital with a non-pressure ulcer at one severity level and it progresses to a higher severity level, two separate codes should be assigned: one code for the site and severity level of the ulcer on admission and a second code for the same ulcer site and the highest severity level reported during the stay.

See Section I.B.14 for pressure ulcer stage documentation by clinicians other than patient's provider.

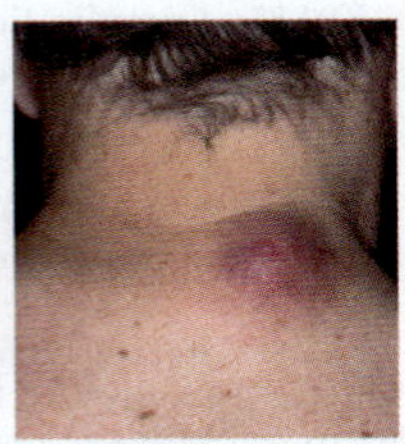

Figure 12-1   Furuncle, also known as a boil, is a staphylococcal infection. The organism enters the body through a hair follicle and so furuncles usually appear in hairy areas of the body. A cluster of furuncles is known as a carbuncle and involves infection into the deep subcutaneous fascia. These usually appear on the back and neck. (**B** from Habif TP, Binnick AN, Meyerson LB: Clinical Dermatology: A Color Guide to Diagnosis and Therapy, S.l., Mosby Elsevier, 2010)

CHAPTER 12

DISEASES OF THE SKIN AND SUBCUTANEOUS TISSUE (L00-L99)

Excludes2   certain conditions originating in the perinatal period (P04-P96)

certain infectious and parasitic diseases (A00-B99)

complications of pregnancy, childbirth and the puerperium (O00-O9A)

congenital malformations, deformations, and chromosomal abnormalities (Q00-Q99)

endocrine, nutritional and metabolic diseases (E00-E88)

lipomelanotic reticulosis (I89.8)

neoplasms (C00-D49)

symptoms, signs and abnormal clinical and laboratory findings, not elsewhere classified (R00-R94)

systemic connective tissue disorders (M30-M36)

viral warts (B07.-)

This chapter contains the following blocks:

L00-L08	Infections of the skin and subcutaneous tissue
L10-L14	Bullous disorders
L20-L30	Dermatitis and eczema
L40-L45	Papulosquamous disorders
L49-L54	Urticaria and erythema
L55-L59	Radiation-related disorders of the skin and subcutaneous tissue
L60-L75	Disorders of skin appendages
L76	Intraoperative and postprocedural complications of skin and subcutaneous tissue
L80-L99	Other disorders of the skin and subcutaneous tissue

INFECTIONS OF THE SKIN AND SUBCUTANEOUS TISSUE (L00-L08)

Use additional code (B95-B97) to identify infectious agent.

Excludes2   hordeolum (H00.0)

infective dermatitis (L30.3)

local infections of skin classified in Chapter 1

lupus panniculitis (L93.2)

panniculitis NOS (M79.3)

panniculitis of neck and back (M54.0-)

Perlèche NOS (K13.0)

Perlèche due to candidiasis (B37.0)

Perlèche due to riboflavin deficiency (E53.0)

pyogenic granuloma (L98.0)

relapsing panniculitis [Weber-Christian] (M35.6)

viral warts (B07.-)

zoster (B02.-)

▶ New   ⏩ Revised   ~~deleted~~ Deleted   Excludes 1   Excludes 2   Includes   Use additional   Code first   Code also   Key words

OGCR Official Guidelines   X Assign placeholder X   ● Use Additional Character(s)   ▶ Manifestation Code   ⓗ Hierarchical Condition Category   **Coding Clinic**

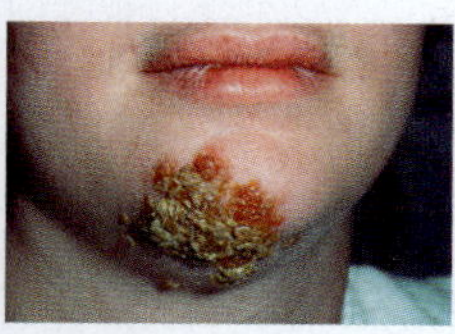

Figure 12-2   Impetigo. A thick, honey-yellow adherent crust covers the entire eroded surface. (From James WD, Elston DM, Berger TG, Andrews GC: Andrews' Diseases of the Skin: Clinical Dermatology, London, Saunders/Elsevier, 2011)

L00   Staphylococcal scalded skin syndrome
Ritter's disease

Use additional code to identify percentage of skin exfoliation (L49.-)

Excludes1   bullous impetigo (L01.03)
pemphigus neonatorum (L01.03)
toxic epidermal necrolysis [Lyell] (L51.2)

● L01   Impetigo
Contagious skin infection caused by a streptococcus or staphylococcus aureus, common skin infections among children

Excludes1   impetigo herpetiformis (L40.1)

● L01.0   Impetigo
Impetigo contagiosa
Impetigo vulgaris

L01.00   **Impetigo, unspecified**
Impetigo NOS

L01.01   **Non-bullous impetigo**

L01.02   **Bockhart's impetigo**
Impetigo follicularis
Perifolliculitis NOS
Superficial pustular perifolliculitis

L01.03   **Bullous impetigo**
Impetigo neonatorum
Pemphigus neonatorum
Neonate = newborn

L01.09   **Other impetigo**
Ulcerative impetigo

L01.1   Impetiginization of other dermatoses

● L02   Cutaneous abscess, furuncle and carbuncle
Use additional code to identify organism (B95-B96)

Excludes2   abscess of anus and rectal regions (K61.-)
abscess of female genital organs (external) (N76.4)
abscess of male genital organs (external) (N48.2, N49.-)

● L02.0   Cutaneous abscess, furuncle and carbuncle of face
Excludes2   abscess of ear, external (H60.0)
abscess of eyelid (H00.0)
abscess of head [any part, except face] (L02.8)
abscess of lacrimal gland (H04.0)
abscess of lacrimal passages (H04.3)
abscess of mouth (K12.2)
abscess of nose (J34.0)
abscess of orbit (H05.0)
submandibular abscess (K12.2)

L02.01   **Cutaneous abscess of face**

L02.02   **Furuncle of face**
Boil of face
Folliculitis of face

L02.03   **Carbuncle of face**

● L02.1   Cutaneous abscess, furuncle and carbuncle of neck
L02.11   **Cutaneous abscess of neck**

L02.12   **Furuncle of neck**
Boil of neck
Folliculitis of neck

L02.13   **Carbuncle of neck**

● L02.2   Cutaneous abscess, furuncle and carbuncle of trunk
Excludes1   non-newborn omphalitis (L08.82)
omphalitis of newborn (P38.-)

Excludes2   abscess of breast (N61.1)
abscess of buttocks (L02.3)
abscess of female external genital organs (N76.4)
abscess of male external genital organs (N48.2, N49.-)
abscess of hip (L02.4)

● L02.21   Cutaneous abscess of trunk
L02.211   **Cutaneous abscess of abdominal wall**

➡ **L02.212**   **Cutaneous abscess of back [any part, except buttock and flank]**

L02.213   **Cutaneous abscess of chest wall**

L02.214   **Cutaneous abscess of groin**

L02.215   **Cutaneous abscess of perineum**

L02.216   **Cutaneous abscess of umbilicus**

▶ **L02.217**   **Cutaneous abscess of flank**

L02.219   **Cutaneous abscess of trunk, unspecified**

● L02.22   Furuncle of trunk
Boil of trunk
Folliculitis of trunk

L02.221   **Furuncle of abdominal wall**

➡ **L02.222**   **Furuncle of back [any part, except buttock and flank]**

L02.223   **Furuncle of chest wall**

L02.224   **Furuncle of groin**

L02.225   **Furuncle of perineum**

L02.226   **Furuncle of umbilicus**

▶ **L02.227**   **Furuncle of flank**

L02.229   **Furuncle of trunk, unspecified**

● L02.23   Carbuncle of trunk
L02.231   **Carbuncle of abdominal wall**

L02.232   **Carbuncle of back [any part, except buttock]**

L02.233   **Carbuncle of chest wall**

L02.234   **Carbuncle of groin**

L02.235   **Carbuncle of perineum**

L02.236   **Carbuncle of umbilicus**

L02.239   **Carbuncle of trunk, unspecified**

● L02.3   Cutaneous abscess, furuncle and carbuncle of buttock
Excludes1   pilonidal cyst with abscess (L05.01)

L02.31   **Cutaneous abscess of buttock**
Cutaneous abscess of gluteal region

L02.32   **Furuncle of buttock**
Boil of buttock
Folliculitis of buttock
Furuncle of gluteal region

L02.33   **Carbuncle of buttock**
Carbuncle of gluteal region

● L02.4   Cutaneous abscess, furuncle and carbuncle of limb
Excludes2   Cutaneous abscess, furuncle and carbuncle of groin (L02.214, L02.224, L02.234)
Cutaneous abscess, furuncle and carbuncle of hand (L02.5-)
Cutaneous abscess, furuncle and carbuncle of foot (L02.6-)

● L02.41   Cutaneous abscess of limb
L02.411   **Cutaneous abscess of right axilla**

L02.412   **Cutaneous abscess of left axilla**

L02.413   **Cutaneous abscess of right upper limb**

L02.414   **Cutaneous abscess of left upper limb**

CHAPTER 12 (L00-L99)

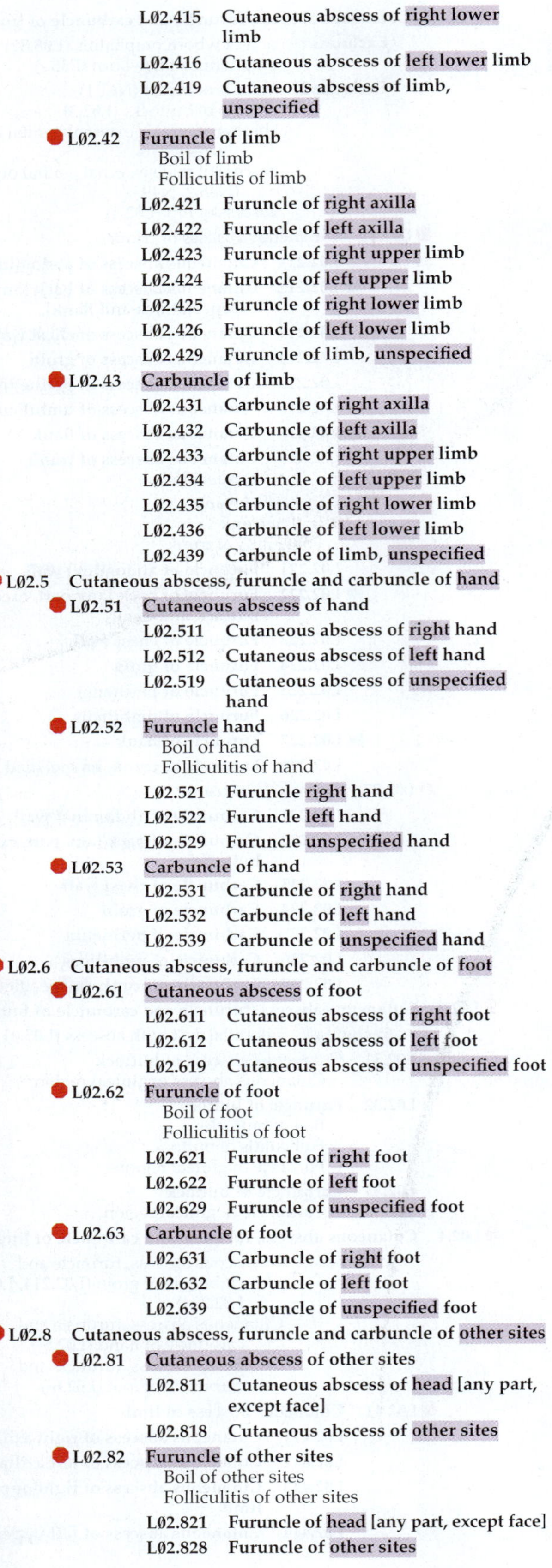

      L02.415   Cutaneous abscess of **right lower limb**

      L02.416   Cutaneous abscess of **left lower limb**

      L02.419   Cutaneous abscess of **limb, unspecified**

● **L02.42**   **Furuncle of limb**
       Boil of limb
       Folliculitis of limb

      L02.421   Furuncle of **right axilla**

      L02.422   Furuncle of **left axilla**

      L02.423   Furuncle of **right upper limb**

      L02.424   Furuncle of **left upper limb**

      L02.425   Furuncle of **right lower limb**

      L02.426   Furuncle of **left lower limb**

      L02.429   Furuncle of **limb, unspecified**

● **L02.43**   **Carbuncle of limb**

      L02.431   Carbuncle of **right axilla**

      L02.432   Carbuncle of **left axilla**

      L02.433   Carbuncle of **right upper limb**

      L02.434   Carbuncle of **left upper limb**

      L02.435   Carbuncle of **right lower limb**

      L02.436   Carbuncle of **left lower limb**

      L02.439   Carbuncle of **limb, unspecified**

● **L02.5**   Cutaneous abscess, furuncle and carbuncle of **hand**

  ● **L02.51**   **Cutaneous abscess of hand**

      L02.511   Cutaneous abscess of **right hand**

      L02.512   Cutaneous abscess of **left hand**

      L02.519   Cutaneous abscess of **unspecified hand**

  ● **L02.52**   **Furuncle hand**
       Boil of hand
       Folliculitis of hand

      L02.521   Furuncle **right hand**

      L02.522   Furuncle **left hand**

      L02.529   Furuncle **unspecified** hand

  ● **L02.53**   **Carbuncle of hand**

      L02.531   Carbuncle of **right hand**

      L02.532   Carbuncle of **left hand**

      L02.539   Carbuncle of **unspecified hand**

● **L02.6**   Cutaneous abscess, furuncle and carbuncle of **foot**

  ● **L02.61**   **Cutaneous abscess of foot**

      L02.611   Cutaneous abscess of **right foot**

      L02.612   Cutaneous abscess of **left foot**

      L02.619   Cutaneous abscess of **unspecified** foot

  ● **L02.62**   **Furuncle of foot**
       Boil of foot
       Folliculitis of foot

      L02.621   Furuncle of **right foot**

      L02.622   Furuncle of **left foot**

      L02.629   Furuncle of **unspecified** foot

  ● **L02.63**   **Carbuncle of foot**

      L02.631   Carbuncle of **right foot**

      L02.632   Carbuncle of **left foot**

      L02.639   Carbuncle of **unspecified** foot

● **L02.8**   Cutaneous abscess, furuncle and carbuncle of **other sites**

  ● **L02.81**   **Cutaneous abscess of other sites**

      L02.811   Cutaneous abscess of **head** [any part, except face]

      L02.818   Cutaneous abscess of **other sites**

  ● **L02.82**   **Furuncle** of other sites
       Boil of other sites
       Folliculitis of other sites

      L02.821   Furuncle of **head** [any part, except face]

      L02.828   Furuncle of **other sites**

Item 12-1   **Onychia** is an inflammation of the tissue surrounding the nail with pus accumulation and loss of the nail, resulting from microscopic pathogens entering through small wounds. **Paronychia** is a nail disease also known as felon or whitlow and is a bacterial or fungal infection.

  ● **L02.83**   **Carbuncle of other sites**

      L02.831   Carbuncle of **head** [any part, except face]

      L02.838   Carbuncle of **other sites**

  ● **L02.9**   Cutaneous abscess, furuncle and carbuncle, **unspecified**

      L02.91   **Cutaneous abscess, unspecified**

      L02.92   **Furuncle, unspecified**
         Boil NOS
         Furunculosis NOS

      L02.93   **Carbuncle, unspecified**

● **L03**   **Cellulitis and acute lymphangitis**

    Excludes2   cellulitis of anal and rectal region (K61.-)
          cellulitis of external auditory canal (H60.1)
          cellulitis of eyelid (H00.0)
          cellulitis of female external genital organs (N76.4)
          cellulitis of lacrimal apparatus (H04.3)
          cellulitis of male external genital organs (N48.2, N49.-)
          cellulitis of mouth (K12.2)
          cellulitis of nose (J34.0)
          eosinophilic cellulitis [Wells] (L98.3)
          febrile neutrophilic dermatosis [Sweet] (L98.2)
          lymphangitis (chronic) (subacute) (I89.1)

  ● **L03.0**   **Cellulitis and acute lymphangitis of finger and toe**
       Infection of nail
       Onychia
       Paronychia
       Perionychia

    ● **L03.01**   **Cellulitis of finger**
         Felon
         Whitlow

      Excludes1   herpetic whitlow (B00.89)

      L03.011   Cellulitis of **right finger**

      L03.012   Cellulitis of **left finger**

      L03.019   Cellulitis of **unspecified finger**

    ● **L03.02**   **Acute lymphangitis of finger**
         Hangnail with lymphangitis of finger

      L03.021   Acute lymphangitis of **right finger**

      L03.022   Acute lymphangitis of **left finger**

      L03.029   Acute lymphangitis of **unspecified finger**

    ● **L03.03**   **Cellulitis of toe**

      L03.031   Cellulitis of **right toe**

      L03.032   Cellulitis of **left toe**

      L03.039   Cellulitis of **unspecified toe**

    ● **L03.04**   **Acute lymphangitis of toe**
         Hangnail with lymphangitis of toe

      L03.041   Acute lymphangitis of **right toe**

      L03.042   Acute lymphangitis of **left toe**

      L03.049   Acute lymphangitis of **unspecified toe**

  ● **L03.1**   Cellulitis and acute lymphangitis of **other parts of limb**

    ● **L03.11**   **Cellulitis of other parts of limb**

      Excludes2   cellulitis of fingers (L03.01-)
           cellulitis of toes (L03.03-)
           groin (L03.314)

      L03.111   Cellulitis of **right axilla**

      L03.112   Cellulitis of **left axilla**

      L03.113   Cellulitis of **right upper limb**

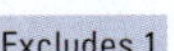

► New   ⇒ Revised   ~~deleted~~ Deleted   Excludes 1   Excludes 2   Includes   Use additional   Code first   Code also   Key words

OGCR Official Guidelines   **X** Assign placeholder X   ● Use Additional Character(s)   ▸ Manifestation Code   Hierarchical Condition Category   **Coding Clinic**

Item 12–2 Cellulitis is an acute spreading bacterial infection below the surface of the skin characterized by redness (erythema), warmth, swelling, pain, fever, chills, and enlarged lymph nodes ("swollen glands").

L03.114   **Cellulitis of left upper limb**
     Coding Clinic: 2019, Q1, P13

L03.115   **Cellulitis of right lower limb**

L03.116   **Cellulitis of left lower limb**

L03.119   **Cellulitis of unspecified part of limb**

● **L03.12   Acute lymphangitis of other parts of limb**

     Excludes2   acute lymphangitis of fingers (L03.2-)
       acute lymphangitis of toes (L03.04-)
       acute lymphangitis of groin (L03.324)

L03.121   **Acute lymphangitis of right axilla**

L03.122   **Acute lymphangitis of left axilla**

L03.123   **Acute lymphangitis of right upper limb**

L03.124   **Acute lymphangitis of left upper limb**

L03.125   **Acute lymphangitis of right lower limb**

L03.126   **Acute lymphangitis of left lower limb**

L03.129   **Acute lymphangitis of unspecified part of limb**

● **L03.2   Cellulitis and acute lymphangitis of face and neck**

   ● **L03.21   Cellulitis and acute lymphangitis of face**

L03.211   **Cellulitis of face**

     Excludes2   abscess of orbit (H05.01-)
       cellulitis of ear (H60.1-)
       cellulitis of eyelid (H00.0-)
       cellulitis of head (L03.81)
       cellulitis of lacrimal apparatus (H04.3)
       cellulitis of lip (K13.0)
       cellulitis of mouth (K12.2)
       cellulitis of nose (internal) (J34.0)
       cellulitis of orbit (H05.01-)
       cellulitis of scalp (L03.81)

L03.212   **Acute lymphangitis of face**

L03.213   **Periorbital cellulitis**
     Preseptal cellulitis
     Coding Clinic: 2016, Q4, P36

   ● **L03.22   Cellulitis and acute lymphangitis of neck**

L03.221   **Cellulitis of neck**

L03.222   **Acute lymphangitis of neck**

● **L03.3   Cellulitis and acute lymphangitis of trunk**

   ● **L03.31   Cellulitis of trunk**

     Excludes2   cellulitis of anal and rectal regions (K61.-)
       cellulitis of breast NOS (N61.0)
       cellulitis of female external genital organs (N76.4)
       cellulitis of male external genital organs (N48.2, N49.-)
       omphalitis of newborn (P38.-)
       puerperal cellulitis of breast (O91.2)

L03.311   **Cellulitis of abdominal wall**

     Excludes2   cellulitis of umbilicus (L03.316)
       cellulitis of groin (L03.314)

L03.312   **Cellulitis of back [any part except buttock]**

L03.313   **Cellulitis of chest wall**

L03.314   **Cellulitis of groin**

L03.315   **Cellulitis of perineum**

L03.316   **Cellulitis of umbilicus**

L03.317   **Cellulitis of buttock**

L03.319   **Cellulitis of trunk, unspecified**

▶ L03.31A   **Cellulitis of flank**

   ● **L03.32   Acute lymphangitis of trunk**

L03.321   **Acute lymphangitis of abdominal wall**

L03.322   **Acute lymphangitis of back [any part except buttock]**

L03.323   **Acute lymphangitis of chest wall**

L03.324   **Acute lymphangitis of groin**

L03.325   **Acute lymphangitis of perineum**

L03.326   **Acute lymphangitis of umbilicus**

L03.327   **Acute lymphangitis of buttock**

L03.329   **Acute lymphangitis of trunk, unspecified**

▶ L03.32A   **Acute lymphangitis of flank**

● **L03.8   Cellulitis and acute lymphangitis of other sites**

   ● **L03.81   Cellulitis of other sites**

L03.811   **Cellulitis of head [any part, except face]**
     Cellulitis of scalp

     Excludes2   cellulitis of face (L03.211)

L03.818   **Cellulitis of other sites**

   ● **L03.89   Acute lymphangitis of other sites**

L03.891   **Acute lymphangitis of head [any part, except face]**

L03.898   **Acute lymphangitis of other sites**

● **L03.9   Cellulitis and acute lymphangitis, unspecified**

L03.90   **Cellulitis, unspecified**

L03.91   **Acute lymphangitis, unspecified**

     Excludes1   lymphangitis NOS (I89.1)

● **L04   Acute lymphadenitis**

Short-term inflammation of lymph nodes which can be regionalized to involve a given area of the lymph system or systemic involving much of the body

     Includes   abscess (acute) of lymph nodes, except mesenteric
       acute lymphadenitis, except mesenteric

     Excludes1   chronic or subacute lymphadenitis, except mesenteric (I88.1)
       enlarged lymph nodes (R59.-)
       human immunodeficiency virus [HIV] disease resulting in generalized lymphadenopathy (B20)
       lymphadenitis NOS (I88.9)
       nonspecific mesenteric lymphadenitis (I88.0)

CHAPTER 12 (L00-L99)

L04.0   **Acute lymphadenitis of face, head and neck**
L04.1   **Acute lymphadenitis of trunk**
L04.2   **Acute lymphadenitis of upper limb**
         Acute lymphadenitis of axilla
         Acute lymphadenitis of shoulder
L04.3   **Acute lymphadenitis of lower limb**
         Acute lymphadenitis of hip
         Excludes2   acute lymphadenitis of groin (L04.1)
L04.8   **Acute lymphadenitis of other sites**
L04.9   **Acute lymphadenitis, unspecified**

Item 12–3   Abscess is a localized collection of pus in tissues or organs and is a sign of infection, resulting in swelling and inflammation.

Item 12–4   Pilonidal cyst, also called a coccygeal cyst, is the result of a disorder called pilonidal disease. The cyst usually contains hair and pus.

● **L05   Pilonidal cyst and sinus**
   ● **L05.0   Pilonidal cyst and sinus with abscess**
      L05.01   **Pilonidal cyst with abscess**
                Pilonidal abscess
                Pilonidal dimple with abscess
                Postanal dimple with abscess
                Excludes2   congenital sacral dimple (Q82.6)
                                 parasacral dimple (Q82.6)
      L05.02   **Pilonidal sinus with abscess**
                Coccygeal fistula with abscess
                Coccygeal sinus with abscess
                Pilonidal fistula with abscess
   ● **L05.9   Pilonidal cyst and sinus without abscess**
      L05.91   **Pilonidal cyst without abscess**
                Pilonidal dimple
                Postanal dimple
                Pilonidal cyst NOS
                Excludes2   congenital sacral dimple (Q82.6)
                                 parasacral dimple (Q82.6)
      L05.92   **Pilonidal sinus without abscess**
                Coccygeal fistula
                Coccygeal sinus without abscess
                Pilonidal fistula

● **L08   Other local infections of skin and subcutaneous tissue**
   L08.0   **Pyoderma**
            Dermatitis gangrenosa
            Purulent dermatitis
            Septic dermatitis
            Suppurative dermatitis
            Excludes1   pyoderma gangrenosum (L88)
                             pyoderma vegetans (L08.81)
   L08.1   **Erythrasma**
   ● **L08.8   Other specified local infections of the skin and subcutaneous tissue**
      L08.81   **Pyoderma vegetans**
                Excludes1   pyoderma gangrenosum (L88)
                                 pyoderma NOS (L08.0)
      L08.82   **Omphalitis not of newborn**
                Excludes1   omphalitis of newborn (P38.-)
      L08.89   **Other specified local infections of the skin and subcutaneous tissue**
   L08.9   **Local infection of the skin and subcutaneous tissue, unspecified**

BULLOUS DISORDERS (L10-L14)

Excludes1   benign familial pemphigus [Hailey-Hailey] (Q82.8)
                 staphylococcal scalded skin syndrome (L00)
                 toxic epidermal necrolysis [Lyell] (L51.2)

● **L10   Pemphigus**
   Excludes1   pemphigus neonatorum (L01.03)
   L10.0   **Pemphigus vulgaris**
   L10.1   **Pemphigus vegetans**
   L10.2   **Pemphigus foliaceous**

Item 12–5   Dermatitis herpetiformis, also known as Duhring's disease, is a systemic disease characterized by small blisters (3 to 5 mm) and occasionally large bullae (> 5 mm).

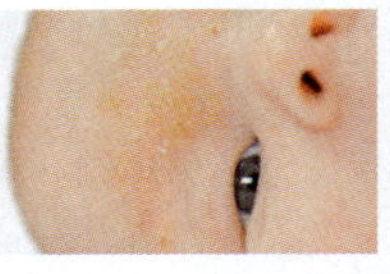

Figure 12-3   Dermatitis herpetiformis. (From Terhorst D: BASICS Dermatologie, München, Elsevier, Urban & Fischer, 2011)

L10.3   **Brazilian pemphigus [fogo selvagem]**
L10.4   **Pemphigus erythematosus**
         Senear-Usher syndrome
L10.5   **Drug-induced pemphigus**
         Use additional code for adverse effect, if applicable, to identify drug (T36-T50 with fifth or sixth character 5)
● **L10.8   Other pemphigus**
   L10.81   **Paraneoplastic pemphigus**
   L10.89   **Other pemphigus**
L10.9   **Pemphigus, unspecified**

● **L11   Other acantholytic disorders**
   L11.0   **Acquired keratosis follicularis**
            Excludes1   keratosis follicularis (congenital) [Darier-White] (Q82.8)
   L11.1   **Transient acantholytic dermatosis [Grover]**
   L11.8   **Other specified acantholytic disorders**
   L11.9   **Acantholytic disorder, unspecified**

● **L12   Pemphigoid**
   Excludes1   herpes gestationis (O26.4-)
                    impetigo herpetiformis (L40.1)
   L12.0   **Bullous pemphigoid**
   L12.1   **Cicatricial pemphigoid**
            Benign mucous membrane pemphigoid
   L12.2   **Chronic bullous disease of childhood**   P
            Juvenile dermatitis herpetiformis
   ● **L12.3   Acquired epidermolysis bullosa**
      Excludes1   epidermolysis bullosa (congenital) (Q81.-)
      L12.30   **Acquired epidermolysis bullosa, unspecified**
      L12.31   **Epidermolysis bullosa due to drug**
                Use additional code for adverse effect, if applicable, to identify drug (T36-T50 with fifth or sixth character 5)
      L12.35   **Other acquired epidermolysis bullosa**
   L12.8   **Other pemphigoid**
   L12.9   **Pemphigoid, unspecified**

● **L13   Other bullous disorders**
   L13.0   **Dermatitis herpetiformis**
            Duhring's disease
            Hydroa herpetiformis
            Excludes1   juvenile dermatitis herpetiformis (L12.2)
                             senile dermatitis herpetiformis (L12.0)
   L13.1   **Subcorneal pustular dermatitis**
            Sneddon-Wilkinson disease
   L13.8   **Other specified bullous disorders**
   L13.9   **Bullous disorder, unspecified**

▶ *L14   Bullous disorders in diseases classified elsewhere*
         Code first underlying disease

Item 12–6   Seborrheic dermatitis is characterized by greasy, scaly, red patches and is associated with oily skin and scalp.

Figure 12-4   Seborrheic dermatitis. (Getty Image)

▶ New   ⇒ Revised   ~~deleted~~ Deleted   Excludes 1   Excludes 2   Includes   Use additional   Code first   Code also   Key words
OGCR Official Guidelines   X Assign placeholder X   ● Use Additional Character(s)   ▶ Manifestation Code   Ⓗⓒ Hierarchical Condition Category   Coding Clinic

DERMATITIS AND ECZEMA (L20-L30)

Note: In this block the terms dermatitis and eczema are used synonymously and interchangeably.

➡ **Excludes2**   chronic (childhood) granulomatous disease (D71.-)
     dermatitis gangrenosa (L08.0)
     dermatitis herpetiformis (L13.0)
     dry skin dermatitis (L85.3)
     factitial dermatitis (L98.1)
     perioral dermatitis (L71.0)
     radiation-related disorders of the skin and subcutaneous tissue (L55-L59)
     stasis dermatitis (I87.2)

● **L20**   **Atopic dermatitis**

   L20.0   **Besnier's prurigo**

●   **L20.8**   **Other atopic dermatitis**

     Excludes2   circumscribed neurodermatitis (L28.0)

     L20.81   **Atopic neurodermatitis**
       Diffuse neurodermatitis

     L20.82   **Flexural eczema**

     L20.83   **Infantile (acute) (chronic) eczema**   **P**

     L20.84   **Intrinsic (allergic) eczema**

     L20.89   **Other atopic dermatitis**

   L20.9   **Atopic dermatitis, unspecified**

● **L21**   **Seborrheic dermatitis**

     Excludes2   infective dermatitis (L30.3)
       seborrheic keratosis (L82.-)

   L21.0   **Seborrhea capitis**
     Cradle cap
     Coding Clinic: 2018, Q1, P6

   L21.1   **Seborrheic infantile dermatitis**   **P**

   L21.8   **Other seborrheic dermatitis**

   L21.9   **Seborrheic dermatitis, unspecified**
     Seborrhea NOS

L22   **Diaper dermatitis**
     Diaper erythema
     Diaper rash
     Psoriasiform diaper rash
     Coding Clinic: 2021, Q4, P18

● **L23**   **Allergic contact dermatitis**

     Excludes1   allergy NOS (T78.40)
       contact dermatitis NOS (L25.9)
       dermatitis NOS (L30.9)

     Excludes2   dermatitis due to substances taken internally (L27.-)
       dermatitis of eyelid (H01.1-)
       diaper dermatitis (L22)
       eczema of external ear (H60.5-)
       irritant contact dermatitis (L24.-)
       perioral dermatitis (L71.0)
       radiation-related disorders of the skin and subcutaneous tissue (L55-L59)

   L23.0   **Allergic contact dermatitis due to metals**
     Allergic contact dermatitis due to chromium
     Allergic contact dermatitis due to nickel

   L23.1   **Allergic contact dermatitis due to adhesives**

   L23.2   **Allergic contact dermatitis due to cosmetics**

   L23.3   **Allergic contact dermatitis due to drugs in contact with skin**

     Use additional code for adverse effect, if applicable, to identify drug (T36-T50 with fifth or sixth character 5)

     Excludes2   dermatitis due to ingested drugs and medicaments (L27.0-L27.1)

   L23.4   **Allergic contact dermatitis due to dyes**

   L23.5   **Allergic contact dermatitis due to other chemical products**
     Allergic contact dermatitis due to cement
     Allergic contact dermatitis due to insecticide
     Allergic contact dermatitis due to plastic
     Allergic contact dermatitis due to rubber

   L23.6   **Allergic contact dermatitis due to food in contact with the skin**

     Excludes2   dermatitis due to ingested food (L27.2)

   L23.7   **Allergic contact dermatitis due to plants, except food**
     Excludes2   allergy NOS due to pollen (J30.1)

●   **L23.8**   **Allergic contact dermatitis due to other agents**

     L23.81   **Allergic contact dermatitis due to animal (cat) (dog) dander**
       Allergic contact dermatitis due to animal (cat) (dog) hair

     L23.89   **Allergic contact dermatitis due to other agents**

   L23.9   **Allergic contact dermatitis, unspecified cause**
     Allergic contact eczema NOS

● **L24**   **Irritant contact dermatitis**

     Excludes1   allergy NOS (T78.40)
       contact dermatitis NOS (L25.9)
       dermatitis NOS (L30.9)

     Excludes2   allergic contact dermatitis (L23.-)
       dermatitis due to substances taken internally (L27.-)
       dermatitis of eyelid (H01.1-)
       diaper dermatitis (L22)
       eczema of external ear (H60.5-)
       perioral dermatitis (L71.0)
       radiation-related disorders of the skin and subcutaneous tissue (L55-L59)

   L24.0   **Irritant contact dermatitis due to detergents**

   L24.1   **Irritant contact dermatitis due to oils and greases**

   L24.2   **Irritant contact dermatitis due to solvents**
     Irritant contact dermatitis due to chlorocompound
     Irritant contact dermatitis due to cyclohexane
     Irritant contact dermatitis due to ester
     Irritant contact dermatitis due to glycol
     Irritant contact dermatitis due to hydrocarbon
     Irritant contact dermatitis due to ketone

   L24.3   **Irritant contact dermatitis due to cosmetics**

   L24.4   **Irritant contact dermatitis due to drugs in contact with skin**
     Use additional code for adverse effect, if applicable, to identify drug (T36-T50 with fifth or sixth character 5)

   L24.5   **Irritant contact dermatitis due to other chemical products**
     Irritant contact dermatitis due to cement
     Irritant contact dermatitis due to insecticide
     Irritant contact dermatitis due to plastic
     Irritant contact dermatitis due to rubber

   L24.6   **Irritant contact dermatitis due to food in contact with skin**
     Excludes2   dermatitis due to ingested food (L27.2)

   L24.7   **Irritant contact dermatitis due to plants, except food**
     Excludes2   allergy NOS to pollen (J30.1)

●   **L24.8**   **Irritant contact dermatitis due to other agents**

     L24.81   **Irritant contact dermatitis due to metals**
       Irritant contact dermatitis due to chromium
       Irritant contact dermatitis due to nickel

     L24.89   **Irritant contact dermatitis due to other agents**
       Irritant contact dermatitis due to dyes

   L24.9   **Irritant contact dermatitis, unspecified cause**
     Irritant contact eczema NOS

Item 12–7 Atopic dermatitis, also known as atopic eczema, infantile eczema, disseminated neuro dermatitis, flexural eczema, and *prurigo diathesique* (Besnier), is characterized by intense itching and is often hereditary.

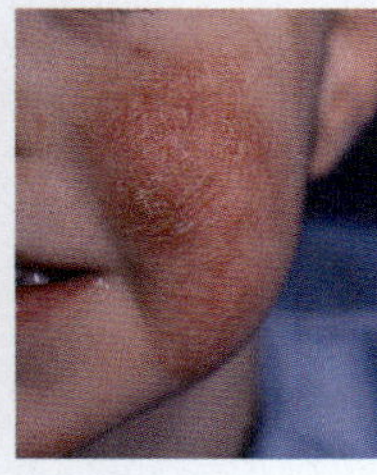

Figure 12-5   Atopic dermatitis. (From Chabner D-E: The Language of Medicine, St. Louis, MO, Saunders/Elsevier, 2007)

CHAPTER 12 (L00-L99)

● **L24.A** **Irritant contact dermatitis due to friction or contact with body fluids**

     Excludes1   virritant contact dermatitis related to stoma or fistula (L24.B-)

     Excludes2   erythema intertrigo (L30.4)

   L24.A0   **Irritant contact dermatitis due to friction or contact with body fluids, unspecified**

   L24.A1   **Irritant contact dermatitis due to saliva**

   L24.A2   **Irritant contact dermatitis due to fecal, urinary or dual incontinence**

     Excludes1   diaper dermatitis (L22)

     Coding Clinic: 2021, Q4, P18

   L24.A9   **Irritant contact dermatitis due friction or contact with other specified body fluids**
      Irritant contact dermatitis related to endotracheal tube
      Wound fluids, exudate

● **L24.B** **Irritant contact dermatitis related to stoma or fistula**

     Use additional code to identify any artificial opening status (Z93.-), if applicable, for contact dermatitis related to stoma secretions

   L24.B0   **Irritant contact dermatitis related to unspecified stoma or fistula**
      Irritant contact dermatitis related to fistula NOS
      Irritant contact dermatitis related to stoma NOS

   L24.B1   **Irritant contact dermatitis related to digestive stoma or fistula**
      Irritant contact dermatitis related to gastrostomy
      Irritant contact dermatitis related to jejunostomy
      Irritant contact dermatitis related to saliva or spit fistula

   L24.B2   **Irritant contact dermatitis related to respiratory stoma or fistula**
      Irritant contact dermatitis related to tracheostomy

   L24.B3   **Irritant contact dermatitis related to fecal or urinary stoma or fistula**
      Irritant contact dermatitis related to colostomy
      Irritant contact dermatitis related to enterocutaneous fistula
      Irritant contact dermatitis related to ileostomy

     Coding Clinic: 2021, Q4, P17,19

● **L25** **Unspecified contact dermatitis**

     Excludes1   allergic contact dermatitis (L23.-)
          allergy NOS (T78.40)
          dermatitis NOS (L30.9)
          irritant contact dermatitis (L24.-)

     Excludes2   dermatitis due to ingested substances (L27.-)
          dermatitis of eyelid (H01.1-)
          eczema of external ear (H60.5-)
          perioral dermatitis (L71.0)
          radiation-related disorders of the skin and subcutaneous tissue (L55-L59)

   L25.0   **Unspecified contact dermatitis due to cosmetics**

   L25.1   **Unspecified contact dermatitis due to drugs in contact with skin**

     Use additional code for adverse effect, if applicable, to identify drug (T36-T50 with fifth or sixth character 5)

     Excludes2   dermatitis due to ingested drugs and medicaments (L27.0-L27.1)

   L25.2   **Unspecified contact dermatitis due to dyes**

   L25.3   **Unspecified contact dermatitis due to other chemical products**
      Unspecified contact dermatitis due to cement
      Unspecified contact dermatitis due to insecticide

   L25.4   **Unspecified contact dermatitis due to food in contact with skin**

     Excludes2   dermatitis due to ingested food (L27.2)

   L25.5   **Unspecified contact dermatitis due to plants, except food**

     Excludes1   nettle rash (L50.9)

     Excludes2   allergy NOS due to pollen (J30.1)

   L25.8   **Unspecified contact dermatitis due to other agents**

   L25.9   **Unspecified contact dermatitis, unspecified cause**
      Contact dermatitis (occupational) NOS
      Contact eczema (occupational) NOS

L26   **Exfoliative dermatitis**
      Hebra's pityriasis

     Excludes1   Ritter's disease (L00)

● **L27** **Dermatitis due to substances taken internally**

     Excludes1   allergy NOS (T78.40)

     Excludes2   adverse food reaction, except dermatitis (T78.0-T78.1)
          contact dermatitis (L23-L25)
          drug photoallergic response (L56.1)
          drug phototoxic response (L56.0)
          urticaria (L50.-)

   L27.0   **Generalized skin eruption due to drugs and medicaments taken internally**

     Use additional code for adverse effect, if applicable, to identify drug (T36-T50 with fifth or sixth character 5)

   L27.1   **Localized skin eruption due to drugs and medicaments taken internally**

     Use additional code for adverse effect, if applicable, to identify drug (T36-T50 with fifth or sixth character 5)

   L27.2   **Dermatitis due to ingested food**

     Excludes2   dermatitis due to food in contact with skin (L23.6, L24.6, L25.4)

   L27.8   **Dermatitis due to other substances taken internally**

   L27.9   **Dermatitis due to unspecified substance taken internally**

● **L28** **Lichen simplex chronicus and prurigo**

   L28.0   **Lichen simplex chronicus**
      Circumscribed neurodermatitis
      Lichen NOS

   L28.1   **Prurigo nodularis**

   L28.2   **Other prurigo**
      Prurigo NOS   Prurigo mitis
      Prurigo Hebra   Urticaria papulosa

● **L29** **Pruritus**

     Excludes1   neurotic excoriation (L98.1)
          psychogenic pruritus (F45.8)

   L29.0   **Pruritus ani**

   L29.1   **Pruritus scroti**

   L29.2   **Pruritus vulvae**

   L29.3   **Anogenital pruritus, unspecified**

   L29.8   **Other pruritus**

     L29.81   **Cholestatic pruritus**

       Code also, if applicable, type of liver disease

       Use Additional code for adverse effect, if applicable, to identify drug (T36-T50 with fifth or sixth character 5)

     L29.89   **Other pruritus**

   L29.9   **Pruritus, unspecified**
      Itch NOS

● **L30** **Other and unspecified dermatitis**

     Excludes2   contact dermatitis (L23-L25)
          dry skin dermatitis (L85.3)
          small plaque parapsoriasis (L41.3)
          stasis dermatitis (I87.2)

   L30.0   **Nummular dermatitis**

   L30.1   **Dyshidrosis [pompholyx]**

   L30.2   **Cutaneous autosensitization**
      Candidid [levurid]   Eczematid
      Dermatophytid

   L30.3   **Infective dermatitis**
      Infectious eczematoid dermatitis

   L30.4   **Erythema intertrigo**

▶ New   ⇒ Revised   ~~deleted~~ Deleted   Excludes 1   Excludes 2   Includes   Use additional   Code first   Code also   Key words

OGCR Official Guidelines   X Assign placeholder X   ● Use Additional Character(s)   ▶ Manifestation Code   Hierarchical Condition Category   **Coding Clinic**

L30.5   **Pityriasis alba**
     Coding Clinic: 2018, Q1, P6

L30.8   **Other specified dermatitis**

L30.9   **Dermatitis, unspecified**
     Eczema NOS

PAPULOSQUAMOUS DISORDERS (L40-L45)

● **L40**   **Psoriasis**

L40.0   **Psoriasis vulgaris**
     Nummular psoriasis   Plaque psoriasis

L40.1   **Generalized pustular psoriasis**
     Impetigo herpetiformis   Von Zumbusch's disease

L40.2   **Acrodermatitis continua**

L40.3   **Pustulosis palmaris et plantaris**

L40.4   **Guttate psoriasis**

● L40.5   **Arthropathic psoriasis**

     L40.50   **Arthropathic psoriasis, unspecified**

     L40.51   **Distal interphalangeal psoriatic arthropathy**

     L40.52   **Psoriatic arthritis mutilans**

     L40.53   **Psoriatic spondylitis**

     L40.54   **Psoriatic juvenile arthropathy**

     L40.59   **Other psoriatic arthropathy**

L40.8   **Other psoriasis**
     Flexural psoriasis

L40.9   **Psoriasis, unspecified**

● **L41**   **Parapsoriasis**

     Excludes1   poikiloderma vasculare atrophicans (L94.5)

L41.0   **Pityriasis lichenoides et varioliformis acuta**
     Mucha-Habermann disease

L41.1   **Pityriasis lichenoides chronica**

L41.3   **Small plaque parapsoriasis**

L41.4   **Large plaque parapsoriasis**

L41.5   **Retiform parapsoriasis**

L41.8   **Other parapsoriasis**

L41.9   **Parapsoriasis, unspecified**

L42   **Pityriasis rosea**

● **L43**   **Lichen planus**

     Excludes1   lichen planopilaris (L66.1-)

L43.0   **Hypertrophic lichen planus**

L43.1   **Bullous lichen planus**

L43.2   **Lichenoid drug reaction**
     Use additional code for adverse effect, if applicable, to
       identify drug (T36-T50 with fifth or sixth character 5)

L43.3   **Subacute (active) lichen planus**
     Lichen planus tropicus

L43.8   **Other lichen planus**

L43.9   **Lichen planus, unspecified**

● **L44**   **Other papulosquamous disorders**

L44.0   **Pityriasis rubra pilaris**

L44.1   **Lichen nitidus**

L44.2   **Lichen striatus**

L44.3   **Lichen ruber moniliformis**

L44.4   **Infantile papular acrodermatitis [Gianotti-Crosti]**   **P**

L44.8   **Other specified papulosquamous disorders**

L44.9   **Papulosquamous disorder, unspecified**

▶ **L45**   *Papulosquamous disorders in diseases classified elsewhere*
     Code first underlying disease

URTICARIA AND ERYTHEMA (L49-L54)

     Excludes1   Lyme disease (A69.2-)
                 rosacea (L71.-)

● **L49**   **Exfoliation due to erythematous conditions according to extent of body surface involved**
     Code first erythematous condition causing exfoliation, such as:
     Ritter's disease (L00)
     (Staphylococcal) scalded skin syndrome (L00)
     Stevens-Johnson syndrome (L51.1)
     Stevens-Johnson syndrome-toxic epidermal necrolysis
       overlap syndrome (L51.3)
     Toxic epidermal necrolysis (L51.2)

L49.0   **Exfoliation due to erythematous condition involving less than 10 percent of body surface**
     Exfoliation due to erythematous condition NOS

L49.1   **Exfoliation due to erythematous condition involving 10-19 percent of body surface**

L49.2   **Exfoliation due to erythematous condition involving 20-29 percent of body surface**

L49.3   **Exfoliation due to erythematous condition involving 30-39 percent of body surface**

L49.4   **Exfoliation due to erythematous condition involving 40-49 percent of body surface**

L49.5   **Exfoliation due to erythematous condition involving 50-59 percent of body surface**

L49.6   **Exfoliation due to erythematous condition involving 60-69 percent of body surface**

L49.7   **Exfoliation due to erythematous condition involving 70-79 percent of body surface**

L49.8   **Exfoliation due to erythematous condition involving 80-89 percent of body surface**

L49.9   **Exfoliation due to erythematous condition involving 90 or more percent of body surface**

● **L50**   **Urticaria**

     Excludes1   allergic contact dermatitis (L23.-)
                 angioneurotic edema (T78.3)
                 giant urticaria (T78.3)
                 hereditary angio-edema (D84.1)
                 Quincke's edema (T78.3)
                 serum urticaria (T80.6-)
                 solar urticaria (L56.3)
                 urticaria neonatorum (P83.8)
                 urticaria papulosa (L28.2)
                 urticaria pigmentosa (D47.01)

L50.0   **Allergic urticaria**

L50.1   **Idiopathic urticaria**

L50.2   **Urticaria due to cold and heat**
     Excludes2   familial cold urticaria (M04.2)

L50.3   **Dermatographic urticaria**

L50.4   **Vibratory urticaria**

L50.5   **Cholinergic urticaria**

L50.6   **Contact urticaria**

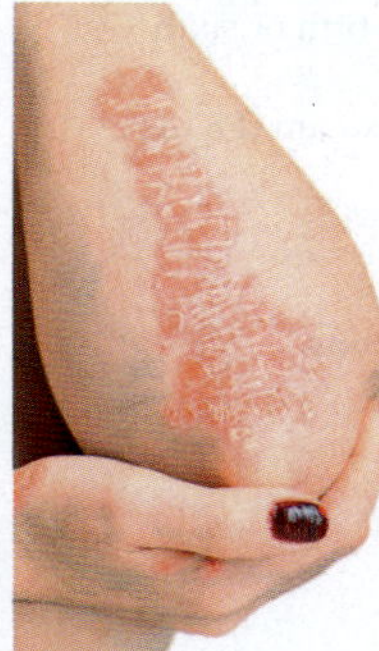

Figure 12-6   Erythematous plaques with silvery scales in a patient with psoriasis. (Getty Image)

Item 12–8 Psoriasis is a chronic, recurrent inflammatory skin disease characterized by small patches covered with thick, silvery scales. **Parapsoriasis** is a treatment-resistant erythroderma. **Pityriasis rosea** is characterized by a herald patch that is a single large lesion and that usually appears on the trunk and is followed by scattered, smaller lesions.

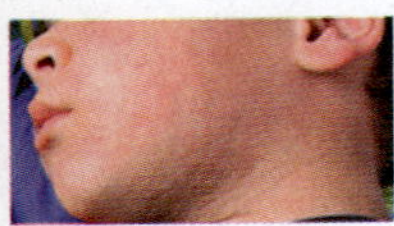

Figure 12-7   Urticaria (hives). *(Courtesy of David Effron, MD.) (Getty Image)*

Item 12–9   Urticaria is a vascular reaction in which wheals surrounded by a red halo appear and cause severe itching. The causes of urticaria or hives are extensive and varied (e.g., food, heat, cold, drugs, stress, infections).

    L50.8   Other urticaria
       Chronic urticaria
       Recurrent periodic urticaria

    L50.9   Urticaria, unspecified

● **L51   Erythema multiforme**
    Use additional code for adverse effect, if applicable, to identify drug (T36-T50 with fifth or sixth character 5)
    Use additional code to identify associated manifestations, such as:
       arthropathy associated with dermatological disorders (M14.8-)
       conjunctival edema (H11.42)
       conjunctivitis (H10.22-)
       corneal scars and opacities (H17.-)
       corneal ulcer (H16.0-)
       edema of eyelid (H02.84-)
       inflammation of eyelid (H01.8-)
       keratoconjunctivitis sicca (H16.22-)
       mechanical lagophthalmos (H02.22-)
       stomatitis (K12.-)
       symblepharon (H11.23-)
    Use additional code to identify percentage of skin exfoliation (L49.-)
    Excludes1   staphylococcal scalded skin syndrome (L00)
               Ritter's disease (L00)

    L51.0   Nonbullous erythema multiforme
    L51.1   Stevens-Johnson syndrome ⓗ
    L51.2   Toxic epidermal necrolysis [Lyell] ⓗ
    L51.3   Stevens-Johnson syndrome-toxic epidermal necrolysis overlap syndrome ⓗ
       SJS-TEN overlap syndrome
    L51.8   Other erythema multiforme
    L51.9   Erythema multiforme, unspecified
       Erythema iris
       Erythema multiforme major NOS
       Erythema multiforme minor NOS
       Herpes iris

   L52   Erythema nodosum
    Excludes1   tuberculous erythema nodosum (A18.4)

● **L53   Other erythematous conditions**
    Excludes1   erythema ab igne (L59.0)
               erythema due to external agents in contact with skin (L23-L25)
               erythema intertrigo (L30.4)

    L53.0   Toxic erythema
       Code first poisoning due to drug or toxin, if applicable (T36-T65 with fifth or sixth character 1-4)
       Use additional code for adverse effect, if applicable, to identify drug (T36-T50 with fifth or sixth character 5)
       Excludes1   neonatal erythema toxicum (P83.1)
    L53.1   Erythema annulare centrifugum
    L53.2   Erythema marginatum
    L53.3   Other chronic figurate erythema
    L53.8   Other specified erythematous conditions
    L53.9   Erythematous condition, unspecified
       Erythema NOS
       Erythroderma NOS

▸ *L54   Erythema in diseases classified elsewhere*
    Code first underlying disease

RADIATION-RELATED DISORDERS OF THE SKIN AND SUBCUTANEOUS TISSUE (L55-L59)

● **L55   Sunburn**
    L55.0   Sunburn of first degree
    L55.1   Sunburn of second degree
    L55.2   Sunburn of third degree
    L55.9   Sunburn, unspecified

● **L56   Other acute skin changes due to ultraviolet radiation**
    Use additional code to identify the source of the ultraviolet radiation (W89, X32)
    L56.0   Drug phototoxic response
       Use additional code for adverse effect, if applicable, to identify drug (T36-T50 with fifth or sixth character 5)
    L56.1   Drug photoallergic response
       Use additional code for adverse effect, if applicable, to identify drug (T36-T50 with fifth or sixth character 5)
    L56.2   Photocontact dermatitis [berloque dermatitis]
    L56.3   Solar urticaria
    L56.4   Polymorphous light eruption
    L56.5   Disseminated superficial actinic porokeratosis (DSAP)
    L56.8   Other specified acute skin changes due to ultraviolet radiation
    L56.9   Acute skin change due to ultraviolet radiation, unspecified

● **L57   Skin changes due to chronic exposure to nonionizing radiation**
    Use additional code to identify the source of the ultraviolet radiation (W89), or other nonionizing radiation (W90)
    L57.0   Actinic keratosis
       Keratosis NOS   Solar keratosis
       Senile keratosis
    L57.1   Actinic reticuloid
    L57.2   Cutis rhomboidalis nuchae
    L57.3   Poikiloderma of Civatte
    L57.4   Cutis laxa senilis
       Elastosis senilis
    L57.5   Actinic granuloma
    L57.8   Other skin changes due to chronic exposure to nonionizing radiation
       Farmer's skin   Solar dermatitis
       Sailor's skin
    L57.9   Skin changes due to chronic exposure to nonionizing radiation, unspecified

● **L58   Radiodermatitis**
    Use additional code to identify the source of the radiation (W88, W90)
    L58.0   Acute radiodermatitis
    L58.1   Chronic radiodermatitis
    L58.9   Radiodermatitis, unspecified

● **L59   Other disorders of skin and subcutaneous tissue related to radiation**
    L59.0   Erythema ab igne [dermatitis ab igne]
    L59.8   Other specified disorders of the skin and subcutaneous tissue related to radiation
       Coding Clinic: 2017, Q1, P34
    L59.9   Disorder of the skin and subcutaneous tissue related to radiation, unspecified

DISORDERS OF SKIN APPENDAGES (L60-L75)

    Excludes1   congenital malformations of integument (Q84.-)

● **L60   Nail disorders**
    Excludes2   clubbing of nails (R68.3)
               onychia and paronychia (L03.0-)
    L60.0   Ingrowing nail
    L60.1   Onycholysis
    L60.2   Onychogryphosis

▶ New   ⇒ Revised   ~~deleted~~ Deleted   Excludes 1   Excludes 2   Includes   Use additional   Code first   Code also   Key words
OGCR Official Guidelines   **X** Assign placeholder X   ● Use Additional Character(s)   ▸ Manifestation Code   ⓗ Hierarchical Condition Category   **Coding Clinic**

L60.3   Nail dystrophy
L60.4   Beau's lines
L60.5   Yellow nail syndrome
L60.8   Other nail disorders
L60.9   Nail disorder, unspecified

L62   *Nail disorders in diseases classified elsewhere*
    Code first underlying disease, such as:
    pachydermoperiostosis (M89.4-)

● **L63**   **Alopecia areata**
L63.0   Alopecia (capitis) totalis
L63.1   Alopecia universalis
L63.2   Ophiasis
L63.8   Other alopecia areata
L63.9   Alopecia areata, unspecified

● **L64**   **Androgenic alopecia**
    Includes   male-pattern baldness
L64.0   **Drug-induced androgenic alopecia**
    Use additional code for adverse effect, if applicable,
    to identify drug (T36-T50 with fifth or sixth
    character 5)
L64.8   **Other androgenic alopecia**
L64.9   **Androgenic alopecia, unspecified**

● **L65**   **Other nonscarring hair loss**
    Use additional code for adverse effect, if applicable, to identify
    drug (T36-T50 with fifth or sixth character 5)
    Excludes1   trichotillomania (F63.3)
L65.0   Telogen effluvium
L65.1   Anagen effluvium
L65.2   Alopecia mucinosa
L65.8   Other specified nonscarring hair loss
L65.9   Nonscarring hair loss, unspecified
    Alopecia NOS

● **L66**   **Cicatricial alopecia [scarring hair loss]**
L66.0   Pseudopelade
L66.1   Lichen planopilaris
    L66.10   Lichen planopilaris, unspecified
    L66.11   Classic lichen planopilaris
       Follicular lichen planus
    L66.12   Frontal fibrosing alopecia
       FFA
    L66.19   Other lichen planopilaris
       Lassueur Graham-Little Piccardi syndrome
L66.2   Folliculitis decalvans
L66.3   Perifolliculitis capitis abscedens
L66.4   Folliculitis ulerythematosa reticulata
L66.8   Other cicatricial alopecia
    Coding Clinic: 2015, Q1, P19
    L66.81   Central centrifugal cicatricial alopecia
       Add CCCA
    L66.89   Other cicatricial alopecia
L66.9   Cicatricial alopecia, unspecified

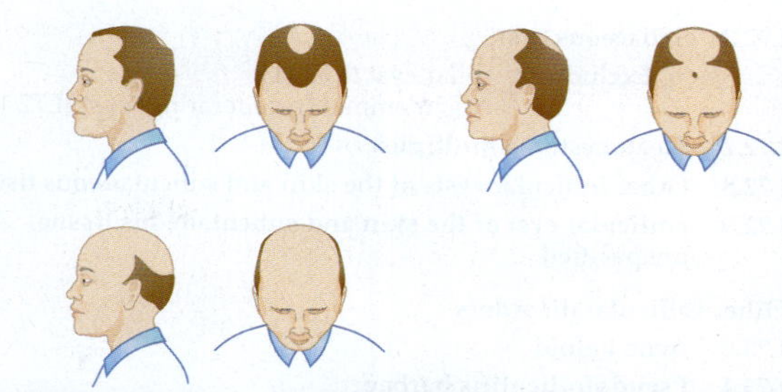

Figure 12-8   Male pattern alopecia.

● **L67**   **Hair color and hair shaft abnormalities**
    Excludes1   monilethrix (Q84.1)
       pili annulati (Q84.1)
       telogen effluvium (L65.0)
L67.0   **Trichorrhexis nodosa**
L67.1   **Variations in hair color**
    Canities
    Greyness, hair (premature)
    Heterochromia of hair
    Poliosis circumscripta, acquired
    Poliosis NOS
L67.8   **Other hair color and hair shaft abnormalities**
    Fragilitas crinium
L67.9   **Hair color and hair shaft abnormality, unspecified**

● **L68**   **Hypertrichosis**
    Includes   excess hair
    Excludes1   congenital hypertrichosis (Q84.2)
       persistent lanugo (Q84.2)
L68.0   **Hirsutism**
    Excessive growth of hair
L68.1   **Acquired hypertrichosis lanuginosa**
L68.2   **Localized hypertrichosis**
L68.3   **Polytrichia**
L68.8   **Other hypertrichosis**
L68.9   **Hypertrichosis, unspecified**

● **L70**   **Acne**
    Excludes2   acne keloid (L73.0)
L70.0   Acne vulgaris
L70.1   Acne conglobata
L70.2   Acne varioliformis
    Acne necrotica miliaris
L70.3   Acne tropica
L70.4   Infantile acne
L70.5   Acné excoriée
    Acné excoriée des jeunes filles
    Picker's acne
L70.8   Other acne
L70.9   Acne, unspecified

● **L71**   **Rosacea**
    Use additional code for adverse effect, if applicable, to identify
    drug (T36-T50 with fifth or sixth character 5)
L71.0   Perioral dermatitis
L71.1   Rhinophyma
L71.8   Other rosacea
    Coding Clinic: 2018, Q4, P15
L71.9   Rosacea, unspecified

● **L72**   **Follicular cysts of skin and subcutaneous tissue**
L72.0   Epidermal cyst
● **L72.1**   Pilar and trichodermal cyst
    L72.11   Pilar cyst
    L72.12   Trichodermal cyst
       Trichilemmal (proliferating) cyst

Item 12–10   **Alopecia** is lack of hair and takes many forms. The most common is male pattern alopecia, also known as **androgenetic alopecia.** **Telogen effluvium** is early and excessive loss of hair resulting from a trauma to the hair follicle (fever, drugs, surgery, etc.).

CHAPTER 12 (L00-L99)

N Newborn Age: 0   **P** Pediatric Age: 0–17   **M** Maternity DX: 9–64   **A** Adult Age: 15–124

L72.3 Sebaceous cyst
> **Excludes2** pilar cyst (L72.11)
> trichilemmal (proliferating) cyst (L72.12)

L72.2 Steatocystoma multiplex

L72.8 Other follicular cysts of the skin and subcutaneous tissue

L72.9 Follicular cyst of the skin and subcutaneous tissue, unspecified

● **L73 Other follicular disorders**

L73.0 Acne keloid

L73.1 Pseudofolliculitis barbae

L73.2 Hidradenitis suppurativa

L73.8 Other specified follicular disorders
Sycosis barbae

L73.9 Follicular disorder, unspecified

● **L74 Eccrine sweat disorders**
> **Excludes2** generalized hyperhidrosis (R61)

L74.0 Miliaria rubra

L74.1 Miliaria crystallina

L74.2 Miliaria profunda
Miliaria tropicalis

L74.3 Miliaria, unspecified

L74.4 Anhidrosis
Hypohidrosis

● **L74.5 Focal hyperhidrosis**

  ● **L74.51 Primary focal hyperhidrosis**

    L74.510 Primary focal hyperhidrosis, axilla

    L74.511 Primary focal hyperhidrosis, face

    L74.512 Primary focal hyperhidrosis, palms

    L74.513 Primary focal hyperhidrosis, soles

    L74.519 Primary focal hyperhidrosis, unspecified

  L74.52 Secondary focal hyperhidrosis
Frey's syndrome

L74.8 Other eccrine sweat disorders

L74.9 Eccrine sweat disorder, unspecified
Sweat gland disorder NOS

● **L75 Apocrine sweat disorders**
> **Excludes1** dyshidrosis (L30.1)
> hidradenitis suppurativa (L73.2)

L75.0 Bromhidrosis

L75.1 Chromhidrosis

L75.2 Apocrine miliaria
Fox-Fordyce disease

L75.8 Other apocrine sweat disorders

L75.9 Apocrine sweat disorder, unspecified
Intraoperative and postprocedural complications of skin and subcutaneous tissue (L76)

INTRAOPERATIVE AND POSTPROCEDURAL COMPLICATIONS OF SKIN AND SUBCUTANEOUS TISSUE (L76)

● **L76 Intraoperative and postprocedural complications of skin and subcutaneous tissue**
Coding Clinic: 2016, Q4, P10

● **L76.0 Intraoperative hemorrhage and hematoma of skin and subcutaneous tissue complicating a procedure**
> **Excludes1** intraoperative hemorrhage and hematoma of skin and subcutaneous tissue due to accidental puncture and laceration during a procedure (L76.1-)

  L76.01 Intraoperative hemorrhage and hematoma of skin and subcutaneous tissue complicating a dermatologic procedure

  L76.02 Intraoperative hemorrhage and hematoma of skin and subcutaneous tissue complicating other procedure

● **L76.1 Accidental puncture and laceration of skin and subcutaneous tissue during a procedure**

  L76.11 Accidental puncture and laceration of skin and subcutaneous tissue during a dermatologic procedure

  L76.12 Accidental puncture and laceration of skin and subcutaneous tissue during other procedure

● **L76.2 Postprocedural hemorrhage of skin and subcutaneous tissue following a procedure**

  L76.21 Postprocedural hemorrhage of skin and subcutaneous tissue following a dermatologic procedure

  L76.22 Postprocedural hemorrhage of skin and subcutaneous tissue following other procedure

● **L76.3 Postprocedural hematoma and seroma of skin and subcutaneous tissue following a procedure**

  L76.31 Postprocedural hematoma of skin and subcutaneous tissue following a dermatologic procedure

  L76.32 Postprocedural hematoma of skin and subcutaneous tissue following other procedure

  L76.33 Postprocedural seroma of skin and subcutaneous tissue following a dermatologic procedure

  L76.34 Postprocedural seroma of skin and subcutaneous tissue following other procedure

● **L76.8 Other intraoperative and postprocedural complications of skin and subcutaneous tissue**
> Use additional code, if applicable, to further specify disorder

  L76.81 Other intraoperative complications of skin and subcutaneous tissue

  L76.82 Other postprocedural complications of skin and subcutaneous tissue
Coding Clinic: 2017, Q3, P6

OTHER DISORDERS OF THE SKIN AND SUBCUTANEOUS TISSUE (L80-L99)

L80 Vitiligo
> **Excludes2** vitiligo of eyelids (H02.73-)
> vitiligo of vulva (N90.89)

● **L81 Other disorders of pigmentation**
> **Excludes1** birthmark NOS (Q82.5)
> Peutz-Jeghers syndrome (Q85.89)
>
> **Excludes2** nevus - see Alphabetical Index

L81.0 Postinflammatory hyperpigmentation

L81.1 Chloasma

L81.2 Freckles

L81.3 Café au lait spots

L81.4 Other melanin hyperpigmentation
Lentigo

L81.5 Leukoderma, not elsewhere classified

L81.6 Other disorders of diminished melanin formation

L81.7 Pigmented purpuric dermatosis
Angioma serpiginosum

L81.8 Other specified disorders of pigmentation
Iron pigmentation
Tattoo pigmentation

L81.9 Disorder of pigmentation, unspecified

● **L82 Seborrheic keratosis**
> **Includes** basal cell papilloma
> dermatosis papulosa nigra
> Leser-Trélat disease
>
> **Excludes2** seborrheic dermatitis (L21.-)

L82.0 Inflamed seborrheic keratosis
Coding Clinic: 2023, Q2, P12; 2021, Q3, P11

L82.1 Other seborrheic keratosis
Seborrheic keratosis NOS

L83 **Acanthosis nigricans**
Confluent and reticulated papillomatosis

L84 **Corns and callosities**
Callus
Clavus

● **L85** **Other epidermal thickening**
Excludes2 hypertrophic disorders of the skin (L91.-)
L85.0 **Acquired ichthyosis**
Excludes1 congenital ichthyosis (Q80.-)
L85.1 **Acquired keratosis [keratoderma] palmaris et plantaris**
Excludes1 inherited keratosis palmaris et plantaris (Q82.8)
L85.2 **Keratosis punctata (palmaris et plantaris)**
L85.3 **Xerosis cutis**
Dry skin dermatitis
L85.8 **Other specified epidermal thickening**
Cutaneous horn
L85.9 **Epidermal thickening, unspecified**

▶ *L86* *Keratoderma in diseases classified elsewhere*
Firm horny papules that have a cobblestone appearance
Code first underlying disease, such as:
Reiter's disease (M02.3-)
Excludes1 gonococcal keratoderma (A54.89)
gonococcal keratosis (A54.89)
keratoderma due to vitamin A deficiency (E50.8)
keratosis due to vitamin A deficiency (E50.8)
xeroderma due to vitamin A deficiency (E50.8)

● **L87** **Transepidermal elimination disorders**
Excludes1 granuloma annulare (perforating) (L92.0)
L87.0 **Keratosis follicularis et parafollicularis in cutem penetrans**
Kyrle disease
Hyperkeratosis follicularis penetrans
L87.1 **Reactive perforating collagenosis**
L87.2 **Elastosis perforans serpiginosa**
L87.8 **Other transepidermal elimination disorders**
L87.9 **Transepidermal elimination disorder, unspecified**

L88 **Pyoderma gangrenosum**
Phagedenic pyoderma
Excludes1 dermatitis gangrenosa (L08.0)

OGCR Section I.B.14.

General Coding Guidelines

Documentation for BMI, *Depth of* Non-pressure ulcers, Pressure Ulcer Stages, **Coma Scale, and** *NIH Stroke Scale*

For the Body Mass Index (BMI), depth of non-pressure chronic ulcers, pressure ulcer stage, **coma scale, and NIH stroke scale (NIHSS) codes,** code assignment may be based on medical record documentation from clinicians who are not the patient's provider (i.e., physician or other qualified healthcare practitioner legally accountable for establishing the patient's diagnosis), since this information is typically documented by other clinicians involved in the care of the patient (e.g., a dietitian often documents the BMI, a nurse often documents the pressure ulcer stages, **and an emergency medical technician often documents the coma scale**). However, the associated diagnosis (such as overweight, obesity, **acute stroke,** or pressure ulcer) must be documented by the patient's provider. If there is conflicting medical record documentation, either from the same clinician or different clinicians, the patient's attending provider should be queried for clarification.

The BMI, **coma scale, and NHSS** codes should only be reported as secondary diagnoses.

● **L89** **Pressure ulcer**
Includes bed sore   pressure area
decubitus ulcer   pressure sore
plaster ulcer
Code first any associated gangrene (I96)
Excludes2 decubitus (trophic) ulcer of cervix (uteri) (N86)
diabetic ulcers (E08.621, E08.622, E09.621, E09.622, E10.621, E10.622, E11.621, E11.622, E13.621, E13.622)
non-pressure chronic ulcer of skin (L97.-)
skin infections (L00-L08)
varicose ulcer (I83.0, I83.2)
Coding Clinic: 2019, Q4, P11; 2018, Q2, P22; 2016, Q4, P124

● **L89.0** **Pressure ulcer of elbow**
● **L89.00** **Pressure ulcer of unspecified elbow**
L89.000 **Pressure ulcer of unspecified elbow, unstageable**
L89.001 **Pressure ulcer of unspecified elbow, stage 1**
Healing pressure ulcer of unspecified elbow, stage 1
Pressure pre-ulcer skin changes limited to persistent focal edema, unspecified elbow
L89.002 **Pressure ulcer of unspecified elbow, stage 2**
Healing pressure ulcer of unspecified elbow, stage 2
Pressure ulcer with abrasion, blister, partial thickness skin loss involving epidermis and/or dermis, unspecified elbow
L89.003 **Pressure ulcer of unspecified elbow, stage 3**
Healing pressure ulcer of unspecified elbow, stage 3
Pressure ulcer with full thickness skin loss involving damage or necrosis of subcutaneous tissue, unspecified elbow
L89.004 **Pressure ulcer of unspecified elbow, stage 4**
Healing pressure ulcer of unspecified elbow, stage 4
Pressure ulcer with necrosis of soft tissues through to underlying muscle, tendon, or bone, unspecified elbow
L89.006 **Pressure-induced deep tissue damage of unspecified elbow**
L89.009 **Pressure ulcer of unspecified elbow, unspecified stage**
Healing pressure ulcer of elbow NOS
Healing pressure ulcer of unspecified elbow, unspecified stage
● **L89.01** **Pressure ulcer of right elbow**
L89.010 **Pressure ulcer of right elbow, unstageable**
L89.011 **Pressure ulcer of right elbow, stage 1**
Healing pressure ulcer of right elbow, stage 1
Pressure pre-ulcer skin changes limited to persistent focal edema, right elbow
L89.012 **Pressure ulcer of right elbow, stage 2**
Healing pressure ulcer of right elbow, stage 2
Pressure ulcer with abrasion, blister, partial thickness skin loss involving epidermis and/or dermis, right elbow

CHAPTER 12 (L00-L99)

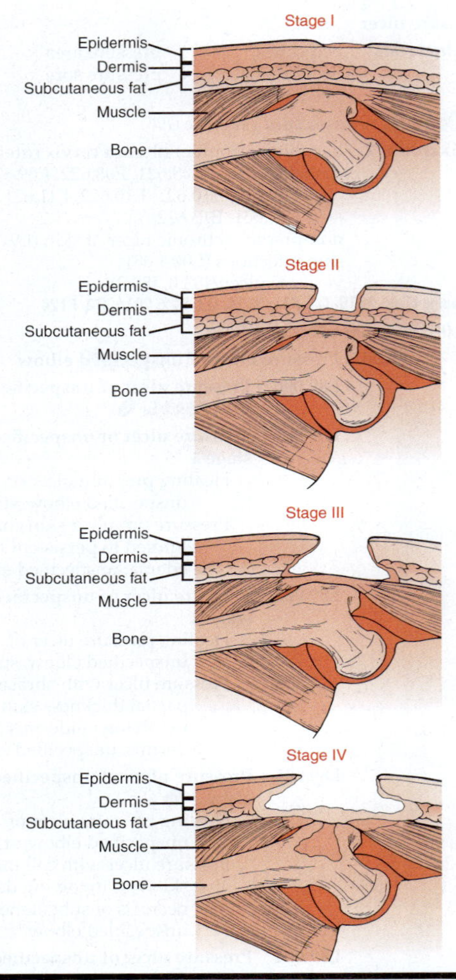

Figure 12-9　Stage I, II, III, and IV of pressure ulcers.

L89.013　Pressure ulcer of right elbow, stage 3 RCC
　　Healing pressure ulcer of right elbow, stage 3
　　Pressure ulcer with full thickness skin loss involving damage or necrosis of subcutaneous tissue, right elbow

L89.014　Pressure ulcer of right elbow, stage 4 RCC
　　Healing pressure ulcer of right elbow, stage 4
　　Pressure ulcer with necrosis of soft tissues through to underlying muscle, tendon, or bone, right elbow

L89.016　Pressure-induced deep tissue damage of right elbow

L89.019　Pressure ulcer of right elbow, unspecified stage
　　Healing pressure ulcer of right elbow NOS

● **L89.02　Pressure ulcer of left elbow**

L89.020　Pressure ulcer of left elbow, unstageable RCC

L89.021　Pressure ulcer of left elbow, stage 1
　　Healing pressure ulcer of left elbow, stage 1
　　Pressure pre-ulcer skin changes limited to persistent focal edema, left elbow

L89.022　Pressure ulcer of left elbow, stage 2
　　Healing pressure ulcer of left elbow, stage 2
　　Pressure ulcer with abrasion, blister, partial thickness skin loss involving epidermis and/or dermis, left elbow

L89.023　Pressure ulcer of left elbow, stage 3 RCC
　　Healing pressure ulcer of left elbow, stage 3
　　Pressure ulcer with full thickness skin loss involving damage or necrosis of subcutaneous tissue, left elbow

L89.024　Pressure ulcer of left elbow, stage 4 RCC
　　Healing pressure ulcer of left elbow, stage 4
　　Pressure ulcer with necrosis of soft tissues through to underlying muscle, tendon, or bone, left elbow

L89.026　Pressure-induced deep tissue damage of left elbow

L89.029　Pressure ulcer of left elbow, unspecified stage
　　Healing pressure ulcer of left elbow NOS

● **L89.1　Pressure ulcer of back**

● **L89.10　Pressure ulcer of unspecified part of back**

L89.100　Pressure ulcer of unspecified part of back, unstageable RCC

L89.101　Pressure ulcer of unspecified part of back, stage 1
　　Healing pressure ulcer of unspecified part of back, stage 1
　　Pressure pre-ulcer skin changes limited to persistent focal edema, unspecified part of back

L89.102　Pressure ulcer of unspecified part of back, stage 2
　　Healing pressure ulcer of unspecified part of back, stage 2
　　Pressure ulcer with abrasion, blister, partial thickness skin loss involving epidermis and/or dermis, unspecified part of back

L89.103　Pressure ulcer of unspecified part of back, stage 3 RCC
　　Healing pressure ulcer of unspecified part of back, stage 3
　　Pressure ulcer with full thickness skin loss involving damage or necrosis of subcutaneous tissue, unspecified part of back

▶ New　　➡ Revised　　~~deleted~~ Deleted　　Excludes 1　　Excludes 2　　Includes　　Use additional　　Code first　　Code also　　Key words
OGCR Official Guidelines　　X Assign placeholder X　　● Use Additional Character(s)　　▶ Manifestation Code　　RCC Hierarchical Condition Category　　**Coding Clinic**

L89.104 **Pressure ulcer of unspecified part of back, stage 4** 🔵
     Healing pressure ulcer of unspecified part of back, stage 4
     Pressure ulcer with necrosis of soft tissues through to underlying muscle, tendon, or bone, unspecified part of back

L89.106 **Pressure-induced deep tissue damage of unspecified part of back**

L89.109 **Pressure ulcer of unspecified part of back, unspecified stage**
     Healing pressure ulcer of unspecified part of back NOS
     Healing pressure ulcer of unspecified part of back, unspecified stage

🔴 **L89.11 Pressure ulcer of right upper back**
     Pressure ulcer of right shoulder blade

L89.110 **Pressure ulcer of right upper back, unstageable** 🔵

L89.111 **Pressure ulcer of right upper back, stage 1**
     Healing pressure ulcer of right upper back, stage 1
     Pressure pre-ulcer skin changes limited to persistent focal edema, right upper back

L89.112 **Pressure ulcer of right upper back, stage 2**
     Healing pressure ulcer of right upper back, stage 2
     Pressure ulcer with abrasion, blister, partial thickness skin loss involving epidermis and/or dermis, right upper back

L89.113 **Pressure ulcer of right upper back, stage 3** 🔵
     Healing pressure ulcer of right upper back, stage 3
     Pressure ulcer with full thickness skin loss involving damage or necrosis of subcutaneous tissue, right upper back

L89.114 **Pressure ulcer of right upper back, stage 4** 🔵
     Healing pressure ulcer of right upper back, stage 4
     Pressure ulcer with necrosis of soft tissues through to underlying muscle, tendon, or bone, right upper back

L89.116 **Pressure-induced deep tissue damage of right upper back**

L89.119 **Pressure ulcer of right upper back, unspecified stage**
     Healing pressure ulcer of right upper back NOS
     Healing pressure ulcer of right upper back, unspecified stage

🔴 **L89.12 Pressure ulcer of left upper back**
     Pressure ulcer of left shoulder blade

L89.120 **Pressure ulcer of left upper back, unstageable** 🔵

L89.121 **Pressure ulcer of left upper back, stage 1**
     Healing pressure ulcer of left upper back, stage 1
     Pressure pre-ulcer skin changes limited to persistent focal edema, left upper back

L89.122 **Pressure ulcer of left upper back, stage 2**
     Healing pressure ulcer of left upper back, stage 2
     Pressure ulcer with abrasion, blister, partial thickness skin loss involving epidermis and/or dermis, left upper back

L89.123 **Pressure ulcer of left upper back, stage 3** 🔵
     Healing pressure ulcer of left upper back, stage 3
     Pressure ulcer with full thickness skin loss involving damage or necrosis of subcutaneous tissue, left upper back

L89.124 **Pressure ulcer of left upper back, stage 4** 🔵
     Healing pressure ulcer of left upper back, stage 4
     Pressure ulcer with necrosis of soft tissues through to underlying muscle, tendon, or bone, left upper back

L89.126 **Pressure-induced deep tissue damage of left upper back**

L89.129 **Pressure ulcer of left upper back, unspecified stage**
     Healing pressure ulcer of left upper back NOS
     Healing pressure ulcer of left upper back, unspecified stage

🔴 **L89.13 Pressure ulcer of right lower back**

L89.130 **Pressure ulcer of right lower back, unstageable** 🔵

L89.131 **Pressure ulcer of right lower back, stage 1**
     Healing pressure ulcer of right lower back, stage 1
     Pressure pre-ulcer skin changes limited to persistent focal edema, right lower back

L89.132 **Pressure ulcer of right lower back, stage 2**
     Healing pressure ulcer of right lower back, stage 2
     Pressure ulcer with abrasion, blister, partial thickness skin loss involving epidermis and/or dermis, right lower back

L89.133 **Pressure ulcer of right lower back, stage 3** 🔵
     Healing pressure ulcer of right lower back, stage 3
     Pressure ulcer with full thickness skin loss involving damage or necrosis of subcutaneous tissue, right lower back

L89.134 **Pressure ulcer of right lower back, stage 4** 🔵
     Healing pressure ulcer of right lower back, stage 4
     Pressure ulcer with necrosis of soft tissues through to underlying muscle, tendon, or bone, right lower back

L89.136 **Pressure-induced deep tissue damage of right lower back**

CHAPTER 12 (L00–L99)

L89.139   Pressure ulcer of right lower back, unspecified stage
    Healing pressure ulcer of right lower back NOS
    Healing pressure ulcer of right lower back, unspecified stage

● **L89.14   Pressure ulcer of left lower back**

L89.140   Pressure ulcer of left lower back, unstageable 🟣

L89.141   Pressure ulcer of left lower back, stage 1
    Healing pressure ulcer of left lower back, stage 1
    Pressure pre-ulcer skin changes limited to persistent focal edema, left lower back

L89.142   Pressure ulcer of left lower back, stage 2
    Healing pressure ulcer of left lower back, stage 2
    Pressure ulcer with abrasion, blister, partial thickness skin loss involving epidermis and/or dermis, left lower back

L89.143   Pressure ulcer of left lower back, stage 3 🟣
    Healing pressure ulcer of left lower back, stage 3
    Pressure ulcer with full thickness skin loss involving damage or necrosis of subcutaneous tissue, left lower back

L89.144   Pressure ulcer of left lower back, stage 4 🟣
    Healing pressure ulcer of left lower back, stage 4
    Pressure ulcer with necrosis of soft tissues through to underlying muscle, tendon, or bone, left lower back

L89.146   Pressure-induced deep tissue damage of left lower back

L89.149   Pressure ulcer of left lower back, unspecified stage
    Healing pressure ulcer of left lower back NOS
    Healing pressure ulcer of left lower back, unspecified stage

● **L89.15   Pressure ulcer of sacral region**
    Pressure ulcer of coccyx
    Pressure ulcer of tailbone
    Coding Clinic: 2021, Q3, P10

L89.150   Pressure ulcer of sacral region, unstageable 🟣

L89.151   Pressure ulcer of sacral region, stage 1
    Healing pressure ulcer of sacral region, stage 1
    Pressure pre-ulcer skin changes limited to persistent focal edema, sacral region

L89.152   Pressure ulcer of sacral region, stage 2
    Healing pressure ulcer of sacral region, stage 2
    Pressure ulcer with abrasion, blister, partial thickness skin loss involving epidermis and/or dermis, sacral region

L89.153   Pressure ulcer of sacral region, stage 3 🟣
    Healing pressure ulcer of sacral region, stage 3
    Pressure ulcer with full thickness skin loss involving damage or necrosis of subcutaneous tissue, sacral region
    Coding Clinic: 2021, Q3, P10

L89.154   Pressure ulcer of sacral region, stage 4 🟣
    Healing pressure ulcer of sacral region, stage 4
    Pressure ulcer with necrosis of soft tissues through to underlying muscle, tendon, or bone, sacral region
    Coding Clinic: 2022, Q2, P9; 2021, Q1, P24

L89.156   Pressure-induced deep tissue damage of sacral region

L89.159   Pressure ulcer of sacral region, unspecified stage
    Healing pressure ulcer of sacral region NOS
    Healing pressure ulcer of sacral region, unspecified stage

● **L89.2   Pressure ulcer of hip**

● **L89.20   Pressure ulcer of unspecified hip**

L89.200   Pressure ulcer of unspecified hip, unstageable 🟣

L89.201   Pressure ulcer of unspecified hip, stage 1
    Healing pressure ulcer of unspecified hip back, stage 1
    Pressure pre-ulcer skin changes limited to persistent focal edema, unspecified hip

L89.202   Pressure ulcer of unspecified hip, stage 2
    Healing pressure ulcer of unspecified hip, stage 2
    Pressure ulcer with abrasion, blister, partial thickness skin loss involving epidermis and/or dermis, unspecified hip

L89.203   Pressure ulcer of unspecified hip, stage 3 🟣
    Healing pressure ulcer of unspecified hip, stage 3
    Pressure ulcer with full thickness skin loss involving damage or necrosis of subcutaneous tissue, unspecified hip

L89.204   Pressure ulcer of unspecified hip, stage 4 🟣
    Healing pressure ulcer of unspecified hip, stage 4
    Pressure ulcer with necrosis of soft tissues through to underlying muscle, tendon, or bone, unspecified hip

L89.206   Pressure-induced deep tissue damage of unspecified hip

L89.209   Pressure ulcer of unspecified hip, unspecified stage
    Healing pressure ulcer of unspecified hip NOS
    Healing pressure ulcer of unspecified hip, unspecified stage

---

▶ New   ⇨ Revised   ~~deleted~~ Deleted   Excludes 1   Excludes 2   Includes   Use additional   Code first   Code also   Key words

OGCR Official Guidelines   X Assign placeholder X   ● Use Additional Character(s)   ❙ Manifestation Code   🟣 Hierarchical Condition Category   **Coding Clinic**

● **L89.21 Pressure ulcer of right hip**

    L89.210 Pressure ulcer of right hip, unstageable 🔖

    L89.211 Pressure ulcer of right hip, stage 1
        Healing pressure ulcer of right hip back, stage 1
        Pressure pre-ulcer skin changes limited to persistent focal edema, right hip

    L89.212 Pressure ulcer of right hip, stage 2
        Healing pressure ulcer of right hip, stage 2
        Pressure ulcer with abrasion, blister, partial thickness skin loss involving epidermis and/or dermis, right hip

    L89.213 Pressure ulcer of right hip, stage 3 🔖
        Healing pressure ulcer of right hip, stage 3
        Pressure ulcer with full thickness skin loss involving damage or necrosis of subcutaneous tissue, right hip

    L89.214 Pressure ulcer of right hip, stage 4 🔖
        Healing pressure ulcer of right hip, stage 4
        Pressure ulcer with necrosis of soft tissues through to underlying muscle, tendon, or bone, right hip

    L89.216 Pressure-induced deep tissue damage of right hip

    L89.219 Pressure ulcer of right hip, unspecified stage
        Healing pressure ulcer of right hip NOS
        Healing pressure ulcer of right hip, unspecified stage

● **L89.22 Pressure ulcer of left hip**

    L89.220 Pressure ulcer of left hip, unstageable 🔖

    L89.221 Pressure ulcer of left hip, stage 1
        Healing pressure ulcer of left hip back, stage 1
        Pressure pre-ulcer skin changes limited to persistent focal edema, left hip

    L89.222 Pressure ulcer of left hip, stage 2
        Healing pressure ulcer of left hip, stage 2
        Pressure ulcer with abrasion, blister, partial thickness skin loss involving epidermis and/or dermis, left hip

    L89.223 Pressure ulcer of left hip, stage 3 🔖
        Healing pressure ulcer of left hip, stage 3
        Pressure ulcer with full thickness skin loss involving damage or necrosis of subcutaneous tissue, left hip

    L89.224 Pressure ulcer of left hip, stage 4 🔖
        Healing pressure ulcer of left hip, stage 4
        Pressure ulcer with necrosis of soft tissues through to underlying muscle, tendon, or bone, left hip

    L89.226 Pressure-induced deep tissue damage of left hip

    L89.229 Pressure ulcer of left hip, unspecified stage
        Healing pressure ulcer of left hip NOS
        Healing pressure ulcer of left hip, unspecified stage

● **L89.3 Pressure ulcer of buttock**

  ● **L89.30 Pressure ulcer of unspecified buttock**

    L89.300 Pressure ulcer of unspecified buttock, unstageable 🔖

    L89.301 Pressure ulcer of unspecified buttock, stage 1
        Healing pressure ulcer of unspecified buttock, stage 1
        Pressure pre-ulcer skin changes limited to persistent focal edema, unspecified buttock

    L89.302 Pressure ulcer of unspecified buttock, stage 2
        Healing pressure ulcer of unspecified buttock, stage 2
        Pressure ulcer with abrasion, blister, partial thickness skin loss involving epidermis and/or dermis, unspecified buttock

    L89.303 Pressure ulcer of unspecified buttock, stage 3 🔖
        Healing pressure ulcer of unspecified buttock, stage 3
        Pressure ulcer with full thickness skin loss involving damage or necrosis of subcutaneous tissue, unspecified buttock

    L89.304 Pressure ulcer of unspecified buttock, stage 4 🔖
        Healing pressure ulcer of unspecified buttock, stage 4
        Pressure ulcer with necrosis of soft tissues through to underlying muscle, tendon, or bone, unspecified buttock

    L89.306 Pressure-induced deep tissue damage of unspecified buttock

    L89.309 Pressure ulcer of unspecified buttock, unspecified stage
        Healing pressure ulcer of unspecified buttock NOS
        Healing pressure ulcer of unspecified buttock, unspecified stage

  ● **L89.31 Pressure ulcer of right buttock**

    L89.310 Pressure ulcer of right buttock, unstageable 🔖

    L89.311 Pressure ulcer of right buttock, stage 1
        Healing pressure ulcer of right buttock, stage 1
        Pressure pre-ulcer skin changes limited to persistent focal edema, right buttock

    L89.312 Pressure ulcer of right buttock, stage 2
        Healing pressure ulcer of right buttock, stage 2
        Pressure ulcer with abrasion, blister, partial thickness skin loss involving epidermis and/or dermis, right buttock

L89.313 **Pressure ulcer of right buttock, stage 3** 🔒
 Healing pressure ulcer of right buttock, stage 3
 Pressure ulcer with full thickness skin loss involving damage or necrosis of subcutaneous tissue, right buttock

L89.314 **Pressure ulcer of right buttock, stage 4** 🔒
 Healing pressure ulcer of right buttock, stage 4
 Pressure ulcer with necrosis of soft tissues through to underlying muscle, tendon, or bone, right buttock

L89.316 **Pressure-induced deep tissue damage of right buttock**

L89.319 **Pressure ulcer of right buttock, unspecified stage**
 Healing pressure ulcer of right buttock NOS
 Healing pressure ulcer of right buttock, unspecified stage

● **L89.32** **Pressure ulcer of left buttock**

L89.320 **Pressure ulcer of left buttock, unstageable** 🔒

L89.321 **Pressure ulcer of left buttock, stage 1**
 Healing pressure ulcer of left buttock, stage 1
 Pressure pre-ulcer skin changes limited to persistent focal edema, left buttock

L89.322 **Pressure ulcer of left buttock, stage 2**
 Healing pressure ulcer of left buttock, stage 2
 Pressure ulcer with abrasion, blister, partial thickness skin loss involving epidermis and/or dermis, left buttock

L89.323 **Pressure ulcer of left buttock, stage 3** 🔒
 Healing pressure ulcer of left buttock, stage 3
 Pressure ulcer with full thickness skin loss involving damage or necrosis of subcutaneous tissue, left buttock

L89.324 **Pressure ulcer of left buttock, stage 4** 🔒
 Healing pressure ulcer of left buttock, stage 4
 Pressure ulcer with necrosis of soft tissues through to underlying muscle, tendon, or bone, left buttock

L89.326 **Pressure-induced deep tissue damage of left buttock**

L89.329 **Pressure ulcer of left buttock, unspecified stage**
 Healing pressure ulcer of left buttock NOS
 Healing pressure ulcer of left buttock, unspecified stage

● **L89.4** **Pressure ulcer of contiguous site of back, buttock and hip**

L89.40 **Pressure ulcer of contiguous site of back, buttock and hip, unspecified stage**
 Healing pressure ulcer of contiguous site of back, buttock and hip NOS
 Healing pressure ulcer of contiguous site of back, buttock and hip, unspecified stage

L89.41 **Pressure ulcer of contiguous site of back, buttock and hip, stage 1**
 Healing pressure ulcer of contiguous site of back, buttock and hip, stage 1
 Pressure pre-ulcer skin changes limited to persistent focal edema, contiguous site of back, buttock and hip

L89.42 **Pressure ulcer of contiguous site of back, buttock and hip, stage 2**
 Healing pressure ulcer of contiguous site of back, buttock and hip, stage 2
 Pressure ulcer with abrasion, blister, partial thickness skin loss involving epidermis and/or dermis, contiguous site of back, buttock and hip

L89.43 **Pressure ulcer of contiguous site of back, buttock and hip, stage 3** 🔒
 Healing pressure ulcer of contiguous site of back, buttock and hip, stage 3
 Pressure ulcer with full thickness skin loss involving damage or necrosis of subcutaneous tissue, contiguous site of back, buttock and hip

L89.44 **Pressure ulcer of contiguous site of back, buttock and hip, stage 4** 🔒
 Healing pressure ulcer of contiguous site of back, buttock and hip, stage 4
 Pressure ulcer with necrosis of soft tissues through to underlying muscle, tendon, or bone, contiguous site of back, buttock and hip

L89.45 **Pressure ulcer of contiguous site of back, buttock and hip, unstageable** 🔒

L89.46 **Pressure-induced deep tissue damage of contiguous site of back, buttock and hip**

● **L89.5** **Pressure ulcer of ankle**

● **L89.50** **Pressure ulcer of unspecified ankle**

L89.500 **Pressure ulcer of unspecified ankle, unstageable** 🔒

L89.501 **Pressure ulcer of unspecified ankle, stage 1**
 Healing pressure ulcer of unspecified ankle, stage 1
 Pressure pre-ulcer skin changes limited to persistent focal edema, unspecified ankle

L89.502 **Pressure ulcer of unspecified ankle, stage 2**
 Healing pressure ulcer of unspecified ankle, stage 2
 Pressure ulcer with abrasion, blister, partial thickness skin loss involving epidermis and/or dermis, unspecified ankle

L89.503 **Pressure ulcer of unspecified ankle, stage 3** 🔒
 Healing pressure ulcer of unspecified ankle, stage 3
 Pressure ulcer with full thickness skin loss involving damage or necrosis of subcutaneous tissue, unspecified ankle

L89.504 **Pressure ulcer of unspecified ankle, stage 4** 🔒
 Healing pressure ulcer of unspecified ankle, stage 4
 Pressure ulcer with necrosis of soft tissues through to underlying muscle, tendon, or bone, unspecified ankle

▶ New   ⇒ Revised   ~~deleted~~ Deleted   Excludes 1   Excludes 2   Includes   Use additional   Code first   Code also   Key words
OGCR Official Guidelines   X Assign placeholder X   ● Use Additional Character(s)   ▶ Manifestation Code   🔒 Hierarchical Condition Category   Coding Clinic

L89.506   **Pressure-induced deep tissue damage of unspecified ankle**

L89.509   **Pressure ulcer of unspecified ankle, unspecified stage**
- Healing pressure ulcer of unspecified ankle NOS
- Healing pressure ulcer of unspecified ankle, unspecified stage

● **L89.51**   **Pressure ulcer of right ankle**

L89.510   **Pressure ulcer of right ankle, unstageable** 🔾

L89.511   **Pressure ulcer of right ankle, stage 1**
- Healing pressure ulcer of right ankle, stage 1
- Pressure pre-ulcer skin changes limited to persistent focal edema, right ankle

L89.512   **Pressure ulcer of right ankle, stage 2**
- Healing pressure ulcer of right ankle, stage 2
- Pressure ulcer with abrasion, blister, partial thickness skin loss involving epidermis and/or dermis, right ankle

L89.513   **Pressure ulcer of right ankle, stage 3** 🔾
- Healing pressure ulcer of right ankle, stage 3
- Pressure ulcer with full thickness skin loss involving damage or necrosis of subcutaneous tissue, right ankle

L89.514   **Pressure ulcer of right ankle, stage 4** 🔾
- Healing pressure ulcer of right ankle, stage 4
- Pressure ulcer with necrosis of soft tissues through to underlying muscle, tendon, or bone, right ankle

L89.516   **Pressure-induced deep tissue damage of right ankle**

L89.519   **Pressure ulcer of right ankle, unspecified stage**
- Healing pressure ulcer of right ankle NOS
- Healing pressure ulcer of right ankle, unspecified stage

● **L89.52**   **Pressure ulcer of left ankle**

L89.520   **Pressure ulcer of left ankle, unstageable**

L89.521   **Pressure ulcer of left ankle, stage 1**
- Healing pressure ulcer of left ankle, stage 1
- Pressure pre-ulcer skin changes limited to persistent focal edema, left ankle

L89.522   **Pressure ulcer of left ankle, stage 2**
- Healing pressure ulcer of left ankle, stage 2
- Pressure ulcer with abrasion, blister, partial thickness skin loss involving epidermis and/or dermis, left ankle

L89.523   **Pressure ulcer of left ankle, stage 3** 🔾
- Healing pressure ulcer of left ankle, stage 3
- Pressure ulcer with full thickness skin loss involving damage or necrosis of subcutaneous tissue, left ankle

L89.524   **Pressure ulcer of left ankle, stage 4** 🔾
- Healing pressure ulcer of left ankle, stage 4
- Pressure ulcer with necrosis of soft tissues through to underlying muscle, tendon, or bone, left ankle

L89.526   **Pressure-induced deep tissue damage of left ankle**

L89.529   **Pressure ulcer of left ankle, unspecified stage**
- Healing pressure ulcer of left ankle NOS
- Healing pressure ulcer of left ankle, unspecified stage

● **L89.6**   **Pressure ulcer of heel**

● **L89.60**   **Pressure ulcer of unspecified heel**

L89.600   **Pressure ulcer of unspecified heel, unstageable** 🔾

L89.601   **Pressure ulcer of unspecified heel, stage 1**
- Healing pressure ulcer of unspecified heel, stage 1
- Pressure pre-ulcer skin changes limited to persistent focal edema, unspecified heel

L89.602   **Pressure ulcer of unspecified heel, stage 2**
- Healing pressure ulcer of unspecified heel, stage 2
- Pressure ulcer with abrasion, blister, partial thickness skin loss involving epidermis and/or dermis, unspecified heel

L89.603   **Pressure ulcer of unspecified heel, stage 3** 🔾
- Healing pressure ulcer of unspecified heel, stage 3
- Pressure ulcer with full thickness skin loss involving damage or necrosis of subcutaneous tissue, unspecified heel

L89.604   **Pressure ulcer of unspecified heel, stage 4** 🔾
- Healing pressure ulcer of unspecified heel, stage 4
- Pressure ulcer with necrosis of soft tissues through to underlying muscle, tendon, or bone, unspecified heel

L89.606   **Pressure-induced deep tissue damage of unspecified heel**

L89.609   **Pressure ulcer of unspecified heel, unspecified stage**
- Healing pressure ulcer of unspecified heel NOS
- Healing pressure ulcer of unspecified heel, unspecified stage

● **L89.61**   **Pressure ulcer of right heel**

    L89.610   **Pressure ulcer of right heel, unstageable** Ⓗ

    L89.611   **Pressure ulcer of right heel, stage 1**
       Healing pressure ulcer of right heel, stage 1
       Pressure pre-ulcer skin changes limited to persistent focal edema, right heel

    L89.612   **Pressure ulcer of right heel, stage 2**
       Healing pressure ulcer of right heel, stage 2
       Pressure ulcer with abrasion, blister, partial thickness skin loss involving epidermis and/or dermis, right heel

    L89.613   **Pressure ulcer of right heel, stage 3** Ⓗ
       Healing pressure ulcer of right heel, stage 3
       Pressure ulcer with full thickness skin loss involving damage or necrosis of subcutaneous tissue, right heel

    L89.614   **Pressure ulcer of right heel, stage 4** Ⓗ
       Healing pressure ulcer of right heel, stage 4
       Pressure ulcer with necrosis of soft tissues through to underlying muscle, tendon, or bone, right heel

    L89.616   **Pressure-induced deep tissue damage of right heel**

    L89.619   **Pressure ulcer of right heel, unspecified stage**
       Healing pressure ulcer of right heel NOS
       Healing pressure ulcer of right heel, unspecified stage

● **L89.62**   **Pressure ulcer of left heel**

    L89.620   **Pressure ulcer of left heel, unstageable** Ⓗ

    L89.621   **Pressure ulcer of left heel, stage 1**
       Healing pressure ulcer of left heel, stage 1
       Pressure pre-ulcer skin changes limited to persistent focal edema, left heel

    L89.622   **Pressure ulcer of left heel, stage 2**
       Healing pressure ulcer of left heel, stage 2
       Pressure ulcer with abrasion, blister, partial thickness skin loss involving epidermis and/or dermis, left heel
       Coding Clinic: 2016, Q4, P142

    L89.623   **Pressure ulcer of left heel, stage 3** Ⓗ
       Healing pressure ulcer of left heel, stage 3
       Pressure ulcer with full thickness skin loss involving damage or necrosis of subcutaneous tissue, left heel
       Coding Clinic: 2016, Q4, P142

    L89.624   **Pressure ulcer of left heel, stage 4** Ⓗ
       Healing pressure ulcer of left heel, stage 4
       Pressure ulcer with necrosis of soft tissues through to underlying muscle, tendon, or bone, left heel

    L89.626   **Pressure-induced deep tissue damage of left heel**

    L89.629   **Pressure ulcer of left heel, unspecified stage**
       Healing pressure ulcer of left heel NOS
       Healing pressure ulcer of left heel, unspecified stage

● **L89.8**   **Pressure ulcer of other site**

● **L89.81**   **Pressure ulcer of head**
       Pressure ulcer of face

    L89.810   **Pressure ulcer of head, unstageable** Ⓗ

    L89.811   **Pressure ulcer of head, stage 1**
       Healing pressure ulcer of head, stage 1
       Pressure pre-ulcer skin changes limited to persistent focal edema, head

    L89.812   **Pressure ulcer of head, stage 2**
       Healing pressure ulcer of head, stage 2
       Pressure ulcer with abrasion, blister, partial thickness skin loss involving epidermis and/or dermis, head

    L89.813   **Pressure ulcer of head, stage 3** Ⓗ
       Healing pressure ulcer of head, stage 3
       Pressure ulcer with full thickness skin loss involving damage or necrosis of subcutaneous tissue, head

    L89.814   **Pressure ulcer of head, stage 4** Ⓗ
       Healing pressure ulcer of head, stage 4
       Pressure ulcer with necrosis of soft tissues through to underlying muscle, tendon, or bone, head

    L89.816   **Pressure-induced deep tissue damage of head**

    L89.819   **Pressure ulcer of head, unspecified stage**
       Healing pressure ulcer of head NOS
       Healing pressure ulcer of head, unspecified stage

● **L89.89**   **Pressure ulcer of other site**

    L89.890   **Pressure ulcer of other site, unstageable** Ⓗ

    L89.891   **Pressure ulcer of other site, stage 1**
       Healing pressure ulcer of other site, stage 1
       Pressure pre-ulcer skin changes limited to persistent focal edema, other site

    L89.892   **Pressure ulcer of other site, stage 2**
       Healing pressure ulcer of other site, stage 2
       Pressure ulcer with abrasion, blister, partial thickness skin loss involving epidermis and/or dermis, other site

    L89.893   **Pressure ulcer of other site, stage 3** Ⓗ
       Healing pressure ulcer of other site, stage 3
       Pressure ulcer with full thickness skin loss involving damage or necrosis of subcutaneous tissue, other site

---

L89.894　**Pressure ulcer of other site, stage 4** 🔵
　　　　　Healing pressure ulcer of other site,
　　　　　　stage 4
　　　　　Pressure ulcer with necrosis of soft
　　　　　　tissues through to underlying
　　　　　　muscle, tendon, or bone, other
　　　　　　site

L89.899　**Pressure ulcer of other site,
　　　　　unspecified stage**
　　　　　Healing pressure ulcer of other site
　　　　　　NOS
　　　　　Healing pressure ulcer of other site,
　　　　　　unspecified stage

🔴 **L89.9　Pressure ulcer of unspecified site**

L89.90　**Pressure ulcer of unspecified site, unspecified
　　　　　stage**
　　　　　Healing pressure ulcer of unspecified site NOS
　　　　　Healing pressure ulcer of unspecified site,
　　　　　　unspecified stage

L89.91　**Pressure ulcer of unspecified site, stage 1**
　　　　　Healing pressure ulcer of unspecified site,
　　　　　　stage 1
　　　　　Pressure pre-ulcer skin changes limited to
　　　　　　persistent focal edema, unspecified site

L89.92　**Pressure ulcer of unspecified site, stage 2**
　　　　　Healing pressure ulcer of unspecified site,
　　　　　　stage 2
　　　　　Pressure ulcer with abrasion, blister, partial
　　　　　　thickness skin loss involving epidermis
　　　　　　and/or dermis, unspecified site

L89.93　**Pressure ulcer of unspecified site, stage 3** 🔵
　　　　　Healing pressure ulcer of unspecified site,
　　　　　　stage 3
　　　　　Pressure ulcer with full thickness skin
　　　　　　loss involving damage or necrosis of
　　　　　　subcutaneous tissue, unspecified site

L89.94　**Pressure ulcer of unspecified site, stage 4** 🔵
　　　　　Healing pressure ulcer of unspecified site,
　　　　　　stage 4
　　　　　Pressure ulcer with necrosis of soft tissues
　　　　　　through to underlying muscle, tendon, or
　　　　　　bone, unspecified site

L89.95　**Pressure ulcer of unspecified site,
　　　　　unstageable** 🔵

L89.96　**Pressure-induced deep tissue damage of
　　　　　unspecified site**

🔴 **L90　Atrophic disorders of skin**

L90.0　**Lichen sclerosus et atrophicus**
　　　　Excludes2　lichen sclerosus of external female genital
　　　　　　　　　　　organs (N90.4)
　　　　　　　　　　lichen sclerosus of external male genital
　　　　　　　　　　　organs (N48.0)

L90.1　**Anetoderma of Schweninger-Buzzi**

L90.2　**Anetoderma of Jadassohn-Pellizzari**

L90.3　**Atrophoderma of Pasini and Pierini**

L90.4　**Acrodermatitis chronica atrophicans**

L90.5　**Scar conditions and fibrosis of skin**
　　　　Adherent scar (skin)
　　　　Cicatrix
　　　　Disfigurement of skin due to scar
　　　　Fibrosis of skin NOS
　　　　Scar NOS
　　　　Excludes2　hypertrophic scar (L91.0)
　　　　　　　　　　keloid scar (L91.0)
　　　　Coding Clinic: 2016, Q2, P5; 2015, Q1, P19

Item 12–11　Scleroderma means hard skin. It is a group of diseases that causes abnormal growth of connective tissues that support the skin and organs. There are two types: localized scleroderma affecting the skin and systemic scleroderma affecting blood vessels and internal organs and the skin.

L90.6　**Striae atrophicae**

L90.8　**Other atrophic disorders of skin**

L90.9　**Atrophic disorder of skin, unspecified**

🔴 **L91　Hypertrophic disorders of skin**

L91.0　**Keloid scar**
　　　　Hypertrophic scar
　　　　Keloid
　　　　Excludes2　acne keloid (L73.0)
　　　　　　　　　　scar NOS (L90.5)

L91.8　**Other hypertrophic disorders of the skin**

L91.9　**Hypertrophic disorder of the skin, unspecified**

🔴 **L92　Granulomatous disorders of skin and subcutaneous tissue**
　　　　Excludes2　actinic granuloma (L57.5)

L92.0　**Granuloma annulare**
　　　　Perforating granuloma annulare

L92.1　**Necrobiosis lipoidica, not elsewhere classified**
　　　　Excludes1　necrobiosis lipoidica associated with
　　　　　　　　　　diabetes mellitus (E08-E13 with .620)

L92.2　**Granuloma faciale [eosinophilic granuloma of skin]**

L92.3　**Foreign body granuloma of the skin and subcutaneous
　　　　tissue**
　　　　Use additional code to identify the type of retained
　　　　　foreign body (Z18.-)

L92.8　**Other granulomatous disorders of the skin and
　　　　subcutaneous tissue**

L92.9　**Granulomatous disorder of the skin and subcutaneous
　　　　tissue, unspecified**
　　　　Excludes2　umbilical granuloma (P83.81)

🔴 **L93　Lupus erythematosus**
　　　　Use additional code for adverse effect, if applicable, to identify
　　　　　drug (T36-T50 with fifth or sixth character 5)
　　　　Excludes1　lupus exedens (A18.4)
　　　　　　　　　　lupus vulgaris (A18.4)
　　　　　　　　　　scleroderma (M34.-)
　　　　　　　　　　systemic lupus erythematosus (M32.-)

L93.0　**Discoid lupus erythematosus**
　　　　Lupus erythematosus NOS

L93.1　**Subacute cutaneous lupus erythematosus**

L93.2　**Other local lupus erythematosus**
　　　　Lupus erythematosus profundus
　　　　Lupus panniculitis

🔴 **L94　Other localized connective tissue disorders**
　　　　Excludes1　systemic connective tissue disorders (M30-M36)

L94.0　**Localized scleroderma [morphea]**
　　　　Circumscribed scleroderma

L94.1　**Linear scleroderma**
　　　　En coup de sabre lesion

L94.2　**Calcinosis cutis**

L94.3　**Sclerodactyly**

L94.4　**Gottron's papules**

L94.5　**Poikiloderma vasculare atrophicans**

L94.6　**Ainhum**

L94.8　**Other specified localized connective tissue disorders**

L94.9　**Localized connective tissue disorder, unspecified**

CHAPTER 12 (L00-L99)

CHAPTER 12 (L00-L99)

● **L95** **Vasculitis limited to skin, not elsewhere classified**

> **Excludes1** angioma serpiginosum (L81.7)
> Henoch(-Schönlein) purpura (D69.0)
> hypersensitivity angiitis (M31.0)
> lupus panniculitis (L93.2)
> panniculitis NOS (M79.3)
> panniculitis of neck and back (M54.0-)
> polyarteritis nodosa (M30.0)
> relapsing panniculitis (M35.6)
> rheumatoid vasculitis (M05.2)
> serum sickness (T80.6-)
> urticaria (L50.-)
> Wegener's granulomatosis (M31.3-)

L95.0 **Livedoid vasculitis**
Atrophie blanche (en plaque)

L95.1 **Erythema elevatum diutinum**

L95.8 **Other vasculitis limited to the skin**

L95.9 **Vasculitis limited to the skin, unspecified**

● **L97** **Non-pressure chronic ulcer of lower limb, not elsewhere classified**

> **Includes** chronic ulcer of skin of lower limb NOS
> non-healing ulcer of skin
> non-infected sinus of skin
> trophic ulcer NOS
> tropical ulcer NOS
> ulcer of skin of lower limb NOS

> *Code first any associated underlying condition, such as:*
> any associated gangrene (I96)
> atherosclerosis of the lower extremities (I70.23-, I70.24-,
>   I70.33-, I70.34-, I70.43-, I70.44-, I70.53-, I70.54-, I70.63-,
>   I70.64-, I70.73-, I70.74-)
> chronic venous hypertension (I87.31-, I87.33-)
> diabetic ulcers (E08.621, E08.622, E09.621, E09.622, E10.621,
>   E10.622, E11.621, E11.622, E13.621, E13.622)
> postphlebitic syndrome (I87.01-, I87.03-)
> postthrombotic syndrome (I87.01-, I87.03-)
> varicose ulcer (I83.0-, I83.2-)

> **Excludes2** pressure ulcer (pressure area) (L89.-)
> skin infections (L00-L08)
> specific infections classified to A00-B99

● **L97.1** **Non-pressure chronic ulcer of thigh**

● **L97.10** **Non-pressure chronic ulcer of unspecified thigh**

L97.101 **Non-pressure chronic ulcer of unspecified thigh limited to breakdown of skin** ℞

L97.102 **Non-pressure chronic ulcer of unspecified thigh with fat layer exposed** ℞

L97.103 **Non-pressure chronic ulcer of unspecified thigh with necrosis of muscle** ℞

L97.104 **Non-pressure chronic ulcer of unspecified thigh with necrosis of bone** ℞

L97.105 **Non-pressure chronic ulcer of unspecified thigh with muscle involvement without evidence of necrosis** ℞

L97.106 **Non-pressure chronic ulcer of unspecified thigh with bone involvement without evidence of necrosis** ℞

L97.108 **Non-pressure chronic ulcer of unspecified thigh with other specified severity** ℞

L97.109 **Non-pressure chronic ulcer of unspecified thigh with unspecified severity** ℞

● **L97.11** **Non-pressure chronic ulcer of right thigh**

L97.111 **Non-pressure chronic ulcer of right thigh limited to breakdown of skin** ℞

L97.112 **Non-pressure chronic ulcer of right thigh with fat layer exposed** ℞

L97.113 **Non-pressure chronic ulcer of right thigh with necrosis of muscle** ℞

L97.114 **Non-pressure chronic ulcer of right thigh with necrosis of bone** ℞

L97.115 **Non-pressure chronic ulcer of right thigh with muscle involvement without evidence of necrosis** ℞

L97.116 **Non-pressure chronic ulcer of right thigh with bone involvement without evidence of necrosis** ℞

L97.118 **Non-pressure chronic ulcer of right thigh with other specified severity** ℞

L97.119 **Non-pressure chronic ulcer of right thigh with unspecified severity** ℞

● **L97.12** **Non-pressure chronic ulcer of left thigh**

L97.121 **Non-pressure chronic ulcer of left thigh limited to breakdown of skin** ℞

L97.122 **Non-pressure chronic ulcer of left thigh with fat layer exposed** ℞

L97.123 **Non-pressure chronic ulcer of left thigh with necrosis of muscle** ℞

L97.124 **Non-pressure chronic ulcer of left thigh with necrosis of bone** ℞

L97.125 **Non-pressure chronic ulcer of left thigh with muscle involvement without evidence of necrosis** ℞

L97.126 **Non-pressure chronic ulcer of left thigh with bone involvement without evidence of necrosis** ℞

L97.128 **Non-pressure chronic ulcer of left thigh with other specified severity** ℞

L97.129 **Non-pressure chronic ulcer of left thigh with unspecified severity** ℞

● **L97.2** **Non-pressure chronic ulcer of calf**
▶ Non-pressure chronic ulcer of shin

● **L97.20** **Non-pressure chronic ulcer of unspecified calf**

L97.201 **Non-pressure chronic ulcer of unspecified calf limited to breakdown of skin** ℞

L97.202 **Non-pressure chronic ulcer of unspecified calf with fat layer exposed** ℞

L97.203 **Non-pressure chronic ulcer of unspecified calf with necrosis of muscle** ℞

L97.204 **Non-pressure chronic ulcer of unspecified calf with necrosis of bone** ℞

L97.205 **Non-pressure chronic ulcer of unspecified calf with muscle involvement without evidence of necrosis** ℞

L97.206 **Non-pressure chronic ulcer of unspecified calf with bone involvement without evidence of necrosis** ℞

L97.208 **Non-pressure chronic ulcer of unspecified calf with other specified severity** ℞

L97.209 **Non-pressure chronic ulcer of unspecified calf with unspecified severity** ℞

● **L97.21** **Non-pressure chronic ulcer of right calf**

L97.211 **Non-pressure chronic ulcer of right calf limited to breakdown of skin** ℞

L97.212 **Non-pressure chronic ulcer of right calf with fat layer exposed** ℞

▶ New ⇒ Revised ~~deleted~~ Deleted Excludes 1 Excludes 2 Includes Use additional Code first Code also Key words

OGCR Official Guidelines X Assign placeholder X ● Use Additional Character(s) ▶ Manifestation Code ℞ Hierarchical Condition Category **Coding Clinic**

L97.213   Non-pressure chronic ulcer of right calf with **necrosis of muscle** 🔖

L97.214   Non-pressure chronic ulcer of right calf with **necrosis of bone** 🔖

L97.215   Non-pressure chronic ulcer of right calf with **muscle involvement** without evidence of necrosis 🔖

L97.216   Non-pressure chronic ulcer of right calf with **bone involvement** without evidence of necrosis 🔖

L97.218   Non-pressure chronic ulcer of right calf with **other specified severity** 🔖

L97.219   Non-pressure chronic ulcer of right calf with **unspecified severity** 🔖
Coding Clinic: 2024, Q1, P16

🔴 **L97.22**   Non-pressure chronic ulcer of **left calf**

L97.221   Non-pressure chronic ulcer of left calf limited to **breakdown of skin** 🔖

L97.222   Non-pressure chronic ulcer of left calf with **fat layer exposed** 🔖

L97.223   Non-pressure chronic ulcer of left calf with **necrosis of muscle** 🔖

L97.224   Non-pressure chronic ulcer of left calf with **necrosis of bone** 🔖

L97.225   Non-pressure chronic ulcer of left calf with **muscle involvement** without evidence of necrosis 🔖

L97.226   Non-pressure chronic ulcer of left calf with **bone involvement** without evidence of necrosis 🔖

L97.228   Non-pressure chronic ulcer of left calf with **other specified severity** 🔖

L97.229   Non-pressure chronic ulcer of left calf with **unspecified severity** 🔖

🔴 **L97.3**   Non-pressure chronic ulcer of **ankle**

🔴 **L97.30**   Non-pressure chronic ulcer of **unspecified** ankle

L97.301   Non-pressure chronic ulcer of unspecified ankle limited to **breakdown of skin** 🔖

L97.302   Non-pressure chronic ulcer of unspecified ankle with **fat layer exposed** 🔖

L97.303   Non-pressure chronic ulcer of unspecified ankle with **necrosis of muscle** 🔖

L97.304   Non-pressure chronic ulcer of unspecified ankle with **necrosis of bone** 🔖

L97.305   Non-pressure chronic ulcer of unspecified ankle with **muscle involvement** without evidence of necrosis 🔖

L97.306   Non-pressure chronic ulcer of unspecified ankle with **bone involvement** without evidence of necrosis 🔖

L97.308   Non-pressure chronic ulcer of unspecified ankle with **other specified severity** 🔖

L97.309   Non-pressure chronic ulcer of unspecified ankle with **unspecified severity** 🔖

🔴 **L97.31**   Non-pressure chronic ulcer of **right ankle**

L97.311   Non-pressure chronic ulcer of right ankle limited to **breakdown of skin** 🔖

L97.312   Non-pressure chronic ulcer of right ankle with **fat layer exposed** 🔖

L97.313   Non-pressure chronic ulcer of right ankle with **necrosis of muscle** 🔖

L97.314   Non-pressure chronic ulcer of right ankle with **necrosis of bone** 🔖

L97.315   Non-pressure chronic ulcer of right ankle with **muscle involvement** without evidence of necrosis 🔖
Coding Clinic: 2017, Q4, P17

L97.316   Non-pressure chronic ulcer of right ankle with **bone involvement** without evidence of necrosis 🔖

L97.318   Non-pressure chronic ulcer of right ankle with **other specified severity** 🔖

L97.319   Non-pressure chronic ulcer of right ankle with **unspecified severity** 🔖

🔴 **L97.32**   Non-pressure chronic ulcer of **left ankle**

L97.321   Non-pressure chronic ulcer of left ankle limited to **breakdown of skin** 🔖

L97.322   Non-pressure chronic ulcer of left ankle with **fat layer exposed** 🔖
Coding Clinic: 2021, Q1, P8

L97.323   Non-pressure chronic ulcer of left ankle with **necrosis of muscle** 🔖

L97.324   Non-pressure chronic ulcer of left ankle with **necrosis of bone** 🔖

L97.325   Non-pressure chronic ulcer of left ankle with **muscle involvement** without evidence of necrosis 🔖

L97.326   Non-pressure chronic ulcer of left ankle with **bone involvement** without evidence of necrosis 🔖

L97.328   Non-pressure chronic ulcer of left ankle with **other specified severity** 🔖

L97.329   Non-pressure chronic ulcer of left ankle with **unspecified severity** 🔖

🔴 **L97.4**   Non-pressure chronic ulcer of **heel and midfoot**
Non-pressure chronic ulcer of plantar surface of midfoot

🔴 **L97.40**   Non-pressure chronic ulcer of **unspecified** heel and midfoot

L97.401   Non-pressure chronic ulcer of unspecified heel and midfoot limited to **breakdown of skin** 🔖

L97.402   Non-pressure chronic ulcer of unspecified heel and midfoot with **fat layer exposed** 🔖

L97.403   Non-pressure chronic ulcer of unspecified heel and midfoot with **necrosis of muscle** 🔖

L97.404   Non-pressure chronic ulcer of unspecified heel and midfoot with **necrosis of bone** 🔖

L97.405   Non-pressure chronic ulcer of unspecified heel and midfoot with **muscle involvement** without evidence of necrosis 🔖

L97.406   Non-pressure chronic ulcer of unspecified heel and midfoot with **bone involvement** without evidence of necrosis 🔖

L97.408   Non-pressure chronic ulcer of unspecified heel and midfoot with **other specified severity** 🔖

L97.409   Non-pressure chronic ulcer of unspecified heel and midfoot with **unspecified severity** 🔖

🔴 **L97.41**   Non-pressure chronic ulcer of **right heel and** midfoot

L97.411   Non-pressure chronic ulcer of right heel and midfoot limited to **breakdown of skin** 🔖

L97.412   Non-pressure chronic ulcer of right heel and midfoot with **fat layer exposed** 🔖

CHAPTER 12 (L00–L99)

L97.413   Non-pressure chronic ulcer of right heel and midfoot with **necrosis of muscle** RCC

L97.414   Non-pressure chronic ulcer of right heel and midfoot with **necrosis of bone** RCC

L97.415   Non-pressure chronic ulcer of right heel and midfoot with **muscle involvement** without evidence of necrosis RCC

L97.416   Non-pressure chronic ulcer of right heel and midfoot with **bone involvement** without evidence of necrosis RCC

L97.418   Non-pressure chronic ulcer of right heel and midfoot with **other specified severity** RCC

L97.419   Non-pressure chronic ulcer of right heel and midfoot with **unspecified severity** RCC

● **L97.42**   Non-pressure chronic ulcer of **left heel and midfoot**

L97.421   Non-pressure chronic ulcer of left heel and midfoot limited to **breakdown of skin** RCC
     Coding Clinic: 2016, Q1, P13

L97.422   Non-pressure chronic ulcer of left heel and midfoot with **fat layer exposed** RCC

L97.423   Non-pressure chronic ulcer of left heel and midfoot with **necrosis of muscle** RCC

L97.424   Non-pressure chronic ulcer of left heel and midfoot with **necrosis of bone** RCC

L97.425   Non-pressure chronic ulcer of left heel and midfoot with **muscle involvement** without evidence of necrosis RCC

L97.426   Non-pressure chronic ulcer of left heel and midfoot with **bone involvement** without evidence of necrosis RCC

L97.428   Non-pressure chronic ulcer of left heel and midfoot with **other specified severity** RCC

L97.429   Non-pressure chronic ulcer of left heel and midfoot with **unspecified severity** RCC

● **L97.5**   Non-pressure chronic ulcer of **other part of foot**
     Non-pressure chronic ulcer of toe

● **L97.50**   Non-pressure chronic ulcer of other part of **unspecified** foot

L97.501   Non-pressure chronic ulcer of other part of unspecified foot limited to **breakdown of skin** RCC

L97.502   Non-pressure chronic ulcer of other part of unspecified foot with **fat layer exposed** RCC

L97.503   Non-pressure chronic ulcer of other part of unspecified foot with **necrosis of muscle** RCC

L97.504   Non-pressure chronic ulcer of other part of unspecified foot with **necrosis of bone** RCC

L97.505   Non-pressure chronic ulcer of other part of unspecified foot with **muscle involvement** without evidence of necrosis RCC

L97.506   Non-pressure chronic ulcer of other part of unspecified foot with **bone involvement** without evidence of necrosis RCC

L97.508   Non-pressure chronic ulcer of other part of unspecified foot with **other specified severity** RCC

L97.509   Non-pressure chronic ulcer of other part of unspecified foot with **unspecified severity** RCC

● **L97.51**   Non-pressure chronic ulcer of other part of **right foot**

L97.511   Non-pressure chronic ulcer of other part of right foot limited to **breakdown of skin** RCC
     Coding Clinic: 2020, Q1, P12

L97.512   Non-pressure chronic ulcer of other part of right foot with **fat layer exposed** RCC

L97.513   Non-pressure chronic ulcer of other part of right foot with **necrosis of muscle** RCC

L97.514   Non-pressure chronic ulcer of other part of right foot with **necrosis of bone** RCC

L97.515   Non-pressure chronic ulcer of other part of right foot with **muscle involvement** without evidence of necrosis RCC

L97.516   Non-pressure chronic ulcer of other part of right foot with **bone involvement** without evidence of necrosis RCC

L97.518   Non-pressure chronic ulcer of other part of right foot with **other specified severity** RCC

L97.519   Non-pressure chronic ulcer of other part of right foot with **unspecified severity** RCC

● **L97.52**   Non-pressure chronic ulcer of other part of **left foot**

L97.521   Non-pressure chronic ulcer of other part of left foot limited to **breakdown of skin** RCC

L97.522   Non-pressure chronic ulcer of other part of left foot with **fat layer exposed** RCC

L97.523   Non-pressure chronic ulcer of other part of left foot with **necrosis of muscle** RCC

L97.524   Non-pressure chronic ulcer of other part of left foot with **necrosis of bone** RCC

L97.525   Non-pressure chronic ulcer of other part of left foot with **muscle involvement** without evidence of necrosis RCC

L97.526   Non-pressure chronic ulcer of other part of left foot with **bone involvement** without evidence of necrosis RCC

L97.528   Non-pressure chronic ulcer of other part of left foot with **other specified severity** RCC

L97.529   Non-pressure chronic ulcer of other part of left foot with **unspecified severity** RCC

● **L97.8**   Non-pressure chronic ulcer of **other part of lower leg**

● **L97.80**   Non-pressure chronic ulcer of other part of **unspecified lower leg**

L97.801   Non-pressure chronic ulcer of other part of unspecified lower leg limited to **breakdown of skin** RCC

L97.802   Non-pressure chronic ulcer of other part of unspecified lower leg with **fat layer exposed** RCC

▶ New   ➡ Revised   ~~deleted~~ Deleted   Excludes 1   Excludes 2   Includes   Use additional   Code first   Code also   Key words
OGCR Official Guidelines   **X** Assign placeholder X   ● Use Additional Character(s)   ▶ Manifestation Code   RCC Hierarchical Condition Category   **Coding Clinic**

L97.803   Non-pressure chronic ulcer of other part of unspecified lower leg with necrosis of muscle

L97.804   Non-pressure chronic ulcer of other part of unspecified lower leg with necrosis of bone

L97.805   Non-pressure chronic ulcer of other part of unspecified lower leg with muscle involvement without evidence of necrosis

L97.806   Non-pressure chronic ulcer of other part of unspecified lower leg with bone involvement without evidence of necrosis

L97.808   Non-pressure chronic ulcer of other part of unspecified lower leg with other specified severity

L97.809   Non-pressure chronic ulcer of other part of unspecified lower leg with unspecified severity

● **L97.81**   Non-pressure chronic ulcer of other part of right lower leg

L97.811   Non-pressure chronic ulcer of other part of right lower leg limited to breakdown of skin

L97.812   Non-pressure chronic ulcer of other part of right lower leg with fat layer exposed

L97.813   Non-pressure chronic ulcer of other part of right lower leg with necrosis of muscle

L97.814   Non-pressure chronic ulcer of other part of right lower leg with necrosis of bone

L97.815   Non-pressure chronic ulcer of other part of right lower leg with muscle involvement without evidence of necrosis

L97.816   Non-pressure chronic ulcer of other part of right lower leg with bone involvement without evidence of necrosis

L97.818   Non-pressure chronic ulcer of other part of right lower leg with other specified severity

L97.819   Non-pressure chronic ulcer of other part of right lower leg with unspecified severity

● **L97.82**   Non-pressure chronic ulcer of other part of left lower leg

L97.821   Non-pressure chronic ulcer of other part of left lower leg limited to breakdown of skin

L97.822   Non-pressure chronic ulcer of other part of left lower leg with fat layer exposed

L97.823   Non-pressure chronic ulcer of other part of left lower leg with necrosis of muscle

L97.824   Non-pressure chronic ulcer of other part of left lower leg with necrosis of bone

L97.825   Non-pressure chronic ulcer of other part of left lower leg with muscle involvement without evidence of necrosis

L97.826   Non-pressure chronic ulcer of other part of left lower leg with bone involvement without evidence of necrosis

L97.828   Non-pressure chronic ulcer of other part of left lower leg with other specified severity

L97.829   Non-pressure chronic ulcer of other part of left lower leg with unspecified severity

● **L97.9**   Non-pressure chronic ulcer of unspecified part of lower leg

● **L97.90**   Non-pressure chronic ulcer of unspecified part of unspecified lower leg

L97.901   Non-pressure chronic ulcer of unspecified part of unspecified lower leg limited to breakdown of skin

L97.902   Non-pressure chronic ulcer of unspecified part of unspecified lower leg with fat layer exposed

L97.903   Non-pressure chronic ulcer of unspecified part of unspecified lower leg with necrosis of muscle

L97.904   Non-pressure chronic ulcer of unspecified part of unspecified lower leg with necrosis of bone

L97.905   Non-pressure chronic ulcer of unspecified part of unspecified lower leg with muscle involvement without evidence of necrosis

L97.906   Non-pressure chronic ulcer of unspecified part of unspecified lower leg with bone involvement without evidence of necrosis

L97.908   Non-pressure chronic ulcer of unspecified part of unspecified lower leg with other specified severity

L97.909   Non-pressure chronic ulcer of unspecified part of unspecified lower leg with unspecified severity

● **L97.91**   Non-pressure chronic ulcer of unspecified part of right lower leg

L97.911   Non-pressure chronic ulcer of unspecified part of right lower leg limited to breakdown of skin

L97.912   Non-pressure chronic ulcer of unspecified part of right lower leg with fat layer exposed

L97.913   Non-pressure chronic ulcer of unspecified part of right lower leg with necrosis of muscle

L97.914   Non-pressure chronic ulcer of unspecified part of right lower leg with necrosis of bone

L97.915   Non-pressure chronic ulcer of unspecified part of right lower leg with muscle involvement without evidence of necrosis

L97.916   Non-pressure chronic ulcer of unspecified part of right lower leg with bone involvement without evidence of necrosis

L97.918   Non-pressure chronic ulcer of unspecified part of right lower leg with other specified severity

L97.919   Non-pressure chronic ulcer of unspecified part of right lower leg with unspecified severity

● **L97.92**   Non-pressure chronic ulcer of unspecified part of left lower leg

L97.921   Non-pressure chronic ulcer of unspecified part of left lower leg limited to breakdown of skin

L97.922   Non-pressure chronic ulcer of unspecified part of left lower leg with fat layer exposed

CHAPTER 12 (L00-L99)

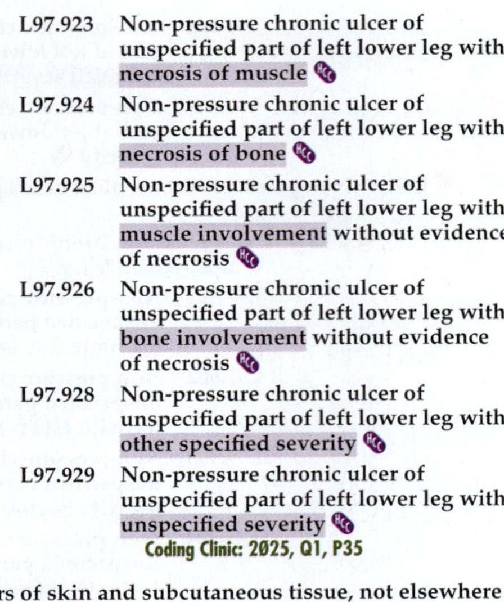

L97.923 Non-pressure chronic ulcer of unspecified part of left lower leg with necrosis of muscle 🗝

L97.924 Non-pressure chronic ulcer of unspecified part of left lower leg with necrosis of bone 🗝

L97.925 Non-pressure chronic ulcer of unspecified part of left lower leg with muscle involvement without evidence of necrosis 🗝

L97.926 Non-pressure chronic ulcer of unspecified part of left lower leg with bone involvement without evidence of necrosis 🗝

L97.928 Non-pressure chronic ulcer of unspecified part of left lower leg with other specified severity 🗝

L97.929 Non-pressure chronic ulcer of unspecified part of left lower leg with unspecified severity 🗝
Coding Clinic: 2025, Q1, P35

● **L98** Other disorders of skin and subcutaneous tissue, not elsewhere classified

L98.0 Pyogenic granuloma
Excludes2 pyogenic granuloma of gingiva (K06.8)
pyogenic granuloma of maxillary alveolar ridge (K04.5)
pyogenic granuloma of oral mucosa (K13.4)

L98.1 Factitial dermatitis
Neurotic excoriation
Excludes1 Excoriation (skin-picking) disorder (F42.4)
Coding Clinic: 2016, Q4, P15

L98.2 Febrile neutrophilic dermatosis [Sweet]

L98.3 Eosinophilic cellulitis [Wells]

● **L98.4** Non-pressure chronic ulcer of skin, not elsewhere classified
Chronic ulcer of skin NOS
Tropical ulcer NOS
Ulcer of skin NOS
Excludes2 pressure ulcer (pressure area) (L89.-)
gangrene (I96) 🗝
skin infections (L00-L08)
specific infections classified to A00-B99
ulcer of lower limb NEC (L97.-)
varicose ulcer (I83.0-I83.93)

● **L98.41** Non-pressure chronic ulcer of buttock

L98.411 Non-pressure chronic ulcer of buttock limited to breakdown of skin 🗝

L98.412 Non-pressure chronic ulcer of buttock with fat layer exposed 🗝

L98.413 Non-pressure chronic ulcer of buttock with necrosis of muscle 🗝

L98.414 Non-pressure chronic ulcer of buttock with necrosis of bone 🗝

L98.415 Non-pressure chronic ulcer of buttock with muscle involvement without evidence of necrosis 🗝

L98.416 Non-pressure chronic ulcer of buttock with bone involvement without evidence of necrosis 🗝

L98.418 Non-pressure chronic ulcer of buttock with other specified severity 🗝

L98.419 Non-pressure chronic ulcer of buttock with unspecified severity 🗝

● **L98.42** Non-pressure chronic ulcer of back

L98.421 Non-pressure chronic ulcer of back limited to breakdown of skin 🗝

L98.422 Non-pressure chronic ulcer of back with fat layer exposed 🗝

L98.423 Non-pressure chronic ulcer of back with necrosis of muscle 🗝

L98.424 Non-pressure chronic ulcer of back with necrosis of bone 🗝

L98.425 Non-pressure chronic ulcer of back with muscle involvement without evidence of necrosis 🗝

L98.426 Non-pressure chronic ulcer of back with bone involvement without evidence of necrosis 🗝

L98.428 Non-pressure chronic ulcer of back with other specified severity 🗝

L98.429 Non-pressure chronic ulcer of back with unspecified severity 🗝

▶ ● **L98.43** Non-pressure chronic ulcer of abdomen

▶ **L98.431** Non-pressure chronic ulcer of abdomen limited to breakdown of skin

▶ **L98.432** Non-pressure chronic ulcer of abdomen with fat layer exposed

▶ **L98.433** Non-pressure chronic ulcer of abdomen with necrosis of muscle

▶ **L98.434** Non-pressure chronic ulcer of abdomen with necrosis of bone

▶ **L98.435** Non-pressure chronic ulcer of abdomen with muscle involvement without evidence of necrosis

▶ **L98.436** Non-pressure chronic ulcer of abdomen with bone involvement without evidence of necrosis

▶ **L98.438** Non-pressure chronic ulcer of abdomen with other specified severity

▶ **L98.439** Non-pressure chronic ulcer of abdomen with unspecified severity

▶ ● **L98.44** Non-pressure chronic ulcer of chest

▶ **L98.441** Non-pressure chronic ulcer of chest limited to breakdown of skin

▶ **L98.442** Non-pressure chronic ulcer of chest with fat layer exposed

▶ **L98.443** Non-pressure chronic ulcer of chest with necrosis of muscle

▶ ● **L98.444** Non-pressure chronic ulcer of chest with necrosis of bone

▶ **L98.445** Non-pressure chronic ulcer of chest with muscle involvement without evidence of necrosis

▶ **L98.446** Non-pressure chronic ulcer of chest with bone involvement without evidence of necrosis

▶ **L98.448** Non-pressure chronic ulcer of chest with other specified severity

▶ **L98.449** Non-pressure chronic ulcer of chest with unspecified severity

▶ ● **L98.45** Non-pressure chronic ulcer of neck

▶ **L98.451** Non-pressure chronic ulcer of neck limited to breakdown of skin

▶ **L98.452** Non-pressure chronic ulcer of neck with fat layer exposed

▶ **L98.453** Non-pressure chronic ulcer of neck with necrosis of muscle

▶ **L98.454** Non-pressure chronic ulcer of neck with necrosis of bone

▶ **L98.455** Non-pressure chronic ulcer of neck with muscle involvement without evidence of necrosis

▶ **L98.456** Non-pressure chronic ulcer of neck with bone involvement without evidence of necrosis

▶ **L98.458** Non-pressure chronic ulcer of neck with other specified severity

▶ **L98.459** Non-pressure chronic ulcer of neck with unspecified severity

▶ New   ⇨ Revised   ~~deleted~~ Deleted   Excludes 1   Excludes 2   Includes   Use additional   Code first   Code also   Key words
OGCR Official Guidelines   X Assign placeholder X   ● Use Additional Character(s)   ▶ Manifestation Code   🗝 Hierarchical Condition Category   Coding Clinic

▶● **L98.46**   Non-pressure chronic ulcer of face

     ▶ **L98.461**   Non-pressure chronic ulcer of face limited to breakdown of skin

     ▶ **L98.462**   Non-pressure chronic ulcer of face with fat layer exposed

     ▶ **L98.463**   Non-pressure chronic ulcer of face with necrosis of muscle

     ▶ **L98.464**   Non-pressure chronic ulcer of face with necrosis of bone

     ▶ **L98.465**   Non-pressure chronic ulcer of face with muscle involvement without evidence of necrosis

     ▶ **L98.466**   Non-pressure chronic ulcer of face with bone involvement without evidence of necrosis

     ▶ **L98.468**   Non-pressure chronic ulcer of face with other specified severity

     ▶ **L98.469**   Non-pressure chronic ulcer of face with unspecified severity

▶● **L98.47**   Non-pressure chronic ulcer of groin

     ▶ **L98.471**   Non-pressure chronic ulcer of groin limited to breakdown of skin

     ▶ **L98.472**   Non-pressure chronic ulcer of groin with fat layer exposed

     ▶ **L98.473**   Non-pressure chronic ulcer of groin with necrosis of muscle

     ▶ **L98.474**   Non-pressure chronic ulcer of groin with necrosis of bone

     ▶ **L98.475**   Non-pressure chronic ulcer of groin with muscle involvement without evidence of necrosis

     ▶ **L98.476**   Non-pressure chronic ulcer of groin with bone involvement without evidence of necrosis

     ▶ **L98.478**   Non-pressure chronic ulcer of groin with other specified severity

     ▶ **L98.479**   Non-pressure chronic ulcer of groin with unspecified severity

● **L98.49**   Non-pressure chronic ulcer of skin of other sites

     Non-pressure chronic ulcer of skin NOS

     L98.491   Non-pressure chronic ulcer of skin of other sites limited to breakdown of skin ℞

     L98.492   Non-pressure chronic ulcer of skin of other sites with fat layer exposed ℞

     L98.493   Non-pressure chronic ulcer of skin of other sites with necrosis of muscle ℞

     L98.494   Non-pressure chronic ulcer of skin of other sites with necrosis of bone ℞

     L98.495   Non-pressure chronic ulcer of skin of other sites with muscle involvement without evidence of necrosis ℞

     L98.496   Non-pressure chronic ulcer of skin of other sites with bone involvement without evidence of necrosis ℞

     L98.498   Non-pressure chronic ulcer of skin of other sites with other specified severity ℞

     L98.499   Non-pressure chronic ulcer of skin of other sites with unspecified severity ℞

L98.5   Mucinosis of the skin

     Focal mucinosis

     Lichen myxedematosus

     Reticular erythematous mucinosis

     Excludes1   focal oral mucinosis (K13.79)

                  myxedema (E03.9)

L98.6   Other infiltrative disorders of the skin and subcutaneous tissue

     Excludes1   hyalinosis cutis et mucosae (E78.89)

L98.7   Excessive and redundant skin and subcutaneous tissue

     Loose or sagging skin following bariatric surgery weight loss

     Loose or sagging skin following dietary weight loss

     Loose or sagging skin, NOS

     Excludes2   acquired excess or redundant skin of eyelid (H02.3-)

                  congenital excess or redundant skin of eyelid (Q10.3)

                  skin changes due to chronic exposure to nonionizing radiation (L57.-)

     Coding Clinic: 2022, Q3, P11; 2016, Q4, P36

L98.8   Other specified disorders of the skin and subcutaneous tissue

     Coding Clinic: 2013, Q2, P32

L98.9   Disorder of the skin and subcutaneous tissue, unspecified

▶● **L98.A**   Non-pressure chronic ulcer of upper limb, not elsewhere classified

     ▶ Chronic ulcer of upper limb NOS

     ▶ Non-healing ulcer of upper limb

     ▶ Ulcer of upper limb NEC

     Excludes2   gangrene (I96)

                  ▶ pressure ulcer (pressure area) (L89.-)

                  ▶ skin infections (L00-L08)

                  ▶ specific infections classified to A00-B99

                  ▶ ulcer of lower limb NEC (L97.-)

                  ▶ varicose ulcer (I83.0-I83.93)

     ▶● **L98.A1**   Non-pressure chronic ulcer of upper arm

         ▶ Non-pressure chronic ulcer of axilla

         ▶● **L98.A11**   Non-pressure chronic ulcer of right upper arm

             ▶ **L98.A111**   Non-pressure chronic ulcer of right upper arm limited to breakdown of skin

             ▶ **L98.A112**   Non-pressure chronic ulcer of right upper arm with fat layer exposed

             ▶ **L98.A113**   Non-pressure chronic ulcer of right upper arm with necrosis of muscle

             ▶ **L98.A114**   Non-pressure chronic ulcer of right upper arm with necrosis of bone

             ▶ **L98.A115**   Non-pressure chronic ulcer of right upper arm with muscle involvement without evidence of necrosis

             ▶ **L98.A116**   Non-pressure chronic ulcer of right upper arm with bone involvement without evidence of necrosis

             ▶ **L98.A118**   Non-pressure chronic ulcer of right upper arm with other specified severity

             ▶ **L98.A119**   Non-pressure chronic ulcer of right upper arm with unspecified severity

         ▶● **L98.A12**   Non-pressure chronic ulcer of left upper arm

             ▶ **L98.A121**   Non-pressure chronic ulcer of left upper arm limited to breakdown of skin

             ▶ **L98.A122**   Non-pressure chronic ulcer of left upper arm with fat layer exposed

             ▶ **L98.A123**   Non-pressure chronic ulcer of left upper arm with necrosis of muscle

L98.A124   Non-pressure chronic ulcer of left upper arm with necrosis of bone

L98.A125   Non-pressure chronic ulcer of left upper arm with muscle involvement without evidence of necrosis

L98.A126   Non-pressure chronic ulcer of left upper arm with bone involvement without evidence of necrosis

L98.A128   Non-pressure chronic ulcer of left upper arm with other specified severity

L98.A129   Non-pressure chronic ulcer of left upper arm with unspecified severity

● L98.A19   Non-pressure chronic ulcer of unspecified upper arm

L98.A191   Non-pressure chronic ulcer of unspecified upper arm limited to breakdown of skin

L98.A192   Non-pressure chronic ulcer of unspecified upper arm with fat layer exposed

L98.A193   Non-pressure chronic ulcer of unspecified upper arm with necrosis of muscle

L98.A194   Non-pressure chronic ulcer of unspecified upper arm with necrosis of bone

L98.A195   Non-pressure chronic ulcer of unspecified upper arm with muscle involvement without evidence of necrosis

L98.A196   Non-pressure chronic ulcer of unspecified upper arm with bone involvement without evidence of necrosis

L98.A198   Non-pressure chronic ulcer of unspecified upper arm with other specified severity

L98.A199   Non-pressure chronic ulcer of unspecified upper arm with unspecified severity

● L98.A2   Non-pressure chronic ulcer of forearm

● L98.A21   Non-pressure chronic ulcer of right forearm

L98.A211   Non-pressure chronic ulcer of right forearm limited to breakdown of skin

L98.A212   Non-pressure chronic ulcer of right forearm with fat layer exposed

L98.A213   Non-pressure chronic ulcer of right forearm with necrosis of muscle

L98.A214   Non-pressure chronic ulcer of right forearm with necrosis of bone

L98.A215   Non-pressure chronic ulcer of right forearm with muscle involvement without evidence of necrosis

L98.A216   Non-pressure chronic ulcer of right forearm with bone involvement without evidence of necrosis

L98.A218   Non-pressure chronic ulcer of right forearm with other specified severity

L98.A219   Non-pressure chronic ulcer of right forearm with unspecified severity

● L98.A22   Non-pressure chronic ulcer of left forearm

L98.A221   Non-pressure chronic ulcer of left forearm limited to breakdown of skin

L98.A222   Non-pressure chronic ulcer of left forearm with fat layer exposed

L98.A223   Non-pressure chronic ulcer of left forearm with necrosis of muscle

L98.A224   Non-pressure chronic ulcer of left forearm with necrosis of bone

L98.A225   Non-pressure chronic ulcer of left forearm with muscle involvement without evidence of necrosis

L98.A226   Non-pressure chronic ulcer of left forearm with bone involvement without evidence of necrosis

L98.A228   Non-pressure chronic ulcer of left forearm with other specified severity

L98.A229   Non-pressure chronic ulcer of left forearm with unspecified severity

● L98.A29   Non-pressure chronic ulcer of unspecified forearm

L98.A291   Non-pressure chronic ulcer of unspecified forearm limited to breakdown of skin

L98.A292   Non-pressure chronic ulcer of unspecified forearm with fat layer exposed

L98.A293   Non-pressure chronic ulcer of unspecified forearm with necrosis of muscle

L98.A294   Non-pressure chronic ulcer of unspecified forearm with necrosis of bone

L98.A295   Non-pressure chronic ulcer of unspecified forearm with muscle involvement without evidence of necrosis

L98.A296   Non-pressure chronic ulcer of unspecified forearm with bone involvement without evidence of necrosis

L98.A298   Non-pressure chronic ulcer of unspecified forearm with other specified severity

L98.A299   Non-pressure chronic ulcer of unspecified forearm with unspecified severity

● L98.A3   Non-pressure chronic ulcer of hand

● L98.A31   Non-pressure chronic ulcer of right hand

L98.A311   Non-pressure chronic ulcer of right hand limited to breakdown of skin

▶ L98.A312   **Non-pressure chronic ulcer of right hand with fat layer exposed**

▶ L98.A313   **Non-pressure chronic ulcer of right hand with necrosis of muscle**

▶ L98.A314   **Non-pressure chronic ulcer of right hand with necrosis of bone**

▶ L98.A315   **Non-pressure chronic ulcer of right hand with muscle involvement without evidence of necrosis**

▶ L98.A316   **Non-pressure chronic ulcer of right hand with bone involvement without evidence of necrosis**

▶ L98.A318   **Non-pressure chronic ulcer of right hand with other specified severity**

▶ L98.A319   **Non-pressure chronic ulcer of right hand with unspecified severity**

▶ ● L98.A32   **Non-pressure chronic ulcer of left hand**

▶ L98.A321   **Non-pressure chronic ulcer of left hand limited to breakdown of skin**

▶ L98.A322   **Non-pressure chronic ulcer of left hand with fat layer exposed**

▶ L98.A323   **Non-pressure chronic ulcer of left hand with necrosis of muscle**

▶ L98.A324   **Non-pressure chronic ulcer of left hand with necrosis of bone**

▶ L98.A325   **Non-pressure chronic ulcer of left hand with muscle involvement without evidence of necrosis**

▶ L98.A326   **Non-pressure chronic ulcer of left hand with bone involvement without evidence of necrosis**

▶ L98.A328   **Non-pressure chronic ulcer of left hand with other specified severity**

▶ L98.A329   **Non-pressure chronic ulcer of left hand with unspecified severity**

▶ ● L98.A39   **Non-pressure chronic ulcer of unspecified hand**

▶ L98.A391   **Non-pressure chronic ulcer of unspecified hand limited to breakdown of skin**

▶ L98.A392   **Non-pressure chronic ulcer of unspecified hand with fat layer exposed**

▶ L98.A393   **Non-pressure chronic ulcer of unspecified hand with necrosis of muscle**

▶ L98.A394   **Non-pressure chronic ulcer of unspecified hand with necrosis of bone**

▶ L98.A395   **Non-pressure chronic ulcer of unspecified hand with muscle involvement without evidence of necrosis**

▶ L98.A396   **Non-pressure chronic ulcer of unspecified hand with bone involvement without evidence of necrosis**

▶ L98.A398   **Non-pressure chronic ulcer of unspecified hand with other specified severity**

▶ L98.A399   **Non-pressure chronic ulcer of unspecified hand with unspecified severity**

▶ **L99**   *Other disorders of skin and subcutaneous tissue in diseases classified elsewhere*

    Code first underlying disease, such as:
      amyloidosis (E85.-)

    Excludes1   skin disorders in diabetes (E08-E13 with .62-)
               skin disorders in gonorrhea (A54.89)
               skin disorders in syphilis (A51.31, A52.79)

CHAPTER 12 (LØØ-L99)

CHAPTER 13

DISEASES OF THE MUSCULOSKELETAL SYSTEM AND CONNECTIVE TISSUE (M00-M99)

OGCR Chapter-Specific Coding Guidelines

13. Chapter 13: Diseases of the Musculoskeletal System and Connective Tissue (M00-M99)

a. Site and laterality

Most of the codes within Chapter 13 have site and laterality designations. The site represents the bone, joint or the muscle involved. For some conditions where more than one bone, joint or muscle is usually involved, such as osteoarthritis, there is a "multiple sites" code available. For categories where no multiple site code is provided and more than one bone, joint or muscle is involved, multiple codes should be used to indicate the different sites involved.

1) Bone versus joint

For certain conditions, the bone may be affected at the upper or lower end (e.g., avascular necrosis of bone, M87, Osteoporosis, M80, M81). Though the portion of the bone affected may be at the joint, the site designation will be the bone, not the joint.

b. Acute traumatic versus chronic or recurrent musculoskeletal conditions

Many musculoskeletal conditions are a result of previous injury or trauma to a site, or are recurrent conditions. Bone, joint or muscle conditions that are the result of a healed injury are usually found in Chapter 13. Recurrent bone, joint or muscle conditions are also usually found in Chapter 13. Any current, acute injury should be coded to the appropriate injury code from Chapter 19. Chronic or recurrent conditions should generally be coded with a code from Chapter 13. If it is difficult to determine from the documentation in the record which code is best to describe a condition, query the provider.

c. Coding of Pathologic Fractures

7th character A is for use as long as the patient is receiving active treatment for the fracture. While the patient may be seen by a new or different provider over the course of treatment for a pathological fracture, assignment of the 7th character is based on whether the patient is undergoing active treatment and not whether the provider is seeing the patient for the first time.

7th character, D is to be used for encounters after the patient has completed active treatment for the fracture and is receiving routine care for the fracture during the healing or recovery phase. The other 7th characters, listed under each subcategory in the Tabular List, are to be used for subsequent encounters for treatment of problems associated with the healing, such as malunions, nonunions, and sequelae.

Care for complications of surgical treatment for fracture repairs during the healing or recovery phase should be coded with the appropriate complication codes.

See Section I.C.19. Coding of traumatic fractures.

d. Osteoporosis

Osteoporosis is a systemic condition, meaning that all bones of the musculoskeletal system are affected. Therefore, site is not a component of the codes under category M81, Osteoporosis without current pathological fracture. The site codes under category M80, Osteoporosis with current pathological fracture, identify the site of the fracture, not the osteoporosis.

1) Osteoporosis without pathological fracture

Category M81, Osteoporosis without current pathological fracture, is for use for patients with osteoporosis who do not currently have a pathologic fracture due to the osteoporosis, even if they have had a fracture in the past. For patients with a history of osteoporosis fractures, status code Z87.310, Personal history of (healed) osteoporosis fracture, should follow the code from M81.

2) Osteoporosis with current pathological fracture

Category M80, Osteoporosis with current pathological fracture, is for patients who have a current pathologic fracture at the time of an encounter. The codes under M80 identify the site of the fracture. A code from category M80, not a traumatic fracture code, should be used for any patient with known osteoporosis who suffers a fracture, even if the patient had a minor fall or trauma, if that fall or trauma would not usually break a normal, healthy bone.

CHAPTER 13

DISEASES OF THE MUSCULOSKELETAL SYSTEM AND CONNECTIVE TISSUE (M00-M99)

Note: Use an external cause code following the code for the musculoskeletal condition, if applicable, to identify the cause of the musculoskeletal condition

Excludes2 arthropathic psoriasis (L40.5-)
certain conditions originating in the perinatal period (P04-P96)
certain infectious and parasitic diseases (A00-B99)
compartment syndrome (traumatic) (T79.A-)
complications of pregnancy, childbirth and the puerperium (O00-O9A)
congenital malformations, deformations, and chromosomal abnormalities (Q00-Q99)
endocrine, nutritional and metabolic diseases (E00-E88)
injury, poisoning and certain other consequences of external causes (S00-T88)
neoplasms (C00-D49)
symptoms, signs and abnormal clinical and laboratory findings, not elsewhere classified (R00-R94)

This chapter contains the following blocks:

M00-M02	Infectious arthropathies
M04	Autoinflammatory syndromes
M05-M14	Inflammatory polyarthropathies
M15-M19	Osteoarthritis
M20-M25	Other joint disorders
M26-M27	Dentofacial anomalies [including malocclusion] and other disorders of jaw
M30-M36	Systemic connective tissue disorders
M40-M43	Deforming dorsopathies
M45-M49	Spondylopathies
M50-M54	Other dorsopathies
M60-M63	Disorders of muscles
M65-M67	Disorders of synovium and tendon
M70-M79	Other soft tissue disorders
M80-M85	Disorders of bone density and structure
M86-M90	Other osteopathies
M91-M94	Chondropathies
M95	Other disorders of the musculoskeletal system and connective tissue
M96	Intraoperative and postprocedural complications and disorders of musculoskeletal system, not elsewhere classified
M97	Periprosthetic fracture around internal prosthetic joint
M99	Biomechanical lesions, not elsewhere classified

Coding Clinic: 2016, Q4, P124

ARTHROPATHIES (M00-M25)

Includes Disorders affecting predominantly peripheral (limb) joints

INFECTIOUS ARTHROPATHIES (M00-M02)

Note: This block comprises arthropathies due to microbiological agents.

Distinction is made between the following types of etiological relationship:

a) direct infection of joint, where organisms invade synovial tissue and microbial antigen is present in the joint;

b) indirect infection, which may be of two types: a reactive arthropathy, where microbial infection of the body is established but neither organisms nor antigens can be identified in the joint, and a postinfective arthropathy, where microbial antigen is present but recovery of an organism is inconstant and evidence of local multiplication is lacking.

● **M00 Pyogenic arthritis**

    Excludes2 infection and inflammatory reaction due to internal joint prosthesis (T84.5-)

● **M00.0 Staphylococcal arthritis and polyarthritis**

    Use additional code (B95.61-B95.8) to identify bacterial agent

    M00.00 Staphylococcal arthritis, unspecified joint

  ● **M00.01** Staphylococcal arthritis, shoulder

    M00.011 Staphylococcal arthritis, right shoulder

    M00.012 Staphylococcal arthritis, left shoulder

    M00.019 Staphylococcal arthritis, unspecified shoulder

  ● **M00.02** Staphylococcal arthritis, elbow

    M00.021 Staphylococcal arthritis, right elbow

    M00.022 Staphylococcal arthritis, left elbow

    M00.029 Staphylococcal arthritis, unspecified elbow

  ● **M00.03** Staphylococcal arthritis, wrist

    Staphylococcal arthritis of carpal bones

    M00.031 Staphylococcal arthritis, right wrist

    M00.032 Staphylococcal arthritis, left wrist

    M00.039 Staphylococcal arthritis, unspecified wrist

  ● **M00.04** Staphylococcal arthritis, hand

    Staphylococcal arthritis of metacarpus and phalanges

    M00.041 Staphylococcal arthritis, right hand

    M00.042 Staphylococcal arthritis, left hand

    M00.049 Staphylococcal arthritis, unspecified hand

  ● **M00.05** Staphylococcal arthritis, hip

    M00.051 Staphylococcal arthritis, right hip

    M00.052 Staphylococcal arthritis, left hip

    M00.059 Staphylococcal arthritis, unspecified hip

  ● **M00.06** Staphylococcal arthritis, knee

    M00.061 Staphylococcal arthritis, right knee

    M00.062 Staphylococcal arthritis, left knee

    M00.069 Staphylococcal arthritis, unspecified knee

  ● **M00.07** Staphylococcal arthritis, ankle and foot

    Staphylococcal arthritis, tarsus, metatarsus and phalanges

    M00.071 Staphylococcal arthritis, right ankle and foot

    M00.072 Staphylococcal arthritis, left ankle and foot

    M00.079 Staphylococcal arthritis, unspecified ankle and foot

    M00.08 Staphylococcal arthritis, vertebrae

    M00.09 Staphylococcal polyarthritis

● **M00.1 Pneumococcal arthritis and polyarthritis**

    M00.10 Pneumococcal arthritis, unspecified joint

  ● **M00.11** Pneumococcal arthritis, shoulder

    M00.111 Pneumococcal arthritis, right shoulder

    M00.112 Pneumococcal arthritis, left shoulder

    M00.119 Pneumococcal arthritis, unspecified shoulder

  ● **M00.12** Pneumococcal arthritis, elbow

    M00.121 Pneumococcal arthritis, right elbow

    M00.122 Pneumococcal arthritis, left elbow

    M00.129 Pneumococcal arthritis, unspecified elbow

  ● **M00.13** Pneumococcal arthritis, wrist

    Pneumococcal arthritis of carpal bones

    M00.131 Pneumococcal arthritis, right wrist

    M00.132 Pneumococcal arthritis, left wrist

    M00.139 Pneumococcal arthritis, unspecified wrist

  ● **M00.14** Pneumococcal arthritis, hand

    Pneumococcal arthritis of metacarpus and phalanges

    M00.141 Pneumococcal arthritis, right hand

    M00.142 Pneumococcal arthritis, left hand

    M00.149 Pneumococcal arthritis, unspecified hand

  ● **M00.15** Pneumococcal arthritis, hip

    M00.151 Pneumococcal arthritis, right hip

    M00.152 Pneumococcal arthritis, left hip

    M00.159 Pneumococcal arthritis, unspecified hip

  ● **M00.16** Pneumococcal arthritis, knee

    M00.161 Pneumococcal arthritis, right knee

    M00.162 Pneumococcal arthritis, left knee

    M00.169 Pneumococcal arthritis, unspecified knee

  ● **M00.17** Pneumococcal arthritis, ankle and foot

    Pneumococcal arthritis, tarsus, metatarsus and phalanges

    M00.171 Pneumococcal arthritis, right ankle and foot

    M00.172 Pneumococcal arthritis, left ankle and foot

    M00.179 Pneumococcal arthritis, unspecified ankle and foot

    M00.18 Pneumococcal arthritis, vertebrae

    M00.19 Pneumococcal polyarthritis

● **M00.2 Other streptococcal arthritis and polyarthritis**

    Use additional code (B95.0-B95.2, B95.4-B95.5) to identify bacterial agent

    M00.20 Other streptococcal arthritis, unspecified joint

  ● **M00.21** Other streptococcal arthritis, shoulder

    M00.211 Other streptococcal arthritis, right shoulder

    M00.212 Other streptococcal arthritis, left shoulder

    M00.219 Other streptococcal arthritis, unspecified shoulder

  ● **M00.22** Other streptococcal arthritis, elbow

    M00.221 Other streptococcal arthritis, right elbow

    M00.222 Other streptococcal arthritis, left elbow

    M00.229 Other streptococcal arthritis, unspecified elbow

● **M00.23**   Other streptococcal arthritis, wrist
Other streptococcal arthritis of carpal bones
    M00.231   Other streptococcal arthritis, right wrist Rcc
    M00.232   Other streptococcal arthritis, left wrist Rcc
    M00.239   Other streptococcal arthritis, unspecified wrist Rcc

● **M00.24**   Other streptococcal arthritis, hand
Other streptococcal arthritis metacarpus and phalanges
    M00.241   Other streptococcal arthritis, right hand Rcc
    M00.242   Other streptococcal arthritis, left hand Rcc
    M00.249   Other streptococcal arthritis, unspecified hand Rcc

● **M00.25**   Other streptococcal arthritis, hip
    M00.251   Other streptococcal arthritis, right hip Rcc
    M00.252   Other streptococcal arthritis, left hip Rcc
    M00.259   Other streptococcal arthritis, unspecified hip Rcc

● **M00.26**   Other streptococcal arthritis, knee
    M00.261   Other streptococcal arthritis, right knee Rcc
    M00.262   Other streptococcal arthritis, left knee Rcc
    M00.269   Other streptococcal arthritis, unspecified knee Rcc

● **M00.27**   Other streptococcal arthritis, ankle and foot
Other streptococcal arthritis, tarsus, metatarsus and phalanges
    M00.271   Other streptococcal arthritis, right ankle and foot Rcc
    M00.272   Other streptococcal arthritis, left ankle and foot Rcc
    M00.279   Other streptococcal arthritis, unspecified ankle and foot Rcc

   M00.28   Other streptococcal arthritis, vertebrae Rcc

   M00.29   Other streptococcal polyarthritis Rcc

● **M00.8**   Arthritis and polyarthritis due to other bacteria
Use additional code (B96) to identify bacteria
   M00.80   Arthritis due to other bacteria, unspecified joint Rcc

● **M00.81**   Arthritis due to other bacteria, shoulder
    M00.811   Arthritis due to other bacteria, right shoulder Rcc
    M00.812   Arthritis due to other bacteria, left shoulder Rcc
    M00.819   Arthritis due to other bacteria, unspecified shoulder Rcc

● **M00.82**   Arthritis due to other bacteria, elbow
    M00.821   Arthritis due to other bacteria, right elbow Rcc
    M00.822   Arthritis due to other bacteria, left elbow Rcc
    M00.829   Arthritis due to other bacteria, unspecified elbow Rcc

● **M00.83**   Arthritis due to other bacteria, wrist
Arthritis due to other bacteria, carpal bones
    M00.831   Arthritis due to other bacteria, right wrist Rcc
    M00.832   Arthritis due to other bacteria, left wrist Rcc
    M00.839   Arthritis due to other bacteria, unspecified wrist Rcc

● **M00.84**   Arthritis due to other bacteria, hand
Arthritis due to other bacteria, metacarpus and phalanges
    M00.841   Arthritis due to other bacteria, right hand Rcc
    M00.842   Arthritis due to other bacteria, left hand Rcc
    M00.849   Arthritis due to other bacteria, unspecified hand Rcc

● **M00.85**   Arthritis due to other bacteria, hip
    M00.851   Arthritis due to other bacteria, right hip Rcc
    M00.852   Arthritis due to other bacteria, left hip Rcc
    M00.859   Arthritis due to other bacteria, unspecified hip Rcc

● **M00.86**   Arthritis due to other bacteria, knee
    M00.861   Arthritis due to other bacteria, right knee Rcc
    M00.862   Arthritis due to other bacteria, left knee Rcc
     Coding Clinic: 2019, Q3, P16
    M00.869   Arthritis due to other bacteria, unspecified knee Rcc

● **M00.87**   Arthritis due to other bacteria, ankle and foot
Arthritis due to other bacteria, tarsus, metatarsus, and phalanges
    M00.871   Arthritis due to other bacteria, right ankle and foot Rcc
    M00.872   Arthritis due to other bacteria, left ankle and foot Rcc
    M00.879   Arthritis due to other bacteria, unspecified ankle and foot Rcc

   M00.88   Arthritis due to other bacteria, vertebrae Rcc

   M00.89   Polyarthritis due to other bacteria Rcc

   M00.9   Pyogenic arthritis, unspecified Rcc
Infective arthritis NOS

● **M01**   Direct infections of joint in infectious and parasitic diseases classified elsewhere
Code first underlying disease, such as:
leprosy [Hansen's disease] (A30.-)
mycoses (B35-B49)
O'nyong-nyong fever (A92.1)
paratyphoid fever (A01.1-A01.4)

   Excludes1   arthropathy in Lyme disease (A69.23)
gonococcal arthritis (A54.42)
meningococcal arthritis (A39.83)
mumps arthritis (B26.85)
postinfective arthropathy (M02.-)
postmeningococcal arthritis (A39.84)
reactive arthritis (M02.3)
rubella arthritis (B06.82)
sarcoidosis arthritis (D86.86)
typhoid fever arthritis (A01.04)
tuberculosis arthritis (A18.01-A18.02)

● **M01.X**   Direct infection of joint in infectious and parasitic diseases classified elsewhere
   ▸ *M01.X0*   Direct infection of unspecified joint in infectious and parasitic diseases classified elsewhere Rcc

● **M01.X1**   Direct infection of shoulder joint in infectious and parasitic diseases classified elsewhere
   ▸ *M01.X11*   Direct infection of right shoulder in infectious and parasitic diseases classified elsewhere Rcc
   ▸ *M01.X12*   Direct infection of left shoulder in infectious and parasitic diseases classified elsewhere Rcc
   ▸ *M01.X19*   Direct infection of unspecified shoulder in infectious and parasitic diseases classified elsewhere Rcc

▶ New   ➡ Revised   ~~deleted~~ Deleted   Excludes 1   Excludes 2   Includes   Use additional   Code first   Code also   Key words
OGCR Official Guidelines   X Assign placeholder X   ● Use Additional Character(s)   ▸ Manifestation Code   Rcc Hierarchical Condition Category   Coding Clinic

● **M01.X2 Direct infection of elbow in infectious and parasitic diseases classified elsewhere**
   ▸ *M01.X21 Direct infection of right elbow in infectious and parasitic diseases classified elsewhere*
   ▸ *M01.X22 Direct infection of left elbow in infectious and parasitic diseases classified elsewhere*
   ▸ *M01.X29 Direct infection of unspecified elbow in infectious and parasitic diseases classified elsewhere*

● **M01.X3 Direct infection of wrist in infectious and parasitic diseases classified elsewhere**
   Direct infection of carpal bones in infectious and parasitic diseases classified elsewhere
   ▸ *M01.X31 Direct infection of right wrist in infectious and parasitic diseases classified elsewhere*
   ▸ *M01.X32 Direct infection of left wrist in infectious and parasitic diseases classified elsewhere*
   ▸ *M01.X39 Direct infection of unspecified wrist in infectious and parasitic diseases classified elsewhere*

● **M01.X4 Direct infection of hand in infectious and parasitic diseases classified elsewhere**
   Direct infection of metacarpus and phalanges in infectious and parasitic diseases classified elsewhere
   ▸ *M01.X41 Direct infection of right hand in infectious and parasitic diseases classified elsewhere*
   ▸ *M01.X42 Direct infection of left hand in infectious and parasitic diseases classified elsewhere*
   ▸ *M01.X49 Direct infection of unspecified hand in infectious and parasitic diseases classified elsewhere*

● **M01.X5 Direct infection of hip in infectious and parasitic diseases classified elsewhere**
   ▸ *M01.X51 Direct infection of right hip in infectious and parasitic diseases classified elsewhere*
   ▸ *M01.X52 Direct infection of left hip in infectious and parasitic diseases classified elsewhere*
   ▸ *M01.X59 Direct infection of unspecified hip in infectious and parasitic diseases classified elsewhere*

● **M01.X6 Direct infection of knee in infectious and parasitic diseases classified elsewhere**
   ▸ *M01.X61 Direct infection of right knee in infectious and parasitic diseases classified elsewhere*
   ▸ *M01.X62 Direct infection of left knee in infectious and parasitic diseases classified elsewhere*
   ▸ *M01.X69 Direct infection of unspecified knee in infectious and parasitic diseases classified elsewhere*

● **M01.X7 Direct infection of ankle and foot in infectious and parasitic diseases classified elsewhere**
   Direct infection of tarsus, metatarsus and phalanges in infectious and parasitic diseases classified elsewhere
   ▸ *M01.X71 Direct infection of right ankle and foot in infectious and parasitic diseases classified elsewhere*

   ▸ *M01.X72 Direct infection of left ankle and foot in infectious and parasitic diseases classified elsewhere*
   ▸ *M01.X79 Direct infection of unspecified ankle and foot in infectious and parasitic diseases classified elsewhere*
   ▸ *M01.X8 Direct infection of vertebrae in infectious and parasitic diseases classified elsewhere*
   ▸ *M01.X9 Direct infection of multiple joints in infectious and parasitic diseases classified elsewhere*

● **M02 Postinfective and reactive arthropathies**
   Code first underlying disease, such as:
       congenital syphilis [Clutton's joints] (A50.5)
       enteritis due to Yersinia enterocolitica (A04.6)
       infective endocarditis (I33.0)
       viral hepatitis (B15-B19)
   Excludes1   Behçet's disease (M35.2)
       direct infections of joint in infectious and parasitic diseases classified elsewhere (M01.-)
       postmeningococcal arthritis (A39.84)
       mumps arthritis (B26.85)
       rubella arthritis (B06.82)
       syphilis arthritis (late) (A52.77)
       rheumatic fever (I00)
       tabetic arthropathy [Charcôt's] (A52.16)

● **M02.0 Arthropathy following intestinal bypass**
   M02.00 Arthropathy following intestinal bypass, unspecified site
   ● **M02.01 Arthropathy following intestinal bypass, shoulder**
       M02.011 Arthropathy following intestinal bypass, right shoulder
       M02.012 Arthropathy following intestinal bypass, left shoulder
       M02.019 Arthropathy following intestinal bypass, unspecified shoulder
   ● **M02.02 Arthropathy following intestinal bypass, elbow**
       M02.021 Arthropathy following intestinal bypass, right elbow
       M02.022 Arthropathy following intestinal bypass, left elbow
       M02.029 Arthropathy following intestinal bypass, unspecified elbow
   ● **M02.03 Arthropathy following intestinal bypass, wrist**
       Arthropathy following intestinal bypass, carpal bones
       M02.031 Arthropathy following intestinal bypass, right wrist
       M02.032 Arthropathy following intestinal bypass, left wrist
       M02.039 Arthropathy following intestinal bypass, unspecified wrist
   ● **M02.04 Arthropathy following intestinal bypass, hand**
       Arthropathy following intestinal bypass, metacarpals and phalanges
       M02.041 Arthropathy following intestinal bypass, right hand
       M02.042 Arthropathy following intestinal bypass, left hand
       M02.049 Arthropathy following intestinal bypass, unspecified hand
   ● **M02.05 Arthropathy following intestinal bypass, hip**
       M02.051 Arthropathy following intestinal bypass, right hip
       M02.052 Arthropathy following intestinal bypass, left hip
       M02.059 Arthropathy following intestinal bypass, unspecified hip

CHAPTER 13 (M00-M99)

- ● **M02.06** Arthropathy following intestinal bypass, knee
    - **M02.061** Arthropathy following intestinal bypass, right knee
    - **M02.062** Arthropathy following intestinal bypass, left knee
    - **M02.069** Arthropathy following intestinal bypass, unspecified knee
- ● **M02.07** Arthropathy following intestinal bypass, ankle and foot
    - Arthropathy following intestinal bypass, tarsus, metatarsus and phalanges
    - **M02.071** Arthropathy following intestinal bypass, right ankle and foot
    - **M02.072** Arthropathy following intestinal bypass, left ankle and foot
    - **M02.079** Arthropathy following intestinal bypass, unspecified ankle and foot
- **M02.08** Arthropathy following intestinal bypass, vertebrae
- **M02.09** Arthropathy following intestinal bypass, multiple sites
- ● **M02.1** Postdysenteric arthropathy
    - **M02.10** Postdysenteric arthropathy, unspecified site
    - ● **M02.11** Postdysenteric arthropathy, shoulder
        - **M02.111** Postdysenteric arthropathy, right shoulder
        - **M02.112** Postdysenteric arthropathy, left shoulder
        - **M02.119** Postdysenteric arthropathy, unspecified shoulder
    - ● **M02.12** Postdysenteric arthropathy, elbow
        - **M02.121** Postdysenteric arthropathy, right elbow
        - **M02.122** Postdysenteric arthropathy, left elbow
        - **M02.129** Postdysenteric arthropathy, unspecified elbow
    - ● **M02.13** Postdysenteric arthropathy, wrist
        - Postdysenteric arthropathy, carpal bones
        - **M02.131** Postdysenteric arthropathy, right wrist
        - **M02.132** Postdysenteric arthropathy, left wrist
        - **M02.139** Postdysenteric arthropathy, unspecified wrist
    - ● **M02.14** Postdysenteric arthropathy, hand
        - Postdysenteric arthropathy, metacarpus and phalanges
        - **M02.141** Postdysenteric arthropathy, right hand
        - **M02.142** Postdysenteric arthropathy, left hand
        - **M02.149** Postdysenteric arthropathy, unspecified hand
    - ● **M02.15** Postdysenteric arthropathy, hip
        - **M02.151** Postdysenteric arthropathy, right hip
        - **M02.152** Postdysenteric arthropathy, left hip
        - **M02.159** Postdysenteric arthropathy, unspecified hip
    - ● **M02.16** Postdysenteric arthropathy, knee
        - **M02.161** Postdysenteric arthropathy, right knee
        - **M02.162** Postdysenteric arthropathy, left knee
        - **M02.169** Postdysenteric arthropathy, unspecified knee
    - ● **M02.17** Postdysenteric arthropathy, ankle and foot
        - Postdysenteric arthropathy, tarsus, metatarsus and phalanges
        - **M02.171** Postdysenteric arthropathy, right ankle and foot
        - **M02.172** Postdysenteric arthropathy, left ankle and foot
        - **M02.179** Postdysenteric arthropathy, unspecified ankle and foot
    - **M02.18** Postdysenteric arthropathy, vertebrae
    - **M02.19** Postdysenteric arthropathy, multiple sites
- ● **M02.2** Postimmunization arthropathy
    - **M02.20** Postimmunization arthropathy, unspecified site
    - ● **M02.21** Postimmunization arthropathy, shoulder
        - **M02.211** Postimmunization arthropathy, right shoulder
        - **M02.212** Postimmunization arthropathy, left shoulder
        - **M02.219** Postimmunization arthropathy, unspecified shoulder
    - ● **M02.22** Postimmunization arthropathy, elbow
        - **M02.221** Postimmunization arthropathy, right elbow
        - **M02.222** Postimmunization arthropathy, left elbow
        - **M02.229** Postimmunization arthropathy, unspecified elbow
    - ● **M02.23** Postimmunization arthropathy, wrist
        - Postimmunization arthropathy, carpal bones
        - **M02.231** Postimmunization arthropathy, right wrist
        - **M02.232** Postimmunization arthropathy, left wrist
        - **M02.239** Postimmunization arthropathy, unspecified wrist
    - ● **M02.24** Postimmunization arthropathy, hand
        - Postimmunization arthropathy, metacarpus and phalanges
        - **M02.241** Postimmunization arthropathy, right hand
        - **M02.242** Postimmunization arthropathy, left hand
        - **M02.249** Postimmunization arthropathy, unspecified hand
    - ● **M02.25** Postimmunization arthropathy, hip
        - **M02.251** Postimmunization arthropathy, right hip
        - **M02.252** Postimmunization arthropathy, left hip
        - **M02.259** Postimmunization arthropathy, unspecified hip
    - ● **M02.26** Postimmunization arthropathy, knee
        - **M02.261** Postimmunization arthropathy, right knee
        - **M02.262** Postimmunization arthropathy, left knee
        - **M02.269** Postimmunization arthropathy, unspecified knee

▶ New   ⇨ Revised   ~~deleted~~ Deleted   Excludes 1   Excludes 2   Includes   Use additional   Code first   Code also   Key words
OGCR Official Guidelines   X Assign placeholder X   ● Use Additional Character(s)   ▶ Manifestation Code   🅷🄲🄲 Hierarchical Condition Category   **Coding Clinic**

● **M02.27 Postimmunization arthropathy, ankle and foot**
   Postimmunization arthropathy, tarsus, metatarsus and phalanges
   M02.271 Postimmunization arthropathy, right ankle and foot
   M02.272 Postimmunization arthropathy, left ankle and foot
   M02.279 Postimmunization arthropathy, unspecified ankle and foot
   M02.28 Postimmunization arthropathy, vertebrae
   M02.29 Postimmunization arthropathy, multiple sites
● M02.3 **Reiter's disease**
   Reactive arthritis
   M02.30 Reiter's disease, unspecified site
● M02.31 Reiter's disease, shoulder
   M02.311 Reiter's disease, right shoulder
   M02.312 Reiter's disease, left shoulder
   M02.319 Reiter's disease, unspecified shoulder
● M02.32 Reiter's disease, elbow
   M02.321 Reiter's disease, right elbow
   M02.322 Reiter's disease, left elbow
   M02.329 Reiter's disease, unspecified elbow
● M02.33 Reiter's disease, wrist
   Reiter's disease, carpal bones
   M02.331 Reiter's disease, right wrist
   M02.332 Reiter's disease, left wrist
   M02.339 Reiter's disease, unspecified wrist
● M02.34 Reiter's disease, hand
   Reiter's disease, metacarpus and phalanges
   M02.341 Reiter's disease, right hand
   M02.342 Reiter's disease, left hand
   M02.349 Reiter's disease, unspecified hand
● M02.35 Reiter's disease, hip
   M02.351 Reiter's disease, right hip
   M02.352 Reiter's disease, left hip
   M02.359 Reiter's disease, unspecified hip
● M02.36 Reiter's disease, knee
   M02.361 Reiter's disease, right knee
   M02.362 Reiter's disease, left knee
   M02.369 Reiter's disease, unspecified knee
● M02.37 Reiter's disease, ankle and foot
   Reiter's disease, tarsus, metatarsus and phalanges
   M02.371 Reiter's disease, right ankle and foot
   M02.372 Reiter's disease, left ankle and foot
   M02.379 Reiter's disease, unspecified ankle and foot

   M02.38 Reiter's disease, vertebrae
   M02.39 Reiter's disease, multiple sites
● M02.8 Other reactive arthropathies
   M02.80 Other reactive arthropathies, unspecified site
● M02.81 Other reactive arthropathies, shoulder
   M02.811 Other reactive arthropathies, right shoulder
   M02.812 Other reactive arthropathies, left shoulder
   M02.819 Other reactive arthropathies, unspecified shoulder
● M02.82 Other reactive arthropathies, elbow
   M02.821 Other reactive arthropathies, right elbow
   M02.822 Other reactive arthropathies, left elbow
   M02.829 Other reactive arthropathies, unspecified elbow
● M02.83 Other reactive arthropathies, wrist
   Other reactive arthropathies, carpal bones
   M02.831 Other reactive arthropathies, right wrist
   M02.832 Other reactive arthropathies, left wrist
   M02.839 Other reactive arthropathies, unspecified wrist
● M02.84 Other reactive arthropathies, hand
   Other reactive arthropathies, metacarpus and phalanges
   M02.841 Other reactive arthropathies, right hand
   M02.842 Other reactive arthropathies, left hand
   M02.849 Other reactive arthropathies, unspecified hand
● M02.85 Other reactive arthropathies, hip
   M02.851 Other reactive arthropathies, right hip
   M02.852 Other reactive arthropathies, left hip
   M02.859 Other reactive arthropathies, unspecified hip
● M02.86 Other reactive arthropathies, knee
   M02.861 Other reactive arthropathies, right knee
   M02.862 Other reactive arthropathies, left knee
   M02.869 Other reactive arthropathies, unspecified knee
● M02.87 Other reactive arthropathies, ankle and foot
   Other reactive arthropathies, tarsus, metatarsus and phalanges
   M02.871 Other reactive arthropathies, right ankle and foot
   M02.872 Other reactive arthropathies, left ankle and foot
   M02.879 Other reactive arthropathies, unspecified ankle and foot
   M02.88 Other reactive arthropathies, vertebrae
   M02.89 Other reactive arthropathies, multiple sites
   M02.9 Reactive arthropathy, unspecified

CHAPTER 13 (M00–M99)

AUTOINFLAMMATORY SYNDROMES (M04)

● **M04 Autoinflammatory syndromes**
     Excludes2   Crohn's disease (K50.-)
     Coding Clinic: 2016, Q4, P37

     M04.1 Periodic fever syndromes Ⓗ
         Familial Mediterranean fever
         Hyperimmunoglobin D syndrome
         Mevalonate kinase deficiency
         Tumor necrosis factor receptor associated periodic
           syndrome [TRAPS]

     M04.2 Cryopyrin-associated periodic syndromes Ⓗ
         Chronic infantile neurological, cutaneous and articular
           syndrome [CINCA]
         Familial cold autoinflammatory syndrome
         Familial cold urticaria
         Muckle-Wells syndrome
         Neonatal onset multisystemic inflammatory disorder
           [NOMID]

     M04.8 Other autoinflammatory syndromes Ⓗ
         Blau syndrome
         Deficiency of interleukin 1 receptor antagonist [DIRA]
         Majeed syndrome
         Periodic fever, aphthous stomatitis, pharyngitis, and
           adenopathy syndrome [PFAPA]
         Pyogenic arthritis, pyoderma gangrenosum, and acne
           syndrome [PAPA]

     M04.9 Autoinflammatory syndrome, unspecified Ⓗ

INFLAMMATORY POLYARTHROPATHIES (M05-M14)

● **M05 Rheumatoid arthritis with rheumatoid factor**
     Excludes1   rheumatic fever (I00)
           juvenile rheumatoid arthritis (M08.-)
           rheumatoid arthritis of spine (M45.-)

  ● **M05.0 Felty's syndrome**
         Rheumatoid arthritis with splenoadenomegaly and
           leukopenia

     M05.00   Felty's syndrome, unspecified site Ⓗ
  ● M05.01   Felty's syndrome, shoulder
         M05.011   Felty's syndrome, right shoulder Ⓗ
         M05.012   Felty's syndrome, left shoulder Ⓗ
         M05.019   Felty's syndrome, unspecified
              shoulder Ⓗ
  ● M05.02   Felty's syndrome, elbow
         M05.021   Felty's syndrome, right elbow Ⓗ
         M05.022   Felty's syndrome, left elbow Ⓗ
         M05.029   Felty's syndrome, unspecified elbow Ⓗ
  ● M05.03   Felty's syndrome, wrist
           Felty's syndrome, carpal bones
         M05.031   Felty's syndrome, right wrist Ⓗ
         M05.032   Felty's syndrome, left wrist Ⓗ
         M05.039   Felty's syndrome, unspecified wrist Ⓗ
  ● M05.04   Felty's syndrome, hand
           Felty's syndrome, metacarpus and phalanges
         M05.041   Felty's syndrome, right hand Ⓗ
         M05.042   Felty's syndrome, left hand Ⓗ
         M05.049   Felty's syndrome, unspecified hand Ⓗ
  ● M05.05   Felty's syndrome, hip
         M05.051   Felty's syndrome, right hip Ⓗ
         M05.052   Felty's syndrome, left hip Ⓗ
         M05.059   Felty's syndrome, unspecified hip Ⓗ

  ● M05.06   Felty's syndrome, knee
         M05.061   Felty's syndrome, right knee Ⓗ
         M05.062   Felty's syndrome, left knee Ⓗ
         M05.069   Felty's syndrome, unspecified knee Ⓗ
  ● M05.07   Felty's syndrome, ankle and foot
           Felty's syndrome, tarsus, metatarsus and
              phalanges
         M05.071   Felty's syndrome, right ankle and
              foot Ⓗ
         M05.072   Felty's syndrome, left ankle and foot Ⓗ
         M05.079   Felty's syndrome, unspecified ankle
              and foot Ⓗ
     M05.09   Felty's syndrome, multiple sites Ⓗ
● M05.1   Rheumatoid lung disease with rheumatoid arthritis
     M05.10   Rheumatoid lung disease with rheumatoid
           arthritis of unspecified site Ⓗ
  ● M05.11   Rheumatoid lung disease with rheumatoid
           arthritis of shoulder
         M05.111   Rheumatoid lung disease with
              rheumatoid arthritis of right
              shoulder Ⓗ
         M05.112   Rheumatoid lung disease with
              rheumatoid arthritis of left shoulder Ⓗ
         M05.119   Rheumatoid lung disease with
              rheumatoid arthritis of unspecified
              shoulder Ⓗ
  ● M05.12   Rheumatoid lung disease with rheumatoid
           arthritis of elbow
         M05.121   Rheumatoid lung disease with
              rheumatoid arthritis of right elbow Ⓗ
         M05.122   Rheumatoid lung disease with
              rheumatoid arthritis of left elbow Ⓗ
         M05.129   Rheumatoid lung disease with
              rheumatoid arthritis of unspecified
              elbow Ⓗ
  ● M05.13   Rheumatoid lung disease with rheumatoid
           arthritis of wrist
           Rheumatoid lung disease with rheumatoid
              arthritis, carpal bones
         M05.131   Rheumatoid lung disease with
              rheumatoid arthritis of right wrist Ⓗ
         M05.132   Rheumatoid lung disease with
              rheumatoid arthritis of left wrist Ⓗ
         M05.139   Rheumatoid lung disease with
              rheumatoid arthritis of unspecified
              wrist Ⓗ
  ● M05.14   Rheumatoid lung disease with rheumatoid
           arthritis of hand
           Rheumatoid lung disease with rheumatoid
              arthritis, metacarpus and phalanges
         M05.141   Rheumatoid lung disease with
              rheumatoid arthritis of right hand Ⓗ
         M05.142   Rheumatoid lung disease with
              rheumatoid arthritis of left hand Ⓗ
         M05.149   Rheumatoid lung disease with
              rheumatoid arthritis of unspecified
              hand Ⓗ
  ● M05.15   Rheumatoid lung disease with rheumatoid
           arthritis of hip
         M05.151   Rheumatoid lung disease with
              rheumatoid arthritis of right hip Ⓗ
         M05.152   Rheumatoid lung disease with
              rheumatoid arthritis of left hip Ⓗ
         M05.159   Rheumatoid lung disease with
              rheumatoid arthritis of unspecified
              hip Ⓗ

Item 13–1   Rheumatoid arthritis (RA) is a chronic systemic inflammatory autoimmune disease of undetermined etiology involving primarily the synovial membranes and articular structures of multiple joints. It can also affect other organs, including the eyes, blood vessels, heart, and lungs. The disease is often progressive. In late stages, deformity, ankylosis, and other **inflammatory polyarthropathies** develop.

▶ New   ⬅ Revised   ~~deleted~~ Deleted   Excludes 1   Excludes 2   Includes   Use additional   Code first   Code also   Key words
OGCR Official Guidelines   X Assign placeholder X   ● Use Additional Character(s)   ▸ Manifestation Code   Ⓗ Hierarchical Condition Category   **Coding Clinic**

● **M05.16** Rheumatoid lung disease with rheumatoid arthritis of knee

 M05.161 Rheumatoid lung disease with rheumatoid arthritis of right knee ◊

 M05.162 Rheumatoid lung disease with rheumatoid arthritis of left knee ◊

 M05.169 Rheumatoid lung disease with rheumatoid arthritis of unspecified knee ◊

● **M05.17** Rheumatoid lung disease with rheumatoid arthritis of ankle and foot

 Rheumatoid lung disease with rheumatoid arthritis, tarsus, metatarsus and phalanges

 M05.171 Rheumatoid lung disease with rheumatoid arthritis of right ankle and foot ◊

 M05.172 Rheumatoid lung disease with rheumatoid arthritis of left ankle and foot ◊

 M05.179 Rheumatoid lung disease with rheumatoid arthritis of unspecified ankle and foot ◊

M05.19 Rheumatoid lung disease with rheumatoid arthritis of multiple sites ◊

● **M05.2** Rheumatoid vasculitis with rheumatoid arthritis

M05.20 Rheumatoid vasculitis with rheumatoid arthritis of unspecified site ◊

● **M05.21** Rheumatoid vasculitis with rheumatoid arthritis of shoulder

 M05.211 Rheumatoid vasculitis with rheumatoid arthritis of right shoulder ◊

 M05.212 Rheumatoid vasculitis with rheumatoid arthritis of left shoulder ◊

 M05.219 Rheumatoid vasculitis with rheumatoid arthritis of unspecified shoulder ◊

● **M05.22** Rheumatoid vasculitis with rheumatoid arthritis of elbow

 M05.221 Rheumatoid vasculitis with rheumatoid arthritis of right elbow ◊

 M05.222 Rheumatoid vasculitis with rheumatoid arthritis of left elbow ◊

 M05.229 Rheumatoid vasculitis with rheumatoid arthritis of unspecified elbow ◊

● **M05.23** Rheumatoid vasculitis with rheumatoid arthritis of wrist

 Rheumatoid vasculitis with rheumatoid arthritis, carpal bones

 M05.231 Rheumatoid vasculitis with rheumatoid arthritis of right wrist ◊

 M05.232 Rheumatoid vasculitis with rheumatoid arthritis of left wrist ◊

 M05.239 Rheumatoid vasculitis with rheumatoid arthritis of unspecified wrist ◊

● **M05.24** Rheumatoid vasculitis with rheumatoid arthritis of hand

 Rheumatoid vasculitis with rheumatoid arthritis, metacarpus and phalanges

 M05.241 Rheumatoid vasculitis with rheumatoid arthritis of right hand ◊

 M05.242 Rheumatoid vasculitis with rheumatoid arthritis of left hand ◊

 M05.249 Rheumatoid vasculitis with rheumatoid arthritis of unspecified hand ◊

● **M05.25** Rheumatoid vasculitis with rheumatoid arthritis of hip

 M05.251 Rheumatoid vasculitis with rheumatoid arthritis of right hip ◊

 M05.252 Rheumatoid vasculitis with rheumatoid arthritis of left hip ◊

 M05.259 Rheumatoid vasculitis with rheumatoid arthritis of unspecified hip ◊

● **M05.26** Rheumatoid vasculitis with rheumatoid arthritis of knee

 M05.261 Rheumatoid vasculitis with rheumatoid arthritis of right knee ◊

 M05.262 Rheumatoid vasculitis with rheumatoid arthritis of left knee ◊

 M05.269 Rheumatoid vasculitis with rheumatoid arthritis of unspecified knee ◊

● **M05.27** Rheumatoid vasculitis with rheumatoid arthritis of ankle and foot

 Rheumatoid vasculitis with rheumatoid arthritis, tarsus, metatarsus and phalanges

 M05.271 Rheumatoid vasculitis with rheumatoid arthritis of right ankle and foot ◊

 M05.272 Rheumatoid vasculitis with rheumatoid arthritis of left ankle and foot ◊

 M05.279 Rheumatoid vasculitis with rheumatoid arthritis of unspecified ankle and foot ◊

M05.29 Rheumatoid vasculitis with rheumatoid arthritis of multiple sites ◊

● **M05.3** Rheumatoid heart disease with rheumatoid arthritis

 Rheumatoid carditis

 Rheumatoid endocarditis

 Rheumatoid myocarditis

 Rheumatoid pericarditis

M05.30 Rheumatoid heart disease with rheumatoid arthritis of unspecified site ◊

● **M05.31** Rheumatoid heart disease with rheumatoid arthritis of shoulder

 M05.311 Rheumatoid heart disease with rheumatoid arthritis of right shoulder ◊

 M05.312 Rheumatoid heart disease with rheumatoid arthritis of left shoulder ◊

 M05.319 Rheumatoid heart disease with rheumatoid arthritis of unspecified shoulder ◊

● **M05.32** Rheumatoid heart disease with rheumatoid arthritis of elbow

 M05.321 Rheumatoid heart disease with rheumatoid arthritis of right elbow ◊

 M05.322 Rheumatoid heart disease with rheumatoid arthritis of left elbow ◊

 M05.329 Rheumatoid heart disease with rheumatoid arthritis of unspecified elbow ◊

● **M05.33** Rheumatoid heart disease with rheumatoid arthritis of wrist

 Rheumatoid heart disease with rheumatoid arthritis, carpal bones

 M05.331 Rheumatoid heart disease with rheumatoid arthritis of right wrist ◊

 M05.332 Rheumatoid heart disease with rheumatoid arthritis of left wrist ◊

 M05.339 Rheumatoid heart disease with rheumatoid arthritis of unspecified wrist ◊

● **M05.34 Rheumatoid heart disease with rheumatoid arthritis of hand**
Rheumatoid heart disease with rheumatoid arthritis, metacarpus and phalanges

M05.341   **Rheumatoid heart disease with rheumatoid arthritis of right hand** ℞

M05.342   **Rheumatoid heart disease with rheumatoid arthritis of left hand** ℞

M05.349   **Rheumatoid heart disease with rheumatoid arthritis of unspecified hand** ℞

● **M05.35 Rheumatoid heart disease with rheumatoid arthritis of hip**

M05.351   **Rheumatoid heart disease with rheumatoid arthritis of right hip** ℞

M05.352   **Rheumatoid heart disease with rheumatoid arthritis of left hip** ℞

M05.359   **Rheumatoid heart disease with rheumatoid arthritis of unspecified hip** ℞

● **M05.36 Rheumatoid heart disease with rheumatoid arthritis of knee**

M05.361   **Rheumatoid heart disease with rheumatoid arthritis of right knee** ℞

M05.362   **Rheumatoid heart disease with rheumatoid arthritis of left knee** ℞

M05.369   **Rheumatoid heart disease with rheumatoid arthritis of unspecified knee** ℞

● **M05.37 Rheumatoid heart disease with rheumatoid arthritis of ankle and foot**
Rheumatoid heart disease with rheumatoid arthritis, tarsus, metatarsus and phalanges

M05.371   **Rheumatoid heart disease with rheumatoid arthritis of right ankle and foot** ℞

M05.372   **Rheumatoid heart disease with rheumatoid arthritis of left ankle and foot** ℞

M05.379   **Rheumatoid heart disease with rheumatoid arthritis of unspecified ankle and foot** ℞

M05.39   **Rheumatoid heart disease with rheumatoid arthritis of multiple sites** ℞

● **M05.4 Rheumatoid myopathy with rheumatoid arthritis**

M05.40   **Rheumatoid myopathy with rheumatoid arthritis of unspecified site** ℞

● **M05.41 Rheumatoid myopathy with rheumatoid arthritis of shoulder**

M05.411   **Rheumatoid myopathy with rheumatoid arthritis of right shoulder** ℞

M05.412   **Rheumatoid myopathy with rheumatoid arthritis of left shoulder** ℞

M05.419   **Rheumatoid myopathy with rheumatoid arthritis of unspecified shoulder** ℞

● **M05.42 Rheumatoid myopathy with rheumatoid arthritis of elbow**

M05.421   **Rheumatoid myopathy with rheumatoid arthritis of right elbow** ℞

M05.422   **Rheumatoid myopathy with rheumatoid arthritis of left elbow** ℞

M05.429   **Rheumatoid myopathy with rheumatoid arthritis of unspecified elbow** ℞

● **M05.43 Rheumatoid myopathy with rheumatoid arthritis of wrist**
Rheumatoid myopathy with rheumatoid arthritis, carpal bones

M05.431   **Rheumatoid myopathy with rheumatoid arthritis of right wrist** ℞

M05.432   **Rheumatoid myopathy with rheumatoid arthritis of left wrist** ℞

M05.439   **Rheumatoid myopathy with rheumatoid arthritis of unspecified wrist** ℞

● **M05.44 Rheumatoid myopathy with rheumatoid arthritis of hand**
Rheumatoid myopathy with rheumatoid arthritis, metacarpus and phalanges

M05.441   **Rheumatoid myopathy with rheumatoid arthritis of right hand** ℞

M05.442   **Rheumatoid myopathy with rheumatoid arthritis of left hand** ℞

M05.449   **Rheumatoid myopathy with rheumatoid arthritis of unspecified hand** ℞

● **M05.45 Rheumatoid myopathy with rheumatoid arthritis of hip**

M05.451   **Rheumatoid myopathy with rheumatoid arthritis of right hip** ℞

M05.452   **Rheumatoid myopathy with rheumatoid arthritis of left hip** ℞

M05.459   **Rheumatoid myopathy with rheumatoid arthritis of unspecified hip** ℞

● **M05.46 Rheumatoid myopathy with rheumatoid arthritis of knee**

M05.461   **Rheumatoid myopathy with rheumatoid arthritis of right knee** ℞

M05.462   **Rheumatoid myopathy with rheumatoid arthritis of left knee** ℞

M05.469   **Rheumatoid myopathy with rheumatoid arthritis of unspecified knee** ℞

● **M05.47 Rheumatoid myopathy with rheumatoid arthritis of ankle and foot**
Rheumatoid myopathy with rheumatoid arthritis, tarsus, metatarsus and phalanges

M05.471   **Rheumatoid myopathy with rheumatoid arthritis of right ankle and foot** ℞

M05.472   **Rheumatoid myopathy with rheumatoid arthritis of left ankle and foot** ℞

M05.479   **Rheumatoid myopathy with rheumatoid arthritis of unspecified ankle and foot** ℞

M05.49   **Rheumatoid myopathy with rheumatoid arthritis of multiple sites** ℞

● **M05.5 Rheumatoid polyneuropathy with rheumatoid arthritis**

M05.50   **Rheumatoid polyneuropathy with rheumatoid arthritis of unspecified site** ℞

● **M05.51 Rheumatoid polyneuropathy with rheumatoid arthritis of shoulder**

M05.511   **Rheumatoid polyneuropathy with rheumatoid arthritis of right shoulder** ℞

M05.512   **Rheumatoid polyneuropathy with rheumatoid arthritis of left shoulder** ℞

M05.519   **Rheumatoid polyneuropathy with rheumatoid arthritis of unspecified shoulder** ℞

▶ New   ⇨ Revised   ~~deleted~~ Deleted   Excludes 1   Excludes 2   Includes   Use additional   Code first   Code also   Key words
OGCR Official Guidelines   X Assign placeholder X   ● Use Additional Character(s)   ▸ Manifestation Code   ℞ Hierarchical Condition Category   Coding Clinic

● **M05.52**   **Rheumatoid polyneuropathy with rheumatoid arthritis of elbow**

     M05.521   Rheumatoid polyneuropathy with rheumatoid arthritis of right elbow

     M05.522   Rheumatoid polyneuropathy with rheumatoid arthritis of left elbow

     M05.529   Rheumatoid polyneuropathy with rheumatoid arthritis of unspecified elbow

● **M05.53**   **Rheumatoid polyneuropathy with rheumatoid arthritis of wrist**

     Rheumatoid polyneuropathy with rheumatoid arthritis, carpal bones

     M05.531   Rheumatoid polyneuropathy with rheumatoid arthritis of right wrist

     M05.532   Rheumatoid polyneuropathy with rheumatoid arthritis of left wrist

     M05.539   Rheumatoid polyneuropathy with rheumatoid arthritis of unspecified wrist

● **M05.54**   **Rheumatoid polyneuropathy with rheumatoid arthritis of hand**

     Rheumatoid polyneuropathy with rheumatoid arthritis, metacarpus and phalanges

     M05.541   Rheumatoid polyneuropathy with rheumatoid arthritis of right hand

     M05.542   Rheumatoid polyneuropathy with rheumatoid arthritis of left hand

     M05.549   Rheumatoid polyneuropathy with rheumatoid arthritis of unspecified hand

● **M05.55**   **Rheumatoid polyneuropathy with rheumatoid arthritis of hip**

     M05.551   Rheumatoid polyneuropathy with rheumatoid arthritis of right hip

     M05.552   Rheumatoid polyneuropathy with rheumatoid arthritis of left hip

     M05.559   Rheumatoid polyneuropathy with rheumatoid arthritis of unspecified hip

● **M05.56**   **Rheumatoid polyneuropathy with rheumatoid arthritis of knee**

     M05.561   Rheumatoid polyneuropathy with rheumatoid arthritis of right knee

     M05.562   Rheumatoid polyneuropathy with rheumatoid arthritis of left knee

     M05.569   Rheumatoid polyneuropathy with rheumatoid arthritis of unspecified knee

● **M05.57**   **Rheumatoid polyneuropathy with rheumatoid arthritis of ankle and foot**

     Rheumatoid polyneuropathy with rheumatoid arthritis, tarsus, metatarsus and phalanges

     M05.571   Rheumatoid polyneuropathy with rheumatoid arthritis of right ankle and foot

     M05.572   Rheumatoid polyneuropathy with rheumatoid arthritis of left ankle and foot

     M05.579   Rheumatoid polyneuropathy with rheumatoid arthritis of unspecified ankle and foot

M05.59   **Rheumatoid polyneuropathy with rheumatoid arthritis of multiple sites**

● **M05.6**   **Rheumatoid arthritis with involvement of other organs and systems**

     M05.60   Rheumatoid arthritis of unspecified site with involvement of other organs and systems

●   **M05.61**   **Rheumatoid arthritis of shoulder with involvement of other organs and systems**

     M05.611   Rheumatoid arthritis of right shoulder with involvement of other organs and systems

     M05.612   Rheumatoid arthritis of left shoulder with involvement of other organs and systems

     M05.619   Rheumatoid arthritis of unspecified shoulder with involvement of other organs and systems

●   **M05.62**   **Rheumatoid arthritis of elbow with involvement of other organs and systems**

     M05.621   Rheumatoid arthritis of right elbow with involvement of other organs and systems

     M05.622   Rheumatoid arthritis of left elbow with involvement of other organs and systems

     M05.629   Rheumatoid arthritis of unspecified elbow with involvement of other organs and systems

●   **M05.63**   **Rheumatoid arthritis of wrist with involvement of other organs and systems**

     Rheumatoid arthritis of carpal bones with involvement of other organs and systems

     M05.631   Rheumatoid arthritis of right wrist with involvement of other organs and systems

     M05.632   Rheumatoid arthritis of left wrist with involvement of other organs and systems

     M05.639   Rheumatoid arthritis of unspecified wrist with involvement of other organs and systems

●   **M05.64**   **Rheumatoid arthritis of hand with involvement of other organs and systems**

     Rheumatoid arthritis of metacarpus and phalanges with involvement of other organs and systems

     M05.641   Rheumatoid arthritis of right hand with involvement of other organs and systems

     M05.642   Rheumatoid arthritis of left hand with involvement of other organs and systems

     M05.649   Rheumatoid arthritis of unspecified hand with involvement of other organs and systems

●   **M05.65**   **Rheumatoid arthritis of hip with involvement of other organs and systems**

     M05.651   Rheumatoid arthritis of right hip with involvement of other organs and systems

     M05.652   Rheumatoid arthritis of left hip with involvement of other organs and systems

     M05.659   Rheumatoid arthritis of unspecified hip with involvement of other organs and systems

CHAPTER 13 (M00-M99)

● **M05.66 Rheumatoid arthritis of knee with involvement of other organs and systems**

M05.661 Rheumatoid arthritis of right knee with involvement of other organs and systems RCC

M05.662 Rheumatoid arthritis of left knee with involvement of other organs and systems RCC

M05.669 Rheumatoid arthritis of unspecified knee with involvement of other organs and systems RCC

● **M05.67 Rheumatoid arthritis of ankle and foot with involvement of other organs and systems**

Rheumatoid arthritis of tarsus, metatarsus and phalanges with involvement of other organs and systems

M05.671 Rheumatoid arthritis of right ankle and foot with involvement of other organs and systems RCC

M05.672 Rheumatoid arthritis of left ankle and foot with involvement of other organs and systems RCC

M05.679 Rheumatoid arthritis of unspecified ankle and foot with involvement of other organs and systems RCC

M05.69 Rheumatoid arthritis of multiple sites with involvement of other organs and systems RCC

● **M05.7 Rheumatoid arthritis with rheumatoid factor without organ or systems involvement**

M05.70 Rheumatoid arthritis with rheumatoid factor of unspecified site without organ or systems involvement RCC

● **M05.71 Rheumatoid arthritis with rheumatoid factor of shoulder without organ or systems involvement**

M05.711 Rheumatoid arthritis with rheumatoid factor of right shoulder without organ or systems involvement RCC

M05.712 Rheumatoid arthritis with rheumatoid factor of left shoulder without organ or systems involvement RCC

M05.719 Rheumatoid arthritis with rheumatoid factor of unspecified shoulder without organ or systems involvement RCC

● **M05.72 Rheumatoid arthritis with rheumatoid factor of elbow without organ or systems involvement**

M05.721 Rheumatoid arthritis with rheumatoid factor of right elbow without organ or systems involvement RCC

M05.722 Rheumatoid arthritis with rheumatoid factor of left elbow without organ or systems involvement RCC

M05.729 Rheumatoid arthritis with rheumatoid factor of unspecified elbow without organ or systems involvement RCC

● **M05.73 Rheumatoid arthritis with rheumatoid factor of wrist without organ or systems involvement**

M05.731 Rheumatoid arthritis with rheumatoid factor of right wrist without organ or systems involvement RCC

M05.732 Rheumatoid arthritis with rheumatoid factor of left wrist without organ or systems involvement RCC

M05.739 Rheumatoid arthritis with rheumatoid factor of unspecified wrist without organ or systems involvement RCC

● **M05.74 Rheumatoid arthritis with rheumatoid factor of hand without organ or systems involvement**

M05.741 Rheumatoid arthritis with rheumatoid factor of right hand without organ or systems involvement RCC

M05.742 Rheumatoid arthritis with rheumatoid factor of left hand without organ or systems involvement RCC

M05.749 Rheumatoid arthritis with rheumatoid factor of unspecified hand without organ or systems involvement RCC

● **M05.75 Rheumatoid arthritis with rheumatoid factor of hip without organ or systems involvement**

M05.751 Rheumatoid arthritis with rheumatoid factor of right hip without organ or systems involvement RCC

M05.752 Rheumatoid arthritis with rheumatoid factor of left hip without organ or systems involvement RCC

M05.759 Rheumatoid arthritis with rheumatoid factor of unspecified hip without organ or systems involvement RCC

● **M05.76 Rheumatoid arthritis with rheumatoid factor of knee without organ or systems involvement**

M05.761 Rheumatoid arthritis with rheumatoid factor of right knee without organ or systems involvement RCC

M05.762 Rheumatoid arthritis with rheumatoid factor of left knee without organ or systems involvement RCC

M05.769 Rheumatoid arthritis with rheumatoid factor of unspecified knee without organ or systems involvement RCC

● **M05.77 Rheumatoid arthritis with rheumatoid factor of ankle and foot without organ or systems involvement**

M05.771 Rheumatoid arthritis with rheumatoid factor of right ankle and foot without organ or systems involvement RCC

M05.772 Rheumatoid arthritis with rheumatoid factor of left ankle and foot without organ or systems involvement RCC

M05.779 Rheumatoid arthritis with rheumatoid factor of unspecified ankle and foot without organ or systems involvement RCC

M05.79 Rheumatoid arthritis with rheumatoid factor of multiple sites without organ or systems involvement RCC

M05.7A Rheumatoid arthritis with rheumatoid factor of other specified site without organ or systems involvement

- **M05.8** Other rheumatoid arthritis with rheumatoid factor
  - **M05.80** Other rheumatoid arthritis with rheumatoid factor of unspecified site
  - **M05.81** Other rheumatoid arthritis with rheumatoid factor of shoulder
    - **M05.811** Other rheumatoid arthritis with rheumatoid factor of right shoulder
    - **M05.812** Other rheumatoid arthritis with rheumatoid factor of left shoulder
    - **M05.819** Other rheumatoid arthritis with rheumatoid factor of unspecified shoulder
  - **M05.82** Other rheumatoid arthritis with rheumatoid factor of elbow
    - **M05.821** Other rheumatoid arthritis with rheumatoid factor of right elbow
    - **M05.822** Other rheumatoid arthritis with rheumatoid factor of left elbow
    - **M05.829** Other rheumatoid arthritis with rheumatoid factor of unspecified elbow
  - **M05.83** Other rheumatoid arthritis with rheumatoid factor of wrist
    - **M05.831** Other rheumatoid arthritis with rheumatoid factor of right wrist
    - **M05.832** Other rheumatoid arthritis with rheumatoid factor of left wrist
    - **M05.839** Other rheumatoid arthritis with rheumatoid factor of unspecified wrist
  - **M05.84** Other rheumatoid arthritis with rheumatoid factor of hand
    - **M05.841** Other rheumatoid arthritis with rheumatoid factor of right hand
    - **M05.842** Other rheumatoid arthritis with rheumatoid factor of left hand
    - **M05.849** Other rheumatoid arthritis with rheumatoid factor of unspecified hand
  - **M05.85** Other rheumatoid arthritis with rheumatoid factor of hip
    - **M05.851** Other rheumatoid arthritis with rheumatoid factor of right hip
    - **M05.852** Other rheumatoid arthritis with rheumatoid factor of left hip
    - **M05.859** Other rheumatoid arthritis with rheumatoid factor of unspecified hip
  - **M05.86** Other rheumatoid arthritis with rheumatoid factor of knee
    - **M05.861** Other rheumatoid arthritis with rheumatoid factor of right knee
    - **M05.862** Other rheumatoid arthritis with rheumatoid factor of left knee
    - **M05.869** Other rheumatoid arthritis with rheumatoid factor of unspecified knee
  - **M05.87** Other rheumatoid arthritis with rheumatoid factor of ankle and foot
    - **M05.871** Other rheumatoid arthritis with rheumatoid factor of right ankle and foot
    - **M05.872** Other rheumatoid arthritis with rheumatoid factor of left ankle and foot
    - **M05.879** Other rheumatoid arthritis with rheumatoid factor of unspecified ankle and foot
  - **M05.89** Other rheumatoid arthritis with rheumatoid factor of multiple sites
  - **M05.8A** Other rheumatoid arthritis with rheumatoid factor of other specified site
  - **M05.9** Rheumatoid arthritis with rheumatoid factor, unspecified
  - ▶**M05.A** Abnormal rheumatoid factor and anti-citrullinated protein antibody with rheumatoidarthritis
    - ▶ *Code first* rheumatoid arthritis with rheumatoid factor by site, if known (M05.00 to M05.8A)

- **M06** Other rheumatoid arthritis
  - **Coding Clinic: 2024, Q1, P17**
  - **M06.0** Rheumatoid arthritis without rheumatoid factor
    - **M06.00** Rheumatoid arthritis without rheumatoid factor, unspecified site
    - **M06.01** Rheumatoid arthritis without rheumatoid factor, shoulder
      - **M06.011** Rheumatoid arthritis without rheumatoid factor, right shoulder
      - **M06.012** Rheumatoid arthritis without rheumatoid factor, left shoulder
      - **M06.019** Rheumatoid arthritis without rheumatoid factor, unspecified shoulder
    - **M06.02** Rheumatoid arthritis without rheumatoid factor, elbow
      - **M06.021** Rheumatoid arthritis without rheumatoid factor, right elbow
      - **M06.022** Rheumatoid arthritis without rheumatoid factor, left elbow
      - **M06.029** Rheumatoid arthritis without rheumatoid factor, unspecified elbow
    - **M06.03** Rheumatoid arthritis without rheumatoid factor, wrist
      - **M06.031** Rheumatoid arthritis without rheumatoid factor, right wrist
      - **M06.032** Rheumatoid arthritis without rheumatoid factor, left wrist
      - **M06.039** Rheumatoid arthritis without rheumatoid factor, unspecified wrist
    - **M06.04** Rheumatoid arthritis without rheumatoid factor, hand
      - **M06.041** Rheumatoid arthritis without rheumatoid factor, right hand
      - **M06.042** Rheumatoid arthritis without rheumatoid factor, left hand
      - **M06.049** Rheumatoid arthritis without rheumatoid factor, unspecified hand
    - **M06.05** Rheumatoid arthritis without rheumatoid factor, hip
      - **M06.051** Rheumatoid arthritis without rheumatoid factor, right hip
      - **M06.052** Rheumatoid arthritis without rheumatoid factor, left hip
      - **M06.059** Rheumatoid arthritis without rheumatoid factor, unspecified hip
    - **M06.06** Rheumatoid arthritis without rheumatoid factor, knee
      - **M06.061** Rheumatoid arthritis without rheumatoid factor, right knee
      - **M06.062** Rheumatoid arthritis without rheumatoid factor, left knee
      - **M06.069** Rheumatoid arthritis without rheumatoid factor, unspecified knee

CHAPTER 13 (M00-M99)

● **M06.07　Rheumatoid arthritis without rheumatoid factor, ankle and foot**
　　M06.071　Rheumatoid arthritis without rheumatoid factor, right ankle and foot ℞
　　M06.072　Rheumatoid arthritis without rheumatoid factor, left ankle and foot ℞
　　M06.079　Rheumatoid arthritis without rheumatoid factor, unspecified ankle and foot ℞
　M06.08　Rheumatoid arthritis without rheumatoid factor, vertebrae ℞
　M06.09　Rheumatoid arthritis without rheumatoid factor, multiple sites ℞
　M06.0A　Rheumatoid arthritis without rheumatoid factor, other specified site
M06.1　Adult-onset Still's disease ℞　　　　　　　　A
　　Excludes1　Still's disease NOS (M08.2-)
● **M06.2　Rheumatoid bursitis**
　M06.20　Rheumatoid bursitis, unspecified site ℞
　● M06.21　Rheumatoid bursitis, shoulder
　　M06.211　Rheumatoid bursitis, right shoulder ℞
　　M06.212　Rheumatoid bursitis, left shoulder ℞
　　M06.219　Rheumatoid bursitis, unspecified shoulder ℞
　● M06.22　Rheumatoid bursitis, elbow
　　M06.221　Rheumatoid bursitis, right elbow ℞
　　M06.222　Rheumatoid bursitis, left elbow ℞
　　M06.229　Rheumatoid bursitis, unspecified elbow ℞
　● M06.23　Rheumatoid bursitis, wrist
　　M06.231　Rheumatoid bursitis, right wrist ℞
　　M06.232　Rheumatoid bursitis, left wrist ℞
　　M06.239　Rheumatoid bursitis, unspecified wrist ℞
　● M06.24　Rheumatoid bursitis, hand
　　M06.241　Rheumatoid bursitis, right hand ℞
　　M06.242　Rheumatoid bursitis, left hand ℞
　　M06.249　Rheumatoid bursitis, unspecified hand ℞
　● M06.25　Rheumatoid bursitis, hip
　　M06.251　Rheumatoid bursitis, right hip ℞
　　M06.252　Rheumatoid bursitis, left hip ℞
　　M06.259　Rheumatoid bursitis, unspecified hip ℞
　● M06.26　Rheumatoid bursitis, knee
　　M06.261　Rheumatoid bursitis, right knee ℞
　　M06.262　Rheumatoid bursitis, left knee ℞
　　M06.269　Rheumatoid bursitis, unspecified knee ℞
　● M06.27　Rheumatoid bursitis, ankle and foot
　　M06.271　Rheumatoid bursitis, right ankle and foot ℞
　　M06.272　Rheumatoid bursitis, left ankle and foot ℞
　　M06.279　Rheumatoid bursitis, unspecified ankle and foot ℞
　M06.28　Rheumatoid bursitis, vertebrae ℞
　M06.29　Rheumatoid bursitis, multiple sites ℞

● **M06.3　Rheumatoid nodule**
　M06.30　Rheumatoid nodule, unspecified site ℞
　● M06.31　Rheumatoid nodule, shoulder
　　M06.311　Rheumatoid nodule, right shoulder ℞
　　M06.312　Rheumatoid nodule, left shoulder ℞
　　M06.319　Rheumatoid nodule, unspecified shoulder ℞
　● M06.32　Rheumatoid nodule, elbow
　　M06.321　Rheumatoid nodule, right elbow ℞
　　M06.322　Rheumatoid nodule, left elbow ℞
　　M06.329　Rheumatoid nodule, unspecified elbow ℞
　● M06.33　Rheumatoid nodule, wrist
　　M06.331　Rheumatoid nodule, right wrist ℞
　　M06.332　Rheumatoid nodule, left wrist ℞
　　M06.339　Rheumatoid nodule, unspecified wrist ℞
　● M06.34　Rheumatoid nodule, hand
　　M06.341　Rheumatoid nodule, right hand ℞
　　M06.342　Rheumatoid nodule, left hand ℞
　　M06.349　Rheumatoid nodule, unspecified hand ℞
　● M06.35　Rheumatoid nodule, hip
　　M06.351　Rheumatoid nodule, right hip ℞
　　M06.352　Rheumatoid nodule, left hip ℞
　　M06.359　Rheumatoid nodule, unspecified hip ℞
　● M06.36　Rheumatoid nodule, knee
　　M06.361　Rheumatoid nodule, right knee ℞
　　M06.362　Rheumatoid nodule, left knee ℞
　　M06.369　Rheumatoid nodule, unspecified knee ℞
　● M06.37　Rheumatoid nodule, ankle and foot
　　M06.371　Rheumatoid nodule, right ankle and foot ℞
　　M06.372　Rheumatoid nodule, left ankle and foot ℞
　　M06.379　Rheumatoid nodule, unspecified ankle and foot ℞
　M06.38　Rheumatoid nodule, vertebrae ℞
　M06.39　Rheumatoid nodule, multiple sites ℞
M06.4　Inflammatory polyarthropathy ℞
　　Excludes1　polyarthritis NOS (M13.0)
　　Coding Clinic: 2025, Q2, P9-10; 2024, Q1, P17
● **M06.8　Other specified rheumatoid arthritis**
　M06.80　Other specified rheumatoid arthritis, unspecified site ℞
　● M06.81　Other specified rheumatoid arthritis, shoulder
　　M06.811　Other specified rheumatoid arthritis, right shoulder ℞
　　M06.812　Other specified rheumatoid arthritis, left shoulder ℞
　　M06.819　Other specified rheumatoid arthritis, unspecified shoulder ℞
　● M06.82　Other specified rheumatoid arthritis, elbow
　　M06.821　Other specified rheumatoid arthritis, right elbow ℞
　　M06.822　Other specified rheumatoid arthritis, left elbow ℞
　　M06.829　Other specified rheumatoid arthritis, unspecified elbow ℞

▶ New　　➡ Revised　　~~deleted~~ Deleted　　Excludes 1　　Excludes 2　　Includes　　Use additional　　Code first　　Code also　　Key words
OGCR Official Guidelines　　X Assign placeholder X　　● Use Additional Character(s)　　▸ Manifestation Code　　℞ Hierarchical Condition Category　　Coding Clinic

- **M06.83** Other specified rheumatoid arthritis, wrist
  - M06.831 Other specified rheumatoid arthritis, right wrist ⚲
  - M06.832 Other specified rheumatoid arthritis, left wrist ⚲
  - M06.839 Other specified rheumatoid arthritis, unspecified wrist ⚲
- **M06.84** Other specified rheumatoid arthritis, hand
  - M06.841 Other specified rheumatoid arthritis, right hand ⚲
  - M06.842 Other specified rheumatoid arthritis, left hand ⚲
  - M06.849 Other specified rheumatoid arthritis, unspecified hand ⚲
- **M06.85** Other specified rheumatoid arthritis, hip
  - M06.851 Other specified rheumatoid arthritis, right hip ⚲
  - M06.852 Other specified rheumatoid arthritis, left hip ⚲
  - M06.859 Other specified rheumatoid arthritis, unspecified hip ⚲
- **M06.86** Other specified rheumatoid arthritis, knee
  - M06.861 Other specified rheumatoid arthritis, right knee ⚲
  - M06.862 Other specified rheumatoid arthritis, left knee ⚲
  - M06.869 Other specified rheumatoid arthritis, unspecified knee ⚲
- **M06.87** Other specified rheumatoid arthritis, ankle and foot
  - M06.871 Other specified rheumatoid arthritis, right ankle and foot ⚲
  - M06.872 Other specified rheumatoid arthritis, left ankle and foot ⚲
  - M06.879 Other specified rheumatoid arthritis, unspecified ankle and foot ⚲
  - M06.88 Other specified rheumatoid arthritis, vertebrae ⚲
  - M06.89 Other specified rheumatoid arthritis, multiple sites ⚲
  - M06.8A Other specified rheumatoid arthritis, other specified site
  - M06.9 Rheumatoid arthritis, unspecified ⚲
    - **Coding Clinic: 2024, Q1, P17**

- **M07 Enteropathic arthropathies**
  - **Code also** associated enteropathy, such as:
    regional enteritis [Crohn's disease] (K50.-)
    ulcerative colitis (K51.-)
  - **Excludes1** psoriatic arthropathies (L40.5-)
  - **M07.6** Enteropathic arthropathies
    - M07.60 Enteropathic arthropathies, unspecified site
    - **M07.61** Enteropathic arthropathies, shoulder
      - M07.611 Enteropathic arthropathies, right shoulder
      - M07.612 Enteropathic arthropathies, left shoulder
      - M07.619 Enteropathic arthropathies, unspecified shoulder
    - **M07.62** Enteropathic arthropathies, elbow
      - M07.621 Enteropathic arthropathies, right elbow
      - M07.622 Enteropathic arthropathies, left elbow
      - M07.629 Enteropathic arthropathies, unspecified elbow

- **M07.63** Enteropathic arthropathies, wrist
  - M07.631 Enteropathic arthropathies, right wrist
  - M07.632 Enteropathic arthropathies, left wrist
  - M07.639 Enteropathic arthropathies, unspecified wrist
- **M07.64** Enteropathic arthropathies, hand
  - M07.641 Enteropathic arthropathies, right hand
  - M07.642 Enteropathic arthropathies, left hand
  - M07.649 Enteropathic arthropathies, unspecified hand
- **M07.65** Enteropathic arthropathies, hip
  - M07.651 Enteropathic arthropathies, right hip
  - M07.652 Enteropathic arthropathies, left hip
  - M07.659 Enteropathic arthropathies, unspecified hip
- **M07.66** Enteropathic arthropathies, knee
  - M07.661 Enteropathic arthropathies, right knee
  - M07.662 Enteropathic arthropathies, left knee
  - M07.669 Enteropathic arthropathies, unspecified knee
- **M07.67** Enteropathic arthropathies, ankle and foot
  - M07.671 Enteropathic arthropathies, right ankle and foot
  - M07.672 Enteropathic arthropathies, left ankle and foot
  - M07.679 Enteropathic arthropathies, unspecified ankle and foot
  - M07.68 Enteropathic arthropathies, vertebrae
  - M07.69 Enteropathic arthropathies, multiple sites

- **M08 Juvenile arthritis**
  - **Code also** any associated underlying condition, such as:
    regional enteritis [Crohn's disease] (K50.-)
    ulcerative colitis (K51.-)
  - **Excludes1** arthropathy in Whipple's disease (M14.8)
    Felty's syndrome (M05.0)
    juvenile dermatomyositis (M33.0-)
    psoriatic juvenile arthropathy (L40.54)
  - **M08.0 Unspecified juvenile rheumatoid arthritis**
    Juvenile rheumatoid arthritis with or without rheumatoid factor
    - M08.00 Unspecified juvenile rheumatoid arthritis of unspecified site ⚲
    - **M08.01** Unspecified juvenile rheumatoid arthritis, shoulder
      - M08.011 Unspecified juvenile rheumatoid arthritis, right shoulder ⚲
      - M08.012 Unspecified juvenile rheumatoid arthritis, left shoulder ⚲
      - M08.019 Unspecified juvenile rheumatoid arthritis, unspecified shoulder ⚲
    - **M08.02** Unspecified juvenile rheumatoid arthritis of elbow
      - M08.021 Unspecified juvenile rheumatoid arthritis, right elbow ⚲
      - M08.022 Unspecified juvenile rheumatoid arthritis, left elbow ⚲
      - M08.029 Unspecified juvenile rheumatoid arthritis, unspecified elbow ⚲

● M08.03　Unspecified juvenile rheumatoid arthritis, wrist
    M08.031　Unspecified juvenile rheumatoid arthritis, right wrist ℞
    M08.032　Unspecified juvenile rheumatoid arthritis, left wrist ℞
    M08.039　Unspecified juvenile rheumatoid arthritis, unspecified wrist ℞
● M08.04　Unspecified juvenile rheumatoid arthritis, hand
    M08.041　Unspecified juvenile rheumatoid arthritis, right hand ℞
    M08.042　Unspecified juvenile rheumatoid arthritis, left hand ℞
    M08.049　Unspecified juvenile rheumatoid arthritis, unspecified hand ℞
● M08.05　Unspecified juvenile rheumatoid arthritis, hip
    M08.051　Unspecified juvenile rheumatoid arthritis, right hip ℞
    M08.052　Unspecified juvenile rheumatoid arthritis, left hip ℞
    M08.059　Unspecified juvenile rheumatoid arthritis, unspecified hip ℞
● M08.06　Unspecified juvenile rheumatoid arthritis, knee
    M08.061　Unspecified juvenile rheumatoid arthritis, right knee ℞
    M08.062　Unspecified juvenile rheumatoid arthritis, left knee ℞
    M08.069　Unspecified juvenile rheumatoid arthritis, unspecified knee ℞
● M08.07　Unspecified juvenile rheumatoid arthritis, ankle and foot
    M08.071　Unspecified juvenile rheumatoid arthritis, right ankle and foot ℞
    M08.072　Unspecified juvenile rheumatoid arthritis, left ankle and foot ℞
    M08.079　Unspecified juvenile rheumatoid arthritis, unspecified ankle and foot ℞
  M08.08　Unspecified juvenile rheumatoid arthritis, vertebrae ℞
  M08.09　Unspecified juvenile rheumatoid arthritis, multiple sites ℞
  M08.0A　Unspecified juvenile rheumatoid arthritis, other specified site
M08.1　Juvenile ankylosing spondylitis ℞
  Excludes1　ankylosing spondylitis in adults (M45.0-)
● M08.2　Juvenile rheumatoid arthritis with systemic onset
  Still's disease NOS
  Excludes1　adult-onset Still's disease (M06.1-)
  M08.20　Juvenile rheumatoid arthritis with systemic onset, unspecified site ℞
● M08.21　Juvenile rheumatoid arthritis with systemic onset, shoulder
    M08.211　Juvenile rheumatoid arthritis with systemic onset, right shoulder ℞
    M08.212　Juvenile rheumatoid arthritis with systemic onset, left shoulder ℞
    M08.219　Juvenile rheumatoid arthritis with systemic onset, unspecified shoulder ℞
● M08.22　Juvenile rheumatoid arthritis with systemic onset, elbow
    M08.221　Juvenile rheumatoid arthritis with systemic onset, right elbow ℞
    M08.222　Juvenile rheumatoid arthritis with systemic onset, left elbow ℞
    M08.229　Juvenile rheumatoid arthritis with systemic onset, unspecified elbow ℞

● M08.23　Juvenile rheumatoid arthritis with systemic onset, wrist
    M08.231　Juvenile rheumatoid arthritis with systemic onset, right wrist ℞
    M08.232　Juvenile rheumatoid arthritis with systemic onset, left wrist ℞
    M08.239　Juvenile rheumatoid arthritis with systemic onset, unspecified wrist ℞
● M08.24　Juvenile rheumatoid arthritis with systemic onset, hand
    M08.241　Juvenile rheumatoid arthritis with systemic onset, right hand ℞
    M08.242　Juvenile rheumatoid arthritis with systemic onset, left hand ℞
    M08.249　Juvenile rheumatoid arthritis with systemic onset, unspecified hand ℞
● M08.25　Juvenile rheumatoid arthritis with systemic onset, hip
    M08.251　Juvenile rheumatoid arthritis with systemic onset, right hip ℞
    M08.252　Juvenile rheumatoid arthritis with systemic onset, left hip ℞
    M08.259　Juvenile rheumatoid arthritis with systemic onset, unspecified hip ℞
● M08.26　Juvenile rheumatoid arthritis with systemic onset, knee
    M08.261　Juvenile rheumatoid arthritis with systemic onset, right knee ℞
    M08.262　Juvenile rheumatoid arthritis with systemic onset, left knee ℞
    M08.269　Juvenile rheumatoid arthritis with systemic onset, unspecified knee ℞
● M08.27　Juvenile rheumatoid arthritis with systemic onset, ankle and foot
    M08.271　Juvenile rheumatoid arthritis with systemic onset, right ankle and foot ℞
    M08.272　Juvenile rheumatoid arthritis with systemic onset, left ankle and foot ℞
    M08.279　Juvenile rheumatoid arthritis with systemic onset, unspecified ankle and foot ℞
  M08.28　Juvenile rheumatoid arthritis with systemic onset, vertebrae ℞
  M08.29　Juvenile rheumatoid arthritis with systemic onset, multiple sites ℞
  M08.2A　Juvenile rheumatoid arthritis with systemic onset, other specified site
M08.3　Juvenile rheumatoid polyarthritis (seronegative)
● M08.4　Pauciarticular juvenile rheumatoid arthritis
  M08.40　Pauciarticular juvenile rheumatoid arthritis, unspecified site ℞
● M08.41　Pauciarticular juvenile rheumatoid arthritis, shoulder
    M08.411　Pauciarticular juvenile rheumatoid arthritis, right shoulder ℞
    M08.412　Pauciarticular juvenile rheumatoid arthritis, left shoulder ℞
    M08.419　Pauciarticular juvenile rheumatoid arthritis, unspecified shoulder ℞
● M08.42　Pauciarticular juvenile rheumatoid arthritis, elbow
    M08.421　Pauciarticular juvenile rheumatoid arthritis, right elbow ℞
    M08.422　Pauciarticular juvenile rheumatoid arthritis, left elbow ℞
    M08.429　Pauciarticular juvenile rheumatoid arthritis, unspecified elbow ℞

▶ New　　➡ Revised　　~~deleted~~ Deleted　　Excludes 1　　Excludes 2　　Includes　　Use additional　　Code first　　Code also　　Key words
OGCR Official Guidelines　　X Assign placeholder X　　● Use Additional Character(s)　　▶ Manifestation Code　　℞ Hierarchical Condition Category　　Coding Clinic

● M08.43　Pauciarticular juvenile rheumatoid arthritis, wrist

　　M08.431　Pauciarticular juvenile rheumatoid arthritis, right wrist 🔵

　　M08.432　Pauciarticular juvenile rheumatoid arthritis, left wrist 🔵

　　M08.439　Pauciarticular juvenile rheumatoid arthritis, unspecified wrist 🔵

● M08.44　Pauciarticular juvenile rheumatoid arthritis, hand

　　M08.441　Pauciarticular juvenile rheumatoid arthritis, right hand 🔵

　　M08.442　Pauciarticular juvenile rheumatoid arthritis, left hand 🔵

　　M08.449　Pauciarticular juvenile rheumatoid arthritis, unspecified hand 🔵

● M08.45　Pauciarticular juvenile rheumatoid arthritis, hip

　　M08.451　Pauciarticular juvenile rheumatoid arthritis, right hip 🔵

　　M08.452　Pauciarticular juvenile rheumatoid arthritis, left hip 🔵

　　M08.459　Pauciarticular juvenile rheumatoid arthritis, unspecified hip 🔵

● M08.46　Pauciarticular juvenile rheumatoid arthritis, knee

　　M08.461　Pauciarticular juvenile rheumatoid arthritis, right knee 🔵

　　M08.462　Pauciarticular juvenile rheumatoid arthritis, left knee 🔵

　　M08.469　Pauciarticular juvenile rheumatoid arthritis, unspecified knee 🔵

● M08.47　Pauciarticular juvenile rheumatoid arthritis, ankle and foot

　　M08.471　Pauciarticular juvenile rheumatoid arthritis, right ankle and foot 🔵

　　M08.472　Pauciarticular juvenile rheumatoid arthritis, left ankle and foot 🔵

　　M08.479　Pauciarticular juvenile rheumatoid arthritis, unspecified ankle and foot 🔵

　　M08.48　Pauciarticular juvenile rheumatoid arthritis, vertebrae 🔵

　　M08.4A　Pauciarticular juvenile rheumatoid arthritis, other specified site

● M08.8　Other juvenile arthritis

　　M08.80　Other juvenile arthritis, unspecified site 🔵

● M08.81　Other juvenile arthritis, shoulder

　　M08.811　Other juvenile arthritis, right shoulder 🔵

　　M08.812　Other juvenile arthritis, left shoulder 🔵

　　M08.819　Other juvenile arthritis, unspecified shoulder 🔵

● M08.82　Other juvenile arthritis, elbow

　　M08.821　Other juvenile arthritis, right elbow 🔵

　　M08.822　Other juvenile arthritis, left elbow 🔵

　　M08.829　Other juvenile arthritis, unspecified elbow 🔵

● M08.83　Other juvenile arthritis, wrist

　　M08.831　Other juvenile arthritis, right wrist 🔵

　　M08.832　Other juvenile arthritis, left wrist 🔵

　　M08.839　Other juvenile arthritis, unspecified wrist 🔵

● M08.84　Other juvenile arthritis, hand

　　M08.841　Other juvenile arthritis, right hand 🔵

　　M08.842　Other juvenile arthritis, left hand 🔵

　　M08.849　Other juvenile arthritis, unspecified hand 🔵

● M08.85　Other juvenile arthritis, hip

　　M08.851　Other juvenile arthritis, right hip 🔵

　　M08.852　Other juvenile arthritis, left hip 🔵

　　M08.859　Other juvenile arthritis, unspecified hip 🔵

● M08.86　Other juvenile arthritis, knee

　　M08.861　Other juvenile arthritis, right knee 🔵

　　M08.862　Other juvenile arthritis, left knee 🔵

　　M08.869　Other juvenile arthritis, unspecified knee 🔵

● M08.87　Other juvenile arthritis, ankle and foot

　　M08.871　Other juvenile arthritis, right ankle and foot 🔵

　　M08.872　Other juvenile arthritis, left ankle and foot 🔵

　　M08.879　Other juvenile arthritis, unspecified ankle and foot 🔵

　　M08.88　Other juvenile arthritis, other specified site 🔵
　　　　　　Other juvenile arthritis, vertebrae

　　M08.89　Other juvenile arthritis, multiple sites 🔵

● M08.9　Juvenile arthritis, unspecified

　　Excludes1　juvenile rheumatoid arthritis, unspecified (M08.0-)

　　M08.90　Juvenile arthritis, unspecified, unspecified site 🔵

● M08.91　Juvenile arthritis, unspecified, shoulder

　　M08.911　Juvenile arthritis, unspecified, right shoulder 🔵

　　M08.912　Juvenile arthritis, unspecified, left shoulder 🔵

　　M08.919　Juvenile arthritis, unspecified, unspecified shoulder 🔵

● M08.92　Juvenile arthritis, unspecified, elbow

　　M08.921　Juvenile arthritis, unspecified, right elbow 🔵

　　M08.922　Juvenile arthritis, unspecified, left elbow 🔵

　　M08.929　Juvenile arthritis, unspecified, unspecified elbow 🔵

● M08.93　Juvenile arthritis, unspecified, wrist

　　M08.931　Juvenile arthritis, unspecified, right wrist 🔵

　　M08.932　Juvenile arthritis, unspecified, left wrist 🔵

　　M08.939　Juvenile arthritis, unspecified, unspecified wrist 🔵

● M08.94　Juvenile arthritis, unspecified, hand

　　M08.941　Juvenile arthritis, unspecified, right hand 🔵

　　M08.942　Juvenile arthritis, unspecified, left hand 🔵

　　M08.949　Juvenile arthritis, unspecified, unspecified hand 🔵

● M08.95　Juvenile arthritis, unspecified, hip

　　M08.951　Juvenile arthritis, unspecified, right hip 🔵

　　M08.952　Juvenile arthritis, unspecified, left hip 🔵

　　M08.959　Juvenile arthritis, unspecified, unspecified hip 🔵

CHAPTER 13 (MØØ-M99)

● M08.96 Juvenile arthritis, unspecified, knee
     M08.961 Juvenile arthritis, unspecified, right knee Ⓗ
     M08.962 Juvenile arthritis, unspecified, left knee Ⓗ
     M08.969 Juvenile arthritis, unspecified, unspecified knee Ⓗ
● M08.97 Juvenile arthritis, unspecified, ankle and foot
     M08.971 Juvenile arthritis, unspecified, right ankle and foot Ⓗ
     M08.972 Juvenile arthritis, unspecified, left ankle and foot Ⓗ
     M08.979 Juvenile arthritis, unspecified, unspecified ankle and foot Ⓗ
     M08.98 Juvenile arthritis, unspecified, vertebrae Ⓗ
     M08.99 Juvenile arthritis, unspecified, multiple sites Ⓗ
     M08.9A Juvenile arthritis, unspecified, other specified site

● **M1A Chronic gout**
   Use additional code to identify:
   Autonomic neuropathy in diseases classified elsewhere (G99.0)
   Calculus of urinary tract in diseases classified elsewhere (N22)
   Cardiomyopathy in diseases classified elsewhere (I43)
   Disorders of external ear in diseases classified elsewhere (H61.1-, H62.8-)
   Disorders of iris and ciliary body in diseases classified elsewhere (H22)
   Glomerular disorders in diseases classified elsewhere (N08)
   Excludes1   gout NOS (M10.-)
   Excludes2   acute gout (M10.-)
   The appropriate 7th character is to be added to each code from category M1A

| 0 | without tophus (tophi) |
| 1 | with tophus (tophi) |

● **M1A.0 Idiopathic chronic gout**
   Chronic gouty bursitis
   Primary chronic gout
   X ● **M1A.00 Idiopathic chronic gout, unspecified site**
   ● M1A.01 Idiopathic chronic gout, shoulder
     ● M1A.011 Idiopathic chronic gout, right shoulder
     ● M1A.012 Idiopathic chronic gout, left shoulder
     ● M1A.019 Idiopathic chronic gout, unspecified shoulder
   ● M1A.02 Idiopathic chronic gout, elbow
     ● M1A.021 Idiopathic chronic gout, right elbow
     ● M1A.022 Idiopathic chronic gout, left elbow
     ● M1A.029 Idiopathic chronic gout, unspecified elbow
   ● M1A.03 Idiopathic chronic gout, wrist
     ● M1A.031 Idiopathic chronic gout, right wrist
     ● M1A.032 Idiopathic chronic gout, left wrist
     ● M1A.039 Idiopathic chronic gout, unspecified wrist
   ● M1A.04 Idiopathic chronic gout, hand
     ● M1A.041 Idiopathic chronic gout, right hand
     ● M1A.042 Idiopathic chronic gout, left hand
     ● M1A.049 Idiopathic chronic gout, unspecified hand

● M1A.05 Idiopathic chronic gout, hip
     ● M1A.051 Idiopathic chronic gout, right hip
     ● M1A.052 Idiopathic chronic gout, left hip
     ● M1A.059 Idiopathic chronic gout, unspecified hip
● M1A.06 Idiopathic chronic gout, knee
     ● M1A.061 Idiopathic chronic gout, right knee
     ● M1A.062 Idiopathic chronic gout, left knee
     ● M1A.069 Idiopathic chronic gout, unspecified knee
● M1A.07 Idiopathic chronic gout, ankle and foot
     ● M1A.071 Idiopathic chronic gout, right ankle and foot
     ● M1A.072 Idiopathic chronic gout, left ankle and foot
     ● M1A.079 Idiopathic chronic gout, unspecified ankle and foot
X ● M1A.08 Idiopathic chronic gout, vertebrae
X ● M1A.09 Idiopathic chronic gout, multiple sites
● **M1A.1 Lead-induced chronic gout**
   Code first toxic effects of lead and its compounds (T56.0-)
   X ● M1A.10 Lead-induced chronic gout, unspecified site
   ● M1A.11 Lead-induced chronic gout, shoulder
     ● M1A.111 Lead-induced chronic gout, right shoulder
     ● M1A.112 Lead-induced chronic gout, left shoulder
     ● M1A.119 Lead-induced chronic gout, unspecified shoulder
   ● M1A.12 Lead-induced chronic gout, elbow
     ● M1A.121 Lead-induced chronic gout, right elbow
     ● M1A.122 Lead-induced chronic gout, left elbow
     ● M1A.129 Lead-induced chronic gout, unspecified elbow
   ● M1A.13 Lead-induced chronic gout, wrist
     ● M1A.131 Lead-induced chronic gout, right wrist
     ● M1A.132 Lead-induced chronic gout, left wrist
     ● M1A.139 Lead-induced chronic gout, unspecified wrist
   ● M1A.14 Lead-induced chronic gout, hand
     ● M1A.141 Lead-induced chronic gout, right hand
     ● M1A.142 Lead-induced chronic gout, left hand
     ● M1A.149 Lead-induced chronic gout, unspecified hand
   ● M1A.15 Lead-induced chronic gout, hip
     ● M1A.151 Lead-induced chronic gout, right hip
     ● M1A.152 Lead-induced chronic gout, left hip
     ● M1A.159 Lead-induced chronic gout, unspecified hip
   ● M1A.16 Lead-induced chronic gout, knee
     ● M1A.161 Lead-induced chronic gout, right knee
     ● M1A.162 Lead-induced chronic gout, left knee
     ● M1A.169 Lead-induced chronic gout, unspecified knee
   ● M1A.17 Lead-induced chronic gout, ankle and foot
     ● M1A.171 Lead-induced chronic gout, right ankle and foot
     ● M1A.172 Lead-induced chronic gout, left ankle and foot
     ● M1A.179 Lead-induced chronic gout, unspecified ankle and foot

▶ New   ▶ Revised   ~~deleted~~ Deleted   Excludes 1   Excludes 2   Includes   Use additional   Code first   Code also   Key words
OGCR Official Guidelines   X Assign placeholder X   ● Use Additional Character(s)   ▶ Manifestation Code   Ⓗ Hierarchical Condition Category   Coding Clinic

X● **M1A.18** Lead-induced chronic gout, vertebrae
X● **M1A.19** Lead-induced chronic gout, multiple sites
● **M1A.2** Drug-induced chronic gout
    Use additional code for adverse effect, if applicable, to identify drug (T36-T50 with fifth or sixth character 5)
X● **M1A.20** Drug-induced chronic gout, unspecified site
● **M1A.21** Drug-induced chronic gout, shoulder
  ● **M1A.211** Drug-induced chronic gout, right shoulder
  ● **M1A.212** Drug-induced chronic gout, left shoulder
  ● **M1A.219** Drug-induced chronic gout, unspecified shoulder
● **M1A.22** Drug-induced chronic gout, elbow
  ● **M1A.221** Drug-induced chronic gout, right elbow
  ● **M1A.222** Drug-induced chronic gout, left elbow
  ● **M1A.229** Drug-induced chronic gout, unspecified elbow
● **M1A.23** Drug-induced chronic gout, wrist
  ● **M1A.231** Drug-induced chronic gout, right wrist
  ● **M1A.232** Drug-induced chronic gout, left wrist
  ● **M1A.239** Drug-induced chronic gout, unspecified wrist
● **M1A.24** Drug-induced chronic gout, hand
  ● **M1A.241** Drug-induced chronic gout, right hand
  ● **M1A.242** Drug-induced chronic gout, left hand
  ● **M1A.249** Drug-induced chronic gout, unspecified hand
● **M1A.25** Drug-induced chronic gout, hip
  ● **M1A.251** Drug-induced chronic gout, right hip
  ● **M1A.252** Drug-induced chronic gout, left hip
  ● **M1A.259** Drug-induced chronic gout, unspecified hip
● **M1A.26** Drug-induced chronic gout, knee
  ● **M1A.261** Drug-induced chronic gout, right knee
  ● **M1A.262** Drug-induced chronic gout, left knee
  ● **M1A.269** Drug-induced chronic gout, unspecified knee
● **M1A.27** Drug-induced chronic gout, ankle and foot
  ● **M1A.271** Drug-induced chronic gout, right ankle and foot
  ● **M1A.272** Drug-induced chronic gout, left ankle and foot
  ● **M1A.279** Drug-induced chronic gout, unspecified ankle and foot
X● **M1A.28** Drug-induced chronic gout, vertebrae
X● **M1A.29** Drug-induced chronic gout, multiple sites
● **M1A.3** Chronic gout due to renal impairment
    Code first associated renal disease
X● **M1A.30** Chronic gout due to renal impairment, unspecified site
● **M1A.31** Chronic gout due to renal impairment, shoulder
  ● **M1A.311** Chronic gout due to renal impairment, right shoulder
  ● **M1A.312** Chronic gout due to renal impairment, left shoulder
  ● **M1A.319** Chronic gout due to renal impairment, unspecified shoulder

● **M1A.32** Chronic gout due to renal impairment, elbow
  ● **M1A.321** Chronic gout due to renal impairment, right elbow
  ● **M1A.322** Chronic gout due to renal impairment, left elbow
  ● **M1A.329** Chronic gout due to renal impairment, unspecified elbow
● **M1A.33** Chronic gout due to renal impairment, wrist
  ● **M1A.331** Chronic gout due to renal impairment, right wrist
  ● **M1A.332** Chronic gout due to renal impairment, left wrist
  ● **M1A.339** Chronic gout due to renal impairment, unspecified wrist
● **M1A.34** Chronic gout due to renal impairment, hand
  ● **M1A.341** Chronic gout due to renal impairment, right hand
  ● **M1A.342** Chronic gout due to renal impairment, left hand
  ● **M1A.349** Chronic gout due to renal impairment, unspecified hand
● **M1A.35** Chronic gout due to renal impairment, hip
  ● **M1A.351** Chronic gout due to renal impairment, right hip
  ● **M1A.352** Chronic gout due to renal impairment, left hip
  ● **M1A.359** Chronic gout due to renal impairment, unspecified hip
● **M1A.36** Chronic gout due to renal impairment, knee
  ● **M1A.361** Chronic gout due to renal impairment, right knee
  ● **M1A.362** Chronic gout due to renal impairment, left knee
  ● **M1A.369** Chronic gout due to renal impairment, unspecified knee
● **M1A.37** Chronic gout due to renal impairment, ankle and foot
  ● **M1A.371** Chronic gout due to renal impairment, right ankle and foot
  ● **M1A.372** Chronic gout due to renal impairment, left ankle and foot
  ● **M1A.379** Chronic gout due to renal impairment, unspecified ankle and foot
X● **M1A.38** Chronic gout due to renal impairment, vertebrae
X● **M1A.39** Chronic gout due to renal impairment, multiple sites
● **M1A.4** Other secondary chronic gout
    Code first associated condition
X● **M1A.40** Other secondary chronic gout, unspecified site
● **M1A.41** Other secondary chronic gout, shoulder
  ● **M1A.411** Other secondary chronic gout, right shoulder
  ● **M1A.412** Other secondary chronic gout, left shoulder
  ● **M1A.419** Other secondary chronic gout, unspecified shoulder
● **M1A.42** Other secondary chronic gout, elbow
  ● **M1A.421** Other secondary chronic gout, right elbow
  ● **M1A.422** Other secondary chronic gout, left elbow
  ● **M1A.429** Other secondary chronic gout, unspecified elbow

CHAPTER 13 (M00-M99)

● M1A.43 Other secondary chronic gout, wrist
  ● M1A.431 Other secondary chronic gout, right wrist
  ● M1A.432 Other secondary chronic gout, left wrist
  ● M1A.439 Other secondary chronic gout, unspecified wrist
● M1A.44 Other secondary chronic gout, hand
  ● M1A.441 Other secondary chronic gout, right hand
  ● M1A.442 Other secondary chronic gout, left hand
  ● M1A.449 Other secondary chronic gout, unspecified hand
● M1A.45 Other secondary chronic gout, hip
  ● M1A.451 Other secondary chronic gout, right hip
  ● M1A.452 Other secondary chronic gout, left hip
  ● M1A.459 Other secondary chronic gout, unspecified hip
● M1A.46 Other secondary chronic gout, knee
  ● M1A.461 Other secondary chronic gout, right knee
  ● M1A.462 Other secondary chronic gout, left knee
  ● M1A.469 Other secondary chronic gout, unspecified knee
● M1A.47 Other secondary chronic gout, ankle and foot
  ● M1A.471 Other secondary chronic gout, right ankle and foot
  ● M1A.472 Other secondary chronic gout, left ankle and foot
  ● M1A.479 Other secondary chronic gout, unspecified ankle and foot
X ● M1A.48 Other secondary chronic gout, vertebrae
X ● M1A.49 Other secondary chronic gout, multiple sites
X M1A.9 Chronic gout, unspecified

● M10 Gout

Accumulation of uric acid that results in swollen, red, hot, painful, stiff joints

Acute gout
Gout attack
Gout flare
Podagra

Use additional code to identify:
Autonomic neuropathy in diseases classified elsewhere (G99.0)
Calculus of urinary tract in diseases classified elsewhere (N22)
Cardiomyopathy in diseases classified elsewhere (I43)
Disorders of external ear in diseases classified elsewhere (H61.1-, H62.8-)
Disorders of iris and ciliary body in diseases classified elsewhere (H22)
Glomerular disorders in diseases classified elsewhere (N08)

Excludes2   chronic gout (M1A.-)

● M10.0 Idiopathic gout
Gouty bursitis
Primary gout
  M10.00 Idiopathic gout, unspecified site
  ● M10.01 Idiopathic gout, shoulder
    M10.011 Idiopathic gout, right shoulder
    M10.012 Idiopathic gout, left shoulder
    M10.019 Idiopathic gout, unspecified shoulder

● M10.02 Idiopathic gout, elbow
  M10.021 Idiopathic gout, right elbow
  M10.022 Idiopathic gout, left elbow
  M10.029 Idiopathic gout, unspecified elbow
● M10.03 Idiopathic gout, wrist
  M10.031 Idiopathic gout, right wrist
  M10.032 Idiopathic gout, left wrist
  M10.039 Idiopathic gout, unspecified wrist
● M10.04 Idiopathic gout, hand
  M10.041 Idiopathic gout, right hand
  M10.042 Idiopathic gout, left hand
  M10.049 Idiopathic gout, unspecified hand
● M10.05 Idiopathic gout, hip
  M10.051 Idiopathic gout, right hip
  M10.052 Idiopathic gout, left hip
  M10.059 Idiopathic gout, unspecified hip
● M10.06 Idiopathic gout, knee
  M10.061 Idiopathic gout, right knee
  M10.062 Idiopathic gout, left knee
  M10.069 Idiopathic gout, unspecified knee
● M10.07 Idiopathic gout, ankle and foot
  M10.071 Idiopathic gout, right ankle and foot
  M10.072 Idiopathic gout, left ankle and foot
  M10.079 Idiopathic gout, unspecified ankle and foot
M10.08 Idiopathic gout, vertebrae
M10.09 Idiopathic gout, multiple sites
● M10.1 Lead-induced gout
Code first toxic effects of lead and its compounds (T56.0-)
  M10.10 Lead-induced gout, unspecified site
● M10.11 Lead-induced gout, shoulder
  M10.111 Lead-induced gout, right shoulder
  M10.112 Lead-induced gout, left shoulder
  M10.119 Lead-induced gout, unspecified shoulder
● M10.12 Lead-induced gout, elbow
  M10.121 Lead-induced gout, right elbow
  M10.122 Lead-induced gout, left elbow
  M10.129 Lead-induced gout, unspecified elbow
● M10.13 Lead-induced gout, wrist
  M10.131 Lead-induced gout, right wrist
  M10.132 Lead-induced gout, left wrist
  M10.139 Lead-induced gout, unspecified wrist
● M10.14 Lead-induced gout, hand
  M10.141 Lead-induced gout, right hand
  M10.142 Lead-induced gout, left hand
  M10.149 Lead-induced gout, unspecified hand
● M10.15 Lead-induced gout, hip
  M10.151 Lead-induced gout, right hip
  M10.152 Lead-induced gout, left hip
  M10.159 Lead-induced gout, unspecified hip
● M10.16 Lead-induced gout, knee
  M10.161 Lead-induced gout, right knee
  M10.162 Lead-induced gout, left knee
  M10.169 Lead-induced gout, unspecified knee
● M10.17 Lead-induced gout, ankle and foot
  M10.171 Lead-induced gout, right ankle and foot
  M10.172 Lead-induced gout, left ankle and foot
  M10.179 Lead-induced gout, unspecified ankle and foot
M10.18 Lead-induced gout, vertebrae
M10.19 Lead-induced gout, multiple sites

● **M10.2**   **Drug-induced gout**
  Use additional code for adverse effect, if applicable, to identify drug (T36-T50 with fifth or sixth character 5)
  M10.20   Drug-induced gout, unspecified site
● M10.21   Drug-induced gout, shoulder
  M10.211   Drug-induced gout, right shoulder
  M10.212   Drug-induced gout, left shoulder
  M10.219   Drug-induced gout, unspecified shoulder
● M10.22   Drug-induced gout, elbow
  M10.221   Drug-induced gout, right elbow
  M10.222   Drug-induced gout, left elbow
  M10.229   Drug-induced gout, unspecified elbow
● M10.23   Drug-induced gout, wrist
  M10.231   Drug-induced gout, right wrist
  M10.232   Drug-induced gout, left wrist
  M10.239   Drug-induced gout, unspecified wrist
● M10.24   Drug-induced gout, hand
  M10.241   Drug-induced gout, right hand
  M10.242   Drug-induced gout, left hand
  M10.249   Drug-induced gout, unspecified hand
● M10.25   Drug-induced gout, hip
  M10.251   Drug-induced gout, right hip
  M10.252   Drug-induced gout, left hip
  M10.259   Drug-induced gout, unspecified hip
● M10.26   Drug-induced gout, knee
  M10.261   Drug-induced gout, right knee
  M10.262   Drug-induced gout, left knee
  M10.269   Drug-induced gout, unspecified knee
● M10.27   Drug-induced gout, ankle and foot
  M10.271   Drug-induced gout, right ankle and foot
  M10.272   Drug-induced gout, left ankle and foot
  M10.279   Drug-induced gout, unspecified ankle and foot
  M10.28   Drug-induced gout, vertebrae
  M10.29   Drug-induced gout, multiple sites
● **M10.3**   **Gout due to renal impairment**
  Code also associated renal disease
  M10.30   Gout due to renal impairment, unspecified site
● M10.31   Gout due to renal impairment, shoulder
  M10.311   Gout due to renal impairment, right shoulder
  M10.312   Gout due to renal impairment, left shoulder
  M10.319   Gout due to renal impairment, unspecified shoulder
● M10.32   Gout due to renal impairment, elbow
  M10.321   Gout due to renal impairment, right elbow
  M10.322   Gout due to renal impairment, left elbow
  M10.329   Gout due to renal impairment, unspecified elbow
● M10.33   Gout due to renal impairment, wrist
  M10.331   Gout due to renal impairment, right wrist
  M10.332   Gout due to renal impairment, left wrist
  M10.339   Gout due to renal impairment, unspecified wrist

● M10.34   Gout due to renal impairment, hand
  M10.341   Gout due to renal impairment, right hand
  M10.342   Gout due to renal impairment, left hand
  M10.349   Gout due to renal impairment, unspecified hand
● M10.35   Gout due to renal impairment, hip
  M10.351   Gout due to renal impairment, right hip
  M10.352   Gout due to renal impairment, left hip
  M10.359   Gout due to renal impairment, unspecified hip
● M10.36   Gout due to renal impairment, knee
  M10.361   Gout due to renal impairment, right knee
  M10.362   Gout due to renal impairment, left knee
  M10.369   Gout due to renal impairment, unspecified knee
● M10.37   Gout due to renal impairment, ankle and foot
  M10.371   Gout due to renal impairment, right ankle and foot
  M10.372   Gout due to renal impairment, left ankle and foot
  M10.379   Gout due to renal impairment, unspecified ankle and foot
  M10.38   Gout due to renal impairment, vertebrae
  M10.39   Gout due to renal impairment, multiple sites
● **M10.4**   **Other secondary gout**
  Code first associated condition
  M10.40   Other secondary gout, unspecified site
● M10.41   Other secondary gout, shoulder
  M10.411   Other secondary gout, right shoulder
  M10.412   Other secondary gout, left shoulder
  M10.419   Other secondary gout, unspecified shoulder
● M10.42   Other secondary gout, elbow
  M10.421   Other secondary gout, right elbow
  M10.422   Other secondary gout, left elbow
  M10.429   Other secondary gout, unspecified elbow
● M10.43   Other secondary gout, wrist
  M10.431   Other secondary gout, right wrist
  M10.432   Other secondary gout, left wrist
  M10.439   Other secondary gout, unspecified wrist
● M10.44   Other secondary gout, hand
  M10.441   Other secondary gout, right hand
  M10.442   Other secondary gout, left hand
  M10.449   Other secondary gout, unspecified hand
● M10.45   Other secondary gout, hip
  M10.451   Other secondary gout, right hip
  M10.452   Other secondary gout, left hip
  M10.459   Other secondary gout, unspecified hip
● M10.46   Other secondary gout, knee
  M10.461   Other secondary gout, right knee
  M10.462   Other secondary gout, left knee
  M10.469   Other secondary gout, unspecified knee

CHAPTER 13 (M00-M99)

● M10.47 Other secondary gout, ankle and foot
  M10.471 Other secondary gout, right ankle and foot
  M10.472 Other secondary gout, left ankle and foot
  M10.479 Other secondary gout, unspecified ankle and foot
 M10.48 Other secondary gout, vertebrae
 M10.49 Other secondary gout, multiple sites
M10.9 Gout, unspecified
  Gout NOS

● M11 Other crystal arthropathies
 ● M11.0 Hydroxyapatite deposition disease
  M11.00 Hydroxyapatite deposition disease, unspecified site
  ● M11.01 Hydroxyapatite deposition disease, shoulder
   M11.011 Hydroxyapatite deposition disease, right shoulder
   M11.012 Hydroxyapatite deposition disease, left shoulder
   M11.019 Hydroxyapatite deposition disease, unspecified shoulder
  ● M11.02 Hydroxyapatite deposition disease, elbow
   M11.021 Hydroxyapatite deposition disease, right elbow
   M11.022 Hydroxyapatite deposition disease, left elbow
   M11.029 Hydroxyapatite deposition disease, unspecified elbow
  ● M11.03 Hydroxyapatite deposition disease, wrist
   M11.031 Hydroxyapatite deposition disease, right wrist
   M11.032 Hydroxyapatite deposition disease, left wrist
   M11.039 Hydroxyapatite deposition disease, unspecified wrist
  ● M11.04 Hydroxyapatite deposition disease, hand
   M11.041 Hydroxyapatite deposition disease, right hand
   M11.042 Hydroxyapatite deposition disease, left hand
   M11.049 Hydroxyapatite deposition disease, unspecified hand
  ● M11.05 Hydroxyapatite deposition disease, hip
   M11.051 Hydroxyapatite deposition disease, right hip
   M11.052 Hydroxyapatite deposition disease, left hip
   M11.059 Hydroxyapatite deposition disease, unspecified hip
  ● M11.06 Hydroxyapatite deposition disease, knee
   M11.061 Hydroxyapatite deposition disease, right knee
   M11.062 Hydroxyapatite deposition disease, left knee
   M11.069 Hydroxyapatite deposition disease, unspecified knee
  ● M11.07 Hydroxyapatite deposition disease, ankle and foot
   M11.071 Hydroxyapatite deposition disease, right ankle and foot
   M11.072 Hydroxyapatite deposition disease, left ankle and foot
   M11.079 Hydroxyapatite deposition disease, unspecified ankle and foot

  M11.08 Hydroxyapatite deposition disease, vertebrae
  M11.09 Hydroxyapatite deposition disease, multiple sites
 ● M11.1 Familial chondrocalcinosis
  M11.10 Familial chondrocalcinosis, unspecified site
  ● M11.11 Familial chondrocalcinosis, shoulder
   M11.111 Familial chondrocalcinosis, right shoulder
   M11.112 Familial chondrocalcinosis, left shoulder
   M11.119 Familial chondrocalcinosis, unspecified shoulder
  ● M11.12 Familial chondrocalcinosis, elbow
   M11.121 Familial chondrocalcinosis, right elbow
   M11.122 Familial chondrocalcinosis, left elbow
   M11.129 Familial chondrocalcinosis, unspecified elbow
  ● M11.13 Familial chondrocalcinosis, wrist
   M11.131 Familial chondrocalcinosis, right wrist
   M11.132 Familial chondrocalcinosis, left wrist
   M11.139 Familial chondrocalcinosis, unspecified wrist
  ● M11.14 Familial chondrocalcinosis, hand
   M11.141 Familial chondrocalcinosis, right hand
   M11.142 Familial chondrocalcinosis, left hand
   M11.149 Familial chondrocalcinosis, unspecified hand
  ● M11.15 Familial chondrocalcinosis, hip
   M11.151 Familial chondrocalcinosis, right hip
   M11.152 Familial chondrocalcinosis, left hip
   M11.159 Familial chondrocalcinosis, unspecified hip
  ● M11.16 Familial chondrocalcinosis, knee
   M11.161 Familial chondrocalcinosis, right knee
   M11.162 Familial chondrocalcinosis, left knee
   M11.169 Familial chondrocalcinosis, unspecified knee
  ● M11.17 Familial chondrocalcinosis, ankle and foot
   M11.171 Familial chondrocalcinosis, right ankle and foot
   M11.172 Familial chondrocalcinosis, left ankle and foot
   M11.179 Familial chondrocalcinosis, unspecified ankle and foot
  M11.18 Familial chondrocalcinosis, vertebrae
  M11.19 Familial chondrocalcinosis, multiple sites
 ● M11.2 Other chondrocalcinosis
  Chondrocalcinosis NOS
  M11.20 Other chondrocalcinosis, unspecified site
  ● M11.21 Other chondrocalcinosis, shoulder
   M11.211 Other chondrocalcinosis, right shoulder
   M11.212 Other chondrocalcinosis, left shoulder
   M11.219 Other chondrocalcinosis, unspecified shoulder
  ● M11.22 Other chondrocalcinosis, elbow
   M11.221 Other chondrocalcinosis, right elbow
   M11.222 Other chondrocalcinosis, left elbow
   M11.229 Other chondrocalcinosis, unspecified elbow

● M11.23   Other chondrocalcinosis, wrist
    M11.231   Other chondrocalcinosis, right wrist
    M11.232   Other chondrocalcinosis, left wrist
    M11.239   Other chondrocalcinosis, unspecified wrist
● M11.24   Other chondrocalcinosis, hand
    M11.241   Other chondrocalcinosis, right hand
    M11.242   Other chondrocalcinosis, left hand
    M11.249   Other chondrocalcinosis, unspecified hand
● M11.25   Other chondrocalcinosis, hip
    M11.251   Other chondrocalcinosis, right hip
    M11.252   Other chondrocalcinosis, left hip
    M11.259   Other chondrocalcinosis, unspecified hip
● M11.26   Other chondrocalcinosis, knee
    M11.261   Other chondrocalcinosis, right knee
    M11.262   Other chondrocalcinosis, left knee
    M11.269   Other chondrocalcinosis, unspecified knee
● M11.27   Other chondrocalcinosis, ankle and foot
    M11.271   Other chondrocalcinosis, right ankle and foot
    M11.272   Other chondrocalcinosis, left ankle and foot
    M11.279   Other chondrocalcinosis, unspecified ankle and foot
    M11.28   Other chondrocalcinosis, vertebrae
    M11.29   Other chondrocalcinosis, multiple sites
● M11.8   Other specified crystal arthropathies
    M11.80   Other specified crystal arthropathies, unspecified site
● M11.81   Other specified crystal arthropathies, shoulder
    M11.811   Other specified crystal arthropathies, right shoulder
    M11.812   Other specified crystal arthropathies, left shoulder
    M11.819   Other specified crystal arthropathies, unspecified shoulder
● M11.82   Other specified crystal arthropathies, elbow
    M11.821   Other specified crystal arthropathies, right elbow
    M11.822   Other specified crystal arthropathies, left elbow
    M11.829   Other specified crystal arthropathies, unspecified elbow
● M11.83   Other specified crystal arthropathies, wrist
    M11.831   Other specified crystal arthropathies, right wrist
    M11.832   Other specified crystal arthropathies, left wrist
    M11.839   Other specified crystal arthropathies, unspecified wrist
● M11.84   Other specified crystal arthropathies, hand
    M11.841   Other specified crystal arthropathies, right hand
    M11.842   Other specified crystal arthropathies, left hand
    M11.849   Other specified crystal arthropathies, unspecified hand

● M11.85   Other specified crystal arthropathies, hip
    M11.851   Other specified crystal arthropathies, right hip
    M11.852   Other specified crystal arthropathies, left hip
    M11.859   Other specified crystal arthropathies, unspecified hip
● M11.86   Other specified crystal arthropathies, knee
    M11.861   Other specified crystal arthropathies, right knee
    M11.862   Other specified crystal arthropathies, left knee
    M11.869   Other specified crystal arthropathies, unspecified knee
● M11.87   Other specified crystal arthropathies, ankle and foot
    M11.871   Other specified crystal arthropathies, right ankle and foot
    M11.872   Other specified crystal arthropathies, left ankle and foot
    M11.879   Other specified crystal arthropathies, unspecified ankle and foot
    M11.88   Other specified crystal arthropathies, vertebrae
    M11.89   Other specified crystal arthropathies, multiple sites
    M11.9   Crystal arthropathy, unspecified
● M12   Other and unspecified arthropathy
    Excludes1   arthrosis (M15-M19)
          cricoarytenoid arthropathy (J38.7)
● M12.0   Chronic postrheumatic arthropathy [Jaccoud]
    M12.00   Chronic postrheumatic arthropathy [Jaccoud], unspecified site 🗫
● M12.01   Chronic postrheumatic arthropathy [Jaccoud], shoulder
    M12.011   Chronic postrheumatic arthropathy [Jaccoud], right shoulder 🗫
    M12.012   Chronic postrheumatic arthropathy [Jaccoud], left shoulder 🗫
    M12.019   Chronic postrheumatic arthropathy [Jaccoud], unspecified shoulder 🗫
● M12.02   Chronic postrheumatic arthropathy [Jaccoud], elbow
    M12.021   Chronic postrheumatic arthropathy [Jaccoud], right elbow 🗫
    M12.022   Chronic postrheumatic arthropathy [Jaccoud], left elbow 🗫
    M12.029   Chronic postrheumatic arthropathy [Jaccoud], unspecified elbow 🗫
● M12.03   Chronic postrheumatic arthropathy [Jaccoud], wrist
    M12.031   Chronic postrheumatic arthropathy [Jaccoud], right wrist 🗫
    M12.032   Chronic postrheumatic arthropathy [Jaccoud], left wrist 🗫
    M12.039   Chronic postrheumatic arthropathy [Jaccoud], unspecified wrist 🗫
● M12.04   Chronic postrheumatic arthropathy [Jaccoud], hand
    M12.041   Chronic postrheumatic arthropathy [Jaccoud], right hand 🗫
    M12.042   Chronic postrheumatic arthropathy [Jaccoud], left hand 🗫
    M12.049   Chronic postrheumatic arthropathy [Jaccoud], unspecified hand 🗫

● **M12.05** Chronic postrheumatic arthropathy [Jaccoud], hip
    M12.051 Chronic postrheumatic arthropathy [Jaccoud], right hip 🕮
    M12.052 Chronic postrheumatic arthropathy [Jaccoud], left hip 🕮
    M12.059 Chronic postrheumatic arthropathy [Jaccoud], unspecified hip 🕮

● **M12.06** Chronic postrheumatic arthropathy [Jaccoud], knee
    M12.061 Chronic postrheumatic arthropathy [Jaccoud], right knee 🕮
    M12.062 Chronic postrheumatic arthropathy [Jaccoud], left knee 🕮
    M12.069 Chronic postrheumatic arthropathy [Jaccoud], unspecified knee 🕮

● **M12.07** Chronic postrheumatic arthropathy [Jaccoud], ankle and foot
    M12.071 Chronic postrheumatic arthropathy [Jaccoud], right ankle and foot 🕮
    M12.072 Chronic postrheumatic arthropathy [Jaccoud], left ankle and foot 🕮
    M12.079 Chronic postrheumatic arthropathy [Jaccoud], unspecified ankle and foot 🕮

M12.08 Chronic postrheumatic arthropathy [Jaccoud], other specified site 🕮
    Chronic postrheumatic arthropathy [Jaccoud], vertebrae

M12.09 Chronic postrheumatic arthropathy [Jaccoud], multiple sites 🕮

● **M12.1** Kaschin-Beck disease
    Osteochondroarthrosis deformans endemica

M12.10 Kaschin-Beck disease, unspecified site

● **M12.11** Kaschin-Beck disease, shoulder
    M12.111 Kaschin-Beck disease, right shoulder
    M12.112 Kaschin-Beck disease, left shoulder
    M12.119 Kaschin-Beck disease, unspecified shoulder

● **M12.12** Kaschin-Beck disease, elbow
    M12.121 Kaschin-Beck disease, right elbow
    M12.122 Kaschin-Beck disease, left elbow
    M12.129 Kaschin-Beck disease, unspecified elbow

● **M12.13** Kaschin-Beck disease, wrist
    M12.131 Kaschin-Beck disease, right wrist
    M12.132 Kaschin-Beck disease, left wrist
    M12.139 Kaschin-Beck disease, unspecified wrist

● **M12.14** Kaschin-Beck disease, hand
    M12.141 Kaschin-Beck disease, right hand
    M12.142 Kaschin-Beck disease, left hand
    M12.149 Kaschin-Beck disease, unspecified hand

● **M12.15** Kaschin-Beck disease, hip
    M12.151 Kaschin-Beck disease, right hip
    M12.152 Kaschin-Beck disease, left hip
    M12.159 Kaschin-Beck disease, unspecified hip

● **M12.16** Kaschin-Beck disease, knee
    M12.161 Kaschin-Beck disease, right knee
    M12.162 Kaschin-Beck disease, left knee
    M12.169 Kaschin-Beck disease, unspecified knee

● **M12.17** Kaschin-Beck disease, ankle and foot
    M12.171 Kaschin-Beck disease, right ankle and foot
    M12.172 Kaschin-Beck disease, left ankle and foot
    M12.179 Kaschin-Beck disease, unspecified ankle and foot

M12.18 Kaschin-Beck disease, vertebrae

M12.19 Kaschin-Beck disease, multiple sites

● **M12.2** Villonodular synovitis (pigmented)

M12.20 Villonodular synovitis (pigmented), unspecified site

● **M12.21** Villonodular synovitis (pigmented), shoulder
    M12.211 Villonodular synovitis (pigmented), right shoulder
    M12.212 Villonodular synovitis (pigmented), left shoulder
    M12.219 Villonodular synovitis (pigmented), unspecified shoulder

● **M12.22** Villonodular synovitis (pigmented), elbow
    M12.221 Villonodular synovitis (pigmented), right elbow
    M12.222 Villonodular synovitis (pigmented), left elbow
    M12.229 Villonodular synovitis (pigmented), unspecified elbow

● **M12.23** Villonodular synovitis (pigmented), wrist
    M12.231 Villonodular synovitis (pigmented), right wrist
    M12.232 Villonodular synovitis (pigmented), left wrist
    M12.239 Villonodular synovitis (pigmented), unspecified wrist

● **M12.24** Villonodular synovitis (pigmented), hand
    M12.241 Villonodular synovitis (pigmented), right hand
    M12.242 Villonodular synovitis (pigmented), left hand
    M12.249 Villonodular synovitis (pigmented), unspecified hand

● **M12.25** Villonodular synovitis (pigmented), hip
    M12.251 Villonodular synovitis (pigmented), right hip
    M12.252 Villonodular synovitis (pigmented), left hip
    M12.259 Villonodular synovitis (pigmented), unspecified hip

● **M12.26** Villonodular synovitis (pigmented), knee
    M12.261 Villonodular synovitis (pigmented), right knee
    M12.262 Villonodular synovitis (pigmented), left knee
    M12.269 Villonodular synovitis (pigmented), unspecified knee

● **M12.27** Villonodular synovitis (pigmented), ankle and foot
    M12.271 Villonodular synovitis (pigmented), right ankle and foot
    M12.272 Villonodular synovitis (pigmented), left ankle and foot
    M12.279 Villonodular synovitis (pigmented), unspecified ankle and foot

M12.28 Villonodular synovitis (pigmented), other specified site
    Villonodular synovitis (pigmented), vertebrae

M12.29 Villonodular synovitis (pigmented), multiple sites

▶ New   ➡ Revised   ~~deleted~~ Deleted   Excludes 1   Excludes 2   Includes   Use additional   Code first   Code also   Key words
OGCR Official Guidelines   **X** Assign placeholder X   ● Use Additional Character(s)   ▶ Manifestation Code   🕮 Hierarchical Condition Category   **Coding Clinic**

● M12.3 **Palindromic rheumatism**
    M12.30 Palindromic rheumatism, unspecified site
● M12.31 Palindromic rheumatism, shoulder
    M12.311 Palindromic rheumatism, right shoulder
    M12.312 Palindromic rheumatism, left shoulder
    M12.319 Palindromic rheumatism, unspecified shoulder
● M12.32 Palindromic rheumatism, elbow
    M12.321 Palindromic rheumatism, right elbow
    M12.322 Palindromic rheumatism, left elbow
    M12.329 Palindromic rheumatism, unspecified elbow
● M12.33 Palindromic rheumatism, wrist
    M12.331 Palindromic rheumatism, right wrist
    M12.332 Palindromic rheumatism, left wrist
    M12.339 Palindromic rheumatism, unspecified wrist
● M12.34 Palindromic rheumatism, hand
    M12.341 Palindromic rheumatism, right hand
    M12.342 Palindromic rheumatism, left hand
    M12.349 Palindromic rheumatism, unspecified hand
● M12.35 Palindromic rheumatism, hip
    M12.351 Palindromic rheumatism, right hip
    M12.352 Palindromic rheumatism, left hip
    M12.359 Palindromic rheumatism, unspecified hip
● M12.36 Palindromic rheumatism, knee
    M12.361 Palindromic rheumatism, right knee
    M12.362 Palindromic rheumatism, left knee
    M12.369 Palindromic rheumatism, unspecified knee
● M12.37 Palindromic rheumatism, ankle and foot
    M12.371 Palindromic rheumatism, right ankle and foot
    M12.372 Palindromic rheumatism, left ankle and foot
    M12.379 Palindromic rheumatism, unspecified ankle and foot
    M12.38 Palindromic rheumatism, other specified site
        Palindromic rheumatism, vertebrae
    M12.39 Palindromic rheumatism, multiple sites
● M12.4 Intermittent hydrarthrosis
    M12.40 Intermittent hydrarthrosis, unspecified site
● M12.41 Intermittent hydrarthrosis, shoulder
    M12.411 Intermittent hydrarthrosis, right shoulder
    M12.412 Intermittent hydrarthrosis, left shoulder
    M12.419 Intermittent hydrarthrosis, unspecified shoulder
● M12.42 Intermittent hydrarthrosis, elbow
    M12.421 Intermittent hydrarthrosis, right elbow
    M12.422 Intermittent hydrarthrosis, left elbow
    M12.429 Intermittent hydrarthrosis, unspecified elbow
● M12.43 Intermittent hydrarthrosis, wrist
    M12.431 Intermittent hydrarthrosis, right wrist
    M12.432 Intermittent hydrarthrosis, left wrist
    M12.439 Intermittent hydrarthrosis, unspecified wrist

● M12.44 Intermittent hydrarthrosis, hand
    M12.441 Intermittent hydrarthrosis, right hand
    M12.442 Intermittent hydrarthrosis, left hand
    M12.449 Intermittent hydrarthrosis, unspecified hand
● M12.45 Intermittent hydrarthrosis, hip
    M12.451 Intermittent hydrarthrosis, right hip
    M12.452 Intermittent hydrarthrosis, left hip
    M12.459 Intermittent hydrarthrosis, unspecified hip
● M12.46 Intermittent hydrarthrosis, knee
    M12.461 Intermittent hydrarthrosis, right knee
    M12.462 Intermittent hydrarthrosis, left knee
    M12.469 Intermittent hydrarthrosis, unspecified knee
● M12.47 Intermittent hydrarthrosis, ankle and foot
    M12.471 Intermittent hydrarthrosis, right ankle and foot
    M12.472 Intermittent hydrarthrosis, left ankle and foot
    M12.479 Intermittent hydrarthrosis, unspecified ankle and foot
    M12.48 Intermittent hydrarthrosis, other site
    M12.49 Intermittent hydrarthrosis, multiple sites
● M12.5 Traumatic arthropathy
    Excludes 1   current injury–see Alphabetic Index
        post-traumatic osteoarthritis of first carpometacarpal joint (M18.2-M18.3)
        post-traumatic osteoarthritis of hip (M16.4-M16.5)
        post-traumatic osteoarthritis of knee (M17.2-M17.3)
        post-traumatic osteoarthritis NOS (M19.1-)
        post-traumatic osteoarthritis of other single joints (M19.1-)
    M12.50 Traumatic arthropathy, unspecified site
● M12.51 Traumatic arthropathy, shoulder
    M12.511 Traumatic arthropathy, right shoulder
    M12.512 Traumatic arthropathy, left shoulder
    M12.519 Traumatic arthropathy, unspecified shoulder
● M12.52 Traumatic arthropathy, elbow
    M12.521 Traumatic arthropathy, right elbow
    M12.522 Traumatic arthropathy, left elbow
    M12.529 Traumatic arthropathy, unspecified elbow
● M12.53 Traumatic arthropathy, wrist
    M12.531 Traumatic arthropathy, right wrist
    M12.532 Traumatic arthropathy, left wrist
    M12.539 Traumatic arthropathy, unspecified wrist
● M12.54 Traumatic arthropathy, hand
    M12.541 Traumatic arthropathy, right hand
    M12.542 Traumatic arthropathy, left hand
    M12.549 Traumatic arthropathy, unspecified hand
● M12.55 Traumatic arthropathy, hip
    M12.551 Traumatic arthropathy, right hip
    M12.552 Traumatic arthropathy, left hip
        Coding Clinic: 2015, Q1, P17
    M12.559 Traumatic arthropathy, unspecified hip

● M12.56 Traumatic arthropathy, knee
    M12.561 Traumatic arthropathy, right knee
    M12.562 Traumatic arthropathy, left knee
    M12.569 Traumatic arthropathy, unspecified knee
● M12.57 Traumatic arthropathy, ankle and foot
    M12.571 Traumatic arthropathy, right ankle and foot
    M12.572 Traumatic arthropathy, left ankle and foot
    M12.579 Traumatic arthropathy, unspecified ankle and foot
M12.58 Traumatic arthropathy, other specified site
    Traumatic arthropathy, vertebrae
M12.59 Traumatic arthropathy, multiple sites
● M12.8 Other specific arthropathies, not elsewhere classified
    Transient arthropathy
M12.80 Other specific arthropathies, not elsewhere classified, unspecified site
● M12.81 Other specific arthropathies, not elsewhere classified, shoulder
    M12.811 Other specific arthropathies, not elsewhere classified, right shoulder
    M12.812 Other specific arthropathies, not elsewhere classified, left shoulder
    M12.819 Other specific arthropathies, not elsewhere classified, unspecified shoulder
● M12.82 Other specific arthropathies, not elsewhere classified, elbow
    M12.821 Other specific arthropathies, not elsewhere classified, right elbow
    M12.822 Other specific arthropathies, not elsewhere classified, left elbow
    M12.829 Other specific arthropathies, not elsewhere classified, unspecified elbow
● M12.83 Other specific arthropathies, not elsewhere classified, wrist
    M12.831 Other specific arthropathies, not elsewhere classified, right wrist
    M12.832 Other specific arthropathies, not elsewhere classified, left wrist
    M12.839 Other specific arthropathies, not elsewhere classified, unspecified wrist
● M12.84 Other specific arthropathies, not elsewhere classified, hand
    M12.841 Other specific arthropathies, not elsewhere classified, right hand
    M12.842 Other specific arthropathies, not elsewhere classified, left hand
    M12.849 Other specific arthropathies, not elsewhere classified, unspecified hand
● M12.85 Other specific arthropathies, not elsewhere classified, hip
    M12.851 Other specific arthropathies, not elsewhere classified, right hip
    M12.852 Other specific arthropathies, not elsewhere classified, left hip
    M12.859 Other specific arthropathies, not elsewhere classified, unspecified hip
● M12.86 Other specific arthropathies, not elsewhere classified, knee
    M12.861 Other specific arthropathies, not elsewhere classified, right knee

    M12.862 Other specific arthropathies, not elsewhere classified, left knee
    M12.869 Other specific arthropathies, not elsewhere classified, unspecified knee
● M12.87 Other specific arthropathies, not elsewhere classified, ankle and foot
    M12.871 Other specific arthropathies, not elsewhere classified, right ankle and foot
    M12.872 Other specific arthropathies, not elsewhere classified, left ankle and foot
    M12.879 Other specific arthropathies, not elsewhere classified, unspecified ankle and foot
M12.88 Other specific arthropathies, not elsewhere classified, other specified site
    Other specific arthropathies, not elsewhere classified, vertebrae
M12.89 Other specific arthropathies, not elsewhere classified, multiple sites
M12.9 Arthropathy, unspecified

● M13 Other arthritis
    Excludes1 arthrosis (M15-M19)
             osteoarthritis (M15-M19)
M13.0 Polyarthritis, unspecified
● M13.1 Monoarthritis, not elsewhere classified
M13.10 Monoarthritis, not elsewhere classified, unspecified site
● M13.11 Monoarthritis, not elsewhere classified, shoulder
    M13.111 Monoarthritis, not elsewhere classified, right shoulder
    M13.112 Monoarthritis, not elsewhere classified, left shoulder
    M13.119 Monoarthritis, not elsewhere classified, unspecified shoulder
● M13.12 Monoarthritis, not elsewhere classified, elbow
    M13.121 Monoarthritis, not elsewhere classified, right elbow
    M13.122 Monoarthritis, not elsewhere classified, left elbow
    M13.129 Monoarthritis, not elsewhere classified, unspecified elbow
● M13.13 Monoarthritis, not elsewhere classified, wrist
    M13.131 Monoarthritis, not elsewhere classified, right wrist
    M13.132 Monoarthritis, not elsewhere classified, left wrist
    M13.139 Monoarthritis, not elsewhere classified, unspecified wrist
● M13.14 Monoarthritis, not elsewhere classified, hand
    M13.141 Monoarthritis, not elsewhere classified, right hand
    M13.142 Monoarthritis, not elsewhere classified, left hand
    M13.149 Monoarthritis, not elsewhere classified, unspecified hand
● M13.15 Monoarthritis, not elsewhere classified, hip
    M13.151 Monoarthritis, not elsewhere classified, right hip
    M13.152 Monoarthritis, not elsewhere classified, left hip
    M13.159 Monoarthritis, not elsewhere classified, unspecified hip

▶ New   ⇒ Revised   ~~deleted~~ Deleted   Excludes 1   Excludes 2   Includes   Use additional   Code first   Code also   Key words
OGCR Official Guidelines   X Assign placeholder X   ● Use Additional Character(s)   ▶ Manifestation Code   HCC Hierarchical Condition Category   Coding Clinic

● **M13.16**   Monoarthritis, not elsewhere classified, knee

    M13.161   Monoarthritis, not elsewhere classified, right knee

    M13.162   Monoarthritis, not elsewhere classified, left knee

    M13.169   Monoarthritis, not elsewhere classified, unspecified knee

● **M13.17**   Monoarthritis, not elsewhere classified, ankle and foot

    M13.171   Monoarthritis, not elsewhere classified, right ankle and foot

    M13.172   Monoarthritis, not elsewhere classified, left ankle and foot

    M13.179   Monoarthritis, not elsewhere classified, unspecified ankle and foot

● **M13.8**   Other specified arthritis

    Allergic arthritis

    Excludes1   osteoarthritis (M15-M19)

    M13.80   Other specified arthritis, unspecified site

       Coding Clinic: 2025, Q2, P9

●   **M13.81**   Other specified arthritis, shoulder

    M13.811   Other specified arthritis, right shoulder

    M13.812   Other specified arthritis, left shoulder

    M13.819   Other specified arthritis, unspecified shoulder

●   **M13.82**   Other specified arthritis, elbow

    M13.821   Other specified arthritis, right elbow

    M13.822   Other specified arthritis, left elbow

    M13.829   Other specified arthritis, unspecified elbow

●   **M13.83**   Other specified arthritis, wrist

    M13.831   Other specified arthritis, right wrist

    M13.832   Other specified arthritis, left wrist

    M13.839   Other specified arthritis, unspecified wrist

●   **M13.84**   Other specified arthritis, hand

    M13.841   Other specified arthritis, right hand

    M13.842   Other specified arthritis, left hand

    M13.849   Other specified arthritis, unspecified hand

●   **M13.85**   Other specified arthritis, hip

    M13.851   Other specified arthritis, right hip

    M13.852   Other specified arthritis, left hip

    M13.859   Other specified arthritis, unspecified hip

●   **M13.86**   Other specified arthritis, knee

    M13.861   Other specified arthritis, right knee

    M13.862   Other specified arthritis, left knee

    M13.869   Other specified arthritis, unspecified knee

●   **M13.87**   Other specified arthritis, ankle and foot

    M13.871   Other specified arthritis, right ankle and foot

    M13.872   Other specified arthritis, left ankle and foot

    M13.879   Other specified arthritis, unspecified ankle and foot

    M13.88   Other specified arthritis, other site

    M13.89   Other specified arthritis, multiple sites

       Coding Clinic: 2025, Q2, P10

● **M14**   Arthropathies in other diseases classified elsewhere

    Excludes1   arthropathy in:

       diabetes mellitus (E08-E13 with .61-)

       hematological disorders (M36.2-M36.3)

       hypersensitivity reactions (M36.4)

       neoplastic disease (M36.1)

       neurosyphillis (A52.16)

       sarcoidosis (D86.86)

    enteropathic arthropathies (M07.0-)

    juvenile psoriatic arthropathy (L40.54)

    lipoid dermatoarthritis (E78.81)

● **M14.6**   Charcôt's joint

    Neuropathic arthropathy

    Excludes1   Charcôt's joint in diabetes mellitus (E08-E13 with .610)

       Charcôt's joint in tabes dorsalis (A52.16)

    M14.60   Charcôt's joint, unspecified site

●   **M14.61**   Charcôt's joint, shoulder

    M14.611   Charcôt's joint, right shoulder

    M14.612   Charcôt's joint, left shoulder

    M14.619   Charcôt's joint, unspecified shoulder

●   **M14.62**   Charcôt's joint, elbow

    M14.621   Charcôt's joint, right elbow

    M14.622   Charcôt's joint, left elbow

    M14.629   Charcôt's joint, unspecified elbow

●   **M14.63**   Charcôt's joint, wrist

    M14.631   Charcôt's joint, right wrist

    M14.632   Charcôt's joint, left wrist

    M14.639   Charcôt's joint, unspecified wrist

●   **M14.64**   Charcôt's joint, hand

    M14.641   Charcôt's joint, right hand

    M14.642   Charcôt's joint, left hand

    M14.649   Charcôt's joint, unspecified hand

●   **M14.65**   Charcôt's joint, hip

    M14.651   Charcôt's joint, right hip

    M14.652   Charcôt's joint, left hip

    M14.659   Charcôt's joint, unspecified hip

●   **M14.66**   Charcôt's joint, knee

    M14.661   Charcôt's joint, right knee

    M14.662   Charcôt's joint, left knee

    M14.669   Charcôt's joint, unspecified knee

●   **M14.67**   Charcôt's joint, ankle and foot

    M14.671   Charcôt's joint, right ankle and foot

    M14.672   Charcôt's joint, left ankle and foot

    M14.679   Charcôt's joint, unspecified ankle and foot

    M14.68   Charcôt's joint, vertebrae

    M14.69   Charcôt's joint, multiple sites

● **M14.8**   Arthropathies in other specified diseases classified elsewhere

    Code first underlying disease, such as:

       amyloidosis (E85.-)

       erythema multiforme (L51.-)

       erythema nodosum (L52)

       hemochromatosis (E83.11-)

       hyperparathyroidism (E21.-)

       hypothyroidism (E00-E03)

       sickle-cell disorders (D57.-)

       thyrotoxicosis [hyperthyroidism] (E05.-)

       Whipple's disease (K90.81)

    ▶ *M14.80*   *Arthropathies in other specified diseases classified elsewhere, unspecified site*

●   **M14.81**   Arthropathies in other specified diseases classified elsewhere, shoulder

    ▶ *M14.811*   *Arthropathies in other specified diseases classified elsewhere, right shoulder*

▶ M14.812　Arthropathies in other specified diseases classified elsewhere, left shoulder

▶ M14.819　Arthropathies in other specified diseases classified elsewhere, unspecified shoulder

● M14.82　Arthropathies in other specified diseases classified elsewhere, elbow

▶ M14.821　Arthropathies in other specified diseases classified elsewhere, right elbow

▶ M14.822　Arthropathies in other specified diseases classified elsewhere, left elbow

▶ M14.829　Arthropathies in other specified diseases classified elsewhere, unspecified elbow

● M14.83　Arthropathies in other specified diseases classified elsewhere, wrist

▶ M14.831　Arthropathies in other specified diseases classified elsewhere, right wrist

▶ M14.832　Arthropathies in other specified diseases classified elsewhere, left wrist

▶ M14.839　Arthropathies in other specified diseases classified elsewhere, unspecified wrist

● M14.84　Arthropathies in other specified diseases classified elsewhere, hand

▶ M14.841　Arthropathies in other specified diseases classified elsewhere, right hand

▶ M14.842　Arthropathies in other specified diseases classified elsewhere, left hand

▶ M14.849　Arthropathies in other specified diseases classified elsewhere, unspecified hand

● M14.85　Arthropathies in other specified diseases classified elsewhere, hip

▶ M14.851　Arthropathies in other specified diseases classified elsewhere, right hip

▶ M14.852　Arthropathies in other specified diseases classified elsewhere, left hip

▶ M14.859　Arthropathies in other specified diseases classified elsewhere, unspecified hip

● M14.86　Arthropathies in other specified diseases classified elsewhere, knee

▶ M14.861　Arthropathies in other specified diseases classified elsewhere, right knee

▶ M14.862　Arthropathies in other specified diseases classified elsewhere, left knee

▶ M14.869　Arthropathies in other specified diseases classified elsewhere, unspecified knee

● M14.87　Arthropathies in other specified diseases classified elsewhere, ankle and foot

▶ M14.871　Arthropathies in other specified diseases classified elsewhere, right ankle and foot

▶ M14.872　Arthropathies in other specified diseases classified elsewhere, left ankle and foot

▶ M14.879　Arthropathies in other specified diseases classified elsewhere, unspecified ankle and foot

▶ M14.88　Arthropathies in other specified diseases classified elsewhere, vertebrae

▶ M14.89　Arthropathies in other specified diseases classified elsewhere, multiple sites

OSTEOARTHRITIS (M15-M19)

Osteoarthritis is the most common degenerative joint disease and form of arthritis that breaks down the cartilage causing pain, swelling, and reduced motion in the joints.

Excludes2　osteoarthritis of spine (M47.-)

● M15　Polyosteoarthritis

Includes　arthritis of multiple sites

Excludes1　bilateral involvement of single joint (M16-M19)

M15.0　Primary generalized (osteo)arthritis

M15.1　Heberden's nodes (with arthropathy)
Interphalangeal distal osteoarthritis

M15.2　Bouchard's nodes (with arthropathy)
Juxtaphalangeal distal osteoarthritis

M15.3　Secondary multiple arthritis
Post-traumatic polyosteoarthritis

M15.4　Erosive (osteo)arthritis

M15.8　Other polyosteoarthritis

M15.9　Polyosteoarthritis, unspecified
Generalized osteoarthritis NOS

● M16　Osteoarthritis of hip

M16.0　Bilateral primary osteoarthritis of hip
Coding Clinic: 2018, Q2, P15; 2016, Q4, P146

● M16.1　Unilateral primary osteoarthritis of hip
Primary osteoarthritis of hip NOS

M16.10　Unilateral primary osteoarthritis, unspecified hip

M16.11　Unilateral primary osteoarthritis, right hip

M16.12　Unilateral primary osteoarthritis, left hip

M16.2　Bilateral osteoarthritis resulting from hip dysplasia

● M16.3　Unilateral osteoarthritis resulting from hip dysplasia
Dysplastic osteoarthritis of hip NOS

M16.30　Unilateral osteoarthritis resulting from hip dysplasia, unspecified hip

M16.31　Unilateral osteoarthritis resulting from hip dysplasia, right hip

M16.32　Unilateral osteoarthritis resulting from hip dysplasia, left hip

M16.4　Bilateral post-traumatic osteoarthritis of hip

● M16.5　Unilateral post-traumatic osteoarthritis of hip
Post-traumatic osteoarthritis of hip NOS

M16.50　Unilateral post-traumatic osteoarthritis, unspecified hip

M16.51　Unilateral post-traumatic osteoarthritis, right hip

M16.52　Unilateral post-traumatic osteoarthritis, left hip

M16.6　Other bilateral secondary osteoarthritis of hip

M16.7　Other unilateral secondary osteoarthritis of hip
Secondary osteoarthritis of hip NOS

M16.9　Osteoarthritis of hip, unspecified

● M17　Osteoarthritis of knee

M17.0　Bilateral primary osteoarthritis of knee

● M17.1　Unilateral primary osteoarthritis of knee
Primary osteoarthritis of knee NOS

M17.10　Unilateral primary osteoarthritis, unspecified knee
Coding Clinic: 2016, Q4, P147

M17.11　Unilateral primary osteoarthritis, right knee

M17.12　Unilateral primary osteoarthritis, left knee
Coding Clinic: 2016, Q4, P146

M17.2　Bilateral post-traumatic osteoarthritis of knee

● M17.3　Unilateral post-traumatic osteoarthritis of knee
Post-traumatic osteoarthritis of knee NOS

M17.30　Unilateral post-traumatic osteoarthritis, unspecified knee

M17.31　Unilateral post-traumatic osteoarthritis, right knee

M17.32　Unilateral post-traumatic osteoarthritis, left knee

M17.4   **Other bilateral secondary osteoarthritis of knee**
M17.5   **Other unilateral secondary osteoarthritis of knee**
    Secondary osteoarthritis of knee NOS
M17.9   **Osteoarthritis of knee, unspecified**
    Coding Clinic: 2016, Q4, P146

● **M18 Osteoarthritis of first carpometacarpal joint**
  M18.0   **Bilateral primary osteoarthritis of first carpometacarpal joints**
  ● M18.1   **Unilateral primary osteoarthritis of first carpometacarpal joint**
    Primary osteoarthritis of first carpometacarpal joint NOS
    M18.10   **Unilateral primary osteoarthritis of first carpometacarpal joint, unspecified hand**
    M18.11   **Unilateral primary osteoarthritis of first carpometacarpal joint, right hand**
    M18.12   **Unilateral primary osteoarthritis of first carpometacarpal joint, left hand**
  M18.2   **Bilateral post-traumatic osteoarthritis of first carpometacarpal joints**
  ● M18.3   **Unilateral post-traumatic osteoarthritis of first carpometacarpal joint**
    Post-traumatic osteoarthritis of first carpometacarpal joint NOS
    M18.30   **Unilateral post-traumatic osteoarthritis of first carpometacarpal joint, unspecified hand**
    M18.31   **Unilateral post-traumatic osteoarthritis of first carpometacarpal joint, right hand**
    M18.32   **Unilateral post-traumatic osteoarthritis of first carpometacarpal joint, left hand**
  M18.4   **Other bilateral secondary osteoarthritis of first carpometacarpal joints**
  ● M18.5   **Other unilateral secondary osteoarthritis of first carpometacarpal joint**
    Secondary osteoarthritis of first carpometacarpal joint NOS
    M18.50   **Other unilateral secondary osteoarthritis of first carpometacarpal joint, unspecified hand**
    M18.51   **Other unilateral secondary osteoarthritis of first carpometacarpal joint, right hand**
    M18.52   **Other unilateral secondary osteoarthritis of first carpometacarpal joint, left hand**
  M18.9   **Osteoarthritis of first carpometacarpal joint, unspecified**

● **M19 Other and unspecified osteoarthritis**
  Excludes1   polyarthritis (M15.-)
  Excludes2   arthrosis of spine (M47.-)
    hallux rigidus (M20.2)
    osteoarthritis of spine (M47.-)
  ● M19.0   **Primary osteoarthritis of other joints**
  ● M19.01   **Primary osteoarthritis, shoulder**
    M19.011   **Primary osteoarthritis, right shoulder**
      Coding Clinic: 2016, Q4, P145
    M19.012   **Primary osteoarthritis, left shoulder**
    M19.019   **Primary osteoarthritis, unspecified shoulder**
  ● M19.02   **Primary osteoarthritis, elbow**
    M19.021   **Primary osteoarthritis, right elbow**
    M19.022   **Primary osteoarthritis, left elbow**
    M19.029   **Primary osteoarthritis, unspecified elbow**
  ● M19.03   **Primary osteoarthritis, wrist**
    M19.031   **Primary osteoarthritis, right wrist**
    M19.032   **Primary osteoarthritis, left wrist**
    M19.039   **Primary osteoarthritis, unspecified wrist**

● M19.04   **Primary osteoarthritis, hand**
  Excludes2   primary osteoarthritis of first carpometacarpal joint (M18.0-, M18.1-)
  M19.041   **Primary osteoarthritis, right hand**
  M19.042   **Primary osteoarthritis, left hand**
  M19.049   **Primary osteoarthritis, unspecified hand**
● M19.07   **Primary osteoarthritis ankle and foot**
  M19.071   **Primary osteoarthritis, right ankle and foot**
  M19.072   **Primary osteoarthritis, left ankle and foot**
  M19.079   **Primary osteoarthritis, unspecified ankle and foot**
M19.09   **Primary osteoarthritis, other specified site**
● M19.1   **Post-traumatic osteoarthritis of other joints**
  ● M19.11   **Post-traumatic osteoarthritis, shoulder**
    M19.111   **Post-traumatic osteoarthritis, right shoulder**
    M19.112   **Post-traumatic osteoarthritis, left shoulder**
    M19.119   **Post-traumatic osteoarthritis, unspecified shoulder**
  ● M19.12   **Post-traumatic osteoarthritis, elbow**
    M19.121   **Post-traumatic osteoarthritis, right elbow**
    M19.122   **Post-traumatic osteoarthritis, left elbow**
    M19.129   **Post-traumatic osteoarthritis, unspecified elbow**
  ● M19.13   **Post-traumatic osteoarthritis, wrist**
    M19.131   **Post-traumatic osteoarthritis, right wrist**
    M19.132   **Post-traumatic osteoarthritis, left wrist**
    M19.139   **Post-traumatic osteoarthritis, unspecified wrist**
  ● M19.14   **Post-traumatic osteoarthritis, hand**
    Excludes2   post-traumatic osteoarthritis of first carpometacarpal joint (M18.2-, M18.3-)
    M19.141   **Post-traumatic osteoarthritis, right hand**
    M19.142   **Post-traumatic osteoarthritis, left hand**
    M19.149   **Post-traumatic osteoarthritis, unspecified hand**
  ● M19.17   **Post-traumatic osteoarthritis, ankle and foot**
    M19.171   **Post-traumatic osteoarthritis, right ankle and foot**
    M19.172   **Post-traumatic osteoarthritis, left ankle and foot**
    M19.179   **Post-traumatic osteoarthritis, unspecified ankle and foot**
  M19.19   **Post-traumatic osteoarthritis, other specified site**
● M19.2   **Secondary osteoarthritis of other joints**
  ● M19.21   **Secondary osteoarthritis, shoulder**
    M19.211   **Secondary osteoarthritis, right shoulder**
    M19.212   **Secondary osteoarthritis, left shoulder**
    M19.219   **Secondary osteoarthritis, unspecified shoulder**
  ● M19.22   **Secondary osteoarthritis, elbow**
    M19.221   **Secondary osteoarthritis, right elbow**
    M19.222   **Secondary osteoarthritis, left elbow**
    M19.229   **Secondary osteoarthritis, unspecified elbow**

CHAPTER 13 (M00–M99)

● **M19.23** Secondary osteoarthritis, wrist
     M19.231 Secondary osteoarthritis, right wrist
     M19.232 Secondary osteoarthritis, left wrist
     M19.239 Secondary osteoarthritis, unspecified wrist

● **M19.24** Secondary osteoarthritis, hand
     M19.241 Secondary osteoarthritis, right hand
     M19.242 Secondary osteoarthritis, left hand
     M19.249 Secondary osteoarthritis, unspecified hand

● **M19.27** Secondary osteoarthritis, ankle and foot
     M19.271 Secondary osteoarthritis, right ankle and foot
     M19.272 Secondary osteoarthritis, left ankle and foot
     M19.279 Secondary osteoarthritis, unspecified ankle and foot

     M19.29 Secondary osteoarthritis, other specified site

● **M19.9** Osteoarthritis, unspecified site
     M19.90 Unspecified osteoarthritis, unspecified site
         Arthrosis NOS
         Arthritis NOS
         Osteoarthritis NOS
         Coding Clinic: 2016, Q4, P147
     M19.91 Primary osteoarthritis, unspecified site
         Primary osteoarthritis NOS
     M19.92 Post-traumatic osteoarthritis, unspecified site
         Post-traumatic osteoarthritis NOS
     M19.93 Secondary osteoarthritis, unspecified site
         Secondary osteoarthritis NOS

OTHER JOINT DISORDERS (M20-M25)

Excludes2   joints of the spine (M40-M54)

● **M20** Acquired deformities of fingers and toes
     Excludes1   acquired absence of fingers and toes (Z89.-)
         congenital absence of fingers and toes (Q71.3-, Q72.3-)
         congenital deformities and malformations of fingers and toes (Q66.-, Q68-Q70, Q74.-)

● **M20.0** Deformity of finger(s)
     Excludes1   clubbing of fingers (R68.3)
         palmar fascial fibromatosis [Dupuytren] (M72.0)
         trigger finger (M65.3)

   ● **M20.00** Unspecified deformity of finger(s)
     M20.001 Unspecified deformity of right finger(s)
     M20.002 Unspecified deformity of left finger(s)
     M20.009 Unspecified deformity of unspecified finger(s)

   ● **M20.01** Mallet finger
     M20.011 Mallet finger of right finger(s)
     M20.012 Mallet finger of left finger(s)
     M20.019 Mallet finger of unspecified finger(s)

   ● **M20.02** Boutonnière deformity
     M20.021 Boutonnière deformity of right finger(s)
     M20.022 Boutonnière deformity of left finger(s)
     M20.029 Boutonnière deformity of unspecified finger(s)

   ● **M20.03** Swan-neck deformity
     M20.031 Swan-neck deformity of right finger(s)
     M20.032 Swan-neck deformity of left finger(s)
     M20.039 Swan-neck deformity of unspecified finger(s)

● **M20.09** Other deformity of finger(s)
     M20.091 Other deformity of right finger(s)
     M20.092 Other deformity of left finger(s)
     M20.099 Other deformity of finger(s), unspecified finger(s)

● **M20.1** Hallux valgus (acquired)
     Excludes2   bunion (M21.6-)
     Coding Clinic: 2016, Q4, P38
     M20.10 Hallux valgus (acquired), unspecified foot
     M20.11 Hallux valgus (acquired), right foot
     M20.12 Hallux valgus (acquired), left foot

● **M20.2** Hallux rigidus
     M20.20 Hallux rigidus, unspecified foot
     M20.21 Hallux rigidus, right foot
     M20.22 Hallux rigidus, left foot

● **M20.3** Hallux varus (acquired)
     M20.30 Hallux varus (acquired), unspecified foot
     M20.31 Hallux varus (acquired), right foot
     M20.32 Hallux varus (acquired), left foot

● **M20.4** Other hammer toe(s) (acquired)
     M20.40 Other hammer toe(s) (acquired), unspecified foot
     M20.41 Other hammer toe(s) (acquired), right foot
     M20.42 Other hammer toe(s) (acquired), left foot

● **M20.5** Other deformities of toe(s) (acquired)
   ● **M20.5X** Other deformities of toe(s) (acquired)
     M20.5X1 Other deformities of toe(s) (acquired), right foot
     M20.5X2 Other deformities of toe(s) (acquired), left foot
     M20.5X9 Other deformities of toe(s) (acquired), unspecified foot

● **M20.6** Acquired deformities of toe(s), unspecified
     M20.60 Acquired deformities of toe(s), unspecified, unspecified foot
     M20.61 Acquired deformities of toe(s), unspecified, right foot
     M20.62 Acquired deformities of toe(s), unspecified, left foot

Item 13-2 Hallux valgus is a sometimes painful structural deformity caused by an inflammation of the bursal sac at the base of the metatarsophalangeal joint (big toe). **Hallus varus** is a deviation of the great toe to the inner side of the foot or away from the next toe.

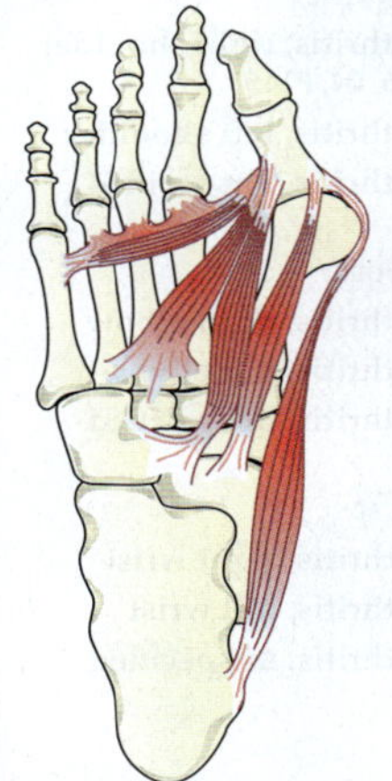

Figure 13-1   Hallux valgus.

● **M21 Other acquired deformities of limbs**

Excludes1 acquired absence of limb (Z89.-)
congenital absence of limbs (Q71-Q73)
congenital deformities and malformations of limbs (Q65-Q66, Q68-Q74)

Excludes2 acquired deformities of fingers or toes (M20.-)
coxa plana (M91.2)

● **M21.0 Valgus deformity, not elsewhere classified**

Excludes1 metatarsus valgus (Q66.6)
talipes calcaneovalgus (Q66.4-)

M21.00 Valgus deformity, not elsewhere classified, unspecified site

● **M21.02 Valgus deformity, not elsewhere classified, elbow**
Cubitus valgus

M21.021 Valgus deformity, not elsewhere classified, right elbow

M21.022 Valgus deformity, not elsewhere classified, left elbow

M21.029 Valgus deformity, not elsewhere classified, unspecified elbow

● **M21.05 Valgus deformity, not elsewhere classified, hip**

M21.051 Valgus deformity, not elsewhere classified, right hip

M21.052 Valgus deformity, not elsewhere classified, left hip

M21.059 Valgus deformity, not elsewhere classified, unspecified hip

● **M21.06 Valgus deformity, not elsewhere classified, knee**
Genu valgum
Knock knee

M21.061 Valgus deformity, not elsewhere classified, right knee

M21.062 Valgus deformity, not elsewhere classified, left knee

M21.069 Valgus deformity, not elsewhere classified, unspecified knee

● **M21.07 Valgus deformity, not elsewhere classified, ankle**

M21.071 Valgus deformity, not elsewhere classified, right ankle

M21.072 Valgus deformity, not elsewhere classified, left ankle

M21.079 Valgus deformity, not elsewhere classified, unspecified ankle

● **M21.1 Varus deformity, not elsewhere classified**

Excludes1 metatarsus varus (Q66.22-)
tibia vara (M92.51-)

M21.10 Varus deformity, not elsewhere classified, unspecified site

● **M21.12 Varus deformity, not elsewhere classified, elbow**
Cubitus varus, elbow

M21.121 Varus deformity, not elsewhere classified, right elbow

M21.122 Varus deformity, not elsewhere classified, left elbow

M21.129 Varus deformity, not elsewhere classified, unspecified elbow

Item 13–3 Cubitus valgus is a deformity of the elbow resulting in an increased carrying angle in which the arm extends at the side and the palm faces forward, which results in the forearm and hand extended at greater than 15 degrees.

Item 13–4 Cubitus varus is a deformity of the elbow resulting in the arm extended at the side and the palm facing forward so that the forearm and hand are held at less than 5 degrees, decreasing the carrying angle.

● **M21.15 Varus deformity, not elsewhere classified, hip**

M21.151 Varus deformity, not elsewhere classified, right hip

M21.152 Varus deformity, not elsewhere classified, left hip

➡ **M21.159 Varus deformity, not elsewhere classified, unspecified hip**

● **M21.16 Varus deformity, not elsewhere classified, knee**
Bow leg
Genu varum

M21.161 Varus deformity, not elsewhere classified, right knee

M21.162 Varus deformity, not elsewhere classified, left knee

M21.169 Varus deformity, not elsewhere classified, unspecified knee

● **M21.17 Varus deformity, not elsewhere classified, ankle**

M21.171 Varus deformity, not elsewhere classified, right ankle

M21.172 Varus deformity, not elsewhere classified, left ankle

M21.179 Varus deformity, not elsewhere classified, unspecified ankle

● **M21.2 Flexion deformity**

M21.20 Flexion deformity, unspecified site

● **M21.21 Flexion deformity, shoulder**

M21.211 Flexion deformity, right shoulder

M21.212 Flexion deformity, left shoulder

M21.219 Flexion deformity, unspecified shoulder

● **M21.22 Flexion deformity, elbow**

M21.221 Flexion deformity, right elbow

M21.222 Flexion deformity, left elbow

M21.229 Flexion deformity, unspecified elbow

● **M21.23 Flexion deformity, wrist**

M21.231 Flexion deformity, right wrist

M21.232 Flexion deformity, left wrist

M21.239 Flexion deformity, unspecified wrist

● **M21.24 Flexion deformity, finger joints**

M21.241 Flexion deformity, right finger joints

M21.242 Flexion deformity, left finger joints

M21.249 Flexion deformity, unspecified finger joints

● **M21.25 Flexion deformity, hip**

M21.251 Flexion deformity, right hip

M21.252 Flexion deformity, left hip

M21.259 Flexion deformity, unspecified hip

● **M21.26 Flexion deformity, knee**

M21.261 Flexion deformity, right knee

M21.262 Flexion deformity, left knee

M21.269 Flexion deformity, unspecified knee

● **M21.27 Flexion deformity, ankle and toes**

M21.271 Flexion deformity, right ankle and toes

M21.272 Flexion deformity, left ankle and toes

M21.279 Flexion deformity, unspecified ankle and toes

● **M21.3 Wrist or foot drop (acquired)**

● **M21.33 Wrist drop (acquired)**

M21.331 Wrist drop, right wrist

M21.332 Wrist drop, left wrist

M21.339 Wrist drop, unspecified wrist

● **M21.37 Foot drop (acquired)**

M21.371 Foot drop, right foot

M21.372 Foot drop, left foot

M21.379 Foot drop, unspecified foot

CHAPTER 13 (MØØ-M99)

● **M21.4**   Flat foot [pes planus] (acquired)

    Excludes1   congenital pes planus (Q66.5-)

    M21.40   Flat foot [pes planus] (acquired), unspecified foot

    M21.41   Flat foot [pes planus] (acquired), right foot

    M21.42   Flat foot [pes planus] (acquired), left foot

● **M21.5**   Acquired clawhand, clubhand, clawfoot and clubfoot

    Excludes1   clubfoot, not specified as acquired (Q66.89)

    ● M21.51   Acquired clawhand

      M21.511   Acquired clawhand, right hand

      M21.512   Acquired clawhand, left hand

      M21.519   Acquired clawhand, unspecified hand

    ● M21.52   Acquired clubhand

      M21.521   Acquired clubhand, right hand

      M21.522   Acquired clubhand, left hand

      M21.529   Acquired clubhand, unspecified hand

    ● M21.53   Acquired clawfoot

      M21.531   Acquired clawfoot, right foot

      M21.532   Acquired clawfoot, left foot

      M21.539   Acquired clawfoot, unspecified foot

    ● M21.54   Acquired clubfoot

      M21.541   Acquired clubfoot, right foot

      M21.542   Acquired clubfoot, left foot

      M21.549   Acquired clubfoot, unspecified foot

● **M21.6**   Other acquired deformities of foot

    Excludes2   deformities of toe (acquired) (M20.1-M20.6-)

    ● M21.61   Bunion

      Coding Clinic: 2016, Q4, P38

      M21.611   Bunion of right foot

      M21.612   Bunion of left foot

      M21.619   Bunion of unspecified foot

    ● M21.62   Bunionette

      Coding Clinic: 2016, Q4, P38

      M21.621   Bunionette of right foot

      M21.622   Bunionette of left foot

      M21.629   Bunionette of unspecified foot

    ● M21.6X   Other acquired deformities of foot

      M21.6X1   Other acquired deformities of right foot

      Coding Clinic: 2023, Q3, P21

      M21.6X2   Other acquired deformities of left foot

      M21.6X9   Other acquired deformities of unspecified foot

● **M21.7**   Unequal limb length (acquired)

    Note: The site used should correspond to the shorter limb.

    M21.70   Unequal limb length (acquired), unspecified site

    ● M21.72   Unequal limb length (acquired), humerus

      M21.721   Unequal limb length (acquired), right humerus

      M21.722   Unequal limb length (acquired), left humerus

      M21.729   Unequal limb length (acquired), unspecified humerus

    ● M21.73   Unequal limb length (acquired), ulna and radius

      M21.731   Unequal limb length (acquired), right ulna

      M21.732   Unequal limb length (acquired), left ulna

      M21.733   Unequal limb length (acquired), right radius

      M21.734   Unequal limb length (acquired), left radius

      M21.739   Unequal limb length (acquired), unspecified ulna and radius

    ● M21.75   Unequal limb length (acquired), femur

      M21.751   Unequal limb length (acquired), right femur

      M21.752   Unequal limb length (acquired), left femur

      M21.759   Unequal limb length (acquired), unspecified femur

    ● M21.76   Unequal limb length (acquired), tibia and fibula

      M21.761   Unequal limb length (acquired), right tibia

      M21.762   Unequal limb length (acquired), left tibia

      M21.763   Unequal limb length (acquired), right fibula

      M21.764   Unequal limb length (acquired), left fibula

      M21.769   Unequal limb length (acquired), unspecified tibia and fibula

● **M21.8**   Other specified acquired deformities of limbs

    Excludes2   coxa plana (M91.2)

    M21.80   Other specified acquired deformities of unspecified limb

    ● M21.82   Other specified acquired deformities of upper arm

      M21.821   Other specified acquired deformities of right upper arm

      M21.822   Other specified acquired deformities of left upper arm

      M21.829   Other specified acquired deformities of unspecified upper arm

    ● M21.83   Other specified acquired deformities of forearm

      M21.831   Other specified acquired deformities of right forearm

      M21.832   Other specified acquired deformities of left forearm

      M21.839   Other specified acquired deformities of unspecified forearm

    ● M21.85   Other specified acquired deformities of thigh

      M21.851   Other specified acquired deformities of right thigh

      M21.852   Other specified acquired deformities of left thigh

      M21.859   Other specified acquired deformities of unspecified thigh

    ● M21.86   Other specified acquired deformities of lower leg

      M21.861   Other specified acquired deformities of right lower leg

      M21.862   Other specified acquired deformities of left lower leg

      M21.869   Other specified acquired deformities of unspecified lower leg

- **M21.9 Unspecified acquired deformity of limb and hand**
  - M21.90   Unspecified acquired deformity of unspecified limb
  - **M21.92   Unspecified acquired deformity of upper arm**
    - M21.921   Unspecified acquired deformity of right upper arm
    - M21.922   Unspecified acquired deformity of left upper arm
    - M21.929   Unspecified acquired deformity of unspecified upper arm
  - **M21.93   Unspecified acquired deformity of forearm**
    - M21.931   Unspecified acquired deformity of right forearm
    - M21.932   Unspecified acquired deformity of left forearm
    - M21.939   Unspecified acquired deformity of unspecified forearm
  - **M21.94   Unspecified acquired deformity of hand**
    - M21.941   Unspecified acquired deformity of hand, right hand
    - M21.942   Unspecified acquired deformity of hand, left hand
    - M21.949   Unspecified acquired deformity of hand, unspecified hand
  - **M21.95   Unspecified acquired deformity of thigh**
    - M21.951   Unspecified acquired deformity of right thigh
    - M21.952   Unspecified acquired deformity of left thigh
    - M21.959   Unspecified acquired deformity of unspecified thigh
  - **M21.96   Unspecified acquired deformity of lower leg**
    - M21.961   Unspecified acquired deformity of right lower leg
    - M21.962   Unspecified acquired deformity of left lower leg
    - M21.969   Unspecified acquired deformity of unspecified lower leg

- **M22   Disorder of patella**
  - **Excludes2**   traumatic dislocation of patella (S83.0-)
  - **M22.0   Recurrent dislocation of patella**
    - M22.00   Recurrent dislocation of patella, unspecified knee
    - M22.01   Recurrent dislocation of patella, right knee
    - M22.02   Recurrent dislocation of patella, left knee
  - **M22.1   Recurrent subluxation of patella**
    - Incomplete dislocation of patella
    - M22.10   Recurrent subluxation of patella, unspecified knee
    - M22.11   Recurrent subluxation of patella, right knee
    - M22.12   Recurrent subluxation of patella, left knee
  - **M22.2   Patellofemoral disorders**
    - **M22.2X   Patellofemoral disorders**
      - M22.2X1   Patellofemoral disorders, right knee
      - M22.2X2   Patellofemoral disorders, left knee
      - M22.2X9   Patellofemoral disorders, unspecified knee
  - **M22.3   Other derangements of patella**
    - **M22.3X   Other derangements of patella**
      - M22.3X1   Other derangements of patella, right knee
      - M22.3X2   Other derangements of patella, left knee
      - M22.3X9   Other derangements of patella, unspecified knee

- **M22.4   Chondromalacia patellae**
  - M22.40   Chondromalacia patellae, unspecified knee
  - M22.41   Chondromalacia patellae, right knee
  - M22.42   Chondromalacia patellae, left knee
- **M22.8   Other disorders of patella**
  - **M22.8X   Other disorders of patella**
    - M22.8X1   Other disorders of patella, right knee
    - M22.8X2   Other disorders of patella, left knee
    - M22.8X9   Other disorders of patella, unspecified knee
- **M22.9   Unspecified disorder of patella**
  - M22.90   Unspecified disorder of patella, unspecified knee
  - M22.91   Unspecified disorder of patella, right knee
  - M22.92   Unspecified disorder of patella, left knee

- **M23   Internal derangement of knee**
  - **Excludes1**   ankylosis (M24.66)
    - deformity of knee (M21.-)
    - osteochondritis dissecans (M93.2)
  - **Excludes2**   current injury - see injury of knee and lower leg (S80-S89)
    - recurrent dislocation or subluxation of joints (M24.4)
    - recurrent dislocation or subluxation of patella (M22.0-M22.1)
  - **Coding Clinic: 2019, Q2, P26**
  - **M23.0   Cystic meniscus**
    - **M23.00   Cystic meniscus, unspecified meniscus**
      - Cystic meniscus, unspecified lateral meniscus
      - Cystic meniscus, unspecified medial meniscus
      - M23.000   Cystic meniscus, unspecified lateral meniscus, right knee
      - M23.001   Cystic meniscus, unspecified lateral meniscus, left knee
      - M23.002   Cystic meniscus, unspecified lateral meniscus, unspecified knee
      - M23.003   Cystic meniscus, unspecified medial meniscus, right knee
      - M23.004   Cystic meniscus, unspecified medial meniscus, left knee
      - M23.005   Cystic meniscus, unspecified medial meniscus, unspecified knee
      - M23.006   Cystic meniscus, unspecified meniscus, right knee
      - M23.007   Cystic meniscus, unspecified meniscus, left knee
      - M23.009   Cystic meniscus, unspecified meniscus, unspecified knee
    - **M23.01   Cystic meniscus, anterior horn of medial meniscus**
      - M23.011   Cystic meniscus, anterior horn of medial meniscus, right knee
      - M23.012   Cystic meniscus, anterior horn of medial meniscus, left knee
      - M23.019   Cystic meniscus, anterior horn of medial meniscus, unspecified knee
    - **M23.02   Cystic meniscus, posterior horn of medial meniscus**
      - M23.021   Cystic meniscus, posterior horn of medial meniscus, right knee
      - M23.022   Cystic meniscus, posterior horn of medial meniscus, left knee
      - M23.029   Cystic meniscus, posterior horn of medial meniscus, unspecified knee

● M23.03   Cystic meniscus, other medial meniscus
  M23.031   Cystic meniscus, other medial meniscus, right knee
  M23.032   Cystic meniscus, other medial meniscus, left knee
  M23.039   Cystic meniscus, other medial meniscus, unspecified knee
● M23.04   Cystic meniscus, anterior horn of lateral meniscus
  M23.041   Cystic meniscus, anterior horn of lateral meniscus, right knee
  M23.042   Cystic meniscus, anterior horn of lateral meniscus, left knee
  M23.049   Cystic meniscus, anterior horn of lateral meniscus, unspecified knee
● M23.05   Cystic meniscus, posterior horn of lateral meniscus
  M23.051   Cystic meniscus, posterior horn of lateral meniscus, right knee
  M23.052   Cystic meniscus, posterior horn of lateral meniscus, left knee
  M23.059   Cystic meniscus, posterior horn of lateral meniscus, unspecified knee
● M23.06   Cystic meniscus, other lateral meniscus
  M23.061   Cystic meniscus, other lateral meniscus, right knee
  M23.062   Cystic meniscus, other lateral meniscus, left knee
  M23.069   Cystic meniscus, other lateral meniscus, unspecified knee

★ (See Plate 34 of the Anatomy Illustrations.)

● M23.2   Derangement of meniscus due to old tear or injury
    Old bucket-handle tear
● M23.20   Derangement of unspecified meniscus due to old tear or injury
    Derangement of unspecified lateral meniscus due to old tear or injury
    Derangement of unspecified medial meniscus due to old tear or injury
  M23.200   Derangement of unspecified lateral meniscus due to old tear or injury, right knee
  M23.201   Derangement of unspecified lateral meniscus due to old tear or injury, left knee
  M23.202   Derangement of unspecified lateral meniscus due to old tear or injury, unspecified knee
  M23.203   Derangement of unspecified medial meniscus due to old tear or injury, right knee
  M23.204   Derangement of unspecified medial meniscus due to old tear or injury, left knee
  M23.205   Derangement of unspecified medial meniscus due to old tear or injury, unspecified knee
  M23.206   Derangement of unspecified meniscus due to old tear or injury, right knee
  M23.207   Derangement of unspecified meniscus due to old tear or injury, left knee
  M23.209   Derangement of unspecified meniscus due to old tear or injury, unspecified knee

● M23.21   Derangement of anterior horn of medial meniscus due to old tear or injury
  M23.211   Derangement of anterior horn of medial meniscus due to old tear or injury, right knee
  M23.212   Derangement of anterior horn of medial meniscus due to old tear or injury, left knee
  M23.219   Derangement of anterior horn of medial meniscus due to old tear or injury, unspecified knee
● M23.22   Derangement of posterior horn of medial meniscus due to old tear or injury
  M23.221   Derangement of posterior horn of medial meniscus due to old tear or injury, right knee
  M23.222   Derangement of posterior horn of medial meniscus due to old tear or injury, left knee
  M23.229   Derangement of posterior horn of medial meniscus due to old tear or injury, unspecified knee
● M23.23   Derangement of other medial meniscus due to old tear or injury
  M23.231   Derangement of other medial meniscus due to old tear or injury, right knee
  M23.232   Derangement of other medial meniscus due to old tear or injury, left knee
  M23.239   Derangement of other medial meniscus due to old tear or injury, unspecified knee
● M23.24   Derangement of anterior horn of lateral meniscus due to old tear or injury
  M23.241   Derangement of anterior horn of lateral meniscus due to old tear or injury, right knee
  M23.242   Derangement of anterior horn of lateral meniscus due to old tear or injury, left knee
  M23.249   Derangement of anterior horn of lateral meniscus due to old tear or injury, unspecified knee
● M23.25   Derangement of posterior horn of lateral meniscus due to old tear or injury
  M23.251   Derangement of posterior horn of lateral meniscus due to old tear or injury, right knee
  M23.252   Derangement of posterior horn of lateral meniscus due to old tear or injury, left knee
  M23.259   Derangement of posterior horn of lateral meniscus due to old tear or injury, unspecified knee
● M23.26   Derangement of other lateral meniscus due to old tear or injury
  M23.261   Derangement of other lateral meniscus due to old tear or injury, right knee
  M23.262   Derangement of other lateral meniscus due to old tear or injury, left knee
  M23.269   Derangement of other lateral meniscus due to old tear or injury, unspecified knee

● **M23.3**   **Other meniscus derangements**
     Degenerate meniscus
     Detached meniscus
     Retained meniscus

● **M23.30**   Other meniscus derangements, unspecified meniscus
     Other meniscus derangements, unspecified lateral meniscus
     Other meniscus derangements, unspecified medial meniscus

     M23.300   Other meniscus derangements, unspecified lateral meniscus, right knee

     M23.301   Other meniscus derangements, unspecified lateral meniscus, left knee

     M23.302   Other meniscus derangements, unspecified lateral meniscus, unspecified knee

     M23.303   Other meniscus derangements, unspecified medial meniscus, right knee

     M23.304   Other meniscus derangements, unspecified medial meniscus, left knee

     M23.305   Other meniscus derangements, unspecified medial meniscus, unspecified knee

     M23.306   Other meniscus derangements, unspecified meniscus, right knee

     M23.307   Other meniscus derangements, unspecified meniscus, left knee

     M23.309   Other meniscus derangements, unspecified meniscus, unspecified knee

● **M23.31**   Other meniscus derangements, anterior horn of medial meniscus

     M23.311   Other meniscus derangements, anterior horn of medial meniscus, right knee

     M23.312   Other meniscus derangements, anterior horn of medial meniscus, left knee

     M23.319   Other meniscus derangements, anterior horn of medial meniscus, unspecified knee

● **M23.32**   Other meniscus derangements, posterior horn of medial meniscus

     M23.321   Other meniscus derangements, posterior horn of medial meniscus, right knee

     M23.322   Other meniscus derangements, posterior horn of medial meniscus, left knee

     M23.329   Other meniscus derangements, posterior horn of medial meniscus, unspecified knee

● **M23.33**   Other meniscus derangements, other medial meniscus

     M23.331   Other meniscus derangements, other medial meniscus, right knee

     M23.332   Other meniscus derangements, other medial meniscus, left knee

     M23.339   Other meniscus derangements, other medial meniscus, unspecified knee

● **M23.34**   Other meniscus derangements, anterior horn of lateral meniscus

     M23.341   Other meniscus derangements, anterior horn of lateral meniscus, right knee

     M23.342   Other meniscus derangements, anterior horn of lateral meniscus, left knee

     M23.349   Other meniscus derangements, anterior horn of lateral meniscus, unspecified knee

● **M23.35**   Other meniscus derangements, posterior horn of lateral meniscus

     M23.351   Other meniscus derangements, posterior horn of lateral meniscus, right knee

     M23.352   Other meniscus derangements, posterior horn of lateral meniscus, left knee

     M23.359   Other meniscus derangements, posterior horn of lateral meniscus, unspecified knee

● **M23.36**   Other meniscus derangements, other lateral meniscus

     M23.361   Other meniscus derangements, other lateral meniscus, right knee

     M23.362   Other meniscus derangements, other lateral meniscus, left knee

     M23.369   Other meniscus derangements, other lateral meniscus, unspecified knee

● **M23.4**   **Loose body in knee**
     M23.40   Loose body in knee, unspecified knee
     M23.41   Loose body in knee, right knee
     M23.42   Loose body in knee, left knee

● **M23.5**   **Chronic instability of knee**
     M23.50   Chronic instability of knee, unspecified knee
     M23.51   Chronic instability of knee, right knee
     M23.52   Chronic instability of knee, left knee

● **M23.6**   Other spontaneous disruption of ligament(s) of knee

 ● **M23.60**   Other spontaneous disruption of unspecified ligament of knee

     M23.601   Other spontaneous disruption of unspecified ligament of right knee

     M23.602   Other spontaneous disruption of unspecified ligament of left knee

     M23.609   Other spontaneous disruption of unspecified ligament of unspecified knee

 ● **M23.61**   Other spontaneous disruption of anterior cruciate ligament of knee

     M23.611   Other spontaneous disruption of anterior cruciate ligament of right knee

     M23.612   Other spontaneous disruption of anterior cruciate ligament of left knee

     M23.619   Other spontaneous disruption of anterior cruciate ligament of unspecified knee

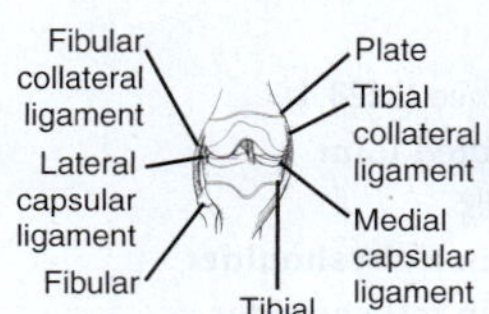

Figure 13-2   Collateral and cruciate ligament of knee. (From DeLee: DeLee and Drez's Orthopaedic Sports Medicine, ed 3, Saunders, 2009)

● **M23.62** Other spontaneous disruption of posterior cruciate ligament of knee
    M23.621 Other spontaneous disruption of posterior cruciate ligament of right knee
    M23.622 Other spontaneous disruption of posterior cruciate ligament of left knee
    M23.629 Other spontaneous disruption of posterior cruciate ligament of unspecified knee

● **M23.63** Other spontaneous disruption of medial collateral ligament of knee
    M23.631 Other spontaneous disruption of medial collateral ligament of right knee
    M23.632 Other spontaneous disruption of medial collateral ligament of left knee
    M23.639 Other spontaneous disruption of medial collateral ligament of unspecified knee

● **M23.64** Other spontaneous disruption of lateral collateral ligament of knee
    M23.641 Other spontaneous disruption of lateral collateral ligament of right knee
    M23.642 Other spontaneous disruption of lateral collateral ligament of left knee
    M23.649 Other spontaneous disruption of lateral collateral ligament of unspecified knee

● **M23.67** Other spontaneous disruption of capsular ligament of knee
    M23.671 Other spontaneous disruption of capsular ligament of right knee
    M23.672 Other spontaneous disruption of capsular ligament of left knee
    M23.679 Other spontaneous disruption of capsular ligament of unspecified knee

● **M23.8** Other internal derangements of knee
    Laxity of ligament of knee
    Snapping knee

● **M23.8X** Other internal derangements of knee
    M23.8X1 Other internal derangements of right knee
    M23.8X2 Other internal derangements of left knee
    M23.8X9 Other internal derangements of unspecified knee

● **M23.9** Unspecified internal derangement of knee
    M23.90 Unspecified internal derangement of unspecified knee
    M23.91 Unspecified internal derangement of right knee
    M23.92 Unspecified internal derangement of left knee

● **M24 Other specific joint derangements**
    Excludes1   current injury - see injury of joint by body region
    Excludes2   ganglion (M67.4)
              snapping knee (M23.8-)
              temporomandibular joint disorders (M26.6-)

● **M24.0** Loose body in joint
    Excludes2   loose body in knee (M23.4)
    M24.00 Loose body in unspecified joint

● **M24.01** Loose body in shoulder
    M24.011 Loose body in right shoulder
    M24.012 Loose body in left shoulder
    M24.019 Loose body in unspecified shoulder

● **M24.02** Loose body in elbow
    M24.021 Loose body in right elbow
    M24.022 Loose body in left elbow
    M24.029 Loose body in unspecified elbow

● **M24.03** Loose body in wrist
    M24.031 Loose body in right wrist
    M24.032 Loose body in left wrist
    M24.039 Loose body in unspecified wrist

● **M24.04** Loose body in finger joints
    M24.041 Loose body in right finger joint(s)
    M24.042 Loose body in left finger joint(s)
    M24.049 Loose body in unspecified finger joint(s)

● **M24.05** Loose body in hip
    M24.051 Loose body in right hip
    M24.052 Loose body in left hip
    M24.059 Loose body in unspecified hip

● **M24.07** Loose body in ankle and toe joints
    M24.071 Loose body in right ankle
    M24.072 Loose body in left ankle
    M24.073 Loose body in unspecified ankle
    M24.074 Loose body in right toe joint(s)
    M24.075 Loose body in left toe joint(s)
    ➡ M24.076 Loose body in unspecified toe joint(s)
    M24.08 Loose body, other site

● **M24.1** Other articular cartilage disorders
    Excludes2   chondrocalcinosis (M11.1-, M11.2-)
              internal derangement of knee (M23.-)
              metastatic calcification (E83.59)
              ochronosis (E70.29)
    M24.10 Other articular cartilage disorders, unspecified site

● **M24.11** Other articular cartilage disorders, shoulder
    M24.111 Other articular cartilage disorders, right shoulder
    M24.112 Other articular cartilage disorders, left shoulder
    M24.119 Other articular cartilage disorders, unspecified shoulder

● **M24.12** Other articular cartilage disorders, elbow
    M24.121 Other articular cartilage disorders, right elbow
    M24.122 Other articular cartilage disorders, left elbow
    M24.129 Other articular cartilage disorders, unspecified elbow

● **M24.13** Other articular cartilage disorders, wrist
    M24.131 Other articular cartilage disorders, right wrist
    M24.132 Other articular cartilage disorders, left wrist
    M24.139 Other articular cartilage disorders, unspecified wrist

● **M24.14** Other articular cartilage disorders, hand
    M24.141 Other articular cartilage disorders, right hand
    M24.142 Other articular cartilage disorders, left hand
    M24.149 Other articular cartilage disorders, unspecified hand

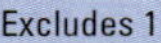

● **M24.15**   Other articular cartilage disorders, hip
    M24.151   Other articular cartilage disorders, right hip
    M24.152   Other articular cartilage disorders, left hip
    M24.159   Other articular cartilage disorders, unspecified hip

● **M24.17**   Other articular cartilage disorders, ankle and foot
    M24.171   Other articular cartilage disorders, right ankle
    M24.172   Other articular cartilage disorders, left ankle
    M24.173   Other articular cartilage disorders, unspecified ankle
    M24.174   Other articular cartilage disorders, right foot
    M24.175   Other articular cartilage disorders, left foot
    M24.176   Other articular cartilage disorders, unspecified foot

   M24.19   Other articular cartilage disorders, other specified site

● **M24.2**   Disorder of ligament
    Instability secondary to old ligament injury
    Ligamentous laxity NOS
    Excludes1   familial ligamentous laxity (M35.7)
    Excludes2   internal derangement of knee (M23.5-M23.8X9)

   M24.20   Disorder of ligament, unspecified site

● **M24.21**   Disorder of ligament, shoulder
    M24.211   Disorder of ligament, right shoulder
    M24.212   Disorder of ligament, left shoulder
    M24.219   Disorder of ligament, unspecified shoulder

● **M24.22**   Disorder of ligament, elbow
    M24.221   Disorder of ligament, right elbow
    M24.222   Disorder of ligament, left elbow
    M24.229   Disorder of ligament, unspecified elbow

● **M24.23**   Disorder of ligament, wrist
    M24.231   Disorder of ligament, right wrist
    M24.232   Disorder of ligament, left wrist
    M24.239   Disorder of ligament, unspecified wrist

● **M24.24**   Disorder of ligament, hand
    M24.241   Disorder of ligament, right hand
    M24.242   Disorder of ligament, left hand
    M24.249   Disorder of ligament, unspecified hand

● **M24.25**   Disorder of ligament, hip
    M24.251   Disorder of ligament, right hip
    M24.252   Disorder of ligament, left hip
    M24.259   Disorder of ligament, unspecified hip

● **M24.27**   Disorder of ligament, ankle and foot
    M24.271   Disorder of ligament, right ankle
    M24.272   Disorder of ligament, left ankle
    M24.273   Disorder of ligament, unspecified ankle
    M24.274   Disorder of ligament, right foot
    M24.275   Disorder of ligament, left foot
    M24.276   Disorder of ligament, unspecified foot

   M24.28   Disorder of ligament, vertebrae
     Coding Clinic: 2023, Q2, P13-14

   M24.29   Disorder of ligament, other specified site

● **M24.3**   Pathological dislocation of joint, not elsewhere classified
    Excludes1   congenital dislocation or displacement of joint - see congenital malformations and deformations of the musculoskeletal system (Q65-Q79)
           current injury - see injury of joints and ligaments by body region
           recurrent dislocation of joint (M24.4-)

   M24.30   Pathological dislocation of unspecified joint, not elsewhere classified

● **M24.31**   Pathological dislocation of shoulder, not elsewhere classified
    M24.311   Pathological dislocation of right shoulder, not elsewhere classified
    M24.312   Pathological dislocation of left shoulder, not elsewhere classified
    M24.319   Pathological dislocation of unspecified shoulder, not elsewhere classified

● **M24.32**   Pathological dislocation of elbow, not elsewhere classified
    M24.321   Pathological dislocation of right elbow, not elsewhere classified
    M24.322   Pathological dislocation of left elbow, not elsewhere classified
    M24.329   Pathological dislocation of unspecified elbow, not elsewhere classified

● **M24.33**   Pathological dislocation of wrist, not elsewhere classified
    M24.331   Pathological dislocation of right wrist, not elsewhere classified
    M24.332   Pathological dislocation of left wrist, not elsewhere classified
    M24.339   Pathological dislocation of unspecified wrist, not elsewhere classified

● **M24.34**   Pathological dislocation of hand, not elsewhere classified
    M24.341   Pathological dislocation of right hand, not elsewhere classified
    M24.342   Pathological dislocation of left hand, not elsewhere classified
    M24.349   Pathological dislocation of unspecified hand, not elsewhere classified

● **M24.35**   Pathological dislocation of hip, not elsewhere classified
    M24.351   Pathological dislocation of right hip, not elsewhere classified
     Coding Clinic: 2022, Q1, P32
    M24.352   Pathological dislocation of left hip, not elsewhere classified
     Coding Clinic: 2022, Q1, P32
    M24.359   Pathological dislocation of unspecified hip, not elsewhere classified

● **M24.36**   Pathological dislocation of knee, not elsewhere classified
    M24.361   Pathological dislocation of right knee, not elsewhere classified
    M24.362   Pathological dislocation of left knee, not elsewhere classified
    M24.369   Pathological dislocation of unspecified knee, not elsewhere classified

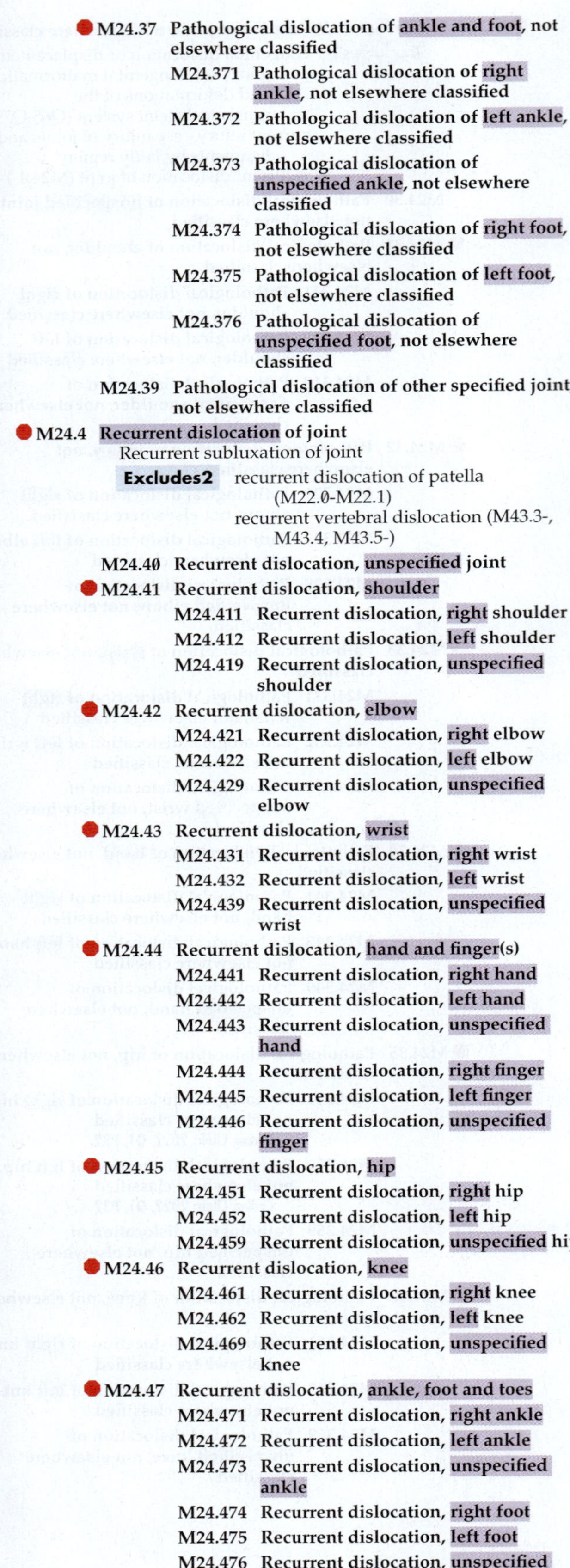

● M24.37   Pathological dislocation of ankle and foot, not elsewhere classified

    M24.371   Pathological dislocation of right ankle, not elsewhere classified

    M24.372   Pathological dislocation of left ankle, not elsewhere classified

    M24.373   Pathological dislocation of unspecified ankle, not elsewhere classified

    M24.374   Pathological dislocation of right foot, not elsewhere classified

    M24.375   Pathological dislocation of left foot, not elsewhere classified

    M24.376   Pathological dislocation of unspecified foot, not elsewhere classified

    M24.39   Pathological dislocation of other specified joint, not elsewhere classified

● M24.4   Recurrent dislocation of joint

    Recurrent subluxation of joint

    Excludes2   recurrent dislocation of patella (M22.0-M22.1)

                recurrent vertebral dislocation (M43.3-, M43.4, M43.5-)

    M24.40   Recurrent dislocation, unspecified joint

● M24.41   Recurrent dislocation, shoulder

    M24.411   Recurrent dislocation, right shoulder

    M24.412   Recurrent dislocation, left shoulder

    M24.419   Recurrent dislocation, unspecified shoulder

● M24.42   Recurrent dislocation, elbow

    M24.421   Recurrent dislocation, right elbow

    M24.422   Recurrent dislocation, left elbow

    M24.429   Recurrent dislocation, unspecified elbow

● M24.43   Recurrent dislocation, wrist

    M24.431   Recurrent dislocation, right wrist

    M24.432   Recurrent dislocation, left wrist

    M24.439   Recurrent dislocation, unspecified wrist

● M24.44   Recurrent dislocation, hand and finger(s)

    M24.441   Recurrent dislocation, right hand

    M24.442   Recurrent dislocation, left hand

    M24.443   Recurrent dislocation, unspecified hand

    M24.444   Recurrent dislocation, right finger

    M24.445   Recurrent dislocation, left finger

    M24.446   Recurrent dislocation, unspecified finger

● M24.45   Recurrent dislocation, hip

    M24.451   Recurrent dislocation, right hip

    M24.452   Recurrent dislocation, left hip

    M24.459   Recurrent dislocation, unspecified hip

● M24.46   Recurrent dislocation, knee

    M24.461   Recurrent dislocation, right knee

    M24.462   Recurrent dislocation, left knee

    M24.469   Recurrent dislocation, unspecified knee

● M24.47   Recurrent dislocation, ankle, foot and toes

    M24.471   Recurrent dislocation, right ankle

    M24.472   Recurrent dislocation, left ankle

    M24.473   Recurrent dislocation, unspecified ankle

    M24.474   Recurrent dislocation, right foot

    M24.475   Recurrent dislocation, left foot

    M24.476   Recurrent dislocation, unspecified foot

    M24.477   Recurrent dislocation, right toe(s)

    M24.478   Recurrent dislocation, left toe(s)

    M24.479   Recurrent dislocation, unspecified toe(s)

    M24.49   Recurrent dislocation, other specified joint

● M24.5   Contracture of joint

    Excludes1   contracture of muscle without contracture of joint (M62.4-)

                contracture of tendon (sheath) without contracture of joint (M62.4-)

                Dupuytren's contracture (M72.0)

    Excludes2   acquired deformities of limbs (M20-M21)

    M24.50   Contracture, unspecified joint

● M24.51   Contracture, shoulder

    M24.511   Contracture, right shoulder

    M24.512   Contracture, left shoulder

    M24.519   Contracture, unspecified shoulder

● M24.52   Contracture, elbow

    M24.521   Contracture, right elbow

    M24.522   Contracture, left elbow

    M24.529   Contracture, unspecified elbow

● M24.53   Contracture, wrist

    M24.531   Contracture, right wrist

    M24.532   Contracture, left wrist

    M24.539   Contracture, unspecified wrist

● M24.54   Contracture, hand

    M24.541   Contracture, right hand

    M24.542   Contracture, left hand

    M24.549   Contracture, unspecified hand

● M24.55   Contracture, hip

    M24.551   Contracture, right hip

       Coding Clinic: 2016, Q2, P6

    M24.552   Contracture, left hip

       Coding Clinic: 2016, Q2, P6

    M24.559   Contracture, unspecified hip

● M24.56   Contracture, knee

    M24.561   Contracture, right knee

       Coding Clinic: 2016, Q2, P6

    M24.562   Contracture, left knee

       Coding Clinic: 2016, Q2, P6

    M24.569   Contracture, unspecified knee

● M24.57   Contracture, ankle and foot

    M24.571   Contracture, right ankle

    M24.572   Contracture, left ankle

    M24.573   Contracture, unspecified ankle

    M24.574   Contracture, right foot

    M24.575   Contracture, left foot

    M24.576   Contracture, unspecified foot

    M24.59   Contracture, other specified joint

● M24.6   Ankylosis of joint

    Excludes1   stiffness of joint without ankylosis (M25.6-)

    Excludes2   spine (M43.2-)

    M24.60   Ankylosis, unspecified joint

● M24.61   Ankylosis, shoulder

    M24.611   Ankylosis, right shoulder

    M24.612   Ankylosis, left shoulder

    M24.619   Ankylosis, unspecified shoulder

Item 13–5   **Ankylosis** or arthrokleisis is a consolidation of a joint due to disease, injury, or surgical procedure. Spondylosis is the degeneration of the vertebral processes and formation of osteophytes and commonly occurs with age. **Spondylitis** or ankylosing spondylitis is a type of arthritis that affects the spine or backbone, causing back pain and stiffness.

▶ New   ⮕ Revised   ~~deleted~~ Deleted   Excludes 1   Excludes 2   Includes   Use additional   Code first   Code also   Key words

OGCR Official Guidelines   **X** Assign placeholder X   ● Use Additional Character(s)   ▌ Manifestation Code   **CC** Hierarchical Condition Category   **Coding Clinic**

● **M24.62** Ankylosis, elbow
    M24.621 Ankylosis, right elbow
    M24.622 Ankylosis, left elbow
    M24.629 Ankylosis, unspecified elbow
● **M24.63** Ankylosis, wrist
    M24.631 Ankylosis, right wrist
    M24.632 Ankylosis, left wrist
    M24.639 Ankylosis, unspecified wrist
● **M24.64** Ankylosis, hand
    M24.641 Ankylosis, right hand
    M24.642 Ankylosis, left hand
    M24.649 Ankylosis, unspecified hand
● **M24.65** Ankylosis, hip
    M24.651 Ankylosis, right hip
    M24.652 Ankylosis, left hip
    M24.659 Ankylosis, unspecified hip
● **M24.66** Ankylosis, knee
    M24.661 Ankylosis, right knee
    M24.662 Ankylosis, left knee
      Coding Clinic: 2025, Q1, P25
    M24.669 Ankylosis, unspecified knee
● **M24.67** Ankylosis, ankle and foot
    M24.671 Ankylosis, right ankle
    M24.672 Ankylosis, left ankle
    M24.673 Ankylosis, unspecified ankle
    M24.674 Ankylosis, right foot
    M24.675 Ankylosis, left foot
    M24.676 Ankylosis, unspecified foot
   M24.69 Ankylosis, other specified joint
   M24.7 Protrusio acetabuli
● **M24.8** Other specific joint derangements, not elsewhere classified
    Excludes2   iliotibial band syndrome (M76.3)
    M24.80 Other specific joint derangements of unspecified joint, not elsewhere classified
●   M24.81 Other specific joint derangements of shoulder, not elsewhere classified
     M24.811 Other specific joint derangements of right shoulder, not elsewhere classified
     M24.812 Other specific joint derangements of left shoulder, not elsewhere classified
     M24.819 Other specific joint derangements of unspecified shoulder, not elsewhere classified
●   M24.82 Other specific joint derangements of elbow, not elsewhere classified
     M24.821 Other specific joint derangements of right elbow, not elsewhere classified
     M24.822 Other specific joint derangements of left elbow, not elsewhere classified
     M24.829 Other specific joint derangements of unspecified elbow, not elsewhere classified
●   M24.83 Other specific joint derangements of wrist, not elsewhere classified
     M24.831 Other specific joint derangements of right wrist, not elsewhere classified
     M24.832 Other specific joint derangements of left wrist, not elsewhere classified
     M24.839 Other specific joint derangements of unspecified wrist, not elsewhere classified

●   M24.84 Other specific joint derangements of hand, not elsewhere classified
     M24.841 Other specific joint derangements of right hand, not elsewhere classified
     M24.842 Other specific joint derangements of left hand, not elsewhere classified
     M24.849 Other specific joint derangements of unspecified hand, not elsewhere classified
●   M24.85 Other specific joint derangements of hip, not elsewhere classified
     Irritable hip
     M24.851 Other specific joint derangements of right hip, not elsewhere classified
     M24.852 Other specific joint derangements of left hip, not elsewhere classified
     M24.859 Other specific joint derangements of unspecified hip, not elsewhere classified
●   M24.87 Other specific joint derangements of ankle and foot, not elsewhere classified
     M24.871 Other specific joint derangements of right ankle, not elsewhere classified
     M24.872 Other specific joint derangements of left ankle, not elsewhere classified
     M24.873 Other specific joint derangements of unspecified ankle, not elsewhere classified
     M24.874 Other specific joint derangements of right foot, not elsewhere classified
     M24.875 Other specific joint derangements left foot, not elsewhere classified
     M24.876 Other specific joint derangements of unspecified foot, not elsewhere classified
    M24.89 Other specific joint derangement of other specified joint, not elsewhere classified
   M24.9 Joint derangement, unspecified
● M25 Other joint disorder, not elsewhere classified
    Excludes2   abnormality of gait and mobility (R26.-)
      acquired deformities of limb (M20-M21)
      calcification of bursa (M71.4-)
      calcification of shoulder (joint) (M75.3)
      calcification of tendon (M65.2-)
      difficulty in walking (R26.2)
      temporomandibular joint disorder (M26.6-)
● **M25.0** Hemarthrosis
    Excludes1   current injury - see injury of joint by body region
      hemophilic arthropathy (M36.2)
    M25.00 Hemarthrosis, unspecified joint
●   M25.01 Hemarthrosis, shoulder
     M25.011 Hemarthrosis, right shoulder
     M25.012 Hemarthrosis, left shoulder
     M25.019 Hemarthrosis, unspecified shoulder
●   M25.02 Hemarthrosis, elbow
     M25.021 Hemarthrosis, right elbow
     M25.022 Hemarthrosis, left elbow
     M25.029 Hemarthrosis, unspecified elbow
●   M25.03 Hemarthrosis, wrist
     M25.031 Hemarthrosis, right wrist
     M25.032 Hemarthrosis, left wrist
     M25.039 Hemarthrosis, unspecified wrist
●   M25.04 Hemarthrosis, hand
     M25.041 Hemarthrosis, right hand
     M25.042 Hemarthrosis, left hand
     M25.049 Hemarthrosis, unspecified hand

● M25.05 Hemarthrosis, hip
    M25.051 Hemarthrosis, right hip
    M25.052 Hemarthrosis, left hip
    M25.059 Hemarthrosis, unspecified hip
● M25.06 Hemarthrosis, knee
    M25.061 Hemarthrosis, right knee
    M25.062 Hemarthrosis, left knee
    M25.069 Hemarthrosis, unspecified knee
● M25.07 Hemarthrosis, ankle and foot
    M25.071 Hemarthrosis, right ankle
    M25.072 Hemarthrosis, left ankle
    M25.073 Hemarthrosis, unspecified ankle
    M25.074 Hemarthrosis, right foot
    M25.075 Hemarthrosis, left foot
    M25.076 Hemarthrosis, unspecified foot
  M25.08 Hemarthrosis, other specified site
      Hemarthrosis, vertebrae
● M25.1 Fistula of joint
  M25.10 Fistula, unspecified joint
● M25.11 Fistula, shoulder
    M25.111 Fistula, right shoulder
    M25.112 Fistula, left shoulder
    M25.119 Fistula, unspecified shoulder
● M25.12 Fistula, elbow
    M25.121 Fistula, right elbow
    M25.122 Fistula, left elbow
    M25.129 Fistula, unspecified elbow
● M25.13 Fistula, wrist
    M25.131 Fistula, right wrist
    M25.132 Fistula, left wrist
    M25.139 Fistula, unspecified wrist
● M25.14 Fistula, hand
    M25.141 Fistula, right hand
    M25.142 Fistula, left hand
    M25.149 Fistula, unspecified hand
● M25.15 Fistula, hip
    M25.151 Fistula, right hip
    M25.152 Fistula, left hip
    M25.159 Fistula, unspecified hip
● M25.16 Fistula, knee
    M25.161 Fistula, right knee
    M25.162 Fistula, left knee
    M25.169 Fistula, unspecified knee
● M25.17 Fistula, ankle and foot
    M25.171 Fistula, right ankle
    M25.172 Fistula, left ankle
    M25.173 Fistula, unspecified ankle
    M25.174 Fistula, right foot
    M25.175 Fistula, left foot
    M25.176 Fistula, unspecified foot
  M25.18 Fistula, other specified site
      Fistula, vertebrae
● M25.2 Flail joint
  M25.20 Flail joint, unspecified joint
● M25.21 Flail joint, shoulder
    M25.211 Flail joint, right shoulder
    M25.212 Flail joint, left shoulder
    M25.219 Flail joint, unspecified shoulder
● M25.22 Flail joint, elbow
    M25.221 Flail joint, right elbow
    M25.222 Flail joint, left elbow
    M25.229 Flail joint, unspecified elbow

● M25.23 Flail joint, wrist
    M25.231 Flail joint, right wrist
    M25.232 Flail joint, left wrist
    M25.239 Flail joint, unspecified wrist
● M25.24 Flail joint, hand
    M25.241 Flail joint, right hand
    M25.242 Flail joint, left hand
    M25.249 Flail joint, unspecified hand
● M25.25 Flail joint, hip
    M25.251 Flail joint, right hip
    M25.252 Flail joint, left hip
    M25.259 Flail joint, unspecified hip
● M25.26 Flail joint, knee
    M25.261 Flail joint, right knee
    M25.262 Flail joint, left knee
    M25.269 Flail joint, unspecified knee
● M25.27 Flail joint, ankle and foot
    M25.271 Flail joint, right ankle and foot
    M25.272 Flail joint, left ankle and foot
    M25.279 Flail joint, unspecified ankle and foot
  M25.28 Flail joint, other site
● M25.3 Other instability of joint
    Excludes1 instability of joint secondary to old
                ligament injury (M24.2-)
              instability of joint secondary to removal
                of joint prosthesis (M96.8-)
    Excludes2 spinal instabilities (M53.2-)
  M25.30 Other instability, unspecified joint
● M25.31 Other instability, shoulder
    M25.311 Other instability, right shoulder
    M25.312 Other instability, left shoulder
    M25.319 Other instability, unspecified
           shoulder
● M25.32 Other instability, elbow
    M25.321 Other instability, right elbow
    M25.322 Other instability, left elbow
    M25.329 Other instability, unspecified elbow
● M25.33 Other instability, wrist
    M25.331 Other instability, right wrist
    M25.332 Other instability, left wrist
    M25.339 Other instability, unspecified wrist
● M25.34 Other instability, hand
    M25.341 Other instability, right hand
    M25.342 Other instability, left hand
    M25.349 Other instability, unspecified hand
● M25.35 Other instability, hip
    M25.351 Other instability, right hip
    M25.352 Other instability, left hip
    M25.359 Other instability, unspecified hip
● M25.36 Other instability, knee
    M25.361 Other instability, right knee
    M25.362 Other instability, left knee
    M25.369 Other instability, unspecified knee
● M25.37 Other instability, ankle and foot
    M25.371 Other instability, right ankle
    M25.372 Other instability, left ankle
    M25.373 Other instability, unspecified ankle
    M25.374 Other instability, right foot
    M25.375 Other instability, left foot
    M25.376 Other instability, unspecified foot
  M25.39 Other instability of joint

● **M25.4 Effusion of joint**
    Excludes1   hydrarthrosis in yaws (A66.6)
                 intermittent hydrarthrosis (M12.4-)
                 other infective (teno)synovitis (M65.1-)
    M25.40 Effusion, unspecified joint
● M25.41 Effusion, shoulder
    M25.411 Effusion, right shoulder
    M25.412 Effusion, left shoulder
    M25.419 Effusion, unspecified shoulder
● M25.42 Effusion, elbow
    M25.421 Effusion, right elbow
    M25.422 Effusion, left elbow
    M25.429 Effusion, unspecified elbow
● M25.43 Effusion, wrist
    M25.431 Effusion, right wrist
    M25.432 Effusion, left wrist
    M25.439 Effusion, unspecified wrist
● M25.44 Effusion, hand
    M25.441 Effusion, right hand
    M25.442 Effusion, left hand
    M25.449 Effusion, unspecified hand
● M25.45 Effusion, hip
    M25.451 Effusion, right hip
    M25.452 Effusion, left hip
    M25.459 Effusion, unspecified hip
● M25.46 Effusion, knee
    M25.461 Effusion, right knee
    M25.462 Effusion, left knee
    M25.469 Effusion, unspecified knee
● M25.47 Effusion, ankle and foot
    M25.471 Effusion, right ankle
    M25.472 Effusion, left ankle
    M25.473 Effusion, unspecified ankle
    M25.474 Effusion, right foot
    M25.475 Effusion, left foot
    M25.476 Effusion, unspecified foot
    M25.48 Effusion, other site
● M25.5 Pain in joint
    Excludes2   pain in hand (M79.64-)
                 pain in fingers (M79.64-)
                 pain in foot (M79.67-)
                 pain in limb (M79.6-)
                 pain in toes (M79.67-)
    M25.50 Pain in unspecified joint
● M25.51 Pain in shoulder
    M25.511 Pain in right shoulder
    M25.512 Pain in left shoulder
    M25.519 Pain in unspecified shoulder
● M25.52 Pain in elbow
    M25.521 Pain in right elbow
    M25.522 Pain in left elbow
    M25.529 Pain in unspecified elbow
● M25.53 Pain in wrist
    M25.531 Pain in right wrist
    M25.532 Pain in left wrist
    M25.539 Pain in unspecified wrist
● M25.54 Pain in joints of hand
    Coding Clinic: 2016, Q4, P38
    M25.541 Pain in joints of right hand
    M25.542 Pain in joints of left hand
    M25.549 Pain in joints of unspecified hand
            Pain in joints of hand NOS

● M25.55 Pain in hip
    M25.551 Pain in right hip
    M25.552 Pain in left hip
    M25.559 Pain in unspecified hip
● M25.56 Pain in knee
    M25.561 Pain in right knee
    M25.562 Pain in left knee
    M25.569 Pain in unspecified knee
● M25.57 Pain in ankle and joints of foot
    M25.571 Pain in right ankle and joints of right foot
    M25.572 Pain in left ankle and joints of left foot
    M25.579 Pain in unspecified ankle and joints of unspecified foot
    M25.59 Pain in other specified joint
● M25.6 Stiffness of joint, not elsewhere classified
    Excludes1   ankylosis of joint (M24.6-)
                 contracture of joint (M24.5-)
    M25.60 Stiffness of unspecified joint, not elsewhere classified
● M25.61 Stiffness of shoulder, not elsewhere classified
    M25.611 Stiffness of right shoulder, not elsewhere classified
    M25.612 Stiffness of left shoulder, not elsewhere classified
    M25.619 Stiffness of unspecified shoulder, not elsewhere classified
● M25.62 Stiffness of elbow, not elsewhere classified
    M25.621 Stiffness of right elbow, not elsewhere classified
    M25.622 Stiffness of left elbow, not elsewhere classified
    M25.629 Stiffness of unspecified elbow, not elsewhere classified
● M25.63 Stiffness of wrist, not elsewhere classified
    M25.631 Stiffness of right wrist, not elsewhere classified
    M25.632 Stiffness of left wrist, not elsewhere classified
    M25.639 Stiffness of unspecified wrist, not elsewhere classified
● M25.64 Stiffness of hand, not elsewhere classified
    M25.641 Stiffness of right hand, not elsewhere classified
    M25.642 Stiffness of left hand, not elsewhere classified
    M25.649 Stiffness of unspecified hand, not elsewhere classified
● M25.65 Stiffness of hip, not elsewhere classified
    M25.651 Stiffness of right hip, not elsewhere classified
    M25.652 Stiffness of left hip, not elsewhere classified
    M25.659 Stiffness of unspecified hip, not elsewhere classified
● M25.66 Stiffness of knee, not elsewhere classified
    M25.661 Stiffness of right knee, not elsewhere classified
    M25.662 Stiffness of left knee, not elsewhere classified
    M25.669 Stiffness of unspecified knee, not elsewhere classified
● M25.67 Stiffness of ankle and foot, not elsewhere classified
    M25.671 Stiffness of right ankle, not elsewhere classified
    M25.672 Stiffness of left ankle, not elsewhere classified

CHAPTER 13 (M00–M99)

M25.673 Stiffness of unspecified ankle, not elsewhere classified

M25.674 Stiffness of right foot, not elsewhere classified

M25.675 Stiffness of left foot, not elsewhere classified

M25.676 Stiffness of unspecified foot, not elsewhere classified

M25.69 Stiffness of other specified joint, not elsewhere classified

● **M25.7 Osteophyte**

M25.70 Osteophyte, unspecified joint

● M25.71 Osteophyte, shoulder

M25.711 Osteophyte, right shoulder

M25.712 Osteophyte, left shoulder

M25.719 Osteophyte, unspecified shoulder

● M25.72 Osteophyte, elbow

M25.721 Osteophyte, right elbow

M25.722 Osteophyte, left elbow

M25.729 Osteophyte, unspecified elbow

● M25.73 Osteophyte, wrist

M25.731 Osteophyte, right wrist

M25.732 Osteophyte, left wrist

M25.739 Osteophyte, unspecified wrist

● M25.74 Osteophyte, hand

M25.741 Osteophyte, right hand

M25.742 Osteophyte, left hand

M25.749 Osteophyte, unspecified hand

● M25.75 Osteophyte, hip

M25.751 Osteophyte, right hip

M25.752 Osteophyte, left hip

M25.759 Osteophyte, unspecified hip

● M25.76 Osteophyte, knee

M25.761 Osteophyte, right knee

M25.762 Osteophyte, left knee

M25.769 Osteophyte, unspecified knee

● M25.77 Osteophyte, ankle and foot

M25.771 Osteophyte, right ankle

M25.772 Osteophyte, left ankle

M25.773 Osteophyte, unspecified ankle

M25.774 Osteophyte, right foot

M25.775 Osteophyte, left foot

M25.776 Osteophyte, unspecified foot

M25.78 Osteophyte, vertebrae

● **M25.8 Other specified joint disorders**

M25.80 Other specified joint disorders, unspecified joint

● M25.81 Other specified joint disorders, shoulder
Coding Clinic: 2022, Q3, P18

M25.811 Other specified joint disorders, right shoulder

M25.812 Other specified joint disorders, left shoulder
Coding Clinic: 2022, Q3, P18

M25.819 Other specified joint disorders, unspecified shoulder

● M25.82 Other specified joint disorders, elbow

M25.821 Other specified joint disorders, right elbow

M25.822 Other specified joint disorders, left elbow

M25.829 Other specified joint disorders, unspecified elbow

● M25.83 Other specified joint disorders, wrist

M25.831 Other specified joint disorders, right wrist

M25.832 Other specified joint disorders, left wrist

M25.839 Other specified joint disorders, unspecified wrist

● M25.84 Other specified joint disorders, hand

M25.841 Other specified joint disorders, right hand

M25.842 Other specified joint disorders, left hand

M25.849 Other specified joint disorders, unspecified hand

● M25.85 Other specified joint disorders, hip

M25.851 Other specified joint disorders, right hip

M25.852 Other specified joint disorders, left hip

M25.859 Other specified joint disorders, unspecified hip

● M25.86 Other specified joint disorders, knee

M25.861 Other specified joint disorders, right knee

M25.862 Other specified joint disorders, left knee

M25.869 Other specified joint disorders, unspecified knee

● M25.87 Other specified joint disorders, ankle and foot

M25.871 Other specified joint disorders, right ankle and foot

M25.872 Other specified joint disorders, left ankle and foot

M25.879 Other specified joint disorders, unspecified ankle and foot

M25.9 Joint disorder, unspecified

DENTOFACIAL ANOMALIES [INCLUDING MALOCCLUSION] AND OTHER DISORDERS OF JAW (M26-M27)

Excludes1 hemifacial atrophy or hypertrophy (Q67.4)
unilateral condylar hyperplasia or hypoplasia (M27.8)

● **M26 Dentofacial anomalies [including malocclusion]**

● **M26.0 Major anomalies of jaw size**

Excludes1 acromegaly (E22.0)
Robin's syndrome (Q87.0)

M26.00 Unspecified anomaly of jaw size

M26.01 Maxillary hyperplasia

M26.02 Maxillary hypoplasia

M26.03 Mandibular hyperplasia

M26.04 Mandibular hypoplasia

M26.05 Macrogenia

M26.06 Microgenia

M26.07 Excessive tuberosity of jaw
Entire maxillary tuberosity

M26.09 Other specified anomalies of jaw size

● **M26.1 Anomalies of jaw-cranial base relationship**

M26.10 Unspecified anomaly of jaw-cranial base relationship

M26.11 Maxillary asymmetry

M26.12 Other jaw asymmetry

M26.19 Other specified anomalies of jaw-cranial base relationship
Coding Clinic: 2020, Q1, P21

● **M26.2 Anomalies of dental arch relationship**

M26.20 Unspecified anomaly of dental arch relationship

● M26.21 Malocclusion, Angle's class

M26.211 Malocclusion, Angle's class I
Neutro-occlusion

M26.212 Malocclusion, Angle's class II
Disto-occlusion Division I
Disto-occlusion Division II

M26.213 Malocclusion, Angle's class III
Mesio-occlusion

M26.219 Malocclusion, Angle's class, unspecified

● **M26.22 Open occlusal relationship**

M26.220 Open anterior occlusal relationship
Anterior open bite

M26.221 Open posterior occlusal relationship
Posterior open bite

M26.23 Excessive horizontal overlap
Excessive horizontal overjet

M26.24 Reverse articulation
Crossbite (anterior) (posterior)

M26.25 Anomalies of interarch distance

M26.29 Other anomalies of dental arch relationship
Midline deviation of dental arch
Overbite (excessive) deep
Overbite (excessive) horizontal
Overbite (excessive) vertical
Posterior lingual occlusion of mandibular teeth

● **M26.3 Anomalies of tooth position of fully erupted tooth or teeth**

Excludes2   embedded and impacted teeth (K01.-)

M26.30 Unspecified anomaly of tooth position of fully erupted tooth or teeth
Abnormal spacing of fully erupted tooth or teeth NOS
Displacement of fully erupted tooth or teeth NOS
Transposition of fully erupted tooth or teeth NOS

M26.31 Crowding of fully erupted teeth

M26.32 Excessive spacing of fully erupted teeth
Diastema of fully erupted tooth or teeth NOS

M26.33 Horizontal displacement of fully erupted tooth or teeth
Tipped tooth or teeth
Tipping of fully erupted tooth

M26.34 Vertical displacement of fully erupted tooth or teeth
Extruded tooth
Infraeruption of tooth or teeth
Supraeruption of tooth or teeth

M26.35 Rotation of fully erupted tooth or teeth

M26.36 Insufficient interocclusal distance of fully erupted teeth (ridge)
Lack of adequate intermaxillary vertical dimension of fully erupted teeth

M26.37 Excessive interocclusal distance of fully erupted teeth
Excessive intermaxillary vertical dimension of fully erupted teeth
Loss of occlusal vertical dimension of fully erupted teeth

M26.39 Other anomalies of tooth position of fully erupted tooth or teeth

M26.4 Malocclusion, unspecified

● **M26.5 Dentofacial functional abnormalities**

Excludes1   bruxism (F45.8)
teeth-grinding NOS (F45.8)

M26.50 Dentofacial functional abnormalities, unspecified

M26.51 Abnormal jaw closure

M26.52 Limited mandibular range of motion

M26.53 Deviation in opening and closing of the mandible

M26.54 Insufficient anterior guidance
Insufficient anterior occlusal guidance

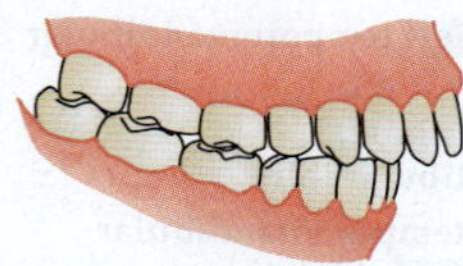

Figure 13-3   Dentofacial malocclusion.

Item 13–6 Hyperplasia is a condition of overdevelopment, whereas **hypoplasia** is a condition of underdevelopment. **Macrogenia** is overdevelopment of the chin, whereas **microgenia** is underdevelopment of the chin.

M26.55 Centric occlusion maximum intercuspation discrepancy

Excludes1   centric occlusion NOS (M26.59)

M26.56 Non-working side interference
Balancing side interference

M26.57 Lack of posterior occlusal support

M26.59 Other dentofacial functional abnormalities
Centric occlusion (of teeth) NOS
Malocclusion due to abnormal swallowing
Malocclusion due to mouth breathing
Malocclusion due to tongue, lip or finger habits

● **M26.6 Temporomandibular joint disorders**

Excludes2   current temporomandibular joint dislocation (S03.0)
current temporomandibular joint sprain (S03.4)

Coding Clinic: 2016, Q4, P38-39

● **M26.60 Temporomandibular joint disorder, unspecified**

M26.601 Right temporomandibular joint disorder, unspecified

M26.602 Left temporomandibular joint disorder, unspecified

M26.603 Bilateral temporomandibular joint disorder, unspecified

M26.609 Unspecified temporomandibular joint disorder, unspecified side
Temporomandibular joint disorder NOS

● **M26.61 Adhesions and ankylosis of temporomandibular joint**

M26.611 Adhesions and ankylosis of right temporomandibular joint

M26.612 Adhesions and ankylosis of left temporomandibular joint

M26.613 Adhesions and ankylosis of bilateral temporomandibular joint

M26.619 Adhesions and ankylosis of temporomandibular joint, unspecified side

● **M26.62 Arthralgia of temporomandibular joint**

M26.621 Arthralgia of right temporomandibular joint

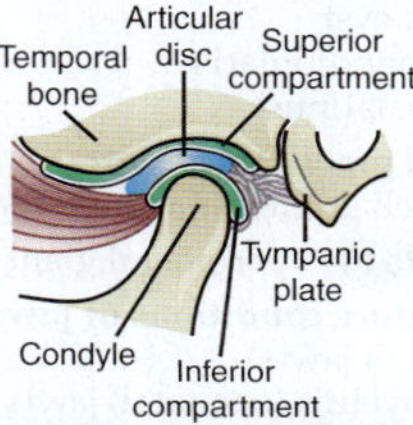

Figure 13-4   Temporomandibular joint.

Item 13–7 Dysfunction of the temporomandibular joint is termed **temporomandibular joint (TMJ) syndrome** and is characterized by pain and tenderness/spasm of the muscles of mastication, joint noise, and in the later stages, limited mandibular movement.

M26.622 Arthralgia of left temporomandibular joint

M26.623 Arthralgia of bilateral temporomandibular joint

M26.629 Arthralgia of temporomandibular joint, unspecified side

● **M26.63 Articular disc disorder of temporomandibular joint**

M26.631 Articular disc disorder of right temporomandibular joint

M26.632 Articular disc disorder of left temporomandibular joint

M26.633 Articular disc disorder of bilateral temporomandibular joint

M26.639 Articular disc disorder of temporomandibular joint, unspecified side

● **M26.64 Arthritis of temporomandibular joint**

M26.641 Arthritis of right temporomandibular joint

M26.642 Arthritis of left temporomandibular joint

M26.643 Arthritis of bilateral temporomandibular joint

M26.649 Arthritis of unspecified temporomandibular joint

● **M26.65 Arthropathy of temporomandibular joint**

M26.651 Arthropathy of right temporomandibular joint

M26.652 Arthropathy of left temporomandibular joint

M26.653 Arthropathy of bilateral temporomandibular joint

M26.659 Arthropathy of unspecified temporomandibular joint

M26.69 Other specified disorders of temporomandibular joint

● **M26.7 Dental alveolar anomalies**

M26.70 Unspecified alveolar anomaly

M26.71 Alveolar maxillary hyperplasia

M26.72 Alveolar mandibular hyperplasia

M26.73 Alveolar maxillary hypoplasia

M26.74 Alveolar mandibular hypoplasia

M26.79 Other specified alveolar anomalies

● **M26.8 Other dentofacial anomalies**

M26.81 Anterior soft tissue impingement
Anterior soft tissue impingement on teeth

M26.82 Posterior soft tissue impingement
Posterior soft tissue impingement on teeth

M26.89 Other dentofacial anomalies

M26.9 Dentofacial anomaly, unspecified

● **M27 Other diseases of jaws**

M27.0 Developmental disorders of jaws
Latent bone cyst of jaw
Stafne's cyst
Torus mandibularis
Torus palatinus

M27.1 Giant cell granuloma, central
Giant cell granuloma NOS

> **Excludes1**   peripheral giant cell granuloma (K06.8)

M27.2 Inflammatory conditions of jaws
Osteitis of jaw(s)
Osteomyelitis (neonatal) jaw(s)
Osteoradionecrosis jaw(s)
Periostitis jaw(s)
Sequestrum of jaw bone

> **Use additional** code (W88-W90, X39.0) to identify radiation, if radiation-induced

> **Excludes2**   osteonecrosis of jaw due to drug (M87.180)

M27.3 Alveolitis of jaws
Alveolar osteitis
Dry socket

● **M27.4 Other and unspecified cysts of jaw**

> **Excludes1**   cysts of oral region (K09.-)
> latent bone cyst of jaw (M27.0)
> Stafne's cyst (M27.0)

M27.40 Unspecified cyst of jaw
Cyst of jaw NOS

M27.49 Other cysts of jaw
Aneurysmal cyst of jaw
Hemorrhagic cyst of jaw
Traumatic cyst of jaw

● **M27.5 Periradicular pathology associated with previous endodontic treatment**

M27.51 Perforation of root canal space due to endodontic treatment

M27.52 Endodontic overfill

M27.53 Endodontic underfill

M27.59 Other periradicular pathology associated with previous endodontic treatment

● **M27.6 Endosseous dental implant failure**

M27.61 Osseointegration failure of dental implant
Hemorrhagic complications of dental implant placement
Iatrogenic osseointegration failure of dental implant
Osseointegration failure of dental implant due to complications of systemic disease
Osseointegration failure of dental implant due to poor bone quality
Pre-integration failure of dental implant NOS
Pre-osseointegration failure of dental implant

M27.62 Post-osseointegration biological failure of dental implant
Failure of dental implant due to lack of attached gingiva
Failure of dental implant due to occlusal trauma (caused by poor prosthetic design)
Failure of dental implant due to parafunctional habits
Failure of dental implant due to periodontal infection (peri–implantitis)
Failure of dental implant due to poor oral hygiene
Iatrogenic post-osseointegration failure of dental implant
Post-osseointegration failure of dental implant due to complications of systemic disease

M27.63 Post-osseointegration mechanical failure of dental implant
Failure of dental prosthesis causing loss of dental implant
Fracture of dental implant

> **Excludes2**   cracked tooth (K03.81)
> fractured dental restorative material with loss of material (K08.531)
> fractured dental restorative material without loss of material (K08.530)
> fractured tooth (S02.5)

M27.69 Other endosseous dental implant failure
Dental implant failure NOS

M27.8 Other specified diseases of jaws
Cherubism
Exostosis
Fibrous dysplasia
Unilateral condylar hyperplasia
Unilateral condylar hypoplasia

> **Excludes1**   jaw pain (R68.84)

M27.9 Disease of jaws, unspecified

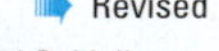 New   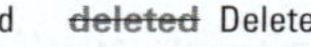 Revised   ~~deleted~~ Deleted   Excludes 1   Excludes 2   Includes   Use additional   Code first   Code also   Key words

OGCR Official Guidelines   X Assign placeholder X   ● Use Additional Character(s)   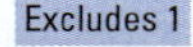 Manifestation Code   Hierarchical Condition Category   **Coding Clinic**

SYSTEMIC CONNECTIVE TISSUE DISORDERS (M30-M36)

Includes   autoimmune disease NOS
collagen (vascular) disease NOS
systemic autoimmune disease
systemic collagen (vascular) disease

Excludes1   autoimmune disease, single organ or single cell-type - code to relevant condition category

● **M30 Polyarteritis nodosa and related conditions**

Excludes1   microscopic polyarteritis (M31.7)

M30.0 Polyarteritis nodosa

M30.1 Polyarteritis with lung involvement [Churg-Strauss]
Allergic granulomatous angiitis
Eosinophilic granulomatosis with polyangiitis [EGPA]
Coding Clinic: 2021, Q1, P23

M30.2 Juvenile polyarteritis

M30.3 Mucocutaneous lymph node syndrome [Kawasaki]

M30.8 Other conditions related to polyarteritis nodosa
Polyangiitis overlap syndrome

● **M31 Other necrotizing vasculopathies**

M31.0 Hypersensitivity angiitis
Goodpasture's syndrome

● **M31.1 Thrombotic microangiopathy**

M31.10 Thrombotic microangiopathy, unspecified

M31.11 Hematopoietic stem cell transplantation-associated thrombotic microangiopathy [HSCT-TMA]
Transplant-associated thrombotic microangiopathy [TA-TMA]
Code first if applicable:
complications of bone marrow transplant (T86.0-)
complications of stem cell transplant (T86.5)
Use Additional code to identify specific organ dysfunction, such as:
acute kidney failure (N17.-)
acute respiratory distress syndrome (J80)
capillary leak syndrome (I78.8)
diffuse alveolar hemorrhage (R04.89)
encephalopathy (metabolic) (septic) (G93.41)
fluid overload, unspecified (E87.70)
graft versus host disease (D89.81-)
hemolytic uremic syndrome (D59.3-)
hepatic failure (K72.-)
hepatic veno-occlusive disease (K76.5)
idiopathic interstitial pneumonia (J84.11-)
sinusoidal obstruction syndrome (K76.5)

M31.19 Other thrombotic microangiopathy
Thrombotic thrombocytopenic purpura

M31.2 Lethal midline granuloma

● **M31.3 Wegener's granulomatosis**
Granulomatosis with polyangiitis
Necrotizing respiratory granulomatosis
Coding Clinic: 2021, Q1, P23

M31.30 Wegener's granulomatosis without renal involvement
Wegener's granulomatosis NOS
Coding Clinic: 2021, Q2, P10

M31.31 Wegener's granulomatosis with renal involvement

M31.4 Aortic arch syndrome [Takayasu]

M31.5 Giant cell arteritis with polymyalgia rheumatica

M31.6 Other giant cell arteritis

M31.7 Microscopic polyangiitis
Microscopic polyarteritis
Excludes1   polyarteritis nodosa (M30.0)
Coding Clinic: 2021, Q1, P23

M31.8 Other specified necrotizing vasculopathies
Hypocomplementemic vasculitis
Septic vasculitis

M31.9 Necrotizing vasculopathy, unspecified

● **M32 Systemic lupus erythematosus (SLE)**
Autoimmune inflammatory connective tissue disease of unknown cause that occurs most often in women

Excludes1   lupus erythematosus (discoid) (NOS) (L93.0)

M32.0 Drug-induced systemic lupus erythematosus
Use additional code for adverse effect, if applicable, to identify drug (T36-T50 with fifth or sixth character 5)

● **M32.1 Systemic lupus erythematosus with organ or system involvement**

M32.10 Systemic lupus erythematosus, organ or system involvement unspecified

M32.11 Endocarditis in systemic lupus erythematosus
Libman-Sacks disease

M32.12 Pericarditis in systemic lupus erythematosus
Lupus pericarditis

M32.13 Lung involvement in systemic lupus erythematosus
Pleural effusion due to systemic lupus erythematosus

M32.14 Glomerular disease in systemic lupus erythematosus
Lupus renal disease NOS

M32.15 Tubulo-interstitial nephropathy in systemic lupus erythematosus

M32.19 Other organ or system involvement in systemic lupus erythematosus
Use additional code(s) to identify organ or system involvement, such as encephalitis (G05.3)

M32.8 Other forms of systemic lupus erythematosus

M32.9 Systemic lupus erythematosus, unspecified
SLE NOS
Systemic lupus erythematosus NOS
Systemic lupus erythematosus without organ involvement

● **M33 Dermatopolymyositis**

● **M33.0 Juvenile dermatomyositis**

M33.00 Juvenile dermatomyositis, organ involvement unspecified

M33.01 Juvenile dermatomyositis with respiratory involvement

M33.02 Juvenile dermatomyositis with myopathy

M33.03 Juvenile dermatomyositis without myopathy

M33.09 Juvenile dermatomyositis with other organ involvement

● **M33.1 Other dermatomyositis**
Adult dermatomyositis

M33.10 Other dermatomyositis, organ involvement unspecified

M33.11 Other dermatomyositis with respiratory involvement

M33.12 Other dermatomyositis with myopathy

M33.13 Other dermatomyositis without myopathy
Dermatomyositis NOS

M33.19 Other dermatomyositis with other organ involvement

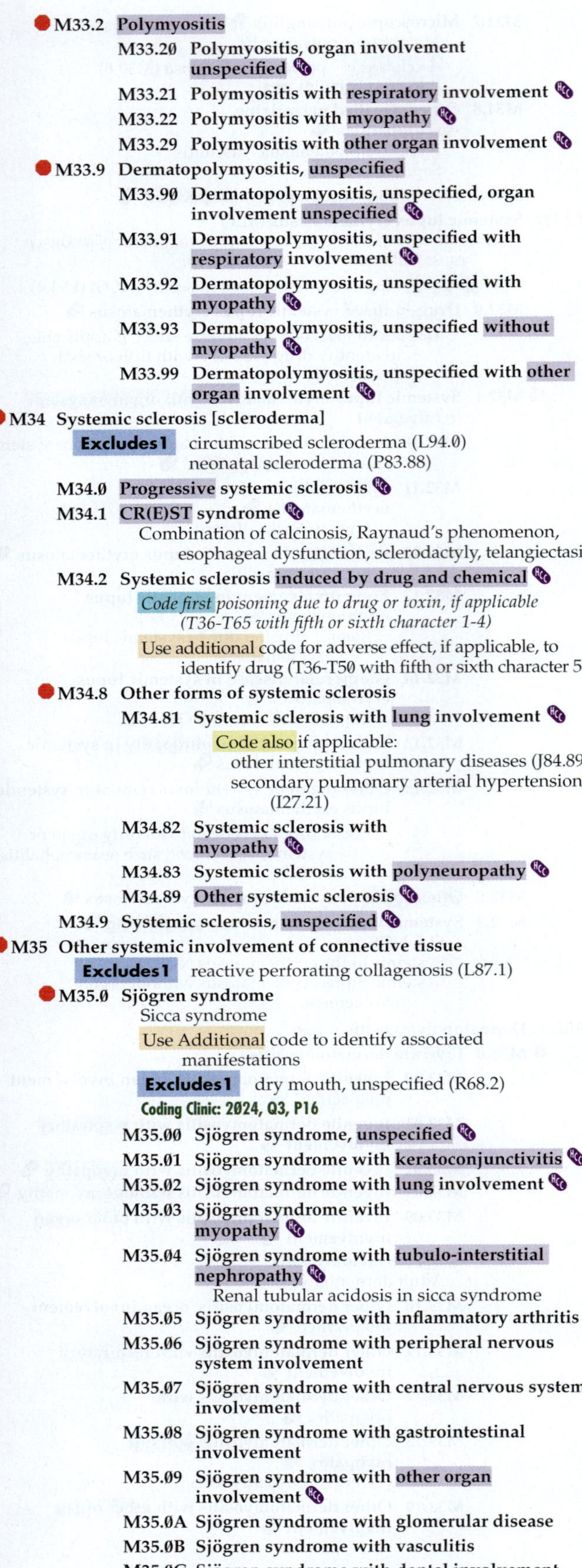

Left column

● **M33.2 Polymyositis**
- **M33.20 Polymyositis, organ involvement unspecified** RCC
- **M33.21 Polymyositis with respiratory involvement** RCC
- **M33.22 Polymyositis with myopathy** RCC
- **M33.29 Polymyositis with other organ involvement** RCC

● **M33.9 Dermatopolymyositis, unspecified**
- **M33.90 Dermatopolymyositis, unspecified, organ involvement unspecified** RCC
- **M33.91 Dermatopolymyositis, unspecified with respiratory involvement** RCC
- **M33.92 Dermatopolymyositis, unspecified with myopathy** RCC
- **M33.93 Dermatopolymyositis, unspecified without myopathy** RCC
- **M33.99 Dermatopolymyositis, unspecified with other organ involvement** RCC

● **M34 Systemic sclerosis [scleroderma]**
- **Excludes1** circumscribed scleroderma (L94.0)
  - neonatal scleroderma (P83.88)

M34.0 Progressive systemic sclerosis RCC

M34.1 CR(E)ST syndrome RCC
- Combination of calcinosis, Raynaud's phenomenon, esophageal dysfunction, sclerodactyly, telangiectasia

M34.2 Systemic sclerosis induced by drug and chemical RCC
- *Code first* poisoning due to drug or toxin, if applicable (T36-T65 with fifth or sixth character 1-4)
- Use additional code for adverse effect, if applicable, to identify drug (T36-T50 with fifth or sixth character 5)

● **M34.8 Other forms of systemic sclerosis**
- **M34.81 Systemic sclerosis with lung involvement** RCC
  - Code also if applicable:
    - other interstitial pulmonary diseases (J84.89)
    - secondary pulmonary arterial hypertension (I27.21)
- **M34.82 Systemic sclerosis with myopathy** RCC
- **M34.83 Systemic sclerosis with polyneuropathy** RCC
- **M34.89 Other systemic sclerosis** RCC

M34.9 Systemic sclerosis, unspecified RCC

● **M35 Other systemic involvement of connective tissue**
- **Excludes1** reactive perforating collagenosis (L87.1)

● **M35.0 Sjögren syndrome**
- Sicca syndrome
- Use Additional code to identify associated manifestations
- **Excludes1** dry mouth, unspecified (R68.2)
- **Coding Clinic: 2024, Q3, P16**
- **M35.00 Sjögren syndrome, unspecified** RCC
- **M35.01 Sjögren syndrome with keratoconjunctivitis** RCC
- **M35.02 Sjögren syndrome with lung involvement** RCC
- **M35.03 Sjögren syndrome with myopathy** RCC
- **M35.04 Sjögren syndrome with tubulo-interstitial nephropathy** RCC
  - Renal tubular acidosis in sicca syndrome
- **M35.05 Sjögren syndrome with inflammatory arthritis**
- **M35.06 Sjögren syndrome with peripheral nervous system involvement**
- **M35.07 Sjögren syndrome with central nervous system involvement**
- **M35.08 Sjögren syndrome with gastrointestinal involvement**
- **M35.09 Sjögren syndrome with other organ involvement** RCC
- **M35.0A Sjögren syndrome with glomerular disease**
- **M35.0B Sjögren syndrome with vasculitis**
- **M35.0C Sjögren syndrome with dental involvement**

Right column

Item 13–8 Polymyalgia rheumatica is a syndrome characterized by aching and morning stiffness and is related to aging and hereditary predisposition.

M35.1 Other overlap syndromes RCC
- Mixed connective tissue disease
- **Excludes1** polyangiitis overlap syndrome (M30.8)

M35.2 Behçet's disease

M35.3 Polymyalgia rheumatica RCC
- **Excludes1** polymyalgia rheumatica with giant cell arteritis (M31.5)

M35.4 Diffuse (eosinophilic) fasciitis

M35.5 Multifocal fibrosclerosis RCC

M35.6 Relapsing panniculitis [Weber-Christian]
- **Excludes1** lupus panniculitis (L93.2)
  - panniculitis NOS (M79.3-)

M35.7 Hypermobility syndrome
- Familial ligamentous laxity
- **Excludes1** ligamentous laxity, NOS (M24.2-)
- **Excludes2** Ehlers-Danlos syndromes (Q79.6-)

● **M35.8 Other specified systemic involvement of connective tissue**
- **Coding Clinic: 2021, Q4, P102; 2021, Q1, P36**
- **M35.81 Multisystem inflammatory syndrome**
  - MIS-A
  - MIS-C
  - Multisystem inflammatory syndrome in adults
  - Multisystem inflammatory syndrome in children
  - Pediatric inflammatory multisystem syndrome
  - PIMS
  - *Code first,* if applicable, COVID-19 (U07.1)
  - Code also any associated complications such as:
    - acute hepatic failure (K72.0-)
    - acute kidney failure (N17.-)
    - acute myocarditis (I40.-)
    - acute respiratory distress syndrome (J80)
    - cardiac arrhythmia (I47-I49.-)
    - pneumonia due to COVID-19 (J12.82)
    - severe sepsis (R65.2-)
    - viral cardiomyopathy (B33.24)
    - viral pericarditis (B33.23)
  - Use additional code, if applicable, for:
    - exposure to COVID-19 or SARS-C
    - personal history of COVID-19 (Z86.16)
    - post COVID-19 condition (U09.9)
  - **Coding Clinic: 2021, Q4, P102; 2021, Q1, P36, 42**
- **M35.89 Other specified systemic involvement of connective tissue**

M35.9 Systemic involvement of connective tissue, unspecified RCC
- Autoimmune disease (systemic) NOS
- Collagen (vascular) disease NOS

● **M36 Systemic disorders of connective tissue in diseases classified elsewhere**
- **Excludes2** arthropathies in diseases classified elsewhere (M14.-)

▸ **M36.0 Dermato(poly)myositis in neoplastic disease** RCC
- *Code first* underlying neoplasm (C00-D49)

▸ **M36.1 Arthropathy in neoplastic disease**
- *Code first* underlying neoplasm, such as:
  - leukemia (C91-C95)
  - malignant histiocytosis (C96.A)
  - multiple myeloma (C90.0)

▸ **M36.2 Hemophilic arthropathy**
- Hemarthrosis in hemophilic arthropathy
- *Code first* underlying disease, such as:
  - factor VIII deficiency (D66)
  - with vascular defect (D68.0-)
  - factor IX deficiency (D67)
  - hemophilia (classical) (D66)
  - hemophilia B (D67)
  - hemophilia C (D68.1)

M36.3 Arthropathy in other blood disorders
▶ *Code first* underlying disease, such as:
▶ disease of blood and blood-forming organs, unspecified (D75.9)
▶ other hemoglobinopathies (D58.2)
▶ thalassemia (D56.-)

M36.4 Arthropathy in hypersensitivity reactions classified elsewhere
Code first underlying disease, such as:
Henoch (-Schönlein) purpura (D69.0)
serum sickness (T80.6-)

M36.8 Systemic disorders of connective tissue in other diseases classified elsewhere
Code first underlying disease, such as:
alkaptonuria (E70.29)
hypogammaglobulinemia (D80.-)
ochronosis (E70.29)

DORSOPATHIES (M40-M54)

DEFORMING DORSOPATHIES (M40-M43)

● **M40 Kyphosis and lordosis**

    Excludes1   congenital kyphosis and lordosis (Q76.4)
                kyphoscoliosis (M41.-)
                postprocedural kyphosis and lordosis (M96.-)

    Code first underlying disease

● **M40.0 Postural kyphosis**

    Excludes1   osteochondrosis of spine (M42.-)

    M40.00 Postural kyphosis, site **unspecified**
    M40.03 Postural kyphosis, **cervicothoracic** region
    M40.04 Postural kyphosis, **thoracic** region
    M40.05 Postural kyphosis, **thoracolumbar** region

● **M40.1 Other secondary kyphosis**

    M40.10 Other secondary kyphosis, site **unspecified**
    M40.12 Other secondary kyphosis, **cervical** region
    M40.13 Other secondary kyphosis, **cervicothoracic** region
    M40.14 Other secondary kyphosis, **thoracic** region
    M40.15 Other secondary kyphosis, **thoracolumbar** region

● **M40.2 Other and unspecified kyphosis**

    ● **M40.20 Unspecified kyphosis**
        M40.202 Unspecified kyphosis, **cervical** region
        M40.203 Unspecified kyphosis, **cervicothoracic** region
        M40.204 Unspecified kyphosis, **thoracic** region
        M40.205 Unspecified kyphosis, **thoracolumbar** region
        M40.209 Unspecified kyphosis, site **unspecified**

    ● **M40.29 Other kyphosis**
        M40.292 Other kyphosis, **cervical** region
        M40.293 Other kyphosis, **cervicothoracic** region
        M40.294 Other kyphosis, **thoracic** region
        M40.295 Other kyphosis, **thoracolumbar** region
        M40.299 Other kyphosis, site **unspecified**

Item 13–9 **Kyphosis** is an abnormal curvature of the spine. **Senile kyphosis** is a result of disc degeneration causing ossification (turning to bone). **Adolescent** or **juvenile** kyphosis is also known as **Scheuermann's disease,** a condition in which the discs of the lower thoracic spine herniate, causing the disc space to narrow and the spine to tilt forward. This condition is attributed to poor posture. **Lordosis or swayback** is an abnormal curvature of the spine resulting in an inward curve of the lumbar spine just above the buttocks. **Scoliosis** causes a sideways curve to the spine. The curves are S- or C-shaped, and it is most commonly acquired in late childhood and early teen years, when growth is fast.

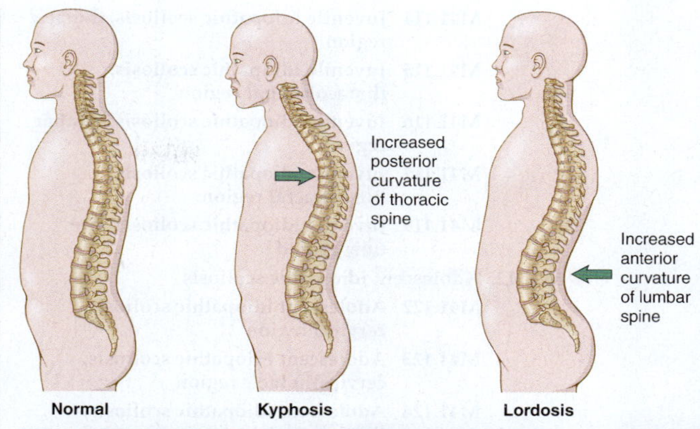

Figure 13-5   Kyphosis, Lordosis, Scoliosis. (From Chabner: The Language of Medicine, ed 8, St. Louis, Saunders, 2007)

● **M40.3 Flatback syndrome**
    M40.30 Flatback syndrome, site **unspecified**
    M40.35 Flatback syndrome, **thoracolumbar** region
    M40.36 Flatback syndrome, **lumbar** region
    M40.37 Flatback syndrome, **lumbosacral** region

● **M40.4 Postural lordosis**
    Abnormal increase in the normal curvature of the lumbar spine (sway back)
    Acquired lordosis
    M40.40 Postural lordosis, site **unspecified**
    M40.45 Postural lordosis, **thoracolumbar** region
    M40.46 Postural lordosis, **lumbar** region
    M40.47 Postural lordosis, **lumbosacral** region

● **M40.5 Lordosis, unspecified**
    M40.50 Lordosis, unspecified, site **unspecified**
    M40.55 Lordosis, unspecified, **thoracolumbar** region
    M40.56 Lordosis, unspecified, **lumbar** region
    M40.57 Lordosis, unspecified, **lumbosacral** region

● **M41 Scoliosis**

    Includes   kyphoscoliosis
    Excludes1   congenital scoliosis NOS (Q67.5)
                congenital scoliosis due to bony malformation (Q76.3)
                postural congenital scoliosis (Q67.5)
                kyphoscoliotic heart disease (I27.1)
    Excludes2   postprocedural scoliosis (M96.89)
                postradiation scoliosis (M96.5)

● **M41.0 Infantile idiopathic scoliosis**
    M41.00 Infantile idiopathic scoliosis, site **unspecified**
    M41.02 Infantile idiopathic scoliosis, **cervical** region
    M41.03 Infantile idiopathic scoliosis, **cervicothoracic** region
    M41.04 Infantile idiopathic scoliosis, **thoracic** region
    M41.05 Infantile idiopathic scoliosis, **thoracolumbar** region
    M41.06 Infantile idiopathic scoliosis, **lumbar** region
    M41.07 Infantile idiopathic scoliosis, **lumbosacral** region
    M41.08 Infantile idiopathic scoliosis, **sacral and sacrococcygeal** region

● **M41.1 Juvenile and adolescent idiopathic scoliosis**
    ● **M41.11 Juvenile idiopathic scoliosis**
        M41.112 Juvenile idiopathic scoliosis, **cervical** region
        M41.113 Juvenile idiopathic scoliosis, **cervicothoracic** region

CHAPTER 13 (MØØ-M99)

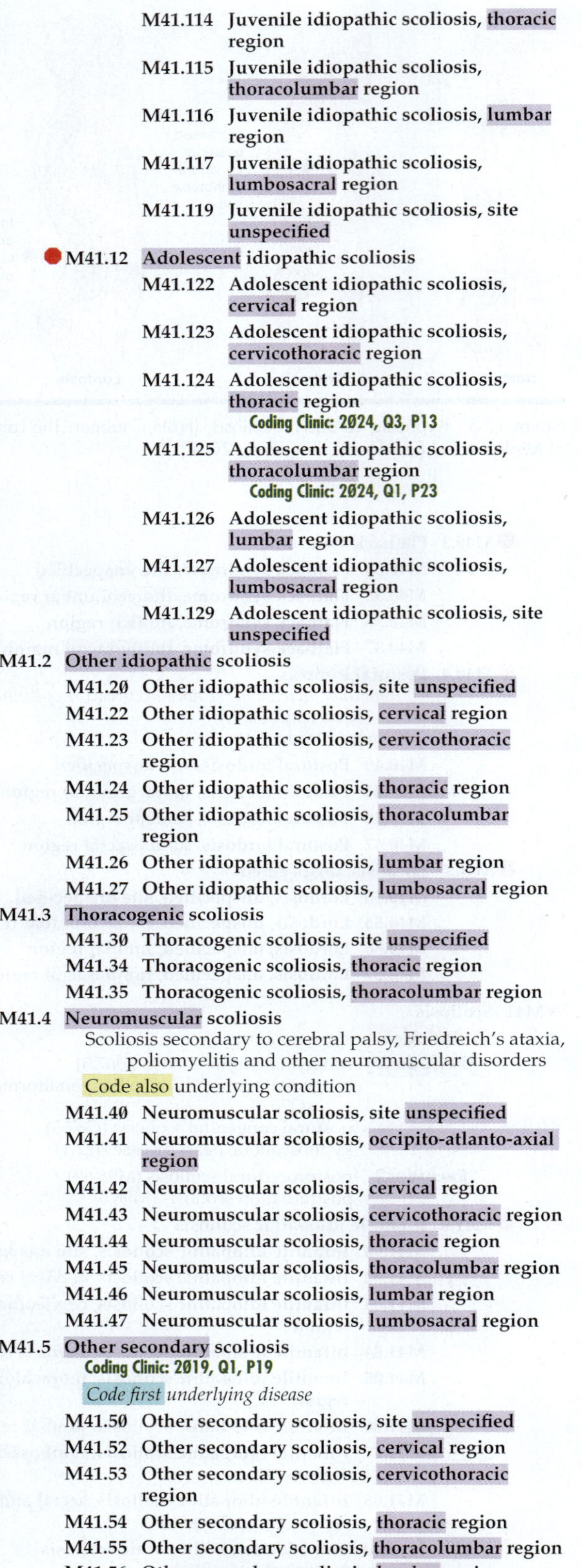

M41.114 Juvenile idiopathic scoliosis, thoracic region

M41.115 Juvenile idiopathic scoliosis, thoracolumbar region

M41.116 Juvenile idiopathic scoliosis, lumbar region

M41.117 Juvenile idiopathic scoliosis, lumbosacral region

M41.119 Juvenile idiopathic scoliosis, site unspecified

● M41.12 Adolescent idiopathic scoliosis

M41.122 Adolescent idiopathic scoliosis, cervical region

M41.123 Adolescent idiopathic scoliosis, cervicothoracic region

M41.124 Adolescent idiopathic scoliosis, thoracic region
Coding Clinic: 2024, Q3, P13

M41.125 Adolescent idiopathic scoliosis, thoracolumbar region
Coding Clinic: 2024, Q1, P23

M41.126 Adolescent idiopathic scoliosis, lumbar region

M41.127 Adolescent idiopathic scoliosis, lumbosacral region

M41.129 Adolescent idiopathic scoliosis, site unspecified

● M41.2 Other idiopathic scoliosis

M41.20 Other idiopathic scoliosis, site unspecified

M41.22 Other idiopathic scoliosis, cervical region

M41.23 Other idiopathic scoliosis, cervicothoracic region

M41.24 Other idiopathic scoliosis, thoracic region

M41.25 Other idiopathic scoliosis, thoracolumbar region

M41.26 Other idiopathic scoliosis, lumbar region

M41.27 Other idiopathic scoliosis, lumbosacral region

● M41.3 Thoracogenic scoliosis

M41.30 Thoracogenic scoliosis, site unspecified

M41.34 Thoracogenic scoliosis, thoracic region

M41.35 Thoracogenic scoliosis, thoracolumbar region

● M41.4 Neuromuscular scoliosis
Scoliosis secondary to cerebral palsy, Friedreich's ataxia, poliomyelitis and other neuromuscular disorders
Code also underlying condition

M41.40 Neuromuscular scoliosis, site unspecified

M41.41 Neuromuscular scoliosis, occipito-atlanto-axial region

M41.42 Neuromuscular scoliosis, cervical region

M41.43 Neuromuscular scoliosis, cervicothoracic region

M41.44 Neuromuscular scoliosis, thoracic region

M41.45 Neuromuscular scoliosis, thoracolumbar region

M41.46 Neuromuscular scoliosis, lumbar region

M41.47 Neuromuscular scoliosis, lumbosacral region

● M41.5 Other secondary scoliosis
Coding Clinic: 2019, Q1, P19
Code first underlying disease

M41.50 Other secondary scoliosis, site unspecified

M41.52 Other secondary scoliosis, cervical region

M41.53 Other secondary scoliosis, cervicothoracic region

M41.54 Other secondary scoliosis, thoracic region

M41.55 Other secondary scoliosis, thoracolumbar region

M41.56 Other secondary scoliosis, lumbar region

M41.57 Other secondary scoliosis, lumbosacral region

● M41.8 Other forms of scoliosis
Coding Clinic: 2022, Q1, P30

M41.80 Other forms of scoliosis, site unspecified

M41.82 Other forms of scoliosis, cervical region

M41.83 Other forms of scoliosis, cervicothoracic region

M41.84 Other forms of scoliosis, thoracic region

M41.85 Other forms of scoliosis, thoracolumbar region

M41.86 Other forms of scoliosis, lumbar region

M41.87 Other forms of scoliosis, lumbosacral region

M41.9 Scoliosis, unspecified
Coding Clinic: 2022, Q1, P30

● M42 Spinal osteochondrosis

● M42.0 Juvenile osteochondrosis of spine
Calvé's disease
Scheuermann's disease
Excludes1 postural kyphosis (M40.0)

M42.00 Juvenile osteochondrosis of spine, site unspecified

M42.01 Juvenile osteochondrosis of spine, occipito-atlanto-axial region

M42.02 Juvenile osteochondrosis of spine, cervical region

M42.03 Juvenile osteochondrosis of spine, cervicothoracic region

M42.04 Juvenile osteochondrosis of spine, thoracic region

M42.05 Juvenile osteochondrosis of spine, thoracolumbar region

M42.06 Juvenile osteochondrosis of spine, lumbar region

M42.07 Juvenile osteochondrosis of spine, lumbosacral region

M42.08 Juvenile osteochondrosis of spine, sacral and sacrococcygeal region

M42.09 Juvenile osteochondrosis of spine, multiple sites in spine

● M42.1 Adult osteochondrosis of spine

M42.10 Adult osteochondrosis of spine, site unspecified A

M42.11 Adult osteochondrosis of spine, occipitoatlanto-axial region A

M42.12 Adult osteochondrosis of spine, cervical region A

M42.13 Adult osteochondrosis of spine, cervicothoracic region A

M42.14 Adult osteochondrosis of spine, thoracic region A

M42.15 Adult osteochondrosis of spine, thoracolumbar region A

M42.16 Adult osteochondrosis of spine, lumbar region A

M42.17 Adult osteochondrosis of spine, lumbosacral region A

M42.18 Adult osteochondrosis of spine, sacral and sacrococcygeal region A

M42.19 Adult osteochondrosis of spine, multiple sites in spine A

M42.9 Spinal osteochondrosis, unspecified

● M43 Other deforming dorsopathies

Excludes1 congenital spondylolysis and spondylolisthesis (Q76.2)
hemivertebra (Q76.3-Q76.4)
Klippel-Feil syndrome (Q76.1)
lumbarization and sacralization (Q76.4)
platyspondylisis (Q76.4)
spina bifida occulta (Q76.0)
spinal curvature in osteoporosis (M80.-)
spinal curvature in Paget's disease of bone [osteitis deformans] (M88.-)

▶ New   ⇨ Revised   ~~deleted~~ Deleted   Excludes 1   Excludes 2   Includes   Use additional   Code first   Code also   Key words
OGCR Official Guidelines   X Assign placeholder X   ● Use Additional Character(s)   ❙ Manifestation Code   Ⓗⓒⓒ Hierarchical Condition Category   **Coding Clinic**

● **M43.0   Spondylolysis**
> **Excludes1**   congenital spondylolysis (Q76.2)
> spondylolisthesis (M43.1)
>
> **Coding Clinic: 2023, Q3, P20**

    M43.00   Spondylolysis, site unspecified
    M43.01   Spondylolysis, occipito-atlanto-axial region
    M43.02   Spondylolysis, cervical region
    M43.03   Spondylolysis, cervicothoracic region
    M43.04   Spondylolysis, thoracic region
    M43.05   Spondylolysis, thoracolumbar region
    M43.06   Spondylolysis, lumbar region
    M43.07   Spondylolysis, lumbosacral region
    M43.08   Spondylolysis, sacral and sacrococcygeal region
    M43.09   Spondylolysis, multiple sites in spine

● **M43.1   Spondylolisthesis**
> **Excludes1**   acute traumatic of lumbosacral region
> (S33.1)
> acute traumatic of sites other than
> lumbosacral - code to Fracture,
> vertebra, by region
> congenital spondylolisthesis (Q76.2)
>
> **Coding Clinic: 2023, Q3, P20**

    M43.10   Spondylolisthesis, site unspecified
    M43.11   Spondylolisthesis, occipito-atlanto-axial region
    M43.12   Spondylolisthesis, cervical region
    M43.13   Spondylolisthesis, cervicothoracic region
    M43.14   Spondylolisthesis, thoracic region

Item 13–10   Spondylolisthesis is a condition caused by the slipping forward of one disc over another.

    M43.15   Spondylolisthesis, thoracolumbar region
    M43.16   Spondylolisthesis, lumbar region
    Coding Clinic: 2024, Q1, P18
    M43.17   Spondylolisthesis, lumbosacral region
    Coding Clinic: 2023, Q3, P20
    M43.18   Spondylolisthesis, sacral and sacrococcygeal region
    M43.19   Spondylolisthesis, multiple sites in spine

● **M43.2   Fusion of spine**
    Ankylosis of spinal joint
> **Excludes1**   ankylosing spondylitis (M45.0-)
> congenital fusion of spine (Q76.4)
>
> **Excludes2**   arthrodesis status (Z98.1)
> pseudoarthrosis after fusion or
> arthrodesis (M96.0)

    M43.20   Fusion of spine, site unspecified
    M43.21   Fusion of spine, occipito-atlanto-axial region
    M43.22   Fusion of spine, cervical region
    M43.23   Fusion of spine, cervicothoracic region
    M43.24   Fusion of spine, thoracic region
    M43.25   Fusion of spine, thoracolumbar region
    M43.26   Fusion of spine, lumbar region
    M43.27   Fusion of spine, lumbosacral region
    M43.28   Fusion of spine, sacral and sacrococcygeal region
    M43.3   Recurrent atlantoaxial dislocation with myelopathy
    M43.4   Other recurrent atlantoaxial dislocation
● **M43.5   Other recurrent vertebral dislocation**
> **Excludes1**   biomechanical lesions NEC (M99.-)

● **M43.5X   Other recurrent vertebral dislocation**
    M43.5X2   Other recurrent vertebral dislocation, cervical region
    M43.5X3   Other recurrent vertebral dislocation, cervicothoracic region
    M43.5X4   Other recurrent vertebral dislocation, thoracic region

    M43.5X5   Other recurrent vertebral dislocation, thoracolumbar region
    M43.5X6   Other recurrent vertebral dislocation, lumbar region
    M43.5X7   Other recurrent vertebral dislocation, lumbosacral region
    M43.5X8   Other recurrent vertebral dislocation, sacral and sacrococcygeal region
    M43.5X9   Other recurrent vertebral dislocation, site unspecified

    M43.6   Torticollis
> **Excludes1**   congenital (sternomastoid) torticollis (Q68.0)
> current injury - see Injury, of spine, by body
> region ocular torticollis (R29.891)
> psychogenic torticollis (F45.8)
> spasmodic torticollis (G24.3)
> torticollis due to birth injury (P15.2)

● **M43.8   Other specified deforming dorsopathies**
> **Excludes2**   kyphosis and lordosis (M40.-)
> scoliosis (M41.-)

  ● **M43.8X   Other specified deforming dorsopathies**
    M43.8X1   Other specified deforming dorsopathies, occipito-atlanto-axial region
    M43.8X2   Other specified deforming dorsopathies, cervical region
    M43.8X3   Other specified deforming dorsopathies, cervicothoracic region
    M43.8X4   Other specified deforming dorsopathies, thoracic region
    M43.8X5   Other specified deforming dorsopathies, thoracolumbar region
    M43.8X6   Other specified deforming dorsopathies, lumbar region
    M43.8X7   Other specified deforming dorsopathies, lumbosacral region
    M43.8X8   Other specified deforming dorsopathies, sacral and sacrococcygeal region
    M43.8X9   Other specified deforming dorsopathies, site unspecified
    M43.9   Deforming dorsopathy, unspecified
    Curvature of spine NOS

SPONDYLOPATHIES (M45-M49)

● **M45   Ankylosing spondylitis**
    Rheumatoid arthritis of spine
> **Excludes1**   arthropathy in Reiter's disease (M02.3-)
> juvenile (ankylosing) spondylitis (M08.1)
>
> **Excludes2**   Behçet's disease (M35.2)

    M45.0   Ankylosing spondylitis of multiple sites in spine
    M45.1   Ankylosing spondylitis of occipito-atlanto-axial region
    M45.2   Ankylosing spondylitis of cervical region
    M45.3   Ankylosing spondylitis of cervicothoracic region
    M45.4   Ankylosing spondylitis of thoracic region
    M45.5   Ankylosing spondylitis of thoracolumbar region
    M45.6   Ankylosing spondylitis lumbar region
    M45.7   Ankylosing spondylitis of lumbosacral region
    M45.8   Ankylosing spondylitis sacral and sacrococcygeal region
    M45.9   Ankylosing spondylitis of unspecified sites in spine
● **M45.A   Non-radiographic axial spondyloarthritis**
    M45.A0   Non-radiographic axial spondyloarthritis of unspecified sites in spine
    M45.A1   Non-radiographic axial spondyloarthritis of occipito-atlanto-axial region
    M45.A2   Non-radiographic axial spondyloarthritis of cervical region
    M45.A3   Non-radiographic axial spondyloarthritis of cervicothoracic region

M45.A4 Non-radiographic axial spondyloarthritis of thoracic region

M45.A5 Non-radiographic axial spondyloarthritis of thoracolumbar region

M45.A6 Non-radiographic axial spondyloarthritis of lumbar region

M45.A7 Non-radiographic axial spondyloarthritis of lumbosacral region

M45.A8 Non-radiographic axial spondyloarthritis of sacral and sacrococcygeal region

M45.AB Non-radiographic axial spondyloarthritis of multiple sites in spine

● M46 Other inflammatory spondylopathies

● M46.0 Spinal enthesopathy
   Disorder of ligamentous or muscular attachments of spine

M46.00 Spinal enthesopathy, site unspecified

M46.01 Spinal enthesopathy, occipito-atlanto-axial region

M46.02 Spinal enthesopathy, cervical region

M46.03 Spinal enthesopathy, cervicothoracic region

M46.04 Spinal enthesopathy, thoracic region

M46.05 Spinal enthesopathy, thoracolumbar region

M46.06 Spinal enthesopathy, lumbar region

M46.07 Spinal enthesopathy, lumbosacral region

M46.08 Spinal enthesopathy, sacral and sacrococcygeal region

M46.09 Spinal enthesopathy, multiple sites in spine

M46.1 Sacroiliitis, not elsewhere classified

● M46.2 Osteomyelitis of vertebra

M46.20 Osteomyelitis of vertebra, site unspecified

M46.21 Osteomyelitis of vertebra, occipito-atlanto-axial region

M46.22 Osteomyelitis of vertebra, cervical region

M46.23 Osteomyelitis of vertebra, cervicothoracic region

M46.24 Osteomyelitis of vertebra, thoracic region

M46.25 Osteomyelitis of vertebra, thoracolumbar region

M46.26 Osteomyelitis of vertebra, lumbar region

M46.27 Osteomyelitis of vertebra, lumbosacral region

M46.28 Osteomyelitis of vertebra, sacral and sacrococcygeal region

● M46.3 Infection of intervertebral disc (pyogenic)
   Use additional code (B95-B97) to identify infectious agent

M46.30 Infection of intervertebral disc (pyogenic), site unspecified

M46.31 Infection of intervertebral disc (pyogenic), occipito-atlanto-axial region

M46.32 Infection of intervertebral disc (pyogenic), cervical region

M46.33 Infection of intervertebral disc (pyogenic), cervicothoracic region

M46.34 Infection of intervertebral disc (pyogenic), thoracic region

M46.35 Infection of intervertebral disc (pyogenic), thoracolumbar region

M46.36 Infection of intervertebral disc (pyogenic), lumbar region

M46.37 Infection of intervertebral disc (pyogenic), lumbosacral region

M46.38 Infection of intervertebral disc (pyogenic), sacral and sacrococcygeal region

M46.39 Infection of intervertebral disc (pyogenic), multiple sites in spine

● M46.4 Discitis, unspecified

M46.40 Discitis, unspecified, site unspecified

M46.41 Discitis, unspecified, occipito-atlanto-axial region

M46.42 Discitis, unspecified, cervical region

M46.43 Discitis, unspecified, cervicothoracic region

M46.44 Discitis, unspecified, thoracic region

M46.45 Discitis, unspecified, thoracolumbar region

M46.46 Discitis, unspecified, lumbar region

M46.47 Discitis, unspecified, lumbosacral region

M46.48 Discitis, unspecified, sacral and sacrococcygeal region

M46.49 Discitis, unspecified, multiple sites in spine

● M46.5 Other infective spondylopathies

M46.50 Other infective spondylopathies, site unspecified

M46.51 Other infective spondylopathies, occipitoatlanto-axial region

M46.52 Other infective spondylopathies, cervical region

M46.53 Other infective spondylopathies, cervicothoracic region

M46.54 Other infective spondylopathies, thoracic region

M46.55 Other infective spondylopathies, thoracolumbar region

M46.56 Other infective spondylopathies, lumbar region

M46.57 Other infective spondylopathies, lumbosacral region

M46.58 Other infective spondylopathies, sacral and sacrococcygeal region

M46.59 Other infective spondylopathies, multiple sites in spine

● M46.8 Other specified inflammatory spondylopathies

M46.80 Other specified inflammatory spondylopathies, site unspecified

M46.81 Other specified inflammatory spondylopathies, occipito-atlanto-axial region

M46.82 Other specified inflammatory spondylopathies, cervical region

M46.83 Other specified inflammatory spondylopathies, cervicothoracic region

M46.84 Other specified inflammatory spondylopathies, thoracic region

M46.85 Other specified inflammatory spondylopathies, thoracolumbar region

M46.86 Other specified inflammatory spondylopathies, lumbar region

M46.87 Other specified inflammatory spondylopathies, lumbosacral region

M46.88 Other specified inflammatory spondylopathies, sacral and sacrococcygeal region

M46.89 Other specified inflammatory spondylopathies, multiple sites in spine

● M46.9 Unspecified inflammatory spondylopathy

M46.90 Unspecified inflammatory spondylopathy, site unspecified

M46.91 Unspecified inflammatory spondylopathy, occipito-atlanto-axial region

M46.92 Unspecified inflammatory spondylopathy, cervical region
   Coding Clinic: 2019, Q3, P10

M46.93 Unspecified inflammatory spondylopathy, cervicothoracic region

M46.94 Unspecified inflammatory spondylopathy, thoracic region

M46.95 Unspecified inflammatory spondylopathy, thoracolumbar region

M46.96   Unspecified inflammatory spondylopathy, lumbar region

M46.97   Unspecified inflammatory spondylopathy, lumbosacral region

M46.98   Unspecified inflammatory spondylopathy, sacral and sacrococcygeal region

M46.99   Unspecified inflammatory spondylopathy, multiple sites in spine

● **M47   Spondylosis**

> **Includes**   arthrosis or osteoarthritis of spine
> degeneration of facet joints

   ● **M47.0   Anterior spinal and vertebral artery compression syndromes**
Coding Clinic: 2019, Q3, P10

     ● **M47.01   Anterior spinal artery compression syndromes**

M47.011   Anterior spinal artery compression syndromes, occipito-atlanto-axial region

M47.012   Anterior spinal artery compression syndromes, cervical region
Coding Clinic: 2023, Q1, P37

M47.013   Anterior spinal artery compression syndromes, cervicothoracic region

M47.014   Anterior spinal artery compression syndromes, thoracic region

M47.015   Anterior spinal artery compression syndromes, thoracolumbar region

M47.016   Anterior spinal artery compression syndromes, lumbar region

M47.019   Anterior spinal artery compression syndromes, site unspecified

     ● **M47.02   Vertebral artery compression syndromes**

M47.021   Vertebral artery compression syndromes, occipito-atlanto-axial region

M47.022   Vertebral artery compression syndromes, cervical region
Coding Clinic: 2023, Q1, P37

M47.029   Vertebral artery compression syndromes, site unspecified

   ● **M47.1   Other spondylosis with myelopathy**
Spondylogenic compression of spinal cord

> **Excludes1**   vertebral subluxation (M43.3-M43.5X9)

M47.10   Other spondylosis with myelopathy, site unspecified

M47.11   Other spondylosis with myelopathy, occipito-atlanto-axial region

M47.12   Other spondylosis with myelopathy, cervical region
Coding Clinic: 2020, Q1, P17

M47.13   Other spondylosis with myelopathy, cervicothoracic region

M47.14   Other spondylosis with myelopathy, thoracic region

M47.15   Other spondylosis with myelopathy, thoracolumbar region

M47.16   Other spondylosis with myelopathy, lumbar region

   ● **M47.2   Other spondylosis with radiculopathy**

M47.20   Other spondylosis with radiculopathy, site unspecified

M47.21   Other spondylosis with radiculopathy, occipito-atlanto-axial region

M47.22   Other spondylosis with radiculopathy, cervical region
Coding Clinic: 2020, Q1, P17

M47.23   Other spondylosis with radiculopathy, cervicothoracic region

M47.24   Other spondylosis with radiculopathy, thoracic region

M47.25   Other spondylosis with radiculopathy, thoracolumbar region

M47.26   Other spondylosis with radiculopathy, lumbar region

M47.27   Other spondylosis with radiculopathy, lumbosacral region

M47.28   Other spondylosis with radiculopathy, sacral and sacrococcygeal region

   ● **M47.8   Other spondylosis**

     ● **M47.81   Spondylosis without myelopathy or radiculopathy**

M47.811   Spondylosis without myelopathy or radiculopathy, occipito-atlanto-axial region

M47.812   Spondylosis without myelopathy or radiculopathy, cervical region
Coding Clinic: 2019, Q3, P10-11; 2018, Q2, P15

M47.813   Spondylosis without myelopathy or radiculopathy, cervicothoracic region

M47.814   Spondylosis without myelopathy or radiculopathy, thoracic region

M47.815   Spondylosis without myelopathy or radiculopathy, thoracolumbar region

M47.816   Spondylosis without myelopathy or radiculopathy, lumbar region

M47.817   Spondylosis without myelopathy or radiculopathy, lumbosacral region

M47.818   Spondylosis without myelopathy or radiculopathy, sacral and sacrococcygeal region

M47.819   Spondylosis without myelopathy or radiculopathy, site unspecified

     ● **M47.89   Other spondylosis**

M47.891   Other spondylosis, occipito-atlanto-axial region

M47.892   Other spondylosis, cervical region

M47.893   Other spondylosis, cervicothoracic region

M47.894   Other spondylosis, thoracic region

M47.895   Other spondylosis, thoracolumbar region

M47.896   Other spondylosis, lumbar region

M47.897   Other spondylosis, lumbosacral region

M47.898   Other spondylosis, sacral and sacrococcygeal region

M47.899   Other spondylosis, site unspecified

   M47.9   Spondylosis, unspecified

● **M48   Other spondylopathies**

   ● **M48.0   Spinal stenosis**
Caudal stenosis

M48.00   Spinal stenosis, site unspecified

M48.01   Spinal stenosis, occipito-atlanto-axial region

M48.02   Spinal stenosis, cervical region
Coding Clinic: 2020, Q1, P17

M48.03   Spinal stenosis, cervicothoracic region

M48.04   Spinal stenosis, thoracic region

M48.05   Spinal stenosis, thoracolumbar region

     ● **M48.06   Spinal stenosis, lumbar region**
Coding Clinic: 2017, Q3, P24

M48.061   Spinal stenosis, lumbar region without neurogenic claudication
Spinal stenosis, lumbar region NOS

M48.062   Spinal stenosis, lumbar region with neurogenic claudication
Coding Clinic: 2017, Q4, P19

M48.07   Spinal stenosis, lumbosacral region

M48.08   Spinal stenosis, sacral and sacrococcygeal region

● **M48.1 Ankylosing hyperostosis [Forestier]**
Diffuse idiopathic skeletal hyperostosis [DISH]

M48.10 Ankylosing hyperostosis [Forestier], site unspecified

M48.11 Ankylosing hyperostosis [Forestier], occipito-atlanto-axial region

M48.12 Ankylosing hyperostosis [Forestier], cervical region

M48.13 Ankylosing hyperostosis [Forestier], cervicothoracic region

M48.14 Ankylosing hyperostosis [Forestier], thoracic region

M48.15 Ankylosing hyperostosis [Forestier], thoracolumbar region

M48.16 Ankylosing hyperostosis [Forestier], lumbar region

M48.17 Ankylosing hyperostosis [Forestier], lumbosacral region

M48.18 Ankylosing hyperostosis [Forestier], sacral and sacrococcygeal region

M48.19 Ankylosing hyperostosis [Forestier], multiple sites in spine

● **M48.2 Kissing spine**

M48.20 Kissing spine, site unspecified

M48.21 Kissing spine, occipito-atlanto-axial region

M48.22 Kissing spine, cervical region

M48.23 Kissing spine, cervicothoracic region

M48.24 Kissing spine, thoracic region

M48.25 Kissing spine, thoracolumbar region

M48.26 Kissing spine, lumbar region

M48.27 Kissing spine, lumbosacral region

● **M48.3 Traumatic spondylopathy**

M48.30 Traumatic spondylopathy, site unspecified

M48.31 Traumatic spondylopathy, occipito-atlanto-axial region

M48.32 Traumatic spondylopathy, cervical region

M48.33 Traumatic spondylopathy, cervicothoracic region

M48.34 Traumatic spondylopathy, thoracic region

M48.35 Traumatic spondylopathy, thoracolumbar region

M48.36 Traumatic spondylopathy, lumbar region

M48.37 Traumatic spondylopathy, lumbosacral region

M48.38 Traumatic spondylopathy, sacral and sacrococcygeal region

● **M48.4 Fatigue fracture of vertebra**
Stress fracture of vertebra

Excludes1 pathological fracture NOS (M84.4-)
pathological fracture of vertebra due to neoplasm (M84.58)
pathological fracture of vertebra due to other diagnosis (M84.68)
pathological fracture of vertebra due to osteoporosis (M80.-)
traumatic fracture of vertebrae (S12.0-S12.3-, S22.0-, S32.0-)

The appropriate 7th character is to be added to each code from subcategory M48.4:

A	initial encounter for fracture
D	subsequent encounter for fracture with routine healing
G	subsequent encounter for fracture with delayed healing
S	sequela of fracture

X● **M48.40 Fatigue fracture of vertebra, site unspecified**

X● **M48.41 Fatigue fracture of vertebra, occipitoatlanto-axial region**

X● **M48.42 Fatigue fracture of vertebra, cervical region**

X● **M48.43 Fatigue fracture of vertebra, cervicothoracic region**

X● **M48.44 Fatigue fracture of vertebra, thoracic region**

X● **M48.45 Fatigue fracture of vertebra, thoracolumbar region**

X● **M48.46 Fatigue fracture of vertebra, lumbar region**

X● **M48.47 Fatigue fracture of vertebra, lumbosacral region**

X● **M48.48 Fatigue fracture of vertebra, sacral and sacrococcygeal region**

● **M48.5 Collapsed vertebra, not elsewhere classified**
Collapsed vertebra NOS
Compression fracture of vertebra NOS
Wedging of vertebra NOS

Excludes1 current injury - see Injury of spine, by body region
fatigue fracture of vertebra (M48.4)
pathological fracture of vertebra due to neoplasm (M84.58)
pathological fracture of vertebra due to other diagnosis (M84.68)
pathological fracture of vertebra due to osteoporosis (M80.-)
pathological fracture NOS (M84.4-)
stress fracture of vertebra (M48.4-)
traumatic fracture of vertebra (S12.-, S22.-, S32.-)

The appropriate 7th character is to be added to each code from subcategory M48.5:

A	initial encounter for fracture
D	subsequent encounter for fracture with routine healing
G	subsequent encounter for fracture with delayed healing
S	sequela of fracture

X● **M48.50 Collapsed vertebra, not elsewhere classified, site unspecified A**

X● **M48.51 Collapsed vertebra, not elsewhere classified, occipito-atlanto-axial region A**

X● **M48.52 Collapsed vertebra, not elsewhere classified, cervical region A**

X● **M48.53 Collapsed vertebra, not elsewhere classified, cervicothoracic region A**

X● **M48.54 Collapsed vertebra, not elsewhere classified, thoracic region A**

X● **M48.55 Collapsed vertebra, not elsewhere classified, thoracolumbar region A**

X● **M48.56 Collapsed vertebra, not elsewhere classified, lumbar region A**

X● **M48.57 Collapsed vertebra, not elsewhere classified, lumbosacral region A**

X● **M48.58 Collapsed vertebra, not elsewhere classified, sacral and sacrococcygeal region A**

● **M48.8 Other specified spondylopathies**
Ossification of posterior longitudinal ligament

● **M48.8X Other specified spondylopathies**

M48.8X1 Other specified spondylopathies, occipito-atlanto-axial region

M48.8X2 Other specified spondylopathies, cervical region

M48.8X3 Other specified spondylopathies, cervicothoracic region

M48.8X4 Other specified spondylopathies, thoracic region

M48.8X5 Other specified spondylopathies, thoracolumbar region

M48.8X6 Other specified spondylopathies, lumbar region

▶ New   ⇨ Revised   ~~deleted~~ Deleted   Excludes 1   Excludes 2   Includes   Use additional   Code first   Code also   Key words
OGCR Official Guidelines   X Assign placeholder X   ● Use Additional Character(s)   ❯ Manifestation Code   Ⓗ Hierarchical Condition Category   Coding Clinic

M48.8X7 **Other specified spondylopathies, lumbosacral region**

M48.8X8 **Other specified spondylopathies, sacral and sacrococcygeal region**

M48.8X9 **Other specified spondylopathies, site unspecified**

M48.9 **Spondylopathy, unspecified**

● **M49 Spondylopathies in diseases classified elsewhere**

Includes   curvature of spine in diseases classified elsewhere
deformity of spine in diseases classified elsewhere
kyphosis in diseases classified elsewhere
scoliosis in diseases classified elsewhere
spondylopathy in diseases classified elsewhere

Code first underlying disease, such as:
brucellosis (A23.-)
Charcot-Marie-Tooth disease (G60.0)
enterobacterial infections (A01-A04)
osteitis fibrosa cystica (E21.0)

Excludes1   curvature of spine in tuberculosis [Pott's] (A18.01)
enteropathic arthropathies (M07.-)
gonococcal spondylitis (A54.41)
neuropathic [tabes dorsalis] spondylitis (A52.11)
neuropathic spondylopathy in syringomyelia (G95.0)
neuropathic spondylopathy in tabes dorsalis (A52.11)
nonsyphilitic neuropathic spondylopathy NEC (G98.0)
spondylitis in syphilis (acquired) (A52.77)
tuberculous spondylitis (A18.01)
typhoid fever spondylitis (A01.05)

● **M49.8 Spondylopathy in diseases classified elsewhere**

▶ *M49.80 Spondylopathy in diseases classified elsewhere, site unspecified*

▶ *M49.81 Spondylopathy in diseases classified elsewhere, occipito-atlanto-axial region*

▶ *M49.82 Spondylopathy in diseases classified elsewhere, cervical region*

▶ *M49.83 Spondylopathy in diseases classified elsewhere, cervicothoracic region*

▶ *M49.84 Spondylopathy in diseases classified elsewhere, thoracic region*

▶ *M49.85 Spondylopathy in diseases classified elsewhere, thoracolumbar region*

▶ *M49.86 Spondylopathy in diseases classified elsewhere, lumbar region*

▶ *M49.87 Spondylopathy in diseases classified elsewhere, lumbosacral region*

▶ *M49.88 Spondylopathy in diseases classified elsewhere, sacral and sacrococcygeal region*

▶ *M49.89 Spondylopathy in diseases classified elsewhere, multiple sites in spine*

OTHER DORSOPATHIES (M50-M54)

Excludes1   current injury - see injury of spine by body region
discitis NOS (M46.4-)

● **M50 Cervical disc disorders**

Includes   cervicothoracic disc disorders with cervicalgia
cervicothoracic disc disorders

Coding Clinic: 2016, Q1, P17

● **M50.0 Cervical disc disorder with myelopathy**

M50.00 **Cervical disc disorder with myelopathy, unspecified cervical region**

M50.01 **Cervical disc disorder with myelopathy, high cervical region**
C2-C3 disc disorder with myelopathy
C3-C4 disc disorder with myelopathy
Coding Clinic: 2016, Q1, P17

● **M50.02 Cervical disc disorder with myelopathy, mid-cervical region**
Coding Clinic: 2016, Q4, P39-40

M50.020 **Cervical disc disorder with myelopathy, mid-cervical region, unspecified level**

M50.021 **Cervical disc disorder at C4-C5 level with myelopathy**
C4-C5 disc disorder with myelopathy

M50.022 **Cervical disc disorder at C5-C6 level with myelopathy**
C5-C6 disc disorder with myelopathy

M50.023 **Cervical disc disorder at C6-C7 level with myelopathy**
C6-C7 disc disorder with myelopathy

M50.03 **Cervical disc disorder with myelopathy, cervicothoracic region**
C7-T1 disc disorder with myelopathy

● **M50.1 Cervical disc disorder with radiculopathy**

Excludes2   brachial radiculitis NOS (M54.13)

M50.10 **Cervical disc disorder with radiculopathy, unspecified cervical region**

M50.11 **Cervical disc disorder with radiculopathy, high cervical region**
C2-C3 disc disorder with radiculopathy
C3 radiculopathy due to disc disorder
C3-C4 disc disorder with radiculopathy
C4 radiculopathy due to disc disorder

● **M50.12 Cervical disc disorder with radiculopathy, mid-cervical region**
Coding Clinic: 2016, Q4, P39-40

M50.120 **Mid-cervical disc disorder, unspecified level**

M50.121 **Cervical disc disorder at C4-C5 level with radiculopathy**
C4-C5 disc disorder with radiculopathy
C5 radiculopathy due to disc disorder

M50.122 **Cervical disc disorder at C5-C6 level with radiculopathy**
C5-C6 disc disorder with radiculopathy
C6 radiculopathy due to disc disorder

M50.123 **Cervical disc disorder at C6-C7 level with radiculopathy**
C6-C7 disc disorder with radiculopathy
C7 radiculopathy due to disc disorder

M50.13 **Cervical disc disorder with radiculopathy, cervicothoracic region**
C7-T1 disc disorder with radiculopathy
C8 radiculopathy due to disc disorder

● **M50.2 Other cervical disc displacement**
Coding Clinic: 2016, Q4, P40

M50.20 **Other cervical disc displacement, unspecified cervical region**

M50.21 **Other cervical disc displacement, high cervical region**
Other C2-C3 cervical disc displacement
Other C3-C4 cervical disc displacement
Coding Clinic: 2021, Q4, P12

● **M50.22 Other cervical disc displacement, mid-cervical region**

M50.220 **Other cervical disc displacement, mid-cervical region, unspecified level**

M50.221 **Other cervical disc displacement at C4-C5 level**
Other C4-C5 cervical disc displacement

M50.222 Other cervical disc displacement at C5-C6 level
 Other C5-C6 cervical disc displacement

M50.223 Other cervical disc displacement at C6-C7 level
 Other C6-C7 cervical disc displacement

M50.23 Other cervical disc displacement, cervicothoracic region
 Other C7-T1 cervical disc displacement

● **M50.3 Other cervical disc degeneration**
 Coding Clinic: 2016, Q4, P40

M50.30 Other cervical disc degeneration, unspecified cervical region

M50.31 Other cervical disc degeneration, high cervical region
 Other C2-C3 cervical disc degeneration
 Other C3-C4 cervical disc degeneration

● **M50.32 Other cervical disc degeneration, mid-cervical region**

M50.320 Other cervical disc degeneration, mid-cervical region, unspecified level

M50.321 Other cervical disc degeneration at C4-C5 level
 Other C4-C5 cervical disc degeneration

M50.322 Other cervical disc degeneration at C5-C6 level
 Other C5-C6 cervical disc degeneration

M50.323 Other cervical disc degeneration at C6-C7 level
 Other C6-C7 cervical disc degeneration

M50.33 Other cervical disc degeneration, cervicothoracic region
 Other C7-T1 cervical disc degeneration

● **M50.8 Other cervical disc disorders**
 Coding Clinic: 2016, Q4, P40

M50.80 Other cervical disc disorders, unspecified cervical region

M50.81 Other cervical disc disorders, high cervical region
 Other C2-C3 cervical disc disorders
 Other C3-C4 cervical disc disorders

● **M50.82 Other cervical disc disorders, mid-cervical region**

M50.820 Other cervical disc disorders, mid-cervical region, unspecified level

M50.821 Other cervical disc disorders at C4-C5 level
 Other C4-C5 cervical disc disorders

M50.822 Other cervical disc disorders at C5-C6 level
 Other C5-C6 cervical disc disorders

M50.823 Other cervical disc disorders at C6-C7 level
 Other C6-C7 cervical disc disorders

M50.83 Other cervical disc disorders, cervicothoracic region
 Other C7-T1 cervical disc disorders

● **M50.9 Cervical disc disorder, unspecified**
 Coding Clinic: 2016, Q4, P40

M50.90 Cervical disc disorder, unspecified, unspecified cervical region

M50.91 Cervical disc disorder, unspecified, high cervical region
 C2-C3 cervical disc disorder, unspecified
 C3-C4 cervical disc disorder, unspecified

● **M50.92 Cervical disc disorder, unspecified, mid-cervical region**

M50.920 Unspecified cervical disc disorder, mid-cervical region, unspecified level

M50.921 Unspecified cervical disc disorder at C4-C5 level
 Unspecified C4-C5 cervical disc disorder

M50.922 Unspecified cervical disc disorder at C5-C6 level
 Unspecified C5-C6 cervical disc disorder

M50.923 Unspecified cervical disc disorder at C6-C7 level
 Unspecified C6-C7 cervical disc disorder

M50.93 Cervical disc disorder, unspecified, cervicothoracic region
 C7-T1 cervical disc disorder, unspecified

● **M51 Thoracic, thoracolumbar, and lumbosacral intervertebral disc disorders**

 Excludes2 cervical and cervicothoracic disc disorders (M50.-)
     sacral and sacrococcygeal disorders (M53.3)

● **M51.0 Thoracic, thoracolumbar and lumbosacral intervertebral disc disorders with myelopathy**

M51.04 Intervertebral disc disorders with myelopathy, thoracic region

M51.05 Intervertebral disc disorders with myelopathy, thoracolumbar region

M51.06 Intervertebral disc disorders with myelopathy, lumbar region

● **M51.1 Thoracic, thoracolumbar and lumbosacral intervertebral disc disorders with radiculopathy**
 Sciatica due to intervertebral disc disorder

 Excludes1 lumbar radiculitis NOS (M54.16)
     sciatica NOS (M54.3)

M51.14 Intervertebral disc disorders with radiculopathy, thoracic region

M51.15 Intervertebral disc disorders with radiculopathy, thoracolumbar region

M51.16 Intervertebral disc disorders with radiculopathy, lumbar region

M51.17 Intervertebral disc disorders with radiculopathy, lumbosacral region

● **M51.2 Other thoracic, thoracolumbar and lumbosacral intervertebral disc displacement**
 Lumbago due to displacement of intervertebral disc

M51.24 Other intervertebral disc displacement, thoracic region

M51.25 Other intervertebral disc displacement, thoracolumbar region

M51.26 Other intervertebral disc displacement, lumbar region

M51.27 Other intervertebral disc displacement, lumbosacral region

● **M51.3 Other thoracic, thoracolumbar and lumbosacral intervertebral disc degeneration**
 Coding Clinic: 2013, Q3, P22

M51.34 Other intervertebral disc degeneration, thoracic region

M51.35 Other intervertebral disc degeneration, thoracolumbar region

M51.36   **Other intervertebral disc degeneration, lumbar region**
    Coding Clinic: 2018, Q2, P15

   M51.360   **Other intervertebral disc degeneration, lumbar region with discogenic back pain only**
     Other intervertebral disc degeneration, lumbar region with axial back pain only

   M51.361   **Other intervertebral disc degeneration, lumbar region with lower extremity pain only**
     Other intervertebral disc degeneration, lumbar region with leg pain only
     Other intervertebral disc degeneration, lumbar region with referred sclerotomal pain only

   M51.362   **Other intervertebral disc degeneration, lumbar region with discogenicback pain and lower extremity pain**
     Other intervertebral disc degeneration, lumbar region with discogenic back pain and leg pain
     Other intervertebral disc degeneration, lumbar region with axial back pain and referred sclerotomal pain

   M51.369   **Other intervertebral disc degeneration, lumbar region without mention of lumbar back pain or lower extremity pain**
     Other intervertebral disc degeneration, lumbar region without mention of lumbar back pain or leg pain
     Other intervertebral disc degeneration, lumbar region, NOS

M51.37   **Other intervertebral disc degeneration, lumbosacral region**
    Coding Clinic: 2022, Q1, P26

   M51.370   **Other intervertebral disc degeneration, lumbosacral region with discogenic back pain only**
     Other intervertebral disc degeneration, lumbosacral region with axial back pain only

   M51.371   **Other intervertebral disc degeneration, lumbosacral region with lower extremity pain only**
     Other intervertebral disc degeneration, lumbosacral region with leg pain only
     Other intervertebral disc degeneration, lumbosacral region with referred sclerotomal pain only

   M51.372   **Other intervertebral disc degeneration, lumbosacral region with discogenic back pain and lower extremity pain**
     Other intervertebral disc degeneration, lumbosacral region with discogenic backpain and leg pain
     Other intervertebral disc degeneration, lumbosacral region with axial back pain and referred sclerotomal pain

   M51.379   **Other intervertebral disc degeneration, lumbosacral region without mention of lumbar back pain or lower extremity pain**
     Other intervertebral disc degeneration, lumbosacral region without mention of lumbar back pain or leg pain
     Other intervertebral disc degeneration, lumbosacral region, NOS

● **M51.4**   **Schmorl's nodes**

   M51.44   **Schmorl's nodes, thoracic region**

   M51.45   **Schmorl's nodes, thoracolumbar region**

   M51.46   **Schmorl's nodes, lumbar region**

   M51.47   **Schmorl's nodes, lumbosacral region**

● **M51.8**   **Other thoracic, thoracolumbar and lumbosacral intervertebral disc disorders**

   M51.84   **Other intervertebral disc disorders, thoracic region**

   M51.85   **Other intervertebral disc disorders, thoracolumbar region**

   M51.86   **Other intervertebral disc disorders, lumbar region**

   M51.87   **Other intervertebral disc disorders, lumbosacral region**

M51.9   **Unspecified thoracic, thoracolumbar and lumbosacral intervertebral disc disorder**

● **M51.A**   **Other lumbar and lumbosacral annulus fibrosus disc defects**

   M51.A0   **Intervertebral annulus fibrosus defect, lumbar region, unspecified size**
     Code first, if applicable, lumbar disc herniation (M51.06, M51.16, M51.26)

   M51.A1   **Intervertebral annulus fibrosus defect, small, lumbar region**
     Code first, if applicable, lumbar disc herniation (M51.06, M51.16, M51.26)

   M51.A2   **Intervertebral annulus fibrosus defect, large, lumbar region**
     Code first, if applicable, lumbar disc herniation (M51.06, M51.16, M51.26)

   M51.A3   **Intervertebral annulus fibrosus defect, lumbosacral region, unspecified size**
     Code first, if applicable, lumbosacral disc herniation (M51.17, M51.27)

   M51.A4   **Intervertebral annulus fibrosus defect, small, lumbosacral region**
     Code first, if applicable, lumbosacral disc herniation (M51.17, M51.27)

   M51.A5   **Intervertebral annulus fibrosus defect, large, lumbosacral region**
     Code first, if applicable, lumbosacral disc herniation (M51.17, M51.27)

● **M53**   **Other and unspecified dorsopathies, not elsewhere classified**

M53.0   **Cervicocranial syndrome**
    Posterior cervical sympathetic syndrome

M53.1   **Cervicobrachial syndrome**
    Excludes2   cervical disc disorder (M50.-)
           thoracic outlet syndrome (G54.0)

● **M53.2**   **Spinal instabilities**

   ● **M53.2X**   **Spinal instabilities**

     M53.2X1   **Spinal instabilities, occipito-atlanto-axial region**

     M53.2X2   **Spinal instabilities, cervical region**

     M53.2X3   **Spinal instabilities, cervicothoracic region**

CHAPTER 13 (M00-M99)

M53.2X4 Spinal instabilities, thoracic region

M53.2X5 Spinal instabilities, thoracolumbar region

M53.2X6 Spinal instabilities, lumbar region

M53.2X7 Spinal instabilities, lumbosacral region

M53.2X8 Spinal instabilities, sacral and sacrococcygeal region

M53.2X9 Spinal instabilities, site unspecified

M53.3 Sacrococcygeal disorders, not elsewhere classified
Coccygodynia

● **M53.8 Other specified dorsopathies**

M53.80 Other specified dorsopathies, site unspecified

M53.81 Other specified dorsopathies, occipito-atlanto-axial region

M53.82 Other specified dorsopathies, cervical region

M53.83 Other specified dorsopathies, cervicothoracic region

M53.84 Other specified dorsopathies, thoracic region

M53.85 Other specified dorsopathies, thoracolumbar region

M53.86 Other specified dorsopathies, lumbar region

M53.87 Other specified dorsopathies, lumbosacral region

M53.88 Other specified dorsopathies, sacral and sacrococcygeal region

M53.9 Dorsopathy, unspecified

● **M54 Dorsalgia**

Excludes1 psychogenic dorsalgia (F45.41)

● **M54.0 Panniculitis affecting regions of neck and back**

Excludes1 lupus panniculitis (L93.2)
panniculitis NOS (M79.3)
relapsing [Weber-Christian] panniculitis (M35.6)

M54.00 Panniculitis affecting regions of neck and back, site unspecified

M54.01 Panniculitis affecting regions of neck and back, occipito-atlanto-axial region

M54.02 Panniculitis affecting regions of neck and back, cervical region

M54.03 Panniculitis affecting regions of neck and back, cervicothoracic region

M54.04 Panniculitis affecting regions of neck and back, thoracic region

M54.05 Panniculitis affecting regions of neck and back, thoracolumbar region

M54.06 Panniculitis affecting regions of neck and back, lumbar region

M54.07 Panniculitis affecting regions of neck and back, lumbosacral region

M54.08 Panniculitis affecting regions of neck and back, sacral and sacrococcygeal region

M54.09 Panniculitis affecting regions, neck and back, multiple sites in spine

● **M54.1 Radiculopathy**
Brachial neuritis or radiculitis NOS
Lumbar neuritis or radiculitis NOS
Lumbosacral neuritis or radiculitis NOS
Thoracic neuritis or radiculitis NOS
Radiculitis NOS

Excludes1 neuralgia and neuritis NOS (M79.2)
radiculopathy with cervical disc disorder (M50.1)
radiculopathy with lumbar and other intervertebral disc disorder (M51.1-)
radiculopathy with spondylosis (M47.2-)

M54.10 Radiculopathy, site unspecified

M54.11 Radiculopathy, occipito-atlanto-axial region

M54.12 Radiculopathy, cervical region

M54.13 Radiculopathy, cervicothoracic region

M54.14 Radiculopathy, thoracic region

M54.15 Radiculopathy, thoracolumbar region

M54.16 Radiculopathy, lumbar region

M54.17 Radiculopathy, lumbosacral region

M54.18 Radiculopathy, sacral and sacrococcygeal region

M54.2 Cervicalgia

Excludes1 cervicalgia due to intervertebral cervical disc disorder (M50.-)

● **M54.3 Sciatica**

Excludes1 intervertebral disc degeneration, lumbar region with lower extremity pain only (M51.361)
intervertebral disc degeneration, lumbosacral region with lower extremity pain only (M51.371)
lesion of sciatic nerve (G57.0)
sciatica due to intervertebral disc disorder (M51.1-)
sciatica with lumbago (M54.4-)

M54.30 Sciatica, unspecified side

M54.31 Sciatica, right side

M54.32 Sciatica, left side

● **M54.4 Lumbago with sciatica**

Excludes1 intervertebral disc degeneration, lumbar region with discogenic back pain and lower extremity pain (M51.362)
intervertebral disc degeneration, lumbosacral region with discogenic back pain and lower extremity pain (M51.372)
lumbago with sciatica due to intervertebral disc disorder (M51.1-)

M54.40 Lumbago with sciatica, unspecified side

M54.41 Lumbago with sciatica, right side

M54.42 Lumbago with sciatica, left side
Coding Clinic: 2016, Q2, P7

● **M54.5 Low back pain**

Excludes1 intervertebral disc degeneration, lumbar region with discogenic back pain only (M51.360)
intervertebral disc degeneration, lumbosacral region with discogenic back pain only (M51.370)
low back strain (S39.012)
lumbago due to intervertebral disc displacement (M51.2-)
lumbago with sciatica (M54.4-)

M54.50 Low back pain, unspecified
Loin pain
Lumbago NOS

M54.51 Vertebrogenic low back pain
Low back vertebral endplate pain
Coding Clinic: 2021, Q4, P22

M54.59 Other low back pain

M54.6 Pain in thoracic spine

Excludes1 pain in thoracic spine due to intervertebral disc disorder (M51.)

● **M54.8 Other dorsalgia**

Excludes1 dorsalgia in thoracic region (M54.6)
low back pain (M54.5-)

M54.81 Occipital neuralgia

M54.89 Other dorsalgia

M54.9 Dorsalgia, unspecified
Backache NOS
Back pain NOS

SOFT TISSUE DISORDERS (M60-M79)

DISORDERS OF MUSCLES (M60-M63)

> **Excludes1**   dermatopolymyositis (M33.-)
> muscular dystrophies and myopathies (G71-G72)
> myopathy in amyloidosis (E85.-)
> myopathy in polyarteritis nodosa (M30.0)
> myopathy in rheumatoid arthritis (M05.32)
> myopathy in scleroderma (M34.-)
> myopathy in Sjögren's syndrome (M35.03)
> myopathy in systemic lupus erythematosus (M32.-)

● **M60   Myositis**

> **Excludes2**   inclusion body myositis [IBM] (G72.41)

● **M60.0   Infective myositis**
> Tropical pyomyositis
> **Use additional** code (B95-B97) to identify infectious agent

   ● **M60.00   Infective myositis, unspecified site**

     M60.000   Infective myositis, unspecified right arm
> Infective myositis, right upper limb NOS

     M60.001   Infective myositis, unspecified left arm
> Infective myositis, left upper limb NOS

     M60.002   Infective myositis, unspecified arm
> Infective myositis, upper limb NOS

     M60.003   Infective myositis, unspecified right leg
> Infective myositis, right lower limb NOS

     M60.004   Infective myositis, unspecified left leg
> Infective myositis, left lower limb NOS

     M60.005   Infective myositis, unspecified leg
> Infective myositis, lower limb NOS

     M60.009   Infective myositis, unspecified site

   ● **M60.01   Infective myositis, shoulder**

     M60.011   Infective myositis, right shoulder

     M60.012   Infective myositis, left shoulder

     M60.019   Infective myositis, unspecified shoulder

   ● **M60.02   Infective myositis, upper arm**

     M60.021   Infective myositis, right upper arm

     M60.022   Infective myositis, left upper arm

     M60.029   Infective myositis, unspecified upper arm

   ● **M60.03   Infective myositis, forearm**

     M60.031   Infective myositis, right forearm

     M60.032   Infective myositis, left forearm

     M60.039   Infective myositis, unspecified forearm

   ● **M60.04   Infective myositis, hand and fingers**

     M60.041   Infective myositis, right hand

     M60.042   Infective myositis, left hand

     M60.043   Infective myositis, unspecified hand

     M60.044   Infective myositis, right finger(s)

     M60.045   Infective myositis, left finger(s)

     M60.046   Infective myositis, unspecified finger(s)

   ● **M60.05   Infective myositis, thigh**

     M60.051   Infective myositis, right thigh

     M60.052   Infective myositis, left thigh

     M60.059   Infective myositis, unspecified thigh

   ● **M60.06   Infective myositis, lower leg**

     M60.061   Infective myositis, right lower leg

     M60.062   Infective myositis, left lower leg

     M60.069   Infective myositis, unspecified lower leg

   ● **M60.07   Infective myositis, ankle, foot and toes**

     M60.070   Infective myositis, right ankle

     M60.071   Infective myositis, left ankle

     M60.072   Infective myositis, unspecified ankle

     M60.073   Infective myositis, right foot

     M60.074   Infective myositis, left foot

     M60.075   Infective myositis, unspecified foot

     M60.076   Infective myositis, right toe(s)

     M60.077   Infective myositis, left toe(s)

     M60.078   Infective myositis, unspecified toe(s)

     M60.08   Infective myositis, other site

     M60.09   Infective myositis, multiple sites

● **M60.1   Interstitial myositis**

     M60.10   Interstitial myositis of unspecified site

   ● **M60.11   Interstitial myositis, shoulder**

     M60.111   Interstitial myositis, right shoulder

     M60.112   Interstitial myositis, left shoulder

     M60.119   Interstitial myositis, unspecified shoulder

   ● **M60.12   Interstitial myositis, upper arm**

     M60.121   Interstitial myositis, right upper arm

     M60.122   Interstitial myositis, left upper arm

     M60.129   Interstitial myositis, unspecified upper arm

   ● **M60.13   Interstitial myositis, forearm**

     M60.131   Interstitial myositis, right forearm

     M60.132   Interstitial myositis, left forearm

     M60.139   Interstitial myositis, unspecified forearm

   ● **M60.14   Interstitial myositis, hand**

     M60.141   Interstitial myositis, right hand

     M60.142   Interstitial myositis, left hand

     M60.149   Interstitial myositis, unspecified hand

   ● **M60.15   Interstitial myositis, thigh**

     M60.151   Interstitial myositis, right thigh

     M60.152   Interstitial myositis, left thigh

     M60.159   Interstitial myositis, unspecified thigh

   ● **M60.16   Interstitial myositis, lower leg**

     M60.161   Interstitial myositis, right lower leg

     M60.162   Interstitial myositis, left lower leg

     M60.169   Interstitial myositis, unspecified lower leg

   ● **M60.17   Interstitial myositis, ankle and foot**

     M60.171   Interstitial myositis, right ankle and foot

     M60.172   Interstitial myositis, left ankle and foot

     M60.179   Interstitial myositis, unspecified ankle and foot

     M60.18   Interstitial myositis, other site

     M60.19   Interstitial myositis, multiple sites

● **M60.2   Foreign body granuloma of soft tissue, not elsewhere classified**
> **Use additional** code to identify the type of retained foreign body (Z18.-)

> **Excludes1**   foreign body granuloma of skin and subcutaneous tissue (L92.3)

     M60.20   Foreign body granuloma of soft tissue, not elsewhere classified, unspecified site

● **M60.21** Foreign body granuloma of soft tissue, not elsewhere classified, shoulder
- **M60.211** Foreign body granuloma of soft tissue, not elsewhere classified, right shoulder
- **M60.212** Foreign body granuloma of soft tissue, not elsewhere classified, left shoulder
- **M60.219** Foreign body granuloma of soft tissue, not elsewhere classified, unspecified shoulder

● **M60.22** Foreign body granuloma of soft tissue, not elsewhere classified, upper arm
- **M60.221** Foreign body granuloma of soft tissue, not elsewhere classified, right upper arm
- **M60.222** Foreign body granuloma of soft tissue, not elsewhere classified, left upper arm
- **M60.229** Foreign body granuloma of soft tissue, not elsewhere classified, unspecified upper arm

● **M60.23** Foreign body granuloma of soft tissue, not elsewhere classified, forearm
- **M60.231** Foreign body granuloma of soft tissue, not elsewhere classified, right forearm
- **M60.232** Foreign body granuloma of soft tissue, not elsewhere classified, left forearm
- **M60.239** Foreign body granuloma of soft tissue, not elsewhere classified, unspecified forearm

● **M60.24** Foreign body granuloma of soft tissue, not elsewhere classified, hand
- **M60.241** Foreign body granuloma of soft tissue, not elsewhere classified, right hand
- **M60.242** Foreign body granuloma of soft tissue, not elsewhere classified, left hand
- **M60.249** Foreign body granuloma of soft tissue, not elsewhere classified, unspecified hand

● **M60.25** Foreign body granuloma of soft tissue, not elsewhere classified, thigh
- **M60.251** Foreign body granuloma of soft tissue, not elsewhere classified, right thigh
- **M60.252** Foreign body granuloma of soft tissue, not elsewhere classified, left thigh
- **M60.259** Foreign body granuloma of soft tissue, not elsewhere classified, unspecified thigh

● **M60.26** Foreign body granuloma of soft tissue, not elsewhere classified, lower leg
- **M60.261** Foreign body granuloma of soft tissue, not elsewhere classified, right lower leg
- **M60.262** Foreign body granuloma of soft tissue, not elsewhere classified, left lower leg
- **M60.269** Foreign body granuloma of soft tissue, not elsewhere classified, unspecified lower leg

● **M60.27** Foreign body granuloma of soft tissue, not elsewhere classified, ankle and foot
- **M60.271** Foreign body granuloma of soft tissue, not elsewhere classified, right ankle and foot
- **M60.272** Foreign body granuloma of soft tissue, not elsewhere classified, left ankle and foot
- **M60.279** Foreign body granuloma of soft tissue, not elsewhere classified, unspecified ankle and foot
- **M60.28** Foreign body granuloma of soft tissue, not elsewhere classified, other site

● **M60.8** Other myositis
- **M60.80** Other myositis, unspecified site
- ● **M60.81** Other myositis shoulder
  - **M60.811** Other myositis, right shoulder
  - **M60.812** Other myositis, left shoulder
  - **M60.819** Other myositis, unspecified shoulder
- ● **M60.82** Other myositis, upper arm
  - **M60.821** Other myositis, right upper arm
  - **M60.822** Other myositis, left upper arm
  - **M60.829** Other myositis, unspecified upper arm
- ● **M60.83** Other myositis, forearm
  - **M60.831** Other myositis, right forearm
  - **M60.832** Other myositis, left forearm
  - **M60.839** Other myositis, unspecified forearm
- ● **M60.84** Other myositis, hand
  - **M60.841** Other myositis, right hand
  - **M60.842** Other myositis, left hand
  - **M60.849** Other myositis, unspecified hand
- ● **M60.85** Other myositis, thigh
  - **M60.851** Other myositis, right thigh
  - **M60.852** Other myositis, left thigh
  - **M60.859** Other myositis, unspecified thigh
- ● **M60.86** Other myositis, lower leg
  - **M60.861** Other myositis, right lower leg
  - **M60.862** Other myositis, left lower leg
  - **M60.869** Other myositis, unspecified lower leg
- ● **M60.87** Other myositis, ankle and foot
  - **M60.871** Other myositis, right ankle and foot
  - **M60.872** Other myositis, left ankle and foot
  - **M60.879** Other myositis, unspecified ankle and foot
- **M60.88** Other myositis, other site
- **M60.89** Other myositis, multiple sites
- **M60.9** Myositis, unspecified

● **M61** Calcification and ossification of muscle
- ● **M61.0** Myositis ossificans traumatica
  - **M61.00** Myositis ossificans traumatica, unspecified site
  - ● **M61.01** Myositis ossificans traumatica, shoulder
    - **M61.011** Myositis ossificans traumatica, right shoulder
    - **M61.012** Myositis ossificans traumatica, left shoulder
    - **M61.019** Myositis ossificans traumatica, unspecified shoulder
  - ● **M61.02** Myositis ossificans traumatica, upper arm
    - **M61.021** Myositis ossificans traumatica, right upper arm
    - **M61.022** Myositis ossificans traumatica, left upper arm
    - **M61.029** Myositis ossificans traumatica, unspecified upper arm
  - ● **M61.03** Myositis ossificans traumatica, forearm
    - **M61.031** Myositis ossificans traumatica, right forearm

M61.032   Myositis ossificans traumatica, left forearm

M61.039   Myositis ossificans traumatica, unspecified forearm

● M61.04   Myositis ossificans traumatica, hand

M61.041   Myositis ossificans traumatica, right hand

M61.042   Myositis ossificans traumatica, left hand

M61.049   Myositis ossificans traumatica, unspecified hand

● M61.05   Myositis ossificans traumatica, thigh

M61.051   Myositis ossificans traumatica, right thigh

M61.052   Myositis ossificans traumatica, left thigh

M61.059   Myositis ossificans traumatica, unspecified thigh

● M61.06   Myositis ossificans traumatica, lower leg

M61.061   Myositis ossificans traumatica, right lower leg

M61.062   Myositis ossificans traumatica, left lower leg

M61.069   Myositis ossificans traumatica, unspecified lower leg

● M61.07   Myositis ossificans traumatica, ankle and foot

M61.071   Myositis ossificans traumatica, right ankle and foot

M61.072   Myositis ossificans traumatica, left ankle and foot

M61.079   Myositis ossificans traumatica, unspecified ankle and foot

M61.08   Myositis ossificans traumatica, other site

M61.09   Myositis ossificans traumatica, multiple sites

● M61.1   Myositis ossificans progressiva
Fibrodysplasia ossificans progressiva

M61.10   Myositis ossificans progressiva, unspecified site

● M61.11   Myositis ossificans progressiva, shoulder

M61.111   Myositis ossificans progressiva, right shoulder

M61.112   Myositis ossificans progressiva, left shoulder

M61.119   Myositis ossificans progressiva, unspecified shoulder

● M61.12   Myositis ossificans progressiva, upper arm

M61.121   Myositis ossificans progressiva, right upper arm

M61.122   Myositis ossificans progressiva, left upper arm

▶ M61.129   Myositis ossificans progressiva, unspecified upper arm

● M61.13   Myositis ossificans progressiva, forearm

M61.131   Myositis ossificans progressiva, right forearm

M61.132   Myositis ossificans progressiva, left forearm

M61.139   Myositis ossificans progressiva, unspecified forearm

● M61.14   Myositis ossificans progressiva, hand and finger(s)

M61.141   Myositis ossificans progressiva, right hand

M61.142   Myositis ossificans progressiva, left hand

M61.143   Myositis ossificans progressiva, unspecified hand

M61.144   Myositis ossificans progressiva, right finger(s)

M61.145   Myositis ossificans progressiva, left finger(s)

M61.146   Myositis ossificans progressiva, unspecified finger(s)

● M61.15   Myositis ossificans progressiva, thigh

M61.151   Myositis ossificans progressiva, right thigh

M61.152   Myositis ossificans progressiva, left thigh

M61.159   Myositis ossificans progressiva, unspecified thigh

● M61.16   Myositis ossificans progressiva, lower leg

M61.161   Myositis ossificans progressiva, right lower leg

M61.162   Myositis ossificans progressiva, left lower leg

M61.169   Myositis ossificans progressiva, unspecified lower leg

● M61.17   Myositis ossificans progressiva, ankle, foot and toe(s)

M61.171   Myositis ossificans progressiva, right ankle

M61.172   Myositis ossificans progressiva, left ankle

M61.173   Myositis ossificans progressiva, unspecified ankle

M61.174   Myositis ossificans progressiva, right foot

M61.175   Myositis ossificans progressiva, left foot

M61.176   Myositis ossificans progressiva, unspecified foot

M61.177   Myositis ossificans progressiva, right toe(s)

M61.178   Myositis ossificans progressiva, left toe(s)

M61.179   Myositis ossificans progressiva, unspecified toe(s)

M61.18   Myositis ossificans progressiva, other site

M61.19   Myositis ossificans progressiva, multiple sites

● M61.2   Paralytic calcification and ossification of muscle
Myositis ossificans associated with quadriplegia or paraplegia

M61.20   Paralytic calcification and ossification of muscle, unspecified site

● M61.21   Paralytic calcification and ossification of muscle, shoulder

M61.211   Paralytic calcification and ossification of muscle, right shoulder

M61.212   Paralytic calcification and ossification of muscle, left shoulder

M61.219   Paralytic calcification and ossification of muscle, unspecified shoulder

● M61.22   Paralytic calcification and ossification of muscle, upper arm

M61.221   Paralytic calcification and ossification of muscle, right upper arm

M61.222   Paralytic calcification and ossification of muscle, left upper arm

M61.229   Paralytic calcification and ossification of muscle, unspecified upper arm

CHAPTER 13 (M00–M99)

● **M61.23** Paralytic calcification and ossification of muscle, forearm
    M61.231 Paralytic calcification and ossification of muscle, right forearm
    M61.232 Paralytic calcification and ossification of muscle, left forearm
    M61.239 Paralytic calcification and ossification of muscle, unspecified forearm

● **M61.24** Paralytic calcification and ossification of muscle, hand
    M61.241 Paralytic calcification and ossification of muscle, right hand
    M61.242 Paralytic calcification and ossification of muscle, left hand
    M61.249 Paralytic calcification and ossification of muscle, unspecified hand

● **M61.25** Paralytic calcification and ossification of muscle, thigh
    M61.251 Paralytic calcification and ossification of muscle, right thigh
    M61.252 Paralytic calcification and ossification of muscle, left thigh
    M61.259 Paralytic calcification and ossification of muscle, unspecified thigh

● **M61.26** Paralytic calcification and ossification of muscle, lower leg
    M61.261 Paralytic calcification and ossification of muscle, right lower leg
    M61.262 Paralytic calcification and ossification of muscle, left lower leg
    M61.269 Paralytic calcification and ossification of muscle, unspecified lower leg

● **M61.27** Paralytic calcification and ossification of muscle, ankle and foot
    M61.271 Paralytic calcification and ossification of muscle, right ankle and foot
    M61.272 Paralytic calcification and ossification of muscle, left ankle and foot
    M61.279 Paralytic calcification and ossification of muscle, unspecified ankle and foot

M61.28 Paralytic calcification and ossification of muscle, other site

M61.29 Paralytic calcification and ossification of muscle, multiple sites

● **M61.3** Calcification and ossification of muscles associated with burns
    Myositis ossificans associated with burns

M61.30 Calcification and ossification of muscles associated with burns, unspecified site

● **M61.31** Calcification and ossification of muscles associated with burns, shoulder
    M61.311 Calcification and ossification of muscles associated with burns, right shoulder
    M61.312 Calcification and ossification of muscles associated with burns, left shoulder
    M61.319 Calcification and ossification of muscles associated with burns, unspecified shoulder

● **M61.32** Calcification and ossification of muscles associated with burns, upper arm
    M61.321 Calcification and ossification of muscles associated with burns, right upper arm
    M61.322 Calcification and ossification of muscles associated with burns, left upper arm
    M61.329 Calcification and ossification of muscles associated with burns, unspecified upper arm

● **M61.33** Calcification and ossification of muscles associated with burns, forearm
    M61.331 Calcification and ossification of muscles associated with burns, right forearm
    M61.332 Calcification and ossification of muscles associated with burns, left forearm
    M61.339 Calcification and ossification of muscles associated with burns, unspecified forearm

● **M61.34** Calcification and ossification of muscles associated with burns, hand
    M61.341 Calcification and ossification of muscles associated with burns, right hand
    M61.342 Calcification and ossification of muscles associated with burns, left hand
    M61.349 Calcification and ossification of muscles associated with burns, unspecified hand

● **M61.35** Calcification and ossification of muscles associated with burns, thigh
    M61.351 Calcification and ossification of muscles associated with burns, right thigh
    M61.352 Calcification and ossification of muscles associated with burns, left thigh
    M61.359 Calcification and ossification of muscles associated with burns, unspecified thigh

● **M61.36** Calcification and ossification of muscles associated with burns, lower leg
    M61.361 Calcification and ossification of muscles associated with burns, right lower leg
    M61.362 Calcification and ossification of muscles associated with burns, left lower leg
    M61.369 Calcification and ossification of muscles associated with burns, unspecified lower leg

● **M61.37** Calcification and ossification of muscles associated with burns, ankle and foot
    M61.371 Calcification and ossification of muscles associated with burns, right ankle and foot
    M61.372 Calcification and ossification of muscles associated with burns, left ankle and foot
    M61.379 Calcification and ossification of muscles associated with burns, unspecified ankle and foot

M61.38 Calcification and ossification of muscles associated with burns, other site

M61.39 Calcification and ossification of muscles associated with burns, multiple sites

● **M61.4** Other calcification of muscle
    Excludes1 calcific tendinitis NOS (M65.2-)
                  calcific tendinitis of shoulder (M75.3)

M61.40 Other calcification of muscle, unspecified site

● **M61.41** Other calcification of muscle, shoulder
    M61.411 Other calcification of muscle, right shoulder
    M61.412 Other calcification of muscle, left shoulder
    M61.419 Other calcification of muscle, unspecified shoulder

● M61.42 Other calcification of muscle, upper arm
    M61.421 Other calcification of muscle, right upper arm
    M61.422 Other calcification of muscle, left upper arm
    M61.429 Other calcification of muscle, unspecified upper arm
● M61.43 Other calcification of muscle, forearm
    M61.431 Other calcification of muscle, right forearm
    M61.432 Other calcification of muscle, left forearm
    M61.439 Other calcification of muscle, unspecified forearm
● M61.44 Other calcification of muscle, hand
    M61.441 Other calcification of muscle, right hand
    M61.442 Other calcification of muscle, left hand
    M61.449 Other calcification of muscle, unspecified hand
● M61.45 Other calcification of muscle, thigh
    M61.451 Other calcification of muscle, right thigh
    M61.452 Other calcification of muscle, left thigh
    M61.459 Other calcification of muscle, unspecified thigh
● M61.46 Other calcification of muscle, lower leg
    M61.461 Other calcification of muscle, right lower leg
    M61.462 Other calcification of muscle, left lower leg
    M61.469 Other calcification of muscle, unspecified lower leg
● M61.47 Other calcification of muscle, ankle and foot
    M61.471 Other calcification of muscle, right ankle and foot
    M61.472 Other calcification of muscle, left ankle and foot
    M61.479 Other calcification of muscle, unspecified ankle and foot
    M61.48 Other calcification of muscle, other site
    M61.49 Other calcification of muscle, multiple sites
● M61.5 Other ossification of muscle
    M61.50 Other ossification of muscle, unspecified site
● M61.51 Other ossification of muscle, shoulder
    M61.511 Other ossification of muscle, right shoulder
    M61.512 Other ossification of muscle, left shoulder
    M61.519 Other ossification of muscle, unspecified shoulder
● M61.52 Other ossification of muscle, upper arm
    M61.521 Other ossification of muscle, right upper arm
    M61.522 Other ossification of muscle, left upper arm
    M61.529 Other ossification of muscle, unspecified upper arm
● M61.53 Other ossification of muscle, forearm
    M61.531 Other ossification of muscle, right forearm
    M61.532 Other ossification of muscle, left forearm
    M61.539 Other ossification of muscle, unspecified forearm

● M61.54 Other ossification of muscle, hand
    M61.541 Other ossification of muscle, right hand
    M61.542 Other ossification of muscle, left hand
    M61.549 Other ossification of muscle, unspecified hand
● M61.55 Other ossification of muscle, thigh
    M61.551 Other ossification of muscle, right thigh
    M61.552 Other ossification of muscle, left thigh
    Coding Clinic: 2024, Q3, P14
    M61.559 Other ossification of muscle, unspecified thigh
● M61.56 Other ossification of muscle, lower leg
    M61.561 Other ossification of muscle, right lower leg
    M61.562 Other ossification of muscle, left lower leg
    M61.569 Other ossification of muscle, unspecified lower leg
● M61.57 Other ossification of muscle, ankle and foot
    M61.571 Other ossification of muscle, right ankle and foot
    M61.572 Other ossification of muscle, left ankle and foot
    M61.579 Other ossification of muscle, unspecified ankle and foot
    M61.58 Other ossification of muscle, other site
    M61.59 Other ossification of muscle, multiple sites
    M61.9 Calcification and ossification of muscle, unspecified

● M62 Other disorders of muscle
    Excludes1 alcoholic myopathy (G72.1)
            cramp and spasm (R25.2)
            drug-induced myopathy (G72.0)
            myalgia (M79.1-)
            stiff-man syndrome (G25.82)
    Excludes2 nontraumatic hematoma of muscle (M79.81)
● M62.0 Separation of muscle (nontraumatic)
    Diastasis of muscle
    Excludes1 diastasis recti complicating pregnancy, labor and delivery (O71.8)
            traumatic separation of muscle - see strain of muscle by body region
    M62.00 Separation of muscle (nontraumatic), unspecified site
● M62.01 Separation of muscle (nontraumatic), shoulder
    M62.011 Separation of muscle (nontraumatic), right shoulder
    M62.012 Separation of muscle (nontraumatic), left shoulder
    M62.019 Separation of muscle (nontraumatic), unspecified shoulder
● M62.02 Separation of muscle (nontraumatic), upper arm
    M62.021 Separation of muscle (nontraumatic), right upper arm
    M62.022 Separation of muscle (nontraumatic), left upper arm
    M62.029 Separation of muscle (nontraumatic), unspecified upper arm
● M62.03 Separation of muscle (nontraumatic), forearm
    M62.031 Separation of muscle (nontraumatic), right forearm
    M62.032 Separation of muscle (nontraumatic), left forearm
    M62.039 Separation of muscle (nontraumatic), unspecified forearm

● M62.04   Separation of muscle (nontraumatic), hand
    M62.041   Separation of muscle (nontraumatic), right hand
    M62.042   Separation of muscle (nontraumatic), left hand
    M62.049   Separation of muscle (nontraumatic), unspecified hand

● M62.05   Separation of muscle (nontraumatic), thigh
    M62.051   Separation of muscle (nontraumatic), right thigh
    M62.052   Separation of muscle (nontraumatic), left thigh
    M62.059   Separation of muscle (nontraumatic), unspecified thigh

● M62.06   Separation of muscle (nontraumatic), lower leg
    M62.061   Separation of muscle (nontraumatic), right lower leg
    M62.062   Separation of muscle (nontraumatic), left lower leg
    M62.069   Separation of muscle (nontraumatic), unspecified lower leg

● M62.07   Separation of muscle (nontraumatic), ankle and foot
    M62.071   Separation of muscle (nontraumatic), right ankle and foot
    M62.072   Separation of muscle (nontraumatic), left ankle and foot
    M62.079   Separation of muscle (nontraumatic), unspecified ankle and foot

    M62.08   Separation of muscle (nontraumatic), other site

● M62.1   Other rupture of muscle (nontraumatic)
    Excludes1   traumatic rupture of muscle - see strain of muscle by body region
    Excludes2   rupture of tendon (M66.-)
    M62.10   Other rupture of muscle (nontraumatic), unspecified site

● M62.11   Other rupture of muscle (nontraumatic), shoulder
    M62.111   Other rupture of muscle (nontraumatic), right shoulder
    M62.112   Other rupture of muscle (nontraumatic), left shoulder
    M62.119   Other rupture of muscle (nontraumatic), unspecified shoulder

● M62.12   Other rupture of muscle (nontraumatic), upper arm
    M62.121   Other rupture of muscle (nontraumatic), right upper arm
    M62.122   Other rupture of muscle (nontraumatic), left upper arm
    M62.129   Other rupture of muscle (nontraumatic), unspecified upper arm

● M62.13   Other rupture of muscle (nontraumatic), forearm
    M62.131   Other rupture of muscle (nontraumatic), right forearm
    M62.132   Other rupture of muscle (nontraumatic), left forearm
    M62.139   Other rupture of muscle (nontraumatic), unspecified forearm

● M62.14   Other rupture of muscle (nontraumatic), hand
    M62.141   Other rupture of muscle (nontraumatic), right hand
    M62.142   Other rupture of muscle (nontraumatic), left hand
    M62.149   Other rupture of muscle (nontraumatic), unspecified hand

● M62.15   Other rupture of muscle (nontraumatic), thigh
    M62.151   Other rupture of muscle (nontraumatic), right thigh
    M62.152   Other rupture of muscle (nontraumatic), left thigh
    M62.159   Other rupture of muscle (nontraumatic), unspecified thigh

● M62.16   Other rupture of muscle (nontraumatic), lower leg
    M62.161   Other rupture of muscle (nontraumatic), right lower leg
    M62.162   Other rupture of muscle (nontraumatic), left lower leg
    M62.169   Other rupture of muscle (nontraumatic), unspecified lower leg

● M62.17   Other rupture of muscle (nontraumatic), ankle and foot
    M62.171   Other rupture of muscle (nontraumatic), right ankle and foot
    M62.172   Other rupture of muscle (nontraumatic), left ankle and foot
    M62.179   Other rupture of muscle (nontraumatic), unspecified ankle and foot

    M62.18   Other rupture of muscle (nontraumatic), other site

● M62.2   Nontraumatic ischemic infarction of muscle
    Excludes1   compartment syndrome (traumatic) (T79.A-)
        nontraumatic compartment syndrome (M79.A-)
        traumatic ischemia of muscle (T79.6)
        rhabdomyolysis (M62.82)
        Volkmann's ischemic contracture (T79.6)

    M62.20   Nontraumatic ischemic infarction of muscle, unspecified site

● M62.21   Nontraumatic ischemic infarction of muscle, shoulder
    M62.211   Nontraumatic ischemic infarction of muscle, right shoulder
    M62.212   Nontraumatic ischemic infarction of muscle, left shoulder
    M62.219   Nontraumatic ischemic infarction of muscle, unspecified shoulder

● M62.22   Nontraumatic ischemic infarction of muscle, upper arm
    M62.221   Nontraumatic ischemic infarction of muscle, right upper arm
    M62.222   Nontraumatic ischemic infarction of muscle, left upper arm
    M62.229   Nontraumatic ischemic infarction of muscle, unspecified upper arm

● M62.23   Nontraumatic ischemic infarction of muscle, forearm
    M62.231   Nontraumatic ischemic infarction of muscle, right forearm
    M62.232   Nontraumatic ischemic infarction of muscle, left forearm
    M62.239   Nontraumatic ischemic infarction of muscle, unspecified forearm

● M62.24   Nontraumatic ischemic infarction of muscle, hand
    M62.241   Nontraumatic ischemic infarction of muscle, right hand
    M62.242   Nontraumatic ischemic infarction of muscle, left hand
    M62.249   Nontraumatic ischemic infarction of muscle, unspecified hand

● **M62.25**   Nontraumatic ischemic infarction of muscle, thigh
     M62.251   Nontraumatic ischemic infarction of muscle, right thigh
     M62.252   Nontraumatic ischemic infarction of muscle, left thigh
     M62.259   Nontraumatic ischemic infarction of muscle, unspecified thigh

● **M62.26**   Nontraumatic ischemic infarction of muscle, lower leg
     M62.261   Nontraumatic ischemic infarction of muscle, right lower leg
     M62.262   Nontraumatic ischemic infarction of muscle, left lower leg
     M62.269   Nontraumatic ischemic infarction of muscle, unspecified lower leg

● **M62.27**   Nontraumatic ischemic infarction of muscle, ankle and foot
     M62.271   Nontraumatic ischemic infarction of muscle, right ankle and foot
     M62.272   Nontraumatic ischemic infarction of muscle, left ankle and foot
     M62.279   Nontraumatic ischemic infarction of muscle, unspecified ankle and foot

M62.28   Nontraumatic ischemic infarction of muscle, other site

M62.3   Immobility syndrome (paraplegic)

M62.4   Contracture of muscle
     Contracture of tendon (sheath)
     Excludes1   contracture of joint (M24.5-)
     M62.40   Contracture of muscle, unspecified site

● **M62.41**   Contracture of muscle, shoulder
     M62.411   Contracture of muscle, right shoulder
     M62.412   Contracture of muscle, left shoulder
     M62.419   Contracture of muscle, unspecified shoulder

● **M62.42**   Contracture of muscle, upper arm
     M62.421   Contracture of muscle, right upper arm
     M62.422   Contracture of muscle, left upper arm
     M62.429   Contracture of muscle, unspecified upper arm

● **M62.43**   Contracture of muscle, forearm
     M62.431   Contracture of muscle, right forearm
     M62.432   Contracture of muscle, left forearm
     M62.439   Contracture of muscle, unspecified forearm

● **M62.44**   Contracture of muscle, hand
     M62.441   Contracture of muscle, right hand
     M62.442   Contracture of muscle, left hand
     M62.449   Contracture of muscle, unspecified hand

● **M62.45**   Contracture of muscle, thigh
     M62.451   Contracture of muscle, right thigh
     M62.452   Contracture of muscle, left thigh
     M62.459   Contracture of muscle, unspecified thigh

● **M62.46**   Contracture of muscle, lower leg
     M62.461   Contracture of muscle, right lower leg
     M62.462   Contracture of muscle, left lower leg
     Coding Clinic: 2023, Q2, P14
     M62.469   Contracture of muscle, unspecified lower leg

● **M62.47**   Contracture of muscle, ankle and foot
     M62.471   Contracture of muscle, right ankle and foot
     M62.472   Contracture of muscle, left ankle and foot
     M62.479   Contracture of muscle, unspecified ankle and foot

M62.48   Contracture of muscle, other site

M62.49   Contracture of muscle, multiple sites

● **M62.5**   Muscle wasting and atrophy, not elsewhere classified
     Disuse atrophy NEC
     Excludes1   neuralgic amyotrophy (G54.5)
                            progressive muscular atrophy (G12.21)
                            sarcopenia (M62.84)
     Excludes2   pelvic muscle wasting (N81.84)
     M62.50   Muscle wasting and atrophy, not elsewhere classified, unspecified site

● **M62.51**   Muscle wasting and atrophy, not elsewhere classified, shoulder
     M62.511   Muscle wasting and atrophy, not elsewhere classified, right shoulder
     M62.512   Muscle wasting and atrophy, not elsewhere classified, left shoulder
     M62.519   Muscle wasting and atrophy, not elsewhere classified, unspecified shoulder

● **M62.52**   Muscle wasting and atrophy, not elsewhere classified, upper arm
     M62.521   Muscle wasting and atrophy, not elsewhere classified, right upper arm
     M62.522   Muscle wasting and atrophy, not elsewhere classified, left upper arm
     M62.529   Muscle wasting and atrophy, not elsewhere classified, unspecified upper arm

● **M62.53**   Muscle wasting and atrophy, not elsewhere classified, forearm
     M62.531   Muscle wasting and atrophy, not elsewhere classified, right forearm
     M62.532   Muscle wasting and atrophy, not elsewhere classified, left forearm
     M62.539   Muscle wasting and atrophy, not elsewhere classified, unspecified forearm

● **M62.54**   Muscle wasting and atrophy, not elsewhere classified, hand
     M62.541   Muscle wasting and atrophy, not elsewhere classified, right hand
     M62.542   Muscle wasting and atrophy, not elsewhere classified, left hand
     M62.549   Muscle wasting and atrophy, not elsewhere classified, unspecified hand

● **M62.55**   Muscle wasting and atrophy, not elsewhere classified, thigh
     M62.551   Muscle wasting and atrophy, not elsewhere classified, right thigh
     M62.552   Muscle wasting and atrophy, not elsewhere classified, left thigh
     M62.559   Muscle wasting and atrophy, not elsewhere classified, unspecified thigh

● **M62.56**   Muscle wasting and atrophy, not elsewhere classified, lower leg
     M62.561   Muscle wasting and atrophy, not elsewhere classified, right lower leg
     M62.562   Muscle wasting and atrophy, not elsewhere classified, left lower leg
     M62.569   Muscle wasting and atrophy, not elsewhere classified, unspecified lower leg

● **M62.57** **Muscle wasting and atrophy, not elsewhere classified, ankle and foot**
　　M62.571 Muscle wasting and atrophy, not elsewhere classified, right ankle and foot
　　M62.572 Muscle wasting and atrophy, not elsewhere classified, left ankle and foot
　　M62.579 Muscle wasting and atrophy, not elsewhere classified, unspecified ankle and foot
　M62.58 Muscle wasting and atrophy, not elsewhere classified, other site
　M62.59 Muscle wasting and atrophy, not elsewhere classified, multiple sites
● **M62.5A** **Muscle wasting and atrophy, not elsewhere classified, back**
　　M62.5A0 Muscle wasting and atrophy, not elsewhere classified, back, cervical
　　M62.5A1 Muscle wasting and atrophy, not elsewhere classified, back, thoracic
　　M62.5A2 Muscle wasting and atrophy, not elsewhere classified, back, lumbosacral
　　M62.5A9 Muscle wasting and atrophy, not elsewhere classified, back, unspecified level

● **M62.8** **Other specified disorders of muscle**
　Excludes2 nontraumatic hematoma of muscle (M79.81)
　M62.81 Muscle weakness (generalized)
　　Excludes1 muscle weakness in sarcopenia (M62.84)
　M62.82 Rhabdomyolysis
　　Excludes1 traumatic rhabdomyolysis (T79.6)
　　Coding Clinic: 2024, Q4, P17; 2019, Q2, P12
● **M62.83** **Muscle spasm**
　　M62.830 Muscle spasm of back
　　M62.831 Muscle spasm of calf
　　　Charley-horse
　　M62.838 Other muscle spasm
　M62.84 Sarcopenia
　　Age-related sarcopenia
　　Code first underlying disease, if applicable, such as:
　　　disorders of myoneural junction and muscle disease in diseases classified elsewhere (G73.-)
　　　other and unspecified myopathies (G72.-)
　　　primary disorders of muscles (G71.-)
　　Coding Clinic: 2016, Q4, P41
　M62.85 Dyfunction of the multifidus muscles, lumbar region
　M62.89 Other specified disorders of muscle
　　Muscle (sheath) hernia
　M62.9 Disorder of muscle, unspecified

● **M63** **Disorders of muscle in diseases classified elsewhere**
　Code first underlying disease, such as:
　　leprosy (A30.-)
　　neoplasm (C49.-, C79.89, D21.-, D48.1-)
　　schistosomiasis (B65.-)
　　trichinellosis (B75)
　Excludes1 myopathy in cysticercosis (B69.81)
　　myopathy in endocrine diseases (G73.7)
　　myopathy in metabolic diseases (G73.7)
　　myopathy in sarcoidosis (D86.87)
　　myopathy in secondary syphilis (A51.49)
　　myopathy in syphilis (late) (A52.78)
　　myopathy in toxoplasmosis (B58.82)
　　myopathy in tuberculosis (A18.09)

● **M63.8** **Disorders of muscle in diuseases classified elsewhere**
　▶ *M63.80* Disorders of muscle in diseases classified elsewhere, unspecified site
● **M63.81** **Disorders of muscle in diseases classified elsewhere, shoulder**
　▶ *M63.811* Disorders of muscle in diseases classified elsewhere, right shoulder
　▶ *M63.812* Disorders of muscle in diseases classified elsewhere, left shoulder
　▶ *M63.819* Disorders of muscle in diseases classified elsewhere, unspecified shoulder
● **M63.82** **Disorders of muscle in diseases classified elsewhere, upper arm**
　▶ *M63.821* Disorders of muscle in diseases classified elsewhere, right upper arm
　▶ *M63.822* Disorders of muscle in diseases classified elsewhere, left upper arm
　▶ *M63.829* Disorders of muscle in diseases classified elsewhere, unspecified upper arm
● **M63.83** **Disorders of muscle in diseases classified elsewhere, forearm**
　▶ *M63.831* Disorders of muscle in diseases classified elsewhere, right forearm
　▶ *M63.832* Disorders of muscle in diseases classified elsewhere, left forearm
　▶ *M63.839* Disorders of muscle in diseases classified elsewhere, unspecified forearm
● **M63.84** **Disorders of muscle in diseases classified elsewhere, hand**
　▶ *M63.841* Disorders of muscle in diseases classified elsewhere, right hand
　▶ *M63.842* Disorders of muscle in diseases classified elsewhere, left hand
　▶ *M63.849* Disorders of muscle in diseases classified elsewhere, unspecified hand
● **M63.85** **Disorders of muscle in diseases classified elsewhere, thigh**
　▶ *M63.851* Disorders of muscle in diseases classified elsewhere, right thigh
　▶ *M63.852* Disorders of muscle in diseases classified elsewhere, left thigh
　▶ *M63.859* Disorders of muscle in diseases classified elsewhere, unspecified thigh
● **M63.86** **Disorders of muscle in diseases classified elsewhere, lower leg**
　▶ *M63.861* Disorders of muscle in diseases classified elsewhere, right lower leg
　▶ *M63.862* Disorders of muscle in diseases classified elsewhere, left lower leg
　▶ *M63.869* Disorders of muscle in diseases classified elsewhere, unspecified lower leg
● **M63.87** **Disorders of muscle in diseases classified elsewhere, ankle and foot**
　▶ *M63.871* Disorders of muscle in diseases classified elsewhere, right ankle and foot
　▶ *M63.872* Disorders of muscle in diseases classified elsewhere, left ankle and foot
　▶ *M63.879* Disorders of muscle in diseases classified elsewhere, unspecified ankle and foot
　▶ *M63.88* Disorders of muscle in diseases classified elsewhere, other site
　▶ *M63.89* Disorders of muscle in diseases classified elsewhere, multiple sites

▶ New　　⇒ Revised　　~~deleted~~ Deleted　　Excludes 1　　Excludes 2　　Includes　　Use additional　　Code first　　Code also　　Key words
OGCR Official Guidelines　　X Assign placeholder X　　● Use Additional Character(s)　　▶ Manifestation Code　　**HCC** Hierarchical Condition Category　　**Coding Clinic**

DISORDERS OF SYNOVIUM AND TENDON (M65-M67)

● **M65   Synovitis and tenosynovitis**

    Excludes1   chronic crepitant synovitis of hand and wrist (M70.0-)

       current injury - see injury of ligament or tendon by body region

       soft tissue disorders related to use, overuse and pressure (M70.-)

  ● **M65.0   Abscess of tendon sheath**

      Use additional code (B95-B96) to identify bacterial agent

     M65.00   Abscess of tendon sheath, **unspecified** site

   ● M65.01   Abscess of tendon sheath, **shoulder**

       M65.011   Abscess of tendon sheath, **right** shoulder

       M65.012   Abscess of tendon sheath, **left** shoulder

       M65.019   Abscess of tendon sheath, **unspecified** shoulder

   ● M65.02   Abscess of tendon sheath, **upper arm**

       M65.021   Abscess of tendon sheath, **right** upper arm

       M65.022   Abscess of tendon sheath, **left** upper arm

       M65.029   Abscess of tendon sheath, **unspecified** upper arm

   ● M65.03   Abscess of tendon sheath, **forearm**

       M65.031   Abscess of tendon sheath, **right** forearm

       M65.032   Abscess of tendon sheath, **left** forearm

       M65.039   Abscess of tendon sheath, **unspecified** forearm

   ● M65.04   Abscess of tendon sheath, **hand**

       M65.041   Abscess of tendon sheath, **right** hand

       M65.042   Abscess of tendon sheath, **left** hand

       M65.049   Abscess of tendon sheath, **unspecified** hand

   ● M65.05   Abscess of tendon sheath, **thigh**

       M65.051   Abscess of tendon sheath, **right** thigh

       M65.052   Abscess of tendon sheath, **left** thigh

       M65.059   Abscess of tendon sheath, **unspecified** thigh

   ● M65.06   Abscess of tendon sheath, **lower leg**

       M65.061   Abscess of tendon sheath, **right** lower leg

       M65.062   Abscess of tendon sheath, **left** lower leg

       M65.069   Abscess of tendon sheath, **unspecified** lower leg

   ● M65.07   Abscess of tendon sheath, **ankle and foot**

       M65.071   Abscess of tendon sheath, **right** ankle and foot

       M65.072   Abscess of tendon sheath, **left** ankle and foot

       M65.079   Abscess of tendon sheath, **unspecified** ankle and foot

     M65.08   Abscess of tendon sheath, **other site**

● M65.1   Other infective (teno)synovitis

     M65.10   Other infective (teno)synovitis, **unspecified** site

   ● M65.11   Other infective (teno)synovitis, **shoulder**

       M65.111   Other infective (teno)synovitis, **right** shoulder

       M65.112   Other infective (teno)synovitis, **left** shoulder

       M65.119   Other infective (teno)synovitis, **unspecified** shoulder

   ● M65.12   Other infective (teno)synovitis, **elbow**

       M65.121   Other infective (teno)synovitis, **right** elbow

       M65.122   Other infective (teno)synovitis, **left** elbow

       M65.129   Other infective (teno)synovitis, **unspecified** elbow

   ● M65.13   Other infective (teno)synovitis, **wrist**

       M65.131   Other infective (teno)synovitis, **right** wrist

       M65.132   Other infective (teno)synovitis, **left** wrist

       M65.139   Other infective (teno)synovitis, **unspecified** wrist

   ● M65.14   Other infective (teno)synovitis, **hand**

       M65.141   Other infective (teno)synovitis, **right** hand

       M65.142   Other infective (teno)synovitis, **left** hand

       M65.149   Other infective (teno)synovitis, **unspecified** hand

   ● M65.15   Other infective (teno)synovitis, **hip**

       M65.151   Other infective (teno)synovitis, **right** hip

       M65.152   Other infective (teno)synovitis, **left** hip

       M65.159   Other infective (teno)synovitis, **unspecified** hip

   ● M65.16   Other infective (teno)synovitis, **knee**

       M65.161   Other infective (teno)synovitis, **right** knee

       M65.162   Other infective (teno)synovitis, **left** knee

       M65.169   Other infective (teno)synovitis, **unspecified** knee

   ● M65.17   Other infective (teno)synovitis, **ankle and foot**

       M65.171   Other infective (teno)synovitis, **right** ankle and foot

       M65.172   Other infective (teno)synovitis, **left** ankle and foot

       M65.179   Other infective (teno)synovitis, **unspecified** ankle and foot

     M65.18   Other infective (teno)synovitis, **other site**

     M65.19   Other infective (teno)synovitis, **multiple sites**

● M65.2   Calcific tendinitis

     Excludes1   tendinitis as classified in M75-M77

        calcified tendinitis of shoulder (M75.3)

     M65.20   Calcific tendinitis, **unspecified** site

   ● M65.22   Calcific tendinitis, **upper arm**

       M65.221   Calcific tendinitis, **right** upper arm

       M65.222   Calcific tendinitis, **left** upper arm

       M65.229   Calcific tendinitis, **unspecified** upper arm

   ● M65.23   Calcific tendinitis, **forearm**

       M65.231   Calcific tendinitis, **right** forearm

       M65.232   Calcific tendinitis, **left** forearm

       M65.239   Calcific tendinitis, **unspecified** forearm

Item 13–11 Synovitis is an inflammation of a synovial membrane resulting in pain on motion and is characterized by fluctuating swelling due to effusion in a synovial sac. **Tenosynovitis** is an inflammation of a tendon sheath and occurs most commonly in the wrists, hands, and feet. Bursitis is inflammation of a bursa (fluid-filled sac) caused by repetitive use, trauma, infection, or systemic inflammatory disease. Bursae act as protectors and facilitate movement between bones and overlapping muscles (deep bursae) or between bones and tendons/skin (superficial bursae).

● M65.24 Calcific tendinitis, hand
    M65.241 Calcific tendinitis, right hand
    M65.242 Calcific tendinitis, left hand
    M65.249 Calcific tendinitis, unspecified hand
● M65.25 Calcific tendinitis, thigh
    M65.251 Calcific tendinitis, right thigh
    M65.252 Calcific tendinitis, left thigh
    M65.259 Calcific tendinitis, unspecified thigh
● M65.26 Calcific tendinitis, lower leg
    M65.261 Calcific tendinitis, right lower leg
    M65.262 Calcific tendinitis, left lower leg
    M65.269 Calcific tendinitis, unspecified lower leg
● M65.27 Calcific tendinitis, ankle and foot
    M65.271 Calcific tendinitis, right ankle and foot
    M65.272 Calcific tendinitis, left ankle and foot
    M65.279 Calcific tendinitis, unspecified ankle and foot
  M65.28 Calcific tendinitis, other site
  M65.29 Calcific tendinitis, multiple sites
● M65.3 Trigger finger
    Nodular tendinous disease
  M65.30 Trigger finger, unspecified finger
● M65.31 Trigger thumb
    M65.311 Trigger thumb, right thumb
    M65.312 Trigger thumb, left thumb
    M65.319 Trigger thumb, unspecified thumb
● M65.32 Trigger finger, index finger
    M65.321 Trigger finger, right index finger
    M65.322 Trigger finger, left index finger
    M65.329 Trigger finger, unspecified index finger
● M65.33 Trigger finger, middle finger
    M65.331 Trigger finger, right middle finger
    M65.332 Trigger finger, left middle finger
    M65.339 Trigger finger, unspecified middle finger
● M65.34 Trigger finger, ring finger
    M65.341 Trigger finger, right ring finger
    M65.342 Trigger finger, left ring finger
    M65.349 Trigger finger, unspecified ring finger
● M65.35 Trigger finger, little finger
    M65.351 Trigger finger, right little finger
    M65.352 Trigger finger, left little finger
    M65.359 Trigger finger, unspecified little finger
  M65.4 Radial styloid tenosynovitis [de Quervain]
● M65.8 Other synovitis and tenosynovitis
  M65.80 Other synovitis and tenosynovitis, unspecified site
● M65.81 Other synovitis and tenosynovitis, shoulder
    M65.811 Other synovitis and tenosynovitis, right shoulder
    M65.812 Other synovitis and tenosynovitis, left shoulder
    M65.819 Other synovitis and tenosynovitis, unspecified shoulder
● M65.82 Other synovitis and tenosynovitis, upper arm
    M65.821 Other synovitis and tenosynovitis, right upper arm
    M65.822 Other synovitis and tenosynovitis, left upper arm
    M65.829 Other synovitis and tenosynovitis, unspecified upper arm

● M65.83 Other synovitis and tenosynovitis, forearm
    M65.831 Other synovitis and tenosynovitis, right forearm
    M65.832 Other synovitis and tenosynovitis, left forearm
    M65.839 Other synovitis and tenosynovitis, unspecified forearm
● M65.84 Other synovitis and tenosynovitis, hand
    M65.841 Other synovitis and tenosynovitis, right hand
    M65.842 Other synovitis and tenosynovitis, left hand
    M65.849 Other synovitis and tenosynovitis, unspecified hand
● M65.85 Other synovitis and tenosynovitis, thigh
    M65.851 Other synovitis and tenosynovitis, right thigh
    M65.852 Other synovitis and tenosynovitis, left thigh
    M65.859 Other synovitis and tenosynovitis, unspecified thigh
● M65.86 Other synovitis and tenosynovitis, lower leg
    M65.861 Other synovitis and tenosynovitis, right lower leg
    M65.862 Other synovitis and tenosynovitis, left lower leg
    M65.869 Other synovitis and tenosynovitis, unspecified lower leg
● M65.87 Other synovitis and tenosynovitis, ankle and foot
    M65.871 Other synovitis and tenosynovitis, right ankle and foot
    M65.872 Other synovitis and tenosynovitis, left ankle and foot
    M65.879 Other synovitis and tenosynovitis, unspecified ankle and foot
  M65.88 Other synovitis and tenosynovitis, other site
  M65.89 Other synovitis and tenosynovitis, multiple sites
  M65.9 Synovitis and tenosynovitis, unspecified
  M65.90 Unspecified synovitis and tenosynovitis, unspecified site
● M65.91 Unspecified synovitis and tenosynovitis, shoulder
    M65.911 Unspecified synovitis and tenosynovitis, right shoulder
    M65.912 Unspecified synovitis and tenosynovitis, left shoulder
    M65.919 Unspecified synovitis and tenosynovitis, unspecified shoulder
● M65.92 Unspecified synovitis and tenosynovitis, upper arm
    M65.921 Unspecified synovitis and tenosynovitis, right upper arm
    M65.922 Unspecified synovitis and tenosynovitis, left upper arm
    M65.929 Unspecified synovitis and tenosynovitis, unspecified upper arm
● M65.93 Unspecified synovitis and tenosynovitis, forearm
    M65.931 Unspecified synovitis and tenosynovitis, right forearm
    M65.932 Unspecified synovitis and tenosynovitis, left forearm
    M65.939 Unspecified synovitis and tenosynovitis, unspecified forearm

● M65.94   Unspecified synovitis and tenosynovitis, hand
     M65.941   Unspecified synovitis and tenosynovitis, right hand
     M65.942   Unspecified synovitis and tenosynovitis, left hand
     M65.949   Unspecified synovitis and tenosynovitis, unspecified hand
● M65.95   Unspecified synovitis and tenosynovitis, thigh
     M65.951   Unspecified synovitis and tenosynovitis, right thigh
     M65.952   Unspecified synovitis and tenosynovitis, left thigh
     M65.959   Unspecified synovitis and tenosynovitis, unspecified thigh
● M65.96   Unspecified synovitis and tenosynovitis, lower leg
     M65.961   Unspecified synovitis and tenosynovitis, right lower leg
     M65.962   Unspecified synovitis and tenosynovitis, left lower leg
     M65.969   Unspecified synovitis and tenosynovitis, unspecified lower leg
● M65.97   Unspecified synovitis and tenosynovitis, ankle and foot
     M65.971   Unspecified synovitis and tenosynovitis, right ankle and foot
     M65.972   Unspecified synovitis and tenosynovitis, left ankle and foot
     M65.979   Unspecified synovitis and tenosynovitis, unspecified ankle and foot
   M65.98   Unspecified synovitis and tenosynovitis, other site
   M65.99   Unspecified synovitis and tenosynovitis, multiple sites

● M66   Spontaneous rupture of synovium and tendon

   Includes   rupture that occurs when a normal force is applied to tissues that are inferred to have less than normal strength

   Excludes2   rotator cuff syndrome (M75.1-)
       rupture where an abnormal force is applied to normal tissue - see injury of tendon by body region

   M66.0   Rupture of popliteal cyst

● M66.1   Rupture of synovium
     Rupture of synovial cyst

   Excludes2   rupture of popliteal cyst (M66.0)

     M66.10   Rupture of synovium, unspecified joint
● M66.11   Rupture of synovium, shoulder
     M66.111   Rupture of synovium, right shoulder
     M66.112   Rupture of synovium, left shoulder
     M66.119   Rupture of synovium, unspecified shoulder
● M66.12   Rupture of synovium, elbow
     M66.121   Rupture of synovium, right elbow
     M66.122   Rupture of synovium, left elbow
     M66.129   Rupture of synovium, unspecified elbow
● M66.13   Rupture of synovium, wrist
     M66.131   Rupture of synovium, right wrist
     M66.132   Rupture of synovium, left wrist
     M66.139   Rupture of synovium, unspecified wrist
● M66.14   Rupture of synovium, hand and fingers
     M66.141   Rupture of synovium, right hand
     M66.142   Rupture of synovium, left hand

     M66.143   Rupture of synovium, unspecified hand
     M66.144   Rupture of synovium, right finger(s)
     M66.145   Rupture of synovium, left finger(s)
     M66.146   Rupture of synovium, unspecified finger(s)
● M66.15   Rupture of synovium, hip
     M66.151   Rupture of synovium, right hip
     M66.152   Rupture of synovium, left hip
     M66.159   Rupture of synovium, unspecified hip
● M66.17   Rupture of synovium, ankle, foot and toes
     M66.171   Rupture of synovium, right ankle
     M66.172   Rupture of synovium, left ankle
     M66.173   Rupture of synovium, unspecified ankle
     M66.174   Rupture of synovium, right foot
     M66.175   Rupture of synovium, left foot
     M66.176   Rupture of synovium, unspecified foot
     M66.177   Rupture of synovium, right toe(s)
     M66.178   Rupture of synovium, left toe(s)
     M66.179   Rupture of synovium, unspecified toe(s)
   M66.18   Rupture of synovium, other site
● M66.2   Spontaneous rupture of extensor tendons
   M66.20   Spontaneous rupture of extensor tendons, unspecified site
● M66.21   Spontaneous rupture of extensor tendons, shoulder
     M66.211   Spontaneous rupture of extensor tendons, right shoulder
     M66.212   Spontaneous rupture of extensor tendons, left shoulder
     M66.219   Spontaneous rupture of extensor tendons, unspecified shoulder
● M66.22   Spontaneous rupture of extensor tendons, upper arm
     M66.221   Spontaneous rupture of extensor tendons, right upper arm
     M66.222   Spontaneous rupture of extensor tendons, left upper arm
     M66.229   Spontaneous rupture of extensor tendons, unspecified upper arm
● M66.23   Spontaneous rupture of extensor tendons, forearm
     M66.231   Spontaneous rupture of extensor tendons, right forearm
     M66.232   Spontaneous rupture of extensor tendons, left forearm
     M66.239   Spontaneous rupture of extensor tendons, unspecified forearm
● M66.24   Spontaneous rupture of extensor tendons, hand
     M66.241   Spontaneous rupture of extensor tendons, right hand
     M66.242   Spontaneous rupture of extensor tendons, left hand
     M66.249   Spontaneous rupture of extensor tendons, unspecified hand
● M66.25   Spontaneous rupture of extensor tendons, thigh
     M66.251   Spontaneous rupture of extensor tendons, right thigh
     M66.252   Spontaneous rupture of extensor tendons, left thigh
     M66.259   Spontaneous rupture of extensor tendons, unspecified thigh

CHAPTER 13 (M00-M99)

● **M66.26** Spontaneous rupture of extensor tendons, lower leg

    M66.261 Spontaneous rupture of extensor tendons, right lower leg

    M66.262 Spontaneous rupture of extensor tendons, left lower leg

    M66.269 Spontaneous rupture of extensor tendons, unspecified lower leg

● **M66.27** Spontaneous rupture of extensor tendons, ankle and foot

    M66.271 Spontaneous rupture of extensor tendons, right ankle and foot

    M66.272 Spontaneous rupture of extensor tendons, left ankle and foot

    M66.279 Spontaneous rupture of extensor tendons, unspecified ankle and foot

  M66.28 Spontaneous rupture of extensor tendons, other site

  M66.29 Spontaneous rupture of extensor tendons, multiple sites

● **M66.3** Spontaneous rupture of flexor tendons

  M66.30 Spontaneous rupture of flexor tendons, unspecified site

● **M66.31** Spontaneous rupture of flexor tendons, shoulder

    M66.311 Spontaneous rupture of flexor tendons, right shoulder

    M66.312 Spontaneous rupture of flexor tendons, left shoulder

    M66.319 Spontaneous rupture of flexor tendons, unspecified shoulder

● **M66.32** Spontaneous rupture of flexor tendons, upper arm

    M66.321 Spontaneous rupture of flexor tendons, right upper arm

    M66.322 Spontaneous rupture of flexor tendons, left upper arm

    M66.329 Spontaneous rupture of flexor tendons, unspecified upper arm

● **M66.33** Spontaneous rupture of flexor tendons, forearm

    M66.331 Spontaneous rupture of flexor tendons, right forearm

    M66.332 Spontaneous rupture of flexor tendons, left forearm

    M66.339 Spontaneous rupture of flexor tendons, unspecified forearm

● **M66.34** Spontaneous rupture of flexor tendons, hand

    M66.341 Spontaneous rupture of flexor tendons, right hand

    M66.342 Spontaneous rupture of flexor tendons, left hand

    M66.349 Spontaneous rupture of flexor tendons, unspecified hand

● **M66.35** Spontaneous rupture of flexor tendons, thigh

    M66.351 Spontaneous rupture of flexor tendons, right thigh

    M66.352 Spontaneous rupture of flexor tendons, left thigh

    M66.359 Spontaneous rupture of flexor tendons, unspecified thigh

● **M66.36** Spontaneous rupture of flexor tendons, lower leg

    M66.361 Spontaneous rupture of flexor tendons, right lower leg

    M66.362 Spontaneous rupture of flexor tendons, left lower leg

    M66.369 Spontaneous rupture of flexor tendons, unspecified lower leg

● **M66.37** Spontaneous rupture of flexor tendons, ankle and foot

    M66.371 Spontaneous rupture of flexor tendons, right ankle and foot

    M66.372 Spontaneous rupture of flexor tendons, left ankle and foot

    M66.379 Spontaneous rupture of flexor tendons, unspecified ankle and foot

  M66.38 Spontaneous rupture of flexor tendons, other site

  M66.39 Spontaneous rupture of flexor tendons, multiple sites

● **M66.8** Spontaneous rupture of other tendons

  M66.80 Spontaneous rupture of other tendons, unspecified site

● **M66.81** Spontaneous rupture of other tendons, shoulder

    M66.811 Spontaneous rupture of other tendons, right shoulder

    M66.812 Spontaneous rupture of other tendons, left shoulder

    M66.819 Spontaneous rupture of other tendons, unspecified shoulder

● **M66.82** Spontaneous rupture of other tendons, upper arm

    M66.821 Spontaneous rupture of other tendons, right upper arm

    M66.822 Spontaneous rupture of other tendons, left upper arm

    M66.829 Spontaneous rupture of other tendons, unspecified upper arm

● **M66.83** Spontaneous rupture of other tendons, forearm

    M66.831 Spontaneous rupture of other tendons, right forearm

    M66.832 Spontaneous rupture of other tendons, left forearm

    M66.839 Spontaneous rupture of other tendons, unspecified forearm

● **M66.84** Spontaneous rupture of other tendons, hand

    M66.841 Spontaneous rupture of other tendons, right hand

    M66.842 Spontaneous rupture of other tendons, left hand

    M66.849 Spontaneous rupture of other tendons, unspecified hand

● **M66.85** Spontaneous rupture of other tendons, thigh

    M66.851 Spontaneous rupture of other tendons, right thigh

    M66.852 Spontaneous rupture of other tendons, left thigh

    M66.859 Spontaneous rupture of other tendons, unspecified thigh

● **M66.86** Spontaneous rupture of other tendons, lower leg

    M66.861 Spontaneous rupture of other tendons, right lower leg

    M66.862 Spontaneous rupture of other tendons, left lower leg

    M66.869 Spontaneous rupture of other tendons, unspecified lower leg

● **M66.87** Spontaneous rupture of other tendons, ankle and foot

    M66.871 Spontaneous rupture of other tendons, right ankle and foot

    M66.872 Spontaneous rupture of other tendons, left ankle and foot

    M66.879 Spontaneous rupture of other tendons, unspecified ankle and foot

M66.88 Spontaneous rupture of other tendons, other sites

M66.89 Spontaneous rupture of other tendons, multiple sites

M66.9 Spontaneous rupture of unspecified tendon
Rupture at musculotendinous junction, nontraumatic

● **M67** **Other disorders of synovium and tendon**

> **Excludes1** palmar fascial fibromatosis [Dupuytren] (M72.0)
> tendinitis NOS (M77.9-)
> xanthomatosis localized to tendons (E78.2)

● **M67.0** **Short Achilles tendon (acquired)**

    M67.00 Short Achilles tendon (acquired), unspecified ankle

    M67.01 Short Achilles tendon (acquired), right ankle

    M67.02 Short Achilles tendon (acquired), left ankle

● **M67.2** **Synovial hypertrophy, not elsewhere classified**

> **Excludes1** villonodular synovitis (pigmented) (M12.2-)

    M67.20 Synovial hypertrophy, not elsewhere classified, unspecified site

●   **M67.21** Synovial hypertrophy, not elsewhere classified, shoulder

      M67.211 Synovial hypertrophy, not elsewhere classified, right shoulder

      M67.212 Synovial hypertrophy, not elsewhere classified, left shoulder

      M67.219 Synovial hypertrophy, not elsewhere classified, unspecified shoulder

●   **M67.22** Synovial hypertrophy, not elsewhere classified, upper arm

      M67.221 Synovial hypertrophy, not elsewhere classified, right upper arm

      M67.222 Synovial hypertrophy, not elsewhere classified, left upper arm

      M67.229 Synovial hypertrophy, not elsewhere classified, unspecified upper arm

●   **M67.23** Synovial hypertrophy, not elsewhere classified, forearm

      M67.231 Synovial hypertrophy, not elsewhere classified, right forearm

      M67.232 Synovial hypertrophy, not elsewhere classified, left forearm

      M67.239 Synovial hypertrophy, not elsewhere classified, unspecified forearm

●   **M67.24** Synovial hypertrophy, not elsewhere classified, hand

      M67.241 Synovial hypertrophy, not elsewhere classified, right hand

      M67.242 Synovial hypertrophy, not elsewhere classified, left hand

      M67.249 Synovial hypertrophy, not elsewhere classified, unspecified hand

●   **M67.25** Synovial hypertrophy, not elsewhere classified, thigh

      M67.251 Synovial hypertrophy, not elsewhere classified, right thigh

      M67.252 Synovial hypertrophy, not elsewhere classified, left thigh

      M67.259 Synovial hypertrophy, not elsewhere classified, unspecified thigh

●   **M67.26** Synovial hypertrophy, not elsewhere classified, lower leg

      M67.261 Synovial hypertrophy, not elsewhere classified, right lower leg

      M67.262 Synovial hypertrophy, not elsewhere classified, left lower leg

      M67.269 Synovial hypertrophy, not elsewhere classified, unspecified lower leg

●   **M67.27** Synovial hypertrophy, not elsewhere classified, ankle and foot

      M67.271 Synovial hypertrophy, not elsewhere classified, right ankle and foot

      M67.272 Synovial hypertrophy, not elsewhere classified, left ankle and foot

      M67.279 Synovial hypertrophy, not elsewhere classified, unspecified ankle and foot

    M67.28 Synovial hypertrophy, not elsewhere classified, other site

    M67.29 Synovial hypertrophy, not elsewhere classified, multiple sites

● **M67.3** **Transient synovitis**
Toxic synovitis

> **Excludes1** palindromic rheumatism (M12.3-)

    M67.30 Transient synovitis, unspecified site

●   **M67.31** Transient synovitis, shoulder

      M67.311 Transient synovitis, right shoulder

      M67.312 Transient synovitis, left shoulder

      M67.319 Transient synovitis, unspecified shoulder

●   **M67.32** Transient synovitis, elbow

      M67.321 Transient synovitis, right elbow

      M67.322 Transient synovitis, left elbow

      M67.329 Transient synovitis, unspecified elbow

●   **M67.33** Transient synovitis, wrist

      M67.331 Transient synovitis, right wrist

      M67.332 Transient synovitis, left wrist

      M67.339 Transient synovitis, unspecified wrist

●   **M67.34** Transient synovitis, hand

      M67.341 Transient synovitis, right hand

      M67.342 Transient synovitis, left hand

      M67.349 Transient synovitis, unspecified hand

●   **M67.35** Transient synovitis, hip

      M67.351 Transient synovitis, right hip

      M67.352 Transient synovitis, left hip

      M67.359 Transient synovitis, unspecified hip

●   **M67.36** Transient synovitis, knee

      M67.361 Transient synovitis, right knee

      M67.362 Transient synovitis, left knee

      M67.369 Transient synovitis, unspecified knee

●   **M67.37** Transient synovitis, ankle and foot

      M67.371 Transient synovitis, right ankle and foot

      M67.372 Transient synovitis, left ankle and foot

      M67.379 Transient synovitis, unspecified ankle and foot

    M67.38 Transient synovitis, other site

    M67.39 Transient synovitis, multiple sites

● **M67.4** **Ganglion**
Ganglion of joint or tendon (sheath)

> **Excludes1** ganglion in yaws (A66.6)
> **Excludes2** cyst of bursa (M71.2-M71.3)
> cyst of synovium (M71.2-M71.3)

    M67.40 Ganglion, unspecified site

●   **M67.41** Ganglion, shoulder

      M67.411 Ganglion, right shoulder

      M67.412 Ganglion, left shoulder

      M67.419 Ganglion, unspecified shoulder

●   **M67.42** Ganglion, elbow

      M67.421 Ganglion, right elbow

      M67.422 Ganglion, left elbow

      M67.429 Ganglion, unspecified elbow

CHAPTER 13 (M00-M99)

● **M67.43 Ganglion, wrist**
   M67.431 Ganglion, right wrist
   M67.432 Ganglion, left wrist
   M67.439 Ganglion, unspecified wrist
● **M67.44 Ganglion, hand**
   M67.441 Ganglion, right hand
   M67.442 Ganglion, left hand
   M67.449 Ganglion, unspecified hand
● **M67.45 Ganglion, hip**
   M67.451 Ganglion, right hip
   M67.452 Ganglion, left hip
   M67.459 Ganglion, unspecified hip
● **M67.46 Ganglion, knee**
   M67.461 Ganglion, right knee
   M67.462 Ganglion, left knee
   M67.469 Ganglion, unspecified knee
● **M67.47 Ganglion, ankle and foot**
   M67.471 Ganglion, right ankle and foot
   M67.472 Ganglion, left ankle and foot
   M67.479 Ganglion, unspecified ankle and foot
  M67.48 Ganglion, other site
  M67.49 Ganglion, multiple sites
● **M67.5 Plica syndrome**
   Plica knee
  M67.50 Plica syndrome, unspecified knee
  M67.51 Plica syndrome, right knee
  M67.52 Plica syndrome, left knee
● **M67.8 Other specified disorders of synovium and tendon**
  M67.80 Other specified disorders of synovium and tendon, unspecified site
● **M67.81 Other specified disorders of synovium and tendon, shoulder**
   M67.811 Other specified disorders of synovium, right shoulder
   M67.812 Other specified disorders of synovium, left shoulder
   M67.813 Other specified disorders of tendon, right shoulder
   M67.814 Other specified disorders of tendon, left shoulder
   M67.819 Other specified disorders of synovium and tendon, unspecified shoulder
● **M67.82 Other specified disorders of synovium and tendon, elbow**
   M67.821 Other specified disorders of synovium, right elbow
   M67.822 Other specified disorders of synovium, left elbow
   M67.823 Other specified disorders of tendon, right elbow
   M67.824 Other specified disorders of tendon, left elbow
   M67.829 Other specified disorders of synovium and tendon, unspecified elbow
● **M67.83 Other specified disorders of synovium and tendon, wrist**
   M67.831 Other specified disorders of synovium, right wrist
   M67.832 Other specified disorders of synovium, left wrist
   M67.833 Other specified disorders of tendon, right wrist
   M67.834 Other specified disorders of tendon, left wrist
   M67.839 Other specified disorders of synovium and tendon, unspecified wrist

● **M67.84 Other specified disorders of synovium and tendon, hand**
   M67.841 Other specified disorders of synovium, right hand
   M67.842 Other specified disorders of synovium, left hand
   M67.843 Other specified disorders of tendon, right hand
   M67.844 Other specified disorders of tendon, left hand
   M67.849 Other specified disorders of synovium and tendon, unspecified hand
● **M67.85 Other specified disorders of synovium and tendon, hip**
   M67.851 Other specified disorders of synovium, right hip
   M67.852 Other specified disorders of synovium, left hip
   M67.853 Other specified disorders of tendon, right hip
   M67.854 Other specified disorders of tendon, left hip
   M67.859 Other specified disorders of synovium and tendon, unspecified hip
● **M67.86 Other specified disorders of synovium and tendon, knee**
   M67.861 Other specified disorders of synovium, right knee
   M67.862 Other specified disorders of synovium, left knee
   M67.863 Other specified disorders of tendon, right knee
   M67.864 Other specified disorders of tendon, left knee
   M67.869 Other specified disorders of synovium and tendon, unspecified knee
● **M67.87 Other specified disorders of synovium and tendon, ankle and foot**
   M67.871 Other specified disorders of synovium, right ankle and foot
   M67.872 Other specified disorders of synovium, left ankle and foot
   M67.873 Other specified disorders of tendon, right ankle and foot
   M67.874 Other specified disorders of tendon, left ankle and foot
   M67.879 Other specified disorders of synovium and tendon, unspecified ankle and foot
  M67.88 Other specified disorders of synovium and tendon, other site
  M67.89 Other specified disorders of synovium and tendon, multiple sites
● **M67.9 Unspecified disorder of synovium and tendon**
  M67.90 Unspecified disorder of synovium and tendon, unspecified site
● **M67.91 Unspecified disorder of synovium and tendon, shoulder**
   M67.911 Unspecified disorder of synovium and tendon, right shoulder
   M67.912 Unspecified disorder of synovium and tendon, left shoulder
   M67.919 Unspecified disorder of synovium and tendon, unspecified shoulder

▶ New ➡ Revised ~~deleted~~ Deleted Excludes 1 Excludes 2 Includes Use additional Code first Code also Key words
OGCR Official Guidelines X Assign placeholder X ● Use Additional Character(s) ▶ Manifestation Code Hierarchical Condition Category Coding Clinic

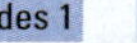
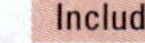
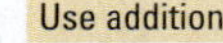
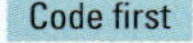

● **M67.92** Unspecified disorder of synovium and tendon, upper arm
    M67.921 Unspecified disorder of synovium and tendon, right upper arm
    M67.922 Unspecified disorder of synovium and tendon, left upper arm
    M67.929 Unspecified disorder of synovium and tendon, unspecified upper arm
● **M67.93** Unspecified disorder of synovium and tendon, forearm
    M67.931 Unspecified disorder of synovium and tendon, right forearm
    M67.932 Unspecified disorder of synovium and tendon, left forearm
    M67.939 Unspecified disorder of synovium and tendon, unspecified forearm
● **M67.94** Unspecified disorder of synovium and tendon, hand
    M67.941 Unspecified disorder of synovium and tendon, right hand
    M67.942 Unspecified disorder of synovium and tendon, left hand
    M67.949 Unspecified disorder of synovium and tendon, unspecified hand
● **M67.95** Unspecified disorder of synovium and tendon, thigh
    M67.951 Unspecified disorder of synovium and tendon, right thigh
    M67.952 Unspecified disorder of synovium and tendon, left thigh
    M67.959 Unspecified disorder of synovium and tendon, unspecified thigh
● **M67.96** Unspecified disorder of synovium and tendon, lower leg
    M67.961 Unspecified disorder of synovium and tendon, right lower leg
    M67.962 Unspecified disorder of synovium and tendon, left lower leg
    M67.969 Unspecified disorder of synovium and tendon, unspecified lower leg
● **M67.97** Unspecified disorder of synovium and tendon, ankle and foot
    M67.971 Unspecified disorder of synovium and tendon, right ankle and foot
    M67.972 Unspecified disorder of synovium and tendon, left ankle and foot
    M67.979 Unspecified disorder of synovium and tendon, unspecified ankle and foot
    M67.98 Unspecified disorder of synovium and tendon, other site
    M67.99 Unspecified disorder of synovium and tendon, multiple sites

OTHER SOFT TISSUE DISORDERS (M70-M79)

● **M70** Soft tissue disorders related to use, overuse and pressure

Includes   soft tissue disorders of occupational origin

Use additional external cause code to identify activity causing disorder (Y93.-)

Excludes1   bursitis NOS (M71.9-)
Excludes2   bursitis of shoulder (M75.5)
             enthesopathies (M76-M77)
             pressure ulcer (pressure area) (L89.-)

● **M70.0** Crepitant synovitis (acute) (chronic) of hand and wrist
    ● **M70.03** Crepitant synovitis (acute) (chronic), wrist
       M70.031 Crepitant synovitis (acute) (chronic), right wrist
       M70.032 Crepitant synovitis (acute) (chronic), left wrist
       M70.039 Crepitant synovitis (acute) (chronic), unspecified wrist

● **M70.04** Crepitant synovitis (acute) (chronic), hand
    M70.041 Crepitant synovitis (acute) (chronic), right hand
    M70.042 Crepitant synovitis (acute) (chronic), left hand
    M70.049 Crepitant synovitis (acute) (chronic), unspecified hand
● **M70.1** Bursitis of hand
    M70.10 Bursitis, unspecified hand
    M70.11 Bursitis, right hand
    M70.12 Bursitis, left hand
● **M70.2** Olecranon bursitis
    M70.20 Olecranon bursitis, unspecified elbow
    M70.21 Olecranon bursitis, right elbow
    M70.22 Olecranon bursitis, left elbow
● **M70.3** Other bursitis of elbow
    M70.30 Other bursitis of elbow, unspecified elbow
    M70.31 Other bursitis of elbow, right elbow
    M70.32 Other bursitis of elbow, left elbow
● **M70.4** Prepatellar bursitis
    M70.40 Prepatellar bursitis, unspecified knee
    M70.41 Prepatellar bursitis, right knee
    M70.42 Prepatellar bursitis, left knee
● **M70.5** Other bursitis of knee
    M70.50 Other bursitis of knee, unspecified knee
    M70.51 Other bursitis of knee, right knee
    M70.52 Other bursitis of knee, left knee
● **M70.6** Trochanteric bursitis
    Trochanteric tendinitis
    M70.60 Trochanteric bursitis, unspecified hip
    M70.61 Trochanteric bursitis, right hip
    M70.62 Trochanteric bursitis, left hip
● **M70.7** Other bursitis of hip
    Ischial bursitis
    M70.70 Other bursitis of hip, unspecified hip
    M70.71 Other bursitis of hip, right hip
    M70.72 Other bursitis of hip, left hip
● **M70.8** Other soft tissue disorders related to use, overuse and pressure
    M70.80 Other soft tissue disorders related to use, overuse and pressure of unspecified site
    ● **M70.81** Other soft tissue disorders related to use, overuse and pressure of shoulder
       M70.811 Other soft tissue disorders related to use, overuse and pressure, right shoulder
       M70.812 Other soft tissue disorders related to use, overuse and pressure, left shoulder
       M70.819 Other soft tissue disorders related to use, overuse and pressure, unspecified shoulder
    ● **M70.82** Other soft tissue disorders related to use, overuse and pressure of upper arm
       M70.821 Other soft tissue disorders related to use, overuse and pressure, right upper arm
       M70.822 Other soft tissue disorders related to use, overuse and pressure, left upper arm
       M70.829 Other soft tissue disorders related to use, overuse and pressure, unspecified upper arms
    ● **M70.83** Other soft tissue disorders related to use, overuse and pressure of forearm
       M70.831 Other soft tissue disorders related to use, overuse and pressure, right forearm

M70.832   Other soft tissue disorders related to use, overuse and pressure, left forearm

M70.839   Other soft tissue disorders related to use, overuse and pressure, unspecified forearm

● M70.84   Other soft tissue disorders related to use, overuse and pressure of hand

M70.841   Other soft tissue disorders related to use, overuse and pressure, right hand

M70.842   Other soft tissue disorders related to use, overuse and pressure, left hand

M70.849   Other soft tissue disorders related to use, overuse and pressure, unspecified hand

● M70.85   Other soft tissue disorders related to use, overuse and pressure of thigh

M70.851   Other soft tissue disorders related to use, overuse and pressure, right thigh

M70.852   Other soft tissue disorders related to use, overuse and pressure, left thigh

M70.859   Other soft tissue disorders related to use, overuse and pressure, unspecified thigh

● M70.86   Other soft tissue disorders related to use, overuse and pressure lower leg

M70.861   Other soft tissue disorders related to use, overuse and pressure, right lower leg

M70.862   Other soft tissue disorders related to use, overuse and pressure, left lower leg

M70.869   Other soft tissue disorders related to use, overuse and pressure, unspecified leg

● M70.87   Other soft tissue disorders related to use, overuse and pressure of ankle and foot

M70.871   Other soft tissue disorders related to use, overuse and pressure, right ankle and foot

M70.872   Other soft tissue disorders related to use, overuse and pressure, left ankle and foot

M70.879   Other soft tissue disorders related to use, overuse and pressure, unspecified ankle and foot

M70.88   Other soft tissue disorders related to use, overuse and pressure other site

M70.89   Other soft tissue disorders related to use, overuse and pressure multiple sites

● M70.9   Unspecified soft tissue disorder related to use, overuse and pressure

M70.90   Unspecified soft tissue disorder related to use, overuse and pressure of unspecified site

● M70.91   Unspecified soft tissue disorder related to use, overuse and pressure of shoulder

M70.911   Unspecified soft tissue disorder related to use, overuse and pressure, right shoulder

M70.912   Unspecified soft tissue disorder related to use, overuse and pressure, left shoulder

M70.919   Unspecified soft tissue disorder related to use, overuse and pressure, unspecified shoulder

● M70.92   Unspecified soft tissue disorder related to use, overuse and pressure of upper arm

M70.921   Unspecified soft tissue disorder related to use, overuse and pressure, right upper arm

M70.922   Unspecified soft tissue disorder related to use, overuse and pressure, left upper arm

M70.929   Unspecified soft tissue disorder related to use, overuse and pressure, unspecified upper arm

● M70.93   Unspecified soft tissue disorder related to use, overuse and pressure of forearm

M70.931   Unspecified soft tissue disorder related to use, overuse and pressure, right forearm

M70.932   Unspecified soft tissue disorder related to use, overuse and pressure, left forearm

M70.939   Unspecified soft tissue disorder related to use, overuse and pressure, unspecified forearm

● M70.94   Unspecified soft tissue disorder related to use, overuse and pressure of hand

M70.941   Unspecified soft tissue disorder related to use, overuse and pressure, right hand

M70.942   Unspecified soft tissue disorder related to use, overuse and pressure, left hand

M70.949   Unspecified soft tissue disorder related to use, overuse and pressure, unspecified hand

● M70.95   Unspecified soft tissue disorder related to use, overuse and pressure of thigh

M70.951   Unspecified soft tissue disorder related to use, overuse and pressure, right thigh

M70.952   Unspecified soft tissue disorder related to use, overuse and pressure, left thigh

M70.959   Unspecified soft tissue disorder related to use, overuse and pressure, unspecified thigh

● M70.96   Unspecified soft tissue disorder related to use, overuse and pressure lower leg

M70.961   Unspecified soft tissue disorder related to use, overuse and pressure, right lower leg

M70.962   Unspecified soft tissue disorder related to use, overuse and pressure, left lower leg

M70.969   Unspecified soft tissue disorder related to use, overuse and pressure, unspecified lower leg

● M70.97   Unspecified soft tissue disorder related to use, overuse and pressure of ankle and foot

M70.971   Unspecified soft tissue disorder related to use, overuse and pressure, right ankle and foot

M70.972   Unspecified soft tissue disorder related to use, overuse and pressure, left ankle and foot

M70.979   Unspecified soft tissue disorder related to use, overuse and pressure, unspecified ankle and foot

M70.98   Unspecified soft tissue disorder related to use, overuse and pressure other

M70.99   Unspecified soft tissue disorder related to use, overuse and pressure multiple sites

● **M71**   **Other bursopathies**

> **Excludes1**   bunion (M20.1)
> bursitis related to use, overuse or pressure (M70.-)
> enthesopathies (M76-M77)

● **M71.0   Abscess of bursa**
> **Use additional** code (B95.-, B96.-) to identify causative organism

     M71.00   Abscess of bursa, unspecified site

● **M71.01**   Abscess of bursa, shoulder
     M71.011   Abscess of bursa, right shoulder
     M71.012   Abscess of bursa, left shoulder
     M71.019   Abscess of bursa, unspecified shoulder

● **M71.02**   Abscess of bursa, elbow
     M71.021   Abscess of bursa, right elbow
     M71.022   Abscess of bursa, left elbow
     M71.029   Abscess of bursa, unspecified elbow

● **M71.03**   Abscess of bursa, wrist
     M71.031   Abscess of bursa, right wrist
     M71.032   Abscess of bursa, left wrist
     M71.039   Abscess of bursa, unspecified wrist

● **M71.04**   Abscess of bursa, hand
     M71.041   Abscess of bursa, right hand
     M71.042   Abscess of bursa, left hand
     M71.049   Abscess of bursa, unspecified hand

● **M71.05**   Abscess of bursa, hip
     M71.051   Abscess of bursa, right hip
     M71.052   Abscess of bursa, left hip
     M71.059   Abscess of bursa, unspecified hip

● **M71.06**   Abscess of bursa, knee
     M71.061   Abscess of bursa, right knee
     M71.062   Abscess of bursa, left knee
     M71.069   Abscess of bursa, unspecified knee

● **M71.07**   Abscess of bursa, ankle and foot
     M71.071   Abscess of bursa, right ankle and foot
     M71.072   Abscess of bursa, left ankle and foot
     M71.079   Abscess of bursa, unspecified ankle and foot

     M71.08   Abscess of bursa, other site
     M71.09   Abscess of bursa, multiple sites

● **M71.1   Other infective bursitis**
> **Use additional** code (B95.-, B96.-) to identify causative organism

     M71.10   Other infective bursitis, unspecified site

● **M71.11**   Other infective bursitis, shoulder
     M71.111   Other infective bursitis, right shoulder
     M71.112   Other infective bursitis, left shoulder
     M71.119   Other infective bursitis, unspecified shoulder

● **M71.12**   Other infective bursitis, elbow
     M71.121   Other infective bursitis, right elbow
     M71.122   Other infective bursitis, left elbow
     M71.129   Other infective bursitis, unspecified elbow

● **M71.13**   Other infective bursitis, wrist
     M71.131   Other infective bursitis, right wrist
     M71.132   Other infective bursitis, left wrist
     M71.139   Other infective bursitis, unspecified wrist

● **M71.14**   Other infective bursitis, hand
     M71.141   Other infective bursitis, right hand
     M71.142   Other infective bursitis, left hand
     M71.149   Other infective bursitis, unspecified hand

● **M71.15**   Other infective bursitis, hip
     M71.151   Other infective bursitis, right hip
     M71.152   Other infective bursitis, left hip
     M71.159   Other infective bursitis, unspecified hip

● **M71.16**   Other infective bursitis, knee
     M71.161   Other infective bursitis, right knee
     M71.162   Other infective bursitis, left knee
     M71.169   Other infective bursitis, unspecified knee

● **M71.17**   Other infective bursitis, ankle and foot
     M71.171   Other infective bursitis, right ankle and foot
     M71.172   Other infective bursitis, left ankle and foot
     M71.179   Other infective bursitis, unspecified ankle and foot

     M71.18   Other infective bursitis, other site
     M71.19   Other infective bursitis, multiple sites

● **M71.2   Synovial cyst of popliteal space [Baker]**
> *Popliteal space = popliteal cavity, popliteal fossa. Depression in the posterior aspect of the knee (behind the knee).*

     Excludes1   synovial cyst of popliteal space with rupture (M66.0)

     M71.20   Synovial cyst of popliteal space [Baker], unspecified knee
     M71.21   Synovial cyst of popliteal space [Baker], right knee
     M71.22   Synovial cyst of popliteal space [Baker], left knee

● **M71.3   Other bursal cyst**
> Synovial cyst NOS

     Excludes1   synovial cyst with rupture (M66.1-)

     M71.30   Other bursal cyst, unspecified site

● **M71.31**   Other bursal cyst, shoulder
     M71.311   Other bursal cyst, right shoulder
     M71.312   Other bursal cyst, left shoulder
     M71.319   Other bursal cyst, unspecified shoulder

● **M71.32**   Other bursal cyst, elbow
     M71.321   Other bursal cyst, right elbow
     M71.322   Other bursal cyst, left elbow
     M71.329   Other bursal cyst, unspecified elbow

● **M71.33**   Other bursal cyst, wrist
     M71.331   Other bursal cyst, right wrist
     M71.332   Other bursal cyst, left wrist
     M71.339   Other bursal cyst, unspecified wrist

● **M71.34**   Other bursal cyst, hand
     M71.341   Other bursal cyst, right hand
     M71.342   Other bursal cyst, left hand
     M71.349   Other bursal cyst, unspecified hand

● **M71.35**   Other bursal cyst, hip
     M71.351   Other bursal cyst, right hip
     M71.352   Other bursal cyst, left hip
     M71.359   Other bursal cyst, unspecified hip

● **M71.37**   Other bursal cyst, ankle and foot
     M71.371   Other bursal cyst, right ankle and foot
     M71.372   Other bursal cyst, left ankle and foot
     M71.379   Other bursal cyst, unspecified ankle and foot

     M71.38   Other bursal cyst, other site
     M71.39   Other bursal cyst, multiple sites

● **M71.4   Calcium deposit in bursa**
     Excludes2   calcium deposit in bursa of shoulder (M75.3)

     M71.40   Calcium deposit in bursa, unspecified site

● **M71.42**   Calcium deposit in bursa, elbow
     M71.421   Calcium deposit in bursa, right elbow
     M71.422   Calcium deposit in bursa, left elbow
     M71.429   Calcium deposit in bursa, unspecified elbow

CHAPTER 13 (M00-M99)

● M71.43   Calcium deposit in bursa, wrist
     M71.431   Calcium deposit in bursa, right wrist
     M71.432   Calcium deposit in bursa, left wrist
     M71.439   Calcium deposit in bursa, unspecified wrist
● M71.44   Calcium deposit in bursa, hand
     M71.441   Calcium deposit in bursa, right hand
     M71.442   Calcium deposit in bursa, left hand
     M71.449   Calcium deposit in bursa, unspecified hand
● M71.45   Calcium deposit in bursa, hip
     M71.451   Calcium deposit in bursa, right hip
     M71.452   Calcium deposit in bursa, left hip
     M71.459   Calcium deposit in bursa, unspecified hip
● M71.46   Calcium deposit in bursa, knee
     M71.461   Calcium deposit in bursa, right knee
     M71.462   Calcium deposit in bursa, left knee
     M71.469   Calcium deposit in bursa, unspecified knee
● M71.47   Calcium deposit in bursa, ankle and foot
     M71.471   Calcium deposit in bursa, right ankle and foot
     M71.472   Calcium deposit in bursa, left ankle and foot
     M71.479   Calcium deposit in bursa, unspecified ankle and foot
     M71.48   Calcium deposit in bursa, other site
     M71.49   Calcium deposit in bursa, multiple sites
● M71.5   Other bursitis, not elsewhere classified
     Excludes1   bursitis NOS (M71.9-)
     Excludes2   bursitis of shoulder (M75.5)
                     bursitis of tibial collateral [Pellegrini-Stieda] (M76.4-)
     M71.50   Other bursitis, not elsewhere classified, unspecified site
● M71.52   Other bursitis, not elsewhere classified, elbow
     M71.521   Other bursitis, not elsewhere classified, right elbow
     M71.522   Other bursitis, not elsewhere classified, left elbow
     M71.529   Other bursitis, not elsewhere classified, unspecified elbow
● M71.53   Other bursitis, not elsewhere classified, wrist
     M71.531   Other bursitis, not elsewhere classified, right wrist
     M71.532   Other bursitis, not elsewhere classified, left wrist
     M71.539   Other bursitis, not elsewhere classified, unspecified wrist
● M71.54   Other bursitis, not elsewhere classified, hand
     M71.541   Other bursitis, not elsewhere classified, right hand
     M71.542   Other bursitis, not elsewhere classified, left hand
     M71.549   Other bursitis, not elsewhere classified, unspecified hand
● M71.55   Other bursitis, not elsewhere classified, hip
     M71.551   Other bursitis, not elsewhere classified, right hip
     M71.552   Other bursitis, not elsewhere classified, left hip
     M71.559   Other bursitis, not elsewhere classified, unspecified hip
● M71.56   Other bursitis, not elsewhere classified, knee
     M71.561   Other bursitis, not elsewhere classified, right knee

     M71.562   Other bursitis, not elsewhere classified, left knee
     M71.569   Other bursitis, not elsewhere classified, unspecified knee
● M71.57   Other bursitis, not elsewhere classified, ankle and foot
     M71.571   Other bursitis, not elsewhere classified, right ankle and foot
     M71.572   Other bursitis, not elsewhere classified, left ankle and foot
     M71.579   Other bursitis, not elsewhere classified, unspecified ankle and foot
     M71.58   Other bursitis, not elsewhere classified, other site
● M71.8   Other specified bursopathies
     M71.80   Other specified bursopathies, unspecified site
● M71.81   Other specified bursopathies, shoulder
     M71.811   Other specified bursopathies, right shoulder
     M71.812   Other specified bursopathies, left shoulder
     M71.819   Other specified bursopathies, unspecified shoulder
● M71.82   Other specified bursopathies, elbow
     M71.821   Other specified bursopathies, right elbow
     M71.822   Other specified bursopathies, left elbow
     M71.829   Other specified bursopathies, unspecified elbow
● M71.83   Other specified bursopathies, wrist
     M71.831   Other specified bursopathies, right wrist
     M71.832   Other specified bursopathies, left wrist
     M71.839   Other specified bursopathies, unspecified wrist
● M71.84   Other specified bursopathies, hand
     M71.841   Other specified bursopathies, right hand
     M71.842   Other specified bursopathies, left hand
     M71.849   Other specified bursopathies, unspecified hand
● M71.85   Other specified bursopathies, hip
     M71.851   Other specified bursopathies, right hip
     M71.852   Other specified bursopathies, left hip
     M71.859   Other specified bursopathies, unspecified hip
● M71.86   Other specified bursopathies, knee
     M71.861   Other specified bursopathies, right knee
     M71.862   Other specified bursopathies, left knee
     M71.869   Other specified bursopathies, unspecified knee
● M71.87   Other specified bursopathies, ankle and foot
     M71.871   Other specified bursopathies, right ankle and foot
     M71.872   Other specified bursopathies, left ankle and foot
     M71.879   Other specified bursopathies, unspecified ankle and foot
     M71.88   Other specified bursopathies, other site
     M71.89   Other specified bursopathies, multiple sites
   M71.9   Bursopathy, unspecified
           Bursitis NOS

▶ New   ⮕ Revised   ~~deleted~~ Deleted   Excludes 1   Excludes 2   Includes   Use additional   Code first   Code also   Key words
OGCR Official Guidelines   X Assign placeholder X   ● Use Additional Character(s)   ▶ Manifestation Code   Hierarchical Condition Category   Coding Clinic

● **M72 Fibroblastic disorders**
    Excludes2 retroperitoneal fibromatosis (D48.3)
  M72.0 Palmar fascial fibromatosis [Dupuytren] **A**
  M72.1 Knuckle pads
  M72.2 Plantar fascial fibromatosis
    Plantar fasciitis
  M72.4 Pseudosarcomatous fibromatosis
    Nodular fasciitis
  M72.6 Necrotizing fasciitis
    Use additional code (B95.-, B96.-) to identify causative
    organism
  M72.8 Other fibroblastic disorders
    Abscess of fascia
    Fasciitis NEC
    Other infective fasciitis
    Use additional code to (B95.-, B96.-) identify causative
    organism
    Excludes1 diffuse (eosinophilic) fasciitis (M35.4)
        necrotizing fasciitis (M72.6)
        nodular fasciitis (M72.4)
        perirenal fasciitis NOS (N13.5)
        perirenal fasciitis with infection (N13.6)
        plantar fasciitis (M72.2)
    Coding Clinic: 2025, Q1, P31
  M72.9 Fibroblastic disorder, unspecified
    Fasciitis NOS
    Fibromatosis NOS

● **M75 Shoulder lesions**
    Excludes2 shoulder-hand syndrome (M89.0-)
  ● **M75.0 Adhesive capsulitis of shoulder**
    Frozen shoulder
    Periarthritis of shoulder
    M75.00 Adhesive capsulitis of unspecified shoulder
    M75.01 Adhesive capsulitis of right shoulder
    M75.02 Adhesive capsulitis of left shoulder
        Coding Clinic: 2015, Q2, P23
  ● **M75.1 Rotator cuff tear or rupture, not specified as traumatic**
    Rotator cuff syndrome
    Supraspinatus syndrome
    Supraspinatus tear or rupture, not specified as
      traumatic
    Excludes1 tear of rotator cuff, traumatic (S46.01-)
    Gradual onset due to repetitive stress to rotator cuff
   ● **M75.10 Unspecified rotator cuff tear or rupture, not
      specified as traumatic**
     **M75.100 Unspecified rotator cuff tear or
        rupture of unspecified shoulder, not
        specified as traumatic**
     **M75.101 Unspecified rotator cuff tear or
        rupture of right shoulder, not
        specified as traumatic**
     **M75.102 Unspecified rotator cuff tear or
        rupture of left shoulder, not specified
        as traumatic**
   ● **M75.11 Incomplete rotator cuff tear or rupture not
      specified as traumatic**
     **M75.110 Incomplete rotator cuff tear or rupture
        of unspecified shoulder, not specified
        as traumatic**
     **M75.111 Incomplete rotator cuff tear or rupture
        of right shoulder, not specified as
        traumatic**
     **M75.112 Incomplete rotator cuff tear or rupture
        of left shoulder, not specified as
        traumatic**
   ● **M75.12 Complete rotator cuff tear or rupture not
      specified as traumatic**
     **M75.120 Complete rotator cuff tear or rupture
        of unspecified shoulder, not specified
        as traumatic**

     **M75.121 Complete rotator cuff tear or rupture
        of right shoulder, not specified as
        traumatic**
     **M75.122 Complete rotator cuff tear or rupture
        of left shoulder, not specified as
        traumatic**
  ● **M75.2 Bicipital tendinitis**
    M75.20 Bicipital tendinitis, unspecified shoulder
    M75.21 Bicipital tendinitis, right shoulder
    M75.22 Bicipital tendinitis, left shoulder
  ● **M75.3 Calcific tendinitis of shoulder**
    Calcified bursa of shoulder
    M75.30 Calcific tendinitis of unspecified shoulder
    M75.31 Calcific tendinitis of right shoulder
    M75.32 Calcific tendinitis of left shoulder
  ● **M75.4 Impingement syndrome of shoulder**
    **M75.40 Impingement syndrome of unspecified
      shoulder**
        Coding Clinic: 2022, Q3, P18-19
    M75.41 Impingement syndrome of right shoulder
    M75.42 Impingement syndrome of left shoulder
  ● **M75.5 Bursitis of shoulder**
    M75.50 Bursitis of unspecified shoulder
    M75.51 Bursitis of right shoulder
    M75.52 Bursitis of left shoulder
  ● **M75.8 Other shoulder lesions**
    M75.80 Other shoulder lesions, unspecified shoulder
    M75.81 Other shoulder lesions, right shoulder
    M75.82 Other shoulder lesions, left shoulder
  ● **M75.9 Shoulder lesion, unspecified**
    **M75.90 Shoulder lesion, unspecified, unspecified
      shoulder**
    M75.91 Shoulder lesion, unspecified, right shoulder
    M75.92 Shoulder lesion, unspecified, left shoulder

● **M76 Enthesopathies, lower limb, excluding foot**
    Excludes2 bursitis due to use, overuse and pressure (M70.-)
        enthesopathies of ankle and foot (M77.5-)
  ● **M76.0 Gluteal tendinitis**
    M76.00 Gluteal tendinitis, unspecified hip
    M76.01 Gluteal tendinitis, right hip
    M76.02 Gluteal tendinitis, left hip
  ● **M76.1 Psoas tendinitis**
    M76.10 Psoas tendinitis, unspecified hip
    M76.11 Psoas tendinitis, right hip
    M76.12 Psoas tendinitis, left hip
  ● **M76.2 Iliac crest spur**
    M76.20 Iliac crest spur, unspecified hip
    M76.21 Iliac crest spur, right hip
    M76.22 Iliac crest spur, left hip
  ● **M76.3 Iliotibial band syndrome**
    M76.30 Iliotibial band syndrome, unspecified leg
    M76.31 Iliotibial band syndrome, right leg
    M76.32 Iliotibial band syndrome, left leg
  ● **M76.4 Tibial collateral bursitis [Pellegrini-Stieda]**
    **M76.40 Tibial collateral bursitis [Pellegrini-Stieda],
      unspecified leg**
    **M76.41 Tibial collateral bursitis [Pellegrini-Stieda],
      right leg**
    **M76.42 Tibial collateral bursitis [Pellegrini-Stieda], left
      leg**
  ● **M76.5 Patellar tendinitis**
    M76.50 Patellar tendinitis, unspecified knee
    M76.51 Patellar tendinitis, right knee
    M76.52 Patellar tendinitis, left knee

CHAPTER 13 (M00-M99)

- **M76.6 Achilles tendinitis**
  - Achilles bursitis
  - M76.60 Achilles tendinitis, unspecified leg
  - M76.61 Achilles tendinitis, right leg
  - M76.62 Achilles tendinitis, left leg
- **M76.7 Peroneal tendinitis**
  - M76.70 Peroneal tendinitis, unspecified leg
  - M76.71 Peroneal tendinitis, right leg
  - M76.72 Peroneal tendinitis, left leg
- **M76.8 Other specified enthesopathies of lower limb, excluding foot**
  - **M76.81 Anterior tibial syndrome**
    - M76.811 Anterior tibial syndrome, right leg
    - M76.812 Anterior tibial syndrome, left leg
    - M76.819 Anterior tibial syndrome, unspecified leg
  - **M76.82 Posterior tibial tendinitis**
    - M76.821 Posterior tibial tendinitis, right leg
    - M76.822 Posterior tibial tendinitis, left leg
    - M76.829 Posterior tibial tendinitis, unspecified leg
  - **M76.89 Other specified enthesopathies of lower limb, excluding foot**
    - M76.891 Other specified enthesopathies of right lower limb, excluding foot
    - M76.892 Other specified enthesopathies of left lower limb, excluding foot
    - M76.899 Other specified enthesopathies of unspecified lower limb, excluding foot
- M76.9 Unspecified enthesopathy, lower limb, excluding foot
- **M77 Other enthesopathies**
  - **Excludes1** bursitis NOS (M71.9-)
  - **Excludes2** bursitis due to use, overuse and pressure (M70.-)
    - osteophyte (M25.7)
    - spinal enthesopathy (M46.0-)
  - **M77.0 Medial epicondylitis**
    - M77.00 Medial epicondylitis, unspecified elbow
    - M77.01 Medial epicondylitis, right elbow
    - M77.02 Medial epicondylitis, left elbow
  - **M77.1 Lateral epicondylitis**
    - Tennis elbow
    - M77.10 Lateral epicondylitis, unspecified elbow
    - M77.11 Lateral epicondylitis, right elbow
    - M77.12 Lateral epicondylitis, left elbow
  - **M77.2 Periarthritis of wrist**
    - M77.20 Periarthritis, unspecified wrist
    - M77.21 Periarthritis, right wrist
    - M77.22 Periarthritis, left wrist
  - **M77.3 Calcaneal spur**
    - M77.30 Calcaneal spur, unspecified foot
    - M77.31 Calcaneal spur, right foot
    - M77.32 Calcaneal spur, left foot
  - **M77.4 Metatarsalgia**
    - **Excludes1** Morton's metatarsalgia (G57.6)
    - M77.40 Metatarsalgia, unspecified foot
    - M77.41 Metatarsalgia, right foot
    - M77.42 Metatarsalgia, left foot
  - **M77.5 Other enthesopathy of foot and ankle**
    - M77.50 Other enthesopathy of unspecified foot and ankle
    - M77.51 Other enthesopathy of right foot and ankle
    - M77.52 Other enthesopathy of left foot and ankle

- M77.8 Other enthesopathies, not elsewhere classified
- M77.9 Enthesopathy, unspecified
  - Bone spur NOS
  - Capsulitis NOS
  - Periarthritis NOS
  - Tendinitis NOS
- **M79 Other and unspecified soft tissue disorders, not elsewhere classified**
  - **Excludes1** psychogenic rheumatism (F45.8)
    - soft tissue pain, psychogenic (F45.41)
  - M79.0 Rheumatism, unspecified
    - **Excludes1** fibromyalgia (M79.7)
      - palindromic rheumatism (M12.3-)
  - **M79.1 Myalgia**
    - Myofascial pain syndrome
    - M79.10 Myalgia, unspecified site
    - M79.11 Myalgia of mastication muscle
    - M79.12 Myalgia of auxiliary muscles, head and neck
    - M79.18 Myalgia, other site
      - **Excludes1** fibromyalgia (M79.7)
        - myositis (M60.-)
  - M79.2 Neuralgia and neuritis, unspecified
    - **Excludes1** brachial radiculitis NOS (M54.1)
      - lumbosacral radiculitis NOS (M54.1)
      - mononeuropathies (G56-G58)
      - radiculitis NOS (M54.1)
      - sciatica (M54.3-M54.4)
  - M79.3 Panniculitis, unspecified
    - **Excludes1** lupus panniculitis (L93.2)
      - neck and back panniculitis (M54.0-)
      - relapsing [Weber-Christian] panniculitis (M35.6)
    - **Coding Clinic: 2024, Q1, P16**
  - M79.4 Hypertrophy of (infrapatellar) fat pad
  - M79.5 Residual foreign body in soft tissue
    - **Excludes1** foreign body granuloma of skin and subcutaneous tissue (L92.3)
      - foreign body granuloma of soft tissue (M60.2-)
  - **M79.6 Pain in limb, hand, foot, fingers and toes**
    - **Excludes2** pain in joint (M25.5-)
    - **M79.60 Pain in limb, unspecified**
      - M79.601 Pain in right arm
        - Pain in right upper limb NOS
      - M79.602 Pain in left arm
        - Pain in left upper limb NOS
      - M79.603 Pain in arm, unspecified
        - Pain in upper limb NOS
      - M79.604 Pain in right leg
        - Pain in right lower limb NOS
      - M79.605 Pain in left leg
        - Pain in left lower limb NOS
      - M79.606 Pain in leg, unspecified
        - Pain in lower limb NOS
      - M79.609 Pain in unspecified limb
        - Pain in limb NOS
    - **M79.62 Pain in upper arm**
      - Pain in axillary region
      - M79.621 Pain in right upper arm
      - M79.622 Pain in left upper arm
      - M79.629 Pain in unspecified upper arm
    - **M79.63 Pain in forearm**
      - M79.631 Pain in right forearm
      - M79.632 Pain in left forearm
      - M79.639 Pain in unspecified forearm

● **M79.64 Pain in hand and fingers**
    M79.641 Pain in right hand
    M79.642 Pain in left hand
    M79.643 Pain in unspecified hand
    M79.644 Pain in right finger(s)
    M79.645 Pain in left finger(s)
    M79.646 Pain in unspecified finger(s)
● **M79.65 Pain in thigh**
    M79.651 Pain in right thigh
    M79.652 Pain in left thigh
    M79.659 Pain in unspecified thigh
● **M79.66 Pain in lower leg**
    M79.661 Pain in right lower leg
    M79.662 Pain in left lower leg
    M79.669 Pain in unspecified lower leg
● **M79.67 Pain in foot and toes**
    M79.671 Pain in right foot
    M79.672 Pain in left foot
    M79.673 Pain in unspecified foot
    M79.674 Pain in right toe(s)
    M79.675 Pain in left toe(s)
    M79.676 Pain in unspecified toe(s)

M79.7 Fibromyalgia
    Fibromyositis
    Fibrositis
    Myofibrositis
● **M79.A Nontraumatic compartment syndrome**
    Code first, if applicable, associated postprocedural complication
    Excludes1 compartment syndrome NOS (T79.A-)
        fibromyalgia (M79.7) nontraumatic
        ischemic infarction of muscle (M62.2-)
        traumatic compartment syndrome (T79.A-)
● **M79.A1 Nontraumatic compartment syndrome of upper extremity**
    Nontraumatic compartment syndrome of
        shoulder, arm, forearm, wrist, hand, and
        fingers
    M79.A11 Nontraumatic compartment syndrome of right upper extremity
    M79.A12 Nontraumatic compartment syndrome of left upper extremity
    M79.A19 Nontraumatic compartment syndrome of unspecified upper extremity
● **M79.A2 Nontraumatic compartment syndrome of lower extremity**
    Nontraumatic compartment syndrome of hip,
        buttock, thigh, leg, foot, and toes
    M79.A21 Nontraumatic compartment syndrome of right lower extremity
    M79.A22 Nontraumatic compartment syndrome of left lower extremity
    M79.A29 Nontraumatic compartment syndrome of unspecified lower extremity
    M79.A3 Nontraumatic compartment syndrome of abdomen
    M79.A9 Nontraumatic compartment syndrome of other sites
● **M79.8 Other specified soft tissue disorders**
    M79.81 Nontraumatic hematoma of soft tissue
        Nontraumatic hematoma of muscle
        Nontraumatic seroma of muscle and soft tissue
    M79.89 Other specified soft tissue disorders
        Polyalgia
M79.9 Soft tissue disorder, unspecified

Osteoporosis

Osteoporosis is a systemic condition, meaning that all bones of the musculoskeletal system are affected. Therefore, site is not a component of the codes under category M81, Osteoporosis without current pathological fracture. The site codes under category M80, Osteoporosis with current pathological fracture, identify the site of the fracture, not the osteoporosis.

1) Osteoporosis without pathological fracture

Category M81, Osteoporosis without current pathological fracture, is for use for patients with osteoporosis who do not currently have a pathologic fracture due to the osteoporosis, even if they have had a fracture in the past. For patients with a history of osteoporosis fractures, status code Z87.310, Personal history of (healed) osteoporosis fracture, should follow the code from M81.

2) Osteoporosis with current pathological fracture

Category M80, Osteoporosis with current pathological fracture, is for patients who have a current pathologic fracture at the time of an encounter. The codes under M80 identify the site of the fracture. A code from category M80, not a traumatic fracture code, should be used for any patient with known osteoporosis who suffers a fracture, even if the patient had a minor fall or trauma, if that fall or trauma would not usually break a normal, healthy bone.

OSTEOPATHIES AND CHONDROPATHIES (M80-M94)

DISORDERS OF BONE DENSITY AND STRUCTURE (M80-M85)

M80 Osteoporosis with current pathological fracture
    Excessive skeletal fragility (porous bone) resulting in bone fractures
    Includes osteoporosis with current fragility fracture
    Use additional code to identify major osseous defect, if applicable (M89.7-)
    Excludes1 collapsed vertebra NOS (M48.5)
        pathological fracture NOS (M84.4)
        wedging of vertebra NOS (M48.5)
    Excludes2 personal history of (healed) osteoporosis fracture (Z87.310)
    Coding Clinic: 2018, Q2, P12

The appropriate 7th character is to be added to each code from category M80:

A	initial encounter for fracture *All encounters involving diagnosis and treatment*
D	subsequent encounter for fracture with routine healing
G	subsequent encounter for fracture with delayed healing *Encounters for attention to casting or fixation devices, medication, and follow-up visits during the healing phase*
K	subsequent encounter for fracture with nonunion *Total failure of fracture healing*
P	subsequent encounter for fracture with malunion *Fracture ends do not heal together correctly.*
S	sequela

● **M80.0 Age-related osteoporosis with current pathological fracture**
    Involutional osteoporosis with current pathological fracture
    Osteoporosis NOS with current pathological fracture
    Postmenopausal osteoporosis with current pathological fracture
    Senile osteoporosis with current pathological fracture
  X ● **M80.00 Age-related osteoporosis with current pathological fracture, unspecified site** A
  ● **M80.01 Age-related osteoporosis with current pathological fracture, shoulder**
    ● **M80.011 Age-related osteoporosis with current pathological fracture, right shoulder** A
    ● **M80.012 Age-related osteoporosis with current pathological fracture, left shoulder** A

CHAPTER 13 (M00-M99)

● **M80.019** Age-related osteoporosis with current pathological fracture, unspecified shoulder A

● **M80.02** Age-related osteoporosis with current pathological fracture, humerus

 ● **M80.021** Age-related osteoporosis with current pathological fracture, right humerus A

 ● **M80.022** Age-related osteoporosis with current pathological fracture, left humerus A

 ● **M80.029** Age-related osteoporosis with current pathological fracture, unspecified humerus A

● **M80.03** Age-related osteoporosis with current pathological fracture, forearm
  Age-related osteoporosis with current pathological fracture of wrist

 ● **M80.031** Age-related osteoporosis with current pathological fracture, right forearm A

 ● **M80.032** Age-related osteoporosis with current pathological fracture, left forearm A

 ● **M80.039** Age-related osteoporosis with current pathological fracture, unspecified forearm A

● **M80.04** Age-related osteoporosis with current pathological fracture, hand

 ● **M80.041** Age-related osteoporosis with current pathological fracture, right hand A

 ● **M80.042** Age-related osteoporosis with current pathological fracture, left hand A

 ● **M80.049** Age-related osteoporosis with current pathological fracture, unspecified hand A

● **M80.05** Age-related osteoporosis with current pathological fracture, femur

  Age-related osteoporosis with current pathological fracture of hip

 ● **M80.051** Age-related osteoporosis with current pathological fracture, right femur A 🅷🅒🅒 A

 ● **M80.052** Age-related osteoporosis with current pathological fracture, left femur A 🅷🅒🅒 A
  Coding Clinic: 2018, Q2, P12

 ● **M80.059** Age-related osteoporosis with current pathological fracture, unspecified femur A 🅷🅒🅒 A

● **M80.06** Age-related osteoporosis with current pathological fracture, lower leg

 ● **M80.061** Age-related osteoporosis with current pathological fracture, right lower leg A

 ● **M80.062** Age-related osteoporosis with current pathological fracture, left lower leg A

 ● **M80.069** Age-related osteoporosis with current pathological fracture, unspecified lower leg A

● **M80.07** Age-related osteoporosis with current pathological fracture, ankle and foot

 ● **M80.071** Age-related osteoporosis with current pathological fracture, right ankle and foot A

 ● **M80.072** Age-related osteoporosis with current pathological fracture, left ankle and foot A

 ● **M80.079** Age-related osteoporosis with current pathological fracture, unspecified ankle and foot A

X ● **M80.08** Age-related osteoporosis with current pathological fracture, vertebra(e) A 🅷🅒🅒 A

M80.0A Age-related osteoporosis with current pathological fracture, other site A

● **M80.0B** Age-related osteoporosis with current pathological fracture, pelvis

 M80.0B1 Age-related osteoporosis with current pathological fracture, right pelvis

 M80.0B2 Age-related osteoporosis with current pathological fracture, left pelvis

 M80.0B9 Age-related osteoporosis with current pathological fracture, unspecified pelvis

● **M80.8** Other osteoporosis with current pathological fracture
  Drug-induced osteoporosis with current pathological fracture
  Idiopathic osteoporosis with current pathological fracture
  Osteoporosis of disuse with current pathological fracture
  Postoophorectomy osteoporosis with current pathological fracture
  Postsurgical malabsorption osteoporosis with current pathological fracture
  Post-traumatic osteoporosis with current pathological fracture
  Use additional code for adverse effect, if applicable, to identify drug (T36-T50 with fifth or sixth character 5)

X ● **M80.80** Other osteoporosis with current pathological fracture, unspecified site A

● **M80.81** Other osteoporosis with pathological fracture, shoulder

 ● **M80.811** Other osteoporosis with current pathological fracture, right shoulder

 ● **M80.812** Other osteoporosis with current pathological fracture, left shoulder

 ● **M80.819** Other osteoporosis with current pathological fracture, unspecified shoulder

● **M80.82** Other osteoporosis with current pathological fracture, humerus

 ● **M80.821** Other osteoporosis with current pathological fracture, right humerus

 ● **M80.822** Other osteoporosis with current pathological fracture, left humerus

 ● **M80.829** Other osteoporosis with current pathological fracture, unspecified humerus

● **M80.83** Other osteoporosis with current pathological fracture, forearm
  Other osteoporosis with current pathological fracture of wrist

 ● **M80.831** Other osteoporosis with current pathological fracture, right forearm

 ● **M80.832** Other osteoporosis with current pathological fracture, left forearm

 ● **M80.839** Other osteoporosis with current pathological fracture, unspecified forearm

● **M80.84** Other osteoporosis with current pathological fracture, hand

 ● **M80.841** Other osteoporosis with current pathological fracture, right hand

 ● **M80.842** Other osteoporosis with current pathological fracture, left hand

 ● **M80.849** Other osteoporosis with current pathological fracture, unspecified hand

● **M80.85** Other osteoporosis with current pathological fracture, femur
  Other osteoporosis with current pathological fracture of hip

 ● **M80.851** Other osteoporosis with current pathological fracture, right femur A 🅷🅒🅒

 ● **M80.852** Other osteoporosis with current pathological fracture, left femur A 🅷🅒🅒

● **M80.859** Other osteoporosis with current pathological fracture, unspecified femur A

● **M80.86** Other osteoporosis with current pathological fracture, lower leg

   ● **M80.861** Other osteoporosis with current pathological fracture, right lower leg

   ● **M80.862** Other osteoporosis with current pathological fracture, left lower leg

   ● **M80.869** Other osteoporosis with current pathological fracture, unspecified lower leg

● **M80.87** Other osteoporosis with current pathological fracture, ankle and foot

   ● **M80.871** Other osteoporosis with current pathological fracture, right ankle and foot

   ● **M80.872** Other osteoporosis with current pathological fracture, left ankle and foot

   ● **M80.879** Other osteoporosis with current pathological fracture, unspecified ankle and foot

X ● **M80.88** Other osteoporosis with current pathological fracture, vertebra(e) A

M80.8A Other osteoporosis with current pathological fracture, other site

● **M80.8B** Other osteoporosis with current pathological fracture, pelvis

   M80.8B1 Other osteoporosis with current pathological fracture, right pelvis

   M80.8B2 Other osteoporosis with current pathological fracture, left pelvis

   M80.8B9 Other osteoporosis with current pathological fracture, unspecified pelvis

● **M81** Osteoporosis without current pathological fracture

Use additional code to identify:
major osseous defect, if applicable (M89.7-)
personal history of (healed) osteoporosis fracture, if applicable (Z87.310)

Excludes1   osteoporosis with current pathological fracture (M80.-)
Sudeck's atrophy (M89.0)

M81.0 Age-related osteoporosis without current pathological fracture   A

Involutional osteoporosis without current pathological fracture
Osteoporosis NOS
Postmenopausal osteoporosis without current pathological fracture
Senile osteoporosis without current pathological fracture

M81.6 Localized osteoporosis [Lequesne]

Excludes1   Sudeck's atrophy (M89.0)

M81.8 Other osteoporosis without current pathological fracture

Drug-induced osteoporosis without current pathological fracture
Idiopathic osteoporosis without current pathological fracture
Osteoporosis of disuse without current pathological fracture
Postoophorectomy osteoporosis without current pathological fracture
Postsurgical malabsorption osteoporosis without current pathological fracture
Post-traumatic osteoporosis without current pathological fracture

Use additional code for adverse effect, if applicable, to identify drug (T36-T50 with fifth or sixth character 5)

● **M83** Adult osteomalacia

Excludes2   infantile and juvenile osteomalacia (E55.0)
renal osteodystrophy (N25.0)
rickets (active) (E55.0)
rickets (active) sequelae (E64.3)
vitamin D-resistant osteomalacia (E83.31)
vitamin D-resistant rickets (active) (E83.31)

M83.0 Puerperal osteomalacia   M

M83.1 Senile osteomalacia   A

M83.2 Adult osteomalacia due to malabsorption   A
Postsurgical malabsorption osteomalacia in adults

M83.3 Adult osteomalacia due to malnutrition   A

M83.4 Aluminum bone disease   A

M83.5 Other drug-induced osteomalacia in adults   A

Use additional code for adverse effect, if applicable, to identify drug (T36-T50 with fifth or sixth character 5)

M83.8 Other adult osteomalacia   A

M83.9 Adult osteomalacia, unspecified   A

● **M84** Disorder of continuity of bone

Excludes2   traumatic fracture of bone-see fracture, by site

● **M84.3** Stress fracture

Fatigue fracture
March fracture
Stress fracture NOS
Stress reaction

Use additional external cause code(s) to identify the cause of the stress fracture

Excludes1   pathological fracture NOS (M84.4.-)
pathological fracture due to osteoporosis (M80.-)
traumatic fracture (S12.-, S22.-, S32.-, S42.-, S52.-, S62.-, S72.-, S82.-, S92.-)

Excludes2   personal history of (healed) stress (fatigue) fracture (Z87.312)
stress fracture of vertebra (M48.4-)

The appropriate 7th character is to be added to each code from subcategory M84.3:

A	initial encounter for fracture
D	subsequent encounter for fracture with routine healing
G	subsequent encounter for fracture with delayed healing
K	subsequent encounter for fracture with nonunion
P	subsequent encounter for fracture with malunion
S	sequela

X ● **M84.30** Stress fracture, unspecified site

● **M84.31** Stress fracture, shoulder

   ● **M84.311** Stress fracture, right shoulder

   ● **M84.312** Stress fracture, left shoulder

   ● **M84.319** Stress fracture, unspecified shoulder

● **M84.32** Stress fracture, humerus

   ● **M84.321** Stress fracture, right humerus

   ● **M84.322** Stress fracture, left humerus

   ● **M84.329** Stress fracture, unspecified humerus

● **M84.33** Stress fracture, ulna and radius

   ● **M84.331** Stress fracture, right ulna

   ● **M84.332** Stress fracture, left ulna

   ● **M84.333** Stress fracture, right radius

   ● **M84.334** Stress fracture, left radius

   ● **M84.339** Stress fracture, unspecified ulna and radius

● **M84.34** Stress fracture, hand and fingers

   ● **M84.341** Stress fracture, right hand

   ● **M84.342** Stress fracture, left hand

   ● **M84.343** Stress fracture, unspecified hand

   ● **M84.344** Stress fracture, right finger(s)

● M84.345   Stress fracture, left finger(s)
  ● M84.346   Stress fracture, unspecified finger(s)
● M84.35   Stress fracture, pelvis and femur
       Stress fracture, hip
  ● M84.350   Stress fracture, pelvis
  ● M84.351   Stress fracture, right femur
  ● M84.352   Stress fracture, left femur
  ● M84.353   Stress fracture, unspecified femur
  ● M84.359   Stress fracture, hip, unspecified
● M84.36   Stress fracture, tibia and fibula
  ● M84.361   Stress fracture, right tibia
  ● M84.362   Stress fracture, left tibia
  ● M84.363   Stress fracture, right fibula
  ● M84.364   Stress fracture, left fibula
  ● M84.369   Stress fracture, unspecified tibia and fibula
● M84.37   Stress fracture, ankle, foot and toes
  ● M84.371   Stress fracture, right ankle
  ● M84.372   Stress fracture, left ankle
  ● M84.373   Stress fracture, unspecified ankle
  ● M84.374   Stress fracture, right foot
  ● M84.375   Stress fracture, left foot
  ● M84.376   Stress fracture, unspecified foot
  ● M84.377   Stress fracture, right toe(s)
  ● M84.378   Stress fracture, left toe(s)
  ● M84.379   Stress fracture, unspecified toe(s)
X ● M84.38   Stress fracture, other site
     Excludes2   stress fracture of vertebra (M48.4-)
● M84.4   Pathological fracture, not elsewhere classified
     Chronic fracture
     Pathological fracture NOS
     Excludes1   collapsed vertebra NEC (M48.5)
                pathological fracture in neoplastic disease (M84.5-)
                pathological fracture in osteoporosis (M80.-)
                pathological fracture in other disease (M84.6-)
                stress fracture (M84.3-)
                traumatic fracture (S12.-, S22.-, S32.-, S42.-, S52.-, S62.-, S72.-, S82.-, S92.-)
     Excludes2   personal history of (healed) pathological fracture (Z87.311)
     The appropriate 7th character is to be added to each code from subcategory M84.4:

A	initial encounter for fracture
D	subsequent encounter for fracture with routine healing
G	subsequent encounter for fracture with delayed healing
K	subsequent encounter for fracture with nonunion
P	subsequent encounter for fracture with malunion
S	sequela

X ● M84.40   Pathological fracture, unspecified site
● M84.41   Pathological fracture, shoulder
  ● M84.411   Pathological fracture, right shoulder
  ● M84.412   Pathological fracture, left shoulder
  ● M84.419   Pathological fracture, unspecified shoulder
● M84.42   Pathological fracture, humerus
  ● M84.421   Pathological fracture, right humerus
  ● M84.422   Pathological fracture, left humerus
  ● M84.429   Pathological fracture, unspecified humerus

● M84.43   Pathological fracture, ulna and radius
  ● M84.431   Pathological fracture, right ulna
  ● M84.432   Pathological fracture, left ulna
  ● M84.433   Pathological fracture, right radius
  ● M84.434   Pathological fracture, left radius
  ● M84.439   Pathological fracture, unspecified ulna and radius
● M84.44   Pathological fracture, hand and fingers
  ● M84.441   Pathological fracture, right hand
  ● M84.442   Pathological fracture, left hand
  ● M84.443   Pathological fracture, unspecified hand
  ● M84.444   Pathological fracture, right finger(s)
  ● M84.445   Pathological fracture, left finger(s)
  ● M84.446   Pathological fracture, unspecified finger(s)
● M84.45   Pathological fracture, femur and pelvis
  ● M84.451   Pathological fracture, right femur A (HCC)
  ● M84.452   Pathological fracture, left femur A (HCC)
  ● M84.453   Pathological fracture, unspecified femur A (HCC)
  ● M84.454   Pathological fracture, pelvis A (HCC)
        Coding Clinic: 2016, Q4, P43
  ● M84.459   Pathological fracture, hip, unspecified A (HCC)
● M84.46   Pathological fracture, tibia and fibula
  ● M84.461   Pathological fracture, right tibia
  ● M84.462   Pathological fracture, left tibia
  ● M84.463   Pathological fracture, right fibula
  ● M84.464   Pathological fracture, left fibula
  ● M84.469   Pathological fracture, unspecified tibia and fibula
● M84.47   Pathological fracture, ankle, foot and toes
  ● M84.471   Pathological fracture, right ankle
  ● M84.472   Pathological fracture, left ankle
  ● M84.473   Pathological fracture, unspecified ankle
  ● M84.474   Pathological fracture, right foot
  ● M84.475   Pathological fracture, left foot
  ● M84.476   Pathological fracture, unspecified foot
  ● M84.477   Pathological fracture, right toe(s)
  ● M84.478   Pathological fracture, left toe(s)
  ● M84.479   Pathological fracture, unspecified toe(s)
X ● M84.48   Pathological fracture, other site

OGCR Section I.C. 13.C.

Coding of Pathologic Fractures

7th character A is for use as long as the patient is receiving active treatment for the fracture. While the patient may be seen by a new or different provider over the course of treatment for a pathological fracture, assignment of the 7th character is based on whether the patient is undergoing active treatment and not whether the provider is seeing the patient for the first time.

7th character, D is to be used for encounters after the patient has completed active treatment for the fracture and is receiving routine care for the fracture during the healing or recovery phase. The other 7th characters, listed under each subcategory in the Tabular List, are to be used for subsequent encounters for treatment of problems associated with the healing, such as malunions, nonunions, and sequelae.

Care for complications of surgical treatment for fracture repairs during the healing or recovery phase should be coded with the appropriate complication codes.

See Section I.C.19. Coding of traumatic fractures.

● **M84.5 Pathological fracture in neoplastic disease**

Code also underlying neoplasm

The appropriate 7th character is to be added to each code from subcategory M84.5:

> A   initial encounter for fracture
> D   subsequent encounter for fracture with routine healing
> G   subsequent encounter for fracture with delayed healing
> K   subsequent encounter for fracture with nonunion
> P   subsequent encounter for fracture with malunion
> S   sequela

X● **M84.50 Pathological fracture in neoplastic disease, unspecified site**

● **M84.51 Pathological fracture in neoplastic disease, shoulder**

  ● **M84.511 Pathological fracture in neoplastic disease, right shoulder**

  ● **M84.512 Pathological fracture in neoplastic disease, left shoulder**

  ● **M84.519 Pathological fracture in neoplastic disease, unspecified shoulder**

● **M84.52 Pathological fracture in neoplastic disease, humerus**

  ● **M84.521 Pathological fracture in neoplastic disease, right humerus**

  ● **M84.522 Pathological fracture in neoplastic disease, left humerus**

  ● **M84.529 Pathological fracture in neoplastic disease, unspecified humerus**

● **M84.53 Pathological fracture in neoplastic disease, ulna and radius**

  ● **M84.531 Pathological fracture in neoplastic disease, right ulna**

  ● **M84.532 Pathological fracture in neoplastic disease, left ulna**

  ● **M84.533 Pathological fracture in neoplastic disease, right radius**

  ● **M84.534 Pathological fracture in neoplastic disease, left radius**

  ● **M84.539 Pathological fracture in neoplastic disease, unspecified ulna and radius**

● **M84.54 Pathological fracture in neoplastic disease, hand**

  ● **M84.541 Pathological fracture in neoplastic disease, right hand**

  ● **M84.542 Pathological fracture in neoplastic disease, left hand**

  ● **M84.549 Pathological fracture in neoplastic disease, unspecified hand**

● **M84.55 Pathological fracture in neoplastic disease, pelvis and femur**

  ● **M84.550 Pathological fracture in neoplastic disease, pelvis**

  ● **M84.551 Pathological fracture in neoplastic disease, right femur A** 🔄

  ● **M84.552 Pathological fracture in neoplastic disease, left femur A** 🔄

  ● **M84.553 Pathological fracture in neoplastic disease, unspecified femur A** 🔄

  ● **M84.559 Pathological fracture in neoplastic disease, hip, unspecified A** 🔄

● **M84.56 Pathological fracture in neoplastic disease, tibia and fibula**

  ● **M84.561 Pathological fracture in neoplastic disease, right tibia**

  ● **M84.562 Pathological fracture in neoplastic disease, left tibia**

  ● **M84.563 Pathological fracture in neoplastic disease, right fibula**

  ● **M84.564 Pathological fracture in neoplastic disease, left fibula**

  ● **M84.569 Pathological fracture in neoplastic disease, unspecified tibia and fibula**

● **M84.57 Pathological fracture in neoplastic disease, ankle and foot**

  ● **M84.571 Pathological fracture in neoplastic disease, right ankle**

  ● **M84.572 Pathological fracture in neoplastic disease, left ankle**

  ● **M84.573 Pathological fracture in neoplastic disease, unspecified ankle**

  ● **M84.574 Pathological fracture in neoplastic disease, right foot**

  ● **M84.575 Pathological fracture in neoplastic disease, left foot**

  ● **M84.576 Pathological fracture in neoplastic disease, unspecified foot**

X● **M84.58 Pathological fracture in neoplastic disease, other specified site**

> Pathological fracture in neoplastic disease, vertebrae

● **M84.6 Pathological fracture in other disease**

Code also underlying condition

Excludes1   pathological fracture in osteoporosis (M80.-)

The appropriate 7th character is to be added to each code from subcategory M84.6:

> A   initial encounter for fracture
> D   subsequent encounter for fracture with routine healing
> G   subsequent encounter for fracture with delayed healing
> K   subsequent encounter for fracture with nonunion
> P   subsequent encounter for fracture with malunion
> S   sequela

X● **M84.60 Pathological fracture in other disease, unspecified site**

● **M84.61 Pathological fracture in other disease, shoulder**

  ● **M84.611 Pathological fracture in other disease, right shoulder**

  ● **M84.612 Pathological fracture in other disease, left shoulder**

  ● **M84.619 Pathological fracture in other disease, unspecified shoulder**

● **M84.62 Pathological fracture in other disease, humerus**

  ● **M84.621 Pathological fracture in other disease, right humerus**

  ● **M84.622 Pathological fracture in other disease, left humerus**

  ● **M84.629 Pathological fracture in other disease, unspecified humerus**

● **M84.63 Pathological fracture in other disease, ulna and radius**

  ● **M84.631 Pathological fracture in other disease, right ulna**

● M84.632   Pathological fracture in other disease, left ulna
● M84.633   Pathological fracture in other disease, right radius
● M84.634   Pathological fracture in other disease, left radius
● M84.639   Pathological fracture in other disease, unspecified ulna and radius
● M84.64   Pathological fracture in other disease, hand
   ● M84.641   Pathological fracture in other disease, right hand
   ● M84.642   Pathological fracture in other disease, left hand
   ● M84.649   Pathological fracture in other disease, unspecified hand
● M84.65   Pathological fracture in other disease, pelvis and femur
   ● M84.650   Pathological fracture in other disease, pelvis
   ● M84.651   Pathological fracture in other disease, right femur A ℞꜀
   ● M84.652   Pathological fracture in other disease, left femur A ℞꜀
   ● M84.653   Pathological fracture in other disease, unspecified femur A ℞꜀
   ● M84.659   Pathological fracture in other disease, hip, unspecified A ℞꜀
● M84.66   Pathological fracture in other disease, tibia and fibula
   ● M84.661   Pathological fracture in other disease, right tibia
   ● M84.662   Pathological fracture in other disease, left tibia
   ● M84.663   Pathological fracture in other disease, right fibula
   ● M84.664   Pathological fracture in other disease, left fibula
   ● M84.669   Pathological fracture in other disease, unspecified tibia and fibula
● M84.67   Pathological fracture in other disease, ankle and foot
   ● M84.671   Pathological fracture in other disease, right ankle
   ● M84.672   Pathological fracture in other disease, left ankle
   ● M84.673   Pathological fracture in other disease, unspecified ankle
   ● M84.674   Pathological fracture in other disease, right foot
   ● M84.675   Pathological fracture in other disease, left foot
   ● M84.676   Pathological fracture in other disease, unspecified foot
X ● M84.68   Pathological fracture in other disease, other site
● M84.7   Nontraumatic fracture, not elsewhere classified
   ● M84.75   **Atypical femoral** fracture

The appropriate 7th character is to be added to each code from M84.75:

> A   initial encounter for fracture
> D   subsequent encounter for fracture with routine healing
> G   subsequent encounter for fracture with delayed healing
> K   subsequent encounter for fracture with nonunion
> P   subsequent encounter for fracture with malunion
> S   sequela

Coding Clinic: 2016, Q4, P41

● M84.750   Atypical femoral fracture, unspecified
● M84.751   Incomplete atypical femoral fracture, right leg
● M84.752   Incomplete atypical femoral fracture, left leg
● M84.753   Incomplete atypical femoral fracture, unspecified leg
● M84.754   Complete transverse atypical femoral fracture, right leg A ℞꜀
● M84.755   Complete transverse atypical femoral fracture, left leg A ℞꜀
● M84.756   Complete transverse atypical femoral fracture, unspecified leg A ℞꜀
● M84.757   Complete oblique atypical femoral fracture, right leg A ℞꜀
● M84.758   Complete oblique atypical femoral fracture, left leg A ℞꜀
● M84.759   Complete oblique atypical femoral fracture, unspecified leg , A ℞꜀
● M84.8   Other disorders of continuity of bone
   M84.80   Other disorders of continuity of bone, unspecified site
   ● M84.81   Other disorders of continuity of bone, shoulder
      M84.811   Other disorders of continuity of bone, right shoulder
      M84.812   Other disorders of continuity of bone, left shoulder
      M84.819   Other disorders of continuity of bone, unspecified shoulder
   ● M84.82   Other disorders of continuity of bone, humerus
      M84.821   Other disorders of continuity of bone, right humerus
      M84.822   Other disorders of continuity of bone, left humerus
      M84.829   Other disorders of continuity of bone, unspecified humerus
   ● M84.83   Other disorders of continuity of bone, ulna and radius
      M84.831   Other disorders of continuity of bone, right ulna
      M84.832   Other disorders of continuity of bone, left ulna
      M84.833   Other disorders of continuity of bone, right radius
      M84.834   Other disorders of continuity of bone, left radius
      M84.839   Other disorders of continuity of bone, unspecified ulna and radius
   ● M84.84   Other disorders of continuity of bone, hand
      M84.841   Other disorders of continuity of bone, right hand
      M84.842   Other disorders of continuity of bone, left hand
      M84.849   Other disorders of continuity of bone, unspecified hand
   ● M84.85   Other disorders of continuity of bone, pelvic region and thigh
      M84.851   Other disorders of continuity of bone, right pelvic region and thigh
      M84.852   Other disorders of continuity of bone, left pelvic region and thigh
      M84.859   Other disorders of continuity of bone, unspecified pelvic region and thigh
   ● M84.86   Other disorders of continuity of bone, tibia and fibula
      M84.861   Other disorders of continuity of bone, right tibia
      M84.862   Other disorders of continuity of bone, left tibia

▶ New   ➡ Revised   ~~deleted~~ Deleted   Excludes 1   Excludes 2   Includes   Use additional   Code first   Code also   Key words

OGCR Official Guidelines   X Assign placeholder X   ● Use Additional Character(s)   ▸ Manifestation Code   ℞꜀ Hierarchical Condition Category   Coding Clinic

M84.863   Other disorders of continuity of bone, **right fibula**

M84.864   Other disorders of continuity of bone, **left fibula**

M84.869   Other disorders of continuity of bone, **unspecified tibia and fibula**

● M84.87   Other disorders of continuity of bone, **ankle and foot**

M84.871   Other disorders of continuity of bone, **right ankle and foot**

M84.872   Other disorders of continuity of bone, **left ankle and foot**

M84.879   Other disorders of continuity of bone, **unspecified ankle and foot**

M84.88   Other disorders of continuity of bone, **other site**

M84.9   Disorder of continuity of bone, **unspecified**

● M85   Other disorders of bone density and structure

Excludes1   osteogenesis imperfecta (Q78.0)
osteopetrosis (Q78.2)
osteopoikilosis (Q78.8)
polyostotic fibrous dysplasia (Q78.1)

● M85.0   Fibrous dysplasia (monostotic)

Excludes2   fibrous dysplasia of jaw (M27.8)

M85.00   Fibrous dysplasia (monostotic), **unspecified site**

● M85.01   Fibrous dysplasia (monostotic), **shoulder**

M85.011   Fibrous dysplasia (monostotic), **right shoulder**

M85.012   Fibrous dysplasia (monostotic), **left shoulder**

M85.019   Fibrous dysplasia (monostotic), **unspecified shoulder**

● M85.02   Fibrous dysplasia (monostotic), **upper arm**

M85.021   Fibrous dysplasia (monostotic), **right upper arm**

M85.022   Fibrous dysplasia (monostotic), **left upper arm**

M85.029   Fibrous dysplasia (monostotic), **unspecified upper arm**

● M85.03   Fibrous dysplasia (monostotic), **forearm**

M85.031   Fibrous dysplasia (monostotic), **right forearm**

M85.032   Fibrous dysplasia (monostotic), **left forearm**

M85.039   Fibrous dysplasia (monostotic), **unspecified forearm**

● M85.04   Fibrous dysplasia (monostotic), **hand**

M85.041   Fibrous dysplasia (monostotic), **right hand**

M85.042   Fibrous dysplasia (monostotic), **left hand**

M85.049   Fibrous dysplasia (monostotic), **unspecified hand**

● M85.05   Fibrous dysplasia (monostotic), **thigh**

M85.051   Fibrous dysplasia (monostotic), **right thigh**

M85.052   Fibrous dysplasia (monostotic), **left thigh**

M85.059   Fibrous dysplasia (monostotic), **unspecified thigh**

● M85.06   Fibrous dysplasia (monostotic), **lower leg**

M85.061   Fibrous dysplasia (monostotic), **right lower leg**

M85.062   Fibrous dysplasia (monostotic), **left lower leg**

M85.069   Fibrous dysplasia (monostotic), **unspecified lower leg**

● M85.07   Fibrous dysplasia (monostotic), **ankle and foot**

M85.071   Fibrous dysplasia (monostotic), **right ankle and foot**

M85.072   Fibrous dysplasia (monostotic), **left ankle and foot**

M85.079   Fibrous dysplasia (monostotic), **unspecified ankle and foot**

M85.08   Fibrous dysplasia (monostotic), **other site**

M85.09   Fibrous dysplasia (monostotic), **multiple sites**

● M85.1   Skeletal fluorosis

M85.10   Skeletal fluorosis, **unspecified site**

● M85.11   Skeletal fluorosis, **shoulder**

M85.111   Skeletal fluorosis, **right shoulder**

M85.112   Skeletal fluorosis, **left shoulder**

M85.119   Skeletal fluorosis, **unspecified shoulder**

● M85.12   Skeletal fluorosis, **upper arm**

M85.121   Skeletal fluorosis, **right upper arm**

M85.122   Skeletal fluorosis, **left upper arm**

M85.129   Skeletal fluorosis, **unspecified upper arm**

● M85.13   Skeletal fluorosis, **forearm**

M85.131   Skeletal fluorosis, **right forearm**

M85.132   Skeletal fluorosis, **left forearm**

M85.139   Skeletal fluorosis, **unspecified forearm**

● M85.14   Skeletal fluorosis, **hand**

M85.141   Skeletal fluorosis, **right hand**

M85.142   Skeletal fluorosis, **left hand**

M85.149   Skeletal fluorosis, **unspecified hand**

● M85.15   Skeletal fluorosis, **thigh**

M85.151   Skeletal fluorosis, **right thigh**

M85.152   Skeletal fluorosis, **left thigh**

M85.159   Skeletal fluorosis, **unspecified thigh**

● M85.16   Skeletal fluorosis, **lower leg**

M85.161   Skeletal fluorosis, **right lower leg**

M85.162   Skeletal fluorosis, **left lower leg**

M85.169   Skeletal fluorosis, **unspecified lower leg**

● M85.17   Skeletal fluorosis, **ankle and foot**

M85.171   Skeletal fluorosis, **right ankle and foot**

M85.172   Skeletal fluorosis, **left ankle and foot**

M85.179   Skeletal fluorosis, **unspecified ankle and foot**

M85.18   Skeletal fluorosis, **other site**

M85.19   Skeletal fluorosis, **multiple sites**

M85.2   Hyperostosis of skull

● M85.3   Osteitis condensans

M85.30   Osteitis condensans, **unspecified site**

● M85.31   Osteitis condensans, **shoulder**

M85.311   Osteitis condensans, **right shoulder**

M85.312   Osteitis condensans, **left shoulder**

M85.319   Osteitis condensans, **unspecified shoulder**

● M85.32   Osteitis condensans, **upper arm**

M85.321   Osteitis condensans, **right upper arm**

M85.322   Osteitis condensans, **left upper arm**

M85.329   Osteitis condensans, **unspecified upper arm**

● M85.33   Osteitis condensans, **forearm**

M85.331   Osteitis condensans, **right forearm**

M85.332   Osteitis condensans, **left forearm**

M85.339   Osteitis condensans, **unspecified forearm**

CHAPTER 13 (M00–M99)

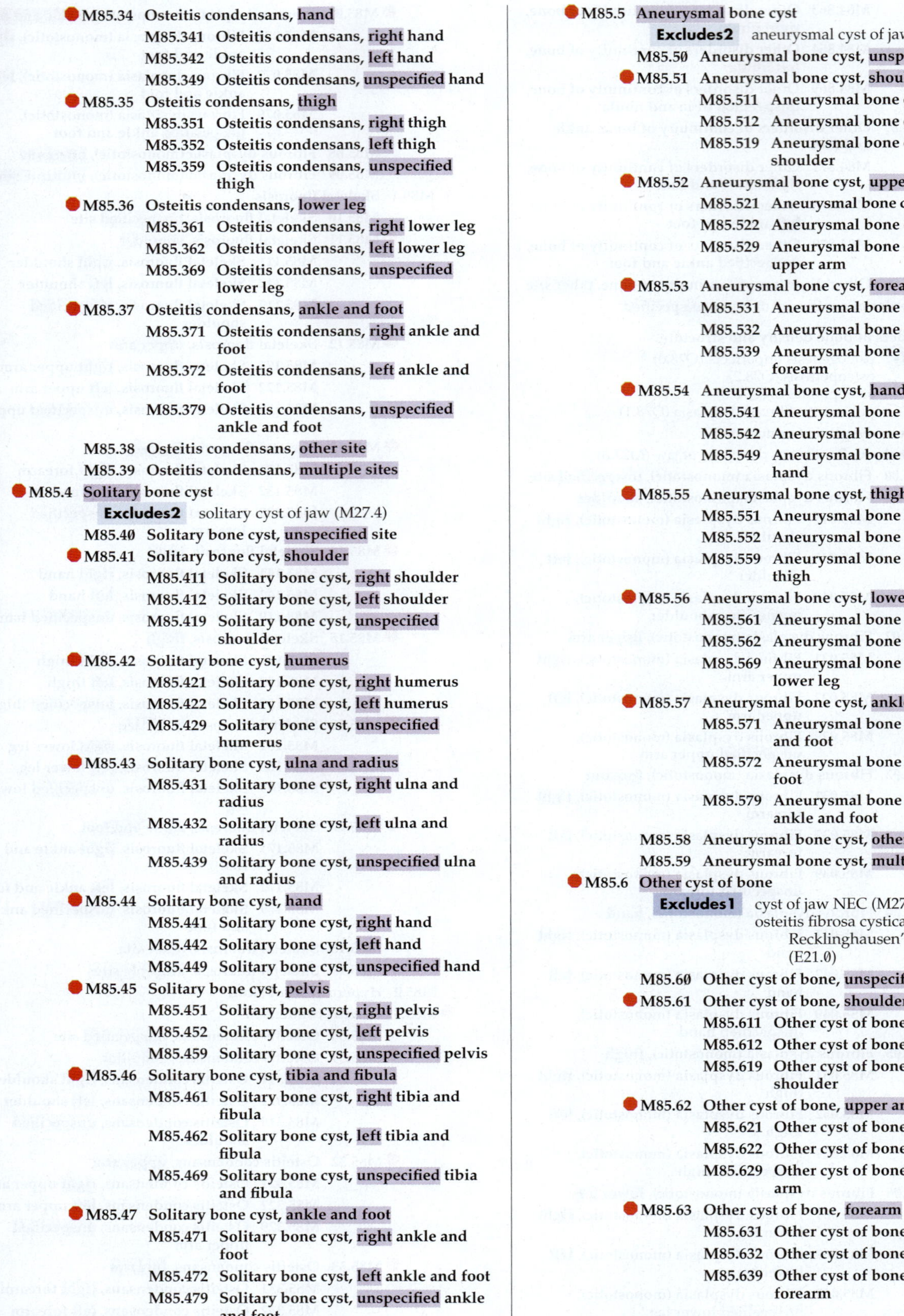

● M85.34   Osteitis condensans, hand
    M85.341   Osteitis condensans, right hand
    M85.342   Osteitis condensans, left hand
    M85.349   Osteitis condensans, unspecified hand
● M85.35   Osteitis condensans, thigh
    M85.351   Osteitis condensans, right thigh
    M85.352   Osteitis condensans, left thigh
    M85.359   Osteitis condensans, unspecified thigh
● M85.36   Osteitis condensans, lower leg
    M85.361   Osteitis condensans, right lower leg
    M85.362   Osteitis condensans, left lower leg
    M85.369   Osteitis condensans, unspecified lower leg
● M85.37   Osteitis condensans, ankle and foot
    M85.371   Osteitis condensans, right ankle and foot
    M85.372   Osteitis condensans, left ankle and foot
    M85.379   Osteitis condensans, unspecified ankle and foot
  M85.38   Osteitis condensans, other site
  M85.39   Osteitis condensans, multiple sites
● M85.4   Solitary bone cyst
    Excludes2   solitary cyst of jaw (M27.4)
  M85.40   Solitary bone cyst, unspecified site
● M85.41   Solitary bone cyst, shoulder
    M85.411   Solitary bone cyst, right shoulder
    M85.412   Solitary bone cyst, left shoulder
    M85.419   Solitary bone cyst, unspecified shoulder
● M85.42   Solitary bone cyst, humerus
    M85.421   Solitary bone cyst, right humerus
    M85.422   Solitary bone cyst, left humerus
    M85.429   Solitary bone cyst, unspecified humerus
● M85.43   Solitary bone cyst, ulna and radius
    M85.431   Solitary bone cyst, right ulna and radius
    M85.432   Solitary bone cyst, left ulna and radius
    M85.439   Solitary bone cyst, unspecified ulna and radius
● M85.44   Solitary bone cyst, hand
    M85.441   Solitary bone cyst, right hand
    M85.442   Solitary bone cyst, left hand
    M85.449   Solitary bone cyst, unspecified hand
● M85.45   Solitary bone cyst, pelvis
    M85.451   Solitary bone cyst, right pelvis
    M85.452   Solitary bone cyst, left pelvis
    M85.459   Solitary bone cyst, unspecified pelvis
● M85.46   Solitary bone cyst, tibia and fibula
    M85.461   Solitary bone cyst, right tibia and fibula
    M85.462   Solitary bone cyst, left tibia and fibula
    M85.469   Solitary bone cyst, unspecified tibia and fibula
● M85.47   Solitary bone cyst, ankle and foot
    M85.471   Solitary bone cyst, right ankle and foot
    M85.472   Solitary bone cyst, left ankle and foot
    M85.479   Solitary bone cyst, unspecified ankle and foot
  M85.48   Solitary bone cyst, other site

● M85.5   Aneurysmal bone cyst
    Excludes2   aneurysmal cyst of jaw (M27.4)
  M85.50   Aneurysmal bone cyst, unspecified site
● M85.51   Aneurysmal bone cyst, shoulder
    M85.511   Aneurysmal bone cyst, right shoulder
    M85.512   Aneurysmal bone cyst, left shoulder
    M85.519   Aneurysmal bone cyst, unspecified shoulder
● M85.52   Aneurysmal bone cyst, upper arm
    M85.521   Aneurysmal bone cyst, right upper arm
    M85.522   Aneurysmal bone cyst, left upper arm
    M85.529   Aneurysmal bone cyst, unspecified upper arm
● M85.53   Aneurysmal bone cyst, forearm
    M85.531   Aneurysmal bone cyst, right forearm
    M85.532   Aneurysmal bone cyst, left forearm
    M85.539   Aneurysmal bone cyst, unspecified forearm
● M85.54   Aneurysmal bone cyst, hand
    M85.541   Aneurysmal bone cyst, right hand
    M85.542   Aneurysmal bone cyst, left hand
    M85.549   Aneurysmal bone cyst, unspecified hand
● M85.55   Aneurysmal bone cyst, thigh
    M85.551   Aneurysmal bone cyst, right thigh
    M85.552   Aneurysmal bone cyst, left thigh
    M85.559   Aneurysmal bone cyst, unspecified thigh
● M85.56   Aneurysmal bone cyst, lower leg
    M85.561   Aneurysmal bone cyst, right lower leg
    M85.562   Aneurysmal bone cyst, left lower leg
    M85.569   Aneurysmal bone cyst, unspecified lower leg
● M85.57   Aneurysmal bone cyst, ankle and foot
    M85.571   Aneurysmal bone cyst, right ankle and foot
    M85.572   Aneurysmal bone cyst, left ankle and foot
    M85.579   Aneurysmal bone cyst, unspecified ankle and foot
  M85.58   Aneurysmal bone cyst, other site
  M85.59   Aneurysmal bone cyst, multiple sites
● M85.6   Other cyst of bone
    Excludes1   cyst of jaw NEC (M27.4)
           osteitis fibrosa cystica generalisata [von Recklinghausen's disease of bone] (E21.0)
  M85.60   Other cyst of bone, unspecified site
● M85.61   Other cyst of bone, shoulder
    M85.611   Other cyst of bone, right shoulder
    M85.612   Other cyst of bone, left shoulder
    M85.619   Other cyst of bone, unspecified shoulder
● M85.62   Other cyst of bone, upper arm
    M85.621   Other cyst of bone, right upper arm
    M85.622   Other cyst of bone, left upper arm
    M85.629   Other cyst of bone, unspecified upper arm
● M85.63   Other cyst of bone, forearm
    M85.631   Other cyst of bone, right forearm
    M85.632   Other cyst of bone, left forearm
    M85.639   Other cyst of bone, unspecified forearm

● **M85.64** Other cyst of bone, **hand**
     M85.641 Other cyst of bone, **right** hand
     M85.642 Other cyst of bone, **left** hand
     M85.649 Other cyst of bone, **unspecified** hand
● **M85.65** Other cyst of bone, **thigh**
     M85.651 Other cyst of bone, **right** thigh
     M85.652 Other cyst of bone, **left** thigh
     M85.659 Other cyst of bone, **unspecified** thigh
● **M85.66** Other cyst of bone, **lower leg**
     M85.661 Other cyst of bone, **right** lower leg
     M85.662 Other cyst of bone, **left** lower leg
     M85.669 Other cyst of bone, **unspecified** lower leg
● **M85.67** Other cyst of bone, **ankle and foot**
     M85.671 Other cyst of bone, **right** ankle and foot
     M85.672 Other cyst of bone, **left** ankle and foot
     M85.679 Other cyst of bone, **unspecified** ankle and foot
     M85.68 Other cyst of bone, **other site**
     M85.69 Other cyst of bone, **multiple sites**
● **M85.8** Other specified disorders of bone density and structure
     Hyperostosis of bones, except skull
     Osteosclerosis, acquired
     Excludes1   diffuse idiopathic skeletal hyperostosis [DISH] (M48.1)
           osteosclerosis congenita (Q77.4)
           osteosclerosis fragilitas (generalista) (Q78.2)
           osteosclerosis myelofibrosis (D75.81)
     M85.80 Other specified disorders of bone density and structure, **unspecified site**
● **M85.81** Other specified disorders of bone density and structure, **shoulder**
     M85.811 Other specified disorders of bone density and structure, **right** shoulder
     M85.812 Other specified disorders of bone density and structure, **left** shoulder
     M85.819 Other specified disorders of bone density and structure, **unspecified** shoulder
● **M85.82** Other specified disorders of bone density and structure, **upper arm**
     M85.821 Other specified disorders of bone density and structure, **right** upper arm
     M85.822 Other specified disorders of bone density and structure, **left** upper arm
     M85.829 Other specified disorders of bone density and structure, **unspecified** upper arm
● **M85.83** Other specified disorders of bone density and structure, **forearm**
     M85.831 Other specified disorders of bone density and structure, **right** forearm
     M85.832 Other specified disorders of bone density and structure, **left** forearm
     M85.839 Other specified disorders of bone density and structure, **unspecified** forearm
● **M85.84** Other specified disorders of bone density and structure, **hand**
     M85.841 Other specified disorders of bone density and structure, **right** hand
     M85.842 Other specified disorders of bone density and structure, **left** hand
     M85.849 Other specified disorders of bone density and structure, **unspecified** hand

● **M85.85** Other specified disorders of bone density and structure, **thigh**
     M85.851 Other specified disorders of bone density and structure, **right** thigh
     M85.852 Other specified disorders of bone density and structure, **left** thigh
     M85.859 Other specified disorders of bone density and structure, **unspecified** thigh
● **M85.86** Other specified disorders of bone density and structure, **lower leg**
     M85.861 Other specified disorders of bone density and structure, **right** lower leg
     M85.862 Other specified disorders of bone density and structure, **left** lower leg
     M85.869 Other specified disorders of bone density and structure, **unspecified** lower leg
● **M85.87** Other specified disorders of bone density and structure, **ankle and foot**
     M85.871 Other specified disorders of bone density and structure, **right** ankle and foot
     M85.872 Other specified disorders of bone density and structure, **left** ankle and foot
     M85.879 Other specified disorders of bone density and structure, **unspecified** ankle and foot
     M85.88 Other specified disorders of bone density and structure, **other site**
     M85.89 Other specified disorders of bone density and structure, **multiple sites**
     M85.9 Disorder of bone density and structure, **unspecified**
       Coding Clinic: 2021, Q3, P11

OTHER OSTEOPATHIES (M86-M90)

     Excludes1   postprocedural osteopathies (M96.-)
● **M86**   **Osteomyelitis**
     Use additional code (B95-B97) to identify infectious agent
     Use additional code to identify major osseous defect, if applicable (M89.7-)
     Excludes1   osteomyelitis due to:
           echinococcus (B67.2)
           gonococcus (A54.43)
           salmonella (A02.24)
     Excludes2   ostemyelitis of:
           orbit (H05.0-)
           petrous bone (H70.2-)
           vertebra (M46.2-)
     Coding Clinic: 2025, Q2, P13
● **M86.0**   **Acute hematogenous osteomyelitis**
     M86.00 Acute hematogenous osteomyelitis, **unspecified site**
● **M86.01** Acute hematogenous osteomyelitis, **shoulder**
     M86.011 Acute hematogenous osteomyelitis, **right shoulder**
     M86.012 Acute hematogenous osteomyelitis, **left shoulder**
     M86.019 Acute hematogenous osteomyelitis, **unspecified shoulder**
● **M86.02** Acute hematogenous osteomyelitis, **humerus**
     M86.021 Acute hematogenous osteomyelitis, **right humerus**
     M86.022 Acute hematogenous osteomyelitis, **left humerus**
     M86.029 Acute hematogenous osteomyelitis, **unspecified humerus**

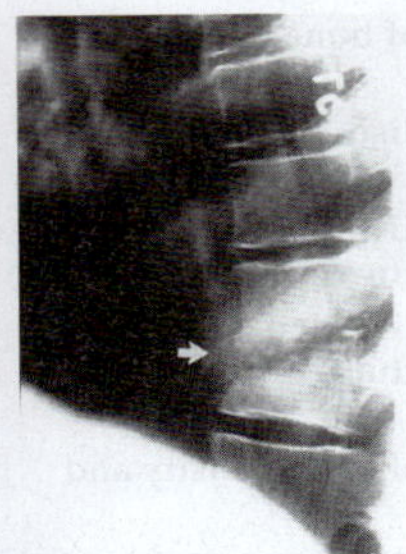

Figure 13-6 Osteomyelitis of the spine. A lateral view of the lower thoracic spine demonstrates destruction of the disk space *(arrow)* as well as destruction of the adjoining vertebral bodies. (From Mettler: Essentials of Radiology, ed 2, Saunders, An Imprint of Elsevier, 2005)

Item 13–12 Osteomyelitis is an inflammation of the bone. **Acute osteomyelitis** is a rapidly destructive, pus-producing infection capable of causing severe bone destruction. **Chronic osteomyelitis** can remain long after the initial acute episode has passed and may lead to a recurrence of the acute phase. **Brodie's abscess** is an encapsulated focal abscess that must be surgically drained. **Periostitis** is an inflammation of the periosteum, a dense membrane composed of fibrous connective tissue that closely wraps all bone, except those with articulating surfaces in joints, which are covered by synovial membranes.

● **M86.03** Acute hematogenous osteomyelitis, radius and ulna
- M86.031 Acute hematogenous osteomyelitis, right radius and ulna
- M86.032 Acute hematogenous osteomyelitis, left radius and ulna
- M86.039 Acute hematogenous osteomyelitis, unspecified radius and ulna

● **M86.04** Acute hematogenous osteomyelitis, hand
- M86.041 Acute hematogenous osteomyelitis, right hand
- M86.042 Acute hematogenous osteomyelitis, left hand
- M86.049 Acute hematogenous osteomyelitis, unspecified hand

● **M86.05** Acute hematogenous osteomyelitis, femur
- M86.051 Acute hematogenous osteomyelitis, right femur
- M86.052 Acute hematogenous osteomyelitis, left femur
- M86.059 Acute hematogenous osteomyelitis, unspecified femur

● **M86.06** Acute hematogenous osteomyelitis, tibia and fibula
- M86.061 Acute hematogenous osteomyelitis, right tibia and fibula
- M86.062 Acute hematogenous osteomyelitis, left tibia and fibula
- M86.069 Acute hematogenous osteomyelitis, unspecified tibia and fibula

● **M86.07** Acute hematogenous osteomyelitis, ankle and foot
- M86.071 Acute hematogenous osteomyelitis, right ankle and foot
- M86.072 Acute hematogenous osteomyelitis, left ankle and foot
- M86.079 Acute hematogenous osteomyelitis, unspecified ankle and foot

- M86.08 Acute hematogenous osteomyelitis, other sites
- M86.09 Acute hematogenous osteomyelitis, multiple sites

● **M86.1** Other acute osteomyelitis
- M86.10 Other acute osteomyelitis, unspecified site

● **M86.11** Other acute osteomyelitis, shoulder
- M86.111 Other acute osteomyelitis, right shoulder
- M86.112 Other acute osteomyelitis, left shoulder
- M86.119 Other acute osteomyelitis, unspecified shoulder

● **M86.12** Other acute osteomyelitis, humerus
- M86.121 Other acute osteomyelitis, right humerus
- M86.122 Other acute osteomyelitis, left humerus
- M86.129 Other acute osteomyelitis, unspecified humerus

● **M86.13** Other acute osteomyelitis, radius and ulna
- M86.131 Other acute osteomyelitis, right radius and ulna
- M86.132 Other acute osteomyelitis, left radius and ulna
- M86.139 Other acute osteomyelitis, unspecified radius and ulna

● **M86.14** Other acute osteomyelitis, hand
- M86.141 Other acute osteomyelitis, right hand
- M86.142 Other acute osteomyelitis, left hand
- M86.149 Other acute osteomyelitis, unspecified hand

● **M86.15** Other acute osteomyelitis, femur
- M86.151 Other acute osteomyelitis, right femur
- M86.152 Other acute osteomyelitis, left femur
- M86.159 Other acute osteomyelitis, unspecified femur

● **M86.16** Other acute osteomyelitis, tibia and fibula
- M86.161 Other acute osteomyelitis, right tibia and fibula
- M86.162 Other acute osteomyelitis, left tibia and fibula
- M86.169 Other acute osteomyelitis, unspecified tibia and fibula

● **M86.17** Other acute osteomyelitis, ankle and foot
- M86.171 Other acute osteomyelitis, right ankle and foot
  Coding Clinic: 2020, Q1, P12
- M86.172 Other acute osteomyelitis, left ankle and foot
- M86.179 Other acute osteomyelitis, unspecified ankle and foot
- M86.18 Other acute osteomyelitis, other site
- M86.19 Other acute osteomyelitis, multiple sites

● **M86.2** Subacute osteomyelitis
- M86.20 Subacute osteomyelitis, unspecified site

● **M86.21** Subacute osteomyelitis, shoulder
- M86.211 Subacute osteomyelitis, right shoulder
- M86.212 Subacute osteomyelitis, left shoulder

CHAPTER 13 (M00–M99)

M86.219   Subacute osteomyelitis, unspecified shoulder

● M86.22   Subacute osteomyelitis, humerus

M86.221   Subacute osteomyelitis, right humerus

M86.222   Subacute osteomyelitis, left humerus

M86.229   Subacute osteomyelitis, unspecified humerus

● M86.23   Subacute osteomyelitis, radius and ulna

M86.231   Subacute osteomyelitis, right radius and ulna

M86.232   Subacute osteomyelitis, left radius and ulna

M86.239   Subacute osteomyelitis, unspecified radius and ulna

● M86.24   Subacute osteomyelitis, hand

M86.241   Subacute osteomyelitis, right hand

M86.242   Subacute osteomyelitis, left hand

M86.249   Subacute osteomyelitis, unspecified hand

● M86.25   Subacute osteomyelitis, femur

M86.251   Subacute osteomyelitis, right femur

M86.252   Subacute osteomyelitis, left femur

M86.259   Subacute osteomyelitis, unspecified femur

● M86.26   Subacute osteomyelitis, tibia and fibula

M86.261   Subacute osteomyelitis, right tibia and fibula

M86.262   Subacute osteomyelitis, left tibia and fibula

M86.269   Subacute osteomyelitis, unspecified tibia and fibula

● M86.27   Subacute osteomyelitis, ankle and foot

M86.271   Subacute osteomyelitis, right ankle and foot

M86.272   Subacute osteomyelitis, left ankle and foot

M86.279   Subacute osteomyelitis, unspecified ankle and foot

M86.28   Subacute osteomyelitis, other site

M86.29   Subacute osteomyelitis, multiple sites

● M86.3   Chronic multifocal osteomyelitis

M86.30   Chronic multifocal osteomyelitis, unspecified site

● M86.31   Chronic multifocal osteomyelitis, shoulder

M86.311   Chronic multifocal osteomyelitis, right shoulder

M86.312   Chronic multifocal osteomyelitis, left shoulder

M86.319   Chronic multifocal osteomyelitis, unspecified shoulder

● M86.32   Chronic multifocal osteomyelitis, humerus

M86.321   Chronic multifocal osteomyelitis, right humerus

M86.322   Chronic multifocal osteomyelitis, left humerus

M86.329   Chronic multifocal osteomyelitis, unspecified humerus

● M86.33   Chronic multifocal osteomyelitis, radius and ulna

M86.331   Chronic multifocal osteomyelitis, right radius and ulna

M86.332   Chronic multifocal osteomyelitis, left radius and ulna

M86.339   Chronic multifocal osteomyelitis, unspecified radius and ulna

● M86.34   Chronic multifocal osteomyelitis, hand

M86.341   Chronic multifocal osteomyelitis, right hand

M86.342   Chronic multifocal osteomyelitis, left hand

M86.349   Chronic multifocal osteomyelitis, unspecified hand

● M86.35   Chronic multifocal osteomyelitis, femur

M86.351   Chronic multifocal osteomyelitis, right femur

M86.352   Chronic multifocal osteomyelitis, left femur

M86.359   Chronic multifocal osteomyelitis, unspecified femur

● M86.36   Chronic multifocal osteomyelitis, tibia and fibula

M86.361   Chronic multifocal osteomyelitis, right tibia and fibula

M86.362   Chronic multifocal osteomyelitis, left tibia and fibula

M86.369   Chronic multifocal osteomyelitis, unspecified tibia and fibula

● M86.37   Chronic multifocal osteomyelitis, ankle and foot

M86.371   Chronic multifocal osteomyelitis, right ankle and foot

M86.372   Chronic multifocal osteomyelitis, left ankle and foot

M86.379   Chronic multifocal osteomyelitis, unspecified ankle and foot

M86.38   Chronic multifocal osteomyelitis, other site

M86.39   Chronic multifocal osteomyelitis, multiple sites

● M86.4   Chronic osteomyelitis with draining sinus

M86.40   Chronic osteomyelitis with draining sinus, unspecified site

● M86.41   Chronic osteomyelitis with draining sinus, shoulder

M86.411   Chronic osteomyelitis with draining sinus, right shoulder

M86.412   Chronic osteomyelitis with draining sinus, left shoulder

M86.419   Chronic osteomyelitis with draining sinus, unspecified shoulder

● M86.42   Chronic osteomyelitis with draining sinus, humerus

M86.421   Chronic osteomyelitis with draining sinus, right humerus

M86.422   Chronic osteomyelitis with draining sinus, left humerus

M86.429   Chronic osteomyelitis with draining sinus, unspecified humerus

● M86.43   Chronic osteomyelitis with draining sinus, radius and ulna

M86.431   Chronic osteomyelitis with draining sinus, right radius and ulna

M86.432   Chronic osteomyelitis with draining sinus, left radius and ulna

M86.439   Chronic osteomyelitis with draining sinus, unspecified radius and ulna

● M86.44   Chronic osteomyelitis with draining sinus, hand

M86.441   Chronic osteomyelitis with draining sinus, right hand

M86.442   Chronic osteomyelitis with draining sinus, left hand

M86.449   Chronic osteomyelitis with draining sinus, unspecified hand

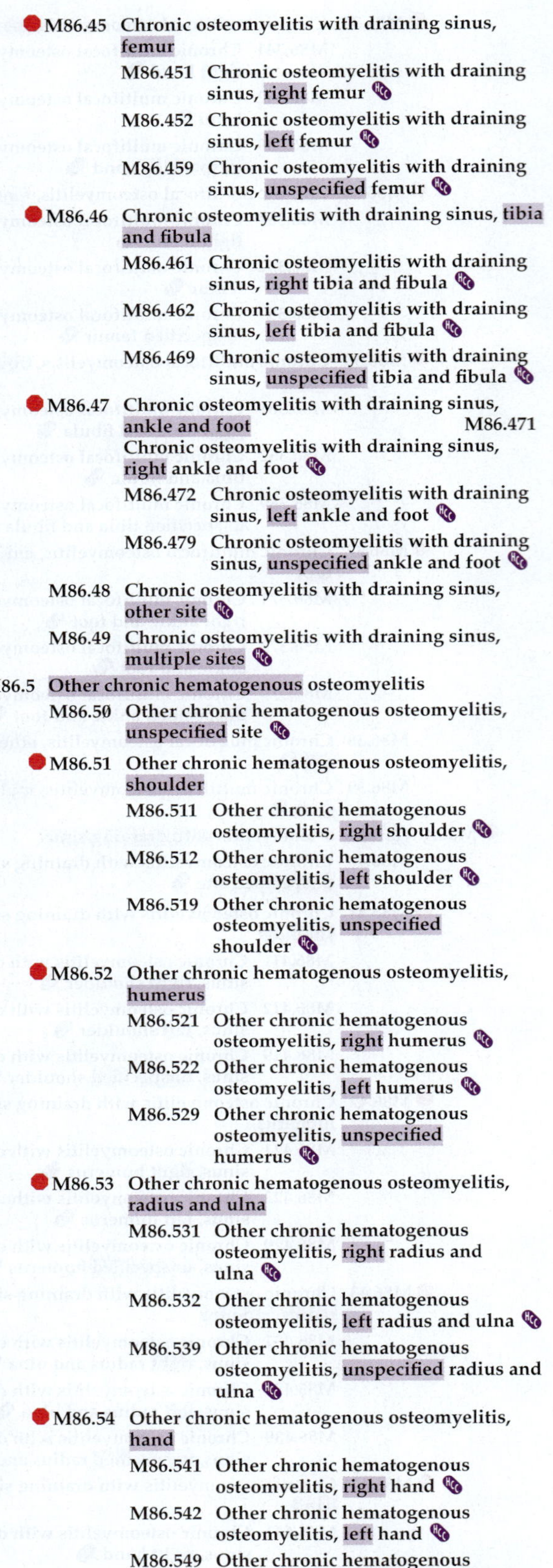

● **M86.45** Chronic osteomyelitis with draining sinus, femur
 M86.451 Chronic osteomyelitis with draining sinus, right femur
 M86.452 Chronic osteomyelitis with draining sinus, left femur
 M86.459 Chronic osteomyelitis with draining sinus, unspecified femur
● **M86.46** Chronic osteomyelitis with draining sinus, tibia and fibula
 M86.461 Chronic osteomyelitis with draining sinus, right tibia and fibula
 M86.462 Chronic osteomyelitis with draining sinus, left tibia and fibula
 M86.469 Chronic osteomyelitis with draining sinus, unspecified tibia and fibula
● **M86.47** Chronic osteomyelitis with draining sinus, ankle and foot
 M86.471 Chronic osteomyelitis with draining sinus, right ankle and foot
 M86.472 Chronic osteomyelitis with draining sinus, left ankle and foot
 M86.479 Chronic osteomyelitis with draining sinus, unspecified ankle and foot
 M86.48 Chronic osteomyelitis with draining sinus, other site
 M86.49 Chronic osteomyelitis with draining sinus, multiple sites
● **M86.5** Other chronic hematogenous osteomyelitis
 M86.50 Other chronic hematogenous osteomyelitis, unspecified site
● **M86.51** Other chronic hematogenous osteomyelitis, shoulder
 M86.511 Other chronic hematogenous osteomyelitis, right shoulder
 M86.512 Other chronic hematogenous osteomyelitis, left shoulder
 M86.519 Other chronic hematogenous osteomyelitis, unspecified shoulder
● **M86.52** Other chronic hematogenous osteomyelitis, humerus
 M86.521 Other chronic hematogenous osteomyelitis, right humerus
 M86.522 Other chronic hematogenous osteomyelitis, left humerus
 M86.529 Other chronic hematogenous osteomyelitis, unspecified humerus
● **M86.53** Other chronic hematogenous osteomyelitis, radius and ulna
 M86.531 Other chronic hematogenous osteomyelitis, right radius and ulna
 M86.532 Other chronic hematogenous osteomyelitis, left radius and ulna
 M86.539 Other chronic hematogenous osteomyelitis, unspecified radius and ulna
● **M86.54** Other chronic hematogenous osteomyelitis, hand
 M86.541 Other chronic hematogenous osteomyelitis, right hand
 M86.542 Other chronic hematogenous osteomyelitis, left hand
 M86.549 Other chronic hematogenous osteomyelitis, unspecified hand

● **M86.55** Other chronic hematogenous osteomyelitis, femur
 M86.551 Other chronic hematogenous osteomyelitis, right femur
 M86.552 Other chronic hematogenous osteomyelitis, left femur
 M86.559 Other chronic hematogenous osteomyelitis, unspecified femur
● **M86.56** Other chronic hematogenous osteomyelitis, tibia and fibula
 M86.561 Other chronic hematogenous osteomyelitis, right tibia and fibula
 M86.562 Other chronic hematogenous osteomyelitis, left tibia and fibula
 M86.569 Other chronic hematogenous osteomyelitis, unspecified tibia and fibula
● **M86.57** Other chronic hematogenous osteomyelitis, ankle and foot
 M86.571 Other chronic hematogenous osteomyelitis, right ankle and foot
 M86.572 Other chronic hematogenous osteomyelitis, left ankle and foot
 M86.579 Other chronic hematogenous osteomyelitis, unspecified ankle and foot
 M86.58 Other chronic hematogenous osteomyelitis, other site
 M86.59 Other chronic hematogenous osteomyelitis, multiple sites
● **M86.6** Other chronic osteomyelitis
 M86.60 Other chronic osteomyelitis, unspecified site
● **M86.61** Other chronic osteomyelitis, shoulder
 M86.611 Other chronic osteomyelitis, right shoulder
 M86.612 Other chronic osteomyelitis, left shoulder
 M86.619 Other chronic osteomyelitis, unspecified shoulder
● **M86.62** Other chronic osteomyelitis, humerus
 M86.621 Other chronic osteomyelitis, right humerus
 M86.622 Other chronic osteomyelitis, left humerus
 M86.629 Other chronic osteomyelitis, unspecified humerus
● **M86.63** Other chronic osteomyelitis, radius and ulna
 M86.631 Other chronic osteomyelitis, right radius and ulna
 M86.632 Other chronic osteomyelitis, left radius and ulna
 M86.639 Other chronic osteomyelitis, unspecified radius and ulna
● **M86.64** Other chronic osteomyelitis, hand
 M86.641 Other chronic osteomyelitis, right hand
 M86.642 Other chronic osteomyelitis, left hand
 M86.649 Other chronic osteomyelitis, unspecified hand
● **M86.65** Other chronic osteomyelitis, thigh
 M86.651 Other chronic osteomyelitis, right thigh
 M86.652 Other chronic osteomyelitis, left thigh
 M86.659 Other chronic osteomyelitis, unspecified thigh

M86.66 Other chronic osteomyelitis, tibia and fibula
    M86.661 Other chronic osteomyelitis, right tibia and fibula
    M86.662 Other chronic osteomyelitis, left tibia and fibula
    M86.669 Other chronic osteomyelitis, unspecified tibia and fibula
M86.67 Other chronic osteomyelitis, ankle and foot
    M86.671 Other chronic osteomyelitis, right ankle and foot
        Coding Clinic: 2016, Q1, P13
    M86.672 Other chronic osteomyelitis, left ankle and foot
    M86.679 Other chronic osteomyelitis, unspecified ankle and foot
  M86.68 Other chronic osteomyelitis, other site
  M86.69 Other chronic osteomyelitis, multiple sites
M86.8 **Other osteomyelitis**
    Brodie's abscess
  M86.8X Other osteomyelitis
    M86.8X0 Other osteomyelitis, multiple sites
    M86.8X1 Other osteomyelitis, shoulder
    M86.8X2 Other osteomyelitis, upper arm
    M86.8X3 Other osteomyelitis, forearm
    M86.8X4 Other osteomyelitis, hand
    M86.8X5 Other osteomyelitis, thigh
    M86.8X6 Other osteomyelitis, lower leg
    M86.8X7 Other osteomyelitis, ankle and foot
    M86.8X8 Other osteomyelitis, other site
        Coding Clinic: 2022, Q1, P31
    M86.8X9 Other osteomyelitis, unspecified sites
M86.9 Osteomyelitis, unspecified
    Infection of bone NOS
    Periostitis without osteomyelitis

M87 Osteonecrosis
  Includes avascular necrosis of bone
  Use additional code to identify major osseous defect, if applicable (M89.7-)
  Excludes1 juvenile osteonecrosis (M91-M92)
    osteochondropathies (M90-M93)
M87.0 **Idiopathic aseptic necrosis of bone**
  M87.00 Idiopathic aseptic necrosis of unspecified bone
  M87.01 Idiopathic aseptic necrosis of shoulder
    Idiopathic aseptic necrosis of clavicle and scapula
    M87.011 Idiopathic aseptic necrosis of right shoulder
    M87.012 Idiopathic aseptic necrosis of left shoulder
    M87.019 Idiopathic aseptic necrosis of unspecified shoulder
  M87.02 Idiopathic aseptic necrosis of humerus
    M87.021 Idiopathic aseptic necrosis of right humerus
    M87.022 Idiopathic aseptic necrosis of left humerus
    M87.029 Idiopathic aseptic necrosis of unspecified humerus

M87.03 Idiopathic aseptic necrosis of radius, ulna and carpus
    M87.031 Idiopathic aseptic necrosis of right radius
    M87.032 Idiopathic aseptic necrosis of left radius
    M87.033 Idiopathic aseptic necrosis of unspecified radius
    M87.034 Idiopathic aseptic necrosis of right ulna
    M87.035 Idiopathic aseptic necrosis of left ulna
    M87.036 Idiopathic aseptic necrosis of unspecified ulna
    M87.037 Idiopathic aseptic necrosis of right carpus
    M87.038 Idiopathic aseptic necrosis of left carpus
    M87.039 Idiopathic aseptic necrosis of unspecified carpus
M87.04 Idiopathic aseptic necrosis of hand and fingers
    Idiopathic aseptic necrosis of metacarpals and phalanges of hands
    M87.041 Idiopathic aseptic necrosis of right hand
    M87.042 Idiopathic aseptic necrosis of left hand
    M87.043 Idiopathic aseptic necrosis of unspecified hand
    M87.044 Idiopathic aseptic necrosis of right finger(s)
    M87.045 Idiopathic aseptic necrosis of left finger(s)
    M87.046 Idiopathic aseptic necrosis of unspecified finger(s)
M87.05 Idiopathic aseptic necrosis of pelvis and femur
    M87.050 Idiopathic aseptic necrosis of pelvis
    M87.051 Idiopathic aseptic necrosis of right femur
    M87.052 Idiopathic aseptic necrosis of left femur
    M87.059 Idiopathic aseptic necrosis of unspecified femur
        Idiopathic aseptic necrosis of hip NOS
M87.06 Idiopathic aseptic necrosis of tibia and fibula
    M87.061 Idiopathic aseptic necrosis of right tibia
    M87.062 Idiopathic aseptic necrosis of left tibia
    M87.063 Idiopathic aseptic necrosis of unspecified tibia
    M87.064 Idiopathic aseptic necrosis of right fibula
    M87.065 Idiopathic aseptic necrosis of left fibula
    M87.066 Idiopathic aseptic necrosis of unspecified fibula
M87.07 Idiopathic aseptic necrosis of ankle, foot and toes
    Idiopathic aseptic necrosis of metatarsus, tarsus, and phalanges of toes
    M87.071 Idiopathic aseptic necrosis of right ankle
    M87.072 Idiopathic aseptic necrosis of left ankle
    M87.073 Idiopathic aseptic necrosis of unspecified ankle

M87.074   Idiopathic aseptic necrosis of right foot 🅡🅒🅒

M87.075   Idiopathic aseptic necrosis of left foot 🅡🅒🅒

M87.076   Idiopathic aseptic necrosis of unspecified foot 🅡🅒🅒

M87.077   Idiopathic aseptic necrosis of right toe(s) 🅡🅒🅒

M87.078   Idiopathic aseptic necrosis of left toe(s) 🅡🅒🅒

M87.079   Idiopathic aseptic necrosis of unspecified toe(s) 🅡🅒🅒

M87.08   Idiopathic aseptic necrosis of bone, other site 🅡🅒🅒

M87.09   Idiopathic aseptic necrosis of bone, multiple sites 🅡🅒🅒

● **M87.1   Osteonecrosis due to drugs**

Use additional code for adverse effect, if applicable, to identify drug (T36-T50 with fifth or sixth character 5)

M87.10   Osteonecrosis due to drugs, unspecified bone 🅡🅒🅒

● M87.11   Osteonecrosis due to drugs, shoulder

M87.111   Osteonecrosis due to drugs, right shoulder 🅡🅒🅒

M87.112   Osteonecrosis due to drugs, left shoulder 🅡🅒🅒

M87.119   Osteonecrosis due to drugs, unspecified shoulder 🅡🅒🅒

● M87.12   Osteonecrosis due to drugs, humerus

M87.121   Osteonecrosis due to drugs, right humerus 🅡🅒🅒

M87.122   Osteonecrosis due to drugs, left humerus 🅡🅒🅒

M87.129   Osteonecrosis due to drugs, unspecified humerus 🅡🅒🅒

● M87.13   Osteonecrosis due to drugs of radius, ulna and carpus

M87.131   Osteonecrosis due to drugs of right radius 🅡🅒🅒

M87.132   Osteonecrosis due to drugs of left radius 🅡🅒🅒

M87.133   Osteonecrosis due to drugs of unspecified radius 🅡🅒🅒

M87.134   Osteonecrosis due to drugs of right ulna 🅡🅒🅒

M87.135   Osteonecrosis due to drugs of left ulna 🅡🅒🅒

M87.136   Osteonecrosis due to drugs of unspecified ulna 🅡🅒🅒

M87.137   Osteonecrosis due to drugs of right carpus 🅡🅒🅒

M87.138   Osteonecrosis due to drugs of left carpus 🅡🅒🅒

M87.139   Osteonecrosis due to drugs of unspecified carpus 🅡🅒🅒

● M87.14   Osteonecrosis due to drugs, hand and fingers

M87.141   Osteonecrosis due to drugs, right hand 🅡🅒🅒

M87.142   Osteonecrosis due to drugs, left hand 🅡🅒🅒

M87.143   Osteonecrosis due to drugs, unspecified hand 🅡🅒🅒

M87.144   Osteonecrosis due to drugs, right finger(s) 🅡🅒🅒

M87.145   Osteonecrosis due to drugs, left finger(s) 🅡🅒🅒

M87.146   Osteonecrosis due to drugs, unspecified finger(s) 🅡🅒🅒

● M87.15   Osteonecrosis due to drugs, pelvis and femur

M87.150   Osteonecrosis due to drugs, pelvis 🅡🅒🅒

M87.151   Osteonecrosis due to drugs, right femur 🅡🅒🅒

M87.152   Osteonecrosis due to drugs, left femur 🅡🅒🅒

M87.159   Osteonecrosis due to drugs, unspecified femur 🅡🅒🅒

● M87.16   Osteonecrosis due to drugs, tibia and fibula

M87.161   Osteonecrosis due to drugs, right tibia 🅡🅒🅒

M87.162   Osteonecrosis due to drugs, left tibia 🅡🅒🅒

M87.163   Osteonecrosis due to drugs, unspecified tibia 🅡🅒🅒

M87.164   Osteonecrosis due to drugs, right fibula 🅡🅒🅒

M87.165   Osteonecrosis due to drugs, left fibula 🅡🅒🅒

M87.166   Osteonecrosis due to drugs, unspecified fibula 🅡🅒🅒

● M87.17   Osteonecrosis due to drugs, ankle, foot and toes

M87.171   Osteonecrosis due to drugs, right ankle 🅡🅒🅒

M87.172   Osteonecrosis due to drugs, left ankle 🅡🅒🅒

M87.173   Osteonecrosis due to drugs, unspecified ankle 🅡🅒🅒

M87.174   Osteonecrosis due to drugs, right foot 🅡🅒🅒

M87.175   Osteonecrosis due to drugs, left foot 🅡🅒🅒

M87.176   Osteonecrosis due to drugs, unspecified foot 🅡🅒🅒

M87.177   Osteonecrosis due to drugs, right toe(s) 🅡🅒🅒

M87.178   Osteonecrosis due to drugs, left toe(s) 🅡🅒🅒

M87.179   Osteonecrosis due to drugs, unspecified toe(s) 🅡🅒🅒

● M87.18   Osteonecrosis due to drugs, other site

M87.180   Osteonecrosis due to drugs, jaw 🅡🅒🅒

M87.188   Osteonecrosis due to drugs, other site 🅡🅒🅒

M87.19   Osteonecrosis due to drugs, multiple sites 🅡🅒🅒

● **M87.2   Osteonecrosis due to previous trauma**

M87.20   Osteonecrosis due to previous trauma, unspecified bone 🅡🅒🅒

● M87.21   Osteonecrosis due to previous trauma, shoulder

M87.211   Osteonecrosis due to previous trauma, right shoulder 🅡🅒🅒

M87.212   Osteonecrosis due to previous trauma, left shoulder 🅡🅒🅒

M87.219   Osteonecrosis due to previous trauma, unspecified shoulder 🅡🅒🅒

● M87.22   Osteonecrosis due to previous trauma, humerus

M87.221   Osteonecrosis due to previous trauma, right humerus 🅡🅒🅒

M87.222   Osteonecrosis due to previous trauma, left humerus 🅡🅒🅒

M87.229   Osteonecrosis due to previous trauma, unspecified humerus 🅡🅒🅒

● M87.23   Osteonecrosis due to previous trauma of radius, ulna and carpus

M87.231   Osteonecrosis due to previous trauma of right radius

M87.232   Osteonecrosis due to previous trauma of left radius

M87.233   Osteonecrosis due to previous trauma of unspecified radius

M87.234   Osteonecrosis due to previous trauma of right ulna

M87.235   Osteonecrosis due to previous trauma of left ulna

M87.236   Osteonecrosis due to previous trauma of unspecified ulna

M87.237   Osteonecrosis due to previous trauma of right carpus

M87.238   Osteonecrosis due to previous trauma of left carpus

M87.239   Osteonecrosis due to previous trauma of unspecified carpus

● M87.24   Osteonecrosis due to previous trauma, hand and fingers

M87.241   Osteonecrosis due to previous trauma, right hand

M87.242   Osteonecrosis due to previous trauma, left hand

M87.243   Osteonecrosis due to previous trauma, unspecified hand

M87.244   Osteonecrosis due to previous trauma, right finger(s)

M87.245   Osteonecrosis due to previous trauma, left finger(s)

M87.246   Osteonecrosis due to previous trauma, unspecified finger(s)

● M87.25   Osteonecrosis due to previous trauma, pelvis and femur

M87.250   Osteonecrosis due to previous trauma, pelvis

M87.251   Osteonecrosis due to previous trauma, right femur

M87.252   Osteonecrosis due to previous trauma, left femur

M87.256   Osteonecrosis due to previous trauma, unspecified femur

● M87.26   Osteonecrosis due to previous trauma, tibia and fibula

M87.261   Osteonecrosis due to previous trauma, right tibia

M87.262   Osteonecrosis due to previous trauma, left tibia

M87.263   Osteonecrosis due to previous trauma, unspecified tibia

M87.264   Osteonecrosis due to previous trauma, right fibula

M87.265   Osteonecrosis due to previous trauma, left fibula

M87.266   Osteonecrosis due to previous trauma, unspecified fibula

● M87.27   Osteonecrosis due to previous trauma, ankle, foot and toes

M87.271   Osteonecrosis due to previous trauma, right ankle

M87.272   Osteonecrosis due to previous trauma, left ankle

M87.273   Osteonecrosis due to previous trauma, unspecified ankle

M87.274   Osteonecrosis due to previous trauma, right foot

M87.275   Osteonecrosis due to previous trauma, left foot

M87.276   Osteonecrosis due to previous trauma, unspecified foot

M87.277   Osteonecrosis due to previous trauma, right toe(s)

M87.278   Osteonecrosis due to previous trauma, left toe(s)

M87.279   Osteonecrosis due to previous trauma, unspecified toe(s)

M87.28   Osteonecrosis due to previous trauma, other site

M87.29   Osteonecrosis due to previous trauma, multiple sites

● M87.3   Other secondary osteonecrosis

M87.30   Other secondary osteonecrosis, unspecified bone

● M87.31   Other secondary osteonecrosis, shoulder

M87.311   Other secondary osteonecrosis, right shoulder

M87.312   Other secondary osteonecrosis, left shoulder

M87.319   Other secondary osteonecrosis, unspecified shoulder

● M87.32   Other secondary osteonecrosis, humerus

M87.321   Other secondary osteonecrosis, right humerus

M87.322   Other secondary osteonecrosis, left humerus

M87.329   Other secondary osteonecrosis, unspecified humerus

● M87.33   Other secondary osteonecrosis of radius, ulna and carpus

M87.331   Other secondary osteonecrosis of right radius

M87.332   Other secondary osteonecrosis of left radius

M87.333   Other secondary osteonecrosis of unspecified radius

M87.334   Other secondary osteonecrosis of right ulna

M87.335   Other secondary osteonecrosis of left ulna

M87.336   Other secondary osteonecrosis of unspecified ulna

M87.337   Other secondary osteonecrosis of right carpus

M87.338   Other secondary osteonecrosis of left carpus

M87.339   Other secondary osteonecrosis of unspecified carpus

● M87.34   Other secondary osteonecrosis, hand and fingers

M87.341   Other secondary osteonecrosis, right hand

M87.342   Other secondary osteonecrosis, left hand

M87.343   Other secondary osteonecrosis, unspecified hand

M87.344   Other secondary osteonecrosis, right finger(s)

M87.345   Other secondary osteonecrosis, left finger(s)

M87.346   Other secondary osteonecrosis, unspecified finger(s)

● M87.35   Other secondary osteonecrosis, pelvis and femur

M87.350   Other secondary osteonecrosis, pelvis

M87.351   Other secondary osteonecrosis, right femur

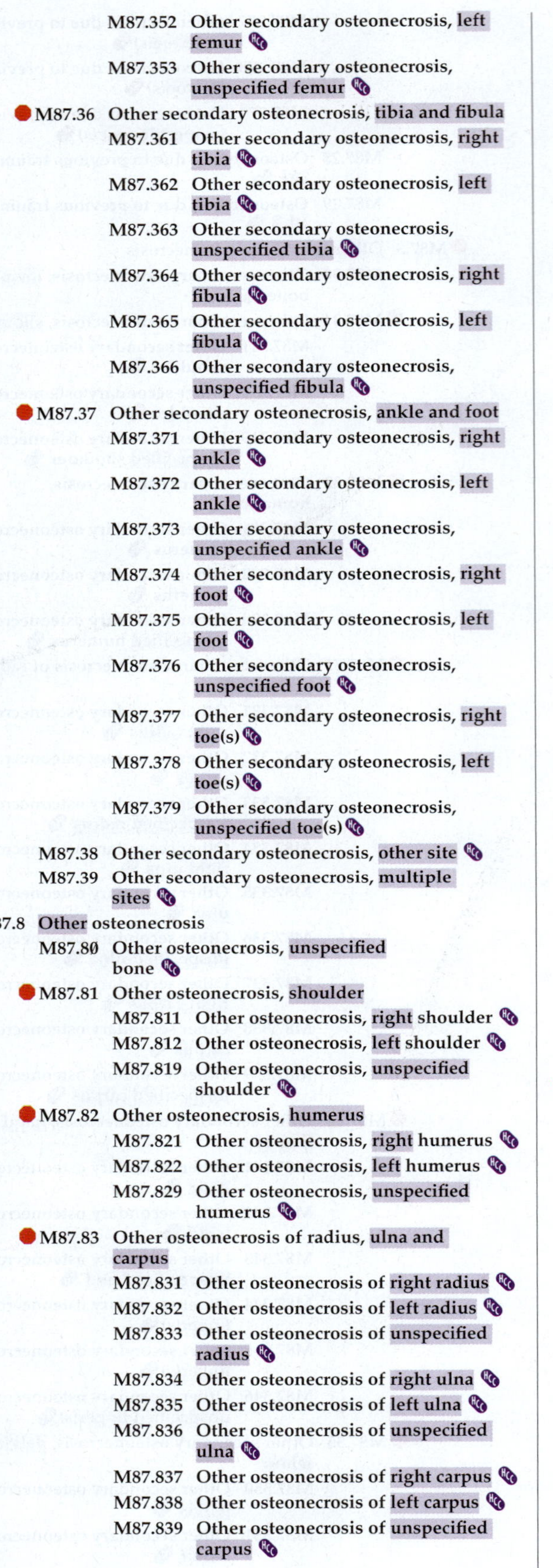

M87.352 Other secondary osteonecrosis, left femur 🅡🅒🅒
M87.353 Other secondary osteonecrosis, unspecified femur 🅡🅒🅒
● M87.36 Other secondary osteonecrosis, tibia and fibula
M87.361 Other secondary osteonecrosis, right tibia 🅡🅒🅒
M87.362 Other secondary osteonecrosis, left tibia 🅡🅒🅒
M87.363 Other secondary osteonecrosis, unspecified tibia 🅡🅒🅒
M87.364 Other secondary osteonecrosis, right fibula 🅡🅒🅒
M87.365 Other secondary osteonecrosis, left fibula 🅡🅒🅒
M87.366 Other secondary osteonecrosis, unspecified fibula 🅡🅒🅒
● M87.37 Other secondary osteonecrosis, ankle and foot
M87.371 Other secondary osteonecrosis, right ankle 🅡🅒🅒
M87.372 Other secondary osteonecrosis, left ankle 🅡🅒🅒
M87.373 Other secondary osteonecrosis, unspecified ankle 🅡🅒🅒
M87.374 Other secondary osteonecrosis, right foot 🅡🅒🅒
M87.375 Other secondary osteonecrosis, left foot 🅡🅒🅒
M87.376 Other secondary osteonecrosis, unspecified foot 🅡🅒🅒
M87.377 Other secondary osteonecrosis, right toe(s) 🅡🅒🅒
M87.378 Other secondary osteonecrosis, left toe(s) 🅡🅒🅒
M87.379 Other secondary osteonecrosis, unspecified toe(s) 🅡🅒🅒
M87.38 Other secondary osteonecrosis, other site 🅡🅒🅒
M87.39 Other secondary osteonecrosis, multiple sites 🅡🅒🅒
● M87.8 Other osteonecrosis
M87.80 Other osteonecrosis, unspecified bone 🅡🅒🅒
● M87.81 Other osteonecrosis, shoulder
M87.811 Other osteonecrosis, right shoulder 🅡🅒🅒
M87.812 Other osteonecrosis, left shoulder 🅡🅒🅒
M87.819 Other osteonecrosis, unspecified shoulder 🅡🅒🅒
● M87.82 Other osteonecrosis, humerus
M87.821 Other osteonecrosis, right humerus 🅡🅒🅒
M87.822 Other osteonecrosis, left humerus 🅡🅒🅒
M87.829 Other osteonecrosis, unspecified humerus 🅡🅒🅒
● M87.83 Other osteonecrosis of radius, ulna and carpus
M87.831 Other osteonecrosis of right radius 🅡🅒🅒
M87.832 Other osteonecrosis of left radius 🅡🅒🅒
M87.833 Other osteonecrosis of unspecified radius 🅡🅒🅒
M87.834 Other osteonecrosis of right ulna 🅡🅒🅒
M87.835 Other osteonecrosis of left ulna 🅡🅒🅒
M87.836 Other osteonecrosis of unspecified ulna 🅡🅒🅒
M87.837 Other osteonecrosis of right carpus 🅡🅒🅒
M87.838 Other osteonecrosis of left carpus 🅡🅒🅒
M87.839 Other osteonecrosis of unspecified carpus 🅡🅒🅒

● M87.84 Other osteonecrosis, hand and fingers
M87.841 Other osteonecrosis, right hand 🅡🅒🅒
M87.842 Other osteonecrosis, left hand 🅡🅒🅒
M87.843 Other osteonecrosis, unspecified hand 🅡🅒🅒
M87.844 Other osteonecrosis, right finger(s) 🅡🅒🅒
M87.845 Other osteonecrosis, left finger(s) 🅡🅒🅒
M87.849 Other osteonecrosis, unspecified finger(s) 🅡🅒🅒
● M87.85 Other osteonecrosis, pelvis and femur
M87.850 Other osteonecrosis, pelvis 🅡🅒🅒
M87.851 Other osteonecrosis, right femur 🅡🅒🅒
M87.852 Other osteonecrosis, left femur 🅡🅒🅒
M87.859 Other osteonecrosis, unspecified femur 🅡🅒🅒
● M87.86 Other osteonecrosis, tibia and fibula
M87.861 Other osteonecrosis, right tibia 🅡🅒🅒
M87.862 Other osteonecrosis, left tibia 🅡🅒🅒
M87.863 Other osteonecrosis, unspecified tibia 🅡🅒🅒
M87.864 Other osteonecrosis, right fibula 🅡🅒🅒
M87.865 Other osteonecrosis, left fibula 🅡🅒🅒
M87.869 Other osteonecrosis, unspecified fibula 🅡🅒🅒
● M87.87 Other osteonecrosis, ankle, foot and toes
M87.871 Other osteonecrosis, right ankle 🅡🅒🅒
M87.872 Other osteonecrosis, left ankle 🅡🅒🅒
M87.873 Other osteonecrosis, unspecified ankle 🅡🅒🅒
M87.874 Other osteonecrosis, right foot 🅡🅒🅒
M87.875 Other osteonecrosis, left foot 🅡🅒🅒
M87.876 Other osteonecrosis, unspecified foot 🅡🅒🅒
M87.877 Other osteonecrosis, right toe(s) 🅡🅒🅒
M87.878 Other osteonecrosis, left toe(s) 🅡🅒🅒
M87.879 Other osteonecrosis, unspecified toe(s) 🅡🅒🅒
M87.88 Other osteonecrosis, other site 🅡🅒🅒
M87.89 Other osteonecrosis, multiple sites 🅡🅒🅒
M87.9 Osteonecrosis, unspecified 🅡🅒🅒
Necrosis of bone NOS

● M88 Osteitis deformans [Paget's disease of bone]
Chronic disorder that results in enlarged and deformed bones. The excessive breakdown and formation of bone tissue causes bones to weaken and results in bone pain, arthritis, deformities, and fractures.
Excludes1   osteitis deformans in neoplastic disease (M90.6)
M88.0 Osteitis deformans of skull
M88.1 Osteitis deformans of vertebrae
● M88.8 Osteitis deformans of other bones
● M88.81 Osteitis deformans of shoulder
M88.811 Osteitis deformans of right shoulder
M88.812 Osteitis deformans of left shoulder
M88.819 Osteitis deformans of unspecified shoulder
● M88.82 Osteitis deformans of upper arm
M88.821 Osteitis deformans of right upper arm
M88.822 Osteitis deformans of left upper arm
M88.829 Osteitis deformans of unspecified upper arm

▶ New   ➡ Revised   ~~deleted~~ Deleted   Excludes 1   Excludes 2   Includes   Use additional   Code first   Code also   Key words
OGCR Official Guidelines   X Assign placeholder X   ● Use Additional Character(s)   ▶ Manifestation Code   🅡🅒🅒 Hierarchical Condition Category   **Coding Clinic**

● **M88.83 Osteitis deformans of forearm**
    M88.831   Osteitis deformans of right forearm
    M88.832   Osteitis deformans of left forearm
    M88.839   Osteitis deformans of unspecified forearm

● **M88.84 Osteitis deformans of hand**
    M88.841   Osteitis deformans of right hand
    M88.842   Osteitis deformans of left hand
    M88.849   Osteitis deformans of unspecified hand

● **M88.85 Osteitis deformans of thigh**
    M88.851   Osteitis deformans of right thigh
    M88.852   Osteitis deformans of left thigh
    M88.859   Osteitis deformans of unspecified thigh

● **M88.86 Osteitis deformans of lower leg**
    M88.861   Osteitis deformans of right lower leg
    M88.862   Osteitis deformans of left lower leg
    M88.869   Osteitis deformans of unspecified lower leg

● **M88.87 Osteitis deformans of ankle and foot**
    M88.871   Osteitis deformans of right ankle and foot
    M88.872   Osteitis deformans of left ankle and foot
    M88.879   Osteitis deformans of unspecified ankle and foot

M88.88 Osteitis deformans of other bones
    Excludes2   osteitis deformans of skull (M88.0)
                  osteitis deformans of vertebrae (M88.1)

M88.89 Osteitis deformans of multiple sites

M88.9 Osteitis deformans of unspecified bone

● **M89 Other disorders of bone**

  ● **M89.0 Algoneurodystrophy**
    Shoulder-hand syndrome
    Sudeck's atrophy
    Excludes1   causalgia, lower limb (G57.7-)
                  causalgia, upper limb (G56.4-)
                  complex regional pain syndrome II, lower limb (G57.7-)
                  complex regional pain syndrome II, upper limb (G56.4-)
                  reflex sympathetic dystrophy (G90.5-)

    M89.00 Algoneurodystrophy, unspecified site

  ● **M89.01 Algoneurodystrophy, shoulder**
    M89.011   Algoneurodystrophy, right shoulder
    M89.012   Algoneurodystrophy, left shoulder
    M89.019   Algoneurodystrophy, unspecified shoulder

  ● **M89.02 Algoneurodystrophy, upper arm**
    M89.021   Algoneurodystrophy, right upper arm
    M89.022   Algoneurodystrophy, left upper arm
    M89.029   Algoneurodystrophy, unspecified upper arm

  ● **M89.03 Algoneurodystrophy, forearm**
    M89.031   Algoneurodystrophy, right forearm
    M89.032   Algoneurodystrophy, left forearm
    M89.039   Algoneurodystrophy, unspecified forearm

  ● **M89.04 Algoneurodystrophy, hand**
    M89.041   Algoneurodystrophy, right hand
    M89.042   Algoneurodystrophy, left hand
    M89.049   Algoneurodystrophy, unspecified hand

● **M89.05 Algoneurodystrophy, thigh**
    M89.051   Algoneurodystrophy, right thigh
    M89.052   Algoneurodystrophy, left thigh
    M89.059   Algoneurodystrophy, unspecified thigh

● **M89.06 Algoneurodystrophy, lower leg**
    M89.061   Algoneurodystrophy, right lower leg
    M89.062   Algoneurodystrophy, left lower leg
    M89.069   Algoneurodystrophy, unspecified lower leg

● **M89.07 Algoneurodystrophy, ankle and foot**
    M89.071   Algoneurodystrophy, right ankle and foot
    M89.072   Algoneurodystrophy, left ankle and foot
    M89.079   Algoneurodystrophy, unspecified ankle and foot

M89.08 Algoneurodystrophy, other site

M89.09 Algoneurodystrophy, multiple sites

● **M89.1 Physeal arrest**
    Arrest of growth plate
    Epiphyseal arrest
    Growth plate arrest

  ● **M89.12 Physeal arrest, humerus**
    M89.121   Complete physeal arrest, right proximal humerus
    M89.122   Complete physeal arrest, left proximal humerus
    M89.123   Partial physeal arrest, right proximal humerus
    M89.124   Partial physeal arrest, left proximal humerus
    M89.125   Complete physeal arrest, right distal humerus
    M89.126   Complete physeal arrest, left distal humerus
    M89.127   Partial physeal arrest, right distal humerus
    M89.128   Partial physeal arrest, left distal humerus
    M89.129   Physeal arrest, humerus, unspecified

  ● **M89.13 Physeal arrest, forearm**
    M89.131   Complete physeal arrest, right distal radius
    M89.132   Complete physeal arrest, left distal radius
    M89.133   Partial physeal arrest, right distal radius
    M89.134   Partial physeal arrest, left distal radius
    M89.138   Other physeal arrest of forearm
    M89.139   Physeal arrest, forearm, unspecified

  ● **M89.15 Physeal arrest, femur**
    M89.151   Complete physeal arrest, right proximal femur
    M89.152   Complete physeal arrest, left proximal femur
    M89.153   Partial physeal arrest, right proximal femur
    M89.154   Partial physeal arrest, left proximal femur
    M89.155   Complete physeal arrest, right distal femur
    M89.156   Complete physeal arrest, left distal femur
    M89.157   Partial physeal arrest, right distal femur

CHAPTER 13 (M00-M99)

M89.158   Partial physeal arrest, left distal femur
M89.159   Physeal arrest, femur, unspecified
● M89.16   Physeal arrest, lower leg
    M89.160   Complete physeal arrest, right proximal tibia
    M89.161   Complete physeal arrest, left proximal tibia
    M89.162   Partial physeal arrest, right proximal tibia
    M89.163   Partial physeal arrest, left proximal tibia
    M89.164   Complete physeal arrest, right distal tibia
    M89.165   Complete physeal arrest, left distal tibia
    M89.166   Partial physeal arrest, right distal tibia
    M89.167   Partial physeal arrest, left distal tibia
    M89.168   Other physeal arrest of lower leg
    M89.169   Physeal arrest, lower leg, unspecified
  M89.18   Physeal arrest, other site
● M89.2   Other disorders of bone development and growth
  M89.20   Other disorders of bone development and growth, unspecified site
  ● M89.21   Other disorders of bone development and growth, shoulder
    M89.211   Other disorders of bone development and growth, right shoulder
    M89.212   Other disorders of bone development and growth, left shoulder
    M89.219   Other disorders of bone development and growth, unspecified shoulder
  ● M89.22   Other disorders of bone development and growth, humerus
    M89.221   Other disorders of bone development and growth, right humerus
    M89.222   Other disorders of bone development and growth, left humerus
    M89.229   Other disorders of bone development and growth, unspecified humerus
  ● M89.23   Other disorders of bone development and growth, ulna and radius
    M89.231   Other disorders of bone development and growth, right ulna
    M89.232   Other disorders of bone development and growth, left ulna
    M89.233   Other disorders of bone development and growth, right radius
    M89.234   Other disorders of bone development and growth, left radius
    M89.239   Other disorders of bone development and growth, unspecified ulna and radius
  ● M89.24   Other disorders of bone development and growth, hand
    M89.241   Other disorders of bone development and growth, right hand
    M89.242   Other disorders of bone development and growth, left hand
    M89.249   Other disorders of bone development and growth, unspecified hand
  ● M89.25   Other disorders of bone development and growth, femur
    M89.251   Other disorders of bone development and growth, right femur
    M89.252   Other disorders of bone development and growth, left femur
    M89.259   Other disorders of bone development and growth, unspecified femur

● M89.26   Other disorders of bone development and growth, tibia and fibula
    M89.261   Other disorders of bone development and growth, right tibia
    M89.262   Other disorders of bone development and growth, left tibia
    M89.263   Other disorders of bone development and growth, right fibula
    M89.264   Other disorders of bone development and growth, left fibula
    M89.269   Other disorders of bone development and growth, unspecified lower leg
● M89.27   Other disorders of bone development and growth, ankle and foot
    M89.271   Other disorders of bone development and growth, right ankle and foot
    M89.272   Other disorders of bone development and growth, left ankle and foot
    M89.279   Other disorders of bone development and growth, unspecified ankle and foot
  M89.28   Other disorders of bone development and growth, other site
  M89.29   Other disorders of bone development and growth, multiple sites
● M89.3   Hypertrophy of bone
  M89.30   Hypertrophy of bone, unspecified site
  ● M89.31   Hypertrophy of bone, shoulder
    M89.311   Hypertrophy of bone, right shoulder
    M89.312   Hypertrophy of bone, left shoulder
    M89.319   Hypertrophy of bone, unspecified shoulder
  ● M89.32   Hypertrophy of bone, humerus
    M89.321   Hypertrophy of bone, right humerus
    M89.322   Hypertrophy of bone, left humerus
    M89.329   Hypertrophy of bone, unspecified humerus
  ● M89.33   Hypertrophy of bone, ulna and radius
    M89.331   Hypertrophy of bone, right ulna
    M89.332   Hypertrophy of bone, left ulna
    M89.333   Hypertrophy of bone, right radius
    M89.334   Hypertrophy of bone, left radius
    M89.339   Hypertrophy of bone, unspecified ulna and radius
  ● M89.34   Hypertrophy of bone, hand
    M89.341   Hypertrophy of bone, right hand
    M89.342   Hypertrophy of bone, left hand
    M89.349   Hypertrophy of bone, unspecified hand
  ● M89.35   Hypertrophy of bone, femur
    M89.351   Hypertrophy of bone, right femur
    M89.352   Hypertrophy of bone, left femur
    M89.359   Hypertrophy of bone, unspecified femur
  ● M89.36   Hypertrophy of bone, tibia and fibula
    M89.361   Hypertrophy of bone, right tibia
    M89.362   Hypertrophy of bone, left tibia
    M89.363   Hypertrophy of bone, right fibula
    M89.364   Hypertrophy of bone, left fibula
    M89.369   Hypertrophy of bone, unspecified tibia and fibula

▶ New   ➡ Revised   ~~deleted~~ Deleted   Excludes 1   Excludes 2   Includes   Use additional   Code first   Code also   Key words
OGCR Official Guidelines   X Assign placeholder X   ● Use Additional Character(s)   ▶ Manifestation Code   Hierarchical Condition Category   Coding Clinic

● **M89.37** Hypertrophy of bone, ankle and foot
    M89.371 Hypertrophy of bone, right ankle and foot
    M89.372 Hypertrophy of bone, left ankle and foot
    M89.379 Hypertrophy of bone, unspecified ankle and foot
  M89.38 Hypertrophy of bone, other site
  M89.39 Hypertrophy of bone, multiple sites

● **M89.4** Other hypertrophic osteoarthropathy
    Marie-Bamberger disease
    Pachydermoperiostosis
  M89.40 Other hypertrophic osteoarthropathy, unspecified site

● **M89.41** Other hypertrophic osteoarthropathy, shoulder
    M89.411 Other hypertrophic osteoarthropathy, right shoulder
    M89.412 Other hypertrophic osteoarthropathy, left shoulder
    M89.419 Other hypertrophic osteoarthropathy, unspecified shoulder

● **M89.42** Other hypertrophic osteoarthropathy, upper arm
    M89.421 Other hypertrophic osteoarthropathy, right upper arm
    M89.422 Other hypertrophic osteoarthropathy, left upper arm
    M89.429 Other hypertrophic osteoarthropathy, unspecified upper arm

● **M89.43** Other hypertrophic osteoarthropathy, forearm
    M89.431 Other hypertrophic osteoarthropathy, right forearm
    M89.432 Other hypertrophic osteoarthropathy, left forearm
    M89.439 Other hypertrophic osteoarthropathy, unspecified forearm

● **M89.44** Other hypertrophic osteoarthropathy, hand
    M89.441 Other hypertrophic osteoarthropathy, right hand
    M89.442 Other hypertrophic osteoarthropathy, left hand
    M89.449 Other hypertrophic osteoarthropathy, unspecified hand

● **M89.45** Other hypertrophic osteoarthropathy, thigh
    M89.451 Other hypertrophic osteoarthropathy, right thigh
    M89.452 Other hypertrophic osteoarthropathy, left thigh
    M89.459 Other hypertrophic osteoarthropathy, unspecified thigh

● **M89.46** Other hypertrophic osteoarthropathy, lower leg
    M89.461 Other hypertrophic osteoarthropathy, right lower leg
    M89.462 Other hypertrophic osteoarthropathy, left lower leg
    M89.469 Other hypertrophic osteoarthropathy, unspecified lower leg

● **M89.47** Other hypertrophic osteoarthropathy, ankle and foot
    M89.471 Other hypertrophic osteoarthropathy, right ankle and foot
    M89.472 Other hypertrophic osteoarthropathy, left ankle and foot
    M89.479 Other hypertrophic osteoarthropathy, unspecified ankle and foot
  M89.48 Other hypertrophic osteoarthropathy, other site
  M89.49 Other hypertrophic osteoarthropathy, multiple sites

● **M89.5** Osteolysis
    Use additional code to identify major osseous defect, if applicable (M89.7-)
    Excludes2   periprosthetic osteolysis of internal prosthetic joint (T84.05-)
  M89.50 Osteolysis, unspecified site

● **M89.51** Osteolysis, shoulder
    M89.511 Osteolysis, right shoulder
    M89.512 Osteolysis, left shoulder
    M89.519 Osteolysis, unspecified shoulder

● **M89.52** Osteolysis, upper arm
    M89.521 Osteolysis, right upper arm
    M89.522 Osteolysis, left upper arm
    M89.529 Osteolysis, unspecified upper arm

● **M89.53** Osteolysis, forearm
    M89.531 Osteolysis, right forearm
    M89.532 Osteolysis, left forearm
    M89.539 Osteolysis, unspecified forearm

● **M89.54** Osteolysis, hand
    M89.541 Osteolysis, right hand
    M89.542 Osteolysis, left hand
    M89.549 Osteolysis, unspecified hand

● **M89.55** Osteolysis, thigh
    M89.551 Osteolysis, right thigh
    M89.552 Osteolysis, left thigh
    M89.559 Osteolysis, unspecified thigh

● **M89.56** Osteolysis, lower leg
    M89.561 Osteolysis, right lower leg
    M89.562 Osteolysis, left lower leg
    M89.569 Osteolysis, unspecified lower leg

● **M89.57** Osteolysis, ankle and foot
    M89.571 Osteolysis, right ankle and foot
    M89.572 Osteolysis, left ankle and foot
    M89.579 Osteolysis, unspecified ankle and foot
  M89.58 Osteolysis, other site
  M89.59 Osteolysis, multiple sites

● **M89.6** Osteopathy after poliomyelitis
    Use additional code (B91) to identify previous poliomyelitis
    Excludes1   postpolio syndrome (G14)
  M89.60 Osteopathy after poliomyelitis, unspecified site ℞

● **M89.61** Osteopathy after poliomyelitis, shoulder
    M89.611 Osteopathy after poliomyelitis, right shoulder ℞
    M89.612 Osteopathy after poliomyelitis, left shoulder ℞
    M89.619 Osteopathy after poliomyelitis, unspecified shoulder ℞

● **M89.62** Osteopathy after poliomyelitis, upper arm
    M89.621 Osteopathy after poliomyelitis, right upper arm ℞
    M89.622 Osteopathy after poliomyelitis, left upper arm ℞
    M89.629 Osteopathy after poliomyelitis, unspecified upper arm ℞

● **M89.63** Osteopathy after poliomyelitis, forearm
    M89.631 Osteopathy after poliomyelitis, right forearm ℞
    M89.632 Osteopathy after poliomyelitis, left forearm ℞
    M89.639 Osteopathy after poliomyelitis, unspecified forearm ℞

CHAPTER 13 (M00-M99)

● **M89.64 Osteopathy after poliomyelitis, hand**
    M89.641 Osteopathy after poliomyelitis, right hand 🔴
    M89.642 Osteopathy after poliomyelitis, left hand 🔴
    M89.649 Osteopathy after poliomyelitis, unspecified hand 🔴
● **M89.65 Osteopathy after poliomyelitis, thigh**
    M89.651 Osteopathy after poliomyelitis, right thigh 🔴
    M89.652 Osteopathy after poliomyelitis, left thigh 🔴
    M89.659 Osteopathy after poliomyelitis, unspecified thigh 🔴
● **M89.66 Osteopathy after poliomyelitis, lower leg**
    M89.661 Osteopathy after poliomyelitis, right lower leg 🔴
    M89.662 Osteopathy after poliomyelitis, left lower leg 🔴
    M89.669 Osteopathy after poliomyelitis, unspecified lower leg 🔴
● **M89.67 Osteopathy after poliomyelitis, ankle and foot**
    M89.671 Osteopathy after poliomyelitis, right ankle and foot 🔴
    M89.672 Osteopathy after poliomyelitis, left ankle and foot 🔴
    M89.679 Osteopathy after poliomyelitis, unspecified ankle and foot 🔴
    M89.68 Osteopathy after poliomyelitis, other site 🔴
    M89.69 Osteopathy after poliomyelitis, multiple sites 🔴

● **M89.7 Major osseous defect**
> *Code first* underlying disease, if known, such as:
> aseptic necrosis of bone (M87.-)
> malignant neoplasm of bone (C40.-)
> osteolysis (M89.5-)
> osteomyelitis (M86.-)
> osteonecrosis (M87.-)
> osteoporosis (M80.-, M81.-)
> periprosthetic osteolysis (T84.05-)

    M89.70 Major osseous defect, unspecified site
● **M89.71 Major osseous defect, shoulder region**
    Major osseous defect clavicle or scapula
    M89.711 Major osseous defect, right shoulder region
    M89.712 Major osseous defect, left shoulder region
    M89.719 Major osseous defect, unspecified shoulder region
● **M89.72 Major osseous defect, humerus**
    M89.721 Major osseous defect, right humerus
    M89.722 Major osseous defect, left humerus
    M89.729 Major osseous defect, unspecified humerus
● **M89.73 Major osseous defect, forearm**
    Major osseous defect of radius and ulna
    M89.731 Major osseous defect, right forearm
    M89.732 Major osseous defect, left forearm
    M89.739 Major osseous defect, unspecified forearm
● **M89.74 Major osseous defect, hand**
    Major osseous defect of carpus, fingers, metacarpus
    M89.741 Major osseous defect, right hand
    M89.742 Major osseous defect, left hand
    M89.749 Major osseous defect, unspecified hand

● **M89.75 Major osseous defect, pelvic region and thigh**
    Major osseous defect of femur and pelvis
    M89.751 Major osseous defect, right pelvic region and thigh
    M89.752 Major osseous defect, left pelvic region and thigh
    M89.759 Major osseous defect, unspecified pelvic region and thigh
● **M89.76 Major osseous defect, lower leg**
    Major osseous defect of fibula and tibia
    M89.761 Major osseous defect, right lower leg
    M89.762 Major osseous defect, left lower leg
    M89.769 Major osseous defect, unspecified lower leg
● **M89.77 Major osseous defect, ankle and foot**
    Major osseous defect of metatarsus, tarsus, toes
    M89.771 Major osseous defect, right ankle and foot
    M89.772 Major osseous defect, left ankle and foot
    M89.779 Major osseous defect, unspecified ankle and foot
    M89.78 Major osseous defect, other site
    M89.79 Major osseous defect, multiple sites
● **M89.8 Other specified disorders of bone**
    Infantile cortical hyperostoses
    Post-traumatic subperiosteal ossification
    Coding Clinic: 2022, Q2, P10
● **M89.8X Other specified disorders of bone**
    M89.8X0 Other specified disorders of bone, multiple sites
    M89.8X1 Other specified disorders of bone, shoulder
    M89.8X2 Other specified disorders of bone, upper arm
    M89.8X3 Other specified disorders of bone, forearm
      Coding Clinic: 2019, Q3, P10
    M89.8X4 Other specified disorders of bone, hand
    M89.8X5 Other specified disorders of bone, thigh
    M89.8X6 Other specified disorders of bone, lower leg
    M89.8X7 Other specified disorders of bone, ankle and foot
    M89.8X8 Other specified disorders of bone, other site
      Coding Clinic: 2025, Q2, P13; 2023, Q2, P19
    M89.8X9 Other specified disorders of bone, unspecified site
    M89.9 Disorder of bone, unspecified

● **M90 Osteopathies in diseases classified elsewhere**
> **Excludes1** osteochondritis, osteomyelitis, and osteopathy (in):
> cryptococcosis (B45.3)
> diabetes mellitus (E08-E13 with .69-)
> gonococcal (A54.43)
> neurogenic syphilis (A52.11)
> renal osteodystrophy (N25.0)
> salmonellosis (A02.24)
> secondary syphilis (A51.46)
> syphilis (late) (A52.77)

● **M90.5 Osteonecrosis in diseases classified elsewhere**
> *Code first* underlying disease, such as:
> caisson disease (T70.3)
> hemoglobinopathy (D50-D64)

▶ *M90.50*   *Osteonecrosis in diseases classified elsewhere, unspecified site* 🔵

● **M90.51**   **Osteonecrosis in diseases classified elsewhere, shoulder**

    ▶ *M90.511*   *Osteonecrosis in diseases classified elsewhere, right shoulder* 🔵

    ▶ *M90.512*   *Osteonecrosis in diseases classified elsewhere, left shoulder* 🔵

    ▶ *M90.519*   *Osteonecrosis in diseases classified elsewhere, unspecified shoulder* 🔵

● **M90.52**   **Osteonecrosis in diseases classified elsewhere, upper arm**

    ▶ *M90.521*   *Osteonecrosis in diseases classified elsewhere, right upper arm* 🔵

    ▶ *M90.522*   *Osteonecrosis in diseases classified elsewhere, left upper arm* 🔵

    ▶ *M90.529*   *Osteonecrosis in diseases classified elsewhere, unspecified upper arm* 🔵

● **M90.53**   **Osteonecrosis in diseases classified elsewhere, forearm**

    ▶ *M90.531*   *Osteonecrosis in diseases classified elsewhere, right forearm* 🔵

    ▶ *M90.532*   *Osteonecrosis in diseases classified elsewhere, left forearm* 🔵

    ▶ *M90.539*   *Osteonecrosis in diseases classified elsewhere, unspecified forearm* 🔵

● **M90.54**   **Osteonecrosis in diseases classified elsewhere, hand**

    ▶ *M90.541*   *Osteonecrosis in diseases classified elsewhere, right hand* 🔵

    ▶ *M90.542*   *Osteonecrosis in diseases classified elsewhere, left hand* 🔵

    ▶ *M90.549*   *Osteonecrosis in diseases classified elsewhere, unspecified hand* 🔵

● **M90.55**   **Osteonecrosis in diseases classified elsewhere, thigh**

    ▶ *M90.551*   *Osteonecrosis in diseases classified elsewhere, right thigh* 🔵

    ▶ *M90.552*   *Osteonecrosis in diseases classified elsewhere, left thigh* 🔵

    ▶ *M90.559*   *Osteonecrosis in diseases classified elsewhere, unspecified thigh* 🔵

● **M90.56**   **Osteonecrosis in diseases classified elsewhere, lower leg**

    ▶ *M90.561*   *Osteonecrosis in diseases classified elsewhere, right lower leg* 🔵

    ▶ *M90.562*   *Osteonecrosis in diseases classified elsewhere, left lower leg* 🔵

    ▶ *M90.569*   *Osteonecrosis in diseases classified elsewhere, unspecified lower leg* 🔵

● **M90.57**   **Osteonecrosis in diseases classified elsewhere, ankle and foot**

    ▶ *M90.571*   *Osteonecrosis in diseases classified elsewhere, right ankle and foot* 🔵

    ▶ *M90.572*   *Osteonecrosis in diseases classified elsewhere, left ankle and foot* 🔵

    ▶ *M90.579*   *Osteonecrosis in diseases classified elsewhere, unspecified ankle and foot* 🔵

▶ *M90.58*   *Osteonecrosis in diseases classified elsewhere, other site* 🔵

▶ *M90.59*   *Osteonecrosis in diseases classified elsewhere, multiple sites* 🔵

● **M90.6**   **Osteitis deformans in neoplastic diseases**

   Osteitis deformans in malignant neoplasm of bone

   Code first the neoplasm (C40.-, C41.-)

   Excludes 1   osteitis deformans [Paget's disease of bone] (M88.-)

▶ *M90.60*   *Osteitis deformans in neoplastic diseases, unspecified site*

● **M90.61**   **Osteitis deformans in neoplastic diseases, shoulder**

    ▶ *M90.611*   *Osteitis deformans in neoplastic diseases, right shoulder*

    ▶ *M90.612*   *Osteitis deformans in neoplastic diseases, left shoulder*

    ▶ *M90.619*   *Osteitis deformans in neoplastic diseases, unspecified shoulder*

● **M90.62**   **Osteitis deformans in neoplastic diseases, upper arm**

    ▶ *M90.621*   *Osteitis deformans in neoplastic diseases, right upper arm*

    ▶ *M90.622*   *Osteitis deformans in neoplastic diseases, left upper arm*

    ▶ *M90.629*   *Osteitis deformans in neoplastic diseases, unspecified upper arm*

● **M90.63**   **Osteitis deformans in neoplastic diseases, forearm**

    ▶ *M90.631*   *Osteitis deformans in neoplastic diseases, right forearm*

    ▶ *M90.632*   *Osteitis deformans in neoplastic diseases, left forearm*

    ▶ *M90.639*   *Osteitis deformans in neoplastic diseases, unspecified forearm*

● **M90.64**   **Osteitis deformans in neoplastic diseases, hand**

    ▶ *M90.641*   *Osteitis deformans in neoplastic diseases, right hand*

    ▶ *M90.642*   *Osteitis deformans in neoplastic diseases, left hand*

    ▶ *M90.649*   *Osteitis deformans in neoplastic diseases, unspecified hand*

● **M90.65**   **Osteitis deformans in neoplastic diseases, thigh**

    ▶ *M90.651*   *Osteitis deformans in neoplastic diseases, right thigh*

    ▶ *M90.652*   *Osteitis deformans in neoplastic diseases, left thigh*

    ▶ *M90.659*   *Osteitis deformans in neoplastic diseases, unspecified thigh*

● **M90.66**   **Osteitis deformans in neoplastic diseases, lower leg**

    ▶ *M90.661*   *Osteitis deformans in neoplastic diseases, right lower leg*

    ▶ *M90.662*   *Osteitis deformans in neoplastic diseases, left lower leg*

    ▶ *M90.669*   *Osteitis deformans in neoplastic diseases, unspecified lower leg*

● **M90.67**   **Osteitis deformans in neoplastic diseases, ankle and foot**

    ▶ *M90.671*   *Osteitis deformans in neoplastic diseases, right ankle and foot*

    ▶ *M90.672*   *Osteitis deformans in neoplastic diseases, left ankle and foot*

    ▶ *M90.679*   *Osteitis deformans in neoplastic diseases, unspecified ankle and foot*

▶ *M90.68*   *Osteitis deformans in neoplastic diseases, other site*

▶ *M90.69*   *Osteitis deformans in neoplastic diseases, multiple sites*

● **M90.8**   **Osteopathy in diseases classified elsewhere**

   Code first underlying disease, such as:
    rickets (E55.0)
    vitamin-D-resistant rickets (E83.31)

▶ *M90.80*   *Osteopathy in diseases classified elsewhere, unspecified site*

● **M90.81**   **Osteopathy in diseases classified elsewhere, shoulder**

    ▶ *M90.811*   *Osteopathy in diseases classified elsewhere, right shoulder*

    ▶ *M90.812*   *Osteopathy in diseases classified elsewhere, left shoulder*

> *M90.819* *Osteopathy in diseases classified elsewhere, unspecified shoulder*
● M90.82 **Osteopathy in diseases classified elsewhere, upper arm**
   M90.821 *Osteopathy in diseases classified elsewhere, right upper arm*
   M90.822 *Osteopathy in diseases classified elsewhere, left upper arm*
   M90.829 *Osteopathy in diseases classified elsewhere, unspecified upper arm*
● M90.83 **Osteopathy in diseases classified elsewhere, forearm**
   M90.831 *Osteopathy in diseases classified elsewhere, right forearm*
   M90.832 *Osteopathy in diseases classified elsewhere, left forearm*
   M90.839 *Osteopathy in diseases classified elsewhere, unspecified forearm*
● M90.84 **Osteopathy in diseases classified elsewhere, hand**
   > *M90.841* *Osteopathy in diseases classified elsewhere, right hand*
   > *M90.842* *Osteopathy in diseases classified elsewhere, left hand*
   > *M90.849* *Osteopathy in diseases classified elsewhere, unspecified hand*
● M90.85 **Osteopathy in diseases classified elsewhere, thigh**
   M90.851 *Osteopathy in diseases classified elsewhere, right thigh*
   M90.852 *Osteopathy in diseases classified elsewhere, left thigh*
   M90.859 *Osteopathy in diseases classified elsewhere, unspecified thigh*
● M90.86 **Osteopathy in diseases classified elsewhere, lower leg**
   M90.861 *Osteopathy in diseases classified elsewhere, right lower leg*
   M90.862 *Osteopathy in diseases classified elsewhere, left lower leg*
   M90.869 *Osteopathy in diseases classified elsewhere, unspecified lower leg*
● M90.87 **Osteopathy in diseases classified elsewhere, ankle and foot**
   M90.871 *Osteopathy in diseases classified elsewhere, right ankle and foot*
   M90.872 *Osteopathy in diseases classified elsewhere, left ankle and foot*
   M90.879 *Osteopathy in diseases classified elsewhere, unspecified ankle and foot*
   > *M90.88* *Osteopathy in diseases classified elsewhere, other site*
   > *M90.89* *Osteopathy in diseases classified elsewhere, multiple sites*

CHONDROPATHIES (M91-M94)

Excludes1 postprocedural chondropathies (M96.-)

● M91 **Juvenile osteochondrosis of hip and pelvis**
   Excludes1 slipped upper femoral epiphysis (nontraumatic) (M93.0-)

M91.0 **Juvenile osteochondrosis of pelvis**
   Osteochondrosis (juvenile) of acetabulum
   Osteochondrosis (juvenile) of iliac crest [Buchanan]
   Osteochondrosis (juvenile) of ischiopubic synchondrosis [van Neck]
   Osteochondrosis (juvenile) of symphysis pubis [Pierson]

● M91.1 **Juvenile osteochondrosis of head of femur [Legg-Calvé-Perthes]**
   M91.10 **Juvenile osteochondrosis of head of femur [Legg-Calvé-Perthes], unspecified leg**
   M91.11 **Juvenile osteochondrosis of head of femur [Legg-Calvé-Perthes], right leg**
   M91.12 **Juvenile osteochondrosis of head of femur [Legg-Calvé-Perthes], left leg**
● M91.2 **Coxa plana**
   Hip deformity due to previous juvenile osteochondrosis
   M91.20 **Coxa plana, unspecified hip**
   M91.21 **Coxa plana, right hip**
   M91.22 **Coxa plana, left hip**
● M91.3 **Pseudocoxalgia**
   M91.30 **Pseudocoxalgia, unspecified hip**
   M91.31 **Pseudocoxalgia, right hip**
   M91.32 **Pseudocoxalgia, left hip**
● M91.4 **Coxa magna**
   M91.40 **Coxa magna, unspecified hip**
   M91.41 **Coxa magna, right hip**
   M91.42 **Coxa magna, left hip**
● M91.8 **Other juvenile osteochondrosis of hip and pelvis**
   Juvenile osteochondrosis after reduction of congenital dislocation of hip
   M91.80 **Other juvenile osteochondrosis of hip and pelvis, unspecified leg**
   M91.81 **Other juvenile osteochondrosis of hip and pelvis, right leg**
   M91.82 **Other juvenile osteochondrosis of hip and pelvis, left leg**
● M91.9 **Juvenile osteochondrosis of hip and pelvis, unspecified**
   M91.90 **Juvenile osteochondrosis of hip and pelvis, unspecified, unspecified leg**
   M91.91 **Juvenile osteochondrosis of hip and pelvis, unspecified, right leg**
   M91.92 **Juvenile osteochondrosis of hip and pelvis, unspecified, left leg**
● M92 **Other juvenile osteochondrosis**
   ● M92.0 **Juvenile osteochondrosis of humerus**
      Osteochondrosis (juvenile) of capitulum of humerus [Panner]
      Osteochondrosis (juvenile) of head of humerus [Haas]
      M92.00 **Juvenile osteochondrosis of humerus, unspecified arm**
      M92.01 **Juvenile osteochondrosis of humerus, right arm**
      M92.02 **Juvenile osteochondrosis of humerus, left arm**
   ● M92.1 **Juvenile osteochondrosis of radius and ulna**
      Osteochondrosis (juvenile) of lower ulna [Burns]
      Osteochondrosis (juvenile) of radial head [Brailsford]
      M92.10 **Juvenile osteochondrosis of radius and ulna, unspecified arm**
      M92.11 **Juvenile osteochondrosis of radius and ulna, right arm**
      M92.12 **Juvenile osteochondrosis of radius and ulna, left arm**
   ● M92.2 **Juvenile osteochondrosis, hand**
      ● M92.20 **Unspecified juvenile osteochondrosis, hand**
         M92.201 **Unspecified juvenile osteochondrosis, right hand**
         M92.202 **Unspecified juvenile osteochondrosis, left hand**
         M92.209 **Unspecified juvenile osteochondrosis, unspecified hand**

● **M92.21** Osteochondrosis (juvenile) of carpal lunate [Kienböck]

   M92.211 Osteochondrosis (juvenile) of carpal lunate [Kienböck], right hand

   M92.212 Osteochondrosis (juvenile) of carpal lunate [Kienböck], left hand

   M92.219 Osteochondrosis (juvenile) of carpal lunate [Kienböck], unspecified hand

● **M92.22** Osteochondrosis (juvenile) of metacarpal heads [Mauclaire]

   M92.221 Osteochondrosis (juvenile) of metacarpal heads [Mauclaire], right hand

   M92.222 Osteochondrosis (juvenile) of metacarpal heads [Mauclaire], left hand

   M92.229 Osteochondrosis (juvenile) of metacarpal heads [Mauclaire], unspecified hand

● **M92.29** Other juvenile osteochondrosis, hand

   M92.291 Other juvenile osteochondrosis, right hand

   M92.292 Other juvenile osteochondrosis, left hand

   M92.299 Other juvenile osteochondrosis, unspecified hand

● **M92.3** Other juvenile osteochondrosis, upper limb

   M92.30 Other juvenile osteochondrosis, unspecified upper limb

   M92.31 Other juvenile osteochondrosis, right upper limb

   M92.32 Other juvenile osteochondrosis, left upper limb

● **M92.4** Juvenile osteochondrosis of patella

   Osteochondrosis (juvenile) of primary patellar center [Köhler]

   Osteochondrosis (juvenile) of secondary patellar center [Sinding Larsen]

   M92.40 Juvenile osteochondrosis of patella, unspecified knee

   M92.41 Juvenile osteochondrosis of patella, right knee

   M92.42 Juvenile osteochondrosis of patella, left knee

● **M92.5** Juvenile osteochondrosis of tibia and fibula

  ● **M92.50** Unspecified juvenile osteochondrosis of tibia and fibula

   M92.501 Unspecified juvenile osteochondrosis, right leg

   M92.502 Unspecified juvenile osteochondrosis, left leg

   M92.503 Unspecified juvenile osteochondrosis, bilateral leg

   M92.509 Unspecified juvenile osteochondrosis, unspecified leg

  ● **M92.51** Juvenile osteochondrosis of proximal tibia

   Blount disease

   Tibia vara

   M92.511 Juvenile osteochondrosis of proximal tibia, right leg

   M92.512 Juvenile osteochondrosis of proximal tibia, left leg

   M92.513 Juvenile osteochondrosis of proximal tibia, bilateral

   M92.519 Juvenile osteochondrosis of proximal tibia, unspecified leg

  ● **M92.52** Juvenile osteochondrosis of tibia tubercle

   Osgood-Schlatter disease

   M92.521 Juvenile osteochondrosis of tibia tubercle, right leg

   M92.522 Juvenile osteochondrosis of tibia tubercle, left leg

   M92.523 Juvenile osteochondrosis of tibia tubercle, bilateral

   M92.529 Juvenile osteochondrosis of tibia tubercle, unspecified leg

  M92.59 Other juvenile osteochondrosis of tibia and fibula

   M92.591 Other juvenile osteochondrosis of tibia and fibula, right leg

   M92.592 Other juvenile osteochondrosis of tibia and fibula, left leg

   M92.593 Other juvenile osteochondrosis of tibia and fibula, bilateral

   M92.599 Other juvenile osteochondrosis of tibia and fibula, unspecified leg

● **M92.6** Juvenile osteochondrosis of tarsus

   Osteochondrosis (juvenile) of calcaneum [Sever]

   Osteochondrosis (juvenile) of os tibiale externum [Haglund]

   Osteochondrosis (juvenile) of talus [Diaz]

   Osteochondrosis (juvenile) of tarsal navicular [Köhler]

  M92.60 Juvenile osteochondrosis of tarsus, unspecified ankle

  M92.61 Juvenile osteochondrosis of tarsus, right ankle

  M92.62 Juvenile osteochondrosis of tarsus, left ankle

● **M92.7** Juvenile osteochondrosis of metatarsus

   Osteochondrosis (juvenile) of fifth metatarsus [Iselin]

   Osteochondrosis (juvenile) of second metatarsus [Freiberg]

  M92.70 Juvenile osteochondrosis of metatarsus, unspecified foot

  M92.71 Juvenile osteochondrosis of metatarsus, right foot

  M92.72 Juvenile osteochondrosis of metatarsus, left foot

M92.8 Other specified juvenile osteochondrosis

M92.9 Juvenile osteochondrosis, unspecified

   Juvenile apophysitis NOS

   Juvenile epiphysitis NOS

   Juvenile osteochondritis NOS

   Juvenile osteochondrosis NOS

● **M93** Other osteochondropathies

  Excludes2 osteochondrosis of spine (M42.-)

● **M93.0** Slipped upper femoral epiphysis (nontraumatic)

   Slipped capital femoral epiphysis (SCFE)

   Slipped upper femoral epiphysis (SUFE)

   Use additional code for associated chondrolysis (M94.3)

  ● **M93.00** Unspecified slipped upper femoral epiphysis (nontraumatic)

   M93.001 Unspecified slipped upper femoral epiphysis (nontraumatic), right hip

   M93.002 Unspecified slipped upper femoral epiphysis (nontraumatic), left hip

   M93.003 Unspecified slipped upper femoral epiphysis (nontraumatic), unspecified hip

   M93.004 Unspecified slipped upper femoral epiphysis (nontraumatic), bilateral hips

  ● **M93.01** Acute slipped upper femoral epiphysis, stable (nontraumatic)

   M93.011 Acute slipped upper femoral epiphysis, stable (nontraumatic), right hip

   M93.012 Acute slipped upper femoral epiphysis, stable (nontraumatic), left hip

M93.013 Acute slipped upper femoral epiphysis, stable (nontraumatic), unspecified hip

M93.014 Acute slipped upper femoral epiphysis, stable (nontraumatic), bilateral hips

● M93.02 Chronic slipped upper femoral epiphysis, stable (nontraumatic)

M93.021 Chronic slipped upper femoral epiphysis, stable (nontraumatic), right hip

M93.022 Chronic slipped upper femoral epiphysis, stable (nontraumatic), left hip

M93.023 Chronic slipped upper femoral epiphysis, stable (nontraumatic), unspecified hip

M93.024 Chronic slipped upper femoral epiphysis, stable (nontraumatic), bilateral hips

● M93.03 Acute on chronic slipped upper femoral epiphysis, stable (nontraumatic)

M93.031 Acute on chronic slipped upper femoral epiphysis, stable (nontraumatic), right hip

M93.032 Acute on chronic slipped upper femoral epiphysis, stable (nontraumatic), left hip

M93.033 Acute on chronic slipped upper femoral epiphysis, stable (nontraumatic), unspecified hip

M93.034 Acute on chronic slipped upper femoral epiphysis, stable (nontraumatic), bilateral hips

● M93.04 Acute slipped upper femoral epiphysis, unstable (nontraumatic)

M93.041 Acute slipped upper femoral epiphysis, unstable (nontraumatic), right hip

M93.042 Acute slipped upper femoral epiphysis, unstable (nontraumatic), left hip

M93.043 Acute slipped upper femoral epiphysis, unstable (nontraumatic), unspecified hip

M93.044 Acute slipped upper femoral epiphysis, unstable (nontraumatic), bilateral hips

● M93.05 Acute on chronic slipped upper femoral epiphysis, unstable (nontraumatic)

M93.051 Acute on chronic slipped upper femoral epiphysis, unstable (nontraumatic), right hip

M93.052 Acute on chronic slipped upper femoral epiphysis, unstable (nontraumatic), left hip

M93.053 Acute on chronic slipped upper femoral epiphysis, unstable (nontraumatic), unspecified hip

M93.054 Acute on chronic slipped upper femoral epiphysis, unstable (nontraumatic), bilateral hips

● M93.06 Acute slipped upper femoral epiphysis, unspecified stability (nontraumatic)

M93.061 Acute slipped upper femoral epiphysis, unspecified stability (nontraumatic), right hip

M93.062 Acute slipped upper femoral epiphysis, unspecified stability (nontraumatic), left hip

M93.063 Acute slipped upper femoral epiphysis, unspecified stability (nontraumatic), unspecified hip

M93.064 Acute slipped upper femoral epiphysis, unspecified stability (nontraumatic), bilateral hips

● M93.07 Acute on chronic slipped upper femoral epiphysis, unspecified stability (nontraumatic)

M93.071 Acute on chronic slipped upper femoral epiphysis, unspecified stability (nontraumatic), right hip

M93.072 Acute on chronic slipped upper femoral epiphysis, unspecified stability (nontraumatic), left hip

M93.073 Acute on chronic slipped upper femoral epiphysis, unspecified stability (nontraumatic), unspecified hip

M93.074 Acute on chronic slipped upper femoral epiphysis, unspecified stability (nontraumatic), bilateral hips

M93.1 Kienböck's disease of adults A

 Adult osteochondrosis of carpal lunates

● M93.2 Osteochondritis dissecans

M93.20 Osteochondritis dissecans of unspecified site

● M93.21 Osteochondritis dissecans of shoulder

M93.211 Osteochondritis dissecans, right shoulder

M93.212 Osteochondritis dissecans, left shoulder

M93.219 Osteochondritis dissecans, unspecified shoulder

● M93.22 Osteochondritis dissecans of elbow

M93.221 Osteochondritis dissecans, right elbow

M93.222 Osteochondritis dissecans, left elbow

M93.229 Osteochondritis dissecans, unspecified elbow

● M93.23 Osteochondritis dissecans of wrist

M93.231 Osteochondritis dissecans, right wrist

M93.232 Osteochondritis dissecans, left wrist

M93.239 Osteochondritis dissecans, unspecified wrist

● M93.24 Osteochondritis dissecans of joints of hand

M93.241 Osteochondritis dissecans, joints of right hand

M93.242 Osteochondritis dissecans, joints of left hand

M93.249 Osteochondritis dissecans, joints of unspecified hand

● M93.25 Osteochondritis dissecans of hip

M93.251 Osteochondritis dissecans, right hip

M93.252 Osteochondritis dissecans, left hip

M93.259 Osteochondritis dissecans, unspecified hip

● M93.26 Osteochondritis dissecans knee

M93.261 Osteochondritis dissecans, right knee

M93.262 Osteochondritis dissecans, left knee

M93.269 Osteochondritis dissecans, unspecified knee

● M93.27 Osteochondritis dissecans of ankle and joints of foot

M93.271 Osteochondritis dissecans, right ankle and joints of right foot

M93.272 Osteochondritis dissecans, left ankle and joints of left foot

M93.279 Osteochondritis dissecans, unspecified ankle and joints of foot

M93.28 Osteochondritis dissecans other site

M93.29 Osteochondritis dissecans multiple sites

● M93.8 Other specified osteochondropathies

M93.80 Other specified osteochondropathies of unspecified site

● M93.81 Other specified osteochondropathies of shoulder

M93.811 Other specified osteochondropathies, right shoulder

M93.812 Other specified osteochondropathies, left shoulder

M93.819 Other specified osteochondropathies, unspecified shoulder

● M93.82 Other specified osteochondropathies of upper arm

M93.821 Other specified osteochondropathies, right upper arm

M93.822 Other specified osteochondropathies, left upper arm

M93.829 Other specified osteochondropathies, unspecified upper arm

● M93.83 Other specified osteochondropathies of forearm

M93.831 Other specified osteochondropathies, right forearm

M93.832 Other specified osteochondropathies, left forearm

M93.839 Other specified osteochondropathies, unspecified forearm

● M93.84 Other specified osteochondropathies of hand

M93.841 Other specified osteochondropathies, right hand

M93.842 Other specified osteochondropathies, left hand

M93.849 Other specified osteochondropathies, unspecified hand

● M93.85 Other specified osteochondropathies of thigh

M93.851 Other specified osteochondropathies, right thigh

M93.852 Other specified osteochondropathies, left thigh

M93.859 Other specified osteochondropathies, unspecified thigh

● M93.86 Other specified osteochondropathies lower leg

M93.861 Other specified osteochondropathies, right lower leg

M93.862 Other specified osteochondropathies, left lower leg

M93.869 Other specified osteochondropathies, unspecified lower leg

● M93.87 Other specified osteochondropathies of ankle and foot

M93.871 Other specified osteochondropathies, right ankle and foot

M93.872 Other specified osteochondropathies, left ankle and foot

M93.879 Other specified osteochondropathies, unspecified ankle and foot

M93.88 Other specified osteochondropathies other

M93.89 Other specified osteochondropathies multiple sites

M93.9 Osteochondropathy, unspecified

Apophysitis NOS
Epiphysitis NOS
Osteochondritis NOS
Osteochondrosis NOS

M93.90 Osteochondropathy, unspecified of unspecified site

● M93.91 Osteochondropathy, unspecified of shoulder

M93.911 Osteochondropathy, unspecified, right shoulder

M93.912 Osteochondropathy, unspecified, left shoulder

M93.919 Osteochondropathy, unspecified, unspecified shoulder

● M93.92 Osteochondropathy, unspecified of upper arm

M93.921 Osteochondropathy, unspecified, right upper arm

M93.922 Osteochondropathy, unspecified, left upper arm

M93.929 Osteochondropathy, unspecified, unspecified upper arm

● M93.93 Osteochondropathy, unspecified of forearm

M93.931 Osteochondropathy, unspecified, right forearm

M93.932 Osteochondropathy, unspecified, left forearm

M93.939 Osteochondropathy, unspecified, unspecified forearm

● M93.94 Osteochondropathy, unspecified of hand

M93.941 Osteochondropathy, unspecified, right hand

M93.942 Osteochondropathy, unspecified, left hand

M93.949 Osteochondropathy, unspecified, unspecified hand

● M93.95 Osteochondropathy, unspecified of thigh

M93.951 Osteochondropathy, unspecified, right thigh

M93.952 Osteochondropathy, unspecified, left thigh

M93.959 Osteochondropathy, unspecified, unspecified thigh

● M93.96 Osteochondropathy, unspecified lower leg

M93.961 Osteochondropathy, unspecified, right lower leg

M93.962 Osteochondropathy, unspecified, left lower leg

M93.969 Osteochondropathy, unspecified, unspecified lower leg

● M93.97 Osteochondropathy, unspecified of ankle and foot

M93.971 Osteochondropathy, unspecified, right ankle and foot

M93.972 Osteochondropathy, unspecified, left ankle and foot

M93.979 Osteochondropathy, unspecified, unspecified ankle and foot

M93.98 Osteochondropathy, unspecified other

M93.99 Osteochondropathy, unspecified multiple sites

● M94 Other disorders of cartilage

M94.0 Chondrocostal junction syndrome [Tietze]

Costochondritis

M94.1 Relapsing polychondritis

● M94.2 Chondromalacia

Excludes1   chondromalacia patellae (M22.4)

M94.20 Chondromalacia, unspecified site

● M94.21 Chondromalacia, shoulder

M94.211 Chondromalacia, right shoulder

M94.212 Chondromalacia, left shoulder

M94.219 Chondromalacia, unspecified shoulder

● M94.22 Chondromalacia, **elbow**
   M94.221 Chondromalacia, **right** elbow
   M94.222 Chondromalacia, **left** elbow
   M94.229 Chondromalacia, **unspecified** elbow
● M94.23 Chondromalacia, **wrist**
   M94.231 Chondromalacia, **right** wrist
   M94.232 Chondromalacia, **left** wrist
   M94.239 Chondromalacia, **unspecified** wrist
● M94.24 Chondromalacia, **joints of hand**
   M94.241 Chondromalacia, joints of **right** hand
   M94.242 Chondromalacia, joints of **left** hand
   M94.249 Chondromalacia, joints of **unspecified** hand
● M94.25 Chondromalacia, **hip**
   M94.251 Chondromalacia, **right** hip
   M94.252 Chondromalacia, **left** hip
   M94.259 Chondromalacia, **unspecified** hip
● M94.26 Chondromalacia, **knee**
   M94.261 Chondromalacia, **right** knee
   M94.262 Chondromalacia, **left** knee
   M94.269 Chondromalacia, **unspecified** knee
● M94.27 Chondromalacia, **ankle and joints of foot**
   M94.271 Chondromalacia, **right** ankle and joints of right foot
   M94.272 Chondromalacia, **left** ankle and joints of left foot
   M94.279 Chondromalacia, **unspecified** ankle and joints of foot
   M94.28 Chondromalacia, **other site**
   M94.29 Chondromalacia, **multiple sites**
● M94.3 **Chondrolysis**
   Code first any associated slipped upper femoral epiphysis (nontraumatic) (M93.0-)
● M94.35 Chondrolysis, **hip**
   M94.351 Chondrolysis, **right** hip
   M94.352 Chondrolysis, **left** hip
   M94.359 Chondrolysis, **unspecified** hip
● M94.8 Other specified disorders of cartilage
  ● M94.8X Other specified disorders of **cartilage**
   M94.8X0 Other specified disorders of cartilage, **multiple sites**
   M94.8X1 Other specified disorders of cartilage, **shoulder**
   M94.8X2 Other specified disorders of cartilage, **upper arm**
   M94.8X3 Other specified disorders of cartilage, **forearm**
   M94.8X4 Other specified disorders of cartilage, **hand**
   M94.8X5 Other specified disorders of cartilage, **thigh**
   M94.8X6 Other specified disorders of cartilage, **lower leg**
   M94.8X7 Other specified disorders of cartilage, **ankle and foot**
   M94.8X8 Other specified disorders of cartilage, **other site**
   M94.8X9 Other specified disorders of cartilage, **unspecified sites**
  M94.9 Disorder of cartilage, **unspecified**

OTHER DISORDERS OF THE MUSCULOSKELETAL SYSTEM AND CONNECTIVE TISSUE (M95)

● M95 Other acquired deformities of musculoskeletal system and connective tissue
  Excludes2 acquired absence of limbs and organs (Z89-Z90)
   acquired deformities of limbs (M20-M21)
   congenital malformations and deformations of the musculoskeletal system (Q65-Q79)
   deforming dorsopathies (M40-M43)
   dentofacial anomalies [including malocclusion] (M26.-)
   postprocedural musculoskeletal disorders (M96.-)
  M95.0 Acquired deformity of **nose**
   Excludes2 deviated nasal septum (J34.2)
● M95.1 **Cauliflower ear**
   Excludes2 other acquired deformities of ear (H61.1)
   M95.10 Cauliflower ear, **unspecified ear**
   M95.11 Cauliflower ear, **right ear**
   M95.12 Cauliflower ear, **left ear**
  M95.2 Other acquired deformity of **head**
   Coding Clinic: 2023, Q1, P31
  M95.3 Acquired deformity of **neck**
  M95.4 Acquired deformity of **chest and rib**
   Coding Clinic: 2022, Q2, P14
  M95.5 Acquired deformity of **pelvis**
   Excludes1 maternal care for known or suspected disproportion (O33.-)
  M95.8 Other specified acquired deformities of musculoskeletal system
  M95.9 Acquired deformity of musculoskeletal system, unspecified

INTRAOPERATIVE AND POSTPROCEDURAL COMPLICATIONS AND DISORDERS OF MUSCULOSKELETAL SYSTEM, NOT ELSEWHERE CLASSIFIED (M96)

● M96 Intraoperative and postprocedural complications and disorders of musculoskeletal system, not elsewhere classified
  Excludes2 arthropathy following intestinal bypass (M02.0-)
   complications of internal orthopedic prosthetic devices, implants and grafts (T84.-)
   disorders associated with osteoporosis (M80)
   periprosthetic fracture around internal prosthetic joint (M97.-)
   presence of functional implants and other devices (Z96-Z97)
  M96.0 Pseudarthrosis after fusion or arthrodesis
  M96.1 Postlaminectomy syndrome, not elsewhere classified
   Coding Clinic: 2024, Q1, P18
  M96.2 Postradiation kyphosis
  M96.3 Postlaminectomy kyphosis
  M96.4 Postsurgical lordosis
  M96.5 Postradiation scoliosis
● M96.6 Fracture of bone following insertion of orthopedic implant, joint prosthesis, or bone plate
   Intraoperative fracture of bone during insertion of orthopedic implant, joint prosthesis, or bone plate
   Excludes2 complication of internal orthopedic devices, implants or grafts (T84.-)
● M96.62 Fracture of **humerus** following insertion of orthopedic implant, joint prosthesis, or bone plate
   M96.621 Fracture of humerus following insertion of orthopedic implant, joint prosthesis, or bone plate, **right arm** Ⓗ

      M96.622   Fracture of humerus following insertion of orthopedic implant, joint prosthesis, or bone plate, **left arm** ℞

      M96.629   Fracture of humerus following insertion of orthopedic implant, joint prosthesis, or bone plate, **unspecified arm** ℞

● M96.63   Fracture of radius or ulna following insertion of orthopedic implant, joint prosthesis, or bone plate

      M96.631   Fracture of radius or ulna following insertion of orthopedic implant, joint prosthesis, or bone plate, **right arm** ℞

      M96.632   Fracture of radius or ulna following insertion of orthopedic implant, joint prosthesis, or bone plate, **left arm** ℞

      M96.639   Fracture of radius or ulna following insertion of orthopedic implant, joint prosthesis, or bone plate, **unspecified arm** ℞

M96.65   Fracture of pelvis following insertion of orthopedic implant, joint prosthesis, or bone plate ℞

● M96.66   Fracture of femur following insertion of orthopedic implant, joint prosthesis, or bone plate

      M96.661   Fracture of femur following insertion of orthopedic implant, joint prosthesis, or bone plate, **right leg** ℞

      M96.662   Fracture of femur following insertion of orthopedic implant, joint prosthesis, or bone plate, **left leg** ℞

      M96.669   Fracture of femur following insertion of orthopedic implant, joint prosthesis, or bone plate, **unspecified leg** ℞

● M96.67   Fracture of tibia or fibula following insertion of orthopedic implant, joint prosthesis, or bone plate

      M96.671   Fracture of tibia or fibula following insertion of orthopedic implant, joint prosthesis, or bone plate, **right leg** ℞

      M96.672   Fracture of tibia or fibula following insertion of orthopedic implant, joint prosthesis, or bone plate, **left leg** ℞

      M96.679   Fracture of tibia or fibula following insertion of orthopedic implant, joint prosthesis, or bone plate, **unspecified leg** ℞

M96.69   Fracture of other bone following insertion of orthopedic implant, joint prosthesis, or bone plate ℞

● **M96.8**   Other intraoperative and postprocedural complications and disorders of musculoskeletal system, not elsewhere classified

      Coding Clinic: 2016, Q4, P10

● M96.81   Intraoperative hemorrhage and hematoma of a musculoskeletal structure complicating a procedure

      Excludes1   intraoperative hemorrhage and hematoma of a musculoskeletal structure due to accidental puncture and laceration during a procedure (M96.82-)

      M96.810   Intraoperative hemorrhage and hematoma of a musculoskeletal structure complicating a **musculoskeletal system procedure**

      M96.811   Intraoperative hemorrhage and hematoma of a musculoskeletal structure complicating **other procedure**

● M96.82   Accidental puncture and laceration of a musculoskeletal structure during a procedure

      M96.820   Accidental puncture and laceration of a musculoskeletal structure during a **musculoskeletal system procedure**

      M96.821   Accidental puncture and laceration of a musculoskeletal structure during **other procedure**

● M96.83   Postprocedural hemorrhage of a musculoskeletal structure following a procedure

      M96.830   Postprocedural hemorrhage of a musculoskeletal structure following a **musculoskeletal system procedure**

      M96.831   Postprocedural hemorrhage of a musculoskeletal structure following **other procedure**

● M96.84   Postprocedural hematoma and seroma of a musculoskeletal structure following a procedure

      M96.840   Postprocedural hematoma of a musculoskeletal structure following a **musculoskeletal system procedure**

      M96.841   Postprocedural hematoma of a musculoskeletal structure following **other procedure**

         Coding Clinic: 2016, Q4, P10

      M96.842   Postprocedural seroma of a musculoskeletal structure following a **musculoskeletal system procedure**

      M96.843   Postprocedural seroma of a musculoskeletal structure following **other procedure**

         Coding Clinic: 2023, Q2, P13

M96.89   Other intraoperative and postprocedural complications and disorders of the musculoskeletal system

      Instability of joint secondary to removal of joint prosthesis

      Use additional code, if applicable, to further specify disorder

      Coding Clinic: 2 2024, Q1, P18, 23; Ø23, Q2, P14; 2022, Q2, P14; 2021, Q1, P5

● **M96.A**   Fracture of ribs, sternum and thorax associated with compression of the chest and cardiopulmonary resuscitation

M96.A1   Fracture of sternum associated with chest compression and cardiopulmonary resuscitation

      Fracture of xiphoid process associated with chest compression and cardiopulmonary resuscitation

M96.A2   Fracture of one rib associated with chest compression and cardiopulmonary resuscitation

M96.A3   Multiple fractures of ribs associated with chest compression and cardiopulmonary resuscitation

      Coding Clinic: 2022, Q4, P32-33

M96.A4   Flail chest associated with chest compression and cardiopulmonary resuscitation

M96.A9   Other fracture associated with chest compression and cardiopulmonary resuscitation

CHAPTER 13 (M00-M99)

PERIPROSTHETIC FRACTURE AROUND INTERNAL PROSTHETIC JOINT (M97)

● **M97 Periprosthetic fracture around internal prosthetic joint**

Code first if known, the specific type and cause of fracture, such as traumatic or pathological

Excludes2 fracture of bone following insertion of orthopedic implant, joint prosthesis or bone plate (M96.6-)

breakage (fracture) of prosthetic joint (T84.01-)

Coding Clinic: 2016, Q4, P42

The appropriate 7th character is to be added to each code from category M97:

> A   initial encounter
> D   subsequent encounter
> S   sequela

● **M97.0 Periprosthetic fracture around internal prosthetic hip joint**

X ● M97.01 Periprosthetic fracture around internal prosthetic right hip joint 🆀
Coding Clinic: 2016, Q4, P43

X ● M97.02 Periprosthetic fracture around internal prosthetic left hip joint 🆀

● **M97.1 Periprosthetic fracture around internal prosthetic knee joint**

X ● M97.11 Periprosthetic fracture around internal prosthetic right knee joint

X ● M97.12 Periprosthetic fracture around internal prosthetic left knee joint

● **M97.2 Periprosthetic fracture around internal prosthetic ankle joint**

X ● M97.21 Periprosthetic fracture around internal prosthetic right ankle joint

X ● M97.22 Periprosthetic fracture around internal prosthetic left ankle joint

● **M97.3 Periprosthetic fracture around internal prosthetic shoulder joint**

X ● M97.31 Periprosthetic fracture around internal prosthetic right shoulder joint

X ● M97.32 Periprosthetic fracture around internal prosthetic left shoulder joint

● **M97.4 Periprosthetic fracture around internal prosthetic elbow joint**

X ● M97.41 Periprosthetic fracture around internal prosthetic right elbow joint

X ● M97.42 Periprosthetic fracture around internal prosthetic left elbow joint

X ● **M97.8 Periprosthetic fracture around other internal prosthetic joint**

Periprosthetic fracture around internal prosthetic finger joint

Periprosthetic fracture around internal prosthetic spinal joint

Periprosthetic fracture around internal prosthetic toe joint

Periprosthetic fracture around internal prosthetic wrist joint

Use additional code to identify the joint (Z96.6-)

X ● **M97.9 Periprosthetic fracture around unspecified internal prosthetic joint**

BIOMECHANICAL LESIONS, NOT ELSEWHERE CLASSIFIED (M99)

● **M99 Biomechanical lesions, not elsewhere classified**

Note: This category should not be used if the condition can be classified elsewhere.

● **M99.0 Segmental and somatic dysfunction**

M99.00 Segmental and somatic dysfunction of head region

M99.01 Segmental and somatic dysfunction of cervical region

M99.02 Segmental and somatic dysfunction of thoracic region

M99.03 Segmental and somatic dysfunction of lumbar region

M99.04 Segmental and somatic dysfunction of sacral region

M99.05 Segmental and somatic dysfunction of pelvic region

M99.06 Segmental and somatic dysfunction of lower extremity

M99.07 Segmental and somatic dysfunction of upper extremity

M99.08 Segmental and somatic dysfunction of rib cage

M99.09 Segmental and somatic dysfunction of abdomen and other regions

● **M99.1 Subluxation complex (vertebral)**

M99.10 Subluxation complex (vertebral) of head region

M99.11 Subluxation complex (vertebral) of cervical region

M99.12 Subluxation complex (vertebral) of thoracic region

M99.13 Subluxation complex (vertebral) of lumbar region

M99.14 Subluxation complex (vertebral) of sacral region

M99.15 Subluxation complex (vertebral) of pelvic region

M99.16 Subluxation complex (vertebral) of lower extremity

M99.17 Subluxation complex (vertebral) of upper extremity

M99.18 Subluxation complex (vertebral) of rib cage

M99.19 Subluxation complex (vertebral) of abdomen and other regions

● **M99.2 Subluxation stenosis of neural canal**

M99.20 Subluxation stenosis of neural canal of head region

M99.21 Subluxation stenosis of neural canal of cervical region

M99.22 Subluxation stenosis of neural canal of thoracic region

M99.23 Subluxation stenosis of neural canal of lumbar region

M99.24 Subluxation stenosis of neural canal of sacral region

M99.25 Subluxation stenosis of neural canal of pelvic region

M99.26 Subluxation stenosis of neural canal of lower extremity

M99.27 Subluxation stenosis of neural canal of upper extremity

M99.28 Subluxation stenosis of neural canal of rib cage

M99.29 Subluxation stenosis of neural canal of abdomen and other regions

● **M99.3 Osseous stenosis of neural canal**

M99.30 Osseous stenosis of neural canal of head region

M99.31 Osseous stenosis of neural canal of cervical region

M99.32 Osseous stenosis of neural canal of thoracic region

M99.33 Osseous stenosis of neural canal of lumbar region

M99.34 Osseous stenosis of neural canal of sacral region

M99.35 Osseous stenosis of neural canal of pelvic region

M99.36 Osseous stenosis of neural canal of lower extremity

M99.37 Osseous stenosis of neural canal of upper extremity

▶ New   ➡ Revised   ~~deleted~~ Deleted   Excludes 1   Excludes 2   Includes   Use additional   Code first   Code also   Key words

OGCR Official Guidelines   X Assign placeholder X   ● Use Additional Character(s)   ▶ Manifestation Code   🆀 Hierarchical Condition Category   **Coding Clinic**

M99.38   Osseous stenosis of neural canal of rib cage
M99.39   Osseous stenosis of neural canal of abdomen and other regions

● **M99.4**   Connective tissue stenosis of neural canal

M99.40   Connective tissue stenosis of neural canal of head region
M99.41   Connective tissue stenosis of neural canal of cervical region
M99.42   Connective tissue stenosis of neural canal of thoracic region
M99.43   Connective tissue stenosis of neural canal of lumbar region
M99.44   Connective tissue stenosis of neural canal of sacral region
M99.45   Connective tissue stenosis of neural canal of pelvic region
M99.46   Connective tissue stenosis of neural canal of lower extremity
M99.47   Connective tissue stenosis of neural canal of upper extremity
M99.48   Connective tissue stenosis of neural canal of rib cage
M99.49   Connective tissue stenosis of neural canal of abdomen and other regions

● **M99.5**   Intervertebral disc stenosis of neural canal

M99.50   Intervertebral disc stenosis of neural canal of head region
M99.51   Intervertebral disc stenosis of neural canal of cervical region
M99.52   Intervertebral disc stenosis of neural canal of thoracic region
M99.53   Intervertebral disc stenosis of neural canal of lumbar region
M99.54   Intervertebral disc stenosis of neural canal of sacral region
M99.55   Intervertebral disc stenosis of neural canal of pelvic region
M99.56   Intervertebral disc stenosis of neural canal of lower extremity
M99.57   Intervertebral disc stenosis of neural canal of upper extremity
M99.58   Intervertebral disc stenosis of neural canal of rib cage
M99.59   Intervertebral disc stenosis of neural canal of abdomen and other regions

● **M99.6**   Osseous and subluxation stenosis of intervertebral foramina

M99.60   Osseous and subluxation stenosis of intervertebral foramina of head region
M99.61   Osseous and subluxation stenosis of intervertebral foramina of cervical region
M99.62   Osseous and subluxation stenosis of intervertebral foramina of thoracic region
M99.63   Osseous and subluxation stenosis of intervertebral foramina of lumbar region
M99.64   Osseous and subluxation stenosis of intervertebral foramina of sacral region
M99.65   Osseous and subluxation stenosis of intervertebral foramina of pelvic region
M99.66   Osseous and subluxation stenosis of intervertebral foramina of lower extremity
M99.67   Osseous and subluxation stenosis of intervertebral foramina of upper extremity
M99.68   Osseous and subluxation stenosis of intervertebral foramina of rib cage
M99.69   Osseous and subluxation stenosis of intervertebral foramina of abdomen and other regions

● **M99.7**   Connective tissue and disc stenosis of intervertebral foramina

M99.70   Connective tissue and disc stenosis of intervertebral foramina of head region
M99.71   Connective tissue and disc stenosis of intervertebral foramina of cervical region
M99.72   Connective tissue and disc stenosis of intervertebral foramina of thoracic region
M99.73   Connective tissue and disc stenosis of intervertebral foramina of lumbar region
M99.74   Connective tissue and disc stenosis of intervertebral foramina of sacral region
M99.75   Connective tissue and disc stenosis of intervertebral foramina of pelvic region
M99.76   Connective tissue and disc stenosis of intervertebral foramina of lower extremity
M99.77   Connective tissue and disc stenosis of intervertebral foramina of upper extremity
M99.78   Connective tissue and disc stenosis of intervertebral foramina of rib cage
M99.79   Connective tissue and disc stenosis of intervertebral foramina of abdomen and other regions

● **M99.8**   Other biomechanical lesions

M99.80   Other biomechanical lesions of head region
M99.81   Other biomechanical lesions of cervical region
M99.82   Other biomechanical lesions of thoracic region
M99.83   Other biomechanical lesions of lumbar region
M99.84   Other biomechanical lesions of sacral region
M99.85   Other biomechanical lesions of pelvic region
M99.86   Other biomechanical lesions of lower extremity
M99.87   Other biomechanical lesions of upper extremity
M99.88   Other biomechanical lesions of rib cage
M99.89   Other biomechanical lesions of abdomen and other regions

M99.9   Biomechanical lesion, unspecified

CHAPTER 14

DISEASES OF THE GENITOURINARY SYSTEM (N00-N99)

OGCR Chapter-Specific Coding Guidelines

14. Chapter 14: Diseases of Genitourinary System (N00-N99)

a. Chronic kidney disease

1) Stages of chronic kidney disease (CKD)

The ICD-10-CM classifies CKD based on severity. The severity of CKD is designated by stages 1-5. Stage 2, code N18.2, equates to mild CKD; stage 3, code N18.3, equates to moderate CKD; and stage 4, code N18.4, equates to severe CKD. Code N18.6, End stage renal disease (ESRD), is assigned when the provider has documented end-stage-renal disease (ESRD).

If both a stage of CKD and ESRD are documented, assign code N18.6 only.

2) Chronic kidney disease and kidney transplant status

Patients who have undergone kidney transplant may still have some form of chronic kidney disease CKD because the kidney transplant may not fully restore kidney function. Therefore, the presence of CKD alone does not constitute a transplant complication. Assign the appropriate N18 code for the patient's stage of CKD and code Z94.0, Kidney transplant status. If a transplant complication such as failure or rejection or other transplant complication is documented, see Section I.C.19.g for information on coding complications of a kidney transplant. If the documentation is unclear as to whether the patient has a complication of the transplant, query the provider.

3) Chronic kidney disease with other conditions

Patients with CKD may also suffer from other serious conditions, most commonly diabetes mellitus and hypertension. The sequencing of the CKD code in relationship to codes for other contributing conditions is based on the conventions in the Tabular List.

See I.C.9. Hypertensive chronic kidney disease.
See I.C.19. Chronic kidney disease and kidney transplant complications.

Item 14-1 Nephritis (inflammation) or **nephropathy** (disease) **with lesion of proliferative glomerulonephritis** results from a streptococcal infection.

Nephritis (inflammation) or **nephropathy** (disease) **with lesion of membranous glomerulonephritis** is characterized by deposits along the epithelial side of the basement membrane.

Nephritis (inflammation) or **nephropathy** (disease) **with lesion of membranoproliferative glomerulonephritis** is characterized by alterations in the basement membranes of the kidney and the glomerular cells.

Nephritis (inflammation) or **nephropathy** (disease) **with lesion of rapidly progressive glomerulonephritis** is characterized by rapid and progressive decline in renal function.

Nephritis (inflammation) or **nephropathy** (disease) **with lesion of renal cortical necrosis** is characterized by death of the cortical tissues.

Nephritis (inflammation) or **nephropathy** (disease) **with lesion of renal medullary necrosis** is characterized by death of the tissues that collect urine.

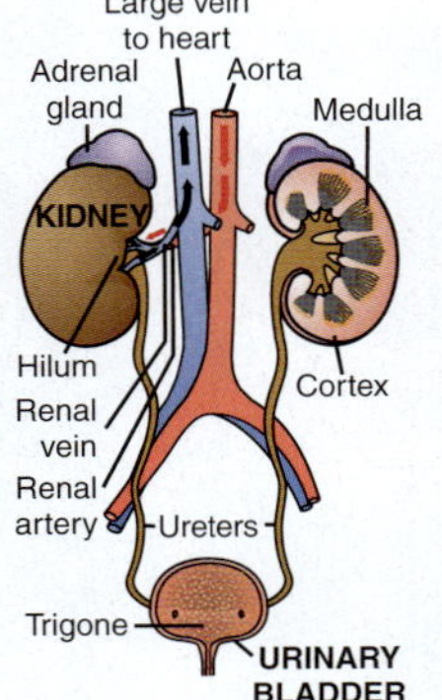

Figure 14-1 Kidneys within the urinary system.

Item 14-2 Glomerulonephritis is nephritis accompanied by inflammation of the glomeruli of the kidney, resulting in the degeneration of the glomeruli and the nephrons.

Acute glomerulonephritis primarily affects children and young adults and is usually a result of a streptococcal infection.

Proliferative glomerulonephritis is the acute form of the disease resulting from a streptococcal infection.

Rapidly progressive glomerulonephritis, also known as **crescentic** or **malignant glomerulonephritis**, is the acute form of the disease, which leads quickly to rapid and progressive decline in renal function.

CHAPTER 14

DISEASES OF THE GENITOURINARY SYSTEM (N00-N99)

Excludes2 certain conditions originating in the perinatal period (P04-P96)
certain infectious and parasitic diseases (A00-B99)
complications of pregnancy, childbirth and the puerperium (O00-O9A)
congenital malformations, deformations and chromosomal abnormalities (Q00-Q99)
endocrine, nutritional and metabolic diseases (E00-E88)
injury, poisoning and certain other consequences of external causes (S00-T88)
neoplasms (C00-D49)
symptoms, signs and abnormal clinical and laboratory findings, not elsewhere classified (R00-R94)

This chapter contains the following blocks:

N00-N08	Glomerular diseases
N10-N16	Renal tubulo-interstitial diseases
N17-N19	Acute kidney failure and chronic kidney disease
N20-N23	Urolithiasis
N25-N29	Other disorders of kidney and ureter
N30-N39	Other diseases of the urinary system
N40-N53	Diseases of male genital organs
N60-N65	Disorders of breast
N70-N77	Inflammatory diseases of female pelvic organs
N80-N98	Noninflammatory disorders of female genital tract
N99	Intraoperative and postprocedural complications and disorders of genitourinary system, not elsewhere classified

GLOMERULAR DISEASES (N00-N08)

Code also any associated kidney failure (N17-N19)

Excludes1 hypertensive chronic kidney disease (I12.-)

● **N00 Acute nephritic syndrome**

Includes acute glomerular disease
acute glomerulonephritis
acute nephritis

Excludes1 acute tubulo-interstitial nephritis (N10)
nephritic syndrome NOS (N05.-)

N00.0 Acute nephritic syndrome with minor glomerular abnormality
Acute nephritic syndrome with minimal change lesion

N00.1 Acute nephritic syndrome with focal and segmental glomerular lesions
Acute nephritic syndrome with focal and segmental hyalinosis
Acute nephritic syndrome with focal and segmental sclerosis
Acute nephritic syndrome with focal glomerulonephritis

N00.2 Acute nephritic syndrome with diffuse membranous glomerulonephritis

N00.3 Acute nephritic syndrome with diffuse mesangial proliferative glomerulonephritis

N00.4 Acute nephritic syndrome with diffuse endocapillary proliferative glomerulonephritis

▶ New ⇒ Revised ~~deleted~~ Deleted Excludes 1 Excludes 2 Includes Use additional Code first Code also Key words

 OGCR Official Guidelines X Assign placeholder X ● Use Additional Character(s) ▶ Manifestation Code 🗞 Hierarchical Condition Category **Coding Clinic**

N00.5 **Acute nephritic syndrome with diffuse mesangiocapillary glomerulonephritis**

Acute nephritic syndrome with membranoproliferative glomerulonephritis, types 1 and 3, or NOS

> **Excludes1** Acute nephritic syndrome with C3 glomerulonephritis (N00.A)
> Acute nephritic syndrome with C3 glomerulopathy (N00.A)

N00.6 **Acute nephritic syndrome with dense deposit disease**

Acute nephritic syndrome with C3 glomerulopathy with dense deposit disease

Acute nephritic syndrome with membranoproliferative glomerulonephritis, type 2

N00.7 **Acute nephritic syndrome with diffuse crescentic glomerulonephritis**

Acute nephritic syndrome with extracapillary glomerulonephritis

N00.8 **Acute nephritic syndrome with other morphologic changes**

Acute nephritic syndrome with proliferative glomerulonephritis NOS

N00.9 **Acute nephritic syndrome with unspecified morphologic changes**

N00.A **Acute nephritic syndrome with C3 glomerulonephritis**

Acute nephritic syndrome with C3 glomerulopathy, NOS

> **Excludes1** Acute nephritic syndrome (with C3 glomerulopathy) with dense deposit disease(N00.6)

● **N01** **Rapidly progressive nephritic syndrome**

> **Includes** rapidly progressive glomerular disease
> rapidly progressive glomerulonephritis
> rapidly progressive nephritis

> **Excludes1** nephritic syndrome NOS (N05.-)

N01.0 **Rapidly progressive nephritic syndrome with minor glomerular abnormality**

Rapidly progressive nephritic syndrome with minimal change lesion

N01.1 **Rapidly progressive nephritic syndrome with focal and segmental glomerular lesions**

Rapidly progressive nephritic syndrome with focal and segmental hyalinosis

Rapidly progressive nephritic syndrome with focal and segmental sclerosis

Rapidly progressive nephritic syndrome with focal glomerulonephritis

N01.2 **Rapidly progressive nephritic syndrome with diffuse membranous glomerulonephritis**

N01.3 **Rapidly progressive nephritic syndrome with diffuse mesangial proliferative glomerulonephritis**

N01.4 **Rapidly progressive nephritic syndrome with diffuse endocapillary proliferative glomerulonephritis**

N01.5 **Rapidly progressive nephritic syndrome with diffuse mesangiocapillary glomerulonephritis**

Rapidly progressive nephritic syndrome with membranoproliferative glomerulonephritis, types 1 and 3, or NOS

> **Excludes1** Rapidly progressive nephritic syndrome with C3 glomerulonephritis (N01.A)
> Rapidly progressive nephritic syndrome with C3 glomerulopathy (N01.A)

N01.6 **Rapidly progressive nephritic syndrome with dense deposit disease**

Rapidly progressive nephritic syndrome with C3 glomerulopathy with dense deposit disease

Rapidly progressive nephritic syndrome with membranoproliferative glomerulonephritis, type 2

N01.7 **Rapidly progressive nephritic syndrome with diffuse crescentic glomerulonephritis**

Rapidly progressive nephritic syndrome with extracapillary glomerulonephritis

N01.8 **Rapidly progressive nephritic syndrome with other morphologic changes**

Rapidly progressive nephritic syndrome with proliferative glomerulonephritis NOS

N01.9 **Rapidly progressive nephritic syndrome with unspecified morphologic changes**

N01.A **Rapidly progressive nephritic syndrome with C3 glomerulonephritis**

Rapidly progressive nephritic syndrome with C3 glomerulopathy, NOS

> **Excludes1** Rapidly progressive nephritic syndrome (with C3 glomerulopathy) with dense deposit disease (N01.6)

● **N02** **Recurrent and persistent hematuria**

> **Excludes1** acute cystitis with hematuria (N30.01)
> hematuria NOS (R31.9)
> hematuria not associated with specified morphologic lesions (R31.-)

N02.0 **Recurrent and persistent hematuria with minor glomerular abnormality**

Recurrent and persistent hematuria with minimal change lesion

N02.1 **Recurrent and persistent hematuria with focal and segmental glomerular lesions**

Recurrent and persistent hematuria with focal and segmental hyalinosis

Recurrent and persistent hematuria with focal and segmental sclerosis

Recurrent and persistent hematuria with focal glomerulonephritis

N02.2 **Recurrent and persistent hematuria with diffuse membranous glomerulonephritis**

N02.3 **Recurrent and persistent hematuria with diffuse mesangial proliferative glomerulonephritis**

N02.4 **Recurrent and persistent hematuria with diffuse endocapillary proliferative glomerulonephritis**

N02.5 **Recurrent and persistent hematuria with diffuse mesangiocapillary glomerulonephritis**

Recurrent and persistent hematuria with membranoproliferative glomerulonephritis, types 1 and 3, or NOS

> **Excludes1** Recurrent and persistent hematuria with C3 glomerulonephritis (N02.A)
> Recurrent and persistent hematuria with C3 glomerulopathy (N02.A)

N02.6 **Recurrent and persistent hematuria with dense deposit disease**

Recurrent and persistent hematuria with C3 glomerulopathy with dense deposit disease

Recurrent and persistent hematuria with membranoproliferative glomerulonephritis, type 2

N02.7 **Recurrent and persistent hematuria with diffuse crescentic glomerulonephritis**

Recurrent and persistent hematuria with extracapillary glomerulonephritis

N02.8 **Recurrent and persistent hematuria with other morphologic changes**

Recurrent and persistent hematuria with proliferative glomerulonephritis NOS

N02.9 **Recurrent and persistent hematuria with unspecified morphologic changes**

Coding Clinic: 2017, Q2, P5

CHAPTER 14 (N00–N99)

Item 14–3 Chronic glomerulonephritis (GN) persists over a period of years, with remissions and exacerbation.

Chronic GN with lesion of proliferative glomerulonephritis results from a streptococcal infection.

Chronic GN with lesion of membranous glomerulonephritis, also known as membranous nephropathy, is characterized by deposits along the epithelial side of the basement membrane.

Chronic GN with lesion of membrano-proliferative glomerulonephritis (MPGN) is a group of disorders characterized by alterations in the basement membranes of the kidney and the glomerular cells.

Chronic GN with lesion of rapidly progressive glomerulonephritis is characterized by necrosis, endothelial proliferation, and mesangial proliferation. The condition is marked by rapid and progressive decline in renal function.

N02.A   **Recurrent and persistent hematuria with C3 glomerulonephritis**

Recurrent and persistent hematuria with C3 glomerulopathy

> **Excludes1**   Recurrent and persistent hematuria (with C3 glomerulopathy) with dense deposit disease (N02.6)

● **N02.B**   **Recurrent and persistent immunoglobulin A nephropathy**

N02.B1   **Recurrent and persistent immunoglobulin A nephropathy with glomerular lesion**

N02.B2   **Recurrent and persistent immunoglobulin A nephropathy with focal and segmentalglomerular lesion**

Recurrent and persistent immunoglobulin A nephropathy with focal and segmentalhyalinosis or sclerosis

N02.B3   **Recurrent and persistent immunoglobulin A nephropathy with diffuse membranoproliferative glomerulonephritis**

N02.B4   **Recurrent and persistent immunoglobulin A nephropathy with diffuse membranous glomerulonephritis**

N02.B5   **Recurrent and persistent immunoglobulin A nephropathy with diffuse mesangialproliferative glomerulonephritis**

N02.B6   **Recurrent and persistent immunoglobulin A nephropathy with diffuse mesangiocapillary glomerulonephritis**

N02.B9   **Other recurrent and persistent immunoglobulin A nephropathy**

● **N03**   **Chronic nephritic syndrome**

> **Includes**   chronic glomerular disease
> chronic glomerulonephritis
> chronic nephritis

> **Excludes1**   chronic tubulo-interstitial nephritis (N11.-)
> diffuse sclerosing glomerulonephritis (N05.8-)
> nephritic syndrome NOS (N05.-)

N03.0   **Chronic nephritic syndrome with minor glomerular abnormality**

Chronic nephritic syndrome with minimal change lesion

N03.1   **Chronic nephritic syndrome with focal and segmental glomerular lesions**

Chronic nephritic syndrome with focal and segmental hyalinosis

Chronic nephritic syndrome with focal and segmental sclerosis

Chronic nephritic syndrome with focal glomerulonephritis

N03.2   **Chronic nephritic syndrome with diffuse membranous glomerulonephritis**

N03.3   **Chronic nephritic syndrome with diffuse mesangial proliferative glomerulonephritis**

N03.4   **Chronic nephritic syndrome with diffuse endocapillary proliferative glomerulonephritis**

N03.5   **Chronic nephritic syndrome with diffuse mesangiocapillary glomerulonephritis**

Chronic nephritic syndrome with membranoproliferative glomerulonephritis, types 1 and 3, or NOS

> **Excludes1**   Chronic nephritic syndrome with C3 glomerulonephritis (N03.A)
> Chronic nephritic syndrome with C3 glomerulopathy (N03.A)

N03.6   **Chronic nephritic syndrome with dense deposit disease**

Chronic nephritic syndrome with C3 glomerulopathy with dense deposit disease

Chronic nephritic syndrome with membranoproliferative glomerulonephritis, type 2

N03.7   **Chronic nephritic syndrome with diffuse crescentic glomerulonephritis**

Chronic nephritic syndrome with extracapillary glomerulonephritis

N03.8   **Chronic nephritic syndrome with other morphologic changes**

Chronic nephritic syndrome with proliferative glomerulonephritis NOS

N03.9   **Chronic nephritic syndrome with unspecified morphologic changes**

N03.A   **Chronic nephritic syndrome with C3 glomerulonephritis**

Chronic nephritic syndrome with C3 glomerulopathy

> **Excludes1**   Chronic nephritic syndrome (with C3 glomerulopathy) with dense deposit disease(N03.6)

● **N04**   **Nephrotic syndrome**

> **Includes**   congenital nephrotic syndrome
> lipoid nephrosis

N04.0   **Nephrotic syndrome with minor glomerular abnormality**

Nephrotic syndrome with minimal change lesion

Coding Clinic: 2024, Q3, P15

N04.1   **Nephrotic syndrome with focal and segmental glomerular lesions**

Nephrotic syndrome with focal and segmental hyalinosis

Nephrotic syndrome with focal and segmental sclerosis

Nephrotic syndrome with focal glomerulonephritis

● **N04.2**   **Nephrotic syndrome with diffuse membranous glomerulonephritis**

N04.20   **Nephrotic syndrome with diffuse membranous glomerulonephritis, unspecified**

Membranous nephropathy NOS with nephrotic syndrome

N04.21   **Primary membranous nephropathy with nephrotic syndrome**

Idiopathic membranous nephropathy with nephrotic syndrome

N04.22   **Secondary membranous nephropathy with nephrotic syndrome**

> *Code first, if applicable, other disease or disorder or poisoning causing membranous nephropathy*

> Use Additional code, if applicable, for adverse effect of drug causing membranous nephropathy

N04.29   **Other nephrotic syndrome with diffuse membranous glomerulonephritis**

N04.3   **Nephrotic syndrome with diffuse mesangial proliferative glomerulonephritis**

N04.4   **Nephrotic syndrome with diffuse endocapillary proliferative glomerulonephritis**

N04.5   **Nephrotic syndrome with diffuse mesangiocapillary glomerulonephritis**

~~Nephrotic syndrome with membranoproliferative glomerulonephritis, types 1 and 3, or NOS~~

> **Excludes1**   Nephrotic syndrome with C3 glomerulonephritis (N04.A)
> Nephrotic syndrome with C3 glomerulopathy (N04.A)

▶ New   ▬▶ Revised   ~~deleted~~ Deleted   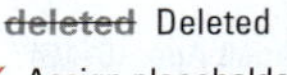 Excludes 1   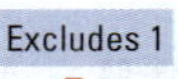 Excludes 2   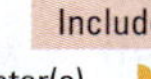 Includes   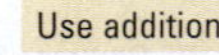 Use additional   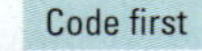 Code first   Code also   Key words

OGCR Official Guidelines   **X** Assign placeholder X   ● Use Additional Character(s)   ▸ Manifestation Code   🔖 Hierarchical Condition Category   **Coding Clinic**

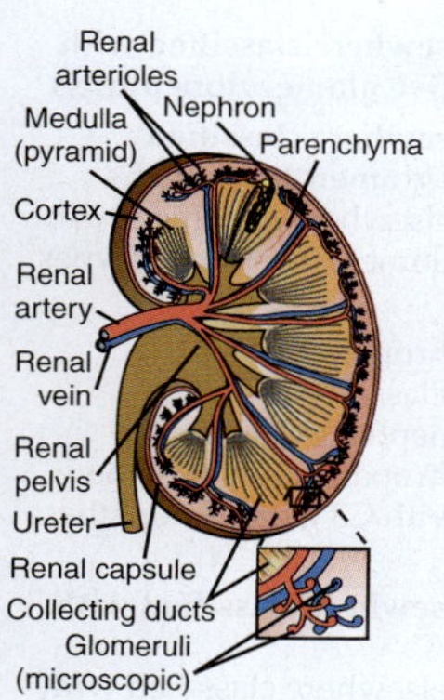

Figure 14-2 Kidney cross section.

Item 14–4 Nephrotic syndrome (NS) is marked by massive proteinuria (protein in the urine) and water retention. Patients with NS are particularly vulnerable to staphylococcal and pneumococcal infections. NS with lesion of proliferative glomerulonephritis results from a streptococcal infection. NS with lesion of membranous glomerulonephritis results in thickening of the capillary walls. NS with lesion of minimal change glomerulonephritis is usually a benign disorder that occurs mostly in children and requires electron microscopy (biopsy) to verify changes in the glomeruli.

N04.6   **Nephrotic syndrome with dense deposit disease**
> Nephrotic syndrome with C3 glomerulopathy with dense deposit disease
> Nephrotic syndrome with membranoproliferative glomerulonephritis, type 2

N04.7   **Nephrotic syndrome with diffuse crescentic glomerulonephritis**
> Nephrotic syndrome with extracapillary glomerulonephritis

N04.8   **Nephrotic syndrome with other morphologic changes**
> Nephrotic syndrome with proliferative glomerulonephritis NOS

N04.9   **Nephrotic syndrome with unspecified morphologic changes**

N04.A   **Nephrotic syndrome with C3 glomerulonephritis**
> Nephrotic syndrome with C3 glomerulopathy
>> **Excludes1**   Nephrotic syndrome (with C3 glomerulopathy) with dense deposit disease (N04.6)

▶ ● **N00.B**   **Acute nephritic syndrome with immune complex membranoproliferative glomerulonephritis**

  ▶ **N00.B1**   **Acute nephritic syndrome with idiopathic immune membranoproliferative glomerulonephritis (IC-MPGN)**

  ▶ **N00.B2**   **Acute nephritic syndrome with secondary immune complex membranoproliferative glomerulonephritis (IC-MPGN)**

● **N05**   **Unspecified nephritic syndrome**
> **Includes**   glomerular disease NOS
> glomerulonephritis NOS
> nephritis NOS
> nephropathy NOS and renal disease NOS with morphological lesion specified in .0-.8
>
> **Excludes1**   nephropathy NOS with no stated morphological lesion (N28.9)
> renal disease NOS with no stated morphological lesion (N28.9)
> tubulo-interstitial nephritis NOS (N12)

N05.0   **Unspecified nephritic syndrome with minor glomerular abnormality**
> Unspecified nephritic syndrome with minimal change lesion

N05.1   **Unspecified nephritic syndrome with focal and segmental glomerular lesions**
> Unspecified nephritic syndrome with focal and segmental hyalinosis
> Unspecified nephritic syndrome with focal and segmental sclerosis
> Unspecified nephritic syndrome with focal glomerulonephritis

N05.2   **Unspecified nephritic syndrome with diffuse membranous glomerulonephritis**

N05.3   **Unspecified nephritic syndrome with diffuse mesangial proliferative glomerulonephritis**

N05.4   **Unspecified nephritic syndrome with diffuse endocapillary proliferative glomerulonephritis**

N05.5   **Unspecified nephritic syndrome with diffuse mesangiocapillary glomerulonephritis**
> Unspecified nephritic syndrome with membranoproliferative glomerulonephritis, types 1 and 3, or NOS
>> **Excludes1**   Unspecified nephritic syndrome with C3 glomerulonephritis (N05.A)
>> Unspecified nephritic syndrome with C3 glomerulopathy (N05.A)

N05.6   **Unspecified nephritic syndrome with dense deposit disease**
> Unspecified nephritic syndrome with C3 glomerulopathy with dense deposit disease
> Unspecified nephritic syndrome with membranoproliferative glomerulonephritis, type 2

N05.7   **Unspecified nephritic syndrome with diffuse crescentic glomerulonephritis**
> Unspecified nephritic syndrome with extracapillary glomerulonephritis

N05.8   **Unspecified nephritic syndrome with other morphologic changes**
> Unspecified nephritic syndrome with proliferative glomerulonephritis NOS

N05.9   **Unspecified nephritic syndrome with unspecified morphologic changes**

N05.A   **Unspecified nephritic syndrome with C3 glomerulonephritis**
> Unspecified nephritic syndrome with C3 glomerulopathy
>> **Excludes1**   Unspecified nephritic syndrome (with C3 glomerulopathy) with dense deposit disease(N05.6)

● **N06**   **Isolated proteinuria with specified morphological lesion**
> **Excludes1**   proteinuria not associated with specific morphologic lesions (R80.0)

N06.0   **Isolated proteinuria with minor glomerular abnormality**
> Isolated proteinuria with minimal change lesion

N06.1   **Isolated proteinuria with focal and segmental glomerular lesions**
> Isolated proteinuria with focal and segmental hyalinosis
> Isolated proteinuria with focal and segmental sclerosis
> Isolated proteinuria with focal glomerulonephritis

N06.2   **Isolated proteinuria with diffuse membranous glomerulonephritis**

  ● **N06.20**   **Isolated proteinuria with diffuse membranous glomerulonephritis, unspecified**
> Membranous nephropathy, NOS
>> **Excludes1**   membranous nephropathy NOS with nephrotic syndrome (N04.20)

  N06.21   **Primary membranous nephropathy with isolated proteinuria**
> Idiopathic membranous nephropathy (with isolated proteinuria)
> Primary membranous nephropathy, NOS
>> **Excludes1**   primary membranous nephropathy with nephrotic syndrome (N04.21)

CHAPTER 14 (N00-N99)

N06.22 Secondary membranous nephropathy with isolated proteinuria
Secondary membranous nephropathy, NOS
Code first, if applicable, other disease or disorder or poisoning causing membranous nephropathy
Use Additional code, if applicable, for adverse effect of drug causing membranous nephropathy
Excludes1 secondary membranous nephropathy with nephrotic syndrome (N04.22)

N06.29 Other isolated proteinuria with diffuse membranous glomerulonephritis

N06.3 Isolated proteinuria with diffuse mesangial proliferative glomerulonephritis

N06.4 Isolated proteinuria with diffuse endocapillary proliferative glomerulonephritis

N06.5 Isolated proteinuria with diffuse mesangiocapillary glomerulonephritis
Isolated proteinuria with membranoproliferative glomerulonephritis, types 1 and 3, or NOS
Excludes1 Isolated proteinuria with C3 glomerulonephritis (N06.A)
Isolated proteinuria with C3 glomerulopathy (N06.A)

N06.6 Isolated proteinuria with dense deposit disease
Isolated proteinuria with C3 glomerulopathy with dense deposit disease
Isolated proteinuria with membranoproliferative glomerulonephritis, type 2

N06.7 Isolated proteinuria with diffuse crescentic glomerulonephritis
Isolated proteinuria with extracapillary glomerulonephritis

N06.8 Isolated proteinuria with other morphologic lesion
Isolated proteinuria with proliferative glomerulonephritis NOS

N06.9 Isolated proteinuria with unspecified morphologic lesion

N06.A Isolated proteinuria with C3 glomerulonephritis
Isolated proteinuria with C3 glomerulopathy
Excludes1 Isolated proteinuria (with C3 glomerulopathy) with dense deposit disease (N06.6)

● **N07 Hereditary nephropathy, not elsewhere classified**
Excludes2 Alport's syndrome (Q87.81-)
hereditary amyloid nephropathy (E85.-)
nail patella syndrome (Q87.2)
non-neuropathic heredofamilial amyloidosis (E85.-)

N07.0 Hereditary nephropathy, not elsewhere classified with minor glomerular abnormality
Hereditary nephropathy, not elsewhere classified with minimal change lesion

N07.1 Hereditary nephropathy, not elsewhere classified with focal and segmental glomerular lesions
Hereditary nephropathy, not elsewhere classified with focal and segmental hyalinosis
Hereditary nephropathy, not elsewhere classified with focal and segmental sclerosis
Hereditary nephropathy, not elsewhere classified with focal glomerulonephritis

N07.2 Hereditary nephropathy, not elsewhere classified with diffuse membranous glomerulonephritis

N07.3 Hereditary nephropathy, not elsewhere classified with diffuse mesangial proliferative glomerulonephritis

N07.4 Hereditary nephropathy, not elsewhere classified with diffuse endocapillary proliferative glomerulonephritis

N07.5 Hereditary nephropathy, not elsewhere classified with diffuse mesangiocapillary glomerulonephritis
Hereditary nephropathy, not elsewhere classified with membranoproliferative glomerulonephritis, types 1 and 3, or NOS
Excludes1 Hereditary nephropathy, not elsewhere classified with C3 glomerulonephritis (N07.A)
Hereditary nephropathy, not elsewhere classified with C3 glomerulopathy (N07.A)

N07.6 Hereditary nephropathy, not elsewhere classified with dense deposit disease
Hereditary nephropathy, not elsewhere classified with C3 glomerulopathy with dense deposit disease
Hereditary nephropathy, not elsewhere classified with membranoproliferative glomerulonephritis, type 2

N07.7 Hereditary nephropathy, not elsewhere classified with diffuse crescentic glomerulonephritis
Hereditary nephropathy, not elsewhere classified with extracapillary glomerulonephritis

N07.8 Hereditary nephropathy, not elsewhere classified with other morphologic lesions
Hereditary nephropathy, not elsewhere classified with proliferative glomerulonephritis NOS

N07.9 Hereditary nephropathy, not elsewhere classified with unspecified morphologic lesions

N07.A Hereditary nephropathy, not elsewhere classified with C3 glomerulonephritis
Hereditary nephropathy, not elsewhere classified with C3 glomerulopathy
Excludes1 Hereditary nephropathy, not elsewhere classified (with C3 glomerulopathy) with dense deposit disease (N07.6)

▶ **N07.B Hereditary nephropathy, not elsewhere classified with APOL1-mediated kidney disease [AMKD]**
AMKD (with glomerulonephritis)
AMKD (with glomerulosclerosis)

N08 Glomerular disorders in diseases classified elsewhere
Glomerulonephritis
Nephritis
Nephropathy
Code first underlying disease, such as:
amyloidosis (E85.-)
congenital syphilis (A50.5)
cryoglobulinemia (D89.1)
disseminated intravascular coagulation (D65)
gout (M1A.-, M10.-)
microscopic polyangiitis (M31.7)
multiple myeloma (C90.0-)
sepsis (A40.0-A41.9)
sickle-cell disease (D57.0-D57.8)
Excludes1 glomerulonephritis, nephritis and nephropathy (in):
antiglomerular basement membrane disease (M31.0)
diabetes (E08-E13 with .21)
gonococcal (A54.21)
Goodpasture's syndrome (M31.0)
hemolytic-uremic syndrome (D59.3)
lupus (M32.14)
mumps (B26.83)
syphilis (A52.75)
systemic lupus erythematosus (M32.14)
Wegener's granulomatosis (M31.31)
pyelonephritis in diseases classified elsewhere (N16)
renal tubulo-interstitial disorders classified elsewhere (N16)

▶ New   ⇨ Revised   ~~deleted~~ Deleted   **Excludes 1**   **Excludes 2**   Includes   Use additional   Code first   Code also   Key words
OGCR Official Guidelines   **X** Assign placeholder X   ● Use Additional Character(s)   ▶ Manifestation Code   Ⓡ Hierarchical Condition Category   **Coding Clinic**

RENAL TUBULO-INTERSTITIAL DISEASES (N10-N16)

Includes   pyelonephritis
Excludes1   pyelou26reteritis cystica (N28.85)

N10   **Acute pyelonephritis**
Acute infectious interstitial nephritis
Acute pyelitis
Acute tubulo-interstitial nephritis
Hemoglobin nephrosis
Myoglobin nephrosis
Use additional code (B95-B97), to identify infectious agent
Coding Clinic: 2019, Q3, P13-14

● **N11**   **Chronic tubulo-interstitial nephritis**
Includes   chronic infectious interstitial nephritis
chronic pyelitis
chronic pyelonephritis
Use additional code (B95-B97), to identify infectious agent

N11.0   **Nonobstructive reflux-associated chronic pyelonephritis**
Pyelonephritis (chronic) associated with (vesicoureteral) reflux
Excludes1   vesicoureteral reflux NOS (N13.70)

N11.1   **Chronic obstructive pyelonephritis**
Pyelonephritis (chronic) associated with anomaly of pelviureteric junction
Pyelonephritis (chronic) associated with anomaly of pyelouereteric junction
Pyelonephritis (chronic) associated with crossing of vessel
Pyelonephritis (chronic) associated with kinking of ureter
Pyelonephritis (chronic) associated with obstruction of ureter
Pyelonephritis (chronic) associated with stricture of pelviureteric junction
Pyelonephritis (chronic) associated with stricture of ureter
Excludes1   calculous pyelonephritis (N20.9)
obstructive uropathy (N13.-)

N11.8   **Other chronic tubulo-interstitial nephritis**
Nonobstructive chronic pyelonephritis NOS

N11.9   **Chronic tubulo-interstitial nephritis, unspecified**
Chronic interstitial nephritis NOS
Chronic pyelitis NOS
Chronic pyelonephritis NOS

N12   **Tubulo-interstitial nephritis, not specified as acute or chronic**
Interstitial nephritis NOS
Pyelitis NOS
Pyelonephritis NOS
Excludes1   calculous pyelonephritis (N20.9)

● **N13**   **Obstructive and reflux uropathy**
Excludes2   calculus of kidney and ureter without hydronephrosis (N20.-)
congenital obstructive defects of renal pelvis and ureter (Q62.0-Q62.3)
hydronephrosis with ureteropelvic junction obstruction (Q62.11)
obstructive pyelonephritis (N11.1)

Item 14–5 Pyelonephritis is an infection of the kidneys and ureters and may be chronic or acute in one or both kidneys.

N13.0   **Hydronephrosis with ureteropelvic junction obstruction**
Hydronephrosis due to acquired occlusion of ureteropelvic junction
Excludes2   Hydronephrosis with ureteropelvic junction obstruction due to calculus (N13.2)
Coding Clinic: 2016, Q4, P43

N13.1   **Hydronephrosis with ureteral stricture, not elsewhere classified**
Excludes1   hydronephrosis with ureteral stricture with infection (N13.6)

N13.2   **Hydronephrosis with renal and ureteral calculous obstruction**
Excludes1   hydronephrosis with renal and ureteral calculous obstruction with infection (N13.6)

● **N13.3**   **Other and unspecified hydronephrosis**
Excludes1   hydronephrosis with infection (N13.6)
N13.30   **Unspecified hydronephrosis**
N13.39   **Other hydronephrosis**

N13.4   **Hydroureter**
Excludes1   congenital hydroureter (Q62.3-)
hydroureter with infection (N13.6)
vesicoureteral-reflux with hydroureter (N13.73-)

N13.5   **Crossing vessel and stricture of ureter without hydronephrosis**
Kinking and stricture of ureter without hydronephrosis
Excludes1   crossing vessel and stricture of ureter without hydronephrosis with infection (N13.6)
Coding Clinic: 2016, Q4, P43

N13.6   **Pyonephrosis**
Conditions in N13.0-N13.5 with infection
Obstructive uropathy with infection
Use additional code (B95-B97), to identify infectious agent
Coding Clinic: 2018, Q2, P21

● **N13.7**   **Vesicoureteral-reflux**
Excludes1   reflux-associated pyelonephritis (N11.0)
N13.70   **Vesicoureteral-reflux, unspecified**
Occurs when urine flows from bladder back into ureters
Vesicoureteral-reflux NOS
N13.71   **Vesicoureteral-reflux without reflux nephropathy**

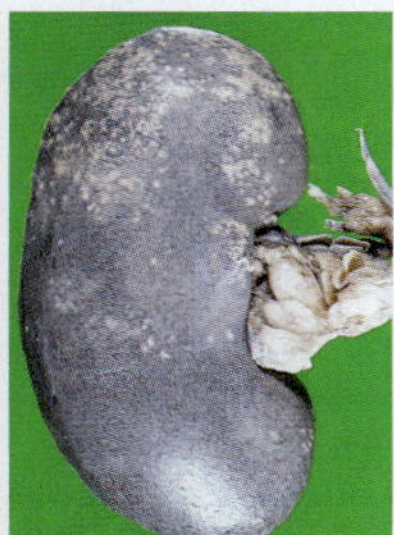

Figure 14-3   Acute pyelonephritis. Cortical surface exhibits grayish white areas of inflammation and abscess formation. (From Frazier MS, Drzymkowski JW: Essentials of Human Diseases and Conditions, St. Louis, Saunders/Elsevier, 2009)

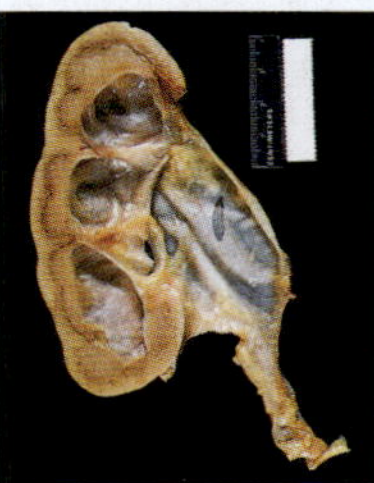

Figure 14-4   Hydronephrosis of the kidney, with marked dilatation of pelvis and calyces and thinning of renal parenchyma. (From Kumar: Robbins and Cotran: Pathologic Basis of Disease, ed 8, Saunders, An Imprint of Elsevier, 2009)

● **N13.72**   **Vesicoureteral-reflux with reflux nephropathy without hydroureter**

    N13.721   **Vesicoureteral-reflux with reflux nephropathy without hydroureter, unilateral**

    N13.722   **Vesicoureteral-reflux with reflux nephropathy without hydroureter, bilateral**

    N13.729   **Vesicoureteral-reflux with reflux nephropathy without hydroureter, unspecified**

● **N13.73**   **Vesicoureteral-reflux with reflux nephropathy with hydroureter**

    N13.731   **Vesicoureteral-reflux with reflux nephropathy with hydroureter, unilateral**

    N13.732   **Vesicoureteral-reflux with reflux nephropathy with hydroureter, bilateral**

    N13.739   **Vesicoureteral-reflux with reflux nephropathy with hydroureter, unspecified**

N13.8   **Other obstructive and reflux uropathy**
Urinary tract obstruction due to specified cause

    Code first, if applicable, any causal condition first, such as:
    enlarged prostate (N40.1)

N13.9   **Obstructive and reflux uropathy, unspecified**
Urinary tract obstruction NOS

● **N14**   **Drug- and heavy-metal-induced tubulo-interstitial and tubular conditions**

    Code first poisoning due to drug or toxin, if applicable (T36-T65 with fifth or sixth character 1-4)

    Use additional code for adverse effect, if applicable, to identify drug (T36-T50 with fifth or sixth character 5)

N14.0   **Analgesic nephropathy**

● **N14.1**   **Nephropathy induced by other drugs, medicaments and biological substances**
    Coding Clinic: 2021, Q3, P9-10

    N14.11   **Contrast-induced nephropathy**
      Contrast medium, radiography nephropathy

      Excludes2   acute kidney failure (N17.-)
      Coding Clinic: 2022, Q4, P33

    N14.19   **Nephropathy induced by other drugs, medicaments and biological substances**

N14.2   **Nephropathy induced by unspecified drug, medicament or biological substance**

N14.3   **Nephropathy induced by heavy metals**

N14.4   **Toxic nephropathy, not elsewhere classified**

● **N15**   **Other renal tubulo-interstitial diseases**

N15.0   **Balkan nephropathy**
Balkan endemic nephropathy

N15.1   **Renal and perinephric abscess**

N15.8   **Other specified renal tubulo-interstitial diseases**

N15.9   **Renal tubulo-interstitial disease, unspecified**
Infection of kidney NOS

    Excludes1   urinary tract infection NOS (N39.0)

N16   **Renal tubulo-interstitial disorders in diseases classified elsewhere**
Pyelonephritis
Tubulo-interstitial nephritis

    Code first underlying disease, such as:
    brucellosis (A23.0-A23.9)
    cryoglobulinemia (D89.1)
    glycogen storage disease (E74.0-)
    leukemia (C91-C95)
    lymphoma (C81-C85.9, C96.0-C96.9)
    multiple myeloma (C90.0-)
    sepsis (A40.0-A41.9)
    Wilson's disease (E83.01)

    Excludes1   diphtheritic pyelonephritis and tubulo-interstitial nephritis (A36.84)
      pyelonephritis and tubulo-interstitial nephritis in candidiasis (B37.49)
      pyelonephritis and tubulo-interstitial nephritis in cystinosis (E72.04)
      pyelonephritis and tubulo-interstitial nephritis in salmonella infection (A02.25)
      pyelonephritis and tubulo-interstitial nephritis in sarcoidosis (D86.84)
      pyelonephritis and tubulo-interstitial nephritis in Sjögren syndrome (M35.04)
      pyelonephritis and tubulo-interstitial nephritis in systemic lupus erythematosus (M32.15)
      pyelonephritis and tubulo-interstitial nephritis in toxoplasmosis (B58.83)
      renal tubular degeneration in diabetes (E08-E13 with .29)
      syphilitic pyelonephritis and tubulo-interstitial nephritis (A52.75)

ACUTE KIDNEY FAILURE AND CHRONIC KIDNEY DISEASE (N17-N19)

    Excludes2   congenital renal failure (P96.0)
      drug- and heavy-metal-induced tubulo-interstitial and tubular conditions (N14.-)
      extrarenal uremia (R39.2)
      hemolytic-uremic syndrome (D59.3-)
      hepatorenal syndrome (K76.7)
      postpartum hepatorenal syndrome (O90.41)
      posttraumatic renal failure (T79.5)
      prerenal uremia (R39.2)
      renal failure complicating abortion or ectopic or molar pregnancy (O00-O07, O08.4)
      renal failure following labor and delivery (O90.41)
      renal failure postprocedural (N99.0)

● **N17**   **Acute kidney failure**

    Code also associated underlying condition

    Excludes1   posttraumatic renal failure (T79.5)
    Coding Clinic: 2025, Q1, P26

N17.0   **Acute kidney failure with tubular necrosis** Ⓗcc
Acute tubular necrosis
Renal tubular necrosis
Tubular necrosis NOS
Coding Clinic: 2024, Q3, P15; 2022, Q4, P33 ; 2021, Q3, P10

N17.1   **Acute kidney failure with acute cortical necrosis** Ⓗcc
Acute cortical necrosis
Cortical necrosis NOS
Renal cortical necrosis

N17.2   **Acute kidney failure with medullary necrosis** Ⓗcc
Medullary [papillary] necrosis NOS
Acute medullary [papillary] necrosis
Renal medullary [papillary] necrosis

N17.8   **Other acute kidney failure** Ⓗcc
Coding Clinic: 2025, Q1, P26-27

N17.9   **Acute kidney failure, unspecified** Ⓗcc
Acute kidney injury (nontraumatic)

    Excludes2   traumatic kidney injury (S37.0-)

    Coding Clinic: 2023, Q3, P5; 2019, Q2, P7,25

▶ New   ⇨ Revised   ~~deleted~~ Deleted   Excludes 1   Excludes 2   Includes   Use additional   Code first   Code also   Key words
OGCR Official Guidelines   X Assign placeholder X   ● Use Additional Character(s)   ▶ Manifestation Code   Ⓗcc Hierarchical Condition Category   **Coding Clinic**

Item 14–6 Decreased blood flow is the usual cause of **acute renal failure** that offers a good prognosis for recovery.
  Chronic renal failure is usually the result of long-standing kidney disease and is a very serious condition that generally results in death.

● **N18** **Chronic kidney disease (CKD)**
  Code first any associated:
    diabetic chronic kidney disease (E08.22, E09.22, E10.22, E11.22, E13.22)
    hypertensive chronic kidney disease (I12.-, I13.-)
  Use additional code to identify kidney transplant status, if applicable, (Z94.0)
  Coding Clinic: 2018, Q4, P89; 2016, Q4, P123

  N18.1 **Chronic kidney disease, stage 1**
  N18.2 **Chronic kidney disease, stage 2 (mild)**
● **N18.3** **Chronic kidney disease, stage 3 (moderate)**
    Coding Clinic: 2022, Q4, P6

    N18.30 **Chronic kidney disease, stage 3 unspecified**
    N18.31 **Chronic kidney disease, stage 3a**
        Coding Clinic: 2025, Q2, P8
    N18.32 **Chronic kidney disease, stage 3b**
  N18.4 **Chronic kidney disease, stage 4 (severe)** 🔣
      Coding Clinic: 2023, Q1, P18; 2022, Q4, P14; 2013, Q1, P24
  N18.5 **Chronic kidney disease, stage 5** 🔣
      Excludes1 chronic kidney disease, stage 5 requiring chronic dialysis (N18.6)
  N18.6 **End stage renal disease** 🔣
      Chronic kidney disease requiring chronic dialysis
      Use additional code to identify dialysis status (Z99.2)
      Coding Clinic: 2022, Q3, P16; 2016, Q3, P23, Q1, P13
  N18.9 **Chronic kidney disease, unspecified**
      Chronic renal disease
      Chronic renal failure NOS
      Chronic renal insufficiency
      Chronic uremia NOS
      Diffuse sclerosing glomerulonephritis NOS
      Coding Clinic: 2018, Q4, P88

  N19 **Unspecified kidney failure**
      Uremia NOS
      Excludes1 acute kidney failure (N17.-)
        chronic kidney disease (N18.-)
        chronic uremia (N18.9)
        extrarenal uremia (R39.2)
        prerenal uremia (R39.2)
        renal insufficiency (acute) (N28.9)
        uremia of newborn (P96.0)

UROLITHIASIS (N20-N23)

● **N20** **Calculus of kidney and ureter**
      Calculous pyelonephritis
      Excludes1 nephrocalcinosis (E83.59)
        that with hydronephrosis (N13.2)
      Coding Clinic: 2019, Q3, P14

  N20.0 **Calculus of kidney**
      Nephrolithiasis NOS   Staghorn calculus
      Renal calculus   Stone in kidney
      Renal stone
      Coding Clinic: 2019, Q3, P13; 2017, Q1, P5
  N20.1 **Calculus of ureter**
      Calculus of the ureteropelvic junction
      Ureteric stone
      Coding Clinic: 2016, Q3, P24

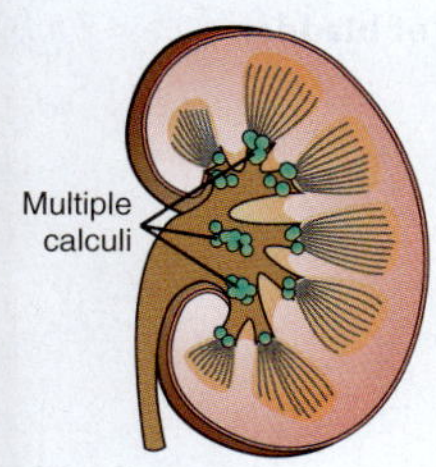

Figure 14-5 Multiple urinary calculi.

  N20.2 **Calculus of kidney with calculus of ureter**
  N20.9 **Urinary calculus, unspecified**
● **N21** **Calculus of lower urinary tract**
      Includes calculus of lower urinary tract with cystitis and urethritis
  N21.0 **Calculus in bladder**
      Calculus in diverticulum of bladder
      Urinary bladder stone
      Excludes2 staghorn calculus (N20.0)
      Coding Clinic: 2015, Q2, P9
  N21.1 **Calculus in urethra**
      Excludes2 calculus of prostate (N42.0)
  N21.8 **Other lower urinary tract calculus**
  N21.9 **Calculus of lower urinary tract, unspecified**
      Excludes1 calculus of urinary tract NOS (N20.9)

  N22 **Calculus of urinary tract in diseases classified elsewhere**
      Code first underlying disease, such as:
        gout (M1A.-, M10.-)
        schistosomiasis (B65.0-B65.9)

  N23 **Unspecified renal colic**

OTHER DISORDERS OF KIDNEY AND URETER (N25-N29)

      Excludes2 disorders of kidney and ureter with urolithiasis (N20-N23)

● **N25** **Disorders resulting from impaired renal tubular function**
  N25.0 **Renal osteodystrophy**
      Azotemic osteodystrophy
      Phosphate-losing tubular disorders
      Renal rickets
      Renal short stature
      Excludes2 metabolic disorders classifiable to E70-E88
  N25.1 **Nephrogenic diabetes insipidus** 🔣
      Excludes1 diabetes insipidus NOS (E23.2)
● **N25.8** **Other disorders resulting from impaired renal tubular function**
    N25.81 **Secondary hyperparathyroidism of renal origin** 🔣
        Excludes1 secondary hyperparathyroidism, non-renal (E21.1)
        Excludes2 metabolic disorders classifiable to E70-E88
    N25.89 **Other disorders resulting from impaired renal tubular function**
        Hypokalemic nephropathy
        Lightwood-Albright syndrome
        Renal tubular acidosis NOS
  N25.9 **Disorder resulting from impaired renal tubular function, unspecified**

● **N26** **Unspecified contracted kidney**
      Excludes1 contracted kidney due to hypertension (I12.-)
        diffuse sclerosing glomerulonephritis (N05.8.-)
        hypertensive nephrosclerosis (arteriolar) (arteriosclerotic) (I12.-)
        small kidney of unknown cause (N27.-)
  N26.1 **Atrophy of kidney (terminal)**
  N26.2 **Page kidney**
  N26.9 **Renal sclerosis, unspecified**

● **N27** **Small kidney of unknown cause**
      Includes oligonephronia
  N27.0 **Small kidney, unilateral**
  N27.1 **Small kidney, bilateral**
  N27.9 **Small kidney, unspecified**

● **N28 Other disorders of kidney and ureter, not elsewhere classified**
  N28.0 Ischemia and infarction of kidney 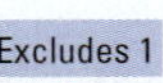
    Renal artery embolism
    Renal artery obstruction
    Renal artery occlusion
    Renal artery thrombosis
    Renal infarct
      Excludes1 atherosclerosis of renal artery (extrarenal
                  part) (I70.1)
                  congenital stenosis of renal artery (Q27.1)
                  Goldblatt's kidney (I70.1)

  N28.1 Cyst of kidney, acquired
    Cyst (multiple) (solitary) of kidney, (acquired)
      Excludes1 cystic kidney disease (congenital) (Q61.-)

● **N28.8 Other specified disorders of kidney and ureter**
      Excludes1 hydroureter (N13.4)
                  ureteric stricture with hydronephrosis
                      (N13.1)
                  ureteric stricture without hydronephrosis
                      (N13.5)

    N28.81 Hypertrophy of kidney
    N28.82 Megaloureter
    N28.83 Nephroptosis
    N28.84 Pyelitis cystica
    N28.85 Pyeloureteritis cystica
    N28.86 Ureteritis cystica
    N28.89 Other specified disorders of kidney and ureter
            Coding Clinic: 2025, Q2, P8; 2023, Q3, P5

  N28.9 Disorder of kidney and ureter, unspecified
    Nephropathy NOS
    Renal disease (acute) NOS
    Renal insufficiency (acute)
      Excludes1 chronic renal insufficiency (N18.9)
                  unspecified nephritic syndrome (N05.-)
            Coding Clinic: 2016, Q1, P13

**N29 Other disorders of kidney and ureter in diseases classified
    elsewhere**
    Code first underlying disease, such as:
      amyloidosis (E85.-)
      nephrocalcinosis (E83.59)
      schistosomiasis (B65.0-B65.9)
      Excludes1 disorders of kidney and ureter in:
                  cystinosis (E72.0)
                  gonorrhea (A54.21)
                  syphilis (A52.75)
                  tuberculosis (A18.11)

OTHER DISEASES OF THE URINARY SYSTEM (N30-N39)
      Excludes2 urinary infection (complicating):
                  abortion or ectopic or molar pregnancy
                      (O00-O07, O08.8)
                  pregnancy, childbirth and the puerperium
                      (O23.-, O75.3, O86.2-)

● **N30 Cystitis**
    Infection of bladder and irritation in lower urinary tract
    Use additional code to identify infectious agent (B95-B97)
      Excludes1 prostatocystitis (N41.3)
  ● **N30.0 Acute cystitis**
      Excludes1 irradiation cystitis (N30.4-)
                  trigonitis (N30.3-)
    N30.00 Acute cystitis without hematuria
    N30.01 Acute cystitis with hematuria
  ● **N30.1 Interstitial cystitis (chronic)**
      Ongoing infection of kidney glomeruli and tubules
    N30.10 Interstitial cystitis (chronic) without hematuria
    N30.11 Interstitial cystitis (chronic) with hematuria

● **N30.2 Other chronic cystitis**
    N30.20 Other chronic cystitis without hematuria
    N30.21 Other chronic cystitis with hematuria
● **N30.3 Trigonitis**
      *Inflammation of triangular area of bladder (where the ureters
          and urethra come together)*
    Urethrotrigonitis
    N30.30 Trigonitis without hematuria
    N30.31 Trigonitis with hematuria
● **N30.4 Irradiation cystitis**
    N30.40 Irradiation cystitis without hematuria
    N30.41 Irradiation cystitis with hematuria
● **N30.8 Other cystitis**
    Abscess of bladder
    N30.80 Other cystitis without hematuria
    N30.81 Other cystitis with hematuria
● **N30.9 Cystitis, unspecified**
    N30.90 Cystitis, unspecified without hematuria
    N30.91 Cystitis, unspecified with hematuria

● **N31 Neuromuscular dysfunction of bladder, not elsewhere classified**
    Use additional code to identify any associated urinary
        incontinence (N39.3-N39.4-)
      Excludes1 cord bladder NOS (G95.89)
                  neurogenic bladder due to cauda equina
                      syndrome (G83.4)
                  neuromuscular dysfunction due to spinal cord
                      lesion (G95.89)
    N31.0 Uninhibited neuropathic bladder, not elsewhere classified
    N31.1 Reflex neuropathic bladder, not elsewhere classified
    N31.2 Flaccid neuropathic bladder, not elsewhere classified
        Atonic (motor) (sensory) neuropathic bladder
        Diminished tone of bladder muscle
        Autonomous neuropathic bladder
        Nonreflex neuropathic bladder
    N31.8 Other neuromuscular dysfunction of bladder
    N31.9 Neuromuscular dysfunction of bladder, unspecified
        Neurogenic bladder dysfunction NOS

● **N32 Other disorders of bladder**
      Excludes2 calculus of bladder (N21.0)
                  cystocele (N81.1-)
                  hernia or prolapse of bladder, female (N81.1-)
    N32.0 Bladder-neck obstruction
        Bladder-neck stenosis (acquired)
      Excludes1 congenital bladder-neck obstruction
                  (Q64.3-)
    N32.1 Vesicointestinal fistula
        Vesicorectal fistula
        Coding Clinic: 2025, Q2, P6
    N32.2 Vesical fistula, not elsewhere classified
      Excludes1 fistula between bladder and female
                  genital tract (N82.0-N82.1)
    N32.3 Diverticulum of bladder
        Formation of sac from a herniation of wall of bladder
      Excludes1 congenital diverticulum of bladder (Q64.6)
                  diverticulitis of bladder (N30.8-)
  ● **N32.8 Other specified disorders of bladder**
    N32.81 Overactive bladder
        Detrusor muscle hyperactivity
      Excludes1 frequent urination due to
                  specified bladder condition-
                  code to condition
    N32.89 Other specified disorders of bladder
        Bladder hemorrhage
        Bladder hypertrophy
        Calcified bladder
        Contracted bladder
    N32.9 Bladder disorder, unspecified

▶ New   ⟹ Revised   ~~deleted~~ Deleted   **Excludes 1**   **Excludes 2**   **Includes**   **Use additional**   **Code first**   **Code also**   **Key words**
OGCR Official Guidelines   **X** Assign placeholder X   ● Use Additional Character(s)   ▶ Manifestation Code   🅗🅒 Hierarchical Condition Category   **Coding Clinic**

N33   Bladder disorders in diseases classified elsewhere

Code first underlying disease, such as:
schistosomiasis (B65.0-B65.9)

Excludes1   bladder disorder in syphilis (A52.76)
bladder disorder in tuberculosis (A18.12)
candidal cystitis (B37.41)
chlamydial cystitis(A56.01)
cystitis in gonorrhea (A54.01)
cystitis in neurogenic bladder (N31.-)
diphtheritic cystitis (A36.85)
syphilitic cystitis (A52.76)
trichomonal cystitis (A59.03)

● **N34   Urethritis and urethral syndrome**

Use additional code (B95-B97), to identify infectious agent

Excludes2   Reiter's disease (M02.3-)
urethritis in diseases with a predominantly sexual
mode of transmission (A50-A64)
urethrotrigonitis (N30.3-)

N34.0   Urethral abscess
Abscess (of) Cowper's gland
Abscess (of) Littré's gland
Abscess (of) urethral (gland)
Periurethral abscess

Excludes1   urethral caruncle (N36.2)

N34.1   Nonspecific urethritis
Nongonococcal urethritis
Nonvenereal urethritis

N34.2   Other urethritis
Inflammation of urethra
Meatitis, urethral
Postmenopausal urethritis
Ulcer of urethra (meatus)
Urethritis NOS

N34.3   Urethral syndrome, unspecified

● **N35   Urethral stricture**

*Narrowing of lumen of urethra caused by scarring due to infection or
injury*

Excludes1   congenital urethral stricture (Q64.3-)
postprocedural urethral stricture (N99.1-)

● **N35.0   Post-traumatic urethral stricture**
Urethral stricture due to injury

Excludes1   postprocedural urethral stricture (N99.1-)

● **N35.01   Post-traumatic urethral stricture, male**

**N35.010   Post-traumatic urethral stricture,
male, meatal**

**N35.011   Post-traumatic bulbous urethral
stricture**

**N35.012   Post-traumatic membranous urethral
stricture**

**N35.013   Post-traumatic anterior urethral
stricture**

**N35.014   Post-traumatic urethral stricture,
male, unspecified**

**N35.016   Post-traumatic urethral stricture,
male, overlapping sites**

● **N35.02   Post-traumatic urethral stricture, female**

N35.021   Urethral stricture due to childbirth

**N35.028   Other post-traumatic urethral
stricture, female**

● **N35.1   Postinfective urethral stricture, not elsewhere classified**

Excludes1   urethral stricture associated with
schistosomiasis (B65.-, N29)
gonococcal urethral stricture (A54.01)
syphilitic urethral stricture (A52.76)

● **N35.11   Postinfective urethral stricture, not elsewhere
classified, male**

**N35.111   Postinfective urethral stricture, not
elsewhere classified, male, meatal**

**N35.112   Postinfective bulbous urethral stricture,
not elsewhere classified, male**

**N35.113   Postinfective membranous urethral
stricture, not elsewhere classified,
male**

**N35.114   Postinfective anterior urethral
stricture, not elsewhere classified,
male**

**N35.116   Postinfective urethral stricture,
not elsewhere classified, male,
overlapping sites**

**N35.119   Postinfective urethral stricture,
not elsewhere classified, male,
unspecified**

**N35.12   Postinfective urethral stricture, not elsewhere
classified, female**

● **N35.8   Other urethral stricture**

Excludes1   postprocedural urethral stricture (N99.1-)

● **N35.81   Other urethral stricture, male**

N35.811   Other urethral stricture, male, meatal

N35.812   Other bulbous urethral stricture, male

**N35.813   Other membranous urethral stricture,
male**

N35.814   Other anterior urethral stricture, male

**N35.816   Other urethral stricture, male,
overlapping sites**

**N35.819   Other urethral stricture, male,
unspecified site**

N35.82   Other urethral stricture, female

● **N35.9   Urethral stricture, unspecified**

● **N35.91   Urethral stricture, unspecified, male**

**N35.911   Unspecified urethral stricture, male,
meatal**

**N35.912   Unspecified bulbous urethral
stricture, male**

**N35.913   Unspecified membranous urethral
stricture, male**

**N35.914   Unspecified anterior urethral
stricture, male**

**N35.916   Unspecified urethral stricture, male,
overlapping sites**

**N35.919   Unspecified urethral stricture, male,
unspecified site**
Pinhole meatus NOS
Urethral stricture NOS

N35.92   Unspecified urethral stricture, female

● **N36   Other disorders of urethra**

N36.0   Urethral fistula
Urethroperineal fistula
Urethrorectal fistula
Urinary fistula NOS

Excludes1   urethroscrotal fistula (N50.89)
urethrovaginal fistula (N82.1)
urethrovesicovaginal fistula (N82.1)

N36.1   Urethral diverticulum

N36.2   Urethral caruncle

● **N36.4   Urethral functional and muscular disorders**

Use additional code to identify associated urinary stress
incontinence (N39.3)

N36.41   Hypermobility of urethra

N36.42   Intrinsic sphincter deficiency (ISD)

**N36.43   Combined hypermobility of urethra and
intrinsic sphincter deficiency**

N36.44   Muscular disorders of urethra
Bladder sphincter dyssynergy

N36.5   Urethral false passage

N36.8   Other specified disorders of urethra

Excludes1   congenital urethrocele (Q64.7)
female urethrocele (N81.0)

Coding Clinic: 2022, Q2, P7

N36.9   Urethral disorder, unspecified

CHAPTER 14 (N00-N99)

N37   Urethral disorders in diseases classified elsewhere
         Code first underlying disease
         Excludes1   urethritis (in):
                         candidal infection (B37.41)
                         chlamydial (A56.01)
                         gonorrhea (A54.01)
                         syphilis (A52.76)
                         trichomonal infection (A59.03)
                         tuberculosis (A18.13)

● N39   Other disorders of urinary system
         Excludes2   hematuria NOS (R31.-)
                         recurrent or persistent hematuria (N02.-)
                         recurrent or persistent hematuria with specified
                             morphological lesion (N02.-)
                         proteinuria NOS (R80.-)

   N39.0   Urinary tract infection, site not specified
            Use additional code (B95-B97), to identify infectious
               agent
            Excludes1   candidiasis of urinary tract (B37.4-)
                            neonatal urinary tract infection (P39.3)
                            pyonephrosis (N13.6)
                            pyuria (R82.81)
                            urinary tract infection of specified site,
                                such as:
                                cystitis (N30.-)
                                urethritis (N34.-)
            Coding Clinic: 2018, Q2, P22; Q1, P16; 2012, Q4, P94

   N39.3   Stress incontinence (female) (male)
            Code also any associated overactive bladder (N32.81)
            Excludes1   mixed incontinence (N39.46)
            Coding Clinic: 2021, Q4, P18

● N39.4   Other specified urinary incontinence
            Code also any associated overactive bladder (N32.81)
            Excludes1   enuresis NOS (R32)
                            functional urinary incontinence (R39.81)
                            urinary incontinence associated with
                                cognitive impairment (R39.81)
                            urinary incontinence NOS (R32)
                            urinary incontinence of nonorganic origin
                                (F98.0)

      N39.41   Urge incontinence
                  Excludes1   mixed incontinence (N39.46)

      N39.42   Incontinence without sensory awareness
                  Insensible (urinary) incontinence

      N39.43   Post-void dribbling

      N39.44   Nocturnal enuresis
                  Excludes2   nocturnal polyuria (R35.81)

      N39.45   Continuous leakage

      N39.46   Mixed incontinence
                  Urge and stress incontinence

   ● N39.49   Other specified urinary incontinence

      N39.490   Overflow incontinence

      N39.491   Coital incontinence
                   Coding Clinic: 2016, Q4, P44

      N39.492   Postural (urinary) incontinence
                   Coding Clinic: 2016, Q4, P44

      N39.498   Other specified urinary incontinence
                   Reflex incontinence
                   Total incontinence

   N39.8   Other specified disorders of urinary system
   N39.9   Disorder of urinary system, unspecified

DISEASES OF MALE GENITAL ORGANS (N40-N53)

★ **(See Plate 5 of the Anatomy Illustrations.)**

● N40   Benign prostatic hyperplasia
         Includes   adenofibromatous hypertrophy of prostate
                        benign hypertrophy of the prostate
                        *Enlargement of prostate gland usually occurring
                            with age and causing obstructed urine flow*
                        benign prostatic hypertrophy
                        BPH
                        enlarged prostate
                        nodular prostate
                        polyp of prostate
         Excludes1   benign neoplasms of prostate (adenoma, benign)
                            (fibroadenoma) (fibroma) (myoma) (D29.1)
                        malignant neoplasm of prostate (C61)

   N40.0   Benign prostatic hyperplasia without lower urinary tract
           symptoms   A
            Enlarged prostate without LUTS
            Enlarged prostate NOS

   N40.1   Benign prostatic hyperplasia with lower urinary tract
           symptoms   A
            Enlarged prostate with LUTS
            Use additional code for associated symptoms, when
               specified:
               incomplete bladder emptying (R39.14)
               nocturia (R35.1)
               straining on urination (R39.16)
               urinary frequency (R35.0)
               urinary hesitancy (R39.11)
               urinary incontinence (N39.4-)
               urinary obstruction (N13.8)
               urinary retention (R33.8)
               urinary urgency (R39.15)
               weak urinary stream (R39.12)
            Coding Clinic: 2018, Q4, P55

   N40.2   Nodular prostate without lower urinary tract
           symptoms   A
            Nodular prostate without LUTS

   N40.3   Nodular prostate with lower urinary tract symptoms   A
            Use additional code for associated symptoms, when
               specified:
               incomplete bladder emptying (R39.14)
               nocturia (R35.1)
               straining on urination (R39.16)
               urinary frequency (R35.0)
               urinary hesitancy (R39.11)
               urinary incontinence (N39.4-)
               urinary obstruction (N13.8)
               urinary retention (R33.8)
               urinary urgency (R39.15)
               weak urinary stream (R39.12)

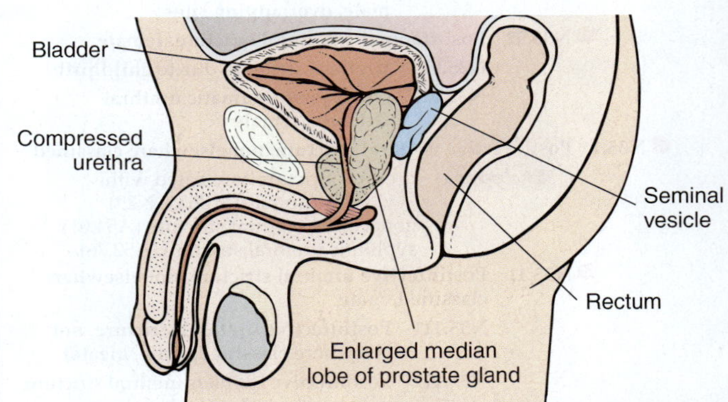

Figure 14-6   Benign prostatic hyperplasia. (From Shiland: Mastering
Healthcare Terminology, ed 3, St. Louis, Mosby, 2010)

► New   ⇒ Revised   ~~deleted~~ Deleted   Excludes 1   Excludes 2   Includes   Use additional   Code first   Code also   Key words
OGCR Official Guidelines   X Assign placeholder X   ● Use Additional Character(s)   ▶ Manifestation Code   ✎ Hierarchical Condition Category   **Coding Clinic**

Item 14–7   **Hydrocele** is a sac of fluid accumulating in the testes membrane.

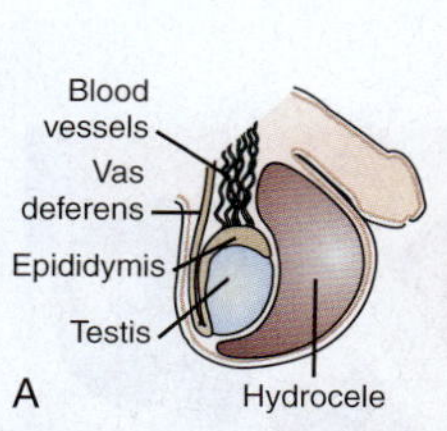

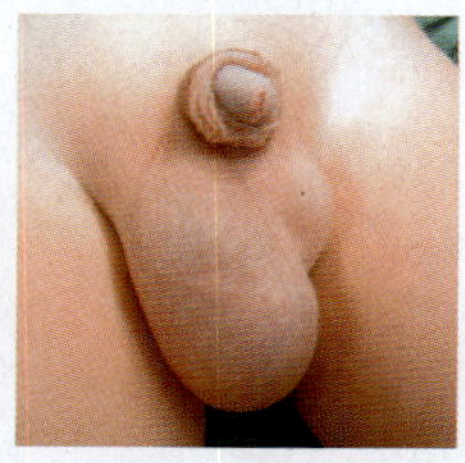

Figure 14-7   **A.** Hydrocele. **B.** Newborn with large right hydrocele. (**B** from Nelson WE, Kliegman R: Nelson Textbook of Pediatrics, Philadelphia, Saunders Elsevier, 2011)

N41   **Inflammatory diseases of prostate**
    Use additional code (B95-B97), to identify infectious agent
    N41.0   **Acute prostatitis**   A
       Coding Clinic: 2024, Q1, P16
    N41.1   **Chronic prostatitis**   A
    N41.2   **Abscess of prostate**   A
    N41.3   **Prostatocystitis**   A
       Coding Clinic: 2024, Q1, P16
    N41.4   **Granulomatous prostatitis**   A
    N41.8   **Other inflammatory diseases of prostate**   A
    N41.9   **Inflammatory disease of prostate, unspecified**   A
       Prostatitis NOS

N42   **Other and unspecified disorders of prostate**
    N42.0   **Calculus of prostate**   A
       Prostatic stone
    N42.1   **Congestion and hemorrhage of prostate**   A
       Excludes1   enlarged prostate (N40.-)
               hematuria (R31.-)
               hyperplasia of prostate (N40.-)
               inflammatory diseases of prostate (N41.-)
    N42.3   **Dysplasia of prostate**
       Coding Clinic: 2016, Q4, P44
       N42.30   **Unspecified dysplasia of prostate**
       N42.31   **Prostatic intraepithelial neoplasia**
           PIN
           Prostatic intraepithelial neoplasia I (PIN I)
           Prostatic intraepithelial neoplasia II (PIN II)
           Excludes1   prostatic intraepithelial neoplasia III (PIN III) (D07.5)
       N42.32   **Atypical small acinar proliferation of prostate**
       N42.39   **Other dysplasia of prostate**
    N42.8   **Other specified disorders of prostate**
       N42.81   **Prostatodynia syndrome**   A
           Painful prostate syndrome
       N42.82   **Prostatosis syndrome**   A
       N42.83   **Cyst of prostate**   A
       N42.89   **Other specified disorders of prostate**   A
    N42.9   **Disorder of prostate, unspecified**   A

N43   **Hydrocele and spermatocele**
    Includes   hydrocele of spermatic cord, testis or tunica vaginalis
    Excludes1   congenital hydrocele (P83.5)
    N43.0   **Encysted hydrocele**
    N43.1   **Infected hydrocele**
       Use additional code (B95-B97), to identify infectious agent
    N43.2   **Other hydrocele**
    N43.3   **Hydrocele, unspecified**
    N43.4   **Spermatocele of epididymis**
       Spermatic cyst
       N43.40   **Spermatocele of epididymis, unspecified**
       N43.41   **Spermatocele of epididymis, single**
       N43.42   **Spermatocele of epididymis, multiple**

N44   **Noninflammatory disorders of testis**
    N44.0   **Torsion of testis**
       N44.00   **Torsion of testis, unspecified**
       N44.01   **Extravaginal torsion of spermatic cord**
       N44.02   **Intravaginal torsion of spermatic cord**
           Torsion of spermatic cord NOS
       N44.03   **Torsion of appendix testis**
       N44.04   **Torsion of appendix epididymis**
    N44.1   **Cyst of tunica albuginea testis**
    N44.2   **Benign cyst of testis**
    N44.8   **Other noninflammatory disorders of the testis**

N45   **Orchitis and epididymitis**
    Orchitis is inflammation of one or both of the testes as a result of mumps or other infection, trauma, or metastasis. **Epididymitis** *is inflammation of the tubular structure that connects the testicle with the vas deferens.*
    Use additional code (B95-B97), to identify infectious agent
    N45.1   **Epididymitis**
    N45.2   **Orchitis**
    N45.3   **Epididymo-orchitis**
    N45.4   **Abscess of epididymis or testis**

N46   **Male infertility**
    Excludes1   vasectomy status (Z98.52)
    N46.0   **Azoospermia**
       Absolute male infertility
       Male infertility due to germinal (cell) aplasia
       Male infertility due to spermatogenic arrest (complete)
       N46.01   **Organic azoospermia**   A
           Azoospermia NOS
       N46.02   **Azoospermia due to extratesticular causes**
           Code also associated cause
           N46.021   **Azoospermia due to drug therapy**   A
           N46.022   **Azoospermia due to infection**   A
           N46.023   **Azoospermia due to obstruction of efferent ducts**   A
           N46.024   **Azoospermia due to radiation**   A
           N46.025   **Azoospermia due to systemic disease**   A
           N46.029   **Azoospermia due to other extratesticular causes**   A
    N46.1   **Oligospermia**
       Male infertility due to germinal cell desquamation
       Male infertility due to hypospermatogenesis
       Male infertility due to incomplete spermatogenic arrest
       N46.11   **Organic oligospermia**   A
           Oligospermia NOS
       N46.12   **Oligospermia due to extratesticular causes**
           Code also associated cause
           N46.121   **Oligospermia due to drug therapy**   A
           N46.122   **Oligospermia due to infection**   A
           N46.123   **Oligospermia due to obstruction of efferent ducts**   A
           N46.124   **Oligospermia due to radiation**   A
           N46.125   **Oligospermia due to systemic disease**   A
           N46.129   **Oligospermia due to other extratesticular causes**   A
    N46.8   **Other male infertility**   A
    N46.9   **Male infertility, unspecified**   A

Item 14–8 Male infertility is the inability of the female sex partner to conceive after one year of unprotected intercourse.

Azoospermia is no sperm ejaculated and **oligospermia** is few sperm ejaculated—both resulting in infertility. Extratesticular causes such as injury, infections, radiation, and chemotherapy may also cause male infertility.

CHAPTER 14 (N00-N99)

● **N47**   **Disorders of prepuce**
     N47.0   **Adherent prepuce, newborn**   **N**
     N47.1   **Phimosis**
     N47.2   **Paraphimosis**
     N47.3   **Deficient foreskin**
     N47.4   **Benign cyst of prepuce**
     N47.5   **Adhesions of prepuce and glans penis**
     N47.6   **Balanoposthitis**
         Use additional code (B95-B97), to identify infectious agent
         Excludes1   balanitis (N48.1)
     N47.7   **Other inflammatory diseases of prepuce**
         Use additional code (B95-B97), to identify infectious agent
     N47.8   **Other disorders of prepuce**

● **N48**   **Other disorders of penis**
     N48.0   **Leukoplakia of penis**
         Balanitis xerotica obliterans
         Kraurosis of penis
         Lichen sclerosus of external male genital organs
         Excludes1   carcinoma in situ of penis (D07.4)
     N48.1   **Balanitis**
         Use additional code (B95-B97), to identify infectious agent
         Excludes1   amebic balanitis (A06.8)
                 balanitis xerotica obliterans (N48.0)
                 candidal balanitis (B37.42)
                 gonococcal balanitis (A54.23)
                 herpesviral [herpes simplex] balanitis (A60.01)
     ● **N48.2**   **Other inflammatory disorders of penis**
         Use additional code (B95-B97), to identify infectious agent
         Excludes1   balanitis (N48.1)
                 balanitis xerotica obliterans (N48.0)
                 balanoposthitis (N47.6)
         N48.21   **Abscess of corpus cavernosum and penis**
         N48.22   **Cellulitis of corpus cavernosum and penis**
         N48.29   **Other inflammatory disorders of penis**
     ● **N48.3**   **Priapism**
         Painful erection
         Code first underlying cause
         N48.30   **Priapism, unspecified**
         N48.31   **Priapism due to trauma**
         N48.32   **Priapism due to disease classified elsewhere**
         N48.33   **Priapism, drug-induced**
         N48.39   **Other priapism**
     N48.5   **Ulcer of penis**
     N48.6   **Induration penis plastica**
         Peyronie's disease
         Plastic induration of penis
     ● **N48.8**   **Other specified disorders of penis**
         N48.81   **Thrombosis of superficial vein of penis**
         N48.82   **Acquired torsion of penis**
             Acquired torsion of penis NOS
             Excludes1   congenital torsion of penis (Q55.63)
         N48.83   **Acquired buried penis**
             Excludes1   congenital hidden penis (Q55.64)
         N48.89   **Other specified disorders of penis**
     N48.9   **Disorder of penis, unspecified**

Item 14–9 Seminal vesiculitis is an inflammation of the seminal vesicle. **Spermatocele** is a benign cystic accumulation of sperm arising from the head of the epididymis. **Torsion of the testis** is a medical emergency occurring most commonly in boys 7 to 12 years of age and results from a congenital abnormality of the covering of the testis allowing the testis to twist within its sac and cutting off the blood supply to the testis.

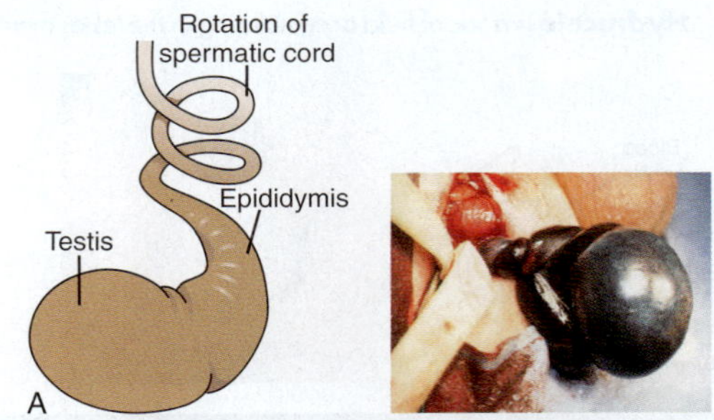

Figure 14-8   **A.** Torsion of testis. **B.** Torsion of the testis. (**B** from Kliegman R, Nelson WE: Nelson Textbook of Pediatrics, Philadelphia, Saunders, 2007)

● **N49**   **Inflammatory disorders of male genital organs, not elsewhere classified**
     Use additional code (B95-B97), to identify infectious agent
     Excludes1   inflammation of penis (N48.1, N48.2-)
                 orchitis and epididymitis (N45.-)
     N49.0   **Inflammatory disorders of seminal vesicle**
         Vesiculitis NOS
     N49.1   **Inflammatory disorders of spermatic cord, tunica vaginalis and vas deferens**
         Vasitis
     N49.2   **Inflammatory disorders of scrotum**
     N49.3   **Fournier gangrene**
     N49.8   **Inflammatory disorders of other specified male genital organs**
         Inflammation of multiple sites in male genital organs
     N49.9   **Inflammatory disorder of unspecified male genital organ**
         Abscess of unspecified male genital organ
         Boil of unspecified male genital organ
         Carbuncle of unspecified male genital organ
         Cellulitis of unspecified male genital organ

● **N50**   **Other and unspecified disorders of male genital organs**
     Excludes2   torsion of testis (N44.0-)
     N50.0   **Atrophy of testis**
     N50.1   **Vascular disorders of male genital organs**
         Hematocele, NOS, of male genital organs
         Hemorrhage of male genital organs
         Thrombosis of male genital organs
     N50.3   **Cyst of epididymis**
     ● **N50.8**   **Other specified disorders of male genital organs**
         Coding Clinic: 2016, Q4, P45
         ● **N50.81**   **Testicular pain**
             N50.811   **Right testicular pain**
             N50.812   **Left testicular pain**
             N50.819   **Testicular pain, unspecified**
         N50.82   **Scrotal pain**
         N50.89   **Other specified disorders of the male genital organs**
             Atrophy of scrotum, seminal vesicle, spermatic cord, tunica vaginalis and vas deferens
             Chylocele, tunica vaginalis (nonfilarial) NOS
             Edema of scrotum, seminal vesicle, spermatic cord, tunica vaginalis and vas deferens
             Hypertrophy of scrotum, seminal vesicle, spermatic cord, tunica vaginalis and vas deferens
             Stricture of spermatic cord, tunica vaginalis, and vas deferens
             Ulcer of scrotum, seminal vesicle, spermatic cord, testis, tunica vaginalis and vas deferens
             Urethroscrotal fistula
     N50.9   **Disorder of male genital organs, unspecified**

N51   **Disorders of male genital organs in diseases classified elsewhere**

Code first underlying disease, such as:
filariasis (B74.0-B74.9)

> **Excludes1**   amebic balanitis (A06.8)
> candidal balanitis (B37.42)
> gonococcal balanitis (A54.23)
> gonococcal prostatitis (A54.22)
> herpesviral [herpes simplex] balanitis (A60.01)
> trichomonal prostatitis (A59.02)
> tuberculous prostatitis (A18.14)

● **N52**   **Male erectile dysfunction**

> **Excludes1**   psychogenic impotence (F52.21)

  ● **N52.0**   **Vasculogenic erectile dysfunction**

     N52.01   **Erectile dysfunction due to arterial insufficiency**   A

     N52.02   **Corporo-venous occlusive erectile dysfunction** A

     N52.03   **Combined arterial insufficiency and corporo-venous occlusive erectile dysfunction**   A

  N52.1   **Erectile dysfunction due to diseases classified elsewhere**   A

> *Code first* underlying disease

  N52.2   **Drug-induced erectile dysfunction**   A

  ● **N52.3**   **Postprocedural erectile dysfunction**

     N52.31   **Erectile dysfunction following radical prostatectomy**   A

     N52.32   **Erectile dysfunction following radical cystectomy**   A

     N52.33   **Erectile dysfunction following urethral surgery**   A

     N52.34   **Erectile dysfunction following simple prostatectomy**   A

     N52.35   **Erectile dysfunction following radiation therapy**   A
> Coding Clinic: 2016, Q4, P45

     N52.36   **Erectile dysfunction following interstitial seed therapy**   A
> Coding Clinic: 2016, Q4, P45

     N52.37   **Erectile dysfunction following prostate ablative therapy**   A
> Erectile dysfunction following cryotherapy
> Erectile dysfunction following other prostate ablative therapies
> Erectile dysfunction following ultrasound ablative therapies
> Coding Clinic: 2016, Q4, P45

     N52.39   **Other and unspecified postprocedural erectile dysfunction**   A

  N52.8   **Other male erectile dysfunction**   A

  N52.9   **Male erectile dysfunction, unspecified**   A
> Impotence NOS

● **N53**   **Other male sexual dysfunction**

> **Excludes1**   psychogenic sexual dysfunction (F52.-)

  ● **N53.1**   **Ejaculatory dysfunction**

> **Excludes1**   premature ejaculation (F52.4)

     N53.11   **Retarded ejaculation**

     N53.12   **Painful ejaculation**

     N53.13   **Anejaculatory orgasm**

     N53.14   **Retrograde ejaculation**

     N53.19   **Other ejaculatory dysfunction**
> Ejaculatory dysfunction NOS

  N53.8   **Other male sexual dysfunction**

  N53.9   **Unspecified male sexual dysfunction**

DISORDERS OF BREAST (N60-N65)

> **Excludes1**   disorders of breast associated with childbirth (O91-O92)

● **N60**   **Benign mammary dysplasia**

Benign lumpiness of breast

> **Includes**   fibrocystic mastopathy

  ● **N60.0**   **Solitary cyst of breast**
> Cyst of breast

     N60.01   **Solitary cyst of right breast**

     N60.02   **Solitary cyst of left breast**

     N60.09   **Solitary cyst of unspecified breast**

  ● **N60.1**   **Diffuse cystic mastopathy**
> Cystic breast
> Fibrocystic disease of breast

> **Excludes1**   diffuse cystic mastopathy with epithelial proliferation (N60.3-)

     N60.11   **Diffuse cystic mastopathy of right breast**   A

     N60.12   **Diffuse cystic mastopathy of left breast**   A

     N60.19   **Diffuse cystic mastopathy of unspecified breast**   A

  ● **N60.2**   **Fibroadenosis of breast**
> Adenofibrosis of breast

> **Excludes2**   fibroadenoma of breast (D24.-)

     N60.21   **Fibroadenosis of right breast**

     N60.22   **Fibroadenosis of left breast**

     N60.29   **Fibroadenosis of unspecified breast**

  ● **N60.3**   **Fibrosclerosis of breast**
> Cystic mastopathy with epithelial proliferation

     N60.31   **Fibrosclerosis of right breast**

     N60.32   **Fibrosclerosis of left breast**

     N60.39   **Fibrosclerosis of unspecified breast**

  ● **N60.4**   **Mammary duct ectasia**

     N60.41   **Mammary duct ectasia of right breast**

     N60.42   **Mammary duct ectasia of left breast**

     N60.49   **Mammary duct ectasia of unspecified breast**

  ● **N60.8**   **Other benign mammary dysplasias**

     N60.81   **Other benign mammary dysplasias of right breast**

     N60.82   **Other benign mammary dysplasias of left breast**

     N60.89   **Other benign mammary dysplasias of unspecified breast**

  ● **N60.9**   **Unspecified benign mammary dysplasia**

     N60.91   **Unspecified benign mammary dysplasia of right breast**

     N60.92   **Unspecified benign mammary dysplasia of left breast**

     N60.99   **Unspecified benign mammary dysplasia of unspecified breast**

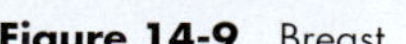

Figure 14-9   Breast.

CHAPTER 14 (N00-N99)

● **N61   Inflammatory disorders of breast**
⇒ **Excludes1**   inflammatory carcinoma of breast (C50.A-)
inflammatory disorder of breast associated with childbirth (O91.-)
neonatal infective mastitis (P39.0)
thrombophlebitis of breast [Mondor's disease] (I80.8)

N61.0   Mastitis without abscess
Infective mastitis (acute) (nonpuerperal) (subacute)
Mastitis (acute) (nonpuerperal) (subacute) NOS
Cellulitis (acute) (nonpuerperal) (subacute) of breast NOS
Cellulitis (acute) (nonpuerperal) (subacute) of nipple NOS

N61.1   Abscess of the breast and nipple
Abscess (acute) (chronic) (nonpuerperal) of areola
Abscess (acute) (chronic) (nonpuerperal) of breast
Carbuncle of breast
Mastitis with abscess

● **N61.2   Granulomatous mastitis**
N61.20   Granulomatous mastitis, unspecified breast
N61.21   Granulomatous mastitis, right breast
N61.22   Granulomatous mastitis, left breast
N61.23   Granulomatous mastitis, bilateral breast

N62   Hypertrophy of breast
Gynecomastia
Hypertrophy of breast NOS
Massive pubertal hypertrophy of breast
Excludes1   breast engorgement of newborn (P83.4)
disproportion of reconstructed breast (N65.1)

● **N63   Unspecified lump in breast**
Nodule(s) NOS in breast

N63.0   Unspecified lump in unspecified breast
● **N63.1   Unspecified lump in the right breast**
N63.10   Unspecified lump in the right breast, unspecified quadrant
Coding Clinic: 2022, Q3, P8
N63.11   Unspecified lump in the right breast, upper outer quadrant
Coding Clinic: 2017, Q4, P19
N63.12   Unspecified lump in the right breast, upper inner quadrant
N63.13   Unspecified lump in the right breast, lower outer quadrant
N63.14   Unspecified lump in the right breast, lower inner quadrant
N63.15   Unspecified lump in the right breast, overlapping quadrants
● **N63.2   Unspecified lump in the left breast**
N63.20   Unspecified lump in the left breast, unspecified quadrant
N63.21   Unspecified lump in the left breast, upper outer quadrant
N63.22   Unspecified lump in the left breast, upper inner quadrant
N63.23   Unspecified lump in the left breast, lower outer quadrant
N63.24   Unspecified lump in the left breast, lower inner quadrant
N63.25   Unspecified lump in the left breast, overlapping quadrants

● **N63.3   Unspecified lump in axillary tail**
N63.31   Unspecified lump in axillary tail of the right breast
N63.32   Unspecified lump in axillary tail of the left breast
● **N63.4   Unspecified lump in breast, subareolar**
N63.41   Unspecified lump in right breast, subareolar
N63.42   Unspecified lump in left breast, subareolar

● **N64   Other disorders of breast**
Excludes2   mechanical complication of breast prosthesis and implant (T85.4-)

N64.0   Fissure and fistula of nipple
N64.1   Fat necrosis of breast
Fat necrosis (segmental) of breast
Code first breast necrosis due to breast graft (T85.898)

N64.2   Atrophy of breast
N64.3   Galactorrhea not associated with childbirth
Excessive or spontaneous flow of milk

N64.4   Mastodynia
● **N64.5   Other signs and symptoms in breast**
Excludes2   abnormal findings on diagnostic imaging of breast (R92.-)
N64.51   Induration of breast
N64.52   Nipple discharge
Excludes1   abnormal findings in nipple discharge (R89.-)
N64.53   Retraction of nipple
N64.59   Other signs and symptoms in breast
● **N64.8   Other specified disorders of breast**
N64.81   Ptosis of breast   A
Excludes1   ptosis of native breast in relation to reconstructed breast (N65.1)
N64.82   Hypoplasia of breast   A
Micromastia
Excludes1   congenital absence of breast (Q83.0)
hypoplasia of native breast in relation to reconstructed breast (N65.1)
N64.89   Other specified disorders of breast
Galactocele
Subinvolution of breast (postlactational)
Coding Clinic: 2019, Q1, P32; 2018, Q1, P4
N64.9   Disorder of breast, unspecified
Coding Clinic: 2018, Q1, P4

● **N65   Deformity and disproportion of reconstructed breast**
N65.0   Deformity of reconstructed breast   A
Contour irregularity in reconstructed breast
Excess tissue in reconstructed breast
Misshapen reconstructed breast
N65.1   Disproportion of reconstructed breast   A
Breast asymmetry between native breast and reconstructed breast
Disproportion between native breast and reconstructed breast

► New   ⇒ Revised   ~~deleted~~ Deleted   Excludes 1   Excludes 2   Includes   Use additional   Code first   Code also   Key words
OGCR Official Guidelines   X Assign placeholder X   ● Use Additional Character(s)   ◗ Manifestation Code   Ⓗ Hierarchical Condition Category   Coding Clinic

INFLAMMATORY DISEASES OF FEMALE PELVIC ORGANS (N70-N77)

Excludes1   inflammatory diseases of female pelvic organs
  complicating:
  abortion or ectopic or molar pregnancy
    (O00-O07, O08.0)
  pregnancy, childbirth and the puerperium
    (O23.-, O75.3, O85, O86.-)

★ **(See Plate 35 of the Anatomy Illustrations.)**

● **N70   Salpingitis and oophoritis**
Oophoritis = inflammation of ovary
Salpingitis = inflammation of falloplan tube

Includes   abscess (of) fallopian tube
  abscess (of) ovary
  pyosalpinx
  salpingo-oophoritis
  tubo-ovarian abscess
  tubo-ovarian inflammatory disease

Use additional code (B95-B97), to identify infectious agent

Excludes1   gonococcal infection (A54.24)
  tuberculous infection (A18.17)

● **N70.0   Acute salpingitis and oophoritis**

N70.01   Acute salpingitis

N70.02   Acute oophoritis

N70.03   Acute salpingitis and oophoritis

● **N70.1   Chronic salpingitis and oophoritis**
Hydrosalpinx

N70.11   Chronic salpingitis

N70.12   Chronic oophoritis

N70.13   Chronic salpingitis and oophoritis

● **N70.9   Salpingitis and oophoritis, unspecified**

N70.91   Salpingitis, unspecified

N70.92   Oophoritis, unspecified

N70.93   Salpingitis and oophoritis, unspecified

● **N71   Inflammatory disease of uterus, except cervix**

Includes   endo (myo) metritis
  metritis
  myometritis
  pyometra
  uterine abscess

Use additional code (B95-B97), to identify infectious agent

Excludes1   hyperplastic endometritis (N85.0-)
  infection of uterus following delivery (O85, O86.-)

N71.0   Acute inflammatory disease of uterus

N71.1   Chronic inflammatory disease of uterus

N71.9   Inflammatory disease of uterus, unspecified

N72   Inflammatory disease of cervix uteri

Includes   cervicitis (with or without erosion or ectropion)
  endocervicitis (with or without erosion or
    ectropion)
  exocervicitis (with or without erosion or ectropion)

Use additional code (B95-B97), to identify infectious agent

Excludes1   erosion and ectropion of cervix without cervicitis
    (N86)

● **N73   Other female pelvic inflammatory diseases**

Use additional code (B95-B97), to identify infectious agent

N73.0   Acute parametritis and pelvic cellulitis
Abscess of broad ligament
Abscess of parametrium
Pelvic cellulitis, female

N73.1   Chronic parametritis and pelvic cellulitis
Any condition in N73.0 specified as chronic

Excludes1   tuberculous parametritis and pelvic
    cellultis (A18.17)

N73.2   Unspecified parametritis and pelvic cellulitis
Any condition in N73.0 unspecified whether acute or
chronic

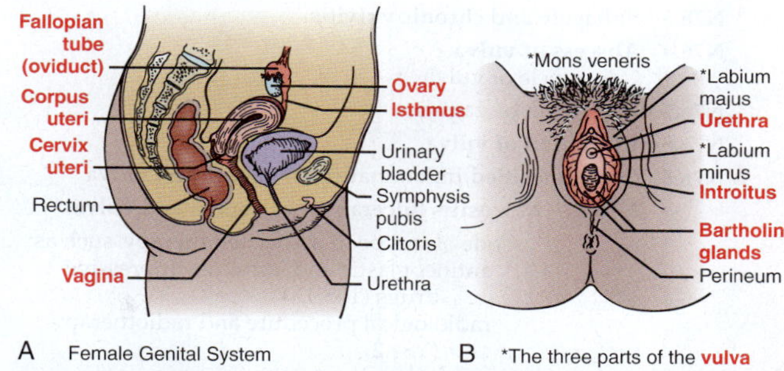

Figure 14-10   A. Female genital system. **B.** External female genital
system. (From Buck CJ: Step-by-Step Medical Coding, ed 2016, St. Louis,
Elsevier, 2016)

Item 14–10 Salpingitis is an infection of one or both fallopian tubes.
Oophoritis is an infection of one or both ovaries.

N73.3   Female acute pelvic peritonitis

N73.4   Female chronic pelvic peritonitis

Excludes1   tuberculous pelvic (female) peritonitis
    (A18.17)

N73.5   Female pelvic peritonitis, unspecified

N73.6   Female pelvic peritoneal adhesions (postinfective)

Excludes2   postprocedural pelvic peritoneal
    adhesions (N99.4)

N73.8   Other specified female pelvic inflammatory diseases

N73.9   Female pelvic inflammatory disease, unspecified
Female pelvic infection or inflammation NOS

**N74   Female pelvic inflammatory disorders in diseases classified
elsewhere**

Code first underlying disease

Excludes1   chlamydial cervicitis (A56.02)
  chlamydial pelvic inflammatory disease (A56.11)
  gonococcal cervicitis (A54.03)
  gonococcal pelvic inflammatory disease (A54.24)
  herpesviral [herpes simplex] cervicitis (A60.03)
  herpesviral [herpes simplex] pelvic inflammatory
    disease (A60.09)
  syphilitic cervicitis (A52.76)
  syphilitic pelvic inflammatory disease (A52.76)
  trichomonal cervicitis (A59.09)
  tuberculous cervicitis (A18.16)
  tuberculous pelvic inflammatory disease (A18.17)

● **N75   Diseases of Bartholin's gland**

N75.0   Cyst of Bartholin's gland
Cysts filled with liquid or semisolid material

N75.1   Abscess of Bartholin's gland
Localized collection of pus
Coding Clinic: 2025, Q1, P22-23

N75.8   Other diseases of Bartholin's gland
Bartholinitis

N75.9   Disease of Bartholin's gland, unspecified

● **N76   Other inflammation of vagina and vulva**

Use additional code (B95-B97), to identify infectious agent

Excludes2   senile (atrophic) vaginitis (N95.2)
  vulvar vestibulitis (N94.810)

N76.0   Acute vaginitis
Acute vulvovaginitis
Vaginitis NOS
Vulvovaginitis NOS

N76.1   Subacute and chronic vaginitis
Chronic vulvovaginitis
Subacute vulvovaginitis

N76.2   Acute vulvitis
Vulvitis NOS

CHAPTER 14 (N00-N99)

N76.3   Subacute and chronic vulvitis

N76.4   Abscess of vulva
> Furuncle of vulva

N76.5   Ulceration of vagina

N76.6   Ulceration of vulva

● **N76.8**   Other specified inflammation of vagina and vulva

    N76.81   Mucositis (ulcerative) of vagina and vulva
> Code also type of associated therapy, such as:
> antineoplastic and immunosuppressive drugs (T45.1X-)
> radiological procedure and radiotherapy (Y84.2)

        Excludes2   gastrointestinal mucositis (ulcerative) (K92.81)
> nasal mucositis (ulcerative) (J34.81)
> oral mucositis (ulcerative) (K12.3-)

    N76.82   Fournier disease of vagina and vulva
> Fournier gangrene of vagina and vulva
> Code also, if applicable, diabetes mellitus (E08-E13 with .9)

        Excludes1   gangrene in diabetes mellitus (E08-E13 with .52)

    N76.89   Other specified inflammation of vagina and vulva

● **N77**   Vulvovaginal ulceration and inflammation in diseases classified elsewhere

  N77.0   Ulceration of vulva in diseases classified elsewhere
> Code first underlying disease, such as:
> Behçet's disease (M35.2)

        Excludes1   ulceration of vulva in gonococcal infection (A54.02)
> ulceration of vulva in herpesviral [herpes simplex] infection (A60.04)
> ulceration of vulva in syphilis (A51.0)
> ulceration of vulva in tuberculosis (A18.18)

  N77.1   Vaginitis, vulvitis and vulvovaginitis in diseases classified elsewhere
> Code first underlying disease, such as:
> pinworm (B80)

        Excludes1   candidial vulvovaginitis (B37.3-)
> chlamydial vulvovaginitis (A56.02)
> gonococcal vulvovaginitis (A54.02)
> herpesviral [herpes simplex] vulvovaginitis (A60.04)
> trichomonal vulvovaginitis (A59.01)
> tuberculous vulvovaginitis (A18.18)
> vulvovaginitis in early syphilis (A51.0)
> vulvovaginitis in late syphilis (A52.76)

NONINFLAMMATORY DISORDERS OF FEMALE GENITAL TRACT (N80-N98)

● **N80**   Endometriosis

● **N80.0**   Endometriosis of uterus
> Endometriosis of the cervix

        Excludes1   stromal endometriosis (D39.0)

  N80.00   Endometriosis of the uterus, unspecified

  N80.01   Superficial endometriosis of the uterus

  N80.02   Deep endometriosis of the uterus
> Deep retrocervical endometriosis

  N80.03   Adenomyosis of the uterus
> Adenomyosis NOS

● **N80.1**   Endometriosis of ovary

  ● **N80.10**   Endometriosis of ovary, unspecified depth

    N80.101   Endometriosis of right ovary, unspecified depth

    N80.102   Endometriosis of left ovary, unspecified depth

    N80.103   Endometriosis of bilateral ovaries, unspecified depth

    N80.109   Endometriosis of ovary, unspecified side, unspecified depth
> Endometriosis of ovary NOS

  ● **N80.11**   Superficial endometriosis of the ovary

    N80.111   Superficial endometriosis of right ovary
> **Coding Clinic: 2022, Q4, P36**

    N80.112   Superficial endometriosis of left ovary

    N80.113   Superficial endometriosis of bilateral ovaries

    N80.119   Superficial endometriosis of ovary, unspecified ovary

  ● **N80.12**   Deep endometriosis of ovary
> Deep ovarian endometriosis
> Endometrioma

    N80.121   Deep endometriosis of right ovary

    N80.122   Deep endometriosis of left ovary

    N80.123   Deep endometriosis of bilateral ovaries

    N80.129   Deep endometriosis of ovary, unspecified ovary

● **N80.2**   Endometriosis of fallopian tube

  ● **N80.20**   Endometriosis of fallopian tube, unspecified depth

    N80.201   Endometriosis of right fallopian tube, unspecified depth

    N80.202   Endometriosis of left fallopian tube, unspecified depth

    N80.203   Endometriosis of bilateral fallopian tubes, unspecified depth

    N80.209   Endometriosis of unspecified fallopian tube, unspecified depth
> Endometriosis fallopian tube NOS

  ● **N80.21**   Superficial endometriosis of fallopian tube

    N80.211   Superficial endometriosis of right fallopian tube

    N80.212   Superficial endometriosis of left fallopian tube

    N80.213   Superficial endometriosis of bilateral fallopian tubes

    N80.219   Superficial endometriosis of unspecified fallopian tube

  ● **N80.22**   Deep endometriosis of the fallopian tube
> Deep endometriosis involving muscular wall of fallopian tube

    N80.221   Deep endometriosis of right fallopian tube

    N80.222   Deep endometriosis of left fallopian tube

    N80.223   Deep endometriosis of bilateral fallopian tubes

    N80.229   Deep endometriosis of unspecified fallopian tube

● **N80.3**   Endometriosis of pelvic peritoneum

  N80.30   Endometriosis of pelvic peritoneum, unspecified
> Endometriosis of the retroperitoneum NOS

  ● **N80.31**   Endometriosis of the anterior cul-de-sac

    N80.311   Superficial endometriosis of the anterior cul-de-sac

    N80.312   Deep endometriosis of the anterior cul-de-sac

    N80.319   Endometriosis of the anterior cul-de-sac, unspecified depth
> Endometriosis of the anterior cul-de-sac NOS

● **N80.32**   Endometriosis of the posterior cul-de-sac

    N80.321   Superficial endometriosis of the posterior cul-de-sac

    N80.322   Deep endometriosis of the posterior cul-de-sac

    N80.329   Endometriosis of the posterior cul-de-sac, unspecified depth
       Endometriosis of the posterior cul-de-sac NOS

● **N80.33**   Superficial endometriosis of the pelvic sidewall

    N80.331   Superficial endometriosis of the right pelvic sidewall

    N80.332   Superficial endometriosis of the left pelvic sidewall

    N80.333   Superficial endometriosis of bilateral pelvic sidewall

    N80.339   Superficial endometriosis of pelvic sidewall, unspecified side

● **N80.34**   Deep endometriosis of the pelvic sidewall

    N80.341   Deep endometriosis of the right pelvic sidewall

    N80.342   Deep endometriosis of the left pelvic sidewall

    N80.343   Deep endometriosis of the bilateral pelvic sidewall

    N80.349   Deep endometriosis of the pelvic sidewall, unspecified side
       Coding Clinic: 2022, Q4, P36

● **N80.35**   Endometriosis of the pelvic sidewall, unspecified depth

    N80.351   Endometriosis of the right pelvic sidewall, unspecified depth

    N80.352   Endometriosis of the left pelvic sidewall, unspecified depth

    N80.353   Endometriosis of bilateral pelvic sidewall, unspecified depth

    N80.359   Endometriosis of pelvic sidewall, unspecified side, unspecified depth
       Endometriosis of the pelvic sidewall NOS

● **N80.36**   Superficial endometriosis of the pelvic brim

    N80.361   Superficial endometriosis of the right pelvic brim

    N80.362   Superficial endometriosis of the left pelvic brim

    N80.363   Superficial endometriosis of bilateral pelvic brim

    N80.369   Superficial endometriosis of the pelvic brim, unspecified side

● **N80.37**   Deep endometriosis of the pelvic brim

    N80.371   Deep endometriosis of the right pelvic brim

    N80.372   Deep endometriosis of the left pelvic brim

    N80.373   Deep endometriosis of bilateral pelvic brim

    N80.379   Deep endometriosis of the pelvic brim, unspecified side

● **N80.38**   Endometriosis of the pelvic brim, unspecified depth

    N80.381   Endometriosis of the right pelvic brim, unspecified depth

    N80.382   Endometriosis of the left pelvic brim, unspecified depth

    N80.383   Endometriosis of bilateral pelvic brim, unspecified depth

    N80.389   Endometriosis of the pelvic brim, unspecified side, unspecified depth
       Endometriosis of the pelvic brim NOS

● **N80.39**   Endometriosis of other pelvic peritoneum

    N80.391   Superficial endometriosis of the pelvic peritoneum, other specified sites

    N80.392   Deep endometriosis of the pelvic peritoneum, other specified sites

    N80.399   Endometriosis of the pelvic peritoneum, other specified sites, unspecified depth

● **N80.3A**   Superficial endometriosis of the uterosacral ligament(s)

    N80.3A1   Superficial endometriosis of the right uterosacral ligament

    N80.3A2   Superficial endometriosis of the left uterosacral ligament

    N80.3A3   Superficial endometriosis of the bilateral uterosacral ligament(s)

    N80.3A9   Superficial endometriosis of the uterosacral ligament(s), unspecified side

● **N80.3B**   Deep endometriosis of the uterosacral ligament(s)

    N80.3B1   Deep endometriosis of the right uterosacral ligament

    N80.3B2   Deep endometriosis of the left uterosacral ligament

    N80.3B3   Deep endometriosis of bilateral uterosacral ligament(s)

    N80.3B9   Deep endometriosis of the uterosacral ligament(s), unspecified side

● **N80.3C**   Endometriosis of the uterosacral ligament(s), unspecified depth

    N80.3C1   Endometriosis of the right uterosacral ligament, unspecified depth

    N80.3C2   Endometriosis of the left uterosacral ligament, unspecified depth

    N80.3C3   Endometriosis of bilateral uterosacral ligament(s), unspecified depth

    N80.3C9   Endometriosis of the uterosacral ligament(s), unspecified side, unspecified depth
       Endometriosis of the uterosacral ligament(s) NOS

● **N80.4**   Endometriosis of rectovaginal septum and vagina

    N80.40   Endometriosis of rectovaginal septum, unspecified involvement of vagina
       Endometriosis of the rectovaginal septum, NOS

    N80.41   Endometriosis of rectovaginal septum without involvement of vagina

    N80.42   Endometriosis of rectovaginal septum with involvement of vagina

● **N80.5**   Endometriosis of intestine

    N80.50   Endometriosis of intestine, unspecified

●   **N80.51**   Endometriosis of the rectum

    N80.511   Superficial endometriosis of the rectum

    N80.512   Deep endometriosis of the rectum
       Deep endometriosis of the rectum, multifocal

    N80.519   Endometriosis of the rectum, unspecified depth
       Endometriosis of the rectum NOS

●   **N80.52**   Endometriosis of the sigmoid colon

    N80.521   Superficial endometriosis of the sigmoid colon

    N80.522   Deep endometriosis of the sigmoid colon

    N80.529   Endometriosis of the sigmoid colon, unspecified depth
       Endometriosis of the sigmoid colon NOS

● **N80.53 Endometriosis of the cecum**
    N80.531   Superficial endometriosis of the cecum
    N80.532   Deep endometriosis of the cecum
    N80.539   Endometriosis of the cecum, unspecified depth
          Endometriosis of the cecum NOS

● **N80.54 Endometriosis of the appendix**
    N80.541   Superficial endometriosis of the appendix
    N80.542   Deep endometriosis of the appendix
    N80.549   Endometriosis of the appendix, unspecified depth
          Endometriosis of the appendix NOS

● **N80.55 Endometriosis of other parts of the colon**
    Endometriosis of descending colon
    Endometriosis of transverse colon
    N80.551   Superficial endometriosis of other parts of the colon
    N80.552   Deep endometriosis of other parts of the colon
    N80.559   Endometriosis of other parts of the colon, unspecified depth
          Endometriosis of colon NOS

N80.6 Endometriosis in cutaneous scar

N80.8 Other endometriosis
    Endometriosis of other sites

N80.9 Endometriosis, unspecified

● **N80.A Endometriosis of bladder and ureters**
    N80.A0   Endometriosis of bladder, unspecified depth
          Endometriosis of bladder NOS
    N80.A1   Superficial endometriosis of bladder
    N80.A2   Deep endometriosis of bladder
●   N80.A4   Superficial endometriosis of ureter
          Extrinsic endometriosis of ureter
          Code also, if applicable, obstructive and reflux uropathy (N13.-)
    N80.A41   Superficial endometriosis of right ureter
    N80.A42   Superficial endometriosis of left ureter
    N80.A43   Superficial endometriosis of bilateral ureters
    N80.A49   Superficial endometriosis of unspecified ureter
●   N80.A5   Deep endometriosis of ureter
          Intrinsic endometriosis of ureter
          Code also, if applicable, obstructive and reflux uropathy (N13.-)
    N80.A51   Deep endometriosis of right ureter
    N80.A52   Deep endometriosis of left ureter
    N80.A53   Deep endometriosis of bilateral ureters
    N80.A59   Deep endometriosis of unspecified ureter
●   N80.A6   Endometriosis of ureter, unspecified depth
          Code also, if applicable, obstructive and reflux uropathy (N13.-)
    N80.A61   Endometriosis of right ureter, unspecified depth
    N80.A62   Endometriosis of left ureter, unspecified depth
    N80.A63   Endometriosis of bilateral ureters, unspecified depth
    N80.A69   Endometriosis of unspecified ureter, unspecified depth

● **N80.B Endometriosis of cardiothoracic space**
    Endometriosis of thorax
    Code also, if applicable:
          catamenial hemothorax (J94.2)
          catamenial pneumothorax (J93.12)
    N80.B1   Endometriosis of pleura
    N80.B2   Endometriosis of lung
●   N80.B3   Endometriosis of diaphragm
    N80.B31   Superficial endometriosis of diaphragm
    N80.B32   Deep endometriosis of diaphragm
    N80.B39   Endometriosis of diaphragm, unspecified depth
          Endometriosis of the diaphragm NOS
    N80.B4   Endometriosis of the pericardial space
    N80.B5   Endometriosis of the mediastinal space
    N80.B6   Endometriosis of cardiothoracic space

N80.C Endometriosis of the abdomen
    N80.C0   Endometriosis of the abdomen, unspecified
          Endometriosis of the abdomen NOS
●   N80.C1   Endometriosis of the anterior abdominal wall
    N80.C10   Endometriosis of the anterior abdominal wall, subcutaneous tissue
    N80.C11   Endometriosis of the anterior abdominal wall, fascia and muscular layers
    N80.C19   Endometriosis of the anterior abdominal wall, unspecified depth
          Endometriosis of the anterior abdominal wall NOS
    N80.C2   Endometriosis of the umbilicus
    N80.C3   Endometriosis of the inguinal canal
    N80.C4   Endometriosis of extra-pelvic abdominal peritoneum
    N80.C9   Endometriosis of other site of abdomen

● **N80.D Endometriosis of the pelvic nerves**
    Endometriosis of the nerves of the retroperitoneum
    N80.D0   Endometriosis of the pelvic nerves, unspecified
          Endometriosis of nerve of the retroperitoneum, NOS
    N80.D1   Endometriosis of the sacral splanchnic nerves
          Endometriosis of the pelvic splanchnic nerves
    N80.D2   Endometriosis of the sacral nerve roots
    N80.D3   Endometriosis of the obturator nerve
    N80.D4   Endometriosis of the sciatic nerve
    N80.D5   Endometriosis of the pudendal nerve
    N80.D6   Endometriosis of the femoral nerve
    N80.D9   Endometriosis of other pelvic nerve
          Endometriosis of the other nerves of the retroperitoneum

● **N81 Female genital prolapse**
    Excludes 1   genital prolapse complicating pregnancy, labor or delivery (O34.5-)
                 prolapse and hernia of ovary and fallopian tube (N83.4-)
                 prolapse of vaginal vault after hysterectomy (N99.3)

N81.0 Urethrocele
    Excludes 1   urethrocele with cystocele (N81.1-)
                 urethrocele with prolapse of uterus (N81.2-N81.4)

Item 14–11 Endometriosis is a condition for which no clear cause has been identified. Endometrial tissue is expelled from the uterus into the abdominal cavity and can implant onto a variety of organs. Classification is based on the site of implant of the endometrial tissue.

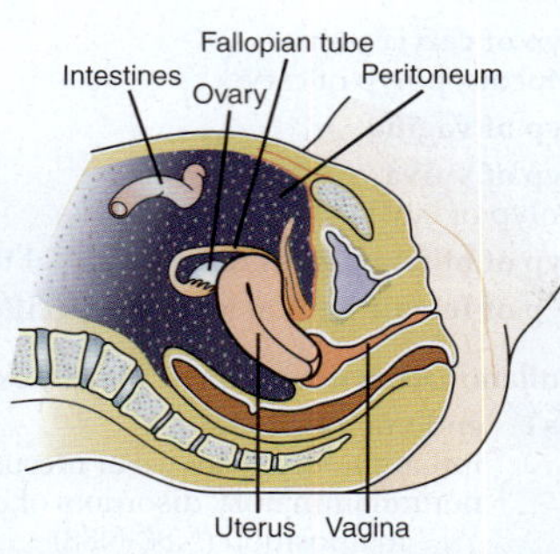

Figure 14-11   Sites of potential endometrial implants.

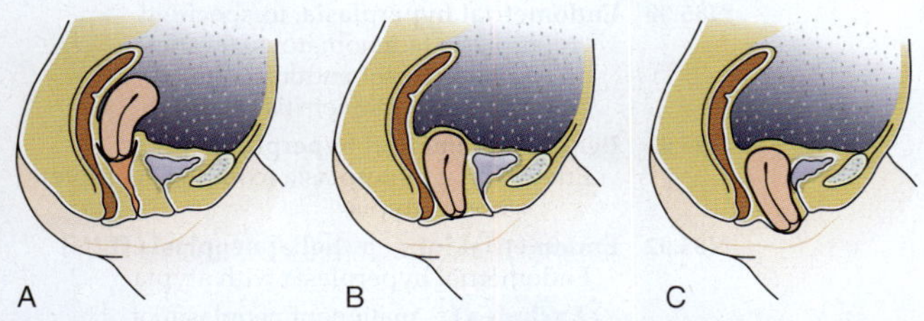

Figure 14-12   Three stages of uterine prolapse. **A.** Uterus is prolapsed. **B.** Vagina and uterus are prolapsed (incomplete uterovaginal prolapse). **C.** Vagina and uterus are completely prolapsed and are exposed through the external genitalia (complete uterovaginal prolapse).

● **N81.1**   **Cystocele**
     Cystocele with urethrocele
     Cystourethrocele
     Excludes1   cystocele with prolapse of uterus (N81.2-N81.4)

    N81.10   **Cystocele, unspecified**
       Prolapse of (anterior) vaginal wall NOS

    N81.11   **Cystocele, midline**

    N81.12   **Cystocele, lateral**
       Paravaginal cystocele

N81.2   **Incomplete uterovaginal prolapse**
     First degree uterine prolapse
     Prolapse of cervix NOS
     Second degree uterine prolapse
     Excludes1   cervical stump prolapse (N81.85)

N81.3   **Complete uterovaginal prolapse**
     Procidentia (uteri) NOS
     Third degree uterine prolapse

N81.4   **Uterovaginal prolapse, unspecified**
     Prolapse of uterus NOS

N81.5   **Vaginal enterocele**
     Excludes1   enterocele with prolapse of uterus (N81.2-N81.4)

N81.6   **Rectocele**
     Prolapse of posterior vaginal wall
     Use additional code for any associated fecal incontinence, if applicable (R15.-)
     Excludes1   rectocele with prolapse of uterus (N81.2-N81.4)
     Excludes2   perineocele (N81.81)
                rectal prolapse (K62.3)

● **N81.8**   **Other female genital prolapse**

    N81.81   **Perineocele**

    N81.82   **Incompetence or weakening of pubocervical tissue**

    N81.83   **Incompetence or weakening of rectovaginal tissue**

    N81.84   **Pelvic muscle wasting**
       Disuse atrophy of pelvic muscles and anal sphincter

    N81.85   **Cervical stump prolapse**

    N81.89   **Other female genital prolapse**
       Deficient perineum
       Old laceration of muscles of pelvic floor

N81.9   **Female genital prolapse, unspecified**

● **N82**   **Fistulae involving female genital tract**
     Excludes1   vesicointestinal fistulae (N32.1)

N82.0   **Vesicovaginal fistula**

N82.1   **Other female urinary-genital tract fistulae**
     Cervicovesical fistula
     Ureterovaginal fistula
     Urethrovaginal fistula
     Uteroureteric fistula
     Uterovesical fistula
     Coding Clinic: 2017, Q3, P4

N82.2   **Fistula of vagina to small intestine**

N82.3   **Fistula of vagina to large intestine**
     Rectovaginal fistula

N82.4   **Other female intestinal-genital tract fistulae**
     Intestinouterine fistula

N82.5   **Female genital tract-skin fistulae**
     Uterus to abdominal wall fistula
     Vaginoperineal fistula

N82.8   **Other female genital tract fistulae**

N82.9   **Female genital tract fistula, unspecified**

● **N83**   **Noninflammatory disorders of ovary, fallopian tube and broad ligament**
     Excludes2   hydrosalpinx (N70.1-)

● **N83.0**   **Follicular cyst of ovary**
     Cyst of graafian follicle
     Hemorrhagic follicular cyst (of ovary)
     Coding Clinic: 2016, Q4, P46

    N83.00   **Follicular cyst of ovary, unspecified side**

    N83.01   **Follicular cyst of right ovary**

    N83.02   **Follicular cyst of left ovary**

● **N83.1**   **Corpus luteum cyst**
     Hemorrhagic corpus luteum cyst
     Coding Clinic: 2016, Q4, P46

    N83.10   **Corpus luteum cyst of ovary, unspecified side**

    N83.11   **Corpus luteum cyst of right ovary**

    N83.12   **Corpus luteum cyst of left ovary**
       Coding Clinic: 2022, Q1, P23

● **N83.2**   **Other and unspecified ovarian cysts**
     Excludes1   developmental ovarian cyst (Q50.1)
                neoplastic ovarian cyst (D27.-)
                polycystic ovarian syndrome (E28.2)
                Stein-Leventhal syndrome (E28.2)
     Coding Clinic: 2016, Q4, P46

    ● **N83.20**   **Unspecified ovarian cysts**
       Coding Clinic: 2022, Q1, P23

       N83.201   **Unspecified ovarian cyst, right side**

       N83.202   **Unspecified ovarian cyst, left side**
          Coding Clinic: 2022, Q1, P23

       N83.209   **Unspecified ovarian cyst, unspecified side**
          Ovarian cyst, NOS

    ● **N83.29**   **Other ovarian cysts**
       Retention cyst of ovary
       Simple cyst of ovary

       N83.291   **Other ovarian cyst, right side**

       N83.292   **Other ovarian cyst, left side**

       N83.299   **Other ovarian cyst, unspecified side**

● **N83.3**   **Acquired atrophy of ovary and fallopian tube**
     Coding Clinic: 2016, Q4, P46

    ● **N83.31**   **Acquired atrophy of ovary**

       N83.311   **Acquired atrophy of right ovary**

       N83.312   **Acquired atrophy of left ovary**

       N83.319   **Acquired atrophy of ovary, unspecified side**
          Acquired atrophy of ovary, NOS

CHAPTER 14 (N00-N99)

● **N83.32** **Acquired atrophy of fallopian tube**

     N83.321 Acquired atrophy of right fallopian tube

     N83.322 Acquired atrophy of left fallopian tube

     N83.329 Acquired atrophy of fallopian tube, unspecified side

        Acquired atrophy of fallopian tube, NOS

● **N83.33** **Acquired atrophy of ovary and fallopian tube**

     N83.331 Acquired atrophy of right ovary and fallopian tube

     N83.332 Acquired atrophy of left ovary and fallopian tube

     N83.339 Acquired atrophy of ovary and fallopian tube, unspecified side

        Acquired atrophy of ovary and fallopian tube, NOS

● **N83.4** **Prolapse and hernia of ovary and fallopian tube**

     Coding Clinic: 2016, Q4, P46

     N83.40 Prolapse and hernia of ovary and fallopian tube, unspecified side

        Prolapse and hernia of ovary and fallopian tube, NOS

     N83.41 Prolapse and hernia of right ovary and fallopian tube

     N83.42 Prolapse and hernia of left ovary and fallopian tube

● **N83.5** **Torsion of ovary, ovarian pedicle and fallopian tube**

     Torsion of accessory tube

     Coding Clinic: 2016, Q4, P46

     ● **N83.51** **Torsion of ovary and ovarian pedicle**

        N83.511 Torsion of right ovary and ovarian pedicle

        N83.512 Torsion of left ovary and ovarian pedicle

        N83.519 Torsion of ovary and ovarian pedicle, unspecified side

           Torsion of ovary and ovarian pedicle, NOS

     ● **N83.52** **Torsion of fallopian tube**

        Torsion of hydatid of Morgagni

        N83.521 Torsion of right fallopian tube

        N83.522 Torsion of left fallopian tube

        N83.529 Torsion of fallopian tube, unspecified side

           Torsion of fallopian tube, NOS

     N83.53 Torsion of ovary, ovarian pedicle and fallopian tube

● **N83.6** **Hematosalpinx**

     Excludes1 hematosalpinx (with) (in):

        hematocolpos (N89.7)

        hematometra (N85.7)

        tubal pregnancy (O00.1-)

● **N83.7** **Hematoma of broad ligament**

● **N83.8** **Other noninflammatory disorders of ovary, fallopian tube and broad ligament**

     Broad ligament laceration syndrome [Allen-Masters]

● **N83.9** **Noninflammatory disorder of ovary, fallopian tube and broad ligament, unspecified**

● **N84** **Polyp of female genital tract**

     Excludes1 adenomatous polyp (D28.-)

        placental polyp (O90.89)

     N84.0 **Polyp of corpus uteri**

        Polyp of endometrium

        Polyp of uterus NOS

        Excludes1 polypoid endometrial hyperplasia (N85.0-)

     N84.1 **Polyp of cervix uteri**

        Mucous polyp of cervix

     N84.2 **Polyp of vagina**

     N84.3 **Polyp of vulva**

        Polyp of labia

     N84.8 **Polyp of other parts of female genital tract**

     N84.9 **Polyp of female genital tract, unspecified**

● **N85** **Other noninflammatory disorders of uterus, except cervix**

     Excludes1 endometriosis (N80.-)

        inflammatory diseases of uterus (N71.-)

        noninflammatory disorders of cervix, except malposition (N86-N88)

        polyp of corpus uteri (N84.0)

        uterine prolapse (N81.-)

     ● **N85.0** **Endometrial hyperplasia**

        N85.00 **Endometrial hyperplasia, unspecified**

           Hyperplasia (adenomatous) (cystic) (glandular) of endometrium

           Hyperplastic endometritis

        N85.01 **Benign endometrial hyperplasia**

           Endometrial hyperplasia (complex) (simple) without atypia

        N85.02 **Endometrial intraepithelial neoplasia [EIN]**

           Endometrial hyperplasia with atypia

           Excludes1 malignant neoplasm of endometrium (with endometrial intraepithelial neoplasia [EIN]) (C54.1)

     N85.2 **Hypertrophy of uterus**

        Bulky or enlarged uterus

        Excludes1 puerperal hypertrophy of uterus (O90.89)

     N85.3 **Subinvolution of uterus**

        Excludes1 puerperal subinvolution of uterus (O90.89)

     N85.4 **Malposition of uterus**

        Anteversion of uterus

        Retroflexion of uterus

        Retroversion of uterus

        Excludes1 malposition of uterus complicating pregnancy, labor or delivery (O34.5-, O65.5)

     N85.5 **Inversion of uterus**

        Excludes1 current obstetric trauma (O71.2)

           postpartum inversion of uterus (O71.2)

     N85.6 **Intrauterine synechiae**

     N85.7 **Hematometra**

        Hematosalpinx with hematometra

        Excludes1 hematometra with hematocolpos (N89.7)

     N85.8 **Other specified noninflammatory disorders of uterus**

        Atrophy of uterus, acquired

        Fibrosis of uterus NOS

     N85.9 **Noninflammatory disorder of uterus, unspecified**

        Disorder of uterus NOS

     N85.A **Isthmocele**

        Isthmocele (non-pregnant state)

        Code also any associated conditions such as:

           abnormal uterine and vaginal bleeding, unspecified (N93.9)

           female infertility of uterine origin (N97.2)

           ➥ pelvic and perineal pain (R10.2-)

        Excludes1 maternal care for cesarean scar defect (isthmocele) (O34.22)

        Coding Clinic: 2022, Q4, P37

N86 **Erosion and ectropion of cervix uteri**

     Decubitus (trophic) ulcer of cervix

     Eversion of cervix

     Excludes1 erosion and ectropion of cervix with cervicitis (N72)

▶ New   ⇨ Revised   ~~deleted~~ Deleted   Excludes 1   Excludes 2   Includes   Use additional   Code first   Code also   Key words

OGCR Official Guidelines   X Assign placeholder X   ● Use Additional Character(s)   ▶ Manifestation Code   Ⓡ Hierarchical Condition Category   Coding Clinic

● **N87**   **Dysplasia of cervix uteri**
> **Excludes1**   abnormal results from cervical cytologic examination without histologic confirmation (R87.61-)
> carcinoma in situ of cervix uteri (D06.-)
> cervical intraepithelial neoplasia III [CIN III] (D06.-)
> HGSIL of cervix (R87.613)
> severe dysplasia of cervix uteri (D06.-)

N87.0   **Mild cervical dysplasia**
Cervical intraepithelial neoplasia I [CIN I]

N87.1   **Moderate cervical dysplasia**
Cervical intraepithelial neoplasia II [CIN II]

N87.9   **Dysplasia of cervix uteri, unspecified**
Anaplasia of cervix
Cervical atypism
Cervical dysplasia NOS

● **N88**   **Other noninflammatory disorders of cervix uteri**
> **Excludes2**   inflammatory disease of cervix (N72)
> polyp of cervix (N84.1)

N88.0   **Leukoplakia of cervix uteri**

N88.1   **Old laceration of cervix uteri**
Adhesions of cervix
> **Excludes1**   current obstetric trauma (O71.3)

N88.2   **Stricture and stenosis of cervix uteri**
> **Excludes1**   stricture and stenosis of cervix uteri complicating labor (O65.5)

N88.3   **Incompetence of cervix uteri**
Investigation and management of (suspected) cervical incompetence in a nonpregnant woman
> **Excludes1**   cervical incompetence complicating pregnancy (O34.3-)

N88.4   **Hypertrophic elongation of cervix uteri**

N88.8   **Other specified noninflammatory disorders of cervix uteri**
> **Excludes1**   current obstetric trauma (O71.3)

N88.9   **Noninflammatory disorder of cervix uteri, unspecified**

● **N89**   **Other noninflammatory disorders of vagina**
> **Excludes1**   abnormal results from vaginal cytologic examination without histologic confirmation (R87.62-)
> carcinoma in situ of vagina (D07.2)
> HGSIL of vagina (R87.623)
> inflammation of vagina (N76.-)
> senile (atrophic) vaginitis (N95.2)
> severe dysplasia of vagina (D07.2)
> trichomonal leukorrhea (A59.00)
> vaginal intraepithelial neoplasia [VAIN], grade III (D07.2)

N89.0   **Mild vaginal dysplasia**
Vaginal intraepithelial neoplasia [VAIN], grade I

N89.1   **Moderate vaginal dysplasia**
Vaginal intraepithelial neoplasia [VAIN], grade II

N89.3   **Dysplasia of vagina, unspecified**

N89.4   **Leukoplakia of vagina**

N89.5   **Stricture and atresia of vagina**
Vaginal adhesions   Vaginal stenosis
> **Excludes1**   congenital atresia or stricture (Q52.4)
> postprocedural adhesions of vagina (N99.2)

N89.6   **Tight hymenal ring**
Rigid hymen   Tight introitus
> **Excludes1**   imperforate hymen (Q52.3)

N89.7   **Hematocolpos**
Hematocolpos with hematometra or hematosalpinx
Coding Clinic: 2016, Q4, P59

N89.8   **Other specified noninflammatory disorders of vagina**
Leukorrhea NOS
Old vaginal laceration
Pessary ulcer of vagina
> **Excludes1**   current obstetric trauma (O70.-, O71.4, O71.7-O71.8)
> old laceration involving muscles of pelvic floor (N81.8)

N89.9   **Noninflammatory disorder of vagina, unspecified**

● **N90**   **Other noninflammatory disorders of vulva and perineum**
> **Excludes1**   anogenital (venereal) warts (A63.0)
> carcinoma in situ of vulva (D07.1)
> condyloma acuminatum (A63.0)
> current obstetric trauma (O70.-, O71.7-O71.8)
> inflammation of vulva (N76.-)
> severe dysplasia of vulva (D07.1)
> vulvar intraepithelial neoplasm III [VIN III] (D07.1)

N90.0   **Mild vulvar dysplasia**
Vulvar intraepithelial neoplasia [VIN], grade I

N90.1   **Moderate vulvar dysplasia**
Vulvar intraepithelial neoplasia [VIN], grade II

N90.3   **Dysplasia of vulva, unspecified**

N90.4   **Leukoplakia of vulva**
Dystrophy of vulva
Kraurosis of vulva
Lichen sclerosus of external female genital organs

N90.5   **Atrophy of vulva**
Stenosis of vulva

● **N90.6**   **Hypertrophy of vulva**
Coding Clinic: 2016, Q4, P46

N90.60   **Unspecified hypertrophy of vulva**
Unspecified hypertrophy of labia

N90.61   **Childhood asymmetric labium majus enlargement**
CALME

N90.69   **Other specified hypertrophy of vulva**
Other specified hypertrophy of labia

N90.7   **Vulvar cyst**

● **N90.8**   **Other specified noninflammatory disorders of vulva and perineum**

● **N90.81**   **Female genital mutilation status**
Female genital cutting status

N90.810   **Female genital mutilation status, unspecified**
Female genital cutting status, unspecified
Female genital mutilation status NOS

N90.811   **Female genital mutilation Type I status**
Clitorectomy status
Female genital cutting Type I status

N90.812   **Female genital mutilation Type II status**
Clitorectomy with excision of labia minora status
Female genital cutting Type II status

N90.813   **Female genital mutilation Type III status**
Female genital cutting Type III status
Infibulation status

N90.818   **Other female genital mutilation status**
Female genital cutting Type IV status
Female genital mutilation Type IV status
Other female genital cutting status

N90.89   **Other specified noninflammatory disorders of vulva and perineum**
Adhesions of vulva
Hypertrophy of clitoris

N90.9   **Noninflammatory disorder of vulva and perineum, unspecified**

CHAPTER 14 (N00-N99)

CHAPTER 14 (N00-N99)

● **N91   Absent, scanty and rare menstruation**
     Excludes1   ovarian dysfunction (E28.-)
   N91.0   Primary amenorrhea
   N91.1   Secondary amenorrhea
   N91.2   Amenorrhea, unspecified
   N91.3   Primary oligomenorrhea
   N91.4   Secondary oligomenorrhea
   N91.5   Oligomenorrhea, unspecified
      Hypomenorrhea NOS

● **N92   Excessive, frequent and irregular menstruation**
     Excludes1   postmenopausal bleeding (N95.0)
                 precocious puberty (menstruation) (E30.1)
   N92.0   Excessive and frequent menstruation with regular cycle
      Heavy periods NOS   Polymenorrhea
      Menorrhagia NOS
   N92.1   Excessive and frequent menstruation with irregular cycle
      Irregular intermenstrual bleeding
      Irregular, shortened intervals between menstrual bleeding
      Menometrorrhagia
      Metrorrhagia
   N92.2   Excessive menstruation at puberty   **P**
      Excessive bleeding associated with onset of menstrual periods
      Pubertal menorrhagia
      Puberty bleeding
   N92.3   Ovulation bleeding
      Regular intermenstrual bleeding
   N92.4   Excessive bleeding in the premenopausal period
      Climacteric menorrhagia or metrorrhagia
      Menopausal menorrhagia or metrorrhagia
      Perimenopausal bleeding
      Perimenopausal menorrhagia or metrorrhagia
      Preclimacteric menorrhagia or metrorrhagia
      Premenopausal menorrhagia or metrorrhagia
   N92.5   Other specified irregular menstruation
   N92.6   Irregular menstruation, unspecified
      Irregular bleeding NOS
      Irregular periods NOS
     Excludes1   irregular menstruation with:
                 lengthened intervals or scanty bleeding (N91.3-N91.5)
                 shortened intervals or excessive bleeding (N92.1)

● **N93   Other abnormal uterine and vaginal bleeding**
     Excludes1   neonatal vaginal hemorrhage (P54.6)
                 precocious puberty (menstruation) (E30.1)
                 pseudomenses (P54.6)
   N93.0   Postcoital and contact bleeding
   N93.1   Pre-pubertal vaginal bleeding
      Coding Clinic: 2016, Q4, P47
   N93.8   Other specified abnormal uterine and vaginal bleeding
      Dysfunctional or functional uterine or vaginal bleeding NOS
   N93.9   Abnormal uterine and vaginal bleeding, unspecified

● **N94   Pain and other conditions associated with female genital organs and menstrual cycle**
   N94.0   Mittelschmerz
      Ovulation pain
  ● **N94.1   Dyspareunia**
      Painful intercourse/coitus
     Excludes1   psychogenic dyspareunia (F52.6)
      Coding Clinic: 2016, Q4, P47
     N94.10   Unspecified dyspareunia
     N94.11   Superficial (introital) dyspareunia
     N94.12   Deep dyspareunia
     N94.19   Other specified dyspareunia

   N94.2   Vaginismus
      Vagina tightness
     Excludes1   psychogenic vaginismus (F52.5)
   N94.3   Premenstrual tension syndrome
      AKA: PMS
     Code also associated menstrual migraine (G43.82-, G43.83-)
     Excludes1   Premenstrual dysphoric disorder (F32.81)
      Coding Clinic: 2016, Q4, P14
   N94.4   Primary dysmenorrhea
      Lifelong painful menstruation
   N94.5   Secondary dysmenorrhea
      Later onset of painful menstruation
   N94.6   Dysmenorrhea, unspecified
     Excludes1   psychogenic dysmenorrhea (F45.8)
  ● **N94.8   Other specified conditions associated with female genital organs and menstrual cycle**
   ● **N94.81   Vulvodynia**
       N94.810   Vulvar vestibulitis
       N94.818   Other vulvodynia
       N94.819   Vulvodynia, unspecified
          Vulvodynia NOS
     N94.89   Other specified conditions associated with female genital organs and menstrual cycle
   N94.9   Unspecified condition associated with female genital organs and menstrual cycle

● **N95   Menopausal and other perimenopausal disorders**
     Menopausal and other perimenopausal disorders due to naturally occurring (age-related) menopause and perimenopause
     Excludes1   excessive bleeding in the premenopausal period (N92.4)
                 menopausal and perimenopausal disorders due to artificial or premature menopause (E89.4-, E28.31-)
                 premature menopause (E28.31-)
     Excludes2   postmenopausal osteoporosis (M81.0-)
                 postmenopausal osteoporosis with current pathological fracture (M80.0-)
                 postmenopausal urethritis (N34.2)
   N95.0   Postmenopausal bleeding
   N95.1   Menopausal and female climacteric states
      Symptoms such as flushing, sleeplessness, headache, lack of concentration, associated with natural (age-related) menopause
     Use additional code for associated symptoms
     Excludes1   asymptomatic menopausal state (Z78.0)
                 symptoms associated with artificial menopause (E89.41)
                 symptoms associated with premature menopause (E28.310)
   N95.2   Postmenopausal atrophic vaginitis
      Senile (atrophic) vaginitis
   N95.8   Other specified menopausal and perimenopausal disorders
   N95.9   Unspecified menopausal and perimenopausal disorder

N96   Recurrent pregnancy loss
     Investigation or care in a nonpregnant woman with history of recurrent pregnancy loss
     Excludes1   recurrent pregnancy loss with current pregnancy (O26.2-)

● **N97   Female infertility**
     Includes   inability to achieve a pregnancy
              sterility, female NOS
     Excludes2   female infertility associated with:
                 hypopituitarism (E23.0)
                 Stein-Leventhal syndrome (E28.2)
                 incompetence of cervix uteri (N88.3)
     Coding Clinic: 2022, Q2, P16

▶ New   ⇒ Revised   ~~deleted~~ Deleted   Excludes 1   Excludes 2   Includes   Use additional   Code first   Code also   Key words
OGCR Official Guidelines   **X** Assign placeholder X   ● Use Additional Character(s)   ▸ Manifestation Code   Hierarchical Condition Category   **Coding Clinic**

N97.0   **Female infertility associated with anovulation**
          Coding Clinic: 2022, Q2, P16

N97.1   **Female infertility of tubal origin**
          Female infertility associated with congenital anomaly
                of tube
          Female infertility due to tubal block
          Female infertility due to tubal occlusion
          Female infertility due to tubal stenosis

N97.2   **Female infertility of uterine origin**
          Female infertility associated with congenital anomaly
                of uterus
          Female infertility due to nonimplantation of ovum

N97.8   **Female infertility of other origin**

N97.9   **Female infertility, unspecified**

● **N98   Complications associated with artificial fertilization**

N98.0   **Infection associated with artificial
          insemination**

N98.1   **Hyperstimulation of ovaries**
          Hyperstimulation of ovaries NOS
          Hyperstimulation of ovaries associated with induced
                ovulation

N98.2   **Complications of attempted introduction of fertilized
          ovum following in vitro fertilization**

N98.3   **Complications of attempted introduction of embryo in
          embryo transfer**

N98.8   **Other complications associated with artificial
          fertilization**

N98.9   **Complication associated with artificial fertilization,
          unspecified**

INTRAOPERATIVE AND POSTPROCEDURAL COMPLICATIONS AND DISORDERS OF GENITOURINARY SYSTEM, NOT ELSEWHERE CLASSIFIED (N99)

● **N99   Intraoperative and postprocedural complications and disorders
          of genitourinary system, not elsewhere classified**
          Excludes2   irradiation cystitis (N30.4-)
                            postoophorectomy osteoporosis with current
                                  pathological fracture (M80.8-)
                            postoophorectomy osteoporosis without current
                                  pathological fracture (M81.8)

N99.0   **Postprocedural (acute) (chronic) kidney failure**
          Use additional code to type of kidney disease

● **N99.1   Postprocedural urethral stricture**
          Postcatheterization urethral stricture

● **N99.11   Postprocedural urethral stricture, male**

N99.110   **Postprocedural urethral stricture,
            male, meatal**

N99.111   **Postprocedural bulbous urethral
            stricture, male**

N99.112   **Postprocedural membranous urethral
            stricture, male**

N99.113   **Postprocedural anterior bulbous
            urethral stricture, male**
            Coding Clinic: 2016, Q4, P48

N99.114   **Postprocedural urethral stricture,
            male, unspecified**

N99.115   **Postprocedural fossa navicularis
            urethral stricture**
            Coding Clinic: 2016, Q4, P47

N99.116   **Postprocedural urethral stricture,
            male, overlapping sites**

N99.12   **Postprocedural urethral stricture, female**

N99.2   **Postprocedural adhesions of vagina**

N99.3   **Prolapse of vaginal vault after hysterectomy**

N99.4   **Postprocedural pelvic peritoneal adhesions**
          Excludes2   pelvic peritoneal adhesions NOS (N73.6)
                            postinfective pelvic peritoneal adhesions
                                  (N73.6)

● **N99.5   Complications of stoma of urinary tract**
          Excludes2   mechanical complication of urinary
                            catheter (T83.0-)

● **N99.51   Complication of cystostomy**

N99.510   **Cystostomy
            hemorrhage** 🔵

N99.511   **Cystostomy infection** 🔵

N99.512   **Cystostomy
            malfunction** 🔵

N99.518   **Other cystostomy
            complication** 🔵

● **N99.52   Complication of incontinent external stoma of
          urinary tract**

N99.520   **Hemorrhage of incontinent external
            stoma of urinary tract** 🔵

N99.521   **Infection of incontinent external
            stoma of urinary tract** 🔵
            Coding Clinic: 2016, Q4, P48

N99.522   **Malfunction of incontinent external
            stoma of urinary tract** 🔵

N99.523   **Herniation of incontinent stoma of
            urinary tract** 🔵
            Coding Clinic: 2016, Q4, P48

N99.524   **Stenosis of incontinent stoma of
            urinary tract** 🔵
            Coding Clinic: 2016, Q4, P48

N99.528   **Other complication of incontinent
            external stoma of urinary tract** 🔵

● **N99.53   Complication of continent stoma of urinary
          tract**

N99.530   **Hemorrhage of continent stoma of
            urinary tract** 🔵

N99.531   **Infection of continent stoma of
            urinary tract** 🔵

N99.532   **Malfunction of continent stoma of
            urinary tract** 🔵

N99.533   **Herniation of continent stoma of
            urinary tract** 🔵
            Coding Clinic: 2016, Q4, P48

N99.534   **Stenosis of continent stoma of urinary
            tract** 🔵
            Coding Clinic: 2016, Q4, P48

N99.538   **Other complication of continent
            stoma of urinary tract** 🔵

● **N99.6   Intraoperative hemorrhage and hematoma of a
          genitourinary system organ or structure complicating a
          procedure**
          Excludes1   intraoperative hemorrhage and
                            hematoma of a genitourinary system
                            organ or structure due to accidental
                            puncture or laceration during a
                            procedure (N99.7-)

N99.61   **Intraoperative hemorrhage and hematoma
          of a genitourinary system organ or structure
          complicating a genitourinary system procedure**

N99.62   **Intraoperative hemorrhage and hematoma
          of a genitourinary system organ or structure
          complicating other procedure**

● **N99.7   Accidental puncture and laceration of a genitourinary
          system organ or structure during a procedure**

N99.71   **Accidental puncture and laceration of a
          genitourinary system organ or structure during
          a genitourinary system procedure**

N99.72   **Accidental puncture and laceration of a
          genitourinary system organ or structure during
          other procedure**

CHAPTER 14 (N00-N99)

● **N99.8** **Other intraoperative and postprocedural complications and disorders of genitourinary system**
    Coding Clinic: 2016, Q4, P10

  N99.81 Other intraoperative complications of genitourinary system

● **N99.82** Postprocedural hemorrhage of a genitourinary system organ or structure following a procedure

    N99.820 Postprocedural hemorrhage of a genitourinary system organ or structure following a genitourinary system procedure
      Coding Clinic: 2025, Q2, P20-21

    N99.821 Postprocedural hemorrhage of a genitourinary system organ or structure following other procedure

  N99.83 Residual ovary syndrome

● **N99.84** Postprocedural hematoma and seroma of a genitourinary system organ or structure following a procedure

    N99.840 Postprocedural hematoma of a genitourinary system organ or structure following a genitourinary system procedure

    N99.841 Postprocedural hematoma of a genitourinary system organ or structure following other procedure

    N99.842 Postprocedural seroma of a genitourinary system organ or structure following a genitourinary system procedure

    N99.843 Postprocedural seroma of a genitourinary system organ or structure following other procedure

  N99.85 Post endometrial ablation syndrome
    Coding Clinic: 2019, Q4, P12

  N99.89 Other postprocedural complications and disorders of genitourinary system

CHAPTER 15

PREGNANCY, CHILDBIRTH, AND THE PUERPERIUM (O00-O9A)

OGCR Chapter-Specific Coding Guidelines

15. Chapter 15: Pregnancy, Childbirth, and the Puerperium (O00-O9A)

a. General Rules for Obstetric Cases

1) Codes from Chapter 15 and sequencing priority

Obstetric cases require codes from Chapter 15, codes in the range O00-O9A, Pregnancy, Childbirth, and the Puerperium. Chapter 15 codes have sequencing priority over codes from other chapters. Additional codes from other chapters may be used in conjunction with Chapter 15 codes to further specify conditions. Should the provider document that the pregnancy is incidental to the encounter, then code Z33.1, Pregnant state, incidental, should be used in place of any Chapter 15 codes. It is the provider's responsibility to state that the condition being treated is not affecting the pregnancy.

2) Chapter 15 codes used only on the maternal record

Chapter 15 codes are to be used only on the maternal record, never on the record of the newborn.

3) Final character for trimester

The majority of codes in Chapter 15 have a final character indicating the trimester of pregnancy. The timeframes for the trimesters are indicated at the beginning of the chapter. If trimester is not a component of a code it is because the condition always occurs in a specific trimester, or the concept of trimester of pregnancy is not applicable. Certain codes have characters for only certain trimesters because the condition does not occur in all trimesters, but it may occur in more than just one.

Assignment of the final character for trimester should be based on the provider's documentation of the trimester (or number of weeks) for the current admission/encounter. This applies to the assignment of trimester for pre-existing conditions as well as those that develop during or are due to the pregnancy. The provider's documentation of the number of weeks may be used to assign the appropriate code identifying the trimester.

Whenever delivery occurs during the current admission, and there is an "in childbirth" option for the obstetric complication being coded, the "in childbirth" code should be assigned.

4) Selection of trimester for inpatient admissions that encompass more than one trimester

In instances when a patient is admitted to a hospital for complications of pregnancy during one trimester and remains in the hospital into a subsequent trimester, the trimester character for the antepartum complication code should be assigned on the basis of the trimester when the complication developed, not the trimester of the discharge. If the complication developed prior to the current admission/encounter or represents a pre-existing condition, the trimester character for the trimester at the time of the admission/encounter should be assigned.

5) Unspecified trimester

Each category that includes codes for trimester has a code for "unspecified trimester." The "unspecified trimester" code should rarely be used, such as when the documentation in the record is insufficient to determine the trimester and it is not possible to obtain clarification.

6) 7th character for Fetus Identification

Where applicable, a 7th character is to be assigned for certain categories (O31, O32, O33.3 - O33.6, O35, O36, O40, O41, O60.1, O60.2, O64, and O69) to identify the fetus for which the complication code applies.

Assign 7th character "0":
- For single gestations
- When the documentation in the record is insufficient to determine the fetus affected and it is not possible to obtain clarification.
- When it is not possible to clinically determine which fetus is affected.

b. Selection of OB Principal or First-listed Diagnosis

1) Routine outpatient prenatal visits

For routine outpatient prenatal visits when no complications are present, a code from category Z34, Encounter for supervision of normal pregnancy, should be used as the first-listed diagnosis. These codes should not be used in conjunction with Chapter 15 codes.

2) Supervision of High-Risk Pregnancy

Codes from category O09, Supervision of high-risk pregnancy, are intended for use only during the prenatal period. For complications during the labor or delivery episode as a result of a high-risk pregnancy, assign the applicable complication codes from Chapter 15. If there are no complications during the labor or delivery episode, assign code O80, Encounter for full-term uncomplicated delivery.

For routine prenatal outpatient visits for patients with high-risk pregnancies, a code from category O09, Supervision of high-risk pregnancy, should be used as the first-listed diagnosis. Secondary Chapter 15 codes may be used in conjunction with these codes if appropriate.

3) Episodes when no delivery occurs

In episodes when no delivery occurs, the principal diagnosis should correspond to the principal complication of the pregnancy which necessitated the encounter. Should more than one complication exist, all of which are treated or monitored, any of the complications codes may be sequenced first.

4) When a delivery occurs

When an obstetric patient is admitted and delivers during that admission, the condition that prompted the admission should be sequenced as the principal diagnosis. If multiple conditions prompted the admission, sequence the one most related to the delivery as the principal diagnosis. A code for any complication of the delivery should be assigned as an additional diagnosis. In cases of cesarean delivery, if the patient was admitted with a condition that resulted in the performance of a cesarean procedure, that condition should be selected as the principal diagnosis. If the reason for the admission was unrelated to the condition resulting in the cesarean delivery, the condition related to the reason for the admission should be selected as the principal diagnosis.

5) Outcome of delivery

A code from category Z37, Outcome of delivery, should be included on every maternal record when a delivery has occurred. These codes are not to be used on subsequent records or on the newborn record.

c. Pre-existing conditions versus conditions due to the pregnancy

Certain categories in Chapter 15 distinguish between conditions of the mother that existed prior to pregnancy (pre-existing) and those that are a direct result of pregnancy. When assigning codes from Chapter 15, it is important to assess if a condition was pre-existing prior to pregnancy or developed during or due to the pregnancy in order to assign the correct code.

Categories that do not distinguish between pre-existing and pregnancy-related conditions may be used for either. It is acceptable to use codes specifically for the puerperium with codes complicating pregnancy and childbirth if a condition arises postpartum during the delivery encounter.

d. Pre-existing hypertension in pregnancy

Category O10, Pre-existing hypertension complicating pregnancy, childbirth and the puerperium, includes codes for hypertensive heart and hypertensive chronic kidney disease. When assigning one of the O10 codes that includes hypertensive heart disease or hypertensive chronic kidney disease, it is necessary to add a secondary code from the appropriate hypertension category to specify the type of heart failure or chronic kidney disease.

See Section I.C.9. Hypertension.

e. Fetal Conditions Affecting the Management of the Mother

1) Codes from categories O35 and O36

Codes from categories O35, Maternal care for known or suspected fetal abnormality and damage, and O36, Maternal care for other fetal problems, are assigned only when the fetal condition is actually responsible for modifying the management of the mother, i.e., by requiring diagnostic studies, additional observation, special care, or termination of pregnancy. The fact that the fetal condition exists does not justify assigning a code from this series to the mother's record.

2) In utero surgery

In cases when surgery is performed on the fetus, a diagnosis code from category O35, Maternal care for known or suspected fetal abnormality and damage, should be assigned identifying the fetal condition. Assign the appropriate procedure code for the procedure performed.

No code from Chapter 16, the perinatal codes, should be used on the mother's record to identify fetal conditions. Surgery performed in utero on a fetus is still to be coded as an obstetric encounter.

f. HIV Infection in Pregnancy, Childbirth, and the Puerperium

During pregnancy, childbirth or the puerperium, a patient admitted because of an HIV-related illness should receive a principal diagnosis from subcategory O98.7-, Human immunodeficiency [HIV] disease complicating pregnancy, childbirth and the puerperium, followed by the code(s) for the HIV-related illness(es).

Patients with asymptomatic HIV infection status admitted during pregnancy, childbirth, or the puerperium should receive codes of O98.7- and Z21, Asymptomatic human immunodeficiency virus [HIV] infection status.

g. Diabetes mellitus in pregnancy

Diabetes mellitus is a significant complicating factor in pregnancy. Pregnant women who are diabetic should be assigned a code from category O24, Diabetes mellitus in pregnancy, childbirth, and the puerperium, first, followed by the appropriate diabetes code(s) (E08-E13) from Chapter 4.

h. Long-term use of insulin and oral hypoglycemics
See Section I.C.4.a.3 for information on the long-term use of insulin and oral hypoglycemic.

i. Gestational (pregnancy induced) diabetes
Gestational (pregnancy induced) diabetes can occur during the second and third trimester of pregnancy in women who were not diabetic prior to pregnancy. Gestational diabetes can cause complications in the pregnancy similar to those of pre-existing diabetes mellitus. It also puts the woman at greater risk of developing diabetes after the pregnancy. Codes for gestational diabetes are in subcategory O24.4, Gestational diabetes mellitus. No other code from category O24, Diabetes mellitus in pregnancy, childbirth, and the puerperium, should be used with a code from O24.4.

The codes under subcategory O24.4 include diet controlled, insulin controlled, and controlled by oral hypoglycemic drugs. If a patient with gestational diabetes is treated with both diet and insulin, only the code for insulin-controlled is required. If a patient with gestational diabetes is treated with both diet and oral hypoglycemic medications, only the code for "controlled by oral hypoglycemic drugs" is required. Code Z79.4, Long-term (current) use of insulin or code Z79.84, Long-term (current) use of oral hypoglycemic drugs, should not be assigned with codes from subcategory O24.4.

An abnormal glucose tolerance in pregnancy is assigned a code from subcategory O99.81, Abnormal glucose complicating pregnancy, childbirth, and the puerperium.

j. Sepsis and septic shock complicating abortion, pregnancy, childbirth and the puerperium
When assigning a Chapter 15 code for sepsis complicating abortion, pregnancy, childbirth, and the puerperium, a code for the specific type of infection should be assigned as an additional diagnosis. If severe sepsis is present, a code from subcategory R65.2, Severe sepsis, and code(s) for associated organ dysfunction(s) should also be assigned as additional diagnoses.

k. Puerperal sepsis
Code O85, Puerperal sepsis, should be assigned with a secondary code to identify the causal organism (e.g., for a bacterial infection, assign a code from category B95-B96, Bacterial infections in conditions classified elsewhere). A code from category A40, Streptococcal sepsis, or A41, Other sepsis, should not be used for puerperal sepsis. If applicable, use additional codes to identify severe sepsis (R65.2-) and any associated acute organ dysfunction.

l. Alcohol, tobacco and drug use during pregnancy, childbirth and the puerperium

1) Alcohol use during pregnancy, childbirth and the puerperium
Codes under subcategory O99.31, Alcohol use complicating pregnancy, childbirth, and the puerperium, should be assigned for any pregnancy case when a mother uses alcohol during the pregnancy or postpartum. A secondary code from category F10, Alcohol-related disorders, should also be assigned to identify manifestations of the alcohol use.

2) Tobacco use during pregnancy, childbirth, and the puerperium
Codes under subcategory O99.33, Smoking (tobacco) complicating pregnancy, childbirth, and the puerperium, should be assigned for any pregnancy case when a mother uses any type of tobacco product during the pregnancy or postpartum. A secondary code from category F17, Nicotine dependence, should also be assigned to identify the type of nicotine dependence.

3) Drug use during pregnancy, childbirth and the puerperium
Codes under subcategory O99.32, Drug use complicating pregnancy, childbirth, and the puerperium, should be assigned for any pregnancy case when a mother uses drugs during the pregnancy or postpartum. This can involve illegal drugs, or inappropriate use or abuse of prescription drugs. Secondary code(s) from categories F11-F16 and F18F19 should also be assigned to identify manifestations of the drug use.

m. Poisoning, toxic effects, adverse effects and underdosing in a pregnant patient
A code from subcategory O9A.2, Injury, poisoning and certain other consequences of external causes complicating pregnancy, childbirth, and the puerperium, should be sequenced first, followed by the appropriate injury, poisoning, toxic effect, adverse effect or underdosing code, and then the additional code(s) that specifies the condition caused by the poisoning, toxic effect, adverse effect or underdosing.
See Section I.C.19. Adverse effects, poisoning, underdosing and toxic effects.

n. Normal Delivery, Code O80

1) Encounter for full-term uncomplicated delivery
Code O80 should be assigned when a woman is admitted for a full-term normal delivery and delivers a single, healthy infant without any complications antepartum, during the delivery, or postpartum during the delivery episode. Code O80 is always a principal diagnosis. It is not to be used if any other code from Chapter 15 is needed to describe a current complication of the antenatal, delivery, or perinatal period. Additional codes from other chapters may be used with code O80 if they are not related to or are in any way complicating the pregnancy.

2) Uncomplicated delivery with resolved antepartum complication
Code O80 may be used if the patient had a complication at some point during the pregnancy, but the complication is not present at the time of the admission for delivery.

3) Outcome of delivery for O80
Z37.0, Single live birth, is the only outcome of delivery code appropriate for use with O80.

o. The Peripartum and Postpartum Periods

1) Peripartum and Postpartum periods
The postpartum period begins immediately after delivery and continues for six weeks following delivery. The peripartum period is defined as the last month of pregnancy to five months postpartum.

2) Peripartum and postpartum complication
A postpartum complication is any complication occurring within the six-week period.

3) Pregnancy-related complications after 6 week period
Chapter 15 codes may also be used to describe pregnancy-related complications after the peripartum or postpartum period if the provider documents that a condition is pregnancy related.

4) Admission for routine postpartum care following delivery outside hospital
When the mother delivers outside the hospital prior to admission and is admitted for routine postpartum care and no complications are noted, code Z39.0, Encounter for care and examination of mother immediately after delivery, should be assigned as the principal diagnosis.

5) Pregnancy associated cardiomyopathy
Pregnancy associated cardiomyopathy, code O90.3, is unique in that it may be diagnosed in the third trimester of pregnancy but may continue to progress months after delivery. For this reason, it is referred to as peripartum cardiomyopathy. Code O90.3 is only for use when the cardiomyopathy develops as a result of pregnancy in a woman who did not have pre-existing heart disease.

p. Code O94, Sequelae of complication of pregnancy, childbirth, and the puerperium

1) Code O94
Code O94, Sequelae of complication of pregnancy, childbirth, and the puerperium, is for use in those cases when an initial complication of a pregnancy develops a sequelae requiring care or treatment at a future date.

2) After the initial postpartum period
This code may be used at any time after the initial postpartum period.

3) Sequencing of Code O94
This code, like all sequela codes, is to be sequenced following the code describing the sequelae of the complication.

q. Termination of Pregnancy and Spontaneous abortions

1) Abortion with Liveborn Fetus
When an attempted termination of pregnancy results in a liveborn fetus assign code Z33.2, Encounter for elective termination of pregnancy and a code from category Z37, Outcome of Delivery.

2) Retained Products of Conception following an abortion
Subsequent encounters for retained products of conception following a spontaneous abortion or elective termination of pregnancy, without complications are assigned O03.4, Incomplete spontaneous, abortion without complication, or codes O07.4, Failed attempted termination of pregnancy without complication. This advice is appropriate even when the patient was discharged previously with a discharge diagnosis of complete abortion. If the patient has a specific complication associated with the spontaneous abortion or elective termination of pregnancy in addition to retained products of conception, assign the appropriate complication in category O03 or O07 instead of code O03.4 or O07.4

3) Complications leading to abortion
Codes from Chapter 15 may be used as additional codes to identify any documented complications of the pregnancy in conjunction with codes in categories in O04, O07 and O08.

r. Abuse in a pregnant patient
For suspected or confirmed cases of abuse of a pregnant patient, a code(s) from subcategories O9A.3, Physical abuse complicating pregnancy, childbirth, and the puerperium, O9A.4, Sexual abuse complicating pregnancy, childbirth, and the puerperium, and O9A.5, Psychological abuse complicating pregnancy, childbirth, and the puerperium, should be sequenced first, followed by the appropriate codes (if applicable) to identify any associated current injury due to physical abuse, sexual abuse, and the perpetrator of abuse.
See Section I.C.19. Adult and child abuse, neglect and other maltreatment.

CHAPTER 15 (O00-O9A)

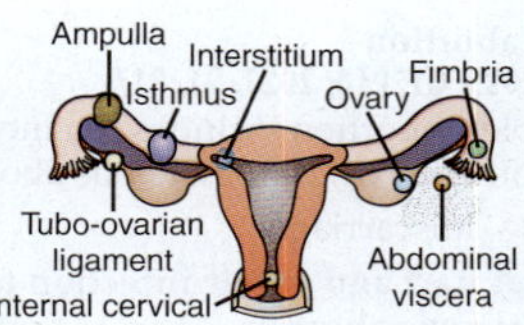

Figure 15-1 Implantation sites of ectopic pregnancy.

Item 15–1 Ectopic pregnancy most often occurs in the fallopian tube. Pregnancy outside the uterus may end in a lifethreatening rupture.

★**(See Plate 4 of the Anatomy Illustrations.)**

CHAPTER 15

PREGNANCY, CHILDBIRTH, AND THE PUERPERIUM (O00-O9A)

Note: CODES FROM THIS CHAPTER ARE FOR USE ONLY ON MATERNAL RECORDS, NEVER ON NEWBORN RECORDS

Codes from this chapter are for use for conditions related to or aggravated by the pregnancy, childbirth, or by the puerperium (maternal causes or obstetric causes)

Trimesters are counted from the first day of the last menstrual period. They are defined as follows:

1st trimester - less than 14 weeks 0 days

2nd trimester - 14 weeks 0 days to less than 28 weeks 0 days

3rd trimester - 28 weeks 0 days until delivery

Use additional code , if applicable, from category Z3A, Weeks of gestation, to identify the specific week of the pregnancy, if known.

Excludes1 supervision of normal pregnancy (Z34.-)

Excludes2 mental and behavioral disorders associated with the puerperium (F53.-)
obstetrical tetanus (A34)
postpartum necrosis of pituitary gland (E23.0)
puerperal osteomalacia (M83.0)

This chapter contains the following blocks:

O00-O08	Pregnancy with abortive outcome
O09	Supervision of high risk pregnancy
O10-O16	Edema, proteinuria and hypertensive disorders in pregnancy, childbirth and the puerperium
O20-O29	Other maternal disorders predominantly related to pregnancy
O30-O48	Maternal care related to the fetus and amniotic cavity and possible delivery problems
O60-O77	Complications of labor and delivery
O80, O82	Encounter for delivery
O85-O92	Complications predominantly related to the puerperium
O94-O9A	Other obstetric conditions, not elsewhere classified

PREGNANCY WITH ABORTIVE OUTCOME (O00-O08)

Excludes1 continuing pregnancy in multiple gestation after abortion of one fetus or more (O31.1-, O31.3-)
Coding Clinic: 2016, Q4, P130

● **O00 Ectopic pregnancy**
Includes ruptured ectopic pregnancy
Use additional code from category O08 to identify any associated complication

● **O00.0 Abdominal pregnancy**
Excludes1 maternal care for viable fetus in abdominal pregnancy (O36.7-)
Coding Clinic: 2016, Q4, P49

    O00.00 **Abdominal pregnancy without intrauterine pregnancy**   M
        Abdominal pregnancy NOS

    O00.01 **Abdominal pregnancy with intrauterine pregnancy**   M

● **O00.1 Tubal pregnancy**
Fallopian pregnancy
Rupture of (fallopian) tube due to pregnancy
Tubal abortion
Coding Clinic: 2016, Q4, P49

  ● **O00.10 Tubal pregnancy without intrauterine pregnancy**
      Tubal pregnancy NOS

      O00.101 **Right tubal pregnancy without intrauterine pregnancy**   M

      O00.102 **Left tubal pregnancy without intrauterine pregnancy**   M

      O00.109 **Unspecified tubal pregnancy without intrauterine pregnancy**   M

  ● **O00.11 Tubal pregnancy with intrauterine pregnancy**

      O00.111 **Right tubal pregnancy with intrauterine pregnancy**   M

      O00.112 **Left tubal pregnancy with intrauterine pregnancy**   M

      O00.119 **Unspecified tubal pregnancy with intrauterine pregnancy**   M

● **O00.2 Ovarian pregnancy**
Coding Clinic: 2016, Q4, P49

  ● **O00.20 Ovarian pregnancy without intrauterine pregnancy**
      Ovarian pregnancy NOS

      O00.201 **Right ovarian pregnancy without intrauterine pregnancy**   M

      O00.202 **Left ovarian pregnancy without intrauterine pregnancy**   M

      O00.209 **Unspecified ovarian pregnancy without intrauterine pregnancy**   M

  ● **O00.21 Ovarian pregnancy with intrauterine pregnancy**

      O00.211 **Right ovarian pregnancy with intrauterine pregnancy**   M

      O00.212 **Left ovarian pregnancy with intrauterine pregnancy**   M

      O00.219 **Unspecified ovarian pregnancy with intrauterine pregnancy**   M

● **O00.8 Other ectopic pregnancy**
Cervical pregnancy
Cornual pregnancy
Intraligamentous pregnancy
Mural pregnancy
Coding Clinic: 2016, Q4, P49

    O00.80 **Other ectopic pregnancy without intrauterine pregnancy**   M
        Other ectopic pregnancy NOS

    O00.81 **Other ectopic pregnancy with intrauterine pregnancy**   M

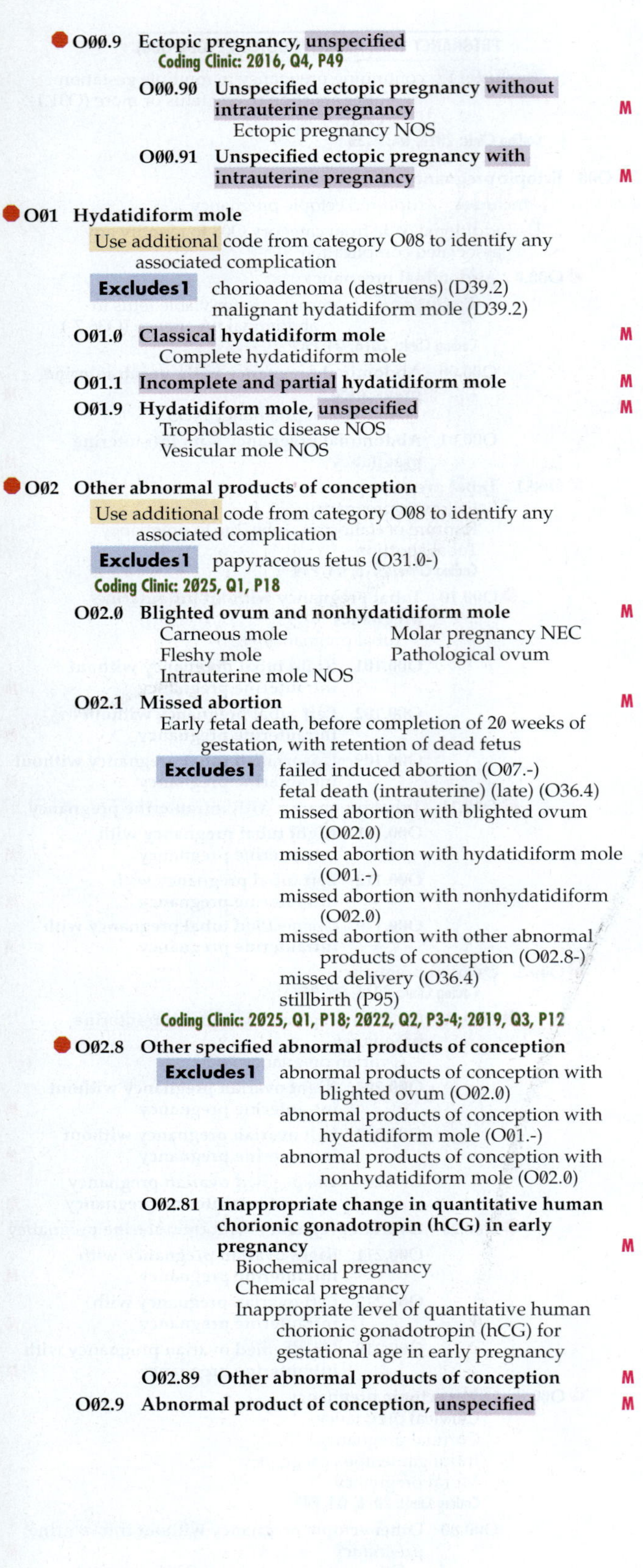

● **O00.9 Ectopic pregnancy, unspecified**
    Coding Clinic: 2016, Q4, P49

    O00.90 Unspecified ectopic pregnancy without intrauterine pregnancy   M
        Ectopic pregnancy NOS

    O00.91 Unspecified ectopic pregnancy with intrauterine pregnancy   M

● **O01 Hydatidiform mole**
    Use additional code from category O08 to identify any associated complication

    Excludes1   chorioadenoma (destruens) (D39.2)
                malignant hydatidiform mole (D39.2)

    O01.0 Classical hydatidiform mole   M
        Complete hydatidiform mole

    O01.1 Incomplete and partial hydatidiform mole   M

    O01.9 Hydatidiform mole, unspecified   M
        Trophoblastic disease NOS
        Vesicular mole NOS

● **O02 Other abnormal products of conception**
    Use additional code from category O08 to identify any associated complication

    Excludes1   papyraceous fetus (O31.0-)

    Coding Clinic: 2025, Q1, P18

    O02.0 Blighted ovum and nonhydatidiform mole   M
        Carneous mole   Molar pregnancy NEC
        Fleshy mole   Pathological ovum
        Intrauterine mole NOS

    O02.1 Missed abortion   M
        Early fetal death, before completion of 20 weeks of gestation, with retention of dead fetus

        Excludes1   failed induced abortion (O07.-)
                    fetal death (intrauterine) (late) (O36.4)
                    missed abortion with blighted ovum (O02.0)
                    missed abortion with hydatidiform mole (O01.-)
                    missed abortion with nonhydatidiform (O02.0)
                    missed abortion with other abnormal products of conception (O02.8-)
                    missed delivery (O36.4)
                    stillbirth (P95)

        Coding Clinic: 2025, Q1, P18; 2022, Q2, P3-4; 2019, Q3, P12

● **O02.8 Other specified abnormal products of conception**
    Excludes1   abnormal products of conception with blighted ovum (O02.0)
                abnormal products of conception with hydatidiform mole (O01.-)
                abnormal products of conception with nonhydatidiform mole (O02.0)

    O02.81 Inappropriate change in quantitative human chorionic gonadotropin (hCG) in early pregnancy   M
        Biochemical pregnancy
        Chemical pregnancy
        Inappropriate level of quantitative human chorionic gonadotropin (hCG) for gestational age in early pregnancy

    O02.89 Other abnormal products of conception   M

    O02.9 Abnormal product of conception, unspecified   M

● **O03 Spontaneous abortion**
    Coding Clinic: 2025, Q1, P18; 2023, Q1, P17
    Note: Incomplete abortion includes retained products of conception following spontaneous abortion.

    Includes   miscarriage

    O03.0 Genital tract and pelvic infection following incomplete spontaneous abortion   M
        Endometritis following incomplete spontaneous abortion
        Oophoritis following incomplete spontaneous abortion
        Parametritis following incomplete spontaneous abortion
        Pelvic peritonitis following incomplete spontaneous abortion
        Salpingitis following incomplete spontaneous abortion
        Salpingo-oophoritis following incomplete spontaneous abortion

        Excludes1   sepsis following incomplete spontaneous abortion (O03.37)
                    urinary tract infection following incomplete spontaneous abortion (O03.38)

    O03.1 Delayed or excessive hemorrhage following incomplete spontaneous abortion   M
        Afibrinogenemia following incomplete spontaneous abortion
        Defibrination syndrome following incomplete spontaneous abortion
        Hemolysis following incomplete spontaneous abortion
        Intravascular coagulation following incomplete spontaneous abortion

    O03.2 Embolism following incomplete spontaneous abortion   M
        Air embolism following incomplete spontaneous abortion
        Amniotic fluid embolism following incomplete spontaneous abortion
        Blood-clot embolism following incomplete spontaneous abortion
        Embolism NOS following incomplete spontaneous abortion
        Fat embolism following incomplete spontaneous abortion
        Pulmonary embolism following incomplete spontaneous abortion
        Pyemic embolism following incomplete spontaneous abortion
        Septic or septicopyemic embolism following incomplete spontaneous abortion
        Soap embolism following incomplete spontaneous abortion

● **O03.3 Other and unspecified complications following incomplete spontaneous abortion**

    O03.30 Unspecified complication following incomplete spontaneous abortion   M

    O03.31 Shock following incomplete spontaneous abortion   M
        Circulatory collapse following incomplete spontaneous abortion
        Shock (postprocedural) following incomplete spontaneous abortion

        Excludes1   shock due to infection following incomplete spontaneous abortion (O03.37)

    O03.32 Renal failure following incomplete spontaneous abortion   M
        Kidney failure (acute) following incomplete spontaneous abortion
        Oliguria following incomplete spontaneous abortion
        Renal shutdown following incomplete spontaneous abortion
        Renal tubular necrosis following incomplete spontaneous abortion
        Uremia following incomplete spontaneous abortion

Item 15–2 A **hydatidiform** mole is an overproduction of placental tissue. The tumor secretes a hormone, chorionic gonadotropic hormone (CGH), that indicates a positive pregnancy test. There is no viable fetus. More than 80% of hydatidiform moles are noncancerous.

O03.33 Metabolic disorder following incomplete spontaneous abortion M

O03.34 Damage to pelvic organs following incomplete spontaneous abortion M

Laceration, perforation, tear or chemical damage of bladder following incomplete spontaneous abortion

Laceration, perforation, tear or chemical damage of bowel following incomplete spontaneous abortion

Laceration, perforation, tear or chemical damage of broad ligament following incomplete spontaneous abortion

Laceration, perforation, tear or chemical damage of cervix following incomplete spontaneous abortion

Laceration, perforation, tear or chemical damage of periurethral tissue following incomplete spontaneous abortion

Laceration, perforation, tear or chemical damage of uterus following incomplete spontaneous abortion

Laceration, perforation, tear or chemical damage of vagina following incomplete spontaneous abortion

O03.35 Other venous complications following incomplete spontaneous abortion M

O03.36 Cardiac arrest following incomplete spontaneous abortion M

O03.37 Sepsis following incomplete spontaneous abortion M

Use additional code to identify infectious agent (B95-B97)

Use additional code to identify severe sepsis, if applicable (R65.2-)

Excludes1   septic or septicopyemic embolism following incomplete spontaneous abortion (O03.2)

O03.38 Urinary tract infection following incomplete spontaneous abortion M

Cystitis following incomplete spontaneous abortion

O03.39 Incomplete spontaneous abortion with other complications M

O03.4 Incomplete spontaneous abortion without complication M
Coding Clinic: 2023, Q1, P17

O03.5 Genital tract and pelvic infection following complete or unspecified spontaneous abortion M

Endometritis following complete or unspecified spontaneous abortion

Oophoritis following complete or unspecified spontaneous abortion

Parametritis following complete or unspecified spontaneous abortion

Pelvic peritonitis following complete or unspecified spontaneous abortion

Salpingitis following complete or unspecified spontaneous abortion

Salpingo-oophoritis following complete or unspecified spontaneous abortion

Excludes1   sepsis following complete or unspecified spontaneous abortion (O03.87)
urinary tract infection following complete or unspecified spontaneous abortion (O03.88)

O03.6 Delayed or excessive hemorrhage following complete or unspecified spontaneous abortion M

Afibrinogenemia following complete or unspecified spontaneous abortion

Defibrination syndrome following complete or unspecified spontaneous abortion

Hemolysis following complete or unspecified spontaneous abortion

Intravascular coagulation following complete or unspecified spontaneous abortion

Coding Clinic: 2022, Q1, P19

O03.7 Embolism following complete or unspecified spontaneous abortion M

Air embolism following complete or unspecified spontaneous abortion

Amniotic fluid embolism following complete or unspecified spontaneous abortion

Blood-clot embolism following complete or unspecified spontaneous abortion

Embolism NOS following complete or unspecified spontaneous abortion

Fat embolism following complete or unspecified spontaneous abortion

Pulmonary embolism following complete or unspecified spontaneous abortion

Pyemic embolism following complete or unspecified spontaneous abortion

Septic or septicopyemic embolism following complete or unspecified spontaneous abortion

Soap embolism following complete or unspecified spontaneous abortion

● **O03.8 Other and unspecified complications following complete or unspecified spontaneous abortion**

O03.80 Unspecified complication following complete or unspecified spontaneous abortion M

O03.81 Shock following complete or unspecified spontaneous abortion M

Circulatory collapse following complete or unspecified spontaneous abortion

Shock (postprocedural) following complete or unspecified spontaneous abortion

Excludes1   shock due to infection following complete or unspecified spontaneous abortion (O03.87)

O03.82 Renal failure following complete or unspecified spontaneous abortion M

Kidney failure (acute) following complete or unspecified spontaneous abortion

Oliguria following complete or unspecified spontaneous abortion

Renal shutdown following complete or unspecified spontaneous abortion

Renal tubular necrosis following complete or unspecified spontaneous abortion

Uremia following complete or unspecified spontaneous abortion

O03.83 Metabolic disorder following complete or unspecified spontaneous abortion M

O03.84 Damage to pelvic organs following complete or unspecified spontaneous abortion M

Laceration, perforation, tear or chemical damage of bladder following complete or unspecified spontaneous abortion

Laceration, perforation, tear or chemical damage of bowel following complete or unspecified spontaneous abortion

Laceration, perforation, tear or chemical damage of broad ligament following complete or unspecified spontaneous abortion

Laceration, perforation, tear or chemical damage of cervix following complete or unspecified spontaneous abortion

Laceration, perforation, tear or chemical damage of periurethral tissue following complete or unspecified spontaneous abortion

Laceration, perforation, tear or chemical damage of uterus following complete or unspecified spontaneous abortion

Laceration, perforation, tear or chemical damage of vagina following complete or unspecified spontaneous abortion

O03.85 Other venous complications following complete or unspecified spontaneous abortion M

CHAPTER 15 (O00-O9A)

O03.86   **Cardiac arrest following complete or unspecified spontaneous abortion**   M

O03.87   **Sepsis following complete or unspecified spontaneous abortion**   M

Use additional code to identify infectious agent (B95-B97)

Use additional code to identify severe sepsis, if applicable (R65.2-)

Excludes1   septic or septicopyemic embolism following complete or unspecified spontaneous abortion (O03.7)

O03.88   **Urinary tract infection following complete or unspecified spontaneous abortion**   M

Cystitis following complete or unspecified spontaneous abortion

O03.89   **Complete or unspecified spontaneous abortion with other complications**   M

O03.9   **Complete or unspecified spontaneous abortion without complication**   M

Miscarriage NOS

Spontaneous abortion NOS

● **O04   Complications following (induced) termination of pregnancy**

Includes   complications following (induced) termination of pregnancy

Excludes2   encounter for elective termination of pregnancy, uncomplicated (Z33.2)

failed attempted termination of pregnancy (O07.-)

Coding Clinic: 2025, Q1, P18; 2023, Q2, P15-16; 2023, Q1, P17

O04.5   **Genital tract and pelvic infection following (induced) termination of pregnancy**   M

Endometritis following (induced) termination of pregnancy

Oophoritis following (induced) termination of pregnancy

Parametritis following (induced) termination of pregnancy

Pelvic peritonitis following (induced) termination of pregnancy

Salpingitis following (induced) termination of pregnancy

Salpingo-oophoritis following (induced) termination of pregnancy

Excludes1   sepsis following (induced) termination of pregnancy (O04.87)

urinary tract infection following (induced) termination of pregnancy (O04.88)

O04.6   **Delayed or excessive hemorrhage following (induced) termination of pregnancy**   M

Afibrinogenemia following (induced) termination of pregnancy

Defibrination syndrome following (induced) termination of pregnancy

Hemolysis following (induced) termination of pregnancy

Intravascular coagulation following (induced) termination of pregnancy

Coding Clinic: 2025, Q1, P18; 2023, Q2, P15-16; 2019, Q3, P12

O04.7   **Embolism following (induced) termination of pregnancy**   M

Air embolism following (induced) termination of pregnancy

Amniotic fluid embolism following (induced) termination of pregnancy

Blood-clot embolism following (induced) termination of pregnancy

Embolism NOS following (induced) termination of pregnancy

Fat embolism following (induced) termination of pregnancy

Pulmonary embolism following (induced) termination of pregnancy

Pyemic embolism following (induced) termination of pregnancy

Septic or septicopyemic embolism following (induced) termination of pregnancy

Soap embolism following (induced) termination of pregnancy

● **O04.8   (Induced) termination of pregnancy with other and unspecified complications**

O04.80   **(Induced) termination of pregnancy with unspecified complications**   M

O04.81   **Shock following (induced) termination of pregnancy**   M

Circulatory collapse following (induced) termination of pregnancy

Shock (postprocedural) following (induced) termination of pregnancy

Excludes1   shock due to infection following (induced) termination of pregnancy (O04.87)

Coding Clinic: 2025, Q1, P18

O04.82   **Renal failure following (induced) termination of pregnancy**   M

Kidney failure (acute) following (induced) termination of pregnancy

Oliguria following (induced) termination of pregnancy

Renal shutdown following (induced) termination of pregnancy

Renal tubular necrosis following (induced) termination of pregnancy

Uremia following (induced) termination of pregnancy

O04.83   **Metabolic disorder following (induced) termination of pregnancy**   M

O04.84   **Damage to pelvic organs following (induced) termination of pregnancy**   M

Laceration, perforation, tear or chemical damage of bladder following (induced) termination of pregnancy

Laceration, perforation, tear or chemical damage of bowel following (induced) termination of pregnancy

Laceration, perforation, tear or chemical damage of broad ligament following (induced) termination of pregnancy

Laceration, perforation, tear or chemical damage of cervix following (induced) termination of pregnancy

Laceration, perforation, tear or chemical damage of periurethral tissue following (induced) termination of pregnancy

Laceration, perforation, tear or chemical damage of uterus following (induced) termination of pregnancy

Laceration, perforation, tear or chemical damage of vagina following (induced) termination of pregnancy

O04.85   **Other venous complications following (induced) termination of pregnancy**   M

O04.86   **Cardiac arrest following (induced) termination of pregnancy**   M

CHAPTER 15 (O00-O9A)

O04.87 **Sepsis following (induced) termination of pregnancy** M

    Use additional code to identify infectious agent (B95-B97)

    Use additional code to identify severe sepsis, if applicable (R65.2-)

    Excludes1 septic or septicopyemic embolism following (induced) termination of pregnancy (O04.7)

O04.88 **Urinary tract infection following (induced) termination of pregnancy** M

    Cystitis following (induced) termination of pregnancy

O04.89 **(Induced) termination of pregnancy with other complications** M

● **O07** **Failed attempted termination of pregnancy**

    Includes failure of attempted induction of termination of pregnancy

        incomplete elective abortion

    Excludes1 incomplete spontaneous abortion (O03.0-)

    Coding Clinic: 2023, Q1, P17

O07.0 **Genital tract and pelvic infection following failed attempted termination of pregnancy** M

    Endometritis following failed attempted termination of pregnancy

    Oophoritis following failed attempted termination of pregnancy

    Parametritis following failed attempted termination of pregnancy

    Pelvic peritonitis following failed attempted termination of pregnancy

    Salpingitis following failed attempted termination of pregnancy

    Salpingo-oophoritis following failed attempted termination of pregnancy

    Excludes1 sepsis following failed attempted termination of pregnancy (O07.37)

        urinary tract infection following failed attempted termination of pregnancy (O07.38)

O07.1 **Delayed or excessive hemorrhage following failed attempted termination of pregnancy** M

    Afibrinogenemia following failed attempted termination of pregnancy

    Defibrination syndrome following failed attempted termination of pregnancy

    Hemolysis following failed attempted termination of pregnancy

    Intravascular coagulation following failed attempted termination of pregnancy

O07.2 **Embolism following failed attempted termination of pregnancy** M

    Air embolism following failed attempted termination of pregnancy

    Amniotic fluid embolism following failed attempted termination of pregnancy

    Blood-clot embolism following failed attempted termination of pregnancy

    Embolism NOS following failed attempted termination of pregnancy

    Fat embolism following failed attempted termination of pregnancy

    Pulmonary embolism following failed attempted termination of pregnancy

    Pyemic embolism following failed attempted termination of pregnancy

    Septic or septicopyemic embolism following failed attempted termination of pregnancy

    Soap embolism following failed attempted termination of pregnancy

● **O07.3** **Failed attempted termination of pregnancy with other and unspecified complications**

O07.30 **Failed attempted termination of pregnancy with unspecified complications** M

O07.31 **Shock following failed attempted termination of pregnancy** M

    Circulatory collapse following failed attempted termination of pregnancy

    Shock (postprocedural) following failed attempted termination of pregnancy

    Excludes1 shock due to infection following failed attempted termination of pregnancy (O07.37)

O07.32 **Renal failure following failed attempted termination of pregnancy** M

    Kidney failure (acute) following failed attempted termination of pregnancy

    Oliguria following failed attempted termination of pregnancy

    Renal shutdown following failed attempted termination of pregnancy

    Renal tubular necrosis following failed attempted termination of pregnancy

    Uremia following failed attempted termination of pregnancy

O07.33 **Metabolic disorder following failed attempted termination of pregnancy** M

O07.34 **Damage to pelvic organs following failed attempted termination of pregnancy** M

    Laceration, perforation, tear or chemical damage of bladder following failed attempted termination of pregnancy

    Laceration, perforation, tear or chemical damage of bowel following failed attempted termination of pregnancy

    Laceration, perforation, tear or chemical damage of broad ligament following failed attempted termination of pregnancy

    Laceration, perforation, tear or chemical damage of cervix following failed attempted termination of pregnancy

    Laceration, perforation, tear or chemical damage of periurethral tissue following failed attempted termination of pregnancy

    Laceration, perforation, tear or chemical damage of uterus following failed attempted termination of pregnancy

    Laceration, perforation, tear or chemical damage of vagina following failed attempted termination of pregnancy

O07.35 **Other venous complications following failed attempted termination of pregnancy** M

O07.36 **Cardiac arrest following failed attempted termination of pregnancy** M

O07.37 **Sepsis following failed attempted termination of pregnancy** M

    Use additional code (B95-B97), to identify infectious agent

    Use additional code (R65.2-) to identify severe sepsis, if applicable

    Excludes1 septic or septicopyemic embolism following failed attempted termination of pregnancy (O07.2)

O07.38 **Urinary tract infection following failed attempted termination of pregnancy** M

    Cystitis following failed attempted termination of pregnancy

O07.39 **Failed attempted termination of pregnancy with other complications** M

O07.4 **Failed attempted termination of pregnancy without complication** M

CHAPTER 15 (O00-O9A)

CHAPTER 15 (O00–O9A)

● **O08 Complications following ectopic and molar pregnancy**

This category is for use with categories O00-O02 to identify any associated complications.

Coding Clinic: 2025, Q1, P18; 2023, Q1, P17

O08.0 Genital tract and pelvic infection following ectopic and molar pregnancy M

Endometritis following ectopic and molar pregnancy
Oophoritis following ectopic and molar pregnancy
Parametritis following ectopic and molar pregnancy
Pelvic peritonitis following ectopic and molar pregnancy
Salpingitis following ectopic and molar pregnancy
Salpingo-oophoritis following ectopic and molar pregnancy

Excludes1 sepsis following ectopic and molar pregnancy (O08.82)
urinary tract infection (O08.83)

O08.1 Delayed or excessive hemorrhage following ectopic and molar pregnancy M

Afibrinogenemia following ectopic and molar pregnancy
Defibrination syndrome following ectopic and molar pregnancy
Hemolysis following ectopic and molar pregnancy
Intravascular coagulation following ectopic and molar pregnancy

Excludes1 delayed or excessive hemorrhage due to incomplete abortion (O03.1)

O08.2 Embolism following ectopic and molar pregnancy M

Air embolism following ectopic and molar pregnancy
Amniotic fluid embolism following ectopic and molar pregnancy
Blood-clot embolism following ectopic and molar pregnancy
Embolism NOS following ectopic and molar pregnancy
Fat embolism following ectopic and molar pregnancy
Pulmonary embolism following ectopic and molar pregnancy
Pyemic embolism following ectopic and molar pregnancy
Septic or septicopyemic embolism following ectopic and molar pregnancy
Soap embolism following ectopic and molar pregnancy

O08.3 Shock following ectopic and molar pregnancy M

Circulatory collapse following ectopic and molar pregnancy
Shock (postprocedural) following ectopic and molar pregnancy

Excludes1 shock due to infection following ectopic and molar pregnancy (O08.82)

O08.4 Renal failure following ectopic and molar pregnancy M

Kidney failure (acute) following ectopic and molar pregnancy
Oliguria following ectopic and molar pregnancy
Renal shutdown following ectopic and molar pregnancy
Renal tubular necrosis following ectopic and molar pregnancy
Uremia following ectopic and molar pregnancy

O08.5 Metabolic disorders following an ectopic and molar pregnancy M

O08.6 Damage to pelvic organs and tissues following an ectopic and molar pregnancy M

Laceration, perforation, tear or chemical damage of bladder following an ectopic and molar pregnancy
Laceration, perforation, tear or chemical damage of bowel following an ectopic and molar pregnancy
Laceration, perforation, tear or chemical damage of broad ligament following an ectopic and molar pregnancy
Laceration, perforation, tear or chemical damage of cervix following an ectopic and molar pregnancy
Laceration, perforation, tear or chemical damage of periurethral tissue following an ectopic and molar pregnancy
Laceration, perforation, tear or chemical damage of uterus following an ectopic and molar pregnancy
Laceration, perforation, tear or chemical damage of vagina following an ectopic and molar pregnancy

O08.7 Other venous complications following an ectopic and molar pregnancy M

● **O08.8 Other complications following an ectopic and molar pregnancy**

O08.81 Cardiac arrest following an ectopic and molar pregnancy M

O08.82 Sepsis following ectopic and molar pregnancy M

Use additional code (B95-B97), to identify infectious agent
Use additional code (R65.2-) to identify severe sepsis, if applicable

Excludes1 septic or septicopyemic embolism following ectopic and molar pregnancy (O08.2)

O08.83 Urinary tract infection following an ectopic and molar pregnancy M

Cystitis following an ectopic and molar pregnancy

O08.89 Other complications following an ectopic and molar pregnancy M

O08.9 Unspecified complication following an ectopic and molar pregnancy M

SUPERVISION OF HIGH RISK PREGNANCY (O09)

● **O09 Supervision of high risk pregnancy**
Coding Clinic: 2016, Q4, P125, 150

● **O09.0 Supervision of pregnancy with history of infertility**

O09.00 Supervision of pregnancy with history of infertility, unspecified trimester M

O09.01 Supervision of pregnancy with history of infertility, first trimester M

O09.02 Supervision of pregnancy with history of infertility, second trimester M

O09.03 Supervision of pregnancy with history of infertility, third trimester M

● **O09.1 Supervision of pregnancy with history of ectopic pregnancy**
Coding Clinic: 2016, Q4, P49-50

O09.10 Supervision of pregnancy with history of ectopic pregnancy, unspecified trimester M

O09.11 Supervision of pregnancy with history of ectopic pregnancy, first trimester M

O09.12 Supervision of pregnancy with history of ectopic pregnancy, second trimester M

O09.13 Supervision of pregnancy with history of ectopic pregnancy, third trimester M

● **O09.A Supervision of pregnancy with history of molar pregnancy**
Coding Clinic: 2016, Q4, P50

O09.A0 Supervision of pregnancy with history of molar pregnancy, unspecified trimester M

O09.A1 Supervision of pregnancy with history of molar pregnancy, first trimester M

▶ New   ➡ Revised   ~~deleted~~ Deleted   Excludes 1   Excludes 2   Includes   Use additional   Code first   Code also   Key words

OGCR Official Guidelines   X Assign placeholder X   ● Use Additional Character(s)   ▶ Manifestation Code   🔗 Hierarchical Condition Category   Coding Clinic

O09.A2 **Supervision of pregnancy with history of molar pregnancy, second trimester**   M

O09.A3 **Supervision of pregnancy with history of molar pregnancy, third trimester**   M

● O09.2 **Supervision of pregnancy with other poor reproductive or obstetric history**

    Excludes2   pregnancy care for patient with history of recurrent pregnancy loss (O26.2-)

   ● O09.21 **Supervision of pregnancy with history of pre-term labor**

     O09.211 **Supervision of pregnancy with history of pre-term labor, first trimester**   M

     O09.212 **Supervision of pregnancy with history of pre-term labor, second trimester**   M

     O09.213 **Supervision of pregnancy with history of pre-term labor, third trimester**   M

     O09.219 **Supervision of pregnancy with history of pre-term labor, unspecified trimester**   M

   ● O09.29 **Supervision of pregnancy with other poor reproductive or obstetric history**

     Supervision of pregnancy with history of neonatal death

     Supervision of pregnancy with history of stillbirth

     O09.291 **Supervision of pregnancy with other poor reproductive or obstetric history, first trimester**   M

     O09.292 **Supervision of pregnancy with other poor reproductive or obstetric history, second trimester**   M

     O09.293 **Supervision of pregnancy with other poor reproductive or obstetric history, third trimester**   M

     O09.299 **Supervision of pregnancy with other poor reproductive or obstetric history, unspecified trimester**   M

● O09.3 **Supervision of pregnancy with insufficient antenatal care**

    Supervision of concealed pregnancy

    Supervision of hidden pregnancy

    O09.30 **Supervision of pregnancy with insufficient antenatal care, unspecified trimester**   M

    O09.31 **Supervision of pregnancy with insufficient antenatal care, first trimester**   M

    O09.32 **Supervision of pregnancy with insufficient antenatal care, second trimester**   M

    O09.33 **Supervision of pregnancy with insufficient antenatal care, third trimester**   M

● O09.4 **Supervision of pregnancy with grand multiparity**

    O09.40 **Supervision of pregnancy with grand multiparity, unspecified trimester**   M

    O09.41 **Supervision of pregnancy with grand multiparity, first trimester**   M

    O09.42 **Supervision of pregnancy with grand multiparity, second trimester**   M

    O09.43 **Supervision of pregnancy with grand multiparity, third trimester**   M

● O09.5 **Supervision of elderly primigravida and multigravida**

    Pregnancy for a female 35 years and older at expected date of delivery

   ● O09.51 **Supervision of elderly primigravida**

     O09.511 **Supervision of elderly primigravida, first trimester**   M

     O09.512 **Supervision of elderly primigravida, second trimester**   M

     O09.513 **Supervision of elderly primigravida, third trimester**   M

     O09.519 **Supervision of elderly primigravida, unspecified trimester**   M

   ● O09.52 **Supervision of elderly multigravida**

     O09.521 **Supervision of elderly multigravida, first trimester**   M

     O09.522 **Supervision of elderly multigravida, second trimester**   M

     O09.523 **Supervision of elderly multigravida, third trimester**   M

      Coding Clinic: 2016, Q4, P150

     O09.529 **Supervision of elderly multigravida, unspecified trimester**   M

● O09.6 **Supervision of young primigravida and multigravida**

    Supervision of pregnancy for a female less than 16 years old at expected date of delivery

   ● O09.61 **Supervision of young primigravida**

     O09.611 **Supervision of young primigravida, first trimester**   M

     O09.612 **Supervision of young primigravida, second trimester**   M

     O09.613 **Supervision of young primigravida, third trimester**   M

     O09.619 **Supervision of young primigravida, unspecified trimester**   M

   ● O09.62 **Supervision of young multigravida**

     O09.621 **Supervision of young multigravida, first trimester**   M

     O09.622 **Supervision of young multigravida, second trimester**   M

     O09.623 **Supervision of young multigravida, third trimester**   M

     O09.629 **Supervision of young multigravida, unspecified trimester**   M

● O09.7 **Supervision of high risk pregnancy due to social problems**

    O09.70 **Supervision of high risk pregnancy due to social problems, unspecified trimester**   M

    O09.71 **Supervision of high risk pregnancy due to social problems, first trimester**   M

    O09.72 **Supervision of high risk pregnancy due to social problems, second trimester**   M

    O09.73 **Supervision of high risk pregnancy due to social problems, third trimester**   M

● O09.8 **Supervision of other high risk pregnancies**

   ● O09.81 **Supervision of pregnancy resulting from assisted reproductive technology**

     Supervision of pregnancy resulting from in-vitro fertilization

     Excludes2   gestational carrier status (Z33.3)

     O09.811 **Supervision of pregnancy resulting from assisted reproductive technology, first trimester**   M

     O09.812 **Supervision of pregnancy resulting from assisted reproductive technology, second trimester**   M

     O09.813 **Supervision of pregnancy resulting from assisted reproductive technology, third trimester**   M

     O09.819 **Supervision of pregnancy resulting from assisted reproductive technology, unspecified trimester**   M

   ● O09.82 **Supervision of pregnancy with history of in utero procedure during previous pregnancy**

     O09.821 **Supervision of pregnancy with history of in utero procedure during previous pregnancy, first trimester**   M

     O09.822 **Supervision of pregnancy with history of in utero procedure during previous pregnancy, second trimester**   M

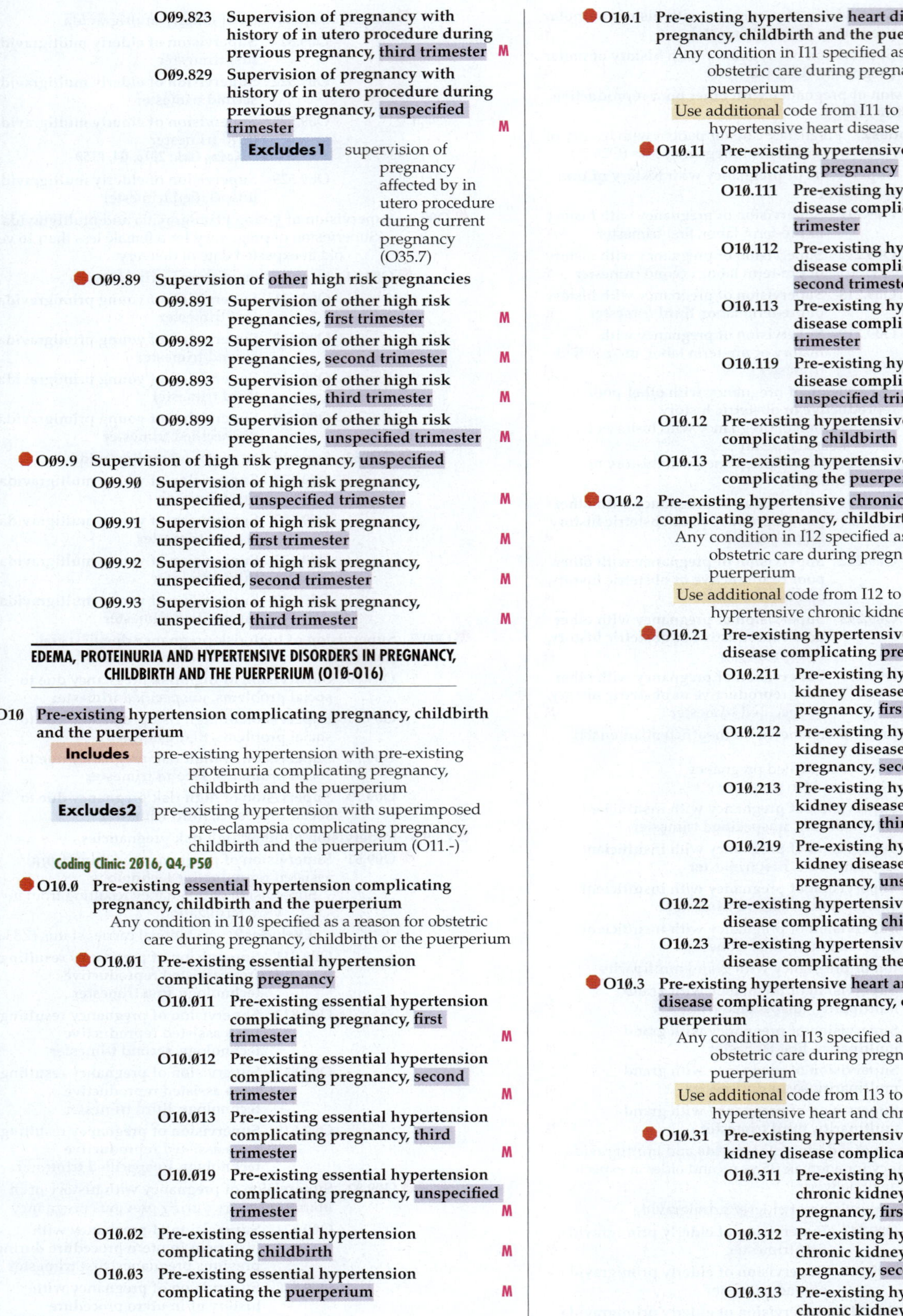

O09.823 Supervision of pregnancy with history of in utero procedure during previous pregnancy, **third trimester** M

O09.829 Supervision of pregnancy with history of in utero procedure during previous pregnancy, **unspecified trimester** M

    Excludes1 supervision of pregnancy affected by in utero procedure during current pregnancy (O35.7)

● **O09.89** Supervision of other high risk pregnancies

O09.891 Supervision of other high risk pregnancies, **first trimester** M

O09.892 Supervision of other high risk pregnancies, **second trimester** M

O09.893 Supervision of other high risk pregnancies, **third trimester** M

O09.899 Supervision of other high risk pregnancies, **unspecified trimester** M

● **O09.9** Supervision of high risk pregnancy, unspecified

O09.90 Supervision of high risk pregnancy, unspecified, **unspecified trimester** M

O09.91 Supervision of high risk pregnancy, unspecified, **first trimester** M

O09.92 Supervision of high risk pregnancy, unspecified, **second trimester** M

O09.93 Supervision of high risk pregnancy, unspecified, **third trimester** M

EDEMA, PROTEINURIA AND HYPERTENSIVE DISORDERS IN PREGNANCY, CHILDBIRTH AND THE PUERPERIUM (O10-O16)

● **O10** Pre-existing hypertension complicating pregnancy, childbirth and the puerperium

    Includes pre-existing hypertension with pre-existing proteinuria complicating pregnancy, childbirth and the puerperium

    Excludes2 pre-existing hypertension with superimposed pre-eclampsia complicating pregnancy, childbirth and the puerperium (O11.-)

Coding Clinic: 2016, Q4, P50

● **O10.0** Pre-existing essential hypertension complicating pregnancy, childbirth and the puerperium

Any condition in I10 specified as a reason for obstetric care during pregnancy, childbirth or the puerperium

● **O10.01** Pre-existing essential hypertension complicating pregnancy

O10.011 Pre-existing essential hypertension complicating pregnancy, **first trimester** M

O10.012 Pre-existing essential hypertension complicating pregnancy, **second trimester** M

O10.013 Pre-existing essential hypertension complicating pregnancy, **third trimester** M

O10.019 Pre-existing essential hypertension complicating pregnancy, **unspecified trimester** M

O10.02 Pre-existing essential hypertension complicating **childbirth** M

O10.03 Pre-existing essential hypertension complicating the **puerperium** M

● **O10.1** Pre-existing hypertensive **heart disease** complicating pregnancy, childbirth and the puerperium

Any condition in I11 specified as a reason for obstetric care during pregnancy, childbirth or the puerperium

    Use additional code from I11 to identify the type of hypertensive heart disease

● **O10.11** Pre-existing hypertensive heart disease complicating **pregnancy**

O10.111 Pre-existing hypertensive heart disease complicating pregnancy, **first trimester** M

O10.112 Pre-existing hypertensive heart disease complicating pregnancy, **second trimester** M

O10.113 Pre-existing hypertensive heart disease complicating pregnancy, **third trimester** M

O10.119 Pre-existing hypertensive heart disease complicating pregnancy, **unspecified trimester** M

O10.12 Pre-existing hypertensive heart disease complicating **childbirth** M

O10.13 Pre-existing hypertensive heart disease complicating the **puerperium** M

● **O10.2** Pre-existing hypertensive chronic kidney disease complicating pregnancy, childbirth and the puerperium

Any condition in I12 specified as a reason for obstetric care during pregnancy, childbirth or the puerperium

    Use additional code from I12 to identify the type of hypertensive chronic kidney disease

● **O10.21** Pre-existing hypertensive chronic kidney disease complicating **pregnancy**

O10.211 Pre-existing hypertensive chronic kidney disease complicating pregnancy, **first trimester** M

O10.212 Pre-existing hypertensive chronic kidney disease complicating pregnancy, **second trimester** M

O10.213 Pre-existing hypertensive chronic kidney disease complicating pregnancy, **third trimester** M

O10.219 Pre-existing hypertensive chronic kidney disease complicating pregnancy, **unspecified trimester** M

O10.22 Pre-existing hypertensive chronic kidney disease complicating **childbirth** M

O10.23 Pre-existing hypertensive chronic kidney disease complicating the **puerperium** M

● **O10.3** Pre-existing hypertensive **heart and chronic kidney disease** complicating pregnancy, childbirth and the puerperium

Any condition in I13 specified as a reason for obstetric care during pregnancy, childbirth or the puerperium

    Use additional code from I13 to identify the type of hypertensive heart and chronic kidney disease

● **O10.31** Pre-existing hypertensive heart and chronic kidney disease complicating **pregnancy**

O10.311 Pre-existing hypertensive heart and chronic kidney disease complicating pregnancy, **first trimester** M

O10.312 Pre-existing hypertensive heart and chronic kidney disease complicating pregnancy, **second trimester** M

O10.313 Pre-existing hypertensive heart and chronic kidney disease complicating pregnancy, **third trimester** M

O10.319 Pre-existing hypertensive heart and chronic kidney disease complicating pregnancy, **unspecified trimester** M

▶ New   ➡ Revised   ~~deleted~~ Deleted   Excludes 1   Excludes 2   Includes   Use additional   Code first   Code also   Key words

OGCR Official Guidelines   **X** Assign placeholder X   ● Use Additional Character(s)   ▶ Manifestation Code   🔍 Hierarchical Condition Category   **Coding Clinic**

O10.32   Pre-existing hypertensive heart and chronic kidney disease complicating childbirth   M

O10.33   Pre-existing hypertensive heart and chronic kidney disease complicating the puerperium   M

● **O10.4**   Pre-existing secondary hypertension complicating pregnancy, childbirth and the puerperium

    Any condition in I15 specified as a reason for obstetric care during pregnancy, childbirth or the puerperium

    Use additional code from I15 to identify the type of secondary hypertension

   ● O10.41   Pre-existing secondary hypertension complicating pregnancy

     O10.411   Pre-existing secondary hypertension complicating pregnancy, first trimester   M

     O10.412   Pre-existing secondary hypertension complicating pregnancy, second trimester   M

     O10.413   Pre-existing secondary hypertension complicating pregnancy, third trimester   M

     O10.419   Pre-existing secondary hypertension complicating pregnancy, unspecified trimester   M

   O10.42   Pre-existing secondary hypertension complicating childbirth   M

   O10.43   Pre-existing secondary hypertension complicating the puerperium   M

● **O10.9**   Unspecified pre-existing hypertension complicating pregnancy, childbirth and the puerperium

   ● O10.91   Unspecified pre-existing hypertension complicating pregnancy

     Coding Clinic: 2025, Q2, P18

     O10.911   Unspecified pre-existing hypertension complicating pregnancy, first trimester   M

     O10.912   Unspecified pre-existing hypertension complicating pregnancy, second trimester   M

     O10.913   Unspecified pre-existing hypertension complicating pregnancy, third trimester   M

     O10.919   Unspecified pre-existing hypertension complicating pregnancy, unspecified trimester   M

   O10.92   Unspecified pre-existing hypertension complicating childbirth   M

   O10.93   Unspecified pre-existing hypertension complicating the puerperium   M

● **O11**   Pre-existing hypertension with pre-eclampsia

   Includes   conditions in O10 complicated by pre-eclampsia
     pre-eclampsia superimposed pre-existing hypertension

   Use additional code from O10 to identify the type of hypertension

   Coding Clinic: 2016, Q4, P50

O11.1   Pre-existing hypertension with pre-eclampsia, first trimester   M

O11.2   Pre-existing hypertension with pre-eclampsia, second trimester   M

O11.3   Pre-existing hypertension with pre-eclampsia, third trimester   M

O11.4   Pre-existing hypertension with pre-eclampsia, complicating childbirth   M

O11.5   Pre-existing hypertension with pre-eclampsia, complicating the puerperium   M

O11.9   Pre-existing hypertension with pre-eclampsia, unspecified trimester   M

● **O12**   Gestational [pregnancy-induced] edema and proteinuria without hypertension

   Coding Clinic: 2016, Q4, P50

   ● O12.0   Gestational edema

     O12.00   Gestational edema, unspecified trimester   M

     O12.01   Gestational edema, first trimester   M

     O12.02   Gestational edema, second trimester   M

     O12.03   Gestational edema, third trimester   M

     O12.04   Gestational edema, complicating childbirth   M

     O12.05   Gestational edema, complicating the puerperium   M

   ● O12.1   Gestational proteinuria

     O12.10   Gestational proteinuria, unspecified trimester   M

     O12.11   Gestational proteinuria, first trimester   M

     O12.12   Gestational proteinuria, second trimester   M

     O12.13   Gestational proteinuria, third trimester   M

     O12.14   Gestational proteinuria, complicating childbirth   M

     O12.15   Gestational proteinuria, complicating the puerperium   M

   ● O12.2   Gestational edema with proteinuria

     O12.20   Gestational edema with proteinuria, unspecified trimester   M

     O12.21   Gestational edema with proteinuria, first trimester   M

     O12.22   Gestational edema with proteinuria, second trimester   M

     O12.23   Gestational edema with proteinuria, third trimester   M

     O12.24   Gestational edema with proteinuria, complicating childbirth   M

     O12.25   Gestational edema with proteinuria, complicating the puerperium   M

● **O13**   Gestational [pregnancy-induced] hypertension without significant proteinuria

   Includes   gestational hypertension NOS
     transient hypertension of pregnancy

   Coding Clinic: 2016, Q4, P50

O13.1   Gestational [pregnancy-induced] hypertension without significant proteinuria, first trimester   M

O13.2   Gestational [pregnancy-induced] hypertension without significant proteinuria, second trimester   M

O13.3   Gestational [pregnancy-induced] hypertension without significant proteinuria, third trimester   M

O13.4   Gestational [pregnancy-induced] hypertension without significant proteinuria, complicating childbirth   M

O13.5   Gestational [pregnancy-induced] hypertension without significant proteinuria, complicating the puerperium   M

O13.9   Gestational [pregnancy-induced] hypertension without significant proteinuria, unspecified trimester   M

● **O14**   Pre-eclampsia

   Excludes1   pre-existing hypertension with pre-eclampsia (O11)

   Coding Clinic: 2016, Q4, P50

   ● O14.0   Mild to moderate pre-eclampsia

     O14.00   Mild to moderate pre-eclampsia, unspecified trimester   M

     O14.02   Mild to moderate pre-eclampsia, second trimester   M

     O14.03   Mild to moderate pre-eclampsia, third trimester   M

     O14.04   Mild to moderate pre-eclampsia, complicating childbirth   M
      Coding Clinic: 2019, Q2, P8

     O14.05   Mild to moderate pre-eclampsia, complicating the puerperium   M

CHAPTER 15 (O00-O9A)

● **O14.1   Severe pre-eclampsia**
     Excludes1   HELLP syndrome (O14.2-)
     H=hemolysis, EL=elevated liver enzymes, LP=low platelet count
     Coding Clinic: 2019, Q3, P12
     O14.10   Severe pre-eclampsia, unspecified trimester   M
     O14.12   Severe pre-eclampsia, second trimester   M
     O14.13   Severe pre-eclampsia, third trimester   M
     O14.14   Severe pre-eclampsia complicating childbirth   M
     O14.15   Severe pre-eclampsia, complicating the puerperium   M

● **O14.2   HELLP syndrome**
     Severe pre-eclampsia with hemolysis, elevated liver enzymes and low platelet count (HELLP)
     O14.20   HELLP syndrome (HELLP), unspecified trimester   M
     O14.22   HELLP syndrome (HELLP), second trimester   M
     O14.23   HELLP syndrome (HELLP), third trimester   M
     O14.24   HELLP syndrome, complicating childbirth   M
     O14.25   HELLP syndrome, complicating the puerperium   M

● **O14.9   Unspecified pre-eclampsia**
     O14.90   Unspecified pre-eclampsia, unspecified trimester   M
     O14.92   Unspecified pre-eclampsia, second trimester   M
     O14.93   Unspecified pre-eclampsia, third trimester   M
     O14.94   Unspecified pre-eclampsia, complicating childbirth   M
     O14.95   Unspecified pre-eclampsia, complicating the puerperium   M

● **O15   Eclampsia**
     Includes   convulsions following conditions in O10-O14 and O16
● **O15.0   Eclampsia complicating pregnancy**
     Coding Clinic: 2016, Q4, P50
     O15.00   Eclampsia complicating pregnancy, unspecified trimester   M
     O15.02   Eclampsia complicating pregnancy, second trimester   M
     O15.03   Eclampsia complicating pregnancy, third trimester   M
     O15.1   Eclampsia complicating labor   M
     O15.2   Eclampsia complicating the puerperium   M
     O15.9   Eclampsia, unspecified as to time period   M
         Eclampsia NOS

● **O16   Unspecified maternal hypertension**
     Coding Clinic: 2016, Q4, P50
     O16.1   Unspecified maternal hypertension, first trimester   M
     O16.2   Unspecified maternal hypertension, second trimester   M
     O16.3   Unspecified maternal hypertension, third trimester   M
     O16.4   Unspecified maternal hypertension, complicating childbirth   M
     O16.5   Unspecified maternal hypertension, complicating the puerperium   M
     O16.9   Unspecified maternal hypertension, unspecified trimester   M

OTHER MATERNAL DISORDERS PREDOMINANTLY RELATED TO PREGNANCY (O20-O29)

     Excludes2   maternal care related to the fetus and amniotic cavity and possible delivery problems (O30-O48)
         maternal diseases classifiable elsewhere but complicating pregnancy, labor and delivery, and the puerperium (O98-O99)

● **O20   Hemorrhage in early pregnancy**
     Includes   hemorrhage before completion of 20 weeks gestation
     Excludes1   pregnancy with abortive outcome (O00-O08)
     O20.0   Threatened abortion   M
         Hemorrhage specified as due to threatened abortion
     O20.8   Other hemorrhage in early pregnancy   M
         Coding Clinic: 2023, Q3, P18
     O20.9   Hemorrhage in early pregnancy, unspecified   M

● **O21   Excessive vomiting in pregnancy**
     O21.0   Mild hyperemesis gravidarum   M
         Hyperemesis gravidarum, mild or unspecified, starting before the end of the 20th week of gestation
     O21.1   Hyperemesis gravidarum with metabolic disturbance   M
         Hyperemesis gravidarum, starting before the end of the 20th week of gestation, with metabolic disturbance such as carbohydrate depletion
         Hyperemesis gravidarum, starting before the end of the 20th week of gestation, with metabolic disturbance such as dehydration
         Hyperemesis gravidarum, starting before the end of the 20th week of gestation, with metabolic disturbance such as electrolyte imbalance
     O21.2   Late vomiting of pregnancy   M
         Excessive vomiting starting after 20 completed weeks of gestation
     O21.8   Other vomiting complicating pregnancy   M
         Vomiting due to diseases classified elsewhere, complicating pregnancy
         Use additional code, to identify cause
     O21.9   Vomiting of pregnancy, unspecified   M

● **O22   Venous complications and hemorrhoids in pregnancy**
     Excludes1   venous complications of:
         abortion NOS (O03.9)
         ectopic or molar pregnancy (O08.7)
         failed attempted abortion (O07.35)
         induced abortion (O04.85)
         spontaneous abortion (O03.89)
     Excludes2   obstetric pulmonary embolism (O88.-)
         venous complications and hemorrhoids of childbirth and the puerperium (O87.-)
● **O22.0   Varicose veins of lower extremity in pregnancy**
     Varicose veins NOS in pregnancy
     O22.00   Varicose veins of lower extremity in pregnancy, unspecified trimester   M
     O22.01   Varicose veins of lower extremity in pregnancy, first trimester   M
     O22.02   Varicose veins of lower extremity in pregnancy, second trimester   M
     O22.03   Varicose veins of lower extremity in pregnancy, third trimester   M
● **O22.1   Genital varices in pregnancy**
     Perineal varices in pregnancy
     Vaginal varices in pregnancy
     Vulval varices in pregnancy
     O22.10   Genital varices in pregnancy, unspecified trimester   M
     O22.11   Genital varices in pregnancy, first trimester

▶ New   ⇨ Revised   ~~deleted~~ Deleted   Excludes 1   Excludes 2   Includes   Use additional   Code first   Code also   Key words
OGCR Official Guidelines   **X** Assign placeholder X   ● Use Additional Character(s)   ▶ Manifestation Code   Hierarchical Condition Category   **Coding Clinic**

O22.12   Genital varices in pregnancy, second trimester M

O22.13   Genital varices in pregnancy, third trimester M

● **O22.2**   **Superficial thrombophlebitis in pregnancy**
Phlebitis in pregnancy NOS
Thrombophlebitis of legs in pregnancy
Thrombosis in pregnancy NOS
Use additional code to identify the superficial thrombophlebitis (I80.0-)

O22.20   **Superficial thrombophlebitis in pregnancy, unspecified trimester** M

O22.21   **Superficial thrombophlebitis in pregnancy, first trimester** M

O22.22   **Superficial thrombophlebitis in pregnancy, second trimester** M

O22.23   **Superficial thrombophlebitis in pregnancy, third trimester** M

● **O22.3**   **Deep phlebothrombosis in pregnancy**
Deep vein thrombosis, antepartum
Use additional code to identify the deep vein thrombosis (I82.4-, I82.5-, I82.62-, I82.72-)
Use additional code, if applicable, for associated long-term (current) use of anticoagulants (Z79.01)

O22.30   **Deep phlebothrombosis in pregnancy, unspecified trimester** M

O22.31   **Deep phlebothrombosis in pregnancy, first trimester** M

O22.32   **Deep phlebothrombosis in pregnancy, second trimester** M

O22.33   **Deep phlebothrombosis in pregnancy, third trimester** M

● **O22.4**   **Hemorrhoids in pregnancy**

O22.40   **Hemorrhoids in pregnancy, unspecified trimester** M

O22.41   **Hemorrhoids in pregnancy, first trimester** M

O22.42   **Hemorrhoids in pregnancy, second trimester** M

O22.43   **Hemorrhoids in pregnancy, third trimester** M

● **O22.5**   **Cerebral venous thrombosis in pregnancy**
Cerebrovenous sinus thrombosis in pregnancy

O22.50   **Cerebral venous thrombosis in pregnancy, unspecified trimester** M

O22.51   **Cerebral venous thrombosis in pregnancy, first trimester** M

O22.52   **Cerebral venous thrombosis in pregnancy, second trimester** M

O22.53   **Cerebral venous thrombosis in pregnancy, third trimester** M

● **O22.8**   **Other venous complications in pregnancy**

● **O22.8X**   **Other venous complications in pregnancy**

O22.8X1   **Other venous complications in pregnancy, first trimester** M

O22.8X2   **Other venous complications in pregnancy, second trimester** M

O22.8X3   **Other venous complications in pregnancy, third trimester** M

O22.8X9   **Other venous complications in pregnancy, unspecified trimester** M

● **O22.9**   **Venous complication in pregnancy, unspecified**
Gestational phlebitis NOS
Gestational phlebopathy NOS
Gestational thrombosis NOS

O22.90   **Venous complication in pregnancy, unspecified, unspecified trimester** M

O22.91   **Venous complication in pregnancy, unspecified, first trimester** M

O22.92   **Venous complication in pregnancy, unspecified, second trimester** M

O22.93   **Venous complication in pregnancy, unspecified, third trimester** M

● **O23**   **Infections of genitourinary tract in pregnancy**
Use additional code to identify organism (B95.-, B96.-)

Excludes2   gonococcal infections complicating pregnancy, childbirth and the puerperium (O98.2)
infections with a predominantly sexual mode of transmission NOS complicating pregnancy, childbirth and the puerperium (O98.3)
syphilis complicating pregnancy, childbirth and the puerperium (O98.1)
tuberculosis of genitourinary system complicating pregnancy, childbirth and the puerperium (O98.0)
venereal disease NOS complicating pregnancy, childbirth and the puerperium (O98.3)

Coding Clinic: 2025, Q1, P22

● **O23.0**   **Infections of kidney in pregnancy**
Pyelonephritis in pregnancy

O23.00   **Infections of kidney in pregnancy, unspecified trimester** M

O23.01   **Infections of kidney in pregnancy, first trimester** M

O23.02   **Infections of kidney in pregnancy, second trimester** M

O23.03   **Infections of kidney in pregnancy, third trimester** M

● **O23.1**   **Infections of bladder in pregnancy**

O23.10   **Infections of bladder in pregnancy, unspecified trimester** M

O23.11   **Infections of bladder in pregnancy, first trimester** M

O23.12   **Infections of bladder in pregnancy, second trimester** M

O23.13   **Infections of bladder in pregnancy, third trimester** M

● **O23.2**   **Infections of urethra in pregnancy**

O23.20   **Infections of urethra in pregnancy, unspecified trimester** M

O23.21   **Infections of urethra in pregnancy, first trimester** M

O23.22   **Infections of urethra in pregnancy, second trimester** M

O23.23   **Infections of urethra in pregnancy, third trimester** M

● **O23.3**   **Infections of other parts of urinary tract in pregnancy**

O23.30   **Infections of other parts of urinary tract in pregnancy, unspecified trimester** M

O23.31   **Infections of other parts of urinary tract in pregnancy, first trimester** M

O23.32   **Infections of other parts of urinary tract in pregnancy, second trimester** M

O23.33   **Infections of other parts of urinary tract in pregnancy, third trimester** M

● **O23.4**   **Unspecified infection of urinary tract in pregnancy**

O23.40   **Unspecified infection of urinary tract in pregnancy, unspecified trimester** M

O23.41   **Unspecified infection of urinary tract in pregnancy, first trimester** M

O23.42   **Unspecified infection of urinary tract in pregnancy, second trimester** M

O23.43   **Unspecified infection of urinary tract in pregnancy, third trimester** M

● **O23.5**   **Infections of the genital tract in pregnancy**

● **O23.51**   **Infection of cervix in pregnancy**

O23.511   **Infections of cervix in pregnancy, first trimester** M

O23.512   **Infections of cervix in pregnancy, second trimester** M

O23.513   **Infections of cervix in pregnancy, third trimester** M

O23.519   **Infections of cervix in pregnancy, unspecified trimester** M

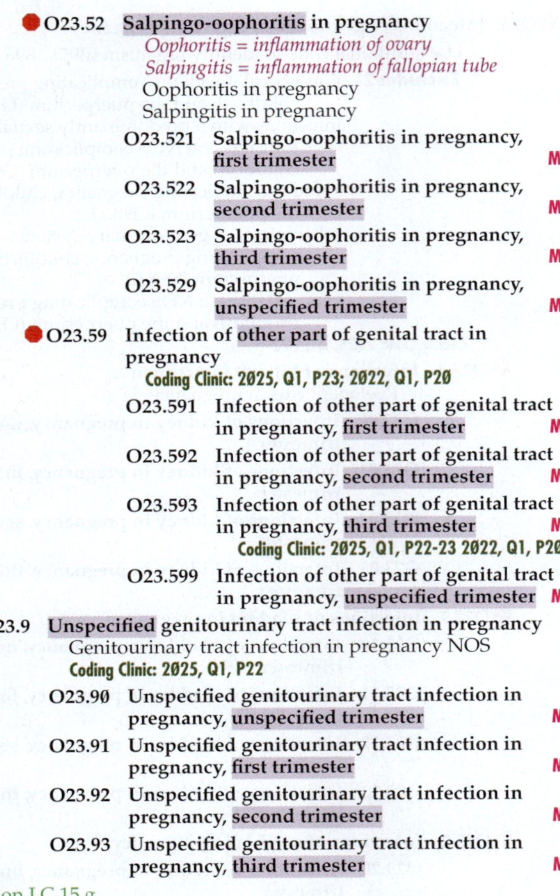

● **O23.52　Salpingo-oophoritis in pregnancy**
Oophoritis = inflammation of ovary
Salpingitis = inflammation of fallopian tube
Oophoritis in pregnancy
Salpingitis in pregnancy

　　O23.521　Salpingo-oophoritis in pregnancy, first trimester　M

　　O23.522　Salpingo-oophoritis in pregnancy, second trimester　M

　　O23.523　Salpingo-oophoritis in pregnancy, third trimester　M

　　O23.529　Salpingo-oophoritis in pregnancy, unspecified trimester　M

● **O23.59　Infection of other part of genital tract in pregnancy**
Coding Clinic: 2025, Q1, P23; 2022, Q1, P20

　　O23.591　Infection of other part of genital tract in pregnancy, first trimester　M

　　O23.592　Infection of other part of genital tract in pregnancy, second trimester　M

　　O23.593　Infection of other part of genital tract in pregnancy, third trimester　M
Coding Clinic: 2025, Q1, P22-23 2022, Q1, P20

　　O23.599　Infection of other part of genital tract in pregnancy, unspecified trimester　M

● **O23.9　Unspecified genitourinary tract infection in pregnancy**
Genitourinary tract infection in pregnancy NOS
Coding Clinic: 2025, Q1, P22

　　O23.90　Unspecified genitourinary tract infection in pregnancy, unspecified trimester　M

　　O23.91　Unspecified genitourinary tract infection in pregnancy, first trimester　M

　　O23.92　Unspecified genitourinary tract infection in pregnancy, second trimester　M

　　O23.93　Unspecified genitourinary tract infection in pregnancy, third trimester　M

OGCR Section I.C.15.g.

Diabetes mellitus in pregnancy
Diabetes mellitus is a significant complicating factor in pregnancy. Pregnant women who are diabetic should be assigned a code from category O24, Diabetes mellitus in pregnancy, childbirth, and the puerperium, first, followed by the appropriate diabetes code(s) (E08-E13) from Chapter 4.

● **O24　Diabetes mellitus in pregnancy, childbirth, and the puerperium**

● **O24.0　Pre-existing type 1 diabetes mellitus, in pregnancy, childbirth and the puerperium**
Juvenile onset diabetes mellitus, in pregnancy, childbirth and the puerperium
Ketosis-prone diabetes mellitus in pregnancy, childbirth and the puerperium
Use additional code from category E10 to further identify any manifestations

● **O24.01　Pre-existing type 1 diabetes mellitus, in pregnancy**

　　O24.011　Pre-existing type 1 diabetes mellitus, in pregnancy, first trimester　M

　　O24.012　Pre-existing type 1 diabetes mellitus, in pregnancy, second trimester　M

　　O24.013　Pre-existing type 1 diabetes mellitus, in pregnancy, third trimester　M

　　O24.019　Pre-existing type 1 diabetes mellitus, in pregnancy, unspecified trimester　M

　　O24.02　Pre-existing type 1 diabetes mellitus, in childbirth　M

　　O24.03　Pre-existing type 1 diabetes mellitus, in the puerperium　M

● **O24.1　Pre-existing type 2 diabetes mellitus, in pregnancy, childbirth and the puerperium**
Insulin-resistant diabetes mellitus in pregnancy, childbirth and the puerperium
Use additional code (for):
from category E11 to further identify any manifestations
long-term (current) use of insulin (Z79.4)
Use additional injectable non-insulin antidiabetic drugs (Z79.85)

● **O24.11　Pre-existing type 2 diabetes mellitus, in pregnancy**

　　O24.111　Pre-existing type 2 diabetes mellitus, in pregnancy, first trimester　M

　　O24.112　Pre-existing type 2 diabetes mellitus, in pregnancy, second trimester　M

　　O24.113　Pre-existing type 2 diabetes mellitus, in pregnancy, third trimester　M

　　O24.119　Pre-existing type 2 diabetes mellitus, in pregnancy, unspecified trimester　M

　　O24.12　Pre-existing type 2 diabetes mellitus, in childbirth　M

　　O24.13　Pre-existing type 2 diabetes mellitus, in the puerperium　M

● **O24.3　Unspecified pre-existing diabetes mellitus in pregnancy, childbirth and the puerperium**
Use additional code (for):
from category E11 to further identify any manifestation
long-term (current) use of insulin (Z79.4)
Use additional injectable non-insulin antidiabetic drugs (Z79.85)

● **O24.31　Unspecified pre-existing diabetes mellitus in pregnancy**

　　O24.311　Unspecified pre-existing diabetes mellitus in pregnancy, first trimester　M

　　O24.312　Unspecified pre-existing diabetes mellitus in pregnancy, second trimester　M

　　O24.313　Unspecified pre-existing diabetes mellitus in pregnancy, third trimester　M

　　O24.319　Unspecified pre-existing diabetes mellitus in pregnancy, unspecified trimester　M

　　O24.32　Unspecified pre-existing diabetes mellitus in childbirth　M

　　O24.33　Unspecified pre-existing diabetes mellitus in the puerperium　M

● **O24.4　Gestational diabetes mellitus**
Diabetes mellitus arising in pregnancy
Gestational diabetes mellitus NOS
Coding Clinic: 2016, Q4, P50, 126

● **O24.41　Gestational diabetes mellitus in pregnancy**

　　O24.410　Gestational diabetes mellitus in pregnancy, diet controlled　M

　　O24.414　Gestational diabetes mellitus in pregnancy, insulin controlled　M

　　O24.415　Gestational diabetes mellitus in pregnancy, controlled by oral hypoglycemic drugs　M
Gestational diabetes mellitus in pregnancy, controlled by oral antidiabetic drugs
Coding Clinic: 2016, Q4, P50

　　O24.419　Gestational diabetes mellitus in pregnancy, unspecified control　M
Coding Clinic: 2015, Q4, P34

▶ New　⇒ Revised　~~deleted~~ Deleted　Excludes 1　Excludes 2　Includes　Use additional　Code first　Code also　Key words
OGCR Official Guidelines　X Assign placeholder X　● Use Additional Character(s)　▶ Manifestation Code　Hierarchical Condition Category　**Coding Clinic**

● **O24.42 Gestational diabetes mellitus in childbirth**
     O24.420   Gestational diabetes mellitus in childbirth, diet controlled   **M**
     O24.424   Gestational diabetes mellitus in childbirth, insulin controlled   **M**
     O24.425   Gestational diabetes mellitus in childbirth, controlled by oral hypoglycemic drugs   **M**
         Gestational diabetes mellitus in childbirth, controlled by oral antidiabetic drugs
         Coding Clinic: 2016, Q4, P50
     O24.429   Gestational diabetes mellitus in childbirth, unspecified control   **M**

OGCR Section I.C.15.i.

> **Gestational (pregnancy induced) diabetes**
>
> Gestational (pregnancy induced) diabetes can occur during the second and third trimester of pregnancy in women who were not diabetic prior to pregnancy. Gestational diabetes can cause complications in the pregnancy similar to those of pre-existing diabetes mellitus. It also puts the woman at greater risk of developing diabetes after the pregnancy. Codes for gestational diabetes are in subcategory O24.4, Gestational diabetes mellitus. No other code from category O24, Diabetes mellitus in pregnancy, childbirth, and the puerperium, should be used with a code from O24.4
>
> The codes under subcategory O24.4 include diet controlled, insulin controlled, **and controlled by oral hypoglycemic drugs.** If a patient with gestational diabetes is treated with both diet and insulin, only the code for insulin-controlled is required. **If a patient with gestational diabetes is treated with both diet and oral hypoglycemic medications, only the code for "controlled by oral hypoglycemic drugs" is required.** Code Z79.4, Long-term (current) use of insulin **or code Z79.84, Long-term (current) use of oral hypoglycemic drugs,** should not be assigned with codes from subcategory O24.4.
>
> An abnormal glucose tolerance in pregnancy is assigned a code from subcategory O99.81, Abnormal glucose complicating pregnancy, childbirth, and the puerperium.

● **O24.43 Gestational diabetes mellitus in the puerperium**
     O24.430   Gestational diabetes mellitus in the puerperium, diet controlled   **M**
     O24.434   Gestational diabetes mellitus in the puerperium, insulin controlled   **M**
     O24.435   Gestational diabetes mellitus in puerperium, controlled by oral hypoglycemic drugs   **M**
         Gestational diabetes mellitus in puerperium, controlled by oral antidiabetic drugs
         Coding Clinic: 2016, Q4, P50
     O24.439   Gestational diabetes mellitus in puerperium, unspecified control   **M**

● **O24.8 Other pre-existing diabetes mellitus in pregnancy, childbirth, and the puerperium**
     Use additional code (for):
         from categories E08, E09 and E13 to further identify any manifestation
         long-term (current) use of insulin (Z79.4)
     Use additional injectable non-insulin antidiabetic drugs (Z79.85)

● **O24.81 Other pre-existing diabetes mellitus in pregnancy**
     O24.811   Other pre-existing diabetes mellitus in pregnancy, first trimester   **M**
     O24.812   Other pre-existing diabetes mellitus in pregnancy, second trimester   **M**
     O24.813   Other pre-existing diabetes mellitus in pregnancy, third trimester   **M**
     O24.819   Other pre-existing diabetes mellitus in pregnancy, unspecified trimester   **M**
     O24.82   Other pre-existing diabetes mellitus in childbirth   **M**
     O24.83   Other pre-existing diabetes mellitus in the puerperium

● **O24.9 Unspecified diabetes mellitus in pregnancy, childbirth and the puerperium**
     Use additional code (for):
         from categories E08, E09 and E13 to further identify any manifestation
         injectable non-insulin antidiabetic drugs (Z79.85)
         long-term (current) use of insulin (Z79.4)
     Unknown whether patient was diabetic before pregnancy occurred

● **O24.91 Unspecified diabetes mellitus in pregnancy**
     O24.911   Unspecified diabetes mellitus in pregnancy, first trimester   **M**
     O24.912   Unspecified diabetes mellitus in pregnancy, second trimester   **M**
     O24.913   Unspecified diabetes mellitus in pregnancy, third trimester   **M**
     O24.919   Unspecified diabetes mellitus in pregnancy, unspecified trimester   **M**
     O24.92   Unspecified diabetes mellitus in childbirth   **M**
     O24.93   Unspecified diabetes mellitus in the puerperium   **M**

● **O25 Malnutrition in pregnancy, childbirth and the puerperium**
● **O25.1 Malnutrition in pregnancy**
     O25.10   Malnutrition in pregnancy, unspecified trimester   **M**
     O25.11   Malnutrition in pregnancy, first trimester   **M**
     O25.12   Malnutrition in pregnancy, second trimester   **M**
     O25.13   Malnutrition in pregnancy, third trimester   **M**
     O25.2   Malnutrition in childbirth   **M**
     O25.3   Malnutrition in the puerperium   **M**

● **O26 Maternal care for other conditions predominantly related to pregnancy**
● **O26.0 Excessive weight gain in pregnancy**
     Excludes2   gestational edema (O12.0, O12.2)
     O26.00   Excessive weight gain in pregnancy, unspecified trimester   **M**
     O26.01   Excessive weight gain in pregnancy, first trimester   **M**
     O26.02   Excessive weight gain in pregnancy, second trimester   **M**
     O26.03   Excessive weight gain in pregnancy, third trimester   **M**

● **O26.1 Low weight gain in pregnancy**
     O26.10   Low weight gain in pregnancy, unspecified trimester   **M**
     O26.11   Low weight gain in pregnancy, first trimester   **M**
     O26.12   Low weight gain in pregnancy, second trimester   **M**
     O26.13   Low weight gain in pregnancy, third trimester   **M**

● **O26.2 Pregnancy care for patient with recurrent pregnancy loss**
     O26.20   Pregnancy care for patient with recurrent pregnancy loss, unspecified trimester   **M**
     O26.21   Pregnancy care for patient with recurrent pregnancy loss, first trimester   **M**
     O26.22   Pregnancy care for patient with recurrent pregnancy loss, second trimester   **M**
     O26.23   Pregnancy care for patient with recurrent pregnancy loss, third trimester   **M**

● **O26.3 Retained intrauterine contraceptive device in pregnancy**
     O26.30   Retained intrauterine contraceptive device in pregnancy, unspecified trimester   **M**
     O26.31   Retained intrauterine contraceptive device in pregnancy, first trimester   **M**
     O26.32   Retained intrauterine contraceptive device in pregnancy, second trimester   **M**
     O26.33   Retained intrauterine contraceptive device in pregnancy, third trimester   **M**

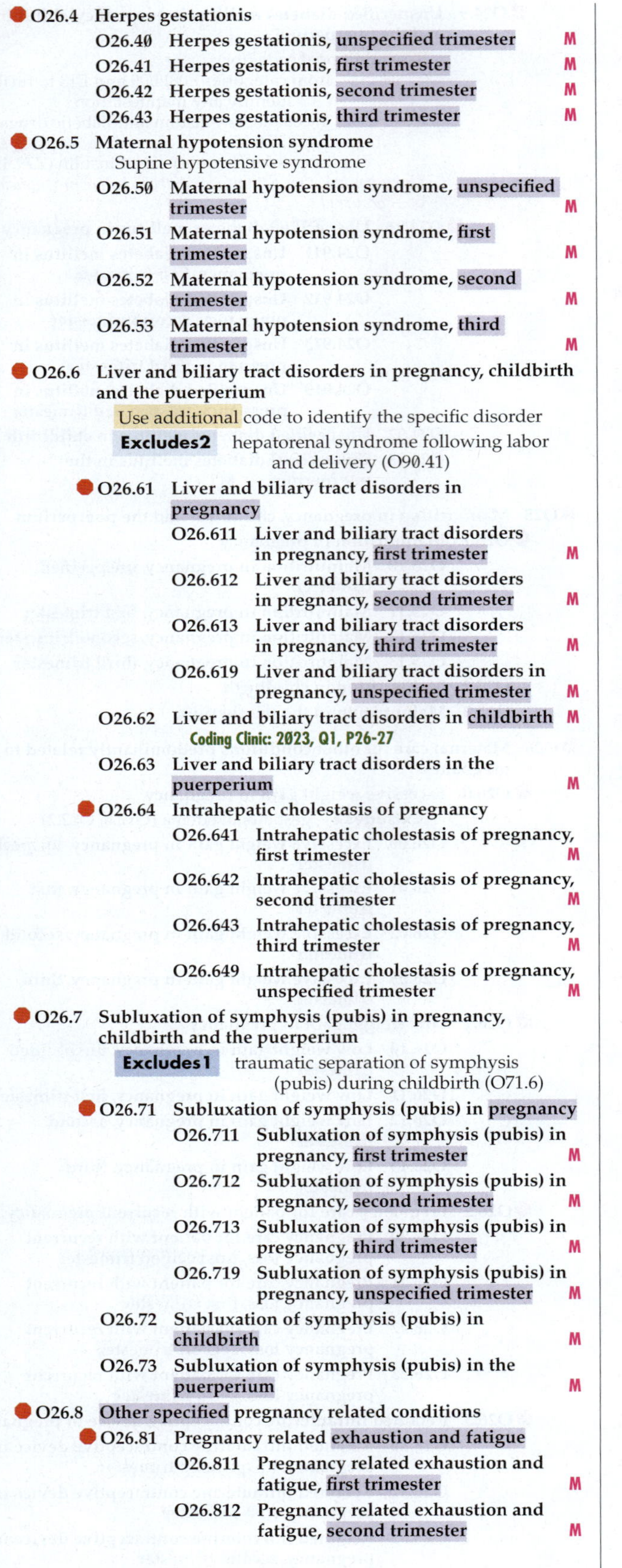

● **O26.4**   **Herpes gestationis**
    O26.40   Herpes gestationis, unspecified trimester   **M**
    O26.41   Herpes gestationis, first trimester   **M**
    O26.42   Herpes gestationis, second trimester   **M**
    O26.43   Herpes gestationis, third trimester   **M**

● **O26.5**   **Maternal hypotension syndrome**
    Supine hypotensive syndrome
    O26.50   Maternal hypotension syndrome, unspecified trimester   **M**
    O26.51   Maternal hypotension syndrome, first trimester   **M**
    O26.52   Maternal hypotension syndrome, second trimester   **M**
    O26.53   Maternal hypotension syndrome, third trimester   **M**

● **O26.6**   **Liver and biliary tract disorders in pregnancy, childbirth and the puerperium**
    Use additional code to identify the specific disorder
    Excludes2   hepatorenal syndrome following labor and delivery (O90.41)

   ● O26.61   **Liver and biliary tract disorders in pregnancy**
      O26.611   Liver and biliary tract disorders in pregnancy, first trimester   **M**
      O26.612   Liver and biliary tract disorders in pregnancy, second trimester   **M**
      O26.613   Liver and biliary tract disorders in pregnancy, third trimester   **M**
      O26.619   Liver and biliary tract disorders in pregnancy, unspecified trimester   **M**

    O26.62   Liver and biliary tract disorders in childbirth   **M**
      Coding Clinic: 2023, Q1, P26-27

    O26.63   Liver and biliary tract disorders in the puerperium   **M**

   ● O26.64   **Intrahepatic cholestasis of pregnancy**
      O26.641   Intrahepatic cholestasis of pregnancy, first trimester   **M**
      O26.642   Intrahepatic cholestasis of pregnancy, second trimester   **M**
      O26.643   Intrahepatic cholestasis of pregnancy, third trimester   **M**
      O26.649   Intrahepatic cholestasis of pregnancy, unspecified trimester   **M**

● **O26.7**   **Subluxation of symphysis (pubis) in pregnancy, childbirth and the puerperium**
    Excludes1   traumatic separation of symphysis (pubis) during childbirth (O71.6)

   ● O26.71   **Subluxation of symphysis (pubis) in pregnancy**
      O26.711   Subluxation of symphysis (pubis) in pregnancy, first trimester   **M**
      O26.712   Subluxation of symphysis (pubis) in pregnancy, second trimester   **M**
      O26.713   Subluxation of symphysis (pubis) in pregnancy, third trimester   **M**
      O26.719   Subluxation of symphysis (pubis) in pregnancy, unspecified trimester   **M**

    O26.72   Subluxation of symphysis (pubis) in childbirth   **M**

    O26.73   Subluxation of symphysis (pubis) in the puerperium   **M**

● **O26.8**   **Other specified pregnancy related conditions**
   ● O26.81   **Pregnancy related exhaustion and fatigue**
      O26.811   Pregnancy related exhaustion and fatigue, first trimester   **M**
      O26.812   Pregnancy related exhaustion and fatigue, second trimester   **M**
      O26.813   Pregnancy related exhaustion and fatigue, third trimester   **M**
      O26.819   Pregnancy related exhaustion and fatigue, unspecified trimester   **M**

   ● O26.82   **Pregnancy related peripheral neuritis**
      O26.821   Pregnancy related peripheral neuritis, first trimester   **M**
      O26.822   Pregnancy related peripheral neuritis, second trimester   **M**
      O26.823   Pregnancy related peripheral neuritis, third trimester   **M**
      O26.829   Pregnancy related peripheral neuritis, unspecified trimester   **M**

   ● O26.83   **Pregnancy related renal disease**
      Use additional code to identify the specific disorder
      O26.831   Pregnancy related renal disease, first trimester   **M**
      O26.832   Pregnancy related renal disease, second trimester   **M**
      O26.833   Pregnancy related renal disease, third trimester   **M**
      O26.839   Pregnancy related renal disease, unspecified trimester   **M**

   ● O26.84   **Uterine size-date discrepancy complicating pregnancy**
      Excludes1   encounter for suspected problem with fetal growth ruled out (Z03.74)
      O26.841   Uterine size-date discrepancy, first trimester   **M**
      O26.842   Uterine size-date discrepancy, second trimester   **M**
      O26.843   Uterine size-date discrepancy, third trimester   **M**
      O26.849   Uterine size-date discrepancy, unspecified trimester   **M**

   ● O26.85   **Spotting complicating pregnancy**
      O26.851   Spotting complicating pregnancy, first trimester   **M**
      O26.852   Spotting complicating pregnancy, second trimester   **M**
      O26.853   Spotting complicating pregnancy, third trimester   **M**
      O26.859   Spotting complicating pregnancy, unspecified trimester   **M**

    O26.86   Pruritic urticarial papules and plaques of pregnancy (PUPPP)   **M**
      Polymorphic eruption of pregnancy

   ● O26.87   **Cervical shortening**
      Excludes1   encounter for suspected cervical shortening ruled out (Z03.75)
      O26.872   Cervical shortening, second trimester   **M**
      O26.873   Cervical shortening, third trimester   **M**
      O26.879   Cervical shortening, unspecified trimester   **M**

   ● O26.89   **Other specified pregnancy related conditions**
      Use Additional code, if applicable, to identify specific condition such as insulin resistance(E88.81-)
      O26.891   Other specified pregnancy related conditions, first trimester   **M**
      O26.892   Other specified pregnancy related conditions, second trimester   **M**

▶ New   ➡ Revised   ~~deleted~~ Deleted   Excludes 1   Excludes 2   Includes   Use additional   Code first   Code also   Key words
OGCR Official Guidelines   X Assign placeholder X   ● Use Additional Character(s)   ▶ Manifestation Code   🔖 Hierarchical Condition Category   **Coding Clinic**

O26.893 **Other specified pregnancy related conditions, third trimester** M
Coding Clinic: 2015, Q3, P40

O26.899 **Other specified pregnancy related conditions, unspecified trimester** M

● O26.9 Pregnancy related conditions, unspecified

O26.90 Pregnancy related conditions, unspecified, unspecified trimester M

O26.91 Pregnancy related conditions, unspecified, first trimester M

O26.92 Pregnancy related conditions, unspecified, second trimester M

O26.93 Pregnancy related conditions, unspecified, third trimester M

● O28 Abnormal findings on antenatal screening of mother

Excludes1 diagnostic findings classified elsewhere - see Alphabetical Index

O28.0 Abnormal **hematological** finding on antenatal screening of mother M

O28.1 Abnormal **biochemical** finding on antenatal screening of mother M

O28.2 Abnormal **cytological** finding on antenatal screening of mother M

O28.3 Abnormal **ultrasonic** finding on antenatal screening of mother M
Coding Clinic: 2016, Q4, P5

O28.4 Abnormal **radiological** finding on antenatal screening of mother M

O28.5 Abnormal **chromosomal and genetic** finding on antenatal screening of mother M

O28.8 Other abnormal findings on antenatal screening of mother M

O28.9 Unspecified abnormal findings on antenatal screening of mother M

● O29 Complications of anesthesia during pregnancy

Includes maternal complications arising from the administration of a general, regional or local anesthetic, analgesic or other sedation during pregnancy

Use additional code, if necessary, to identify the complication

Excludes2 complications of anesthesia during labor and delivery (O74.-)
complications of anesthesia during the puerperium (O89.-)

● O29.0 Pulmonary complications of anesthesia during pregnancy

● O29.01 **Aspiration pneumonitis** due to anesthesia during pregnancy
Inhalation of stomach contents or secretions NOS due to anesthesia during pregnancy
Mendelson's syndrome due to anesthesia during pregnancy

O29.011 Aspiration pneumonitis due to anesthesia during pregnancy, **first trimester** M

O29.012 Aspiration pneumonitis due to anesthesia during pregnancy, **second trimester** M

O29.013 Aspiration pneumonitis due to anesthesia during pregnancy, **third trimester** M

O29.019 Aspiration pneumonitis due to anesthesia during pregnancy, **unspecified trimester** M

● O29.02 **Pressure collapse of lung** due to anesthesia during pregnancy

O29.021 Pressure collapse of lung due to anesthesia during pregnancy, **first trimester** M

O29.022 Pressure collapse of lung due to anesthesia during pregnancy, **second trimester** M

O29.023 Pressure collapse of lung due to anesthesia during pregnancy, **third trimester** M

O29.029 Pressure collapse of lung due to anesthesia during pregnancy, **unspecified trimester** M

● O29.09 Other pulmonary complications of anesthesia during pregnancy

O29.091 Other pulmonary complications of anesthesia during pregnancy, **first trimester** M

O29.092 Other pulmonary complications of anesthesia during pregnancy, **second trimester** M

O29.093 Other pulmonary complications of anesthesia during pregnancy, **third trimester** M

O29.099 Other pulmonary complications of anesthesia during pregnancy, **unspecified trimester** M

● O29.1 Cardiac complications of anesthesia during pregnancy

● O29.11 Cardiac arrest due to anesthesia during pregnancy

O29.111 Cardiac arrest due to anesthesia during pregnancy, **first trimester** M

O29.112 Cardiac arrest due to anesthesia during pregnancy, **second trimester** M

O29.113 Cardiac arrest due to anesthesia during pregnancy, **third trimester** M

O29.119 Cardiac arrest due to anesthesia during pregnancy, **unspecified trimester** M

● O29.12 Cardiac failure due to anesthesia during pregnancy

O29.121 Cardiac failure due to anesthesia during pregnancy, **first trimester** M

O29.122 Cardiac failure due to anesthesia during pregnancy, **second trimester** M

O29.123 Cardiac failure due to anesthesia during pregnancy, **third trimester** M

O29.129 Cardiac failure due to anesthesia during pregnancy, **unspecified trimester** M

● O29.19 Other cardiac complications of anesthesia during pregnancy

O29.191 Other cardiac complications of anesthesia during pregnancy, **first trimester** M

O29.192 Other cardiac complications of anesthesia during pregnancy, **second trimester** M

O29.193 Other cardiac complications of anesthesia during pregnancy, **third trimester** M

O29.199 Other cardiac complications of anesthesia during pregnancy, **unspecified trimester** M

● O29.2 **Central nervous system** complications of anesthesia during pregnancy

● O29.21 **Cerebral anoxia** due to anesthesia during pregnancy

O29.211 Cerebral anoxia due to anesthesia during pregnancy, **first trimester** M

O29.212 Cerebral anoxia due to anesthesia during pregnancy, **second trimester** M

O29.213 Cerebral anoxia due to anesthesia during pregnancy, **third trimester** M

O29.219 Cerebral anoxia due to anesthesia during pregnancy, **unspecified trimester** M

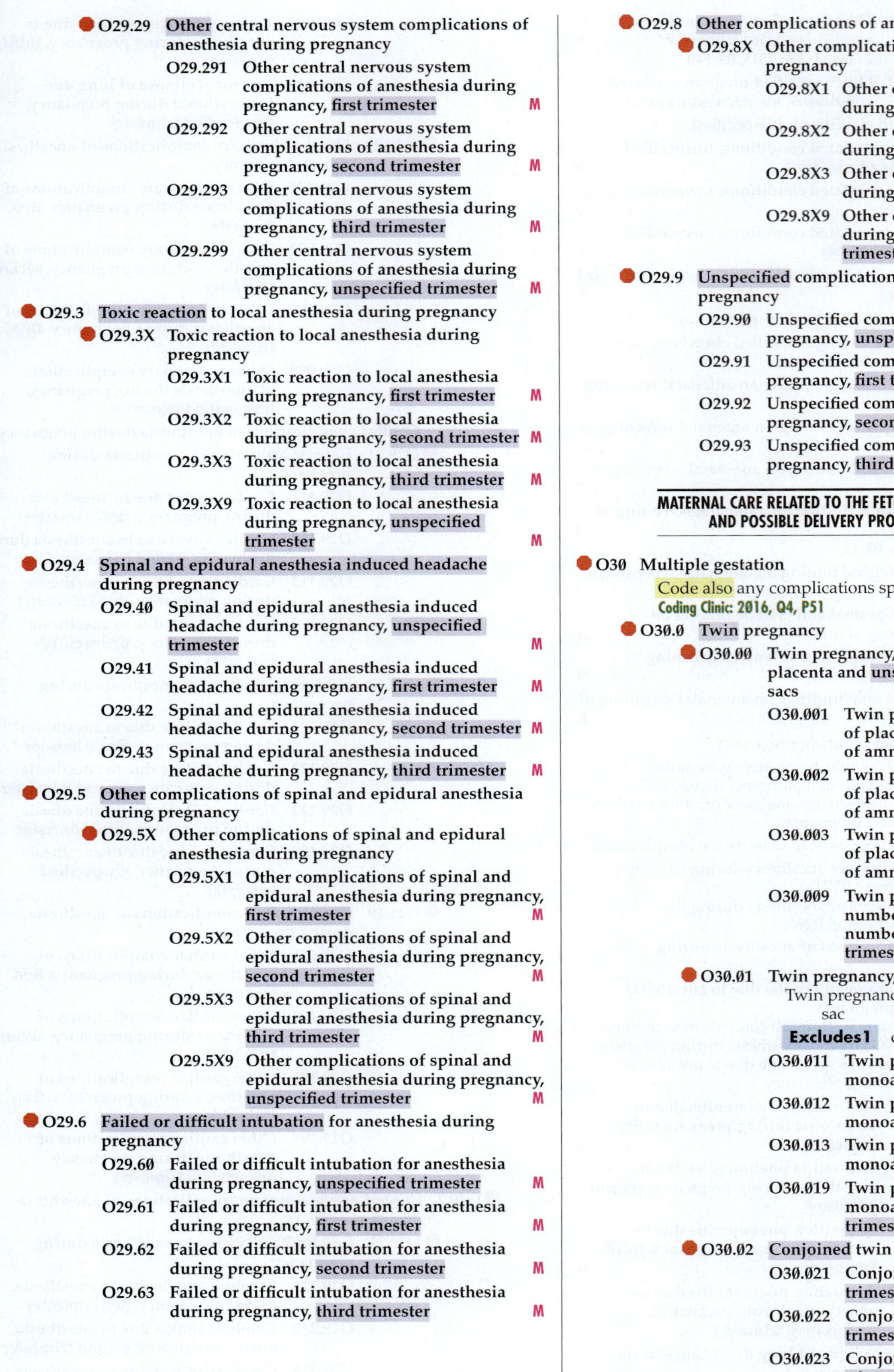

● **O29.29** Other central nervous system complications of anesthesia during pregnancy

O29.291 Other central nervous system complications of anesthesia during pregnancy, first trimester **M**

O29.292 Other central nervous system complications of anesthesia during pregnancy, second trimester **M**

O29.293 Other central nervous system complications of anesthesia during pregnancy, third trimester **M**

O29.299 Other central nervous system complications of anesthesia during pregnancy, unspecified trimester **M**

● **O29.3** Toxic reaction to local anesthesia during pregnancy

● **O29.3X** Toxic reaction to local anesthesia during pregnancy

O29.3X1 Toxic reaction to local anesthesia during pregnancy, first trimester **M**

O29.3X2 Toxic reaction to local anesthesia during pregnancy, second trimester **M**

O29.3X3 Toxic reaction to local anesthesia during pregnancy, third trimester **M**

O29.3X9 Toxic reaction to local anesthesia during pregnancy, unspecified trimester **M**

● **O29.4** Spinal and epidural anesthesia induced headache during pregnancy

O29.40 Spinal and epidural anesthesia induced headache during pregnancy, unspecified trimester **M**

O29.41 Spinal and epidural anesthesia induced headache during pregnancy, first trimester **M**

O29.42 Spinal and epidural anesthesia induced headache during pregnancy, second trimester **M**

O29.43 Spinal and epidural anesthesia induced headache during pregnancy, third trimester **M**

● **O29.5** Other complications of spinal and epidural anesthesia during pregnancy

● **O29.5X** Other complications of spinal and epidural anesthesia during pregnancy

O29.5X1 Other complications of spinal and epidural anesthesia during pregnancy, first trimester **M**

O29.5X2 Other complications of spinal and epidural anesthesia during pregnancy, second trimester **M**

O29.5X3 Other complications of spinal and epidural anesthesia during pregnancy, third trimester **M**

O29.5X9 Other complications of spinal and epidural anesthesia during pregnancy, unspecified trimester **M**

● **O29.6** Failed or difficult intubation for anesthesia during pregnancy

O29.60 Failed or difficult intubation for anesthesia during pregnancy, unspecified trimester **M**

O29.61 Failed or difficult intubation for anesthesia during pregnancy, first trimester **M**

O29.62 Failed or difficult intubation for anesthesia during pregnancy, second trimester **M**

O29.63 Failed or difficult intubation for anesthesia during pregnancy, third trimester **M**

● **O29.8** Other complications of anesthesia during pregnancy

● **O29.8X** Other complications of anesthesia during pregnancy

O29.8X1 Other complications of anesthesia during pregnancy, first trimester **M**

O29.8X2 Other complications of anesthesia during pregnancy, second trimester **M**

O29.8X3 Other complications of anesthesia during pregnancy, third trimester **M**

O29.8X9 Other complications of anesthesia during pregnancy, unspecified trimester **M**

● **O29.9** Unspecified complication of anesthesia during pregnancy

O29.90 Unspecified complication of anesthesia during pregnancy, unspecified trimester **M**

O29.91 Unspecified complication of anesthesia during pregnancy, first trimester **M**

O29.92 Unspecified complication of anesthesia during pregnancy, second trimester **M**

O29.93 Unspecified complication of anesthesia during pregnancy, third trimester **M**

MATERNAL CARE RELATED TO THE FETUS AND AMNIOTIC CAVITY AND POSSIBLE DELIVERY PROBLEMS (O30–O48)

● **O30** Multiple gestation

Code also any complications specific to multiple gestation
Coding Clinic: 2016, Q4, P51

● **O30.0** Twin pregnancy

● **O30.00** Twin pregnancy, unspecified number of placenta and unspecified number of amniotic sacs

O30.001 Twin pregnancy, unspecified number of placenta and unspecified number of amniotic sacs, first trimester **M**

O30.002 Twin pregnancy, unspecified number of placenta and unspecified number of amniotic sacs, second trimester **M**

O30.003 Twin pregnancy, unspecified number of placenta and unspecified number of amniotic sacs, third trimester **M**

O30.009 Twin pregnancy, unspecified number of placenta and unspecified number of amniotic sacs, unspecified trimester **M**

● **O30.01** Twin pregnancy, monochorionic/monoamniotic
Twin pregnancy, one placenta, one amniotic sac

Excludes1 conjoined twins (O30.02-)

O30.011 Twin pregnancy, monochorionic/monoamniotic, first trimester **M**

O30.012 Twin pregnancy, monochorionic/monoamniotic, second trimester **M**

O30.013 Twin pregnancy, monochorionic/monoamniotic, third trimester **M**

O30.019 Twin pregnancy, monochorionic/monoamniotic, unspecified trimester **M**

● **O30.02** Conjoined twin pregnancy

O30.021 Conjoined twin pregnancy, first trimester **M**

O30.022 Conjoined twin pregnancy, second trimester **M**

O30.023 Conjoined twin pregnancy, third trimester **M**

O30.029 Conjoined twin pregnancy, unspecified trimester **M**

▶ New   ⇒ Revised   ~~deleted~~ Deleted   Excludes 1   Excludes 2   Includes   Use additional   Code first   Code also   Key words
OGCR Official Guidelines   **X** Assign placeholder X   ● Use Additional Character(s)   ▶ Manifestation Code   Hierarchical Condition Category   **Coding Clinic**

● **O30.03**   Twin pregnancy, monochorionic/diamniotic
     Twin pregnancy, one placenta, two amniotic sacs

   O30.031   Twin pregnancy, monochorionic/diamniotic, first trimester   **M**

   O30.032   Twin pregnancy, monochorionic/diamniotic, second trimester   **M**

   O30.033   Twin pregnancy, monochorionic/diamniotic, third trimester   **M**

   O30.039   Twin pregnancy, monochorionic/diamniotic, unspecified trimester   **M**

● **O30.04**   Twin pregnancy, dichorionic/diamniotic
     Twin pregnancy, two placentae, two amniotic sacs

   O30.041   Twin pregnancy, dichorionic/diamniotic, first trimester   **M**

   O30.042   Twin pregnancy, dichorionic/diamniotic, second trimester   **M**

   O30.043   Twin pregnancy, dichorionic/diamniotic, third trimester   **M**

   O30.049   Twin pregnancy, dichorionic/diamniotic, unspecified trimester   **M**

● **O30.09**   Twin pregnancy, unable to determine number of placenta and number of amniotic sacs

   O30.091   Twin pregnancy, unable to determine number of placenta and number of amniotic sacs, first trimester   **M**

   O30.092   Twin pregnancy, unable to determine number of placenta and number of amniotic sacs, second trimester   **M**

   O30.093   Twin pregnancy, unable to determine number of placenta and number of amniotic sacs, third trimester   **M**

   O30.099   Twin pregnancy, unable to determine number of placenta and number of amniotic sacs, unspecified trimester   **M**

● **O30.1**   Triplet pregnancy

● **O30.10**   Triplet pregnancy, unspecified number of placenta and unspecified number of amniotic sacs

   O30.101   Triplet pregnancy, unspecified number of placenta and unspecified number of amniotic sacs, first trimester   **M**

   O30.102   Triplet pregnancy, unspecified number of placenta and unspecified number of amniotic sacs, second trimester   **M**

   O30.103   Triplet pregnancy, unspecified number of placenta and unspecified number of amniotic sacs, third trimester   **M**
     Coding Clinic: 2016, Q2, P8

   O30.109   Triplet pregnancy, unspecified number of placenta and unspecified number of amniotic sacs, unspecified trimester   **M**

● **O30.11**   Triplet pregnancy with two or more monochorionic fetuses

   O30.111   Triplet pregnancy with two or more monochorionic fetuses, first trimester   **M**

   O30.112   Triplet pregnancy with two or more monochorionic fetuses, second trimester   **M**

   O30.113   Triplet pregnancy with two or more monochorionic fetuses, third trimester   **M**

   O30.119   Triplet pregnancy with two or more monochorionic fetuses, unspecified trimester   **M**

● **O30.12**   Triplet pregnancy with two or more monoamniotic fetuses

   O30.121   Triplet pregnancy with two or more monoamniotic fetuses, first trimester   **M**

   O30.122   Triplet pregnancy with two or more monoamniotic fetuses, second trimester   **M**

   O30.123   Triplet pregnancy with two or more monoamniotic fetuses, third trimester   **M**

   O30.129   Triplet pregnancy with two or more monoamniotic fetuses, unspecified trimester   **M**

● **O30.13**   Triplet pregnancy, trichorionic/triamniotic

   O30.131   Triplet pregnancy, trichorionic/triamniotic, first trimester   **M**

   O30.132   Triplet pregnancy, trichorionic/triamniotic, second trimester   **M**

   O30.133   Triplet pregnancy, trichorionic/triamniotic, third trimester   **M**

   O30.139   Triplet pregnancy, trichorionic/triamniotic, unspecified trimester   **M**

● **O30.19**   Triplet pregnancy, unable to determine number of placenta and number of amniotic sacs

   O30.191   Triplet pregnancy, unable to determine number of placenta and number of amniotic sacs, first trimester   **M**

   O30.192   Triplet pregnancy, unable to determine number of placenta and number of amniotic sacs, second trimester   **M**

   O30.193   Triplet pregnancy, unable to determine number of placenta and number of amniotic sacs, third trimester   **M**

   O30.199   Triplet pregnancy, unable to determine number of placenta and number of amniotic sacs, unspecified trimester   **M**

● **O30.2**   Quadruplet pregnancy

● **O30.20**   Quadruplet pregnancy, unspecified number of placenta and unspecified number of amniotic sacs

   O30.201   Quadruplet pregnancy, unspecified number of placenta and unspecified number of amniotic sacs, first trimester   **M**

   O30.202   Quadruplet pregnancy, unspecified number of placenta and unspecified number of amniotic sacs, second trimester   **M**

   O30.203   Quadruplet pregnancy, unspecified number of placenta and unspecified number of amniotic sacs, third trimester   **M**

   O30.209   Quadruplet pregnancy, unspecified number of placenta and unspecified number of amniotic sacs, unspecified trimester   **M**

● **O30.21**   Quadruplet pregnancy with two or more monochorionic fetuses

   O30.211   Quadruplet pregnancy with two or more monochorionic fetuses, first trimester   **M**

   O30.212   Quadruplet pregnancy with two or more monochorionic fetuses, second trimester   **M**

O30.213　Quadruplet pregnancy with two or more monochorionic fetuses, **third trimester** M

O30.219　Quadruplet pregnancy with two or more monochorionic fetuses, unspecified trimester M

● O30.22　Quadruplet pregnancy with **two or more monoamniotic fetuses**

O30.221　Quadruplet pregnancy with two or more monoamniotic fetuses, **first trimester** M

O30.222　Quadruplet pregnancy with two or more monoamniotic fetuses, **second trimester** M

O30.223　Quadruplet pregnancy with two or more monoamniotic fetuses, **third trimester** M

O30.229　Quadruplet pregnancy with two or more monoamniotic fetuses, unspecified trimester M

● O30.23　Quadruplet pregnancy, quadrachorionic/quadra-amniotic

O30.231　Quadruplet pregnancy, quadrachorionic/quadra-amniotic, first trimester M

O30.232　Quadruplet pregnancy, quadrachorionic/quadra-amniotic, second trimester M

O30.233　Quadruplet pregnancy, quadrachorionic/quadra-amniotic, third trimester M

O30.239　Quadruplet pregnancy, quadrachorionic/quadra-amniotic, unspecifiedtrimester M

● O30.29　Quadruplet pregnancy, **unable to determine number of placenta and number of amniotic sacs**

O30.291　Quadruplet pregnancy, unable to determine number of placenta and number of amniotic sacs, **first trimester** M

O30.292　Quadruplet pregnancy, unable to determine number of placenta and number of amniotic sacs, **second trimester** M

O30.293　Quadruplet pregnancy, unable to determine number of placenta and number of amniotic sacs, **third trimester** M

O30.299　Quadruplet pregnancy, unable to determine number of placenta and number of amniotic sacs, **unspecified trimester**

● O30.8　Other specified multiple gestation
Multiple gestation pregnancy greater then quadruplets

● O30.80　Other specified multiple gestation, **unspecified number of placenta and unspecified number of amniotic sacs**

O30.801　Other specified multiple gestation, unspecified number of placenta and unspecified number of amniotic sacs, **first trimester** M

O30.802　Other specified multiple gestation, unspecified number of placenta and unspecified number of amniotic sacs, **second trimester** M

O30.803　Other specified multiple gestation, unspecified number of placenta and unspecified number of amniotic sacs, **third trimester** M

O30.809　Other specified multiple gestation, unspecified number of placenta and unspecified number of amniotic sacs, **unspecified trimester** M

● O30.81　Other specified multiple gestation with **two or more monochorionic fetuses**

O30.811　Other specified multiple gestation with two or more monochorionic fetuses, **first trimester** M

O30.812　Other specified multiple gestation with two or more monochorionic fetuses, **second trimester** M

O30.813　Other specified multiple gestation with two or more monochorionic fetuses, **third trimester** M

O30.819　Other specified multiple gestation with two or more monochorionic fetuses, **unspecified trimester** M

● O30.82　Other specified multiple gestation with **two or more monoamniotic fetuses**

O30.821　Other specified multiple gestation with two or more monoamniotic fetuses, **first trimester** M

O30.822　Other specified multiple gestation with two or more monoamniotic fetuses, **second trimester** M

O30.823　Other specified multiple gestation with two or more monoamniotic fetuses, **third trimester** M

O30.829　Other specified multiple gestation with two or more monoamniotic fetuses, **unspecified trimester** M

● O30.83　Other specified multiple gestation, number of chorions and amnions are both equalto the number of fetuses
Pentachorionic, penta-amniotic pregnancy (quintuplets)
Hexachorionic, hexa-amniotic pregnancy (sextuplets)
Heptachorionic, hepta-amniotic pregnancy (septuplets)

O30.831　Other specified multiple gestation, number of chorions and amnions are both equal to the number of fetuses, first trimester M

O30.832　Other specified multiple gestation, number of chorions and amnions are both equal to the number of fetuses, second trimester M

O30.833　Other specified multiple gestation, number of chorions and amnions are both equal to the number of fetuses, third trimester M

O30.839　Other specified multiple gestation, number of chorions and amnions are both equal to the number of fetuses, unspecified trimester M

● O30.89　Other specified multiple gestation, **unable to determine** number of placenta and number of amniotic sacs

O30.891　Other specified multiple gestation, unable to determine number of placenta and number of amniotic sacs, **first trimester** M

O30.892　Other specified multiple gestation, unable to determine number of placenta and number of amniotic sacs, **second trimester** M

O30.893　Other specified multiple gestation, unable to determine number of placenta and number of amniotic sacs, **third trimester** M

O30.899　Other specified multiple gestation, unable to determine number of placenta and number of amniotic sacs, **unspecified trimester** M

▶ New　⇒ Revised　~~deleted~~ Deleted　Excludes 1　Excludes 2　Includes　Use additional　Code first　Code also　Key words
OGCR Official Guidelines　X Assign placeholder X　● Use Additional Character(s)　▶ Manifestation Code　HCC Hierarchical Condition Category　Coding Clinic

● **O30.9 Multiple gestation, unspecified**
Multiple pregnancy NOS

    O30.90 Multiple gestation, unspecified, unspecified trimester **M**

    O30.91 Multiple gestation, unspecified, first trimester **M**

    O30.92 Multiple gestation, unspecified, second trimester **M**

    O30.93 Multiple gestation, unspecified, third trimester **M**

● **O31 Complications specific to multiple gestation**

    Excludes2   delayed delivery of second twin, triplet, etc. (O63.2)
                malpresentation of one fetus or more (O32.9)
                placental transfusion syndromes (O43.0-)

    Coding Clinic: 2012, Q4, P107

One of the following 7th characters is to be assigned to each code under category O31. 7th character 0 is for single gestations and multiple gestations where the fetus is unspecified. 7th characters 1 through 9 are for cases of multiple gestations to identify the fetus for which the code applies. The appropriate code from category O30, Multiple gestation, must also be assigned when assigning a code from category O31 that has a 7th character of 1 through 9.

0	not applicable or unspecified
1	fetus 1
2	fetus 2
3	fetus 3
4	fetus 4
5	fetus 5
9	other fetus

● **O31.0 Papyraceous fetus**
Fetus compressus

    X● O31.00 Papyraceous fetus, unspecified trimester **M**

    X● O31.01 Papyraceous fetus, first trimester **M**

    X● O31.02 Papyraceous fetus, second trimester **M**

    X● O31.03 Papyraceous fetus, third trimester **M**

● **O31.1 Continuing pregnancy after spontaneous abortion of one fetus or more**

    X● O31.10 Continuing pregnancy after spontaneous abortion of one fetus or more, unspecified trimester **M**

    X● O31.11 Continuing pregnancy after spontaneous abortion of one fetus or more, first trimester **M**

    X● O31.12 Continuing pregnancy after spontaneous abortion of one fetus or more, second trimester **M**

    X● O31.13 Continuing pregnancy after spontaneous abortion of one fetus or more, third trimester **M**

● **O31.2 Continuing pregnancy after intrauterine death of one fetus or more**

    X● O31.20 Continuing pregnancy after intrauterine death of one fetus or more, unspecified trimester **M**

    X● O31.21 Continuing pregnancy after intrauterine death of one fetus or more, first trimester **M**

    X● O31.22 Continuing pregnancy after intrauterine death of one fetus or more, second trimester **M**

    X● O31.23 Continuing pregnancy after intrauterine death of one fetus or more, third trimester **M**

● **O31.3 Continuing pregnancy after elective fetal reduction of one fetus or more**
Continuing pregnancy after selective termination of one fetus or more

    X● O31.30 Continuing pregnancy after elective fetal reduction of one fetus or more, unspecified trimester **M**

    X● O31.31 Continuing pregnancy after elective fetal reduction of one fetus or more, first trimester **M**

    X● O31.32 Continuing pregnancy after elective fetal reduction of one fetus or more, second trimester **M**

    X● O31.33 Continuing pregnancy after elective fetal reduction of one fetus or more, third trimester **M**

● **O31.8 Other complications specific to multiple gestation**

    ● O31.8X Other complications specific to multiple gestation

       ● O31.8X1 Other complications specific to multiple gestation, first trimester **M**

       ● O31.8X2 Other complications specific to multiple gestation, second trimester **M**

       ● O31.8X3 Other complications specific to multiple gestation, third trimester **M**

       ● O31.8X9 Other complications specific to multiple gestation, unspecified trimester **M**

● **O32 Maternal care for malpresentation of fetus**

    Includes   the listed conditions as a reason for observation, hospitalization or other obstetric care of the mother, or for cesarean delivery before onset of labor

    Excludes1   malpresentation of fetus with obstructed labor (O64.-)

    Coding Clinic: 2012, Q4, P107

One of the following 7th characters is to be assigned to each code under category O32. 7th character 0 is for single gestations and multiple gestations where the fetus is unspecified. 7th characters 1 through 9 are for cases of multiple gestations to identify the fetus for which the code applies. The appropriate code from category O30, Multiple gestation, must also be assigned when assigning a code from category O32 that has a 7th character of 1 through 9.

0	not applicable or unspecified
1	fetus 1
2	fetus 2
3	fetus 3
4	fetus 4
5	fetus 5
9	other fetus

X● **O32.0 Maternal care for unstable lie** **M**

X● **O32.1 Maternal care for breech presentation** **M**
Maternal care for buttocks presentation
Maternal care for complete breech
Maternal care for frank breech

    Excludes1   footling presentation (O32.8)
                incomplete breech (O32.8)

X● **O32.2 Maternal care for transverse and oblique lie** **M**
Maternal care for oblique presentation
Maternal care for transverse presentation

X● **O32.3 Maternal care for face, brow and chin presentation** **M**

X● **O32.4 Maternal care for high head at term** **M**
Maternal care for failure of head to enter pelvic brim

X● **O32.6 Maternal care for compound presentation** **M**

X● **O32.8 Maternal care for other malpresentation of fetus** **M**
Maternal care for footling presentation
Maternal care for incomplete breech

X● **O32.9 Maternal care for malpresentation of fetus, unspecified** **M**

● **O33**   **Maternal care for disproportion**

    Includes   the listed conditions as a reason for observation, hospitalization or other obstetric care of the mother, or for cesarean delivery before onset of labor

    Excludes1   disproportion with obstructed labor (O65-O66)

O33.0   **Maternal care for disproportion due to deformity of maternal pelvic bones**   M

    Maternal care for disproportion due to pelvic deformity causing disproportion NOS

O33.1   **Maternal care for disproportion due to generally contracted pelvis**   M

    Maternal care for disproportion due to contracted pelvis NOS causing disproportion

O33.2   **Maternal care for disproportion due to inlet contraction of pelvis**   M

    Maternal care for disproportion due to inlet contraction (pelvis) causing disproportion

X ● **O33.3**   **Maternal care for disproportion due to outlet contraction of pelvis**   M

    Maternal care for disproportion due to mid-cavity contraction (pelvis)

    Maternal care for disproportion due to outlet contraction (pelvis)

One of the following 7th characters is to be assigned to code O33.3. 7th character 0 is for single gestations and multiple gestations where the fetus is unspecified. 7th characters 1 through 9 are for cases of multiple gestations to identify the fetus for which the code applies. The appropriate code from category O30, Multiple gestation, must also be assigned when assigning code O33.3 with a 7th character of 1 through 9.

0	not applicable or unspecified
1	fetus 1
2	fetus 2
3	fetus 3
4	fetus 4
5	fetus 5
9	other fetus

X ● **O33.4**   **Maternal care for disproportion of mixed maternal and fetal origin**   M

One of the following 7th characters is to be assigned to code O33.4. 7th character 0 is for single gestations and multiple gestations where the fetus is unspecified. 7th characters 1 through 9 are for cases of multiple gestations to identify the fetus for which the code applies. The appropriate code from category O30, Multiple gestation, must also be assigned when assigning code O33.4 with a 7th character of 1 through 9.

0	not applicable or unspecified
1	fetus 1
2	fetus 2
3	fetus 3
4	fetus 4
5	fetus 5
9	other fetus

X ● **O33.5**   **Maternal care for disproportion due to unusually large fetus**   M

    Maternal care for disproportion due to disproportion of fetal origin with normally formed fetus

    Maternal care for disproportion due to fetal disproportion NOS

One of the following 7th characters is to be assigned to code O33.5. 7th character 0 is for single gestations and multiple gestations where the fetus is unspecified. 7th characters 1 through 9 are for cases of multiple gestations to identify the fetus for which the code applies. The appropriate code from category O30, Multiple gestation, must also be assigned when assigning code O33.5 with a 7th character of 1 through 9.

0	not applicable or unspecified
1	fetus 1
2	fetus 2
3	fetus 3
4	fetus 4
5	fetus 5
9	other fetus

X ● **O33.6**   **Maternal care for disproportion due to hydrocephalic fetus**   M

One of the following 7th characters is to be assigned to code O33.6. 7th character 0 is for single gestations and multiple gestations where the fetus is unspecified. 7th characters 1 through 9 are for cases of multiple gestations to identify the fetus for which the code applies. The appropriate code from category O30, Multiple gestation, must also be assigned when assigning code O33.6 with a 7th character of 1 through 9.

0	not applicable or unspecified
1	fetus 1
2	fetus 2
3	fetus 3
4	fetus 4
5	fetus 5
9	other fetus

X ● **O33.7**   **Maternal care for disproportion due to other fetal deformities**   M

    Maternal care for disproportion due to fetal ascites

    Maternal care for disproportion due to fetal hydrops

    Maternal care for disproportion due to fetal meningomyelocele

    Maternal care for disproportion due to fetal sacral teratoma

    Maternal care for disproportion due to fetal tumor

    Excludes1   obstructed labor due to other fetal deformities (O66.3)

Coding Clinic: 2016, Q4, P51

One of the following 7th characters is to be assigned to code O33.7. 7th character 0 is for single gestations and multiple gestations where the fetus is unspecified. 7th characters 1 through 9 are for cases of multiple gestations to identify the fetus for which the code applies. The appropriate code from category O30, Multiple gestation, must also be assigned when assigning code O33.7 with a 7th character of 1 through 9.

0	not applicable or unspecified
1	fetus 1
2	fetus 2
3	fetus 3
4	fetus 4
5	fetus 5
9	other fetus

▶ New   ⇒ Revised   ~~deleted~~ Deleted   Excludes 1   Excludes 2   Includes   Use additional   Code first   Code also   Key words

OGCR Official Guidelines   X Assign placeholder X   ● Use Additional Character(s)   ▶ Manifestation Code   🅗🅒 Hierarchical Condition Category   **Coding Clinic**

O33.8   **Maternal care for disproportion of other origin**   M

O33.9   **Maternal care for disproportion, unspecified**   M
     Maternal care for disproportion due to cephalopelvic disproportion NOS
     Maternal care for disproportion due to fetopelvic disproportion NOS

● **O34**   **Maternal care for abnormality of pelvic organs**

   Includes   the listed conditions as a reason for hospitalization or other obstetric care of the mother, or for cesarean delivery before onset of labor

   Code first any associated obstructed labor (O65.5)

   Use additional code for specific condition

● **O34.0**   **Maternal care for congenital malformation of uterus**
     Maternal care for double uterus
     Maternal care for uterus bicornis

   O34.00   **Maternal care for unspecified congenital malformation of uterus, unspecified trimester**   M

   O34.01   **Maternal care for unspecified congenital malformation of uterus, first trimester**   M

   O34.02   **Maternal care for unspecified congenital malformation of uterus, second trimester**   M

   O34.03   **Maternal care for unspecified congenital malformation of uterus, third trimester**   M

● **O34.1**   **Maternal care for benign tumor of corpus uteri**

   Excludes2   maternal care for benign tumor of cervix (O34.4-)
     maternal care for malignant neoplasm of uterus (O9A.1-)

   O34.10   **Maternal care for benign tumor of corpus uteri, unspecified trimester**   M

   O34.11   **Maternal care for benign tumor of corpus uteri, first trimester**   M

   O34.12   **Maternal care for benign tumor of corpus uteri, second trimester**   M

   O34.13   **Maternal care for benign tumor of corpus uteri, third trimester**   M

● **O34.2**   **Maternal care due to uterine scar from previous surgery**
     Coding Clinic: 2016, Q4, P76

   ● **O34.21**   **Maternal care for scar from previous cesarean delivery**
     Coding Clinic: 2016, Q4, P51

     O34.211   **Maternal care for low transverse scar from previous cesarean delivery**   M

     O34.212   **Maternal care for vertical scar from previous cesarean delivery**   M
       Maternal care for classical scar from previous cesarean delivery

     O34.218   **Maternal care for other type scar from previous cesarean delivery**   M
       Mid-transverse T incision

     O34.219   **Maternal care for unspecified type scar from previous cesarean delivery**   M

   O34.22   **Maternal care for cesarean scar defect (isthmocele)**   M

   O34.29   **Maternal care due to uterine scar from other previous surgery**   M
     Maternal care due to uterine scar from other transmural uterine incision

● **O34.3**   **Maternal care for cervical incompetence**
     Maternal care for cerclage with or without cervical incompetence
     Maternal care for Shirodkar suture with or without cervical incompetence

   O34.30   **Maternal care for cervical incompetence, unspecified trimester**   M

   O34.31   **Maternal care for cervical incompetence, first trimester**   M

   O34.32   **Maternal care for cervical incompetence, second trimester**   M

   O34.33   **Maternal care for cervical incompetence, third trimester**   M

● **O34.4**   **Maternal care for other abnormalities of cervix**

   O34.40   **Maternal care for other abnormalities of cervix, unspecified trimester**   M

   O34.41   **Maternal care for other abnormalities of cervix, first trimester**   M

   O34.42   **Maternal care for other abnormalities of cervix, second trimester**   M

   O34.43   **Maternal care for other abnormalities of cervix, third trimester**   M

● **O34.5**   **Maternal care for other abnormalities of gravid uterus**

   ● **O34.51**   **Maternal care for incarceration of gravid uterus**

     O34.511   **Maternal care for incarceration of gravid uterus, first trimester**   M

     O34.512   **Maternal care for incarceration of gravid uterus, second trimester**   M

     O34.513   **Maternal care for incarceration of gravid uterus, third trimester**   M

     O34.519   **Maternal care for incarceration of gravid uterus, unspecified trimester**   M

   ● **O34.52**   **Maternal care for prolapse of gravid uterus**

     O34.521   **Maternal care for prolapse of gravid uterus, first trimester**   M

     O34.522   **Maternal care for prolapse of gravid uterus, second trimester**   M

     O34.523   **Maternal care for prolapse of gravid uterus, third trimester**   M

     O34.529   **Maternal care for prolapse of gravid uterus, unspecified trimester**   M

   ● **O34.53**   **Maternal care for retroversion of gravid uterus**

     O34.531   **Maternal care for retroversion of gravid uterus, first trimester**   M

     O34.532   **Maternal care for retroversion of gravid uterus, second trimester**   M

     O34.533   **Maternal care for retroversion of gravid uterus, third trimester**   M

     O34.539   **Maternal care for retroversion of gravid uterus, unspecified trimester**   M

   ● **O34.59**   **Maternal care for other abnormalities of gravid uterus**

     O34.591   **Maternal care for other abnormalities of gravid uterus, first trimester**   M

     O34.592   **Maternal care for other abnormalities of gravid uterus, second trimester**   M

     O34.593   **Maternal care for other abnormalities of gravid uterus, third trimester**   M

     O34.599   **Maternal care for other abnormalities of gravid uterus, unspecified trimester**   M

● **O34.6**   **Maternal care for abnormality of vagina**

   Excludes2   maternal care for vaginal varices in pregnancy (O22.1-)

   O34.60   **Maternal care for abnormality of vagina, unspecified trimester**   M

   O34.61   **Maternal care for abnormality of vagina, first trimester**   M

   O34.62   **Maternal care for abnormality of vagina, second trimester**   M

   O34.63   **Maternal care for abnormality of vagina, third trimester**   M

CHAPTER 15 (O00-O9A)

● **O34.7** Maternal care for abnormality of vulva and perineum

> **Excludes2**   maternal care for perineal and vulval varices in pregnancy (O22.1-)

O34.70   Maternal care for abnormality of vulva and perineum, unspecified trimester   M

O34.71   Maternal care for abnormality of vulva and perineum, first trimester   M

O34.72   Maternal care for abnormality of vulva and perineum, second trimester   M

O34.73   Maternal care for abnormality of vulva and perineum, third trimester   M

● **O34.8** Maternal care for other abnormalities of pelvic organs

O34.80   Maternal care for other abnormalities of pelvic organs, unspecified trimester   M

O34.81   Maternal care for other abnormalities of pelvic organs, first trimester   M

O34.82   Maternal care for other abnormalities of pelvic organs, second trimester   M

O34.83   Maternal care for other abnormalities of pelvic organs, third trimester   M

● **O34.9** Maternal care for abnormality of pelvic organ, unspecified

O34.90   Maternal care for abnormality of pelvic organ, unspecified, unspecified trimester   M

O34.91   Maternal care for abnormality of pelvic organ, unspecified, first trimester   M

O34.92   Maternal care for abnormality of pelvic organ, unspecified, second trimester   M

O34.93   Maternal care for abnormality of pelvic organ, unspecified, third trimester   M

● **O35** Maternal care for known or suspected fetal abnormality and damage

> **Includes**   the listed conditions in the fetus as a reason for hospitalization or other obstetric care to the mother, or for termination of pregnancy

Code also any associated maternal condition

> **Excludes1**   encounter for suspected maternal and fetal conditions ruled out (Z03.7-)

One of the following 7th characters is to be assigned to each code under category O35. 7th character 0 is for single gestations and multiple gestations where the fetus is unspecified. 7th characters 1 through 9 are for cases of multiple gestations to identify the fetus for which the code applies. The appropriate code from category O30, Multiple gestation, must also be assigned when assigning a code from category O35 that has a 7th character of 1 through 9.

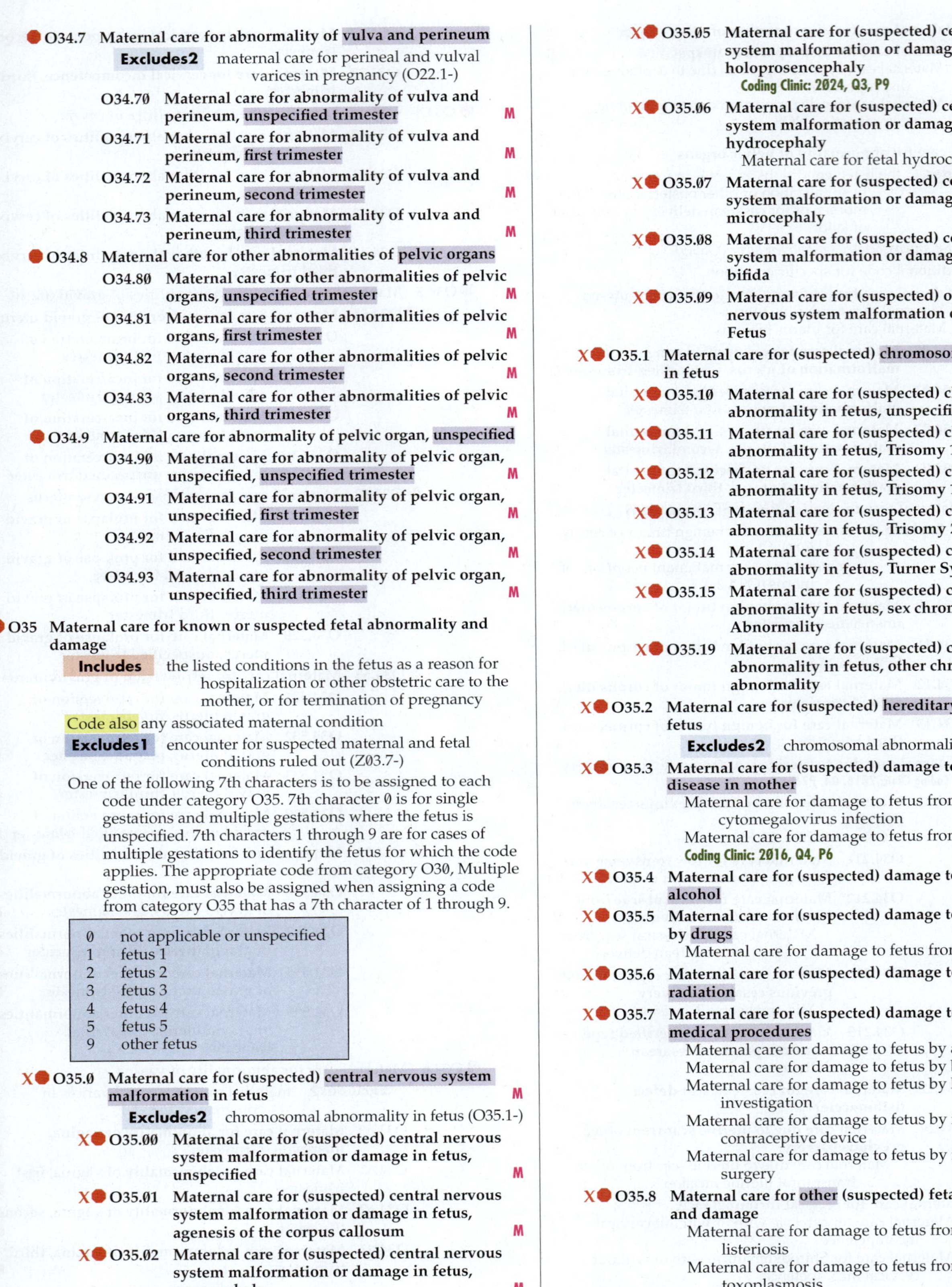

X ● **O35.0** Maternal care for (suspected) central nervous system malformation in fetus   M

> **Excludes2**   chromosomal abnormality in fetus (O35.1-)

X ● O35.00   Maternal care for (suspected) central nervous system malformation or damage in fetus, unspecified   M

X ● O35.01   Maternal care for (suspected) central nervous system malformation or damage in fetus, agenesis of the corpus callosum   M

X ● O35.02   Maternal care for (suspected) central nervous system malformation or damage in fetus, anencephaly   M

X ● O35.03   Maternal care for (suspected) central nervous system malformation or damage in fetus, choroid plexus cysts   M

X ● O35.04   Maternal care for (suspected) central nervous system malformation or damage in fetus, encephalocele   M

X ● O35.05   Maternal care for (suspected) central nervous system malformation or damage in fetus, holoprosencephaly   M
Coding Clinic: 2024, Q3, P9

X ● O35.06   Maternal care for (suspected) central nervous system malformation or damage in fetus, hydrocephaly   M
Maternal care for fetal hydrocephalus

X ● O35.07   Maternal care for (suspected) central nervous system malformation or damage in fetus, microcephaly   M

X ● O35.08   Maternal care for (suspected) central nervous system malformation or damage in fetus, spina bifida   M

X ● O35.09   Maternal care for (suspected) other central nervous system malformation or damage in Fetus   M

X ● **O35.1** Maternal care for (suspected) chromosomal abnormality in fetus   M

X ● O35.10   Maternal care for (suspected) chromosomal abnormality in fetus, unspecified   M

X ● O35.11   Maternal care for (suspected) chromosomal abnormality in fetus, Trisomy 13   M

X ● O35.12   Maternal care for (suspected) chromosomal abnormality in fetus, Trisomy 18   M

X ● O35.13   Maternal care for (suspected) chromosomal abnormality in fetus, Trisomy 21   M

X ● O35.14   Maternal care for (suspected) chromosomal abnormality in fetus, Turner Syndrome   M

X ● O35.15   Maternal care for (suspected) chromosomal abnormality in fetus, sex chromosome Abnormality   M

X ● O35.19   Maternal care for (suspected) chromosomal abnormality in fetus, other chromosomal abnormality   M

X ● **O35.2** Maternal care for (suspected) hereditary disease in fetus   M

> **Excludes2**   chromosomal abnormality in fetus (O35.1-)

X ● **O35.3** Maternal care for (suspected) damage to fetus from viral disease in mother   M
Maternal care for damage to fetus from maternal cytomegalovirus infection
Maternal care for damage to fetus from maternal rubella
Coding Clinic: 2016, Q4, P6

X ● **O35.4** Maternal care for (suspected) damage to fetus from alcohol   M

X ● **O35.5** Maternal care for (suspected) damage to fetus by drugs   M
Maternal care for damage to fetus from drug addiction

X ● **O35.6** Maternal care for (suspected) damage to fetus by radiation   M

X ● **O35.7** Maternal care for (suspected) damage to fetus by other medical procedures   M
Maternal care for damage to fetus by amniocentesis
Maternal care for damage to fetus by biopsy procedures
Maternal care for damage to fetus by hematological investigation
Maternal care for damage to fetus by intrauterine contraceptive device
Maternal care for damage to fetus by intrauterine surgery

X ● **O35.8** Maternal care for other (suspected) fetal abnormality and damage   M
Maternal care for damage to fetus from maternal listeriosis
Maternal care for damage to fetus from maternal toxoplasmosis

X ● **O35.9** Maternal care for (suspected) fetal abnormality and damage, unspecified   M

X ● **O35.A** Maternal care for other (suspected) fetal abnormality and damage, fetal facial anomalies   M

X ● **O35.B** Maternal care for other (suspected) fetal abnormality and damage, fetal cardiac anomalies   M

X ● **O35.C** Maternal care for other (suspected) fetal abnormality and damage, fetal pulmonary anomalies   M

X ● **O35.D** Maternal care for other (suspected) fetal abnormality and damage, fetal gastrointestinal anomalies   M

X ● **O35.E** Maternal care for other (suspected) fetal abnormality and damage, fetal genitourinary anomalies   M

X ● **O35.F** Maternal care for other (suspected) fetal abnormality and damage, fetal musculoskeletal anomalies of trunk   M

     Excludes2 maternal care for other (suspected) fetal abnormality and damage, fetal lower extremities anomalies (O35.H)
maternal care for other (suspected) fetal abnormality and damage, fetal upper extremities anomalies (O35.G)

X ● **O35.G** Maternal care for other (suspected) fetal abnormality and damage, fetal upper extremities anomalies   M

X ● **O35.H** Maternal care for other (suspected) fetal abnormality and damage, fetal lower extremities Anomalies   M

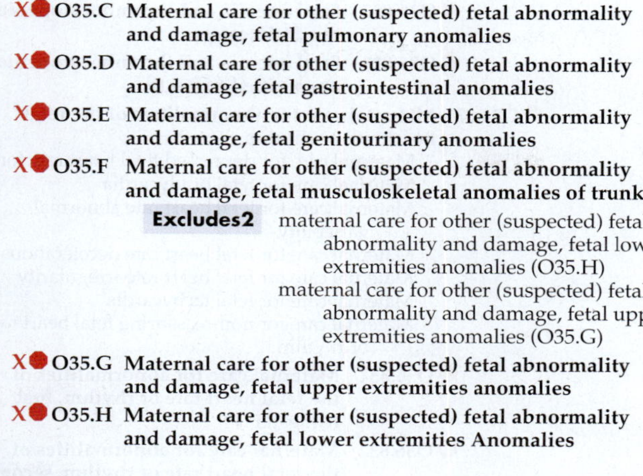

OGCR Section I.C.15.e.l.

Fetal Conditions Affecting the Management of the Mother

1) Code from categories O35 and O36

Codes from categories O35, Maternal care for known or suspected fetal abnormality and damage, and O36, Maternal care for other fetal problems, are assigned only when the fetal condition is actually responsible for modifying the management of the mother, i.e., by requiring diagnostic studies, additional observation, special care, or termination of pregnancy. The fact that the fetal condition exists does not justify assigning a code from this series to the mother's record.

2) In utero surgery

In cases when surgery is performed on the fetus, a diagnosis code from category O35, Maternal care for known or suspected fetal abnormality and damage, should be assigned identifying the fetal condition. Assign the appropriate procedure code for the procedure performed.

No code from Chapter 16, the perinatal codes, should be used on the mother's record to identify fetal conditions. Surgery performed in utero on a fetus is still to be coded as an obstetric encounter.

● **O36** Maternal care for other fetal problems

     Includes the listed conditions in the fetus as a reason for hospitalization or other obstetric care of the mother, or for termination of pregnancy

     Excludes1 encounter for suspected maternal and fetal conditions ruled out (Z03.7-)
placental transfusion syndromes (O43.0-)

     Excludes2 labor and delivery complicated by fetal stress (O77.-)

One of the following 7th characters is to be assigned to each code under category O36. 7th character 0 is for single gestations and multiple gestations where the fetus is unspecified. 7th characters 1 through 9 are for cases of multiple gestations to identify the fetus for which the code applies. The appropriate code from category O30, Multiple gestation, must also be assigned when assigning a code from category O36 that has a 7th character of 1 through 9.

0	not applicable or unspecified
1	fetus 1
2	fetus 2
3	fetus 3
4	fetus 4
5	fetus 5
9	other fetus

Coding Clinic: 2015, Q3, P40

● **O36.0** Maternal care for rhesus isoimmunization
Maternal care for Rh incompatibility (with hydrops fetalis)

     ● **O36.01** Maternal care for anti-D [Rh] antibodies

         ● **O36.011** Maternal care for anti-D [Rh] antibodies, first trimester   M

         ● **O36.012** Maternal care for anti-D [Rh] antibodies, second trimester   M

         ● **O36.013** Maternal care for anti-D [Rh] antibodies, third trimester   M

         ● **O36.019** Maternal care for anti-D [Rh] antibodies, unspecified trimester   M

     ● **O36.09** Maternal care for other rhesus isoimmunization

         ● **O36.091** Maternal care for other rhesus isoimmunization, first trimester   M

         ● **O36.092** Maternal care for other rhesus isoimmunization, second trimester   M

         ● **O36.093** Maternal care for other rhesus isoimmunization, third trimester   M
Coding Clinic: 2015, Q3, P40

         ● **O36.099** Maternal care for other rhesus isoimmunization, unspecified trimester   M

● **O36.1** Maternal care for other isoimmunization
Maternal care for ABO isoimmunization

     ● **O36.11** Maternal care for Anti-A sensitization
Maternal care for isoimmunization NOS (with hydrops fetalis)

         ● **O36.111** Maternal care for Anti-A sensitization, first trimester   M

         ● **O36.112** Maternal care for Anti-A sensitization, second trimester   M

         ● **O36.113** Maternal care for Anti-A sensitization, third trimester   M

         ● **O36.119** Maternal care for Anti-A sensitization, unspecified trimester   M

     ● **O36.19** Maternal care for other isoimmunization
Maternal care for Anti-B sensitization

         ● **O36.191** Maternal care for other isoimmunization, first trimester   M

         ● **O36.192** Maternal care for other isoimmunization, second trimester   M

         ● **O36.193** Maternal care for other isoimmunization, third trimester   M

         ● **O36.199** Maternal care for other isoimmunization, unspecified trimester   M

● **O36.2** Maternal care for hydrops fetalis
Maternal care for hydrops fetalis NOS
Maternal care for hydrops fetalis not associated with isoimmunization

     Excludes1 hydrops fetalis associated with ABO isoimmunization (O36.1-)
hydrops fetalis associated with rhesus isoimmunization (O36.0-)

     ● **O36.20** Maternal care for hydrops fetalis, unspecified trimester   M

     ● **O36.21** Maternal care for hydrops fetalis, first trimester   M

     ● **O36.22** Maternal care for hydrops fetalis, second trimester   M

     ● **O36.23** Maternal care for hydrops fetalis, third trimester   M

● **O36.4** Maternal care for intrauterine death   M
Maternal care for intrauterine fetal death NOS
Maternal care for intrauterine fetal death after completion of 20 weeks of gestation
Maternal care for late fetal death
Maternal care for missed delivery

     Excludes1 missed abortion (O02.1)
stillbirth (P95)
Coding Clinic: 2022, Q2, P3-4

● **O36.5** Maternal care for known or suspected poor fetal growth

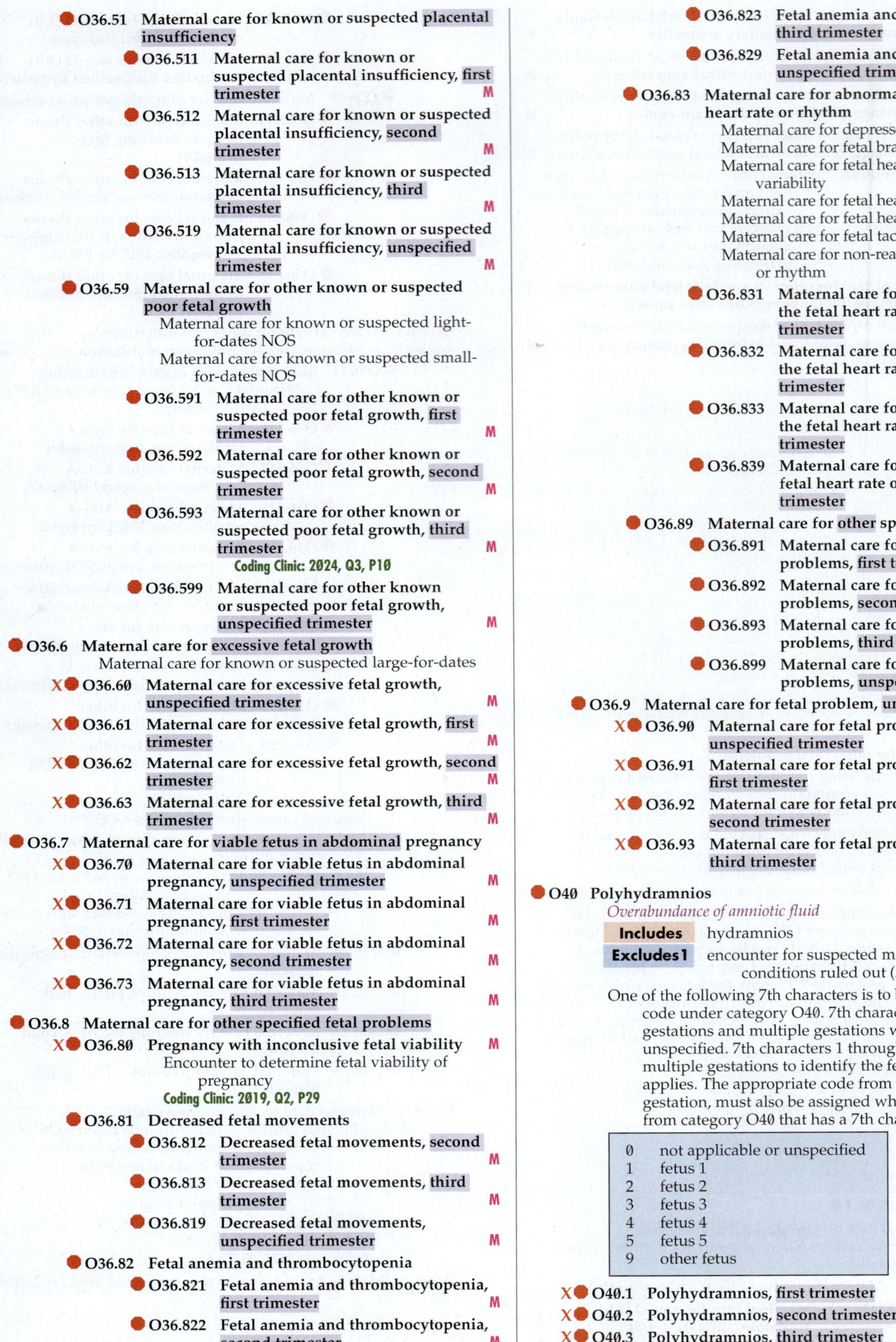

● **O36.51** Maternal care for known or suspected placental insufficiency
  ● **O36.511** Maternal care for known or suspected placental insufficiency, first trimester   M
  ● **O36.512** Maternal care for known or suspected placental insufficiency, second trimester   M
  ● **O36.513** Maternal care for known or suspected placental insufficiency, third trimester   M
  ● **O36.519** Maternal care for known or suspected placental insufficiency, unspecified trimester   M
● **O36.59** Maternal care for other known or suspected poor fetal growth
  Maternal care for known or suspected light-for-dates NOS
  Maternal care for known or suspected small-for-dates NOS
  ● **O36.591** Maternal care for other known or suspected poor fetal growth, first trimester   M
  ● **O36.592** Maternal care for other known or suspected poor fetal growth, second trimester   M
  ● **O36.593** Maternal care for other known or suspected poor fetal growth, third trimester   M
    Coding Clinic: 2024, Q3, P10
  ● **O36.599** Maternal care for other known or suspected poor fetal growth, unspecified trimester   M
● **O36.6** Maternal care for excessive fetal growth
  Maternal care for known or suspected large-for-dates
  X ● **O36.60** Maternal care for excessive fetal growth, unspecified trimester   M
  X ● **O36.61** Maternal care for excessive fetal growth, first trimester   M
  X ● **O36.62** Maternal care for excessive fetal growth, second trimester   M
  X ● **O36.63** Maternal care for excessive fetal growth, third trimester   M
● **O36.7** Maternal care for viable fetus in abdominal pregnancy
  X ● **O36.70** Maternal care for viable fetus in abdominal pregnancy, unspecified trimester   M
  X ● **O36.71** Maternal care for viable fetus in abdominal pregnancy, first trimester   M
  X ● **O36.72** Maternal care for viable fetus in abdominal pregnancy, second trimester   M
  X ● **O36.73** Maternal care for viable fetus in abdominal pregnancy, third trimester   M
● **O36.8** Maternal care for other specified fetal problems
  X ● **O36.80** Pregnancy with inconclusive fetal viability   M
    Encounter to determine fetal viability of pregnancy
    Coding Clinic: 2019, Q2, P29
  ● **O36.81** Decreased fetal movements
    ● **O36.812** Decreased fetal movements, second trimester   M
    ● **O36.813** Decreased fetal movements, third trimester   M
    ● **O36.819** Decreased fetal movements, unspecified trimester   M
  ● **O36.82** Fetal anemia and thrombocytopenia
    ● **O36.821** Fetal anemia and thrombocytopenia, first trimester   M
    ● **O36.822** Fetal anemia and thrombocytopenia, second trimester   M
    ● **O36.823** Fetal anemia and thrombocytopenia, third trimester   M
    ● **O36.829** Fetal anemia and thrombocytopenia, unspecified trimester   M
  ● **O36.83** Maternal care for abnormalities of the fetal heart rate or rhythm
    Maternal care for depressed fetal heart rate tones
    Maternal care for fetal bradycardia
    Maternal care for fetal heart rate abnormal variability
    Maternal care for fetal heart rate decelerations
    Maternal care for fetal heart rate irregularity
    Maternal care for fetal tachycardia
    Maternal care for non-reassuring fetal heart rate or rhythm
    ● **O36.831** Maternal care for abnormalities of the fetal heart rate or rhythm, first trimester   M
    ● **O36.832** Maternal care for abnormalities of the fetal heart rate or rhythm, second trimester   M
    ● **O36.833** Maternal care for abnormalities of the fetal heart rate or rhythm, third trimester   M
    ● **O36.839** Maternal care for abnormalities of the fetal heart rate or rhythm, unspecified trimester   M
  ● **O36.89** Maternal care for other specified fetal problems
    ● **O36.891** Maternal care for other specified fetal problems, first trimester   M
    ● **O36.892** Maternal care for other specified fetal problems, second trimester   M
    ● **O36.893** Maternal care for other specified fetal problems, third trimester   M
    ● **O36.899** Maternal care for other specified fetal problems, unspecified trimester   M
● **O36.9** Maternal care for fetal problem, unspecified
  X ● **O36.90** Maternal care for fetal problem, unspecified, unspecified trimester   M
  X ● **O36.91** Maternal care for fetal problem, unspecified, first trimester   M
  X ● **O36.92** Maternal care for fetal problem, unspecified, second trimester   M
  X ● **O36.93** Maternal care for fetal problem, unspecified, third trimester   M

● **O40** Polyhydramnios
Overabundance of amniotic fluid

Includes	hydramnios
Excludes1	encounter for suspected maternal and fetal conditions ruled out (Z03.7-)

One of the following 7th characters is to be assigned to each code under category O40. 7th character 0 is for single gestations and multiple gestations where the fetus is unspecified. 7th characters 1 through 9 are for cases of multiple gestations to identify the fetus for which the code applies. The appropriate code from category O30, Multiple gestation, must also be assigned when assigning a code from category O40 that has a 7th character of 1 through 9.

0	not applicable or unspecified
1	fetus 1
2	fetus 2
3	fetus 3
4	fetus 4
5	fetus 5
9	other fetus

X ● **O40.1** Polyhydramnios, first trimester   M
X ● **O40.2** Polyhydramnios, second trimester   M
X ● **O40.3** Polyhydramnios, third trimester   M
X ● **O40.9** Polyhydramnios, unspecified trimester   M

▶ New   ⇨ Revised   ~~deleted~~ Deleted   Excludes 1   Excludes 2   Includes   Use additional   Code first   Code also   Key words
OGCR Official Guidelines   X Assign placeholder X   ● Use Additional Character(s)   ▸ Manifestation Code   Ⓗⓒ Hierarchical Condition Category   Coding Clinic

● O41   Other disorders of amniotic fluid and membranes

    Excludes1   encounter for suspected maternal and fetal conditions ruled out (Z03.7-)

    One of the following 7th characters is to be assigned to each code under category O41. 7th character 0 is for single gestations and multiple gestations where the fetus is unspecified. 7th characters 1 through 9 are for cases of multiple gestations to identify the fetus for which the code applies. The appropriate code from category O30, Multiple gestation, must also be assigned when assigning a code from category O41 that has a 7th character of 1 through 9.

0	not applicable or unspecified
1	fetus 1
2	fetus 2
3	fetus 3
4	fetus 4
5	fetus 5
9	other fetus

● O41.0   Oligohydramnios

    Scant volume of amniotic fluid

    Oligohydramnios without rupture of membranes

    X ● O41.00   Oligohydramnios, unspecified trimester   M

    X ● O41.01   Oligohydramnios, first trimester   M

    X ● O41.02   Oligohydramnios, second trimester   M

    X ● O41.03   Oligohydramnios, third trimester   M

● O41.1   Infection of amniotic sac and membranes

    ● O41.10   Infection of amniotic sac and membranes, unspecified

      ● O41.101   Infection of amniotic sac and membranes, unspecified, first trimester   M

      ● O41.102   Infection of amniotic sac and membranes, unspecified, second trimester   M

      ● O41.103   Infection of amniotic sac and membranes, unspecified, third trimester   M

      ● O41.109   Infection of amniotic sac and membranes, unspecified, unspecified trimester   M

    ● O41.12   Chorioamnionitis

      Coding Clinic: 2019, Q2, P34-35

      ● O41.121   Chorioamnionitis, first trimester   M

      ● O41.122   Chorioamnionitis, second trimester   M

      ● O41.123   Chorioamnionitis, third trimester   M

      ● O41.129   Chorioamnionitis, unspecified trimester   M

    ● O41.14   Placentitis

      ● O41.141   Placentitis, first trimester   M

      ● O41.142   Placentitis, second trimester   M

      ● O41.143   Placentitis, third trimester   M

      ● O41.149   Placentitis, unspecified trimester   M

● O41.8   Other specified disorders of amniotic fluid and membranes

    ● O41.8X   Other specified disorders of amniotic fluid and membranes

      ● O41.8X1   Other specified disorders of amniotic fluid and membranes, first trimester   M

      ● O41.8X2   Other specified disorders of amniotic fluid and membranes, second trimester   M

      ● O41.8X3   Other specified disorders of amniotic fluid and membranes, third trimester   M

      Coding Clinic: 2024, Q1, P14

      ● O41.8X9   Other specified disorders of amniotic fluid and membranes, unspecified trimester   M

● O41.9   Disorder of amniotic fluid and membranes, unspecified

    X ● O41.90   Disorder of amniotic fluid and membranes, unspecified, unspecified trimester   M

    X ● O41.91   Disorder of amniotic fluid and membranes, unspecified, first trimester   M

    X ● O41.92   Disorder of amniotic fluid and membranes, unspecified, second trimester   M

    X ● O41.93   Disorder of amniotic fluid and membranes, unspecified, third trimester   M

● O42   Premature rupture of membranes

    Coding Clinic: 2023, Q3, P17

    ● O42.0   Premature rupture of membranes, onset of labor within 24 hours of rupture

      O42.00   Premature rupture of membranes, onset of labor within 24 hours of rupture, unspecified weeks of gestation   M

      ● O42.01   Preterm premature rupture of membranes, onset of labor within 24 hours of rupture

        Premature rupture of membranes before 37 completed weeks of gestation

        O42.011   Preterm premature rupture of membranes, onset of labor within 24 hours of rupture, first trimester   M

        O42.012   Preterm premature rupture of membranes, onset of labor within 24 hours of rupture, second trimester   M

        O42.013   Preterm premature rupture of membranes, onset of labor within 24 hours of rupture, third trimester   M

        O42.019   Preterm premature rupture of membranes, onset of labor within 24 hours of rupture, unspecified trimester   M

      O42.02   Full-term premature rupture of membranes, onset of labor within 24 hours of rupture   M

        Premature rupture of membranes at or after 37 completed weeks of gestation, onset of labor within 24 hours of rupture

    ● O42.1   Premature rupture of membranes, onset of labor more than 24 hours following rupture

      O42.10   Premature rupture of membranes, onset of labor more than 24 hours following rupture, unspecified weeks of gestation   M

      ● O42.11   Preterm premature rupture of membranes, onset of labor more than 24 hours following rupture

        Premature rupture of membranes before 37 completed weeks of gestation

        O42.111   Preterm premature rupture of membranes, onset of labor more than 24 hours following rupture, first trimester   M

        O42.112   Preterm premature rupture of membranes, onset of labor more than 24 hours following rupture, second trimester   M

        O42.113   Preterm premature rupture of membranes, onset of labor more than 24 hours following rupture, third trimester   M

        O42.119   Preterm premature rupture of membranes, onset of labor more than 24 hours following rupture, unspecified trimester   M

      O42.12   Full-term premature rupture of membranes, onset of labor more than 24 hours following rupture   M

        Premature rupture of membranes at or after 37 completed weeks of gestation, onset of labor more than 24 hours following rupture

CHAPTER 15 (O00-O9A)

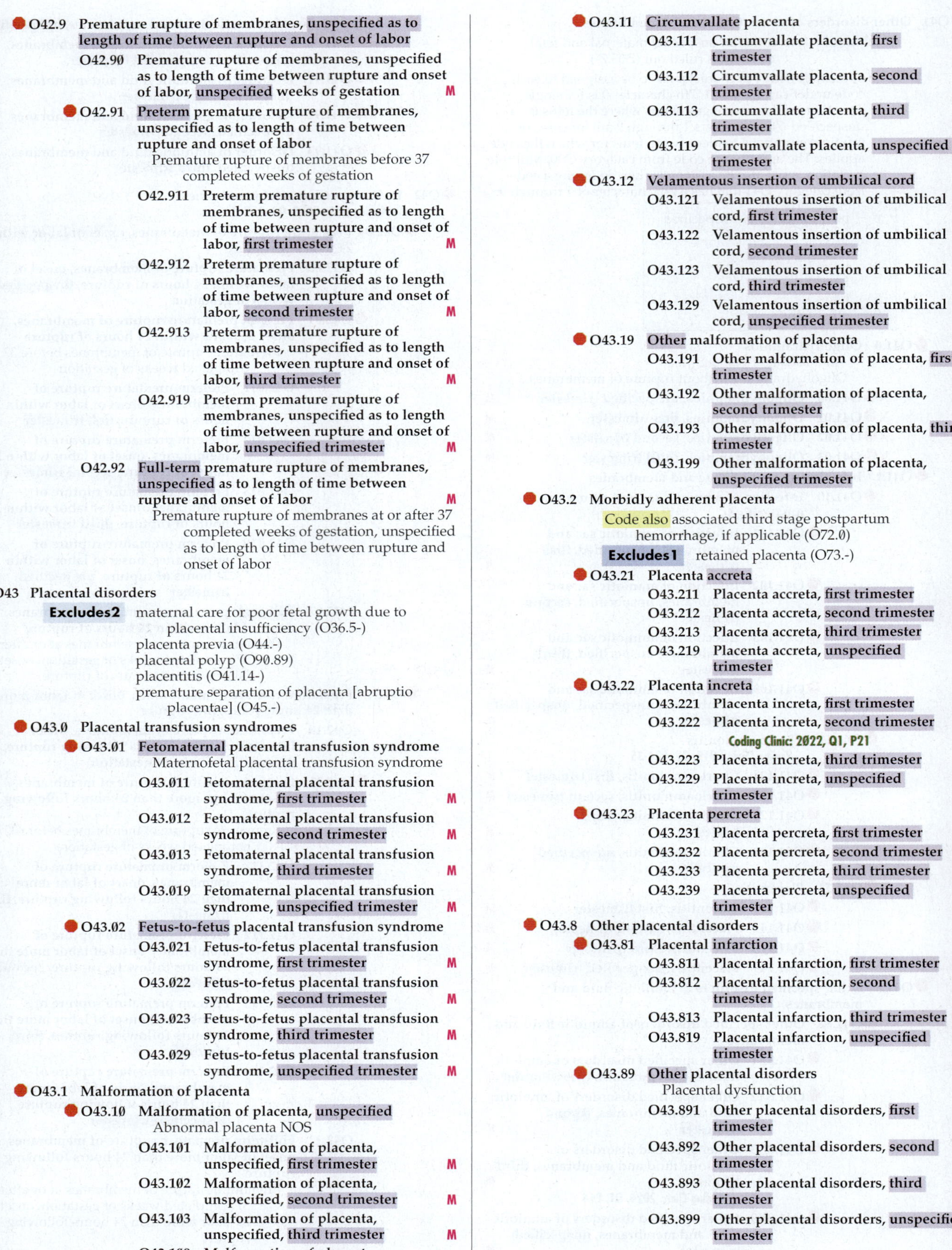

● **O42.9**   **Premature rupture of membranes, unspecified as to length of time between rupture and onset of labor**

     O42.90   Premature rupture of membranes, unspecified as to length of time between rupture and onset of labor, unspecified weeks of gestation   M

     ● O42.91   Preterm premature rupture of membranes, unspecified as to length of time between rupture and onset of labor
        Premature rupture of membranes before 37 completed weeks of gestation

        O42.911   Preterm premature rupture of membranes, unspecified as to length of time between rupture and onset of labor, first trimester   M

        O42.912   Preterm premature rupture of membranes, unspecified as to length of time between rupture and onset of labor, second trimester   M

        O42.913   Preterm premature rupture of membranes, unspecified as to length of time between rupture and onset of labor, third trimester   M

        O42.919   Preterm premature rupture of membranes, unspecified as to length of time between rupture and onset of labor, unspecified trimester   M

     O42.92   Full-term premature rupture of membranes, unspecified as to length of time between rupture and onset of labor   M
        Premature rupture of membranes at or after 37 completed weeks of gestation, unspecified as to length of time between rupture and onset of labor

● **O43**   **Placental disorders**

     Excludes2   maternal care for poor fetal growth due to placental insufficiency (O36.5-)
          placenta previa (O44.-)
          placental polyp (O90.89)
          placentitis (O41.14-)
          premature separation of placenta [abruptio placentae] (O45.-)

     ● **O43.0**   **Placental transfusion syndromes**

        ● **O43.01**   **Fetomaternal placental transfusion syndrome**
          Maternofetal placental transfusion syndrome

          O43.011   Fetomaternal placental transfusion syndrome, first trimester   M

          O43.012   Fetomaternal placental transfusion syndrome, second trimester   M

          O43.013   Fetomaternal placental transfusion syndrome, third trimester   M

          O43.019   Fetomaternal placental transfusion syndrome, unspecified trimester   M

        ● **O43.02**   **Fetus-to-fetus placental transfusion syndrome**

          O43.021   Fetus-to-fetus placental transfusion syndrome, first trimester   M

          O43.022   Fetus-to-fetus placental transfusion syndrome, second trimester   M

          O43.023   Fetus-to-fetus placental transfusion syndrome, third trimester   M

          O43.029   Fetus-to-fetus placental transfusion syndrome, unspecified trimester   M

     ● **O43.1**   **Malformation of placenta**

        ● **O43.10**   **Malformation of placenta, unspecified**
          Abnormal placenta NOS

          O43.101   Malformation of placenta, unspecified, first trimester   M

          O43.102   Malformation of placenta, unspecified, second trimester   M

          O43.103   Malformation of placenta, unspecified, third trimester   M

          O43.109   Malformation of placenta, unspecified, unspecified trimester   M

     ● **O43.11**   **Circumvallate placenta**

          O43.111   Circumvallate placenta, first trimester   M

          O43.112   Circumvallate placenta, second trimester   M

          O43.113   Circumvallate placenta, third trimester   M

          O43.119   Circumvallate placenta, unspecified trimester   M

     ● **O43.12**   **Velamentous insertion of umbilical cord**

          O43.121   Velamentous insertion of umbilical cord, first trimester   M

          O43.122   Velamentous insertion of umbilical cord, second trimester   M

          O43.123   Velamentous insertion of umbilical cord, third trimester   M

          O43.129   Velamentous insertion of umbilical cord, unspecified trimester   M

     ● **O43.19**   **Other malformation of placenta**

          O43.191   Other malformation of placenta, first trimester   M

          O43.192   Other malformation of placenta, second trimester   M

          O43.193   Other malformation of placenta, third trimester   M

          O43.199   Other malformation of placenta, unspecified trimester   M

● **O43.2**   **Morbidly adherent placenta**

     Code also associated third stage postpartum hemorrhage, if applicable (O72.0)

     Excludes1   retained placenta (O73.-)

     ● **O43.21**   **Placenta accreta**

          O43.211   Placenta accreta, first trimester   M

          O43.212   Placenta accreta, second trimester   M

          O43.213   Placenta accreta, third trimester   M

          O43.219   Placenta accreta, unspecified trimester   M

     ● **O43.22**   **Placenta increta**

          O43.221   Placenta increta, first trimester   M

          O43.222   Placenta increta, second trimester   M
            Coding Clinic: 2022, Q1, P21

          O43.223   Placenta increta, third trimester   M

          O43.229   Placenta increta, unspecified trimester   M

     ● **O43.23**   **Placenta percreta**

          O43.231   Placenta percreta, first trimester   M

          O43.232   Placenta percreta, second trimester   M

          O43.233   Placenta percreta, third trimester   M

          O43.239   Placenta percreta, unspecified trimester   M

● **O43.8**   **Other placental disorders**

     ● **O43.81**   **Placental infarction**

          O43.811   Placental infarction, first trimester   M

          O43.812   Placental infarction, second trimester   M

          O43.813   Placental infarction, third trimester   M

          O43.819   Placental infarction, unspecified trimester   M

     ● **O43.89**   **Other placental disorders**
          Placental dysfunction

          O43.891   Other placental disorders, first trimester   M

          O43.892   Other placental disorders, second trimester   M

          O43.893   Other placental disorders, third trimester   M

          O43.899   Other placental disorders, unspecified trimester   M

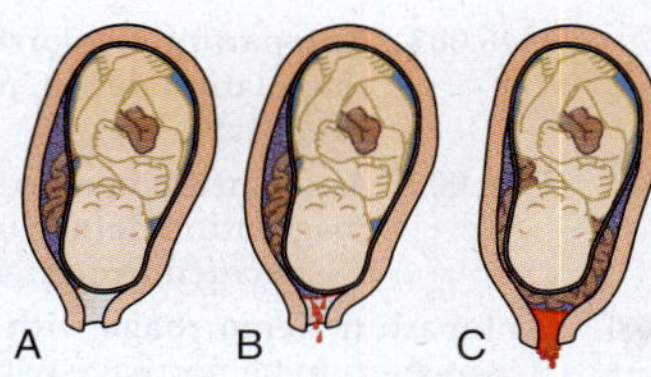

Figure 15-2   A. Marginal placento previa. **B.** Partial placenta previa. **C.** Total placento previa.

Item 15–3   Placenta previa is a condition in which the opening of the cervix is obstructed by the displaced placenta. The three types, marginal, partial, and total, are varying degrees of placenta displacement. Placenta abruption is the premature breaking away of the placenta from the site of the uterine implant before the delivery of the fetus.

● **O43.9   Unspecified** placental disorder
 O43.90   Unspecified placental disorder, **unspecified trimester**   M
 O43.91   Unspecified placental disorder, **first trimester**   M
 O43.92   Unspecified placental disorder, **second trimester**   M
 O43.93   Unspecified placental disorder, **third trimester** M

● **O44   Placenta previa**
  Coding Clinic: 2016, Q4, P52
 ● **O44.0   Complete placenta previa NOS or without hemorrhage**
   Placenta previa NOS
  O44.00   Complete placenta previa NOS or without hemorrhage, **unspecified trimester**   M
  O44.01   Complete placenta previa NOS or without hemorrhage, **first trimester**   M
  O44.02   Complete placenta previa NOS or without hemorrhage, **second trimester**   M
  O44.03   Complete placenta previa NOS or without hemorrhage, **third trimester**   M
 ● **O44.1   Complete placenta previa with hemorrhage**
   Excludes1   labor and delivery complicated by hemorrhage from vasa previa (O69.4)
  O44.10   Complete placenta previa with hemorrhage, **unspecified trimester**   M
  O44.11   Complete placenta previa with hemorrhage, **first trimester**   M
  O44.12   Complete placenta previa with hemorrhage, **second trimester**   M
  O44.13   Complete placenta previa with hemorrhage, **third trimester**   M
 ● **O44.2   Partial placenta previa without hemorrhage**
   Marginal placenta previa, NOS or without hemorrhage
  O44.20   Partial placenta previa NOS or without hemorrhage, **unspecified trimester**   M
  O44.21   Partial placenta previa NOS or without hemorrhage, **first trimester**   M
  O44.22   Partial placenta previa NOS or without hemorrhage, **second trimester**   M
  O44.23   Partial placenta previa NOS or without hemorrhage, **third trimester**   M
 ● **O44.3   Partial placenta previa with hemorrhage**
   Marginal placenta previa with hemorrhage
  O44.30   Partial placenta previa with hemorrhage, **unspecified trimester**   M
  O44.31   Partial placenta previa with hemorrhage, **first trimester**   M
  O44.32   Partial placenta previa with hemorrhage, **second trimester**   M
  O44.33   Partial placenta previa with hemorrhage, **third trimester**   M

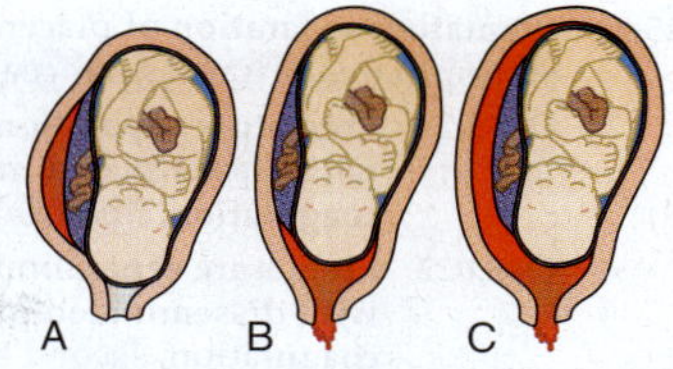

Figure 15-3   Abruptio placentae is classified according to the grade of separation of the placenta from the uterine wall. **A.** Mild separation in which hemorrhage is internal. **B.** Moderate separation in which there is external hemorrhage. **C.** Severe separation in which there is external hemorrhage and extreme separation.

 ● **O44.4   Low lying placenta NOS or without hemorrhage**
   Low implantation of placenta NOS or without hemorrhage
  O44.40   Low lying placenta NOS or without hemorrhage, **unspecified trimester**   M
  O44.41   Low lying placenta NOS or without hemorrhage, **first trimester**   M
  O44.42   Low lying placenta NOS or without hemorrhage, **second trimester**   M
  O44.43   Low lying placenta NOS or without hemorrhage, **third trimester**   M
 ● **O44.5   Low lying placenta with hemorrhage**
   Low implantation of placenta with hemorrhage
  O44.50   Low lying placenta with hemorrhage, **unspecified trimester**   M
  O44.51   Low lying placenta with hemorrhage, **first trimester**   M
  O44.52   Low lying placenta with hemorrhage, **second trimester**   M
  O44.53   Low lying placenta with hemorrhage, **third trimester**   M
● **O45   Premature separation of placenta [abruptio placentae]**
 ● **O45.0   Premature separation of placenta with coagulation defect**
  ● **O45.00   Premature separation of placenta with coagulation defect, unspecified**
   O45.001   Premature separation of placenta with coagulation defect, unspecified, **first trimester**   M
   O45.002   Premature separation of placenta with coagulation defect, unspecified, **second trimester**   M
   O45.003   Premature separation of placenta with coagulation defect, unspecified, **third trimester**   M
   O45.009   Premature separation of placenta with coagulation defect, unspecified, **unspecified trimester**   M
  ● **O45.01   Premature separation of placenta with afibrinogenemia**
    Premature separation of placenta with hypofibrinogenemia
   O45.011   Premature separation of placenta with afibrinogenemia, **first trimester**   M
   O45.012   Premature separation of placenta with afibrinogenemia, **second trimester**   M
   O45.013   Premature separation of placenta with afibrinogenemia, **third trimester**   M
   O45.019   Premature separation of placenta with afibrinogenemia, **unspecified trimester**   M

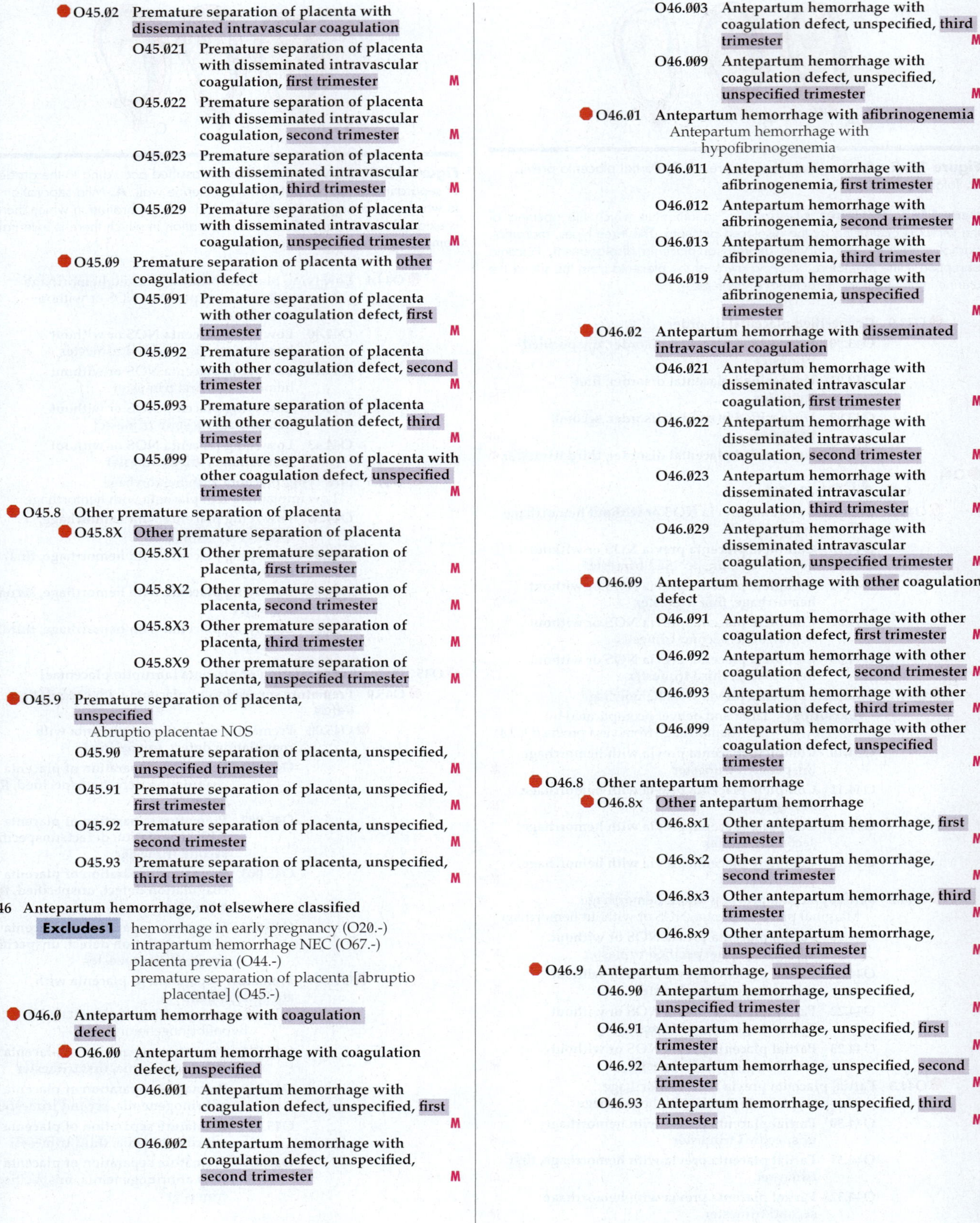

● O45.02   Premature separation of placenta with disseminated intravascular coagulation

    O45.021   Premature separation of placenta with disseminated intravascular coagulation, first trimester   **M**

    O45.022   Premature separation of placenta with disseminated intravascular coagulation, second trimester   **M**

    O45.023   Premature separation of placenta with disseminated intravascular coagulation, third trimester   **M**

    O45.029   Premature separation of placenta with disseminated intravascular coagulation, unspecified trimester   **M**

● O45.09   Premature separation of placenta with other coagulation defect

    O45.091   Premature separation of placenta with other coagulation defect, first trimester   **M**

    O45.092   Premature separation of placenta with other coagulation defect, second trimester   **M**

    O45.093   Premature separation of placenta with other coagulation defect, third trimester   **M**

    O45.099   Premature separation of placenta with other coagulation defect, unspecified trimester   **M**

● O45.8   Other premature separation of placenta

   ● O45.8X   Other premature separation of placenta

    O45.8X1   Other premature separation of placenta, first trimester   **M**

    O45.8X2   Other premature separation of placenta, second trimester   **M**

    O45.8X3   Other premature separation of placenta, third trimester   **M**

    O45.8X9   Other premature separation of placenta, unspecified trimester   **M**

● O45.9   Premature separation of placenta, unspecified

    Abruptio placentae NOS

    O45.90   Premature separation of placenta, unspecified, unspecified trimester   **M**

    O45.91   Premature separation of placenta, unspecified, first trimester   **M**

    O45.92   Premature separation of placenta, unspecified, second trimester   **M**

    O45.93   Premature separation of placenta, unspecified, third trimester   **M**

● O46   Antepartum hemorrhage, not elsewhere classified

   Excludes 1   hemorrhage in early pregnancy (O20.-)
    intrapartum hemorrhage NEC (O67.-)
    placenta previa (O44.-)
    premature separation of placenta [abruptio placentae] (O45.-)

● O46.0   Antepartum hemorrhage with coagulation defect

   ● O46.00   Antepartum hemorrhage with coagulation defect, unspecified

    O46.001   Antepartum hemorrhage with coagulation defect, unspecified, first trimester   **M**

    O46.002   Antepartum hemorrhage with coagulation defect, unspecified, second trimester   **M**

    O46.003   Antepartum hemorrhage with coagulation defect, unspecified, third trimester   **M**

    O46.009   Antepartum hemorrhage with coagulation defect, unspecified, unspecified trimester   **M**

● O46.01   Antepartum hemorrhage with afibrinogenemia
    Antepartum hemorrhage with hypofibrinogenemia

    O46.011   Antepartum hemorrhage with afibrinogenemia, first trimester   **M**

    O46.012   Antepartum hemorrhage with afibrinogenemia, second trimester   **M**

    O46.013   Antepartum hemorrhage with afibrinogenemia, third trimester   **M**

    O46.019   Antepartum hemorrhage with afibrinogenemia, unspecified trimester   **M**

● O46.02   Antepartum hemorrhage with disseminated intravascular coagulation

    O46.021   Antepartum hemorrhage with disseminated intravascular coagulation, first trimester   **M**

    O46.022   Antepartum hemorrhage with disseminated intravascular coagulation, second trimester   **M**

    O46.023   Antepartum hemorrhage with disseminated intravascular coagulation, third trimester   **M**

    O46.029   Antepartum hemorrhage with disseminated intravascular coagulation, unspecified trimester   **M**

● O46.09   Antepartum hemorrhage with other coagulation defect

    O46.091   Antepartum hemorrhage with other coagulation defect, first trimester   **M**

    O46.092   Antepartum hemorrhage with other coagulation defect, second trimester   **M**

    O46.093   Antepartum hemorrhage with other coagulation defect, third trimester   **M**

    O46.099   Antepartum hemorrhage with other coagulation defect, unspecified trimester   **M**

● O46.8   Other antepartum hemorrhage

   ● O46.8x   Other antepartum hemorrhage

    O46.8x1   Other antepartum hemorrhage, first trimester   **M**

    O46.8x2   Other antepartum hemorrhage, second trimester   **M**

    O46.8x3   Other antepartum hemorrhage, third trimester   **M**

    O46.8x9   Other antepartum hemorrhage, unspecified trimester   **M**

● O46.9   Antepartum hemorrhage, unspecified

    O46.90   Antepartum hemorrhage, unspecified, unspecified trimester   **M**

    O46.91   Antepartum hemorrhage, unspecified, first trimester   **M**

    O46.92   Antepartum hemorrhage, unspecified, second trimester   **M**

    O46.93   Antepartum hemorrhage, unspecified, third trimester   **M**

CHAPTER 15 (O00-O9A)

● **O47 False labor**

    Includes   Braxton Hicks contractions
                  threatened labor

    Excludes1   preterm labor (O60.-)

  ● **O47.0 False labor before 37 completed weeks of gestation**

      O47.00 False labor before 37 completed weeks of gestation, unspecified trimester   M

      O47.02 False labor before 37 completed weeks of gestation, second trimester   M

      O47.03 False labor before 37 completed weeks of gestation, third trimester   M

  O47.1 False labor at or after 37 completed weeks of gestation   M
      Coding Clinic: 2021, Q1, P10

  O47.9 False labor, unspecified   M

● **O48 Late pregnancy**

  O48.0 Post-term pregnancy   M
      Pregnancy over 40 completed weeks to 42 completed weeks gestation
      Coding Clinic: 2022, Q2 P3-4

  O48.1 Prolonged pregnancy   M
      Pregnancy which has advanced beyond 42 completed weeks gestation
      Coding Clinic: 2022, Q2 P3-4

COMPLICATIONS OF LABOR AND DELIVERY (O60-O77)

● **O60 Preterm labor**

    Includes   onset (spontaneous) of labor before 37 completed weeks of gestation

    Excludes1   false labor (O47.0-)
                  threatened labor NOS (O47.0-)

  ● **O60.0 Preterm labor without delivery**

      O60.00 Preterm labor without delivery, unspecified trimester   M

      O60.02 Preterm labor without delivery, second trimester   M

      O60.03 Preterm labor without delivery, third trimester   M

  ● **O60.1 Preterm labor with preterm delivery**

      One of the following 7th characters is to be assigned to each code under subcategory O60.1. 7th character 0 is for single gestations and multiple gestations where the fetus is unspecified. 7th characters 1 through 9 are for cases of multiple gestations to identify the fetus for which the code applies. The appropriate code from category O30, Multiple gestation, must also be assigned when assigning a code from subcategory O60.1 that has a 7th character of 1 through 9.

0	not applicable or unspecified
1	fetus 1
2	fetus 2
3	fetus 3
4	fetus 4
5	fetus 5
9	other fetus

      Coding Clinic: 2016, Q2, P11

    X● **O60.10 Preterm labor with preterm delivery, unspecified trimester**   M
        Preterm labor with delivery NOS

    X● **O60.12 Preterm labor second trimester with preterm delivery second trimester**   M

    X● **O60.13 Preterm labor second trimester with preterm delivery third trimester**   M

    X● **O60.14 Preterm labor third trimester with preterm delivery third trimester**   M
      Coding Clinic: 2016, Q2, P10

  ● **O60.2 Term delivery with preterm labor**

      One of the following 7th characters is to be assigned to each code under subcategory O60.2. 7th character 0 is for single gestations and multiple gestations where the fetus is unspecified. 7th characters 1 through 9 are for cases of multiple gestations to identify the fetus for which the code applies. The appropriate code from category O30, Multiple gestation, must also be assigned when assigning a code from subcategory O60.2 that has a 7th character of 1 through 9.

0	not applicable or unspecified
1	fetus 1
2	fetus 2
3	fetus 3
4	fetus 4
5	fetus 5
9	other fetus

    X● **O60.20 Term delivery with preterm labor, unspecified trimester**   M

    X● **O60.22 Term delivery with preterm labor, second trimester**   M

    X● **O60.23 Term delivery with preterm labor, third trimester**   M

● **O61 Failed induction of labor**

  O61.0 Failed medical induction of labor   M
      Failed induction (of labor) by oxytocin
      Failed induction (of labor) by prostaglandins

  O61.1 Failed instrumental induction of labor   M
      Failed mechanical induction (of labor)
      Failed surgical induction (of labor)

  O61.8 Other failed induction of labor   M

  O61.9 Failed induction of labor, unspecified   M

● **O62 Abnormalities of forces of labor**

  O62.0 Primary inadequate contractions   M
      Failure of cervical dilatation
      Primary hypotonic uterine dysfunction
      Uterine inertia during latent phase of labor
      Coding Clinic: 2024, Q1, P13

  O62.1 Secondary uterine inertia   M
      Arrested active phase of labor
      Secondary hypotonic uterine dysfunction

  O62.2 Other uterine inertia   M
      Atony of uterus without hemorrhage
      Atony of uterus NOS
      Desultory labor
      Hypotonic uterine dysfunction NOS
      Irregular labor
      Poor contractions
      Slow slope active phase of labor
      Uterine inertia NOS

    Excludes1   atony of uterus with hemorrhage (postpartum) (O72.1)
                  postpartum atony of uterus without hemorrhage (O75.89)

  O62.3 Precipitate labor   M

  O62.4 Hypertonic, incoordinate, and prolonged uterine contractions   M
      Cervical spasm
      Contraction ring dystocia
      Dyscoordinate labor
      Hour-glass contraction of uterus
      Hypertonic uterine dysfunction
      Incoordinate uterine action
      Tetanic contractions
      Uterine dystocia NOS
      Uterine spasm

    Excludes1   dystocia (fetal) (maternal) NOS (O66.9)

  O62.8 Other abnormalities of forces of labor   M

  O62.9 Abnormality of forces of labor, unspecified   M

CHAPTER 15 (O00-O9A)

CHAPTER 15 (O00-O9A)

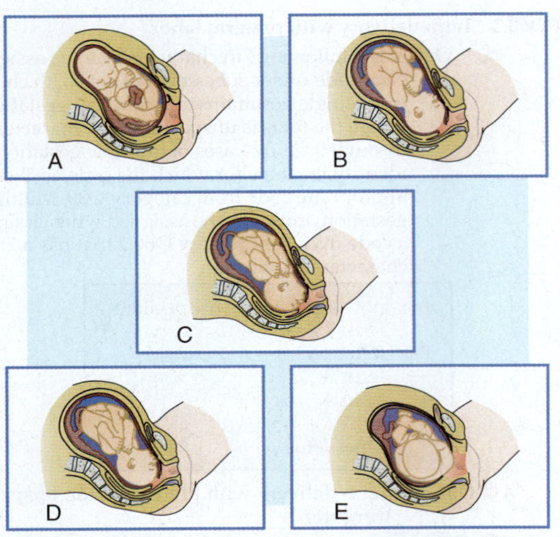

Figure 15-4 Five types of malposition and malpresentation of the fetus:
A. Breech. **B.** Vertex. **C.** Face. **D.** Brow. **E.** Shoulder.

● **O63**   **Long labor**

    O63.0   Prolonged first stage (of labor)   M

    O63.1   Prolonged second stage (of labor)   M

    O63.2   Delayed delivery of second twin, triplet, etc.   M

    O63.9   Long labor, unspecified   M
          Prolonged labor NOS

● **O64**   **Obstructed labor due to malposition and malpresentation of fetus**

    One of the following 7th characters is to be assigned to each code under category O64. 7th character 0 is for single gestations and multiple gestations where the fetus is unspecified. 7th characters 1 through 9 are for cases of multiple gestations to identify the fetus for which the code applies. The appropriate code from category O30, Multiple gestation, must also be assigned when assigning a code from category O64 that has a 7th character of 1 through 9.

0	not applicable or unspecified
1	fetus 1
2	fetus 2
3	fetus 3
4	fetus 4
5	fetus 5
9	other fetus

X ●   **O64.0**   Obstructed labor due to incomplete rotation of fetal head   M
        Deep transverse arrest
        Obstructed labor due to persistent occipitoiliac (position)
        Obstructed labor due to persistent occipitoposterior (position)
        Obstructed labor due to persistent occipitosacral (position)
        Obstructed labor due to persistent occipitotransverse (position)

X ●   **O64.1**   Obstructed labor due to breech presentation   M
        Obstructed labor due to buttocks presentation
        Obstructed labor due to complete breech presentation
        Obstructed labor due to frank breech presentation

X ●   **O64.2**   Obstructed labor due to face presentation   M
        Obstructed labor due to chin presentation

X ●   **O64.3**   Obstructed labor due to brow presentation   M

X ●   **O64.4**   Obstructed labor due to shoulder presentation   M
        Prolapsed arm
        Excludes1   impacted shoulders (O66.0)
                shoulder dystocia (O66.0)

X ●   **O64.5**   Obstructed labor due to compound presentation   M

X ●   **O64.8**   Obstructed labor due to other malposition and malpresentation   M
        Obstructed labor due to footling presentation
        Obstructed labor due to incomplete breech presentation

X ●   **O64.9**   Obstructed labor due to malposition and malpresentation, unspecified   M

● **O65**   **Obstructed labor due to maternal pelvic abnormality**

    O65.0   Obstructed labor due to deformed pelvis   M

    O65.1   Obstructed labor due to generally contracted pelvis   M

    O65.2   Obstructed labor due to pelvic inlet contraction   M

    O65.3   Obstructed labor due to pelvic outlet and mid-cavity contraction   M

    O65.4   Obstructed labor due to fetopelvic disproportion, unspecified   M
        Excludes1   dystocia due to abnormality of fetus (O66.2-O66.3)

    O65.5   Obstructed labor due to abnormality of maternal pelvic organs   M
        Obstructed labor due to conditions listed in O34.-
        Use additional code to identify abnormality of pelvic organs O34.-

    O65.8   Obstructed labor due to other maternal pelvic abnormalities   M

    O65.9   Obstructed labor due to maternal pelvic abnormality, unspecified   M

● **O66**   **Other obstructed labor**

    O66.0   Obstructed labor due to shoulder dystocia   M
        Impacted shoulders

    O66.1   Obstructed labor due to locked twins   M

    O66.2   Obstructed labor due to unusually large fetus   M

    O66.3   Obstructed labor due to other abnormalities of fetus   M
        Dystocia due to fetal ascites
        Dystocia due to fetal hydrops
        Dystocia due to fetal meningomyelocele
        Dystocia due to fetal sacral teratoma
        Dystocia due to fetal tumor
        Dystocia due to hydrocephalic fetus
        Use additional code to identify cause of obstruction

●   **O66.4**   **Failed trial of labor**

    O66.40   Failed trial of labor, unspecified   M

    O66.41   Failed attempted vaginal birth after previous cesarean delivery   M
        Code first rupture of uterus, if applicable (O71.0-, O71.1)

    O66.5   Attempted application of vacuum extractor and forceps   M
        Attempted application of vacuum or forceps, with subsequent delivery by forceps or cesarean delivery

    O66.6   Obstructed labor due to other multiple fetuses   M

    O66.8   Other specified obstructed labor   M
        Use additional code to identify cause of obstruction

    O66.9   Obstructed labor, unspecified   M
        Dystocia NOS
        Fetal dystocia NOS
        Maternal dystocia NOS

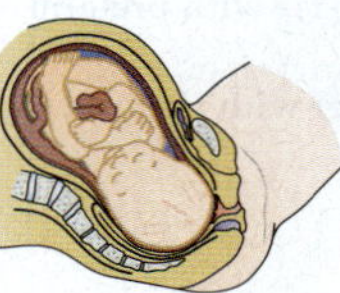

Figure 15-5 Hydrocephalic fetus causing disproportion.

▶ New   ⇥ Revised   ~~deleted~~ Deleted   Excludes 1   Excludes 2   Includes   Use additional   Code first   Code also   Key words

OGCR Official Guidelines   X Assign placeholder X   ● Use Additional Character(s)   ▶ Manifestation Code   🗣 Hierarchical Condition Category   Coding Clinic

● **O67** **Labor and delivery complicated by intrapartum hemorrhage, not elsewhere classified**

> **Excludes1**   antepartum hemorrhage NEC (O46.-)
> placenta previa (O44.-)
> premature separation of placenta [abruptio placentae] (O45.-)

> **Excludes2**   postpartum hemorrhage (O72.-)

O67.0 **Intrapartum hemorrhage with coagulation defect**   **M**
Intrapartum hemorrhage (excessive) associated with afibrinogenemia
Intrapartum hemorrhage (excessive) associated with disseminated intravascular coagulation
Intrapartum hemorrhage (excessive) associated with hyperfibrinolysis
Intrapartum hemorrhage (excessive) associated with hypofibrinogenemia

O67.8 **Other intrapartum hemorrhage**   **M**
Excessive intrapartum hemorrhage

O67.9 **Intrapartum hemorrhage, unspecified**   **M**

O68 **Labor and delivery complicated by abnormality of fetal acid-base balance**   **M**
Fetal acidemia complicating labor and delivery
Fetal acidosis complicating labor and delivery
Fetal alkalosis complicating labor and delivery
Fetal metabolic acidemia complicating labor and delivery

> **Excludes1**   fetal stress NOS (O77.9)
> labor and delivery complicated by electrocardiographic evidence of fetal stress (O77.8)
> labor and delivery complicated by ultrasonic evidence of fetal stress (O77.8)

> **Excludes2**   abnormality in fetal heart rate or rhythm (O76)
> labor and delivery complicated by meconium in amniotic fluid (O77.0)

● **O69** **Labor and delivery complicated by umbilical cord complications**
One of the following 7th characters is to be assigned to each code under category O69. 7th character 0 is for single gestations and multiple gestations where the fetus is unspecified. 7th characters 1 through 9 are for cases of multiple gestations to identify the fetus for which the code applies. The appropriate code from category O30, Multiple gestation, must also be assigned when assigning a code from category O69 that has a 7th character of 1 through 9.

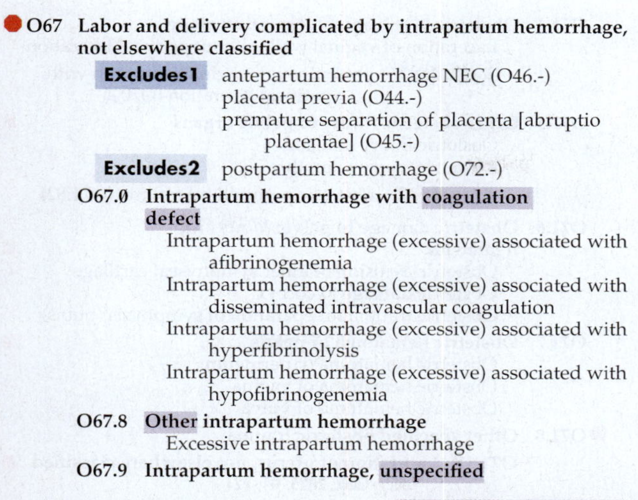

X ● **O69.0** **Labor and delivery complicated by prolapse of cord**   **M**

X ● **O69.1** **Labor and delivery complicated by cord around neck, with compression**   **M**

> **Excludes1**   labor and delivery complicated by cord around neck, without compression (O69.81)

X ● **O69.2** **Labor and delivery complicated by other cord entanglement, with compression**   **M**
Labor and delivery complicated by compression of cord NOS
Labor and delivery complicated by entanglement of cords of twins in monoamniotic sac
Labor and delivery complicated by knot in cord

> **Excludes1**   labor and delivery complicated by other cord entanglement, without compression (O69.82)

X ● **O69.3** **Labor and delivery complicated by short cord**   **M**

X ● **O69.4** **Labor and delivery complicated by vasa previa**   **M**
Labor and delivery complicated by hemorrhage from vasa previa

X ● **O69.5** **Labor and delivery complicated by vascular lesion of cord**   **M**
Labor and delivery complicated by cord bruising
Labor and delivery complicated by cord hematoma
Labor and delivery complicated by thrombosis of umbilical vessels

● **O69.8** **Labor and delivery complicated by other cord complications**

X ● **O69.81** **Labor and delivery complicated by cord around neck, without compression**   **M**

X ● **O69.82** **Labor and delivery complicated by other cord entanglement, without compression**   **M**

X ● **O69.89** **Labor and delivery complicated by other cord complications**   **M**
Coding Clinic: 2023, Q2, P29

X ● **O69.9** **Labor and delivery complicated by cord complication, unspecified**   **M**

● **O70** **Perineal laceration during delivery**

> **Includes**   episiotomy extended by laceration
> **Excludes1**   obstetric high vaginal laceration alone (O71.4)

O70.0 **First degree perineal laceration during delivery**   **M**
Perineal laceration, rupture or tear involving fourchette during delivery
Perineal laceration, rupture or tear involving labia during delivery
Perineal laceration, rupture or tear involving skin during delivery
Perineal laceration, rupture or tear involving vagina during delivery
Perineal laceration, rupture or tear involving vulva during delivery
Slight perineal laceration, rupture or tear during delivery

O70.1 **Second degree perineal laceration during delivery**   **M**
Perineal laceration, rupture or tear during delivery as in O70.0, also involving pelvic floor
Perineal laceration, rupture or tear during delivery as in O70.0, also involving perineal muscles
Perineal laceration, rupture or tear during delivery as in O70.0, also involving vaginal muscles

> **Excludes1**   perineal laceration involving anal sphincter (O70.2-)

Coding Clinic: 2016, Q4, P53; Q2, P34

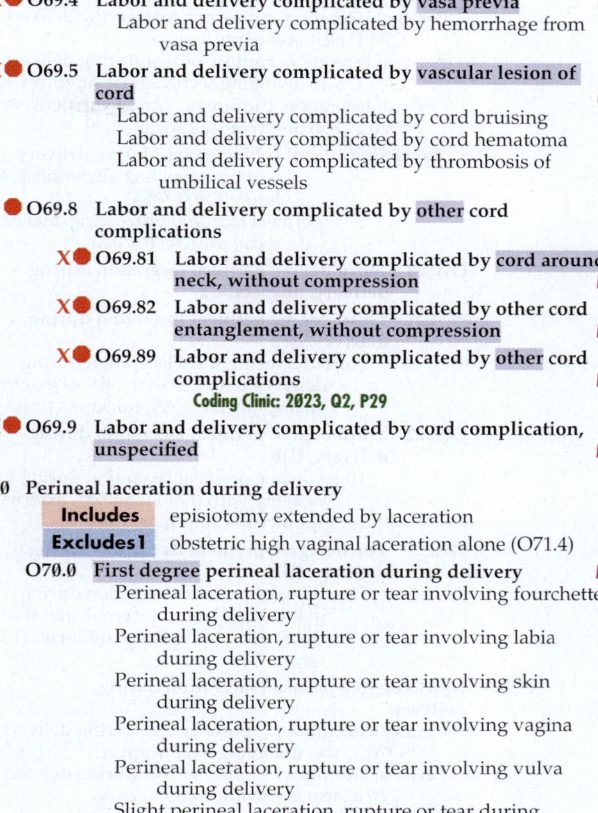

Figure 15-6   Perineal lacerations: **A.** First-degree is laceration of superficial tissues. **B.** Second-degree is limited to the pelvic floor and may involve the perineal or vaginal muscles. **C.** Third-degree involves the anal sphincter. **D.** Fourth-degree involves anal or rectal mucosa.

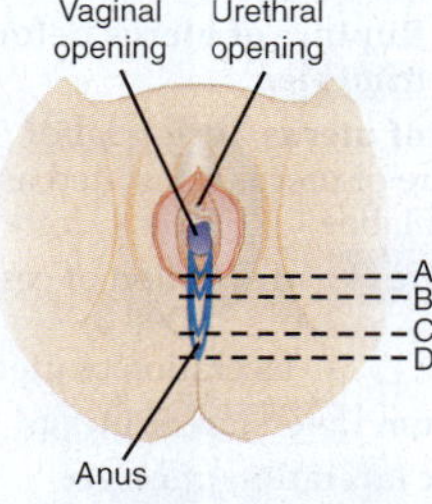

CHAPTER 15 (O00-O9A)

● **O70.2** **Third degree perineal laceration during delivery**
Perineal laceration, rupture or tear during delivery as in O70.1, also involving anal sphincter
Perineal laceration, rupture or tear during delivery as in O70.1, also involving rectovaginal septum
Perineal laceration, rupture or tear during delivery as in O70.1, also involving sphincter NOS

Excludes1   anal sphincter tear during delivery without third degree perineal laceration (O70.4)
perineal laceration involving anal or rectal mucosa (O70.3)

O70.20   **Third degree perineal laceration during delivery, unspecified**   M

O70.21   **Third degree perineal laceration during delivery, IIIa**   M
Third degree perineal laceration during delivery with less than 50% of external anal sphincter (EAS) thickness torn

O70.22   **Third degree perineal laceration during delivery, IIIb**   M
Third degree perineal laceration during delivery with more than 50% external anal sphincter (EAS) thickness torn

O70.23   **Third degree perineal laceration during delivery, IIIc**   M
Third degree perineal laceration during delivery with both external anal sphincter (EAS) and internal anal sphincter (IAS) torn

O70.3   **Fourth degree perineal laceration during delivery**   M
Perineal laceration, rupture or tear during delivery as in O70.2, also involving anal mucosa
Perineal laceration, rupture or tear during delivery as in O70.2, also involving rectal mucosa

O70.4   **Anal sphincter tear complicating delivery, not associated with third degree laceration**   M
➡ **Excludes1**   anal sphincter tear with third degree perineal laceration (O70.2-)

O70.9   **Perineal laceration during delivery, unspecified**   M

● **O71**   **Other obstetric trauma**
Includes   obstetric damage from instruments

● **O71.0**   **Rupture of uterus (spontaneous) before onset of labor**
Excludes1   disruption of (current) cesarean delivery wound (O90.0)
laceration of uterus, NEC (O71.81)

O71.00   **Rupture of uterus before onset of labor, unspecified trimester**   M

O71.02   **Rupture of uterus before onset of labor, second trimester**   M

O71.03   **Rupture of uterus before onset of labor, third trimester**   M

O71.1   **Rupture of uterus during labor**   M
Rupture of uterus not stated as occurring before onset of labor
Excludes1   disruption of cesarean delivery wound (O90.0)
laceration of uterus, NEC (O71.81)

O71.2   **Postpartum inversion of uterus**   M

O71.3   **Obstetric laceration of cervix**   M
Annular detachment of cervix

O71.4   **Obstetric high vaginal laceration alone**   M
Laceration of vaginal wall without perineal laceration
Excludes1   obstetric high vaginal laceration with perineal laceration (O70.-)

O71.5   **Other obstetric injury to pelvic organs**   M
Obstetric injury to bladder
Obstetric injury to urethra
Excludes2   obstetric periurethral trauma (O71.82)

O71.6   **Obstetric damage to pelvic joints and ligaments**   M
Obstetric avulsion of inner symphyseal cartilage
Obstetric damage to coccyx
Obstetric traumatic separation of symphysis (pubis)

O71.7   **Obstetric hematoma of pelvis**   M
Obstetric hematoma of perineum
Obstetric hematoma of vagina
Obstetric hematoma of vulva

● **O71.8**   **Other specified obstetric trauma**
O71.81   **Laceration of uterus, not elsewhere classified**   M
Coding Clinic: 2025, Q1, P21

O71.82   **Other specified trauma to perineum and vulva**   M
Obstetric periurethral trauma

O71.89   **Other specified obstetric trauma**   M

O71.9   **Obstetric trauma, unspecified**   M

● **O72**   **Postpartum hemorrhage**
Includes   hemorrhage after delivery of fetus or infant

O72.0   **Third-stage hemorrhage**   M
Hemorrhage associated with retained, trapped or adherent placenta
Retained placenta NOS
Code also type of adherent placenta (O43.2-)

O72.1   **Other immediate postpartum hemorrhage**   M
Hemorrhage following delivery of placenta
Postpartum hemorrhage (atonic) NOS
Uterine atony with hemorrhage
Excludes1   uterine atony NOS (O62.2)
uterine atony without hemorrhage (O62.2)
postpartum atony of uterus without hemorrhage (O75.89)
Coding Clinic: 2023, Q2, P15

O72.2   **Delayed and secondary postpartum hemorrhage**   M
Hemorrhage associated with retained portions of placenta or membranes after the first 24 hours following delivery of placenta
Retained products of conception NOS, following delivery

O72.3   **Postpartum coagulation defects**   M
Postpartum afibrinogenemia
Postpartum fibrinolysis

● **O73**   **Retained placenta and membranes, without hemorrhage**
Excludes1   placenta accreta (O43.21-)
placenta increta (O43.22-)
placenta percreta (O43.23-)

O73.0   **Retained placenta without hemorrhage**   M
Adherent placenta, without hemorrhage
Trapped placenta without hemorrhage

O73.1   **Retained portions of placenta and membranes, without hemorrhage**   M
Retained products of conception following delivery, without hemorrhage

▶ New   ➡ Revised   ~~deleted~~ Deleted   **Excludes 1**   **Excludes 2**   **Includes**   **Use additional**   **Code first**   **Code also**   **Key words**
OGCR Official Guidelines   X Assign placeholder X   ● Use Additional Character(s)   ▶ Manifestation Code   🐾 Hierarchical Condition Category   **Coding Clinic**

● **O74** **Complications of anesthesia during labor and delivery**

> **Includes**   maternal complications arising from the administration of a general, regional or local anesthetic, analgesic or other sedation during labor and delivery

> **Use additional** code, if applicable, to identify specific complication

O74.0 **Aspiration pneumonitis** due to anesthesia during labor and delivery   M
> Inhalation of stomach contents or secretions NOS due to anesthesia during labor and delivery
> Mendelson's syndrome due to anesthesia during labor and delivery

O74.1 **Other pulmonary** complications of anesthesia during labor and delivery   M

O74.2 **Cardiac** complications of anesthesia during labor and delivery   M

O74.3 **Central nervous system** complications of anesthesia during labor and delivery   M

O74.4 **Toxic reaction** to local anesthesia during labor and delivery   M

O74.5 **Spinal and epidural anesthesia-induced headache** during labor and delivery   M

O74.6 **Other complications of spinal and epidural anesthesia** during labor and delivery   M

O74.7 **Failed or difficult intubation** for anesthesia during labor and delivery   M

O74.8 **Other complications** of anesthesia during labor and delivery   M

O74.9 **Complication of anesthesia during labor and delivery, unspecified**   M

● **O75** **Other complications of labor and delivery, not elsewhere classified**

> **Excludes2**   puerperal (postpartum) infection (O86.-)
> puerperal (postpartum) sepsis (O85)

O75.0 **Maternal distress during labor and delivery**   M

O75.1 **Shock during or following labor and delivery**   M
> Obstetric shock following labor and delivery

O75.2 **Pyrexia during labor, not elsewhere classified**   M

O75.3 **Other infection during labor**   M
> Sepsis during labor
> **Use additional** code (B95-B97), to identify infectious agent
> **Coding Clinic: 2025, Q1, P22-23**

O75.4 **Other complications of obstetric surgery and procedures**   M
> Cardiac arrest following obstetric surgery or procedures
> Cardiac failure following obstetric surgery or procedures
> Cerebral anoxia following obstetric surgery or procedures
> Pulmonary edema following obstetric surgery or procedures
> **Use additional** code to identify specific complication
> **Excludes2**   complications of anesthesia during labor and delivery (O74.-)
> disruption of obstetrical (surgical) wound (O90.0-O90.1)
> hematoma of obstetrical (surgical) wound (O90.2)
> infection of obstetrical (surgical) wound (O86.0-)
> **Coding Clinic: 2025, Q1, P21**

O75.5 **Delayed delivery after artificial rupture of membranes**   M

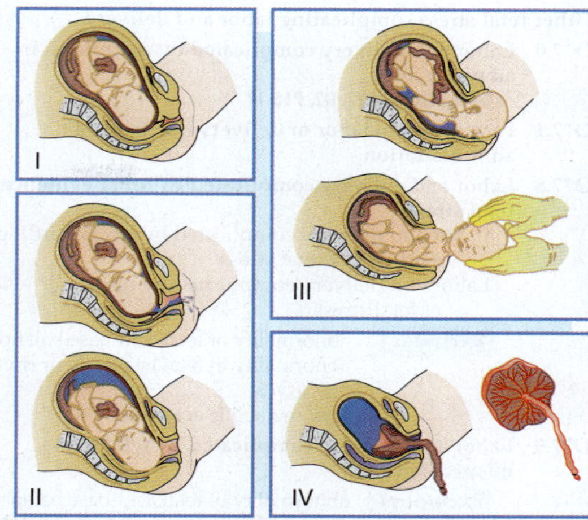

Figure 15-7 The four stages of normal delivery: **I.** Lightening, which occurs 2 to 4 weeks before birth, at which time the fetus turns with head toward the vagina. **II.** Regular contractions begin, the amniotic sac ruptures, and dilation is complete. **III.** Delivery of the head and rotation. **IV.** Expulsion of placenta.

● **O75.8** **Other specified complications of labor and delivery**

O75.81 **Maternal exhaustion complicating labor and delivery**   M

O75.82 **Onset (spontaneous) of labor after 37 completed weeks of gestation but before 39 completed weeks gestation, with delivery by (planned) cesarean section**   M
> Delivery by (planned) cesarean section occurring after 37 completed weeks of gestation but before 39 completed weeks gestation due to (spontaneous) onset of labor
> *Code first to specify reason for planned cesarean section such as:*
> cephalopelvic disproportion (normally formed fetus) (O33.9)
> previous cesarean delivery (O34.21-)
> **Coding Clinic: 2022, Q2, P3-4**

O75.89 **Other specified complications of labor and delivery**   M

O75.9 **Complication of labor and delivery, unspecified**   M

O76 **Abnormality in fetal heart rate and rhythm complicating labor and delivery**   M
> Depressed fetal heart rate tones complicating labor and delivery
> Fetal bradycardia complicating labor and delivery
> Fetal heart rate decelerations complicating labor and delivery
> Fetal heart rate irregularity complicating labor and delivery
> Fetal heart rate abnormal variability complicating labor and delivery
> Fetal tachycardia complicating labor and delivery
> Non-reassuring fetal heart rate or rhythm complicating labor and delivery
> **Excludes1**   fetal stress NOS (O77.9)
> labor and delivery complicated by electrocardiographic evidence of fetal stress (O77.8)
> labor and delivery complicated by ultrasonic evidence of fetal stress (O77.8)
> **Excludes2**   fetal metabolic acidemia (O68)
> other fetal stress (O77.0-O77.1)

CHAPTER 15 (O00-O9A)

● **O77 Other fetal stress complicating labor and delivery**

O77.0 Labor and delivery complicated by meconium in amniotic fluid M
Coding Clinic: 2022, Q2, P16-17

O77.1 Fetal stress in labor or delivery due to drug administration M

O77.8 Labor and delivery complicated by other evidence of fetal stress M
Labor and delivery complicated by electrocardiographic evidence of fetal stress
Labor and delivery complicated by ultrasonic evidence of fetal stress

> **Excludes1** abnormality of fetal acid-base balance (O68)
> abnormality in fetal heart rate or rhythm (O76)
> fetal metabolic acidemia (O68)

O77.9 Labor and delivery complicated by fetal stress, unspecified M

> **Excludes1** abnormality of fetal acid-base balance (O68)
> abnormality in fetal heart rate or rhythm (O76)
> fetal metabolic acidemia (O68)

OGCR Section I.C., Chapter 15.n.

Normal Delivery, Code O80

1) Encounter for full-term uncomplicated delivery

Code O80 should be assigned when a woman is admitted for a full-term normal delivery and delivers a single, healthy infant without any complications antepartum, during the delivery, or postpartum during the delivery episode. Code O80 is always a principal diagnosis. It is not to be used if any other code from Chapter 15 is needed to describe a current complication of the antenatal, delivery, or perinatal period. Additional codes from other chapters may be used with code O80 if they are not related to or are in any way complicating the pregnancy.

2) Uncomplicated delivery with resolved antepartum complication

Code O80 may be used if the patient had a complication at some point during the pregnancy, but the complication is not present at the time of the admission for delivery.

3) Outcome of delivery for O80

Z37.0, Single live brith, is the only outcome of delivery code appropriate for use with O80.

ENCOUNTER FOR DELIVERY (O80-O82)

O80 Encounter for full-term uncomplicated delivery M
Delivery requiring minimal or no assistance, with or without episiotomy, without fetal manipulation [e.g., rotation version] or instrumentation [forceps] of a spontaneous, cephalic, vaginal, full-term, single, live-born infant. This code is for use as a single diagnosis code and is not to be used with any other code from Chapter 15.

Use additional code to indicate outcome of delivery (Z37.0)
Coding Clinic: 2016, Q4, P124, 150

O82 Encounter for cesarean delivery without indication M
Use additional code to indicate outcome of delivery (Z37.0)

COMPLICATIONS PREDOMINANTLY RELATED TO THE PUERPERIUM (O85-O92)

> **Excludes2** mental and behavioral disorders associated with the puerperium (F53.-)
> obstetrical tetanus (A34)
> puerperal osteomalacia (M83.0)

O85 Puerperal sepsis M
Postpartum sepsis
Puerperal peritonitis
Puerperal pyemia

Use additional code (B95-B97), to identify infectious agent
Use additional code (R65.2-) to identify severe sepsis, if applicable

> **Excludes1** fever of unknown origin following delivery (O86.4)
> obstetric pyemic and septic embolism (O88.3-)
> puerperal septic thrombophlebitis (O86.81)

> **Excludes2** genital tract infection following delivery (O86.1-)
> sepsis during labor (O75.3)
> urinary tract infection following delivery (O86.2-)

Coding Clinic: 2022, Q2, P5; 2018, Q4, P23

● **O86 Other puerperal infections**
Use additional code (B95-B97), to identify infectious agent

> **Excludes2** infection during labor (O75.3)
> obstetrical tetanus (A34)

● **O86.0 Infection of obstetric surgical wound**
Infected cesarean delivery wound following delivery
Infected perineal repair following delivery

> **Excludes1** complications of procedures, not elsewhere classified (T81.44)
> postprocedural fever NOS (R50.82)
> postprocedural retroperitoneal abscess (K68.11)

O86.00 Infection of obstetric surgical wound, unspecified M

O86.01 Infection of obstetric surgical wound, superficial incisional site M
Subcutaneous abscess following an obstetrical procedure
Stitch abscess following an obstetrical procedure

O86.02 Infection of obstetric surgical wound, deep incisional site M
Intramuscular abscess following an obstetrical procedure
Sub-fascial abscess following an obstetrical procedure
Coding Clinic: 2018, Q4, P23

O86.03 Infection of obstetric surgical wound, organ and space site M
Intraabdominal abscess following an obstetrical procedure
Subphrenic abscess following an obstetrical procedure

O86.04 Sepsis following an obstetrical procedure M
Use additional code to identify the sepsis

O86.09 Infection of obstetric surgical wound, other surgical site M

● **O86.1 Other infection of genital tract following delivery**

O86.11 Cervicitis following delivery M

O86.12 Endometritis following delivery M

O86.13 Vaginitis following delivery M

O86.19 Other infection of genital tract following delivery M

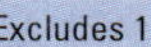 New   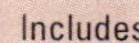 Revised   ~~deleted~~ Deleted   Excludes 1   Excludes 2   Includes   Use additional   Code first   Code also   Key words
OGCR Official Guidelines   X Assign placeholder X   ● Use Additional Character(s)   ▶ Manifestation Code   Hierarchical Condition Category   Coding Clinic

● **O86.2** **Urinary tract infection following delivery**

    O86.20 **Urinary tract infection following delivery, unspecified** — M
        Puerperal urinary tract infection NOS
        Coding Clinic: 2022, Q2, P5

    O86.21 **Infection of kidney following delivery** — M

    O86.22 **Infection of bladder following delivery** — M
        Infection of urethra following delivery

    O86.29 **Other urinary tract infection following delivery** — M

● **O86.4** **Pyrexia of unknown origin following delivery** — M
    Puerperal infection NOS following delivery
    Puerperal pyrexia NOS following delivery
    Excludes2   pyrexia during labor (O75.2)

● **O86.8** **Other specified puerperal infections**

    O86.81 **Puerperal septic thrombophlebitis** — M

    O86.89 **Other specified puerperal infections** — M

● **O87** **Venous complications and hemorrhoids in the puerperium**

    Includes   venous complications in labor, delivery and the puerperium

    Excludes2   obstetric embolism (O88.-)
        puerperal septic thrombophlebitis (O86.81)
        venous complications in pregnancy (O22.-)

O87.0 **Superficial thrombophlebitis in the puerperium** — M
    Puerperal phlebitis NOS
    Puerperal thrombosis NOS
    Use additional code, if applicable, to identify the superficial vein thrombosis, such as thrombosis of superficial vessels of lower extremities (I80.0-)

O87.1 **Deep phlebothrombosis in the puerperium** — M
    Deep vein thrombosis, postpartum
    Pelvic thrombophlebitis, postpartum
    Use additional code to identify the deep vein thrombosis (I82.4-, I82.5-, I82.62-, I82.72-)
    Use additional code, if applicable, for associated long-term (current) use of anticoagulants (Z79.01)

O87.2 **Hemorrhoids in the puerperium** — M

O87.3 **Cerebral venous thrombosis in the puerperium** — M
    Cerebrovenous sinus thrombosis in the puerperium

O87.4 **Varicose veins of lower extremity in the puerperium** — M

O87.8 **Other venous complications in the puerperium** — M
    Genital varices in the puerperium

O87.9 **Venous complication in the puerperium, unspecified** — M
    Puerperal phlebopathy NOS

O88 **Obstetric embolism**

    Excludes1   embolism complicating abortion NOS (O03.2)
        embolism complicating ectopic or molar pregnancy (O08.2)
        embolism complicating failed attempted abortion (O07.2)
        embolism complicating induced abortion (O04.7)
        embolism complicating spontaneous abortion (O03.2, O03.7)

● **O88.0** **Obstetric air embolism**

    ● **O88.01** **Obstetric air embolism in pregnancy**

        O88.011 **Air embolism in pregnancy, first trimester** — M

        O88.012 **Air embolism in pregnancy, second trimester** — M

        O88.013 **Air embolism in pregnancy, third trimester** — M

        O88.019 **Air embolism in pregnancy, unspecified trimester** — M

    O88.02 **Air embolism in childbirth** — M

    O88.03 **Air embolism in the puerperium** — M

● **O88.1** **Amniotic fluid embolism**
    Anaphylactoid syndrome in pregnancy

    ● **O88.11** **Amniotic fluid embolism in pregnancy**

        O88.111 **Amniotic fluid embolism in pregnancy, first trimester** — M

        O88.112 **Amniotic fluid embolism in pregnancy, second trimester** — M

        O88.113 **Amniotic fluid embolism in pregnancy, third trimester** — M

        O88.119 **Amniotic fluid embolism in pregnancy, unspecified trimester** — M

    O88.12 **Amniotic fluid embolism in childbirth** — M

    O88.13 **Amniotic fluid embolism in the puerperium** — M

● **O88.2** **Obstetric thromboembolism**

    ● **O88.21** **Thromboembolism in pregnancy**
        Obstetric (pulmonary) embolism NOS

        O88.211 **Thromboembolism in pregnancy, first trimester** — M

        O88.212 **Thromboembolism in pregnancy, second trimester** — M

        O88.213 **Thromboembolism in pregnancy, third trimester** — M

        O88.219 **Thromboembolism in pregnancy, unspecified trimester** — M

    O88.22 **Thromboembolism in childbirth** — M

    O88.23 **Thromboembolism in the puerperium** — M
        Puerperal (pulmonary) embolism NOS

● **O88.3** **Obstetric pyemic and septic embolism**

    ● **O88.31** **Pyemic and septic embolism in pregnancy**

        O88.311 **Pyemic and septic embolism in pregnancy, first trimester** — M

        O88.312 **Pyemic and septic embolism in pregnancy, second trimester** — M

        O88.313 **Pyemic and septic embolism in pregnancy, third trimester** — M

        O88.319 **Pyemic and septic embolism in pregnancy, unspecified trimester** — M

    O88.32 **Pyemic and septic embolism in childbirth** — M

    O88.33 **Pyemic and septic embolism in the puerperium** — M

● **O88.8** **Other obstetric embolism**
    Obstetric fat embolism

    ● **O88.81** **Other embolism in pregnancy**

        O88.811 **Other embolism in pregnancy, first trimester** — M

        O88.812 **Other embolism in pregnancy, second trimester** — M

        O88.813 **Other embolism in pregnancy, third trimester** — M

        O88.819 **Other embolism in pregnancy, unspecified trimester** — M

    O88.82 **Other embolism in childbirth** — M

    O88.83 **Other embolism in the puerperium** — M

● **O89** **Complications of anesthesia during the puerperium**

    Includes   maternal complications arising from the administration of a general, regional or local anesthetic, analgesic or other sedation during the puerperium

    Use additional code, if applicable, to identify specific complication

● **O89.0** **Pulmonary complications of anesthesia during the puerperium**

    O89.01 **Aspiration pneumonitis due to anesthesia during the puerperium** — M
        Inhalation of stomach contents or secretions NOS due to anesthesia during the puerperium
        Mendelson's syndrome due to anesthesia during the puerperium

    O89.09 **Other pulmonary complications of anesthesia during the puerperium** — M

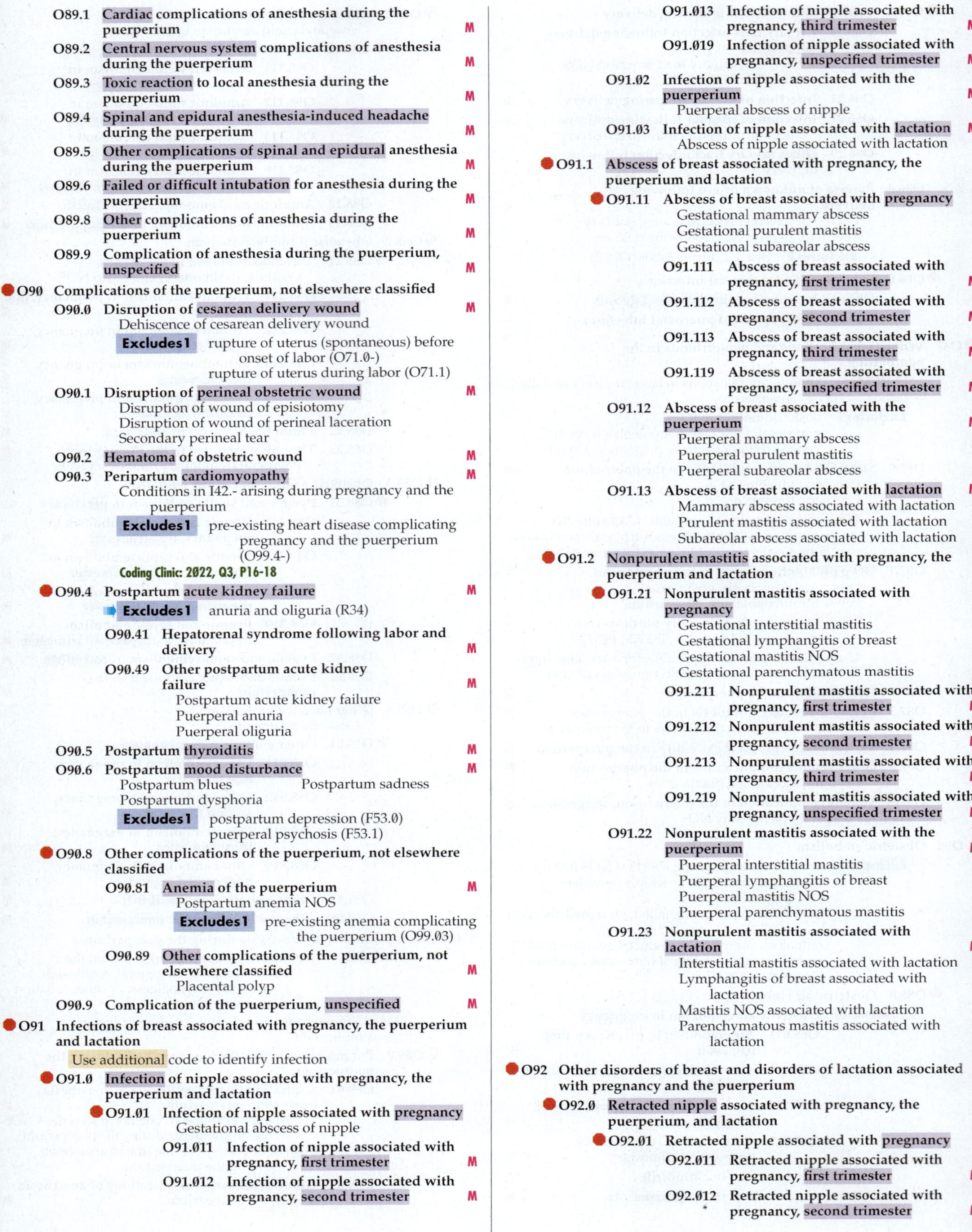

CHAPTER 15 (O00-O9A)

O89.1 **Cardiac complications of anesthesia during the puerperium** M

O89.2 **Central nervous system complications of anesthesia during the puerperium** M

O89.3 **Toxic reaction to local anesthesia during the puerperium** M

O89.4 **Spinal and epidural anesthesia-induced headache during the puerperium** M

O89.5 **Other complications of spinal and epidural anesthesia during the puerperium** M

O89.6 **Failed or difficult intubation for anesthesia during the puerperium** M

O89.8 **Other complications of anesthesia during the puerperium** M

O89.9 **Complication of anesthesia during the puerperium, unspecified** M

● O90 **Complications of the puerperium, not elsewhere classified**

O90.0 **Disruption of cesarean delivery wound** M
Dehiscence of cesarean delivery wound
Excludes1 rupture of uterus (spontaneous) before onset of labor (O71.0-)
rupture of uterus during labor (O71.1)

O90.1 **Disruption of perineal obstetric wound** M
Disruption of wound of episiotomy
Disruption of wound of perineal laceration
Secondary perineal tear

O90.2 **Hematoma of obstetric wound** M

O90.3 **Peripartum cardiomyopathy** M
Conditions in I42.- arising during pregnancy and the puerperium
Excludes1 pre-existing heart disease complicating pregnancy and the puerperium (O99.4-)
Coding Clinic: 2022, Q3, P16-18

● O90.4 **Postpartum acute kidney failure** M
➡ **Excludes1** anuria and oliguria (R34)

O90.41 **Hepatorenal syndrome following labor and delivery** M

O90.49 **Other postpartum acute kidney failure** M
Postpartum acute kidney failure
Puerperal anuria
Puerperal oliguria

O90.5 **Postpartum thyroiditis** M

O90.6 **Postpartum mood disturbance** M
Postpartum blues   Postpartum sadness
Postpartum dysphoria
Excludes1 postpartum depression (F53.0)
puerperal psychosis (F53.1)

● O90.8 **Other complications of the puerperium, not elsewhere classified**

O90.81 **Anemia of the puerperium** M
Postpartum anemia NOS
Excludes1 pre-existing anemia complicating the puerperium (O99.03)

O90.89 **Other complications of the puerperium, not elsewhere classified** M
Placental polyp

O90.9 **Complication of the puerperium, unspecified** M

● O91 **Infections of breast associated with pregnancy, the puerperium and lactation**
Use additional code to identify infection

● O91.0 **Infection of nipple associated with pregnancy, the puerperium and lactation**

● O91.01 **Infection of nipple associated with pregnancy**
Gestational abscess of nipple

O91.011 **Infection of nipple associated with pregnancy, first trimester** M

O91.012 **Infection of nipple associated with pregnancy, second trimester** M

O91.013 **Infection of nipple associated with pregnancy, third trimester** M

O91.019 **Infection of nipple associated with pregnancy, unspecified trimester** M

O91.02 **Infection of nipple associated with the puerperium** M
Puerperal abscess of nipple

O91.03 **Infection of nipple associated with lactation** M
Abscess of nipple associated with lactation

● O91.1 **Abscess of breast associated with pregnancy, the puerperium and lactation**

● O91.11 **Abscess of breast associated with pregnancy**
Gestational mammary abscess
Gestational purulent mastitis
Gestational subareolar abscess

O91.111 **Abscess of breast associated with pregnancy, first trimester** M

O91.112 **Abscess of breast associated with pregnancy, second trimester** M

O91.113 **Abscess of breast associated with pregnancy, third trimester** M

O91.119 **Abscess of breast associated with pregnancy, unspecified trimester** M

O91.12 **Abscess of breast associated with the puerperium** M
Puerperal mammary abscess
Puerperal purulent mastitis
Puerperal subareolar abscess

O91.13 **Abscess of breast associated with lactation** M
Mammary abscess associated with lactation
Purulent mastitis associated with lactation
Subareolar abscess associated with lactation

● O91.2 **Nonpurulent mastitis associated with pregnancy, the puerperium and lactation**

● O91.21 **Nonpurulent mastitis associated with pregnancy**
Gestational interstitial mastitis
Gestational lymphangitis of breast
Gestational mastitis NOS
Gestational parenchymatous mastitis

O91.211 **Nonpurulent mastitis associated with pregnancy, first trimester** M

O91.212 **Nonpurulent mastitis associated with pregnancy, second trimester** M

O91.213 **Nonpurulent mastitis associated with pregnancy, third trimester** M

O91.219 **Nonpurulent mastitis associated with pregnancy, unspecified trimester** M

O91.22 **Nonpurulent mastitis associated with the puerperium** M
Puerperal interstitial mastitis
Puerperal lymphangitis of breast
Puerperal mastitis NOS
Puerperal parenchymatous mastitis

O91.23 **Nonpurulent mastitis associated with lactation** M
Interstitial mastitis associated with lactation
Lymphangitis of breast associated with lactation
Mastitis NOS associated with lactation
Parenchymatous mastitis associated with lactation

● O92 **Other disorders of breast and disorders of lactation associated with pregnancy and the puerperium**

● O92.0 **Retracted nipple associated with pregnancy, the puerperium, and lactation**

● O92.01 **Retracted nipple associated with pregnancy**

O92.011 **Retracted nipple associated with pregnancy, first trimester** M

O92.012 **Retracted nipple associated with pregnancy, second trimester** M

▶ New   ➡ Revised   ~~deleted~~ Deleted   Excludes 1   Excludes 2   Includes   Use additional   Code first   Code also   Key words
OGCR Official Guidelines   X Assign placeholder X   ● Use Additional Character(s)   ▶ Manifestation Code   Hierarchical Condition Category   Coding Clinic

O92.013   Retracted nipple associated with pregnancy, third trimester   **M**

O92.019   Retracted nipple associated with pregnancy, unspecified trimester   **M**

O92.02   Retracted nipple associated with the puerperium   **M**

O92.03   Retracted nipple associated with lactation   **M**

● **O92.1 Cracked nipple associated with pregnancy, the puerperium, and lactation**
   Fissure of nipple, gestational or puerperal

   ● **O92.11 Cracked nipple associated with pregnancy**

     O92.111   Cracked nipple associated with pregnancy, first trimester   **M**

     O92.112   Cracked nipple associated with pregnancy, second trimester   **M**

     O92.113   Cracked nipple associated with pregnancy, third trimester   **M**

     O92.119   Cracked nipple associated with pregnancy, unspecified trimester   **M**

   O92.12   Cracked nipple associated with the puerperium   **M**

   O92.13   Cracked nipple associated with lactation   **M**

● **O92.2 Other and unspecified disorders of breast associated with pregnancy and the puerperium**

   O92.20   Unspecified disorder of breast associated with pregnancy and the puerperium   **M**

   O92.29   Other disorders of breast associated with pregnancy and the puerperium   **M**

O92.3   **Agalactia**   **M**
   Primary agalactia

   Excludes1   elective agalactia (O92.5)
               secondary agalactia (O92.5)
               therapeutic agalactia (O92.5)

O92.4   **Hypogalactia**   **M**

O92.5   **Suppressed lactation**   **M**
   Elective agalactia   Therapeutic agalactia
   Secondary agalactia

   Excludes1   primary agalactia (O92.3)

O92.6   **Galactorrhea**   **M**

● O92.7   **Other and unspecified disorders of lactation**

   O92.70   Unspecified disorders of lactation   **M**

   O92.79   Other disorders of lactation   **M**
         Puerperal galactocele

OTHER OBSTETRIC CONDITIONS, NOT ELSEWHERE CLASSIFIED (O94-O9A)

O94   **Sequelae of complication of pregnancy, childbirth, and the puerperium**   **M**

   Note: This category is to be used to indicate conditions in O00-O77.-, O85-O94 and O98-O9A.- as the cause of late effects. The "sequelae" include conditions specified as such, or as late effects, which may occur at any time after the puerperium.

   Code first condition resulting from (sequela) of complication of pregnancy, childbirth, and the puerperium
     Coding Clinic: 2022, Q3, P17-18

O98   **Maternal infectious and parasitic diseases classifiable elsewhere but complicating pregnancy, childbirth and the puerperium**

   Includes   the listed conditions when complicating the pregnant state, when aggravated by the pregnancy, or as a reason for obstetric care

   Use additional code (Chapter 1), to identify specific infectious or parasitic disease

   Excludes2   herpes gestationis (O26.4-)
               infectious carrier state (O99.82-, O99.83-)
               obstetrical tetanus (A34)
               puerperal infection (O86.-)
               puerperal sepsis (O85)
               when the reason for maternal care is that the disease is known or suspected to have affected the fetus (O35-O36)

● **O98.0 Tuberculosis complicating pregnancy, childbirth and the puerperium**
   Conditions in A15-A19

   ● **O98.01 Tuberculosis complicating pregnancy**

     O98.011   Tuberculosis complicating pregnancy, first trimester   **M**

     O98.012   Tuberculosis complicating pregnancy, second trimester   **M**

     O98.013   Tuberculosis complicating pregnancy, third trimester   **M**

     O98.019   Tuberculosis complicating pregnancy, unspecified trimester   **M**

   O98.02   Tuberculosis complicating childbirth   **M**

   O98.03   Tuberculosis complicating the puerperium   **M**

● **O98.1 Syphilis complicating pregnancy, childbirth and the puerperium**
   Conditions in A50-A53

   ● **O98.11 Syphilis complicating pregnancy**

     O98.111   Syphilis complicating pregnancy, first trimester   **M**

     O98.112   Syphilis complicating pregnancy, second trimester   **M**

     O98.113   Syphilis complicating pregnancy, third trimester   **M**

     O98.119   Syphilis complicating pregnancy, unspecified trimester   **M**

   O98.12   Syphilis complicating childbirth   **M**

   O98.13   Syphilis complicating the puerperium   **M**

● **O98.2 Gonorrhea complicating pregnancy, childbirth and the puerperium**
   Conditions in A54.-

   ● **O98.21 Gonorrhea complicating pregnancy**

     O98.211   Gonorrhea complicating pregnancy, first trimester   **M**

     O98.212   Gonorrhea complicating pregnancy, second trimester   **M**

     O98.213   Gonorrhea complicating pregnancy, third trimester   **M**

     O98.219   Gonorrhea complicating pregnancy, unspecified trimester   **M**

   O98.22   Gonorrhea complicating childbirth   **M**

   O98.23   Gonorrhea complicating the puerperium   **M**

● **O98.3 Other infections with a predominantly sexual mode of transmission complicating pregnancy, childbirth and the puerperium**
   Conditions in A55-A64

   ● **O98.31 Other infections with a predominantly sexual mode of transmission complicating pregnancy**

     O98.311   Other infections with a predominantly sexual mode of transmission complicating pregnancy, first trimester   **M**

     O98.312   Other infections with a predominantly sexual mode of transmission complicating pregnancy, second trimester   **M**

     O98.313   Other infections with a predominantly sexual mode of transmission complicating pregnancy, third trimester   **M**

     O98.319   Other infections with a predominantly sexual mode of transmission complicating pregnancy, unspecified trimester   **M**

   O98.32   Other infections with a predominantly sexual mode of transmission complicating childbirth   **M**
     Coding Clinic: 2020, Q1, P20

   O98.33   Other infections with a predominantly sexual mode of transmission complicating the puerperium   **M**

CHAPTER 15 (O00-O9A)

● O98.4 **Viral hepatitis** complicating pregnancy, childbirth and the puerperium
Conditions in B15-B19

  ● O98.41 Viral hepatitis complicating **pregnancy**

    O98.411   Viral hepatitis complicating pregnancy, **first trimester**   M

    O98.412   Viral hepatitis complicating pregnancy, **second trimester**   M

    O98.413   Viral hepatitis complicating pregnancy, **third trimester**   M

    O98.419   Viral hepatitis complicating pregnancy, **unspecified trimester**   M

    O98.42   Viral hepatitis complicating **childbirth**   M

    O98.43   Viral hepatitis complicating the **puerperium**   M

● O98.5 **Other viral diseases** complicating pregnancy, childbirth and the puerperium
Conditions in A80-B09, B25-B34, R87.81-, R87.82-

  Excludes:1   human immunodeficiency virus [HIV] disease complicating pregnancy, childbirth and the puerperium (O98.7-)

  ● O98.51 Other viral diseases complicating **pregnancy**

    O98.511   Other viral diseases complicating pregnancy, **first trimester**   M

    O98.512   Other viral diseases complicating pregnancy, **second trimester**   M
      Coding Clinic: 2016, Q4, P5-6

    O98.513   Other viral diseases complicating pregnancy, **third trimester**   M
      Coding Clinic: 2016, Q4, P6

    O98.519   Other viral diseases complicating pregnancy, **unspecified trimester**   M

    O98.52   Other viral diseases complicating **childbirth**   M

    O98.53   Other viral diseases complicating the **puerperium**   M

● O98.6 **Protozoal diseases** complicating pregnancy, childbirth and the puerperium
Conditions in B50-B64

  ● O98.61 Protozoal diseases complicating **pregnancy**

    O98.611   Protozoal diseases complicating pregnancy, **first trimester**   M

    O98.612   Protozoal diseases complicating pregnancy, **second trimester**   M

    O98.613   Protozoal diseases complicating pregnancy, **third trimester**   M

    O98.619   Protozoal diseases complicating pregnancy, **unspecified trimester**   M

    O98.62   Protozoal diseases complicating **childbirth**   M

    O98.63   Protozoal diseases complicating the **puerperium**   M

● O98.7 **Human immunodeficiency virus [HIV] disease** complicating pregnancy, childbirth and the puerperium

  Use additional code to identify the type of HIV disease:
  Acquired immune deficiency syndrome (AIDS) (B20)
  Asymptomatic HIV status (Z21)
  HIV positive NOS (Z21)
  Symptomatic HIV disease (B20)

● O98.71 Human immunodeficiency virus [HIV] disease complicating **pregnancy**

  O98.711   Human immunodeficiency virus [HIV] disease complicating pregnancy, **first trimester**   M

  O98.712   Human immunodeficiency virus [HIV] disease complicating pregnancy, **second trimester**   M

  O98.713   Human immunodeficiency virus [HIV] disease complicating pregnancy, **third trimester**   M

  O98.719   Human immunodeficiency virus [HIV] disease complicating pregnancy, **unspecified trimester**   M

  O98.72   Human immunodeficiency virus [HIV] disease complicating **childbirth**   M

  O98.73   Human immunodeficiency virus [HIV] disease complicating the **puerperium**   M

● O98.8 **Other maternal infectious** and parasitic diseases complicating pregnancy, childbirth and the puerperium

  ● O98.81 Other maternal infectious and parasitic diseases complicating **pregnancy**

    O98.811   Other maternal infectious and parasitic diseases complicating pregnancy, **first trimester**   M

    O98.812   Other maternal infectious and parasitic diseases complicating pregnancy, **second trimester**   M

    O98.813   Other maternal infectious and parasitic diseases complicating pregnancy, **third trimester**   M

    O98.819   Other maternal infectious and parasitic diseases complicating pregnancy, **unspecified trimester**   M

    O98.82   Other maternal infectious and parasitic diseases complicating **childbirth**   M
      Coding Clinic: 2020, Q1, P10

    O98.83   Other maternal infectious and parasitic diseases complicating the **puerperium**   M
      Coding Clinic: 2022, Q2, P5

● O98.9 **Unspecified maternal infectious and parasitic disease** complicating pregnancy, childbirth and the puerperium

  ● O98.91 **Unspecified** maternal infectious and parasitic disease complicating **pregnancy**

    O98.911   Unspecified maternal infectious and parasitic disease complicating pregnancy, **first trimester**   M

    O98.912   Unspecified maternal infectious and parasitic disease complicating pregnancy, **second trimester**   M

    O98.913   Unspecified maternal infectious and parasitic disease complicating pregnancy, **third trimester**   M

O98.919   Unspecified maternal infectious and parasitic disease complicating pregnancy, **unspecified trimester**   **M**

O98.92   Unspecified maternal infectious and parasitic disease complicating **childbirth**   **M**

O98.93   Unspecified maternal infectious and parasitic disease complicating the **puerperium**   **M**

● **O99   Other maternal diseases classifiable elsewhere but complicating pregnancy, childbirth and the puerperium**

     Includes: conditions which complicate the pregnant state, are aggravated by the pregnancy or are a main reason for obstetric care

     Use additional code to identify specific condition

     Excludes2   when the reason for maternal care is that the condition is known or suspected to have affected the fetus (O35-O36)

     Coding Clinic: 2018, Q4, P8-9

● **O99.0   Anemia complicating pregnancy, childbirth and the puerperium**

     Conditions in D50-D64

     Excludes1   anemia arising in the puerperium (O90.81)
              postpartum anemia NOS (O90.81)

     ● **O99.01   Anemia complicating pregnancy**

         O99.011   Anemia complicating pregnancy, **first trimester**   **M**

         O99.012   Anemia complicating pregnancy, second trimester   **M**

         O99.013   Anemia complicating pregnancy, third trimester   **M**

         O99.019   Anemia complicating pregnancy, unspecified trimester   **M**

     O99.02   Anemia complicating **childbirth**   **M**

     O99.03   Anemia complicating the **puerperium**   **M**

         Excludes1   postpartum anemia not pre-existing prior to delivery (O90.81)

● **O99.1   Other diseases of the blood and blood-forming organs and certain disorders involving the immune mechanism complicating pregnancy, childbirth and the puerperium**

     Conditions in D65-D89

     Excludes1   hemorrhage with coagulation defects (O45.-, O46.0-, O67.0, O72.3)

     ● **O99.11   Other diseases of the blood and blood-forming organs and certain disorders involving the immune mechanism complicating pregnancy**

         O99.111   Other diseases of the blood and blood-forming organs and certain disorders involving the immune mechanism complicating pregnancy, first trimester   **M**

         O99.112   Other diseases of the blood and blood-forming organs and certain disorders involving the immune mechanism complicating pregnancy, second trimester   **M**

         O99.113   Other diseases of the blood and blood-forming organs and certain disorders involving the immune mechanism complicating pregnancy, third trimester   **M**

         O99.119   Other diseases of the blood and blood-forming organs and certain disorders involving the immune mechanism complicating pregnancy, **unspecified trimester**   **M**

O99.12   Other diseases of the blood and blood-forming organs and certain disorders involving the immune mechanism complicating **childbirth**   **M**

O99.13   Other diseases of the blood and blood-forming organs and certain disorders involving the immune mechanism complicating the **puerperium**   **M**

● **O99.2   Endocrine, nutritional and metabolic diseases complicating pregnancy, childbirth and the puerperium**

     Conditions in E00-E89

     Excludes2   diabetes mellitus (O24.-)
              malnutrition (O25.-)
              postpartum thyroiditis (O90.5)

● **O99.21   Obesity complicating pregnancy, childbirth, and the puerperium**

     Use additional code to identify the type of obesity (E66.-)

     O99.210   Obesity complicating pregnancy, unspecified trimester   **M**

     O99.211   Obesity complicating pregnancy, **first** trimester   **M**

     O99.212   Obesity complicating pregnancy, second trimester   **M**

     O99.213   Obesity complicating pregnancy, third trimester   **M**

     O99.214   Obesity complicating **childbirth**   **M**

         Coding Clinic: 2021, Q2, P10-11; 2018, Q4, P80

     O99.215   Obesity complicating the puerperium   **M**

● **O99.28   Other endocrine, nutritional and metabolic diseases complicating pregnancy, childbirth and the puerperium**

     O99.280   Endocrine, nutritional and metabolic diseases complicating pregnancy, unspecified trimester   **M**

     O99.281   Endocrine, nutritional and metabolic diseases complicating pregnancy, **first** trimester   **M**

     O99.282   Endocrine, nutritional and metabolic diseases complicating pregnancy, second trimester   **M**

     O99.283   Endocrine, nutritional and metabolic diseases complicating pregnancy, third trimester   **M**

     O99.284   Endocrine, nutritional and metabolic diseases complicating **childbirth**   **M**

     O99.285   Endocrine, nutritional and metabolic diseases complicating the puerperium   **M**

         Coding Clinic: 2021, Q1, P9

● **O99.3   Mental disorders and diseases of the nervous system complicating pregnancy, childbirth and the puerperium**

     ● **O99.31   Alcohol use complicating pregnancy, childbirth, and the puerperium**

     Use additional code(s) from F10 to identify manifestations of the alcohol use

     O99.310   Alcohol use complicating pregnancy, unspecified trimester   **M**

     O99.311   Alcohol use complicating pregnancy, first trimester   **M**

     O99.312   Alcohol use complicating pregnancy, second trimester   **M**

     O99.313   Alcohol use complicating pregnancy, third trimester   **M**

     O99.314   Alcohol use complicating **childbirth**   **M**

     O99.315   Alcohol use complicating the puerperium   **M**

CHAPTER 15 (O00-O9A)

CHAPTER 15 (O00-O9A)

● **O99.32 Drug use complicating pregnancy, childbirth, and the puerperium**
  Use additional code(s) from F11-F16 and F18-F19 to identify manifestations of the drug use
  - **O99.320 Drug use complicating pregnancy, unspecified trimester** M
  - **O99.321 Drug use complicating pregnancy, first trimester** M
  - **O99.322 Drug use complicating pregnancy, second trimester** M
  - **O99.323 Drug use complicating pregnancy, third trimester** M
  - **O99.324 Drug use complicating childbirth** M
  - **O99.325 Drug use complicating the puerperium** M

● **O99.33 Tobacco use disorder complicating pregnancy, childbirth, and the puerperium**
  Smoking complicating pregnancy, childbirth, and the puerperium
  Use additional code from category F17 to identify type of tobacco nicotine dependence
  - **O99.330 Smoking (tobacco) complicating pregnancy, unspecified trimester** M
  - **O99.331 Smoking (tobacco) complicating pregnancy, first trimester** M
  - **O99.332 Smoking (tobacco) complicating pregnancy, second trimester** M
  - **O99.333 Smoking (tobacco) complicating pregnancy, third trimester** M
  - **O99.334 Smoking (tobacco) complicating childbirth** M
  - **O99.335 Smoking (tobacco) complicating the puerperium** M

● **O99.34 Other mental disorders complicating pregnancy, childbirth, and the puerperium**
  Conditions in F01-F09, F20-F52 and F54-F99
  Excludes2 postpartum mood disturbance (O90.6)
  postnatal psychosis (F53.1)
  puerperal psychosis (F53.1)
  Coding Clinic: 2018, Q4, P9
  - **O99.340 Other mental disorders complicating pregnancy, unspecified trimester** M
  - **O99.341 Other mental disorders complicating pregnancy, first trimester** M
  - **O99.342 Other mental disorders complicating pregnancy, second trimester** M
  - **O99.343 Other mental disorders complicating pregnancy, third trimester** M
  - **O99.344 Other mental disorders complicating childbirth** M
  - **O99.345 Other mental disorders complicating the puerperium** M
  Coding Clinic: 2018, Q4, P8-9

● **O99.35 Diseases of the nervous system complicating pregnancy, childbirth, and the puerperium**
  Conditions in G00-G99
  Excludes2 pregnancy related peripheral neuritis (O26.8-)
  - **O99.350 Diseases of the nervous system complicating pregnancy, unspecified trimester** M
  - **O99.351 Diseases of the nervous system complicating pregnancy, first trimester** M
  - **O99.352 Diseases of the nervous system complicating pregnancy, second trimester** M
  - **O99.353 Diseases of the nervous system complicating pregnancy, third trimester** M
  - **O99.354 Diseases of the nervous system complicating childbirth** M
  - **O99.355 Diseases of the nervous system complicating the puerperium** M

● **O99.4 Diseases of the circulatory system complicating pregnancy, childbirth and the puerperium**
  Conditions in I00-I99
  Excludes1 peripartum cardiomyopathy (O90.3)
  Excludes2 hypertensive disorders (O10-O16)
  obstetric embolism (O88.-)
  venous complications and cerebrovenous sinus thrombosis in labor, childbirth and the puerperium (O87.-)
  venous complications and cerebrovenous sinus thrombosis in pregnancy (O22.-)

● **O99.41 Diseases of the circulatory system complicating pregnancy**
  Coding Clinic: 2016, Q2, P8
  - **O99.411 Diseases of the circulatory system complicating pregnancy, first trimester** M
  - **O99.412 Diseases of the circulatory system complicating pregnancy, second trimester** M
  - **O99.413 Diseases of the circulatory system complicating pregnancy, third trimester** M
  - **O99.419 Diseases of the circulatory system complicating pregnancy, unspecified trimester** M
  - **O99.42 Diseases of the circulatory system complicating childbirth** M
  - **O99.43 Diseases of the circulatory system complicating the puerperium** M

● **O99.5 Diseases of the respiratory system complicating pregnancy, childbirth and the puerperium**
  Conditions in J00-J99
● **O99.51 Diseases of the respiratory system complicating pregnancy**
  - **O99.511 Diseases of the respiratory system complicating pregnancy, first trimester** M
  - **O99.512 Diseases of the respiratory system complicating pregnancy, second trimester** M
  - **O99.513 Diseases of the respiratory system complicating pregnancy, third trimester** M
  - **O99.519 Diseases of the respiratory system complicating pregnancy, unspecified trimester** M
  - **O99.52 Diseases of the respiratory system complicating childbirth** M
  - **O99.53 Diseases of the respiratory system complicating the puerperium** M

● **O99.6　Diseases of the digestive system complicating pregnancy, childbirth and the puerperium**
Conditions in K00-K93

　　Excludes2　hemorrhoids in pregnancy (O22.4-)
　　　　liver and biliary tract disorders in pregnancy, childbirth and the puerperium (O26.6-)

　● **O99.61　Diseases of the digestive system complicating pregnancy**

　　　O99.611　Diseases of the digestive system complicating pregnancy, first trimester　　M

　　　O99.612　Diseases of the digestive system complicating pregnancy, second trimester　　M

　　　O99.613　Diseases of the digestive system complicating pregnancy, third trimester　　M

　　　O99.619　Diseases of the digestive system complicating pregnancy, unspecified trimester　　M

　　O99.62　Diseases of the digestive system complicating childbirth　　M

　　O99.63　Diseases of the digestive system complicating the puerperium　　M

● **O99.7　Diseases of the skin and subcutaneous tissue complicating pregnancy, childbirth and the puerperium**
Conditions in L00-L99

　　Excludes2　herpes gestationis (O26.4)
　　　　pruritic urticarial papules and plaques of pregnancy (PUPPP) (O26.86)

　● **O99.71　Diseases of the skin and subcutaneous tissue complicating pregnancy**

　　　O99.711　Diseases of the skin and subcutaneous tissue complicating pregnancy, first trimester　　M

　　　O99.712　Diseases of the skin and subcutaneous tissue complicating pregnancy, second trimester　　M

　　　O99.713　Diseases of the skin and subcutaneous tissue complicating pregnancy, third trimester　　M

　　　O99.719　Diseases of the skin and subcutaneous tissue complicating pregnancy, unspecified trimester　　M

　　O99.72　Diseases of the skin and subcutaneous tissue complicating childbirth　　M

　　O99.73　Diseases of the skin and subcutaneous tissue complicating the puerperium　　M

● **O99.8　Other specified diseases and conditions complicating pregnancy, childbirth and the puerperium**
Conditions in D00-D48, H00-H95, M00-N99, and Q00-Q99

Use additional code to identify condition

　　Excludes2　genitourinary infections in pregnancy (O23.-)
　　　　infection of genitourinary tract following delivery (O86.1-O86.4)
　　　　malignant neoplasm complicating pregnancy, childbirth and the puerperium (O9A.1-)
　　　　maternal care for known or suspected abnormality of maternal pelvic organs (O34.-)
　　　　postpartum acute kidney failure (O90.49)
　　　　traumatic injuries in pregnancy (O9A.2-)

● **O99.81　Abnormal glucose complicating pregnancy, childbirth and the puerperium**

　　Excludes1　gestational diabetes (O24.4-)

　　O99.810　Abnormal glucose complicating pregnancy　　M

　　O99.814　Abnormal glucose complicating childbirth　　M

　　O99.815　Abnormal glucose complicating the puerperium　　M

● **O99.82　Streptococcus B carrier state complicating pregnancy, childbirth and the puerperium**

　　Excludes1　Carrier of streptococcus group B (GBS) in a nonpregnant woman (Z22.330)

　　O99.820　Streptococcus B carrier state complicating pregnancy　　M

　　O99.824　Streptococcus B carrier state complicating childbirth　　M
　　　　Coding Clinic: 2019, Q2, P9

　　O99.825　Streptococcus B carrier state complicating the puerperium　　M

● **O99.83　Other infection carrier state complicating pregnancy, childbirth and the puerperium**

Use additional code to identify the carrier state (Z22.-)

　　O99.830　Other infection carrier state complicating pregnancy　　M

　　O99.834　Other infection carrier state complicating childbirth　　M

　　O99.835　Other infection carrier state complicating the puerperium　　M

● **O99.84　Bariatric surgery status complicating pregnancy, childbirth and the puerperium**
Gastric banding status complicating pregnancy, childbirth and the puerperium
Gastric bypass status for obesity complicating pregnancy, childbirth and the puerperium
Obesity surgery status complicating pregnancy, childbirth and the puerperium

　　O99.840　Bariatric surgery status complicating pregnancy, unspecified trimester　　M

　　O99.841　Bariatric surgery status complicating pregnancy, first trimester　　M

　　O99.842　Bariatric surgery status complicating pregnancy, second trimester　　M

　　O99.843　Bariatric surgery status complicating pregnancy, third trimester　　M

　　O99.844　Bariatric surgery status complicating childbirth　　M

　　O99.845　Bariatric surgery status complicating the puerperium　　M

● **O99.89　Other specified diseases and conditions complicating pregnancy, childbirth and the puerperium**　　M

　　O99.891　Other specified diseases and conditions complicating pregnancy　　M

　　O99.892　Other specified diseases and conditions complicating childbirth　　M
　　　　Coding Clinic: 2023, Q3, P17

　　O99.893　Other specified diseases and conditions complicating puerperium　　M

● **O9A**   **Maternal malignant neoplasms, traumatic injuries and abuse classifiable elsewhere but complicating pregnancy, childbirth and the puerperium**

   ● **O9A.1**   **Malignant neoplasm complicating pregnancy, childbirth and the puerperium**

     Conditions in C00-C96

     Use additional code to identify neoplasm

     Excludes2   maternal care for benign tumor of corpus uteri (O34.1-)

           maternal care for benign tumor of cervix (O34.4-)

     ● **O9A.11**   **Malignant neoplasm complicating pregnancy**

       O9A.111   Malignant neoplasm complicating pregnancy, first trimester   **M**

       O9A.112   Malignant neoplasm complicating pregnancy, second trimester   **M**

       O9A.113   Malignant neoplasm complicating pregnancy, third trimester   **M**

       O9A.119   Malignant neoplasm complicating pregnancy, unspecified trimester   **M**

     O9A.12   Malignant neoplasm complicating childbirth   **M**

     O9A.13   Malignant neoplasm complicating the puerperium   **M**

       Coding Clinic: 2015, Q3, P19

   ● **O9A.2**   **Injury, poisoning and certain other consequences of external causes complicating pregnancy, childbirth and the puerperium**

     Conditions in S00-T88, except T74 and T76

     Use additional code(s) to identify the injury or poisoning

     Excludes2   physical, sexual and psychological abuse complicating pregnancy, childbirth and the puerperium (O9A.3-, O9A.4-, O9A.5-)

     ● **O9A.21**   **Injury, poisoning and certain other consequences of external causes complicating pregnancy**

       O9A.211   Injury, poisoning and certain other consequences of external causes complicating pregnancy, first trimester   **M**

       O9A.212   Injury, poisoning and certain other consequences of external causes complicating pregnancy, second trimester   **M**

       O9A.213   Injury, poisoning and certain other consequences of external causes complicating pregnancy, third trimester   **M**

       O9A.219   Injury, poisoning and certain other consequences of external causes complicating pregnancy, unspecified trimester   **M**

     O9A.22   Injury, poisoning and certain other consequences of external causes complicating childbirth   **M**

     O9A.23   Injury, poisoning and certain other consequences of external causes complicating the puerperium   **M**

   ● **O9A.3**   **Physical abuse complicating pregnancy, childbirth and the puerperium**

     Conditions in T74.11 or T76.11

     Use additional code (if applicable):

       to identify any associated current injury due to physical abuse

       to identify the perpetrator of abuse (Y07.-)

     Excludes2   sexual abuse complicating pregnancy, childbirth and the puerperium (O9A.4)

     ● **O9A.31**   **Physical abuse complicating pregnancy**

       O9A.311   Physical abuse complicating pregnancy, first trimester   **M**

       O9A.312   Physical abuse complicating pregnancy, second trimester   **M**

       O9A.313   Physical abuse complicating pregnancy, third trimester   **M**

       O9A.319   Physical abuse complicating pregnancy, unspecified trimester   **M**

     O9A.32   Physical abuse complicating childbirth   **M**

     O9A.33   Physical abuse complicating the puerperium   **M**

   ● **O9A.4**   **Sexual abuse complicating pregnancy, childbirth and the puerperium**

     Conditions in T74.21 or T76.21

     Use additional code (if applicable):

       to identify any associated current injury due to sexual abuse

       to identify the perpetrator of abuse (Y07.-)

     ● **O9A.41**   **Sexual abuse complicating pregnancy**

       O9A.411   Sexual abuse complicating pregnancy, first trimester   **M**

       O9A.412   Sexual abuse complicating pregnancy, second trimester   **M**

       O9A.413   Sexual abuse complicating pregnancy, third trimester   **M**

       O9A.419   Sexual abuse complicating pregnancy, unspecified trimester   **M**

     O9A.42   Sexual abuse complicating childbirth   **M**

     O9A.43   Sexual abuse complicating the puerperium   **M**

   ● **O9A.5**   **Psychological abuse complicating pregnancy, childbirth and the puerperium**

     Conditions in T74.31 or T76.31

     Use additional code to identify the perpetrator of abuse (Y07.-)

     ● **O9A.51**   **Psychological abuse complicating pregnancy**

       O9A.511   Psychological abuse complicating pregnancy, first trimester   **M**

       O9A.512   Psychological abuse complicating pregnancy, second trimester   **M**

       O9A.513   Psychological abuse complicating pregnancy, third trimester   **M**

       O9A.519   Psychological abuse complicating pregnancy, unspecified trimester   **M**

     O9A.52   Psychological abuse complicating childbirth   **M**

     O9A.53   Psychological abuse complicating the puerperium   **M**

CHAPTER 16

CERTAIN CONDITIONS ORIGINATING IN THE PERINATAL PERIOD (P00-P96)

OGCR Chapter-Specific Coding Guidelines

16. Chapter 16: Certain Conditions Originating in the Perinatal Period (P00-P96)

For coding and reporting purposes the perinatal period is defined as before birth through the 28th day following birth. The following guidelines are provided for reporting purposes

a. General Perinatal Rules

1) Use of Chapter 16 Codes

Codes in this chapter are never for use on the maternal record. Codes from Chapter 15, the obstetric chapter, are never permitted on the newborn record. Chapter 16 codes may be used throughout the life of the patient if the condition is still present.

2) Principal Diagnosis for Birth Record

When coding the birth episode in a newborn record, assign a code from category Z38, Liveborn infants according to place of birth and type of delivery, as the principal diagnosis. A code from category Z38 is assigned only once, to a newborn at the time of birth. If a newborn is transferred to another institution, a code from category Z38 should not be used at the receiving hospital.

A code from category Z38 is used only on the newborn record, not on the mother's record.

3) Use of Codes from other Chapters with Codes from Chapter 16

Codes from other chapters may be used with codes from chapter 16 if the codes from the other chapters provide more specific detail. Codes for signs and symptoms may be assigned when a definitive diagnosis has not been established. If the reason for the encounter is a perinatal condition, the code from Chapter 16 should be sequenced first.

4) Use of Chapter 16 Codes after the Perinatal Period

Should a condition originate in the perinatal period, and continue throughout the life of the patient, the perinatal code should continue to be used regardless of the patient's age.

5) Birth process or community acquired conditions

If a newborn has a condition that may be either due to the birth process or community acquired and the documentation does not indicate which it is, the default is due to the birth process and the code from Chapter 16 should be used. If the condition is community-acquired, a code from Chapter 16 should not be assigned.

6) Code all clinically significant conditions

All clinically significant conditions noted on routine newborn examination should be coded. A condition is clinically significant if it requires:

- clinical evaluation; or
- therapeutic treatment; or
- diagnostic procedures; or
- extended length of hospital stay; or
- increased nursing care and/or monitoring; or
- has implications for future health care needs

Note: The perinatal guidelines listed above are the same as the general coding guidelines for "additional diagnoses", except for the final point regarding implications for future health care needs. Codes should be assigned for conditions that have been specified by the provider as having implications for future health care needs.

b. Observation and Evaluation of Newborns for Suspected Conditions Not Found

1) Use of Z05 codes

Assign a code from category Z05, Observation and evaluation of newborns and infants for suspected conditions ruled out, to identify those instances when a healthy newborn is evaluated for a suspected condition that is determined after study not to be present. Do not use a code from category Z05 when the patient has identified signs or symptoms of a suspected problem; in such cases code the sign or symptom.

2) Z05 on Other than the Birth Record

A code from category Z05 may also be assigned as a principal or first-listed code for readmissions or encounters when the code from category Z38 code no longer applies. Codes from category Z05 are for use only for healthy newborns and infants for which no condition after study is found to be present.

3) Z05 on a birth record

A code from category Z05 is to be used as a secondary code after the code from category Z38, Liveborn infants according to place of birth and type of delivery.

c. Coding Additional Perinatal Diagnoses

1) Assigning codes for conditions that require treatment

Assign codes for conditions that require treatment or further investigation, prolong the length of stay, or require resource utilization.

2) Codes for conditions specified as having implications for future health care needs

Assign codes for conditions that have been specified by the provider as having implications for future health care needs.

Note: This guideline should not be used for adult patients.

d. Prematurity and Fetal Growth Retardation

Providers utilize different criteria in determining prematurity. A code for prematurity should not be assigned unless it is documented. Assignment of codes in categories P05, Disorders of newborn related to slow fetal growth and fetal malnutrition, and P07, Disorders of newborn related to short gestation and low birth weight, not elsewhere classified, should be based on the recorded birth weight and estimated gestational age.

When both birth weight and gestational age are available, two codes from category P07 should be assigned, with the code for birth weight sequenced before the code for gestational age.

e. Low birth weight and immaturity status

Codes from category P07, Disorders of newborn related to short gestation and low birth weight, not elsewhere classified, are for use for a child or adult who was premature or had a low birth weight as a newborn and this is affecting the patient's current health status.

See Section I.C.21. Factors influencing health status and contact with health services, Status.

f. Bacterial Sepsis of Newborn

Category P36, Bacterial sepsis of newborn, includes congenital sepsis. If a perinate is documented as having sepsis without documentation of congenital or community acquired, the default is congenital and a code from category P36 should be assigned. If the P36 code includes the causal organism, an additional code from category B95, Streptococcus, Staphylococcus, and Enterococcus as the cause of diseases classified elsewhere, or B96, Other bacterial agents as the cause of diseases classified elsewhere, should not be assigned. If the P36 code does not include the causal organism, assign an additional code from category B96. If applicable, use additional codes to identify severe sepsis (R65.2-) and any associated acute organ dysfunction.

g. Stillbirth

Code P95, Stillbirth, is only for use in institutions that maintain separate records for stillbirths. No other code should be used with P95. Code P95 should not be used on the mother's record.

CHAPTER 16 (P00-P96)

CHAPTER 16

CERTAIN CONDITIONS ORIGINATING IN THE PERINATAL PERIOD (P00-P96)

Note: Codes from this chapter are for use on newborn records only, never on maternal records.

Includes conditions that have their origin in the fetal or perinatal period (before birth through the first 28 days after birth) even if morbidity occurs later

Excludes2 congenital malformations, deformations and chromosomal abnormalities (Q00-Q99)
endocrine, nutritional and metabolic diseases (E00-E88)
injury, poisoning and certain other consequences of external causes (S00-T88)
neoplasms (C00-D49)
tetanus neonatorum (A33)

This chapter contains the following blocks:

P00-P04	Newborn affected by maternal factors and by complications of pregnancy, labor, and delivery
P05-P08	Disorders of newborns related to length of gestation and fetal growth
P09	Abnormal findings on neonatal screening
P10-P15	Birth trauma
P19-P29	Respiratory and cardiovascular disorders specific to the perinatal period
P35-P39	Infections specific to the perinatal period
P50-P61	Hemorrhagic and hematological disorders of newborn
P70-P74	Transitory endocrine and metabolic disorders specific to newborn
P76-P78	Digestive system disorders of newborn
P80-P83	Conditions involving the integument and temperature regulation of newborn
P84	Other problems with newborn
P90-P96	Other disorders originating in the perinatal period

NEWBORN AFFECTED BY MATERNAL FACTORS AND BY COMPLICATIONS OF PREGNANCY, LABOR, AND DELIVERY (P00–P04)

Note: These codes are for use when the listed maternal conditions are specified as the cause of confirmed morbidity or potential morbidity which have their origin in the perinatal period (before birth through the first 28 days after birth).

● **P00** **Newborn affected by maternal conditions that may be unrelated to present pregnancy**

Code first any current condition in newborn

Excludes2 encounter for observation of newborn for suspected diseases and conditions ruled out (Z05.-)
newborn affected by maternal complications of pregnancy (P01.-)
newborn affected by maternal endocrine and metabolic disorders (P70–P74)
newborn affected by noxious substances transmitted via placenta or breast milk (P04.-)

Coding Clinic: 2016, Q4, P54

P00.0 **Newborn affected by maternal hypertensive disorders**
Newborn affected by maternal conditions classifiable to O10-O11, O13-O16

P00.1 **Newborn affected by maternal renal and urinary tract diseases**
Newborn affected by maternal conditions classifiable to N00-N39

P00.2 **Newborn affected by maternal infectious and parasitic diseases**
Newborn affected by maternal infectious disease classifiable to A00-B99, J09 and J10

    Excludes1 maternal genital tract or other localized infections (P00.8)

    Excludes2 infections specific to the perinatal period (P35-P39)

       newborn affected by (positive) maternal group B streptococcus (GBS) colonization (P00.82)

Coding Clinic: 2019, Q2, P10; 2015, Q3, P21

P00.3 **Newborn affected by other maternal circulatory and respiratory diseases**
Newborn affected by maternal conditions classifiable to I00-I99, J00-J99, Q20-Q34 and not included in P00.0, P00.2

P00.4 **Newborn affected by maternal nutritional disorders**
Newborn affected by maternal disorders classifiable to E40-E64
Maternal malnutrition NOS

P00.5 **Newborn affected by maternal injury**
Newborn affected by maternal conditions classifiable to O9A.2-

P00.6 **Newborn affected by surgical procedure on mother**
Newborn affected by amniocentesis

    Excludes1 Cesarean delivery for present delivery (P03.4)
damage to placenta from amniocentesis, cesarean delivery or surgical induction (P02.1)
previous surgery to uterus or pelvic organs (P03.89)

    Excludes2 newborn affected by complication of (fetal) intrauterine procedure (P96.5)

P00.7 **Newborn affected by other medical procedures on mother, not elsewhere classified**
Newborn affected by radiation to mother

    Excludes1 damage to placenta from amniocentesis, cesarean delivery or surgical induction (P02.1)
newborn affected by other complications of labor and delivery (P03.-)

● **P00.8** **Newborn affected by other maternal conditions**

P00.81 **Newborn affected by periodontal disease in mother**

P00.82 **Newborn affected by (positive) maternal group B streptococcus (GBS) colonization**
Contact with positive maternal group B streptococcus
Coding Clinic: 2021, Q4, P23

P00.89 **Newborn affected by other maternal conditions**
Newborn affected by conditions classifiable to T80-T88
Newborn affected by maternal genital tract or other localized infections
Newborn affected by maternal systemic lupus erythematosus
Use additional code to identify infectious agent, if known

    Excludes2 newborn affected by positive maternal group B streptococcus (GBS) colonization (P00.82)

Coding Clinic: 2019, Q2, P9

P00.9 **Newborn affected by unspecified maternal condition**

● **P01** **Newborn affected by maternal complications of pregnancy**

Code first any current condition in newborn

    Excludes2 encounter for observation of newborn for suspected diseases and conditions ruled out (Z05.-)

Coding Clinic: 2016, Q4, P54

P01.0 **Newborn affected by incompetent cervix**

P01.1 **Newborn affected by premature rupture of membranes**

▶ New   ⇒ Revised   ~~deleted~~ Deleted   Excludes 1   Excludes 2   Includes   Use additional   Code first   Code also   Key words

OGCR Official Guidelines   X Assign placeholder X   ● Use Additional Character(s)   ❘ Manifestation Code   Hierarchical Condition Category   Coding Clinic

P01.2   **Newborn affected by oligohydramnios**
  Excludes1   oligohydramnios due to premature rupture of membranes (P01.1)

P01.3   **Newborn affected by polyhydramnios**
  Excess of amniotic fluid, usually > 2000 mL
  Newborn affected by hydramnios

P01.4   **Newborn affected by ectopic pregnancy**
  Newborn affected by abdominal pregnancy

P01.5   **Newborn affected by multiple pregnancy**
  Newborn affected by triplet (pregnancy)
  Newborn affected by twin (pregnancy)

P01.6   **Newborn affected by maternal death**

P01.7   **Newborn affected by malpresentation before labor**
  Newborn affected by breech presentation before labor
  Newborn affected by external version before labor
  Newborn affected by face presentation before labor
  Newborn affected by transverse lie before labor
  Newborn affected by unstable lie before labor
  Coding Clinic: 2025, Q1, P23

P01.8   **Newborn affected by other maternal complications of pregnancy**

P01.9   **Newborn affected by maternal complication of pregnancy, unspecified**

● **P02**   **Newborn affected by complications of placenta, cord and membranes**
  Code first any current condition in newborn
  Excludes2   encounter for observation of newborn for suspected diseases and conditions ruled out (Z05.-)
  Coding Clinic: 2016, Q4, P54

P02.0   **Newborn affected by placenta previa**

P02.1   **Newborn affected by other forms of placental separation and hemorrhage**
  Newborn affected by abruptio placenta
  Newborn affected by accidental hemorrhage
  Newborn affected by antepartum hemorrhage
  Newborn affected by damage to placenta from amniocentesis, cesarean delivery or surgical induction
  Newborn affected by maternal blood loss
  Newborn affected by premature separation of placenta

● **P02.2**   **Newborn affected by other and unspecified morphological and functional abnormalities of placenta**

  P02.20   **Newborn affected by unspecified morphological and functional abnormalities of placenta**

  P02.29   **Newborn affected by other morphological and functional abnormalities of placenta**
    Newborn affected by placental dysfunction
    Newborn affected by placental infarction
    Newborn affected by placental insufficiency

P02.3   **Newborn affected by placental transfusion syndromes**
  Newborn affected by placental and cord abnormalities resulting in twin-to-twin or other transplacental transfusion

P02.4   **Newborn affected by prolapsed cord**

P02.5   **Newborn affected by other compression of umbilical cord**
  Newborn affected by umbilical cord (tightly) around neck
  Newborn affected by entanglement of umbilical cord
  Newborn affected by knot in umbilical cord
  Coding Clinic: 2022, Q1, P22

● **P02.6**   **Newborn affected by other and unspecified conditions of umbilical cord**

  P02.60   **Newborn affected by unspecified conditions of umbilical cord**

  P02.69   **Newborn affected by other conditions of umbilical cord**
    Newborn affected by short umbilical cord
    Newborn affected by vasa previa
    Excludes1   newborn affected by single umbilical artery (Q27.0)

● **P02.7**   **Newborn affected by chorioamnionitis**
  Inflammation of chorion and amnion

  P02.70   **Newborn affected by fetal inflammatory response syndrome** ⬮
    Newborn affected by FIRS

  P02.78   **Newborn affected by other conditions from chorioamnionitis**
    Newborn affected by amnionitis
    Newborn affected by membranitis
    Newborn affected by placentitis

P02.8   **Newborn affected by other abnormalities of membranes**

P02.9   **Newborn affected by abnormality of membranes, unspecified**

● **P03**   **Newborn affected by other complications of labor and delivery**
  Code first any current condition in newborn
  Excludes2   encounter for observation of newborn for suspected diseases and conditions ruled out (Z05.-)
  Coding Clinic: 2016, Q4, P54

P03.0   **Newborn affected by breech delivery and extraction**

P03.1   **Newborn affected by other malpresentation, malposition and disproportion during labor and delivery**
  Newborn affected by contracted pelvis
  Newborn affected by conditions classifiable to O64-O66
  Newborn affected by persistent occipitoposterior
  Newborn affected by transverse lie

P03.2   **Newborn affected by forceps delivery**

P03.3   **Newborn affected by delivery by vacuum extractor [ventouse]**

P03.4   **Newborn affected by Cesarean delivery**

P03.5   **Newborn affected by precipitate delivery**
  Newborn affected by rapid second stage

P03.6   **Newborn affected by abnormal uterine contractions**
  Newborn affected by conditions classifiable to O62.-, except O62.3
  Newborn affected by hypertonic labor
  Newborn affected by uterine inertia

● **P03.8**   **Newborn affected by other specified complications of labor and delivery**

  ● **P03.81**   **Newborn affected by abnormality in fetal (intrauterine) heart rate or rhythm**
    Excludes1   neonatal cardiac dysrhythmia (P29.1-)

    P03.810   **Newborn affected by abnormality in fetal (intrauterine) heart rate or rhythm before the onset of labor**

    P03.811   **Newborn affected by abnormality in fetal (intrauterine) heart rate or rhythm during labor**

    P03.819   **Newborn affected by abnormality in fetal (intrauterine) heart rate or rhythm, unspecified as to time of onset**

  P03.82   **Meconium passage during delivery**
    Excludes1   meconium aspiration (P24.00, P24.01)
    meconium staining (P96.83)

  P03.89   **Newborn affected by other specified complications of labor and delivery**
    Newborn affected by abnormality of maternal soft tissues
    Newborn affected by conditions classifiable to O60-O75 and by procedures used in labor and delivery not included in P02.- and P03.0-P03.6
    Newborn affected by induction of labor

P03.9   **Newborn affected by complication of labor and delivery, unspecified**

CHAPTER 16 (P00-P96)

● **P04** **Newborn affected by noxious substances transmitted via placenta or breast milk**

  Code first any current condition in newborn, if applicable

  Includes nonteratogenic effects of substances transmitted via placenta

  Excludes2 congenital malformations (Q00-Q99)
     encounter for observation of newborn for suspected diseases and conditions ruled out (Z05.-)
     neonatal jaundice from excessive hemolysis due to drugs or toxins transmitted from mother (P58.4)
     newborn in contact with and (suspected) exposures hazardous to health not transmitted via placenta or breast milk (Z77.-)

  Coding Clinic: 2016, Q4, P54

 P04.0 **Newborn affected by maternal anesthesia and analgesia in pregnancy, labor and delivery**
   Newborn affected by reactions and intoxications from maternal opiates and tranquilizers administered for procedures during pregnancy or labor and delivery

  Excludes2 newborn affected by other maternal medication (P04.1-)

● **P04.1** **Newborn affected by other maternal medication**
  Code first , if applicable, withdrawal symptoms from maternal use of drugs of addiction (P96.1)
   withdrawal symptoms from therapeutic use of drugs in newborn (P96.2)

  Excludes1 dysmorphism due to warfarin (Q86.2)
     fetal hydantoin syndrome (Q86.1)

  Excludes2 maternal anesthesia and analgesia in pregnancy, labor and delivery (P04.0)
     maternal use of drugs of addiction (P04.4-)

  P04.11 **Newborn affected by maternal antineoplastic chemotherapy**

  P04.12 **Newborn affected by maternal cytotoxic drugs**

  P04.13 **Newborn affected by maternal use of anticonvulsants**

  P04.14 **Newborn affected by maternal use of opiates**

  P04.15 **Newborn affected by maternal use of antidepressants**

  P04.16 **Newborn affected by maternal use of amphetamines**

  P04.17 **Newborn affected by maternal use of sedative-hypnotics**

  P04.1A **Newborn affected by maternal use of anxiolytics**

  P04.18 **Newborn affected by other maternal medication**

  P04.19 **Newborn affected by maternal use of unspecified medication**
  Coding Clinic: 2016, Q4, P55

 P04.2 **Newborn affected by maternal use of tobacco**
   Newborn affected by exposure in utero to tobacco smoke

  Excludes2 newborn exposure to environmental tobacco smoke (P96.81)

 P04.3 **Newborn affected by maternal use of alcohol**

  Excludes1 fetal alcohol syndrome (Q86.0)

● **P04.4** **Newborn affected by maternal use of drugs of addiction**

  P04.40 **Newborn affected by maternal use of unspecified drugs of addiction**

  P04.41 **Newborn affected by maternal use of cocaine**

  P04.42 **Newborn affected by maternal use of hallucinogens**

    Excludes2 newborn affected by other maternal medication (P04.1-)

  P04.49 **Newborn affected by maternal use of other drugs of addiction**

    Excludes2 newborn affected by maternal anesthesia and analgesia (P04.0)
      withdrawal symptoms from maternal use of drugs of addiction (P96.1)

 P04.5 **Newborn affected by maternal use of nutritional chemical substances**

 P04.6 **Newborn affected by maternal exposure to environmental chemical substances**

● **P04.8** **Newborn affected by other maternal noxious substances**

  P04.81 **Newborn affected by maternal use of cannabis**

  P04.89 **Newborn affected by other maternal noxious substances**

 P04.9 **Newborn affected by maternal noxious substance, unspecified**

OGCR Section I.C.16.d.

 Prematurity and Fetal Growth Retardation

 Providers utilize different criteria in determining prematurity. A code for prematurity should not be assigned unless it is documented. Assignment of codes in categories P05, Disorders of newborn related to slow fetal growth and fetal malnutrition, and P07, Disorders of newborn related to short gestation and low birth weight, not elsewhere classified, should be based on the recorded birth weight and estimated gestational age.

 When both birth weight and gestational age are available, two codes from category P07 should be assigned, with the code for birth weight sequenced before the code for gestational age.

DISORDERS OF NEWBORN RELATED TO LENGTH OF GESTATION AND FETAL GROWTH (P05-P08)

● **P05** **Disorders of newborn related to slow fetal growth and fetal malnutrition**
  Coding Clinic: 2016, Q4, P56

 ● **P05.0** **Newborn light for gestational age**
   Newborn light-for-dates
   Weight below but length above 10th percentile for gestational age

  P05.00 **Newborn light for gestational age, unspecified weight**

  P05.01 **Newborn light for gestational age, less than 500 grams**

  P05.02 **Newborn light for gestational age, 500-749 grams**

  P05.03 **Newborn light for gestational age, 750-999 grams**

  P05.04 **Newborn light for gestational age, 1000-1249 grams**

  P05.05 **Newborn light for gestational age, 1250-1499 grams**

  P05.06 **Newborn light for gestational age, 1500-1749 grams**

  P05.07 **Newborn light for gestational age, 1750-1999 grams**

  P05.08 **Newborn light for gestational age, 2000-2499 grams**

  P05.09 **Newborn light for gestational age, 2500 grams and over**
   Newborn light for gestational age, other
   Coding Clinic: 2016, Q4, P55

● **P05.1**   **Newborn small for gestational age**
Newborn small-and-light-for-dates
Newborn small-for-dates
Weight and length below 10th percentile for gestational age

    P05.10   Newborn small for gestational age, unspecified weight

    P05.11   Newborn small for gestational age, less than 500 grams

    P05.12   Newborn small for gestational age, 500-749 grams

    P05.13   Newborn small for gestational age, 750-999 grams

    P05.14   Newborn small for gestational age, 1000-1249 grams

    P05.15   Newborn small for gestational age, 1250-1499 grams

    P05.16   Newborn small for gestational age, 1500-1749 grams

    P05.17   Newborn small for gestational age, 1750-1999 grams

    P05.18   Newborn small for gestational age, 2000-2499 grams

    P05.19   Newborn small for gestational age, other
Newborn small for gestational age, 2500 grams and over
Coding Clinic: 2016, Q4, P55

P05.2   **Newborn affected by fetal (intrauterine) malnutrition not light or small for gestational age**
Infant, not light or small for gestational age, showing signs of fetal malnutrition, such as dry, peeling skin and loss of subcutaneous tissue

    Excludes1   newborn affected by fetal malnutrition with light for gestational age (P05.0-)
newborn affected by fetal malnutrition with small for gestational age (P05.1-)

P05.9   **Newborn affected by slow intrauterine growth, unspecified**
Newborn affected by fetal growth retardation NOS

● **P07**   **Disorders of newborn related to short gestation and low birth weight, not elsewhere classified**
Note: When both birth weight and gestational age of the newborn are available, both should be coded with birth weight sequenced before gestational age.

    Includes   the listed conditions, without further specification, as the cause of morbidity or additional care, in newborn

● **P07.0**   **Extremely low birth weight newborn**
Newborn birth weight 999 g. or less

    Excludes1   low birth weight due to slow fetal growth and fetal malnutrition (P05.-)

    P07.00   Extremely low birth weight newborn, unspecified weight

    P07.01   Extremely low birth weight newborn, less than 500 grams

    P07.02   Extremely low birth weight newborn, 500-749 grams

    P07.03   Extremely low birth weight newborn, 750-999 grams

● **P07.1**   **Other low birth weight newborn**
Newborn birth weight 1000-2499 g.

    Excludes1   low birth weight due to slow fetal growth and fetal malnutrition (P05.-)

    P07.10   Other low birth weight newborn, unspecified weight

    P07.14   Other low birth weight newborn, 1000-1249 grams

    P07.15   Other low birth weight newborn, 1250-1499 grams

    P07.16   Other low birth weight newborn, 1500-1749 grams

    P07.17   Other low birth weight newborn, 1750-1999 grams

    P07.18   Other low birth weight newborn, 2000-2499 grams

● **P07.2**   **Extreme immaturity of newborn**
Less than 28 completed weeks (less than 196 completed days) of gestation

    P07.20   Extreme immaturity of newborn, unspecified weeks of gestation
Gestational age less than 28 completed weeks NOS

    P07.21   Extreme immaturity of newborn, gestational age less than 23 completed weeks
Extreme immaturity of newborn, gestational age less than 23 weeks, 0 days

    P07.22   Extreme immaturity of newborn, gestational age 23 completed weeks
Extreme immaturity of newborn, gestational age 23 weeks, 0 days through 23 weeks, 6 days

    P07.23   Extreme immaturity of newborn, gestational age 24 completed weeks
Extreme immaturity of newborn, gestational age 24 weeks, 0 days through 24 weeks, 6 days

    P07.24   Extreme immaturity of newborn, gestational age 25 completed weeks
Extreme immaturity of newborn, gestational age 25 weeks, 0 days through 25 weeks, 6 days

    P07.25   Extreme immaturity of newborn, gestational age 26 completed weeks
Extreme immaturity of newborn, gestational age 26 weeks, 0 days through 26 weeks, 6 days

    P07.26   Extreme immaturity of newborn, gestational age 27 completed weeks
Extreme immaturity of newborn, gestational age 27 weeks, 0 days through 27 weeks, 6 days

● **P07.3**   **Preterm [premature] newborn [other]**
28 completed weeks or more but less than 37 completed weeks (196 completed days but less than 259 completed days) of gestation
Prematurity NOS

    P07.30   Preterm newborn, unspecified weeks of gestation

    P07.31   Preterm newborn, gestational age 28 completed weeks
Preterm newborn, gestational age 28 weeks, 0 days through 28 weeks, 6 days

    P07.32   Preterm newborn, gestational age 29 completed weeks
Preterm newborn, gestational age 29 weeks, 0 days through 29 weeks, 6 days

    P07.33   Preterm newborn, gestational age 30 completed weeks
Preterm newborn, gestational age 30 weeks, 0 days through 30 weeks, 6 days

    P07.34   Preterm newborn, gestational age 31 completed weeks
Preterm newborn, gestational age 31 weeks, 0 days through 31 weeks, 6 days

    P07.35   Preterm newborn, gestational age 32 completed weeks
Preterm newborn, gestational age 32 weeks, 0 days through 32 weeks, 6 days

    P07.36   Preterm newborn, gestational age 33 completed weeks
Preterm newborn, gestational age 33 weeks, 0 days through 33 weeks, 6 days

CHAPTER 16 (P00-P96)

P07.37 **Preterm newborn, gestational age 34 completed weeks**
Preterm newborn, gestational age 34 weeks, 0 days through 34 weeks, 6 days
Coding Clinic: 2017, Q2, P7

P07.38 **Preterm newborn, gestational age 35 completed weeks**
Preterm newborn, gestational age 35 weeks, 0 days through 35 weeks, 6 days

P07.39 **Preterm newborn, gestational age 36 completed weeks**
Preterm newborn, gestational age 36 weeks, 0 days through 36 weeks, 6 days
Coding Clinic: 2017, Q3, P26

● **P08** **Disorders of newborn related to long gestation and high birth weight**
Note: When both birth weight and gestational age of the newborn are available, priority of assignment should be given to birth weight.
Includes the listed conditions, without further specification, as causes of morbidity or additional care, in newborn

P08.0 **Exceptionally large newborn baby**
Usually implies a birth weight of 4500 g. or more
Excludes1 syndrome of infant of diabetic mother (P70.1)
syndrome of infant of mother with gestational diabetes (P70.0)

P08.1 **Other heavy for gestational age newborn**
Other newborn heavy- or large-for-dates regardless of period of gestation
Usually implies a birth weight of 4000 g. to 4499 g.
Excludes1 newborn with a birth weight of 4500 or more (P08.0)
syndrome of infant of diabetic mother (P70.1)
syndrome of infant of mother with gestational diabetes (P70.0)

● **P08.2** **Late newborn, not heavy for gestational age**

P08.21 **Post-term newborn**
Newborn with gestation period over 40 completed weeks to 42 completed weeks

P08.22 **Prolonged gestation of newborn**
Newborn with gestation period over 42 completed weeks (294 days or more), not heavy- or large-for-dates
Postmaturity NOS

ABNORMAL FINDINGS ON NEONATAL SCREENING (P09)

● **P09** **Abnormal findings on neonatal screening**
Includes: Abnormal findings on state mandated newborn screens
Failed newborn screening
Excludes2 nonspecific serologic evidence of human immunodeficiency virus [HIV] (R75)

P09.1 **Abnormal findings on neonatal screening for inborn errors of metabolism**

P09.2 **Abnormal findings on neonatal screening for congenital endocrine disease**
Abnormal findings on neonatal screening for congenital adrenal hyperplasia
Abnormal findings on neonatal screening for hypothyroidism screen

P09.3 **Abnormal findings on neonatal screening for congenital hematologic disorders**
Abnormal findings for hemoglobinopathy screening
Abnormal findings on red cell membrane defects screen
Abnormal findings on sickle cell screen

P09.4 **Abnormal findings on neonatal screening for cystic fibrosis**

P09.5 **Abnormal findings on neonatal screening for critical congenital heart disease**
Neonatal congenital heart disease screening failure

➡ **P09.6** **Abnormal findings on neonatal screening hearing screening**
Excludes2 encounter for hearing examination following failed hearing screening (Z01.110)

P09.8 **Other abnormal findings on neonatal screening**

P09.9 **Abnormal findings on neonatal screening, unspecified**

BIRTH TRAUMA (P10-P15)

● **P10** **Intracranial laceration and hemorrhage due to birth injury**
Excludes1 intracranial hemorrhage of newborn NOS (P52.9)
intracranial hemorrhage of newborn due to anoxia or hypoxia (P52.-)
nontraumatic intracranial hemorrhage of newborn (P52.-)

P10.0 **Subdural hemorrhage due to birth injury**
Subdural hematoma (localized) due to birth injury
Excludes1 subdural hemorrhage accompanying tentorial tear (P10.4)

P10.1 **Cerebral hemorrhage due to birth injury**

P10.2 **Intraventricular hemorrhage due to birth injury**

P10.3 **Subarachnoid hemorrhage due to birth injury**

P10.4 **Tentorial tear due to birth injury**
Pertaining to tentorium of cerebellum (extension of dura mater that separates cerebellum from inferior portion of occipital lobes)

P10.8 **Other intracranial lacerations and hemorrhages due to birth injury**

P10.9 **Unspecified intracranial laceration and hemorrhage due to birth injury**

● **P11** **Other birth injuries to central nervous system**

P11.0 **Cerebral edema due to birth injury**

P11.1 **Other specified brain damage due to birth injury**

P11.2 **Unspecified brain damage due to birth injury**

P11.3 **Birth injury to facial nerve**
Facial palsy due to birth injury

P11.4 **Birth injury to other cranial nerves**

P11.5 **Birth injury to spine and spinal cord**
Fracture of spine due to birth injury

P11.9 **Birth injury to central nervous system, unspecified**

● **P12** **Birth injury to scalp**

P12.0 **Cephalhematoma due to birth injury**

P12.1 **Chignon (from vacuum extraction) due to birth injury**

P12.2 **Epicranial subaponeurotic hemorrhage due to birth injury**
Subgaleal hemorrhage

P12.3 **Bruising of scalp due to birth injury**

P12.4 **Injury of scalp of newborn due to monitoring equipment**
Sampling incision of scalp of newborn
Scalp clip (electrode) injury of newborn

● **P12.8** **Other birth injuries to scalp**

P12.81 **Caput succedaneum**

P12.89 **Other birth injuries to scalp**

P12.9 **Birth injury to scalp, unspecified**

● **P13** **Birth injury to skeleton**
Excludes2 birth injury to spine (P11.5)

P13.0 **Fracture of skull due to birth injury**

P13.1 **Other birth injuries to skull**
Excludes1 cephalhematoma (P12.0)

P13.2 **Birth injury to femur**

P13.3 **Birth injury to other long bones**

▶ New   ➡ Revised   ~~deleted~~ Deleted   Excludes 1   Excludes 2   Includes   Use additional   Code first   Code also   Key words
OGCR Official Guidelines   **X** Assign placeholder X   ● Use Additional Character(s)   ▶ Manifestation Code   Hierarchical Condition Category   **Coding Clinic**

Item 16–1 The **peripheral nervous system** consists of 31 pairs of spinal nerves, 12 pairs of cranial nerves, and the autonomic nerves, which are divided into the parasympathetic and sympathetic nerves. The cranial nerves are: olfactory (I), optic (II), oculomotor (III), trochlear (IV), trigeminal (V), abducens (VI), facial (VII), vestibulocochlear (VIII), glossopharyngeal (IX), vagus (X), accessory (XI), and hypoglossal (XII).

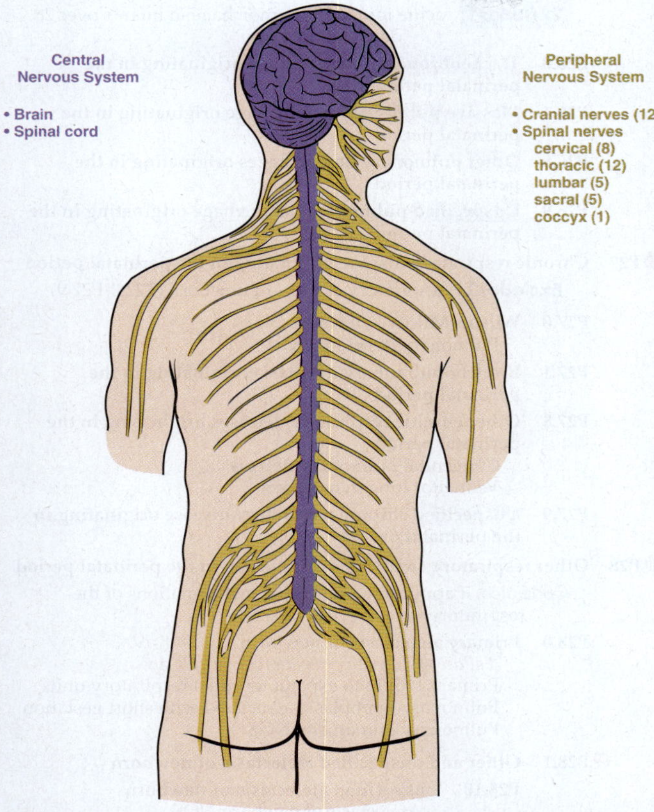

Figure 16-1 The central nervous system consists of the brain and spinal cord. The peripheral nervous system consists of nerves that lie outside the skull and spinal cord. (From Stoy: Mosby's EMT-Basic Textbook, ed 2, St. Louis, Mosby, 2007)

P13.4   **Fracture of clavicle due to birth injury**

P13.8   **Birth injuries to other parts of skeleton**

P13.9   **Birth injury to skeleton, unspecified**

● **P14**   **Birth injury to peripheral nervous system**

P14.0   **Erb's paralysis due to birth injury**

P14.1   **Klumpke's paralysis due to birth injury**

P14.2   **Phrenic nerve paralysis due to birth injury**

P14.3   **Other brachial plexus birth injuries**

P14.8   **Birth injuries to other parts of peripheral nervous system**

P14.9   **Birth injury to peripheral nervous system, unspecified**

● **P15**   **Other birth injuries**

P15.0   **Birth injury to liver**
Rupture of liver due to birth injury

P15.1   **Birth injury to spleen**
Rupture of spleen due to birth injury

P15.2   **Sternomastoid injury due to birth injury**

P15.3   **Birth injury to eye**
Subconjunctival hemorrhage due to birth injury
Traumatic glaucoma due to birth injury

P15.4   **Birth injury to face**
Facial congestion due to birth injury

P15.5   **Birth injury to external genitalia**

P15.6   **Subcutaneous fat necrosis due to birth injury**

P15.8   **Other specified birth injuries**

P15.9   **Birth injury, unspecified**

RESPIRATORY AND CARDIOVASCULAR DISORDERS SPECIFIC TO THE PERINATAL PERIOD (P19-P29)

● **P19**   **Metabolic acidemia in newborn**

   Includes   metabolic acidemia in newborn

P19.0   **Metabolic acidemia in newborn first noted before onset of labor**

P19.1   **Metabolic acidemia in newborn first noted during labor**

P19.2   **Metabolic acidemia noted at birth**

P19.9   **Metabolic acidemia in newborn, unspecified**

● **P22**   **Respiratory distress of newborn**
   Coding Clinic: 2019, Q2, P29

P22.0   **Respiratory distress syndrome of newborn**
Cardiorespiratory distress syndrome of newborn
Hyaline membrane disease
Idiopathic respiratory distress syndrome [IRDS or RDS] of newborn
Pulmonary hypoperfusion syndrome
Respiratory distress syndrome, type I

   Excludes2   respiratory arrest of newborn (P28.81)
respiratory failure of newborn NOS (P28.5)

   Coding Clinic: 2019, Q2, P29

P22.1   **Transient tachypnea of newborn**
Idiopathic tachypnea of newborn
Respiratory distress syndrome, type II
Wet lung syndrome

P22.8   **Other respiratory distress of newborn**

   Excludes1   respiratory arrest of newborn (P28.81)
respiratory failure of newborn NOS (P28.5)

P22.9   **Respiratory distress of newborn, unspecified**

   Excludes1   respiratory arrest of newborn (P28.81)
respiratory failure of newborn NOS (P28.5)

● **P23**   **Congenital pneumonia**

   Includes   infective pneumonia acquired in utero or during birth

   Excludes1   neonatal pneumonia resulting from aspiration (P24.-)

P23.0   **Congenital pneumonia due to viral agent**
Use additional code (B97) to identify organism

   Excludes1   congenital rubella pneumonitis (P35.0)

P23.1   **Congenital pneumonia due to Chlamydia**

P23.2   **Congenital pneumonia due to staphylococcus**

P23.3   **Congenital pneumonia due to streptococcus, group B**

P23.4   **Congenital pneumonia due to Escherichia coli**

P23.5   **Congenital pneumonia due to Pseudomonas**

P23.6   **Congenital pneumonia due to other bacterial agents**
Congenital pneumonia due to Hemophilus influenzae
Congenital pneumonia due to Klebsiella pneumoniae
Congenital pneumonia due to Mycoplasma
Congenital pneumonia due to Streptococcus, except group B
Use additional code (B95-B96) to identify organism

P23.8   **Congenital pneumonia due to other organisms**

P23.9   **Congenital pneumonia, unspecified**

● **P24**   **Neonatal aspiration**

   Includes   aspiration in utero and during delivery

● **P24.0**   **Meconium aspiration**

   Excludes1   meconium passage (without aspiration) during delivery (P03.82)
meconium staining (P96.83)

P24.00   **Meconium aspiration without respiratory symptoms**
Meconium aspiration NOS

CHAPTER 16 (P00-P96)

P24.01 **Meconium aspiration with respiratory symptoms**
Meconium aspiration pneumonia
Meconium aspiration pneumonitis
Meconium aspiration syndrome NOS
 code to identify any secondary pulmonary hypertension, if applicable (I27.2-)

● **P24.1** **Neonatal aspiration of (clear) amniotic fluid and mucus**
Neonatal aspiration of liquor (amnii)

P24.10 **Neonatal aspiration of (clear) amniotic fluid and mucus without respiratory symptoms**
Neonatal aspiration of amniotic fluid and mucus NOS

P24.11 **Neonatal aspiration of (clear) amniotic fluid and mucus with respiratory symptoms**
Neonatal aspiration of amniotic fluid and mucus with pneumonia
Neonatal aspiration of amniotic fluid and mucus with pneumonitis
Use additional code to identify any secondary pulmonary hypertension, if applicable (I27.2-)

● **P24.2** **Neonatal aspiration of blood**

P24.20 **Neonatal aspiration of blood without respiratory symptoms**
Neonatal aspiration of blood NOS

P24.21 **Neonatal aspiration of blood with respiratory symptoms**
Neonatal aspiration of blood with pneumonia
Neonatal aspiration of blood with pneumonitis
Use additional code to identify any secondary pulmonary hypertension, if applicable (I27.2-)

● **P24.3** **Neonatal aspiration of milk and regurgitated food**
Neonatal aspiration of stomach contents

P24.30 **Neonatal aspiration of milk and regurgitated food without respiratory symptoms**
Neonatal aspiration of milk and regurgitated food NOS

P24.31 **Neonatal aspiration of milk and regurgitated food with respiratory symptoms**
Neonatal aspiration of milk and regurgitated food with pneumonia
Neonatal aspiration of milk and regurgitated food with pneumonitis
Use additional code to identify any secondary pulmonary hypertension, if applicable (I27.2-)

● **P24.8** **Other neonatal aspiration**

P24.80 **Other neonatal aspiration without respiratory symptoms**
Neonatal aspiration NEC

P24.81 **Other neonatal aspiration with respiratory symptoms**
Neonatal aspiration pneumonia NEC
Neonatal aspiration with pneumonitis NEC
Neonatal aspiration with pneumonia NOS
Neonatal aspiration with pneumonitis NOS
Use additional code to identify any secondary pulmonary hypertension, if applicable (I27.2-)

P24.9 **Neonatal aspiration, unspecified**

● **P25** **Interstitial emphysema and related conditions originating in the perinatal period**

P25.0 **Interstitial emphysema originating in the perinatal period**

P25.1 **Pneumothorax originating in the perinatal period**

P25.2 **Pneumomediastinum originating in the perinatal period**

P25.3 **Pneumopericardium originating in the perinatal period**

P25.8 **Other conditions related to interstitial emphysema originating in the perinatal period**

● **P26** **Pulmonary hemorrhage originating in the perinatal period**
Excludes1 acute idiopathic hemorrhage in infants over 28 days old (R04.81)

P26.0 **Tracheobronchial hemorrhage originating in the perinatal period**

P26.1 **Massive pulmonary hemorrhage originating in the perinatal period**

P26.8 **Other pulmonary hemorrhages originating in the perinatal period**

P26.9 **Unspecified pulmonary hemorrhage originating in the perinatal period**

● **P27** **Chronic respiratory disease originating in the perinatal period**
Excludes2 respiratory distress of newborn (P22.0-P22.9)

P27.0 **Wilson-Mikity syndrome**
Pulmonary dysmaturity

P27.1 **Bronchopulmonary dysplasia originating in the perinatal period**

P27.8 **Other chronic respiratory diseases originating in the perinatal period**
Congenital pulmonary fibrosis
Ventilator lung in newborn

P27.9 **Unspecified chronic respiratory disease originating in the perinatal period**

● **P28** **Other respiratory conditions originating in the perinatal period**
, if applicable, congenital malformations of the respiratory system (Q30-Q34)

P28.0 **Primary atelectasis of newborn**
Failure of lungs to expand properly at birth
Primary failure to expand terminal respiratory units
Pulmonary hypoplasia associated with short gestation
Pulmonary immaturity NOS

● **P28.1** **Other and unspecified atelectasis of newborn**

P28.10 **Unspecified atelectasis of newborn**
Atelectasis of newborn NOS

P28.11 **Resorption atelectasis without respiratory distress syndrome**
Excludes1 resorption atelectasis with respiratory distress syndrome (P22.0)

P28.19 **Other atelectasis of newborn**
Partial atelectasis of newborn
Secondary atelectasis of newborn

P28.2 **Cyanotic attacks of newborn**
Excludes1 apnea of newborn (P28.3- - P28.4-)

● **P28.3** **Primary sleep apnea of newborn**
Sleep apnea of newborn NOS
Excludes2 other apnea of newborn (P28.4-)

P28.30 **Primary sleep apnea of newborn, unspecified**
Transient oxygen desaturation spells of newborn during sleep

P28.31 **Primary central sleep apnea of newborn**

P28.32 **Primary obstructive sleep apnea of newborn**

P28.33 **Primary mixed sleep apnea of newborn**

P28.39 **Other primary sleep apnea of newborn**

▶ New   ↪ Revised   ~~deleted~~ Deleted   Excludes 1   Excludes 2   Includes   Use additional   Code first   Code also   Key words
OGCR Official Guidelines   X Assign placeholder X   ● Use Additional Character(s)   ▮ Manifestation Code   Hierarchical Condition Category   **Coding Clinic**

● **P28.4** **Other apnea of newborn**
Excludes2 primary sleep apnea of newborn (P28.3-)

P28.40 **Unspecified apnea of newborn**
Apnea of newborn, NOS
Transient oxygen desaturation spells of newborn

P28.41 **Central neonatal apnea of newborn**

P28.42 **Obstructive apnea of newborn**

P28.43 **Mixed neonatal apnea of newborn**

P28.49 **Other apnea of newborn**
Apnea of prematurity

P28.5 **Respiratory failure of newborn**
Excludes2 respiratory arrest of newborn (P28.81)
respiratory distress of newborn (P22.0)
Coding Clinic: 2019, Q2, P29

● **P28.8** **Other specified respiratory conditions of newborn**

P28.81 **Respiratory arrest of newborn**
Coding Clinic: 2017, Q2, P6

P28.89 **Other specified respiratory conditions of newborn**
Congenital laryngeal stridor
Sniffles in newborn
Snuffles in newborn
Excludes1 early congenital syphilitic rhinitis (A50.05)

P28.9 **Respiratory condition of newborn, unspecified**
Respiratory depression in newborn
Code also associated underlying condition

● **P29** **Cardiovascular disorders originating in the perinatal period**
Excludes2 congenital malformations of the circulatory system (Q20-Q28)

P29.0 **Neonatal cardiac failure**

● **P29.1** **Neonatal cardiac dysrhythmia**

P29.11 **Neonatal tachycardia**

P29.12 **Neonatal bradycardia**

P29.2 **Neonatal hypertension**

● **P29.3** **Persistent fetal circulation**

P29.30 **Pulmonary hypertension of newborn**
Persistent pulmonary hypertension of newborn

P29.38 **Other persistent fetal circulation**
Delayed closure of ductus arteriosus

P29.4 **Transient myocardial ischemia in newborn**

● **P29.8** **Other cardiovascular disorders originating in the perinatal period**

P29.81 **Cardiac arrest of newborn**

P29.89 **Other cardiovascular disorders originating in the perinatal period**

P29.9 **Cardiovascular disorder originating in the perinatal period, unspecified**

INFECTIONS SPECIFIC TO THE PERINATAL PERIOD (P35-P39)

Infections acquired in utero, during birth via the umbilicus, or during the first 28 days after birth

Excludes2 asymptomatic human immunodeficiency virus [HIV] infection status (Z21)
congenital gonococcal infection (A54.-)
congenital pneumonia (P23.-)
congenital syphilis (A50.-)
human immunodeficiency virus [HIV] disease (B20)
infant botulism (A48.51)
infectious diseases not specific to the perinatal period (A00-B99, J09, J10.-)
intestinal infectious disease (A00-A09)
laboratory evidence of human immunodeficiency virus [HIV] (R75)
tetanus neonatorum (A33)

● **P35** **Congenital viral diseases**
Includes infections acquired in utero or during birth

P35.0 **Congenital rubella syndrome**
Congenital rubella pneumonitis

P35.1 **Congenital cytomegalovirus infection**
Viruses transmitted by multiple routes that cause mild/ subclinical infection

P35.2 **Congenital herpesviral [herpes simplex] infection**

P35.3 **Congenital viral hepatitis**

P35.4 **Congenital Zika virus disease**
Use additional code to identify manifestations of congenital Zika virus disease
Coding Clinic: 2018, Q4, P26

P35.8 **Other congenital viral diseases**
Congenital varicella [chickenpox]
Coding Clinic: 2016, Q4, P7

P35.9 **Congenital viral disease, unspecified**

● **P36** **Bacterial sepsis of newborn**
Includes congenital sepsis
Use additional code(s), if applicable, to identify severe sepsis (R65.2-) and associated acute organ dysfunction(s)

P36.0 **Sepsis of newborn due to streptococcus, group B**

● **P36.1** **Sepsis of newborn due to other and unspecified streptococci**

P36.10 **Sepsis of newborn due to unspecified streptococci**

P36.19 **Sepsis of newborn due to other streptococci**

P36.2 **Sepsis of newborn due to Staphylococcus aureus**

● **P36.3** **Sepsis of newborn due to other and unspecified staphylococci**

P36.30 **Sepsis of newborn due to unspecified staphylococci**

P36.39 **Sepsis of newborn due to other staphylococci**

P36.4 **Sepsis of newborn due to Escherichia coli**

P36.5 **Sepsis of newborn due to anaerobes**

P36.8 **Other bacterial sepsis of newborn**
Use additional code from category B96 to identify organism

P36.9 **Bacterial sepsis of newborn, unspecified**

● **P37** **Other congenital infectious and parasitic diseases**
Excludes2 congenital syphilis (A50.-)
infectious neonatal diarrhea (A00-A09)
necrotizing enterocolitis in newborn (P77.-)
noninfectious neonatal diarrhea (P78.3)
ophthalmia neonatorum due to gonococcus (A54.31)
tetanus neonatorum (A33)

P37.0 **Congenital tuberculosis**

P37.1 **Congenital toxoplasmosis**
Parasitic infection, often causing mild flu-like illness
Hydrocephalus due to congenital toxoplasmosis

P37.2 **Neonatal (disseminated) listeriosis**
Acquired transplacentally or during/after parturition in which symptoms are those of sepsis

P37.3 **Congenital falciparum malaria**

P37.4 **Other congenital malaria**

P37.5 **Neonatal candidiasis**

P37.8 **Other specified congenital infectious and parasitic diseases**

P37.9 **Congenital infectious or parasitic disease, unspecified**

● **P38** **Omphalitis of newborn**
Inflammation of umbilicus
Excludes1 omphalitis not of newborn (L08.82)
tetanus omphalitis (A33)
umbilical hemorrhage of newborn (P51.-)

P38.1 **Omphalitis with mild hemorrhage**

P38.9 **Omphalitis without hemorrhage**
Omphalitis of newborn NOS

CHAPTER 16 (P00-P96)

● **P39 Other infections specific to the perinatal period**
Use additional code to identify organism or specific infection

P39.0 Neonatal infective mastitis
> **Excludes1** breast engorgement of newborn (P83.4)
> noninfective mastitis of newborn (P83.4)

P39.1 Neonatal conjunctivitis and dacryocystitis
Neonatal chlamydial conjunctivitis
Ophthalmia neonatorum NOS
Neonate = newborn
> **Excludes1** gonococcal conjunctivitis (A54.31)

P39.2 Intra-amniotic infection affecting newborn, not elsewhere classified

P39.3 Neonatal urinary tract infection

P39.4 Neonatal skin infection
Neonatal pyoderma
> **Excludes1** pemphigus neonatorum (L00)
> staphylococcal scalded skin syndrome (L00)

P39.8 Other specified infections specific to the perinatal period

P39.9 Infection specific to the perinatal period, unspecified

HEMORRHAGIC AND HEMATOLOGICAL DISORDERS OF NEWBORN (P50-P61)

> **Excludes1** congenital stenosis and stricture of bile ducts (Q44.3)
> Crigler-Najjar syndrome (E80.5)
> Dubin-Johnson syndrome (E80.6)
> Gilbert syndrome (E80.4)
> hereditary hemolytic anemias (D55-D58)

● **P50 Newborn affected by intrauterine (fetal) blood loss**
> **Excludes1** congenital anemia from intrauterine (fetal) blood loss (P61.3)

P50.0 Newborn affected by intrauterine (fetal) blood loss from vasa previa

P50.1 Newborn affected by intrauterine (fetal) blood loss from ruptured cord

P50.2 Newborn affected by intrauterine (fetal) blood loss from placenta

P50.3 Newborn affected by hemorrhage into co-twin

P50.4 Newborn affected by hemorrhage into maternal circulation

P50.5 Newborn affected by intrauterine (fetal) blood loss from cut end of co-twin's cord

P50.8 Newborn affected by other intrauterine (fetal) blood loss

P50.9 Newborn affected by intrauterine (fetal) blood loss, unspecified
Newborn affected by fetal hemorrhage NOS

● **P51 Umbilical hemorrhage of newborn**
> **Excludes1** omphalitis with mild hemorrhage (P38.1)
> umbilical hemorrhage from cut end of co-twins cord (P50.5)

P51.0 Massive umbilical hemorrhage of newborn

P51.8 Other umbilical hemorrhages of newborn
Slipped umbilical ligature NOS

P51.9 Umbilical hemorrhage of newborn, unspecified

● **P52 Intracranial nontraumatic hemorrhage of newborn**
> **Includes** intracranial hemorrhage due to anoxia or hypoxia
> **Excludes1** intracranial hemorrhage due to birth injury (P10.-)
> intracranial hemorrhage due to other injury (S06.-)

P52.0 Intraventricular (nontraumatic) hemorrhage, grade 1, of newborn
Subependymal hemorrhage (without intraventricular extension)
Bleeding into germinal matrix

P52.1 Intraventricular (nontraumatic) hemorrhage, grade 2, of newborn
Subependymal hemorrhage with intraventricular extension
Bleeding into ventricle

P52.2 Intraventricular (nontraumatic) hemorrhage, grade 3 and grade 4, of newborn

P52.21 Intraventricular (nontraumatic) hemorrhage, grade 3, of newborn
Subependymal hemorrhage with intraventricular extension with enlargement of ventricle

P52.22 Intraventricular (nontraumatic) hemorrhage, grade 4, of newborn
Bleeding into cerebral cortex
Subependymal hemorrhage with intracerebral extension

P52.3 Unspecified intraventricular (nontraumatic) hemorrhage of newborn

P52.4 Intracerebral (nontraumatic) hemorrhage of newborn

P52.5 Subarachnoid (nontraumatic) hemorrhage of newborn

P52.6 Cerebellar (nontraumatic) and posterior fossa hemorrhage of newborn

P52.8 Other intracranial (nontraumatic) hemorrhages of newborn

P52.9 Intracranial (nontraumatic) hemorrhage of newborn, unspecified

P53 Hemorrhagic disease of newborn
Vitamin K deficiency of newborn

● **P54 Other neonatal hemorrhages**
> **Excludes1** newborn affected by (intrauterine) blood loss (P50.-)
> pulmonary hemorrhage originating in the perinatal period (P26.-)

P54.0 Neonatal hematemesis
Vomiting of blood
> **Excludes1** neonatal hematemesis due to swallowed maternal blood (P78.2)

P54.1 Neonatal melena
Dark-colored feces stained with blood pigments
> **Excludes1** neonatal melena due to swallowed maternal blood (P78.2)

P54.2 Neonatal rectal hemorrhage

P54.3 Other neonatal gastrointestinal hemorrhage

P54.4 Neonatal adrenal hemorrhage

P54.5 Neonatal cutaneous hemorrhage
Neonatal bruising
Neonatal ecchymoses
Neonatal petechiae
Neonatal superficial hematomata
> **Excludes2** bruising of scalp due to birth injury (P12.3)
> cephalhematoma due to birth injury (P12.0)

P54.6 Neonatal vaginal hemorrhage
Neonatal pseudomenses

P54.8 Other specified neonatal hemorrhages

P54.9 Neonatal hemorrhage, unspecified

● **P55 Hemolytic disease of newborn**
AKA erythroblastosis fetalis and is due to Rh isoimmunization, result of Rh blood factor incompatibilities between mother (Rh negative) and fetus (Rh positive)

P55.0 Rh isoimmunization of newborn

P55.1 ABO isoimmunization of newborn
Coding Clinic: 2015, Q3, P20

P55.8 Other hemolytic diseases of newborn

P55.9 Hemolytic disease of newborn, unspecified

● **P56 Hydrops fetalis due to hemolytic disease**
Caused by maternal sensitization to fetal blood group antigen
> **Excludes1** hydrops fetalis NOS (P83.2)

P56.0 Hydrops fetalis due to isoimmunization

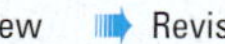 New   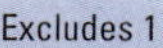 Revised   ~~deleted~~ Deleted   Excludes 1   Excludes 2   Includes   Use additional   Code first   Code also   Key words
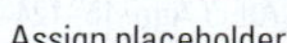 OGCR Official Guidelines   X Assign placeholder X   ● Use Additional Character(s)   ▶ Manifestation Code   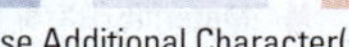 Hierarchical Condition Category   Coding Clinic

● **P56.9   Hydrops fetalis due to other and unspecified hemolytic disease**

　　　　P56.90   Hydrops fetalis due to unspecified hemolytic disease

　　　　P56.99   Hydrops fetalis due to other hemolytic disease

● **P57   Kernicterus**
　　High levels of bilirubin in blood, with severe neural symptoms

　　P57.0   Kernicterus due to isoimmunization

　　P57.8   Other specified kernicterus
　　　　　Excludes1   Crigler-Najjar syndrome (E80.5)

　　P57.9   Kernicterus, unspecified

● **P58   Neonatal jaundice due to other excessive hemolysis**
　　　　Excludes1   jaundice due to isoimmunization (P55-P57)

　　P58.0   Neonatal jaundice due to bruising

　　P58.1   Neonatal jaundice due to bleeding

　　P58.2   Neonatal jaundice due to infection

　　P58.3   Neonatal jaundice due to polycythemia

● **P58.4   Neonatal jaundice due to drugs or toxins transmitted from mother or given to newborn**
　　　　Code first poisoning due to drug or toxin, if applicable (T36-T65 with fifth or sixth character 1-4)
　　　　Use additional code for adverse effect, if applicable, to identify drug (T36-T50 with fifth or sixth character 5)

　　　　P58.41   Neonatal jaundice due to drugs or toxins transmitted from mother

　　　　P58.42   Neonatal jaundice due to drugs or toxins given to newborn

　　P58.5   Neonatal jaundice due to swallowed maternal blood

　　P58.8   Neonatal jaundice due to other specified excessive hemolysis

　　P58.9   Neonatal jaundice due to excessive hemolysis, unspecified

● **P59   Neonatal jaundice from other and unspecified causes**
　　　　Excludes1   jaundice due to inborn errors of metabolism (E70-E88)
　　　　　　kernicterus (P57.-)

　　P59.0   Neonatal jaundice associated with preterm delivery
　　　　Hyperbilirubinemia of prematurity
　　　　Jaundice due to delayed conjugation associated with preterm delivery
　　　　Coding Clinic: 2025, Q1, P24

　　P59.1   Inspissated bile syndrome

● **P59.2   Neonatal jaundice from other and unspecified hepatocellular damage**
　　　　Excludes1   congenital viral hepatitis (P35.3)

　　　　P59.20   Neonatal jaundice from unspecified hepatocellular damage

　　　　P59.29   Neonatal jaundice from other hepatocellular damage
　　　　　　Neonatal giant cell hepatitis
　　　　　　Neonatal (idiopathic) hepatitis

　　P59.3   Neonatal jaundice from breast milk inhibitor

　　P59.8   Neonatal jaundice from other specified causes

　　P59.9   Neonatal jaundice, unspecified
　　　　Neonatal physiological jaundice (intense)(prolonged) NOS
　　　　Coding Clinic: 2015, Q3, P20

P60   Disseminated intravascular coagulation of newborn
　　　　Defibrination syndrome of newborn

● **P61   Other perinatal hematological disorders**
　　　　Excludes1   transient hypogammaglobulinemia of infancy (D80.7)

　　P61.0   Transient neonatal thrombocytopenia
　　　　Lack of sufficient numbers of circulating throm bocytes (platelets)
　　　　Neonatal thrombocytopenia due to exchange transfusion
　　　　Neonatal thrombocytopenia due to idiopathic maternal thrombocytopenia
　　　　Neonatal thrombocytopenia due to isoimmunization

　　P61.1   Polycythemia neonatorum
　　　　Neonate = newborn

　　P61.2   Anemia of prematurity

　　P61.3   Congenital anemia from fetal blood loss

　　P61.4   Other congenital anemias, not elsewhere classified
　　　　Congenital anemia NOS

　　P61.5   Transient neonatal neutropenia
　　　　Low levels of granulocytic neutrophilic white blood cells
　　　　　Excludes1   congenital neutropenia (nontransient) (D70.0)

　　P61.6   Other transient neonatal disorders of coagulation

　　P61.8   Other specified perinatal hematological disorders

　　P61.9   Perinatal hematological disorder, unspecified

TRANSITORY ENDOCRINE AND METABOLIC DISORDERS SPECIFIC TO NEWBORN (P70-P74)

　　Includes   transitory endocrine and metabolic disturbances caused by the infant's response to maternal endocrine and metabolic factors, or its adjustment to extrauterine environment

● **P70   Transitory disorders of carbohydrate metabolism specific to newborn**

　　P70.0   Syndrome of infant of mother with gestational diabetes
　　　　Newborn (with hypoglycemia) affected by maternal gestational diabetes
　　　　　Excludes1   newborn (with hypoglycemia) affected by maternal (pre-existing) diabetes mellitus (P70.1)
　　　　　　syndrome of infant of a diabetic mother (P70.1)

　　P70.1   Syndrome of infant of a diabetic mother
　　　　Newborn (with hypoglycemia) affected by maternal (pre-existing) diabetes mellitus
　　　　　Excludes1   newborn (with hypoglycemia) affected by maternal gestational diabetes (P70.0)
　　　　　　syndrome of infant of mother with gestational diabetes (P70.0)

　　P70.2   Neonatal diabetes mellitus

　　P70.3   Iatrogenic neonatal hypoglycemia

　　P70.4   Other neonatal hypoglycemia
　　　　Transitory neonatal hypoglycemia

　　P70.8   Other transitory disorders of carbohydrate metabolism of newborn

　　P70.9   Transitory disorder of carbohydrate metabolism of newborn, unspecified

● **P71   Transitory neonatal disorders of calcium and magnesium metabolism**

　　P71.0   Cow's milk hypocalcemia in newborn

　　P71.1   Other neonatal hypocalcemia
　　　　　Excludes1   neonatal hypoparathyroidism (P71.4)

　　P71.2   Neonatal hypomagnesemia

　　P71.3   Neonatal tetany without calcium or magnesium deficiency
　　　　Neonatal tetany NOS

　　P71.4   Transitory neonatal hypoparathyroidism

CHAPTER 16 (P00-P96)

P71.8   **Other** transitory neonatal disorders of calcium and magnesium metabolism
Coding Clinic: 2016, Q4, P55

P71.9   Transitory neonatal disorder of calcium and magnesium metabolism, **unspecified**

● **P72**   Other transitory neonatal **endocrine** disorders
     Excludes1   congenital hypothyroidism with or without goiter (E03.0-E03.1)
           dyshormogenetic goiter (E07.1)
           Pendred's syndrome (E07.1)

P72.0   **Neonatal goiter, not elsewhere classified**
Transitory congenital goiter with normal functioning

P72.1   **Transitory neonatal hyperthyroidism**
Neonatal thyrotoxicosis

P72.2   **Other transitory neonatal disorders of thyroid function, not elsewhere classified**
Transitory neonatal hypothyroidism

P72.8   **Other specified transitory neonatal endocrine disorders**

P72.9   Transitory neonatal endocrine disorder, **unspecified**

● **P74**   Other transitory neonatal **electrolyte** and metabolic disturbances

P74.0   **Late metabolic acidosis of newborn**
     Excludes1   (fetal) metabolic acidosis of newborn (P19)

P74.1   **Dehydration of newborn**

● **P74.2**   **Disturbances of sodium balance of newborn**
Coding Clinic: 2018, Q2, P6

     P74.21   **Hypernatremia of newborn**

     P74.22   **Hyponatremia of newborn**

● **P74.3**   **Disturbances of potassium balance of newborn**

     P74.31   **Hyperkalemia of newborn**

     P74.32   **Hypokalemia of newborn**

● **P74.4**   **Other transitory electrolyte disturbances of newborn**

     P74.41   **Alkalosis of newborn**
         Hyperbicarbonatemia

     ● **P74.42**   **Disturbances of chlorine balance of newborn**

         P74.421   **Hyperchloremia of newborn**
Hyperchloremic metabolic acidosis
           Excludes2   late metabolic acidosis of the newborn (P74.0)

         P74.422   **Hypochloremia of newborn**

     P74.49   **Other transitory electrolyte disturbance of newborn**

P74.5   Transitory **tyrosinemia** of newborn

P74.6   Transitory **hyperammonemia** of newborn

P74.8   **Other transitory metabolic disturbances of newborn**
Amino-acid metabolic disorders described as transitory

P74.9   **Transitory metabolic disturbance of newborn, unspecified**

DIGESTIVE SYSTEM DISORDERS OF NEWBORN (P76-P78)

● **P76**   Other intestinal obstruction of newborn

P76.0   **Meconium plug syndrome**
Fetal stool obstruction in large intestine, present at birth; may be symptom of organic disease.
Meconium ileus NOS
     Excludes1   meconium ileus in cystic fibrosis (E84.11)

P76.1   **Transitory ileus of newborn**
Temporary obstruction of ileus (small intestine)
     Excludes1   Hirschsprung's disease (Q43.1)

P76.2   **Intestinal obstruction due to inspissated milk**
Being thickened, dried, or made less fluid

P76.8   **Other specified intestinal obstruction of newborn**
     Excludes1   intestinal obstruction classifiable to K56.-

P76.9   Intestinal obstruction of newborn, **unspecified**

● **P77**   Necrotizing enterocolitis of newborn

P77.1   **Stage 1 necrotizing enterocolitis in newborn**
Necrotizing enterocolitis without pneumatosis, without perforation

P77.2   **Stage 2 necrotizing enterocolitis in newborn**
Necrotizing enterocolitis with pneumatosis, without perforation

P77.3   **Stage 3 necrotizing enterocolitis in newborn**
Necrotizing enterocolitis with perforation
Necrotizing enterocolitis with pneumatosis and perforation

P77.9   **Necrotizing enterocolitis in newborn, unspecified**
Necrotizing enterocolitis in newborn, NOS

● **P78**   Other perinatal digestive system disorders
     Excludes1   cystic fibrosis (E84.0-E84.9)
           neonatal gastrointestinal hemorrhages (P54.0-P54.3)

P78.0   **Perinatal intestinal perforation**
Meconium peritonitis

P78.1   **Other neonatal peritonitis**
Neonatal peritonitis NOS

P78.2   **Neonatal hematemesis and melena due to swallowed maternal blood**

P78.3   **Noninfective neonatal diarrhea**
Neonatal diarrhea NOS

● **P78.8**   **Other specified perinatal digestive system disorders**

     P78.81   **Congenital cirrhosis (of liver)**

     P78.82   **Peptic ulcer of newborn**

     P78.83   **Newborn esophageal reflux**
Neonatal esophageal reflux

     P78.84   **Gestational alloimmune liver disease**
GALD
Neonatal hemochromatosis
           Excludes1   hemochromatosis (E83.11-)

     P78.89   **Other specified perinatal digestive system disorders**

P78.9   Perinatal digestive system disorder, **unspecified**

CONDITIONS INVOLVING THE INTEGUMENT AND TEMPERATURE REGULATION OF NEWBORN (P80-P83)

● **P80**   Hypothermia of newborn

P80.0   **Cold injury syndrome**
Severe and usually chronic hypothermia associated with a pink flushed appearance, edema and neurological and biochemical abnormalities.
     Excludes1   mild hypothermia of newborn (P80.8)

P80.8   **Other hypothermia of newborn**
Mild hypothermia of newborn

P80.9   Hypothermia of newborn, **unspecified**

● **P81**   Other disturbances of temperature regulation of newborn

P81.0   **Environmental hyperthermia of newborn**

P81.8   **Other specified disturbances of temperature regulation of newborn**

P81.9   **Disturbance of temperature regulation of newborn, unspecified**
Fever of newborn NOS

● **P83**   Other conditions of integument specific to newborn
     Excludes1   congenital malformations of skin and integument (Q80-Q84)
           hydrops fetalis due to hemolytic disease (P56.-)
           neonatal skin infection (P39.4)
           staphylococcal scalded skin syndrome (L00)
     Excludes2   cradle cap (L21.0)
           diaper [napkin] dermatitis (L22)

P83.0   **Sclerema neonatorum**
Neonate = newborn

P83.1   **Neonatal erythema toxicum**
Benign, generalized, transient pustules that become firm vesicles

P83.2   **Hydrops fetalis not due to hemolytic disease**
     Severe, life-threatening problem of severe edema (swelling) as a result of too much fluid leaving blood and entering tissue
     Hydrops fetalis NOS

● **P83.3**   **Other and unspecified edema specific to newborn**
     P83.30   Unspecified edema specific to newborn
     P83.39   Other edema specific to newborn

P83.4   **Breast engorgement of newborn**
     Noninfective mastitis of newborn

P83.5   **Congenital hydrocele**

P83.6   **Umbilical polyp of newborn**

● **P83.8**   **Other specified conditions of integument specific to newborn**
     P83.81   **Umbilical granuloma**
         Excludes2   Granulomatous disorder of the skin and subcutaneous tissue, unspecified (L92.9)
     P83.88   **Other specified conditions of integument specific to newborn**
         Bronze baby syndrome
         Neonatal scleroderma
         Urticaria neonatorum

P83.9   **Condition of the integument specific to newborn, unspecified**

OTHER PROBLEMS WITH NEWBORN (P84)

P84   **Other problems with newborn**
     Acidemia of newborn
     Acidosis of newborn
     Anoxia of newborn NOS
     Asphyxia of newborn NOS
     Hypercapnia of newborn
     Hypoxemia of newborn
     Hypoxia of newborn NOS
     Mixed metabolic and respiratory acidosis of newborn
     Excludes1   intracranial hemorrhage due to anoxia or hypoxia (P52.-)
         hypoxic ischemic encephalopathy [HIE] (P91.6-)
         late metabolic acidosis of newborn (P74.0)

OTHER DISORDERS ORIGINATING IN THE PERINATAL PERIOD (P90-P96)

P90   **Convulsions of newborn**
     Excludes1   benign myoclonic epilepsy in infancy (G40.3-)
         benign neonatal convulsions (familial) (G40.3-)

● **P91**   **Other disturbances of cerebral status of newborn**
     P91.0   **Neonatal cerebral ischemia**
         Excludes1   Neonatal cerebral infarction (P91.82-)
     P91.1   **Acquired periventricular cysts of newborn**
     P91.2   **Neonatal cerebral leukomalacia**
         Degeneration of white matter adjacent to cerebral ventricles following cerebral hypoxia or brain ischemia in neonates
         Periventricular leukomalacia
     P91.3   **Neonatal cerebral irritability**
     P91.4   **Neonatal cerebral depression**
     P91.5   **Neonatal coma**
●   **P91.6**   **Hypoxic ischemic encephalopathy [HIE]**
         Excludes1   Neonatal cerebral depression (P91.4)
         Neonatal cerebral irritability (P91.3)
         Neonatal coma (P91.5)
     P91.60   **Hypoxic ischemic encephalopathy [HIE], unspecified**
     P91.61   **Mild hypoxic ischemic encephalopathy [HIE]**

P91.62   **Moderate hypoxic ischemic encephalopathy [HIE]**

P91.63   **Severe hypoxic ischemic encephalopathy [HIE]**

● **P91.8**   **Other specified disturbances of cerebral status of newborn**
     ● **P91.81**   **Neonatal encephalopathy**
         P91.811   **Neonatal encephalopathy in diseases classified elsewhere**
             Code first underlying condition, if known, such as:
             congenital cirrhosis (of liver) (P78.81)
             intracranial nontraumatic hemorrhage of newborn (P52.-)
             kernicterus (P57.-)
         P91.819   **Neonatal encephalopathy, unspecified**
     ● **P91.82**   **Neonatal cerebral infarction**
         Neonatal stroke
         Perinatal arterial ischemic stroke
         Perinatal cerebral infarction
         Excludes1   cerebral infarction (I63.-)
         Excludes2   intracranial hemorrhage of newborn (P52.-)
         P91.821   **Neonatal cerebral infarction, right side of brain**
         P91.822   **Neonatal cerebral infarction, left side of brain**
         P91.823   **Neonatal cerebral infarction, bilateral**
         P91.829   **Neonatal cerebral infarction, unspecified side**
     P91.88   **Other specified disturbances of cerebral status of newborn**

P91.9   **Disturbance of cerebral status of newborn, unspecified**

● **P92**   **Feeding problems of newborn**
     Excludes2   feeding problems in child over 28 days old (R63.3-)
     Coding Clinic: 2017, Q1, P28; 2016, Q3, P19
     ● **P92.0**   **Vomiting of newborn**
         Excludes1   vomiting of child over 28 days old (R11.-)
         P92.01   **Bilious vomiting of newborn**
             Excludes1   bilious vomiting in child over 28 days old (R11.14)
         P92.09   **Other vomiting of newborn**
             Excludes1   regurgitation of food in newborn (P92.1)
     P92.1   **Regurgitation and rumination of newborn**
     P92.2   **Slow feeding of newborn**
     P92.3   **Underfeeding of newborn**
     P92.4   **Overfeeding of newborn**
     P92.5   **Neonatal difficulty in feeding at breast**
         Coding Clinic: 2017, Q1, P28; 2016, Q3, P19
     P92.6   **Failure to thrive in newborn**
         Excludes1   failure to thrive in child over 28 days old (R62.51)
     P92.8   **Other feeding problems of newborn**
     P92.9   **Feeding problem of newborn, unspecified**

CHAPTER 16 (P00-P96)

● **P93** **Reactions and intoxications due to drugs administered to newborn**

> **Includes**   reactions and intoxications due to drugs administered to fetus affecting newborn
>
> **Excludes1**   jaundice due to drugs or toxins transmitted from mother or given to newborn (P58.4-)
> reactions and intoxications from maternal opiates, tranquilizers and other medication (P04.0-P04.1, P04.4-)
> withdrawal symptoms from maternal use of drugs of addiction (P96.1)
> withdrawal symptoms from therapeutic use of drugs in newborn (P96.2)

P93.0   **Grey baby syndrome**
> Grey syndrome from chloramphenicol administration in newborn

P93.8   **Other reactions and intoxications due to drugs administered to newborn**
> **Use additional** code for adverse effect, if applicable, to identify drug (T36-T50 with fifth or sixth character 5)

● **P94** **Disorders of muscle tone of newborn**

P94.0   **Transient neonatal myasthenia gravis**
> **Excludes1**   myasthenia gravis (G70.0)

P94.1   **Congenital hypertonia**

P94.2   **Congenital hypotonia**
> Floppy baby syndrome, unspecified

P94.8   **Other disorders of muscle tone of newborn**

P94.9   **Disorder of muscle tone of newborn, unspecified**

OGCR Section I.C.16.g.

> Stillbirth
> Code P95, Stillbirth, is only for use for institutions that maintain separate records for stillbirths. No other code should be used with P95. Code P95 should not be used on the mother's record.

P95 **Stillbirth**
> Deadborn fetus NOS
> Fetal death of unspecified cause
> Stillbirth NOS
>
> **Excludes1**   maternal care for intrauterine death (O36.4)
> missed abortion (O02.1)
> outcome of delivery, stillbirth (Z37.1, Z37.3, Z37.4, Z37.7)

● **P96** **Other conditions originating in the perinatal period**

P96.0   **Congenital renal failure**
> Uremia of newborn

P96.1   **Neonatal withdrawal symptoms from maternal use of drugs of addiction**
> Drug withdrawal syndrome in infant of dependent mother
> Neonatal abstinence syndrome
>
> **Excludes1**   reactions and intoxications from maternal opiates and tranquilizers administered during labor and delivery (P04.0)

P96.2   **Withdrawal symptoms from therapeutic use of drugs in newborn**

P96.3   **Wide cranial sutures of newborn**
> Neonatal craniotabes

P96.5   **Complication to newborn due to (fetal) intrauterine procedure**
> **Excludes2**   newborn affected by amniocentesis (P00.6)

● **P96.8** **Other specified conditions originating in the perinatal period**

P96.81   **Exposure to (parental) (environmental) tobacco smoke in the perinatal period**
> **Excludes2**   newborn affected by in utero exposure to tobacco (P04.2)
> exposure to environmental tobacco smoke after the perinatal period (Z77.22)

P96.82   **Delayed separation of umbilical cord**

P96.83   **Meconium staining**
> **Excludes1**   meconium aspiration (P24.00, P24.01)
> meconium passage during delivery (P03.82)

P96.89   **Other specified conditions originating in the perinatal period**
> **Use additional** code to specify condition

P96.9   **Condition originating in the perinatal period, unspecified**
> Congenital debility NOS

CHAPTER 17

CONGENITAL MALFORMATIONS, DEFORMATIONS, AND CHROMOSOMAL ABNORMALITIES (Q00-Q99)

OGCR Chapter-Specific Coding Guidelines

17. **Chapter 17: Congenital malformations, deformations, and chromosomal abnormalities (Q00-Q99)**
Assign an appropriate code(s) from categories Q00-Q99, Congenital malformations, deformations, and chromosomal abnormalities when a malformation/deformation or chromosomal abnormality is documented. A malformation/deformation/ or chromosomal abnormality may be the principal/first-listed diagnosis on a record or a secondary diagnosis.

When a malformation/deformation/or chromosomal abnormality does not have a unique code assignment, assign additional code(s) for any manifestations that may be present.

When the code assignment specifically identifies the malformation/deformation/or chromosomal abnormality, manifestations that are an inherent component of the anomaly should not be coded separately. Additional codes should be assigned for manifestations that are not an inherent component.

Codes from Chapter 17 may be used throughout the life of the patient. If a congenital malformation or deformity has been corrected, a personal history code should be used to identify the history of the malformation or deformity. Although present at birth, malformation/deformation/or chromosomal abnormality may not be identified until later in life. Whenever the condition is diagnosed by the physician, it is appropriate to assign a code from codes Q00-Q99.

For the birth admission, the appropriate code from category Z38, Liveborn infants, according to place of birth and type of delivery, should be sequenced as the principal diagnosis, followed by any congenital anomaly codes, Q00-Q99.

CHAPTER 17

CONGENITAL MALFORMATIONS, DEFORMATIONS, AND CHROMOSOMAL ABNORMALITIES (Q00-Q99)

Note: Codes from this chapter are not for use on maternal records

Excludes2 inborn errors of metabolism (E70-E88)

This chapter contains the following blocks:

Q00-Q07	Congenital malformations of the nervous system
Q10-Q18	Congenital malformations of eye, ear, face and neck
Q20-Q28	Congenital malformations of the circulatory system
Q30-Q34	Congenital malformations of the respiratory system
Q35-Q37	Cleft lip and cleft palate
Q38-Q45	Other congenital malformations of the digestive system
Q50-Q56	Congenital malformations of genital organs
Q60-Q64	Congenital malformations of the urinary system
Q65-Q79	Congenital malformations and deformations of the musculoskeletal system
Q80-Q89	Other congenital malformations
Q90-Q99	Chromosomal abnormalities, not elsewhere classified
▶ QA0	Genetic disorders, not elsewhere classified

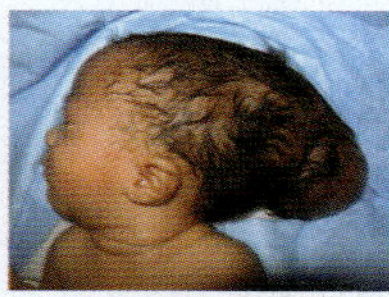

Figure 17-1   An infant with a large occipital encephalocele. The large skin-covered encephalocele is visible. (From Swaiman KF, Ashwal S, Ferriero DM: Pediatric Neurology: Principles and Practice, Philadelphia, Saunders, 2012)

CONGENITAL MALFORMATIONS OF THE NERVOUS SYSTEM (Q00–Q07)

● **Q00**   **Anencephaly and similar malformations**
   Q00.0   **Anencephaly** 🔍
     Absence of skull with cerebral hemispheres missing or reduced to small masses attached to base of cranium
     Acephaly
     Acrania
     Amyelencephaly
     Hemianencephaly
     Hemicephaly

   Q00.1   **Craniorachischisis** 🔍
     Developmental anomaly consisting of fissure of cranium and vertebral column

   Q00.2   **Iniencephaly** 🔍
     Developmental anomaly characterized by enlargement of foramen magnum and absence of laminae and spinous processes of cervical, dorsal

● **Q01**   **Encephalocele**
   Sac-like protrusions of brain and membranes visible through an opening in skull

   Includes   Arnold-Chiari syndrome, type III
     encephalocystocele
     encephalomyelocele
     hydroencephalocele
     hydromeningocele, cranial
     meningocele, cerebral
     meningoencephalocele

   Excludes1   Meckel-Gruber syndrome (Q61.9)

   Q01.0   **Frontal encephalocele** 🔍
   Q01.1   **Nasofrontal encephalocele** 🔍
   Q01.2   **Occipital encephalocele** 🔍
   Q01.8   **Encephalocele of other sites** 🔍
   Q01.9   **Encephalocele, unspecified** 🔍

● **Q02**   **Microcephaly** 🔍
   Head size measures significantly below normal based on standardized charts

   Includes   hydromicrocephaly
     micrencephalon

   Code first, if applicable, congenital Zika virus disease

   Excludes1   Meckel-Gruber syndrome (Q61.9)

   Coding Clinic: 2018, Q4, P26; 2016, Q4, P7

● **Q03**   **Congenital hydrocephalus**
   Accumulation of cerebrospinal fluid in ventricles resulting in swelling and enlargement

   Includes   hydrocephalus in newborn

   Excludes1   Arnold-Chiari syndrome, type II (Q07.0-)
     acquired hydrocephalus (G91.-)
     hydrocephalus due to congenital toxoplasmosis (P37.1)
     hydrocephalus with spina bifida (Q05.0-Q05.4)

   Q03.0   **Malformations of aqueduct of Sylvius** 🔍
     Anomaly of aqueduct of Sylvius
     Obstruction of aqueduct of Sylvius, congenital
     Stenosis of aqueduct of Sylvius

   Q03.1   **Atresia of foramina of Magendie and Luschka** 🔍
     Dandy-Walker syndrome

   Q03.8   **Other congenital hydrocephalus** 🔍
   Q03.9   **Congenital hydrocephalus, unspecified** 🔍

CHAPTER 17 (Q00-Q99)

● **Q04   Other congenital malformations of brain**
> **Excludes1**   cyclopia (Q87.0)
> macrocephaly (Q75.3)

Q04.0   Congenital malformations of corpus callosum 🄷
Agenesis of corpus callosum

Q04.1   Arhinencephaly 🄷
Congenital absence of olfactory bulbs, tract, or nerves

Q04.2   Holoprosencephaly 🄷
Failure of cleavage of forebrain (prosencephalon) resulting in incomplete or absent cortical separation and deficits in midline facial development

Q04.3   Other reduction deformities of brain 🄷
Absence of part of brain
Agenesis of part of brain
Cerebral cortex are not fully formed, brain surface is smooth
Agyria
Aplasia of part of brain
Hydranencephaly
Hypoplasia of part of brain
Lissencephaly
Congenital malformation or absence of convolutions of cerebral cortex
Microgyria
Malformation of brain characterized by excessive number of small convolutions (gyri) on surface
Pachygyria
Reduction in number of sulci of cerebrum
> **Excludes1**   congenital malformations of corpus callosum (Q04.0)

Q04.4   Septo-optic dysplasia of brain 🄷

Q04.5   Megalencephaly 🄷
Abnormally large brain

Q04.6   Congenital cerebral cysts 🄷
Porencephaly   Schizencephaly
> **Excludes1**   acquired porencephalic cyst (G93.0)

Q04.8   Other specified congenital malformations of brain 🄷
Arnold-Chiari syndrome, type IV
Macrogyria

Q04.9   Congenital malformation of brain, unspecified 🄷
Congenital anomaly NOS of brain
Congenital deformity NOS of brain
Congenital disease or lesion NOS of brain
Multiple anomalies NOS of brain, congenital

● **Q05   Spina bifida**
Developmental anomaly characterized by defective closure of vertebral arch, through which spinal cord and meninges may protrude
> **Includes**   hydromeningocele (spinal)
> meningocele (spinal)
> meningomyelocele
> myelocele
> myelomeningocele
> rachischisis
> spina bifida (aperta)(cystica)
> syringomyelocele

Use additional code for any associated paraplegia (paraparesis) (G82.2-)
> **Excludes1**   Arnold-Chiari syndrome, type II (Q07.0-)
> spina bifida occulta (Q76.0)

Q05.0   Cervical spina bifida with hydrocephalus 🄷

Q05.1   Thoracic spina bifida with hydrocephalus 🄷
Dorsal spina bifida with hydrocephalus
Thoracolumbar spina bifida with hydrocephalus

Q05.2   Lumbar spina bifida with hydrocephalus 🄷
Lumbosacral spina bifida with hydrocephalus

Q05.3   Sacral spina bifida with hydrocephalus 🄷

Q05.4   Unspecified spina bifida with hydrocephalus 🄷

Q05.5   Cervical spina bifida without hydrocephalus 🄷

Q05.6   Thoracic spina bifida without hydrocephalus 🄷
Dorsal spina bifida NOS
Thoracolumbar spina bifida NOS

Q05.7   Lumbar spina bifida without hydrocephalus 🄷
Lumbosacral spina bifida NOS

Q05.8   Sacral spina bifida without hydrocephalus 🄷

Q05.9   Spina bifida, unspecified 🄷

● **Q06   Other congenital malformations of spinal cord**

Q06.0   Amyelia 🄷
Congenital absence of spinal cord

Q06.1   Hypoplasia and dysplasia of spinal cord 🄷
Underdevelopment of spinal cord
Atelomyelia
Congenitally incomplete development of spinal cord
Myelatelia
Myelodysplasia of spinal cord
Defective development of spinal cord, especially lower segments

Q06.2   Diastematomyelia 🄷
Congenital anomaly, associated with spina bifida, in which spinal cord is split into halves and surrounded by dural sac

Q06.3   Other congenital cauda equina malformations 🄷

Q06.4   Hydromyelia 🄷
Dilation of central canal of spinal cord with increased fluid accumulation
Hydrorachis

Q06.8   Other specified congenital malformations of spinal cord 🄷

Q06.9   Congenital malformation of spinal cord, unspecified 🄷
Congenital anomaly NOS of spinal cord
Congenital deformity NOS of spinal cord
Congenital disease or lesion NOS of spinal cord

● **Q07   Other congenital malformations of nervous system**
> **Excludes2**   congenital central alveolar hypoventilation syndrome (G47.35)
> familial dysautonomia [Riley-Day] (G90.1)
> neurofibromatosis (nonmalignant) (Q85.0-)

● **Q07.0   Arnold-Chiari syndrome**
Herniation of cerebellar tonsils and vermis through foramen magnum into spinal canal
Arnold-Chiari syndrome, type II
> **Excludes1**   Arnold-Chiari syndrome, type III (Q01.-)
> Arnold-Chiari syndrome, type IV (Q04.8)

Q07.00   Arnold-Chiari syndrome without spina bifida or hydrocephalus 🄷

Q07.01   Arnold-Chiari syndrome with spina bifida 🄷

Q07.02   Arnold-Chiari syndrome with hydrocephalus 🄷

Q07.03   Arnold-Chiari syndrome with spina bifida and hydrocephalus 🄷

Q07.8   Other specified congenital malformations of nervous system 🄷
Agenesis of nerve
Displacement of brachial plexus
Jaw-winking syndrome
Marcus Gunn's syndrome

Q07.9   Congenital malformation of nervous system, unspecified 🄷
Congenital anomaly NOS of nervous system
Congenital deformity NOS of nervous system
Congenital disease or lesion NOS of nervous system

CHAPTER 17 (Q00-QA0.8)

CONGENITAL MALFORMATIONS OF EYE, EAR, FACE AND NECK (Q10-Q18)

Excludes2   cleft lip and cleft palate (Q35-Q37)
congenital malformation of cervical spine (Q05.0,
Q05.5, Q67.5, Q76.0-Q76.4)
congenital malformation of larynx (Q31.-)
congenital malformation of lip NEC (Q38.0)
congenital malformation of nose (Q30.-)
congenital malformation of parathyroid gland
(Q89.2)
congenital malformation of thyroid gland (Q89.2)

● **Q10** **Congenital malformations of eyelid, lacrimal apparatus and orbit**

Excludes1   cryptophthalmos NOS (Q11.2)
cryptophthalmos syndrome (Q87.0)

Q10.0 **Congenital ptosis**
*Prolapse or drooping of upper eyelid from paralysis of third
nerve or from sympathetic innervations*

Q10.1 **Congenital ectropion**
Outward turning of eyelid

Q10.2 **Congenital entropion**
Inward turning of eyelid

Q10.3 **Other congenital malformations of eyelid**
Ablepharon
Blepharophimosis, congenital
Coloboma of eyelid
Congenital absence or agenesis of cilia
Congenital absence or agenesis of eyelid
Congenital accessory eyelid
Congenital accessory eye muscle
Congenital malformation of eyelid NOS

Q10.4 **Absence and agenesis of lacrimal apparatus**
Congenital absence of punctum lacrimale

Q10.5 **Congenital stenosis and stricture of lacrimal duct**

Q10.6 **Other congenital malformations of lacrimal apparatus**
Congenital malformation of lacrimal apparatus NOS

Q10.7 **Congenital malformation of orbit**

● **Q11** **Anophthalmos, microphthalmos and macrophthalmos**
Absence of eye and optic pit

Q11.0 **Cystic eyeball**

Q11.1 **Other anophthalmos**
Anophthalmos NOS
Agenesis of eye
Absence of eye
Aplasia of eye

Q11.2 **Microphthalmos**
Partial absence of eye and optic pit
Cryptophthalmos NOS
Dysplasia of eye
Hypoplasia of eye
Rudimentary eye

Excludes1   cryptophthalmos syndrome (Q87.0)

Q11.3 **Macrophthalmos**
Congenital enlargement of eyes

Excludes1   macrophthalmos in congenital glaucoma
(Q15.0)

● **Q12** **Congenital lens malformations**

Q12.0 **Congenital cataract**

Q12.1 **Congenital displaced lens**

Q12.2 **Coloboma of lens**

Q12.3 **Congenital aphakia**

Q12.4 **Spherophakia**
Smaller, more spherical optic lens than normal

Q12.8 **Other congenital lens malformations**
Microphakia

Q12.9 **Congenital lens malformation, unspecified**

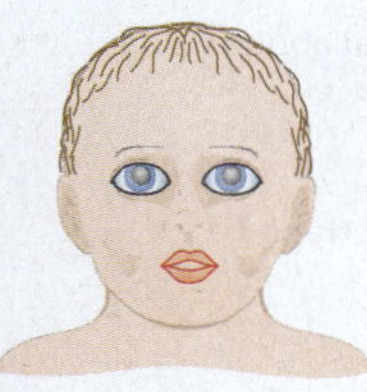

Figure 17-2 Bilateral congenital
hydrophthalmia, in which the eyes
are very large in comparison to the
other facial features due to glaucoma.

● **Q13** **Congenital malformations of anterior segment of eye**

Q13.0 **Coloboma of iris**
Coloboma NOS

Q13.1 **Absence of iris**
Aniridia
Use additional code for associated glaucoma (H42)

Q13.2 **Other congenital malformations of iris**
Anisocoria, congenital
Atresia of pupil
Congenital malformation of iris NOS
Corectopia

Q13.3 **Congenital corneal opacity**

Q13.4 **Other congenital corneal malformations**
Congenital malformation of cornea NOS
Microcornea
Peter's anomaly

Q13.5 **Blue sclera**
Condition of unusual blueness of sclera; not harmful

● **Q13.8** **Other congenital malformations of anterior segment of eye**

Q13.81 **Rieger anomaly**
Axenfeld-Rieger syndrome
Code also any other associated congenital
malformations such as cardiac defects
Use additional code for associated glaucoma
(H42)

Q13.89 **Other congenital malformations of anterior
segment of eye**

Q13.9 **Congenital malformation of anterior segment of eye,
unspecified**

● **Q14** **Congenital malformations of posterior segment of eye**

Excludes2   optic nerve hypoplasia (H47.03-)

Q14.0 **Congenital malformation of vitreous humor**
Congenital vitreous opacity

Q14.1 **Congenital malformation of retina**
Congenital retinal aneurysm

Q14.2 **Congenital malformation of optic disc**
Coloboma of optic disc

Q14.3 **Congenital malformation of choroid**

Q14.8 **Other congenital malformations of posterior segment of
eye**
Coloboma of the fundus

Q14.9 **Congenital malformation of posterior segment of eye,
unspecified**

● **Q15** **Other congenital malformations of eye**

Excludes1   congenital nystagmus (H55.01)
ocular albinism (E70.31-)
optic nerve hypoplasia (H47.03-)
retinitis pigmentosa (H35.52)

Q15.0 **Congenital glaucoma**
Axenfeld's anomaly
Buphthalmos
*Congenital syndrome characterized by enlargement of the
eye with symptoms of glaucoma.*
Glaucoma of childhood
Glaucoma of newborn
Hydrophthalmos
Keratoglobus, congenital, with glaucoma
Macrocornea with glaucoma
Macrophthalmos in congenital glaucoma
Megalocornea with glaucoma

Q15.8 **Other specified congenital malformations of eye**

Q15.9 **Congenital malformation of eye, unspecified**
Congenital anomaly of eye
Congenital deformity of eye

● **Q16** **Congenital malformations of ear causing impairment of hearing**

Excludes1   congenital deafness (H90.-)

Q16.0 **Congenital absence of (ear) auricle**

Q16.1 **Congenital absence, atresia and stricture of auditory
canal (external)**
Congenital atresia or stricture of osseous meatus

Q16.2 **Absence of eustachian tube**

Q16.3 Congenital malformation of ear ossicles
Congenital fusion of ear ossicles

Q16.4 Other congenital malformations of middle ear
Congenital malformation of middle ear NOS

Q16.5 Congenital malformation of inner ear
Congenital anomaly of membranous labyrinth
Congenital anomaly of organ of Corti

Q16.9 Congenital malformation of ear causing impairment of hearing, unspecified
Congenital absence of ear NOS

● **Q17 Other congenital malformations of ear**
> **Excludes1** congenital malformations of ear with impairment of hearing (Q16.0-Q16.9)
> preauricular sinus (Q18.1)

Q17.0 Accessory auricle
Accessory tragus
Polyotia
Preauricular appendage or tag
Supernumerary ear
Supernumerary lobule

Q17.1 Macrotia
Enlarged ears

Q17.2 Microtia
An abnormally small or underdeveloped external ear

Q17.3 Other misshapen ear
Pointed ear

Q17.4 Misplaced ear
Low-set ears
> **Excludes1** cervical auricle (Q18.2)

Q17.5 Prominent ear
Bat ear

Q17.8 Other specified congenital malformations of ear
Congenital absence of lobe of ear

Q17.9 Congenital malformation of ear, unspecified
Congenital anomaly of ear NOS

● **Q18 Other congenital malformations of face and neck**
> **Excludes1** cleft lip and cleft palate (Q35-Q37)
> conditions classified to Q67.0-Q67.4
> congenital malformations of skull and face bones (Q75.-)
> cyclopia (Q87.0)
> dentofacial anomalies [including malocclusion] (M26.-)
> malformation syndromes affecting facial appearance (Q87.0)
> persistent thyroglossal duct (Q89.2)

Q18.0 Sinus, fistula and cyst of branchial cleft
Branchial vestige
Brachial remnants (cysts, fistula, skin tags) that are developmental anomalies

Q18.1 Preauricular sinus and cyst
Fistula of auricle, congenital
Cervicoaural fistula
Abnormal passage in neck originating from first branchial cleft

Q18.2 Other branchial cleft malformations
Branchial cleft malformation NOS
Cervical auricle
Otocephaly

Q18.3 Webbing of neck
Pterygium colli
Thick fold of skin on side of neck

Q18.4 Macrostomia
Results from failure of union of maxillary and mandibular processes, results in abnormally large mouth

Q18.5 Microstomia

Q18.6 Macrocheilia
Excessive size of lips
Hypertrophy of lip, congenital

Q18.7 Microcheilia
Abnormal smallness of lips

Q18.8 Other specified congenital malformations of face and neck
Medial cyst of face and neck
Medial fistula of face and neck
Medial sinus of face and neck

Q18.9 Congenital malformation of face and neck, unspecified
Congenital anomaly NOS of face and neck

CONGENITAL MALFORMATIONS OF THE CIRCULATORY SYSTEM (Q20-Q28)

● **Q20 Congenital malformations of cardiac chambers and connections**
> **Excludes1** dextrocardia with situs inversus (Q89.3)
> mirror-image atrial arrangement with situs inversus (Q89.3)

Q20.0 Common arterial trunk
Persistent truncus arteriosus
> **Excludes1** aortic septal defect (Q21.4)

Q20.1 Double outlet right ventricle
Taussig-Bing syndrome

Q20.2 Double outlet left ventricle

Q20.3 Discordant ventriculoarterial connection
Dextrotransposition of aorta
Transposition of great vessels (complete)

Q20.4 Double inlet ventricle
Common ventricle
Cor triloculare biatriatum
Single ventricle

Q20.5 Discordant atrioventricular connection
Corrected transposition
Levotransposition
Ventricular inversion

Q20.6 Isomerism of atrial appendages
Isomerism of atrial appendages with asplenia or polysplenia

Q20.8 Other congenital malformations of cardiac chambers and connections
Cor binoculare

Q20.9 Congenital malformation of cardiac chambers and connections, unspecified

● **Q21 Congenital malformations of cardiac septa**
> **Excludes1** acquired cardiac septal defect (I51.0)

Q21.0 Ventricular septal defect
Roger's disease

Q21.1 Atrial septal defect
> **Excludes 2** ostium primum atrial septal defect (type I) (Q21.20)

Q21.10 Atrial septal defect, unspecified

Q21.11 Secundum atrial septal defect
Fenestrated atrial septum
Patent or persistent ostium secundum defect (type II)

Q21.12 Patent foramen ovale
Persistent foramen ovale

Q21.13 Coronary sinus atrial septal defect
Coronary sinus defect
Unroofed coronary sinus

Q21.14 Superior sinus venosus atrial septal defect
Superior vena cava type atrial septal defect

Q21.15 Inferior sinus venosus atrial septal defect
Inferior vena cava type atrial septal defect

Q21.16 Sinus venosus atrial septal defect, unspecified
Sinus venosus defect, NOS

Q21.19 Other specified atrial septal defect
Common atrium
Other specified atrial septal abnormality

Q21.2 Atrioventricular septal defect
Atrioventricular canal defect
Endocardial cushion defect
Ostium primum atrial septal defect (type I)

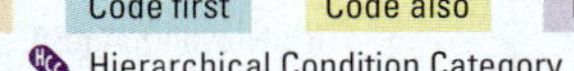

Q21.20 **Atrioventricular septal defect, unspecified as to partial or complete**
Atrioventricular canal, NOS
Endocardial cushion defect NOS
Ostium primum atrial septal defect (type I) NOS

Q21.21 **Partial atrioventricular septal defect**
Incomplete atrioventricular canal
Incomplete atrioventricular septal defect
Incomplete endocardial cushion defect
Ostium primum atrial septal defect (type I)
with separate atrioventricular valves
Partial atrioventricular canal
Partial endocardial cushion defect

Q21.22 **Transitional atrioventricular septal defect**
Intermediate atrioventricular canal
Intermediate atrioventricular septal defect
Intermediate endocardial cushion defect
Ostium primum atrial septal defect (type I)
with separate atrioventricular valves and
a small or restrictive inlet VSD
Transitional atrioventricular canal
Transitional endocardial cushion defect

Q21.23 **Complete atrioventricular septal defect**
Common atrioventricular canal
Common atrioventricular septal defect
Common endocardial cushion defect
Ostium primum atrial septal defect (type I)
with common atrioventricular valve and a
moderate or larger inlet VSD

Q21.3 **Tetralogy of Fallot**
Ventricular septal defect with pulmonary stenosis or
atresia, dextroposition of aorta and hypertrophy of
right ventricle.

Q21.4 **Aortopulmonary septal defect**
Aortic septal defect
Aortopulmonary window

Q21.8 **Other congenital malformations of cardiac septa**
Eisenmenger's defect
Pentalogy of Fallot
Code also, if applicable:
Eisenmenger's complex (I27.83)
Eisenmenger's syndrome (I27.83)

Q21.9 **Congenital malformation of cardiac septum, unspecified**
Septal (heart) defect NOS

● **Q22** **Congenital malformations of pulmonary and tricuspid valves**

Q22.0 **Pulmonary valve atresia**

Q22.1 **Congenital pulmonary valve stenosis**

Q22.2 **Congenital pulmonary valve insufficiency**
Congenital pulmonary valve regurgitation

Q22.3 **Other congenital malformations of pulmonary valve**
Congenital malformation of pulmonary valve NOS
Supernumerary cusps of pulmonary valve

Q22.4 **Congenital tricuspid stenosis**
Congenital tricuspid atresia

Q22.5 **Ebstein's anomaly**
Malformation of tricuspid valve

Q22.6 **Hypoplastic right heart syndrome**

Q22.8 **Other congenital malformations of tricuspid valve**

Q22.9 **Congenital malformation of tricuspid valve, unspecified**

● **Q23** **Congenital malformations of aortic and mitral valves**

Q23.0 **Congenital stenosis of aortic valve**
Congenital aortic atresia
Congenital aortic stenosis NOS

Excludes1   congenital stenosis of aortic valve in
hypoplastic left heart syndrome
(Q23.4)
congenital subaortic stenosis (Q24.4)
supravalvular aortic stenosis (congenital)
(Q25.3)

Q23.1 **Congenital insufficiency of aortic valve**
Congenital aortic insufficiency

Q23.2 **Congenital mitral stenosis**
Congenital mitral atresia

Q23.3 **Congenital mitral insufficiency**

Q23.4 **Hypoplastic left heart syndrome**

Q23.8 **Other congenital malformations of aortic and mitral valves**

Q23.81 **Bicuspid aortic valve**
Congenital bicuspid aortic valve
Unicuspid (congenital) aortic valve (at birth)
Code also, if applicable, acquired aortic valve
disorders, such as:
aortic (valve) insufficiency (nonrheumatic)
(I35.1)
aortic (valve) stenosis (nonrheumatic) (I35.0)
aortic (valve) stenosis with insufficiency
(nonrheumatic) (I35.2)
Coding Clinic: 2024, Q4, P26

Q23.82 **Congenital mitral valve cleft leaflet**
Cleft mitral valve leaflet at birth

Q23.88 **Other congenital malformations of aortic and mitral valves**

Q23.9 **Congenital malformation of aortic and mitral valves, unspecified**

● **Q24** **Other congenital malformations of heart**
Excludes1   endocardial fibroelastosis (I42.4)

Q24.0 **Dextrocardia**
Heart is located in right hemithorax
Excludes1   dextrocardia with situs inversus (Q89.3)
isomerism of atrial appendages (with
asplenia or polysplenia) (Q20.6)
mirror-image atrial arrangement with
situs inversus (Q89.3)

Q24.1 **Levocardia**
Normal position of heart but related structures on wrong side

Q24.2 **Cor triatriatum**
Congenital heart defect; left atrium is subdivided

Q24.3 **Pulmonary infundibular stenosis**
Subvalvular pulmonic stenosis

Q24.4 **Congenital subaortic stenosis**

Q24.5 **Malformation of coronary vessels**
Congenital coronary (artery) aneurysm

Q24.6 **Congenital heart block**

Q24.8 **Other specified congenital malformations of heart**
Congenital diverticulum of left ventricle
Congenital malformation of myocardium
Congenital malformation of pericardium
Malposition of heart
Uhl's disease

Q24.9 **Congenital malformation of heart, unspecified**
Congenital anomaly of heart
Congenital disease of heart

● **Q25** **Congenital malformations of great arteries**

Q25.0 **Patent ductus arteriosus**
Fetal blood vessel connecting left pulmonary artery directly to descending aorta
Patent ductus Botallo
Persistent ductus arteriosus

Q25.1 **Coarctation of aorta**
Coarctation of aorta (preductal) (postductal)
Stenosis of aorta
Coding Clinic: 2016, Q4, P56-57

● **Q25.2** **Atresia of aorta**
Coding Clinic: 2016, Q4, P56

Q25.21 **Interruption of aortic arch**
Atresia of aortic arch

Q25.29 **Other atresia of aorta**
Atresia of aorta

Q25.3 **Supravalvular aortic stenosis**
Excludes1   congenital aortic stenosis NOS (Q23.0)
congenital stenosis of aortic valve (Q23.0)

CHAPTER 17 (Q00-Q99)

CHAPTER 17 (Q00–QA0.8)

● **Q25.4   Other congenital malformations of aorta**

     Excludes1   hypoplasia of aorta in hypoplastic left heart syndrome (Q23.4)

     Coding Clinic: 2016, Q4, P57

     Q25.40   Congenital malformation of aorta unspecified

     Q25.41   Absence and aplasia of aorta

     Q25.42   Hypoplasia of aorta

     Q25.43   Congenital aneurysm of aorta
        Congenital aneurysm of aortic root
        Congenital aneurysm of aortic sinus

     Q25.44   Congenital dilation of aorta

     Q25.45   Double aortic arch
        Vascular ring of aorta

     Q25.46   Tortuous aortic arch
        Persistent convolutions of aortic arch

     Q25.47   Right aortic arch
        Persistent right aortic arch

     Q25.48   Anomalous origin of subclavian artery

     Q25.49   Other congenital malformations of aorta
        Aortic arch
        Bovine arch

Q25.5   Atresia of pulmonary artery

Q25.6   Stenosis of pulmonary artery
     Supravalvular pulmonary stenosis

● **Q25.7   Other congenital malformations of pulmonary artery**

     Q25.71   Coarctation of pulmonary artery

     Q25.72   Congenital pulmonary arteriovenous malformation
        Congenital pulmonary arteriovenous aneurysm

     Q25.79   Other congenital malformations of pulmonary artery
        Aberrant pulmonary artery
        Agenesis of pulmonary artery
        Congenital aneurysm of pulmonary artery
        Congenital anomaly of pulmonary artery
        Hypoplasia of pulmonary artery

Q25.8   Other congenital malformations of other great arteries

Q25.9   Congenital malformation of great arteries, unspecified

● **Q26   Congenital malformations of great veins**

Q26.0   Congenital stenosis of vena cava
     Congenital stenosis of vena cava (inferior)(superior)

Q26.1   Persistent left superior vena cava

Q26.2   Total anomalous pulmonary venous connection
     Total anomalous pulmonary venous return [TAPVR], subdiaphragmatic
     Total anomalous pulmonary venous return [TAPVR], supradiaphragmatic

Q26.3   Partial anomalous pulmonary venous connection
     Partial anomalous pulmonary venous return

Q26.4   Anomalous pulmonary venous connection, unspecified

Q26.5   Anomalous portal venous connection

Q26.6   Portal vein-hepatic artery fistula

Q26.8   Other congenital malformations of great veins
     Absence of vena cava (inferior) (superior)
     Azygos continuation of inferior vena cava
     Persistent left posterior cardinal vein
     Scimitar syndrome

Q26.9   Congenital malformation of great vein, unspecified
     Congenital anomaly of vena cava (inferior) (superior) NOS

● **Q27   Other congenital malformations of peripheral vascular system**

     Excludes2   anomalies of cerebral and precerebral vessels (Q28.0-Q28.3)
        anomalies of coronary vessels (Q24.5)
        anomalies of pulmonary artery (Q25.5-Q25.7)
        congenital retinal aneurysm (Q14.1)
        hemangioma and lymphangioma (D18.-)

Q27.0   Congenital absence and hypoplasia of umbilical artery
     Single umbilical artery

Q27.1   Congenital renal artery stenosis

Q27.2   Other congenital malformations of renal artery
     Congenital malformation of renal artery NOS
     Multiple renal arteries

● **Q27.3   Arteriovenous malformation (peripheral)**
     Arteriovenous aneurysm

     Excludes1   acquired arteriovenous aneurysm (I77.0)

     Excludes2   arteriovenous malformation of cerebral vessels (Q28.2)
        arteriovenous malformation of precerebral vessels (Q28.0)

     Q27.30   Arteriovenous malformation, site unspecified

     Q27.31   Arteriovenous malformation of vessel of upper limb

     Q27.32   Arteriovenous malformation of vessel of lower limb

     Q27.33   Arteriovenous malformation of digestive system vessel

     Q27.34   Arteriovenous malformation of renal vessel

     Q27.39   Arteriovenous malformation, other site

Q27.4   Congenital phlebectasia

Q27.8   Other specified congenital malformations of peripheral vascular system
     Absence of peripheral vascular system
     Atresia of peripheral vascular system
     Congenital aneurysm (peripheral)
     Congenital stricture, artery
     Congenital varix

     Excludes1   arteriovenous malformation (Q27.3-)

Q27.9   Congenital malformation of peripheral vascular system, unspecified
     Anomaly of artery or vein NOS

● **Q28   Other congenital malformations of circulatory system**

     Excludes1   congenital aneurysm NOS (Q27.8)
        congenital coronary aneurysm (Q24.5)
        ruptured cerebral arteriovenous malformation (I60.8)
        ruptured malformation of precerebral vessels (I72.0)

     Excludes2   congenital peripheral aneurysm (Q27.8)
        congenital pulmonary aneurysm (Q25.79)
        congenital retinal aneurysm (Q14.1)

Q28.0   Arteriovenous malformation of precerebral vessels
     Congenital arteriovenous precerebral aneurysm (nonruptured)

Q28.1   Other malformations of precerebral vessels
     Congenital malformation of precerebral vessels NOS
     Congenital precerebral aneurysm (nonruptured)

Q28.2   Arteriovenous malformation of cerebral vessels
     Arteriovenous malformation of brain NOS
     Congenital arteriovenous cerebral aneurysm (nonruptured)

Q28.3   Other malformations of cerebral vessels
     Congenital cerebral aneurysm (nonruptured)
     Congenital malformation of cerebral vessels NOS
     Developmental venous anomaly

Q28.8 Other specified congenital malformations of circulatory system
Congenital aneurysm, specified site NEC
Spinal vessel anomaly
▶ **Excludes2**   disorders of pyrophosphate metabolism (E83.82-)

Q28.9 Congenital malformation of circulatory system, unspecified

CONGENITAL MALFORMATIONS OF THE RESPIRATORY SYSTEM (Q30-Q34)

● **Q30 Congenital malformations of nose**
Excludes1   congenital deviation of nasal septum (Q67.4)

Q30.0 Choanal atresia
Atresia of nares (anterior) (posterior)
Congenital stenosis of nares (anterior) (posterior)

Q30.1 Agenesis and underdevelopment of nose
Congenital absent of nose

Q30.2 Fissured, notched and cleft nose

Q30.3 Congenital perforated nasal septum

Q30.8 Other congenital malformations of nose
Accessory nose
Congenital anomaly of nasal sinus wall
Coding Clinic: 2022, Q2, P17

Q30.9 Congenital malformation of nose, unspecified

● **Q31 Congenital malformations of larynx**
Excludes1   congenital laryngeal stridor NOS (P28.89)

Q31.0 Web of larynx
Glottic web of larynx
Subglottic web of larynx
Web of larynx NOS

Q31.1 Congenital subglottic stenosis

Q31.2 Laryngeal hypoplasia

Q31.3 Laryngocele

Q31.5 Congenital laryngomalacia

Q31.8 Other congenital malformations of larynx
Absence of larynx
Agenesis of larynx
Atresia of larynx
Congenital cleft thyroid cartilage
Congenital fissure of epiglottis
Congenital stenosis of larynx NEC
Posterior cleft of cricoid cartilage

Q31.9 Congenital malformation of larynx, unspecified

● **Q32 Congenital malformations of trachea and bronchus**
Excludes1   congenital bronchiectasis (Q33.4)

Q32.0 Congenital tracheomalacia

Q32.1 Other congenital malformations of trachea
Atresia of trachea
Congenital anomaly of tracheal cartilage
Congenital dilatation of trachea
Congenital malformation of trachea
Congenital stenosis of trachea
Congenital tracheocele

Q32.2 Congenital bronchomalacia

Q32.3 Congenital stenosis of bronchus

Q32.4 Other congenital malformations of bronchus
Absence of bronchus
Agenesis of bronchus
Atresia of bronchus
Congenital diverticulum of bronchus
Congenital malformation of bronchus NOS

● **Q33 Congenital malformations of lung**

Q33.0 Congenital cystic lung
Congenital cystic lung disease
Congenital honeycomb lung
Congenital polycystic lung disease
Excludes1   cystic fibrosis (E84.0)
cystic lung disease, acquired or unspecified (J98.4)

Q33.1 Accessory lobe of lung
Azygos lobe (fissured), lung

Q33.2 Sequestration of lung

Q33.3 Agenesis of lung
Congenital absence of lung (lobe)

Q33.4 Congenital bronchiectasis

Q33.5 Ectopic tissue in lung

Q33.6 Congenital hypoplasia and dysplasia of lung
Excludes1   pulmonary hypoplasia associated with short gestation (P28.0)

Q33.8 Other congenital malformations of lung

Q33.9 Congenital malformation of lung, unspecified

● **Q34 Other congenital malformations of respiratory system**
Excludes2   congenital central alveolar hypoventilation syndrome (G47.35)

Q34.0 Anomaly of pleura

Q34.1 Congenital cyst of mediastinum

Q34.8 Other specified congenital malformations of respiratory system
Atresia of nasopharynx

Q34.9 Congenital malformation of respiratory system, unspecified
Congenital absence of respiratory system
Congenital anomaly of respiratory system NOS

CLEFT LIP AND CLEFT PALATE (Q35-Q37)

Use additional code to identify associated malformation of the nose (Q30.2)
Excludes2   Robin's syndrome (Q87.0)

● **Q35 Cleft palate**
Includes   fissure of palate
palatoschisis
Excludes1   cleft palate with cleft lip (Q37.-)

Q35.1 Cleft hard palate

Q35.3 Cleft soft palate

Q35.5 Cleft hard palate with cleft soft palate

Q35.7 Cleft uvula

Q35.9 Cleft palate, unspecified
Cleft palate NOS

● **Q36 Cleft lip**
Includes   cheiloschisis
congenital fissure of lip
harelip
labium leporinum
Excludes1   cleft lip with cleft palate (Q37.-)

Q36.0 Cleft lip, bilateral

Q36.1 Cleft lip, median

Q36.9 Cleft lip, unilateral
Cleft lip NOS

● **Q37 Cleft palate with cleft lip**
Includes   cheilopalatoschisis

Q37.0 Cleft hard palate with bilateral cleft lip

Q37.1 Cleft hard palate with unilateral cleft lip
Cleft hard palate with cleft lip NOS

Q37.2 Cleft soft palate with bilateral cleft lip

Q37.3 Cleft soft palate with unilateral cleft lip
Cleft soft palate with cleft lip NOS

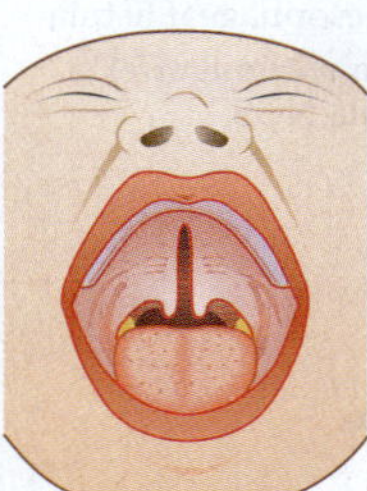

Figure 17-3   Cleft palate.

CHAPTER 17 (Q00-QA0.8)

Q37.4	Cleft hard and soft palate with bilateral cleft lip
Q37.5	Cleft hard and soft palate with unilateral cleft lip
	Cleft hard and soft palate with cleft lip NOS
Q37.8	Unspecified cleft palate with bilateral cleft lip
Q37.9	Unspecified cleft palate with unilateral cleft lip
	Cleft palate with cleft lip NOS

OTHER CONGENITAL MALFORMATIONS OF THE DIGESTIVE SYSTEM (Q38-Q45)

● **Q38   Other congenital malformations of tongue, mouth and pharynx**

    Excludes1   dentofacial anomalies (M26.-)
            macrostomia (Q18.4)
            microstomia (Q18.5)

Q38.0   Congenital malformations of lips, not elsewhere classified
    Congenital fistula of lip
    Congenital malformation of lip NOS
    Van der Woude's syndrome

      Excludes1   cleft lip (Q36.-)
              cleft lip with cleft palate (Q37.-)
              macrocheilia (Q18.6)
              microcheilia (Q18.7)

Q38.1   Ankyloglossia
    Restricted movement of tongue resulting in speech difficulty
    Tongue tie

Q38.2   Macroglossia
    Excessive size of tongue
    Congenital hypertrophy of tongue

Q38.3   Other congenital malformations of tongue
    Aglossia
    Bifid tongue
    Congenital adhesion of tongue
    Congenital fissure of tongue
    Congenital malformation of tongue NOS
    Double tongue
    Hypoglossia
    Hypoplasia of tongue
    Microglossia

Q38.4   Congenital malformations of salivary glands and ducts
    Atresia of salivary glands and ducts
    Congenital absence of salivary glands and ducts
    Congenital accessory salivary glands and ducts
    Congenital fistula of salivary gland

Q38.5   Congenital malformations of palate, not elsewhere classified
    Congenital absence of uvula
    Congenital malformation of palate NOS
    Congenital high arched palate

      Excludes1   cleft palate (Q35.-)
              cleft palate with cleft lip (Q37.-)

Q38.6   Other congenital malformations of mouth
    Congenital malformation of mouth NOS

Q38.7   Congenital pharyngeal pouch
    Congenital diverticulum of pharynx

      Excludes1   pharyngeal pouch syndrome (D82.1)

Q38.8   Other congenital malformations of pharynx
    Congenital malformation of pharynx NOS
    Imperforate pharynx

● **Q39   Congenital malformations of esophagus**

Q39.0   Atresia of esophagus without fistula
    Atresia of esophagus NOS

Q39.1   Atresia of esophagus with tracheo-esophageal fistula
    Atresia of esophagus with broncho-esophageal fistula

Q39.2   Congenital tracheo-esophageal fistula without atresia
    Congenital tracheo-esophageal fistula NOS

Q39.3   Congenital stenosis and stricture of esophagus

Q39.4   Esophageal web

Q39.5   Congenital dilatation of esophagus
    Congenital cardiospasm

Q39.6   Congenital diverticulum of esophagus
    Congenital esophageal pouch

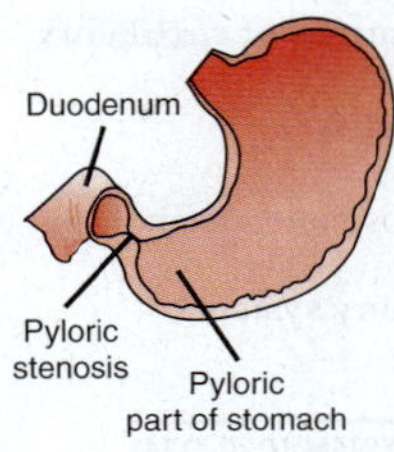

Figure 17-4   Pyloric stenosis.

Q39.8   Other congenital malformations of esophagus
    Congenital absence of esophagus
    Congenital displacement of esophagus
    Congenital duplication of esophagus

Q39.9   Congenital malformation of esophagus, unspecified

● **Q40   Other congenital malformations of upper alimentary tract**

Q40.0   Congenital hypertrophic pyloric stenosis
    Congenital or infantile constriction
    Congenital or infantile hypertrophy
    Congenital or infantile spasm
    Congenital or infantile stenosis
    Congenital or infantile stricture

Q40.1   Congenital hiatus hernia
    Congenital displacement of cardia through esophageal hiatus

      Excludes1   congenital diaphragmatic hernia (Q79.0)

Q40.2   Other specified congenital malformations of stomach
    Congenital displacement of stomach
    Congenital diverticulum of stomach
    Congenital hourglass stomach
    Congenital duplication of stomach
    Megalogastria
    Microgastria

Q40.3   Congenital malformation of stomach, unspecified

Q40.8   Other specified congenital malformations of upper alimentary tract

Q40.9   Congenital malformation of upper alimentary tract, unspecified
    Congenital anomaly of upper alimentary tract
    Congenital deformity of upper alimentary tract

● **Q41   Congenital absence, atresia and stenosis of small intestine**

    Includes   congenital obstruction, occlusion or stricture of small intestine or intestine NOS

    Excludes1   cystic fibrosis with intestinal manifestation (E84.11)
            meconium ileus NOS (without cystic fibrosis) (P76.0)

Q41.0   Congenital absence, atresia and stenosis of duodenum

Q41.1   Congenital absence, atresia and stenosis of jejunum
    Apple peel syndrome
    Imperforate jejunum

Q41.2   Congenital absence, atresia and stenosis of ileum

Q41.8   Congenital absence, atresia and stenosis of other specified parts of small intestine

Q41.9   Congenital absence, atresia and stenosis of small intestine, part unspecified
    Congenital absence, atresia and stenosis of intestine NOS

● **Q42   Congenital absence, atresia and stenosis of large intestine**

    Includes   congenital obstruction, occlusion and stricture of large intestine

Q42.0   Congenital absence, atresia and stenosis of rectum with fistula

Q42.1   Congenital absence, atresia and stenosis of rectum without fistula
    Imperforate rectum

Q42.2   Congenital absence, atresia and stenosis of anus with fistula

▶ New   ⇒ Revised   ~~deleted~~ Deleted   Excludes 1   Excludes 2   Includes   Use additional   Code first   Code also   Key words
OGCR Official Guidelines   X Assign placeholder X   ● Use Additional Character(s)   ▶ Manifestation Code   Hierarchical Condition Category   **Coding Clinic**

Q42.3 **Congenital absence, atresia and stenosis of anus without fistula**
Imperforate anus

Q42.8 **Congenital absence, atresia and stenosis of other parts of large intestine**

Q42.9 **Congenital absence, atresia and stenosis of large intestine, part unspecified**

● Q43 **Other congenital malformations of intestine**

Q43.0 **Meckel's diverticulum (displaced) (hypertrophic)**
Congenital abnormality in which a pouch remains on the lower end of the small intestine
Persistent omphalomesenteric duct
Persistent vitelline duct

Q43.1 **Hirschsprung's disease**
Developmental disorder of enteric nervous system characterized by absence of ganglion cells in distal colon resulting in functional obstruction
Aganglionosis
Congenital (aganglionic) megacolon

Q43.2 **Other congenital functional disorders of colon**
Congenital dilatation of colon

Q43.3 **Congenital malformations of intestinal fixation**
Congenital omental, anomalous adhesions [bands]
Congenital peritoneal adhesions [bands]
Incomplete rotation of cecum and colon
Insufficient rotation of cecum and colon
Jackson's membrane
Malrotation of colon
Rotation failure of cecum and colon
Universal mesentery

Q43.4 **Duplication of intestine**

Q43.5 **Ectopic anus**
Anal opening in abnormal location

Q43.6 **Congenital fistula of rectum and anus**
Excludes1   congenital fistula of anus with absence, atresia and stenosis (Q42.2)
congenital fistula of rectum with absence, atresia and stenosis (Q42.0)
congenital rectovaginal fistula (Q52.2)
congenital urethrorectal fistula (Q64.73)
pilonidal fistula or sinus (L05.-)

Q43.7 **Persistent cloaca**
Malformation in which rectum, vagina, and urinary tract form one channel; AKA congenital cloaca
Cloaca NOS

Q43.8 **Other specified congenital malformations of intestine**
Congenital blind loop syndrome
Congenital diverticulitis, colon
Congenital diverticulum, intestine
Dolichocolon
Megaloappendix
Megaloduodenum
Microcolon
Transposition of appendix
Transposition of colon
Transposition of intestine

Q43.9 **Congenital malformation of intestine, unspecified**

● Q44 **Congenital malformations of gallbladder, bile ducts and liver**

Q44.0 **Agenesis, aplasia and hypoplasia of gallbladder**
Congenital absence of gallbladder

Q44.1 **Other congenital malformations of gallbladder**
Congenital malformation of gallbladder NOS
Intrahepatic gallbladder

Q44.2 **Atresia of bile ducts**

Q44.3 **Congenital stenosis and stricture of bile ducts**

Q44.4 **Choledochal cyst**

Q44.5 **Other congenital malformations of bile ducts**
Accessory hepatic duct
Biliary duct duplication
Congenital malformation of bile duct NOS
Cystic duct duplication

Q44.6 **Cystic disease of liver**
Fibrocystic disease of liver

● Q44.7 **Other congenital malformations of liver**
Code also associated underlying condition

Q44.70 **Other congenital malformation of liver, unspecified**
Congenital malformation of liver, NOS

Q44.71 **Alagille syndrome**
Alagille-Watson syndrome

Q44.79 **Other congenital malformations of liver**
Accessory liver
Congenital absence of liver
Congenital hepatomegaly

● Q45 **Other congenital malformations of digestive system**
Excludes2   congenital diaphragmatic hernia (Q79.0)
congenital hiatus hernia (Q40.1)

Q45.0 **Agenesis, aplasia and hypoplasia of pancreas**
Congenital absence of pancreas

Q45.1 **Annular pancreas**

Q45.2 **Congenital pancreatic cyst**

Q45.3 **Other congenital malformations of pancreas and pancreatic duct**
Accessory pancreas
Congenital malformation of pancreas or pancreatic duct NOS
Excludes1   congenital diabetes mellitus (E10.-)
cystic fibrosis (E84.0-E84.9)
fibrocystic disease of pancreas (E84.-)
neonatal diabetes mellitus (P70.2)

Q45.8 **Other specified congenital malformations of digestive system**
Absence (complete) (partial) of alimentary tract NOS
Duplication of digestive system
Malposition, congenital of digestive system

Q45.9 **Congenital malformation of digestive system, unspecified**
Congenital anomaly of digestive system
Congenital deformity of digestive system

CONGENITAL MALFORMATIONS OF GENITAL ORGANS (Q50-Q56)

Excludes1   androgen insensitivity syndrome (E34.5-)
syndromes associated with anomalies in the number and form of chromosomes (Q90-Q99)

● Q50 **Congenital malformations of ovaries, fallopian tubes and broad ligaments**

● Q50.0 **Congenital absence of ovary**
Excludes1   Turner's syndrome (Q96.-)

Q50.01 **Congenital absence of ovary, unilateral**

Q50.02 **Congenital absence of ovary, bilateral**

Q50.1 **Developmental ovarian cyst**

Q50.2 **Congenital torsion of ovary**

● Q50.3 **Other congenital malformations of ovary**

Q50.31 **Accessory ovary**

Q50.32 **Ovarian streak**
Inadequate ovaries with absent follicular and hormonal function
46, XX with streak gonads

Q50.39 **Other congenital malformation of ovary**
Congenital malformation of ovary NOS

Q50.4 **Embryonic cyst of fallopian tube**
Fimbrial cyst

Q50.5 Embryonic cyst of broad ligament
Epoophoron cyst
Parovarian cyst

Q50.6 Other congenital malformations of fallopian tube and broad ligament
Absence of fallopian tube and broad ligament
Accessory fallopian tube and broad ligament
Atresia of fallopian tube and broad ligament
Congenital malformation of fallopian tube or broad ligament NOS

● **Q51 Congenital malformations of uterus and cervix**

Q51.0 Agenesis and aplasia of uterus
Congenital absence of uterus

● **Q51.1 Doubling of uterus with doubling of cervix and vagina**

Q51.10 Doubling of uterus with doubling of cervix and vagina without obstruction
Doubling of uterus with doubling of cervix and vagina NOS

Q51.11 Doubling of uterus with doubling of cervix and vagina with obstruction

● **Q51.2 Other doubling of uterus**
Doubling of uterus NOS
Septate uterus

Q51.21 Complete doubling of uterus
Complete septate uterus

Q51.22 Partial doubling of uterus
Partial septate uterus

Q51.28 Other and unspecified doubling of uterus
Septate uterus NOS

Q51.3 Bicornate uterus
Bicornate uterus, complete or partial
Birth defect in which uterus has two separate "horns" that form top of uterus

Q51.4 Unicornate uterus
Unicornate uterus with or without a separate uterine horn
Uterus with only one functioning horn
Uterus with half being undeveloped

Q51.5 Agenesis and aplasia of cervix
Congenital absence of cervix

Q51.6 Embryonic cyst of cervix

Q51.7 Congenital fistulae between uterus and digestive and urinary tracts

● **Q51.8 Other congenital malformations of uterus and cervix**

● **Q51.81 Other congenital malformations of uterus**

Q51.810 Arcuate uterus
Arcuatus uterus

Q51.811 Hypoplasia of uterus

Q51.818 Other congenital malformations of uterus
Müllerian anomaly of uterus NEC

● **Q51.82 Other congenital malformations of cervix**

Q51.820 Cervical duplication

Q51.821 Hypoplasia of cervix

Q51.828 Other congenital malformations of cervix

Q51.9 Congenital malformation of uterus and cervix, unspecified

● **Q52 Other congenital malformations of female genitalia**

Q52.0 Congenital absence of vagina
Vaginal agenesis, total or partial

● **Q52.1 Doubling of vagina**

Excludes1   doubling of vagina with doubling of uterus and cervix (Q51.1-)

Q52.10 Doubling of vagina, unspecified
Septate vagina NOS

Q52.11 Transverse vaginal septum

● **Q52.12 Longitudinal vaginal septum**
Coding Clinic: 2016, Q4, P58

Q52.120 Longitudinal vaginal septum, nonobstructing

Q52.121 Longitudinal vaginal septum, obstructing, right side

Q52.122 Longitudinal vaginal septum, obstructing, left side

Q52.123 Longitudinal vaginal septum, microperforate, right side

Q52.124 Longitudinal vaginal septum, microperforate, left side
Coding Clinic: 2016, Q4, P59

Q52.129 Other and unspecified longitudinal vaginal septum

Q52.2 Congenital rectovaginal fistula
Excludes1   cloaca (Q43.7)

Q52.3 Imperforate hymen
Membrane (hymen) completely closes vaginal orifice

Q52.4 Other congenital malformations of vagina
Canal of Nuck cyst, congenital
Congenital malformation of vagina NOS
Embryonic vaginal cyst
Gartner's duct cyst
Coding Clinic: 2022, Q2, P16

Q52.5 Fusion of labia

Q52.6 Congenital malformation of clitoris

● **Q52.7 Other and unspecified congenital malformations of vulva**

Q52.70 Unspecified congenital malformations of vulva
Congenital malformation of vulva NOS

Q52.71 Congenital absence of vulva

Q52.79 Other congenital malformations of vulva
Congenital cyst of vulva

Q52.8 Other specified congenital malformations of female genitalia

Q52.9 Congenital malformation of female genitalia, unspecified

● **Q53 Undescended and ectopic testicle**

● **Q53.0 Ectopic testis**

Q53.00 Ectopic testis, unspecified

Q53.01 Ectopic testis, unilateral

Q53.02 Ectopic testes, bilateral

● **Q53.1 Undescended testicle, unilateral**

Q53.10 Unspecified undescended testicle, unilateral

● **Q53.11 Abdominal testis, unilateral**

Q53.111 Unilateral intraabdominal testis

Q53.112 Unilateral inguinal testis

Q53.12 Ectopic perineal testis, unilateral

Q53.13 Unilateral high scrotal testis

● **Q53.2 Undescended testicle, bilateral**

Item 17–1 Testes form in the abdomen of the male and only descend into the scrotum during normal embryonic development. "Ectopic" testes are out of their normal place or "retained" (left behind) in the abdomen. Crypto (hidden) orchism (testicle) is a major risk factor for testicular cancer.

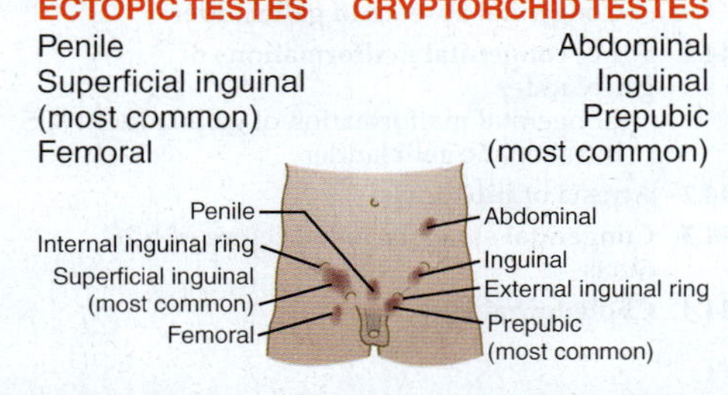

Figure 17-5 Undescended testes and the positions of the testes in various types of cryptorchidism or abnormal paths of descent.

▶ New   ⇨ Revised   ~~deleted~~ Deleted   Excludes 1   Excludes 2   Includes   Use additional   Code first   Code also   Key words

    OGCR Official Guidelines   X Assign placeholder X   ● Use Additional Character(s)   ▶ Manifestation Code   Hierarchical Condition Category   Coding Clinic

Q53.20 Undescended testicle, **unspecified**, bilateral

● Q53.21 **Abdominal** testis, bilateral

    Q53.211 Bilateral **intraabdominal** testes

    Q53.212 Bilateral **inguinal** testes

Q53.22 Ectopic **perineal** testis, bilateral

Q53.23 **Bilateral high scrotal** testes

Q53.9 **Undescended testicle, unspecified**
    Cryptorchism NOS

● **Q54 Hypospadias**
    Birth defect of male; urethra opens in abnormal location on shaft

    Excludes 1 epispadias (Q64.0)

Q54.0 **Hypospadias, balanic**
    Hypospadias, coronal
    Hypospadias, glandular

Q54.1 **Hypospadias, penile**

Q54.2 **Hypospadias, penoscrotal**

Q54.3 **Hypospadias, perineal**

Q54.4 **Congenital chordee**
    Chordee without hypospadias

Q54.8 **Other hypospadias**
    Hypospadias with intersex state

Q54.9 **Hypospadias, unspecified**

● **Q55 Other congenital malformations of male genital organs**

    Excludes 1 congenital hydrocele (P83.5)
        hypospadias (Q54.-)

Q55.0 **Absence and aplasia of testis**
    Monorchism

Q55.1 **Hypoplasia of testis and scrotum**
    Fusion of testes

● Q55.2 **Other and unspecified congenital malformations of testis and scrotum**

    Q55.20 **Unspecified congenital malformations of testis and scrotum**
        Congenital malformation of testis or scrotum NOS

    Q55.21 **Polyorchism**
        Developmental anomaly characterized by presence of more than two testes

    Q55.22 **Retractile testis**

    Q55.23 **Scrotal transposition**

    Q55.29 **Other congenital malformations of testis and scrotum**

Q55.3 **Atresia of vas deferens**
    Code first any associated cystic fibrosis (E84.-)

Q55.4 **Other congenital malformations of vas deferens, epididymis, seminal vesicles and prostate**
    Absence or aplasia of prostate
    Absence or aplasia of spermatic cord
    Congenital malformation of vas deferens, epididymis, seminal vesicles or prostate NOS

Q55.5 **Congenital absence and aplasia of penis**

● Q55.6 **Other congenital malformations of penis**

    Q55.61 **Curvature of penis (lateral)**

    Q55.62 **Hypoplasia of penis**
        Underdevelopment penis
        Micropenis

    Q55.63 **Congenital torsion of penis**

        Excludes 1 acquired torsion of penis (N48.82)

    Q55.64 **Hidden penis**
        Buried penis
        Concealed penis

        Excludes 1 acquired buried penis (N48.83)

    Q55.69 **Other congenital malformation of penis**
        Congenital malformation of penis NOS

Q55.7 **Congenital vasocutaneous fistula**
    Abnormal opening between vas deferens and skin

Q55.8 **Other specified congenital malformations of male genital organs**

Q55.9 **Congenital malformation of male genital organ, unspecified**
    Congenital anomaly of male genital organ
    Congenital deformity of male genital organ

● **Q56 Indeterminate sex and pseudohermaphroditism**
    Internal reproductive organs are opposite external physical characteristics.

    Excludes 1 46,XX true hermaphrodite (Q99.1)
        androgen insensitivity syndrome (E34.5-)
        chimera 46,XX/46,XY true hermaphrodite (Q99.0)
        female pseudohermaphroditism with adrenocortical disorder (E25.-)
        pseudohermaphroditism with specified chromosomal anomaly (Q96-Q99)
        pure gonadal dysgenesis (Q99.1)

Q56.0 **Hermaphroditism, not elsewhere classified**
    Ovotestis

Q56.1 **Male pseudohermaphroditism, not elsewhere classified**
    46, XY with streak gonads
    Male pseudohermaphroditism NOS

Q56.2 **Female pseudohermaphroditism, not elsewhere classified**
    Female pseudohermaphroditism NOS

Q56.3 **Pseudohermaphroditism, unspecified**

Q56.4 **Indeterminate sex, unspecified**
    Ambiguous genitalia

CONGENITAL MALFORMATIONS OF THE URINARY SYSTEM (Q60-Q64)

● **Q60 Renal agenesis and other reduction defects of kidney**

    Includes congenital absence of kidney
        congenital atrophy of kidney
        infantile atrophy of kidney

Q60.0 **Renal agenesis, unilateral**

Q60.1 **Renal agenesis, bilateral**

Q60.2 **Renal agenesis, unspecified**

Q60.3 **Renal hypoplasia, unilateral**

Q60.4 **Renal hypoplasia, bilateral**

Q60.5 **Renal hypoplasia, unspecified**

Q60.6 **Potter's syndrome**

● **Q61 Cystic kidney disease**
    Cysts that develop in failing kidney due to end-stage renal disease

    Excludes 1 acquired cyst of kidney (N28.1)
        Potter's syndrome (Q60.6)

● Q61.0 **Congenital renal cyst**

    Q61.00 **Congenital renal cyst, unspecified**
        Cyst of kidney NOS (congenital)

    Q61.01 **Congenital single renal cyst**

    Q61.02 **Congenital multiple renal cysts**

● Q61.1 **Polycystic kidney, infantile type**
    Polycystic kidney, autosomal recessive

    Q61.11 **Cystic dilatation of collecting ducts**

    Q61.19 **Other polycystic kidney, infantile type**

Q61.2 **Polycystic kidney, adult type**
    Polycystic kidney, autosomal dominant

Q61.3 **Polycystic kidney, unspecified**
    Coding Clinic: 2016, Q3, P23

Q61.4 **Renal dysplasia**
    Multicystic dysplastic kidney
    Multicystic kidney (development)
    Multicystic kidney disease
    Multicystic renal dysplasia

    Excludes 1 polycystic kidney disease (Q61.11-Q61.3)

Q61.5 **Medullary cystic kidney**
    Nephronophthisis
    Sponge kidney NOS

Q61.8 Other cystic kidney diseases
Fibrocystic kidney
Fibrocystic renal degeneration or disease

Q61.9 Cystic kidney disease, unspecified
Meckel-Gruber syndrome

● **Q62 Congenital obstructive defects of renal pelvis and congenital malformations of ureter**

Q62.0 Congenital hydronephrosis

● **Q62.1 Congenital occlusion of ureter**
Atresia and stenosis of ureter

Q62.10 Congenital occlusion of ureter, unspecified

Q62.11 Congenital occlusion of ureteropelvic junction

Q62.12 Congenital occlusion of ureterovesical orifice

Q62.2 Congenital megaureter
Congenital dilatation of ureter

● **Q62.3 Other obstructive defects of renal pelvis and ureter**

Q62.31 Congenital ureterocele, orthotopic

Q62.32 Cecoureterocele
Ectopic ureterocele

Q62.39 Other obstructive defects of renal pelvis and ureter
Ureteropelvic junction obstruction NOS

Q62.4 Agenesis of ureter
Congenital absence ureter

Q62.5 Duplication of ureter
Accessory ureter
Double ureter

● **Q62.6 Malposition of ureter**

Q62.60 Malposition of ureter, unspecified

Q62.61 Deviation of ureter

Q62.62 Displacement of ureter

Q62.63 Anomalous implantation of ureter
Ectopia of ureter
Ectopic ureter

Q62.69 Other malposition of ureter

Q62.7 Congenital vesico-uretero-renal reflux

Q62.8 Other congenital malformations of ureter
Anomaly of ureter NOS

● **Q63 Other congenital malformations of kidney**
Excludes1 congenital nephrotic syndrome (N04.-)

Q63.0 Accessory kidney

Q63.1 Lobulated, fused and horseshoe kidney

Q63.2 Ectopic kidney
Congenital displaced kidney
Malrotation of kidney

Q63.3 Hyperplastic and giant kidney
Compensatory hypertrophy of kidney

Q63.8 Other specified congenital malformations of kidney
Congenital renal calculi

Q63.9 Congenital malformation of kidney, unspecified

● **Q64 Other congenital malformations of urinary system**

Q64.0 Epispadias
Urethral opening somewhere on dorsum of penis
Excludes1 hypospadias (Q54.-)

● **Q64.1 Exstrophy of urinary bladder**
Bladder is exposed, inside out, and protrudes through abdominal wall

Q64.10 Exstrophy of urinary bladder, unspecified
Ectopia vesicae

Q64.11 Supravesical fissure of urinary bladder

Q64.12 Cloacal exstrophy of urinary bladder

Q64.19 Other exstrophy of urinary bladder
Extroversion of bladder

Q64.2 Congenital posterior urethral valves

● **Q64.3 Other atresia and stenosis of urethra and bladder neck**

Q64.31 Congenital bladder neck obstruction
Congenital obstruction of vesicourethral orifice

Q64.32 Congenital stricture of urethra

Q64.33 Congenital stricture of urinary meatus

Q64.39 Other atresia and stenosis of urethra and bladder neck
Atresia and stenosis of urethra and bladder neck NOS

Q64.4 Malformation of urachus
Cyst of urachus
Patent urachus
Prolapse of urachus

Q64.5 Congenital absence of bladder and urethra

Q64.6 Congenital diverticulum of bladder

● **Q64.7 Other and unspecified congenital malformations of bladder and urethra**
Excludes1 congenital prolapse of bladder (mucosa) (Q79.4)

Q64.70 Unspecified congenital malformation of bladder and urethra
Malformation of bladder or urethra NOS

Q64.71 Congenital prolapse of urethra

Q64.72 Congenital prolapse of urinary meatus

Q64.73 Congenital urethrorectal fistula

Q64.74 Double urethra

Q64.75 Double urinary meatus

Q64.79 Other congenital malformations of bladder and urethra

Q64.8 Other specified congenital malformations of urinary system

Q64.9 Congenital malformation of urinary system, unspecified
Congenital anomaly NOS of urinary system
Congenital deformity NOS of urinary system

CONGENITAL MALFORMATIONS AND DEFORMATIONS OF THE MUSCULOSKELETAL SYSTEM (Q65-Q79)

● **Q65 Congenital deformities of hip**
Excludes1 clicking hip (R29.4)

● **Q65.0 Congenital dislocation of hip, unilateral**

Q65.00 Congenital dislocation of unspecified hip, unilateral

Q65.01 Congenital dislocation of right hip, unilateral

Q65.02 Congenital dislocation of left hip, unilateral

Q65.1 Congenital dislocation of hip, bilateral

Q65.2 Congenital dislocation of hip, unspecified

● **Q65.3 Congenital partial dislocation of hip, unilateral**

Q65.30 Congenital partial dislocation of unspecified hip, unilateral

Q65.31 Congenital partial dislocation of right hip, unilateral

Q65.32 Congenital partial dislocation of left hip, unilateral

Q65.4 Congenital partial dislocation of hip, bilateral

Q65.5 Congenital partial dislocation of hip, unspecified

Q65.6 Congenital unstable hip
Congenital dislocatable hip

● **Q65.8 Other congenital deformities of hip**

Q65.81 Congenital coxa valga

Q65.82 Congenital coxa vara

Q65.89 Other specified congenital deformities of hip
Anteversion of femoral neck
Congenital acetabular dysplasia

Q65.9 Congenital deformity of hip, unspecified

Item 17–2 Equinus foot is a term referring to the hoof of a horse. The deformity is usually congenital or spastic. **Talipes equinovarus** is referred to as clubfoot. The foot tends to be smaller than normal, with the heel pointing downward and the forefoot turning inward. The heel cord (Achilles tendon) is tight, causing the heel to be drawn up toward the leg.

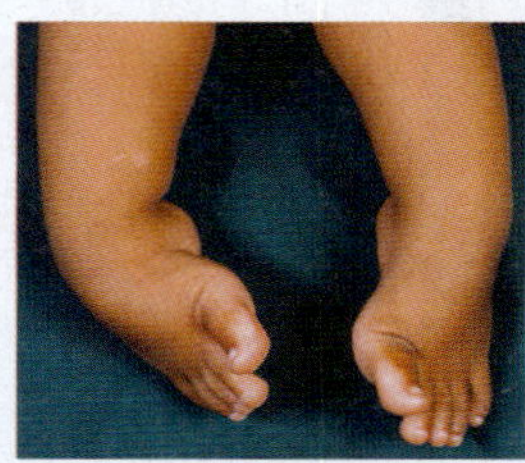

Figure 17-6 Supination and cavus deformity of forefoot. (From Kliegman R, Nelson WE: Nelson Textbook of Pediatrics, Philadelphia, Saunders, 2007)

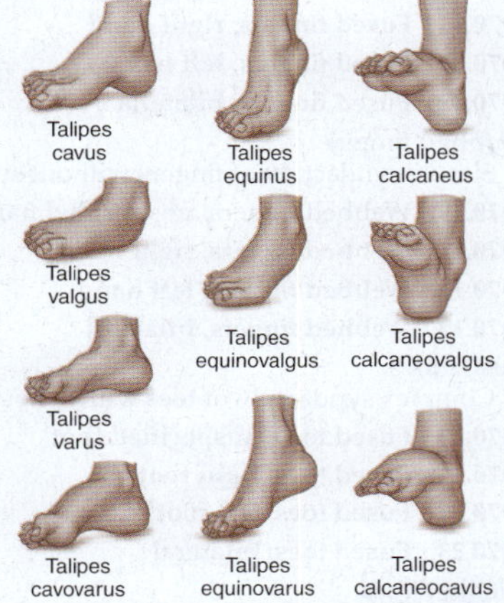

Figure 17-7 Talipes. (From Dorland: Dorland's Illustrated Medical Dictionary, ed 31, Saunders, 2007, p 1893)

● **Q66 Congenital deformities of feet**

    Excludes1 reduction defects of feet (Q72.-)
            valgus deformities (acquired) (M21.0-)
            varus deformities (acquired) (M21.1-)

● **Q66.0 Congenital talipes equinovarus**
    Heel is turned inward from midline and foot is plantar flexed; AKA clubfoot

    Q66.00 Congenital talipes equinovarus, unspecified foot

    Q66.01 Congenital talipes equinovarus, right foot

    Q66.02 Congenital talipes equinovarus, left foot

● **Q66.1 Congenital talipes calcaneovarus**
    Deformity of foot in which heel is turned toward midline of body and anterior of foot is elevated

    Q66.10 Congenital talipes calcaneovarus, unspecified foot

    Q66.11 Congenital talipes calcaneovarus, right foot

    Q66.12 Congenital talipes calcaneovarus, left foot

● **Q66.2 Congenital metatarsus (primus) varus**
    Angulation of first metatarsal bone toward midline of body
    Coding Clinic: 2016, Q4, P59

    ● **Q66.21** Congenital metatarsus primus varus

        Q66.211 Congenital metatarsus primus varus, right foot

        Q66.212 Congenital metatarsus primus varus, left foot

        Q66.219 Congenital metatarsus primus varus, unspecified foot

    ● **Q66.22** Congenital metatarsus adductus
        Congenital metatarsus varus

        Q66.221 Congenital metatarsus adductus, right foot

        Q66.222 Congenital metatarsus adductus, left foot

        Q66.229 Congenital metatarsus adductus, unspecified foot

● **Q66.3 Other congenital varus deformities of feet**
    Hallux varus, congenital

    Q66.30 Other congenital varus deformities of feet, unspecified foot

    Q66.31 Other congenital varus deformities of feet, right foot

    Q66.32 Other congenital varus deformities of feet, left foot

● **Q66.4 Congenital talipes calcaneovalgus**

    Q66.40 Congenital talipes calcaneovalgus, unspecified foot

    Q66.41 Congenital talipes calcaneovalgus, right foot

    Q66.42 Congenital talipes calcaneovalgus, left foot

● **Q66.5 Congenital pes planus**
    Congenital flat foot
    Congenital rigid flat foot
    Congenital spastic (everted) flat foot

    Excludes1 pes planus, acquired (M21.4)

    Q66.50 Congenital pes planus, unspecified foot

    Q66.51 Congenital pes planus, right foot

    Q66.52 Congenital pes planus, left foot

Q66.6 Other congenital valgus deformities of feet
    Inward angulation
    Congenital metatarsus valgus

● **Q66.7 Congenital pes cavus**

    Q66.70 Congenital pes cavus, unspecified foot

    Q66.71 Congenital pes cavus, right foot

    Q66.72 Congenital pes cavus, left foot

● **Q66.8 Other congenital deformities of feet**

    Q66.80 Congenital vertical talus deformity, unspecified foot

    Q66.81 Congenital vertical talus deformity, right foot

    Q66.82 Congenital vertical talus deformity, left foot

    Q66.89 Other specified congenital deformities of feet
        Congenital asymmetric talipes
        Congenital clubfoot NOS
        Congenital talipes NOS
        Congenital tarsal coalition
        Hammer toe, congenital

● **Q66.9 Congenital deformity of feet, unspecified**

    Q66.90 Congenital deformity of feet, unspecified, unspecified foot

    Q66.91 Congenital deformity of feet, unspecified, right foot

    Q66.92 Congenital deformity of feet, unspecified, left foot

● **Q67 Congenital musculoskeletal deformities of head, face, spine and chest**

    Excludes1 congenital malformation syndromes classified to Q87.-
            Potter's syndrome (Q60.6)

Q67.0 Congenital facial asymmetry

Q67.1 Congenital compression facies

Q67.2 Dolichocephaly
    Long head dimension

    Excludes1 sagittal craniosynostosis (Q75.01)

Q67.3 Plagiocephaly
    Asymmetric shape of head resulting from irregular closure of cranial sutures

    Excludes1 coronal craniosynostosis (Q75.02-)
            lambdoid craniosynostosis (Q75.04-)

CHAPTER 17 (Q00-Q99)

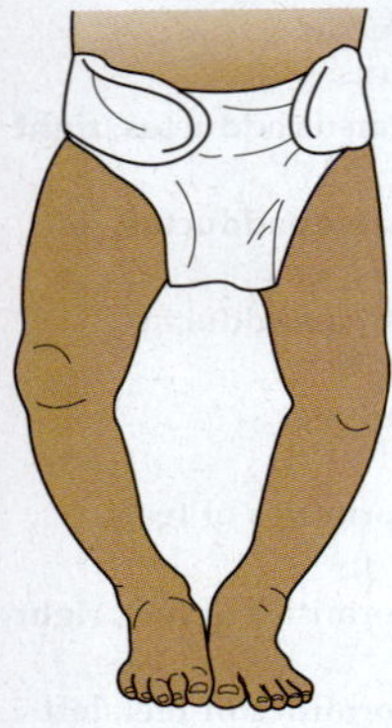

Figure 17-8   Mild to moderate inbowing of the lower leg. (From Lissauer T, Clayden G: Illustrated Textbook of Paediatrics, Edinburgh, Mosby, 2011)

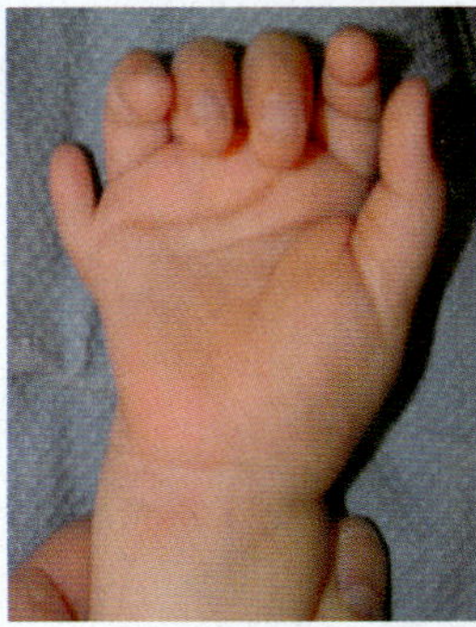

Figure 17-9   Thumb and index finger. (From Chung K: Hand and Upper Extremity Reconstruction, 1e, Saunders, 2008)

Q67.4   **Other congenital deformities of skull, face and jaw**
Congenital depressions in skull
Congenital hemifacial atrophy or hypertrophy
Deviation of nasal septum, congenital
Squashed or bent nose, congenital
> **Excludes1**   dentofacial anomalies [including malocclusion] (M26.-)
> syphilitic saddle nose (A50.5)

Q67.5   **Congenital deformity of spine**
Congenital postural scoliosis
Congenital scoliosis NOS
> **Excludes1**   infantile idiopathic scoliosis (M41.0)
> scoliosis due to congenital bony malformation (Q76.3)

Q67.6   **Pectus excavatum**
Congenital funnel chest
Funnel-shaped chest depression

Q67.7   **Pectus carinatum**
Congenital pigeon chest

Q67.8   **Other congenital deformities of chest**
Congenital deformity of chest wall NOS

● **Q68**   **Other congenital musculoskeletal deformities**
> **Excludes1**   reduction defects of limb(s) (Q71-Q73)
> **Excludes2**   congenital myotonic chondrodystrophy (G71.13)

Q68.0   **Congenital deformity of sternocleidomastoid muscle**
Congenital contracture of sternocleidomastoid (muscle)
Congenital (sternomastoid) torticollis
Sternomastoid tumor (congenital)

Q68.1   **Congenital deformity of finger(s) and hand**
Congenital clubfinger
Spade-like hand (congenital)

Q68.2   **Congenital deformity of knee**
Congenital dislocation of knee
Congenital genu recurvatum
Hyperextension of knee resulting from hypermobility

Q68.3   **Congenital bowing of femur**
> **Excludes1**   anteversion of femur (neck) (Q65.89)

Q68.4   **Congenital bowing of tibia and fibula**

Q68.5   **Congenital bowing of long bones of leg, unspecified**

Q68.6   **Discoid meniscus**

Q68.8   **Other specified congenital musculoskeletal deformities**
Congenital deformity of clavicle
Congenital deformity of elbow
Congenital deformity of forearm
Congenital deformity of scapula
Congenital deformity of wrist
Congenital dislocation of elbow
Congenital dislocation of shoulder
Congenital dislocation of wrist

● **Q69**   **Polydactyly**
AKA hyperdactyly, consists of supernumerary fingers or toes

Q69.0   **Accessory finger(s)**

Q69.1   **Accessory thumb(s)**

Q69.2   **Accessory toe(s)**
Accessory hallux

Q69.9   **Polydactyly, unspecified**
Supernumerary digit(s) NOS

● **Q70**   **Syndactyly**
Webbing between distal phalanges of adjacent digits

● **Q70.0**   **Fused fingers**
Complex syndactyly of fingers with synostosis
   Q70.00   Fused fingers, **unspecified** hand
   Q70.01   Fused fingers, **right** hand
   Q70.02   Fused fingers, **left** hand
   Q70.03   Fused fingers, **bilateral**

● **Q70.1**   **Webbed fingers**
Simple syndactyly of fingers without synostosis
   Q70.10   Webbed fingers, **unspecified** hand
   Q70.11   Webbed fingers, **right** hand
   Q70.12   Webbed fingers, **left** hand
   Q70.13   Webbed fingers, **bilateral**

● **Q70.2**   **Fused toes**
Complex syndactyly of toes with synostosis
   Q70.20   Fused toes, **unspecified** foot
   Q70.21   Fused toes, **right** foot
   Q70.22   Fused toes, **left** foot
   Q70.23   Fused toes, **bilateral**

● **Q70.3**   **Webbed toes**
Simple syndactyly of toes without synostosis
   Q70.30   Webbed toes, **unspecified** foot
   Q70.31   Webbed toes, **right** foot
   Q70.32   Webbed toes, **left** foot
   Q70.33   Webbed toes, **bilateral**

Q70.4   **Polysyndactyly, unspecified**
> **Excludes1**   specified syndactyly of hand and feet - code to specified conditions (Q70.0- -Q70.3-)

Extra and webbed digits

Q70.9   **Syndactyly, unspecified**
Symphalangy NOS

● **Q71**   **Reduction defects of upper limb**

● **Q71.0**   **Congenital complete absence of upper limb**
   Q71.00   Congenital complete absence of **unspecified** upper limb
   Q71.01   Congenital complete absence of **right** upper limb
   Q71.02   Congenital complete absence of **left** upper limb
   Q71.03   Congenital complete absence of upper limb, **bilateral**

● **Q71.1**   **Congenital absence of upper arm and forearm with hand present**
   Q71.10   Congenital absence of **unspecified** upper arm and forearm with hand present
   Q71.11   Congenital absence of **right** upper arm and forearm with hand present
   Q71.12   Congenital absence of **left** upper arm and forearm with hand present
   Q71.13   Congenital absence of upper arm and forearm with hand present, **bilateral**

▶ New   ⇒ Revised   ~~deleted~~ Deleted   Excludes 1   Excludes 2   Includes   Use additional   Code first   Code also   Key words
OGCR Official Guidelines   X Assign placeholder X   ● Use Additional Character(s)   ◗ Manifestation Code   **HCC** Hierarchical Condition Category   **Coding Clinic**

● **Q71.2** Congenital absence of both forearm and hand

    Q71.20 Congenital absence of both forearm and hand, unspecified upper limb

    Q71.21 Congenital absence of both forearm and hand, right upper limb

    Q71.22 Congenital absence of both forearm and hand, left upper limb

    Q71.23 Congenital absence of both forearm and hand, bilateral

● **Q71.3** Congenital absence of hand and finger

    Q71.30 Congenital absence of unspecified hand and finger

    Q71.31 Congenital absence of right hand and finger

    Q71.32 Congenital absence of left hand and finger

    Q71.33 Congenital absence of hand and finger, bilateral

● **Q71.4** Longitudinal reduction defect of radius

    Clubhand (congenital)

    Radial clubhand

    Q71.40 Longitudinal reduction defect of unspecified radius

    Q71.41 Longitudinal reduction defect of right radius

    Q71.42 Longitudinal reduction defect of left radius

    Q71.43 Longitudinal reduction defect of radius, bilateral

● **Q71.5** Longitudinal reduction defect of ulna

    Q71.50 Longitudinal reduction defect of unspecified ulna

    Q71.51 Longitudinal reduction defect of right ulna

    Q71.52 Longitudinal reduction defect of left ulna

    Q71.53 Longitudinal reduction defect of ulna, bilateral

● **Q71.6** Lobster-claw hand

    Q71.60 Lobster-claw hand, unspecified hand

    Q71.61 Lobster-claw right hand

    Q71.62 Lobster-claw left hand

    Q71.63 Lobster-claw hand, bilateral

● **Q71.8** Other reduction defects of upper limb

    ● **Q71.81** Congenital shortening of upper limb

        Q71.811 Congenital shortening of right upper limb

        Q71.812 Congenital shortening of left upper limb

        Q71.813 Congenital shortening of upper limb, bilateral

        Q71.819 Congenital shortening of unspecified upper limb

    ● **Q71.89** Other reduction defects of upper limb

        Q71.891 Other reduction defects of right upper limb

        Q71.892 Other reduction defects of left upper limb

        Q71.893 Other reduction defects of upper limb, bilateral

        Q71.899 Other reduction defects of unspecified upper limb

● **Q71.9** Unspecified reduction defect of upper limb

    Q71.90 Unspecified reduction defect of unspecified upper limb

    Q71.91 Unspecified reduction defect of right upper limb

    Q71.92 Unspecified reduction defect of left upper limb

    Q71.93 Unspecified reduction defect of upper limb, bilateral

● **Q72** Reduction defects of lower limb

    ● **Q72.0** Congenital complete absence of lower limb

        Q72.00 Congenital complete absence of unspecified lower limb

        Q72.01 Congenital complete absence of right lower limb

    Q72.02 Congenital complete absence of left lower limb

    Q72.03 Congenital complete absence of lower limb, bilateral

● **Q72.1** Congenital absence of thigh and lower leg with foot present

    Q72.10 Congenital absence of unspecified thigh and lower leg with foot present

    Q72.11 Congenital absence of right thigh and lower leg with foot present

    Q72.12 Congenital absence of left thigh and lower leg with foot present

    Q72.13 Congenital absence of thigh and lower leg with foot present, bilateral

● **Q72.2** Congenital absence of both lower leg and foot

    Q72.20 Congenital absence of both lower leg and foot, unspecified lower limb

    Q72.21 Congenital absence of both lower leg and foot, right lower limb

    Q72.22 Congenital absence of both left lower leg and foot, left lower limb

    Q72.23 Congenital absence of both lower leg and foot, bilateral

● **Q72.3** Congenital absence of foot and toe(s)

    Q72.30 Congenital absence of unspecified foot and toe(s)

    Q72.31 Congenital absence of right foot and toe(s)

    Q72.32 Congenital absence of left foot and toe(s)

    Q72.33 Congenital absence of foot and toe(s), bilateral

● **Q72.4** Longitudinal reduction defect of femur

    Proximal femoral focal deficiency

    Q72.40 Longitudinal reduction defect of unspecified femur

    Q72.41 Longitudinal reduction defect of right femur

    Q72.42 Longitudinal reduction defect of left femur

    Q72.43 Longitudinal reduction defect of femur, bilateral

● **Q72.5** Longitudinal reduction defect of tibia

    Q72.50 Longitudinal reduction defect of unspecified tibia

    Q72.51 Longitudinal reduction defect of right tibia

    Q72.52 Longitudinal reduction defect of left tibia

    Q72.53 Longitudinal reduction defect of tibia, bilateral

● **Q72.6** Longitudinal reduction defect of fibula

    Q72.60 Longitudinal reduction defect of unspecified fibula

    Q72.61 Longitudinal reduction defect of right fibula

    Q72.62 Longitudinal reduction defect of left fibula

    Q72.63 Longitudinal reduction defect of fibula, bilateral

● **Q72.7** Split foot

    Q72.70 Split foot, unspecified lower limb

    Q72.71 Split foot, right lower limb

    Q72.72 Split foot, left lower limb

    Q72.73 Split foot, bilateral

● **Q72.8** Other reduction defects of lower limb

    ● **Q72.81** Congenital shortening of lower limb

        Q72.811 Congenital shortening of right lower limb

        Q72.812 Congenital shortening of left lower limb

        Q72.813 Congenital shortening of lower limb, bilateral

        Q72.819 Congenital shortening of unspecified lower limb

CHAPTER 17 (Q00–Q99)

CHAPTER 17 (Q00–QA0.8)

● **Q72.89**   **Other reduction defects of lower limb**
    Q72.891   Other reduction defects of **right** lower limb
    Q72.892   Other reduction defects of **left** lower limb
    Q72.893   Other reduction defects of lower limb, **bilateral**
    Q72.899   Other reduction defects of **unspecified** lower limb

● **Q72.9**   **Unspecified** reduction defect of lower limb
    Q72.90   Unspecified reduction defect of **unspecified** lower limb
    Q72.91   Unspecified reduction defect of **right** limb
    Q72.92   Unspecified reduction defect of **left** lower limb
    Q72.93   Unspecified reduction defect of lower limb, **bilateral**

● **Q73**   **Reduction defects of unspecified limb**
   Q73.0   **Congenital absence of unspecified limb(s)**
     Amelia NOS
   Q73.1   **Phocomelia, unspecified limb(s)**
     Phocomelia NOS
     Absence/shortening of long bones primarily as a result of thalidomide
   Q73.8   **Other reduction defects of unspecified limb(s)**
     Longitudinal reduction deformity of unspecified limb(s)
     Ectromelia of limb NOS
     Gross hypoplasia or aplasia of one or more long bones of limb(s)
     Hemimelia of limb NOS
     Absence of one-half of long bone
     Reduction defect of limb NOS

● **Q74**   **Other congenital malformations of limb(s)**
   Excludes1   polydactyly (Q69.-)
            reduction defect of limb (Q71-Q73)
            syndactyly (Q70.-)
   Q74.0   **Other congenital malformations of upper limb(s), including shoulder girdle**
     Accessory carpal bones
     Cleidocranial dysostosis
     Congenital pseudarthrosis of clavicle
     Macrodactylia (fingers)
     Madelung's deformity
     Radioulnar synostosis
     Sprengel's deformity
     Triphalangeal thumb
   Q74.1   **Congenital malformation of knee**
     Congenital absence of patella
     Congenital dislocation of patella
     Congenital genu valgum
     Congenital genu varum
     Rudimentary patella
     Excludes1   congenital dislocation of knee (Q68.2)
               congenital genu recurvatum (Q68.2)
               nail patella syndrome (Q87.2)
   Q74.2   **Other congenital malformations of lower limb(s), including pelvic girdle**
     Congenital fusion of sacroiliac joint
     Congenital malformation of ankle joint
     Congenital malformation of sacroiliac joint
     Excludes1   anteversion of femur (neck) (Q65.89)
   Q74.3   **Arthrogryposis multiplex congenita**
   Q74.8   **Other specified congenital malformations of limb(s)**
   Q74.9   **Unspecified congenital malformation of limb(s)**
     Congenital anomaly of limb(s) NOS

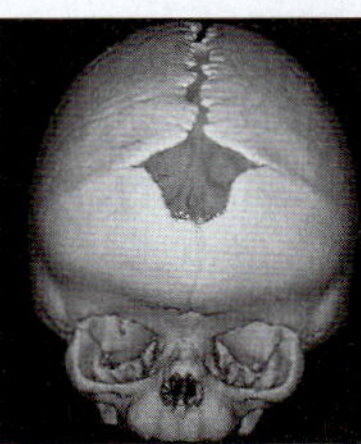

Figure 17-10   Generalized craniosynostosis without symptoms or signs of increased intracranial pressure. (From Goetz C: Textbook of Clinical Neurology, St. Louis, MO, Elsevier, 2007)

Item 17–3   **Anencephalus** is a congenital deformity of the cranial vault. **Craniosynostosis**, also known as craniostenosis and stenocephaly, signifies any form of congenital deformity of the skull that results from the premature closing of the sutures of the skull. **Iniencephaly** is a deformity in which the head and neck are flexed backward to a great extent and the head is very large in comparison to the shortened body.

● **Q75**   **Other congenital malformations of skull and face bones**
   Excludes1   congenital malformation of face NOS (Q18.-)
            congenital malformation syndromes classified to Q87.-
            dentofacial anomalies [including malocclusion] (M26.-)
            musculoskeletal deformities of head and face (Q67.0-Q67.4)
            skull defects associated with congenital anomalies of brain such as:
               anencephaly (Q00.0)
               encephalocele (Q01.-)
               hydrocephalus (Q03.-)
               microcephaly (Q02)
   ● **Q75.0**   **Craniosynostosis**
     Premature closure of sutures of skull
     ● **Q75.00**   **Craniosynostosis, unspecified**
       Craniosynostosis NOS
       Q75.001   **Craniosynostosis, unspecified, unilateral**
       Q75.002   **Craniosynostosis, unspecified, bilateral**
       Q75.009   **Craniosynostosis, unspecified**
         Imperfect fusion of skull
     ● **Q75.01**   **Sagittal craniosynostosis**
       Non-deformational dolichocephaly
       Non-deformational scaphocephaly
       Excludes1   plagiocephaly (Q67.3)
     ● **Q75.02**   **Coronal craniosynostosis**
       Non-deformational anterior plagiocephaly
       Excludes1   dolichocephaly (Q67.2)
       Q75.021   **Coronal craniosynostosis, unilateral**
         Non-deformational anterior plagiocephaly
       Q75.022   **Coronal craniosynostosis, bilateral**
         Non-deformational brachycephaly
       Q75.029   **Coronal craniosynostosis, unspecified**
     ● **Q75.03**   **Metopic craniosynostosis**
       Trigonocephaly
     ● **Q75.04**   **Lambdoid craniosynostosis**
       Non-deformational posterior plagiocephaly
       Excludes1   dolichocephaly (Q67.2)
       Q75.041   **Lambdoid craniosynostosis, unilateral**
       Q75.042   **Lambdoid craniosynostosis, bilateral**
       Q75.049   **Lambdoid craniosynostosis, unspecified**

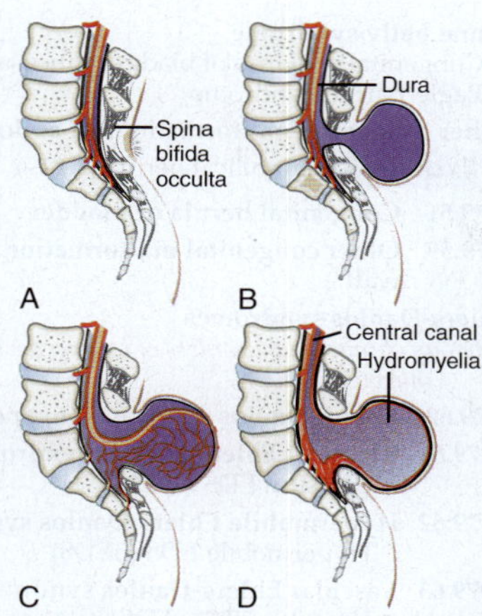

Figure 17-11   **A.** Spina bifida occulta. **B.** Meningocele.
C. Myelomeningocele. **D.** Myelocystocele (syringomyelocele)
or hydromyelia.

Item 17–4   Spina bifida is a midline spinal defect in which one or more vertebrae fail to fuse, leaving an opening in the vertebral canal. When the defect is not visible, it is called spina bifida occulta, and when it is visible, it is called spina bifida cystica.

● **Q75.Ø5   Multi-suture craniosynostosis**
   Q75.Ø51   Cloverleaf skull
     Kleeblattschaedel skull
   Q75.Ø52   Pansynostosis
   Q75.Ø58   Other multi-suture craniosynostosis
     Excludes1   coronal craniosynostosis, bilateral (Q75.Ø22)
           lambdoid craniosynostosis, bilateral (Q75.Ø42)

   Q75.Ø8   Other single-suture craniosynostosis

Q75.1   Craniofacial dysostosis
Congenital deformity of head
Crouzon's disease

Q75.2   Hypertelorism

Q75.3   Macrocephaly
Unusually large size of head; AKA megalocephaly

Q75.4   Mandibulofacial dysostosis
Franceschetti syndrome
Treacher Collins syndrome

Q75.5   Oculomandibular dysostosis
Ossification of occular and mandibular bones

Q75.8   Other specified congenital malformations of skull and face bones
Absence of skull bone, congenital
Congenital deformity of forehead
Platybasia

Q75.9   Congenital malformation of skull and face bones, unspecified
Congenital anomaly of face bones NOS
Congenital anomaly of skull NOS

● **Q76   Congenital malformations of spine and bony thorax**
   Excludes1   congenital musculoskeletal deformities of spine and chest (Q67.5-Q67.8)

Q76.Ø   Spina bifida occulta
   Excludes1   meningocele (spinal) (Q05.-)
           spina bifida (aperta) (cystica) (Q05.-)

Q76.1   Klippel-Feil syndrome
Cervical fusion syndrome

Q76.2   Congenital spondylolisthesis
Congenital spondylolysis
   Excludes1   spondylolisthesis (acquired) (M43.1-)
           spondylolysis (acquired) (M43.0-)

Q76.3   Congenital scoliosis due to congenital bony malformation
Hemivertebra fusion or failure of segmentation with scoliosis
Coding Clinic: 2022, Q4, P41

● **Q76.4   Other congenital malformations of spine, not associated with scoliosis**
   ● **Q76.41   Congenital kyphosis**
     Abnormal increase in convexity curvature of thoracic spinal column; AKA humpback
     Q76.411   Congenital kyphosis, occipito-atlanto-axial region
     Q76.412   Congenital kyphosis, cervical region
     Q76.413   Congenital kyphosis, cervicothoracic region
     Q76.414   Congenital kyphosis, thoracic region
     Q76.415   Congenital kyphosis, thoracolumbar region
     Q76.419   Congenital kyphosis, unspecified region

   ● **Q76.42   Congenital lordosis**
     An abnormal increase in curvature of lumbar spine (sway back)
     Q76.425   Congenital lordosis, thoracolumbar region
     Q76.426   Congenital lordosis, lumbar region
     Q76.427   Congenital lordosis, lumbosacral region
     Q76.428   Congenital lordosis, sacral and sacrococcygeal region
     Q76.429   Congenital lordosis, unspecified region

   Q76.49   Other congenital malformations of spine, not associated with scoliosis
     Congenital absence of vertebra NOS
     Congenital fusion of spine NOS
     Congenital malformation of lumbosacral (joint) (region) NOS
     Congenital malformation of spine NOS
     Hemivertebra NOS
     Malformation of spine NOS
     Platyspondylisis NOS
     Supernumerary vertebra NOS

Q76.5   Cervical rib
Supernumerary rib in cervical region

Q76.6   Other congenital malformations of ribs
Accessory rib
Congenital absence of rib
Congenital fusion of ribs
Congenital malformation of ribs NOS
   Excludes1   short rib syndrome (Q77.2)

Q76.7   Congenital malformation of sternum
Congenital absence of sternum
Sternum bifidum

Q76.8   Other congenital malformations of bony thorax

Q76.9   Congenital malformation of bony thorax, unspecified

● **Q77   Osteochondrodysplasia with defects of growth of tubular bones and spine**
   Excludes1   mucopolysaccharidosis (E76.0-E76.3)
   Excludes2   congenital myotonic chondrodystrophy (G71.13)

Q77.Ø   Achondrogenesis
Hypochondrogenesis

Q77.1   Thanatophoric short stature

Q77.2   Short rib syndrome
Asphyxiating thoracic dysplasia [Jeune]

Q77.3 Chondrodysplasia punctata
Benign cartilaginous neoplasms
➡ **Excludes1** rhizomelic chondrodysplasia punctata
(E71.540)

Q77.4 Achondroplasia
*Disturbance of epiphyseal chondroblastic growth and
maturation, results in dwarfism*
Hypochondroplasia
Osteosclerosis congenita

Q77.5 Diastrophic dysplasia

Q77.6 Chondroectodermal dysplasia
*Defective development of skin, hair, teeth, with polydactyly
and defect of cardiac septum*
Ellis-van Creveld syndrome

Q77.7 Spondyloepiphyseal dysplasia

**Q77.8 Other osteochondrodysplasia with defects of growth of
tubular bones and spine**

**Q77.9 Osteochondrodysplasia with defects of growth of
tubular bones and spine, unspecified**

● **Q78 Other osteochondrodysplasias**
*Disorder of development of bone and cartilage; common cause of
dwarfism*
Excludes2 congenital myotonic chondrodystrophy (G71.13)

Q78.0 Osteogenesis imperfecta
Fragilitas ossium
Osteopsathyrosis

Q78.1 Polyostotic fibrous dysplasia
Albright(-McCune)(-Sternberg) syndrome

Q78.2 Osteopetrosis
Abnormally dense bone; AKA marble bones disease, ivory bones
Albers-Schönberg syndrome
Osteosclerosis NOS

Q78.3 Progressive diaphyseal dysplasia
Camurati-Engelmann syndrome

Q78.4 Enchondromatosis
Thinning of overlying cortex of bone and distorted length
Maffucci's syndrome
Ollier's disease

Q78.5 Metaphyseal dysplasia
*Disturbance in enchondral bone growth, causing ends of
shafts to remain larger than normal in circumference*
Pyle's syndrome

Q78.6 Multiple congenital exostoses
Diaphyseal aclasis

Q78.8 Other specified osteochondrodysplasias
Osteopoikilosis

Q78.9 Osteochondrodysplasia, unspecified
Chondrodystrophy NOS
*AKA skeletal dysplasia (dwarfism) caused by genetic
mutations affecting hyaline cartilage capping long
bones and vertebrae*
Osteodystrophy NOS

● **Q79 Congenital malformations of musculoskeletal system, not
elsewhere classified**
Excludes2 congenital (sternomastoid) torticollis (Q68.0)

Q79.0 Congenital diaphragmatic hernia
Excludes1 congenital hiatus hernia (Q40.1)

Q79.1 Other congenital malformations of diaphragm
Absence of diaphragm
Congenital malformation of diaphragm NOS
Eventration of diaphragm

Q79.2 Exomphalos
*Abdominal hernia in which part of intestine protrudes at
umbilicus; AKA exomphalos and exumbilication*
Omphalocele
Excludes1 umbilical hernia (K42.-)

Q79.3 Gastroschisis
*Congenital fissure of anterior abdominal wall often with
protrusion of small/large intestine*

Q79.4 Prune belly syndrome
Congenital prolapse of bladder mucosa
Eagle-Barrett syndrome

● **Q79.5 Other congenital malformations of abdominal wall**
Excludes1 umbilical hernia (K42.-)

Q79.51 Congenital hernia of bladder

**Q79.59 Other congenital malformations of abdominal
wall**

● **Q79.6 Ehlers-Danlos syndromes**
*Group of inherited disorders of connective tissue; AKA cutis
hyperelastica*

Q79.60 Ehlers-Danlos syndrome, unspecified

Q79.61 Classical Ehlers-Danlos syndrome
Classical EDS (cEDS)

Q79.62 Hypermobile Ehlers-Danlos syndrome
Hypermobile EDS (hEDS)

Q79.63 Vascular Ehlers-Danlos syndrome
Vascular EDS (vEDS)

Q79.69 Other Ehlers-Danlos syndromes

Q79.8 Other congenital malformations of musculoskeletal system
Absence of muscle
Absence of tendon
Accessory muscle
Amyotrophia congenita
Congenital constricting bands
Congenital shortening of tendon
Poland syndrome

**Q79.9 Congenital malformation of musculoskeletal system,
unspecified**
Congenital anomaly of musculoskeletal system NOS
Congenital deformity of musculoskeletal system NOS

OTHER CONGENITAL MALFORMATIONS (Q80-Q89)

● **Q80 Congenital ichthyosis**
*Characterized by increased keratinization, resulting in
noninflammatory scaling of skin*
Excludes1 Refsum's disease (G60.1)

Q80.0 Ichthyosis vulgaris

Q80.1 X-linked ichthyosis

Q80.2 Lamellar ichthyosis
Collodion baby

Q80.3 Congenital bullous ichthyosiform erythroderma

Q80.4 Harlequin fetus

Q80.8 Other congenital ichthyosis

Q80.9 Congenital ichthyosis, unspecified

● **Q81 Epidermolysis bullosa**
Loosening of epidermis

Q81.0 Epidermolysis bullosa simplex
Excludes1 Cockayne's syndrome (Q87.19)

Q81.1 Epidermolysis bullosa letalis
Herlitz' syndrome

Q81.2 Epidermolysis bullosa dystrophica

Q81.8 Other epidermolysis bullosa

Q81.9 Epidermolysis bullosa, unspecified

● **Q82 Other congenital malformations of skin**
Excludes1 acrodermatitis enteropathica (E83.2)
congenital erythropoietic porphyria (E80.0)
pilonidal cyst or sinus (L05.-)
Sturge-Weber (-Dimitri) syndrome (Q85.89)

Q82.0 Hereditary lymphedema
*Characterized by swelling of subcutaneous tissue caused by
obstruction of lymphatic vessels and resulting edema of
lymph fluid*

Q82.1 Xeroderma pigmentosum
*Extreme sensitivity to ultraviolet rays that most commonly
affects the eyes and skin, but may also involve the
nervous system*

Q82.2 Congenital cutaneous mastocytosis
Characterized by infiltrates of mast cells in tissues/organs
Congenital diffuse cutaneous mastocytosis
Congenital maculopapular cutaneous mastocytosis
Congenital urticaria pigmentosa

> **Excludes1**   cutaneous mastocytosis NOS (D47.01)
> diffuse cutaneous mastocytosis (with onset after newborn period) (D47.01)
> malignant mastocytosis (C96.2-)
> systemic mastocytosis (D47.02)
> urticaria pigmentosa (non-congenital) (with onset after newborn period) (D47.01)

Q82.3 Incontinentia pigmenti
Characterized by hypopigmented cutaneous in adults and early childhood

Q82.4 Ectodermal dysplasia (anhidrotic)
Absence/deficiency of tissues/structures, including teeth, hair, nails, and certain glands

> **Excludes1**   Ellis-van Creveld syndrome (Q77.6)

Q82.5 Congenital non-neoplastic nevus
Birthmark NOS
Flammeus Nevus
Portwine Nevus
Sanguineous Nevus
Strawberry Nevus
Vascular Nevus NOS
Verrucous Nevus

> **Excludes2**   Café au lait spots (L81.3)
> lentigo (L81.4)
> nevus NOS (D22.-)
> araneus nevus (I78.1)
> melanocytic nevus (D22.-)
> pigmented nevus (D22.-)
> spider nevus (I78.1)
> stellar nevus (I78.1)

Coding Clinic: 2024, Q3, P5

Q82.6 Congenital sacral dimple
Parasacral dimple

> **Excludes2**   pilonidal cyst with abscess (L05.01)
> pilonidal cyst without abscess (L05.91)

Coding Clinic: 2016, Q4, P60

Q82.8 Other specified congenital malformations of skin
Abnormal palmar creases
Accessory skin tags
Benign familial pemphigus [Hailey-Hailey]
Congenital poikiloderma
Cutis laxa (hyperelastica)
Dermatoglyphic anomalies
Inherited keratosis palmaris et plantaris
Keratosis follicularis [Darier-White]

> **Excludes1**   Ehlers-Danlos syndromes (Q79.6-)

> ▶ **Excludes2**   disorders of pyrophosphate metabolism (E83.82-)

Coding Clinic: 2016, Q1, P17

Q82.9 Congenital malformation of skin, unspecified

● **Q83 Congenital malformations of breast**

> **Excludes2**   absence of pectoral muscle (Q79.8)
> hypoplasia of breast (N64.82)
> micromastia (N64.82)

Q83.0 Congenital absence of breast with absent nipple

Q83.1 Accessory breast
Supernumerary breast

Q83.2 Absent nipple

Q83.3 Accessory nipple
Supernumerary nipple

Q83.8 Other congenital malformations of breast

Q83.9 Congenital malformation of breast, unspecified

● **Q84 Other congenital malformations of integument**

Q84.0 Congenital alopecia
Congenital atrichosis

Q84.1 Congenital morphological disturbances of hair, not elsewhere classified
Beaded hair
Monilethrix
Pili annulati

> **Excludes1**   Menkes' kinky hair syndrome (E83.09)

Q84.2 Other congenital malformations of hair
Congenital hypertrichosis
Congenital malformation of hair NOS
Persistent lanugo

Q84.3 Anonychia
Absence of nail

> **Excludes1**   nail patella syndrome (Q87.2)

Q84.4 Congenital leukonychia
Opaque, whitish discoloration of nails; AKA leukopathia unguium

Q84.5 Enlarged and hypertrophic nails
Congenital onychauxis
Pachyonychia

Q84.6 Other congenital malformations of nails
Congenital clubnail
Congenital koilonychia
Congenital malformation of nail NOS

Q84.8 Other specified congenital malformations of integument
Aplasia cutis congenita

Q84.9 Congenital malformation of integument, unspecified
Congenital anomaly of integument NOS
Congenital deformity of integument NOS

● **Q85 Phakomatoses, not elsewhere classified**

> **Excludes1**   ataxia telangiectasia [Louis-Bar] (G11.3)
> familial dysautonomia [Riley-Day] (G90.1)

● **Q85.0 Neurofibromatosis (nonmalignant)**
Developmental changes in nervous system and other structures, with formation of neurofibromas

Q85.00 Neurofibromatosis, unspecified 🆁🅲🅲

Q85.01 Neurofibromatosis, type 1 🆁🅲🅲
Von Recklinghausen disease

Q85.02 Neurofibromatosis, type 2 🆁🅲🅲
Acoustic neurofibromatosis

Q85.03 Schwannomatosis 🆁🅲🅲

Q85.09 Other neurofibromatosis 🆁🅲🅲

Q85.1 Tuberous sclerosis 🆁🅲🅲
Bourneville's disease
Epiloia

● **Q85.8 Other phakomatoses, not elsewhere classified** 🆁🅲🅲

> **Excludes1**   Meckel-Gruber syndrome (Q61.9)

Coding Clinic: 2021, Q3, P12

Q85.81 PTEN hamartoma tumor syndrome
PHTS
PTEN related Cowden syndrome
> **Code also**, if applicable, genetic susceptibility to malignant neoplasm (Z15.0-)

Coding Clinic: 2022, Q4, P41

Q85.82 Other Cowden syndrome

Q85.83 Von Hippel-Lindau syndrome
> **Code also** manifestations
> **Coding Clinic: 2023, Q2, P16**

Q85.89 Other phakomatoses, not elsewhere classified
Peutz-Jeghers syndrome
Sturge-Weber(-Dimitri) syndrome

Q85.9 Phakomatosis, unspecified 🆁🅲🅲
Hamartosis NOS

● **Q86 Congenital malformation syndromes due to known exogenous causes, not elsewhere classified**

> **Excludes2**   iodine-deficiency-related hypothyroidism (E00-E02)
> nonteratogenic effects of substances transmitted via placenta or breast milk (P04.-)

Q86.0 Fetal alcohol syndrome (dysmorphic)

Q86.1 Fetal hydantoin syndrome
Meadow's syndrome

CHAPTER 17 (Q00-QA0.8)

Q86.2   **Dysmorphism due to warfarin**

Q86.8   **Other congenital malformation syndromes due to known exogenous causes**

● **Q87**   **Other specified congenital malformation syndromes affecting multiple systems**

Use additional code(s) to identify all associated manifestations

Q87.0   **Congenital malformation syndromes predominantly affecting facial appearance**
> Acrocephalopolysyndactyly
> Acrocephalosyndactyly [Apert]
> Cryptophthalmos syndrome
> Cyclopia
> Goldenhar syndrome
> Moebius syndrome
> Oro-facial-digital syndrome
> Robin syndrome
> Whistling face

● Q87.1   **Congenital malformation syndromes predominantly associated with short stature**

Q87.11   **Prader-Willi syndrome**
Coding Clinic: 2024, Q4, P11

Q87.19   **Other congenital malformation syndromes predominantly associated with short stature**
> Aarskog syndrome
> Cockayne syndrome
> De Lange syndrome
> Dubowitz syndrome
> Noonan syndrome
> Robinow-Silverman-Smith syndrome
> Russell-Silver syndrome
> Seckel syndrome

Excludes1   Ellis-van Creveld syndrome (Q77.6)
Smith-Lemli-Opitz syndrome (E78.72)

Q87.2   **Congenital malformation syndromes predominantly involving limbs**
> Holt-Oram syndrome
> Klippel-Trenaunay-Weber syndrome
> Nail patella syndrome
> Rubinstein-Taybi syndrome
> Sirenomelia syndrome
> Thrombocytopenia with absent radius [TAR] syndrome
> VATER syndrome

Q87.3   **Congenital malformation syndromes involving early overgrowth**
> Beckwith-Wiedemann syndrome
> Sotos' syndrome
> Weaver syndrome

● Q87.4   **Marfan's syndrome**

Q87.40   **Marfan's syndrome, unspecified**

● Q87.41   **Marfan syndrome with cardiovascular manifestations**

Q87.410   **Marfan syndrome with aortic dilation**

Q87.418   **Marfan syndrome with other cardiovascular manifestations**

Q87.42   **Marfan syndrome with ocular manifestations**

Q87.43   **Marfan syndrome with skeletal manifestation**

Q87.5   **Other congenital malformation syndromes with other skeletal changes**

● Q87.8   **Other specified congenital malformation syndromes, not elsewhere classified**

Excludes1   Zellweger syndrome (E71.510)

Q87.81   **Alport syndrome**
Progressive sensorineural hearing loss, progressive pyelonephritis or glomerulonephritis, and ocular defects

Use additional code to identify stage of chronic kidney disease (N18.1-N18.6)

Q87.82   **Arterial tortuosity syndrome**
Coding Clinic: 2016, Q4, P60-61

Q87.83   **Bardet-Biedl syndrome**

Q87.84   **Laurence-Moon syndrome**

Q87.85   **MED13L syndrome**
> Asadollahi-Rauch syndrome
> Mediator complex subunit 13L syndrome

Code also, if applicable, any associated manifestations such as:
> autism spectrum disorder (F84.0-)
> congenital malformations of cardiac septa (Q21.-)
> epilepsy and recurrent seizures (G40.-)
> intellectual disability (F70-F79)

Q87.86   **Kleefstra syndrome**

▶ Q87.87   **Hao-Fountain Syndrome**
> ▶HAFOUS

▶ Use Additional code, if applicable, for associated conditions such as:
> ▶autism spectrum disorder (F84.0)
> ▶developmental speech disorder (F80.-)
> ▶epilepsy, by specific type (G40.-)
> ▶intellectual disabilities (F70-F79)
> ▶pervasive developmental disorders (F84.-)

▶ Q87.88   **CTNNB1 syndrome**

Use Additional code, if applicable, for associated conditions such as:
> ▶cerebral palsy (G80.-)
> ▶congenital heart malformations (Q20.0-Q24.9)
> ▶developmental disorder of speech and language (F80.-)
> ▶exudative retinopathy (H35.02-)
> ▶intellectual disability (F70-F79)
> ▶microcephaly (Q02)

Q87.89   **Other specified congenital malformation syndromes, not elsewhere classified**

● **Q89**   **Other congenital malformations, not elsewhere classified**

● Q89.0   **Congenital absence and malformations of spleen**

Excludes1   isomerism of atrial appendages (with asplenia or polysplenia) (Q20.6)

Q89.01   **Asplenia (congenital)**
Coding Clinic: 2025, Q1, P24-25

Q89.09   **Congenital malformations of spleen**
> Congenital splenomegaly

Q89.1   **Congenital malformations of adrenal gland**

Excludes1   adrenogenital disorders (E25.-)
congenital adrenal hyperplasia (E25.0)

Q89.2   **Congenital malformations of other endocrine glands**
> Congenital malformation of parathyroid or thyroid gland
> Persistent thyroglossal duct
> Thyroglossal cyst

Excludes1   congenital goiter (E03.0)
congenital hypothyroidism (E03.1)

Q89.3   **Situs inversus**
Lateral transposition of viscera of thorax and abdomen
> Dextrocardia with situs inversus
> Mirror-image atrial arrangement with situs inversus
> Situs inversus or transversus abdominalis
> Situs inversus or transversus thoracis
> Transposition of abdominal viscera
> Transposition of thoracic viscera

Excludes1   dextrocardia NOS (Q24.0)

Q89.4   **Conjoined twins**
> Craniopagus
> Dicephaly
> Pygopagus
> Thoracopagus

Q89.7   **Multiple congenital malformations, not elsewhere classified**
> Multiple congenital anomalies NOS
> Multiple congenital deformities NOS

Excludes1   congenital malformation syndromes affecting multiple systems (Q87.-)

▶ New   ➡ Revised   ~~deleted~~ Deleted   Excludes 1   Excludes 2   Includes   Use additional   Code first   Code also   Key words

OGCR Official Guidelines   X Assign placeholder X   ● Use Additional Character(s)   ▶ Manifestation Code   Hierarchical Condition Category   **Coding Clinic**

● **Q89.8   Other specified congenital malformations**
  Use additional code(s) to identify all associated
  manifestations
  Coding Clinic: 2021, Q3, P12

▶ **Q89.81   Kabuki syndrome**
  ▶ Kabuki syndrome, type 1, due to KMT2D
    mutation
  ▶ Kabuki syndrome, type 2, due to KDM6A
    mutation
  ▶ Niikawa-Kuroki syndrome

▶ **Q89.89   Other specified congenital malformations**

Q89.9   Congenital malformation, unspecified
  Congenital anomaly NOS
  Congenital deformity NOS

CHROMOSOMAL ABNORMALITIES, NOT ELSEWHERE CLASSIFIED (Q90-Q99)

  Excludes2   mitochondrial metabolic disorders (E88.4-)

● **Q90   Down syndrome**
  Code also associated physical condition(s), such as
    atrioventricular septal defect (Q21.2-)
  Use additional code(s) to identify any associated and degree of
    intellectual disabilities (F70-F79)

  Q90.0   Trisomy 21, nonmosaicism (meiotic nondisjunction)
    *Trisomy 21, nondisjunction, accounts for 95% of Downs
      syndrome cases*

  Q90.1   Trisomy 21, mosaicism (mitotic nondisjunction)

  Q90.2   Trisomy 21, translocation

  Q90.9   Down syndrome, unspecified
    Trisomy 21 NOS

● **Q91   Trisomy 18 and Trisomy 13**
  Q91.0   Trisomy 18, nonmosaicism (meiotic nondisjunction)
  Q91.1   Trisomy 18, mosaicism (mitotic nondisjunction)
  Q91.2   Trisomy 18, translocation
  Q91.3   Trisomy 18, unspecified
  Q91.4   Trisomy 13, nonmosaicism (meiotic nondisjunction)
  Q91.5   Trisomy 13, mosaicism (mitotic nondisjunction)
  Q91.6   Trisomy 13, translocation
  Q91.7   Trisomy 13, unspecified

● **Q92   Other trisomies and partial trisomies of the autosomes, not
  elsewhere classified**
  Includes   unbalanced translocations and insertions
  Excludes1   trisomies of chromosomes 13, 18, 21 (Q90-Q91)

  **Q92.0   Whole chromosome trisomy, nonmosaicism (meiotic
    nondisjunction)**

  **Q92.1   Whole chromosome trisomy, mosaicism (mitotic
    nondisjunction)**

  Q92.2   Partial trisomy
    Less than whole arm duplicated
    Whole arm or more duplicated
    Excludes1   partial trisomy due to unbalanced
      translocation (Q92.5)

  Q92.5   Duplications with other complex rearrangements
    Partial trisomy due to unbalanced translocations
    Code also any associated deletions due to unbalanced
      translocations, inversions and insertions (Q93.7)

● **Q92.6   Marker chromosomes**
    Trisomies due to dicentrics
    Trisomies due to extra rings
    Trisomies due to isochromosomes
    Individual with marker heterochromatin

  Q92.61   Marker chromosomes in normal individual

  Q92.62   Marker chromosomes in abnormal individual

  Q92.7   Triploidy and polyploidy

  **Q92.8   Other specified trisomies and partial trisomies of
    autosomes**
    Duplications identified by fluorescence in situ
      hybridization (FISH)
    Duplications identified by in situ hybridization (ISH)
    Duplications seen only at prometaphase

  Q92.9   Trisomy and partial trisomy of autosomes, unspecified

● **Q93   Monosomies and deletions from the autosomes, not elsewhere
  classified**

  **Q93.0   Whole chromosome monosomy, nonmosaicism (meiotic
    nondisjunction)**

  **Q93.1   Whole chromosome monosomy, mosaicism (mitotic
    nondisjunction)**

  **Q93.2   Chromosome replaced with ring, dicentric or
    isochromosome**

  Q93.3   Deletion of short arm of chromosome 4
    Wolff-Hirschorn syndrome

  Q93.4   Deletion of short arm of chromosome 5
    Cri-du-chat syndrome

● **Q93.5   Other deletions of part of a chromosome**

  Q93.51   Angelman syndrome

  Q93.52   Phelan-McDermid syndrome
    22q13.3 deletion syndrome
    Use additional code(s) to identify any
      associated conditions, such as:
    autism spectrum disorder (F84.0)
    degree of intellectual disabilities (F70-F79)
    epilepsy and recurrent seizures (G40.-)
    lymphedema (I89.0)

  Q93.59   Other deletions of part of a chromosome

  **Q93.7   Deletions with other complex
    rearrangements**
    Deletions due to unbalanced translocations, inversions
      and insertions
    Code also any associated duplications due to
      unbalanced translocations, inversions and
      insertions (Q92.5)

● **Q93.8   Other deletions from the autosomes**

  Q93.81   Velo-cardio-facial syndrome
    Deletion 22q11.2
    Coding Clinic: 2019, Q3, P14

  Q93.82   Williams syndrome

  Q93.88   Other microdeletions Miller-Dieker syndrome
    Smith-Magenis syndrome

  Q93.89   Other deletions from the autosomes
    Deletions identified by fluorescence in situ
      hybridization (FISH)
    Deletions identified by in situ hybridization
      (ISH)
    Deletions seen only at prometaphase

  Q93.9   Deletion from autosomes, unspecified

● **Q95   Balanced rearrangements and structural markers, not elsewhere
  classified**
  Includes   Robertsonian and balanced reciprocal
    translocations and insertions

  **Q95.0   Balanced translocation and insertion in normal
    individual**

  Q95.1   Chromosome inversion in normal individual

  **Q95.2   Balanced autosomal rearrangement in abnormal
    individual**

  **Q95.3   Balanced sex/autosomal rearrangement in abnormal
    individual**

  Q95.5   Individual with autosomal fragile site

  Q95.8   Other balanced rearrangements and structural markers

  **Q95.9   Balanced rearrangement and structural marker,
    unspecified**

● **Q96   Turner's syndrome**
  *Caused by missing or incomplete X chromosome affecting growth and
    sexual development*
  Excludes1   Noonan syndrome (Q87.19)

  Q96.0   Karyotype 45, X

  Q96.1   Karyotype 46, X iso (Xq)
    Karyotype 46, isochromosome Xq

  **Q96.2   Karyotype 46, X with abnormal sex chromosome, except
    iso (Xq)**
    Karyotype 46, X with abnormal sex chromosome, except
      isochromosome Xq

CHAPTER 17 (Q00-Q99)

CHAPTER 17 (Q00–QA0.8)

Q96.3   Mosaicism, 45, X/46, XX or XY

Q96.4   Mosaicism, 45, X/other cell line(s) with abnormal sex chromosome

Q96.8   Other variants of Turner's syndrome

Q96.9   Turner's syndrome, unspecified

● Q97   Other sex chromosome abnormalities, female phenotype, not elsewhere classified

     Excludes1   Turner's syndrome (Q96.-)

Q97.0   Karyotype 47, XXX

Q97.1   Female with more than three X chromosomes

Q97.2   Mosaicism, lines with various numbers of X chromosomes

Q97.3   Female with 46, XY karyotype

Q97.8   Other specified sex chromosome abnormalities, female phenotype

Q97.9   Sex chromosome abnormality, female phenotype, unspecified

● Q98   Other sex chromosome abnormalities, male phenotype, not elsewhere classified

Q98.0   Klinefelter syndrome karyotype 47, XXY

Q98.1   Klinefelter syndrome, male with more than two X chromosomes

Q98.3   Other male with 46, XX karyotype

Q98.4   Klinefelter syndrome, unspecified

Q98.5   Karyotype 47, XYY

Q98.6   Male with structurally abnormal sex chromosome

Q98.7   Male with sex chromosome mosaicism

Q98.8   Other specified sex chromosome abnormalities, male phenotype

Q98.9   Sex chromosome abnormality, male phenotype, unspecified

● Q99   Other chromosome abnormalities, not elsewhere classified

Q99.0   Chimera 46, XX/46, XY
       Chimera 46, XX/46, XY true hermaphrodite

Q99.1   46, XX true hermaphrodite
       46, XX with streak gonads
       46, XY with streak gonads
       Pure gonadal dysgenesis

Q99.2   Fragile X chromosome
       Fragile X syndrome

● Q99.8   Other specified chromosome abnormalities

   ▶ ● Q99.81   Usher syndrome

      ▶ Use Additional code to identify any auditory and visual manifestations

     ▶ Q99.811   Usher syndrome, type 1

     ▶ Q99.812   Usher syndrome, type 2

     ▶ Q99.813   Usher syndrome, type 3

     ▶ Q99.818   Other Usher syndrome
       ▶ Usher syndrome, type 4

     ▶ Q99.819   Usher syndrome, unspecified

   ▶ Q99.89   Other specified chromosome abnormalities

Q99.9   Chromosomal abnormality, unspecified

GENETIC DISORDERS, NOT ELSEWHERE CLASSIFIED (QA0)

▶ ● QA0   Neurodevelopmental disorders related to specific genetic pathogenic variants

   Code also, if applicable, any associated conditions, such as:
     ▶ attention-deficit hyperactivity disorders (F90.-)
     ▶ autism spectrum disorder (F84.0)
     ▶ developmental and epileptic encephalopathy (G93.45)
     ▶ epilepsy, by specific type (G40.-)
     ▶ intellectual disabilities (F70-F79)
     ▶ pervasive developmental disorders (F84.-)

▶ ● QA0.0   Neurodevelopmental disorders related to pathogenic variants in specific genes

   ▶ QA0.01   Neurodevelopmental disorders related to pathogenic variants in certain specific genes

     ▶ ● QA0.010   Neurodevelopmental disorders, related to pathogenic variants in ion channel genes

       ▶ QA0.0101   SCN2A-related neurodevelopmental disorder

       ▶ QA0.0102   CACNA1A-related neurodevelopmental disorder

       ▶ QA0.0109   Neurodevelopmental disorder related to pathogenic variant in other ion channel gene
         ▶ SCN8A-related neurodevelopmental disorder

     ▶ QA0.011   Neurodevelopmental disorders, related to pathogenic variants in glutamate receptor genes

     ▶ QA0.012   Neurodevelopmental disorders, related to pathogenic variants in other receptor genes

     ▶ ● QA0.013   Neurodevelopmental disorders, related to pathogenic variants in other transporter and solute carrier genes

       ▶ QA0.0131   SLC6A1-related disorder
         ▶ GABA transporter 1 deficiency

       ▶ QA0.0139   Neurodevelopmental disorder, related to pathogenic variant in other transporter or solute carrier gene

     ▶ ● QA0.014   Neurodevelopmental disorders, related to pathogenic variants in synapserelated genes

       ▶ QA0.0141   Syntaxin-binding protein 1-related disorder
         ▶ STXBP1-related disorders

       ▶ QA0.0142   DLG4-related synaptopathy

       ▶ QA0.0149   Neurodevelopmental disorder, related to pathogenic variant in other synapse related gene
         ▶ Other genetic synaptopathy

     ▶ ● QA0.015   Neurodevelopmental disorders, related to genes associated with transcription and gene expression

       ▶ QA0.0151   FOXG1 syndrome
         ▶ FOXG1-related disorder
         ▶ FOXG1-related encephalopathy
         ▶ FOXG1-related neurodevelopmental disorder

       ▶ QA0.0159   Neurodevelopmental disorder, related to other genes associated with transcription and gene expression

   ▶ QA0.8   Other neurodevelopmental disorders related to pathogenic variants in other specific genes

CHAPTER 18

SYMPTOMS, SIGNS, AND ABNORMAL CLINICAL AND LABORATORY FINDINGS, NOT ELSEWHERE CLASSIFIED (R00–R99)

OGCR Chapter-Specific Coding Guidelines

18. **Chapter 18: Symptoms, signs, and abnormal clinical and laboratory findings, not elsewhere classified (R00-R99)**
Chapter 18 includes symptoms, signs, abnormal results of clinical or other investigative procedures, and ill-defined conditions regarding which no diagnosis classifiable elsewhere is recorded. Signs and symptoms that point to a specific diagnosis have been assigned to a category in other chapters of the classification.

a. Use of symptom codes
Codes that describe symptoms and signs are acceptable for reporting purposes when a related definitive diagnosis has not been established (confirmed) by the provider.

b. Use of a symptom code with a definitive diagnosis code
Codes for signs and symptoms may be reported in addition to a related definitive diagnosis when the sign or symptom is not routinely associated with that diagnosis, such as the various signs and symptoms associated with complex syndromes. The definitive diagnosis code should be sequenced before the symptom code.

Signs or symptoms that are associated routinely with a disease process should not be assigned as additional codes, unless otherwise instructed by the classification.

c. Combination codes that include symptoms
ICD-10-CM contains a number of combination codes that identify both the definitive diagnosis and common symptoms of that diagnosis. When using one of these combination codes, an additional code should not be assigned for the symptom.

d. Repeated falls
Code R29.6, Repeated falls, is for use for encounters when a patient has recently fallen and the reason for the fall is being investigated.

Code Z91.81, History of falling, is for use when a patient has fallen in the past and is at risk for future falls. When appropriate, both codes R29.6 and Z91.81 may be assigned together.

e. Coma scale
The coma scale codes (R40.2-) can be used in conjunction with traumatic brain injury codes, acute cerebrovascular disease or sequelae of cerebrovascular disease codes. These codes are primarily for use by trauma registries, but they may be used in any setting where this information is collected. The coma scale may also be used to assess the status of the central nervous system for other non-trauma conditions, such as monitoring patients in the intensive care unit regardless of medical condition. The coma scale codes should be sequenced after the diagnosis code(s).

These codes, one from each subcategory, are needed to complete the scale. The 7th character indicates when the scale was recorded. The 7th character should match for all three codes.

At a minimum, report the initial score documented on presentation at your facility. This may be a score from the emergency medicine technician (EMT) or in the emergency department. If desired, a facility may choose to capture multiple coma scale scores.

Assign code R40.24, Glasgow coma scale, total score, when only the total score is documented in the medical record and not the individual score(s).

Do not report codes for individual or total Glasgow coma scale scores for a patient with a medically induced coma or a sedated patient.

See Section I.B.14 for coma scale documentation by clinicians other than patient's provider.

f. Functional quadriplegia
GUIDELINE HAS BEEN DELETED EFFECTIVE OCTOBER 1, 2017

g. SIRS due to Non-Infectious Process
The systemic inflammatory response syndrome (SIRS) can develop as a result of certain non-infectious disease processes, such as trauma, malignant neoplasm, or pancreatitis. When SIRS is documented with a noninfectious condition, and no subsequent infection is documented, the code for the underlying condition, such as an injury, should be assigned, followed by code R65.10, Systemic inflammatory response syndrome (SIRS) of non-infectious origin without acute organ dysfunction, or code R65.11, Systemic inflammatory response syndrome (SIRS) of non-infectious origin with acute organ dysfunction. If an associated acute organ dysfunction is documented, the appropriate code(s) for the specific type of organ dysfunction(s) should be assigned in addition to code R65.11. If acute organ dysfunction is documented, but it cannot be determined if the acute organ dysfunction is associated with SIRS or due to another condition (e.g., directly due to the trauma), the provider should be queried.

h. Death NOS
Code R99, Ill-defined and unknown cause of mortality, is only for use in the very limited circumstance when a patient who has already died is brought into an emergency department or other healthcare facility and is pronounced dead upon arrival. It does not represent the discharge disposition of death.

i. NIHSS Stroke Scale
The NIH stroke scale (NIHSS) codes (R29.7- -) can be used in conjunction with acute stroke codes (I63) to identify the patient's neurological status and the severity of the stroke. The stroke scale codes should be sequenced after the acute stroke diagnosis code(s).

At a minimum, report the initial score documented. If desired, a facility may choose to capture multiple stroke scale scores.

See Section I.B.14 for NIHSS stroke scale documentation by clinicians other than patient's provider.

CHAPTER 18

SYMPTOMS, SIGNS, AND ABNORMAL CLINICAL AND LABORATORY FINDINGS, NOT ELSEWHERE CLASSIFIED (R00-R99)

Note: This chapter includes symptoms, signs, abnormal results of clinical or other investigative procedures, and ill-defined conditions regarding which no diagnosis classifiable elsewhere is recorded.

Signs and symptoms that point rather definitely to a given diagnosis have been assigned to a category in other chapters of the classification. In general, categories in this chapter include the less well-defined conditions and symptoms that, without the necessary study of the case to establish a final diagnosis, point perhaps equally to two or more diseases or to two or more systems of the body. Practically all categories in the chapter could be designated "not otherwise specified", "unknown etiology" or "transient". The Alphabetical Index should be consulted to determine which symptoms and signs are to be allocated here and which to other chapters. The residual subcategories, numbered .8, are generally provided for other relevant symptoms that cannot be allocated elsewhere in the classification.

The conditions and signs or symptoms included in categories R00-R94 consist of:
(a) cases for which no more specific diagnosis can be made even after all the facts bearing on the case have been investigated;
(b) signs or symptoms existing at the time of initial encounter that proved to be transient and whose causes could not be determined;
(c) provisional diagnosis in a patient who failed to return for further investigation or care;
(d) cases referred elsewhere for investigation or treatment before the diagnosis was made;
(e) cases in which a more precise diagnosis was not available for any other reason;
(f) certain symptoms, for which supplementary information is provided, that represent important problems in medical care in their own right.

Excludes2   abnormal findings on antenatal screening of mother (O28.-)
certain conditions originating in the perinatal period (P04-P96)
signs and symptoms classified in the body system chapters
signs and symptoms of breast (N63, N64.5)

This chapter contains the following blocks:

R00-R09	Symptoms and signs involving the circulatory and respiratory systems
R10-R19	Symptoms and signs involving the digestive system and abdomen
R20-R23	Symptoms and signs involving the skin and subcutaneous tissue
R25-R29	Symptoms and signs involving the nervous and musculoskeletal systems
R30-R39	Symptoms and signs involving the genitourinary system
R40-R46	Symptoms and signs involving cognition, perception, emotional state and behavior
R47-R49	Symptoms and signs involving speech and voice
R50-R69	General symptoms and signs
R70-R79	Abnormal findings on examination of blood, without diagnosis
R80-R82	Abnormal findings on examination of urine, without diagnosis
R83-R89	Abnormal findings on examination of other body fluids, substances and tissues, without diagnosis
R90-R94	Abnormal findings on diagnostic imaging and in function studies, without diagnosis
R97	Abnormal tumor markers
R99	Ill-defined and unknown cause of mortality

SYMPTOMS AND SIGNS INVOLVING THE CIRCULATORY AND RESPIRATORY SYSTEMS (R00-R09)

● **R00**   **Abnormalities of heart beat**

  Excludes1   abnormalities originating in the perinatal period (P29.1-)
inappropriate sinus tachycardia, so stated (I47.11)

  Excludes2   specified arrhythmias (I47-I49)

  R00.0   **Tachycardia, unspecified**
Rapid heart rate >100 beats
Rapid heart beat
Sinoauricular tachycardia NOS
Sinus [sinusal] tachycardia NOS

    Excludes1   neonatal tachycardia (P29.11)
paroxysmal tachycardia (I47.-)

Coding Clinic: 2022, Q4, P47

  R00.1   **Bradycardia, unspecified**
Slow heart rate, <60
Sinoatrial bradycardia
Sinus bradycardia
Slow heart beat
Vagal bradycardia
Use additional code for adverse effect, if applicable, to identify drug (T36-T50 with fifth or sixth character 5)

    Excludes1   neonatal bradycardia (P29.12)

  R00.2   **Palpitations**
Awareness of heart beat

  R00.8   **Other abnormalities of heart beat**

  R00.9   **Unspecified abnormalities of heart beat**

▶ New   ⇒ Revised   ~~deleted~~ Deleted   Excludes 1   Excludes 2   Includes   Use additional   Code first   Code also   Key words
OGCR Official Guidelines   **X** Assign placeholder X   ● Use Additional Character(s)   ▶ Manifestation Code   Ⓗ Hierarchical Condition Category   Coding Clinic

● **R01** **Cardiac murmurs and other cardiac sounds**
  Excludes1 cardiac murmurs and sounds originating in the perinatal period (P29.8)
 R01.0 **Benign and innocent cardiac murmurs**
   Functional cardiac murmur
 R01.1 **Cardiac murmur, unspecified**
   Cardiac bruit NOS
   Heart murmur NOS
   Systolic murmur NOS
 R01.2 **Other cardiac sounds**
   Cardiac dullness, increased or decreased
   Precordial friction

OGCR **Section I.C.9.a.7.**

Hypertension, Transient

Assign code R03.0, Elevated blood pressure reading without diagnosis of hypertension, unless patient has an established diagnosis of hypertension. Assign code O13.-, Gestational [pregnancy-induced] hypertension with significant proteinuria, or O14.-, Pre-eclampsia, for transient hypertension of pregnancy.

● **R03** **Abnormal blood-pressure reading, without diagnosis**
 R03.0 **Elevated blood-pressure reading, without diagnosis of hypertension**
   Note: This category is to be used to record an episode of elevated blood pressure in a patient in whom no formal diagnosis of hypertension has been made, or as an isolated incidental finding.
 R03.1 **Nonspecific low blood-pressure reading**
  Excludes1 hypotension (I95.-)
    maternal hypotension syndrome (O26.5-)
    neurogenic orthostatic hypotension (G90.3)

● **R04** **Hemorrhage from respiratory passages**
 R04.0 **Epistaxis**
   Hemorrhage from nose
   Nosebleed
   Coding Clinic: 2023, Q2, P28; 2018, Q4, P38
 R04.1 **Hemorrhage from throat**
  Excludes2 hemoptysis (R04.2)
 R04.2 **Hemoptysis**
   Blood-stained sputum
   Cough with hemorrhage
● **R04.8** **Hemorrhage from other sites in respiratory passages**
  R04.81 **Acute idiopathic pulmonary hemorrhage in infants** P
   AIPHI
   Acute idiopathic hemorrhage in infants over 28 days old
   Excludes1 perinatal pulmonary hemorrhage (P26.-)
    von Willebrand's disease (D68.0-)
  R04.89 **Hemorrhage from other sites in respiratory passages**
   Pulmonary hemorrhage NOS
 R04.9 **Hemorrhage from respiratory passages, unspecified**

● **R05** **Cough**
  Excludes1 paroxysmal cough due to Bordetella pertussis (A37.0-)
    smoker's cough (J41.0)
  Excludes2 cough with hemorrhage (R04.2))
 R05.1 **Acute cough**
 R05.2 **Subacute cough**
 R05.3 **Chronic cough**
   Persistent cough
   Refractory cough
   Unexplained cough

 R05.4 **Cough syncope**
   Code first syncope and collapse (R55)
 R05.8 **Other specified cough**
 R05.9 **Cough, unspecified**

● **R06** **Abnormalities of breathing**
  Excludes1 acute respiratory distress syndrome (J80)
    respiratory arrest (R09.2)
    respiratory arrest of newborn (P28.81)
    respiratory distress syndrome of newborn (P22.-)
    respiratory failure (J96.-)
    respiratory failure of newborn (P28.5)
● **R06.0** **Dyspnea**
  Excludes1 tachypnea NOS (R06.82)
    transient tachypnea of newborn (P22.1)
  R06.00 **Dyspnea, unspecified**
   Coding Clinic: 2017, Q1, P26-27
  R06.01 **Orthopnea**
  R06.02 **Shortness of breath**
  R06.03 **Acute respiratory distress**
  R06.09 **Other forms of dyspnea**
 R06.1 **Stridor**
   Harsh, high-pitched breath sound
  Excludes1 congenital laryngeal stridor (P28.89)
    laryngismus (stridulus) (J38.5)
 R06.2 **Wheezing**
  Excludes1 Asthma (J45.-)
   Coding Clinic: 2016, Q2, P34
 R06.3 **Periodic breathing**
   Cheyne-Stokes breathing
   An abnormal pattern of breathing with gradually increasing and decreasing tidal volume with some periods of apnea
 R06.4 **Hyperventilation**
  Excludes1 psychogenic hyperventilation (F45.8)
 R06.5 **Mouth breathing**
  Excludes2 dry mouth NOS (R68.2)
 R06.6 **Hiccough**
  Excludes1 psychogenic hiccough (F45.8)
 R06.7 **Sneezing**
● **R06.8** **Other abnormalities of breathing**
  R06.81 **Apnea, not elsewhere classified**
   Apnea NOS
   Excludes1 apnea (of) newborn (P28.4-)
    sleep apnea (G47.3-)
    sleep apnea of newborn (primary) (P28.3-)
  R06.82 **Tachypnea, not elsewhere classified**
   Tachypnea NOS
   Excludes1 transitory tachypnea of newborn (P22.1)
  R06.83 **Snoring**
  R06.89 **Other abnormalities of breathing**
   Breath-holding (spells)
   Sighing
 R06.9 **Unspecified abnormalities of breathing**

● **R07** **Pain in throat and chest**
  Excludes1 epidemic myalgia (B33.0)
  Excludes2 jaw pain R68.84
    pain in breast (N64.4)
 R07.0 **Pain in throat**
  Excludes1 chronic sore throat (J31.2)
    sore throat (acute) NOS (J02.9)
  Excludes2 dysphagia (R13.1-)
    pain in neck (M54.2)
 R07.1 **Chest pain on breathing**
   Painful respiration
 R07.2 **Precordial pain**

CHAPTER 18 (R00-R99)

● **R07.8**   **Other chest pain**
    R07.81   **Pleurodynia**
        Pleurodynia NOS
        Excludes1   epidemic pleurodynia (B33.0)
        Coding Clinic: 2024, Q3, P16-17
    R07.82   **Intercostal pain**
    R07.89   **Other chest pain**
        Anterior chest-wall pain NOS
        Coding Clinic: 2024, Q3, P17; 2021, Q1, P42
  R07.9   **Chest pain, unspecified**

● **R09**   **Other symptoms and signs involving the circulatory and respiratory system**
    Excludes1   acute respiratory distress syndrome (J80)
        respiratory arrest of newborn (P28.81)
        respiratory distress syndrome of newborn (P22.0)
        respiratory failure (J96.-)
        respiratory failure of newborn (P28.5)

● **R09.0**   **Asphyxia and hypoxemia**
    Excludes1   asphyxia due to carbon monoxide (T58.-)
        asphyxia due to foreign body in respiratory tract (T17.-)
        birth (intrauterine) asphyxia (P84)
        hyperventilation (R06.4)
        traumatic asphyxia (T71.-)
    Excludes2   hypercapnia (R06.89)
    R09.01   **Asphyxia**
    R09.02   **Hypoxemia**
        Coding Clinic: 2019, Q3, P15

  R09.1   **Pleurisy**
    Occurs when double membrane (pleura) lining chest cavity and lung surface becomes inflamed, causing sharp pain on inspiration/expiration
    Excludes1   pleurisy with effusion (J90)

  R09.2   **Respiratory arrest**
    Cardiorespiratory failure
    Excludes1   cardiac arrest (I46.-)
        respiratory arrest of newborn (P28.81)
        respiratory distress of newborn (P22.0)
        respiratory failure (J96.-)
        respiratory failure of newborn (P28.5)
        respiratory insufficiency (R06.89)
        respiratory insufficiency of newborn (P28.5)

  R09.3   **Abnormal sputum**
    Abnormal amount of sputum
    Abnormal color of sputum
    Abnormal odor of sputum
    Excessive sputum
    Excludes1   blood-stained sputum (R04.2)

● **R09.8**   **Other specified symptoms and signs involving the circulatory and respiratory systems**
    R09.81   **Nasal congestion**
    R09.82   **Postnasal drip**
    R09.89   **Other specified symptoms and signs involving the circulatory and respiratory systems**
        Bruit (arterial)
        Abnormal chest percussion
        Friction sounds in chest
        Chest tympany
        Choking sensation
        Rales
        Wet rattling, clicking, crackling sounds on auscultation
        Weak pulse
        Excludes2   foreign body in throat (T17.2-)
            wheezing (R06.2)
        Coding Clinic: 2021, Q1, P42

● **R09.A**   **Foreign body sensation of the circulatory and respiratory system**
    R09.A0   **Foreign body sensation, unspecified**
    R09.A1   **Foreign body sensation, nose**
    R09.A2   **Foreign body sensation, throat**
        Foreign body sensation globus
    R09.A9   **Foreign body sensation, other site**

SYMPTOMS AND SIGNS INVOLVING THE DIGESTIVE SYSTEM AND ABDOMEN (R10-R19)

  Excludes2   congenital or infantile pylorospasm (Q40.0)
    gastrointestinal hemorrhage (K92.0-K92.2)
    intestinal obstruction (K56.-)
    newborn gastrointestinal hemorrhage (P54.0-P54.3)
    newborn intestinal obstruction (P76.-)
    pylorospasm (K31.3)
    signs and symptoms involving the urinary system (R30-R39)
    symptoms referable to female genital organs (N94.-)
    symptoms referable to male genital organs (N48-N50)

● **R10**   **Abdominal and pelvic pain**
    Excludes1   renal colic (N23)
    ▶ **Excludes2**   costovertebral (angle) tenderness (R39.85)
        dorsalgia (M54.-)
        flatulence and related conditions (R14.-)

  R10.0   **Acute abdomen**
    Severe abdominal pain (generalized) (with abdominal rigidity)
    Excludes1   abdominal rigidity NOS (R19.3)
        generalized abdominal pain NOS (R10.84)
        localized abdominal pain (R10.1-R10.3-)

● **R10.1**   **Pain localized to upper abdomen**
    ▶ **Excludes2**   pain localized to flank (R10.A-)
        ▶ pelvic and perineal pain (R10.2-)
    R10.10   **Upper abdominal pain, unspecified**
    R10.11   **Right upper quadrant pain**
    R10.12   **Left upper quadrant pain**
    R10.13   **Epigastric pain**
        Dyspepsia
        Excludes1   functional dyspepsia (K30)

● **R10.2**   **Pelvic and perineal pain**
    Excludes1   vulvodynia (N94.81)
    ▶ **Excludes2**   pain localized to other parts of lower abdomen (R10.3-)
        ▶ pain localized to upper abdomen (R10.1-)
    ▶ **R10.20**   **Pelvic and perineal pain unspecified side**
    ▶ **R10.21**   **Pelvic and perineal pain right side**
    ▶ **R10.22**   **Pelvic and perineal pain left side**
    ▶ **R10.23**   **Pelvic and perineal pain bilateral**
    ▶ **R10.24**   **Suprapubic pain**

● **R10.3**   **Pain localized to other parts of lower abdomen**
    ▶ **Excludes2**   pain localized to flank (R10.A-)
        ▶ pelvic and perineal pain (R10.2-)
    R10.30   **Lower abdominal pain, unspecified**
    R10.31   **Right lower quadrant pain**
    R10.32   **Left lower quadrant pain**
    R10.33   **Periumbilical pain**

● **R10.8**   **Other abdominal pain**
  ● **R10.81**   **Abdominal tenderness**
    Abdominal tenderness NOS
    ▶ **Excludes2**   pain localized to other parts of lower abdomen (R10.3-)
        ▶ pain localized to upper abdomen (R10.1-)
    R10.811   **Right upper quadrant abdominal tenderness**
    R10.812   **Left upper quadrant abdominal tenderness**
    R10.813   **Right lower quadrant abdominal tenderness**
    R10.814   **Left lower quadrant abdominal tenderness**
    R10.815   **Periumbilic abdominal tenderness**
    R10.816   **Epigastric abdominal tenderness**
    R10.817   **Generalized abdominal tenderness**
    R10.819   **Abdominal tenderness, unspecified site**

▶ New   ⇒ Revised   ~~deleted~~ Deleted   Excludes 1   Excludes 2   Includes   Use additional   Code first   Code also   Key words
OGCR Official Guidelines   **X** Assign placeholder X   ● Use Additional Character(s)   ▌ Manifestation Code   Hierarchical Condition Category   Coding Clinic

● **R10.82**   **Rebound abdominal tenderness**
   ▶ **Excludes2**   pain localized to other parts of lower abdomen (R10.3-)
      ▶ pain localized to upper abdomen (R10.1-)

    R10.821   **Right upper quadrant rebound abdominal tenderness**

    R10.822   **Left upper quadrant rebound abdominal tenderness**

    R10.823   **Right lower quadrant rebound abdominal tenderness**

    R10.824   **Left lower quadrant rebound abdominal tenderness**

    R10.825   **Periumbilic rebound abdominal tenderness**

    R10.826   **Epigastric rebound abdominal tenderness**

    R10.827   **Generalized rebound abdominal tenderness**

    R10.829   **Rebound abdominal tenderness, unspecified site**

R10.83   **Colic**   P
    Colic NOS
    Infantile colic
     Excludes1   colic in adult and child over 12 months old (R10.84)

R10.84   **Generalized abdominal pain**
     Excludes1   generalized abdominal pain associated with acute abdomen (R10.0)

▶ **R10.85**   **Abdominal pain of multiple sites**
   ▶ **Excludes1**   abdominal rigidity NOS (R19.3)
      ▶ generalized abdominal pain associated with acute abdomen (R10.0)
      ▶ generalized abdominal pain NOS (R10.84)
      ▶ localized abdominal pain (R10.1-R10.4-)

▶ **R10.8A**   **Flank tenderness**
   ▶ **R10.8A1**   **Right flank tenderness**
   ▶ **R10.8A2**   **Left flank tenderness**
   ▶ **R10.8A3**   **Suprapubic tenderness**
   ▶ **R10.8A9**   **Flank tenderness, unspecified**
      ▶ Flank tenderness NOS

R10.9   **Unspecified abdominal pain**

▶● **R10.A**   **Pain localized to flank**
   ▶ Lateral abdomen pain
   ▶ Lateral flank pain
   ▶ Latus region pain
   ▶ **Excludes2**   pain localized to other parts of lower abdomen (R10.3-)
      ▶ pain localized to upper abdomen (R10.1-)

▶ **R10.A0**   **Flank pain, unspecified side**
▶ **R10.A1**   **Flank pain, right side**
▶ **R10.A2**   **Flank pain, left side**
▶ **R10.A3**   **Flank pain, bilateral**

● **R11**   **Nausea and vomiting**
    Excludes1   cyclical vomiting associated with migraine (G43.A-)
       excessive vomiting in pregnancy (O21.-)
       hematemesis (K92.0)
       neonatal hematemesis (P54.0)
       newborn vomiting (P92.0-)
       psychogenic vomiting (F50.89)
       vomiting associated with bulimia nervosa (F50.2-)
       vomiting following gastrointestinal surgery (K91.0)
    Coding Clinic: 2017, Q1, P27

● **R11.0**   **Nausea**
    Nausea NOS
    Nausea without vomiting

● **R11.1**   **Vomiting**

    R11.10   **Vomiting, unspecified**
       Vomiting NOS

    R11.11   **Vomiting without nausea**

    R11.12   **Projectile vomiting**

    R11.13   **Vomiting of fecal matter**

    R11.14   **Bilious vomiting**
       Bilious emesis

    R11.15   **Cyclical vomiting syndrome unrelated to migraine**
       Cyclic vomiting syndrome NOS
       Persistent vomiting
     Excludes1   cyclical vomiting in migraine (G43.A-)
     Excludes2   bulimia nervosa (F50.20)
       diabetes mellitus due to underlying condition (E08.-)

  ▶ **R11.16**   **Cannabis hyperemesis syndrome**
   ▶ Cannabinoid hyperemesis syndrome
   ▶ Code also
      ▶ cannabis abuse (F12.1-)
      ▶ cannabis dependence (F12.2-)
      ▶ cannabis use, unspecified (F12.92-, F12.93, F12.95-, F12.98-, F12.99)
      ▶ manifestations, such as:
         ▶ dehydration (E86.0)
         ▶ electrolyte imbalance (E87.8)

R11.2   **Nausea with vomiting, unspecified**
    Persistent nausea with vomiting NOS
    Coding Clinic: 2020, Q1, P8

R12   **Heartburn**
    Excludes1   dyspepsia NOS (R10.13)
       functional dyspepsia (K30)

● **R13**   **Aphagia and dysphagia**

    R13.0   **Aphagia**
       Inability to swallow
     Excludes1   psychogenic aphagia (F50.9)

● **R13.1**   **Dysphagia**
    Difficulty swallowing
    Code first, *if applicable, dysphagia following cerebrovascular disease (I69. with final characters -91)*
     Excludes1   psychogenic dysphagia (F45.8)

    R13.10   **Dysphagia, unspecified**
       Difficulty in swallowing NOS

    R13.11   **Dysphagia, oral phase**
    R13.12   **Dysphagia, oropharyngeal phase**
    R13.13   **Dysphagia, pharyngeal phase**
    R13.14   **Dysphagia, pharyngoesophageal phase**
    R13.19   **Other dysphagia**
       Cervical dysphagia
       Neurogenic dysphagia

● **R14**   **Flatulence and related conditions**
    Excludes1   psychogenic aerophagy (F45.8)

    R14.0   **Abdominal distension (gaseous)**
       Bloating
       Tympanites (abdominal) (intestinal)

    R14.1   **Gas pain**
    R14.2   **Eructation**
    Belching air from stomach through mouth

    R14.3   **Flatulence**

● **R15**   **Fecal incontinence**
    Includes   encopresis NOS
    Excludes1   fecal incontinence of nonorganic origin (F98.1)

    R15.0   **Incomplete defecation**
     ~~**Excludes1**   constipation (K59.0-)~~
       ~~fecal impaction (K56.41)~~
   ▶ **Excludes2**   constipation (K59.0-)
      ▶ fecal impaction (K56.41)

    R15.1   **Fecal smearing**
       Fecal soiling

R15.2   Fecal urgency

R15.9   Full incontinence of feces
Fecal incontinence NOS

● **R16**   Hepatomegaly and splenomegaly, not elsewhere classified
Enlargement of liver or spleen

R16.0   Hepatomegaly, not elsewhere classified
Hepatomegaly NOS

R16.1   Splenomegaly, not elsewhere classified
Splenomegaly NOS 9

R16.2   Hepatomegaly with splenomegaly, not elsewhere classified
Hepatosplenomegaly NOS

R17   Unspecified jaundice
> **Excludes1**   neonatal jaundice (P55, P57-P59)

● **R18**   Ascites
> **Includes**   fluid in peritoneal cavity
> **Excludes1**   ascites in alcoholic cirrhosis (K70.31)
> ascites in alcoholic hepatitis (K70.11)
> ascites in toxic liver disease with chronic active hepatitis (K71.51)

R18.0   Malignant ascites
> *Code first malignancy, such as:*
> malignant neoplasm of ovary (C56.-)
> secondary malignant neoplasm of retroperitoneum and peritoneum (C78.6)

R18.8   Other ascites
Ascites NOS
Peritoneal effusion (chronic)
Coding Clinic: 2018, Q1, P4

● **R19**   Other symptoms and signs involving the digestive system and abdomen
> **Excludes1**   acute abdomen (R10.0)

● **R19.0**   Intra-abdominal and pelvic swelling, mass and lump
> **Excludes1**   abdominal distension (gaseous) (R14.-)
> ascites (R18.-)

R19.00   Intra-abdominal and pelvic swelling, mass and lump, unspecified site

R19.01   Right upper quadrant abdominal swelling, mass and lump

R19.02   Left upper quadrant abdominal swelling, mass and lump

R19.03   Right lower quadrant abdominal swelling, mass and lump

R19.04   Left lower quadrant abdominal swelling, mass and lump

R19.05   Periumbilic swelling, mass or lump
Diffuse or generalized umbilical swelling or mass

R19.06   Epigastric swelling, mass or lump

R19.07   Generalized intra-abdominal and pelvic swelling, mass and lump
Diffuse or generalized intra-abdominal swelling or mass NOS
Diffuse or generalized pelvic swelling or mass NOS

R19.09   Other intra-abdominal and pelvic swelling, mass and lump

● **R19.1**   Abnormal bowel sounds

R19.11   Absent bowel sounds

R19.12   Hyperactive bowel sounds

R19.15   Other abnormal bowel sounds
Abnormal bowel sounds NOS

R19.2   Visible peristalsis
Hyperperistalsis

● **R19.3**   Abdominal rigidity
> **Excludes1**   abdominal rigidity with severe abdominal pain (R10.0)

R19.30   Abdominal rigidity, unspecified site

R19.31   Right upper quadrant abdominal rigidity

R19.32   Left upper quadrant abdominal rigidity

R19.33   Right lower quadrant abdominal rigidity

R19.34   Left lower quadrant abdominal rigidity

R19.35   Periumbilic abdominal rigidity

R19.36   Epigastric abdominal rigidity

R19.37   Generalized abdominal rigidity

R19.4   Change in bowel habit
> **Excludes1**   constipation (K59.0-)
> functional diarrhea (K59.1)

R19.5   Other fecal abnormalities
Abnormal stool color
Bulky stools
Mucus in stools
Occult blood in feces
Occult blood in stools
> **Excludes1**   melena (K92.1)
> neonatal melena (P54.1)

Coding Clinic: 2021, Q1, P10; 2019, Q1, P32

R19.6   Halitosis

R19.7   Diarrhea, unspecified
Diarrhea NOS
> **Excludes1**   functional diarrhea (K59.1)
> neonatal diarrhea (P78.3)
> psychogenic diarrhea (F45.8)

Coding Clinic: 2021, Q3, P4

R19.8   Other specified symptoms and signs involving the digestive system and abdomen

SYMPTOMS AND SIGNS INVOLVING THE SKIN AND SUBCUTANEOUS TISSUE (R20-R23)

> **Excludes2**   symptoms relating to breast (N64.4-N64.5)

● **R20**   Disturbances of skin sensation
> **Excludes1**   dissociative anesthesia and sensory loss (F44.6)
> psychogenic disturbances (F45.8)

R20.0   Anesthesia of skin
Loss of sensation

R20.1   Hypoesthesia of skin
Unpleasant abnormal sensation

R20.2   Paresthesia of skin
Abnormal touch sensation, including burning, prickling, often in absence of external stimulus
Formication   Tingling skin
Pins and needles
> **Excludes1**   acroparesthesia (I73.8)

R20.3   Hyperesthesia

R20.8   Other disturbances of skin sensation

R20.9   Unspecified disturbances of skin sensation

R21   Rash and other nonspecific skin eruption
> **Includes**   rash NOS
> **Excludes1**   specified type of rash- code to condition
> vesicular eruption (R23.8)

● **R22**   Localized swelling, mass and lump of skin and subcutaneous tissue
> **Includes**   subcutaneous nodules (localized) (superficial)
> **Excludes1**   abnormal findings on diagnostic imaging (R90-R93)
> edema (R60.-)
> enlarged lymph nodes (R59.-)
> localized adiposity (E65)
> swelling of joint (M25.4-)

R22.0   Localized swelling, mass and lump, head

R22.1   Localized swelling, mass and lump, neck

R22.2   Localized swelling, mass and lump, trunk
> **Excludes1**   intra-abdominal or pelvic mass and lump (R19.0-)
> intra-abdominal or pelvic swelling (R19.0-)
> **Excludes2**   breast mass and lump (N63)

Coding Clinic: 2022, Q3, P8

● **R22.3**   Localized swelling, mass and lump, upper limb

R22.30   Localized swelling, mass and lump, unspecified upper limb

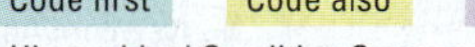

R22.31   Localized swelling, mass and lump, right upper limb

R22.32   Localized swelling, mass and lump, left upper limb

R22.33   Localized swelling, mass and lump, upper limb, bilateral

● **R22.4**   Localized swelling, mass and lump, lower limb

R22.40   Localized swelling, mass and lump, unspecified lower limb

R22.41   Localized swelling, mass and lump, right lower limb

R22.42   Localized swelling, mass and lump, left lower limb

R22.43   Localized swelling, mass and lump, lower limb, bilateral

R22.9   Localized swelling, mass and lump, unspecified

● **R23**   Other skin changes

R23.0   Cyanosis

    Excludes1   acrocyanosis (I73.8)
      cyanotic attacks of newborn (P28.2)

R23.1   Pallor
   Clammy skin

R23.2   Flushing
   Excessive blushing
   Code first, if applicable, menopausal and female climacteric states (N95.1)

R23.3   Spontaneous ecchymoses
   Small hemorrhagic spot of skin; AKA black and blue spot
   Petechiae

    Excludes1   ecchymoses of newborn (P54.5)
      purpura (D69.-)

R23.4   Changes in skin texture
   Desquamation of skin   Scaling of skin
   Induration of skin

    Excludes1   epidermal thickening NOS (L85.9)

R23.8   Other skin changes

R23.9   Unspecified skin changes

SYMPTOMS AND SIGNS INVOLVING THE NERVOUS AND MUSCULOSKELETAL SYSTEMS (R25-R29)

● **R25**   Abnormal involuntary movements

    Excludes1   specific movement disorders (G20-G26)
      stereotyped movement disorders (F98.4)
      tic disorders (F95.-)

R25.0   Abnormal head movements

R25.1   Tremor, unspecified

    Excludes1   chorea NOS (G25.5)
      essential tremor (G25.0)
      hysterical tremor (F44.4)
      intention tremor (G25.2)

R25.2   Cramp and spasm

    Excludes2   carpopedal spasm (R29.0)
      charley-horse (M62.831)
      infantile spasms (G40.4-)
      muscle spasm of back (M62.830)
      muscle spasm of calf (M62.831)

R25.3   Fasciculation
   Twitching NOS

R25.8   Other abnormal involuntary movements

R25.9   Unspecified abnormal involuntary movements

● **R26**   Abnormalities of gait and mobility

    Excludes1   ataxia NOS (R27.0)
      hereditary ataxia (G11.-)
      locomotor (syphilitic) ataxia (A52.11)
      immobility syndrome (paraplegic) (M62.3)

R26.0   Ataxic gait
   Staggering gait
   Coding Clinic: 2022, Q2, P12

R26.1   Paralytic gait
   Spastic gait

R26.2   Difficulty in walking, not elsewhere classified

    Excludes1   falling (R29.6)
      unsteadiness on feet (R26.81)
   Coding Clinic: 2016, Q2, P7

● **R26.8**   Other abnormalities of gait and mobility

R26.81   Unsteadiness on feet

R26.89   Other abnormalities of gait and mobility

R26.9   Unspecified abnormalities of gait and mobility

● **R27**   Other lack of coordination

    Excludes1   ataxic gait (R26.0)
      hereditary ataxia (G11.-)
      vertigo NOS (R42)

R27.0   Ataxia, unspecified

    Excludes1   ataxia following cerebrovascular disease (I69. with final characters -93)

   Coding Clinic: 2022, Q3, P10

R27.8   Other lack of coordination

R27.9   Unspecified lack of coordination

● **R29**   Other symptoms and signs involving the nervous and musculoskeletal systems

R29.0   Tetany
   Hyperexcitability of nerves and muscles characterized by spasm, twitching, and cramps
   Carpopedal spasm

    Excludes1   hysterical tetany (F44.5)
      neonatal tetany (P71.3)
      parathyroid tetany (E20.9)
      post-thyroidectomy tetany (E89.2)

R29.1   Meningismus

R29.2   Abnormal reflex

    Excludes2   abnormal pupillary reflex (H57.0)
      hyperactive gag reflex (J39.2)
      vasovagal reaction or syncope (R55)

R29.3   Abnormal posture

R29.4   Clicking hip

    Excludes1   congenital deformities of hip (Q65.-)

R29.5   Transient paralysis
   Code first any associated spinal cord injury (S14.0, S14.1-, S24.0, S24.1-, S34.0-, S34.1-)

    Excludes1   transient ischemic attack (G45.9)

R29.6   Repeated falls
   Falling
   Tendency to fall

    Excludes2   at risk for falling (Z91.81)
      history of falling (Z91.81)

OGCR   Section I.C.18.d.

Repeated falls

Code R29.6, Repeated falls, is for use for encounters when a patient has recently fallen and the reason for the fall is being investigated.

Code Z91.81, History of falling, is for use when a patient has fallen in the past and is at risk for future falls. When appropriate, both codes R29.6 and Z91.81 may be assigned together.

Coding Clinic: 2016, Q2, P7

● **R29.7**   National Institutes of Health Stroke Scale (NIHSS) score
   Code first the type of cerebral infarction (I63.-)
   Coding Clinic: 2016, Q4, P61, 127

● **R29.70**   NIHSS score 0-9

R29.700   NIHSS score 0

R29.701   NIHSS score 1

R29.702   NIHSS score 2

R29.703   NIHSS score 3

R29.704   NIHSS score 4

R29.705   NIHSS score 5

R29.706   NIHSS score 6

R29.707   NIHSS score 7

R29.708   NIHSS score 8

R29.709   NIHSS score 9

● **R29.71**   NIHSS score 10-19
    R29.710   NIHSS score 10
    R29.711   NIHSS score 11
    R29.712   NIHSS score 12
    R29.713   NIHSS score 13
    R29.714   NIHSS score 14
    R29.715   NIHSS score 15
    R29.716   NIHSS score 16
    R29.717   NIHSS score 17
    R29.718   NIHSS score 18
    R29.719   NIHSS score 19

● **R29.72**   NIHSS score 20-29
    R29.720   NIHSS score 20
    R29.721   NIHSS score 21
    R29.722   NIHSS score 22
    R29.723   NIHSS score 23
    R29.724   NIHSS score 24
    R29.725   NIHSS score 25
    R29.726   NIHSS score 26
    R29.727   NIHSS score 27
    R29.728   NIHSS score 28
    R29.729   NIHSS score 29

OGCR   Section I.C.18.i.

> **NIHSS Stroke Scale**
>
> The NIH stroke scale (NIHSS) codes (R29.7- -) can be used in conjunction with acute stroke codes (I63) to identify the patient's neurological status and the severity of the stroke. The stroke scale codes should be sequenced after the acute stroke diagnosis code(s).
>
> At a minimum, report the initial score documented. If desired, a facility may choose to capture multiple stroke scale scores.

● **R29.73**   NIHSS score 30-39
    R29.730   NIHSS score 30
       Coding Clinic: 2016, Q4, P62
    R29.731   NIHSS score 31
    R29.732   NIHSS score 32
    R29.733   NIHSS score 33
    R29.734   NIHSS score 34
    R29.735   NIHSS score 35
    R29.736   NIHSS score 36
    R29.737   NIHSS score 37
    R29.738   NIHSS score 38
    R29.739   NIHSS score 39

● **R29.74**   NIHSS score 40-42
    R29.740   NIHSS score 40
    R29.741   NIHSS score 41
    R29.742   NIHSS score 42

● **R29.8**   Other symptoms and signs involving the nervous and musculoskeletal systems

● **R29.81**   Other symptoms and signs involving the nervous system
    R29.810   **Facial weakness**
       Facial droop
       Excludes1   Bell's palsy (G51.0) facial weakness following cerebrovascular disease (I69. with final characters -92)
       Coding Clinic: 2022, Q3, P9
    R29.818   **Other symptoms and signs involving the nervous system**

● **R29.89**   Other symptoms and signs involving the musculoskeletal system
    Excludes2   pain in limb (M79.6-)
    R29.890   **Loss of height**
       Excludes1   osteoporosis (M80-M81)

    R29.891   **Ocular torticollis**
       Excludes1   congenital (sternomastoid) torticollis Q68.0
       psychogenic torticollis (F45.8)
       spasmodic torticollis (G24.3)
       torticollis due to birth injury (P15.8)
       torticollis NOS M43.6
    R29.898   **Other symptoms and signs involving the musculoskeletal system**

● **R29.9**   Unspecified symptoms and signs involving the nervous and musculoskeletal systems
    R29.90   Unspecified symptoms and signs involving the nervous system
    R29.91   Unspecified symptoms and signs involving the musculoskeletal system

---

SYMPTOMS AND SIGNS INVOLVING THE GENITOURINARY SYSTEM (R30-R39)

● **R30**   **Pain associated with micturition**
    Excludes1   psychogenic pain associated with micturition (F45.8)
    R30.0   **Dysuria**
       Painful urination
       Strangury
    R30.1   **Vesical tenesmus**
       Straining to urinate, with sensation of a full bladder even when empty
    R30.9   **Painful micturition, unspecified**
       Painful urination NOS

● **R31**   **Hematuria**
    Excludes1   hematuria included with underlying conditions, such as:
       acute cystitis with hematuria (N30.01)
       recurrent and persistent hematuria in glomerular diseases (N02.-)
    R31.0   **Gross hematuria**
       Coding Clinic: 2025, Q2, P21; 2017, Q1, P17
    R31.1   **Benign essential microscopic hematuria**
   ● **R31.2**   **Other microscopic hematuria**
       Coding Clinic: 2016, Q4, P62
       R31.21   **Asymptomatic microscopic hematuria**
          AMH
       R31.29   **Other microscopic hematuria**
    R31.9   **Hematuria, unspecified**
       Coding Clinic: 2025, Q2, P21; 2017, Q1, P6

R32   **Unspecified urinary incontinence**
    Enuresis NOS
    Excludes1   functional urinary incontinence (R39.81)
       nonorganic enuresis (F98.0)
       stress incontinence and other specified urinary incontinence (N39.3-N39.4-)
       urinary incontinence associated with cognitive impairment (R39.81)
    Coding Clinic: 2021, Q4, P18

● **R33**   **Retention of urine**
    Excludes1   psychogenic retention of urine (F45.8)
    R33.0   **Drug induced retention of urine**
       Use additional code for adverse effect, if applicable, to identify drug (T36-T50 with fifth or sixth character 5)
    R33.8   **Other retention of urine**
       Code first, if applicable, any causal condition, such as:
       enlarged prostate (N40.1)
       Coding Clinic: 2018, Q4, P55
    R33.9   **Retention of urine, unspecified**

R34 Anuria and oliguria

> **Excludes1** anuria and oliguria complicating abortion or ectopic or molar pregnancy (O00-O07, O08.4)
> anuria and oliguria complicating pregnancy (O26.83-)
> anuria and oliguria complicating the puerperium (O90.49)

● R35 Polyuria

Passage of excessive volume of urine

Code first, if applicable, any causal condition, such as:
enlarged prostate (N40.1)

> **Excludes1** psychogenic polyuria (F45.8)

R35.0 Frequency of micturition

Discharge or passage of urine; AKA uresis

R35.1 Nocturia

Urinary frequency at night

● R35.8 Other polyuria

R35.81 Nocturnal polyuria

> **Excludes2** nocturnal enuresis (N39.44)

R35.89 Other polyuria
Polyuria NOS

● R36 Urethral discharge

R36.0 Urethral discharge without blood

R36.1 Hematospermia

Presence of blood in semen

R36.9 Urethral discharge, unspecified
Penile discharge NOS
Urethrorrhea

R37 Sexual dysfunction, unspecified

● R39 Other and unspecified symptoms and signs involving the genitourinary system

R39.0 Extravasation of urine

Leakage, discharge

● R39.1 Other difficulties with micturition

Code first, if applicable, any causal condition, such as:
enlarged prostate (N40.1)

R39.11 Hesitancy of micturition

R39.12 Poor urinary stream
➡ Weak urinary stream

R39.13 Splitting of urinary stream

R39.14 Feeling of incomplete bladder emptying

R39.15 Urgency of urination

> **Excludes1** urge incontinence (N39.41, N39.46)

R39.16 Straining to void

● R39.19 Other difficulties with micturition
Coding Clinic: 2016, Q4, P63

R39.191 Need to immediately re-void

R39.192 Position dependent micturition

R39.198 Other difficulties with micturition

R39.2 Extrarenal uremia
Prerenal uremia

> **Excludes1** uremia NOS (N19)

● R39.8 Other symptoms and signs involving the genitourinary system

R39.81 Functional urinary incontinence
Urinary incontinence due to cognitive impairment, or severe physical disability or immobility

> **Excludes1** stress incontinence and other specified urinary incontinence (N39.3-N39.4-)
> urinary incontinence NOS (R32)

R39.82 Chronic bladder pain
Coding Clinic: 2016, Q4, P64

R39.83 Unilateral non-palpable testicle

R39.84 Bilateral non-palpable testicles

▶● R39.85 Costovertebral (angle) tenderness

> **▶ Excludes2** abdominal and pelvic pain (R10.-)

▶ R39.851 Costovertebral (angle) tenderness, right side

▶ R39.852 Costovertebral (angle) tenderness, left side

▶ R39.853 Costovertebral (angle) tenderness, bilateral

▶ R39.859 Costovertebral (angle) tenderness, unspecified side

R39.89 Other symptoms and signs involving the genitourinary system
Coding Clinic: 2016, Q4, P64

R39.9 Unspecified symptoms and signs involving the genitourinary system

SYMPTOMS AND SIGNS INVOLVING COGNITION, PERCEPTION, EMOTIONAL STATE AND BEHAVIOR (R40-R46)

> **Excludes2** symptoms and signs constituting part of a pattern of mental disorder (F01-F99)

Coding Clinic: 2015, Q4, P40

● R40 Somnolence, stupor and coma

> **Excludes1** neonatal coma (P91.5)
> somnolence, stupor and coma in diabetes (E08-E13)
> somnolence, stupor and coma in hepatic failure (K72.-)
> somnolence, stupor and coma in hypoglycemia (nondiabetic) (E15)

R40.0 Somnolence
Drowsiness

> **Excludes1** coma (R40.2-)

R40.1 Stupor

Lowered level of consciousness
Catatonic stupor
Semicoma

> **Excludes1** catatonic schizophrenia (F20.2)
> coma (R40.2-)
> ➡ depressive stupor (F31.-, F32.-, F33.-)
> dissociative stupor (F44.2)
> manic stupor (F30.2)

OGCR Section I.C.18.e.

Coma scale

The coma scale codes (R40.2-) can be used in conjunction with traumatic brain injury codes, acute cerebrovascular disease or sequelae of cerebrovascular disease codes. These codes are primarily for use by trauma registries, but they may be used in any setting where this information is collected. The coma scale may also be used to assess the status of the central nervous system for other non-trauma conditions, such as monitoring patients in the intensive care unit regardless of medical condition. The coma scale codes should be sequenced after the diagnosis code(s).

These codes, one from each subcategory, are needed to complete the scale. The 7th character indicates when the scale was recorded. The 7th character should match for all three codes.

At a minimum, report the initial score documented on presentation at your facility. This may be a score from the emergency medicine technician (EMT) or in the emergency department. If desired, a facility may choose to capture multiple coma scale scores.

Assign code R40.24, Glasgow coma scale, total score, when only the total score is documented in the medical record and not the individual score(s).

● R40.2 Coma

Code first any associated:
fracture of skull (S02.-)
intracranial injury (S06.-)

Note: One code from each subcategory R40.21-R40-23 is required to complete the coma scale
Coding Clinic: 2021, Q4, P112; 2016, Q4, P127

R40.20 Unspecified coma 🔁
Coma NOS
Unconsciousness NOS
Coding Clinic: 2021, Q4, P112

● **R40.21**   **Coma scale, eyes open**

The following appropriate 7th character is to be added to subcategory R40.21-:

0	unspecified time
1	in the field [EMT or ambulance]
2	at arrival to emergency department
3	at hospital admission
4	24 hours or more after hospital admission

Coding Clinic: 2021, Q4, P112; 2017, Q4, P25; 2015, Q2, P18

● **R40.211**   **Coma scale, eyes open, never** 🅷
Coma scale eye opening score of 1

● **R40.212**   **Coma scale, eyes open, to pain** 🅷
Coma scale eye opening score of 2

● **R40.213**   **Coma scale, eyes open, to sound**
Coma scale eye opening score of 3

● **R40.214**   **Coma scale, eyes open, spontaneous**
Coma scale eye opening score of 4

● **R40.22**   **Coma scale, best verbal response**

The following appropriate 7th character is to be added to subcategory R40.22-:

0	unspecified time
1	in the field [EMT or ambulance]
2	at arrival to emergency department
3	at hospital admission
4	24 hours or more after hospital admission

Coding Clinic: 2021, Q4, P112; 2017, Q4, P25; 2015, Q2, P18

● **R40.221**   **Coma scale, best verbal response, none** 🅷
Coma scale verbal score of 1

● **R40.222**   **Coma scale, best verbal response, incomprehensible words** 🅷
Coma scale verbal score of 2
Incomprehensible sounds (2-5 years of age)
Moans/grunts to pain; restless (< 2 years old)

● **R40.223**   **Coma scale, best verbal response, inappropriate words**
Coma scale verbal score of 3
Inappropriate crying or screaming (< 2 years of age)
Screaming (2-5 years of age)

● **R40.224**   **Coma scale, best verbal response, confused conversation**
Coma scale verbal score of 4
Inappropriate words (2-5 years of age)
Irritable cries (< 2 years of age)

● **R40.225**   **Coma scale, best verbal response, oriented**
Coma scale verbal score of 5
Cooing or babbling or crying appropriately (< 2 years of age)
Uses appropriate words (2- 5 years of age)

● **R40.23**   **Coma scale, best motor response**

The following appropriate 7th character is to be added to subcategory R40.23-:

0	unspecified time
1	in the field [EMT or ambulance]
2	at arrival to emergency department
3	at hospital admission
4	24 hours or more after hospital admission

Coding Clinic: 2017, Q4, P25; 2015, Q2, P18

● **R40.231**   **Coma scale, best motor response, none** 🅷
Coma scale motor score of 1

Glasgow Coma Scale

Eye Opening Response	
• Spontaneous--open with blinking at baseline	4 points
• To verbal stimuli, command, speech	3 points
• To pain only (not applied to face)	2 points
• No response	1 point
Verbal Response	
• Oriented	5 points
• Confused conversation, but able to answer questions	4 points
• Inappropriate words	3 points
• Incomprehensible speech	2 points
• No response	1 point
Motor Response	
• Obeys commands for movement	6 points
• Purposeful movement to painful stimulus	5 points
• Withdraws in response to pain	4 points
• Flexion in response to pain (decorticate posturing)	3 points
• Extension response in response to pain (decerebrate posturing)	2 points
• No response	1 point

Categorization:
Coma: No eye opening, no ability to follow commands, no word verbalizations (3-8)

Head Injury Classification:
Severe Head Injury--GCS score of 8 or less
Moderate Head Injury--GCS score of 9 to 12
Mild head injury--GCS score of 13 to 15

(Adapted from: Advanced Trauma Life Support: Course for Physicians, American College of Surgeons, 1993).
http://www.bt.cdc.gov/masscasulatires/gscale.asp

Figure 18-1

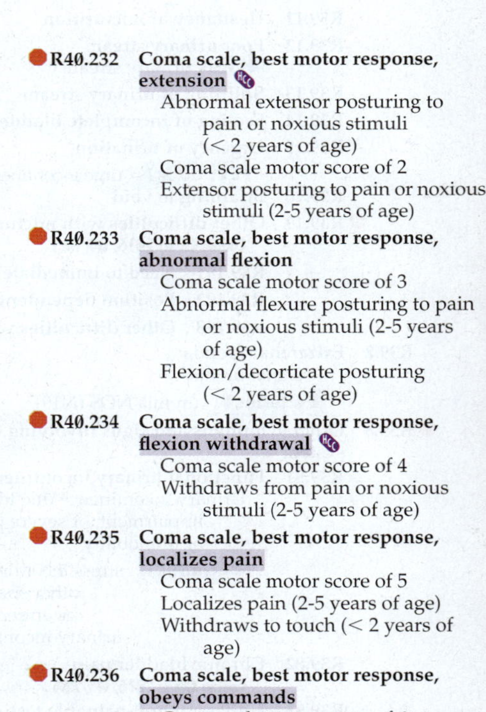

● **R40.232**   **Coma scale, best motor response, extension** 🅷
Abnormal extensor posturing to pain or noxious stimuli (< 2 years of age)
Coma scale motor score of 2
Extensor posturing to pain or noxious stimuli (2-5 years of age)

● **R40.233**   **Coma scale, best motor response, abnormal flexion**
Coma scale motor score of 3
Abnormal flexure posturing to pain or noxious stimuli (2-5 years of age)
Flexion/decorticate posturing (< 2 years of age)

● **R40.234**   **Coma scale, best motor response, flexion withdrawal** 🅷
Coma scale motor score of 4
Withdraws from pain or noxious stimuli (2-5 years of age)

● **R40.235**   **Coma scale, best motor response, localizes pain**
Coma scale motor score of 5
Localizes pain (2-5 years of age)
Withdraws to touch (< 2 years of age)

● **R40.236**   **Coma scale, best motor response, obeys commands**
Coma scale motor score of 6
Normal or spontaneous movement (< 2 years of age)
Obeys commands (2-5 years of age)

▶ New   ➡ Revised   ~~deleted~~ Deleted   Excludes 1   Excludes 2   Includes   Use additional   Code first   Code also   Key words
OGCR Official Guidelines   **X** Assign placeholder X   ● Use Additional Character(s)   ▶ Manifestation Code   🅷 Hierarchical Condition Category   **Coding Clinic**

● **R40.24   Glasgow coma scale, total score**
Note: Assign a code from subcategory R40.24, when only the total coma score is documented
The following appropriate 7th character is to be added to subcategory R40.24-:

0	unspecified time
1	in the field [EMT or ambulance]
2	at arrival to emergency department
3	at hospital admission
4	24 hours or more after hospital admission

Coding Clinic: 2016, Q4, P64; 2015, Q2, P18

● **R40.241   Glasgow coma scale score 13-15**
● **R40.242   Glasgow coma scale score 9-12**
● **R40.243   Glasgow coma scale score 3-8**
● **R40.244   Other coma, without documented Glasgow coma scale score, or with partial score reported**

R40.2A   Nontraumatic coma due to underlying condition
Secondary coma
Code first underlying condition

▶ **Excludes1**   coma scale, best motor response (R40.24.-)
▶ coma scale, best verbal response (R40.22.-)
▶ coma scale, eyes open (R40.21.-)
▶ Glasgow coma scale, total score (R40.23.-)

Coding Clinic: 2023, Q4, P42

R40.3   Persistent vegetative state
R40.4   Transient alteration of awareness

● **R41   Other symptoms and signs involving cognitive functions and awareness**
Excludes1   dissociative [conversion] disorders (F44.-)
mild cognitive impairment, of uncertain or unknown etiology (G31.84)

R41.0   Disorientation, unspecified
Confusion NOS   Delirium NOS
Excludes1   delirium due to known physiological condition (F05)

Coding Clinic: 2022, Q2, P11; 2019, Q2, P34; 2016, Q4, P71

R41.1   Anterograde amnesia
R41.2   Retrograde amnesia
R41.3   Other amnesia
Amnesia NOS
Memory loss NOS

Excludes1   amnestic disorder due to known physiologic condition (F04)
amnestic syndrome due to psychoactive substance use (F10-F19 with 5th character .6)
mild memory disturbance due to known physiological condition (F06.8)
transient global amnesia (G45.4)

R41.4   Neurologic neglect syndrome
Asomatognosia   Left-sided neglect
Hemi-akinesia   Sensory neglect
Hemi-inattention   Visuospatial neglect
Hemispatial neglect

Excludes1   visuospatial deficit (R41.842)

● **R41.8   Other symptoms and signs involving cognitive functions and awareness**
R41.81   Age-related cognitive decline   **A**
Senility NOS

R41.82   Altered mental status, unspecified
Change in mental status NOS
Excludes1   altered level of consciousness (R40.-)
altered mental status due to known condition - code to condition
delirium NOS (R41.0)

Coding Clinic: 2012, Q4, P98

R41.83   Borderline intellectual functioning
IQ level 71 to 84
Excludes1   intellectual disabilities (F70-F79)

● **R41.84   Other specified cognitive deficit**
Code first the underlying condition, if known, such as:
schizophrenia (F20.-)
Excludes1   cognitive deficits as sequelae of cerebrovascular disease (I69.01-, I69.11-, I69.21-, I69.31-, I69.81-, I69.91-)

R41.840   Attention and concentration deficit
Excludes1   attention-deficit hyperactivity disorders (F90.-)

R41.841   Cognitive communication deficit
R41.842   Visuospatial deficit
R41.843   Psychomotor deficit
R41.844   Frontal lobe and executive function deficit

R41.85   Anosognosia
R41.89   Other symptoms and signs involving cognitive functions and awareness

R41.9   Unspecified symptoms and signs involving cognitive functions and awareness
Unspecified neurocognitive disorder

R42   Dizziness and giddiness
Light-headedness
Vertigo NOS
Excludes1   vertiginous syndromes (H81.-)
vertigo from infrasound (T75.23)
Coding Clinic: 2015, Q4, P40

● **R43   Disturbances of smell and taste**
R43.0   Anosmia
Absence of sense of smell; AKA anosphresia and olfactory anesthesia

R43.1   Parosmia
R43.2   Parageusia
Perversion of sense of taste or bad taste in mouth; AKA dysgeusia

R43.8   Other disturbances of smell and taste
Mixed disturbance of smell and taste
R43.9   Unspecified disturbances of smell and taste

● **R44   Other symptoms and signs involving general sensations and perceptions**
Excludes1   alcoholic hallucinations (F10.151, F10.251, F10.951)
hallucinations in drug psychosis (F11-F19 with fifth to sixth characters 51)
hallucinations in mood disorders with psychotic symptoms (F30.2, F31.5, F32.3, F33.3)
hallucinations in schizophrenia, schizotypal and delusional disorders (F20-F29)

Excludes2   disturbances of skin sensation (R20.-)
R44.0   Auditory hallucinations
R44.1   Visual hallucinations
R44.2   Other hallucinations
R44.3   Hallucinations, unspecified
Coding Clinic: 2022, Q2, P11

CHAPTER 18 (R00-R99)

R44.8   **Other symptoms and signs involving general sensations and perceptions**

R44.9   **Unspecified symptoms and signs involving general sensations and perceptions**

● **R45**   **Symptoms and signs involving emotional state**

R45.0   **Nervousness**
    Nervous tension

R45.1   **Restlessness and agitation**

R45.2   **Unhappiness**

R45.3   **Demoralization and apathy**
    Excludes1   anhedonia (R45.84)

R45.4   **Irritability and anger**

R45.5   **Hostility**

R45.6   **Violent behavior**

R45.7   **State of emotional shock and stress, unspecified**

● R45.8   **Other symptoms and signs involving emotional state**

    R45.81   **Low self-esteem**

    R45.82   **Worries**

    R45.83   **Excessive crying of child, adolescent or adult**
      Excludes1   excessive crying of infant (baby) R68.11

    R45.84   **Anhedonia**
      Total loss of feeling of pleasure in pleasurable acts

    ● R45.85   **Homicidal and suicidal ideations**
      Excludes1   suicide attempt (T14.91)

      R45.850   **Homicidal ideations**

      R45.851   **Suicidal ideations**
        Coding Clinic: 2022, Q1, P29

    R45.86   **Emotional lability**

    R45.87   **Impulsiveness**

    R45.88   **Nonsuicidal self-harm**
      Nonsuicidal self-injury
      Nonsuicidal self-mutilation
      Self-inflicted injury without suicidal intent
      Code also injury, if known
      Coding Clinic: 2021, Q4, P27

    R45.89   **Other symptoms and signs involving emotional state**
      Flat affect
      Loneliness

● **R46**   **Symptoms and signs involving appearance and behavior**
    Excludes1   appearance and behavior in schizophrenia, schizotypal and delusional disorders (F20-F29)
      mental and behavioral disorders (F01-F99)

R46.0   **Very low level of personal hygiene**

R46.1   **Bizarre personal appearance**

R46.2   **Strange and inexplicable behavior**

R46.3   **Overactivity**

R46.4   **Slowness and poor responsiveness**
    Excludes1   stupor (R40.1)

R46.5   **Suspiciousness and marked evasiveness**

R46.6   **Undue concern and preoccupation with stressful events**

R46.7   **Verbosity and circumstantial detail obscuring reason for contact**

● R46.8   **Other symptoms and signs involving appearance and behavior**

    R46.81   **Obsessive-compulsive behavior**
      Excludes1   obsessive-compulsive disorder (F42.-)

    R46.89   **Other symptoms and signs involving appearance and behavior**

SYMPTOMS AND SIGNS INVOLVING SPEECH AND VOICE (R47-R49)

● **R47**   **Speech disturbances, not elsewhere classified**
    Excludes1   autism (F84.0)
      cluttering (F80.81)
      specific developmental disorders of speech and language (F80.-)
      stuttering (F80.81)

● R47.0   **Dysphasia and aphasia**

    R47.01   **Aphasia**
      Excludes1   aphasia following cerebrovascular disease (I69. with final characters -20)
      progressive isolated aphasia (G31.01)
      Coding Clinic: 2022, Q3, P9

    R47.02   **Dysphasia**
      Impairment in comprehension of speech, caused by left-sided brain damage
      Excludes1   dysphasia following cerebrovascular disease (I69. with final characters -21)

R47.1   **Dysarthria and anarthria**
    Motor speech disorder
    Excludes1   dysarthria following cerebrovascular disease (I69. with final characters -22)
    Coding Clinic: 2022, Q3, P9

● R47.8   **Other speech disturbances**
    Excludes1   dysarthria following cerebrovascular disease (I69. with final characters -28)

    R47.81   **Slurred speech**

    R47.82   **Fluency disorder in conditions classified elsewhere**
      Stuttering in conditions classified elsewhere
      Code first underlying disease or condition, such as:
      Parkinson's disease (G20.-)
      Excludes1   adult onset fluency disorder (F98.5)
      childhood onset fluency disorder (F80.81)
      fluency disorder (stuttering) following cerebrovascular disease (I69. with final characters -23)

    R47.89   **Other speech disturbances**

R47.9   **Unspecified speech disturbances**

● **R48**   **Dyslexia and other symbolic dysfunctions, not elsewhere classified**
    Excludes1   specific developmental disorders of scholastic skills (F81.-)

R48.0   **Dyslexia and alexia**

R48.1   **Agnosia**
    Loss of ability to recognize objects, persons, sounds, shapes, or smells
    Astereognosis (astereognosis)
    Autotopagnosia
    Excludes1   visual object agnosia (R48.3)

R48.2   **Apraxia**
    Loss of ability to execute or carry out learned purposeful movements
    Excludes1   apraxia following cerebrovascular disease (I69. with final characters -90)

R48.3   **Visual agnosia**
    Prosopagnosia
    Simultanagnosia (asimultagnosia)

R48.8 Other symbolic dysfunctions
Acalculia
Difficulty performing simple mathematical tasks resulting from neurological injury
Agraphia
Coding Clinic: 2017, Q1, P27

R48.9 Unspecified symbolic dysfunctions

● **R49 Voice and resonance disorders**
Excludes1   psychogenic voice and resonance disorders (F44.4)

R49.0 Dysphonia
Hoarseness

R49.1 Aphonia
Loss of voice

● **R49.2 Hypernasality and hyponasality**
R49.21 Hypernasality
R49.22 Hyponasality

R49.8 Other voice and resonance disorders

R49.9 Unspecified voice and resonance disorder
Change in voice NOS
Resonance disorder NOS

GENERAL SYMPTOMS AND SIGNS (R50-R69)

● **R50 Fever of other and unknown origin**
Excludes1   chills without fever (R68.83)
febrile convulsions (R56.0-)
fever of unknown origin during labor (O75.2)
fever of unknown origin in newborn (P81.9)
hypothermia due to illness (R68.0)
malignant hyperthermia due to anesthesia (T88.3)
puerperal pyrexia NOS (O86.4)

R50.2 Drug induced fever
Use additional code for adverse effect, if applicable, to identify drug (T36-T50 with fifth or sixth character 5)
Excludes1   postvaccination (postimmunization) fever (R50.83)

● **R50.8 Other specified fever**
R50.81 Fever presenting with conditions classified elsewhere
Code first underlying condition when associated fever is present, such as with:
leukemia (C91-C95)
neutropenia (D70.-)
sickle-cell disease (D57.-)
Coding Clinic: 2023, Q4, P7; 2019, Q2, P25

R50.82 Postprocedural fever
Excludes1   postprocedural infection (T81.44)
posttransfusion fever (R50.84)
postvaccination (postimmunization) fever (R50.83)

R50.83 Postvaccination fever
Postimmunization fever

R50.84 Febrile nonhemolytic transfusion reaction
FNHTR
Posttransfusion fever

R50.9 Fever, unspecified
Fever NOS
Fever of unknown origin [FUO]
Fever with chills
Fever with rigors
Hyperpyrexia NOS
Persistent fever
Pyrexia NOS

● **R51 Headache**
Excludes2   atypical face pain (G50.1)
migraine and other headache syndromes (G43-G44)
trigeminal neuralgia (G50.0)

R51.0 Headache with orthostatic component, not elsewhere classified
Headache with positional component, not elsewhere classified

R51.9 Headache, unspecified
Facial pain NOS

R52 Pain, unspecified
Acute pain NOS
Generalized pain NOS
Excludes1   acute and chronic pain, not elsewhere classified (G89.-)
localized pain, unspecified type - code to pain by site, such as:
abdomen pain (R10.-)
back pain (M54.9)
breast pain (N64.4)
chest pain (R07.1-R07.9)
ear pain (H92.0-)
eye pain (H57.1)
headache (R51.9)
joint pain (M25.5-)
limb pain (M79.6-)
lumbar region pain (M54.5-)
pelvic and perineal pain (R10.2-)
shoulder pain (M25.51-)
spine pain (M54.-)
throat pain (R07.0)
tongue pain (K14.6)
tooth pain (K08.8)
renal colic (N23)
pain disorders exclusively related to psychological factors (F45.41)

● **R53 Malaise and fatigue**
R53.0 Neoplastic (malignant) related fatigue
Code first associated neoplasm

R53.1 Weakness
Asthenia NOS
Excludes1   age-related weakness (R54)
muscle weakness (generalized) (M62.81)
sarcopenia (M62.84)
senile asthenia (R54)
Coding Clinic: 2021, Q4, P103; 2017, Q1, P7

R53.2 Functional quadriplegia
Complete immobility due to severe physical disability or frailty
Excludes1   frailty NOS (R54)
hysterical paralysis (F44.4)
immobility syndrome (M62.3)
neurologic quadriplegia (G82.5-)
quadriplegia (G82.50)
Coding Clinic: 2022, Q4, P15; 2016, Q2, P6

● **R53.8 Other malaise and fatigue**
Excludes1   combat exhaustion and fatigue (F43.0)
congenital debility (P96.9)
exhaustion and fatigue due to excessive exertion (T73.3)
exhaustion and fatigue due to exposure (T73.2)
exhaustion and fatigue due to heat (T67.-)
exhaustion and fatigue due to pregnancy (O26.8-)
exhaustion and fatigue due to recurrent depressive episode (F33.-)
exhaustion and fatigue due to senile debility (R54)

CHAPTER 18 (R00-R99)

R53.81   Other malaise
Chronic debility
Debility NOS
General physical deterioration
Malaise NOS
Nervous debility
Excludes1   age-related physical debility (R54)
Coding Clinic: 2021, Q1, P43

R53.82   Chronic fatigue, unspecified
Excludes1
chronic fatigue syndrome (G93.32)
myalgic encephalomyelitis (G93.32)
other post infection and related fatigue syndromes (G93.39)
postviral fatigue syndrome (G93.31)

R53.83   Other fatigue
Fatigue NOS   Lethargy
Lack of energy   Tiredness
Excludes2   exhaustion and fatigue due to depressive episode (F32.-)
Coding Clinic: 2017, Q1, P7

R54   Age-related physical debility   A
Frailty   Senile asthenia
Old age   Senile debility
Senescence
Excludes1   age-related cognitive decline (R41.81)
sarcopenia (M62.84)
senile psychosis (F03.-)
senility NOS (R41.81)

R55   Syncope and collapse
Blackout
Fainting
Vasovagal attack
Excludes1   cardiogenic shock (R57.0)
carotid sinus syncope (G90.01)
heat syncope (T67.1)
neurocirculatory asthenia (F45.8)
neurogenic orthostatic hypotension (G90.3)
orthostatic hypotension (I95.1)
postprocedural shock (T81.1-)
psychogenic syncope (F48.8)
shock NOS (R57.9)
shock complicating or following abortion or ectopic or molar pregnancy (O00-O07, O08.3)
shock complicating or following labor and delivery (O75.1)
Stokes-Adams attack (I45.9)
unconsciousness NOS (R40.2-)

● R56   Convulsions, not elsewhere classified
Excludes1   dissociative convulsions and seizures (F44.5)
epileptic convulsions and seizures (G40.-)
newborn convulsions and seizures (P90)

● R56.0   Febrile convulsions
R56.00   Simple febrile convulsions HCC
Febrile convulsion NOS
Febrile seizure NOS

R56.01   Complex febrile convulsions HCC
Atypical febrile seizure
Complex febrile seizure
Complicated febrile seizure
Excludes1   status epilepticus (G40.901)

R56.1   Post traumatic seizures HCC
Excludes1   post traumatic epilepsy (G40.-)

R56.9   Unspecified convulsions HCC
Convulsion disorder   Recurrent convulsions
Fit NOS   Seizure(s) (convulsive) NOS
Coding Clinic: 2022, Q4, P46; 2021, Q1, P3; 2019, Q4, P18

● R57   Shock, not elsewhere classified
Excludes1   anaphylactic shock NOS (T78.2)
anaphylactic reaction or shock due to adverse food reaction (T78.0-)
anaphylactic shock due to adverse effect of correct drug or medicament properly administered (T88.6)
anaphylactic shock due to serum (T80.5-)
electric shock (T75.4)
obstetric shock (O75.1)
postprocedural shock (T81.1-)
psychic shock (F43.0)
shock complicating or following ectopic or molar pregnancy (O00-O07, O08.3)
shock due to anesthesia (T88.2)
shock due to lightning (T75.01)
traumatic shock (T79.4)
toxic shock syndrome (A48.3)

R57.0   Cardiogenic shock HCC
Excludes2   septic shock (R65.21)

R57.1   Hypovolemic shock HCC
Decreased blood volume (loss)
Coding Clinic: 2019, Q2, P7-8

R57.8   Other shock HCC
R57.9   Shock, unspecified HCC
Failure of peripheral circulation NOS
Resulting in significant blood pressure drop

R58   Hemorrhage, not elsewhere classified
Hemorrhage NOS
Excludes1   hemorrhage included with underlying conditions, such as:
acute duodenal ulcer with hemorrhage (K26.0)
acute gastritis with bleeding (K29.01)
ulcerative enterocolitis with rectal bleeding (K51.01)

● R59   Enlarged lymph nodes
Includes   swollen glands
Excludes1   lymphadenitis NOS (I88.9)
acute lymphadenitis (L04.-)
chronic lymphadenitis (I88.1)
mesenteric (acute) (chronic) lymphadenitis (I88.0)

R59.0   Localized enlarged lymph nodes
R59.1   Generalized enlarged lymph nodes
Lymphadenopathy NOS
R59.9   Enlarged lymph nodes, unspecified

● R60   Edema, not elsewhere classified
Excludes1   angioneurotic edema (T78.3)
ascites (R18.-)
cerebral edema (G93.6)
cerebral edema due to birth injury (P11.0)
edema of larynx (J38.4)
edema of nasopharynx (J39.2)
edema of pharynx (J39.2)
gestational edema (O12.0-)
hereditary edema (Q82.0)
hydrops fetalis NOS (P83.2)
hydrothorax (J94.8)
hydrops fetalis NOS (P83.2)
newborn edema (P83.3)
pulmonary edema (J81.-)

R60.0   Localized edema
R60.1   Generalized edema
Excludes2   nutritional edema (E40-E46)
R60.9   Edema, unspecified
Fluid retention NOS

R61   Generalized hyperhidrosis
> Excessive sweating
> Night sweats
> Secondary hyperhidrosis
>> *Code first*, if applicable, menopausal and female climacteric states (N95.1)
>
> **Excludes1**   focal (primary) (secondary) hyperhidrosis (L74.5-)
>> Frey's syndrome (L74.52)
>> localized (primary) (secondary) hyperhidrosis (L74.5-)

● **R62   Lack of expected normal physiological development in childhood and adults**
> **Excludes1**   delayed puberty (E30.0)
>> gonadal dysgenesis (Q99.1)
>> hypopituitarism (E23.0)

R62.0   Delayed milestone in childhood   P
> Delayed attainment of expected physiological developmental stage
> Late talker
> Late walker

● **R62.5   Other and unspecified lack of expected normal physiological development in childhood**
> **Excludes1**   HIV disease resulting in failure to thrive (B20)
>> physical retardation due to malnutrition (E45)

R62.50   Unspecified lack of expected normal physiological development in childhood
> Infantilism NOS

R62.51   Failure to thrive (child)   P
> Failure to gain weight
> ▶ Faltering growth
>> **Excludes1**   failure to thrive in child under 28 days old (P92.6)
>
> **Coding Clinic: 2018, Q4, P82**

R62.52   Short stature (child)
> Lack of growth   Short stature NOS
> Physical retardation
>> **Excludes1**   short stature due to endocrine disorder (E34.3-)

R62.59   Other lack of expected normal physiological development in childhood

R62.7   Adult failure to thrive   A

● **R63   Symptoms and signs concerning food and fluid intake**
> **Excludes1**   bulimia NOS (F50.2-)

R63.0   Anorexia
> Loss of appetite
>> **Excludes1**   anorexia nervosa (F50.0-)
>> loss of appetite of nonorganic origin (F50.89)

R63.1   Polydipsia
> Excessive thirst

R63.2   Polyphagia
> Excessive eating   Hyperalimentation NOS

● **R63.3   Feeding difficulties**
> **Excludes2**   eating disorders (F50.-)
>> feeding problems of newborn (P92.-)
>> infant feeding disorder of nonorganic origin (F98.2-)

R63.30   Feeding difficulties, unspecified   P

R63.31   Pediatric feeding disorder, acute
> Pediatric feeding dysfunction, acute
> *Code also*, if applicable, associated conditions such as:
>> aspiration pneumonia (J69.0)
>> dysphagia (R13.1-)
>> gastro-esophageal reflux disease (K21.-)
>> malnutrition (E40-E46)

R63.32   Pediatric feeding disorder, chronic   P
> Pediatric feeding dysfunction, chronic
> *Code also*, if applicable, associated conditions such as:
>> aspiration pneumonia (J69.0)
>> dysphagia (R13.1-)
>> gastro-esophageal reflux disease (K21.-)
>> malnutrition (E40-E46)

R63.39   Other feeding difficulties
> Feeding problem (elderly) (infant) NOS
> Picky eater
>
> **Coding Clinic: 2017, Q1, P27; 2016, Q3, P19**

R63.4   Abnormal weight loss

R63.5   Abnormal weight gain
> **Excludes1**   excessive weight gain in pregnancy (O26.0-)
>> obesity (E66.-)

R63.6   Underweight
> **Use additional** code to identify body mass index (BMI), if known (Z68.-)
>
> **Excludes1**   abnormal weight loss (R63.4)
>> anorexia nervosa (F50.0-)
>> malnutrition (E40-E46)

R63.8   Other symptoms and signs concerning food and fluid intake

R64   Cachexia 🔲
> **Excludes1**   abnormal weight loss (R63.4)
>> cachexia due to underlying condition (E88.A)
>> nutritional marasmus (E41)
>
> **Coding Clinic: 2017, Q3, P25**

● **R65   Symptoms and signs specifically associated with systemic inflammation and infection**

● **R65.1   Systemic inflammatory response syndrome (SIRS) of non-infectious origin**
> *Code first* underlying condition, such as:
>> heatstroke (T67.0-)
>> injury and trauma (S00-T88)
>
> **Excludes1**   sepsis - code to infection
>> severe sepsis (R65.2)
>
> **Coding Clinic: 2019, Q2, P38**

R65.10   Systemic inflammatory response syndrome (SIRS) of non-infectious origin without acute organ dysfunction 🔲
> Systemic inflammatory response syndrome (SIRS) NOS
>
> **Coding Clinic: 2019, Q2, P25, 38**

R65.11   Systemic inflammatory response syndrome (SIRS) of non-infectious origin with acute organ dysfunction 🔲
> **Use additional** code to identify specific acute organ dysfunction, such as:
>> acute kidney failure (N17.-)
>> acute respiratory failure (J96.0-)
>> critical illness myopathy (G72.81)
>> critical illness polyneuropathy (G62.81)
>> disseminated intravascular coagulopathy [DIC] (D65)
>> encephalopathy (metabolic) (septic) (G93.41)
>> hepatic failure (K72.0-)

OGCR   Section I.C.18.g.

> **SIRS due to Non-Infectious Process**
>
> The systemic inflammatory response syndrome (SIRS) can develop as a result of certain non-infectious disease processes, such as trauma, malignant neoplasm, or pancreatitis. When SIRS is documented with a noninfectious condition, and no subsequent infection is documented, the code for the underlying condition, such as an injury, should be assigned, followed by code R65.10, Systemic inflammatory response syndrome (SIRS) of non-infectious origin without acute organ dysfunction, or code R65.11, Systemic inflammatory response syndrome (SIRS) of non-infectious origin with acute organ dysfunction. If an associated acute organ dysfunction is documented, the appropriate code(s) for the specific type of organ dysfunction(s) should be assigned in addition to code R65.11. If acute organ dysfunction is documented, but it cannot be determined if the acute organ dysfunction is associated with SIRS or due to another condition (e.g., directly due to the trauma), the provider should be queried.

CHAPTER 18 (R00-R99)

● **R65.2** **Severe sepsis**
Infection with associated acute organ dysfunction
Sepsis with acute organ dysfunction
Sepsis with multiple organ dysfunction
Systemic inflammatory response syndrome due to infectious process with acute organ dysfunction

Code first *underlying infection, such as:*
infection following a procedure (T81.44)
infections following infusion, transfusion and therapeutic injection (T80.2-)
puerperal sepsis (O85)
sepsis following complete or unspecified spontaneous abortion (O03.87)
sepsis following ectopic and molar pregnancy (O08.82)
sepsis following incomplete spontaneous abortion (O03.37)
sepsis following (induced) termination of pregnancy (O04.87)
sepsis NOS (A41.9)

Use additional code to identify specific acute organ dysfunction, such as:
acute kidney failure (N17.-)
acute respiratory failure (J96.0-)
critical illness myopathy (G72.81)
critical illness polyneuropathy (G62.81)
disseminated intravascular coagulopathy [DIC] (D65)
encephalopathy (metabolic) (septic) (G93.41)
hepatic failure (K72.0-)
Coding Clinic: 2017, Q4, P99; 2016, Q3, P8

R65.20 **Severe sepsis without septic shock** 🔵
Severe sepsis NOS
Coding Clinic: 2019, Q1, P14; 2018, Q4, P90; 2016, Q3, P14

R65.21 **Severe sepsis with septic shock** 🔵
▶ **Excludes1**   postprocedural septic shock (T81.12-)

● **R68** **Other general symptoms and signs**
R68.0 **Hypothermia, not associated with low environmental temperature**
Excludes1   hypothermia NOS (accidental) (T68)
hypothermia due to anesthesia (T88.51)
hypothermia due to low environmental temperature (T68)
newborn hypothermia (P80.-)

● **R68.1** **Nonspecific symptoms peculiar to infancy**
Excludes1   colic, infantile (R10.83)
neonatal cerebral irritability (P91.3)
teething syndrome (K00.7)

R68.11 **Excessive crying of infant (baby)** P
Excludes1   excessive crying of child, adolescent, or adult (R45.83)

R68.12 **Fussy infant (baby)** P
Irritable infant

R68.13 **Apparent life threatening event in infant (ALTE)** P
Apparent life threatening event in newborn
Brief resolved unexplained event (BRUE)
Code first *confirmed diagnosis, if known*
Use additional code(s) for associated signs and symptoms if no confirmed diagnosis established, or if signs and symptoms are not associated routinely with confirmed diagnosis, or provide additional information for cause of ALTE

R68.19 **Other nonspecific symptoms peculiar to infancy** P

R68.2 **Dry mouth, unspecified**
Excludes1   dry mouth due to dehydration (E86.0)
dry mouth due to Sjögren syndrome (M35.0-)
Excludes2   salivary gland hyposecretion (K11.7)

R68.3 **Clubbing of fingers**
Clubbing of nails
Excludes1   congenital clubfinger (Q68.1)

● **R68.8** **Other general symptoms and signs**
R68.81 **Early satiety**
R68.82 **Decreased libido**   A
Decreased sexual desire

R68.83 **Chills (without fever)**
Chills NOS
Excludes1   chills with fever (R50.9)

R68.84 **Jaw pain**
Mandibular pain
Maxilla pain
Excludes1   temporomandibular joint arthralgia (M26.62-)

R68.89 **Other general symptoms and signs**

R69 **Illness, unspecified**
➡ Unknown and unspecified causes of morbidity

ABNORMAL FINDINGS ON EXAMINATION OF BLOOD, WITHOUT DIAGNOSIS (R70-R79)

Excludes2   abnormal findings on antenatal screening of mother (O28.-)
abnormalities of lipids (E78.-)
abnormalities of platelets and thrombocytes (D69.-)
abnormalities of white blood cells classified elsewhere (D70-D72)
coagulation hemorrhagic disorders (D65-D68)
diagnostic abnormal findings classified elsewhere —*see* Alphabetical Index
hemorrhagic and hematological disorders of newborn (P50-P61)

● **R70** **Elevated erythrocyte sedimentation rate and abnormality of plasma viscosity**
R70.0 **Elevated erythrocyte sedimentation rate**
R70.1 **Abnormal plasma viscosity**

● **R71** **Abnormality of red blood cells**
Excludes1   anemias (D50-D64)
anemia of premature infant (P61.2)
benign (familial) polycythemia (D75.0)
congenital anemias (P61.2-P61.4)
newborn anemia due to isoimmunization (P55.-)
polycythemia neonatorum (P61.1)
polycythemia NOS (D75.1)
polycythemia vera (D45)
secondary polycythemia (D75.1)

R71.0 **Precipitous drop in hematocrit**
Drop (precipitous) in hemoglobin
Drop in hematocrit
Blood volume that has decreased red blood cells

R71.8 **Other abnormality of red blood cells**
Abnormal red-cell morphology NOS
Abnormal red-cell volume NOS
Anisocytosis
Red blood cells of unequal size
Poikilocytosis
Red blood cells of abnormal shape

● **R73** **Elevated blood glucose level**
Excludes1   diabetes mellitus (E08-E13)
diabetes mellitus in pregnancy, childbirth and the puerperium (O24.-)
neonatal disorders (P70.0-P70.2)
postsurgical hypoinsulinemia (E89.1)

● **R73.0** **Abnormal glucose**
Excludes1   abnormal glucose in pregnancy (O99.81-)
diabetes mellitus (E08-E13)
dysmetabolic syndrome X (E88.81-)
gestational diabetes (O24.4-)
glycosuria (R81)
hypoglycemia (E16.2)
type 1 diabetes mellitus, presymptomatic (E10.A-)

CHAPTER 18 (R00-R99)

▶ New   ➡ Revised   ~~deleted~~ Deleted   Excludes 1   Excludes 2   Includes   Use additional   Code first   Code also   Key words
OGCR Official Guidelines   X Assign placeholder X   ● Use Additional Character(s)   ▸ Manifestation Code   🔵 Hierarchical Condition Category   **Coding Clinic**

R73.01 Impaired fasting glucose
 Elevated fasting glucose

R73.02 Impaired glucose tolerance (oral)
 Elevated glucose tolerance

R73.03 Prediabetes
 Latent diabetes
 Coding Clinic: 2016, Q4, P65

R73.09 Other abnormal glucose
 Abnormal glucose NOS
 Abnormal non-fasting glucose tolerance
 Coding Clinic: 2024, Q3, P11; 2016, Q4, P65

R73.9 Hyperglycemia, unspecified

● **R74 Abnormal serum enzyme levels**

● **R74.0 Nonspecific elevation of levels of transaminase and lactic acid dehydrogenase [LDH]**

R74.01 Elevation of levels of liver transaminase levels
 Elevation of levels of alanine transaminase (ALT)
 Elevation of levels of aspartate transaminase (AST)

R74.02 Elevation of levels of lactic acid dehydrogenase [LDH]

R74.8 Abnormal levels of other serum enzymes
 Abnormal level of acid phosphatase
 Abnormal level of alkaline phosphatase
 Abnormal level of amylase
 Abnormal level of lipase [triacylglycerol lipase]
 Coding Clinic: 2019, Q2, P6

R74.9 Abnormal serum enzyme level, unspecified

R75 Inconclusive laboratory evidence of human immunodeficiency virus [HIV]
 Nonconclusive HIV-test finding in infants

 Excludes1 asymptomatic human immunodeficiency virus [HIV] infection status (Z21)
   human immunodeficiency virus [HIV] disease (B20)

● **R76 Other abnormal immunological findings in serum**

R76.0 Raised antibody titer

 Excludes1 isoimmunization in pregnancy (O36.0-O36.1)
   isoimmunization affecting newborn (P55.-)

 Coding Clinic: 2021, Q1, P7

● **R76.1 Nonspecific reaction to test for tuberculosis**

R76.11 Nonspecific reaction to tuberculin skin test without active tuberculosis
 Abnormal result of Mantoux test
 PPD positive
 Tuberculin (skin test) positive
 Tuberculin (skin test) reactor

 Excludes1 nonspecific reaction to cell mediated immunity measurement of gamma interferon antigen response without active tuberculosis (R76.12)

R76.12 Nonspecific reaction to cell mediated immunity measurement of gamma interferon antigen response without active tuberculosis
 Nonspecific reaction to QuantiFERON-TB test (QFT) without active tuberculosis

 Excludes1 nonspecific reaction to tuberculin skin test without active tuberculosis (R76.11)
   positive tuberculin skin test (R76.11)

● **R76.8 Other specified abnormal immunological findings in serum**
 ~~Raised level of immunoglobulins NOS~~
 Coding Clinic: 2021, Q1, P7

▶ **R76.81 Abnormal rheumatoid factor and anti-citrullinated protein antibody without rheumatoid arthritis**
 ▶Abnormal anti-CCP
 ▶Abnormal anti-cyclic citrullinated protein antibody and rheumatoid factor

 ▶ **Excludes1** rheumatoid arthritis with rheumatoid factor (M05.-)

▶ **R76.89 Other specified abnormal immunological findings in serum**
 ▶Raised level of immunoglobulins NOS

R76.9 Abnormal immunological finding in serum, unspecified

● **R77 Other abnormalities of plasma proteins**

 Excludes1 disorders of plasma-protein metabolism (E88.0-)

R77.0 Abnormality of albumin

R77.1 Abnormality of globulin
 Hyperglobulinemia NOS

R77.2 Abnormality of alphafetoprotein

R77.8 Other specified abnormalities of plasma proteins
 Coding Clinic: 2019, Q2, P6

R77.9 Abnormality of plasma protein, unspecified
 Coding Clinic: 2019, Q2, P6

● **R78 Findings of drugs and other substances, not normally found in blood**
 Use additional code to identify any retained foreign body, if applicable (Z18.-)

 Excludes2 mental or behavioral disorders due to psychoactive substance use (F10-F19)

R78.0 Finding of alcohol in blood
 Use additional external cause code (Y90.-), for detail regarding alcohol level.

R78.1 Finding of opiate drug in blood

R78.2 Finding of cocaine in blood

R78.3 Finding of hallucinogen in blood

R78.4 Finding of other drugs of addictive potential in blood

R78.5 Finding of other psychotropic drug in blood

R78.6 Finding of steroid agent in blood

● **R78.7 Finding of abnormal level of heavy metals in blood**

R78.71 Abnormal lead level in blood

 Excludes1 lead poisoning (T56.0-)

R78.79 Finding of abnormal level of heavy metals in blood

● **R78.8 Finding of other specified substances, not normally found in blood**

R78.81 Bacteremia
 Blood poisoning/bacteremia

 Excludes1 sepsis-code to specified infection
 Coding Clinic: 2025, Q1, P21

R78.89 Finding of other specified substances, not normally found in blood
 Finding of abnormal level of lithium in blood

R78.9 Finding of unspecified substance, not normally found in blood

CHAPTER 18 (R00-R99)

● **R79   Other abnormal findings of blood chemistry**

Use additional code to identify any retained foreign body, if applicable (Z18.-)

Excludes1   asymptomatic hyperuricemia (E79.0)
hyperglycemia NOS (R73.9)
hypoglycemia NOS (E16.2)
neonatal hypoglycemia (P70.3-P70.4)
specific findings indicating disorder of amino-acid metabolism (E70-E72)
specific findings indicating disorder of carbohydrate metabolism (E73-E74)
specific findings indicating disorder of lipid metabolism (E75.-)

R79.0   Abnormal level of blood mineral
Abnormal blood level of cobalt
Abnormal blood level of copper
Abnormal blood level of iron
Abnormal blood level of magnesium
Abnormal blood level of mineral NEC
Abnormal blood level of zinc

Excludes1   abnormal level of lithium (R78.89)
disorders of mineral metabolism (E83.-)
neonatal hypomagnesemia (P71.2)
nutritional mineral deficiency (E58-E61)

R79.1   Abnormal coagulation profile
Abnormal or prolonged bleeding time
Abnormal or prolonged coagulation time
Abnormal or prolonged partial thromboplastin time [PTT]
Abnormal or prolonged prothrombin time [PT]
Low von Willebrand factor

Excludes1   coagulation defects (D68.-)

Excludes2   abnormality of fluid, electrolyte or acid-base balance (E86-E87)

● **R79.8   Other specified abnormal findings of blood chemistry**

R79.81   Abnormal blood-gas level

R79.82   Elevated C-reactive protein (CRP)

R79.83   Abnormal findings of blood amino-acid level
Homocysteinemia

Excludes1   disorders of amino-acid metabolism (E70-E72)

Coding Clinic: 2021, Q4, P28

R79.89   Other specified abnormal findings of blood chemistry
Coding Clinic: 2019, Q2, P6

R79.9   Abnormal finding of blood chemistry, unspecified

ABNORMAL FINDINGS ON EXAMINATION OF URINE, WITHOUT DIAGNOSIS (R80-R82)

Excludes1   abnormal findings on antenatal screening of mother (O28.-)
diagnostic abnormal findings classified elsewhere - see Alphabetical Index
specific findings indicating disorder of amino-acid metabolism (E70-E72)
specific findings indicating disorder of carbohydrate metabolism (E73-E74)

● **R80   Proteinuria**

Excludes1   gestational proteinuria (O12.1-)

R80.0   Isolated proteinuria
Idiopathic proteinuria

Excludes1   isolated proteinuria with specific morphological lesion (N06.-)

R80.1   Persistent proteinuria, unspecified

R80.2   Orthostatic proteinuria, unspecified
Postural proteinuria

R80.3   Bence Jones proteinuria

R80.8   Other proteinuria

R80.9   Proteinuria, unspecified
Albuminuria NOS

R81   Glycosuria

Excludes1   renal glycosuria (E74.818)

● **R82   Other and unspecified abnormal findings in urine**

Includes   chromoabnormalities in urine

Use additional code to identify any retained foreign body, if applicable (Z18.-)

Excludes2   hematuria (R31.-)

R82.0   Chyluria
White milky urine

Excludes1   filarial chyluria (B74.-)

R82.1   Myoglobinuria
Presence of myoglobin (iron containing protein) in urine

R82.2   Biliuria
Presence of bile pigments/salts in urine

R82.3   Hemoglobinuria
Presence of hemoglobin in urine

Excludes1   hemoglobinuria due to hemolysis from external causes NEC (D59.6)
hemoglobinuria due to paroxysmal nocturnal [Marchiafava-Micheli] (D59.5)

R82.4   Acetonuria
Ketonuria

R82.5   Elevated urine levels of drugs, medicaments and biological substances
Elevated urine levels of catecholamines
Elevated urine levels of indoleacetic acid
Elevated urine levels of 17-ketosteroids
Elevated urine levels of steroids

R82.6   Abnormal urine levels of substances chiefly nonmedicinal as to source
Abnormal urine level of heavy metals

● **R82.7   Abnormal findings on microbiological examination of urine**

Excludes1   colonization status (Z22.-)
Coding Clinic: 2016, Q4, P65

R82.71   Bacteriuria

R82.79   Other abnormal findings on microbiological examination of urine
Positive culture findings of urine

● **R82.8   Abnormal findings on cytological and histological examination of urine**

R82.81   Pyuria
Sterile pyuria
Coding Clinic: 2019, Q4, P16

R82.89   Other abnormal findings on cytological and histological examination of urine

● **R82.9   Other and unspecified abnormal findings in urine**

R82.90   Unspecified abnormal findings in urine

R82.91   Other chromoabnormalities of urine
Chromoconversion (dipstick)
Idiopathic dipstick converts positive for blood with no cellular forms in sediment

Excludes1   hemoglobinuria (R82.3)
myoglobinuria (R82.1)

● **R82.99   Other abnormal findings in urine**

R82.991   Hypocitraturia

R82.992   Hyperoxaluria

Excludes1   ~~Primary hyperoxaluria (E72.53)~~
▶ Primary hyperoxaluria (E72.53-)
▶ Secondary hyperoxaluria (E72.54-)

R82.993   Hyperuricosuria

R82.994   Hypercalciuria
Idiopathic hypercalciuria

R82.998   Other abnormal findings in urine
Cells and casts in urine
Crystalluria
Melanuria

▶ New   ⇨ Revised   ~~deleted~~ Deleted   Excludes 1   Excludes 2   Includes   Use additional   Code first   Code also   Key words
OGCR Official Guidelines   X Assign placeholder X   ● Use Additional Character(s)   ▌ Manifestation Code   ⊛ Hierarchical Condition Category   Coding Clinic

ABNORMAL FINDINGS ON EXAMINATION OF OTHER BODY FLUIDS, SUBSTANCES AND TISSUES, WITHOUT DIAGNOSIS (R83-R89)

Excludes1   abnormal findings on antenatal screening of mother (O28.-)

diagnostic abnormal findings classified elsewhere - see Alphabetical Index

Excludes2   abnormal findings on examination of blood, without diagnosis (R70-R79)

abnormal findings on examination of urine, without diagnosis (R80-R82)

abnormal tumor markers (R97.-)

● **R83 Abnormal findings in cerebrospinal fluid**

R83.0 Abnormal level of enzymes in cerebrospinal fluid

R83.1 Abnormal level of hormones in cerebrospinal fluid

R83.2 Abnormal level of other drugs, medicaments and biological substances in cerebrospinal fluid

R83.3 Abnormal level of substances chiefly nonmedicinal as to source in cerebrospinal fluid

R83.4 Abnormal immunological findings in cerebrospinal fluid

R83.5 Abnormal microbiological findings in cerebrospinal fluid

Positive culture findings in cerebrospinal fluid

Excludes1   colonization status (Z22.-)

R83.6 Abnormal cytological findings in cerebrospinal fluid

R83.8 Other abnormal findings in cerebrospinal fluid

Abnormal chromosomal findings in cerebrospinal fluid

R83.9 Unspecified abnormal finding in cerebrospinal fluid

● **R84 Abnormal findings in specimens from respiratory organs and thorax**

Includes   abnormal findings in bronchial washings

abnormal findings in nasal secretions

abnormal findings in pleural fluid

abnormal findings in sputum

abnormal findings in throat scrapings

Excludes1   blood-stained sputum (R04.2)

R84.0 Abnormal level of enzymes in specimens from respiratory organs and thorax

R84.1 Abnormal level of hormones in specimens from respiratory organs and thorax

R84.2 Abnormal level of other drugs, medicaments and biological substances in specimens from respiratory organs and thorax

R84.3 Abnormal level of substances chiefly nonmedicinal as to source in specimens from respiratory organs and thorax

R84.4 Abnormal immunological findings in specimens from respiratory organs and thorax

R84.5 Abnormal microbiological findings in specimens from respiratory organs and thorax

Positive culture findings in specimens from respiratory organs and thorax

Excludes1   colonization status (Z22.-)

R84.6 Abnormal cytological findings in specimens from respiratory organs and thorax

R84.7 Abnormal histological findings in specimens from respiratory organs and thorax

R84.8 Other abnormal findings in specimens from respiratory organs and thorax

Abnormal chromosomal findings in specimens from respiratory organs and thorax

R84.9 Unspecified abnormal finding in specimens from respiratory organs and thorax

● **R85 Abnormal findings in specimens from digestive organs and abdominal cavity**

Includes   abnormal findings in peritoneal fluid

abnormal findings in saliva

Excludes1   cloudy peritoneal dialysis effluent (R88.0)

fecal abnormalities (R19.5)

R85.0 Abnormal level of enzymes in specimens from digestive organs and abdominal cavity

R85.1 Abnormal level of hormones in specimens from digestive organs and abdominal cavity

R85.2 Abnormal level of other drugs, medicaments and biological substances in specimens from digestive organs and abdominal cavity

R85.3 Abnormal level of substances chiefly nonmedicinal as to source in specimens from digestive organs and abdominal cavity

R85.4 Abnormal immunological findings in specimens from digestive organs and abdominal cavity

R85.5 Abnormal microbiological findings in specimens from digestive organs and abdominal cavity

Positive culture findings in specimens from digestive organs and abdominal cavity

Excludes1   colonization status (Z22.-)

● **R85.6 Abnormal cytological findings in specimens from digestive organs and abdominal cavity**

● **R85.61 Abnormal cytologic smear of anus**

Excludes1   abnormal cytological findings in specimens from other digestive organs and abdominal cavity (R85.69)

carcinoma in situ of anus (histologically confirmed) (D01.3)

anal intraepithelial neoplasia I [AIN I] (K62.82)

anal intraepithelial neoplasia II [AIN II] (K62.82)

anal intraepithelial neoplasia III [AIN III] (D01.3)

dysplasia (mild) (moderate) of anus (histologically confirmed) (K62.82)

severe dysplasia of anus (histologically confirmed) (D01.3)

Excludes2   anal high risk human papillomavirus (HPV) DNA test positive (R85.81)

anal low risk human papillomavirus (HPV) DNA test positive (R85.82)

R85.610 Atypical squamous cells of undetermined significance on cytologic smear of anus (ASC-US)

R85.611 Atypical squamous cells cannot exclude high grade squamous intraepithelial lesion on cytologic smear of anus (ASC-H)

R85.612 Low grade squamous intraepithelial lesion on cytologic smear of anus (LGSIL)

R85.613 High grade squamous intraepithelial lesion on cytologic smear of anus (HGSIL)

R85.614 Cytologic evidence of malignancy on smear of anus

R85.615 Unsatisfactory cytologic smear of anus

Inadequate sample of cytologic smear of anus

R85.616 Satisfactory anal smear but lacking transformation zone

R85.618 Other abnormal cytological findings on specimens from anus

R85.619 Unspecified abnormal cytological findings in specimens from anus

Abnormal anal cytology NOS

Atypical glandular cells of anus NOS

R85.69 Abnormal cytological findings in specimens from other digestive organs and abdominal cavity

R85.7   **Abnormal histological findings in specimens from digestive organs and abdominal cavity**

● R85.8   **Other abnormal findings in specimens from digestive organs and abdominal cavity**

    R85.81   **Anal high risk human papillomavirus (HPV) DNA test positive**

       Excludes1   anogenital warts due to human papillomavirus (HPV) (A63.0)

           condyloma acuminatum (A63.0)

    R85.82   **Anal low risk human papillomavirus (HPV) DNA test positive**

       Use additional code for associated human papillomavirus (B97.7)

    R85.89   **Other abnormal findings in specimens from digestive organs and abdominal cavity**

       Abnormal chromosomal findings in specimens from digestive organs and abdominal cavity

    R85.9   **Unspecified abnormal finding in specimens from digestive organs and abdominal cavity**

● R86   **Abnormal findings in specimens from male genital organs**

    Includes   abnormal findings in prostatic secretions

       abnormal findings in semen, seminal fluid

       abnormal spermatozoa

    Excludes1   azoospermia (N46.0-)

        oligospermia (N46.1-)

    R86.0   **Abnormal level of enzymes in specimens from male genital organs**

    R86.1   **Abnormal level of hormones in specimens from male genital organs**

    R86.2   **Abnormal level of other drugs, medicaments and biological substances in specimens from male genital organs**

    R86.3   **Abnormal level of substances chiefly nonmedicinal as to source in specimens from male genital organs**

    R86.4   **Abnormal immunological findings in specimens from male genital organs**

    R86.5   **Abnormal microbiological findings in specimens from male genital organs**

       Positive culture findings in specimens from male genital organs

       Excludes1   colonization status (Z22.-)

    R86.6   **Abnormal cytological findings in specimens from male genital organs**

    R86.7   **Abnormal histological findings in specimens from male genital organs**

    R86.8   **Other abnormal findings in specimens from male genital organs**

       Abnormal chromosomal findings in specimens from male genital organs

    R86.9   **Unspecified abnormal finding in specimens from male genital organs**

● R87   **Abnormal findings in specimens from female genital organs**

    Includes   abnormal findings in secretion and smears from cervix uteri

       abnormal findings in secretion and smears from vagina

       abnormal findings in secretion and smears from vulva

    R87.0   **Abnormal level of enzymes in specimens from female genital organs**

    R87.1   **Abnormal level of hormones in specimens from female genital organs**

    R87.2   **Abnormal level of other drugs, medicaments and biological substances in specimens from female genital organs**

    R87.3   **Abnormal level of substances chiefly nonmedicinal as to source in specimens from female genital organs**

    R87.4   **Abnormal immunological findings in specimens from female genital organs**

R87.5   **Abnormal microbiological findings in specimens from female genital organs**

    Positive culture findings in specimens from female genital organs

    Excludes1   colonization status (Z22.-)

● R87.6   **Abnormal cytological findings in specimens from female genital organs**

● R87.61   **Abnormal cytological findings in specimens from cervix uteri**

    Excludes1   abnormal cytological findings in specimens from other female genital organs (R87.69)

       abnormal cytological findings in specimens from vagina (R87.62-)

       carcinoma in situ of cervix uteri (histologically confirmed) (D06.-)

       cervical intraepithelial neoplasia I [CIN I] (N87.0)

       cervical intraepithelial neoplasia II [CIN II] (N87.1)

       cervical intraepithelial neoplasia III [CIN III] (D06.-)

       dysplasia (mild) (moderate) of cervix uteri (histologically confirmed) (N87.-)

       severe dysplasia of cervix uteri (histologically confirmed) (D06.-)

    Excludes2   cervical high risk human papillomavirus (HPV) DNA test positive (R87.810)

       cervical low risk human papillomavirus (HPV) DNA test positive (R87.820)

    R87.610   **Atypical squamous cells of undetermined significance on cytologic smear of cervix (ASC-US)**

    R87.611   **Atypical squamous cells cannot exclude high grade squamous intraepithelial lesion on cytologic smear of cervix (ASC-H)**

    R87.612   **Low grade squamous intraepithelial lesion on cytologic smear of cervix (LGSIL)**

    R87.613   **High grade squamous intraepithelial lesion on cytologic smear of cervix (HGSIL)**

    R87.614   **Cytologic evidence of malignancy on smear of cervix**

    R87.615   **Unsatisfactory cytologic smear of cervix**

       Inadequate sample of cytologic smear of cervix

    R87.616   **Satisfactory cervical smear but lacking transformation zone**

    R87.618   **Other abnormal cytological findings on specimens from cervix uteri**

    R87.619   **Unspecified abnormal cytological findings in specimens from cervix uteri**

       Abnormal cervical cytology NOS

       Abnormal Papanicolaou smear of cervix NOS

       Abnormal thin preparation smear of cervix NOS

       ⇒ Atypical endocervical cells of cervix NOS

       Atypical endometrial cells of cervix NOS

       Atypical glandular cells of cervix NOS

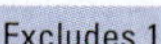

● **R87.62   Abnormal cytological findings in specimens from vagina**

Use additional code to identify acquired absence of uterus and cervix, if applicable (Z90.71-)

Excludes1   abnormal cytological findings in specimens from cervix uteri (R87.61-)
abnormal cytological findings in specimens from other female genital organs (R87.69)
carcinoma in situ of vagina (histologically confirmed) (D07.2)
vaginal intraepithelial neoplasia I [VAIN I] (N89.0)
vaginal intraepithelial neoplasia II [VAIN II] (N89.1)
vaginal intraepithelial neoplasia III [VAIN III] (D07.2)
dysplasia (mild) (moderate) of vagina (histologically confirmed) (N89.-)
severe dysplasia of vagina (histologically confirmed) (D07.2)

Excludes2   vaginal high risk human papillomavirus (HPV) DNA test positive (R87.811)
vaginal low risk human papillomavirus (HPV) DNA test positive (R87.821)

R87.620   **Atypical squamous cells of undetermined significance on cytologic smear of vagina (ASC-US)**

R87.621   **Atypical squamous cells cannot exclude high grade squamous intraepithelial lesion on cytologic smear of vagina (ASC-H)**

R87.622   **Low grade squamous intraepithelial lesion on cytologic smear of vagina (LGSIL)**

R87.623   **High grade squamous intraepithelial lesion on cytologic smear of vagina (HGSIL)**

R87.624   **Cytologic evidence of malignancy on smear of vagina**

R87.625   **Unsatisfactory cytologic smear of vagina**
Inadequate sample of cytologic smear of vagina

R87.628   **Other abnormal cytological findings on specimens from vagina**

R87.629   **Unspecified abnormal cytological findings in specimens from vagina**
Abnormal Papanicolaou smear of vagina NOS
Abnormal thin preparation smear of vagina NOS
Abnormal vaginal cytology NOS
Atypical endocervical cells of vagina NOS
Atypical endometrial cells of vagina NOS
Atypical glandular cells of vagina NOS

R87.69   **Abnormal cytological findings in specimens from other female genital organs**
Abnormal cytological findings in specimens from female genital organs NOS

Excludes1   dysplasia of vulva (histologically confirmed) (N90.0-N90.3)

R87.7   **Abnormal histological findings in specimens from female genital organs**

Excludes1   carcinoma in situ (histologically confirmed) of female genital organs (D06-D07.3)
cervical intraepithelial neoplasia I [CIN I] (N87.0)
cervical intraepithelial neoplasia II [CIN II] (N87.1)
cervical intraepithelial neoplasia III [CIN III] (D06.-)
dysplasia (mild) (moderate) of cervix uteri (histologically confirmed) (N87.-)
dysplasia (mild) (moderate) of vagina (histologically confirmed) (N89.-)
vaginal intraepithelial neoplasia I [VAIN I] (N89.0)
vaginal intraepithelial neoplasia II [VAIN II] (N89.1)
vaginal intraepithelial neoplasia III [VAIN III] (D07.2)
severe dysplasia of cervix uteri (histologically confirmed) (D06.-)
severe dysplasia of vagina (histologically confirmed) (D07.2)

● **R87.8   Other abnormal findings in specimens from female genital organs**

● **R87.81   High risk human papillomavirus (HPV) DNA test positive from female genital organs**

Excludes1   anogenital warts due to human papillomavirus (HPV) (A63.0)
condyloma acuminatum (A63.0)

R87.810   **Cervical high risk human papillomavirus (HPV) DNA test positive**

R87.811   **Vaginal high risk human papillomavirus (HPV) DNA test positive**

● **R87.82   Low risk human papillomavirus (HPV) DNA test positive from female genital organs**

Use additional code for associated human papillomavirus (B97.7)

R87.820   **Cervical low risk human papillomavirus (HPV) DNA test positive**

R87.821   **Vaginal low risk human papillomavirus (HPV) DNA test positive**

R87.89   **Other abnormal findings in specimens from female genital organs**
Abnormal chromosomal findings in specimens from female genital organs

R87.9   **Unspecified abnormal finding in specimens from female genital organs**

● **R88   Abnormal findings in other body fluids and substances**

R88.0   **Cloudy (hemodialysis) (peritoneal) dialysis effluent**

R88.8   **Abnormal findings in other body fluids and substances**

● **R89   Abnormal findings in specimens from other organs, systems and tissues**

Includes   abnormal findings in nipple discharge
abnormal findings in synovial fluid
abnormal findings in wound secretions

R89.0   **Abnormal level of enzymes in specimens from other organs, systems and tissues**

R89.1   **Abnormal level of hormones in specimens from other organs, systems and tissues**

R89.2   **Abnormal level of other drugs, medicaments and biological substances in specimens from other organs, systems and tissues**

CHAPTER 18 (R00-R99)

R89.3   Abnormal level of substances chiefly nonmedicinal as to source in specimens from other organs, systems and tissues

R89.4   Abnormal immunological findings in specimens from other organs, systems and tissues

R89.5   Abnormal microbiological findings in specimens from other organs, systems and tissues
> Positive culture findings in specimens from other organs, systems and tissues
>> **Excludes1**   colonization status (Z22.-)

R89.6   Abnormal cytological findings in specimens from other organs, systems and tissues

R89.7   Abnormal histological findings in specimens from other organs, systems and tissues
> **Coding Clinic: 2025, Q2, P5**

R89.8   Other abnormal findings in specimens from other organs, systems and tissues
> Abnormal chromosomal findings in specimens from other organs, systems and tissues

R89.9   Unspecified abnormal finding in specimens from other organs, systems and tissues

---

ABNORMAL FINDINGS ON DIAGNOSTIC IMAGING AND IN FUNCTION STUDIES, WITHOUT DIAGNOSIS (R90-R94)

Includes   nonspecific abnormal findings on diagnostic imaging by computerized axial tomography [CAT scan]
nonspecific abnormal findings on diagnostic imaging by magnetic resonance imaging [MRI][NMR]
nonspecific abnormal findings on diagnostic imaging by positron emission tomography [PET scan]
nonspecific abnormal findings on diagnostic imaging by thermography
nonspecific abnormal findings on diagnostic imaging by ultrasound [echogram]
nonspecific abnormal findings on diagnostic imaging by X-ray examination

Excludes1   abnormal findings on antenatal screening of mother (O28.-)
diagnostic abnormal findings classified elsewhere - see Alphabetical Index

● R90   Abnormal findings on diagnostic imaging of central nervous system

    R90.0   Intracranial space-occupying lesion found on diagnostic imaging of central nervous system

    ● R90.8   Other abnormal findings on diagnostic imaging of central nervous system

       R90.81   Abnormal echoencephalogram

       R90.82   White matter disease, unspecified

       R90.89   Other abnormal findings on diagnostic imaging of central nervous system
> Other cerebrovascular abnormality found on diagnostic imaging of central nervous system

● R91   Abnormal findings on diagnostic imaging of lung

    R91.1   Solitary pulmonary nodule
> Coin lesion lung
> Solitary pulmonary nodule, subsegmental branch of the bronchial tree

    R91.8   Other nonspecific abnormal finding of lung field
> Lung mass NOS found on diagnostic imaging of lung
> Pulmonary infiltrate NOS
> Shadow, lung

● R92   Abnormal and inconclusive findings on diagnostic imaging of breast

    R92.0   Mammographic microcalcification found on diagnostic imaging of breast
>> **Excludes2**   mammographic calcification (calculus) found on diagnostic imaging of breast (R92.1)

    R92.1   Mammographic calcification found on diagnostic imaging of breast
> Mammographic calculus found on diagnostic imaging of breast

    R92.2   Inconclusive mammogram
> Inconclusive mammogram NEC
> Inconclusive mammography NEC
> **Coding Clinic: 2015, Q1, P24**

    ● R92.3   Mammographic density found on imaging of breast
> Code also, if applicable, inconclusive mammogram (R92.2)

       R92.30   Dense breasts, unspecified
> Dense breasts NOS
> Low density

       ● R92.31   Mammographic fatty tissue density of breast
> Breast Imaging Reporting and Data System (BI-RADS): A
> Breast Imaging Reporting and Data System (BI-RADS): 1

          R92.311   Mammographic fatty tissue density, right breast

          R92.312   Mammographic fatty tissue density, left breast

          R92.313   Mammographic fatty tissue density, bilateral breasts

       ● R92.32   Mammographic fibroglandular density of breast
> Breast Imaging Reporting and Data System (BI-RADS): B
> Breast Imaging Reporting and Data System (BI-RADS): 2

          R92.321   Mammographic fibroglandular density, right breast

          R92.322   Mammographic fibroglandular density, left breast

          R92.323   Mammographic fibroglandular density, bilateral breasts

       ● R92.33   Mammographic heterogeneous density of breast
> Breast Imaging Reporting and Data System (BI-RADS): C
> Breast Imaging Reporting and Data System (BI-RADS): 3

          R92.331   Mammographic heterogeneous density, right breast

          R92.332   Mammographic heterogeneous density, left breast

          R92.333   Mammographic heterogeneous density, bilateral breasts
> **Coding Clinic: 2023, Q4, P44**

       ● R92.34   Mammographic extreme density of breast
> Breast Imaging Reporting and Data System (BI-RADS): D
> Breast Imaging Reporting and Data System (BI-RADS): 4

          R92.341   Mammographic extreme density, right breast

          R92.342   Mammographic extreme density, left breast

          R92.343   Mammographic extreme density, bilateral breasts

    R92.8   Other abnormal and inconclusive findings on diagnostic imaging of breast

● **R93** **Abnormal findings on diagnostic imaging of other body structures**

    R93.0 **Abnormal findings on diagnostic imaging of skull and head, not elsewhere classified**

        Excludes1   intracranial space-occupying lesion found on diagnostic imaging (R90.0)

    R93.1 **Abnormal findings on diagnostic imaging of heart and coronary circulation**
        Abnormal echocardiogram NOS
        Abnormal heart shadow

    R93.2 **Abnormal findings on diagnostic imaging of liver and biliary tract**
        Nonvisualization of gallbladder

    R93.3 **Abnormal findings on diagnostic imaging of other parts of digestive tract**

●   **R93.4** **Abnormal findings on diagnostic imaging of urinary organs**

        Excludes2   hypertrophy of kidney (N28.81)

        Coding Clinic: 2016, Q4, P66

      R93.41 **Abnormal radiologic findings on diagnostic imaging of renal pelvis, ureter, or bladder**
        Filling defect of bladder found on diagnostic imaging
        Filling defect of renal pelvis found on diagnostic imaging
        Filling defect of ureter found on diagnostic imaging

●   **R93.42** **Abnormal radiologic findings on diagnostic imaging of kidney**

      R93.421 **Abnormal radiologic findings on diagnostic imaging of right kidney**

      R93.422 **Abnormal radiologic findings on diagnostic imaging of left kidney**

      R93.429 **Abnormal radiologic findings on diagnostic imaging of unspecified kidney**

    R93.49 **Abnormal radiologic findings on diagnostic imaging of other urinary organs**

    R93.5 **Abnormal findings on diagnostic imaging of other abdominal regions, including retroperitoneum**

    R93.6 **Abnormal findings on diagnostic imaging of limbs**

        Excludes2   abnormal finding in skin and subcutaneous tissue (R93.8-)

        Coding Clinic: 2020, Q1, P14

    R93.7 **Abnormal findings on diagnostic imaging of other parts of musculoskeletal system**

        Excludes2   abnormal findings on diagnostic imaging of skull (R93.0)

Item 18–1 The **peripheral nervous system** consists of 31 pairs of spinal nerves, 12 pairs of cranial nerves, and the autonomic nerves, which are divided into the parasympathetic and sympathetic nerves. The cranial nerves are: olfactory (I), optic (II), oculomotor (III), trochlear (IV), trigeminal (V), abducens (VI), facial (VII), vestibulocochlear (VIII), glossopharyngeal (IX), vagus (X), accessory (XI), and hypoglossal (XII).

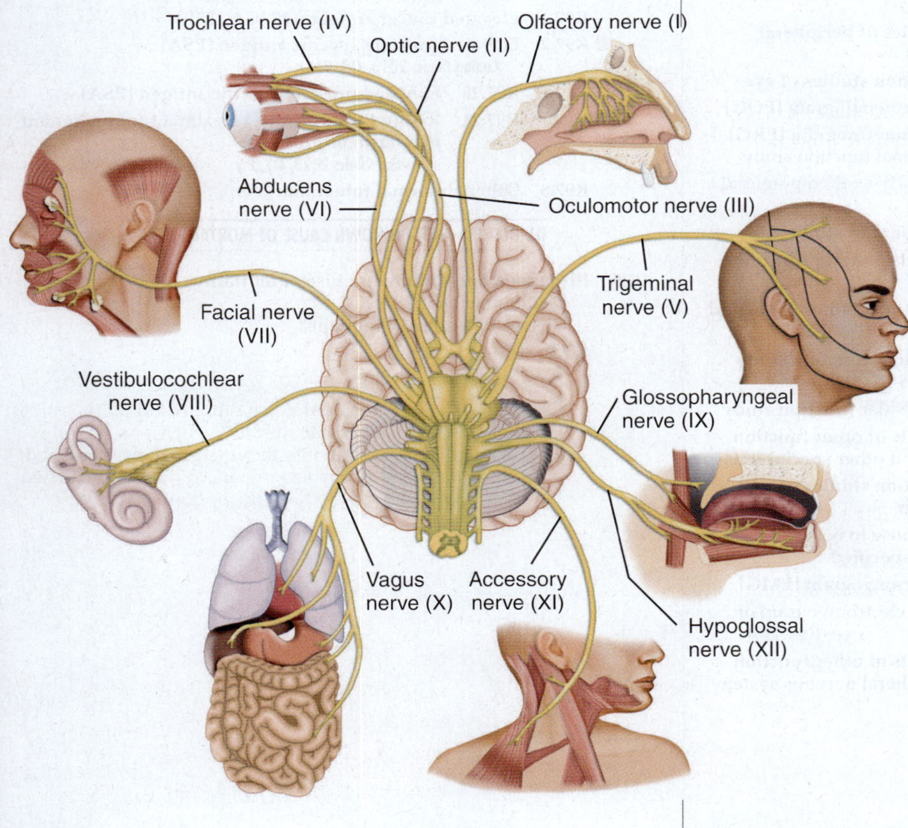

Figure 18-2 Cranial nerves. (From Patton and Thibodeau: Anatomy and physiology, ed 7, St. Louis, Mosby, 2009)

● **R93.8** **Abnormal findings on diagnostic imaging of other specified body structures**

  ● **R93.81** **Abnormal radiologic findings on diagnostic imaging of testis**

    R93.811 **Abnormal radiologic findings on diagnostic imaging of right testicle**

    R93.812 **Abnormal radiologic findings on diagnostic imaging of left testicle**

    R93.813 **Abnormal radiologic findings on diagnostic imaging of testicles, bilateral**

    R93.819 **Abnormal radiologic findings on diagnostic imaging of unspecified testicle**

  R93.89 **Abnormal findings on diagnostic imaging of other specified body structures**
    Abnormal finding by radioisotope localization of placenta
    Abnormal radiological finding in skin and subcutaneous tissue
    Mediastinal shift

R93.9 **Diagnostic imaging inconclusive due to excess body fat of patient**

● **R94** **Abnormal results of function studies**
  Includes   abnormal results of radionuclide [radioisotope] uptake studies
    abnormal results of scintigraphy

● **R94.0** **Abnormal results of function studies of central nervous system**

  R94.01 **Abnormal electroencephalogram [EEG]**

  R94.02 **Abnormal brain scan**

  R94.09 **Abnormal results of other function studies of central nervous system**

● **R94.1** **Abnormal results of function studies of peripheral nervous system and special senses**

  ● **R94.11** **Abnormal results of function studies of eye**

    R94.110 **Abnormal electro-oculogram [EOG]**

    R94.111 **Abnormal electroretinogram [ERG]**
      Abnormal retinal function study

    R94.112 **Abnormal visually evoked potential [VEP]**

    R94.113 **Abnormal oculomotor study**

    R94.118 **Abnormal results of other function studies of eye**

  ● **R94.12** **Abnormal results of function studies of ear and other special senses**

    R94.120 **Abnormal auditory function study**
      Coding Clinic: 2016, Q3, P17

    R94.121 **Abnormal vestibular function study**

    R94.128 **Abnormal results of other function studies of ear and other special senses**

  ● **R94.13** **Abnormal results of function studies of peripheral nervous system**

    R94.130 **Abnormal response to nerve stimulation, unspecified**

    R94.131 **Abnormal electromyogram [EMG]**
      Excludes1   electromyogram of eye (R94.113)

    R94.138 **Abnormal results of other function studies of peripheral nervous system**

R94.2 **Abnormal results of pulmonary function studies**
    Reduced ventilatory capacity
    Reduced vital capacity

● **R94.3** **Abnormal results of cardiovascular function studies**

  R94.30 **Abnormal result of cardiovascular function study, unspecified**

  R94.31 **Abnormal electrocardiogram [ECG] [EKG]**
      Excludes1   long QT syndrome (I45.81)

  R94.39 **Abnormal result of other cardiovascular function study**
      Abnormal electrophysiological intracardiac studies
      Abnormal phonocardiogram
      Abnormal vectorcardiogram
      Coding Clinic: 2023, Q1, P25

R94.4 **Abnormal results of kidney function studies**
    Abnormal renal function test

R94.5 **Abnormal results of liver function studies**

R94.6 **Abnormal results of thyroid function studies**

R94.7 **Abnormal results of other endocrine function studies**
      Excludes2   abnormal glucose (R73.0-)

R94.8 **Abnormal results of function studies of other organs and systems**
    Abnormal basal metabolic rate [BMR]
    Abnormal bladder function test
    Abnormal splenic function test

ABNORMAL TUMOR MARKERS (R97)

● **R97** **Abnormal tumor markers**
    Elevated tumor associated antigens [TAA]
    Elevated tumor specific antigens [TSA]

  R97.0 **Elevated carcinoembryonic antigen [CEA]**

  R97.1 **Elevated cancer antigen 125 [CA 125]**

  ● **R97.2** **Elevated prostate specific antigen [PSA]**
      Coding Clinic: 2016, Q4, P66

    R97.20 **Elevated prostate specific antigen [PSA]**   A

    R97.21 **Rising PSA following treatment for malignant neoplasm of prostate**   A
      Coding Clinic: 2023, Q2, P5

  R97.8 **Other abnormal tumor markers**

ILL-DEFINED AND UNKNOWN CAUSE OF MORTALITY (R99)

R99 **Ill-defined and unknown cause of mortality**
    Death (unexplained) NOS
    Unspecified cause of mortality
  OGCR **Section I.C.18.h.**

    Death NOS

    Code R99, Ill-defined and unknown cause of mortality, is only for use in the very limited circumstance when a patient who has already died is brought into the emergency department or other healthcare facility and is pronounced dead upon arrival. It does not represent the discharge disposition of death.

CHAPTER 19

INJURY, POISONING AND CERTAIN OTHER CONSEQUENCES OF EXTERNAL CAUSES (S00-T88)

OGCR Chapter-Specific Coding Guidelines

19. Chapter 19: Injury, poisoning, and certain other consequences of external causes (S00-T88)

a. Application of 7th Characters in Chapter 19

Most categories in Chapter 19 have a 7th character requirement for each applicable code. Most categories in this chapter have three 7th character values (with the exception of fractures): A, initial encounter, D, subsequent encounter and S, sequela. Categories for traumatic fractures have additional 7th character values. While the patient may be seen by a new or different provider over the course of treatment for an injury, assignment of the 7th character is based on whether the patient is undergoing active treatment and not whether the provider is seeing the patient for the first time.

For complication codes, active treatment refers to treatment for the condition described by the code, even though it may be related to an earlier precipitating problem. For example, code T84.50XA, Infection and inflammatory reaction due to unspecified internal joint prosthesis, initial encounter, is used when active treatment is provided for the infection, even though the condition relates to the prosthetic device, implant or graft that was placed at a previous encounter.

7th character "A", initial encounter is used for each encounter where the patient is receiving active treatment for the condition.

7th character "D" subsequent encounter is used for encounters after the patient has completed active treatment of the condition and is receiving routine care for the condition during the healing or recovery phase.

The aftercare Z codes should not be used for aftercare for conditions such as injuries or poisonings, where 7th characters are provided to identify subsequent care. For example, for aftercare of an injury, assign the acute injury code with the 7th character "D" (subsequent encounter).

7th character "S", sequela, is for use for complications or conditions that arise as a direct result of a condition, such as scar formation after a burn. The scars are sequelae of the burn. When using 7th character "S", it is necessary to use both the injury code that precipitated the sequela and the code for the sequela itself. The "S" is added only to the injury code, not the sequela code. The 7th character "S" identifies the injury responsible for the sequela. The specific type of sequela (e.g. scar) is sequenced first, followed by the injury code.

See Section I.B.10. Sequelae, (Late Effects).

b. Coding of Injuries

When coding injuries, assign separate codes for each injury unless a combination code is provided, in which case the combination code is assigned. Codes from category T07, Unspecified multiple injuries should not be assigned in the inpatient setting unless information for a more specific code is not available. Traumatic injury codes (S00-T14.9) are not to be used for normal, healing surgical wounds or to identify complications of surgical wounds.

The code for the most serious injury, as determined by the provider and the focus of treatment, is sequenced first.

1) Superficial injuries

Superficial injuries such as abrasions or contusions are not coded when associated with more severe injuries of the same site.

2) Primary injury with damage to nerves/blood vessels

When a primary injury results in minor damage to peripheral nerves or blood vessels, the primary injury is sequenced first with additional code(s) for injuries to nerves and spinal cord (such as category S04), and/or injury to blood vessels (such as category S15). When the primary injury is to the blood vessels or nerves, that injury should be sequenced first.

c. Coding of Traumatic Fractures

The principles of multiple coding of injuries should be followed in coding fractures. Fractures of specified sites are coded individually by site in accordance with both the provisions within categories S02, S12, S22, S32, S42, S49, S52, S59, S62, S72, S79, S82, S89, S92 and the level of detail furnished by medical record content.

A fracture not indicated as open or closed should be coded to closed. A fracture not indicated whether displaced or not displaced should be coded to displaced.

More specific guidelines are as follows:

1) Initial vs. Subsequent Encounter for Fractures

Traumatic fractures are coded using the appropriate 7th character for initial encounter (A, B, C) for each encounter where the patient is receiving active treatment for the fracture. The appropriate 7th character for initial encounter should also be assigned for a patient who delayed seeking treatment for the fracture or nonunion.

Fractures are coded using the appropriate 7th character for subsequent care for encounters after the patient has completed active treatment of the fracture and is receiving routine care for the fracture during the healing or recovery phase.

Care for complications of surgical treatment for fracture repairs during the healing or recovery phase should be coded with the appropriate complication codes.

Care of complications of fractures, such as malunion and nonunion, should be reported with the appropriate 7th character for subsequent care with nonunion (K, M, N,) or subsequent care with malunion (P, Q, R).

Malunion/nonunion: The appropriate 7th character for initial encounter should also be assigned for a patient who delayed seeking treatment for the fracture or nonunion.

The open fracture designations in the assignment of the 7th character for fractures of the forearm, femur and lower leg, including ankle are based on the Gustilo open fracture classification. When the Gustilo classification type is not specified for an open fracture, the 7th character for open fracture type I or II should be assigned (B, E, H, M, Q).

A code from category M80, not a traumatic fracture code, should be used for any patient with known osteoporosis who suffers a fracture, even if the patient had a minor fall or trauma, if that fall or trauma would not usually break a normal, healthy bone.

See Section I.C.13. Osteoporosis.

The aftercare Z codes should not be used for aftercare for traumatic fractures. For aftercare of a traumatic fracture, assign the acute fracture code with the appropriate 7th character.

2) Multiple fractures sequencing

Multiple fractures are sequenced in accordance with the severity of the fracture.

d. Coding of Burns and Corrosions

The ICD-10-CM makes a distinction between burns and corrosions. The burn codes are for thermal burns, except sunburns, that come from a heat source, such as a fire or hot appliance. The burn codes are also for burns resulting from electricity and radiation. Corrosions are burns due to chemicals. The guidelines are the same for burns and corrosions.

Current burns (T20-T25) are classified by depth, extent and by agent (X code). Burns are classified by depth as first degree (erythema), second degree (blistering), and third degree (full-thickness involvement). Burns of the eye and internal organs (T26-T28) are classified by site, but not by degree.

1) Sequencing of burn and related condition codes

Sequence first the code that reflects the highest degree of burn when more than one burn is present.

    a. When the reason for the admission or encounter is for treatment of external multiple burns, sequence first the code that reflects the burn of the highest degree.

    b. When a patient has both internal and external burns, the circumstances of admission govern the selection of the principal diagnosis or first-listed diagnosis.

    c. When a patient is admitted for burn injuries and other related conditions such as smoke inhalation and/or respiratory failure, the circumstances of admission govern the selection of the principal or first-listed diagnosis.

2) Burns of the same *anatomic* site
Classify burns of the same anatomic site and on the same side but of different degrees to the subcategory identifying the highest degree recorded in the diagnosis (e.g., for second- and third-degree burns of right thigh, assign only code T24.311-).

3) Non-healing burns
Non-healing burns are coded as acute burns.
Necrosis of burned skin should be coded as a non-healed burn.

4) Infected Burn
For any documented infected burn site, use an additional code for the infection.

5) Assign separate codes for each burn site
When coding burns, assign separate codes for each burn site. Category T30, Burn and corrosion, body region unspecified is extremely vague and should rarely be used.
Codes for burns of "multiple sites" should only be assigned when the medical record documentation does not specify the individual sites.

6) Burns and Corrosions Classified According to Extent of Body Surface Involved
Assign codes from category T31, Burns classified according to extent of body surface involved, or T32, Corrosions classified according to extent of body surface involved, when the site of the burn is not specified or when there is a need for additional data. It is advisable to use category T31 as additional coding when needed to provide data for evaluating burn mortality, such as that needed by burn units. It is also advisable to use category T31 as an additional code for reporting purposes when there is mention of a third-degree burn involving 20 percent or more of the body surface.
Categories T31 and T32 are based on the classic "rule of nines" in estimating body surface involved: head and neck are assigned nine percent, each arm nine percent, each leg 18 percent, the anterior trunk 18 percent, posterior trunk 18 percent, and genitalia one percent. Providers may change these percentage assignments where necessary to accommodate infants and children who have proportionately larger heads than adults, and patients who have large buttocks, thighs, or abdomen that involve burns.

7) Encounters for treatment of sequela of burns
Encounters for the treatment of the late effects of burns or corrosions (i.e., scars or joint contractures) should be coded with a burn or corrosion code with the 7th character "S" for sequela.

8) Sequelae with a late effect code and current burn
When appropriate, both a code for a current burn or corrosion with 7th character "A" or "D" and a burn or corrosion code with 7th character "S" may be assigned on the same record (when both a current burn and sequelae of an old burn exist). Burns and corrosions do not heal at the same rate and a current healing wound may still exist with sequela of a healed burn or corrosion.
See Section I.B.10. Sequela, (Late Effects).

9) Use of an external cause code with burns and corrosions
An external cause code should be used with burns and corrosions to identify the source and intent of the burn, as well as the place where it occurred.

e. Adverse Effects, Poisoning , Underdosing and Toxic Effects
Codes in categories T36-T65 are combination codes that include the substance that was taken as well as the intent. No additional external cause code is required for poisonings, toxic effects, adverse effects and underdosing codes.

1) Do not code directly from the Table of Drugs
Do not code directly from the Table of Drugs and Chemicals. Always refer back to the Tabular List.

2) Use as many codes as necessary to describe
Use as many codes as necessary to describe completely all drugs, medicinal or biological substances.

3) If the same code would describe the causative agent
If the same code would describe the causative agent for more than one adverse reaction, poisoning, toxic effect or underdosing, assign the code only once.

4) If two or more drugs, medicinal or biological substances
If two or more drugs, medicinal or biological substances are reported, code each individually unless a combination code is listed in the Table of Drugs and Chemicals.

5) The occurrence of drug toxicity is classified in ICD-10-CM as follows:

(a) Adverse Effect
When coding an adverse effect of a drug that has been correctly prescribed and properly administered, assign the appropriate code for the nature of the adverse effect followed by the appropriate code for the adverse effect of the drug (T36-T50). The code for the drug should have a 5th or 6th character "5" (for example T36.0X5-) Examples of the nature of an adverse effect are tachycardia, delirium, gastrointestinal hemorrhaging, vomiting, hypokalemia, hepatitis, renal failure, or respiratory failure.

(b) Poisoning
When coding a poisoning or reaction to the improper use of a medication (e.g., overdose, wrong substance given or taken in error, wrong route of administration), first assign the appropriate code from categories T36-T50. The poisoning codes have an associated intent as their 5th or 6th character (accidental, intentional self-harm, assault and undetermined). If the intent of the poisoning is unknown or unspecified, code the intent as accidental intent. The undetermined intent is only for use if the documentation in the record specifies that the intent cannot be determined. Use additional code(s) for all manifestations of poisonings.
If there is also a diagnosis of abuse or dependence of the substance, the abuse or dependence is assigned as an additional code.
Examples of poisoning include:

   (i) Error was made in drug prescription
      Errors made in drug prescription or in the administration of the drug by provider, nurse, patient, or other person.

   (ii) Overdose of a drug intentionally taken If an overdose of a drug was intentionally taken or administered and resulted in drug toxicity, it would be coded as a poisoning.

   (iii) Nonprescribed drug taken with correctly prescribed and properly administered drug. If a nonprescribed drug or medicinal agent was taken in combination with a correctly prescribed and properly administered drug, any drug toxicity or other reaction resulting from the interaction of the two drugs would be classified as a poisoning.

   (iv) Interaction of drug(s) and alcohol. When a reaction results from the interaction of a drug(s) and alcohol, this would be classified as poisoning.
See Section I.C.4. if poisoning is the result of insulin pump malfunctions.

(c) Underdosing
Underdosing refers to taking less of a medication than is prescribed by a provider or a manufacturer's instruction. Discontinuing the use of a prescribed medication on the patient's own initiative (not directed by the patient's provider) is also classified as an underdosing. For underdosing, assign the code from categories T36-T50 (fifth or sixth character "6").

Codes for underdosing should never be assigned as principal or first-listed codes. If a patient has a relapse or exacerbation of the medical condition for which the drug is prescribed because of the reduction in dose, then the medical condition itself should be coded.

Noncompliance (Z91.12-, Z91.13- and Z91.14-) or complication of care (Y63.6-Y63.9) codes are to be used with an underdosing code to indicate intent, if known.

(d) Toxic Effects

When a harmful substance is ingested or comes in contact with a person, this is classified as a toxic effect. The toxic effect codes are in categories T51-T65.

Toxic effect codes have an associated intent: accidental, intentional self-harm, assault and undetermined.

f. Adult and child abuse, neglect and other maltreatment

Sequence first the appropriate code from categories T74 (Adult and child abuse, neglect and other maltreatment, confirmed) or T76 (Adult and child abuse, neglect and other maltreatment, suspected) for abuse, neglect and other maltreatment, followed by any accompanying mental health or injury code(s).

If the documentation in the medical record states abuse or neglect it is coded as confirmed (T74.-). It is coded as suspected if it is documented as suspected (T76.-).

For cases of confirmed abuse or neglect an external cause code from the assault section (X92-Y09) should be added to identify the cause of any physical injuries. A perpetrator code (Y07) should be added when the perpetrator of the abuse is known. For suspected cases of abuse or neglect, do not report external cause or perpetrator code.

If a suspected case of abuse, neglect or mistreatment is ruled out during an encounter code Z04.71, Encounter for examination and observation following alleged physical adult abuse, ruled out, or code Z04.72, Encounter for examination and observation following alleged child physical abuse, ruled out, should be used, not a code from T76.

If a suspected case of alleged rape or sexual abuse is ruled out during an encounter code Z04.41, Encounter for examination and observation following alleged adult rape or code Z04.42, Encounter for examination and observation following alleged child rape, should be used, not a code from T76.

If a suspected case of forced sexual exploitation or forced labor exploitation is ruled out during an encounter, code Z04.81, Encounter for examination and observation of victim following forced sexual exploitation, or code Z04.82, Encounter for examination and observation of victim following forced labor exploitation, should be used, not a code from T76.

See Section I.C.15. Abuse in a pregnant patient.

g. Complications of care

1) General guidelines for complications of care

(a) Documentation of complications of care

See Section I.B.16. for information on documentation of complications of care.

2) Pain due to medical devices

Pain associated with devices, implants or grafts left in a surgical site (for example painful hip prosthesis) is assigned to the appropriate code(s) found in Chapter 19, Injury, poisoning, and certain other consequences of external causes. Specific codes for pain due to medical devices are found in the T code section of the ICD-10-CM. Use additional code(s) from category G89 to identify acute or chronic pain due to presence of the device, implant or graft (G89.18 or G89.28).

3) Transplant complications

(a) Transplant complications other than kidney

Codes under category T86, Complications of transplanted organs and tissues, are for use for both complications and rejection of transplanted organs. A transplant complication code is only assigned if the complication affects the function of the transplanted organ. Two codes are required to fully describe a transplant complication: the appropriate code from category T86 and a secondary code that identifies the complication.

Pre-existing conditions or conditions that develop after the transplant are not coded as complications unless they affect the function of the transplanted organs.

See I.C.21. for transplant organ removal status.

See I.C.2. for malignant neoplasm associated with transplanted organ.

(b) Kidney transplant complications

Patients who have undergone kidney transplant may still have some form of chronic kidney disease (CKD) because the kidney transplant may not fully restore kidney function. Code T86.1- should be assigned for documented complications of a kidney transplant, such as transplant failure or rejection or other transplant complication. Code T86.1- should not be assigned for post kidney transplant patients who have chronic kidney (CKD) unless a transplant complication such as transplant failure or rejection is documented. If the documentation is unclear as to whether the patient has a complication of the transplant, query the provider.

Conditions that affect the function of the transplanted kidney, other than CKD, should be assigned a code from subcategory T86.1, Complications of transplanted organ, Kidney, and a secondary code that identifies the complication.

For patients with CKD following a kidney transplant, but who do not have a complication such as failure or rejection, *see Section I.C.14. Chronic kidney disease and kidney transplant status.*

4) Complication codes that include the external cause

As with certain other T codes, some of the complications of care codes have the external cause included in the code. The code includes the nature of the complication as well as the type of procedure that caused the complication. No external cause code indicating the type of procedure is necessary for these codes.

5) Complications of care codes within the body system chapters

Intraoperative and postprocedural complication codes are found within the body system chapters with codes specific to the organs and structures of that body system. These codes should be sequenced first, followed by a code(s) for the specific complication, if applicable.

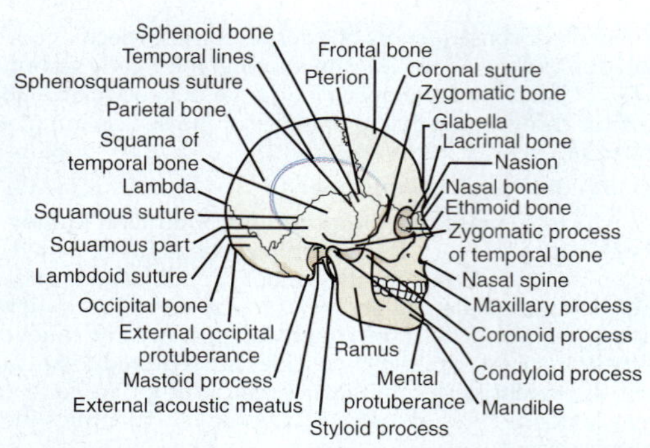

Figure 19-1 Lateral view of skull.

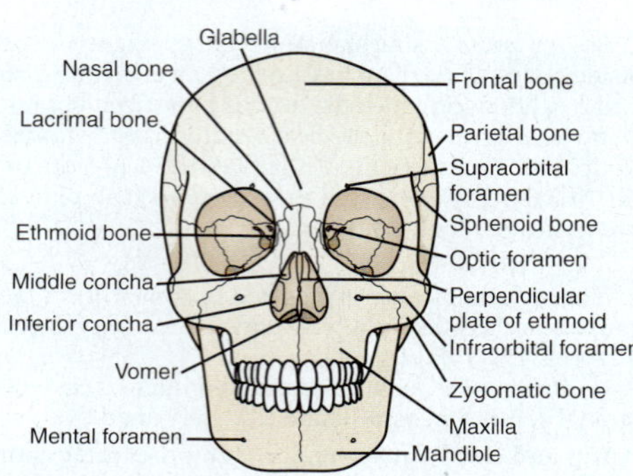

Figure 19-2 Frontal view of skull.

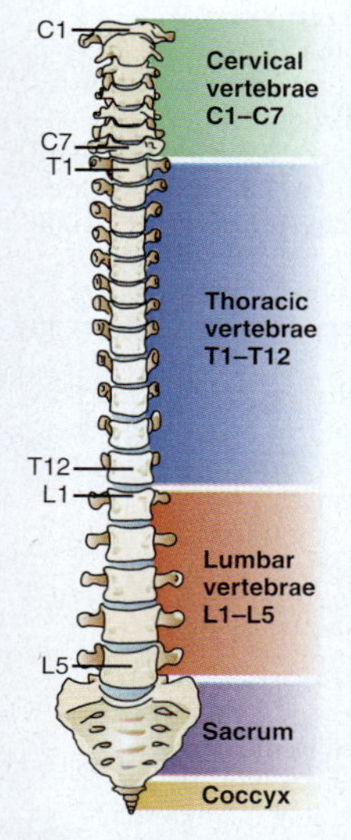

Figure 19-3 Anterior view of vertebral column.

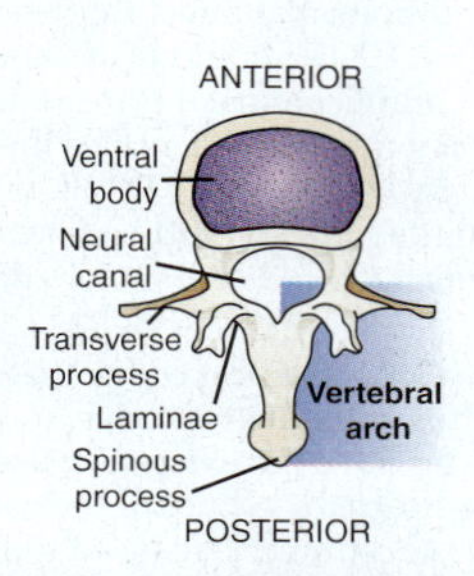

Figure 19-4 Vertebra viewed from above.

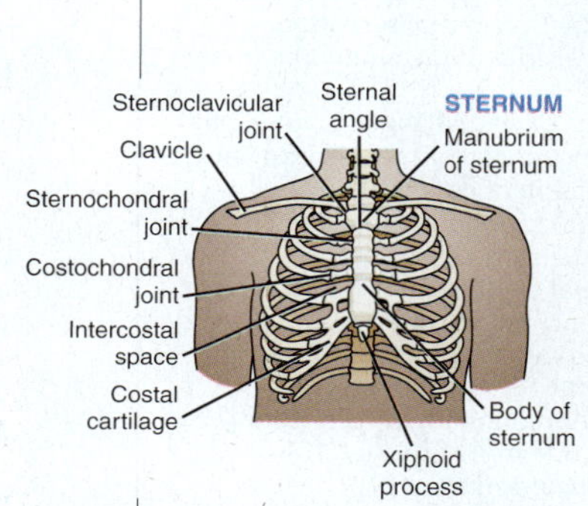

Figure 19-5 Anterior view of rib cage.

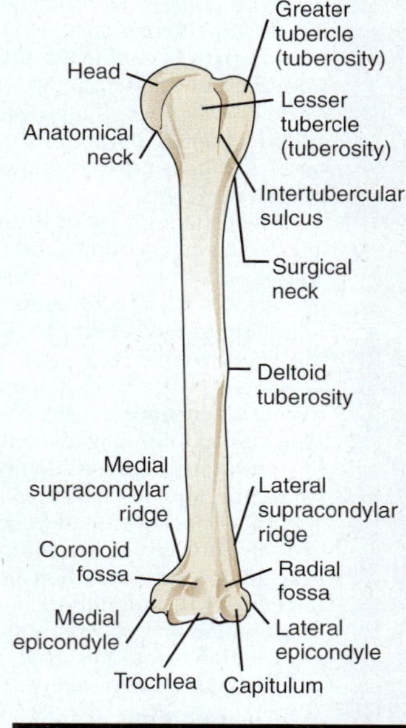

Figure 19-6 Anterior aspect of left humerus.

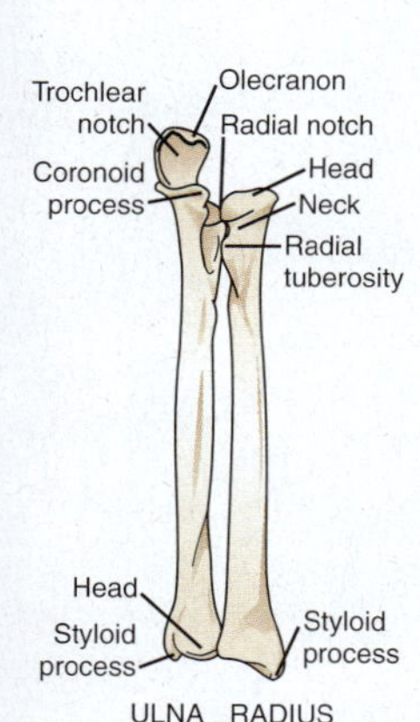

Figure 19-7 Anterior aspect of left radius and ulna.

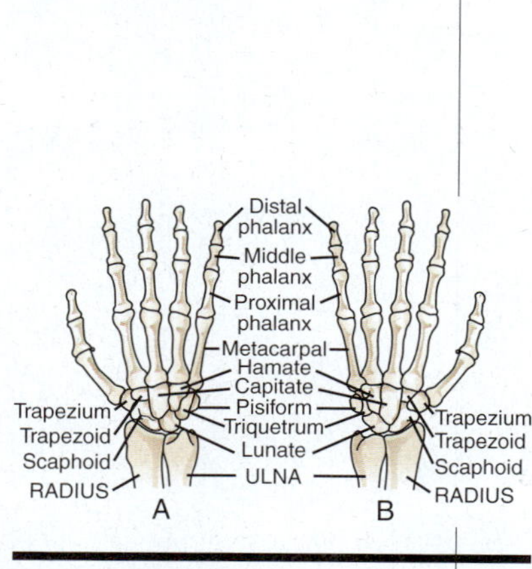

Figure 19-8 Right hand and wrist: **A.** Dorsal surface. **B.** Palmar surface.

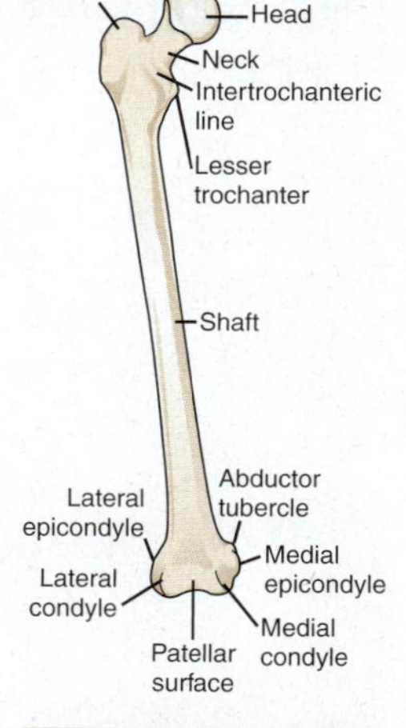

Figure 19-9 Anterior aspect of right femur.

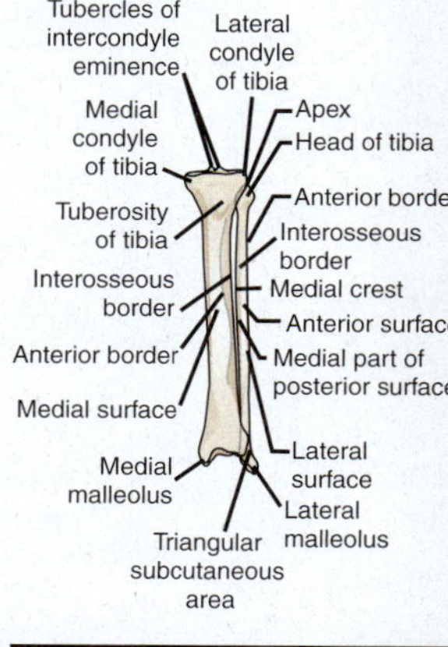

Figure 19-10 Anterior aspect of left tibia and fibula.

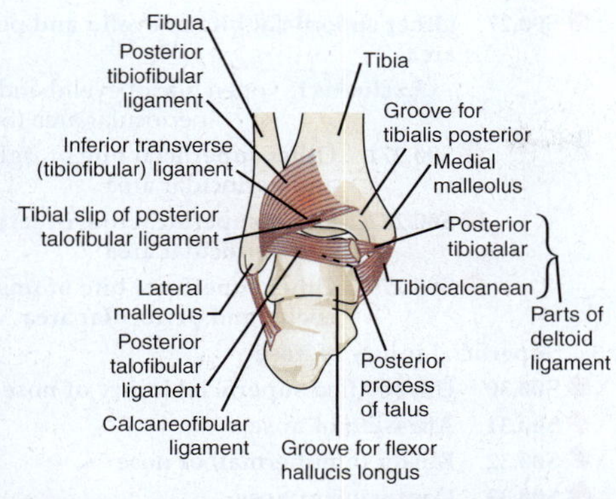

Figure 19-11   Posterior aspect of the left ankle joint.

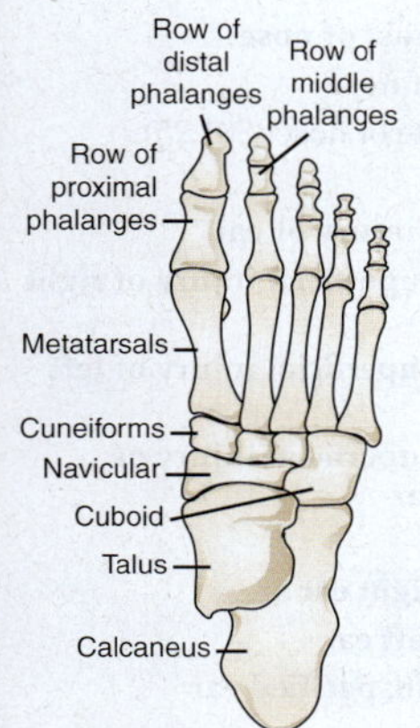

Figure 19-12   Right foot viewed from above.

CHAPTER 19

INJURY, POISONING AND CERTAIN OTHER CONSEQUENCES OF EXTERNAL CAUSES (S00-T88)

Note: Use secondary code(s) from Chapter 20, External causes of morbidity, to indicate cause of injury. Codes within the T section that include the external cause do not require an additional external cause code.

Use additional code to identify any retained foreign body, if applicable (Z18.-)

Excludes1   birth trauma (P10-P15)
obstetric trauma (O70-O71)

Note: The chapter uses the S-section for coding different types of injuries related to single body regions and the T-section to cover injuries to unspecified body regions as well as poisoning and certain other consequences of external causes.

This chapter contains the following blocks:

S00-S09	Injuries to the head
S10-S19	Injuries to the neck
S20-S29	Injuries to the thorax
S30-S39	Injuries to the abdomen, lower back, lumbar spine, pelvis and external genitals
S40-S49	Injuries to the shoulder and upper arm
S50-S59	Injuries to the elbow and forearm
S60-S69	Injuries to the wrist, hand, and fingers
S70-S79	Injuries to the hip and thigh
S80-S89	Injuries to the knee and lower leg
S90-S99	Injuries to the ankle and foot

T07	Injuries involving multiple body regions
T14	Injury of unspecified body region
T15-T19	Effects of foreign body entering through natural orifice
T20-T25	Burns and corrosions of external body surface, specified by site
T26-T28	Burns and corrosions confined to eye and internal organs
T30-T32	Burns and corrosions of multiple and unspecified body regions
T33-T34	Frostbite
T36-T50	Poisoning by, adverse effect of and underdosing of drugs, medicaments and biological substances
T51-T65	Toxic effects of substances chiefly nonmedicinal as to source
T66-T78	Other and unspecified effects of external causes
T79	Certain early complications of trauma
T80-T88	Complications of surgical and medical care, not elsewhere classified

INJURIES TO THE HEAD (S00-S09)

Includes   injuries of ear
injuries of eye
injuries of face [any part]
injuries of gum
injuries of jaw
injuries of oral cavity
injuries of palate
injuries of periocular area
injuries of scalp
injuries of temporomandibular joint area
injuries of tongue
injuries of tooth

Code also for any associated infection

Excludes2   burns and corrosions (T20-T32)
effects of foreign body in ear (T16)
effects of foreign body in larynx (T17.3)
effects of foreign body in mouth NOS (T18.0)
effects of foreign body in nose (T17.0-T17.1)
effects of foreign body in pharynx (T17.2)
effects of foreign body on external eye (T15.-)
frostbite (T33-T34)
insect bite or sting, venomous (T63.4)

● **S00**   **Superficial injury of head**

Excludes1   diffuse cerebral contusion (S06.2-)
focal cerebral contusion (S06.3-)
injury of eye and orbit (S05.-)
open wound of head (S01.-)

The appropriate 7th character is to be added to each code from category S00

A	initial encounter	
	All encounters involving diagnosis and treatment	
D	subsequent encounter	
	Encounters during the healing phase	
S	sequela	

● **S00.0**   **Superficial injury of scalp**

X ● **S00.00**   **Unspecified** superficial injury of scalp

X ● **S00.01**   **Abrasion** of scalp

X ● **S00.02**   **Blister (nonthermal)** of scalp

X ● **S00.03**   **Contusion** of scalp
Bruise of scalp
Hematoma of scalp

X ● **S00.04**   **External constriction** of part of scalp

X ● **S00.05**   **Superficial foreign body** of scalp
Splinter in the scalp

X ● **S00.06**   **Insect bite (nonvenomous)** of scalp

X ● **S00.07**   **Other superficial bite** of scalp
Excludes1   open bite of scalp (S01.05)

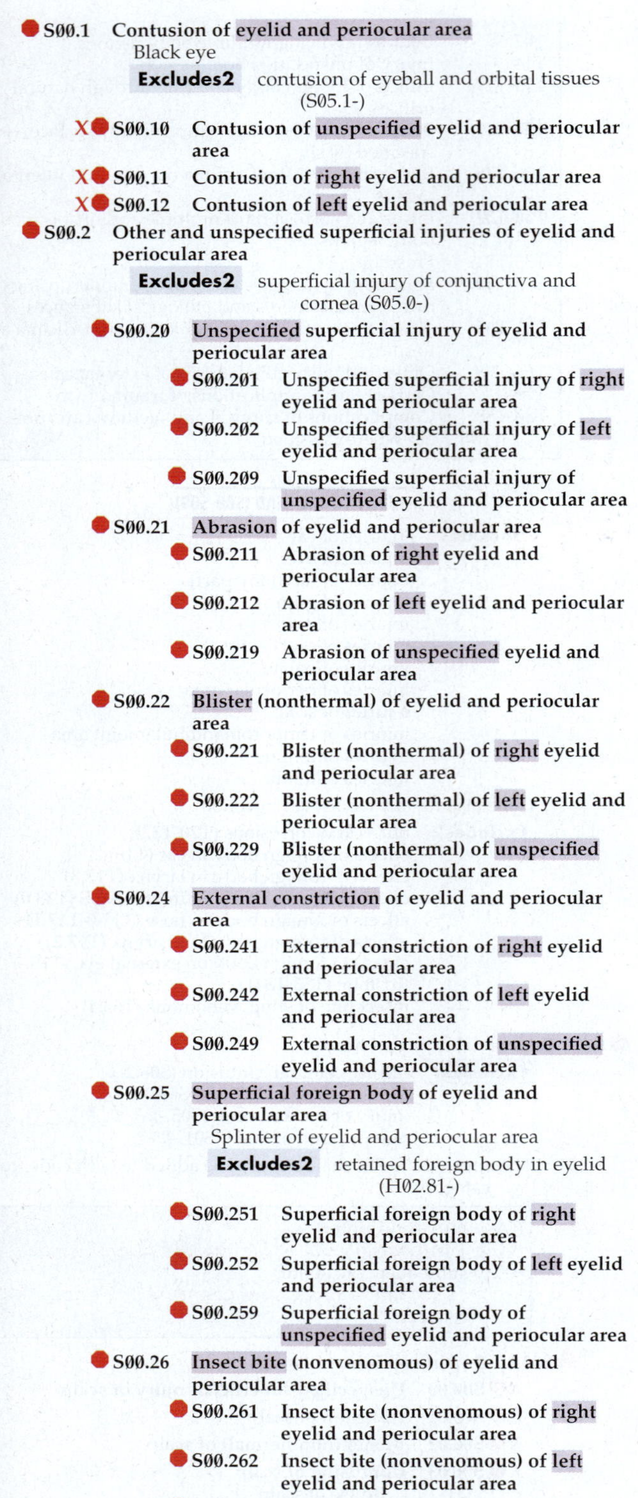

● **S00.1** Contusion of eyelid and periocular area
Black eye

     Excludes2   contusion of eyeball and orbital tissues (S05.1-)

X● **S00.10** Contusion of unspecified eyelid and periocular area

X● **S00.11** Contusion of right eyelid and periocular area

X● **S00.12** Contusion of left eyelid and periocular area

● **S00.2** Other and unspecified superficial injuries of eyelid and periocular area

     Excludes2   superficial injury of conjunctiva and cornea (S05.0-)

● **S00.20** Unspecified superficial injury of eyelid and periocular area

   ● **S00.201** Unspecified superficial injury of right eyelid and periocular area

   ● **S00.202** Unspecified superficial injury of left eyelid and periocular area

   ● **S00.209** Unspecified superficial injury of unspecified eyelid and periocular area

● **S00.21** Abrasion of eyelid and periocular area

   ● **S00.211** Abrasion of right eyelid and periocular area

   ● **S00.212** Abrasion of left eyelid and periocular area

   ● **S00.219** Abrasion of unspecified eyelid and periocular area

● **S00.22** Blister (nonthermal) of eyelid and periocular area

   ● **S00.221** Blister (nonthermal) of right eyelid and periocular area

   ● **S00.222** Blister (nonthermal) of left eyelid and periocular area

   ● **S00.229** Blister (nonthermal) of unspecified eyelid and periocular area

● **S00.24** External constriction of eyelid and periocular area

   ● **S00.241** External constriction of right eyelid and periocular area

   ● **S00.242** External constriction of left eyelid and periocular area

   ● **S00.249** External constriction of unspecified eyelid and periocular area

● **S00.25** Superficial foreign body of eyelid and periocular area
Splinter of eyelid and periocular area

     Excludes2   retained foreign body in eyelid (H02.81-)

   ● **S00.251** Superficial foreign body of right eyelid and periocular area

   ● **S00.252** Superficial foreign body of left eyelid and periocular area

   ● **S00.259** Superficial foreign body of unspecified eyelid and periocular area

● **S00.26** Insect bite (nonvenomous) of eyelid and periocular area

   ● **S00.261** Insect bite (nonvenomous) of right eyelid and periocular area

   ● **S00.262** Insect bite (nonvenomous) of left eyelid and periocular area

   ● **S00.269** Insect bite (nonvenomous) of unspecified eyelid and periocular area

● **S00.27** Other superficial bite of eyelid and periocular area

     Excludes1   open bite of eyelid and periocular area (S01.15)

   ● **S00.271** Other superficial bite of right eyelid and periocular area

   ● **S00.272** Other superficial bite of left eyelid and periocular area

   ● **S00.279** Other superficial bite of unspecified eyelid and periocular area

● **S00.3** Superficial injury of nose

X● **S00.30** Unspecified superficial injury of nose

X● **S00.31** Abrasion of nose

X● **S00.32** Blister (nonthermal) of nose

X● **S00.33** Contusion of nose
Bruise of nose
Hematoma of nose

X● **S00.34** External constriction of nose

X● **S00.35** Superficial foreign body of nose
Splinter in the nose

X● **S00.36** Insect bite (nonvenomous) of nose

X● **S00.37** Other superficial bite of nose

     Excludes1   open bite of nose (S01.25)

● **S00.4** Superficial injury of ear

● **S00.40** Unspecified superficial injury of ear

   ● **S00.401** Unspecified superficial injury of right ear

   ● **S00.402** Unspecified superficial injury of left ear

   ● **S00.409** Unspecified superficial injury of unspecified ear

● **S00.41** Abrasion of ear

   ● **S00.411** Abrasion of right ear

   ● **S00.412** Abrasion of left ear

   ● **S00.419** Abrasion of unspecified ear

● **S00.42** Blister (nonthermal) of ear

   ● **S00.421** Blister (nonthermal) of right ear

   ● **S00.422** Blister (nonthermal) of left ear

   ● **S00.429** Blister (nonthermal) of unspecified ear

● **S00.43** Contusion of ear
Bruise of ear
Hematoma of ear

   ● **S00.431** Contusion of right ear

   ● **S00.432** Contusion of left ear

   ● **S00.439** Contusion of unspecified ear

● **S00.44** External constriction of ear

   ● **S00.441** External constriction of right ear

   ● **S00.442** External constriction of left ear

   ● **S00.449** External constriction of unspecified ear

● **S00.45** Superficial foreign body of ear
Splinter in the ear

   ● **S00.451** Superficial foreign body of right ear

   ● **S00.452** Superficial foreign body of left ear

   ● **S00.459** Superficial foreign body of unspecified ear

● **S00.46** Insect bite (nonvenomous) of ear

   ● **S00.461** Insect bite (nonvenomous) of right ear

   ● **S00.462** Insect bite (nonvenomous) of left ear

   ● **S00.469** Insect bite (nonvenomous) of unspecified ear

▶ New   ➡ Revised   ~~deleted~~ Deleted   Excludes 1   Excludes 2   Includes   Use additional   Code first   Code also   Key words
OGCR Official Guidelines   X Assign placeholder X   ● Use Additional Character(s)   ▶ Manifestation Code   Hierarchical Condition Category   **Coding Clinic**

● **S00.47**   Other superficial bite of ear
     Excludes1   open bite of ear (S01.35)
   ● **S00.471**   Other superficial bite of right ear
   ● **S00.472**   Other superficial bite of left ear
   ● **S00.479**   Other superficial bite of unspecified ear

● **S00.5**   Superficial injury of lip and oral cavity
   ● **S00.50**   Unspecified superficial injury of lip and oral cavity
     ● **S00.501**   Unspecified superficial injury of lip
     ● **S00.502**   Unspecified superficial injury of oral cavity
   ● **S00.51**   Abrasion of lip and oral cavity
     ● **S00.511**   Abrasion of lip
     ● **S00.512**   Abrasion of oral cavity
   ● **S00.52**   Blister (nonthermal) of lip and oral cavity
     ● **S00.521**   Blister (nonthermal) of lip
     ● **S00.522**   Blister (nonthermal) of oral cavity
   ● **S00.53**   Contusion of lip and oral cavity
     ● **S00.531**   Contusion of lip
        Bruise of lip
        Hematoma of lip
     ● **S00.532**   Contusion of oral cavity
        Bruise of oral cavity
        Hematoma of oral cavity
   ● **S00.54**   External constriction of lip and oral cavity
     ● **S00.541**   External constriction of lip
     ● **S00.542**   External constriction of oral cavity
   ● **S00.55**   Superficial foreign body of lip and oral cavity
     ● **S00.551**   Superficial foreign body of lip
        Splinter of lip and oral cavity
     ● **S00.552**   Superficial foreign body of oral cavity
        Splinter of lip and oral cavity
   ● **S00.56**   Insect bite (nonvenomous) of lip and oral cavity
     ● **S00.561**   Insect bite (nonvenomous) of lip
     ● **S00.562**   Insect bite (nonvenomous) of oral cavity
   ● **S00.57**   Other superficial bite of lip and oral cavity
     ● **S00.571**   Other superficial bite of lip
        Excludes1   open bite of lip (S01.551)
     ● **S00.572**   Other superficial bite of oral cavity
        Excludes1   open bite of oral cavity (S01.552)

● **S00.8**   Superficial injury of other parts of head
     Superficial injuries of face [any part]
   X ● **S00.80**   Unspecified superficial injury of other part of head
   X ● **S00.81**   Abrasion of other part of head
   X ● **S00.82**   Blister (nonthermal) of other part of head
   X ● **S00.83**   Contusion of other part of head
        Bruise of other part of head
        Hematoma of other part of head
   X ● **S00.84**   External constriction of other part of head
   X ● **S00.85**   Superficial foreign body of other part of head
        Splinter in other part of head
   X ● **S00.86**   Insect bite (nonvenomous) of other part of head
   X ● **S00.87**   Other superficial bite of other part of head
        Excludes1   open bite of other part of head (S01.85)

● **S00.9**   Superficial injury of unspecified part of head
   X ● **S00.90**   Unspecified superficial injury of unspecified part of head
   X ● **S00.91**   Abrasion of unspecified part of head
   X ● **S00.92**   Blister (nonthermal) of unspecified part of head

   X ● **S00.93**   Contusion of unspecified part of head
        Bruise of head
        Hematoma of head
   X ● **S00.94**   External constriction of unspecified part of head
   X ● **S00.95**   Superficial foreign body of unspecified part of head
        Splinter of head
   X ● **S00.96**   Insect bite (nonvenomous) of unspecified part of head
   X ● **S00.97**   Other superficial bite of unspecified part of head
        Excludes1   open bite of head (S01.95)

● **S01**   Open wound of head
   Code also any associated:
     injury of cranial nerve (S04.-)
     injury of muscle and tendon of head (S09.1-)
     intracranial injury (S06.-)
     wound infection
   Excludes1   open skull fracture (S02.- with 7th character B)
   Excludes2   injury of eye and orbit (S05.-)
        traumatic amputation of part of head (S08.-)
   The appropriate 7th character is to be added to each code from category S01

     A   initial encounter
     D   subsequent encounter
     S   sequela

   ● **S01.0**   Open wound of scalp
     Excludes1   avulsion of scalp (S08.0-)
   X ● **S01.00**   Unspecified open wound of scalp
   X ● **S01.01**   Laceration without foreign body of scalp
   X ● **S01.02**   Laceration with foreign body of scalp
        Coding Clinic: 2015, Q1, P5-7
   X ● **S01.03**   Puncture wound without foreign body of scalp
   X ● **S01.04**   Puncture wound with foreign body of scalp
   X ● **S01.05**   Open bite of scalp
        Bite of scalp NOS
        Excludes1   superficial bite of scalp (S00.06, S00.07-)

   ● **S01.1**   Open wound of eyelid and periocular area
     Open wound of eyelid and periocular area with or without involvement of lacrimal passages
     ● **S01.10**   Unspecified open wound of eyelid and periocular area
       ● **S01.101**   Unspecified open wound of right eyelid and periocular area
       ● **S01.102**   Unspecified open wound of left eyelid and periocular area
       ● **S01.109**   Unspecified open wound of unspecified eyelid and periocular area
     ● **S01.11**   Laceration without foreign body of eyelid and periocular area
       ● **S01.111**   Laceration without foreign body of right eyelid and periocular area
       ● **S01.112**   Laceration without foreign body of left eyelid and periocular area
       ● **S01.119**   Laceration without foreign body of unspecified eyelid and periocular area
     ● **S01.12**   Laceration with foreign body of eyelid and periocular area
       ● **S01.121**   Laceration with foreign body of right eyelid and periocular area
       ● **S01.122**   Laceration with foreign body of left eyelid and periocular area
       ● **S01.129**   Laceration with foreign body of unspecified eyelid and periocular area

- ● S01.13 Puncture wound without foreign body of eyelid and periocular area
  - ● S01.131 Puncture wound without foreign body of right eyelid and periocular area
  - ● S01.132 Puncture wound without foreign body of left eyelid and periocular area
  - ● S01.139 Puncture wound without foreign body of unspecified eyelid and periocular area
- ● S01.14 Puncture wound with foreign body of eyelid and periocular area
  - ● S01.141 Puncture wound with foreign body of right eyelid and periocular area
  - ● S01.142 Puncture wound with foreign body of left eyelid and periocular area
  - ● S01.149 Puncture wound with foreign body of unspecified eyelid and periocular area
- ● S01.15 Open bite of eyelid and periocular area
  - Bite of eyelid and periocular area NOS
  - **Excludes1** superficial bite of eyelid and periocular area (S00.26, S00.27)
  - ● S01.151 Open bite of right eyelid and periocular area
  - ● S01.152 Open bite of left eyelid and periocular area
  - ● S01.159 Open bite of unspecified eyelid and periocular area
- ● S01.2 Open wound of nose
  - X ● S01.20 Unspecified open wound of nose
  - X ● S01.21 Laceration without foreign body of nose
    - Coding Clinic: 2015, Q1, P5-6
  - X ● S01.22 Laceration with foreign body of nose
  - X ● S01.23 Puncture wound without foreign body of nose
  - X ● S01.24 Puncture wound with foreign body of nose
  - X ● S01.25 Open bite of nose
    - Bite of nose NOS
    - **Excludes1** superficial bite of nose (S00.36, S00.37)
- ● S01.3 Open wound of ear
  - ● S01.30 Unspecified open wound of ear
    - ● S01.301 Unspecified open wound of right ear
    - ● S01.302 Unspecified open wound of left ear
    - ● S01.309 Unspecified open wound of unspecified ear
  - ● S01.31 Laceration without foreign body of ear
    - ● S01.311 Laceration without foreign body of right ear
    - ● S01.312 Laceration without foreign body of left ear
    - ● S01.319 Laceration without foreign body of unspecified ear
  - ● S01.32 Laceration with foreign body of ear
    - ● S01.321 Laceration with foreign body of right ear
    - ● S01.322 Laceration with foreign body of left ear
    - ● S01.329 Laceration with foreign body of unspecified ear
  - ● S01.33 Puncture wound without foreign body of ear
    - ● S01.331 Puncture wound without foreign body of right ear
    - ● S01.332 Puncture wound without foreign body of left ear
    - ● S01.339 Puncture wound without foreign body of unspecified ear
- ● S01.34 Puncture wound with foreign body of ear
  - ● S01.341 Puncture wound with foreign body of right ear
  - ● S01.342 Puncture wound with foreign body of left ear
  - ● S01.349 Puncture wound with foreign body of unspecified ear
- ● S01.35 Open bite of ear
  - Bite of ear NOS
  - **Excludes1** superficial bite of ear (S00.46, S00.47)
  - ● S01.351 Open bite of right ear
  - ● S01.352 Open bite of left ear
  - ● S01.359 Open bite of unspecified ear
- ● S01.4 Open wound of cheek and temporomandibular area
  - ● S01.40 Unspecified open wound of cheek and temporomandibular area
    - ● S01.401 Unspecified open wound of right cheek and temporomandibular area
    - ● S01.402 Unspecified open wound of left cheek and temporomandibular area
    - ● S01.409 Unspecified open wound of unspecified cheek and temporomandibular area
  - ● S01.41 Laceration without foreign body of cheek and temporomandibular area
    - ● S01.411 Laceration without foreign body of right cheek and temporomandibular area
      - Coding Clinic: 2015, Q1, P5-7
    - ● S01.412 Laceration without foreign body of left cheek and temporomandibular area
    - ● S01.419 Laceration without foreign body of unspecified cheek and temporomandibular area
  - ● S01.42 Laceration with foreign body of cheek and temporomandibular area
    - ● S01.421 Laceration with foreign body of right cheek and temporomandibular area
    - ● S01.422 Laceration with foreign body of left cheek and temporomandibular area
    - ● S01.429 Laceration with foreign body of unspecified cheek and temporomandibular area
  - ● S01.43 Puncture wound without foreign body of cheek and temporomandibular area
    - ● S01.431 Puncture wound without foreign body of right cheek and temporomandibular area
    - ● S01.432 Puncture wound without foreign body of left cheek and temporomandibular area
    - ● S01.439 Puncture wound without foreign body of unspecified cheek and temporomandibular area
  - ● S01.44 Puncture wound with foreign body of cheek and temporomandibular area
    - ● S01.441 Puncture wound with foreign body of right cheek and temporomandibular area
    - ● S01.442 Puncture wound with foreign body of left cheek and temporomandibular area
    - ● S01.449 Puncture wound with foreign body of unspecified cheek and temporomandibular area

▶ New ⇨ Revised ~~deleted~~ Deleted Excludes 1 Excludes 2 Includes Use additional Code first Code also Key words

OGCR Official Guidelines X Assign placeholder X ● Use Additional Character(s) ▶ Manifestation Code 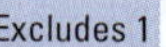 Hierarchical Condition Category Coding Clinic

- S01.45 **Open bite of cheek and temporomandibular area**
  Bite of cheek and temporomandibular area NOS
  Excludes2 superficial bite of cheek and temporomandibular area (S00.86, S00.87)
  - S01.451 **Open bite of right cheek and temporomandibular area**
  - S01.452 **Open bite of left cheek and temporomandibular area**
  - S01.459 **Open bite of unspecified cheek and temporomandibular area**
- S01.5 **Open wound of lip and oral cavity**
  Excludes2 tooth dislocation (S03.2)
  tooth fracture (S02.5)
  - S01.50 **Unspecified open wound of lip and oral cavity**
    - S01.501 **Unspecified open wound of lip**
    - S01.502 **Unspecified open wound of oral cavity**
  - S01.51 **Laceration of lip and oral cavity without foreign body**
    - S01.511 **Laceration without foreign body of lip**
    - S01.512 **Laceration without foreign body of oral cavity**
  - S01.52 **Laceration of lip and oral cavity with foreign body**
    - S01.521 **Laceration with foreign body of lip**
    - S01.522 **Laceration with foreign body of oral cavity**
  - S01.53 **Puncture wound of lip and oral cavity without foreign body**
    - S01.531 **Puncture wound without foreign body of lip**
    - S01.532 **Puncture wound without foreign body of oral cavity**
  - S01.54 **Puncture wound of lip and oral cavity with foreign body**
    - S01.541 **Puncture wound with foreign body of lip**
    - S01.542 **Puncture wound with foreign body of oral cavity**
  - S01.55 **Open bite of lip and oral cavity**
    - S01.551 **Open bite of lip**
      Bite of lip NOS
      Excludes1 superficial bite of lip (S00.571)
    - S01.552 **Open bite of oral cavity**
      Bite of oral cavity NOS
      Excludes1 superficial bite of oral cavity (S00.572)
- S01.8 **Open wound of other parts of head**
  - X S01.80 **Unspecified open wound of other part of head**
  - X S01.81 **Laceration without foreign body of other part of head**
  - X S01.82 **Laceration with foreign body of other part of head**
  - X S01.83 **Puncture wound without foreign body of other part of head**
  - X S01.84 **Puncture wound with foreign body of other part of head**
  - X S01.85 **Open bite of other part of head**
    Bite of other part of head NOS
    Excludes1 superficial bite of other part of head (S00.87)

- S01.9 **Open wound of unspecified part of head**
  - X S01.90 **Unspecified open wound of unspecified part of head**
  - X S01.91 **Laceration without foreign body of unspecified part of head**
  - X S01.92 **Laceration with foreign body of unspecified part of head**
  - X S01.93 **Puncture wound without foreign body of unspecified part of head**
  - X S01.94 **Puncture wound with foreign body of unspecified part of head**
  - X S01.95 **Open bite of unspecified part of head**
    Bite of head NOS
    Excludes1 superficial bite of head NOS (S00.97)

- S02 **Fracture of skull and facial bones**
  Note: A fracture not indicated as open or closed should be coded to closed
  The appropriate 7th character is to be added to each code from category S02

A	initial encounter for closed fracture
B	initial encounter for open fracture
D	subsequent encounter for fracture with routine healing
G	subsequent encounter for fracture with delayed healing
K	subsequent encounter for fracture with nonunion
S	sequela

  Code also any associated intracranial injury (S06.-)
  - X S02.0 **Fracture of vault of skull A, B, S** 🔵
    Fracture of frontal bone
    Fracture of parietal bone
  - S02.1 **Fracture of base of skull**
    Excludes2 lateral orbital wall (S02.84-)
    medial orbital wall (S02.83-)
    orbital floor (S02.3-)
    Coding Clinic: 2016, Q4, P66
    - S02.10 **Unspecified fracture of base of skull**
      - S02.101 **Fracture of base of skull, right side A, B, S** 🔵
      - S02.102 **Fracture of base of skull, left side A, B, S** 🔵
      - S02.109 **Fracture of base of skull, unspecified side A, B, S** 🔵
    - S02.11 **Fracture of occiput**
      - S02.110 **Type I occipital condyle fracture, unspecified side A, B, S** 🔵
      - S02.111 **Type II occipital condyle fracture, unspecified side A, B, S** 🔵
      - S02.112 **Type III occipital condyle fracture, unspecified side A, B, S** 🔵
      - S02.113 **Unspecified occipital condyle fracture A, B, S** 🔵
      - S02.118 **Other fracture of occiput, unspecified side A, B, S** 🔵
      - S02.119 **Unspecified fracture of occiput A, B, S** 🔵
      - S02.11A **Type I occipital condyle fracture, right side A, B, S** 🔵
      - S02.11B **Type I occipital condyle fracture, left side A, B, S** 🔵
      - S02.11C **Type II occipital condyle fracture, right side A, B, S** 🔵
      - S02.11D **Type II occipital condyle fracture, left side A, B, S** 🔵

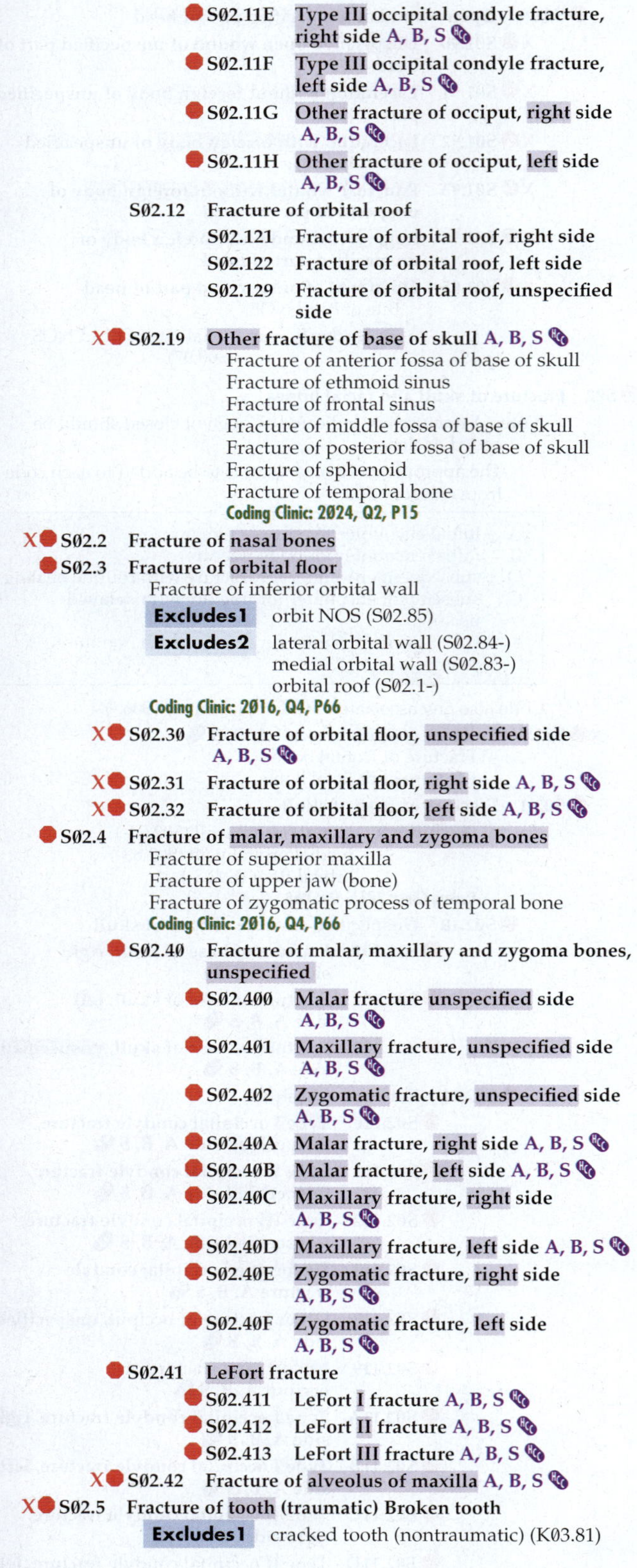

● **S02.11E** Type III occipital condyle fracture, right side A, B, S ℞

● **S02.11F** Type III occipital condyle fracture, left side A, B, S ℞

● **S02.11G** Other fracture of occiput, right side A, B, S ℞

● **S02.11H** Other fracture of occiput, left side A, B, S ℞

S02.12 Fracture of orbital roof

   S02.121 Fracture of orbital roof, right side

   S02.122 Fracture of orbital roof, left side

   S02.129 Fracture of orbital roof, unspecified side

X ● **S02.19** Other fracture of base of skull A, B, S ℞
> Fracture of anterior fossa of base of skull
> Fracture of ethmoid sinus
> Fracture of frontal sinus
> Fracture of middle fossa of base of skull
> Fracture of posterior fossa of base of skull
> Fracture of sphenoid
> Fracture of temporal bone
> **Coding Clinic: 2024, Q2, P15**

X ● **S02.2** Fracture of nasal bones

● **S02.3** Fracture of orbital floor
> Fracture of inferior orbital wall
>
> **Excludes1**   orbit NOS (S02.85)
>
> **Excludes2**   lateral orbital wall (S02.84-)
>   medial orbital wall (S02.83-)
>   orbital roof (S02.1-)
>
> **Coding Clinic: 2016, Q4, P66**

X ● **S02.30** Fracture of orbital floor, unspecified side A, B, S ℞

X ● **S02.31** Fracture of orbital floor, right side A, B, S ℞

X ● **S02.32** Fracture of orbital floor, left side A, B, S ℞

● **S02.4** Fracture of malar, maxillary and zygoma bones
> Fracture of superior maxilla
> Fracture of upper jaw (bone)
> Fracture of zygomatic process of temporal bone
> **Coding Clinic: 2016, Q4, P66**

● **S02.40** Fracture of malar, maxillary and zygoma bones, unspecified

   ● **S02.400** Malar fracture unspecified side A, B, S ℞

   ● **S02.401** Maxillary fracture, unspecified side A, B, S ℞

   ● **S02.402** Zygomatic fracture, unspecified side A, B, S ℞

   ● **S02.40A** Malar fracture, right side A, B, S ℞

   ● **S02.40B** Malar fracture, left side A, B, S ℞

   ● **S02.40C** Maxillary fracture, right side A, B, S ℞

   ● **S02.40D** Maxillary fracture, left side A, B, S ℞

   ● **S02.40E** Zygomatic fracture, right side A, B, S ℞

   ● **S02.40F** Zygomatic fracture, left side A, B, S ℞

● **S02.41** LeFort fracture

   ● **S02.411** LeFort I fracture A, B, S ℞

   ● **S02.412** LeFort II fracture A, B, S ℞

   ● **S02.413** LeFort III fracture A, B, S ℞

X ● **S02.42** Fracture of alveolus of maxilla A, B, S ℞

X ● **S02.5** Fracture of tooth (traumatic) Broken tooth
> **Excludes1**   cracked tooth (nontraumatic) (K03.81)

● **S02.6** Fracture of mandible
> Fracture of lower jaw (bone)
> **Coding Clinic: 2016, Q4, P66**

● **S02.60** Fracture of mandible of unspecified site

   ● **S02.600** Fracture of unspecified part of body of mandible, unspecified side A, B, S ℞

   ● **S02.601** Fracture of unspecified part of body of right mandible A, B, S ℞

   ● **S02.602** Fracture of unspecified part of body of left mandible A, B, S ℞

   ● **S02.609** Fracture of mandible, unspecified A, B, S ℞

● **S02.61** Fracture of condylar process of mandible

   ● **S02.610** Fracture of condylar process of mandible, unspecified side A, B, S ℞

   ● **S02.611** Fracture of condylar process of right mandible A, B, S ℞
> **Coding Clinic: 2021, Q1, P6**

   ● **S02.612** Fracture of condylar process of left mandible A, B, S ℞

● **S02.62** Fracture of subcondylar process of mandible

   ● **S02.620** Fracture of subcondylar process of mandible, unspecified side A, B, S ℞

   ● **S02.621** Fracture of subcondylar process of right mandible A, B, S ℞

   ● **S02.622** Fracture of subcondylar process of left mandible A, B, S ℞

● **S02.63** Fracture of coronoid process of mandible

   ● **S02.630** Fracture of coronoid process of mandible, unspecified side A, B, S ℞

   ● **S02.631** Fracture of coronoid process of right mandible A, B, S ℞

   ● **S02.632** Fracture of coronoid process of left mandible A, B, S ℞

● **S02.64** Fracture of ramus of mandible

   ● **S02.640** Fracture of ramus of mandible, unspecified side A, B, S ℞

   ● **S02.641** Fracture of ramus of right mandible A, B, S ℞

   ● **S02.642** Fracture of ramus of left mandible A, B, S ℞

● **S02.65** Fracture of angle of mandible

   ● **S02.650** Fracture of angle of mandible, unspecified side A, B, S ℞

   ● **S02.651** Fracture of angle of right mandible A, B, S ℞

   ● **S02.652** Fracture of angle of left mandible A, B, S ℞

X ● **S02.66** Fracture of symphysis of mandible A, B, S ℞
> **Coding Clinic: 2021, Q1, P6**

● **S02.67** Fracture of alveolus of mandible

   ● **S02.670** Fracture of alveolus of mandible, unspecified side A, B, S ℞

   ● **S02.671** Fracture of alveolus of right mandible A, B, S ℞

   ● **S02.672** Fracture of alveolus of left mandible A, B, S ℞

X ● **S02.69** Fracture of mandible of other specified site A, B, S ℞

● **S02.8** Fractures of other specified skull and facial bones
> Fracture of palate
>
> **Excludes2**   lateral orbital wall (S02.84-)
>   medial orbital wall (S02.83-)
>
> **Coding Clinic: 2016, Q4, P66**

X ● **S02.80** Fracture of other specified skull and facial bones, unspecified side A, B, S ℞

▶ New   ⮕ Revised   ~~deleted~~ Deleted   Excludes 1   Excludes 2   Includes   Use additional   Code first   Code also   Key words

OGCR Official Guidelines   X Assign placeholder X   ● Use Additional Character(s)   ▸ Manifestation Code   ℞ Hierarchical Condition Category   **Coding Clinic**

X● **S02.81**   Fracture of other specified skull and facial bones, right side A, B, S

X● **S02.82**   Fracture of other specified skull and facial bones, left side A, B, S

● **S02.83** Fracture of medial orbital wall

     Excludes2   orbital floor (S02.3-)
                        orbital roof (S02.12-)

     S02.831   Fracture of medial orbital wall, right side

     S02.832   Fracture of medial orbital wall, left side

     S02.839   Fracture of medial orbital wall, unspecified side

● **S02.84** Fracture of lateral orbital wall

     Excludes2   orbital floor (S02.3-)
                        orbital roof (S02.12-)

     S02.841   Fracture of lateral orbital wall, right side

     S02.842   Fracture of lateral orbital wall, left side

     S02.849   Fracture of lateral orbital wall, unspecified side

     S02.85 Fracture of orbit, unspecified
           Fracture of orbit NOS
           Fracture of orbit wall NOS

           Excludes1   lateral orbital wall (S02.84-)
                              medial orbital wall (S02.83-)
                              orbital floor (S02.3-)
                              orbital roof (S02.12-)

● **S02.9**   Fracture of unspecified skull and facial bones

     X● **S02.91**   Unspecified fracture of skull A, B, S

     X● **S02.92**   Unspecified fracture of facial bones A, B, S

● **S03**   Dislocation and sprain of joints and ligaments of head

     Includes   avulsion of joint (capsule) or ligament of head
                    laceration of cartilage, joint (capsule) or ligament of head
                    sprain of cartilage, joint (capsule) or ligament of head
                    traumatic hemarthrosis of joint or ligament of head
                    traumatic rupture of joint or ligament of head
                    traumatic subluxation of joint or ligament of head
                    traumatic tear of joint or ligament of head

     Code also any associated open wound

     Excludes2   Strain of muscle or tendon of head (S09.1)

     The appropriate 7th character is to be added to each code from category S03

     A   initial encounter
     D   subsequent encounter
     S   sequela

● **S03.0**   Dislocation of jaw
           Dislocation of jaw (cartilage) (meniscus)
           Dislocation of mandible
           Dislocation of temporomandibular (joint)
           Coding Clinic: 2016, Q4, P67

     X● **S03.00**   Dislocation of jaw, unspecified side

     X● **S03.01**   Dislocation of jaw, right side

     X● **S03.02**   Dislocation of jaw, left side

     X● **S03.03**   Dislocation of jaw, bilateral side

X● **S03.1**   Dislocation of septal cartilage of nose

X● **S03.2**   Dislocation of tooth

● **S03.4**   Sprain of jaw
           Sprain of temporomandibular (joint) (ligament)
           Coding Clinic: 2016, Q4, P67

CHAPTER 19 (S00–T88)

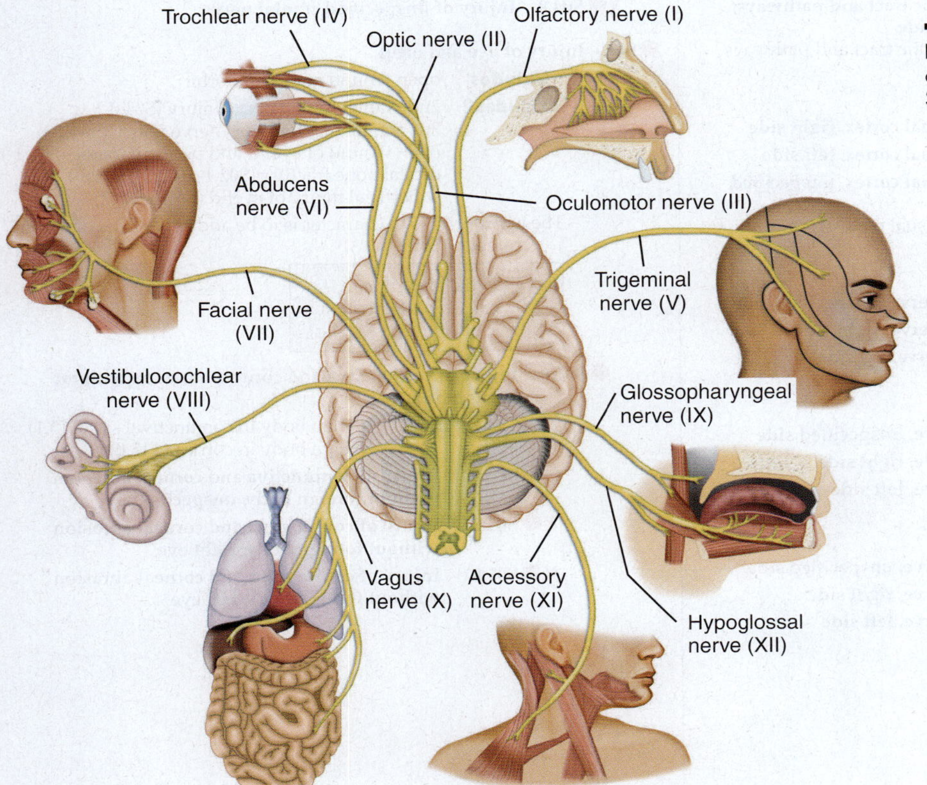

Figure 19-13 Cranial nerves. (From Patton and Thibodeau: Anatomy and physiology, ed 7, St. Louis, Mosby, 2009)

X● S03.40   Sprain of jaw, unspecified side
X● S03.41   Sprain of jaw, right side
X● S03.42   Sprain of jaw, left side
X● S03.43   Sprain of jaw, bilateral side
X● S03.8   Sprain of joints and ligaments of other parts of head
X● S03.9   Sprain of joints and ligaments of unspecified parts of head

● S04   **Injury of cranial nerve**
The selection of side should be based on the side of the body being affected

Code first any associated intracranial injury (S06.-)

Code also any associated:
   open wound of head (S01.-)
   skull fracture (S02.-)

The appropriate 7th character is to be added to each code from category S04

> A   initial encounter
> D   subsequent encounter
> S   sequela

● S04.0   **Injury of optic nerve and pathways**
Use additional code to identify any visual field defect or blindness (H53.4-, H54.-)

   ● S04.01   **Injury of optic nerve**
     Injury of 2nd cranial nerve
     ● S04.011   Injury of optic nerve, right eye
     ● S04.012   Injury of optic nerve, left eye
     ● S04.019   Injury of optic nerve, unspecified eye
       Injury of optic nerve NOS

X● S04.02   **Injury of optic chiasm**

   ● S04.03   **Injury of optic tract and pathways**
     Injury of optic radiation
     ● S04.031   Injury of optic tract and pathways, right side
     ● S04.032   Injury of optic tract and pathways, left side
     ● S04.039   Injury of optic tract and pathways, unspecified side
       Injury of optic tract and pathways NOS

   ● S04.04   **Injury of visual cortex**
     ● S04.041   Injury of visual cortex, right side
     ● S04.042   Injury of visual cortex, left side
     ● S04.049   Injury of visual cortex, unspecified side
       Injury of visual cortex NOS

● S04.1   **Injury of oculomotor nerve**
Injury of 3rd cranial nerve
X● S04.10   Injury of oculomotor nerve, unspecified side
X● S04.11   Injury of oculomotor nerve, right side
X● S04.12   Injury of oculomotor nerve, left side

● S04.2   **Injury of trochlear nerve**
Injury of 4th cranial nerve
X● S04.20   Injury of trochlear nerve, unspecified side
X● S04.21   Injury of trochlear nerve, right side
X● S04.22   Injury of trochlear nerve, left side

● S04.3   **Injury of trigeminal nerve**
Injury of 5th cranial nerve
X● S04.30   Injury of trigeminal nerve, unspecified side
X● S04.31   Injury of trigeminal nerve, right side
X● S04.32   Injury of trigeminal nerve, left side

● S04.4   **Injury of abducent nerve**
Injury of 6th cranial nerve
X● S04.40   Injury of abducent nerve, unspecified side
X● S04.41   Injury of abducent nerve, right side
X● S04.42   Injury of abducent nerve, left side

● S04.5   **Injury of facial nerve**
Injury of 7th cranial nerve
X● S04.50   Injury of facial nerve, unspecified side
X● S04.51   Injury of facial nerve, right side
X● S04.52   Injury of facial nerve, left side

● S04.6   **Injury of acoustic nerve**
Injury of auditory nerve
Injury of 8th cranial nerve
X● S04.60   Injury of acoustic nerve, unspecified side
X● S04.61   Injury of acoustic nerve, right side
X● S04.62   Injury of acoustic nerve, left side

● S04.7   **Injury of accessory nerve**
Injury of 11th cranial nerve
X● S04.70   Injury of accessory nerve, unspecified side
X● S04.71   Injury of accessory nerve, right side
X● S04.72   Injury of accessory nerve, left side

● S04.8   **Injury of other cranial nerves**
   ● S04.81   **Injury of olfactory [1st] nerve**
     ● S04.811   Injury of olfactory [1st] nerve, right side
     ● S04.812   Injury of olfactory [1st] nerve, left side
     ● S04.819   Injury of olfactory [1st] nerve, unspecified side

   ● S04.89   **Injury of other cranial nerves**
     Injury of vagus [10th] nerve
     ● S04.891   Injury of other cranial nerves, right side
     ● S04.892   Injury of other cranial nerves, left side
     ● S04.899   Injury of other cranial nerves, unspecified side

X● S04.9   **Injury of unspecified cranial nerve**

● S05   **Injury of eye and orbit**
Includes   open wound of eye and orbit
Excludes2   2nd cranial [optic] nerve injury (S04.0-)
     3rd cranial [oculomotor] nerve injury (S04.1-)
     open wound of eyelid and periocular area (S01.1-)
     orbital bone fracture (S02.1-, S02.3-, S02.8-)
     superficial injury of eyelid (S00.1-S00.2)

The appropriate 7th character is to be added to each code from category S05

> A   initial encounter
> D   subsequent encounter
> S   sequela

● S05.0   **Injury of conjunctiva and corneal abrasion without foreign body**
Excludes1   foreign body in conjunctival sac (T15.1)
     foreign body in cornea (T15.0)
X● S05.00   Injury of conjunctiva and corneal abrasion without foreign body, unspecified eye
X● S05.01   Injury of conjunctiva and corneal abrasion without foreign body, right eye
X● S05.02   Injury of conjunctiva and corneal abrasion without foreign body, left eye

● **S05.1**   **Contusion of eyeball and orbital tissues**
Traumatic hyphema
    Excludes2   black eye NOS (S00.1)
              contusion of eyelid and periocular area (S00.1)

X ● **S05.10**   **Contusion of eyeball and orbital tissues, unspecified eye**

X ● **S05.11**   **Contusion of eyeball and orbital tissues, right eye**

X ● **S05.12**   **Contusion of eyeball and orbital tissues, left eye**

● **S05.2**   **Ocular laceration and rupture with prolapse or loss of intraocular tissue**

X ● **S05.20**   **Ocular laceration and rupture with prolapse or loss of intraocular tissue, unspecified eye**

X ● **S05.21**   **Ocular laceration and rupture with prolapse or loss of intraocular tissue, right eye**

X ● **S05.22**   **Ocular laceration and rupture with prolapse or loss of intraocular tissue, left eye**

● **S05.3**   **Ocular laceration without prolapse or loss of intraocular tissue**
Laceration of eye NOS

X ● **S05.30**   **Ocular laceration without prolapse or loss of intraocular tissue, unspecified eye**

X ● **S05.31**   **Ocular laceration without prolapse or loss of intraocular tissue, right eye**

X ● **S05.32**   **Ocular laceration without prolapse or loss of intraocular tissue, left eye**

● **S05.4**   **Penetrating wound of orbit with or without foreign body**
    Excludes2   retained (old) foreign body following penetrating wound in orbit (H05.5-)

X ● **S05.40**   **Penetrating wound of orbit with or without foreign body, unspecified eye**

X ● **S05.41**   **Penetrating wound of orbit with or without foreign body, right eye**

X ● **S05.42**   **Penetrating wound of orbit with or without foreign body, left eye**

● **S05.5**   **Penetrating wound with foreign body of eyeball**
    Excludes2   retained (old) intraocular foreign body (H44.6-, H44.7)

X ● **S05.50**   **Penetrating wound with foreign body of unspecified eyeball**

X ● **S05.51**   **Penetrating wound with foreign body of right eyeball**

X ● **S05.52**   **Penetrating wound with foreign body of left eyeball**

● **S05.6**   **Penetrating wound without foreign body of eyeball**
Ocular penetration NOS

X ● **S05.60**   **Penetrating wound without foreign body of unspecified eyeball**

X ● **S05.61**   **Penetrating wound without foreign body of right eyeball**

X ● **S05.62**   **Penetrating wound without foreign body of left eyeball**

● **S05.7**   **Avulsion of eye**
Traumatic enucleation

X ● **S05.70**   **Avulsion of unspecified eye**

X ● **S05.71**   **Avulsion of right eye**

X ● **S05.72**   **Avulsion of left eye**

● **S05.8**   **Other injuries of eye and orbit**
Lacrimal duct injury

● **S05.8X**   **Other injuries of eye and orbit**

● **S05.8X1**   **Other injuries of right eye and orbit**

● **S05.8X2**   **Other injuries of left eye and orbit**

● **S05.8X9**   **Other injuries of unspecified eye and orbit**

● **S05.9**   **Unspecified injury of eye and orbit**
Injury of eye NOS

X ● **S05.90**   **Unspecified injury of unspecified eye and orbit**

X ● **S05.91**   **Unspecified injury of right eye and orbit**

X ● **S05.92**   **Unspecified injury of left eye and orbit**

● **S06**   **Intracranial injury**
    Includes   traumatic brain injury
    Code also any associated:
      open wound of head (S01.-)
      skull fracture (S02.-)
    Excludes1   head injury NOS (S09.90)
The appropriate 7th character is to be added to each code from category S06

A	initial encounter
D	subsequent encounter
S	sequela

Note: 7th characters D and S do not apply to codes in category S06 with 6th character 7 - death due to brain injury prior to regaining consciousness, or 8 - death due to other cause prior to regaining consciousness.
Coding Clinic: 2015, Q4, P40

● **S06.0**   **Concussion**
Commotio cerebri
    Excludes1   concussion with other intracranial injuries classified in subcategories S06.1- to S06.6- , and S06.81- to S06.82-, code to specified intracranial injury
Coding Clinic: 2016, Q4, P67

● **S06.0X**   **Concussion**

● **S06.0X0**   **Concussion without loss of consciousness S**

● **S06.0X1**   **Concussion with loss of consciousness of 30 minutes or less S**
Concussion with brief loss of consciousness

● **S06.0X9**   **Concussion with loss of consciousness of unspecified duration S**
Coding Clinic: 2016, Q4, P68

● **S06.0XA**   **Concussion with loss of consciousness status unknown**
Concussion NOS

● **S06.1**   **Traumatic cerebral edema**
Diffuse traumatic cerebral edema
Focal traumatic cerebral edema
Coding Clinic: 2016, Q4, P67

● **S06.1X**   **Traumatic cerebral edema**

● **S06.1X0**   **Traumatic cerebral edema without loss of consciousness A, S**
Coding Clinic: 2015, Q1, P12

● **S06.1X1**   **Traumatic cerebral edema with loss of consciousness of 30 minutes or less A, S**
Traumatic cerebral edema with brief loss of consciousness

● **S06.1X2**   **Traumatic cerebral edema with loss of consciousness of 31 minutes to 59 minutes A, S**

● **S06.1X3**   **Traumatic cerebral edema with loss of consciousness of 1 hour to 5 hours 59 minutes A, S**

● **S06.1X4**   **Traumatic cerebral edema with loss of consciousness of 6 hours to 24 hours A, S**

● **S06.1X5**   **Traumatic cerebral edema with loss of consciousness greater than 24 hours with return to pre-existing conscious level A, S**

● **S06.1X6**   **Traumatic cerebral edema with loss of consciousness greater than 24 hours without return to pre-existing conscious level with patient surviving A, S**

CHAPTER 19 (S00–T88)

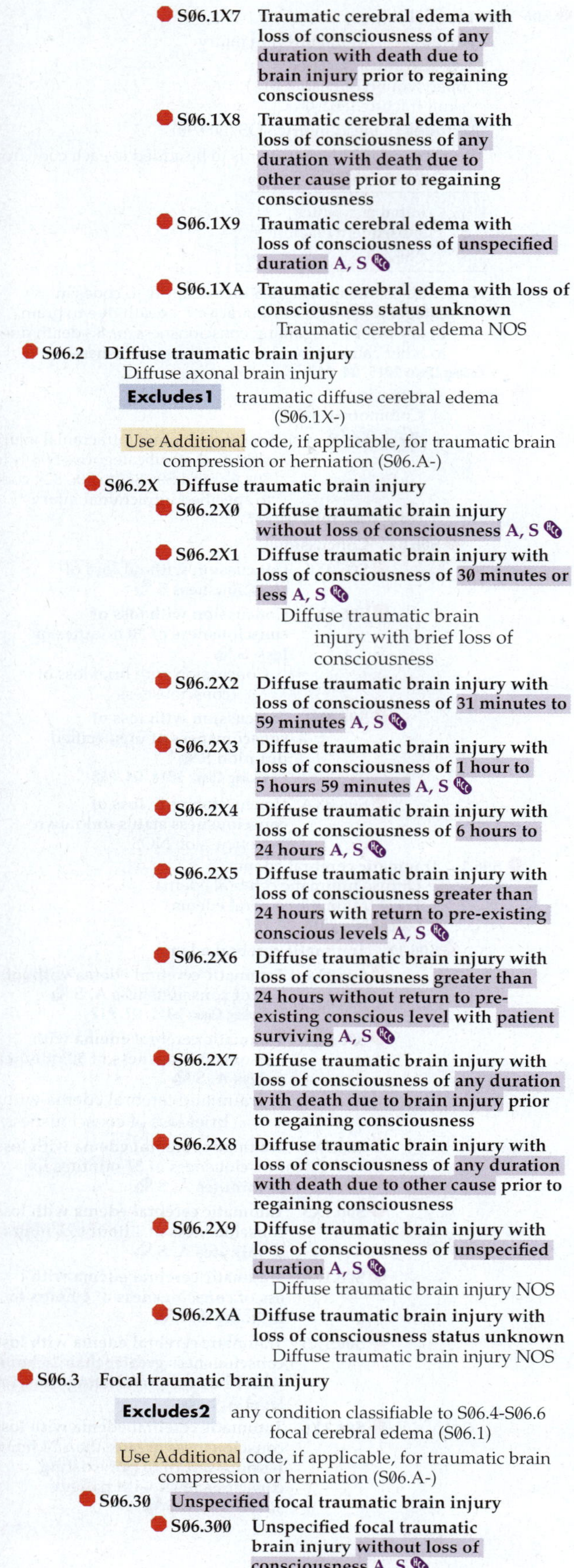

- **S06.1X7**   Traumatic cerebral edema with loss of consciousness of any duration with death due to brain injury prior to regaining consciousness
- **S06.1X8**   Traumatic cerebral edema with loss of consciousness of any duration with death due to other cause prior to regaining consciousness
- **S06.1X9**   Traumatic cerebral edema with loss of consciousness of unspecified duration A, S
- **S06.1XA**   Traumatic cerebral edema with loss of consciousness status unknown
  Traumatic cerebral edema NOS

- **S06.2**   **Diffuse traumatic brain injury**
  Diffuse axonal brain injury

  Excludes1   traumatic diffuse cerebral edema (S06.1X-)

  Use Additional code, if applicable, for traumatic brain compression or herniation (S06.A-)

  - **S06.2X**   **Diffuse traumatic brain injury**
    - **S06.2X0**   Diffuse traumatic brain injury without loss of consciousness A, S
    - **S06.2X1**   Diffuse traumatic brain injury with loss of consciousness of 30 minutes or less A, S
      Diffuse traumatic brain injury with brief loss of consciousness
    - **S06.2X2**   Diffuse traumatic brain injury with loss of consciousness of 31 minutes to 59 minutes A, S
    - **S06.2X3**   Diffuse traumatic brain injury with loss of consciousness of 1 hour to 5 hours 59 minutes A, S
    - **S06.2X4**   Diffuse traumatic brain injury with loss of consciousness of 6 hours to 24 hours A, S
    - **S06.2X5**   Diffuse traumatic brain injury with loss of consciousness greater than 24 hours with return to pre-existing conscious levels A, S
    - **S06.2X6**   Diffuse traumatic brain injury with loss of consciousness greater than 24 hours without return to pre-existing conscious level with patient surviving A, S
    - **S06.2X7**   Diffuse traumatic brain injury with loss of consciousness of any duration with death due to brain injury prior to regaining consciousness
    - **S06.2X8**   Diffuse traumatic brain injury with loss of consciousness of any duration with death due to other cause prior to regaining consciousness
    - **S06.2X9**   Diffuse traumatic brain injury with loss of consciousness of unspecified duration A, S
      Diffuse traumatic brain injury NOS
    - **S06.2XA**   Diffuse traumatic brain injury with loss of consciousness status unknown
      Diffuse traumatic brain injury NOS

- **S06.3**   **Focal traumatic brain injury**

  Excludes2   any condition classifiable to S06.4-S06.6 focal cerebral edema (S06.1)

  Use Additional code, if applicable, for traumatic brain compression or herniation (S06.A-)

  - **S06.30**   **Unspecified focal traumatic brain injury**
    - **S06.300**   Unspecified focal traumatic brain injury without loss of consciousness A, S

- **S06.301**   Unspecified focal traumatic brain injury with loss of consciousness of 30 minutes or less A, S
  Unspecified focal traumatic brain injury with brief loss of consciousness
- **S06.302**   Unspecified focal traumatic brain injury with loss of consciousness of 31 minutes to 59 minutes A, S
- **S06.303**   Unspecified focal traumatic brain injury with loss of consciousness of 1 hour to 5 hours 59 minutes A, S
- **S06.304**   Unspecified focal traumatic brain injury with loss of consciousness of 6 hours to 24 hours A, S
- **S06.305**   Unspecified focal traumatic brain injury with loss of consciousness greater than 24 hours with return to pre-existing conscious level A, S
- **S06.306**   Unspecified focal traumatic brain injury with loss of consciousness greater than 24 hours without return to pre-existing conscious level with patient surviving A, S
- **S06.307**   Unspecified focal traumatic brain injury with loss of consciousness of any duration with death due to brain injury prior to regaining consciousness
- **S06.308**   Unspecified focal traumatic brain injury with loss of consciousness of any duration with death due to other cause prior to regaining consciousness
- **S06.309**   Unspecified focal traumatic brain injury with loss of consciousness of unspecified duration A, S
- **S06.30A**   Unspecified focal traumatic brain injury with loss of consciousness status unknown
  Unspecified focal traumatic brain injury NOS

- **S06.31**   **Contusion and laceration of right cerebrum**
  - **S06.310**   Contusion and laceration of right cerebrum without loss of consciousness A, S
  - **S06.311**   Contusion and laceration of right cerebrum with loss of consciousness of 30 minutes or less A, S
    Contusion and laceration of right cerebrum with brief loss of consciousness
  - **S06.312**   Contusion and laceration of right cerebrum with loss of consciousness of 31 minutes to 59 minutes A, S
  - **S06.313**   Contusion and laceration of right cerebrum with loss of consciousness of 1 hour to 5 hours 59 minutes A, S
  - **S06.314**   Contusion and laceration of right cerebrum with loss of consciousness of 6 hours to 24 hours A, S
  - **S06.315**   Contusion and laceration of right cerebrum with loss of consciousness greater than 24 hours with return to pre-existing conscious level A, S

▶ New   ⇒ Revised   ~~deleted~~ Deleted   Excludes 1   Excludes 2   Includes   Use additional   Code first   Code also   Key words
OGCR Official Guidelines   X Assign placeholder X   ● Use Additional Character(s)   ▶ Manifestation Code   Hierarchical Condition Category   Coding Clinic

● S06.316   Contusion and laceration of right cerebrum with loss of consciousness greater than 24 hours without return to pre-existing conscious level with patient surviving A, S

● S06.317   Contusion and laceration of right cerebrum with loss of consciousness of any duration with death due to brain injury prior to regaining consciousness

● S06.318   Contusion and laceration of right cerebrum with loss of consciousness of any duration with death due to other cause prior to regaining consciousness

● S06.319   Contusion and laceration of right cerebrum with loss of consciousness of unspecified duration A, S

● S06.31A   Contusion and laceration of right cerebrum with loss of consciousness status unknown

     Contusion and laceration of right cerebrum NOS

● S06.32   Contusion and laceration of left cerebrum

● S06.320   Contusion and laceration of left cerebrum without loss of consciousness A, S

● S06.321   Contusion and laceration of left cerebrum with loss of consciousness of 30 minutes or less A, S

     Contusion and laceration of left cerebrum with brief loss of consciousness

● S06.322   Contusion and laceration of left cerebrum with loss of consciousness of 31 minutes to 59 minutes A, S

● S06.323   Contusion and laceration of left cerebrum with loss of consciousness of 1 hour to 5 hours 59 minutes A, S

● S06.324   Contusion and laceration of left cerebrum with loss of consciousness of 6 hours to 24 hours A, S

● S06.325   Contusion and laceration of left cerebrum with loss of consciousness greater than 24 hours with return to pre-existing conscious level A, S

● S06.326   Contusion and laceration of left cerebrum with loss of consciousness greater than 24 hours without return to pre-existing conscious level with patient surviving A, S

● S06.327   Contusion and laceration of left cerebrum with loss of consciousness of any duration with death due to brain injury prior to regaining consciousness

● S06.328   Contusion and laceration of left cerebrum with loss of consciousness of any duration with death due to other cause prior to regaining consciousness

● S06.329   Contusion and laceration of left cerebrum with loss of consciousness of unspecified duration A, S

● S06.32A   Contusion and laceration of left cerebrum with loss of consciousness status unknown

     Contusion and laceration of left cerebrum NOS

● S06.33   Contusion and laceration of cerebrum, unspecified

● S06.330   Contusion and laceration of cerebrum, unspecified, without loss of consciousness A, S

● S06.331   Contusion and laceration of cerebrum, unspecified, with loss of consciousness of 30 minutes or less A, S

     Contusion and laceration of cerebrum, unspecified, with brief loss of consciousness

● S06.332   Contusion and laceration of cerebrum, unspecified, with loss of consciousness of 31 minutes to 59 minutes A, S

● S06.333   Contusion and laceration of cerebrum, unspecified, with loss of consciousness of 1 hour to 5 hours 59 minutes A, S

● S06.334   Contusion and laceration of cerebrum, unspecified, with loss of consciousness of 6 hours to 24 hours A, S

● S06.335   Contusion and laceration of cerebrum, unspecified, with loss of consciousness greater than 24 hours with return to pre-existing conscious level A, S

● S06.336   Contusion and laceration of cerebrum, unspecified, with loss of consciousness greater than 24 hours without return to pre-existing conscious level with patient surviving A, S

● S06.337   Contusion and laceration of cerebrum, unspecified, with loss of consciousness of any duration with death due to brain injury prior to regaining consciousness

● S06.338   Contusion and laceration of cerebrum, unspecified, with loss of consciousness of any duration with death due to other cause prior to regaining consciousness

● S06.339   Contusion and laceration of cerebrum, unspecified, with loss of consciousness of unspecified duration A, S

● S06.33A   Contusion and laceration of cerebrum, unspecified, with loss of consciousness status unknown

     Contusion and laceration of cerebrum NOS

● S06.34   Traumatic hemorrhage of right cerebrum

     Traumatic intracerebral hemorrhage and hematoma of right cerebrum

● S06.340   Traumatic hemorrhage of right cerebrum without loss of consciousness A, S

     Coding Clinic: 2015, Q1, P12

● S06.341   Traumatic hemorrhage of right cerebrum with loss of consciousness of 30 minutes or less A, S

     Traumatic hemorrhage of right cerebrum with brief loss of consciousness

● S06.342   Traumatic hemorrhage of right cerebrum with loss of consciousness of 31 minutes to 59 minutes A, S

● S06.343   Traumatic hemorrhage of right cerebrum with loss of consciousness of 1 hours to 5 hours 59 minutes A, S

CHAPTER 19 (S00-T88)

● **S06.344**   Traumatic hemorrhage of right cerebrum with loss of consciousness of 6 hours to 24 hours A, S ♥

● **S06.345**   Traumatic hemorrhage of right cerebrum with loss of consciousness greater than 24 hours with return to pre-existing conscious level A, S ♥

● **S06.346**   Traumatic hemorrhage of right cerebrum with loss of consciousness greater than 24 hours without return to pre-existing conscious level with patient surviving A, S ♥

● **S06.347**   Traumatic hemorrhage of right cerebrum with loss of consciousness of any duration with death due to brain injury prior to regaining consciousness

● **S06.348**   Traumatic hemorrhage of right cerebrum with loss of consciousness of any duration with death due to other cause prior to regaining consciousness

● **S06.349**   Traumatic hemorrhage of right cerebrum with loss of consciousness of unspecified duration A, S ♥

● **S06.34A**   Traumatic hemorrhage of right cerebrum with loss of consciousness status unknown
     Traumatic hemorrhage of right cerebrum NOS

● **S06.35**   Traumatic hemorrhage of left cerebrum
     Traumatic intracerebral hemorrhage and hematoma of left cerebrum

● **S06.350**   Traumatic hemorrhage of left cerebrum without loss of consciousness A, S ♥

● **S06.351**   Traumatic hemorrhage of left cerebrum with loss of consciousness of 30 minutes or less A, S ♥
     Traumatic hemorrhage of left cerebrum with brief loss of consciousness

● **S06.352**   Traumatic hemorrhage of left cerebrum with loss of consciousness of 31 minutes to 59 minutes A, S ♥

● **S06.353**   Traumatic hemorrhage of left cerebrum with loss of consciousness of 1 hours to 5 hours 59 minutes A, S ♥

● **S06.354**   Traumatic hemorrhage of left cerebrum with loss of consciousness of 6 hours to 24 hours A, S ♥

● **S06.355**   Traumatic hemorrhage of left cerebrum with loss of consciousness greater than 24 hours with return to pre-existing conscious level A, S ♥

● **S06.356**   Traumatic hemorrhage of left cerebrum with loss of consciousness greater than 24 hours without return to pre-existing conscious level with patient surviving A, S ♥

● **S06.357**   Traumatic hemorrhage of left cerebrum with loss of consciousness of any duration with death due to brain injury prior to regaining consciousness

● **S06.358**   Traumatic hemorrhage of left cerebrum with loss of consciousness of any duration with death due to other cause prior to regaining consciousness

● **S06.359**   Traumatic hemorrhage of left cerebrum with loss of consciousness of unspecified duration A, S ♥

● **S06.35A**   Traumatic hemorrhage of left cerebrum with loss of consciousness status unknown
     Traumatic hemorrhage of left cerebrum NOS

● **S06.36**   Traumatic hemorrhage of cerebrum, unspecified
     Traumatic intracerebral hemorrhage and hematoma, unspecified

● **S06.360**   Traumatic hemorrhage of cerebrum, unspecified, without loss of consciousness A, S ♥

● **S06.361**   Traumatic hemorrhage of cerebrum, unspecified, with loss of consciousness of 30 minutes or less A, S ♥
     Traumatic hemorrhage of cerebrum, unspecified, with brief loss of consciousness

● **S06.362**   Traumatic hemorrhage of cerebrum, unspecified, with loss of consciousness of 31 minutes to 59 minutes A, S ♥

● **S06.363**   Traumatic hemorrhage of cerebrum, unspecified, with loss of consciousness of 1 hours to 5 hours 59 minutes A, S ♥

● **S06.364**   Traumatic hemorrhage of cerebrum, unspecified, with loss of consciousness of 6 hours to 24 hours A, S ♥

● **S06.365**   Traumatic hemorrhage of cerebrum, unspecified, with loss of consciousness greater than 24 hours with return to pre-existing conscious level A, S ♥

● **S06.366**   Traumatic hemorrhage of cerebrum, unspecified, with loss of consciousness greater than 24 hours without return to pre-existing conscious level with patient surviving A, S ♥

● **S06.367**   Traumatic hemorrhage of cerebrum, unspecified, with loss of consciousness of any duration with death due to brain injury prior to regaining consciousness

● **S06.368**   Traumatic hemorrhage of cerebrum, unspecified, with loss of consciousness of any duration with death due to other cause prior to regaining consciousness

● **S06.369**   Traumatic hemorrhage of cerebrum, unspecified, with loss of consciousness of unspecified duration A, S ♥

● **S06.36A**   Traumatic hemorrhage of cerebrum, unspecified, with loss of consciousness status unknown
     Traumatic hemorrhage of cerebrum NOS

● **S06.37**   Contusion, laceration, and hemorrhage of cerebellum

● **S06.370**   Contusion, laceration, and hemorrhage of cerebellum without loss of consciousness A, S ♥

● **S06.371**   Contusion, laceration, and hemorrhage of cerebellum with loss of consciousness of 30 minutes or less A, S ♥
     Contusion, laceration, and hemorrhage of cerebellum with brief loss of consciousness

● **S06.372**   Contusion, laceration, and hemorrhage of cerebellum with loss of consciousness of 31 minutes to 59 minutes A, S ♥

▶ New   ➡ Revised   ~~deleted~~ Deleted   Excludes 1   Excludes 2   Includes   Use additional   Code first   Code also   Key words
OGCR Official Guidelines   **X** Assign placeholder X   ● Use Additional Character(s)   ▶ Manifestation Code   ♥ Hierarchical Condition Category   **Coding Clinic**

● **S06.373**   Contusion, laceration, and hemorrhage of cerebellum with loss of consciousness of 1 hour to 5 hours 59 minutes A, S

● **S06.374**   Contusion, laceration, and hemorrhage of cerebellum with loss of consciousness of 6 hours to 24 hours A, S

● **S06.375**   Contusion, laceration, and hemorrhage of cerebellum with loss of consciousness greater than 24 hours with return to pre-existing conscious level A, S

● **S06.376**   Contusion, laceration, and hemorrhage of cerebellum with loss of consciousness greater than 24 hours without return to pre-existing conscious level with patient surviving A, S

● **S06.377**   Contusion, laceration, and hemorrhage of cerebellum with loss of consciousness of any duration with death due to brain injury prior to regaining consciousness

● **S06.378**   Contusion, laceration, and hemorrhage of cerebellum with loss of consciousness of any duration with death due to other cause prior to regaining consciousness

● **S06.379**   Contusion, laceration, and hemorrhage of cerebellum with loss of consciousness of unspecified duration A, S

● **S06.37A**   Contusion, laceration, and hemorrhage of cerebellum with loss of consciousness status unknown
> Contusion, laceration, and hemorrhage of cerebellum NOS

● **S06.38**   Contusion, laceration, and hemorrhage of brainstem

● **S06.380**   Contusion, laceration, and hemorrhage of brainstem without loss of consciousness A, S

● **S06.381**   Contusion, laceration, and hemorrhage of brainstem with loss of consciousness of 30 minutes or less A, S
> Contusion, laceration, and hemorrhage of brainstem with brief loss of consciousness

● **S06.382**   Contusion, laceration, and hemorrhage of brainstem with loss of consciousness of 31 minutes to 59 minutes A, S

● **S06.383**   Contusion, laceration, and hemorrhage of brainstem with loss of consciousness of 1 hour to 5 hours 59 minutes A, S

● **S06.384**   Contusion, laceration, and hemorrhage of brainstem with loss of consciousness of 6 hours to 24 hours A, S

● **S06.385**   Contusion, laceration, and hemorrhage of brainstem with loss of consciousness greater than 24 hours with return to pre-existing conscious level A, S

● **S06.386**   Contusion, laceration, and hemorrhage of brainstem with loss of consciousness greater than 24 hours without return to pre-existing conscious level with patient surviving A, S

● **S06.387**   Contusion, laceration, and hemorrhage of brainstem with loss of consciousness of any duration with death due to brain injury prior to regaining consciousness

● **S06.388**   Contusion, laceration, and hemorrhage of brainstem with loss of consciousness of any duration with death due to other cause prior to regaining consciousness

● **S06.389**   Contusion, laceration, and hemorrhage of brainstem with loss of consciousness of unspecified duration A, S

● **S06.38A**   Contusion, laceration, and hemorrhage of brainstem with loss of consciousness status unknown
> Contusion, laceration, and hemorrhage of brainstem NOS

● **S06.4**   **Epidural hemorrhage**
> *Situated outside dura mater*
> Extradural hemorrhage NOS
> *Intracranial hemorrhage due to trauma*
> Extradural hemorrhage (traumatic)

● **S06.4X**   Epidural hemorrhage

● **S06.4X0**   Epidural hemorrhage without loss of consciousness A, S

● **S06.4X1**   Epidural hemorrhage with loss of consciousness of 30 minutes or less A, S
> Epidural hemorrhage with brief loss of consciousness

● **S06.4X2**   Epidural hemorrhage with loss of consciousness of 31 minutes to 59 minutes A, S

● **S06.4X3**   Epidural hemorrhage with loss of consciousness of 1 hour to 5 hours 59 minutes A, S

● **S06.4X4**   Epidural hemorrhage with loss of consciousness of 6 hours to 24 hours A, S

● **S06.4X5**   Epidural hemorrhage with loss of consciousness greater than 24 hours with return to pre-existing conscious level A, S

● **S06.4X6**   Epidural hemorrhage with loss of consciousness greater than 24 hours without return to pre-existing conscious level with patient surviving A, S

● **S06.4X7**   Epidural hemorrhage with loss of consciousness of any duration with death due to brain injury prior to regaining consciousness

● **S06.4X8**   Epidural hemorrhage with loss of consciousness of any duration with death due to other causes prior to regaining consciousness

● **S06.4X9**   Epidural hemorrhage with loss of consciousness of unspecified duration A, S

● **S06.4XA**   Epidural hemorrhage with loss of consciousness status unknown
> Epidural hemorrhage NOS

● **S06.5**   **Traumatic subdural hemorrhage**
> **Use Additional** code, if applicable, for traumatic brain compression or herniation (S06.A-)
> **Coding Clinic: 2024, Q2, P15**

● **S06.5X**   Traumatic subdural hemorrhage

● **S06.5X0**   Traumatic subdural hemorrhage without loss of consciousness A, S
> **Coding Clinic: 2021, Q1, P4; 2018, Q2, P13; 2015, Q3, P37**

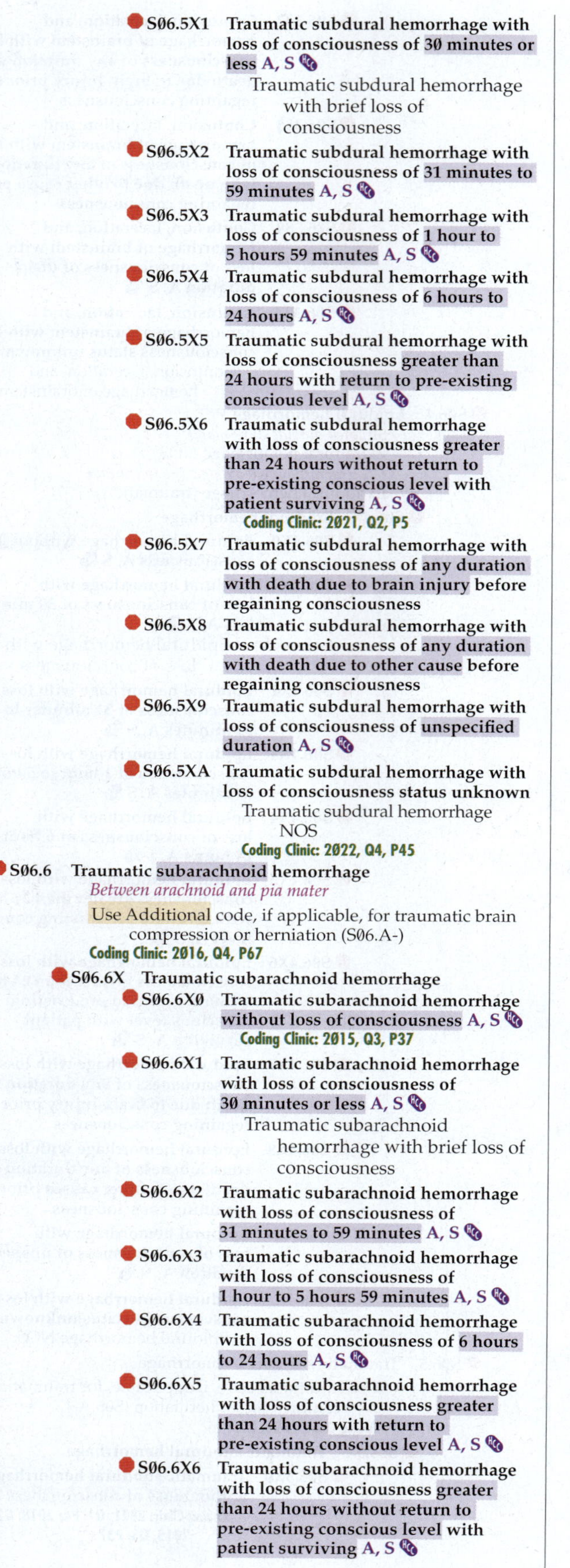

● **S06.5X1**   Traumatic subdural hemorrhage with loss of consciousness of 30 minutes or less **A, S** 🔴
    Traumatic subdural hemorrhage with brief loss of consciousness

● **S06.5X2**   Traumatic subdural hemorrhage with loss of consciousness of 31 minutes to 59 minutes **A, S** 🔴

● **S06.5X3**   Traumatic subdural hemorrhage with loss of consciousness of 1 hour to 5 hours 59 minutes **A, S** 🔴

● **S06.5X4**   Traumatic subdural hemorrhage with loss of consciousness of 6 hours to 24 hours **A, S** 🔴

● **S06.5X5**   Traumatic subdural hemorrhage with loss of consciousness greater than 24 hours with return to pre-existing conscious level **A, S** 🔴

● **S06.5X6**   Traumatic subdural hemorrhage with loss of consciousness greater than 24 hours without return to pre-existing conscious level with patient surviving **A, S** 🔴
    Coding Clinic: 2021, Q2, P5

● **S06.5X7**   Traumatic subdural hemorrhage with loss of consciousness of any duration with death due to brain injury before regaining consciousness

● **S06.5X8**   Traumatic subdural hemorrhage with loss of consciousness of any duration with death due to other cause before regaining consciousness

● **S06.5X9**   Traumatic subdural hemorrhage with loss of consciousness of unspecified duration **A, S** 🔴

● **S06.5XA**   Traumatic subdural hemorrhage with loss of consciousness status unknown
    Traumatic subdural hemorrhage NOS
    Coding Clinic: 2022, Q4, P45

● **S06.6**   **Traumatic subarachnoid hemorrhage**
    Between arachnoid and pia mater
    Use Additional code, if applicable, for traumatic brain compression or herniation (S06.A-)
    Coding Clinic: 2016, Q4, P67

● **S06.6X**   **Traumatic subarachnoid hemorrhage**

● **S06.6X0**   Traumatic subarachnoid hemorrhage without loss of consciousness **A, S** 🔴
    Coding Clinic: 2015, Q3, P37

● **S06.6X1**   Traumatic subarachnoid hemorrhage with loss of consciousness of 30 minutes or less **A, S** 🔴
    Traumatic subarachnoid hemorrhage with brief loss of consciousness

● **S06.6X2**   Traumatic subarachnoid hemorrhage with loss of consciousness of 31 minutes to 59 minutes **A, S** 🔴

● **S06.6X3**   Traumatic subarachnoid hemorrhage with loss of consciousness of 1 hour to 5 hours 59 minutes **A, S** 🔴

● **S06.6X4**   Traumatic subarachnoid hemorrhage with loss of consciousness of 6 hours to 24 hours **A, S** 🔴

● **S06.6X5**   Traumatic subarachnoid hemorrhage with loss of consciousness greater than 24 hours with return to pre-existing conscious level **A, S** 🔴

● **S06.6X6**   Traumatic subarachnoid hemorrhage with loss of consciousness greater than 24 hours without return to pre-existing conscious level with patient surviving **A, S** 🔴

    Coding Clinic: 2021, Q2, P5

● **S06.6X7**   Traumatic subarachnoid hemorrhage with loss of consciousness of any duration with death due to brain injury prior to regaining consciousness

● **S06.6X8**   Traumatic subarachnoid hemorrhage with loss of consciousness of any duration with death due to other cause prior to regaining consciousness

● **S06.6X9**   Traumatic subarachnoid hemorrhage with loss of consciousness of unspecified duration **A, S** 🔴

● **S06.6XA**   Traumatic subarachnoid hemorrhage with loss of consciousness status unknown
    Traumatic subarachnoid hemorrhage NOS
    Coding Clinic: 2022, Q4, P45

● **S06.8**   **Other specified intracranial injuries**

● **S06.81**   **Injury of right internal carotid artery, intracranial portion, not elsewhere classified**
    Coding Clinic: 2016, Q4, P67

● **S06.810**   Injury of right internal carotid artery, intracranial portion, not elsewhere classified without loss of consciousness **A, S** 🔴

● **S06.811**   Injury of right internal carotid artery, intracranial portion, not elsewhere classified with loss of consciousness of 30 minutes or less **A, S** 🔴
    Injury of right internal carotid artery, intracranial portion, not elsewhere classified with brief loss of consciousness

● **S06.812**   Injury of right internal carotid artery, intracranial portion, not elsewhere classified with loss of consciousness of 31 minutes to 59 minutes **A, S** 🔴

● **S06.813**   Injury of right internal carotid artery, intracranial portion, not elsewhere classified with loss of consciousness of 1 hour to 5 hours 59 minutes **A, S** 🔴

● **S06.814**   Injury of right internal carotid artery, intracranial portion, not elsewhere classified with loss of consciousness of 6 hours to 24 hours **A, S** 🔴

● **S06.815**   Injury of right internal carotid artery, intracranial portion, not elsewhere classified with loss of consciousness greater than 24 hours with return to pre-existing conscious level **A, S** 🔴

● **S06.816**   Injury of right internal carotid artery, intracranial portion, not elsewhere classified with loss of consciousness greater than 24 hours without return to pre-existing conscious level with patient surviving **A, S** 🔴

● **S06.817**   Injury of right internal carotid artery, intracranial portion, not elsewhere classified with loss of consciousness of any duration with death due to brain injury prior to regaining consciousness

● **S06.818**   Injury of right internal carotid artery, intracranial portion, not elsewhere classified with loss of consciousness of any duration with death due to other cause prior to regaining consciousness

● **S06.819**   **Injury of right internal carotid artery, intracranial portion, not elsewhere classified with loss of consciousness of unspecified duration** A, S

● **S06.81A**   **Injury of right internal carotid artery, intracranial portion, not elsewhere classified with loss of consciousness status unknown**
    Injury of right internal carotid artery, intracranial portion, not elsewhere classified NOS

● **S06.82**   **Injury of left internal carotid artery, intracranial portion, not elsewhere classified**
    Coding Clinic: 2016, Q4, P67

● **S06.820**   **Injury of left internal carotid artery, intracranial portion, not elsewhere classified without loss of consciousness** A, S

● **S06.821**   **Injury of left internal carotid artery, intracranial portion, not elsewhere classified with loss of consciousness of 30 minutes or less** A, S
    Injury of left internal carotid artery, intracranial portion, not elsewhere classified with brief loss of consciousness

● **S06.822**   **Injury of left internal carotid artery, intracranial portion, not elsewhere classified with loss of consciousness of 31 minutes to 59 minutes** A, S

● **S06.823**   **Injury of left internal carotid artery, intracranial portion, not elsewhere classified with loss of consciousness of 1 hour to 5 hours 59 minutes** A, S

● **S06.824**   **Injury of left internal carotid artery, intracranial portion, not elsewhere classified with loss of consciousness of 6 hours to 24 hours** A, S

● **S06.825**   **Injury of left internal carotid artery, intracranial portion, not elsewhere classified with loss of consciousness greater than 24 hours with return to pre-existing conscious level**

● **S06.826**   **Injury of left internal carotid artery, intracranial portion, not elsewhere classified with loss of consciousness greater than 24 hours without return to pre-existing conscious level with patient surviving** A, S

● **S06.827**   **Injury of left internal carotid artery, intracranial portion, not elsewhere classified with loss of consciousness of any duration with death due to brain injury prior to regaining consciousness**

● **S06.828**   **Injury of left internal carotid artery, intracranial portion, not elsewhere classified with loss of consciousness of any duration with death due to other cause prior to regaining consciousness**

● **S06.829**   **Injury of left internal carotid artery, intracranial portion, not elsewhere classified with loss of consciousness of unspecified duration** A, S

● **S06.82A**   **Injury of left internal carotid artery, intracranial portion, not elsewhere classified with loss of consciousness status unknown**
    Injury of left internal carotid artery, intracranial portion, not elsewhere classified NOS

● **S06.89**   **Other specified intracranial injury**
    Excludes1   concussion (S06.0X-)

● **S06.890**   **Other specified intracranial injury without loss of consciousness** A, S
    Coding Clinic: 2024, Q2, P16

● **S06.891**   **Other specified intracranial injury with loss of consciousness of 30 minutes or less** A, S
    Other specified intracranial injury with brief loss of consciousness

● **S06.892**   **Other specified intracranial injury with loss of consciousness of 31 minutes to 59 minutes** A, S

● **S06.893**   **Other specified intracranial injury with loss of consciousness of 1 hour to 5 hours 59 minutes** A, S

● **S06.894**   **Other specified intracranial injury with loss of consciousness of 6 hours to 24 hours** A, S

● **S06.895**   **Other specified intracranial injury with loss of consciousness greater than 24 hours with return to pre-existing conscious level** A, S

● **S06.896**   **Other specified intracranial injury with loss of consciousness greater than 24 hours without return to pre-existing conscious level with patient surviving** A, S

● **S06.897**   **Other specified intracranial injury with loss of consciousness of any duration with death due to brain injury prior to regaining consciousness**

● **S06.898**   **Other specified intracranial injury with loss of consciousness of any duration with death due to other cause prior to regaining consciousness**

● **S06.899**   **Other specified intracranial injury with loss of consciousness of unspecified duration** A, S

● **S06.89A**   **Other specified intracranial injury with loss of consciousness status unknown**

● **S06.8A**   **Primary blast injury of brain, not elsewhere classified**
    Code also, if applicable, focal traumatic brain injury (S06.3-)
    Excludes2   traumatic cerebral edema (S06.1)

● **S06.8A0**   **Primary blast injury of brain, not elsewhere classified without loss of consciousness**

● **S06.8A1**   **Primary blast injury of brain, not elsewhere classified with loss of consciousness of 30 minutes or less**
    Primary blast injury of brain, not elsewhere classified with brief loss of consciousness

● **S06.8A2**   **Primary blast injury of brain, not elsewhere classified with loss of consciousness of 31 minutes to 59 minutes**

● **S06.8A3**   **Primary blast injury of brain, not elsewhere classified with loss of consciousness of 1 hour to 5 hours 59 minutes**

● **S06.8A4**   **Primary blast injury of brain, not elsewhere classified with loss of consciousness of 6 hours to 24 hours**

● **S06.8A5** Primary blast injury of brain, not elsewhere classified with loss of consciousness greater than 24 hours with return to pre-existing conscious level

● **S06.8A6** Primary blast injury of brain, not elsewhere classified with loss of consciousness greater than 24 hours without return to pre-existing conscious level with patient surviving

● **S06.8A7** Primary blast injury of brain, not elsewhere classified with loss of consciousness of any duration with death due to brain injury prior to regaining consciousness

● **S06.8A8** Primary blast injury of brain, not elsewhere classified with loss of consciousness of any duration with death due to other cause prior to regaining consciousness

● **S06.8AA** Primary blast injury of brain, not elsewhere classified with loss of consciousness status unknown
     Primary blast injury of brain NOS

● **S06.8A9** Primary blast injury of brain, not elsewhere classified with loss of consciousness of unspecified duration

● **S06.9**   **Unspecified intracranial injury**
   Brain injury NOS
   Head injury NOS with loss of consciousness
   Traumatic brain injury NOS

    Excludes1   conditions classifiable to S06.0- to S06.8- code to specified intracranial injury head injury NOS (S09.90)

● **S06.9X**   **Unspecified intracranial injury**

  ● **S06.9X0**   Unspecified intracranial injury without loss of consciousness A, S

  ● **S06.9X1**   Unspecified intracranial injury with loss of consciousness of 30 minutes or less A, S
      Unspecified intracranial injury with brief loss of consciousness

  ● **S06.9X2**   Unspecified intracranial injury with loss of consciousness of 31 minutes to 59 minutes A, S

  ● **S06.9X3**   Unspecified intracranial injury with loss of consciousness of 1 hour to 5 hours 59 minutes A, S

  ● **S06.9X4**   Unspecified intracranial injury with loss of consciousness of 6 hours to 24 hours A, S

  ● **S06.9X5**   Unspecified intracranial injury with loss of consciousness greater than 24 hours with return to pre-existing conscious level A, S

  ● **S06.9X6**   Unspecified intracranial injury with loss of consciousness greater than 24 hours without return to pre-existing conscious level with patient surviving A, S

  ● **S06.9X7**   Unspecified intracranial injury with loss of consciousness of any duration with death due to brain injury prior to regaining consciousness

  ● **S06.9X8**   Unspecified intracranial injury with loss of consciousness of any duration with death due to other cause prior to regaining consciousness

  ● **S06.9X9**   Unspecified intracranial injury with loss of consciousness of unspecified duration A, S

● **S06.9XA**   Unspecified intracranial injury with loss of consciousness status unknown

● **S06.A**   **Traumatic brain compression and herniation**
   Traumatic cerebral compression
   Code first the underlying traumatic brain injury, such as:
     diffuse traumatic brain injury (S06.2-)
     focal traumatic brain injury (S06.3-)
     traumatic subdural hemorrhage (S06.5-)
     traumatic subarachnoid hemorrhage (S06.6-)

   S06.A0   Traumatic brain compression without herniation
     Traumatic brain compression NOS
     Traumatic cerebral compression NOS

   S06.A1   Traumatic brain compression with herniation
     Traumatic brain herniation
     Traumatic brainstem compression with herniation
     Traumatic cerebellar compression with herniation
     Traumatic cerebral compression with herniation

● **S07**   **Crushing injury of head**
   Use additional code for all associated injuries, such as:
     intracranial injuries (S06.-)
     skull fractures (S02.-)

   The appropriate 7th character is to be added to each code from category S07

> A   initial encounter
> D   subsequent encounter
> S   sequela

X ● **S07.0**   Crushing injury of face
X ● **S07.1**   Crushing injury of skull
X ● **S07.8**   Crushing injury of other parts of head
X ● **S07.9**   Crushing injury of head, part unspecified

● **S08**   **Avulsion and traumatic amputation of part of head**
   An amputation not identified as partial or complete should be coded to complete

   The appropriate 7th character is to be added to each code from category S08

> A   initial encounter
> D   subsequent encounter
> S   sequela

X ● **S08.0**   **Avulsion of scalp**

● **S08.1**   **Traumatic amputation of ear**

  ● **S08.11**   Complete traumatic amputation of ear
    ● **S08.111**   Complete traumatic amputation of right ear
    ● **S08.112**   Complete traumatic amputation of left ear
    ● **S08.119**   Complete traumatic amputation of unspecified ear

  ● **S08.12**   Partial traumatic amputation of ear
    ● **S08.121**   Partial traumatic amputation of right ear
    ● **S08.122**   Partial traumatic amputation of left ear
    ● **S08.129**   Partial traumatic amputation of unspecified ear

● **S08.8**   **Traumatic amputation of other parts of head**
  ● **S08.81**   Traumatic amputation of nose
    ● **S08.811**   Complete traumatic amputation of nose
    ● **S08.812**   Partial traumatic amputation of nose
X ● **S08.89**   Traumatic amputation of other parts of head

● S09 Other and unspecified injuries of head

The appropriate 7th character is to be added to each code from category S09

> A initial encounter
> D subsequent encounter
> S sequela

X ● S09.0 Injury of blood vessels of head, not elsewhere classified
> **Excludes1** injury of cerebral blood vessels (S06.-)
>   injury of precerebral blood vessels (S15.-)

● S09.1 Injury of muscle and tendon of head
> Code also any associated open wound (S01.-)
> **Excludes2** sprain to joints and ligament of head (S03.9)

X ● S09.10 Unspecified injury of muscle and tendon of head
> Injury of muscle and tendon of head NOS

X ● S09.11 Strain of muscle and tendon of head

X ● S09.12 Laceration of muscle and tendon of head

X ● S09.19 Other specified injury of muscle and tendon of head

● S09.2 Traumatic rupture of ear drum
> **Excludes1** traumatic rupture of ear drum due to blast injury (S09.31-)

X ● S09.20 Traumatic rupture of unspecified ear drum

X ● S09.21 Traumatic rupture of right ear drum

X ● S09.22 Traumatic rupture of left ear drum

● S09.3 Other specified and unspecified injury of middle and inner ear
> **Excludes1** injury to ear NOS (S09.91-)
> **Excludes2** injury to external ear (S00.4-, S01.3-, S08.1-)

● S09.30 Unspecified injury of middle and inner ear

 ● S09.301 Unspecified injury of right middle and inner ear

 ● S09.302 Unspecified injury of left middle and inner ear

 ● S09.309 Unspecified injury of unspecified middle and inner ear

● S09.31 Primary blast injury of ear
> Blast injury of ear NOS

 ● S09.311 Primary blast injury of right ear

 ● S09.312 Primary blast injury of left ear

 ● S09.313 Primary blast injury of ear, bilateral

 ● S09.319 Primary blast injury of unspecified ear

● S09.39 Other specified injury of middle and inner ear
> Secondary blast injury to ear

 ● S09.391 Other specified injury of right middle and inner ear

 ● S09.392 Other specified injury of left middle and inner ear

 ● S09.399 Other specified injury of unspecified middle and inner ear

X ● S09.8 Other specified injuries of head

● S09.9 Unspecified injury of face and head

X ● S09.90 Unspecified injury of head
> Head injury NOS
> **Excludes1** brain injury NOS (S06.9-)
>   head injury NOS with loss of consciousness (S06.9-)
>   intracranial injury NOS (S06.9-)

X ● S09.91 Unspecified injury of ear
> Injury of ear NOS

X ● S09.92 Unspecified injury of nose
> Injury of nose NOS

X ● S09.93 Unspecified injury of face
> Injury of face NOS

INJURIES TO THE NECK (S10–S19)

> **Includes** injuries of nape
>   injuries of supraclavicular region
>   injuries of throat
> **Excludes2** burns and corrosions (T20-T32)
>   effects of foreign body in esophagus (T18.1)
>   effects of foreign body in larynx (T17.3)
>   effects of foreign body in pharynx (T17.2)
>   effects of foreign body in trachea (T17.4)
>   frostbite (T33-T34)
>   insect bite or sting, venomous (T63.4)

● S10 Superficial injury of neck

The appropriate 7th character is to be added to each code from category S10

> A initial encounter
> D subsequent encounter
> S sequela

X ● S10.0 Contusion of throat
> Contusion of cervical esophagus
> Contusion of larynx
> Contusion of pharynx
> Contusion of trachea

● S10.1 Other and unspecified superficial injuries of throat

X ● S10.10 Unspecified superficial injuries of throat

X ● S10.11 Abrasion of throat

X ● S10.12 Blister (nonthermal) of throat

X ● S10.14 External constriction of part of throat

X ● S10.15 Superficial foreign body of throat
> Splinter in the throat

X ● S10.16 Insect bite (nonvenomous) of throat

X ● S10.17 Other superficial bite of throat
> **Excludes1** open bite of throat (S11.85)

● S10.8 Superficial injury of other specified parts of neck

X ● S10.80 Unspecified superficial injury of other specified part of neck

X ● S10.81 Abrasion of other specified part of neck

X ● S10.82 Blister (nonthermal) of other specified part of neck

X ● S10.83 Contusion of other specified part of neck

X ● S10.84 External constriction of other specified part of neck

X ● S10.85 Superficial foreign body of other specified part of neck
> Splinter in other part of neck

X ● S10.86 Insect bite of other specified part of neck

X ● S10.87 Other superficial bite of other specified part of neck
> **Excludes1** open bite of other specified parts of neck (S11.85)

● S10.9 Superficial injury of unspecified part of neck

X ● S10.90 Unspecified superficial injury of unspecified part of neck

X ● S10.91 Abrasion of unspecified part of neck

X ● S10.92 Blister (nonthermal) of unspecified part of neck

X ● S10.93 Contusion of unspecified part of neck

X ● S10.94 External constriction of unspecified part of neck

X ● S10.95 Superficial foreign body of unspecified part of neck

X ● S10.96 Insect bite of unspecified part of neck

X ● S10.97 Other superficial bite of unspecified part of neck

CHAPTER 19 (S00–T88)

● **S11**   **Open wound of neck**
    Code also any associated:
      spinal cord injury (S14.0, S14.1-)
      wound infection
    Excludes2   open fracture of vertebra (S12.- with 7th character B)
    The appropriate 7th character is to be added to each code from category S11

> A   initial encounter
> D   subsequent encounter
> S   sequela

  ● **S11.0**   **Open wound of larynx and trachea**
    ● **S11.01**   **Open wound of larynx**
      Excludes2   open wound of vocal cord (S11.03)
      ● **S11.011**   **Laceration without foreign body of larynx**
      ● **S11.012**   **Laceration with foreign body of larynx**
      ● **S11.013**   **Puncture wound without foreign body of larynx**
      ● **S11.014**   **Puncture wound with foreign body of larynx**
      ● **S11.015**   **Open bite of larynx**
        Bite of larynx NOS
      ● **S11.019**   **Unspecified open wound of larynx**
    ● **S11.02**   **Open wound of trachea**
      Open wound of cervical trachea
      Open wound of trachea NOS
      Excludes2   open wound of thoracic trachea (S27.5-)
      ● **S11.021**   **Laceration without foreign body of trachea**
      ● **S11.022**   **Laceration with foreign body of trachea**
      ● **S11.023**   **Puncture wound without foreign body of trachea**
      ● **S11.024**   **Puncture wound with foreign body of trachea**
      ● **S11.025**   **Open bite of trachea**
        Bite of trachea NOS
      ● **S11.029**   **Unspecified open wound of trachea**
    ● **S11.03**   **Open wound of vocal cord**
      ● **S11.031**   **Laceration without foreign body of vocal cord**
      ● **S11.032**   **Laceration with foreign body of vocal cord**
      ● **S11.033**   **Puncture wound without foreign body of vocal cord**
      ● **S11.034**   **Puncture wound with foreign body of vocal cord**
      ● **S11.035**   **Open bite of vocal cord**
        Bite of vocal cord NOS
      ● **S11.039**   **Unspecified open wound of vocal cord**
  ● **S11.1**   **Open wound of thyroid gland**
    X ● **S11.10**   **Unspecified open wound of thyroid gland**
    X ● **S11.11**   **Laceration without foreign body of thyroid gland**
    X ● **S11.12**   **Laceration with foreign body of thyroid gland**
    X ● **S11.13**   **Puncture wound without foreign body of thyroid gland**
    X ● **S11.14**   **Puncture wound with foreign body of thyroid gland**
    X ● **S11.15**   **Open bite of thyroid gland**
      Bite of thyroid gland NOS

● **S11.2**   **Open wound of pharynx and cervical esophagus**
    Excludes1   open wound of esophagus NOS (S27.8-)
  X ● **S11.20**   **Unspecified open wound of pharynx and cervical esophagus**
  X ● **S11.21**   **Laceration without foreign body of pharynx and cervical esophagus**
  X ● **S11.22**   **Laceration with foreign body of pharynx and cervical esophagus**
  X ● **S11.23**   **Puncture wound without foreign body of pharynx and cervical esophagus**
  X ● **S11.24**   **Puncture wound with foreign body of pharynx and cervical esophagus**
  X ● **S11.25**   **Open bite of pharynx and cervical esophagus**
    Bite of pharynx and cervical esophagus NOS
● **S11.8**   **Open wound of other specified parts of neck**
  X ● **S11.80**   **Unspecified open specified wound of other part of neck**
  X ● **S11.81**   **Laceration without foreign body of other specified part of neck**
  X ● **S11.82**   **Laceration with foreign body of other specified part of neck**
  X ● **S11.83**   **Puncture wound without foreign body of other specified part of neck**
  X ● **S11.84**   **Puncture wound with foreign body of other specified part of neck**
  X ● **S11.85**   **Open bite of other specified part of neck**
    Bite of other part of neck NOS
    Excludes1   superficial bite of other specified part of neck (S10.87)
  X ● **S11.89**   **Other open wound of other part of neck**
● **S11.9**   **Open wound of unspecified part of neck**
  X ● **S11.90**   **Unspecified open wound of unspecified part of neck**
  X ● **S11.91**   **Laceration without foreign body of unspecified part of neck**
  X ● **S11.92**   **Laceration with foreign body of unspecified part of neck**
  X ● **S11.93**   **Puncture wound without foreign body of unspecified part of neck**
  X ● **S11.94**   **Puncture wound with foreign body of unspecified part of neck**
  X ● **S11.95**   **Open bite of unspecified part of neck**
    Bite of neck NOS
    Excludes1   superficial bite of neck (S10.97)

● **S12**   **Fracture of cervical vertebra and other parts of neck**
    Note: A fracture not indicated as displaced or nondisplaced should be coded to displaced
    A fracture not indicated as open or closed should be coded to closed
    Includes   fracture of cervical neural arch
      fracture of cervical spine
      fracture of cervical spinous process
      fracture of cervical transverse process
      fracture of cervical vertebral arch
      fracture of neck
    Code first any associated cervical spinal cord injury (S14.0, S14.1-)
    The appropriate 7th character is to be added to all codes from subcategories S12.0-S12.6

> A   initial encounter for closed fracture
> B   initial encounter for open fracture
> D   subsequent encounter for fracture with routine healing
> G   subsequent encounter for fracture with delayed healing
> K   subsequent encounter for fracture with nonunion
> S   sequela

▶ New   ⇒ Revised   ~~deleted~~ Deleted   Excludes 1   Excludes 2   Includes   Use additional   Code first   Code also   Key words
OGCR Official Guidelines   X Assign placeholder X   ● Use Additional Character(s)   ▶ Manifestation Code   Ⓗ Hierarchical Condition Category   Coding Clinic

● **S12.0**   **Fracture of first cervical vertebra**
Atlas
- ● **S12.00**   Unspecified fracture of first cervical vertebra
  - ● **S12.000**   Unspecified displaced fracture of first cervical vertebra **A, B** 🔎
  - ● **S12.001**   Unspecified nondisplaced fracture of first cervical vertebra **A, B** 🔎
- **X** ● **S12.01**   Stable burst fracture of first cervical vertebra **A, B** 🔎
- **X** ● **S12.02**   Unstable burst fracture of first cervical vertebra **A, B** 🔎
- ● **S12.03**   Posterior arch fracture of first cervical vertebra
  - ● **S12.030**   Displaced posterior arch fracture of first cervical vertebra **A, B** 🔎
  - ● **S12.031**   Nondisplaced posterior arch fracture of first cervical vertebra **A, B** 🔎
- ● **S12.04**   Lateral mass fracture of first cervical vertebra
  - ● **S12.040**   Displaced lateral mass fracture of first cervical vertebra **A, B** 🔎
  - ● **S12.041**   Nondisplaced lateral mass fracture of first cervical vertebra **A, B** 🔎
- ● **S12.09**   Other fracture of first cervical vertebra
  - ● **S12.090**   Other displaced fracture of first cervical vertebra **A, B** 🔎
  - ● **S12.091**   Other nondisplaced fracture of first cervical vertebra **A, B** 🔎

● **S12.1**   **Fracture of second cervical vertebra**
Axis
- ● **S12.10**   Unspecified fracture of second cervical vertebra
  - ● **S12.100**   Unspecified displaced fracture of second cervical vertebra **A, B** 🔎
    Coding Clinic: 2024, Q2, P23
  - ● **S12.101**   Unspecified nondisplaced fracture of second cervical vertebra **A, B** 🔎
- ● **S12.11**   Type II dens fracture
  - ● **S12.110**   Anterior displaced Type II dens fracture **A, B** 🔎
  - ● **S12.111**   Posterior displaced Type II dens fracture **A, B** 🔎
  - ● **S12.112**   Nondisplaced Type II dens fracture **A, B** 🔎
- ● **S12.12**   Other dens fracture
  - ● **S12.120**   Other displaced dens fracture **A, B** 🔎
  - ● **S12.121**   Other nondisplaced dens fracture **A, B** 🔎
- ● **S12.13**   Unspecified traumatic spondylolisthesis of second cervical vertebra
  - ● **S12.130**   Unspecified traumatic displaced spondylolisthesis of second cervical vertebra **A, B** 🔎
  - ● **S12.131**   Unspecified traumatic nondisplaced spondylolisthesis of second cervical vertebra **A, B** 🔎
- **X** ● **S12.14**   Type III traumatic spondylolisthesis of second cervical vertebra **A, B** 🔎
- ● **S12.15**   Other traumatic spondylolisthesis of second cervical vertebra
  - ● **S12.150**   Other traumatic displaced spondylolisthesis of second cervical vertebra **A, B** 🔎
  - ● **S12.151**   Other traumatic nondisplaced spondylolisthesis of second cervical vertebra **A, B** 🔎
- ● **S12.19**   Other fracture of second cervical vertebra
  - ● **S12.190**   Other displaced fracture of second cervical vertebra **A, B** 🔎
  - ● **S12.191**   Other nondisplaced fracture of second cervical vertebra **A, B** 🔎

● **S12.2**   **Fracture of third cervical vertebra**
- ● **S12.20**   Unspecified fracture of third cervical vertebra
  - ● **S12.200**   Unspecified displaced fracture of third cervical vertebra **A, B** 🔎
  - ● **S12.201**   Unspecified nondisplaced fracture of third cervical vertebra **A, B** 🔎
- ● **S12.23**   Unspecified traumatic spondylolisthesis of third cervical vertebra
  - ● **S12.230**   Unspecified traumatic displaced spondylolisthesis of third cervical vertebra **A, B** 🔎
  - ● **S12.231**   Unspecified traumatic nondisplaced spondylolisthesis of third cervical vertebra **A, B** 🔎
- **X** ● **S12.24**   Type III traumatic spondylolisthesis of third cervical vertebra **A, B** 🔎
- ● **S12.25**   Other traumatic spondylolisthesis of third cervical vertebra
  - ● **S12.250**   Other traumatic displaced spondylolisthesis of third cervical vertebra **A, B** 🔎
  - ● **S12.251**   Other traumatic nondisplaced spondylolisthesis of third cervical vertebra **A, B** 🔎
- ● **S12.29**   Other fracture of third cervical vertebra
  - ● **S12.290**   Other displaced fracture of third cervical vertebra **A, B** 🔎
  - ● **S12.291**   Other nondisplaced fracture of third cervical vertebra **A, B** 🔎

● **S12.3**   **Fracture of fourth cervical vertebra**
- ● **S12.30**   Unspecified fracture of fourth cervical vertebra
  - ● **S12.300**   Unspecified displaced fracture of fourth cervical vertebra **A, B** 🔎
  - ● **S12.301**   Unspecified nondisplaced fracture of fourth cervical vertebra **A, B** 🔎
- ● **S12.33**   Unspecified traumatic spondylolisthesis of fourth cervical vertebra
  - ● **S12.330**   Unspecified traumatic displaced spondylolisthesis of fourth cervical vertebra **A, B** 🔎
  - ● **S12.331**   Unspecified traumatic nondisplaced spondylolisthesis of fourth cervical vertebra **A, B** 🔎
- **X** ● **S12.34**   Type III traumatic spondylolisthesis of fourth cervical vertebra **A, B** 🔎
- ● **S12.35**   Other traumatic spondylolisthesis of fourth cervical vertebra
  - ● **S12.350**   Other traumatic displaced spondylolisthesis of fourth cervical vertebra **A, B** 🔎
  - ● **S12.351**   Other traumatic nondisplaced spondylolisthesis of fourth cervical vertebra **A, B** 🔎
- ● **S12.39**   Other fracture of fourth cervical vertebra
  - ● **S12.390**   Other displaced fracture of fourth cervical vertebra **A, B** 🔎
  - ● **S12.391**   Other nondisplaced fracture of fourth cervical vertebra **A, B** 🔎

● **S12.4**   **Fracture of fifth cervical vertebra**
- ● **S12.40**   Unspecified fracture of fifth cervical vertebra
  - ● **S12.400**   Unspecified displaced fracture of fifth cervical vertebra **A, B** 🔎
  - ● **S12.401**   Unspecified nondisplaced fracture of fifth cervical vertebra **A, B** 🔎
- ● **S12.43**   Unspecified traumatic spondylolisthesis of fifth cervical vertebra
  - ● **S12.430**   Unspecified traumatic displaced spondylolisthesis of fifth cervical vertebra **A, B** 🔎
  - ● **S12.431**   Unspecified traumatic nondisplaced spondylolisthesis of fifth cervical vertebra **A, B** 🔎

CHAPTER 19 (S00-T88)

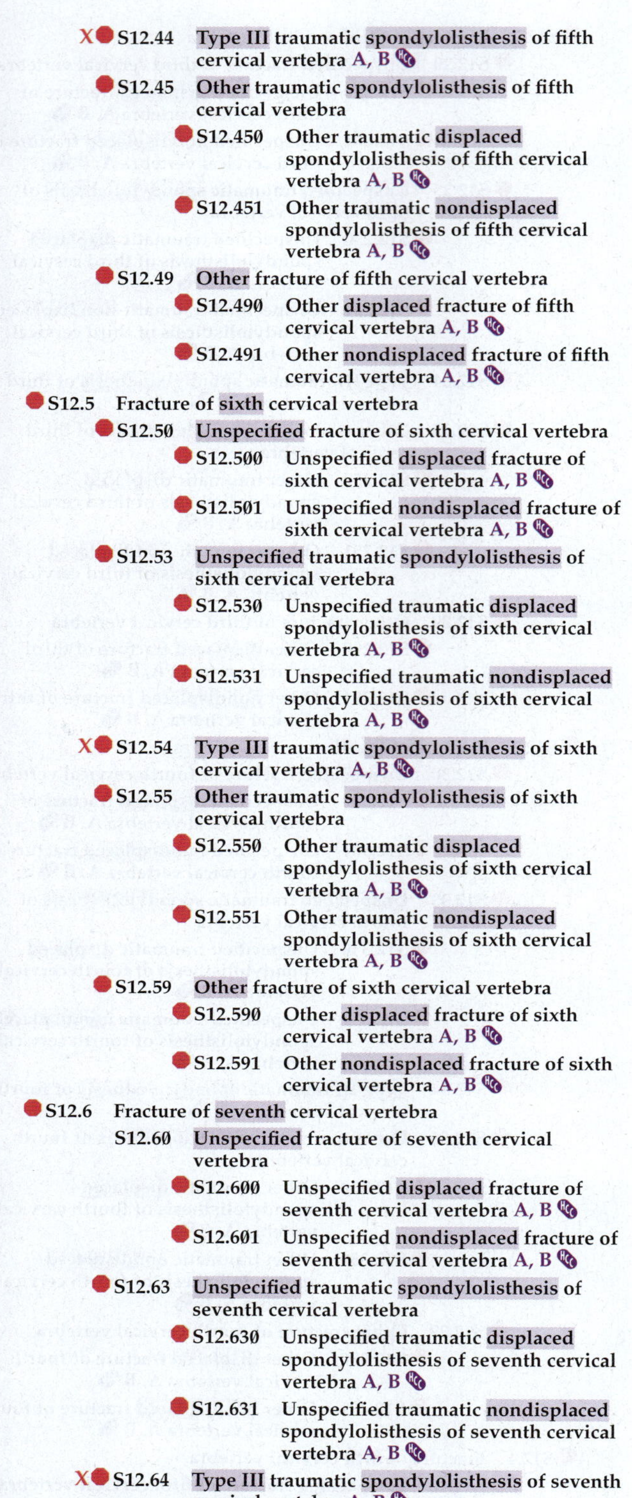

X ● **S12.44**   **Type III traumatic spondylolisthesis of fifth cervical vertebra A, B** 🅡🅒

● **S12.45**   **Other traumatic spondylolisthesis of fifth cervical vertebra**

    ● **S12.450**   **Other traumatic displaced spondylolisthesis of fifth cervical vertebra A, B** 🅡🅒

    ● **S12.451**   **Other traumatic nondisplaced spondylolisthesis of fifth cervical vertebra A, B** 🅡🅒

● **S12.49**   **Other fracture of fifth cervical vertebra**

    ● **S12.490**   **Other displaced fracture of fifth cervical vertebra A, B** 🅡🅒

    ● **S12.491**   **Other nondisplaced fracture of fifth cervical vertebra A, B** 🅡🅒

● **S12.5**   **Fracture of sixth cervical vertebra**

    ● **S12.50**   **Unspecified fracture of sixth cervical vertebra**

       ● **S12.500**   **Unspecified displaced fracture of sixth cervical vertebra A, B** 🅡🅒

       ● **S12.501**   **Unspecified nondisplaced fracture of sixth cervical vertebra A, B** 🅡🅒

    ● **S12.53**   **Unspecified traumatic spondylolisthesis of sixth cervical vertebra**

       ● **S12.530**   **Unspecified traumatic displaced spondylolisthesis of sixth cervical vertebra A, B** 🅡🅒

       ● **S12.531**   **Unspecified traumatic nondisplaced spondylolisthesis of sixth cervical vertebra A, B** 🅡🅒

X ● **S12.54**   **Type III traumatic spondylolisthesis of sixth cervical vertebra A, B** 🅡🅒

    ● **S12.55**   **Other traumatic spondylolisthesis of sixth cervical vertebra**

       ● **S12.550**   **Other traumatic displaced spondylolisthesis of sixth cervical vertebra A, B** 🅡🅒

       ● **S12.551**   **Other traumatic nondisplaced spondylolisthesis of sixth cervical vertebra A, B** 🅡🅒

    ● **S12.59**   **Other fracture of sixth cervical vertebra**

       ● **S12.590**   **Other displaced fracture of sixth cervical vertebra A, B** 🅡🅒

       ● **S12.591**   **Other nondisplaced fracture of sixth cervical vertebra A, B** 🅡🅒

● **S12.6**   **Fracture of seventh cervical vertebra**

    S12.60   **Unspecified fracture of seventh cervical vertebra**

       ● **S12.600**   **Unspecified displaced fracture of seventh cervical vertebra A, B** 🅡🅒

       ● **S12.601**   **Unspecified nondisplaced fracture of seventh cervical vertebra A, B** 🅡🅒

    ● **S12.63**   **Unspecified traumatic spondylolisthesis of seventh cervical vertebra**

       ● **S12.630**   **Unspecified traumatic displaced spondylolisthesis of seventh cervical vertebra A, B** 🅡🅒

       ● **S12.631**   **Unspecified traumatic nondisplaced spondylolisthesis of seventh cervical vertebra A, B** 🅡🅒

X ● **S12.64**   **Type III traumatic spondylolisthesis of seventh cervical vertebra A, B** 🅡🅒

● **S12.65**   **Other traumatic spondylolisthesis of seventh cervical vertebra**

    ● **S12.650**   **Other traumatic displaced spondylolisthesis of seventh cervical vertebra A, B** 🅡🅒

    ● **S12.651**   **Other traumatic nondisplaced spondylolisthesis of seventh cervical vertebra A, B** 🅡🅒

● **S12.69**   **Other fracture of seventh cervical vertebra**

    ● **S12.690**   **Other displaced fracture of seventh cervical vertebra A, B** 🅡🅒

    ● **S12.691**   **Other nondisplaced fracture of seventh cervical vertebra A, B** 🅡🅒

X ● **S12.8**   **Fracture of other parts of neck A** 🅡🅒
    ➡ Fracture of hyoid bone   ➡ Fracture of thyroid cartilage
    ➡ Fracture of larynx   ➡ Fracture of trachea

    The appropriate 7th character is to be added to code S12.8

A	initial encounter
D	subsequent encounter
S	sequela

X ● **S12.9**   **Fracture of neck, unspecified A** 🅡🅒
    Fracture of neck NOS
    Fracture of cervical spine NOS
    Fracture of cervical vertebra NOS

    The appropriate 7th character is to be added to code S12.9

A	initial encounter
D	subsequent encounter
S	sequela

● **S13**   **Dislocation and sprain of joints and ligaments at neck level**

    Includes   avulsion of joint or ligament at neck level
       laceration of cartilage, joint or ligament at neck level
       sprain of cartilage, joint or ligament at neck level
       traumatic hemarthrosis of joint or ligament at neck level
       traumatic rupture of joint or ligament at neck level
       traumatic subluxation of joint or ligament at neck level
       traumatic tear of joint or ligament at neck level

    Code also any associated open wound

    Excludes2   strain of muscle or tendon at neck level (S16.1)

    The appropriate 7th character is to be added to each code from category S13

A	initial encounter
D	subsequent encounter
S	sequela

X ● **S13.0**   **Traumatic rupture of cervical intervertebral disc**

    Excludes1   rupture or displacement (nontraumatic) of cervical intervertebral disc NOS (M50.-)

● **S13.1**   **Subluxation and dislocation of cervical vertebrae**

    Code also any associated:
       open wound of neck (S11.-)
       spinal cord injury (S14.1-)

    Excludes2   fracture of cervical vertebrae (S12.0-S12.3-)

    ● **S13.10**   **Subluxation and dislocation of unspecified cervical vertebrae**

       ● **S13.100**   **Subluxation of unspecified cervical vertebrae**

       ● **S13.101**   **Dislocation of unspecified cervical vertebrae**

- **S13.11 Subluxation and dislocation of C0/C1 cervical vertebrae**
  Subluxation and dislocation of atlantooccipital joint
  Subluxation and dislocation of atloidooccipital joint
  Subluxation and dislocation of occipitoatloid joint
  - **S13.110 Subluxation of C0/C1 cervical vertebrae**
  - **S13.111 Dislocation of C0/C1 cervical vertebrae**
- **S13.12 Subluxation and dislocation of C1/C2 cervical vertebrae**
  Subluxation and dislocation of atlantoaxial joint
  - **S13.120 Subluxation of C1/C2 cervical vertebrae**
  - **S13.121 Dislocation of C1/C2 cervical vertebrae**
- **S13.13 Subluxation and dislocation of C2/C3 cervical vertebrae**
  - **S13.130 Subluxation of C2/C3 cervical vertebrae**
  - **S13.131 Dislocation of C2/C3 cervical vertebrae**
- **S13.14 Subluxation and dislocation of C3/C4 cervical vertebrae**
  - **S13.140 Subluxation of C3/C4 cervical vertebrae**
  - **S13.141 Dislocation of C3/C4 cervical vertebrae**
- **S13.15 Subluxation and dislocation of C4/C5 cervical vertebrae**
  - **S13.150 Subluxation of C4/C5 cervical vertebrae**
  - **S13.151 Dislocation of C4/C5 cervical vertebrae**
- **S13.16 Subluxation and dislocation of C5/C6 cervical vertebrae**
  - **S13.160 Subluxation of C5/C6 cervical vertebrae**
  - **S13.161 Dislocation of C5/C6 cervical vertebrae**
- **S13.17 Subluxation and dislocation of C6/C7 cervical vertebrae**
  - **S13.170 Subluxation of C6/C7 cervical vertebrae**
  - **S13.171 Dislocation of C6/C7 cervical vertebrae**
- **S13.18 Subluxation and dislocation of C7/T1 cervical vertebrae**
  - **S13.180 Subluxation of C7/T1 cervical vertebrae**
  - **S13.181 Dislocation of C7/T1 cervical vertebrae**
- **S13.2 Dislocation of other and unspecified parts of neck**
  - X **S13.20 Dislocation of unspecified parts of neck**
  - X **S13.29 Dislocation of other parts of neck**
- X **S13.4 Sprain of ligaments of cervical spine**
  Sprain of anterior longitudinal (ligament), cervical
  Sprain of atlanto-axial (joints)
  Sprain of atlanto-occipital (joints)
  Whiplash injury of cervical spine
- X **S13.5 Sprain of thyroid region**
  Sprain of cricoarytenoid (joint) (ligament)
  Sprain of cricothyroid (joint) (ligament)
  Sprain of thyroid cartilage
- X **S13.8 Sprain of joints and ligaments of other parts of neck**
- X **S13.9 Sprain of joints and ligaments of unspecified parts of neck**

- **S14 Injury of nerves and spinal cord at neck level**
  Note: Code to highest level of cervical cord injury
  Code also any associated:
     fracture of cervical vertebra (S12.0--S12.6.-)
     open wound of neck (S11.-)
     transient paralysis (R29.5)
  The appropriate 7th character is to be added to each code from category S14

A	initial encounter
D	subsequent encounter
S	sequela

  - X **S14.0 Concussion and edema of cervical spinal cord A, D, S**
    Coding Clinic: 2024, Q2, P24
  - **S14.1 Other and unspecified injuries of cervical spinal cord**
    - **S14.10 Unspecified injury of cervical spinal cord**
      - **S14.101 Unspecified injury at C1 level of cervical spinal cord A, D, S**
      - **S14.102 Unspecified injury at C2 level of cervical spinal cord A, D, S**
      - **S14.103 Unspecified injury at C3 level of cervical spinal cord A, D, S**
      - **S14.104 Unspecified injury at C4 level of cervical spinal cord A, D, S**
      - **S14.105 Unspecified injury at C5 level of cervical spinal cord A, D, S**
      - **S14.106 Unspecified injury at C6 level of cervical spinal cord A, D, S**
      - **S14.107 Unspecified injury at C7 level of cervical spinal cord A, D, S**
      - **S14.108 Unspecified injury at C8 level of cervical spinal cord A, D, S**
      - **S14.109 Unspecified injury at unspecified level of cervical spinal cord A, D, S**
        Injury of cervical spinal cord NOS
    - **S14.11 Complete lesion of cervical spinal cord**
      - **S14.111 Complete lesion at C1 level of cervical spinal cord A, D, S**
      - **S14.112 Complete lesion at C2 level of cervical spinal cord A, D, S**
      - **S14.113 Complete lesion at C3 level of cervical spinal cord A, D, S**
      - **S14.114 Complete lesion at C4 level of cervical spinal cord A, D, S**
      - **S14.115 Complete lesion at C5 level of cervical spinal cord A, D, S**
      - **S14.116 Complete lesion at C6 level of cervical spinal cord A, D, S**
      - **S14.117 Complete lesion at C7 level of cervical spinal cord A, D, S**
      - **S14.118 Complete lesion at C8 level of cervical spinal cord A, D, S**
      - **S14.119 Complete lesion at unspecified level of cervical spinal cord A, D, S**
    - **S14.12 Central cord syndrome of cervical spinal cord**
      - **S14.121 Central cord syndrome at C1 level of cervical spinal cord A, D, S**
      - **S14.122 Central cord syndrome at C2 level of cervical spinal cord A, D, S**
      - **S14.123 Central cord syndrome at C3 level of cervical spinal cord A, D, S**
        Coding Clinic: 2024, Q2, P23
      - **S14.124 Central cord syndrome at C4 level of cervical spinal cord A, D, S**
      - **S14.125 Central cord syndrome at C5 level of cervical spinal cord A, D, S**
      - **S14.126 Central cord syndrome at C6 level of cervical spinal cord A, D, S**
      - **S14.127 Central cord syndrome at C7 level of cervical spinal cord A, D, S**

CHAPTER 19 (S00-T88)

CHAPTER 19 (S00-T88)

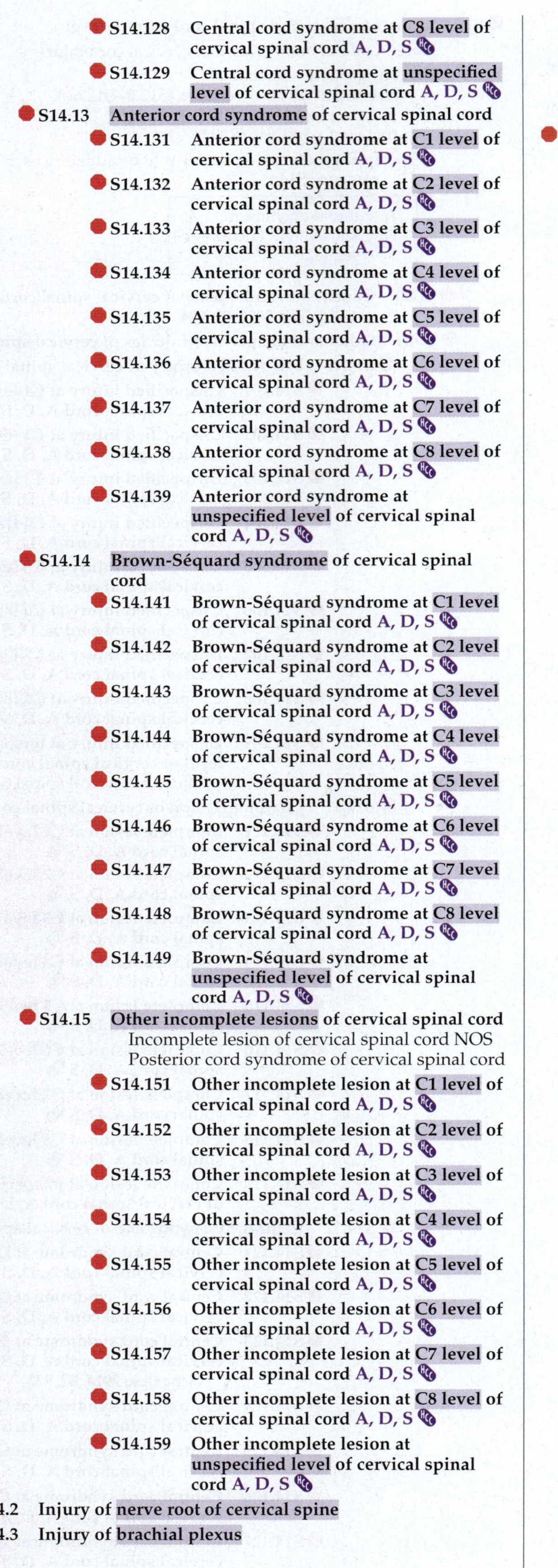

● **S14.128** Central cord syndrome at C8 level of cervical spinal cord A, D, S

● **S14.129** Central cord syndrome at unspecified level of cervical spinal cord A, D, S

● **S14.13** Anterior cord syndrome of cervical spinal cord

● **S14.131** Anterior cord syndrome at C1 level of cervical spinal cord A, D, S

● **S14.132** Anterior cord syndrome at C2 level of cervical spinal cord A, D, S

● **S14.133** Anterior cord syndrome at C3 level of cervical spinal cord A, D, S

● **S14.134** Anterior cord syndrome at C4 level of cervical spinal cord A, D, S

● **S14.135** Anterior cord syndrome at C5 level of cervical spinal cord A, D, S

● **S14.136** Anterior cord syndrome at C6 level of cervical spinal cord A, D, S

● **S14.137** Anterior cord syndrome at C7 level of cervical spinal cord A, D, S

● **S14.138** Anterior cord syndrome at C8 level of cervical spinal cord A, D, S

● **S14.139** Anterior cord syndrome at unspecified level of cervical spinal cord A, D, S

● **S14.14** Brown-Séquard syndrome of cervical spinal cord

● **S14.141** Brown-Séquard syndrome at C1 level of cervical spinal cord A, D, S

● **S14.142** Brown-Séquard syndrome at C2 level of cervical spinal cord A, D, S

● **S14.143** Brown-Séquard syndrome at C3 level of cervical spinal cord A, D, S

● **S14.144** Brown-Séquard syndrome at C4 level of cervical spinal cord A, D, S

● **S14.145** Brown-Séquard syndrome at C5 level of cervical spinal cord A, D, S

● **S14.146** Brown-Séquard syndrome at C6 level of cervical spinal cord A, D, S

● **S14.147** Brown-Séquard syndrome at C7 level of cervical spinal cord A, D, S

● **S14.148** Brown-Séquard syndrome at C8 level of cervical spinal cord A, D, S

● **S14.149** Brown-Séquard syndrome at unspecified level of cervical spinal cord A, D, S

● **S14.15** Other incomplete lesions of cervical spinal cord
Incomplete lesion of cervical spinal cord NOS
Posterior cord syndrome of cervical spinal cord

● **S14.151** Other incomplete lesion at C1 level of cervical spinal cord A, D, S

● **S14.152** Other incomplete lesion at C2 level of cervical spinal cord A, D, S

● **S14.153** Other incomplete lesion at C3 level of cervical spinal cord A, D, S

● **S14.154** Other incomplete lesion at C4 level of cervical spinal cord A, D, S

● **S14.155** Other incomplete lesion at C5 level of cervical spinal cord A, D, S

● **S14.156** Other incomplete lesion at C6 level of cervical spinal cord A, D, S

● **S14.157** Other incomplete lesion at C7 level of cervical spinal cord A, D, S

● **S14.158** Other incomplete lesion at C8 level of cervical spinal cord A, D, S

● **S14.159** Other incomplete lesion at unspecified level of cervical spinal cord A, D, S

X ● **S14.2** Injury of nerve root of cervical spine

X ● **S14.3** Injury of brachial plexus

X ● **S14.4** Injury of peripheral nerves of neck

X ● **S14.5** Injury of cervical sympathetic nerves

X ● **S14.8** Injury of other specified nerves of neck

X ● **S14.9** Injury of unspecified nerves of neck

● **S15** Injury of blood vessels at neck level
Code also any associated open wound (S11.-)
The appropriate 7th character is to be added to each code from category S15

> A initial encounter
> D subsequent encounter
> S sequela

● **S15.0** Injury of carotid artery of neck
Injury of carotid artery (common) (external) (internal, extracranial portion)
Injury of carotid artery NOS

Excludes1 injury of internal carotid artery, intracranial portion (S06.8)

● **S15.00** Unspecified injury of carotid artery

● **S15.001** Unspecified injury of right carotid artery

● **S15.002** Unspecified injury of left carotid artery

● **S15.009** Unspecified injury of unspecified carotid artery

● **S15.01** Minor laceration of carotid artery
Incomplete transection of carotid artery
Laceration of carotid artery NOS
Superficial laceration of carotid artery

● **S15.011** Minor laceration of right carotid artery

● **S15.012** Minor laceration of left carotid artery

● **S15.019** Minor laceration of unspecified carotid artery

● **S15.02** Major laceration of carotid artery
Complete transection of carotid artery
Traumatic rupture of carotid artery

● **S15.021** Major laceration of right carotid artery

● **S15.022** Major laceration of left carotid artery

● **S15.029** Major laceration of unspecified carotid artery

● **S15.09** Other specified injury of carotid artery

● **S15.091** Other specified injury of right carotid artery

● **S15.092** Other specified injury of left carotid artery

● **S15.099** Other specified injury of unspecified carotid artery

● **S15.1** Injury of vertebral artery

● **S15.10** Unspecified injury of vertebral artery

● **S15.101** Unspecified injury of right vertebral artery

● **S15.102** Unspecified injury of left vertebral artery

● **S15.109** Unspecified injury of unspecified vertebral artery

● **S15.11** Minor laceration of vertebral artery
Incomplete transection of vertebral artery
Laceration of vertebral artery NOS
Superficial laceration of vertebral artery

● **S15.111** Minor laceration of right vertebral artery

● **S15.112** Minor laceration of left vertebral artery

● **S15.119** Minor laceration of unspecified vertebral artery

▶ New   ⇒ Revised   ~~deleted~~ Deleted   Excludes 1   Excludes 2   Includes   Use additional   Code first   Code also   Key words
OGCR Official Guidelines   X Assign placeholder X   ● Use Additional Character(s)   ▸ Manifestation Code   ⊕ Hierarchical Condition Category   **Coding Clinic**

● **S15.12** **Major laceration of vertebral artery**
Complete transection of vertebral artery
Traumatic rupture of vertebral artery
  ● **S15.121** Major laceration of **right** vertebral artery
  ● **S15.122** Major laceration of **left** vertebral artery
  ● **S15.129** Major laceration of **unspecified** vertebral artery

● **S15.19** Other specified injury of vertebral artery
  ● **S15.191** Other specified injury of **right** vertebral artery
  ● **S15.192** Other specified injury of **left** vertebral artery
  ● **S15.199** Other specified injury of **unspecified** vertebral artery

● **S15.2** Injury of external jugular vein
  ● **S15.20** **Unspecified** injury of external jugular vein
    ● **S15.201** Unspecified injury of **right** external jugular vein
    ● **S15.202** Unspecified injury of **left** external jugular vein
    ● **S15.209** Unspecified injury of **unspecified** external jugular vein

  ● **S15.21** **Minor laceration of external jugular vein**
Incomplete transection of external jugular vein
Laceration of external jugular vein NOS
Superficial laceration of external jugular vein
    ● **S15.211** Minor laceration of **right** external jugular vein
    ● **S15.212** Minor laceration of **left** external jugular vein
    ● **S15.219** Minor laceration of **unspecified** external jugular vein

  ● **S15.22** **Major laceration of external jugular vein**
Complete transection of external jugular vein
Traumatic rupture of external jugular vein
    ● **S15.221** Major laceration of **right** external jugular vein
    ● **S15.222** Major laceration of **left** external jugular vein
    ● **S15.229** Major laceration of **unspecified** external jugular vein

  ● **S15.29** Other specified injury of external jugular vein
    ● **S15.291** Other specified injury of **right** external jugular vein
    ● **S15.292** Other specified injury of **left** external jugular vein
    ● **S15.299** Other specified injury of **unspecified** external jugular vein

● **S15.3** Injury of internal jugular vein
  ● **S15.30** **Unspecified** injury of internal jugular vein
    ● **S15.301** Unspecified injury of **right** internal jugular vein
    ● **S15.302** Unspecified injury of **left** internal jugular vein
    ● **S15.309** Unspecified injury of **unspecified** internal jugular vein

  ● **S15.31** **Minor laceration of internal jugular vein**
Incomplete transection of internal jugular vein
Laceration of internal jugular vein NOS
Superficial laceration of internal jugular vein
    ● **S15.311** Minor laceration of **right** internal jugular vein
    ● **S15.312** Minor laceration of **left** internal jugular vein
    ● **S15.319** Minor laceration of **unspecified** internal jugular vein

● **S15.32** **Major laceration of internal jugular vein**
Complete transection of internal jugular vein
Traumatic rupture of internal jugular vein
  ● **S15.321** Major laceration of **right** internal jugular vein
  ● **S15.322** Major laceration of **left** internal jugular vein
  ● **S15.329** Major laceration of **unspecified** internal jugular vein

● **S15.39** Other specified injury of internal jugular vein
  ● **S15.391** Other specified injury of **right** internal jugular vein
  ● **S15.392** Other specified injury of **left** internal jugular vein
  ● **S15.399** Other specified injury of **unspecified** internal jugular vein

X ● **S15.8** Injury of **other** specified blood vessels at neck level
X ● **S15.9** Injury of **unspecified** blood vessel at neck level

● **S16** Injury of muscle, fascia and tendon at neck level
Code also any associated open wound (S11.-)
Excludes2 sprain of joint or ligament at neck level (S13.9)
The appropriate 7th character is to be added to each code from category S16

> A initial encounter
> D subsequent encounter
> S sequela

X ● **S16.1** **Strain** of muscle, fascia and tendon at neck level
X ● **S16.2** **Laceration** of muscle, fascia and tendon at neck level
X ● **S16.8** **Other** specified injury of muscle, fascia and tendon at neck level
X ● **S16.9** **Unspecified** injury of muscle, fascia and tendon at neck level

● **S17** Crushing injury of neck
Use additional code for all associated injuries, such as:
injury of blood vessels (S15.-)
open wound of neck (S11.-)
spinal cord injury (S14.0, S14.1-)
vertebral fracture (S12.0--S12.3-)
The appropriate 7th character is to be added to each code from category S17

> A initial encounter
> D subsequent encounter
> S sequela

X ● **S17.0** Crushing injury of **larynx and trachea**
X ● **S17.8** Crushing injury of **other** specified parts of neck
X ● **S17.9** Crushing injury of neck, part **unspecified**

● **S19** Other and unspecified injuries of neck
The appropriate 7th character is to be added to each code from category S19

> A initial encounter
> D subsequent encounter
> S sequela

● **S19.8** **Other** specified injuries of neck
  X ● **S19.80** Other specified injuries of **unspecified** part of neck
  X ● **S19.81** Other specified injuries of **larynx**
  X ● **S19.82** Other specified injuries of **cervical trachea**
    Excludes2 other specified injury of thoracic trachea (S27.5-)
  X ● **S19.83** Other specified injuries of **vocal cord**
  X ● **S19.84** Other specified injuries of **thyroid gland**

CHAPTER 19 (S00-T88)

X ● **S19.85** Other specified injuries of **pharynx and cervical esophagus**
　　　　Coding Clinic: 2022, Q1, P27

X ● **S19.89** Other specified injuries of other specified part of neck

X ● **S19.9** Unspecified injury of neck

INJURIES TO THE THORAX (S20-S29)

Includes injuries of breast
　　　　　injuries of chest (wall)
　　　　　injuries of interscapular area

Excludes2 burns and corrosions (T20-T32)
　　　　　effects of foreign body in bronchus (T17.5)
　　　　　effects of foreign body in esophagus (T18.1)
　　　　　effects of foreign body in lung (T17.8)
　　　　　effects of foreign body in trachea (T17.4)
　　　　　frostbite (T33-T34)
　　　　　injuries of axilla
　　　　　injuries of clavicle
　　　　　injuries of scapular region
　　　　　injuries of shoulder
　　　　　insect bite or sting, venomous (T63.4)

● **S20** Superficial injury of thorax

The appropriate 7th character is to be added to each code from category S20

> A　initial encounter
> D　subsequent encounter
> S　sequela

● **S20.0** Contusion of breast

X ● **S20.00** Contusion of breast, **unspecified** breast

X ● **S20.01** Contusion of **right** breast

X ● **S20.02** Contusion of **left** breast

● **S20.1** Other and unspecified superficial injuries of breast

● **S20.10** **Unspecified** superficial injuries of breast

● **S20.101** Unspecified superficial injuries of breast, **right** breast

● **S20.102** Unspecified superficial injuries of breast, **left** breast

● **S20.109** Unspecified superficial injuries of breast, **unspecified** breast

● **S20.11** **Abrasion** of breast

● **S20.111** Abrasion of breast, **right** breast

● **S20.112** Abrasion of breast, **left** breast

● **S20.119** Abrasion of breast, **unspecified** breast

● **S20.12** **Blister** (nonthermal) of breast

● **S20.121** Blister (nonthermal) of breast, **right** breast

● **S20.122** Blister (nonthermal) of breast, **left** breast

● **S20.129** Blister (nonthermal) of breast, **unspecified** breast

● **S20.14** **External constriction** of part of breast

● **S20.141** External constriction of part of breast, **right** breast

● **S20.142** External constriction of part of breast, **left** breast

● **S20.149** External constriction of part of breast, **unspecified** breast

● **S20.15** **Superficial foreign body** of breast
　　　　Splinter in the breast

● **S20.151** Superficial foreign body of breast, **right** breast

● **S20.152** Superficial foreign body of breast, **left** breast

● **S20.159** Superficial foreign body of breast, **unspecified** breast

● **S20.16** Insect bite (nonvenomous) of breast

● **S20.161** Insect bite (nonvenomous) of breast, **right** breast

● **S20.162** Insect bite (nonvenomous) of breast, **left** breast

● **S20.169** Insect bite (nonvenomous) of breast, **unspecified** breast

● **S20.17** Other superficial bite of breast

　　　　Excludes1 open bite of breast (S21.05-)

● **S20.171** Other superficial bite of breast, **right** breast

● **S20.172** Other superficial bite of breast, **left** breast

● **S20.179** Other superficial bite of breast, **unspecified** breast

● **S20.2** Contusion of thorax

X ● **S20.20** Contusion of thorax, **unspecified**

● **S20.21** Contusion of **front wall** of thorax

● **S20.211** Contusion of **right** front wall of thorax

● **S20.212** Contusion of **left** front wall of thorax

● **S20.213** Contusion of bilateral front wall of thorax

● **S20.214** Contusion of middle front wall of thorax

● **S20.219** Contusion of **unspecified** front wall of thorax

● **S20.22** Contusion of **back wall** of thorax

● **S20.221** Contusion of **right** back wall of thorax

● **S20.222** Contusion of **left** back wall of thorax

● **S20.223** Contusion of bilateral back wall of thorax

● **S20.224** Contusion of middle back wall of thorax

● **S20.229** Contusion of **unspecified** back wall of thorax

● **S20.3** Other and unspecified superficial injuries of **front wall** of thorax

● **S20.30** **Unspecified** superficial injuries of front wall of thorax

● **S20.301** Unspecified superficial injuries of **right** front wall of thorax

● **S20.302** Unspecified superficial injuries of **left** front wall of thorax

● **S20.303** Unspecified superficial injuries of bilateral front wall of thorax

● **S20.304** Unspecified superficial injuries of middle front wall of thorax

● **S20.309** Unspecified superficial injuries of **unspecified** front wall of thorax

● **S20.31** **Abrasion** of front wall of thorax

● **S20.311** Abrasion of **right** front wall of thorax

● **S20.312** Abrasion of **left** front wall of thorax

● **S20.313** Abrasion of bilateral front wall of thorax

● **S20.314** Abrasion of middle front wall of thorax

● **S20.319** Abrasion of **unspecified** front wall of thorax

● **S20.32** **Blister** (nonthermal) of front wall of thorax

● **S20.321** Blister (nonthermal) of **right** front wall of thorax

● **S20.322** Blister (nonthermal) of **left** front wall of thorax

S20.323   Blister (nonthermal) of bilateral front wall of thorax

S20.324   Blister (nonthermal) of middle front wall of thorax

● S20.329   Blister (nonthermal) of unspecified front wall of thorax

● S20.34   External constriction of front wall of thorax

● S20.341   External constriction of right front wall of thorax

● S20.342   External constriction of left front wall of thorax

S20.343   External constriction of bilateral front wall of thorax

S20.344   External constriction of middle front wall of thorax

● S20.349   External constriction of unspecified front wall of thorax

● S20.35   Superficial foreign body of front wall of thorax
Splinter in front wall of thorax

● S20.351   Superficial foreign body of right front wall of thorax

● S20.352   Superficial foreign body of left front wall of thorax

S20.353   Superficial foreign body of bilateral front wall of thorax

S20.354   Superficial foreign body of middle front wall of thorax

● S20.359   Superficial foreign body of unspecified front wall of thorax

● S20.36   Insect bite (nonvenomous) of front wall of thorax

● S20.361   Insect bite (nonvenomous) of right front wall of thorax

● S20.362   Insect bite (nonvenomous) of left front wall of thorax

S20.363   Insect bite (nonvenomous) of bilateral front wall of thorax

S20.364   Insect bite (nonvenomous) of middle front wall of thorax

● S20.369   Insect bite (nonvenomous) of unspecified front wall of thorax

● S20.37   Other superficial bite of front wall of thorax

    Excludes1   open bite of front wall of thorax (S21.14)

● S20.371   Other superficial bite of right front wall of thorax

● S20.372   Other superficial bite of left front wall of thorax

S20.373   Other superficial bite of bilateral front wall of thorax

S20.374   Other superficial bite of middle front wall of thorax

● S20.379   Other superficial bite of unspecified front wall of thorax

● S20.4   Other and unspecified superficial injuries of back wall of thorax

● S20.40   Unspecified superficial injuries of back wall of thorax

● S20.401   Unspecified superficial injuries of right back wall of thorax

● S20.402   Unspecified superficial injuries of left back wall of thorax

● S20.409   Unspecified superficial injuries of unspecified back wall of thorax

● S20.41   Abrasion of back wall of thorax

● S20.411   Abrasion of right back wall of thorax

● S20.412   Abrasion of left back wall of thorax

● S20.419   Abrasion of unspecified back wall of thorax

● S20.42   Blister (nonthermal) of back wall of thorax

● S20.421   Blister (nonthermal) of right back wall of thorax

● S20.422   Blister (nonthermal) of left back wall of thorax

● S20.429   Blister (nonthermal) of unspecified back wall of thorax

● S20.44   External constriction of back wall of thorax

● S20.441   External constriction of right back wall of thorax

● S20.442   External constriction of left back wall of thorax

● S20.449   External constriction of unspecified back wall of thorax

● S20.45   Superficial foreign body of back wall of thorax
Splinter of back wall of thorax

● S20.451   Superficial foreign body of right back wall of thorax

● S20.452   Superficial foreign body of left back wall of thorax

● S20.459   Superficial foreign body of unspecified back wall of thorax

● S20.46   Insect bite (nonvenomous) of back wall of thorax

● S20.461   Insect bite (nonvenomous) of right back wall of thorax

● S20.462   Insect bite (nonvenomous) of left back wall of thorax

● S20.469   Insect bite (nonvenomous) of unspecified back wall of thorax

● S20.47   Other superficial bite of back wall of thorax

    Excludes1   open bite of back wall of thorax (S21.24)

● S20.471   Other superficial bite of right back wall of thorax

● S20.472   Other superficial bite of left back wall of thorax

● S20.479   Other superficial bite of unspecified back wall of thorax

● S20.9   Superficial injury of unspecified parts of thorax

    Excludes1   contusion of thorax NOS (S20.20)

X ● S20.90   Unspecified superficial injury of unspecified parts of thorax
Superficial injury of thoracic wall NOS

X ● S20.91   Abrasion of unspecified parts of thorax

X ● S20.92   Blister (nonthermal) of unspecified parts of thorax

X ● S20.94   External constriction of unspecified parts of thorax

X ● S20.95   Superficial foreign body of unspecified parts of thorax
Splinter in thorax NOS

X ● S20.96   Insect bite (nonvenomous) of unspecified parts of thorax

X ● S20.97   Other superficial bite of unspecified parts of thorax

    Excludes1   open bite of thorax NOS (S21.95)

CHAPTER 19 (S00-T88)

● **S21   Open wound of thorax**

Code also any associated injury such as:
  injury of heart (S26.-)
  injury of intrathoracic organs (S27.-)
  rib fracture (S22.3-, S22.4-)
  spinal cord injury (S24.0-, S24.1-)
  traumatic hemothorax (S27.1)
  traumatic hemopneumothorax (S27.3)
  traumatic pneumothorax (S27.0)
  wound infection

Excludes1   traumatic amputation (partial) of thorax (S28.1)

The appropriate 7th character is to be added to each code from category S21

> A   initial encounter
> D   subsequent encounter
> S   sequela

● **S21.0   Open wound of breast**

● **S21.00   Unspecified open wound of breast**

● S21.001   Unspecified open wound of **right** breast

● S21.002   Unspecified open wound of **left** breast

● S21.009   Unspecified open wound of **unspecified** breast

● **S21.01   Laceration without foreign body of breast**

● S21.011   Laceration without foreign body of **right** breast

● S21.012   Laceration without foreign body of **left** breast

● S21.019   Laceration without foreign body of **unspecified** breast

● **S21.02   Laceration with foreign body of breast**

● S21.021   Laceration with foreign body of **right** breast

● S21.022   Laceration with foreign body of **left** breast

● S21.029   Laceration with foreign body of **unspecified** breast

● **S21.03   Puncture wound without foreign body of breast**

● S21.031   Puncture wound without foreign body of **right** breast

● S21.032   Puncture wound without foreign body of **left** breast

● S21.039   Puncture wound without foreign body of **unspecified** breast

● **S21.04   Puncture wound with foreign body of breast**

● S21.041   Puncture wound with foreign body of **right** breast

● S21.042   Puncture wound with foreign body of **left** breast

● S21.049   Puncture wound with foreign body of **unspecified** breast

● **S21.05   Open bite of breast**
  Bite of breast NOS

Excludes1   superficial bite of breast (S20.17)

● S21.051   Open bite of **right** breast

● S21.052   Open bite of **left** breast

● S21.059   Open bite of **unspecified** breast

Item 19–1 Pneumothorax is a collection of gas (positive air pressure) in the pleural space, resulting in the lung collapsing. A **tension pneumothorax** is life-threatening and is a result of air in the pleural space causing a displacement in the mediastinal structures and cardiopulmonary function compromise. A **traumatic pneumothorax** results from blunt or penetrating injury that disrupts the parietal/visceral pleura. **Hemothorax** is blood or bloody fluid in the pleural cavity as a result of traumatic blood vessel rupture or inflammation of the lungs from pneumonia.

● **S21.1   Open wound of front wall of thorax without penetration into thoracic cavity**
  Open wound of chest without penetration into thoracic cavity

● **S21.10   Unspecified open wound of front wall of thorax without penetration into thoracic cavity**

● S21.101   Unspecified open wound of **right** front wall of thorax without penetration into thoracic cavity

● S21.102   Unspecified open wound of **left** front wall of thorax without penetration into thoracic cavity

● S21.109   Unspecified open wound of **unspecified** front wall of thorax without penetration into thoracic cavity

● **S21.11   Laceration without foreign body of front wall of thorax without penetration into thoracic cavity**

● S21.111   Laceration without foreign body of **right** front wall of thorax without penetration into thoracic cavity

● S21.112   Laceration without foreign body of **left** front wall of thorax without penetration into thoracic cavity

● S21.119   Laceration without foreign body of **unspecified** front wall of thorax without penetration into thoracic cavity

● **S21.12   Laceration with foreign body of front wall of thorax without penetration into thoracic cavity**

● S21.121   Laceration with foreign body of **right** front wall of thorax without penetration into thoracic cavity

● S21.122   Laceration with foreign body of **left** front wall of thorax without penetration into thoracic cavity

● S21.129   Laceration with foreign body of **unspecified** front wall of thorax without penetration into thoracic cavity

● **S21.13   Puncture wound without foreign body of front wall of thorax without penetration into thoracic cavity**

● S21.131   Puncture wound without foreign body of **right** front wall of thorax without penetration into thoracic cavity

● S21.132   Puncture wound without foreign body of **left** front wall of thorax without penetration into thoracic cavity

● S21.139   Puncture wound without foreign body of **unspecified** front wall of thorax without penetration into thoracic cavity

● **S21.14   Puncture wound with foreign body of front wall of thorax without penetration into thoracic cavity**

● S21.141   Puncture wound with foreign body of **right** front wall of thorax without penetration into thoracic cavity

● S21.142   Puncture wound with foreign body of **left** front wall of thorax without penetration into thoracic cavity

● S21.149   Puncture wound with foreign body of **unspecified** front wall of thorax without penetration into thoracic cavity

● **S21.15   Open bite of front wall of thorax without penetration into thoracic cavity**
  Bite of front wall of thorax NOS

Excludes1   superficial bite of front wall of thorax (S20.37)

▶ New   ➡ Revised   ~~deleted~~ Deleted | Excludes 1 | Excludes 2 | Includes | Use additional | Code first | Code also | Key words |

OGCR Official Guidelines   **X** Assign placeholder X   ● Use Additional Character(s)   ▶ Manifestation Code   Hierarchical Condition Category   **Coding Clinic**

- ● **S21.151** Open bite of **right** front wall of thorax without penetration into thoracic cavity
- ● **S21.152** Open bite of **left** front wall of thorax without penetration into thoracic cavity
- ● **S21.159** Open bite of **unspecified** front wall of thorax without penetration into thoracic cavity
- ● **S21.2** **Open wound of back wall of thorax without penetration into thoracic cavity**
  - ● **S21.20** **Unspecified** open wound of back wall of thorax without penetration into thoracic cavity
    - ● **S21.201** Unspecified open wound of **right** back wall of thorax without penetration into thoracic cavity
    - ● **S21.202** Unspecified open wound of **left** back wall of thorax without penetration into thoracic cavity
    - ● **S21.209** Unspecified open wound of **unspecified** back wall of thorax without penetration into thoracic cavity
  - ● **S21.21** **Laceration without foreign body** of back wall of thorax without penetration into thoracic cavity
    - ● **S21.211** Laceration without foreign body of **right** back wall of thorax without penetration into thoracic cavity
    - ● **S21.212** Laceration without foreign body of **left** back wall of thorax without penetration into thoracic cavity
    - ● **S21.219** Laceration without foreign body of **unspecified** back wall of thorax without penetration into thoracic cavity
  - ● **S21.22** **Laceration with foreign body** of back wall of thorax without penetration into thoracic cavity
    - ● **S21.221** Laceration with foreign body of **right** back wall of thorax without penetration into thoracic cavity
    - ● **S21.222** Laceration with foreign body of **left** back wall of thorax without penetration into thoracic cavity
    - ● **S21.229** Laceration with foreign body of **unspecified** back wall of thorax without penetration into thoracic cavity
  - ● **S21.23** **Puncture wound without foreign body** of back wall of thorax without penetration into thoracic cavity
    - ● **S21.231** Puncture wound without foreign body of **right** back wall of thorax without penetration into thoracic cavity
    - ● **S21.232** Puncture wound without foreign body of **left** back wall of thorax without penetration into thoracic cavity
    - ● **S21.239** Puncture wound without foreign body of **unspecified** back wall of thorax without penetration into thoracic cavity
  - ● **S21.24** **Puncture wound with foreign body** of back wall of thorax without penetration into thoracic cavity
    - ● **S21.241** Puncture wound with foreign body of **right** back wall of thorax without penetration into thoracic cavity
    - ● **S21.242** Puncture wound with foreign body of **left** back wall of thorax without penetration into thoracic cavity
    - ● **S21.249** Puncture wound with foreign body of **unspecified** back wall of thorax without penetration into thoracic cavity
- ● **S21.25** **Open bite** of back wall of thorax without penetration into thoracic cavity

  Bite of back wall of thorax NOS

  Excludes1 superficial bite of back wall of thorax (S20.47)
  - ● **S21.251** Open bite of **right** back wall of thorax without penetration into thoracic cavity
  - ● **S21.252** Open bite of **left** back wall of thorax without penetration into thoracic cavity
  - ● **S21.259** Open bite of **unspecified** back wall of thorax without penetration into thoracic cavity
- ● **S21.3** **Open wound of front wall of thorax with penetration into thoracic cavity**

  Open wound of chest with penetration into thoracic cavity
  - ● **S21.30** **Unspecified** open wound of front wall of thorax with penetration into thoracic cavity
    - ● **S21.301** Unspecified open wound of **right** front wall of thorax with penetration into thoracic cavity
    - ● **S21.302** Unspecified open wound of **left** front wall of thorax with penetration into thoracic cavity
    - ● **S21.309** Unspecified open wound of **unspecified** front wall of thorax with penetration into thoracic cavity
  - ● **S21.31** **Laceration without foreign body** of front wall of thorax with penetration into thoracic cavity
    - ● **S21.311** Laceration without foreign body of **right** front wall of thorax with penetration into thoracic cavity
    - ● **S21.312** Laceration without foreign body of **left** front wall of thorax with penetration into thoracic cavity
    - ● **S21.319** Laceration without foreign body of **unspecified** front wall of thorax with penetration into thoracic cavity
  - ● **S21.32** **Laceration with foreign body** of front wall of thorax with penetration into thoracic cavity
    - ● **S21.321** Laceration with foreign body of **right** front wall of thorax with penetration into thoracic cavity
    - ● **S21.322** Laceration with foreign body of **left** front wall of thorax with penetration into thoracic cavity
    - ● **S21.329** Laceration with foreign body of **unspecified** front wall of thorax with penetration into thoracic cavity
  - ● **S21.33** **Puncture wound without foreign body** of front wall of thorax with penetration into thoracic cavity
    - ● **S21.331** Puncture wound without foreign body of **right** front wall of thorax with penetration into thoracic cavity
    - ● **S21.332** Puncture wound without foreign body of **left** front wall of thorax with penetration into thoracic cavity
    - ● **S21.339** Puncture wound without foreign body of **unspecified** front wall of thorax with penetration into thoracic cavity

CHAPTER 19 (S00-T88)

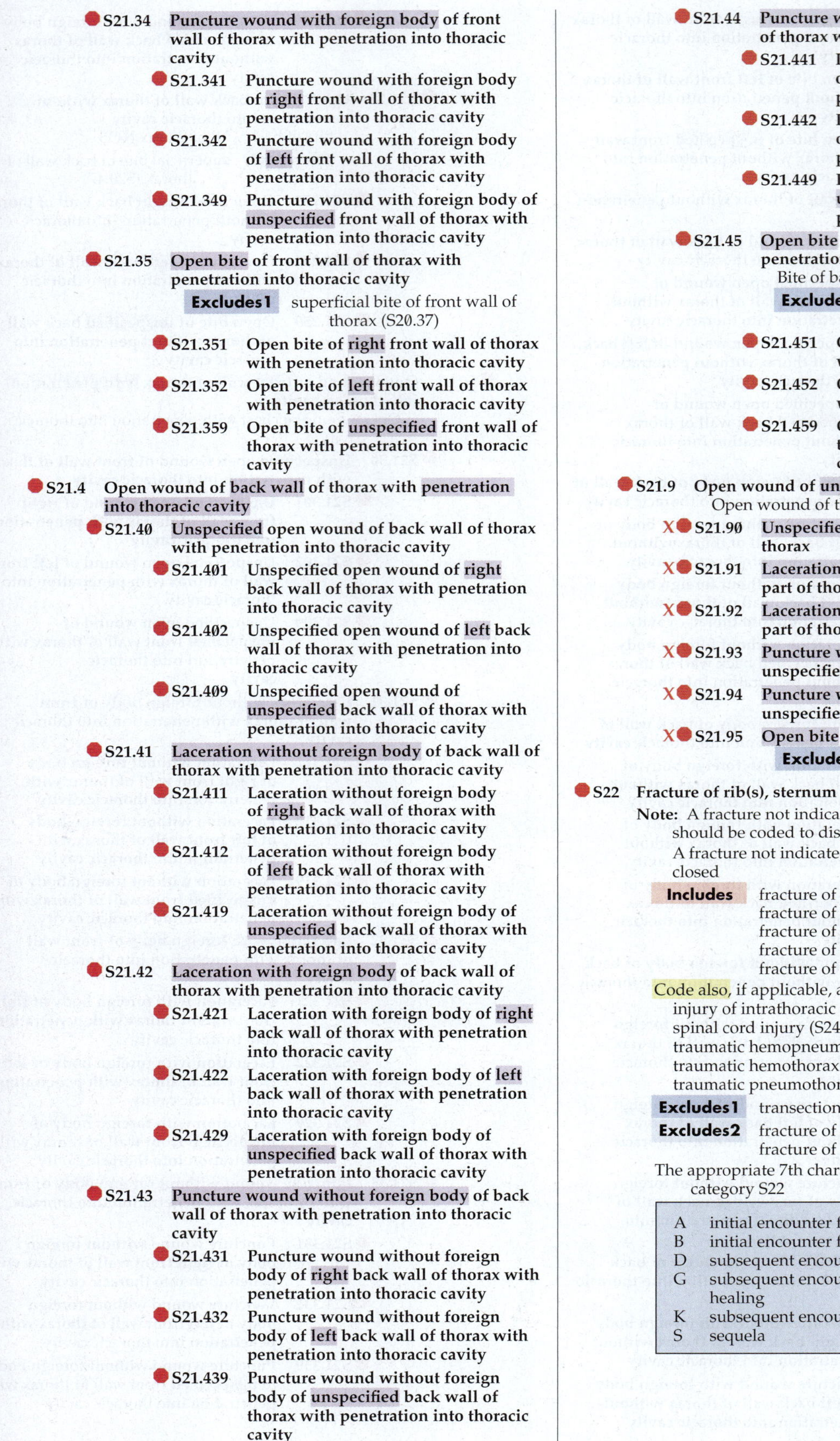

● S21.34 **Puncture wound with foreign body** of front wall of thorax with penetration into thoracic cavity

    ● S21.341   Puncture wound with foreign body of right front wall of thorax with penetration into thoracic cavity

    ● S21.342   Puncture wound with foreign body of left front wall of thorax with penetration into thoracic cavity

    ● S21.349   Puncture wound with foreign body of unspecified front wall of thorax with penetration into thoracic cavity

● S21.35 **Open bite** of front wall of thorax with penetration into thoracic cavity

    Excludes1   superficial bite of front wall of thorax (S20.37)

    ● S21.351   Open bite of right front wall of thorax with penetration into thoracic cavity

    ● S21.352   Open bite of left front wall of thorax with penetration into thoracic cavity

    ● S21.359   Open bite of unspecified front wall of thorax with penetration into thoracic cavity

● S21.4   Open wound of **back wall** of thorax with **penetration** into thoracic cavity

    ● S21.40   **Unspecified** open wound of back wall of thorax with penetration into thoracic cavity

       ● S21.401   Unspecified open wound of right back wall of thorax with penetration into thoracic cavity

       ● S21.402   Unspecified open wound of left back wall of thorax with penetration into thoracic cavity

       ● S21.409   Unspecified open wound of unspecified back wall of thorax with penetration into thoracic cavity

    ● S21.41   **Laceration without foreign body** of back wall of thorax with penetration into thoracic cavity

       ● S21.411   Laceration without foreign body of right back wall of thorax with penetration into thoracic cavity

       ● S21.412   Laceration without foreign body of left back wall of thorax with penetration into thoracic cavity

       ● S21.419   Laceration without foreign body of unspecified back wall of thorax with penetration into thoracic cavity

    ● S21.42   **Laceration with foreign body** of back wall of thorax with penetration into thoracic cavity

       ● S21.421   Laceration with foreign body of right back wall of thorax with penetration into thoracic cavity

       ● S21.422   Laceration with foreign body of left back wall of thorax with penetration into thoracic cavity

       ● S21.429   Laceration with foreign body of unspecified back wall of thorax with penetration into thoracic cavity

    ● S21.43   **Puncture wound without foreign body** of back wall of thorax with penetration into thoracic cavity

       ● S21.431   Puncture wound without foreign body of right back wall of thorax with penetration into thoracic cavity

       ● S21.432   Puncture wound without foreign body of left back wall of thorax with penetration into thoracic cavity

       ● S21.439   Puncture wound without foreign body of unspecified back wall of thorax with penetration into thoracic cavity

● S21.44   **Puncture wound with foreign body** of back wall of thorax with penetration into thoracic cavity

    ● S21.441   Puncture wound with foreign body of right back wall of thorax with penetration into thoracic cavity

    ● S21.442   Puncture wound with foreign body of left back wall of thorax with penetration into thoracic cavity

    ● S21.449   Puncture wound with foreign body of unspecified back wall of thorax with penetration into thoracic cavity

● S21.45   **Open bite** of back wall of thorax with penetration into thoracic cavity

    Bite of back wall of thorax NOS

    Excludes1   superficial bite of back wall of thorax (S20.47)

    ● S21.451   Open bite of right back wall of thorax with penetration into thoracic cavity

    ● S21.452   Open bite of left back wall of thorax with penetration into thoracic cavity

    ● S21.459   Open bite of unspecified back wall of thorax with penetration into thoracic cavity

● S21.9   Open wound of **unspecified** part of thorax

    Open wound of thoracic wall NOS

    X ● S21.90   **Unspecified** open wound of unspecified part of thorax

    X ● S21.91   Laceration without foreign body of unspecified part of thorax

    X ● S21.92   Laceration with foreign body of unspecified part of thorax

    X ● S21.93   Puncture wound without foreign body of unspecified part of thorax

    X ● S21.94   Puncture wound with foreign body of unspecified part of thorax

    X ● S21.95   Open bite of unspecified part of thorax

       Excludes1   superficial bite of thorax (S20.97)

● S22   **Fracture of rib(s), sternum and thoracic spine**

    Note: A fracture not indicated as displaced or nondisplaced should be coded to displaced

       A fracture not indicated as open or closed should be coded to closed

    Includes   fracture of thoracic neural arch
         fracture of thoracic spinous process
         fracture of thoracic transverse process
         fracture of thoracic vertebra
         fracture of thoracic vertebral arch

    Code also, if applicable, any associated condition such as:
       injury of intrathoracic organ (S27.-)
       spinal cord injury (S24.0-, S24.1-)
       traumatic hemopneumothorax (S27.2)
       traumatic hemothorax (S27.1-)
       traumatic pneumothorax (S27.0)

    Excludes1   transection of thorax (S28.1)

    Excludes2   fracture of clavicle (S42.0-)
              fracture of scapula (S42.1-)

    The appropriate 7th character is to be added to each code from category S22

A	initial encounter for closed fracture
B	initial encounter for open fracture
D	subsequent encounter for fracture with routine healing
G	subsequent encounter for fracture with delayed healing
K	subsequent encounter for fracture with nonunion
S	sequela

- ● S22.0   Fracture of thoracic vertebra
  - ● S22.00   Fracture of unspecified thoracic vertebra
    - ● S22.000   Wedge compression fracture of unspecified thoracic vertebra A, B ℞
    - ● S22.001   Stable burst fracture of unspecified thoracic vertebra A, B ℞
    - ● S22.002   Unstable burst fracture of unspecified thoracic vertebra A, B ℞
    - ● S22.008   Other fracture of unspecified thoracic vertebra A, B ℞
    - ● S22.009   Unspecified fracture of unspecified thoracic vertebra A, B ℞
  - ● S22.01   Fracture of first thoracic vertebra
    - ● S22.010   Wedge compression fracture of first thoracic vertebra A, B ℞
    - ● S22.011   Stable burst fracture of first thoracic vertebra A, B ℞
    - ● S22.012   Unstable burst fracture of first thoracic vertebra A, B ℞
    - ● S22.018   Other fracture of first thoracic vertebra A, B ℞
    - ● S22.019   Unspecified fracture of first thoracic vertebra A, B ℞
  - ● S22.02   Fracture of second thoracic vertebra
    - ● S22.020   Wedge compression fracture of second thoracic vertebra A, B ℞
    - ● S22.021   Stable burst fracture of second thoracic vertebra A, B ℞
    - ● S22.022   Unstable burst fracture of second thoracic vertebra A, B ℞
    - ● S22.028   Other fracture of second thoracic vertebra A, B ℞
    - ● S22.029   Unspecified fracture of second thoracic vertebra A, B ℞
  - ● S22.03   Fracture of third thoracic vertebra
    - ● S22.030   Wedge compression fracture of third thoracic vertebra A, B ℞
    - ● S22.031   Stable burst fracture of third thoracic vertebra A, B ℞
    - ● S22.032   Unstable burst fracture of third thoracic vertebra A, B ℞
    - ● S22.038   Other fracture of third thoracic vertebra A, B ℞
    - ● S22.039   Unspecified fracture of third thoracic vertebra A, B ℞
  - ● S22.04   Fracture of fourth thoracic vertebra
    - ● S22.040   Wedge compression fracture of fourth thoracic vertebra A, B ℞
    - ● S22.041   Stable burst fracture of fourth thoracic vertebra A, B ℞
    - ● S22.042   Unstable burst fracture of fourth thoracic vertebra A, B ℞
    - ● S22.048   Other fracture of fourth thoracic vertebra A, B ℞
    - ● S22.049   Unspecified fracture of fourth thoracic vertebra A, B ℞
  - ● S22.05   Fracture of T5-T6 vertebra
    - ● S22.050   Wedge compression fracture of T5-T6 vertebra A, B ℞
    - ● S22.051   Stable burst fracture of T5-T6 vertebra A, B ℞
    - ● S22.052   Unstable burst fracture of T5-T6 vertebra A, B ℞
    - ● S22.058   Other fracture of T5-T6 vertebra A, B ℞
    - ● S22.059   Unspecified fracture of T5-T6 vertebra A, B ℞
  - ● S22.06   Fracture of T7-T8 vertebra
    - ● S22.060   Wedge compression fracture of T7-T8 vertebra A, B ℞
    - ● S22.061   Stable burst fracture of T7-T8 vertebra A, B ℞
    - ● S22.062   Unstable burst fracture of T7-T8 vertebra A, B ℞
    - ● S22.068   Other fracture of T7-T8 thoracic vertebra A, B ℞
    - ● S22.069   Unspecified fracture of T7-T8 vertebra A, B ℞
  - ● S22.07   Fracture of T9-T10 vertebra
    - ● S22.070   Wedge compression fracture of T9-T10 vertebra A, B ℞
    - ● S22.071   Stable burst fracture of T9-T10 vertebra A, B ℞
    - ● S22.072   Unstable burst fracture of T9-T10 vertebra A, B ℞
    - ● S22.078   Other fracture of T9-T10 vertebra A, B ℞
    - ● S22.079   Unspecified fracture of T9-T10 vertebra A, B ℞
  - ● S22.08   Fracture of T11-T12 vertebra
    - ● S22.080   Wedge compression fracture of T11-T12 vertebra A, B ℞
    - ● S22.081   Stable burst fracture of T11-T12 vertebra A, B ℞
    - ● S22.082   Unstable burst fracture of T11-T12 vertebra A, B ℞
    - ● S22.088   Other fracture of T11-T12 vertebra A, B ℞
    - ● S22.089   Unspecified fracture of T11-T12 vertebra A, B ℞
      - **Coding Clinic: 2024, Q4, P19**
- ● S22.2   Fracture of sternum
  - X ● S22.20   Unspecified fracture of sternum
  - X ● S22.21   Fracture of manubrium
  - X ● S22.22   Fracture of body of sternum
  - X ● S22.23   Sternal manubrial dissociation
  - X ● S22.24   Fracture of xiphoid process
- ● S22.3   Fracture of one rib
  - X ● S22.31   Fracture of one rib, right side
  - X ● S22.32   Fracture of one rib, left side
  - X ● S22.39   Fracture of one rib, unspecified side
- ● S22.4   Multiple fractures of ribs
  - Fractures of two or more ribs
  - **Excludes1**   flail chest (S22.5-)
  - X ● S22.41   Multiple fractures of ribs, right side
  - X ● S22.42   Multiple fractures of ribs, left side
  - X ● S22.43   Multiple fractures of ribs, bilateral
  - X ● S22.49   Multiple fractures of ribs, unspecified side
- X ● S22.5   Flail chest
  - *Unstable chest due to sternum and/or rib fracture*
- X ● S22.9   Fracture of bony thorax, part unspecified

● **S23 Dislocation and sprain of joints and ligaments of thorax**

Includes   avulsion of joint or ligament of thorax
laceration of cartilage, joint or ligament of thorax
sprain of cartilage, joint or ligament of thorax
traumatic hemarthrosis of joint or ligament of thorax
traumatic rupture of joint or ligament of thorax
traumatic subluxation of joint or ligament of thorax
traumatic tear of joint or ligament of thorax

Code also any associated: open wound

Excludes2   dislocation, sprain of sternoclavicular joint (S43.2, S43.6)
strain of muscle or tendon of thorax (S29.01-)

The appropriate 7th character is to be added to each code from category S23

> A   initial encounter
> D   subsequent encounter
> S   sequela

X ● **S23.0 Traumatic rupture of thoracic intervertebral disc**

Excludes1   rupture or displacement (nontraumatic) of thoracic intervertebral disc NOS (M51.- with fifth character 4)

● **S23.1 Subluxation and dislocation of thoracic vertebra**

Code also any associated
open wound of thorax (S21.-)
spinal cord injury (S24.0-, S24.1-)

Excludes2   fracture of thoracic vertebrae (S22.0-)

    ● **S23.10 Subluxation and dislocation of unspecified thoracic vertebra**

       ● **S23.100 Subluxation of unspecified thoracic vertebra**

       ● **S23.101 Dislocation of unspecified thoracic vertebra**

    ● **S23.11 Subluxation and dislocation of T1/T2 thoracic vertebra**

       ● **S23.110 Subluxation of T1/T2 thoracic vertebra**

       ● **S23.111 Dislocation of T1/T2 thoracic vertebra**

    ● **S23.12 Subluxation and dislocation of T2/T3-T3/T4 thoracic vertebra**

       ● **S23.120 Subluxation of T2/T3 thoracic vertebra**

       ● **S23.121 Dislocation of T2/T3 thoracic vertebra**

       ● **S23.122 Subluxation of T3/T4 thoracic vertebra**

       ● **S23.123 Dislocation of T3/T4 thoracic vertebra**

    ● **S23.13 Subluxation and dislocation of T4/T5-T5/T6 thoracic vertebra**

       ● **S23.130 Subluxation of T4/T5 thoracic vertebra**

       ● **S23.131 Dislocation of T4/T5 thoracic vertebra**

       ● **S23.132 Subluxation of T5/T6 thoracic vertebra**

       ● **S23.133 Dislocation of T5/T6 thoracic vertebra**

    ● **S23.14 Subluxation and dislocation of T6/T7-T7/T8 thoracic vertebra**

       ● **S23.140 Subluxation of T6/T7 thoracic vertebra**

       ● **S23.141 Dislocation of T6/T7 thoracic vertebra**

       ● **S23.142 Subluxation of T7/T8 thoracic vertebra**

       ● **S23.143 Dislocation of T7/T8 thoracic vertebra**

    ● **S23.15 Subluxation and dislocation of T8/T9-T9/T10 thoracic vertebra**

       ● **S23.150 Subluxation of T8/T9 thoracic vertebra**

       ● **S23.151 Dislocation of T8/T9 thoracic vertebra**

       ● **S23.152 Subluxation of T9/T10 thoracic vertebra**

       ● **S23.153 Dislocation of T9/T10 thoracic vertebra**

    ● **S23.16 Subluxation and dislocation of T10/T11-T11/T12 thoracic vertebra**

       ● **S23.160 Subluxation of T10/T11 thoracic vertebra**

       ● **S23.161 Dislocation of T10/T11 thoracic vertebra**

       ● **S23.162 Subluxation of T11/T12 thoracic vertebra**

       ● **S23.163 Dislocation of T11/T12 thoracic vertebra**

    ● **S23.17 Subluxation and dislocation of T12/L1 thoracic vertebra**

       ● **S23.170 Subluxation of T12/L1 thoracic vertebra**

       ● **S23.171 Dislocation of T12/L1 thoracic vertebra**

● **S23.2 Dislocation of other and unspecified parts of thorax**

X ● **S23.20 Dislocation of unspecified part of thorax**

X ● **S23.29 Dislocation of other parts of thorax**

X ● **S23.3 Sprain of ligaments of thoracic spine**

● **S23.4 Sprain of ribs and sternum**

X ● **S23.41 Sprain of ribs**

● **S23.42 Sprain of sternum**

       ● **S23.420 Sprain of sternoclavicular (joint) (ligament)**

       ● **S23.421 Sprain of chondrosternal joint**

       ● **S23.428 Other sprain of sternum**

       ● **S23.429 Unspecified sprain of sternum**

X ● **S23.8 Sprain of other specified parts of thorax**

X ● **S23.9 Sprain of unspecified parts of thorax**

● **S24 Injury of nerves and spinal cord at thorax level**

Note: Code to highest level of thoracic spinal cord injury.

Injuries to the spinal cord (S24.0 and S24.1) refer to the cord level and not bone level injury, and can affect nerve roots at and below the level given.

Code also any associated:
fracture of thoracic vertebra (S22.0-)
open wound of thorax (S21.-)
transient paralysis (R29.5)

Excludes2   injury of brachial plexus (S14.3)

The appropriate 7th character is to be added to each code from category S24

> A   initial encounter
> D   subsequent encounter
> S   sequela

X ● **S24.0 Concussion and edema of thoracic spinal cord** A, D, S 

● **S24.1 Other and unspecified injuries of thoracic spinal cord**

    ● **S24.10 Unspecified injury of thoracic spinal cord**

       ● **S24.101 Unspecified injury at T1 level of thoracic spinal cord** A, D, S

       ● **S24.102 Unspecified injury at T2-T6 level of thoracic spinal cord** A, D, S

       ● **S24.103 Unspecified injury at T7-T10 level of thoracic spinal cord** A, D, S

       ● **S24.104 Unspecified injury at T11-T12 level of thoracic spinal cord** A, D, S

       ● **S24.109 Unspecified injury at unspecified level of thoracic spinal cord** A, D, S
          Injury of thoracic spinal cord NOS

    ● **S24.11 Complete lesion of thoracic spinal cord**

       ● **S24.111 Complete lesion at T1 level of thoracic spinal cord** A, D, S

       ● **S24.112 Complete lesion at T2-T6 level of thoracic spinal cord** A, D, S

▶ New   ➡ Revised   ~~deleted~~ Deleted   Excludes 1   Excludes 2   Includes   Use additional   Code first   Code also   Key words
OGCR Official Guidelines   X Assign placeholder X   ● Use Additional Character(s)   ▸ Manifestation Code   Hierarchical Condition Category   **Coding Clinic**

- ● **S24.113** Complete lesion at **T7-T10 level of** thoracic spinal cord A, D, S
- ● **S24.114** Complete lesion at **T11-T12 level of** thoracic spinal cord A, D, S
- ● **S24.119** Complete lesion at **unspecified level** of thoracic spinal cord A, D, S
- ● **S24.13** Anterior cord syndrome of thoracic spinal cord
  - ● **S24.131** Anterior cord syndrome at **T1 level of** thoracic spinal cord A, D, S
  - ● **S24.132** Anterior cord syndrome at **T2-T6 level** of thoracic spinal cord A, D, S
  - ● **S24.133** Anterior cord syndrome at **T7-T10** level of thoracic spinal cord A, D, S
  - ● **S24.134** Anterior cord syndrome at **T11-T12** level of thoracic spinal cord A, D, S
  - ● **S24.139** Anterior cord syndrome at **unspecified level** of thoracic spinal cord A, D, S
- ● **S24.14** Brown-Séquard syndrome of thoracic spinal cord
  - ● **S24.141** Brown-Séquard syndrome at **T1 level** of thoracic spinal cord A, D, S
  - ● **S24.142** Brown-Séquard syndrome at **T2-T6** level of thoracic spinal cord A, D, S
  - ● **S24.143** Brown-Séquard syndrome at **T7-T10** level of thoracic spinal cord A, D, S
  - ● **S24.144** Brown-Séquard syndrome at **T11-T12** level of thoracic spinal cord A, D, S
  - ● **S24.149** Brown-Séquard syndrome at **unspecified level** of thoracic spinal cord A, D, S
- ● **S24.15** Other incomplete lesions of thoracic spinal cord
  Incomplete lesion of thoracic spinal cord NOS
  Posterior cord syndrome of thoracic spinal cord
  - ● **S24.151** Other incomplete lesion at **T1 level of** thoracic spinal cord A, D, S
  - ● **S24.152** Other incomplete lesion at **T2-T6** level of thoracic spinal cord A, D, S
  - ● **S24.153** Other incomplete lesion at **T7-T10** level of thoracic spinal cord A, D, S
  - ● **S24.154** Other incomplete lesion at **T11-T12** level of thoracic spinal cord A, D, S
  - ● **S24.159** Other incomplete lesion at **unspecified level** of thoracic spinal cord A, D, S
- X ● **S24.2** Injury of nerve root of thoracic spine
- X ● **S24.3** Injury of peripheral nerves of thorax
- X ● **S24.4** Injury of thoracic sympathetic nervous system
  Injury of cardiac plexus
  Injury of esophageal plexus
  Injury of pulmonary plexus
  Injury of stellate ganglion
  Injury of thoracic sympathetic ganglion
- X ● **S24.8** Injury of other specified nerves of thorax
- X ● **S24.9** Injury of unspecified nerve of thorax
- ● **S25** Injury of blood vessels of thorax

  The appropriate 7th character is to be added to each code from category S25

A	initial encounter
D	subsequent encounter
S	sequela

  Code also any associated open wound (S21.-)

- ● **S25.0** Injury of thoracic aorta
  Injury of aorta NOS
  - X ● **S25.00** Unspecified injury of thoracic aorta

- X ● **S25.01** Minor laceration of thoracic aorta
  Incomplete transection of thoracic aorta
  Laceration of thoracic aorta NOS
  Superficial laceration of thoracic aorta
- X ● **S25.02** Major laceration of thoracic aorta
  Complete transection of thoracic aorta
  Traumatic rupture of thoracic aorta
- X ● **S25.09** Other specified injury of thoracic aorta
- ● **S25.1** Injury of innominate or subclavian artery
  - ● **S25.10** Unspecified injury of innominate or subclavian artery
    - ● **S25.101** Unspecified injury of **right** innominate or subclavian artery
    - ● **S25.102** Unspecified injury of **left** innominate or subclavian artery
    - ● **S25.109** Unspecified injury of **unspecified** innominate or subclavian artery
  - ● **S25.11** Minor laceration of innominate or subclavian artery
    Incomplete transection of innominate or subclavian artery
    Laceration of innominate or subclavian artery NOS
    Superficial laceration of innominate or subclavian artery
    - ● **S25.111** Minor laceration of **right** innominate or subclavian artery
    - ● **S25.112** Minor laceration of **left** innominate or subclavian artery
    - ● **S25.119** Minor laceration of **unspecified** innominate or subclavian artery
  - ● **S25.12** Major laceration of innominate or subclavian artery
    Complete transection of innominate or subclavian artery
    Traumatic rupture of innominate or subclavian artery
    - ● **S25.121** Major laceration of **right** innominate or subclavian artery
    - ● **S25.122** Major laceration of **left** innominate or subclavian artery
    - ● **S25.129** Major laceration of **unspecified** innominate or subclavian artery
  - ● **S25.19** Other specified injury of innominate or subclavian artery
    - ● **S25.191** Other specified injury of **right** innominate or subclavian artery
    - ● **S25.192** Other specified injury of **left** innominate or subclavian artery
    - ● **S25.199** Other specified injury of **unspecified** innominate or subclavian artery
- ● **S25.2** Injury of superior vena cava
  Injury of vena cava NOS
  - X ● **S25.20** Unspecified injury of superior vena cava
  - X ● **S25.21** Minor laceration of superior vena cava
    Incomplete transection of superior vena cava
    Laceration of superior vena cava NOS
    Superficial laceration of superior vena cava
  - X ● **S25.22** Major laceration of superior vena cava
    Complete transection of superior vena cava
    Traumatic rupture of superior vena cava
  - X ● **S25.29** Other specified injury of superior vena cava
- ● **S25.3** Injury of innominate or subclavian vein
  - ● **S25.30** Unspecified injury of innominate or subclavian vein
    - ● **S25.301** Unspecified injury of **right** innominate or subclavian vein
    - ● **S25.302** Unspecified injury of **left** innominate or subclavian vein
    - ● **S25.309** Unspecified injury of **unspecified** innominate or subclavian vein

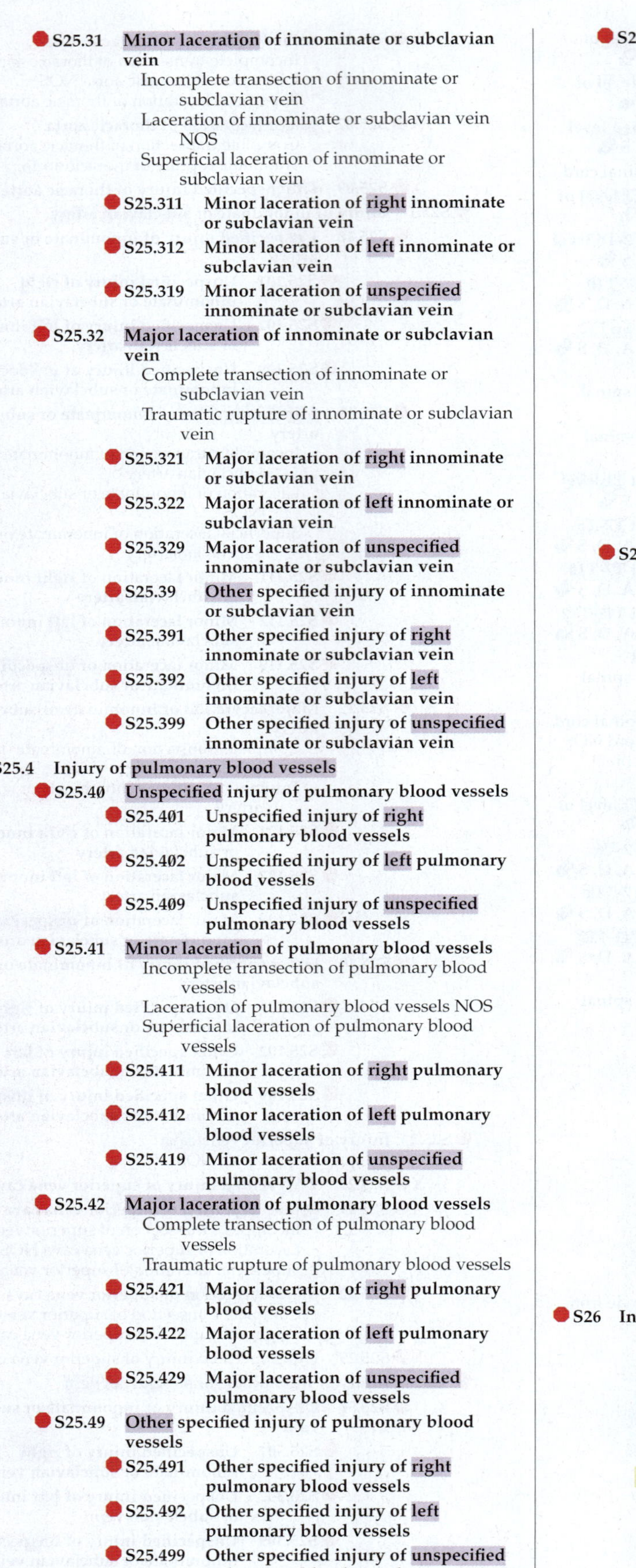

CHAPTER 19 (S00-T88)

● S25.31   **Minor laceration** of innominate or subclavian vein
　　Incomplete transection of innominate or subclavian vein
　　Laceration of innominate or subclavian vein NOS
　　Superficial laceration of innominate or subclavian vein

　● S25.311   Minor laceration of **right** innominate or subclavian vein
　● S25.312   Minor laceration of **left** innominate or subclavian vein
　● S25.319   Minor laceration of **unspecified** innominate or subclavian vein

● S25.32   **Major laceration** of innominate or subclavian vein
　　Complete transection of innominate or subclavian vein
　　Traumatic rupture of innominate or subclavian vein

　● S25.321   Major laceration of **right** innominate or subclavian vein
　● S25.322   Major laceration of **left** innominate or subclavian vein
　● S25.329   Major laceration of **unspecified** innominate or subclavian vein
　● S25.39   Other specified injury of innominate or subclavian vein
　● S25.391   Other specified injury of **right** innominate or subclavian vein
　● S25.392   Other specified injury of **left** innominate or subclavian vein
　● S25.399   Other specified injury of **unspecified** innominate or subclavian vein

● S25.4   Injury of **pulmonary blood vessels**
● S25.40   **Unspecified** injury of pulmonary blood vessels
　● S25.401   Unspecified injury of **right** pulmonary blood vessels
　● S25.402   Unspecified injury of **left** pulmonary blood vessels
　● S25.409   Unspecified injury of **unspecified** pulmonary blood vessels

● S25.41   **Minor laceration** of pulmonary blood vessels
　　Incomplete transection of pulmonary blood vessels
　　Laceration of pulmonary blood vessels NOS
　　Superficial laceration of pulmonary blood vessels

　● S25.411   Minor laceration of **right** pulmonary blood vessels
　● S25.412   Minor laceration of **left** pulmonary blood vessels
　● S25.419   Minor laceration of **unspecified** pulmonary blood vessels

● S25.42   **Major laceration** of pulmonary blood vessels
　　Complete transection of pulmonary blood vessels
　　Traumatic rupture of pulmonary blood vessels

　● S25.421   Major laceration of **right** pulmonary blood vessels
　● S25.422   Major laceration of **left** pulmonary blood vessels
　● S25.429   Major laceration of **unspecified** pulmonary blood vessels

● S25.49   Other specified injury of pulmonary blood vessels
　● S25.491   Other specified injury of **right** pulmonary blood vessels
　● S25.492   Other specified injury of **left** pulmonary blood vessels
　● S25.499   Other specified injury of **unspecified** pulmonary blood vessels

● S25.5   Injury of **intercostal blood vessels**
● S25.50   **Unspecified** injury of intercostal blood vessels
　● S25.501   Unspecified injury of intercostal blood vessels, **right** side
　● S25.502   Unspecified injury of intercostal blood vessels, **left** side
　● S25.509   Unspecified injury of intercostal blood vessels, **unspecified** side

● S25.51   **Laceration** of intercostal blood vessels
　● S25.511   Laceration of intercostal blood vessels, **right** side
　● S25.512   Laceration of intercostal blood vessels, **left** side
　● S25.519   Laceration of intercostal blood vessels, **unspecified** side

● S25.59   Other specified injury of intercostal blood vessels
　● S25.591   Other specified injury of intercostal blood vessels, **right** side
　● S25.592   Other specified injury of intercostal blood vessels, **left** side
　● S25.599   Other specified injury of intercostal blood vessels, **unspecified** side

● S25.8   Injury of other blood vessels of thorax
　　Injury of azygos vein
　　Injury of mammary artery or vein

● S25.80   **Unspecified** injury of other blood vessels of thorax
　● S25.801   Unspecified injury of other blood vessels of thorax, **right** side
　● S25.802   Unspecified injury of other blood vessels of thorax, **left** side
　● S25.809   Unspecified injury of other blood vessels of thorax, **unspecified** side
　● S25.81   **Laceration** of other blood vessels of thorax
　● S25.811   Laceration of other blood vessels of thorax, **right** side
　● S25.812   Laceration of other blood vessels of thorax, **left** side
　● S25.819   Laceration of other blood vessels of thorax, **unspecified** side

● S25.89   Other specified injury of other blood vessels of thorax
　● S25.891   Other specified injury of other blood vessels of thorax, **right** side
　● S25.892   Other specified injury of other blood vessels of thorax, **left** side
　● S25.899   Other specified injury of other blood vessels of thorax, **unspecified** side
　● S25.9   Injury of **unspecified blood vessel** of thorax

X ● S25.90   **Unspecified** injury of unspecified blood vessel of thorax
X ● S25.91   **Laceration** of unspecified blood vessel of thorax
X ● S25.99   Other specified injury of unspecified blood vessel of thorax

● S26   **Injury of heart**
　The appropriate 7th character is to be added to each code from category S26

A	initial encounter
D	subsequent encounter
S	sequela

Code also any associated:
　open wound of thorax (S21.-)
　traumatic hemopneumothorax (S27.2)
　traumatic hemothorax (S27.1)
　traumatic pneumothorax (S27.0)

▶ New　⇨ Revised　~~deleted~~ Deleted　Excludes 1　Excludes 2　Includes　Use additional　Code first　Code also　Key words
OGCR Official Guidelines　X Assign placeholder X　● Use Additional Character(s)　▸ Manifestation Code　🔵 Hierarchical Condition Category　**Coding Clinic**

Item 19–2 Pneumothorax is a collection of gas (positive air pressure) in the pleural space resulting in the lung collapsing. A **tension pneumothorax** is life-threatening and is a result of air in the pleural space causing a displacement in the mediastinal structures and cardiopulmonary function compromise. A **traumatic pneumothorax** results from blunt or penetrating injury that disrupts the parietal/visceral pleura. **Hemothorax** is blood or bloody fluid in the pleural cavity as a result of traumatic blood vessel rupture or inflammation of the lungs from pneumonia.

● **S26.0　Injury of heart with hemopericardium**
　　Hemopericardium: effusion of blood within pericardium
　X ● **S26.00　Unspecified** injury of heart with hemopericardium
　X ● **S26.01　Contusion** of heart with hemopericardium
　　● **S26.02　Laceration** of heart with hemopericardium
　　　● **S26.020　Mild laceration** of heart with hemopericardium
　　　　　Laceration of heart without penetration of heart chamber
　　　● **S26.021　Moderate laceration** of heart with hemopericardium
　　　　　Laceration of heart with penetration of heart chamber
　　　● **S26.022　Major laceration** of heart with hemopericardium
　　　　　Laceration of heart with penetration of multiple heart chambers
　X ● **S26.09　Other** injury of heart with hemopericardium
● **S26.1　Injury of heart without hemopericardium**
　　Hemopericardium: effusion of blood within pericardium
　X ● **S26.10　Unspecified** injury of heart without hemopericardium
　X ● **S26.11　Contusion** of heart without hemopericardium
　X ● **S26.12　Laceration** of heart without hemopericardium
　X ● **S26.19　Other** injury of heart without hemopericardium
● **S26.9　Injury of heart, unspecified with or without hemopericardium**
　　Hemopericardium: effusion of blood within pericardium
　X ● **S26.90　Unspecified** injury of heart, unspecified with or without hemopericardium
　X ● **S26.91　Contusion** of heart, unspecified with or without hemopericardium
　X ● **S26.92　Laceration** of heart, unspecified with or without hemopericardium
　　　Laceration of heart NOS
　X ● **S26.99　Other** injury of heart, unspecified with or without hemopericardium

● **S27　Injury of other and unspecified intrathoracic organs**
　　Code also any associated open wound of thorax (S21.-)
　　Excludes2　injury of cervical esophagus (S10-S19)
　　　　　injury of trachea (cervical) (S10-S19)
　　The appropriate 7th character is to be added to each code from category S27

A	initial encounter
D	subsequent encounter
S	sequela

　X ● **S27.0　Traumatic pneumothorax**
　　　Excludes1　spontaneous pneumothorax (J93.-)
　X ● **S27.1　Traumatic hemothorax**
　X ● **S27.2　Traumatic hemopneumothorax**
　　● **S27.3　Other and unspecified injuries of lung**
　　　● **S27.30　Unspecified injury of lung**
　　　　● **S27.301　Unspecified** injury of lung, **unilateral**
　　　　● **S27.302　Unspecified** injury of lung, **bilateral**
　　　　● **S27.309　Unspecified** injury of lung, **unspecified**

　　● **S27.31　Primary blast injury of lung**
　　　　Blast injury of lung NOS
　　　● **S27.311　Primary blast injury of lung, unilateral**
　　　● **S27.312　Primary blast injury of lung, bilateral**
　　　● **S27.319　Primary blast injury of lung, unspecified**
　　● **S27.32　Contusion of lung**
　　　● **S27.321　Contusion** of lung, **unilateral**
　　　● **S27.322　Contusion** of lung, **bilateral**
　　　● **S27.329　Contusion** of lung, **unspecified**
　　● **S27.33　Laceration of lung**
　　　● **S27.331　Laceration** of lung, **unilateral**
　　　● **S27.332　Laceration** of lung, **bilateral**
　　　● **S27.339　Laceration** of lung, **unspecified**
　　● **S27.39　Other injuries of lung**
　　　　Secondary blast injury of lung
　　　● **S27.391　Other injuries** of lung, **unilateral**
　　　● **S27.392　Other injuries** of lung, **bilateral**
　　　● **S27.399　Other injuries** of lung, **unspecified**
● **S27.4　Injury of bronchus**
　● **S27.40　Unspecified injury of bronchus**
　　　● **S27.401　Unspecified injury** of bronchus, **unilateral**
　　　● **S27.402　Unspecified injury** of bronchus, **bilateral**
　　　● **S27.409　Unspecified injury** of bronchus, **unspecified**
　● **S27.41　Primary blast injury of bronchus**
　　　Blast injury of bronchus NOS
　　　● **S27.411　Primary blast injury** of bronchus, **unilateral**
　　　● **S27.412　Primary blast injury** of bronchus, **bilateral**
　　　● **S27.419　Primary blast injury** of bronchus, **unspecified**
　● **S27.42　Contusion of bronchus**
　　　● **S27.421　Contusion** of bronchus, **unilateral**
　　　● **S27.422　Contusion** of bronchus, **bilateral**
　　　● **S27.429　Contusion** of bronchus, **unspecified**
　● **S27.43　Laceration of bronchus**
　　　● **S27.431　Laceration** of bronchus, **unilateral**
　　　● **S27.432　Laceration** of bronchus, **bilateral**
　　　● **S27.439　Laceration** of bronchus, **unspecified**
　● **S27.49　Other injury of bronchus**
　　　Secondary blast injury of bronchus
　　　● **S27.491　Other injury** of bronchus, **unilateral**
　　　● **S27.492　Other injury** of bronchus, **bilateral**
　　　● **S27.499　Other injury** of bronchus, **unspecified**
● **S27.5　Injury of thoracic trachea**
　X ● **S27.50　Unspecified** injury of thoracic trachea
　X ● **S27.51　Primary blast injury** of thoracic trachea
　　　Blast injury of thoracic trachea NOS
　X ● **S27.52　Contusion** of thoracic trachea
　X ● **S27.53　Laceration** of thoracic trachea
　X ● **S27.59　Other injury** of thoracic trachea
　　　Secondary blast injury of thoracic trachea
● **S27.6　Injury of pleura**
　X ● **S27.60　Unspecified** injury of pleura
　X ● **S27.63　Laceration** of pleura
　X ● **S27.69　Other injury** of pleura
● **S27.8　Injury of other specified intrathoracic organs**
　● **S27.80　Injury of diaphragm**
　　　● **S27.802　Contusion** of diaphragm
　　　● **S27.803　Laceration** of diaphragm
　　　● **S27.808　Other injury** of diaphragm
　　　● **S27.809　Unspecified injury** of diaphragm

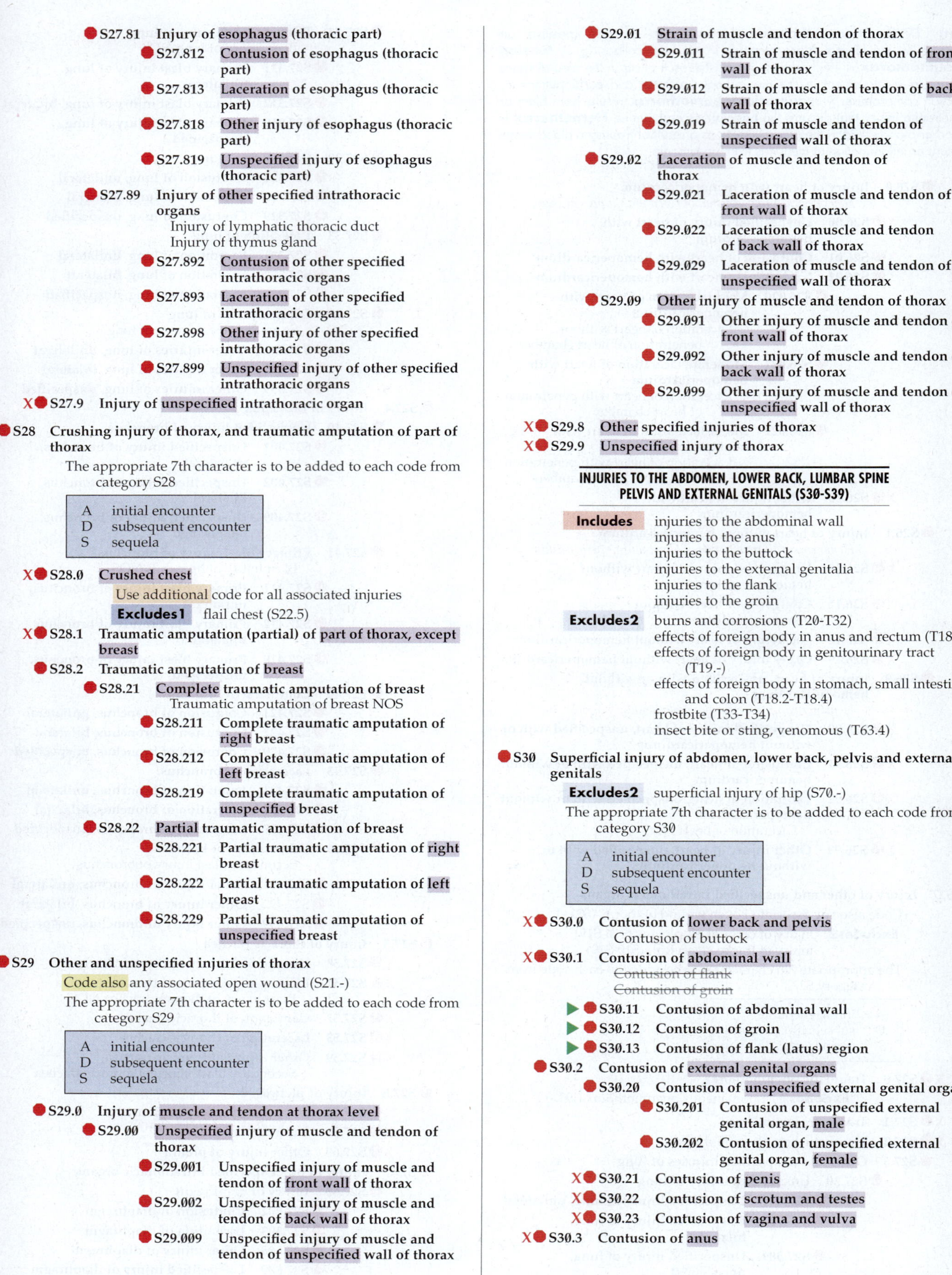

CHAPTER 19 (S00–T88)

- S27.81   Injury of esophagus (thoracic part)
  - S27.812   Contusion of esophagus (thoracic part)
  - S27.813   Laceration of esophagus (thoracic part)
  - S27.818   Other injury of esophagus (thoracic part)
  - S27.819   Unspecified injury of esophagus (thoracic part)
- S27.89   Injury of other specified intrathoracic organs
  - Injury of lymphatic thoracic duct
  - Injury of thymus gland
  - S27.892   Contusion of other specified intrathoracic organs
  - S27.893   Laceration of other specified intrathoracic organs
  - S27.898   Other injury of other specified intrathoracic organs
  - S27.899   Unspecified injury of other specified intrathoracic organs
- X S27.9   Injury of unspecified intrathoracic organ

- S28   Crushing injury of thorax, and traumatic amputation of part of thorax

  The appropriate 7th character is to be added to each code from category S28

  > A   initial encounter
  > D   subsequent encounter
  > S   sequela

  - X S28.0   Crushed chest
    - Use additional code for all associated injuries
    - Excludes1   flail chest (S22.5)
  - X S28.1   Traumatic amputation (partial) of part of thorax, except breast
  - S28.2   Traumatic amputation of breast
    - S28.21   Complete traumatic amputation of breast
      - Traumatic amputation of breast NOS
      - S28.211   Complete traumatic amputation of right breast
      - S28.212   Complete traumatic amputation of left breast
      - S28.219   Complete traumatic amputation of unspecified breast
    - S28.22   Partial traumatic amputation of breast
      - S28.221   Partial traumatic amputation of right breast
      - S28.222   Partial traumatic amputation of left breast
      - S28.229   Partial traumatic amputation of unspecified breast

- S29   Other and unspecified injuries of thorax

  Code also any associated open wound (S21.-)

  The appropriate 7th character is to be added to each code from category S29

  > A   initial encounter
  > D   subsequent encounter
  > S   sequela

  - S29.0   Injury of muscle and tendon at thorax level
    - S29.00   Unspecified injury of muscle and tendon of thorax
      - S29.001   Unspecified injury of muscle and tendon of front wall of thorax
      - S29.002   Unspecified injury of muscle and tendon of back wall of thorax
      - S29.009   Unspecified injury of muscle and tendon of unspecified wall of thorax
    - S29.01   Strain of muscle and tendon of thorax
      - S29.011   Strain of muscle and tendon of front wall of thorax
      - S29.012   Strain of muscle and tendon of back wall of thorax
      - S29.019   Strain of muscle and tendon of unspecified wall of thorax
    - S29.02   Laceration of muscle and tendon of thorax
      - S29.021   Laceration of muscle and tendon of front wall of thorax
      - S29.022   Laceration of muscle and tendon of back wall of thorax
      - S29.029   Laceration of muscle and tendon of unspecified wall of thorax
    - S29.09   Other injury of muscle and tendon of thorax
      - S29.091   Other injury of muscle and tendon of front wall of thorax
      - S29.092   Other injury of muscle and tendon of back wall of thorax
      - S29.099   Other injury of muscle and tendon of unspecified wall of thorax
  - X S29.8   Other specified injuries of thorax
  - X S29.9   Unspecified injury of thorax

INJURIES TO THE ABDOMEN, LOWER BACK, LUMBAR SPINE PELVIS AND EXTERNAL GENITALS (S30-S39)

Includes   injuries to the abdominal wall
injuries to the anus
injuries to the buttock
injuries to the external genitalia
injuries to the flank
injuries to the groin

Excludes2   burns and corrosions (T20-T32)
effects of foreign body in anus and rectum (T18.5)
effects of foreign body in genitourinary tract (T19.-)
effects of foreign body in stomach, small intestine and colon (T18.2-T18.4)
frostbite (T33-T34)
insect bite or sting, venomous (T63.4)

- S30   Superficial injury of abdomen, lower back, pelvis and external genitals

  Excludes2   superficial injury of hip (S70.-)

  The appropriate 7th character is to be added to each code from category S30

  > A   initial encounter
  > D   subsequent encounter
  > S   sequela

  - X S30.0   Contusion of lower back and pelvis
    - Contusion of buttock
  - X S30.1   Contusion of abdominal wall
    - ~~Contusion of flank~~
    - ~~Contusion of groin~~
    - ▶ S30.11   Contusion of abdominal wall
    - ▶ S30.12   Contusion of groin
    - ▶ S30.13   Contusion of flank (latus) region
  - S30.2   Contusion of external genital organs
    - S30.20   Contusion of unspecified external genital organ
      - S30.201   Contusion of unspecified external genital organ, male
      - S30.202   Contusion of unspecified external genital organ, female
    - X S30.21   Contusion of penis
    - X S30.22   Contusion of scrotum and testes
    - X S30.23   Contusion of vagina and vulva
  - X S30.3   Contusion of anus

▶ New   ⇨ Revised   ~~deleted~~ Deleted   Excludes 1   Excludes 2   Includes   Use additional   Code first   Code also   Key words
OGCR Official Guidelines   X Assign placeholder X   ● Use Additional Character(s)   ▶ Manifestation Code   Hierarchical Condition Category   Coding Clinic

● **S30.8** **Other superficial injuries of abdomen, lower back, pelvis and external genitals**
  ● **S30.81** **Abrasion of abdomen, lower back, pelvis and external genitals**
    ● **S30.810** Abrasion of lower back and pelvis
    ● **S30.811** Abrasion of abdominal wall
    ● **S30.812** Abrasion of penis
    ● **S30.813** Abrasion of scrotum and testes
    ● **S30.814** Abrasion of vagina and vulva
    ● **S30.815** Abrasion of unspecified external genital organs, male
    ● **S30.816** Abrasion of unspecified external genital organs, female
    ● **S30.817** Abrasion of anus
    ▶ ● **S30.81A** Abrasion of flank
  ● **S30.82** **Blister (nonthermal) of abdomen, lower back, pelvis and external genitals**
    ● **S30.820** Blister (nonthermal) of lower back and pelvis
    ● **S30.821** Blister (nonthermal) of abdominal wall
    ● **S30.822** Blister (nonthermal) of penis
    ● **S30.823** Blister (nonthermal) of scrotum and testes
    ● **S30.824** Blister (nonthermal) of vagina and vulva
    ● **S30.825** Blister (nonthermal) of unspecified external genital organs, male
    ● **S30.826** Blister (nonthermal) of unspecified external genital organs, female
    ● **S30.827** Blister (nonthermal) of anus
    ▶ ● **S30.82A** Blister (nonthermal) of flank
  ● **S30.84** **External constriction of abdomen, lower back, pelvis and external genitals**
    ● **S30.840** External constriction of lower back and pelvis
    ● **S30.841** External constriction of abdominal wall
    ● **S30.842** External constriction of penis
      Hair tourniquet syndrome of penis
      Use additional cause code to identify the constricting item (W49.0-)
    ● **S30.843** External constriction of scrotum and testes
    ● **S30.844** External constriction of vagina and vulva
    ● **S30.845** External constriction of unspecified external genital organs, male
    ● **S30.846** External constriction of unspecified external genital organs, female
    ▶ ● **S30.84A** External constriction of flank
  ● **S30.85** **Superficial foreign body of abdomen, lower back, pelvis and external genitals**
      Splinter in the abdomen, lower back, pelvis and external genitals
    ● **S30.850** Superficial foreign body of lower back and pelvis
    ● **S30.851** Superficial foreign body of abdominal wall
    ● **S30.852** Superficial foreign body of penis
    ● **S30.853** Superficial foreign body of scrotum and testes
    ● **S30.854** Superficial foreign body of vagina and vulva

    ● **S30.855** Superficial foreign body of unspecified external genital organs, male
    ● **S30.856** Superficial foreign body of unspecified external genital organs, female
    ● **S30.857** Superficial foreign body of anus
    ▶ ● **S30.85A** Superficial foreign body of flank
  ● **S30.86** **Insect bite (nonvenomous) of abdomen, lower back, pelvis and external genitals**
    ● **S30.860** Insect bite (nonvenomous) of lower back and pelvis
    ● **S30.861** Insect bite (nonvenomous) of abdominal wall
    ● **S30.862** Insect bite (nonvenomous) of penis
    ● **S30.863** Insect bite (nonvenomous) of scrotum and testes
    ● **S30.864** Insect bite (nonvenomous) of vagina and vulva
    ● **S30.865** Insect bite (nonvenomous) of unspecified external genital organs, male
    ● **S30.866** Insect bite (nonvenomous) of unspecified external genital organs, female
    ● **S30.867** Insect bite (nonvenomous) of anus
    ▶ ● **S30.86A** Insect bite (nonvenomous) of flank
  ● **S30.87** **Other superficial bite of abdomen, lower back, pelvis and external genitals**
    Excludes1   open bite of abdomen, lower back, pelvis and external genitals (S31.05, S31.15, S31.25, S31.35, S31.45, S31.55)
    ● **S30.870** Other superficial bite of lower back and pelvis
    ● **S30.871** Other superficial bite of abdominal wall
    ● **S30.872** Other superficial bite of penis
    ● **S30.873** Other superficial bite of scrotum and testes
    ● **S30.874** Other superficial bite of vagina and vulva
    ● **S30.875** Other superficial bite of unspecified external genital organs, male
    ● **S30.876** Other superficial bite of unspecified external genital organs, female
    ● **S30.877** Other superficial bite of anus
    ▶ ● **S30.87A** Other superficial bite of flank
  ● **S30.9** **Unspecified superficial injury of abdomen, lower back, pelvis and external genitals**
    X ● **S30.91** Unspecified superficial injury of lower back and pelvis
    X ● **S30.92** Unspecified superficial injury of abdominal wall
    X ● **S30.93** Unspecified superficial injury of penis
    X ● **S30.94** Unspecified superficial injury of scrotum and testes
    X ● **S30.95** Unspecified superficial injury of vagina and vulva
    X ● **S30.96** Unspecified superficial injury of unspecified external genital organs, male
    X ● **S30.97** Unspecified superficial injury of unspecified external genital organs, female
    X ● **S30.98** Unspecified superficial injury of anus
    ▶ X ● **S30.9A** Unspecified superficial injury of flank

CHAPTER 19 (S00-T88)

● **S31 Open wound of abdomen, lower back, pelvis and external genitals**

Code also any associated:
spinal cord injury (S24.0, S24.1-, S34.0-, S34.1-)
wound infection

Excludes1 traumatic amputation of part of abdomen, lower back and pelvis (S38.2-, S38.3)

Excludes2 open wound of hip (S71.00-S71.02)
open fracture of pelvis (S32.1--S32.9 with 7th character B)

The appropriate 7th character is to be added to each code from category S31

> A   initial encounter
> D   subsequent encounter
> S   sequela

● **S31.0 Open wound of lower back and pelvis**

● **S31.00 Unspecified open wound of lower back and pelvis**

● **S31.000 Unspecified open wound of lower back and pelvis without penetration into retroperitoneum**
Unspecified open wound of lower back and pelvis NOS

● **S31.001 Unspecified open wound of lower back and pelvis with penetration into retroperitoneum**

● **S31.01 Laceration without foreign body of lower back and pelvis**

● **S31.010 Laceration without foreign body of lower back and pelvis without penetration into retroperitoneum**
Laceration without foreign body of lower back and pelvis NOS

● **S31.011 Laceration without foreign body of lower back and pelvis with penetration into retroperitoneum**

● **S31.02 Laceration with foreign body of lower back and pelvis**

● **S31.020 Laceration with foreign body of lower back and pelvis without penetration into retroperitoneum**
Laceration with foreign body of lower back and pelvis NOS

● **S31.021 Laceration with foreign body of lower back and pelvis with penetration into retroperitoneum**

● **S31.03 Puncture wound without foreign body of lower back and pelvis**

● **S31.030 Puncture wound without foreign body of lower back and pelvis without penetration into retroperitoneum**
Puncture wound without foreign body of lower back and pelvis NOS

● **S31.031 Puncture wound without foreign body of lower back and pelvis with penetration into retroperitoneum**

● **S31.04 Puncture wound with foreign body of lower back and pelvis**

● **S31.040 Puncture wound with foreign body of lower back and pelvis without penetration into retroperitoneum**
Puncture wound with foreign body of lower back and pelvis NOS

● **S31.041 Puncture wound with foreign body of lower back and pelvis with penetration into retroperitoneum**

● **S31.05 Open bite of lower back and pelvis**
Bite of lower back and pelvis NOS

Excludes1 superficial bite of lower back and pelvis (S30.860, S30.870)

● **S31.050 Open bite of lower back and pelvis without penetration into retroperitoneum**
Open bite of lower back and pelvis NOS

● **S31.051 Open bite of lower back and pelvis with penetration into retroperitoneum**

● **S31.1 Open wound of abdominal wall without penetration into peritoneal cavity**
Open wound of abdominal wall NOS

Excludes2 open wound of abdominal wall with penetration into peritoneal cavity (S31.6-)

● **S31.10 Unspecified open wound of abdominal wall without penetration into peritoneal cavity**

● **S31.100 Unspecified open wound of abdominal wall, right upper quadrant without penetration into peritoneal cavity**

● **S31.101 Unspecified open wound of abdominal wall, left upper quadrant without penetration into peritoneal cavity**

● **S31.102 Unspecified open wound of abdominal wall, epigastric region without penetration into peritoneal cavity**

● **S31.103 Unspecified open wound of abdominal wall, right lower quadrant without penetration into peritoneal cavity**

● **S31.104 Unspecified open wound of abdominal wall, left lower quadrant without penetration into peritoneal cavity**

● **S31.105 Unspecified open wound of abdominal wall, periumbilic region without penetration into peritoneal cavity**

▶● **S31.106 Unspecified open wound of abdominal wall, right flank without penetration into peritoneal cavity**

▶● **S31.107 Unspecified open wound of abdominal wall, left flank without penetration into peritoneal cavity**

● **S31.109 Unspecified open wound of abdominal wall, unspecified quadrant without penetration into peritoneal cavity**
Unspecified open wound of abdominal wall NOS

▶● **S31.10A Unspecified open wound of abdominal wall, unspecified flank without penetration into peritoneal cavity**
▶Open wound of abdominal wall of flank NOS without penetration into peritoneal cavity

● **S31.11 Laceration without foreign body of abdominal wall without penetration into peritoneal cavity**

● **S31.110 Laceration without foreign body of abdominal wall, right upper quadrant without penetration into peritoneal cavity**

● **S31.111 Laceration without foreign body of abdominal wall, left upper quadrant without penetration into peritoneal cavity**

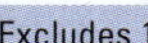

▶ New   ⇒ Revised   ~~deleted~~ Deleted   Excludes 1   Excludes 2   Includes   Use additional   Code first   Code also   Key words
OGCR Official Guidelines   X Assign placeholder X   ● Use Additional Character(s)   ▶ Manifestation Code   Hierarchical Condition Category   Coding Clinic

● S31.112   Laceration without foreign body of abdominal wall, epigastric region without penetration into peritoneal cavity

● S31.113   Laceration without foreign body of abdominal wall, right lower quadrant without penetration into peritoneal cavity

● S31.114   Laceration without foreign body of abdominal wall, left lower quadrant without penetration into peritoneal cavity

● S31.115   Laceration without foreign body of abdominal wall, periumbilic region without penetration into peritoneal cavity

▶ ● S31.116   Laceration without foreign body of abdominal wall, right flank without penetration into peritoneal cavity

▶ ● S31.117   Laceration without foreign body of abdominal wall, left flank without penetration into peritoneal cavity

● S31.119   Laceration without foreign body of abdominal wall, unspecified quadrant without penetration into peritoneal cavity

▶ ● SS31.11A   Laceration without foreign body of abdominal wall, unspecified flank without penetration into peritoneal cavity
    ▶ Laceration without foreign body of flank NOS without penetration into peritoneal cavity [new]

● S31.12   **Laceration with foreign body of abdominal wall without penetration into peritoneal cavity**

● S31.120   Laceration of abdominal wall with foreign body, right upper quadrant without penetration into peritoneal cavity

● S31.121   Laceration of abdominal wall with foreign body, left upper quadrant without penetration into peritoneal cavity

● S31.122   Laceration of abdominal wall with foreign body, epigastric region without penetration into peritoneal cavity

● S31.123   Laceration of abdominal wall with foreign body, right lower quadrant without penetration into peritoneal cavity

● S31.124   Laceration of abdominal wall with foreign body, left lower quadrant without penetration into peritoneal cavity

● S31.125   Laceration of abdominal wall with foreign body, periumbilic region without penetration into peritoneal cavity

▶ ● S31.126   Laceration with foreign body of abdominal wall, right flank without penetration into peritoneal cavity

▶ ● S31.127   Laceration with foreign body of abdominal wall, left flank without penetration into peritoneal cavity

● S31.129   Laceration of abdominal wall with foreign body, unspecified quadrant without penetration into peritoneal cavity

▶ ● S31.12A   Laceration with foreign body of abdominal wall unspecified flank without penetration into peritoneal cavity
    ▶ Laceration with foreign body of abdominal wall of flank NOS without penetration into peritoneal cavity

● S31.13   **Puncture wound of abdominal wall without foreign body without penetration into peritoneal cavity**

● S31.130   Puncture wound of abdominal wall without foreign body, right upper quadrant without penetration into peritoneal cavity

● S31.131   Puncture wound of abdominal wall without foreign body, left upper quadrant without penetration into peritoneal cavity

● S31.132   Puncture wound of abdominal wall without foreign body, epigastric region without penetration into peritoneal cavity

● S31.133   Puncture wound of abdominal wall without foreign body, right lower quadrant without penetration into peritoneal cavity

● S31.134   Puncture wound of abdominal wall without foreign body, left lower quadrant without penetration into peritoneal cavity

● S31.135   Puncture wound of abdominal wall without foreign body, periumbilic region without penetration into peritoneal cavity

▶ ● S31.136   Puncture wound of abdominal wall without foreign body, right flank without penetration into peritoneal cavity

▶ ● S31.137   Puncture wound of abdominal wall without foreign body, left flank without penetration into peritoneal cavity

● S31.139   Puncture wound of abdominal wall without foreign body, unspecified quadrant without penetration into peritoneal cavity

▶ ● S31.13A   Puncture wound of abdominal wall without foreign body, unspecified flank without penetration into peritoneal cavity
    ▶ Puncture wound of abdominal wall of flank NOS without foreign body

● S31.14   **Puncture wound of abdominal wall with foreign body without penetration into peritoneal cavity**

● S31.140   Puncture wound of abdominal wall with foreign body, right upper quadrant without penetration into peritoneal cavity

● S31.141   Puncture wound of abdominal wall with foreign body, left upper quadrant without penetration into peritoneal cavity

● S31.142   Puncture wound of abdominal wall with foreign body, epigastric region without penetration into peritoneal cavity

● S31.143   Puncture wound of abdominal wall with foreign body, right lower quadrant without penetration into peritoneal cavity

- ● **S31.144** Puncture wound of abdominal wall with foreign body, left lower quadrant without penetration into peritoneal cavity
- ● **S31.145** Puncture wound of abdominal wall with foreign body, periumbilic region without penetration into peritoneal cavity
- ▶● **S31.146** Puncture wound of abdominal wall with foreign body, right flank without penetration into peritoneal cavity
- ▶● **S31.147** Puncture wound of abdominal wall with foreign body, left flank without penetration into peritoneal cavity
- ● **S31.149** Puncture wound of abdominal wall with foreign body, unspecified quadrant without penetration into peritoneal cavity
- ▶● **S31.14A** Puncture wound of abdominal wall with foreign body, unspecified flank without penetration into peritoneal cavity
  - ▶ Puncture wound of abdominal wall with foreign body of flank NOS without penetration into peritoneal cavity
- ● **S31.15** **Open bite of abdominal wall without penetration into peritoneal cavity**
  Bite of abdominal wall NOS

  Excludes1   superficial bite of abdominal wall (S30.871)

  - ● **S31.150** Open bite of abdominal wall, right upper quadrant without penetration into peritoneal cavity
  - ● **S31.151** Open bite of abdominal wall, left upper quadrant without penetration into peritoneal cavity
  - ● **S31.152** Open bite of abdominal wall, epigastric region without penetration into peritoneal cavity
  - ● **S31.153** Open bite of abdominal wall, right lower quadrant without penetration into peritoneal cavity
  - ● **S31.154** Open bite of abdominal wall, left lower quadrant without penetration into peritoneal cavity
  - ● **S31.155** Open bite of abdominal wall, periumbilic region without penetration into peritoneal cavity
  - ▶● **S31.156** Open bite of abdominal wall, right flank without penetration into peritoneal cavity
  - ▶● **S31.157** Open bite of abdominal wall, left flank without penetration into peritoneal cavity
  - ● **S31.159** Open bite of abdominal wall, unspecified quadrant without penetration into peritoneal cavity
  - ▶● **S31.15A** Open bite of abdominal wall, unspecified flank without penetration into peritoneal cavity
    - ▶ Open bite of abdominal wall of flank NOS without penetration into peritoneal cavity
- ● **S31.2** **Open wound of penis**
  - X● **S31.20** **Unspecified open wound of penis**
  - X● **S31.21** **Laceration without foreign body of penis**
  - X● **S31.22** **Laceration with foreign body of penis**
  - X● **S31.23** **Puncture wound without foreign body of penis**
  - X● **S31.24** **Puncture wound with foreign body of penis**
  - X● **S31.25** **Open bite of penis**
    Bite of penis NOS

    Excludes1   superficial bite of penis (S30.862, S30.872)

- ● **S31.3** **Open wound of scrotum and testes**
  - X● **S31.30** Unspecified open wound of scrotum and testes
  - X● **S31.31** Laceration without foreign body of scrotum and testes
  - X● **S31.32** Laceration with foreign body of scrotum and testes
  - X● **S31.33** Puncture wound without foreign body of scrotum and testes
  - X● **S31.34** Puncture wound with foreign body of scrotum and testes
  - X● **S31.35** Open bite of scrotum and testes
    Bite of scrotum and testes NOS

    Excludes1   superficial bite of scrotum and testes (S30.863, S30.873)

- ● **S31.4** **Open wound of vagina and vulva**

  Excludes1   injury to vagina and vulva during delivery (O70.-, O71.4)

  - X● **S31.40** Unspecified open wound of vagina and vulva
  - X● **S31.41** Laceration without foreign body of vagina and vulva
  - X● **S31.42** Laceration with foreign body of vagina and vulva
  - X● **S31.43** Puncture wound without foreign body of vagina and vulva
  - X● **S31.44** Puncture wound with foreign body of vagina and vulva
  - X● **S31.45** Open bite of vagina and vulva
    Bite of vagina and vulva NOS

    Excludes1   superficial bite of vagina and vulva (S30.864, S30.874)

- ● **S31.5** **Open wound of unspecified external genital organs**

  Excludes1   traumatic amputation of external genital organs (S38.21, S38.22)

  - ● **S31.50** Unspecified open wound of unspecified external genital organs
    - ● **S31.501** Unspecified open wound of unspecified external genital organs, male
    - ● **S31.502** Unspecified open wound of unspecified external genital organs, female
  - ● **S31.51** Laceration without foreign body of unspecified external genital organs
    - ● **S31.511** Laceration without foreign body of unspecified external genital organs, male
    - ● **S31.512** Laceration without foreign body of unspecified external genital organs, female
  - ● **S31.52** Laceration with foreign body of unspecified external genital organs
    - ● **S31.521** Laceration with foreign body of unspecified external genital organs, male
    - ● **S31.522** Laceration with foreign body of unspecified external genital organs, female
  - ● **S31.53** Puncture wound without foreign body of unspecified external genital organs
    - ● **S31.531** Puncture wound without foreign body of unspecified external genital organs, male
    - ● **S31.532** Puncture wound without foreign body of unspecified external genital organs, female
  - ● **S31.54** Puncture wound with foreign body of unspecified external genital organs
    - ● **S31.541** Puncture wound with foreign body of unspecified external genital organs, male

● **S31.542**   **Puncture wound with foreign body of unspecified external genital organs, female**

● **S31.55**   **Open bite of unspecified external genital organs**

Bite of unspecified external genital organs NOS

Excludes1   superficial bite of unspecified external genital organs (S30.865, S30.866, S30.875, S30.876)

● **S31.551**   **Open bite of unspecified external genital organs, male**

● **S31.552**   **Open bite of unspecified external genital organs, female**

● **S31.6**   **Open wound of abdominal wall with penetration into peritoneal cavity**

Coding Clinic: 2023, Q3, P9

● **S31.60**   **Unspecified open wound of abdominal wall with penetration into peritoneal cavity**

● **S31.600**   **Unspecified open wound of abdominal wall, right upper quadrant with penetration into peritoneal cavity**

● **S31.601**   **Unspecified open wound of abdominal wall, left upper quadrant with penetration into peritoneal cavity**

● **S31.602**   **Unspecified open wound of abdominal wall, epigastric region with penetration into peritoneal cavity**

● **S31.603**   **Unspecified open wound of abdominal wall, right lower quadrant with penetration into peritoneal cavity**

● **S31.604**   **Unspecified open wound of abdominal wall, left lower quadrant with penetration into peritoneal cavity**

● **S31.605**   **Unspecified open wound of abdominal wall, periumbilic region with penetration into peritoneal cavity**

▶ ● **S31.606**   **Unspecified open wound of abdominal wall, right flank with penetration into peritoneal cavity**

▶ ● **S31.607**   **Unspecified open wound of abdominal wall, left flank with penetration into peritoneal cavity**

● **S31.609**   **Unspecified open wound of abdominal wall, unspecified quadrant with penetration into peritoneal cavity**

▶ ● **S31.60A**   **Unspecified open wound of abdominal wall, unspecified flank with penetration into peritoneal cavity**

▶ Unspecified open wound of abdominal wall of flank NOS, with penetration into peritoneal cavity

● **S31.61**   **Laceration without foreign body of abdominal wall with penetration into peritoneal cavity**

● **S31.610**   **Laceration without foreign body of abdominal wall, right upper quadrant with penetration into peritoneal cavity**

● **S31.611**   **Laceration without foreign body of abdominal wall, left upper quadrant with penetration into peritoneal cavity**

● **S31.612**   **Laceration without foreign body of abdominal wall, epigastric region with penetration into peritoneal cavity**

● **S31.613**   **Laceration without foreign body of abdominal wall, right lower quadrant with penetration into peritoneal cavity**

Coding Clinic: 2015, Q4, P37

● **S31.614**   **Laceration without foreign body of abdominal wall, left lower quadrant with penetration into peritoneal cavity**

● **S31.615**   **Laceration without foreign body of abdominal wall, periumbilic region with penetration into peritoneal cavity**

▶ ● **S31.616**   **Laceration without foreign body of abdominal wall, right flank with penetration into peritoneal cavity**

▶ ● **S31.617**   **Laceration without foreign body of abdominal wall, left flank with penetration into peritoneal cavity**

● **S31.619**   **Laceration without foreign body of abdominal wall, unspecified quadrant with penetration into peritoneal cavity**

▶ ● **S31.61A**   **Laceration without foreign body of abdominal wall, unspecified flank with penetration into peritoneal cavity**

▶ Laceration without foreign body of abdominal wall of flank NOS, with penetration into peritoneal cavity

● **S31.62**   **Laceration with foreign body of abdominal wall with penetration into peritoneal cavity**

● **S31.620**   **Laceration with foreign body of abdominal wall, right upper quadrant with penetration into peritoneal cavity**

● **S31.621**   **Laceration with foreign body of abdominal wall, left upper quadrant with penetration into peritoneal cavity**

● **S31.622**   **Laceration with foreign body of abdominal wall, epigastric region with penetration into peritoneal cavity**

● **S31.623**   **Laceration with foreign body of abdominal wall, right lower quadrant with penetration into peritoneal cavity**

● **S31.624**   **Laceration with foreign body of abdominal wall, left lower quadrant with penetration into peritoneal cavity**

● **S31.625**   **Laceration with foreign body of abdominal wall, periumbilic region with penetration into peritoneal cavity**

▶ ● **S31.626**   **Laceration with foreign body of abdominal wall, right flank with penetration into peritoneal cavity**

▶ ● **S31.627**   **Laceration with foreign body of abdominal wall, left flank with penetration into peritoneal cavity**

● **S31.629**   **Laceration with foreign body of abdominal wall, unspecified quadrant with penetration into peritoneal cavity**

▶ ● **S31.62A**   **Laceration with foreign body of abdominal wall, unspecified flank with penetration into peritoneal cavity**

▶ Laceration with foreign body of abdominal wall, flank NOS, with penetration into peritoneal cavity

CHAPTER 19 (S00–T88)

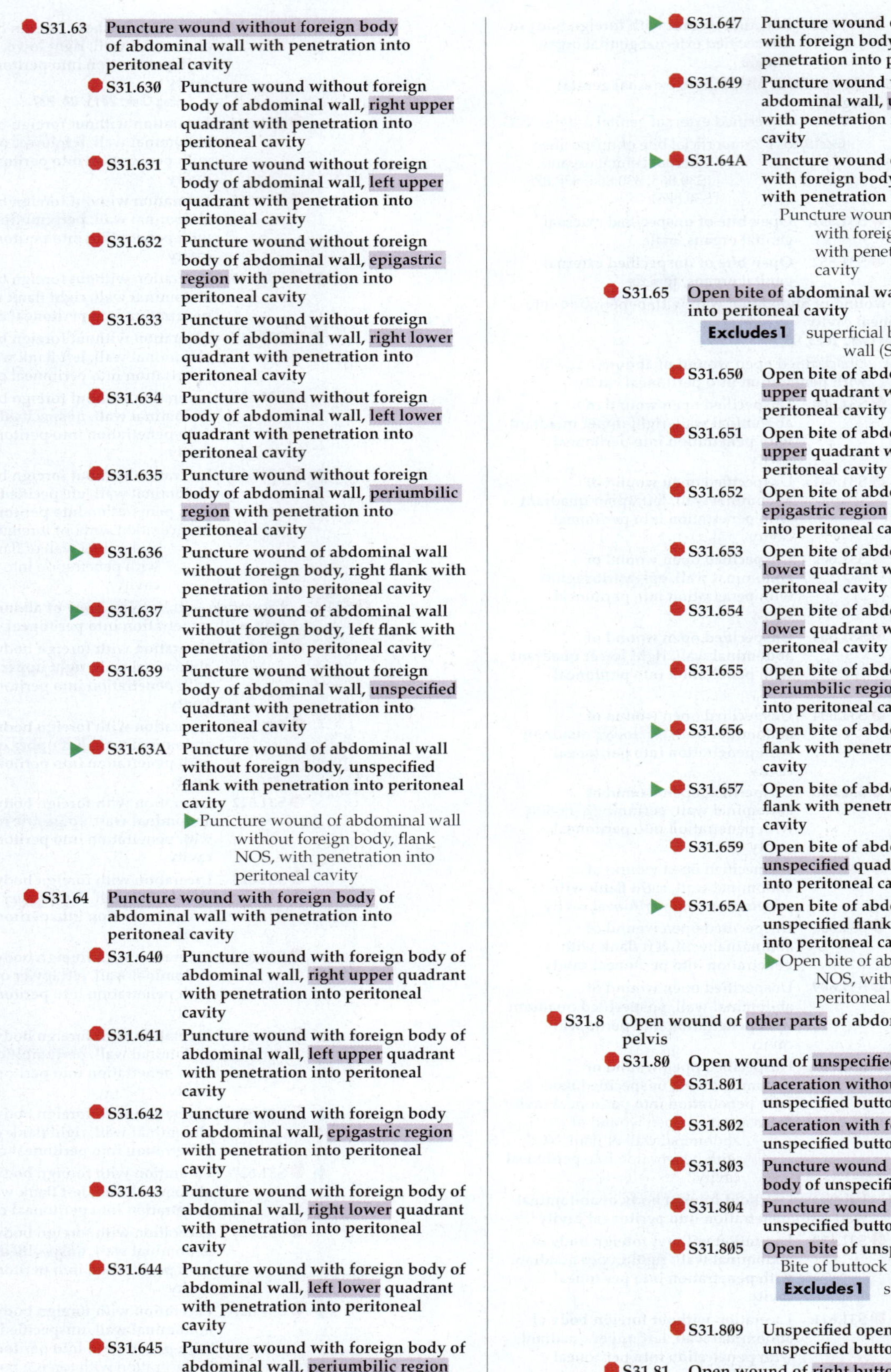

● **S31.63** Puncture wound without foreign body of abdominal wall with penetration into peritoneal cavity

● **S31.630** Puncture wound without foreign body of abdominal wall, right upper quadrant with penetration into peritoneal cavity

● **S31.631** Puncture wound without foreign body of abdominal wall, left upper quadrant with penetration into peritoneal cavity

● **S31.632** Puncture wound without foreign body of abdominal wall, epigastric region with penetration into peritoneal cavity

● **S31.633** Puncture wound without foreign body of abdominal wall, right lower quadrant with penetration into peritoneal cavity

● **S31.634** Puncture wound without foreign body of abdominal wall, left lower quadrant with penetration into peritoneal cavity

● **S31.635** Puncture wound without foreign body of abdominal wall, periumbilic region with penetration into peritoneal cavity

▶ ● **S31.636** Puncture wound of abdominal wall without foreign body, right flank with penetration into peritoneal cavity

▶ ● **S31.637** Puncture wound of abdominal wall without foreign body, left flank with penetration into peritoneal cavity

● **S31.639** Puncture wound without foreign body of abdominal wall, unspecified quadrant with penetration into peritoneal cavity

▶ ● **S31.63A** Puncture wound of abdominal wall without foreign body, unspecified flank with penetration into peritoneal cavity
▶ Puncture wound of abdominal wall without foreign body, flank NOS, with penetration into peritoneal cavity

● **S31.64** Puncture wound with foreign body of abdominal wall with penetration into peritoneal cavity

● **S31.640** Puncture wound with foreign body of abdominal wall, right upper quadrant with penetration into peritoneal cavity

● **S31.641** Puncture wound with foreign body of abdominal wall, left upper quadrant with penetration into peritoneal cavity

● **S31.642** Puncture wound with foreign body of abdominal wall, epigastric region with penetration into peritoneal cavity

● **S31.643** Puncture wound with foreign body of abdominal wall, right lower quadrant with penetration into peritoneal cavity

● **S31.644** Puncture wound with foreign body of abdominal wall, left lower quadrant with penetration into peritoneal cavity

● **S31.645** Puncture wound with foreign body of abdominal wall, periumbilic region with penetration into peritoneal cavity

▶ ● **S31.646** Puncture wound of abdominal wall with foreign body, right flank with penetration into peritoneal cavity

▶ ● **S31.647** Puncture wound of abdominal wall with foreign body, left flank with penetration into peritoneal cavity

● **S31.649** Puncture wound with foreign body of abdominal wall, unspecified quadrant with penetration into peritoneal cavity

▶ ● **S31.64A** Puncture wound of abdominal wall with foreign body, unspecified flank with penetration into peritoneal cavity
Puncture wound of abdominal wall with foreign body, flank NOS, with penetration into peritoneal cavity

● **S31.65** Open bite of abdominal wall with penetration into peritoneal cavity
Excludes1   superficial bite of abdominal wall (S30.861, S30.871)

● **S31.650** Open bite of abdominal wall, right upper quadrant with penetration into peritoneal cavity

● **S31.651** Open bite of abdominal wall, left upper quadrant with penetration into peritoneal cavity

● **S31.652** Open bite of abdominal wall, epigastric region with penetration into peritoneal cavity

● **S31.653** Open bite of abdominal wall, right lower quadrant with penetration into peritoneal cavity

● **S31.654** Open bite of abdominal wall, left lower quadrant with penetration into peritoneal cavity

● **S31.655** Open bite of abdominal wall, periumbilic region with penetration into peritoneal cavity

▶ ● **S31.656** Open bite of abdominal wall, right flank with penetration into peritoneal cavity

▶ ● **S31.657** Open bite of abdominal wall, left flank with penetration into peritoneal cavity

● **S31.659** Open bite of abdominal wall, unspecified quadrant with penetration into peritoneal cavity

▶ ● **S31.65A** Open bite of abdominal wall, unspecified flank with penetration into peritoneal cavity
▶ Open bite of abdominal wall, flank NOS, with penetration into peritoneal cavity

● **S31.8** Open wound of other parts of abdomen, lower back and pelvis

● **S31.80** Open wound of unspecified buttock

● **S31.801** Laceration without foreign body of unspecified buttock

● **S31.802** Laceration with foreign body of unspecified buttock

● **S31.803** Puncture wound without foreign body of unspecified buttock

● **S31.804** Puncture wound with foreign body of unspecified buttock

● **S31.805** Open bite of unspecified buttock
Bite of buttock NOS
Excludes1   superficial bite of buttock (S30.870)

● **S31.809** Unspecified open wound of unspecified buttock

● **S31.81** Open wound of right buttock

● **S31.811** Laceration without foreign body of right buttock

● **S31.812** Laceration with foreign body of right buttock

▶ New ▶ Revised ~~deleted~~ Deleted Excludes 1 Excludes 2 Includes Use additional Code first Code also Key words
OGCR Official Guidelines **X** Assign placeholder X ● Use Additional Character(s) ▸ Manifestation Code ℟ Hierarchical Condition Category **Coding Clinic**

● **S31.813**   **Puncture wound without foreign body of right buttock**

● **S31.814**   **Puncture wound with foreign body of right buttock**

● **S31.815**   **Open bite of right buttock**
Bite of right buttock NOS
Excludes1   superficial bite of buttock (S30.870)

● **S31.819**   **Unspecified open wound of right buttock**

● **S31.82**   **Open wound of left buttock**

● **S31.821**   **Laceration without foreign body of left buttock**

● **S31.822**   **Laceration with foreign body of left buttock**

● **S31.823**   **Puncture wound without foreign body of left buttock**

● **S31.824**   **Puncture wound with foreign body of left buttock**

● **S31.825**   **Open bite of left buttock**
Bite of left buttock NOS
Excludes1   superficial bite of buttock (S30.870)

● **S31.829**   **Unspecified open wound of left buttock**

● **S31.83**   **Open wound of anus**

● **S31.831**   **Laceration without foreign body of anus**

● **S31.832**   **Laceration with foreign body of anus**

● **S31.833**   **Puncture wound without foreign body of anus**

● **S31.834**   **Puncture wound with foreign body of anus**

● **S31.835**   **Open bite of anus**
Bite of anus NOS
Excludes1   superficial bite of anus (S30.877)

● **S31.839**   **Unspecified open wound of anus**

● **S32**   **Fracture of lumbar spine and pelvis**
Note: A fracture not indicated as displaced or nondisplaced should be coded to displaced

A fracture not indicated as opened or closed should be coded to closed

Includes   fracture of lumbosacral neural arch
fracture of lumbosacral spinous process
fracture of lumbosacral transverse process
fracture of lumbosacral vertebra
fracture of lumbosacral vertebral arch

Code first any associated spinal cord and spinal nerve injury (S34.-)

Excludes1   transection of abdomen (S38.3)

Excludes2   fracture of hip NOS (S72.0-)

The appropriate 7th character is to be added to each code from category S32

A   initial encounter for closed fracture
B   initial encounter for open fracture
D   subsequent encounter for fracture with routine healing
G   subsequent encounter for fracture with delayed healing
K   subsequent encounter for fracture with nonunion
S   sequela

● **S32.0**   **Fracture of lumbar vertebra**
Fracture of lumbar spine NOS

● **S32.00**   **Fracture of unspecified lumbar vertebra**

● **S32.000**   **Wedge compression fracture of unspecified lumbar vertebra** A, B

● **S32.001**   **Stable burst fracture of unspecified lumbar vertebra** A, B

● **S32.002**   **Unstable burst fracture of unspecified lumbar vertebra** A, B

● **S32.008**   **Other fracture of unspecified lumbar vertebra** A, B

● **S32.009**   **Unspecified fracture of unspecified lumbar vertebra** A, B

● **S32.01**   **Fracture of first lumbar vertebra**

● **S32.010**   **Wedge compression fracture of first lumbar vertebra** A, B

● **S32.011**   **Stable burst fracture of first lumbar vertebra** A, B

● **S32.012**   **Unstable burst fracture of first lumbar vertebra** A, B

● **S32.018**   **Other fracture of first lumbar vertebra** A, B

● **S32.019**   **Unspecified fracture of first lumbar vertebra** A, B

● **S32.02**   **Fracture of second lumbar vertebra**

● **S32.020**   **Wedge compression fracture of second lumbar vertebra** A, B

● **S32.021**   **Stable burst fracture of second lumbar vertebra** A, B

● **S32.022**   **Unstable burst fracture of second lumbar vertebra** A, B

● **S32.028**   **Other fracture of second lumbar vertebra** A, B

● **S32.029**   **Unspecified fracture of second lumbar vertebra** A, B

● **S32.03**   **Fracture of third lumbar vertebra**

● **S32.030**   **Wedge compression fracture of third lumbar vertebra** A, B

● **S32.031**   **Stable burst fracture of third lumbar vertebra** A, B

● **S32.032**   **Unstable burst fracture of third lumbar vertebra** A, B

● **S32.038**   **Other fracture of third lumbar vertebra** A, B

● **S32.039**   **Unspecified fracture of third lumbar vertebra** A, B

● **S32.04**   **Fracture of fourth lumbar vertebra**

● **S32.040**   **Wedge compression fracture of fourth lumbar vertebra** A, B

● **S32.041**   **Stable burst fracture of fourth lumbar vertebra** A, B

● **S32.042**   **Unstable burst fracture of fourth lumbar vertebra** A, B

● **S32.048**   **Other fracture of fourth lumbar vertebra** A, B

● **S32.049**   **Unspecified fracture of fourth lumbar vertebra** A, B

● **S32.05**   **Fracture of fifth lumbar vertebra**

● **S32.050**   **Wedge compression fracture of fifth lumbar vertebra** A, B

● **S32.051**   **Stable burst fracture of fifth lumbar vertebra** A, B

● **S32.052**   **Unstable burst fracture of fifth lumbar vertebra** A, B

● **S32.058**   **Other fracture of fifth lumbar vertebra** A, B

● **S32.059**   **Unspecified fracture of fifth lumbar vertebra** A, B

● **S32.1**   **Fracture of sacrum**
For vertical fractures, code to most medial fracture extension

Use two codes if both a vertical and transverse fracture are present

Code also any associated fracture of pelvic ring (S32.8-)

X ● **S32.10**   **Unspecified fracture of sacrum** A, B

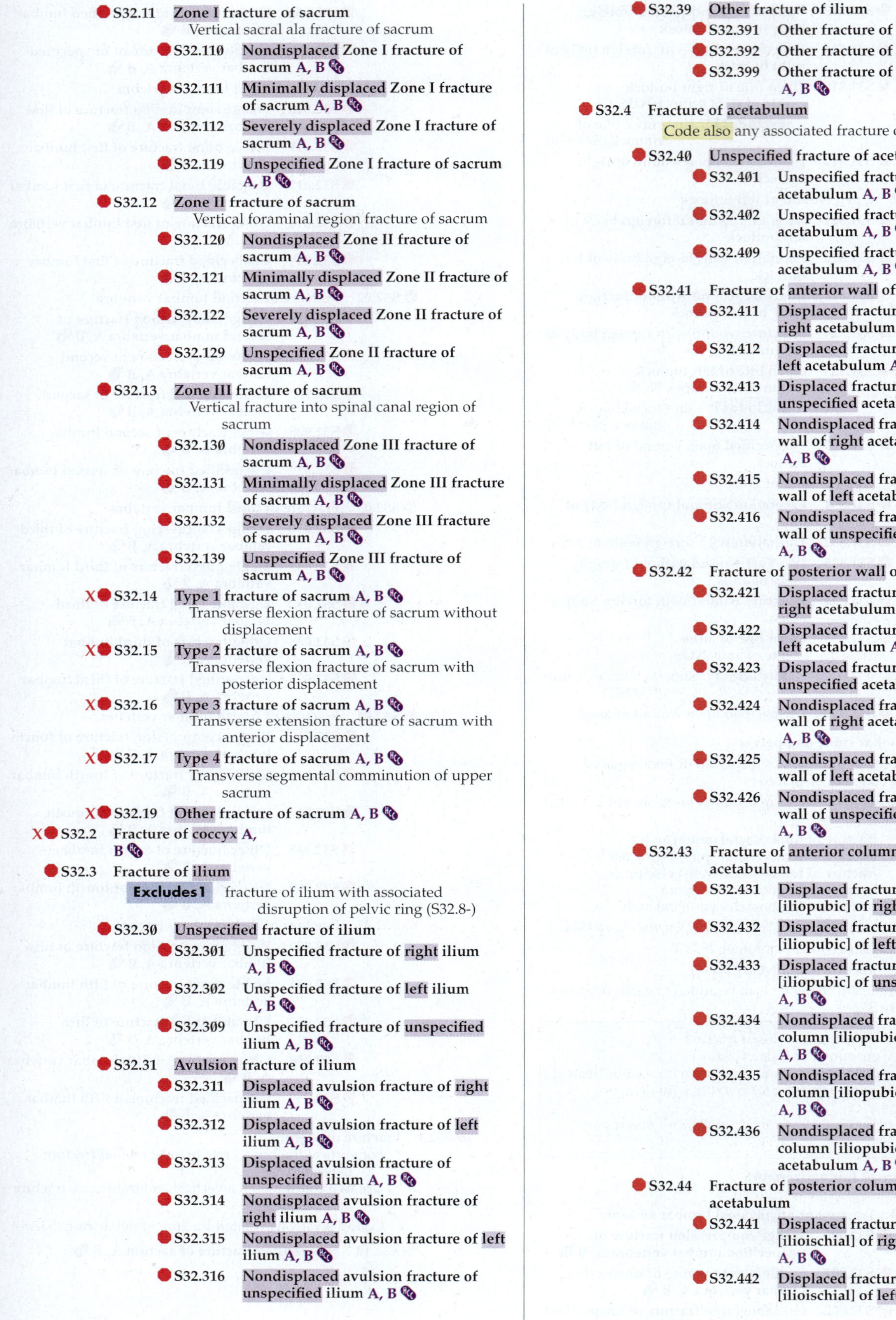

● **S32.11**   **Zone I fracture of sacrum**
Vertical sacral ala fracture of sacrum
   ● **S32.110**   **Nondisplaced Zone I fracture of sacrum A, B** 🐾
   ● **S32.111**   **Minimally displaced Zone I fracture of sacrum A, B** 🐾
   ● **S32.112**   **Severely displaced Zone I fracture of sacrum A, B** 🐾
   ● **S32.119**   **Unspecified Zone I fracture of sacrum A, B** 🐾

● **S32.12**   **Zone II fracture of sacrum**
Vertical foraminal region fracture of sacrum
   ● **S32.120**   **Nondisplaced Zone II fracture of sacrum A, B** 🐾
   ● **S32.121**   **Minimally displaced Zone II fracture of sacrum A, B** 🐾
   ● **S32.122**   **Severely displaced Zone II fracture of sacrum A, B** 🐾
   ● **S32.129**   **Unspecified Zone II fracture of sacrum A, B** 🐾

● **S32.13**   **Zone III fracture of sacrum**
Vertical fracture into spinal canal region of sacrum
   ● **S32.130**   **Nondisplaced Zone III fracture of sacrum A, B** 🐾
   ● **S32.131**   **Minimally displaced Zone III fracture of sacrum A, B** 🐾
   ● **S32.132**   **Severely displaced Zone III fracture of sacrum A, B** 🐾
   ● **S32.139**   **Unspecified Zone III fracture of sacrum A, B** 🐾

X ● **S32.14**   **Type 1 fracture of sacrum A, B** 🐾
Transverse flexion fracture of sacrum without displacement
X ● **S32.15**   **Type 2 fracture of sacrum A, B** 🐾
Transverse flexion fracture of sacrum with posterior displacement
X ● **S32.16**   **Type 3 fracture of sacrum A, B** 🐾
Transverse extension fracture of sacrum with anterior displacement
X ● **S32.17**   **Type 4 fracture of sacrum A, B** 🐾
Transverse segmental comminution of upper sacrum
X ● **S32.19**   **Other fracture of sacrum A, B** 🐾

X ● **S32.2**   **Fracture of coccyx A, B** 🐾

● **S32.3**   **Fracture of ilium**
> **Excludes1**   fracture of ilium with associated disruption of pelvic ring (S32.8-)
   ● **S32.30**   **Unspecified fracture of ilium**
    ● **S32.301**   **Unspecified fracture of right ilium A, B** 🐾
    ● **S32.302**   **Unspecified fracture of left ilium A, B** 🐾
    ● **S32.309**   **Unspecified fracture of unspecified ilium A, B** 🐾
   ● **S32.31**   **Avulsion fracture of ilium**
    ● **S32.311**   **Displaced avulsion fracture of right ilium A, B** 🐾
    ● **S32.312**   **Displaced avulsion fracture of left ilium A, B** 🐾
    ● **S32.313**   **Displaced avulsion fracture of unspecified ilium A, B** 🐾
    ● **S32.314**   **Nondisplaced avulsion fracture of right ilium A, B** 🐾
    ● **S32.315**   **Nondisplaced avulsion fracture of left ilium A, B** 🐾
    ● **S32.316**   **Nondisplaced avulsion fracture of unspecified ilium A, B** 🐾

   ● **S32.39**   **Other fracture of ilium**
    ● **S32.391**   **Other fracture of right ilium A, B** 🐾
    ● **S32.392**   **Other fracture of left ilium A, B** 🐾
    ● **S32.399**   **Other fracture of unspecified ilium A, B** 🐾

● **S32.4**   **Fracture of acetabulum**
> Code also any associated fracture of pelvic ring (S32.8-)
   ● **S32.40**   **Unspecified fracture of acetabulum**
    ● **S32.401**   **Unspecified fracture of right acetabulum A, B** 🐾
    ● **S32.402**   **Unspecified fracture of left acetabulum A, B** 🐾
    ● **S32.409**   **Unspecified fracture of unspecified acetabulum A, B** 🐾

   ● **S32.41**   **Fracture of anterior wall of acetabulum**
    ● **S32.411**   **Displaced fracture of anterior wall of right acetabulum A, B** 🐾
    ● **S32.412**   **Displaced fracture of anterior wall of left acetabulum A, B** 🐾
    ● **S32.413**   **Displaced fracture of anterior wall of unspecified acetabulum A, B** 🐾
    ● **S32.414**   **Nondisplaced fracture of anterior wall of right acetabulum A, B** 🐾
    ● **S32.415**   **Nondisplaced fracture of anterior wall of left acetabulum A, B** 🐾
    ● **S32.416**   **Nondisplaced fracture of anterior wall of unspecified acetabulum A, B** 🐾

   ● **S32.42**   **Fracture of posterior wall of acetabulum**
    ● **S32.421**   **Displaced fracture of posterior wall of right acetabulum A, B** 🐾
    ● **S32.422**   **Displaced fracture of posterior wall of left acetabulum A, B** 🐾
    ● **S32.423**   **Displaced fracture of posterior wall of unspecified acetabulum A, B** 🐾
    ● **S32.424**   **Nondisplaced fracture of posterior wall of right acetabulum A, B** 🐾
    ● **S32.425**   **Nondisplaced fracture of posterior wall of left acetabulum A, B** 🐾
    ● **S32.426**   **Nondisplaced fracture of posterior wall of unspecified acetabulum A, B** 🐾

   ● **S32.43**   **Fracture of anterior column [iliopubic] of acetabulum**
    ● **S32.431**   **Displaced fracture of anterior column [iliopubic] of right acetabulum A, B** 🐾
    ● **S32.432**   **Displaced fracture of anterior column [iliopubic] of left acetabulum A, B** 🐾
    ● **S32.433**   **Displaced fracture of anterior column [iliopubic] of unspecified acetabulum A, B** 🐾
    ● **S32.434**   **Nondisplaced fracture of anterior column [iliopubic] of right acetabulum A, B** 🐾
    ● **S32.435**   **Nondisplaced fracture of anterior column [iliopubic] of left acetabulum A, B** 🐾
    ● **S32.436**   **Nondisplaced fracture of anterior column [iliopubic] of unspecified acetabulum A, B** 🐾

   ● **S32.44**   **Fracture of posterior column [ilioischial] of acetabulum**
    ● **S32.441**   **Displaced fracture of posterior column [ilioischial] of right acetabulum A, B** 🐾
    ● **S32.442**   **Displaced fracture of posterior column [ilioischial] of left acetabulum A, B** 🐾

● S32.443   Displaced fracture of posterior column [ilioischial] of unspecified acetabulum A, B ℞

● S32.444   Nondisplaced fracture of posterior column [ilioischial] of right acetabulum A, B ℞

● S32.445   Nondisplaced fracture of posterior column [ilioischial] of left acetabulum A, B ℞

● S32.446   Nondisplaced fracture of posterior column [ilioischial] of unspecified acetabulum A, B ℞

● S32.45   Transverse fracture of acetabulum

● S32.451   Displaced transverse fracture of right acetabulum A, B ℞

● S32.452   Displaced transverse fracture of left acetabulum A, B ℞

● S32.453   Displaced transverse fracture of unspecified acetabulum A, B ℞

● S32.454   Nondisplaced transverse fracture of right acetabulum A, B ℞

● S32.455   Nondisplaced transverse fracture of left acetabulum A, B ℞

● S32.456   Nondisplaced transverse fracture of unspecified acetabulum A, B ℞

● S32.46   Associated transverse-posterior fracture of acetabulum

● S32.461   Displaced associated transverse-posterior fracture of right acetabulum A, B ℞

● S32.462   Displaced associated transverse-posterior fracture of left acetabulum A, B ℞

● S32.463   Displaced associated transverse-posterior fracture of unspecified acetabulum A, B ℞

● S32.464   Nondisplaced associated transverse-posterior fracture of right acetabulum A, B ℞

● S32.465   Nondisplaced associated transverse-posterior fracture of left acetabulum A, B ℞

● S32.466   Nondisplaced associated transverse-posterior fracture of unspecified acetabulum A, B ℞

● S32.47   Fracture of medial wall of acetabulum

● S32.471   Displaced fracture of medial wall of right acetabulum A, B ℞

● S32.472   Displaced fracture of medial wall of left acetabulum A, B ℞

● S32.473   Displaced fracture of medial wall of unspecified acetabulum A, B ℞

● S32.474   Nondisplaced fracture of medial wall of right acetabulum A, B ℞

● S32.475   Nondisplaced fracture of medial wall of left acetabulum A, B ℞

● S32.476   Nondisplaced fracture of medial wall of unspecified acetabulum A, B ℞

● S32.48   Dome fracture of acetabulum

● S32.481   Displaced dome fracture of right acetabulum A, B ℞

● S32.482   Displaced dome fracture of left acetabulum A, B ℞

● S32.483   Displaced dome fracture of unspecified acetabulum A, B ℞

● S32.484   Nondisplaced dome fracture of right acetabulum A, B ℞

● S32.485   Nondisplaced dome fracture of left acetabulum A, B ℞

● S32.486   Nondisplaced dome fracture of unspecified acetabulum A, B ℞

● S32.49   Other fracture of acetabulum

● S32.491   Other fracture of right acetabulum A, B ℞

● S32.492   Other fracture of left acetabulum A, B ℞

● S32.499   Other fracture of unspecified acetabulum A, B ℞

● S32.5   Fracture of pubis

    Excludes1   fracture of pubis with associated disruption of pelvic ring (S32.8-)

● S32.50   Unspecified fracture of pubis

● S32.501   Unspecified fracture of right pubis A, B ℞

● S32.502   Unspecified fracture of left pubis A, B ℞

● S32.509   Unspecified fracture of unspecified pubis A, B ℞

● S32.51   Fracture of superior rim of pubis

● S32.511   Fracture of superior rim of right pubis A, B ℞

● S32.512   Fracture of superior rim of left pubis A, B ℞

● S32.519   Fracture of superior rim of unspecified pubis A, B ℞

● S32.59   Other specified fracture of pubis

● S32.591   Other specified fracture of right pubis A, B ℞

● S32.592   Other specified fracture of left pubis A, B ℞

● S32.599   Other specified fracture of unspecified pubis A, B ℞

● S32.6   Fracture of ischium

    Excludes1   fracture of ischium with associated disruption of pelvic ring (S32.8-)

● S32.60   Unspecified fracture of ischium

● S32.601   Unspecified fracture of right ischium A, B ℞

● S32.602   Unspecified fracture of left ischium A, B ℞

● S32.609   Unspecified fracture of unspecified ischium A, B ℞

● S32.61   Avulsion fracture of ischium

● S32.611   Displaced avulsion fracture of right ischium A, B ℞

● S32.612   Displaced avulsion fracture of left ischium A, B ℞

● S32.613   Displaced avulsion fracture of unspecified ischium A, B ℞

● S32.614   Nondisplaced avulsion fracture of right ischium A, B ℞

● S32.615   Nondisplaced avulsion fracture of left ischium A, B ℞

● S32.616   Nondisplaced avulsion fracture of unspecified ischium A, B ℞

● S32.69   Other specified fracture of ischium

● S32.691   Other specified fracture of right ischium A, B ℞

● S32.692   Other specified fracture of left ischium A, B ℞

● S32.699   Other specified fracture of unspecified ischium A, B ℞

● **S32.8   Fracture of other parts of pelvis**
  Code also any associated:
    fracture of acetabulum (S32.4-)
    sacral fracture (S32.1-)
  ● **S32.81   Multiple fractures of pelvis with disruption of pelvic ring**
      Multiple pelvic fractures with disruption of pelvic circle
    ● **S32.810   Multiple fractures of pelvis with stable disruption of pelvic ring** A, B ⓗ
    ● **S32.811   Multiple fractures of pelvis with unstable disruption of pelvic ring** A, B ⓗ
  X ● **S32.82   Multiple fractures of pelvis without disruption of pelvic ring** A, B ⓗ
      Multiple pelvic fractures without disruption of pelvic circle
  X ● **S32.89   Fracture of other parts of pelvis** A, B ⓗ
X ● **S32.9   Fracture of unspecified parts of lumbosacral spine and pelvis** A, B ⓗ
    Fracture of lumbosacral spine NOS
    Fracture of pelvis NOS
    Coding Clinic: 2012, Q4, P93

● **S33   Dislocation and sprain of joints and ligaments of lumbar spine and pelvis**
  Includes   avulsion of joint or ligament of lumbar spine and pelvis
    laceration of cartilage, joint or ligament of lumbar spine and pelvis
    sprain of cartilage, joint or ligament of lumbar spine and pelvis
    traumatic hemarthrosis of joint or ligament of lumbar spine and pelvis
    traumatic rupture of joint or ligament of lumbar spine and pelvis
    traumatic subluxation of joint or ligament of lumbar spine and pelvis
    traumatic tear of joint or ligament of lumbar spine and pelvis
  Code also any associated open wound
  Excludes1   nontraumatic rupture or displacement of lumbar intervertebral disc NOS (M51.-)
    obstetric damage to pelvic joints and ligaments (O71.6)
  Excludes2   dislocation and sprain of joints and ligaments of hip (S73.-)
    strain of muscle of lower back and pelvis (S39.01-)

  The appropriate 7th character is to be added to each code from category S33

A	initial encounter
D	subsequent encounter
S	sequela

X ● **S33.0   Traumatic rupture of lumbar intervertebral disc**
    Excludes1   rupture or displacement (nontraumatic) of lumbar intervertebral disc NOS (M51.- with fifth character 6)
● **S33.1   Subluxation and dislocation of lumbar vertebra**
    Code also any associated:
      open wound of abdomen, lower back and pelvis (S31)
      spinal cord injury (S24.0, S24.1-, S34.0-, S34.1-)
    Excludes2   fracture of lumbar vertebrae (S32.0-)
  ● **S33.10   Subluxation and dislocation of unspecified lumbar vertebra**
    ● **S33.100   Subluxation of unspecified lumbar vertebra**
    ● **S33.101   Dislocation of unspecified lumbar vertebra**

  ● **S33.11   Subluxation and dislocation of L1/L2 lumbar vertebra**
    ● **S33.110   Subluxation of L1/L2 lumbar vertebra**
    ● **S33.111   Dislocation of L1/L2 lumbar vertebra**
  ● **S33.12   Subluxation and dislocation of L2/L3 lumbar vertebra**
    ● **S33.120   Subluxation of L2/L3 lumbar vertebra**
    ● **S33.121   Dislocation of L2/L3 lumbar vertebra**
  ● **S33.13   Subluxation and dislocation of L3/L4 lumbar vertebra**
    ● **S33.130   Subluxation of L3/L4 lumbar vertebra**
    ● **S33.131   Dislocation of L3/L4 lumbar vertebra**
  ● **S33.14   Subluxation and dislocation of L4/L5 lumbar vertebra**
    ● **S33.140   Subluxation of L4/L5 lumbar vertebra**
    ● **S33.141   Dislocation of L4/L5 lumbar vertebra**
X ● **S33.2   Dislocation of sacroiliac and sacrococcygeal joint**
● **S33.3   Dislocation of other and unspecified parts of lumbar spine and pelvis**
  X ● **S33.30   Dislocation of unspecified parts of lumbar spine and pelvis**
  X ● **S33.39   Dislocation of other parts of lumbar spine and pelvis**
X ● **S33.4   Traumatic rupture of symphysis pubis**
X ● **S33.5   Sprain of ligaments of lumbar spine**
X ● **S33.6   Sprain of sacroiliac joint**
X ● **S33.8   Sprain of other parts of lumbar spine and pelvis**
X ● **S33.9   Sprain of unspecified parts of lumbar spine and pelvis**

● **S34   Injury of lumbar and sacral spinal cord and nerves at abdomen, lower back and pelvis level**
  Note: Code to highest level of lumbar cord injury
    Injuries to the spinal cord (S34.0 and S34.1) refer to the cord level and not bone level injury, and can affect nerve roots at and below the level given.
  The appropriate 7th character is to be added to each code from category S34

A	initial encounter
D	subsequent encounter
S	sequela

  Code also any associated:
    fracture of vertebra (S22.0-, S32.0-)
    open wound of abdomen, lower back and pelvis (S31.-)
    transient paralysis (R29.5)
● **S34.0   Concussion and edema of lumbar and sacral spinal cord**
  X ● **S34.01   Concussion and edema of lumbar spinal cord** A, D, S ⓗ
  X ● **S34.02   Concussion and edema of sacral spinal cord** A, D, S ⓗ
      Concussion and edema of conus medullaris
● **S34.1   Other and unspecified injury of lumbar and sacral spinal cord**
  ● **S34.10   Unspecified injury to lumbar spinal cord**
    ● **S34.101   Unspecified injury to L_1 level of lumbar spinal cord** A, D, S ⓗ
        Unspecified injury to lumbar spinal cord level 1
    ● **S34.102   Unspecified injury to L_2 level of lumbar spinal cord** A, D, S ⓗ
        Unspecified injury to lumbar spinal cord level 2
    ● **S34.103   Unspecified injury to L_3 level of lumbar spinal cord** A, D, S ⓗ
        Unspecified injury to lumbar spinal cord level 3
    ● **S34.104   Unspecified injury to L_4 level of lumbar spinal cord** A, D, S ⓗ
        Unspecified injury to lumbar spinal cord level 4

▶ New   ➤ Revised   ~~deleted~~ Deleted   Excludes 1   Excludes 2   Includes   Use additional   Code first   Code also   Key words
OGCR Official Guidelines   X Assign placeholder X   ● Use Additional Character(s)   ▶ Manifestation Code   ⓗ Hierarchical Condition Category   **Coding Clinic**

● **S34.105** **Unspecified injury to L₅ level of lumbar spinal cord A, D, S** 🔒
  Unspecified injury to lumbar spinal cord level 5

● **S34.109** **Unspecified injury to unspecified level of lumbar spinal cord A, D, S** 🔒

● **S34.11** **Complete lesion of lumbar spinal cord**

● **S34.111** **Complete lesion of L₁ level of lumbar spinal cord A, D, S** 🔒
  Complete lesion of lumbar spinal cord level 1

● **S34.112** **Complete lesion of L₂ level of lumbar spinal cord A, D, S** 🔒
  Complete lesion of lumbar spinal cord level 2

● **S34.113** **Complete lesion of L₃ level of lumbar spinal cord A, D, S** 🔒
  Complete lesion of lumbar spinal cord level 3

● **S34.114** **Complete lesion of L₄ level of lumbar spinal cord A, D, S** 🔒
  Complete lesion of lumbar spinal cord level 4

● **S34.115** **Complete lesion of L₅ level of lumbar spinal cord A, D, S** 🔒
  Complete lesion of lumbar spinal cord level 5

● **S34.119** **Complete lesion of unspecified level of lumbar spinal cord A, D, S** 🔒

● **S34.12** **Incomplete lesion of lumbar spinal cord**

● **S34.121** **Incomplete lesion of L₁ level of lumbar spinal cord A, D, S** 🔒
  Incomplete lesion of lumbar spinal cord level 1

● **S34.122** **Incomplete lesion of L₂ level of lumbar spinal cord A, D, S** 🔒
  Incomplete lesion of lumbar spinal cord level 2

● **S34.123** **Incomplete lesion of L₃ level of lumbar spinal cord A, D, S** 🔒
  Incomplete lesion of lumbar spinal cord level 3

● **S34.124** **Incomplete lesion of L₄ level of lumbar spinal cord A, D, S** 🔒
  Incomplete lesion of lumbar spinal cord level 4

● **S34.125** **Incomplete lesion of L₅ level of lumbar spinal cord A, D, S** 🔒
  Incomplete lesion of lumbar spinal cord level 5

● **S34.129** **Incomplete lesion of unspecified level of lumbar spinal cord A, D, S** 🔒

● **S34.13** **Other and unspecified injury to sacral spinal cord**
  Other injury to conus medullaris

● **S34.131** **Complete lesion of sacral spinal cord A, D, S** 🔒
  Complete lesion of conus medullaris

● **S34.132** **Incomplete lesion of sacral spinal cord A, D, S** 🔒
  Incomplete lesion of conus medullaris

● **S34.139** **Unspecified injury to sacral spinal cord A, D, S** 🔒
  Unspecified injury of conus medullaris

● **S34.2** **Injury of nerve root of lumbar and sacral spine**

X ● **S34.21** **Injury of nerve root of lumbar spine**

X ● **S34.22** **Injury of nerve root of sacral spine**

X ● **S34.3** **Injury of cauda equina A, D, S** 🔒

X ● **S34.4** **Injury of lumbosacral plexus**

X ● **S34.5** **Injury of lumbar, sacral and pelvic sympathetic nerves**
  Injury of celiac ganglion or plexus
  Injury of hypogastric plexus
  Injury of mesenteric plexus (inferior) (superior)
  Injury of splanchnic nerve

X ● **S34.6** **Injury of peripheral nerve(s) at abdomen, lower back and pelvis level**

X ● **S34.8** **Injury of other nerves at abdomen, lower back and pelvis level**

X ● **S34.9** **Injury of unspecified nerves at abdomen, lower back and pelvis level**

● **S35** **Injury of blood vessels at abdomen, lower back and pelvis level**
  The appropriate 7th character is to be added to each code from category S35

> A initial encounter
> D subsequent encounter
> S sequela

Code also any associated open wound (S31.-)

● **S35.0** **Injury of abdominal aorta**
  Excludes1 injury of aorta NOS (S25.0)

X ● **S35.00** **Unspecified injury of abdominal aorta**

X ● **S35.01** **Minor laceration of abdominal aorta**
  Incomplete transection of abdominal aorta
  Laceration of abdominal aorta NOS
  Superficial laceration of abdominal aorta

X ● **S35.02** **Major laceration of abdominal aorta**
  Complete transection of abdominal aorta
  Traumatic rupture of abdominal aorta

X ● **S35.09** **Other injury of abdominal aorta**

● **S35.1** **Injury of inferior vena cava**
  Injury of hepatic vein
  Excludes1 injury of vena cava NOS (S25.2)

X ● **S35.10** **Unspecified injury of inferior vena cava**

X ● **S35.11** **Minor laceration of inferior vena cava**
  Incomplete transection of inferior vena cava
  Laceration of inferior vena cava NOS
  Superficial laceration of inferior vena cava

X ● **S35.12** **Major laceration of inferior vena cava**
  Complete transection of inferior vena cava
  Traumatic rupture of inferior vena cava

X ● **S35.19** **Other injury of inferior vena cava**

● **S35.2** **Injury of celiac or mesenteric artery and branches**

● **S35.21** **Injury of celiac artery**

● **S35.211** **Minor laceration of celiac artery**
  Incomplete transection of celiac artery
  Laceration of celiac artery NOS
  Superficial laceration of celiac artery

● **S35.212** **Major laceration of celiac artery**
  Complete transection of celiac artery
  Traumatic rupture of celiac artery

● **S35.218** **Other injury of celiac artery**

● **S35.219** **Unspecified injury of celiac artery**

● **S35.22** **Injury of superior mesenteric artery**

● **S35.221** **Minor laceration of superior mesenteric artery**
  Incomplete transection of superior mesenteric artery
  Laceration of superior mesenteric artery NOS
  Superficial laceration of superior mesenteric artery

● **S35.222** **Major laceration of superior mesenteric artery**
  Complete transection of superior mesenteric artery
  Traumatic rupture of superior mesenteric artery

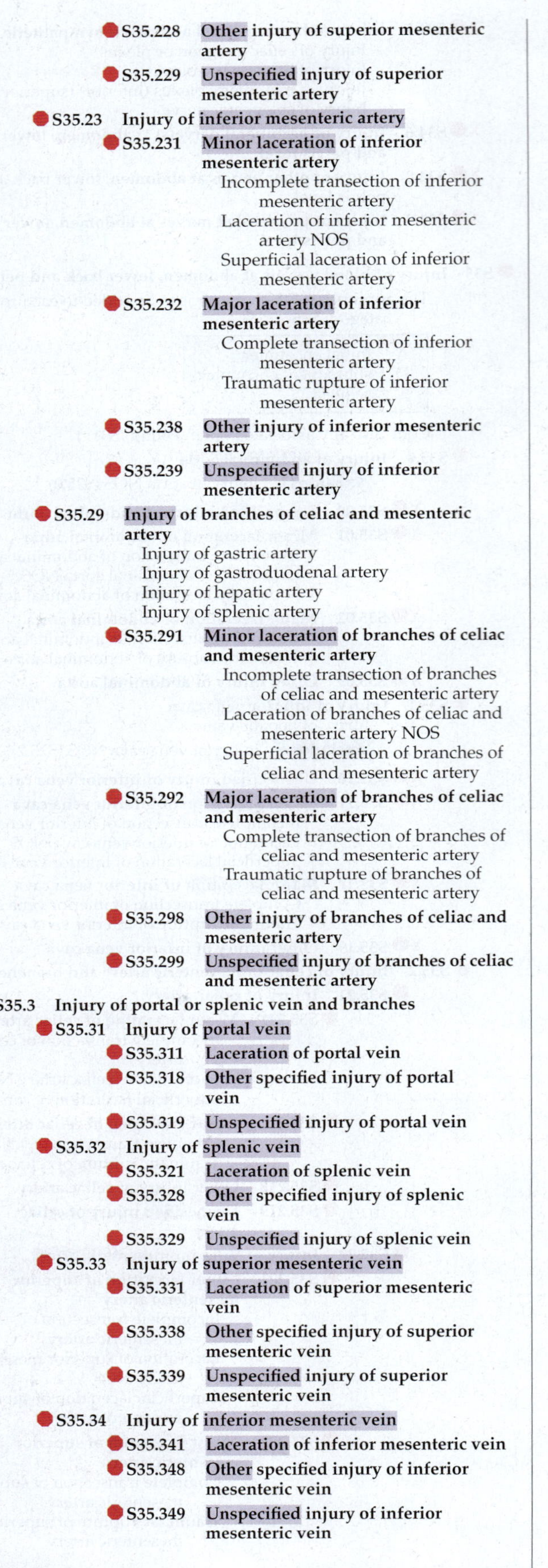

● **S35.228** Other injury of superior mesenteric artery

● **S35.229** Unspecified injury of superior mesenteric artery

● **S35.23** Injury of inferior mesenteric artery

● **S35.231** Minor laceration of inferior mesenteric artery
Incomplete transection of inferior mesenteric artery
Laceration of inferior mesenteric artery NOS
Superficial laceration of inferior mesenteric artery

● **S35.232** Major laceration of inferior mesenteric artery
Complete transection of inferior mesenteric artery
Traumatic rupture of inferior mesenteric artery

● **S35.238** Other injury of inferior mesenteric artery

● **S35.239** Unspecified injury of inferior mesenteric artery

● **S35.29** Injury of branches of celiac and mesenteric artery
Injury of gastric artery
Injury of gastroduodenal artery
Injury of hepatic artery
Injury of splenic artery

● **S35.291** Minor laceration of branches of celiac and mesenteric artery
Incomplete transection of branches of celiac and mesenteric artery
Laceration of branches of celiac and mesenteric artery NOS
Superficial laceration of branches of celiac and mesenteric artery

● **S35.292** Major laceration of branches of celiac and mesenteric artery
Complete transection of branches of celiac and mesenteric artery
Traumatic rupture of branches of celiac and mesenteric artery

● **S35.298** Other injury of branches of celiac and mesenteric artery

● **S35.299** Unspecified injury of branches of celiac and mesenteric artery

● **S35.3** Injury of portal or splenic vein and branches

● **S35.31** Injury of portal vein

● **S35.311** Laceration of portal vein

● **S35.318** Other specified injury of portal vein

● **S35.319** Unspecified injury of portal vein

● **S35.32** Injury of splenic vein

● **S35.321** Laceration of splenic vein

● **S35.328** Other specified injury of splenic vein

● **S35.329** Unspecified injury of splenic vein

● **S35.33** Injury of superior mesenteric vein

● **S35.331** Laceration of superior mesenteric vein

● **S35.338** Other specified injury of superior mesenteric vein

● **S35.339** Unspecified injury of superior mesenteric vein

● **S35.34** Injury of inferior mesenteric vein

● **S35.341** Laceration of inferior mesenteric vein

● **S35.348** Other specified injury of inferior mesenteric vein

● **S35.349** Unspecified injury of inferior mesenteric vein

● **S35.4** Injury of renal blood vessels

● **S35.40** Unspecified injury of renal blood vessel

● **S35.401** Unspecified injury of right renal artery

● **S35.402** Unspecified injury of left renal artery

● **S35.403** Unspecified injury of unspecified renal artery

● **S35.404** Unspecified injury of right renal vein

● **S35.405** Unspecified injury of left renal vein

● **S35.406** Unspecified injury of unspecified renal vein

● **S35.41** Laceration of renal blood vessel

● **S35.411** Laceration of right renal artery

● **S35.412** Laceration of left renal artery

● **S35.413** Laceration of unspecified renal artery

● **S35.414** Laceration of right renal vein

● **S35.415** Laceration of left renal vein

● **S35.416** Laceration of unspecified renal vein

● **S35.49** Other specified injury of renal blood vessel

● **S35.491** Other specified injury of right renal artery

● **S35.492** Other specified injury of left renal artery

● **S35.493** Other specified injury of unspecified renal artery

● **S35.494** Other specified injury of right renal vein

● **S35.495** Other specified injury of left renal vein

● **S35.496** Other specified injury of unspecified renal vein

● **S35.5** Injury of iliac blood vessels

X ● **S35.50** Injury of unspecified iliac blood vessel(s)

● **S35.51** Injury of iliac artery or vein
Injury of hypogastric artery or vein

● **S35.511** Injury of right iliac artery

● **S35.512** Injury of left iliac artery

● **S35.513** Injury of unspecified iliac artery

● **S35.514** Injury of right iliac vein

● **S35.515** Injury of left iliac vein

● **S35.516** Injury of unspecified iliac vein

● **S35.53** Injury of uterine artery or vein

● **S35.531** Injury of right uterine artery

● **S35.532** Injury of left uterine artery

● **S35.533** Injury of unspecified uterine artery

● **S35.534** Injury of right uterine vein

● **S35.535** Injury of left uterine vein

● **S35.536** Injury of unspecified uterine vein

X ● **S35.59** Injury of other iliac blood vessels

● **S35.8** Injury of other blood vessels at abdomen, lower back and pelvis level
Injury of ovarian artery or vein

● **S35.8X** Injury of other blood vessels at abdomen, lower back and pelvis level

● **S35.8X1** Laceration of other blood vessels at abdomen, lower back and pelvis level

● **S35.8X8** Other specified injury of other blood vessels at abdomen, lower back and pelvis level

● **S35.8X9** Unspecified injury of other blood vessels at abdomen, lower back and pelvis level

● S35.9 **Injury of unspecified blood vessel at abdomen, lower back and pelvis level**
 X ● S35.90 Unspecified injury of unspecified blood vessel at abdomen, lower back and pelvis level
 X ● S35.91 Laceration of unspecified blood vessel at abdomen, lower back and pelvis level
 X ● S35.99 Other specified injury of unspecified blood vessel at abdomen, lower back and pelvis level

● S36 **Injury of intra-abdominal organs**
 The appropriate 7th character is to be added to each code from category S36

> A initial encounter
> D subsequent encounter
> S sequela

 Code also any associated open wound (S31.-)

● S36.0 **Injury of spleen**
 X ● S36.00 Unspecified injury of spleen
 ● S36.02 Contusion of spleen
  ● S36.020 **Minor contusion of spleen**
   Contusion of spleen less than 2 cm
  ● S36.021 **Major contusion of spleen**
   Contusion of spleen greater than 2 cm
  ● S36.029 **Unspecified contusion of spleen**
   Coding Clinic: 2015, Q2, P36, Q1, P11
 ● S36.03 Laceration of spleen
  ● S36.030 **Superficial (capsular) laceration of spleen**
   Laceration of spleen less than 1 cm
   Minor laceration of spleen
  ● S36.031 **Moderate laceration of spleen**
   Laceration of spleen 1 to 3 cm
   Coding Clinic: 2022, Q1, P23; 2015, Q2, P36, Q1, P11
  ● S36.032 **Major laceration of spleen**
   Avulsion of spleen
   Laceration of spleen greater than 3 cm
   Massive laceration of spleen
   Multiple moderate lacerations of spleen
   Stellate laceration of spleen
  ● S36.039 **Unspecified laceration of spleen**
 X ● S36.09 Other injury of spleen
● S36.1 **Injury of liver and gallbladder and bile duct**
 ● S36.11 Injury of liver
  Coding Clinic: 2024, Q1, P25
  ● S36.112 **Contusion of liver**
  ● S36.113 **Laceration of liver, unspecified degree**
  ● S36.114 **Minor laceration of liver**
   Laceration involving capsule only, or, without significant involvement of hepatic parenchyma [i.e., less than 1 cm deep]
  ● S36.115 **Moderate laceration of liver**
   Laceration involving parenchyma but without major disruption of parenchyma [i.e., less than 10 cm long and less than 3 cm deep]
  ● S36.116 **Major laceration of liver**
   Laceration with significant disruption of hepatic parenchyma [i.e., greater than 10 cm long and 3 cm deep]
   Multiple moderate lacerations, with or without hematoma
   Stellate laceration of liver

  ● S36.118 **Other injury of liver**
  ● S36.119 **Unspecified injury of liver**
   Coding Clinic: 2015, Q2, P17
 ● S36.12 Injury of gallbladder
  ● S36.122 **Contusion of gallbladder**
  ● S36.123 **Laceration of gallbladder**
  ● S36.128 **Other injury of gallbladder**
  ● S36.129 **Unspecified injury of gallbladder**
 X ● S36.13 Injury of bile duct
● S36.2 **Injury of pancreas**
 ● S36.20 Unspecified injury of pancreas
  ● S36.200 **Unspecified injury of head of pancreas**
  ● S36.201 **Unspecified injury of body of pancreas**
  ● S36.202 **Unspecified injury of tail of pancreas**
  ● S36.209 **Unspecified injury of unspecified part of pancreas**
 ● S36.22 Contusion of pancreas
  ● S36.220 **Contusion of head of pancreas**
  ● S36.221 **Contusion of body of pancreas**
  ● S36.222 **Contusion of tail of pancreas**
  ● S36.229 **Contusion of unspecified part of pancreas**
 ● S36.23 Laceration of pancreas, unspecified degree
  ● S36.230 **Laceration of head of pancreas, unspecified degree**
  ● S36.231 **Laceration of body of pancreas, unspecified degree**
  ● S36.232 **Laceration of tail of pancreas, unspecified degree**
  ● S36.239 **Laceration of unspecified part of pancreas, unspecified degree**
 ● S36.24 Minor laceration of pancreas
  ● S36.240 **Minor laceration of head of pancreas**
  ● S36.241 **Minor laceration of body of pancreas**
  ● S36.242 **Minor laceration of tail of pancreas**
  ● S36.249 **Minor laceration of unspecified part of pancreas**
 ● S36.25 Moderate laceration of pancreas
  ● S36.250 **Moderate laceration of head of pancreas**
  ● S36.251 **Moderate laceration of body of pancreas**
  ● S36.252 **Moderate laceration of tail of pancreas**
  ● S36.259 **Moderate laceration of unspecified part of pancreas**
 ● S36.26 Major laceration of pancreas
  ● S36.260 **Major laceration of head of pancreas**
  ● S36.261 **Major laceration of body of pancreas**
  ● S36.262 **Major laceration of tail of pancreas**
  ● S36.269 **Major laceration of unspecified part of pancreas**
 ● S36.29 Other injury of pancreas
  ● S36.290 **Other injury of head of pancreas**
  ● S36.291 **Other injury of body of pancreas**
  ● S36.292 **Other injury of tail of pancreas**
  ● S36.299 **Other injury of unspecified part of pancreas**
● S36.3 **Injury of stomach**
 X ● S36.30 Unspecified injury of stomach
 X ● S36.32 Contusion of stomach
 X ● S36.33 Laceration of stomach
 X ● S36.39 Other injury of stomach

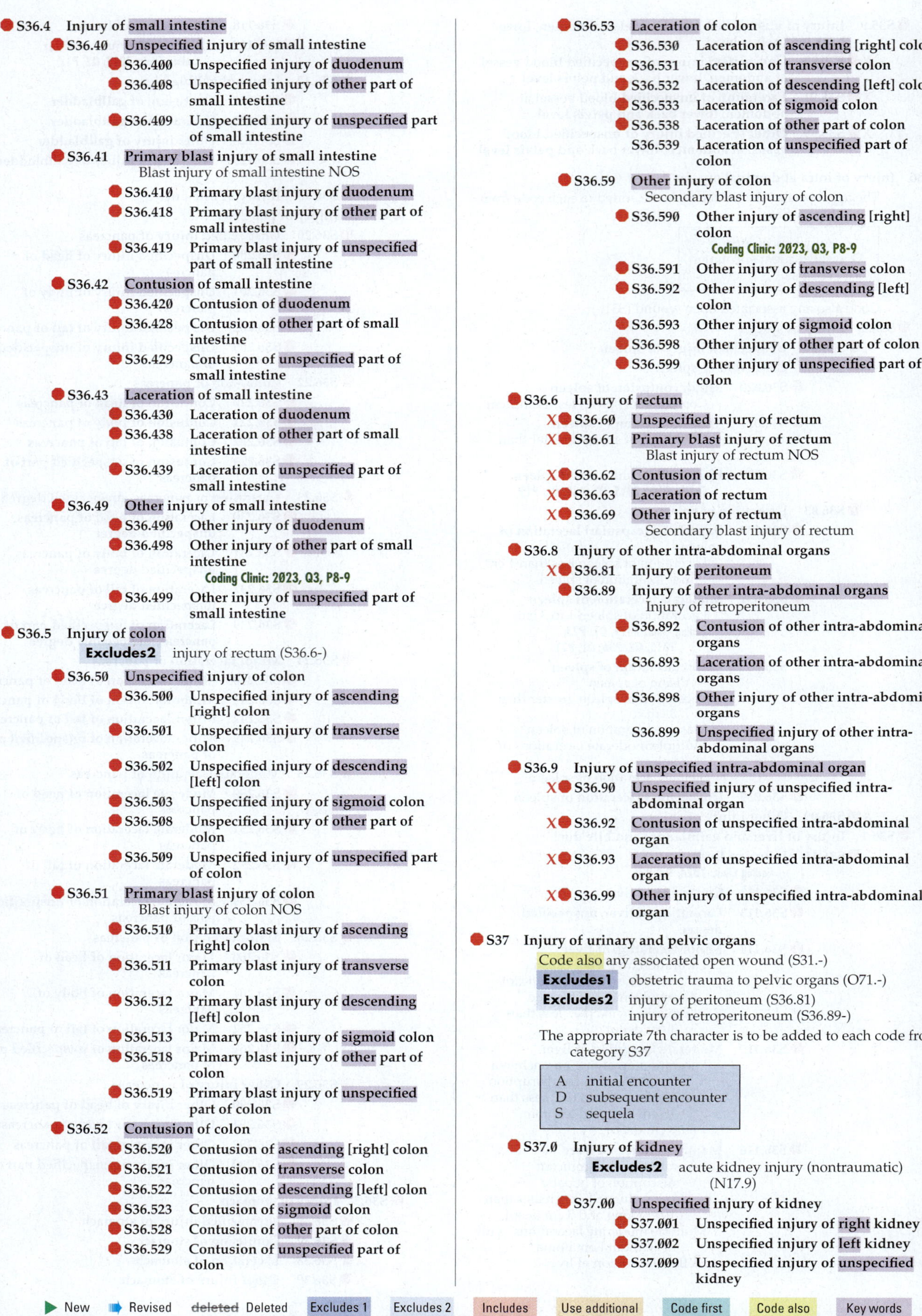

- ● **S36.4**   **Injury of small intestine**
  - ● **S36.40**   Unspecified injury of small intestine
    - ● **S36.400**   Unspecified injury of duodenum
    - ● **S36.408**   Unspecified injury of other part of small intestine
    - ● **S36.409**   Unspecified injury of unspecified part of small intestine
  - ● **S36.41**   Primary blast injury of small intestine
    Blast injury of small intestine NOS
    - ● **S36.410**   Primary blast injury of duodenum
    - ● **S36.418**   Primary blast injury of other part of small intestine
    - ● **S36.419**   Primary blast injury of unspecified part of small intestine
  - ● **S36.42**   Contusion of small intestine
    - ● **S36.420**   Contusion of duodenum
    - ● **S36.428**   Contusion of other part of small intestine
    - ● **S36.429**   Contusion of unspecified part of small intestine
  - ● **S36.43**   Laceration of small intestine
    - ● **S36.430**   Laceration of duodenum
    - ● **S36.438**   Laceration of other part of small intestine
    - ● **S36.439**   Laceration of unspecified part of small intestine
  - ● **S36.49**   Other injury of small intestine
    - ● **S36.490**   Other injury of duodenum
    - ● **S36.498**   Other injury of other part of small intestine
      Coding Clinic: 2023, Q3, P8-9
    - ● **S36.499**   Other injury of unspecified part of small intestine
- ● **S36.5**   **Injury of colon**
  - **Excludes2**   injury of rectum (S36.6-)
  - ● **S36.50**   Unspecified injury of colon
    - ● **S36.500**   Unspecified injury of ascending [right] colon
    - ● **S36.501**   Unspecified injury of transverse colon
    - ● **S36.502**   Unspecified injury of descending [left] colon
    - ● **S36.503**   Unspecified injury of sigmoid colon
    - ● **S36.508**   Unspecified injury of other part of colon
    - ● **S36.509**   Unspecified injury of unspecified part of colon
  - ● **S36.51**   Primary blast injury of colon
    Blast injury of colon NOS
    - ● **S36.510**   Primary blast injury of ascending [right] colon
    - ● **S36.511**   Primary blast injury of transverse colon
    - ● **S36.512**   Primary blast injury of descending [left] colon
    - ● **S36.513**   Primary blast injury of sigmoid colon
    - ● **S36.518**   Primary blast injury of other part of colon
    - ● **S36.519**   Primary blast injury of unspecified part of colon
  - ● **S36.52**   Contusion of colon
    - ● **S36.520**   Contusion of ascending [right] colon
    - ● **S36.521**   Contusion of transverse colon
    - ● **S36.522**   Contusion of descending [left] colon
    - ● **S36.523**   Contusion of sigmoid colon
    - ● **S36.528**   Contusion of other part of colon
    - ● **S36.529**   Contusion of unspecified part of colon

- ● **S36.53**   Laceration of colon
  - ● **S36.530**   Laceration of ascending [right] colon
  - ● **S36.531**   Laceration of transverse colon
  - ● **S36.532**   Laceration of descending [left] colon
  - ● **S36.533**   Laceration of sigmoid colon
  - ● **S36.538**   Laceration of other part of colon
  - **S36.539**   Laceration of unspecified part of colon
- ● **S36.59**   Other injury of colon
  Secondary blast injury of colon
  - ● **S36.590**   Other injury of ascending [right] colon
    Coding Clinic: 2023, Q3, P8-9
  - ● **S36.591**   Other injury of transverse colon
  - ● **S36.592**   Other injury of descending [left] colon
  - ● **S36.593**   Other injury of sigmoid colon
  - ● **S36.598**   Other injury of other part of colon
  - ● **S36.599**   Other injury of unspecified part of colon
- ● **S36.6**   **Injury of rectum**
  - X ● **S36.60**   Unspecified injury of rectum
  - X ● **S36.61**   Primary blast injury of rectum
    Blast injury of rectum NOS
  - X ● **S36.62**   Contusion of rectum
  - X ● **S36.63**   Laceration of rectum
  - X ● **S36.69**   Other injury of rectum
    Secondary blast injury of rectum
- ● **S36.8**   **Injury of other intra-abdominal organs**
  - X ● **S36.81**   Injury of peritoneum
  - ● **S36.89**   Injury of other intra-abdominal organs
    Injury of retroperitoneum
    - ● **S36.892**   Contusion of other intra-abdominal organs
    - ● **S36.893**   Laceration of other intra-abdominal organs
    - ● **S36.898**   Other injury of other intra-abdominal organs
    - **S36.899**   Unspecified injury of other intra-abdominal organs
- ● **S36.9**   **Injury of unspecified intra-abdominal organ**
  - X ● **S36.90**   Unspecified injury of unspecified intra-abdominal organ
  - X ● **S36.92**   Contusion of unspecified intra-abdominal organ
  - X ● **S36.93**   Laceration of unspecified intra-abdominal organ
  - X ● **S36.99**   Other injury of unspecified intra-abdominal organ
- ● **S37**   **Injury of urinary and pelvic organs**
  - Code also any associated open wound (S31.-)
  - **Excludes1**   obstetric trauma to pelvic organs (O71.-)
  - **Excludes2**   injury of peritoneum (S36.81)
    injury of retroperitoneum (S36.89-)
  - The appropriate 7th character is to be added to each code from category S37

A	initial encounter
D	subsequent encounter
S	sequela

  - ● **S37.0**   **Injury of kidney**
    - **Excludes2**   acute kidney injury (nontraumatic) (N17.9)
    - ● **S37.00**   Unspecified injury of kidney
      - ● **S37.001**   Unspecified injury of right kidney
      - ● **S37.002**   Unspecified injury of left kidney
      - ● **S37.009**   Unspecified injury of unspecified kidney

▶ New   ⇒ Revised   ~~deleted~~ Deleted   Excludes 1   Excludes 2   Includes   Use additional   Code first   Code also   Key words
OGCR Official Guidelines   X Assign placeholder X   ● Use Additional Character(s)   ▶ Manifestation Code   Hierarchical Condition Category   **Coding Clinic**

● **S37.01**   **Minor contusion of kidney**
     Contusion of kidney less than 2 cm
     Contusion of kidney NOS
   ● **S37.011**   Minor contusion of **right** kidney
   ● **S37.012**   Minor contusion of **left** kidney
   ● **S37.019**   Minor contusion of **unspecified** kidney
● **S37.02**   **Major contusion of kidney**
     Contusion of kidney greater than 2 cm
   ● **S37.021**   Major contusion of **right** kidney
   ● **S37.022**   Major contusion of **left** kidney
   ● **S37.029**   Major contusion of **unspecified** kidney
● **S37.03**   **Laceration of kidney, unspecified degree**
   ● **S37.031**   Laceration of **right** kidney, unspecified degree
   ● **S37.032**   Laceration of **left** kidney, unspecified degree
   ● **S37.039**   Laceration of **unspecified** kidney, unspecified degree
● **S37.04**   **Minor laceration of kidney**
     Laceration of kidney less than 1 cm
   ● **S37.041**   Minor laceration of **right** kidney
   ● **S37.042**   Minor laceration of **left** kidney
   ● **S37.049**   Minor laceration of **unspecified** kidney
● **S37.05**   **Moderate laceration of kidney**
     Laceration of kidney 1 to 3 cm
   ● **S37.051**   Moderate laceration of **right** kidney
   ● **S37.052**   Moderate laceration of **left** kidney
   ● **S37.059**   Moderate laceration of **unspecified** kidney
● **S37.06**   **Major laceration of kidney**
     Avulsion of kidney
     Laceration of kidney greater than 3 cm
     Massive laceration of kidney
     Multiple moderate lacerations of kidney
     Stellate laceration of kidney
   ● **S37.061**   Major laceration of **right** kidney
   ● **S37.062**   Major laceration of **left** kidney
   ● **S37.069**   Major laceration of **unspecified** kidney
● **S37.09**   **Other injury of kidney**
   ● **S37.091**   Other injury of **right** kidney
   ● **S37.092**   Other injury of **left** kidney
   ● **S37.099**   Other injury of **unspecified** kidney
● **S37.1**   **Injury of ureter**
  X ● **S37.10**   **Unspecified injury of ureter**
  X ● **S37.12**   **Contusion of ureter**
  X ● **S37.13**   **Laceration of ureter**
  X ● **S37.19**   **Other injury of ureter**
● **S37.2**   **Injury of bladder**
  X ● **S37.20**   **Unspecified injury of bladder**
  X ● **S37.22**   **Contusion of bladder**
  X ● **S37.23**   **Laceration of bladder**
  X ● **S37.29**   **Other injury of bladder**
● **S37.3**   **Injury of urethra**
  X ● **S37.30**   **Unspecified injury of urethra**
  X ● **S37.32**   **Contusion of urethra**
  X ● **S37.33**   **Laceration of urethra**
  X ● **S37.39**   **Other injury of urethra**
● **S37.4**   **Injury of ovary**
   ● **S37.40**   **Unspecified injury of ovary**
     ● **S37.401**   Unspecified injury of ovary, **unilateral**
     ● **S37.402**   Unspecified injury of ovary, **bilateral**
     ● **S37.409**   Unspecified injury of ovary, **unspecified**

● **S37.42**   **Contusion of ovary**
   ● **S37.421**   Contusion of ovary, **unilateral**
   ● **S37.422**   Contusion of ovary, **bilateral**
   ● **S37.429**   Contusion of ovary, **unspecified**
● **S37.43**   **Laceration of ovary**
   ● **S37.431**   Laceration of ovary, **unilateral**
   ● **S37.432**   Laceration of ovary, **bilateral**
   ● **S37.439**   Laceration of ovary, **unspecified**
● **S37.49**   **Other injury of ovary**
   ● **S37.491**   Other injury of ovary, **unilateral**
   ● **S37.492**   Other injury of ovary, **bilateral**
   ● **S37.499**   Other injury of ovary, **unspecified**
● **S37.5**   **Injury of fallopian tube**
   ● **S37.50**   **Unspecified injury of fallopian tube**
     ● **S37.501**   Unspecified injury of fallopian tube, **unilateral**
     ● **S37.502**   Unspecified injury of fallopian tube, **bilateral**
     ● **S37.509**   Unspecified injury of fallopian tube, **unspecified**
   ● **S37.51**   **Primary blast injury of fallopian tube**
     Blast injury of fallopian tube NOS
     ● **S37.511**   Primary blast injury of fallopian tube, **unilateral**
     ● **S37.512**   Primary blast injury of fallopian tube, **bilateral**
     ● **S37.519**   Primary blast injury of fallopian tube, **unspecified**
   ● **S37.52**   **Contusion of fallopian tube**
     ● **S37.521**   Contusion of fallopian tube, **unilateral**
     ● **S37.522**   Contusion of fallopian tube, **bilateral**
     ● **S37.529**   Contusion of fallopian tube, **unspecified**
   ● **S37.53**   **Laceration of fallopian tube**
     ● **S37.531**   Laceration of fallopian tube, **unilateral**
     ● **S37.532**   Laceration of fallopian tube, **bilateral**
     ● **S37.539**   Laceration of fallopian tube, **unspecified**
   ● **S37.59**   **Other injury of fallopian tube**
     Secondary blast injury of fallopian tube
     ● **S37.591**   Other injury of fallopian tube, **unilateral**
     ● **S37.592**   Other injury of fallopian tube, **bilateral**
     ● **S37.599**   Other injury of fallopian tube, **unspecified**
● **S37.6**   **Injury of uterus**
   Excludes1   injury to gravid uterus (O9A.2-)
                     injury to uterus during delivery (O71.-)
  X ● **S37.60**   **Unspecified injury of uterus**
  X ● **S37.62**   **Contusion of uterus**
  X ● **S37.63**   **Laceration of uterus**
  X ● **S37.69**   **Other injury of uterus**
● **S37.8**   **Injury of other urinary and pelvic organs**
   ● **S37.81**   **Injury of adrenal gland**
     ● **S37.812**   Contusion of adrenal gland
     ● **S37.813**   Laceration of adrenal gland
     ● **S37.818**   Other injury of adrenal gland
     ● **S37.819**   Unspecified injury of adrenal gland
   ● **S37.82**   **Injury of prostate**
     ● **S37.822**   Contusion of prostate
     ● **S37.823**   Laceration of prostate
     ● **S37.828**   Other injury of prostate
     ● **S37.829**   Unspecified injury of prostate

CHAPTER 19 (S00-T88)

- ● **S37.89**   Injury of other urinary and pelvic organ
  - ● **S37.892**   Contusion of other urinary and pelvic organ
  - ● **S37.893**   Laceration of other urinary and pelvic organ
  - ● **S37.898**   Other injury of other urinary and pelvic organ
  - ● **S37.899**   Unspecified injury of other urinary and pelvic organ
- ● **S37.9**   Injury of unspecified urinary and pelvic organ
  - **X** ● **S37.90**   Unspecified injury of unspecified urinary and pelvic organ
  - **X** ● **S37.92**   Contusion of unspecified urinary and pelvic organ
  - **X** ● **S37.93**   Laceration of unspecified urinary and pelvic organ
  - **X** ● **S37.99**   Other injury of unspecified urinary and pelvic organ

- ● **S38**   Crushing injury and traumatic amputation of abdomen, lower back, pelvis and external genitals

  An amputation not identified as partial or complete should be coded to complete

  The appropriate 7th character is to be added to each code from category S38

  > A   initial encounter
  > D   subsequent encounter
  > S   sequela

  - ● **S38.0**   Crushing injury of external genital organs

    Use additional code for any associated injuries
    - ● **S38.00**   Crushing injury of unspecified external genital organs
      - ● **S38.001**   Crushing injury of unspecified external genital organs, male
      - ● **S38.002**   Crushing injury of unspecified external genital organs, female
    - **X** ● **S38.01**   Crushing injury of penis
    - **X** ● **S38.02**   Crushing injury of scrotum and testis
    - **X** ● **S38.03**   Crushing injury of vulva
  - **X** ● **S38.1**   Crushing injury of abdomen, lower back, and pelvis

    Use additional code for all associated injuries, such as:
    fracture of thoracic or lumbar spine and pelvis (S22.0-, S32.-)
    injury to intra-abdominal organs (S36.-)
    injury to urinary and pelvic organs (S37.-)
    open wound of abdominal wall (S31.-)
    spinal cord injury (S34.0, S34.1-)

    Excludes2   crushing injury of external genital organs (S38.0-)
  - ● **S38.2**   Traumatic amputation of external genital organs
    - ● **S38.21**   Traumatic amputation of female external genital organs

      Traumatic amputation of clitoris
      Traumatic amputation of labium (majus) (minus)
      Traumatic amputation of vulva
      - ● **S38.211**   Complete traumatic amputation of female external genital organs
      - ● **S38.212**   Partial traumatic amputation of female external genital organs
    - ● **S38.22**   Traumatic amputation of penis
      - ● **S38.221**   Complete traumatic amputation of penis
      - ● **S38.222**   Partial traumatic amputation of penis

- ● **S38.23**   Traumatic amputation of scrotum and testis
  - ● **S38.231**   Complete traumatic amputation of scrotum and testis
  - ● **S38.232**   Partial traumatic amputation of scrotum and testis
- **X** ● **S38.3**   Transection (partial) of abdomen

- ● **S39**   Other and unspecified injuries of abdomen, lower back, pelvis and external genitals

  Code also any associated open wound (S31.-)

  Excludes2   sprain of joints and ligaments of lumbar spine and pelvis (S33.-)

  The appropriate 7th character is to be added to each code from category S39

  > A   initial encounter
  > D   subsequent encounter
  > S   sequela

  - ● **S39.0**   Injury of muscle, fascia and tendon of abdomen, lower back and pelvis
    - ● **S39.00**   Unspecified injury of muscle, fascia and tendon of abdomen, lower back and pelvis
      - ● **S39.001**   Unspecified injury of muscle, fascia and tendon of abdomen
      - ● **S39.002**   Unspecified injury of muscle, fascia and tendon of lower back
      - ● **S39.003**   Unspecified injury of muscle, fascia and tendon of pelvis
    - ● **S39.01**   Strain of muscle, fascia and tendon of abdomen, lower back and pelvis
      - ● **S39.011**   Strain of muscle, fascia and tendon of abdomen
      - ● **S39.012**   Strain of muscle, fascia and tendon of lower back

        Coding Clinic: 2016, Q4, P74
      - ● **S39.013**   Strain of muscle, fascia and tendon of pelvis
    - ● **S39.02**   Laceration of muscle, fascia and tendon of abdomen, lower back and pelvis
      - ● **S39.021**   Laceration of muscle, fascia and tendon of abdomen
      - ● **S39.022**   Laceration of muscle, fascia and tendon of lower back
      - ● **S39.023**   Laceration of muscle, fascia and tendon of pelvis
    - ● **S39.09**   Other injury of muscle, fascia and tendon of abdomen, lower back and pelvis
      - ● **S39.091**   Other injury of muscle, fascia and tendon of abdomen
      - ● **S39.092**   Other injury of muscle, fascia and tendon of lower back
      - ● **S39.093**   Other injury of muscle, fascia and tendon of pelvis
  - ● **S39.8**   Other specified injuries of abdomen, lower back, pelvis and external genitals
    - **X** ● **S39.81**   Other specified injuries of abdomen
    - **X** ● **S39.82**   Other specified injuries of lower back
    - **X** ● **S39.83**   Other specified injuries of pelvis
    - ● **S39.84**   Other specified injuries of external genitals
      - ● **S39.840**   Fracture of corpus cavernosum penis
      - ● **S39.848**   Other specified injuries of external genitals
  - ● **S39.9**   Unspecified injury of abdomen, lower back, pelvis and external genitals
    - **X** ● **S39.91**   Unspecified injury of abdomen
    - **X** ● **S39.92**   Unspecified injury of lower back
    - **X** ● **S39.93**   Unspecified injury of pelvis
    - **X** ● **S39.94**   Unspecified injury of external genitals

▶ New   ⇨ Revised   ~~deleted~~ Deleted   Excludes 1   Excludes 2   Includes   Use additional   Code first   Code also   Key words

OGCR Official Guidelines   **X** Assign placeholder X   ● Use Additional Character(s)   ❭ Manifestation Code   Hierarchical Condition Category   **Coding Clinic**

INJURIES TO THE SHOULDER AND UPPER ARM (S40-S49)

Includes	injuries of axilla injuries of scapular region
Excludes2	burns and corrosions (T20-T32)
	frostbite (T33-T34)
	injuries of elbow (S50-S59)
	insect bite or sting, venomous (T63.4)

- **S40 Superficial injury of shoulder and upper arm**

  The appropriate 7th character is to be added to each code from category S40

A	initial encounter
D	subsequent encounter
S	sequela

  - **S40.0 Contusion of shoulder and upper arm**
    - **S40.01 Contusion of shoulder**
      - S40.011 Contusion of right shoulder
      - S40.012 Contusion of left shoulder
      - S40.019 Contusion of unspecified shoulder
    - **S40.02 Contusion of upper arm**
      - S40.021 Contusion of right upper arm
      - S40.022 Contusion of left upper arm
      - S40.029 Contusion of unspecified upper arm
  - **S40.2 Other superficial injuries of shoulder**
    - **S40.21 Abrasion of shoulder**
      - S40.211 Abrasion of right shoulder
      - S40.212 Abrasion of left shoulder
      - S40.219 Abrasion of unspecified shoulder
    - **S40.22 Blister (nonthermal) of shoulder**
      - S40.221 Blister (nonthermal) of right shoulder
      - S40.222 Blister (nonthermal) of left shoulder
      - S40.229 Blister (nonthermal) of unspecified shoulder
    - **S40.24 External constriction of shoulder**
      - S40.241 External constriction of right shoulder
      - S40.242 External constriction of left shoulder
      - S40.249 External constriction of unspecified shoulder
    - **S40.25 Superficial foreign body of shoulder**
      Splinter in the shoulder
      - S40.251 Superficial foreign body of right shoulder
      - S40.252 Superficial foreign body of left shoulder
      - S40.259 Superficial foreign body of unspecified shoulder
    - **S40.26 Insect bite (nonvenomous) of shoulder**
      - S40.261 Insect bite (nonvenomous) of right shoulder
      - S40.262 Insect bite (nonvenomous) of left shoulder
      - S40.269 Insect bite (nonvenomous) of unspecified shoulder
    - **S40.27 Other superficial bite of shoulder**
      | **Excludes1** | open bite of shoulder (S41.05) |
      - S40.271 Other superficial bite of right shoulder
      - S40.272 Other superficial bite of left shoulder
      - S40.279 Other superficial bite of unspecified shoulder
  - **S40.8 Other superficial injuries of upper arm**
    - **S40.81 Abrasion of upper arm**
      - S40.811 Abrasion of right upper arm
      - S40.812 Abrasion of left upper arm
      - S40.819 Abrasion of unspecified upper arm
    - **S40.82 Blister (nonthermal) of upper arm**
      - S40.821 Blister (nonthermal) of right upper arm
      - S40.822 Blister (nonthermal) of left upper arm
      - S40.829 Blister (nonthermal) of unspecified upper arm
    - **S40.84 External constriction of upper arm**
      - S40.841 External constriction of right upper arm
      - S40.842 External constriction of left upper arm
      - S40.849 External constriction of unspecified upper arm
    - **S40.85 Superficial foreign body of upper arm**
      Splinter in the upper arm
      - S40.851 Superficial foreign body of right upper arm
      - S40.852 Superficial foreign body of left upper arm
      - S40.859 Superficial foreign body of unspecified upper arm
    - **S40.86 Insect bite (nonvenomous) of upper arm**
      - S40.861 Insect bite (nonvenomous) of right upper arm
      - S40.862 Insect bite (nonvenomous) of left upper arm
      - S40.869 Insect bite (nonvenomous) of unspecified upper arm
    - **S40.87 Other superficial bite of upper arm**
      | **Excludes1** | open bite of upper arm (S41.14) |
      | **Excludes2** | other superficial bite of shoulder (S40.27-) |
      - S40.871 Other superficial bite of right upper arm
      - S40.872 Other superficial bite of left upper arm
      - S40.879 Other superficial bite of unspecified upper arm
  - **S40.9 Unspecified superficial injury of shoulder and upper arm**
    - **S40.91 Unspecified superficial injury of shoulder**
      - S40.911 Unspecified superficial injury of right shoulder
      - S40.912 Unspecified superficial injury of left shoulder
      - S40.919 Unspecified superficial injury of unspecified shoulder
    - **S40.92 Unspecified superficial injury of upper arm**
      - S40.921 Unspecified superficial injury of right upper arm
      - S40.922 Unspecified superficial injury of left upper arm
      - S40.929 Unspecified superficial injury of unspecified upper arm

- **S41 Open wound of shoulder and upper arm**

  Code also any associated wound infection

  | **Excludes1** | traumatic amputation of shoulder and upper arm (S48.-) |
  | **Excludes2** | open fracture of shoulder and upper arm (S42.- with 7th character B or C) |

  The appropriate 7th character is to be added to each code from category S41

A	initial encounter
D	subsequent encounter
S	sequela

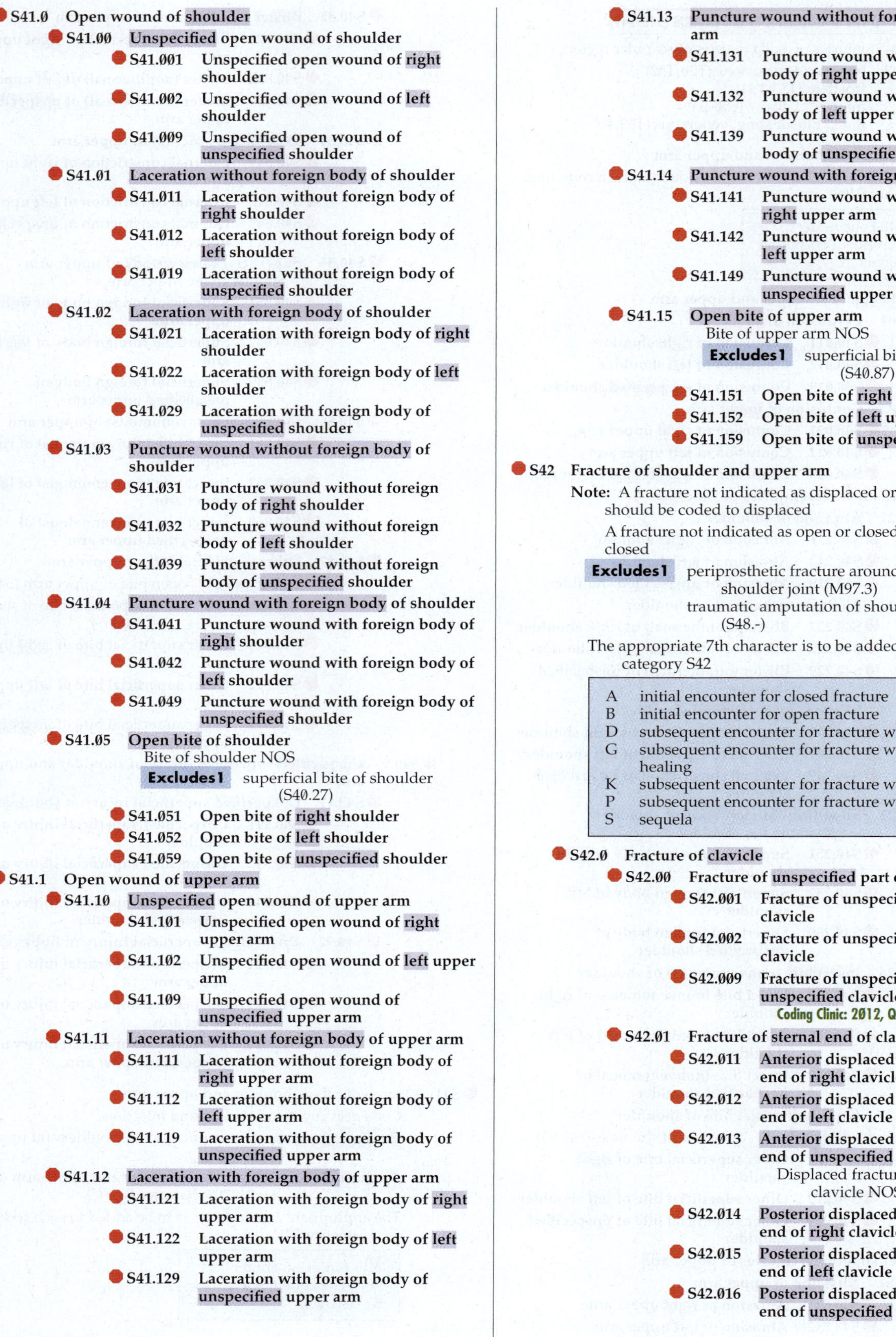

- ● **S41.0   Open wound of shoulder**
  - ● **S41.00   Unspecified open wound of shoulder**
    - ● **S41.001   Unspecified open wound of right shoulder**
    - ● **S41.002   Unspecified open wound of left shoulder**
    - ● **S41.009   Unspecified open wound of unspecified shoulder**
  - ● **S41.01   Laceration without foreign body of shoulder**
    - ● **S41.011   Laceration without foreign body of right shoulder**
    - ● **S41.012   Laceration without foreign body of left shoulder**
    - ● **S41.019   Laceration without foreign body of unspecified shoulder**
  - ● **S41.02   Laceration with foreign body of shoulder**
    - ● **S41.021   Laceration with foreign body of right shoulder**
    - ● **S41.022   Laceration with foreign body of left shoulder**
    - ● **S41.029   Laceration with foreign body of unspecified shoulder**
  - ● **S41.03   Puncture wound without foreign body of shoulder**
    - ● **S41.031   Puncture wound without foreign body of right shoulder**
    - ● **S41.032   Puncture wound without foreign body of left shoulder**
    - ● **S41.039   Puncture wound without foreign body of unspecified shoulder**
  - ● **S41.04   Puncture wound with foreign body of shoulder**
    - ● **S41.041   Puncture wound with foreign body of right shoulder**
    - ● **S41.042   Puncture wound with foreign body of left shoulder**
    - ● **S41.049   Puncture wound with foreign body of unspecified shoulder**
  - ● **S41.05   Open bite of shoulder**
    Bite of shoulder NOS
    > **Excludes1**   superficial bite of shoulder (S40.27)
    - ● **S41.051   Open bite of right shoulder**
    - ● **S41.052   Open bite of left shoulder**
    - ● **S41.059   Open bite of unspecified shoulder**
- ● **S41.1   Open wound of upper arm**
  - ● **S41.10   Unspecified open wound of upper arm**
    - ● **S41.101   Unspecified open wound of right upper arm**
    - ● **S41.102   Unspecified open wound of left upper arm**
    - ● **S41.109   Unspecified open wound of unspecified upper arm**
  - ● **S41.11   Laceration without foreign body of upper arm**
    - ● **S41.111   Laceration without foreign body of right upper arm**
    - ● **S41.112   Laceration without foreign body of left upper arm**
    - ● **S41.119   Laceration without foreign body of unspecified upper arm**
  - ● **S41.12   Laceration with foreign body of upper arm**
    - ● **S41.121   Laceration with foreign body of right upper arm**
    - ● **S41.122   Laceration with foreign body of left upper arm**
    - ● **S41.129   Laceration with foreign body of unspecified upper arm**
  - ● **S41.13   Puncture wound without foreign body of upper arm**
    - ● **S41.131   Puncture wound without foreign body of right upper arm**
    - ● **S41.132   Puncture wound without foreign body of left upper arm**
    - ● **S41.139   Puncture wound without foreign body of unspecified upper arm**
  - ● **S41.14   Puncture wound with foreign body of upper arm**
    - ● **S41.141   Puncture wound with foreign body of right upper arm**
    - ● **S41.142   Puncture wound with foreign body of left upper arm**
    - ● **S41.149   Puncture wound with foreign body of unspecified upper arm**
  - ● **S41.15   Open bite of upper arm**
    Bite of upper arm NOS
    > **Excludes1**   superficial bite of upper arm (S40.87)
    - ● **S41.151   Open bite of right upper arm**
    - ● **S41.152   Open bite of left upper arm**
    - ● **S41.159   Open bite of unspecified upper arm**

- ● **S42   Fracture of shoulder and upper arm**

  Note: A fracture not indicated as displaced or nondisplaced should be coded to displaced

  A fracture not indicated as open or closed should be coded to closed

  > **Excludes1**   periprosthetic fracture around internal prosthetic shoulder joint (M97.3)
  >
  > traumatic amputation of shoulder and upper arm (S48.-)

  The appropriate 7th character is to be added to all codes from category S42

A	initial encounter for closed fracture
B	initial encounter for open fracture
D	subsequent encounter for fracture with routine healing
G	subsequent encounter for fracture with delayed healing
K	subsequent encounter for fracture with nonunion
P	subsequent encounter for fracture with malunion
S	sequela

  - ● **S42.0   Fracture of clavicle**
    - ● **S42.00   Fracture of unspecified part of clavicle**
      - ● **S42.001   Fracture of unspecified part of right clavicle**
      - ● **S42.002   Fracture of unspecified part of left clavicle**
      - ● **S42.009   Fracture of unspecified part of unspecified clavicle**
        Coding Clinic: 2012, Q4, P3
    - ● **S42.01   Fracture of sternal end of clavicle**
      - ● **S42.011   Anterior displaced fracture of sternal end of right clavicle**
      - ● **S42.012   Anterior displaced fracture of sternal end of left clavicle**
      - ● **S42.013   Anterior displaced fracture of sternal end of unspecified clavicle**
        Displaced fracture of sternal end of clavicle NOS
      - ● **S42.014   Posterior displaced fracture of sternal end of right clavicle**
      - ● **S42.015   Posterior displaced fracture of sternal end of left clavicle**
      - ● **S42.016   Posterior displaced fracture of sternal end of unspecified clavicle**

- ● S42.017   Nondisplaced fracture of sternal end of right clavicle
- ● S42.018   Nondisplaced fracture of sternal end of left clavicle
- ● S42.019   Nondisplaced fracture of sternal end of unspecified clavicle
- ● S42.02   Fracture of shaft of clavicle
  - ● S42.021   Displaced fracture of shaft of right clavicle
  - ● S42.022   Displaced fracture of shaft of left clavicle
  - ● S42.023   Displaced fracture of shaft of unspecified clavicle
  - ● S42.024   Nondisplaced fracture of shaft of right clavicle
  - ● S42.025   Nondisplaced fracture of shaft of left clavicle
  - ● S42.026   Nondisplaced fracture of shaft of unspecified clavicle
- ● S42.03   Fracture of lateral end of clavicle

  Fracture of acromial end of clavicle
  - ● S42.031   Displaced fracture of lateral end of right clavicle
  - ● S42.032   Displaced fracture of lateral end of left clavicle
  - ● S42.033   Displaced fracture of lateral end of unspecified clavicle
  - ● S42.034   Nondisplaced fracture of lateral end of right clavicle
  - ● S42.035   Nondisplaced fracture of lateral end of left clavicle
  - ● S42.036   Nondisplaced fracture of lateral end of unspecified clavicle
- ● S42.1   Fracture of scapula
  - ● S42.10   Fracture of unspecified part of scapula
    - ● S42.101   Fracture of unspecified part of scapula, right shoulder
    - ● S42.102   Fracture of unspecified part of scapula, left shoulder
    - ● S42.109   Fracture of unspecified part of scapula, unspecified shoulder
  - ● S42.11   Fracture of body of scapula
    - ● S42.111   Displaced fracture of body of scapula, right shoulder
    - ● S42.112   Displaced fracture of body of scapula, left shoulder
    - ● S42.113   Displaced fracture of body of scapula, unspecified shoulder
    - ● S42.114   Nondisplaced fracture of body of scapula, right shoulder
    - ● S42.115   Nondisplaced fracture of body of scapula, left shoulder
    - ● S42.116   Nondisplaced fracture of body of scapula, unspecified shoulder
  - ● S42.12   Fracture of acromial process
    - ● S42.121   Displaced fracture of acromial process, right shoulder
    - ● S42.122   Displaced fracture of acromial process, left shoulder
    - ● S42.123   Displaced fracture of acromial process, unspecified shoulder
    - ● S42.124   Nondisplaced fracture of acromial process, right shoulder
    - ● S42.125   Nondisplaced fracture of acromial process, left shoulder
    - ● S42.126   Nondisplaced fracture, of acromial process, unspecified shoulder

- ● S42.13   Fracture of coracoid process
  - ● S42.131   Displaced fracture of coracoid process, right shoulder
  - ● S42.132   Displaced fracture of coracoid process, left shoulder
  - ● S42.133   Displaced fracture of coracoid process, unspecified shoulder
  - ● S42.134   Nondisplaced fracture of coracoid process, right shoulder
  - ● S42.135   Nondisplaced fracture of coracoid process, left shoulder
  - ● S42.136   Nondisplaced fracture of coracoid process, unspecified shoulder
- ● S42.14   Fracture of glenoid cavity of scapula
  - ● S42.141   Displaced fracture of glenoid cavity of scapula, right shoulder
  - ● S42.142   Displaced fracture of glenoid cavity of scapula, left shoulder
  - ● S42.143   Displaced fracture of glenoid cavity of scapula, unspecified shoulder
  - ● S42.144   Nondisplaced fracture of glenoid cavity of scapula, right shoulder
  - ● S42.145   Nondisplaced fracture of glenoid cavity of scapula, left shoulder
  - ● S42.146   Nondisplaced fracture of glenoid cavity of scapula, unspecified shoulder
- ● S42.15   Fracture of neck of scapula
  - ● S42.151   Displaced fracture of neck of scapula, right shoulder
  - ● S42.152   Displaced fracture of neck of scapula, left shoulder
  - ● S42.153   Displaced fracture of neck of scapula, unspecified shoulder
  - ● S42.154   Nondisplaced fracture of neck of scapula, right shoulder
  - ● S42.155   Nondisplaced fracture of neck of scapula, left shoulder
  - ● S42.156   Nondisplaced fracture of neck of scapula, unspecified shoulder
- ● S42.19   Fracture of other part of scapula
  - ● S42.191   Fracture of other part of scapula, right shoulder
  - ● S42.192   Fracture of other part of scapula, left shoulder
  - ● S42.199   Fracture of other part of scapula, unspecified shoulder
- ● S42.2   Fracture of upper end of humerus

  Fracture of proximal end of humerus

  Excludes2   fracture of shaft of humerus (S42.3-)
  physeal fracture of upper end of humerus (S49.0-)
  - ● S42.20   Unspecified fracture of upper end of humerus
    - ● S42.201   Unspecified fracture of upper end of right humerus
    - ● S42.202   Unspecified fracture of upper end of left humerus
    - ● S42.209   Unspecified fracture of upper end of unspecified humerus

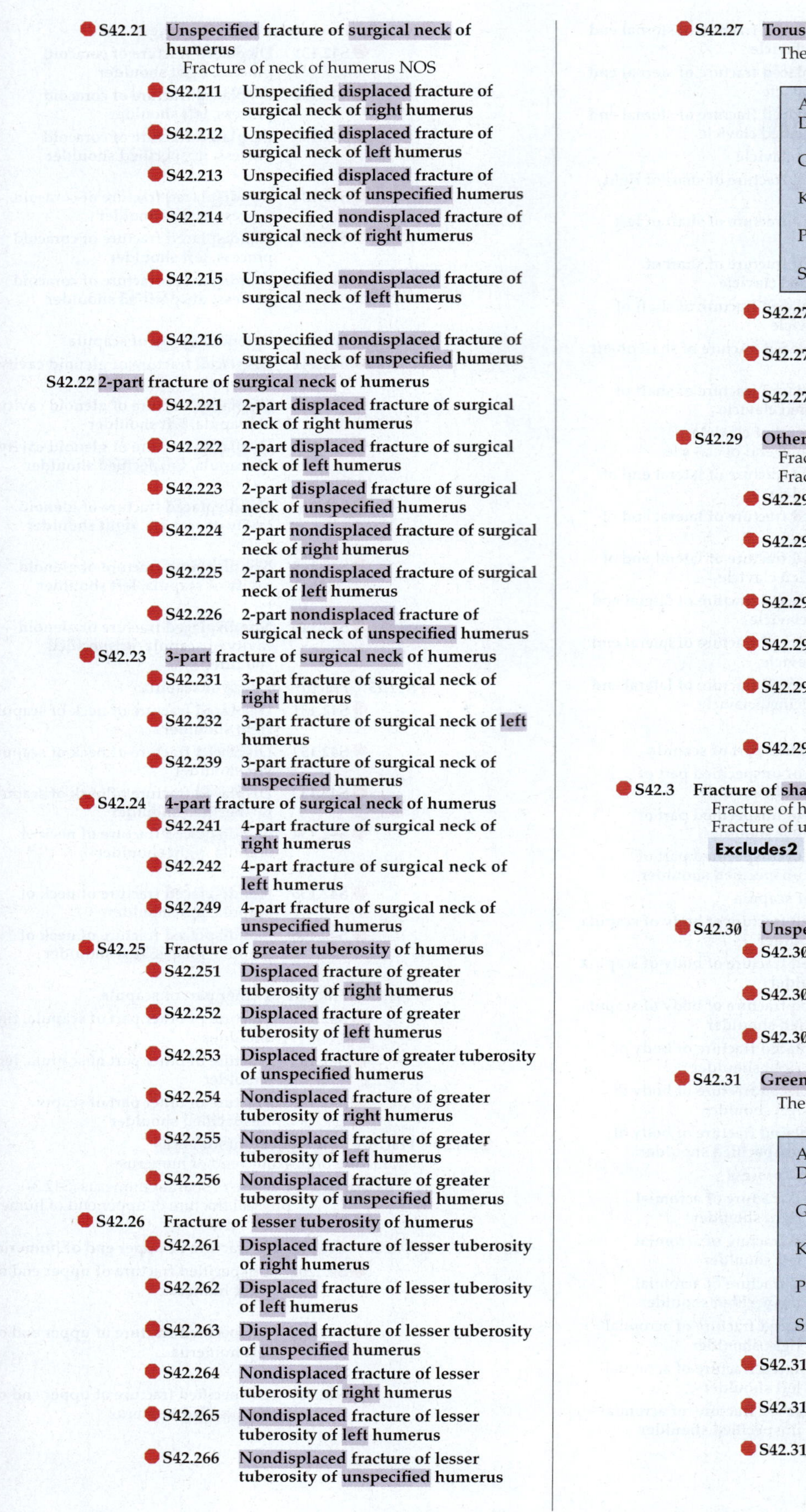

● **S42.21** **Unspecified** fracture of **surgical neck** of **humerus**
Fracture of neck of humerus NOS

  ● **S42.211** Unspecified **displaced** fracture of surgical neck of **right humerus**

  ● **S42.212** Unspecified **displaced** fracture of surgical neck of **left humerus**

  ● **S42.213** Unspecified **displaced** fracture of surgical neck of **unspecified humerus**

  ● **S42.214** Unspecified **nondisplaced** fracture of surgical neck of **right humerus**

  ● **S42.215** Unspecified **nondisplaced** fracture of surgical neck of **left humerus**

  ● **S42.216** Unspecified **nondisplaced** fracture of surgical neck of **unspecified humerus**

● S42.22 **2-part** fracture of **surgical neck** of **humerus**

  ● **S42.221** **2-part displaced** fracture of surgical neck of **right humerus**

  ● **S42.222** **2-part displaced** fracture of surgical neck of **left humerus**

  ● **S42.223** **2-part displaced** fracture of surgical neck of **unspecified humerus**

  ● **S42.224** **2-part nondisplaced** fracture of surgical neck of **right humerus**

  ● **S42.225** **2-part nondisplaced** fracture of surgical neck of **left humerus**

  ● **S42.226** **2-part nondisplaced** fracture of surgical neck of **unspecified humerus**

● S42.23 **3-part** fracture of **surgical neck** of **humerus**

  ● **S42.231** **3-part** fracture of surgical neck of **right humerus**

  ● **S42.232** **3-part** fracture of surgical neck of **left humerus**

  ● **S42.239** **3-part** fracture of surgical neck of **unspecified humerus**

● S42.24 **4-part** fracture of **surgical neck** of **humerus**

  ● **S42.241** **4-part** fracture of surgical neck of **right humerus**

  ● **S42.242** **4-part** fracture of surgical neck of **left humerus**

  ● **S42.249** **4-part** fracture of surgical neck of **unspecified humerus**

● **S42.25** Fracture of **greater tuberosity** of **humerus**

  ● **S42.251** **Displaced** fracture of greater tuberosity of **right humerus**

  ● **S42.252** **Displaced** fracture of greater tuberosity of **left humerus**

  ● **S42.253** **Displaced** fracture of greater tuberosity of **unspecified humerus**

  ● **S42.254** **Nondisplaced** fracture of greater tuberosity of **right humerus**

  ● **S42.255** **Nondisplaced** fracture of greater tuberosity of **left humerus**

  ● **S42.256** **Nondisplaced** fracture of greater tuberosity of **unspecified humerus**

● **S42.26** Fracture of **lesser tuberosity** of **humerus**

  ● **S42.261** **Displaced** fracture of lesser tuberosity of **right humerus**

  ● **S42.262** **Displaced** fracture of lesser tuberosity of **left humerus**

  ● **S42.263** **Displaced** fracture of lesser tuberosity of **unspecified humerus**

  ● **S42.264** **Nondisplaced** fracture of lesser tuberosity of **right humerus**

  ● **S42.265** **Nondisplaced** fracture of lesser tuberosity of **left humerus**

  ● **S42.266** **Nondisplaced** fracture of lesser tuberosity of **unspecified humerus**

● **S42.27** **Torus fracture** of **upper end** of **humerus**
The appropriate 7th character is to be added to all codes in subcategory S42.27

A	initial encounter for closed fracture
D	subsequent encounter for fracture with routine healing
G	subsequent encounter for fracture with delayed healing
K	subsequent encounter for fracture with nonunion
P	subsequent encounter for fracture with malunion
S	sequela

  ● **S42.271** **Torus** fracture of upper end of **right humerus**

  ● **S42.272** **Torus** fracture of upper end of **left humerus**

  ● **S42.279** **Torus** fracture of upper end of **unspecified humerus**

● **S42.29** **Other** fracture of **upper end** of **humerus**
Fracture of anatomical neck of humerus
Fracture of articular head of humerus

  ● **S42.291** **Other displaced** fracture of upper end of **right humerus**

  ● **S42.292** **Other displaced** fracture of upper end of **left humerus**
Coding Clinic: 2024, Q2, P24

  ● **S42.293** **Other displaced** fracture of upper end of **unspecified humerus**

  ● **S42.294** **Other nondisplaced** fracture of upper end of **right humerus**

  ● **S42.295** **Other nondisplaced** fracture of upper end of **left humerus**
Coding Clinic: 2019, Q1, P19

  ● **S42.296** **Other nondisplaced** fracture of upper end of **unspecified humerus**

● **S42.3** Fracture of **shaft** of **humerus**
Fracture of humerus NOS
Fracture of upper arm NOS

  Excludes2   physeal fractures of upper end of humerus (S49.0-)
          physeal fractures of lower end of humerus (S49.1-)

● **S42.30** **Unspecified** fracture of **shaft** of **humerus**

  ● **S42.301** **Unspecified** fracture of shaft of humerus, **right arm**

  ● **S42.302** **Unspecified** fracture of shaft of humerus, **left arm**

  ● **S42.309** **Unspecified** fracture of shaft of humerus, **unspecified arm**

● **S42.31** **Greenstick fracture** of **shaft** of **humerus**
The appropriate 7th character is to be added to all codes in subcategory S42.3

A	initial encounter for closed fracture
D	subsequent encounter for fracture with routine healing
G	subsequent encounter for fracture with delayed healing
K	subsequent encounter for fracture with nonunion
P	subsequent encounter for fracture with malunion
S	sequela

  ● **S42.311** **Greenstick** fracture of shaft of humerus, **right arm**

  ● **S42.312** **Greenstick** fracture of shaft of humerus, **left arm**

  ● **S42.319** **Greenstick** fracture of shaft of humerus, **unspecified arm**

● **S42.32**   **Transverse** fracture of shaft of humerus
- ● **S42.321**   Displaced transverse fracture of shaft of humerus, **right arm**
- ● **S42.322**   Displaced transverse fracture of shaft of humerus, **left arm**
- ● **S42.323**   Displaced transverse fracture of shaft of humerus, **unspecified arm**
- ● **S42.324**   Nondisplaced transverse fracture of shaft of humerus, **right arm**
- ● **S42.325**   Nondisplaced transverse fracture of shaft of humerus, **left arm**
- ● **S42.326**   Nondisplaced transverse fracture of shaft of humerus, **unspecified arm**

● **S42.33**   **Oblique** fracture of shaft of humerus
- ● **S42.331**   Displaced oblique fracture of shaft of humerus, **right arm**
- ● **S42.332**   Displaced oblique fracture of shaft of humerus, **left arm**
- ● **S42.333**   Displaced oblique fracture of shaft of humerus, **unspecified arm**
- ● **S42.334**   Nondisplaced oblique fracture of shaft of humerus, **right arm**
- ● **S42.335**   Nondisplaced oblique fracture of shaft of humerus, **left arm**
- ● **S42.336**   Nondisplaced oblique fracture of shaft of humerus, **unspecified arm**

● **S42.34**   **Spiral** fracture of shaft of humerus
- ● **S42.341**   Displaced spiral fracture of shaft of humerus, **right arm**
- ● **S42.342**   Displaced spiral fracture of shaft of humerus, **left arm**
- ● **S42.343**   Displaced spiral fracture of shaft of humerus, **unspecified arm**
- ● **S42.344**   Nondisplaced spiral fracture of shaft of humerus, **right arm**
- ● **S42.345**   Nondisplaced spiral fracture of shaft of humerus, **left arm**
- ● **S42.346**   Nondisplaced spiral fracture of shaft of humerus, **unspecified arm**

● **S42.35**   **Comminuted** fracture of shaft of humerus
- ● **S42.351**   Displaced comminuted fracture of shaft of humerus, **right arm**
- ● **S42.352**   Displaced comminuted fracture of shaft of humerus, **left arm**
- ● **S42.353**   Displaced comminuted fracture of shaft of humerus, **unspecified arm**
- ● **S42.354**   Nondisplaced comminuted fracture of shaft of humerus, **right arm**
- ● **S42.355**   Nondisplaced comminuted fracture of shaft of humerus, **left arm**
- ● **S42.356**   Nondisplaced comminuted fracture of shaft of humerus, **unspecified arm**

● **S42.36**   **Segmental** fracture of shaft of humerus
- ● **S42.361**   Displaced segmental fracture of shaft of humerus, **right arm**
- ● **S42.362**   Displaced segmental fracture of shaft of humerus, **left arm**
- ● **S42.363**   Displaced segmental fracture of shaft of humerus, **unspecified arm**
- ● **S42.364**   Nondisplaced segmental fracture of shaft of humerus, **right arm**
- ● **S42.365**   Nondisplaced segmental fracture of shaft of humerus, **left arm**
- ● **S42.366**   Nondisplaced segmental fracture of shaft of humerus, **unspecified arm**

● **S42.39**   **Other** fracture of shaft of humerus
- ● **S42.391**   Other fracture of shaft of **right** humerus
- ● **S42.392**   Other fracture of shaft of **left** humerus

● **S42.399**   Other fracture of shaft of **unspecified** humerus

● **S42.4**   Fracture of **lower** end of humerus
Fracture of distal end of humerus
> **Excludes2**   fracture of shaft of humerus (S42.3-)
> physeal fracture of lower end of humerus (S49.1-)

● **S42.40**   **Unspecified** fracture of lower end of humerus
Fracture of elbow NOS
- ● **S42.401**   Unspecified fracture of lower end of **right** humerus
- ● **S42.402**   Unspecified fracture of lower end of **left** humerus
- ● **S42.409**   Unspecified fracture of lower end of **unspecified** humerus

● **S42.41**   Simple supracondylar fracture **without** intercondylar fracture of humerus
- ● **S42.411**   Displaced simple supracondylar fracture without intercondylar fracture of **right** humerus
- ● **S42.412**   Displaced simple supracondylar fracture without intercondylar fracture of **left** humerus
- ● **S42.413**   Displaced simple supracondylar fracture without intercondylar fracture of **unspecified** humerus
- ● **S42.414**   Nondisplaced simple supracondylar fracture without intercondylar fracture of **right** humerus
- ● **S42.415**   Nondisplaced simple supracondylar fracture without intercondylar fracture of **left** humerus
- ● **S42.416**   Nondisplaced simple supracondylar fracture without intercondylar fracture of **unspecified** humerus

● **S42.42**   Comminuted supracondylar fracture **without** intercondylar fracture of humerus
- ● **S42.421**   Displaced comminuted supracondylar fracture without intercondylar fracture of **right** humerus
- ● **S42.422**   Displaced comminuted supracondylar fracture without intercondylar fracture of **left** humerus
- ● **S42.423**   Displaced comminuted supracondylar fracture without intercondylar fracture of **unspecified** humerus
- ● **S42.424**   Nondisplaced comminuted supracondylar fracture without intercondylar fracture of **right** humerus
- ● **S42.425**   Nondisplaced comminuted supracondylar fracture without intercondylar fracture of **left** humerus
- ● **S42.426**   Nondisplaced comminuted supracondylar fracture without intercondylar fracture of **unspecified** humerus

● **S42.43**   Fracture (avulsion) of **lateral epicondyle** of humerus
- ● **S42.431**   Displaced fracture (avulsion) of lateral epicondyle of **right** humerus
- ● **S42.432**   Displaced fracture (avulsion) of lateral epicondyle of **left** humerus
- ● **S42.433**   Displaced fracture (avulsion) of lateral epicondyle of **unspecified** humerus
- ● **S42.434**   Nondisplaced fracture (avulsion) of lateral epicondyle of **right** humerus
- ● **S42.435**   Nondisplaced fracture (avulsion) of lateral epicondyle of **left** humerus
- ● **S42.436**   Nondisplaced fracture (avulsion) of lateral epicondyle of **unspecified** humerus

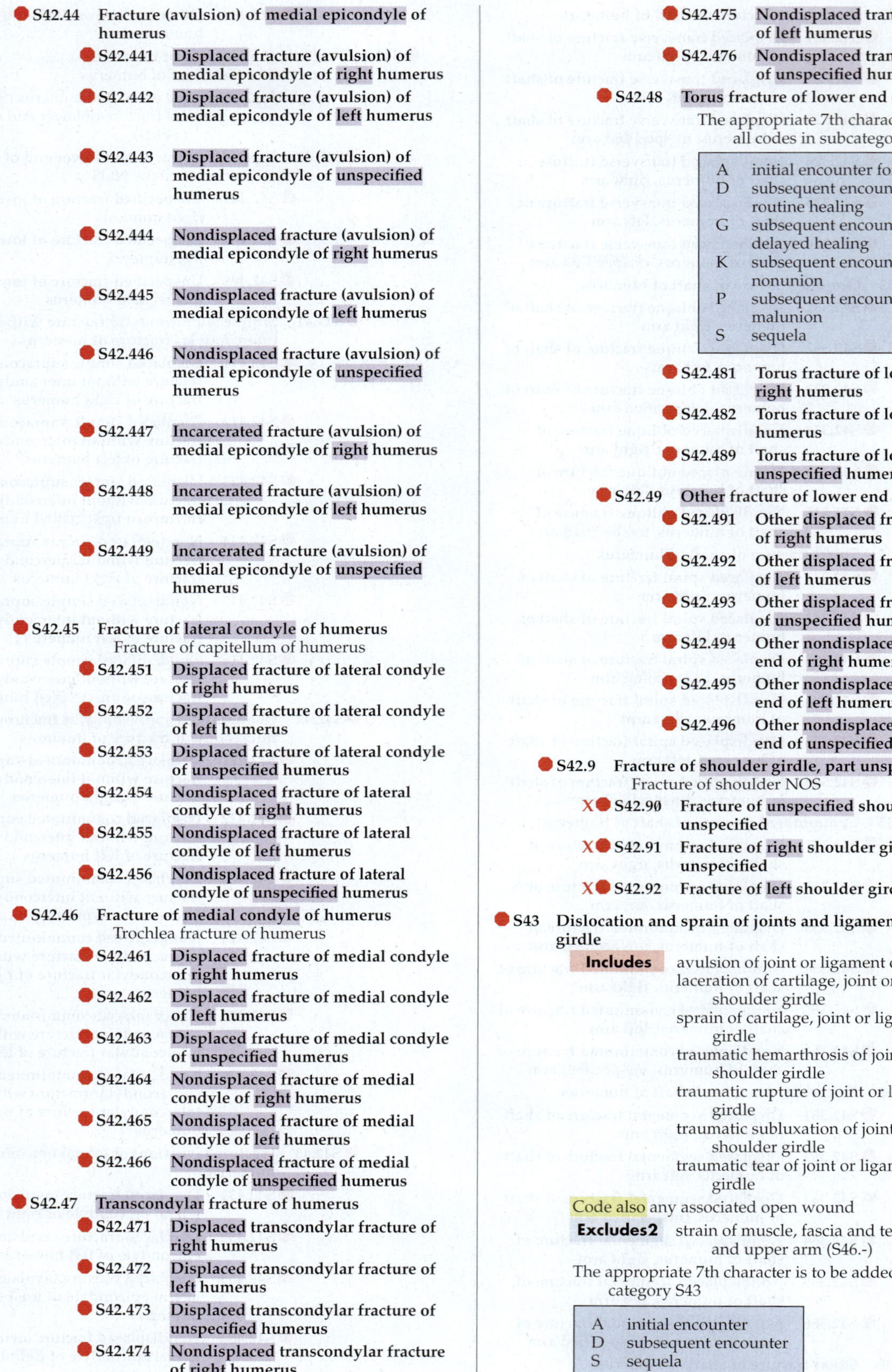

● **S42.44**   Fracture (avulsion) of medial epicondyle of humerus

  ● **S42.441**   Displaced fracture (avulsion) of medial epicondyle of right humerus

  ● **S42.442**   Displaced fracture (avulsion) of medial epicondyle of left humerus

  ● **S42.443**   Displaced fracture (avulsion) of medial epicondyle of unspecified humerus

  ● **S42.444**   Nondisplaced fracture (avulsion) of medial epicondyle of right humerus

  ● **S42.445**   Nondisplaced fracture (avulsion) of medial epicondyle of left humerus

  ● **S42.446**   Nondisplaced fracture (avulsion) of medial epicondyle of unspecified humerus

  ● **S42.447**   Incarcerated fracture (avulsion) of medial epicondyle of right humerus

  ● **S42.448**   Incarcerated fracture (avulsion) of medial epicondyle of left humerus

  ● **S42.449**   Incarcerated fracture (avulsion) of medial epicondyle of unspecified humerus

● **S42.45**   Fracture of lateral condyle of humerus
Fracture of capitellum of humerus

  ● **S42.451**   Displaced fracture of lateral condyle of right humerus

  ● **S42.452**   Displaced fracture of lateral condyle of left humerus

  ● **S42.453**   Displaced fracture of lateral condyle of unspecified humerus

  ● **S42.454**   Nondisplaced fracture of lateral condyle of right humerus

  ● **S42.455**   Nondisplaced fracture of lateral condyle of left humerus

  ● **S42.456**   Nondisplaced fracture of lateral condyle of unspecified humerus

● **S42.46**   Fracture of medial condyle of humerus
Trochlea fracture of humerus

  ● **S42.461**   Displaced fracture of medial condyle of right humerus

  ● **S42.462**   Displaced fracture of medial condyle of left humerus

  ● **S42.463**   Displaced fracture of medial condyle of unspecified humerus

  ● **S42.464**   Nondisplaced fracture of medial condyle of right humerus

  ● **S42.465**   Nondisplaced fracture of medial condyle of left humerus

  ● **S42.466**   Nondisplaced fracture of medial condyle of unspecified humerus

● **S42.47**   Transcondylar fracture of humerus

  ● **S42.471**   Displaced transcondylar fracture of right humerus

  ● **S42.472**   Displaced transcondylar fracture of left humerus

  ● **S42.473**   Displaced transcondylar fracture of unspecified humerus

  ● **S42.474**   Nondisplaced transcondylar fracture of right humerus

  ● **S42.475**   Nondisplaced transcondylar fracture of left humerus

  ● **S42.476**   Nondisplaced transcondylar fracture of unspecified humerus

● **S42.48**   Torus fracture of lower end of humerus
The appropriate 7th character is to be added to all codes in subcategory S42.48

A	initial encounter for closed fracture
D	subsequent encounter for fracture with routine healing
G	subsequent encounter for fracture with delayed healing
K	subsequent encounter for fracture with nonunion
P	subsequent encounter for fracture with malunion
S	sequela

  ● **S42.481**   Torus fracture of lower end of right humerus

  ● **S42.482**   Torus fracture of lower end of left humerus

  ● **S42.489**   Torus fracture of lower end of unspecified humerus

● **S42.49**   Other fracture of lower end of humerus

  ● **S42.491**   Other displaced fracture of lower end of right humerus

  ● **S42.492**   Other displaced fracture of lower end of left humerus

  ● **S42.493**   Other displaced fracture of lower end of unspecified humerus

  ● **S42.494**   Other nondisplaced fracture of lower end of right humerus

  ● **S42.495**   Other nondisplaced fracture of lower end of left humerus

  ● **S42.496**   Other nondisplaced fracture of lower end of unspecified humerus

● **S42.9**   Fracture of shoulder girdle, part unspecified
Fracture of shoulder NOS

  X ● **S42.90**   Fracture of unspecified shoulder girdle, part unspecified

  X ● **S42.91**   Fracture of right shoulder girdle, part unspecified

  X ● **S42.92**   Fracture of left shoulder girdle, part unspecified

● **S43**   Dislocation and sprain of joints and ligaments of shoulder girdle

Includes   avulsion of joint or ligament of shoulder girdle
laceration of cartilage, joint or ligament of shoulder girdle
sprain of cartilage, joint or ligament of shoulder girdle
traumatic hemarthrosis of joint or ligament of shoulder girdle
traumatic rupture of joint or ligament of shoulder girdle
traumatic subluxation of joint or ligament of shoulder girdle
traumatic tear of joint or ligament of shoulder girdle

Code also any associated open wound

Excludes2   strain of muscle, fascia and tendon of shoulder and upper arm (S46.-)

The appropriate 7th character is to be added to each code from category S43

A	initial encounter
D	subsequent encounter
S	sequela

● **S43.0** **Subluxation and dislocation of shoulder joint**
 Dislocation of glenohumeral joint
 Subluxation of glenohumeral joint
 ● **S43.00** **Unspecified subluxation and dislocation of shoulder joint**
  Dislocation of humerus NOS
  Subluxation of humerus NOS
  ● **S43.001** Unspecified subluxation of right shoulder joint
  ● **S43.002** Unspecified subluxation of left shoulder joint
  ● **S43.003** Unspecified subluxation of unspecified shoulder joint
  ● **S43.004** Unspecified dislocation of right shoulder joint
  ● **S43.005** Unspecified dislocation of left shoulder joint
  ● **S43.006** Unspecified dislocation of unspecified shoulder joint
 ● **S43.01** **Anterior subluxation and dislocation of humerus**
  ● **S43.011** Anterior subluxation of right humerus
  ● **S43.012** Anterior subluxation of left humerus
  ● **S43.013** Anterior subluxation of unspecified humerus
  ● **S43.014** Anterior dislocation of right humerus
  ● **S43.015** Anterior dislocation of left humerus
  ● **S43.016** Anterior dislocation of unspecified humerus
 ● **S43.02** **Posterior subluxation and dislocation of humerus**
  ● **S43.021** Posterior subluxation of right humerus
  ● **S43.022** Posterior subluxation of left humerus
  ● **S43.023** Posterior subluxation of unspecified humerus
  ● **S43.024** Posterior dislocation of right humerus
  ● **S43.025** Posterior dislocation of left humerus
  ● **S43.026** Posterior dislocation of unspecified humerus
 ● **S43.03** **Inferior subluxation and dislocation of humerus**
  ● **S43.031** Inferior subluxation of right humerus
  ● **S43.032** Inferior subluxation of left humerus
  ● **S43.033** Inferior subluxation of unspecified humerus
  ● **S43.034** Inferior dislocation of right humerus
  ● **S43.035** Inferior dislocation of left humerus
  ● **S43.036** Inferior dislocation of unspecified humerus
 ● **S43.08** **Other subluxation and dislocation of shoulder joint**
  ● **S43.081** Other subluxation of right shoulder joint
  ● **S43.082** Other subluxation of left shoulder joint
  ● **S43.083** Other subluxation of unspecified shoulder joint
  ● **S43.084** Other dislocation of right shoulder joint
  ● **S43.085** Other dislocation of left shoulder joint
  ● **S43.086** Other dislocation of unspecified shoulder joint
● **S43.1** **Subluxation and dislocation of acromioclavicular joint**
 ● **S43.10** **Unspecified dislocation of acromioclavicular joint**
  ● **S43.101** Unspecified dislocation of right acromioclavicular joint

  ● **S43.102** Unspecified dislocation of left acromioclavicular joint
  ● **S43.109** Unspecified dislocation of unspecified acromioclavicular joint
 ● **S43.11** **Subluxation of acromioclavicular joint**
  ● **S43.111** Subluxation of right acromioclavicular joint
  ● **S43.112** Subluxation of left acromioclavicular joint
  ● **S43.119** Subluxation of unspecified acromioclavicular joint
 ● **S43.12** **Dislocation of acromioclavicular joint, 100%-200% displacement**
  ● **S43.121** Dislocation of right acromioclavicular joint, 100%-200% displacement
  ● **S43.122** Dislocation of left acromioclavicular joint, 100%-200% displacement
  ● **S43.129** Dislocation of unspecified acromioclavicular joint, 100%-200% displacement
 ● **S43.13** **Dislocation of acromioclavicular joint, greater than 200% displacement**
  ● **S43.131** Dislocation of right acromioclavicular joint, greater than 200% displacement
  ● **S43.132** Dislocation of left acromioclavicular joint, greater than 200% displacement
  ● **S43.139** Dislocation of unspecified acromioclavicular joint, greater than 200% displacement
 ● **S43.14** **Inferior dislocation of acromioclavicular joint**
  ● **S43.141** Inferior dislocation of right acromioclavicular joint
  ● **S43.142** Inferior dislocation of left acromioclavicular joint
  ● **S43.149** Inferior dislocation of unspecified acromioclavicular joint
 ● **S43.15** **Posterior dislocation of acromioclavicular joint**
  ● **S43.151** Posterior dislocation of right acromioclavicular joint
  ● **S43.152** Posterior dislocation of left acromioclavicular joint
  ● **S43.159** Posterior dislocation of unspecified acromioclavicular joint
● **S43.2** **Subluxation and dislocation of sternoclavicular joint**
 ● **S43.20** **Unspecified subluxation and dislocation of sternoclavicular joint**
  ● **S43.201** Unspecified subluxation of right sternoclavicular joint
  ● **S43.202** Unspecified subluxation of left sternoclavicular joint
  ● **S43.203** Unspecified subluxation of unspecified sternoclavicular joint
  ● **S43.204** Unspecified dislocation of right sternoclavicular joint
  ● **S43.205** Unspecified dislocation of left sternoclavicular joint
  ● **S43.206** Unspecified dislocation of unspecified sternoclavicular joint
 ● **S43.21** **Anterior subluxation and dislocation of sternoclavicular joint**
  ● **S43.211** Anterior subluxation of right sternoclavicular joint
  ● **S43.212** Anterior subluxation of left sternoclavicular joint
  ● **S43.213** Anterior subluxation of unspecified sternoclavicular joint
  ● **S43.214** Anterior dislocation of right sternoclavicular joint
  ● **S43.215** Anterior dislocation of left sternoclavicular joint
  ● **S43.216** Anterior dislocation of unspecified sternoclavicular joint

CHAPTER 19 (S00-T88)

● **S43.22** Posterior subluxation and dislocation of sternoclavicular joint

   ● **S43.221** Posterior subluxation of right sternoclavicular joint

   ● **S43.222** Posterior subluxation of left sternoclavicular joint

   ● **S43.223** Posterior subluxation of unspecified sternoclavicular joint

   ● **S43.224** Posterior dislocation of right sternoclavicular joint

   ● **S43.225** Posterior dislocation of left sternoclavicular joint

   ● **S43.226** Posterior dislocation of unspecified sternoclavicular joint

● **S43.3** Subluxation and dislocation of other and unspecified parts of shoulder girdle

  ● **S43.30** Subluxation and dislocation of unspecified parts of shoulder girdle

    Dislocation of shoulder girdle NOS
    Subluxation of shoulder girdle NOS

   ● **S43.301** Subluxation of unspecified parts of right shoulder girdle

   ● **S43.302** Subluxation of unspecified parts of left shoulder girdle

   ● **S43.303** Subluxation of unspecified parts of unspecified shoulder girdle

   ● **S43.304** Dislocation of unspecified parts of right shoulder girdle

   ● **S43.305** Dislocation of unspecified parts of left shoulder girdle

   ● **S43.306** Dislocation of unspecified parts of unspecified shoulder girdle

  ● **S43.31** Subluxation and dislocation of scapula

   ● **S43.311** Subluxation of right scapula

   ● **S43.312** Subluxation of left scapula

   ● **S43.313** Subluxation of unspecified scapula

   ● **S43.314** Dislocation of right scapula

   ● **S43.315** Dislocation of left scapula

   ● **S43.316** Dislocation of unspecified scapula

  ● **S43.39** Subluxation and dislocation of other parts of shoulder girdle

   ● **S43.391** Subluxation of other parts of right shoulder girdle

   ● **S43.392** Subluxation of other parts of left shoulder girdle

   ● **S43.393** Subluxation of other parts of unspecified shoulder girdle

   ● **S43.394** Dislocation of other parts of right shoulder girdle

   ● **S43.395** Dislocation of other parts of left shoulder girdle

   ● **S43.396** Dislocation of other parts of unspecified shoulder girdle

● **S43.4** Sprain of shoulder joint

  ● **S43.40** Unspecified sprain of shoulder joint

   ● **S43.401** Unspecified sprain of right shoulder joint

   ● **S43.402** Unspecified sprain of left shoulder joint

   ● **S43.409** Unspecified sprain of unspecified shoulder joint

  ● **S43.41** Sprain of coracohumeral (ligament)

   ● **S43.411** Sprain of right coracohumeral (ligament)

   ● **S43.412** Sprain of left coracohumeral (ligament)

   ● **S43.419** Sprain of unspecified coracohumeral (ligament)

● **S43.42** Sprain of rotator cuff capsule

   Encounters during the healing phase

   Excludes1 rotator cuff syndrome (complete) (incomplete), not specified as traumatic (M75.1-)

   Excludes2 injury of tendon of rotator cuff (S46.0-)

   ● **S43.421** Sprain of right rotator cuff capsule

   ● **S43.422** Sprain of left rotator cuff capsule

   ● **S43.429** Sprain of unspecified rotator cuff capsule

  ● **S43.43** Superior glenoid labrum lesion

    SLAP lesion

    Coding Clinic: 2019, Q2, P27

   ● **S43.431** Superior glenoid labrum lesion of right shoulder

   ● **S43.432** Superior glenoid labrum lesion of left shoulder

    Coding Clinic: 2024, Q2, P24

   ● **S43.439** Superior glenoid labrum lesion of unspecified shoulder

  ● **S43.49** Other sprain of shoulder joint

   ● **S43.491** Other sprain of right shoulder joint

   ● **S43.492** Other sprain of left shoulder joint

   ● **S43.499** Other sprain of unspecified shoulder joint

● **S43.5** Sprain of acromioclavicular joint

   Sprain of acromioclavicular ligament

  X ● **S43.50** Sprain of unspecified acromioclavicular joint

  X ● **S43.51** Sprain of right acromioclavicular joint

  X ● **S43.52** Sprain of left acromioclavicular joint

● **S43.6** Sprain of sternoclavicular joint

  X ● **S43.60** Sprain of unspecified sternoclavicular joint

  X ● **S43.61** Sprain of right sternoclavicular joint

  X ● **S43.62** Sprain of left sternoclavicular joint

● **S43.8** Sprain of other specified parts of shoulder girdle

  X ● **S43.80** Sprain of other specified parts of unspecified shoulder girdle

  X ● **S43.81** Sprain of other specified parts of right shoulder girdle

  X ● **S43.82** Sprain of other specified parts of left shoulder girdle

● **S43.9** Sprain of unspecified parts of shoulder girdle

  X ● **S43.90** Sprain of unspecified parts of unspecified shoulder girdle

    Sprain of shoulder girdle NOS

  X ● **S43.91** Sprain of unspecified parts of right shoulder girdle

  X ● **S43.92** Sprain of unspecified parts of left shoulder girdle

● **S44** Injury of nerves at shoulder and upper arm level

   Code also any associated open wound (S41.-)

   Excludes2 injury of brachial plexus (S14.3-)

   The appropriate 7th character is to be added to each code from category S44

A	initial encounter
D	subsequent encounter
S	sequela

● **S44.0** Injury of ulnar nerve at upper arm level

   Excludes1 ulnar nerve NOS (S54.0)

  X ● **S44.00** Injury of ulnar nerve at upper arm level, unspecified arm

  X ● **S44.01** Injury of ulnar nerve at upper arm level, right arm

  X ● **S44.02** Injury of ulnar nerve at upper arm level, left arm

● **S44.1** Injury of median nerve at upper arm level

   Excludes1 median nerve NOS (S54.1)

X ● **S44.10**   Injury of median nerve at upper arm level, unspecified arm

X ● **S44.11**   Injury of median nerve at upper arm level, right arm

X ● **S44.12**   Injury of median nerve at upper arm level, left arm

● **S44.2**   Injury of radial nerve at upper arm level

> **Excludes1**   radial nerve NOS (S54.2)

X ● **S44.20**   Injury of radial nerve at upper arm level, unspecified arm

X ● **S44.21**   Injury of radial nerve at upper arm level, right arm

X ● **S44.22**   Injury of radial nerve at upper arm level, left arm

● **S44.3**   Injury of axillary nerve

X ● **S44.30**   Injury of axillary nerve, unspecified arm

X ● **S44.31**   Injury of axillary nerve, right arm

X ● **S44.32**   Injury of axillary nerve, left arm

● **S44.4**   Injury of musculocutaneous nerve

X ● **S44.40**   Injury of musculocutaneous nerve, unspecified arm

X ● **S44.41**   Injury of musculocutaneous nerve, right arm

X ● **S44.42**   Injury of musculocutaneous nerve, left arm

● **S44.5**   Injury of cutaneous sensory nerve at shoulder and upper arm level

X ● **S44.50**   Injury of cutaneous sensory nerve at shoulder and upper arm level, unspecified arm

X ● **S44.51**   Injury of cutaneous sensory nerve at shoulder and upper arm level, right arm

X ● **S44.52**   Injury of cutaneous sensory nerve at shoulder and upper arm level, left arm

● **S44.8**   Injury of other nerves at shoulder and upper arm level

● **S44.8X**   Injury of other nerves at shoulder and upper arm level

● **S44.8X1**   Injury of other nerves at shoulder and upper arm level, right arm

● **S44.8X2**   Injury of other nerves at shoulder and upper arm level, left arm

● **S44.8X9**   Injury of other nerves at shoulder and upper arm level, unspecified arm

● **S44.9**   Injury of unspecified nerve at shoulder and upper arm level

X ● **S44.90**   Injury of unspecified nerve at shoulder and upper arm level, unspecified arm

X ● **S44.91**   Injury of unspecified nerve at shoulder and upper arm level, right arm

X ● **S44.92**   Injury of unspecified nerve at shoulder and upper arm level, left arm

● **S45**   Injury of blood vessels at shoulder and upper arm level

> Code also any associated open wound (S41.-)
>
> **Excludes2**   injury of subclavian artery (S25.1)
> injury of subclavian vein (S25.3)

The appropriate 7th character is to be added to each code from category S45

> A   initial encounter
> D   subsequent encounter
> S   sequela

● **S45.0**   Injury of axillary artery

● **S45.00**   Unspecified injury of axillary artery

● **S45.001**   Unspecified injury of axillary artery, right side

● **S45.002**   Unspecified injury of axillary artery, left side

● **S45.009**   Unspecified injury of axillary artery, unspecified side

● **S45.01**   Laceration of axillary artery

● **S45.011**   Laceration of axillary artery, right side

● **S45.012**   Laceration of axillary artery, left side

● **S45.019**   Laceration of axillary artery, unspecified side

● **S45.09**   Other specified injury of axillary artery

● **S45.091**   Other specified injury of axillary artery, right side

● **S45.092**   Other specified injury of axillary artery, left side

● **S45.099**   Other specified injury of axillary artery, unspecified side

● **S45.1**   Injury of brachial artery

● **S45.10**   Unspecified injury of brachial artery

● **S45.101**   Unspecified injury of brachial artery, right side

● **S45.102**   Unspecified injury of brachial artery, left side

● **S45.109**   Unspecified injury of brachial artery, unspecified side

● **S45.11**   Laceration of brachial artery

● **S45.111**   Laceration of brachial artery, right side

● **S45.112**   Laceration of brachial artery, left side

● **S45.119**   Laceration of brachial artery, unspecified side

● **S45.19**   Other specified injury of brachial artery

● **S45.191**   Other specified injury of brachial artery, right side

● **S45.192**   Other specified injury of brachial artery, left side

● **S45.199**   Other specified injury of brachial artery, unspecified side

● **S45.2**   Injury of axillary or brachial vein

● **S45.20**   Unspecified injury of axillary or brachial vein

● **S45.201**   Unspecified injury of axillary or brachial vein, right side

● **S45.202**   Unspecified injury of axillary or brachial vein, left side

● **S45.209**   Unspecified injury of axillary or brachial vein, unspecified side

● **S45.21**   Laceration of axillary or brachial vein

● **S45.211**   Laceration of axillary or brachial vein, right side

● **S45.212**   Laceration of axillary or brachial vein, left side

● **S45.219**   Laceration of axillary or brachial vein, unspecified side

● **S45.29**   Other specified injury of axillary or brachial vein

● **S45.291**   Other specified injury of axillary or brachial vein, right side

● **S45.292**   Other specified injury of axillary or brachial vein, left side

● **S45.299**   Other specified injury of axillary or brachial vein, unspecified side

● **S45.3**   Injury of superficial vein at shoulder and upper arm level

● **S45.30**   Unspecified injury of superficial vein at shoulder and upper arm level

● **S45.301**   Unspecified injury of superficial vein at shoulder and upper arm level, right arm

● **S45.302**   Unspecified injury of superficial vein at shoulder and upper arm level, left arm

● **S45.309**   Unspecified injury of superficial vein at shoulder and upper arm level, unspecified arm

● **S45.31** **Laceration** of superficial vein at shoulder and upper arm level
   ● **S45.311** Laceration of superficial vein at shoulder and upper arm level, **right** arm
   ● **S45.312** Laceration of superficial vein at shoulder and upper arm level, **left** arm
   ● **S45.319** Laceration of superficial vein at shoulder and upper arm level, **unspecified** arm
● **S45.39** Other specified injury of superficial vein at shoulder and upper arm level
   ● **S45.391** Other specified injury of superficial vein at shoulder and upper arm level, **right arm**
   ● **S45.392** Other specified injury of superficial vein at shoulder and upper arm level, **left arm**
   ● **S45.399** Other specified injury of superficial vein at shoulder and upper arm level, **unspecified arm**
● **S45.8** Injury of **other specified blood vessels** at shoulder and upper arm level
   ● **S45.80** **Unspecified** injury of other specified blood vessels at shoulder and upper arm level
      ● **S45.801** Unspecified injury of other specified blood vessels at shoulder and upper arm level, **right arm**
      ● **S45.802** Unspecified injury of other specified blood vessels at shoulder and upper arm level, **left arm**
      ● **S45.809** Unspecified injury of other specified blood vessels at shoulder and upper arm level, **unspecified arm**
   ● **S45.81** **Laceration** of other specified blood vessels at shoulder and upper arm level
      ● **S45.811** Laceration of other specified blood vessels at shoulder and upper arm level, **right arm**
      ● **S45.812** Laceration of other specified blood vessels at shoulder and upper arm level, **left arm**
      ● **S45.819** Laceration of other specified blood vessels at shoulder and upper arm level, **unspecified arm**
   ● **S45.89** **Other specified injury** of other specified blood vessels at shoulder and upper arm level
      ● **S45.891** Other specified injury of other specified blood vessels at shoulder and upper arm level, **right arm**
      ● **S45.892** Other specified injury of other specified blood vessels at shoulder and upper arm level, **left arm**
      ● **S45.899** Other specified injury of other specified blood vessels at shoulder and upper arm level, **unspecified arm**
● **S45.9** Injury of **unspecified blood vessel** at shoulder and upper arm level
   ● **S45.90** **Unspecified** injury of unspecified blood vessel at shoulder and upper arm level
      ● **S45.901** Unspecified injury of unspecified blood vessel at shoulder and upper arm level, **right arm**
      ● **S45.902** Unspecified injury of unspecified blood vessel at shoulder and upper arm level, **left arm**

● **S45.909** Unspecified injury of unspecified blood vessel at shoulder and upper arm level, **unspecified arm**
   ● **S45.91** **Laceration** of unspecified blood vessel at shoulder and upper arm level
      ● **S45.911** Laceration of unspecified blood vessel at shoulder and upper arm level, **right arm**
      ● **S45.912** Laceration of unspecified blood vessel at shoulder and upper arm level, **left arm**
      ● **S45.919** Laceration of unspecified blood vessel at shoulder and upper arm level, **unspecified arm**
   ● **S45.99** **Other** specified injury of unspecified blood vessel at shoulder and upper arm level
      ● **S45.991** Other specified injury of unspecified blood vessel at shoulder and upper arm level, **right arm**
      ● **S45.992** Other specified injury of unspecified blood vessel at shoulder and upper arm level, **left arm**
      ● **S45.999** Other specified injury of unspecified blood vessel at shoulder and upper arm level, **unspecified arm**

● **S46** **Injury of muscle, fascia and tendon at shoulder and upper arm level**
   Code also any associated open wound (S41.-)
   Excludes2 injury of muscle, fascia and tendon at elbow (S56.-)
               sprain of joints and ligaments of shoulder girdle (S43.9)

   The appropriate 7th character is to be added to each code from category S46

A	initial encounter
D	subsequent encounter
S	sequela

   ● **S46.0** Injury of muscle(s) and tendon(s) of the **rotator cuff of** shoulder
      ● **S46.00** **Unspecified** injury of muscle(s) and tendon(s) of the rotator cuff of shoulder
         ● **S46.001** Unspecified injury of muscle(s) and tendon(s) of the rotator cuff of **right** shoulder
         ● **S46.002** Unspecified injury of muscle(s) and tendon(s) of the rotator cuff of **left** shoulder
         ● **S46.009** Unspecified injury of muscle(s) and tendon(s) of the rotator cuff of **unspecified** shoulder
      ● **S46.01** **Strain** of muscle(s) and tendon(s) of the rotator cuff of shoulder
         Acute onset due to trauma to rotator cuff muscle/ tendon
         ● **S46.011** Strain of muscle(s) and tendon(s) of the rotator cuff of **right** shoulder
         ● **S46.012** Strain of muscle(s) and tendon(s) of the rotator cuff of **left** shoulder
         ● **S46.019** Strain of muscle(s) and tendon(s) of the rotator cuff of **unspecified** shoulder
      ● **S46.02** **Laceration** of muscle(s) and tendon(s) of the rotator cuff of shoulder
         ● **S46.021** Laceration of muscle(s) and tendon(s) of the rotator cuff of **right** shoulder
         ● **S46.022** Laceration of muscle(s) and tendon(s) of the rotator cuff of **left** shoulder
         ● **S46.029** Laceration of muscle(s) and tendon(s) of the rotator cuff of **unspecified** shoulder

▶ New   ⇒ Revised   ~~deleted~~ Deleted   Excludes 1   Excludes 2   Includes   Use additional   Code first   Code also   Key words
OGCR Official Guidelines   X Assign placeholder X   ● Use Additional Character(s)   ▌ Manifestation Code   ⬟ Hierarchical Condition Category   **Coding Clinic**

- ● **S46.09**   Other injury of muscle(s) and tendon(s) of the rotator cuff of shoulder
  - ● **S46.091**   Other injury of muscle(s) and tendon(s) of the rotator cuff of right shoulder
  - ● **S46.092**   Other injury of muscle(s) and tendon(s) of the rotator cuff of left shoulder
  - ● **S46.099**   Other injury of muscle(s) and tendon(s) of the rotator cuff of unspecified shoulder
- ● **S46.1**   Injury of muscle, fascia and tendon of long head of biceps
  - ● **S46.10**   Unspecified injury of muscle, fascia and tendon of long head of biceps
    - ● **S46.101**   Unspecified injury of muscle, fascia and tendon of long head of biceps, right arm
    - ● **S46.102**   Unspecified injury of muscle, fascia and tendon of long head of biceps, left arm
    - ● **S46.109**   Unspecified injury of muscle, fascia and tendon of long head of biceps, unspecified arm
  - ● **S46.11**   Strain of muscle, fascia and tendon of long head of biceps
    - **Coding Clinic: 2019, Q2, P27**
    - ● **S46.111**   Strain of muscle, fascia and tendon of long head of biceps, right arm
    - ● **S46.112**   Strain of muscle, fascia and tendon of long head of biceps, left arm
    - ● **S46.119**   Strain of muscle, fascia and tendon of long head of biceps, unspecified arm
  - ● **S46.12**   Laceration of muscle, fascia and tendon of long head of biceps
    - ● **S46.121**   Laceration of muscle, fascia and tendon of long head of biceps, right arm
    - ● **S46.122**   Laceration of muscle, fascia and tendon of long head of biceps, left arm
    - ● **S46.129**   Laceration of muscle, fascia and tendon of long head of biceps, unspecified arm
  - ● **S46.19**   Other injury of muscle, fascia and tendon of long head of biceps
    - ● **S46.191**   Other injury of muscle, fascia and tendon of long head of biceps, right arm
    - ● **S46.192**   Other injury of muscle, fascia and tendon of long head of biceps, left arm
    - ● **S46.199**   Other injury of muscle, fascia and tendon of long head of biceps, unspecified arm
- ● **S46.2**   Injury of muscle, fascia and tendon of other parts of biceps
  - ● **S46.20**   Unspecified injury of muscle, fascia and tendon of other parts of biceps
    - ● **S46.201**   Unspecified injury of muscle, fascia and tendon of other parts of biceps, right arm
    - ● **S46.202**   Unspecified injury of muscle, fascia and tendon of other parts of biceps, left arm
    - ● **S46.209**   Unspecified injury of muscle, fascia and tendon of other parts of biceps, unspecified arm
  - ● **S46.21**   Strain of muscle, fascia and tendon of other parts of biceps
    - ● **S46.211**   Strain of muscle, fascia and tendon of other parts of biceps, right arm

- ● **S46.212**   Strain of muscle, fascia and tendon of other parts of biceps, left arm
- ● **S46.219**   Strain of muscle, fascia and tendon of other parts of biceps, unspecified arm
  - ● **S46.22**   Laceration of muscle, fascia and tendon of other parts of biceps
    - ● **S46.221**   Laceration of muscle, fascia and tendon of other parts of biceps, right arm
    - ● **S46.222**   Laceration of muscle, fascia and tendon of other parts of biceps, left arm
    - ● **S46.229**   Laceration of muscle, fascia and tendon of other parts of biceps, unspecified arm
  - ● **S46.29**   Other injury of muscle, fascia and tendon of other parts of biceps
    - ● **S46.291**   Other injury of muscle, fascia and tendon of other parts of biceps, right arm
    - ● **S46.292**   Other injury of muscle, fascia and tendon of other parts of biceps, left arm
    - ● **S46.299**   Other injury of muscle, fascia and tendon of other parts of biceps, unspecified arm
- ● **S46.3**   Injury of muscle, fascia and tendon of triceps
  - ● **S46.30**   Unspecified injury of muscle, fascia and tendon of triceps
    - ● **S46.301**   Unspecified injury of muscle, fascia and tendon of triceps, right arm
    - ● **S46.302**   Unspecified injury of muscle, fascia and tendon of triceps, left arm
    - ● **S46.309**   Unspecified injury of muscle, fascia and tendon of triceps, unspecified arm
  - ● **S46.31**   Strain of muscle, fascia and tendon of triceps
    - ● **S46.311**   Strain of muscle, fascia and tendon of triceps, right arm
    - ● **S46.312**   Strain of muscle, fascia and tendon of triceps, left arm
    - ● **S46.319**   Strain of muscle, fascia and tendon of triceps, unspecified arm
  - ● **S46.32**   Laceration of muscle, fascia and tendon of triceps
    - ● **S46.321**   Laceration of muscle, fascia and tendon of triceps, right arm
    - ● **S46.322**   Laceration of muscle, fascia and tendon of triceps, left arm
    - ● **S46.329**   Laceration of muscle, fascia and tendon of triceps, unspecified arm
  - ● **S46.39**   Other injury of muscle, fascia and tendon of triceps
    - ● **S46.391**   Other injury of muscle, fascia and tendon of triceps, right arm
    - ● **S46.392**   Other injury of muscle, fascia and tendon of triceps, left arm
    - ● **S46.399**   Other injury of muscle, fascia and tendon of triceps, unspecified arm
- ● **S46.8**   Injury of other muscles, fascia and tendons at shoulder and upper arm level
  - ● **S46.80**   Unspecified injury of other muscles, fascia and tendons at shoulder and upper arm level
    - ● **S46.801**   Unspecified injury of other muscles, fascia and tendons at shoulder and upper arm level, right arm
    - ● **S46.802**   Unspecified injury of other muscles, fascia and tendons at shoulder and upper arm level, left arm
    - ● **S46.809**   Unspecified injury of other muscles, fascia and tendons at shoulder and upper arm level, unspecified arm

CHAPTER 19 (S00–T88)

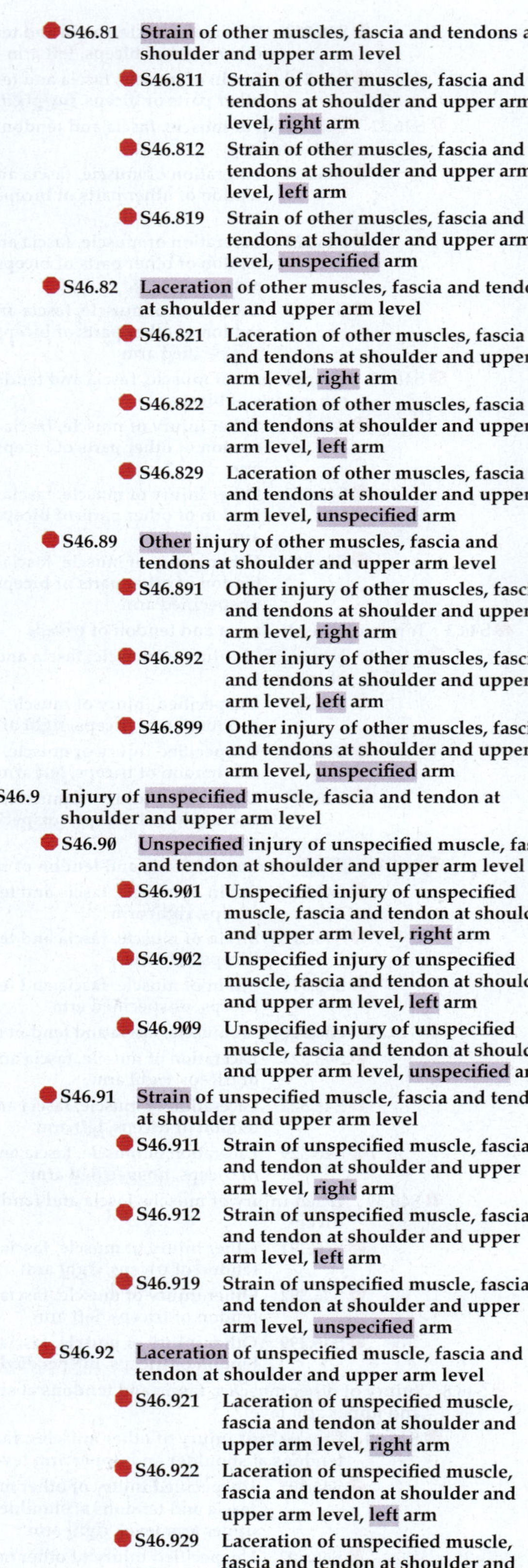

● S46.81 **Strain** of other muscles, fascia and tendons at shoulder and upper arm level

  ● S46.811 Strain of other muscles, fascia and tendons at shoulder and upper arm level, **right arm**

  ● S46.812 Strain of other muscles, fascia and tendons at shoulder and upper arm level, **left arm**

  ● S46.819 Strain of other muscles, fascia and tendons at shoulder and upper arm level, **unspecified arm**

● S46.82 **Laceration** of other muscles, fascia and tendons at shoulder and upper arm level

  ● S46.821 Laceration of other muscles, fascia and tendons at shoulder and upper arm level, **right arm**

  ● S46.822 Laceration of other muscles, fascia and tendons at shoulder and upper arm level, **left arm**

  ● S46.829 Laceration of other muscles, fascia and tendons at shoulder and upper arm level, **unspecified arm**

● S46.89 **Other injury** of other muscles, fascia and tendons at shoulder and upper arm level

  ● S46.891 Other injury of other muscles, fascia and tendons at shoulder and upper arm level, **right arm**

  ● S46.892 Other injury of other muscles, fascia and tendons at shoulder and upper arm level, **left arm**

  ● S46.899 Other injury of other muscles, fascia and tendons at shoulder and upper arm level, **unspecified arm**

● S46.9 Injury of **unspecified** muscle, fascia and tendon at shoulder and upper arm level

  ● S46.90 **Unspecified** injury of unspecified muscle, fascia and tendon at shoulder and upper arm level

    ● S46.901 Unspecified injury of unspecified muscle, fascia and tendon at shoulder and upper arm level, **right arm**

    ● S46.902 Unspecified injury of unspecified muscle, fascia and tendon at shoulder and upper arm level, **left arm**

    ● S46.909 Unspecified injury of unspecified muscle, fascia and tendon at shoulder and upper arm level, **unspecified** arm

  ● S46.91 **Strain** of unspecified muscle, fascia and tendon at shoulder and upper arm level

    ● S46.911 Strain of unspecified muscle, fascia and tendon at shoulder and upper arm level, **right arm**

    ● S46.912 Strain of unspecified muscle, fascia and tendon at shoulder and upper arm level, **left arm**

    ● S46.919 Strain of unspecified muscle, fascia and tendon at shoulder and upper arm level, **unspecified** arm

  ● S46.92 **Laceration** of unspecified muscle, fascia and tendon at shoulder and upper arm level

    ● S46.921 Laceration of unspecified muscle, fascia and tendon at shoulder and upper arm level, **right arm**

    ● S46.922 Laceration of unspecified muscle, fascia and tendon at shoulder and upper arm level, **left arm**

    ● S46.929 Laceration of unspecified muscle, fascia and tendon at shoulder and upper arm level, **unspecified arm**

● S46.99 **Other injury** of unspecified muscle, fascia and tendon at shoulder and upper arm level

  ● S46.991 Other injury of unspecified muscle, fascia and tendon at shoulder and upper arm level, **right arm**

  ● S46.992 Other injury of unspecified muscle, fascia and tendon at shoulder and upper arm level, **left arm**

  ● S46.999 Other injury of unspecified muscle, fascia and tendon at shoulder and upper arm level, **unspecified arm**

● S47 **Crushing injury** of shoulder and upper arm

  Use additional code for all associated injuries

  Excludes2   crushing injury of elbow (S57.0-)

  The appropriate 7th character is to be added to each code from category S47

A	initial encounter
D	subsequent encounter
S	sequela

X ● S47.1 Crushing injury of **right** shoulder and upper arm

X ● S47.2 Crushing injury of **left** shoulder and upper arm

X ● S47.9 Crushing injury of shoulder and upper arm, **unspecified** arm

● S48 **Traumatic amputation** of shoulder and upper arm

  An amputation not identified as partial or complete should be coded to complete

  Excludes1   traumatic amputation at elbow level (S58.0)

  The appropriate 7th character is to be added to each code from category S48

A	initial encounter
D	subsequent encounter
S	sequela

  ● S48.0 **Traumatic amputation at shoulder joint**

    ● S48.01 **Complete** traumatic amputation at shoulder joint

      ● S48.011 Complete traumatic amputation at **right** shoulder joint A, S 🅗

      ● S48.012 Complete traumatic amputation at **left** shoulder joint A, S 🅗

      ● S48.019 Complete traumatic amputation at **unspecified** shoulder joint A, S 🅗

    ● S48.02 **Partial** traumatic amputation at shoulder joint

      ● S48.021 Partial traumatic amputation at **right** shoulder joint A, S 🅗

      ● S48.022 Partial traumatic amputation at **left** shoulder joint A, S 🅗

      ● S48.029 Partial traumatic amputation at **unspecified** shoulder joint A, S 🅗

  ● S48.1 Traumatic amputation at level **between shoulder and elbow**

    ● S48.11 **Complete** traumatic amputation at level between shoulder and elbow

      ● S48.111 Complete traumatic amputation at level between **right** shoulder and elbow A, S 🅗

      ● S48.112 Complete traumatic amputation at level between **left** shoulder and elbow A, S 🅗

      ● S48.119 Complete traumatic amputation at level between **unspecified** shoulder and elbow A, S 🅗

● **S48.12** **Partial** traumatic amputation at level between shoulder and elbow
   ● **S48.121** Partial traumatic amputation at level between **right** shoulder and elbow A, S
   ● **S48.122** Partial traumatic amputation at level between **left** shoulder and elbow A, S
   ● **S48.129** Partial traumatic amputation at level between **unspecified** shoulder and elbow A, S

● **S48.9** Traumatic amputation of shoulder and upper arm, level **unspecified**
  ● **S48.91** **Complete** traumatic amputation of shoulder and upper arm, level unspecified
   ● **S48.911** Complete traumatic amputation of **right** shoulder and upper arm, level unspecified A, S
   ● **S48.912** Complete traumatic amputation of **left** shoulder and upper arm, level unspecified A, S
   ● **S48.919** Complete traumatic amputation of **unspecified** shoulder and upper arm, level unspecified A, S
  ● **S48.92** **Partial** traumatic amputation of shoulder and upper arm, level unspecified
   ● **S48.921** Partial traumatic amputation of **right** shoulder and upper arm, level unspecified A, S
   ● **S48.922** Partial traumatic amputation of **left** shoulder and upper arm, level unspecified A, S
   ● **S48.929** Partial traumatic amputation of **unspecified** shoulder and upper arm, level unspecified A, S

● **S49** Other and unspecified injuries of shoulder and upper arm

The appropriate 7th character is to be added to each code from subcategories S49.0 and S49.1

> A   initial encounter for closed fracture
> D   subsequent encounter for fracture with routine healing
> G   subsequent encounter for fracture with delayed healing
> K   subsequent encounter for fracture with nonunion
> P   subsequent encounter for fracture with malunion
> S   sequela

  ● **S49.0** **Physeal** fracture of **upper end of humerus**
  ● **S49.00** **Unspecified** physeal fracture of upper end of humerus
   ● **S49.001** Unspecified physeal fracture of upper end of humerus, **right** arm
   ● **S49.002** Unspecified physeal fracture of upper end of humerus, **left** arm
   ● **S49.009** Unspecified physeal fracture of upper end of humerus, **unspecified** arm
  ● **S49.01** **Salter-Harris Type I** physeal fracture of upper end of humerus
   ● **S49.011** Salter-Harris Type I physeal fracture of upper end of humerus, **right** arm
   ● **S49.012** Salter-Harris Type I physeal fracture of upper end of humerus, **left** arm
   ● **S49.019** Salter-Harris Type I physeal fracture of upper end of humerus, **unspecified** arm
  ● **S49.02** **Salter-Harris Type II** physeal fracture of upper end of humerus
   ● **S49.021** Salter-Harris Type II physeal fracture of upper end of humerus, **right** arm

Item 19–3 **SALTER-HARRIS TYPE 1:** epiphysis is completely separated from end of bone, or metaphysic growth plate remains attached to epiphysis

SALTER-HARRIS TYPE 2: epiphysis and growth plate are partially separated from metaphysis, which is cracked—most common type

SALTER-HARRIS TYPE 3: fracture occurring through epiphysis and separates part of epiphysis and growth plate from metaphysis fracture, usually at distal end of tibia

SALTER-HARRIS TYPE 4: fracture runs through epiphysis, across growth plate, into metaphysic, surgery is required to restore joint surface to normal and align growth plate

   ● **S49.022** Salter-Harris Type II physeal fracture of upper end of humerus, **left** arm –
   ● **S49.029** Salter-Harris Type II physeal fracture of upper end of humerus, **unspecified** arm
  ● **S49.03** **Salter-Harris Type III** physeal fracture of upper end of humerus
   ● **S49.031** Salter-Harris Type III physeal fracture of upper end of humerus, **right** arm
   ● **S49.032** Salter-Harris Type III physeal fracture of upper end of humerus, **left** arm
   ● **S49.039** Salter-Harris Type III physeal fracture of upper end of humerus, **unspecified** arm
  ● **S49.04** **Salter-Harris Type IV** physeal fracture of upper end of humerus
   ● **S49.041** Salter-Harris Type IV physeal fracture of upper end of humerus, **right** arm
   ● **S49.042** Salter-Harris Type IV physeal fracture of upper end of humerus, **left** arm
   ● **S49.049** Salter-Harris Type IV physeal fracture of upper end of humerus, **unspecified** arm
  ● **S49.09** **Other** physeal fracture of upper end of humerus
   ● **S49.091** Other physeal fracture of upper end of humerus, **right** arm
   ● **S49.092** Other physeal fracture of upper end of humerus, **left** arm
   ● **S49.099** Other physeal fracture of upper end of humerus, **unspecified** arm
  ● **S49.1** Physeal fracture of **lower end of humerus**
  ● **S49.10** **Unspecified** physeal fracture of lower end of humerus
   ● **S49.101** Unspecified physeal fracture of lower end of humerus, **right** arm
   ● **S49.102** Unspecified physeal fracture of lower end of humerus, **left** arm
   ● **S49.109** Unspecified physeal fracture of lower end of humerus, **unspecified** arm
  ● **S49.11** **Salter-Harris Type I** physeal fracture of lower end of humerus
   ● **S49.111** Salter-Harris Type I physeal fracture of lower end of humerus, **right** arm
   ● **S49.112** Salter-Harris Type I physeal fracture of lower end of humerus, **left** arm
   ● **S49.119** Salter-Harris Type I physeal fracture of lower end of humerus, **unspecified** arm
  ● **S49.12** **Salter-Harris Type II** physeal fracture of lower end of humerus
   ● **S49.121** Salter-Harris Type II physeal fracture of lower end of humerus, **right** arm
   ● **S49.122** Salter-Harris Type II physeal fracture of lower end of humerus, **left** arm
   ● **S49.129** Salter-Harris Type II physeal fracture of lower end of humerus, **unspecified** arm

CHAPTER 19 (S00-T88)

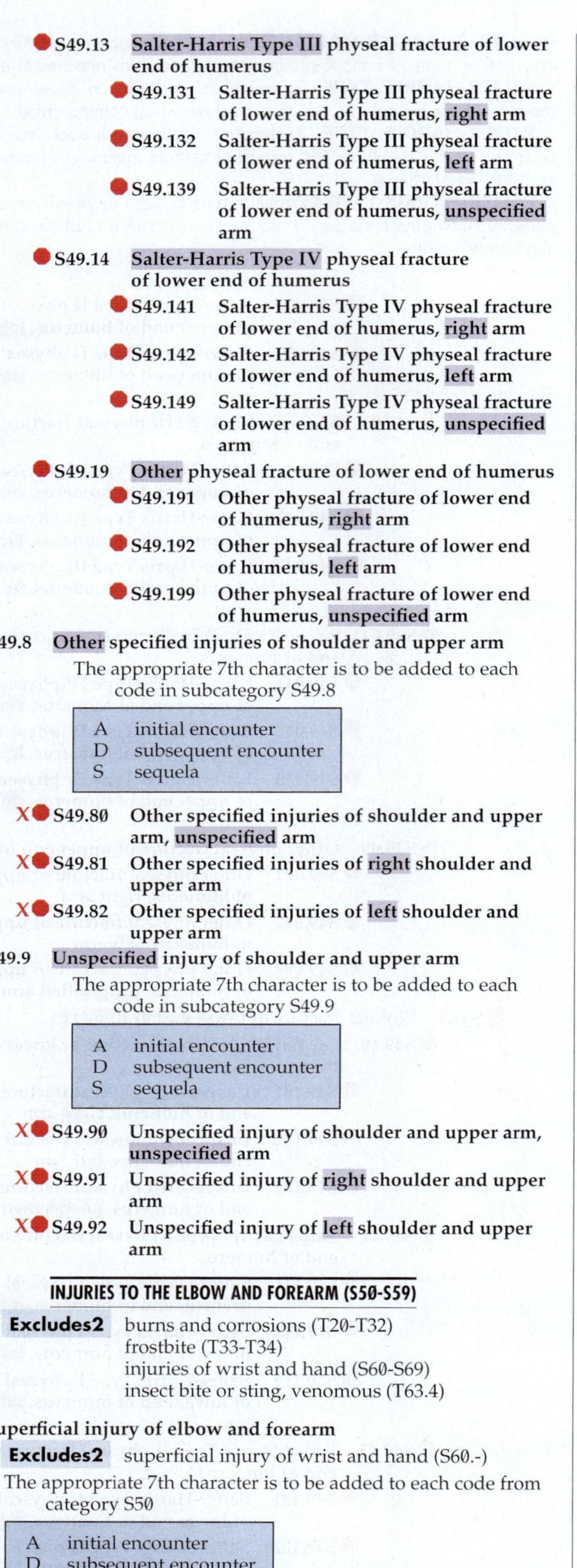

S49.13   Salter-Harris Type III physeal fracture of lower end of humerus

- **S49.131**   Salter-Harris Type III physeal fracture of lower end of humerus, right arm
- **S49.132**   Salter-Harris Type III physeal fracture of lower end of humerus, left arm
- **S49.139**   Salter-Harris Type III physeal fracture of lower end of humerus, unspecified arm

S49.14   Salter-Harris Type IV physeal fracture of lower end of humerus

- **S49.141**   Salter-Harris Type IV physeal fracture of lower end of humerus, right arm
- **S49.142**   Salter-Harris Type IV physeal fracture of lower end of humerus, left arm
- **S49.149**   Salter-Harris Type IV physeal fracture of lower end of humerus, unspecified arm

S49.19   Other physeal fracture of lower end of humerus

- **S49.191**   Other physeal fracture of lower end of humerus, right arm
- **S49.192**   Other physeal fracture of lower end of humerus, left arm
- **S49.199**   Other physeal fracture of lower end of humerus, unspecified arm

S49.8   Other specified injuries of shoulder and upper arm

The appropriate 7th character is to be added to each code in subcategory S49.8

A	initial encounter
D	subsequent encounter
S	sequela

- X **S49.80**   Other specified injuries of shoulder and upper arm, unspecified arm
- X **S49.81**   Other specified injuries of right shoulder and upper arm
- X **S49.82**   Other specified injuries of left shoulder and upper arm

S49.9   Unspecified injury of shoulder and upper arm

The appropriate 7th character is to be added to each code in subcategory S49.9

A	initial encounter
D	subsequent encounter
S	sequela

- X **S49.90**   Unspecified injury of shoulder and upper arm, unspecified arm
- X **S49.91**   Unspecified injury of right shoulder and upper arm
- X **S49.92**   Unspecified injury of left shoulder and upper arm

---

INJURIES TO THE ELBOW AND FOREARM (S50-S59)

Excludes2   burns and corrosions (T20-T32)
frostbite (T33-T34)
injuries of wrist and hand (S60-S69)
insect bite or sting, venomous (T63.4)

S50   Superficial injury of elbow and forearm

Excludes2   superficial injury of wrist and hand (S60.-)

The appropriate 7th character is to be added to each code from category S50

A	initial encounter
D	subsequent encounter
S	sequela

S50.0   Contusion of elbow

- X **S50.00**   Contusion of unspecified elbow
- X **S50.01**   Contusion of right elbow
- X **S50.02**   Contusion of left elbow

S50.1   Contusion of forearm

- X **S50.10**   Contusion of unspecified forearm
- X **S50.11**   Contusion of right forearm
- X **S50.12**   Contusion of left forearm

S50.3   Other superficial injuries of elbow

- **S50.31**   Abrasion of elbow
  - **S50.311**   Abrasion of right elbow
  - **S50.312**   Abrasion of left elbow
  - **S50.319**   Abrasion of unspecified elbow
- **S50.32**   Blister (nonthermal) of elbow
  - **S50.321**   Blister (nonthermal) of right elbow
  - **S50.322**   Blister (nonthermal) of left elbow
  - **S50.329**   Blister (nonthermal) of unspecified elbow
- **S50.34**   External constriction of elbow
  - **S50.341**   External constriction of right elbow
  - **S50.342**   External constriction of left elbow
  - **S50.349**   External constriction of unspecified elbow
- **S50.35**   Superficial foreign body of elbow
  Splinter in the elbow
  - **S50.351**   Superficial foreign body of right elbow
  - **S50.352**   Superficial foreign body of left elbow
  - **S50.359**   Superficial foreign body of unspecified elbow
- **S50.36**   Insect bite (nonvenomous) of elbow
  - **S50.361**   Insect bite (nonvenomous) of right elbow
  - **S50.362**   Insect bite (nonvenomous) of left elbow
  - **S50.369**   Insect bite (nonvenomous) of unspecified elbow
- **S50.37**   Other superficial bite of elbow
  - **Excludes1**   open bite of elbow (S51.04)
  - **S50.371**   Other superficial bite of right elbow
  - **S50.372**   Other superficial bite of left elbow
  - **S50.379**   Other superficial bite of unspecified elbow

S50.8   Other superficial injuries of forearm

- **S50.81**   Abrasion of forearm
  - **S50.811**   Abrasion of right forearm
  - **S50.812**   Abrasion of left forearm
  - **S50.819**   Abrasion of unspecified forearm
- **S50.82**   Blister (nonthermal) of forearm
  - **S50.821**   Blister (nonthermal) of right forearm
  - **S50.822**   Blister (nonthermal) of left forearm
  - **S50.829**   Blister (nonthermal) of unspecified forearm
- **S50.84**   External constriction of forearm
  - **S50.841**   External constriction of right forearm
  - **S50.842**   External constriction of left forearm
  - **S50.849**   External constriction of unspecified forearm
- **S50.85**   Superficial foreign body of forearm
  Splinter in the forearm
  - **S50.851**   Superficial foreign body of right forearm
  - **S50.852**   Superficial foreign body of left forearm
  - **S50.859**   Superficial foreign body of unspecified forearm

▶ New   ⇨ Revised   ~~deleted~~ Deleted   Excludes 1   Excludes 2   Includes   Use additional   Code first   Code also   Key words
OGCR Official Guidelines   X Assign placeholder X   ● Use Additional Character(s)   ▶ Manifestation Code   Hierarchical Condition Category   Coding Clinic

● **S50.86**   **Insect bite (nonvenomous) of forearm**
    ● **S50.861**   Insect bite (nonvenomous) of right forearm
    ● **S50.862**   Insect bite (nonvenomous) of left forearm
    ● **S50.869**   Insect bite (nonvenomous) of unspecified forearm
● **S50.87**   **Other superficial bite of forearm**
    Excludes1   open bite of forearm (S51.84)
    ● **S50.871**   Other superficial bite of right forearm
    ● **S50.872**   Other superficial bite of left forearm
    ● **S50.879**   Other superficial bite of unspecified forearm
● **S50.9**   **Unspecified superficial injury of elbow and forearm**
   ● **S50.90**   **Unspecified superficial injury of elbow**
    ● **S50.901**   Unspecified superficial injury of right elbow
    ● **S50.902**   Unspecified superficial injury of left elbow
    ● **S50.909**   Unspecified superficial injury of unspecified elbow
   ● **S50.91**   **Unspecified superficial injury of forearm**
    ● **S50.911**   Unspecified superficial injury of right forearm
    ● **S50.912**   Unspecified superficial injury of left forearm
    ● **S50.919**   Unspecified superficial injury of unspecified forearm

● **S51**   **Open wound of elbow and forearm**
    Code also any associated wound infection
    Excludes1   open fracture of elbow and forearm (S52.- with open fracture 7th character)
                traumatic amputation of elbow and forearm (S58.-)
    Excludes2   open wound of wrist and hand (S61.-)
    The appropriate 7th character is to be added to each code from category S51

> A   initial encounter
> D   subsequent encounter
> S   sequela

   ● **S51.0**   **Open wound of elbow**
    ● **S51.00**   **Unspecified open wound of elbow**
     ● **S51.001**   Unspecified open wound of right elbow
        Coding Clinic: 2012, Q4, P108
     ● **S51.002**   Unspecified open wound of left elbow
     ● **S51.009**   Unspecified open wound of unspecified elbow
        Open wound of elbow NOS
    ● **S51.01**   **Laceration without foreign body of elbow**
     ● **S51.011**   Laceration without foreign body of right elbow
     ● **S51.012**   Laceration without foreign body of left elbow
     ● **S51.019**   Laceration without foreign body of unspecified elbow
    ● **S51.02**   **Laceration with foreign body of elbow**
     ● **S51.021**   Laceration with foreign body of right elbow
     ● **S51.022**   Laceration with foreign body of left elbow
     ● **S51.029**   Laceration with foreign body of unspecified elbow

● **S51.03**   **Puncture wound without foreign body of elbow**
    ● **S51.031**   Puncture wound without foreign body of right elbow
    ● **S51.032**   Puncture wound without foreign body of left elbow
    ● **S51.039**   Puncture wound without foreign body of unspecified elbow
● **S51.04**   **Puncture wound with foreign body of elbow**
    ● **S51.041**   Puncture wound with foreign body of right elbow
    ● **S51.042**   Puncture wound with foreign body of left elbow
    ● **S51.049**   Puncture wound with foreign body of unspecified elbow
● **S51.05**   **Open bite of elbow**
    Bite of elbow NOS
    Excludes1   superficial bite of elbow (S50.36, S50.37)
    ● **S51.051**   Open bite, right elbow
    ● **S51.052**   Open bite, left elbow
    ● **S51.059**   Open bite, unspecified elbow
● **S51.8**   **Open wound of forearm**
    Excludes2   open wound of elbow (S51.0-)
   ● **S51.80**   **Unspecified open wound of forearm**
    ● **S51.801**   Unspecified open wound of right forearm
    ● **S51.802**   Unspecified open wound of left forearm
    ● **S51.809**   Unspecified open wound of unspecified forearm
        Open wound of forearm NOS
   ● **S51.81**   **Laceration without foreign body of forearm**
    ● **S51.811**   Laceration without foreign body of right forearm
    ● **S51.812**   Laceration without foreign body of left forearm
    ● **S51.819**   Laceration without foreign body of unspecified forearm
   ● **S51.82**   **Laceration with foreign body of forearm**
    ● **S51.821**   Laceration with foreign body of right forearm
    ● **S51.822**   Laceration with foreign body of left forearm
    ● **S51.829**   Laceration with foreign body of unspecified forearm
   ● **S51.83**   **Puncture wound without foreign body of forearm**
    ● **S51.831**   Puncture wound without foreign body of right forearm
    ● **S51.832**   Puncture wound without foreign body of left forearm
    ● **S51.839**   Puncture wound without foreign body of unspecified forearm
   ● **S51.84**   **Puncture wound with foreign body of forearm**
    ● **S51.841**   Puncture wound with foreign body of right forearm
    ● **S51.842**   Puncture wound with foreign body of left forearm
    ● **S51.849**   Puncture wound with foreign body of unspecified forearm
   ● **S51.85**   **Open bite of forearm**
    Bite of forearm NOS
    Excludes1   superficial bite of forearm (S50.86, S50.87)
    ● **S51.851**   Open bite of right forearm
    ● **S51.852**   Open bite of left forearm
    ● **S51.859**   Open bite of unspecified forearm

CHAPTER 19 (S00-T88)

● **S52 Fracture of forearm**

Note: A fracture not identified as displaced or nondisplaced should be coded to displaced

A fracture not designated as open or closed should be coded to closed

The open fracture designations are based on the Gustilo open fracture classification

Excludes1 traumatic amputation of forearm (S58.-)

Excludes2 fracture at wrist and hand level (S62.-)

periprosthetic fracture around internal prosthetic elbow joint (M97.4)

The appropriate 7th character is to be added to all codes from category S52

A	initial encounter for closed fracture
B	initial encounter for open fracture type I or II
	initial encounter for open fracture NOS
C	initial encounter for open fracture type IIIA, IIIB, or IIIC
D	subsequent encounter for closed fracture with routine healing
E	subsequent encounter for open fracture type I or II with routine healing
F	subsequent encounter for open fracture type IIIA, IIIB, or IIIC with routine healing
G	subsequent encounter for closed fracture with delayed healing
H	subsequent encounter for open fracture type I or II with delayed healing
J	subsequent encounter for open fracture type IIIA, IIIB, or IIIC with delayed healing
K	subsequent encounter for closed fracture with nonunion
M	subsequent encounter for open fracture type I or II with nonunion
N	subsequent encounter for open fracture type IIIA, IIIB, or IIIC with nonunion
P	subsequent encounter for closed fracture with malunion
Q	subsequent encounter for open fracture type I or II with malunion
R	subsequent encounter for open fracture type IIIA, IIIB, or IIIC with malunion
S	sequela

Coding Clinic: 2016, Q1, P33

● **S52.0 Fracture of upper end of ulna**

Fracture of proximal end of ulna

Excludes2 fracture of elbow NOS (S42.40-)

fractures of shaft of ulna (S52.2-)

● **S52.00 Unspecified fracture of upper end of ulna**

● S52.001 Unspecified fracture of upper end of right ulna

● S52.002 Unspecified fracture of upper end of left ulna

● S52.009 Unspecified fracture of upper end of unspecified ulna

● **S52.01 Torus fracture of upper end of ulna**

The appropriate 7th character is to be added to all codes in subcategory S52.01

A	initial encounter for closed fracture
D	subsequent encounter for fracture with routine healing
G	subsequent encounter for fracture with delayed healing
K	subsequent encounter for fracture with nonunion
P	subsequent encounter for fracture with malunion
S	sequela

● S52.011 Torus fracture of upper end of right ulna

● S52.012 Torus fracture of upper end of left ulna

● S52.019 Torus fracture of upper end of unspecified ulna

● **S52.02 Fracture of olecranon process without intraarticular extension of ulna**

● S52.021 Displaced fracture of olecranon process without intraarticular extension of right ulna

● S52.022 Displaced fracture of olecranon process without intraarticular extension of left ulna

● S52.023 Displaced fracture of olecranon process without intraarticular extension of unspecified ulna

● S52.024 Nondisplaced fracture of olecranon process without intraarticular extension of right ulna

● S52.025 Nondisplaced fracture of olecranon process without intraarticular extension of left ulna

● S52.026 Nondisplaced fracture of olecranon process without intraarticular extension of unspecified ulna

● **S52.03 Fracture of olecranon process with intraarticular extension of ulna**

● S52.031 Displaced fracture of olecranon process with intraarticular extension of right ulna

● S52.032 Displaced fracture of olecranon process with intraarticular extension of left ulna

● S52.033 Displaced fracture of olecranon process with intraarticular extension of unspecified ulna

● S52.034 Nondisplaced fracture of olecranon process with intraarticular extension of right ulna

● S52.035 Nondisplaced fracture of olecranon process with intraarticular extension of left ulna

● S52.036 Nondisplaced fracture of olecranon process with intraarticular extension of unspecified ulna

● **S52.04 Fracture of coronoid process of ulna**

● S52.041 Displaced fracture of coronoid process of right ulna

● S52.042 Displaced fracture of coronoid process of left ulna

● S52.043 Displaced fracture of coronoid process of unspecified ulna

● S52.044 Nondisplaced fracture of coronoid process of right ulna

● S52.045 Nondisplaced fracture of coronoid process of left ulna

● S52.046 Nondisplaced fracture of coronoid process of unspecified ulna

● **S52.09 Other fracture of upper end of ulna**

● S52.091 Other fracture of upper end of right ulna

● S52.092 Other fracture of upper end of left ulna

● S52.099 Other fracture of upper end of unspecified ulna

▶ New   ⇒ Revised   ~~deleted~~ Deleted   Excludes 1   Excludes 2   Includes   Use additional   Code first   Code also   Key words

OGCR Official Guidelines   X Assign placeholder X   ● Use Additional Character(s)   ▶ Manifestation Code   Hierarchical Condition Category   **Coding Clinic**

● **S52.1**   **Fracture of upper end of radius**
    Fracture of proximal end of radius
    Excludes2   physeal fractures of upper end of radius
          (S59.2-)
          fracture of shaft of radius (S52.3-)

   ● **S52.10**   **Unspecified fracture of upper end of radius**
      ● **S52.101**   Unspecified fracture of upper end of right radius
      ● **S52.102**   Unspecified fracture of upper end of left radius
      ● **S52.109**   Unspecified fracture of upper end of unspecified radius

   ● **S52.11**   **Torus fracture of upper end of radius**
      The appropriate 7th character is to be added to all codes in subcategory S52.11

> A   initial encounter for closed fracture
> D   subsequent encounter for fracture with routine healing
> G   subsequent encounter for fracture with delayed healing
> K   subsequent encounter for fracture with nonunion
> P   subsequent encounter for fracture with malunion
> S   sequela

      ● **S52.111**   Torus fracture of upper end of right radius
      ● **S52.112**   Torus fracture of upper end of left radius
      ● **S52.119**   Torus fracture of upper end of unspecified radius

   ● **S52.12**   **Fracture of head of radius**
      ● **S52.121**   Displaced fracture of head of right radius
      ● **S52.122**   Displaced fracture of head of left radius
      ● **S52.123**   Displaced fracture of head of unspecified radius
      ● **S52.124**   Nondisplaced fracture of head of right radius
      ● **S52.125**   Nondisplaced fracture of head of left radius
      ● **S52.126**   Nondisplaced fracture of head of unspecified radius

   ● **S52.13**   **Fracture of neck of radius**
      ● **S52.131**   Displaced fracture of neck of right radius
      ● **S52.132**   Displaced fracture of neck of left radius
      ● **S52.133**   Displaced fracture of neck of unspecified radius
      ● **S52.134**   Nondisplaced fracture of neck of right radius
      ● **S52.135**   Nondisplaced fracture of neck of left radius
      ● **S52.136**   Nondisplaced fracture of neck of unspecified radius

   ● **S52.18**   **Other fracture of upper end of radius**
      ● **S52.181**   Other fracture of upper end of right radius
      ● **S52.182**   Other fracture of upper end of left radius
      ● **S52.189**   Other fracture of upper end of unspecified radius

● **S52.2**   **Fracture of shaft of ulna**
   ● **S52.20**   **Unspecified fracture of shaft of ulna**
      Fracture of ulna NOS
      ● **S52.201**   Unspecified fracture of shaft of right ulna
      ● **S52.202**   Unspecified fracture of shaft of left ulna
      ● **S52.209**   Unspecified fracture of shaft of unspecified ulna

   ● **S52.21**   **Greenstick fracture of shaft of ulna**
      The appropriate 7th character is to be added to all codes in subcategory S52.21

> A   initial encounter for closed fracture
> D   subsequent encounter for fracture with routine healing
> G   subsequent encounter for fracture with delayed healing
> K   subsequent encounter for fracture with nonunion
> P   subsequent encounter for fracture with malunion
> S   sequela

      ● **S52.211**   Greenstick fracture of shaft of right ulna
      ● **S52.212**   Greenstick fracture of shaft of left ulna
      ● **S52.219**   Greenstick fracture of shaft of unspecified ulna

   ● **S52.22**   **Transverse fracture of shaft of ulna**
      ● **S52.221**   Displaced transverse fracture of shaft of right ulna
      ● **S52.222**   Displaced transverse fracture of shaft of left ulna
      ● **S52.223**   Displaced transverse fracture of shaft of unspecified ulna
      ● **S52.224**   Nondisplaced transverse fracture of shaft of right ulna
      ● **S52.225**   Nondisplaced transverse fracture of shaft of left ulna
      ● **S52.226**   Nondisplaced transverse fracture of shaft of unspecified ulna

   ● **S52.23**   **Oblique fracture of shaft of ulna**
      ● **S52.231**   Displaced oblique fracture of shaft of right ulna
      ● **S52.232**   Displaced oblique fracture of shaft of left ulna
      ● **S52.233**   Displaced oblique fracture of shaft of unspecified ulna
      ● **S52.234**   Nondisplaced oblique fracture of shaft of right ulna
      ● **S52.235**   Nondisplaced oblique fracture of shaft of left ulna
      ● **S52.236**   Nondisplaced oblique fracture of shaft of unspecified ulna

   ● **S52.24**   **Spiral fracture of shaft of ulna**
      ● **S52.241**   Displaced spiral fracture of shaft of ulna, right arm
      ● **S52.242**   Displaced spiral fracture of shaft of ulna, left arm
      ● **S52.243**   Displaced spiral fracture of shaft of ulna, unspecified arm
      ● **S52.244**   Nondisplaced spiral fracture of shaft of ulna, right arm
      ● **S52.245**   Nondisplaced spiral fracture of shaft of ulna, left arm
      ● **S52.246**   Nondisplaced spiral fracture of shaft of ulna, unspecified arm

CHAPTER 19 (S00–T88)

⬤ S52.25 **Comminuted** fracture of shaft of ulna
- ⬤ S52.251 Displaced comminuted fracture of shaft of ulna, **right arm**
- ⬤ S52.252 Displaced comminuted fracture of shaft of ulna, **left arm**
- ⬤ S52.253 Displaced comminuted fracture of shaft of ulna, **unspecified arm**
- ⬤ S52.254 Nondisplaced comminuted fracture of shaft of ulna, **right arm**
- ⬤ S52.255 Nondisplaced comminuted fracture of shaft of ulna, **left arm**
- ⬤ S52.256 Nondisplaced comminuted fracture of shaft of ulna, **unspecified arm**

⬤ S52.26 **Segmental** fracture of shaft of ulna
- ⬤ S52.261 Displaced segmental fracture of shaft of ulna, **right arm**
- ⬤ S52.262 Displaced segmental fracture of shaft of ulna, **left arm**
- ⬤ S52.263 Displaced segmental fracture of shaft of ulna, **unspecified arm**
- ⬤ S52.264 Nondisplaced segmental fracture of shaft of ulna, **right arm**
- ⬤ S52.265 Nondisplaced segmental fracture of shaft of ulna, **left arm**
- ⬤ S52.266 Nondisplaced segmental fracture of shaft of ulna, **unspecified arm**

⬤ S52.27 **Monteggia's** fracture of ulna
  Fracture of upper shaft of ulna with dislocation of radial head
- ⬤ S52.271 Monteggia's fracture of **right** ulna
- ⬤ S52.272 Monteggia's fracture of **left** ulna
- ⬤ S52.279 Monteggia's fracture of **unspecified** ulna

⬤ S52.28 **Bent bone** of ulna
- ⬤ S52.281 Bent bone of **right** ulna
- ⬤ S52.282 Bent bone of **left** ulna
- ⬤ S52.283 Bent bone of **unspecified** ulna

⬤ S52.29 **Other** fracture of shaft of ulna
- ⬤ S52.291 Other fracture of shaft of **right** ulna
- ⬤ S52.292 Other fracture of shaft of **left** ulna
- ⬤ S52.299 Other fracture of shaft of **unspecified** ulna

⬤ S52.3 Fracture of **shaft of radius**

⬤ S52.30 **Unspecified** fracture of shaft of radius
- ⬤ S52.301 Unspecified fracture of shaft of **right** radius
- ⬤ S52.302 Unspecified fracture of shaft of **left** radius
- ⬤ S52.309 Unspecified fracture of shaft of **unspecified** radius

⬤ S52.31 **Greenstick** fracture of shaft of radius
  The appropriate 7th character is to be added to all codes in subcategory S52.31

> A   initial encounter for closed fracture
> D   subsequent encounter for fracture with routine healing
> G   subsequent encounter for fracture with delayed healing
> K   subsequent encounter for fracture with nonunion
> P   subsequent encounter for fracture with malunion
> S   sequela

- ⬤ S52.311 Greenstick fracture of shaft of radius, **right arm**
- ⬤ S52.312 Greenstick fracture of shaft of radius, **left arm**
- ⬤ S52.319 Greenstick fracture of shaft of radius, **unspecified arm**

⬤ S52.32 **Transverse** fracture of shaft of radius
- ⬤ S52.321 Displaced transverse fracture of shaft of **right** radius
- ⬤ S52.322 Displaced transverse fracture of shaft of **left** radius
- ⬤ S52.323 Displaced transverse fracture of shaft of **unspecified** radius
- ⬤ S52.324 Nondisplaced transverse fracture of shaft of **right** radius
- ⬤ S52.325 Nondisplaced transverse fracture of shaft of **left** radius
- ⬤ S52.326 Nondisplaced transverse fracture of shaft of **unspecified** radius

⬤ S52.33 **Oblique** fracture of shaft of radius
- ⬤ S52.331 Displaced oblique fracture of shaft of **right** radius
- ⬤ S52.332 Displaced oblique fracture of shaft of **left** radius
- ⬤ S52.333 Displaced oblique fracture of shaft of **unspecified** radius
- ⬤ S52.334 Nondisplaced oblique fracture of shaft of **right** radius
- ⬤ S52.335 Nondisplaced oblique fracture of shaft of **left** radius
- ⬤ S52.336 Nondisplaced oblique fracture of shaft of **unspecified** radius

⬤ S52.34 **Spiral** fracture of shaft of radius
- ⬤ S52.341 Displaced spiral fracture of shaft of radius, **right arm**
- ⬤ S52.342 Displaced spiral fracture of shaft of radius, **left arm**
- ⬤ S52.343 Displaced spiral fracture of shaft of radius, **unspecified arm**
- ⬤ S52.344 Nondisplaced spiral fracture of shaft of radius, **right arm**
- ⬤ S52.345 Nondisplaced spiral fracture of shaft of radius, **left arm**
- ⬤ S52.346 Nondisplaced spiral fracture of shaft of radius, **unspecified arm**

⬤ S52.35 **Comminuted** fracture of shaft of radius
- ⬤ S52.351 Displaced comminuted fracture of shaft of radius, **right arm**
- ⬤ S52.352 Displaced comminuted fracture of shaft of radius, **left arm**
- ⬤ S52.353 Displaced comminuted fracture of shaft of radius, **unspecified arm**
- ⬤ S52.354 Nondisplaced comminuted fracture of shaft of radius, **right arm**
- ⬤ S52.355 Nondisplaced comminuted fracture of shaft of radius, **left arm**
- ⬤ S52.356 Nondisplaced comminuted fracture of shaft of radius, **unspecified arm**

⬤ S52.36 **Segmental** fracture of shaft of radius
- ⬤ S52.361 Displaced segmental fracture of shaft of radius, **right arm**
- ⬤ S52.362 Displaced segmental fracture of shaft of radius, **left arm**
- ⬤ S52.363 Displaced segmental fracture of shaft of radius, **unspecified arm**
- ⬤ S52.364 Nondisplaced segmental fracture of shaft of radius, **right arm**
- ⬤ S52.365 Nondisplaced segmental fracture of shaft of radius, **left arm**
- ⬤ S52.366 Nondisplaced segmental fracture of shaft of radius, **unspecified arm**

⬤ S52.37 **Galeazzi's** fracture
  Fracture of lower shaft of radius with radioulnar joint dislocation
- ⬤ S52.371 Galeazzi's fracture of **right** radius

- ● S52.372   Galeazzi's fracture of **left** radius
- ● S52.379   Galeazzi's fracture of **unspecified** radius
- ● S52.38   **Bent bone** of radius
  - ● S52.381   Bent bone of **right** radius
  - ● S52.382   Bent bone of **left** radius
  - ● S52.389   Bent bone of **unspecified** radius
- ● S52.39   **Other fracture** of shaft of radius
  - ● S52.391   Other fracture of shaft of radius, **right** arm
  - ● S52.392   Other fracture of shaft of radius, **left** arm
  - ● S52.399   Other fracture of shaft of radius, **unspecified** arm
- ● S52.5   Fracture of **lower end** of radius
  Fracture of distal end of radius

  Excludes2   physeal fractures of lower end of radius (S59.2-)

  - ● S52.50   **Unspecified** fracture of the lower end of radius
    - ● S52.501   Unspecified fracture of the lower end of **right** radius
    - ● S52.502   Unspecified fracture of the lower end of **left** radius
    - ● S52.509   Unspecified fracture of the lower end of **unspecified** radius
  - ● S52.51   Fracture of **radial styloid** process
    - ● S52.511   **Displaced** fracture of **right** radial styloid process
    - ● S52.512   **Displaced** fracture of **left** radial styloid process
    - ● S52.513   **Displaced** fracture of **unspecified** radial styloid process
    - ● S52.514   **Nondisplaced** fracture of **right** radial styloid process
    - ● S52.515   **Nondisplaced** fracture of **left** radial styloid process
    - ● S52.516   **Nondisplaced** fracture of **unspecified** radial styloid process
  - ● S52.52   **Torus** fracture of lower end of radius

    The appropriate 7th character is to be added to all codes in subcategory S52.52

A	initial encounter for closed fracture
D	subsequent encounter for fracture with routine healing
G	subsequent encounter for fracture with delayed healing
K	subsequent encounter for fracture with nonunion
P	subsequent encounter for fracture with malunion
S	sequela

    - ● S52.521   Torus fracture of lower end of **right** radius
    - ● S52.522   Torus fracture of lower end of **left** radius
    - ● S52.529   Torus fracture of lower end of **unspecified** radius
  - ● S52.53   **Colles'** fracture
    - ● S52.531   Colles' fracture of **right** radius
    - ● S52.532   Colles' fracture of **left** radius
      Coding Clinic: 2016, Q2, P5
    - ● S52.539   Colles' fracture of **unspecified** radius
  - ● S52.54   **Smith's** fracture
    - ● S52.541   Smith's fracture of **right** radius
    - ● S52.542   Smith's fracture of **left** radius
    - ● S52.549   Smith's fracture of **unspecified** radius
  - ● S52.55   **Other extraarticular** fracture of lower end of radius
    - ● S52.551   Other extraarticular fracture of lower end of **right** radius
    - ● S52.552   Other extraarticular fracture of lower end of **left** radius
    - ● S52.559   Other extraarticular fracture of lower end of **unspecified** radius
  - ● S52.56   **Barton's** fracture
    - ● S52.561   Barton's fracture of **right** radius
    - ● S52.562   Barton's fracture of **left** radius
    - ● S52.569   Barton's fracture of **unspecified** radius
  - ● S52.57   **Other intraarticular** fracture of lower end of radius
    - ● S52.571   Other intraarticular fracture of lower end of **right** radius
    - ● S52.572   Other intraarticular fracture of lower end of **left** radius
    - ● S52.579   Other intraarticular fracture of lower end of **unspecified** radius
  - ● S52.59   **Other fractures** of lower end of radius
    - ● S52.591   Other fractures of lower end of **right** radius
      Coding Clinic: 2019, Q3, P10
    - ● S52.592   Other fractures of lower end of **left** radius
    - ● S52.599   Other fractures of lower end of **unspecified** radius
- ● S52.6   Fracture of **lower end** of ulna
  - ● S52.60   **Unspecified** fracture of lower end of ulna
    - ● S52.601   Unspecified fracture of lower end of **right** ulna
    - ● S52.602   Unspecified fracture of lower end of **left** ulna
    - ● S52.609   Unspecified fracture of lower end of **unspecified** ulna
  - ● S52.61   Fracture of **ulna styloid** process
    - ● S52.611   **Displaced** fracture of **right** ulna styloid process
    - ● S52.612   **Displaced** fracture of **left** ulna styloid process
    - ● S52.613   **Displaced** fracture of **unspecified** ulna styloid process
    - ● S52.614   **Nondisplaced** fracture of **right** ulna styloid process
    - ● S52.615   **Nondisplaced** fracture of **left** ulna styloid process
    - ● S52.616   **Nondisplaced** fracture of **unspecified** ulna styloid process
  - ● S52.62   **Torus** fracture of lower end of ulna

    The appropriate 7th character is to be added to all codes in subcategory S52.62

A	initial encounter for closed fracture
D	subsequent encounter for fracture with routine healing
G	subsequent encounter for fracture with delayed healing
K	subsequent encounter for fracture with nonunion
P	subsequent encounter for fracture with malunion
S	sequela

    - ● S52.621   Torus fracture of lower end of **right** ulna
    - ● S52.622   Torus fracture of lower end of **left** ulna
    - ● S52.629   Torus fracture of lower end of **unspecified** ulna

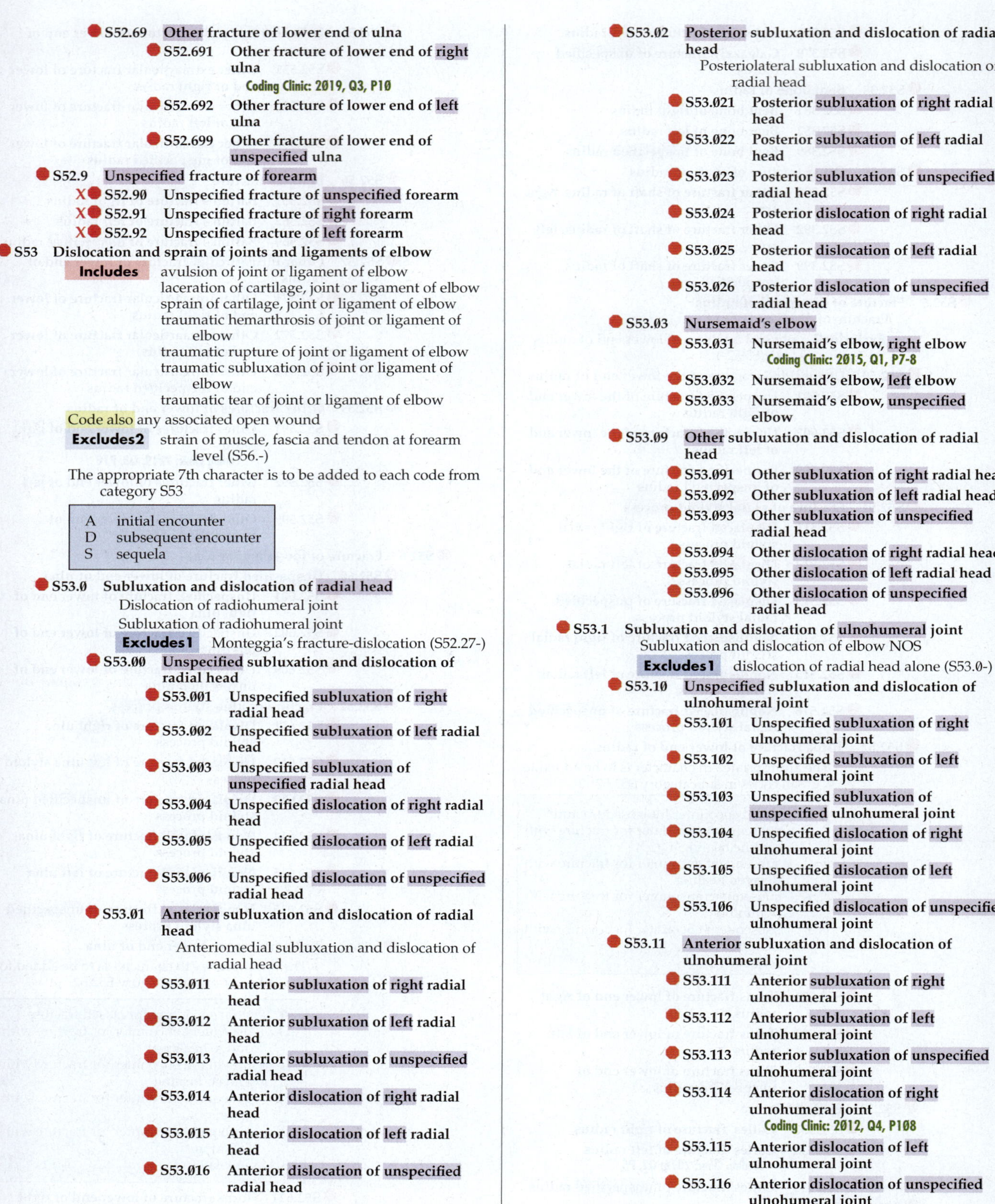

- ● **S52.69**   **Other fracture of lower end of ulna**
  - ● **S52.691**   **Other fracture of lower end of right ulna**
    - **Coding Clinic: 2019, Q3, P10**
  - ● **S52.692**   **Other fracture of lower end of left ulna**
  - ● **S52.699**   **Other fracture of lower end of unspecified ulna**
- ● **S52.9**   **Unspecified fracture of forearm**
  - X ● **S52.90**   **Unspecified fracture of unspecified forearm**
  - X ● **S52.91**   **Unspecified fracture of right forearm**
  - X ● **S52.92**   **Unspecified fracture of left forearm**
- ● **S53**   **Dislocation and sprain of joints and ligaments of elbow**
  - **Includes**   avulsion of joint or ligament of elbow
    laceration of cartilage, joint or ligament of elbow
    sprain of cartilage, joint or ligament of elbow
    traumatic hemarthrosis of joint or ligament of elbow
    traumatic rupture of joint or ligament of elbow
    traumatic subluxation of joint or ligament of elbow
    traumatic tear of joint or ligament of elbow
  - **Code also** any associated open wound
  - **Excludes2**   strain of muscle, fascia and tendon at forearm level (S56.-)

  The appropriate 7th character is to be added to each code from category S53

A	initial encounter
D	subsequent encounter
S	sequela

  - ● **S53.0**   **Subluxation and dislocation of radial head**
    Dislocation of radiohumeral joint
    Subluxation of radiohumeral joint
    - **Excludes1**   Monteggia's fracture-dislocation (S52.27-)
    - ● **S53.00**   **Unspecified subluxation and dislocation of radial head**
      - ● **S53.001**   **Unspecified subluxation of right radial head**
      - ● **S53.002**   **Unspecified subluxation of left radial head**
      - ● **S53.003**   **Unspecified subluxation of unspecified radial head**
      - ● **S53.004**   **Unspecified dislocation of right radial head**
      - ● **S53.005**   **Unspecified dislocation of left radial head**
      - ● **S53.006**   **Unspecified dislocation of unspecified radial head**
    - ● **S53.01**   **Anterior subluxation and dislocation of radial head**
      Anteriomedial subluxation and dislocation of radial head
      - ● **S53.011**   **Anterior subluxation of right radial head**
      - ● **S53.012**   **Anterior subluxation of left radial head**
      - ● **S53.013**   **Anterior subluxation of unspecified radial head**
      - ● **S53.014**   **Anterior dislocation of right radial head**
      - ● **S53.015**   **Anterior dislocation of left radial head**
      - ● **S53.016**   **Anterior dislocation of unspecified radial head**
  - ● **S53.02**   **Posterior subluxation and dislocation of radial head**
    Posteriolateral subluxation and dislocation of radial head
    - ● **S53.021**   **Posterior subluxation of right radial head**
    - ● **S53.022**   **Posterior subluxation of left radial head**
    - ● **S53.023**   **Posterior subluxation of unspecified radial head**
    - ● **S53.024**   **Posterior dislocation of right radial head**
    - ● **S53.025**   **Posterior dislocation of left radial head**
    - ● **S53.026**   **Posterior dislocation of unspecified radial head**
  - ● **S53.03**   **Nursemaid's elbow**
    - ● **S53.031**   **Nursemaid's elbow, right elbow**
      - **Coding Clinic: 2015, Q1, P7-8**
    - ● **S53.032**   **Nursemaid's elbow, left elbow**
    - ● **S53.033**   **Nursemaid's elbow, unspecified elbow**
  - ● **S53.09**   **Other subluxation and dislocation of radial head**
    - ● **S53.091**   **Other subluxation of right radial head**
    - ● **S53.092**   **Other subluxation of left radial head**
    - ● **S53.093**   **Other subluxation of unspecified radial head**
    - ● **S53.094**   **Other dislocation of right radial head**
    - ● **S53.095**   **Other dislocation of left radial head**
    - ● **S53.096**   **Other dislocation of unspecified radial head**
- ● **S53.1**   **Subluxation and dislocation of ulnohumeral joint**
  Subluxation and dislocation of elbow NOS
  - **Excludes1**   dislocation of radial head alone (S53.0-)
  - ● **S53.10**   **Unspecified subluxation and dislocation of ulnohumeral joint**
    - ● **S53.101**   **Unspecified subluxation of right ulnohumeral joint**
    - ● **S53.102**   **Unspecified subluxation of left ulnohumeral joint**
    - ● **S53.103**   **Unspecified subluxation of unspecified ulnohumeral joint**
    - ● **S53.104**   **Unspecified dislocation of right ulnohumeral joint**
    - ● **S53.105**   **Unspecified dislocation of left ulnohumeral joint**
    - ● **S53.106**   **Unspecified dislocation of unspecified ulnohumeral joint**
  - ● **S53.11**   **Anterior subluxation and dislocation of ulnohumeral joint**
    - ● **S53.111**   **Anterior subluxation of right ulnohumeral joint**
    - ● **S53.112**   **Anterior subluxation of left ulnohumeral joint**
    - ● **S53.113**   **Anterior subluxation of unspecified ulnohumeral joint**
    - ● **S53.114**   **Anterior dislocation of right ulnohumeral joint**
      - **Coding Clinic: 2012, Q4, P108**
    - ● **S53.115**   **Anterior dislocation of left ulnohumeral joint**
    - ● **S53.116**   **Anterior dislocation of unspecified ulnohumeral joint**

● S53.12   **Posterior** subluxation and dislocation of ulnohumeral joint
    ● S53.121   Posterior **subluxation** of **right** ulnohumeral joint
    ● S53.122   Posterior **subluxation** of **left** ulnohumeral joint
    ● S53.123   Posterior **subluxation** of **unspecified** ulnohumeral joint
    ● S53.124   Posterior **dislocation** of **right** ulnohumeral joint
    ● S53.125   Posterior **dislocation** of **left** ulnohumeral joint
    ● S53.126   Posterior **dislocation** of **unspecified** ulnohumeral joint

● S53.13   **Medial** subluxation and dislocation of ulnohumeral joint
    ● S53.131   Medial **subluxation** of **right** ulnohumeral joint
    ● S53.132   Medial **subluxation** of **left** ulnohumeral joint
    ● S53.133   Medial **subluxation** of **unspecified** ulnohumeral joint
    ● S53.134   Medial **dislocation** of **right** ulnohumeral joint
    ● S53.135   Medial **dislocation** of **left** ulnohumeral joint
    ● S53.136   Medial **dislocation** of **unspecified** ulnohumeral joint

● S53.14   **Lateral** subluxation and dislocation of ulnohumeral joint
    ● S53.141   Lateral **subluxation** of **right** ulnohumeral joint
    ● S53.142   Lateral **subluxation** of **left** ulnohumeral joint
    ● S53.143   Lateral **subluxation** of **unspecified** ulnohumeral joint
    ● S53.144   Lateral **dislocation** of **right** ulnohumeral joint
    ● S53.145   Lateral **dislocation** of **left** ulnohumeral joint
    ● S53.146   Lateral **dislocation** of **unspecified** ulnohumeral joint

● S53.19   **Other** subluxation and dislocation of ulnohumeral joint
    ● S53.191   Other **subluxation** of **right** ulnohumeral joint
    ● S53.192   Other **subluxation** of **left** ulnohumeral joint
    ● S53.193   Other **subluxation** of **unspecified** ulnohumeral joint
    ● S53.194   Other **dislocation** of **right** ulnohumeral joint
    ● S53.195   Other **dislocation** of **left** ulnohumeral joint
    ● S53.196   Other **dislocation** of **unspecified** ulnohumeral joint

● S53.2   **Traumatic rupture of** **radial collateral ligament**
    Excludes1   sprain of radial collateral ligament NOS (S53.43-)
   X ● S53.20   Traumatic rupture of **unspecified** radial collateral ligament
   X ● S53.21   Traumatic rupture of **right** radial collateral ligament
   X ● S53.22   Traumatic rupture of **left** radial collateral ligament

● S53.3   Traumatic rupture of **ulnar collateral ligament**
    Excludes1   sprain of ulnar collateral ligament (S53.44-)
   X ● S53.30   Traumatic rupture of **unspecified** ulnar collateral ligament
   X ● S53.31   Traumatic rupture of **right** ulnar collateral ligament
   X ● S53.32   Traumatic rupture of **left** ulnar collateral ligament

● S53.4   Sprain of elbow
    Excludes2   traumatic rupture of radial collateral ligament (S53.2-)
                 traumatic rupture of ulnar collateral ligament (S53.3-)
   ● S53.40   **Unspecified** sprain of elbow
    ● S53.401   Unspecified sprain of **right** elbow
    ● S53.402   Unspecified sprain of **left** elbow
    ● S53.409   Unspecified sprain of **unspecified** elbow
        Sprain of elbow NOS
   ● S53.41   **Radiohumeral (joint) sprain**
    ● S53.411   Radiohumeral (joint) sprain of **right** elbow
    ● S53.412   Radiohumeral (joint) sprain of **left** elbow
    ● S53.419   Radiohumeral (joint) sprain of **unspecified** elbow
   ● S53.42   **Ulnohumeral (joint) sprain**
    ● S53.421   Ulnohumeral (joint) sprain of **right** elbow
    ● S53.422   Ulnohumeral (joint) sprain of **left** elbow
    ● S53.429   Ulnohumeral (joint) sprain of **unspecified** elbow
   ● S53.43   **Radial collateral ligament** sprain
    ● S53.431   Radial collateral ligament sprain of **right** elbow
    ● S53.432   Radial collateral ligament sprain of **left** elbow
    ● S53.439   Radial collateral ligament sprain of **unspecified** elbow
   ● S53.44   **Ulnar collateral ligament** sprain
    ● S53.441   Ulnar collateral ligament sprain of **right** elbow
    ● S53.442   Ulnar collateral ligament sprain of **left** elbow
    ● S53.449   Ulnar collateral ligament sprain of **unspecified** elbow
   ● S53.49   **Other** sprain of elbow
    ● S53.491   Other sprain of **right** elbow
    ● S53.492   Other sprain of **left** elbow
    ● S53.499   Other sprain of **unspecified** elbow

● S54   **Injury of nerves at forearm level**
    Code also any associated open wound (S51.-)
    Excludes2   injury of nerves at wrist and hand level (S64.-)
    The appropriate 7th character is to be added to each code from category S54

> A   initial encounter
> D   subsequent encounter
> S   sequela

● S54.0   **Injury of ulnar nerve at forearm level**
    Injury of ulnar nerve NOS
   X ● S54.00   Injury of ulnar nerve at forearm level, **unspecified arm**
   X ● S54.01   Injury of ulnar nerve at forearm level, **right arm**
   X ● S54.02   Injury of ulnar nerve at forearm level, **left arm**

CHAPTER 19 (S00-T88)

CHAPTER 19 (S00-T88)

● **S54.1** **Injury of median nerve at forearm level**
Injury of median nerve NOS
   X ● **S54.10** Injury of median nerve at forearm level, **unspecified arm**
   X ● **S54.11** Injury of median nerve at forearm level, **right arm**
   X ● **S54.12** Injury of median nerve at forearm level, **left arm**

● **S54.2** **Injury of radial nerve at forearm level**
Injury of radial nerve NOS
   X ● **S54.20** Injury of radial nerve at forearm level, **unspecified arm**
   X ● **S54.21** Injury of radial nerve at forearm level, **right arm**
   X ● **S54.22** Injury of radial nerve at forearm level, **left arm**

● **S54.3** **Injury of cutaneous sensory nerve at forearm level**
   X ● **S54.30** Injury of cutaneous sensory nerve at forearm level, **unspecified arm**
   X ● **S54.31** Injury of cutaneous sensory nerve at forearm level, **right arm**
   X ● **S54.32** Injury of cutaneous sensory nerve at forearm level, **left arm**

● **S54.8** **Injury of other nerves at forearm level**
   ● **S54.8X** Injury of other nerves at forearm level
     ● **S54.8X1** Injury of other nerves at forearm level, **right arm**
     ● **S54.8X2** Injury of other nerves at forearm level, **left arm**
     ● **S54.8X9** Injury of other nerves at forearm level, **unspecified arm**

● **S54.9** **Injury of unspecified nerve at forearm level**
   X ● **S54.90** Injury of unspecified nerve at forearm level, **unspecified arm**
   X ● **S54.91** Injury of unspecified nerve at forearm level, **right arm**
   X ● **S54.92** Injury of unspecified nerve at forearm level, **left arm**

● **S55** **Injury of blood vessels at forearm level**
Code also any associated open wound (S51.-)
Excludes2   injury of blood vessels at wrist and hand level (S65.-)
         injury of brachial vessels (S45.1-S45.2)

The appropriate 7th character is to be added to each code from category S55

> A   initial encounter
> D   subsequent encounter
> S   sequela

● **S55.0** **Injury of ulnar artery at forearm level**
   ● **S55.00** **Unspecified** injury of ulnar artery at forearm level
     ● **S55.001** Unspecified injury of ulnar artery at forearm level, **right arm**
     ● **S55.002** Unspecified injury of ulnar artery at forearm level, **left arm**
     ● **S55.009** Unspecified injury of ulnar artery at forearm level, **unspecified arm**
   ● **S55.01** **Laceration** of ulnar artery at forearm level
     ● **S55.011** Laceration of ulnar artery at forearm level, **right arm**
     ● **S55.012** Laceration of ulnar artery at forearm level, **left arm**
     ● **S55.019** Laceration of ulnar artery at forearm level, **unspecified arm**
   ● **S55.09** **Other** specified injury of ulnar artery at forearm level
     ● **S55.091** Other specified injury of ulnar artery at forearm level, **right arm**

● **S55.092** Other specified injury of ulnar artery at forearm level, **left arm**
● **S55.099** Other specified injury of ulnar artery at forearm level, **unspecified arm**

● **S55.1** **Injury of radial artery at forearm level**
   ● **S55.10** **Unspecified** injury of radial artery at forearm level
     ● **S55.101** Unspecified injury of radial artery at forearm level, **right arm**
     ● **S55.102** Unspecified injury of radial artery at forearm level, **left arm**
     ● **S55.109** Unspecified injury of radial artery at forearm level, **unspecified arm**
   ● **S55.11** **Laceration** of radial artery at forearm level
     ● **S55.111** Laceration of radial artery at forearm level, **right arm**
     ● **S55.112** Laceration of radial artery at forearm level, **left arm**
     ● **S55.119** Laceration of radial artery at forearm level, **unspecified arm**
   ● **S55.19** **Other** specified injury of radial artery at forearm level
     ● **S55.191** Other specified injury of radial artery at forearm level, **right arm**
     ● **S55.192** Other specified injury of radial artery at forearm level, **left arm**
     ● **S55.199** Other specified injury of radial artery at forearm level, **unspecified arm**

● **S55.2** **Injury of vein at forearm level**
   ● **S55.20** **Unspecified** injury of vein at forearm level
     ● **S55.201** Unspecified injury of vein at forearm level, **right arm**
     ● **S55.202** Unspecified injury of vein at forearm level, **left arm**
     ● **S55.209** Unspecified injury of vein at forearm level, **unspecified arm**
   ● **S55.21** **Laceration** of vein at forearm level
     ● **S55.211** Laceration of vein at forearm level, **right arm**
     ● **S55.212** Laceration of vein at forearm level, **left arm**
     ● **S55.219** Laceration of vein at forearm level, **unspecified arm**
   ● **S55.29** **Other** specified injury of vein at forearm level
     ● **S55.291** Other specified injury of vein at forearm level, **right arm**
     ● **S55.292** Other specified injury of vein at forearm level, **left arm**
     ● **S55.299** Other specified injury of vein at forearm level, **unspecified arm**

● **S55.8** **Injury of other blood vessels at forearm level**
   ● **S55.80** **Unspecified** injury of other blood vessels at forearm level
     ● **S55.801** Unspecified injury of other blood vessels at forearm level, **right arm**
     ● **S55.802** Unspecified injury of other blood vessels at forearm level, **left arm**
     ● **S55.809** Unspecified injury of other blood vessels at forearm level, **unspecified arm**
   ● **S55.81** **Laceration** of other blood vessels at forearm level
     ● **S55.811** Laceration of other blood vessels at forearm level, **right arm**
     ● **S55.812** Laceration of other blood vessels at forearm level, **left arm**
     ● **S55.819** Laceration of other blood vessels at forearm level, **unspecified arm**

● **S55.89**   **Other specified injury of other blood vessels at forearm level**
  ● **S55.891**   Other specified injury of other blood vessels at forearm level, **right** arm
  ● **S55.892**   Other specified injury of other blood vessels at forearm level, **left** arm
  ● **S55.899**   Other specified injury of other blood vessels at forearm level, **unspecified** arm

● **S55.9**   Injury of unspecified blood vessel at forearm level
 ● **S55.90**   Unspecified injury of unspecified blood vessel at forearm level
  ● **S55.901**   Unspecified injury of unspecified blood vessel at forearm level, **right** arm
  ● **S55.902**   Unspecified injury of unspecified blood vessel at forearm level, **left** arm
  ● **S55.909**   Unspecified injury of unspecified blood vessel at forearm level, **unspecified** arm
 ● **S55.91**   Laceration of unspecified blood vessel at forearm level
  ● **S55.911**   Laceration of **unspecified** blood vessel at forearm level, **right** arm
  ● **S55.912**   Laceration of **unspecified** blood vessel at forearm level, **left** arm
  ● **S55.919**   Laceration of **unspecified** blood vessel at forearm level, unspecified arm
 ● **S55.99**   Other specified injury of unspecified blood vessel at forearm level
  ● **S55.991**   Other specified injury of **unspecified** blood vessel at forearm level, **right** arm
  ● **S55.992**   Other specified injury of **unspecified** blood vessel at forearm level, **left** arm
  ● **S55.999**   Other specified injury of **unspecified** blood vessel at forearm level, **unspecified** arm

● **S56**   **Injury of muscle, fascia and tendon at forearm level**

  Code also any associated open wound (S51.-)

  Excludes2   injury of muscle, fascia and tendon at or below wrist (S66.-)
        sprain of joints and ligaments of elbow (S53.4-)

  The appropriate 7th character is to be added to each code from category S56

A	initial encounter
D	subsequent encounter
S	sequela

● **S56.0**   **Injury of flexor muscle, fascia and tendon of thumb at forearm level**
 ● **S56.00**   Unspecified injury of flexor muscle, fascia and tendon of thumb at forearm level
  ● **S56.001**   Unspecified injury of flexor muscle, fascia and tendon of **right** thumb at forearm level
  ● **S56.002**   Unspecified injury of flexor muscle, fascia and tendon of **left** thumb at forearm level
  ● **S56.009**   Unspecified injury of flexor muscle, fascia and tendon of **unspecified** thumb at forearm level
 ● **S56.01**   Strain of flexor muscle, fascia and tendon of thumb at forearm level
  ● **S56.011**   Strain of flexor muscle, fascia and tendon of **right** thumb at forearm level
  ● **S56.012**   Strain of flexor muscle, fascia and tendon of **left** thumb at forearm level
  ● **S56.019**   Strain of flexor muscle, fascia and tendon of **unspecified** thumb at forearm level

● **S56.02**   Laceration of flexor muscle, fascia and tendon of thumb at forearm level
  ● **S56.021**   Laceration of flexor muscle, fascia and tendon of **right** thumb at forearm level
  ● **S56.022**   Laceration of flexor muscle, fascia and tendon of **left** thumb at forearm level
  ● **S56.029**   Laceration of flexor muscle, fascia and tendon of **unspecified** thumb at forearm level
 ● **S56.09**   Other injury of flexor muscle, fascia and tendon of thumb at forearm level
  ● **S56.091**   Other injury of flexor muscle, fascia and tendon of **right** thumb at forearm level
  ● **S56.092**   Other injury of flexor muscle, fascia and tendon of **left** thumb at forearm level
  ● **S56.099**   Other injury of flexor muscle, fascia and tendon of **unspecified** thumb at forearm level

● **S56.1**   Injury of flexor muscle, fascia and tendon of **other and unspecified finger** at forearm level
 ● **S56.10**   **Unspecified** injury of flexor muscle, fascia and tendon of other and unspecified finger at forearm level
  ● **S56.101**   Unspecified injury of flexor muscle, fascia and tendon of **right index** finger at forearm level
  ● **S56.102**   Unspecified injury of flexor muscle, fascia and tendon of **left index** finger at forearm level
  ● **S56.103**   Unspecified injury of flexor muscle, fascia and tendon of **right middle** finger at forearm level
  ● **S56.104**   Unspecified injury of flexor muscle, fascia and tendon of **left middle** finger at forearm level
  ● **S56.105**   Unspecified injury of flexor muscle, fascia and tendon of **right ring** finger at forearm level
  ● **S56.106**   Unspecified injury of flexor muscle, fascia and tendon of **left ring** finger at forearm level
  ● **S56.107**   Unspecified injury of flexor muscle, fascia and tendon of **right little** finger at forearm level
  ● **S56.108**   Unspecified injury of flexor muscle, fascia and tendon of **left little** finger at forearm level
  ● **S56.109**   Unspecified injury of flexor muscle, fascia and tendon of **unspecified** finger at forearm level
 ● **S56.11**   **Strain** of flexor muscle, fascia and tendon of other and unspecified finger at forearm level
  ● **S56.111**   Strain of flexor muscle, fascia and tendon of **right index** finger at forearm level
  ● **S56.112**   Strain of flexor muscle, fascia and tendon of **left index** finger at forearm level
  ● **S56.113**   Strain of flexor muscle, fascia and tendon of **right middle** finger at forearm level
  ● **S56.114**   Strain of flexor muscle, fascia and tendon of **left middle** finger at forearm level
  ● **S56.115**   Strain of flexor muscle, fascia and tendon of **right ring** finger at forearm level
  ● **S56.116**   Strain of flexor muscle, fascia and tendon of **left ring** finger at forearm level

● **S56.117** Strain of flexor muscle, fascia and tendon of right little finger at forearm level

● **S56.118** Strain of flexor muscle, fascia and tendon of left little finger at forearm level

● **S56.119** Strain of flexor muscle, fascia and tendon of finger of unspecified finger at forearm level

● **S56.12** Laceration of flexor muscle, fascia and tendon of other and unspecified finger at forearm level

● **S56.121** Laceration of flexor muscle, fascia and tendon of right index finger at forearm level

● **S56.122** Laceration of flexor muscle, fascia and tendon of left index finger at forearm level

● **S56.123** Laceration of flexor muscle, fascia and tendon of right middle finger at forearm level

● **S56.124** Laceration of flexor muscle, fascia and tendon of left middle finger at forearm level

● **S56.125** Laceration of flexor muscle, fascia and tendon of right ring finger at forearm level

● **S56.126** Laceration of flexor muscle, fascia and tendon of left ring finger at forearm level

● **S56.127** Laceration of flexor muscle, fascia and tendon of right little finger at forearm level

● **S56.128** Laceration of flexor muscle, fascia and tendon of left little finger at forearm level

● **S56.129** Laceration of flexor muscle, fascia and tendon of unspecified finger at forearm level

● **S56.19** Other injury of flexor muscle, fascia and tendon of other and unspecified finger at forearm level

● **S56.191** Other injury of flexor muscle, fascia and tendon of right index finger at forearm level

● **S56.192** Other injury of flexor muscle, fascia and tendon of left index finger at forearm level

● **S56.193** Other injury of flexor muscle, fascia and tendon of right middle finger at forearm level

● **S56.194** Other injury of flexor muscle, fascia and tendon of left middle finger at forearm level

● **S56.195** Other injury of flexor muscle, fascia and tendon of right ring finger at forearm level

● **S56.196** Other injury of flexor muscle, fascia and tendon of left ring finger at forearm level

● **S56.197** Other injury of flexor muscle, fascia and tendon of right little finger at forearm level

● **S56.198** Other injury of flexor muscle, fascia and tendon of left little finger at forearm level

● **S56.199** Other injury of flexor muscle, fascia and tendon of unspecified finger at forearm level

● **S56.2** Injury of other flexor muscle, fascia and tendon at forearm level

● **S56.20** Unspecified injury of other flexor muscle, fascia and tendon at forearm level

● **S56.201** Unspecified injury of other flexor muscle, fascia and tendon at forearm level, right arm

● **S56.202** Unspecified injury of other flexor muscle, fascia and tendon at forearm level, left arm

● **S56.209** Unspecified injury of other flexor muscle, fascia and tendon at forearm level, unspecified arm

● **S56.21** Strain of other flexor muscle, fascia and tendon at forearm level

● **S56.211** Strain of other flexor muscle, fascia and tendon at forearm level, right arm

● **S56.212** Strain of other flexor muscle, fascia and tendon at forearm level, left arm

● **S56.219** Strain of other flexor muscle, fascia and tendon at forearm level, unspecified arm

● **S56.22** Laceration of other flexor muscle, fascia and tendon at forearm level

● **S56.221** Laceration of other flexor muscle, fascia and tendon at forearm level, right arm

● **S56.222** Laceration of other flexor muscle, fascia and tendon at forearm level, left arm

● **S56.229** Laceration of other flexor muscle, fascia and tendon at forearm level, unspecified arm

● **S56.29** Other injury of other flexor muscle, fascia and tendon at forearm level

● **S56.291** Other injury of other flexor muscle, fascia and tendon at forearm level, right arm

● **S56.292** Other injury of other flexor muscle, fascia and tendon at forearm level, left arm

● **S56.299** Other injury of other flexor muscle, fascia and tendon at forearm level, unspecified arm

● **S56.3** Injury of extensor or abductor muscles, fascia and tendons of thumb at forearm level

● **S56.30** Unspecified injury of extensor or abductor muscles, fascia and tendons of thumb at forearm level

● **S56.301** Unspecified injury of extensor or abductor muscles, fascia and tendons of right thumb at forearm level

● **S56.302** Unspecified injury of extensor or abductor muscles, fascia and tendons of left thumb at forearm level

● **S56.309** Unspecified injury of extensor or abductor muscles, fascia and tendons of unspecified thumb at forearm level

● **S56.31** Strain of extensor or abductor muscles, fascia and tendons of thumb at forearm level

● **S56.311** Strain of extensor or abductor muscles, fascia and tendons of right thumb at forearm level

● **S56.312** Strain of extensor or abductor muscles, fascia and tendons of left thumb at forearm level

● **S56.319** Strain of extensor or abductor muscles, fascia and tendons of unspecified thumb at forearm level

▶ New　　⟹ Revised　　~~deleted~~ Deleted　　Excludes 1　　Excludes 2　　Includes　　Use additional　　Code first　　Code also　　Key words

OGCR Official Guidelines　　**X** Assign placeholder X　　● Use Additional Character(s)　　▸ Manifestation Code　　**HCC** Hierarchical Condition Category　　**Coding Clinic**

- S56.32 Laceration of extensor or abductor muscles, fascia and tendons of thumb at forearm level
  - S56.321 Laceration of extensor or abductor muscles, fascia and tendons of right thumb at forearm level
  - S56.322 Laceration of extensor or abductor muscles, fascia and tendons of left thumb at forearm level
  - S56.329 Laceration of extensor or abductor muscles, fascia and tendons of unspecified thumb at forearm level
- S56.39 Other injury of extensor or abductor muscles, fascia and tendons of thumb at forearm level
  - S56.391 Other injury of extensor or abductor muscles, fascia and tendons of right thumb at forearm level
  - S56.392 Other injury of extensor or abductor muscles, fascia and tendons of left thumb at forearm level
  - S56.399 Other injury of extensor or abductor muscles, fascia and tendons of unspecified thumb at forearm level
- S56.4 Injury of extensor muscle, fascia and tendon of other and unspecified finger at forearm level
  - S56.40 Unspecified injury of extensor muscle, fascia and tendon of other and unspecified finger at forearm level
    - S56.401 Unspecified injury of extensor muscle, fascia and tendon of right index finger at forearm level
    - S56.402 Unspecified injury of extensor muscle, fascia and tendon of left index finger at forearm level
    - S56.403 Unspecified injury of extensor muscle, fascia and tendon of right middle finger at forearm level
    - S56.404 Unspecified injury of extensor muscle, fascia and tendon of left middle finger at forearm level
    - S56.405 Unspecified injury of extensor muscle, fascia and tendon of right ring finger at forearm level
    - S56.406 Unspecified injury of extensor muscle, fascia and tendon of left ring finger at forearm level
    - S56.407 Unspecified injury of extensor muscle, fascia and tendon of right little finger at forearm level
    - S56.408 Unspecified injury of extensor muscle, fascia and tendon of left little finger at forearm level
    - S56.409 Unspecified injury of extensor muscle, fascia and tendon of unspecified finger at forearm level
  - S56.41 Strain of extensor muscle, fascia and tendon of other and unspecified finger at forearm level
    - S56.411 Strain of extensor muscle, fascia and tendon of right index finger at forearm level
    - S56.412 Strain of extensor muscle, fascia and tendon of left index finger at forearm level
    - S56.413 Strain of extensor muscle, fascia and tendon of right middle finger at forearm level
    - S56.414 Strain of extensor muscle, fascia and tendon of left middle finger at forearm level
    - S56.415 Strain of extensor muscle, fascia and tendon of right ring finger at forearm level
    - S56.416 Strain of extensor muscle, fascia and tendon of left ring finger at forearm level
    - S56.417 Strain of extensor muscle, fascia and tendon of right little finger at forearm level
    - S56.418 Strain of extensor muscle, fascia and tendon of left little finger at forearm level
    - S56.419 Strain of extensor muscle, fascia and tendon of finger, unspecified finger at forearm level
  - S56.42 Laceration of extensor muscle, fascia and tendon of other and unspecified finger at forearm level
    - S56.421 Laceration of extensor muscle, fascia and tendon of right index finger at forearm level
    - S56.422 Laceration of extensor muscle, fascia and tendon of left index finger at forearm level
    - S56.423 Laceration of extensor muscle, fascia and tendon of right middle finger at forearm level
    - S56.424 Laceration of extensor muscle, fascia and tendon of left middle finger at forearm level
    - S56.425 Laceration of extensor muscle, fascia and tendon of right ring finger at forearm level
    - S56.426 Laceration of extensor muscle, fascia and tendon of left ring finger at forearm level
    - S56.427 Laceration of extensor muscle, fascia and tendon of right little finger at forearm level
    - S56.428 Laceration of extensor muscle, fascia and tendon of left little finger at forearm level
    - S56.429 Laceration of extensor muscle, fascia and tendon of unspecified finger at forearm level
  - S56.49 Other injury of extensor muscle, fascia and tendon of other and unspecified finger at forearm level
    - S56.491 Other injury of extensor muscle, fascia and tendon of right index finger at forearm level
    - S56.492 Other injury of extensor muscle, fascia and tendon of left index finger at forearm level
    - S56.493 Other injury of extensor muscle, fascia and tendon of right middle finger at forearm level
    - S56.494 Other injury of extensor muscle, fascia and tendon of left middle finger at forearm level
    - S56.495 Other injury of extensor muscle, fascia and tendon of right ring finger at forearm level
    - S56.496 Other injury of extensor muscle, fascia and tendon of left ring finger at forearm level
    - S56.497 Other injury of extensor muscle, fascia and tendon of right little finger at forearm level
    - S56.498 Other injury of extensor muscle, fascia and tendon of left little finger at forearm level
    - S56.499 Other injury of extensor muscle, fascia and tendon of unspecified finger at forearm level

CHAPTER 19 (S00-T88)

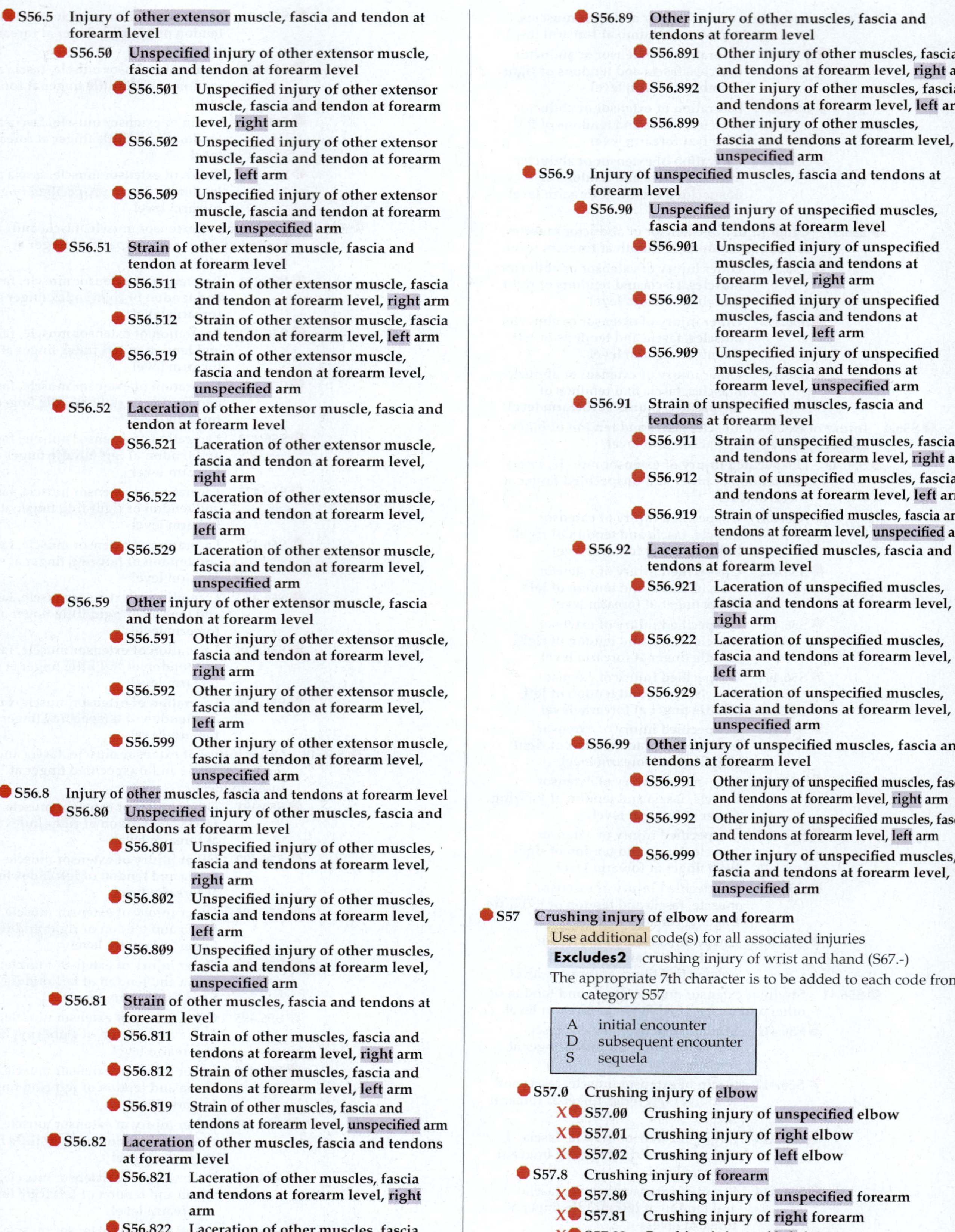

● **S56.5**   Injury of other extensor muscle, fascia and tendon at forearm level
   ● **S56.50**   Unspecified injury of other extensor muscle, fascia and tendon at forearm level
     ● **S56.501**   Unspecified injury of other extensor muscle, fascia and tendon at forearm level, right arm
     ● **S56.502**   Unspecified injury of other extensor muscle, fascia and tendon at forearm level, left arm
     ● **S56.509**   Unspecified injury of other extensor muscle, fascia and tendon at forearm level, unspecified arm
   ● **S56.51**   Strain of other extensor muscle, fascia and tendon at forearm level
     ● **S56.511**   Strain of other extensor muscle, fascia and tendon at forearm level, right arm
     ● **S56.512**   Strain of other extensor muscle, fascia and tendon at forearm level, left arm
     ● **S56.519**   Strain of other extensor muscle, fascia and tendon at forearm level, unspecified arm
   ● **S56.52**   Laceration of other extensor muscle, fascia and tendon at forearm level
     ● **S56.521**   Laceration of other extensor muscle, fascia and tendon at forearm level, right arm
     ● **S56.522**   Laceration of other extensor muscle, fascia and tendon at forearm level, left arm
     ● **S56.529**   Laceration of other extensor muscle, fascia and tendon at forearm level, unspecified arm
   ● **S56.59**   Other injury of other extensor muscle, fascia and tendon at forearm level
     ● **S56.591**   Other injury of other extensor muscle, fascia and tendon at forearm level, right arm
     ● **S56.592**   Other injury of other extensor muscle, fascia and tendon at forearm level, left arm
     ● **S56.599**   Other injury of other extensor muscle, fascia and tendon at forearm level, unspecified arm
● **S56.8**   Injury of other muscles, fascia and tendons at forearm level
   ● **S56.80**   Unspecified injury of other muscles, fascia and tendons at forearm level
     ● **S56.801**   Unspecified injury of other muscles, fascia and tendons at forearm level, right arm
     ● **S56.802**   Unspecified injury of other muscles, fascia and tendons at forearm level, left arm
     ● **S56.809**   Unspecified injury of other muscles, fascia and tendons at forearm level, unspecified arm
   ● **S56.81**   Strain of other muscles, fascia and tendons at forearm level
     ● **S56.811**   Strain of other muscles, fascia and tendons at forearm level, right arm
     ● **S56.812**   Strain of other muscles, fascia and tendons at forearm level, left arm
     ● **S56.819**   Strain of other muscles, fascia and tendons at forearm level, unspecified arm
   ● **S56.82**   Laceration of other muscles, fascia and tendons at forearm level
     ● **S56.821**   Laceration of other muscles, fascia and tendons at forearm level, right arm
     ● **S56.822**   Laceration of other muscles, fascia and tendons at forearm level, left arm
     ● **S56.829**   Laceration of other muscles, fascia and tendons at forearm level, unspecified arm

   ● **S56.89**   Other injury of other muscles, fascia and tendons at forearm level
     ● **S56.891**   Other injury of other muscles, fascia and tendons at forearm level, right arm
     ● **S56.892**   Other injury of other muscles, fascia and tendons at forearm level, left arm
     ● **S56.899**   Other injury of other muscles, fascia and tendons at forearm level, unspecified arm
● **S56.9**   Injury of unspecified muscles, fascia and tendons at forearm level
   ● **S56.90**   Unspecified injury of unspecified muscles, fascia and tendons at forearm level
     ● **S56.901**   Unspecified injury of unspecified muscles, fascia and tendons at forearm level, right arm
     ● **S56.902**   Unspecified injury of unspecified muscles, fascia and tendons at forearm level, left arm
     ● **S56.909**   Unspecified injury of unspecified muscles, fascia and tendons at forearm level, unspecified arm
   ● **S56.91**   Strain of unspecified muscles, fascia and tendons at forearm level
     ● **S56.911**   Strain of unspecified muscles, fascia and tendons at forearm level, right arm
     ● **S56.912**   Strain of unspecified muscles, fascia and tendons at forearm level, left arm
     ● **S56.919**   Strain of unspecified muscles, fascia and tendons at forearm level, unspecified arm
   ● **S56.92**   Laceration of unspecified muscles, fascia and tendons at forearm level
     ● **S56.921**   Laceration of unspecified muscles, fascia and tendons at forearm level, right arm
     ● **S56.922**   Laceration of unspecified muscles, fascia and tendons at forearm level, left arm
     ● **S56.929**   Laceration of unspecified muscles, fascia and tendons at forearm level, unspecified arm
   ● **S56.99**   Other injury of unspecified muscles, fascia and tendons at forearm level
     ● **S56.991**   Other injury of unspecified muscles, fascia and tendons at forearm level, right arm
     ● **S56.992**   Other injury of unspecified muscles, fascia and tendons at forearm level, left arm
     ● **S56.999**   Other injury of unspecified muscles, fascia and tendons at forearm level, unspecified arm

● **S57**   **Crushing injury of elbow and forearm**
   Use additional code(s) for all associated injuries
   Excludes2   crushing injury of wrist and hand (S67.-)
   The appropriate 7th character is to be added to each code from category S57

> A   initial encounter
> D   subsequent encounter
> S   sequela

● **S57.0**   Crushing injury of elbow
   X ● **S57.00**   Crushing injury of unspecified elbow
   X ● **S57.01**   Crushing injury of right elbow
   X ● **S57.02**   Crushing injury of left elbow
● **S57.8**   Crushing injury of forearm
   X ● **S57.80**   Crushing injury of unspecified forearm
   X ● **S57.81**   Crushing injury of right forearm
   X ● **S57.82**   Crushing injury of left forearm

▶ New   ▶ Revised   ~~deleted~~ Deleted   Excludes 1   Excludes 2   Includes   Use additional   Code first   Code also   Key words
OGCR Official Guidelines   X Assign placeholder X   ● Use Additional Character(s)   ▶ Manifestation Code   Hierarchical Condition Category   Coding Clinic

● **S58 Traumatic amputation of elbow and forearm**
An amputation not identified as partial or complete should be coded to complete

Excludes1 traumatic amputation of wrist and hand (S68.-)

The appropriate 7th character is to be added to each code from category S58

> A   initial encounter
> D   subsequent encounter
> S   sequela

● **S58.0 Traumatic amputation at elbow level**
  ● **S58.01 Complete traumatic amputation at elbow level**
    ● S58.011 Complete traumatic amputation at elbow level, right arm A, S
    ● S58.012 Complete traumatic amputation at elbow level, left arm A, S
    ● S58.019 Complete traumatic amputation at elbow level, unspecified arm A, S
  ● **S58.02 Partial traumatic amputation at elbow level**
    ● S58.021 Partial traumatic amputation at elbow level, right arm A, S
    ● S58.022 Partial traumatic amputation at elbow level, left arm A, S
    ● S58.029 Partial traumatic amputation at elbow level, unspecified arm A, S

● **S58.1 Traumatic amputation at level between elbow and wrist**
  ● **S58.11 Complete traumatic amputation at level between elbow and wrist**
    ● S58.111 Complete traumatic amputation at level between elbow and wrist, right arm A, S
    ● S58.112 Complete traumatic amputation at level between elbow and wrist, left arm A, S
    ● S58.119 Complete traumatic amputation at level between elbow and wrist, unspecified arm A, S
  ● **S58.12 Partial traumatic amputation at level between elbow and wrist**
    ● S58.121 Partial traumatic amputation at level between elbow and wrist, right arm A, S
    ● S58.122 Partial traumatic amputation at level between elbow and wrist, left arm A, S
    ● S58.129 Partial traumatic amputation at level between elbow and wrist, unspecified arm A, S

● **S58.9 Traumatic amputation of forearm, level unspecified**
Excludes1 traumatic amputation of wrist (S68.-)
  ● **S58.91 Complete traumatic amputation of forearm, level unspecified**
    ● S58.911 Complete traumatic amputation of right forearm, level unspecified A, S
    ● S58.912 Complete traumatic amputation of left forearm, level unspecified A, S
    ● S58.919 Complete traumatic amputation of unspecified forearm, level unspecified A, S
  ● **S58.92 Partial traumatic amputation of forearm, level unspecified**
    ● S58.921 Partial traumatic amputation of right forearm, level unspecified A, S
    ● S58.922 Partial traumatic amputation of left forearm, level unspecified A, S
    ● S58.929 Partial traumatic amputation of unspecified forearm, level unspecified A, S

● **S59 Other and unspecified injuries of elbow and forearm**

Excludes2 other and unspecified injuries of wrist and hand (S69.-)

The appropriate 7th character is to be added to each code from subcategories S59.0, S59.1, and S59.2

> A   initial encounter for closed fracture
> D   subsequent encounter for fracture with routine healing
> G   subsequent encounter for fracture with delayed healing
> K   subsequent encounter for fracture with nonunion
> P   subsequent encounter for fracture with malunion
> S   sequela

● **S59.0 Physeal fracture of lower end of ulna**
  ● **S59.00 Unspecified physeal fracture of lower end of ulna**
    ● S59.001 Unspecified physeal fracture of lower end of ulna, right arm
    ● S59.002 Unspecified physeal fracture of lower end of ulna, left arm
    ● S59.009 Unspecified physeal fracture of lower end of ulna, unspecified arm
  ● **S59.01 Salter-Harris Type I physeal fracture of lower end of ulna**
    ● S59.011 Salter-Harris Type I physeal fracture of lower end of ulna, right arm
    ● S59.012 Salter-Harris Type I physeal fracture of lower end of ulna, left arm
    ● S59.019 Salter-Harris Type I physeal fracture of lower end of ulna, unspecified arm
  ● **S59.02 Salter-Harris Type II physeal fracture of lower end of ulna**
    ● S59.021 Salter-Harris Type II physeal fracture of lower end of ulna, right arm
    ● S59.022 Salter-Harris Type II physeal fracture of lower end of ulna, left arm
    ● S59.029 Salter-Harris Type II physeal fracture of lower end of ulna, unspecified arm
  ● **S59.03 Salter-Harris Type III physeal fracture of lower end of ulna**
    ● S59.031 Salter-Harris Type III physeal fracture of lower end of ulna, right arm
    ● S59.032 Salter-Harris Type III physeal fracture of lower end of ulna, left arm
    ● S59.039 Salter-Harris Type III physeal fracture of lower end of ulna, unspecified arm
  ● **S59.04 Salter-Harris Type IV physeal fracture of lower end of ulna**
    ● S59.041 Salter-Harris Type IV physeal fracture of lower end of ulna, right arm
    ● S59.042 Salter-Harris Type IV physeal fracture of lower end of ulna, left arm
    ● S59.049 Salter-Harris Type IV physeal fracture of lower end of ulna, unspecified arm
  ● **S59.09 Other physeal fracture of lower end of ulna**
    ● S59.091 Other physeal fracture of lower end of ulna, right arm
    ● S59.092 Other physeal fracture of lower end of ulna, left arm
    ● S59.099 Other physeal fracture of lower end of ulna, unspecified arm

Item 19–4   SALTER-HARRIS TYPE 1: epiphysis is completely separated from end of bone, or metaphysic growth plate remains attached to epiphysis
SALTER-HARRIS TYPE 2: epiphysis and growth plate are partially separated from metaphysis, which is cracked—most common type
SALTER-HARRIS TYPE 3: fracture occurring through epiphysis and separates part of epiphysis and growth plate from metaphysis fracture, usually at distal end of tibia
SALTER-HARRIS TYPE 4: fracture runs through epiphysis, across growth plate, into metaphysic, surgery is required to restore joint surface to normal and align growth plate

CHAPTER 19 (S00–T88)

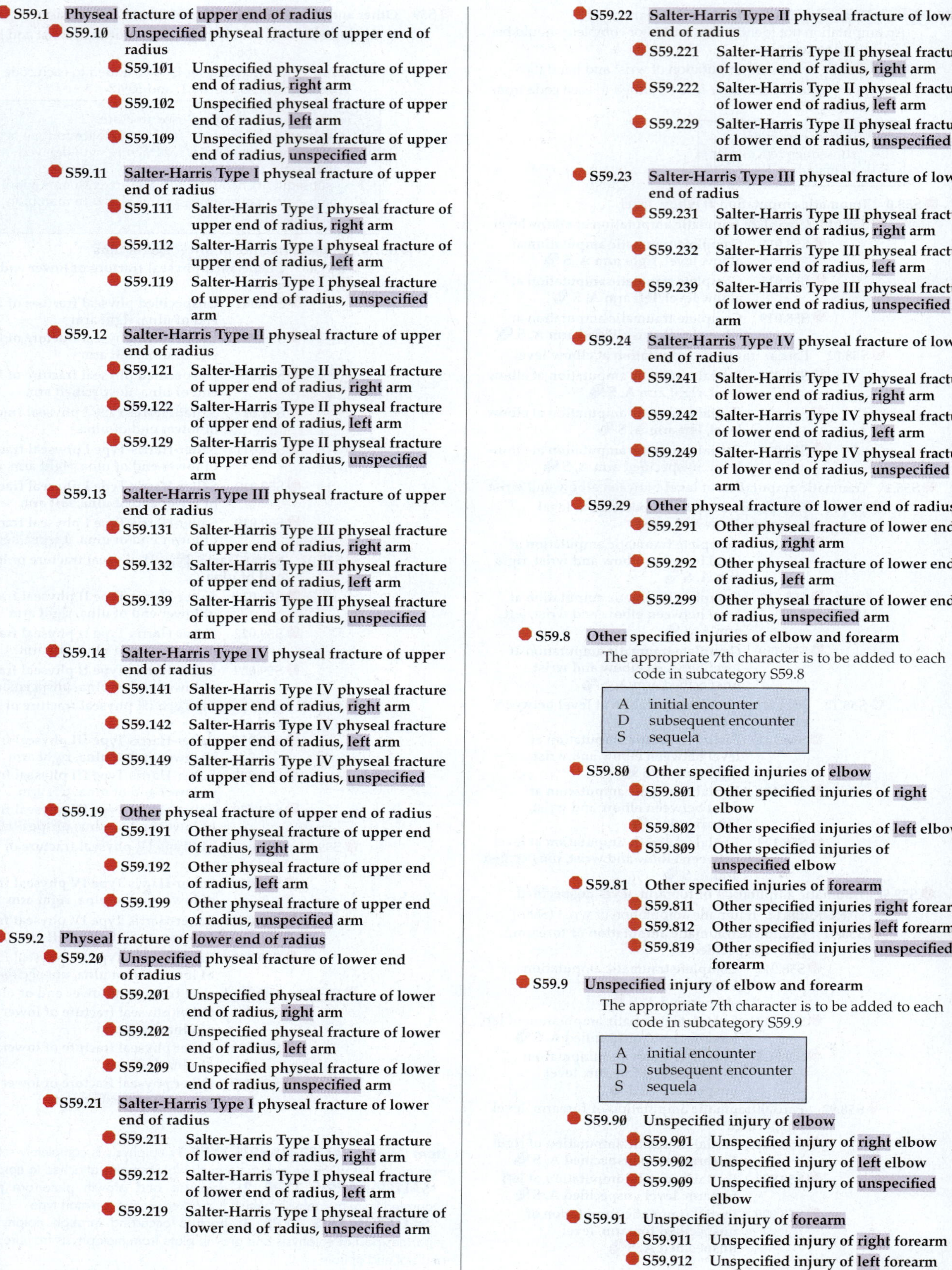

- ● S59.1   **Physeal fracture of upper end of radius**
  - ● S59.10   **Unspecified** physeal fracture of upper end of radius
    - ● S59.101   Unspecified physeal fracture of upper end of radius, **right arm**
    - ● S59.102   Unspecified physeal fracture of upper end of radius, **left arm**
    - ● S59.109   Unspecified physeal fracture of upper end of radius, **unspecified arm**
  - ● S59.11   **Salter-Harris Type I physeal fracture of upper end of radius**
    - ● S59.111   Salter-Harris Type I physeal fracture of upper end of radius, **right arm**
    - ● S59.112   Salter-Harris Type I physeal fracture of upper end of radius, **left arm**
    - ● S59.119   Salter-Harris Type I physeal fracture of upper end of radius, **unspecified arm**
  - ● S59.12   **Salter-Harris Type II physeal fracture of upper end of radius**
    - ● S59.121   Salter-Harris Type II physeal fracture of upper end of radius, **right arm**
    - ● S59.122   Salter-Harris Type II physeal fracture of upper end of radius, **left arm**
    - ● S59.129   Salter-Harris Type II physeal fracture of upper end of radius, **unspecified arm**
  - ● S59.13   **Salter-Harris Type III physeal fracture of upper end of radius**
    - ● S59.131   Salter-Harris Type III physeal fracture of upper end of radius, **right arm**
    - ● S59.132   Salter-Harris Type III physeal fracture of upper end of radius, **left arm**
    - ● S59.139   Salter-Harris Type III physeal fracture of upper end of radius, **unspecified arm**
  - ● S59.14   **Salter-Harris Type IV physeal fracture of upper end of radius**
    - ● S59.141   Salter-Harris Type IV physeal fracture of upper end of radius, **right arm**
    - ● S59.142   Salter-Harris Type IV physeal fracture of upper end of radius, **left arm**
    - ● S59.149   Salter-Harris Type IV physeal fracture of upper end of radius, **unspecified arm**
  - ● S59.19   **Other physeal fracture of upper end of radius**
    - ● S59.191   Other physeal fracture of upper end of radius, **right arm**
    - ● S59.192   Other physeal fracture of upper end of radius, **left arm**
    - ● S59.199   Other physeal fracture of upper end of radius, **unspecified arm**
- ● S59.2   **Physeal fracture of lower end of radius**
  - ● S59.20   **Unspecified** physeal fracture of lower end of radius
    - ● S59.201   Unspecified physeal fracture of lower end of radius, **right arm**
    - ● S59.202   Unspecified physeal fracture of lower end of radius, **left arm**
    - ● S59.209   Unspecified physeal fracture of lower end of radius, **unspecified arm**
  - ● S59.21   **Salter-Harris Type I physeal fracture of lower end of radius**
    - ● S59.211   Salter-Harris Type I physeal fracture of lower end of radius, **right arm**
    - ● S59.212   Salter-Harris Type I physeal fracture of lower end of radius, **left arm**
    - ● S59.219   Salter-Harris Type I physeal fracture of lower end of radius, **unspecified arm**

- ● S59.22   **Salter-Harris Type II physeal fracture of lower end of radius**
  - ● S59.221   Salter-Harris Type II physeal fracture of lower end of radius, **right arm**
  - ● S59.222   Salter-Harris Type II physeal fracture of lower end of radius, **left arm**
  - ● S59.229   Salter-Harris Type II physeal fracture of lower end of radius, **unspecified arm**
- ● S59.23   **Salter-Harris Type III physeal fracture of lower end of radius**
  - ● S59.231   Salter-Harris Type III physeal fracture of lower end of radius, **right arm**
  - ● S59.232   Salter-Harris Type III physeal fracture of lower end of radius, **left arm**
  - ● S59.239   Salter-Harris Type III physeal fracture of lower end of radius, **unspecified arm**
- ● S59.24   **Salter-Harris Type IV physeal fracture of lower end of radius**
  - ● S59.241   Salter-Harris Type IV physeal fracture of lower end of radius, **right arm**
  - ● S59.242   Salter-Harris Type IV physeal fracture of lower end of radius, **left arm**
  - ● S59.249   Salter-Harris Type IV physeal fracture of lower end of radius, **unspecified arm**
- ● S59.29   **Other physeal fracture of lower end of radius**
  - ● S59.291   Other physeal fracture of lower end of radius, **right arm**
  - ● S59.292   Other physeal fracture of lower end of radius, **left arm**
  - ● S59.299   Other physeal fracture of lower end of radius, **unspecified arm**
- ● S59.8   Other specified injuries of elbow and forearm

  The appropriate 7th character is to be added to each code in subcategory S59.8

  > A   initial encounter
  > D   subsequent encounter
  > S   sequela

  - ● S59.80   **Other specified injuries of elbow**
    - ● S59.801   Other specified injuries of **right** elbow
    - ● S59.802   Other specified injuries of **left** elbow
    - ● S59.809   Other specified injuries of **unspecified** elbow
  - ● S59.81   **Other specified injuries of forearm**
    - ● S59.811   Other specified injuries **right** forearm
    - ● S59.812   Other specified injuries **left** forearm
    - ● S59.819   Other specified injuries **unspecified** forearm
- ● S59.9   Unspecified injury of elbow and forearm

  The appropriate 7th character is to be added to each code in subcategory S59.9

  > A   initial encounter
  > D   subsequent encounter
  > S   sequela

  - ● S59.90   **Unspecified injury of elbow**
    - ● S59.901   Unspecified injury of **right** elbow
    - ● S59.902   Unspecified injury of **left** elbow
    - ● S59.909   Unspecified injury of **unspecified** elbow
  - ● S59.91   **Unspecified injury of forearm**
    - ● S59.911   Unspecified injury of **right** forearm
    - ● S59.912   Unspecified injury of **left** forearm
    - ● S59.919   Unspecified injury of **unspecified** forearm

INJURIES TO THE WRIST, HAND AND FINGERS (S60-S69)

Excludes2　burns and corrosions (T20-T32)
frostbite (T33-T34)
insect bite or sting, venomous (T63.4)

● **S60**　**Superficial injury of wrist, hand and fingers**
The appropriate 7th character is to be added to each code from category S60

> A　initial encounter
> D　subsequent encounter
> S　sequela

● **S60.0**　**Contusion of finger without damage to nail**
　Excludes1　contusion involving nail (matrix) (S60.1)
X ● **S60.00**　Contusion of **unspecified** finger without damage to nail
　　Contusion of finger(s) NOS
● **S60.01**　Contusion of **thumb** without damage to nail
　● **S60.011**　Contusion of **right** thumb without damage to nail
　● **S60.012**　Contusion of **left** thumb without damage to nail
　● **S60.019**　Contusion of **unspecified** thumb without damage to nail
● **S60.02**　Contusion of **index** finger without damage to nail
　● **S60.021**　Contusion of **right** index finger without damage to nail
　● **S60.022**　Contusion of **left** index finger without damage to nail
　● **S60.029**　Contusion of **unspecified** index finger without damage to nail
● **S60.03**　Contusion of **middle** finger without damage to nail
　● **S60.031**　Contusion of **right** middle finger without damage to nail
　● **S60.032**　Contusion of **left** middle finger without damage to nail
　● **S60.039**　Contusion of **unspecified** middle finger without damage to nail
● **S60.04**　Contusion of **ring** finger without damage to nail
　● **S60.041**　Contusion of **right** ring finger without damage to nail
　● **S60.042**　Contusion of **left** ring finger without damage to nail
　● **S60.049**　Contusion of **unspecified** ring finger without damage to nail
● **S60.05**　Contusion of **little** finger without damage to nail
　● **S60.051**　Contusion of **right** little finger without damage to nail
　● **S60.052**　Contusion of **left** little finger without damage to nail
　● **S60.059**　Contusion of **unspecified** little finger without damage to nail
● **S60.1**　**Contusion of finger with damage to nail**
X ● **S60.10**　Contusion of **unspecified** finger with damage to nail
● **S60.11**　Contusion of **thumb** with damage to nail
　● **S60.111**　Contusion of **right** thumb with damage to nail
　● **S60.112**　Contusion of **left** thumb with damage to nail
　● **S60.119**　Contusion of **unspecified** thumb with damage to nail

● **S60.12**　Contusion of **index** finger with damage to nail
　● **S60.121**　Contusion of **right** index finger with damage to nail
　● **S60.122**　Contusion of **left** index finger with damage to nail
　● **S60.129**　Contusion of **unspecified** index finger with damage to nail
● **S60.13**　Contusion of **middle** finger with damage to nail
　● **S60.131**　Contusion of **right** middle finger with damage to nail
　● **S60.132**　Contusion of **left** middle finger with damage to nail
　● **S60.139**　Contusion of **unspecified** middle finger with damage to nail
● **S60.14**　Contusion of **ring** finger with damage to nail
　● **S60.141**　Contusion of **right** ring finger with damage to nail
　● **S60.142**　Contusion of **left** ring finger with damage to nail
　● **S60.149**　Contusion of **unspecified** ring finger with damage to nail
● **S60.15**　Contusion of **little** finger with damage to nail
　● **S60.151**　Contusion of **right** little finger with damage to nail
　● **S60.152**　Contusion of **left** little finger with damage to nail
　● **S60.159**　Contusion of **unspecified** little finger with damage to nail
● **S60.2**　Contusion of **wrist and hand**
　Excludes2　contusion of fingers (S60.0-, S60.1-)
● **S60.21**　Contusion of **wrist**
　● **S60.211**　Contusion of **right** wrist
　● **S60.212**　Contusion of **left** wrist
　● **S60.219**　Contusion of **unspecified** wrist
● **S60.22**　Contusion of **hand**
　● **S60.221**　Contusion of **right** hand
　● **S60.222**　Contusion of **left** hand
　● **S60.229**　Contusion of **unspecified** hand
● **S60.3**　Other superficial injuries of **thumb**
● **S60.31**　**Abrasion** of thumb
　● **S60.311**　Abrasion of **right** thumb
　● **S60.312**　Abrasion of **left** thumb
　● **S60.319**　Abrasion of **unspecified** thumb
● **S60.32**　**Blister** (nonthermal) of thumb
　● **S60.321**　Blister (nonthermal) of **right** thumb
　● **S60.322**　Blister (nonthermal) of **left** thumb
　● **S60.329**　Blister (nonthermal) of **unspecified** thumb
● **S60.34**　**External constriction** of thumb
　Hair tourniquet syndrome of thumb
　Use additional cause code to identify the constricting item (W49.0-)
　● **S60.341**　External constriction of **right** thumb
　● **S60.342**　External constriction of **left** thumb
　● **S60.349**　External constriction of **unspecified** thumb
● **S60.35**　**Superficial foreign body** of thumb
　Splinter in the thumb
　● **S60.351**　Superficial foreign body of **right** thumb
　● **S60.352**　Superficial foreign body of **left** thumb
　● **S60.359**　Superficial foreign body of **unspecified** thumb

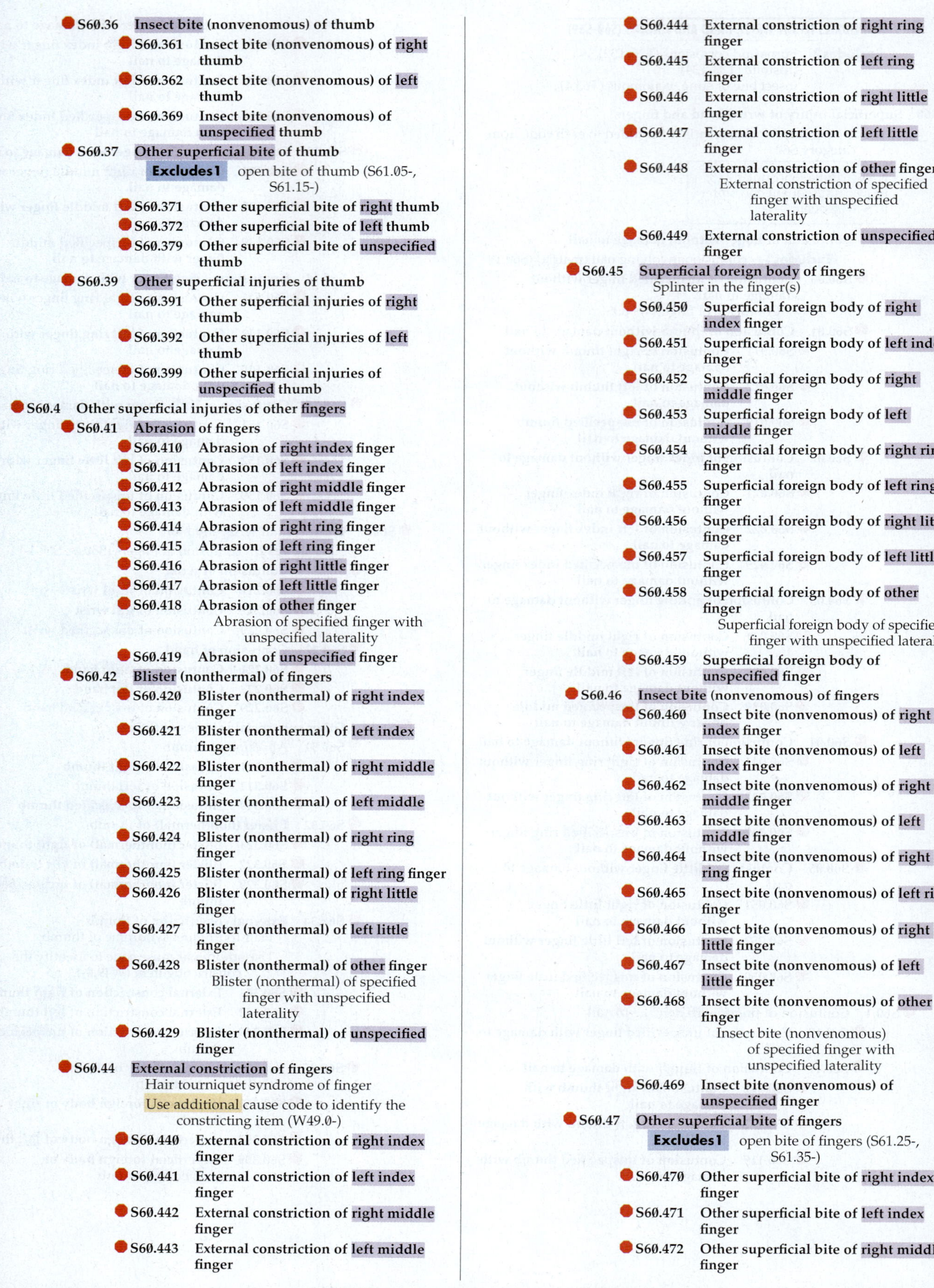

● **S60.36**   **Insect bite (nonvenomous) of thumb**
   ● S60.361   Insect bite (nonvenomous) of right thumb
   ● S60.362   Insect bite (nonvenomous) of left thumb
   ● S60.369   Insect bite (nonvenomous) of unspecified thumb
● **S60.37**   **Other superficial bite of thumb**
   Excludes1   open bite of thumb (S61.05-, S61.15-)
   ● S60.371   Other superficial bite of right thumb
   ● S60.372   Other superficial bite of left thumb
   ● S60.379   Other superficial bite of unspecified thumb
● **S60.39**   **Other superficial injuries of thumb**
   ● S60.391   Other superficial injuries of right thumb
   ● S60.392   Other superficial injuries of left thumb
   ● S60.399   Other superficial injuries of unspecified thumb

● **S60.4**   **Other superficial injuries of other fingers**
   ● **S60.41**   **Abrasion of fingers**
     ● S60.410   Abrasion of right index finger
     ● S60.411   Abrasion of left index finger
     ● S60.412   Abrasion of right middle finger
     ● S60.413   Abrasion of left middle finger
     ● S60.414   Abrasion of right ring finger
     ● S60.415   Abrasion of left ring finger
     ● S60.416   Abrasion of right little finger
     ● S60.417   Abrasion of left little finger
     ● S60.418   Abrasion of other finger
       Abrasion of specified finger with unspecified laterality
     ● S60.419   Abrasion of unspecified finger
   ● **S60.42**   **Blister (nonthermal) of fingers**
     ● S60.420   Blister (nonthermal) of right index finger
     ● S60.421   Blister (nonthermal) of left index finger
     ● S60.422   Blister (nonthermal) of right middle finger
     ● S60.423   Blister (nonthermal) of left middle finger
     ● S60.424   Blister (nonthermal) of right ring finger
     ● S60.425   Blister (nonthermal) of left ring finger
     ● S60.426   Blister (nonthermal) of right little finger
     ● S60.427   Blister (nonthermal) of left little finger
     ● S60.428   Blister (nonthermal) of other finger
       Blister (nonthermal) of specified finger with unspecified laterality
     ● S60.429   Blister (nonthermal) of unspecified finger
   ● **S60.44**   **External constriction of fingers**
     Hair tourniquet syndrome of finger
     Use additional cause code to identify the constricting item (W49.0-)
     ● S60.440   External constriction of right index finger
     ● S60.441   External constriction of left index finger
     ● S60.442   External constriction of right middle finger
     ● S60.443   External constriction of left middle finger

     ● S60.444   External constriction of right ring finger
     ● S60.445   External constriction of left ring finger
     ● S60.446   External constriction of right little finger
     ● S60.447   External constriction of left little finger
     ● S60.448   External constriction of other finger
       External constriction of specified finger with unspecified laterality
     ● S60.449   External constriction of unspecified finger
   ● **S60.45**   **Superficial foreign body of fingers**
     Splinter in the finger(s)
     ● S60.450   Superficial foreign body of right index finger
     ● S60.451   Superficial foreign body of left index finger
     ● S60.452   Superficial foreign body of right middle finger
     ● S60.453   Superficial foreign body of left middle finger
     ● S60.454   Superficial foreign body of right ring finger
     ● S60.455   Superficial foreign body of left ring finger
     ● S60.456   Superficial foreign body of right little finger
     ● S60.457   Superficial foreign body of left little finger
     ● S60.458   Superficial foreign body of other finger
       Superficial foreign body of specified finger with unspecified laterality
     ● S60.459   Superficial foreign body of unspecified finger
   ● **S60.46**   **Insect bite (nonvenomous) of fingers**
     ● S60.460   Insect bite (nonvenomous) of right index finger
     ● S60.461   Insect bite (nonvenomous) of left index finger
     ● S60.462   Insect bite (nonvenomous) of right middle finger
     ● S60.463   Insect bite (nonvenomous) of left middle finger
     ● S60.464   Insect bite (nonvenomous) of right ring finger
     ● S60.465   Insect bite (nonvenomous) of left ring finger
     ● S60.466   Insect bite (nonvenomous) of right little finger
     ● S60.467   Insect bite (nonvenomous) of left little finger
     ● S60.468   Insect bite (nonvenomous) of other finger
       Insect bite (nonvenomous) of specified finger with unspecified laterality
     ● S60.469   Insect bite (nonvenomous) of unspecified finger
   ● **S60.47**   **Other superficial bite of fingers**
     Excludes1   open bite of fingers (S61.25-, S61.35-)
     ● S60.470   Other superficial bite of right index finger
     ● S60.471   Other superficial bite of left index finger
     ● S60.472   Other superficial bite of right middle finger

- **S60.473** Other superficial bite of left middle finger
- **S60.474** Other superficial bite of right ring finger
- **S60.475** Other superficial bite of left ring finger
- **S60.476** Other superficial bite of right little finger
- **S60.477** Other superficial bite of left little finger
- **S60.478** Other superficial bite of other finger
  - Other superficial bite of specified finger with unspecified laterality
- **S60.479** Other superficial bite of unspecified finger
- **S60.5** Other superficial injuries of hand
  - **Excludes2** superficial injuries of fingers (S60.3-, S60.4-)
  - **S60.51** Abrasion of hand
    - **S60.511** Abrasion of right hand
    - **S60.512** Abrasion of left hand
    - **S60.519** Abrasion of unspecified hand
  - **S60.52** Blister (nonthermal) of hand
    - **S60.521** Blister (nonthermal) of right hand
    - **S60.522** Blister (nonthermal) of left hand
    - **S60.529** Blister (nonthermal) of unspecified hand
  - **S60.54** External constriction of hand
    - **S60.541** External constriction of right hand
    - **S60.542** External constriction of left hand
    - **S60.549** External constriction of unspecified hand
  - **S60.55** Superficial foreign body of hand
    - Splinter in the hand
    - **S60.551** Superficial foreign body of right hand
    - **S60.552** Superficial foreign body of left hand
    - **S60.559** Superficial foreign body of unspecified hand
  - **S60.56** Insect bite (nonvenomous) of hand
    - **S60.561** Insect bite (nonvenomous) of right hand
    - **S60.562** Insect bite (nonvenomous) of left hand
    - **S60.569** Insect bite (nonvenomous) of unspecified hand
  - **S60.57** Other superficial bite of hand
    - **Excludes1** open bite of hand (S61.45-)
    - **S60.571** Other superficial bite of hand of right hand
    - **S60.572** Other superficial bite of hand of left hand
    - **S60.579** Other superficial bite of hand of unspecified hand
- **S60.8** Other superficial injuries of wrist
  - **S60.81** Abrasion of wrist
    - **S60.811** Abrasion of right wrist
    - **S60.812** Abrasion of left wrist
    - **S60.819** Abrasion of unspecified wrist
  - **S60.82** Blister (nonthermal) of wrist
    - **S60.821** Blister (nonthermal) of right wrist
    - **S60.822** Blister (nonthermal) of left wrist
    - **S60.829** Blister (nonthermal) of unspecified wrist

- **S60.84** External constriction of wrist
  - **S60.841** External constriction of right wrist
  - **S60.842** External constriction of left wrist
  - **S60.849** External constriction of unspecified wrist
- **S60.85** Superficial foreign body of wrist
  - Splinter in the wrist
  - **S60.851** Superficial foreign body of right wrist
  - **S60.852** Superficial foreign body of left wrist
  - **S60.859** Superficial foreign body of unspecified wrist
- **S60.86** Insect bite (nonvenomous) of wrist
  - **S60.861** Insect bite (nonvenomous) of right wrist
  - **S60.862** Insect bite (nonvenomous) of left wrist
  - **S60.869** Insect bite (nonvenomous) of unspecified wrist
- **S60.87** Other superficial bite of wrist
  - **Excludes1** open bite of wrist (S61.55)
  - **S60.871** Other superficial bite of right wrist
  - **S60.872** Other superficial bite of left wrist
  - **S60.879** Other superficial bite of unspecified wrist
- **S60.9** Unspecified superficial injury of wrist, hand and fingers
  - **S60.91** Unspecified superficial injury of wrist
    - **S60.911** Unspecified superficial injury of right wrist
    - **S60.912** Unspecified superficial injury of left wrist
    - **S60.919** Unspecified superficial injury of unspecified wrist
  - **S60.92** Unspecified superficial injury of hand
    - **S60.921** Unspecified superficial injury of right hand
    - **S60.922** Unspecified superficial injury of left hand
    - **S60.929** Unspecified superficial injury of unspecified hand
  - **S60.93** Unspecified superficial injury of thumb
    - **S60.931** Unspecified superficial injury of right thumb
    - **S60.932** Unspecified superficial injury of left thumb
    - **S60.939** Unspecified superficial injury of unspecified thumb
  - **S60.94** Unspecified superficial injury of other fingers
    - **S60.940** Unspecified superficial injury of right index finger
    - **S60.941** Unspecified superficial injury of left index finger
    - **S60.942** Unspecified superficial injury of right middle finger
    - **S60.943** Unspecified superficial injury of left middle finger
    - **S60.944** Unspecified superficial injury of right ring finger
    - **S60.945** Unspecified superficial injury of left ring finger
    - **S60.946** Unspecified superficial injury of right little finger
    - **S60.947** Unspecified superficial injury of left little finger
    - **S60.948** Unspecified superficial injury of other finger
      - Unspecified superficial injury of specified finger with unspecified laterality
    - **S60.949** Unspecified superficial injury of unspecified finger

● **S61 Open wound of wrist, hand and fingers**
  Code also any associated wound infection
  Excludes1 open fracture of wrist, hand and finger (S62.-
        with 7th character B)
      traumatic amputation of wrist and hand (S68.-)
  The appropriate 7th character is to be added to each code from
      category S61

> A initial encounter
> D subsequent encounter
> S sequela

● **S61.0 Open wound of thumb without damage to nail**
  Excludes1 open wound of thumb with damage to
        nail (S61.1-)
  ● **S61.00 Unspecified open wound of thumb without
        damage to nail**
    ● **S61.001 Unspecified open wound of right
          thumb without damage to nail**
    ● **S61.002 Unspecified open wound of left
          thumb without damage to nail**
    ● **S61.009 Unspecified open wound of
          unspecified thumb without damage to
          nail**
  ● **S61.01 Laceration without foreign body of thumb
        without damage to nail**
    ● **S61.011 Laceration without foreign body of
          right thumb without damage to nail**
    ● **S61.012 Laceration without foreign body of
          left thumb without damage to nail**
    ● **S61.019 Laceration without foreign body of
          unspecified thumb without damage to
          nail**
  ● **S61.02 Laceration with foreign body of thumb without
        damage to nail**
    ● **S61.021 Laceration with foreign body of right
          thumb without damage to nail**
    ● **S61.022 Laceration with foreign body of left
          thumb without damage to nail**
    ● **S61.029 Laceration with foreign body of
          unspecified thumb without damage to
          nail**
  ● **S61.03 Puncture wound without foreign body of
        thumb without damage to nail**
    ● **S61.031 Puncture wound without foreign
          body of right thumb without damage
          to nail**
    ● **S61.032 Puncture wound without foreign
          body of left thumb without damage to
          nail**
    ● **S61.039 Puncture wound without foreign
          body of unspecified thumb without
          damage to nail**
  ● **S61.04 Puncture wound with foreign body of thumb
        without damage to nail**
    ● **S61.041 Puncture wound with foreign body of
          right thumb without damage to nail**
    ● **S61.042 Puncture wound with foreign body of
          left thumb without damage to nail**
    ● **S61.049 Puncture wound with foreign body of
          unspecified thumb without damage to
          nail**
  ● **S61.05 Open bite of thumb without damage to nail**
      Bite of thumb NOS
    Excludes1 superficial bite of thumb
          (S60.36-, S60.37-)
    ● **S61.051 Open bite of right thumb without
          damage to nail**
    ● **S61.052 Open bite of left thumb without
          damage to nail**
    ● **S61.059 Open bite of unspecified thumb
          without damage to nail**

● **S61.1 Open wound of thumb with damage to nail**
  ● **S61.10 Unspecified open wound of thumb with
        damage to nail**
    ● **S61.101 Unspecified open wound of right
          thumb with damage to nail**
    ● **S61.102 Unspecified open wound of left
          thumb with damage to nail**
    ● **S61.109 Unspecified open wound of
          unspecified thumb with damage to
          nail**
  ● **S61.11 Laceration without foreign body of thumb with
        damage to nail**
    ● **S61.111 Laceration without foreign body of
          right thumb with damage to nail**
    ● **S61.112 Laceration without foreign body of
          left thumb with damage to nail**
    ● **S61.119 Laceration without foreign body of
          unspecified thumb with damage to
          nail**
  ● **S61.12 Laceration with foreign body of thumb with
        damage to nail**
    ● **S61.121 Laceration with foreign body of right
          thumb with damage to nail**
    ● **S61.122 Laceration with foreign body of left
          thumb with damage to nail**
    ● **S61.129 Laceration with foreign body of
          unspecified thumb with damage to
          nail**
  ● **S61.13 Puncture wound without foreign body of
        thumb with damage to nail**
    ● **S61.131 Puncture wound without foreign
          body of right thumb with damage to
          nail**
    ● **S61.132 Puncture wound without foreign
          body of left thumb with damage to
          nail**
    ● **S61.139 Puncture wound without foreign
          body of unspecified thumb with
          damage to nail**
  ● **S61.14 Puncture wound with foreign body of thumb
        with damage to nail**
    ● **S61.141 Puncture wound with foreign body of
          right thumb with damage to nail**
    ● **S61.142 Puncture wound with foreign body of
          left thumb with damage to nail**
    ● **S61.149 Puncture wound with foreign body
          of unspecified thumb with damage to
          nail**
  ● **S61.15 Open bite of thumb with damage to nail**
      Bite of thumb with damage to nail NOS
    Excludes1 superficial bite of thumb
          (S60.36-, S60.37-)
    ● **S61.151 Open bite of right thumb with
          damage to nail**
    ● **S61.152 Open bite of left thumb with damage
          to nail**
    ● **S61.159 Open bite of unspecified thumb with
          damage to nail**
● **S61.2 Open wound of other finger without damage to nail**
  Excludes1 open wound of finger involving nail
        (matrix) (S61.3-)
  Excludes2 open wound of thumb without damage
        to nail (S61.0-)
  ● **S61.20 Unspecified open wound of other finger
        without damage to nail**
    ● **S61.200 Unspecified open wound of right
          index finger without damage to nail**
    ● **S61.201 Unspecified open wound of left index
          finger without damage to nail**
    ● **S61.202 Unspecified open wound of right
          middle finger without damage to nail**

● S61.203 Unspecified open wound of left middle finger without damage to nail

● S61.204 Unspecified open wound of right ring finger without damage to nail

● S61.205 Unspecified open wound of left ring finger without damage to nail

● S61.206 Unspecified open wound of right little finger without damage to nail

● S61.207 Unspecified open wound of left little finger without damage to nail

● S61.208 Unspecified open wound of other finger without damage to nail

Unspecified open wound of specified finger with unspecified laterality without damage to nail

● S61.209 Unspecified open wound of unspecified finger without damage to nail

● S61.21 Laceration without foreign body of finger without damage to nail

● S61.210 Laceration without foreign body of right index finger without damage to nail

● S61.211 Laceration without foreign body of left index finger without damage to nail

● S61.212 Laceration without foreign body of right middle finger without damage to nail

● S61.213 Laceration without foreign body of left middle finger without damage to nail

● S61.214 Laceration without foreign body of right ring finger without damage to nail

● S61.215 Laceration without foreign body of left ring finger without damage to nail

● S61.216 Laceration without foreign body of right little finger without damage to nail

● S61.217 Laceration without foreign body of left little finger without damage to nail

● S61.218 Laceration without foreign body of other finger without damage to nail

Laceration without foreign body of specified finger with unspecified laterality without damage to nail

● S61.219 Laceration without foreign body of unspecified finger without damage to nail

● S61.22 Laceration with foreign body of finger without damage to nail

● S61.220 Laceration with foreign body of right index finger without damage to nail

● S61.221 Laceration with foreign body of left index finger without damage to nail

● S61.222 Laceration with foreign body of right middle finger without damage to nail

● S61.223 Laceration with foreign body of left middle finger without damage to nail

● S61.224 Laceration with foreign body of right ring finger without damage to nail

● S61.225 Laceration with foreign body of left ring finger without damage to nail

● S61.226 Laceration with foreign body of right little finger without damage to nail

● S61.227 Laceration with foreign body of left little finger without damage to nail

● S61.228 Laceration with foreign body of other finger without damage to nail

Laceration with foreign body of specified finger with unspecified laterality without damage to nail

● S61.229 Laceration with foreign body of unspecified finger without damage to nail

● S61.23 Puncture wound without foreign body of finger without damage to nail

● S61.230 Puncture wound without foreign body of right index finger without damage to nail

● S61.231 Puncture wound without foreign body of left index finger without damage to nail

● S61.232 Puncture wound without foreign body of right middle finger without damage to nail

● S61.233 Puncture wound without foreign body of left middle finger without damage to nail

● S61.234 Puncture wound without foreign body of right ring finger without damage to nail

● S61.235 Puncture wound without foreign body of left ring finger without damage to nail

● S61.236 Puncture wound without foreign body of right little finger without damage to nail

● S61.237 Puncture wound without foreign body of left little finger without damage to nail

● S61.238 Puncture wound without foreign body of other finger without damage to nail

Puncture wound without foreign body of specified finger with unspecified laterality without damage to nail

● S61.239 Puncture wound without foreign body of unspecified finger without damage to nail

● S61.24 Puncture wound with foreign body of finger without damage to nail

● S61.240 Puncture wound with foreign body of right index finger without damage to nail

● S61.241 Puncture wound with foreign body of left index finger without damage to nail

● S61.242 Puncture wound with foreign body of right middle finger without damage to nail

● S61.243 Puncture wound with foreign body of left middle finger without damage to nail

● S61.244 Puncture wound with foreign body of right ring finger without damage to nail

● S61.245 Puncture wound with foreign body of left ring finger without damage to nail

● S61.246 Puncture wound with foreign body of right little finger without damage to nail

● S61.247 Puncture wound with foreign body of left little finger without damage to nail

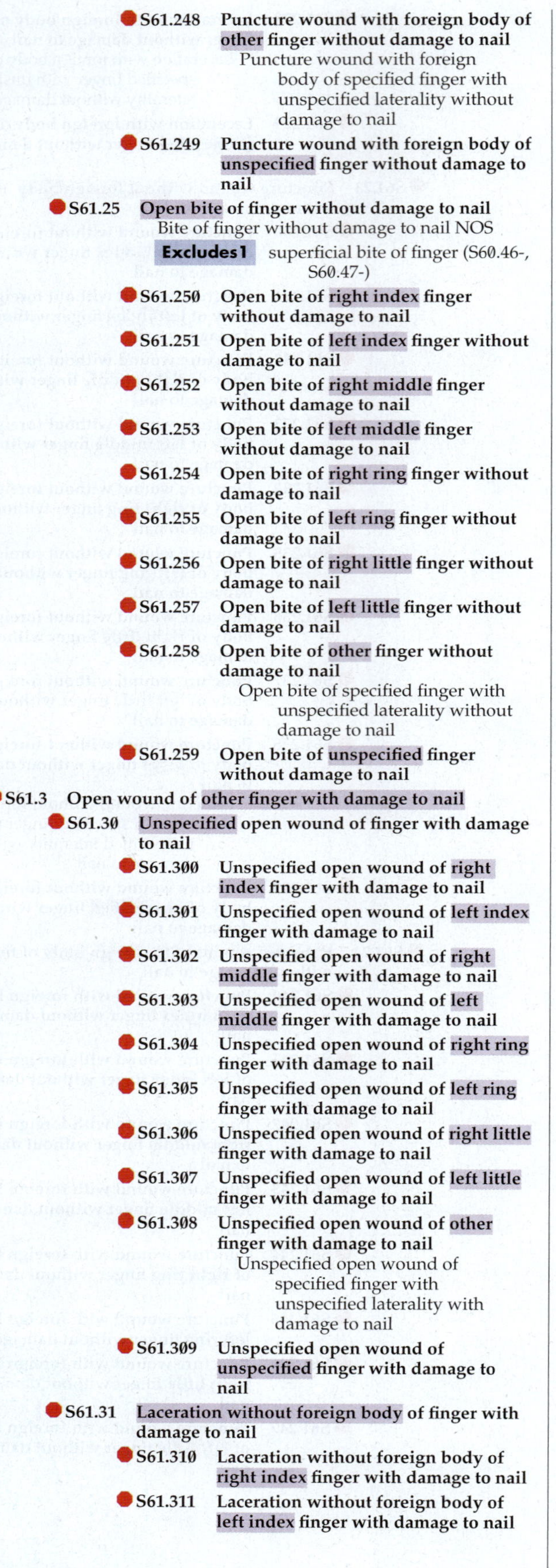

● S61.248   **Puncture wound with foreign body of other finger without damage to nail**
Puncture wound with foreign body of specified finger with unspecified laterality without damage to nail

● S61.249   **Puncture wound with foreign body of unspecified finger without damage to nail**

● S61.25   **Open bite of finger without damage to nail**
Bite of finger without damage to nail NOS

    Excludes1   superficial bite of finger (S60.46-, S60.47-)

● S61.250   **Open bite of right index finger without damage to nail**

● S61.251   **Open bite of left index finger without damage to nail**

● S61.252   **Open bite of right middle finger without damage to nail**

● S61.253   **Open bite of left middle finger without damage to nail**

● S61.254   **Open bite of right ring finger without damage to nail**

● S61.255   **Open bite of left ring finger without damage to nail**

● S61.256   **Open bite of right little finger without damage to nail**

● S61.257   **Open bite of left little finger without damage to nail**

● S61.258   **Open bite of other finger without damage to nail**
Open bite of specified finger with unspecified laterality without damage to nail

● S61.259   **Open bite of unspecified finger without damage to nail**

● S61.3   **Open wound of other finger with damage to nail**

● S61.30   **Unspecified open wound of finger with damage to nail**

● S61.300   **Unspecified open wound of right index finger with damage to nail**

● S61.301   **Unspecified open wound of left index finger with damage to nail**

● S61.302   **Unspecified open wound of right middle finger with damage to nail**

● S61.303   **Unspecified open wound of left middle finger with damage to nail**

● S61.304   **Unspecified open wound of right ring finger with damage to nail**

● S61.305   **Unspecified open wound of left ring finger with damage to nail**

● S61.306   **Unspecified open wound of right little finger with damage to nail**

● S61.307   **Unspecified open wound of left little finger with damage to nail**

● S61.308   **Unspecified open wound of other finger with damage to nail**
Unspecified open wound of specified finger with unspecified laterality with damage to nail

● S61.309   **Unspecified open wound of unspecified finger with damage to nail**

● S61.31   **Laceration without foreign body of finger with damage to nail**

● S61.310   **Laceration without foreign body of right index finger with damage to nail**

● S61.311   **Laceration without foreign body of left index finger with damage to nail**

● S61.312   **Laceration without foreign body of right middle finger with damage to nail**

● S61.313   **Laceration without foreign body of left middle finger with damage to nail**

● S61.314   **Laceration without foreign body of right ring finger with damage to nail**

● S61.315   **Laceration without foreign body of left ring finger with damage to nail**

● S61.316   **Laceration without foreign body of right little finger with damage to nail**

● S61.317   **Laceration without foreign body of left little finger with damage to nail**

● S61.318   **Laceration without foreign body of other finger with damage to nail**
Laceration without foreign body of specified finger with unspecified laterality with damage to nail

● S61.319   **Laceration without foreign body of unspecified finger with damage to nail**

● S61.32   **Laceration with foreign body of finger with damage to nail**

● S61.320   **Laceration with foreign body of right index finger with damage to nail**

● S61.321   **Laceration with foreign body of left index finger with damage to nail**

● S61.322   **Laceration with foreign body of right middle finger with damage to nail**

● S61.323   **Laceration with foreign body of left middle finger with damage to nail**

● S61.324   **Laceration with foreign body of right ring finger with damage to nail**

● S61.325   **Laceration with foreign body of left ring finger with damage to nail**

● S61.326   **Laceration with foreign body of right little finger with damage to nail**

● S61.327   **Laceration with foreign body of left little finger with damage to nail**

● S61.328   **Laceration with foreign body of other finger with damage to nail**
Laceration with foreign body of specified finger with unspecified laterality with damage to nail

● S61.329   **Laceration with foreign body of unspecified finger with damage to nail**

● S61.33   **Puncture wound without foreign body of finger with damage to nail**

● S61.330   **Puncture wound without foreign body of right index finger with damage to nail**

● S61.331   **Puncture wound without foreign body of left index finger with damage to nail**

● S61.332   **Puncture wound without foreign body of right middle finger with damage to nail**

● S61.333   **Puncture wound without foreign body of left middle finger with damage to nail**

● S61.334   **Puncture wound without foreign body of right ring finger with damage to nail**

● S61.335   **Puncture wound without foreign body of left ring finger with damage to nail**

● S61.336   **Puncture wound without foreign body of right little finger with damage to nail**

▶ New   ➡ Revised   ~~deleted~~ Deleted   Excludes 1   Excludes 2   Includes   Use additional   Code first   Code also   Key words
OGCR Official Guidelines   X Assign placeholder X   ● Use Additional Character(s)   ▶ Manifestation Code   Hierarchical Condition Category   **Coding Clinic**

- ● S61.337   Puncture wound without foreign body of left little finger with damage to nail
- ● S61.338   Puncture wound without foreign body of other finger with damage to nail
  - Puncture wound without foreign body of specified finger with unspecified laterality with damage to nail
- ● S61.339   Puncture wound without foreign body of unspecified finger with damage to nail
- ● **S61.34**   Puncture wound with foreign body of finger with damage to nail
  - ● S61.340   Puncture wound with foreign body of right index finger with damage to nail
  - ● S61.341   Puncture wound with foreign body of left index finger with damage to nail
  - ● S61.342   Puncture wound with foreign body of right middle finger with damage to nail
  - ● S61.343   Puncture wound with foreign body of left middle finger with damage to nail
  - ● S61.344   Puncture wound with foreign body of right ring finger with damage to nail
  - ● S61.345   Puncture wound with foreign body of left ring finger with damage to nail
  - ● S61.346   Puncture wound with foreign body of right little finger with damage to nail
  - ● S61.347   Puncture wound with foreign body of left little finger with damage to nail
  - ● S61.348   Puncture wound with foreign body of other finger with damage to nail
    - Puncture wound with foreign body of specified finger with unspecified laterality with damage to nail
  - ● S61.349   Puncture wound with foreign body of unspecified finger with damage to nail
- ● **S61.35**   Open bite of finger with damage to nail
  - Bite of finger with damage to nail NOS
  - **Excludes1**   superficial bite of finger (S60.46-, S60.47-)
  - ● S61.350   Open bite of right index finger with damage to nail
  - ● S61.351   Open bite of left index finger with damage to nail
  - ● S61.352   Open bite of right middle finger with damage to nail
  - ● S61.353   Open bite of left middle finger with damage to nail
  - ● S61.354   Open bite of right ring finger with damage to nail
  - ● S61.355   Open bite of left ring finger with damage to nail
  - ● S61.356   Open bite of right little finger with damage to nail
  - ● S61.357   Open bite of left little finger with damage to nail
  - ● S61.358   Open bite of other finger with damage to nail
    - Open bite of specified finger with unspecified laterality with damage to nail
  - ● S61.359   Open bite of unspecified finger with damage to nail

- ● **S61.4**   Open wound of hand
  - ● **S61.40**   Unspecified open wound of hand
    - ● S61.401   Unspecified open wound of right hand
    - ● S61.402   Unspecified open wound of left hand
    - ● S61.409   Unspecified open wound of unspecified hand
  - ● **S61.41**   Laceration without foreign body of hand
    - ● S61.411   Laceration without foreign body of right hand
    - ● S61.412   Laceration without foreign body of left hand
    - ● S61.419   Laceration without foreign body of unspecified hand
  - ● **S61.42**   Laceration with foreign body of hand
    - ● S61.421   Laceration with foreign body of right hand
    - ● S61.422   Laceration with foreign body of left hand
    - ● S61.429   Laceration with foreign body of unspecified hand
  - ● **S61.43**   Puncture wound without foreign body of hand
    - ● S61.431   Puncture wound without foreign body of right hand
    - ● S61.432   Puncture wound without foreign body of left hand
    - ● S61.439   Puncture wound without foreign body of unspecified hand
  - ● **S61.44**   Puncture wound with foreign body of hand
    - ● S61.441   Puncture wound with foreign body of right hand
    - ● S61.442   Puncture wound with foreign body of left hand
    - ● S61.449   Puncture wound with foreign body of unspecified hand
  - ● **S61.45**   Open bite of hand
    - Bite of hand NOS
    - **Excludes1**   superficial bite of hand (S60.56-, S60.57-)
    - ● S61.451   Open bite of right hand
    - ● S61.452   Open bite of left hand
    - ● S61.459   Open bite of unspecified hand
- ● **S61.5**   Open wound of wrist
  - ● **S61.50**   Unspecified open wound of wrist
    - ● S61.501   Unspecified open wound of right wrist
    - ● S61.502   Unspecified open wound of left wrist
    - ● S61.509   Unspecified open wound of unspecified wrist
  - ● **S61.51**   Laceration without foreign body of wrist
    - ● S61.511   Laceration without foreign body of right wrist
    - ● S61.512   Laceration without foreign body of left wrist
    - ● S61.519   Laceration without foreign body of unspecified wrist
  - ● **S61.52**   Laceration with foreign body of wrist
    - ● S61.521   Laceration with foreign body of right wrist
    - ● S61.522   Laceration with foreign body of left wrist
    - ● S61.529   Laceration with foreign body of unspecified wrist

CHAPTER 19 (S00–T88)

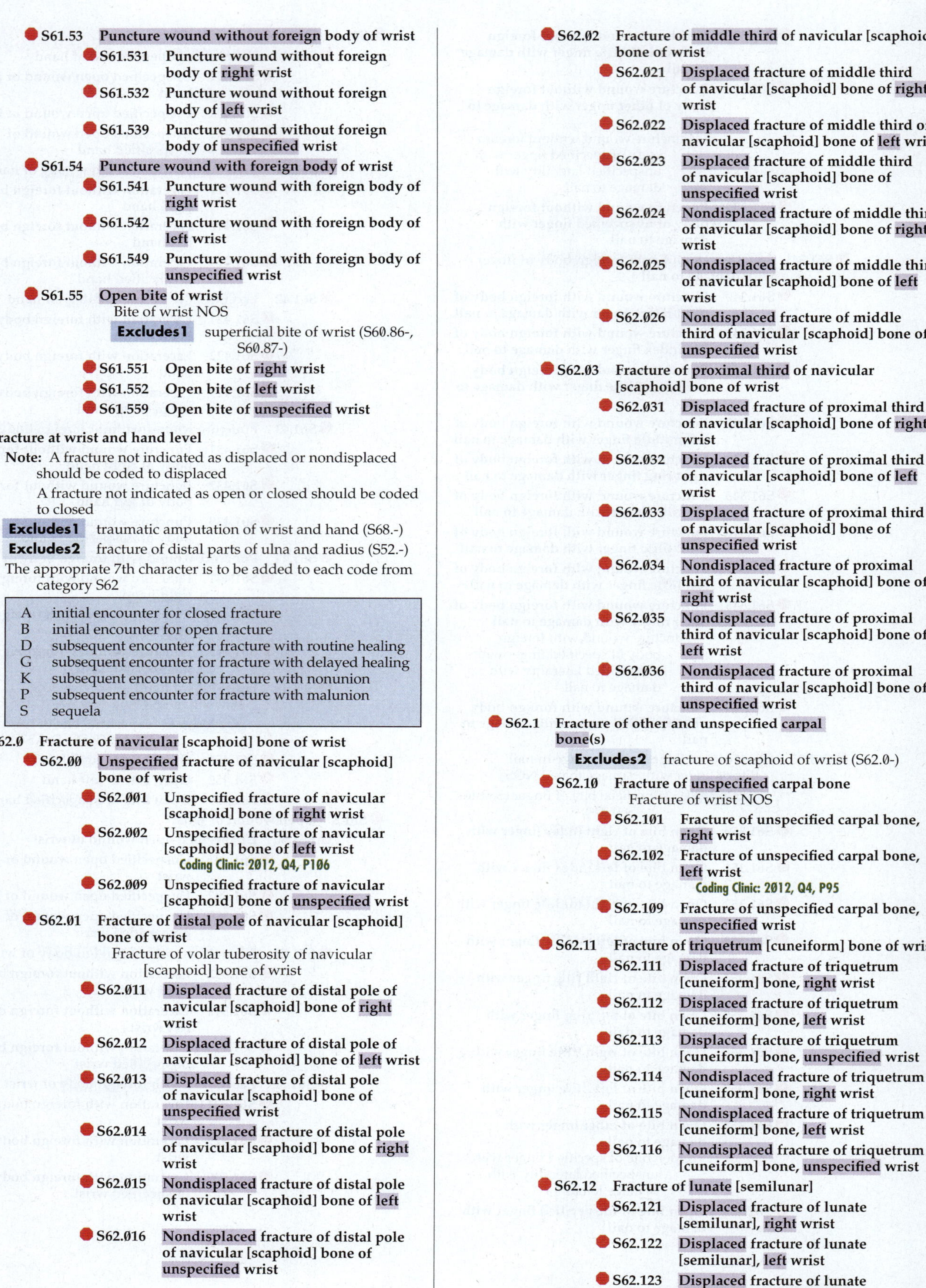

● **S61.53** Puncture wound without foreign body of wrist
  ● **S61.531** Puncture wound without foreign body of right wrist
  ● **S61.532** Puncture wound without foreign body of left wrist
  ● **S61.539** Puncture wound without foreign body of unspecified wrist
● **S61.54** Puncture wound with foreign body of wrist
  ● **S61.541** Puncture wound with foreign body of right wrist
  ● **S61.542** Puncture wound with foreign body of left wrist
  ● **S61.549** Puncture wound with foreign body of unspecified wrist
● **S61.55** Open bite of wrist
  Bite of wrist NOS
  Excludes1 superficial bite of wrist (S60.86-, S60.87-)
  ● **S61.551** Open bite of right wrist
  ● **S61.552** Open bite of left wrist
  ● **S61.559** Open bite of unspecified wrist

● **S62** Fracture at wrist and hand level
  Note: A fracture not indicated as displaced or nondisplaced should be coded to displaced
  A fracture not indicated as open or closed should be coded to closed
  Excludes1 traumatic amputation of wrist and hand (S68.-)
  Excludes2 fracture of distal parts of ulna and radius (S52.-)
  The appropriate 7th character is to be added to each code from category S62

A	initial encounter for closed fracture
B	initial encounter for open fracture
D	subsequent encounter for fracture with routine healing
G	subsequent encounter for fracture with delayed healing
K	subsequent encounter for fracture with nonunion
P	subsequent encounter for fracture with malunion
S	sequela

  ● **S62.0** Fracture of navicular [scaphoid] bone of wrist
    ● **S62.00** Unspecified fracture of navicular [scaphoid] bone of wrist
      ● **S62.001** Unspecified fracture of navicular [scaphoid] bone of right wrist
      ● **S62.002** Unspecified fracture of navicular [scaphoid] bone of left wrist
        Coding Clinic: 2012, Q4, P106
      ● **S62.009** Unspecified fracture of navicular [scaphoid] bone of unspecified wrist
    ● **S62.01** Fracture of distal pole of navicular [scaphoid] bone of wrist
      Fracture of volar tuberosity of navicular [scaphoid] bone of wrist
      ● **S62.011** Displaced fracture of distal pole of navicular [scaphoid] bone of right wrist
      ● **S62.012** Displaced fracture of distal pole of navicular [scaphoid] bone of left wrist
      ● **S62.013** Displaced fracture of distal pole of navicular [scaphoid] bone of unspecified wrist
      ● **S62.014** Nondisplaced fracture of distal pole of navicular [scaphoid] bone of right wrist
      ● **S62.015** Nondisplaced fracture of distal pole of navicular [scaphoid] bone of left wrist
      ● **S62.016** Nondisplaced fracture of distal pole of navicular [scaphoid] bone of unspecified wrist

● **S62.02** Fracture of middle third of navicular [scaphoid] bone of wrist
  ● **S62.021** Displaced fracture of middle third of navicular [scaphoid] bone of right wrist
  ● **S62.022** Displaced fracture of middle third of navicular [scaphoid] bone of left wrist
  ● **S62.023** Displaced fracture of middle third of navicular [scaphoid] bone of unspecified wrist
  ● **S62.024** Nondisplaced fracture of middle third of navicular [scaphoid] bone of right wrist
  ● **S62.025** Nondisplaced fracture of middle third of navicular [scaphoid] bone of left wrist
  ● **S62.026** Nondisplaced fracture of middle third of navicular [scaphoid] bone of unspecified wrist
● **S62.03** Fracture of proximal third of navicular [scaphoid] bone of wrist
  ● **S62.031** Displaced fracture of proximal third of navicular [scaphoid] bone of right wrist
  ● **S62.032** Displaced fracture of proximal third of navicular [scaphoid] bone of left wrist
  ● **S62.033** Displaced fracture of proximal third of navicular [scaphoid] bone of unspecified wrist
  ● **S62.034** Nondisplaced fracture of proximal third of navicular [scaphoid] bone of right wrist
  ● **S62.035** Nondisplaced fracture of proximal third of navicular [scaphoid] bone of left wrist
  ● **S62.036** Nondisplaced fracture of proximal third of navicular [scaphoid] bone of unspecified wrist
● **S62.1** Fracture of other and unspecified carpal bone(s)
  Excludes2 fracture of scaphoid of wrist (S62.0-)
  ● **S62.10** Fracture of unspecified carpal bone
    Fracture of wrist NOS
    ● **S62.101** Fracture of unspecified carpal bone, right wrist
    ● **S62.102** Fracture of unspecified carpal bone, left wrist
      Coding Clinic: 2012, Q4, P95
    ● **S62.109** Fracture of unspecified carpal bone, unspecified wrist
  ● **S62.11** Fracture of triquetrum [cuneiform] bone of wrist
    ● **S62.111** Displaced fracture of triquetrum [cuneiform] bone, right wrist
    ● **S62.112** Displaced fracture of triquetrum [cuneiform] bone, left wrist
    ● **S62.113** Displaced fracture of triquetrum [cuneiform] bone, unspecified wrist
    ● **S62.114** Nondisplaced fracture of triquetrum [cuneiform] bone, right wrist
    ● **S62.115** Nondisplaced fracture of triquetrum [cuneiform] bone, left wrist
    ● **S62.116** Nondisplaced fracture of triquetrum [cuneiform] bone, unspecified wrist
  ● **S62.12** Fracture of lunate [semilunar]
    ● **S62.121** Displaced fracture of lunate [semilunar], right wrist
    ● **S62.122** Displaced fracture of lunate [semilunar], left wrist
    ● **S62.123** Displaced fracture of lunate [semilunar], unspecified wrist

- ● **S62.124** Nondisplaced fracture of lunate [semilunar], **right** wrist
- ● **S62.125** Nondisplaced fracture of lunate [semilunar], **left** wrist
- ● **S62.126** Nondisplaced fracture of lunate [semilunar], **unspecified** wrist
- ● **S62.13** Fracture of capitate [os magnum] bone
  - ● **S62.131** Displaced fracture of capitate [os magnum] bone, **right** wrist
  - ● **S62.132** Displaced fracture of capitate [os magnum] bone, **left** wrist
  - ● **S62.133** Displaced fracture of capitate [os magnum] bone, **unspecified** wrist
  - ● **S62.134** Nondisplaced fracture of capitate [os magnum] bone, **right** wrist
  - ● **S62.135** Nondisplaced fracture of capitate [os magnum] bone, **left** wrist
  - ● **S62.136** Nondisplaced fracture of capitate [os magnum] bone, **unspecified** wrist
- ● **S62.14** Fracture of body of hamate [unciform] bone
  Fracture of hamate [unciform] bone NOS
  - ● **S62.141** Displaced fracture of body of hamate [unciform] bone, **right** wrist
  - ● **S62.142** Displaced fracture of body of hamate [unciform] bone, **left** wrist
  - ● **S62.143** Displaced fracture of body of hamate [unciform] bone, **unspecified** wrist
  - ● **S62.144** Nondisplaced fracture of body of hamate [unciform] bone, **right** wrist
  - ● **S62.145** Nondisplaced fracture of body of hamate [unciform] bone, **left** wrist
  - ● **S62.146** Nondisplaced fracture of body of hamate [unciform] bone, **unspecified** wrist
- ● **S62.15** Fracture of hook process of hamate [unciform] bone
  Fracture of unciform process of hamate [unciform] bone
  - ● **S62.151** Displaced fracture of hook process of hamate [unciform] bone, **right** wrist
  - ● **S62.152** Displaced fracture of hook process of hamate [unciform] bone, **left** wrist
  - ● **S62.153** Displaced fracture of hook process of hamate [unciform] bone, **unspecified** wrist
  - ● **S62.154** Nondisplaced fracture of hook process of hamate [unciform] bone, **right** wrist
  - ● **S62.155** Nondisplaced fracture of hook process of hamate [unciform] bone, **left** wrist
  - ● **S62.156** Nondisplaced fracture of hook process of hamate [unciform] bone, **unspecified** wrist
- ● **S62.16** Fracture of pisiform
  - ● **S62.161** Displaced fracture of pisiform, **right** wrist
  - ● **S62.162** Displaced fracture of pisiform, **left** wrist
  - ● **S62.163** Displaced fracture of pisiform, **unspecified** wrist
  - ● **S62.164** Nondisplaced fracture of pisiform, **right** wrist
  - ● **S62.165** Nondisplaced fracture of pisiform, **left** wrist
  - ● **S62.166** Nondisplaced fracture of pisiform, **unspecified** wrist
- ● **S62.17** Fracture of trapezium [larger multangular]
  - ● **S62.171** Displaced fracture of trapezium [larger multangular], **right** wrist
  - ● **S62.172** Displaced fracture of trapezium [larger multangular], **left** wrist
- ● **S62.173** Displaced fracture of trapezium [larger multangular], **unspecified** wrist
- ● **S62.174** Nondisplaced fracture of trapezium [larger multangular], **right** wrist
- ● **S62.175** Nondisplaced fracture of trapezium [larger multangular], **left** wrist
- ● **S62.176** Nondisplaced fracture of trapezium [larger multangular], **unspecified** wrist
- ● **S62.18** Fracture of trapezoid [smaller multangular]
  - ● **S62.181** Displaced fracture of trapezoid [smaller multangular], **right** wrist
  - ● **S62.182** Displaced fracture of trapezoid [smaller multangular], **left** wrist
  - ● **S62.183** Displaced fracture of trapezoid [smaller multangular], **unspecified** wrist
  - ● **S62.184** Nondisplaced fracture of trapezoid [smaller multangular], **right** wrist
  - ● **S62.185** Nondisplaced fracture of trapezoid [smaller multangular], **left** wrist
  - ● **S62.186** Nondisplaced fracture of trapezoid [smaller multangular], **unspecified** wrist
- ● **S62.2** Fracture of first metacarpal bone
  - ● **S62.20** Unspecified fracture of first metacarpal bone
    - ● **S62.201** Unspecified fracture of first metacarpal bone, **right** hand
    - ● **S62.202** Unspecified fracture of first metacarpal bone, **left** hand
    - ● **S62.209** Unspecified fracture of first metacarpal bone, **unspecified** hand
  - ● **S62.21** Bennett's fracture
    - ● **S62.211** Bennett's fracture, **right** hand
    - ● **S62.212** Bennett's fracture, **left** hand
    - ● **S62.213** Bennett's fracture, **unspecified** hand
  - ● **S62.22** Rolando's fracture
    - ● **S62.221** Displaced Rolando's fracture, **right** hand
    - ● **S62.222** Displaced Rolando's fracture, **left** hand
    - ● **S62.223** Displaced Rolando's fracture, **unspecified** hand
    - ● **S62.224** Nondisplaced Rolando's fracture, **right** hand
    - ● **S62.225** Nondisplaced Rolando's fracture, **left** hand
    - ● **S62.226** Nondisplaced Rolando's fracture, **unspecified** hand
  - ● **S62.23** Other fracture of base of first metacarpal bone
    - ● **S62.231** Other displaced fracture of base of first metacarpal bone, **right** hand
    - ● **S62.232** Other displaced fracture of base of first metacarpal bone, **left** hand
    - ● **S62.233** Other displaced fracture of base of first metacarpal bone, **unspecified** hand
    - ● **S62.234** Other nondisplaced fracture of base of first metacarpal bone, **right** hand
    - ● **S62.235** Other nondisplaced fracture of base of first metacarpal bone, **left** hand
    - ● **S62.236** Other nondisplaced fracture of base of first metacarpal bone, **unspecified** hand
  - ● **S62.24** Fracture of shaft of first metacarpal bone
    - ● **S62.241** Displaced fracture of shaft of first metacarpal bone, **right** hand
    - ● **S62.242** Displaced fracture of shaft of first metacarpal bone, **left** hand

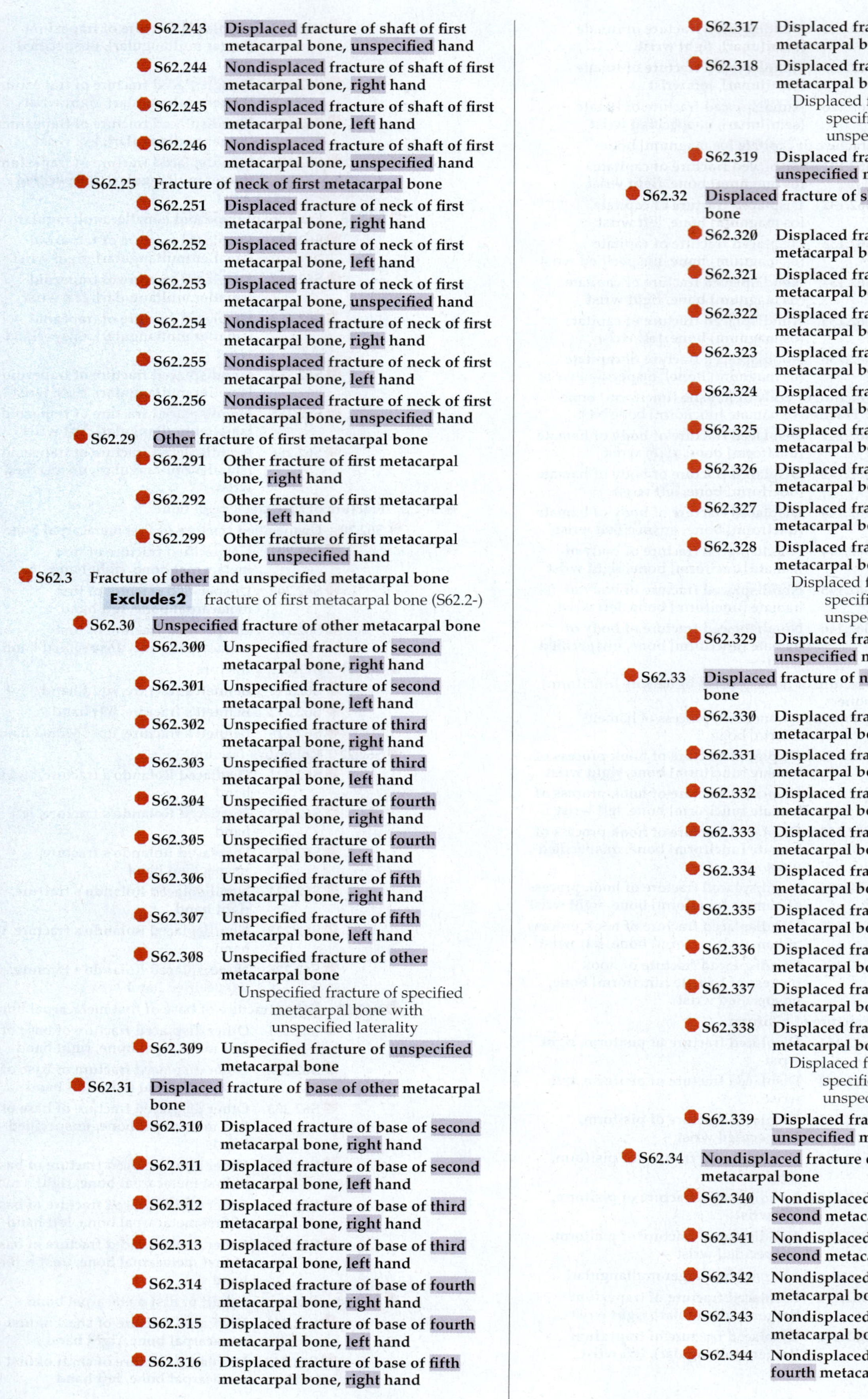

CHAPTER 19 (S00–T88)

● S62.243   **Displaced** fracture of shaft of first metacarpal bone, **unspecified** hand

● S62.244   **Nondisplaced** fracture of shaft of first metacarpal bone, right hand

● S62.245   **Nondisplaced** fracture of shaft of first metacarpal bone, left hand

● S62.246   **Nondisplaced** fracture of shaft of first metacarpal bone, **unspecified** hand

● S62.25   Fracture of neck of first metacarpal bone

● S62.251   **Displaced** fracture of neck of first metacarpal bone, right hand

● S62.252   **Displaced** fracture of neck of first metacarpal bone, left hand

● S62.253   **Displaced** fracture of neck of first metacarpal bone, **unspecified** hand

● S62.254   **Nondisplaced** fracture of neck of first metacarpal bone, right hand

● S62.255   **Nondisplaced** fracture of neck of first metacarpal bone, left hand

● S62.256   **Nondisplaced** fracture of neck of first metacarpal bone, **unspecified** hand

● S62.29   Other fracture of first metacarpal bone

● S62.291   Other fracture of first metacarpal bone, right hand

● S62.292   Other fracture of first metacarpal bone, left hand

● S62.299   Other fracture of first metacarpal bone, unspecified hand

● S62.3   Fracture of other and unspecified metacarpal bone

   Excludes2   fracture of first metacarpal bone (S62.2-)

● S62.30   Unspecified fracture of other metacarpal bone

● S62.300   Unspecified fracture of second metacarpal bone, right hand

● S62.301   Unspecified fracture of second metacarpal bone, left hand

● S62.302   Unspecified fracture of third metacarpal bone, right hand

● S62.303   Unspecified fracture of third metacarpal bone, left hand

● S62.304   Unspecified fracture of fourth metacarpal bone, right hand

● S62.305   Unspecified fracture of fourth metacarpal bone, left hand

● S62.306   Unspecified fracture of fifth metacarpal bone, right hand

● S62.307   Unspecified fracture of fifth metacarpal bone, left hand

● S62.308   Unspecified fracture of other metacarpal bone

   Unspecified fracture of specified metacarpal bone with unspecified laterality

● S62.309   Unspecified fracture of unspecified metacarpal bone

● S62.31   **Displaced** fracture of base of other metacarpal bone

● S62.310   Displaced fracture of base of second metacarpal bone, right hand

● S62.311   Displaced fracture of base of second metacarpal bone, left hand

● S62.312   Displaced fracture of base of third metacarpal bone, right hand

● S62.313   Displaced fracture of base of third metacarpal bone, left hand

● S62.314   Displaced fracture of base of fourth metacarpal bone, right hand

● S62.315   Displaced fracture of base of fourth metacarpal bone, left hand

● S62.316   Displaced fracture of base of fifth metacarpal bone, right hand

● S62.317   Displaced fracture of base of fifth metacarpal bone, left hand

● S62.318   Displaced fracture of base of other metacarpal bone

   Displaced fracture of base of specified metacarpal bone with unspecified laterality

● S62.319   Displaced fracture of base of unspecified metacarpal bone

● S62.32   **Displaced** fracture of shaft of other metacarpal bone

● S62.320   Displaced fracture of shaft of second metacarpal bone, right hand

● S62.321   Displaced fracture of shaft of second metacarpal bone, left hand

● S62.322   Displaced fracture of shaft of third metacarpal bone, right hand

● S62.323   Displaced fracture of shaft of third metacarpal bone, left hand

● S62.324   Displaced fracture of shaft of fourth metacarpal bone, right hand

● S62.325   Displaced fracture of shaft of fourth metacarpal bone, left hand

● S62.326   Displaced fracture of shaft of fifth metacarpal bone, right hand

● S62.327   Displaced fracture of shaft of fifth metacarpal bone, left hand

● S62.328   Displaced fracture of shaft of other metacarpal bone

   Displaced fracture of shaft of specified metacarpal bone with unspecified laterality

● S62.329   Displaced fracture of shaft of unspecified metacarpal bone

● S62.33   **Displaced** fracture of neck of other metacarpal bone

● S62.330   Displaced fracture of neck of second metacarpal bone, right hand

● S62.331   Displaced fracture of neck of second metacarpal bone, left hand

● S62.332   Displaced fracture of neck of third metacarpal bone, right hand

● S62.333   Displaced fracture of neck of third metacarpal bone, left hand

● S62.334   Displaced fracture of neck of fourth metacarpal bone, right hand

● S62.335   Displaced fracture of neck of fourth metacarpal bone, left hand

● S62.336   Displaced fracture of neck of fifth metacarpal bone, right hand

● S62.337   Displaced fracture of neck of fifth metacarpal bone, left hand

● S62.338   Displaced fracture of neck of other metacarpal bone

   Displaced fracture of neck of specified metacarpal bone with unspecified laterality

● S62.339   Displaced fracture of neck of unspecified metacarpal bone

● S62.34   **Nondisplaced** fracture of base of other metacarpal bone

● S62.340   Nondisplaced fracture of base of second metacarpal bone, right hand

● S62.341   Nondisplaced fracture of base of second metacarpal bone, left hand

● S62.342   Nondisplaced fracture of base of third metacarpal bone, right hand

● S62.343   Nondisplaced fracture of base of third metacarpal bone, left hand

● S62.344   Nondisplaced fracture of base of fourth metacarpal bone, right hand

● **S62.345** Nondisplaced fracture of base of fourth metacarpal bone, left hand

● **S62.346** Nondisplaced fracture of base of fifth metacarpal bone, right hand

● **S62.347** Nondisplaced fracture of base of fifth metacarpal bone, left hand

● **S62.348** Nondisplaced fracture of base of other metacarpal bone
Nondisplaced fracture of base of specified metacarpal bone with unspecified laterality

● **S62.349** Nondisplaced fracture of base of unspecified metacarpal bone

● **S62.35** Nondisplaced fracture of shaft of other metacarpal bone

● **S62.350** Nondisplaced fracture of shaft of second metacarpal bone, right hand

● **S62.351** Nondisplaced fracture of shaft of second metacarpal bone, left hand

● **S62.352** Nondisplaced fracture of shaft of third metacarpal bone, right hand

● **S62.353** Nondisplaced fracture of shaft of third metacarpal bone, left hand

● **S62.354** Nondisplaced fracture of shaft of fourth metacarpal bone, right hand

● **S62.355** Nondisplaced fracture of shaft of fourth metacarpal bone, left hand

● **S62.356** Nondisplaced fracture of shaft of fifth metacarpal bone, right hand

● **S62.357** Nondisplaced fracture of shaft of fifth metacarpal bone, left hand

● **S62.358** Nondisplaced fracture of shaft of other metacarpal bone
Nondisplaced fracture of shaft of specified metacarpal bone with unspecified laterality

● **S62.359** Nondisplaced fracture of shaft of unspecified metacarpal bone

● **S62.36** Nondisplaced fracture of neck of other metacarpal bone

● **S62.360** Nondisplaced fracture of neck of second metacarpal bone, right hand

● **S62.361** Nondisplaced fracture of neck of second metacarpal bone, left hand

● **S62.362** Nondisplaced fracture of neck of third metacarpal bone, right hand

● **S62.363** Nondisplaced fracture of neck of third metacarpal bone, left hand

● **S62.364** Nondisplaced fracture of neck of fourth metacarpal bone, right hand

● **S62.365** Nondisplaced fracture of neck of fourth metacarpal bone, left hand

● **S62.366** Nondisplaced fracture of neck of fifth metacarpal bone, right hand

● **S62.367** Nondisplaced fracture of neck of fifth metacarpal bone, left hand

● **S62.368** Nondisplaced fracture of neck of other metacarpal bone
Nondisplaced fracture of neck of specified metacarpal bone with unspecified laterality

● **S62.369** Nondisplaced fracture of neck of unspecified metacarpal bone

● **S62.39** Other fracture of other metacarpal bone

● **S62.390** Other fracture of second metacarpal bone, right hand

● **S62.391** Other fracture of second metacarpal bone, left hand

● **S62.392** Other fracture of third metacarpal bone, right hand

● **S62.393** Other fracture of third metacarpal bone, left hand

● **S62.394** Other fracture of fourth metacarpal bone, right hand

● **S62.395** Other fracture of fourth metacarpal bone, left hand

● **S62.396** Other fracture of fifth metacarpal bone, right hand

● **S62.397** Other fracture of fifth metacarpal bone, left hand

● **S62.398** Other fracture of other metacarpal bone
Other fracture of specified metacarpal bone with unspecified laterality

● **S62.399** Other fracture of unspecified metacarpal bone

● **S62.5** Fracture of thumb

● **S62.50** Fracture of unspecified phalanx of thumb

● **S62.501** Fracture of unspecified phalanx of right thumb

● **S62.502** Fracture of unspecified phalanx of left thumb

● **S62.509** Fracture of unspecified phalanx of unspecified thumb

● **S62.51** Fracture of proximal phalanx of thumb

● **S62.511** Displaced fracture of proximal phalanx of right thumb

● **S62.512** Displaced fracture of proximal phalanx of left thumb

● **S62.513** Displaced fracture of proximal phalanx of unspecified thumb

● **S62.514** Nondisplaced fracture of proximal phalanx of right thumb

● **S62.515** Nondisplaced fracture of proximal phalanx of left thumb

● **S62.516** Nondisplaced fracture of proximal phalanx of unspecified thumb

● **S62.52** Fracture of distal phalanx of thumb

● **S62.521** Displaced fracture of distal phalanx of right thumb

● **S62.522** Displaced fracture of distal phalanx of left thumb

● **S62.523** Displaced fracture of distal phalanx of unspecified thumb

● **S62.524** Nondisplaced fracture of distal phalanx of right thumb

● **S62.525** Nondisplaced fracture of distal phalanx of left thumb

● **S62.526** Nondisplaced fracture of distal phalanx of unspecified thumb

● **S62.6** Fracture of other and unspecified finger(s)

Excludes2 fracture of thumb (S62.5-)

● **S62.60** Fracture of unspecified phalanx of finger

● **S62.600** Fracture of unspecified phalanx of right index finger

● **S62.601** Fracture of unspecified phalanx of left index finger

● **S62.602** Fracture of unspecified phalanx of right middle finger

● **S62.603** Fracture of unspecified phalanx of left middle finger

● **S62.604** Fracture of unspecified phalanx of right ring finger

● **S62.605** Fracture of unspecified phalanx of left ring finger

● **S62.606** Fracture of unspecified phalanx of right little finger

● **S62.607** Fracture of unspecified phalanx of left little finger

CHAPTER 19 (S00-T88)

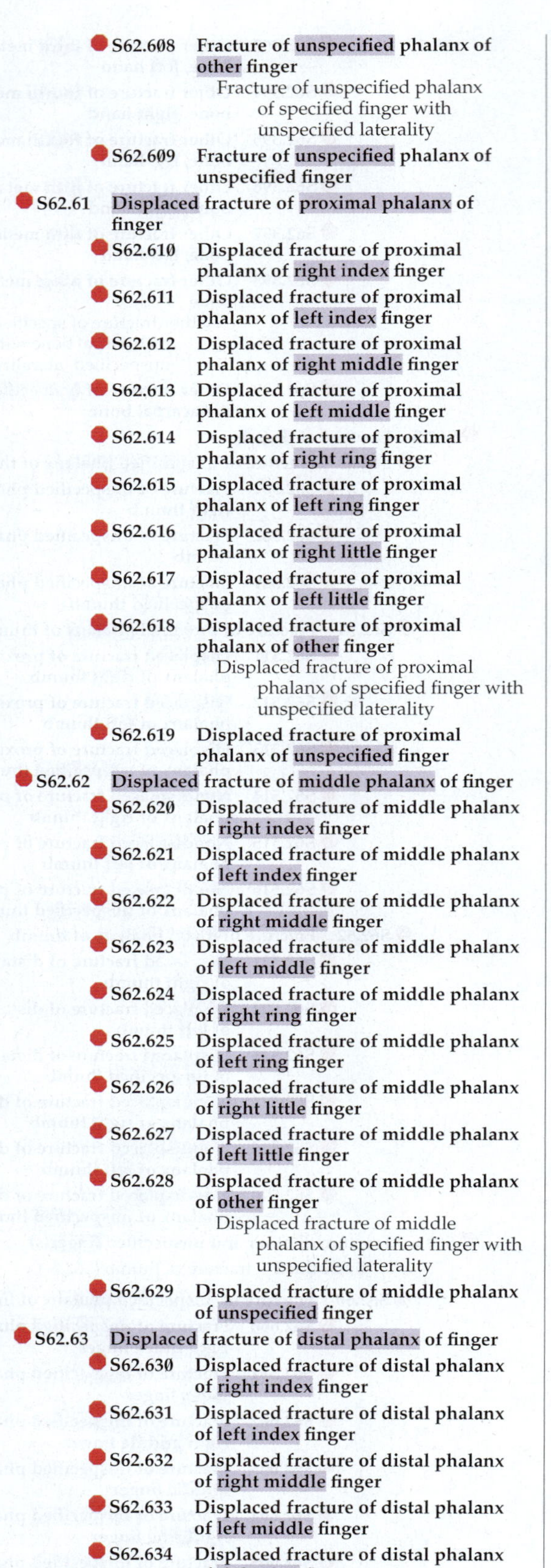

- S62.608   Fracture of unspecified phalanx of other finger
  - Fracture of unspecified phalanx of specified finger with unspecified laterality
- S62.609   Fracture of unspecified phalanx of unspecified finger
- S62.61   Displaced fracture of proximal phalanx of finger
  - S62.610   Displaced fracture of proximal phalanx of right index finger
  - S62.611   Displaced fracture of proximal phalanx of left index finger
  - S62.612   Displaced fracture of proximal phalanx of right middle finger
  - S62.613   Displaced fracture of proximal phalanx of left middle finger
  - S62.614   Displaced fracture of proximal phalanx of right ring finger
  - S62.615   Displaced fracture of proximal phalanx of left ring finger
  - S62.616   Displaced fracture of proximal phalanx of right little finger
  - S62.617   Displaced fracture of proximal phalanx of left little finger
  - S62.618   Displaced fracture of proximal phalanx of other finger
    - Displaced fracture of proximal phalanx of specified finger with unspecified laterality
  - S62.619   Displaced fracture of proximal phalanx of unspecified finger
- S62.62   Displaced fracture of middle phalanx of finger
  - S62.620   Displaced fracture of middle phalanx of right index finger
  - S62.621   Displaced fracture of middle phalanx of left index finger
  - S62.622   Displaced fracture of middle phalanx of right middle finger
  - S62.623   Displaced fracture of middle phalanx of left middle finger
  - S62.624   Displaced fracture of middle phalanx of right ring finger
  - S62.625   Displaced fracture of middle phalanx of left ring finger
  - S62.626   Displaced fracture of middle phalanx of right little finger
  - S62.627   Displaced fracture of middle phalanx of left little finger
  - S62.628   Displaced fracture of middle phalanx of other finger
    - Displaced fracture of middle phalanx of specified finger with unspecified laterality
  - S62.629   Displaced fracture of middle phalanx of unspecified finger
- S62.63   Displaced fracture of distal phalanx of finger
  - S62.630   Displaced fracture of distal phalanx of right index finger
  - S62.631   Displaced fracture of distal phalanx of left index finger
  - S62.632   Displaced fracture of distal phalanx of right middle finger
  - S62.633   Displaced fracture of distal phalanx of left middle finger
  - S62.634   Displaced fracture of distal phalanx of right ring finger
  - S62.635   Displaced fracture of distal phalanx of left ring finger
  - S62.636   Displaced fracture of distal phalanx of right little finger

- S62.637   Displaced fracture of distal phalanx of left little finger
- S62.638   Displaced fracture of distal phalanx of other finger
  - Displaced fracture of distal phalanx of specified finger with unspecified laterality
- S62.639   Displaced fracture of distal phalanx of unspecified finger
- S62.64   Nondisplaced fracture of proximal phalanx of finger
  - S62.640   Nondisplaced fracture of proximal phalanx of right index finger
  - S62.641   Nondisplaced fracture of proximal phalanx of left index finger
  - S62.642   Nondisplaced fracture of proximal phalanx of right middle finger
  - S62.643   Nondisplaced fracture of proximal phalanx of left middle finger
  - S62.644   Nondisplaced fracture of proximal phalanx of right ring finger
  - S62.645   Nondisplaced fracture of proximal phalanx of left ring finger
  - S62.646   Nondisplaced fracture of proximal phalanx of right little finger
  - S62.647   Nondisplaced fracture of proximal phalanx of left little finger
  - S62.648   Nondisplaced fracture of proximal phalanx of other finger
    - Nondisplaced fracture of proximal phalanx of specified finger with unspecified laterality
  - S62.649   Nondisplaced fracture of proximal phalanx of unspecified finger
- S62.65   Nondisplaced fracture of middle phalanx of finger
  - S62.650   Nondisplaced fracture of middle phalanx of right index finger
  - S62.651   Nondisplaced fracture of middle phalanx of left index finger
  - S62.652   Nondisplaced fracture of middle phalanx of right middle finger
  - S62.653   Nondisplaced fracture of middle phalanx of left middle finger

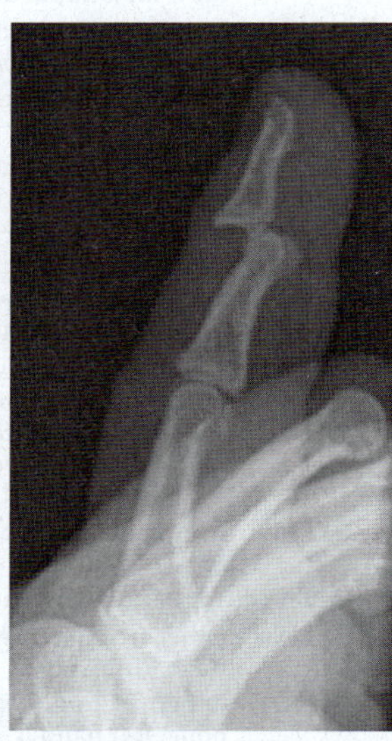

Figure 19-14   Dorsal dislocation of the distal phalanx of the index finger. (From Hardy M, Snaith B: Musculoskeletal Trauma: A Guide to Assessment and Diagnosis, 1e, Elsevier, 2011)

- **S62.654**   Nondisplaced fracture of middle phalanx of right ring finger
- **S62.655**   Nondisplaced fracture of middle phalanx of left ring finger
- **S62.656**   Nondisplaced fracture of middle phalanx of right little finger
- **S62.657**   Nondisplaced fracture of middle phalanx of left little finger
- **S62.658**   Nondisplaced fracture of middle phalanx of other finger
  - Nondisplaced fracture of middle phalanx of specified finger with unspecified laterality
- **S62.659**   Nondisplaced fracture of middle phalanx of unspecified finger
- **S62.66**   Nondisplaced fracture of distal phalanx of finger
  - **S62.660**   Nondisplaced fracture of distal phalanx of right index finger
  - **S62.661**   Nondisplaced fracture of distal phalanx of left index finger
  - **S62.662**   Nondisplaced fracture of distal phalanx of right middle finger
  - **S62.663**   Nondisplaced fracture of distal phalanx of left middle finger
  - **S62.664**   Nondisplaced fracture of distal phalanx of right ring finger
  - **S62.665**   Nondisplaced fracture of distal phalanx of left ring finger
  - **S62.666**   Nondisplaced fracture of distal phalanx of right little finger
  - **S62.667**   Nondisplaced fracture of distal phalanx of left little finger
  - **S62.668**   Nondisplaced fracture of distal phalanx of other finger
    - Nondisplaced fracture of distal phalanx of specified finger with unspecified laterality
  - **S62.669**   Nondisplaced fracture of distal phalanx of unspecified finger
- **S62.9**   Unspecified fracture of hand
  - **X** **S62.90**   Unspecified fracture of unspecified hand
  - **X** **S62.91**   Unspecified fracture of right hand
  - **X** **S62.92**   Unspecified fracture of left hand

- **S63**   **Dislocation and sprain of joints and ligaments at wrist and hand level**

  Includes   avulsion of joint or ligament at wrist and hand level

  laceration of cartilage, joint or ligament at wrist and hand level

  sprain of cartilage, joint or ligament at wrist and hand level

  traumatic hemarthrosis of joint or ligament at wrist and hand level

  traumatic rupture of joint or ligament at wrist and hand level

  traumatic subluxation of joint or ligament at wrist and hand level

  traumatic tear of joint or ligament at wrist and hand level

  Code also any associated open wound

  Excludes2   strain of muscle, fascia and tendon of wrist and hand (S66.-)

  The appropriate 7th character is to be added to each code from category S63

A	initial encounter
D	subsequent encounter
S	sequela

- **S63.0**   Subluxation and dislocation of wrist and hand joints
  - **S63.00**   Unspecified subluxation and dislocation of wrist and hand
    - Dislocation of carpal bone NOS
    - Dislocation of distal end of radius NOS
    - Subluxation of carpal bone NOS
    - Subluxation of distal end of radius NOS
    - **S63.001**   Unspecified subluxation of right wrist and hand
    - **S63.002**   Unspecified subluxation of left wrist and hand
    - **S63.003**   Unspecified subluxation of unspecified wrist and hand
    - **S63.004**   Unspecified dislocation of right wrist and hand
    - **S63.005**   Unspecified dislocation of left wrist and hand
    - **S63.006**   Unspecified dislocation of unspecified wrist and hand
  - **S63.01**   Subluxation and dislocation of distal radioulnar joint
    - **S63.011**   Subluxation of distal radioulnar joint of right wrist
    - **S63.012**   Subluxation of distal radioulnar joint of left wrist
    - **S63.013**   Subluxation of distal radioulnar joint of unspecified wrist
    - **S63.014**   Dislocation of distal radioulnar joint of right wrist
    - **S63.015**   Dislocation of distal radioulnar joint of left wrist
    - **S63.016**   Dislocation of distal radioulnar joint of unspecified wrist
  - **S63.02**   Subluxation and dislocation of radiocarpal joint
    - **S63.021**   Subluxation of radiocarpal joint of right wrist
    - **S63.022**   Subluxation of radiocarpal joint of left wrist
    - **S63.023**   Subluxation of radiocarpal joint of unspecified wrist
    - **S63.024**   Dislocation of radiocarpal joint of right wrist
    - **S63.025**   Dislocation of radiocarpal joint of left wrist
    - **S63.026**   Dislocation of radiocarpal joint of unspecified wrist
  - **S63.03**   Subluxation and dislocation of midcarpal joint
    - **S63.031**   Subluxation of midcarpal joint of right wrist
    - **S63.032**   Subluxation of midcarpal joint of left wrist
    - **S63.033**   Subluxation of midcarpal joint of unspecified wrist
    - **S63.034**   Dislocation of midcarpal joint of right wrist
    - **S63.035**   Dislocation of midcarpal joint of left wrist
    - **S63.036**   Dislocation of midcarpal joint of unspecified wrist
  - **S63.04**   Subluxation and dislocation of carpometacarpal joint of thumb

    Excludes2   interphalangeal subluxation and dislocation of thumb (S63.1-)

    - **S63.041**   Subluxation of carpometacarpal joint of right thumb
    - **S63.042**   Subluxation of carpometacarpal joint of left thumb
    - **S63.043**   Subluxation of carpometacarpal joint of unspecified thumb

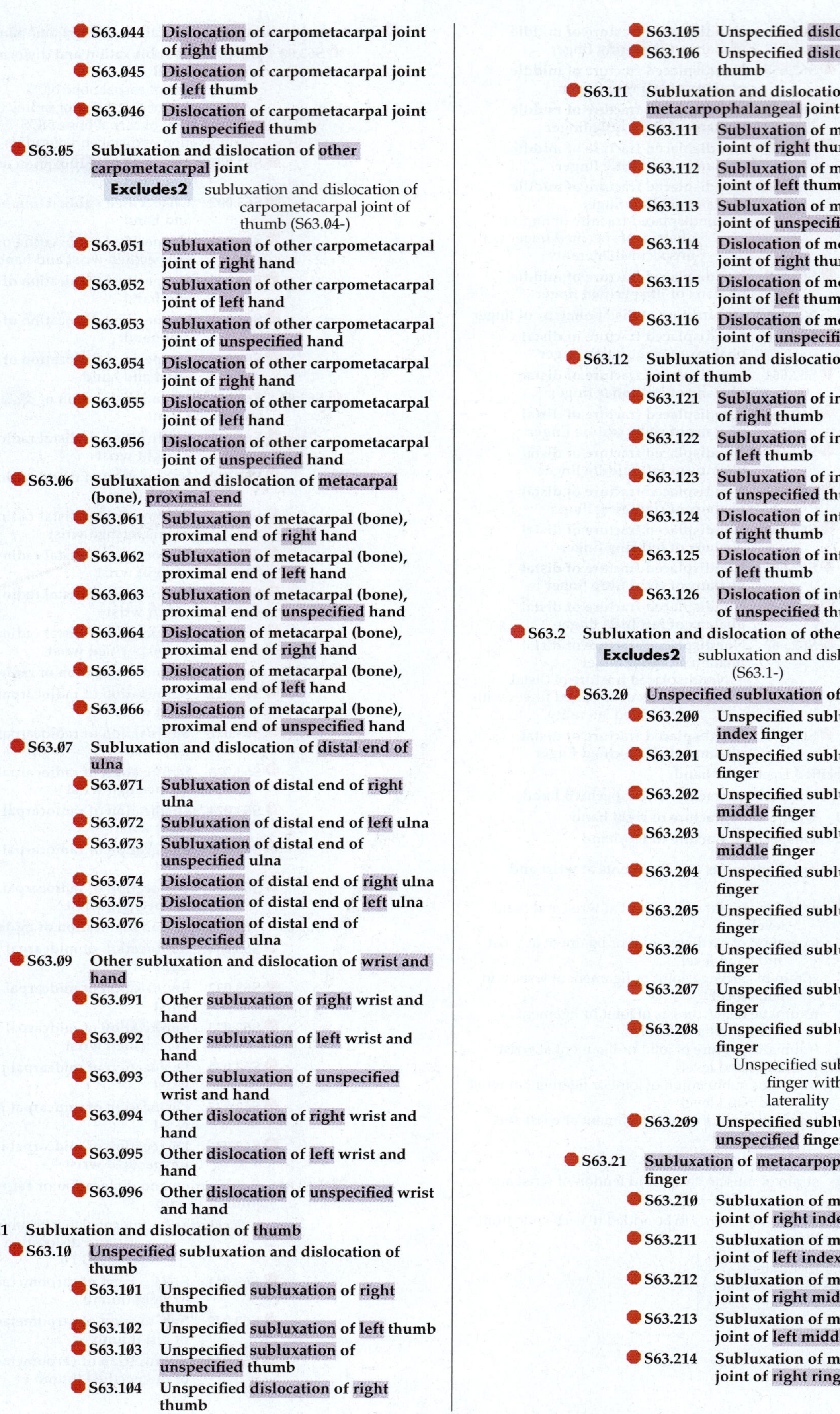

● S63.044 **Dislocation of carpometacarpal joint of right thumb**

● S63.045 **Dislocation of carpometacarpal joint of left thumb**

● S63.046 **Dislocation of carpometacarpal joint of unspecified thumb**

● S63.05 **Subluxation and dislocation of other carpometacarpal joint**

> **Excludes2** subluxation and dislocation of carpometacarpal joint of thumb (S63.04-)

● S63.051 **Subluxation of other carpometacarpal joint of right hand**

● S63.052 **Subluxation of other carpometacarpal joint of left hand**

● S63.053 **Subluxation of other carpometacarpal joint of unspecified hand**

● S63.054 **Dislocation of other carpometacarpal joint of right hand**

● S63.055 **Dislocation of other carpometacarpal joint of left hand**

● S63.056 **Dislocation of other carpometacarpal joint of unspecified hand**

● S63.06 **Subluxation and dislocation of metacarpal (bone), proximal end**

● S63.061 **Subluxation of metacarpal (bone), proximal end of right hand**

● S63.062 **Subluxation of metacarpal (bone), proximal end of left hand**

● S63.063 **Subluxation of metacarpal (bone), proximal end of unspecified hand**

● S63.064 **Dislocation of metacarpal (bone), proximal end of right hand**

● S63.065 **Dislocation of metacarpal (bone), proximal end of left hand**

● S63.066 **Dislocation of metacarpal (bone), proximal end of unspecified hand**

● S63.07 **Subluxation and dislocation of distal end of ulna**

● S63.071 **Subluxation of distal end of right ulna**

● S63.072 **Subluxation of distal end of left ulna**

● S63.073 **Subluxation of distal end of unspecified ulna**

● S63.074 **Dislocation of distal end of right ulna**

● S63.075 **Dislocation of distal end of left ulna**

● S63.076 **Dislocation of distal end of unspecified ulna**

● S63.09 **Other subluxation and dislocation of wrist and hand**

● S63.091 **Other subluxation of right wrist and hand**

● S63.092 **Other subluxation of left wrist and hand**

● S63.093 **Other subluxation of unspecified wrist and hand**

● S63.094 **Other dislocation of right wrist and hand**

● S63.095 **Other dislocation of left wrist and hand**

● S63.096 **Other dislocation of unspecified wrist and hand**

● S63.1 **Subluxation and dislocation of thumb**

● S63.10 **Unspecified subluxation and dislocation of thumb**

● S63.101 **Unspecified subluxation of right thumb**

● S63.102 **Unspecified subluxation of left thumb**

● S63.103 **Unspecified subluxation of unspecified thumb**

● S63.104 **Unspecified dislocation of right thumb**

● S63.105 **Unspecified dislocation of left thumb**

● S63.106 **Unspecified dislocation of unspecified thumb**

● S63.11 **Subluxation and dislocation of metacarpophalangeal joint of thumb**

● S63.111 **Subluxation of metacarpophalangeal joint of right thumb**

● S63.112 **Subluxation of metacarpophalangeal joint of left thumb**

● S63.113 **Subluxation of metacarpophalangeal joint of unspecified thumb**

● S63.114 **Dislocation of metacarpophalangeal joint of right thumb**

● S63.115 **Dislocation of metacarpophalangeal joint of left thumb**

● S63.116 **Dislocation of metacarpophalangeal joint of unspecified thumb**

● S63.12 **Subluxation and dislocation of interphalangeal joint of thumb**

● S63.121 **Subluxation of interphalangeal joint of right thumb**

● S63.122 **Subluxation of interphalangeal joint of left thumb**

● S63.123 **Subluxation of interphalangeal joint of unspecified thumb**

● S63.124 **Dislocation of interphalangeal joint of right thumb**

● S63.125 **Dislocation of interphalangeal joint of left thumb**

● S63.126 **Dislocation of interphalangeal joint of unspecified thumb**

● S63.2 **Subluxation and dislocation of other finger(s)**

> **Excludes2** subluxation and dislocation of thumb (S63.1-)

● S63.20 **Unspecified subluxation of other finger**

● S63.200 **Unspecified subluxation of right index finger**

● S63.201 **Unspecified subluxation of left index finger**

● S63.202 **Unspecified subluxation of right middle finger**

● S63.203 **Unspecified subluxation of left middle finger**

● S63.204 **Unspecified subluxation of right ring finger**

● S63.205 **Unspecified subluxation of left ring finger**

● S63.206 **Unspecified subluxation of right little finger**

● S63.207 **Unspecified subluxation of left little finger**

● S63.208 **Unspecified subluxation of other finger**

Unspecified subluxation of specified finger with unspecified laterality

● S63.209 **Unspecified subluxation of unspecified finger**

● S63.21 **Subluxation of metacarpophalangeal joint of finger**

● S63.210 **Subluxation of metacarpophalangeal joint of right index finger**

● S63.211 **Subluxation of metacarpophalangeal joint of left index finger**

● S63.212 **Subluxation of metacarpophalangeal joint of right middle finger**

● S63.213 **Subluxation of metacarpophalangeal joint of left middle finger**

● S63.214 **Subluxation of metacarpophalangeal joint of right ring finger**

▶ New   ⇒ Revised   ~~deleted~~ Deleted   Excludes 1   Excludes 2   Includes   Use additional   Code first   Code also   Key words
OGCR Official Guidelines   X Assign placeholder X   ● Use Additional Character(s)   ▶ Manifestation Code   Hierarchical Condition Category   Coding Clinic

- S63.215 Subluxation of metacarpophalangeal joint of left ring finger
- S63.216 Subluxation of metacarpophalangeal joint of right little finger
- S63.217 Subluxation of metacarpophalangeal joint of left little finger
- S63.218 Subluxation of metacarpophalangeal joint of other finger

  Subluxation of metacarpophalangeal joint of specified finger with unspecified laterality
- S63.219 Subluxation of metacarpophalangeal joint of unspecified finger
- S63.22 **Subluxation of unspecified interphalangeal joint of finger**
  - S63.220 Subluxation of unspecified interphalangeal joint of right index finger
  - S63.221 Subluxation of unspecified interphalangeal joint of left index finger
  - S63.222 Subluxation of unspecified interphalangeal joint of right middle finger
  - S63.223 Subluxation of unspecified interphalangeal joint of left middle finger
  - S63.224 Subluxation of unspecified interphalangeal joint of right ring finger
  - S63.225 Subluxation of unspecified interphalangeal joint of left ring finger
  - S63.226 Subluxation of unspecified interphalangeal joint of right little finger
  - S63.227 Subluxation of unspecified interphalangeal joint of left little finger
  - S63.228 Subluxation of unspecified interphalangeal joint of other finger

    Subluxation of unspecified interphalangeal joint of specified finger with unspecified laterality
  - S63.229 Subluxation of unspecified interphalangeal joint of unspecified finger
- S63.23 **Subluxation of proximal interphalangeal joint of finger**
  - S63.230 Subluxation of proximal interphalangeal joint of right index finger
  - S63.231 Subluxation of proximal interphalangeal joint of left index finger
  - S63.232 Subluxation of proximal interphalangeal joint of right middle finger
  - S63.233 Subluxation of proximal interphalangeal joint of left middle finger
  - S63.234 Subluxation of proximal interphalangeal joint of right ring finger
  - S63.235 Subluxation of proximal interphalangeal joint of left ring finger
  - S63.236 Subluxation of proximal interphalangeal joint of right little finger

- S63.237 Subluxation of proximal interphalangeal joint of left little finger
- S63.238 Subluxation of proximal interphalangeal joint of other finger

  Subluxation of proximal interphalangeal joint of specified finger with unspecified laterality
- S63.239 Subluxation of proximal interphalangeal joint of unspecified finger
- S63.24 **Subluxation of distal interphalangeal joint of finger**
  - S63.240 Subluxation of distal interphalangeal joint of right index finger
  - S63.241 Subluxation of distal interphalangeal joint of left index finger
  - S63.242 Subluxation of distal interphalangeal joint of right middle finger
  - S63.243 Subluxation of distal interphalangeal joint of left middle finger
  - S63.244 Subluxation of distal interphalangeal joint of right ring finger
  - S63.245 Subluxation of distal interphalangeal joint of left ring finger
  - S63.246 Subluxation of distal interphalangeal joint of right little finger
  - S63.247 Subluxation of distal interphalangeal joint of left little finger
  - S63.248 Subluxation of distal interphalangeal joint of other finger

    Subluxation of distal interphalangeal joint of specified finger with unspecified laterality
  - S63.249 Subluxation of distal interphalangeal joint of unspecified finger
- S63.25 **Unspecified dislocation of other finger**
  - S63.250 Unspecified dislocation of right index finger
  - S63.251 Unspecified dislocation of left index finger
  - S63.252 Unspecified dislocation of right middle finger
  - S63.253 Unspecified dislocation of left middle finger
  - S63.254 Unspecified dislocation of right ring finger
  - S63.255 Unspecified dislocation of left ring finger
  - S63.256 Unspecified dislocation of right little finger
  - S63.257 Unspecified dislocation of left little finger
  - S63.258 Unspecified dislocation of other finger

    Unspecified dislocation of specified finger with unspecified laterality
  - S63.259 Unspecified dislocation of unspecified finger

    Unspecified dislocation of unspecified finger with unspecified laterality
- S63.26 **Dislocation of metacarpophalangeal joint of finger**
  - S63.260 Dislocation of metacarpophalangeal joint of right index finger
  - S63.261 Dislocation of metacarpophalangeal joint of left index finger
  - S63.262 Dislocation of metacarpophalangeal joint of right middle finger

● S63.263　Dislocation of metacarpophalangeal joint of **left middle finger**

● S63.264　Dislocation of metacarpophalangeal joint of **right ring finger**

● S63.265　Dislocation of metacarpophalangeal joint of **left ring finger**

● S63.266　Dislocation of metacarpophalangeal joint of **right little finger**

● S63.267　Dislocation of metacarpophalangeal joint of **left little finger**

● S63.268　Dislocation of metacarpophalangeal joint of **other finger**
　　　　　　Dislocation of metacarpophalangeal joint of specified finger with unspecified laterality

● S63.269　Dislocation of metacarpophalangeal joint of **unspecified finger**

● S63.27　**Dislocation of unspecified interphalangeal** joint of finger

● S63.270　Dislocation of unspecified interphalangeal joint of **right index finger**

● S63.271　Dislocation of unspecified interphalangeal joint of **left index finger**

● S63.272　Dislocation of unspecified interphalangeal joint of **right middle finger**

● S63.273　Dislocation of unspecified interphalangeal joint of **left middle finger**

● S63.274　Dislocation of unspecified interphalangeal joint of **right ring finger**

● S63.275　Dislocation of unspecified interphalangeal joint of **left ring finger**

● S63.276　Dislocation of unspecified interphalangeal joint of **right little finger**

● S63.277　Dislocation of unspecified interphalangeal joint of **left little finger**

● S63.278　Dislocation of unspecified interphalangeal joint of **other finger**
　　　　　　Dislocation of unspecified interphalangeal joint of specified finger with unspecified laterality

● S63.279　Dislocation of unspecified interphalangeal joint of **unspecified finger**
　　　　　　Dislocation of unspecified interphalangeal joint of unspecified finger without specified laterality

● S63.28　**Dislocation of proximal interphalangeal** joint of finger

● S63.280　Dislocation of proximal interphalangeal joint of **right index finger**

● S63.281　Dislocation of proximal interphalangeal joint of **left index finger**

● S63.282　Dislocation of proximal interphalangeal joint of **right middle finger**

● S63.283　Dislocation of proximal interphalangeal joint of **left middle finger**

● S63.284　Dislocation of proximal interphalangeal joint of **right ring finger**

● S63.285　Dislocation of proximal interphalangeal joint of **left ring finger**

● S63.286　Dislocation of proximal interphalangeal joint of **right little finger**

● S63.287　Dislocation of proximal interphalangeal joint of **left little finger**

● S63.288　Dislocation of proximal interphalangeal joint of **other finger**
　　　　　　Dislocation of proximal interphalangeal joint of specified finger with unspecified laterality

● S63.289　Dislocation of proximal interphalangeal joint of **unspecified finger**

● S63.29　**Dislocation of distal interphalangeal** joint of finger

● S63.290　Dislocation of distal interphalangeal joint of **right index finger**

● S63.291　Dislocation of distal interphalangeal joint of **left index finger**

● S63.292　Dislocation of distal interphalangeal joint of **right middle finger**

● S63.293　Dislocation of distal interphalangeal joint of **left middle finger**

● S63.294　Dislocation of distal interphalangeal joint of **right ring finger**

● S63.295　Dislocation of distal interphalangeal joint of **left ring finger**

● S63.296　Dislocation of distal interphalangeal joint of **right little finger**

● S63.297　Dislocation of distal interphalangeal joint of **left little finger**

● S63.298　Dislocation of distal interphalangeal joint of **other finger**
　　　　　　Dislocation of distal interphalangeal joint of specified finger with unspecified laterality

● S63.299　Dislocation of distal interphalangeal joint of **unspecified finger**

● S63.3　Traumatic rupture of **ligament of wrist**

● S63.30　Traumatic rupture of **unspecified** ligament of wrist

● S63.301　Traumatic rupture of unspecified ligament of **right wrist**

● S63.302　Traumatic rupture of unspecified ligament of **left wrist**

● S63.309　Traumatic rupture of unspecified ligament of **unspecified** wrist

● S63.31　Traumatic rupture of **collateral ligament of** wrist

● S63.311　Traumatic rupture of collateral ligament of **right** wrist

● S63.312　Traumatic rupture of collateral ligament of **left** wrist

● S63.319　Traumatic rupture of collateral ligament of **unspecified** wrist

● S63.32　Traumatic rupture of **radiocarpal ligament**

● S63.321　Traumatic rupture of **right radiocarpal** ligament

● S63.322　Traumatic rupture of **left radiocarpal** ligament

● S63.329　Traumatic rupture of **unspecified** radiocarpal ligament

● **S63.33** Traumatic rupture of ulnocarpal (palmar) ligament
  ● **S63.331** Traumatic rupture of right ulnocarpal (palmar) ligament
  ● **S63.332** Traumatic rupture of left ulnocarpal (palmar) ligament
  ● **S63.339** Traumatic rupture of unspecified ulnocarpal (palmar) ligament
● **S63.39** Traumatic rupture of other ligament of wrist
  ● **S63.391** Traumatic rupture of other ligament of right wrist
  ● **S63.392** Traumatic rupture of other ligament of left wrist
  ● **S63.399** Traumatic rupture of other ligament of unspecified wrist
● **S63.4** **Traumatic rupture of ligament of finger at metacarpophalangeal and interphalangeal joint(s)**
  ● **S63.40** Traumatic rupture of unspecified ligament of finger at metacarpophalangeal and interphalangeal joint
    ● **S63.400** Traumatic rupture of unspecified ligament of right index finger at metacarpophalangeal and interphalangeal joint
    ● **S63.401** Traumatic rupture of unspecified ligament of left index finger at metacarpophalangeal and interphalangeal joint
    ● **S63.402** Traumatic rupture of unspecified ligament of right middle finger at metacarpophalangeal and interphalangeal joint
    ● **S63.403** Traumatic rupture of unspecified ligament of left middle finger at metacarpophalangeal and interphalangeal joint
    ● **S63.404** Traumatic rupture of unspecified ligament of right ring finger at metacarpophalangeal and interphalangeal joint
    ● **S63.405** Traumatic rupture of unspecified ligament of left ring finger at metacarpophalangeal and interphalangeal joint
    ● **S63.406** Traumatic rupture of unspecified ligament of right little finger at metacarpophalangeal and interphalangeal joint
    ● **S63.407** Traumatic rupture of unspecified ligament of left little finger at metacarpophalangeal and interphalangeal joint
    ● **S63.408** Traumatic rupture of unspecified ligament of other finger at metacarpophalangeal and interphalangeal joint
      Traumatic rupture of unspecified ligament of specified finger with unspecified laterality at metacarpophalangeal and interphalangeal joint
    ● **S63.409** Traumatic rupture of unspecified ligament of unspecified finger at metacarpophalangeal and interphalangeal joint
  ● **S63.41** Traumatic rupture of collateral ligament of finger at metacarpophalangeal and interphalangeal joint
    ● **S63.410** Traumatic rupture of collateral ligament of right index finger at metacarpophalangeal and interphalangeal joint
    ● **S63.411** Traumatic rupture of collateral ligament of left index finger at metacarpophalangeal and interphalangeal joint
    ● **S63.412** Traumatic rupture of collateral ligament of right middle finger at metacarpophalangeal and interphalangeal joint
    ● **S63.413** Traumatic rupture of collateral ligament of left middle finger at metacarpophalangeal and interphalangeal joint
    ● **S63.414** Traumatic rupture of collateral ligament of right ring finger at metacarpophalangeal and interphalangeal joint
    ● **S63.415** Traumatic rupture of collateral ligament of left ring finger at metacarpophalangeal and interphalangeal joint
    ● **S63.416** Traumatic rupture of collateral ligament of right little finger at metacarpophalangeal and interphalangeal joint
    ● **S63.417** Traumatic rupture of collateral ligament of left little finger at metacarpophalangeal and interphalangeal joint
    ● **S63.418** Traumatic rupture of collateral ligament of other finger at metacarpophalangeal and interphalangeal joint
      Traumatic rupture of collateral ligament of specified finger with unspecified laterality at metacarpophalangeal and interphalangeal joint
    ● **S63.419** Traumatic rupture of collateral ligament of unspecified finger at metacarpophalangeal and interphalangeal joint
  ● **S63.42** Traumatic rupture of palmar ligament of finger at metacarpophalangeal and interphalangeal joint
    ● **S63.420** Traumatic rupture of palmar ligament of right index finger at metacarpophalangeal and interphalangeal joint
    ● **S63.421** Traumatic rupture of palmar ligament of left index finger at metacarpophalangeal and interphalangeal joint
    ● **S63.422** Traumatic rupture of palmar ligament of right middle finger at metacarpophalangeal and interphalangeal joint
    ● **S63.423** Traumatic rupture of palmar ligament of left middle finger at metacarpophalangeal and interphalangeal joint
    ● **S63.424** Traumatic rupture of palmar ligament of right ring finger at metacarpophalangeal and interphalangeal joint
    ● **S63.425** Traumatic rupture of palmar ligament of left ring finger at metacarpophalangeal and interphalangeal joint
    ● **S63.426** Traumatic rupture of palmar ligament of right little finger at metacarpophalangeal and interphalangeal joint

🔴 **S63.427** Traumatic rupture of palmar ligament of **left little** finger at metacarpophalangeal and interphalangeal joint

🔴 **S63.428** Traumatic rupture of palmar ligament of **other** finger at metacarpophalangeal and interphalangeal joint
　　Traumatic rupture of palmar ligament of specified finger with unspecified laterality at metacarpophalangeal and interphalangeal joint

🔴 **S63.429** Traumatic rupture of palmar ligament of **unspecified** finger at metacarpophalangeal and interphalangeal joint

🔴 **S63.43** Traumatic rupture of **volar plate** of finger at metacarpophalangeal and interphalangeal joint

🔴 **S63.430** Traumatic rupture of volar plate of **right index** finger at metacarpophalangeal and interphalangeal joint

🔴 **S63.431** Traumatic rupture of volar plate of **left index** finger at metacarpophalangeal and interphalangeal joint

🔴 **S63.432** Traumatic rupture of volar plate of **right middle** finger at metacarpophalangeal and interphalangeal joint

🔴 **S63.433** Traumatic rupture of volar plate of **left middle** finger at metacarpophalangeal and interphalangeal joint

🔴 **S63.434** Traumatic rupture of volar plate of **right ring** finger at metacarpophalangeal and interphalangeal joint

🔴 **S63.435** Traumatic rupture of volar plate of **left ring** finger at metacarpophalangeal and interphalangeal joint

🔴 **S63.436** Traumatic rupture of volar plate of **right little** finger at metacarpophalangeal and interphalangeal joint

🔴 **S63.437** Traumatic rupture of volar plate of **left little** finger at metacarpophalangeal and interphalangeal joint

🔴 **S63.438** Traumatic rupture of volar plate of **other** finger at metacarpophalangeal and interphalangeal joint
　　Traumatic rupture of volar plate of specified finger with unspecified laterality at metacarpophalangeal and interphalangeal joint

🔴 **S63.439** Traumatic rupture of volar plate of **unspecified** finger at metacarpophalangeal and interphalangeal joint

🔴 **S63.49** Traumatic rupture of **other** ligament of finger at metacarpophalangeal and interphalangeal joint

🔴 **S63.490** Traumatic rupture of other ligament of **right index** finger at metacarpophalangeal and interphalangeal joint

🔴 **S63.491** Traumatic rupture of other ligament of **left index** finger at metacarpophalangeal and interphalangeal joint

🔴 **S63.492** Traumatic rupture of other ligament of **right middle** finger at metacarpophalangeal and interphalangeal joint

🔴 **S63.493** Traumatic rupture of other ligament of **left middle** finger at metacarpophalangeal and interphalangeal joint

🔴 **S63.494** Traumatic rupture of other ligament of **right ring** finger at metacarpophalangeal and interphalangeal joint

🔴 **S63.495** Traumatic rupture of other ligament of **left ring** finger at metacarpophalangeal and interphalangeal joint

🔴 **S63.496** Traumatic rupture of other ligament of **right little** finger at metacarpophalangeal and interphalangeal joint

🔴 **S63.497** Traumatic rupture of other ligament of **left little** finger at metacarpophalangeal and interphalangeal joint

🔴 **S63.498** Traumatic rupture of other ligament of **other** finger at metacarpophalangeal and interphalangeal joint
　　Traumatic rupture of ligament of specified finger with unspecified laterality at metacarpophalangeal and interphalangeal joint

🔴 **S63.499** Traumatic rupture of other ligament of **unspecified** finger at metacarpophalangeal and interphalangeal joint

🔴 **S63.5** Other and unspecified sprain of **wrist**

🔴 **S63.50** **Unspecified** sprain of wrist

🔴 **S63.501** Unspecified sprain of **right** wrist

🔴 **S63.502** Unspecified sprain of **left** wrist

🔴 **S63.509** Unspecified sprain of **unspecified** wrist

🔴 **S63.51** Sprain of **carpal** (joint)

🔴 **S63.511** Sprain of carpal joint of **right** wrist

🔴 **S63.512** Sprain of carpal joint of **left** wrist

🔴 **S63.519** Sprain of carpal joint of **unspecified** wrist

🔴 **S63.52** Sprain of **radiocarpal** joint

> **Excludes1** traumatic rupture of radiocarpal ligament (S63.32-)

🔴 **S63.521** Sprain of radiocarpal joint of **right** wrist

🔴 **S63.522** Sprain of radiocarpal joint of **left** wrist

🔴 **S63.529** Sprain of radiocarpal joint of **unspecified** wrist

🔴 **S63.59** **Other** specified sprain of wrist

🔴 **S63.591** Other specified sprain of **right** wrist

🔴 **S63.592** Other specified sprain of **left** wrist

🔴 **S63.599** Other specified sprain of **unspecified** wrist

🔴 **S63.6** Other and unspecified sprain of **finger(s)**

> **Excludes1** traumatic rupture of ligament of finger at metacarpophalangeal and interphalangeal joint(s) (S63.4-)

🔴 **S63.60** **Unspecified** sprain of thumb

🔴 **S63.601** Unspecified sprain of **right** thumb

🔴 **S63.602** Unspecified sprain of **left** thumb

🔴 **S63.609** Unspecified sprain of **unspecified** thumb

● **S63.61** **Unspecified sprain of other and unspecified finger(s)**
   ● **S63.610** Unspecified sprain of **right index** finger
   ● **S63.611** Unspecified sprain of **left index** finger
   ● **S63.612** Unspecified sprain of **right middle** finger
   ● **S63.613** Unspecified sprain of **left middle** finger
   ● **S63.614** Unspecified sprain of **right ring** finger
   ● **S63.615** Unspecified sprain of **left ring** finger
   ● **S63.616** Unspecified sprain of **right little** finger
   ● **S63.617** Unspecified sprain of **left little** finger
   ● **S63.618** Unspecified sprain of **other** finger
       Unspecified sprain of specified finger with unspecified laterality
   ● **S63.619** Unspecified sprain of **unspecified** finger

● **S63.62** **Sprain of interphalangeal joint of thumb**
   ● **S63.621** Sprain of interphalangeal joint of **right thumb**
   ● **S63.622** Sprain of interphalangeal joint of **left thumb**
   ● **S63.629** Sprain of interphalangeal joint of **unspecified thumb**

● **S63.63** **Sprain of interphalangeal joint of other and unspecified finger(s)**
   ● **S63.630** Sprain of interphalangeal joint of **right index** finger
   ● **S63.631** Sprain of interphalangeal joint of **left index** finger
   ● **S63.632** Sprain of interphalangeal joint of **right middle** finger
   ● **S63.633** Sprain of interphalangeal joint of **left middle** finger
   ● **S63.634** Sprain of interphalangeal joint of **right ring** finger
   ● **S63.635** Sprain of interphalangeal joint of **left ring** finger
   ● **S63.636** Sprain of interphalangeal joint of **right little** finger
   ● **S63.637** Sprain of interphalangeal joint of **left little** finger
   ● **S63.638** Sprain of interphalangeal joint of **other** finger
   ● **S63.639** Sprain of interphalangeal joint of **unspecified** finger

● **S63.64** **Sprain of metacarpophalangeal joint of thumb**
   ● **S63.641** Sprain of metacarpophalangeal joint of **right thumb**
   ● **S63.642** Sprain of metacarpophalangeal joint of **left thumb**
   ● **S63.649** Sprain of metacarpophalangeal joint of **unspecified thumb**

● **S63.65** **Sprain of metacarpophalangeal joint of other and unspecified finger(s)**
   ● **S63.650** Sprain of metacarpophalangeal joint of **right index** finger
   ● **S63.651** Sprain of metacarpophalangeal joint of **left index** finger
   ● **S63.652** Sprain of metacarpophalangeal joint of **right middle** finger
   ● **S63.653** Sprain of metacarpophalangeal joint of **left middle** finger
   ● **S63.654** Sprain of metacarpophalangeal joint of **right ring** finger

● **S63.655** Sprain of metacarpophalangeal joint of **left ring** finger
   ● **S63.656** Sprain of metacarpophalangeal joint of **right little** finger
   ● **S63.657** Sprain of metacarpophalangeal joint of **left little** finger
   ● **S63.658** Sprain of metacarpophalangeal joint of **other** finger
       Sprain of metacarpophalangeal joint of specified finger with unspecified laterality
   ● **S63.659** Sprain of metacarpophalangeal joint of **unspecified** finger

● **S63.68** **Other sprain of thumb**
   ● **S63.681** Other sprain of **right thumb**
   ● **S63.682** Other sprain of **left thumb**
   ● **S63.689** Other sprain of **unspecified thumb**

● **S63.69** **Other sprain of other and unspecified finger(s)**
   ● **S63.690** Other sprain of **right index** finger
   ● **S63.691** Other sprain of **left index** finger
   ● **S63.692** Other sprain of **right middle** finger
   ● **S63.693** Other sprain of **left middle** finger
   ● **S63.694** Other sprain of **right ring** finger
   ● **S63.695** Other sprain of **left ring** finger
   ● **S63.696** Other sprain of **right little** finger
   ● **S63.697** Other sprain of **left little** finger
   ● **S63.698** Other sprain of **other** finger
       Other sprain of specified finger with unspecified laterality
   ● **S63.699** Other sprain of **unspecified** finger

● **S63.8** **Sprain of other part of wrist and hand**
  ● **S63.8X** **Sprain of other part of wrist and hand**
   ● **S63.8X1** Sprain of other part of **right** wrist and hand
   ● **S63.8X2** Sprain of other part of **left** wrist and hand
   ● **S63.8X9** Sprain of other part of **unspecified** wrist and hand

● **S63.9** **Sprain of unspecified part of wrist and hand**
  X● **S63.90** Sprain of unspecified part of **unspecified** wrist and hand
  X● **S63.91** Sprain of unspecified part of **right** wrist and hand
  X● **S63.92** Sprain of unspecified part of **left** wrist and hand

● **S64** **Injury of nerves at wrist and hand level**
    The appropriate 7th character is to be added to each code from category S64

A	initial encounter
D	subsequent encounter
S	sequela

    Code also any associated open wound (S61.-)

● **S64.0** **Injury of ulnar nerve at wrist and hand level**
  X● **S64.00** Injury of ulnar nerve at wrist and hand level of **unspecified** arm
  X● **S64.01** Injury of ulnar nerve at wrist and hand level of **right** arm
  X● **S64.02** Injury of ulnar nerve at wrist and hand level of **left** arm

● **S64.1** **Injury of median nerve at wrist and hand level**
  X● **S64.10** Injury of median nerve at wrist and hand level of **unspecified** arm
  X● **S64.11** Injury of median nerve at wrist and hand level of **right** arm
  X● **S64.12** Injury of median nerve at wrist and hand level of **left** arm

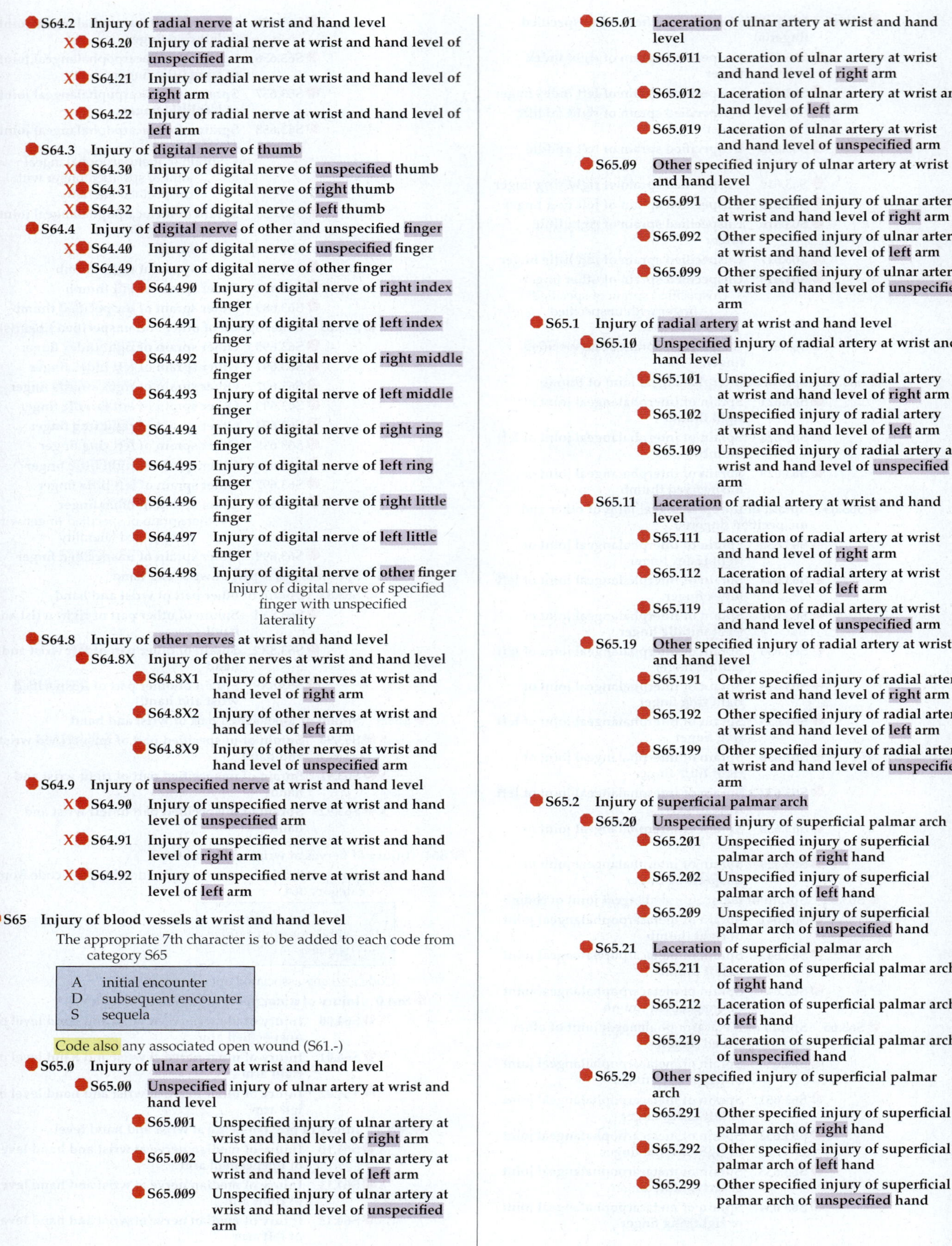

CHAPTER 19 (S00-T88)

● **S64.2** Injury of radial nerve at wrist and hand level
   X ● **S64.20** Injury of radial nerve at wrist and hand level of unspecified arm
   X ● **S64.21** Injury of radial nerve at wrist and hand level of right arm
   X ● **S64.22** Injury of radial nerve at wrist and hand level of left arm

● **S64.3** Injury of digital nerve of thumb
   X ● **S64.30** Injury of digital nerve of unspecified thumb
   X ● **S64.31** Injury of digital nerve of right thumb
   X ● **S64.32** Injury of digital nerve of left thumb

● **S64.4** Injury of digital nerve of other and unspecified finger
   X ● **S64.40** Injury of digital nerve of unspecified finger
   ● **S64.49** Injury of digital nerve of other finger
     ● **S64.490** Injury of digital nerve of right index finger
     ● **S64.491** Injury of digital nerve of left index finger
     ● **S64.492** Injury of digital nerve of right middle finger
     ● **S64.493** Injury of digital nerve of left middle finger
     ● **S64.494** Injury of digital nerve of right ring finger
     ● **S64.495** Injury of digital nerve of left ring finger
     ● **S64.496** Injury of digital nerve of right little finger
     ● **S64.497** Injury of digital nerve of left little finger
     ● **S64.498** Injury of digital nerve of other finger
       Injury of digital nerve of specified finger with unspecified laterality

● **S64.8** Injury of other nerves at wrist and hand level
   ● **S64.8X** Injury of other nerves at wrist and hand level
     ● **S64.8X1** Injury of other nerves at wrist and hand level of right arm
     ● **S64.8X2** Injury of other nerves at wrist and hand level of left arm
     ● **S64.8X9** Injury of other nerves at wrist and hand level of unspecified arm

● **S64.9** Injury of unspecified nerve at wrist and hand level
   X ● **S64.90** Injury of unspecified nerve at wrist and hand level of unspecified arm
   X ● **S64.91** Injury of unspecified nerve at wrist and hand level of right arm
   X ● **S64.92** Injury of unspecified nerve at wrist and hand level of left arm

● **S65** Injury of blood vessels at wrist and hand level
   The appropriate 7th character is to be added to each code from category S65

     A   initial encounter
     D   subsequent encounter
     S   sequela

   Code also any associated open wound (S61.-)

● **S65.0** Injury of ulnar artery at wrist and hand level
   ● **S65.00** Unspecified injury of ulnar artery at wrist and hand level
     ● **S65.001** Unspecified injury of ulnar artery at wrist and hand level of right arm
     ● **S65.002** Unspecified injury of ulnar artery at wrist and hand level of left arm
     ● **S65.009** Unspecified injury of ulnar artery at wrist and hand level of unspecified arm

● **S65.01** Laceration of ulnar artery at wrist and hand level
   ● **S65.011** Laceration of ulnar artery at wrist and hand level of right arm
   ● **S65.012** Laceration of ulnar artery at wrist and hand level of left arm
   ● **S65.019** Laceration of ulnar artery at wrist and hand level of unspecified arm

● **S65.09** Other specified injury of ulnar artery at wrist and hand level
   ● **S65.091** Other specified injury of ulnar artery at wrist and hand level of right arm
   ● **S65.092** Other specified injury of ulnar artery at wrist and hand level of left arm
   ● **S65.099** Other specified injury of ulnar artery at wrist and hand level of unspecified arm

● **S65.1** Injury of radial artery at wrist and hand level
   ● **S65.10** Unspecified injury of radial artery at wrist and hand level
     ● **S65.101** Unspecified injury of radial artery at wrist and hand level of right arm
     ● **S65.102** Unspecified injury of radial artery at wrist and hand level of left arm
     ● **S65.109** Unspecified injury of radial artery at wrist and hand level of unspecified arm

   ● **S65.11** Laceration of radial artery at wrist and hand level
     ● **S65.111** Laceration of radial artery at wrist and hand level of right arm
     ● **S65.112** Laceration of radial artery at wrist and hand level of left arm
     ● **S65.119** Laceration of radial artery at wrist and hand level of unspecified arm

   ● **S65.19** Other specified injury of radial artery at wrist and hand level
     ● **S65.191** Other specified injury of radial artery at wrist and hand level of right arm
     ● **S65.192** Other specified injury of radial artery at wrist and hand level of left arm
     ● **S65.199** Other specified injury of radial artery at wrist and hand level of unspecified arm

● **S65.2** Injury of superficial palmar arch
   ● **S65.20** Unspecified injury of superficial palmar arch
     ● **S65.201** Unspecified injury of superficial palmar arch of right hand
     ● **S65.202** Unspecified injury of superficial palmar arch of left hand
     ● **S65.209** Unspecified injury of superficial palmar arch of unspecified hand

   ● **S65.21** Laceration of superficial palmar arch
     ● **S65.211** Laceration of superficial palmar arch of right hand
     ● **S65.212** Laceration of superficial palmar arch of left hand
     ● **S65.219** Laceration of superficial palmar arch of unspecified hand

   ● **S65.29** Other specified injury of superficial palmar arch
     ● **S65.291** Other specified injury of superficial palmar arch of right hand
     ● **S65.292** Other specified injury of superficial palmar arch of left hand
     ● **S65.299** Other specified injury of superficial palmar arch of unspecified hand

▶ New   ⇨ Revised   ~~deleted~~ Deleted   Excludes 1   Excludes 2   Includes   Use additional   Code first   Code also   Key words
OGCR Official Guidelines   X Assign placeholder X   ● Use Additional Character(s)   ▸ Manifestation Code   HCC Hierarchical Condition Category   **Coding Clinic**

● S65.3   Injury of deep palmar arch
  ● S65.30   Unspecified injury of deep palmar arch
    ● S65.301   Unspecified injury of deep palmar arch of **right** hand
    ● S65.302   Unspecified injury of deep palmar arch of **left** hand
    ● S65.309   Unspecified injury of deep palmar arch of **unspecified** hand
  ● S65.31   Laceration of deep palmar arch
    ● S65.311   Laceration of deep palmar arch of **right** hand
    ● S65.312   Laceration of deep palmar arch of **left** hand
    ● S65.319   Laceration of deep palmar arch of **unspecified** hand
  ● S65.39   Other specified injury of deep palmar arch
    ● S65.391   Other specified injury of deep palmar arch of **right** hand
    ● S65.392   Other specified injury of deep palmar arch of **left** hand
    ● S65.399   Other specified injury of deep palmar arch of **unspecified** hand
● S65.4   Injury of blood vessel of **thumb**
  ● S65.40   Unspecified injury of blood vessel of thumb
    ● S65.401   Unspecified injury of blood vessel of **right** thumb
    ● S65.402   Unspecified injury of blood vessel of **left** thumb
    ● S65.409   Unspecified injury of blood vessel of **unspecified** thumb
  ● S65.41   Laceration of blood vessel of thumb
    ● S65.411   Laceration of blood vessel of **right** thumb
    ● S65.412   Laceration of blood vessel of **left** thumb
    ● S65.419   Laceration of blood vessel of **unspecified** thumb
  ● S65.49   Other specified injury of blood vessel of thumb
    ● S65.491   Other specified injury of blood vessel of **right** thumb
    ● S65.492   Other specified injury of blood vessel of **left** thumb
    ● S65.499   Other specified injury of blood vessel of **unspecified** thumb
● S65.5   Injury of blood vessel of other and unspecified **finger**
  ● S65.50   Unspecified injury of blood vessel of other and unspecified finger
    ● S65.500   Unspecified injury of blood vessel of **right** index finger
    ● S65.501   Unspecified injury of blood vessel of **left** index finger
    ● S65.502   Unspecified injury of blood vessel of **right** middle finger
    ● S65.503   Unspecified injury of blood vessel of **left** middle finger
    ● S65.504   Unspecified injury of blood vessel of **right** ring finger
    ● S65.505   Unspecified injury of blood vessel of **left** ring finger
    ● S65.506   Unspecified injury of blood vessel of **right** little finger
    ● S65.507   Unspecified injury of blood vessel of **left** little finger
    ● S65.508   Unspecified injury of blood vessel of **other** finger
          Unspecified injury of blood vessel of specified finger with unspecified laterality
    ● S65.509   Unspecified injury of blood vessel of **unspecified** finger

● S65.51   Laceration of blood vessel of other and unspecified finger
    ● S65.510   Laceration of blood vessel of **right** index finger
    ● S65.511   Laceration of blood vessel of **left** index finger
    ● S65.512   Laceration of blood vessel of **right** middle finger
    ● S65.513   Laceration of blood vessel of **left** middle finger
    ● S65.514   Laceration of blood vessel of **right** ring finger
    ● S65.515   Laceration of blood vessel of **left ring** finger
    ● S65.516   Laceration of blood vessel of **right** little finger
    ● S65.517   Laceration of blood vessel of **left little** finger
    ● S65.518   Laceration of blood vessel of **other** finger
          Laceration of blood vessel of specified finger with unspecified laterality
    ● S65.519   Laceration of blood vessel of **unspecified** finger
  ● S65.59   Other specified injury of blood vessel of other and unspecified finger
    ● S65.590   Other specified injury of blood vessel of **right** index finger
    ● S65.591   Other specified injury of blood vessel of **left** index finger
    ● S65.592   Other specified injury of blood vessel of **right** middle finger
    ● S65.593   Other specified injury of blood vessel of **left** middle finger
    ● S65.594   Other specified injury of blood vessel of **right** ring finger
    ● S65.595   Other specified injury of blood vessel of **left** ring finger
    ● S65.596   Other specified injury of blood vessel of **right** little finger
    ● S65.597   Other specified injury of blood vessel of **left** little finger
    ● S65.598   Other specified injury of blood vessel of **other** finger
          Other specified injury of blood vessel of specified finger with unspecified laterality
    ● S65.599   Other specified injury of blood vessel of **unspecified** finger
● S65.8   Injury of other blood vessels at wrist and hand level
  ● S65.80   Unspecified injury of other blood vessels at wrist and hand level
    ● S65.801   Unspecified injury of other blood vessels at wrist and hand level of **right** arm
    ● S65.802   Unspecified injury of other blood vessels at wrist and hand level of **left** arm
    ● S65.809   Unspecified injury of other blood vessels at wrist and hand level of **unspecified** arm
  ● S65.81   Laceration of other blood vessels at wrist and hand level
    ● S65.811   Laceration of other blood vessels at wrist and hand level of **right** arm
    ● S65.812   Laceration of other blood vessels at wrist and hand level of **left** arm
    ● S65.819   Laceration of other blood vessels at wrist and hand level of **unspecified** arm

CHAPTER 19 (SØØ-T88)

● **S65.89**   **Other** specified injury of other blood vessels at wrist and hand level
    ● **S65.891**   Other specified injury of other blood vessels at wrist and hand level of **right** arm
    ● **S65.892**   Other specified injury of other blood vessels at wrist and hand level of **left** arm
    ● **S65.899**   Other specified injury of other blood vessels at wrist and hand level of **unspecified** arm
● **S65.9**   Injury of **unspecified blood vessel** at wrist and hand level
   ● **S65.90**   **Unspecified** injury of unspecified blood vessel at wrist and hand level
    ● **S65.901**   Unspecified injury of unspecified blood vessel at wrist and hand level of **right** arm
    ● **S65.902**   Unspecified injury of unspecified blood vessel at wrist and hand level of **left** arm
    ● **S65.909**   Unspecified injury of unspecified blood vessel at wrist and hand level of **unspecified** arm
   ● **S65.91**   Laceration of **unspecified** blood vessel at wrist and hand level
    ● **S65.911**   Laceration of unspecified blood vessel at wrist and hand level of **right** arm
    ● **S65.912**   Laceration of unspecified blood vessel at wrist and hand level of **left** arm
    ● **S65.919**   Laceration of unspecified blood vessel at wrist and hand level of **unspecified** arm
   ● **S65.99**   Other specified injury of unspecified blood vessel at wrist and hand level
    ● **S65.991**   Other specified injury of **unspecified** blood vessel at wrist and hand of **right** arm
    ● **S65.992**   Other specified injury of **unspecified** blood vessel at wrist and hand of **left** arm
    ● **S65.999**   Other specified injury of **unspecified** blood vessel at wrist and hand of **unspecified** arm

● **S66**   Injury of muscle, fascia and tendon at wrist and hand level
   Code also any associated open wound (S61.-)
   Excludes2   sprain of joints and ligaments of wrist and hand (S63.-)

The appropriate 7th character is to be added to each code from category S66

A	initial encounter
D	subsequent encounter
S	sequela

● **S66.0**   Injury of **long flexor** muscle, fascia and tendon of **thumb** at wrist and hand level
   ● **S66.00**   **Unspecified** injury of long flexor muscle, fascia and tendon of thumb at wrist and hand level
    ● **S66.001**   Unspecified injury of long flexor muscle, fascia and tendon of **right** thumb at wrist and hand level
    ● **S66.002**   Unspecified injury of long flexor muscle, fascia and tendon of **left** thumb at wrist and hand level
    ● **S66.009**   Unspecified injury of long flexor muscle, fascia and tendon of **unspecified** thumb at wrist and hand level

● **S66.01**   **Strain** of long flexor muscle, fascia and tendon of thumb at wrist and hand level
    ● **S66.011**   Strain of long flexor muscle, fascia and tendon of **right** thumb at wrist and hand level
    ● **S66.012**   Strain of long flexor muscle, fascia and tendon of **left** thumb at wrist and hand level
    ● **S66.019**   Strain of long flexor muscle, fascia and tendon of **unspecified** thumb at wrist and hand level
● **S66.02**   Laceration of long flexor muscle, fascia and tendon of thumb at wrist and hand level
    ● **S66.021**   Laceration of long flexor muscle, fascia and tendon of **right** thumb at wrist and hand level
    ● **S66.022**   Laceration of long flexor muscle, fascia and tendon of **left** thumb at wrist and hand level
    ● **S66.029**   Laceration of long flexor muscle, fascia and tendon of **unspecified** thumb at wrist and hand level
● **S66.09**   Other specified injury of long flexor muscle, fascia and tendon of thumb at wrist and hand level
    ● **S66.091**   Other specified injury of long flexor muscle, fascia and tendon of **right** thumb at wrist and hand level
    ● **S66.092**   Other specified injury of long flexor muscle, fascia and tendon of **left** thumb at wrist and hand level
    ● **S66.099**   Other specified injury of long flexor muscle, fascia and tendon of **unspecified** thumb at wrist and hand level
● **S66.1**   Injury of **flexor** muscle, fascia and tendon of other and unspecified **finger** at wrist and hand level
   Excludes2   injury of long flexor muscle, fascia and tendon of thumb at wrist and hand level (S66.0-)
   ● **S66.10**   **Unspecified** injury of flexor muscle, fascia and tendon of other and unspecified finger at wrist and hand level
    ● **S66.100**   Unspecified injury of flexor muscle, fascia and tendon of **right index** finger at wrist and hand level
    ● **S66.101**   Unspecified injury of flexor muscle, fascia and tendon of **left index** finger at wrist and hand level
    ● **S66.102**   Unspecified injury of flexor muscle, fascia and tendon of **right middle** finger at wrist and hand level
    ● **S66.103**   Unspecified injury of flexor muscle, fascia and tendon of **left middle** finger at wrist and hand level
    ● **S66.104**   Unspecified injury of flexor muscle, fascia and tendon of **right ring** finger at wrist and hand level
    ● **S66.105**   Unspecified injury of flexor muscle, fascia and tendon of **left ring** finger at wrist and hand level
    ● **S66.106**   Unspecified injury of flexor muscle, fascia and tendon of **right little** finger at wrist and hand level
    ● **S66.107**   Unspecified injury of flexor muscle, fascia and tendon of **left little** finger at wrist and hand level

- **S66.108** **Unspecified** injury of flexor muscle, fascia and tendon of **other** finger at wrist and hand level

  Unspecified injury of flexor muscle, fascia and tendon of specified finger with unspecified laterality at wrist and hand level

- **S66.109** **Unspecified** injury of flexor muscle, fascia and tendon of **unspecified** finger at wrist and hand level

- **S66.11** **Strain** of flexor muscle, fascia and tendon of other and unspecified finger at wrist and hand level

  - **S66.110** Strain of flexor muscle, fascia and tendon of **right index** finger at wrist and hand level

  - **S66.111** Strain of flexor muscle, fascia and tendon of **left index** finger at wrist and hand level

  - **S66.112** Strain of flexor muscle, fascia and tendon of **right middle** finger at wrist and hand level

  - **S66.113** Strain of flexor muscle, fascia and tendon of **left middle** finger at wrist and hand level

  - **S66.114** Strain of flexor muscle, fascia and tendon of **right ring** finger at wrist and hand level

  - **S66.115** Strain of flexor muscle, fascia and tendon of **left ring** finger at wrist and hand level

  - **S66.116** Strain of flexor muscle, fascia and tendon of **right little** finger at wrist and hand level

  - **S66.117** Strain of flexor muscle, fascia and tendon of **left little** finger at wrist and hand level

  - **S66.118** Strain of flexor muscle, fascia and tendon of **other** finger at wrist and hand level

    Strain of flexor muscle, fascia and tendon of specified finger with unspecified laterality at wrist and hand level

  - **S66.119** Strain of flexor muscle, fascia and tendon of **unspecified** finger at wrist and hand level

- **S66.12** **Laceration** of flexor muscle, fascia and tendon of other and unspecified finger at wrist and hand level

  - **S66.120** Laceration of flexor muscle, fascia and tendon of **right index** finger at wrist and hand level

  - **S66.121** Laceration of flexor muscle, fascia and tendon of **left index** finger at wrist and hand level

  - **S66.122** Laceration of flexor muscle, fascia and tendon of **right middle** finger at wrist and hand level

  - **S66.123** Laceration of flexor muscle, fascia and tendon of **left middle** finger at wrist and hand level

  - **S66.124** Laceration of flexor muscle, fascia and tendon of **right ring** finger at wrist and hand level

  - **S66.125** Laceration of flexor muscle, fascia and tendon of **left ring** finger at wrist and hand level

- **S66.126** Laceration of flexor muscle, fascia and tendon of **right little** finger at wrist and hand level

- **S66.127** Laceration of flexor muscle, fascia and tendon of **left little** finger at wrist and hand level

- **S66.128** Laceration of flexor muscle, fascia and tendon of **other** finger at wrist and hand level

  Laceration of flexor muscle, fascia and tendon of specified finger with unspecified laterality at wrist and hand level

- **S66.129** Laceration of flexor muscle, fascia and tendon of **unspecified** finger at wrist and hand level

- **S66.19** **Other** injury of flexor muscle, fascia and tendon of other and unspecified finger at wrist and hand level

  - **S66.190** Other injury of flexor muscle, fascia and tendon of **right index** finger at wrist and hand level

  - **S66.191** Other injury of flexor muscle, fascia and tendon of **left index** finger at wrist and hand level

  - **S66.192** Other injury of flexor muscle, fascia and tendon of **right middle** finger at wrist and hand level

  - **S66.193** Other injury of flexor muscle, fascia and tendon of **left middle** finger at wrist and hand level

  - **S66.194** Other injury of flexor muscle, fascia and tendon of **right ring** finger at wrist and hand level

  - **S66.195** Other injury of flexor muscle, fascia and tendon of **left ring** finger at wrist and hand level

  - **S66.196** Other injury of flexor muscle, fascia and tendon of **right little** finger at wrist and hand level

  - **S66.197** Other injury of flexor muscle, fascia and tendon of **left little** finger at wrist and hand level

  - **S66.198** Other injury of flexor muscle, fascia and tendon of **other** finger at wrist and hand level

    Other injury of flexor muscle, fascia and tendon of specified finger with unspecified laterality at wrist and hand level

  - **S66.199** Other injury of flexor muscle, fascia and tendon of **unspecified** finger at wrist and hand level

- **S66.2** Injury of **extensor** muscle, fascia and tendon of **thumb** at wrist and hand level

  - **S66.20** **Unspecified** injury of extensor muscle, fascia and tendon of thumb at wrist and hand level

    - **S66.201** Unspecified injury of extensor muscle, fascia and tendon of **right** thumb at wrist and hand level

    - **S66.202** Unspecified injury of extensor muscle, fascia and tendon of **left** thumb at wrist and hand level

    - **S66.209** Unspecified injury of extensor muscle, fascia and tendon of **unspecified** thumb at wrist and hand level

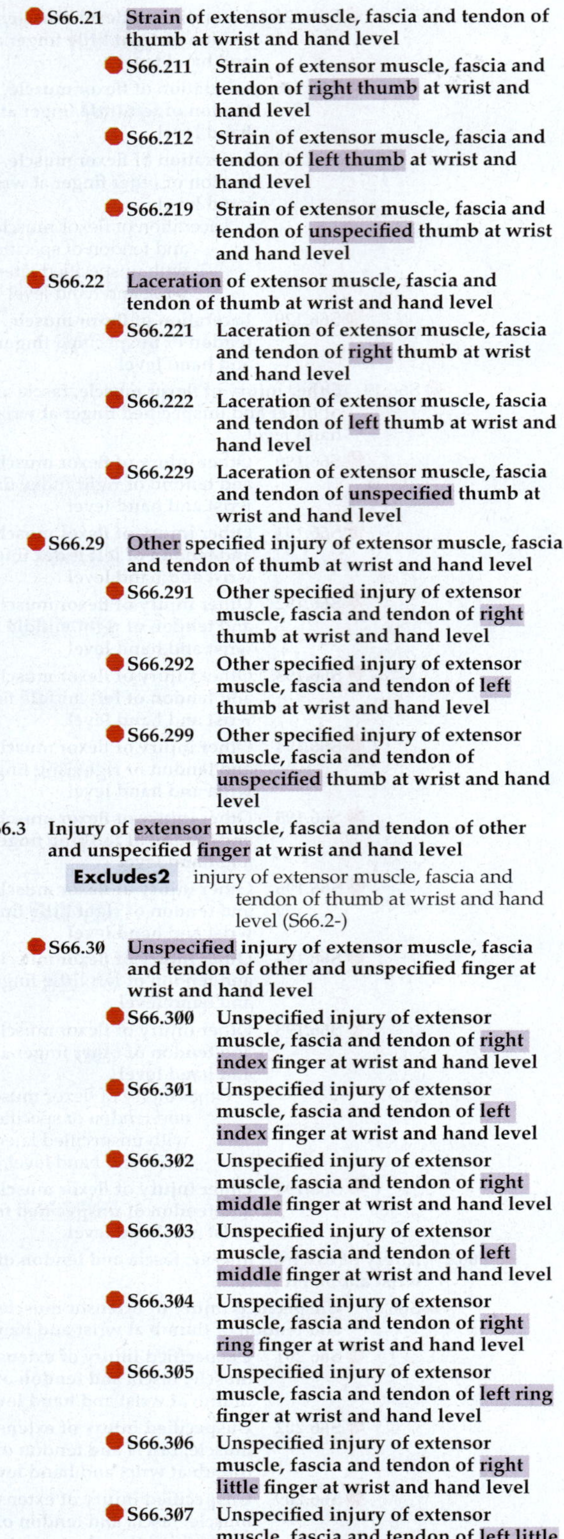

● S66.21 **Strain** of extensor muscle, fascia and tendon of thumb at wrist and hand level
- ● S66.211 Strain of extensor muscle, fascia and tendon of **right thumb** at wrist and hand level
- ● S66.212 Strain of extensor muscle, fascia and tendon of **left thumb** at wrist and hand level
- ● S66.219 Strain of extensor muscle, fascia and tendon of **unspecified** thumb at wrist and hand level

● S66.22 **Laceration** of extensor muscle, fascia and tendon of thumb at wrist and hand level
- ● S66.221 Laceration of extensor muscle, fascia and tendon of **right** thumb at wrist and hand level
- ● S66.222 Laceration of extensor muscle, fascia and tendon of **left** thumb at wrist and hand level
- ● S66.229 Laceration of extensor muscle, fascia and tendon of **unspecified** thumb at wrist and hand level

● S66.29 **Other** specified injury of extensor muscle, fascia and tendon of thumb at wrist and hand level
- ● S66.291 Other specified injury of extensor muscle, fascia and tendon of **right** thumb at wrist and hand level
- ● S66.292 Other specified injury of extensor muscle, fascia and tendon of **left** thumb at wrist and hand level
- ● S66.299 Other specified injury of extensor muscle, fascia and tendon of **unspecified** thumb at wrist and hand level

● S66.3 Injury of **extensor** muscle, fascia and tendon of other and unspecified **finger** at wrist and hand level

Excludes2 injury of extensor muscle, fascia and tendon of thumb at wrist and hand level (S66.2-)

● S66.30 **Unspecified** injury of extensor muscle, fascia and tendon of other and unspecified finger at wrist and hand level
- ● S66.300 Unspecified injury of extensor muscle, fascia and tendon of **right index** finger at wrist and hand level
- ● S66.301 Unspecified injury of extensor muscle, fascia and tendon of **left index** finger at wrist and hand level
- ● S66.302 Unspecified injury of extensor muscle, fascia and tendon of **right middle** finger at wrist and hand level
- ● S66.303 Unspecified injury of extensor muscle, fascia and tendon of **left middle** finger at wrist and hand level
- ● S66.304 Unspecified injury of extensor muscle, fascia and tendon of **right ring** finger at wrist and hand level
- ● S66.305 Unspecified injury of extensor muscle, fascia and tendon of **left ring** finger at wrist and hand level
- ● S66.306 Unspecified injury of extensor muscle, fascia and tendon of **right little** finger at wrist and hand level
- ● S66.307 Unspecified injury of extensor muscle, fascia and tendon of **left little** finger at wrist and hand level

- ● S66.308 Unspecified injury of extensor muscle, fascia and tendon of **other** finger at wrist and hand level
  Unspecified injury of extensor muscle, fascia and tendon of specified finger with unspecified laterality at wrist and hand level
- ● S66.309 Unspecified injury of extensor muscle, fascia and tendon of **unspecified** finger at wrist and hand level

● S66.31 **Strain** of extensor muscle, fascia and tendon of other and unspecified finger at wrist and hand level
- ● S66.310 Strain of extensor muscle, fascia and tendon of **right index** finger at wrist and hand level
- ● S66.311 Strain of extensor muscle, fascia and tendon of **left index** finger at wrist and hand level
- ● S66.312 Strain of extensor muscle, fascia and tendon of **right middle** finger at wrist and hand level
- ● S66.313 Strain of extensor muscle, fascia and tendon of **left middle** finger at wrist and hand level
- ● S66.314 Strain of extensor muscle, fascia and tendon of **right ring** finger at wrist and hand level
- ● S66.315 Strain of extensor muscle, fascia and tendon of **left ring** finger at wrist and hand level
- ● S66.316 Strain of extensor muscle, fascia and tendon of **right little** finger at wrist and hand level
- ● S66.317 Strain of extensor muscle, fascia and tendon of **left little** finger at wrist and hand level
- ● S66.318 Strain of extensor muscle, fascia and tendon of **other** finger at wrist and hand level
  Strain of extensor muscle, fascia and tendon of specified finger with unspecified laterality at wrist and hand level
- ● S66.319 Strain of extensor muscle, fascia and tendon of **unspecified** finger at wrist and hand level

● S66.32 **Laceration** of extensor muscle, fascia and tendon of other and unspecified finger at wrist and hand level
- ● S66.320 Laceration of extensor muscle, fascia and tendon of **right index** finger at wrist and hand level
- ● S66.321 Laceration of extensor muscle, fascia and tendon of **left index** finger at wrist and hand level
- ● S66.322 Laceration of extensor muscle, fascia and tendon of **right middle** finger at wrist and hand level
- ● S66.323 Laceration of extensor muscle, fascia and tendon of **left middle** finger at wrist and hand level
- ● S66.324 Laceration of extensor muscle, fascia and tendon of **right ring** finger at wrist and hand level
- ● S66.325 Laceration of extensor muscle, fascia and tendon of **left ring** finger at wrist and hand level

● **S66.326** Laceration of extensor muscle, fascia and tendon of right little finger at wrist and hand level

● **S66.327** Laceration of extensor muscle, fascia and tendon of left little finger at wrist and hand level

● **S66.328** Laceration of extensor muscle, fascia and tendon of other finger at wrist and hand level

     Laceration of extensor muscle, fascia and tendon of specified finger with unspecified laterality at wrist and hand level

● **S66.329** Laceration of extensor muscle, fascia and tendon of unspecified finger at wrist and hand level

● **S66.39** Other injury of extensor muscle, fascia and tendon of other and unspecified finger at wrist and hand level

● **S66.390** Other injury of extensor muscle, fascia and tendon of right index finger at wrist and hand level

● **S66.391** Other injury of extensor muscle, fascia and tendon of left index finger at wrist and hand level

● **S66.392** Other injury of extensor muscle, fascia and tendon of right middle finger at wrist and hand level

● **S66.393** Other injury of extensor muscle, fascia and tendon of left middle finger at wrist and hand level

● **S66.394** Other injury of extensor muscle, fascia and tendon of right ring finger at wrist and hand level

● **S66.395** Other injury of extensor muscle, fascia and tendon of left ring finger at wrist and hand level

● **S66.396** Other injury of extensor muscle, fascia and tendon of right little finger at wrist and hand level

● **S66.397** Other injury of extensor muscle, fascia and tendon of left little finger at wrist and hand level

● **S66.398** Other injury of extensor muscle, fascia and tendon of other finger at wrist and hand level

     Other injury of extensor muscle, fascia and tendon of specified finger with unspecified laterality at wrist and hand level

● **S66.399** Other injury of extensor muscle, fascia and tendon of unspecified finger at wrist and hand level

● **S66.4** Injury of intrinsic muscle, fascia and tendon of thumb at wrist and hand level

● **S66.40** Unspecified injury of intrinsic muscle, fascia and tendon of thumb at wrist and hand level

● **S66.401** Unspecified injury of intrinsic muscle, fascia and tendon of right thumb at wrist and hand level

● **S66.402** Unspecified injury of intrinsic muscle, fascia and tendon of left thumb at wrist and hand level

● **S66.409** Unspecified injury of intrinsic muscle, fascia and tendon of unspecified thumb at wrist and hand level

● **S66.41** Strain of intrinsic muscle, fascia and tendon of thumb at wrist and hand level

● **S66.411** Strain of intrinsic muscle, fascia and tendon of right thumb at wrist and hand level

● **S66.412** Strain of intrinsic muscle, fascia and tendon of left thumb at wrist and hand level

● **S66.419** Strain of intrinsic muscle, fascia and tendon of unspecified thumb at wrist and hand level

● **S66.42** Laceration of intrinsic muscle, fascia and tendon of thumb at wrist and hand level

● **S66.421** Laceration of intrinsic muscle, fascia and tendon of right thumb at wrist and hand level

● **S66.422** Laceration of intrinsic muscle, fascia and tendon of left thumb at wrist and hand level

● **S66.429** Laceration of intrinsic muscle, fascia and tendon of unspecified thumb at wrist and hand level

● **S66.49** Other specified injury of intrinsic muscle, fascia and tendon of thumb at wrist and hand level

● **S66.491** Other specified injury of intrinsic muscle, fascia and tendon of right thumb at wrist and hand level

● **S66.492** Other specified injury of intrinsic muscle, fascia and tendon of left thumb at wrist and hand level

● **S66.499** Other specified injury of intrinsic muscle, fascia and tendon of unspecified thumb at wrist and hand level

● **S66.5** Injury of intrinsic muscle, fascia and tendon of other and unspecified finger at wrist and hand level

     Excludes2   injury of intrinsic muscle, fascia and tendon of thumb at wrist and hand level (S66.4-)

● **S66.50** Unspecified injury of intrinsic muscle, fascia and tendon of other and unspecified finger at wrist and hand level

● **S66.500** Unspecified injury of intrinsic muscle, fascia and tendon of right index finger at wrist and hand level

● **S66.501** Unspecified injury of intrinsic muscle, fascia and tendon of left index finger at wrist and hand level

● **S66.502** Unspecified injury of intrinsic muscle, fascia and tendon of right middle finger at wrist and hand level

● **S66.503** Unspecified injury of intrinsic muscle, fascia and tendon of left middle finger at wrist and hand level

● **S66.504** Unspecified injury of intrinsic muscle, fascia and tendon of right ring finger at wrist and hand level

● **S66.505** Unspecified injury of intrinsic muscle, fascia and tendon of left ring finger at wrist and hand level

● **S66.506** Unspecified injury of intrinsic muscle, fascia and tendon of right little finger at wrist and hand level

● **S66.507** Unspecified injury of intrinsic muscle, fascia and tendon of left little finger at wrist and hand level

CHAPTER 19 (S00–T88)

● **S66.508** Unspecified injury of intrinsic muscle, fascia and tendon of **other** finger at wrist and hand level
  Unspecified injury of intrinsic muscle, fascia and tendon of specified finger with unspecified laterality at wrist and hand level

● **S66.509** Unspecified injury of intrinsic muscle, fascia and tendon of **unspecified** finger at wrist and hand level

● **S66.51** Strain of intrinsic muscle, fascia and tendon of other and unspecified finger at wrist and hand level

● **S66.510** Strain of intrinsic muscle, fascia and tendon of **right index** finger at wrist and hand level

● **S66.511** Strain of intrinsic muscle, fascia and tendon of **left index** finger at wrist and hand level

● **S66.512** Strain of intrinsic muscle, fascia and tendon of **right middle** finger at wrist and hand level

● **S66.513** Strain of intrinsic muscle, fascia and tendon of **left middle** finger at wrist and hand level

● **S66.514** Strain of intrinsic muscle, fascia and tendon of **right ring** finger at wrist and hand level

● **S66.515** Strain of intrinsic muscle, fascia and tendon of **left ring** finger at wrist and hand level

● **S66.516** Strain of intrinsic muscle, fascia and tendon of **right little** finger at wrist and hand level

● **S66.517** Strain of intrinsic muscle, fascia and tendon of **left little** finger at wrist and hand level

● **S66.518** Strain of intrinsic muscle, fascia and tendon of **other** finger at wrist and hand level
  Strain of intrinsic muscle, fascia and tendon of specified finger with unspecified laterality at wrist and hand level

● **S66.519** Strain of intrinsic muscle, fascia and tendon of **unspecified** finger at wrist and hand level

● **S66.52** Laceration of intrinsic muscle, fascia and tendon of other and unspecified finger at wrist and hand level

● **S66.520** Laceration of intrinsic muscle, fascia and tendon of **right index** finger at wrist and hand level

● **S66.521** Laceration of intrinsic muscle, fascia and tendon of **left index** finger at wrist and hand level

● **S66.522** Laceration of intrinsic muscle, fascia and tendon of **right middle** finger at wrist and hand level

● **S66.523** Laceration of intrinsic muscle, fascia and tendon of **left middle** finger at wrist and hand level

● **S66.524** Laceration of intrinsic muscle, fascia and tendon of **right ring** finger at wrist and hand level

● **S66.525** Laceration of intrinsic muscle, fascia and tendon of **left ring** finger at wrist and hand level

● **S66.526** Laceration of intrinsic muscle, fascia and tendon of **right little** finger at wrist and hand level

● **S66.527** Laceration of intrinsic muscle, fascia and tendon of **left little** finger at wrist and hand level

● **S66.528** Laceration of intrinsic muscle, fascia and tendon of **other** finger at wrist and hand level
  Laceration of intrinsic muscle, fascia and tendon of specified finger with unspecified laterality at wrist and hand level

● **S66.529** Laceration of intrinsic muscle, fascia and tendon of **unspecified** finger at wrist and hand level

● **S66.59** Other injury of intrinsic muscle, fascia and tendon of other and unspecified finger at wrist and hand level

● **S66.590** Other injury of intrinsic muscle, fascia and tendon of **right index** finger at wrist and hand level

● **S66.591** Other injury of intrinsic muscle, fascia and tendon of **left index** finger at wrist and hand level

● **S66.592** Other injury of intrinsic muscle, fascia and tendon of **right middle** finger at wrist and hand level

● **S66.593** Other injury of intrinsic muscle, fascia and tendon of **left middle** finger at wrist and hand level

● **S66.594** Other injury of intrinsic muscle, fascia and tendon of **right ring** finger at wrist and hand level

● **S66.595** Other injury of intrinsic muscle, fascia and tendon of **left ring** finger at wrist and hand level

● **S66.596** Other injury of intrinsic muscle, fascia and tendon of **right little** finger at wrist and hand level

● **S66.597** Other injury of intrinsic muscle, fascia and tendon of **left little** finger at wrist and hand level

● **S66.598** Other injury of intrinsic muscle, fascia and tendon of **other** finger at wrist and hand level
  Other injury of intrinsic muscle, fascia and tendon of specified finger with unspecified laterality at wrist and hand level

● **S66.599** Other injury of intrinsic muscle, fascia and tendon of **unspecified** finger at wrist and hand level

● **S66.8** Injury of **other specified** muscles, fascia and tendons at wrist and hand level

● **S66.80** Unspecified injury of other specified muscles, fascia and tendons at wrist and hand level

● **S66.801** Unspecified injury of other specified muscles, fascia and tendons at wrist and hand level, **right hand**

● **S66.802** Unspecified injury of other specified muscles, fascia and tendons at wrist and hand level, **left hand**

● **S66.809** Unspecified injury of other specified muscles, fascia and tendons at wrist and hand level, **unspecified hand**

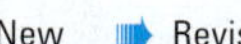

● **S66.81** **Strain** of other specified muscles, fascia and tendons at wrist and hand level
  ● **S66.811** Strain of other specified muscles, fascia and tendons at wrist and hand level, **right** hand
  ● **S66.812** Strain of other specified muscles, fascia and tendons at wrist and hand level, **left** hand
  ● **S66.819** Strain of other specified muscles, fascia and tendons at wrist and hand level, **unspecified** hand
● **S66.82** **Laceration** of other specified muscles, fascia and tendons at wrist and hand level
  ● **S66.821** Laceration of other specified muscles, fascia and tendons at wrist and hand level, **right** hand
  ● **S66.822** Laceration of other specified muscles, fascia and tendons at wrist and hand level, **left** hand
  ● **S66.829** Laceration of other specified muscles, fascia and tendons at wrist and hand level, **unspecified** hand
● **S66.89** **Other injury** of other specified muscles, fascia and tendons at wrist and hand level
  ● **S66.891** Other injury of other specified muscles, fascia and tendons at wrist and hand level, **right** hand
  ● **S66.892** Other injury of other specified muscles, fascia and tendons at wrist and hand level, **left** hand
  ● **S66.899** Other injury of other specified muscles, fascia and tendons at wrist and hand level, **unspecified** hand
● **S66.9** Injury of **unspecified** muscle, fascia and tendon at wrist and hand level
  ● **S66.90** **Unspecified injury** of unspecified muscle, fascia and tendon at wrist and hand level
    ● **S66.901** Unspecified injury of unspecified muscle, fascia and tendon at wrist and hand level, **right** hand
    ● **S66.902** Unspecified injury of unspecified muscle, fascia and tendon at wrist and hand level, **left** hand
    ● **S66.909** Unspecified injury of unspecified muscle, fascia and tendon at wrist and hand level, **unspecified** hand
  ● **S66.91** **Strain** of unspecified muscle, fascia and tendon at wrist and hand level
    ● **S66.911** Strain of unspecified muscle, fascia and tendon at wrist and hand level, **right** hand
    ● **S66.912** Strain of unspecified muscle, fascia and tendon at wrist and hand level, **left** hand
    ● **S66.919** Strain of unspecified muscle, fascia and tendon at wrist and hand level, **unspecified** hand
  ● **S66.92** **Laceration** of unspecified muscle, fascia and tendon at wrist and hand level
    ● **S66.921** Laceration of unspecified muscle, fascia and tendon at wrist and hand level, **right** hand
    ● **S66.922** Laceration of unspecified muscle, fascia and tendon at wrist and hand level, **left** hand
    ● **S66.929** Laceration of unspecified muscle, fascia and tendon at wrist and hand level, **unspecified** hand

● **S66.99** **Other injury** of unspecified muscle, fascia and tendon at wrist and hand level
  ● **S66.991** Other injury of unspecified muscle, fascia and tendon at wrist and hand level, **right** hand
  ● **S66.992** Other injury of unspecified muscle, fascia and tendon at wrist and hand level, **left** hand
  ● **S66.999** Other injury of unspecified muscle, fascia and tendon at wrist and hand level, **unspecified** hand
● **S67** **Crushing injury of wrist, hand and fingers**

Use additional code for all associated injuries, such as:
fracture of wrist and hand (S62.-)
open wound of wrist and hand (S61.-)

The appropriate 7th character is to be added to each code from category S67

> A   initial encounter
> D   subsequent encounter
> S   sequela

● **S67.0** Crushing injury of **thumb**
  X ● **S67.00** Crushing injury of **unspecified** thumb
  X ● **S67.01** Crushing injury of **right** thumb
  X ● **S67.02** Crushing injury of **left** thumb
● **S67.1** Crushing injury of other and unspecified **finger(s)**
  Excludes2 crushing injury of thumb (S67.0-)
  X ● **S67.10** Crushing injury of **unspecified** finger(s)
  ● **S67.19** Crushing injury of other finger(s)
    ● **S67.190** Crushing injury of **right index** finger
    ● **S67.191** Crushing injury of **left index** finger
    ● **S67.192** Crushing injury of **right middle** finger
    ● **S67.193** Crushing injury of **left middle** finger
    ● **S67.194** Crushing injury of **right ring** finger
    ● **S67.195** Crushing injury of **left ring** finger
    ● **S67.196** Crushing injury of **right little** finger
    ● **S67.197** Crushing injury of **left little** finger
    ● **S67.198** Crushing injury of **other** finger
      Crushing injury of specified finger with unspecified laterality
● **S67.2** Crushing injury of **hand**
  Excludes2 crushing injury of fingers (S67.1-)
               crushing injury of thumb (S67.0-)
  X ● **S67.20** Crushing injury of **unspecified** hand
  X ● **S67.21** Crushing injury of **right** hand
  X ● **S67.22** Crushing injury of **left** hand
● **S67.3** Crushing injury of **wrist**
  X ● **S67.30** Crushing injury of **unspecified** wrist
  X ● **S67.31** Crushing injury of **right** wrist
  X ● **S67.32** Crushing injury of **left** wrist
● **S67.4** Crushing injury of **wrist and hand**
  Excludes1 crushing injury of hand alone (S67.2-)
               crushing injury of wrist alone (S67.3-)
  Excludes2 crushing injury of fingers (S67.1-)
               crushing injury of thumb (S67.0-)
  X ● **S67.40** Crushing injury of **unspecified** wrist and hand
  X ● **S67.41** Crushing injury of **right** wrist and hand
  X ● **S67.42** Crushing injury of **left** wrist and hand

CHAPTER 19 (S00-T88)

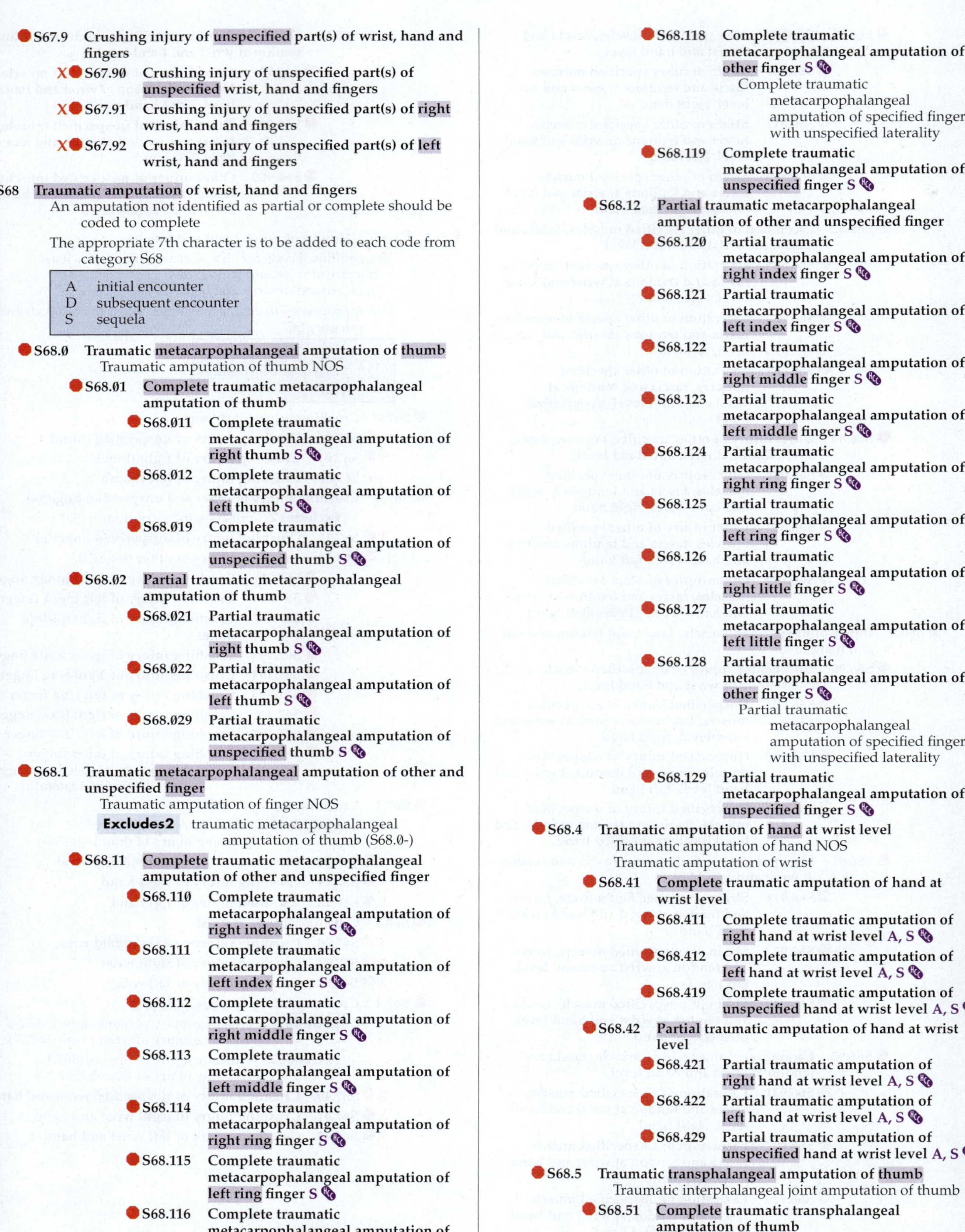

● **S67.9**　**Crushing injury of unspecified part(s) of wrist, hand and fingers**
　X ● **S67.90**　Crushing injury of unspecified part(s) of unspecified wrist, hand and fingers
　X ● **S67.91**　Crushing injury of unspecified part(s) of right wrist, hand and fingers
　X ● **S67.92**　Crushing injury of unspecified part(s) of left wrist, hand and fingers

● **S68**　**Traumatic amputation of wrist, hand and fingers**
　An amputation not identified as partial or complete should be coded to complete

　The appropriate 7th character is to be added to each code from category S68

> | | |
> |---|---|
> | A | initial encounter |
> | D | subsequent encounter |
> | S | sequela |

● **S68.0**　**Traumatic metacarpophalangeal amputation of thumb**
　Traumatic amputation of thumb NOS
　● **S68.01**　Complete traumatic metacarpophalangeal amputation of thumb
　　● **S68.011**　Complete traumatic metacarpophalangeal amputation of right thumb S ℞
　　● **S68.012**　Complete traumatic metacarpophalangeal amputation of left thumb S ℞
　　● **S68.019**　Complete traumatic metacarpophalangeal amputation of unspecified thumb S ℞
　● **S68.02**　Partial traumatic metacarpophalangeal amputation of thumb
　　● **S68.021**　Partial traumatic metacarpophalangeal amputation of right thumb S ℞
　　● **S68.022**　Partial traumatic metacarpophalangeal amputation of left thumb S ℞
　　● **S68.029**　Partial traumatic metacarpophalangeal amputation of unspecified thumb S ℞

● **S68.1**　**Traumatic metacarpophalangeal amputation of other and unspecified finger**
　Traumatic amputation of finger NOS
　Excludes2　traumatic metacarpophalangeal amputation of thumb (S68.0-)
　● **S68.11**　Complete traumatic metacarpophalangeal amputation of other and unspecified finger
　　● **S68.110**　Complete traumatic metacarpophalangeal amputation of right index finger S ℞
　　● **S68.111**　Complete traumatic metacarpophalangeal amputation of left index finger S ℞
　　● **S68.112**　Complete traumatic metacarpophalangeal amputation of right middle finger S ℞
　　● **S68.113**　Complete traumatic metacarpophalangeal amputation of left middle finger S ℞
　　● **S68.114**　Complete traumatic metacarpophalangeal amputation of right ring finger S ℞
　　● **S68.115**　Complete traumatic metacarpophalangeal amputation of left ring finger S ℞
　　● **S68.116**　Complete traumatic metacarpophalangeal amputation of right little finger S ℞
　　● **S68.117**　Complete traumatic metacarpophalangeal amputation of left little finger S ℞
　　● **S68.118**　Complete traumatic metacarpophalangeal amputation of other finger S ℞
　　　Complete traumatic metacarpophalangeal amputation of specified finger with unspecified laterality
　　● **S68.119**　Complete traumatic metacarpophalangeal amputation of unspecified finger S ℞
　● **S68.12**　Partial traumatic metacarpophalangeal amputation of other and unspecified finger
　　● **S68.120**　Partial traumatic metacarpophalangeal amputation of right index finger S ℞
　　● **S68.121**　Partial traumatic metacarpophalangeal amputation of left index finger S ℞
　　● **S68.122**　Partial traumatic metacarpophalangeal amputation of right middle finger S ℞
　　● **S68.123**　Partial traumatic metacarpophalangeal amputation of left middle finger S ℞
　　● **S68.124**　Partial traumatic metacarpophalangeal amputation of right ring finger S ℞
　　● **S68.125**　Partial traumatic metacarpophalangeal amputation of left ring finger S ℞
　　● **S68.126**　Partial traumatic metacarpophalangeal amputation of right little finger S ℞
　　● **S68.127**　Partial traumatic metacarpophalangeal amputation of left little finger S ℞
　　● **S68.128**　Partial traumatic metacarpophalangeal amputation of other finger S ℞
　　　Partial traumatic metacarpophalangeal amputation of specified finger with unspecified laterality
　　● **S68.129**　Partial traumatic metacarpophalangeal amputation of unspecified finger S ℞

● **S68.4**　**Traumatic amputation of hand at wrist level**
　Traumatic amputation of hand NOS
　Traumatic amputation of wrist
　● **S68.41**　Complete traumatic amputation of hand at wrist level
　　● **S68.411**　Complete traumatic amputation of right hand at wrist level A, S ℞
　　● **S68.412**　Complete traumatic amputation of left hand at wrist level A, S ℞
　　● **S68.419**　Complete traumatic amputation of unspecified hand at wrist level A, S ℞
　● **S68.42**　Partial traumatic amputation of hand at wrist level
　　● **S68.421**　Partial traumatic amputation of right hand at wrist level A, S ℞
　　● **S68.422**　Partial traumatic amputation of left hand at wrist level A, S ℞
　　● **S68.429**　Partial traumatic amputation of unspecified hand at wrist level A, S ℞

● **S68.5**　**Traumatic transphalangeal amputation of thumb**
　Traumatic interphalangeal joint amputation of thumb
　● **S68.51**　Complete traumatic transphalangeal amputation of thumb
　　● **S68.511**　Complete traumatic transphalangeal amputation of right thumb S ℞
　　● **S68.512**　Complete traumatic transphalangeal amputation of left thumb S ℞

● **S68.519** Complete traumatic transphalangeal amputation of unspecified thumb S ℞

● **S68.52** Partial traumatic transphalangeal amputation of thumb

● **S68.521** Partial traumatic transphalangeal amputation of right thumb S ℞

● **S68.522** Partial traumatic transphalangeal amputation of left thumb S ℞

● **S68.529** Partial traumatic transphalangeal amputation of unspecified thumb S ℞

● **S68.6** Traumatic transphalangeal amputation of other and unspecified finger

● **S68.61** Complete traumatic transphalangeal amputation of other and unspecified finger(s)

● **S68.610** Complete traumatic transphalangeal amputation of right index finger S ℞

● **S68.611** Complete traumatic transphalangeal amputation of left index finger S ℞

● **S68.612** Complete traumatic transphalangeal amputation of right middle finger S ℞

● **S68.613** Complete traumatic transphalangeal amputation of left middle finger S ℞

● **S68.614** Complete traumatic transphalangeal amputation of right ring finger S ℞

● **S68.615** Complete traumatic transphalangeal amputation of left ring finger S ℞

● **S68.616** Complete traumatic transphalangeal amputation of right little finger S ℞

● **S68.617** Complete traumatic transphalangeal amputation of left little finger S ℞

● **S68.618** Complete traumatic transphalangeal amputation of other finger S ℞
Complete traumatic transphalangeal amputation of specified finger with unspecified laterality

● **S68.619** Complete traumatic transphalangeal amputation of unspecified finger S ℞

● **S68.62** Partial traumatic transphalangeal amputation of other and unspecified finger

● **S68.620** Partial traumatic transphalangeal amputation of right index finger S ℞

● **S68.621** Partial traumatic transphalangeal amputation of left index finger S ℞

● **S68.622** Partial traumatic transphalangeal amputation of right middle finger S ℞

● **S68.623** Partial traumatic transphalangeal amputation of left middle finger S ℞

● **S68.624** Partial traumatic transphalangeal amputation of right ring finger S ℞

● **S68.625** Partial traumatic transphalangeal amputation of left ring finger S ℞

● **S68.626** Partial traumatic transphalangeal amputation of right little finger S ℞

● **S68.627** Partial traumatic transphalangeal amputation of left little finger S ℞

● **S68.628** Partial traumatic transphalangeal amputation of other finger S ℞
Partial traumatic transphalangeal amputation of specified finger with unspecified laterality

● **S68.629** Partial traumatic transphalangeal amputation of unspecified finger S ℞

● **S68.7** Traumatic transmetacarpal amputation of hand

● **S68.71** Complete traumatic transmetacarpal amputation of hand

● **S68.711** Complete traumatic transmetacarpal amputation of right hand A, S ℞

● **S68.712** Complete traumatic transmetacarpal amputation of left hand A, S ℞

● **S68.719** Complete traumatic transmetacarpal amputation of unspecified hand A, S ℞

● **S68.72** Partial traumatic transmetacarpal amputation of hand

● **S68.721** Partial traumatic transmetacarpal amputation of right hand A, S ℞

● **S68.722** Partial traumatic transmetacarpal amputation of left hand A, S ℞

● **S68.729** Partial traumatic transmetacarpal amputation of unspecified hand A, S ℞

● **S69** Other and unspecified injuries of wrist, hand and finger(s)
The appropriate 7th character is to be added to each code from category S69

A	initial encounter
D	subsequent encounter
S	sequela

● **S69.8** Other specified injuries of wrist, hand and finger(s)

X● **S69.80** Other specified injuries of unspecified wrist, hand and finger(s)

X● **S69.81** Other specified injuries of right wrist, hand and finger(s)

X● **S69.82** Other specified injuries of left wrist, hand and finger(s)

● **S69.9** Unspecified injury of wrist, hand and finger(s)

X● **S69.90** Unspecified injury of unspecified wrist, hand and finger(s)

X● **S69.91** Unspecified injury of right wrist, hand and finger(s)

X● **S69.92** Unspecified injury of left wrist, hand and finger(s)

INJURIES TO THE HIP AND THIGH (S70-S79)

Excludes2   burns and corrosions (T20-T32)
frostbite (T33-T34)
snake bite (T63.0-)
venomous insect bite or sting (T63.4-)

● **S70** Superficial injury of hip and thigh
The appropriate 7th character is to be added to each code from category S70

A	initial encounter
D	subsequent encounter
S	sequela

● **S70.0** Contusion of hip

X● **S70.00** Contusion of unspecified hip

X● **S70.01** Contusion of right hip

X● **S70.02** Contusion of left hip

● **S70.1** Contusion of thigh

X● **S70.10** Contusion of unspecified thigh

X● **S70.11** Contusion of right thigh

X● **S70.12** Contusion of left thigh

● **S70.2** Other superficial injuries of hip

● **S70.21** Abrasion of hip

● **S70.211** Abrasion, right hip

● **S70.212** Abrasion, left hip

● **S70.219** Abrasion, unspecified hip

● **S70.22** Blister (nonthermal) of hip

● **S70.221** Blister (nonthermal), right hip

● **S70.222** Blister (nonthermal), left hip

● **S70.229** Blister (nonthermal), unspecified hip

● **S70.24** External constriction of hip

● **S70.241** External constriction, right hip

● **S70.242** External constriction, left hip

● **S70.249** External constriction, unspecified hip

CHAPTER 19 (S00-T88)

● **S70.25** **Superficial foreign body of hip**
Splinter in the hip
 ● **S70.251** Superficial foreign body, **right** hip
 ● **S70.252** Superficial foreign body, **left** hip
 ● **S70.259** Superficial foreign body, **unspecified** hip
● **S70.26** **Insect bite (nonvenomous) of hip**
 ● **S70.261** Insect bite (nonvenomous), **right** hip
 ● **S70.262** Insect bite (nonvenomous), **left** hip
 ● **S70.269** Insect bite (nonvenomous), **unspecified** hip
● **S70.27** **Other superficial bite of hip**
 Excludes1 open bite of hip (S71.05-)
 ● **S70.271** Other superficial bite of hip, **right** hip
 ● **S70.272** Other superficial bite of hip, **left** hip
 ● **S70.279** Other superficial bite of hip, **unspecified** hip
● **S70.3** **Other superficial injuries of thigh**
 ● **S70.31** **Abrasion of thigh**
  ● **S70.311** Abrasion, **right** thigh
  ● **S70.312** Abrasion, **left** thigh
  ● **S70.319** Abrasion, **unspecified** thigh
 ● **S70.32** **Blister (nonthermal) of thigh**
  ● **S70.321** Blister (nonthermal), **right** thigh
  ● **S70.322** Blister (nonthermal), **left** thigh
  ● **S70.329** Blister (nonthermal), **unspecified** thigh
 ● **S70.34** **External constriction of thigh**
  ● **S70.341** External constriction, **right** thigh
  ● **S70.342** External constriction, **left** thigh
  ● **S70.349** External constriction, **unspecified** thigh
 ● **S70.35** **Superficial foreign body of thigh**
  Splinter in the thigh
  ● **S70.351** Superficial foreign body, **right** thigh
  ● **S70.352** Superficial foreign body, **left** thigh
  ● **S70.359** Superficial foreign body, **unspecified** thigh
 ● **S70.36** **Insect bite (nonvenomous) of thigh**
  ● **S70.361** Insect bite (nonvenomous), **right** thigh
  ● **S70.362** Insect bite (nonvenomous), **left** thigh
  ● **S70.369** Insect bite (nonvenomous), **unspecified** thigh
 ● **S70.37** **Other superficial bite of thigh**
  Excludes1 open bite of thigh (S71.15)
  ● **S70.371** Other superficial bite of **right** thigh
  ● **S70.372** Other superficial bite of **left** thigh
  ● **S70.379** Other superficial bite of **unspecified** thigh
● **S70.9** **Unspecified superficial injury of hip and thigh**
 ● **S70.91** **Unspecified superficial injury of hip**
  ● **S70.911** Unspecified superficial injury of **right** hip
  ● **S70.912** Unspecified superficial injury of **left** hip
  ● **S70.919** Unspecified superficial injury of **unspecified** hip
 ● **S70.92** **Unspecified superficial injury of thigh**
  ● **S70.921** Unspecified superficial injury of **right** thigh
  ● **S70.922** Unspecified superficial injury of **left** thigh
  ● **S70.929** Unspecified superficial injury of **unspecified** thigh

● **S71** **Open wound of hip and thigh**
Code also any associated wound infection
 Excludes1 open fracture of hip and thigh (S72.-)
     traumatic amputation of hip and thigh (S78.-)
 Excludes2 bite of venomous animal (T63.-)
     open wound of ankle, foot and toes (S91.-)
     open wound of knee and lower leg (S81.-)
The appropriate 7th character is to be added to each code from category S71

 A initial encounter
 D subsequent encounter
 S sequela

● **S71.0** **Open wound of hip**
 ● **S71.00** **Unspecified open wound of hip**
  ● **S71.001** Unspecified open wound, **right** hip
  ● **S71.002** Unspecified open wound, **left** hip
  ● **S71.009** Unspecified open wound, **unspecified** hip
 ● **S71.01** **Laceration without foreign body of hip**
  ● **S71.011** Laceration without foreign body, **right** hip
  ● **S71.012** Laceration without foreign body, **left** hip
  ● **S71.019** Laceration without foreign body, **unspecified** hip
 ● **S71.02** **Laceration with foreign body of hip**
  ● **S71.021** Laceration with foreign body, **right** hip
  ● **S71.022** Laceration with foreign body, **left** hip
  ● **S71.029** Laceration with foreign body, **unspecified** hip
 ● **S71.03** **Puncture wound without foreign body of hip**
  ● **S71.031** Puncture wound without foreign body, **right** hip
  ● **S71.032** Puncture wound without foreign body, **left** hip
  ● **S71.039** Puncture wound without foreign body, **unspecified** hip
 ● **S71.04** **Puncture wound with foreign body of hip**
  ● **S71.041** Puncture wound with foreign body, **right** hip
  ● **S71.042** Puncture wound with foreign body, **left** hip
  ● **S71.049** Puncture wound with foreign body, **unspecified** hip
 ● **S71.05** **Open bite of hip**
  Bite of hip NOS
  Excludes1 superficial bite of hip (S70.26, S70.27)
  ● **S71.051** Open bite, **right** hip
  ● **S71.052** Open bite, **left** hip
  ● **S71.059** Open bite, **unspecified** hip
● **S71.1** **Open wound of thigh**
 ● **S71.10** **Unspecified open wound of thigh**
  ● **S71.101** Unspecified open wound, **right** thigh
  ● **S71.102** Unspecified open wound, **left** thigh
  ● **S71.109** Unspecified open wound, **unspecified** thigh
 ● **S71.11** **Laceration without foreign body of thigh**
  ● **S71.111** Laceration without foreign body, **right** thigh
  ● **S71.112** Laceration without foreign body, **left** thigh
  ● **S71.119** Laceration without foreign body, **unspecified** thigh

● **S71.12**   Laceration with foreign body of thigh
- ● **S71.121**   Laceration with foreign body, right thigh
- ● **S71.122**   Laceration with foreign body, left thigh
- ● **S71.129**   Laceration with foreign body, unspecified thigh

● **S71.13**   Puncture wound without foreign body of thigh
- ● **S71.131**   Puncture wound without foreign body, right thigh
- ● **S71.132**   Puncture wound without foreign body, left thigh
  - **Coding Clinic: 2023, Q3, P12**
- ● **S71.139**   Puncture wound without foreign body, unspecified thigh

● **S71.14**   Puncture wound with foreign body of thigh
- ● **S71.141**   Puncture wound with foreign body, right thigh
- ● **S71.142**   Puncture wound with foreign body, left thigh
- ● **S71.149**   Puncture wound with foreign body, unspecified thigh

● **S71.15**   Open bite of thigh
    Bite of thigh NOS
> **Excludes1**   superficial bite of thigh (S70.37-)
- ● **S71.151**   Open bite, right thigh
- ● **S71.152**   Open bite, left thigh
- ● **S71.159**   Open bite, unspecified thigh

● **S72**   **Fracture of femur**
    Note: A fracture not indicated as displaced or nondisplaced should be coded to displaced

    A fracture not indicated as open or closed should be coded to closed

    The open fracture designations are based on the Gustilo open fracture classification

> **Excludes1**   traumatic amputation of hip and thigh (S78.-)
> **Excludes2**   fracture of lower leg and ankle (S82.-)
>   fracture of foot (S92.-)
>   periprosthetic fracture of prosthetic implant of hip (M97.0-)

The appropriate 7th character is to be added to all codes from category S72

A	initial encounter for closed fracture
B	initial encounter for open fracture type I or II initial encounter for open fracture NOS
C	initial encounter for open fracture type IIIA, IIIB, or IIIC
D	subsequent encounter for closed fracture with routine healing
E	subsequent encounter for open fracture type I or II with routine healing
F	subsequent encounter for open fracture type IIIA, IIIB, or IIIC with routine healing
G	subsequent encounter for closed fracture with delayed healing
H	subsequent encounter for open fracture type I or II with delayed healing
J	subsequent encounter for open fracture type IIIA, IIIB, or IIIC with delayed healing
K	subsequent encounter for closed fracture with nonunion
M	subsequent encounter for open fracture type I or II with nonunion
N	subsequent encounter for open fracture type IIIA, IIIB, or IIIC with nonunion
P	subsequent encounter for closed fracture with malunion
Q	subsequent encounter for open fracture type I or II with malunion
R	subsequent encounter for open fracture type IIIA, IIIB, or IIIC with malunion
S	sequela

● **S72.0**   Fracture of head and neck of femur
> **Excludes2**   physeal fracture of lower end of femur (S79.1-)
>   physeal fracture of upper end of femur (S79.0-)

- ● **S72.00**   Fracture of unspecified part of neck of femur
      Fracture of hip NOS
      Fracture of neck of femur NOS
  - ● **S72.001**   Fracture of unspecified part of neck of right femur A, B, C
  - ● **S72.002**   Fracture of unspecified part of neck of left femur A, B, C
    - **Coding Clinic: 2015, Q4, P37, Q1, P17**
  - ● **S72.009**   Fracture of unspecified part of neck of unspecified femur A, B, C

- ● **S72.01**   Unspecified intracapsular fracture of femur
      Subcapital fracture of femur
  - ● **S72.011**   Unspecified intracapsular fracture of right femur A, B, C
  - ● **S72.012**   Unspecified intracapsular fracture of left femur A, B, C
  - ● **S72.019**   Unspecified intracapsular fracture of unspecified femur A, B, C

- ● **S72.02**   Fracture of epiphysis (separation) (upper) of femur
      Transepiphyseal fracture of femur
      Fracture and separation across growth plate
  > **Excludes1**   capital femoral epiphyseal fracture (pediatric) of femur (S79.01-)
  >   Salter-Harris Type I physeal fracture of upper end of femur (S79.01-)
  - ● **S72.021**   Displaced fracture of epiphysis (separation) (upper) of right femur A, B, C
  - ● **S72.022**   Displaced fracture of epiphysis (separation) (upper) of left femur A, B, C
  - ● **S72.023**   Displaced fracture of epiphysis (separation) (upper) of unspecified femur A, B, C
  - ● **S72.024**   Nondisplaced fracture of epiphysis (separation) (upper) of right femur A, B, C
  - ● **S72.025**   Nondisplaced fracture of epiphysis (separation) (upper) of left femur A, B, C
  - ● **S72.026**   Nondisplaced fracture of epiphysis (separation) (upper) of unspecified femur A, B, C

- ● **S72.03**   Midcervical fracture of femur
      Transcervical fracture of femur NOS
  - ● **S72.031**   Displaced midcervical fracture of right femur A, B, C
  - ● **S72.032**   Displaced midcervical fracture of left femur A, B, C
  - ● **S72.033**   Displaced midcervical fracture of unspecified femur A, B, C
  - ● **S72.034**   Nondisplaced midcervical fracture of right femur A, B, C
  - ● **S72.035**   Nondisplaced midcervical fracture of left femur A, B, C
  - ● **S72.036**   Nondisplaced midcervical fracture of unspecified femur A, B, C

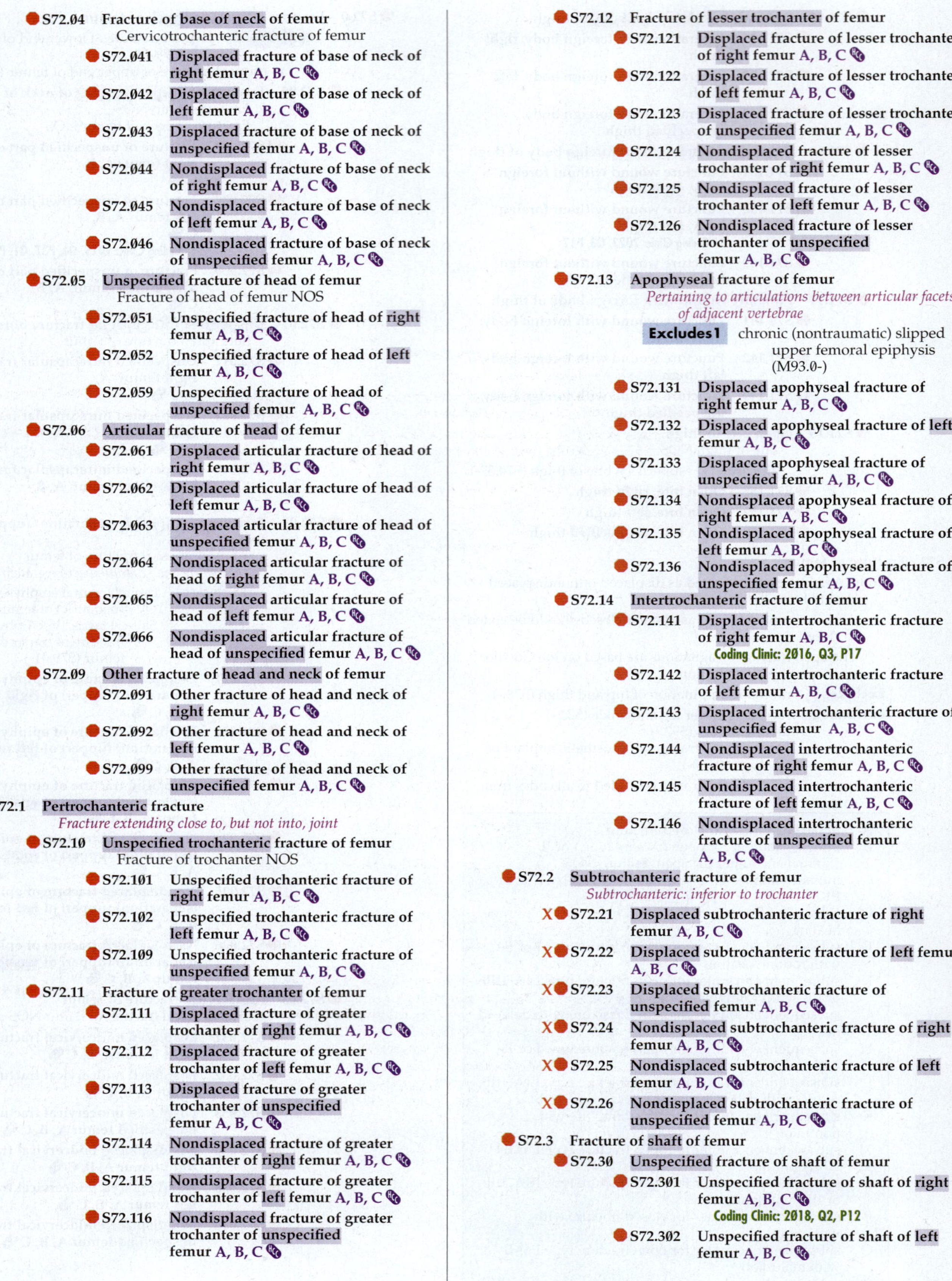

- ● **S72.04** Fracture of base of neck of femur
  Cervicotrochanteric fracture of femur
  - ● **S72.041** Displaced fracture of base of neck of right femur A, B, C ⓡ
  - ● **S72.042** Displaced fracture of base of neck of left femur A, B, C ⓡ
  - ● **S72.043** Displaced fracture of base of neck of unspecified femur A, B, C ⓡ
  - ● **S72.044** Nondisplaced fracture of base of neck of right femur A, B, C ⓡ
  - ● **S72.045** Nondisplaced fracture of base of neck of left femur A, B, C ⓡ
  - ● **S72.046** Nondisplaced fracture of base of neck of unspecified femur A, B, C ⓡ
- ● **S72.05** Unspecified fracture of head of femur
  Fracture of head of femur NOS
  - ● **S72.051** Unspecified fracture of head of right femur A, B, C ⓡ
  - ● **S72.052** Unspecified fracture of head of left femur A, B, C ⓡ
  - ● **S72.059** Unspecified fracture of head of unspecified femur A, B, C ⓡ
- ● **S72.06** Articular fracture of head of femur
  - ● **S72.061** Displaced articular fracture of head of right femur A, B, C ⓡ
  - ● **S72.062** Displaced articular fracture of head of left femur A, B, C ⓡ
  - ● **S72.063** Displaced articular fracture of head of unspecified femur A, B, C ⓡ
  - ● **S72.064** Nondisplaced articular fracture of head of right femur A, B, C ⓡ
  - ● **S72.065** Nondisplaced articular fracture of head of left femur A, B, C ⓡ
  - ● **S72.066** Nondisplaced articular fracture of head of unspecified femur A, B, C ⓡ
- ● **S72.09** Other fracture of head and neck of femur
  - ● **S72.091** Other fracture of head and neck of right femur A, B, C ⓡ
  - ● **S72.092** Other fracture of head and neck of left femur A, B, C ⓡ
  - ● **S72.099** Other fracture of head and neck of unspecified femur A, B, C ⓡ
- ● **S72.1** Pertrochanteric fracture
  Fracture extending close to, but not into, joint
  - ● **S72.10** Unspecified trochanteric fracture of femur
    Fracture of trochanter NOS
    - ● **S72.101** Unspecified trochanteric fracture of right femur A, B, C ⓡ
    - ● **S72.102** Unspecified trochanteric fracture of left femur A, B, C ⓡ
    - ● **S72.109** Unspecified trochanteric fracture of unspecified femur A, B, C ⓡ
  - ● **S72.11** Fracture of greater trochanter of femur
    - ● **S72.111** Displaced fracture of greater trochanter of right femur A, B, C ⓡ
    - ● **S72.112** Displaced fracture of greater trochanter of left femur A, B, C ⓡ
    - ● **S72.113** Displaced fracture of greater trochanter of unspecified femur A, B, C ⓡ
    - ● **S72.114** Nondisplaced fracture of greater trochanter of right femur A, B, C ⓡ
    - ● **S72.115** Nondisplaced fracture of greater trochanter of left femur A, B, C ⓡ
    - ● **S72.116** Nondisplaced fracture of greater trochanter of unspecified femur A, B, C ⓡ

- ● **S72.12** Fracture of lesser trochanter of femur
  - ● **S72.121** Displaced fracture of lesser trochanter of right femur A, B, C ⓡ
  - ● **S72.122** Displaced fracture of lesser trochanter of left femur A, B, C ⓡ
  - ● **S72.123** Displaced fracture of lesser trochanter of unspecified femur A, B, C ⓡ
  - ● **S72.124** Nondisplaced fracture of lesser trochanter of right femur A, B, C ⓡ
  - ● **S72.125** Nondisplaced fracture of lesser trochanter of left femur A, B, C ⓡ
  - ● **S72.126** Nondisplaced fracture of lesser trochanter of unspecified femur A, B, C ⓡ
- ● **S72.13** Apophyseal fracture of femur
  Pertaining to articulations between articular facets of adjacent vertebrae

  > **Excludes1** chronic (nontraumatic) slipped upper femoral epiphysis (M93.0-)

  - ● **S72.131** Displaced apophyseal fracture of right femur A, B, C ⓡ
  - ● **S72.132** Displaced apophyseal fracture of left femur A, B, C ⓡ
  - ● **S72.133** Displaced apophyseal fracture of unspecified femur A, B, C ⓡ
  - ● **S72.134** Nondisplaced apophyseal fracture of right femur A, B, C ⓡ
  - ● **S72.135** Nondisplaced apophyseal fracture of left femur A, B, C ⓡ
  - ● **S72.136** Nondisplaced apophyseal fracture of unspecified femur A, B, C ⓡ
- ● **S72.14** Intertrochanteric fracture of femur
  - ● **S72.141** Displaced intertrochanteric fracture of right femur A, B, C ⓡ
    Coding Clinic: 2016, Q3, P17
  - ● **S72.142** Displaced intertrochanteric fracture of left femur A, B, C ⓡ
  - ● **S72.143** Displaced intertrochanteric fracture of unspecified femur A, B, C ⓡ
  - ● **S72.144** Nondisplaced intertrochanteric fracture of right femur A, B, C ⓡ
  - ● **S72.145** Nondisplaced intertrochanteric fracture of left femur A, B, C ⓡ
  - ● **S72.146** Nondisplaced intertrochanteric fracture of unspecified femur A, B, C ⓡ
- ● **S72.2** Subtrochanteric fracture of femur
  Subtrochanteric: inferior to trochanter
  - X ● **S72.21** Displaced subtrochanteric fracture of right femur A, B, C ⓡ
  - X ● **S72.22** Displaced subtrochanteric fracture of left femur A, B, C ⓡ
  - X ● **S72.23** Displaced subtrochanteric fracture of unspecified femur A, B, C ⓡ
  - X ● **S72.24** Nondisplaced subtrochanteric fracture of right femur A, B, C ⓡ
  - X ● **S72.25** Nondisplaced subtrochanteric fracture of left femur A, B, C ⓡ
  - X ● **S72.26** Nondisplaced subtrochanteric fracture of unspecified femur A, B, C ⓡ
- ● **S72.3** Fracture of shaft of femur
  - ● **S72.30** Unspecified fracture of shaft of femur
    - ● **S72.301** Unspecified fracture of shaft of right femur A, B, C ⓡ
      Coding Clinic: 2018, Q2, P12
    - ● **S72.302** Unspecified fracture of shaft of left femur A, B, C ⓡ

- ● S72.309   Unspecified fracture of shaft of unspecified femur A, B, C 🔗
- ● S72.32   Transverse fracture of shaft of femur
  - ● S72.321   Displaced transverse fracture of shaft of right femur A, B, C 🔗
  - ● S72.322   Displaced transverse fracture of shaft of left femur A, B, C 🔗
  - ● S72.323   Displaced transverse fracture of shaft of unspecified femur A, B, C 🔗
  - ● S72.324   Nondisplaced transverse fracture of shaft of right femur A, B, C 🔗
  - ● S72.325   Nondisplaced transverse fracture of shaft of left femur A, B, C 🔗
  - ● S72.326   Nondisplaced transverse fracture of shaft of unspecified femur A, B, C 🔗
- ● S72.33   Oblique fracture of shaft of femur
  - ● S72.331   Displaced oblique fracture of shaft of right femur A, B, C 🔗
  - ● S72.332   Displaced oblique fracture of shaft of left femur A, B, C 🔗
  - ● S72.333   Displaced oblique fracture of shaft of unspecified femur A, B, C 🔗
  - ● S72.334   Nondisplaced oblique fracture of shaft of right femur A, B, C 🔗
  - ● S72.335   Nondisplaced oblique fracture of shaft of left femur A, B, C 🔗
  - ● S72.336   Nondisplaced oblique fracture of shaft of unspecified femur A, B, C 🔗
- ● S72.34   Spiral fracture of shaft of femur
  - ● S72.341   Displaced spiral fracture of shaft of right femur A, B, C 🔗
  - ● S72.342   Displaced spiral fracture of shaft of left femur A, B, C 🔗
  - ● S72.343   Displaced spiral fracture of shaft of unspecified femur A, B, C 🔗
  - ● S72.344   Nondisplaced spiral fracture of shaft of right femur A, B, C 🔗
  - ● S72.345   Nondisplaced spiral fracture of shaft of left femur A, B, C 🔗
  - ● S72.346   Nondisplaced spiral fracture of shaft of unspecified femur A, B, C 🔗
- ● S72.35   Comminuted fracture of shaft of femur
  - ● S72.351   Displaced comminuted fracture of shaft of right femur A, B, C 🔗
  - ● S72.352   Displaced comminuted fracture of shaft of left femur A, B, C 🔗
  - ● S72.353   Displaced comminuted fracture of shaft of unspecified femur A, B, C 🔗
  - ● S72.354   Nondisplaced comminuted fracture of shaft of right femur A, B, C 🔗
  - ● S72.355   Nondisplaced comminuted fracture of shaft of left femur A, B, C 🔗
  - ● S72.356   Nondisplaced comminuted fracture of shaft of unspecified femur A, B, C 🔗
- ● S72.36   Segmental fracture of shaft of femur
  - ● S72.361   Displaced segmental fracture of shaft of right femur A, B, C 🔗
  - ● S72.362   Displaced segmental fracture of shaft of left femur A, B, C 🔗
  - ● S72.363   Displaced segmental fracture of shaft of unspecified femur A, B, C 🔗
  - ● S72.364   Nondisplaced segmental fracture of shaft of right femur A, B, C 🔗
  - ● S72.365   Nondisplaced segmental fracture of shaft of left femur A, B, C 🔗
  - ● S72.366   Nondisplaced segmental fracture of shaft of unspecified femur A, B, C 🔗

- ● S72.39   Other fracture of shaft of femur
  - ● S72.391   Other fracture of shaft of right femur A, B, C 🔗
  - ● S72.392   Other fracture of shaft of left femur A, B, C 🔗
  - ● S72.399   Other fracture of shaft of unspecified femur A, B, C 🔗
- ● S72.4   Fracture of lower end of femur
  Fracture of distal end of femur
  Excludes2   fracture of shaft of femur (S72.3-)
  physeal fracture of lower end of femur (S79.1-)
  - ● S72.40   Unspecified fracture of lower end of femur
    - ● S72.401   Unspecified fracture of lower end of right femur A, B, C 🔗
      Coding Clinic: 2016, Q4, P43
    - ● S72.402   Unspecified fracture of lower end of left femur A, B, C 🔗
    - ● S72.409   Unspecified fracture of lower end of unspecified femur A, B, C 🔗
  - ● S72.41   Unspecified condyle fracture of lower end of femur
    Condyle fracture of femur NOS
    - ● S72.411   Displaced unspecified condyle fracture of lower end of right femur A, B, C 🔗
    - ● S72.412   Displaced unspecified condyle fracture of lower end of left femur A, B, C 🔗
    - ● S72.413   Displaced unspecified condyle fracture of lower end of unspecified femur A, B, C 🔗
    - ● S72.414   Nondisplaced unspecified condyle fracture of lower end of right femur A, B, C 🔗
    - ● S72.415   Nondisplaced unspecified condyle fracture of lower end of left femur A, B, C 🔗
    - ● S72.416   Nondisplaced unspecified condyle fracture of lower end of unspecified femur A, B, C 🔗
  - ● S72.42   Fracture of lateral condyle of femur
    - ● S72.421   Displaced fracture of lateral condyle of right femur A, B, C 🔗
    - ● S72.422   Displaced fracture of lateral condyle of left femur A, B, C 🔗
    - ● S72.423   Displaced fracture of lateral condyle of unspecified femur A, B, C 🔗
    - ● S72.424   Nondisplaced fracture of lateral condyle of right femur A, B, C 🔗
    - ● S72.425   Nondisplaced fracture of lateral condyle of left femur A, B, C 🔗
    - ● S72.426   Nondisplaced fracture of lateral condyle of unspecified femur A, B, C 🔗
  - ● S72.43   Fracture of medial condyle of femur
    - ● S72.431   Displaced fracture of medial condyle of right femur A, B, C 🔗
    - ● S72.432   Displaced fracture of medial condyle of left femur A, B, C 🔗
    - ● S72.433   Displaced fracture of medial condyle of unspecified femur A, B, C 🔗
    - ● S72.434   Nondisplaced fracture of medial condyle of right femur A, B, C 🔗
    - ● S72.435   Nondisplaced fracture of medial condyle of left femur A, B, C 🔗
    - ● S72.436   Nondisplaced fracture of medial condyle of unspecified femur A, B, C 🔗

CHAPTER 19 (S00-T88)

● **S72.44 Fracture of lower epiphysis (separation) of femur**
> **Excludes1** Salter-Harris Type I physeal fracture of lower end of femur (S79.11-)

● **S72.441 Displaced fracture of lower epiphysis (separation) of right femur A, B, C** 🅒🅒

● **S72.442 Displaced fracture of lower epiphysis (separation) of left femur A, B, C** 🅒🅒

● **S72.443 Displaced fracture of lower epiphysis (separation) of unspecified femur A, B, C** 🅒🅒

● **S72.444 Nondisplaced fracture of lower epiphysis (separation) of right femur A, B, C** 🅒🅒

● **S72.445 Nondisplaced fracture of lower epiphysis (separation) of left femur A, B, C** 🅒🅒

● **S72.446 Nondisplaced fracture of lower epiphysis (separation) of unspecified femur A, B, C** 🅒🅒

● **S72.45 Supracondylar fracture without intracondylar extension of lower end of femur**
Supracondylar fracture of lower end of femur NOS
> **Excludes1** supracondylar fracture with intracondylar extension of lower end of femur (S72.46-)

● **S72.451 Displaced supracondylar fracture without intracondylar extension of lower end of right femur A, B, C** 🅒🅒

● **S72.452 Displaced supracondylar fracture without intracondylar extension of lower end of left femur A, B, C** 🅒🅒

● **S72.453 Displaced supracondylar fracture without intracondylar extension of lower end of unspecified femur A, B, C** 🅒🅒

● **S72.454 Nondisplaced supracondylar fracture without intracondylar extension of lower end of right femur A, B, C** 🅒🅒

● **S72.455 Nondisplaced supracondylar fracture without intracondylar extension of lower end of left femur A, B, C** 🅒🅒

● **S72.456 Nondisplaced supracondylar fracture without intracondylar extension of lower end of unspecified femur A, B, C** 🅒🅒

● **S72.46 Supracondylar fracture with intracondylar extension of lower end of femur**
> **Excludes1** supracondylar fracture without intracondylar extension of lower end of femur (S72.45-)

● **S72.461 Displaced supracondylar fracture with intracondylar extension of lower end of right femur A, B, C** 🅒🅒

● **S72.462 Displaced supracondylar fracture with intracondylar extension of lower end of left femur A, B, C** 🅒🅒

● **S72.463 Displaced supracondylar fracture with intracondylar extension of lower end of unspecified femur A, B, C** 🅒🅒

● **S72.464 Nondisplaced supracondylar fracture with intracondylar extension of lower end of right femur A, B, C** 🅒🅒

● **S72.465 Nondisplaced supracondylar fracture with intracondylar extension of lower end of left femur A, B, C** 🅒🅒

● **S72.466 Nondisplaced supracondylar fracture with intracondylar extension of lower end of unspecified femur A, B, C** 🅒🅒

● **S72.47 Torus fracture of lower end of femur**
The appropriate 7th character is to be added to all codes in subcategory S72.47

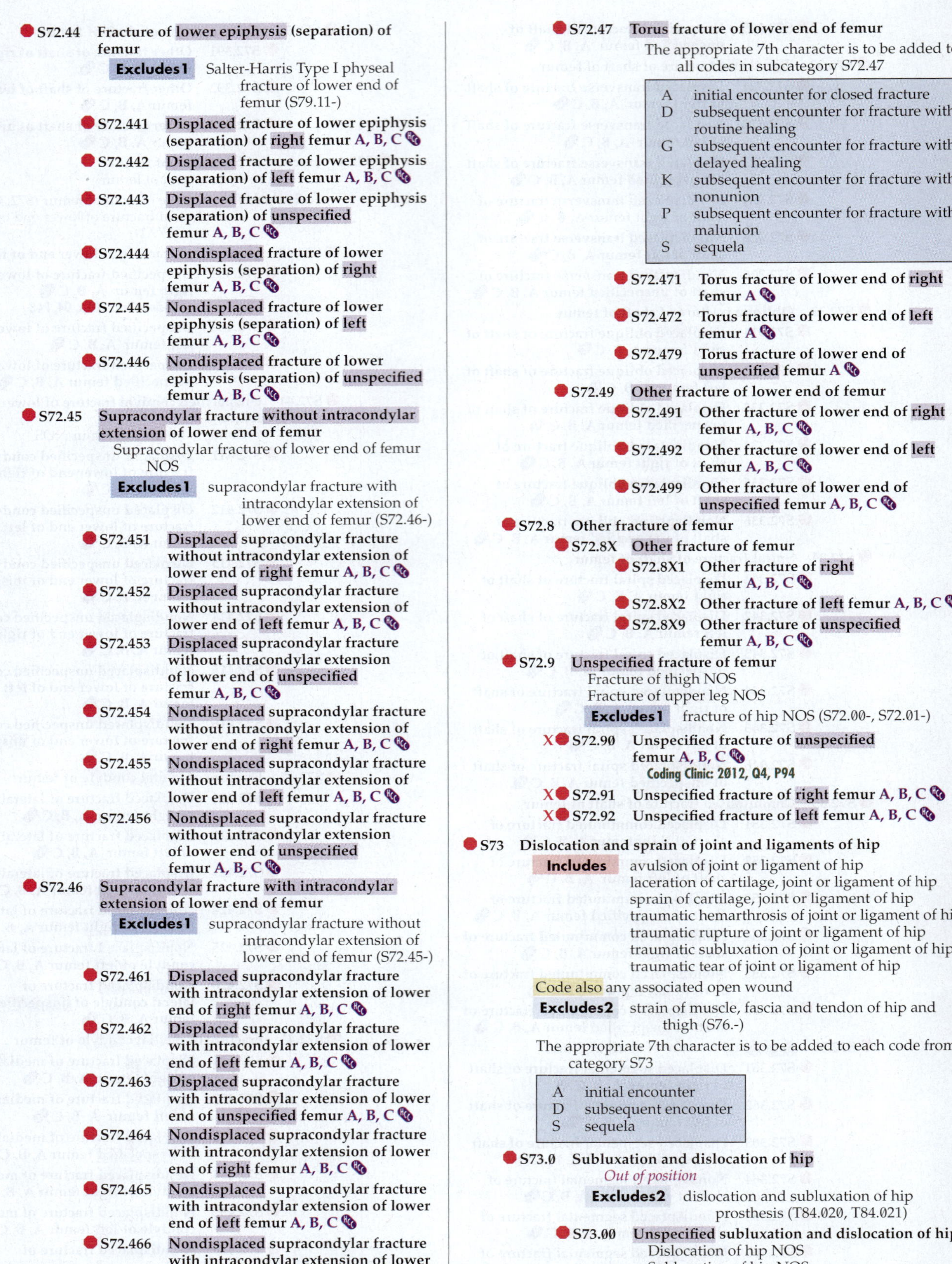

● **S72.471 Torus fracture of lower end of right femur A** 🅒🅒

● **S72.472 Torus fracture of lower end of left femur A** 🅒🅒

● **S72.479 Torus fracture of lower end of unspecified femur A** 🅒🅒

● **S72.49 Other fracture of lower end of femur**

● **S72.491 Other fracture of lower end of right femur A, B, C** 🅒🅒

● **S72.492 Other fracture of lower end of left femur A, B, C** 🅒🅒

● **S72.499 Other fracture of lower end of unspecified femur A, B, C** 🅒🅒

● **S72.8 Other fracture of femur**

● **S72.8X Other fracture of femur**

● **S72.8X1 Other fracture of right femur A, B, C** 🅒🅒

● **S72.8X2 Other fracture of left femur A, B, C** 🅒🅒

● **S72.8X9 Other fracture of unspecified femur A, B, C** 🅒🅒

● **S72.9 Unspecified fracture of femur**
Fracture of thigh NOS
Fracture of upper leg NOS
> **Excludes1** fracture of hip NOS (S72.00-, S72.01-)

X ● **S72.90 Unspecified fracture of unspecified femur A, B, C** 🅒🅒
Coding Clinic: 2012, Q4, P94

X ● **S72.91 Unspecified fracture of right femur A, B, C** 🅒🅒

X ● **S72.92 Unspecified fracture of left femur A, B, C** 🅒🅒

● **S73 Dislocation and sprain of joint and ligaments of hip**
> **Includes** avulsion of joint or ligament of hip
> laceration of cartilage, joint or ligament of hip
> sprain of cartilage, joint or ligament of hip
> traumatic hemarthrosis of joint or ligament of hip
> traumatic rupture of joint or ligament of hip
> traumatic subluxation of joint or ligament of hip
> traumatic tear of joint or ligament of hip

Code also any associated open wound
> **Excludes2** strain of muscle, fascia and tendon of hip and thigh (S76.-)

The appropriate 7th character is to be added to each code from category S73

A initial encounter
D subsequent encounter
S sequela

● **S73.0 Subluxation and dislocation of hip**
Out of position
> **Excludes2** dislocation and subluxation of hip prosthesis (T84.020, T84.021)

● **S73.00 Unspecified subluxation and dislocation of hip**
Dislocation of hip NOS
Subluxation of hip NOS

● **S73.001 Unspecified subluxation of right hip A** 🅒🅒

- ● S73.002   Unspecified subluxation of left hip A ⓡ
- ● S73.003   Unspecified subluxation of unspecified hip A ⓡ
- ● S73.004   Unspecified dislocation of right hip A ⓡ
- ● S73.005   Unspecified dislocation of left hip A ⓡ
- ● S73.006   Unspecified dislocation of unspecified hip A ⓡ
- ● S73.01   Posterior subluxation and dislocation of hip
  - ● S73.011   Posterior subluxation of right hip A ⓡ
  - ● S73.012   Posterior subluxation of left hip A ⓡ
  - ● S73.013   Posterior subluxation of unspecified hip A ⓡ
  - ● S73.014   Posterior dislocation of right hip A ⓡ
  - ● S73.015   Posterior dislocation of left hip A ⓡ
  - ● S73.016   Posterior dislocation of unspecified hip A ⓡ
- ● S73.02   Obturator subluxation and dislocation of hip
  - ● S73.021   Obturator subluxation of right hip A ⓡ
  - ● S73.022   Obturator subluxation of left hip A ⓡ
  - ● S73.023   Obturator subluxation of unspecified hip A ⓡ
  - ● S73.024   Obturator dislocation of right hip A ⓡ
  - ● S73.025   Obturator dislocation of left hip A ⓡ
  - ● S73.026   Obturator dislocation of unspecified hip A ⓡ
- ● S73.03   Other anterior subluxation and dislocation of hip
  - ● S73.031   Other anterior subluxation of right hip A ⓡ
  - ● S73.032   Other anterior subluxation of left hip A ⓡ
  - ● S73.033   Other anterior subluxation of unspecified hip A ⓡ
  - ● S73.034   Other anterior dislocation of right hip A ⓡ
  - ● S73.035   Other anterior dislocation of left hip A ⓡ
  - ● S73.036   Other anterior dislocation of unspecified hip A ⓡ
- ● S73.04   Central subluxation and dislocation of hip
  - ● S73.041   Central subluxation of right hip A ⓡ
  - ● S73.042   Central subluxation of left hip A ⓡ
  - ● S73.043   Central subluxation of unspecified hip A ⓡ
  - ● S73.044   Central dislocation of right hip A ⓡ
  - ● S73.045   Central dislocation of left hip A ⓡ
  - ● S73.046   Central dislocation of unspecified hip A ⓡ
- ● S73.1   Sprain of hip
  - ● S73.10   Unspecified sprain of hip
    - ● S73.101   Unspecified sprain of right hip
    - ● S73.102   Unspecified sprain of left hip
    - ● S73.109   Unspecified sprain of unspecified hip
  - ● S73.11   Iliofemoral ligament sprain of hip
    - ● S73.111   Iliofemoral ligament sprain of right hip
    - ● S73.112   Iliofemoral ligament sprain of left hip
    - ● S73.119   Iliofemoral ligament sprain of unspecified hip

- ● S73.12   Ischiocapsular (ligament) sprain of hip
  - ● S73.121   Ischiocapsular ligament sprain of right hip
  - ● S73.122   Ischiocapsular ligament sprain of left hip
  - ● S73.129   Ischiocapsular ligament sprain of unspecified hip
- ● S73.19   Other sprain of hip
  - ● S73.191   Other sprain of right hip
  - ● S73.192   Other sprain of left hip
  - ● S73.199   Other sprain of unspecified hip

- ● S74   **Injury of nerves at hip and thigh level**
  - Code also any associated open wound (S71.-)
  - **Excludes2**   injury of nerves at ankle and foot level (S94.-)
    injury of nerves at lower leg level (S84.-)
  - The appropriate 7th character is to be added to each code from category S74

A	initial encounter
D	subsequent encounter
S	sequela

  - ● S74.0   Injury of sciatic nerve at hip and thigh level
    - ✕ ● S74.00   Injury of sciatic nerve at hip and thigh level, unspecified leg
    - ✕ ● S74.01   Injury of sciatic nerve at hip and thigh level, right leg
    - ✕ ● S74.02   Injury of sciatic nerve at hip and thigh level, left leg
  - ● S74.1   Injury of femoral nerve at hip and thigh level
    - ✕ ● S74.10   Injury of femoral nerve at hip and thigh level, unspecified leg
    - ✕ ● S74.11   Injury of femoral nerve at hip and thigh level, right leg
    - ✕ ● S74.12   Injury of femoral nerve at hip and thigh level, left leg
  - ● S74.2   Injury of cutaneous sensory nerve at hip and thigh level
    - ✕ ● S74.20   Injury of cutaneous sensory nerve at hip and thigh level, unspecified leg
    - ➡ ✕ ● S74.21   Injury of cutaneous sensory nerve at hip and thigh level, right leg
    - ✕ ● S74.22   Injury of cutaneous sensory nerve at hip and thigh level, left leg
  - ● S74.8   Injury of other nerves at hip and thigh level
    - ● S74.8X   Injury of other nerves at hip and thigh level
      - ● S74.8X1   Injury of other nerves at hip and thigh level, right leg
      - ● S74.8X2   Injury of other nerves at hip and thigh level, left leg
      - ● S74.8X9   Injury of other nerves at hip and thigh level, unspecified leg
  - ● S74.9   Injury of unspecified nerve at hip and thigh level
    - ✕ ● S74.90   Injury of unspecified nerve at hip and thigh level, unspecified leg
    - ✕ ● S74.91   Injury of unspecified nerve at hip and thigh level, right leg
    - ✕ ● S74.92   Injury of unspecified nerve at hip and thigh level, left leg

- ● S75   **Injury of blood vessels at hip and thigh level**
  - Code also any associated open wound (S71.-)
  - **Excludes2**   injury of blood vessels at lower leg level (S85.-)
    injury of popliteal artery (S85.0)
  - The appropriate 7th character is to be added to each code from category S75

A	initial encounter
D	subsequent encounter
S	sequela

CHAPTER 19 (S00-T88)

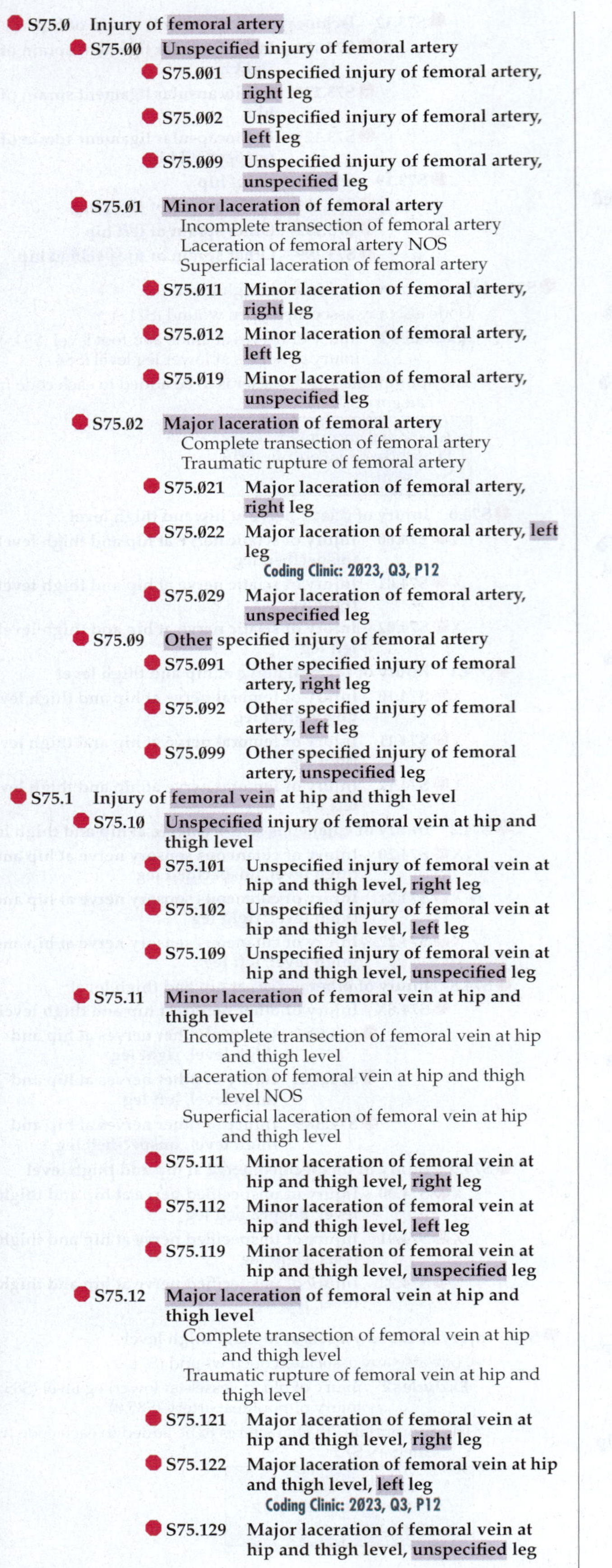

- ● **S75.0**   **Injury of femoral artery**
  - ● **S75.00**   **Unspecified injury of femoral artery**
    - ● **S75.001**   Unspecified injury of femoral artery, right leg
    - ● **S75.002**   Unspecified injury of femoral artery, left leg
    - ● **S75.009**   Unspecified injury of femoral artery, unspecified leg
  - ● **S75.01**   **Minor laceration of femoral artery**
    Incomplete transection of femoral artery
    Laceration of femoral artery NOS
    Superficial laceration of femoral artery
    - ● **S75.011**   Minor laceration of femoral artery, right leg
    - ● **S75.012**   Minor laceration of femoral artery, left leg
    - ● **S75.019**   Minor laceration of femoral artery, unspecified leg
  - ● **S75.02**   **Major laceration of femoral artery**
    Complete transection of femoral artery
    Traumatic rupture of femoral artery
    - ● **S75.021**   Major laceration of femoral artery, right leg
    - ● **S75.022**   Major laceration of femoral artery, left leg
      Coding Clinic: 2023, Q3, P12
    - ● **S75.029**   Major laceration of femoral artery, unspecified leg
  - ● **S75.09**   **Other specified injury of femoral artery**
    - ● **S75.091**   Other specified injury of femoral artery, right leg
    - ● **S75.092**   Other specified injury of femoral artery, left leg
    - ● **S75.099**   Other specified injury of femoral artery, unspecified leg
- ● **S75.1**   **Injury of femoral vein at hip and thigh level**
  - ● **S75.10**   **Unspecified injury of femoral vein at hip and thigh level**
    - ● **S75.101**   Unspecified injury of femoral vein at hip and thigh level, right leg
    - ● **S75.102**   Unspecified injury of femoral vein at hip and thigh level, left leg
    - ● **S75.109**   Unspecified injury of femoral vein at hip and thigh level, unspecified leg
  - ● **S75.11**   **Minor laceration of femoral vein at hip and thigh level**
    Incomplete transection of femoral vein at hip and thigh level
    Laceration of femoral vein at hip and thigh level NOS
    Superficial laceration of femoral vein at hip and thigh level
    - ● **S75.111**   Minor laceration of femoral vein at hip and thigh level, right leg
    - ● **S75.112**   Minor laceration of femoral vein at hip and thigh level, left leg
    - ● **S75.119**   Minor laceration of femoral vein at hip and thigh level, unspecified leg
  - ● **S75.12**   **Major laceration of femoral vein at hip and thigh level**
    Complete transection of femoral vein at hip and thigh level
    Traumatic rupture of femoral vein at hip and thigh level
    - ● **S75.121**   Major laceration of femoral vein at hip and thigh level, right leg
    - ● **S75.122**   Major laceration of femoral vein at hip and thigh level, left leg
      Coding Clinic: 2023, Q3, P12
    - ● **S75.129**   Major laceration of femoral vein at hip and thigh level, unspecified leg
- ● **S75.19**   **Other specified injury of femoral vein at hip and thigh level**
  - ● **S75.191**   Other specified injury of femoral vein at hip and thigh level, right leg
  - ● **S75.192**   Other specified injury of femoral vein at hip and thigh level, left leg
  - ● **S75.199**   Other specified injury of femoral vein at hip and thigh level, unspecified leg
- ● **S75.2**   **Injury of greater saphenous vein at hip and thigh level**
  Excludes1   greater saphenous vein NOS (S85.3)
  - ● **S75.20**   **Unspecified injury of greater saphenous vein at hip and thigh level**
    - ● **S75.201**   Unspecified injury of greater saphenous vein at hip and thigh level, right leg
    - ● **S75.202**   Unspecified injury of greater saphenous vein at hip and thigh level, left leg
    - ● **S75.209**   Unspecified injury of greater saphenous vein at hip and thigh level, unspecified leg
  - ● **S75.21**   **Minor laceration of greater saphenous vein at hip and thigh level**
    Incomplete transection of greater saphenous vein at hip and thigh level
    Laceration of greater saphenous vein at hip and thigh level NOS
    Superficial laceration of greater saphenous vein at hip and thigh level
    - ● **S75.211**   Minor laceration of greater saphenous vein at hip and thigh level, right leg
    - ● **S75.212**   Minor laceration of greater saphenous vein at hip and thigh level, left leg
    - ● **S75.219**   Minor laceration of greater saphenous vein at hip and thigh level, unspecified leg
  - ● **S75.22**   **Major laceration of greater saphenous vein at hip and thigh level**
    Complete transection of greater saphenous vein at hip and thigh level
    Traumatic rupture of greater saphenous vein at hip and thigh level
    - ● **S75.221**   Major laceration of greater saphenous vein at hip and thigh level, right leg
    - ● **S75.222**   Major laceration of greater saphenous vein at hip and thigh level, left leg
    - ● **S75.229**   Major laceration of greater saphenous vein at hip and thigh level, unspecified leg
  - ● **S75.29**   **Other specified injury of greater saphenous vein at hip and thigh level**
    - ● **S75.291**   Other specified injury of greater saphenous vein at hip and thigh level, right leg
    - ● **S75.292**   Other specified injury of greater saphenous vein at hip and thigh level, left leg
    - ● **S75.299**   Other specified injury of greater saphenous vein at hip and thigh level, unspecified leg
- ● **S75.8**   **Injury of other blood vessels at hip and thigh level**
  - ● **S75.80**   **Unspecified injury of other blood vessels at hip and thigh level**
    - ● **S75.801**   Unspecified injury of other blood vessels at hip and thigh level, right leg
    - ● **S75.802**   Unspecified injury of other blood vessels at hip and thigh level, left leg
    - ● **S75.809**   Unspecified injury of other blood vessels at hip and thigh level, unspecified leg

- ● S75.81   Laceration of other blood vessels at hip and thigh level
  - ● S75.811   Laceration of other blood vessels at hip and thigh level, right leg
  - ● S75.812   Laceration of other blood vessels at hip and thigh level, left leg
  - ● S75.819   Laceration of other blood vessels at hip and thigh level, unspecified leg
- ● S75.89   Other specified injury of other blood vessels at hip and thigh level
  - ● S75.891   Other specified injury of other blood vessels at hip and thigh level, right leg
  - ● S75.892   Other specified injury of other blood vessels at hip and thigh level, left leg
  - ● S75.899   Other specified injury of other blood vessels at hip and thigh level, unspecified leg
- ● S75.9   Injury of unspecified blood vessel at hip and thigh level
  - ● S75.90   Unspecified injury of unspecified blood vessel at hip and thigh level
    - ● S75.901   Unspecified injury of unspecified blood vessel at hip and thigh level, right leg
    - ● S75.902   Unspecified injury of unspecified blood vessel at hip and thigh level, left leg
    - ● S75.909   Unspecified injury of unspecified blood vessel at hip and thigh level, unspecified leg
  - ● S75.91   Laceration of unspecified blood vessel at hip and thigh level
    - ● S75.911   Laceration of unspecified blood vessel at hip and thigh level, right leg
    - ● S75.912   Laceration of unspecified blood vessel at hip and thigh level, left leg
    - ● S75.919   Laceration of unspecified blood vessel at hip and thigh level, unspecified leg
  - ● S75.99   Other specified injury of unspecified blood vessel at hip and thigh level
    - ● S75.991   Other specified injury of unspecified blood vessel at hip and thigh level, right leg
    - ● S75.992   Other specified injury of unspecified blood vessel at hip and thigh level, left leg
    - ● S75.999   Other specified injury of unspecified blood vessel at hip and thigh level, unspecified leg

- ● S76   **Injury of muscle, fascia and tendon at hip and thigh level**

  Code also any associated open wound (S71.-)

  Excludes2   injury of muscle, fascia and tendon at lower leg level (S86)

         sprain of joint and ligament of hip (S73.1)

  The appropriate 7th character is to be added to each code from category S76

A	initial encounter
D	subsequent encounter
S	sequela

  - ● S76.0   Injury of muscle, fascia and tendon of hip
    - ● S76.00   Unspecified injury of muscle, fascia and tendon of hip
      - ● S76.001   Unspecified injury of muscle, fascia and tendon of right hip
      - ● S76.002   Unspecified injury of muscle, fascia and tendon of left hip
      - ● S76.009   Unspecified injury of muscle, fascia and tendon of unspecified hip
    - ● S76.01   Strain of muscle, fascia and tendon of hip
      - ● S76.011   Strain of muscle, fascia and tendon of right hip
      - ● S76.012   Strain of muscle, fascia and tendon of left hip
      - ● S76.019   Strain of muscle, fascia and tendon of unspecified hip
    - ● S76.02   Laceration of muscle, fascia and tendon of hip
      - ● S76.021   Laceration of muscle, fascia and tendon of right hip
      - ● S76.022   Laceration of muscle, fascia and tendon of left hip
      - ● S76.029   Laceration of muscle, fascia and tendon of unspecified hip
    - ● S76.09   Other specified injury of muscle, fascia and tendon of hip
      - ● S76.091   Other specified injury of muscle, fascia and tendon of right hip
      - ● S76.092   Other specified injury of muscle, fascia and tendon of left hip
      - ● S76.099   Other specified injury of muscle, fascia and tendon of unspecified hip
  - ● S76.1   Injury of quadriceps muscle, fascia and tendon

    Injury of patellar ligament (tendon)

    - ● S76.10   Unspecified injury of quadriceps muscle, fascia and tendon
      - ● S76.101   Unspecified injury of right quadriceps muscle, fascia and tendon
      - ● S76.102   Unspecified injury of left quadriceps muscle, fascia and tendon
      - ● S76.109   Unspecified injury of unspecified quadriceps muscle, fascia and tendon
    - ● S76.11   Strain of quadriceps muscle, fascia and tendon
      - ● S76.111   Strain of right quadriceps muscle, fascia and tendon
      - ● S76.112   Strain of left quadriceps muscle, fascia and tendon
      - ● S76.119   Strain of unspecified quadriceps muscle, fascia and tendon
    - ● S76.12   Laceration of quadriceps muscle, fascia and tendon
      - ● S76.121   Laceration of right quadriceps muscle, fascia and tendon
      - ● S76.122   Laceration of left quadriceps muscle, fascia and tendon
      - ● S76.129   Laceration of unspecified quadriceps muscle, fascia and tendon
    - ● S76.19   Other specified injury of quadriceps muscle, fascia and tendon
      - ● S76.191   Other specified injury of right quadriceps muscle, fascia and tendon
      - ● S76.192   Other specified injury of left quadriceps muscle, fascia and tendon
      - ● S76.199   Other specified injury of unspecified quadriceps muscle, fascia and tendon
  - ● S76.2   Injury of adductor muscle, fascia and tendon of thigh
    - ● S76.20   Unspecified injury of adductor muscle, fascia and tendon of thigh
      - ● S76.201   Unspecified injury of adductor muscle, fascia and tendon of right thigh
      - ● S76.202   Unspecified injury of adductor muscle, fascia and tendon of left thigh
      - ● S76.209   Unspecified injury of adductor muscle, fascia and tendon of unspecified thigh

CHAPTER 19 (S00–T88)

● S76.21   **Strain** of adductor muscle, fascia and tendon of thigh
   ● S76.211   Strain of adductor muscle, fascia and tendon of **right** thigh
   ● S76.212   Strain of adductor muscle, fascia and tendon of **left** thigh
   ● S76.219   Strain of adductor muscle, fascia and tendon of **unspecified** thigh
● S76.22   **Laceration** of adductor muscle, fascia and tendon of thigh
   ● S76.221   Laceration of adductor muscle, fascia and tendon of **right** thigh
   ● S76.222   Laceration of adductor muscle, fascia and tendon of **left** thigh
   ● S76.229   Laceration of adductor muscle, fascia and tendon of **unspecified** thigh
● S76.29   **Other** injury of adductor muscle, fascia and tendon of thigh
   ● S76.291   Other injury of adductor muscle, fascia and tendon of **right** thigh
   ● S76.292   Other injury of adductor muscle, fascia and tendon of **left** thigh
   ● S76.299   Other injury of adductor muscle, fascia and tendon of **unspecified** thigh

● S76.3   Injury of muscle, fascia and tendon of the **posterior** muscle group at thigh level
  ● S76.30   **Unspecified** injury of muscle, fascia and tendon of the posterior muscle group at thigh level
   ● S76.301   Unspecified injury of muscle, fascia and tendon of the posterior muscle group at thigh level, **right** thigh
   ● S76.302   Unspecified injury of muscle, fascia and tendon of the posterior muscle group at thigh level, **left** thigh
   ● S76.309   Unspecified injury of muscle, fascia and tendon of the posterior muscle group at thigh level, **unspecified thigh**
  ● S76.31   **Strain** of muscle, fascia and tendon of the posterior muscle group at thigh level
   ● S76.311   Strain of muscle, fascia and tendon of the posterior muscle group at thigh level, **right** thigh
   ● S76.312   Strain of muscle, fascia and tendon of the posterior muscle group at thigh level, **left** thigh
   ● S76.319   Strain of muscle, fascia and tendon of the posterior muscle group at thigh level, **unspecified** thigh
  ● S76.32   **Laceration** of muscle, fascia and tendon of the posterior muscle group at thigh level
   ● S76.321   Laceration of muscle, fascia and tendon of the posterior muscle group at thigh level, **right** thigh
   ● S76.322   Laceration of muscle, fascia and tendon of the posterior muscle group at thigh level, **left** thigh
   ● S76.329   Laceration of muscle, fascia and tendon of the posterior muscle group at thigh level, **unspecified** thigh
  ● S76.39   **Other** specified injury of muscle, fascia and tendon of the posterior muscle group at thigh level
   ● S76.391   Other specified injury of muscle, fascia and tendon of the posterior muscle group at thigh level, **right** thigh
   ● S76.392   Other specified injury of muscle, fascia and tendon of the posterior muscle group at thigh level, **left** thigh
   ● S76.399   Other specified injury of muscle, fascia and tendon of the posterior muscle group at thigh level, **unspecified thigh**

● S76.8   Injury of other specified muscles, fascia and tendons at thigh level
  ● S76.80   **Unspecified** injury of other specified muscles, fascia and tendons at thigh level
   ● S76.801   Unspecified injury of other specified muscles, fascia and tendons at thigh level, **right** thigh
   ● S76.802   Unspecified injury of other specified muscles, fascia and tendons at thigh level, **left** thigh
   ● S76.809   Unspecified injury of other specified muscles, fascia and tendons at thigh level, **unspecified** thigh
  ● S76.81   **Strain** of other specified specified muscles, fascia and tendons at thigh level
   ● S76.811   Strain of other specified muscles, fascia and tendons at thigh level, **right** thigh
   ● S76.812   Strain of other specified muscles, fascia and tendons at thigh level, **left** thigh
   ● S76.819   Strain of other specified muscles, fascia and tendons at thigh level, **unspecified** thigh
  ● S76.82   **Laceration** of other specified muscles, fascia and tendons at thigh level
   ● S76.821   Laceration of other specified muscles, fascia and tendons at thigh level, **right** thigh
   ● S76.822   Laceration of other specified muscles, fascia and tendons at thigh level, **left** thigh
   ● S76.829   Laceration of other specified muscles, fascia and tendons at thigh level, **unspecified** thigh
  ● S76.89   **Other** injury of other specified muscles, fascia and tendons at thigh level
   ● S76.891   Other injury of other specified muscles, fascia and tendons at thigh level, **right** thigh
   ● S76.892   Other injury of other specified muscles, fascia and tendons at thigh level, **left** thigh
   ● S76.899   Other injury of other specified muscles, fascia and tendons at thigh level, **unspecified** thigh

● S76.9   Injury of **unspecified** muscles, fascia and tendons at thigh level
  ● S76.90   **Unspecified** injury of unspecified muscles, fascia and tendons at thigh level
   ● S76.901   Unspecified injury of unspecified muscles, fascia and tendons at thigh level, **right** thigh
   ● S76.902   Unspecified injury of unspecified muscles, fascia and tendons at thigh level, **left** thigh
   ● S76.909   Unspecified injury of unspecified muscles, fascia and tendons at thigh level, **unspecified** thigh
  ● S76.91   **Strain** of unspecified muscles, fascia and tendons at thigh level
   ● S76.911   Strain of unspecified muscles, fascia and tendons at thigh level, **right** thigh
   ● S76.912   Strain of unspecified muscles, fascia and tendons at thigh level, **left** thigh
   ● S76.919   Strain of unspecified muscles fascia and tendons at thigh level, **unspecified** thigh

CHAPTER 19 (S00-T88)

● **S76.92** Laceration of unspecified muscles, fascia and tendons at thigh level
   ● **S76.921** Laceration of unspecified muscles, fascia and tendons at thigh level, **right** thigh
   ● **S76.922** Laceration of unspecified muscles, fascia and tendons at thigh level, **left** thigh
   ● **S76.929** Laceration of unspecified muscles, fascia and tendons at thigh level, **unspecified** thigh
  ● **S76.99** Other specified injury of unspecified muscles, fascia and tendons at thigh level
   ● **S76.991** Other specified injury of unspecified muscles, fascia and tendons at thigh level, **right** thigh
   ● **S76.992** Other specified injury of unspecified muscles, fascia and tendons at thigh level, **left** thigh
   ● **S76.999** Other specified injury of unspecified muscles, fascia and tendons at thigh level, **unspecified** thigh

● **S77** Crushing injury of hip and thigh
Use additional code(s) for all associated injuries
Excludes2   crushing injury of ankle and foot (S97.-)
           crushing injury of lower leg (S87.-)
The appropriate 7th character is to be added to each code from category S77

A	initial encounter
D	subsequent encounter
S	sequela

  ● **S77.0** Crushing injury of hip
   X● **S77.00** Crushing injury of **unspecified** hip
   X● **S77.01** Crushing injury of **right** hip
   X● **S77.02** Crushing injury of **left** hip
  ● **S77.1** Crushing injury of thigh
   X● **S77.10** Crushing injury of **unspecified** thigh
   X● **S77.11** Crushing injury of **right** thigh
   X● **S77.12** Crushing injury of **left** thigh
  ● **S77.2** Crushing injury of hip with thigh
   X● **S77.20** Crushing injury of **unspecified** hip with thigh
   X● **S77.21** Crushing injury of **right** hip with thigh
   X● **S77.22** Crushing injury of **left** hip with thigh

● **S78** Traumatic amputation of hip and thigh
An amputation not identified as partial or complete should be coded to complete
Excludes1   traumatic amputation of knee (S88.0-)
The appropriate 7th character is to be added to each code from category S78

A	initial encounter
D	subsequent encounter
S	sequela

  ● **S78.0** Traumatic amputation at hip joint
   ● **S78.01** Complete traumatic amputation at hip joint
    ● **S78.011** Complete traumatic amputation at **right** hip joint A, D, S
    ● **S78.012** Complete traumatic amputation at **left** hip joint A, D, S
    ● **S78.019** Complete traumatic amputation at **unspecified** hip joint A, D, S
   ● **S78.02** Partial traumatic amputation at hip joint
    ● **S78.021** Partial traumatic amputation at **right** hip joint A, D, S
    ● **S78.022** Partial traumatic amputation at **left** hip joint A, D, S
    ● **S78.029** Partial traumatic amputation at **unspecified** hip joint A, D, S

● **S78.1** Traumatic amputation at level between hip and knee
Excludes1   traumatic amputation of knee (S88.0-)
  ● **S78.11** Complete traumatic amputation at level between hip and knee
   ● **S78.111** Complete traumatic amputation at level between **right** hip and knee A, D, S
   ● **S78.112** Complete traumatic amputation at level between **left** hip and knee A, D, S
   ● **S78.119** Complete traumatic amputation at level between **unspecified** hip and knee A, D, S
  ● **S78.12** Partial traumatic amputation at level between hip and knee
   ● **S78.121** Partial traumatic amputation at level between **right** hip and knee A, D, S
   ● **S78.122** Partial traumatic amputation at level between **left** hip and knee A, D, S
   ● **S78.129** Partial traumatic amputation at level between **unspecified** hip and knee A, D, S

● **S78.9** Traumatic amputation of hip and thigh, **level** unspecified
  ● **S78.91** Complete traumatic amputation of hip and thigh, level unspecified
   ● **S78.911** Complete traumatic amputation of **right** hip and thigh, level unspecified A, D, S
   ● **S78.912** Complete traumatic amputation of **left** hip and thigh, level unspecified A, D, S
   ● **S78.919** Complete traumatic amputation of **unspecified** hip and thigh, level unspecified A, D, S
  ● **S78.92** Partial traumatic amputation of hip and thigh, level unspecified
   ● **S78.921** Partial traumatic amputation of **right** hip and thigh, level unspecified A, D, S
   ● **S78.922** Partial traumatic amputation of **left** hip and thigh, level unspecified A, D, S
   ● **S78.929** Partial traumatic amputation of **unspecified** hip and thigh, level unspecified A, D, S

● **S79** Other and unspecified injuries of hip and thigh
Note: A fracture not indicated as open or closed should be coded to closed
The appropriate 7th character is to be added to each code from subcategories S79.0 and S79.1

A	initial encounter for closed fracture
D	subsequent encounter for fracture with routine healing
G	subsequent encounter for fracture with delayed healing
K	subsequent encounter for fracture with nonunion
P	subsequent encounter for fracture with malunion
S	sequela

Item 19–5   SALTER-HARRIS TYPE 1: epiphysis is completely separated from end of bone, or metaphysic growth plate remains attached to epiphysis
   SALTER-HARRIS TYPE 2: epiphysis and growth plate are partially separated from metaphysis, which is cracked—most common type
   SALTER-HARRIS TYPE 3: fracture occurring through epiphysis and separates part of epiphysis and growth plate from metaphysis fracture, usually at distal end of tibia
   SALTER-HARRIS TYPE 4: fracture runs through epiphysis, across growth plate, into metaphysic; surgery is required to restore joint surface to normal and align growth plate

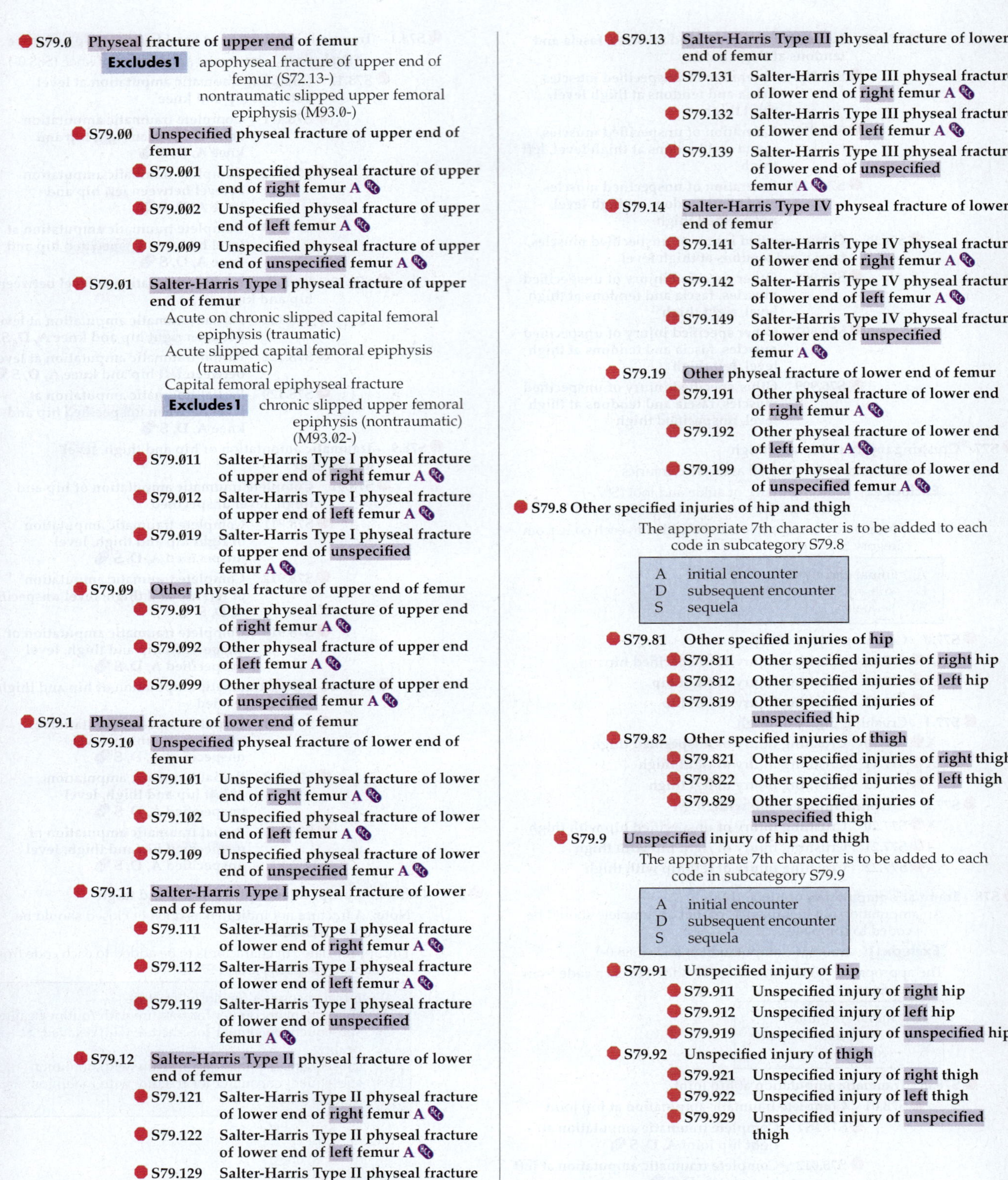

● **S79.0** Physeal fracture of **upper end** of femur
  Excludes1 apophyseal fracture of upper end of femur (S72.13-)
  nontraumatic slipped upper femoral epiphysis (M93.0-)

● **S79.00** **Unspecified** physeal fracture of upper end of femur
  ● **S79.001** Unspecified physeal fracture of upper end of **right** femur **A**
  ● **S79.002** Unspecified physeal fracture of upper end of **left** femur **A**
  ● **S79.009** Unspecified physeal fracture of upper end of **unspecified** femur **A**

● **S79.01** **Salter-Harris Type I** physeal fracture of upper end of femur
  Acute on chronic slipped capital femoral epiphysis (traumatic)
  Acute slipped capital femoral epiphysis (traumatic)
  Capital femoral epiphyseal fracture
  Excludes1 chronic slipped upper femoral epiphysis (nontraumatic) (M93.02-)
  ● **S79.011** Salter-Harris Type I physeal fracture of upper end of **right** femur **A**
  ● **S79.012** Salter-Harris Type I physeal fracture of upper end of **left** femur **A**
  ● **S79.019** Salter-Harris Type I physeal fracture of upper end of **unspecified** femur **A**

● **S79.09** Other physeal fracture of upper end of femur
  ● **S79.091** Other physeal fracture of upper end of **right** femur **A**
  ● **S79.092** Other physeal fracture of upper end of **left** femur **A**
  ● **S79.099** Other physeal fracture of upper end of **unspecified** femur **A**

● **S79.1** Physeal fracture of **lower end** of femur
● **S79.10** **Unspecified** physeal fracture of lower end of femur
  ● **S79.101** Unspecified physeal fracture of lower end of **right** femur **A**
  ● **S79.102** Unspecified physeal fracture of lower end of **left** femur **A**
  ● **S79.109** Unspecified physeal fracture of lower end of **unspecified** femur **A**

● **S79.11** **Salter-Harris Type I** physeal fracture of lower end of femur
  ● **S79.111** Salter-Harris Type I physeal fracture of lower end of **right** femur **A**
  ● **S79.112** Salter-Harris Type I physeal fracture of lower end of **left** femur **A**
  ● **S79.119** Salter-Harris Type I physeal fracture of lower end of **unspecified** femur **A**

● **S79.12** **Salter-Harris Type II** physeal fracture of lower end of femur
  ● **S79.121** Salter-Harris Type II physeal fracture of lower end of **right** femur **A**
  ● **S79.122** Salter-Harris Type II physeal fracture of lower end of **left** femur **A**
  ● **S79.129** Salter-Harris Type II physeal fracture of lower end of **unspecified** femur **A**

● **S79.13** **Salter-Harris Type III** physeal fracture of lower end of femur
  ● **S79.131** Salter-Harris Type III physeal fracture of lower end of **right** femur **A**
  ● **S79.132** Salter-Harris Type III physeal fracture of lower end of **left** femur **A**
  ● **S79.139** Salter-Harris Type III physeal fracture of lower end of **unspecified** femur **A**

● **S79.14** **Salter-Harris Type IV** physeal fracture of lower end of femur
  ● **S79.141** Salter-Harris Type IV physeal fracture of lower end of **right** femur **A**
  ● **S79.142** Salter-Harris Type IV physeal fracture of lower end of **left** femur **A**
  ● **S79.149** Salter-Harris Type IV physeal fracture of lower end of **unspecified** femur **A**

● **S79.19** Other physeal fracture of lower end of femur
  ● **S79.191** Other physeal fracture of lower end of **right** femur **A**
  ● **S79.192** Other physeal fracture of lower end of **left** femur **A**
  ● **S79.199** Other physeal fracture of lower end of **unspecified** femur **A**

● **S79.8 Other specified injuries of hip and thigh**
  The appropriate 7th character is to be added to each code in subcategory S79.8
A	initial encounter
D	subsequent encounter
S	sequela

● **S79.81** Other specified injuries of **hip**
  ● **S79.811** Other specified injuries of **right** hip
  ● **S79.812** Other specified injuries of **left** hip
  ● **S79.819** Other specified injuries of **unspecified** hip

● **S79.82** Other specified injuries of **thigh**
  ● **S79.821** Other specified injuries of **right** thigh
  ● **S79.822** Other specified injuries of **left** thigh
  ● **S79.829** Other specified injuries of **unspecified** thigh

● **S79.9** **Unspecified** injury of hip and thigh
  The appropriate 7th character is to be added to each code in subcategory S79.9
A	initial encounter
D	subsequent encounter
S	sequela

● **S79.91** Unspecified injury of **hip**
  ● **S79.911** Unspecified injury of **right** hip
  ● **S79.912** Unspecified injury of **left** hip
  ● **S79.919** Unspecified injury of **unspecified** hip

● **S79.92** Unspecified injury of **thigh**
  ● **S79.921** Unspecified injury of **right** thigh
  ● **S79.922** Unspecified injury of **left** thigh
  ● **S79.929** Unspecified injury of **unspecified** thigh

▶ New   ➡ Revised   ~~deleted~~ Deleted   Excludes 1   Excludes 2   Includes   Use additional   Code first   Code also   Key words
OGCR Official Guidelines   X Assign placeholder X   ● Use Additional Character(s)   ▶ Manifestation Code   Hierarchical Condition Category   **Coding Clinic**

CHAPTER 19 (S00-T88)

INJURIES TO THE KNEE AND LOWER LEG (S80-S89)

Excludes2   burns and corrosions (T20-T32)
           frostbite (T33-T34)
           injuries of ankle and foot, except fracture of ankle
              and malleolus (S90-S99)
           insect bite or sting, venomous (T63.4)

● **S80** **Superficial injury of knee and lower leg**

Excludes2   superficial injury of ankle and foot (S90.-)

The appropriate 7th character is to be added to each code from
category S80

A	initial encounter
D	subsequent encounter
S	sequela

● **S80.0** **Contusion of knee**
  X● **S80.00** Contusion of **unspecified** knee
  X● **S80.01** Contusion of **right** knee
  X● **S80.02** Contusion of **left** knee
● **S80.1** **Contusion of lower leg**
  X● **S80.10** Contusion of **unspecified** lower leg
  X● **S80.11** Contusion of **right** lower leg
  X● **S80.12** Contusion of **left** lower leg
● **S80.2** **Other superficial injuries of knee**
  ● **S80.21** **Abrasion of knee**
    ● **S80.211** Abrasion, **right** knee
    ● **S80.212** Abrasion, **left** knee
    ● **S80.219** Abrasion, **unspecified** knee
  ● **S80.22** **Blister (nonthermal) of knee**
    ● **S80.221** Blister (nonthermal), **right** knee
    ● **S80.222** Blister (nonthermal), **left** knee
    ● **S80.229** Blister (nonthermal), **unspecified** knee
  ● **S80.24** **External constriction of knee**
    ● **S80.241** External constriction, **right** knee
    ● **S80.242** External constriction, **left** knee
    ● **S80.249** External constriction, **unspecified** knee
  ● **S80.25** **Superficial foreign body of knee**
    Splinter in the knee
    ● **S80.251** Superficial foreign body, **right** knee
    ● **S80.252** Superficial foreign body, **left** knee
    ● **S80.259** Superficial foreign body, **unspecified** knee
  ● **S80.26** **Insect bite (nonvenomous) of knee**
    ● **S80.261** Insect bite (nonvenomous), **right** knee
    ● **S80.262** Insect bite (nonvenomous), **left** knee
    ● **S80.269** Insect bite (nonvenomous), **unspecified** knee
  ● **S80.27** **Other superficial bite of knee**
    Excludes1   open bite of knee (S81.05-)
    ● **S80.271** Other superficial bite of **right** knee
    ● **S80.272** Other superficial bite of **left** knee
    ● **S80.279** Other superficial bite of **unspecified** knee
● **S80.8** **Other superficial injuries of lower leg**
  ● **S80.81** **Abrasion of lower leg**
    ● **S80.811** Abrasion, **right** lower leg
    ● **S80.812** Abrasion, **left** lower leg
    ● **S80.819** Abrasion, **unspecified** lower leg
  ● **S80.82** **Blister (nonthermal) of lower leg**
    ● **S80.821** Blister (nonthermal), **right** lower leg
    ● **S80.822** Blister (nonthermal), **left** lower leg
    ● **S80.829** Blister (nonthermal), **unspecified** lower leg
  ● **S80.84** **External constriction of lower leg**
    ● **S80.841** External constriction, **right** lower leg
    ● **S80.842** External constriction, **left** lower leg
    ● **S80.849** External constriction, **unspecified** lower leg

  ● **S80.85** **Superficial foreign body of lower leg**
    Splinter in the lower leg
    ● **S80.851** Superficial foreign body, **right** lower leg
    ● **S80.852** Superficial foreign body, **left** lower leg
    ● **S80.859** Superficial foreign body, **unspecified** lower leg
  ● **S80.86** **Insect bite (nonvenomous) of lower leg**
    ● **S80.861** Insect bite (nonvenomous), **right** lower leg
    ● **S80.862** Insect bite (nonvenomous), **left** lower leg
    ● **S80.869** Insect bite (nonvenomous), **unspecified** lower leg
  ● **S80.87** **Other superficial bite of lower leg**
    Excludes1   open bite of lower leg (S81.85-)
    ● **S80.871** Other superficial bite, **right** lower leg
    ● **S80.872** Other superficial bite, **left** lower leg
    ● **S80.879** Other superficial bite, **unspecified** lower leg
● **S80.9** **Unspecified superficial injury of knee and lower leg**
  ● **S80.91** **Unspecified superficial injury of knee**
    ● **S80.911** Unspecified superficial injury of **right** knee
    ● **S80.912** Unspecified superficial injury of **left** knee
    ● **S80.919** Unspecified superficial injury of **unspecified** knee
  ● **S80.92** **Unspecified superficial injury of lower leg**
    ● **S80.921** Unspecified superficial injury of **right** lower leg
    ● **S80.922** Unspecified superficial injury of **left** lower leg
    ● **S80.929** Unspecified superficial injury of **unspecified** lower leg

● **S81** **Open wound of knee and lower leg**
Code also any associated wound infection
Excludes1   open fracture of knee and lower leg (S82.-)
                traumatic amputation of lower leg (S88.-)
Excludes2   open wound of ankle and foot (S91.-)

The appropriate 7th character is to be added to each code from
category S81

A	initial encounter
D	subsequent encounter
S	sequela

● **S81.0** **Open wound of knee**
  ● **S81.00** **Unspecified open wound of knee**
    ● **S81.001** Unspecified open wound, **right** knee
    ● **S81.002** Unspecified open wound, **left** knee
    ● **S81.009** Unspecified open wound, **unspecified** knee
  ● **S81.01** **Laceration without foreign body of knee**
    ● **S81.011** Laceration without foreign body, **right** knee
    ● **S81.012** Laceration without foreign body, **left** knee
    ● **S81.019** Laceration without foreign body, **unspecified** knee
  ● **S81.02** **Laceration with foreign body of knee**
    ● **S81.021** Laceration with foreign body, **right** knee
    ● **S81.022** Laceration with foreign body, **left** knee
    ● **S81.029** Laceration with foreign body, **unspecified** knee

- ● S81.03   Puncture wound without foreign body of knee
  - ● S81.031   Puncture wound without foreign body, right knee
    - *Coding Clinic: 2025, Q1, P31*
  - ● S81.032   Puncture wound without foreign body, left knee
  - ● S81.039   Puncture wound without foreign body, unspecified knee
- ● S81.04   Puncture wound with foreign body of knee
  - ● S81.041   Puncture wound with foreign body, right knee
  - ● S81.042   Puncture wound with foreign body, left knee
  - ● S81.049   Puncture wound with foreign body, unspecified knee
- ● S81.05   Open bite of knee
  - Bite of knee NOS
  - **Excludes1**   superficial bite of knee (S80.27-)
  - ● S81.051   Open bite, right knee
  - ● S81.052   Open bite, left knee
  - ● S81.059   Open bite, unspecified knee
- ● S81.8   Open wound of lower leg
  - ● S81.80   Unspecified open wound of lower leg
    - ● S81.801   Unspecified open wound, right lower leg
    - ● S81.802   Unspecified open wound, left lower leg
    - ● S81.809   Unspecified open wound, unspecified lower leg
  - ● S81.81   Laceration without foreign body of lower leg
    - ● S81.811   Laceration without foreign body, right lower leg
    - ● S81.812   Laceration without foreign body, left lower leg
    - ● S81.819   Laceration without foreign body, unspecified lower leg
  - ● S81.82   Laceration with foreign body of lower leg
    - ● S81.821   Laceration with foreign body, right lower leg
    - ● S81.822   Laceration with foreign body, left lower leg
    - ● S81.829   Laceration with foreign body, unspecified lower leg
  - ● S81.83   Puncture wound without foreign body of lower leg
    - ● S81.831   Puncture wound without foreign body, right lower leg
    - ● S81.832   Puncture wound without foreign body, left lower leg
    - ● S81.839   Puncture wound without foreign body, unspecified lower leg
  - ● S81.84   Puncture wound with foreign body of lower leg
    - ● S81.841   Puncture wound with foreign body, right lower leg
      - *Coding Clinic: 2016, Q3, P46*
    - ● S81.842   Puncture wound with foreign body, left lower leg
    - ● S81.849   Puncture wound with foreign body, unspecified lower leg
  - ● S81.85   Open bite of lower leg
    - Bite of lower leg NOS
    - **Excludes1**   superficial bite of lower leg (S80.86-, S80.87-)
    - ● S81.851   Open bite, right lower leg
    - ● S81.852   Open bite, left lower leg
    - ● S81.859   Open bite, unspecified lower leg

- ● S82   Fracture of lower leg, including ankle
  - **Note:** A fracture not indicated as displaced or nondisplaced should be coded to displaced
  - A fracture not indicated as open or closed should be coded to closed
  - The open fracture designations are based on the Gustilo open fracture classification
  - **Includes**   fracture of malleolus
  - **Excludes1**   traumatic amputation of lower leg (S88.-)
  - **Excludes2**   fracture of foot, except ankle (S92.-)
    - periprosthetic fracture around internal prosthetic ankle joint (M97.2)
    - periprosthetic fracture around internal of prosthetic implant of knee joint (M97.1-)
  - The appropriate 7th character is to be added to all codes from category S82

A	initial encounter for closed fracture
B	initial encounter for open fracture type I or II initial encounter for open fracture NOS
C	initial encounter for open fracture type IIIA, IIIB, or IIIC
D	subsequent encounter for closed fracture with routine healing
E	subsequent encounter for open fracture type I or II with routine healing
F	subsequent encounter for open fracture type IIIA, IIIB, or IIIC with routine healing
G	subsequent encounter for closed fracture with delayed healing
H	subsequent encounter for open fracture type I or II with delayed healing
J	subsequent encounter for open fracture type IIIA, IIIB, or IIIC with delayed healing
K	subsequent encounter for closed fracture with nonunion
M	subsequent encounter for open fracture type I or II with nonunion
N	subsequent encounter for open fracture type IIIA, IIIB, or IIIC with nonunion
P	subsequent encounter for closed fracture with malunion
Q	subsequent encounter for open fracture type I or II with malunion
R	subsequent encounter for open fracture type IIIA, IIIB, or IIIC with malunion
S	sequela

- ● S82.0   Fracture of patella
  - *Knee cap*
  - ● S82.00   Unspecified fracture of patella
    - ● S82.001   Unspecified fracture of right patella
    - ● S82.002   Unspecified fracture of left patella
    - ● S82.009   Unspecified fracture of unspecified patella
  - ● S82.01   Osteochondral fracture of patella
    - ● S82.011   Displaced osteochondral fracture of right patella
    - ● S82.012   Displaced osteochondral fracture of left patella
    - ● S82.013   Displaced osteochondral fracture of unspecified patella
    - ● S82.014   Nondisplaced osteochondral fracture of right patella
    - ● S82.015   Nondisplaced osteochondral fracture of left patella
    - ● S82.016   Nondisplaced osteochondral fracture of unspecified patella
  - ● S82.02   Longitudinal fracture of patella
    - ● S82.021   Displaced longitudinal fracture of right patella
    - ● S82.022   Displaced longitudinal fracture of left patella

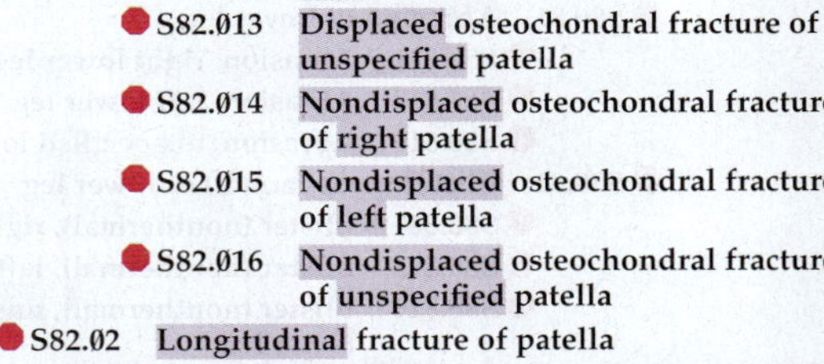

● S82.023 Displaced longitudinal fracture of unspecified patella
● S82.024 Nondisplaced longitudinal fracture of right patella
● S82.025 Nondisplaced longitudinal fracture of left patella
● S82.026 Nondisplaced longitudinal fracture of unspecified patella

● S82.03 Transverse fracture of patella
● S82.031 Displaced transverse fracture of right patella
● S82.032 Displaced transverse fracture of left patella
● S82.033 Displaced transverse fracture of unspecified patella
● S82.034 Nondisplaced transverse fracture of right patella
● S82.035 Nondisplaced transverse fracture of left patella
● S82.036 Nondisplaced transverse fracture of unspecified patella

● S82.04 Comminuted fracture of patella
● S82.041 Displaced comminuted fracture of right patella
● S82.042 Displaced comminuted fracture of left patella
● S82.043 Displaced comminuted fracture of unspecified patella
● S82.044 Nondisplaced comminuted fracture of right patella
● S82.045 Nondisplaced comminuted fracture of left patella
● S82.046 Nondisplaced comminuted fracture of unspecified patella

● S82.09 Other fracture of patella
● S82.091 Other fracture of right patella
● S82.092 Other fracture of left patella
● S82.099 Other fracture of unspecified patella

● S82.1 Fracture of upper end of tibia
Fracture of proximal end of tibia

Excludes2 fracture of shaft of tibia (S82.2-)
physeal fracture of upper end of tibia (S89.0-)

● S82.10 Unspecified fracture of upper end of tibia
● S82.101 Unspecified fracture of upper end of right tibia
● S82.102 Unspecified fracture of upper end of left tibia
● S82.109 Unspecified fracture of upper end of unspecified tibia

● S82.11 Fracture of tibial spine
● S82.111 Displaced fracture of right tibial spine
● S82.112 Displaced fracture of left tibial spine
● S82.113 Displaced fracture of unspecified tibial spine
● S82.114 Nondisplaced fracture of right tibial spine
● S82.115 Nondisplaced fracture of left tibial spine
● S82.116 Nondisplaced fracture of unspecified tibial spine

● S82.12 Fracture of lateral condyle of tibia
● S82.121 Displaced fracture of lateral condyle of right tibia
● S82.122 Displaced fracture of lateral condyle of left tibia
● S82.123 Displaced fracture of lateral condyle of unspecified tibia
● S82.124 Nondisplaced fracture of lateral condyle of right tibia

● S82.125 Nondisplaced fracture of lateral condyle of left tibia
● S82.126 Nondisplaced fracture of lateral condyle of unspecified tibia

● S82.13 Fracture of medial condyle of tibia
● S82.131 Displaced fracture of medial condyle of right tibia
● S82.132 Displaced fracture of medial condyle of left tibia
● S82.133 Displaced fracture of medial condyle of unspecified tibia
● S82.134 Nondisplaced fracture of medial condyle of right tibia
● S82.135 Nondisplaced fracture of medial condyle of left tibia
● S82.136 Nondisplaced fracture of medial condyle of unspecified tibia

● S82.14 Bicondylar fracture of tibia
Fracture of tibial plateau NOS
● S82.141 Displaced bicondylar fracture of right tibia
● S82.142 Displaced bicondylar fracture of left tibia
● S82.143 Displaced bicondylar fracture of unspecified tibia
● S82.144 Nondisplaced bicondylar fracture of right tibia
● S82.145 Nondisplaced bicondylar fracture of left tibia
● S82.146 Nondisplaced bicondylar fracture of unspecified tibia

● S82.15 Fracture of tibial tuberosity
● S82.151 Displaced fracture of right tibial tuberosity
● S82.152 Displaced fracture of left tibial tuberosity
● S82.153 Displaced fracture of unspecified tibial tuberosity
● S82.154 Nondisplaced fracture of right tibial tuberosity
● S82.155 Nondisplaced fracture of left tibial tuberosity
● S82.156 Nondisplaced fracture of unspecified tibial tuberosity

● S82.16 Torus fracture of upper end of tibia
The appropriate 7th character is to be added to all codes in subcategory S82.16

A	initial encounter for closed fracture
D	subsequent encounter for fracture with routine healing
G	subsequent encounter for fracture with delayed healing
K	subsequent encounter for fracture with nonunion
P	subsequent encounter for fracture with malunion
S	sequela

● S82.161 Torus fracture of upper end of right tibia
● S82.162 Torus fracture of upper end of left tibia
● S82.169 Torus fracture of upper end of unspecified tibia

● S82.19 Other fracture of upper end of tibia
● S82.191 Other fracture of upper end of right tibia
● S82.192 Other fracture of upper end of left tibia
● S82.199 Other fracture of upper end of unspecified tibia

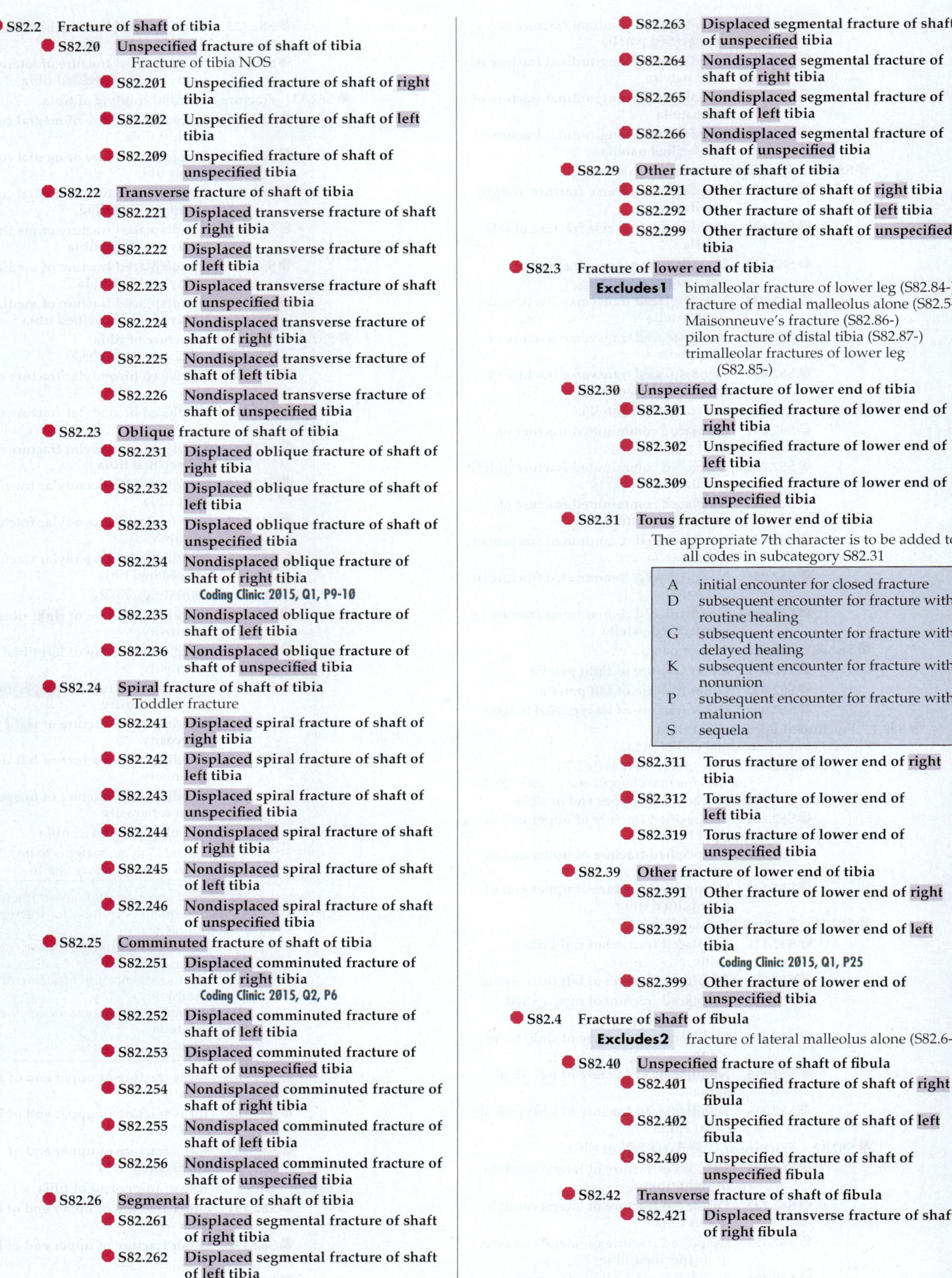

● **S82.2**   **Fracture of shaft of tibia**
  ● **S82.20**   **Unspecified fracture of shaft of tibia**
    Fracture of tibia NOS
    ● **S82.201**   **Unspecified fracture of shaft of right tibia**
    ● **S82.202**   **Unspecified fracture of shaft of left tibia**
    ● **S82.209**   **Unspecified fracture of shaft of unspecified tibia**
  ● **S82.22**   **Transverse fracture of shaft of tibia**
    ● **S82.221**   **Displaced transverse fracture of shaft of right tibia**
    ● **S82.222**   **Displaced transverse fracture of shaft of left tibia**
    ● **S82.223**   **Displaced transverse fracture of shaft of unspecified tibia**
    ● **S82.224**   **Nondisplaced transverse fracture of shaft of right tibia**
    ● **S82.225**   **Nondisplaced transverse fracture of shaft of left tibia**
    ● **S82.226**   **Nondisplaced transverse fracture of shaft of unspecified tibia**
  ● **S82.23**   **Oblique fracture of shaft of tibia**
    ● **S82.231**   **Displaced oblique fracture of shaft of right tibia**
    ● **S82.232**   **Displaced oblique fracture of shaft of left tibia**
    ● **S82.233**   **Displaced oblique fracture of shaft of unspecified tibia**
    ● **S82.234**   **Nondisplaced oblique fracture of shaft of right tibia**
      Coding Clinic: 2015, Q1, P9-10
    ● **S82.235**   **Nondisplaced oblique fracture of shaft of left tibia**
    ● **S82.236**   **Nondisplaced oblique fracture of shaft of unspecified tibia**
  ● **S82.24**   **Spiral fracture of shaft of tibia**
    Toddler fracture
    ● **S82.241**   **Displaced spiral fracture of shaft of right tibia**
    ● **S82.242**   **Displaced spiral fracture of shaft of left tibia**
    ● **S82.243**   **Displaced spiral fracture of shaft of unspecified tibia**
    ● **S82.244**   **Nondisplaced spiral fracture of shaft of right tibia**
    ● **S82.245**   **Nondisplaced spiral fracture of shaft of left tibia**
    ● **S82.246**   **Nondisplaced spiral fracture of shaft of unspecified tibia**
  ● **S82.25**   **Comminuted fracture of shaft of tibia**
    ● **S82.251**   **Displaced comminuted fracture of shaft of right tibia**
      Coding Clinic: 2015, Q2, P6
    ● **S82.252**   **Displaced comminuted fracture of shaft of left tibia**
    ● **S82.253**   **Displaced comminuted fracture of shaft of unspecified tibia**
    ● **S82.254**   **Nondisplaced comminuted fracture of shaft of right tibia**
    ● **S82.255**   **Nondisplaced comminuted fracture of shaft of left tibia**
    ● **S82.256**   **Nondisplaced comminuted fracture of shaft of unspecified tibia**
  ● **S82.26**   **Segmental fracture of shaft of tibia**
    ● **S82.261**   **Displaced segmental fracture of shaft of right tibia**
    ● **S82.262**   **Displaced segmental fracture of shaft of left tibia**
    ● **S82.263**   **Displaced segmental fracture of shaft of unspecified tibia**
    ● **S82.264**   **Nondisplaced segmental fracture of shaft of right tibia**
    ● **S82.265**   **Nondisplaced segmental fracture of shaft of left tibia**
    ● **S82.266**   **Nondisplaced segmental fracture of shaft of unspecified tibia**
  ● **S82.29**   **Other fracture of shaft of tibia**
    ● **S82.291**   **Other fracture of shaft of right tibia**
    ● **S82.292**   **Other fracture of shaft of left tibia**
    ● **S82.299**   **Other fracture of shaft of unspecified tibia**
● **S82.3**   **Fracture of lower end of tibia**
  Excludes1   bimalleolar fracture of lower leg (S82.84-)
    fracture of medial malleolus alone (S82.5-)
    Maisonneuve's fracture (S82.86-)
    pilon fracture of distal tibia (S82.87-)
    trimalleolar fractures of lower leg (S82.85-)
  ● **S82.30**   **Unspecified fracture of lower end of tibia**
    ● **S82.301**   **Unspecified fracture of lower end of right tibia**
    ● **S82.302**   **Unspecified fracture of lower end of left tibia**
    ● **S82.309**   **Unspecified fracture of lower end of unspecified tibia**
  ● **S82.31**   **Torus fracture of lower end of tibia**
    The appropriate 7th character is to be added to all codes in subcategory S82.31

A	initial encounter for closed fracture
D	subsequent encounter for fracture with routine healing
G	subsequent encounter for fracture with delayed healing
K	subsequent encounter for fracture with nonunion
P	subsequent encounter for fracture with malunion
S	sequela

    ● **S82.311**   **Torus fracture of lower end of right tibia**
    ● **S82.312**   **Torus fracture of lower end of left tibia**
    ● **S82.319**   **Torus fracture of lower end of unspecified tibia**
  ● **S82.39**   **Other fracture of lower end of tibia**
    ● **S82.391**   **Other fracture of lower end of right tibia**
    ● **S82.392**   **Other fracture of lower end of left tibia**
      Coding Clinic: 2015, Q1, P25
    ● **S82.399**   **Other fracture of lower end of unspecified tibia**
● **S82.4**   **Fracture of shaft of fibula**
  Excludes2   fracture of lateral malleolus alone (S82.6-)
  ● **S82.40**   **Unspecified fracture of shaft of fibula**
    ● **S82.401**   **Unspecified fracture of shaft of right fibula**
    ● **S82.402**   **Unspecified fracture of shaft of left fibula**
    ● **S82.409**   **Unspecified fracture of shaft of unspecified fibula**
  ● **S82.42**   **Transverse fracture of shaft of fibula**
    ● **S82.421**   **Displaced transverse fracture of shaft of right fibula**

▶ New   ⇒ Revised   ~~deleted~~ Deleted   Excludes 1   Excludes 2   Includes   Use additional   Code first   Code also   Key words
OGCR Official Guidelines   X Assign placeholder X   ● Use Additional Character(s)   ▶ Manifestation Code   🔒 Hierarchical Condition Category   **Coding Clinic**

- S82.422 **Displaced transverse fracture of shaft of left fibula**
- S82.423 **Displaced transverse fracture of shaft of unspecified fibula**
- S82.424 **Nondisplaced transverse fracture of shaft of right fibula**
- S82.425 **Nondisplaced transverse fracture of shaft of left fibula**
- S82.426 **Nondisplaced transverse fracture of shaft of unspecified fibula**
- S82.43 **Oblique fracture of shaft of fibula**
  - S82.431 **Displaced oblique fracture of shaft of right fibula**
  - S82.432 **Displaced oblique fracture of shaft of left fibula**
  - S82.433 **Displaced oblique fracture of shaft of unspecified fibula**
  - S82.434 **Nondisplaced oblique fracture of shaft of right fibula**
  - S82.435 **Nondisplaced oblique fracture of shaft of left fibula**
  - S82.436 **Nondisplaced oblique fracture of shaft of unspecified fibula**
- S82.44 **Spiral fracture of shaft of fibula**
  - S82.441 **Displaced spiral fracture of shaft of right fibula**
  - S82.442 **Displaced spiral fracture of shaft of left fibula**
  - S82.443 **Displaced spiral fracture of shaft of unspecified fibula**
  - S82.444 **Nondisplaced spiral fracture of shaft of right fibula**
  - S82.445 **Nondisplaced spiral fracture of shaft of left fibula**
  - S82.446 **Nondisplaced spiral fracture of shaft of unspecified fibula**
- S82.45 **Comminuted fracture of shaft of fibula**
  - S82.451 **Displaced comminuted fracture of shaft of right fibula**
  - S82.452 **Displaced comminuted fracture of shaft of left fibula**
  - S82.453 **Displaced comminuted fracture of shaft of unspecified fibula**
  - S82.454 **Nondisplaced comminuted fracture of shaft of right fibula**
  - S82.455 **Nondisplaced comminuted fracture of shaft of left fibula**
  - S82.456 **Nondisplaced comminuted fracture of shaft of unspecified fibula**
- S82.46 **Segmental fracture of shaft of fibula**
  - S82.461 **Displaced segmental fracture of shaft of right fibula**
  - S82.462 **Displaced segmental fracture of shaft of left fibula**
  - S82.463 **Displaced segmental fracture of shaft of unspecified fibula**
  - S82.464 **Nondisplaced segmental fracture of shaft of right fibula**
  - S82.465 **Nondisplaced segmental fracture of shaft of left fibula**
  - S82.466 **Nondisplaced segmental fracture of shaft of unspecified fibula**
- S82.49 **Other fracture of shaft of fibula**
  - S82.491 **Other fracture of shaft of right fibula**
  - S82.492 **Other fracture of shaft of left fibula**
  - S82.499 **Other fracture of shaft of unspecified fibula**

- S82.5 **Fracture of medial malleolus**
  - **Excludes1** pilon fracture of distal tibia (S82.87-)
      Salter-Harris type III of lower end of tibia (S89.13-)
      Salter-Harris type IV of lower end of tibia (S89.14-)
  - X S82.51 **Displaced fracture of medial malleolus of right tibia**
  - X S82.52 **Displaced fracture of medial malleolus of left tibia**
  - X S82.53 **Displaced fracture of medial malleolus of unspecified tibia**
  - X S82.54 **Nondisplaced fracture of medial malleolus of right tibia**
  - X S82.55 **Nondisplaced fracture of medial malleolus of left tibia**
  - X S82.56 **Nondisplaced fracture of medial malleolus of unspecified tibia**
- S82.6 **Fracture of lateral malleolus**
  - **Excludes1** pilon fracture of distal tibia (S82.87-)
  - X S82.61 **Displaced fracture of lateral malleolus of right fibula**
  - X S82.62 **Displaced fracture of lateral malleolus of left fibula**
  - X S82.63 **Displaced fracture of lateral malleolus of unspecified fibula**
  - X S82.64 **Nondisplaced fracture of lateral malleolus of right fibula**
  - X S82.65 **Nondisplaced fracture of lateral malleolus of left fibula**
  - X S82.66 **Nondisplaced fracture of lateral malleolus of unspecified fibula**
- S82.8 **Other fractures of lower leg**
  - S82.81 **Torus fracture of upper end of fibula**

    The appropriate 7th character is to be added to all codes in subcategory S82.81

A	initial encounter for closed fracture
D	subsequent encounter for fracture with routine healing
G	subsequent encounter for fracture with delayed healing
K	subsequent encounter for fracture with nonunion
P	subsequent encounter for fracture with malunion
S	sequela

  - S82.811 **Torus fracture of upper end of right fibula**
  - S82.812 **Torus fracture of upper end of left fibula**
  - S82.819 **Torus fracture of upper end of unspecified fibula**
  - S82.82 **Torus fracture of lower end of fibula**

    The appropriate 7th character is to be added to all codes in subcategory S82.82

A	initial encounter for closed fracture
D	subsequent encounter for fracture with routine healing
G	subsequent encounter for fracture with delayed healing
K	subsequent encounter for fracture with nonunion
P	subsequent encounter for fracture with malunion
S	sequela

  - S82.821 **Torus fracture of lower end of right fibula**
  - S82.822 **Torus fracture of lower end of left fibula**
  - S82.829 **Torus fracture of lower end of unspecified fibula**

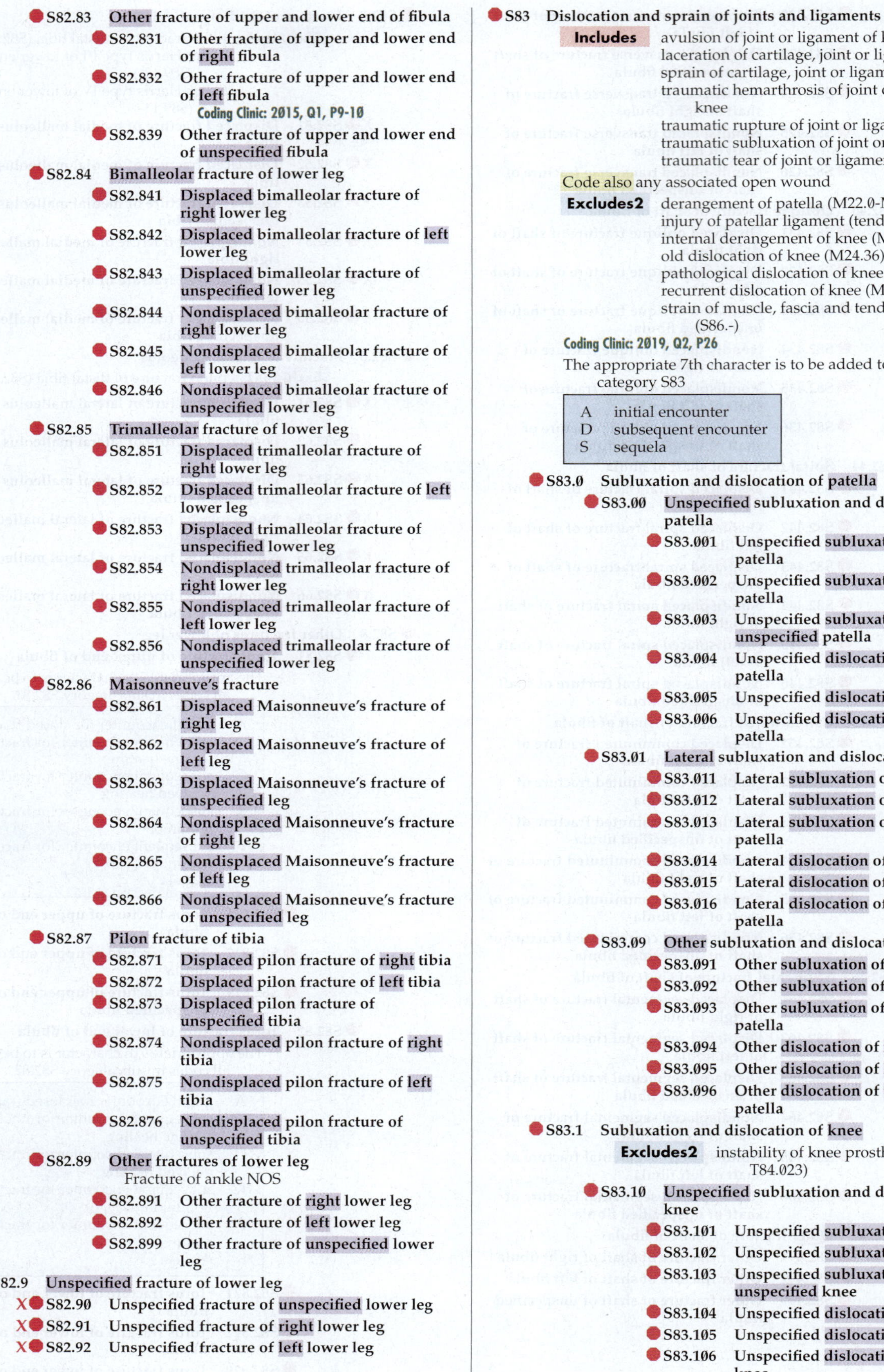

● **S82.83**   **Other fracture of upper and lower end of fibula**
- ● **S82.831**   Other fracture of upper and lower end of **right** fibula
- ● **S82.832**   Other fracture of upper and lower end of **left** fibula
  - **Coding Clinic: 2015, Q1, P9-10**
- ● **S82.839**   Other fracture of upper and lower end of **unspecified** fibula

● **S82.84**   **Bimalleolar fracture of lower leg**
- ● **S82.841**   Displaced bimalleolar fracture of **right** lower leg
- ● **S82.842**   Displaced bimalleolar fracture of **left** lower leg
- ● **S82.843**   Displaced bimalleolar fracture of **unspecified** lower leg
- ● **S82.844**   Nondisplaced bimalleolar fracture of **right** lower leg
- ● **S82.845**   Nondisplaced bimalleolar fracture of **left** lower leg
- ● **S82.846**   Nondisplaced bimalleolar fracture of **unspecified** lower leg

● **S82.85**   **Trimalleolar fracture of lower leg**
- ● **S82.851**   Displaced trimalleolar fracture of **right** lower leg
- ● **S82.852**   Displaced trimalleolar fracture of **left** lower leg
- ● **S82.853**   Displaced trimalleolar fracture of **unspecified** lower leg
- ● **S82.854**   Nondisplaced trimalleolar fracture of **right** lower leg
- ● **S82.855**   Nondisplaced trimalleolar fracture of **left** lower leg
- ● **S82.856**   Nondisplaced trimalleolar fracture of **unspecified** lower leg

● **S82.86**   **Maisonneuve's fracture**
- ● **S82.861**   Displaced Maisonneuve's fracture of **right** leg
- ● **S82.862**   Displaced Maisonneuve's fracture of **left** leg
- ● **S82.863**   Displaced Maisonneuve's fracture of **unspecified** leg
- ● **S82.864**   Nondisplaced Maisonneuve's fracture of **right** leg
- ● **S82.865**   Nondisplaced Maisonneuve's fracture of **left** leg
- ● **S82.866**   Nondisplaced Maisonneuve's fracture of **unspecified** leg

● **S82.87**   **Pilon fracture of tibia**
- ● **S82.871**   Displaced pilon fracture of **right** tibia
- ● **S82.872**   Displaced pilon fracture of **left** tibia
- ● **S82.873**   Displaced pilon fracture of **unspecified** tibia
- ● **S82.874**   Nondisplaced pilon fracture of **right** tibia
- ● **S82.875**   Nondisplaced pilon fracture of **left** tibia
- ● **S82.876**   Nondisplaced pilon fracture of **unspecified** tibia

● **S82.89**   **Other fractures of lower leg**
  - Fracture of ankle NOS
- ● **S82.891**   Other fracture of **right** lower leg
- ● **S82.892**   Other fracture of **left** lower leg
- ● **S82.899**   Other fracture of **unspecified** lower leg

● **S82.9**   **Unspecified fracture of lower leg**
- X ● **S82.90**   Unspecified fracture of **unspecified** lower leg
- X ● **S82.91**   Unspecified fracture of **right** lower leg
- X ● **S82.92**   Unspecified fracture of **left** lower leg

● **S83**   **Dislocation and sprain of joints and ligaments of knee**

Includes	avulsion of joint or ligament of knee
	laceration of cartilage, joint or ligament of knee
	sprain of cartilage, joint or ligament of knee
	traumatic hemarthrosis of joint or ligament of knee
	traumatic rupture of joint or ligament of knee
	traumatic subluxation of joint or ligament of knee
	traumatic tear of joint or ligament of knee

Code also any associated open wound

Excludes2	derangement of patella (M22.0-M22.3)
	injury of patellar ligament (tendon) (S76.1-)
	internal derangement of knee (M23.-)
	old dislocation of knee (M24.36)
	pathological dislocation of knee (M24.36)
	recurrent dislocation of knee (M22.0)
	strain of muscle, fascia and tendon of lower leg (S86.-)

Coding Clinic: 2019, Q2, P26

The appropriate 7th character is to be added to each code from category S83

A	initial encounter
D	subsequent encounter
S	sequela

● **S83.0**   **Subluxation and dislocation of patella**
- ● **S83.00**   **Unspecified subluxation and dislocation of patella**
  - ● **S83.001**   Unspecified subluxation of right patella
  - ● **S83.002**   Unspecified subluxation of left patella
  - ● **S83.003**   Unspecified subluxation of unspecified patella
  - ● **S83.004**   Unspecified dislocation of right patella
  - ● **S83.005**   Unspecified dislocation of left patella
  - ● **S83.006**   Unspecified dislocation of unspecified patella
- ● **S83.01**   **Lateral subluxation and dislocation of patella**
  - ● **S83.011**   Lateral subluxation of right patella
  - ● **S83.012**   Lateral subluxation of left patella
  - ● **S83.013**   Lateral subluxation of unspecified patella
  - ● **S83.014**   Lateral dislocation of right patella
  - ● **S83.015**   Lateral dislocation of left patella
  - ● **S83.016**   Lateral dislocation of unspecified patella
- ● **S83.09**   **Other subluxation and dislocation of patella**
  - ● **S83.091**   Other subluxation of right patella
  - ● **S83.092**   Other subluxation of left patella
  - ● **S83.093**   Other subluxation of unspecified patella
  - ● **S83.094**   Other dislocation of right patella
  - ● **S83.095**   Other dislocation of left patella
  - ● **S83.096**   Other dislocation of unspecified patella

● **S83.1**   **Subluxation and dislocation of knee**

Excludes2	instability of knee prosthesis (T84.022, T84.023)

- ● **S83.10**   **Unspecified subluxation and dislocation of knee**
  - ● **S83.101**   Unspecified subluxation of right knee
  - ● **S83.102**   Unspecified subluxation of left knee
  - ● **S83.103**   Unspecified subluxation of unspecified knee
  - ● **S83.104**   Unspecified dislocation of right knee
  - ● **S83.105**   Unspecified dislocation of left knee
  - ● **S83.106**   Unspecified dislocation of unspecified knee

- **S83.11** **Anterior subluxation and dislocation of proximal end of tibia**
  Posterior subluxation and dislocation of distal end of femur
  - **S83.111** Anterior subluxation of proximal end of tibia, right knee
  - **S83.112** Anterior subluxation of proximal end of tibia, left knee
  - **S83.113** Anterior subluxation of proximal end of tibia, unspecified knee
  - **S83.114** Anterior dislocation of proximal end of tibia, right knee
  - **S83.115** Anterior dislocation of proximal end of tibia, left knee
  - **S83.116** Anterior dislocation of proximal end of tibia, unspecified knee
- **S83.12** **Posterior subluxation and dislocation of proximal end of tibia**
  Anterior dislocation of distal end of femur
  - **S83.121** Posterior subluxation of proximal end of tibia, right knee
  - **S83.122** Posterior subluxation of proximal end of tibia, left knee
  - **S83.123** Posterior subluxation of proximal end of tibia, unspecified knee
  - **S83.124** Posterior dislocation of proximal end of tibia, right knee
  - **S83.125** Posterior dislocation of proximal end of tibia, left knee
  - **S83.126** Posterior dislocation of proximal end of tibia, unspecified knee
- **S83.13** **Medial subluxation and dislocation of proximal end of tibia**
  - **S83.131** Medial subluxation of proximal end of tibia, right knee
  - **S83.132** Medial subluxation of proximal end of tibia, left knee
  - **S83.133** Medial subluxation of proximal end of tibia, unspecified knee
  - **S83.134** Medial dislocation of proximal end of tibia, right knee
  - **S83.135** Medial dislocation of proximal end of tibia, left knee
  - **S83.136** Medial dislocation of proximal end of tibia, unspecified knee
- **S83.14** **Lateral subluxation and dislocation of proximal end of tibia**
  - **S83.141** Lateral subluxation of proximal end of tibia, right knee
  - **S83.142** Lateral subluxation of proximal end of tibia, left knee
  - **S83.143** Lateral subluxation of proximal end of tibia, unspecified knee
  - **S83.144** Lateral dislocation of proximal end of tibia, right knee
  - **S83.145** Lateral dislocation of proximal end of tibia, left knee
  - **S83.146** Lateral dislocation of proximal end of tibia, unspecified knee
- **S83.19** **Other subluxation and dislocation of knee**
  - **S83.191** Other subluxation of right knee
  - **S83.192** Other subluxation of left knee
  - **S83.193** Other subluxation of unspecified knee
  - **S83.194** Other dislocation of right knee
  - **S83.195** Other dislocation of left knee
  - **S83.196** Other dislocation of unspecified knee

- **S83.2** **Tear of meniscus**, current injury
  - **Excludes1** old bucket-handle tear (M23.2)
  - **S83.20** **Tear of unspecified meniscus, current injury**
    Tear of meniscus of knee NOS
    - **S83.200** Bucket-handle tear of unspecified meniscus, current injury, right knee
    - **S83.201** Bucket-handle tear of unspecified meniscus, current injury, left knee
    - **S83.202** Bucket-handle tear of unspecified meniscus, current injury, unspecified knee
    - **S83.203** Other tear of unspecified meniscus, current injury, right knee
    - **S83.204** Other tear of unspecified meniscus, current injury, left knee
    - **S83.205** Other tear of unspecified meniscus, current injury, unspecified knee
    - **S83.206** Unspecified tear of unspecified meniscus, current injury, right knee
    - **S83.207** Unspecified tear of unspecified meniscus, current injury, left knee
    - **S83.209** Unspecified tear of unspecified meniscus, current injury, unspecified knee
  - **S83.21** **Bucket-handle tear of medial meniscus, current injury**
    - **S83.211** Bucket-handle tear of medial meniscus, current injury, right knee
    - **S83.212** Bucket-handle tear of medial meniscus, current injury, left knee
    - **S83.219** Bucket-handle tear of medial meniscus, current injury, unspecified knee
  - **S83.22** **Peripheral tear of medial meniscus, current injury**
    - **S83.221** Peripheral tear of medial meniscus, current injury, right knee
    - **S83.222** Peripheral tear of medial meniscus, current injury, left knee
    - **S83.229** Peripheral tear of medial meniscus, current injury, unspecified knee
  - **S83.23** **Complex tear of medial meniscus, current injury**
    - **S83.231** Complex tear of medial meniscus, current injury, right knee
    - **S83.232** Complex tear of medial meniscus, current injury, left knee
      Coding Clinic: 2019, Q2, P26
    - **S83.239** Complex tear of medial meniscus, current injury, unspecified knee
  - **S83.24** **Other tear of medial meniscus, current injury**
    - **S83.241** Other tear of medial meniscus, current injury, right knee
    - **S83.242** Other tear of medial meniscus, current injury, left knee
    - **S83.249** Other tear of medial meniscus, current injury, unspecified knee
  - **S83.25** **Bucket-handle tear of lateral meniscus, current injury**
    - **S83.251** Bucket-handle tear of lateral meniscus, current injury, right knee
    - **S83.252** Bucket-handle tear of lateral meniscus, current injury, left knee
    - **S83.259** Bucket-handle tear of lateral meniscus, current injury, unspecified knee
  - **S83.26** **Peripheral tear of lateral meniscus, current injury**
    - **S83.261** Peripheral tear of lateral meniscus, current injury, right knee
    - **S83.262** Peripheral tear of lateral meniscus, current injury, left knee

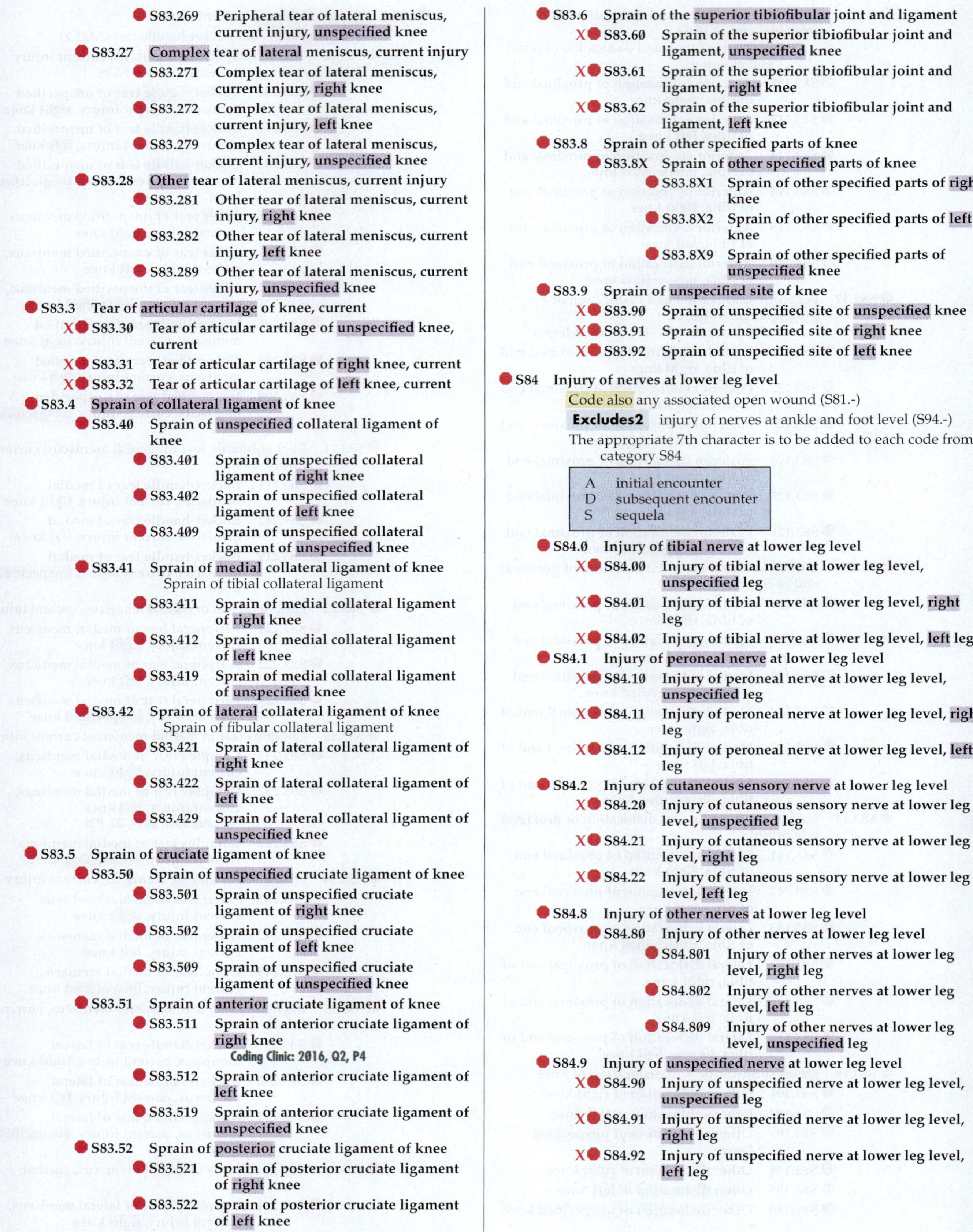

● S83.269   Peripheral tear of lateral meniscus, current injury, unspecified knee
● S83.27   Complex tear of lateral meniscus, current injury
   ● S83.271   Complex tear of lateral meniscus, current injury, right knee
   ● S83.272   Complex tear of lateral meniscus, current injury, left knee
   ● S83.279   Complex tear of lateral meniscus, current injury, unspecified knee
● S83.28   Other tear of lateral meniscus, current injury
   ● S83.281   Other tear of lateral meniscus, current injury, right knee
   ● S83.282   Other tear of lateral meniscus, current injury, left knee
   ● S83.289   Other tear of lateral meniscus, current injury, unspecified knee
● S83.3   Tear of articular cartilage of knee, current
  X ● S83.30   Tear of articular cartilage of unspecified knee, current
  X ● S83.31   Tear of articular cartilage of right knee, current
  X ● S83.32   Tear of articular cartilage of left knee, current
● S83.4   Sprain of collateral ligament of knee
  ● S83.40   Sprain of unspecified collateral ligament of knee
   ● S83.401   Sprain of unspecified collateral ligament of right knee
   ● S83.402   Sprain of unspecified collateral ligament of left knee
   ● S83.409   Sprain of unspecified collateral ligament of unspecified knee
  ● S83.41   Sprain of medial collateral ligament of knee
     Sprain of tibial collateral ligament
   ● S83.411   Sprain of medial collateral ligament of right knee
   ● S83.412   Sprain of medial collateral ligament of left knee
   ● S83.419   Sprain of medial collateral ligament of unspecified knee
  ● S83.42   Sprain of lateral collateral ligament of knee
     Sprain of fibular collateral ligament
   ● S83.421   Sprain of lateral collateral ligament of right knee
   ● S83.422   Sprain of lateral collateral ligament of left knee
   ● S83.429   Sprain of lateral collateral ligament of unspecified knee
● S83.5   Sprain of cruciate ligament of knee
  ● S83.50   Sprain of unspecified cruciate ligament of knee
   ● S83.501   Sprain of unspecified cruciate ligament of right knee
   ● S83.502   Sprain of unspecified cruciate ligament of left knee
   ● S83.509   Sprain of unspecified cruciate ligament of unspecified knee
  ● S83.51   Sprain of anterior cruciate ligament of knee
   ● S83.511   Sprain of anterior cruciate ligament of right knee
     Coding Clinic: 2016, Q2, P4
   ● S83.512   Sprain of anterior cruciate ligament of left knee
   ● S83.519   Sprain of anterior cruciate ligament of unspecified knee
  ● S83.52   Sprain of posterior cruciate ligament of knee
   ● S83.521   Sprain of posterior cruciate ligament of right knee
   ● S83.522   Sprain of posterior cruciate ligament of left knee
   ● S83.529   Sprain of posterior cruciate ligament of unspecified knee

● S83.6   Sprain of the superior tibiofibular joint and ligament
  X ● S83.60   Sprain of the superior tibiofibular joint and ligament, unspecified knee
  X ● S83.61   Sprain of the superior tibiofibular joint and ligament, right knee
  X ● S83.62   Sprain of the superior tibiofibular joint and ligament, left knee
● S83.8   Sprain of other specified parts of knee
  ● S83.8X   Sprain of other specified parts of knee
   ● S83.8X1   Sprain of other specified parts of right knee
   ● S83.8X2   Sprain of other specified parts of left knee
   ● S83.8X9   Sprain of other specified parts of unspecified knee
● S83.9   Sprain of unspecified site of knee
  X ● S83.90   Sprain of unspecified site of unspecified knee
  X ● S83.91   Sprain of unspecified site of right knee
  X ● S83.92   Sprain of unspecified site of left knee

● S84   Injury of nerves at lower leg level
  Code also any associated open wound (S81.-)
  Excludes2   injury of nerves at ankle and foot level (S94.-)
  The appropriate 7th character is to be added to each code from category S84

> A   initial encounter
> D   subsequent encounter
> S   sequela

● S84.0   Injury of tibial nerve at lower leg level
  X ● S84.00   Injury of tibial nerve at lower leg level, unspecified leg
  X ● S84.01   Injury of tibial nerve at lower leg level, right leg
  X ● S84.02   Injury of tibial nerve at lower leg level, left leg
● S84.1   Injury of peroneal nerve at lower leg level
  X ● S84.10   Injury of peroneal nerve at lower leg level, unspecified leg
  X ● S84.11   Injury of peroneal nerve at lower leg level, right leg
  X ● S84.12   Injury of peroneal nerve at lower leg level, left leg
● S84.2   Injury of cutaneous sensory nerve at lower leg level
  X ● S84.20   Injury of cutaneous sensory nerve at lower leg level, unspecified leg
  X ● S84.21   Injury of cutaneous sensory nerve at lower leg level, right leg
  X ● S84.22   Injury of cutaneous sensory nerve at lower leg level, left leg
● S84.8   Injury of other nerves at lower leg level
  ● S84.80   Injury of other nerves at lower leg level
   ● S84.801   Injury of other nerves at lower leg level, right leg
   ● S84.802   Injury of other nerves at lower leg level, left leg
   ● S84.809   Injury of other nerves at lower leg level, unspecified leg
● S84.9   Injury of unspecified nerve at lower leg level
  X ● S84.90   Injury of unspecified nerve at lower leg level, unspecified leg
  X ● S84.91   Injury of unspecified nerve at lower leg level, right leg
  X ● S84.92   Injury of unspecified nerve at lower leg level, left leg

● **S85   Injury of blood vessels at lower leg level**
     Code also any associated open wound (S81.-)
     Excludes2   injury of blood vessels at ankle and foot level
           (S95.-)

     The appropriate 7th character is to be added to each code from
       category S85

       A   initial encounter
       D   subsequent encounter
       S   sequela

● **S85.0   Injury of popliteal artery**
   ● **S85.00   Unspecified injury of popliteal artery**
     ● **S85.001   Unspecified injury of popliteal artery, right leg**
     ● **S85.002   Unspecified injury of popliteal artery, left leg**
     ● **S85.009   Unspecified injury of popliteal artery, unspecified leg**
   ● **S85.01   Laceration of popliteal artery**
     ● **S85.011   Laceration of popliteal artery, right leg**
     ● **S85.012   Laceration of popliteal artery, left leg**
     ● **S85.019   Laceration of popliteal artery, unspecified leg**
   ● **S85.09   Other specified injury of popliteal artery**
     ● **S85.091   Other specified injury of popliteal artery, right leg**
     ● **S85.092   Other specified injury of popliteal artery, left leg**
     ● **S85.099   Other specified injury of popliteal artery, unspecified leg**
● **S85.1   Injury of tibial artery**
   ● **S85.10   Unspecified injury of unspecified tibial artery**
       Injury of tibial artery NOS
     ● **S85.101   Unspecified injury of unspecified tibial artery, right leg**
     ● **S85.102   Unspecified injury of unspecified tibial artery, left leg**
     ● **S85.109   Unspecified injury of unspecified tibial artery, unspecified leg**
   ● **S85.11   Laceration of unspecified tibial artery**
     ● **S85.111   Laceration of unspecified tibial artery, right leg**
     ● **S85.112   Laceration of unspecified tibial artery, left leg**
     ● **S85.119   Laceration of unspecified tibial artery, unspecified leg**
   ● **S85.12   Other specified injury of unspecified tibial artery**
     ● **S85.121   Other specified injury of unspecified tibial artery, right leg**
     ● **S85.122   Other specified injury of unspecified tibial artery, left leg**
     ● **S85.129   Other specified injury of unspecified tibial artery, unspecified leg**
   ● **S85.13   Unspecified injury of anterior tibial artery**
     ● **S85.131   Unspecified injury of anterior tibial artery, right leg**
     ● **S85.132   Unspecified injury of anterior tibial artery, left leg**
     ● **S85.139   Unspecified injury of anterior tibial artery, unspecified leg**
   ● **S85.14   Laceration of anterior tibial artery**
     ● **S85.141   Laceration of anterior tibial artery, right leg**
     ● **S85.142   Laceration of anterior tibial artery, left leg**
     ● **S85.149   Laceration of anterior tibial artery, unspecified leg**

   ● **S85.15   Other specified injury of anterior tibial artery**
     ● **S85.151   Other specified injury of anterior tibial artery, right leg**
     ● **S85.152   Other specified injury of anterior tibial artery, left leg**
     ● **S85.159   Other specified injury of anterior tibial artery, unspecified leg**
   ● **S85.16   Unspecified injury of posterior tibial artery**
     ● **S85.161   Unspecified injury of posterior tibial artery, right leg**
     ● **S85.162   Unspecified injury of posterior tibial artery, left leg**
     ● **S85.169   Unspecified injury of posterior tibial artery, unspecified leg**
   ● **S85.17   Laceration of posterior tibial artery**
     ● **S85.171   Laceration of posterior tibial artery, right leg**
     ● **S85.172   Laceration of posterior tibial artery, left leg**
     ● **S85.179   Laceration of posterior tibial artery, unspecified leg**
   ● **S85.18   Other specified injury of posterior tibial artery**
     ● **S85.181   Other specified injury of posterior tibial artery, right leg**
     ● **S85.182   Other specified injury of posterior tibial artery, left leg**
     ● **S85.189   Other specified injury of posterior tibial artery, unspecified leg**
● **S85.2   Injury of peroneal artery**
   ● **S85.20   Unspecified injury of peroneal artery**
     ● **S85.201   Unspecified injury of peroneal artery, right leg**
     ● **S85.202   Unspecified injury of peroneal artery, left leg**
     ● **S85.209   Unspecified injury of peroneal artery, unspecified leg**
   ● **S85.21   Laceration of peroneal artery**
     ● **S85.211   Laceration of peroneal artery, right leg**
     ● **S85.212   Laceration of peroneal artery, left leg**
     ● **S85.219   Laceration of peroneal artery, unspecified leg**
   ● **S85.29   Other specified injury of peroneal artery**
     ● **S85.291   Other specified injury of peroneal artery, right leg**
     ● **S85.292   Other specified injury of peroneal artery, left leg**
     ● **S85.299   Other specified injury of peroneal artery, unspecified leg**
● **S85.3   Injury of greater saphenous vein at lower leg level**
     Injury of greater saphenous vein NOS
     Injury of saphenous vein NOS
   ● **S85.30   Unspecified injury of greater saphenous vein at lower leg level**
     ● **S85.301   Unspecified injury of greater saphenous vein at lower leg level, right leg**
     ● **S85.302   Unspecified injury of greater saphenous vein at lower leg level, left leg**
     ● **S85.309   Unspecified injury of greater saphenous vein at lower leg level, unspecified leg**
   ● **S85.31   Laceration of greater saphenous vein at lower leg level**
     ● **S85.311   Laceration of greater saphenous vein at lower leg level, right leg**
     ● **S85.312   Laceration of greater saphenous vein at lower leg level, left leg**
     ● **S85.319   Laceration of greater saphenous vein at lower leg level, unspecified leg**

CHAPTER 19 (S00–T88)

● S85.39   Other specified injury of greater saphenous vein at lower leg level
- ● S85.391   Other specified injury of greater saphenous vein at lower leg level, right leg
- ● S85.392   Other specified injury of greater saphenous vein at lower leg level, left leg
- ● S85.399   Other specified injury of greater saphenous vein at lower leg level, unspecified leg

● S85.4   Injury of lesser saphenous vein at lower leg level
- ● S85.40   Unspecified injury of lesser saphenous vein at lower leg level
  - ● S85.401   Unspecified injury of lesser saphenous vein at lower leg level, right leg
  - ● S85.402   Unspecified injury of lesser saphenous vein at lower leg level, left leg
  - ● S85.409   Unspecified injury of lesser saphenous vein at lower leg level, unspecified leg
- ● S85.41   Laceration of lesser saphenous vein at lower leg level
  - ● S85.411   Laceration of lesser saphenous vein at lower leg level, right leg
  - ● S85.412   Laceration of lesser saphenous vein at lower leg level, left leg
  - ● S85.419   Laceration of lesser saphenous vein at lower leg level, unspecified leg
- ● S85.49   Other specified injury of lesser saphenous vein at lower leg level
  - ● S85.491   Other specified injury of lesser saphenous vein at lower leg level, right leg
  - ● S85.492   Other specified injury of lesser saphenous vein at lower leg level, left leg
  - ● S85.499   Other specified injury of lesser saphenous vein at lower leg level, unspecified leg

● S85.5   Injury of popliteal vein
- ● S85.50   Unspecified injury of popliteal vein
  - ● S85.501   Unspecified injury of popliteal vein, right leg
  - ● S85.502   Unspecified injury of popliteal vein, left leg
  - ● S85.509   Unspecified injury of popliteal vein, unspecified leg
- ● S85.51   Laceration of popliteal vein
  - ● S85.511   Laceration of popliteal vein, right leg
  - ● S85.512   Laceration of popliteal vein, left leg
  - ● S85.519   Laceration of popliteal vein, unspecified leg
- ● S85.59   Other specified injury of popliteal vein
  - ● S85.591   Other specified injury of popliteal vein, right leg
  - ● S85.592   Other specified injury of popliteal vein, left leg
  - ● S85.599   Other specified injury of popliteal vein, unspecified leg

● S85.8   Injury of other blood vessels at lower leg level
- ● S85.80   Unspecified injury of other blood vessels at lower leg level
  - ● S85.801   Unspecified injury of other blood vessels at lower leg level, right leg
  - ● S85.802   Unspecified injury of other blood vessels at lower leg level, left leg
  - ● S85.809   Unspecified injury of other blood vessels at lower leg level, unspecified leg

● S85.81   Laceration of other blood vessels at lower leg level
- ● S85.811   Laceration of other blood vessels at lower leg level, right leg
- ● S85.812   Laceration of other blood vessels at lower leg level, left leg
- ● S85.819   Laceration of other blood vessels at lower leg level, unspecified leg

● S85.89   Other specified injury of other blood vessels at lower leg level
- ● S85.891   Other specified injury of other blood vessels at lower leg level, right leg
- ● S85.892   Other specified injury of other blood vessels at lower leg level, left leg
- ● S85.899   Other specified injury of other blood vessels at lower leg level, unspecified leg

● S85.9   Injury of unspecified blood vessel at lower leg level
- ● S85.90   Unspecified injury of unspecified blood vessel at lower leg level
  - ● S85.901   Unspecified injury of unspecified blood vessel at lower leg level, right leg
  - ● S85.902   Unspecified injury of unspecified blood vessel at lower leg level, left leg
  - ● S85.909   Unspecified injury of unspecified blood vessel at lower leg level, unspecified leg
- ● S85.91   Laceration of unspecified blood vessel at lower leg level
  - ● S85.911   Laceration of unspecified blood vessel at lower leg level, right leg
  - ● S85.912   Laceration of unspecified blood vessel at lower leg level, left leg
  - ● S85.919   Laceration of unspecified blood vessel at lower leg level, unspecified leg
- ● S85.99   Other specified injury of unspecified blood vessel at lower leg level
  - ● S85.991   Other specified injury of unspecified blood vessel at lower leg level, right leg
  - ● S85.992   Other specified injury of unspecified blood vessel at lower leg level, left leg
  - ● S85.999   Other specified injury of unspecified blood vessel at lower leg level, unspecified leg

● S86   **Injury of muscle, fascia and tendon at lower leg level**
Code also any associated open wound (S81.-)

Excludes2   injury of muscle, fascia and tendon at ankle (S96.-)
injury of patellar ligament (tendon) (S76.1-)
sprain of joints and ligaments of knee (S83.-)

The appropriate 7th character is to be added to each code from category S86

A	initial encounter
D	subsequent encounter
S	sequela

● S86.0   Injury of Achilles tendon
- ● S86.00   Unspecified injury of Achilles tendon
  - ● S86.001   Unspecified injury of right Achilles tendon
  - ● S86.002   Unspecified injury of left Achilles tendon
  - ● S86.009   Unspecified injury of unspecified Achilles tendon
- ● S86.01   Strain of Achilles tendon
  - ● S86.011   Strain of right Achilles tendon
  - ● S86.012   Strain of left Achilles tendon
  - ● S86.019   Strain of unspecified Achilles tendon

● **S86.02** **Laceration** of Achilles tendon
  ● S86.021 Laceration of right Achilles tendon
  ● S86.022 Laceration of left Achilles tendon
  ● S86.029 Laceration of unspecified Achilles tendon
● **S86.09** Other specified injury of Achilles tendon
  ● S86.091 Other specified injury of right Achilles tendon
  ● S86.092 Other specified injury of left Achilles tendon
  ● S86.099 Other specified injury of unspecified Achilles tendon
● **S86.1** Injury of other muscle(s) and tendon(s) of posterior muscle group at lower leg level
  ● **S86.10** Unspecified injury of other muscle(s) and tendon(s) of posterior muscle group at lower leg level
    ● S86.101 Unspecified injury of other muscle(s) and tendon(s) of posterior muscle group at lower leg level, right leg
    ● S86.102 Unspecified injury of other muscle(s) and tendon(s) of posterior muscle group at lower leg level, left leg
    ● S86.109 Unspecified injury of other muscle(s) and tendon(s) of posterior muscle group at lower leg level, unspecified leg
  ● **S86.11** Strain of other muscle(s) and tendon(s) of posterior muscle group at lower leg level
    ● S86.111 Strain of other muscle(s) and tendon(s) of posterior muscle group at lower leg level, right leg
    ● S86.112 Strain of other muscle(s) and tendon(s) of posterior muscle group at lower leg level, left leg
    ● S86.119 Strain of other muscle(s) and tendon(s) of posterior muscle group at lower leg level, unspecified leg
  ● **S86.12** Laceration of other muscle(s) and tendon(s) of posterior muscle group at lower leg level
    ● S86.121 Laceration of other muscle(s) and tendon(s) of posterior muscle group at lower leg level, right leg
    ● S86.122 Laceration of other muscle(s) and tendon(s) of posterior muscle group at lower leg level, left leg
    ● S86.129 Laceration of other muscle(s) and tendon(s) of posterior muscle group at lower leg level, unspecified leg
  ● **S86.19** Other injury of other muscle(s) and tendon(s) of posterior muscle group at lower leg level
    ● S86.191 Other injury of other muscle(s) and tendon(s) of posterior muscle group at lower leg level, right leg
    ● S86.192 Other injury of other muscle(s) and tendon(s) of posterior muscle group at lower leg level, left leg
    ● S86.199 Other injury of other muscle(s) and tendon(s) of posterior muscle group at lower leg level, unspecified leg
● **S86.2** Injury of muscle(s) and tendon(s) of anterior muscle group at lower leg level
  ● **S86.20** Unspecified injury of muscle(s) and tendon(s) of anterior muscle group at lower leg level
    ● S86.201 Unspecified injury of muscle(s) and tendon(s) of anterior muscle group at lower leg level, right leg
    ● S86.202 Unspecified injury of muscle(s) and tendon(s) of anterior muscle group at lower leg level, left leg

    ● S86.209 Unspecified injury of muscle(s) and tendon(s) of anterior muscle group at lower leg level, unspecified leg
  ● **S86.21** Strain of muscle(s) and tendon(s) of anterior muscle group at lower leg level
    ● S86.211 Strain of muscle(s) and tendon(s) of anterior muscle group at lower leg level, right leg
    ● S86.212 Strain of muscle(s) and tendon(s) of anterior muscle group at lower leg level, left leg
    ● S86.219 Strain of muscle(s) and tendon(s) of anterior muscle group at lower leg level, unspecified leg
  ● **S86.22** Laceration of muscle(s) and tendon(s) of anterior muscle group at lower leg level
    ● S86.221 Laceration of muscle(s) and tendon(s) of anterior muscle group at lower leg level, right leg
    ● S86.222 Laceration of muscle(s) and tendon(s) of anterior muscle group at lower leg level, left leg
    ● S86.229 Laceration of muscle(s) and tendon(s) of anterior muscle group at lower leg level, unspecified leg
  ● **S86.29** Other injury of muscle(s) and tendon(s) of anterior muscle group at lower leg level
    ● S86.291 Other injury of muscle(s) and tendon(s) of anterior muscle group at lower leg level, right leg
    ● S86.292 Other injury of muscle(s) and tendon(s) of anterior muscle group at lower leg level, left leg
    ● S86.299 Other injury of muscle(s) and tendon(s) of anterior muscle group at lower leg level, unspecified leg
● **S86.3** Injury of muscle(s) and tendon(s) of peroneal muscle group at lower leg level
  ● **S86.30** Unspecified injury of muscle(s) and tendon(s) of peroneal muscle group at lower leg level
    ● S86.301 Unspecified injury of muscle(s) and tendon(s) of peroneal muscle group at lower leg level, right leg
    ● S86.302 Unspecified injury of muscle(s) and tendon(s) of peroneal muscle group at lower leg level, left leg
    ● S86.309 Unspecified injury of muscle(s) and tendon(s) of peroneal muscle group at lower leg level, unspecified leg
  ● **S86.31** Strain of muscle(s) and tendon(s) of peroneal muscle group at lower leg level
    ● S86.311 Strain of muscle(s) and tendon(s) of peroneal muscle group at lower leg level, right leg
    ● S86.312 Strain of muscle(s) and tendon(s) of peroneal muscle group at lower leg level, left leg
    ● S86.319 Strain of muscle(s) and tendon(s) of peroneal muscle group at lower leg level, unspecified leg
  ● **S86.32** Laceration of muscle(s) and tendon(s) of peroneal muscle group at lower leg level
    ● S86.321 Laceration of muscle(s) and tendon(s) of peroneal muscle group at lower leg level, right leg
    ● S86.322 Laceration of muscle(s) and tendon(s) of peroneal muscle group at lower leg level, left leg
    ● S86.329 Laceration of muscle(s) and tendon(s) of peroneal muscle group at lower leg level, unspecified leg

CHAPTER 19 (S00-T88)

- ● **S86.39** Other injury of muscle(s) and tendon(s) of peroneal muscle group at lower leg level
  - ● **S86.391** Other injury of muscle(s) and tendon(s) of peroneal muscle group at lower leg level, **right leg**
  - ● **S86.392** Other injury of muscle(s) and tendon(s) of peroneal muscle group at lower leg level, **left leg**
  - ● **S86.399** Other injury of muscle(s) and tendon(s) of peroneal muscle group at lower leg level, **unspecified leg**
- ● **S86.8** Injury of other muscles and tendons at lower leg level
  - ● **S86.80** Unspecified injury of other muscles and tendons at lower leg level
    - ● **S86.801** Unspecified injury of other muscle(s) and tendon(s) at lower leg level, **right leg**
    - ● **S86.802** Unspecified injury of other muscle(s) and tendon(s) at lower leg level, **left leg**
    - ● **S86.809** Unspecified injury of other muscle(s) and tendon(s) at lower leg level, **unspecified leg**
  - ● **S86.81** Strain of other muscles and tendons at lower leg level
    - ● **S86.811** Strain of other muscle(s) and tendon(s) at lower leg level, **right leg**
    - ● **S86.812** Strain of other muscle(s) and tendon(s) at lower leg level, **left leg**
    - ● **S86.819** Strain of other muscle(s) and tendon(s) at lower leg level, **unspecified leg**
  - ● **S86.82** Laceration of other muscles and tendons at lower leg level
    - ● **S86.821** Laceration of other muscle(s) and tendon(s) at lower leg level, **right leg**
    - ● **S86.822** Laceration of other muscle(s) and tendon(s) at lower leg level, **left leg**
    - ● **S86.829** Laceration of other muscle(s) and tendon(s) at lower leg level, **unspecified leg**
  - ● **S86.89** Other injury of other muscles and tendons at lower leg level
    - ● **S86.891** Other injury of other muscle(s) and tendon(s) at lower leg level, **right leg**
    - ● **S86.892** Other injury of other muscle(s) and tendon(s) at lower leg level, **left leg**
    - ● **S86.899** Other injury of other muscle(s) and tendon(s) at lower leg level, **unspecified leg**
- ● **S86.9** Injury of **unspecified** muscle and tendon at lower leg level
  - ● **S86.90** Unspecified injury of unspecified muscle and tendon at lower leg level
    - ● **S86.901** Unspecified injury of unspecified muscle(s) and tendon(s) at lower leg level, **right leg**
    - ● **S86.902** Unspecified injury of unspecified muscle(s) and tendon(s) at lower leg level, **left leg**
    - ● **S86.909** Unspecified injury of unspecified muscle(s) and tendon(s) at lower leg level, **unspecified leg**
  - ● **S86.91** Strain of unspecified muscle and tendon at lower leg level
    - ● **S86.911** Strain of unspecified muscle(s) and tendon(s) at lower leg level, **right leg**
    - ● **S86.912** Strain of unspecified muscle(s) and tendon(s) at lower leg level, **left leg**
    - ● **S86.919** Strain of unspecified muscle(s) and tendon(s) at lower leg level, **unspecified leg**
- ● **S86.92** Laceration of unspecified muscle and tendon at lower leg level
  - ● **S86.921** Laceration of unspecified muscle(s) and tendon(s) at lower leg level, **right leg**
  - ● **S86.922** Laceration of unspecified muscle(s) and tendon(s) at lower leg level, **left leg**
  - ● **S86.929** Laceration of unspecified muscle(s) and tendon(s) at lower leg level, **unspecified leg**
- ● **S86.99** Other injury of unspecified muscle and tendon at lower leg level
  - ● **S86.991** Other injury of unspecified muscle(s) and tendon(s) at lower leg level, **right leg**
  - ● **S86.992** Other injury of unspecified muscle(s) and tendon(s) at lower leg level, **left leg**
  - ● **S86.999** Other injury of unspecified muscle(s) and tendon(s) at lower leg level, **unspecified leg**

● **S87** Crushing injury of lower leg

Use additional code(s) for all associated injuries

Excludes2 crushing injury of ankle and foot (S97.-)

The appropriate 7th character is to be added to each code from category S87

A	initial encounter
D	subsequent encounter
S	sequela

- ● **S87.0** Crushing injury of knee
  - X ● **S87.00** Crushing injury of **unspecified** knee
  - X ● **S87.01** Crushing injury of **right** knee
  - X ● **S87.02** Crushing injury of **left** knee
- ● **S87.8** Crushing injury of **lower leg**
  - X ● **S87.80** Crushing injury of **unspecified** lower leg
  - X ● **S87.81** Crushing injury of **right** lower leg
  - X ● **S87.82** Crushing injury of **left** lower leg

● **S88** **Traumatic amputation** of lower leg

An amputation not identified as partial or complete should be coded to complete

Excludes1 traumatic amputation of ankle and foot (S98.-)

The appropriate 7th character is to be added to each code from category S88

A	initial encounter
D	subsequent encounter
S	sequela

- ● **S88.0** Traumatic amputation at **knee level**
  - ● **S88.01** Complete traumatic amputation at knee level
    - ● **S88.011** Complete traumatic amputation at knee level, **right lower leg** A, D, S ⬗
      Coding Clinic: 2023, Q1, P28-29
    - ● **S88.012** Complete traumatic amputation at knee level, **left lower leg** A, D, S ⬗
      Coding Clinic: 2023, Q1, P28-29
    - ● **S88.019** Complete traumatic amputation at knee level, **unspecified lower leg** A, D, S ⬗
  - ● **S88.02** Partial traumatic amputation at knee level
    - ● **S88.021** Partial traumatic amputation at knee level, **right lower leg** A, D, S ⬗
    - ● **S88.022** Partial traumatic amputation at knee level, **left lower leg** A, D, S ⬗
    - ● **S88.029** Partial traumatic amputation at knee level, **unspecified lower leg** A, D, S ⬗

● **S88.1**   Traumatic amputation at level between knee and ankle
  ● **S88.11**   Complete traumatic amputation at level between knee and ankle
    ● **S88.111**   Complete traumatic amputation at level between knee and ankle, right lower leg A, D, S
    ● **S88.112**   Complete traumatic amputation at level between knee and ankle, left lower leg A, D, S
    ● **S88.119**   Complete traumatic amputation at level between knee and ankle, unspecified lower leg A, D, S
  ● **S88.12**   Partial traumatic amputation at level between knee and ankle
    ● **S88.121**   Partial traumatic amputation at level between knee and ankle, right lower leg A, D, S
    ● **S88.122**   Partial traumatic amputation at level between knee and ankle, left lower leg A, D, S
    ● **S88.129**   Partial traumatic amputation at level between knee and ankle, unspecified lower leg A, D, S
● **S88.9**   Traumatic amputation of lower leg, level unspecified
  ● **S88.91**   Complete traumatic amputation of lower leg, level unspecified
    ● **S88.911**   Complete traumatic amputation of right lower leg, level unspecified A, D, S
    ● **S88.912**   Complete traumatic amputation of left lower leg, level unspecified A, D, S
    ● **S88.919**   Complete traumatic amputation of unspecified lower leg, level unspecified A, D, S
  ● **S88.92**   Partial traumatic amputation of lower leg, level unspecified
    ● **S88.921**   Partial traumatic amputation of right lower leg, level unspecified A, D, S
    ● **S88.922**   Partial traumatic amputation of left lower leg, level unspecified A, D, S
    ● **S88.929**   Partial traumatic amputation of unspecified lower leg, level unspecified A, D, S

● **S89**   Other and unspecified injuries of lower leg
  Note: A fracture not indicated as open or closed should be coded to closed
  Excludes2   other and unspecified injuries of ankle and foot (S99.-)

  The appropriate 7th character is to be added to each code from subcategories S89.0, S89.1, S89.2, and S89.3

> A   initial encounter for closed fracture
> D   subsequent encounter for fracture with routine healing
> G   subsequent encounter for fracture with delayed healing
> K   subsequent encounter for fracture with nonunion
> P   subsequent encounter for fracture with malunion
> S   sequela

  ● **S89.0**   Physeal fracture of upper end of tibia
    ● **S89.00**   Unspecified physeal fracture of upper end of tibia
      ● **S89.001**   Unspecified physeal fracture of upper end of right tibia
      ● **S89.002**   Unspecified physeal fracture of upper end of left tibia
      ● **S89.009**   Unspecified physeal fracture of upper end of unspecified tibia

    ● **S89.01**   Salter-Harris Type I physeal fracture of upper end of tibia
      ● **S89.011**   Salter-Harris Type I physeal fracture of upper end of right tibia
      ● **S89.012**   Salter-Harris Type I physeal fracture of upper end of left tibia
      ● **S89.019**   Salter-Harris Type I physeal fracture of upper end of unspecified tibia
    ● **S89.02**   Salter-Harris Type II physeal fracture of upper end of tibia
      ● **S89.021**   Salter-Harris Type II physeal fracture of upper end of right tibia
      ● **S89.022**   Salter-Harris Type II physeal fracture of upper end of left tibia
      ● **S89.029**   Salter-Harris Type II physeal fracture of upper end of unspecified tibia
    ● **S89.03**   Salter-Harris Type III physeal fracture of upper end of tibia
      ● **S89.031**   Salter-Harris Type III physeal fracture of upper end of right tibia
      ● **S89.032**   Salter-Harris Type III physeal fracture of upper end of left tibia
      ● **S89.039**   Salter-Harris Type III physeal fracture of upper end of unspecified tibia
    ● **S89.04**   Salter-Harris Type IV physeal fracture of upper end of tibia
      ● **S89.041**   Salter-Harris Type IV physeal fracture of upper end of right tibia
      ● **S89.042**   Salter-Harris Type IV physeal fracture of upper end of left tibia
      ● **S89.049**   Salter-Harris Type IV physeal fracture of upper end of unspecified tibia
    ● **S89.09**   Other physeal fracture of upper end of tibia
      ● **S89.091**   Other physeal fracture of upper end of right tibia
      ● **S89.092**   Other physeal fracture of upper end of left tibia
      ● **S89.099**   Other physeal fracture of upper end of unspecified tibia
  ● **S89.1**   Physeal fracture of lower end of tibia
    ● **S89.10**   Unspecified physeal fracture of lower end of tibia
      ● **S89.101**   Unspecified physeal fracture of lower end of right tibia
      ● **S89.102**   Unspecified physeal fracture of lower end of left tibia
      ● **S89.109**   Unspecified physeal fracture of lower end of unspecified tibia
    ● **S89.11**   Salter-Harris Type I physeal fracture of lower end of tibia
      ● **S89.111**   Salter-Harris Type I physeal fracture of lower end of right tibia
      ● **S89.112**   Salter-Harris Type I physeal fracture of lower end of left tibia
      ● **S89.119**   Salter-Harris Type I physeal fracture of lower end of unspecified tibia
    ● **S89.12**   Salter-Harris Type II physeal fracture of lower end of tibia
      ● **S89.121**   Salter-Harris Type II physeal fracture of lower end of right tibia
      ● **S89.122**   Salter-Harris Type II physeal fracture of lower end of left tibia
      ● **S89.129**   Salter-Harris Type II physeal fracture of lower end of unspecified tibia
    ● **S89.13**   Salter-Harris Type III physeal fracture of lower end of tibia
      Excludes1   fracture of medial malleolus (adult) (S82.5-)
      ● **S89.131**   Salter-Harris Type III physeal fracture of lower end of right tibia

CHAPTER 19 (S00–T88)

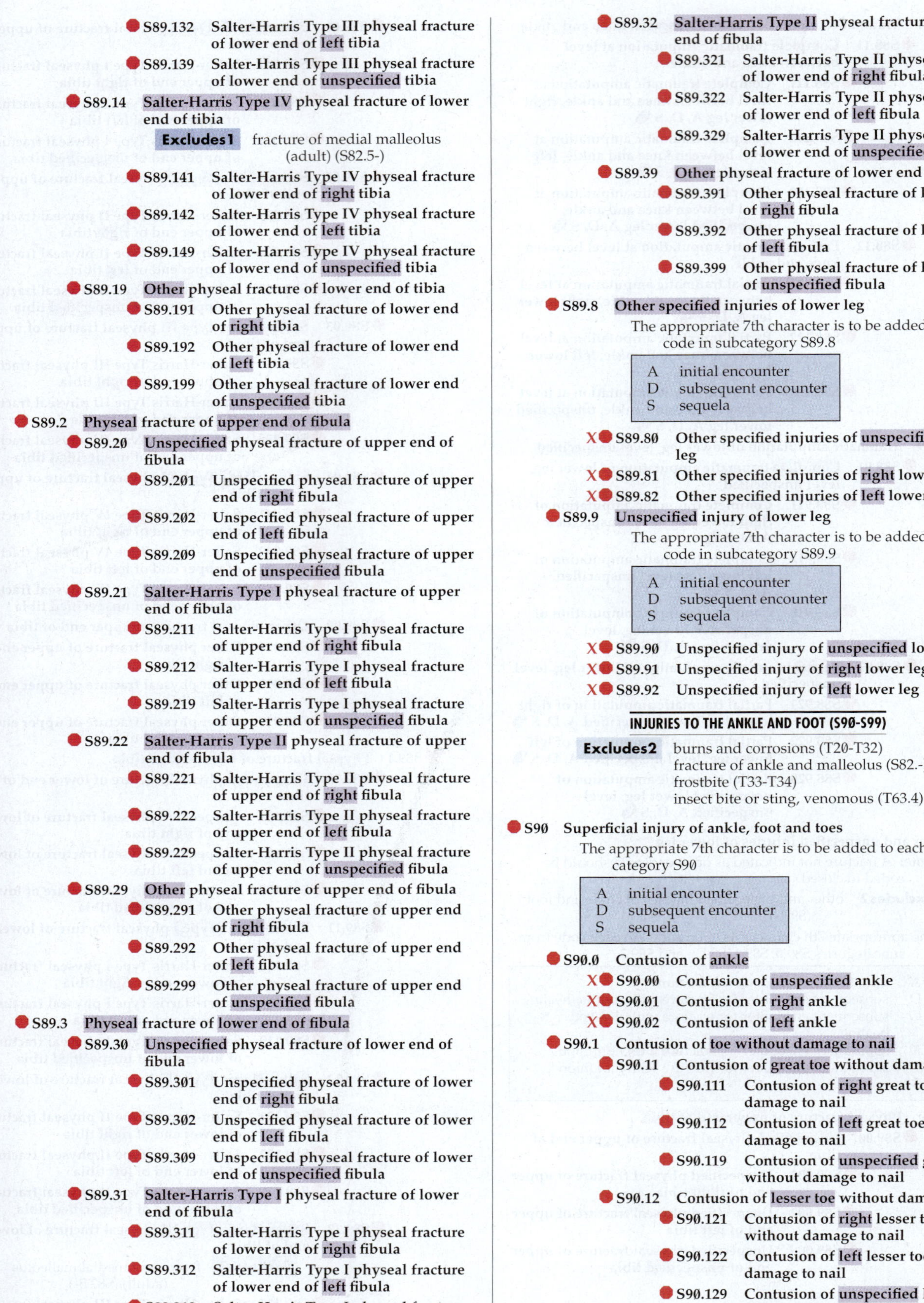

CHAPTER 19 (S00-T88)

● S89.132   Salter-Harris Type III physeal fracture of lower end of **left** tibia

● S89.139   Salter-Harris Type III physeal fracture of lower end of **unspecified** tibia

● S89.14   **Salter-Harris Type IV physeal fracture of lower end of tibia**

    Excludes1   fracture of medial malleolus (adult) (S82.5-)

● S89.141   Salter-Harris Type IV physeal fracture of lower end of **right** tibia

● S89.142   Salter-Harris Type IV physeal fracture of lower end of **left** tibia

● S89.149   Salter-Harris Type IV physeal fracture of lower end of **unspecified** tibia

● S89.19   Other physeal fracture of lower end of tibia

● S89.191   Other physeal fracture of lower end of **right** tibia

● S89.192   Other physeal fracture of lower end of **left** tibia

● S89.199   Other physeal fracture of lower end of **unspecified** tibia

● S89.2   Physeal fracture of **upper end** of fibula

● S89.20   **Unspecified** physeal fracture of upper end of fibula

● S89.201   Unspecified physeal fracture of upper end of **right** fibula

● S89.202   Unspecified physeal fracture of upper end of **left** fibula

● S89.209   Unspecified physeal fracture of upper end of **unspecified** fibula

● S89.21   **Salter-Harris Type I** physeal fracture of upper end of fibula

● S89.211   Salter-Harris Type I physeal fracture of upper end of **right** fibula

● S89.212   Salter-Harris Type I physeal fracture of upper end of **left** fibula

● S89.219   Salter-Harris Type I physeal fracture of upper end of **unspecified** fibula

● S89.22   **Salter-Harris Type II** physeal fracture of upper end of fibula

● S89.221   Salter-Harris Type II physeal fracture of upper end of **right** fibula

● S89.222   Salter-Harris Type II physeal fracture of upper end of **left** fibula

● S89.229   Salter-Harris Type II physeal fracture of upper end of **unspecified** fibula

● S89.29   Other physeal fracture of upper end of fibula

● S89.291   Other physeal fracture of upper end of **right** fibula

● S89.292   Other physeal fracture of upper end of **left** fibula

● S89.299   Other physeal fracture of upper end of **unspecified** fibula

● S89.3   Physeal fracture of **lower end** of fibula

● S89.30   **Unspecified** physeal fracture of lower end of fibula

● S89.301   Unspecified physeal fracture of lower end of **right** fibula

● S89.302   Unspecified physeal fracture of lower end of **left** fibula

● S89.309   Unspecified physeal fracture of lower end of **unspecified** fibula

● S89.31   **Salter-Harris Type I physeal fracture of lower end of fibula**

● S89.311   Salter-Harris Type I physeal fracture of upper end of **right** fibula

● S89.312   Salter-Harris Type I physeal fracture of lower end of **left** fibula

● S89.319   Salter-Harris Type I physeal fracture of lower end of **unspecified** fibula

● S89.32   **Salter-Harris Type II physeal fracture of lower end of fibula**

● S89.321   Salter-Harris Type II physeal fracture of lower end of **right** fibula

● S89.322   Salter-Harris Type II physeal fracture of lower end of **left** fibula

● S89.329   Salter-Harris Type II physeal fracture of lower end of **unspecified** fibula

● S89.39   Other physeal fracture of lower end of fibula

● S89.391   Other physeal fracture of lower end of **right** fibula

● S89.392   Other physeal fracture of lower end of **left** fibula

● S89.399   Other physeal fracture of lower end of **unspecified** fibula

● S89.8   Other specified injuries of lower leg

    The appropriate 7th character is to be added to each code in subcategory S89.8

A	initial encounter
D	subsequent encounter
S	sequela

X ● S89.80   Other specified injuries of **unspecified** lower leg

X ● S89.81   Other specified injuries of **right** lower leg

X ● S89.82   Other specified injuries of **left** lower leg

● S89.9   Unspecified injury of lower leg

    The appropriate 7th character is to be added to each code in subcategory S89.9

A	initial encounter
D	subsequent encounter
S	sequela

X ● S89.90   Unspecified injury of **unspecified** lower leg

X ● S89.91   Unspecified injury of **right** lower leg

X ● S89.92   Unspecified injury of **left** lower leg

INJURIES TO THE ANKLE AND FOOT (S90-S99)

    Excludes2   burns and corrosions (T20-T32)
       fracture of ankle and malleolus (S82.-)
       frostbite (T33-T34)
       insect bite or sting, venomous (T63.4)

● S90   Superficial injury of ankle, foot and toes

    The appropriate 7th character is to be added to each code from category S90

A	initial encounter
D	subsequent encounter
S	sequela

● S90.0   Contusion of ankle

X ● S90.00   Contusion of **unspecified** ankle

X ● S90.01   Contusion of **right** ankle

X ● S90.02   Contusion of **left** ankle

● S90.1   Contusion of toe without damage to nail

● S90.11   Contusion of **great** toe without damage to nail

● S90.111   Contusion of **right** great toe without damage to nail

● S90.112   Contusion of **left** great toe without damage to nail

● S90.119   Contusion of **unspecified** great toe without damage to nail

● S90.12   Contusion of **lesser** toe without damage to nail

● S90.121   Contusion of **right** lesser toe(s) without damage to nail

● S90.122   Contusion of **left** lesser toe(s) without damage to nail

● S90.129   Contusion of **unspecified** lesser toe(s) without damage to nail
       Contusion of toe NOS

● **S90.2**   **Contusion of toe with damage to nail**
  ● **S90.21**   **Contusion of great toe with damage to nail**
    ● **S90.211**   Contusion of right great toe with damage to nail
    ● **S90.212**   Contusion of left great toe with damage to nail
    ● **S90.219**   Contusion of unspecified great toe with damage to nail
  ● **S90.22**   **Contusion of lesser toe with damage to nail**
    ● **S90.221**   Contusion of right lesser toe(s) with damage to nail
    ● **S90.222**   Contusion of left lesser toe(s) with damage to nail
    ● **S90.229**   Contusion of unspecified lesser toe(s) with damage to nail
● **S90.3**   **Contusion of foot**
  Excludes2   contusion of toes (S90.1-, S90.2-)
  X● **S90.30**   **Contusion of unspecified foot**
          Contusion of foot NOS
  X● **S90.31**   **Contusion of right foot**
  X● **S90.32**   **Contusion of left foot**
● **S90.4**   **Other superficial injuries of toe**
  ● **S90.41**   **Abrasion of toe**
    ● **S90.411**   Abrasion, right great toe
    ● **S90.412**   Abrasion, left great toe
    ● **S90.413**   Abrasion, unspecified great toe
    ● **S90.414**   Abrasion, right lesser toe(s)
    ● **S90.415**   Abrasion, left lesser toe(s)
    ● **S90.416**   Abrasion, unspecified lesser toe(s)
  ● **S90.42**   **Blister (nonthermal) of toe**
    ● **S90.421**   Blister (nonthermal), right great toe
    ● **S90.422**   Blister (nonthermal), left great toe
    ● **S90.423**   Blister (nonthermal), unspecified great toe
    ● **S90.424**   Blister (nonthermal), right lesser toe(s)
    ● **S90.425**   Blister (nonthermal), left lesser toe(s)
    ● **S90.426**   Blister (nonthermal), unspecified lesser toe(s)
  ● **S90.44**   **External constriction of toe**
          Hair tourniquet syndrome of toe
    ● **S90.441**   External constriction, right great toe
    ● **S90.442**   External constriction, left great toe
    ● **S90.443**   External constriction, unspecified great toe
    ● **S90.444**   External constriction, right lesser toe(s)
    ● **S90.445**   External constriction, left lesser toe(s)
    ● **S90.446**   External constriction, unspecified lesser toe(s)
  ● **S90.45**   **Superficial foreign body of toe**
          Splinter in the toe
    ● **S90.451**   Superficial foreign body, right great toe
    ● **S90.452**   Superficial foreign body, left great toe
    ● **S90.453**   Superficial foreign body, unspecified great toe
    ● **S90.454**   Superficial foreign body, right lesser toe(s)
    ● **S90.455**   Superficial foreign body, left lesser toe(s)
    ● **S90.456**   Superficial foreign body, unspecified lesser toe(s)
  ● **S90.46**   **Insect bite (nonvenomous) of toe**
    ● **S90.461**   Insect bite (nonvenomous), right great toe
    ● **S90.462**   Insect bite (nonvenomous), left great toe

● **S90.463**   Insect bite (nonvenomous), unspecified great toe
● **S90.464**   Insect bite (nonvenomous), right lesser toe(s)
● **S90.465**   Insect bite (nonvenomous), left lesser toe(s)
● **S90.466**   Insect bite (nonvenomous), unspecified lesser toe(s)
  ● **S90.47**   **Other superficial bite of toe**
      Excludes1   open bite of toe (S91.15-, S91.25-)
    ● **S90.471**   Other superficial bite of right great toe
    ● **S90.472**   Other superficial bite of left great toe
    ● **S90.473**   Other superficial bite of unspecified great toe
    ● **S90.474**   Other superficial bite of right lesser toe(s)
    ● **S90.475**   Other superficial bite of left lesser toe(s)
    ● **S90.476**   Other superficial bite of unspecified lesser toe(s)
● **S90.5**   **Other superficial injuries of ankle**
  ● **S90.51**   **Abrasion of ankle**
    ● **S90.511**   Abrasion, right ankle
    ● **S90.512**   Abrasion, left ankle
    ● **S90.519**   Abrasion, unspecified ankle
  ● **S90.52**   **Blister (nonthermal) of ankle**
    ● **S90.521**   Blister (nonthermal), right ankle
    ● **S90.522**   Blister (nonthermal), left ankle
    ● **S90.529**   Blister (nonthermal), unspecified ankle
  ● **S90.54**   **External constriction of ankle**
    ● **S90.541**   External constriction, right ankle
    ● **S90.542**   External constriction, left ankle
    ● **S90.549**   External constriction, unspecified ankle
  ● **S90.55**   **Superficial foreign body of ankle**
          Splinter in the ankle
    ● **S90.551**   Superficial foreign body, right ankle
    ● **S90.552**   Superficial foreign body, left ankle
    ● **S90.559**   Superficial foreign body, unspecified ankle
  ● **S90.56**   **Insect bite (nonvenomous) of ankle**
    ● **S90.561**   Insect bite (nonvenomous), right ankle
    ● **S90.562**   Insect bite (nonvenomous), left ankle
    ● **S90.569**   Insect bite (nonvenomous), unspecified ankle
  ● **S90.57**   **Other superficial bite of ankle**
      Excludes1   open bite of ankle (S91.05-)
    ● **S90.571**   Other superficial bite of ankle, right ankle
    ● **S90.572**   Other superficial bite of ankle, left ankle
    ● **S90.579**   Other superficial bite of ankle, unspecified ankle
● **S90.8**   **Other superficial injuries of foot**
  ● **S90.81**   **Abrasion of foot**
    ● **S90.811**   Abrasion, right foot
    ● **S90.812**   Abrasion, left foot
    ● **S90.819**   Abrasion, unspecified foot
  ● **S90.82**   **Blister (nonthermal) of foot**
    ● **S90.821**   Blister (nonthermal), right foot
    ● **S90.822**   Blister (nonthermal), left foot
    ● **S90.829**   Blister (nonthermal), unspecified foot
  ● **S90.84**   **External constriction of foot**
    ● **S90.841**   External constriction, right foot

CHAPTER 19 (S00-T88)

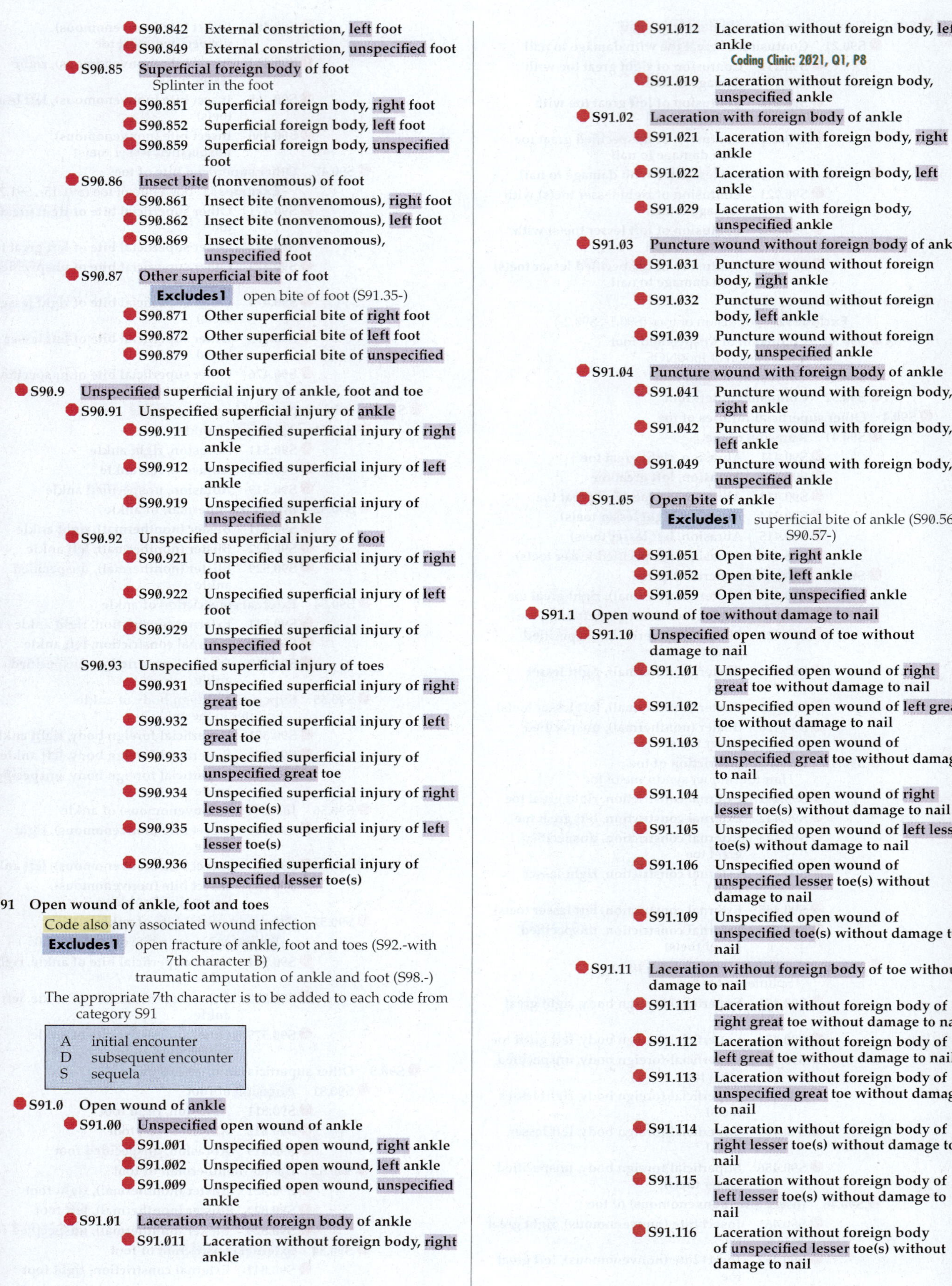

● S90.842   External constriction, left foot
● S90.849   External constriction, unspecified foot
● S90.85   **Superficial foreign body of foot**
            Splinter in the foot
● S90.851   Superficial foreign body, right foot
● S90.852   Superficial foreign body, left foot
● S90.859   Superficial foreign body, unspecified foot
● S90.86   **Insect bite (nonvenomous) of foot**
● S90.861   Insect bite (nonvenomous), right foot
● S90.862   Insect bite (nonvenomous), left foot
● S90.869   Insect bite (nonvenomous), unspecified foot
● S90.87   **Other superficial bite of foot**
            Excludes1   open bite of foot (S91.35-)
● S90.871   Other superficial bite of right foot
● S90.872   Other superficial bite of left foot
● S90.879   Other superficial bite of unspecified foot
● S90.9   **Unspecified superficial injury of ankle, foot and toe**
  ● S90.91   **Unspecified superficial injury of ankle**
  ● S90.911   Unspecified superficial injury of right ankle
  ● S90.912   Unspecified superficial injury of left ankle
  ● S90.919   Unspecified superficial injury of unspecified ankle
  ● S90.92   **Unspecified superficial injury of foot**
  ● S90.921   Unspecified superficial injury of right foot
  ● S90.922   Unspecified superficial injury of left foot
  ● S90.929   Unspecified superficial injury of unspecified foot
  S90.93   **Unspecified superficial injury of toes**
  ● S90.931   Unspecified superficial injury of right great toe
  ● S90.932   Unspecified superficial injury of left great toe
  ● S90.933   Unspecified superficial injury of unspecified great toe
  ● S90.934   Unspecified superficial injury of right lesser toe(s)
  ● S90.935   Unspecified superficial injury of left lesser toe(s)
  ● S90.936   Unspecified superficial injury of unspecified lesser toe(s)

● **S91   Open wound of ankle, foot and toes**
    Code also any associated wound infection
    Excludes1   open fracture of ankle, foot and toes (S92.-with 7th character B)
                   traumatic amputation of ankle and foot (S98.-)
    The appropriate 7th character is to be added to each code from category S91

    | A | initial encounter |
    | D | subsequent encounter |
    | S | sequela |

  ● S91.0   **Open wound of ankle**
    ● S91.00   **Unspecified open wound of ankle**
    ● S91.001   Unspecified open wound, right ankle
    ● S91.002   Unspecified open wound, left ankle
    ● S91.009   Unspecified open wound, unspecified ankle
    ● S91.01   **Laceration without foreign body of ankle**
    ● S91.011   Laceration without foreign body, right ankle

● S91.012   Laceration without foreign body, left ankle
              Coding Clinic: 2021, Q1, P8
● S91.019   Laceration without foreign body, unspecified ankle
● S91.02   **Laceration with foreign body of ankle**
● S91.021   Laceration with foreign body, right ankle
● S91.022   Laceration with foreign body, left ankle
● S91.029   Laceration with foreign body, unspecified ankle
● S91.03   **Puncture wound without foreign body of ankle**
● S91.031   Puncture wound without foreign body, right ankle
● S91.032   Puncture wound without foreign body, left ankle
● S91.039   Puncture wound without foreign body, unspecified ankle
● S91.04   **Puncture wound with foreign body of ankle**
● S91.041   Puncture wound with foreign body, right ankle
● S91.042   Puncture wound with foreign body, left ankle
● S91.049   Puncture wound with foreign body, unspecified ankle
● S91.05   **Open bite of ankle**
            Excludes1   superficial bite of ankle (S90.56-, S90.57-)
● S91.051   Open bite, right ankle
● S91.052   Open bite, left ankle
● S91.059   Open bite, unspecified ankle
● **S91.1   Open wound of toe without damage to nail**
  ● S91.10   **Unspecified open wound of toe without damage to nail**
  ● S91.101   Unspecified open wound of right great toe without damage to nail
  ● S91.102   Unspecified open wound of left great toe without damage to nail
  ● S91.103   Unspecified open wound of unspecified great toe without damage to nail
  ● S91.104   Unspecified open wound of right lesser toe(s) without damage to nail
  ● S91.105   Unspecified open wound of left lesser toe(s) without damage to nail
  ● S91.106   Unspecified open wound of unspecified lesser toe(s) without damage to nail
  ● S91.109   Unspecified open wound of unspecified toe(s) without damage to nail
  ● S91.11   **Laceration without foreign body of toe without damage to nail**
  ● S91.111   Laceration without foreign body of right great toe without damage to nail
  ● S91.112   Laceration without foreign body of left great toe without damage to nail
  ● S91.113   Laceration without foreign body of unspecified great toe without damage to nail
  ● S91.114   Laceration without foreign body of right lesser toe(s) without damage to nail
  ● S91.115   Laceration without foreign body of left lesser toe(s) without damage to nail
  ● S91.116   Laceration without foreign body of unspecified lesser toe(s) without damage to nail

▶ New   ➡ Revised   ~~deleted~~ Deleted   Excludes 1   Excludes 2   Includes   Use additional   Code first   Code also   Key words
OGCR Official Guidelines   X Assign placeholder X   ● Use Additional Character(s)   ▶ Manifestation Code   🔗 Hierarchical Condition Category   **Coding Clinic**

● **S91.119** Laceration without foreign body of unspecified toe without damage to nail

● **S91.12** Laceration with foreign body of toe without damage to nail

    ● **S91.121** Laceration with foreign body of right great toe without damage to nail

    ● **S91.122** Laceration with foreign body of left great toe without damage to nail

    ● **S91.123** Laceration with foreign body of unspecified great toe without damage to nail

    ● **S91.124** Laceration with foreign body of right lesser toe(s) without damage to nail

    ● **S91.125** Laceration with foreign body of left lesser toe(s) without damage to nail

    ● **S91.126** Laceration with foreign body of unspecified lesser toe(s) without damage to nail

    ● **S91.129** Laceration with foreign body of unspecified toe(s) without damage to nail

● **S91.13** Puncture wound without foreign body of toe without damage to nail

    ● **S91.131** Puncture wound without foreign body of right great toe without damage to nail

    ● **S91.132** Puncture wound without foreign body of left great toe without damage to nail

    ● **S91.133** Puncture wound without foreign body of unspecified great toe without damage to nail

    ● **S91.134** Puncture wound without foreign body of right lesser toe(s) without damage to nail

    ● **S91.135** Puncture wound without foreign body of left lesser toe(s) without damage to nail

    ● **S91.136** Puncture wound without foreign body of unspecified lesser toe(s) without damage to nail

    ● **S91.139** Puncture wound without foreign body of unspecified toe(s) without damage to nail

● **S91.14** Puncture wound with foreign body of toe without damage to nail

    ● **S91.141** Puncture wound with foreign body of right great toe without damage to nail

    ● **S91.142** Puncture wound with foreign body of left great toe without damage to nail

    ● **S91.143** Puncture wound with foreign body of unspecified great toe without damage to nail

    ● **S91.144** Puncture wound with foreign body of right lesser toe(s) without damage to nail

    ● **S91.145** Puncture wound with foreign body of left lesser toe(s) without damage to nail

    ● **S91.146** Puncture wound with foreign body of unspecified lesser toe(s) without damage to nail

    ● **S91.149** Puncture wound with foreign body of unspecified toe(s) without damage to nail

● **S91.15** Open bite of toe without damage to nail
    Bite of toe NOS

    Excludes1   superficial bite of toe (S90.46-, S90.47-)

    ● **S91.151** Open bite of right great toe without damage to nail

    ● **S91.152** Open bite of left great toe without damage to nail

    ● **S91.153** Open bite of unspecified great toe without damage to nail

    ● **S91.154** Open bite of right lesser toe(s) without damage to nail

    ● **S91.155** Open bite of left lesser toe(s) without damage to nail

    ● **S91.156** Open bite of unspecified lesser toe(s) without damage to nail

    ● **S91.159** Open bite of unspecified toe(s) without damage to nail

● **S91.2** Open wound of toe with damage to nail

● **S91.20** Unspecified open wound of toe with damage to nail

    ● **S91.201** Unspecified open wound of right great toe with damage to nail

    ● **S91.202** Unspecified open wound of left great toe with damage to nail

    ● **S91.203** Unspecified open wound of unspecified great toe with damage to nail

    ● **S91.204** Unspecified open wound of right lesser toe(s) with damage to nail

    ● **S91.205** Unspecified open wound of left lesser toe(s) with damage to nail

    ● **S91.206** Unspecified open wound of unspecified lesser toe(s) with damage to nail

    ● **S91.209** Unspecified open wound of unspecified toe(s) with damage to nail

● **S91.21** Laceration without foreign body of toe with damage to nail

    ● **S91.211** Laceration without foreign body of right great toe with damage to nail

    ● **S91.212** Laceration without foreign body of left great toe with damage to nail

    ● **S91.213** Laceration without foreign body of unspecified great toe with damage to nail

    ● **S91.214** Laceration without foreign body of right lesser toe(s) with damage to nail

    ● **S91.215** Laceration without foreign body of left lesser toe(s) with damage to nail

    ● **S91.216** Laceration without foreign body of unspecified lesser toe(s) with damage to nail

    ● **S91.219** Laceration without foreign body of unspecified toe(s) with damage to nail

● **S91.22** Laceration with foreign body of toe with damage to nail

    ● **S91.221** Laceration with foreign body of right great toe with damage to nail

    ● **S91.222** Laceration with foreign body of left great toe with damage to nail

    ● **S91.223** Laceration with foreign body of unspecified great toe with damage to nail

    ● **S91.224** Laceration with foreign body of right lesser toe(s) with damage to nail

    ● **S91.225** Laceration with foreign body of left lesser toe(s) with damage to nail

    ● **S91.226** Laceration with foreign body of unspecified lesser toe(s) with damage to nail

    ● **S91.229** Laceration with foreign body of unspecified toe(s) with damage to nail

CHAPTER 19 (S00-T88)

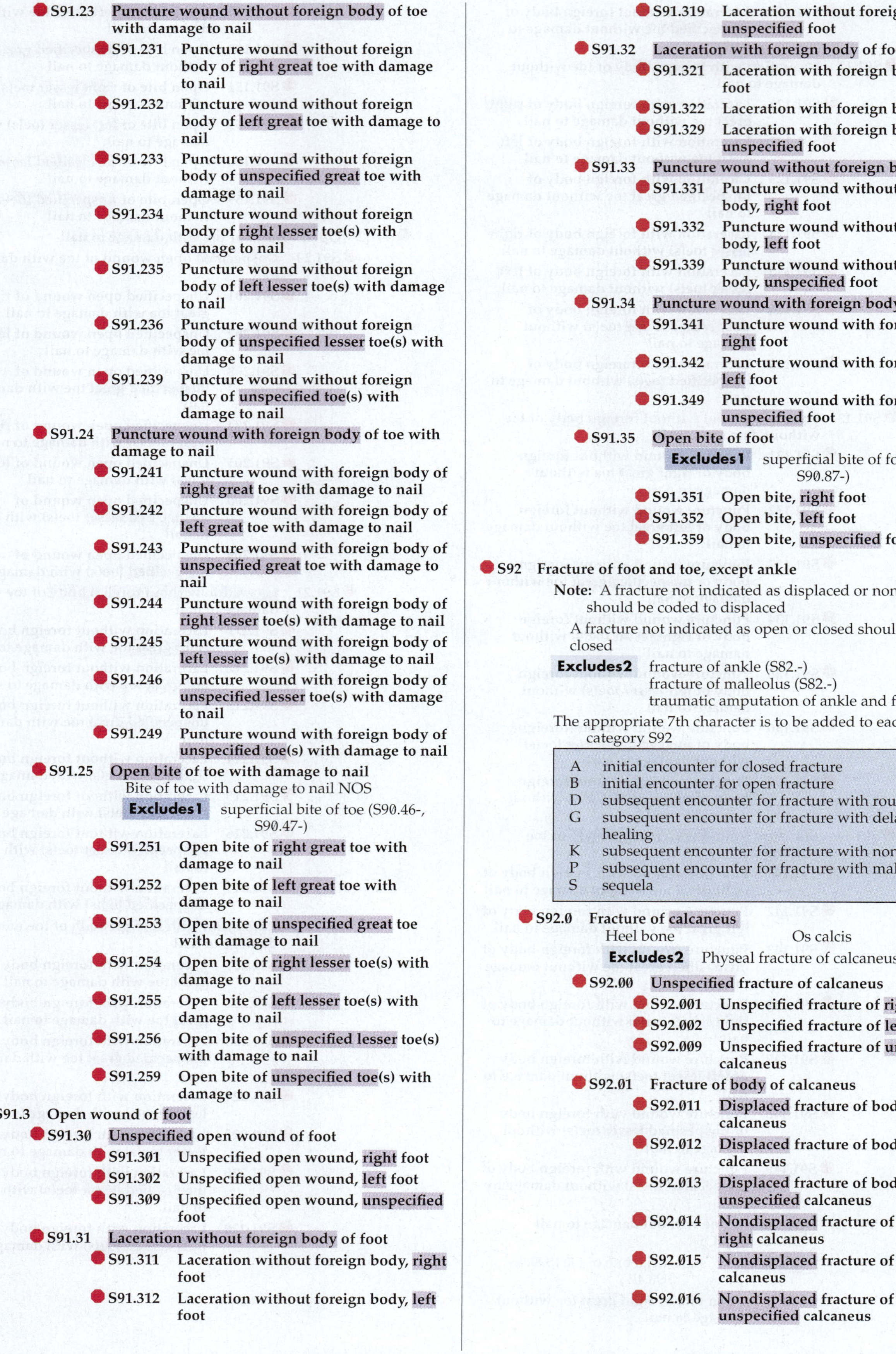

- 🔴 **S91.23** **Puncture** wound without **foreign body** of **toe** with damage to nail
  - 🔴 S91.231 Puncture wound without foreign body of **right great toe** with damage to nail
  - 🔴 S91.232 Puncture wound without foreign body of **left great toe** with damage to nail
  - 🔴 S91.233 Puncture wound without foreign body of **unspecified great toe** with damage to nail
  - 🔴 S91.234 Puncture wound without foreign body of **right lesser toe(s)** with damage to nail
  - 🔴 S91.235 Puncture wound without foreign body of **left lesser toe(s)** with damage to nail
  - 🔴 S91.236 Puncture wound without foreign body of **unspecified lesser toe(s)** with damage to nail
  - 🔴 S91.239 Puncture wound without foreign body of **unspecified toe(s)** with damage to nail
- 🔴 **S91.24** **Puncture** wound with **foreign body** of **toe** with damage to nail
  - 🔴 S91.241 Puncture wound with foreign body of **right great** toe with damage to nail
  - 🔴 S91.242 Puncture wound with foreign body of **left great** toe with damage to nail
  - 🔴 S91.243 Puncture wound with foreign body of **unspecified great** toe with damage to nail
  - 🔴 S91.244 Puncture wound with foreign body of **right lesser toe(s)** with damage to nail
  - 🔴 S91.245 Puncture wound with foreign body of **left lesser toe(s)** with damage to nail
  - 🔴 S91.246 Puncture wound with foreign body of **unspecified lesser toe(s)** with damage to nail
  - 🔴 S91.249 Puncture wound with foreign body of **unspecified toe(s)** with damage to nail
- 🔴 **S91.25** **Open bite** of **toe** with damage to nail
  Bite of toe with damage to nail NOS
  > **Excludes1** superficial bite of toe (S90.46-, S90.47-)
  - 🔴 S91.251 Open bite of **right great** toe with damage to nail
  - 🔴 S91.252 Open bite of **left great** toe with damage to nail
  - 🔴 S91.253 Open bite of **unspecified great** toe with damage to nail
  - 🔴 S91.254 Open bite of **right lesser toe(s)** with damage to nail
  - 🔴 S91.255 Open bite of **left lesser toe(s)** with damage to nail
  - 🔴 S91.256 Open bite of **unspecified lesser toe(s)** with damage to nail
  - 🔴 S91.259 Open bite of **unspecified toe(s)** with damage to nail
- 🔴 **S91.3** **Open wound** of **foot**
  - 🔴 **S91.30** **Unspecified** open wound of foot
    - 🔴 S91.301 Unspecified open wound, **right** foot
    - 🔴 S91.302 Unspecified open wound, **left** foot
    - 🔴 S91.309 Unspecified open wound, **unspecified** foot
  - 🔴 **S91.31** **Laceration** without foreign body of foot
    - 🔴 S91.311 Laceration without foreign body, **right** foot
    - 🔴 S91.312 Laceration without foreign body, **left** foot

- 🔴 S91.319 Laceration without foreign body, **unspecified** foot
- 🔴 **S91.32** **Laceration** with foreign body of foot
  - 🔴 S91.321 Laceration with foreign body, **right** foot
  - 🔴 S91.322 Laceration with foreign body, **left** foot
  - 🔴 S91.329 Laceration with foreign body, **unspecified** foot
- 🔴 **S91.33** **Puncture** wound without **foreign body** of foot
  - 🔴 S91.331 Puncture wound without foreign body, **right** foot
  - 🔴 S91.332 Puncture wound without foreign body, **left** foot
  - 🔴 S91.339 Puncture wound without foreign body, **unspecified** foot
- 🔴 **S91.34** **Puncture** wound with **foreign body** of foot
  - 🔴 S91.341 Puncture wound with foreign body, **right** foot
  - 🔴 S91.342 Puncture wound with foreign body, **left** foot
  - 🔴 S91.349 Puncture wound with foreign body, **unspecified** foot
- 🔴 **S91.35** **Open bite** of foot
  > **Excludes1** superficial bite of foot (S90.86-, S90.87-)
  - 🔴 S91.351 Open bite, **right** foot
  - 🔴 S91.352 Open bite, **left** foot
  - 🔴 S91.359 Open bite, **unspecified** foot

- 🔴 **S92** **Fracture** of **foot** and **toe, except ankle**
  > **Note:** A fracture not indicated as displaced or nondisplaced should be coded to displaced
  >
  > A fracture not indicated as open or closed should be coded to closed
  > **Excludes2** fracture of ankle (S82.-)
  > fracture of malleolus (S82.-)
  > traumatic amputation of ankle and foot (S98.-)
  >
  > The appropriate 7th character is to be added to each code from category S92

A	initial encounter for closed fracture
B	initial encounter for open fracture
D	subsequent encounter for fracture with routine healing
G	subsequent encounter for fracture with delayed healing
K	subsequent encounter for fracture with nonunion
P	subsequent encounter for fracture with malunion
S	sequela

  - 🔴 **S92.0** **Fracture** of **calcaneus**
    Heel bone   Os calcis
    > **Excludes2** Physeal fracture of calcaneus (S99.0-)
    - 🔴 **S92.00** **Unspecified** fracture of calcaneus
      - 🔴 S92.001 Unspecified fracture of **right** calcaneus
      - 🔴 S92.002 Unspecified fracture of **left** calcaneus
      - 🔴 S92.009 Unspecified fracture of **unspecified** calcaneus
    - 🔴 **S92.01** **Fracture** of **body** of calcaneus
      - 🔴 S92.011 Displaced fracture of body of **right** calcaneus
      - 🔴 S92.012 Displaced fracture of body of **left** calcaneus
      - 🔴 S92.013 Displaced fracture of body of **unspecified** calcaneus
      - 🔴 S92.014 Nondisplaced fracture of body of **right** calcaneus
      - 🔴 S92.015 Nondisplaced fracture of body of **left** calcaneus
      - 🔴 S92.016 Nondisplaced fracture of body of **unspecified** calcaneus

▶ New   ⇒ Revised   ~~deleted~~ Deleted   Excludes 1   Excludes 2   Includes   Use additional   Code first   Code also   Key words

OGCR Official Guidelines   X Assign placeholder X   🔴 Use Additional Character(s)   ▶ Manifestation Code   🔮 Hierarchical Condition Category   **Coding Clinic**

- ● **S92.02** Fracture of anterior process of calcaneus
  - ● **S92.021** Displaced fracture of anterior process of right calcaneus
  - ● **S92.022** Displaced fracture of anterior process of left calcaneus
  - ● **S92.023** Displaced fracture of anterior process of unspecified calcaneus
  - ● **S92.024** Nondisplaced fracture of anterior process of right calcaneus
  - ● **S92.025** Nondisplaced fracture of anterior process of left calcaneus
  - ● **S92.026** Nondisplaced fracture of anterior process of unspecified calcaneus
- ● **S92.03** Avulsion fracture of tuberosity of calcaneus
  - ● **S92.031** Displaced avulsion fracture of tuberosity of right calcaneus
  - ● **S92.032** Displaced avulsion fracture of tuberosity of left calcaneus
  - ● **S92.033** Displaced avulsion fracture of tuberosity of unspecified calcaneus
  - ● **S92.034** Nondisplaced avulsion fracture of tuberosity of right calcaneus
  - ● **S92.035** Nondisplaced avulsion fracture of tuberosity of left calcaneus
  - ● **S92.036** Nondisplaced avulsion fracture of tuberosity of unspecified calcaneus
- ● **S92.04** Other fracture of tuberosity of calcaneus
  - ● **S92.041** Displaced other fracture of tuberosity of right calcaneus
  - ● **S92.042** Displaced other fracture of tuberosity of left calcaneus
  - ● **S92.043** Displaced other fracture of tuberosity of unspecified calcaneus
  - ● **S92.044** Nondisplaced other fracture of tuberosity of right calcaneus
  - ● **S92.045** Nondisplaced other fracture of tuberosity of left calcaneus
  - ● **S92.046** Nondisplaced other fracture of tuberosity of unspecified calcaneus
- ● **S92.05** Other extraarticular fracture of calcaneus
  - ● **S92.051** Displaced other extraarticular fracture of right calcaneus
  - ● **S92.052** Displaced other extraarticular fracture of left calcaneus
  - ● **S92.053** Displaced other extraarticular fracture of unspecified calcaneus
  - ● **S92.054** Nondisplaced other extraarticular fracture of right calcaneus
  - ● **S92.055** Nondisplaced other extraarticular fracture of left calcaneus
  - ● **S92.056** Nondisplaced other extraarticular fracture of unspecified calcaneus
- ● **S92.06** Intraarticular fracture of calcaneus
  - ● **S92.061** Displaced intraarticular fracture of right calcaneus
  - ● **S92.062** Displaced intraarticular fracture of left calcaneus
  - ● **S92.063** Displaced intraarticular fracture of unspecified calcaneus
  - ● **S92.064** Nondisplaced intraarticular fracture of right calcaneus
  - ● **S92.065** Nondisplaced intraarticular fracture of left calcaneus
  - ● **S92.066** Nondisplaced intraarticular fracture of unspecified calcaneus
- ● **S92.1** Fracture of talus
  Astragalus
  - ● **S92.10** Unspecified fracture of talus
    - ● **S92.101** Unspecified fracture of right talus
    - ● **S92.102** Unspecified fracture of left talus
    - ● **S92.109** Unspecified fracture of unspecified talus

- ● **S92.11** Fracture of neck of talus
  - ● **S92.111** Displaced fracture of neck of right talus
  - ● **S92.112** Displaced fracture of neck of left talus
  - ● **S92.113** Displaced fracture of neck of unspecified talus
  - ● **S92.114** Nondisplaced fracture of neck of right talus
  - ● **S92.115** Nondisplaced fracture of neck of left talus
  - ● **S92.116** Nondisplaced fracture of neck of unspecified talus
- ● **S92.12** Fracture of body of talus
  - ● **S92.121** Displaced fracture of body of right talus
  - ● **S92.122** Displaced fracture of body of left talus
  - ● **S92.123** Displaced fracture of body of unspecified talus
  - ● **S92.124** Nondisplaced fracture of body of right talus
  - ● **S92.125** Nondisplaced fracture of body of left talus
  - ● **S92.126** Nondisplaced fracture of body of unspecified talus
- ● **S92.13** Fracture of posterior process of talus
  - ● **S92.131** Displaced fracture of posterior process of right talus
  - ● **S92.132** Displaced fracture of posterior process of left talus
  - ● **S92.133** Displaced fracture of posterior process of unspecified talus
  - ● **S92.134** Nondisplaced fracture of posterior process of right talus
  - ● **S92.135** Nondisplaced fracture of posterior process of left talus
  - ● **S92.136** Nondisplaced fracture of posterior process of unspecified talus
- ● **S92.14** Dome fracture of talus
  - **Excludes1** osteochondritis dissecans (M93.2)
  - ● **S92.141** Displaced dome fracture of right talus
  - ● **S92.142** Displaced dome fracture of left talus
  - ● **S92.143** Displaced dome fracture of unspecified talus
  - ● **S92.144** Nondisplaced dome fracture of right talus
  - ● **S92.145** Nondisplaced dome fracture of left talus
  - ● **S92.146** Nondisplaced dome fracture of unspecified talus
- ● **S92.15** Avulsion fracture (chip fracture) of talus
  - ● **S92.151** Displaced avulsion fracture (chip fracture) of right talus
  - ● **S92.152** Displaced avulsion fracture (chip fracture) of left talus
  - ● **S92.153** Displaced avulsion fracture (chip fracture) of unspecified talus
  - ● **S92.154** Nondisplaced avulsion fracture (chip fracture) of right talus
  - ● **S92.155** Nondisplaced avulsion fracture (chip fracture) of left talus
  - ● **S92.156** Nondisplaced avulsion fracture (chip fracture) of unspecified talus
- ● **S92.19** Other fracture of talus
  - ● **S92.191** Other fracture of right talus
  - ● **S92.192** Other fracture of left talus
  - ● **S92.199** Other fracture of unspecified talus

● **S92.2**   Fracture of other and unspecified tarsal bone(s)
  ● **S92.20**   Fracture of unspecified tarsal bone(s)
    ● **S92.201**   Fracture of unspecified tarsal bone(s) of right foot
    ● **S92.202**   Fracture of unspecified tarsal bone(s) of left foot
    ● **S92.209**   Fracture of unspecified tarsal bone(s) of unspecified foot
  ● **S92.21**   Fracture of cuboid bone
    ● **S92.211**   Displaced fracture of cuboid bone of right foot
    ● **S92.212**   Displaced fracture of cuboid bone of left foot
    ● **S92.213**   Displaced fracture of cuboid bone of unspecified foot
    ● **S92.214**   Nondisplaced fracture of cuboid bone of right foot
    ● **S92.215**   Nondisplaced fracture of cuboid bone of left foot
    ● **S92.216**   Nondisplaced fracture of cuboid bone of unspecified foot
  ● **S92.22**   Fracture of lateral cuneiform
    ● **S92.221**   Displaced fracture of lateral cuneiform of right foot
    ● **S92.222**   Displaced fracture of lateral cuneiform of left foot
    ● **S92.223**   Displaced fracture of lateral cuneiform of unspecified foot
    ● **S92.224**   Nondisplaced fracture of lateral cuneiform of right foot
    ● **S92.225**   Nondisplaced fracture of lateral cuneiform of left foot
    ● **S92.226**   Nondisplaced fracture of lateral cuneiform of unspecified foot
  ● **S92.23**   Fracture of intermediate cuneiform
    ● **S92.231**   Displaced fracture of intermediate cuneiform of right foot
    ● **S92.232**   Displaced fracture of intermediate cuneiform of left foot
    ● **S92.233**   Displaced fracture of intermediate cuneiform of unspecified foot
    ● **S92.234**   Nondisplaced fracture of intermediate cuneiform of right foot
    ● **S92.235**   Nondisplaced fracture of intermediate cuneiform of left foot
    ● **S92.236**   Nondisplaced fracture of intermediate cuneiform of unspecified foot
  ● **S92.24**   Fracture of medial cuneiform
    ● **S92.241**   Displaced fracture of medial cuneiform of right foot
    ● **S92.242**   Displaced fracture of medial cuneiform of left foot
    ● **S92.243**   Displaced fracture of medial cuneiform of unspecified foot
    ● **S92.244**   Nondisplaced fracture of medial cuneiform of right foot
    ● **S92.245**   Nondisplaced fracture of medial cuneiform of left foot
    ● **S92.246**   Nondisplaced fracture of medial cuneiform of unspecified foot
  ● **S92.25**   Fracture of navicular [scaphoid] of foot
    ● **S92.251**   Displaced fracture of navicular [scaphoid] of right foot
    ● **S92.252**   Displaced fracture of navicular [scaphoid] of left foot
    ● **S92.253**   Displaced fracture of navicular [scaphoid] of unspecified foot

    ● **S92.254**   Nondisplaced fracture of navicular [scaphoid] of right foot
    ● **S92.255**   Nondisplaced fracture of navicular [scaphoid] of left foot
    ● **S92.256**   Nondisplaced fracture of navicular [scaphoid] of unspecified foot
● **S92.3**   Fracture of metatarsal bone(s)
    Excludes2   Physeal fracture of metatarsal (S99.1-)
  ● **S92.30**   Fracture of unspecified metatarsal bone(s)
    ● **S92.301**   Fracture of unspecified metatarsal bone(s), right foot
    ● **S92.302**   Fracture of unspecified metatarsal bone(s), left foot
    ● **S92.309**   Fracture of unspecified metatarsal bone(s), unspecified foot
  ● **S92.31**   Fracture of first metatarsal bone
    ● **S92.311**   Displaced fracture of first metatarsal bone, right foot
    ● **S92.312**   Displaced fracture of first metatarsal bone, left foot
    ● **S92.313**   Displaced fracture of first metatarsal bone, unspecified foot
    ● **S92.314**   Nondisplaced fracture of first metatarsal bone, right foot
    ● **S92.315**   Nondisplaced fracture of first metatarsal bone, left foot
    ● **S92.316**   Nondisplaced fracture of first metatarsal bone, unspecified foot
  ● **S92.32**   Fracture of second metatarsal bone
    ● **S92.321**   Displaced fracture of second metatarsal bone, right foot
    ● **S92.322**   Displaced fracture of second metatarsal bone, left foot
    ● **S92.323**   Displaced fracture of second metatarsal bone, unspecified foot
    ● **S92.324**   Nondisplaced fracture of second metatarsal bone, right foot
    ● **S92.325**   Nondisplaced fracture of second metatarsal bone, left foot
    ● **S92.326**   Nondisplaced fracture of second metatarsal bone, unspecified foot
  ● **S92.33**   Fracture of third metatarsal bone
    Coding Clinic: 2018, Q1, P3
    ● **S92.331**   Displaced fracture of third metatarsal bone, right foot
    ● **S92.332**   Displaced fracture of third metatarsal bone, left foot
    ● **S92.333**   Displaced fracture of third metatarsal bone, unspecified foot
    ● **S92.334**   Nondisplaced fracture of third metatarsal bone, right foot
    ● **S92.335**   Nondisplaced fracture of third metatarsal bone, left foot
    ● **S92.336**   Nondisplaced fracture of third metatarsal bone, unspecified foot
  ● **S92.34**   Fracture of fourth metatarsal bone
    ● **S92.341**   Displaced fracture of fourth metatarsal bone, right foot
    ● **S92.342**   Displaced fracture of fourth metatarsal bone, left foot
    ● **S92.343**   Displaced fracture of fourth metatarsal bone, unspecified foot
    ● **S92.344**   Nondisplaced fracture of fourth metatarsal bone, right foot
    ● **S92.345**   Nondisplaced fracture of fourth metatarsal bone, left foot
    ● **S92.346**   Nondisplaced fracture of fourth metatarsal bone, unspecified foot

▶ New   ⇨ Revised   ~~deleted~~ Deleted   Excludes 1   Excludes 2   Includes   Use additional   Code first   Code also   Key words
OGCR Official Guidelines   X Assign placeholder X   ● Use Additional Character(s)   ▶ Manifestation Code   HCC Hierarchical Condition Category   Coding Clinic

- **S92.35**   Fracture of fifth metatarsal bone
  - **S92.351**   Displaced fracture of fifth metatarsal bone, right foot
  - **S92.352**   Displaced fracture of fifth metatarsal bone, left foot
  - **S92.353**   Displaced fracture of fifth metatarsal bone, unspecified foot
  - **S92.354**   Nondisplaced fracture of fifth metatarsal bone, right foot
  - **S92.355**   Nondisplaced fracture of fifth metatarsal bone, left foot
  - **S92.356**   Nondisplaced fracture of fifth metatarsal bone, unspecified foot
- **S92.4**   Fracture of great toe

  Excludes2   Physeal fracture of phalanx of toe (S99.2-)
  - **S92.40**   Unspecified fracture of great toe
    - **S92.401**   Displaced unspecified fracture of right great toe
    - **S92.402**   Displaced unspecified fracture of left great toe
    - **S92.403**   Displaced unspecified fracture of unspecified great toe
    - **S92.404**   Nondisplaced unspecified fracture of right great toe
    - **S92.405**   Nondisplaced unspecified fracture of left great toe
    - **S92.406**   Nondisplaced unspecified fracture of unspecified great toe
  - **S92.41**   Fracture of proximal phalanx of great toe
    - **S92.411**   Displaced fracture of proximal phalanx of right great toe
    - **S92.412**   Displaced fracture of proximal phalanx of left great toe
    - **S92.413**   Displaced fracture of proximal phalanx of unspecified great toe
    - **S92.414**   Nondisplaced fracture of proximal phalanx of right great toe
    - **S92.415**   Nondisplaced fracture of proximal phalanx of left great toe
    - **S92.416**   Nondisplaced fracture of proximal phalanx of unspecified great toe
  - **S92.42**   Fracture of distal phalanx of great toe
    - **S92.421**   Displaced fracture of distal phalanx of right great toe
    - **S92.422**   Displaced fracture of distal phalanx of left great toe
    - **S92.423**   Displaced fracture of distal phalanx of unspecified great toe
    - **S92.424**   Nondisplaced fracture of distal phalanx of right great toe
    - **S92.425**   Nondisplaced fracture of distal phalanx of left great toe
    - **S92.426**   Nondisplaced fracture of distal phalanx of unspecified great toe
  - **S92.49**   Other fracture of great toe
    - **S92.491**   Other fracture of right great toe
    - **S92.492**   Other fracture of left great toe
    - **S92.499**   Other fracture of unspecified great toe
- **S92.5**   Fracture of lesser toe(s)

  Excludes2   Physeal fracture of phalanx of toe (S99.2-)
  - **S92.50**   Unspecified fracture of lesser toe(s)
    - **S92.501**   Displaced unspecified fracture of right lesser toe(s)
    - **S92.502**   Displaced unspecified fracture of left lesser toe(s)
    - **S92.503**   Displaced unspecified fracture of unspecified lesser toe(s)
    - **S92.504**   Nondisplaced unspecified fracture of right lesser toe(s)
    - **S92.505**   Nondisplaced unspecified fracture of left lesser toe(s)
    - **S92.506**   Nondisplaced unspecified fracture of unspecified lesser toe(s)
  - **S92.51**   Fracture of proximal phalanx of lesser toe(s)
    - **S92.511**   Displaced fracture of proximal phalanx of right lesser toe(s)
    - **S92.512**   Displaced fracture of proximal phalanx of left lesser toe(s)
    - **S92.513**   Displaced fracture of proximal phalanx of unspecified lesser toe(s)
    - **S92.514**   Nondisplaced fracture of proximal phalanx of right lesser toe(s)
    - **S92.515**   Nondisplaced fracture of proximal phalanx of left lesser toe(s)
    - **S92.516**   Nondisplaced fracture of proximal phalanx of unspecified lesser toe(s)
  - **S92.52**   Fracture of middle phalanx of lesser toe(s)
    - **S92.521**   Displaced fracture of middle phalanx of right lesser toe(s)
    - **S92.522**   Displaced fracture of middle phalanx of left lesser toe(s)
    - **S92.523**   Displaced fracture of middle phalanx of unspecified lesser toe(s)
    - **S92.524**   Nondisplaced fracture of middle phalanx of right lesser toe(s)
    - **S92.525**   Nondisplaced fracture of middle phalanx of left lesser toe(s)
    - **S92.526**   Nondisplaced fracture of middle phalanx of unspecified lesser toe(s)
  - **S92.53**   Fracture of distal phalanx of lesser toe(s)
    - **S92.531**   Displaced fracture of distal phalanx of right lesser toe(s)
    - **S92.532**   Displaced fracture of distal phalanx of left lesser toe(s)
    - **S92.533**   Displaced fracture of distal phalanx of unspecified lesser toe(s)
    - **S92.534**   Nondisplaced fracture of distal phalanx of right lesser toe(s)
    - **S92.535**   Nondisplaced fracture of distal phalanx of left lesser toe(s)
    - **S92.536**   Nondisplaced fracture of distal phalanx of unspecified lesser toe(s)
  - **S92.59**   Other fracture of lesser toe(s)
    - **S92.591**   Other fracture of right lesser toe(s)
    - **S92.592**   Other fracture of left lesser toe(s)
    - **S92.599**   Other fracture of unspecified lesser toe(s)
- **S92.8**   Other fracture of foot, except ankle
  - **S92.81**   Other fracture of foot

    Sesamoid fracture of foot

    Coding Clinic: 2016, Q4, P68
    - **S92.811**   Other fracture of right foot
    - **S92.812**   Other fracture of left foot
    - **S92.819**   Other fracture of unspecified foot
- **S92.9**   Unspecified fracture of foot and toe
  - **S92.90**   Unspecified fracture of foot
    - **S92.901**   Unspecified fracture of right foot
    - **S92.902**   Unspecified fracture of left foot
    - **S92.909**   Unspecified fracture of unspecified foot
  - **S92.91**   Unspecified fracture of toe
    - **S92.911**   Unspecified fracture of right toe(s)
    - **S92.912**   Unspecified fracture of left toe(s)
    - **S92.919**   Unspecified fracture of unspecified toe(s)

CHAPTER 19 (S00–T88)

● **S93**   **Dislocation and sprain of joints and ligaments at ankle, foot and toe level**

    Includes   avulsion of joint or ligament of ankle, foot and toe
        laceration of cartilage, joint or ligament of ankle, foot and toe
        sprain of cartilage, joint or ligament of ankle, foot and toe
        traumatic hemarthrosis of joint or ligament of ankle, foot and toe
        traumatic rupture of joint or ligament of ankle, foot and toe
        traumatic subluxation of joint or ligament of ankle, foot and toe
        traumatic tear of joint or ligament of ankle, foot and toe

    Code also any associated open wound

    Excludes2   strain of muscle and tendon of ankle and foot (S96.-)

    The appropriate 7th character is to be added to each code from category S93

      A   initial encounter
      D   subsequent encounter
      S   sequela

● **S93.0**   **Subluxation and dislocation of ankle joint**
    Subluxation and dislocation of astragalus
    Subluxation and dislocation of fibula, lower end
    Subluxation and dislocation of talus
    Subluxation and dislocation of tibia, lower end

  X ● **S93.01**   **Subluxation of right ankle joint**
  X ● **S93.02**   **Subluxation of left ankle joint**
  X ● **S93.03**   **Subluxation of unspecified ankle joint**
  X ● **S93.04**   **Dislocation of right ankle joint**
  X ● **S93.05**   **Dislocation of left ankle joint**
  X ● **S93.06**   **Dislocation of unspecified ankle joint**

● **S93.1**   **Subluxation and dislocation of toe**
  ● **S93.10**   **Unspecified subluxation and dislocation of toe**
    Dislocation of toe NOS
    Subluxation of toe NOS

    ● **S93.101**   **Unspecified subluxation of right toe(s)**
    ● **S93.102**   **Unspecified subluxation of left toe(s)**
    ● **S93.103**   **Unspecified subluxation of unspecified toe(s)**
    ● **S93.104**   **Unspecified dislocation of right toe(s)**
    ● **S93.105**   **Unspecified dislocation of left toe(s)**
    ● **S93.106**   **Unspecified dislocation of unspecified toe(s)**

  ● **S93.11**   **Dislocation of interphalangeal joint**
    ● **S93.111**   **Dislocation of interphalangeal joint of right great toe**
    ● **S93.112**   **Dislocation of interphalangeal joint of left great toe**
    ● **S93.113**   **Dislocation of interphalangeal joint of unspecified great toe**
    ● **S93.114**   **Dislocation of interphalangeal joint of right lesser toe(s)**
    ● **S93.115**   **Dislocation of interphalangeal joint of left lesser toe(s)**
    ● **S93.116**   **Dislocation of interphalangeal joint of unspecified lesser toe(s)**
    ● **S93.119**   **Dislocation of interphalangeal joint of unspecified toe(s)**

  ● **S93.12**   **Dislocation of metatarsophalangeal joint**
    ● **S93.121**   **Dislocation of metatarsophalangeal joint of right great toe**
    ● **S93.122**   **Dislocation of metatarsophalangeal joint of left great toe**
    ● **S93.123**   **Dislocation of metatarsophalangeal joint of unspecified great toe**
    ● **S93.124**   **Dislocation of metatarsophalangeal joint of right lesser toe(s)**

    ● **S93.125**   **Dislocation of metatarsophalangeal joint of left lesser toe(s)**
    ● **S93.126**   **Dislocation of metatarsophalangeal joint of unspecified lesser toe(s)**
    ● **S93.129**   **Dislocation of metatarsophalangeal joint of unspecified toe(s)**

  ● **S93.13**   **Subluxation of interphalangeal joint**
    ● **S93.131**   **Subluxation of interphalangeal joint of right great toe**
    ● **S93.132**   **Subluxation of interphalangeal joint of left great toe**
    ● **S93.133**   **Subluxation of interphalangeal joint of unspecified great toe**
    ● **S93.134**   **Subluxation of interphalangeal joint of right lesser toe(s)**
    ● **S93.135**   **Subluxation of interphalangeal joint of left lesser toe(s)**
    ● **S93.136**   **Subluxation of interphalangeal joint of unspecified lesser toe(s)**
    ● **S93.139**   **Subluxation of interphalangeal joint of unspecified toe(s)**

  ● **S93.14**   **Subluxation of metatarsophalangeal joint**
    ● **S93.141**   **Subluxation of metatarsophalangeal joint of right great toe**
    ● **S93.142**   **Subluxation of metatarsophalangeal joint of left great toe**
    ● **S93.143**   **Subluxation of metatarsophalangeal joint of unspecified great toe**
    ● **S93.144**   **Subluxation of metatarsophalangeal joint of right lesser toe(s)**
    ● **S93.145**   **Subluxation of metatarsophalangeal joint of left lesser toe(s)**
    ● **S93.146**   **Subluxation of metatarsophalangeal joint of unspecified lesser toe(s)**
    ● **S93.149**   **Subluxation of metatarsophalangeal joint of unspecified toe(s)**

● **S93.3**   **Subluxation and dislocation of foot**
    Excludes2   dislocation of toe (S93.1-)
  ● **S93.30**   **Unspecified subluxation and dislocation of foot**
    Dislocation of foot NOS
    Subluxation of foot NOS

    ● **S93.301**   **Unspecified subluxation of right foot**
    ● **S93.302**   **Unspecified subluxation of left foot**
    ● **S93.303**   **Unspecified subluxation of unspecified foot**
    ● **S93.304**   **Unspecified dislocation of right foot**
    ● **S93.305**   **Unspecified dislocation of left foot**
    ● **S93.306**   **Unspecified dislocation of unspecified foot**

  ● **S93.31**   **Subluxation and dislocation of tarsal joint**
    ● **S93.311**   **Subluxation of tarsal joint of right foot**
    ● **S93.312**   **Subluxation of tarsal joint of left foot**
    ● **S93.313**   **Subluxation of tarsal joint of unspecified foot**
    ● **S93.314**   **Dislocation of tarsal joint of right foot**
    ● **S93.315**   **Dislocation of tarsal joint of left foot**
    ● **S93.316**   **Dislocation of tarsal joint of unspecified foot**

  ● **S93.32**   **Subluxation and dislocation of tarsometatarsal joint**
    ● **S93.321**   **Subluxation of tarsometatarsal joint of right foot**
    ● **S93.322**   **Subluxation of tarsometatarsal joint of left foot**
    ● **S93.323**   **Subluxation of tarsometatarsal joint of unspecified foot**
    ● **S93.324**   **Dislocation of tarsometatarsal joint of right foot**

     ● S93.325   Dislocation of tarsometatarsal joint of left foot
     ● S93.326   Dislocation of tarsometatarsal joint of unspecified foot
  ● S93.33   Other subluxation and dislocation of foot
     ● S93.331   Other subluxation of right foot
     ● S93.332   Other subluxation of left foot
     ● S93.333   Other subluxation of unspecified foot
     ● S93.334   Other dislocation of right foot
     ● S93.335   Other dislocation of left foot
     ● S93.336   Other dislocation of unspecified foot
● **S93.4**   Sprain of ankle
     Injury to ligaments when one or more is stretched/torn
     Excludes2   injury of Achilles tendon (S86.0-)
  ● S93.40   Sprain of unspecified ligament of ankle
     Sprain of ankle NOS
     Sprained ankle NOS
     ● S93.401   Sprain of unspecified ligament of right ankle
     ● S93.402   Sprain of unspecified ligament of left ankle
     ● S93.409   Sprain of unspecified ligament of unspecified ankle
  ● S93.41   Sprain of calcaneofibular ligament
     ● S93.411   Sprain of calcaneofibular ligament of right ankle
     ● S93.412   Sprain of calcaneofibular ligament of left ankle
     ● S93.419   Sprain of calcaneofibular ligament of unspecified ankle
  ● S93.42   Sprain of deltoid ligament
     ● S93.421   Sprain of deltoid ligament of right ankle
     ● S93.422   Sprain of deltoid ligament of left ankle
     ● S93.429   Sprain of deltoid ligament of unspecified ankle
  ● S93.43   Sprain of tibiofibular ligament
     ● S93.431   Sprain of tibiofibular ligament of right ankle
     ● S93.432   Sprain of tibiofibular ligament of left ankle
     ● S93.439   Sprain of tibiofibular ligament of unspecified ankle
  ● S93.49   Sprain of other ligament of ankle
     Sprain of internal collateral ligament
     Sprain of talofibular ligament
     ● S93.491   Sprain of other ligament of right ankle
     ● S93.492   Sprain of other ligament of left ankle
     ● S93.499   Sprain of other ligament of unspecified ankle
● **S93.5**   Sprain of toe
  ● S93.50   Unspecified sprain of toe
     ● S93.501   Unspecified sprain of right great toe
     ● S93.502   Unspecified sprain of left great toe
     ● S93.503   Unspecified sprain of unspecified great toe
     ● S93.504   Unspecified sprain of right lesser toe(s)
     ● S93.505   Unspecified sprain of left lesser toe(s)
     ● S93.506   Unspecified sprain of unspecified lesser toe(s)
     ● S93.509   Unspecified sprain of unspecified toe(s)
  ● S93.51   Sprain of interphalangeal joint of toe
     ● S93.511   Sprain of interphalangeal joint of right great toe
     ● S93.512   Sprain of interphalangeal joint of left great toe
     ● S93.513   Sprain of interphalangeal joint of unspecified great toe
     ● S93.514   Sprain of interphalangeal joint of right lesser toe(s)

     ● S93.515   Sprain of interphalangeal joint of left lesser toe(s)
     ● S93.516   Sprain of interphalangeal joint of unspecified lesser toe(s)
     ● S93.519   Sprain of interphalangeal joint of unspecified toe(s)
  ● S93.52   Sprain of metatarsophalangeal joint of toe
     ● S93.521   Sprain of metatarsophalangeal joint of right great toe
     ● S93.522   Sprain of metatarsophalangeal joint of left great toe
     ● S93.523   Sprain of metatarsophalangeal joint of unspecified great toe
     ● S93.524   Sprain of metatarsophalangeal joint of right lesser toe(s)
     ● S93.525   Sprain of metatarsophalangeal joint of left lesser toe(s)
     ● S93.526   Sprain of metatarsophalangeal joint of unspecified lesser toe(s)
     ● S93.529   Sprain of metatarsophalangeal joint of unspecified toe(s)
● **S93.6**   Sprain of foot
     Excludes2   sprain of metatarsophalangeal joint of toe (S93.52-)
                sprain of toe (S93.5-)
  ● S93.60   Unspecified sprain of foot
     ● S93.601   Unspecified sprain of right foot
     ● S93.602   Unspecified sprain of left foot
     ● S93.609   Unspecified sprain of unspecified foot
  ● S93.61   Sprain of tarsal ligament of foot
     ● S93.611   Sprain of tarsal ligament of right foot
     ● S93.612   Sprain of tarsal ligament of left foot
     ● S93.619   Sprain of tarsal ligament of unspecified foot
  ● S93.62   Sprain of tarsometatarsal ligament of foot
     ● S93.621   Sprain of tarsometatarsal ligament of right foot
     ● S93.622   Sprain of tarsometatarsal ligament of left foot
     ● S93.629   Sprain of tarsometatarsal ligament of unspecified foot
  ● S93.69   Other sprain of foot
     ● S93.691   Other sprain of right foot
     ● S93.692   Other sprain of left foot
     ● S93.699   Other sprain of unspecified foot
● **S94**   Injury of nerves at ankle and foot level
     The appropriate 7th character is to be added to each code from category S94

A	initial encounter
D	subsequent encounter
S	sequela

     Code also any associated open wound (S91.-)
● **S94.0**   Injury of lateral plantar nerve
     X ● S94.00   Injury of lateral plantar nerve, unspecified leg
     X ● S94.01   Injury of lateral plantar nerve, right leg
     X ● S94.02   Injury of lateral plantar nerve, left leg
● **S94.1**   Injury of medial plantar nerve
     X ● S94.10   Injury of medial plantar nerve, unspecified leg
     X ● S94.11   Injury of medial plantar nerve, right leg
     X ● S94.12   Injury of medial plantar nerve, left leg
● **S94.2**   Injury of deep peroneal nerve at ankle and foot level
     Injury of terminal, lateral branch of deep peroneal nerve
     X ● S94.20   Injury of deep peroneal nerve at ankle and foot level, unspecified leg
     X ● S94.21   Injury of deep peroneal nerve at ankle and foot level, right leg
     X ● S94.22   Injury of deep peroneal nerve at ankle and foot level, left leg

CHAPTER 19 (S00–T88)

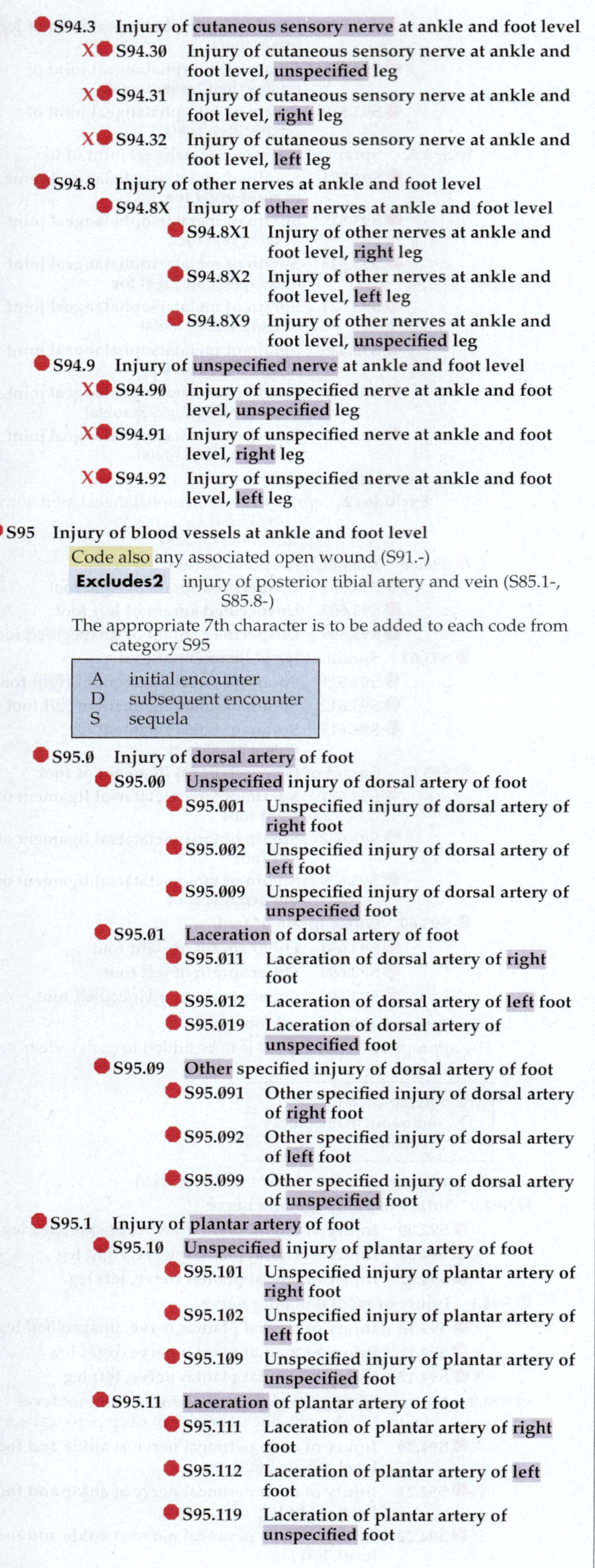

- ● **S94.3**   Injury of cutaneous sensory nerve at ankle and foot level
  - X ● **S94.30**   Injury of cutaneous sensory nerve at ankle and foot level, unspecified leg
  - X ● **S94.31**   Injury of cutaneous sensory nerve at ankle and foot level, right leg
  - X ● **S94.32**   Injury of cutaneous sensory nerve at ankle and foot level, left leg
- ● **S94.8**   Injury of other nerves at ankle and foot level
  - ● **S94.8X**   Injury of other nerves at ankle and foot level
    - ● **S94.8X1**   Injury of other nerves at ankle and foot level, right leg
    - ● **S94.8X2**   Injury of other nerves at ankle and foot level, left leg
    - ● **S94.8X9**   Injury of other nerves at ankle and foot level, unspecified leg
- ● **S94.9**   Injury of unspecified nerve at ankle and foot level
  - X ● **S94.90**   Injury of unspecified nerve at ankle and foot level, unspecified leg
  - X ● **S94.91**   Injury of unspecified nerve at ankle and foot level, right leg
  - X ● **S94.92**   Injury of unspecified nerve at ankle and foot level, left leg

- ● **S95**   Injury of blood vessels at ankle and foot level

  Code also any associated open wound (S91.-)

  Excludes2   injury of posterior tibial artery and vein (S85.1-, S85.8-)

  The appropriate 7th character is to be added to each code from category S95

  > A   initial encounter
  > D   subsequent encounter
  > S   sequela

  - ● **S95.0**   Injury of dorsal artery of foot
    - ● **S95.00**   Unspecified injury of dorsal artery of foot
      - ● **S95.001**   Unspecified injury of dorsal artery of right foot
      - ● **S95.002**   Unspecified injury of dorsal artery of left foot
      - ● **S95.009**   Unspecified injury of dorsal artery of unspecified foot
    - ● **S95.01**   Laceration of dorsal artery of foot
      - ● **S95.011**   Laceration of dorsal artery of right foot
      - ● **S95.012**   Laceration of dorsal artery of left foot
      - ● **S95.019**   Laceration of dorsal artery of unspecified foot
    - ● **S95.09**   Other specified injury of dorsal artery of foot
      - ● **S95.091**   Other specified injury of dorsal artery of right foot
      - ● **S95.092**   Other specified injury of dorsal artery of left foot
      - ● **S95.099**   Other specified injury of dorsal artery of unspecified foot
  - ● **S95.1**   Injury of plantar artery of foot
    - ● **S95.10**   Unspecified injury of plantar artery of foot
      - ● **S95.101**   Unspecified injury of plantar artery of right foot
      - ● **S95.102**   Unspecified injury of plantar artery of left foot
      - ● **S95.109**   Unspecified injury of plantar artery of unspecified foot
    - ● **S95.11**   Laceration of plantar artery of foot
      - ● **S95.111**   Laceration of plantar artery of right foot
      - ● **S95.112**   Laceration of plantar artery of left foot
      - ● **S95.119**   Laceration of plantar artery of unspecified foot

- ● **S95.19**   Other specified injury of plantar artery of foot
  - ● **S95.191**   Other specified injury of plantar artery of right foot
  - ● **S95.192**   Other specified injury of plantar artery of left foot
  - ● **S95.199**   Other specified injury of plantar artery of unspecified foot
- ● **S95.2**   Injury of dorsal vein of foot
  - ● **S95.20**   Unspecified injury of dorsal vein of foot
    - ● **S95.201**   Unspecified injury of dorsal vein of right foot
    - ● **S95.202**   Unspecified injury of dorsal vein of left foot
    - ● **S95.209**   Unspecified injury of dorsal vein of unspecified foot
  - ● **S95.21**   Laceration of dorsal vein of foot
    - ● **S95.211**   Laceration of dorsal vein of right foot
    - ● **S95.212**   Laceration of dorsal vein of left foot
    - ● **S95.219**   Laceration of dorsal vein of unspecified foot
  - ● **S95.29**   Other specified injury of dorsal vein of foot
    - ● **S95.291**   Other specified injury of dorsal vein of right foot
    - ● **S95.292**   Other specified injury of dorsal vein of left foot
    - ● **S95.299**   Other specified injury of dorsal vein of unspecified foot
- ● **S95.8**   Injury of other blood vessels at ankle and foot level
  - ● **S95.80**   Unspecified injury of other blood vessels at ankle and foot level
    - ● **S95.801**   Unspecified injury of other blood vessels at ankle and foot level, right leg
    - ● **S95.802**   Unspecified injury of other blood vessels at ankle and foot level, left leg
    - ● **S95.809**   Unspecified injury of other blood vessels at ankle and foot level, unspecified leg
  - ● **S95.81**   Laceration of other blood vessels at ankle and foot level
    - ● **S95.811**   Laceration of other blood vessels at ankle and foot level, right leg
    - ● **S95.812**   Laceration of other blood vessels at ankle and foot level, left leg
    - ● **S95.819**   Laceration of other blood vessels at ankle and foot level, unspecified leg
  - ● **S95.89**   Other specified injury of other blood vessels at ankle and foot level
    - ● **S95.891**   Other specified injury of other blood vessels at ankle and foot level, right leg
    - ● **S95.892**   Other specified injury of other blood vessels at ankle and foot level, left leg
    - ● **S95.899**   Other specified injury of other blood vessels at ankle and foot level, unspecified leg
- ● **S95.9**   Injury of unspecified blood vessel at ankle and foot level
  - ● **S95.90**   Unspecified injury of unspecified blood vessel at ankle and foot level
    - ● **S95.901**   Unspecified injury of unspecified blood vessel at ankle and foot level, right leg
    - ● **S95.902**   Unspecified injury of unspecified blood vessel at ankle and foot level, left leg
    - ● **S95.909**   Unspecified injury of unspecified blood vessel at ankle and foot level, unspecified leg

▶ New   ⇒ Revised   ~~deleted~~ Deleted   Excludes 1   Excludes 2   Includes   Use additional   Code first   Code also   Key words
OGCR Official Guidelines   X Assign placeholder X   ● Use Additional Character(s)   ▮ Manifestation Code   Hierarchical Condition Category   **Coding Clinic**

● **S95.91** Laceration of unspecified blood vessel at ankle and foot level

  ● **S95.911** Laceration of unspecified blood vessel at ankle and foot level, right leg

  ● **S95.912** Laceration of unspecified blood vessel at ankle and foot level, left leg

  ● **S95.919** Laceration of unspecified blood vessel at ankle and foot level, unspecified leg

● **S95.99** Other specified injury of unspecified blood vessel at ankle and foot level

  ● **S95.991** Other specified injury of unspecified blood vessel at ankle and foot level, right leg

  ● **S95.992** Other specified injury of unspecified blood vessel at ankle and foot level, left leg

  ● **S95.999** Other specified injury of unspecified blood vessel at ankle and foot level, unspecified leg

● **S96** Injury of muscle and tendon at ankle and foot level

Code also any associated open wound (S91.-)

Excludes2   injury of Achilles tendon (S86.0-)
         sprain of joints and ligaments of ankle and foot (S93.-)

The appropriate 7th character is to be added to each code from category S96

A	initial encounter
D	subsequent encounter
S	sequela

● **S96.0** Injury of muscle and tendon of long flexor muscle of toe at ankle and foot level

  ● **S96.00** Unspecified injury of muscle and tendon of long flexor muscle of toe at ankle and foot level

    ● **S96.001** Unspecified injury of muscle and tendon of long flexor muscle of toe at ankle and foot level, right foot

    ● **S96.002** Unspecified injury of muscle and tendon of long flexor muscle of toe at ankle and foot level, left foot

    ● **S96.009** Unspecified injury of muscle and tendon of long flexor muscle of toe at ankle and foot level, unspecified foot

  ● **S96.01** Strain of muscle and tendon of long flexor muscle of toe at ankle and foot level

    ● **S96.011** Strain of muscle and tendon of long flexor muscle of toe at ankle and foot level, right foot

    ● **S96.012** Strain of muscle and tendon of long flexor muscle of toe at ankle and foot level, left foot

    ● **S96.019** Strain of muscle and tendon of long flexor muscle of toe at ankle and foot level, unspecified foot

  ● **S96.02** Laceration of muscle and tendon of long flexor muscle of toe at ankle and foot level

    ● **S96.021** Laceration of muscle and tendon of long flexor muscle of toe at ankle and foot level, right foot

    ● **S96.022** Laceration of muscle and tendon of long flexor muscle of toe at ankle and foot level, left foot

    ● **S96.029** Laceration of muscle and tendon of long flexor muscle of toe at ankle and foot level, unspecified foot

  ● **S96.09** Other injury of muscle and tendon of long flexor muscle of toe at ankle and foot level

    ● **S96.091** Other injury of muscle and tendon of long flexor muscle of toe at ankle and foot level, right foot

    ● **S96.092** Other injury of muscle and tendon of long flexor muscle of toe at ankle and foot level, left foot

    ● **S96.099** Other injury of muscle and tendon of long flexor muscle of toe at ankle and foot level, unspecified foot

● **S96.1** Injury of muscle and tendon of long extensor muscle of toe at ankle and foot level

  ● **S96.10** Unspecified injury of muscle and tendon of long extensor muscle of toe at ankle and foot level

    ● **S96.101** Unspecified injury of muscle and tendon of long extensor muscle of toe at ankle and foot level, right foot

    ● **S96.102** Unspecified injury of muscle and tendon of long extensor muscle of toe at ankle and foot level, left foot

    ● **S96.109** Unspecified injury of muscle and tendon of long extensor muscle of toe at ankle and foot level, unspecified foot

  ● **S96.11** Strain of muscle and tendon of long extensor muscle of toe at ankle and foot level

    ● **S96.111** Strain of muscle and tendon of long extensor muscle of toe at ankle and foot level, right foot

    ● **S96.112** Strain of muscle and tendon of long extensor muscle of toe at ankle and foot level, left foot

    ● **S96.119** Strain of muscle and tendon of long extensor muscle of toe at ankle and foot level, unspecified foot

  ● **S96.12** Laceration of muscle and tendon of long extensor muscle of toe at ankle and foot level

    ● **S96.121** Laceration of muscle and tendon of long extensor muscle of toe at ankle and foot level, right foot

    ● **S96.122** Laceration of muscle and tendon of long extensor muscle of toe at ankle and foot level, left foot

    ● **S96.129** Laceration of muscle and tendon of long extensor muscle of toe at ankle and foot level, unspecified foot

  ● **S96.19** Other specified injury of muscle and tendon of long extensor muscle of toe at ankle and foot level

    ● **S96.191** Other specified injury of muscle and tendon of long extensor muscle of toe at ankle and foot level, right foot

    ● **S96.192** Other specified injury of muscle and tendon of long extensor muscle of toe at ankle and foot level, left foot

    ● **S96.199** Other specified injury of muscle and tendon of long extensor muscle of toe at ankle and foot level, unspecified foot

● **S96.2** Injury of intrinsic muscle and tendon at ankle and foot level

  ● **S96.20** Unspecified injury of intrinsic muscle and tendon at ankle and foot level

    ● **S96.201** Unspecified injury of intrinsic muscle and tendon at ankle and foot level, right foot

    ● **S96.202** Unspecified injury of intrinsic muscle and tendon at ankle and foot level, left foot

    ● **S96.209** Unspecified injury of intrinsic muscle and tendon at ankle and foot level, unspecified foot

  ● **S96.21** Strain of intrinsic muscle and tendon at ankle and foot level

    ● **S96.211** Strain of intrinsic muscle and tendon at ankle and foot level, right foot

S96.212   Strain of intrinsic muscle and tendon at ankle and foot level, **left** foot

S96.219   Strain of intrinsic muscle and tendon at ankle and foot level, **unspecified** foot

S96.22   **Laceration** of intrinsic muscle and tendon at ankle and foot level

S96.221   Laceration of intrinsic muscle and tendon at ankle and foot level, **right** foot

S96.222   Laceration of intrinsic muscle and tendon at left ankle and foot level, **left** foot

S96.229   Laceration of intrinsic muscle and tendon at ankle and foot level, **unspecified** foot

S96.29   **Other** specified injury of intrinsic muscle and tendon at ankle and foot level

S96.291   Other specified injury of intrinsic muscle and tendon at ankle and foot level, **right** foot

S96.292   Other specified injury of intrinsic muscle and tendon at ankle and foot level, **left** foot

S96.299   Other specified injury of intrinsic muscle and tendon at ankle and foot level, **unspecified** foot

S96.8   Injury of **other** specified muscles and tendons at ankle and foot level

S96.80   **Unspecified** injury of other specified muscles and tendons at ankle and foot level

S96.801   Unspecified injury of other specified muscles and tendons at ankle and foot level, **right** foot

S96.802   Unspecified injury of other specified muscles and tendons at ankle and foot level, **left** foot

S96.809   Unspecified injury of other specified muscles and tendons at ankle and foot level, **unspecified** foot

S96.81   **Strain** of other specified muscles and tendons at ankle and foot level

S96.811   Strain of other specified muscles and tendons at ankle and foot level, **right** foot

S96.812   Strain of other specified muscles and tendons at ankle and foot level, **left** foot

S96.819   Strain of other specified muscles and tendons at ankle and foot level, **unspecified** foot

S96.82   **Laceration** of other specified muscles and tendons at ankle and foot level

S96.821   Laceration of other specified muscles and tendons at ankle and foot level, **right** foot

S96.822   Laceration of other specified muscles and tendons at ankle and foot level, **left** foot

S96.829   Laceration of other specified muscles and tendons at ankle and foot level, **unspecified** foot

S96.89   **Other** specified injury of other specified muscles and tendons at ankle and foot level

S96.891   Other specified injury of other specified muscles and tendons at ankle and foot level, **right** foot

S96.892   Other specified injury of other specified muscles and tendons at ankle and foot level, **left** foot

S96.899   Other specified injury of other specified muscles and tendons at ankle and foot level, **unspecified** foot

S96.9   Injury of **unspecified** muscle and tendon at ankle and foot level

S96.90   **Unspecified** injury of unspecified muscle and tendon at ankle and foot level

S96.901   Unspecified injury of unspecified muscle and tendon at ankle and foot level, **right** foot

S96.902   Unspecified injury of unspecified muscle and tendon at ankle and foot level, **left** foot

S96.909   Unspecified injury of unspecified muscle and tendon at ankle and foot level, **unspecified** foot

S96.91   **Strain** of unspecified muscle and tendon at ankle and foot level

S96.911   Strain of unspecified muscle and tendon at ankle and foot level, **right** foot

S96.912   Strain of unspecified muscle and tendon at ankle and foot level, **left** foot

S96.919   Strain of unspecified muscle and tendon at ankle and foot level, **unspecified** foot

S96.92   **Laceration** of unspecified muscle and tendon at ankle and foot level

S96.921   Laceration of unspecified muscle and tendon at ankle and foot level, **right** foot

S96.922   Laceration of unspecified muscle and tendon at ankle and foot level, **left** foot

S96.929   Laceration of unspecified muscle and tendon at ankle and foot level, **unspecified** foot

S96.99   **Other** specified injury of unspecified muscle and tendon at ankle and foot level

S96.991   Other specified injury of unspecified muscle and tendon at ankle and foot level, **right** foot

S96.992   Other specified injury of unspecified muscle and tendon at ankle and foot level, **left** foot

S96.999   Other specified injury of unspecified muscle and tendon at ankle and foot level, **unspecified** foot

S97   **Crushing injury of ankle and foot**

Use additional code(s) for all associated injuries

The appropriate 7th character is to be added to each code from category S97

A	initial encounter
D	subsequent encounter
S	sequela

S97.0   **Crushing injury of ankle**

X S97.00   Crushing injury of **unspecified** ankle

X S97.01   Crushing injury of **right** ankle

X S97.02   Crushing injury of **left** ankle

S97.1   **Crushing injury of toe**

S97.10   Crushing injury of **unspecified** toe(s)

S97.101   Crushing injury of unspecified **right** toe(s)

S97.102   Crushing injury of unspecified **left** toe(s)

S97.109   Crushing injury of **unspecified** toe(s)
Crushing injury of toe NOS

● S97.11   Crushing injury of great toe
   ● S97.111   Crushing injury of right great toe
   ● S97.112   Crushing injury of left great toe
   ● S97.119   Crushing injury of unspecified great toe
● S97.12   Crushing injury of lesser toe(s)
   ● S97.121   Crushing injury of right lesser toe(s)
   ● S97.122   Crushing injury of left lesser toe(s)
   ● S97.129   Crushing injury of lesser toe(s), unspecified toe(s)
● S97.8   Crushing injury of foot
   X ● S97.80   Crushing injury of foot, unspecified side
      Crushing injury of foot NOS
   X ● S97.81   Crushing injury of right foot
   X ● S97.82   Crushing injury of left foot

● S98   Traumatic amputation of ankle and foot
An amputation not identified as partial or complete should be coded to complete

The appropriate 7th character is to be added to each code from category S98

> A   initial encounter
> D   subsequent encounter
> S   sequela

● S98.0   Traumatic amputation of foot at ankle level
   ● S98.01   Complete traumatic amputation of foot at ankle level
      ● S98.011   Complete traumatic amputation of right foot at ankle level A, D, S
      ● S98.012   Complete traumatic amputation of left foot at ankle level A, D, S
      ● S98.019   Complete traumatic amputation of unspecified foot at ankle level A, D, S
   ● S98.02   Partial traumatic amputation of foot at ankle level
      ● S98.021   Partial traumatic amputation of right foot at ankle level A, D, S
      ● S98.022   Partial traumatic amputation of left foot at ankle level A, D, S
      ● S98.029   Partial traumatic amputation of unspecified foot at ankle level A, D, S

● S98.1   Traumatic amputation of one toe
   ● S98.11   Complete traumatic amputation of great toe
      ● S98.111   Complete traumatic amputation of right great toe A, D, S
      ● S98.112   Complete traumatic amputation of left great toe A, D, S
      ● S98.119   Complete traumatic amputation of unspecified great toe A, D, S
   ● S98.12   Partial traumatic amputation of great toe
      ● S98.121   Partial traumatic amputation of right great toe A, D, S
      ● S98.122   Partial traumatic amputation of left great toe A, D, S
      ● S98.129   Partial traumatic amputation of unspecified great toe A, D, S
   ● S98.13   Complete traumatic amputation of one lesser toe
      Traumatic amputation of toe NOS
      ● S98.131   Complete traumatic amputation of one right lesser toe A, D, S

      ● S98.132   Complete traumatic amputation of one left lesser toe A, D, S
      ● S98.139   Complete traumatic amputation of one unspecified lesser toe A, D, S
   ● S98.14   Partial traumatic amputation of one lesser toe
      ● S98.141   Partial traumatic amputation of one right lesser toe A, D, S
      ● S98.142   Partial traumatic amputation of one left lesser toe A, D, S
      ● S98.149   Partial traumatic amputation of one unspecified lesser toe A, D, S
● S98.2   Traumatic amputation of two or more lesser toes
   ● S98.21   Complete traumatic amputation of two or more lesser toes
      ● S98.211   Complete traumatic amputation of two or more right lesser toes A, D, S
      ● S98.212   Complete traumatic amputation of two or more left lesser toes A, D, S
      ● S98.219   Complete traumatic amputation of two or more unspecified lesser toes A, D, S
   ● S98.22   Partial traumatic amputation of two or more lesser toes
      ● S98.221   Partial traumatic amputation of two or more right lesser toes A, D, S
      ● S98.222   Partial traumatic amputation of two or more left lesser toes A, D, S
      ● S98.229   Partial traumatic amputation of two or more unspecified lesser toes A, D, S
● S98.3   Traumatic amputation of midfoot
   ● S98.31   Complete traumatic amputation of midfoot
      ● S98.311   Complete traumatic amputation of right midfoot A, D, S
      ● S98.312   Complete traumatic amputation of left midfoot A, D, S
      ● S98.319   Complete traumatic amputation of unspecified midfoot A, D, S
   ● S98.32   Partial traumatic amputation of midfoot
      ● S98.321   Partial traumatic amputation of right midfoot A, D, S
      ● S98.322   Partial traumatic amputation of left midfoot A, D, S
      ● S98.329   Partial traumatic amputation of unspecified midfoot A, D, S
● S98.9   Traumatic amputation of foot, level unspecified
   ● S98.91   Complete traumatic amputation of foot, level unspecified
      ● S98.911   Complete traumatic amputation of right foot, level unspecified A, D, S
      ● S98.912   Complete traumatic amputation of left foot, level unspecified A, D, S
      ● S98.919   Complete traumatic amputation of unspecified foot, level unspecified A, D, S
   ● S98.92   Partial traumatic amputation of foot, level unspecified
      ● S98.921   Partial traumatic amputation of right foot, level unspecified A, D, S
      ● S98.922   Partial traumatic amputation of left foot, level unspecified A, D, S
      ● S98.929   Partial traumatic amputation of unspecified foot, level unspecified A, D, S

CHAPTER 19 (S00–T88)

● **S99 Other and unspecified injuries of ankle and foot**
Coding Clinic: 2016, Q4, P68

● **S99.0 Physeal fracture of calcaneus**

The appropriate 7th character is to be added to each code from subcategories S99.0

A	initial encounter for closed fracture
B	initial encounter for open fracture
D	subsequent encounter for fracture with routine healing
G	subsequent encounter for fracture with delayed healing
K	subsequent encounter for fracture with nonunion
P	subsequent encounter for fracture with malunion
S	sequela

● **S99.00 Unspecified physeal fracture of calcaneus**

  ● **S99.001 Unspecified physeal fracture of right calcaneus**

  ● **S99.002 Unspecified physeal fracture of left calcaneus**

  ● **S99.009 Unspecified physeal fracture of unspecified calcaneus**

● **S99.01 Salter-Harris Type I physeal fracture of calcaneus**
Coding Clinic: 2016, Q4, P69

  ● **S99.011 Salter-Harris Type I physeal fracture of right calcaneus**

  ● **S99.012 Salter-Harris Type I physeal fracture of left calcaneus**

  ● **S99.019 Salter-Harris Type I physeal fracture of unspecified calcaneus**

● **S99.02 Salter-Harris Type II physeal fracture of calcaneus**
Coding Clinic: 2016, Q4, P69

  ● **S99.021 Salter-Harris Type II physeal fracture of right calcaneus**

  ● **S99.022 Salter-Harris Type II physeal fracture of left calcaneus**

  ● **S99.029 Salter-Harris Type II physeal fracture of unspecified calcaneus**

● **S99.03 Salter-Harris Type III physeal fracture of calcaneus**
Coding Clinic: 2016, Q4, P69

  ● **S99.031 Salter-Harris Type III physeal fracture of right calcaneus**

  ● **S99.032 Salter-Harris Type III physeal fracture of left calcaneus**

  ● **S99.039 Salter-Harris Type III physeal fracture of unspecified calcaneus**

● **S99.04 Salter-Harris Type IV physeal fracture of calcaneus**
Coding Clinic: 2016, Q4, P69

  ● **S99.041 Salter-Harris Type IV physeal fracture of right calcaneus**

  ● **S99.042 Salter-Harris Type IV physeal fracture of left calcaneus**

  ● **S99.049 Salter-Harris Type IV physeal fracture of unspecified calcaneus**

● **S99.09 Other physeal fracture of calcaneus**
Coding Clinic: 2016, Q4, P69

  ● **S99.091 Other physeal fracture of right calcaneus**

  ● **S99.092 Other physeal fracture of left calcaneus**

  ● **S99.099 Other physeal fracture of unspecified calcaneus**

● **S99.1 Physeal fracture of metatarsal**

The appropriate 7th character is to be added to each code from subcategories S99.1

A	initial encounter for closed fracture
B	initial encounter for open fracture
D	subsequent encounter for fracture with routine healing
G	subsequent encounter for fracture with delayed healing
K	subsequent encounter for fracture with nonunion
P	subsequent encounter for fracture with malunion
S	sequela

● **S99.10 Unspecified physeal fracture of metatarsal**

  ● **S99.101 Unspecified physeal fracture of right metatarsal**

  ● **S99.102 Unspecified physeal fracture of left metatarsal**

  ● **S99.109 Unspecified physeal fracture of unspecified metatarsal**

● **S99.11 Salter-Harris Type I physeal fracture of metatarsal**
Coding Clinic: 2016, Q4, P69

  ● **S99.111 Salter-Harris Type I physeal fracture of right metatarsal**

  ● **S99.112 Salter-Harris Type I physeal fracture of left metatarsal**
Coding Clinic: 2018, Q1, P3

  ● **S99.119 Salter-Harris Type I physeal fracture of unspecified metatarsal**

● **S99.12 Salter-Harris Type II physeal fracture of metatarsal**
Coding Clinic: 2016, Q4, P69

  ● **S99.121 Salter-Harris Type II physeal fracture of right metatarsal**

  ● **S99.122 Salter-Harris Type II physeal fracture of left metatarsal**

  ● **S99.129 Salter-Harris Type II physeal fracture of unspecified metatarsal**

● **S99.13 Salter-Harris Type III physeal fracture of metatarsal**
Coding Clinic: 2016, Q4, P69

  ● **S99.131 Salter-Harris Type III physeal fracture of right metatarsal**

  ● **S99.132 Salter-Harris Type III physeal fracture of left metatarsal**

  ● **S99.139 Salter-Harris Type III physeal fracture of unspecified metatarsal**

● **S99.14 Salter-Harris Type IV physeal fracture of metatarsal**
Coding Clinic: 2016, Q4, P69

  ● **S99.141 Salter-Harris Type IV physeal fracture of right metatarsal**

  ● **S99.142 Salter-Harris Type IV physeal fracture of left metatarsal**

  ● **S99.149 Salter-Harris Type IV physeal fracture of unspecified metatarsal**

● **S99.19 Other physeal fracture of metatarsal**
Coding Clinic: 2016, Q4, P69

  ● **S99.191 Other physeal fracture of right metatarsal**

  ● **S99.192 Other physeal fracture of left metatarsal**

  ● **S99.199 Other physeal fracture of unspecified metatarsal**

▶ New   ➡ Revised   ~~deleted~~ Deleted   Excludes 1   Excludes 2   Includes   Use additional   Code first   Code also   Key words
OGCR Official Guidelines   X Assign placeholder X   ● Use Additional Character(s)   ▶ Manifestation Code   HCC Hierarchical Condition Category   Coding Clinic

● **S99.2   Physeal fracture of phalanx of toe**

The appropriate 7th character is to be added to each code from subcategories S99.2

A	initial encounter for closed fracture
B	initial encounter for open fracture
D	subsequent encounter for fracture with routine healing
G	subsequent encounter for fracture with delayed healing
K	subsequent encounter for fracture with nonunion
P	subsequent encounter for fracture with malunion
S	sequela

● **S99.20   Unspecified physeal fracture of phalanx of toe**
  ● **S99.201   Unspecified physeal fracture of phalanx of right toe**
  ● **S99.202   Unspecified physeal fracture of phalanx of right toe**
  ● **S99.209   Unspecified physeal fracture of phalanx of unspecified toe**
● **S99.21   Salter-Harris Type I physeal fracture of phalanx of toe**
      Coding Clinic: 2016, Q4, P69
  ● **S99.211   Salter-Harris Type I physeal fracture of phalanx of right toe**
  ● **S99.212   Salter-Harris Type I physeal fracture of phalanx of left toe**
  ● **S99.219   Salter-Harris Type I physeal fracture of phalanx of unspecified toe**
● **S99.22   Salter-Harris Type II physeal fracture of phalanx of toe**
      Coding Clinic: 2016, Q4, P69
  ● **S99.221   Salter-Harris Type II physeal fracture of phalanx of right toe**
  ● **S99.222   Salter-Harris Type II physeal fracture of phalanx of left toe**
  ● **S99.229   Salter-Harris Type II physeal fracture of phalanx of unspecified toe**
● **S99.23   Salter-Harris Type III physeal fracture of phalanx of toe**
      Coding Clinic: 2016, Q4, P69
  ● **S99.231   Salter-Harris Type III physeal fracture of phalanx of right toe**
  ● **S99.232   Salter-Harris Type III physeal fracture of phalanx of left toe**
  ● **S99.239   Salter-Harris Type III physeal fracture of phalanx of unspecified toe**
● **S99.24   Salter-Harris Type IV physeal fracture of phalanx of toe**
      Coding Clinic: 2016, Q4, P69
  ● **S99.241   Salter-Harris Type IV physeal fracture of phalanx of right toe**
  ● **S99.242   Salter-Harris Type IV physeal fracture of phalanx of left toe**
  ● **S99.249   Salter-Harris Type IV physeal fracture of phalanx of unspecified toe**
● **S99.29   Other physeal fracture of phalanx of toe**
      Coding Clinic: 2016, Q4, P69
  ● **S99.291   Other physeal fracture of phalanx of right toe**
  ● **S99.292   Other physeal fracture of phalanx of left toe**
  ● **S99.299   Other physeal fracture of phalanx of unspecified toe**

● **S99.8   Other specified injuries of ankle and foot**

The appropriate 7th character is to be added to each code from subcategory S99.8

A	initial encounter
D	subsequent encounter
S	sequela

● **S99.81   Other specified injuries of ankle**
  ● **S99.811   Other specified injuries of right ankle**
  ● **S99.812   Other specified injuries of left ankle**
  ● **S99.819   Other specified injuries of unspecified ankle**
● **S99.82   Other specified injuries of foot**
  ● **S99.821   Other specified injuries of right foot**
  ● **S99.822   Other specified injuries of left foot**
  ● **S99.829   Other specified injuries of unspecified foot**
● **S99.9   Unspecified injury of ankle and foot**

The appropriate 7th character is to be added to each code from subcategory S99.9

A	initial encounter
D	subsequent encounter
S	sequela

● **S99.91   Unspecified injury of ankle**
  ● **S99.911   Unspecified injury of right ankle**
  ● **S99.912   Unspecified injury of left ankle**
  ● **S99.919   Unspecified injury of unspecified ankle**
● **S99.92   Unspecified injury of foot**
  ● **S99.921   Unspecified injury of right foot**
  ● **S99.922   Unspecified injury of left foot**
  ● **S99.929   Unspecified injury of unspecified foot**

INJURY, POISONING AND CERTAIN OTHER CONSEQUENCES OF EXTERNAL CAUSES (T07-T88)

INJURIES INVOLVING MULTIPLE BODY REGIONS (T07)

Excludes1   burns and corrosions (T20-T32)
            frostbite (T33-T34)
            insect bite or sting, venomous (T63.4)
            sunburn (L55.-)

X ● **T07   Unspecified multiple injuries**

The appropriate 7th character is to be added to code T07

A	initial encounter
D	subsequent encounter
S	sequela

Excludes1   injury NOS (T14.90)

INJURY OF UNSPECIFIED BODY REGION (T14)

● **T14   Injury of unspecified body region**

The appropriate 7th character is to be added to each code from category T14

A	initial encounter
D	subsequent encounter
S	sequela

Excludes1   multiple unspecified injuries (T07)

X ● **T14.8   Other injury of unspecified body region**
      Abrasion NOS   Skin injury NOS
      Contusion NOS   Vascular injury NOS
      Crush injury NOS   Wound NOS
      Fracture NOS
● **T14.9   Unspecified injury**
  X ● **T14.90   Injury, unspecified**
          Injury NOS
  X ● **T14.91   Suicide attempt A, D, S**
          Attempted suicide NOS

EFFECTS OF FOREIGN BODY ENTERING THROUGH NATURAL ORIFICE (T15-T19)

Use additional code, if known, for foreign body entering into or through a natural orifice (W44.-)

Excludes2   foreign body accidentally left in operation wound (T81.5-)

foreign body in penetrating wound - see open wound by body region

residual foreign body in soft tissue (M79.5)

splinter, without open wound - see superficial injury by body region

● **T15   Foreign body on external eye**

Excludes2   foreign body in penetrating wound of orbit and eye ball (S05.4-, S05.5-)

open wound of eyelid and periocular area (S01.1-)

retained foreign body in eyelid (H02.8-)

retained (old) foreign body in penetrating wound of orbit and eye ball (H05.5-, H44.6-, H44.7-)

superficial foreign body of eyelid and periocular area (S00.25-)

The appropriate 7th character is to be added to each code from category T15

> A   initial encounter
> D   subsequent encounter
> S   sequela

● **T15.0 Foreign body in cornea**

X ● T15.00   Foreign body in cornea, **unspecified** eye

X ● T15.01   Foreign body in cornea, **right** eye

X ● T15.02   Foreign body in cornea, **left** eye

● **T15.1 Foreign body in conjunctival sac**

X ● T15.10   Foreign body in conjunctival sac, **unspecified** eye

X ● T15.11   Foreign body in conjunctival sac, **right** eye

X ● T15.12   Foreign body in conjunctival sac, **left** eye

● **T15.8 Foreign body in other and multiple parts of external eye**

Foreign body in lacrimal punctum

X ● T15.80   Foreign body in other and multiple parts of external eye, **unspecified** eye

X ● T15.81   Foreign body in other and multiple parts of external eye, **right** eye

X ● T15.82   Foreign body in other and multiple parts of external eye, **left** eye

● **T15.9 Foreign body on external eye, part unspecified**

X ● T15.90   Foreign body on external eye, part unspecified, **unspecified** eye

X ● T15.91   Foreign body on external eye, part unspecified, **right** eye

X ● T15.92   Foreign body on external eye, part unspecified, **left** eye

● **T16   Foreign body in ear**

Includes   foreign body in auditory canal

The appropriate 7th character is to be added to each code from category T16

> A   initial encounter
> D   subsequent encounter
> S   sequela

X ● T16.1   Foreign body in **right** ear

X ● T16.2   Foreign body in **left** ear

X ● T16.9   Foreign body in ear, **unspecified** ear

● **T17   Foreign body in respiratory tract**

The appropriate 7th character is to be added to each code from category T17

> A   initial encounter
> D   subsequent encounter
> S   sequela

X ● T17.0   Foreign body in **nasal sinus**

X ● T17.1   Foreign body in **nostril**

Foreign body in nose NOS

● **T17.2 Foreign body in pharynx**

Foreign body in nasopharynx

Foreign body in throat NOS

● **T17.20 Unspecified foreign body in pharynx**

● T17.200   **Unspecified foreign body in pharynx causing asphyxiation**

● T17.208   **Unspecified foreign body in pharynx causing other injury**

● **T17.21 Gastric contents in pharynx**

Aspiration of gastric contents into pharynx

Vomitus in pharynx

● T17.210   **Gastric contents in pharynx causing asphyxiation**

● T17.218   **Gastric contents in pharynx causing other injury**

● **T17.22 Food in pharynx**

Bones in pharynx

Seeds in pharynx

● T17.220   **Food in pharynx causing asphyxiation**

● T17.228   **Food in pharynx causing other injury**

● **T17.29 Other foreign object in pharynx**

● T17.290   **Other foreign object in pharynx causing asphyxiation**

● T17.298   **Other foreign object in pharynx causing other injury**

● **T17.3 Foreign body in larynx**

● **T17.30 Unspecified foreign body in larynx**

● T17.300   **Unspecified foreign body in larynx causing asphyxiation**

● T17.308   **Unspecified foreign body in larynx causing other injury**

● **T17.31 Gastric contents in larynx**

Aspiration of gastric contents into larynx

Vomitus in larynx

● T17.310   **Gastric contents in larynx causing asphyxiation**

● T17.318   **Gastric contents in larynx causing other injury**

● **T17.32 Food in larynx**

Bones in larynx

Seeds in larynx

● T17.320   **Food in larynx causing asphyxiation**

● T17.328   **Food in larynx causing other injury**

● **T17.39 Other foreign object in larynx**

● T17.390   **Other foreign object in larynx causing asphyxiation**

● T17.398   **Other foreign object in larynx causing other injury**

● **T17.4 Foreign body in trachea**

● **T17.40 Unspecified foreign body in trachea**

● T17.400   **Unspecified foreign body in trachea causing asphyxiation**

● T17.408   **Unspecified foreign body in trachea causing other injury**

● **T17.41 Gastric contents in trachea**

Aspiration of gastric contents into trachea

Vomitus in trachea

● T17.410   **Gastric contents in trachea causing asphyxiation**

● T17.418   **Gastric contents in trachea causing other injury**

● **T17.42 Food in trachea**

Bones in trachea

Seeds in trachea

● T17.420   **Food in trachea causing asphyxiation**

● T17.428   **Food in trachea causing other injury**

● **T17.49 Other foreign object in trachea**

● T17.490   **Other foreign object in trachea causing asphyxiation**

● T17.498   **Other foreign object in trachea causing other injury**

▶ New   ◀ Revised   ~~deleted~~ Deleted   Excludes 1   Excludes 2   Includes   Use additional   Code first   Code also   Key words

OGCR Official Guidelines   X Assign placeholder X   ● Use Additional Character(s)   ▶ Manifestation Code   **HCc** Hierarchical Condition Category   **Coding Clinic**

● **T17.5**   Foreign body in bronchus
  ● **T17.50**   Unspecified foreign body in bronchus
    ● **T17.500**   Unspecified foreign body in bronchus causing asphyxiation
    ● **T17.508**   Unspecified foreign body in bronchus causing other injury
  ● **T17.51**   Gastric contents in bronchus
          Aspiration of gastric contents into bronchus
          Vomitus in bronchus
    ● **T17.510**   Gastric contents in bronchus causing asphyxiation
    ● **T17.518**   Gastric contents in bronchus causing other injury
  ● **T17.52**   Food in bronchus
          Bones in bronchus
          Seeds in bronchus
    ● **T17.520**   Food in bronchus causing asphyxiation
    ● **T17.528**   Food in bronchus causing other injury
  ● **T17.59**   Other foreign object in bronchus
    ● **T17.590**   Other foreign object in bronchus causing asphyxiation
    ● **T17.598**   Other foreign object in bronchus causing other injury
● **T17.8**   Foreign body in other parts of respiratory tract
        Foreign body in bronchioles
        Foreign body in lung
  ● **T17.80**   Unspecified foreign body in other parts of respiratory tract
    ● **T17.800**   Unspecified foreign body in other parts of respiratory tract causing asphyxiation
    ● **T17.808**   Unspecified foreign body in other parts of respiratory tract causing other injury
  ● **T17.81**   Gastric contents in other parts of respiratory tract
          Aspiration of gastric contents into other parts of respiratory tract
          Vomitus in other parts of respiratory tract
    ● **T17.810**   Gastric contents in other parts of respiratory tract causing asphyxiation
    ● **T17.818**   Gastric contents in other parts of respiratory tract causing other injury
  ● **T17.82**   Food in other parts of respiratory tract
          Bones in other parts of respiratory tract
          Seeds in other parts of respiratory tract
    ● **T17.820**   Food in other parts of respiratory tract causing asphyxiation
    ● **T17.828**   Food in other parts of respiratory tract causing other injury
  ● **T17.89**   Other foreign object in other parts of respiratory tract
    ● **T17.890**   Other foreign object in other parts of respiratory tract causing asphyxiation
    ● **T17.898**   Other foreign object in other parts of respiratory tract causing other injury
● **T17.9**   Foreign body in respiratory tract, part unspecified
  ● **T17.90**   Unspecified foreign body in respiratory tract, part unspecified
    ● **T17.900**   Unspecified foreign body in respiratory tract, part unspecified causing asphyxiation
    ● **T17.908**   Unspecified foreign body in respiratory tract, part unspecified causing other injury
  ● **T17.91**   Gastric contents in respiratory tract, part unspecified
          Aspiration of gastric contents into respiratory tract, part unspecified
          Vomitus in trachea respiratory tract, part unspecified

  ● **T17.910**   Gastric contents in respiratory tract, part unspecified causing asphyxiation
  ● **T17.918**   Gastric contents in respiratory tract, part unspecified causing other injury
● **T17.92**   Food in respiratory tract, part unspecified
        Bones in respiratory tract, part unspecified
        Seeds in respiratory tract, part unspecified
  ● **T17.920**   Food in respiratory tract, part unspecified causing asphyxiation
  ● **T17.928**   Food in respiratory tract, part unspecified causing other injury
● **T17.99**   Other foreign object in respiratory tract, part unspecified
  ● **T17.990**   Other foreign object in respiratory tract, part unspecified in causing asphyxiation
          Coding Clinic: 2019, Q3, P15
  ● **T17.998**   Other foreign object in respiratory tract, part unspecified causing other injury

● **T18**   Foreign body in alimentary tract
      Excludes2   foreign body in pharynx (T17.2-)
      The appropriate 7th character is to be added to each code from category T18

> A   initial encounter
> D   subsequent encounter
> S   sequela

X● **T18.0**   Foreign body in mouth
X● **T18.1**   Foreign body in esophagus
      Excludes2   foreign body in respiratory tract (T17.-)
  ● **T18.10**   Unspecified foreign body in esophagus
    ● **T18.100**   Unspecified foreign body in esophagus causing compression of trachea
            Unspecified foreign body in esophagus causing obstruction of respiration
    ● **T18.108**   Unspecified foreign body in esophagus causing other injury
  ● **T18.11**   Gastric contents in esophagus
          Vomitus in esophagus
    ● **T18.110**   Gastric contents in esophagus causing compression of trachea
            Gastric contents in esophagus causing obstruction of respiration
    ● **T18.118**   Gastric contents in esophagus causing other injury
  ● **T18.12**   Food in esophagus
          Bones in esophagus
          Seeds in esophagus
    ● **T18.120**   Food in esophagus causing compression of trachea
            Food in esophagus causing obstruction of respiration
    ● **T18.128**   Food in esophagus causing other injury
  ● **T18.19**   Other foreign object in esophagus
    ● **T18.190**   Other foreign object in esophagus causing compression of trachea
            Other foreign body in esophagus causing obstruction of respiration
            Coding Clinic: 2015, Q1, P24
    ● **T18.198**   Other foreign object in esophagus causing other injury
            Coding Clinic: 2015, Q1, P24
X● **T18.2**   Foreign body in stomach
X● **T18.3**   Foreign body in small intestine
X● **T18.4**   Foreign body in colon

X● **T18.5** **Foreign body in anus and rectum**
Foreign body in rectosigmoid (junction)

X● **T18.8** **Foreign body in other parts of alimentary tract**

X● **T18.9** **Foreign body of alimentary tract, part unspecified**
Foreign body in digestive system NOS
Swallowed foreign body NOS

● **T19** **Foreign body in genitourinary tract**

Excludes2 complications due to implanted mesh (T83.7-)
mechanical complications of contraceptive device (intrauterine) (vaginal) (T83.3-)
presence of contraceptive device (intrauterine) (vaginal) (Z97.5)

The appropriate 7th character is to be added to each code from category T19

A	initial encounter
D	subsequent encounter
S	sequela

X● **T19.0** **Foreign body in urethra**

X● **T19.1** **Foreign body in bladder**

X● **T19.2** **Foreign body in vulva and vagina**

X● **T19.3** **Foreign body in uterus**

X● **T19.4** **Foreign body in penis**

X● **T19.8** **Foreign body in other parts of genitourinary tract**

X● **T19.9** **Foreign body in genitourinary tract, part unspecified**

BURNS AND CORROSIONS (T20-T32)

Includes   burns (thermal) from electrical heating appliances
burns (thermal) from electricity
burns (thermal) from flame
burns (thermal) from friction
burns (thermal) from hot air and hot gases
burns (thermal) from hot objects
burns (thermal) from lightning
burns (thermal) from radiation chemical
burn [corrosion] (external) (internal) scalds

Excludes2 erythema [dermatitis] ab igne (L59.0)
radiation-related disorders of the skin and subcutaneous tissue (L55-L59)
sunburn (L55.-)

OGCR Section I.C.19.d.

Burns and Corrosions

The ICD-10-CM makes a distinction between burn and corrosions. The burn codes are for thermal burns, except sunburns, that come from a heat source, such as a fire or hot appliance. The burn codes are also for burns resulting from electricity and radiation. Corrosions are burns due to chemicals. The guidelines for burns and corrosions are the same.

Current burns (T20-T25) are classified by depth, extent and by agent (X code). Burns are classified by depth as first degree (erythema), second degree (blistering), and third degree (full-thickness involvement). Burns of the eye and internal organs (T26-T28) are classified by site, but not by degree.

1) Sequencing of burn and related condition codes

Sequence first the code that reflects the highest degree of burn when more than one burn is present.

a. When the reason for the admission or encounter is for treatment of external multiple burns, sequence first the code that reflects the burn of the highest degree.

b. When a patient has both internal and external burns, the circumstances of admission govern the selection of the principal diagnosis or first-listed diagnosis.

c. When a patient is admitted for burn injuries and other related conditions such as smoke inhalation and/or respiratory failure, the circumstances of admission govern the selection of the principal or first-listed diagnosis.

2) Burns of the same local site

Classify burns of the same local site (three-character category level, T20-T28) but of different degrees to the subcategory identifying the highest degree recorded in the diagnosis.

BURNS AND CORROSIONS OF EXTERNAL BODY SURFACE, SPECIFIED BY SITE (T20-T25)

Includes   burns and corrosions of first degree [erythema]
burns and corrosions of second degree [blisters] [epidermal loss]
burns and corrosions of third degree [deep necrosis of underlying tissue] [full-thickness skin loss]

Use additional code from category T31 or T32 to identify extent of body surface involved

● **T20** **Burn and corrosion of head, face, and neck**

Excludes2 burn and corrosion of ear drum (T28.41, T28.91)
burn and corrosion of eye and adnexa (T26.-)
burn and corrosion of mouth and pharynx (T28.0)

The appropriate 7th character is to be added to each code from category T20

A	initial encounter
D	subsequent encounter
S	sequela

● **T20.0** **Burn of unspecified degree of head, face, and neck**

Use additional external cause code to identify the source, place and intent of the burn (X00-X19, X75-X77, X96-X98, Y92)

X● **T20.00** **Burn of unspecified degree of head, face, and neck, unspecified site**

● **T20.01** **Burn of unspecified degree of ear [any part, except ear drum]**

Excludes2 burn of ear drum (T28.41-)

● **T20.011** **Burn of unspecified degree of right ear [any part, except ear drum]**

● **T20.012** **Burn of unspecified degree of left ear [any part, except ear drum]**

● **T20.019** **Burn of unspecified degree of unspecified ear [any part, except ear drum]**

X● **T20.02** **Burn of unspecified degree of lip(s)**

X● **T20.03** **Burn of unspecified degree of chin**

X● **T20.04** **Burn of unspecified degree of nose (septum)**

X● **T20.05** **Burn of unspecified degree of scalp [any part]**

X● **T20.06** **Burn of unspecified degree of forehead and cheek**

X● **T20.07** **Burn of unspecified degree of neck**

X● **T20.09** **Burn of unspecified degree of multiple sites of head, face, and neck**

● **T20.1** **Burn of first degree of head, face, and neck**

Use additional external cause code to identify the source, place and intent of the burn (X00-X19, X75-X77, X96-X98, Y92)

X● **T20.10** **Burn of first degree of head, face, and neck, unspecified site**

● **T20.11** **Burn of first degree of ear [any part, except ear drum]**

Excludes2 burn of ear drum (T28.41-)

● **T20.111** **Burn of first degree of right ear [any part, except ear drum]**

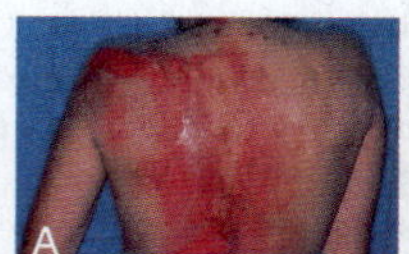 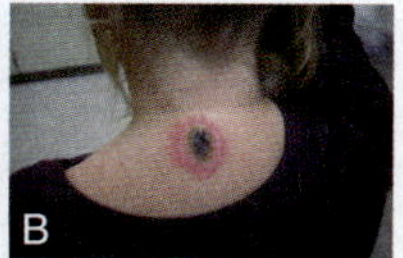

Figure 19-15   **A.** Second-degree burn. **B.** Third-degree burn. (A. From Black J, Hawks J: Medical-Surgical Nursing: Clinical Management for Positive Outcomes, 8e, Saunders, 2008. B. From Marx J, Hockberger R, Walls R: Rosen's Emergency Medicine - Concepts and Clinical Practice, 7e, Mosby, 2009)

▶ New   ➡ Revised   ~~deleted~~ Deleted   Excludes 1   Excludes 2   Includes   Use additional   Code first   Code also   Key words
OGCR Official Guidelines   X Assign placeholder X   ● Use Additional Character(s)   ▶ Manifestation Code   ⦿ Hierarchical Condition Category   **Coding Clinic**

● T20.112   Burn of first degree of **left** ear [any part, except ear drum]

● T20.119   Burn of first degree of **unspecified** ear [any part, except ear drum]

X● T20.12   Burn of first degree of **lip(s)**

X● T20.13   Burn of first degree of **chin**

X● T20.14   Burn of first degree of **nose** (septum)

X● T20.15   Burn of first degree of **scalp** [any part]

X● T20.16   Burn of first degree of **forehead and cheek**

X● T20.17   Burn of first degree of **neck**

X● T20.19   Burn of first degree of **multiple sites** of head, face, and neck

● T20.2   Burn of **second degree** of head, face, and neck

Use additional external cause code to identify the source, place and intent of the burn (X00-X19, X75-X77, X96-X98, Y92)

X● T20.20   Burn of second degree of head, face, and neck, **unspecified** site

● T20.21   Burn of second degree of **ear** [any part, except ear drum]

Excludes2   burn of ear drum (T28.41-)

● T20.211   Burn of second degree of **right** ear [any part, except ear drum]

● T20.212   Burn of second degree of **left** ear [any part, except ear drum]

● T20.219   Burn of second degree of **unspecified** ear [any part, except ear drum]

X● T20.22   Burn of second degree of **lip(s)**

X● T20.23   Burn of second degree of **chin**

X● T20.24   Burn of second degree of **nose** (septum)

X● T20.25   Burn of second degree of **scalp** [any part]
Coding Clinic: 2015, Q1, P19

X● T20.26   Burn of second degree of **forehead and cheek**

X● T20.27   Burn of second degree of **neck**

X● T20.29   Burn of second degree of **multiple sites** of head, face, and neck

● T20.3   Burn of **third degree** of head, face, and neck

Use additional external cause code to identify the source, place and intent of the burn (X00-X19, X75-X77, X96-X98, Y92)

X● T20.30   Burn of third degree of head, face, and neck, **unspecified** site

● T20.31   Burn of third degree of **ear** [any part, except ear drum]

Excludes2   burn of ear drum (T28.41-)

● T20.311   Burn of third degree of **right** ear [any part, except ear drum]

● T20.312   Burn of third degree of **left** ear [any part, except ear drum]
Coding Clinic: 2015, Q1, P18

● T20.319   Burn of third degree of **unspecified** ear [any part, except ear drum]

X● T20.32   Burn of third degree of **lip(s)**

X● T20.33   Burn of third degree of **chin**

X● T20.34   Burn of third degree of **nose** (septum)

X● T20.35   Burn of third degree of **scalp** [any part]

X● T20.36   Burn of third degree of **forehead and cheek**

X● T20.37   Burn of third degree of **neck**

X● T20.39   Burn of third degree of **multiple sites** of head, face, and neck

● T20.4   Corrosion of **unspecified degree** of head, face, and neck

Code first (T51-T65) *to identify chemical and intent*

Use additional external cause code to identify place (Y92)

X● T20.40   Corrosion of unspecified degree of head, face, and neck, **unspecified site**

● T20.41   Corrosion of unspecified degree of **ear** [any part, except ear drum]

Excludes2   corrosion of ear drum (T28.91-)

● T20.411   Corrosion of unspecified degree of **right** ear [any part, except ear drum]

● T20.412   Corrosion of unspecified degree of **left** ear [any part, except ear drum]

● T20.419   Corrosion of unspecified degree of **unspecified** ear [any part, except ear drum]

X● T20.42   Corrosion of unspecified degree of **lip(s)**

X● T20.43   Corrosion of unspecified degree of **chin**

X● T20.44   Corrosion of unspecified degree of **nose** (septum)

X● T20.45   Corrosion of unspecified degree of **scalp** [any part]

X● T20.46   Corrosion of unspecified degree of **forehead and cheek**

X● T20.47   Corrosion of unspecified degree of **neck**

X● T20.49   Corrosion of unspecified degree of **multiple sites** of head, face, and neck

● T20.5   Corrosion of **first degree** of head, face, and neck

Code first (T51-T65) *to identify chemical and intent*

Use additional external cause code to identify place (Y92)

X● T20.50   Corrosion of first degree of head, face, and neck, **unspecified site**

● T20.51   Corrosion of first degree of **ear** [any part, except ear drum]

Excludes2   corrosion of ear drum (T28.91-)

● T20.511   Corrosion of first degree of **right** ear [any part, except ear drum]

● T20.512   Corrosion of first degree of **left** ear [any part, except ear drum]

● T20.519   Corrosion of first degree of **unspecified** ear [any part, except ear drum]

X● T20.52   Corrosion of first degree of **lip(s)**

X● T20.53   Corrosion of first degree of **chin**

X● T20.54   Corrosion of first degree of **nose** (septum)

X● T20.55   Corrosion of first degree of **scalp** [any part]

X● T20.56   Corrosion of first degree of **forehead and cheek**

X● T20.57   Corrosion of first degree of **neck**

X● T20.59   Corrosion of first degree of **multiple sites** of head, face, and neck

● T20.6   Corrosion of **second degree** of head, face, and neck

Code first (T51-T65) *to identify chemical and intent*

Use additional external cause code to identify place (Y92)

X● T20.60   Corrosion of second degree of head, face, and neck, **unspecified site**

● T20.61   Corrosion of second degree of **ear** [any part, except ear drum]

Excludes2   corrosion of ear drum (T28.91-)

● T20.611   Corrosion of second degree of **right** ear [any part, except ear drum]

● T20.612   Corrosion of second degree of **left** ear [any part, except ear drum]

● T20.619   Corrosion of second degree of **unspecified** ear [any part, except ear drum]

X● T20.62   Corrosion of second degree of **lip(s)**

X● T20.63   Corrosion of second degree of **chin**

X● T20.64   Corrosion of second degree of **nose** (septum)

X● T20.65   Corrosion of second degree of **scalp** [any part]

X● T20.66   Corrosion of second degree of **forehead and cheek**

CHAPTER 19 (S00-T88)

CHAPTER 19 (S00-T88)

X ● T20.67   Corrosion of second degree of neck
X ● T20.69   Corrosion of second degree of multiple sites of head, face, and neck
● T20.7   Corrosion of third degree of head, face, and neck
    Code first (T51-T65) to identify chemical and intent
    Use additional external cause code to identify place (Y92)
X ● T20.70   Corrosion of third degree of head, face, and neck, unspecified site
● T20.71   Corrosion of third degree of ear [any part, except ear drum]
      Excludes2   corrosion of ear drum (T28.91-)
● T20.711   Corrosion of third degree of right ear [any part, except ear drum]
● T20.712   Corrosion of third degree of left ear [any part, except ear drum]
● T20.719   Corrosion of third degree of unspecified ear [any part, except ear drum]
X ● T20.72   Corrosion of third degree of lip(s)
X ● T20.73   Corrosion of third degree of chin
X ● T20.74   Corrosion of third degree of nose (septum)
X ● T20.75   Corrosion of third degree of scalp [any part]
X ● T20.76   Corrosion of third degree of forehead and cheek
X ● T20.77   Corrosion of third degree of neck
X ● T20.79   Corrosion of third degree of multiple sites of head, face, and neck

● T21   Burn and corrosion of trunk
    Includes   burns and corrosion of hip region
    Excludes2   burns and corrosion of axilla (T22.- with fifth character 4)
      burns and corrosion of scapular region (T22.- with fifth character 6)
      burns and corrosion of shoulder (T22.- with fifth character 5)
    The appropriate 7th character is to be added to each code from category T21

    A   initial encounter
    D   subsequent encounter
    S   sequela

● T21.0   Burn of unspecified degree of trunk
    Use additional external cause code to identify the source, place and intent of the burn (X00-X19, X75-X77, X96-X98, Y92)
X ● T21.00   Burn of unspecified degree of trunk, unspecified site
X ● T21.01   Burn of unspecified degree of chest wall
    Burn of unspecified degree of breast
X ● T21.02   Burn of unspecified degree of abdominal wall
    Burn of unspecified degree of flank
    Burn of unspecified degree of groin
X ● T21.03   Burn of unspecified degree of upper back
    Burn of unspecified degree of interscapular region
X ● T21.04   Burn of unspecified degree of lower back
X ● T21.05   Burn of unspecified degree of buttock
    Burn of unspecified degree of anus
X ● T21.06   Burn of unspecified degree of male genital region
    Burn of unspecified degree of penis
    Burn of unspecified degree of scrotum
    Burn of unspecified degree of testis

X ● T21.07   Burn of unspecified degree of female genital region
    Burn of unspecified degree of labium (majus) (minus)
    Burn of unspecified degree of perineum
    Burn of unspecified degree of vulva
      Excludes2   burn of vagina (T28.3)
X ● T21.09   Burn of unspecified degree of other site of trunk
● T21.1   Burn of first degree of trunk
    Use additional external cause code to identify the source, place and intent of the burn (X00-X19, X75-X77, X96-X98, Y92)
X ● T21.10   Burn of first degree of trunk, unspecified site
X ● T21.11   Burn of first degree of chest wall
    Burn of first degree of breast
X ● T21.12   Burn of first degree of abdominal wall
    Burn of first degree of flank
    Burn of first degree of groin
X ● T21.13   Burn of first degree of upper back
    Burn of first degree of interscapular region
X ● T21.14   Burn of first degree of lower back
X ● T21.15   Burn of first degree of buttock
    Burn of first degree of anus
X ● T21.16   Burn of first degree of male genital region
    Burn of first degree of penis
    Burn of first degree of scrotum
    Burn of first degree of testis
X ● T21.17   Burn of first degree of female genital region
    Burn of first degree of labium (majus) (minus)
    Burn of first degree of perineum
    Burn of first degree of vulva
      Excludes2   burn of vagina (T28.3)
X ● T21.19   Burn of first degree of other site of trunk
● T21.2   Burn of second degree of trunk
    Use additional external cause code to identify the source, place and intent of the burn (X00-X19, X75-X77, X96-X98, Y92)
X ● T21.20   Burn of second degree of trunk, unspecified site
X ● T21.21   Burn of second degree of chest wall
    Burn of second degree of breast
X ● T21.22   Burn of second degree of abdominal wall
    Burn of second degree of flank
    Burn of second degree of groin
X ● T21.23   Burn of second degree of upper back
    Burn of second degree of interscapular region
X ● T21.24   Burn of second degree of lower back
X ● T21.25   Burn of second degree of buttock
    Burn of second degree of anus
X ● T21.26   Burn of second degree of male genital region
    Burn of second degree of penis
    Burn of second degree of scrotum
    Burn of second degree of testis
X ● T21.27   Burn of second degree of female genital region
    Burn of second degree of labium (majus) (minus)
    Burn of second degree of perineum
    Burn of second degree of vulva
      Excludes2   burn of vagina (T28.3)
X ● T21.29   Burn of second degree of other site of trunk
● T21.3   Burn of third degree of trunk
    Use additional external cause code to identify the source, place and intent of the burn (X00-X19, X75-X77, X96-X98, Y92)
X ● T21.30   Burn of third degree of trunk, unspecified site
X ● T21.31   Burn of third degree of chest wall
    Burn of third degree of breast
    Coding Clinic: 2016, Q2, P6

X● **T21.32**　**Burn of third degree of abdominal wall**
　　Burn of third degree of flank
　　Burn of third degree of groin

X● **T21.33**　**Burn of third degree of upper back**
　　Burn of third degree of interscapular region

X● **T21.34**　**Burn of third degree of lower back**

X● **T21.35**　**Burn of third degree of buttock**
　　Burn of third degree of anus

X● **T21.36**　**Burn of third degree of male genital region**
　　Burn of third degree of penis
　　Burn of third degree of scrotum
　　Burn of third degree of testis

X● **T21.37**　**Burn of third degree of female genital region**
　　Burn of third degree of labium (majus) (minus)
　　Burn of third degree of perineum
　　Burn of third degree of vulva

　　Excludes2　　burn of vagina (T28.3)

X● **T21.39**　**Burn of third degree of other site of trunk**

● **T21.4**　**Corrosion of unspecified degree of trunk**

　　Code first (T51-T65) *to identify chemical and intent*
　　Use additional external cause code to identify place (Y92)

X● **T21.40**　**Corrosion of unspecified degree of trunk, unspecified site**

X● **T21.41**　**Corrosion of unspecified degree of chest wall**
　　Corrosion of unspecified degree of breast

X● **T21.42**　**Corrosion of unspecified degree of abdominal wall**
　　Corrosion of unspecified degree of flank
　　Corrosion of unspecified degree of groin

X● **T21.43**　**Corrosion of unspecified degree of upper back**
　　Corrosion of unspecified degree of interscapular region

X● **T21.44**　**Corrosion of unspecified degree of lower back**

X● **T21.45**　**Corrosion of unspecified degree of buttock**
　　Corrosion of unspecified degree of anus

X● **T21.46**　**Corrosion of unspecified degree of male genital region**
　　Corrosion of unspecified degree of penis
　　Corrosion of unspecified degree of scrotum
　　Corrosion of unspecified degree of testis

X● **T21.47**　**Corrosion of unspecified degree of female genital region**
　　Corrosion of unspecified degree of labium (majus) (minus)
　　Corrosion of unspecified degree of perineum
　　Corrosion of unspecified degree of vulva

　　Excludes2　　corrosion of vagina (T28.8)

X● **T21.49**　**Corrosion of unspecified degree of other site of trunk**

● **T21.5**　**Corrosion of first degree of trunk**

　　Code first (T51-T65) *to identify chemical and intent*
　　Use additional external cause code to identify place (Y92)

X● **T21.50**　**Corrosion of first degree of trunk, unspecified site**

X● **T21.51**　**Corrosion of first degree of chest wall**
　　Corrosion of first degree of breast

X● **T21.52**　**Corrosion of first degree of abdominal wall**
　　Corrosion of first degree of flank
　　Corrosion of first degree of groin

X● **T21.53**　**Corrosion of first degree of upper back**
　　Corrosion of first degree of interscapular region

X● **T21.54**　**Corrosion of first degree of lower back**

X● **T21.55**　**Corrosion of first degree of buttock**
　　Corrosion of first degree of anus

X● **T21.56**　**Corrosion of first degree of male genital region**
　　Corrosion of first degree of penis
　　Corrosion of first degree of scrotum
　　Corrosion of first degree of testis

X● **T21.57**　**Corrosion of first degree of female genital region**
　　Corrosion of first degree of labium (majus) (minus)
　　Corrosion of first degree of perineum
　　Corrosion of first degree of vulva

　　Excludes2　　corrosion of vagina (T28.8)

X● **T21.59**　**Corrosion of first degree of other site of trunk**

● **T21.6**　**Corrosion of second degree of trunk**

　　Code first (T51-T65) *to identify chemical and intent*
　　Use additional external cause code to identify place (Y92)

X● **T21.60**　**Corrosion of second degree of trunk, unspecified site**

X● **T21.61**　**Corrosion of second degree of chest wall**
　　Corrosion of second degree of breast

X● **T21.62**　**Corrosion of second degree of abdominal wall**
　　Corrosion of second degree of flank
　　Corrosion of second degree of groin

X● **T21.63**　**Corrosion of second degree of upper back**
　　Corrosion of second degree of interscapular region

X● **T21.64**　**Corrosion of second degree of lower back**

X● **T21.65**　**Corrosion of second degree of buttock**
　　Corrosion of second degree of anus

X● **T21.66**　**Corrosion of second degree of male genital region**
　　Corrosion of second degree of penis
　　Corrosion of second degree of scrotum
　　Corrosion of second degree of testis

X● **T21.67**　**Corrosion of second degree of female genital region**
　　Corrosion of second degree of labium (majus) (minus)
　　Corrosion of second degree of perineum
　　Corrosion of second degree of vulva

　　Excludes2　　corrosion of vagina (T28.8)

X● **T21.69**　**Corrosion of second degree of other site of trunk**

● **T21.7**　**Corrosion of third degree of trunk**

　　Code first (T51-T65) *to identify chemical and intent*
　　Use additional external cause code to identify place (Y92)

X● **T21.70**　**Corrosion of third degree of trunk, unspecified site**

X● **T21.71**　**Corrosion of third degree of chest wall**
　　Corrosion of third degree of breast

X● **T21.72**　**Corrosion of third degree of abdominal wall**
　　Corrosion of third degree of flank
　　Corrosion of third degree of groin

X● **T21.73**　**Corrosion of third degree of upper back**
　　Corrosion of third degree of interscapular region

X● **T21.74**　**Corrosion of third degree of lower back**

X● **T21.75**　**Corrosion of third degree of buttock**
　　Corrosion of third degree of anus

X● **T21.76**　**Corrosion of third degree of male genital region**
　　Corrosion of third degree of penis
　　Corrosion of third degree of scrotum
　　Corrosion of third degree of testis

X● **T21.77**　**Corrosion of third degree of female genital region**
　　Corrosion of third degree of labium (majus) (minus)
　　Corrosion of third degree of perineum
　　Corrosion of third degree of vulva

　　Excludes2　　corrosion of vagina (T28.8)

X● **T21.79**　**Corrosion of third degree of other site of trunk**

● **T22**   **Burn and corrosion of shoulder and upper limb, except wrist and hand**

> **Excludes2**   burn and corrosion of interscapular region (T21.-)
> burn and corrosion of wrist and hand (T23.-)

> The appropriate 7th character is to be added to each code from category T22

> | | |
> |---|---|
> | A | initial encounter |
> | D | subsequent encounter |
> | S | sequela |

● **T22.0**   **Burn of unspecified degree of shoulder and upper limb, except wrist and hand**

> **Use additional** external cause code to identify the source, place and intent of the burn (X00-X19, X75-X77, X96-X98, Y92)

   X ● **T22.00**   Burn of unspecified degree of shoulder and upper limb, except wrist and hand, **unspecified site**

   ● **T22.01**   Burn of unspecified degree of **forearm**

     ● **T22.011**   Burn of unspecified degree of **right** forearm

     ● **T22.012**   Burn of unspecified degree of **left** forearm

     ● **T22.019**   Burn of unspecified degree of **unspecified** forearm

   ● **T22.02**   Burn of unspecified degree of **elbow**

     ● **T22.021**   Burn of unspecified degree of **right** elbow

     ● **T22.022**   Burn of unspecified degree of **left** elbow

     ● **T22.029**   Burn of unspecified degree of **unspecified** elbow

   ● **T22.03**   Burn of unspecified degree of **upper arm**

     ● **T22.031**   Burn of unspecified degree of **right** upper arm

     ● **T22.032**   Burn of unspecified degree of **left** upper arm

     ● **T22.039**   Burn of unspecified degree of **unspecified** upper arm

   ● **T22.04**   Burn of unspecified degree of **axilla**

     ● **T22.041**   Burn of unspecified degree of **right** axilla

     ● **T22.042**   Burn of unspecified degree of **left** axilla

     ● **T22.049**   Burn of unspecified degree of **unspecified** axilla

   ● **T22.05**   Burn of unspecified degree of **shoulder**

     ● **T22.051**   Burn of unspecified degree of **right** shoulder

     ● **T22.052**   Burn of unspecified degree of **left** shoulder

     ● **T22.059**   Burn of unspecified degree of **unspecified** shoulder

   ● **T22.06**   Burn of unspecified degree of **scapular region**

     ● **T22.061**   Burn of unspecified degree of **right** scapular region

     ● **T22.062**   Burn of unspecified degree of **left** scapular region

     ● **T22.069**   Burn of unspecified degree of **unspecified** scapular region

   ● **T22.09**   Burn of unspecified degree of **multiple sites** of shoulder and upper limb, except wrist and hand

     ● **T22.091**   Burn of unspecified degree of multiple sites of **right** shoulder and upper limb, except wrist and hand

     ● **T22.092**   Burn of unspecified degree of multiple sites of **left** shoulder and upper limb, except wrist and hand

     ● **T22.099**   Burn of unspecified degree of multiple sites of **unspecified** shoulder and upper limb, except wrist and hand

● **T22.1**   **Burn of first degree of shoulder and upper limb, except wrist and hand**

> **Use additional** external cause code to identify the source, place and intent of the burn (X00-X19, X75-X77, X96-X98, Y92)

   X ● **T22.10**   Burn of first degree of shoulder and upper limb, except wrist and hand, **unspecified site**

   ● **T22.11**   Burn of first degree of **forearm**

     ● **T22.111**   Burn of first degree of **right** forearm

     ● **T22.112**   Burn of first degree of **left** forearm

     ● **T22.119**   Burn of first degree of **unspecified** forearm

   ● **T22.12**   Burn of first degree of **elbow**

     ● **T22.121**   Burn of first degree of **right** elbow

     ● **T22.122**   Burn of first degree of **left** elbow

     ● **T22.129**   Burn of first degree of **unspecified** elbow

   ● **T22.13**   Burn of first degree of **upper arm**

     ● **T22.131**   Burn of first degree of **right** upper arm

     ● **T22.132**   Burn of first degree of **left** upper arm

     ● **T22.139**   Burn of first degree of **unspecified** upper arm

   ● **T22.14**   Burn of first degree of **axilla**

     ● **T22.141**   Burn of first degree of **right** axilla

     ● **T22.142**   Burn of first degree of **left** axilla

     ● **T22.149**   Burn of first degree of **unspecified** axilla

   ● **T22.15**   Burn of first degree of **shoulder**

     ● **T22.151**   Burn of first degree of **right** shoulder

     ● **T22.152**   Burn of first degree of **left** shoulder

     ● **T22.159**   Burn of first degree of **unspecified** shoulder

   ● **T22.16**   Burn of first degree of **scapular region**

     ● **T22.161**   Burn of first degree of **right** scapular region

     ● **T22.162**   Burn of first degree of **left** scapular region

     ● **T22.169**   Burn of first degree of **unspecified** scapular region

   ● **T22.19**   Burn of first degree of **multiple sites** of shoulder and upper limb, except wrist and hand

     ● **T22.191**   Burn of first degree of multiple sites of **right** shoulder and upper limb, except wrist and hand

     ● **T22.192**   Burn of first degree of multiple sites of **left** shoulder and upper limb, except wrist and hand

     ● **T22.199**   Burn of first degree of multiple sites of **unspecified** shoulder and upper limb, except wrist and hand

● **T22.2**   **Burn of second degree of shoulder and upper limb, except wrist and hand**

> **Use additional** external cause code to identify the source, place and intent of the burn (X00-X19, X75-X77, X96-X98, Y92)

   X ● **T22.20**   Burn of second degree of shoulder and upper limb, except wrist and hand, **unspecified site**

   ● **T22.21**   Burn of second degree of **forearm**

     ● **T22.211**   Burn of second degree of **right** forearm

     ● **T22.212**   Burn of second degree of **left** forearm

     ● **T22.219**   Burn of second degree of **unspecified** forearm

CHAPTER 19 (S00-T88)

▶ New   ⇒ Revised   ~~deleted~~ Deleted   Excludes 1   Excludes 2   Includes   Use additional   Code first   Code also   Key words

OGCR Official Guidelines   X Assign placeholder X   ● Use Additional Character(s)   ▸ Manifestation Code   Hierarchical Condition Category   Coding Clinic

● **T22.22**   Burn of second degree of elbow
    ● **T22.221**   Burn of second degree of right elbow
    ● **T22.222**   Burn of second degree of left elbow
    ● **T22.229**   Burn of second degree of unspecified elbow
● **T22.23**   Burn of second degree of upper arm
    ● **T22.231**   Burn of second degree of right upper arm
    ● **T22.232**   Burn of second degree of left upper arm
    ● **T22.239**   Burn of second degree of unspecified upper arm
● **T22.24**   Burn of second degree of axilla
    ● **T22.241**   Burn of second degree of right axilla
    ● **T22.242**   Burn of second degree of left axilla
    ● **T22.249**   Burn of second degree of unspecified axilla
● **T22.25**   Burn of second degree of shoulder
    ● **T22.251**   Burn of second degree of right shoulder
    ● **T22.252**   Burn of second degree of left shoulder
    ● **T22.259**   Burn of second degree of unspecified shoulder
● **T22.26**   Burn of second degree of scapular region
    ● **T22.261**   Burn of second degree of right scapular region
    ● **T22.262**   Burn of second degree of left scapular region
    ● **T22.269**   Burn of second degree of unspecified scapular region
● **T22.29**   Burn of second degree of multiple sites of shoulder and upper limb, except wrist and hand
    ● **T22.291**   Burn of second degree of multiple sites of right shoulder and upper limb, except wrist and hand
    ● **T22.292**   Burn of second degree of multiple sites of left shoulder and upper limb, except wrist and hand
    ● **T22.299**   Burn of second degree of multiple sites of unspecified shoulder and upper limb, except wrist and hand
● **T22.3**   Burn of third degree of shoulder and upper limb, except wrist and hand
    Use additional external cause code to identify the source, place and intent of the burn (X00-X19, X75-X77, X96-X98, Y92)
   X ● **T22.30**   Burn of third degree of shoulder and upper limb, except wrist and hand, unspecified site
    ● **T22.31**   Burn of third degree of forearm
     ● **T22.311**   Burn of third degree of right forearm
     ● **T22.312**   Burn of third degree of left forearm
     ● **T22.319**   Burn of third degree of unspecified forearm
    ● **T22.32**   Burn of third degree of elbow
     ● **T22.321**   Burn of third degree of right elbow
     ● **T22.322**   Burn of third degree of left elbow
     ● **T22.329**   Burn of third degree of unspecified elbow
    ● **T22.33**   Burn of third degree of upper arm
     ● **T22.331**   Burn of third degree of right upper arm
     ● **T22.332**   Burn of third degree of left upper arm
     ● **T22.339**   Burn of third degree of unspecified upper arm

● **T22.34**   Burn of third degree of axilla
    ● **T22.341**   Burn of third degree of right axilla
    ● **T22.342**   Burn of third degree of left axilla
    ● **T22.349**   Burn of third degree of unspecified axilla
● **T22.35**   Burn of third degree of shoulder
    ● **T22.351**   Burn of third degree of right shoulder
    ● **T22.352**   Burn of third degree of left shoulder
    ● **T22.359**   Burn of third degree of unspecified shoulder
● **T22.36**   Burn of third degree of scapular region
    ● **T22.361**   Burn of third degree of right scapular region
    ● **T22.362**   Burn of third degree of left scapular region
    ● **T22.369**   Burn of third degree of unspecified scapular region
● **T22.39**   Burn of third degree of multiple sites of shoulder and upper limb, except wrist and hand
    ● **T22.391**   Burn of third degree of multiple sites of right shoulder and upper limb, except wrist and hand
    ● **T22.392**   Burn of third degree of multiple sites of left shoulder and upper limb, except wrist and hand
    ● **T22.399**   Burn of third degree of multiple sites of unspecified shoulder and upper limb, except wrist and hand
● **T22.4**   Corrosion of unspecified degree of shoulder and upper limb, except wrist and hand
    Code first (T51-T65) *to identify chemical and intent*
    Use additional external cause code to identify place (Y92)
   X ● **T22.40**   Corrosion of unspecified degree of shoulder and upper limb, except wrist and hand, unspecified site
    ● **T22.41**   Corrosion of unspecified degree of forearm
     ● **T22.411**   Corrosion of unspecified degree of right forearm
     ● **T22.412**   Corrosion of unspecified degree of left forearm
     ● **T22.419**   Corrosion of unspecified degree of unspecified forearm
    ● **T22.42**   Corrosion of unspecified degree of elbow
     ● **T22.421**   Corrosion of unspecified degree of right elbow
     ● **T22.422**   Corrosion of unspecified degree of left elbow
     ● **T22.429**   Corrosion of unspecified degree of unspecified elbow
    ● **T22.43**   Corrosion of unspecified degree of upper arm
     ● **T22.431**   Corrosion of unspecified degree of right upper arm
     ● **T22.432**   Corrosion of unspecified degree of left upper arm
     ● **T22.439**   Corrosion of unspecified degree of unspecified upper arm
    ● **T22.44**   Corrosion of unspecified degree of axilla
     ● **T22.441**   Corrosion of unspecified degree of right axilla
     ● **T22.442**   Corrosion of unspecified degree of left axilla
     ● **T22.449**   Corrosion of unspecified degree of unspecified axilla

CHAPTER 19 (S00-T88)

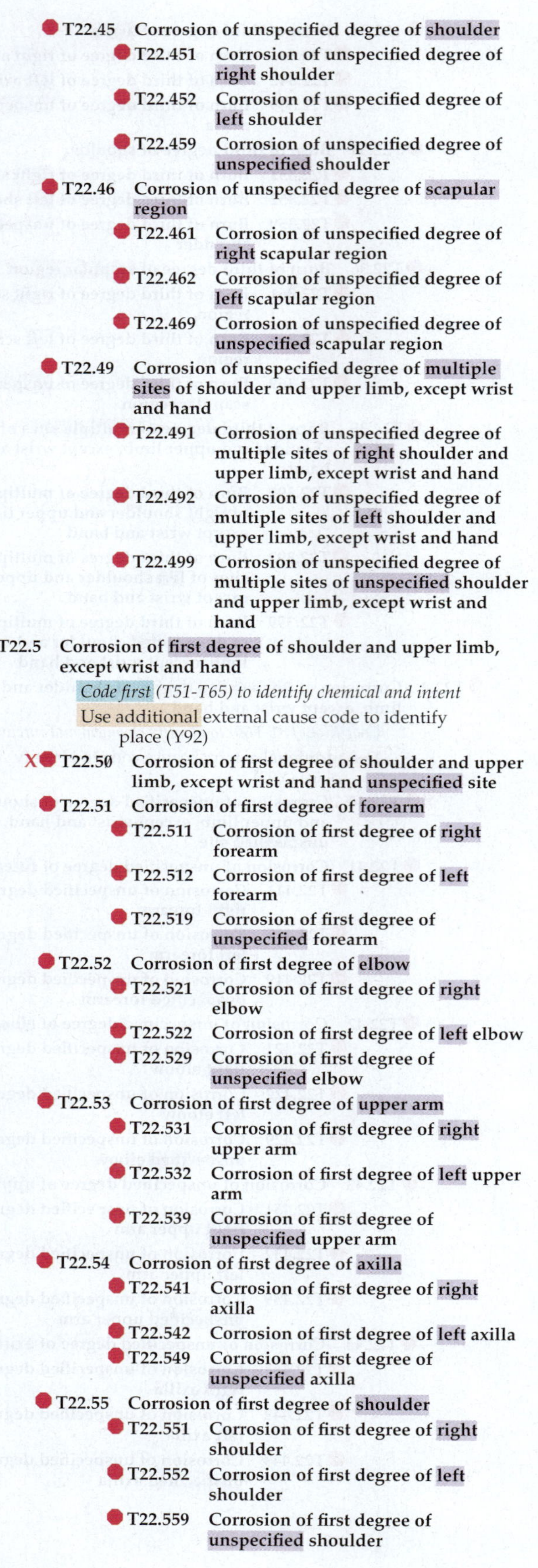

● **T22.45** Corrosion of unspecified degree of shoulder
   ● **T22.451** Corrosion of unspecified degree of right shoulder
   ● **T22.452** Corrosion of unspecified degree of left shoulder
   ● **T22.459** Corrosion of unspecified degree of unspecified shoulder
● **T22.46** Corrosion of unspecified degree of scapular region
   ● **T22.461** Corrosion of unspecified degree of right scapular region
   ● **T22.462** Corrosion of unspecified degree of left scapular region
   ● **T22.469** Corrosion of unspecified degree of unspecified scapular region
● **T22.49** Corrosion of unspecified degree of multiple sites of shoulder and upper limb, except wrist and hand
   ● **T22.491** Corrosion of unspecified degree of multiple sites of right shoulder and upper limb, except wrist and hand
   ● **T22.492** Corrosion of unspecified degree of multiple sites of left shoulder and upper limb, except wrist and hand
   ● **T22.499** Corrosion of unspecified degree of multiple sites of unspecified shoulder and upper limb, except wrist and hand
● **T22.5** Corrosion of first degree of shoulder and upper limb, except wrist and hand

Code first (T51-T65) to identify chemical and intent

Use additional external cause code to identify place (Y92)

X ● **T22.50** Corrosion of first degree of shoulder and upper limb, except wrist and hand unspecified site
● **T22.51** Corrosion of first degree of forearm
   ● **T22.511** Corrosion of first degree of right forearm
   ● **T22.512** Corrosion of first degree of left forearm
   ● **T22.519** Corrosion of first degree of unspecified forearm
● **T22.52** Corrosion of first degree of elbow
   ● **T22.521** Corrosion of first degree of right elbow
   ● **T22.522** Corrosion of first degree of left elbow
   ● **T22.529** Corrosion of first degree of unspecified elbow
● **T22.53** Corrosion of first degree of upper arm
   ● **T22.531** Corrosion of first degree of right upper arm
   ● **T22.532** Corrosion of first degree of left upper arm
   ● **T22.539** Corrosion of first degree of unspecified upper arm
● **T22.54** Corrosion of first degree of axilla
   ● **T22.541** Corrosion of first degree of right axilla
   ● **T22.542** Corrosion of first degree of left axilla
   ● **T22.549** Corrosion of first degree of unspecified axilla
● **T22.55** Corrosion of first degree of shoulder
   ● **T22.551** Corrosion of first degree of right shoulder
   ● **T22.552** Corrosion of first degree of left shoulder
   ● **T22.559** Corrosion of first degree of unspecified shoulder

● **T22.56** Corrosion of first degree of scapular region
   ● **T22.561** Corrosion of first degree of right scapular region
   ● **T22.562** Corrosion of first degree of left scapular region
   ● **T22.569** Corrosion of first degree of unspecified scapular region
● **T22.59** Corrosion of first degree of multiple sites of shoulder and upper limb, except wrist and hand
   ● **T22.591** Corrosion of first degree of multiple sites of right shoulder and upper limb, except wrist and hand
   ● **T22.592** Corrosion of first degree of multiple sites of left shoulder and upper limb, except wrist and hand
   ● **T22.599** Corrosion of first degree of multiple sites of unspecified shoulder and upper limb, except wrist and hand
● **T22.6** Corrosion of second degree of shoulder and upper limb, except wrist and hand

Code first (T51-T65) to identify chemical and intent

Use additional external cause code to identify place (Y92)

X ● **T22.60** Corrosion of second degree of shoulder and upper limb, except wrist and hand, unspecified site
● **T22.61** Corrosion of second degree of forearm
   ● **T22.611** Corrosion of second degree of right forearm
   ● **T22.612** Corrosion of second degree of left forearm
   ● **T22.619** Corrosion of second degree of unspecified forearm
● **T22.62** Corrosion of second degree of elbow
   ● **T22.621** Corrosion of second degree of right elbow
   ● **T22.622** Corrosion of second degree of left elbow
   ● **T22.629** Corrosion of second degree of unspecified elbow
● **T22.63** Corrosion of second degree of upper arm
   ● **T22.631** Corrosion of second degree of right upper arm
   ● **T22.632** Corrosion of second degree of left upper arm
   ● **T22.639** Corrosion of second degree of unspecified upper arm
● **T22.64** Corrosion of second degree of axilla
   ● **T22.641** Corrosion of second degree of right axilla
   ● **T22.642** Corrosion of second degree of left axilla
   ● **T22.649** Corrosion of second degree of unspecified axilla
● **T22.65** Corrosion of second degree of shoulder
   ● **T22.651** Corrosion of second degree of right shoulder
   ● **T22.652** Corrosion of second degree of left shoulder
   ● **T22.659** Corrosion of second degree of unspecified shoulder
● **T22.66** Corrosion of second degree of scapular region
   ● **T22.661** Corrosion of second degree of right scapular region
   ● **T22.662** Corrosion of second degree of left scapular region
   ● **T22.669** Corrosion of second degree of unspecified scapular region

● **T22.69** Corrosion of second degree of multiple sites of shoulder and upper limb, except wrist and hand

  ● **T22.691** Corrosion of second degree of multiple sites of right shoulder and upper limb, except wrist and hand

  ● **T22.692** Corrosion of second degree of multiple sites of left shoulder and upper limb, except wrist and hand

  ● **T22.699** Corrosion of second degree of multiple sites of unspecified shoulder and upper limb, except wrist and hand

● **T22.7** Corrosion of third degree of shoulder and upper limb, except wrist and hand

Code first (T51-T65) to identify chemical and intent

Use additional external cause code to identify place (Y92)

X ● **T22.70** Corrosion of third degree of shoulder and upper limb, except wrist and hand, unspecified site

● **T22.71** Corrosion of third degree of forearm

  ● **T22.711** Corrosion of third degree of right forearm

  ● **T22.712** Corrosion of third degree of left forearm

  ● **T22.719** Corrosion of third degree of unspecified forearm

● **T22.72** Corrosion of third degree of elbow

  ● **T22.721** Corrosion of third degree of right elbow

  ● **T22.722** Corrosion of third degree of left elbow

  ● **T22.729** Corrosion of third degree of unspecified elbow

● **T22.73** Corrosion of third degree of upper arm

  ● **T22.731** Corrosion of third degree of right upper arm

  ● **T22.732** Corrosion of third degree of left upper arm

  ● **T22.739** Corrosion of third degree of unspecified upper arm

● **T22.74** Corrosion of third degree of axilla

  ● **T22.741** Corrosion of third degree of right axilla

  ● **T22.742** Corrosion of third degree of left axilla

  ● **T22.749** Corrosion of third degree of unspecified axilla

● **T22.75** Corrosion of third degree of shoulder

  ● **T22.751** Corrosion of third degree of right shoulder

  ● **T22.752** Corrosion of third degree of left shoulder

  ● **T22.759** Corrosion of third degree of unspecified shoulder

● **T22.76** Corrosion of third degree of scapular region

  ● **T22.761** Corrosion of third degree of right scapular region

  ● **T22.762** Corrosion of third degree of left scapular region

  ● **T22.769** Corrosion of third degree of unspecified scapular region

● **T22.79** Corrosion of third degree of multiple sites of shoulder and upper limb, except wrist and hand

  ● **T22.791** Corrosion of third degree of multiple sites of right shoulder and upper limb, except wrist and hand

  ● **T22.792** Corrosion of third degree of multiple sites of left shoulder and upper limb, except wrist and hand

  ● **T22.799** Corrosion of third degree of multiple sites of unspecified shoulder and upper limb, except wrist and hand

● **T23** Burn and corrosion of wrist and hand

The appropriate 7th character is to be added to each code from category T23

A	initial encounter
D	subsequent encounter
S	sequela

● **T23.0** Burn of unspecified degree of wrist and hand

Use additional external cause code to identify the source, place and intent of the burn (X00-X19, X75-X77, X96-X98, Y92)

  ● **T23.00** Burn of unspecified degree of hand, unspecified site

  ● **T23.001** Burn of unspecified degree of right hand, unspecified site

  ● **T23.002** Burn of unspecified degree of left hand, unspecified site

  ● **T23.009** Burn of unspecified degree of unspecified hand, unspecified site

  ● **T23.01** Burn of unspecified degree of thumb (nail)

  ● **T23.011** Burn of unspecified degree of right thumb (nail)

  ● **T23.012** Burn of unspecified degree of left thumb (nail)

  ● **T23.019** Burn of unspecified degree of unspecified thumb (nail)

  ● **T23.02** Burn of unspecified degree of single finger (nail) except thumb

  ● **T23.021** Burn of unspecified degree of single right finger (nail) except thumb

  ● **T23.022** Burn of unspecified degree of single left finger (nail) except thumb

  ● **T23.029** Burn of unspecified degree of unspecified single finger (nail) except thumb

  ● **T23.03** Burn of unspecified degree of multiple fingers (nail), not including thumb

  ● **T23.031** Burn of unspecified degree of multiple right fingers (nail), not including thumb

  ● **T23.032** Burn of unspecified degree of multiple left fingers (nail), not including thumb

  ● **T23.039** Burn of unspecified degree of unspecified multiple fingers (nail), not including thumb

  ● **T23.04** Burn of unspecified degree of multiple fingers (nail), including thumb

  ● **T23.041** Burn of unspecified degree of multiple right fingers (nail), including thumb

  ● **T23.042** Burn of unspecified degree of multiple left fingers (nail), including thumb

  ● **T23.049** Burn of unspecified degree of unspecified multiple fingers (nail), including thumb

  ● **T23.05** Burn of unspecified degree of palm

  ● **T23.051** Burn of unspecified degree of right palm

  ● **T23.052** Burn of unspecified degree of left palm

  ● **T23.059** Burn of unspecified degree of unspecified palm

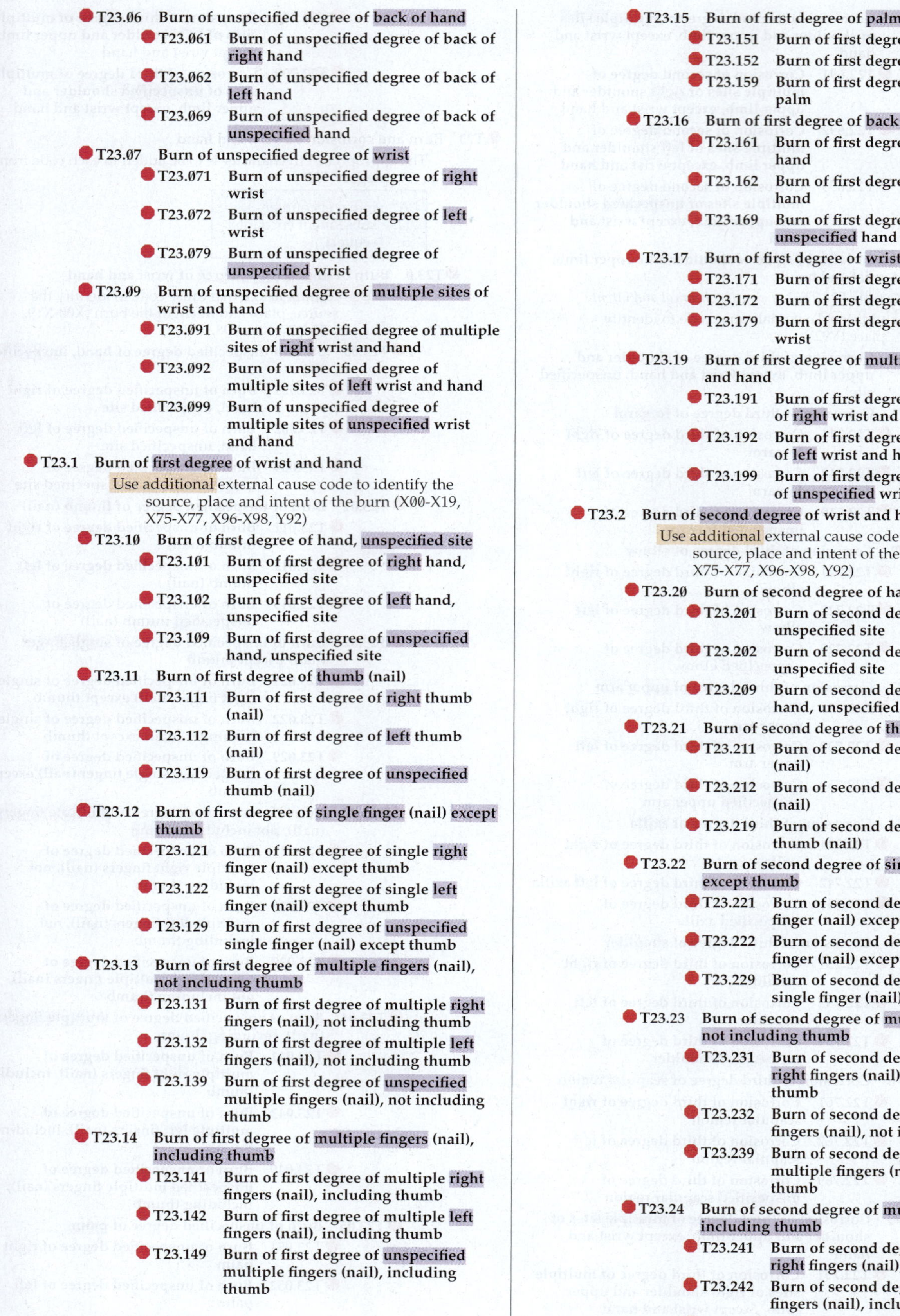

● T23.06   Burn of unspecified degree of back of hand
- ● T23.061   Burn of unspecified degree of back of right hand
- ● T23.062   Burn of unspecified degree of back of left hand
- ● T23.069   Burn of unspecified degree of back of unspecified hand

● T23.07   Burn of unspecified degree of wrist
- ● T23.071   Burn of unspecified degree of right wrist
- ● T23.072   Burn of unspecified degree of left wrist
- ● T23.079   Burn of unspecified degree of unspecified wrist

● T23.09   Burn of unspecified degree of multiple sites of wrist and hand
- ● T23.091   Burn of unspecified degree of multiple sites of right wrist and hand
- ● T23.092   Burn of unspecified degree of multiple sites of left wrist and hand
- ● T23.099   Burn of unspecified degree of multiple sites of unspecified wrist and hand

● T23.1   Burn of first degree of wrist and hand

Use additional external cause code to identify the source, place and intent of the burn (X00-X19, X75-X77, X96-X98, Y92)

- ● T23.10   Burn of first degree of hand, unspecified site
  - ● T23.101   Burn of first degree of right hand, unspecified site
  - ● T23.102   Burn of first degree of left hand, unspecified site
  - ● T23.109   Burn of first degree of unspecified hand, unspecified site
- ● T23.11   Burn of first degree of thumb (nail)
  - ● T23.111   Burn of first degree of right thumb (nail)
  - ● T23.112   Burn of first degree of left thumb (nail)
  - ● T23.119   Burn of first degree of unspecified thumb (nail)
- ● T23.12   Burn of first degree of single finger (nail) except thumb
  - ● T23.121   Burn of first degree of single right finger (nail) except thumb
  - ● T23.122   Burn of first degree of single left finger (nail) except thumb
  - ● T23.129   Burn of first degree of unspecified single finger (nail) except thumb
- ● T23.13   Burn of first degree of multiple fingers (nail), not including thumb
  - ● T23.131   Burn of first degree of multiple right fingers (nail), not including thumb
  - ● T23.132   Burn of first degree of multiple left fingers (nail), not including thumb
  - ● T23.139   Burn of first degree of unspecified multiple fingers (nail), not including thumb
- ● T23.14   Burn of first degree of multiple fingers (nail), including thumb
  - ● T23.141   Burn of first degree of multiple right fingers (nail), including thumb
  - ● T23.142   Burn of first degree of multiple left fingers (nail), including thumb
  - ● T23.149   Burn of first degree of unspecified multiple fingers (nail), including thumb

● T23.15   Burn of first degree of palm
- ● T23.151   Burn of first degree of right palm
- ● T23.152   Burn of first degree of left palm
- ● T23.159   Burn of first degree of unspecified palm

● T23.16   Burn of first degree of back of hand
- ● T23.161   Burn of first degree of back of right hand
- ● T23.162   Burn of first degree of back of left hand
- ● T23.169   Burn of first degree of back of unspecified hand

● T23.17   Burn of first degree of wrist
- ● T23.171   Burn of first degree of right wrist
- ● T23.172   Burn of first degree of left wrist
- ● T23.179   Burn of first degree of unspecified wrist

● T23.19   Burn of first degree of multiple sites of wrist and hand
- ● T23.191   Burn of first degree of multiple sites of right wrist and hand
- ● T23.192   Burn of first degree of multiple sites of left wrist and hand
- ● T23.199   Burn of first degree of multiple sites of unspecified wrist and hand

● T23.2   Burn of second degree of wrist and hand

Use additional external cause code to identify the source, place and intent of the burn (X00-X19, X75-X77, X96-X98, Y92)

- ● T23.20   Burn of second degree of hand, unspecified site
  - ● T23.201   Burn of second degree of right hand, unspecified site
  - ● T23.202   Burn of second degree of left hand, unspecified site
  - ● T23.209   Burn of second degree of unspecified hand, unspecified site
- ● T23.21   Burn of second degree of thumb (nail)
  - ● T23.211   Burn of second degree of right thumb (nail)
  - ● T23.212   Burn of second degree of left thumb (nail)
  - ● T23.219   Burn of second degree of unspecified thumb (nail)
- ● T23.22   Burn of second degree of single finger (nail) except thumb
  - ● T23.221   Burn of second degree of single right finger (nail) except thumb
  - ● T23.222   Burn of second degree of single left finger (nail) except thumb
  - ● T23.229   Burn of second degree of unspecified single finger (nail) except thumb
- ● T23.23   Burn of second degree of multiple fingers (nail), not including thumb
  - ● T23.231   Burn of second degree of multiple right fingers (nail), not including thumb
  - ● T23.232   Burn of second degree of multiple left fingers (nail), not including thumb
  - ● T23.239   Burn of second degree of unspecified multiple fingers (nail), not including thumb
- ● T23.24   Burn of second degree of multiple fingers (nail), including thumb
  - ● T23.241   Burn of second degree of multiple right fingers (nail), including thumb
  - ● T23.242   Burn of second degree of multiple left fingers (nail), including thumb
  - ● T23.249   Burn of second degree of unspecified multiple fingers (nail), including thumb

● T23.25 Burn of second degree of palm
  ● T23.251 Burn of second degree of right palm
  ● T23.252 Burn of second degree of left palm
  ● T23.259 Burn of second degree of unspecified palm
● T23.26 Burn of second degree of back of hand
  ● T23.261 Burn of second degree of back of right hand
  ● T23.262 Burn of second degree of back of left hand
  ● T23.269 Burn of second degree of back of unspecified hand
● T23.27 Burn of second degree of wrist
  ● T23.271 Burn of second degree of right wrist
  ● T23.272 Burn of second degree of left wrist
  ● T23.279 Burn of second degree of unspecified wrist
● T23.29 Burn of second degree of multiple sites of wrist and hand
  ● T23.291 Burn of second degree of multiple sites of right wrist and hand
  ● T23.292 Burn of second degree of multiple sites of left wrist and hand
  ● T23.299 Burn of second degree of multiple sites of unspecified wrist and hand
● T23.3 Burn of third degree of wrist and hand
  Use additional external cause code to identify the source, place and intent of the burn (X00-X19, X75-X77, X96-X98, Y92)
  ● T23.30 Burn of third degree of hand, unspecified site
    ● T23.301 Burn of third degree of right hand, unspecified site
      Coding Clinic: 2015, Q1, P19
    ● T23.302 Burn of third degree of left hand, unspecified site
      Coding Clinic: 2016, Q2, P5
    ● T23.309 Burn of third degree of unspecified hand, unspecified site
  ● T23.31 Burn of third degree of thumb (nail)
    ● T23.311 Burn of third degree of right thumb (nail)
    ● T23.312 Burn of third degree of left thumb (nail)
    ● T23.319 Burn of third degree of unspecified thumb (nail)
  ● T23.32 Burn of third degree of single finger (nail) except thumb
    ● T23.321 Burn of third degree of single right finger (nail) except thumb
    ● T23.322 Burn of third degree of single left finger (nail) except thumb
    ● T23.329 Burn of third degree of unspecified single finger (nail) except thumb
  ● T23.33 Burn of third degree of multiple fingers (nail), not including thumb
    ● T23.331 Burn of third degree of multiple right fingers (nail), not including thumb
    ● T23.332 Burn of third degree of multiple left fingers (nail), not including thumb
    ● T23.339 Burn of third degree of unspecified multiple fingers (nail), not including thumb
  ● T23.34 Burn of third degree of multiple fingers (nail), including thumb
    ● T23.341 Burn of third degree of multiple right fingers (nail), including thumb
    ● T23.342 Burn of third degree of multiple left fingers (nail), including thumb

  ● T23.349 Burn of third degree of unspecified multiple fingers (nail), including thumb
● T23.35 Burn of third degree of palm
  ● T23.351 Burn of third degree of right palm
  ● T23.352 Burn of third degree of left palm
  ● T23.359 Burn of third degree of unspecified palm
● T23.36 Burn of third degree of back of hand
  ● T23.361 Burn of third degree of back of right hand
  ● T23.362 Burn of third degree of back of left hand
  ● T23.369 Burn of third degree of back of unspecified hand
● T23.37 Burn of third degree of wrist
  ● T23.371 Burn of third degree of right wrist
  ● T23.372 Burn of third degree of left wrist
  ● T23.379 Burn of third degree of unspecified wrist
● T23.39 Burn of third degree of multiple sites of wrist and hand
  ● T23.391 Burn of third degree of multiple sites of right wrist and hand
  ● T23.392 Burn of third degree of multiple sites of left wrist and hand
  ● T23.399 Burn of third degree of multiple sites of unspecified wrist and hand
● T23.4 Corrosion of unspecified degree of wrist and hand
  Code first (T51-T65) to identify chemical and intent
  Use additional external cause code to identify place (Y92)
  ● T23.40 Corrosion of unspecified degree of hand, unspecified site
    ● T23.401 Corrosion of unspecified degree of right hand, unspecified site
    ● T23.402 Corrosion of unspecified degree of left hand, unspecified site
    ● T23.409 Corrosion of unspecified degree of unspecified hand, unspecified site
  ● T23.41 Corrosion of unspecified degree of thumb (nail)
    ● T23.411 Corrosion of unspecified degree of right thumb (nail)
    ● T23.412 Corrosion of unspecified degree of left thumb (nail)
    ● T23.419 Corrosion of unspecified degree of unspecified thumb (nail)
  ● T23.42 Corrosion of unspecified degree of single finger (nail) except thumb
    ● T23.421 Corrosion of unspecified degree of single right finger (nail) except thumb
    ● T23.422 Corrosion of unspecified degree of single left finger (nail) except thumb
    ● T23.429 Corrosion of unspecified degree of unspecified single finger (nail) except thumb
  ● T23.43 Corrosion of unspecified degree of multiple fingers (nail), not including thumb
    ● T23.431 Corrosion of unspecified degree of multiple right fingers (nail), not including thumb
    ● T23.432 Corrosion of unspecified degree of multiple left fingers (nail), not including thumb
    ● T23.439 Corrosion of unspecified degree of unspecified multiple fingers (nail), not including thumb

CHAPTER 19 (S00-T88)

● T23.44   Corrosion of unspecified degree of multiple fingers (nail), including thumb
- ● T23.441   Corrosion of unspecified degree of multiple right fingers (nail), including thumb
- ● T23.442   Corrosion of unspecified degree of multiple left fingers (nail), including thumb
- ● T23.449   Corrosion of unspecified degree of unspecified multiple fingers (nail), including thumb

● T23.45   Corrosion of unspecified degree of palm
- ● T23.451   Corrosion of unspecified degree of right palm
- ● T23.452   Corrosion of unspecified degree of left palm
- ● T23.459   Corrosion of unspecified degree of unspecified palm

● T23.46   Corrosion of unspecified degree of back of hand
- ● T23.461   Corrosion of unspecified degree of back of right hand
- ● T23.462   Corrosion of unspecified degree of back of left hand
- ● T23.469   Corrosion of unspecified degree of back of unspecified hand

● T23.47   Corrosion of unspecified degree of wrist
- ● T23.471   Corrosion of unspecified degree of right wrist
- ● T23.472   Corrosion of unspecified degree of left wrist
- ● T23.479   Corrosion of unspecified degree of unspecified wrist

● T23.49   Corrosion of unspecified degree of multiple sites of wrist and hand
- ● T23.491   Corrosion of unspecified degree of multiple sites of right wrist and hand
- ● T23.492   Corrosion of unspecified degree of multiple sites of left wrist and hand
- ● T23.499   Corrosion of unspecified degree of multiple sites of unspecified wrist and hand

● T23.5   Corrosion of first degree of wrist and hand

Code first (T51-T65) to identify chemical and intent

Use additional external cause code to identify place (Y92)

● T23.50   Corrosion of first degree of hand, unspecified site
- ● T23.501   Corrosion of first degree of right hand, unspecified site
- ● T23.502   Corrosion of first degree of left hand, unspecified site
- ● T23.509   Corrosion of first degree of unspecified hand, unspecified site

● T23.51   Corrosion of first degree of thumb (nail)
- ● T23.511   Corrosion of first degree of right thumb (nail)
- ● T23.512   Corrosion of first degree of left thumb (nail)
- ● T23.519   Corrosion of first degree of unspecified thumb (nail)

● T23.52   Corrosion of first degree of single finger (nail) except thumb
- ● T23.521   Corrosion of first degree of single right finger (nail) except thumb
- ● T23.522   Corrosion of first degree of single left finger (nail) except thumb
- ● T23.529   Corrosion of first degree of unspecified single finger (nail) except thumb

● T23.53   Corrosion of first degree of multiple fingers (nail), not including thumb
- ● T23.531   Corrosion of first degree of multiple right fingers (nail), not including thumb
- ● T23.532   Corrosion of first degree of multiple left fingers (nail), not including thumb
- ● T23.539   Corrosion of first degree of unspecified multiple fingers (nail), not including thumb

● T23.54   Corrosion of first degree of multiple fingers (nail), including thumb
- ● T23.541   Corrosion of first degree of multiple right fingers (nail), including thumb
- ● T23.542   Corrosion of first degree of multiple left fingers (nail), including thumb
- ● T23.549   Corrosion of first degree of unspecified multiple fingers (nail), including thumb

● T23.55   Corrosion of first degree of palm
- ● T23.551   Corrosion of first degree of right palm
- ● T23.552   Corrosion of first degree of left palm
- ● T23.559   Corrosion of first degree of unspecified palm

● T23.56   Corrosion of first degree of back of hand
- ● T23.561   Corrosion of first degree of back of right hand
- ● T23.562   Corrosion of first degree of back of left hand
- ● T23.569   Corrosion of first degree of back of unspecified hand

● T23.57   Corrosion of first degree of wrist
- ● T23.571   Corrosion of first degree of right wrist
- ● T23.572   Corrosion of first degree of left wrist
- ● T23.579   Corrosion of first degree of unspecified wrist

● T23.59   Corrosion of first degree of multiple sites of wrist and hand
- ● T23.591   Corrosion of first degree of multiple sites of right wrist and hand
- ● T23.592   Corrosion of first degree of multiple sites of left wrist and hand
- ● T23.599   Corrosion of first degree of multiple sites of unspecified wrist and hand

● T23.6   Corrosion of second degree of wrist and hand

Code first (T51-T65) to identify chemical and intent

Use additional external cause code to identify place (Y92)

● T23.60   Corrosion of second degree of hand, unspecified site
- ● T23.601   Corrosion of second degree of right hand, unspecified site
- ● T23.602   Corrosion of second degree of left hand, unspecified site
- ● T23.609   Corrosion of second degree of unspecified hand, unspecified site

● T23.61   Corrosion of second degree of thumb (nail)
- ● T23.611   Corrosion of second degree of right thumb (nail)

● **T23.612** Corrosion of second degree of left thumb (nail)

● **T23.619** Corrosion of second degree of unspecified thumb (nail)

● **T23.62** Corrosion of second degree of single finger (nail) except thumb

● **T23.621** Corrosion of second degree of single right finger (nail) except thumb

● **T23.622** Corrosion of second degree of single left finger (nail) except thumb

● **T23.629** Corrosion of second degree of unspecified single finger (nail) except thumb

● **T23.63** Corrosion of second degree of multiple fingers (nail), not including thumb

● **T23.631** Corrosion of second degree of multiple right fingers (nail), not including thumb

● **T23.632** Corrosion of second degree of multiple left fingers (nail), not including thumb

● **T23.639** Corrosion of second degree of unspecified multiple fingers (nail), not including thumb

● **T23.64** Corrosion of second degree of multiple fingers (nail), including thumb

● **T23.641** Corrosion of second degree of multiple right fingers (nail), including thumb

● **T23.642** Corrosion of second degree of multiple left fingers (nail), including thumb

● **T23.649** Corrosion of second degree of unspecified multiple fingers (nail), including thumb

● **T23.65** Corrosion of second degree of palm

● **T23.651** Corrosion of second degree of right palm

● **T23.652** Corrosion of second degree of left palm

● **T23.659** Corrosion of second degree of unspecified palm

● **T23.66** Corrosion of second degree of back of hand

● **T23.661** Corrosion of second degree back of right hand

● **T23.662** Corrosion of second degree back of left hand

● **T23.669** Corrosion of second degree back of unspecified hand

● **T23.67** Corrosion of second degree of wrist

● **T23.671** Corrosion of second degree of right wrist

● **T23.672** Corrosion of second degree of left wrist

● **T23.679** Corrosion of second degree of unspecified wrist

● **T23.69** Corrosion of second degree of multiple sites of wrist and hand

● **T23.691** Corrosion of second degree of multiple sites of right wrist and hand

● **T23.692** Corrosion of second degree of multiple sites of left wrist and hand

● **T23.699** Corrosion of second degree of multiple sites of unspecified wrist and hand

● **T23.7** Corrosion of third degree of wrist and hand

Code first (T51-T65) *to identify chemical and intent*

Use additional external cause code to identify place (Y92)

● **T23.70** Corrosion of third degree of hand, unspecified site

● **T23.701** Corrosion of third degree of right hand, unspecified site

● **T23.702** Corrosion of third degree of left hand, unspecified site

● **T23.709** Corrosion of third degree of unspecified hand, unspecified site

● **T23.71** Corrosion of third degree of thumb (nail)

● **T23.711** Corrosion of third degree of right thumb (nail)

● **T23.712** Corrosion of third degree of left thumb (nail)

● **T23.719** Corrosion of third degree of unspecified thumb (nail)

● **T23.72** Corrosion of third degree of single finger (nail) except thumb

● **T23.721** Corrosion of third degree of single right finger (nail) except thumb

● **T23.722** Corrosion of third degree of single left finger (nail) except thumb

● **T23.729** Corrosion of third degree of unspecified single finger (nail) except thumb

● **T23.73** Corrosion of third degree of multiple fingers (nail), not including thumb

● **T23.731** Corrosion of third degree of multiple right fingers (nail), not including thumb

● **T23.732** Corrosion of third degree of multiple left fingers (nail), not including thumb

● **T23.739** Corrosion of third degree of unspecified multiple fingers (nail), not including thumb

● **T23.74** Corrosion of third degree of multiple fingers (nail), including thumb

● **T23.741** Corrosion of third degree of multiple right fingers (nail), including thumb

● **T23.742** Corrosion of third degree of multiple left fingers (nail), including thumb

● **T23.749** Corrosion of third degree of unspecified multiple fingers (nail), including thumb

● **T23.75** Corrosion of third degree of palm

● **T23.751** Corrosion of third degree of right palm

● **T23.752** Corrosion of third degree of left palm

● **T23.759** Corrosion of third degree of unspecified palm

● **T23.76** Corrosion of third degree of back of hand

● **T23.761** Corrosion of third degree of back of right hand

● **T23.762** Corrosion of third degree of back of left hand

● **T23.769** Corrosion of third degree of back of unspecified hand

● **T23.77** Corrosion of third degree of wrist

● **T23.771** Corrosion of third degree of right wrist

● **T23.772** Corrosion of third degree of left wrist

● **T23.779** Corrosion of third degree of unspecified wrist

CHAPTER 19 (S00-T88)

● **T23.79** Corrosion of third degree of multiple sites of wrist and hand
   ● **T23.791** Corrosion of third degree of multiple sites of right wrist and hand
   ● **T23.792** Corrosion of third degree of multiple sites of left wrist and hand
   ● **T23.799** Corrosion of third degree of multiple sites of unspecified wrist and hand

● **T24** Burn and corrosion of lower limb, except ankle and foot

    Excludes2   burn and corrosion of ankle and foot (T25.-)
                  burn and corrosion of hip region (T21.-)

    The appropriate 7th character is to be added to each code from category T24

> A   initial encounter
> D   subsequent encounter
> S   sequela

● **T24.0** Burn of unspecified degree of lower limb, except ankle and foot

    Use additional external cause code to identify the source, place and intent of the burn (X00-X19, X75-X77, X96-X98, Y92)

  ● **T24.00** Burn of unspecified degree of unspecified site of lower limb, except ankle and foot
    ● **T24.001** Burn of unspecified degree of unspecified site of right lower limb, except ankle and foot
    ● **T24.002** Burn of unspecified degree of unspecified site of left lower limb, except ankle and foot
    ● **T24.009** Burn of unspecified degree of unspecified site of unspecified lower limb, except ankle and foot
  ● **T24.01** Burn of unspecified degree of thigh
    ● **T24.011** Burn of unspecified degree of right thigh
    ● **T24.012** Burn of unspecified degree of left thigh
    ● **T24.019** Burn of unspecified degree of unspecified thigh
  ● **T24.02** Burn of unspecified degree of knee
    ● **T24.021** Burn of unspecified degree of right knee
    ● **T24.022** Burn of unspecified degree of left knee
    ● **T24.029** Burn of unspecified degree of unspecified knee
  ● **T24.03** Burn of unspecified degree of lower leg
    ● **T24.031** Burn of unspecified degree of right lower leg
    ● **T24.032** Burn of unspecified degree of left lower leg
    ● **T24.039** Burn of unspecified degree of unspecified lower leg
  ● **T24.09** Burn of unspecified degree of multiple sites of lower limb, except ankle and foot
    ● **T24.091** Burn of unspecified degree of multiple sites of right lower limb, except ankle and foot
    ● **T24.092** Burn of unspecified degree of multiple sites of left lower limb, except ankle and foot
    ● **T24.099** Burn of unspecified degree of multiple sites of unspecified lower limb, except ankle and foot

● **T24.1** Burn of first degree of lower limb, except ankle and foot

    Use additional external cause code to identify the source, place and intent of the burn (X00-X19, X75-X77, X96-X98, Y92)

  ● **T24.10** Burn of first degree of unspecified site of lower limb, except ankle and foot
    ● **T24.101** Burn of first degree of unspecified site of right lower limb, except ankle and foot
    ● **T24.102** Burn of first degree of unspecified site of left lower limb, except ankle and foot
    ● **T24.109** Burn of first degree of unspecified site of unspecified lower limb, except ankle and foot
  ● **T24.11** Burn of first degree of thigh
    ● **T24.111** Burn of first degree of right thigh
    ● **T24.112** Burn of first degree of left thigh
    ● **T24.119** Burn of first degree of unspecified thigh
  ● **T24.12** Burn of first degree of knee
    ● **T24.121** Burn of first degree of right knee
    ● **T24.122** Burn of first degree of left knee
    ● **T24.129** Burn of first degree of unspecified knee
  ● **T24.13** Burn of first degree of lower leg
    ● **T24.131** Burn of first degree of right lower leg
    ● **T24.132** Burn of first degree of left lower leg
    ● **T24.139** Burn of first degree of unspecified lower leg
  ● **T24.19** Burn of first degree of multiple sites of lower limb, except ankle and foot
    ● **T24.191** Burn of first degree of multiple sites of right lower limb, except ankle and foot
    ● **T24.192** Burn of first degree of multiple sites of left lower limb, except ankle and foot
    ● **T24.199** Burn of first degree of multiple sites of unspecified lower limb, except ankle and foot

● **T24.2** Burn of second degree of lower limb, except ankle and foot

    Use additional external cause code to identify the source, place and intent of the burn (X00-X19, X75-X77, X96-X98, Y92)

  ● **T24.20** Burn of second degree of unspecified site of lower limb, except ankle and foot
    ● **T24.201** Burn of second degree of unspecified site of right lower limb, except ankle and foot
    ● **T24.202** Burn of second degree of unspecified site of left lower limb, except ankle and foot
    ● **T24.209** Burn of second degree of unspecified site of unspecified lower limb, except ankle and foot
  ● **T24.21** Burn of second degree of thigh
    ● **T24.211** Burn of second degree of right thigh
    ● **T24.212** Burn of second degree of left thigh
    ● **T24.219** Burn of second degree of unspecified thigh
  ● **T24.22** Burn of second degree of knee
    ● **T24.221** Burn of second degree of right knee
    ● **T24.222** Burn of second degree of left knee
    ● **T24.229** Burn of second degree of unspecified knee

● **T24.23** Burn of second degree of lower leg
 ● **T24.231** Burn of second degree of right lower leg
 ● **T24.232** Burn of second degree of left lower leg
 ● **T24.239** Burn of second degree of unspecified lower leg
● **T24.29** Burn of second degree of multiple sites of lower limb, except ankle and foot
 ● **T24.291** Burn of second degree of multiple sites of right lower limb, except ankle and foot
 ● **T24.292** Burn of second degree of multiple sites of left lower limb, except ankle and foot
 ● **T24.299** Burn of second degree of multiple sites of unspecified lower limb, except ankle and foot
● **T24.3** Burn of third degree of lower limb, except ankle and foot

> Use additional external cause code to identify the source, place and intent of the burn (X00-X19, X75-X77, X96-X98, Y92)

 ● **T24.30** Burn of third degree of unspecified site of lower limb, except ankle and foot
 ● **T24.301** Burn of third degree of unspecified site of right lower limb, except ankle and foot
 ● **T24.302** Burn of third degree of unspecified site of left lower limb, except ankle and foot
 ● **T24.309** Burn of third degree of unspecified site of unspecified lower limb, except ankle and foot
 ● **T24.31** Burn of third degree of thigh
 ● **T24.311** Burn of third degree of right thigh
 ● **T24.312** Burn of third degree of left thigh
 ● **T24.319** Burn of third degree of unspecified thigh
 ● **T24.32** Burn of third degree of knee
 ● **T24.321** Burn of third degree of right knee
 ● **T24.322** Burn of third degree of left knee
 ● **T24.329** Burn of third degree of unspecified knee
 ● **T24.33** Burn of third degree of lower leg
 ● **T24.331** Burn of third degree of right lower leg
 ● **T24.332** Burn of third degree of left lower leg
 ● **T24.339** Burn of third degree of unspecified lower leg
 ● **T24.39** Burn of third degree of multiple sites of lower limb, except ankle and foot
 ● **T24.391** Burn of third degree of multiple sites of right lower limb, except ankle and foot
 Coding Clinic: 2016, Q2, P5
 ● **T24.392** Burn of third degree of multiple sites of left lower limb, except ankle and foot
 ● **T24.399** Burn of third degree of multiple sites of unspecified lower limb, except ankle and foot

● **T24.4** Corrosion of unspecified degree of lower limb, except ankle and foot

> Code first (T51-T65) to identify chemical and intent

> Use additional external cause code to identify place (Y92)

 ● **T24.40** Corrosion of unspecified degree of unspecified site of lower limb, except ankle and foot
 ● **T24.401** Corrosion of unspecified degree of unspecified site of right lower limb, except ankle and foot
 ● **T24.402** Corrosion of unspecified degree of unspecified site of left lower limb, except ankle and foot
 ● **T24.409** Corrosion of unspecified degree of unspecified site of unspecified lower limb, except ankle and foot
 ● **T24.41** Corrosion of unspecified degree of thigh
 ● **T24.411** Corrosion of unspecified degree of right thigh
 ● **T24.412** Corrosion of unspecified degree of left thigh
 ● **T24.419** Corrosion of unspecified degree of unspecified thigh
 ● **T24.42** Corrosion of unspecified degree of knee
 ● **T24.421** Corrosion of unspecified degree of right knee
 ● **T24.422** Corrosion of unspecified degree of left knee
 ● **T24.429** Corrosion of unspecified degree of unspecified knee
 ● **T24.43** Corrosion of unspecified degree of lower leg
 ● **T24.431** Corrosion of unspecified degree of right lower leg
 ● **T24.432** Corrosion of unspecified degree of left lower leg
 ● **T24.439** Corrosion of unspecified degree of unspecified lower leg
 ● **T24.49** Corrosion of unspecified degree of multiple sites of lower limb, except ankle and foot
 ● **T24.491** Corrosion of unspecified degree of multiple sites of right lower limb, except ankle and foot
 ● **T24.492** Corrosion of unspecified degree of multiple sites of left lower limb, except ankle and foot
 ● **T24.499** Corrosion of unspecified degree of multiple sites of unspecified lower limb, except ankle and foot
● **T24.5** Corrosion of first degree of lower limb, except ankle and foot

> Code first (T51-T65) to identify chemical and intent

> Use additional external cause code to identify place (Y92)

 ● **T24.50** Corrosion of first degree of unspecified site of lower limb, except ankle and foot
 ● **T24.501** Corrosion of first degree of unspecified site of right lower limb, except ankle and foot
 ● **T24.502** Corrosion of first degree of unspecified site of left lower limb, except ankle and foot
 ● **T24.509** Corrosion of first degree of unspecified site of unspecified lower limb, except ankle and foot

● **T24.51**   Corrosion of first degree of thigh
   ● **T24.511**   Corrosion of first degree of right thigh
   ● **T24.512**   Corrosion of first degree of left thigh
   ● **T24.519**   Corrosion of first degree of unspecified thigh
● **T24.52**   Corrosion of first degree of knee
   ● **T24.521**   Corrosion of first degree of right knee
   ● **T24.522**   Corrosion of first degree of left knee
   ● **T24.529**   Corrosion of first degree of unspecified knee
● **T24.53**   Corrosion of first degree of lower leg
   ● **T24.531**   Corrosion of first degree of right lower leg
   ● **T24.532**   Corrosion of first degree of left lower leg
   ● **T24.539**   Corrosion of first degree of unspecified lower leg
● **T24.59**   Corrosion of first degree of multiple sites of lower limb, except ankle and foot
   ● **T24.591**   Corrosion of first degree of multiple sites of right lower limb, except ankle and foot
   ● **T24.592**   Corrosion of first degree of multiple sites of left lower limb, except ankle and foot
   ● **T24.599**   Corrosion of first degree of multiple sites of unspecified lower limb, except ankle and foot
● **T24.6**   Corrosion of second degree of lower limb, except ankle and foot

> *Code first* (T51-T65) *to identify chemical and intent*
> Use additional external cause code to identify place (Y92)

   ● **T24.60**   Corrosion of second degree of unspecified site of lower limb, except ankle and foot
     ● **T24.601**   Corrosion of second degree of unspecified site of right lower limb, except ankle and foot
     ● **T24.602**   Corrosion of second degree of unspecified site of left lower limb, except ankle and foot
     ● **T24.609**   Corrosion of second degree of unspecified site of unspecified lower limb, except ankle and foot
   ● **T24.61**   Corrosion of second degree of thigh
     ● **T24.611**   Corrosion of second degree of right thigh
     ● **T24.612**   Corrosion of second degree of left thigh
     ● **T24.619**   Corrosion of second degree of unspecified thigh
   ● **T24.62**   Corrosion of second degree of knee
     ● **T24.621**   Corrosion of second degree of right knee
     ● **T24.622**   Corrosion of second degree of left knee
     ● **T24.629**   Corrosion of second degree of unspecified knee
   ● **T24.63**   Corrosion of second degree of lower leg
     ● **T24.631**   Corrosion of second degree of right lower leg
     ● **T24.632**   Corrosion of second degree of left lower leg
     ● **T24.639**   Corrosion of second degree of unspecified lower leg

   ● **T24.69**   Corrosion of second degree of multiple sites of lower limb, except ankle and foot
     ● **T24.691**   Corrosion of second degree of multiple sites of right lower limb, except ankle and foot
     ● **T24.692**   Corrosion of second degree of multiple sites of left lower limb, except ankle and foot
     ● **T24.699**   Corrosion of second degree of multiple sites of unspecified lower limb, except ankle and foot
● **T24.7**   Corrosion of third degree of lower limb, except ankle and foot

> *Code first* (T51-T65) *to identify chemical and intent*
> Use additional external cause code to identify place (Y92)

   ● **T24.70**   Corrosion of third degree of unspecified site of lower limb, except ankle and foot
     ● **T24.701**   Corrosion of third degree of unspecified site of right lower limb, except ankle and foot
     ● **T24.702**   Corrosion of third degree of unspecified site of left lower limb, except ankle and foot
     ● **T24.709**   Corrosion of third degree of unspecified site of unspecified lower limb, except ankle and foot
   ● **T24.71**   Corrosion of third degree of thigh
     ● **T24.711**   Corrosion of third degree of right thigh
     ● **T24.712**   Corrosion of third degree of left thigh
     ● **T24.719**   Corrosion of third degree of unspecified thigh
   ● **T24.72**   Corrosion of third degree of knee
     ● **T24.721**   Corrosion of third degree of right knee
     ● **T24.722**   Corrosion of third degree of left knee
     ● **T24.729**   Corrosion of third degree of unspecified knee
   ● **T24.73**   Corrosion of third degree of lower leg
     ● **T24.731**   Corrosion of third degree of right lower leg
     ● **T24.732**   Corrosion of third degree of left lower leg
     ● **T24.739**   Corrosion of third degree of unspecified lower leg
   ● **T24.79**   Corrosion of third degree of multiple sites of lower limb, except ankle and foot
     ● **T24.791**   Corrosion of third degree of multiple sites of right lower limb, except ankle and foot
     ● **T24.792**   Corrosion of third degree of multiple sites of left lower limb, except ankle and foot
     ● **T24.799**   Corrosion of third degree of multiple sites of unspecified lower limb, except ankle and foot

● **T25**   Burn and corrosion of ankle and foot

> The appropriate 7th character is to be added to each code from category T25
>
> | | |
> |---|---|
> | A | initial encounter |
> | D | subsequent encounter |
> | S | sequela |

● **T25.0**   Burn of unspecified degree of ankle and foot

> Use additional external cause code to identify the source, place and intent of the burn (X00-X19, X75-X77, X96-X98, Y92)

▶ New   ➡ Revised   ~~deleted~~ Deleted   Excludes 1   Excludes 2   Includes   Use additional   Code first   Code also   Key words
OGCR Official Guidelines   X Assign placeholder X   ● Use Additional Character(s)   ▌ Manifestation Code   HCC Hierarchical Condition Category   Coding Clinic

● **T25.01**   Burn of unspecified degree of ankle
   ● **T25.011**   Burn of unspecified degree of right ankle
   ● **T25.012**   Burn of unspecified degree of left ankle
   ● **T25.019**   Burn of unspecified degree of unspecified ankle
● **T25.02**   Burn of unspecified degree of foot
   Excludes2   burn of unspecified degree of toe(s) (nail) (T25.03-)
   ● **T25.021**   Burn of unspecified degree of right foot
   ● **T25.022**   Burn of unspecified degree of left foot
   ● **T25.029**   Burn of unspecified degree of unspecified foot
● **T25.03**   Burn of unspecified degree of toe(s) (nail)
   ● **T25.031**   Burn of unspecified degree of right toe(s) (nail)
   ● **T25.032**   Burn of unspecified degree of left toe(s) (nail)
   ● **T25.039**   Burn of unspecified degree of unspecified toe(s) (nail)
● **T25.09**   Burn of unspecified degree of multiple sites of ankle and foot
   ● **T25.091**   Burn of unspecified degree of multiple sites of right ankle and foot
   ● **T25.092**   Burn of unspecified degree of multiple sites of left ankle and foot
   ● **T25.099**   Burn of unspecified degree of multiple sites of unspecified ankle and foot

● **T25.1**   Burn of first degree of ankle and foot
   Use additional external cause code to identify the source, place and intent of the burn (X00-X19, X75-X77, X96-X98, Y92)
   ● **T25.11**   Burn of first degree of ankle
     ● **T25.111**   Burn of first degree of right ankle
     ● **T25.112**   Burn of first degree of left ankle
     ● **T25.119**   Burn of first degree of unspecified ankle
   ● **T25.12**   Burn of first degree of foot
     Excludes2   burn of first degree of toe(s) (nail) (T25.13-)
     ● **T25.121**   Burn of first degree of right foot
     ● **T25.122**   Burn of first degree of left foot
     ● **T25.129**   Burn of first degree of unspecified foot
   ● **T25.13**   Burn of first degree of toe(s) (nail)
     ● **T25.131**   Burn of first degree of right toe(s) (nail)
     ● **T25.132**   Burn of first degree of left toe(s) (nail)
     ● **T25.139**   Burn of first degree of unspecified toe(s) (nail)
   ● **T25.19**   Burn of first degree of multiple sites of ankle and foot
     ● **T25.191**   Burn of first degree of multiple sites of right ankle and foot
     ● **T25.192**   Burn of first degree of multiple sites of left ankle and foot
     ● **T25.199**   Burn of first degree of multiple sites of unspecified ankle and foot

● **T25.2**   Burn of second degree of ankle and foot
   Use additional external cause code to identify the source, place and intent of the burn (X00-X19, X75-X77, X96-X98, Y92)
   ● **T25.21**   Burn of second degree of ankle
     ● **T25.211**   Burn of second degree of right ankle
     ● **T25.212**   Burn of second degree of left ankle

     ● **T25.219**   Burn of second degree of unspecified ankle
   ● **T25.22**   Burn of second degree of foot
     Excludes2   burn of second degree of toe(s) (nail) (T25.23-)
     ● **T25.221**   Burn of second degree of right foot
     ● **T25.222**   Burn of second degree of left foot
     ● **T25.229**   Burn of second degree of unspecified foot
   ● **T25.23**   Burn of second degree of toe(s) (nail)
     ● **T25.231**   Burn of second degree of right toe(s) (nail)
     ● **T25.232**   Burn of second degree of left toe(s) (nail)
     ● **T25.239**   Burn of second degree of unspecified toe(s) (nail)
   ● **T25.29**   Burn of second degree of multiple sites of ankle and foot
     ● **T25.291**   Burn of second degree of multiple sites of right ankle and foot
     ● **T25.292**   Burn of second degree of multiple sites of left ankle and foot
     ● **T25.299**   Burn of second degree of multiple sites of unspecified ankle and foot

● **T25.3**   Burn of third degree of ankle and foot
   Use additional external cause code to identify the source, place and intent of the burn (X00-X19, X75-X77, X96-X98, Y92)
   ● **T25.31**   Burn of third degree of ankle
     ● **T25.311**   Burn of third degree of right ankle
     ● **T25.312**   Burn of third degree of left ankle
     ● **T25.319**   Burn of third degree of unspecified ankle
   ● **T25.32**   Burn of third degree of foot
     Excludes2   burn of third degree of toe(s) (nail) (T25.33-)
     ● **T25.321**   Burn of third degree of right foot
     ● **T25.322**   Burn of third degree of left foot
     ● **T25.329**   Burn of third degree of unspecified foot
   ● **T25.33**   Burn of third degree of toe(s) (nail)
     ● **T25.331**   Burn of third degree of right toe(s) (nail)
     ● **T25.332**   Burn of third degree of left toe(s) (nail)
     ● **T25.339**   Burn of third degree of unspecified toe(s) (nail)
   ● **T25.39**   Burn of third degree of multiple sites of ankle and foot
     ● **T25.391**   Burn of third degree of multiple sites of right ankle and foot
     ● **T25.392**   Burn of third degree of multiple sites of left ankle and foot
     ● **T25.399**   Burn of third degree of multiple sites of unspecified ankle and foot

● **T25.4**   Corrosion of unspecified degree of ankle and foot
   Code first (T51-T65) *to identify chemical and intent*
   Use additional external cause code to identify place (Y92)
   ● **T25.41**   Corrosion of unspecified degree of ankle
     ● **T25.411**   Corrosion of unspecified degree of right ankle
     ● **T25.412**   Corrosion of unspecified degree of left ankle
     ● **T25.419**   Corrosion of unspecified degree of unspecified ankle

CHAPTER 19 (S00-T88)

- **T25.42**   Corrosion of unspecified degree of foot
  - **Excludes2**   corrosion of unspecified degree of toe(s) (nail) (T25.43-)
  - **T25.421**   Corrosion of unspecified degree of right foot
  - **T25.422**   Corrosion of unspecified degree of left foot
  - **T25.429**   Corrosion of unspecified degree of unspecified foot
- **T25.43**   Corrosion of unspecified degree of toe(s) (nail)
  - **T25.431**   Corrosion of unspecified degree of right toe(s) (nail)
  - **T25.432**   Corrosion of unspecified degree of left toe(s) (nail)
  - **T25.439**   Corrosion of unspecified degree of unspecified toe(s) (nail)
- **T25.49**   Corrosion of unspecified degree of multiple sites of ankle and foot
  - **T25.491**   Corrosion of unspecified degree of multiple sites of right ankle and foot
  - **T25.492**   Corrosion of unspecified degree of multiple sites of left ankle and foot
  - **T25.499**   Corrosion of unspecified degree of multiple sites of unspecified ankle and foot
- **T25.5**   Corrosion of first degree of ankle and foot
  - *Code first* (T51-T65) *to identify chemical and intent*
  - Use additional external cause code to identify place (Y92)
  - **T25.51**   Corrosion of first degree of ankle
    - **T25.511**   Corrosion of first degree of right ankle
    - **T25.512**   Corrosion of first degree of left ankle
    - **T25.519**   Corrosion of first degree of unspecified ankle
  - **T25.52**   Corrosion of first degree of foot
    - **Excludes2**   corrosion of first degree of toe(s) (nail) (T25.53-)
    - **T25.521**   Corrosion of first degree of right foot
    - **T25.522**   Corrosion of first degree of left foot
    - **T25.529**   Corrosion of first degree of unspecified foot
  - **T25.53**   Corrosion of first degree of toe(s) (nail)
    - **T25.531**   Corrosion of first degree of right toe(s) (nail)
    - **T25.532**   Corrosion of first degree of left toe(s) (nail)
    - **T25.539**   Corrosion of first degree of unspecified toe(s) (nail)
  - **T25.59**   Corrosion of first degree of multiple sites of ankle and foot
    - **T25.591**   Corrosion of first degree of multiple sites of right ankle and foot
    - **T25.592**   Corrosion of first degree of multiple sites of left ankle and foot
    - **T25.599**   Corrosion of first degree of multiple sites of unspecified ankle and foot
- **T25.6**   Corrosion of second degree of ankle and foot
  - *Code first* (T51-T65) *to identify chemical and intent*
  - Use additional external cause code to identify place (Y92)
  - **T25.61**   Corrosion of second degree of ankle
    - **T25.611**   Corrosion of second degree of right ankle
    - **T25.612**   Corrosion of second degree of left ankle
    - **T25.619**   Corrosion of second degree of unspecified ankle

- **T25.62**   Corrosion of second degree of foot
  - **Excludes2**   corrosion of second degree of toe(s) (nail) (T25.63-)
  - **T25.621**   Corrosion of second degree of right foot
  - **T25.622**   Corrosion of second degree of left foot
  - **T25.629**   Corrosion of second degree of unspecified foot
- **T25.63**   Corrosion of second degree of toe(s) (nail)
  - **T25.631**   Corrosion of second degree of right toe(s) (nail)
  - **T25.632**   Corrosion of second degree of left toe(s) (nail)
  - **T25.639**   Corrosion of second degree of unspecified toe(s) (nail)
- **T25.69**   Corrosion of second degree of multiple sites of ankle and foot
  - **T25.691**   Corrosion of second degree of right ankle and foot
  - **T25.692**   Corrosion of second degree of left ankle and foot
  - **T25.699**   Corrosion of second degree of unspecified ankle and foot
- **T25.7**   Corrosion of third degree of ankle and foot
  - *Code first* (T51-T65) *to identify chemical and intent*
  - Use additional external cause code to identify place (Y92)
  - **T25.71**   Corrosion of third degree of ankle
    - **T25.711**   Corrosion of third degree of right ankle
    - **T25.712**   Corrosion of third degree of left ankle
    - **T25.719**   Corrosion of third degree of unspecified ankle
  - **T25.72**   Corrosion of third degree of foot
    - **Excludes2**   corrosion of third degree of toe(s) (nail) (T25.73-)
    - **T25.721**   Corrosion of third degree of right foot
    - **T25.722**   Corrosion of third degree of left foot
    - **T25.729**   Corrosion of third degree of unspecified foot
  - **T25.73**   Corrosion of third degree of toe(s) (nail)
    - **T25.731**   Corrosion of third degree of right toe(s) (nail)
    - **T25.732**   Corrosion of third degree of left toe(s) (nail)
    - **T25.739**   Corrosion of third degree of unspecified toe(s) (nail)
  - **T25.79**   Corrosion of third degree of multiple sites of ankle and foot
    - **T25.791**   Corrosion of third degree of multiple sites of right ankle and foot
    - **T25.792**   Corrosion of third degree of multiple sites of left ankle and foot
    - **T25.799**   Corrosion of third degree of multiple sites of unspecified ankle and foot

---

BURNS AND CORROSIONS CONFINED TO EYE AND INTERNAL ORGANS (T26-T28)

- **T26**   Burn and corrosion confined to eye and adnexa

  The appropriate 7th character is to be added to each code from category T26

A	initial encounter
D	subsequent encounter
S	sequela

  - **T26.0**   Burn of eyelid and periocular area
    - Use additional external cause code to identify the source, place and intent of the burn (X00-X19, X75-X77, X96-X98, Y92)

X● **T26.00** Burn of unspecified eyelid and periocular area
X● **T26.01** Burn of right eyelid and periocular area
X● **T26.02** Burn of left eyelid and periocular area
● **T26.1** Burn of cornea and conjunctival sac
    Use additional external cause code to identify the source, place and intent of the burn (X00-X19, X75-X77, X96-X98, Y92)
    X● **T26.10** Burn of cornea and conjunctival sac, unspecified eye
    X● **T26.11** Burn of cornea and conjunctival sac, right eye
    X● **T26.12** Burn of cornea and conjunctival sac, left eye
● **T26.2** Burn with resulting rupture and destruction of eyeball
    Use additional external cause code to identify the source, place and intent of the burn (X00-X19, X75-X77, X96-X98, Y92)
    X● **T26.20** Burn with resulting rupture and destruction of unspecified eyeball
    X● **T26.21** Burn with resulting rupture and destruction of right eyeball
    X● **T26.22** Burn with resulting rupture and destruction of left eyeball
● **T26.3** Burns of other specified parts of eye and adnexa
    Use additional external cause code to identify the source, place and intent of the burn (X00-X19, X75-X77, X96-X98, Y92)
    X● **T26.30** Burns of other specified parts of unspecified eye and adnexa
    X● **T26.31** Burns of other specified parts of right eye and adnexa
    X● **T26.32** Burns of other specified parts of left eye and adnexa
● **T26.4** Burn of eye and adnexa, part unspecified
    Use additional external cause code to identify the source, place and intent of the burn (X00-X19, X75-X77, X96-X98, Y92)
    X● **T26.40** Burn of unspecified eye and adnexa, part unspecified
    X● **T26.41** Burn of right eye and adnexa, part unspecified
    X● **T26.42** Burn of left eye and adnexa, part unspecified
● **T26.5** Corrosion of eyelid and periocular area
    Code first (T51-T65) to identify chemical and intent
    Use additional external cause code to identify place (Y92)
    X● **T26.50** Corrosion of unspecified eyelid and periocular area
    X● **T26.51** Corrosion of right eyelid and periocular area
    X● **T26.52** Corrosion of left eyelid and periocular area
● **T26.6** Corrosion of cornea and conjunctival sac
    Code first (T51-T65) to identify chemical and intent
    Use additional external cause code to identify place (Y92)
    X● **T26.60** Corrosion of cornea and conjunctival sac, unspecified eye
    X● **T26.61** Corrosion of cornea and conjunctival sac, right eye
    X● **T26.62** Corrosion of cornea and conjunctival sac, left eye
● **T26.7** Corrosion with resulting rupture and destruction of eyeball
    Code first (T51-T65) to identify chemical and intent
    Use additional external cause code to identify place (Y92)
    X● **T26.70** Corrosion with resulting rupture and destruction of unspecified eyeball
    X● **T26.71** Corrosion with resulting rupture and destruction of right eyeball
    X● **T26.72** Corrosion with resulting rupture and destruction of left eyeball

● **T26.8** Corrosions of other specified parts of eye and adnexa
    Code first (T51-T65) to identify chemical and intent
    Use additional external cause code to identify place (Y92)
    X● **T26.80** Corrosions of other specified parts of unspecified eye and adnexa
    X● **T26.81** Corrosions of other specified parts of right eye and adnexa
    X● **T26.82** Corrosions of other specified parts of left eye and adnexa
● **T26.9** Corrosion of eye and adnexa, part unspecified
    Code first (T51-T65) to identify chemical and intent
    Use additional external cause code to identify place (Y92)
    X● **T26.90** Corrosion of unspecified eye and adnexa, part unspecified
    X● **T26.91** Corrosion of right eye and adnexa, part unspecified
    X● **T26.92** Corrosion of left eye and adnexa, part unspecified
● **T27** Burn and corrosion of respiratory tract
    Use additional external cause code to identify the source and intent of the burn (X00-X19, X75-X77, X96-X98)
    Use additional external cause code to identify place (Y92)
    The appropriate 7th character is to be added to each code from category T27

> A   initial encounter
> D   subsequent encounter
> S   sequela

X● **T27.0** Burn of larynx and trachea
X● **T27.1** Burn involving larynx and trachea with lung
X● **T27.2** Burn of other parts of respiratory tract
    Burn of thoracic cavity
X● **T27.3** Burn of respiratory tract, part unspecified
X● **T27.4** Corrosion of larynx and trachea
    Code first (T51-T65) to identify chemical and intent
X● **T27.5** Corrosion involving larynx and trachea with lung
    Code first (T51-T65) to identify chemical and intent
X● **T27.6** Corrosion of other parts of respiratory tract
    Code first (T51-T65) to identify chemical and intent
X● **T27.7** Corrosion of respiratory tract, part unspecified
    Code first (T51-T65) to identify chemical and intent

● **T28** Burn and corrosion of other internal organs
    Use additional external cause code to identify the source and intent of the burn (X00-X19, X75-X77, X96-X98)
    Use additional external cause code to identify place (Y92)
    The appropriate 7th character is to be added to each code from category T28

> A   initial encounter
> D   subsequent encounter
> S   sequela

X● **T28.0** Burn of mouth and pharynx
X● **T28.1** Burn of esophagus
X● **T28.2** Burn of other parts of alimentary tract
X● **T28.3** Burn of internal genitourinary organs
X● **T28.4** Burns of other and unspecified internal organs
    X● **T28.40** Burn of unspecified internal organ
    ● **T28.41** Burn of ear drum
       ● **T28.411** Burn of right ear drum
       ● **T28.412** Burn of left ear drum
       ● **T28.419** Burn of unspecified ear drum
    X● **T28.49** Burn of other internal organ
X● **T28.5** Corrosion of mouth and pharynx
    Code first (T51-T65) to identify chemical and intent

X ● **T28.6   Corrosion of esophagus**
  Code first (T51-T65) *to identify chemical and intent*
X ● **T28.7   Corrosion of other parts of alimentary tract**
  Code first (T51-T65) *to identify chemical and intent*
X ● **T28.8   Corrosion of internal genitourinary organs**
  Code first (T51-T65) *to identify chemical and intent*
● **T28.9   Corrosions of other and unspecified internal organs**
  Code first (T51-T65) *to identify chemical and intent*
 X ● **T28.90   Corrosions of unspecified internal organs**
 ● **T28.91   Corrosions of ear drum**
  ● **T28.911   Corrosions of right ear drum**
  ● **T28.912   Corrosions of left ear drum**
  ● **T28.919   Corrosions of unspecified ear drum**
 X ● **T28.99   Corrosions of other internal organs**

OGCR Section I.C.19.d.5.
Assign separate code for each burn site
When coding burns, assign separate codes for each burn site. Category T30, Burn and corrosion, body region unspecified is extremely vague and should rarely be used.

BURNS AND CORROSIONS OF MULTIPLE AND UNSPECIFIED BODY REGIONS (T30-T32)

● **T30   Burn and corrosion, body region unspecified**
 T30.0   Burn of unspecified body region, unspecified degree
  This code is not for inpatient use. Code to specified site and degree of burns
  Burn NOS
  Multiple burns NOS
 T30.4   Corrosion of unspecified body region, unspecified degree
  This code is not for inpatient use. Code to specified site and degree of corrosion
  Corrosion NOS
  Multiple corrosion NOS

● **T31   Burns classified according to extent of body surface involved**
 Note: This category is to be used as the primary code only when the site of the burn is unspecified. It should be used as a supplementary code with categories T20-T25 when the site is specified.
 T31.0   Burns involving less than 10% of body surface
● **T31.1   Burns involving 10-19% of body surface**
 T31.10   Burns involving 10-19% of body surface with 0% to 9% third degree burns
  Burns involving 10-19% of body surface NOS
 T31.11   Burns involving 10-19% of body surface with 10-19% third degree burns 🐾

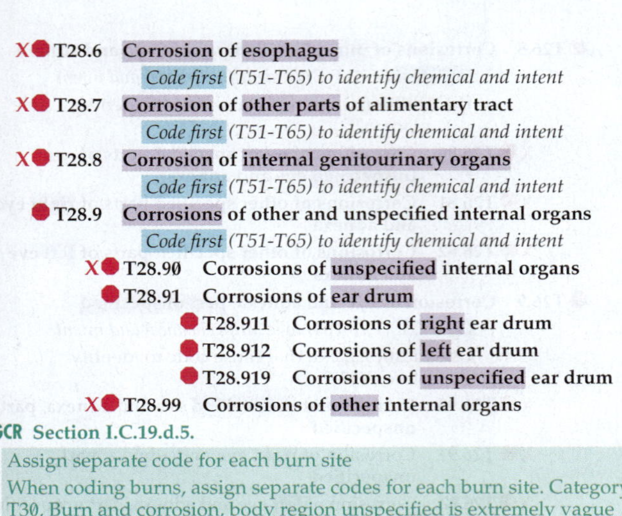

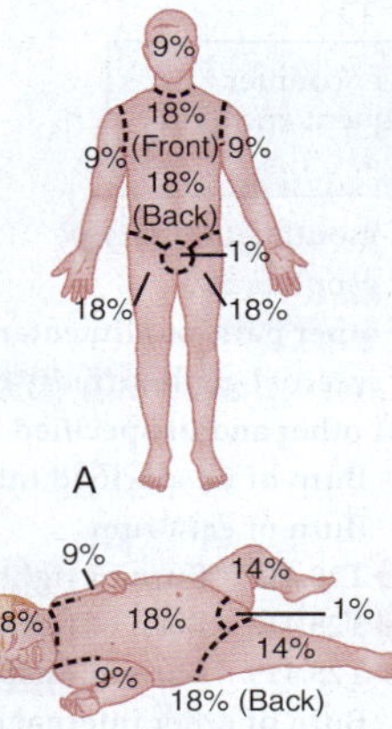

Figure 19-16   Rule of nines: percentages of total body area. (From Marx: Rosen's Emergency Medicine: Concepts and Clinical Practice, ed 6, Mosby, 2006)

● **T31.2   Burns involving 20-29% of body surface**
 T31.20   Burns involving 20-29% of body surface with 0% to 9% third degree burns
  Burns involving 20-29% of body surface NOS
 T31.21   Burns involving 20-29% of body surface with 10-19% third degree burns 🐾
 T31.22   Burns involving 20-29% of body surface with 20-29% third degree burns 🐾
● **T31.3   Burns involving 30-39% of body surface**
 T31.30   Burns involving 30-39% of body surface with 0% to 9% third degree burns
  Burns involving 30-39% of body surface NOS
 T31.31   Burns involving 30-39% of body surface with 10-19% third degree burns 🐾
 T31.32   Burns involving 30-39% of body surface with 20-29% third degree burns 🐾
 T31.33   Burns involving 30-39% of body surface with 30-39% third degree burns 🐾
● **T31.4   Burns involving 40-49% of body surface**
 T31.40   Burns involving 40-49% of body surface with 0% to 9% third degree burns
  Burns involving 40-49% of body surface NOS
 T31.41   Burns involving 40-49% of body surface with 10-19% third degree burns 🐾
 T31.42   Burns involving 40-49% of body surface with 20-29% third degree burns 🐾
 T31.43   Burns involving 40-49% of body surface with 30-39% third degree burns 🐾
 T31.44   Burns involving 40-49% of body surface with 40-49% third degree burns 🐾
● **T31.5   Burns involving 50-59% of body surface**
 T31.50   Burns involving 50-59% of body surface with 0% to 9% third degree burns
  Burns involving 50-59% of body surface NOS
 T31.51   Burns involving 50-59% of body surface with 10-19% third degree burns 🐾
 T31.52   Burns involving 50-59% of body surface with 20-29% third degree burns 🐾
 T31.53   Burns involving 50-59% of body surface with 30-39% third degree burns 🐾
 T31.54   Burns involving 50-59% of body surface with 40-49% third degree burns 🐾
 T31.55   Burns involving 50-59% of body surface with 50-59% third degree burns 🐾
● **T31.6   Burns involving 60-69% of body surface**
 T31.60   Burns involving 60-69% of body surface with 0% to 9% third degree burns
  Burns involving 60-69% of body surface NOS
 T31.61   Burns involving 60-69% of body surface with 10-19% third degree burns 🐾
 T31.62   Burns involving 60-69% of body surface with 20-29% third degree burns 🐾
 T31.63   Burns involving 60-69% of body surface with 30-39% third degree burns 🐾
 T31.64   Burns involving 60-69% of body surface with 40-49% third degree burns 🐾
 T31.65   Burns involving 60-69% of body surface with 50-59% third degree burns 🐾
 T31.66   Burns involving 60-69% of body surface with 60-69% third degree burns 🐾
● **T31.7   Burns involving 70-79% of body surface**
 T31.70   Burns involving 70-79% of body surface with 0% to 9% third degree burns
  Burns involving 70-79% of body surface NOS
 T31.71   Burns involving 70-79% of body surface with 10-19% third degree burns 🐾
 T31.72   Burns involving 70-79% of body surface with 20-29% third degree burns 🐾
 T31.73   Burns involving 70-79% of body surface with 30-39% third degree burns 🐾

T31.74 Burns involving 70-79% of body surface with 40-49% third degree burns ⚤

T31.75 Burns involving 70-79% of body surface with 50-59% third degree burns ⚤

T31.76 Burns involving 70-79% of body surface with 60-69% third degree burns ⚤

T31.77 Burns involving 70-79% of body surface with 70-79% third degree burns ⚤

● **T31.8 Burns involving 80-89% of body surface**

T31.80 Burns involving 80-89% of body surface with 0% to 9% third degree burns
Burns involving 80-89% of body surface NOS

T31.81 Burns involving 80-89% of body surface with 10-19% third degree burns ⚤

T31.82 Burns involving 80-89% of body surface with 20-29% third degree burns ⚤

T31.83 Burns involving 80-89% of body surface with 30-39% third degree burns ⚤

T31.84 Burns involving 80-89% of body surface with 40-49% third degree burns ⚤

T31.85 Burns involving 80-89% of body surface with 50-59% third degree burns ⚤

T31.86 Burns involving 80-89% of body surface with 60-69% third degree burns ⚤

T31.87 Burns involving 80-89% of body surface with 70-79% third degree burns ⚤

T31.88 Burns involving 80-89% of body surface with 80-89% third degree burns ⚤

● **T31.9 Burns involving 90% or more of body surface**

T31.90 Burns involving 90% or more of body surface with 0% to 9% third degree burns
Burns involving 90% or more of body surface NOS

T31.91 Burns involving 90% or more of body surface with 10-19% third degree burns ⚤

T31.92 Burns involving 90% or more of body surface with 20-29% third degree burns ⚤

T31.93 Burns involving 90% or more of body surface with 30-39% third degree burns ⚤

T31.94 Burns involving 90% or more of body surface with 40-49% third degree burns ⚤

T31.95 Burns involving 90% or more of body surface with 50-59% third degree burns ⚤

T31.96 Burns involving 90% or more of body surface with 60-69% third degree burns ⚤

T31.97 Burns involving 90% or more of body surface with 70-79% third degree burns ⚤

T31.98 Burns involving 90% or more of body surface with 80-89% third degree burns ⚤

T31.99 Burns involving 90% or more of body surface with 90% or more third degree burns ⚤

● **T32 Corrosions** classified according to **extent of body surface involved**

Note: This category is to be used as the primary code only when the site of the corrosion is unspecified. It may be used as a supplementary code with categories T20-T25 when the site is specified.

T32.0 Corrosions involving less than 10% of body surface

● **T32.1 Corrosions involving 10-19% of body surface**

T32.10 Corrosions involving 10-19% of body surface with 0% to 9% third degree corrosion
Corrosions involving 10-19% of body surface NOS

T32.11 Corrosions involving 10-19% of body surface with 10-19% third degree corrosion ⚤

● **T32.2 Corrosions involving 20-29% of body surface**

T32.20 Corrosions involving 20-29% of body surface with 0% to 9% third degree corrosion

T32.21 Corrosions involving 20-29% of body surface with 10-19% third degree corrosion ⚤

T32.22 Corrosions involving 20-29% of body surface with 20-29% third degree corrosion ⚤

● **T32.3 Corrosions involving 30-39% of body surface**

T32.30 Corrosions involving 30-39% of body surface with 0% to 9% third degree corrosion

T32.31 Corrosions involving 30-39% of body surface with 10-19% third degree corrosion ⚤

T32.32 Corrosions involving 30-39% of body surface with 20-29% third degree corrosion ⚤

T32.33 Corrosions involving 30-39% of body surface with 30-39% third degree corrosion ⚤

● **T32.4 Corrosions involving 40-49% of body surface**

T32.40 Corrosions involving 40-49% of body surface with 0% to 9% third degree corrosion

T32.41 Corrosions involving 40-49% of body surface with 10-19% third degree corrosion ⚤

T32.42 Corrosions involving 40-49% of body surface with 20-29% third degree corrosion ⚤

T32.43 Corrosions involving 40-49% of body surface with 30-39% third degree corrosion ⚤

T32.44 Corrosions involving 40-49% of body surface with 40-49% third degree corrosion ⚤

● **T32.5 Corrosions involving 50-59% of body surface**

T32.50 Corrosions involving 50-59% of body surface with 0% to 9% third degree corrosion

T32.51 Corrosions involving 50-59% of body surface with 10-19% third degree corrosion ⚤

T32.52 Corrosions involving 50-59% of body surface with 20-29% third degree corrosion ⚤

T32.53 Corrosions involving 50-59% of body surface with 30-39% third degree corrosion ⚤

T32.54 Corrosions involving 50-59% of body surface with 40-49% third degree corrosion ⚤

T32.55 Corrosions involving 50-59% of body surface with 50-59% third degree corrosion ⚤

● **T32.6 Corrosions involving 60-69% of body surface**

T32.60 Corrosions involving 60-69% of body surface with 0% to 9% third degree corrosion

T32.61 Corrosions involving 60-69% of body surface with 10-19% third degree corrosion ⚤

T32.62 Corrosions involving 60-69% of body surface with 20-29% third degree corrosion ⚤

T32.63 Corrosions involving 60-69% of body surface with 30-39% third degree corrosion ⚤

T32.64 Corrosions involving 60-69% of body surface with 40-49% third degree corrosion ⚤

T32.65 Corrosions involving 60-69% of body surface with 50-59% third degree corrosion ⚤

T32.66 Corrosions involving 60-69% of body surface with 60-69% third degree corrosion ⚤

● **T32.7 Corrosions involving 70-79% of body surface**

T32.70 Corrosions involving 70-79% of body surface with 0% to 9% third degree corrosion

T32.71 Corrosions involving 70-79% of body surface with 10-19% third degree corrosion ⚤

T32.72 Corrosions involving 70-79% of body surface with 20-29% third degree corrosion ⚤

T32.73 Corrosions involving 70-79% of body surface with 30-39% third degree corrosion ⚤

T32.74 Corrosions involving 70-79% of body surface with 40-49% third degree corrosion ⚤

T32.75 Corrosions involving 70-79% of body surface with 50-59% third degree corrosion ⚤

T32.76 Corrosions involving 70-79% of body surface with 60-69% third degree corrosion ⚤

T32.77 Corrosions involving 70-79% of body surface with 70-79% third degree corrosion ⚤

CHAPTER 19 (S00–T88)

● **T32.8**   **Corrosions involving 80-89% of body surface**

    T32.80   Corrosions involving 80-89% of body surface with 0% to 9% third degree corrosion

    T32.81   Corrosions involving 80-89% of body surface with 10-19% third degree corrosion ⓗⓒⓒ

    T32.82   Corrosions involving 80-89% of body surface with 20-29% third degree corrosion ⓗⓒⓒ

    T32.83   Corrosions involving 80-89% of body surface with 30-39% third degree corrosion ⓗⓒⓒ

    T32.84   Corrosions involving 80-89% of body surface with 40-49% third degree corrosion ⓗⓒⓒ

    T32.85   Corrosions involving 80-89% of body surface with 50-59% third degree corrosion ⓗⓒⓒ

    T32.86   Corrosions involving 80-89% of body surface with 60-69% third degree corrosion ⓗⓒⓒ

    T32.87   Corrosions involving 80-89% of body surface with 70-79% third degree corrosion ⓗⓒⓒ

    T32.88   Corrosions involving 80-89% of body surface with 80-89% third degree corrosion ⓗⓒⓒ

● **T32.9**   **Corrosions involving 90% or more of body surface**

    T32.90   Corrosions involving 90% or more of body surface with 0% to 9% third degree corrosion

    T32.91   Corrosions involving 90% or more of body surface with 10-19% third degree corrosion ⓗⓒⓒ

    T32.92   Corrosions involving 90% or more of body surface with 20-29% third degree corrosion ⓗⓒⓒ

    T32.93   Corrosions involving 90% or more of body surface with 30-39% third degree corrosion ⓗⓒⓒ

    T32.94   Corrosions involving 90% or more of body surface with 40-49% third degree corrosion ⓗⓒⓒ

    T32.95   Corrosions involving 90% or more of body surface with 50-59% third degree corrosion ⓗⓒⓒ

    T32.96   Corrosions involving 90% or more of body surface with 60-69% third degree corrosion ⓗⓒⓒ

    T32.97   Corrosions involving 90% or more of body surface with 70-79% third degree corrosion ⓗⓒⓒ

    T32.98   Corrosions involving 90% or more of body surface with 80-89% third degree corrosion ⓗⓒⓒ

    T32.99   Corrosions involving 90% or more of body surface with 90% or more third degree corrosion ⓗⓒⓒ

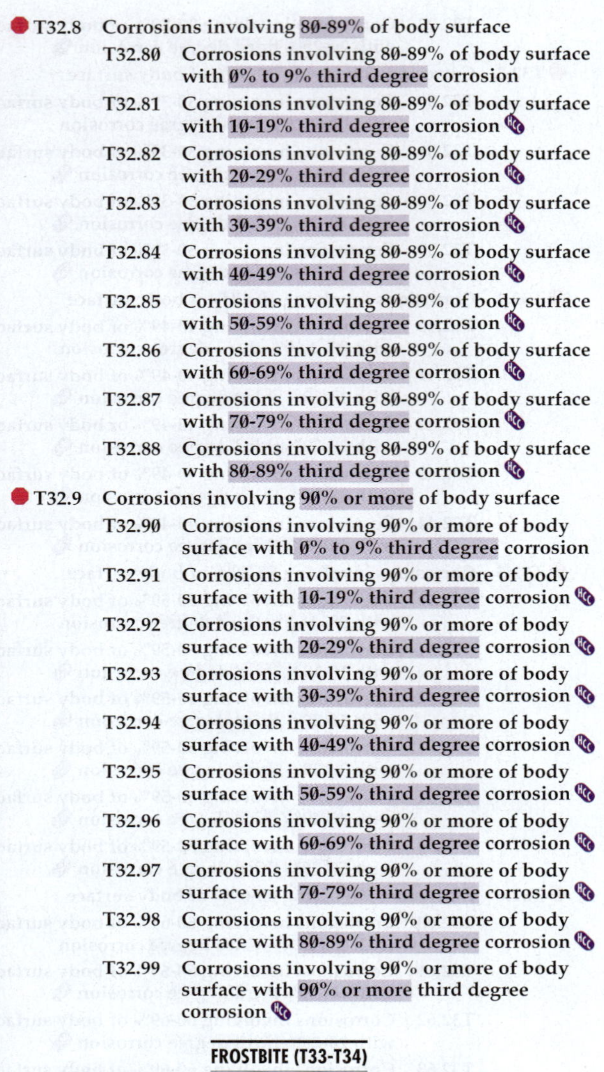

FROSTBITE (T33-T34)

Excludes2   hypothermia and other effects of reduced temperature (T68, T69.-)

● **T33**   **Superficial frostbite**

   Includes   frostbite with partial thickness skin loss

   The appropriate 7th character is to be added to each code from category T33

    A   initial encounter
    D   subsequent encounter
    S   sequela

● **T33.0**   **Superficial frostbite of head**

   ● **T33.01**   Superficial frostbite of ear

     ● **T33.011**   Superficial frostbite of right ear

     ● **T33.012**   Superficial frostbite of left ear

     ● **T33.019**   Superficial frostbite of unspecified ear

   X● **T33.02**   Superficial frostbite of nose

   X● **T33.09**   Superficial frostbite of other part of head

X● **T33.1**   **Superficial frostbite of neck**

X● **T33.2**   **Superficial frostbite of thorax**

X● **T33.3**   **Superficial frostbite of abdominal wall, lower back and pelvis**

● **T33.4**   **Superficial frostbite of arm**

   Excludes2   superficial frostbite of wrist and hand (T33.5-)

   X● **T33.40**   Superficial frostbite of unspecified arm

   X● **T33.41**   Superficial frostbite of right arm

   X● **T33.42**   Superficial frostbite of left arm

● **T33.5**   **Superficial frostbite of wrist, hand, and fingers**

   ● **T33.51**   Superficial frostbite of wrist

     ● **T33.511**   Superficial frostbite of right wrist

     ● **T33.512**   Superficial frostbite of left wrist

     ● **T33.519**   Superficial frostbite of unspecified wrist

   ● **T33.52**   Superficial frostbite of hand

     Excludes2   superficial frostbite of fingers (T33.53-)

     ● **T33.521**   Superficial frostbite of right hand

     ● **T33.522**   Superficial frostbite of left hand

     ● **T33.529**   Superficial frostbite of unspecified hand

   ● **T33.53**   Superficial frostbite of finger(s)

     ● **T33.531**   Superficial frostbite of right finger(s)

     ● **T33.532**   Superficial frostbite of left finger(s)

     ● **T33.539**   Superficial frostbite of unspecified finger(s)

● **T33.6**   **Superficial frostbite of hip and thigh**

   X● **T33.60**   Superficial frostbite of unspecified hip and thigh

   X● **T33.61**   Superficial frostbite of right hip and thigh

   X● **T33.62**   Superficial frostbite of left hip and thigh

● **T33.7**   **Superficial frostbite of knee and lower leg**

   Excludes2   superficial frostbite of ankle and foot (T33.8-)

   X● **T33.70**   Superficial frostbite of unspecified knee and lower leg

   X● **T33.71**   Superficial frostbite of right knee and lower leg

   X● **T33.72**   Superficial frostbite of left knee and lower leg

● **T33.8**   **Superficial frostbite of ankle, foot, and toe(s)**

   ● **T33.81**   Superficial frostbite of ankle

     ● **T33.811**   Superficial frostbite of right ankle

     ● **T33.812**   Superficial frostbite of left ankle

     ● **T33.819**   Superficial frostbite of unspecified ankle

   ● **T33.82**   Superficial frostbite of foot

     ● **T33.821**   Superficial frostbite of right foot

     ● **T33.822**   Superficial frostbite of left foot

     ● **T33.829**   Superficial frostbite of unspecified foot

   ● **T33.83**   Superficial frostbite of toe(s)

     ● **T33.831**   Superficial frostbite of right toe(s)

     ● **T33.832**   Superficial frostbite of left toe(s)

     ● **T33.839**   Superficial frostbite of unspecified toe(s)

● **T33.9**   **Superficial frostbite of other and unspecified sites**

   X● **T33.90**   Superficial frostbite of unspecified sites

     Superficial frostbite NOS

   X● **T33.99**   Superficial frostbite of other sites

     Superficial frostbite of leg NOS

     Superficial frostbite of trunk NOS

● **T34**   **Frostbite with tissue necrosis**

   The appropriate 7th character is to be added to each code from category T34

    A   initial encounter
    D   subsequent encounter
    S   sequela

● **T34.0** Frostbite with tissue necrosis of head
 ● **T34.01** Frostbite with tissue necrosis of ear
  ● **T34.011** Frostbite with tissue necrosis of right ear
  ● **T34.012** Frostbite with tissue necrosis of left ear
  ● **T34.019** Frostbite with tissue necrosis of unspecified ear
 X ● **T34.02** Frostbite with tissue necrosis of nose
 X ● **T34.09** Frostbite with tissue necrosis of other part of head
X ● **T34.1** Frostbite with tissue necrosis of neck
X ● **T34.2** Frostbite with tissue necrosis of thorax
X ● **T34.3** Frostbite with tissue necrosis of abdominal wall, lower back and pelvis
● **T34.4** Frostbite with tissue necrosis of arm
 Excludes2 frostbite with tissue necrosis of wrist and hand (T34.5-)
 X ● **T34.40** Frostbite with tissue necrosis of unspecified arm
 X ● **T34.41** Frostbite with tissue necrosis of right arm
 X ● **T34.42** Frostbite with tissue necrosis of left arm
● **T34.5** Frostbite with tissue necrosis of wrist, hand, and finger(s)
 ● **T34.51** Frostbite with tissue necrosis of wrist
  ● **T34.511** Frostbite with tissue necrosis of right wrist
  ● **T34.512** Frostbite with tissue necrosis of left wrist
  ● **T34.519** Frostbite with tissue necrosis of unspecified wrist
 ● **T34.52** Frostbite with tissue necrosis of hand
  Excludes2 frostbite with tissue necrosis of finger(s) (T34.53-)
  ● **T34.521** Frostbite with tissue necrosis of right hand
  ● **T34.522** Frostbite with tissue necrosis of left hand
  ● **T34.529** Frostbite with tissue necrosis of unspecified hand
 ● **T34.53** Frostbite with tissue necrosis of finger(s)
  ● **T34.531** Frostbite with tissue necrosis of right finger(s)
  ● **T34.532** Frostbite with tissue necrosis of left finger(s)
  ● **T34.539** Frostbite with tissue necrosis of unspecified finger(s)
● **T34.6** Frostbite with tissue necrosis of hip and thigh
 X ● **T34.60** Frostbite with tissue necrosis of unspecified hip and thigh
 X ● **T34.61** Frostbite with tissue necrosis of right hip and thigh
 X ● **T34.62** Frostbite with tissue necrosis of left hip and thigh
● **T34.7** Frostbite with tissue necrosis of knee and lower leg
 Excludes2 frostbite with tissue necrosis of ankle and foot (T34.8-)
 X ● **T34.70** Frostbite with tissue necrosis of unspecified knee and lower leg
 X ● **T34.71** Frostbite with tissue necrosis of right knee and lower leg
 X ● **T34.72** Frostbite with tissue necrosis of left knee and lower leg
● **T34.8** Frostbite with tissue necrosis of ankle, foot, and toe(s)
 ● **T34.81** Frostbite with tissue necrosis of ankle
  ● **T34.811** Frostbite with tissue necrosis of right ankle

● **T34.812** Frostbite with tissue necrosis of left ankle
● **T34.819** Frostbite with tissue necrosis of unspecified ankle
● **T34.82** Frostbite with tissue necrosis of foot
 ● **T34.821** Frostbite with tissue necrosis of right foot
 ● **T34.822** Frostbite with tissue necrosis of left foot
 ● **T34.829** Frostbite with tissue necrosis of unspecified foot
● **T34.83** Frostbite with tissue necrosis of toe(s)
 ● **T34.831** Frostbite with tissue necrosis of right toe(s)
 ● **T34.832** Frostbite with tissue necrosis of left toe(s)
 ● **T34.839** Frostbite with tissue necrosis of unspecified toe(s)
● **T34.9** Frostbite with tissue necrosis of other and unspecified sites
 X ● **T34.90** Frostbite with tissue necrosis of unspecified sites
  Frostbite with tissue necrosis NOS
 X ● **T34.99** Frostbite with tissue necrosis of other sites
  Frostbite with tissue necrosis of leg NOS
  Frostbite with tissue necrosis of trunk NOS

OGCR See Section I.C.19.e.

Adverse Effects, Poisoning, Underdosing and Toxic Effects

Codes in categories T36-T65 are combination codes that include the substance that was taken as well as the intent. No additional external cause code is required for poisonings, toxic effects, adverse effects and underdosing codes.

POISONING BY, ADVERSE EFFECTS OF AND UNDERDOSING OF DRUGS MEDICAMENTS AND BIOLOGICAL SUBSTANCES (T36-T50)

Includes adverse effect of correct substance properly administered
 poisoning by overdose of substance
 poisoning by wrong substance given or taken in error
 underdosing by (inadvertently) (deliberately) taking less substance than prescribed or instructed

Code first, for adverse effects, the nature of the adverse effect, such as:
 adverse effect NOS (T88.7)
 aspirin gastritis (K29.-)
 blood disorders (D56-D76)
 contact dermatitis (L23-L25)
 dermatitis due to substances taken internally (L27.-)
 nephropathy (N14.0-N14.2)

Note: The drug giving rise to the adverse effect should be identified by use of codes from categories T36-T50 with fifth or sixth character 5.

Use additional code(s) to specify:
 manifestations of poisoning
 underdosing or failure in dosage during medical and surgical care (Y63.6, Y63.8-Y63.9)
 underdosing of medication regimen (Z91.12-, Z91.13-)

Excludes1 toxic reaction to local anesthesia in pregnancy (O29.3-)

Excludes2 abuse and dependence of psychoactive substances (F10-F19)
 abuse of non-dependence-producing substances (F55.-)
 drug reaction and poisoning affecting newborn (P00-P96)
 immunodeficiency due to drugs (D84.821)
 pathological drug intoxication (inebriation) (F10-F19)

CHAPTER 19 (S00-T88)

● **T36   Poisoning by, adverse effect of and underdosing of systemic antibiotics**

> **Excludes1**   antineoplastic antibiotics (T45.1-)
> locally applied antibiotic NEC (T49.0)
> topically used antibiotic for ear, nose and throat (T49.6)
> topically used antibiotic for eye (T49.5)

> The appropriate 7th character is to be added to each code from category T36

> > A   initial encounter
> > D   subsequent encounter
> > S   sequela

● **T36.0   Poisoning by, adverse effect of and underdosing of penicillins**

  ● **T36.0X   Poisoning by, adverse effect of and underdosing of penicillins**

    ● **T36.0X1   Poisoning by penicillins, accidental (unintentional)**
       Poisoning by penicillins NOS

    ● **T36.0X2   Poisoning by penicillins, intentional self-harm A, S** ℗

    ● **T36.0X3   Poisoning by penicillins, assault**

    ● **T36.0X4   Poisoning by penicillins, undetermined**

    ● **T36.0X5   Adverse effect of penicillins**

    ● **T36.0X6   Underdosing of penicillins**

● **T36.1   Poisoning by, adverse effect of and underdosing of cephalosporins and other betalactam antibiotics**

  ● **T36.1X   Poisoning by, adverse effect of and underdosing of cephalosporins and other beta-lactam antibiotics**

    ● **T36.1X1   Poisoning by cephalosporins and other beta-lactam antibiotics, accidental (unintentional)**
       Poisoning by cephalosporins and other beta-lactam antibiotics NOS

    ● **T36.1X2   Poisoning by cephalosporins and other beta-lactam antibiotics, intentional self-harm A, S** ℗

    ● **T36.1X3   Poisoning by cephalosporins and other beta-lactam antibiotics, assault**

    ● **T36.1X4   Poisoning by cephalosporins and other beta-lactam antibiotics, undetermined**

    ● **T36.1X5   Adverse effect of cephalosporins and other beta-lactam antibiotics**

    ● **T36.1X6   Underdosing of cephalosporins and other beta-lactam antibiotics**

● **T36.2   Poisoning by, adverse effect of and underdosing of chloramphenicol group**

  ● **T36.2X   Poisoning by, adverse effect of and underdosing of chloramphenicol group**

    ● **T36.2X1   Poisoning by chloramphenicol group, accidental (unintentional)**
       Poisoning by chloramphenicol group NOS

    ● **T36.2X2   Poisoning by chloramphenicol group, intentional self-harm A, S** ℗

    ● **T36.2X3   Poisoning by chloramphenicol group, assault**

    ● **T36.2X4   Poisoning by chloramphenicol group, undetermined**

    ● **T36.2X5   Adverse effect of chloramphenicol group**

    ● **T36.2X6   Underdosing of chloramphenicol group**

● **T36.3   Poisoning by, adverse effect of and underdosing of macrolides**

  ● **T36.3X   Poisoning by, adverse effect of and underdosing of macrolides**

    ● **T36.3X1   Poisoning by macrolides, accidental (unintentional)**
       Poisoning by macrolides NOS

    ● **T36.3X2   Poisoning by macrolides, intentional self-harm A, S** ℗

    ● **T36.3X3   Poisoning by macrolides, assault**

    ● **T36.3X4   Poisoning by macrolides, undetermined**

    ● **T36.3X5   Adverse effect of macrolides**

    ● **T36.3X6   Underdosing of macrolides**

● **T36.4   Poisoning by, adverse effect of and underdosing of tetracyclines**

  ● **T36.4X   Poisoning by, adverse effect of and underdosing of tetracyclines**

    ● **T36.4X1   Poisoning by tetracyclines, accidental (unintentional)**
       Poisoning by tetracyclines NOS

    ● **T36.4X2   Poisoning by tetracyclines, intentional self-harm A, S** ℗

    ● **T36.4X3   Poisoning by tetracyclines, assault**

    ● **T36.4X4   Poisoning by tetracyclines, undetermined**

    ● **T36.4X5   Adverse effect of tetracyclines**

    ● **T36.4X6   Underdosing of tetracyclines**

● **T36.5   Poisoning by, adverse effect of and underdosing of aminoglycosides**
   Poisoning by, adverse effect of and underdosing of streptomycin

  ● **T36.5X   Poisoning by, adverse effect of and underdosing of aminoglycosides**

    ● **T36.5X1   Poisoning by aminoglycosides, accidental (unintentional)**
       Poisoning by aminoglycosides NOS

    ● **T36.5X2   Poisoning by aminoglycosides, intentional self-harm A, S** ℗

    ● **T36.5X3   Poisoning by aminoglycosides, assault**

    ● **T36.5X4   Poisoning by aminoglycosides, undetermined**

    ● **T36.5X5   Adverse effect of aminoglycosides**

    ● **T36.5X6   Underdosing of aminoglycosides**

● **T36.6   Poisoning by, adverse effect of and underdosing of rifampicins**

  ● **T36.6X   Poisoning by, adverse effect of and underdosing of rifampicins**

    ● **T36.6X1   Poisoning by rifampicins, accidental (unintentional)**
       Poisoning by rifampicins NOS

    ● **T36.6X2   Poisoning by rifampicins, intentional self-harm A, S** ℗

    ● **T36.6X3   Poisoning by rifampicins, assault**

    ● **T36.6X4   Poisoning by rifampicins, undetermined**

    ● **T36.6X5   Adverse effect of rifampicins**

    ● **T36.6X6   Underdosing of rifampicins**

● **T36.7   Poisoning by, adverse effect of and underdosing of antifungal antibiotics, systemically used**

  ● **T36.7X   Poisoning by, adverse effect of and underdosing of antifungal antibiotics, systemically used**

    ● **T36.7X1   Poisoning by antifungal antibiotics, systemically used, accidental (unintentional)**
       Poisoning by antifungal antibiotics, systemically used NOS

    ● **T36.7X2   Poisoning by antifungal antibiotics, systemically used, intentional self-harm A, S** ℗

    ● **T36.7X3   Poisoning by antifungal antibiotics, systemically used, assault**

    ● **T36.7X4   Poisoning by antifungal antibiotics, systemically used, undetermined**

● **T36.7X5**   **Adverse effect** of antifungal antibiotics, systemically used
● **T36.7X6**   **Underdosing** of antifungal antibiotics, systemically used
● **T36.8**   Poisoning by, adverse effect of and underdosing of other systemic antibiotics
    ● **T36.8X**   Poisoning by, adverse effect of and underdosing of other systemic antibiotics
      ● **T36.8X1**   Poisoning by other systemic antibiotics, **accidental (unintentional)**
        Poisoning by other systemic antibiotics NOS
      ● **T36.8X2**   Poisoning by other systemic antibiotics, **intentional self-harm A, S**
      ● **T36.8X3**   Poisoning by other systemic antibiotics, **assault**
      ● **T36.8X4**   Poisoning by other systemic antibiotics, **undetermined**
      ● **T36.8X5**   **Adverse effect** of other systemic antibiotics
        Coding Clinic: 2017, Q1, P39
      ● **T36.8X6**   **Underdosing** of other systemic antibiotics
● **T36.9**   Poisoning by, adverse effect of and underdosing of unspecified systemic antibiotic
    X ● **T36.91**   Poisoning by unspecified systemic antibiotic, **accidental (unintentional)**
      Poisoning by systemic antibiotic NOS
    X ● **T36.92**   Poisoning by unspecified systemic antibiotic, **intentional self-harm A, S**
    X ● **T36.93**   Poisoning by unspecified systemic antibiotic, **assault**
    X ● **T36.94**   Poisoning by unspecified systemic antibiotic, **undetermined**
    X ● **T36.95**   **Adverse effect** of unspecified systemic antibiotic
    X ● **T36.96**   **Underdosing** of unspecified systemic antibiotic
▶ ● **T36.A**   Poisoning by, adverse effect of and underdosing of fluoroquinolone antibiotics
    ▶ ● **T36.AX**   Poisoning by, adverse effect of and underdosing of fluoroquinolone antibiotics
      ▶ X ● **T36.AX1**   Poisoning by fluoroquinolone antibiotics, **accidental (unintentional)**
        Poisoning by fluoroquinolone antibiotics NOS
      ▶ X ● **T36.AX2**   Poisoning by fluoroquinolone antibiotics, **intentional self-harm**
      ▶ X ● **T36.AX3**   Poisoning by fluoroquinolone antibiotics, **assault**
      ▶ X ● **T36.AX4**   Poisoning by fluoroquinolone antibiotics, **undetermined**
      ▶ X ● **T36.AX5**   **Adverse effect** of fluoroquinolone antibiotics
      ▶ X ● **T36.AX6**   **Underdosing** of fluoroquinolone antibiotics

● **T37**   Poisoning by, adverse effect of and underdosing of other systemic anti-infectives and antiparasitics
    Excludes1   anti-infectives topically used for ear, nose and throat (T49.6-)
      anti-infectives topically used for eye (T49.5-)
      locally applied anti-infectives NEC (T49.0-)

The appropriate 7th character is to be added to each code from category T37

> A   initial encounter
> D   subsequent encounter
> S   sequela

● **T37.0**   Poisoning by, adverse effect of and underdosing of sulfonamides
    ● **T37.0X**   Poisoning by, adverse effect of and underdosing of sulfonamides

● **T37.0X1**   Poisoning by sulfonamides, **accidental (unintentional)**
    Poisoning by sulfonamides NOS
● **T37.0X2**   Poisoning by sulfonamides, **intentional self-harm A, S**
● **T37.0X3**   Poisoning by sulfonamides, **assault**
● **T37.0X4**   Poisoning by sulfonamides, **undetermined**
● **T37.0X5**   **Adverse effect** of sulfonamides
● **T37.0X6**   **Underdosing** of sulfonamides
● **T37.1**   Poisoning by, adverse effect of and underdosing of antimycobacterial drugs
    Excludes1   rifampicins (T36.6-) streptomycin (T36.5-)
    ● **T37.1X**   Poisoning by, adverse effect of and underdosing of antimycobacterial drugs
      ● **T37.1X1**   Poisoning by antimycobacterial drugs, **accidental (unintentional)**
        Poisoning by antimycobacterial drugs NOS
      ● **T37.1X2**   Poisoning by antimycobacterial drugs, **intentional self-harm A, S**
      ● **T37.1X3**   Poisoning by antimycobacterial drugs, **assault**
      ● **T37.1X4**   Poisoning by antimycobacterial drugs, **undetermined**
      ● **T37.1X5**   **Adverse effect** of antimycobacterial drugs
      ● **T37.1X6**   **Underdosing** of antimycobacterial drugs
● **T37.2**   Poisoning by, adverse effect of and underdosing of antimalarials and drugs acting on other blood protozoa
    Excludes1   hydroxyquinoline derivatives (T37.8-)
    ● **T37.2X**   Poisoning by, adverse effect of and underdosing of antimalarials and drugs acting on other blood protozoa
      ● **T37.2X1**   Poisoning by antimalarials and drugs acting on other blood protozoa, **accidental (unintentional)**
        Poisoning by antimalarials and drugs acting on other blood protozoa NOS
      ● **T37.2X2**   Poisoning by antimalarials and drugs acting on other blood protozoa, **intentional self-harm A, S**
      ● **T37.2X3**   Poisoning by antimalarials and drugs acting on other blood protozoa, **assault**
      ● **T37.2X4**   Poisoning by antimalarials and drugs acting on other blood protozoa, **undetermined**
      ● **T37.2X5**   **Adverse effect** of antimalarials and drugs acting on other blood protozoa
      ● **T37.2X6**   **Underdosing** of antimalarials and drugs acting on other blood protozoa
● **T37.3**   Poisoning by, adverse effect of and underdosing of other antiprotozoal drugs
    ● **T37.3X**   Poisoning by, adverse effect of and underdosing of other antiprotozoal drugs
      ● **T37.3X1**   Poisoning by other antiprotozoal drugs, **accidental (unintentional)**
        Poisoning by other antiprotozoal drugs NOS
      ● **T37.3X2**   Poisoning by other antiprotozoal drugs, **intentional self-harm A, S**
      ● **T37.3X3**   Poisoning by other antiprotozoal drugs, **assault**
      ● **T37.3X4**   Poisoning by other antiprotozoal drugs, **undetermined**
      ● **T37.3X5**   **Adverse effect** of other antiprotozoal drugs
      ● **T37.3X6**   **Underdosing** of other antiprotozoal drugs

● **T37.4** Poisoning by, adverse effect of and underdosing of anthelminthics
  ● **T37.4X** Poisoning by, adverse effect of and underdosing of anthelminthics
    ● **T37.4X1** Poisoning by anthelminthics, accidental (unintentional)
      Poisoning by anthelminthics NOS
    ● **T37.4X2** Poisoning by anthelminthics, intentional self-harm A, S
    ● **T37.4X3** Poisoning by anthelminthics, assault
    ● **T37.4X4** Poisoning by anthelminthics, undetermined
    ● **T37.4X5** Adverse effect of anthelminthics
    ● **T37.4X6** Underdosing of anthelminthics
● **T37.5** Poisoning by, adverse effect of and underdosing of antiviral drugs
  Excludes1 amantadine (T42.8-)
    cytarabine (T45.1-)
  ● **T37.5X** Poisoning by, adverse effect of and underdosing of antiviral drugs
    ● **T37.5X1** Poisoning by antiviral drugs, accidental (unintentional)
      Poisoning by antiviral drugs NOS
    ● **T37.5X2** Poisoning by antiviral drugs, intentional self-harm A, S
    ● **T37.5X3** Poisoning by antiviral drugs, assault
    ● **T37.5X4** Poisoning by antiviral drugs, undetermined
    ● **T37.5X5** Adverse effect of antiviral drugs
    ● **T37.5X6** Underdosing of antiviral drugs
● **T37.8** Poisoning by, adverse effect of and underdosing of other specified systemic anti-infectives and antiparasitics
  Poisoning by, adverse effect of and underdosing of hydroxyquinoline derivatives
  Excludes1 antimalarial drugs (T37.2-)
  ● **T37.8X** Poisoning by, adverse effect of and underdosing of other specified systemic anti-infectives and antiparasitics
    ● **T37.8X1** Poisoning by other specified systemic anti-infectives and antiparasitics, accidental (unintentional)
      Poisoning by other specified systemic anti-infectives and antiparasitics NOS
    ● **T37.8X2** Poisoning by other specified systemic anti-infectives and antiparasitics, intentional self-harm A, S
    ● **T37.8X3** Poisoning by other specified systemic anti-infectives and antiparasitics, assault
    ● **T37.8X4** Poisoning by other specified systemic anti-infectives and antiparasitics, undetermined
    ● **T37.8X5** Adverse effect of other specified systemic anti-infectives and antiparasitics
    ● **T37.8X6** Underdosing of other specified systemic anti-infectives and antiparasitics
● **T37.9** Poisoning by, adverse effect of and underdosing of unspecified systemic anti-infective and antiparasitics
  X ● **T37.91** Poisoning by unspecified systemic anti-infective and antiparasitics, accidental (unintentional)
    Poisoning by, adverse effect of and underdosing of systemic anti-infective and antiparasitics NOS
  X ● **T37.92** Poisoning by unspecified systemic anti-infective and antiparasitics, intentional self-harm A, S
  X ● **T37.93** Poisoning by unspecified systemic anti-infective and antiparasitics, assault

  X ● **T37.94** Poisoning by unspecified systemic anti-infective and antiparasitics, undetermined
  X ● **T37.95** Adverse effect of unspecified systemic anti-infective and antiparasitic
  X ● **T37.96** Underdosing of unspecified systemic anti-infectives and antiparasitics
● **T38** Poisoning by, adverse effect of and underdosing of hormones and their synthetic substitutes and antagonists, not elsewhere classified
  Excludes1 mineralocorticoids and their antagonists (T50.0-)
    oxytocic hormones (T48.0-)
    parathyroid hormones and derivatives (T50.9-)
  The appropriate 7th character is to be added to each code from category T38

  A   initial encounter
  D   subsequent encounter
  S   sequela

● **T38.0** Poisoning by, adverse effect of and underdosing of glucocorticoids and synthetic analogues
  Excludes1 glucocorticoids, topically used (T49.-)
  ● **T38.0X** Poisoning by, adverse effect of and underdosing of glucocorticoids and synthetic analogues
    ● **T38.0X1** Poisoning by glucocorticoids and synthetic analogues, accidental (unintentional)
      Poisoning by glucocorticoids and synthetic analogues NOS
    ● **T38.0X2** Poisoning by glucocorticoids and synthetic analogues, intentional self-harm A, S
    ● **T38.0X3** Poisoning by glucocorticoids and synthetic analogues, assault
    ● **T38.0X4** Poisoning by glucocorticoids and synthetic analogues, undetermined
    ● **T38.0X5** Adverse effect of glucocorticoids and synthetic analogues
    ● **T38.0X6** Underdosing of glucocorticoids and synthetic analogues
● **T38.1** Poisoning by, adverse effect of and underdosing of thyroid hormones and substitutes
  ● **T38.1X** Poisoning by, adverse effect of and underdosing of thyroid hormones and substitutes
    ● **T38.1X1** Poisoning by thyroid hormones and substitutes, accidental (unintentional)
      Poisoning by thyroid hormones and substitutes NOS
    ● **T38.1X2** Poisoning by thyroid hormones and substitutes, intentional self-harm A, S
    ● **T38.1X3** Poisoning by thyroid hormones and substitutes, assault
    ● **T38.1X4** Poisoning by thyroid hormones and substitutes, undetermined
    ● **T38.1X5** Adverse effect of thyroid hormones and substitutes
    ● **T38.1X6** Underdosing of thyroid hormones and substitutes
● **T38.2** Poisoning by, adverse effect of and underdosing of antithyroid drugs
  ● **T38.2X** Poisoning by, adverse effect of and underdosing of antithyroid drugs
    ● **T38.2X1** Poisoning by antithyroid drugs, accidental (unintentional)
      Poisoning by antithyroid drugs NOS
    ● **T38.2X2** Poisoning by antithyroid drugs, intentional self-harm A, S
    ● **T38.2X3** Poisoning by antithyroid drugs, assault

● T38.2X4   **Poisoning by antithyroid drugs, undetermined**
● T38.2X5   **Adverse effect of antithyroid drugs**
● T38.2X6   **Underdosing of antithyroid drugs**
● **T38.3   Poisoning by, adverse effect of and underdosing of insulin and oral hypoglycemic [antidiabetic] drugs**
● **T38.3X   Poisoning by, adverse effect of and underdosing of insulin and oral hypoglycemic [antidiabetic] drugs**
● T38.3X1   **Poisoning by insulin and oral hypoglycemic [antidiabetic] drugs, accidental (unintentional)**
Poisoning by insulin and oral hypoglycemic [antidiabetic] drugs NOS
● T38.3X2   **Poisoning by insulin and oral hypoglycemic [antidiabetic] drugs, intentional self-harm**
● T38.3X3   **Poisoning by insulin and oral hypoglycemic [antidiabetic] drugs, assault A, S** 🔖
● T38.3X4   **Poisoning by insulin and oral hypoglycemic [antidiabetic] drugs, undetermined**
● T38.3X5   **Adverse effect of insulin and oral hypoglycemic [antidiabetic] drugs**
● T38.3X6   **Underdosing of insulin and oral hypoglycemic [antidiabetic] drugs**
● **T38.4   Poisoning by, adverse effect of and underdosing of oral contraceptives**
Poisoning by, adverse effect of and underdosing of multiple- and single-ingredient oral contraceptive preparations
● **T38.4X   Poisoning by, adverse effect of and underdosing of oral contraceptives**
● T38.4X1   **Poisoning by oral contraceptives, accidental (unintentional)**
Poisoning by oral contraceptives NOS
● T38.4X2   **Poisoning by oral contraceptives, intentional self-harm A, S** 🔖
● T38.4X3   **Poisoning by oral contraceptives, assault**
● T38.4X4   **Poisoning by oral contraceptives, undetermined**
● T38.4X5   **Adverse effect of oral contraceptives**
● T38.4X6   **Underdosing of oral contraceptives**
● **T38.5   Poisoning by, adverse effect of and underdosing of other estrogens and progestogens**
Poisoning by, adverse effect of and underdosing of estrogens and progestogens mixtures and substitutes
● **T38.5X   Poisoning by, adverse effect of and underdosing of other estrogens and progestogens**
● T38.5X1   **Poisoning by other estrogens and progestogens, accidental (unintentional)**
Poisoning by other estrogens and progestogens NOS
● T38.5X2   **Poisoning by other estrogens and progestogens, intentional self-harm A, S** 🔖
● T38.5X3   **Poisoning by other estrogens and progestogens, assault**
● T38.5X4   **Poisoning by other estrogens and progestogens, undetermined**
● T38.5X5   **Adverse effect of other estrogens and progestogens**
● T38.5X6   **Underdosing of other estrogens and progestogens**

● **T38.6   Poisoning by, adverse effect of and underdosing of antigonadotrophins, antiestrogens, antiandrogens, not elsewhere classified**
Poisoning by, adverse effect of and underdosing of tamoxifen
● **T38.6X   Poisoning by, adverse effect of and underdosing of antigonadotrophins, antiestrogens, antiandrogens, not elsewhere classified**
● T38.6X1   **Poisoning by antigonadotrophins, antiestrogens, antiandrogens, not elsewhere classified, accidental (unintentional)**
Poisoning by antigonadotrophins, antiestrogens, antiandrogens, not elsewhere classified NOS
● T38.6X2   **Poisoning by antigonadotrophins, antiestrogens, antiandrogens, not elsewhere classified, intentional self-harm A, S** 🔖
● T38.6X3   **Poisoning by antigonadotrophins, antiestrogens, antiandrogens, not elsewhere classified, assault**
● T38.6X4   **Poisoning by antigonadotrophins, antiestrogens, antiandrogens, not elsewhere classified, undetermined**
● T38.6X5   **Adverse effect of antigonadotrophins, antiestrogens, antiandrogens, not elsewhere classified**
● T38.6X6   **Underdosing of antigonadotrophins, antiestrogens, antiandrogens, not elsewhere classified**
● **T38.7   Poisoning by, adverse effect of and underdosing of androgens and anabolic congeners**
● **T38.7X   Poisoning by, adverse effect of and underdosing of androgens and anabolic congeners**
● T38.7X1   **Poisoning by androgens and anabolic congeners, accidental (unintentional)**
Poisoning by androgens and anabolic congeners NOS
● T38.7X2   **Poisoning by androgens and anabolic congeners, intentional self-harm A, S** 🔖
● T38.7X3   **Poisoning by androgens and anabolic congeners, assault**
● T38.7X4   **Poisoning by androgens and anabolic congeners, undetermined**
● T38.7X5   **Adverse effect of androgens and anabolic congeners**
● T38.7X6   **Underdosing of androgens and anabolic congeners**
● **T38.8   Poisoning by, adverse effect of and underdosing of other and unspecified hormones and synthetic substitutes**
● **T38.80   Poisoning by, adverse effect of and underdosing of unspecified hormones and synthetic substitutes**
● T38.801   **Poisoning by unspecified hormones and synthetic substitutes, accidental (unintentional)**
Poisoning by unspecified hormones and synthetic substitutes NOS
● T38.802   **Poisoning by unspecified hormones and synthetic substitutes, intentional self-harm A, S** 🔖
● T38.803   **Poisoning by unspecified hormones and synthetic substitutes, assault**
● T38.804   **Poisoning by unspecified hormones and synthetic substitutes, undetermined**
● T38.805   **Adverse effect of unspecified hormones and synthetic substitutes**
● T38.806   **Underdosing of unspecified hormones and synthetic substitutes**

CHAPTER 19 (S00-T88)

CHAPTER 19 (S00–T88)

● **T38.81** Poisoning by, adverse effect of and underdosing of anterior pituitary [adenohypophyseal] hormones

  ● **T38.811** Poisoning by anterior pituitary [adenohypophyseal] hormones, accidental (unintentional)
    Poisoning by anterior pituitary [adenohypophyseal] hormones NOS

  ● **T38.812** Poisoning by anterior pituitary [adenohypophyseal] hormones, intentional self-harm **A, S** 🅗🅒🅒

  ● **T38.813** Poisoning by anterior pituitary [adenohypophyseal] hormones, assault

  ● **T38.814** Poisoning by anterior pituitary [adenohypophyseal] hormones, undetermined

  ● **T38.815** Adverse effect of anterior pituitary [adenohypophyseal] hormones

  ● **T38.816** Underdosing of anterior pituitary [adenohypophyseal] hormones

● **T38.89** Poisoning by, adverse effect of and underdosing of other hormones and synthetic substitutes

  ● **T38.891** Poisoning by other hormones and synthetic substitutes, accidental (unintentional)
    Poisoning by other hormones and synthetic substitutes NOS

  ● **T38.892** Poisoning by other hormones and synthetic substitutes, intentional self-harm **A, S** 🅗🅒🅒

  ● **T38.893** Poisoning by other hormones and synthetic substitutes, assault

  ● **T38.894** Poisoning by other hormones and synthetic substitutes, undetermined

  ● **T38.895** Adverse effect of other hormones and synthetic substitutes

  ● **T38.896** Underdosing of other hormones and synthetic substitutes

● **T38.9** Poisoning by, adverse effect of and underdosing of other and unspecified hormone antagonists

● **T38.90** Poisoning by, adverse effect of and underdosing of unspecified hormone antagonists

  ● **T38.901** Poisoning by unspecified hormone antagonists, accidental (unintentional)
    Poisoning by unspecified hormone antagonists NOS

  ● **T38.902** Poisoning by unspecified hormone antagonists, intentional self-harm **A, S** 🅗🅒🅒

  ● **T38.903** Poisoning by unspecified hormone antagonists, assault

  ● **T38.904** Poisoning by unspecified hormone antagonists, undetermined

  ● **T38.905** Adverse effect of unspecified hormone antagonists

  ● **T38.906** Underdosing of unspecified hormone antagonists

● **T38.99** Poisoning by, adverse effect of and underdosing of other hormone antagonists

  ● **T38.991** Poisoning by other hormone antagonists, accidental (unintentional)
    Poisoning by other hormone antagonists NOS

  ● **T38.992** Poisoning by other hormone antagonists, intentional self-harm **A, S** 🅗🅒🅒

  ● **T38.993** Poisoning by other hormone antagonists, assault

● **T38.994** Poisoning by other hormone antagonists, undetermined

● **T38.995** Adverse effect of other hormone antagonists

● **T38.996** Underdosing of other hormone antagonists

● **T39** Poisoning by, adverse effect of and underdosing of nonopioid analgesics, antipyretics and antirheumatics

The appropriate 7th character is to be added to each code from category T39

  A   initial encounter
  D   subsequent encounter
  S   sequela

● **T39.0** Poisoning by, adverse effect of and underdosing of salicylates

● **T39.01** Poisoning by, adverse effect of and underdosing of aspirin
  Poisoning by, adverse effect of and underdosing of acetylsalicylic acid

  ● **T39.011** Poisoning by aspirin, accidental (unintentional)

  ● **T39.012** Poisoning by aspirin, intentional self-harm **A, S** 🅗🅒🅒

  ● **T39.013** Poisoning by aspirin, assault

  ● **T39.014** Poisoning by aspirin, undetermined

  ● **T39.015** Adverse effect of aspirin
    Coding Clinic: 2016, Q1, P15

  ● **T39.016** Underdosing of aspirin

● **T39.09** Poisoning by, adverse effect of and underdosing of other salicylates

  ● **T39.091** Poisoning by salicylates, accidental (unintentional)
    Poisoning by salicylates NOS

  ● **T39.092** Poisoning by salicylates, intentional self-harm **A, S** 🅗🅒🅒

  ● **T39.093** Poisoning by salicylates, assault

  ● **T39.094** Poisoning by salicylates, undetermined

  ● **T39.095** Adverse effect of salicylates

  ● **T39.096** Underdosing of salicylates

● **T39.1** Poisoning by, adverse effect of and underdosing of 4-Aminophenol derivatives

● **T39.1X** Poisoning by, adverse effect of and underdosing of 4-Aminophenol derivatives

  ● **T39.1X1** Poisoning by 4-Aminophenol derivatives, accidental (unintentional)
    Poisoning by 4-Aminophenol derivatives NOS

  ● **T39.1X2** Poisoning by 4-Aminophenol derivatives, intentional self-harm **A, S** 🅗🅒🅒

  ● **T39.1X3** Poisoning by 4-Aminophenol derivatives, assault

  ● **T39.1X4** Poisoning by 4-Aminophenol derivatives, undetermined

  ● **T39.1X5** Adverse effect of 4-Aminophenol derivatives

  ● **T39.1X6** Underdosing of 4-Aminophenol derivatives

● **T39.2** Poisoning by, adverse effect of and underdosing of pyrazolone derivatives

● **T39.2X** Poisoning by, adverse effect of and underdosing of pyrazolone derivatives

  ● **T39.2X1** Poisoning by pyrazolone derivatives, accidental (unintentional)
    Poisoning by pyrazolone derivatives NOS

  ● **T39.2X2** Poisoning by pyrazolone derivatives, intentional self-harm **A, S** 🅗🅒🅒

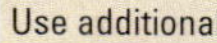

▶ New   ⇒ Revised   ~~deleted~~ Deleted   Excludes 1   Excludes 2   Includes   Use additional   Code first   Code also   Key words

OGCR Official Guidelines   **X** Assign placeholder X   ● Use Additional Character(s)   ▶ Manifestation Code   🅗🅒🅒 Hierarchical Condition Category   **Coding Clinic**

- ● **T39.2X3** Poisoning by pyrazolone derivatives, **assault**
- ● **T39.2X4** Poisoning by pyrazolone derivatives, **undetermined**
- ● **T39.2X5** **Adverse effect** of pyrazolone derivatives
- ● **T39.2X6** **Underdosing** of pyrazolone derivatives
- ● **T39.3** Poisoning by, adverse effect of and underdosing of other nonsteroidal anti-inflammatory drugs [NSAID]
  - ● **T39.31** Poisoning by, adverse effect of and underdosing of propionic acid derivatives
    Poisoning by, adverse effect of and underdosing of fenoprofen
    Poisoning by, adverse effect of and underdosing of flurbiprofen
    Poisoning by, adverse effect of and underdosing of ibuprofen
    Poisoning by, adverse effect of and underdosing of ketoprofen
    Poisoning by, adverse effect of and underdosing of naproxen
    Poisoning by, adverse effect of and underdosing of oxaprozin
    - ● **T39.311** Poisoning by propionic acid derivatives, **accidental (unintentional)**
    - ● **T39.312** Poisoning by propionic acid derivatives, **intentional self-harm** A, S ®
    - ● **T39.313** Poisoning by propionic acid derivatives, **assault**
    - ● **T39.314** Poisoning by propionic acid derivatives, **undetermined**
    - ● **T39.315** **Adverse effect** of propionic acid derivatives
    - ● **T39.316** **Underdosing** of propionic acid derivatives
  - ● **T39.39** Poisoning by, adverse effect of and underdosing of other nonsteroidal anti-inflammatory drugs [NSAID]
    - ● **T39.391** Poisoning by other nonsteroidal anti-inflammatory drugs [NSAID], **accidental (unintentional)**
      Poisoning by other nonsteroidal anti-inflammatory drugs NOS
    - ● **T39.392** Poisoning by other nonsteroidal anti-inflammatory drugs [NSAID], **intentional self-harm** A, S ®
    - ● **T39.393** Poisoning by other nonsteroidal anti-inflammatory drugs [NSAID], **assault**
    - ● **T39.394** Poisoning by other nonsteroidal anti-inflammatory drugs [NSAID], **undetermined**
    - ● **T39.395** **Adverse effect** of other nonsteroidal anti-inflammatory drugs [NSAID]
    - ● **T39.396** **Underdosing** of other nonsteroidal anti-inflammatory drugs [NSAID]
- ● **T39.4** Poisoning by, adverse effect of and underdosing of antirheumatics, not elsewhere classified

  Excludes1 poisoning by, adverse effect of and underdosing of glucocorticoids (T38.0-)
  poisoning by, adverse effect of and underdosing of salicylates (T39.0-)

  - ● **T39.4X** Poisoning by, adverse effect of and underdosing of antirheumatics, not elsewhere classified
    - ● **T39.4X1** Poisoning by antirheumatics, not elsewhere classified, **accidental (unintentional)**
      Poisoning by antirheumatics, not elsewhere classified NOS

- ● **T39.4X2** Poisoning by antirheumatics, not elsewhere classified, **intentional self-harm** A, S ®
- ● **T39.4X3** Poisoning by antirheumatics, not elsewhere classified, **assault**
- ● **T39.4X4** Poisoning by antirheumatics, not elsewhere classified, **undetermined**
- ● **T39.4X5** **Adverse effect** of antirheumatics, not elsewhere classified
- ● **T39.4X6** **Underdosing** of antirheumatics, not elsewhere classified
- ● **T39.8** Poisoning by, adverse effect of and underdosing of other nonopioid analgesics and antipyretics, not elsewhere classified
  - ● **T39.8X** Poisoning by, adverse effect of and underdosing of other nonopioid analgesics and antipyretics, not elsewhere classified
    - ● **T39.8X1** Poisoning by other nonopioid analgesics and antipyretics, not elsewhere classified, **accidental (unintentional)**
      Poisoning by other nonopioid analgesics and antipyretics, not elsewhere classified NOS
    - ● **T39.8X2** Poisoning by other nonopioid analgesics and antipyretics, not elsewhere classified, **intentional self-harm** A, S ®
    - ● **T39.8X3** Poisoning by other nonopioid analgesics and antipyretics, not elsewhere classified, **assault**
    - ● **T39.8X4** Poisoning by other nonopioid analgesics and antipyretics, not elsewhere classified, **undetermined**
    - ● **T39.8X5** **Adverse effect** of other nonopioid analgesics and antipyretics, not elsewhere classified
    - ● **T39.8X6** **Underdosing** of other nonopioid analgesics and antipyretics, not elsewhere classified
- ● **T39.9** Poisoning by, adverse effect of and underdosing of unspecified nonopioid analgesic, antipyretic and antirheumatic
  - X ● **T39.91** Poisoning by unspecified nonopioid analgesic, antipyretic and antirheumatic, **accidental (unintentional)**
    Poisoning by nonopioid analgesic, antipyretic and antirheumatic NOS
  - X ● **T39.92** Poisoning by unspecified nonopioid analgesic, antipyretic and antirheumatic, **intentional self-harm** A, S ®
  - X ● **T39.93** Poisoning by unspecified nonopioid analgesic, antipyretic and antirheumatic, **assault**
  - X ● **T39.94** Poisoning by unspecified nonopioid analgesic, antipyretic and antirheumatic, **undetermined**
  - X ● **T39.95** **Adverse effect** of unspecified nonopioid analgesic, antipyretic and antirheumatic
  - X ● **T39.96** **Underdosing** of unspecified nonopioid analgesic, antipyretic and antirheumatic
- ● **T40** Poisoning by, adverse effect of and underdosing of narcotics and psychodysleptics [hallucinogens]

  Excludes2 drug dependence and related mental and behavioral disorders due to psychoactive substance use (F10.-F19.-)

  The appropriate 7th character is to be added to each code from category T40

A	initial encounter
D	subsequent encounter
S	sequela

  - ● **T40.0** Poisoning by, adverse effect of and underdosing of opium

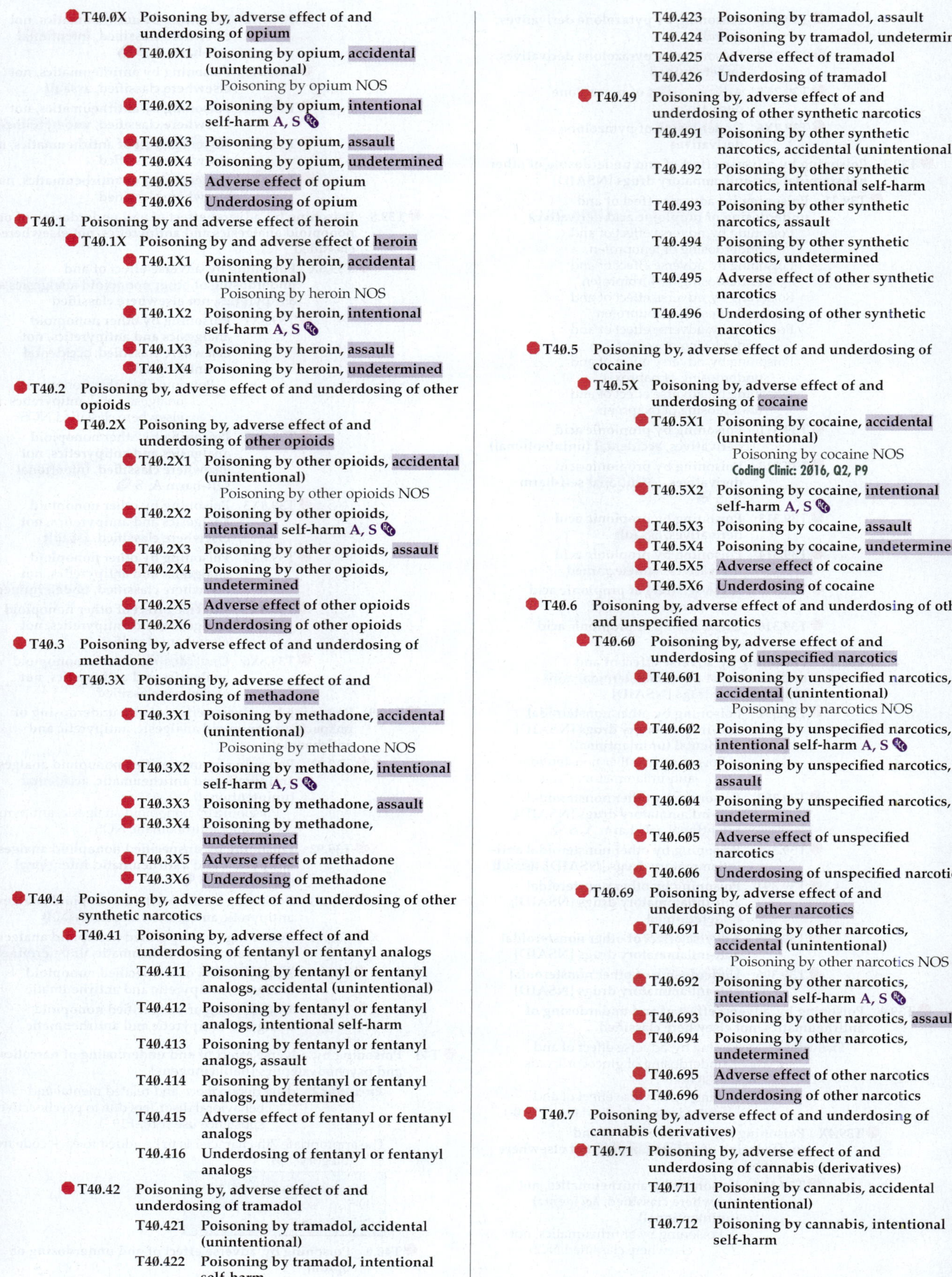

CHAPTER 19 (S00-T88)

● **T40.0X**   Poisoning by, adverse effect of and underdosing of opium
- ● **T40.0X1**   Poisoning by opium, accidental (unintentional)
  - Poisoning by opium NOS
- ● **T40.0X2**   Poisoning by opium, intentional self-harm A, S
- ● **T40.0X3**   Poisoning by opium, assault
- ● **T40.0X4**   Poisoning by opium, undetermined
- ● **T40.0X5**   Adverse effect of opium
- ● **T40.0X6**   Underdosing of opium

● **T40.1**   Poisoning by and adverse effect of heroin
- ● **T40.1X**   Poisoning by and adverse effect of heroin
  - ● **T40.1X1**   Poisoning by heroin, accidental (unintentional)
    - Poisoning by heroin NOS
  - ● **T40.1X2**   Poisoning by heroin, intentional self-harm A, S
  - ● **T40.1X3**   Poisoning by heroin, assault
  - ● **T40.1X4**   Poisoning by heroin, undetermined

● **T40.2**   Poisoning by, adverse effect of and underdosing of other opioids
- ● **T40.2X**   Poisoning by, adverse effect of and underdosing of other opioids
  - ● **T40.2X1**   Poisoning by other opioids, accidental (unintentional)
    - Poisoning by other opioids NOS
  - ● **T40.2X2**   Poisoning by other opioids, intentional self-harm A, S
  - ● **T40.2X3**   Poisoning by other opioids, assault
  - ● **T40.2X4**   Poisoning by other opioids, undetermined
  - ● **T40.2X5**   Adverse effect of other opioids
  - ● **T40.2X6**   Underdosing of other opioids

● **T40.3**   Poisoning by, adverse effect of and underdosing of methadone
- ● **T40.3X**   Poisoning by, adverse effect of and underdosing of methadone
  - ● **T40.3X1**   Poisoning by methadone, accidental (unintentional)
    - Poisoning by methadone NOS
  - ● **T40.3X2**   Poisoning by methadone, intentional self-harm A, S
  - ● **T40.3X3**   Poisoning by methadone, assault
  - ● **T40.3X4**   Poisoning by methadone, undetermined
  - ● **T40.3X5**   Adverse effect of methadone
  - ● **T40.3X6**   Underdosing of methadone

● **T40.4**   Poisoning by, adverse effect of and underdosing of other synthetic narcotics
- ● **T40.41**   Poisoning by, adverse effect of and underdosing of fentanyl or fentanyl analogs
  - **T40.411**   Poisoning by fentanyl or fentanyl analogs, accidental (unintentional)
  - **T40.412**   Poisoning by fentanyl or fentanyl analogs, intentional self-harm
  - **T40.413**   Poisoning by fentanyl or fentanyl analogs, assault
  - **T40.414**   Poisoning by fentanyl or fentanyl analogs, undetermined
  - **T40.415**   Adverse effect of fentanyl or fentanyl analogs
  - **T40.416**   Underdosing of fentanyl or fentanyl analogs
- ● **T40.42**   Poisoning by, adverse effect of and underdosing of tramadol
  - **T40.421**   Poisoning by tramadol, accidental (unintentional)
  - **T40.422**   Poisoning by tramadol, intentional self-harm

T40.423   Poisoning by tramadol, assault
T40.424   Poisoning by tramadol, undetermined
T40.425   Adverse effect of tramadol
T40.426   Underdosing of tramadol

● **T40.49**   Poisoning by, adverse effect of and underdosing of other synthetic narcotics
- **T40.491**   Poisoning by other synthetic narcotics, accidental (unintentional)
- **T40.492**   Poisoning by other synthetic narcotics, intentional self-harm
- **T40.493**   Poisoning by other synthetic narcotics, assault
- **T40.494**   Poisoning by other synthetic narcotics, undetermined
- **T40.495**   Adverse effect of other synthetic narcotics
- **T40.496**   Underdosing of other synthetic narcotics

● **T40.5**   Poisoning by, adverse effect of and underdosing of cocaine
- ● **T40.5X**   Poisoning by, adverse effect of and underdosing of cocaine
  - ● **T40.5X1**   Poisoning by cocaine, accidental (unintentional)
    - Poisoning by cocaine NOS
    - **Coding Clinic: 2016, Q2, P9**
  - ● **T40.5X2**   Poisoning by cocaine, intentional self-harm A, S
  - ● **T40.5X3**   Poisoning by cocaine, assault
  - ● **T40.5X4**   Poisoning by cocaine, undetermined
  - ● **T40.5X5**   Adverse effect of cocaine
  - ● **T40.5X6**   Underdosing of cocaine

● **T40.6**   Poisoning by, adverse effect of and underdosing of other and unspecified narcotics
- ● **T40.60**   Poisoning by, adverse effect of and underdosing of unspecified narcotics
  - ● **T40.601**   Poisoning by unspecified narcotics, accidental (unintentional)
    - Poisoning by narcotics NOS
  - ● **T40.602**   Poisoning by unspecified narcotics, intentional self-harm A, S
  - ● **T40.603**   Poisoning by unspecified narcotics, assault
  - ● **T40.604**   Poisoning by unspecified narcotics, undetermined
  - ● **T40.605**   Adverse effect of unspecified narcotics
  - ● **T40.606**   Underdosing of unspecified narcotics
- ● **T40.69**   Poisoning by, adverse effect of and underdosing of other narcotics
  - ● **T40.691**   Poisoning by other narcotics, accidental (unintentional)
    - Poisoning by other narcotics NOS
  - ● **T40.692**   Poisoning by other narcotics, intentional self-harm A, S
  - ● **T40.693**   Poisoning by other narcotics, assault
  - ● **T40.694**   Poisoning by other narcotics, undetermined
  - ● **T40.695**   Adverse effect of other narcotics
  - ● **T40.696**   Underdosing of other narcotics

● **T40.7**   Poisoning by, adverse effect of and underdosing of cannabis (derivatives)
- ● **T40.71**   Poisoning by, adverse effect of and underdosing of cannabis (derivatives)
  - **T40.711**   Poisoning by cannabis, accidental (unintentional)
  - **T40.712**   Poisoning by cannabis, intentional self-harm

► New   ➡ Revised   ~~deleted~~ Deleted   Excludes 1   Excludes 2   Includes   Use additional   Code first   Code also   Key words

OGCR Official Guidelines   X Assign placeholder X   ● Use Additional Character(s)   ◗ Manifestation Code   Hierarchical Condition Category   **Coding Clinic**

● T40.713   Poisoning by cannabis, assault

T40.714   Poisoning by cannabis, undetermined

T40.715   Adverse effect of cannabis

T40.716   Underdosing of cannabis

● T40.72   Poisoning by, adverse effect of and underdosing of synthetic cannabinoids

T40.721   Poisoning by synthetic cannabinoids, accidental (unintentional)

T40.722   Poisoning by synthetic cannabinoids, intentional self-harm

T40.723   Poisoning by synthetic cannabinoids, assault

T40.724   Poisoning by synthetic cannabinoids, undetermined

T40.725   Adverse effect of synthetic cannabinoids

T40.726   Underdosing of synthetic cannabinoids

● T40.8   Poisoning by and adverse effect of lysergide [LSD]

● T40.8X   Poisoning by and adverse effect of lysergide [LSD]

● T40.8X1   Poisoning by lysergide [LSD], accidental (unintentional)
Poisoning by lysergide [LSD] NOS

● T40.8X2   Poisoning by lysergide [LSD], intentional self-harm A, S 🔗

● T40.8X3   Poisoning by lysergide [LSD], assault

● T40.8X4   Poisoning by lysergide [LSD], undetermined

● T40.9   Poisoning by, adverse effect of and underdosing of other and unspecified psychodysleptics [hallucinogens]

● T40.90   Poisoning by, adverse effect of and underdosing of unspecified psychodysleptics [hallucinogens]

● T40.901   Poisoning by unspecified psychodysleptics [hallucinogens], accidental (unintentional)

● T40.902   Poisoning by unspecified psychodysleptics [hallucinogens], intentional self-harm A, S 🔗

● T40.903   Poisoning by unspecified psychodysleptics [hallucinogens], assault

● T40.904   Poisoning by unspecified psychodysleptics [hallucinogens], undetermined

● T40.905   Adverse effect of unspecified psychodysleptics [hallucinogens]

● T40.906   Underdosing of unspecified psychodysleptics [hallucinogens]

● T40.99   Poisoning by, adverse effect of and underdosing of other psychodysleptics [hallucinogens]

● T40.991   Poisoning by other psychodysleptics [hallucinogens], accidental (unintentional)
Poisoning by other psychodysleptics [hallucinogens] NOS

● T40.992   Poisoning by other psychodysleptics [hallucinogens], intentional self-harm A, S 🔗

● T40.993   Poisoning by other psychodysleptics [hallucinogens], assault

● T40.994   Poisoning by other psychodysleptics [hallucinogens], undetermined

● T40.995   Adverse effect of other psychodysleptics [hallucinogens]

● T40.996   Underdosing of other psychodysleptics [hallucinogens]

● T41   Poisoning by, adverse effect of and underdosing of anesthetics and therapeutic gases

Excludes1   benzodiazepines (T42.4-)
cocaine (T40.5-)
complications of anesthesia during pregnancy (O29.-)
complications of anesthesia during labor and delivery (O74.-)
complications of anesthesia during the puerperium (O89.-) opioids (T40.0-T40.2-)

The appropriate 7th character is to be added to each code from category T41

A	initial encounter
D	subsequent encounter
S	sequela

● T41.0   Poisoning by, adverse effect of and underdosing of inhaled anesthetics

Excludes1   oxygen (T41.5-)

● T41.0X   Poisoning by, adverse effect of and underdosing of inhaled anesthetics

● T41.0X1   Poisoning by inhaled anesthetics, accidental (unintentional)
Poisoning by inhaled anesthetics NOS

● T41.0X2   Poisoning by inhaled anesthetics, intentional self-harm A, S 🔗

● T41.0X3   Poisoning by inhaled anesthetics, assault

● T41.0X4   Poisoning by inhaled anesthetics, undetermined

● T41.0X5   Adverse effect of inhaled anesthetics

● T41.0X6   Underdosing of inhaled anesthetics

● T41.1   Poisoning by, adverse effect of and underdosing of intravenous anesthetics
Poisoning by, adverse effect of and underdosing of thiobarbiturates

● T41.1X   Poisoning by, adverse effect of and underdosing of intravenous anesthetics

● T41.1X1   Poisoning by intravenous anesthetics, accidental (unintentional)
Poisoning by intravenous anesthetics NOS

● T41.1X2   Poisoning by intravenous anesthetics, intentional self-harm A, S 🔗

● T41.1X3   Poisoning by intravenous anesthetics, assault

● T41.1X4   Poisoning by intravenous anesthetics, undetermined

● T41.1X5   Adverse effect of intravenous anesthetics

● T41.1X6   Underdosing of intravenous anesthetics

● T41.2   Poisoning by, adverse effect of and underdosing of other and unspecified general anesthetics

● T41.20   Poisoning by, adverse effect of and underdosing of unspecified general anesthetics

● T41.201   Poisoning by unspecified general anesthetics, accidental (unintentional)
Poisoning by general anesthetics NOS

● T41.202   Poisoning by unspecified general anesthetics, intentional self-harm A, S 🔗

● T41.203   Poisoning by unspecified general anesthetics, assault

● T41.204   Poisoning by unspecified general anesthetics, undetermined

● T41.205   Adverse effect of unspecified general anesthetics
Coding Clinic: 2016, Q4, P73

● T41.206   Underdosing of unspecified general anesthetics

CHAPTER 19 (S00-T88)

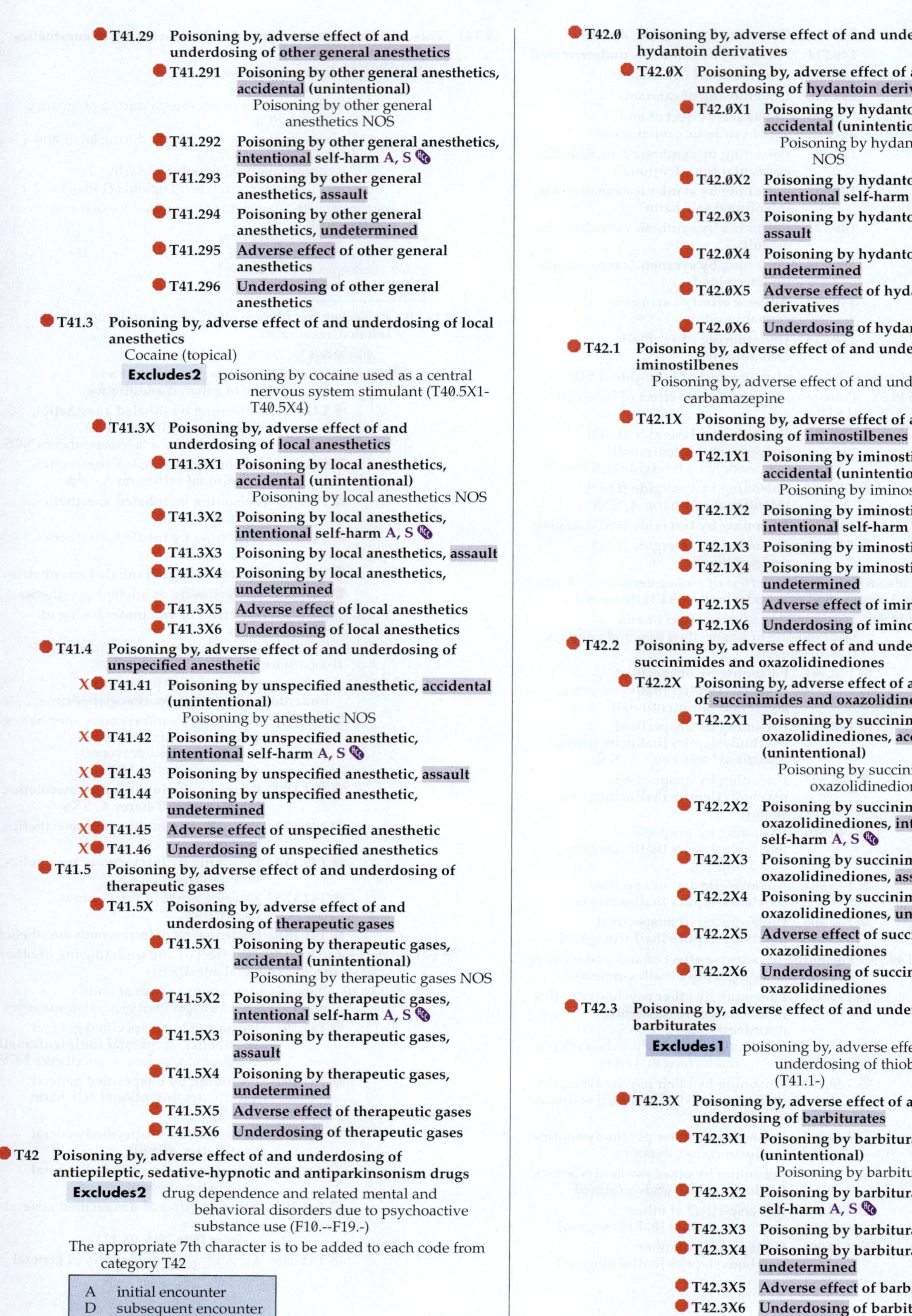

● T41.29 Poisoning by, adverse effect of and underdosing of other general anesthetics
- ● T41.291 Poisoning by other general anesthetics, accidental (unintentional)
  Poisoning by other general anesthetics NOS
- ● T41.292 Poisoning by other general anesthetics, intentional self-harm A, S ⓡ
- ● T41.293 Poisoning by other general anesthetics, assault
- ● T41.294 Poisoning by other general anesthetics, undetermined
- ● T41.295 Adverse effect of other general anesthetics
- ● T41.296 Underdosing of other general anesthetics

● T41.3 Poisoning by, adverse effect of and underdosing of local anesthetics
  Cocaine (topical)
  Excludes2 poisoning by cocaine used as a central nervous system stimulant (T40.5X1-T40.5X4)
- ● T41.3X Poisoning by, adverse effect of and underdosing of local anesthetics
  - ● T41.3X1 Poisoning by local anesthetics, accidental (unintentional)
    Poisoning by local anesthetics NOS
  - ● T41.3X2 Poisoning by local anesthetics, intentional self-harm A, S ⓡ
  - ● T41.3X3 Poisoning by local anesthetics, assault
  - ● T41.3X4 Poisoning by local anesthetics, undetermined
  - ● T41.3X5 Adverse effect of local anesthetics
  - ● T41.3X6 Underdosing of local anesthetics

● T41.4 Poisoning by, adverse effect of and underdosing of unspecified anesthetic
- X ● T41.41 Poisoning by unspecified anesthetic, accidental (unintentional)
    Poisoning by anesthetic NOS
- X ● T41.42 Poisoning by unspecified anesthetic, intentional self-harm A, S ⓡ
- X ● T41.43 Poisoning by unspecified anesthetic, assault
- X ● T41.44 Poisoning by unspecified anesthetic, undetermined
- X ● T41.45 Adverse effect of unspecified anesthetic
- X ● T41.46 Underdosing of unspecified anesthetics

● T41.5 Poisoning by, adverse effect of and underdosing of therapeutic gases
- ● T41.5X Poisoning by, adverse effect of and underdosing of therapeutic gases
  - ● T41.5X1 Poisoning by therapeutic gases, accidental (unintentional)
    Poisoning by therapeutic gases NOS
  - ● T41.5X2 Poisoning by therapeutic gases, intentional self-harm A, S ⓡ
  - ● T41.5X3 Poisoning by therapeutic gases, assault
  - ● T41.5X4 Poisoning by therapeutic gases, undetermined
  - ● T41.5X5 Adverse effect of therapeutic gases
  - ● T41.5X6 Underdosing of therapeutic gases

● T42 Poisoning by, adverse effect of and underdosing of antiepileptic, sedative-hypnotic and antiparkinsonism drugs
  Excludes2 drug dependence and related mental and behavioral disorders due to psychoactive substance use (F10.--F19.-)
  The appropriate 7th character is to be added to each code from category T42
A	initial encounter
D	subsequent encounter
S	sequela

● T42.0 Poisoning by, adverse effect of and underdosing of hydantoin derivatives
- ● T42.0X Poisoning by, adverse effect of and underdosing of hydantoin derivatives
  - ● T42.0X1 Poisoning by hydantoin derivatives, accidental (unintentional)
    Poisoning by hydantoin derivatives NOS
  - ● T42.0X2 Poisoning by hydantoin derivatives, intentional self-harm A, S ⓡ
  - ● T42.0X3 Poisoning by hydantoin derivatives, assault
  - ● T42.0X4 Poisoning by hydantoin derivatives, undetermined
  - ● T42.0X5 Adverse effect of hydantoin derivatives
  - ● T42.0X6 Underdosing of hydantoin derivatives

● T42.1 Poisoning by, adverse effect of and underdosing of iminostilbenes
  Poisoning by, adverse effect of and underdosing of carbamazepine
- ● T42.1X Poisoning by, adverse effect of and underdosing of iminostilbenes
  - ● T42.1X1 Poisoning by iminostilbenes, accidental (unintentional)
    Poisoning by iminostilbenes NOS
  - ● T42.1X2 Poisoning by iminostilbenes, intentional self-harm A, S ⓡ
  - ● T42.1X3 Poisoning by iminostilbenes, assault
  - ● T42.1X4 Poisoning by iminostilbenes, undetermined
  - ● T42.1X5 Adverse effect of iminostilbenes
  - ● T42.1X6 Underdosing of iminostilbenes

● T42.2 Poisoning by, adverse effect of and underdosing of succinimides and oxazolidinediones
- ● T42.2X Poisoning by, adverse effect of and underdosing of succinimides and oxazolidinediones
  - ● T42.2X1 Poisoning by succinimides and oxazolidinediones, accidental (unintentional)
    Poisoning by succinimides and oxazolidinediones NOS
  - ● T42.2X2 Poisoning by succinimides and oxazolidinediones, intentional self-harm A, S ⓡ
  - ● T42.2X3 Poisoning by succinimides and oxazolidinediones, assault
  - ● T42.2X4 Poisoning by succinimides and oxazolidinediones, undetermined
  - ● T42.2X5 Adverse effect of succinimides and oxazolidinediones
  - ● T42.2X6 Underdosing of succinimides and oxazolidinediones

● T42.3 Poisoning by, adverse effect of and underdosing of barbiturates
  Excludes1 poisoning by, adverse effect of and underdosing of thiobarbiturates (T41.1-)
- ● T42.3X Poisoning by, adverse effect of and underdosing of barbiturates
  - ● T42.3X1 Poisoning by barbiturates, accidental (unintentional)
    Poisoning by barbiturates NOS
  - ● T42.3X2 Poisoning by barbiturates, intentional self-harm A, S ⓡ
  - ● T42.3X3 Poisoning by barbiturates, assault
  - ● T42.3X4 Poisoning by barbiturates, undetermined
  - ● T42.3X5 Adverse effect of barbiturates
  - ● T42.3X6 Underdosing of barbiturates

▶ New   ⇨ Revised   ~~deleted~~ Deleted   Excludes 1   Excludes 2   Includes   Use additional   Code first   Code also   Key words
OGCR Official Guidelines   X Assign placeholder X   ● Use Additional Character(s)   ▸ Manifestation Code   ⓡ Hierarchical Condition Category   **Coding Clinic**

● **T42.4**   Poisoning by, adverse effect of and underdosing of benzodiazepines

  ● **T42.4X**   Poisoning by, adverse effect of and underdosing of benzodiazepines

    ● **T42.4X1**   Poisoning by benzodiazepines, accidental (unintentional)
         Poisoning by benzodiazepines NOS

    ● **T42.4X2**   Poisoning by benzodiazepines, intentional self-harm A, S ✍

    ● **T42.4X3**   Poisoning by benzodiazepines, assault

    ● **T42.4X4**   Poisoning by benzodiazepines, undetermined

    ● **T42.4X5**   Adverse effect of benzodiazepines

    ● **T42.4X6**   Underdosing of benzodiazepines

● **T42.5**   Poisoning by, adverse effect of and underdosing of mixed antiepileptics

  ● **T42.5X**   Poisoning by, adverse effect of and underdosing of antiepileptics

    ● **T42.5X1**   Poisoning by mixed antiepileptics, accidental (unintentional)
         Poisoning by mixed antiepileptics NOS

    ● **T42.5X2**   Poisoning by mixed antiepileptics, intentional self-harm A, S ✍

    ● **T42.5X3**   Poisoning by mixed antiepileptics, assault

    ● **T42.5X4**   Poisoning by mixed antiepileptics, undetermined

    ● **T42.5X5**   Adverse effect of mixed antiepileptics

    ● **T42.5X6**   Underdosing of mixed antiepileptics

● **T42.6**   Poisoning by, adverse effect of and underdosing of other antiepileptic and sedative-hypnotic drugs
     Poisoning by, adverse effect of and underdosing of methaqualone
     Poisoning by, adverse effect of and underdosing of valproic acid

     Excludes1   poisoning by, adverse effect of and underdosing of carbamazepine (T42.1-)

  ● **T42.6X**   Poisoning by, adverse effect of and underdosing of other antiepileptic and sedative-hypnotic drugs

    ● **T42.6X1**   Poisoning by other antiepileptic and sedative-hypnotic drugs, accidental (unintentional)
         Poisoning by other antiepileptic and sedative-hypnotic drugs NOS

    ● **T42.6X2**   Poisoning by other antiepileptic and sedative-hypnotic drugs, intentional self-harm A, S ✍

    ● **T42.6X3**   Poisoning by other antiepileptic and sedative-hypnotic drugs, assault

    ● **T42.6X4**   Poisoning by other antiepileptic and sedative-hypnotic drugs, undetermined

    ● **T42.6X5**   Adverse effect of other antiepileptic and sedative-hypnotic drugs

    ● **T42.6X6**   Underdosing of other antiepileptic and sedative-hypnotic drugs

● **T42.7**   Poisoning by, adverse effect of and underdosing of unspecified antiepileptic and sedative-hypnotic drugs

  X ● **T42.71**   Poisoning by unspecified antiepileptic and sedative-hypnotic drugs, accidental (unintentional)
         Poisoning by antiepileptic and sedative-hypnotic drugs NOS

  X ● **T42.72**   Poisoning by unspecified antiepileptic and sedative-hypnotic drugs, intentional self-harm A, S ✍

  X ● **T42.73**   Poisoning by unspecified antiepileptic and sedative-hypnotic drugs, assault

  X ● **T42.74**   Poisoning by unspecified antiepileptic and sedative-hypnotic drugs, undetermined

  X ● **T42.75**   Adverse effect of unspecified antiepileptic and sedative-hypnotic drugs

  X ● **T42.76**   Underdosing of unspecified antiepileptic and sedative-hypnotic drugs

● **T42.8**   Poisoning by, adverse effect of and underdosing of antiparkinsonism drugs and other central muscle-tone depressants
     Poisoning by, adverse effect of and underdosing of amantadine

  ● **T42.8X**   Poisoning by, adverse effect of and underdosing of antiparkinsonism drugs and other central muscle-tone depressants

    ● **T42.8X1**   Poisoning by antiparkinsonism drugs and other central muscle-tone depressants, accidental (unintentional)
         Poisoning by antiparkinsonism drugs and other central muscle-tone depressants NOS

    ● **T42.8X2**   Poisoning by antiparkinsonism drugs and other central muscle-tone depressants, intentional self-harm A, S ✍

    ● **T42.8X3**   Poisoning by antiparkinsonism drugs and other central muscle-tone depressants, assault

    ● **T42.8X4**   Poisoning by antiparkinsonism drugs and other central muscle-tone depressants, undetermined

    ● **T42.8X5**   Adverse effect of antiparkinsonism drugs and other central muscle-tone depressants

    ● **T42.8X6**   Underdosing of antiparkinsonism drugs and other central muscle-tone depressants

● **T43**   Poisoning by, adverse effect of and underdosing of psychotropic drugs, not elsewhere classified

     Excludes1   appetite depressants (T50.5-)
         barbiturates (T42.3-)
         benzodiazepines (T42.4-)
         methaqualone (T42.6-)
         psychodysleptics [hallucinogens] (T40.7-T40.9-)

     Excludes2   drug dependence and related mental and behavioral disorders due to psychoactive substance use (F10.--F19.-)

     The appropriate 7th character is to be added to each code from category T43

> A   initial encounter
> D   subsequent encounter
> S   sequela

● **T43.0**   Poisoning by, adverse effect of and underdosing of tricyclic and tetracyclic antidepressants

  ● **T43.01**   Poisoning by, adverse effect of and underdosing of tricyclic antidepressants

    ● **T43.011**   Poisoning by tricyclic antidepressants, accidental (unintentional)
         Poisoning by tricyclic antidepressants NOS

    ● **T43.012**   Poisoning by tricyclic antidepressants, intentional self-harm A, S ✍

    ● **T43.013**   Poisoning by tricyclic antidepressants, assault

    ● **T43.014**   Poisoning by tricyclic antidepressants, undetermined

    ● **T43.015**   Adverse effect of tricyclic antidepressants

    ● **T43.016**   Underdosing of tricyclic antidepressants

CHAPTER 19 (S00-T88)

● **T43.02**   Poisoning by, adverse effect of and underdosing of tetracyclic antidepressants

● **T43.021**   Poisoning by tetracyclic antidepressants, accidental (unintentional)
Poisoning by tetracyclic antidepressants NOS

● **T43.022**   Poisoning by tetracyclic antidepressants, intentional self-harm A, S

● **T43.023**   Poisoning by tetracyclic antidepressants, assault

● **T43.024**   Poisoning by tetracyclic antidepressants, undetermined

● **T43.025**   Adverse effect of tetracyclic antidepressants

● **T43.026**   Underdosing of tetracyclic antidepressants

● **T43.1**   Poisoning by, adverse effect of and underdosing of monoamine-oxidase-inhibitor antidepressants

● **T43.1X**   Poisoning by, adverse effect of and underdosing of monoamine-oxidase-inhibitor antidepressants

● **T43.1X1**   Poisoning by monoamine-oxidase-inhibitor antidepressants, accidental (unintentional)
Poisoning by monoamine-oxidase-inhibitor antidepressants NOS

● **T43.1X2**   Poisoning by monoamine-oxidase-inhibitor antidepressants, intentional self-harm A, S

● **T43.1X3**   Poisoning by monoamine-oxidase-inhibitor antidepressants, assault

● **T43.1X4**   Poisoning by monoamine-oxidase-inhibitor antidepressants, undetermined

● **T43.1X5**   Adverse effect of monoamine-oxidase-inhibitor antidepressants

● **T43.1X6**   Underdosing of monoamine-oxidase-inhibitor antidepressants

● **T43.2**   Poisoning by, adverse effect of and underdosing of other and unspecified antidepressants

● **T43.20**   Poisoning by, adverse effect of and underdosing of unspecified antidepressants

● **T43.201**   Poisoning by unspecified antidepressants, accidental (unintentional)
Poisoning by antidepressants NOS

● **T43.202**   Poisoning by unspecified antidepressants, intentional self-harm A, S

● **T43.203**   Poisoning by unspecified antidepressants, assault

● **T43.204**   Poisoning by unspecified antidepressants, undetermined

● **T43.205**   Adverse effect of unspecified antidepressants
Antidepressant discontinuation syndrome

● **T43.206**   Underdosing of unspecified antidepressants

● **T43.21**   Poisoning by, adverse effect of and underdosing of selective serotonin and norepinephrine reuptake inhibitors
Poisoning by, adverse effect of and underdosing of SSNRI antidepressants

● **T43.211**   Poisoning by selective serotonin and norepinephrine reuptake inhibitors, accidental (unintentional)

● **T43.212**   Poisoning by selective serotonin and norepinephrine reuptake inhibitors, intentional self-harm A, S

● **T43.213**   Poisoning by selective serotonin and norepinephrine reuptake inhibitors, assault

● **T43.214**   Poisoning by selective serotonin and norepinephrine reuptake inhibitors, undetermined

● **T43.215**   Adverse effect of selective serotonin and norepinephrine reuptake inhibitors

● **T43.216**   Underdosing of selective serotonin and norepinephrine reuptake inhibitors

● **T43.22**   Poisoning by, adverse effect of and underdosing of selective serotonin reuptake inhibitors
Poisoning by, adverse effect of and underdosing of SSRI antidepressants

● **T43.221**   Poisoning by selective serotonin reuptake inhibitors, accidental (unintentional)

● **T43.222**   Poisoning by selective serotonin reuptake inhibitors, intentional self-harm A, S

● **T43.223**   Poisoning by selective serotonin reuptake inhibitors, assault

● **T43.224**   Poisoning by selective serotonin reuptake inhibitors, undetermined

● **T43.225**   Adverse effect of selective serotonin reuptake inhibitors
Coding Clinic: 2024, Q4, P17; 2022, Q2, P11

● **T43.226**   Underdosing of selective serotonin reuptake inhibitors

● **T43.29**   Poisoning by, adverse effect of and underdosing of other antidepressants

● **T43.291**   Poisoning by other antidepressants, accidental (unintentional)
Poisoning by other antidepressants NOS

● **T43.292**   Poisoning by other antidepressants, intentional self-harm A, S

● **T43.293**   Poisoning by other antidepressants, assault

● **T43.294**   Poisoning by other antidepressants, undetermined

● **T43.295**   Adverse effect of other antidepressants

● **T43.296**   Underdosing of other antidepressants

● **T43.3**   Poisoning by, adverse effect of and underdosing of phenothiazine antipsychotics and neuroleptics

● **T43.3X**   Poisoning by, adverse effect of and underdosing of phenothiazine antipsychotics and neuroleptics

● **T43.3X1**   Poisoning by phenothiazine antipsychotics and neuroleptics, accidental (unintentional)
Poisoning by phenothiazine antipsychotics and neuroleptics NOS

● **T43.3X2**   Poisoning by phenothiazine antipsychotics and neuroleptics, intentional self-harm A, S

● **T43.3X3**   Poisoning by phenothiazine antipsychotics and neuroleptics, assault

● **T43.3X4**   Poisoning by phenothiazine antipsychotics and neuroleptics, undetermined

● **T43.3X5**   Adverse effect of phenothiazine antipsychotics and neuroleptics

● **T43.3X6**   Underdosing of phenothiazine antipsychotics and neuroleptics

▶ New   ⇒ Revised   ~~deleted~~ Deleted   Excludes 1   Excludes 2   Includes   Use additional   Code first   Code also   Key words
OGCR Official Guidelines   X Assign placeholder X   ● Use Additional Character(s)   ▶ Manifestation Code   Hierarchical Condition Category   Coding Clinic

● **T43.4**   Poisoning by, adverse effect of and underdosing of butyrophenone and thiothixene neuroleptics

  ● **T43.4X**   Poisoning by, adverse effect of and underdosing of butyrophenone and thiothixene neuroleptics

    ● **T43.4X1**   Poisoning by butyrophenone and thiothixene neuroleptics, accidental (unintentional)
       Poisoning by butyrophenone and thiothixene neuroleptics NOS

    ● **T43.4X2**   Poisoning by butyrophenone and thiothixene neuroleptics, intentional self-harm A, S

    ● **T43.4X3**   Poisoning by butyrophenone and thiothixene neuroleptics, assault

    ● **T43.4X4**   Poisoning by butyrophenone and thiothixene neuroleptics, undetermined

    ● **T43.4X5**   Adverse effect of butyrophenone and thiothixene neuroleptics

    ● **T43.4X6**   Underdosing of butyrophenone and thiothixene neuroleptics

● **T43.5**   Poisoning by, adverse effect of and underdosing of other and unspecified antipsychotics and neuroleptics

  Excludes1   poisoning by, adverse effect of and underdosing of rauwolfia (T46.5-)

  ● **T43.50**   Poisoning by, adverse effect of and underdosing of unspecified antipsychotics and neuroleptics

    ● **T43.501**   Poisoning by unspecified antipsychotics and neuroleptics, accidental (unintentional)
       Poisoning by antipsychotics and neuroleptics NOS

    ● **T43.502**   Poisoning by unspecified antipsychotics and neuroleptics, intentional self-harm A, S

    ● **T43.503**   Poisoning by unspecified antipsychotics and neuroleptics, assault

    ● **T43.504**   Poisoning by unspecified antipsychotics and neuroleptics, undetermined

    ● **T43.505**   Adverse effect of unspecified antipsychotics and neuroleptics
       Coding Clinic: 2022, Q4, P24

    ● **T43.506**   Underdosing of unspecified antipsychotics and neuroleptics

  ● **T43.59**   Poisoning by, adverse effect of and underdosing of other antipsychotics and neuroleptics

    ● **T43.591**   Poisoning by other antipsychotics and neuroleptics, accidental (unintentional)
       Poisoning by other antipsychotics and neuroleptics NOS

    ● **T43.592**   Poisoning by other antipsychotics and neuroleptics, intentional self-harm A, S
       Coding Clinic: 2017, Q1, P40

    ● **T43.593**   Poisoning by other antipsychotics and neuroleptics, assault

    ● **T43.594**   Poisoning by other antipsychotics and neuroleptics, undetermined

    ● **T43.595**   Adverse effect of other antipsychotics and neuroleptics
       Coding Clinic: 2022, Q2, P11

    ● **T43.596**   Underdosing of other antipsychotics and neuroleptics

● **T43.6**   Poisoning by, adverse effect of and underdosing of psychostimulants

  Excludes1   poisoning by, adverse effect of and underdosing of cocaine (T40.5-)

  ● **T43.60**   Poisoning by, adverse effect of and underdosing of unspecified psychostimulant

    ● **T43.601**   Poisoning by unspecified psychostimulants, accidental (unintentional)
       Poisoning by psychostimulants NOS

    ● **T43.602**   Poisoning by unspecified psychostimulants, intentional self-harm A, S

    ● **T43.603**   Poisoning by unspecified psychostimulants, assault

    ● **T43.604**   Poisoning by unspecified psychostimulants, undetermined

    ● **T43.605**   Adverse effect of unspecified psychostimulants

    ● **T43.606**   Underdosing of unspecified psychostimulants

  ● **T43.61**   Poisoning by, adverse effect of and underdosing of caffeine

    ● **T43.611**   Poisoning by caffeine, accidental (unintentional)
       Poisoning by caffeine NOS

    ● **T43.612**   Poisoning by caffeine, intentional self-harm A, S

    ● **T43.613**   Poisoning by caffeine, assault

    ● **T43.614**   Poisoning by caffeine, undetermined

    ● **T43.615**   Adverse effect of caffeine

    ● **T43.616**   Underdosing of caffeine

  ● **T43.62**   Poisoning by, adverse effect of and underdosing of amphetamines

    ● **T43.621**   Poisoning by amphetamines, accidental (unintentional)
       Poisoning by amphetamines NOS
       Coding Clinic: 2021, Q3, P8

    ● **T43.622**   Poisoning by amphetamines, intentional self-harm A, S

    ● **T43.623**   Poisoning by amphetamines, assault

    ● **T43.624**   Poisoning by amphetamines, undetermined

    ● **T43.625**   Adverse effect of amphetamines

    ● **T43.626**   Underdosing of amphetamines

  ● **T43.63**   Poisoning by, adverse effect of and underdosing of methylphenidate

    ● **T43.631**   Poisoning by methylphenidate, accidental (unintentional)
       Poisoning by methylphenidate NOS

    ● **T43.632**   Poisoning by methylphenidate, intentional self-harm A, S

    ● **T43.633**   Poisoning by methylphenidate, assault

    ● **T43.634**   Poisoning by methylphenidate, undetermined

    ● **T43.635**   Adverse effect of methylphenidate

    ● **T43.636**   Underdosing of methylphenidate

  ● **T43.64**   Poisoning by ecstasy
     Poisoning by MDMA
     Poisoning by 3,4-methylenedioxymethamphetamine

    ● **T43.641**   Poisoning by ecstasy, accidental (unintentional)
       Poisoning by ecstasy NOS
       Coding Clinic: 2018, Q4, P31

    ● **T43.642**   Poisoning by ecstasy, intentional self-harm A, S

    ● **T43.643**   Poisoning by ecstasy, assault

    ● **T43.644**   Poisoning by ecstasy, undetermined

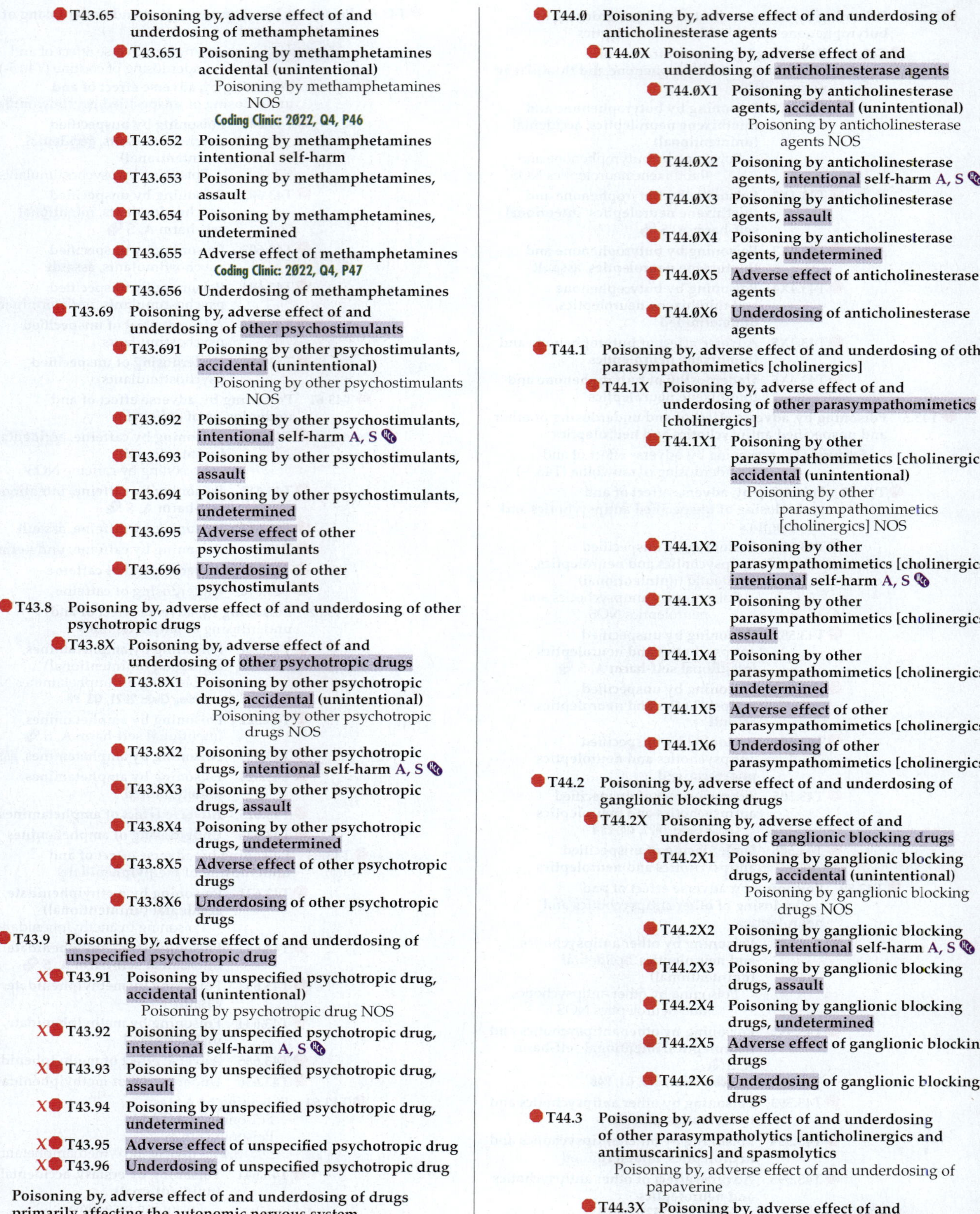

● **T43.65**   **Poisoning by, adverse effect of and underdosing of methamphetamines**

   ● **T43.651**   **Poisoning by methamphetamines accidental (unintentional)**
       Poisoning by methamphetamines NOS
       Coding Clinic: 2022, Q4, P46

   ● **T43.652**   **Poisoning by methamphetamines intentional self-harm**

   ● **T43.653**   **Poisoning by methamphetamines, assault**

   ● **T43.654**   **Poisoning by methamphetamines, undetermined**

   ● **T43.655**   **Adverse effect of methamphetamines**
       Coding Clinic: 2022, Q4, P47

   ● **T43.656**   **Underdosing of methamphetamines**

● **T43.69**   **Poisoning by, adverse effect of and underdosing of other psychostimulants**

   ● **T43.691**   **Poisoning by other psychostimulants, accidental (unintentional)**
       Poisoning by other psychostimulants NOS

   ● **T43.692**   **Poisoning by other psychostimulants, intentional self-harm A, S**

   ● **T43.693**   **Poisoning by other psychostimulants, assault**

   ● **T43.694**   **Poisoning by other psychostimulants, undetermined**

   ● **T43.695**   **Adverse effect of other psychostimulants**

   ● **T43.696**   **Underdosing of other psychostimulants**

● **T43.8**   **Poisoning by, adverse effect of and underdosing of other psychotropic drugs**

  ● **T43.8X**   **Poisoning by, adverse effect of and underdosing of other psychotropic drugs**

   ● **T43.8X1**   **Poisoning by other psychotropic drugs, accidental (unintentional)**
       Poisoning by other psychotropic drugs NOS

   ● **T43.8X2**   **Poisoning by other psychotropic drugs, intentional self-harm A, S**

   ● **T43.8X3**   **Poisoning by other psychotropic drugs, assault**

   ● **T43.8X4**   **Poisoning by other psychotropic drugs, undetermined**

   ● **T43.8X5**   **Adverse effect of other psychotropic drugs**

   ● **T43.8X6**   **Underdosing of other psychotropic drugs**

● **T43.9**   **Poisoning by, adverse effect of and underdosing of unspecified psychotropic drug**

  X ● **T43.91**   **Poisoning by unspecified psychotropic drug, accidental (unintentional)**
       Poisoning by psychotropic drug NOS

  X ● **T43.92**   **Poisoning by unspecified psychotropic drug, intentional self-harm A, S**

  X ● **T43.93**   **Poisoning by unspecified psychotropic drug, assault**

  X ● **T43.94**   **Poisoning by unspecified psychotropic drug, undetermined**

  X ● **T43.95**   **Adverse effect of unspecified psychotropic drug**

  X ● **T43.96**   **Underdosing of unspecified psychotropic drug**

● **T44**   **Poisoning by, adverse effect of and underdosing of drugs primarily affecting the autonomic nervous system**

    The appropriate 7th character is to be added to each code from category T44

     A   initial encounter
     D   subsequent encounter
     S   sequela

● **T44.0**   **Poisoning by, adverse effect of and underdosing of anticholinesterase agents**

  ● **T44.0X**   **Poisoning by, adverse effect of and underdosing of anticholinesterase agents**

   ● **T44.0X1**   **Poisoning by anticholinesterase agents, accidental (unintentional)**
       Poisoning by anticholinesterase agents NOS

   ● **T44.0X2**   **Poisoning by anticholinesterase agents, intentional self-harm A, S**

   ● **T44.0X3**   **Poisoning by anticholinesterase agents, assault**

   ● **T44.0X4**   **Poisoning by anticholinesterase agents, undetermined**

   ● **T44.0X5**   **Adverse effect of anticholinesterase agents**

   ● **T44.0X6**   **Underdosing of anticholinesterase agents**

● **T44.1**   **Poisoning by, adverse effect of and underdosing of other parasympathomimetics [cholinergics]**

  ● **T44.1X**   **Poisoning by, adverse effect of and underdosing of other parasympathomimetics [cholinergics]**

   ● **T44.1X1**   **Poisoning by other parasympathomimetics [cholinergics], accidental (unintentional)**
       Poisoning by other parasympathomimetics [cholinergics] NOS

   ● **T44.1X2**   **Poisoning by other parasympathomimetics [cholinergics], intentional self-harm A, S**

   ● **T44.1X3**   **Poisoning by other parasympathomimetics [cholinergics], assault**

   ● **T44.1X4**   **Poisoning by other parasympathomimetics [cholinergics], undetermined**

   ● **T44.1X5**   **Adverse effect of other parasympathomimetics [cholinergics]**

   ● **T44.1X6**   **Underdosing of other parasympathomimetics [cholinergics]**

● **T44.2**   **Poisoning by, adverse effect of and underdosing of ganglionic blocking drugs**

  ● **T44.2X**   **Poisoning by, adverse effect of and underdosing of ganglionic blocking drugs**

   ● **T44.2X1**   **Poisoning by ganglionic blocking drugs, accidental (unintentional)**
       Poisoning by ganglionic blocking drugs NOS

   ● **T44.2X2**   **Poisoning by ganglionic blocking drugs, intentional self-harm A, S**

   ● **T44.2X3**   **Poisoning by ganglionic blocking drugs, assault**

   ● **T44.2X4**   **Poisoning by ganglionic blocking drugs, undetermined**

   ● **T44.2X5**   **Adverse effect of ganglionic blocking drugs**

   ● **T44.2X6**   **Underdosing of ganglionic blocking drugs**

● **T44.3**   **Poisoning by, adverse effect of and underdosing of other parasympatholytics [anticholinergics and antimuscarinics] and spasmolytics**
    Poisoning by, adverse effect of and underdosing of papaverine

  ● **T44.3X**   **Poisoning by, adverse effect of and underdosing of other parasympatholytics [anticholinergics and antimuscarinics] and spasmolytics**

● T44.3X1 **Poisoning by other parasympatholytics [anticholinergics and antimuscarinics] and spasmolytics, accidental (unintentional)**
     Poisoning by other parasympatholytics [anticholinergics and antimuscarinics] and spasmolytics NOS

● T44.3X2 **Poisoning by other parasympatholytics [anticholinergics and antimuscarinics] and spasmolytics, intentional self-harm A, S**

● T44.3X3 **Poisoning by other parasympatholytics [anticholinergics and antimuscarinics] and spasmolytics, assault**

● T44.3X4 **Poisoning by other parasympatholytics [anticholinergics and antimuscarinics] and spasmolytics, undetermined**

● T44.3X5 **Adverse effect of other parasympatholytics [anticholinergics and antimuscarinics] and spasmolytics**

● T44.3X6 **Underdosing of other parasympatholytics [anticholinergics and antimuscarinics] and spasmolytics**

● T44.4 **Poisoning by, adverse effect of and underdosing of predominantly alpha-adrenoreceptor agonists**
     Poisoning by, adverse effect of and underdosing of metaraminol

● T44.4X **Poisoning by, adverse effect of and underdosing of predominantly alpha-adrenoreceptor agonists**

● T44.4X1 **Poisoning by predominantly alpha-adrenoreceptor agonists, accidental (unintentional)**
     Poisoning by predominantly alpha-adrenoreceptor agonists NOS

● T44.4X2 **Poisoning by predominantly alpha-adrenoreceptor agonists, intentional self-harm A, S**

● T44.4X3 **Poisoning by predominantly alpha-adrenoreceptor agonists, assault**

● T44.4X4 **Poisoning by predominantly alpha-adrenoreceptor agonists, undetermined**

● T44.4X5 **Adverse effect of predominantly alpha-adrenoreceptor agonists**

● T44.4X6 **Underdosing of predominantly alpha-adrenoreceptor agonists**

● T44.5 **Poisoning by, adverse effect of and underdosing of predominantly beta-adrenoreceptor agonists**

Excludes1   poisoning by, adverse effect of and underdosing of beta-adrenoreceptor agonists used in asthma therapy (T48.6-)

● T44.5X **Poisoning by, adverse effect of and underdosing of predominantly beta-adrenoreceptor agonists**

● T44.5X1 **Poisoning by predominantly beta-adrenoreceptor agonists, accidental (unintentional)**
     Poisoning by predominantly beta-adrenoreceptor agonists NOS

● T44.5X2 **Poisoning by predominantly beta-adrenoreceptor agonists, intentional self-harm A, S**

● T44.5X3 **Poisoning by predominantly beta-adrenoreceptor agonists, assault**

● T44.5X4 **Poisoning by predominantly beta-adrenoreceptor agonists, undetermined**

● T44.5X5 **Adverse effect of predominantly beta-adrenoreceptor agonists**

● T44.5X6 **Underdosing of predominantly beta-adrenoreceptor agonists**

● T44.6 **Poisoning by, adverse effect of and underdosing of alpha-adrenoreceptor antagonists**

Excludes1   poisoning by, adverse effect of and underdosing of ergot alkaloids (T48.0)

● T44.6X **Poisoning by, adverse effect of and underdosing of alpha-adrenoreceptor antagonists**

● T44.6X1 **Poisoning by alpha-adrenoreceptor antagonists, accidental (unintentional)**
     Poisoning by alpha-adrenoreceptor antagonists NOS

● T44.6X2 **Poisoning by alpha-adrenoreceptor antagonists, intentional self-harm A, S**

● T44.6X3 **Poisoning by alpha-adrenoreceptor antagonists, assault**

● T44.6X4 **Poisoning by alpha-adrenoreceptor antagonists, undetermined**

● T44.6X5 **Adverse effect of alpha-adrenoreceptor antagonists**

● T44.6X6 **Underdosing of alpha-adrenoreceptor antagonists**

● T44.7 **Poisoning by, adverse effect of and underdosing of beta-adrenoreceptor antagonists**

● T44.7X **Poisoning by, adverse effect of and underdosing of beta-adrenoreceptor antagonists**

● T44.7X1 **Poisoning by beta-adrenoreceptor antagonists, accidental (unintentional)**
     Poisoning by beta-adrenoreceptor antagonists NOS

● T44.7X2 **Poisoning by beta-adrenoreceptor antagonists, intentional self-harm A, S**

● T44.7X3 **Poisoning by beta-adrenoreceptor antagonists, assault**

● T44.7X4 **Poisoning by beta-adrenoreceptor antagonists, undetermined**

● T44.7X5 **Adverse effect of beta-adrenoreceptor antagonists**

● T44.7X6 **Underdosing of beta-adrenoreceptor antagonists**

● T44.8 **Poisoning by, adverse effect of and underdosing of centrally-acting and adrenergic-neuron-blocking agents**

Excludes2   poisoning by, adverse effect of and underdosing of clonidine (T46.5)
     poisoning by, adverse effect of and underdosing of guanethidine (T46.5)

● T44.8X **Poisoning by, adverse effect of and underdosing of centrally-acting and adrenergic-neuron-blocking agents**

● T44.8X1 **Poisoning by centrally-acting and adrenergic-neuron-blocking agents, accidental (unintentional)**
     Poisoning by centrally-acting and adrenergic-neuron-blocking agents NOS

● T44.8X2 **Poisoning by centrally-acting and adrenergic-neuron-blocking agents, intentional self-harm A, S**

● T44.8X3 **Poisoning by centrally-acting and adrenergic-neuron-blocking agents, assault**

● T44.8X4 **Poisoning by centrally-acting and adrenergic-neuron-blocking agents, undetermined**

CHAPTER 19 (S00–T88)

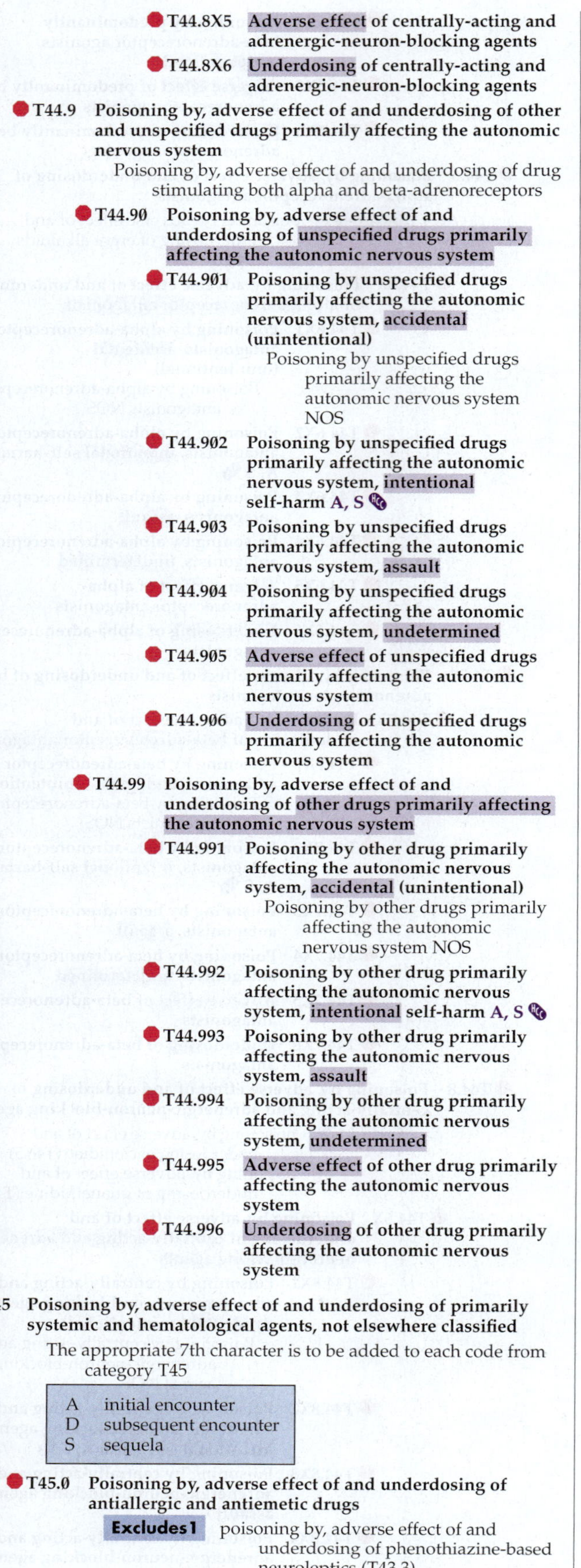

CHAPTER 19 (S00-T88)

● T44.8X5　**Adverse effect** of centrally-acting and adrenergic-neuron-blocking agents

● T44.8X6　**Underdosing** of centrally-acting and adrenergic-neuron-blocking agents

● T44.9　Poisoning by, adverse effect of and underdosing of other and unspecified drugs primarily affecting the autonomic nervous system

　　Poisoning by, adverse effect of and underdosing of drug stimulating both alpha and beta-adrenoreceptors

　● T44.90　Poisoning by, adverse effect of and underdosing of **unspecified drugs primarily affecting the autonomic nervous system**

　　● T44.901　Poisoning by unspecified drugs primarily affecting the autonomic nervous system, **accidental (unintentional)**

　　　　Poisoning by unspecified drugs primarily affecting the autonomic nervous system NOS

　　● T44.902　Poisoning by unspecified drugs primarily affecting the autonomic nervous system, **intentional self-harm** A, S 🕮

　　● T44.903　Poisoning by unspecified drugs primarily affecting the autonomic nervous system, **assault**

　　● T44.904　Poisoning by unspecified drugs primarily affecting the autonomic nervous system, **undetermined**

　　● T44.905　**Adverse effect** of unspecified drugs primarily affecting the autonomic nervous system

　　● T44.906　**Underdosing** of unspecified drugs primarily affecting the autonomic nervous system

　● T44.99　Poisoning by, adverse effect of and underdosing of **other drugs primarily affecting the autonomic nervous system**

　　● T44.991　Poisoning by other drug primarily affecting the autonomic nervous system, **accidental (unintentional)**

　　　　Poisoning by other drugs primarily affecting the autonomic nervous system NOS

　　● T44.992　Poisoning by other drug primarily affecting the autonomic nervous system, **intentional self-harm** A, S 🕮

　　● T44.993　Poisoning by other drug primarily affecting the autonomic nervous system, **assault**

　　● T44.994　Poisoning by other drug primarily affecting the autonomic nervous system, **undetermined**

　　● T44.995　**Adverse effect** of other drug primarily affecting the autonomic nervous system

　　● T44.996　**Underdosing** of other drug primarily affecting the autonomic nervous system

● T45　Poisoning by, adverse effect of and underdosing of primarily systemic and hematological agents, not elsewhere classified

　　The appropriate 7th character is to be added to each code from category T45

A	initial encounter
D	subsequent encounter
S	sequela

　● T45.0　Poisoning by, adverse effect of and underdosing of antiallergic and antiemetic drugs

　　Excludes1　poisoning by, adverse effect of and underdosing of phenothiazine-based neuroleptics (T43.3)

● T45.0X　Poisoning by, adverse effect of and underdosing of **antiallergic and antiemetic drugs**

　● T45.0X1　Poisoning by antiallergic and antiemetic drugs, **accidental (unintentional)**

　　　Poisoning by antiallergic and antiemetic drugs NOS

　● T45.0X2　Poisoning by antiallergic and antiemetic drugs, **intentional self-harm** A, S 🕮

　● T45.0X3　Poisoning by antiallergic and antiemetic drugs, **assault**

　● T45.0X4　Poisoning by antiallergic and antiemetic drugs, **undetermined**

　● T45.0X5　**Adverse effect** of antiallergic and antiemetic drugs

　● T45.0X6　**Underdosing** of antiallergic and antiemetic drugs

● T45.1　Poisoning by, adverse effect of and underdosing of antineoplastic and immunosuppressive drugs

　Excludes1　poisoning by, adverse effect of and underdosing of immune checkpoint inhibitors and immunostimulant drugs (T45.A)

　Coding Clinic: 2023, Q2, P10

● T45.1X　Poisoning by, adverse effect of and underdosing of **antineoplastic and immunosuppressive drugs**

　● T45.1X1　Poisoning by antineoplastic and immunosuppressive drugs, **accidental (unintentional)**

　　　Poisoning by antineoplastic and immunosuppressive drugs NOS

　● T45.1X2　Poisoning by antineoplastic and immunosuppressive drugs, **intentional self-harm** A, S 🕮

　● T45.1X3　Poisoning by antineoplastic and immunosuppressive drugs, **assault**

　● T45.1X4　Poisoning by antineoplastic and immunosuppressive drugs, **undetermined**

　● T45.1X5　**Adverse effect** of antineoplastic and immunosuppressive drugs

　　Coding Clinic: 2024, Q1, P25; 2021, Q3, P4; 2019, Q2, P25, 28; Q1, P17, 21

　● T45.1X6　**Underdosing** of antineoplastic and immunosuppressive drugs

● T45.2　Poisoning by, adverse effect of and underdosing of vitamins

　Excludes2　poisoning by, adverse effect of and underdosing of nicotinic acid (derivatives) (T46.7)
　　poisoning by, adverse effect of and underdosing of iron (T45.4)
　　poisoning by, adverse effect of and underdosing of vitamin K (T45.7)

● T45.2X　Poisoning by, adverse effect of and underdosing of **vitamins**

　● T45.2X1　Poisoning by vitamins, **accidental (unintentional)**

　　　Poisoning by vitamins NOS

　● T45.2X2　Poisoning by vitamins, **intentional self-harm** A, S 🕮

　● T45.2X3　Poisoning by vitamins, **assault**

　● T45.2X4　Poisoning by vitamins, **undetermined**

　● T45.2X5　**Adverse effect** of vitamins

　● T45.2X6　**Underdosing** of vitamins

　　Excludes1　vitamin deficiencies (E50-E56)

▶ New　　➡ Revised　　~~deleted~~ Deleted　　Excludes 1　　Excludes 2　　Includes　　Use additional　　Code first　　Code also　　Key words
OGCR Official Guidelines　　X Assign placeholder X　　● Use Additional Character(s)　　▌ Manifestation Code　　🕮 Hierarchical Condition Category　　**Coding Clinic**

- ● **T45.3** Poisoning by, adverse effect of and underdosing of enzymes
  - ● **T45.3X** Poisoning by, adverse effect of and underdosing of enzymes
    - ● **T45.3X1** Poisoning by enzymes, accidental (unintentional)
      Poisoning by enzymes NOS
    - ● **T45.3X2** Poisoning by enzymes, intentional self-harm **A, S** 🔷
    - ● **T45.3X3** Poisoning by enzymes, assault
    - ● **T45.3X4** Poisoning by enzymes, undetermined
    - ● **T45.3X5** Adverse effect of enzymes
    - ● **T45.3X6** Underdosing of enzymes
- ● **T45.4** Poisoning by, adverse effect of and underdosing of iron and its compounds
  - ● **T45.4X** Poisoning by, adverse effect of and underdosing of iron and its compounds
    - ● **T45.4X1** Poisoning by iron and its compounds, accidental (unintentional)
      Poisoning by iron and its compounds NOS
    - ● **T45.4X2** Poisoning by iron and its compounds, intentional self-harm **A, S** 🔷
    - ● **T45.4X3** Poisoning by iron and its compounds, assault
    - ● **T45.4X4** Poisoning by iron and its compounds, undetermined
    - ● **T45.4X5** Adverse effect of iron and its compounds
    - ● **T45.4X6** Underdosing of iron and its compounds
      > **Excludes1**   iron deficiency (E61.1)
- ● **T45.5** Poisoning by, adverse effect of and underdosing of anticoagulants and antithrombotic drugs
  - ● **T45.51** Poisoning by, adverse effect of and underdosing of anticoagulants
    - ● **T45.511** Poisoning by anticoagulants, accidental (unintentional)
      Poisoning by anticoagulants NOS
    - ● **T45.512** Poisoning by anticoagulants, intentional self-harm **A, S** 🔷
    - ● **T45.513** Poisoning by anticoagulants, assault
    - ● **T45.514** Poisoning by anticoagulants, undetermined
    - ● **T45.515** Adverse effect of anticoagulants
      Coding Clinic: 2021, Q1, P5; 2016, Q1, P14; 2013, Q2, P35
    - ● **T45.516** Underdosing of anticoagulants
  - ● **T45.52** Poisoning by, adverse effect of and underdosing of antithrombotic drugs
    Poisoning by, adverse effect of and underdosing of antiplatelet drugs
    > **Excludes2**   poisoning by, adverse effect of and underdosing of aspirin (T39.01-)
    > poisoning by, adverse effect of and underdosing of acetylsalicylic acid (T39.01-)
    - ● **T45.521** Poisoning by antithrombotic drugs, accidental (unintentional)
      Poisoning by antithrombotic drug NOS
    - ● **T45.522** Poisoning by antithrombotic drugs, intentional self-harm **A, S** 🔷
    - ● **T45.523** Poisoning by antithrombotic drugs, assault
    - ● **T45.524** Poisoning by antithrombotic drugs, undetermined
    - ● **T45.525** Adverse effect of antithrombotic drugs
      Coding Clinic: 2016, Q1, P15
    - ● **T45.526** Underdosing of antithrombotic drugs
- ● **T45.6** Poisoning by, adverse effect of and underdosing of fibrinolysis-affecting drugs
  - ● **T45.60** Poisoning by, adverse effect of and underdosing of unspecified fibrinolysis-affecting drugs
    - ● **T45.601** Poisoning by unspecified fibrinolysis-affecting drugs, accidental (unintentional)
      Poisoning by fibrinolysis-affecting drug NOS
    - ● **T45.602** Poisoning by unspecified fibrinolysis-affecting drugs, intentional self-harm **A, S** 🔷
    - ● **T45.603** Poisoning by unspecified fibrinolysis-affecting drugs, assault
    - ● **T45.604** Poisoning by unspecified fibrinolysis-affecting drugs, undetermined
    - ● **T45.605** Adverse effect of unspecified fibrinolysis-affecting drugs
    - ● **T45.606** Underdosing of unspecified fibrinolysis-affecting drugs
  - ● **T45.61** Poisoning by, adverse effect of and underdosing of thrombolytic drugs
    - ● **T45.611** Poisoning by thrombolytic drug, accidental (unintentional)
      Poisoning by thrombolytic drug NOS
    - ● **T45.612** Poisoning by thrombolytic drug, intentional self-harm **A, S** 🔷
    - ● **T45.613** Poisoning by thrombolytic drug, assault
    - ● **T45.614** Poisoning by thrombolytic drug, undetermined
    - ● **T45.615** Adverse effect of thrombolytic drugs
      Coding Clinic: 2017, Q2, P10
    - ● **T45.616** Underdosing of thrombolytic drug
  - ● **T45.62** Poisoning by, adverse effect of and underdosing of hemostatic drugs
    - ● **T45.621** Poisoning by hemostatic drug, accidental (unintentional)
      Poisoning by hemostatic drug NOS
    - ● **T45.622** Poisoning by hemostatic drug, intentional self-harm **A, S** 🔷
    - ● **T45.623** Poisoning by hemostatic drug, assault
    - ● **T45.624** Poisoning by hemostatic drug, undetermined
    - ● **T45.625** Adverse effect of hemostatic drug
    - ● **T45.626** Underdosing of hemostatic drugs
  - ● **T45.69** Poisoning by, adverse effect of and underdosing of other fibrinolysis-affecting drugs
    - ● **T45.691** Poisoning by other fibrinolysis-affecting drugs, accidental (unintentional)
      Poisoning by other fibrinolysis-affecting drug NOS
    - ● **T45.692** Poisoning by other fibrinolysis-affecting drugs, intentional self-harm **A, S** 🔷
    - ● **T45.693** Poisoning by other fibrinolysis-affecting drugs, assault
    - ● **T45.694** Poisoning by other fibrinolysis-affecting drugs, undetermined
    - ● **T45.695** Adverse effect of other fibrinolysis-affecting drugs
    - ● **T45.696** Underdosing of other fibrinolysis-affecting drugs

● **T45.7** **Poisoning by, adverse effect of and underdosing of anticoagulant antagonists, vitamin K and other coagulants**
  ● **T45.7X** **Poisoning by, adverse effect of and underdosing of anticoagulant antagonists, vitamin K and other coagulants**
    ● **T45.7X1** **Poisoning by anticoagulant antagonists, vitamin K and other coagulants, accidental (unintentional)**
      Poisoning by anticoagulant antagonists, vitamin K and other coagulants NOS
    ● **T45.7X2** **Poisoning by anticoagulant antagonists, vitamin K and other coagulants, intentional self-harm A, S** 🔖
    ● **T45.7X3** **Poisoning by anticoagulant antagonists, vitamin K and other coagulants, assault**
    ● **T45.7X4** **Poisoning by anticoagulant antagonists, vitamin K and other coagulants, undetermined**
    ● **T45.7X5** **Adverse effect of anticoagulant antagonists, vitamin K and other coagulants**
    ● **T45.7X6** **Underdosing of anticoagulant antagonist, vitamin K and other coagulants**
      Excludes1 vitamin K deficiency (E56.1)

● **T45.8** **Poisoning by, adverse effect of and underdosing of other primarily systemic and hematological agents**
  Poisoning by, adverse effect of and underdosing of liver preparations and other antianemic agents
  Poisoning by, adverse effect of and underdosing of natural blood and blood products
  Poisoning by, adverse effect of and underdosing of plasma substitute
    Excludes2 poisoning by, adverse effect of and underdosing of immunoglobulin (T50.Z1)
      poisoning by, adverse effect of and underdosing of iron (T45.4)
      transfusion reactions (T80.-)
  ● **T45.8X** **Poisoning by, adverse effect of and underdosing of other primarily systemic and hematological agents**
    ● **T45.8X1** **Poisoning by other primarily systemic and hematological agents, accidental (unintentional)**
      Poisoning by other primarily systemic and hematological agents NOS
    ● **T45.8X2** **Poisoning by other primarily systemic and hematological agents, intentional self-harm A, S** 🔖
    ● **T45.8X3** **Poisoning by other primarily systemic and hematological agents, assault**
    ● **T45.8X4** **Poisoning by other primarily systemic and hematological agents, undetermined**
    ● **T45.8X5** **Adverse effect of other primarily systemic and hematological agents**
      Coding Clinic: 2016, Q4, P42
    ● **T45.8X6** **Underdosing of other primarily systemic and hematological agents**

● **T45.9** **Poisoning by, adverse effect of and underdosing of unspecified primarily systemic and hematological agent**
  X ● **T45.91** **Poisoning by unspecified primarily systemic and hematological agent, accidental (unintentional)**
    Poisoning by primarily systemic and hematological agent NOS
  X ● **T45.92** **Poisoning by unspecified primarily systemic and hematological agent, intentional self-harm A, S** 🔖
  X ● **T45.93** **Poisoning by unspecified primarily systemic and hematological agent, assault**
  X ● **T45.94** **Poisoning by unspecified primarily systemic and hematological agent, undetermined**
  X ● **T45.95** **Adverse effect of unspecified primarily systemic and hematological agent**
  X ● **T45.96** **Underdosing of unspecified primarily systemic and hematological agent**

● **T45.A** **Poisoning by, adverse effect of and underdosing of immune checkpoint inhibitors and immunostimulant drugs**
    Excludes1 poisoning by, adverse effect of and underdosing of antineoplastic and immunosuppressive drug (T45.1)
  ● **T45.AX** **Poisoning by, adverse effect of and underdosing of immune checkpoint inhibitors and immunostimulant drugs**
    T45.AX1 **Poisoning by immune checkpoint inhibitors and immunostimulant drugs, accidental (unintentional)**
      Poisoning by immune checkpoint inhibitors and immunosuppressive drugs NOS
    T45.AX2 **Poisoning by immune checkpoint inhibitors and immunostimulant drugs, intentional self-harm**
    T45.AX3 **Poisoning by immune checkpoint inhibitors and immunostimulant drugs, assault**
    T45.AX4 **Poisoning by immune checkpoint inhibitors and immunostimulant drugs, undetermined**
    T45.AX5 **Adverse effect of immune checkpoint inhibitors and immunostimulant drugs**
    T45.AX6 **Underdosing of immune checkpoint inhibitors and immunostimulant drugs**

● **T46** **Poisoning by, adverse effect of and underdosing of agents primarily affecting the cardiovascular system**
    Excludes1 poisoning by, adverse effect of and underdosing of metaraminol (T44.4)
  The appropriate 7th character is to be added to each code from category T46

A	initial encounter
D	subsequent encounter
S	sequela

● **T46.0** **Poisoning by, adverse effect of and underdosing of cardiac-stimulant glycosides and drugs of similar action**
  ● **T46.0X** **Poisoning by, adverse effect of and underdosing of cardiac-stimulant glycosides and drugs of similar action**
    ● **T46.0X1** **Poisoning by cardiac-stimulant glycosides and drugs of similar action, accidental (unintentional)**
      Poisoning by cardiac-stimulant glycosides and drugs of similar action NOS

● **T46.0X2** Poisoning by cardiac-stimulant glycosides and drugs of similar action, intentional self-harm A, S

● **T46.0X3** Poisoning by cardiac-stimulant glycosides and drugs of similar action, assault

● **T46.0X4** Poisoning by cardiac-stimulant glycosides and drugs of similar action, undetermined

● **T46.0X5** Adverse effect of cardiac-stimulant glycosides and drugs of similar action

● **T46.0X6** Underdosing of cardiac-stimulant glycosides and drugs of similar action

● **T46.1** Poisoning by, adverse effect of and underdosing of calcium-channel blockers

　● **T46.1X** Poisoning by, adverse effect of and underdosing of calcium-channel blockers

　　● **T46.1X1** Poisoning by calcium-channel blockers, accidental (unintentional)
　　　　Poisoning by calcium-channel blockers NOS

　　● **T46.1X2** Poisoning by calcium-channel blockers, intentional self-harm A, S

　　● **T46.1X3** Poisoning by calcium-channel blockers, assault

　　● **T46.1X4** Poisoning by calcium-channel blockers, undetermined

　　● **T46.1X5** Adverse effect of calcium-channel blockers

　　● **T46.1X6** Underdosing of calcium-channel blockers

● **T46.2** Poisoning by, adverse effect of and underdosing of other antidysrhythmic drugs, not elsewhere classified

　　Excludes1　poisoning by, adverse effect of and underdosing of beta-adrenoreceptor antagonists (T44.7-)

　● **T46.2X** Poisoning by, adverse effect of and underdosing of other antidysrhythmic drugs

　　● **T46.2X1** Poisoning by other antidysrhythmic drugs, accidental (unintentional)
　　　　Poisoning by other antidysrhythmic drugs NOS

　　● **T46.2X2** Poisoning by other antidysrhythmic drugs, intentional self-harm A, S

　　● **T46.2X3** Poisoning by other antidysrhythmic drugs, assault

　　● **T46.2X4** Poisoning by other antidysrhythmic drugs, undetermined

　　● **T46.2X5** Adverse effect of other antidysrhythmic drugs

　　● **T46.2X6** Underdosing of other antidysrhythmic drugs

● **T46.3** Poisoning by, adverse effect of and underdosing of coronary vasodilators
　　Poisoning by, adverse effect of and underdosing of dipyridamole

　　Excludes1　poisoning by, adverse effect of and underdosing of calcium-channel blockers (T46.1)

　● **T46.3X** Poisoning by, adverse effect of and underdosing of coronary vasodilators

　　● **T46.3X1** Poisoning by coronary vasodilators, accidental (unintentional)
　　　　Poisoning by coronary vasodilators NOS

　　● **T46.3X2** Poisoning by coronary vasodilators, intentional self-harm A, S

　　● **T46.3X3** Poisoning by coronary vasodilators, assault

　　● **T46.3X4** Poisoning by coronary vasodilators, undetermined

　　● **T46.3X5** Adverse effect of coronary vasodilators

　　● **T46.3X6** Underdosing of coronary vasodilators

● **T46.4** Poisoning by, adverse effect of and underdosing of angiotensin-converting-enzyme inhibitors

　● **T46.4X** Poisoning by, adverse effect of and underdosing of angiotensin-converting-enzyme inhibitors

　　● **T46.4X1** Poisoning by angiotensin-converting-enzyme inhibitors, accidental (unintentional)
　　　　Poisoning by angiotensin-converting-enzyme inhibitors NOS

　　● **T46.4X2** Poisoning by angiotensin-converting-enzyme inhibitors, intentional self-harm A, S

　　● **T46.4X3** Poisoning by angiotensin-converting-enzyme inhibitors, assault

　　● **T46.4X4** Poisoning by angiotensin-converting-enzyme inhibitors, undetermined

　　● **T46.4X5** Adverse effect of angiotensin-converting-enzyme inhibitors

　　● **T46.4X6** Underdosing of angiotensin-converting-enzyme inhibitors

● **T46.5** Poisoning by, adverse effect of and underdosing of other antihypertensive drugs

　　Excludes2　poisoning by, adverse effect of and underdosing of beta-adrenoreceptor antagonists (T44.7)
　　　　poisoning by, adverse effect of and underdosing of calcium-channel blockers (T46.1)
　　　　poisoning by, adverse effect of and underdosing of diuretics (T50.0-T50.2)

　● **T46.5X** Poisoning by, adverse effect of and underdosing of other antihypertensive drugs

　　● **T46.5X1** Poisoning by other antihypertensive drugs, accidental (unintentional)
　　　　Poisoning by other antihypertensive drugs NOS

　　● **T46.5X2** Poisoning by other antihypertensive drugs, intentional self-harm A, S

　　● **T46.5X3** Poisoning by other antihypertensive drugs, assault

　　● **T46.5X4** Poisoning by other antihypertensive drugs, undetermined

　　● **T46.5X5** Adverse effect of other antihypertensive drugs

　　● **T46.5X6** Underdosing of other antihypertensive drugs
　　　　Coding Clinic: 2022, Q1, P36

● **T46.6** Poisoning by, adverse effect of and underdosing of antihyperlipidemic and antiarteriosclerotic drugs

　● **T46.6X** Poisoning by, adverse effect of and underdosing of antihyperlipidemic and antiarteriosclerotic drugs

　　● **T46.6X1** Poisoning by antihyperlipidemic and antiarteriosclerotic drugs, accidental (unintentional)
　　　　Poisoning by antihyperlipidemic and antiarteriosclerotic drugs NOS

　　● **T46.6X2** Poisoning by antihyperlipidemic and antiarteriosclerotic drugs, intentional self-harm A, S

CHAPTER 19 (S00-T88)

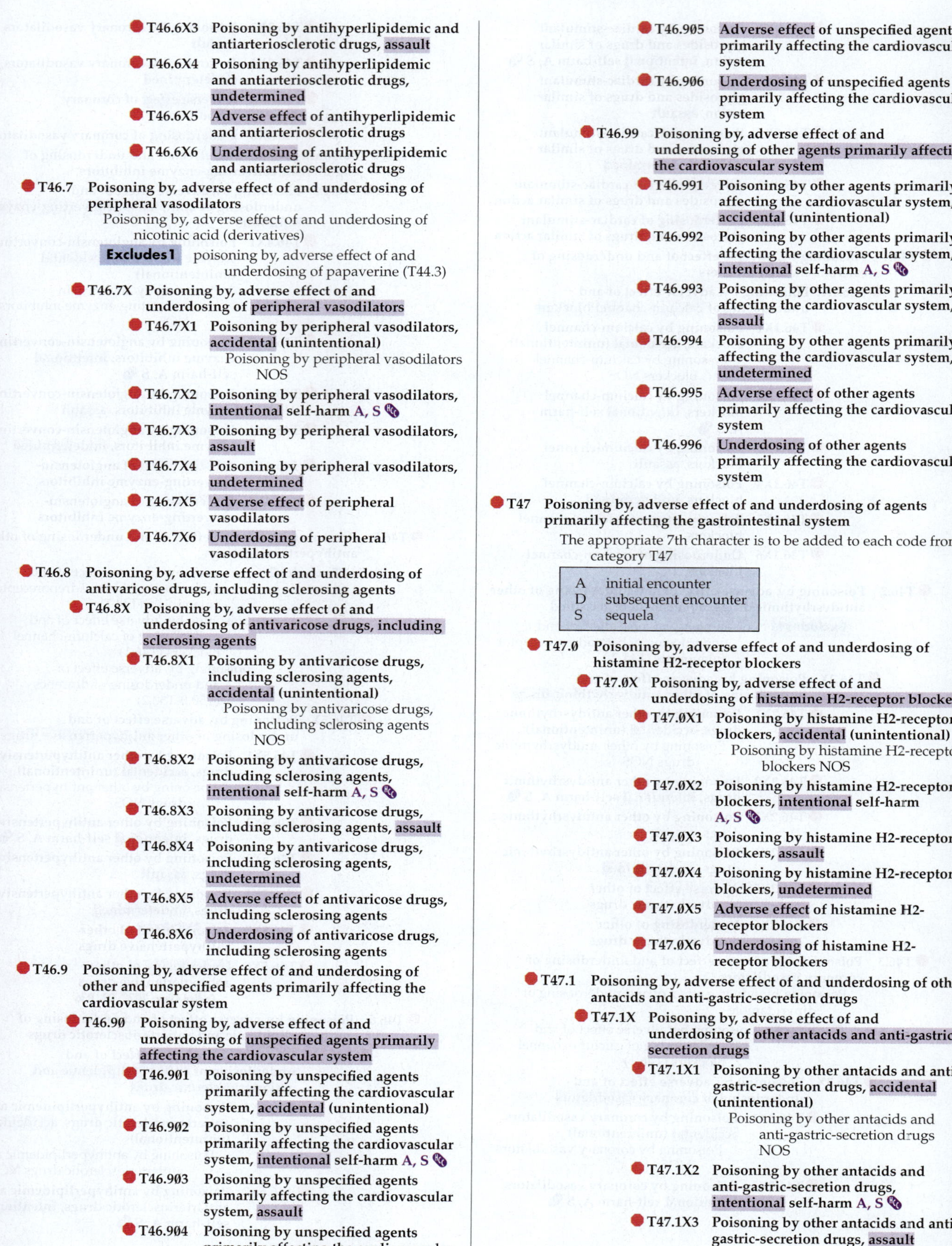

● **T46.6X3** Poisoning by antihyperlipidemic and antiarteriosclerotic drugs, assault

● **T46.6X4** Poisoning by antihyperlipidemic and antiarteriosclerotic drugs, undetermined

● **T46.6X5** Adverse effect of antihyperlipidemic and antiarteriosclerotic drugs

● **T46.6X6** Underdosing of antihyperlipidemic and antiarteriosclerotic drugs

● **T46.7** Poisoning by, adverse effect of and underdosing of peripheral vasodilators
  Poisoning by, adverse effect of and underdosing of nicotinic acid (derivatives)

  Excludes1 poisoning by, adverse effect of and underdosing of papaverine (T44.3)

● **T46.7X** Poisoning by, adverse effect of and underdosing of peripheral vasodilators

  ● **T46.7X1** Poisoning by peripheral vasodilators, accidental (unintentional)
    Poisoning by peripheral vasodilators NOS

  ● **T46.7X2** Poisoning by peripheral vasodilators, intentional self-harm A, S

  ● **T46.7X3** Poisoning by peripheral vasodilators, assault

  ● **T46.7X4** Poisoning by peripheral vasodilators, undetermined

  ● **T46.7X5** Adverse effect of peripheral vasodilators

  ● **T46.7X6** Underdosing of peripheral vasodilators

● **T46.8** Poisoning by, adverse effect of and underdosing of antivaricose drugs, including sclerosing agents

● **T46.8X** Poisoning by, adverse effect of and underdosing of antivaricose drugs, including sclerosing agents

  ● **T46.8X1** Poisoning by antivaricose drugs, including sclerosing agents, accidental (unintentional)
    Poisoning by antivaricose drugs, including sclerosing agents NOS

  ● **T46.8X2** Poisoning by antivaricose drugs, including sclerosing agents, intentional self-harm A, S

  ● **T46.8X3** Poisoning by antivaricose drugs, including sclerosing agents, assault

  ● **T46.8X4** Poisoning by antivaricose drugs, including sclerosing agents, undetermined

  ● **T46.8X5** Adverse effect of antivaricose drugs, including sclerosing agents

  ● **T46.8X6** Underdosing of antivaricose drugs, including sclerosing agents

● **T46.9** Poisoning by, adverse effect of and underdosing of other and unspecified agents primarily affecting the cardiovascular system

● **T46.90** Poisoning by, adverse effect of and underdosing of unspecified agents primarily affecting the cardiovascular system

  ● **T46.901** Poisoning by unspecified agents primarily affecting the cardiovascular system, accidental (unintentional)

  ● **T46.902** Poisoning by unspecified agents primarily affecting the cardiovascular system, intentional self-harm A, S

  ● **T46.903** Poisoning by unspecified agents primarily affecting the cardiovascular system, assault

  ● **T46.904** Poisoning by unspecified agents primarily affecting the cardiovascular system, undetermined

● **T46.905** Adverse effect of unspecified agents primarily affecting the cardiovascular system

● **T46.906** Underdosing of unspecified agents primarily affecting the cardiovascular system

● **T46.99** Poisoning by, adverse effect of and underdosing of other agents primarily affecting the cardiovascular system

  ● **T46.991** Poisoning by other agents primarily affecting the cardiovascular system, accidental (unintentional)

  ● **T46.992** Poisoning by other agents primarily affecting the cardiovascular system, intentional self-harm A, S

  ● **T46.993** Poisoning by other agents primarily affecting the cardiovascular system, assault

  ● **T46.994** Poisoning by other agents primarily affecting the cardiovascular system, undetermined

  ● **T46.995** Adverse effect of other agents primarily affecting the cardiovascular system

  ● **T46.996** Underdosing of other agents primarily affecting the cardiovascular system

● **T47** Poisoning by, adverse effect of and underdosing of agents primarily affecting the gastrointestinal system
  The appropriate 7th character is to be added to each code from category T47

A	initial encounter
D	subsequent encounter
S	sequela

● **T47.0** Poisoning by, adverse effect of and underdosing of histamine H2-receptor blockers

● **T47.0X** Poisoning by, adverse effect of and underdosing of histamine H2-receptor blockers

  ● **T47.0X1** Poisoning by histamine H2-receptor blockers, accidental (unintentional)
    Poisoning by histamine H2-receptor blockers NOS

  ● **T47.0X2** Poisoning by histamine H2-receptor blockers, intentional self-harm A, S

  ● **T47.0X3** Poisoning by histamine H2-receptor blockers, assault

  ● **T47.0X4** Poisoning by histamine H2-receptor blockers, undetermined

  ● **T47.0X5** Adverse effect of histamine H2-receptor blockers

  ● **T47.0X6** Underdosing of histamine H2-receptor blockers

● **T47.1** Poisoning by, adverse effect of and underdosing of other antacids and anti-gastric-secretion drugs

● **T47.1X** Poisoning by, adverse effect of and underdosing of other antacids and anti-gastric-secretion drugs

  ● **T47.1X1** Poisoning by other antacids and anti-gastric-secretion drugs, accidental (unintentional)
    Poisoning by other antacids and anti-gastric-secretion drugs NOS

  ● **T47.1X2** Poisoning by other antacids and anti-gastric-secretion drugs, intentional self-harm A, S

  ● **T47.1X3** Poisoning by other antacids and anti-gastric-secretion drugs, assault

● **T47.1X4** Poisoning by other antacids and anti-gastric-secretion drugs, undetermined

■ **T47.1X5** Adverse effect of other antacids and anti-gastric-secretion drugs

■ **T47.1X6** Underdosing of other antacids and anti-gastric-secretion drugs

● **T47.2** Poisoning by, adverse effect of and underdosing of stimulant laxatives

● **T47.2X** Poisoning by, adverse effect of and underdosing of stimulant laxatives

● **T47.2X1** Poisoning by stimulant laxatives, accidental (unintentional)
Poisoning by stimulant laxatives NOS

● **T47.2X2** Poisoning by stimulant laxatives, intentional self-harm A, S

● **T47.2X3** Poisoning by stimulant laxatives, assault

● **T47.2X4** Poisoning by stimulant laxatives, undetermined

■ **T47.2X5** Adverse effect of stimulant laxatives

■ **T47.2X6** Underdosing of stimulant laxatives

● **T47.3** Poisoning by, adverse effect of and underdosing of saline and osmotic laxatives

● **T47.3X** Poisoning by and adverse effect of saline and osmotic laxatives

● **T47.3X1** Poisoning by saline and osmotic laxatives, accidental (unintentional)
Poisoning by saline and osmotic laxatives NOS

● **T47.3X2** Poisoning by saline and osmotic laxatives, intentional self-harm

● **T47.3X3** Poisoning by saline and osmotic laxatives, assault A, S

● **T47.3X4** Poisoning by saline and osmotic laxatives, undetermined

■ **T47.3X5** Adverse effect of saline and osmotic laxatives

■ **T47.3X6** Underdosing of saline and osmotic laxatives

● **T47.4** Poisoning by, adverse effect of and underdosing of other laxatives

● **T47.4X** Poisoning by, adverse effect of and underdosing of other laxatives

● **T47.4X1** Poisoning by other laxatives, accidental (unintentional)
Poisoning by other laxatives NOS

● **T47.4X2** Poisoning by other laxatives, intentional self-harm A, S

● **T47.4X3** Poisoning by other laxatives, assault

● **T47.4X4** Poisoning by other laxatives, undetermined

■ **T47.4X5** Adverse effect of other laxatives

■ **T47.4X6** Underdosing of other laxatives

● **T47.5** Poisoning by, adverse effect of and underdosing of digestants

● **T47.5X** Poisoning by, adverse effect of and underdosing of digestants

● **T47.5X1** Poisoning by digestants, accidental (unintentional)
Poisoning by digestants NOS

● **T47.5X2** Poisoning by digestants, intentional self-harm A, S

● **T47.5X3** Poisoning by digestants, assault

● **T47.5X4** Poisoning by digestants, undetermined

■ **T47.5X5** Adverse effect of digestants

■ **T47.5X6** Underdosing of digestants

● **T47.6** Poisoning by, adverse effect of and underdosing of antidiarrheal drugs

Excludes2 poisoning by, adverse effect of and underdosing of systemic antibiotics and other anti-infectives (T36-T37)

● **T47.6X** Poisoning by, adverse effect of and underdosing of antidiarrheal drugs

● **T47.6X1** Poisoning by antidiarrheal drugs, accidental (unintentional)
Poisoning by antidiarrheal drugs NOS

● **T47.6X2** Poisoning by antidiarrheal drugs, intentional self-harm A, S

● **T47.6X3** Poisoning by antidiarrheal drugs, assault

● **T47.6X4** Poisoning by antidiarrheal drugs, undetermined

■ **T47.6X5** Adverse effect of antidiarrheal drugs

■ **T47.6X6** Underdosing of antidiarrheal drugs

● **T47.7** Poisoning by, adverse effect of and underdosing of emetics

● **T47.7X** Poisoning by, adverse effect of and underdosing of emetics

● **T47.7X1** Poisoning by emetics, accidental (unintentional)
Poisoning by emetics NOS

● **T47.7X2** Poisoning by emetics, intentional self-harm A, S

● **T47.7X3** Poisoning by emetics, assault

● **T47.7X4** Poisoning by emetics, undetermined

■ **T47.7X5** Adverse effect of emetics

■ **T47.7X6** Underdosing of emetics

● **T47.8** Poisoning by, adverse effect of and underdosing of other agents primarily affecting gastrointestinal system

● **T47.8X** Poisoning by, adverse effect of and underdosing of other agents primarily affecting gastrointestinal system

● **T47.8X1** Poisoning by other agents primarily affecting gastrointestinal system, accidental (unintentional)
Poisoning by other agents primarily affecting gastrointestinal system NOS

● **T47.8X2** Poisoning by other agents primarily affecting gastrointestinal system, intentional self-harm A, S

● **T47.8X3** Poisoning by other agents primarily affecting gastrointestinal system, assault

● **T47.8X4** Poisoning by other agents primarily affecting gastrointestinal system, undetermined

■ **T47.8X5** Adverse effect of other agents primarily affecting gastrointestinal system

■ **T47.8X6** Underdosing of other agents primarily affecting gastrointestinal system

● **T47.9** Poisoning by, adverse effect of and underdosing of unspecified agents primarily affecting the gastrointestinal system

X ● **T47.91** Poisoning by unspecified agents primarily affecting the gastrointestinal system, accidental (unintentional)
Poisoning by agents primarily affecting the gastrointestinal system NOS

X ● **T47.92** Poisoning by unspecified agents primarily affecting the gastrointestinal system, intentional self-harm A, S

X ● **T47.93** Poisoning by unspecified agents primarily affecting the gastrointestinal system, assault

X ● T47.94   Poisoning by unspecified agents primarily affecting the gastrointestinal system, undetermined

X ● T47.95   Adverse effect of unspecified agents primarily affecting the gastrointestinal system

X ● T47.96   Underdosing of unspecified agents primarily affecting the gastrointestinal system

● T48   Poisoning by, adverse effect of and underdosing of agents primarily acting on smooth and skeletal muscles and the respiratory system

The appropriate 7th character is to be added to each code from category T48

> A   initial encounter
> D   subsequent encounter
> S   sequela

● T48.0   Poisoning by, adverse effect of and underdosing of oxytocic drugs

Excludes1   poisoning by, adverse effect of and underdosing of estrogens, progestogens and antagonists (T38.4-T38.6)

● T48.0X   Poisoning by, adverse effect of and underdosing of oxytocic drugs

● T48.0X1   Poisoning by oxytocic drugs, accidental (unintentional)
Poisoning by oxytocic drugs NOS

● T48.0X2   Poisoning by oxytocic drugs, intentional self-harm A, S 🏥

● T48.0X3   Poisoning by oxytocic drugs, assault

● T48.0X4   Poisoning by oxytocic drugs, undetermined

● T48.0X5   Adverse effect of oxytocic drugs

● T48.0X6   Underdosing of oxytocic drugs

● T48.1   Poisoning by, adverse effect of and underdosing of skeletal muscle relaxants [neuromuscular blocking agents]

● T48.1X   Poisoning by, adverse effect of and underdosing of skeletal muscle relaxants [neuromuscular blocking agents]

● T48.1X1   Poisoning by skeletal muscle relaxants [neuromuscular blocking agents], accidental (unintentional)
Poisoning by skeletal muscle relaxants [neuromuscular blocking agents] NOS

● T48.1X2   Poisoning by skeletal muscle relaxants [neuromuscular blocking agents], intentional self-harm A, S 🏥

● T48.1X3   Poisoning by skeletal muscle relaxants [neuromuscular blocking agents], assault

● T48.1X4   Poisoning by skeletal muscle relaxants [neuromuscular blocking agents], undetermined

● T48.1X5   Adverse effect of skeletal muscle relaxants [neuromuscular blocking agents]

● T48.1X6   Underdosing of skeletal muscle relaxants [neuromuscular blocking agents]

● T48.2   Poisoning by, adverse effect of and underdosing of other and unspecified drugs acting on muscles

● T48.20   Poisoning by, adverse effect of and underdosing of unspecified drugs acting on muscles

● T48.201   Poisoning by unspecified drugs acting on muscles, accidental (unintentional)
Poisoning by unspecified drugs acting on muscles NOS

● T48.202   Poisoning by unspecified drugs acting on muscles, intentional self-harm A, S 🏥

● T48.203   Poisoning by unspecified drugs acting on muscles, assault

● T48.204   Poisoning by unspecified drugs acting on muscles, undetermined

● T48.205   Adverse effect of unspecified drugs acting on muscles

● T48.206   Underdosing of unspecified drugs acting on muscles

● T48.29   Poisoning by, adverse effect of and underdosing of other drugs acting on muscles

● T48.291   Poisoning by other drugs acting on muscles, accidental (unintentional)
Poisoning by other drugs acting on muscles NOS

● T48.292   Poisoning by other drugs acting on muscles, intentional self-harm A, S 🏥

● T48.293   Poisoning by other drugs acting on muscles, assault

● T48.294   Poisoning by other drugs acting on muscles, undetermined

● T48.295   Adverse effect of other drugs acting on muscles

● T48.296   Underdosing of other drugs acting on muscles

● T48.3   Poisoning by, adverse effect of and underdosing of antitussives

● T48.3X   Poisoning by, adverse effect of and underdosing of antitussives

● T48.3X1   Poisoning by antitussives, accidental (unintentional)
Poisoning by antitussives NOS

● T48.3X2   Poisoning by antitussives, intentional self-harm A, S 🏥

● T48.3X3   Poisoning by antitussives, assault

● T48.3X4   Poisoning by antitussives, undetermined

● T48.3X5   Adverse effect of antitussives

● T48.3X6   Underdosing of antitussives

● T48.4   Poisoning by, adverse effect of and underdosing of expectorants

● T48.4X   Poisoning by, adverse effect of and underdosing of expectorants

● T48.4X1   Poisoning by expectorants, accidental (unintentional)
Poisoning by expectorants NOS

● T48.4X2   Poisoning by expectorants, intentional self-harm A, S 🏥

● T48.4X3   Poisoning by expectorants, assault

● T48.4X4   Poisoning by expectorants, undetermined

● T48.4X5   Adverse effect of expectorants

● T48.4X6   Underdosing of expectorants

● T48.5   Poisoning by, adverse effect of and underdosing of other anti-common-cold drugs
Poisoning by, adverse effect of and underdosing of decongestants

Excludes2   poisoning by, adverse effect of and underdosing of antipyretics, NEC (T39.9-)
poisoning by, adverse effect of and underdosing of non-steroidal antiinflammatory drugs (T39.3-)
poisoning by, adverse effect of and underdosing of salicylates (T39.0-)

▶ New   ⇨ Revised   ~~deleted~~ Deleted   Excludes 1   Excludes 2   Includes   Use additional   Code first   Code also   Key words
OGCR Official Guidelines   X Assign placeholder X   ● Use Additional Character(s)   ▸ Manifestation Code   🏥 Hierarchical Condition Category   Coding Clinic

● **T48.5X** **Poisoning by, adverse effect of and underdosing of other anti-common-cold drugs**
    ● **T48.5X1** **Poisoning by other anti-common-cold drugs, accidental (unintentional)**
       Poisoning by other anti-common-cold drugs NOS
    ● **T48.5X2** **Poisoning by other anti-common-cold drugs, intentional self-harm A, S**
    ● **T48.5X3** **Poisoning by other anti-common-cold drugs, assault**
    ● **T48.5X4** **Poisoning by other anti-common-cold drugs, undetermined**
    ● **T48.5X5** **Adverse effect of other anti-common-cold drugs**
    ● **T48.5X6** **Underdosing of other anti-common-cold drugs**

● **T48.6** **Poisoning by, adverse effect of and underdosing of antiasthmatics, not elsewhere classified**
    Poisoning by, adverse effect of and underdosing of beta-adrenoreceptor agonists used in asthma therapy
    Excludes 1   poisoning by, adverse effect of and underdosing of beta-adrenoreceptor agonists not used in asthma therapy (T44.5)
               poisoning by, adverse effect of and underdosing of anterior pituitary [adenohypophyseal] hormones (T38.8)

    ● **T48.6X** **Poisoning by, adverse effect of and underdosing of antiasthmatics**
       ● **T48.6X1** **Poisoning by antiasthmatics, accidental (unintentional)**
          Poisoning by antiasthmatics NOS
       ● **T48.6X2** **Poisoning by antiasthmatics, intentional self-harm A, S**
       ● **T48.6X3** **Poisoning by antiasthmatics, assault**
       ● **T48.6X4** **Poisoning by antiasthmatics, undetermined**
       ● **T48.6X5** **Adverse effect of antiasthmatics**
       ● **T48.6X6** **Underdosing of antiasthmatics**

● **T48.9** **Poisoning by, adverse effect of and underdosing of other and unspecified agents primarily acting on the respiratory system**
    ● **T48.90** **Poisoning by, adverse effect of and underdosing of unspecified agents primarily acting on the respiratory system**
       ● **T48.901** **Poisoning by unspecified agents primarily acting on the respiratory system, accidental (unintentional)**
       ● **T48.902** **Poisoning by unspecified agents primarily acting on the respiratory system, intentional self-harm A, S**
       ● **T48.903** **Poisoning by unspecified agents primarily acting on the respiratory system, assault**
       ● **T48.904** **Poisoning by unspecified agents primarily acting on the respiratory system, undetermined**
       ● **T48.905** **Adverse effect of unspecified agents primarily acting on the respiratory system**
       ● **T48.906** **Underdosing of unspecified agents primarily acting on the respiratory system**

● **T48.99** **Poisoning by, adverse effect of and underdosing of other agents primarily acting on the respiratory system**
    ● **T48.991** **Poisoning by other agents primarily acting on the respiratory system, accidental (unintentional)**
    ● **T48.992** **Poisoning by other agents primarily acting on the respiratory system, intentional self-harm A, S**
    ● **T48.993** **Poisoning by other agents primarily acting on the respiratory system, assault**
    ● **T48.994** **Poisoning by other agents primarily acting on the respiratory system, undetermined**
    ● **T48.995** **Adverse effect of other agents primarily acting on the respiratory system**
    ● **T48.996** **Underdosing of other agents primarily acting on the respiratory system**

● **T49** **Poisoning by, adverse effect of and underdosing of topical agents primarily affecting skin and mucous membrane and by ophthalmological, otorhinorlaryngological and dental drugs**
    Includes   poisoning by, adverse effect of and underdosing of glucocorticoids, topically used
    The appropriate 7th character is to be added to each code from category T49

A	initial encounter
D	subsequent encounter
S	sequela

● **T49.0** **Poisoning by, adverse effect of and underdosing of local antifungal, anti-infective and anti-inflammatory drugs**
    ● **T49.0X** **Poisoning by, adverse effect of and underdosing of local antifungal, anti-infective and anti-inflammatory drugs**
       ● **T49.0X1** **Poisoning by local antifungal, anti-infective and anti-inflammatory drugs, accidental (unintentional)**
          Poisoning by local antifungal, anti-infective and anti-inflammatory drugs NOS
       ● **T49.0X2** **Poisoning by local antifungal, anti-infective and anti-inflammatory drugs, intentional self-harm A, S**
       ● **T49.0X3** **Poisoning by local antifungal, anti-infective and anti-inflammatory drugs, assault**
       ● **T49.0X4** **Poisoning by local antifungal, anti-infective and anti-inflammatory drugs, undetermined**
       ● **T49.0X5** **Adverse effect of local antifungal, anti-infective and anti-inflammatory drugs**
       ● **T49.0X6** **Underdosing of local antifungal, anti-infective and anti-inflammatory drugs**

● **T49.1** **Poisoning by, adverse effect of and underdosing of antipruritics**
    ● **T49.1X** **Poisoning by, adverse effect of and underdosing of antipruritics**
       ● **T49.1X1** **Poisoning by antipruritics, accidental (unintentional)**
          Poisoning by antipruritics NOS
       ● **T49.1X2** **Poisoning by antipruritics, intentional self-harm A, S**
       ● **T49.1X3** **Poisoning by antipruritics, assault**
       ● **T49.1X4** **Poisoning by antipruritics, undetermined**
       ● **T49.1X5** **Adverse effect of antipruritics**
       ● **T49.1X6** **Underdosing of antipruritics**

CHAPTER 19 (S00-T88)

● **T49.2** Poisoning by, adverse effect of and underdosing of local astringents and local detergents

  ● **T49.2X** Poisoning by, adverse effect of and underdosing of local astringents and local detergents

    ● **T49.2X1** Poisoning by local astringents and local detergents, accidental (unintentional)
      Poisoning by local astringents and local detergents NOS

    ● **T49.2X2** Poisoning by local astringents and local detergents, intentional self-harm A, S

    ● **T49.2X3** Poisoning by local astringents and local detergents, assault

    ● **T49.2X4** Poisoning by local astringents and local detergents, undetermined

    ● **T49.2X5** Adverse effect of local astringents and local detergents

    ● **T49.2X6** Underdosing of local astringents and local detergents

● **T49.3** Poisoning by, adverse effect of and underdosing of emollients, demulcents and protectants

  ● **T49.3X** Poisoning by, adverse effect of and underdosing of emollients, demulcents and protectants

    ● **T49.3X1** Poisoning by emollients, demulcents and protectants, accidental (unintentional)
      Poisoning by emollients, demulcents and protectants NOS

    ● **T49.3X2** Poisoning by emollients, demulcents and protectants, intentional self-harm A, S

    ● **T49.3X3** Poisoning by emollients, demulcents and protectants, assault

    ● **T49.3X4** Poisoning by emollients, demulcents and protectants, undetermined

    ● **T49.3X5** Adverse effect of emollients, demulcents and protectants

    ● **T49.3X6** Underdosing of emollients, demulcents and protectants

● **T49.4** Poisoning by, adverse effect of and underdosing of keratolytics, keratoplastics, and other hair treatment drugs and preparations

  ● **T49.4X** Poisoning by, adverse effect of and underdosing of keratolytics, keratoplastics, and other hair treatment drugs and preparations

    ● **T49.4X1** Poisoning by keratolytics, keratoplastics, and other hair treatment drugs and preparations, accidental (unintentional)
      Poisoning by keratolytics, keratoplastics, and other hair treatment drugs and preparations NOS

    ● **T49.4X2** Poisoning by keratolytics, keratoplastics, and other hair treatment drugs and preparations, intentional self-harm A, S

    ● **T49.4X3** Poisoning by keratolytics, keratoplastics, and other hair treatment drugs and preparations, assault

    ● **T49.4X4** Poisoning by keratolytics, keratoplastics, and other hair treatment drugs and preparations, undetermined

    ● **T49.4X5** Adverse effect of keratolytics, keratoplastics, and other hair treatment drugs and preparations

    ● **T49.4X6** Underdosing of keratolytics, keratoplastics, and other hair treatment drugs and preparations

● **T49.5** Poisoning by, adverse effect of and underdosing of ophthalmological drugs and preparations

  ● **T49.5X** Poisoning by, adverse effect of and underdosing of ophthalmological drugs and preparations

    ● **T49.5X1** Poisoning by ophthalmological drugs and preparations, accidental (unintentional)
      Poisoning by ophthalmological drugs and preparations NOS

    ● **T49.5X2** Poisoning by ophthalmological drugs and preparations, intentional self-harm A, S

    ● **T49.5X3** Poisoning by ophthalmological drugs and preparations, assault

    ● **T49.5X4** Poisoning by ophthalmological drugs and preparations, undetermined

    ● **T49.5X5** Adverse effect of ophthalmological drugs and preparations

    ● **T49.5X6** Underdosing of ophthalmological drugs and preparations

● **T49.6** Poisoning by, adverse effect of and underdosing of otorhinolaryngological drugs and preparations

  ● **T49.6X** Poisoning by, adverse effect of and underdosing of otorhinolaryngological drugs and preparations

    ● **T49.6X1** Poisoning by otorhinolaryngological drugs and preparations, accidental (unintentional)
      Poisoning by otorhinolaryngological drugs and preparations NOS

    ● **T49.6X2** Poisoning by otorhinolaryngological drugs and preparations, intentional self-harm A, S

    ● **T49.6X3** Poisoning by otorhinolaryngological drugs and preparations, assault

    ● **T49.6X4** Poisoning by otorhinolaryngological drugs and preparations, undetermined

    ● **T49.6X5** Adverse effect of otorhinolaryngological drugs and preparations

    ● **T49.6X6** Underdosing of otorhinolaryngological drugs and preparations

● **T49.7** Poisoning by, adverse effect of and underdosing of dental drugs, topically applied

  ● **T49.7X** Poisoning by, adverse effect of and underdosing of dental drugs, topically applied

    ● **T49.7X1** Poisoning by dental drugs, topically applied, accidental (unintentional)
      Poisoning by dental drugs, topically applied NOS

    ● **T49.7X2** Poisoning by dental drugs, topically applied, intentional self-harm A, S

    ● **T49.7X3** Poisoning by dental drugs, topically applied, assault

    ● **T49.7X4** Poisoning by dental drugs, topically applied, undetermined

    ● **T49.7X5** Adverse effect of dental drugs, topically applied

    ● **T49.7X6** Underdosing of dental drugs, topically applied

● **T49.8** Poisoning by, adverse effect of and underdosing of other topical agents
  Poisoning by, adverse effect of and underdosing of spermicides

  ● **T49.8X** Poisoning by, adverse effect of and underdosing of other topical agents

    ● **T49.8X1** Poisoning by other topical agents, accidental (unintentional)
      Poisoning by other topical agents NOS

CHAPTER 19 (S00–T88)

● T49.8X2 Poisoning by other topical agents, intentional self-harm A, S 🔃

● T49.8X3 Poisoning by other topical agents, assault

● T49.8X4 Poisoning by other topical agents, undetermined

● T49.8X5 Adverse effect of other topical agents

● T49.8X6 Underdosing of other topical agents

● T49.9 Poisoning by, adverse effect of and underdosing of unspecified topical agent

X ● T49.91 Poisoning by unspecified topical agent, accidental (unintentional)

X ● T49.92 Poisoning by unspecified topical agent, intentional self-harm A, S 🔃

X ● T49.93 Poisoning by unspecified topical agent, assault

X ● T49.94 Poisoning by unspecified topical agent, undetermined

X ● T49.95 Adverse effect of unspecified topical agent

X ● T49.96 Underdosing of unspecified topical agent

● T50 Poisoning by, adverse effect of and underdosing of diuretics and other and unspecified drugs, medicaments and biological substances

The appropriate 7th character is to be added to each code from category T50

A	initial encounter
D	subsequent encounter
S	sequela

● T50.0 Poisoning by, adverse effect of and underdosing of mineralocorticoids and their antagonists

● T50.0X Poisoning by, adverse effect of and underdosing of mineralocorticoids and their antagonists

● T50.0X1 Poisoning by mineralocorticoids and their antagonists, accidental (unintentional)
Poisoning by mineralocorticoids and their antagonists NOS

● T50.0X2 Poisoning by mineralocorticoids and their antagonists, intentional self-harm A, S 🔃

● T50.0X3 Poisoning by mineralocorticoids and their antagonists, assault

● T50.0X4 Poisoning by mineralocorticoids and their antagonists, undetermined

● T50.0X5 Adverse effect of mineralocorticoids and their antagonists

● T50.0X6 Underdosing of mineralocorticoids and their antagonists

● T50.1 Poisoning by, adverse effect of and underdosing of loop [high-ceiling] diuretics

● T50.1X Poisoning by, adverse effect of and underdosing of loop [high-ceiling] diuretics

● T50.1X1 Poisoning by loop [high-ceiling] diuretics, accidental (unintentional)
Poisoning by loop [high-ceiling] diuretics NOS

● T50.1X2 Poisoning by loop [high-ceiling] diuretics, intentional self-harm A, S 🔃

● T50.1X3 Poisoning by loop [high-ceiling] diuretics, assault

● T50.1X4 Poisoning by loop [high-ceiling] diuretics, undetermined

● T50.1X5 Adverse effect of loop [high-ceiling] diuretics

● T50.1X6 Underdosing of loop [high-ceiling] diuretics

● T50.2 Poisoning by, adverse effect of and underdosing of carbonic-anhydrase inhibitors, benzothiadiazides and other diuretics
Poisoning by, adverse effect of and underdosing of acetazolamide

● T50.2X Poisoning by, adverse effect of and underdosing of carbonic-anhydrase inhibitors, benzothiadiazides and other diuretics

● T50.2X1 Poisoning by carbonic-anhydrase inhibitors, benzothiadiazides and other diuretics, accidental (unintentional)
Poisoning by carbonic-anhydrase inhibitors, benzothiadiazides and other diuretics NOS

● T50.2X2 Poisoning by carbonic-anhydrase inhibitors, benzothiadiazides and other diuretics, intentional self-harm A, S 🔃

● T50.2X3 Poisoning by carbonic-anhydrase inhibitors, benzothiadiazides and other diuretics, assault

● T50.2X4 Poisoning by carbonic-anhydrase inhibitors, benzothiadiazides and other diuretics, undetermined

● T50.2X5 Adverse effect of carbonic-anhydrase inhibitors, benzothiadiazides and other diuretics

● T50.2X6 Underdosing of carbonic-anhydrase inhibitors, benzothiadiazides and other diuretics

● T50.3 Poisoning by, adverse effect of and underdosing of electrolytic, caloric and water-balance agents
Poisoning by, adverse effect of and underdosing of oral rehydration salts

● T50.3X Poisoning by, adverse effect of and underdosing of electrolytic, caloric and water-balance agents

● T50.3X1 Poisoning by electrolytic, caloric and water-balance agents, accidental (unintentional)
Poisoning by electrolytic, caloric and water-balance agents NOS

● T50.3X2 Poisoning by electrolytic, caloric and water-balance agents, intentional self-harm A, S 🔃

● T50.3X3 Poisoning by electrolytic, caloric and water-balance agents, assault

● T50.3X4 Poisoning by electrolytic, caloric and water-balance agents, undetermined

● T50.3X5 Adverse effect of electrolytic, caloric and water-balance agents
Coding Clinic: 2022, Q2, P11

● T50.3X6 Underdosing of electrolytic, caloric and water-balance agents

● T50.4 Poisoning by, adverse effect of and underdosing of drugs affecting uric acid metabolism

● T50.4X Poisoning by, adverse effect of and underdosing of drugs affecting uric acid metabolism

● T50.4X1 Poisoning by drugs affecting uric acid metabolism, accidental (unintentional)
Poisoning by drugs affecting uric acid metabolism NOS

● T50.4X2 Poisoning by drugs affecting uric acid metabolism, intentional self-harm A, S 🔃

● T50.4X3 Poisoning by drugs affecting uric acid metabolism, assault

● T50.4X4 Poisoning by drugs affecting uric acid metabolism, undetermined

● T50.4X5 Adverse effect of drugs affecting uric acid metabolism

● T50.4X6 Underdosing of drugs affecting uric acid metabolism

CHAPTER 19 (S00–T88)

- ● T50.5   Poisoning by, adverse effect of and underdosing of appetite depressants
  - ● T50.5X   Poisoning by, adverse effect of and underdosing of appetite depressants
    - ● T50.5X1   Poisoning by appetite depressants, accidental (unintentional)
      Poisoning by appetite depressants NOS
    - ● T50.5X2   Poisoning by appetite depressants, intentional self-harm A, S 🅷
    - ● T50.5X3   Poisoning by appetite depressants, assault
    - ● T50.5X4   Poisoning by appetite depressants, undetermined
    - ● T50.5X5   Adverse effect of appetite depressants
    - ● T50.5X6   Underdosing of appetite depressants
- ● T50.6   Poisoning by, adverse effect of and underdosing of antidotes and chelating agents
  Poisoning by, adverse effect of and underdosing of alcohol deterrents
  - ● T50.6X   Poisoning by, adverse effect of and underdosing of antidotes and chelating agents
    - ● T50.6X1   Poisoning by antidotes and chelating agents, accidental (unintentional)
      Poisoning by antidotes and chelating agents NOS
    - ● T50.6X2   Poisoning by antidotes and chelating agents, intentional self-harm A, S 🅷
    - ● T50.6X3   Poisoning by antidotes and chelating agents, assault
    - ● T50.6X4   Poisoning by antidotes and chelating agents, undetermined
    - ● T50.6X5   Adverse effect of antidotes and chelating agents
    - ● T50.6X6   Underdosing of antidotes and chelating agents
- ● T50.7   Poisoning by, adverse effect of and underdosing of analeptics and opioid receptor antagonists
  - ● T50.7X   Poisoning by, adverse effect of and underdosing of analeptics and opioid receptor antagonists
    - ● T50.7X1   Poisoning by analeptics and opioid receptor antagonists, accidental (unintentional)
      Poisoning by analeptics and opioid receptor antagonists NOS
    - ● T50.7X2   Poisoning by analeptics and opioid receptor antagonists, intentional self-harm A, S 🅷
    - ● T50.7X3   Poisoning by analeptics and opioid receptor antagonists, assault
    - ● T50.7X4   Poisoning by analeptics and opioid receptor antagonists, undetermined
    - ● T50.7X5   Adverse effect of analeptics and opioid receptor antagonists
    - ● T50.7X6   Underdosing of analeptics and opioid receptor antagonists
- ● T50.8   Poisoning by, adverse effect of and underdosing of diagnostic agents
  - ● T50.8X   Poisoning by, adverse effect of and underdosing of diagnostic agents
    - ● T50.8X1   Poisoning by diagnostic agents, accidental (unintentional)
      Poisoning by diagnostic agents NOS
    - ● T50.8X2   Poisoning by diagnostic agents, intentional self-harm A, S 🅷

- ● T50.8X3   Poisoning by diagnostic agents, assault
- ● T50.8X4   Poisoning by diagnostic agents, undetermined
- ● T50.8X5   Adverse effect of diagnostic agents
  Coding Clinic: 2023, Q3, P4-5; 2022, Q4, P33; 2021, Q3, P9-10
- ● T50.8X6   Underdosing of diagnostic agents
- ● T50.A   Poisoning by, adverse effect of and underdosing of bacterial vaccines
  - ● T50.A1   Poisoning by, adverse effect of and underdosing of pertussis vaccine, including combinations with a pertussis component
    - ● T50.A11   Poisoning by pertussis vaccine, including combinations with a pertussis component, accidental (unintentional)
    - ● T50.A12   Poisoning by pertussis vaccine, including combinations with a pertussis component, intentional self-harm A, S 🅷
    - ● T50.A13   Poisoning by pertussis vaccine, including combinations with a pertussis component, assault
    - ● T50.A14   Poisoning by pertussis vaccine, including combinations with a pertussis component, undetermined
    - ● T50.A15   Adverse effect of pertussis vaccine, including combinations with a pertussis component
    - ● T50.A16   Underdosing of pertussis vaccine, including combinations with a pertussis component
  - ● T50.A2   Poisoning by, adverse effect of and underdosing of mixed bacterial vaccines without a pertussis component
    - ● T50.A21   Poisoning by mixed bacterial vaccines without a pertussis component, accidental (unintentional)
    - ● T50.A22   Poisoning by mixed bacterial vaccines without a pertussis component, intentional self-harm A, S 🅷
    - ● T50.A23   Poisoning by mixed bacterial vaccines without a pertussis component, assault
    - ● T50.A24   Poisoning by mixed bacterial vaccines without a pertussis component, undetermined
    - ● T50.A25   Adverse effect of mixed bacterial vaccines without a pertussis component
    - ● T50.A26   Underdosing of mixed bacterial vaccines without a pertussis component
  - ● T50.A9   Poisoning by, adverse effect of and underdosing of other bacterial vaccines
    - ● T50.A91   Poisoning by other bacterial vaccines, accidental (unintentional)
    - ● T50.A92   Poisoning by other bacterial vaccines, intentional self-harm A, S 🅷
    - ● T50.A93   Poisoning by other bacterial vaccines, assault
    - ● T50.A94   Poisoning by other bacterial vaccines, undetermined
    - ● T50.A95   Adverse effect of other bacterial vaccines
    - ● T50.A96   Underdosing of other bacterial vaccines

▶ New   ➡ Revised   ~~deleted~~ Deleted   Excludes 1   Excludes 2   Includes   Use additional   Code first   Code also   Key words
OGCR Official Guidelines   X Assign placeholder X   ● Use Additional Character(s)   ▶ Manifestation Code   🅷 Hierarchical Condition Category   Coding Clinic

● **T50.B** Poisoning by, adverse effect of and underdosing of viral vaccines
     ● **T50.B1** Poisoning by, adverse effect of and underdosing of smallpox vaccines
         ● **T50.B11** Poisoning by smallpox vaccines, accidental (unintentional)
         ● **T50.B12** Poisoning by smallpox vaccines, intentional self-harm A, S
         ● **T50.B13** Poisoning by smallpox vaccines, assault
         ● **T50.B14** Poisoning by smallpox vaccines, undetermined
         ● **T50.B15** Adverse effect of smallpox vaccines
         ● **T50.B16** Underdosing of smallpox vaccines
     ● **T50.B9** Poisoning by, adverse effect of and underdosing of other viral vaccines
         ● **T50.B91** Poisoning by other viral vaccines, accidental (unintentional)
         ● **T50.B92** Poisoning by other viral vaccines, intentional self-harm A, S
         ● **T50.B93** Poisoning by other viral vaccines, assault
         ● **T50.B94** Poisoning by other viral vaccines, undetermined
         ● **T50.B95** Adverse effect of other viral vaccines
            Coding Clinic: 2021, Q1, P43-44
         ● **T50.B96** Underdosing of other viral vaccines
● **T50.Z** Poisoning by, adverse effect of and underdosing of other vaccines and biological substances
     ● **T50.Z1** Poisoning by, adverse effect of and underdosing of immunoglobulin
         ● **T50.Z11** Poisoning by immunoglobulin, accidental (unintentional)
         ● **T50.Z12** Poisoning by immunoglobulin, intentional self-harm A, S
         ● **T50.Z13** Poisoning by immunoglobulin, assault
         ● **T50.Z14** Poisoning by immunoglobulin, undetermined
         ● **T50.Z15** Adverse effect of immunoglobulin
         ● **T50.Z16** Underdosing of immunoglobulin
     ● **T50.Z9** Poisoning by, adverse effect of and underdosing of other vaccines and biological substances
         ● **T50.Z91** Poisoning by other vaccines and biological substances, accidental (unintentional)
         ● **T50.Z92** Poisoning by other vaccines and biological substances, intentional self-harm A, S
         ● **T50.Z93** Poisoning by other vaccines and biological substances, assault
         ● **T50.Z94** Poisoning by other vaccines and biological substances, undetermined
         ● **T50.Z95** Adverse effect of other vaccines and biological substances
            Coding Clinic: 2020, Q1, P19
         ● **T50.Z96** Underdosing of other vaccines and biological substances
● **T50.9** Poisoning by, adverse effect of and underdosing of other and unspecified drugs, medicaments and biological substances
     ● **T50.90** Poisoning by, adverse effect of and underdosing of unspecified drugs, medicaments and biological substances
         ● **T50.901** Poisoning by unspecified drugs, medicaments and biological substances, accidental (unintentional)
            Coding Clinic: 2015, Q1, P21

         ● **T50.902** Poisoning by unspecified drugs, medicaments and biological substances, intentional self-harm A, S
         ● **T50.903** Poisoning by unspecified drugs, medicaments and biological substances, assault
         ● **T50.904** Poisoning by unspecified drugs, medicaments and biological substances, undetermined
         ● **T50.905** Adverse effect of unspecified drugs, medicaments and biological substances
         ● **T50.906** Underdosing of unspecified drugs, medicaments and biological substances
     ● **T50.91** Poisoning by, adverse effect of and underdosing of multiple unspecified drugs, medicaments and biological substances
         Multiple drug ingestion NOS
         Code also any specific drugs, medicaments and biological substances
         ● **T50.911** Poisoning by multiple unspecified drugs, medicaments and biological substances, accidental (unintentional)
         ● **T50.912** Poisoning by multiple unspecified drugs, medicaments and biological substances, intentional self-harm
         ● **T50.913** Poisoning by multiple unspecified drugs, medicaments and biological substances, assault
         ● **T50.914** Poisoning by multiple unspecified drugs, medicaments and biological substances, undetermined
         ● **T50.915** Adverse effect of multiple unspecified drugs, medicaments and biological substances
         ● **T50.916** Underdosing of multiple unspecified drugs, medicaments and biological substances
     ● **T50.99** Poisoning by, adverse effect of and underdosing of other drugs, medicaments and biological substances
         ● **T50.991** Poisoning by other drugs, medicaments and biological substances, accidental (unintentional)
         ● **T50.992** Poisoning by other drugs, medicaments and biological substances, intentional self-harm A, S
         ● **T50.993** Poisoning by other drugs, medicaments and biological substances, assault
         ● **T50.994** Poisoning by other drugs, medicaments and biological substances, undetermined
         ● **T50.995** Adverse effect of other drugs, medicaments and biological substances
            Coding Clinic: 2023, Q3, P4-5
         ● **T50.996** Underdosing of other drugs, medicaments and biological substances

TOXIC EFFECTS OF SUBSTANCES CHIEFLY NONMEDICINAL AS TO SOURCE (T51-T65)

Note: When no intent is indicated code to accidental. Undetermined intent is only for use when there is specific documentation in the record that the intent of the toxic effect cannot be determined.

Use additional code(s): for all associated manifestations of toxic effect, such as:
respiratory conditions due to external agents (J60-J70)
personal history of foreign body fully removed (Z87.821)
to identify any retained foreign body, if applicable (Z18.-)

Excludes1   contact with and (suspected) exposure to toxic substances (Z77.-)

● **T51**   **Toxic effect of alcohol**

The appropriate 7th character is to be added to each code from category T51

> A   initial encounter
> D   subsequent encounter
> S   sequela

● **T51.0**   **Toxic effect of ethanol**
Toxic effect of ethyl alcohol

    Excludes2   acute alcohol intoxication or 'hangover' effects (F10.129, F10.229, F10.929)
drunkenness (F10.129, F10.229, F10.929)
pathological alcohol intoxication (F10.129, F10.229, F10.929)

● **T51.0X**   **Toxic effect of ethanol**

● **T51.0X1**   **Toxic effect of ethanol, accidental (unintentional)**
Toxic effect of ethanol NOS

● **T51.0X2**   **Toxic effect of ethanol, intentional self-harm A, S** Ⓗⓒ

● **T51.0X3**   **Toxic effect of ethanol, assault**

● **T51.0X4**   **Toxic effect of ethanol, undetermined**

● **T51.1**   **Toxic effect of methanol**
Toxic effect of methyl alcohol

● **T51.1X**   **Toxic effect of methanol**

● **T51.1X1**   **Toxic effect of methanol, accidental (unintentional)**
Toxic effect of methanol NOS

● **T51.1X2**   **Toxic effect of methanol, intentional self-harm A, S** Ⓗⓒ

● **T51.1X3**   **Toxic effect of methanol, assault**

● **T51.1X4**   **Toxic effect of methanol, undetermined**

● **T51.2**   **Toxic effect of 2-Propanol**
Toxic effect of isopropyl alcohol

● **T51.2X**   **Toxic effect of 2-Propanol**

● **T51.2X1**   **Toxic effect of 2-Propanol, accidental (unintentional)**
Toxic effect of 2-Propanol NOS

● **T51.2X2**   **Toxic effect of 2-Propanol, intentional self-harm A, S** Ⓗⓒ

● **T51.2X3**   **Toxic effect of 2-Propanol, assault**

● **T51.2X4**   **Toxic effect of 2-Propanol, undetermined**

● **T51.3**   **Toxic effect of fusel oil**
Toxic effect of amyl alcohol
Toxic effect of butyl [1-butanol] alcohol
Toxic effect of propyl [1-propanol] alcohol

● **T51.3X**   **Toxic effect of fusel oil**

● **T51.3X1**   **Toxic effect of fusel oil, accidental (unintentional)**
Toxic effect of fusel oil NOS

● **T51.3X2**   **Toxic effect of fusel oil, intentional self-harm A, S** Ⓗⓒ

● **T51.3X3**   **Toxic effect of fusel oil, assault**

● **T51.3X4**   **Toxic effect of fusel oil, undetermined**

● **T51.8**   **Toxic effect of other alcohols**

● **T51.8X**   **Toxic effect of other alcohols**

● **T51.8X1**   **Toxic effect of other alcohols, accidental (unintentional)**
Toxic effect of other alcohols NOS

● **T51.8X2**   **Toxic effect of other alcohols, intentional self-harm A, S** Ⓗⓒ

● **T51.8X3**   **Toxic effect of other alcohols, assault**

● **T51.8X4**   **Toxic effect of other alcohols, undetermined**

● **T51.9**   **Toxic effect of unspecified alcohol**

X ● **T51.91**   **Toxic effect of unspecified alcohol, accidental (unintentional)**

X ● **T51.92**   **Toxic effect of unspecified alcohol, intentional self-harm A, S** Ⓗⓒ

X ● **T51.93**   **Toxic effect of unspecified alcohol, assault**

X ● **T51.94**   **Toxic effect of unspecified alcohol, undetermined**

● **T52**   **Toxic effect of organic solvents**

    Excludes1   halogen derivatives of aliphatic and aromatic hydrocarbons (T53.-)

The appropriate 7th character is to be added to each code from category T52

> A   initial encounter
> D   subsequent encounter
> S   sequela

● **T52.0**   **Toxic effects of petroleum products**
Toxic effects of gasoline [petrol]
Toxic effects of kerosene [paraffin oil]
Toxic effects of paraffin wax
Toxic effects of ether petroleum
Toxic effects of naphtha petroleum
Toxic effects of spirit petroleum

● **T52.0X**   **Toxic effects of petroleum products**

● **T52.0X1**   **Toxic effect of petroleum products, accidental (unintentional)**
Toxic effects of petroleum products NOS

● **T52.0X2**   **Toxic effect of petroleum products, intentional self-harm A, S** Ⓗⓒ

● **T52.0X3**   **Toxic effect of petroleum products, assault**

● **T52.0X4**   **Toxic effect of petroleum products, undetermined**

● **T52.1**   **Toxic effects of benzene**

    Excludes1   homologues of benzene (T52.2)
nitroderivatives and aminoderivatives of benzene and its homologues (T65.3)

● **T52.1X**   **Toxic effects of benzene**

● **T52.1X1**   **Toxic effect of benzene, accidental (unintentional)**
Toxic effects of benzene NOS

● **T52.1X2**   **Toxic effect of benzene, intentional self-harm A, S** Ⓗⓒ

● **T52.1X3**   **Toxic effect of benzene, assault**

● **T52.1X4**   **Toxic effect of benzene, undetermined**

● **T52.2**   **Toxic effects of homologues of benzene**
Toxic effects of toluene [methylbenzene]
Toxic effects of xylene [dimethylbenzene]

● **T52.2X**   **Toxic effects of homologues of benzene**

● **T52.2X1**   **Toxic effect of homologues of benzene, accidental (unintentional)**
Toxic effects of homologues of benzene NOS

● **T52.2X2**   **Toxic effect of homologues of benzene, intentional self-harm A, S** Ⓗⓒ

● **T52.2X3** Toxic effect of homologues of benzene, assault

● **T52.2X4** Toxic effect of homologues of benzene, undetermined

● **T52.3** Toxic effects of glycols

  ● **T52.3X** Toxic effects of glycols

    ● **T52.3X1** Toxic effect of glycols, accidental (unintentional)
      Toxic effects of glycols NOS

    ● **T52.3X2** Toxic effect of glycols, intentional self-harm A, S ℞

    ● **T52.3X3** Toxic effect of glycols, assault

    ● **T52.3X4** Toxic effect of glycols, undetermined

● **T52.4** Toxic effects of ketones

  ● **T52.4X** Toxic effects of ketones

    ● **T52.4X1** Toxic effect of ketones, accidental (unintentional)
      Toxic effects of ketones NOS

    ● **T52.4X2** Toxic effect of ketones, intentional self-harm A, S ℞

    ● **T52.4X3** Toxic effect of ketones, assault

    ● **T52.4X4** Toxic effect of ketones, undetermined

● **T52.8** Toxic effects of other organic solvents

  ● **T52.8X** Toxic effects of other organic solvents

    ● **T52.8X1** Toxic effect of other organic solvents, accidental (unintentional)
      Toxic effects of other organic solvents NOS

    ● **T52.8X2** Toxic effect of other organic solvents, intentional self-harm A, S ℞

    ● **T52.8X3** Toxic effect of other organic solvents, assault

    ● **T52.8X4** Toxic effect of other organic solvents, undetermined

● **T52.9** Toxic effects of unspecified organic solvent

  X ● **T52.91** Toxic effect of unspecified organic solvent, accidental (unintentional)

  X ● **T52.92** Toxic effect of unspecified organic solvent, intentional self-harm A, S ℞

  X ● **T52.93** Toxic effect of unspecified organic solvent, assault

  X ● **T52.94** Toxic effect of unspecified organic solvent, undetermined

● **T53** Toxic effect of halogen derivatives of aliphatic and aromatic hydrocarbons

  The appropriate 7th character is to be added to each code from category T53

A	initial encounter
D	subsequent encounter
S	sequela

● **T53.0** Toxic effects of carbon tetrachloride
  Toxic effects of tetrachloromethane

  ● **T53.0X** Toxic effects of carbon tetrachloride

    ● **T53.0X1** Toxic effect of carbon tetrachloride, accidental (unintentional)
      Toxic effects of carbon tetrachloride NOS

    ● **T53.0X2** Toxic effect of carbon tetrachloride, intentional self-harm A, S ℞

    ● **T53.0X3** Toxic effect of carbon tetrachloride, assault

    ● **T53.0X4** Toxic effect of carbon tetrachloride, undetermined

● **T53.1** Toxic effects of chloroform
  Toxic effects of trichloromethane

  ● **T53.1X** Toxic effects of chloroform

    ● **T53.1X1** Toxic effect of chloroform, accidental (unintentional)
      Toxic effects of chloroform NOS

    ● **T53.1X2** Toxic effect of chloroform, intentional self-harm A, S ℞

    ● **T53.1X3** Toxic effect of chloroform, assault

    ● **T53.1X4** Toxic effect of chloroform, undetermined

● **T53.2** Toxic effects of trichloroethylene
  Toxic effects of trichloroethene

  ● **T53.2X** Toxic effects of trichloroethylene

    ● **T53.2X1** Toxic effect of trichloroethylene, accidental (unintentional)
      Toxic effects of trichloroethylene NOS

    ● **T53.2X2** Toxic effect of trichloroethylene, intentional self-harm A, S ℞

    ● **T53.2X3** Toxic effect of trichloroethylene, assault

    ● **T53.2X4** Toxic effect of trichloroethylene, undetermined

● **T53.3** Toxic effects of tetrachloroethylene
  Toxic effects of perchloroethylene
  Toxic effect of tetrachloroethene

  ● **T53.3X** Toxic effects of tetrachloroethylene

    ● **T53.3X1** Toxic effect of tetrachloroethylene, accidental (unintentional)
      Toxic effects of tetrachloroethylene NOS

    ● **T53.3X2** Toxic effect of tetrachloroethylene, intentional self-harm A, S ℞

    ● **T53.3X3** Toxic effect of tetrachloroethylene, assault

    ● **T53.3X4** Toxic effect of tetrachloroethylene, undetermined

● **T53.4** Toxic effects of dichloromethane
  Toxic effects of methylene chloride

  ● **T53.4X** Toxic effects of dichloromethane

    ● **T53.4X1** Toxic effect of dichloromethane, accidental (unintentional)
      Toxic effects of dichloromethane NOS

    ● **T53.4X2** Toxic effect of dichloromethane, intentional self-harm A, S ℞

    ● **T53.4X3** Toxic effect of dichloromethane, assault

    ● **T53.4X4** Toxic effect of dichloromethane, undetermined

● **T53.5** Toxic effects of chlorofluorocarbons

  ● **T53.5X** Toxic effects of chlorofluorocarbons

    ● **T53.5X1** Toxic effect of chlorofluorocarbons, accidental (unintentional)
      Toxic effects of chlorofluorocarbons NOS

    ● **T53.5X2** Toxic effect of chlorofluorocarbons, intentional self-harm A, S ℞

    ● **T53.5X3** Toxic effect of chlorofluorocarbons, assault

    ● **T53.5X4** Toxic effect of chlorofluorocarbons, undetermined

● **T53.6** Toxic effects of other halogen derivatives of aliphatic hydrocarbons

  ● **T53.6X** Toxic effects of other halogen derivatives of aliphatic hydrocarbons

    ● **T53.6X1** Toxic effect of other halogen derivatives of aliphatic hydrocarbons, accidental (unintentional)
      Toxic effects of other halogen derivatives of aliphatic hydrocarbons NOS

    ● **T53.6X2** Toxic effect of other halogen derivatives of aliphatic hydrocarbons, intentional self-harm A, S ℞

    ● **T53.6X3** Toxic effect of other halogen derivatives of aliphatic hydrocarbons, assault

CHAPTER 19 (SØØ-T88)

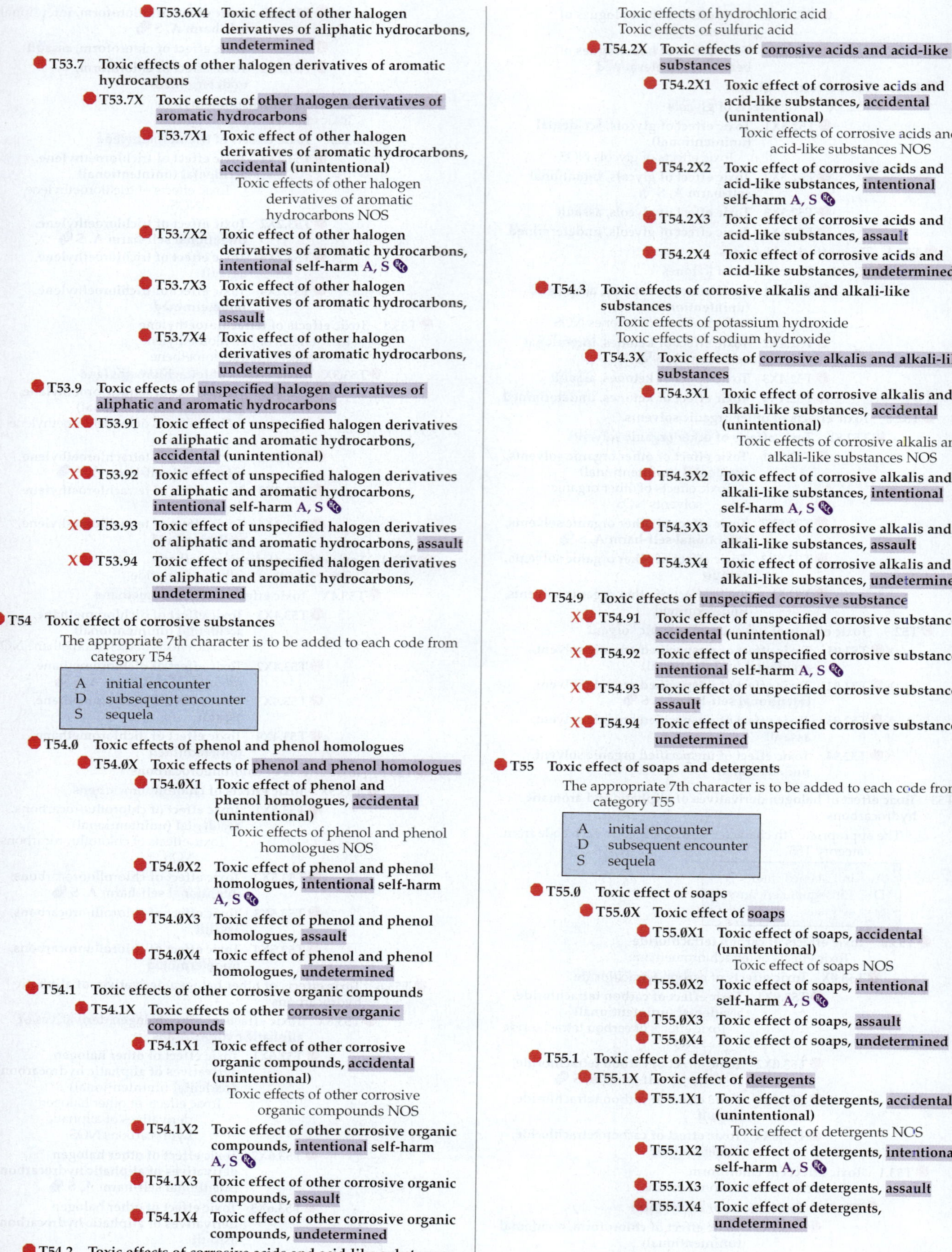

● **T53.6X4** Toxic effect of other halogen derivatives of aliphatic hydrocarbons, undetermined

● **T53.7** Toxic effects of other halogen derivatives of aromatic hydrocarbons

● **T53.7X** Toxic effects of other halogen derivatives of aromatic hydrocarbons

● **T53.7X1** Toxic effect of other halogen derivatives of aromatic hydrocarbons, accidental (unintentional)
  Toxic effects of other halogen derivatives of aromatic hydrocarbons NOS

● **T53.7X2** Toxic effect of other halogen derivatives of aromatic hydrocarbons, intentional self-harm A, S

● **T53.7X3** Toxic effect of other halogen derivatives of aromatic hydrocarbons, assault

● **T53.7X4** Toxic effect of other halogen derivatives of aromatic hydrocarbons, undetermined

● **T53.9** Toxic effects of unspecified halogen derivatives of aliphatic and aromatic hydrocarbons

X ● **T53.91** Toxic effect of unspecified halogen derivatives of aliphatic and aromatic hydrocarbons, accidental (unintentional)

X ● **T53.92** Toxic effect of unspecified halogen derivatives of aliphatic and aromatic hydrocarbons, intentional self-harm A, S

X ● **T53.93** Toxic effect of unspecified halogen derivatives of aliphatic and aromatic hydrocarbons, assault

X ● **T53.94** Toxic effect of unspecified halogen derivatives of aliphatic and aromatic hydrocarbons, undetermined

● **T54** Toxic effect of corrosive substances

The appropriate 7th character is to be added to each code from category T54

> A   initial encounter
> D   subsequent encounter
> S   sequela

● **T54.0** Toxic effects of phenol and phenol homologues

● **T54.0X** Toxic effects of phenol and phenol homologues

● **T54.0X1** Toxic effect of phenol and phenol homologues, accidental (unintentional)
  Toxic effects of phenol and phenol homologues NOS

● **T54.0X2** Toxic effect of phenol and phenol homologues, intentional self-harm A, S

● **T54.0X3** Toxic effect of phenol and phenol homologues, assault

● **T54.0X4** Toxic effect of phenol and phenol homologues, undetermined

● **T54.1** Toxic effects of other corrosive organic compounds

● **T54.1X** Toxic effects of other corrosive organic compounds

● **T54.1X1** Toxic effect of other corrosive organic compounds, accidental (unintentional)
  Toxic effects of other corrosive organic compounds NOS

● **T54.1X2** Toxic effect of other corrosive organic compounds, intentional self-harm A, S

● **T54.1X3** Toxic effect of other corrosive organic compounds, assault

● **T54.1X4** Toxic effect of other corrosive organic compounds, undetermined

● **T54.2** Toxic effects of corrosive acids and acid-like substances

Toxic effects of hydrochloric acid
Toxic effects of sulfuric acid

● **T54.2X** Toxic effects of corrosive acids and acid-like substances

● **T54.2X1** Toxic effects of corrosive acids and acid-like substances, accidental (unintentional)
  Toxic effects of corrosive acids and acid-like substances NOS

● **T54.2X2** Toxic effect of corrosive acids and acid-like substances, intentional self-harm A, S

● **T54.2X3** Toxic effect of corrosive acids and acid-like substances, assault

● **T54.2X4** Toxic effect of corrosive acids and acid-like substances, undetermined

● **T54.3** Toxic effects of corrosive alkalis and alkali-like substances

Toxic effects of potassium hydroxide
Toxic effects of sodium hydroxide

● **T54.3X** Toxic effects of corrosive alkalis and alkali-like substances

● **T54.3X1** Toxic effect of corrosive alkalis and alkali-like substances, accidental (unintentional)
  Toxic effects of corrosive alkalis and alkali-like substances NOS

● **T54.3X2** Toxic effect of corrosive alkalis and alkali-like substances, intentional self-harm A, S

● **T54.3X3** Toxic effect of corrosive alkalis and alkali-like substances, assault

● **T54.3X4** Toxic effect of corrosive alkalis and alkali-like substances, undetermined

● **T54.9** Toxic effects of unspecified corrosive substance

X ● **T54.91** Toxic effect of unspecified corrosive substance, accidental (unintentional)

X ● **T54.92** Toxic effect of unspecified corrosive substance, intentional self-harm A, S

X ● **T54.93** Toxic effect of unspecified corrosive substance, assault

X ● **T54.94** Toxic effect of unspecified corrosive substance, undetermined

● **T55** Toxic effect of soaps and detergents

The appropriate 7th character is to be added to each code from category T55

> A   initial encounter
> D   subsequent encounter
> S   sequela

● **T55.0** Toxic effect of soaps

● **T55.0X** Toxic effect of soaps

● **T55.0X1** Toxic effect of soaps, accidental (unintentional)
  Toxic effect of soaps NOS

● **T55.0X2** Toxic effect of soaps, intentional self-harm A, S

● **T55.0X3** Toxic effect of soaps, assault

● **T55.0X4** Toxic effect of soaps, undetermined

● **T55.1** Toxic effect of detergents

● **T55.1X** Toxic effect of detergents

● **T55.1X1** Toxic effect of detergents, accidental (unintentional)
  Toxic effect of detergents NOS

● **T55.1X2** Toxic effect of detergents, intentional self-harm A, S

● **T55.1X3** Toxic effect of detergents, assault

● **T55.1X4** Toxic effect of detergents, undetermined

▶ New   ◀ Revised   ~~deleted~~ Deleted   Excludes 1   Excludes 2   Includes   Use additional   Code first   Code also   Key words
OGCR Official Guidelines   X Assign placeholder X   ● Use Additional Character(s)   ▶ Manifestation Code   Hierarchical Condition Category   **Coding Clinic**

● **T56   Toxic effect of metals**

    Includes   toxic effects of fumes and vapors of metals
            toxic effects of metals from all sources, except
            medicinal substances

    Use additional code to identify any retained metal foreign
        body, if applicable (Z18.0-, T18.1-)

    Excludes1   arsenic and its compounds (T57.0)
             manganese and its compounds (T57.2)

    The appropriate 7th character is to be added to each code from
    category T56

      A   initial encounter
      D   subsequent encounter
      S   sequela

● **T56.0   Toxic effects of lead and its compounds**

    ● **T56.0X   Toxic effects of lead and its compounds**

       ● **T56.0X1   Toxic effect of lead and
                its compounds, accidental
                (unintentional)**
                  Toxic effects of lead and its
                  compounds NOS

       ● **T56.0X2   Toxic effect of lead and its
                compounds, intentional
                self-harm A, S** 🔞

       ● **T56.0X3   Toxic effect of lead and its
                compounds, assault**

       ● **T56.0X4   Toxic effect of lead and its
                compounds, undetermined**

● **T56.1   Toxic effects of mercury and its compounds**

    ● **T56.1X   Toxic effects of mercury and its compounds**

       ● **T56.1X1   Toxic effect of mercury and
                its compounds, accidental
                (unintentional)**
                  Toxic effects of mercury and its
                  compounds NOS

       ● **T56.1X2   Toxic effect of mercury and its
                compounds, intentional
                self-harm A, S** 🔞

       ● **T56.1X3   Toxic effect of mercury and its
                compounds, assault**

       ● **T56.1X4   Toxic effect of mercury and its
                compounds, undetermined**

● **T56.2   Toxic effects of chromium and its compounds**

    ● **T56.2X   Toxic effects of chromium and its compounds**

       ● **T56.2X1   Toxic effect of chromium and
                its compounds, accidental
                (unintentional)**
                  Toxic effects of chromium and its
                  compounds NOS

       ● **T56.2X2   Toxic effect of chromium and its
                compounds, intentional self-harm
                A, S** 🔞

       ● **T56.2X3   Toxic effect of chromium and its
                compounds, assault**

       ● **T56.2X4   Toxic effect of chromium and its
                compounds, undetermined**

● **T56.3   Toxic effects of cadmium and its compounds**

    ● **T56.3X   Toxic effects of cadmium and its compounds**

       ● **T56.3X1   Toxic effect of cadmium and
                its compounds, accidental
                (unintentional)**
                  Toxic effects of cadmium and its
                  compounds NOS

       ● **T56.3X2   Toxic effect of cadmium and its
                compounds, intentional self-harm
                A, S** 🔞

       ● **T56.3X3   Toxic effect of cadmium and its
                compounds, assault**

       ● **T56.3X4   Toxic effect of cadmium and its
                compounds, undetermined**

● **T56.4   Toxic effects of copper and its compounds**

    ● **T56.4X   Toxic effects of copper and its compounds**

       ● **T56.4X1   Toxic effect of copper and
                its compounds, accidental
                (unintentional)**
                  Toxic effects of copper and its
                  compounds NOS

       ● **T56.4X2   Toxic effect of copper and its
                compounds, intentional
                self-harm A, S** 🔞

       ● **T56.4X3   Toxic effect of copper and its
                compounds, assault**

       ● **T56.4X4   Toxic effect of copper and its
                compounds, undetermined**

● **T56.5   Toxic effects of zinc and its compounds**

    ● **T56.5X   Toxic effects of zinc and its compounds**

       ● **T56.5X1   Toxic effect of zinc and
                its compounds, accidental
                (unintentional)**
                  Toxic effects of zinc and its
                  compounds NOS

       ● **T56.5X2   Toxic effect of zinc and its
                compounds, intentional
                self-harm A, S** 🔞

       ● **T56.5X3   Toxic effect of zinc and its
                compounds, assault**

       ● **T56.5X4   Toxic effect of zinc and its
                compounds, undetermined**

● **T56.6   Toxic effects of tin and its compounds**

    ● **T56.6X   Toxic effects of tin and its compounds**

       ● **T56.6X1   Toxic effect of tin and its compounds,
                accidental (unintentional)**
                  Toxic effects of tin and its
                  compounds NOS

       ● **T56.6X2   Toxic effect of tin and its compounds,
                intentional self-harm A, S** 🔞

       ● **T56.6X3   Toxic effect of tin and its compounds,
                assault**

       ● **T56.6X4   Toxic effect of tin and its compounds,
                undetermined**

● **T56.7   Toxic effects of beryllium and its compounds**

    ● **T56.7X   Toxic effects of beryllium and its compounds**

       ● **T56.7X1   Toxic effect of beryllium and
                its compounds, accidental
                (unintentional)**
                  Toxic effects of beryllium and its
                  compounds NOS

       ● **T56.7X2   Toxic effect of beryllium and its
                compounds, intentional self-harm
                A, S** 🔞

       ● **T56.7X3   Toxic effect of beryllium and its
                compounds, assault**

       ● **T56.7X4   Toxic effect of beryllium and its
                compounds, undetermined**

● **T56.8   Toxic effects of other metals**

    ● **T56.81   Toxic effect of thallium**

       ● **T56.811   Toxic effect of thallium, accidental
                (unintentional)**
                  Toxic effect of thallium NOS

       ● **T56.812   Toxic effect of thallium, intentional
                self-harm A, S** 🔞

       ● **T56.813   Toxic effect of thallium, assault**

       ● **T56.814   Toxic effect of thallium,
                undetermined**

    ● **T56.82   Toxic effect of gadolinium**

          Excludes1   adverse effect of diagnostic
                      agents (T50.8X5-)

       **T56.821   Toxic effect of gadolinium, accidental
                (unintentional)**
                  Toxic effect of gadolinium NOS

CHAPTER 19 (S00–T88)

CHAPTER 19 (S00-T88)

T56.822 Toxic effect of gadolinium, intentional self-harm

T56.823 Toxic effect of gadolinium, assault

T56.824 Toxic effect of gadolinium, undetermined

● T56.89 Toxic effects of other metals

● T56.891 Toxic effect of other metals, accidental (unintentional)
Toxic effects of other metals NOS

● T56.892 Toxic effect of other metals, intentional self-harm A, S ⓗ

● T56.893 Toxic effect of other metals, assault

● T56.894 Toxic effect of other metals, undetermined

● T56.9 Toxic effects of unspecified metal

X ● T56.91 Toxic effect of unspecified metal, accidental (unintentional)

X ● T56.92 Toxic effect of unspecified metal, intentional self-harm A, S ⓗ

X ● T56.93 Toxic effect of unspecified metal, assault

X ● T56.94 Toxic effect of unspecified metal, undetermined

● T57 Toxic effect of other inorganic substances

The appropriate 7th character is to be added to each code from category T57

A	initial encounter
D	subsequent encounter
S	sequela

● T57.0 Toxic effect of arsenic and its compounds

● T57.0X Toxic effect of arsenic and its compounds

● T57.0X1 Toxic effect of arsenic and its compounds, accidental (unintentional)
Toxic effect of arsenic and its compounds NOS

● T57.0X2 Toxic effect of arsenic and its compounds, intentional self-harm A, S ⓗ

● T57.0X3 Toxic effect of arsenic and its compounds, assault

● T57.0X4 Toxic effect of arsenic and its compounds, undetermined

● T57.1 Toxic effect of phosphorus and its compounds

Excludes1 organophosphate insecticides (T60.0)

● T57.1X Toxic effect of phosphorus and its compounds

● T57.1X1 Toxic effect of phosphorus and its compounds, accidental (unintentional)
Toxic effect of phosphorus and its compounds NOS

● T57.1X2 Toxic effect of phosphorus and its compounds, intentional self-harm A, S ⓗ

● T57.1X3 Toxic effect of phosphorus and its compounds, assault

● T57.1X4 Toxic effect of phosphorus and its compounds, undetermined

● T57.2 Toxic effect of manganese and its compounds

● T57.2X Toxic effect of manganese and its compounds

● T57.2X1 Toxic effect of manganese and its compounds, accidental (unintentional)
Toxic effect of manganese and its compounds NOS

● T57.2X2 Toxic effect of manganese and its compounds, intentional self-harm A, S ⓗ

● T57.2X3 Toxic effect of manganese and its compounds, assault

● T57.2X4 Toxic effect of manganese and its compounds, undetermined

● T57.3 Toxic effect of hydrogen cyanide

● T57.3X Toxic effect of hydrogen cyanide

● T57.3X1 Toxic effect of hydrogen cyanide, accidental (unintentional)
Toxic effect of hydrogen cyanide NOS

● T57.3X2 Toxic effect of hydrogen cyanide, intentional self-harm A, S ⓗ

● T57.3X3 Toxic effect of hydrogen cyanide, assault

● T57.3X4 Toxic effect of hydrogen cyanide, undetermined

● T57.8 Toxic effect of other specified inorganic substances

● T57.8X Toxic effect of other specified inorganic substances

● T57.8X1 Toxic effect of other specified inorganic substances, accidental (unintentional)
Toxic effect of other specified inorganic substances NOS

● T57.8X2 Toxic effect of other specified inorganic substances, intentional self-harm A, S ⓗ

● T57.8X3 Toxic effect of other specified inorganic substances, assault

● T57.8X4 Toxic effect of other specified inorganic substances, undetermined

● T57.9 Toxic effect of unspecified inorganic substance

X ● T57.91 Toxic effect of unspecified inorganic substance, accidental (unintentional)

X ● T57.92 Toxic effect of unspecified inorganic substance, intentional self-harm A, S ⓗ

X ● T57.93 Toxic effect of unspecified inorganic substance, assault

X ● T57.94 Toxic effect of unspecified inorganic substance, undetermined

● T58 Toxic effect of carbon monoxide

Includes asphyxiation from carbon monoxide
toxic effect of carbon monoxide from all sources

The appropriate 7th character is to be added to each code from category T58

A	initial encounter
D	subsequent encounter
S	sequela

● T58.0 Toxic effect of carbon monoxide from motor vehicle exhaust
Toxic effect of exhaust gas from gas engine
Toxic effect of exhaust gas from motor pump

X ● T58.01 Toxic effect of carbon monoxide from motor vehicle exhaust, accidental (unintentional)

X ● T58.02 Toxic effect of carbon monoxide from motor vehicle exhaust, intentional self-harm A, S ⓗ

X ● T58.03 Toxic effect of carbon monoxide from motor vehicle exhaust, assault

X ● T58.04 Toxic effect of carbon monoxide from motor vehicle exhaust, undetermined

● T58.1 Toxic effect of carbon monoxide from utility gas
Toxic effect of acetylene
Toxic effect of gas NOS used for lighting, heating, cooking
Toxic effect of water gas

X ● T58.11 Toxic effect of carbon monoxide from utility gas, accidental (unintentional)

X ● T58.12 Toxic effect of carbon monoxide from utility gas, intentional self-harm A, S ⓗ

X ● T58.13 Toxic effect of carbon monoxide from utility gas, assault

X ● T58.14 Toxic effect of carbon monoxide from utility gas, undetermined

● **T58.2** **Toxic effect of carbon monoxide from incomplete combustion of other domestic fuels**
Toxic effect of carbon monoxide from incomplete combustion of coal, coke, kerosene, wood
  ● **T58.2X** **Toxic effect of carbon monoxide from incomplete combustion of other domestic fuels**
    ● **T58.2X1** Toxic effect of carbon monoxide from incomplete combustion of other domestic fuels, **accidental (unintentional)**
    ● **T58.2X2** Toxic effect of carbon monoxide from incomplete combustion of other domestic fuels, **intentional self-harm** A, S 🔄
    ● **T58.2X3** Toxic effect of carbon monoxide from incomplete combustion of other domestic fuels, **assault**
    ● **T58.2X4** Toxic effect of carbon monoxide from incomplete combustion of other domestic fuels, **undetermined**
● **T58.8** **Toxic effect of carbon monoxide from other source**
Toxic effect of carbon monoxide from blast furnace gas
Toxic effect of carbon monoxide from fuels in industrial use
Toxic effect of carbon monoxide from kiln vapor
  ● **T58.8X** **Toxic effect of carbon monoxide from other source**
    ● **T58.8X1** Toxic effect of carbon monoxide from other source, **accidental (unintentional)**
    ● **T58.8X2** Toxic effect of carbon monoxide from other source, **intentional self-harm** A, S 🔄
    ● **T58.8X3** Toxic effect of carbon monoxide from other source, **assault**
    ● **T58.8X4** Toxic effect of carbon monoxide from other source, **undetermined**
● **T58.9** **Toxic effect of carbon monoxide from unspecified source**
  X ● **T58.91** Toxic effect of carbon monoxide from unspecified source, **accidental (unintentional)**
  X ● **T58.92** Toxic effect of carbon monoxide from unspecified source, **intentional self-harm** A, S 🔄
  X ● **T58.93** Toxic effect of carbon monoxide from unspecified source, **assault**
  X ● **T58.94** Toxic effect of carbon monoxide from unspecified source, **undetermined**

● **T59** **Toxic effect of other gases, fumes and vapors**

Includes	aerosol propellants
Excludes 1	chlorofluorocarbons (T53.5)

The appropriate 7th character is to be added to each code from category T59.

A	initial encounter
D	subsequent encounter
S	sequela

● **T59.0** **Toxic effect of nitrogen oxides**
  ● **T59.0X** **Toxic effect of nitrogen oxides**
    ● **T59.0X1** Toxic effect of nitrogen oxides, **accidental (unintentional)**
Toxic effect of nitrogen oxides NOS
    ● **T59.0X2** Toxic effect of nitrogen oxides, **intentional self-harm** A, S 🔄
    ● **T59.0X3** Toxic effect of nitrogen oxides, **assault**
    ● **T59.0X4** Toxic effect of nitrogen oxides, **undetermined**

● **T59.1** **Toxic effect of sulfur dioxide**
  ● **T59.1X** **Toxic effect of sulfur dioxide**
    ● **T59.1X1** Toxic effect of sulfur dioxide, **accidental (unintentional)**
Toxic effect of sulfur dioxide NOS
    ● **T59.1X2** Toxic effect of sulfur dioxide, **intentional self-harm** A, S 🔄
    ● **T59.1X3** Toxic effect of sulfur dioxide, **assault**
    ● **T59.1X4** Toxic effect of sulfur dioxide, **undetermined**
● **T59.2** **Toxic effect of formaldehyde**
  ● **T59.2X** **Toxic effect of formaldehyde**
    ● **T59.2X1** Toxic effect of formaldehyde, **accidental (unintentional)**
Toxic effect of formaldehyde NOS
    ● **T59.2X2** Toxic effect of formaldehyde, **intentional self-harm** A, S 🔄
    ● **T59.2X3** Toxic effect of formaldehyde, **assault**
    ● **T59.2X4** Toxic effect of formaldehyde, **undetermined**
● **T59.3** **Toxic effect of lacrimogenic gas**
Toxic effect of tear gas
  ● **T59.3X** **Toxic effect of lacrimogenic gas**
    ● **T59.3X1** Toxic effect of lacrimogenic gas, **accidental (unintentional)**
Toxic effect of lacrimogenic gas NOS
    ● **T59.3X2** Toxic effect of lacrimogenic gas, **intentional self-harm** A, S 🔄
    ● **T59.3X3** Toxic effect of lacrimogenic gas, **assault**
    ● **T59.3X4** Toxic effect of lacrimogenic gas, **undetermined**
● **T59.4** **Toxic effect of chlorine gas**
  ● **T59.4X** **Toxic effect of chlorine gas**
    ● **T59.4X1** Toxic effect of chlorine gas, **accidental (unintentional)**
Toxic effect of chlorine gas NOS
    ● **T59.4X2** Toxic effect of chlorine gas, **intentional self-harm** A, S 🔄
    ● **T59.4X3** Toxic effect of chlorine gas, **assault**
    ● **T59.4X4** Toxic effect of chlorine gas, **undetermined**
● **T59.5** **Toxic effect of fluorine gas and hydrogen fluoride**
  ● **T59.5X** **Toxic effect of fluorine gas and hydrogen fluoride**
    ● **T59.5X1** Toxic effect of fluorine gas and hydrogen fluoride, **accidental (unintentional)**
Toxic effect of fluorine gas and hydrogen fluoride NOS
    ● **T59.5X2** Toxic effect of fluorine gas and hydrogen fluoride, **intentional self-harm** A, S 🔄
    ● **T59.5X3** Toxic effect of fluorine gas and hydrogen fluoride, **assault**
    ● **T59.5X4** Toxic effect of fluorine gas and hydrogen fluoride, **undetermined**
● **T59.6** **Toxic effect of hydrogen sulfide**
  ● **T59.6X** **Toxic effect of hydrogen sulfide**
    ● **T59.6X1** Toxic effect of hydrogen sulfide, **accidental (unintentional)**
Toxic effect of hydrogen sulfide NOS
    ● **T59.6X2** Toxic effect of hydrogen sulfide, **intentional self-harm** A, S 🔄
    ● **T59.6X3** Toxic effect of hydrogen sulfide, **assault**
    ● **T59.6X4** Toxic effect of hydrogen sulfide, **undetermined**

CHAPTER 19 (S00-T88)

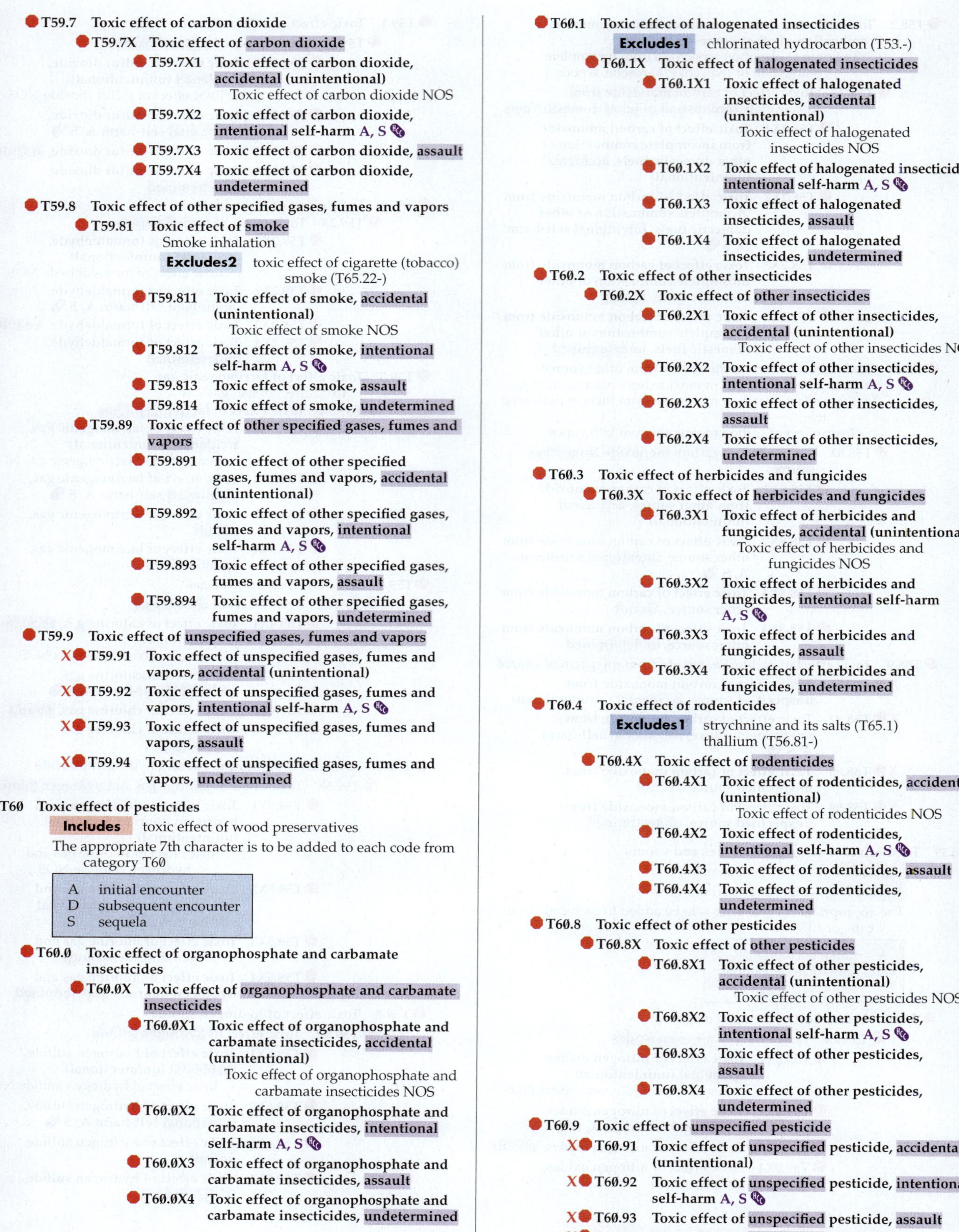

- ● T59.7   Toxic effect of carbon dioxide
  - ● T59.7X   Toxic effect of carbon dioxide
    - ● T59.7X1   Toxic effect of carbon dioxide, accidental (unintentional)
      Toxic effect of carbon dioxide NOS
    - ● T59.7X2   Toxic effect of carbon dioxide, intentional self-harm A, S ℞
    - ● T59.7X3   Toxic effect of carbon dioxide, assault
    - ● T59.7X4   Toxic effect of carbon dioxide, undetermined
- ● T59.8   Toxic effect of other specified gases, fumes and vapors
  - ● T59.81   Toxic effect of smoke
    Smoke inhalation
    Excludes2   toxic effect of cigarette (tobacco) smoke (T65.22-)
    - ● T59.811   Toxic effect of smoke, accidental (unintentional)
      Toxic effect of smoke NOS
    - ● T59.812   Toxic effect of smoke, intentional self-harm A, S ℞
    - ● T59.813   Toxic effect of smoke, assault
    - ● T59.814   Toxic effect of smoke, undetermined
  - ● T59.89   Toxic effect of other specified gases, fumes and vapors
    - ● T59.891   Toxic effect of other specified gases, fumes and vapors, accidental (unintentional)
    - ● T59.892   Toxic effect of other specified gases, fumes and vapors, intentional self-harm A, S ℞
    - ● T59.893   Toxic effect of other specified gases, fumes and vapors, assault
    - ● T59.894   Toxic effect of other specified gases, fumes and vapors, undetermined
- ● T59.9   Toxic effect of unspecified gases, fumes and vapors
  - X ● T59.91   Toxic effect of unspecified gases, fumes and vapors, accidental (unintentional)
  - X ● T59.92   Toxic effect of unspecified gases, fumes and vapors, intentional self-harm A, S ℞
  - X ● T59.93   Toxic effect of unspecified gases, fumes and vapors, assault
  - X ● T59.94   Toxic effect of unspecified gases, fumes and vapors, undetermined

- ● T60   Toxic effect of pesticides
  Includes   toxic effect of wood preservatives
  The appropriate 7th character is to be added to each code from category T60

A	initial encounter
D	subsequent encounter
S	sequela

  - ● T60.0   Toxic effect of organophosphate and carbamate insecticides
    - ● T60.0X   Toxic effect of organophosphate and carbamate insecticides
      - ● T60.0X1   Toxic effect of organophosphate and carbamate insecticides, accidental (unintentional)
        Toxic effect of organophosphate and carbamate insecticides NOS
      - ● T60.0X2   Toxic effect of organophosphate and carbamate insecticides, intentional self-harm A, S ℞
      - ● T60.0X3   Toxic effect of organophosphate and carbamate insecticides, assault
      - ● T60.0X4   Toxic effect of organophosphate and carbamate insecticides, undetermined

- ● T60.1   Toxic effect of halogenated insecticides
  Excludes1   chlorinated hydrocarbon (T53.-)
  - ● T60.1X   Toxic effect of halogenated insecticides
    - ● T60.1X1   Toxic effect of halogenated insecticides, accidental (unintentional)
      Toxic effect of halogenated insecticides NOS
    - ● T60.1X2   Toxic effect of halogenated insecticides, intentional self-harm A, S ℞
    - ● T60.1X3   Toxic effect of halogenated insecticides, assault
    - ● T60.1X4   Toxic effect of halogenated insecticides, undetermined
- ● T60.2   Toxic effect of other insecticides
  - ● T60.2X   Toxic effect of other insecticides
    - ● T60.2X1   Toxic effect of other insecticides, accidental (unintentional)
      Toxic effect of other insecticides NOS
    - ● T60.2X2   Toxic effect of other insecticides, intentional self-harm A, S ℞
    - ● T60.2X3   Toxic effect of other insecticides, assault
    - ● T60.2X4   Toxic effect of other insecticides, undetermined
- ● T60.3   Toxic effect of herbicides and fungicides
  - ● T60.3X   Toxic effect of herbicides and fungicides
    - ● T60.3X1   Toxic effect of herbicides and fungicides, accidental (unintentional)
      Toxic effect of herbicides and fungicides NOS
    - ● T60.3X2   Toxic effect of herbicides and fungicides, intentional self-harm A, S ℞
    - ● T60.3X3   Toxic effect of herbicides and fungicides, assault
    - ● T60.3X4   Toxic effect of herbicides and fungicides, undetermined
- ● T60.4   Toxic effect of rodenticides
  Excludes1   strychnine and its salts (T65.1)
  thallium (T56.81-)
  - ● T60.4X   Toxic effect of rodenticides
    - ● T60.4X1   Toxic effect of rodenticides, accidental (unintentional)
      Toxic effect of rodenticides NOS
    - ● T60.4X2   Toxic effect of rodenticides, intentional self-harm A, S ℞
    - ● T60.4X3   Toxic effect of rodenticides, assault
    - ● T60.4X4   Toxic effect of rodenticides, undetermined
- ● T60.8   Toxic effect of other pesticides
  - ● T60.8X   Toxic effect of other pesticides
    - ● T60.8X1   Toxic effect of other pesticides, accidental (unintentional)
      Toxic effect of other pesticides NOS
    - ● T60.8X2   Toxic effect of other pesticides, intentional self-harm A, S ℞
    - ● T60.8X3   Toxic effect of other pesticides, assault
    - ● T60.8X4   Toxic effect of other pesticides, undetermined
- ● T60.9   Toxic effect of unspecified pesticide
  - X ● T60.91   Toxic effect of unspecified pesticide, accidental (unintentional)
  - X ● T60.92   Toxic effect of unspecified pesticide, intentional self-harm A, S ℞
  - X ● T60.93   Toxic effect of unspecified pesticide, assault
  - X ● T60.94   Toxic effect of unspecified pesticide, undetermined

● **T61** Toxic effect of noxious substances eaten as seafood

  Excludes1 allergic reaction to food, such as:
      anaphylactic reaction or shock due to adverse
       food reaction (T78.0-)
      bacterial foodborne intoxications (A05.-)
      dermatitis (L23.6, L25.4, L27.2)
      food protein-induced enterocolitis syndrome
       (K52.21)
      food protein-induced enteropathy (K52.22)
      gastroenteritis (noninfective) (K52.29)
      toxic effect of aflatoxin and other mycotoxins
       (T64)
      toxic effect of cyanides (T65.0-)
      toxic effect of harmful algae bloom (T65.82-)
      toxic effect of hydrogen cyanide (T57.3-)
      toxic effect of mercury (T56.1-)
      toxic effect of red tide (T65.82-)

  The appropriate 7th character is to be added to each code from
  category T61

   A initial encounter
   D subsequent encounter
   S sequela

 ● **T61.0** **Ciguatera fish poisoning**
  X● **T61.01** Ciguatera fish poisoning, accidental
     (unintentional)
  X● **T61.02** Ciguatera fish poisoning, intentional self-harm
     A, S 🔲
  X● **T61.03** Ciguatera fish poisoning, assault
  X● **T61.04** Ciguatera fish poisoning, undetermined

 ● **T61.1** **Scombroid fish poisoning**
    Histamine-like syndrome
  X● **T61.11** Scombroid fish poisoning, accidental
     (unintentional)
  X● **T61.12** Scombroid fish poisoning, intentional
     self-harm A, S 🔲
  X● **T61.13** Scombroid fish poisoning, assault
  X● **T61.14** Scombroid fish poisoning, undetermined

 ● **T61.7** **Other fish and shellfish poisoning**
  ● **T61.77** **Other fish poisoning**
   ● **T61.771** Other fish poisoning, accidental
      (unintentional)
   ● **T61.772** Other fish poisoning, intentional
      self-harm A, S 🔲
   ● **T61.773** Other fish poisoning, assault
   ● **T61.774** Other fish poisoning, undetermined
  ● **T61.78** **Other shellfish poisoning**
   ● **T61.781** Other shellfish poisoning, accidental
      (unintentional)
   ● **T61.782** Other shellfish poisoning, intentional
      self-harm A, S 🔲
   ● **T61.783** Other shellfish poisoning, assault
   ● **T61.784** Other shellfish poisoning,
      undetermined

 ● **T61.8** **Toxic effect of other seafood**
  ● **T61.8X** **Toxic effect of other seafood**
   ● **T61.8X1** Toxic effect of other seafood,
      accidental (unintentional)
   ● **T61.8X2** Toxic effect of other seafood,
      intentional self-harm A, S 🔲
   ● **T61.8X3** Toxic effect of other seafood, assault
   ● **T61.8X4** Toxic effect of other seafood,
      undetermined

 ● **T61.9** **Toxic effect of unspecified seafood**
  X● **T61.91** Toxic effect of unspecified seafood, accidental
     (unintentional)
  X● **T61.92** Toxic effect of unspecified seafood, intentional
     self-harm A, S 🔲

  X● **T61.93** Toxic effect of unspecified seafood, assault
  X● **T61.94** Toxic effect of unspecified seafood,
     undetermined

● **T62** Toxic effect of other noxious substances eaten as food

  Excludes1 allergic reaction to food, such as:
      anaphylactic shock (reaction) due to adverse
       food reaction (T78.0-)
      dermatitis (L23.6, L25.4, L27.2)
      food protein-induced enterocolitis syndrome
       (K52.21)
      food protein-induced enteropathy (K52.22)
      gastroenteritis (noninfective) (K52.29)
      bacterial food borne intoxications (A05.-)
     toxic effect of aflatoxin and other mycotoxins
       (T64)
     toxic effect of cyanides (T65.0-)
     toxic effect of hydrogen cyanide (T57.3-)
     toxic effect of mercury (T56.1-)

  The appropriate 7th character is to be added to each code from
  category T62

   A initial encounter
   D subsequent encounter
   S sequela

 ● **T62.0** **Toxic effect of ingested mushrooms**
  ● **T62.0X** **Toxic effect of ingested mushrooms**
   ● **T62.0X1** Toxic effect of ingested mushrooms,
      accidental (unintentional)
      Toxic effect of ingested mushrooms
       NOS
   ● **T62.0X2** Toxic effect of ingested mushrooms,
      intentional self-harm A, S 🔲
   ● **T62.0X3** Toxic effect of ingested mushrooms,
      assault
   ● **T62.0X4** Toxic effect of ingested mushrooms,
      undetermined

 ● **T62.1** **Toxic effect of ingested berries**
  ● **T62.1X** **Toxic effect of ingested berries**
   ● **T62.1X1** Toxic effect of ingested berries,
      accidental (unintentional)
      Toxic effect of ingested berries NOS
   ● **T62.1X2** Toxic effect of ingested berries,
      intentional self-harm A, S 🔲
   ● **T62.1X3** Toxic effect of ingested berries,
      assault
   ● **T62.1X4** Toxic effect of ingested berries,
      undetermined

 ● **T62.2** **Toxic effect of other ingested (parts of) plant(s)**
  ● **T62.2X** **Toxic effect of other ingested (parts of) plant(s)**
   ● **T62.2X1** Toxic effect of other ingested (parts
      of) plant(s), accidental (unintentional)
      Toxic effect of other ingested (parts
       of) plant(s) NOS
   ● **T62.2X2** Toxic effect of other ingested (parts
      of) plant(s), intentional self-harm
      A, S 🔲
   ● **T62.2X3** Toxic effect of other ingested (parts
      of) plant(s), assault
   ● **T62.2X4** Toxic effect of other ingested (parts
      of) plant(s), undetermined

 ● **T62.8** **Toxic effect of other specified noxious substances eaten
   as food**
  ● **T62.8X** **Toxic effect of other specified noxious
    substances eaten as food**
   ● **T62.8X1** Toxic effect of other specified noxious
      substances eaten as food, accidental
      (unintentional)
      Toxic effect of other specified
       noxious substances eaten as
       food NOS

CHAPTER 19 (S00–T88)

CHAPTER 19 (S00-T88)

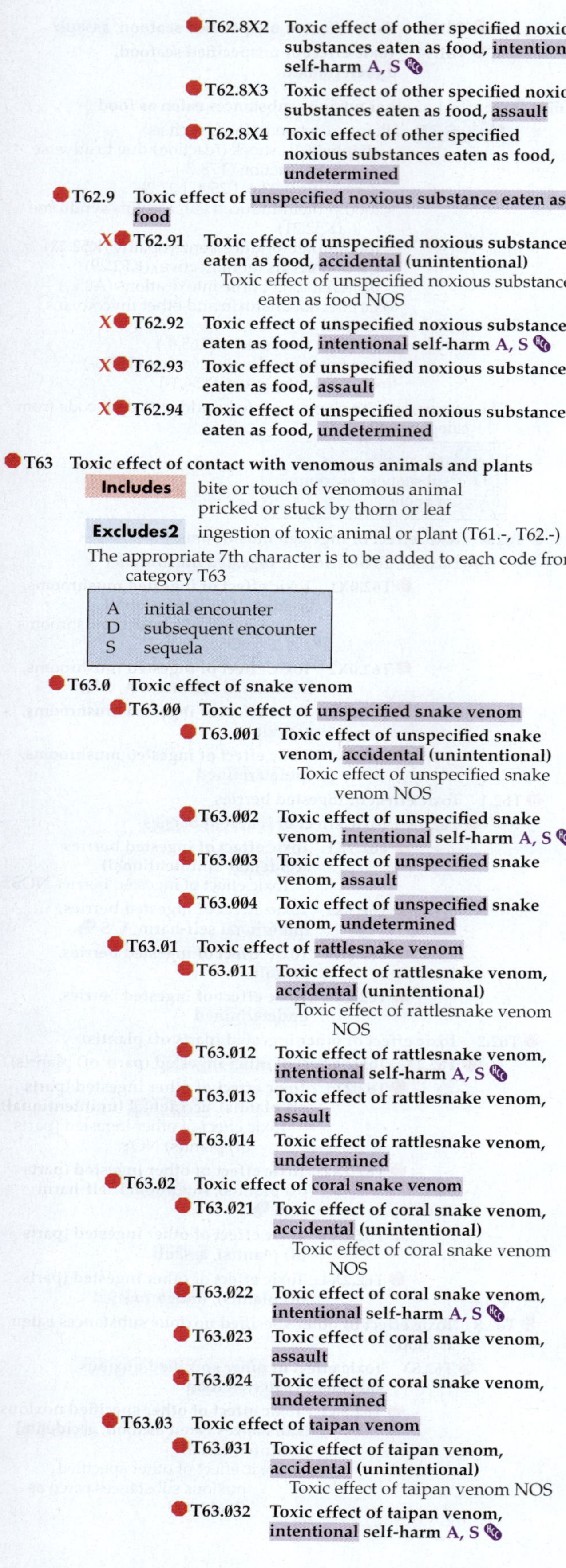

● T62.8X2 Toxic effect of other specified noxious substances eaten as food, intentional self-harm A, S

● T62.8X3 Toxic effect of other specified noxious substances eaten as food, assault

● T62.8X4 Toxic effect of other specified noxious substances eaten as food, undetermined

● T62.9 Toxic effect of unspecified noxious substance eaten as food

X ● T62.91 Toxic effect of unspecified noxious substance eaten as food, accidental (unintentional)
     Toxic effect of unspecified noxious substance eaten as food NOS

X ● T62.92 Toxic effect of unspecified noxious substance eaten as food, intentional self-harm A, S

X ● T62.93 Toxic effect of unspecified noxious substance eaten as food, assault

X ● T62.94 Toxic effect of unspecified noxious substance eaten as food, undetermined

● T63 Toxic effect of contact with venomous animals and plants

Includes   bite or touch of venomous animal
     pricked or stuck by thorn or leaf

Excludes2   ingestion of toxic animal or plant (T61.-, T62.-)

The appropriate 7th character is to be added to each code from category T63

     A   initial encounter
     D   subsequent encounter
     S   sequela

● T63.0 Toxic effect of snake venom

● T63.00 Toxic effect of unspecified snake venom

● T63.001 Toxic effect of unspecified snake venom, accidental (unintentional)
     Toxic effect of unspecified snake venom NOS

● T63.002 Toxic effect of unspecified snake venom, intentional self-harm A, S

● T63.003 Toxic effect of unspecified snake venom, assault

● T63.004 Toxic effect of unspecified snake venom, undetermined

● T63.01 Toxic effect of rattlesnake venom

● T63.011 Toxic effect of rattlesnake venom, accidental (unintentional)
     Toxic effect of rattlesnake venom NOS

● T63.012 Toxic effect of rattlesnake venom, intentional self-harm A, S

● T63.013 Toxic effect of rattlesnake venom, assault

● T63.014 Toxic effect of rattlesnake venom, undetermined

● T63.02 Toxic effect of coral snake venom

● T63.021 Toxic effect of coral snake venom, accidental (unintentional)
     Toxic effect of coral snake venom NOS

● T63.022 Toxic effect of coral snake venom, intentional self-harm A, S

● T63.023 Toxic effect of coral snake venom, assault

● T63.024 Toxic effect of coral snake venom, undetermined

● T63.03 Toxic effect of taipan venom

● T63.031 Toxic effect of taipan venom, accidental (unintentional)
     Toxic effect of taipan venom NOS

● T63.032 Toxic effect of taipan venom, intentional self-harm A, S

● T63.033 Toxic effect of taipan venom, assault

● T63.034 Toxic effect of taipan venom, undetermined

● T63.04 Toxic effect of cobra venom

● T63.041 Toxic effect of cobra venom, accidental (unintentional)
     Toxic effect of cobra venom NOS

● T63.042 Toxic effect of cobra venom, intentional self-harm A, S

● T63.043 Toxic effect of cobra venom, assault

● T63.044 Toxic effect of cobra venom, undetermined

● T63.06 Toxic effect of venom of other North and South American snake

● T63.061 Toxic effect of venom of other North and South American snake, accidental (unintentional)
     Toxic effect of venom of other North and South American snake NOS

● T63.062 Toxic effect of venom of other North and South American snake, intentional self-harm A, S

● T63.063 Toxic effect of venom of other North and South American snake, assault

● T63.064 Toxic effect of venom of other North and South American snake, undetermined

● T63.07 Toxic effect of venom of other Australian snake

● T63.071 Toxic effect of venom of other Australian snake, accidental (unintentional)
     Toxic effect of venom of other Australian snake NOS

● T63.072 Toxic effect of venom of other Australian snake, intentional self-harm A, S

● T63.073 Toxic effect of venom of other Australian snake, assault

● T63.074 Toxic effect of venom of other Australian snake, undetermined

● T63.08 Toxic effect of venom of other African and Asian snake

● T63.081 Toxic effect of venom of other African and Asian snake, accidental (unintentional)
     Toxic effect of venom of other African and Asian snake NOS

● T63.082 Toxic effect of venom of other African and Asian snake, intentional self-harm A, S

● T63.083 Toxic effect of venom of other African and Asian snake, assault

● T63.084 Toxic effect of venom of other African and Asian snake, undetermined

● T63.09 Toxic effect of venom of other snake

● T63.091 Toxic effect of venom of other snake, accidental (unintentional)
     Toxic effect of venom of other snake NOS

● T63.092 Toxic effect of venom of other snake, intentional self-harm A, S

● T63.093 Toxic effect of venom of other snake, assault

● T63.094 Toxic effect of venom of other snake, undetermined

● T63.1 Toxic effect of venom of other reptiles

● T63.11 Toxic effect of venom of gila monster

● T63.111 Toxic effect of venom of gila monster, accidental (unintentional)
     Toxic effect of venom of gila monster NOS

● T63.112 Toxic effect of venom of gila monster, intentional self-harm A, S ℞
● T63.113 Toxic effect of venom of gila monster, assault
● T63.114 Toxic effect of venom of gila monster, undetermined
● T63.12 Toxic effect of venom of other venomous lizard
  ● T63.121 Toxic effect of venom of other venomous lizard, accidental (unintentional)
    Toxic effect of venom of other venomous lizard NOS
  ● T63.122 Toxic effect of venom of other venomous lizard, intentional self-harm A, S ℞
  ● T63.123 Toxic effect of venom of other venomous lizard, assault
  ● T63.124 Toxic effect of venom of other venomous lizard, undetermined
● T63.19 Toxic effect of venom of other reptiles
  ● T63.191 Toxic effect of venom of other reptiles, accidental (unintentional)
    Toxic effect of venom of other reptiles NOS
  ● T63.192 Toxic effect of venom of other reptiles, intentional self-harm A, S ℞
  ● T63.193 Toxic effect of venom of other reptiles, assault
  ● T63.194 Toxic effect of venom of other reptiles, undetermined
● T63.2 Toxic effect of venom of scorpion
● T63.2X Toxic effect of venom of scorpion
  ● T63.2X1 Toxic effect of venom of scorpion, accidental (unintentional)
    Toxic effect of venom of scorpion NOS
  ● T63.2X2 Toxic effect of venom of scorpion, intentional self-harm A, S ℞
  ● T63.2X3 Toxic effect of venom of scorpion, assault
  ● T63.2X4 Toxic effect of venom of scorpion, undetermined
● T63.3 Toxic effect of venom of spider
● T63.30 Toxic effect of unspecified spider venom
  ● T63.301 Toxic effect of unspecified spider venom, accidental (unintentional)
  ● T63.302 Toxic effect of unspecified spider venom, intentional self-harm A, S ℞
  ● T63.303 Toxic effect of unspecified spider venom, assault
  ● T63.304 Toxic effect of unspecified spider venom, undetermined
● T63.31 Toxic effect of venom of black widow spider
  ● T63.311 Toxic effect of venom of black widow spider, accidental (unintentional)
  ● T63.312 Toxic effect of venom of black widow spider, intentional self-harm A, S ℞
  ● T63.313 Toxic effect of venom of black widow spider, assault
  ● T63.314 Toxic effect of venom of black widow spider, undetermined
● T63.32 Toxic effect of venom of tarantula
  ● T63.321 Toxic effect of venom of tarantula, accidental (unintentional)
  ● T63.322 Toxic effect of venom of tarantula, intentional self-harm A, S ℞
  ● T63.323 Toxic effect of venom of tarantula, assault
  ● T63.324 Toxic effect of venom of tarantula, undetermined

● T63.33 Toxic effect of venom of brown recluse spider
  ● T63.331 Toxic effect of venom of brown recluse spider, accidental (unintentional)
  ● T63.332 Toxic effect of venom of brown recluse spider, intentional self-harm A, S ℞
  ● T63.333 Toxic effect of venom of brown recluse spider, assault
  ● T63.334 Toxic effect of venom of brown recluse spider, undetermined
● T63.39 Toxic effect of venom of other spider
  ● T63.391 Toxic effect of venom of other spider, accidental (unintentional)
  ● T63.392 Toxic effect of venom of other spider, intentional self-harm A, S ℞
  ● T63.393 Toxic effect of venom of other spider, assault
  ● T63.394 Toxic effect of venom of other spider, undetermined
● T63.4 Toxic effect of venom of other arthropods
Use additional code, if applicable, for anaphylactic shock (T78.2)
● T63.41 Toxic effect of venom of centipedes and venomous millipedes
  ● T63.411 Toxic effect of venom of centipedes and venomous millipedes, accidental (unintentional)
  ● T63.412 Toxic effect of venom of centipedes and venomous millipedes, intentional self-harm A, S ℞
  ● T63.413 Toxic effect of venom of centipedes and venomous millipedes, assault
  ● T63.414 Toxic effect of venom of centipedes and venomous millipedes, undetermined
● T63.42 Toxic effect of venom of ants
  ● T63.421 Toxic effect of venom of ants, accidental (unintentional)
  ● T63.422 Toxic effect of venom of ants, intentional self-harm A, S ℞
  ● T63.423 Toxic effect of venom of ants, assault
  ● T63.424 Toxic effect of venom of ants, undetermined
● T63.43 Toxic effect of venom of caterpillars
  ● T63.431 Toxic effect of venom of caterpillars, accidental (unintentional)
  ● T63.432 Toxic effect of venom of caterpillars, intentional self-harm A, S ℞
  ● T63.433 Toxic effect of venom of caterpillars, assault
  ● T63.434 Toxic effect of venom of caterpillars, undetermined
● T63.44 Toxic effect of venom of bees
  ● T63.441 Toxic effect of venom of bees, accidental (unintentional)
  ● T63.442 Toxic effect of venom of bees, intentional self-harm A, S ℞
  ● T63.443 Toxic effect of venom of bees, assault
  ● T63.444 Toxic effect of venom of bees, undetermined
● T63.45 Toxic effect of venom of hornets
  ● T63.451 Toxic effect of venom of hornets, accidental (unintentional)
  ● T63.452 Toxic effect of venom of hornets, intentional self-harm A, S ℞
  ● T63.453 Toxic effect of venom of hornets, assault
  ● T63.454 Toxic effect of venom of hornets, undetermined

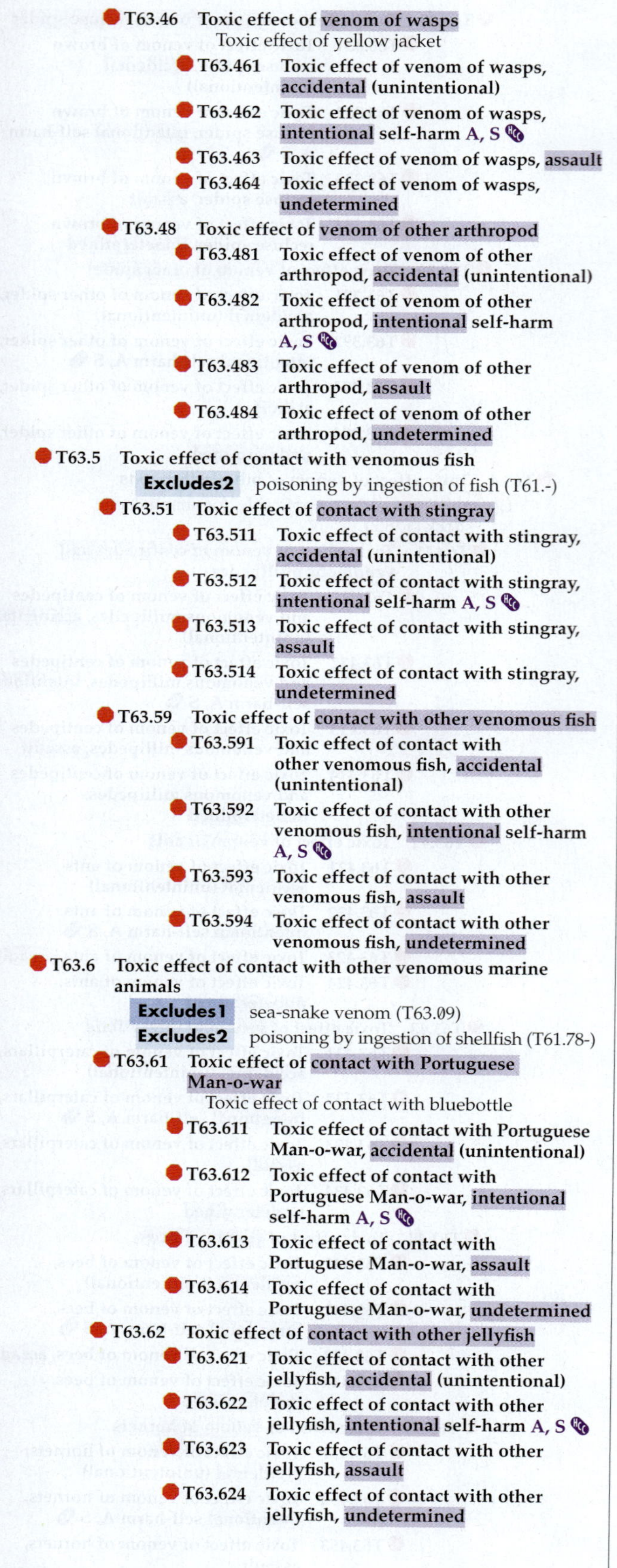

● **T63.46** Toxic effect of venom of wasps
Toxic effect of yellow jacket
  ● **T63.461** Toxic effect of venom of wasps, accidental (unintentional)
  ● **T63.462** Toxic effect of venom of wasps, intentional self-harm A, S
  ● **T63.463** Toxic effect of venom of wasps, assault
  ● **T63.464** Toxic effect of venom of wasps, undetermined
● **T63.48** Toxic effect of venom of other arthropod
  ● **T63.481** Toxic effect of venom of other arthropod, accidental (unintentional)
  ● **T63.482** Toxic effect of venom of other arthropod, intentional self-harm A, S
  ● **T63.483** Toxic effect of venom of other arthropod, assault
  ● **T63.484** Toxic effect of venom of other arthropod, undetermined
● **T63.5** Toxic effect of contact with venomous fish
  Excludes2   poisoning by ingestion of fish (T61.-)
  ● **T63.51** Toxic effect of contact with stingray
    ● **T63.511** Toxic effect of contact with stingray, accidental (unintentional)
    ● **T63.512** Toxic effect of contact with stingray, intentional self-harm A, S
    ● **T63.513** Toxic effect of contact with stingray, assault
    ● **T63.514** Toxic effect of contact with stingray, undetermined
  ● **T63.59** Toxic effect of contact with other venomous fish
    ● **T63.591** Toxic effect of contact with other venomous fish, accidental (unintentional)
    ● **T63.592** Toxic effect of contact with other venomous fish, intentional self-harm A, S
    ● **T63.593** Toxic effect of contact with other venomous fish, assault
    ● **T63.594** Toxic effect of contact with other venomous fish, undetermined
● **T63.6** Toxic effect of contact with other venomous marine animals
  Excludes1   sea-snake venom (T63.09)
  Excludes2   poisoning by ingestion of shellfish (T61.78-)
  ● **T63.61** Toxic effect of contact with Portuguese Man-o-war
    Toxic effect of contact with bluebottle
    ● **T63.611** Toxic effect of contact with Portuguese Man-o-war, accidental (unintentional)
    ● **T63.612** Toxic effect of contact with Portuguese Man-o-war, intentional self-harm A, S
    ● **T63.613** Toxic effect of contact with Portuguese Man-o-war, assault
    ● **T63.614** Toxic effect of contact with Portuguese Man-o-war, undetermined
  ● **T63.62** Toxic effect of contact with other jellyfish
    ● **T63.621** Toxic effect of contact with other jellyfish, accidental (unintentional)
    ● **T63.622** Toxic effect of contact with other jellyfish, intentional self-harm A, S
    ● **T63.623** Toxic effect of contact with other jellyfish, assault
    ● **T63.624** Toxic effect of contact with other jellyfish, undetermined

● **T63.63** Toxic effect of contact with sea anemone
  ● **T63.631** Toxic effect of contact with sea anemone, accidental (unintentional)
  ● **T63.632** Toxic effect of contact with sea anemone, intentional self-harm A, S
  ● **T63.633** Toxic effect of contact with sea anemone, assault
  ● **T63.634** Toxic effect of contact with sea anemone, undetermined
● **T63.69** Toxic effect of contact with other venomous marine animals
  ● **T63.691** Toxic effect of contact with other venomous marine animals, accidental (unintentional)
  ● **T63.692** Toxic effect of contact with other venomous marine animals, intentional self-harm A, S
  ● **T63.693** Toxic effect of contact with other venomous marine animals, assault
  ● **T63.694** Toxic effect of contact with other venomous marine animals, undetermined
● **T63.7** Toxic effect of contact with venomous plant
  ● **T63.71** Toxic effect of contact with venomous marine plant
    ● **T63.711** Toxic effect of contact with venomous marine plant, accidental (unintentional)
    ● **T63.712** Toxic effect of contact with venomous marine plant, intentional self-harm A, S
    ● **T63.713** Toxic effect of contact with venomous marine plant, assault
    ● **T63.714** Toxic effect of contact with venomous marine plant, undetermined
  ● **T63.79** Toxic effect of contact with other venomous plant
    ● **T63.791** Toxic effect of contact with other venomous plant, accidental (unintentional)
    ● **T63.792** Toxic effect of contact with other venomous plant, intentional self-harm A, S
    ● **T63.793** Toxic effect of contact with other venomous plant, assault
    ● **T63.794** Toxic effect of contact with other venomous plant, undetermined
● **T63.8** Toxic effect of contact with other venomous animals
  ● **T63.81** Toxic effect of contact with venomous frog
    Excludes1   contact with nonvenomous frog (W62.0)
    ● **T63.811** Toxic effect of contact with venomous frog, accidental (unintentional)
    ● **T63.812** Toxic effect of contact with venomous frog, intentional self-harm A, S
    ● **T63.813** Toxic effect of contact with venomous frog, assault
    ● **T63.814** Toxic effect of contact with venomous frog, undetermined
  ● **T63.82** Toxic effect of contact with venomous toad
    Excludes1   contact with nonvenomous toad (W62.1)
    ● **T63.821** Toxic effect of contact with venomous toad, accidental (unintentional)
    ● **T63.822** Toxic effect of contact with venomous toad, intentional self-harm A, S

▶ New   ⇒ Revised   ~~deleted~~ Deleted   Excludes 1   Excludes 2   Includes   Use additional   Code first   Code also   Key words
OGCR Official Guidelines   **X** Assign placeholder X   ● Use Additional Character(s)   ▶ Manifestation Code   Hierarchical Condition Category   **Coding Clinic**

● T63.823   Toxic effect of contact with venomous toad, assault
● T63.824   Toxic effect of contact with venomous toad, undetermined
● T63.83   Toxic effect of contact with other venomous amphibian

Excludes1   contact with nonvenomous amphibian (W62.9)

● T63.831   Toxic effect of contact with other venomous amphibian, accidental (unintentional)
● T63.832   Toxic effect of contact with other venomous amphibian, intentional self-harm A, S
● T63.833   Toxic effect of contact with other venomous amphibian, assault
● T63.834   Toxic effect of contact with other venomous amphibian, undetermined
● T63.89   Toxic effect of contact with other venomous animals
● T63.891   Toxic effect of contact with other venomous animals, accidental (unintentional)
● T63.892   Toxic effect of contact with other venomous animals, intentional self-harm A, S
● T63.893   Toxic effect of contact with other venomous animals, assault
● T63.894   Toxic effect of contact with other venomous animals, undetermined
● T63.9   Toxic effect of contact with unspecified venomous animal
X ● T63.91   Toxic effect of contact with unspecified venomous animal, accidental (unintentional)
X ● T63.92   Toxic effect of contact with unspecified venomous animal, intentional self-harm A, S
X ● T63.93   Toxic effect of contact with unspecified venomous animal, assault
X ● T63.94   Toxic effect of contact with unspecified venomous animal, undetermined

● T64   **Toxic effect of aflatoxin and other mycotoxin food contaminants**

The appropriate 7th character is to be added to each code from category T64

> A   initial encounter
> D   subsequent encounter
> S   sequela

● T64.0   Toxic effect of aflatoxin
X ● T64.01   Toxic effect of aflatoxin, accidental (unintentional)
X ● T64.02   Toxic effect of aflatoxin, intentional self-harm A, S
X ● T64.03   Toxic effect of aflatoxin, assault
X ● T64.04   Toxic effect of aflatoxin, undetermined
● T64.8   Toxic effect of other mycotoxin food contaminants
X ● T64.81   Toxic effect of other mycotoxin food contaminants, accidental (unintentional)
X ● T64.82   Toxic effect of other mycotoxin food contaminants, intentional self-harm A, S
X ● T64.83   Toxic effect of other mycotoxin food contaminants, assault
X ● T64.84   Toxic effect of other mycotoxin food contaminants, undetermined

● T65   **Toxic effect of other and unspecified substances**

The appropriate 7th character is to be added to each code from category T65

> A   initial encounter
> D   subsequent encounter
> S   sequela

● T65.0   Toxic effect of cyanides

Excludes1   hydrogen cyanide (T57.3-)

● T65.0X   Toxic effect of cyanides
● T65.0X1   Toxic effect of cyanides, accidental (unintentional)
Toxic effect of cyanides NOS
● T65.0X2   Toxic effect of cyanides, intentional self-harm A, S
● T65.0X3   Toxic effect of cyanides, assault
● T65.0X4   Toxic effect of cyanides, undetermined
● T65.1   Toxic effect of strychnine and its salts
● T65.1X   Toxic effect of strychnine and its salts
● T65.1X1   Toxic effect of strychnine and its salts, accidental (unintentional)
Toxic effect of strychnine and its salts NOS
● T65.1X2   Toxic effect of strychnine and its salts, intentional self-harm A, S
● T65.1X3   Toxic effect of strychnine and its salts, assault
● T65.1X4   Toxic effect of strychnine and its salts, undetermined
● T65.2   Toxic effect of tobacco and nicotine

Excludes2   nicotine dependence (F17.-)

● T65.21   Toxic effect of chewing tobacco
● T65.211   Toxic effect of chewing tobacco, accidental (unintentional)
Toxic effect of chewing tobacco NOS
● T65.212   Toxic effect of chewing tobacco, intentional self-harm A, S
● T65.213   Toxic effect of chewing tobacco, assault
● T65.214   Toxic effect of chewing tobacco, undetermined
● T65.22   Toxic effect of tobacco cigarettes
Toxic effect of tobacco smoke

Use additional code for exposure to second hand tobacco smoke (Z57.31, Z77.22)

● T65.221   Toxic effect of tobacco cigarettes, accidental (unintentional)
Toxic effect of tobacco cigarettes NOS
● T65.222   Toxic effect of tobacco cigarettes, intentional self-harm A, S
● T65.223   Toxic effect of tobacco cigarettes, assault
● T65.224   Toxic effect of tobacco cigarettes, undetermined
● T65.29   Toxic effect of other tobacco and nicotine
● T65.291   Toxic effect of other tobacco and nicotine, accidental (unintentional)
Toxic effect of other tobacco and nicotine NOS
● T65.292   Toxic effect of other tobacco and nicotine, intentional self-harm A, S
● T65.293   Toxic effect of other tobacco and nicotine, assault
● T65.294   Toxic effect of other tobacco and nicotine, undetermined

● **T65.3** **Toxic effect of nitroderivatives and aminoderivatives of benzene and its homologues**
Toxic effect of aniline [benzenamine]
Toxic effect of nitrobenzene
Toxic effect of trinitrotoluene

● **T65.3X** **Toxic effect of nitroderivatives and aminoderivatives of benzene and its homologues**

● **T65.3X1** **Toxic effect of nitroderivatives and aminoderivatives of benzene and its homologues, accidental (unintentional)**
Toxic effect of nitroderivatives and aminoderivatives of benzene and its homologues NOS

● **T65.3X2** **Toxic effect of nitroderivatives and aminoderivatives of benzene and its homologues, intentional self-harm A, S** 🅗🅒

● **T65.3X3** **Toxic effect of nitroderivatives and aminoderivatives of benzene and its homologues, assault**

● **T65.3X4** **Toxic effect of nitroderivatives and aminoderivatives of benzene and its homologues, undetermined**

● **T65.4** **Toxic effect of carbon disulfide**

● **T65.4X** **Toxic effect of carbon disulfide**

● **T65.4X1** **Toxic effect of carbon disulfide, accidental (unintentional)**
Toxic effect of carbon disulfide NOS

● **T65.4X2** **Toxic effect of carbon disulfide, intentional self-harm A, S** 🅗🅒

● **T65.4X3** **Toxic effect of carbon disulfide, assault**

● **T65.4X4** **Toxic effect of carbon disulfide, undetermined**

● **T65.5** **Toxic effect of nitroglycerin and other nitric acids and esters**
Toxic effect of 1,2,3-Propanetriol trinitrate

● **T65.5X** **Toxic effect of nitroglycerin and other nitric acids and esters**

● **T65.5X1** **Toxic effect of nitroglycerin and other nitric acids and esters, accidental (unintentional)**
Toxic effect of nitroglycerin and other nitric acids and esters NOS

● **T65.5X2** **Toxic effect of nitroglycerin and other nitric acids and esters, intentional self-harm A, S** 🅗🅒

● **T65.5X3** **Toxic effect of nitroglycerin and other nitric acids and esters, assault**

● **T65.5X4** **Toxic effect of nitroglycerin and other nitric acids and esters, undetermined**

● **T65.6** **Toxic effect of paints and dyes, not elsewhere classified**

● **T65.6X** **Toxic effect of paints and dyes, not elsewhere classified**

● **T65.6X1** **Toxic effect of paints and dyes, not elsewhere classified, accidental (unintentional)**
Toxic effect of paints and dyes NOS

● **T65.6X2** **Toxic effect of paints and dyes, not elsewhere classified, intentional self-harm A, S** 🅗🅒

● **T65.6X3** **Toxic effect of paints and dyes, not elsewhere classified, assault**

● **T65.6X4** **Toxic effect of paints and dyes, not elsewhere classified, undetermined**

● **T65.8** **Toxic effect of other specified substances**

● **T65.81** **Toxic effect of latex**

● **T65.811** **Toxic effect of latex, accidental (unintentional)**
Toxic effect of latex NOS

● **T65.812** **Toxic effect of latex, intentional self-harm A, S** 🅗🅒

● **T65.813** **Toxic effect of latex, assault**

● **T65.814** **Toxic effect of latex, undetermined**

● **T65.82** **Toxic effect of harmful algae and algae toxins**
Toxic effect of (harmful) algae bloom NOS
Toxic effect of blue-green algae bloom
Toxic effect of brown tide
Toxic effect of cyanobacteria bloom
Toxic effect of Florida red tide
Toxic effect of pfiesteria piscicida
Toxic effect of red tide

● **T65.821** **Toxic effect of harmful algae and algae toxins, accidental (unintentional)**
Toxic effect of harmful algae and algae toxins NOS

● **T65.822** **Toxic effect of harmful algae and algae toxins, intentional self-harm A, S** 🅗🅒

● **T65.823** **Toxic effect of harmful algae and algae toxins, assault**

● **T65.824** **Toxic effect of harmful algae and algae toxins, undetermined**

● **T65.83** **Toxic effect of fiberglass**

● **T65.831** **Toxic effect of fiberglass, accidental (unintentional)**
Toxic effect of fiberglass NOS

● **T65.832** **Toxic effect of fiberglass, intentional self-harm A, S** 🅗🅒

● **T65.833** **Toxic effect of fiberglass, assault**

● **T65.834** **Toxic effect of fiberglass, undetermined**

▶ **T65.84** **Toxic effect of xylazine**
▶ Use Additional code(s) for all associated manifestations, such as:
▶ cellulitis and acute lymphangitis (L03.-)
▶ cutaneous abscess, furuncle and carbuncle (L02.-)
▶ non-pressure chronic ulcer of lower limb, not elsewhere classified (L97.-)
▶ non-pressure chronic ulcer of skin, not elsewhere classified (L98.4-)

▶ ● **T65.841** **Toxic effect of xylazine, accidental (unintentional)**
Toxic effect of xylazine NOS

▶ ● **T65.842** **Toxic effect of xylazine, intentional self-harm**

▶ ● **T65.843** **Toxic effect of xylazine, assault**

▶ ● **T65.844** **Toxic effect of xylazine, undetermined**

● **T65.89** **Toxic effect of other specified substances**

● **T65.891** **Toxic effect of other specified substances, accidental (unintentional)**
Toxic effect of other specified substances NOS
Coding Clinic: 2018, Q1, P5

● **T65.892** **Toxic effect of other specified substances, intentional self-harm A, S** 🅗🅒

● **T65.893** **Toxic effect of other specified substances, assault**

● **T65.894** **Toxic effect of other specified substances, undetermined**

● **T65.9** **Toxic effect of unspecified substance**

X ● **T65.91** **Toxic effect of unspecified substance, accidental (unintentional)**
Poisoning NOS

X ● **T65.92** **Toxic effect of unspecified substance, intentional self-harm A, S** 🅗🅒

X ● **T65.93** **Toxic effect of unspecified substance, assault**

X ● **T65.94** **Toxic effect of unspecified substance, undetermined**

▶ New   ⇨ Revised   ~~deleted~~ Deleted   Excludes 1   Excludes 2   Includes   Use additional   Code first   Code also   Key words
OGCR Official Guidelines   X Assign placeholder X   ● Use Additional Character(s)   ▶ Manifestation Code   🅗🅒 Hierarchical Condition Category   **Coding Clinic**

OTHER AND UNSPECIFIED EFFECTS OF EXTERNAL CAUSES (T66-T78)

● **T66**   **Radiation sickness, unspecified**

    Excludes1   specified adverse effects of radiation, such as:
       burns (T20-T31)
       leukemia (C91-C95)
       radiation gastroenteritis and colitis (K52.0)
       radiation pneumonitis (J70.0)
       radiation related disorders of the skin and
         subcutaneous tissue (L55-L59)
       sunburn (L55.-)

    The appropriate 7th character is to be added to code T66

A	initial encounter
D	subsequent encounter
S	sequela

● **T67**   **Effects of heat and light**

    Excludes1   erythema [dermatitis] ab igne (L59.0)
       malignant hyperpyrexia due to anesthesia (T88.3)
       radiation-related disorders of the skin and
         subcutaneous tissue (L55-L59)

    Excludes2   burns (T20-T31)
       sunburn (L55.-)
       sweat disorder due to heat (L74-L75)

    The appropriate 7th character is to be added to each code from
       category T67

A	initial encounter
D	subsequent encounter
S	sequela

X ● **T67.0**   **Heatstroke and sunstroke**

    Use additional code(s) to identify any associated
      complications of heatstroke, such as:
      coma and stupor (R40.-)
      rhabdomyolysis (M62.82)
      systemic inflammatory response syndrome (R65.1-)
    Coding Clinic: 2019, Q4, P18

    X ● **T67.01**   **Heatstroke and sunstroke**
       Heat apoplexy
       Heat pyrexia
       Siriasis
       Thermoplegia

    X ● **T67.02**   **Exertional heatstroke**
       Coding Clinic: 2019, Q4, P18

    X ● **T67.09**   **Other heatstroke and sunstroke**

X ● **T67.1**   **Heat syncope**
     Heat collapse

X ● **T67.2**   **Heat cramp**

X ● **T67.3**   **Heat exhaustion, anhydrotic**
     Heat prostration due to water depletion

    Excludes1   heat exhaustion due to salt depletion
         (T67.4)

X ● **T67.4**   **Heat exhaustion due to salt depletion**
     Heat prostration due to salt (and water) depletion

X ● **T67.5**   **Heat exhaustion, unspecified**
     Heat prostration NOS

X ● **T67.6**   **Heat fatigue, transient**

X ● **T67.7**   **Heat edema**

X ● **T67.8**   **Other effects of heat and light**

X ● **T67.9**   **Effect of heat and light, unspecified**

X ● **T68**   **Hypothermia**
     Accidental hypothermia
     Hypothermia NOS

    Use additional code to identify source of exposure:
      Exposure to excessive cold of man-made origin (W93)
      Exposure to excessive cold of natural origin (X31)

    Excludes1   hypothermia following anesthesia (T88.51)
       hypothermia not associated with low
         environmental temperature (R68.0)
       hypothermia of newborn (P80.-)

    Excludes2   frostbite (T33-T34)

    The appropriate 7th character is to be added to code T68

A	initial encounter
D	subsequent encounter
S	sequela

● **T69**   **Other effects of reduced temperature**

    Use additional code to identify source of exposure:
      Exposure to excessive cold of man-made origin (W93)
      Exposure to excessive cold of natural origin (X31)

    Excludes2   frostbite (T33-T34)

    The appropriate 7th character is to be added to each code from
       category T69

A	initial encounter
D	subsequent encounter
S	sequela

   ● **T69.0**   **Immersion hand and foot**

     ● **T69.01**   **Immersion hand**

       ● **T69.011**   **Immersion hand, right hand**
       ● **T69.012**   **Immersion hand, left hand**
       ● **T69.019**   **Immersion hand, unspecified hand**

     ● **T69.02**   **Immersion foot**
       Trench foot

       ● **T69.021**   **Immersion foot, right foot**
       ● **T69.022**   **Immersion foot, left foot**
       ● **T69.029**   **Immersion foot, unspecified foot**

X ● **T69.1**   **Chilblains**

X ● **T69.8**   **Other specified effects of reduced temperature**

X ● **T69.9**   **Effect of reduced temperature, unspecified**

● **T70**   **Effects of air pressure and water pressure**

    The appropriate 7th character is to be added to each code from
       category T70

A	initial encounter
D	subsequent encounter
S	sequela

X ● **T70.0**   **Otitic barotrauma**
     Aero-otitis media
     Effects of change in ambient atmospheric pressure or
       water pressure on ears

X ● **T70.1**   **Sinus barotrauma**
     Aerosinusitis
     Effects of change in ambient atmospheric pressure on
       sinuses

   ● **T70.2**   **Other and unspecified effects of high altitude**

     Excludes2   polycythemia due to high altitude (D75.1)

    X ● **T70.20**   **Unspecified effects of high altitude**

    X ● **T70.29**   **Other effects of high altitude**
       Alpine sickness
       Anoxia due to high altitude
       Barotrauma NOS
       Hypobaropathy
       Mountain sickness

X ● **T70.3**   **Caisson disease [decompression sickness]**
     Compressed-air disease
     Diver's palsy or paralysis

CHAPTER 19 (S00-T88)

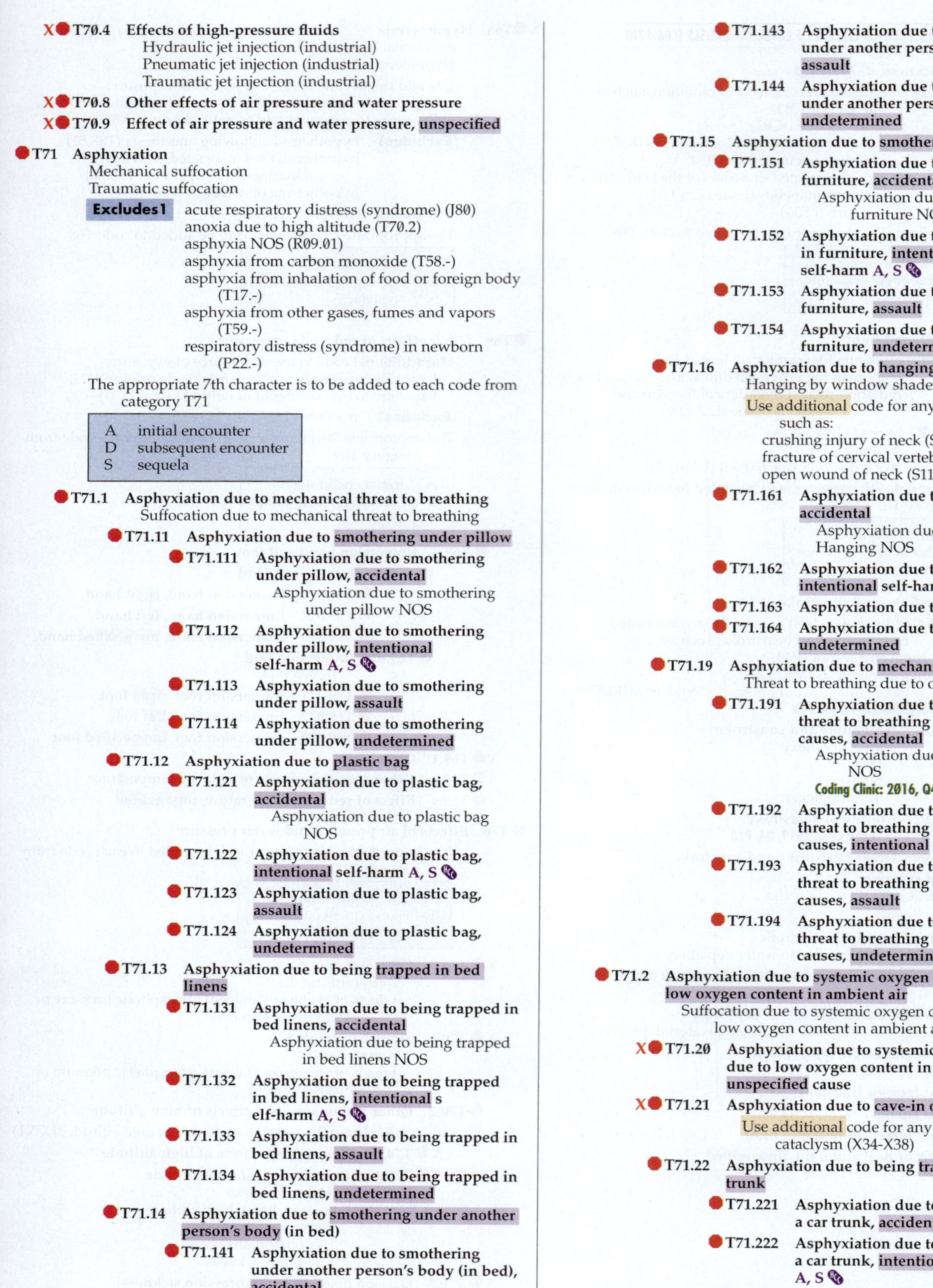

X ● **T70.4**   **Effects of high-pressure fluids**
     Hydraulic jet injection (industrial)
     Pneumatic jet injection (industrial)
     Traumatic jet injection (industrial)

X ● **T70.8**   **Other effects of air pressure and water pressure**

X ● **T70.9**   **Effect of air pressure and water pressure, unspecified**

● **T71**   **Asphyxiation**
     Mechanical suffocation
     Traumatic suffocation

     Excludes1   acute respiratory distress (syndrome) (J80)
                anoxia due to high altitude (T70.2)
                asphyxia NOS (R09.01)
                asphyxia from carbon monoxide (T58.-)
                asphyxia from inhalation of food or foreign body
                    (T17.-)
                asphyxia from other gases, fumes and vapors
                    (T59.-)
                respiratory distress (syndrome) in newborn
                    (P22.-)

     The appropriate 7th character is to be added to each code from
     category T71

       A   initial encounter
       D   subsequent encounter
       S   sequela

● **T71.1**   **Asphyxiation due to mechanical threat to breathing**
     Suffocation due to mechanical threat to breathing

  ● **T71.11**   **Asphyxiation due to smothering under pillow**

    ● **T71.111**   **Asphyxiation due to smothering
                under pillow, accidental**
                Asphyxiation due to smothering
                  under pillow NOS

    ● **T71.112**   **Asphyxiation due to smothering
                under pillow, intentional
                self-harm A, S** 🄷

    ● **T71.113**   **Asphyxiation due to smothering
                under pillow, assault**

    ● **T71.114**   **Asphyxiation due to smothering
                under pillow, undetermined**

  ● **T71.12**   **Asphyxiation due to plastic bag**

    ● **T71.121**   **Asphyxiation due to plastic bag,
                accidental**
                Asphyxiation due to plastic bag
                  NOS

    ● **T71.122**   **Asphyxiation due to plastic bag,
                intentional self-harm A, S** 🄷

    ● **T71.123**   **Asphyxiation due to plastic bag,
                assault**

    ● **T71.124**   **Asphyxiation due to plastic bag,
                undetermined**

  ● **T71.13**   **Asphyxiation due to being trapped in bed
          linens**

    ● **T71.131**   **Asphyxiation due to being trapped in
                bed linens, accidental**
                Asphyxiation due to being trapped
                  in bed linens NOS

    ● **T71.132**   **Asphyxiation due to being trapped
                in bed linens, intentional s
                elf-harm A, S** 🄷

    ● **T71.133**   **Asphyxiation due to being trapped in
                bed linens, assault**

    ● **T71.134**   **Asphyxiation due to being trapped in
                bed linens, undetermined**

  ● **T71.14**   **Asphyxiation due to smothering under another
          person's body (in bed)**

    ● **T71.141**   **Asphyxiation due to smothering
                under another person's body (in bed),
                accidental**
                Asphyxiation due to smothering
                  under another person's body
                  (in bed) NOS

● **T71.143**   **Asphyxiation due to smothering
           under another person's body (in bed),
           assault**

● **T71.144**   **Asphyxiation due to smothering
           under another person's body (in bed),
           undetermined**

  ● **T71.15**   **Asphyxiation due to smothering in furniture**

    ● **T71.151**   **Asphyxiation due to smothering in
                furniture, accidental**
                Asphyxiation due to smothering in
                  furniture NOS

    ● **T71.152**   **Asphyxiation due to smothering
                in furniture, intentional
                self-harm A, S** 🄷

    ● **T71.153**   **Asphyxiation due to smothering in
                furniture, assault**

    ● **T71.154**   **Asphyxiation due to smothering in
                furniture, undetermined**

  ● **T71.16**   **Asphyxiation due to hanging**
          Hanging by window shade cord
          Use additional code for any associated injuries,
             such as:
          crushing injury of neck (S17.-)
          fracture of cervical vertebrae (S12.0-S12.2-)
          open wound of neck (S11.-)

    ● **T71.161**   **Asphyxiation due to hanging,
                accidental**
                Asphyxiation due to hanging NOS
                Hanging NOS

    ● **T71.162**   **Asphyxiation due to hanging,
                intentional self-harm A, S** 🄷

    ● **T71.163**   **Asphyxiation due to hanging, assault**

    ● **T71.164**   **Asphyxiation due to hanging,
                undetermined**

  ● **T71.19**   **Asphyxiation due to mechanical**
          Threat to breathing due to other causes

    ● **T71.191**   **Asphyxiation due to mechanical
                threat to breathing due to other
                causes, accidental**
                Asphyxiation due to other causes
                  NOS
                Coding Clinic: 2016, Q4, P76

    ● **T71.192**   **Asphyxiation due to mechanical
                threat to breathing due to other
                causes, intentional self-harm A, S** 🄷

    ● **T71.193**   **Asphyxiation due to mechanical
                threat to breathing due to other
                causes, assault**

    ● **T71.194**   **Asphyxiation due to mechanical
                threat to breathing due to other
                causes, undetermined**

● **T71.2**   **Asphyxiation due to systemic oxygen deficiency due to
     low oxygen content in ambient air**
     Suffocation due to systemic oxygen deficiency due to
       low oxygen content in ambient air

X ● **T71.20**   **Asphyxiation due to systemic oxygen deficiency
             due to low oxygen content in ambient air due to
             unspecified cause**

X ● **T71.21**   **Asphyxiation due to cave-in or falling earth**
             Use additional code for any associated
               cataclysm (X34-X38)

  ● **T71.22**   **Asphyxiation due to being trapped in a car
          trunk**

    ● **T71.221**   **Asphyxiation due to being trapped in
                a car trunk, accidental**

    ● **T71.222**   **Asphyxiation due to being trapped in
                a car trunk, intentional self-harm
                A, S** 🄷

    ● **T71.223**   **Asphyxiation due to being trapped in
                a car trunk, assault**

    ● **T71.224**   **Asphyxiation due to being trapped in
                a car trunk, undetermined**

T71.23 Asphyxiation due to being trapped in a (discarded) refrigerator

     T71.231 Asphyxiation due to being trapped in a (discarded) refrigerator, accidental

     T71.232 Asphyxiation due to being trapped in a (discarded) refrigerator, intentional self-harm A, S

     T71.233 Asphyxiation due to being trapped in a (discarded) refrigerator, assault

     T71.234 Asphyxiation due to being trapped in a (discarded) refrigerator, undetermined

X **T71.29** Asphyxiation due to being trapped in other low oxygen environment

X **T71.9** Asphyxiation due to unspecified cause

     Suffocation (by strangulation) due to unspecified cause

     Suffocation NOS

     Systemic oxygen deficiency due to low oxygen content in ambient air due to unspecified cause

     Systemic oxygen deficiency due to mechanical threat to breathing due to unspecified cause

     Traumatic asphyxia NOS

T73 Effects of other deprivation

     The appropriate 7th character is to be added to each code from category T73

> A   initial encounter
> D   subsequent encounter
> S   sequela

X **T73.0** Starvation

     Deprivation of food

X **T73.1** Deprivation of water

X **T73.2** Exhaustion due to exposure

X **T73.3** Exhaustion due to excessive exertion

     Exhaustion due to overexertion

X **T73.8** Other effects of deprivation

X **T73.9** Effect of deprivation, unspecified

T74 Adult and child abuse, neglect and other maltreatment, confirmed

     Use additional code, if applicable, to identify any associated current injury

     Use additional external cause code to identify perpetrator, if known (Y07.-)

     Excludes1 abuse and maltreatment in pregnancy (O9A.3-, O9A.4-, O9A.5-)

               adult and child maltreatment, suspected (T76.-)

     The appropriate 7th character is to be added to each code from category T74

> A   initial encounter
> D   subsequent encounter
> S   sequela

T74.0 Neglect or abandonment, confirmed

     X **T74.01** Adult neglect or abandonment, confirmed   A

     X **T74.02** Child neglect or abandonment, confirmed   P

T74.1 Physical abuse, confirmed

     Excludes2 sexual abuse (T74.2-)

     X **T74.11** Adult physical abuse, confirmed   A

     X **T74.12** Child physical abuse, confirmed   P

         Excludes2 shaken infant syndrome (T74.4)

T74.2 Sexual abuse, confirmed

     Rape, confirmed

     Sexual assault, confirmed

     X **T74.21** Adult sexual abuse, confirmed   A

     X **T74.22** Child sexual abuse, confirmed   P

T74.3 Psychological abuse, confirmed

     Bullying and intimidation, confirmed

     Intimidation through social media, confirmed

     Target of threatened harm, confirmed

     Target of threatened physical violence, confirmed

     Target of threatened sexual abuse, confirmed

     X **T74.31** Adult psychological abuse, confirmed   A

     X **T74.32** Child psychological abuse, confirmed   P

X **T74.4** Shaken infant syndrome   P

T74.5 Forced sexual exploitation, confirmed

     X **T74.51** Adult forced sexual exploitation, confirmed   P

     X **T74.52** Child sexual exploitation, confirmed   P

T74.6 Forced labor exploitation, confirmed

     X **T74.61** Adult forced labor exploitation, confirmed   P

     X **T74.62** Child forced labor exploitation, confirmed   P

T74.9 Unspecified maltreatment, confirmed

     X **T74.91** Unspecified adult maltreatment, confirmed   A

     X **T74.92** Unspecified child maltreatment, confirmed   P

T74.A Financial abuse, confirmed

     T74.A1 Adult financial abuse, confirmed

     T74.A2 Child financial abuse, confirmed

T75 Other and unspecified effects of other external causes

     Excludes1 adverse effects NEC (T78.-)

     Excludes2 burns (electric) (T20-T31)

     The appropriate 7th character is to be added to each code from category T75

> A   initial encounter
> D   subsequent encounter
> S   sequela

T75.0 Effects of lightning

     Struck by lightning

     X **T75.00** Unspecified effects of lightning

         Struck by lightning NOS

     X **T75.01** Shock due to being struck by lightning

     X **T75.09** Other effects of lightning

         Use additional code for other effects of lightning

X **T75.1** Unspecified effects of drowning and nonfatal submersion

     Immersion

     Excludes1 specified effects of drowning code to effects

     Coding Clinic: 2023, Q1, P26

T75.2 Effects of vibration

     X **T75.20** Unspecified effects of vibration

     X **T75.21** Pneumatic hammer syndrome

     X **T75.22** Traumatic vasospastic syndrome

     X **T75.23** Vertigo from infrasound

         Excludes1 vertigo NOS (R42)

     X **T75.29** Other effects of vibration

X **T75.3** Motion sickness

     Airsickness   Travel sickness

     Seasickness

     Use additional external cause code to identify vehicle or type of motion (Y92.81-)

X **T75.4** Electrocution

     Shock from electric current

     Shock from electroshock gun (taser)

T75.8 Other specified effects of external causes

     X **T75.81** Effects of abnormal gravitation [G] forces

     X **T75.82** Effects of weightlessness

     ▶ X **T75.83** Effects of war theater

         ▶ Use Additional code to identify associated manifestations

         ▶ X **T75.830** Gulf war illness

             ▶ Gulf war syndrome

         ▶ X **T75.838** Effects of other war theater

     X **T75.89** Other specified effects of external causes

CHAPTER 19 (S00-T88)

● **T76** **Adult and child abuse, neglect and other maltreatment, suspected**

    Use additional code, if applicable, to identify any associated current injury

    Excludes1　adult and child maltreatment, confirmed (T74.-)
        suspected abuse and maltreatment in pregnancy (O9A.3-, O9A.4-, O9A.5-)
        suspected adult physical abuse, ruled out (Z04.71)
        suspected adult sexual abuse, ruled out (Z04.41)
        suspected child physical abuse, ruled out (Z04.72)
        suspected child sexual abuse, ruled out (Z04.42)

    The appropriate 7th character is to be added to each code from category T76

A	initial encounter
D	subsequent encounter
S	sequela

Coding Clinic: 2016, Q4, P129

● **T76.0**　Neglect or abandonment, suspected
    X● **T76.01**　**Adult** neglect or abandonment, suspected　**A**
    X● **T76.02**　**Child** neglect or abandonment, suspected　**P**

● **T76.1**　Physical abuse, suspected
    X● **T76.11**　**Adult** physical abuse, suspected　**A**
    X● **T76.12**　**Child** physical abuse, suspected　**P**
        Coding Clinic: 2019, Q2, P12

● **T76.2**　Sexual abuse, suspected
    Rape, suspected
      Excludes1　alleged abuse, ruled out (Z04.7)
    X● **T76.21**　**Adult** sexual abuse, suspected　**A**
    X● **T76.22**　**Child** sexual abuse, suspected　**P**

● **T76.3**　Psychological abuse, suspected
    Bullying and intimidation, suspected
    Intimidation through social media, suspected
    Target of threatened harm, suspected
    Target of threatened physical violence, suspected
    Target of threatened sexual abuse, suspected
    X● **T76.31**　**Adult** psychological abuse, suspected　**A**
    X● **T76.32**　**Child** psychological abuse, suspected　**P**

● **T76.5**　Forced sexual exploitation, suspected
    X● **T76.51**　**Adult** forced sexual exploitation, suspected　**P**
    X● **T76.52**　**Child** sexual exploitation, suspected　**P**

● **T76.6**　Forced labor exploitation, suspected
    X● **T76.61**　**Adult** forced labor exploitation, suspected　**P**
    X● **T76.62**　**Child** forced labor exploitation, suspected　**P**

● **T76.9**　Unspecified maltreatment, suspected
    X● **T76.91**　Unspecified **adult** maltreatment, suspected　**A**
    X● **T76.92**　Unspecified **child** maltreatment, suspected　**P**

● **T76.A**　Financial abuse, suspected
    X● **T76.A1**　**Adult** financial abuse, suspected
    X● **T76.A2**　**Child** financial abuse, suspected

● **T78**　**Adverse effects, not elsewhere classified**
    Excludes2　complications of surgical and medical care NEC (T80-T88)

    The appropriate 7th character is to be added to each code from category T78

A	initial encounter
D	subsequent encounter
S	sequela

● **T78.0**　Anaphylactic reaction due to food
    Anaphylactic reaction due to adverse food reaction
    Anaphylactic shock or reaction due to nonpoisonous foods
    Anaphylactoid reaction due to food
    X● **T78.00**　Anaphylactic reaction due to **unspecified** food
    X● **T78.01**　Anaphylactic reaction due to **peanuts**

X● **T78.02**　Anaphylactic reaction due to **shellfish (crustaceans)**
X● **T78.03**　Anaphylactic reaction due to **other fish**
X● **T78.04**　Anaphylactic reaction due to **fruits and vegetables**
X● **T78.05**　Anaphylactic reaction due to **tree nuts and seeds**
    Excludes2　anaphylactic reaction due to peanuts (T78.01)
X● **T78.06**　Anaphylactic reaction due to **food additives**
X● **T78.07**　Anaphylactic reaction due to **milk and dairy products**
    ▶ ● **T78.070**　Anaphylactic reaction due to milk and dairy products with tolerance to baked milk
      ▶ **Excludes1**　Anaphylactic reaction due to milk and dairy products with reactivity to baked milk (T78.071)
    ▶ **T78.071**　Anaphylactic reaction due to milk and dairy products with reactivity to baked milk
      ▶ **Excludes1**　Anaphylactic reaction due to milk and dairy products with tolerance to baked milk (T78.070)
    ▶ **T78.079**　Anaphylactic reaction due to milk and dairy products, unspecified
X● **T78.08**　Anaphylactic reaction due to **eggs**
    ▶ **T78.080**　Anaphylactic reaction due to egg with tolerance to baked egg
      ▶ **Excludes1**　Anaphylactic reaction due to egg with reactivity to baked egg (T78.081)
    ▶ **T78.081**　Anaphylactic reaction due to egg with reactivity to baked egg
      ▶ **Excludes1**　Anaphylactic reaction due to egg with tolerance to baked egg(T78.080)
    ▶ **T78.089**　Anaphylactic reaction due to eggs, unspecified
X● **T78.09**　Anaphylactic reaction due to **other food products**

X● **T78.1**　Other adverse food reactions, not elsewhere classified
    Use additional code to identify the type of reaction, if applicable
    Excludes1　anaphylactic reaction or shock due to adverse food reaction (T78.0-)
        anaphylactic reaction due to food (T78.0-)
        bacterial food borne intoxications (A05.-)
    Excludes2　allergic and dietetic gastroenteritis and colitis (K52.29)
        allergic rhinitis due to food (J30.5)
        dermatitis due to food in contact with skin (L23.6, L24.6, L25.4)
        dermatitis due to ingested food (L27.2)
        food protein-induced enterocolitis syndrome (K52.21)
        food protein-induced enteropathy (K52.22)

▶ New　➡ Revised　~~deleted~~ Deleted　Excludes 1　Excludes 2　Includes　Use additional　Code first　Code also　Key words
OGCR Official Guidelines　X Assign placeholder X　● Use Additional Character(s)　▶ Manifestation Code　HCC Hierarchical Condition Category　**Coding Clinic**

▶● **T78.11 Other adverse food reactions due to milk and dairy products**

   ▶**T78.11Ø Other adverse food reactions due to milk and dairy products with tolerance to baked milk**

      ▶**Excludes1** Other adverse food reaction due to milk and dairy products with reactivity to baked milk (T78.111)

   ▶**T78.111 Other adverse food reaction due to milk and dairy products with reactivity to baked milk**

      ▶**Excludes1** Other adverse food reaction due to milk and dairy products with tolerance to baked milk (T78.110)

   ▶**T78.119 Other adverse food reaction due to milk and dairy products with baked milk tolerance/reactivity, unspecified**

▶● **T78.12 Other adverse food reaction due to eggs**

   ▶**T78.12Ø Other adverse food reaction due to egg with tolerance to baked egg**

      ▶**Excludes1** Other adverse food reaction due to egg with reactivity to baked egg (T78.121)

   ▶**T78.121 Other adverse food reaction due to egg with reactivity to baked egg**

      ▶**Excludes1** Other adverse food reaction due to egg with tolerance to baked egg (T78.120)

   ▶**T78.129 Other adverse food reaction due to egg with baked egg tolerance/reactivity, unspecified**

   ▶**T78.19 Other adverse food reactions, not elsewhere classified**

X● **T78.2 Anaphylactic shock, unspecified**
Occurs when allergic response triggers large quantities of histamines, prostaglandins, leukotrienes resulting in systemic vasodilation

Allergic shock
Anaphylactic reaction
Anaphylaxis

   Excludes1 anaphylactic reaction or shock due to adverse effect of correct medicinal substance properly administered (T88.6)
anaphylactic reaction or shock due to adverse food reaction (T78.0-)
anaphylactic reaction or shock due to serum (T80.5-)

X● **T78.3 Angioneurotic edema**
Allergic angioedema
Giant urticaria
Vascular disorder resulting from abnormalities of autonomic nervous system fibers supplying blood vessels
Quincke's edema

   Excludes1 serum urticaria (T80.6-)
urticaria (L50.-)

● **T78.4 Other and unspecified allergy**

   Excludes1 specified types of allergic reaction such as:
allergic diarrhea (K52.29)
allergic gastroenteritis and colitis (K52.29)
dermatitis (L23-L25, L27.-)
food protein-induced enterocolitis syndrome (K52.21)
food protein-induced enteropathy (K52.22)
hay fever (J30.1)

X● **T78.4Ø Allergy, unspecified**
Allergic reaction NOS
Hypersensitivity NOS

X● **T78.41 Arthus phenomenon**
Arthus reaction

X● **T78.49 Other allergy**
Coding Clinic: 2021, Q1, P42

X● **T78.8 Other adverse effects, not elsewhere classified**

CERTAIN EARLY COMPLICATIONS OF TRAUMA (T79)

● **T79 Certain early complications of trauma, not elsewhere classified**

   Excludes2 acute respiratory distress syndrome (J80)
complications occurring during or following medical procedures (T80-T88)
complications of surgical and medical care NEC (T80-T88)
newborn respiratory distress syndrome (P22.0)

The appropriate 7th character is to be added to each code from category T79

   A   initial encounter
   D   subsequent encounter
   S   sequela

X● **T79.Ø Air embolism (traumatic) A**

   Excludes1 air embolism complicating abortion or ectopic or molar pregnancy (O00-O07, O08.2)
air embolism complicating pregnancy, childbirth and the puerperium (O88.0)
air embolism following infusion, transfusion, and therapeutic injection (T80.0)
air embolism following procedure NEC (T81.7-)

   Coding Clinic: 2024, Q2, P16

X● **T79.1 Fat embolism (traumatic) A**

   Excludes1 fat embolism complicating:
abortion or ectopic or molar pregnancy (O00-O07, O08.2)
pregnancy, childbirth and the puerperium (O88.8)

X● **T79.2 Traumatic secondary and recurrent hemorrhage and seroma A**

X● **T79.4 Traumatic shock A**
Shock (immediate) (delayed) following injury

   Excludes1 anaphylactic shock due to adverse food reaction (T78.0-)
anaphylactic shock due to correct medicinal substance properly administered (T88.6)
anaphylactic shock due to serum (T80.5-)
anaphylactic shock NOS (T78.2)
electric shock (T75.4)
nontraumatic shock NEC (R57.-)
obstetric shock (O75.1)
postprocedural shock (T81.1-)
septic shock (R65.21)
shock complicating abortion or ectopic or molar pregnancy (O00-O07, O08.3)
shock due to anesthesia (T88.2)
shock due to lightning (T75.01)
shock NOS (R57.9)

CHAPTER 19 (SØØ-T88)

X ● T79.5 Traumatic anuria A ^{RCC}
Crush syndrome
Renal failure following crushing

X ● T79.6 Traumatic ischemia of muscle A ^{RCC}
Traumatic rhabdomyolysis
Volkmann's ischemic contracture
> **Excludes2** anterior tibial syndrome (M76.8)
> compartment syndrome (traumatic)
>   (T79.A-)
> nontraumatic ischemia of muscle (M62.2-)

**X ● T79.7 Traumatic subcutaneous emphysema
A** ^{RCC}
> **Excludes2** emphysema NOS (J43)
> emphysema (subcutaneous) resulting
>   from a procedure (T81.82)

X ● T79.8 Other early complications of trauma A ^{RCC}
Coding Clinic: 2024, Q2, P16

X ● T79.9 Unspecified early complication of trauma A ^{RCC}

● T79.A Traumatic compartment syndrome
> **Excludes1** fibromyalgia (M79.7)
> nontraumatic compartment syndrome
>   (M79.A-)
>
> **Excludes2** traumatic ischemic infarction of muscle
>   (T79.6)

X ● T79.A0 Compartment syndrome, unspecified

Compartment syndrome NOS

**● T79.A1 Traumatic compartment syndrome of upper
extremity**
Traumatic compartment syndrome of shoulder,
   arm, forearm, wrist, hand, and fingers

**● T79.A11 Traumatic compartment syndrome of
right upper extremity A** ^{RCC}

**● T79.A12 Traumatic compartment syndrome
of left upper extremity A** ^{RCC}

**● T79.A19 Traumatic compartment syndrome of
unspecified upper extremity A** ^{RCC}

**● T79.A2 Traumatic compartment syndrome of lower
extremity**
Traumatic compartment syndrome of hip,
   buttock, thigh, leg, foot, and toes

**● T79.A21 Traumatic compartment syndrome
of right lower extremity A** ^{RCC}

**● T79.A22 Traumatic compartment syndrome
of left lower extremity A** ^{RCC}

**● T79.A29 Traumatic compartment syndrome of
unspecified lower extremity**

**X ● T79.A3 Traumatic compartment syndrome of
abdomen A** ^{RCC}

**X ● T79.A9 Traumatic compartment syndrome of
other sites A** ^{RCC}

COMPLICATIONS OF SURGICAL AND MEDICAL CARE
NOT ELSEWHERE CLASSIFIED (T80-T88)

Use additional code for adverse effect, if applicable, to identify
   drug (T36-T50 with fifth or sixth character 5)
Use additional code(s) to identify the specified condition
   resulting from the complication.
Use additional code to identify devices involved and details of
   circumstances (Y62-Y82)
> **Excludes2** any encounters with medical care for
>   postprocedural conditions in which no
>   complications are present, such as:
> artificial opening status (Z93.-)
> closure of external stoma (Z43.-)
> fitting and adjustment of external prosthetic
>   device (Z44.-)
> burns and corrosions from local applications and
>   irradiation (T20-T32)
> complications of surgical procedures during
>   pregnancy, childbirth and the puerperium
>   (O00-O9A)
> mechanical complication of respirator [ventilator]
>   (J95.850)
> poisoning and toxic effects of drugs and
>   chemicals (T36-T65 with fifth or sixth
>   character 1-4 or 6)
> postprocedural fever (R50.82)
> specified complications classified elsewhere, such
>   as:
> cerebrospinal fluid leak from spinal puncture
>   (G97.0)
> colostomy malfunction (K94.0-)
> disorders of fluid and electrolyte imbalance
>   (E86-E87)
> functional disturbances following cardiac
>   surgery (I97.0-I97.1)
> intraoperative and postprocedural
>   complications of specified body systems
>   (D78.-, E36.-, E89.-, G97.3-, G97.4, H59.3-,
>   H59.-, H95.2-, H95.3, I97.4-, I97.5, J95.6-,
>   J95.7, K91.6-, L76.-, M96.-, N99.-)
> ostomy complications (J95.0-, K94.-, N99.5-)
> postgastric surgery syndromes (K91.1)
> postlaminectomy syndrome NEC (M96.1)
> postmastectomy lymphedema syndrome (I97.2)
> postsurgical blind-loop syndrome (K91.2)
> ventilator associated pneumonia (J95.851)

**● T80 Complications following infusion, transfusion and therapeutic
injection**
> **Includes** complications following perfusion
> **Excludes2** bone marrow transplant rejection (T86.01)
> febrile nonhemolytic transfusion reaction (R50.84)
> fluid overload due to transfusion (E87.71)
> posttransfusion purpura (D69.51)
> transfusion associated circulatory overload
>   (TACO) (E87.71)
> transfusion (red blood cell) associated
>   hemochromatosis (E83.111)
> transfusion related acute lung injury (TRALI)
>   (J95.84)

The appropriate 7th character is to be added to each code from
   category T80

> A   initial encounter
> D   subsequent encounter
> S   sequela

**X ● T80.0 Air embolism following infusion, transfusion and
therapeutic injection**

X ● **T80.1 Vascular complications** following infusion, transfusion and therapeutic injection

> Use additional code to identify the vascular complication
>
> **Excludes2** extravasation of vesicant agent (T80.81-)
> infiltration of vesicant agent (T80.81-)
> vascular complications specified as due to prosthetic devices, implants and grafts (T82.8- T83.8-, T84.8-, T85.8-)
> postprocedural vascular complications (T81.7-)

● **T80.2 Infections** following infusion, transfusion and therapeutic injection

> Use additional code to identify the specific infection, such as:
> sepsis (A41.9)
>
> Use additional code (R65.2-) to identify severe sepsis, if applicable
>
> **Excludes2** infections specified as due to prosthetic devices, implants and grafts (T82.6-T82.7, T83.5-T83.6, T84.5-T84.7, T85.7)
> postprocedural infections (T81.44)
>
> **Coding Clinic: 2018, Q4, P89**

● **T80.21 Infection** due to central venous catheter

> Infection due to pulmonary artery catheter (Swan-Ganz catheter)
>
> **Coding Clinic: 2019, Q1, P13-14; 2018, Q4, P89**

● **T80.211 Bloodstream** infection due to central venous catheter

> Catheter-related bloodstream infection (CRBSI) NOS
> Central line-associated bloodstream infection (CLABSI)
> Bloodstream infection due to Hickman catheter
> Bloodstream infection due to peripherally inserted central catheter (PICC)
> Bloodstream infection due to portacath (port-a-cath)
> Bloodstream infection due to pulmonary artery catheter
> Bloodstream infection due to triple lumen catheter
> Bloodstream infection due to umbilical venous catheter
>
> **Coding Clinic: 2018, Q4, P89**

● **T80.212 Local infection** due to central venous catheter

> Exit or insertion site infection
> Local infection due to Hickman catheter
> Local infection due to peripherally inserted central catheter (PICC)
> Local infection due to portacath (port-a-cath)
> Local infection due to pulmonary artery catheter
> Local infection due to triple lumen catheter
> Local infection due to umbilical venous catheter
> Port or reservoir infection
> Tunnel infection

● **T80.218 Other infection** due to central venous catheter

> Other central line-associated infection
> Other infection due to Hickman catheter
> Other infection due to peripherally inserted central catheter (PICC)
> Other infection due to portacath (port-a-cath)
> Other infection due to pulmonary artery catheter
> Other infection due to triple lumen catheter
> Other infection due to umbilical venous catheter

● **T80.219 Unspecified infection** due to central venous catheter

> Central line-associated infection NOS
> Unspecified infection due to Hickman catheter
> Unspecified infection due to peripherally inserted central catheter (PICC)
> Unspecified infection due to portacath (port-a-cath)
> Unspecified infection due to pulmonary artery catheter
> Unspecified infection due to triple lumen catheter
> Unspecified infection due to umbilical venous catheter

X ● **T80.22 Acute infection** following transfusion, infusion, or injection of blood and blood products

X ● **T80.29 Infection** following other infusion, transfusion and therapeutic injection

● **T80.3 ABO incompatibility** reaction due to transfusion of blood or blood products

> **Excludes1** minor blood group antigens reactions (Duffy) (E) (K) (Kell) (Kidd) (Lewis) (M) (N) (P) (S) (T80.A-)

X ● **T80.30 ABO incompatibility reaction** due to transfusion of blood or blood products, unspecified

> ABO incompatibility blood transfusion NOS
> Reaction to ABO incompatibility from transfusion NOS

● **T80.31 ABO incompatibility** with **hemolytic transfusion reaction**

● **T80.310 ABO incompatibility** with **acute hemolytic transfusion reaction**

> ABO incompatibility with hemolytic transfusion reaction less than 24 hours after transfusion
> Acute hemolytic transfusion reaction (AHTR) due to ABO incompatibility

● **T80.311 ABO incompatibility** with **delayed hemolytic transfusion reaction**

> ABO incompatibility with hemolytic transfusion reaction 24 hours or more after transfusion
> Delayed hemolytic transfusion reaction (DHTR) due to ABO incompatibility

● **T80.319**   **ABO incompatibility with hemolytic transfusion reaction, unspecified**
    ABO incompatibility with hemolytic transfusion reaction at unspecified time after transfusion
    Hemolytic transfusion reaction (HTR) due to ABO incompatibility NOS

X ● **T80.39**   **Other ABO incompatibility reaction due to transfusion of blood or blood products**
    Delayed serologic transfusion reaction (DSTR) from ABO incompatibility
    Other ABO incompatible blood transfusion
    Other reaction to ABO incompatible blood transfusion

● **T80.4**   **Rh incompatibility reaction due to transfusion of blood or blood products**
    Reaction due to incompatibility of Rh antigens (C) (c) (D) (E) (e)

X ● **T80.40**   **Rh incompatibility reaction due to transfusion of blood or blood products, unspecified**
    Reaction due to Rh factor in transfusion NOS
    Rh incompatible blood transfusion NOS

● **T80.41**   **Rh incompatibility with hemolytic transfusion reaction**

   ● **T80.410**   **Rh incompatibility with acute hemolytic transfusion reaction**
     Acute hemolytic transfusion reaction (AHTR) due to Rh incompatibility
     Rh incompatibility with hemolytic transfusion reaction less than 24 hours after transfusion

   ● **T80.411**   **Rh incompatibility with delayed hemolytic transfusion reaction**
     Delayed hemolytic transfusion reaction (DHTR) due to Rh incompatibility
     Rh incompatibility with hemolytic transfusion reaction 24 hours or more after transfusion

   ● **T80.419**   **Rh incompatibility with hemolytic transfusion reaction, unspecified**
     Rh incompatibility with hemolytic transfusion reaction at unspecified time after transfusion
     Hemolytic transfusion reaction (HTR) due to Rh incompatibility NOS

X ● **T80.49**   **Other Rh incompatibility reaction due to transfusion of blood or blood products**
    Delayed serologic transfusion reaction (DSTR) from Rh incompatibility
    Other reaction to Rh incompatible blood transfusion

● **T80.5**   **Anaphylactic reaction due to serum**
    Allergic reaction due to serum
    Anaphylactic shock due to serum
    Anaphylactoid reaction due to serum
    Anaphylaxis due to serum

   Excludes1   ABO incompatibility reaction due to transfusion of blood or blood products (T80.3-)
    allergic reaction or shock NOS (T78.2)
    anaphylactic reaction or shock NOS (T78.2)
    anaphylactic reaction or shock due to adverse effect of correct medicinal substance properly administered (T88.6)
    other serum reaction (T80.6-)

X ● **T80.51**   **Anaphylactic reaction due to administration of blood and blood products**

X ● **T80.52**   **Anaphylactic reaction due to vaccination**
    Coding Clinic: 2021, Q1, P43

X ● **T80.59**   **Anaphylactic reaction due to other serum**

● **T80.6**   **Other serum reactions**
    Intoxication by serum   Serum sickness
    Protein sickness   Serum urticaria
    Serum rash

   Excludes2   serum hepatitis (B16-B19)

X ● **T80.61**   **Other serum reaction due to administration of blood and blood products**

X ● **T80.62**   **Other serum reaction due to vaccination**
    Coding Clinic: 2021, Q1, P42

X ● **T80.69**   **Other serum reaction due to other serum**
    Code also, if applicable, arthropathy in hypersensitivity reactions classified elsewhere (M36.4)

● **T80.8**   **Other complications following infusion, transfusion and therapeutic injection**

● **T80.81**   **Extravasation of vesicant agent**
    Infiltration of vesicant agent

   ● **T80.810**   **Extravasation of vesicant antineoplastic chemotherapy**
     Infiltration of vesicant antineoplastic chemotherapy

   ● **T80.818**   **Extravasation of other vesicant agent**
     Infiltration of other vesicant agent

T80.82   **Complication of immune effector cellular therapy**
    Complication of chimeric antigen receptor (CAR-T) cell therapy
    Complication of IEC therapy

   Excludes2   adverse effect of immune checkpoint inhibitors and immunostimulant drugs (T45.AX5)
    complication of bone marrow transplant (T86.0)
    complication of stem cell transplant (T86.5)

   Use additional code to identify the specific complication, such as:
    cytokine release syndrome (D89.83-)
    immune effector cell-associated neurotoxicity syndrome (G92.0-)

X ● **T80.89**   **Other complications following infusion, transfusion and therapeutic injection**
    Delayed serologic transfusion reaction (DSTR), unspecified incompatibility
    Use additional code to identify graft-versus-host reaction, if applicable, (D89.81-)

● **T80.9**   **Unspecified complication following infusion, transfusion and therapeutic injection**

X ● **T80.90**   **Unspecified complication following infusion and therapeutic injection**

● **T80.91**   **Hemolytic transfusion reaction, unspecified incompatibility**

   Excludes1   ABO incompatibility with hemolytic transfusion reaction (T80.31-)
    Non-ABO incompatibility with hemolytic transfusion reaction (T80.A1-)
    Rh incompatibility with hemolytic transfusion reaction (T80.41-)

   ● **T80.910**   **Acute hemolytic transfusion reaction, unspecified incompatibility**

   ● **T80.911**   **Delayed hemolytic transfusion reaction, unspecified incompatibility**

   ● **T80.919**   **Hemolytic transfusion reaction, unspecified incompatibility, unspecified as acute or delayed**
     Hemolytic transfusion reaction NOS

X ● **T80.92**   **Unspecified transfusion reaction**
    Transfusion reaction NOS

▶ New   ◀ Revised   ~~deleted~~ Deleted   Excludes 1   Excludes 2   Includes   Use additional   Code first   Code also   Key words
OGCR Official Guidelines   X Assign placeholder X   ● Use Additional Character(s)   ▶ Manifestation Code   HCC Hierarchical Condition Category   Coding Clinic

● **T80.A**   **Non-ABO incompatibility reaction due to transfusion of blood or blood products**
> Reaction due to incompatibility of minor antigens (Duffy) (Kell) (Kidd) (Lewis) (M) (N) (P) (S)

✕● **T80.A0**   **Non-ABO incompatibility reaction due to transfusion of blood or blood products, unspecified**
> Non-ABO antigen incompatibility reaction from transfusion NOS

● **T80.A1**   **Non-ABO incompatibility with hemolytic transfusion reaction**

● **T80.A10**   **Non-ABO incompatibility with acute hemolytic transfusion reaction**
> Acute hemolytic transfusion reaction (AHTR) due to non-ABO incompatibility
>
> Non-ABO incompatibility with hemolytic transfusion reaction less than 24 hours after transfusion

● **T80.A11**   **Non-ABO incompatibility with delayed hemolytic transfusion reaction**
> Delayed hemolytic transfusion reaction (DHTR) due to non-ABO incompatibility
>
> Non-ABO incompatibility with hemolytic transfusion reaction 24 or more hours after transfusion

● **T80.A19**   **Non-ABO incompatibility with hemolytic transfusion reaction, unspecified**
> Hemolytic transfusion reaction (HTR) due to non-ABO incompatibility NOS
>
> Non-ABO incompatibility with hemolytic transfusion reaction at unspecified time after transfusion

✕● **T80.A9**   **Other non-ABO incompatibility reaction due to transfusion of blood or blood products**
> Delayed serologic transfusion reaction (DSTR) from non-ABO incompatibility
>
> Other reaction to non-ABO incompatible blood transfusion

● **T81**   **Complications of procedures, not elsewhere classified**
> Use additional code for adverse effect, if applicable, to identify drug (T36-T50 with fifth or sixth character 5)

> **Excludes2**   complications following immunization (T88.0-T88.1)
> complications following infusion, transfusion and therapeutic injection (T80.-)
> complications of transplanted organs and tissue (T86.-)
> poisoning and toxic effects of drugs and chemicals (T36-T65 with fifth or sixth character 1-4)
> specified complications classified elsewhere, such as:
> complication of prosthetic devices, implants and grafts (T82-T85)
> dermatitis due to drugs and medicaments (L23.3, L24.4, L25.1, L27.0-L27.1)
> endosseous dental implant failure (M27.6-)
> floppy iris syndrome (IFIS) (intraoperative) H21.81
> intraoperative and postprocedural complications of specific body system (D78.-, E36.-, E89.-, G97.3-, G97.4, H59.3-, H59.-, H95.2-, H95.3, I97.4-, I97.5, J95, K91.-, L76.-, M96.-, N99.-)
> ostomy complications (J95.0-, K94.-, N99.5-)
> plateau iris syndrome (post-iridectomy) (postprocedural) H21.82

Coding Clinic: 2019, Q2, P21-22; 2016, Q4, P29

The appropriate 7th character is to be added to each code from category T81

A	initial encounter
D	subsequent encounter
S	sequela

● **T81.1**   **Postprocedural shock**
> Shock during or resulting from a procedure, not elsewhere classified

> **Excludes1**   anaphylactic shock NOS (T78.2)
> anaphylactic shock due to correct substance properly administered (T88.6)
> anaphylactic shock due to serum (T80.5-)
> electric shock (T75.4)
> obstetric shock (O75.1)
> septic shock (R65.21)
> shock due to anesthesia (T88.2)
> shock following abortion or ectopic or molar pregnancy (O00-O07, O08.3)
> traumatic shock (T79.4)

✕● **T81.10**   **Postprocedural shock unspecified**
> Collapse NOS during or resulting from a procedure, not elsewhere classified
> Postprocedural failure of peripheral circulation
> Postprocedural shock NOS

✕● **T81.11**   **Postprocedural cardiogenic shock A** 🔖

✕● **T81.12**   **Postprocedural septic shock A** 🔖
> Postprocedural endotoxic shock resulting from a procedure, not elsewhere classified
> Postprocedural gram-negative shock resulting from a procedure, not elsewhere classified
> *Code first* underlying infection
> Use additional code, to identify any associated acute organ dysfunction, if applicable

✕● **T81.19**   **Other postprocedural shock**
> Postprocedural hypovolemic shock
> **Coding Clinic: 2021, Q1, P14**

● **T81.3**   **Disruption of wound, not elsewhere classified**
> Disruption of any suture materials or other closure methods

> **Excludes1**   breakdown (mechanical) of permanent sutures (T85.612)
> displacement of permanent sutures (T85.622)
> disruption of cesarean delivery wound (O90.0)
> disruption of perineal obstetric wound (O90.1)
> mechanical complication of permanent sutures NEC (T85.692)

✕● **T81.30**   **Disruption of wound, unspecified**
> Disruption of wound NOS

✕● **T81.31**   **Disruption of external operation (surgical) wound, not elsewhere classified**

> **Excludes1**   dehiscence of amputation stump (T87.81)
> Dehiscence of operation wound NOS
> Disruption of operation wound NOS
> Disruption or dehiscence of closure of cornea
> Disruption or dehiscence of closure of mucosa
> Disruption or dehiscence of closure of skin and subcutaneous tissue
> Full-thickness skin disruption or dehiscence
> Superficial disruption or dehiscence of operation wound
> **Coding Clinic: 2015, Q1, P20**

✕● **T81.32**   **Disruption of internal operation (surgical) wound, not elsewhere classified**
> **Coding Clinic: 2017, Q3, P4**

● **T81.320**   **Disruption or dehiscence of gastrointestinal tract anastomosis, repair, or closure**
> **Coding Clinic: 2024, Q4, P30**

● **T81.321**   **Disruption or dehiscence of closure of internal operation (surgical) wound of abdominal wall muscle or fascia**

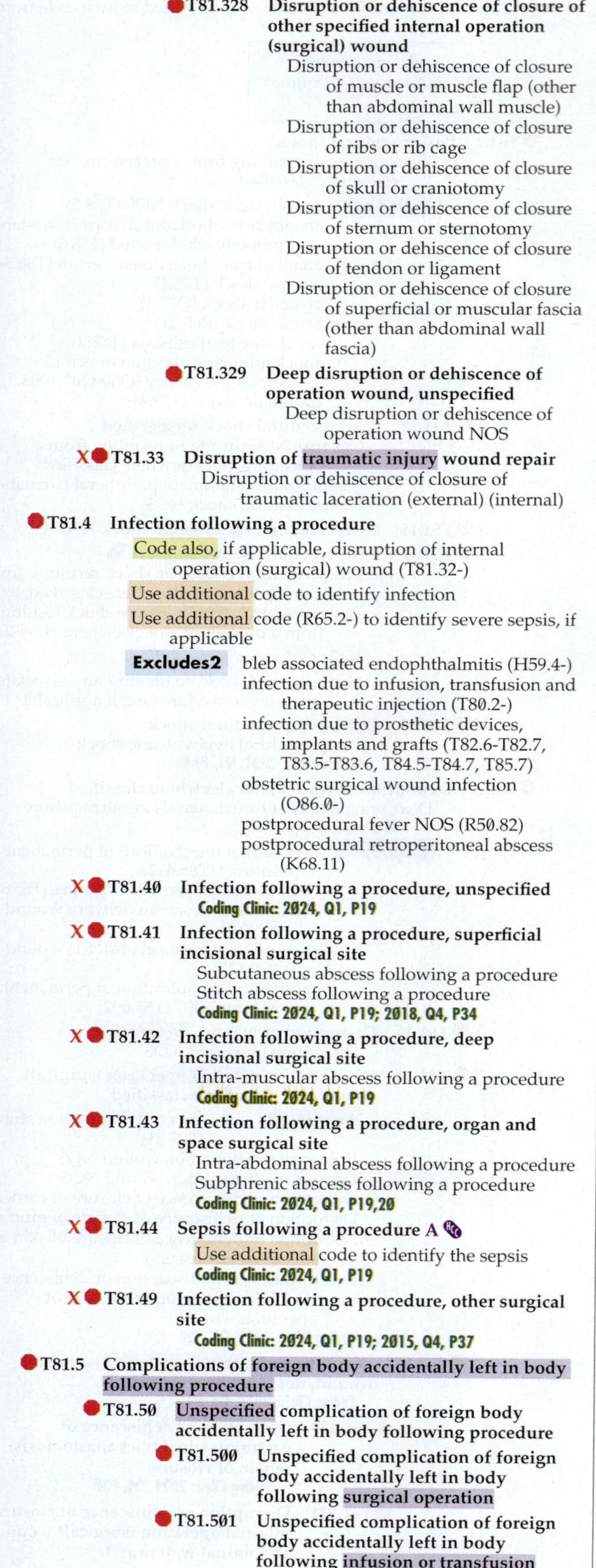

● **T81.328** **Disruption or dehiscence of closure of other specified internal operation (surgical) wound**
Disruption or dehiscence of closure of muscle or muscle flap (other than abdominal wall muscle)
Disruption or dehiscence of closure of ribs or rib cage
Disruption or dehiscence of closure of skull or craniotomy
Disruption or dehiscence of closure of sternum or sternotomy
Disruption or dehiscence of closure of tendon or ligament
Disruption or dehiscence of closure of superficial or muscular fascia (other than abdominal wall fascia)

● **T81.329** **Deep disruption or dehiscence of operation wound, unspecified**
Deep disruption or dehiscence of operation wound NOS

X ● **T81.33** **Disruption of traumatic injury wound repair**
Disruption or dehiscence of closure of traumatic laceration (external) (internal)

● **T81.4** **Infection following a procedure**
Code also, if applicable, disruption of internal operation (surgical) wound (T81.32-)
Use additional code to identify infection
Use additional code (R65.2-) to identify severe sepsis, if applicable

Excludes2 bleb associated endophthalmitis (H59.4-)
infection due to infusion, transfusion and therapeutic injection (T80.2-)
infection due to prosthetic devices, implants and grafts (T82.6-T82.7, T83.5-T83.6, T84.5-T84.7, T85.7)
obstetric surgical wound infection (O86.0-)
postprocedural fever NOS (R50.82)
postprocedural retroperitoneal abscess (K68.11)

X ● **T81.40** **Infection following a procedure, unspecified**
Coding Clinic: 2024, Q1, P19

X ● **T81.41** **Infection following a procedure, superficial incisional surgical site**
Subcutaneous abscess following a procedure
Stitch abscess following a procedure
Coding Clinic: 2024, Q1, P19; 2018, Q4, P34

X ● **T81.42** **Infection following a procedure, deep incisional surgical site**
Intra-muscular abscess following a procedure
Coding Clinic: 2024, Q1, P19

X ● **T81.43** **Infection following a procedure, organ and space surgical site**
Intra-abdominal abscess following a procedure
Subphrenic abscess following a procedure
Coding Clinic: 2024, Q1, P19,20

X ● **T81.44** **Sepsis following a procedure** A
Use additional code to identify the sepsis
Coding Clinic: 2024, Q1, P19

X ● **T81.49** **Infection following a procedure, other surgical site**
Coding Clinic: 2024, Q1, P19; 2015, Q4, P37

● **T81.5** **Complications of foreign body accidentally left in body following procedure**

● **T81.50** **Unspecified complication of foreign body accidentally left in body following procedure**

● **T81.500** **Unspecified complication of foreign body accidentally left in body following surgical operation**

● **T81.501** **Unspecified complication of foreign body accidentally left in body following infusion or transfusion**

● **T81.502** **Unspecified complication of foreign body accidentally left in body following kidney dialysis** A, D, S

● **T81.503** **Unspecified complication of foreign body accidentally left in body following injection or immunization**

● **T81.504** **Unspecified complication of foreign body accidentally left in body following endoscopic examination**

● **T81.505** **Unspecified complication of foreign body accidentally left in body following heart catheterization**

● **T81.506** **Unspecified complication of foreign body accidentally left in body following aspiration, puncture or other catheterization**

● **T81.507** **Unspecified complication of foreign body accidentally left in body following removal of catheter or packing**

● **T81.508** **Unspecified complication of foreign body accidentally left in body following other procedure**

● **T81.509** **Unspecified complication of foreign body accidentally left in body following unspecified procedure**

● **T81.51** **Adhesions due to foreign body accidentally left in body following procedure**

● **T81.510** **Adhesions due to foreign body accidentally left in body following surgical operation**

● **T81.511** **Adhesions due to foreign body accidentally left in body following infusion or transfusion**

● **T81.512** **Adhesions due to foreign body accidentally left in body following kidney dialysis** A, D, S

● **T81.513** **Adhesions due to foreign body accidentally left in body following injection or immunization**

● **T81.514** **Adhesions due to foreign body accidentally left in body following endoscopic examination**

● **T81.515** **Adhesions due to foreign body accidentally left in body following heart catheterization**

● **T81.516** **Adhesions due to foreign body accidentally left in body following aspiration, puncture or other catheterization**

● **T81.517** **Adhesions due to foreign body accidentally left in body following removal of catheter or packing**

● **T81.518** **Adhesions due to foreign body accidentally left in body following other procedure**

● **T81.519** **Adhesions due to foreign body accidentally left in body following unspecified procedure**

● **T81.52** **Obstruction due to foreign body accidentally left in body following procedure**

● **T81.520** **Obstruction due to foreign body accidentally left in body following surgical operation**

● **T81.521** **Obstruction due to foreign body accidentally left in body following infusion or transfusion**

● **T81.522** **Obstruction due to foreign body accidentally left in body following kidney dialysis** A, D, S

● **T81.523** **Obstruction due to foreign body accidentally left in body following injection or immunization**

● T81.524   Obstruction due to foreign body accidentally left in body following endoscopic examination

● T81.525   Obstruction due to foreign body accidentally left in body following heart catheterization

● T81.526   Obstruction due to foreign body accidentally left in body following aspiration, puncture or other catheterization

● T81.527   Obstruction due to foreign body accidentally left in body following removal of catheter or packing

● T81.528   Obstruction due to foreign body accidentally left in body following other procedure

● T81.529   Obstruction due to foreign body accidentally left in body following unspecified procedure

● T81.53   Perforation due to foreign body accidentally left in body following procedure

● T81.530   Perforation due to foreign body accidentally left in body following surgical operation

● T81.531   Perforation due to foreign body accidentally left in body following infusion or transfusion

● T81.532   Perforation due to foreign body accidentally left in body following kidney dialysis **A, D, S** ⬤

● T81.533   Perforation due to foreign body accidentally left in body following injection or immunization

● T81.534   Perforation due to foreign body accidentally left in body following endoscopic examination

● T81.535   Perforation due to foreign body accidentally left in body following heart catheterization

● T81.536   Perforation due to foreign body accidentally left in body following aspiration, puncture or other catheterization

● T81.537   Perforation due to foreign body accidentally left in body following removal of catheter or packing

● T81.538   Perforation due to foreign body accidentally left in body following other procedure

● T81.539   Perforation due to foreign body accidentally left in body following unspecified procedure

● T81.59   Other complications of foreign body accidentally left in body following procedure

    Excludes2   obstruction or perforation due to prosthetic devices and implants intentionally left in body (T82.0-T82.5, T83.0-T83.4, T83.7, T84.0-T84.4, T85.0-T85.6)

● T81.590   Other complications of foreign body accidentally left in body following surgical operation
    Coding Clinic: 2025, Q2, P10

● T81.591   Other complications of foreign body accidentally left in body following infusion or transfusion

● T81.592   Other complications of foreign body accidentally left in body following kidney dialysis **A, D, S** ⬤

● T81.593   Other complications of foreign body accidentally left in body following injection or immunization

● T81.594   Other complications of foreign body accidentally left in body following endoscopic examination

● T81.595   Other complications of foreign body accidentally left in body following heart catheterization

● T81.596   Other complications of foreign body accidentally left in body following aspiration, puncture or other catheterization

● T81.597   Other complications of foreign body accidentally left in body following removal of catheter or packing

● T81.598   Other complications of foreign body accidentally left in body following other procedure

● T81.599   Other complications of foreign body accidentally left in body following unspecified procedure

● T81.6   Acute reaction to foreign substance accidentally left during a procedure

    Excludes2   complications of foreign body accidentally left in body cavity or operation wound following procedure (T81.5-)

X ● T81.60   Unspecified acute reaction to foreign substance accidentally left during a procedure

X ● T81.61   Aseptic peritonitis due to foreign substance accidentally left during a procedure
    Chemical peritonitis

X ● T81.69   Other acute reaction to foreign substance accidentally left during a procedure

● T81.7   Vascular complications following a procedure, not elsewhere classified
    Air embolism following procedure NEC
    Phlebitis or thrombophlebitis resulting from a procedure

    Excludes1   embolism complicating abortion or ectopic or molar pregnancy (O00-O07, O08.2)
       embolism complicating pregnancy, childbirth and the puerperium (O88.-)
       traumatic embolism (T79.0)

    Excludes2   embolism due to prosthetic devices, implants and grafts (T82.8, T83.81, T84.8-, T85.1-)
       embolism following infusion, transfusion and therapeutic injection (T80.0)

    Coding Clinic: 2019, Q2, P23

● T81.71   Complication of artery following a procedure, not elsewhere classified
    Coding Clinic: 2019, Q2, P22

● T81.710   Complication of mesenteric artery following a procedure, not elsewhere classified

● T81.711   Complication of renal artery following a procedure, not elsewhere classified

● T81.718   Complication of other artery following a procedure, not elsewhere classified
    Coding Clinic: 2024, Q4, P19; 2019, Q2, P22-23

● T81.719   Complication of unspecified artery following a procedure, not elsewhere classified
    Coding Clinic: 2024, Q4, P56

X ● T81.72   Complication of vein following a procedure, not elsewhere classified
    Coding Clinic: 2019, Q2, P22

CHAPTER 19 (S00-T88)

● **T81.8** **Other complications of procedures, not elsewhere classified**

Excludes2   hypothermia following anesthesia (T88.51)
malignant hyperpyrexia due to anesthesia (T88.3)

X ● **T81.81** **Complication of inhalation therapy**

X ● **T81.82** **Emphysema (subcutaneous) resulting from a procedure**

X ● **T81.83** **Persistent postprocedural fistula**
Code also, if applicable, disruption of internal operation (surgical) wound (T81.32-)
Use additional code, if known, for site of fistula such as:
anal fistula (K60.3-)
anorectal fistula (K60.5-)
bladder fistula (N32.2)
other female intestinal-genital tract fistulae (N82.4)
Coding Clinic: 2024, Q3, P4; 2023, Q1, P30; 2017, Q3, P3-5

X ● **T81.89** **Other complications of procedures, not elsewhere classified**
Use additional code to specify complication, such as:
postprocedural delirium (F05)

X ● **T81.9** **Unspecified complication of procedure**

● **T82** **Complications of cardiac and vascular prosthetic devices, implants and grafts**

Excludes2   failure and rejection of transplanted organs and tissue (T86.-)

The appropriate 7th character is to be added to each code from category T82

A   initial encounter
D   subsequent encounter
S   sequela

● **T82.0** **Mechanical complication of heart valve prosthesis**
Mechanical complication of artificial heart valve

Excludes1   mechanical complication of biological heart valve graft (T82.22-)

X ● **T82.01** **Breakdown (mechanical) of heart valve prosthesis**

X ● **T82.02** **Displacement of heart valve prosthesis**
Malposition of heart valve prosthesis

X ● **T82.03** **Leakage of heart valve prosthesis**

X ● **T82.09** **Other mechanical complication of heart valve prosthesis**
Obstruction (mechanical) of heart valve prosthesis
Perforation of heart valve prosthesis
Protrusion of heart valve prosthesis

● **T82.1** **Mechanical complication of cardiac electronic device**

● **T82.11** **Breakdown (mechanical) of cardiac electronic device**

● **T82.110** **Breakdown (mechanical) of cardiac electrode**

● **T82.111** **Breakdown (mechanical) of cardiac pulse generator (battery)**

● **T82.118** **Breakdown (mechanical) of other cardiac electronic device**

● **T82.119** **Breakdown (mechanical) of unspecified cardiac electronic device**

● **T82.12** **Displacement of cardiac electronic device**
Malposition of cardiac electronic device

● **T82.120** **Displacement of cardiac electrode**

● **T82.121** **Displacement of cardiac pulse generator (battery)**

● **T82.128** **Displacement of other cardiac electronic device**

● **T82.129** **Displacement of unspecified cardiac electronic device**

● **T82.19** **Other mechanical complication of cardiac electronic device**
Leakage of cardiac electronic device
Obstruction of cardiac electronic device
Perforation of cardiac electronic device
Protrusion of cardiac electronic device

● **T82.190** **Other mechanical complication of cardiac electrode**

● **T82.191** **Other mechanical complication of cardiac pulse generator (battery)**

● **T82.198** **Other mechanical complication of other cardiac electronic device**

● **T82.199** **Other mechanical complication of unspecified cardiac device**

● **T82.2** **Mechanical complication of coronary artery bypass graft and biological heart valve graft**

Excludes1   mechanical complication of artificial heart valve prosthesis (T82.0-)

● **T82.21** **Mechanical complication of coronary artery bypass graft**

● **T82.211** **Breakdown (mechanical) of coronary artery bypass graft**

● **T82.212** **Displacement of coronary artery bypass graft**
Malposition of coronary artery bypass graft

● **T82.213** **Leakage of coronary artery bypass graft**

● **T82.218** **Other mechanical complication of coronary artery bypass graft**
Obstruction, mechanical of coronary artery bypass graft
Perforation of coronary artery bypass graft
Protrusion of coronary artery bypass graft

● **T82.22** **Mechanical complication of biological heart valve graft**

● **T82.221** **Breakdown (mechanical) of biological heart valve graft**

● **T82.222** **Displacement of biological heart valve graft**
Malposition of biological heart valve graft

● **T82.223** **Leakage of biological heart valve graft**

● **T82.228** **Other mechanical complication of biological heart valve graft**
Obstruction, mechanical of biological heart valve graft
Perforation of biological heart valve graft
Protrusion of biological heart valve graft

● **T82.3** **Mechanical complication of other vascular grafts**

● **T82.31** **Breakdown (mechanical) of other vascular grafts**

● **T82.310** **Breakdown (mechanical) of aortic (bifurcation) graft (replacement) A** �️

● **T82.311** **Breakdown (mechanical) of carotid arterial graft (bypass) A** �️

● **T82.312** **Breakdown (mechanical) of femoral arterial graft (bypass) A** �️

● **T82.318** **Breakdown (mechanical) of other vascular grafts A** �️

● **T82.319** **Breakdown (mechanical) of unspecified vascular grafts A** �️

● **T82.32** **Displacement of other vascular grafts**
Malposition of other vascular grafts

● **T82.320** **Displacement of aortic (bifurcation) graft (replacement) A** �️

● **T82.321** **Displacement of carotid arterial graft (bypass) A** �️

● T82.322   Displacement of femoral arterial graft (bypass) A ℞

● T82.328   Displacement of other vascular grafts A ℞

● T82.329   Displacement of unspecified vascular grafts A ℞

● **T82.33**   **Leakage of other vascular grafts**

● T82.330   Leakage of aortic (bifurcation) graft (replacement) A ℞

● T82.331   Leakage of carotid arterial graft (bypass) A ℞

● T82.332   Leakage of femoral arterial graft (bypass) A ℞

● T82.338   Leakage of other vascular grafts A ℞

● T82.339   Leakage of unspecified vascular graft A ℞

● **T82.39**   **Other mechanical complication of other vascular grafts**

Obstruction (mechanical) of other vascular grafts

Perforation of other vascular grafts

Protrusion of other vascular grafts

● T82.390   Other mechanical complication of aortic (bifurcation) graft (replacement) A ℞

● T82.391   Other mechanical complication of carotid arterial graft (bypass) A ℞

● T82.392   Other mechanical complication of femoral arterial graft (bypass) A ℞

● T82.398   Other mechanical complication of other vascular grafts A ℞

● T82.399   Other mechanical complication of unspecified vascular grafts A ℞

● **T82.4**   **Mechanical complication of vascular dialysis catheter**

Mechanical complication of hemodialysis catheter

Excludes1   mechanical complication of intraperitoneal dialysis catheter (T85.62)

X ● **T82.41**   **Breakdown (mechanical) of vascular dialysis catheter A, D, S ℞**

X ● **T82.42**   **Displacement of vascular dialysis catheter A, D, S ℞**

Malposition of vascular dialysis catheter

X ● **T82.43**   **Leakage of vascular dialysis catheter A, D, S ℞**

X ● **T82.49**   **Other complication of vascular dialysis catheter A, D, S ℞**

Obstruction (mechanical) of vascular dialysis catheter

Perforation of vascular dialysis catheter

Protrusion of vascular dialysis catheter

● **T82.5**   **Mechanical complication of other cardiac and vascular devices and implants**

Excludes2   mechanical complication of epidural and subdural infusion catheter (T85.61)

● **T82.51**   **Breakdown (mechanical) of other cardiac and vascular devices and implants**

● T82.510   Breakdown (mechanical) of surgically created arteriovenous fistula A ℞

● T82.511   Breakdown (mechanical) of surgically created arteriovenous shunt A ℞

● T82.512   Breakdown (mechanical) of artificial heart A ℞

● T82.513   Breakdown (mechanical) of balloon (counterpulsation) device A ℞

● T82.514   Breakdown (mechanical) of infusion catheter A ℞

● T82.515   Breakdown (mechanical) of umbrella device A ℞

● T82.518   Breakdown (mechanical) of other cardiac and vascular devices and implants A ℞

● T82.519   Breakdown (mechanical) of unspecified cardiac and vascular devices and implants

● **T82.52**   **Displacement of other cardiac and vascular devices and implants**

Malposition of other cardiac and vascular devices and implants

● T82.520   Displacement of surgically created arteriovenous fistula A ℞

● T82.521   Displacement of surgically created arteriovenous shunt A ℞

● T82.522   Displacement of artificial heart A ℞

● T82.523   Displacement of balloon (counterpulsation) device A ℞

● T82.524   Displacement of infusion catheter A ℞

Coding Clinic: 2019, Q3, P15

● T82.525   Displacement of umbrella device A ℞

● T82.528   Displacement of other cardiac and vascular devices and implants A ℞

● T82.529   Displacement of unspecified cardiac and vascular devices and implants

● **T82.53**   **Leakage of other cardiac and vascular devices and implants**

● T82.530   Leakage of surgically created arteriovenous fistula A ℞

● T82.531   Leakage of surgically created arteriovenous shunt A ℞

● T82.532   Leakage of artificial heart A ℞

● T82.533   Leakage of balloon (counterpulsation) device A ℞

● T82.534   Leakage of infusion catheter A ℞

● T82.535   Leakage of umbrella device A ℞

● T82.538   Leakage of other cardiac and vascular devices and implants A ℞

● T82.539   Leakage of unspecified cardiac and vascular devices and implants

● **T82.59**   **Other mechanical complication of other cardiac and vascular devices and implants**

Obstruction (mechanical) of other cardiac and vascular devices and implants

Perforation of other cardiac and vascular devices and implants

Protrusion of other cardiac and vascular devices and implants

● T82.590   Other mechanical complication of surgically created arteriovenous fistula A ℞

● T82.591   Other mechanical complication of surgically created arteriovenous shunt A ℞

● T82.592   Other mechanical complication of artificial heart A ℞

● T82.593   Other mechanical complication of balloon (counterpulsation) device A ℞

● T82.594   Other mechanical complication of infusion catheter A ℞

● T82.595   Other mechanical complication of umbrella device A ℞

● T82.598   Other mechanical complication of other cardiac and vascular devices and implants A ℞

● T82.599   Other mechanical complication of unspecified cardiac and vascular devices and implants

X ● **T82.6**   **Infection and inflammatory reaction due to cardiac valve prosthesis A ℞**

Use additional code to identify infection

Coding Clinic: 2025, Q1, P19-20

X ● **T82.7**   **Infection and inflammatory reaction due to other cardiac and vascular devices, implants and grafts A ℞**

Use additional code to identify infection

Coding Clinic: 2019, Q1, P13-14; 2018, Q4, P89

● **T82.8** **Other specified complications** of cardiac and vascular prosthetic devices, implants and grafts

  ● **T82.81** **Embolism** due to cardiac and vascular prosthetic devices, implants and grafts
     Coding Clinic: 2016, Q4, P70

    ● **T82.817** **Embolism** due to **cardiac** prosthetic devices, implants and grafts
       Coding Clinic: 2016, Q4, P70; 2015, Q1, P20

    ● **T82.818** **Embolism** due to **vascular** prosthetic devices, implants and grafts A

  ● **T82.82** **Fibrosis** due to cardiac and vascular prosthetic devices, implants and grafts
     Coding Clinic: 2016, Q4, P70

    ● **T82.827** **Fibrosis** due to **cardiac** prosthetic devices, implants and grafts

    ● **T82.828** **Fibrosis** due to **vascular** prosthetic devices, implants and grafts A

  ● **T82.83** **Hemorrhage** due to cardiac and vascular prosthetic devices, implants and grafts
     Coding Clinic: 2016, Q4, P70

    ● **T82.837** **Hemorrhage** due to **cardiac** prosthetic devices, implants and grafts

    ● **T82.838** **Hemorrhage** due to **vascular** prosthetic devices, implants and grafts A

  ● **T82.84** **Pain** due to cardiac and vascular prosthetic devices, implants and grafts
     Coding Clinic: 2016, Q4, P70

    ● **T82.847** **Pain** due to **cardiac** prosthetic devices, implants and grafts

    ● **T82.848** **Pain** due to **vascular** prosthetic devices, implants and grafts A

  ● **T82.85** **Stenosis** due to cardiac and vascular prosthetic devices, implants and grafts

    ● **T82.855** **Stenosis** of **coronary artery stent**
      In-stent stenosis (restenosis) of coronary artery stent
      Restenosis of coronary artery stent
      Coding Clinic: 2025, Q1, P20; 2021, Q3, P6-7; 2016, Q4, P70

    ● **T82.856** **Stenosis** of **peripheral vascular stent** A
      In-stent stenosis (restenosis) of peripheral vascular stent
      Restenosis of peripheral vascular stent
      Coding Clinic: 2016, Q4, P70

    ● **T82.857** **Stenosis** of other **cardiac** prosthetic devices, implants and grafts
      Coding Clinic: 2025, Q1, P19; 2016, Q4, P70

    ● **T82.858** **Stenosis** of other **vascular** prosthetic devices, implants and grafts A
      Coding Clinic: 2016, Q4, P70

  ● **T82.86** **Thrombosis** of cardiac and vascular prosthetic devices, implants and grafts

    ● **T82.867** **Thrombosis** due to **cardiac** prosthetic devices, implants and grafts

    ● **T82.868** **Thrombosis** due to **vascular** prosthetic devices, implants and grafts A
      Coding Clinic: 2023, Q2, P7

  ● **T82.89** **Other specified complication** of cardiac and vascular prosthetic devices, implants and grafts

    ● **T82.897** **Other specified complication of cardiac** prosthetic devices, implants and grafts
      Coding Clinic: 2019, Q2, P32-33

    ● **T82.898** Other specified complication of **vascular** prosthetic devices, implants and grafts A

X ● **T82.9** **Unspecified** complication of cardiac and vascular prosthetic device, implant and graft

● **T83** **Complications of genitourinary prosthetic devices, implants and grafts**

  Excludes2   failure and rejection of transplanted organs and tissue (T86.-)

The appropriate 7th character is to be added to each code from category T83

  A   initial encounter
  D   subsequent encounter
  S   sequela

  Coding Clinic: 2016, Q4, P70-71

● **T83.0** **Mechanical complication of urinary catheter**
  Excludes2   complications of stoma of urinary tract (N99.5-)
  Coding Clinic: 2016, Q4, P70

  ● **T83.01** **Breakdown (mechanical) of urinary catheter**

    ● **T83.010** **Breakdown (mechanical) of cystostomy catheter** A

    ● **T83.011** **Breakdown (mechanical) of indwelling urethral catheter** A

    ● **T83.012** **Breakdown (mechanical) of nephrostomy catheter** A

    ● **T83.018** **Breakdown (mechanical) of other urinary catheter** A
      Breakdown (mechanical) of Hopkins catheter
      Breakdown (mechanical) of ileostomy catheter
      Breakdown (mechanical) urostomy catheter

  ● **T83.02** **Displacement of urinary catheter**
    Malposition of urinary catheter

    ● **T83.020** **Displacement of cystostomy catheter** A

    ● **T83.021** **Displacement of indwelling urethral catheter** A

    ● **T83.022** **Displacement of nephrostomy catheter** A

    ● **T83.028** **Displacement of other urinary catheter** A
      0Displacement of Hopkins catheter
      Displacement of ileostomy catheter
      Displacement of urostomy catheter

  ● **T83.03** **Leakage of urinary catheter**

    ● **T83.030** **Leakage of cystostomy catheter** A
      Coding Clinic: 2021, Q4, P19

    ● **T83.031** **Leakage of indwelling urethral catheter** A

    ● **T83.032** **Leakage of nephrostomy catheter** A

    ● **T83.038** **Leakage of other urinary catheter** A
      Leakage of Hopkins catheter
      Leakage of ileostomy catheter
      Leakage of urostomy catheter

  ● **T83.09** **Other mechanical complication of urinary catheter**
    Obstruction (mechanical) of urinary catheter
    Perforation of urinary catheter
    Protrusion of urinary catheter

    ● **T83.090** **Other mechanical complication of cystostomy catheter** A

    ● **T83.091** **Other mechanical complication of indwelling urethral catheter** A

    ● **T83.092** **Other mechanical complication of nephrostomy catheter** A

    ● **T83.098** **Other mechanical complication of other urinary catheter** A
      Other mechanical complication of Hopkins catheter
      Other mechanical complication of ileostomy catheter
      Other mechanical complication of urostomy catheter

● **T83.1 Mechanical complication of other urinary devices and implants**
     Coding Clinic: 2016, Q4, P70

● **T83.11 Breakdown (mechanical) of other urinary devices and implants**

   ● **T83.110 Breakdown (mechanical) of urinary electronic stimulator device A** Ⓡ

     Excludes2 Breakdown (mechanical) of electrode (lead) for sacral nerve neurostimulator (T85.111)
     Breakdown (mechanical) of implanted electronic sacral neurostimulator, pulse generator or receiver (T85.113)

   ● **T83.111 Breakdown (mechanical) of implanted urinary sphincter A** Ⓡ

   ● **T83.112 Breakdown (mechanical) of indwelling ureteral stent A** Ⓡ

   ● **T83.113 Breakdown (mechanical) of other urinary stents A** Ⓡ
     Breakdown (mechanical) of ileal conduit stent
     Breakdown (mechanical) of nephroureteral stent

   ● **T83.118 Breakdown (mechanical) of other urinary devices and implants A** Ⓡ

● **T83.12 Displacement of other urinary devices and implants**
     Malposition of other urinary devices and implants

   ● **T83.120 Displacement of urinary electronic stimulator device A** Ⓡ

     Excludes2 Displacement of electrode (lead) for sacral nerve neurostimulator (T85.121)
     Displacement of implanted electronic sacral neurostimulator, pulse generator or receiver (T85.123)

   ● **T83.121 Displacement of implanted urinary sphincter A** Ⓡ

   ● **T83.122 Displacement of indwelling ureteral stent A** Ⓡ

   ● **T83.123 Displacement of other urinary stents A** Ⓡ
     Displacement of ileal conduit stent
     Displacement of nephroureteral stent

   ● **T83.128 Displacement of other urinary devices and implants A** Ⓡ

● **T83.19 Other mechanical complication of other urinary devices and implants**
     Leakage of other urinary devices and implants
     Obstruction (mechanical) of other urinary devices and implants
     Perforation of other urinary devices and implants
     Protrusion of other urinary devices and implants

   ● **T83.190 Other mechanical complication of urinary electronic stimulator device A** Ⓡ

     Excludes2 Other mechanical complication of electrode (lead) for sacral nerve neurostimulator (T85.191)
     Other mechanical complication of implanted electronic sacral neurostimulator, pulse generator or receiver (T85.193)

   ● **T83.191 Other mechanical complication of implanted urinary sphincter A** Ⓡ

   ● **T83.192 Other mechanical complication of indwelling ureteral stent A** Ⓡ

   ● **T83.193 Other mechanical complication of other urinary stent A** Ⓡ
     Other mechanical complication of ileal conduit stent
     Other mechanical complication of nephroureteral stent

   ● **T83.198 Other mechanical complication of other urinary devices and implants A** Ⓡ

● **T83.2 Mechanical complication of graft of urinary organ**
     Coding Clinic: 2016, Q4, P70

   X ● **T83.21 Breakdown (mechanical) of graft of urinary organ A** Ⓡ

   X ● **T83.22 Displacement of graft of urinary organ A** Ⓡ
     Malposition of graft of urinary organ

   X ● **T83.23 Leakage of graft of urinary organ A** Ⓡ

   X ● **T83.24 Erosion of graft of urinary organ A** Ⓡ
     Coding Clinic: 2016, Q4, P70

   X ● **T83.25 Exposure of graft of urinary organ A** Ⓡ
     Coding Clinic: 2016, Q4, P70

   X ● **T83.29 Other mechanical complication of graft of urinary organ A** Ⓡ
     Obstruction (mechanical) of graft of urinary organ
     Perforation of graft of urinary organ
     Protrusion of graft of urinary organ

● **T83.3 Mechanical complication of intrauterine contraceptive device**

   X ● **T83.31 Breakdown (mechanical) of intrauterine contraceptive device**

   X ● **T83.32 Displacement of intrauterine contraceptive device**
     Malposition of intrauterine contraceptive device
     Missing string of intrauterine contraceptive device

   X ● **T83.39 Other mechanical complication of intrauterine contraceptive device**
     Leakage of intrauterine contraceptive device
     Obstruction (mechanical) of intrauterine contraceptive device
     Perforation of intrauterine contraceptive device
     Protrusion of intrauterine contraceptive device

● **T83.4 Mechanical complication of other prosthetic devices, implants and grafts of genital tract**
     Coding Clinic: 2016, Q4, P71

   ● **T83.41 Breakdown (mechanical) of other prosthetic devices, implants and grafts of genital tract**

CHAPTER 19 (S00–T88)

● **T83.410** **Breakdown (mechanical) of implanted penile prosthesis** A 🅡🅒
    Breakdown (mechanical) of penile prosthesis cylinder
    Breakdown (mechanical) of penile prosthesis pump
    Breakdown (mechanical) of penile prosthesis reservoir

● **T83.411** **Breakdown (mechanical) of implanted testicular prosthesis** A 🅡🅒

● **T83.418** **Breakdown (mechanical) of other prosthetic devices, implants and grafts of genital tract** A 🅡🅒

● **T83.42** **Displacement of other prosthetic devices, implants and grafts of genital tract**
    Malposition of other prosthetic devices, implants and grafts of genital tract

● **T83.420** **Displacement of implanted penile prosthesis** A 🅡🅒
    Displacement of penile prosthesis cylinder
    Displacement of penile prosthesis pump
    Displacement of penile prosthesis reservoir

● **T83.421** **Displacement of implanted testicular prosthesis** A 🅡🅒

● **T83.428** **Displacement of other prosthetic devices, implants and grafts of genital tract** A 🅡🅒
    Coding Clinic: 2018, Q1, P6

● **T83.49** **Other mechanical complication of other prosthetic devices, implants and grafts of genital tract**
    Leakage of other prosthetic devices, implants and grafts of genital tract
    Obstruction, mechanical of other prosthetic devices, implants and grafts of genital tract
    Perforation of other prosthetic devices, implants and grafts of genital tract
    Protrusion of other prosthetic devices, implants and grafts of genital tract

● **T83.490** **Other mechanical complication of implanted penile prosthesis** A 🅡🅒
    Other mechanical complication of penile prosthesis cylinder
    Other mechanical complication of penile prosthesis pump
    Other mechanical complication of penile prosthesis reservoir

● **T83.491** **Other mechanical complication of implanted testicular prosthesis** A 🅡🅒

● **T83.498** **Other mechanical complication of other prosthetic devices, implants and grafts of genital tract** A 🅡🅒

● **T83.5** **Infection and inflammatory reaction due to prosthetic device, implant and graft in urinary system**
    Use additional code to identify infection
    Coding Clinic: 2016, Q4, P71

● **T83.51** **Infection and inflammatory reaction due to urinary catheter**
    Excludes2   complications of stoma of urinary tract (N99.5-)

● **T83.510** **Infection and inflammatory reaction due to cystostomy catheter** A 🅡🅒

● **T83.511** **Infection and inflammatory reaction due to indwelling urethral catheter** A 🅡🅒
    Coding Clinic: 2022, Q2, P7

● **T83.512** **Infection and inflammatory reaction due to nephrostomy catheter** A 🅡🅒

● **T83.518** **Infection and inflammatory reaction due to other urinary catheter** A 🅡🅒
    Infection and inflammatory reaction due to Hopkins catheter
    Infection and inflammatory reaction due to ileostomy catheter
    Infection and inflammatory reaction due to urostomy catheter

● **T83.59** **Infection and inflammatory reaction due to prosthetic device, implant and graft in urinary system**

● **T83.590** **Infection and inflammatory reaction due to implanted urinary neurostimulation device** A 🅡🅒
    Excludes2   Infection and inflammatory reaction due to electrode lead of sacral nerve neurostimulator (T85.732)
        Infection and inflammatory reaction due to pulse generator or receiver of sacral nerve neurostimulator (T85.734)

● **T83.591** **Infection and inflammatory reaction due to implanted urinary sphincter** A 🅡🅒

● **T83.592** **Infection and inflammatory reaction due to indwelling ureteral stent** A 🅡🅒

● **T83.593** **Infection and inflammatory reaction due to other urinary stents** A 🅡🅒
    Infection and inflammatory reaction due to ileal conduit stents
    Infection and inflammatory reaction due to nephroureteral stent

● **T83.598** **Infection and inflammatory reaction due to other prosthetic device, implant and graft in urinary system** A 🅡🅒

● **T83.6** **Infection and inflammatory reaction due to prosthetic device, implant and graft in genital tract**
    Use additional code to identify infection
    Coding Clinic: 2016, Q4, P71

● **T83.61** **Infection and inflammatory reaction due to implanted penile prosthesis** A 🅡🅒
    Infection and inflammatory reaction due to penile prosthesis cylinder
    Infection and inflammatory reaction due to penile prosthesis pump
    Infection and inflammatory reaction due to penile prosthesis reservoir

● **T83.62** **Infection and inflammatory reaction due to implanted testicular prosthesis** A 🅡🅒

● **T83.69** **Infection and inflammatory reaction due to other prosthetic device, implant and graft in genital tract** A 🅡🅒

● **T83.7** **Complications due to implanted mesh and other prosthetic materials**
    Coding Clinic: 2016, Q4, P71

● **T83.71** **Erosion of implanted mesh and other prosthetic materials to surrounding organ or tissue**
    Coding Clinic: 2016, Q4, P71

● **T83.711** **Erosion of implanted vaginal mesh to surrounding organ or tissue** A 🅡🅒
    Erosion of implanted vaginal mesh into pelvic floor muscles
    Coding Clinic: 2016, Q4, P71

● **T83.712**   **Erosion of implanted urethral mesh to surrounding organ or tissue A** 🔒
     Erosion of implanted female urethral sling
     Erosion of implanted male urethral sling
     Erosion of implanted urethral mesh into pelvic floor muscles

● **T83.713**   **Erosion of implanted urethral bulking agent to surrounding organ or tissue A** 🔒

● **T83.714**   **Erosion of implanted ureteral bulking agent to surrounding organ or tissue A** 🔒

● **T83.718**   **Erosion of other implanted mesh to organ or tissue A** 🔒
     Coding Clinic: 2016, Q4, P71

● **T83.719**   **Erosion of other prosthetic materials to surrounding organ or tissue A** 🔒
     Coding Clinic: 2016, Q4, P71

● **T83.72**   **Exposure of implanted mesh and other prosthetic materials into surrounding organ or tissue**
     Extrusion of implanted mesh
     Coding Clinic: 2016, Q4, P71

● **T83.721**   **Exposure of implanted vaginal mesh into vagina A** 🔒
     Exposure of implanted vaginal mesh through vaginal wall

● **T83.722**   **Exposure of implanted urethral mesh into urethra A** 🔒
     Exposure of implanted female urethral sling
     Exposure of implanted male urethral sling
     Exposure of implanted urethral mesh through urethral wall

● **T83.723**   **Exposure of implanted urethral bulking agent into urethra A** 🔒

● **T83.724**   **Exposure of implanted ureteral bulking agent into ureter A** 🔒

● **T83.728**   **Exposure of other implanted mesh into organ or tissue A** 🔒
     Coding Clinic: 2016, Q4, P71

● **T83.729**   **Exposure of other prosthetic materials into organ or tissue A** 🔒
     Coding Clinic: 2016, Q4, P71

X ● **T83.79**   **Other specified complications due to other genitourinary prosthetic materials A** 🔒

● **T83.8**   **Other specified complications of genitourinary prosthetic devices, implants and grafts**

X ● **T83.81**   **Embolism due to genitourinary prosthetic devices, implants and grafts A** 🔒

X ● **T83.82**   **Fibrosis due to genitourinary prosthetic devices, implants and grafts A** 🔒

X ● **T83.83**   **Hemorrhage due to genitourinary prosthetic devices, implants and grafts A** 🔒
     Coding Clinic: 2025, Q2, P21

X ● **T83.84**   **Pain due to genitourinary prosthetic devices, implants and grafts A** 🔒

X ● **T83.85**   **Stenosis due to genitourinary prosthetic devices, implants and grafts A** 🔒

X ● **T83.86**   **Thrombosis due to genitourinary prosthetic devices, implants and grafts A** 🔒
     Coding Clinic: 2024, Q3, P6

X ● **T83.89**   **Other specified complication of genitourinary prosthetic devices, implants and grafts A** 🔒
     Coding Clinic: 2022, Q3, P13

X ● **T83.9**   **Unspecified complication of genitourinary prosthetic device, implant and graft A** 🔒

● **T84**   **Complications of internal orthopedic prosthetic devices, implants and grafts**
     Excludes2   failure and rejection of transplanted organs and tissues (T86.-)
         fracture of bone following insertion of orthopedic implant, joint prosthesis or bone plate (M96.6)
     The appropriate 7th character is to be added to each code from category T84

> A   initial encounter
> D   subsequent encounter
> S   sequela

● **T84.0**   **Mechanical complication of internal joint prosthesis**

   ● **T84.01**   **Broken internal joint prosthesis**
     Breakage (fracture) of prosthetic joint
     Broken prosthetic joint implant
     Excludes1   periprosthetic joint implant fracture (M97.-)
     Coding Clinic: 2016, Q4, P42

● **T84.010**   **Broken internal right hip prosthesis A** 🔒

● **T84.011**   **Broken internal left hip prosthesis A** 🔒

● **T84.012**   **Broken internal right knee prosthesis A** 🔒

● **T84.013**   **Broken internal left knee prosthesis A** 🔒

● **T84.018**   **Broken internal joint prosthesis, other site A** 🔒
     Use additional code to identify the joint (Z96.6-)

● **T84.019**   **Broken internal joint prosthesis, unspecified site A** 🔒

● **T84.02**   **Dislocation of internal joint prosthesis**
     Instability of internal joint prosthesis
     Subluxation of internal joint prosthesis

● **T84.020**   **Dislocation of internal right hip prosthesis A** 🔒

● **T84.021**   **Dislocation of internal left hip prosthesis A** 🔒
     Coding Clinic: 2019, Q2, P27

● **T84.022**   **Instability of internal right knee prosthesis A** 🔒

● **T84.023**   **Instability of internal left knee prosthesis A** 🔒

● **T84.028**   **Dislocation of other internal joint prosthesis A** 🔒
     Use additional code to identify the joint (Z96.6-)

● **T84.029**   **Dislocation of unspecified internal joint prosthesis A** 🔒

● **T84.03**   **Mechanical loosening of internal prosthetic joint**
     Aseptic loosening of prosthetic joint

● **T84.030**   **Mechanical loosening of internal right hip prosthetic joint A** 🔒

● **T84.031**   **Mechanical loosening of internal left hip prosthetic joint A** 🔒

● **T84.032**   **Mechanical loosening of internal right knee prosthetic joint A** 🔒

● **T84.033**   **Mechanical loosening of internal left knee prosthetic joint A** 🔒

● **T84.038**   **Mechanical loosening of other internal prosthetic joint A** 🔒
     Use additional code to identify the joint (Z96.6-)

● **T84.039**   **Mechanical loosening of unspecified internal prosthetic joint A** 🔒

CHAPTER 19 (S00-T88)

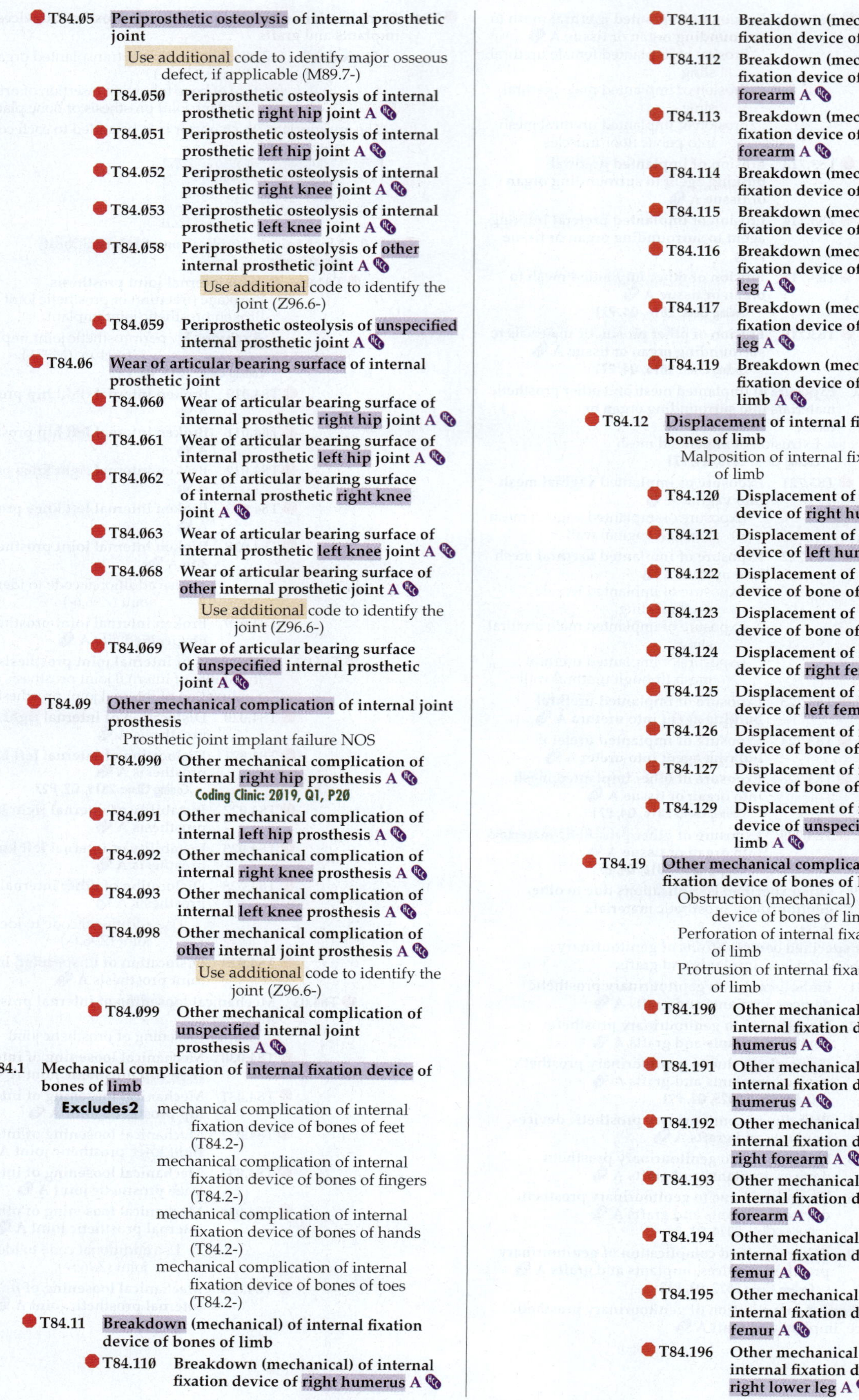

● **T84.05** **Periprosthetic osteolysis** of internal prosthetic joint

> **Use additional** code to identify major osseous defect, if applicable (M89.7-)

  ● **T84.050** Periprosthetic osteolysis of internal prosthetic **right hip joint** A

  ● **T84.051** Periprosthetic osteolysis of internal prosthetic **left hip joint** A

  ● **T84.052** Periprosthetic osteolysis of internal prosthetic **right knee joint** A

  ● **T84.053** Periprosthetic osteolysis of internal prosthetic **left knee joint** A

  ● **T84.058** Periprosthetic osteolysis of **other internal prosthetic joint** A

> **Use additional** code to identify the joint (Z96.6-)

  ● **T84.059** Periprosthetic osteolysis of **unspecified internal prosthetic joint** A

● **T84.06** **Wear of articular bearing surface** of internal prosthetic joint

  ● **T84.060** Wear of articular bearing surface of internal prosthetic **right hip joint** A

  ● **T84.061** Wear of articular bearing surface of internal prosthetic **left hip joint** A

  ● **T84.062** Wear of articular bearing surface of internal prosthetic **right knee joint** A

  ● **T84.063** Wear of articular bearing surface of internal prosthetic **left knee joint** A

  ● **T84.068** Wear of articular bearing surface of **other internal prosthetic joint** A

> **Use additional** code to identify the joint (Z96.6-)

  ● **T84.069** Wear of articular bearing surface of **unspecified internal prosthetic joint** A

● **T84.09** **Other mechanical complication** of internal joint prosthesis

> Prosthetic joint implant failure NOS

  ● **T84.090** Other mechanical complication of internal **right hip prosthesis** A
> **Coding Clinic: 2019, Q1, P20**

  ● **T84.091** Other mechanical complication of internal **left hip prosthesis** A

  ● **T84.092** Other mechanical complication of internal **right knee prosthesis** A

  ● **T84.093** Other mechanical complication of internal **left knee prosthesis** A

  ● **T84.098** Other mechanical complication of **other internal joint prosthesis** A

> **Use additional** code to identify the joint (Z96.6-)

  ● **T84.099** Other mechanical complication of **unspecified internal joint prosthesis** A

● **T84.1** Mechanical complication of **internal fixation device** of bones of limb

> **Excludes2**   mechanical complication of internal fixation device of bones of feet (T84.2-)
> mechanical complication of internal fixation device of bones of fingers (T84.2-)
> mechanical complication of internal fixation device of bones of hands (T84.2-)
> mechanical complication of internal fixation device of bones of toes (T84.2-)

  ● **T84.11** **Breakdown (mechanical)** of internal fixation device of bones of limb

    ● **T84.110** Breakdown (mechanical) of internal fixation device of **right humerus** A

● **T84.111** Breakdown (mechanical) of internal fixation device of **left humerus** A

● **T84.112** Breakdown (mechanical) of internal fixation device of bone of **right forearm** A

● **T84.113** Breakdown (mechanical) of internal fixation device of bone of **left forearm** A

● **T84.114** Breakdown (mechanical) of internal fixation device of **right femur** A

● **T84.115** Breakdown (mechanical) of internal fixation device of **left femur** A

● **T84.116** Breakdown (mechanical) of internal fixation device of bone of **right lower leg** A

● **T84.117** Breakdown (mechanical) of internal fixation device of bone of **left lower leg** A

● **T84.119** Breakdown (mechanical) of internal fixation device of **unspecified** bone of limb A

● **T84.12** **Displacement of internal fixation device** of bones of limb

> Malposition of internal fixation device of bones of limb

  ● **T84.120** Displacement of internal fixation device of **right humerus** A

  ● **T84.121** Displacement of internal fixation device of **left humerus** A

  ● **T84.122** Displacement of internal fixation device of bone of **right forearm** A

  ● **T84.123** Displacement of internal fixation device of bone of **left forearm** A

  ● **T84.124** Displacement of internal fixation device of **right femur** A

  ● **T84.125** Displacement of internal fixation device of **left femur** A

  ● **T84.126** Displacement of internal fixation device of bone of **right lower leg** A

  ● **T84.127** Displacement of internal fixation device of bone of **left lower leg** A

  ● **T84.129** Displacement of internal fixation device of **unspecified** bone of limb A

● **T84.19** **Other mechanical complication** of internal fixation device of bones of limb

> Obstruction (mechanical) of internal fixation device of bones of limb
> Perforation of internal fixation device of bones of limb
> Protrusion of internal fixation device of bones of limb

  ● **T84.190** Other mechanical complication of internal fixation device of **right humerus** A

  ● **T84.191** Other mechanical complication of internal fixation device of **left humerus** A

  ● **T84.192** Other mechanical complication of internal fixation device of bone of **right forearm** A

  ● **T84.193** Other mechanical complication of internal fixation device of bone of **left forearm** A

  ● **T84.194** Other mechanical complication of internal fixation device of **right femur** A

  ● **T84.195** Other mechanical complication of internal fixation device of **left femur** A

  ● **T84.196** Other mechanical complication of internal fixation device of bone of **right lower leg** A

▶ New   ➡ Revised   ~~deleted~~ Deleted   Excludes 1   Excludes 2   Includes   Use additional   Code first   Code also   Key words
OGCR Official Guidelines   **X** Assign placeholder X   ● Use Additional Character(s)   ▶ Manifestation Code   Hierarchical Condition Category   **Coding Clinic**

● T84.197   Other mechanical complication of internal fixation device of bone of left lower leg A ℞

● T84.199   Other mechanical complication of internal fixation device of unspecified bone of limb A ℞

● **T84.2   Mechanical complication of internal fixation device of other bones**

   ● **T84.21   Breakdown (mechanical) of internal fixation device of other bones**

      ● T84.210   Breakdown (mechanical) of internal fixation device of bones of hand and fingers A ℞

      ● T84.213   Breakdown (mechanical) of internal fixation device of bones of foot and toes A ℞

      ● T84.216   Breakdown (mechanical) of internal fixation device of vertebrae A ℞

      ● T84.218   Breakdown (mechanical) of internal fixation device of other bones A ℞

   ● **T84.22   Displacement of internal fixation device of other bones**

      Malposition of internal fixation device of other bones

      ● T84.220   Displacement of internal fixation device of bones of hand and fingers A ℞

      ● T84.223   Displacement of internal fixation device of bones of foot and toes A ℞

      ● T84.226   Displacement of internal fixation device of vertebrae A ℞

      ● T84.228   Displacement of internal fixation device of other bones A ℞

   ● **T84.29   Other mechanical complication of internal fixation device of other bones**

      Obstruction (mechanical) of internal fixation device of other bones

      Perforation of internal fixation device of other bones

      Protrusion of internal fixation device of other bones

      ● T84.290   Other mechanical complication of internal fixation device of bones of hand and fingers A ℞

      ● T84.293   Other mechanical complication of internal fixation device of bones of foot and toes A ℞

      ● T84.296   Other mechanical complication of internal fixation device of vertebrae A ℞
         Coding Clinic: 2024, Q2, P12

      ● T84.298   Other mechanical complication of internal fixation device of other bones A ℞

● **T84.3   Mechanical complication of other bone devices, implants and grafts**

   Excludes2   other complications of bone graft (T86.83-)

   ● **T84.31   Breakdown (mechanical) of other bone devices, implants and grafts**

      ● T84.310   Breakdown (mechanical) of electronic bone stimulator A ℞

      ● T84.318   Breakdown (mechanical) of other bone devices, implants and grafts A ℞

   ● **T84.32   Displacement of other bone devices, implants and grafts**

      Malposition of other bone devices, implants and grafts

      ● T84.320   Displacement of electronic bone stimulator A ℞

      ● T84.328   Displacement of other bone devices, implants and grafts A ℞

● **T84.39   Other mechanical complication of other bone devices, implants and grafts**

   Obstruction (mechanical) of other bone devices, implants and grafts

   Perforation of other bone devices, implants and grafts

   Protrusion of other bone devices, implants and grafts

   ● T84.390   Other mechanical complication of electronic bone stimulator A ℞

   ● T84.398   Other mechanical complication of other bone devices, implants and grafts A ℞

● **T84.4   Mechanical complication of other internal orthopedic devices, implants and grafts**

   ● **T84.41   Breakdown (mechanical) of other internal orthopedic devices, implants and grafts**

      ● T84.410   Breakdown (mechanical) of muscle and tendon graft A ℞

      ● T84.418   Breakdown (mechanical) of other internal orthopedic devices, implants and grafts A ℞

   ● **T84.42   Displacement of other internal orthopedic devices, implants and grafts**

      Malposition of other internal orthopedic devices, implants and grafts

      ● T84.420   Displacement of muscle and tendon graft A ℞

      ● T84.428   Displacement of other internal orthopedic devices, implants and grafts A ℞

   ● **T84.49   Other mechanical complication of other internal orthopedic devices, implants and grafts**

      Mechanical complication of other internal orthopedic devices, implants and grafts NOS

      Obstruction (mechanical) of other internal orthopedic devices, implants and grafts

      Perforation of other internal orthopedic devices, implants and grafts

      Protrusion of other internal orthopedic devices, implants and grafts

      ● T84.490   Other mechanical complication of muscle and tendon graft A ℞

      ● T84.498   Other mechanical complication of other internal orthopedic devices, implants and grafts A ℞

● **T84.5   Infection and inflammatory reaction due to internal joint prosthesis**

   Use additional code to identify infection
   Coding Clinic: 2015, Q1, P16

   X ● **T84.50**   Infection and inflammatory reaction due to unspecified internal joint prosthesis A ℞
      Coding Clinic: 2015, Q1, P3

   X ● **T84.51**   Infection and inflammatory reaction due to internal right hip prosthesis A ℞
      Coding Clinic: 2015, Q4, P36

   X ● **T84.52**   Infection and inflammatory reaction due to internal left hip prosthesis A ℞
      Coding Clinic: 2015, Q1, P16-17

   X ● **T84.53**   Infection and inflammatory reaction due to internal right knee prosthesis A ℞

   X ● **T84.54**   Infection and inflammatory reaction due to internal left knee prosthesis A ℞
      Coding Clinic: 2019, Q3, P16

   X ● **T84.59**   Infection and inflammatory reaction due to other internal joint prosthesis A ℞

● **T84.6   Infection and inflammatory reaction due to internal fixation device**

   Use additional code to identify infection

   X ● **T84.60**   Infection and inflammatory reaction due to internal fixation device of unspecified site A ℞

● **T84.61** Infection and inflammatory reaction due to internal fixation device of **arm**
    ● **T84.610** Infection and inflammatory reaction due to internal fixation device of **right humerus** A ℞
    ● **T84.611** Infection and inflammatory reaction due to internal fixation device of **left humerus** A ℞
    ● **T84.612** Infection and inflammatory reaction due to internal fixation device of **right radius** A ℞
    ● **T84.613** Infection and inflammatory reaction due to internal fixation device of **left radius** A ℞
    ● **T84.614** Infection and inflammatory reaction due to internal fixation device of **right ulna** A ℞
    ● **T84.615** Infection and inflammatory reaction due to internal fixation device of **left ulna** A ℞
    ● **T84.619** Infection and inflammatory reaction due to internal fixation device of **unspecified bone of arm** A ℞

● **T84.62** Infection and inflammatory reaction due to internal fixation device of **leg**
    ● **T84.620** Infection and inflammatory reaction due to internal fixation device of **right femur** A ℞
    ● **T84.621** Infection and inflammatory reaction due to internal fixation device of **left femur** A ℞
    ● **T84.622** Infection and inflammatory reaction due to internal fixation device of **right tibia** A ℞
    ● **T84.623** Infection and inflammatory reaction due to internal fixation device of **left tibia** A ℞
    ● **T84.624** Infection and inflammatory reaction due to internal fixation device of **right fibula** A ℞
    ● **T84.625** Infection and inflammatory reaction due to internal fixation device of **left fibula** A ℞
    ● **T84.629** Infection and inflammatory reaction due to internal fixation device of **unspecified bone of leg** A ℞

X ● **T84.63** Infection and inflammatory reaction due to internal fixation device of **spine** A ℞

X ● **T84.69** Infection and inflammatory reaction due to internal fixation device of **other site** A ℞

● **T84.7** Infection and inflammatory reaction due to other **internal orthopedic prosthetic devices, implants and grafts** A ℞
    Use additional code to identify infection

● **T84.8** Other specified complications of internal orthopedic prosthetic devices, implants and grafts
X ● **T84.81** **Embolism** due to internal orthopedic prosthetic devices, implants and grafts A ℞
X ● **T84.82** **Fibrosis** due to internal orthopedic prosthetic devices, implants and grafts A ℞
    Coding Clinic: 2025, Q1, P25
X ● **T84.83** **Hemorrhage** due to internal orthopedic prosthetic devices, implants and grafts A ℞
X ● **T84.84** **Pain** due to internal orthopedic prosthetic devices, implants and grafts A ℞
    Coding Clinic: 2024, Q2, P13
X ● **T84.85** **Stenosis** due to internal orthopedic prosthetic devices, implants and grafts A ℞
X ● **T84.86** **Thrombosis** due to internal orthopedic prosthetic devices, implants and grafts A ℞
X ● **T84.89** **Other** specified complication of internal orthopedic prosthetic devices, implants and grafts A ℞

X ● **T84.9** **Unspecified** complication of internal orthopedic prosthetic device, implant and graft A ℞

● **T85** Complications of other internal prosthetic devices, implants and grafts
    Excludes2 failure and rejection of transplanted organs and tissue (T86.-)
    The appropriate 7th character is to be added to each code from category T85

A	initial encounter
D	subsequent encounter
S	sequela

    Coding Clinic: 2016, Q4, P71

● **T85.0** Mechanical complication of **ventricular intracranial (communicating) shunt**
X ● **T85.01** **Breakdown (mechanical)** of ventricular intracranial (communicating) shunt A ℞
X ● **T85.02** **Displacement** of ventricular intracranial (communicating) shunt A ℞
    Malposition of ventricular intracranial (communicating) shunt
X ● **T85.03** **Leakage** of ventricular intracranial (communicating) shunt A ℞
X ● **T85.09** **Other** mechanical complication of ventricular intracranial (communicating) shunt A ℞
    Obstruction (mechanical) of ventricular intracranial (communicating) shunt
    Perforation of ventricular intracranial (communicating) shunt
    Protrusion of ventricular intracranial (communicating) shunt

● **T85.1** Mechanical complication of **implanted electronic stimulator of nervous system**
    Coding Clinic: 2016, Q4, P71
● **T85.11** **Breakdown (mechanical)** of implanted electronic stimulator of nervous system
    ● **T85.110** Breakdown (mechanical) of implanted electronic neurostimulator of **brain electrode (lead)** A ℞
    ● **T85.111** Breakdown (mechanical) of implanted electronic neurostimulator of **peripheral nerve electrode (lead)** A ℞
        Breakdown of electrode (lead) for cranial nerve neurostimulators
        Breakdown of electrode (lead) for gastric neurostimulator
        Breakdown of electrode (lead) for sacral nerve neurostimulator
        Breakdown of electrode (lead) for vagal nerve neurostimulators
    ● **T85.112** Breakdown (mechanical) of implanted electronic neurostimulator of **spinal cord electrode (lead)** A ℞
    ● **T85.113** Breakdown (mechanical) of implanted electronic neurostimulator, **generator** A ℞
        Breakdown (mechanical) of implanted electronic neurostimulator generator, brain, peripheral, gastric, spinal
        Breakdown (mechanical) of implanted electronic sacral neurostimulator, pulse generator or receiver
    ● **T85.118** Breakdown (mechanical) of **other** implanted electronic stimulator of nervous system A ℞

● **T85.12** **Displacement** of implanted electronic stimulator of nervous system
    Malposition of implanted electronic stimulator of nervous system
    ● **T85.120** Displacement of implanted electronic neurostimulator of **brain electrode (lead)** A ℞

▶ New   ⇨ Revised   ~~deleted~~ Deleted   Excludes 1   Excludes 2   Includes   Use additional   Code first   Code also   Key words
OGCR Official Guidelines   X Assign placeholder X   ● Use Additional Character(s)   ⟩ Manifestation Code   ℞ Hierarchical Condition Category   Coding Clinic

● **T85.121** **Displacement of implanted electronic neurostimulator of peripheral nerve electrode (lead) A**
Displacement of electrode (lead) for cranial nerve neurostimulators
Displacement of electrode (lead) for gastric neurostimulator
Displacement of electrode (lead) for sacral nerve neurostimulator
Displacement of electrode (lead) for vagal nerve neurostimulators

● **T85.122** **Displacement of implanted electronic neurostimulator of spinal cord electrode (lead) A**

● **T85.123** **Displacement of implanted electronic neurostimulator, generator A**
Displacement of implanted electronic neurostimulator generator, brain, peripheral, gastric, spinal
Displacement of implanted electronic sacral neurostimulator, pulse generator or receiver

● **T85.128** **Displacement of other implanted electronic stimulator of nervous system A**

● **T85.19** **Other mechanical complication of implanted electronic stimulator of nervous system**
Leakage of implanted electronic stimulator of nervous system
Obstruction (mechanical) of implanted electronic stimulator of nervous system
Perforation of implanted electronic stimulator of nervous system
Protrusion of implanted electronic stimulator of nervous system

● **T85.190** **Other mechanical complication of implanted electronic neurostimulator of brain electrode (lead) A**

● **T85.191** **Other mechanical complication of implanted electronic neurostimulator of peripheral nerve electrode (lead) A**
Other mechanical complication of electrode (lead) for cranial nerve neurostimulators
Other mechanical complication of electrode (lead) for gastric neurostimulator
Other mechanical complication of electrode (lead) for sacral nerve neurostimulator
Other mechanical complication of electrode (lead) for vagal nerve neurostimulators

● **T85.192** **Other mechanical complication of implanted electronic neurostimulator of spinal cord electrode (lead) A**

● **T85.193** **Other mechanical complication of implanted electronic neurostimulator, generator A**
Other mechanical complication of implanted electronic neurostimulator generator, brain, peripheral, gastric, spinal
Other mechanical complication of implanted electronic sacral neurostimulator, pulse generator or receiver

● **T85.199** **Other mechanical complication of other implanted electronic stimulator of nervous system A**

● **T85.2** **Mechanical complication of intraocular lens**
X● **T85.21** **Breakdown (mechanical) of intraocular lens**
X● **T85.22** **Displacement of intraocular lens**
Malposition of intraocular lens
X● **T85.29** **Other mechanical complication of intraocular lens**
Obstruction (mechanical) of intraocular lens
Perforation of intraocular lens
Protrusion of intraocular lens

● **T85.3** **Mechanical complication of other ocular prosthetic devices, implants and grafts**
> **Excludes2**   other complications of corneal graft (T86.84-)

● **T85.31** **Breakdown (mechanical) of other ocular prosthetic devices, implants and grafts**
● **T85.310** **Breakdown (mechanical) of prosthetic orbit of right eye**
● **T85.311** **Breakdown (mechanical) of prosthetic orbit of left eye**
● **T85.318** **Breakdown (mechanical) of other ocular prosthetic devices, implants and grafts**

● **T85.32** **Displacement of other ocular prosthetic devices, implants and grafts**
Malposition of other ocular prosthetic devices, implants and grafts
● **T85.320** **Displacement of prosthetic orbit of right eye**
● **T85.321** **Displacement of prosthetic orbit of left eye**
● **T85.328** **Displacement of other ocular prosthetic devices, implants and grafts**

● **T85.39** **Other mechanical complication of other ocular prosthetic devices, implants and grafts**
Obstruction (mechanical) of other ocular prosthetic devices, implants and grafts
Perforation of other ocular prosthetic devices, implants and grafts
Protrusion of other ocular prosthetic devices, implants and grafts
● **T85.390** **Other mechanical complication of prosthetic orbit of right eye**
● **T85.391** **Other mechanical complication of prosthetic orbit of left eye**
● **T85.398** **Other mechanical complication of other ocular prosthetic devices, implants and grafts**

● **T85.4** **Mechanical complication of breast prosthesis and implant**
X● **T85.41** **Breakdown (mechanical) of breast prosthesis and implant**
X● **T85.42** **Displacement of breast prosthesis and implant**
Malposition of breast prosthesis and implant
X● **T85.43** **Leakage of breast prosthesis and implant**
X● **T85.44** **Capsular contracture of breast implant**
X● **T85.49** **Other mechanical complication of breast prosthesis and implant**
Obstruction (mechanical) of breast prosthesis and implant
Perforation of breast prosthesis and implant
Protrusion of breast prosthesis and implant

● **T85.5** **Mechanical complication of gastrointestinal prosthetic devices, implants and grafts**
● **T85.51** **Breakdown (mechanical) of gastrointestinal prosthetic devices, implants and grafts**
● **T85.510** **Breakdown (mechanical) of bile duct prosthesis**
● **T85.511** **Breakdown (mechanical) of esophageal anti-reflux device**
● **T85.518** **Breakdown (mechanical) of other gastrointestinal prosthetic devices, implants and grafts**

● **T85.52 Displacement of gastrointestinal prosthetic devices, implants and grafts**
  Malposition of gastrointestinal prosthetic devices, implants and grafts
  - ● **T85.520 Displacement of bile duct prosthesis**
  - ● **T85.521 Displacement of esophageal anti-reflux device**
  - ● **T85.528 Displacement of other gastrointestinal prosthetic devices, implants and grafts**
- ● **T85.59 Other mechanical complication of gastrointestinal prosthetic devices, implants and**
  Obstruction, mechanical of gastrointestinal prosthetic devices, implants and grafts
  Perforation of gastrointestinal prosthetic devices, implants and grafts
  Protrusion of gastrointestinal prosthetic devices, implants and grafts
  - ● **T85.590 Other mechanical complication of bile duct prosthesis**
  - ● **T85.591 Other mechanical complication of esophageal anti-reflux device**
  - ● **T85.598 Other mechanical complication of other gastrointestinal prosthetic devices, implants and grafts**
- ● **T85.6 Mechanical complication of other specified internal and external prosthetic devices, implants and grafts**
  Coding Clinic: 2016, Q4, P71
  - ● **T85.61 Breakdown (mechanical) of other specified internal prosthetic devices, implants and grafts**
    - ● **T85.610 Breakdown (mechanical) of cranial or spinal infusion catheter**
      Breakdown (mechanical) of epidural infusion catheter
      Breakdown (mechanical) of intrathecal infusion catheter
      Breakdown (mechanical) of subarachnoid infusion catheter
      Breakdown (mechanical) of subdural infusion catheter
    - ● **T85.611 Breakdown (mechanical) of intraperitoneal dialysis catheter A, D, S** 🅡🅒
      | **Excludes1** | mechanical complication of vascular dialysis catheter (T82.4-) |
    - ● **T85.612 Breakdown (mechanical) of permanent sutures**
      | **Excludes1** | mechanical complication of permanent (wire) suture used in bone repair (T84.1-T84.2) |
    - ● **T85.613 Breakdown (mechanical) of artificial skin graft and decellularized allodermis**
      Failure of artificial skin graft and decellularized allodermis
      Non-adherence of artificial skin graft and decellularized allodermis
      Poor incorporation of artificial skin graft and decellularized allodermis
      Shearing of artificial skin graft and decellularized allodermis
    - ● **T85.614 Breakdown (mechanical) of insulin pump**
    - ● **T85.615 Breakdown (mechanical) of other nervous system device, implant or graft A** 🅡🅒
      Breakdown (mechanical) of intrathecal infusion pump

- ● **T85.618 Breakdown (mechanical) of other specified internal prosthetic devices, implants and grafts**
- ● **T85.62 Displacement of other specified internal prosthetic devices, implants and grafts**
  Malposition of other specified internal prosthetic devices, implants and grafts
  - ● **T85.620 Displacement of cranial or spinal infusion catheter**
    Displacement of epidural infusion catheter
    Displacement of intrathecal infusion catheter
    Displacement of subarachnoid infusion catheter
    Displacement of subdural infusion catheter
  - ● **T85.621 Displacement of intraperitoneal dialysis catheter A, D, S** 🅡🅒
    | **Excludes1** | mechanical complication of vascular dialysis catheter (T82.4-) |
  - ● **T85.622 Displacement of permanent sutures**
    | **Excludes1** | mechanical complication of permanent (wire) suture used in bone repair (T84.1-T84.2) |
  - ● **T85.623 Displacement of artificial skin graft and decellularized allodermis**
    Dislodgement of artificial skin graft and decellularized allodermis
  - ● **T85.624 Displacement of insulin pump**
  - ● **T85.625 Displacement of other nervous system device, implant or graft A** 🅡🅒
    Displacement of intrathecal infusion pump
  - ● **T85.628 Displacement of other specified internal prosthetic devices, implants and grafts**
    Coding Clinic: 2015, Q1, P15
- ● **T85.63 Leakage of other specified internal prosthetic devices, implants and grafts**
  - ● **T85.630 Leakage of cranial or spinal infusion catheter**
    Leakage of epidural infusion catheter
    Leakage of intrathecal infusion catheter
    Leakage of subdural infusion catheter
    Leakage of subarachnoid infusion catheter
    Coding Clinic: 2022, Q3, P24
  - ● **T85.631 Leakage of intraperitoneal dialysis catheter A, D, S** 🅡🅒
    | **Excludes1** | mechanical complication of vascular dialysis catheter (T82.4) |
  - ● **T85.633 Leakage of insulin pump**
  - ● **T85.635 Leakage of other nervous system device, implant or graft A** 🅡🅒
    Leakage of intrathecal infusion pump
  - ● **T85.638 Leakage of other specified internal prosthetic devices, implants and grafts**

▶ New ⇨ Revised ~~deleted~~ Deleted Excludes 1 Excludes 2 Includes Use additional Code first Code also Key words
OGCR Official Guidelines X Assign placeholder X ● Use Additional Character(s) ▶ Manifestation Code 🅡🅒 Hierarchical Condition Category **Coding Clinic**

● **T85.69   Other mechanical complication** of other
specified internal prosthetic devices, implants
and grafts
Obstruction, mechanical of other specified
internal prosthetic devices, implants and
grafts
Perforation of other specified internal
prosthetic devices, implants and grafts
Protrusion of other specified internal prosthetic
devices, implants and grafts

● **T85.690   Other mechanical complication of
cranial or spinal infusion catheter**
Other mechanical complication of
epidural infusion catheter
Other mechanical complication of
intrathecal infusion catheter
Other mechanical complication
of subarachnoid infusion
catheter
Other mechanical complication of
subdural infusion catheter

● **T85.691   Other mechanical complication of
intraperitoneal dialysis catheter**
A, D, S 🔲
    Excludes1 mechanical
complication of
vascular dialysis
catheter (T82.4)

● **T85.692   Other mechanical complication of
permanent sutures**
    Excludes1 mechanical
complication of
permanent (wire)
suture used
in bone repair
(T84.1-T84.2)

● **T85.693   Other mechanical complication of
artificial skin graft and decellularized
allodermis**

● **T85.694   Other mechanical complication of
insulin pump**

● **T85.695   Other mechanical complication of
other nervous system device, implant
or graft A** 🔲
Other mechanical complication of
intrathecal infusion pump

● **T85.698   Other mechanical complication of
other specified internal
prosthetic devices, implants and
grafts**
Mechanical complication of
nonabsorbable surgical material
NOS

● **T85.7   Infection and inflammatory reaction due to other
internal prosthetic devices, implants and grafts**
Use additional code to identify infection
Coding Clinic: 2016, Q4, P72

X ● **T85.71   Infection and inflammatory reaction due to
peritoneal dialysis catheter A, D,
S** 🔲

X ● **T85.72   Infection and inflammatory reaction due to
insulin pump A** 🔲

● **T85.73   Infection and inflammatory reaction due to
nervous system devices, implants and
graft**

● **T85.730   Infection and inflammatory reaction
due to ventricular intracranial
(communicating) shunt A** 🔲

● **T85.731   Infection and inflammatory reaction
due to implanted electronic
neurostimulator of brain, electrode
(lead) A** 🔲

● **T85.732   Infection and inflammatory reaction
due to implanted electronic
neurostimulator of peripheral nerve,
electrode (lead) A** 🔲
Infection and inflammatory reaction
due to electrode (lead)
for cranial nerve
neurostimulators
Infection and inflammatory reaction
due to electrode (lead) for
gastric neurostimulator
Infection and inflammatory reaction
due to electrode (lead) for sacral
nerve neurostimulator
Infection and inflammatory reaction
due to electrode (lead) for vagal
nerve neurostimulators

● **T85.733   Infection and inflammatory reaction
due to implanted electronic
neurostimulator of spinal cord,
electrode (lead) A** 🔲

● **T85.734   Infection and inflammatory reaction
due to implanted electronic
neurostimulator, generator A** 🔲
Generator pocket infection

● **T85.735   Infection and inflammatory reaction
due to cranial or spinal infusion
catheter A** 🔲
Infection and inflammatory reaction
due to epidural catheter
Infection and inflammatory reaction
due to intrathecal infusion
catheter
Infection and inflammatory reaction
due to subarachnoid catheter
Infection and inflammatory reaction
due to subdural catheter

● **T85.738   Infection and inflammatory reaction
due to other nervous system device,
implant or graft A** 🔲
Infection and inflammatory reaction
due to intrathecal infusion
pump

X ● **T85.79   Infection and inflammatory reaction due to
other internal prosthetic devices, implants and
grafts A** 🔲
Coding Clinic: 2023, Q2, P28; 2022, Q2, P8; 2016, Q4, P72

● **T85.8   Other specified complications of internal prosthetic
devices, implants and grafts, not elsewhere
classified**
Coding Clinic: 2016, Q4, P72

● **T85.81   Embolism due to internal prosthetic devices,
implants and grafts, not elsewhere classified**

● **T85.810   Embolism due to nervous system
prosthetic devices, implants and
grafts A** 🔲

● **T85.818   Embolism due to other internal
prosthetic devices, implants and
grafts**

● **T85.82   Fibrosis due to internal prosthetic devices,
implants and grafts, not elsewhere classified**

● **T85.820   Fibrosis due to nervous system
prosthetic devices, implants and
grafts A** 🔲

● **T85.828   Fibrosis due to other internal
prosthetic devices, implants and
grafts**

● **T85.83   Hemorrhage due to internal prosthetic devices,
implants and grafts, not elsewhere classified**

● **T85.830   Hemorrhage due to nervous system
prosthetic devices, implants and
grafts A** 🔲

● **T85.838   Hemorrhage due to other internal
prosthetic devices, implants and
grafts**

CHAPTER 19 (S00-T88)

● **T85.84** **Pain** due to internal prosthetic devices, implants and grafts, not elsewhere classified
- ● **T85.840** **Pain** due to **nervous system** prosthetic devices, implants and grafts **A** 🅡
- ● **T85.848** **Pain** due to **other** internal prosthetic devices, implants and grafts

● **T85.85** **Stenosis** due to internal prosthetic devices, implants and grafts, not elsewhere classified
- ● **T85.850** **Stenosis** due to **nervous system** prosthetic devices, implants and grafts **A** 🅡
- ● **T85.858** **Stenosis** due to **other** internal prosthetic devices, implants and grafts

● **T85.86** **Thrombosis** due to internal prosthetic devices, implants and grafts, not elsewhere classified
- ● **T85.860** **Thrombosis** due to **nervous system** prosthetic devices, implants and grafts **A** 🅡
- ● **T85.868** **Thrombosis** due to **other** internal prosthetic devices, implants and grafts
  Coding Clinic: 2024, Q2, P7

● **T85.89** **Other specified** complication of internal prosthetic devices, implants and grafts, not elsewhere classified
  Coding Clinic: 2024, Q2, P8; 2016, Q4, P72
- ● **T85.890** **Other specified** complication of **nervous system** prosthetic devices, implants and grafts **A** 🅡
- ● **T85.898** **Other specified** complication of **other** internal prosthetic devices, implants and grafts
  Coding Clinic: 2024, Q2, P8

X ● **T85.9** **Unspecified** complication of internal prosthetic device, implant and graft
  Complication of internal prosthetic device, implant and graft NOS

OGCR **Section I.C.19.g.3.**

Organ Transplant Complications

Transplant Complications

(a) Transplant complications other than kidney

Codes under category T86, Complications of transplanted organs and tissues, are for use for both complications and rejection of transplanted organs. A transplant complication code is only assigned if the complication affects the function of the transplanted organ. Two codes are required to fully describe a transplant complication: the appropriate code from category T86 and a secondary code that identifies the complication.

Pre-existing conditions or conditions that develop after the transplant are not coded as complications unless they affect the function of the transplanted organs.

See I.C.21 for transplant organ removal status.

See I.C.2 for malignant neoplasm associated with transplanted organ.

● **T86** **Complications of transplanted organs and tissue**
  Use additional code to identify other transplant complications, such as:
     graft-versus-host disease (D89.81-)
     malignancy associated with organ transplant (C80.2)
     post-transplant lymphoproliferative disorders (PTLD) (D47.Z1)

- ● **T86.0** **Complications of bone marrow transplant**
  - **T86.00** **Unspecified** complication of bone marrow transplant 🅡
  - **T86.01** Bone marrow transplant **rejection** 🅡
  - **T86.02** Bone marrow transplant **failure** 🅡
  - **T86.03** Bone marrow transplant **infection** 🅡
  - **T86.09** **Other** complications of bone marrow transplant 🅡
    Coding Clinic: 2023, Q3, P20

- ● **T86.1** **Complications of kidney transplant**
  - **T86.10** **Unspecified** complication of kidney transplant
  - **T86.11** Kidney transplant **rejection**
  - **T86.12** Kidney transplant **failure**
    Coding Clinic: 2013, Q1, P24
  - **T86.13** Kidney transplant **infection**
    Use additional code to specify infection
  - **T86.19** **Other** complication of kidney transplant
    Coding Clinic: 2019, Q2, P7

- ● **T86.2** **Complications of heart transplant**
  - **Excludes1** complication of:
       artificial heart device (T82.5-)
       heart-lung transplant (T86.3-)
  - **T86.20** **Unspecified** complication of heart transplant 🅡
  - **T86.21** Heart transplant **rejection** 🅡
  - **T86.22** Heart transplant **failure** 🅡
  - **T86.23** Heart transplant **infection** 🅡
    Use additional code to specify infection
  - ● **T86.29** **Other** complications of heart transplant
    - **T86.290** **Cardiac allograft vasculopathy** 🅡
      - **Excludes1** atherosclerosis of coronary arteries (I25.75-, I25.76-, I25.81-)
    - **T86.298** **Other** complications of heart transplant 🅡

- ● **T86.3** **Complications of heart-lung transplant**
  - **T86.30** **Unspecified** complication of heart-lung transplant 🅡
  - **T86.31** Heart-lung transplant **rejection** 🅡
  - **T86.32** Heart-lung transplant **failure** 🅡
  - **T86.33** Heart-lung transplant **infection** 🅡
    Use additional code to specify infection
  - **T86.39** **Other** complications of heart-lung transplant 🅡

- ● **T86.4** **Complications of liver transplant**
  - **T86.40** **Unspecified** complication of liver transplant 🅡
  - **T86.41** Liver transplant **rejection** 🅡
  - **T86.42** Liver transplant **failure** 🅡
  - **T86.43** Liver transplant **infection** 🅡
    Use additional code to identify infection, such as:
       Cytomegalovirus (CMV) infection (B25.-)
  - **T86.49** **Other** complications of liver transplant 🅡

- ● **T86.5** **Complications of stem cell transplant** 🅡
  Complications from stem cells from peripheral blood
  Complications from stem cells from umbilical cord

- ● **T86.8** **Complications of other transplanted organs and tissues**
  - ● **T86.81** **Complications of lung transplant**
    - **Excludes1** complication of heart-lung transplant (T86.3-)
    - **T86.810** Lung transplant **rejection** 🅡
    - **T86.811** Lung transplant **failure** 🅡
    - **T86.812** Lung transplant **infection** 🅡
      Use additional code to specify infection
    - **T86.818** **Other** complications of lung transplant 🅡
      Coding Clinic: 2019, Q2, P7
    - **T86.819** **Unspecified** complication of lung transplant 🅡
  - ● **T86.82** **Complications of skin graft (allograft) (autograft)**
    - **Excludes2** complication of artificial skin graft (T85.693)
    - **T86.820** Skin graft (allograft) **rejection**
    - **T86.821** Skin graft (allograft) (autograft) **failure**

▶ New   ⇨ Revised   ~~deleted~~ Deleted   Excludes 1   Excludes 2   Includes   Use additional   Code first   Code also   Key words
OGCR Official Guidelines   **X** Assign placeholder X   ● Use Additional Character(s)   ▸ Manifestation Code   🅡 Hierarchical Condition Category   **Coding Clinic**

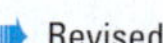
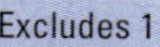
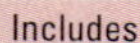
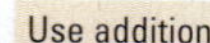
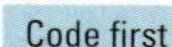

T86.822   **Skin graft (allograft) (autograft) infection**
    Use additional code to specify infection

T86.828   **Other complications of skin graft (allograft) (autograft)**

T86.829   **Unspecified complication of skin graft (allograft) (autograft)**

● T86.83   **Complications of bone graft**
    Excludes2   mechanical complications of bone graft (T84.3-)

T86.830   **Bone graft rejection**

T86.831   **Bone graft failure**

T86.832   **Bone graft infection**
    Use additional code to specify infection

T86.838   **Other complications of bone graft**
    Coding Clinic: 2023, Q1, P31

T86.839   **Unspecified complication of bone graft**

● T86.84   **Complications of corneal transplant**
    Excludes2   mechanical complications of corneal graft (T85.3-)

   ● T86.840   **Corneal transplant rejection**

     T86.8401   **Corneal transplant rejection, right eye**

     T86.8402   **Corneal transplant rejection, left eye**

     T86.8403   **Corneal transplant rejection, bilateral**

     T86.8409   **Corneal transplant rejection, unspecified eye**

   ● T86.841   **Corneal transplant failure**

     T86.8411   **Corneal transplant failure, right eye**

     T86.8412   **Corneal transplant failure, left eye**

     T86.8413   **Corneal transplant failure, bilateral**

     T86.8419   **Corneal transplant failure, unspecified eye**

   ● T86.842   **Corneal transplant infection** ℞
    Use additional code to specify infection

     T86.8421   **Corneal transplant infection, right eye**

     T86.8422   **Corneal transplant infection, left eye**

     T86.8423   **Corneal transplant infection, bilateral**

     T86.8429   **Corneal transplant infection, unspecified eye**

   ● T86.848   **Other complications of corneal transplant**

     T86.8481   **Other complications of corneal transplant, right eye**

     T86.8482   **Other complications of corneal transplant, left eye**

     T86.8483   **Other complications of corneal transplant, bilateral**

     T86.8489   **Other complications of corneal transplant, unspecified eye**

   ● T86.849   **Unspecified complication of corneal transplant**

     T86.8491   **Unspecified complication of corneal transplant, right eye**

     T86.8492   **Unspecified complication of corneal transplant, left eye**

     T86.8493   **Unspecified complication of corneal transplant, bilateral**

     T86.8499   **Unspecified complication of corneal transplant, unspecified eye**

● T86.85   **Complication of intestine transplant**

     T86.850   **Intestine transplant rejection** ℞

     T86.851   **Intestine transplant failure** ℞

     T86.852   **Intestine transplant infection** ℞
    Use additional code to specify infection

     T86.858   **Other complications of intestine transplant** ℞

     T86.859   **Unspecified complication of intestine transplant** ℞

● T86.89   **Complications of other transplanted tissue**
    Transplant failure or rejection of pancreas

     T86.890   **Other transplanted tissue rejection**

     T86.891   **Other transplanted tissue failure**

     T86.892   **Other transplanted tissue infection**
    Use additional code to specify infection

     T86.898   **Other complications of other transplanted tissue**

     T86.899   **Unspecified complication of other transplanted tissue**

● T86.9   **Complication of unspecified transplanted organ and tissue**

     T86.90   **Unspecified complication of unspecified transplanted organ and tissue**

     T86.91   **Unspecified transplanted organ and tissue rejection**

     T86.92   **Unspecified transplanted organ and tissue failure**

     T86.93   **Unspecified transplanted organ and tissue infection**
    Use additional code to specify infection

     T86.99   **Other complications of unspecified transplanted organ and tissue**

● T87   **Complications peculiar to reattachment and amputation**

   ● T87.0   **Complications of reattached (part of) upper extremity**

     ● T87.0X   **Complications of reattached (part of) upper extremity**

       T87.0X1   **Complications of reattached (part of) right upper extremity** ℞

       T87.0X2   **Complications of reattached (part of) left upper extremity** ℞

       T87.0X9   **Complications of reattached (part of) unspecified upper extremity** ℞

   ● T87.1   **Complications of reattached (part of) lower extremity**

     ● T87.1X   **Complications of reattached (part of) lower extremity**

       T87.1X1   **Complications of reattached (part of) right lower extremity** ℞

       T87.1X2   **Complications of reattached (part of) left lower extremity** ℞

       T87.1X9   **Complications of reattached (part of) unspecified lower extremity** ℞

   T87.2   **Complications of other reattached body part** ℞

   ● T87.3   **Neuroma of amputation stump**

     T87.30   **Neuroma of amputation stump, unspecified extremity** ℞

T87.31　Neuroma of amputation stump, **right upper** extremity (HCC)

T87.32　Neuroma of amputation stump, **left upper** extremity (HCC)

T87.33　Neuroma of amputation stump, **right lower** extremity (HCC)

T87.34　Neuroma of amputation stump, **left lower** extremity (HCC)

● T87.4　Infection of amputation stump

T87.40　Infection of amputation stump, **unspecified** extremity (HCC)

T87.41　Infection of amputation stump, **right upper** extremity (HCC)

T87.42　Infection of amputation stump, **left upper** extremity (HCC)

T87.43　Infection of amputation stump, **right lower** extremity (HCC)

T87.44　Infection of amputation stump, **left lower** extremity (HCC)

● T87.5　Necrosis of amputation stump

T87.50　Necrosis of amputation stump, **unspecified** extremity (HCC)

T87.51　Necrosis of amputation stump, **right upper** extremity (HCC)

T87.52　Necrosis of amputation stump, **left upper** extremity (HCC)

T87.53　Necrosis of amputation stump, **right lower** extremity (HCC)

T87.54　Necrosis of amputation stump, **left lower** extremity (HCC)

● T87.8　Other complications of amputation stump

T87.81　**Dehiscence** of amputation stump (HCC)

T87.89　**Other complications** of amputation stump (HCC)
Amputation stump contracture
Amputation stump contracture of next proximal joint
Amputation stump flexion
Amputation stump edema
Amputation stump hematoma

> **Excludes2**　phantom limb syndrome (G54.6-G54.7)

Coding Clinic: 2022, Q3, P11

T87.9　**Unspecified** complications of amputation stump (HCC)

● T88　Other complications of surgical and medical care, not elsewhere classified

> **Excludes2**　complication following infusion, transfusion and therapeutic injection (T80.-)
> complication following procedure NEC (T81.-)
> complications of anesthesia in labor and delivery (O74.-)
> complications of anesthesia in pregnancy (O29.-)
> complications of anesthesia in puerperium (O89.-)
> complications of devices, implants and grafts (T82-T85)
> complications of obstetric surgery and procedure (O75.4)
> dermatitis due to drugs and medicaments (L23.3, L24.4, L25.1, L27.0-L27.1)
> poisoning and toxic effects of drugs and chemicals (T36-T65 with fifth or sixth character 1-4)
> specified complications classified elsewhere

The appropriate 7th character is to be added to each code from category T88

A	initial encounter
D	subsequent encounter
S	sequela

X ● T88.0　Infection following immunization
Sepsis following immunization
Coding Clinic: 2019, Q1, P14;2018, Q4, P90

X ● T88.1　Other complications following immunization, not elsewhere classified
Generalized vaccinia
Rash following immunization

> **Excludes1**　vaccinia not from vaccine (B08.011)
> **Excludes2**　anaphylactic shock due to serum (T80.5-)
> other serum reactions (T80.6-)
> postimmunization arthropathy (M02.2)
> postimmunization encephalitis (G04.02)
> postimmunization fever (R50.83)

X ● T88.2　Shock due to anesthesia

> **Use additional** code for adverse effect, if applicable, to identify drug (T41.- with fifth or sixth character 5)
> **Excludes1**　complications of anesthesia (in):
> labor and delivery (O74.-)
> pregnancy (O29.-)
> puerperium (O89.-)
> postprocedural shock NOS (T81.1-)

X ● T88.3　Malignant hyperthermia due to anesthesia

> **Use additional** code for adverse effect, if applicable, to identify drug (T41.- with fifth or sixth character 5)

X ● T88.4　Failed or difficult intubation

● T88.5　Other complications of anesthesia

> **Use additional** code for adverse effect, if applicable, to identify drug (T41.- with fifth or sixth character 5)

Coding Clinic: 2016, Q4, P72

X ● T88.51　Hypothermia following anesthesia

X ● T88.52　Failed moderate sedation during procedure
Failed conscious sedation during procedure

> **Excludes2**　personal history of failed moderate sedation (Z92.83)

X ● T88.53　Unintended awareness under general anesthesia during procedure

> **Excludes2**　personal history of unintended awareness under general anesthesia (Z92.84)

Coding Clinic: 2016, Q4, P72-73

X ● T88.59　Other complications of anesthesia

X ● T88.6　Anaphylactic reaction due to adverse effect of correct drug or medicament properly administered
Anaphylactic shock due to adverse effect of correct drug or medicament properly administered
Anaphylactoid reaction NOS

> **Use additional** code for adverse effect, if applicable, to identify drug (T36-T50 with fifth or sixth character 5)
> **Excludes1**　anaphylactic reaction due to serum (T80.5-)
> anaphylactic shock or reaction due to adverse food reaction (T78.0-)

Coding Clinic: 2020, Q1, P18

X ● T88.7　Unspecified adverse effect of drug or medicament
Drug hypersensitivity NOS
Drug reaction NOS

> **Use additional** code for adverse effect, if applicable, to identify drug (T36-T50 with fifth or sixth character 5)
> **Excludes1**　specified adverse effects of drugs and medicaments (A00-R94 and T80-T88.6, T88.8)

X ● T88.8　Other specified complications of surgical and medical care, not elsewhere classified

> **Use additional** code to identify the complication

Coding Clinic: 2022, Q2, P8

X ● T88.9　Complication of surgical and medical care, **unspecified**

CHAPTER 20

EXTERNAL CAUSES OF MORBIDITY
(V00-Y99)

OGCR Chapter-Specific Coding Guidelines

20. Chapter 20: External Causes of Morbidity (V00-Y99)
The external causes of morbidity codes should never be sequenced as the first-listed or principal diagnosis.

External cause codes are intended to provide data for injury research and evaluation of injury prevention strategies. These codes capture how the injury or health condition happened (cause), the intent (unintentional or accidental; or intentional, such as suicide or assault), the place where the event occurred the activity of the patient at the time of the event, and the person's status (e.g., civilian, military).

There is no national requirement for mandatory ICD-10-CM external cause code reporting. Unless a provider is subject to a state-based external cause code reporting mandate or these codes are required by a particular payer, reporting of ICD-10-CM codes in Chapter 20, External Causes of Morbidity, is not required. In the absence of a mandatory reporting requirement, providers are encouraged to voluntarily report external cause codes, as they provide valuable data for injury research and evaluation of injury prevention strategies.

a. General External Cause Coding Guidelines

1) Used with any code in the range of A00.0-T88.9, Z00-Z99
An external cause code may be used with any code in the range of A00.0-T88.9, Z00-Z99, classification that represents a health condition due to an external cause. Though they are most applicable to injuries, they are also valid for use with such things as infections or diseases due to an external source, and other health conditions, such as a heart attack that occurs during strenuous physical activity.

2) External cause code used for length of treatment
Assign the external cause code, with the appropriate 7th character (initial encounter, subsequent encounter or sequela) for each encounter for which the injury or condition is being treated.

Most categories in Chapter 20 have a 7th character requirement for each applicable code. Most categories in this chapter have three 7th character values: A, initial encounter, D, subsequent encounter and S, sequela. While the patient may be seen by a new or different provider over the course of treatment for an injury or condition, assignment of the 7th character for external cause should match the 7th character of the code assigned for the associated injury or condition for the encounter.

3) Use the full range of external cause codes
Use the full range of external cause codes to completely describe the cause, the intent, the place of occurrence and if applicable, the activity of the patient at the time of the event, and the patient's status, for all injuries, and other health conditions due to an external cause.

4) Assign as many external cause codes as necessary
Assign as many external cause codes as necessary to fully explain each cause. If only one external code can be recorded, assign the code most related to the principal diagnosis.

5) The selection of the appropriate external cause code
The selection of the appropriate external cause code is guided by the Alphabetic Index of External Causes and by Inclusion and Exclusion notes in the Tabular List.

6) External cause code can never be a principal diagnosis
An external cause code can never be a principal (first-listed) diagnosis.

7) Combination external cause codes
Certain of the external cause codes are combination codes that identify sequential events that result in an injury, such as a fall which results in striking against an object. The injury may be due to either event or both. The combination external cause code used should correspond to the sequence of events regardless of which caused the most serious injury.

8) No external cause code needed in certain circumstances
No external cause code from Chapter 20 is needed if the external cause and intent are included in a code from another chapter (e.g., T36.0X1- Poisoning by penicillins, accidental (unintentional)).

b. Place of Occurrence Guideline
Codes from category Y92, Place of occurrence of the external cause, are secondary codes for use after other external cause codes to identify the location of the patient at the time of injury or other condition.

Generally, a place of occurrence code is assigned only once, at the initial encounter for treatment. However, in the rare instance that a new injury occurs during hospitalization, an additional place of occurrence code may be assigned. No 7th characters are used for Y92. Only one code from Y92 should be recorded on a medical record.

Do not use place of occurrence code Y92.9 if the place is not stated or is not applicable.

c. Activity Code
Assign a code from category Y93, Activity code, to describe the activity of the patient at the time the injury or other health condition occurred.

An activity code is used only once, at the initial encounter for treatment. Only one code from Y93 should be recorded on a medical record.

The activity codes are not applicable to poisonings, adverse effects, misadventures or sequela.

Do not assign Y93.9, Unspecified activity, if the activity is not stated.

A code from category Y93 is appropriate for use with external cause and intent codes if identifying the activity provides additional information about the event.

d. Place of Occurrence, Activity, and Status Codes Used with Other External Cause Code
When applicable, place of occurrence, activity, and external cause status codes are sequenced after the main external cause code(s). Regardless of the number of external cause codes assigned, there should be only one place of occurrence code, one activity code, and one external cause status code assigned to an encounter.

e. If the Reporting Format Limits the Number of External Cause Codes

If the reporting format limits the number of external cause codes that can be used in reporting clinical data, report the code for the cause/intent most related to the principal diagnosis. If the format permits capture of additional external cause codes, the cause/intent, including medical misadventures, of the additional events should be reported rather than the codes for place, activity, or external status.

f. Multiple External Cause Coding Guidelines

More than one external cause code is required to fully describe the external cause of an illness or injury. The assignment of external cause codes should be sequenced in the following priority:

If two or more events cause separate injuries, an external cause code should be assigned for each cause. The first-listed external cause code will be selected in the following order:

External codes for child and adult abuse take priority over all other external cause codes.

See Section I.C.19., Child and Adult abuse guidelines.

External codes for terrorism events take priority over all other external cause codes except child and adult abuse.

External cause codes for cataclysmic events take priority over all other external cause codes except child and adult abuse and terrorism.

External cause codes for transport accidents take priority over all other external cause codes except cataclysmic events, child and adult abuse and terrorism.

Activity and external cause status codes are assigned following all causal (intent) external cause codes.

The first-listed external cause code should correspond to the cause of the most serious diagnosis due to an assault, accident, or self-harm, following the order of hierarchy listed above.

g. Child and Adult Abuse Guideline

Adult and child abuse, neglect and maltreatment are classified as assault. Any of the assault codes may be used to indicate the external cause of any injury resulting from the confirmed abuse.

For confirmed cases of abuse, neglect and maltreatment, when the perpetrator is known, a code from Y07, Perpetrator of maltreatment and neglect, should accompany any other assault codes.

See Section I.C.19. Adult and child abuse, neglect and other maltreatment

h. Unknown or Undetermined Intent Guideline

If the intent (accident, self-harm, assault) of the cause of an injury or other condition is unknown or unspecified, code the intent as accidental intent. All transport accident categories assume accidental intent.

1) Use of undetermined intent

External cause codes for events of undetermined intent are only for use if the documentation in the record specifies that the intent cannot be determined.

i. Sequelae (Late Effects) of External Cause Guidelines

1) Sequelae external cause codes

Sequela are reported using the external cause code with the 7th character "S" for sequela. These codes should be used with any report of a late effect or sequela resulting from a previous injury.

See Section I.B.10. Sequela, (Late Effects).

2) Sequela external cause code with a related current injury

A sequela external cause code should never be used with a related current nature of injury code.

3) Use of sequela external cause codes for subsequent visits

Use a late effect external cause code for subsequent visits when a late effect of the initial injury is being treated. Do not use a late effect external cause code for subsequent visits for follow-up care (e.g., to assess healing, to receive rehabilitative therapy) of the injury when no late effect of the injury has been documented.

j. Terrorism Guidelines

1) Cause of injury identified by the Federal Government (FBI) as terrorism

When the cause of an injury is identified by the Federal Government (FBI) as terrorism, the first-listed external cause code should be a code from category Y38, Terrorism. The definition of terrorism employed by the FBI is found at the inclusion note at the beginning of category Y38. Use additional code for place of occurrence (Y92.-). More than one Y38 code may be assigned if the injury is the result of more than one mechanism of terrorism.

2) Cause of an injury is suspected to be the result of terrorism

When the cause of an injury is suspected to be the result of terrorism a code from category Y38 should not be assigned. Suspected cases should be classified as assault.

3) Code Y38.9, Terrorism, secondary effects

Assign code Y38.9, Terrorism, secondary effects, for conditions occurring subsequent to the terrorist event. This code should not be assigned for conditions that are due to the initial terrorist act.

It is acceptable to assign code Y38.9 with another code from Y38 if there is an injury due to the initial terrorist event and an injury that is a subsequent result of the terrorist event.

k. External cause status

A code from category Y99, External cause status, should be assigned whenever any other external cause code is assigned for an encounter, including an Activity code, except for the events noted below. Assign a code from category Y99, External cause status, to indicate the work status of the person at the time the event occurred. The status code indicates whether the event occurred during military activity, whether a non-military person was at work, whether an individual including a student or volunteer was involved in a non-work activity at the time of the causal event.

A code from Y99, External cause status, should be assigned, when applicable, with other external cause codes, such as transport accidents and falls. The external cause status codes are not applicable to poisonings, adverse effects, misadventures or late effects.

Do not assign a code from category Y99 if no other external cause codes (cause, activity) are applicable for the encounter.

An external cause status code is used only once, at the initial encounter for treatment. Only one code from Y99 should be recorded on a medical record.

Do not assign code Y99.9, Unspecified external cause status, if the status is not stated.

CHAPTER 20

EXTERNAL CAUSES OF MORBIDITY (V00-Y99)

Note: This chapter permits the classification of environmental events and circumstances as the cause of injury, and other adverse effects. Where a code from this section is applicable, it is intended that it shall be used secondary to a code from another chapter of the Classification indicating the nature of the condition. Most often, the condition will be classifiable to Chapter 19, Injury, poisoning and certain other consequences of external causes (S00-T88). Other conditions that may be stated to be due to external causes are classified in Chapters 1 to 18. For these conditions, codes from Chapter 20 should be used to provide additional information as to the cause of the condition.

This chapter contains the following blocks:

V00-X58	Accidents
V00-V99	Transport accidents
V00-V09	Pedestrian injured in transport accident
V10-V19	Pedal cycle rider injured in transport accident
V20-V29	Motorcycle rider injured in transport accident
V30-V39	Occupant of three-wheeled motor vehicle injured in transport accident
V40-V49	Car occupant injured in transport accident
V50-V59	Occupant of pick-up truck or van injured in transport accident
V60-V69	Occupant of heavy transport vehicle injured in transport accident
V70-V79	Bus occupant injured in transport accident
V80-V89	Other land transport accidents
V90-V94	Water transport accidents
V95-V97	Air and space transport accidents
V98-V99	Other and unspecified transport accidents
W00-X58	Other external causes of accidental injury
W00-W19	Slipping, tripping, stumbling and falls
W20-W49	Exposure to inanimate mechanical forces
W50-W64	Exposure to animate mechanical forces
W65-W74	Accidental non-transport drowning and submersion
W85-W99	Exposure to electric current, radiation and extreme ambient air temperature and pressure
X00-X08	Exposure to smoke, fire and flames
X10-X19	Contact with heat and hot substances
X30-X39	Exposure to forces of nature
X50	Overexertion and strenuous or repetitive movements
X52, X58	Accidental exposure to other specified factors
X71-X83	Intentional self-harm
X92-Y09	Assault
Y21-Y33	Event of undetermined intent
Y35-Y38	Legal intervention, operations of war, military operations, and terrorism
Y62-Y84	Complications of medical and surgical care
Y62-Y69	Misadventures to patients during surgical and medical care
Y70-Y82	Medical devices associated with adverse incidents in diagnostic and therapeutic use
Y83-Y84	Surgical and other medical procedures as the cause of abnormal reaction of the patient, or of later complication, without mention of misadventure at the time of the procedure
Y90-Y99	Supplementary factors related to causes of morbidity classified elsewhere

ACCIDENTS (V00-X58)

TRANSPORT ACCIDENTS (V00-V99)

Note: This section is structured in 12 groups. Those relating to land transport accidents (V00-V89) reflect the victim's mode of transport and are subdivided to identify the victim's 'counterpart' or the type of event. The vehicle of which the injured person is an occupant is identified in the first two characters since it is seen as the most important factor to identify for prevention purposes. A transport accident is one in which the vehicle involved must be moving or running or in use for transport purposes at the time of the accident.

Use additional code to identify:
Airbag injury (W22.1)
Type of street or road (Y92.4-)
Use of cellular telephone and other electronic equipment at the time of the transport accident (Y93.C-)

Excludes1 agricultural vehicles in stationary use or maintenance (W31.-)
assault by crashing of motor vehicle (Y03.-)
automobile or motor cycle in stationary use or maintenance - code to type of accident
crashing of motor vehicle, undetermined intent (Y32)
intentional self-harm by crashing of motor vehicle (X82)

Excludes2 transport accidents due to cataclysm (X34-X38)

Note: Definitions related to transport accidents:

(a) A transport accident (V00-V99) is any accident involving a device designed primarily for, or used at the time primarily for, conveying persons or good from one place to another.

(b) A public highway [trafficway] or street is the entire width between property lines (or other boundary lines) of land open to the public as a matter of right or custom for purposes of moving persons or property from one place to another. A roadway is that part of the public highway designed, improved and customarily used for vehicular traffic.

(c) A traffic accident is any vehicle accident occurring on the public highway [i.e., originating on, terminating on, or involving a vehicle partially on the highway]. A vehicle accident is assumed to have occurred on the public highway unless another place is specified, except in the case of accidents involving only off-road motor vehicles, which are classified as nontraffic accidents unless the contrary is stated.

(d) A nontraffic accident is any vehicle accident that occurs entirely in any place other than a public highway.

(e) A pedestrian is any person involved in an accident who was not at the time of the accident riding in or on a motor vehicle, railway train, streetcar or animal-drawn or other vehicle, or on a pedal cycle or animal. This includes, a person changing a tire, working on a parked car, or a person on foot. It also includes the user of a pedestrian conveyance such as a baby stroller, ice-skates, skis, sled, roller skates, a skateboard, nonmotorized or motorized wheelchair, motorized mobility scooter, or nonmotorized scooter.

(f) A driver is an occupant of a transport vehicle who is operating or intending to operate it.

(g) A passenger is any occupant of a transport vehicle other than the driver, except a person traveling on the outside of the vehicle.

(h) A person on the outside of a vehicle is any person being transported by a vehicle but not occupying the space normally reserved for the driver or passengers, or the space intended for the transport of property. This includes a person travelling on the bodywork, bumper, fender, roof, running board or step of a vehicle, as well as, hanging on the outside of the vehicle.

(i) A pedal cycle is any land transport vehicle operated solely by nonmotorized pedals including a bicycle or tricycle.

(j) A pedal cyclist is any person riding a pedal cycle or in a sidecar or trailer attached to a pedal cycle.

(k) A motorcycle is a two-wheeled motor vehicle with one or two riding saddles and sometimes with a third wheel for the support of a sidecar. The sidecar is considered part of the motorcycle. This includes a moped, motor scooter, or motorized bicycle.

(l) A motorcycle rider is any person riding a motorcycle or in a sidecar or trailer attached to the motorcycle.

(m) A three-wheeled motor vehicle is a motorized tricycle designed primarily for on-road use. This includes a motor-driven tricycle, a motorized rickshaw, or a three-wheeled motor car.

(n) A car [automobile] is a four-wheeled motor vehicle designed primarily for carrying up to 7 persons. A trailer being towed by the car is considered part of the car. It does not include a van or minivan—see definition (o)

(o) A pick-up truck or van is a four or six-wheeled motor vehicle designed for carrying passengers as well as property or cargo weighing less than the local limit for classification as a heavy goods vehicle, and not requiring a special driver's license. This includes a minivan and a sport-utility vehicle (SUV).

(p) A heavy transport vehicle is a motor vehicle designed primarily for carrying property, meeting local criteria for classification as a heavy goods vehicle in terms of weight and requiring a special driver's license.

(q) A bus (coach) is a motor vehicle designed or adapted primarily for carrying more than 10 passengers, and requiring a special driver's license.

(r) A railway train or railway vehicle is any device, with or without freight or passenger cars coupled to it, designed for traffic on a railway track. This includes subterranean (subways) or elevated trains.

(s) A streetcar is a device designed and used primarily for transporting passengers within a municipality, running on rails, usually subject to normal traffic control signals, and operated principally on a right-of-way that forms part of the roadway. This includes a tram or trolley that runs on rails. A trailer being towed by a streetcar is considered part of the streetcar.

(t) A special vehicle mainly used on industrial premises is a motor vehicle designed primarily for use within the buildings and premises of industrial or commercial establishments. This includes battery-powered airport passenger vehicles or baggage/mail trucks, forklifts, coal-cars in a coal mine, logging cars and trucks used in mines or quarries.

(u) A special vehicle mainly used in agriculture is a motor vehicle designed specifically for use in farming and agriculture (horticulture), to work the land, tend and harvest crops and transport materials on the farm. This includes harvesters, farm machinery and tractor and trailers.

(v) A special construction vehicle is a motor vehicle designed specifically for use on construction and demolition sites. This includes bulldozers, diggers, earth levellers, dump trucks, backhoes, front-end loaders, pavers, and mechanical shovels.

(w) A special all-terrain vehicle is a motor vehicle of special design to enable it to negotiate over rough or soft terrain, snow or sand. Examples of special design are high construction, special wheels and tires, tracks, and support on a cushion of air. This includes snow mobiles, all-terrain vehicles (ATV), and dune buggies. It does not include passenger vehicle designated as sport utility vehicles (SUV).

(x) A watercraft is any device designed for transporting passengers or goods on water. This includes motor or sail boats, ships, and hovercraft.

(y) An aircraft is any device for transporting passengers or goods in the air. This includes hot-air balloons, gliders, helicopters and airplanes.

(z) A military vehicle is any motorized vehicle operating on a public roadway owned by the military and being operated by a member of the military.

PEDESTRIAN INJURED IN TRANSPORT ACCIDENT (V00-V09)

Includes   person changing tire on transport vehicle
person examining engine of vehicle broken down in (on side of) road

Excludes1   fall due to non-transport collision with other person (W03)
pedestrian on foot falling (slipping) on ice and snow (W00.-)
struck or bumped by another person (W51)

● **V00** **Pedestrian conveyance accident**

Use additional place of occurrence and activity external cause codes, if known (Y92.-, Y93.-)

Excludes1   collision with another person without fall (W51)
fall due to person on foot colliding with another person on foot (W03)
fall from non-moving wheelchair, nonmotorized scooter and motorized mobility scooter without collision (W05.-)
pedestrian (conveyance) collision with other land transport vehicle (V01-V09)
pedestrian on foot falling (slipping) on ice and snow (W00.-)

The appropriate 7th character is to be added to each code from category V00

A	initial encounter
D	subsequent encounter
S	sequela

● **V00.0** **Pedestrian on foot injured in collision with pedestrian conveyance**

X● **V00.01** **Pedestrian on foot injured in collision with roller-skater**

X● **V00.02** **Pedestrian on foot injured in collision with skateboarder**

● **V00.03** **Pedestrian on foot injured in collision with standing micro-mobility pedestrian conveyance**

    V00.031 **Pedestrian on foot injured in collision with rider of standing electric scooter**

    V00.038 **Pedestrian on foot injured in collision with rider of other standing micro-mobility pedestrian conveyance**
Pedestrian on foot injured in collision with rider of hoverboard
Pedestrian on foot injured in collision with rider of segway

X● **V00.09** **Pedestrian on foot injured in collision with other pedestrian conveyance**

● **V00.1** **Rolling-type pedestrian conveyance accident**

Excludes1   accident with baby stroller (V00.82-)
accident with wheelchair (powered) (V00.81-)
accident with motorized mobility scooter (V00.83-)

● **V00.11** **In-line roller-skate accident**

● **V00.111** **Fall from in-line roller-skates**

● **V00.112** **In-line roller-skater colliding with stationary object**

● **V00.118** **Other in-line roller-skate accident**

Excludes1   roller-skater collision with other land transport vehicle (V01-V09 with 5th character 1)

▶ New   ➡ Revised   ~~deleted~~ Deleted   Excludes 1   Excludes 2   Includes   Use additional   Code first   Code also   Key words
OGCR Official Guidelines   **X** Assign placeholder X   ● Use Additional Character(s)   ▶ Manifestation Code   Hierarchical Condition Category   **Coding Clinic**

- ● **V00.12**   Non-in-line roller-skate accident
  - ● **V00.121**   Fall from non-in-line roller-skates
  - ● **V00.122**   Non-in-line roller-skater colliding with stationary object
  - ● **V00.128**   Other non-in-line roller-skating accident
    - **Excludes1**   roller-skater collision with other land transport vehicle (V01-V09 with 5th character 1)
- ● **V00.13**   Skateboard accident
  - ● **V00.131**   Fall from skateboard
  - ● **V00.132**   Skateboarder colliding with stationary object
  - ● **V00.138**   Other skateboard accident
    - **Excludes1**   skateboarder collision with other land transport vehicle (V01-V09 with 5th character 2)
- ● **V00.14**   Scooter (nonmotorized) accident
  - **Excludes1**   motor scooter accident (V20-V29)
  - ● **V00.141**   Fall from scooter (nonmotorized)
  - ● **V00.142**   Scooter (nonmotorized) colliding with stationary object
  - ● **V00.148**   Other scooter (nonmotorized) accident
    - **Excludes1**   scooter (non-motorized) collision with other land transport vehicle (V01-V09 with fifth character 9)
- ● **V00.15**   Heelies accident
  - Rolling shoe
  - Wheeled shoe
  - Wheelies accident
  - ● **V00.151**   Fall from heelies
  - ● **V00.152**   Heelies colliding with stationary object
  - ● **V00.158**   Other heelies accident
- ● **V00.18**   Accident on other rolling-type pedestrian conveyance
  - ● **V00.181**   Fall from other rolling-type pedestrian conveyance
  - ● **V00.182**   Pedestrian on other rolling-type pedestrian conveyance colliding with stationary object
  - ● **V00.188**   Other accident on other rolling-type pedestrian conveyance
- ● **V00.2**   Gliding-type pedestrian conveyance accident
  - ● **V00.21**   Ice-skates accident
    - ● **V00.211**   Fall from ice-skates
    - ● **V00.212**   Ice-skater colliding with stationary object
    - ● **V00.218**   Other ice-skates accident
      - **Excludes1**   ice-skater collision with other land transport vehicle (V01-V09 with 5th character 9)
  - ● **V00.22**   Sled accident
    - ● **V00.221**   Fall from sled
    - ● **V00.222**   Sledder colliding with stationary object
    - ● **V00.228**   Other sled accident
      - **Excludes1**   sled collision with other land transport vehicle (V01-V09 with 5th character 9)
  - ● **V00.28**   Other gliding-type pedestrian conveyance accident
    - ● **V00.281**   Fall from other gliding-type pedestrian conveyance
    - ● **V00.282**   Pedestrian on other gliding-type pedestrian conveyance colliding with stationary object
    - ● **V00.288**   Other accident on other gliding-type pedestrian conveyance
      - **Excludes1**   gliding-type pedestrian conveyance collision with other land transport vehicle (V01-V09 with 5th character 9)
- ● **V00.3**   Flat-bottomed pedestrian conveyance accident
  - ● **V00.31**   Snowboard accident
    - ● **V00.311**   Fall from snowboard
    - ● **V00.312**   Snowboarder colliding with stationary object
    - ● **V00.318**   Other snowboard accident
      - **Excludes1**   snowboarder collision with other land transport vehicle (V01-V09 with 5th character 9)
  - ● **V00.32**   Snow-ski accident
    - ● **V00.321**   Fall from snow-skis
      - **Coding Clinic: 2015, Q1, P12**
    - ● **V00.322**   Snow-skier colliding with stationary object
    - ● **V00.328**   Other snow-ski accident
      - **Excludes1**   snow-skier collision with other land transport vehicle (V01-V09 with 5th character 9)
  - ● **V00.38**   Other flat-bottomed pedestrian conveyance accident
    - ● **V00.381**   Fall from other flat-bottomed pedestrian conveyance
    - ● **V00.382**   Pedestrian on other flat-bottomed pedestrian conveyance colliding with stationary object
    - ● **V00.388**   Other accident on other flat-bottomed pedestrian conveyance
- ● **V00.8**   Accident on other pedestrian conveyance
  - ● **V00.81**   Accident with wheelchair (powered)
    - ● **V00.811**   Fall from moving wheelchair (powered)
      - **Excludes1**   fall from non-moving wheelchair (W05.0)
    - ● **V00.812**   Wheelchair (powered) colliding with stationary object
    - ● **V00.818**   Other accident with wheelchair (powered)
  - ● **V00.82**   Accident with baby stroller
    - ● **V00.821**   Fall from baby stroller
    - ● **V00.822**   Baby stroller colliding with stationary object
    - ● **V00.828**   Other accident with baby stroller

● **V00.83**   **Accident with motorized mobility scooter**
    ● **V00.831**   **Fall from motorized mobility scooter**
       Excludes1   fall from non-moving motorized mobility scooter (W05.2)
    ● **V00.832**   **Motorized mobility scooter colliding with stationary object**
    ● **V00.838**   **Other accident with motorized mobility scooter**
● **V00.84**   **Accident with standing micro-mobility pedestrian conveyance**
    V00.841   **Fall from standing electric scooter**
    V00.842   **Pedestrian on standing electric scooter colliding with stationary object**
    V00.848   **Other accident with standing micro-mobility pedestrian conveyance**
       Accident with hoverboard
       Accident with segway
● **V00.89**   **Accident on other pedestrian conveyance**
    ● **V00.891**   **Fall from other pedestrian conveyance**
    ● **V00.892**   **Pedestrian on other pedestrian conveyance colliding with stationary object**
    ● **V00.898**   **Other accident on other pedestrian conveyance**
       Excludes1   other pedestrian (conveyance) collision with other land transport vehicle (V01-V09 with 5th character 9)

● **V01**   **Pedestrian injured in collision with pedal cycle**

The appropriate 7th character is to be added to each code from category V01

> A   initial encounter
> D   subsequent encounter
> S   sequela

● **V01.0**   **Pedestrian injured in collision with pedal cycle in nontraffic accident**
    X ● **V01.00**   **Pedestrian on foot injured in collision with pedal cycle in nontraffic accident**
       Pedestrian NOS injured in collision with pedal cycle in nontraffic accident
    X ● **V01.01**   **Pedestrian on roller-skates injured in collision with pedal cycle in nontraffic accident**
    X ● **V01.02**   **Pedestrian on skateboard injured in collision with pedal cycle in nontraffic accident**
    ● **V01.03**   **Pedestrian on standing micro-mobility pedestrian conveyance injured in collision with pedal cycle in nontraffic accident**
       V01.031   **Pedestrian on standing electric scooter injured in collision with pedal cycle in nontraffic accident**
       V01.038   **Pedestrian on other standing micro-mobility pedestrian conveyance injured in collision with pedal cycle in nontraffic accident**
          Pedestrian on hoverboard injured in collision with pedal cycle in nontraffic accident
          Pedestrian on segway injured in collision with pedal cycle in nontraffic accident

X ● **V01.09**   **Pedestrian with other conveyance injured in collision with pedal cycle in nontraffic accident**
    Pedestrian with baby stroller injured in collision with pedal cycle in nontraffic accident
    Pedestrian in wheelchair (powered) injured in collision with pedal cycle in nontraffic accident
    Pedestrian in motorized mobility scooter injured in collision with pedal cycle in nontraffic accident
    Pedestrian on ice-skates injured in collision with pedal cycle in nontraffic accident
    Pedestrian on nonmotorized scooter injured in collision with pedal cycle in nontraffic accident
    Pedestrian on sled injured in collision with pedal cycle in nontraffic accident
    Pedestrian on snowboard injured in collision with pedal cycle in nontraffic accident
    Pedestrian on snow-skis injured in collision with pedal cycle in nontraffic accident

● **V01.1**   **Pedestrian injured in collision with pedal cycle in traffic accident**
    X ● **V01.10**   **Pedestrian on foot injured in collision with pedal cycle in traffic accident**
       Pedestrian NOS injured in collision with pedal cycle in traffic accident
    X ● **V01.11**   **Pedestrian on roller-skates injured in collision with pedal cycle in traffic accident**
    X ● **V01.12**   **Pedestrian on skateboard injured in collision with pedal cycle in traffic accident**
    ● **V01.13**   **Pedestrian on standing micro-mobility pedestrian conveyance injured in collision with pedal cycle in traffic accident**
       V01.131   **Pedestrian on standing electric scooter injured in collision with pedal cycle in traffic accident**
       V01.138   **Pedestrian on other standing micro-mobility pedestrian conveyance injured in collision with pedal cycle in traffic accident**
          Pedestrian on hoverboard injured in collision with pedal cycle in traffic accident
          Pedestrian on segway injured in collision with pedal cycle in traffic accident
    X ● **V01.19**   **Pedestrian with other conveyance injured in collision with pedal cycle in traffic accident**
    Pedestrian with baby stroller injured in collision with pedal cycle in traffic accident
    Pedestrian in wheelchair (powered) injured in collision with pedal cycle in traffic accident
    Pedestrian in motorized mobility scooter injured in collision with pedal cycle in traffic accident
    Pedestrian on ice-skates injured in collision with pedal cycle in traffic accident
    Pedestrian on nonmotorized scooter injured in collision with pedal cycle in traffic accident
    Pedestrian on sled injured in collision with pedal cycle in traffic accident
    Pedestrian on snowboard injured in collision with pedal cycle in traffic accident
    Pedestrian on snow-skis injured in collision with pedal cycle in traffic accident

● **V01.9**   **Pedestrian injured in collision with pedal cycle, unspecified whether traffic or nontraffic accident**

X ● **V01.90**   **Pedestrian on foot injured in collision with pedal cycle, unspecified whether traffic or nontraffic accident**
Pedestrian NOS injured in collision with pedal cycle, unspecified whether traffic or nontraffic accident

X ● **V01.91**   **Pedestrian on roller-skates injured in collision with pedal cycle, unspecified whether traffic or nontraffic accident**

X ● **V01.92**   **Pedestrian on skateboard injured in collision with pedal cycle, unspecified whether traffic or nontraffic accident**

● **V01.93**   **Pedestrian on standing micro-mobility pedestrian conveyance injured in collision with pedal cycle, unspecified whether traffic or nontraffic accident**

    V01.931   Pedestrian on standing electric scooter injured in collision with pedal cycle, unspecified whether traffic or nontraffic accident

    V01.938   Pedestrian on other standing micro-mobility pedestrian conveyance injured in collision with pedal cycle, unspecified whether traffic or nontraffic accident
Pedestrian on hoverboard injured in collision with pedal cycle, unspecified whether traffic or nontraffic accident
Pedestrian on segway injured in collision with pedal cycle, unspecified whether traffic or nontraffic accident

X ● **V01.99**   **Pedestrian with other conveyance injured in collision with pedal cycle, unspecified whether traffic or nontraffic accident**
Pedestrian with baby stroller injured in collision with pedal cycle, unspecified whether traffic or nontraffic accident
Pedestrian in wheelchair (powered) injured in collision with pedal cycle, unspecified whether traffic or nontraffic accident
Pedestrian in motorized mobility scooter injured in collision with pedal cycle, unspecified whether traffic or nontraffic accident
Pedestrian on ice-skates injured in collision with pedal cycle unspecified, whether traffic or nontraffic accident
Pedestrian on nonmotorized scooter injured in collision with pedal cycle, unspecified whether traffic or nontraffic accident
Pedestrian on sled injured in collision with pedal cycle unspecified, whether traffic or nontraffic accident
Pedestrian on snowboard injured in collision with pedal cycle, unspecified whether traffic or nontraffic accident
Pedestrian on snow-skis injured in collision with pedal cycle, unspecified whether traffic or nontraffic accident

● **V02**   **Pedestrian injured in collision with two- or three-wheeled motor vehicle**

The appropriate 7th character is to be added to each code from category V02

> A   initial encounter
> D   subsequent encounter
> S   sequela

● **V02.0**   **Pedestrian injured in collision with two- or three-wheeled motor vehicle in nontraffic accident**

X ● **V02.00**   **Pedestrian on foot injured in collision with two- or three-wheeled motor vehicle in nontraffic accident**
Pedestrian NOS injured in collision with two- or three-wheeled motor vehicle in nontraffic accident

X ● **V02.01**   **Pedestrian on roller-skates injured in collision with two- or three-wheeled motor vehicle in nontraffic accident**

X ● **V02.02**   **Pedestrian on skateboard injured in collision with two- or three-wheeled motor vehicle in nontraffic accident**

● **V02.03**   **Pedestrian on standing micro-mobility pedestrian conveyance injured in collision with two- or three-wheeled motor vehicle in nontraffic accident**

    V02.031   Pedestrian on standing electric scooter injured in collision with two- or three-wheeled motor vehicle in nontraffic accident

    V02.038   Pedestrian on other standing micro-mobility pedestrian conveyance injured in collision with two- or three-wheeled motor vehicle in nontraffic accident
Pedestrian on hoverboard injured in collision with two-or three wheeled motor vehicle in nontraffic accident
Pedestrian on segway injured in collision with two- or three-wheeled motor vehicle in nontraffic accident

X ● **V02.09**   **Pedestrian with other conveyance injured in collision with two- or three-wheeled motor vehicle in nontraffic accident**
Pedestrian with baby stroller injured in collision with two- or three-wheeled motor vehicle in nontraffic accident
Pedestrian on ice-skates injured in collision with two- or three-wheeled motor vehicle in nontraffic accident
Pedestrian in wheelchair (powered) injured in collision with two- or three-wheeled motor vehicle in nontraffic accident
Pedestrian in motorized mobility scooter injured in collision with two- or three-wheeled motor vehicle in nontraffic accident
Pedestrian on nonmotorized scooter injured in collision with two- or three-wheeled motor vehicle in nontraffic accident
Pedestrian on sled injured in collision with two- or three-wheeled motor vehicle in nontraffic accident
Pedestrian on snowboard injured in collision with two- or three-wheeled motor vehicle in nontraffic accident
Pedestrian on snow-skis injured in collision with two- or three-wheeled motor vehicle in nontraffic accident

CHAPTER 20 (V00-Y99)

● **V02.1** **Pedestrian injured in collision with two- or three-wheeled motor vehicle in traffic accident**

X ● **V02.10** Pedestrian on foot injured in collision with two- or three-wheeled motor vehicle in traffic accident
  Pedestrian NOS injured in collision with two- or three-wheeled motor vehicle in traffic accident

X ● **V02.11** Pedestrian on roller-skates injured in collision with two- or three-wheeled motor vehicle in traffic accident

X ● **V02.12** Pedestrian on skateboard injured in collision with two- or three-wheeled motor vehicle in traffic accident

● **V02.13** Pedestrian on standing micro-mobility pedestrian conveyance injured in collision with two- or three-wheeled motor vehicle in traffic accident

V02.131 Pedestrian on standing electric scooter injured in collision with two- or three-wheeled motor vehicle in traffic accident

V02.138 Pedestrian on other standing micro-mobility pedestrian conveyance injured in collision with two- or three-wheeled motor vehicle in traffic accident
  Pedestrian on hoverboard injured in collision with two-or three wheeled motor vehicle in traffic accident
  Pedestrian on segway injured in collision with two- or three-wheeled motor vehicle in traffic accident

X ● **V02.19** Pedestrian with other conveyance injured in collision with two- or three-wheeled motor vehicle in traffic accident
  Pedestrian with baby stroller injured in collision with two- or three-wheeled motor vehicle in traffic accident
  Pedestrian in wheelchair (powered) injured in collision with two- or three-wheeled motor vehicle in traffic accident
  Pedestrian in motorized mobility scooter injured in collision with two- or three-wheeled motor vehicle in traffic accident
  Pedestrian on ice-skates injured in collision with two- or three-wheeled motor vehicle in traffic accident
  Pedestrian on nonmotorized scooter injured in collision with two- or three-wheeled motor vehicle in traffic accident
  Pedestrian on sled injured in collision with two- or three-wheeled motor vehicle in traffic accident
  Pedestrian on snowboard injured in collision with two- or three-wheeled motor vehicle in traffic accident
  Pedestrian on snow-skis injured in collision with two- or three-wheeled motor vehicle in traffic accident

● **V02.9** **Pedestrian injured in collision with two- or three-wheeled motor vehicle, unspecified whether traffic or nontraffic accident**

X ● **V02.90** Pedestrian on foot injured in collision with two- or three-wheeled motor vehicle, unspecified whether traffic or nontraffic accident
  Pedestrian NOS injured in collision with two- or three-wheeled motor vehicle, unspecified whether traffic or nontraffic accident

X ● **V02.91** Pedestrian on roller-skates injured in collision with two- or three-wheeled motor vehicle, unspecified whether traffic or nontraffic accident

X ● **V02.92** Pedestrian on skateboard injured in collision with two- or three-wheeled motor vehicle, unspecified whether traffic or nontraffic accident

● **V02.93** Pedestrian on standing micro-mobility pedestrian conveyance injured in collision with two-or three-wheeled motor vehicle, unspecified whether traffic or nontraffic accident

V02.931 Pedestrian on standing electric scooter injured in collision with two- or three wheeled motor vehicle, unspecified whether traffic or nontraffic accident

V02.938 Pedestrian on other standing micro-mobility pedestrian conveyance injured in collision with two- or three wheeled motor vehicle, unspecified whether traffic or nontraffic accident
  Pedestrian on hoverboard injured in collision with two-three-wheeled motor vehicle, unspecified whether traffic or nontraffic accident
  Pedestrian on segway injured in collision with two- or three wheeled motor vehicle, unspecified whether traffic or nontraffic accident

X ● **V02.99** Pedestrian with other conveyance injured in collision with two- or three-wheeled motor vehicle, unspecified whether traffic or nontraffic accident
  Pedestrian with baby stroller injured in collision with two- or three-wheeled motor vehicle, unspecified whether traffic or nontraffic accident
  Pedestrian in wheelchair (powered) injured in collision with two- or three-wheeled motor vehicle, unspecified whether traffic or nontraffic accident
  Pedestrian in motorized mobility scooter injured in collision with two- or three-wheeled motor vehicle, unspecified whether traffic or nontraffic accident
  Pedestrian on ice-skates injured in collision with two- or three-wheeled motor vehicle, unspecified whether traffic or nontraffic accident
  Pedestrian on nonmotorized scooter injured in collision with two- or three-wheeled motor vehicle, unspecified whether traffic or nontraffic accident
  Pedestrian on sled injured in collision with two- or three-wheeled motor vehicle, unspecified whether traffic or nontraffic accident
  Pedestrian on snowboard injured in collision with two- or three-wheeled motor vehicle, unspecified whether traffic or nontraffic accident
  Pedestrian on snow-skis injured in collision with two- or three-wheeled motor vehicle, unspecified whether traffic or nontraffic accident

● **V03 Pedestrian injured in collision with car, pick-up truck or van**

 The appropriate 7th character is to be added to each code from category V03

  A initial encounter
  D subsequent encounter
  S sequela

● **V03.0 Pedestrian injured in collision with car, pick-up truck or van in nontraffic accident**

X ● **V03.00 Pedestrian on foot injured in collision with car, pick-up truck or van in nontraffic accident**
  Pedestrian NOS injured in collision with car, pick-up truck or van in nontraffic accident

X ● **V03.01 Pedestrian on roller-skates injured in collision with car, pick-up truck or van in nontraffic accident**

X ● **V03.02 Pedestrian on skateboard injured in collision with car, pick-up truck or van in nontraffic accident**

● **V03.03 Pedestrian on standing micro-mobility pedestrian conveyance injured in collision with car, pick-up or van in nontraffic accident**

 V03.031 Pedestrian on standing electric scooter injured in collision with car, pick-up or van in nontraffic accident

 V03.038 Pedestrian on other standing micro-mobility pedestrian conveyance injured in collision with car, pick-up or van in nontraffic accident
  Pedestrian on hoverboard injured in collision with car, pick-up or van in nontraffic accident
  Pedestrian on segway injured in collision with car, pick-up or van in nontraffic accident

X ● **V03.09 Pedestrian with other conveyance injured in collision with car, pick-up truck or van in nontraffic accident**
  Pedestrian with baby stroller injured in collision with car, pick-up truck or van in nontraffic accident
  Pedestrian in wheelchair (powered) injured in collision with car, pick-up truck or van in nontraffic accident
  Pedestrian in motorized mobility scooter injured in collision with car, pick-up truck or van in nontraffic accident
  Pedestrian on ice-skates injured in collision with car, pick-up truck or van in nontraffic accident
  Pedestrian on nonmotorized scooter injured in collision with car, pick-up truck or van in nontraffic accident
  Pedestrian on sled injured in collision with car, pick-up truck or van in nontraffic accident
  Pedestrian on snowboard injured in collision with car, pick-up truck or van in nontraffic accident
  Pedestrian on snow-skis injured in collision with car, pick-up truck or van in nontraffic accident

● **V03.1 Pedestrian injured in collision with car, pick-up truck or van in traffic accident**

X ● **V03.10 Pedestrian on foot injured in collision with car, pick-up truck or van in traffic accident**
  Pedestrian NOS injured in collision with car, pick-up truck or van in traffic accident

X ● **V03.11 Pedestrian on roller-skates injured in collision with car, pick-up truck or van in traffic accident**

X ● **V03.12 Pedestrian on skateboard injured in collision with car, pick-up truck or van in traffic accident**

● **V03.13 Pedestrian on standing micro-mobility pedestrian conveyance injured in collision with car, pick-up or van in traffic accident**

 V03.131 Pedestrian on standing electric scooter injured in collision with car, pick-up or van in traffic accident

 V03.138 Pedestrian on other standing micro-mobility pedestrian conveyance injured in collision with car, pick-up or van in traffic accident
  Pedestrian on hoverboard injured in collision with car, pick-up or van in traffic accident
  Pedestrian on segway injured in collision with car, pick-up or van in traffic accident

X ● **V03.19 Pedestrian with other conveyance injured in collision with car, pick-up truck or van in traffic accident**
  Pedestrian with baby stroller injured in collision with car, pick-up truck or van in traffic accident
  Pedestrian in wheelchair (powered) injured in collision with car, pick-up truck or van in traffic accident
  Pedestrian in motorized mobility scooter injured in collision with car, pick-up truck or van in traffic accident
  Pedestrian on ice-skates injured in collision with car, pick-up truck or van in traffic accident
  Pedestrian on nonmotorized scooter injured in collision with car, pick-up truck or van in traffic accident
  Pedestrian on sled injured in collision with car, pick-up truck or van in traffic accident
  Pedestrian on snowboard injured in collision with car, pick-up truck or van in traffic accident
  Pedestrian on snow-skis injured in collision with car, pick-up truck or van in traffic accident

● **V03.9 Pedestrian injured in collision with car, pick-up truck or van, unspecified whether traffic or nontraffic accident**

X ● **V03.90 Pedestrian on foot injured in collision with car, pick-up truck or van, unspecified whether traffic or nontraffic accident**
  Pedestrian NOS injured in collision with car, pick-up truck or van, unspecified whether traffic or nontraffic accident

X ● **V03.91 Pedestrian on roller-skates injured in collision with car, pick-up truck or van, unspecified whether traffic or nontraffic accident**

X ● **V03.92 Pedestrian on skateboard injured in collision with car, pick-up truck or van, unspecified whether traffic or nontraffic accident**

CHAPTER 20 (V00–Y99)

● V03.93　**Pedestrian on standing micro-mobility pedestrian conveyance injured in collision with car, pick-up or van, unspecified whether traffic or nontraffic accident**

　　V03.931　**Pedestrian on standing electric scooter injured in collision with car, pick-up or van, unspecified whether traffic or nontraffic accident**

　　V03.938　**Pedestrian on other standing micro-mobility pedestrian conveyance injured in collision with car, pick-up or van, unspecified whether traffic or nontraffic accident**
　　　　　Pedestrian on hoverboard injured in collision with car, pick-up or van, unspecified whether traffic or nontraffic accident
　　　　　Pedestrian on segway injured in collision with car, pick-up or van, unspecified whether traffic or nontraffic accident

X ● V03.99　**Pedestrian with other conveyance injured in collision with car, pick-up truck or van, unspecified whether traffic or nontraffic accident**
　　　Pedestrian with baby stroller injured in collision with car, pick-up truck or van, unspecified whether traffic or nontraffic accident
　　　Pedestrian in wheelchair (powered) injured in collision with car, pick-up truck or van, unspecified whether traffic or nontraffic accident
　　　Pedestrian in motorized mobility scooter injured in collision with car, pick-up truck or van, unspecified whether traffic or nontraffic accident
　　　Pedestrian on ice-skates injured in collision with car, pick-up truck or van, unspecified whether traffic or nontraffic accident
　　　Pedestrian on nonmotorized scooter injured in collision with car, pick-up truck or van, unspecified whether traffic or nontraffic accident
　　　Pedestrian on sled injured in collision with car, pick-up truck or van in nontraffic accident
　　　Pedestrian on snowboard injured in collision with car, pick-up truck or van, unspecified whether traffic or nontraffic accident
　　　Pedestrian on snow-skis injured in collision with car, pick-up truck or van, unspecified whether traffic or nontraffic accident

● V04　**Pedestrian injured in collision with heavy transport vehicle or bus**

　　Excludes1　pedestrian injured in collision with military vehicle (V09.01, V09.21)

　　The appropriate 7th character is to be added to each code from category V04

A	initial encounter
D	subsequent encounter
S	sequela

● V04.0　**Pedestrian injured in collision with heavy transport vehicle or bus in nontraffic accident**

X ● V04.00　**Pedestrian on foot injured in collision with heavy transport vehicle or bus in nontraffic accident**
　　　Pedestrian NOS injured in collision with heavy transport vehicle or bus in nontraffic accident

X ● V04.01　**Pedestrian on roller-skates injured in collision with heavy transport vehicle or bus in nontraffic accident**

X ● V04.02　**Pedestrian on skateboard injured in collision with heavy transport vehicle or bus in nontraffic accident**

● V04.03　**Pedestrian on standing micro-mobility pedestrian conveyance injured in collision with heavy transport vehicle or bus in nontraffic accident**

　　V04.031　**Pedestrian on standing electric scooter injured in collision with heavy transport vehicle or bus in nontraffic accident**

　　V04.038　**Pedestrian on other standing micro-mobility pedestrian conveyance injured in collision with heavy transport vehicle or bus in nontraffic accident**
　　　　　Pedestrian on hoverboard injured in collision with heavy transport vehicle or bus in nontraffic accident
　　　　　Pedestrian on segway injured in collision with heavy transport vehicle or bus in nontraffic accident

X ● V04.09　**Pedestrian with other conveyance injured in collision with heavy transport vehicle or bus in nontraffic accident**
　　　Pedestrian with baby stroller injured in collision with heavy transport vehicle or bus in nontraffic accident
　　　Pedestrian in wheelchair (powered) injured in collision with heavy transport vehicle or bus in nontraffic accident
　　　Pedestrian in motorized mobility scooter injured in collision with heavy transport vehicle or bus in nontraffic accident
　　　Pedestrian on ice-skates injured in collision with heavy transport vehicle or bus in nontraffic accident
　　　Pedestrian on nonmotorized scooter injured in collision with heavy transport vehicle or bus in nontraffic accident
　　　Pedestrian on sled injured in collision with heavy transport vehicle or bus in nontraffic accident
　　　Pedestrian on snowboard injured in collision with heavy transport vehicle or bus in nontraffic accident
　　　Pedestrian on snow-skis injured in collision with heavy transport vehicle or bus in nontraffic accident

● V04.1　**Pedestrian injured in collision with heavy transport vehicle or bus in traffic accident**

X ● V04.10　**Pedestrian on foot injured in collision with heavy transport vehicle or bus in traffic accident**
　　　Pedestrian NOS injured in collision with heavy transport vehicle or bus in traffic accident

X ● V04.11　**Pedestrian on roller-skates injured in collision with heavy transport vehicle or bus in traffic accident**

X ● V04.12　**Pedestrian on skateboard injured in collision with heavy transport vehicle or bus in traffic accident**

● V04.13　**Pedestrian on standing micro-mobility pedestrian conveyance injured in collision with heavy transport vehicle or bus in traffic accident**

　　V04.131　**Pedestrian on standing electric scooter injured in collision with heavy transport vehicle or bus in traffic accident**

V04.138   **Pedestrian on other standing micro-mobility pedestrian conveyance injured in collision with heavy transport vehicle or bus in traffic accident**
> Pedestrian on hoverboard injured in collision with heavy transport vehicle or bus in traffic accident
> Pedestrian on segway injured in collision with heavy transport vehicle or bus in traffic accident

X ● **V04.19   Pedestrian with other conveyance injured in collision with heavy transport vehicle or bus in traffic accident**
> Pedestrian with baby stroller injured in collision with heavy transport vehicle or bus in traffic accident
> Pedestrian in wheelchair (powered) injured in collision with heavy transport vehicle or bus in traffic accident
> Pedestrian in motorized mobility scooter injured in collision with heavy transport vehicle or bus in traffic accident
> Pedestrian on ice-skates injured in collision with heavy transport vehicle or bus in traffic accident
> Pedestrian on nonmotorized scooter injured in collision with heavy transport vehicle or bus in traffic accident
> Pedestrian on sled injured in collision with heavy transport vehicle or bus in traffic accident
> Pedestrian on snowboard injured in collision with heavy transport vehicle or bus in traffic accident
> Pedestrian on snow-skis injured in collision with heavy transport vehicle or bus in traffic accident

● **V04.9   Pedestrian injured in collision with heavy transport vehicle or bus, unspecified whether traffic or nontraffic accident**

X ● **V04.90   Pedestrian on foot injured in collision with heavy transport vehicle or bus, unspecified whether traffic or nontraffic accident**
> Pedestrian NOS injured in collision with heavy transport vehicle or bus, unspecified whether traffic or nontraffic accident

X ● **V04.91   Pedestrian on roller-skates injured in collision with heavy transport vehicle or bus, unspecified whether traffic or nontraffic accident**

X ● **V04.92   Pedestrian on skateboard injured in collision with heavy transport vehicle or bus, unspecified whether traffic or nontraffic accident**

● **V04.93   Pedestrian on standing micro-mobility pedestrian conveyance injured in collision with heavy transport vehicle or bus, unspecified whether traffic or nontraffic accident**

V04.931   **Pedestrian on standing electric scooter injured in collision with heavy transport vehicle or bus, unspecified whether traffic or nontraffic accident**

V04.938   **Pedestrian on other standing micro-mobility pedestrian conveyance injured in collision with heavy transport vehicle or bus, unspecified whether traffic or nontraffic accident**
> Pedestrian on hoverboard injured in collision with heavy transport vehicle or bus, unspecified whether traffic or nontraffic accident
> Pedestrian on segway injured in collision with heavy transport vehicle or bus, unspecified whether traffic or nontraffic accident

X ● **V04.99   Pedestrian with other conveyance injured in collision with heavy transport vehicle or bus, unspecified whether traffic or nontraffic accident**
> Pedestrian with baby stroller injured in collision with heavy transport vehicle or bus, unspecified whether traffic or nontraffic accident
> Pedestrian in wheelchair (powered) injured in collision with heavy transport vehicle or bus, unspecified whether traffic or nontraffic accident
> Pedestrian in motorized mobility scooter injured in collision with heavy transport vehicle or bus, unspecified whether traffic or nontraffic accident
> Pedestrian on ice-skates injured in collision with heavy transport vehicle or bus, unspecified whether traffic or nontraffic accident
> Pedestrian on nonmotorized scooter injured in collision with heavy transport vehicle or bus, unspecified whether traffic or nontraffic accident
> Pedestrian on sled injured in collision with heavy transport vehicle or bus, unspecified whether traffic or nontraffic accident
> Pedestrian on snowboard injured in collision with heavy transport vehicle or bus, unspecified whether traffic or nontraffic accident
> Pedestrian on snow-skis injured in collision with heavy transport vehicle or bus, unspecified whether traffic or nontraffic accident

● **V05   Pedestrian injured in collision with railway train or railway vehicle**

The appropriate 7th character is to be added to each code from category V05

A	initial encounter
D	subsequent encounter
S	sequela

● **V05.0   Pedestrian injured in collision with railway train or railway vehicle in nontraffic accident**

X ● **V05.00   Pedestrian on foot injured in collision with railway train or railway vehicle in nontraffic accident**
> Pedestrian NOS injured in collision with railway train or railway vehicle in nontraffic accident

X ● **V05.01   Pedestrian on roller-skates injured in collision with railway train or railway vehicle in nontraffic accident**

X ● **V05.02   Pedestrian on skateboard injured in collision with railway train or railway vehicle in nontraffic accident**

● **V05.03   Pedestrian on standing micro-mobility pedestrian conveyance injured in collision with railway train or railway vehicle in nontraffic accident**

V05.031   **Pedestrian on standing electric scooter injured in collision with railway train or railway vehicle in nontraffic accident**

V05.038   **Pedestrian on other standing micro-mobility pedestrian conveyance injured in collision with railway train or railway vehicle in nontraffic accident**
> Pedestrian on hoverboard injured in collision with railway train or railway vehicle in nontraffic accident
> Pedestrian on segway injured in collision with railway train or railway vehicle in nontraffic accident

CHAPTER 20 (V00–Y99)

CHAPTER 20 (V00-Y99)

X● **V05.09** **Pedestrian with other conveyance injured in collision with railway train or railway vehicle in nontraffic accident**
Pedestrian with baby stroller injured in collision with railway train or railway vehicle in nontraffic accident
Pedestrian in wheelchair (powered) injured in collision with railway train or railway vehicle in nontraffic accident
Pedestrian in motorized mobility scooter injured in collision with railway train or railway vehicle in nontraffic accident
Pedestrian on ice-skates injured in collision with railway train or railway vehicle in nontraffic accident
Pedestrian on nonmotorized scooter injured in collision with railway train or railway vehicle in nontraffic accident
Pedestrian on sled injured in collision with railway train or railway vehicle in nontraffic accident
Pedestrian on snowboard injured in collision with railway train or railway vehicle in nontraffic accident
Pedestrian on snow-skis injured in collision with railway train or railway vehicle in nontraffic accident

● **V05.1**   **Pedestrian injured in collision with railway train or railway vehicle in traffic accident**

X● **V05.10**   **Pedestrian on foot injured in collision with railway train or railway vehicle in traffic accident**
Pedestrian NOS injured in collision with railway train or railway vehicle in traffic accident

X● **V05.11**   **Pedestrian on roller-skates injured in collision with railway train or railway vehicle in traffic accident**

X● **V05.12**   **Pedestrian on skateboard injured in collision with railway train or railway vehicle in traffic accident**

● **V05.13**   **Pedestrian on standing micro-mobility pedestrian conveyance injured in collision with railway train or railway vehicle in traffic accident**

V05.131   **Pedestrian on standing electric scooter injured in collision with railway train or railway vehicle in traffic accident**

V05.138   **Pedestrian on other standing micro-mobility pedestrian conveyance injured in collision with railway train or railway vehicle in traffic accident**
Pedestrian on hoverboard injured in collision with railway train or railway vehicle in traffic accident
Pedestrian on segway injured in collision with railway train or railway vehicle in traffic accident

X● **V05.19** **Pedestrian with other conveyance injured in collision with railway train or railway vehicle in traffic accident**
Pedestrian with baby stroller injured in collision with railway train or railway vehicle in traffic accident
Pedestrian in wheelchair (powered) injured in collision with railway train or railway vehicle in traffic accident
Pedestrian in motorized mobility scooter injured in collision with railway train or railway vehicle in traffic accident
Pedestrian on ice-skates injured in collision with railway train or railway vehicle in traffic accident
Pedestrian on nonmotorized scooter injured in collision with railway train or railway vehicle in traffic accident
Pedestrian on sled injured in collision with railway train or railway vehicle in traffic accident
Pedestrian on snowboard injured in collision with railway train or railway vehicle in traffic accident
Pedestrian on snow-skis injured in collision with railway train or railway vehicle in traffic accident

● **V05.9**   **Pedestrian injured in collision with railway train or railway vehicle, unspecified whether traffic or nontraffic accident**

X● **V05.90**   **Pedestrian on foot injured in collision with railway train or railway vehicle, unspecified whether traffic or nontraffic accident**
Pedestrian NOS injured in collision with railway train or railway vehicle, unspecified whether traffic or nontraffic accident

X● **V05.91**   **Pedestrian on roller-skates injured in collision with railway train or railway vehicle, unspecified whether traffic or nontraffic accident**

X● **V05.92**   **Pedestrian on skateboard injured in collision with railway train or railway vehicle, unspecified whether traffic or nontraffic accident**

● **V05.93**   **Pedestrian on standing micro-mobility pedestrian conveyance injured in collision with railway train or railway vehicle, unspecified whether traffic or nontraffic accident**

V05.931   **Pedestrian on standing electric scooter injured in collision with railway train or railway vehicle, unspecified whether traffic or nontraffic accident**

V05.938   **Pedestrian on other standing micro-mobility pedestrian conveyance injured in collision with railway train or railway vehicle, unspecified whether traffic or nontraffic accident**
Pedestrian on hoverboard injured in collision with railway train or railway vehicle, unspecified whether traffic or nontraffic accident
Pedestrian on segway injured in collision with railway train or railway vehicle, unspecified whether traffic or nontraffic accident

▶ New   ➡ Revised   ~~deleted~~ Deleted   Excludes 1   Excludes 2   Includes   Use additional   Code first   Code also   Key words
OGCR Official Guidelines   X Assign placeholder X   ● Use Additional Character(s)   ▶ Manifestation Code   🏵 Hierarchical Condition Category   **Coding Clinic**

X⬤ **V05.99 Pedestrian with** other **conveyance injured in collision with railway train or railway vehicle, unspecified whether traffic or nontraffic accident**

    Pedestrian with baby stroller injured in collision with railway train or railway vehicle, unspecified whether traffic or nontraffic

    Pedestrian in wheelchair (powered) injured in collision with railway train or railway vehicle, unspecified whether traffic or nontraffic

    Pedestrian in motorized mobility scooter injured in collision with railway train or railway vehicle, unspecified whether traffic or nontraffic

    Pedestrian on ice-skates injured in collision with railway train or railway vehicle, unspecified whether traffic or nontraffic

    Pedestrian on nonmotorized scooter injured in collision with railway train or railway vehicle, unspecified whether traffic or nontraffic

    Pedestrian on sled injured in collision with railway train or railway vehicle, unspecified whether traffic or nontraffic

    Pedestrian on snowboard injured in collision with railway train or railway vehicle, unspecified whether traffic or nontraffic

    Pedestrian on snow-skis injured in collision with railway train or railway vehicle, unspecified whether traffic or nontraffic

⬤ **V06 Pedestrian injured in collision with other nonmotor vehicle**

    Includes   collision with animal-drawn vehicle, animal being ridden, nonpowered streetcar

    Excludes1   pedestrian injured in collision with pedestrian conveyance (V00.0-)

The appropriate 7th character is to be added to each code from category V06

    A   initial encounter
    D   subsequent encounter
    S   sequela

⬤ **V06.0 Pedestrian injured in collision with other nonmotor vehicle in** nontraffic accident

X⬤ **V06.00 Pedestrian on** foot **injured in collision with other nonmotor vehicle in nontraffic accident**

    Pedestrian NOS injured in collision with other nonmotor vehicle in nontraffic accident

X⬤ **V06.01 Pedestrian on** roller-skates **injured in collision with other nonmotor vehicle in nontraffic accident**

X⬤ **V06.02 Pedestrian on** skateboard **injured in collision with other nonmotor vehicle in nontraffic accident**

⬤ **V06.03 Pedestrian on standing micro-mobility pedestrian conveyance injured in collision with other nonmotor vehicle in nontraffic accident**

    V06.031 Pedestrian on standing electric scooter injured in collision with other nonmotor vehicle in nontraffic accident

    V06.038 Pedestrian on other standing micro-mobility pedestrian conveyance injured in collision with other nonmotor vehicle in nontraffic accident

        Pedestrian on hoverboard injured in collision with other nonmotor vehicle in nontraffic accident

        Pedestrian on segway injured in collision with other nonmotor vehicle in nontraffic accident

X⬤ **V06.09 Pedestrian with** other **conveyance injured in collision with other nonmotor vehicle in nontraffic accident**

    Pedestrian with baby stroller injured in collision with other nonmotor vehicle in nontraffic accident

    Pedestrian in wheelchair (powered) injured in collision with other nonmotor vehicle in nontraffic accident

    Pedestrian in motorized mobility scooter injured in collision with other nonmotor vehicle in nontraffic accident

    Pedestrian on ice-skates injured in collision with other nonmotor vehicle in nontraffic accident

    Pedestrian on nonmotorized scooter injured in collision with other nonmotor vehicle in nontraffic accident

    Pedestrian on sled injured in collision with other nonmotor vehicle in nontraffic accident

    Pedestrian on snowboard injured in collision with other nonmotor vehicle in nontraffic accident

    Pedestrian on snow-skis injured in collision with other nonmotor vehicle in nontraffic accident

⬤ **V06.1 Pedestrian injured in collision with other nonmotor vehicle in** traffic accident

X⬤ **V06.10 Pedestrian on** foot **injured in collision with other nonmotor vehicle in traffic accident**

    Pedestrian NOS injured in collision with other nonmotor vehicle in traffic accident

X⬤ **V06.11 Pedestrian on** roller-skates **injured in collision with other nonmotor vehicle in traffic accident**

X⬤ **V06.12 Pedestrian on** skateboard **injured in collision with other nonmotor vehicle in traffic accident**

⬤ **V06.13 Pedestrian on standing micro-mobility pedestrian conveyance injured in collision with other nonmotor vehicle in traffic accident**

    V06.131 Pedestrian on standing electric scooter injured in collision with other nonmotor vehicle in traffic accident

    V06.138 Pedestrian on other standing micro-mobility pedestrian conveyance injured in collision with other nonmotor vehicle in traffic accident

        Pedestrian on hoverboard injured in collision with other nonmotor vehicle in traffic accident

        Pedestrian on segway injured in collision with other nonmotor vehicle in traffic accident

X⬤ **V06.19 Pedestrian with** other **conveyance injured in collision with other nonmotor vehicle in traffic accident**

    Pedestrian with baby stroller injured in collision with other nonmotor vehicle in nontraffic accident

    Pedestrian in wheelchair (powered) injured in collision with other nonmotor vehicle in traffic accident

    Pedestrian in motorized mobility scooter injured in collision with other nonmotor vehicle in traffic accident

    Pedestrian on ice-skates injured in collision with other nonmotor vehicle in traffic accident

    Pedestrian on nonmotorized scooter injured in collision with other nonmotor vehicle in traffic accident

    Pedestrian on sled injured in collision with other nonmotor vehicle in traffic accident

    Pedestrian on snowboard injured in collision with other nonmotor vehicle in traffic accident

    Pedestrian on snow-skis injured in collision with other nonmotor vehicle in traffic accident

CHAPTER 20 (V00-Y99)

● **V06.9** **Pedestrian injured in collision with other nonmotor vehicle, unspecified whether traffic or nontraffic accident**

X● **V06.90** **Pedestrian on foot injured in collision with other nonmotor vehicle, unspecified whether traffic or nontraffic accident**
Pedestrian NOS injured in collision with other nonmotor vehicle, unspecified whether traffic or nontraffic accident

X● **V06.91** **Pedestrian on roller-skates injured in collision with other nonmotor vehicle, unspecified whether traffic or nontraffic accident**

X● **V06.92** **Pedestrian on skateboard injured in collision with other nonmotor vehicle, unspecified whether traffic or nontraffic accident**

● **V06.93** **Pedestrian on standing micro-mobility pedestrian conveyance injured in collision with other nonmotor vehicle, unspecified whether traffic or nontraffic accident**

V06.931 **Pedestrian on standing electric scooter injured in collision with other nonmotor vehicle, unspecified whether traffic or nontraffic accident**

V06.938 **Pedestrian on other standing micro-mobility pedestrian conveyance injured in collision with other nonmotor vehicle, unspecified whether traffic or nontraffic accident**
Pedestrian on hoverboard injured in collision with other nonmotor vehicle, unspecified whether traffic or nontraffic accident
Pedestrian on segway injured in collision with other nonmotor vehicle, unspecified whether traffic or nontraffic accident

X● **V06.99** **Pedestrian with other conveyance injured in collision with other nonmotor vehicle, unspecified whether traffic or nontraffic accident**
Pedestrian with baby stroller injured in collision with other nonmotor vehicle, unspecified whether traffic or nontraffic accident
Pedestrian in wheelchair (powered) injured in collision with other nonmotor vehicle, unspecified whether traffic or nontraffic accident
Pedestrian in motorized mobility scooter injured in collision with other nonmotor vehicle, unspecified whether traffic or nontraffic accident
Pedestrian on ice-skates injured in collision with other nonmotor vehicle, unspecified whether traffic or nontraffic accident
Pedestrian on nonmotorized scooter injured in collision with other nonmotor vehicle, unspecified whether traffic or nontraffic accident
Pedestrian on sled injured in collision with other nonmotor vehicle, unspecified whether traffic or nontraffic accident
Pedestrian on snowboard injured in collision with other nonmotor vehicle, unspecified whether traffic or nontraffic accident
Pedestrian on snow-skis injured in collision with other nonmotor vehicle, unspecified whether traffic or nontraffic accident

● **V09** **Pedestrian injured in other and unspecified transport accidents**
The appropriate 7th character is to be added to each code from category V09

A	initial encounter
D	subsequent encounter
S	sequela

● **V09.0** **Pedestrian injured in nontraffic accident involving other and unspecified motor vehicles**

X● **V09.00** **Pedestrian injured in nontraffic accident involving unspecified motor vehicles**

X● **V09.01** **Pedestrian injured in nontraffic accident involving military vehicle**

X● **V09.09** **Pedestrian injured in nontraffic accident involving other motor vehicles**
Pedestrian injured in nontraffic accident by special vehicle

X● **V09.1** **Pedestrian injured in unspecified nontraffic accident**

● **V09.2** **Pedestrian injured in traffic accident involving other and unspecified motor vehicles**

X● **V09.20** **Pedestrian injured in traffic accident involving unspecified motor vehicles**

X● **V09.21** **Pedestrian injured in traffic accident involving military vehicle**

X● **V09.29** **Pedestrian injured in traffic accident involving other motor vehicles**

X● **V09.3** **Pedestrian injured in unspecified traffic accident**

X● **V09.9** **Pedestrian injured in unspecified transport accident**

PEDAL CYCLE RIDER INJURED IN TRANSPORT ACCIDENT (V10-V19)

Includes   any non-motorized vehicle, excluding an animal-drawn vehicle, or a sidecar or trailer attached to the pedal cycle

Excludes2   rupture of pedal cycle tire (W37.0)

● **V10** **Pedal cycle rider injured in collision with pedestrian or animal**
Excludes1   pedal cycle rider collision with animal-drawn vehicle or animal being ridden (V16.-)
The appropriate 7th character is to be added to each code from category V10

A	initial encounter
D	subsequent encounter
S	sequela

X● **V10.0** **Pedal cycle driver injured in collision with pedestrian or animal in nontraffic accident**

X● **V10.1** **Pedal cycle passenger injured in collision with pedestrian or animal in nontraffic accident**

X● **V10.2** **Unspecified pedal cyclist injured in collision with pedestrian or animal in nontraffic accident**

X● **V10.3** **Person boarding or alighting a pedal cycle injured in collision with pedestrian or animal**

X● **V10.4** **Pedal cycle driver injured in collision with pedestrian or animal in traffic accident**

X● **V10.5** **Pedal cycle passenger injured in collision with pedestrian or animal in traffic accident**

X● **V10.9** **Unspecified pedal cyclist injured in collision with pedestrian or animal in traffic accident**

▶ New   ➡ Revised   ~~deleted~~ Deleted   Excludes 1   Excludes 2   Includes   Use additional   Code first   Code also   Key words
OGCR Official Guidelines   X Assign placeholder X   ● Use Additional Character(s)   ▶ Manifestation Code   Ⓗ Hierarchical Condition Category   **Coding Clinic**

● **V11** **Pedal cycle rider injured in collision with other pedal cycle**

The appropriate 7th character is to be added to each code from category V11

A	initial encounter
D	subsequent encounter
S	sequela

X● **V11.0** **Pedal cycle driver** injured in collision with other pedal cycle in **nontraffic accident**

X● **V11.1** **Pedal cycle passenger** injured in collision with other pedal cycle in **nontraffic accident**

X● **V11.2** **Unspecified pedal cyclist** injured in collision with other pedal cycle in **nontraffic accident**

X● **V11.3** **Person boarding or alighting** a pedal cycle injured in collision with other pedal cycle

X● **V11.4** **Pedal cycle driver** injured in collision with other pedal cycle in **traffic accident**

X● **V11.5** **Pedal cycle passenger** injured in collision with other pedal cycle in **traffic accident**

X● **V11.9** **Unspecified pedal cyclist** injured in collision with other pedal cycle in **traffic accident**

● **V12** **Pedal cycle rider injured in collision with two- or three-wheeled motor vehicle**

The appropriate 7th character is to be added to each code from category V12

A	initial encounter
D	subsequent encounter
S	sequela

X● **V12.0** **Pedal cycle driver** injured in collision with two- or three-wheeled motor vehicle in **nontraffic accident**

X● **V12.1** **Pedal cycle passenger** injured in collision with two- or three-wheeled motor vehicle in **nontraffic accident**

X● **V12.2** **Unspecified pedal cyclist** injured in collision with two- or three-wheeled motor vehicle in **nontraffic accident**

X● **V12.3** **Person boarding or alighting** a pedal cycle injured in collision with two- or three-wheeled motor vehicle

X● **V12.4** **Pedal cycle driver** injured in collision with two- or three-wheeled motor vehicle in **traffic accident**

X● **V12.5** **Pedal cycle passenger** injured in collision with two- or three-wheeled motor vehicle in **traffic accident**

X● **V12.9** **Unspecified pedal cyclist** injured in collision with two- or three-wheeled motor vehicle in **traffic accident**

● **V13** **Pedal cycle rider injured in collision with car, pick-up truck or van**

The appropriate 7th character is to be added to each code from category V13

A	initial encounter
D	subsequent encounter
S	sequela

X● **V13.0** **Pedal cycle driver** injured in collision with car, pick-up truck or van in **nontraffic accident**

X● **V13.1** **Pedal cycle passenger** injured in collision with car, pick-up truck or van in **nontraffic accident**

X● **V13.2** **Unspecified pedal cyclist** injured in collision with car, pick-up truck or van in **nontraffic accident**

X● **V13.3** **Person boarding or alighting** a pedal cycle injured in collision with car, pick-up truck or van

X● **V13.4** **Pedal cycle driver** injured in collision with car, pick-up truck or van in **traffic accident**

X● **V13.5** **Pedal cycle passenger** injured in collision with car, pick-up truck or van in **traffic accident**

X● **V13.9** **Unspecified pedal cyclist** injured in collision with car, pick-up truck or van in **traffic accident**

● **V14** **Pedal cycle rider injured in collision with heavy transport vehicle or bus**

Excludes1 pedal cycle rider injured in collision with military vehicle (V19.81)

The appropriate 7th character is to be added to each code from category V14

A	initial encounter
D	subsequent encounter
S	sequela

X● **V14.0** **Pedal cycle driver** injured in collision with heavy transport vehicle or bus in **nontraffic accident**

X● **V14.1** **Pedal cycle passenger** injured in collision with heavy transport vehicle or bus in **nontraffic accident**

X● **V14.2** **Unspecified pedal cyclist** injured in collision with heavy transport vehicle or bus in **nontraffic accident**

X● **V14.3** **Person boarding or alighting** a pedal cycle injured in collision with heavy transport vehicle or bus

X● **V14.4** **Pedal cycle driver** injured in collision with heavy transport vehicle or bus in **traffic accident**

X● **V14.5** **Pedal cycle passenger** injured in collision with heavy transport vehicle or bus in **traffic accident**

X● **V14.9** **Unspecified pedal cyclist** injured in collision with heavy transport vehicle or bus in **traffic accident**

● **V15** **Pedal cycle rider injured in collision with railway train or railway vehicle**

The appropriate 7th character is to be added to each code from category V15

A	initial encounter
D	subsequent encounter
S	sequela

X● **V15.0** **Pedal cycle driver** injured in collision with railway train or railway vehicle in **nontraffic accident**

X● **V15.1** **Pedal cycle passenger** injured in collision with railway train or railway vehicle in **nontraffic accident**

X● **V15.2** **Unspecified pedal cyclist** injured in collision with railway train or railway vehicle in **nontraffic accident**

X● **V15.3** **Person boarding or alighting** a pedal cycle injured in collision with railway train or railway vehicle

X● **V15.4** **Pedal cycle driver** injured in collision with railway train or railway vehicle in **traffic accident**

X● **V15.5** **Pedal cycle passenger** injured in collision with railway train or railway vehicle in **traffic accident**

X● **V15.9** **Unspecified pedal cyclist** injured in collision with railway train or railway vehicle in **traffic accident**

● **V16** **Pedal cycle rider injured in collision with other nonmotor vehicle**

Includes collision with animal-drawn vehicle, animal being ridden, streetcar

The appropriate 7th character is to be added to each code from category V16

A	initial encounter
D	subsequent encounter
S	sequela

X● **V16.0** **Pedal cycle driver** injured in collision with other nonmotor vehicle in **nontraffic accident**

X● **V16.1** **Pedal cycle passenger** injured in collision with other nonmotor vehicle in **nontraffic accident**

X● **V16.2** **Unspecified pedal cyclist** injured in collision with other nonmotor vehicle in **nontraffic accident**

X● **V16.3** **Person boarding or alighting** a pedal cycle injured in collision with other nonmotor vehicle in nontraffic accident

X● **V16.4** **Pedal cycle driver** injured in collision with other nonmotor vehicle in **traffic accident**

CHAPTER 20 (V00-Y99)

X ● **V16.5**   Pedal cycle passenger injured in collision with other nonmotor vehicle in traffic accident

X ● **V16.9**   Unspecified pedal cyclist injured in collision with other nonmotor vehicle in traffic accident

● **V17**   Pedal cycle rider injured in collision with fixed or stationary object

> The appropriate 7th character is to be added to each code from category V17

> | A | initial encounter |
> |---|---|
> | D | subsequent encounter |
> | S | sequela |

X ● **V17.0**   Pedal cycle driver injured in collision with fixed or stationary object in nontraffic accident

X ● **V17.1**   Pedal cycle passenger injured in collision with fixed or stationary object in nontraffic accident

X ● **V17.2**   Unspecified pedal cyclist injured in collision with fixed or stationary object in nontraffic accident

X ● **V17.3**   Person boarding or alighting a pedal cycle injured in collision with fixed or stationary object

X ● **V17.4**   Pedal cycle driver injured in collision with fixed or stationary object in traffic accident

X ● **V17.5**   Pedal cycle passenger injured in collision with fixed or stationary object in traffic accident

X ● **V17.9**   Unspecified pedal cyclist injured in collision with fixed or stationary object in traffic accident

● **V18**   Pedal cycle rider injured in noncollision transport accident

> **Includes**   fall or thrown from pedal cycle (without antecedent collision)
> overturning pedal cycle NOS
> overturning pedal cycle without collision

> The appropriate 7th character is to be added to each code from category V18

> | A | initial encounter |
> |---|---|
> | D | subsequent encounter |
> | S | sequela |

X ● **V18.0**   Pedal cycle driver injured in noncollision transport accident in nontraffic accident

X ● **V18.1**   Pedal cycle passenger injured in noncollision transport accident in nontraffic accident

X ● **V18.2**   Unspecified pedal cyclist injured in noncollision transport accident in nontraffic accident

X ● **V18.3**   Person boarding or alighting a pedal cycle injured in noncollision transport accident

X ● **V18.4**   Pedal cycle driver injured in noncollision transport accident in traffic accident

X ● **V18.5**   Pedal cycle passenger injured in noncollision transport accident in traffic accident

X ● **V18.9**   Unspecified pedal cyclist injured in noncollision transport accident in traffic accident

● **V19**   Pedal cycle rider injured in other and unspecified transport accidents

> The appropriate 7th character is to be added to each code from category V19

> | A | initial encounter |
> |---|---|
> | D | subsequent encounter |
> | S | sequela |

● **V19.0**   Pedal cycle driver injured in collision with other and unspecified motor vehicles in nontraffic accident

X ● **V19.00**   Pedal cycle driver injured in collision with unspecified motor vehicles in nontraffic accident

X ● **V19.09**   Pedal cycle driver injured in collision with other motor vehicles in nontraffic accident

● **V19.1**   Pedal cycle passenger injured in collision with other and unspecified motor vehicles in nontraffic accident

X ● **V19.10**   Pedal cycle passenger injured in collision with unspecified motor vehicles in nontraffic accident

X ● **V19.19**   Pedal cycle passenger injured in collision with other motor vehicles in nontraffic accident

● **V19.2**   Unspecified pedal cyclist injured in collision with other and unspecified motor vehicles in nontraffic accident

X ● **V19.20**   Unspecified pedal cyclist injured in collision with unspecified motor vehicles in nontraffic accident

> Pedal cycle collision NOS, nontraffic

X ● **V19.29**   Unspecified pedal cyclist injured in collision with other motor vehicles in nontraffic accident

X ● **V19.3**   Pedal cyclist (driver) (passenger) injured in unspecified nontraffic accident

> Pedal cycle accident NOS, nontraffic
> Pedal cyclist injured in nontraffic accident NOS

● **V19.4**   Pedal cycle driver injured in collision with other and unspecified motor vehicles in traffic accident

X ● **V19.40**   Pedal cycle driver injured in collision with unspecified motor vehicles in traffic accident

X ● **V19.49**   Pedal cycle driver injured in collision with other motor vehicles in traffic accident

● **V19.5**   Pedal cycle passenger injured in collision with other and unspecified motor vehicles in traffic accident

X ● **V19.50**   Pedal cycle passenger injured in collision with unspecified motor vehicles in traffic accident

X ● **V19.59**   Pedal cycle passenger injured in collision with other motor vehicles in traffic accident

● **V19.6**   Unspecified pedal cyclist injured in collision with other and unspecified motor vehicles in traffic accident

X ● **V19.60**   Unspecified pedal cyclist injured in collision with unspecified motor vehicles in traffic accident

> Pedal cycle collision NOS (traffic)

X ● **V19.69**   Unspecified pedal cyclist injured in collision with other motor vehicles in traffic accident

● **V19.8**   Pedal cyclist (driver) (passenger) injured in other specified transport accidents

X ● **V19.81**   Pedal cyclist (driver) (passenger) injured in transport accident with military vehicle

X ● **V19.88**   Pedal cyclist (driver) (passenger) injured in other specified transport accidents

X ● **V19.9**   Pedal cyclist (driver) (passenger) injured in unspecified traffic accident

> Pedal cycle accident NOS

MOTORCYCLE RIDER INJURED IN TRANSPORT ACCIDENT (V20-V29)

> **Includes**   electric bicycle
> e-bike
> e-bicycle
> moped motorcycle with sidecar motorized bicycle
> motor scooter

> **Excludes1**   three-wheeled motor vehicle (V30-V39)

● **V20**   Motorcycle rider injured in collision with pedestrian or animal

> **Excludes1**   motorcycle rider collision with animal-drawn vehicle or animal being ridden (V26.-)

> The appropriate 7th character is to be added to each code from category V20

> | A | initial encounter |
> |---|---|
> | D | subsequent encounter |
> | S | sequela |

X ● **V20.0**   Motorcycle driver injured in collision with pedestrian or animal in nontraffic accident

X ● **V20.01**   Electric (assisted) bicycle driver injured in collision with pedestrian or animal in nontraffic accident

X ● **V20.09**   Other motorcycle driver injured in collision with pedestrian or animal in nontraffic accident

X● **V20.1** Motorcycle passenger injured in collision with pedestrian or animal in nontraffic accident

X● **V20.11** Electric (assisted) bicycle passenger injured in collision with pedestrian or animal in nontraffic accident

X● **V20.19** Other motorcycle passenger injured in collision with pedestrian or animal in nontraffic accident

X● **V20.2** Unspecified motorcycle rider injured in collision with pedestrian or animal in nontraffic accident

X● **V20.21** Unspecified electric (assisted) bicycle rider injured in collision with pedestrian or animal in nontraffic accident

X● **V20.29** Unspecified rider of other motorcycle injured in collision with pedestrian or animal in nontraffic accident

X● **V20.3** Person boarding or alighting a motorcycle injured in collision with pedestrian or animal

X● **V20.31** Person boarding or alighting an electric (assisted) bicycle injured in collision with pedestrian or animal

X● **V20.39** Person boarding or alighting other motorcycle injured in collision with pedestrian or animal

X● **V20.4** Motorcycle driver injured in collision with pedestrian or animal in traffic accident

X● **V20.41** Electric (assisted) bicycle driver injured in collision with pedestrian or animal in traffic accident

X● **V20.49** Other motorcycle driver injured in collision with pedestrian or animal in traffic accident

X● **V20.5** Motorcycle passenger injured in collision with pedestrian or animal in traffic accident

X● **V20.51** Electric (assisted) bicycle passenger injured in collision with pedestrian or animal in traffic accident

X● **V20.59** Other motorcycle passenger injured in collision with pedestrian or animal in traffic accident

X● **V20.9** Unspecified motorcycle rider injured in collision with pedestrian or animal in traffic accident

X● **V20.91** Unspecified electric (assisted) bicycle rider injured in collision with pedestrian or animal in traffic accident

X● **V20.99** Unspecified rider of other motorcycle injured in collision with pedestrian or animal in traffic accident

● **V21** Motorcycle rider injured in collision with pedal cycle

The appropriate 7th character is to be added to each code from category V21

A	initial encounter
D	subsequent encounter
S	sequela

X● **V21.0** Motorcycle driver injured in collision with pedal cycle in nontraffic accident

X● **V21.01** Electric (assisted) bicycle driver injured in collision with pedal cycle in nontraffic accident

X● **V21.09** Other motorcycle driver injured in collision with pedal cycle in nontraffic accident

X● **V21.1** Motorcycle passenger injured in collision with pedal cycle in nontraffic accident

X● **V21.11** Electric (assisted) bicycle passenger injured in collision with pedal cycle in nontraffic accident

X● **V21.19** Other motorcycle passenger injured in collision with pedal cycle in nontraffic accident

X● **V21.2** Unspecified motorcycle rider injured in collision with pedal cycle in nontraffic accident

X● **V21.21** Unspecified electric (assisted) bicycle rider injured in collision with pedal cycle in nontraffic accident

X● **V21.29** Unspecified rider of other motorcycle injured in collision with pedal cycle in nontraffic accident

X● **V21.3** Person boarding or alighting a motorcycle injured in collision with pedal cycle

X● **V21.31** Person boarding or alighting an electric (assisted) bicycle injured in collision with pedal cycle

X● **V21.39** Person boarding or alighting other motorcycle injured in collision with pedal cycle

X● **V21.4** Motorcycle driver injured in collision with pedal cycle in traffic accident

X● **V21.41** Electric (assisted) bicycle driver injured in collision with pedal cycle in traffic accident

X● **V21.49** Other motorcycle driver injured in collision with pedal cycle in traffic accident

X● **V21.5** Motorcycle passenger injured in collision with pedal cycle in traffic accident

X● **V21.51** Electric (assisted) bicycle passenger injured in collision with pedal cycle in traffic accident

X● **V21.59** Other motorcycle passenger injured in collision with pedal cycle in traffic accident

X● **V21.9** Unspecified motorcycle rider injured in collision with pedal cycle in traffic accident

X● **V21.91** Unspecified electric (assisted) bicycle rider injured in collision with pedal cycle in traffic accident

X● **V21.99** Unspecified rider of other motorcycle injured in collision with pedal cycle in traffic accident

● **V22** Motorcycle rider injured in collision with two- or three-wheeled motor vehicle

The appropriate 7th character is to be added to each code from category V22

A	initial encounter
D	subsequent encounter
S	sequela

X● **V22.0** Motorcycle driver injured in collision with two- or three-wheeled motor vehicle in nontraffic accident

X● **V22.01** Electric (assisted) bicycle driver injured in collision with two- or three-wheeled motor vehicle in nontraffic accident

X● **V22.09** Other motorcycle driver injured in collision with two- or three-wheeled motor vehicle in nontraffic accident

X● **V22.1** Motorcycle passenger injured in collision with two- or three-wheeled motor vehicle in nontraffic accident

X● **V22.11** Electric (assisted) bicycle passenger injured in collision with two- or three-wheeled motor vehicle in nontraffic accident

X● **V22.19** Other motorcycle passenger injured in collision with two- or three-wheeled motor vehicle in nontraffic accident

X● **V22.2** Unspecified motorcycle rider injured in collision with two- or three-wheeled motor vehicle in nontraffic accident

X● **V22.21** Unspecified electric (assisted) bicycle rider injured in collision with two- or three-wheeled motor vehicle in nontraffic accident

X● **V22.29** Unspecified rider of other motorcycle injured in collision with two- or three-wheeled motor vehicle in nontraffic accident

X● **V22.3** Person boarding or alighting a motorcycle injured in collision with two- or three-wheeled motor vehicle

X● **V22.31** Person boarding or alighting an electric (assisted) bicycle injured in collision with two- or three-wheeled motor vehicle

X● **V22.39** Person boarding or alighting other motorcycle injured in collision with two- or three-wheeled motor vehicle

X● **V22.4** Motorcycle driver injured in collision with two- or three-wheeled motor vehicle in traffic accident

X● **V22.41** Electric (assisted) bicycle driver injured in collision with two- or three-wheeled motor vehicle in traffic accident

X● **V22.49** Other motorcycle driver injured in collision with two- or three-wheeled motor vehicle in traffic accident

X● **V22.5** Motorcycle passenger injured in collision with two- or three-wheeled motor vehicle in traffic accident

X● **V22.51** Electric (assisted) bicycle passenger injured in collision with two- or three-wheeled motor vehicle in traffic accident

X● **V22.59** Other motorcycle passenger injured in collision with two- or three-wheeled motor vehicle in traffic accident

X● **V22.9** Unspecified motorcycle rider injured in collision with two- or three-wheeled motor vehicle in traffic accident

X● **V22.91** Unspecified electric (assisted) bicycle rider injured in collision with two- or three-wheeled motor vehicle in traffic accident

X● **V22.99** Unspecified rider of other motorcycle injured in collision with two- or three-wheeled motor vehicle in traffic accident

● **V23** Motorcycle rider injured in collision with car, pick-up truck or van

The appropriate 7th character is to be added to each code from category V23

A	initial encounter
D	subsequent encounter
S	sequela

X● **V23.0** Motorcycle driver injured in collision with car, pick-up truck or van in nontraffic accident

X● **V23.01** Electric (assisted) bicycle driver injured in collision with car, pick-up truck or van in nontraffic accident

X● **V23.09** Other motorcycle driver injured in collision with car, pick-up truck or van in nontraffic accident

X● **V23.1** Motorcycle passenger injured in collision with car, pick-up truck or van in nontraffic accident

X● **V23.11** Electric (assisted) bicycle passenger injured in collision with car, pick-up truck or van in nontraffic accident

X● **V23.19** Other motorcycle passenger injured in collision with car, pick-up truck or van in nontraffic accident

X● **V23.2** Unspecified motorcycle rider injured in collision with car, pick-up truck or van in nontraffic accident

X● **V23.21** Unspecified electric (assisted) bicycle rider injured in collision with car, pick-up truck or van in nontraffic accident

X● **V23.29** Unspecified rider of other motorcycle injured in collision with car, pick-up truck or van in nontraffic accident

X● **V23.3** Person boarding or alighting a motorcycle injured in collision with car, pick-up truck or van

X● **V23.31** Person boarding or alighting an electric (assisted) bicycle injured in collision with car, pick-up truck or van

X● **V23.39** Person boarding or alighting other motorcycle injured in collision with car, pick-up truck or van

X● **V23.4** Motorcycle driver injured in collision with car, pick-up truck or van in traffic accident

X● **V23.41** Electric (assisted) bicycle driver injured in collision with car, pick-up truck or van in traffic accident

X● **V23.49** Other motorcycle driver injured in collision with car, pick-up truck or van in traffic accident

X● **V23.5** Motorcycle passenger injured in collision with car, pick-up truck or van in traffic accident

X● **V23.51** Electric (assisted) bicycle passenger injured in collision with car, pick-up truck or van in traffic accident

X● **V23.59** Other motorcycle passenger injured in collision with car, pick-up truck or van in traffic accident

X● **V23.9** Unspecified motorcycle rider injured in collision with car, pick-up truck or van in traffic accident

X● **V23.91** Unspecified electric (assisted) bicycle rider injured in collision with car, pick-up truck or van in traffic accident

X● **V23.99** Unspecified rider of other motorcycle injured in collision with car, pick-up truck or van in traffic accident

● **V24** Motorcycle rider injured in collision with heavy transport vehicle or bus

Excludes1 motorcycle rider injured in collision with military vehicle (V29.818)

The appropriate 7th character is to be added to each code from category V24

A	initial encounter
D	subsequent encounter
S	sequela

X● **V24.0** Motorcycle driver injured in collision with heavy transport vehicle or bus in nontraffic accident

X● **V24.01** Electric (assisted) bicycle driver injured in collision with heavy transport vehicle or bus in nontraffic accident

X● **V24.09** Other motorcycle driver injured in collision with heavy transport vehicle or bus in nontraffic accident

X● **V24.1** Motorcycle passenger injured in collision with heavy transport vehicle or bus in nontraffic accident

X● **V24.11** Electric (assisted) bicycle passenger injured in collision with heavy transport vehicle or bus in nontraffic accident

X● **V24.19** Other motorcycle passenger injured in collision with heavy transport vehicle or bus in nontraffic accident

X● **V24.2** Unspecified motorcycle rider injured in collision with heavy transport vehicle or bus in nontraffic accident

X● **V24.21** Unspecified electric (assisted) bicycle rider injured in collision with heavy transport vehicle or bus in nontraffic accident

X● **V24.29** Unspecified rider of other motorcycle injured in collision with heavy transport vehicle or bus in nontraffic accident

X● **V24.3** Person boarding or alighting a motorcycle injured in collision with heavy transport vehicle or bus

X● **V24.31** Person boarding or alighting an electric (assisted) bicycle injured in collision with heavy transport vehicle or bus

X● **V24.39** Person boarding or alighting other motorcycle injured in collision with heavy transport vehicle or bus

X● **V24.4** Motorcycle driver injured in collision with heavy transport vehicle or bus in traffic accident

X● **V24.41** Electric (assisted) bicycle driver injured in collision with heavy transport vehicle or bus in traffic accident

X● **V24.49** Other motorcycle driver injured in collision with heavy transport vehicle or bus in traffic accident

X● **V24.5** Motorcycle passenger injured in collision with heavy transport vehicle or bus in traffic accident

X● **V24.51** Electric (assisted) bicycle passenger injured in collision with heavy transport vehicle or bus in traffic accident

X● **V24.59** Other motorcycle passenger injured in collision with heavy transport vehicle or bus in traffic accident

X● **V24.9** **Unspecified** motorcycle rider injured in collision with heavy transport vehicle or bus in traffic accident

    X● **V24.91** Unspecified electric (assisted) bicycle rider injured in collision with heavy transport vehicle or bus in traffic accident

    X● **V24.99** Unspecified rider of other motorcycle injured in collision with heavy transport vehicle or bus in traffic accident

● **V25** Motorcycle rider injured in collision with railway train or railway vehicle

    The appropriate 7th character is to be added to each code from category V25

> A   initial encounter
> D   subsequent encounter
> S   sequela

X● **V25.0** Motorcycle **driver** injured in collision with railway train or railway vehicle in **nontraffic accident**

    X● **V25.01** Electric (assisted) bicycle driver injured in collision with railway train or railway vehicle in nontraffic accident

    X● **V25.09** Other motorcycle driver injured in collision with railway train or railway vehicle in nontraffic accident

X● **V25.1** Motorcycle **passenger** injured in collision with railway train or railway vehicle in **nontraffic accident**

    X● **V25.11** Electric (assisted) bicycle passenger injured in collision with railway train or railway vehicle in nontraffic accident

    X● **V25.19** Other motorcycle passenger injured in collision with railway train or railway vehicle in nontraffic accident

X● **V25.2** **Unspecified** motorcycle rider injured in collision with railway train or railway vehicle in **nontraffic accident**

    X● **V25.21** Unspecified electric (assisted) bicycle rider injured in collision with railway train or railway vehicle in nontraffic accident

    X● **V25.29** Unspecified rider of other motorcycle injured in collision with railway train or railway vehicle in nontraffic accident

X● **V25.3** Person **boarding or alighting** a motorcycle injured in collision with railway train or railway vehicle

    X● **V25.31** Person boarding or alighting an electric (assisted) bicycle injured in collision with railway train or railway vehicle

    X● **V25.39** Person boarding or alighting other motorcycle injured in collision with railway train or railway vehicle

X● **V25.4** Motorcycle **driver** injured in collision with railway train or railway vehicle in **traffic accident**

    X● **V25.41** Electric (assisted) bicycle driver injured in collision with railway train or railway vehicle in traffic accident

    X● **V25.49** Other motorcycle driver injured in collision with railway train or railway vehicle in traffic accident

X● **V25.5** Motorcycle **passenger** injured in collision with railway train or railway vehicle in **traffic accident**

    X● **V25.51** Electric (assisted) bicycle passenger injured in collision with railway train or railway vehicle in traffic accident

    X● **V25.59** Other motorcycle passenger injured in collision with railway train or railway vehicle in traffic accident

X● **V25.9** **Unspecified** motorcycle rider injured in collision with railway train or railway vehicle in **traffic accident**

    X● **V25.91** Unspecified electric (assisted) bicycle rider injured in collision with railway train or railway vehicle in traffic accident

    X● **V25.99** Unspecified rider of other motorcycle injured in collision with railway train or railway vehicle in traffic accident

● **V26** Motorcycle rider injured in collision with other nonmotor vehicle

> **Includes** collision with animal-drawn vehicle, animal being ridden, streetcar

    The appropriate 7th character is to be added to each code from category V26

> A   initial encounter
> D   subsequent encounter
> S   sequela

X● **V26.0** Motorcycle **driver** injured in collision with other nonmotor vehicle in **nontraffic accident**

    X● **V26.01** Electric (assisted) bicycle driver injured in collision with other nonmotor vehicle in nontraffic accident

    X● **V26.09** Other motorcycle driver injured in collision with other nonmotor vehicle in nontraffic accident

X● **V26.1** Motorcycle **passenger** injured in collision with other nonmotor vehicle in **nontraffic accident**

    X● **V26.11** Electric (assisted) bicycle passenger injured in collision with other nonmotor vehicle in nontraffic accident

    X● **V26.19** Other motorcycle passenger injured in collision with other nonmotor vehicle in nontraffic accident

X● **V26.2** **Unspecified** motorcycle rider injured in collision with other nonmotor vehicle in **nontraffic accident**

    X● **V26.21** Unspecified electric (assisted) bicycle rider injured in collision with other nonmotor vehicle in nontraffic accident

    X● **V26.29** Unspecified rider of other motorcycle injured in collision with other nonmotor vehicle in nontraffic accident

X● **V26.3** Person **boarding or alighting** a motorcycle injured in collision with other nonmotor vehicle

    X● **V26.31** Person boarding or alighting an electric (assisted) bicycle injured in collision with other nonmotor vehicle

    X● **V26.39** Person boarding or alighting other motorcycle injured in collision with other nonmotor vehicle

X● **V26.4** Motorcycle **driver** injured in collision with other nonmotor vehicle in **traffic accident**

    X● **V26.41** Electric (assisted) bicycle driver injured in collision with other nonmotor vehicle in traffic accident

    X● **V26.49** Other motorcycle driver injured in collision with other nonmotor vehicle in traffic accident

X● **V26.5** Motorcycle **passenger** injured in collision with other nonmotor vehicle in **traffic accident**

    X● **V26.51** Electric (assisted) bicycle passenger injured in collision with other nonmotor vehicle in traffic accident

    X● **V26.59** Other motorcycle passenger injured in collision with other nonmotor vehicle in traffic accident

X● **V26.9** **Unspecified** motorcycle rider injured in collision with other nonmotor vehicle in **traffic accident**

    X● **V26.91** Unspecified electric (assisted) bicycle rider injured in collision with other nonmotor vehicle in traffic accident

    X● **V26.99** Unspecified rider of other motorcycle injured in collision with other nonmotor vehicle in traffic accident

CHAPTER 20 (V00-Y99)

● **V27   Motorcycle rider injured in collision with fixed or stationary object**

The appropriate 7th character is to be added to each code from category V27

> A   initial encounter
> D   subsequent encounter
> S   sequela

X● **V27.0   Motorcycle driver injured in collision with fixed or stationary object in nontraffic accident**

    X● **V27.01   Electric (assisted) bicycle driver injured in collision with fixed or stationary object in nontraffic accident**

    X● **V27.09   Other motorcycle driver injured in collision with fixed or stationary object in nontraffic accident**

X● **V27.1   Motorcycle passenger injured in collision with fixed or stationary object in nontraffic accident**

    X● **V27.11   Electric (assisted) bicycle passenger injured in collision with fixed or stationary object in nontraffic accident**

    X● **V27.19   Other motorcycle passenger injured in collision with fixed or stationary object in nontraffic accident**

X● **V27.2   Unspecified motorcycle rider injured in collision with fixed or stationary object in nontraffic accident**

    X● **V27.21   Unspecified electric (assisted) bicycle rider injured in collision with fixed or stationary object in nontraffic accident**

    X● **V27.29   Unspecified rider of other motorcycle injured in collision with fixed or stationary object in nontraffic accident**

X● **V27.3   Person boarding or alighting a motorcycle injured in collision with fixed or stationary object**

    X● **V27.31   Person boarding or alighting an electric (assisted) bicycle injured in collision with fixed or stationary object**

    X● **V27.39   Person boarding or alighting other motorcycle injured in collision with fixed or stationary object**

X● **V27.4   Motorcycle driver injured in collision with fixed or stationary object in traffic accident**

    X● **V27.41   Electric (assisted) bicycle driver injured in collision with fixed or stationary object in traffic accident**

    X● **V27.49   Other motorcycle driver injured in collision with fixed or stationary object in traffic accident**

X● **V27.5   Motorcycle passenger injured in collision with fixed or stationary object in traffic accident**

    X● **V27.51   Electric (assisted) bicycle passenger injured in collision with fixed or stationary object in traffic accident**

    X● **V27.59   Other motorcycle passenger injured in collision with fixed or stationary object in traffic accident**

X● **V27.9   Unspecified motorcycle rider injured in collision with fixed or stationary object in traffic accident**

    X● **V27.91   Unspecified electric (assisted) bicycle rider injured in collision with fixed or stationary object in traffic accident**

    X● **V27.99   Unspecified rider of other motorcycle injured in collision with fixed or stationary object in traffic accident**

● **V28   Motorcycle rider injured in noncollision transport accident**

> **Includes**   fall or thrown from motorcycle (without antecedent collision)
> overturning motorcycle NOS
> overturning motorcycle without collision

The appropriate 7th character is to be added to each code from category V28

> A   initial encounter
> D   subsequent encounter
> S   sequela

X● **V28.0   Motorcycle driver injured in noncollision transport accident in nontraffic accident**

    X● **V28.01   Electric (assisted) bicycle driver injured in noncollision transport accident in nontraffic accident**

    X● **V28.09   Other motorcycle driver injured in noncollision transport accident in nontraffic accident**

X● **V28.1   Motorcycle passenger injured in noncollision transport accident in nontraffic accident**

    X● **V28.11   Electric (assisted) bicycle passenger injured in noncollision transport accident in nontraffic accident**

    X● **V28.19   Other motorcycle passenger injured in noncollision transport accident in nontraffic accident**

X● **V28.2   Unspecified motorcycle rider injured in noncollision transport accident in nontraffic accident**

    X● **V28.21   Unspecified electric (assisted) bicycle rider injured in noncollision transport accident in nontraffic accident**

    X● **V28.29   Unspecified rider of other motorcycle injured in noncollision transport accident in nontraffic accident**

X● **V28.3   Person boarding or alighting a motorcycle injured in noncollision transport accident**

    X● **V28.31   Person boarding or alighting an electric (assisted) bicycle injured in noncollision transport accident**

    X● **V28.39   Person boarding or alighting other motorcycle injured in noncollision transport accident**

X● **V28.4   Motorcycle driver injured in noncollision transport accident in traffic accident**

    X● **V28.41   Electric (assisted) bicycle driver injured in noncollision transport accident in traffic accident**

    X● **V28.49   Other motorcycle driver injured in noncollision transport accident in traffic accident**

X● **V28.5   Motorcycle passenger injured in noncollision transport accident in traffic accident**

    X● **V28.51   Electric (assisted) bicycle passenger injured in noncollision transport accident in traffic accident**

    X● **V28.59   Other motorcycle passenger injured in noncollision transport accident in traffic accident**

X● **V28.9   Unspecified motorcycle rider injured in noncollision transport accident in traffic accident**

    X● **V28.91   Unspecified electric (assisted) bicycle rider injured in noncollision transport accident in traffic accident**

    X● **V28.99   Unspecified rider of other motorcycle injured in noncollision transport accident in traffic accident**

● **V29 Motorcycle rider injured in other and unspecified transport accidents**

> The appropriate 7th character is to be added to each code from category V29

> | A | initial encounter |
> | D | subsequent encounter |
> | S | sequela |

Coding Clinic: 2015, Q3, P20

● **V29.0 Motorcycle driver injured in collision with other and unspecified motor vehicles in nontraffic accident**

  ● **V29.00 Motorcycle driver injured in collision with unspecified motor vehicles in nontraffic accident**

    ● V29.001 Electric (assisted) bicycle driver injured in collision with unspecified motor vehicles in nontraffic accident

    ● V29.008 Other motorcycle driver injured in collision with unspecified motor vehicles in nontraffic accident

  ● **V29.09 Motorcycle driver injured in collision with other motor vehicles in nontraffic accident**

    ● V29.091 Electric (assisted) bicycle driver injured in collision with other motor vehicles in nontraffic accident

    ● V29.098 Other motorcycle driver injured in collision with other motor vehicles in nontraffic accident

● **V29.1 Motorcycle passenger injured in collision with other and unspecified motor vehicles in nontraffic accident**

  ● **V29.10 Motorcycle passenger injured in collision with unspecified motor vehicles in nontraffic accident**

    ● V29.101 Electric (assisted) bicycle passenger injured in collision with unspecified motor vehicles in nontraffic accident

    ● V29.108 Other motorcycle passenger injured in collision with unspecified motor vehicles in nontraffic accident

  ● **V29.19 Motorcycle passenger injured in collision with other motor vehicles in nontraffic accident**

    ● V29.191 Electric (assisted) bicycle passenger injured in collision with other motor vehicles in nontraffic accident

    ● V29.198 Other motorcycle passenger injured in collision with other motor vehicles in nontraffic accident

● **V29.2 Unspecified motorcycle rider injured in collision with other and unspecified motor vehicles in nontraffic accident**

  ● **V29.20 Unspecified motorcycle rider injured in collision with unspecified motor vehicles in nontraffic accident**
> Motorcycle collision NOS, nontraffic

    ● V29.201 Unspecified electric (assisted) bicycle rider injured in collision with unspecified motor vehicles in nontraffic accident

    ● V29.208 Unspecified rider of other motorcycle injured in collision with unspecified motor vehicles in nontraffic accident
> Motorcycle collision NOS, nontraffic

  ● **V29.29 Unspecified motorcycle rider injured in collision with other motor vehicles in nontraffic accident**

    ● V29.291 Unspecified electric (assisted) bicycle rider injured in collision with other motor vehicles in nontraffic accident

    ● V29.298 Unspecified rider of other motorcycle injured in collision with other motor vehicles in nontraffic accident

X ● **V29.3 Motorcycle rider (driver) (passenger) injured in unspecified nontraffic accident**
> Motorcycle accident NOS, nontraffic
> Motorcycle rider injured in nontraffic accident NOS

  X ● **V29.31 Electric (assisted) bicycle (driver) (passenger) injured in unspecified nontraffic accident**

  X ● **V29.39 Other motorcycle (driver) (passenger) injured in unspecified nontraffic accident**
> Motorcycle accident NOS, nontraffic
> Motorcycle rider injured in nontraffic accident NOS

● **V29.4 Motorcycle driver injured in collision with other and unspecified motor vehicles in traffic accident**

  ● **V29.40 Motorcycle driver injured in collision with unspecified motor vehicles in traffic accident**

    ● V29.401 Electric (assisted) bicycle driver injured in collision with unspecified motor vehicles in traffic accident

    ● V29.408 Other motorcycle driver injured in collision with unspecified motor vehicles in traffic accident

  ● **V29.49 Motorcycle driver injured in collision with other motor vehicles in traffic accident**

    ● V29.491 Electric (assisted) bicycle driver injured in collision with other motor vehicles in traffic accident

    ● V29.498 Other motorcycle driver injured in collision with other motor vehicles in traffic accident

● **V29.5 Motorcycle passenger injured in collision with other and unspecified motor vehicles in traffic accident**

  ● **V29.50 Motorcycle passenger injured in collision with unspecified motor vehicles in traffic accident**

    ● V29.501 Electric (assisted) bicycle passenger injured in collision with unspecified motor vehicles in traffic accident

    ● V29.508 Other motorcycle passenger injured in collision with unspecified motor vehicles in traffic accident

  ● **V29.59 Motorcycle passenger injured in collision with other motor vehicles in traffic accident**

    ● V29.591 Electric (assisted) bicycle passenger injured in collision with other motor vehicles in traffic accident

    ● V29.598 Other motorcycle passenger injured in collision with other motor vehicles in traffic accident

● **V29.6 Unspecified motorcycle rider injured in collision with other and unspecified motor vehicles in traffic accident**

  ● **V29.60 Unspecified motorcycle rider injured in collision with unspecified motor vehicles in traffic accident**
> Motorcycle collision NOS (traffic)

    ● V29.601 Unspecified electric (assisted) bicycle rider injured in collision with unspecified motor vehicles in traffic accident

    ● V29.608 Unspecified rider of other motorcycle injured in collision with unspecified motor vehicles in traffic accident
> Motorcycle collision NOS (traffic)

  ● **V29.69 Unspecified motorcycle rider injured in collision with other motor vehicles in traffic accident**

    ● V29.691 Unspecified electric (assisted) bicycle rider injured in collision with other motor vehicles in traffic accident

    ● V29.698 Unspecified rider of other motorcycle injured in collision with other motor vehicles in traffic accident

CHAPTER 20 (V00–Y99)

● **V29.8** Motorcycle rider (driver) (passenger) injured in other specified transport accidents

● **V29.81** Motorcycle rider (driver) (passenger) injured in transport accident with military vehicle

● **V29.811** Electric (assisted) bicycle rider (driver) (passenger) injured in transport accident with military vehicle

● **V29.818** Rider (driver) (passenger) of other motorcycle injured in transport accident with military vehicle

● **V29.88** Motorcycle rider (driver) (passenger) injured in other specified transport accidents

● **V29.881** Electric (assisted) bicycle rider (driver) (passenger) injured in other specified transport accidents

● **V29.888** Rider (driver) (passenger) of other motorcycle injured in other specified transport accidents

X ● **V29.9** Motorcycle rider (driver) (passenger) injured in unspecified traffic accident
Motorcycle accident NOS

X ● **V29.91** Electric (assisted) bicycle rider (driver) (passenger) injured in unspecified traffic accident

X ● **V29.99** Rider (driver) (passenger) of other motorcycle injured in unspecified traffic accident
Motorcycle accident NOS

OCCUPANT OF THREE-WHEELED MOTOR VEHICLE INJURED IN TRANSPORT ACCIDENT (V30-V39)

Includes　motorized tricycle
motorized rickshaw
three-wheeled motor car

Excludes1　all-terrain vehicles (V86.-)
motorcycle with sidecar (V20-V29)
vehicle designed primarily for off-road use (V86.-)

● **V30** Occupant of three-wheeled motor vehicle injured in collision with pedestrian or animal

Excludes1　three-wheeled motor vehicle collision with animal-drawn vehicle or animal being ridden (V36.-)

The appropriate 7th character is to be added to each code from category V30

A	initial encounter
D	subsequent encounter
S	sequela

X ● **V30.0** Driver of three-wheeled motor vehicle injured in collision with pedestrian or animal in nontraffic accident

X ● **V30.1** Passenger in three-wheeled motor vehicle injured in collision with pedestrian or animal in nontraffic accident

X ● **V30.2** Person on outside of three-wheeled motor vehicle injured in collision with pedestrian or animal in nontraffic accident

X ● **V30.3** Unspecified occupant of three-wheeled motor vehicle injured in collision with pedestrian or animal in nontraffic accident

X ● **V30.4** Person boarding or alighting a three-wheeled motor vehicle injured in collision with pedestrian or animal

X ● **V30.5** Driver of three-wheeled motor vehicle injured in collision with pedestrian or animal in traffic accident

X ● **V30.6** Passenger in three-wheeled motor vehicle injured in collision with pedestrian or animal in traffic accident

X ● **V30.7** Person on outside of three-wheeled motor vehicle injured in collision with pedestrian or animal in traffic accident

X ● **V30.9** Unspecified occupant of three-wheeled motor vehicle injured in collision with pedestrian or animal in traffic accident

● **V31** Occupant of three-wheeled motor vehicle injured in collision with pedal cycle

The appropriate 7th character is to be added to each code from category V31

A	initial encounter
D	subsequent encounter
S	sequela

X ● **V31.0** Driver of three-wheeled motor vehicle injured in collision with pedal cycle in nontraffic accident

X ● **V31.1** Passenger in three-wheeled motor vehicle injured in collision with pedal cycle in nontraffic accident

X ● **V31.2** Person on outside of three-wheeled motor vehicle injured in collision with pedal cycle in nontraffic accident

X ● **V31.3** Unspecified occupant of three-wheeled motor vehicle injured in collision with pedal cycle in nontraffic accident

X ● **V31.4** Person boarding or alighting a three-wheeled motor vehicle injured in collision with pedal cycle

X ● **V31.5** Driver of three-wheeled motor vehicle injured in collision with pedal cycle in traffic accident

X ● **V31.6** Passenger in three-wheeled motor vehicle injured in collision with pedal cycle in traffic accident

X ● **V31.7** Person on outside of three-wheeled motor vehicle injured in collision with pedal cycle in traffic accident

X ● **V31.9** Unspecified occupant of three-wheeled motor vehicle injured in collision with pedal cycle in traffic accident

● **V32** Occupant of three-wheeled motor vehicle injured in collision with two- or three-wheeled motor vehicle

The appropriate 7th character is to be added to each code from category V32

A	initial encounter
D	subsequent encounter
S	sequela

X ● **V32.0** Driver of three-wheeled motor vehicle injured in collision with two- or three-wheeled motor vehicle in nontraffic accident

X ● **V32.1** Passenger in three-wheeled motor vehicle injured in collision with two- or three-wheeled motor vehicle in nontraffic accident

X ● **V32.2** Person on outside of three-wheeled motor vehicle injured in collision with two- or three-wheeled motor vehicle in nontraffic accident

X ● **V32.3** Unspecified occupant of three-wheeled motor vehicle injured in collision with two- or three-wheeled motor vehicle in nontraffic accident

X ● **V32.4** Person boarding or alighting a three-wheeled motor vehicle injured in collision with two- or three-wheeled motor vehicle

X ● **V32.5** Driver of three-wheeled motor vehicle injured in collision with two- or three-wheeled motor vehicle in traffic accident

X ● **V32.6** Passenger in three-wheeled motor vehicle injured in collision with two- or three-wheeled motor vehicle in traffic accident

X ● **V32.7** Person on outside of three-wheeled motor vehicle injured in collision with two- or three-wheeled motor vehicle in traffic accident

X ● **V32.9** Unspecified occupant of three-wheeled motor vehicle injured in collision with two- or three-wheeled motor vehicle in traffic accident

● **V33** Occupant of three-wheeled motor vehicle injured in collision with car, pick-up truck or van

The appropriate 7th character is to be added to each code from category V33

> A initial encounter
> D subsequent encounter
> S sequela

X ● **V33.0** Driver of three-wheeled motor vehicle injured in collision with car, pick-up truck or van in nontraffic accident

X ● **V33.1** Passenger in three-wheeled motor vehicle injured in collision with car, pick-up truck or van in nontraffic accident

X ● **V33.2** Person on outside of three-wheeled motor vehicle injured in collision with car, pick-up truck or van in nontraffic accident

X ● **V33.3** Unspecified occupant of three-wheeled motor vehicle injured in collision with car, pick-up truck or van in nontraffic accident

X ● **V33.4** Person boarding or alighting a three-wheeled motor vehicle injured in collision with car, pick-up truck or van

X ● **V33.5** Driver of three-wheeled motor vehicle injured in collision with car, pick-up truck or van in traffic accident

X ● **V33.6** Passenger in three-wheeled motor vehicle injured in collision with car, pick-up truck or van in traffic accident

X ● **V33.7** Person on outside of three-wheeled motor vehicle injured in collision with car, pick-up truck or van in traffic accident

X ● **V33.9** Unspecified occupant of three-wheeled motor vehicle injured in collision with car, pick-up truck or van in traffic accident

● **V34** Occupant of three-wheeled motor vehicle injured in collision with heavy transport vehicle or bus

Excludes1 occupant of three-wheeled motor vehicle injured in collision with military vehicle (V39.81)

The appropriate 7th character is to be added to each code from category V34

> A initial encounter
> D subsequent encounter
> S sequela

X ● **V34.0** Driver of three-wheeled motor vehicle injured in collision with heavy transport vehicle or bus in nontraffic accident

X ● **V34.1** Passenger in three-wheeled motor vehicle injured in collision with heavy transport vehicle or bus in nontraffic accident

X ● **V34.2** Person on outside of three-wheeled motor vehicle injured in collision with heavy transport vehicle or bus in nontraffic accident

X ● **V34.3** Unspecified occupant of three-wheeled motor vehicle injured in collision with heavy transport vehicle or bus in nontraffic accident

X ● **V34.4** Person boarding or alighting a three-wheeled motor vehicle injured in collision with heavy transport vehicle or bus

X ● **V34.5** Driver of three-wheeled motor vehicle injured in collision with heavy transport vehicle or bus in traffic accident

X ● **V34.6** Passenger in three-wheeled motor vehicle injured in collision with heavy transport vehicle or bus in traffic accident

X ● **V34.7** Person on outside of three-wheeled motor vehicle injured in collision with heavy transport vehicle or bus in traffic accident

X ● **V34.9** Unspecified occupant of three-wheeled motor vehicle injured in collision with heavy transport vehicle or bus in traffic accident

● **V35** Occupant of three-wheeled motor vehicle injured in collision with railway train or railway vehicle

The appropriate 7th character is to be added to each code from category V35

> A initial encounter
> D subsequent encounter
> S sequela

X ● **V35.0** Driver of three-wheeled motor vehicle injured in collision with railway train or railway vehicle in nontraffic accident

X ● **V35.1** Passenger in three-wheeled motor vehicle injured in collision with railway train or railway vehicle in nontraffic accident

X ● **V35.2** Person on outside of three-wheeled motor vehicle injured in collision with railway train or railway vehicle in nontraffic accident

X ● **V35.3** Unspecified occupant of three-wheeled motor vehicle injured in collision with railway train or railway vehicle in nontraffic accident

X ● **V35.4** Person boarding or alighting a three-wheeled motor vehicle injured in collision with railway train or railway vehicle

X ● **V35.5** Driver of three-wheeled motor vehicle injured in collision with railway train or railway vehicle in traffic accident

X ● **V35.6** Passenger in three-wheeled motor vehicle injured in collision with railway train or railway vehicle in traffic accident

X ● **V35.7** Person on outside of three-wheeled motor vehicle injured in collision with railway train or railway vehicle in traffic accident

X ● **V35.9** Unspecified occupant of three-wheeled motor vehicle injured in collision with railway train or railway vehicle in traffic accident

● **V36** Occupant of three-wheeled motor vehicle injured in collision with other nonmotor vehicle

Includes collision with animal-drawn vehicle, animal being ridden, streetcar

The appropriate 7th character is to be added to each code from category V36

> A initial encounter
> D subsequent encounter
> S sequela

X ● **V36.0** Driver of three-wheeled motor vehicle injured in collision with other nonmotor vehicle in nontraffic accident

X ● **V36.1** Passenger in three-wheeled motor vehicle injured in collision with other nonmotor vehicle in nontraffic accident

X ● **V36.2** Person on outside of three-wheeled motor vehicle injured in collision with other nonmotor vehicle in nontraffic accident

X ● **V36.3** Unspecified occupant of three-wheeled motor vehicle injured in collision with other nonmotor vehicle in nontraffic accident

X ● **V36.4** Person boarding or alighting a three-wheeled motor vehicle injured in collision with other nonmotor vehicle

X ● **V36.5** Driver of three-wheeled motor vehicle injured in collision with other nonmotor vehicle in traffic accident

X ● **V36.6** Passenger in three-wheeled motor vehicle injured in collision with other nonmotor vehicle in traffic accident

X ● **V36.7** Person on outside of three-wheeled motor vehicle injured in collision with other nonmotor vehicle in traffic accident

X ● **V36.9** Unspecified occupant of three-wheeled motor vehicle injured in collision with other nonmotor vehicle in traffic accident

CHAPTER 20 (V00-Y99)

● **V37　Occupant of three-wheeled motor vehicle injured in collision with fixed or stationary object**

The appropriate 7th character is to be added to each code from category V37

A	initial encounter
D	subsequent encounter
S	sequela

X● **V37.0　Driver** of three-wheeled motor vehicle injured in collision with fixed or stationary object in **nontraffic accident**

X● **V37.1　Passenger** in three-wheeled motor vehicle injured in collision with fixed or stationary object in **nontraffic accident**

X● **V37.2　Person on outside** of three-wheeled motor vehicle injured in collision with fixed or stationary object in **nontraffic accident**

X● **V37.3　Unspecified** occupant of three-wheeled motor vehicle injured in collision with fixed or stationary object in **nontraffic accident**

X● **V37.4　Person boarding or alighting** a three-wheeled motor vehicle injured in collision with fixed or stationary object

X● **V37.5　Driver** of three-wheeled motor vehicle injured in collision with fixed or stationary object in **traffic accident**

X● **V37.6　Passenger** in three-wheeled motor vehicle injured in collision with fixed or stationary object in **traffic accident**

X● **V37.7　Person on outside** of three-wheeled motor vehicle injured in collision with fixed or stationary object in **traffic accident**

X● **V37.9　Unspecified** occupant of three-wheeled motor vehicle injured in collision with fixed or stationary object in **traffic accident**

● **V38　Occupant of three-wheeled motor vehicle injured in noncollision transport accident**

Includes　fall or thrown from three-wheeled motor vehicle
overturning of three-wheeled motor vehicle NOS
overturning of three-wheeled motor vehicle without collision

The appropriate 7th character is to be added to each code from category V38

A	initial encounter
D	subsequent encounter
S	sequela

X● **V38.0　Driver** of three-wheeled motor vehicle injured in noncollision transport accident in **nontraffic accident**

X● **V38.1　Passenger** in three-wheeled motor vehicle injured in noncollision transport accident in **nontraffic accident**

X● **V38.2　Person on outside** of three-wheeled motor vehicle injured in noncollision transport accident in **nontraffic accident**

X● **V38.3　Unspecified** occupant of three-wheeled motor vehicle injured in noncollision transport accident in **nontraffic accident**

X● **V38.4　Person boarding or alighting** a three-wheeled motor vehicle injured in noncollision transport accident

X● **V38.5　Driver** of three-wheeled motor vehicle injured in noncollision transport accident in **traffic accident**

X● **V38.6　Passenger** in three-wheeled motor vehicle injured in noncollision transport accident in **traffic accident**

X● **V38.7　Person on outside** of three-wheeled motor vehicle injured in noncollision transport accident in **traffic accident**

X● **V38.9　Unspecified** occupant of three-wheeled motor vehicle injured in noncollision transport accident in **traffic accident**

● **V39　Occupant of three-wheeled motor vehicle injured in other and unspecified transport accidents**

The appropriate 7th character is to be added to each code from category V39

A	initial encounter
D	subsequent encounter
S	sequela

● **V39.0　Driver** of three-wheeled motor vehicle injured in collision with other and unspecified motor vehicles in **nontraffic accident**

X● **V39.00　Driver** of three-wheeled motor vehicle injured in collision with **unspecified** motor vehicles in nontraffic accident

X● **V39.09　Driver** of three-wheeled motor vehicle injured in collision with **other** motor vehicles in nontraffic accident

● **V39.1　Passenger** in three-wheeled motor vehicle injured in collision with other and unspecified motor vehicles in **nontraffic accident**

X● **V39.10　Passenger** in three-wheeled motor vehicle injured in collision with **unspecified** motor vehicles in nontraffic accident

X● **V39.19　Passenger** in three-wheeled motor vehicle injured in collision with **other** motor vehicles in nontraffic accident

● **V39.2　Unspecified** occupant of three-wheeled motor vehicle injured in collision with other and unspecified motor vehicles in **nontraffic accident**

X● **V39.20　Unspecified** occupant of three-wheeled motor vehicle injured in collision with **unspecified** motor vehicles in nontraffic accident
Collision NOS involving three-wheeled motor vehicle, nontraffic

X● **V39.29　Unspecified** occupant of three-wheeled motor vehicle injured in collision with **other** motor vehicles in nontraffic accident

X● **V39.3　Occupant (driver) (passenger)** of three-wheeled motor vehicle injured in **unspecified nontraffic accident**
Accident NOS involving three-wheeled motor vehicle, nontraffic
Occupant of three-wheeled motor vehicle injured in nontraffic accident NOS

● **V39.4　Driver** of three-wheeled motor vehicle injured in collision with other and unspecified motor vehicles in **traffic accident**

X● **V39.40　Driver** of three-wheeled motor vehicle injured in collision with **unspecified** motor vehicles in traffic accident

X● **V39.49　Driver** of three-wheeled motor vehicle injured in collision with **other** motor vehicles in traffic accident

● **V39.5　Passenger** in three-wheeled motor vehicle injured in collision with other and unspecified motor vehicles in **traffic accident**

X● **V39.50　Passenger** in three-wheeled motor vehicle injured in collision with **unspecified** motor vehicles in traffic accident

X● **V39.59　Passenger** in three-wheeled motor vehicle injured in collision with **other** motor vehicles in traffic accident

● **V39.6　Unspecified** occupant of three-wheeled motor vehicle injured in collision with other and unspecified motor vehicles in **traffic accident**

X● **V39.60　Unspecified** occupant of three-wheeled motor vehicle injured in collision with **unspecified** motor vehicles in traffic accident
Collision NOS involving three-wheeled motor vehicle (traffic)

X● **V39.69　Unspecified** occupant of three-wheeled motor vehicle injured in collision with **other** motor vehicles in traffic accident

▶ New　　◀ Revised　　~~deleted~~ Deleted　　Excludes 1　　Excludes 2　　Includes　　Use additional　　Code first　　Code also　　Key words
OGCR Official Guidelines　　X Assign placeholder X　　● Use Additional Character(s)　　▶ Manifestation Code　　Hierarchical Condition Category　　**Coding Clinic**

● V39.8   Occupant (driver) (passenger) of three-wheeled motor vehicle injured in other specified transport accidents
   X● V39.81   Occupant (driver) (passenger) of three-wheeled motor vehicle injured in transport accident with military vehicle
   X● V39.89   Occupant (driver) (passenger) of three-wheeled motor vehicle injured in other specified transport accidents
X● V39.9   Occupant (driver) (passenger) of three-wheeled motor vehicle injured in unspecified traffic accident
     Accident NOS involving three-wheeled motor vehicle

CAR OCCUPANT INJURED IN TRANSPORT ACCIDENT (V40-V49)

Includes	a four-wheeled motor vehicle designed primarily for carrying passengers automobile (pulling a trailer or camper)
Excludes1	bus (V50-V59) minibus (V50-V59) minivan (V50-V59) motorcoach (V70-V79) pick-up truck (V50-V59) sport utility vehicle (SUV) (V50-V59)

● V40   Car occupant injured in collision with pedestrian or animal

Excludes1	car collision with animal-drawn vehicle or animal being ridden (V46.-)

The appropriate 7th character is to be added to each code from category V40

A	initial encounter
D	subsequent encounter
S	sequela

X● V40.0   Car driver injured in collision with pedestrian or animal in nontraffic accident
X● V40.1   Car passenger injured in collision with pedestrian or animal in nontraffic accident
X● V40.2   Person on outside of car injured in collision with pedestrian or animal in nontraffic accident
X● V40.3   Unspecified car occupant injured in collision with pedestrian or animal in nontraffic accident
X● V40.4   Person boarding or alighting a car injured in collision with pedestrian or animal
X● V40.5   Car driver injured in collision with pedestrian or animal in traffic accident
X● V40.6   Car passenger injured in collision with pedestrian or animal in traffic accident
X● V40.7   Person on outside of car injured in collision with pedestrian or animal in traffic accident
X● V40.9   Unspecified car occupant injured in collision with pedestrian or animal in traffic accident

● V41   Car occupant injured in collision with pedal cycle

The appropriate 7th character is to be added to each code from category V41

A	initial encounter
D	subsequent encounter
S	sequela

X● V41.0   Car driver injured in collision with pedal cycle in nontraffic accident
X● V41.1   Car passenger injured in collision with pedal cycle in nontraffic accident
X● V41.2   Person on outside of car injured in collision with pedal cycle in nontraffic accident
X● V41.3   Unspecified car occupant injured in collision with pedal cycle in nontraffic accident
X● V41.4   Person boarding or alighting a car injured in collision with pedal cycle
X● V41.5   Car driver injured in collision with pedal cycle in traffic accident
X● V41.6   Car passenger injured in collision with pedal cycle in traffic accident

X● V41.7   Person on outside of car injured in collision with pedal cycle in traffic accident
X● V41.9   Unspecified car occupant injured in collision with pedal cycle in traffic accident

● V42   Car occupant injured in collision with two- or three-wheeled motor vehicle

The appropriate 7th character is to be added to each code from category V42

A	initial encounter
D	subsequent encounter
S	sequela

X● V42.0   Car driver injured in collision with two- or three-wheeled motor vehicle in nontraffic accident
X● V42.1   Car passenger injured in collision with two- or three-wheeled motor vehicle in nontraffic accident
X● V42.2   Person on outside of car injured in collision with two- or three-wheeled motor vehicle in nontraffic accident
X● V42.3   Unspecified car occupant injured in collision with two- or three-wheeled motor vehicle in nontraffic accident
X● V42.4   Person boarding or alighting a car injured in collision with two- or three-wheeled motor vehicle
X● V42.5   Car driver injured in collision with two- or three-wheeled motor vehicle in traffic accident
X● V42.6   Car passenger injured in collision with two- or three-wheeled motor vehicle in traffic accident
X● V42.7   Person on outside of car injured in collision with two- or three-wheeled motor vehicle in traffic accident
X● V42.9   Unspecified car occupant injured in collision with two- or three-wheeled motor vehicle in traffic accident

● V43   Car occupant injured in collision with car, pick-up truck or van

The appropriate 7th character is to be added to each code from category V43

A	initial encounter
D	subsequent encounter
S	sequela

● V43.0   Car driver injured in collision with car, pick-up truck or van in nontraffic accident
   X● V43.01   Car driver injured in collision with sport utility vehicle in nontraffic accident
   X● V43.02   Car driver injured in collision with other type car in nontraffic accident
   X● V43.03   Car driver injured in collision with pick-up truck in nontraffic accident
   X● V43.04   Car driver injured in collision with van in nontraffic accident
● V43.1   Car passenger injured in collision with car, pick-up truck or van in nontraffic accident
   X● V43.11   Car passenger injured in collision with sport utility vehicle in nontraffic accident
   X● V43.12   Car passenger injured in collision with other type car in nontraffic accident
   X● V43.13   Car passenger injured in collision with pick-up truck in nontraffic accident
   X● V43.14   Car passenger injured in collision with van in nontraffic accident
● V43.2   Person on outside of car injured in collision with car, pick-up truck or van in nontraffic accident
   X● V43.21   Person on outside of car injured in collision with sport utility vehicle in nontraffic accident
   X● V43.22   Person on outside of car injured in collision with other type car in nontraffic accident
   X● V43.23   Person on outside of car injured in collision with pick-up truck in nontraffic accident
   X● V43.24   Person on outside of car injured in collision with van in nontraffic accident

CHAPTER 20 (V00-Y99)

●V43.3　Unspecified car occupant injured in collision with car, pick-up truck or van in nontraffic accident
- X●V43.31　Unspecified car occupant injured in collision with sport utility vehicle in nontraffic accident
- X●V43.32　Unspecified car occupant injured in collision with other type car in nontraffic accident
- X●V43.33　Unspecified car occupant injured in collision with pick-up truck in nontraffic accident
- X●V43.34　Unspecified car occupant injured in collision with van in nontraffic accident

●V43.4　Person boarding or alighting a car injured in collision with car, pick-up truck or van
- X●V43.41　Person boarding or alighting a car injured in collision with sport utility vehicle
- X●V43.42　Person boarding or alighting a car injured in collision with other type car
- X●V43.43　Person boarding or alighting a car injured in collision with pick-up truck
- X●V43.44　Person boarding or alighting a car injured in collision with van

●V43.5　Car driver injured in collision with car, pick-up truck or van in traffic accident
- X●V43.51　Car driver injured in collision with sport utility vehicle in traffic accident
- X●V43.52　Car driver injured in collision with other type car in traffic accident
- X●V43.53　Car driver injured in collision with pick-up truck in traffic accident
- X●V43.54　Car driver injured in collision with van in traffic accident

●V43.6　Car passenger injured in collision with car, pick-up truck or van in traffic accident
- X●V43.61　Car passenger injured in collision with sport utility vehicle in traffic accident
  - **Coding Clinic: 2015, Q1, P5-7**
- X●V43.62　Car passenger injured in collision with other type car in traffic accident
- X●V43.63　Car passenger injured in collision with pick-up truck in traffic accident
- X●V43.64　Car passenger injured in collision with van in traffic accident

●V43.7　Person on outside of car injured in collision with car, pick-up truck or van in traffic accident
- X●V43.71　Person on outside of car injured in collision with sport utility vehicle in traffic accident
- X●V43.72　Person on outside of car injured in collision with other type car in traffic accident
- X●V43.73　Person on outside of car injured in collision with pick-up truck in traffic accident
- X●V43.74　Person on outside of car injured in collision with van in traffic accident

●V43.9　Unspecified car occupant injured in collision with car, pick-up truck or van in traffic accident
- X●V43.91　Unspecified car occupant injured in collision with sport utility vehicle in traffic accident
- X●V43.92　Unspecified car occupant injured in collision with other type car in traffic accident
- X●V43.93　Unspecified car occupant injured in collision with pick-up truck in traffic accident
- X●V43.94　Unspecified car occupant injured in collision with van in traffic accident

●V44　Car occupant injured in collision with heavy transport vehicle or bus

> **Excludes1**　car occupant injured in collision with military vehicle (V49.81)

The appropriate 7th character is to be added to each code from category V44

A	initial encounter
D	subsequent encounter
S	sequela

- X●V44.0　Car driver injured in collision with heavy transport vehicle or bus in nontraffic accident
- X●V44.1　Car passenger injured in collision with heavy transport vehicle or bus in nontraffic accident
- X●V44.2　Person on outside of car injured in collision with heavy transport vehicle or bus in nontraffic accident
- X●V44.3　Unspecified car occupant injured in collision with heavy transport vehicle or bus in nontraffic accident
- X●V44.4　Person boarding or alighting a car injured in collision with heavy transport vehicle or bus
- X●V44.5　Car driver injured in collision with heavy transport vehicle or bus in traffic accident
- X●V44.6　Car passenger injured in collision with heavy transport vehicle or bus in traffic accident
- X●V44.7　Person on outside of car injured in collision with heavy transport vehicle or bus in traffic accident
- X●V44.9　Unspecified car occupant injured in collision with heavy transport vehicle or bus in traffic accident

●V45　Car occupant injured in collision with railway train or railway vehicle

The appropriate 7th character is to be added to each code from category V45

A	initial encounter
D	subsequent encounter
S	sequela

- X●V45.0　Car driver injured in collision with railway train or railway vehicle in nontraffic accident
- X●V45.1　Car passenger injured in collision with railway train or railway vehicle in nontraffic accident
- X●V45.2　Person on outside of car injured in collision with railway train or railway vehicle in nontraffic accident
- X●V45.3　Unspecified car occupant injured in collision with railway train or railway vehicle in nontraffic accident
- X●V45.4　Person boarding or alighting a car injured in collision with railway train or railway vehicle
- X●V45.5　Car driver injured in collision with railway train or railway vehicle in traffic accident
- X●V45.6　Car passenger injured in collision with railway train or railway vehicle in traffic accident
- X●V45.7　Person on outside of car injured in collision with railway train or railway vehicle in traffic accident
- X●V45.9　Unspecified car occupant injured in collision with railway train or railway vehicle in traffic accident

●V46　Car occupant injured in collision with other nonmotor vehicle

> **Includes**　collision with animal-drawn vehicle, animal being ridden, streetcar

The appropriate 7th character is to be added to each code from category V46

A	initial encounter
D	subsequent encounter
S	sequela

- X●V46.0　Car driver injured in collision with other nonmotor vehicle in nontraffic accident
- X●V46.1　Car passenger injured in collision with other nonmotor vehicle in nontraffic accident

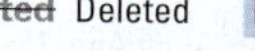
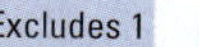
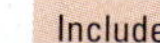
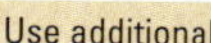
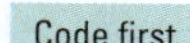

X ● **V46.2**   Person on outside of car injured in collision with other nonmotor vehicle in nontraffic accident

X ● **V46.3**   Unspecified car occupant injured in collision with other nonmotor vehicle in nontraffic accident

X ● **V46.4**   Person boarding or alighting a car injured in collision with other nonmotor vehicle

X ● **V46.5**   Car driver injured in collision with other nonmotor vehicle in traffic accident

X ● **V46.6**   Car passenger injured in collision with other nonmotor vehicle in traffic accident

X ● **V46.7**   Person on outside of car injured in collision with other nonmotor vehicle in traffic accident

X ● **V46.9**   Unspecified car occupant injured in collision with other nonmotor vehicle in traffic accident

● **V47**   Car occupant injured in collision with fixed or stationary object

The appropriate 7th character is to be added to each code from category V47

A	initial encounter
D	subsequent encounter
S	sequela

Coding Clinic: 2016, Q4, P73

X ● **V47.0**   Car driver injured in collision with fixed or stationary object in nontraffic accident

X ● **V47.1**   Car passenger injured in collision with fixed or stationary object in nontraffic accident

X ● **V47.2**   Person on outside of car injured in collision with fixed or stationary object in nontraffic accident

X ● **V47.3**   Unspecified car occupant injured in collision with fixed or stationary object in nontraffic accident

X ● **V47.4**   Person boarding or alighting a car injured in collision with fixed or stationary object

X ● **V47.5**   Car driver injured in collision with fixed or stationary object in traffic accident

X ● **V47.6**   Car passenger injured in collision with fixed or stationary object in traffic accident

X ● **V47.7**   Person on outside of car injured in collision with fixed or stationary object in traffic accident

X ● **V47.9**   Unspecified car occupant injured in collision with fixed or stationary object in traffic accident

● **V48**   Car occupant injured in noncollision transport accident

Includes   overturning car NOS
overturning car without collision

The appropriate 7th character is to be added to each code from category V48

A	initial encounter
D	subsequent encounter
S	sequela

X ● **V48.0**   Car driver injured in noncollision transport accident in nontraffic accident

X ● **V48.1**   Car passenger injured in noncollision transport accident in nontraffic accident

X ● **V48.2**   Person on outside of car injured in noncollision transport accident in nontraffic accident

X ● **V48.3**   Unspecified car occupant injured in noncollision transport accident in nontraffic accident

X ● **V48.4**   Person boarding or alighting a car injured in noncollision transport accident

X ● **V48.5**   Car driver injured in noncollision transport accident in traffic accident

X ● **V48.6**   Car passenger injured in noncollision transport accident in traffic accident

X ● **V48.7**   Person on outside of car injured in noncollision transport accident in traffic accident

X ● **V48.9**   Unspecified car occupant injured in noncollision transport accident in traffic accident

● **V49**   Car occupant injured in other and unspecified transport accidents

The appropriate 7th character is to be added to each code from category V49

A	initial encounter
D	subsequent encounter
S	sequela

● **V49.0**   Driver injured in collision with other and unspecified motor vehicles in nontraffic accident

X ● **V49.00**   Driver injured in collision with unspecified motor vehicles in nontraffic accident

X ● **V49.09**   Driver injured in collision with other motor vehicles in nontraffic accident

● **V49.1**   Passenger injured in collision with other and unspecified motor vehicles in nontraffic accident

X ● **V49.10**   Passenger injured in collision with unspecified motor vehicles in nontraffic accident

X ● **V49.19**   Passenger injured in collision with other motor vehicles in nontraffic accident

● **V49.2**   Unspecified car occupant injured in collision with other and unspecified motor vehicles in nontraffic accident

X ● **V49.20**   Unspecified car occupant injured in collision with unspecified motor vehicles in nontraffic accident
Car collision NOS, nontraffic

X ● **V49.29**   Unspecified car occupant injured in collision with other motor vehicles in nontraffic accident

X ● **V49.3**   Car occupant (driver) (passenger) injured in unspecified nontraffic accident
Car accident NOS, nontraffic
Car occupant injured in nontraffic accident NOS

● **V49.4**   Driver injured in collision with other and unspecified motor vehicles in traffic accident

X ● **V49.40**   Driver injured in collision with unspecified motor vehicles in traffic accident

X ● **V49.49**   Driver injured in collision with other motor vehicles in traffic accident

● **V49.5**   Passenger injured in collision with other and unspecified motor vehicles in traffic accident

X ● **V49.50**   Passenger injured in collision with unspecified motor vehicles in traffic accident

X ● **V49.59**   Passenger injured in collision with other motor vehicles in traffic accident

● **V49.6**   Unspecified car occupant injured in collision with other and unspecified motor vehicles in traffic accident

X ● **V49.60**   Unspecified car occupant injured in collision with unspecified motor vehicles in traffic accident
Car collision NOS (traffic)

X ● **V49.69**   Unspecified car occupant injured in collision with other motor vehicles in traffic accident

● **V49.8**   Car occupant (driver) (passenger) injured in other specified transport accidents

X ● **V49.81**   Car occupant (driver) (passenger) injured in transport accident with military vehicle

X ● **V49.88**   Car occupant (driver) (passenger) injured in other specified transport accidents

X ● **V49.9**   Car occupant (driver) (passenger) injured in unspecified traffic accident
Car accident NOS
Coding Clinic: 2015, Q1, P11

CHAPTER 20 (V00-Y99)

OCCUPANT OF PICK-UP TRUCK OR VAN INJURED IN TRANSPORT ACCIDENT (V50-V59)

Includes   a four- or six-wheel motor vehicle designed primarily for carrying passengers and property but weighing less than the local limit for classification as a heavy goods vehicle
minibus
minivan
sport utility vehicle (SUV)
truck
van

Excludes1   heavy transport vehicle (V60-V69)

● **V50 Occupant of pick-up truck or van injured in collision with pedestrian or animal**

Excludes1   pick-up truck or van collision with animal-drawn vehicle or animal being ridden (V56.-)

The appropriate 7th character is to be added to each code from category V50

A	initial encounter	
D	subsequent encounter	
S	sequela	

X● **V50.0 Driver** of pick-up truck or van injured in collision with pedestrian or animal in nontraffic accident

X● **V50.1 Passenger** in pick-up truck or van injured in collision with pedestrian or animal in nontraffic accident

X● **V50.2 Person on outside** of pick-up truck or van injured in collision with pedestrian or animal in nontraffic accident

X● **V50.3 Unspecified** occupant of pick-up truck or van injured in collision with pedestrian or animal in nontraffic accident

X● **V50.4 Person boarding or alighting** a pick-up truck or van injured in collision with pedestrian or animal

X● **V50.5 Driver** of pick-up truck or van injured in collision with pedestrian or animal in traffic accident

X● **V50.6 Passenger** in pick-up truck or van injured in collision with pedestrian or animal in traffic accident

X● **V50.7 Person on outside** of pick-up truck or van injured in collision with pedestrian or animal in traffic accident

X● **V50.9 Unspecified** occupant of pick-up truck or van injured in collision with pedestrian or animal in traffic accident

● **V51 Occupant of pick-up truck or van injured in collision with pedal cycle**

The appropriate 7th character is to be added to each code from category V51

A	initial encounter	
D	subsequent encounter	
S	sequela	

X● **V51.0 Driver** of pick-up truck or van injured in collision with pedal cycle in nontraffic accident

X● **V51.1 Passenger** in pick-up truck or van injured in collision with pedal cycle in nontraffic accident

X● **V51.2 Person on outside** of pick-up truck or van injured in collision with pedal cycle in nontraffic accident

X● **V51.3 Unspecified** occupant of pick-up truck or van injured in collision with pedal cycle in nontraffic accident

X● **V51.4 Person boarding or alighting** a pick-up truck or van injured in collision with pedal cycle

X● **V51.5 Driver** of pick-up truck or van injured in collision with pedal cycle in traffic accident

X● **V51.6 Passenger** in pick-up truck or van injured in collision with pedal cycle in traffic accident

X● **V51.7 Person on outside** of pick-up truck or van injured in collision with pedal cycle in traffic accident

X● **V51.9 Unspecified** occupant of pick-up truck or van injured in collision with pedal cycle in traffic accident

● **V52 Occupant of pick-up truck or van injured in collision with two- or three-wheeled motor vehicle**

The appropriate 7th character is to be added to each code from category V52

A	initial encounter	
D	subsequent encounter	
S	sequela	

X● **V52.0 Driver** of pick-up truck or van injured in collision with two- or three-wheeled motor vehicle in nontraffic accident

X● **V52.1 Passenger** in pick-up truck or van injured in collision with two- or three-wheeled motor vehicle in nontraffic accident

X● **V52.2 Person on outside** of pick-up truck or van injured in collision with two- or three-wheeled motor vehicle in nontraffic accident

X● **V52.3 Unspecified** occupant of pick-up truck or van injured in collision with two- or three-wheeled motor vehicle in nontraffic accident

X● **V52.4 Person boarding or alighting** a pick-up truck or van injured in collision with two- or three-wheeled motor vehicle

X● **V52.5 Driver** of pick-up truck or van injured in collision with two- or three-wheeled motor vehicle in traffic accident

X● **V52.6 Passenger** in pick-up truck or van injured in collision with two- or three-wheeled motor vehicle in traffic accident

X● **V52.7 Person on outside** of pick-up truck or van injured in collision with two- or three-wheeled motor vehicle in traffic accident

X● **V52.9 Unspecified** occupant of pick-up truck or van injured in collision with two- or three-wheeled motor vehicle in traffic accident

● **V53 Occupant of pick-up truck or van injured in collision with car, pick-up truck or van**

The appropriate 7th character is to be added to each code from category V53

A	initial encounter	
D	subsequent encounter	
S	sequela	

X● **V53.0 Driver** of pick-up truck or van injured in collision with car, pick-up truck or van in nontraffic accident

X● **V53.1 Passenger** in pick-up truck or van injured in collision with car, pick-up truck or van in nontraffic accident

X● **V53.2 Person on outside** of pick-up truck or van injured in collision with car, pick-up truck or van in nontraffic accident

X● **V53.3 Unspecified** occupant of pick-up truck or van injured in collision with car, pick-up truck or van in nontraffic accident

X● **V53.4 Person boarding or alighting** a pick-up truck or van injured in collision with car, pick-up truck or van

X● **V53.5 Driver** of pick-up truck or van injured in collision with car, pick-up truck or van in traffic accident

X● **V53.6 Passenger** in pick-up truck or van injured in collision with car, pick-up truck or van in traffic accident

X● **V53.7 Person on outside** of pick-up truck or van injured in collision with car, pick-up truck or van in traffic accident

X● **V53.9 Unspecified** occupant of pick-up truck or van injured in collision with car, pick-up truck or van in traffic accident

► New   ◄ Revised   ~~deleted~~ Deleted   Excludes 1   Excludes 2   Includes   Use additional   Code first   Code also   Key words
OGCR Official Guidelines   X Assign placeholder X   ● Use Additional Character(s)   ► Manifestation Code   HCC Hierarchical Condition Category   **Coding Clinic**

● **V54**   **Occupant of pick-up truck or van injured in collision with heavy transport vehicle or bus**

> **Excludes1**   occupant of pick-up truck or van injured in collision with military vehicle (V59.81)

> The appropriate 7th character is to be added to each code from category V54

> | A | initial encounter |
> | D | subsequent encounter |
> | S | sequela |

X● **V54.0**   Driver of pick-up truck or van injured in collision with heavy transport vehicle or bus in nontraffic accident

X● **V54.1**   Passenger in pick-up truck or van injured in collision with heavy transport vehicle or bus in nontraffic accident

X● **V54.2**   Person on outside of pick-up truck or van injured in collision with heavy transport vehicle or bus in nontraffic accident

X● **V54.3**   Unspecified occupant of pick-up truck or van injured in collision with heavy transport vehicle or bus in nontraffic accident

X● **V54.4**   Person boarding or alighting a pick-up truck or van injured in collision with heavy transport vehicle or bus

X● **V54.5**   Driver of pick-up truck or van injured in collision with heavy transport vehicle or bus in traffic accident

X● **V54.6**   Passenger in pick-up truck or van injured in collision with heavy transport vehicle or bus in traffic accident

X● **V54.7**   Person on outside of pick-up truck or van injured in collision with heavy transport vehicle or bus in traffic accident

X● **V54.9**   Unspecified occupant of pick-up truck or van injured in collision with heavy transport vehicle or bus in traffic accident

● **V55**   **Occupant of pick-up truck or van injured in collision with railway train or railway vehicle**

> The appropriate 7th character is to be added to each code from category V55

> | A | initial encounter |
> | D | subsequent encounter |
> | S | sequela |

X● **V55.0**   Driver of pick-up truck or van injured in collision with railway train or railway vehicle in nontraffic accident

X● **V55.1**   Passenger in pick-up truck or van injured in collision with railway train or railway vehicle in nontraffic accident

X● **V55.2**   Person on outside of pick-up truck or van injured in collision with railway train or railway vehicle in nontraffic accident

X● **V55.3**   Unspecified occupant of pick-up truck or van injured in collision with railway train or railway vehicle in nontraffic accident

X● **V55.4**   Person boarding or alighting a pick-up truck or van injured in collision with railway train or railway vehicle

X● **V55.5**   Driver of pick-up truck or van injured in collision with railway train or railway vehicle in traffic accident

X● **V55.6**   Passenger in pick-up truck or van injured in collision with railway train or railway vehicle in traffic accident

X● **V55.7**   Person on outside of pick-up truck or van injured in collision with railway train or railway vehicle in traffic accident

X● **V55.9**   Unspecified occupant of pick-up truck or van injured in collision with railway train or railway vehicle in traffic accident

● **V56**   **Occupant of pick-up truck or van injured in collision with other nonmotor vehicle**

> **Includes**   collision with animal-drawn vehicle, animal being ridden, streetcar

> The appropriate 7th character is to be added to each code from category V56

> | A | initial encounter |
> | D | subsequent encounter |
> | S | sequela |

X● **V56.0**   Driver of pick-up truck or van injured in collision with other nonmotor vehicle in nontraffic accident

X● **V56.1**   Passenger in pick-up truck or van injured in collision with other nonmotor vehicle in nontraffic accident

X● **V56.2**   Person on outside of pick-up truck or van injured in collision with other nonmotor vehicle in nontraffic accident

X● **V56.3**   Unspecified occupant of pick-up truck or van injured in collision with other nonmotor vehicle in nontraffic accident

X● **V56.4**   Person boarding or alighting a pick-up truck or van injured in collision with other nonmotor vehicle

X● **V56.5**   Driver of pick-up truck or van injured in collision with other nonmotor vehicle in traffic accident

X● **V56.6**   Passenger in pick-up truck or van injured in collision with other nonmotor vehicle in traffic accident

X● **V56.7**   Person on outside of pick-up truck or van injured in collision with other nonmotor vehicle in traffic accident

X● **V56.9**   Unspecified occupant of pick-up truck or van injured in collision with other nonmotor vehicle in traffic accident

● **V57**   **Occupant of pick-up truck or van injured in collision with fixed or stationary object**

> The appropriate 7th character is to be added to each code from category V57

> | A | initial encounter |
> | D | subsequent encounter |
> | S | sequela |

X● **V57.0**   Driver of pick-up truck or van injured in collision with fixed or stationary object in nontraffic accident

X● **V57.1**   Passenger in pick-up truck or van injured in collision with fixed or stationary object in nontraffic accident

X● **V57.2**   Person on outside of pick-up truck or van injured in collision with fixed or stationary object in nontraffic accident

X● **V57.3**   Unspecified occupant of pick-up truck or van injured in collision with fixed or stationary object in nontraffic accident

X● **V57.4**   Person boarding or alighting a pick-up truck or van injured in collision with fixed or stationary object

X● **V57.5**   Driver of pick-up truck or van injured in collision with fixed or stationary object in traffic accident

X● **V57.6**   Passenger in pick-up truck or van injured in collision with fixed or stationary object in traffic accident

X● **V57.7**   Person on outside of pick-up truck or van injured in collision with fixed or stationary object in traffic accident

X● **V57.9**   Unspecified occupant of pick-up truck or van injured in collision with fixed or stationary object in traffic accident

CHAPTER 20 (V00-Y99)

● **V58 Occupant of pick-up truck or van injured in noncollision transport accident**

> **Includes**   overturning pick-up truck or van NOS
>   overturning pick-up truck or van without collision

The appropriate 7th character is to be added to each code from category V58

> A   initial encounter
> D   subsequent encounter
> S   sequela

X● **V58.0** Driver of pick-up truck or van injured in noncollision transport accident in nontraffic accident

X● **V58.1** Passenger in pick-up truck or van injured in noncollision transport accident in nontraffic accident

X● **V58.2** Person on outside of pick-up truck or van injured in noncollision transport accident in nontraffic accident

X● **V58.3** Unspecified occupant of pick-up truck or van injured in noncollision transport accident in nontraffic accident

X● **V58.4** Person boarding or alighting a pick-up truck or van injured in noncollision transport accident

X● **V58.5** Driver of pick-up truck or van injured in noncollision transport accident in traffic accident

X● **V58.6** Passenger in pick-up truck or van injured in noncollision transport accident in traffic accident

X● **V58.7** Person on outside of pick-up truck or van injured in noncollision transport accident in traffic accident

X● **V58.9** Unspecified occupant of pick-up truck or van injured in noncollision transport accident in traffic accident

● **V59 Occupant of pick-up truck or van injured in other and unspecified transport accidents**

The appropriate 7th character is to be added to each code from category V59

> A   initial encounter
> D   subsequent encounter
> S   sequela

● **V59.0** Driver of pick-up truck or van injured in collision with other and unspecified motor vehicles in nontraffic accident

   X● **V59.00** Driver of pick-up truck or van injured in collision with unspecified motor vehicles in nontraffic accident

   X● **V59.09** Driver of pick-up truck or van injured in collision with other motor vehicles in nontraffic accident

● **V59.1** Passenger in pick-up truck or van injured in collision with other and unspecified motor vehicles in nontraffic accident

   X● **V59.10** Passenger in pick-up truck or van injured in collision with unspecified motor vehicles in nontraffic accident

   X● **V59.19** Passenger in pick-up truck or van injured in collision with other motor vehicles in nontraffic accident

● **V59.2** Unspecified occupant of pick-up truck or van injured in collision with other and unspecified motor vehicles in nontraffic accident

   X● **V59.20** Unspecified occupant of pick-up truck or van injured in collision with unspecified motor vehicles in nontraffic accident
> Collision NOS involving pick-up truck or van, nontraffic

   X● **V59.29** Unspecified occupant of pick-up truck or van injured in collision with other motor vehicles in nontraffic accident

X● **V59.3** Occupant (driver) (passenger) of pick-up truck or van injured in unspecified nontraffic accident
> Accident NOS involving pick-up truck or van, nontraffic
> Occupant of pick-up truck or van injured in nontraffic accident NOS

● **V59.4** Driver of pick-up truck or van injured in collision with other and unspecified motor vehicles in traffic accident

   X● **V59.40** Driver of pick-up truck or van injured in collision with unspecified motor vehicles in traffic accident

   X● **V59.49** Driver of pick-up truck or van injured in collision with other motor vehicles in traffic accident

● **V59.5** Passenger in pick-up truck or van injured in collision with other and unspecified motor vehicles in traffic accident

   X● **V59.50** Passenger in pick-up truck or van injured in collision with unspecified motor vehicles in traffic accident

   X● **V59.59** Passenger in pick-up truck or van injured in collision with other motor vehicles in traffic accident

● **V59.6** Unspecified occupant of pick-up truck or van injured in collision with other and unspecified motor vehicles in traffic accident

   X● **V59.60** Unspecified occupant of pick-up truck or van injured in collision with unspecified motor vehicles in traffic accident
> Collision NOS involving pick-up truck or van (traffic)

   X● **V59.69** Unspecified occupant of pick-up truck or van injured in collision with other motor vehicles in traffic accident

● **V59.8** Occupant (driver) (passenger) of pick-up truck or van injured in other specified transport accidents

   X● **V59.81** Occupant (driver) (passenger) of pick-up truck or van injured in transport accident with military vehicle

   X● **V59.88** Occupant (driver) (passenger) of pick-up truck or van injured in other specified transport accidents

X● **V59.9** Occupant (driver) (passenger) of pick-up truck or van injured in unspecified traffic accident
> Accident NOS involving pick-up truck or van

OCCUPANT OF HEAVY TRANSPORT VEHICLE INJURED IN TRANSPORT ACCIDENT (V60-V69)

> **Includes**   18 wheeler
>   armored car
>   panel truck
>
> **Excludes1**   bus
>   motorcoach

● **V60 Occupant of heavy transport vehicle injured in collision with pedestrian or animal**

> **Excludes1**   heavy transport vehicle collision with animal-drawn vehicle or animal being ridden (V66.-)

The appropriate 7th character is to be added to each code from category V60

> A   initial encounter
> D   subsequent encounter
> S   sequela

X● **V60.0** Driver of heavy transport vehicle injured in collision with pedestrian or animal in nontraffic accident

X● **V60.1** Passenger in heavy transport vehicle injured in collision with pedestrian or animal in nontraffic accident

X● **V60.2** Person on outside of heavy transport vehicle injured in collision with pedestrian or animal in nontraffic accident

X● **V60.3** Unspecified occupant of heavy transport vehicle injured in collision with pedestrian or animal in nontraffic accident

X● **V60.4** Person boarding or alighting a heavy transport vehicle injured in collision with pedestrian or animal

X● **V60.5** Driver of heavy transport vehicle injured in collision with pedestrian or animal in traffic accident

---

▶ New   ⬛ Revised   ~~deleted~~ Deleted   Excludes 1   Excludes 2   Includes   Use additional   Code first   Code also   Key words

OGCR Official Guidelines   X Assign placeholder X   ● Use Additional Character(s)   ▶ Manifestation Code   Hierarchical Condition Category   **Coding Clinic** 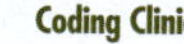

X● **V60.6** **Passenger** in heavy transport vehicle injured in collision with pedestrian or animal in traffic accident

X● **V60.7** **Person on outside** of heavy transport vehicle injured in collision with pedestrian or animal in traffic accident

X● **V60.9** **Unspecified** occupant of heavy transport vehicle injured in collision with pedestrian or animal in traffic accident

● **V61** **Occupant** of heavy transport vehicle injured in collision with pedal cycle

The appropriate 7th character is to be added to each code from category V61

A	initial encounter
D	subsequent encounter
S	sequela

X● **V61.0** **Driver** of heavy transport vehicle injured in collision with pedal cycle in nontraffic accident

X● **V61.1** **Passenger** in heavy transport vehicle injured in collision with pedal cycle in nontraffic accident

X● **V61.2** **Person on outside** of heavy transport vehicle injured in collision with pedal cycle in nontraffic accident

X● **V61.3** **Unspecified** occupant of heavy transport vehicle injured in collision with pedal cycle in nontraffic accident

X● **V61.4** **Person boarding or alighting** a heavy transport vehicle injured in collision with pedal cycle while boarding or alighting

X● **V61.5** **Driver** of heavy transport vehicle injured in collision with pedal cycle in traffic accident

X● **V61.6** **Passenger** in heavy transport vehicle injured in collision with pedal cycle in traffic accident

X● **V61.7** **Person on outside** of heavy transport vehicle injured in collision with pedal cycle in traffic accident

X● **V61.9** **Unspecified** occupant of heavy transport vehicle injured in collision with pedal cycle in traffic accident

● **V62** **Occupant** of heavy transport vehicle injured in collision with two- or three-wheeled motor vehicle

The appropriate 7th character is to be added to each code from category V62

A	initial encounter
D	subsequent encounter
S	sequela

X● **V62.0** **Driver** of heavy transport vehicle injured in collision with two- or three-wheeled motor vehicle in nontraffic accident

X● **V62.1** **Passenger** in heavy transport vehicle injured in collision with two- or three-wheeled motor vehicle in nontraffic accident

X● **V62.2** **Person on outside** of heavy transport vehicle injured in collision with two- or three-wheeled motor vehicle in nontraffic accident

X● **V62.3** **Unspecified** occupant of heavy transport vehicle injured in collision with two- or three-wheeled motor vehicle in nontraffic accident

X● **V62.4** **Person boarding or alighting** a heavy transport vehicle injured in collision with two- or three-wheeled motor vehicle

X● **V62.5** **Driver** of heavy transport vehicle injured in collision with two- or three-wheeled motor vehicle in traffic accident

X● **V62.6** **Passenger** in heavy transport vehicle injured in collision with two- or three-wheeled motor vehicle in traffic accident

X● **V62.7** **Person on outside** of heavy transport vehicle injured in collision with two- or three-wheeled motor vehicle in traffic accident

X● **V62.9** **Unspecified** occupant of heavy transport vehicle injured in collision with two- or three-wheeled motor vehicle in traffic accident

● **V63** **Occupant** of heavy transport vehicle injured in collision with car, pick-up truck or van

The appropriate 7th character is to be added to each code from category V63

A	initial encounter
D	subsequent encounter
S	sequela

X● **V63.0** **Driver** of heavy transport vehicle injured in collision with car, pick-up truck or van in nontraffic accident

X● **V63.1** **Passenger** in heavy transport vehicle injured in collision with car, pick-up truck or van in nontraffic accident

X● **V63.2** **Person on outside** of heavy transport vehicle injured in collision with car, pick-up truck or van in nontraffic accident

X● **V63.3** **Unspecified** occupant of heavy transport vehicle injured in collision with car, pick-up truck or van in nontraffic accident

X● **V63.4** **Person boarding or alighting** a heavy transport vehicle injured in collision with car, pick-up truck or van

X● **V63.5** **Driver** of heavy transport vehicle injured in collision with car, pick-up truck or van in traffic accident

X● **V63.6** **Passenger** in heavy transport vehicle injured in collision with car, pick-up truck or van in traffic accident

X● **V63.7** **Person on outside** of heavy transport vehicle injured in collision with car, pick-up truck or van in traffic accident

X● **V63.9** **Unspecified** occupant of heavy transport vehicle injured in collision with car, pick-up truck or van in traffic accident

● **V64** **Occupant** of heavy transport vehicle injured in collision with heavy transport vehicle or bus

Excludes1   occupant of heavy transport vehicle injured in collision with military vehicle (V69.81)

The appropriate 7th character is to be added to each code from category V64

A	initial encounter
D	subsequent encounter
S	sequela

X● **V64.0** **Driver** of heavy transport vehicle injured in collision with heavy transport vehicle or bus in nontraffic accident

X● **V64.1** **Passenger** in heavy transport vehicle injured in collision with heavy transport vehicle or bus in nontraffic accident

X● **V64.2** **Person on outside** of heavy transport vehicle injured in collision with heavy transport vehicle or bus in nontraffic accident

X● **V64.3** **Unspecified** occupant of heavy transport vehicle injured in collision with heavy transport vehicle or bus in nontraffic accident

X● **V64.4** **Person boarding or alighting** a heavy transport vehicle injured in collision with heavy transport vehicle or bus while boarding or alighting

X● **V64.5** **Driver** of heavy transport vehicle injured in collision with heavy transport vehicle or bus in traffic accident

X● **V64.6** **Passenger** in heavy transport vehicle injured in collision with heavy transport vehicle or bus in traffic accident

X● **V64.7** **Person on outside** of heavy transport vehicle injured in collision with heavy transport vehicle or bus in traffic accident

X● **V64.9** **Unspecified** occupant of heavy transport vehicle injured in collision with heavy transport vehicle or bus in traffic accident

CHAPTER 20 (V00-Y99)

CHAPTER 20 (V00-Y99)

● V65   **Occupant of heavy transport vehicle injured in collision with railway train or railway vehicle**

The appropriate 7th character is to be added to each code from category V65

> A   initial encounter
> D   subsequent encounter
> S   sequela

X● **V65.0**   **Driver** of heavy transport vehicle injured in collision with railway train or railway vehicle in nontraffic accident

X● **V65.1**   **Passenger** in heavy transport vehicle injured in collision with railway train or railway vehicle in nontraffic accident

X● **V65.2**   **Person on outside** of heavy transport vehicle injured in collision with railway train or railway vehicle in nontraffic accident

X● **V65.3**   **Unspecified** occupant of heavy transport vehicle injured in collision with railway train or railway vehicle in nontraffic accident

X● **V65.4**   **Person boarding or alighting** a heavy transport vehicle injured in collision with railway train or railway vehicle

X● **V65.5**   **Driver** of heavy transport vehicle injured in collision with railway train or railway vehicle in traffic accident

X● **V65.6**   **Passenger** in heavy transport vehicle injured in collision with railway train or railway vehicle in traffic accident

X● **V65.7**   **Person on outside** of heavy transport vehicle injured in collision with railway train or railway vehicle in traffic accident

X● **V65.9**   **Unspecified** occupant of heavy transport vehicle injured in collision with railway train or railway vehicle in traffic accident

● V66   **Occupant of heavy transport vehicle injured in collision with other nonmotor vehicle**

> **Includes**   collision with animal-drawn vehicle, animal being ridden, streetcar

The appropriate 7th character is to be added to each code from category V66

> A   initial encounter
> D   subsequent encounter
> S   sequela

X● **V66.0**   **Driver** of heavy transport vehicle injured in collision with other nonmotor vehicle in nontraffic accident

X● **V66.1**   **Passenger** in heavy transport vehicle injured in collision with other nonmotor vehicle in nontraffic accident

X● **V66.2**   **Person on outside** of heavy transport vehicle injured in collision with other nonmotor vehicle in nontraffic accident

X● **V66.3**   **Unspecified** occupant of heavy transport vehicle injured in collision with other nonmotor vehicle in nontraffic accident

X● **V66.4**   **Person boarding or alighting** a heavy transport vehicle injured in collision with other nonmotor vehicle

X● **V66.5**   **Driver** of heavy transport vehicle injured in collision with other nonmotor vehicle in traffic accident

X● **V66.6**   **Passenger** in heavy transport vehicle injured in collision with other nonmotor vehicle in traffic accident

X● **V66.7**   **Person on outside** of heavy transport vehicle injured in collision with other nonmotor vehicle in traffic accident

X● **V66.9**   **Unspecified** occupant of heavy transport vehicle injured in collision with other nonmotor vehicle in traffic accident

● V67   **Occupant of heavy transport vehicle injured in collision with fixed or stationary object**

The appropriate 7th character is to be added to each code from category V67

> A   initial encounter
> D   subsequent encounter
> S   sequela

X● **V67.0**   **Driver** of heavy transport vehicle injured in collision with fixed or stationary object in nontraffic accident

X● **V67.1**   **Passenger** in heavy transport vehicle injured in collision with fixed or stationary object in nontraffic accident

X● **V67.2**   **Person on outside** of heavy transport vehicle injured in collision with fixed or stationary object in nontraffic accident

X● **V67.3**   **Unspecified** occupant of heavy transport vehicle injured in collision with fixed or stationary object in nontraffic accident

X● **V67.4**   **Person boarding or alighting** a heavy transport vehicle injured in collision with fixed or stationary object

X● **V67.5**   **Driver** of heavy transport vehicle injured in collision with fixed or stationary object in traffic accident

X● **V67.6**   **Passenger** in heavy transport vehicle injured in collision with fixed or stationary object in traffic accident

X● **V67.7**   **Person on outside** of heavy transport vehicle injured in collision with fixed or stationary object in traffic accident

X● **V67.9**   **Unspecified** occupant of heavy transport vehicle injured in collision with fixed or stationary object in traffic accident

● V68   **Occupant of heavy transport vehicle injured in noncollision transport accident**

> **Includes**   overturning heavy transport vehicle NOS
> overturning heavy transport vehicle without collision

The appropriate 7th character is to be added to each code from category V68

> A   initial encounter
> D   subsequent encounter
> S   sequela

X● **V68.0**   **Driver** of heavy transport vehicle injured in noncollision transport accident in nontraffic accident

X● **V68.1**   **Passenger** in heavy transport vehicle injured in noncollision transport accident in nontraffic accident

X● **V68.2**   **Person on outside** of heavy transport vehicle injured in noncollision transport accident in nontraffic accident

X● **V68.3**   **Unspecified** occupant of heavy transport vehicle injured in noncollision transport accident in nontraffic accident

X● **V68.4**   **Person boarding or alighting** a heavy transport vehicle injured in noncollision transport accident

X● **V68.5**   **Driver** of heavy transport vehicle injured in noncollision transport accident in traffic accident

X● **V68.6**   **Passenger** in heavy transport vehicle injured in noncollision transport accident in traffic accident

X● **V68.7**   **Person on outside** of heavy transport vehicle injured in noncollision transport accident in traffic accident

X● **V68.9**   **Unspecified** occupant of heavy transport vehicle injured in noncollision transport accident in traffic accident

● **V69** **Occupant of heavy transport vehicle injured in other and unspecified transport accidents**

The appropriate 7th character is to be added to each code from category V69

A	initial encounter
D	subsequent encounter
S	sequela

● **V69.0** **Driver of heavy transport vehicle injured in collision with other and unspecified motor vehicles in nontraffic accident**

X ● **V69.00** Driver of heavy transport vehicle injured in collision with unspecified motor vehicles in nontraffic accident

X ● **V69.09** Driver of heavy transport vehicle injured in collision with other motor vehicles in nontraffic accident

● **V69.1** **Passenger in heavy transport vehicle injured in collision with other and unspecified motor vehicles in nontraffic accident**

X ● **V69.10** Passenger in heavy transport vehicle injured in collision with unspecified motor vehicles in nontraffic accident

X ● **V69.19** Passenger in heavy transport vehicle injured in collision with other motor vehicles in nontraffic accident

● **V69.2** **Unspecified occupant of heavy transport vehicle injured in collision with other and unspecified motor vehicles in nontraffic accident**

X ● **V69.20** Unspecified occupant of heavy transport vehicle injured in collision with unspecified motor vehicles in nontraffic accident

    Collision NOS involving heavy transport vehicle, nontraffic

X ● **V69.29** Unspecified occupant of heavy transport vehicle injured in collision with other motor vehicles in nontraffic accident

X ● **V69.3** **Occupant (driver) (passenger) of heavy transport vehicle injured in unspecified nontraffic accident**

    Accident NOS involving heavy transport vehicle, nontraffic

    Occupant of heavy transport vehicle injured in nontraffic accident NOS

● **V69.4** **Driver of heavy transport vehicle injured in collision with other and unspecified motor vehicles in traffic accident**

X ● **V69.40** Driver of heavy transport vehicle injured in collision with unspecified motor vehicles in traffic accident

X ● **V69.49** Driver of heavy transport vehicle injured in collision with other motor vehicles in traffic accident

● **V69.5** **Passenger in heavy transport vehicle injured in collision with other and unspecified motor vehicles in traffic accident**

X ● **V69.50** Passenger in heavy transport vehicle injured in collision with unspecified motor vehicles in traffic accident

X ● **V69.59** Passenger in heavy transport vehicle injured in collision with other motor vehicles in traffic accident

● **V69.6** **Unspecified occupant of heavy transport vehicle injured in collision with other and unspecified motor vehicles in traffic accident**

X ● **V69.60** Unspecified occupant of heavy transport vehicle injured in collision with unspecified motor vehicles in traffic accident

    Collision NOS involving heavy transport vehicle (traffic)

X ● **V69.69** Unspecified occupant of heavy transport vehicle injured in collision with other motor vehicles in traffic accident

● **V69.8** **Occupant (driver) (passenger) of heavy transport vehicle injured in other specified transport accidents**

X ● **V69.81** Occupant (driver) (passenger) of heavy transport vehicle injured in transport accidents with military vehicle

X ● **V69.88** Occupant (driver) (passenger) of heavy transport vehicle injured in other specified transport accidents

X ● **V69.9** **Occupant (driver) (passenger) of heavy transport vehicle injured in unspecified traffic accident**

    Accident NOS involving heavy transport vehicle

BUS OCCUPANT INJURED IN TRANSPORT ACCIDENT (V70-V79)

Includes	motorcoach
Excludes1	minibus (V50-V59)

● **V70** **Bus occupant injured in collision with pedestrian or animal**

Excludes1   bus collision with animal-drawn vehicle or animal being ridden (V76.-)

The appropriate 7th character is to be added to each code from category V70

A	initial encounter
D	subsequent encounter
S	sequela

X ● **V70.0** **Driver of bus injured in collision with pedestrian or animal in nontraffic accident**

X ● **V70.1** **Passenger on bus injured in collision with pedestrian or animal in nontraffic accident**

X ● **V70.2** **Person on outside of bus injured in collision with pedestrian or animal in nontraffic accident**

X ● **V70.3** **Unspecified occupant of bus injured in collision with pedestrian or animal in nontraffic accident**

X ● **V70.4** **Person boarding or alighting from bus injured in collision with pedestrian or animal**

X ● **V70.5** **Driver of bus injured in collision with pedestrian or animal in traffic accident**

X ● **V70.6** **Passenger on bus injured in collision with pedestrian or animal in traffic accident**

X ● **V70.7** **Person on outside of bus injured in collision with pedestrian or animal in traffic accident**

X ● **V70.9** **Unspecified occupant of bus injured in collision with pedestrian or animal in traffic accident**

● **V71** **Bus occupant injured in collision with pedal cycle**

The appropriate 7th character is to be added to each code from category V71

A	initial encounter
D	subsequent encounter
S	sequela

X ● **V71.0** **Driver of bus injured in collision with pedal cycle in nontraffic accident**

X ● **V71.1** **Passenger on bus injured in collision with pedal cycle in nontraffic accident**

X ● **V71.2** **Person on outside of bus injured in collision with pedal cycle in nontraffic accident**

X ● **V71.3** **Unspecified occupant of bus injured in collision with pedal cycle in nontraffic accident**

X ● **V71.4** **Person boarding or alighting from bus injured in collision with pedal cycle**

X ● **V71.5** **Driver of bus injured in collision with pedal cycle in traffic accident**

X ● **V71.6** **Passenger on bus injured in collision with pedal cycle in traffic accident**

X ● **V71.7** **Person on outside of bus injured in collision with pedal cycle in traffic accident**

X ● **V71.9** **Unspecified occupant of bus injured in collision with pedal cycle in traffic accident**

● **V72** **Bus occupant injured in collision with two- or three-wheeled motor vehicle**

The appropriate 7th character is to be added to each code from category V72

> A   initial encounter
> D   subsequent encounter
> S   sequela

X● **V72.0** Driver of bus injured in collision with two- or three-wheeled motor vehicle in nontraffic accident

X● **V72.1** Passenger on bus injured in collision with two- or three-wheeled motor vehicle in nontraffic accident

X● **V72.2** Person on outside of bus injured in collision with two- or three-wheeled motor vehicle in nontraffic accident

X● **V72.3** Unspecified occupant of bus injured in collision with two- or three-wheeled motor vehicle in nontraffic accident

X● **V72.4** Person boarding or alighting from bus injured in collision with two- or three-wheeled motor vehicle

X● **V72.5** Driver of bus injured in collision with two- or three-wheeled motor vehicle in traffic accident

X● **V72.6** Passenger on bus injured in collision with two- or three-wheeled motor vehicle in traffic accident

X● **V72.7** Person on outside of bus injured in collision with two- or three-wheeled motor vehicle in traffic accident

X● **V72.9** Unspecified occupant of bus injured in collision with two- or three-wheeled motor vehicle in traffic accident

● **V73** **Bus occupant injured in collision with car, pick-up truck or van**

The appropriate 7th character is to be added to each code from category V73

> A   initial encounter
> D   subsequent encounter
> S   sequela

X● **V73.0** Driver of bus injured in collision with car, pick-up truck or van in nontraffic accident

X● **V73.1** Passenger on bus injured in collision with car, pick-up truck or van in nontraffic accident

X● **V73.2** Person on outside of bus injured in collision with car, pick-up truck or van in nontraffic accident

X● **V73.3** Unspecified occupant of bus injured in collision with car, pick-up truck or van in nontraffic accident

X● **V73.4** Person boarding or alighting from bus injured in collision with car, pick-up truck or van

X● **V73.5** Driver of bus injured in collision with car, pick-up truck or van in traffic accident

X● **V73.6** Passenger on bus injured in collision with car, pick-up truck or van in traffic accident

X● **V73.7** Person on outside of bus injured in collision with car, pick-up truck or van in traffic accident

X● **V73.9** Unspecified occupant of bus injured in collision with car, pick-up truck or van in traffic accident

● **V74** **Bus occupant injured in collision with heavy transport vehicle or bus**

> **Excludes1**   bus occupant injured in collision with military vehicle (V79.81)

The appropriate 7th character is to be added to each code from category V74

> A   initial encounter
> D   subsequent encounter
> S   sequela

X● **V74.0** Driver of bus injured in collision with heavy transport vehicle or bus in nontraffic accident

X● **V74.1** Passenger on bus injured in collision with heavy transport vehicle or bus in nontraffic accident

X● **V74.2** Person on outside of bus injured in collision with heavy transport vehicle or bus in nontraffic accident

X● **V74.3** Unspecified occupant of bus injured in collision with heavy transport vehicle or bus in nontraffic accident

X● **V74.4** Person boarding or alighting from bus injured in collision with heavy transport vehicle or bus

X● **V74.5** Driver of bus injured in collision with heavy transport vehicle or bus in traffic accident

X● **V74.6** Passenger on bus injured in collision with heavy transport vehicle or bus in traffic accident

X● **V74.7** Person on outside of bus injured in collision with heavy transport vehicle or bus in traffic accident

X● **V74.9** Unspecified occupant of bus injured in collision with heavy transport vehicle or bus in traffic accident

● **V75** **Bus occupant injured in collision with railway train or railway vehicle**

The appropriate 7th character is to be added to each code from category V75

> A   initial encounter
> D   subsequent encounter
> S   sequela

X● **V75.0** Driver of bus injured in collision with railway train or railway vehicle in nontraffic accident

X● **V75.1** Passenger on bus injured in collision with railway train or railway vehicle in nontraffic accident

X● **V75.2** Person on outside of bus injured in collision with railway train or railway vehicle in nontraffic accident

X● **V75.3** Unspecified occupant of bus injured in collision with railway train or railway vehicle in nontraffic accident

X● **V75.4** Person boarding or alighting from bus injured in collision with railway train or railway vehicle

X● **V75.5** Driver of bus injured in collision with railway train or railway vehicle in traffic accident

X● **V75.6** Passenger on bus injured in collision with railway train or railway vehicle in traffic accident

X● **V75.7** Person on outside of bus injured in collision with railway train or railway vehicle in traffic accident

X● **V75.9** Unspecified occupant of bus injured in collision with railway train or railway vehicle in traffic accident

● **V76** **Bus occupant injured in collision with other nonmotor vehicle**

> **Includes**   collision with animal-drawn vehicle, animal being ridden, streetcar

The appropriate 7th character is to be added to each code from category V76

> A   initial encounter
> D   subsequent encounter
> S   sequela

X● **V76.0** Driver of bus injured in collision with other nonmotor vehicle in nontraffic accident

X● **V76.1** Passenger on bus injured in collision with other nonmotor vehicle in nontraffic accident

X● **V76.2** Person on outside of bus injured in collision with other nonmotor vehicle in nontraffic accident

X● **V76.3** Unspecified occupant of bus injured in collision with other nonmotor vehicle in nontraffic accident

X● **V76.4** Person boarding or alighting from bus injured in collision with other nonmotor vehicle

X● **V76.5** Driver of bus injured in collision with other nonmotor vehicle in traffic accident

X● **V76.6** Passenger on bus injured in collision with other nonmotor vehicle in traffic accident

X● **V76.7** Person on outside of bus injured in collision with other nonmotor vehicle in traffic accident

X● **V76.9** Unspecified occupant of bus injured in collision with other nonmotor vehicle in traffic accident

● **V77   Bus occupant injured in collision with fixed or stationary object**

The appropriate 7th character is to be added to each code from category V77

A	initial encounter
D	subsequent encounter
S	sequela

X● **V77.0**   Driver of bus injured in collision with fixed or stationary object in nontraffic accident

X● **V77.1**   Passenger on bus injured in collision with fixed or stationary object in nontraffic accident

X● **V77.2**   Person on outside of bus injured in collision with fixed or stationary object in nontraffic accident

X● **V77.3**   Unspecified occupant of bus injured in collision with fixed or stationary object in nontraffic accident

X● **V77.4**   Person boarding or alighting from bus injured in collision with fixed or stationary object

X● **V77.5**   Driver of bus injured in collision with fixed or stationary object in traffic accident

X● **V77.6**   Passenger on bus injured in collision with fixed or stationary object in traffic accident

X● **V77.7**   Person on outside of bus injured in collision with fixed or stationary object in traffic accident

X● **V77.9**   Unspecified occupant of bus injured in collision with fixed or stationary object in traffic accident

● **V78   Bus occupant injured in noncollision transport accident**

Includes   overturning bus NOS
overturning bus without collision

The appropriate 7th character is to be added to each code from category V78

A	initial encounter
D	subsequent encounter
S	sequela

X● **V78.0**   Driver of bus injured in noncollision transport accident in nontraffic accident

X● **V78.1**   Passenger on bus injured in noncollision transport accident in nontraffic accident

X● **V78.2**   Person on outside of bus injured in noncollision transport accident in nontraffic accident

X● **V78.3**   Unspecified occupant of bus injured in noncollision transport accident in nontraffic accident

X● **V78.4**   Person boarding or alighting from bus injured in noncollision transport accident

X● **V78.5**   Driver of bus injured in noncollision transport accident in traffic accident

X● **V78.6**   Passenger on bus injured in noncollision transport accident in traffic accident

X● **V78.7**   Person on outside of bus injured in noncollision transport accident in traffic accident

X● **V78.9**   Unspecified occupant of bus injured in noncollision transport accident in traffic accident

● **V79   Bus occupant injured in other and unspecified transport accidents**

The appropriate 7th character is to be added to each code from category V79

A	initial encounter
D	subsequent encounter
S	sequela

● **V79.0**   Driver of bus injured in collision with other and unspecified motor vehicles in nontraffic accident

X● **V79.00**   Driver of bus injured in collision with unspecified motor vehicles in nontraffic accident

X● **V79.09**   Driver of bus injured in collision with other motor vehicles in nontraffic accident

● **V79.1**   Passenger on bus injured in collision with other and unspecified motor vehicles in nontraffic accident

X● **V79.10**   Passenger on bus injured in collision with unspecified motor vehicles in nontraffic accident

X● **V79.19**   Passenger on bus injured in collision with other motor vehicles in nontraffic accident

● **V79.2**   Unspecified bus occupant injured in collision with other and unspecified motor vehicles in nontraffic accident

X● **V79.20**   Unspecified bus occupant injured in collision with unspecified motor vehicles in nontraffic accident

Bus collision NOS, nontraffic

X● **V79.29**   Unspecified bus occupant injured in collision with other motor vehicles in nontraffic accident

X● **V79.3**   Bus occupant (driver) (passenger) injured in unspecified nontraffic accident

Bus accident NOS, nontraffic
Bus occupant injured in nontraffic accident NOS

● **V79.4**   Driver of bus injured in collision with other and unspecified motor vehicles in traffic accident

X● **V79.40**   Driver of bus injured in collision with unspecified motor vehicles in traffic accident

X● **V79.49**   Driver of bus injured in collision with other motor vehicles in traffic accident

● **V79.5**   Passenger on bus injured in collision with other and unspecified motor vehicles in traffic accident

X● **V79.50**   Passenger on bus injured in collision with unspecified motor vehicles in traffic accident

X● **V79.59**   Passenger on bus injured in collision with other motor vehicles in traffic accident

● **V79.6**   Unspecified bus occupant injured in collision with other and unspecified motor vehicles in traffic accident

X● **V79.60**   Unspecified bus occupant injured in collision with unspecified motor vehicles in traffic accident

Bus collision NOS (traffic)

X● **V79.69**   Unspecified bus occupant injured in collision with other motor vehicles in traffic accident

● **V79.8**   Bus occupant (driver) (passenger) injured in other specified transport accidents

X● **V79.81**   Bus occupant (driver) (passenger) injured in transport accidents with military vehicle

X● **V79.88**   Bus occupant (driver) (passenger) injured in other specified transport accidents

X● **V79.9**   Bus occupant (driver) (passenger) injured in unspecified traffic accident

Bus accident NOS

OTHER LAND TRANSPORT ACCIDENTS (V80-V89)

● **V80   Animal-rider or occupant of animal-drawn vehicle injured in transport accident**

The appropriate 7th character is to be added to each code from category V80

A	initial encounter
D	subsequent encounter
S	sequela

● **V80.0**   Animal-rider or occupant of animal drawn vehicle injured by fall from or being thrown from animal or animal-drawn vehicle in noncollision accident

● **V80.01**   Animal-rider injured by fall from or being thrown from animal in noncollision accident

● **V80.010**   Animal-rider injured by fall from or being thrown from horse in noncollision accident

● **V80.018**   Animal-rider injured by fall from or being thrown from other animal in noncollision accident

X ● **V80.02** **Occupant** of animal-drawn vehicle injured by fall from or being thrown from animal-drawn vehicle in noncollision accident
Overturning animal-drawn vehicle NOS
Overturning animal-drawn vehicle without collision

● **V80.1** Animal-rider or occupant of animal-drawn vehicle injured in collision with pedestrian or animal

Excludes1 animal-rider or animal-drawn vehicle collision with animal-drawn vehicle or animal being ridden (V80.7)

X ● **V80.11** **Animal-rider** injured in collision with pedestrian or animal

X ● **V80.12** **Occupant** of animal-drawn vehicle injured in collision with pedestrian or animal

● **V80.2** Animal-rider or occupant of animal-drawn vehicle injured in collision with pedal cycle

X ● **V80.21** **Animal-rider** injured in collision with pedal cycle

X ● **V80.22** Occupant of animal-drawn vehicle injured in collision with pedal cycle

● **V80.3** Animal-rider or occupant of animal-drawn vehicle injured in collision with two- or three-wheeled motor vehicle

X ● **V80.31** **Animal-rider** injured in collision with two- or three-wheeled motor vehicle

X ● **V80.32** **Occupant** of animal-drawn vehicle injured in collision with two- or three-wheeled motor vehicle

● **V80.4** Animal-rider or occupant of animal-drawn vehicle injured in collision with car, pick-up truck, van, heavy transport vehicle or bus

Excludes1 animal-rider injured in collision with military vehicle (V80.910)
occupant of animal-drawn vehicle injured in collision with military vehicle (V80.920)

X ● **V80.41** **Animal-rider** injured in collision with car, pick-up truck, van, heavy transport vehicle or bus

X ● **V80.42** **Occupant** of animal-drawn vehicle injured in collision with car, pick-up truck, van, heavy transport vehicle or bus

● **V80.5** Animal-rider or occupant of animal-drawn vehicle injured in collision with other specified motor vehicle

X ● **V80.51** **Animal-rider** injured in collision with other specified motor vehicle

X ● **V80.52** **Occupant** of animal-drawn vehicle injured in collision with other specified motor vehicle

● **V80.6** Animal-rider or occupant of animal-drawn vehicle injured in collision with railway train or railway vehicle

X ● **V80.61** **Animal-rider** injured in collision with railway train or railway vehicle

X ● **V80.62** **Occupant** of animal-drawn vehicle injured in collision with railway train or railway vehicle

● **V80.7** Animal-rider or occupant of animal-drawn vehicle injured in collision with other nonmotor vehicles

● **V80.71** Animal-rider or occupant of animal-drawn vehicle injured in collision with animal being ridden

● **V80.710** **Animal-rider** injured in collision with other animal being ridden

● **V80.711** **Occupant** of animal-drawn vehicle injured in collision with animal being ridden

● **V80.72** Animal-rider or occupant of animal-drawn vehicle injured in collision with other animal-drawn vehicle

● **V80.720** **Animal-rider** injured in collision with animal-drawn vehicle

● **V80.721** **Occupant** of animal-drawn vehicle injured in collision with other animal-drawn vehicle

● **V80.73** Animal-rider or occupant of animal-drawn vehicle injured in collision with streetcar

● **V80.730** **Animal-rider** injured in collision with streetcar

● **V80.731** Occupant of animal-drawn vehicle injured in collision with streetcar

● **V80.79** Animal-rider or occupant of animal-drawn vehicle injured in collision with other nonmotor vehicles

● **V80.790** **Animal-rider** injured in collision with other nonmotor vehicles

● **V80.791** Occupant of animal-drawn vehicle injured in collision with other nonmotor vehicles

● **V80.8** Animal-rider or occupant of animal-drawn vehicle injured in collision with fixed or stationary object

X ● **V80.81** Animal-rider injured in collision with fixed or stationary object

X ● **V80.82** Occupant of animal-drawn vehicle injured in collision with fixed or stationary object

● **V80.9** Animal-rider or occupant of animal-drawn vehicle injured in other and unspecified transport accidents

● **V80.91** Animal-rider injured in other and unspecified transport accidents

● **V80.910** Animal-rider injured in transport accident with military vehicle

● **V80.918** Animal-rider injured in other transport accident

● **V80.919** Animal-rider injured in unspecified transport accident
Animal rider accident NOS

● **V80.92** Occupant of animal-drawn vehicle injured in other and unspecified transport accidents

● **V80.920** Occupant of animal-drawn vehicle injured in transport accident with military vehicle

● **V80.928** Occupant of animal-drawn vehicle injured in other transport accident

● **V80.929** Occupant of animal-drawn vehicle injured in unspecified transport accident
Animal-drawn vehicle accident NOS

● **V81** Occupant of railway train or railway vehicle injured in transport accident

Includes derailment of railway train or railway vehicle
person on outside of train

Excludes1 streetcar (V82.-)

The appropriate 7th character is to be added to each code from category V81

A	initial encounter
D	subsequent encounter
S	sequela

X ● **V81.0** Occupant of railway train or railway vehicle injured in collision with motor vehicle in nontraffic accident

Excludes1 occupant of railway train or railway vehicle injured due to collision with military vehicle (V81.83)

X ● **V81.1** Occupant of railway train or railway vehicle injured in collision with motor vehicle in traffic accident

Excludes1 occupant of railway train or railway vehicle injured due to collision with military vehicle (V81.83)

X ● **V81.2** Occupant of railway train or railway vehicle injured in collision with or hit by rolling stock

X ● **V81.3** Occupant of railway train or railway vehicle injured in collision with other object
Railway collision NOS

X ● **V81.4** Person injured while boarding or alighting from railway train or railway vehicle

▶ New   ⇨ Revised   ~~deleted~~ Deleted   Excludes 1   Excludes 2   Includes   Use additional   Code first   Code also   Key words
OGCR Official Guidelines   X Assign placeholder X   ● Use Additional Character(s)   ▶ Manifestation Code   Ⓗ Hierarchical Condition Category   Coding Clinic

X● **V81.5** **Occupant of railway train or railway vehicle injured by fall in railway train or railway vehicle**

X● **V81.6** **Occupant of railway train or railway vehicle injured by fall from railway train or railway vehicle**

X● **V81.7** **Occupant of railway train or railway vehicle injured in derailment without antecedent collision**

● **V81.8** **Occupant of railway train or railway vehicle injured in other specified railway accidents**

  X● **V81.81** **Occupant of railway train or railway vehicle injured due to explosion or fire on train**

  X● **V81.82** **Occupant of railway train or railway vehicle injured due to object falling onto train**
    Occupant of railway train or railway vehicle injured due to falling earth onto train
    Occupant of railway train or railway vehicle injured due to falling rocks onto train
    Occupant of railway train or railway vehicle injured due to falling snow onto train
    Occupant of railway train or railway vehicle injured due to falling trees onto train

  X● **V81.83** **Occupant of railway train or railway vehicle injured due to collision with military vehicle**

  X● **V81.89** **Occupant of railway train or railway vehicle injured due to other specified railway accident**

X● **V81.9** **Occupant of railway train or railway vehicle injured in unspecified railway accident**
    Railway accident NOS

● **V82** **Occupant of powered streetcar injured in transport accident**

  Includes   interurban electric car
               person on outside of streetcar
               tram (car)
               trolley (car)

  Excludes1   bus (V70-V79)
               motorcoach (V70-V79)
               nonpowered streetcar (V76.-)
               train (V81.-)

The appropriate 7th character is to be added to each code from category V82

A	initial encounter
D	subsequent encounter
S	sequela

X● **V82.0** **Occupant of streetcar injured in collision with motor vehicle in nontraffic accident**

X● **V82.1** **Occupant of streetcar injured in collision with motor vehicle in traffic accident**

X● **V82.2** **Occupant of streetcar injured in collision with or hit by rolling stock**

X● **V82.3** **Occupant of streetcar injured in collision with other object**
    Excludes1   collision with animal-drawn vehicle or animal being ridden (V82.8)

X● **V82.4** **Person injured while boarding or alighting from streetcar**

X● **V82.5** **Occupant of streetcar injured by fall in streetcar**
    Excludes1   fall in streetcar:
        while boarding or alighting (V82.4)
        with antecedent collision (V82.0-V82.3)

X● **V82.6** **Occupant of streetcar injured by fall from streetcar**
    Excludes1   fall from streetcar:
        while boarding or alighting (V82.4)
        with antecedent collision (V82.0-V82.3)

X● **V82.7** **Occupant of streetcar injured in derailment without antecedent collision**
    Excludes1   occupant of streetcar injured in derailment with antecedent collision (V82.0-V82.3)

X● **V82.8** **Occupant of streetcar injured in other specified transport accidents**
    Streetcar collision with military vehicle
    Streetcar collision with train or nonmotor vehicles

X● **V82.9** **Occupant of streetcar injured in unspecified traffic accident**
    Streetcar accident NOS

● **V83** **Occupant of special vehicle mainly used on industrial premises injured in transport accident**

  Includes   battery-powered airport passenger vehicle
               battery-powered truck (baggage) (mail)
               coal-car in mine
               forklift (truck)
               logging car
               self-propelled industrial truck
               station baggage truck (powered)
               tram, truck, or tub (powered) in mine or quarry

  Excludes1   special construction vehicles (V85.-)
               special industrial vehicle in stationary use or maintenance (W31.-)

The appropriate 7th character is to be added to each code from category V83

A	initial encounter
D	subsequent encounter
S	sequela

X● **V83.0** **Driver of special industrial vehicle injured in traffic accident**

X● **V83.1** **Passenger of special industrial vehicle injured in traffic accident**

X● **V83.2** **Person on outside of special industrial vehicle injured in traffic accident**

X● **V83.3** **Unspecified occupant of special industrial vehicle injured in traffic accident**

X● **V83.4** **Person injured while boarding or alighting from special industrial vehicle**

X● **V83.5** **Driver of special industrial vehicle injured in nontraffic accident**

X● **V83.6** **Passenger of special industrial vehicle injured in nontraffic accident**

X● **V83.7** **Person on outside of special industrial vehicle injured in nontraffic accident**

X● **V83.9** **Unspecified occupant of special industrial vehicle injured in nontraffic accident**
    Special-industrial-vehicle accident NOS

● **V84** **Occupant of special vehicle mainly used in agriculture injured in transport accident**

  Includes   self-propelled farm machinery
               tractor (and trailer)

  Excludes1   animal-powered farm machinery accident (W30.8-)
               contact with combine harvester (W30.0)
               special agricultural vehicle in stationary use or maintenance (W30.-)

The appropriate 7th character is to be added to each code from category V84

A	initial encounter
D	subsequent encounter
S	sequela

X● **V84.0** **Driver of special agricultural vehicle injured in traffic accident**

X● **V84.1** **Passenger of special agricultural vehicle injured in traffic accident**

X● **V84.2** **Person on outside of special agricultural vehicle injured in traffic accident**

X● **V84.3** **Unspecified occupant of special agricultural vehicle injured in traffic accident**

X● **V84.4** **Person injured while boarding or alighting from special agricultural vehicle**

X● **V84.5** **Driver of special agricultural vehicle injured in nontraffic accident**

X● **V84.6** **Passenger of special agricultural vehicle injured in nontraffic accident**

CHAPTER 20 (V00-Y99)

X● **V84.7** **Person on outside of special agricultural vehicle injured in nontraffic accident**

X● **V84.9** **Unspecified occupant of special agricultural vehicle injured in nontraffic accident**
Special-agricultural vehicle accident NOS

● **V85** **Occupant of special construction vehicle injured in transport accident**

Includes	bulldozer
	digger
	dump truck
	earth-leveller
	mechanical shovel
	road-roller

Excludes1	special industrial vehicle (V83.-)
	special construction vehicle in stationary use or maintenance (W31.-)

The appropriate 7th character is to be added to each code from category V85

A	initial encounter
D	subsequent encounter
S	sequela

X● **V85.0** **Driver of special construction vehicle injured in traffic accident**

X● **V85.1** **Passenger of special construction vehicle injured in traffic accident**

X● **V85.2** **Person on outside of special construction vehicle injured in traffic accident**

X● **V85.3** **Unspecified occupant of special construction vehicle injured in traffic accident**

X● **V85.4** **Person injured while boarding or alighting from special construction vehicle**

X● **V85.5** **Driver of special construction vehicle injured in nontraffic accident**

X● **V85.6** **Passenger of special construction vehicle injured in nontraffic accident**

X● **V85.7** **Person on outside of special construction vehicle injured in nontraffic accident**

X● **V85.9** **Unspecified occupant of special construction vehicle injured in nontraffic accident**
Special-construction-vehicle accident NOS

● **V86** **Occupant of special all-terrain or other off-road motor vehicle, injured in transport accident**

Excludes1	special all-terrain vehicle in stationary use or maintenance (W31.-)
	sport-utility vehicle (V50-V59)
	three-wheeled motor vehicle designed for on-road use (V30-V39)

The appropriate 7th character is to be added to each code from category V86

A	initial encounter
D	subsequent encounter
S	sequela

● **V86.0** **Driver of special all-terrain or other off-road motor vehicle injured in traffic accident**

X● **V86.01** **Driver of ambulance or fire engine injured in traffic accident**

X● **V86.02** **Driver of snowmobile injured in traffic accident**

X● **V86.03** **Driver of dune buggy injured in traffic accident**

X● **V86.04** **Driver of military vehicle injured in traffic accident**

X● **V86.05** **Driver of 3- or 4-wheeled all-terrain vehicle (ATV) injured in traffic accident**

X● **V86.06** **Driver of dirt bike or motor/cross bike injured in traffic accident**

X● **V86.09** **Driver of other off-road special all-terrain or other off-road vehicle injured in traffic accident**
Driver of go cart injured in traffic accident
Driver of golf cart injured in traffic accident

● **V86.1** **Passenger of special all-terrain or other off-road motor vehicle injured in traffic accident**

X● **V86.11** **Passenger of ambulance or fire engine injured in traffic accident**

X● **V86.12** **Passenger of snowmobile injured in traffic accident**

X● **V86.13** **Passenger of dune buggy injured in traffic accident**

X● **V86.14** **Passenger of military vehicle injured in traffic accident**

X● **V86.15** **Passenger of 3- or 4-wheeled all-terrain vehicle (ATV) injured in traffic accident**

X● **V86.16** **Passenger of dirt bike or motor/cross bike injured in traffic accident**

X● **V86.19** **Passenger of other off-road special all-terrain or other off-road off-road motor vehicle injured in traffic accident**
Passenger of go cart injured in traffic accident
Passenger of golf cart injured in traffic accident

● **V86.2** **Person on outside of special all-terrain or other off-road motor vehicle injured in traffic accident**

X● **V86.21** **Person on outside of ambulance or fire engine injured in traffic accident**

X● **V86.22** **Person on outside of snowmobile injured in traffic accident**

X● **V86.23** **Person on outside of dune buggy injured in traffic accident**

X● **V86.24** **Person on outside of military vehicle injured in traffic accident**

X● **V86.25** **Person on outside of 3- or 4-wheeled all-terrain vehicle (ATV) injured in traffic accident**

X● **V86.26** **Person on outside of dirt bike or motor/cross bike injured in traffic accident**

X● **V86.29** **Person on outside of other special all-terrain or other off-road motor vehicle injured in traffic accident**
Person on outside of go cart in traffic accident
Person on outside of golf cart injured in traffic accident

● **V86.3** **Unspecified occupant of special all-terrain or other off-road motor vehicle injured in traffic accident**

X● **V86.31** **Unspecified occupant of ambulance or fire engine injured in traffic accident**

X● **V86.32** **Unspecified occupant of snowmobile injured in traffic accident**

X● **V86.33** **Unspecified occupant of dune buggy injured in traffic accident**

X● **V86.34** **Unspecified occupant of military vehicle injured in traffic accident**

X● **V86.35** **Unspecified occupant of 3- or 4-wheeled all-terrain vehicle (ATV) injured in traffic accident**

X● **V86.36** **Unspecified occupant of dirt bike or motor/cross bike injured in traffic accident**

X● **V86.39** **Unspecified occupant of other special all-terrain or other off-road motor vehicle injured in traffic accident**
Unspecified occupant of go cart injured in traffic accident
Unspecified occupant of golf cart injured in traffic accident

● **V86.4** **Person injured while boarding or alighting from special all-terrain or other off-road motor vehicle**

X● **V86.41** **Person injured while boarding or alighting from ambulance or fire engine**

X● **V86.42** **Person injured while boarding or alighting from snowmobile**

X● **V86.43** **Person injured while boarding or alighting from dune buggy**

X● **V86.44** **Person injured while boarding or alighting from military vehicle**

X● **V86.45** **Person injured while boarding or alighting from a 3- or 4-wheeled all-terrain vehicle (ATV)**

X ● **V86.46**   Person injured while boarding or alighting from a dirt bike or motor/cross bike

X ● **V86.49**   Person injured while boarding or alighting from other special all-terrain or other off-road motor vehicle

    Person injured while boarding or alighting from go cart

    Person injured while boarding or alighting from golf cart

● **V86.5**   Driver of special all-terrain or other off-road motor vehicle injured in nontraffic accident

X ● **V86.51**   Driver of ambulance or fire engine injured in nontraffic accident

X ● **V86.52**   Driver of snowmobile injured in nontraffic accident

X ● **V86.53**   Driver of dune buggy injured in nontraffic accident

X ● **V86.54**   Driver of military vehicle injured in nontraffic accident

X ● **V86.55**   Driver of 3- or 4-wheeled all-terrain vehicle (ATV) injured in nontraffic accident

X ● **V86.56**   Driver of dirt bike or motor/cross bike injured in nontraffic accident

X ● **V86.59**   Driver of other off-road special all-terrain or other off-road motor vehicle injured in nontraffic accident

    Driver of go cart injured in nontraffic accident

    Driver of golf cart injured in nontraffic accident

● **V86.6**   Passenger of special all-terrain or other off-road motor vehicle injured in nontraffic accident

X ● **V86.61**   Passenger of ambulance or fire engine injured in nontraffic accident

X ● **V86.62**   Passenger of snowmobile injured in nontraffic accident

X ● **V86.63**   Passenger of dune buggy injured in nontraffic accident

X ● **V86.64**   Passenger of military vehicle injured in nontraffic accident

X ● **V86.65**   Passenger of 3- or 4-wheeled all-terrain vehicle (ATV) injured in nontraffic accident

X ● **V86.66**   Passenger of dirt bike or motor/cross bike injured in nontraffic accident

X ● **V86.69**   Passenger of other special all-terrain or other off-road vehicle injured in nontraffic accident

    Passenger of go cart injured in nontraffic accident

    Passenger of golf cart injured in nontraffic accident

● **V86.7**   Person on outside of special all-terrain or other off-road motor vehicle injured in nontraffic accident

X ● **V86.71**   Person on outside of ambulance or fire engine injured in nontraffic accident

X ● **V86.72**   Person on outside of snowmobile injured in nontraffic accident

X ● **V86.73**   Person on outside of dune buggy injured in nontraffic accident

X ● **V86.74**   Person on outside of military vehicle injured in nontraffic accident

X ● **V86.75**   Person on outside of 3- or 4-wheeled all-terrain vehicle (ATV) injured in nontraffic accident

X ● **V86.76**   Person on outside of dirt bike or motor/cross bike injured in nontraffic accident

X ● **V86.79**   Person on outside of other special all-terrain or other off-road motor vehicles injured in nontraffic accident

    Person on outside of go cart injured in nontraffic accident

    Person on outside of golf cart injured in nontraffic accident

● **V86.9**   Unspecified occupant of special all-terrain or other off-road motor vehicle injured in nontraffic accident

X ● **V86.91**   Unspecified occupant of ambulance or fire engine injured in nontraffic accident

X ● **V86.92**   Unspecified occupant of snowmobile injured in nontraffic accident

X ● **V86.93**   Unspecified occupant of dune buggy injured in nontraffic accident

X ● **V86.94**   Unspecified occupant of military vehicle injured in nontraffic accident

X ● **V86.95**   Unspecified occupant of 3- or 4-wheeled all-terrain vehicle (ATV) injured in nontraffic accident

X ● **V86.96**   Unspecified occupant of dirt bike or motor/cross bike injured in nontraffic accident

X ● **V86.99**   Unspecified occupant of other special all-terrain or other off-road motor vehicle injured in nontraffic accident

    Off-road motor-vehicle accident NOS

    Other motor-vehicle accident NOS

    Unspecified occupant of go cart injured in nontraffic accident

    Unspecified occupant of golf cart injured in nontraffic accident

    Unspecified occupant of race car injured in nontraffic accident

● **V87**   Traffic accident of specified type but victim's mode of transport unknown

    Excludes1   collision involving:

        pedal cycle (V10-V19)

        pedestrian (V01-V09)

    The appropriate 7th character is to be added to each code from category V87

    A   initial encounter
    D   subsequent encounter
    S   sequela

X ● **V87.0**   Person injured in collision between car and two- or three-wheeled powered vehicle (traffic)

X ● **V87.1**   Person injured in collision between other motor vehicle and two- or three-wheeled motor vehicle (traffic)

X ● **V87.2**   Person injured in collision between car and pick-up truck or van (traffic)

X ● **V87.3**   Person injured in collision between car and bus (traffic)

X ● **V87.4**   Person injured in collision between car and heavy transport vehicle (traffic)

X ● **V87.5**   Person injured in collision between heavy transport vehicle and bus (traffic)

X ● **V87.6**   Person injured in collision between railway train or railway vehicle and car (traffic)

X ● **V87.7**   Person injured in collision between other specified motor vehicles (traffic)

X ● **V87.8**   Person injured in other specified noncollision transport accidents involving motor vehicle (traffic)

X ● **V87.9**   Person injured in other specified (collision) (noncollision) transport accidents involving nonmotor vehicle (traffic)

● **V88**   Nontraffic accident of specified type but victim's mode of transport unknown

    Excludes1   collision involving:

        pedal cycle (V10-V19)

        pedestrian (V01-V09)

    The appropriate 7th character is to be added to each code from category V88

    A   initial encounter
    D   subsequent encounter
    S   sequela

X ● **V88.0**   Person injured in collision between car and two- or three-wheeled motor vehicle, nontraffic

X ● **V88.1**   Person injured in collision between other motor vehicle and two- or three-wheeled motor vehicle, nontraffic

X ● **V88.2**   Person injured in collision between car and pick-up truck or van, nontraffic

CHAPTER 20 (V00-Y99)

X ● V88.3   Person injured in collision between car and bus, nontraffic

X ● V88.4   Person injured in collision between car and heavy transport vehicle, nontraffic

X ● V88.5   Person injured in collision between heavy transport vehicle and bus, nontraffic

X ● V88.6   Person injured in collision between railway train or railway vehicle and car, nontraffic

X ● V88.7   Person injured in collision between other specified motor vehicle, nontraffic

X ● V88.8   Person injured in other specified noncollision transport accidents involving motor vehicle, nontraffic

X ● V88.9   Person injured in other specified (collision) (noncollision) transport accidents involving nonmotor vehicle, nontraffic

● V89   Motor- or nonmotor-vehicle accident, type of vehicle unspecified

The appropriate 7th character is to be added to each code from category V89

> A   initial encounter
> D   subsequent encounter
> S   sequela

X ● V89.0   Person injured in unspecified motor-vehicle accident, nontraffic
Motor-vehicle accident NOS, nontraffic

X ● V89.1   Person injured in unspecified nonmotor-vehicle accident, nontraffic
Nonmotor-vehicle accident NOS (nontraffic)

X ● V89.2   Person injured in unspecified motor-vehicle accident, traffic
Motor-vehicle accident [MVA] NOS
Road (traffic) accident [RTA] NOS

X ● V89.3   Person injured in unspecified nonmotor-vehicle accident, traffic
Nonmotor-vehicle traffic accident NOS

X ● V89.9   Person injured in unspecified vehicle accident
Collision NOS

WATER TRANSPORT ACCIDENTS (V90-V94)

● V90   Drowning and submersion due to accident to watercraft

Excludes1   civilian water transport accident involving military watercraft (V94.81-)
fall into water not from watercraft (W16.-)
military watercraft accident in military or war operations (Y36.0-, Y37.0-)
water-transport–related drowning or submersion without accident to watercraft (V92.-)

The appropriate 7th character is to be added to each code from category V90

> A   initial encounter
> D   subsequent encounter
> S   sequela

● V90.0   Drowning and submersion due to watercraft overturning

X ● V90.00   Drowning and submersion due to merchant ship overturning

X ● V90.01   Drowning and submersion due to passenger ship overturning
Drowning and submersion due to ferry-boat overturning
Drowning and submersion due to liner overturning

X ● V90.02   Drowning and submersion due to fishing boat overturning

X ● V90.03   Drowning and submersion due to other powered watercraft overturning
Drowning and submersion due to hovercraft (on open water) overturning
Drowning and submersion due to jet ski overturning

X ● V90.04   Drowning and submersion due to sailboat overturning

X ● V90.05   Drowning and submersion due to canoe or kayak overturning

X ● V90.06   Drowning and submersion due to (nonpowered) inflatable craft overturning

X ● V90.08   Drowning and submersion due to other unpowered watercraft overturning
Drowning and submersion due to windsurfer overturning

X ● V90.09   Drowning and submersion due to unspecified watercraft overturning
Drowning and submersion due to boat NOS overturning
Drowning and submersion due to ship NOS overturning
Drowning and submersion due to watercraft NOS overturning

● V90.1   Drowning and submersion due to watercraft sinking

X ● V90.10   Drowning and submersion due to merchant ship sinking

X ● V90.11   Drowning and submersion due to passenger ship sinking
Drowning and submersion due to ferry-boat sinking
Drowning and submersion due to liner sinking

X ● V90.12   Drowning and submersion due to fishing boat sinking

X ● V90.13   Drowning and submersion due to other powered watercraft sinking
Drowning and submersion due to hovercraft (on open water) sinking
Drowning and submersion due to jet ski sinking

X ● V90.14   Drowning and submersion due to sailboat sinking

X ● V90.15   Drowning and submersion due to canoe or kayak sinking

X ● V90.16   Drowning and submersion due to (nonpowered) inflatable craft sinking

X ● V90.18   Drowning and submersion due to other unpowered watercraft sinking

X ● V90.19   Drowning and submersion due to unspecified watercraft sinking
Drowning and submersion due to boat NOS sinking
Drowning and submersion due to ship NOS sinking
Drowning and submersion due to watercraft NOS sinking

● V90.2   Drowning and submersion due to falling or jumping from burning watercraft

X ● V90.20   Drowning and submersion due to falling or jumping from burning merchant ship

X ● V90.21   Drowning and submersion due to falling or jumping from burning passenger ship
Drowning and submersion due to falling or jumping from burning ferry-boat
Drowning and submersion due to falling or jumping from burning liner

X ● V90.22   Drowning and submersion due to falling or jumping from burning fishing boat

X ● V90.23   Drowning and submersion due to falling or jumping from other burning powered watercraft
Drowning and submersion due to falling and jumping from burning hovercraft (on open water)
Drowning and submersion due to falling and jumping from burning jet ski

X ● V90.24   Drowning and submersion due to falling or jumping from burning sailboat

X ● V90.25   Drowning and submersion due to falling or jumping from burning canoe or kayak

X⬤ **V90.26** **Drowning and submersion due to falling or jumping from burning (nonpowered) inflatable craft**

X⬤ **V90.27** **Drowning and submersion due to falling or jumping from burning water-skis**

X⬤ **V90.28** **Drowning and submersion due to falling or jumping from other burning unpowered watercraft**
　　Drowning and submersion due to falling and jumping from burning surf-board
　　Drowning and submersion due to falling and jumping from burning windsurfer

X⬤ **V90.29** **Drowning and submersion due to falling or jumping from unspecified burning watercraft**
　　Drowning and submersion due to falling or jumping from burning boat NOS
　　Drowning and submersion due to falling or jumping from burning ship NOS
　　Drowning and submersion due to falling or jumping from burning watercraft NOS

⬤ **V90.3** **Drowning and submersion due to falling or jumping from crushed watercraft**

X⬤ **V90.30** **Drowning and submersion due to falling or jumping from crushed merchant ship**

X⬤ **V90.31** **Drowning and submersion due to falling or jumping from crushed passenger ship**
　　Drowning and submersion due to falling and jumping from crushed ferry-boat
　　Drowning and submersion due to falling and jumping from crushed liner

X⬤ **V90.32** **Drowning and submersion due to falling or jumping from crushed fishing boat**

X⬤ **V90.33** **Drowning and submersion due to falling or jumping from other crushed powered watercraft**
　　Drowning and submersion due to falling and jumping from crushed hovercraft
　　Drowning and submersion due to falling and jumping from crushed jet ski

X⬤ **V90.34** **Drowning and submersion due to falling or jumping from crushed sailboat**

X⬤ **V90.35** **Drowning and submersion due to falling or jumping from crushed canoe or kayak**

X⬤ **V90.36** **Drowning and submersion due to falling or jumping from crushed (nonpowered) inflatable craft**

X⬤ **V90.37** **Drowning and submersion due to falling or jumping from crushed water-skis**

X⬤ **V90.38** **Drowning and submersion due to falling or jumping from other crushed unpowered watercraft**
　　Drowning and submersion due to falling and jumping from crushed surf-board
　　Drowning and submersion due to falling and jumping from crushed windsurfer

X⬤ **V90.39** **Drowning and submersion due to falling or jumping from crushed unspecified watercraft**
　　Drowning and submersion due to falling and jumping from crushed boat NOS
　　Drowning and submersion due to falling and jumping from crushed ship NOS
　　Drowning and submersion due to falling and jumping from crushed watercraft NOS

⬤ **V90.8** **Drowning and submersion due to other accident to watercraft**

X⬤ **V90.80** **Drowning and submersion due to other accident to merchant ship**

X⬤ **V90.81** **Drowning and submersion due to other accident to passenger ship**
　　Drowning and submersion due to other accident to ferry-boat
　　Drowning and submersion due to other accident to liner

X⬤ **V90.82** **Drowning and submersion due to other accident to fishing boat**

X⬤ **V90.83** **Drowning and submersion due to other accident to other powered watercraft**
　　Drowning and submersion due to other accident to hovercraft (on open water)
　　Drowning and submersion due to other accident to jet ski

X⬤ **V90.84** **Drowning and submersion due to other accident to sailboat**

X⬤ **V90.85** **Drowning and submersion due to other accident to canoe or kayak**

X⬤ **V90.86** **Drowning and submersion due to other accident to (nonpowered) inflatable craft**

X⬤ **V90.87** **Drowning and submersion due to other accident to water-skis**

X⬤ **V90.88** **Drowning and submersion due to other accident to other unpowered watercraft**
　　Drowning and submersion due to other accident to surf-board
　　Drowning and submersion due to other accident to windsurfer

X⬤ **V90.89** **Drowning and submersion due to other accident to unspecified watercraft**
　　Drowning and submersion due to other accident to boat NOS
　　Drowning and submersion due to other accident to ship NOS
　　Drowning and submersion due to other accident to watercraft NOS

⬤ **V91** **Other injury due to accident to watercraft**

Includes   any injury except drowning and submersion as a result of an accident to watercraft

Excludes1   civilian water transport accident involving military watercraft (V94.81-)
military watercraft accident in military or war operations (Y36, Y37.-)

Excludes2   drowning and submersion due to accident to watercraft (V90.-)

The appropriate 7th character is to be added to each code from category V91

A	initial encounter
D	subsequent encounter
S	sequela

⬤ **V91.0** **Burn due to watercraft on fire**

Excludes1   burn from localized fire or explosion on board ship without accident to watercraft (V93.-)

X⬤ **V91.00** **Burn due to merchant ship on fire**

X⬤ **V91.01** **Burn due to passenger ship on fire**
　　Burn due to ferry-boat on fire
　　Burn due to liner on fire

X⬤ **V91.02** **Burn due to fishing boat on fire**

X⬤ **V91.03** **Burn due to other powered watercraft on fire**
　　Burn due to hovercraft (on open water) on fire
　　Burn due to jet ski on fire

X⬤ **V91.04** **Burn due to sailboat on fire**

X⬤ **V91.05** **Burn due to canoe or kayak on fire**

X⬤ **V91.06** **Burn due to (nonpowered) inflatable craft on fire**

X⬤ **V91.07** **Burn due to water-skis on fire**

X⬤ **V91.08** **Burn due to other unpowered watercraft on fire**

X⬤ **V91.09** **Burn due to unspecified watercraft on fire**
　　Burn due to boat NOS on fire
　　Burn due to ship NOS on fire
　　Burn due to watercraft NOS on fire

● **V91.1   Crushed between watercraft and other watercraft or other object due to collision**
　　Crushed by lifeboat after abandoning ship in a collision
　　Note: Select the specified type of watercraft that the victim was on at the time of the collision.

X ● **V91.10   Crushed between merchant ship and other watercraft or other object due to collision**

X ● **V91.11   Crushed between passenger ship and other watercraft or other object due to collision**
　　Crushed between ferry-boat and other watercraft or other object due to collision
　　Crushed between liner and other watercraft or other object due to collision

X ● **V91.12   Crushed between fishing boat and other watercraft or other object due to collision**

X ● **V91.13   Crushed between other powered watercraft and other watercraft or other object due to collision**
　　Crushed between hovercraft (on open water) and other watercraft or other object due to collision
　　Crushed between jet ski and other watercraft or other object due to collision

X ● **V91.14   Crushed between sailboat and other watercraft or other object due to collision**

X ● **V91.15   Crushed between canoe or kayak and other watercraft or other object due to collision**

X ● **V91.16   Crushed between (nonpowered) inflatable craft and other watercraft or other object due to collision**

X ● **V91.18   Crushed between other unpowered watercraft and other watercraft or other object due to collision**
　　Crushed between surfboard and other watercraft or other object due to collision
　　Crushed between windsurfer and other watercraft or other object due to collision

X ● **V91.19   Crushed between unspecified watercraft and other watercraft or other object due to collision**
　　Crushed between boat NOS and other watercraft or other object due to collision
　　Crushed between ship NOS and other watercraft or other object due to collision
　　Crushed between watercraft NOS and other watercraft or other object due to collision

● **V91.2   Fall due to collision between watercraft and other watercraft or other object**
　　Fall while remaining on watercraft after collision
　　Note: Select the specified type of watercraft that the victim was on at the time of the collision.
　　Excludes1   crushed between watercraft and other watercraft and other object due to collision (V91.1-)
　　　　drowning and submersion due to falling from crushed watercraft (V90.3-)

X ● **V91.20   Fall due to collision between merchant ship and other watercraft or other object**

X ● **V91.21   Fall due to collision between passenger ship and other watercraft or other object**
　　Fall due to collision between ferry-boat and other watercraft or other object
　　Fall due to collision between liner and other watercraft or other object

X ● **V91.22   Fall due to collision between fishing boat and other watercraft or other object**

X ● **V91.23   Fall due to collision between other powered watercraft and other watercraft or other object**
　　Fall due to collision between hovercraft (on open water) and other watercraft or other object
　　Fall due to collision between jet ski and other watercraft or other object

X ● **V91.24   Fall due to collision between sailboat and other watercraft or other object**

X ● **V91.25   Fall due to collision between canoe or kayak and other watercraft or other object**

X ● **V91.26   Fall due to collision between (nonpowered) inflatable craft and other watercraft or other object**

X ● **V91.29   Fall due to collision between unspecified watercraft and other watercraft or other object**
　　Fall due to collision between boat NOS and other watercraft or other object
　　Fall due to collision between ship NOS and other watercraft or other object
　　Fall due to collision between watercraft NOS and other watercraft or other object

● **V91.3   Hit or struck by falling object due to accident to watercraft**
　　Hit or struck by falling object (part of damaged watercraft or other object) after falling or jumping from damaged watercraft
　　Excludes2   drowning or submersion due to fall or jumping from damaged watercraft (V90.2-, V90.3-)

X ● **V91.30   Hit or struck by falling object due to accident to merchant ship**

X ● **V91.31   Hit or struck by falling object due to accident to passenger ship**
　　Hit or struck by falling object due to accident to ferry-boat
　　Hit or struck by falling object due to accident to liner

X ● **V91.32   Hit or struck by falling object due to accident to fishing boat**

X ● **V91.33   Hit or struck by falling object due to accident to other powered watercraft**
　　Hit or struck by falling object due to accident to hovercraft (on open water)
　　Hit or struck by falling object due to accident to jet ski

X ● **V91.34   Hit or struck by falling object due to accident to sailboat**

X ● **V91.35   Hit or struck by falling object due to accident to canoe or kayak**

X ● **V91.36   Hit or struck by falling object due to accident to (nonpowered) inflatable craft**

X ● **V91.37   Hit or struck by falling object due to accident to water-skis**
　　Hit by water-skis after jumping off of waterskis

X ● **V91.38   Hit or struck by falling object due to accident to other unpowered watercraft**
　　Hit or struck by surf-board after falling off damaged surf-board
　　Hit or struck by object after falling off damaged windsurfer

X ● **V91.39   Hit or struck by falling object due to accident to unspecified watercraft**
　　Hit or struck by falling object due to accident to boat NOS
　　Hit or struck by falling object due to accident to ship NOS
　　Hit or struck by falling object due to accident to watercraft NOS

● **V91.8   Other injury due to other accident to watercraft**

X ● **V91.80   Other injury due to other accident to merchant ship**

X ● **V91.81   Other injury due to other accident to passenger ship**
　　Other injury due to other accident to ferry-boat
　　Other injury due to other accident to liner

X ● **V91.82   Other injury due to other accident to fishing boat**

X ● **V91.83   Other injury due to other accident to other powered watercraft**
　　Other injury due to other accident to hovercraft (on open water)
　　Other injury due to other accident to jet ski

X● **V91.84** **Other injury due to other accident to sailboat**
X● **V91.85** **Other injury due to other accident to canoe or kayak**
X● **V91.86** **Other injury due to other accident to (nonpowered) inflatable craft**
X● **V91.87** **Other injury due to other accident to water-skis**
X● **V91.88** **Other injury due to other accident to other unpowered watercraft**
    Other injury due to other accident to surf-board
    Other injury due to other accident to windsurfer
X● **V91.89** **Other injury due to other accident to unspecified watercraft**
    Other injury due to other accident to boat NOS
    Other injury due to other accident to ship NOS
    Other injury due to other accident to watercraft NOS

● **V92** **Drowning and submersion due to accident on board watercraft, without accident to watercraft**

    Excludes1   civilian water transport accident involving military watercraft (V94.81-)
       drowning or submersion due to accident to watercraft (V90-V91)
       drowning or submersion of diver who voluntarily jumps from boat not involved in an accident (W16.711, W16.721)
       fall into water without watercraft (W16.-)
       military watercraft accident in military or war operations (Y36, Y37)

The appropriate 7th character is to be added to each code from category V92

    A   initial encounter
    D   subsequent encounter
    S   sequela

● **V92.0** **Drowning and submersion due to fall off watercraft**
    Drowning and submersion due to fall from gangplank of watercraft
    Drowning and submersion due to fall overboard watercraft

    Excludes2   hitting head on object or bottom of body of water due to fall from watercraft (V94.0-)

X● **V92.00** **Drowning and submersion due to fall off merchant ship**
X● **V92.01** **Drowning and submersion due to fall off passenger ship**
    Drowning and submersion due to fall off ferry-boat
    Drowning and submersion due to fall off liner
X● **V92.02** **Drowning and submersion due to fall off fishing boat**
X● **V92.03** **Drowning and submersion due to fall off other powered watercraft**
    Drowning and submersion due to fall off hovercraft (on open water)
    Drowning and submersion due to fall off jet ski
X● **V92.04** **Drowning and submersion due to fall off sailboat**
X● **V92.05** **Drowning and submersion due to fall off canoe or kayak**
X● **V92.06** **Drowning and submersion due to fall off (nonpowered) inflatable craft**
X● **V92.07** **Drowning and submersion due to fall off water-skis**

    Excludes1   drowning and submersion due to falling off burning water-skis (V90.27)
       drowning and submersion due to falling off crushed water-skis (V90.37)
       hit by boat while water-skiing NOS (V94.-)

X● **V92.08** **Drowning and submersion due to fall off other unpowered watercraft**
    Drowning and submersion due to fall off surf-board
    Drowning and submersion due to fall off windsurfer

    Excludes1   drowning and submersion due to fall off burning unpowered watercraft (V90.28)
       drowning and submersion due to fall off crushed unpowered watercraft (V90.38)
       drowning and submersion due to fall off damaged unpowered watercraft (V90.88)
       drowning and submersion due to rider of nonpowered watercraft being hit by other watercraft (V94.-)
       other injury due to rider of nonpowered watercraft being hit by other watercraft (V94.-)

X● **V92.09** **Drowning and submersion due to fall off unspecified watercraft**
    Drowning and submersion due to fall off boat NOS
    Drowning and submersion due to fall off ship NOS
    Drowning and submersion due to fall off watercraft NOS

● **V92.1** **Drowning and submersion due to being thrown overboard by motion of watercraft**

    Excludes1   drowning and submersion due to fall off surf-board (V92.08)
       drowning and submersion due to fall off water-skis (V92.07)
       drowning and submersion due to fall off windsurfer (V92.08)

X● **V92.10** **Drowning and submersion due to being thrown overboard by motion of merchant ship**
X● **V92.11** **Drowning and submersion due to being thrown overboard by motion of passenger ship**
    Drowning and submersion due to being thrown overboard by motion of ferry-boat
    Drowning and submersion due to being thrown overboard by motion of liner
X● **V92.12** **Drowning and submersion due to being thrown overboard by motion of fishing boat**
X● **V92.13** **Drowning and submersion due to being thrown overboard by motion of other powered watercraft**
    Drowning and submersion due to being thrown overboard by motion of hovercraft
X● **V92.14** **Drowning and submersion due to being thrown overboard by motion of sailboat**
X● **V92.15** **Drowning and submersion due to being thrown overboard by motion of canoe or kayak**
X● **V92.16** **Drowning and submersion due to being thrown overboard by motion of (nonpowered) inflatable craft**
X● **V92.19** **Drowning and submersion due to being thrown overboard by motion of unspecified watercraft**
    Drowning and submersion due to being thrown overboard by motion of boat NOS
    Drowning and submersion due to being thrown overboard by motion of ship NOS
    Drowning and submersion due to being thrown overboard by motion of watercraft NOS

● **V92.2 Drowning and submersion due to being washed overboard from watercraft**

Code first any associated cataclysm (X37.0-)

X● **V92.20 Drowning and submersion due to being washed overboard from merchant ship**

X● **V92.21 Drowning and submersion due to being washed overboard from passenger ship**

Drowning and submersion due to being washed overboard from ferry-boat

Drowning and submersion due to being washed overboard from liner

X● **V92.22 Drowning and submersion due to being washed overboard from fishing boat**

X● **V92.23 Drowning and submersion due to being washed overboard from other powered watercraft**

Drowning and submersion due to being washed overboard from hovercraft (on open water)

Drowning and submersion due to being washed overboard from jet ski

X● **V92.24 Drowning and submersion due to being washed overboard from sailboat**

X● **V92.25 Drowning and submersion due to being washed overboard from canoe or kayak**

X● **V92.26 Drowning and submersion due to being washed overboard from (nonpowered) inflatable craft**

X● **V92.27 Drowning and submersion due to being washed overboard from water-skis**

Excludes1   drowning and submersion due to fall off water-skis (V92.07)

X● **V92.28 Drowning and submersion due to being washed overboard from other unpowered watercraft**

Drowning and submersion due to being washed overboard from surf-board

Drowning and submersion due to being washed overboard from windsurfer

X● **V92.29 Drowning and submersion due to being washed overboard from unspecified watercraft**

Drowning and submersion due to being washed overboard from boat NOS

Drowning and submersion due to being washed overboard from ship NOS

Drowning and submersion due to being washed overboard from watercraft NOS

● **V93 Other injury due to accident on board watercraft, without accident to watercraft**

Excludes1   civilian water transport accident involving military watercraft (V94.81-)

other injury due to accident to watercraft (V91.-)

military watercraft accident in military or war operations (Y36, Y37.-)

Excludes2   drowning and submersion due to accident on board watercraft, without accident to watercraft (V92.-)

The appropriate 7th character is to be added to each code from category V93

A	initial encounter
D	subsequent encounter
S	sequela

● **V93.0 Burn due to localized fire on board watercraft**

Excludes1   burn due to watercraft on fire (V91.0-)

X● **V93.00 Burn due to localized fire on board merchant vessel**

X● **V93.01 Burn due to localized fire on board passenger vessel**

Burn due to localized fire on board ferry-boat

Burn due to localized fire on board liner

X● **V93.02 Burn due to localized fire on board fishing boat**

X● **V93.03 Burn due to localized fire on board other powered watercraft**

Burn due to localized fire on board hovercraft

Burn due to localized fire on board jet ski

X● **V93.04 Burn due to localized fire on board sailboat**

X● **V93.09 Burn due to localized fire on board unspecified watercraft**

Burn due to localized fire on board boat NOS

Burn due to localized fire on board ship NOS

Burn due to localized fire on board watercraft NOS

● **V93.1 Other burn on board watercraft**

Burn due to source other than fire on board watercraft

Excludes1   burn due to watercraft on fire (V91.0-)

X● **V93.10 Other burn on board merchant vessel**

X● **V93.11 Other burn on board passenger vessel**

Other burn on board ferry-boat

Other burn on board liner

X● **V93.12 Other burn on board fishing boat**

X● **V93.13 Other burn on board other powered watercraft**

Other burn on board hovercraft

Other burn on board jet ski

X● **V93.14 Other burn on board sailboat**

X● **V93.19 Other burn on board unspecified watercraft**

Other burn on board boat NOS

Other burn on board ship NOS

Other burn on board watercraft NOS

● **V93.2 Heat exposure on board watercraft**

Excludes1   exposure to man-made heat not aboard watercraft (W92)

exposure to natural heat while on board watercraft (X30)

exposure to sunlight while on board watercraft (X32)

Excludes2   burn due to fire on board watercraft (V93.0-)

X● **V93.20 Heat exposure on board merchant ship**

X● **V93.21 Heat exposure on board passenger ship**

Heat exposure on board ferry-boat

Heat exposure on board liner

X● **V93.22 Heat exposure on board fishing boat**

X● **V93.23 Heat exposure on board other powered watercraft**

Heat exposure on board hovercraft

X● **V93.24 Heat exposure on board sailboat**

X● **V93.29 Heat exposure on board unspecified watercraft**

Heat exposure on board boat NOS

Heat exposure on board ship NOS

Heat exposure on board watercraft NOS

● **V93.3 Fall on board watercraft**

Excludes1   fall due to collision of watercraft (V91.2-)

X● **V93.30 Fall on board merchant ship**

X● **V93.31 Fall on board passenger ship**

Fall on board ferry-boat

Fall on board liner

X● **V93.32 Fall on board fishing boat**

X● **V93.33 Fall on board other powered watercraft**

Fall on board hovercraft (on open water)

Fall on board jet ski

X● **V93.34 Fall on board sailboat**

X● **V93.35 Fall on board canoe or kayak**

X● **V93.36 Fall on board (nonpowered) inflatable craft**

X● **V93.38 Fall on board other unpowered watercraft**

X● **V93.39 Fall on board unspecified watercraft**

Fall on board boat NOS

Fall on board ship NOS

Fall on board watercraft NOS

- **● V93.4　Struck by falling object on board watercraft**
  Hit by falling object on board watercraft
  > **Excludes1**　struck by falling object due to accident to watercraft (V91.3)
  - X● **V93.40　Struck by falling object on merchant ship**
  - X● **V93.41　Struck by falling object on passenger ship**
    Struck by falling object on ferry-boat
    Struck by falling object on liner
  - X● **V93.42　Struck by falling object on fishing boat**
  - X● **V93.43　Struck by falling object on other powered watercraft**
    Struck by falling object on hovercraft
  - X● **V93.44　Struck by falling object on sailboat**
  - X● **V93.48　Struck by falling object on other unpowered watercraft**
  - X● **V93.49　Struck by falling object on unspecified watercraft**
- ● **V93.5　Explosion on board watercraft**
  Boiler explosion on steamship
  > **Excludes2**　fire on board watercraft (V93.0-)
  - X● **V93.50　Explosion on board merchant ship**
  - X● **V93.51　Explosion on board passenger ship**
    Explosion on board ferry-boat
    Explosion on board liner
  - X● **V93.52　Explosion on board fishing boat**
  - X● **V93.53　Explosion on board other powered watercraft**
    Explosion on board hovercraft
    Explosion on board jet ski
  - X● **V93.54　Explosion on board sailboat**
  - X● **V93.59　Explosion on board unspecified watercraft**
    Explosion on board boat NOS
    Explosion on board ship NOS
    Explosion on board watercraft NOS
- ● **V93.6　Machinery accident on board watercraft**
  > **Excludes1**　machinery explosion on board watercraft (V93.4-)
  > machinery fire on board watercraft (V93.0-)
  - X● **V93.60　Machinery accident on board merchant ship**
  - X● **V93.61　Machinery accident on board passenger ship**
    Machinery accident on board ferry-boat
    Machinery accident on board liner
  - X● **V93.62　Machinery accident on board fishing boat**
  - X● **V93.63　Machinery accident on board other powered watercraft**
    Machinery accident on board hovercraft
  - X● **V93.64　Machinery accident on board sailboat**
  - X● **V93.69　Machinery accident on board unspecified watercraft**
    Machinery accident on board boat NOS
    Machinery accident on board ship NOS
    Machinery accident on board watercraft NOS
- ● **V93.8　Other injury due to other accident on board watercraft**
  Accidental poisoning by gases or fumes on watercraft
  - X● **V93.80　Other injury due to other accident on board merchant ship**
  - X● **V93.81　Other injury due to other accident on board passenger ship**
    Other injury due to other accident on board ferry-boat
    Other injury due to other accident on board liner
  - X● **V93.82　Other injury due to other accident on board fishing boat**
  - X● **V93.83　Other injury due to other accident on board other powered watercraft**
    Other injury due to other accident on board hovercraft
    Other injury due to other accident on board jet ski
  - X● **V93.84　Other injury due to other accident on board sailboat**

- X● **V93.85　Other injury due to other accident on board canoe or kayak**
- X● **V93.86　Other injury due to other accident on board (nonpowered) inflatable craft**
- X● **V93.87　Other injury due to other accident on board water-skis**
  Hit or struck by object while waterskiing
- X● **V93.88　Other injury due to other accident on board other unpowered watercraft**
  Hit or struck by object while surfing
  Hit or struck by object while on board windsurfer
- X● **V93.89　Other injury due to other accident on board unspecified watercraft**
  Other injury due to other accident on board boat NOS
  Other injury due to other accident on board ship NOS
  Other injury due to other accident on board watercraft NOS

- ● **V94　Other and unspecified water transport accidents**
  > **Excludes1**　military watercraft accidents in military or war operations (Y36, Y37)

  The appropriate 7th character is to be added to each code from category V94

A	initial encounter
D	subsequent encounter
S	sequela

  - X● **V94.0　Hitting object or bottom of body of water due to fall from watercraft**
    > **Excludes2**　drowning and submersion due to fall from watercraft (V92.0-)
  - ● **V94.1　Bather struck by watercraft**
    Swimmer hit by watercraft
    - X● **V94.11　Bather struck by powered watercraft**
    - X● **V94.12　Bather struck by nonpowered watercraft**
  - ● **V94.2　Rider of nonpowered watercraft struck by other watercraft**
    - X● **V94.21　Rider of nonpowered watercraft struck by other nonpowered watercraft**
      Canoer hit by other nonpowered watercraft
      Surfer hit by other nonpowered watercraft
      Windsurfer hit by other nonpowered watercraft
    - X● **V94.22　Rider of nonpowered watercraft struck by powered watercraft**
      Canoer hit by motorboat
      Surfer hit by motorboat
      Windsurfer hit by motorboat
  - ● **V94.3　Injury to rider of (inflatable) watercraft being pulled behind other watercraft**
    - X● **V94.31　Injury to rider of (inflatable) recreational watercraft being pulled behind other watercraft**
      Injury to rider of inner-tube pulled behind motor boat
    - X● **V94.32　Injury to rider of non-recreational watercraft being pulled behind other watercraft**
      Injury to occupant of dingy being pulled behind boat or ship
      Injury to occupant of life-raft being pulled behind boat or ship
  - X● **V94.4　Injury to barefoot water-skier**
    Injury to person being pulled behind boat or ship
  - ● **V94.8　Other water transport accident**
    - ● **V94.81　Water transport accident involving military watercraft**
      - ● **V94.810　Civilian watercraft involved in water transport accident with military watercraft**
        Passenger on civilian watercraft injured due to accident with military watercraft

● V94.811   Civilian in water injured by military watercraft
● V94.818   Other water transport accident involving military watercraft

X ● V94.89   Other water transport accident

X ● V94.9   **Unspecified** water transport accident
Water transport accident NOS

AIR AND SPACE TRANSPORT ACCIDENTS (V95-V97)

Excludes1   military aircraft accidents in military or war operations (Y36, Y37)

● V95   **Accident to powered aircraft causing injury to occupant**
The appropriate 7th character is to be added to each code from category V95

A	initial encounter
D	subsequent encounter
S	sequela

● V95.0   Helicopter accident injuring occupant
X ● V95.00   **Unspecified** helicopter accident injuring occupant
X ● V95.01   Helicopter **crash** injuring occupant
X ● V95.02   **Forced landing** of helicopter injuring occupant
X ● V95.03   Helicopter **collision** injuring occupant
Helicopter collision with any object, fixed, movable or moving
X ● V95.04   Helicopter **fire** injuring occupant
X ● V95.05   Helicopter **explosion** injuring occupant
X ● V95.09   **Other** helicopter accident injuring occupant

● V95.1   Ultralight, microlight or powered-glider accident injuring occupant
X ● V95.10   **Unspecified** ultralight, microlight or powered-glider accident injuring occupant
X ● V95.11   Ultralight, microlight or powered-glider **crash** injuring occupant
X ● V95.12   **Forced landing** of ultralight, microlight or powered-glider injuring occupant
X ● V95.13   Ultralight, microlight or powered-glider **collision** injuring occupant
Ultralight, microlight or powered-glider collision with any object, fixed, movable or moving
X ● V95.14   Ultralight, microlight or powered-glider **fire** injuring occupant
X ● V95.15   Ultralight, microlight or powered-glider **explosion** injuring occupant
X ● V95.19   **Other** ultralight, microlight or powered-glider accident injuring occupant

● V95.2   Other private fixed-wing aircraft accident injuring occupant
X ● V95.20   **Unspecified** accident to other private fixed-wing aircraft, injuring occupant
X ● V95.21   Other private fixed-wing aircraft **crash** injuring occupant
X ● V95.22   **Forced landing** of other private fixed-wing aircraft injuring occupant
X ● V95.23   Other private fixed-wing aircraft **collision** injuring occupant
Other private fixed-wing aircraft collision with any object, fixed, movable or moving
X ● V95.24   Other private fixed-wing aircraft **fire** injuring occupant
X ● V95.25   Other private fixed-wing aircraft **explosion** injuring occupant
X ● V95.29   **Other** accident to other private fixed-wing aircraft injuring occupant

● V95.3   **Commercial fixed-wing aircraft** accident injuring occupant
X ● V95.30   **Unspecified** accident to commercial fixed-wing aircraft injuring occupant
X ● V95.31   Commercial fixed-wing aircraft **crash** injuring occupant
X ● V95.32   **Forced landing** of commercial fixed-wing aircraft injuring occupant
X ● V95.33   Commercial fixed-wing aircraft **collision** injuring occupant
Commercial fixed-wing aircraft collision with any object, fixed, movable or moving
X ● V95.34   Commercial fixed-wing aircraft **fire** injuring occupant
X ● V95.35   Commercial fixed-wing aircraft **explosion** injuring occupant
X ● V95.39   **Other** accident to commercial fixed-wing aircraft injuring occupant

● V95.4   **Spacecraft** accident injuring occupant
X ● V95.40   **Unspecified** spacecraft accident injuring occupant
X ● V95.41   Spacecraft **crash** injuring occupant
X ● V95.42   **Forced landing** of spacecraft injuring occupant
X ● V95.43   Spacecraft **collision** injuring occupant
Spacecraft collision with any object, fixed, moveable or moving
X ● V95.44   Spacecraft **fire** injuring occupant
X ● V95.45   Spacecraft **explosion** injuring occupant
X ● V95.49   **Other** spacecraft accident injuring occupant

X ● V95.8   Other powered aircraft accidents injuring occupant
X ● V95.9   **Unspecified** aircraft accident injuring occupant
Aircraft accident NOS
Air transport accident NOS

● V96   **Accident to nonpowered aircraft causing injury to occupant**
The appropriate 7th character is to be added to each code from category V96

A	initial encounter
D	subsequent encounter
S	sequela

● V96.0   Balloon accident injuring occupant
X ● V96.00   **Unspecified** balloon accident injuring occupant
X ● V96.01   Balloon **crash** injuring occupant
X ● V96.02   **Forced landing** of balloon injuring occupant
X ● V96.03   Balloon **collision** injuring occupant
Balloon collision with any object, fixed, moveable or moving
X ● V96.04   Balloon **fire** injuring occupant
X ● V96.05   Balloon **explosion** injuring occupant
X ● V96.09   **Other** balloon accident injuring occupant

● V96.1   Hang-glider accident injuring occupant
X ● V96.10   **Unspecified** hang-glider accident injuring occupant
X ● V96.11   Hang-glider **crash** injuring occupant
X ● V96.12   **Forced landing** of hang-glider injuring occupant
X ● V96.13   Hang-glider **collision** injuring occupant
Hang-glider collision with any object, fixed, moveable or moving
X ● V96.14   Hang-glider **fire** injuring occupant
X ● V96.15   Hang-glider **explosion** injuring occupant
X ● V96.19   **Other** hang-glider accident injuring occupant

● V96.2   Glider (nonpowered) accident injuring occupant
X ● V96.20   **Unspecified** glider (nonpowered) accident injuring occupant
X ● V96.21   Glider (nonpowered) **crash** injuring occupant
X ● V96.22   **Forced landing** of glider (nonpowered) injuring occupant

---

▶ New   ⇨ Revised   ~~deleted~~ Deleted   Excludes 1   Excludes 2   Includes   Use additional   Code first   Code also   Key words
OGCR Official Guidelines   X Assign placeholder X   ● Use Additional Character(s)   ▶ Manifestation Code   Hierarchical Condition Category   **Coding Clinic**

X● **V96.23**   **Glider (nonpowered) collision injuring occupant**
    Glider (nonpowered) collision with any object, fixed, moveable or moving

X● **V96.24**   **Glider (nonpowered) fire injuring occupant**

X● **V96.25**   **Glider (nonpowered) explosion injuring occupant**

X● **V96.29**   **Other glider (nonpowered) accident injuring occupant**

X● **V96.8**   **Other nonpowered-aircraft accidents injuring occupant**
    Kite carrying a person accident injuring occupant

X● **V96.9**   **Unspecified nonpowered-aircraft accident injuring occupant**
    Nonpowered-aircraft accident NOS

● **V97**   **Other specified air transport accidents**
    The appropriate 7th character is to be added to each code from category V97

    A   initial encounter
    D   subsequent encounter
    S   sequela

X● **V97.0**   **Occupant of aircraft injured in other specified air transport accidents**
    Fall in, on or from aircraft in air transport accident
    Excludes1   accident while boarding or alighting aircraft (V97.1)

X● **V97.1**   **Person injured while boarding or alighting from aircraft**

● **V97.2**   **Parachutist accident**

X● **V97.21**   **Parachutist entangled in object**
    Parachutist landing in tree

X● **V97.22**   **Parachutist injured on landing**

X● **V97.29**   **Other parachutist accident**

● **V97.3**   **Person on ground injured in air transport accident**

X● **V97.31**   **Hit by object falling from aircraft**
    Hit by crashing aircraft
    Injured by aircraft hitting house
    Injured by aircraft hitting car

X● **V97.32**   **Injured by rotating propeller**

X● **V97.33**   **Sucked into jet engine**

X● **V97.39**   **Other injury to person on ground due to air transport accident**

● **V97.8**   **Other air transport accidents, not elsewhere classified**
    Excludes1   aircraft accident NOS (V95.9)
       exposure to changes in air pressure during ascent or descent (W94.-)

● **V97.81**   **Air transport accident involving military aircraft**

● **V97.810**   **Civilian aircraft involved in air transport accident with military aircraft**
    Passenger in civilian aircraft injured due to accident with military aircraft

● **V97.811**   **Civilian injured by military aircraft**

● **V97.818**   **Other air transport accident involving military aircraft**

X● **V97.89**   **Other air transport accidents, not elsewhere classified**
    Injury from machinery on aircraft

OTHER AND UNSPECIFIED TRANSPORT ACCIDENTS (V98-V99)

Excludes1   vehicle accident, type of vehicle unspecified (V89.-)

● **V98**   **Other specified transport accidents**
    The appropriate 7th character is to be added to each code from category V98

    A   initial encounter
    D   subsequent encounter
    S   sequela

X● **V98.0**   **Accident to, on or involving cable-car, not on rails**
    Caught or dragged by cable-car, not on rails
    Fall or jump from cable-car, not on rails
    Object thrown from or in cable-car, not on rails

X● **V98.1**   **Accident to, on or involving land-yacht**

X● **V98.2**   **Accident to, on or involving ice yacht**

X● **V98.3**   **Accident to, on or involving ski lift**
    Accident to, on or involving ski chair-lift
    Accident to, on or involving ski-lift with gondola

X● **V98.8**   **Other specified transport accidents**

X● **V99**   **Unspecified transport accident**
    The appropriate 7th character is to be added to code V99

    A   initial encounter
    D   subsequent encounter
    S   sequela

OTHER EXTERNAL CAUSES OF ACCIDENTAL INJURY (W00-X58)

SLIPPING, TRIPPING, STUMBLING AND FALLS (W00-W19)

Excludes1   assault involving a fall (Y01-Y02)
    fall from animal (V80.-)
    fall (in) (from) machinery (in operation) (W28-W31)
    fall (in) (from) transport vehicle (V01-V99)
    intentional self-harm involving a fall (X80-X81)

Excludes2   at risk for fall (history of fall) Z91.81
    fall (in) (from) burning building (X00.-)
    fall into fire (X00-X04, X08)

● **W00**   **Fall due to ice and snow**
    Includes   pedestrian on foot falling (slipping) on ice and snow
    Excludes1   fall on (from) ice and snow involving pedestrian conveyance (V00.-)
       fall from stairs and steps not due to ice and snow (W10.-)

    The appropriate 7th character is to be added to each code from category W00

    A   initial encounter
    D   subsequent encounter
    S   sequela

X● **W00.0**   **Fall on same level due to ice and snow**
    Coding Clinic: 2016, Q2, P5

X● **W00.1**   **Fall from stairs and steps due to ice and snow**

X● **W00.2**   **Other fall from one level to another due to ice and snow**

X● **W00.9**   **Unspecified fall due to ice and snow**

● **W01**   **Fall on same level from slipping, tripping and stumbling**
    Includes   fall on moving sidewalk
    Excludes1   fall due to bumping (striking) against object (W18.0-)
       fall in shower or bathtub (W18.2-)
       fall on same level NOS (W18.30)
       fall on same level from slipping, tripping and stumbling due to ice or snow (W00.0)
       fall off or from toilet (W18.1-)
       slipping, tripping and stumbling NOS (W18.40)
       slipping, tripping and stumbling without falling (W18.4-)

    The appropriate 7th character is to be added to each code from category W01

    A   initial encounter
    D   subsequent encounter
    S   sequela

X● **W01.0**   **Fall on same level from slipping, tripping and stumbling without subsequent striking against object**
    Falling over animal

● **W01.1**   **Fall on same level from slipping, tripping and stumbling with subsequent striking against object**

CHAPTER 20 (V00-Y99)

CHAPTER 20 (V00–Y99)

X ● W01.10 **Fall on same level from slipping, tripping and stumbling with subsequent striking against unspecified object**

● W01.11 **Fall on same level from slipping, tripping and stumbling with subsequent striking against sharp object**

  ● W01.110 **Fall on same level from slipping, tripping and stumbling with subsequent striking against sharp glass**

  ● W01.111 **Fall on same level from slipping, tripping and stumbling with subsequent striking against power tool or machine**

  ● W01.118 **Fall on same level from slipping, tripping and stumbling with subsequent striking against other sharp object**

  ● W01.119 **Fall on same level from slipping, tripping and stumbling with subsequent striking against unspecified sharp object**

● W01.19 **Fall on same level from slipping, tripping and stumbling with subsequent striking against other object**

  ● W01.190 **Fall on same level from slipping, tripping and stumbling with subsequent striking against furniture**
    Coding Clinic: 2021, Q1, P5

  ● W01.198 **Fall on same level from slipping, tripping and stumbling with subsequent striking against other object**

X ● W03 **Other fall on same level due to collision with another person**
Fall due to non-transport collision with other person

Excludes1 collision with another person without fall (W51)
crushed or pushed by a crowd or human stampede (W52)
fall involving pedestrian conveyance (V00-V09)
fall due to ice or snow (W00)
fall on same level NOS (W18.30)

The appropriate 7th character is to be added to code W03

A	initial encounter
D	subsequent encounter
S	sequela

Coding Clinic: 2015, Q1, P9-10; 2012, Q4, P108

X ● W04 **Fall while being carried or supported by other persons**
Accidentally dropped while being carried

The appropriate 7th character is to be added to code W04

A	initial encounter
D	subsequent encounter
S	sequel

● W05 **Fall from non-moving wheelchair, nonmotorized scooter and motorized mobility scooter**

Excludes1 fall from moving wheelchair (powered) (V00.811)
fall from moving motorized mobility scooter (V00.831)
fall from nonmotorized scooter (V00.141)

The appropriate 7th character is to be added to each code from category W05

A	initial encounter
D	subsequent encounter
S	sequela

X ● W05.0 **Fall from non-moving wheelchair**
Coding Clinic: 2019, Q2, P27

X ● W05.1 **Fall from non-moving nonmotorized scooter**

X ● W05.2 **Fall from non-moving motorized mobility scooter**

X ● W06 **Fall from bed**

The appropriate 7th character is to be added to code W06

A	initial encounter
D	subsequent encounter
S	sequela

X ● W07 **Fall from chair**

The appropriate 7th character is to be added to code W07

A	initial encounter
D	subsequent encounter
S	sequela

X ● W08 **Fall from other furniture**

The appropriate 7th character is to be added to code W08

A	initial encounter
D	subsequent encounter
S	sequela

● W09 **Fall on and from playground equipment**

Excludes1 fall involving recreational machinery (W31)

The appropriate 7th character is to be added to each code from category W09

A	initial encounter
D	subsequent encounter
S	sequela

X ● W09.0 **Fall on or from playground slide**

X ● W09.1 **Fall from playground swing**

X ● W09.2 **Fall on or from jungle gym**

X ● W09.8 **Fall on or from other playground equipment**

● W10 **Fall on and from stairs and steps**

Excludes1 fall from stairs and steps due to ice and snow (W00.1)

The appropriate 7th character is to be added to each code from category W10

A	initial encounter
D	subsequent encounter
S	sequela

X ● W10.0 **Fall (on) (from) escalator**

X ● W10.1 **Fall (on) (from) sidewalk curb**

X ● W10.2 **Fall (on) (from) incline**
Fall (on) (from) ramp

X ● W10.8 **Fall (on) (from) other stairs and steps**

X ● W10.9 **Fall (on) (from) unspecified stairs and steps**

X ● W11 **Fall on and from ladder**

The appropriate 7th character is to be added to code W11

A	initial encounter
D	subsequent encounter
S	sequela

X ● W12 **Fall on and from scaffolding**

The appropriate 7th character is to be added to code W12

A	initial encounter
D	subsequent encounter
S	sequela

● W13 **Fall from, out of or through building or structure**

The appropriate 7th character is to be added to each code from category W13

A	initial encounter
D	subsequent encounter
S	sequela

▶ New   ➡ Revised   ~~deleted~~ Deleted   Excludes 1   Excludes 2   Includes   Use additional   Code first   Code also   Key words
OGCR Official Guidelines   X Assign placeholder X   ● Use Additional Character(s)   ▶ Manifestation Code   HCC Hierarchical Condition Category   Coding Clinic

X● **W13.0 Fall from, out of or through balcony**
Fall from, out of or through railing

X● **W13.1 Fall from, out of or through bridge**

X● **W13.2 Fall from, out of or through roof**

X● **W13.3 Fall through floor**

X● **W13.4 Fall from, out of or through window**
> **Excludes2** fall with subsequent striking against sharp glass (W01.110-)

X● **W13.8 Fall from, out of or through other building or structure**
Fall from, out of or through viaduct
Fall from, out of or through wall
Fall from, out of or through flag-pole

X● **W13.9 Fall from, out of or through building, not otherwise specified**
> **Excludes1** collapse of a building or structure (W20.-)
> fall or jump from burning building or structure (X00.-)

X● **W14 Fall from tree**
The appropriate 7th character is to be added to code W14

A	initial encounter
D	subsequent encounter
S	sequela

X● **W15 Fall from cliff**
The appropriate 7th character is to be added to code W15

A	initial encounter
D	subsequent encounter
S	sequela

● **W16 Fall, jump or diving into water**
> **Excludes1** accidental non-watercraft drowning and submersion not involving fall (W65-W74)
> effects of air pressure from diving (W94.-)
> fall into water from watercraft (V90-V94)
> hitting an object or against bottom when falling from watercraft (V94.0)
>
> **Excludes2** striking or hitting diving board (W21.4)

The appropriate 7th character is to be added to each code from category W16

A	initial encounter
D	subsequent encounter
S	sequela

● **W16.0 Fall into swimming pool**
Fall into swimming pool NOS
> **Excludes1** fall into empty swimming pool (W17.3)

● **W16.01 Fall into swimming pool striking water surface**

● **W16.011 Fall into swimming pool striking water surface causing drowning and submersion**
> **Excludes1** drowning and submersion while in swimming pool without fall (W67)

● **W16.012 Fall into swimming pool striking water surface causing other injury**

● **W16.02 Fall into swimming pool striking bottom**

● **W16.021 Fall into swimming pool striking bottom causing drowning and submersion**
> **Excludes1** drowning and submersion while in swimming pool without fall (W67)

● **W16.022 Fall into swimming pool striking bottom causing other injury**

● **W16.03 Fall into swimming pool striking wall**

● **W16.031 Fall into swimming pool striking wall causing drowning and submersion**
> **Excludes1** drowning and submersion while in swimming pool without fall (W67)

● **W16.032 Fall into swimming pool striking wall causing other injury**

● **W16.1 Fall into natural body of water**
Fall into lake
Fall into open sea
Fall into river
Fall into stream

● **W16.11 Fall into natural body of water striking water surface**

● **W16.111 Fall into natural body of water striking water surface causing drowning and submersion**
> **Excludes1** drowning and submersion while in natural body of water without fall (W69)

● **W16.112 Fall into natural body of water striking water surface causing other injury**

● **W16.12 Fall into natural body of water striking bottom**

● **W16.121 Fall into natural body of water striking bottom causing drowning and submersion**
> **Excludes1** drowning and submersion while in natural body of water without fall (W69)

● **W16.122 Fall into natural body of water striking bottom causing other injury**

● **W16.13 Fall into natural body of water striking side**

● **W16.131 Fall into natural body of water striking side causing drowning and submersion**
> **Excludes1** drowning and submersion while in natural body of water without fall (W69)

● **W16.132 Fall into natural body of water striking side causing other injury**

● **W16.2 Fall in (into) filled bathtub or bucket of water**

● **W16.21 Fall in (into) filled bathtub**
> **Excludes1** fall into empty bathtub (W18.2)

● **W16.211 Fall in (into) filled bathtub causing drowning and submersion**
> **Excludes1** drowning and submersion while in filled bathtub without fall (W65)

● **W16.212 Fall in (into) filled bathtub causing other injury**

● **W16.22 Fall in (into) bucket of water**

● **W16.221 Fall in (into) bucket of water causing drowning and submersion**

● **W16.222 Fall in (into) bucket of water causing other injury**

CHAPTER 20 (V00-Y99)

● **W16.3**   **Fall into other water**
Fall into fountain
Fall into reservoir

● **W16.31**   **Fall into other water striking water surface**

● **W16.311**   **Fall into other water striking water surface causing drowning and submersion**

    Excludes1   drowning and submersion while in other water without fall (W73)

● **W16.312**   **Fall into other water striking water surface causing other injury**

● **W16.32**   **Fall into other water striking bottom**

● **W16.321**   **Fall into other water striking bottom causing drowning and submersion**

    Excludes1   drowning and submersion while in other water without fall (W73)

● **W16.322**   **Fall into other water striking bottom causing other injury**

● **W16.33**   **Fall into other water striking wall**

● **W16.331**   **Fall into other water striking wall causing drowning and submersion**

    Excludes1   drowning and submersion while in other water without fall (W73)

● **W16.332**   **Fall into other water striking wall causing other injury**

● **W16.4**   **Fall into unspecified water**

X ● **W16.41**   **Fall into unspecified water causing drowning and submersion**

X ● **W16.42**   **Fall into unspecified water causing other injury**

● **W16.5**   **Jumping or diving into swimming pool**

● **W16.51**   **Jumping or diving into swimming pool striking water surface**

● **W16.511**   **Jumping or diving into swimming pool striking water surface causing drowning and submersion**

    Excludes1   drowning and submersion while in swimming pool without jumping or diving (W67)

● **W16.512**   **Jumping or diving into swimming pool striking water surface causing other injury**

● **W16.52**   **Jumping or diving into swimming pool striking bottom**

● **W16.521**   **Jumping or diving into swimming pool striking bottom causing drowning and submersion**

    Excludes1   drowning and submersion while in swimming pool without jumping or diving (W67)

● **W16.522**   **Jumping or diving into swimming pool striking bottom causing other injury**

● **W16.53**   **Jumping or diving into swimming pool striking wall**

● **W16.531**   **Jumping or diving into swimming pool striking wall causing drowning and submersion**

    Excludes1   drowning and submersion while in swimming pool without jumping or diving (W67)

● **W16.532**   **Jumping or diving into swimming pool striking wall causing other injury**

● **W16.6**   **Jumping or diving into natural body of water**
Jumping or diving into lake
Jumping or diving into open sea
Jumping or diving into river
Jumping or diving into stream

● **W16.61**   **Jumping or diving into natural body of water striking water surface**

● **W16.611**   **Jumping or diving into natural body of water striking water surface causing drowning and submersion**

    Excludes1   drowning and submersion while in natural body of water without jumping or diving (W69)

● **W16.612**   **Jumping or diving into natural body of water striking water surface causing other injury**

● **W16.62**   **Jumping or diving into natural body of water striking bottom**

● **W16.621**   **Jumping or diving into natural body of water striking bottom causing drowning and submersion**

    Excludes1   drowning and submersion while in natural body of water without jumping or diving (W69)

● **W16.622**   **Jumping or diving into natural body of water striking bottom causing other injury**

● **W16.7**   **Jumping or diving from boat**

    Excludes1   fall from boat into water - see watercraft accident (V90-V94)

● **W16.71**   **Jumping or diving from boat striking water surface**

● **W16.711**   **Jumping or diving from boat striking water surface causing drowning and submersion**

● **W16.712**   **Jumping or diving from boat striking water surface causing other injury**

● **W16.72**   **Jumping or diving from boat striking bottom**

● **W16.721**   **Jumping or diving from boat striking bottom causing drowning and submersion**

● **W16.722**   **Jumping or diving from boat striking bottom causing other injury**

● **W16.8 Jumping or diving into other water**
Jumping or diving into fountain
Jumping or diving into reservoir

  ● **W16.81 Jumping or diving into other water striking water surface**

    ● **W16.811 Jumping or diving into other water striking water surface causing drowning and submersion**
Excludes1   drowning and submersion while in other water without jumping or diving (W73)

    ● **W16.812 Jumping or diving into other water striking water surface causing other injury**

  ● **W16.82 Jumping or diving into other water striking bottom**

    ● **W16.821 Jumping or diving into other water striking bottom causing drowning and submersion**
Excludes1   drowning and submersion while in other water without jumping or diving (W73)

    ● **W16.822 Jumping or diving into other water striking bottom causing other injury**

  ● **W16.83 Jumping or diving into other water striking wall**

    ● **W16.831 Jumping or diving into other water striking wall causing drowning and submersion**
Excludes1   drowning and submersion while in other water without jumping or diving (W73)

    ● **W16.832 Jumping or diving into other water striking wall causing other injury**

● **W16.9 Jumping or diving into unspecified water**

  X ● **W16.91 Jumping or diving into unspecified water causing drowning and submersion**

  X ● **W16.92 Jumping or diving into unspecified water causing other injury**

● **W17 Other fall from one level to another**
The appropriate 7th character is to be added to each code from category W17

A	initial encounter
D	subsequent encounter
S	sequela

X ● **W17.0 Fall into well**

X ● **W17.1 Fall into storm drain or manhole**

X ● **W17.2 Fall into hole**
Fall into pit

X ● **W17.3 Fall into empty swimming pool**
Excludes1   fall into filled swimming pool (W16.0-)

X ● **W17.4 Fall from dock**

● **W17.8 Other fall from one level to another**

  X ● **W17.81 Fall down embankment (hill)**

  X ● **W17.82 Fall from (out of) grocery cart**
Fall due to grocery cart tipping over

  X ● **W17.89 Other fall from one level to another**
Fall from cherry picker
Fall from lifting device
Fall from mobile elevated work platform [MEWP]
Fall from sky lift
Coding Clinic: 2015, Q2, P6

● **W18 Other slipping, tripping and stumbling and falls**
The appropriate 7th character is to be added to each code from category W18

A	initial encounter
D	subsequent encounter
S	sequela

● **W18.0 Fall due to bumping against object**
Striking against object with subsequent fall
Excludes1   fall on same level due to slipping, tripping, or stumbling with subsequent striking against object (W01.1-)

  X ● **W18.00 Striking against unspecified object with subsequent fall**

  X ● **W18.01 Striking against sports equipment with subsequent fall**

  X ● **W18.02 Striking against glass with subsequent fall**

  X ● **W18.09 Striking against other object with subsequent fall**

● **W18.1 Fall from or off toilet**

  X ● **W18.11 Fall from or off toilet without subsequent striking against object**
Fall from (off) toilet NOS

  X ● **W18.12 Fall from or off toilet with subsequent striking against object**

X ● **W18.2 Fall in (into) shower or empty bathtub**
Excludes1   fall in full bathtub causing drowning or submersion (W16.21-)

● **W18.3 Other and unspecified fall on same level**

  X ● **W18.30 Fall on same level, unspecified**

  X ● **W18.31 Fall on same level due to stepping on an object**
Fall on same level due to stepping on an animal
Excludes1   slipping, tripping and stumbling without fall due to stepping on animal (W18.41)

  X ● **W18.39 Other fall on same level**

● **W18.4 Slipping, tripping and stumbling without falling**
Excludes1   collision with another person without fall (W51)

  X ● **W18.40 Slipping, tripping and stumbling without falling, unspecified**

  X ● **W18.41 Slipping, tripping and stumbling without falling due to stepping on object**
Slipping, tripping and stumbling without falling due to stepping on animal
Excludes1   slipping, tripping and stumbling with fall due to stepping on animal (W18.31)

  X ● **W18.42 Slipping, tripping and stumbling without falling due to stepping into hole or opening**

  X ● **W18.43 Slipping, tripping and stumbling without falling due to stepping from one level to another**

  X ● **W18.49 Other slipping, tripping and stumbling without falling**

X ● **W19 Unspecified fall**
Accidental fall NOS
The appropriate 7th character is to be added to code W19

A	initial encounter
D	subsequent encounter
S	sequela

CHAPTER 20 (V00–Y99)

EXPOSURE TO INANIMATE MECHANICAL FORCES (W20-W49)

Excludes1   assault (X92-Y09)
contact or collision with animals or persons (W50-W64)
exposure to inanimate mechanical forces involving military or war operations (Y36.-, Y37.-)
intentional self-harm (X71-X83)
Coding Clinic: 2022, Q4, P45; 2021, Q2, P5; 2016, Q4, P129; 2012, Q4, P95

● **W20   Struck by thrown, projected or falling object**
Code first any associated:
cataclysm (X34-X39)
lightning strike (T75.00)
Excludes1   falling object in machinery accident (W24, W28-W31)
falling object in transport accident (V01-V99)
object set in motion by explosion (W35-W40)
object set in motion by firearm (W32-W34)
struck by thrown sports equipment (W21.-)

The appropriate 7th character is to be added to each code from category W20

> A   initial encounter
> D   subsequent encounter
> S   sequela

X● **W20.0   Struck by falling object in cave-in**
Excludes2   asphyxiation due to cave-in (T71.21)
X● **W20.1   Struck by object due to collapse of building**
Excludes1   struck by object due to collapse of burning building (X00.2, X02.2)
X● **W20.8   Other cause of strike by thrown, projected or falling object**
Excludes1   struck by thrown sports equipment (W21.-)

● **W21   Striking against or struck by sports equipment**
Excludes1   assault with sports equipment (Y08.0-)
striking against or struck by sports equipment with subsequent fall (W18.01)

The appropriate 7th character is to be added to each code from category W21

> A   initial encounter
> D   subsequent encounter
> S   sequela

● **W21.0   Struck by hit or thrown ball**
X● **W21.00   Struck by hit or thrown ball, unspecified type**
X● **W21.01   Struck by football**
X● **W21.02   Struck by soccer ball**
X● **W21.03   Struck by baseball**
X● **W21.04   Struck by golf ball**
X● **W21.05   Struck by basketball**
X● **W21.06   Struck by volleyball**
X● **W21.07   Struck by softball**
X● **W21.09   Struck by other hit or thrown ball**
● **W21.1   Struck by bat, racquet or club**
X● **W21.11   Struck by baseball bat**
X● **W21.12   Struck by tennis racquet**
X● **W21.13   Struck by golf club**
X● **W21.19   Struck by other bat, racquet or club**
● **W21.2   Struck by hockey stick or puck**
● **W21.21   Struck by hockey stick**
● **W21.210   Struck by ice hockey stick**
● **W21.211   Struck by field hockey stick**

● **W21.22   Struck by hockey puck**
● **W21.220   Struck by ice hockey puck**
● **W21.221   Struck by field hockey puck**
● **W21.3   Struck by sports foot wear**
X● **W21.31   Struck by shoe cleats**
Stepped on by shoe cleats
X● **W21.32   Struck by skate blades**
Skated over by skate blades
X● **W21.39   Struck by other sports foot wear**
X● **W21.4   Striking against diving board**
Use additional code for subsequent falling into water, if applicable (W16.-)
● **W21.8   Striking against or struck by other sports equipment**
X● **W21.81   Striking against or struck by football helmet**
X● **W21.89   Striking against or struck by other sports equipment**
X● **W21.9   Striking against or struck by unspecified sports equipment**

● **W22   Striking against or struck by other objects**
Excludes1   striking against or struck by object with subsequent fall (W18.09)

The appropriate 7th character is to be added to each code from category W22

> A   initial encounter
> D   subsequent encounter
> S   sequela

● **W22.0   Striking against stationary object**
Excludes1   striking against stationary sports equipment (W21.8)
X● **W22.01   Walked into wall**
X● **W22.02   Walked into lamppost**
X● **W22.03   Walked into furniture**
● **W22.04   Striking against wall of swimming pool**
● **W22.041   Striking against wall of swimming pool causing drowning and submersion**
Excludes1   drowning and submersion while swimming without striking against wall (W67)
● **W22.042   Striking against wall of swimming pool causing other injury**
X● **W22.09   Striking against other stationary object**
● **W22.1   Striking against or struck by automobile airbag**
X● **W22.10   Striking against or struck by unspecified automobile airbag**
X● **W22.11   Striking against or struck by driver side automobile airbag**
X● **W22.12   Striking against or struck by front passenger side automobile airbag**
X● **W22.19   Striking against or struck by other automobile airbag**
X● **W22.8   Striking against or struck by other objects**
Striking against or struck by object NOS
Excludes1   struck by thrown, projected or falling object (W20.-)

● W23 Caught, crushed, jammed or pinched in or between objects

> **Excludes1**   injury caused by cutting or piercing instruments (W25-W27)
>
> injury caused by firearms malfunction (W32.1, W33.1-, W34.1-)
>
> injury caused by lifting and transmission devices (W24.-)
>
> injury caused by machinery (W28-W31)
>
> injury caused by nonpowered hand tools (W27.-)
>
> injury caused by transport vehicle being used as a means of transportation (V01-V99)
>
> injury caused by struck by thrown, projected or falling object (W20.-)

The appropriate 7th character is to be added to each code from category W23

A	initial encounter
D	subsequent encounter
S	sequela

X ● W23.0 Caught, crushed, jammed, or pinched between moving objects

X ● W23.1 Caught, crushed, jammed, or pinched between stationary objects

X ● W23.2 Caught, crushed, jammed or pinched between a moving and stationary object

● W24 Contact with lifting and transmission devices, not elsewhere classified

> **Excludes1**   transport accidents (V01-V99)

The appropriate 7th character is to be added to each code from category W24

A	initial encounter
D	subsequent encounter
S	sequela

X ● W24.0 Contact with lifting devices, not elsewhere classified
> Contact with chain hoist
> Contact with drive belt
> Contact with pulley (block)

X ● W24.1 Contact with transmission devices, not elsewhere classified
> Contact with transmission belt or cable

X ● W25 Contact with sharp glass

> *Code first* any associated:
> injury due to flying glass from explosion or firearm discharge (W32-W40)
> transport accident (V00-V99)

> **Excludes1**   fall on same level due to slipping, tripping and stumbling with subsequent striking against sharp glass (W01.110-)
>
> striking against sharp glass with subsequent fall (W18.02-)

> **Excludes2**   glass embedded in skin (W45.-)

The appropriate 7th character is to be added to code W25

A	initial encounter
D	subsequent encounter
S	sequela

● W26 Contact with other sharp objects

> **Excludes2**   sharp object(s) embedded in skin (W45.-)

The appropriate 7th character is to be added to each code from category W26

A	initial encounter
D	subsequent encounter
S	sequela

Coding Clinic: 2016, Q4, P73

X ● W26.0 Contact with knife
> **Excludes1**   contact with electric knife (W29.1)

X ● W26.1 Contact with sword or dagger

X ● W26.2 Contact with edge of stiff paper
> Paper cut
> **Coding Clinic: 2016, Q4, P73**

X ● W26.8 Contact with other sharp object(s), not elsewhere classified
> Contact with tin can lid
> **Coding Clinic: 2016, Q4, P73**

X ● W26.9 Contact with unspecified sharp object(s)
> **Coding Clinic: 2016, Q4, P73**

● W27 Contact with nonpowered hand tool

The appropriate 7th character is to be added to each code from category W27

A	initial encounter
D	subsequent encounter
S	sequela

X ● W27.0 Contact with workbench tool
> Contact with auger
> Contact with axe
> Contact with chisel
> Contact with handsaw
> Contact with screwdriver

X ● W27.1 Contact with garden tool
> Contact with hoe
> Contact with nonpowered lawn mower
> Contact with pitchfork
> Contact with rake

X ● W27.2 Contact with scissors

X ● W27.3 Contact with needle (sewing)
> **Excludes1**   contact with hypodermic needle (W46.-)

X ● W27.4 Contact with kitchen utensil
> Contact with fork
> Contact with ice-pick
> Contact with can-opener NOS

X ● W27.5 Contact with paper-cutter

X ● W27.8 Contact with other nonpowered hand tool
> Contact with nonpowered sewing machine
> Contact with shovel

X ● W28 Contact with powered lawn mower
> Powered lawn mower (commercial) (residential)
> **Excludes1**   contact with nonpowered lawn mower (W27.1)
> **Excludes2**   exposure to electric current (W86.-)

The appropriate 7th character is to be added to code W28

A	initial encounter
D	subsequent encounter
S	sequela

● W29 Contact with other powered hand tools and household machinery

> **Excludes1**   contact with commercial machinery (W31.82)
> contact with hot household appliance (X15)
> contact with nonpowered hand tool (W27.-)
> exposure to electric current (W86)

The appropriate 7th character is to be added to each code from category W29

A	initial encounter
D	subsequent encounter
S	sequela

X ● W29.0 Contact with powered kitchen appliance
> Contact with blender
> Contact with can-opener
> Contact with garbage disposal
> Contact with mixer

X ● W29.1 Contact with electric knife

X ● W29.2 Contact with other powered household machinery
> Contact with electric fan
> Contact with powered dryer (clothes) (powered) (spin)
> Contact with washing-machine
> Contact with sewing machine

N Newborn Age: 0   **P** Pediatric Age: 0–17   **M** Maternity DX: 9–64   **A** Adult Age: 15–124

X● **W29.3**   **Contact with powered garden and outdoor hand tools and machinery**
     Contact with chainsaw
     Contact with edger
     Contact with garden cultivator (tiller)
     Contact with hedge trimmer
     Contact with other powered garden tool
       Excludes1   contact with powered lawn mower (W28)

X● **W29.4**   **Contact with nail gun**

X● **W29.8**   **Contact with other powered hand tools and household machinery**
     Contact with do-it-yourself tool NOS

● **W30**   **Contact with agricultural machinery**
     Includes   animal-powered farm machine
     Excludes1   agricultural transport vehicle accident (V01-V99)
           explosion of grain store (W40.8)
           exposure to electric current (W86.-)

The appropriate 7th character is to be added to each code from category W30

     A   initial encounter
     D   subsequent encounter
     S   sequela

X● **W30.0**   **Contact with combine harvester**
     Contact with reaper
     Contact with thresher

X● **W30.1**   **Contact with power take-off devices (PTO)**

X● **W30.2**   **Contact with hay derrick**

X● **W30.3**   **Contact with grain storage elevator**
       Excludes1   explosion of grain store (W40.8)

● **W30.8**   **Contact with other specified agricultural machinery**

   X● **W30.81**   **Contact with agricultural transport vehicle in stationary use**
       Contact with agricultural transport vehicle under repair, not on public roadway
         Excludes1   agricultural transport vehicle accident (V01-V99)

   X● **W30.89**   **Contact with other specified agricultural machinery**

X● **W30.9**   **Contact with unspecified agricultural machinery**
     Contact with farm machinery NOS

● **W31**   **Contact with other and unspecified machinery**
     Excludes1   contact with agricultural machinery (W30.-)
           contact with machinery in transport under own power or being towed by a vehicle (V01-V99)
           exposure to electric current (W86)

The appropriate 7th character is to be added to each code from category W31

     A   initial encounter
     D   subsequent encounter
     S   sequela

X● **W31.0**   **Contact with mining and earth-drilling machinery**
     Contact with bore or drill (land) (seabed)
     Contact with shaft hoist
     Contact with shaft lift
     Contact with undercutter

X● **W31.1**   **Contact with metalworking machines**
     Contact with abrasive wheel
     Contact with forging machine
     Contact with lathe
     Contact with mechanical shears
     Contact with metal drilling machine
     Contact with milling machine
     Contact with power press
     Contact with rolling-mill
     Contact with metal sawing machine

X● **W31.2**   **Contact with powered woodworking and forming machines**
     Contact with band saw
     Contact with bench saw
     Contact with circular saw
     Contact with molding machine
     Contact with overhead plane
     Contact with powered saw
     Contact with radial saw
     Contact with sander
       Excludes1   nonpowered woodworking tools (W27.0)

X● **W31.3**   **Contact with prime movers**
     Contact with gas turbine
     Contact with internal combustion engine
     Contact with steam engine
     Contact with water driven turbine

● **W31.8**   **Contact with other specified machinery**

   X● **W31.81**   **Contact with recreational machinery**
       Contact with roller-coaster

   X● **W31.82**   **Contact with other commercial machinery**
       Contact with commercial electric fan
       Contact with commercial kitchen appliances
       Contact with commercial powered dryer (clothes) (powered) (spin)
       Contact with commercial washing-machine
       Contact with commercial sewing machine
         Excludes1   contact with household machinery (W29.-)
                contact with powered lawn mower (W28)

   X● **W31.83**   **Contact with special construction vehicle in stationary use**
       Contact with special construction vehicle under repair, not on public roadway
         Excludes1   special construction vehicle accident (V01-V99)

   X● **W31.89**   **Contact with other specified machinery**

X● **W31.9**   **Contact with unspecified machinery**
     Contact with machinery NOS

● **W32**   **Accidental handgun discharge and malfunction**
     Includes   accidental discharge and malfunction of gun for single hand use
           accidental discharge and malfunction of pistol
           accidental discharge and malfunction of revolver
           handgun discharge and malfunction NOS
     Excludes1   accidental airgun discharge and malfunction (W34.010, W34.110)
           accidental BB gun discharge and malfunction (W34.010, W34.110)
           accidental pellet gun discharge and malfunction (W34.010, W34.110)
           accidental shotgun discharge and malfunction (W33.01, W33.11)
           assault by handgun discharge (X93)
           handgun discharge involving legal intervention (Y35.0-)
           handgun discharge involving military or war operations (Y36.4-)
           intentional self-harm by handgun discharge (X72)
           Very pistol discharge and malfunction (W34.09, W34.19)

The appropriate 7th character is to be added to each code from category W32

     A   initial encounter
     D   subsequent encounter
     S   sequela

X● **W32.0**   **Accidental handgun discharge**

X● **W32.1**   **Accidental handgun malfunction**
     Injury due to explosion of handgun (parts)
     Injury due to malfunction of mechanism or component of handgun
     Injury due to recoil of handgun
     Powder burn from handgun

▶ New   ➡ Revised   ~~deleted~~ Deleted   Excludes 1   Excludes 2   Includes   Use additional   Code first   Code also   Key words
OGCR Official Guidelines   X Assign placeholder X   ● Use Additional Character(s)   ▶ Manifestation Code   HCC Hierarchical Condition Category   Coding Clinic

● **W33 Accidental rifle, shotgun and larger firearm discharge and malfunction**

Includes	rifle, shotgun and larger firearm discharge and malfunction NOS
Excludes1	accidental airgun discharge and malfunction (W34.010, W34.110)
	accidental BB gun discharge and malfunction (W34.010, W34.110)
	accidental handgun discharge and malfunction (W32.-)
	accidental pellet gun discharge and malfunction (W34.010, W34.110)
	assault by rifle, shotgun and larger firearm discharge (X94)
	firearm discharge involving legal intervention (Y35.0-)
	firearm discharge involving military or war operations (Y36.4-)
	intentional self-harm by rifle, shotgun and larger firearm discharge (X73)

The appropriate 7th character is to be added to each code from category W33

A	initial encounter
D	subsequent encounter
S	sequela

● **W33.0 Accidental rifle, shotgun and larger firearm discharge**

X● **W33.00 Accidental discharge of unspecified larger firearm**
Discharge of unspecified larger firearm NOS

X● **W33.01 Accidental discharge of shotgun**
Discharge of shotgun NOS

X● **W33.02 Accidental discharge of hunting rifle**
Discharge of hunting rifle NOS

X● **W33.03 Accidental discharge of machine gun**
Discharge of machine gun NOS

X● **W33.09 Accidental discharge of other larger firearm**
Discharge of other larger firearm NOS

● **W33.1 Accidental rifle, shotgun and larger firearm malfunction**
Injury due to explosion of rifle, shotgun and larger firearm (parts)
Injury due to malfunction of mechanism or component of rifle, shotgun and larger firearm
Injury due to piercing, cutting, crushing or pinching due to (by) slide trigger mechanism, scope or other gun part
Injury due to recoil of rifle, shotgun and larger firearm
Powder burn from rifle, shotgun and larger firearm

X● **W33.10 Accidental malfunction of unspecified larger firearm**
Malfunction of unspecified larger firearm NOS

X● **W33.11 Accidental malfunction of shotgun**
Malfunction of shotgun NOS

X● **W33.12 Accidental malfunction of hunting rifle**
Malfunction of hunting rifle NOS

X● **W33.13 Accidental malfunction of machine gun**
Malfunction of machine gun NOS

X● **W33.19 Accidental malfunction of other larger firearm**
Malfunction of other larger firearm NOS

● **W34 Accidental discharge and malfunction from other and unspecified firearms and guns**

The appropriate 7th character is to be added to each code from category W34

A	initial encounter
D	subsequent encounter
S	sequela

● **W34.0 Accidental discharge from other and unspecified firearms and guns**

X● **W34.00 Accidental discharge from unspecified firearms or gun**
Discharge from firearm NOS
Gunshot wound NOS
Shot NOS
Coding Clinic: 2015, Q1, P17

● **W34.01 Accidental discharge of gas, air or spring-operated guns**

● **W34.010 Accidental discharge of airgun**
Accidental discharge of BB gun
Accidental discharge of pellet gun

● **W34.011 Accidental discharge of paintball gun**
Accidental injury due to paintball discharge

● **W34.018 Accidental discharge of other gas, air or spring-operated gun**

X● **W34.09 Accidental discharge from other specified firearms**
Accidental discharge from Very pistol [flare]

● **W34.1 Accidental malfunction from other and unspecified firearms and guns**

X● **W34.10 Accidental malfunction from unspecified firearms or gun**
Firearm malfunction NOS

● **W34.11 Accidental malfunction of gas, air or spring-operated guns**

● **W34.110 Accidental malfunction of airgun**
Accidental malfunction of BB gun
Accidental malfunction of pellet gun

● **W34.111 Accidental malfunction of paintball gun**
Accidental injury due to paintball gun malfunction

● **W34.118 Accidental malfunction of other gas, air or spring-operated gun**

X● **W34.19 Accidental malfunction from other specified firearms**
Accidental malfunction from Very pistol [flare]

X● **W35 Explosion and rupture of boiler**

Excludes1	explosion and rupture of boiler on watercraft (V93.4)

The appropriate 7th character is to be added to code W35

A	initial encounter
D	subsequent encounter
S	sequela

● **W36 Explosion and rupture of gas cylinder**

The appropriate 7th character is to be added to each code from category W36

A	initial encounter
D	subsequent encounter
S	sequela

X● **W36.1 Explosion and rupture of aerosol can**

X● **W36.2 Explosion and rupture of air tank**

X● **W36.3 Explosion and rupture of pressurized-gas tank**

X● **W36.8 Explosion and rupture of other gas cylinder**

X● **W36.9 Explosion and rupture of unspecified gas cylinder**

● **W37 Explosion and rupture of pressurized tire, pipe or hose**

The appropriate 7th character is to be added to each code from category W37

A	initial encounter
D	subsequent encounter
S	sequela

X● **W37.0 Explosion of bicycle tire**

X● **W37.8 Explosion and rupture of other pressurized tire, pipe or hose**

CHAPTER 20 (V00–Y99)

X ● W38 Explosion and rupture of other specified pressurized devices
The appropriate 7th character is to be added to code W38

> A   initial encounter
> D   subsequent encounter
> S   sequela

X ● W39 Discharge of firework
The appropriate 7th character is to be added to code W39

> A   initial encounter
> D   subsequent encounter
> S   sequela

● W40 Explosion of other materials
> **Excludes1**   assault by explosive material (X96)
> explosion involving legal intervention (Y35.1-)
> explosion involving military or war operations (Y36.0-, Y36.2-)
> intentional self-harm by explosive material (X75)

The appropriate 7th character is to be added to each code from category W40

> A   initial encounter
> D   subsequent encounter
> S   sequela

X ● W40.0 Explosion of blasting material
Explosion of blasting cap
Explosion of detonator
Explosion of dynamite
Explosion of explosive (any) used in blasting operations

X ● W40.1 Explosion of explosive gases
Explosion of acetylene
Explosion of butane
Explosion of coal gas
Explosion in mine NOS
Explosion of explosive gas
Explosion of fire damp
Explosion of gasoline fumes
Explosion of methane
Explosion of propane

X ● W40.8 Explosion of other specified explosive materials
Explosion in dump NOS
Explosion in factory NOS
Explosion in grain store
Explosion in munitions
> **Excludes1**   explosion involving legal intervention (Y35.1-)
> explosion involving military or war operations (Y36.0-, Y36.2-)

X ● W40.9 Explosion of unspecified explosive materials
Explosion NOS

● W42 Exposure to noise
The appropriate 7th character is to be added to each code from category W42

> A   initial encounter
> D   subsequent encounter
> S   sequela

X ● W42.0 Exposure to supersonic waves
X ● W42.9 Exposure to other noise
Exposure to sound waves NOS

● W44 Foreign body entering into or through a natural orifice
> **Excludes2**   contact with other sharp objects (W26)
> contact with sharp glass (W25)
> foreign body or object entering through skin (W45)

The appropriate 7th character is to be added to each code from category W44

> A   initial encounter
> D   subsequent encounter
> S   sequela

X ● W44.A Battery entering into or through a natural orifice

W44.A0 Battery unspecified, entering into or through a natural orifice

W44.A1 Button battery entering into or through a natural orifice

W44.A9 Other batteries entering into or through a natural orifice
➡ Cylindrical battery entering into or through a natural orifice

X ● W44.B Plastic entering into or through a natural orifice

W44.B0 Plastic object unspecified, entering into or through a natural orifice

W44.B1 Plastic bead entering into or through a natural orifice
> **Excludes2**   Plastic jewelry entering into or through a natural orifice (W44.B4)

W44.B2 Plastic coin entering into or through a natural orifice

W44.B3 Plastic toy and toy part entering into or through a natural orifice

W44.B4 Plastic jewelry entering into or through a natural orifice
> **Excludes2**   Plastic bead entering into or through a natural orifice (W44.B1)

W44.B5 Plastic bottle entering into or through a natural orifice

W44.B9 Other plastic object entering into or through a natural orifice

X ● W44.C Glass entering into or through a natural orifice

W44.C0 Glass unspecified, entering into or through a natural orifice

W44.C1 Sharp glass entering into or through a natural orifice
Glass shard entering into or through a natural orifice

W44.C2 Intact glass entering into or through a natural orifice
Intact glass bottle entering into or through a natural orifice

X ● W44.D Magnetic metal entering into or through a natural orifice

W44.D0 Magnetic metal object unspecified, entering into or through a natural orifice

W44.D1 Magnetic metal bead entering into or through a natural orifice

W44.D2 Magnetic metal coin entering into or through a natural orifice

W44.D3 Magnetic metal toy entering into or through a natural orifice

W44.D4 Magnetic metal jewelry entering into or through a natural orifice

W44.D9 Other magnetic metal objects entering into or through a natural orifice

X ● W44.E Non-magnetic metal entering into or through a natural orifice

W44.E0 Non-magnetic metal object unspecified, entering into or through a natural orifice

W44.E1 Non-magnetic metal bead entering into or through a natural orifice

W44.E2 Non-magnetic metal coin entering into or through a natural orifice

CHAPTER 20 (V00-Y99)

W44.E3 Non-magnetic metal toy entering into or through a natural orifice

W44.E4 Non-magnetic metal jewelry entering into or through a natural orifice

W44.E9 Other non-magnetic metal objects entering into or through a natural orifice
> Bottle cap entering into or through a natural orifice
> Can lid entering into or through a natural orifice
> Pull tab entering into or through a natural orifice

X● W44.F Objects of natural or organic material entering into or through a natural orifice

W44.F0 Objects of natural or organic material unspecified, entering into or through anatural orifice

W44.F1 Bezoar entering into or through a natural orifice

W44.F2 Rubber band entering into or through a natural orifice

W44.F3 Food entering into or through a natural orifice

W44.F4 Insect entering into or through a natural orifice

W44.F9 Other object of natural or organic material, entering into or through a natural orifice

X● W44.G Other non-organic objects entering into or through a natural orifice

W44.G0 Other non-organic objects unspecified, entering into or through a natural orifice

W44.G1 Audio device entering into or through a natural orifice
> Ear buds
> Hearing aids

W44.G2 Combination metal and plastic toy and toy part entering into or through natural orifice

W44.G3 Combination metal and plastic jewelry entering into or through a natural orifice

W44.G9 Other non-organic objects entering into or through a natural orifice

X● W44.H Other sharp object entering into or through a natural orifice

W44.H0 Other sharp object unspecified, entering into or through a natural orifice

W44.H1 Needle entering into or through a natural orifice
> Dart entering into or through a natural orifice
> Hypodermic needle entering into or through a natural orifice
> Safety pin entering into or through a natural orifice
> Sewing needle entering into or through a natural orifice

W44.H2 Knife, sword or dagger entering into or through a natural orifice

▶ W44.H9 Other sharp object entering into or through a natural orifice
> ▶ Shard pottery entering into or through a natural orifice

W44.8 Other foreign body entering into or through a natural orifice

W44.9 Unspecified foreign body entering into or through a natural orifice
> Foreign body NOS entering into or through a natural orifice

● W45 Foreign body or object entering through skin

Includes   foreign body or object embedded in skin
nail embedded in skin

Excludes2   contact with hand tools (nonpowered) (powered) (W27-W29)
contact with other sharp object(s) (W26.-)
contact with sharp glass (W25.-)
struck by objects (W20-W22)

The appropriate 7th character is to be added to each code from category W45

A	initial encounter
D	subsequent encounter
S	sequela

X● W45.0 Nail entering through skin

▶ X● W45.3 Fishing hook entering through skin

X● W45.8 Other foreign body or object entering through skin
> Splinter in skin NOS

● W46 Contact with hypodermic needle

The appropriate 7th character is to be added to each code from category W46

A	initial encounter
D	subsequent encounter
S	sequela

X● W46.0 Contact with hypodermic needle
> Hypodermic needle stick NOS

X● W46.1 Contact with contaminated hypodermic needle

● W49 Exposure to other inanimate mechanical forces

Includes   exposure to abnormal gravitational [G] forces
exposure to inanimate mechanical forces NEC

Excludes1   exposure to inanimate mechanical forces involving military or war operations (Y36.-, Y37.-)

The appropriate 7th character is to be added to each code from category W49

A	initial encounter
D	subsequent encounter
S	sequela

● W49.0 Item causing external constriction

X● W49.01 Hair causing external constriction

X● W49.02 String or thread causing external constriction

X● W49.03 Rubber band causing external constriction

X● W49.04 Ring or other jewelry causing external constriction

X● W49.09 Other item causing external constriction

X● W49.9 Exposure to other inanimate mechanical forces

EXPOSURE TO ANIMATE MECHANICAL FORCES (W50-W64)

Excludes1   toxic effect of contact with venomous animals and plants (T63.-)

● W50 Accidental hit, strike, kick, twist, bite or scratch by another person

Includes   hit, strike, kick, twist, bite, or scratch by another person NOS

Excludes1   assault by bodily force (Y04)
struck by objects (W20-W22)

The appropriate 7th character is to be added to each code from category W50

A	initial encounter
D	subsequent encounter
S	sequela

X● W50.0 Accidental hit or strike by another person
> Hit or strike by another person NOS

X● W50.1 Accidental kick by another person
> Kick by another person NOS

X● W50.2 Accidental twist by another person
> Twist by another person NOS
> **Coding Clinic: 2015, Q1, P8**

X● W50.3 Accidental bite by another person
> Human bite
> Bite by another person NOS

X● W50.4 Accidental scratch by another person
> Scratch by another person NOS

CHAPTER 20 (V00-Y99)

X ● **W51   Accidental striking against or bumped into by another person**

> **Excludes1**   assault by striking against or bumping into by another person (Y04.2)
> fall due to collision with another person (W03)

> The appropriate 7th character is to be added to code W51
>
> | | |
> |---|---|
> | A | initial encounter |
> | D | subsequent encounter |
> | S | sequela |

X ● **W52   Crushed, pushed or stepped on by crowd or human stampede**

> Crushed, pushed or stepped on by crowd or human stampede with or without fall

> The appropriate 7th character is to be added to code W52
>
> | | |
> |---|---|
> | A | initial encounter |
> | D | subsequent encounter |
> | S | sequela |

● **W53   Contact with rodent**

> **Includes**   contact with saliva, feces or urine of rodent

> The appropriate 7th character is to be added to each code from category W53
>
> | | |
> |---|---|
> | A | initial encounter |
> | D | subsequent encounter |
> | S | sequela |

   ● **W53.0   Contact with mouse**
     X ● **W53.01   Bitten by mouse**
     X ● **W53.09   Other contact with mouse**
   ● **W53.1   Contact with rat**
     X ● **W53.11   Bitten by rat**
     X ● **W53.19   Other contact with rat**
   ● **W53.2   Contact with squirrel**
     X ● **W53.21   Bitten by squirrel**
     X ● **W53.29   Other contact with squirrel**
   ● **W53.8   Contact with other rodent**
     X ● **W53.81   Bitten by other rodent**
     X ● **W53.89   Other contact with other rodent**

● **W54   Contact with dog**

> **Includes**   contact with saliva, feces or urine of dog

> The appropriate 7th character is to be added to each code from category W54
>
> | | |
> |---|---|
> | A | initial encounter |
> | D | subsequent encounter |
> | S | sequela |

   X ● **W54.0   Bitten by dog**
   X ● **W54.1   Struck by dog**
     Knocked over by dog
   X ● **W54.8   Other contact with dog**

● **W55   Contact with other mammals**

> **Includes**   contact with saliva, feces or urine of mammal
>
> **Excludes1**   animal being ridden - see transport accidents
> bitten or struck by dog (W54)
> bitten or struck by rodent (W53.-)
> contact with marine mammals (W56.X-)

> The appropriate 7th character is to be added to each code from category W55
>
> | | |
> |---|---|
> | A | initial encounter |
> | D | subsequent encounter |
> | S | sequela |

   ● **W55.0   Contact with cat**
     X ● **W55.01   Bitten by cat**
     X ● **W55.03   Scratched by cat**
     X ● **W55.09   Other contact with cat**
   ● **W55.1   Contact with horse**
     X ● **W55.11   Bitten by horse**
     X ● **W55.12   Struck by horse**
     X ● **W55.19   Other contact with horse**
   ● **W55.2   Contact with cow**
     Contact with bull
     X ● **W55.21   Bitten by cow**
     X ● **W55.22   Struck by cow**
      Gored by bull
     X ● **W55.29   Other contact with cow**
   ● **W55.3   Contact with other hoof stock**
     Contact with goats
     Contact with sheep
     X ● **W55.31   Bitten by other hoof stock**
     X ● **W55.32   Struck by other hoof stock**
      Gored by goat
      Gored by ram
     X ● **W55.39   Other contact with other hoof stock**
   ● **W55.4   Contact with pig**
     X ● **W55.41   Bitten by pig**
     X ● **W55.42   Struck by pig**
     X ● **W55.49   Other contact with pig**
   ● **W55.5   Contact with raccoon**
     X ● **W55.51   Bitten by raccoon**
     X ● **W55.52   Struck by raccoon**
     X ● **W55.59   Other contact with raccoon**
   ● **W55.8   Contact with other mammals**
     X ● **W55.81   Bitten by other mammals**
     X ● **W55.82   Struck by other mammals**
     X ● **W55.89   Other contact with other mammals**

● **W56   Contact with nonvenomous marine animal**

> **Excludes1**   contact with venomous marine animal (T63.-)

> The appropriate 7th character is to be added to each code from category W56
>
> | | |
> |---|---|
> | A | initial encounter |
> | D | subsequent encounter |
> | S | sequela |

   ● **W56.0   Contact with dolphin**
     X ● **W56.01   Bitten by dolphin**
     X ● **W56.02   Struck by dolphin**
     X ● **W56.09   Other contact with dolphin**
   ● **W56.1   Contact with sea lion**
     X ● **W56.11   Bitten by sea lion**
     X ● **W56.12   Struck by sea lion**
     X ● **W56.19   Other contact with sea lion**
   ● **W56.2   Contact with orca**
     Contact with killer whale
     X ● **W56.21   Bitten by orca**
     X ● **W56.22   Struck by orca**
     X ● **W56.29   Other contact with orca**
   ● **W56.3   Contact with other marine mammals**
     X ● **W56.31   Bitten by other marine mammals**
     X ● **W56.32   Struck by other marine mammals**
     X ● **W56.39   Other contact with other marine mammals**
   ● **W56.4   Contact with shark**
     X ● **W56.41   Bitten by shark**
     X ● **W56.42   Struck by shark**
     X ● **W56.49   Other contact with shark**
   ● **W56.5   Contact with other fish**
     X ● **W56.51   Bitten by other fish**
     X ● **W56.52   Struck by other fish**
     X ● **W56.59   Other contact with other fish**

▶ New   ⇨ Revised   ~~deleted~~ Deleted   Excludes 1   Excludes 2   Includes   Use additional   Code first   Code also   Key words

OGCR Official Guidelines   **X** Assign placeholder X   ● Use Additional Character(s)   ⬦ Manifestation Code   **Hc** Hierarchical Condition Category   **Coding Clinic**

● **W56.8 Contact with other nonvenomous marine animals**
    X● **W56.81 Bitten by other nonvenomous marine animals**
    X● **W56.82 Struck by other nonvenomous marine animals**
    X● **W56.89 Other contact with other nonvenomous marine animals**

X● **W57 Bitten or stung by nonvenomous insect and other nonvenomous arthropods**
    Excludes1   contact with venomous insects and arthropods (T63.2-, T63.3-, T63.4-)

The appropriate 7th character is to be added to code W57

A	initial encounter
D	subsequent encounter
S	sequela

● **W58 Contact with crocodile or alligator**
The appropriate 7th character is to be added to each code from category W58

A	initial encounter
D	subsequent encounter
S	sequela

   ● **W58.0 Contact with alligator**
    X● **W58.01 Bitten by alligator**
    X● **W58.02 Struck by alligator**
    X● **W58.03 Crushed by alligator**
    X● **W58.09 Other contact with alligator**
   ● **W58.1 Contact with crocodile**
    X● **W58.11 Bitten by crocodile**
    X● **W58.12 Struck by crocodile**
    X● **W58.13 Crushed by crocodile**
    X● **W58.19 Other contact with crocodile**

● **W59 Contact with other nonvenomous reptiles**
    Excludes1   contact with venomous reptile (T63.0-, T63.1-)
The appropriate 7th character is to be added to each code from category W59

A	initial encounter
D	subsequent encounter
S	sequela

   ● **W59.0 Contact with nonvenomous lizards**
    X● **W59.01 Bitten by nonvenomous lizards**
    X● **W59.02 Struck by nonvenomous lizards**
    X● **W59.09 Other contact with nonvenomous lizards**
       Exposure to nonvenomous lizards
   ● **W59.1 Contact with nonvenomous snakes**
    X● **W59.11 Bitten by nonvenomous snake**
    X● **W59.12 Struck by nonvenomous snake**
    X● **W59.13 Crushed by nonvenomous snake**
    X● **W59.19 Other contact with nonvenomous snake**
   ● **W59.2 Contact with turtles**
    Excludes1   contact with tortoises (W59.8-)
    X● **W59.21 Bitten by turtle**
    X● **W59.22 Struck by turtle**
    X● **W59.29 Other contact with turtle**
       Exposure to turtles
   ● **W59.8 Contact with other nonvenomous reptiles**
    X● **W59.81 Bitten by other nonvenomous reptiles**
    X● **W59.82 Struck by other nonvenomous reptiles**
    X● **W59.83 Crushed by other nonvenomous reptiles**
    X● **W59.89 Other contact with other nonvenomous reptiles**

X● **W60 Contact with nonvenomous plant thorns and spines and sharp leaves**
    Excludes1   contact with venomous plants (T63.X7-)
The appropriate 7th character is to be added to code W60

A	initial encounter
D	subsequent encounter
S	sequela

● **W61 Contact with birds (domestic) (wild)**
    Includes   contact with excreta of birds
The appropriate 7th character is to be added to each code from category W61

A	initial encounter
D	subsequent encounter
S	sequela

   ● **W61.0 Contact with parrot**
    X● **W61.01 Bitten by parrot**
    X● **W61.02 Struck by parrot**
    X● **W61.09 Other contact with parrot**
       Exposure to parrots
   ● **W61.1 Contact with macaw**
    X● **W61.11 Bitten by macaw**
    X● **W61.12 Struck by macaw**
    X● **W61.19 Other contact with macaw**
       Exposure to macaws
   ● **W61.2 Contact with other psittacines**
    X● **W61.21 Bitten by other psittacines**
    X● **W61.22 Struck by other psittacines**
    X● **W61.29 Other contact with other psittacines**
       Exposure to other psittacines
   ● **W61.3 Contact with chicken**
    X● **W61.32 Struck by chicken**
    X● **W61.33 Pecked by chicken**
    X● **W61.39 Other contact with chicken**
       Exposure to chickens
   ● **W61.4 Contact with turkey**
    X● **W61.42 Struck by turkey**
    X● **W61.43 Pecked by turkey**
    X● **W61.49 Other contact with turkey**
   ● **W61.5 Contact with goose**
    X● **W61.51 Bitten by goose**
    X● **W61.52 Struck by goose**
    X● **W61.59 Other contact with goose**
   ● **W61.6 Contact with duck**
    X● **W61.61 Bitten by duck**
    X● **W61.62 Struck by duck**
    X● **W61.69 Other contact with duck**
   ● **W61.9 Contact with other birds**
    X● **W61.91 Bitten by other birds**
    X● **W61.92 Struck by other birds**
    X● **W61.99 Other contact with other birds**
       Contact with bird NOS

● **W62 Contact with nonvenomous amphibians**
    Excludes1   contact with venomous amphibians (T63.81-T63.83)
The appropriate 7th character is to be added to each code from category W62

A	initial encounter
D	subsequent encounter
S	sequela

   X● **W62.0 Contact with nonvenomous frogs**
   X● **W62.1 Contact with nonvenomous toads**
   X● **W62.9 Contact with other nonvenomous amphibians**

CHAPTER 20 (V00–Y99)

X⬤ W64   Exposure to other animate mechanical forces

> **Includes**   exposure to nonvenomous animal NOS
>
> **Excludes1**   contact with venomous animal (T63.-)

The appropriate 7th character is to be added to code W64

> A   initial encounter
> D   subsequent encounter
> S   sequela

ACCIDENTAL NON-TRANSPORT DROWNING AND SUBMERSION (W65-W74)

> **Excludes1**   accidental drowning and submersion due to fall into water (W16.-)
>
> accidental drowning and submersion due to water transport accident (V90.-, V92.-)
>
> **Excludes2**   accidental drowning and submersion due to cataclysm (X34-X39)

X⬤ W65   Accidental drowning and submersion while in bathtub

> **Excludes1**   accidental drowning and submersion due to fall in (into) bathtub (W16.211)

The appropriate 7th character is to be added to code W65

> A   initial encounter
> D   subsequent encounter
> S   sequela

X⬤ W67   Accidental drowning and submersion while in swimming pool

> **Excludes1**   accidental drowning and submersion due to fall into swimming pool (W16.011, W16.021, W16.031)
>
> accidental drowning and submersion due to striking into wall of swimming pool (W22.041)

Coding Clinic: 2023, Q1, P26

The appropriate 7th character is to be added to code W67

> A   initial encounter
> D   subsequent encounter
> S   sequela

X⬤ W69   Accidental drowning and submersion while in natural water

Accidental drowning and submersion while in lake
Accidental drowning and submersion while in open sea
Accidental drowning and submersion while in river
Accidental drowning and submersion while in stream

> **Excludes1**   accidental drowning and submersion due to fall into natural body of water (W16.111, W16.121, W16.131)

The appropriate 7th character is to be added to code W69

> A   initial encounter
> D   subsequent encounter
> S   sequela

X⬤ W73   Other specified cause of accidental non-transport drowning and submersion

Accidental drowning and submersion while in quenching tank
Accidental drowning and submersion while in reservoir

> **Excludes1**   accidental drowning and submersion due to fall into other water (W16.311, W16.321, W16.331)

The appropriate 7th character is to be added to code W73

> A   initial encounter
> D   subsequent encounter
> S   sequela

X⬤ W74   Unspecified cause of accidental drowning and submersion

Drowning NOS

The appropriate 7th character is to be added to code W74

> A   initial encounter
> D   subsequent encounter
> S   sequela

EXPOSURE TO ELECTRIC CURRENT, RADIATION AND EXTREME AMBIENT AIR TEMPERATURE AND PRESSURE (W85-W99)

> **Excludes1**   exposure to:
>
> failure in dosage of radiation or temperature during surgical and medical care (Y63.2-Y63.5)
> lightning (T75.0-)
> natural cold (X31)
> natural heat (X30)
> natural radiation NOS (X39)
> radiological procedure and radiotherapy (Y84.2)
> sunlight (X32)

X⬤ W85   Exposure to electric transmission lines

Broken power line

The appropriate 7th character is to be added to code W85

> A   initial encounter
> D   subsequent encounter
> S   sequela

⬤ W86   Exposure to other specified electric current

The appropriate 7th character is to be added to each code from category W86

> A   initial encounter
> D   subsequent encounter
> S   sequela

X⬤ W86.0   Exposure to domestic wiring and appliances

X⬤ W86.1   Exposure to industrial wiring, appliances and electrical machinery

Exposure to conductors
Exposure to control apparatus
Exposure to electrical equipment and machinery
Exposure to transformers

X⬤ W86.8   Exposure to other electric current

Exposure to wiring and appliances in or on farm (not farmhouse)
Exposure to wiring and appliances outdoors
Exposure to wiring and appliances in or on public building
Exposure to wiring and appliances in or on residential institutions
Exposure to wiring and appliances in or on schools

⬤ W88   Exposure to ionizing radiation

> **Excludes1**   exposure to sunlight (X32)

The appropriate 7th character is to be added to each code from category W88

> A   initial encounter
> D   subsequent encounter
> S   sequela

X⬤ W88.0   Exposure to X-rays

X⬤ W88.1   Exposure to radioactive isotopes

X⬤ W88.8   Exposure to other ionizing radiation

⬤ W89   Exposure to man-made visible and ultraviolet light

> **Includes**   exposure to welding light (arc)
>
> **Excludes2**   exposure to sunlight (X32)

The appropriate 7th character is to be added to each code from category W89

> A   initial encounter
> D   subsequent encounter
> S   sequela

X⬤ W89.0   Exposure to welding light (arc)

X⬤ W89.1   Exposure to tanning bed

X⬤ W89.8   Exposure to other man-made visible and ultraviolet light

X⬤ W89.9   Exposure to unspecified man-made visible and ultraviolet light

▶ New   ⬌ Revised   ~~deleted~~ Deleted   Excludes 1   Excludes 2   Includes   Use additional   Code first   Code also   Key words

OGCR Official Guidelines   X Assign placeholder X   ⬤ Use Additional Character(s)   ▶ Manifestation Code   HCC Hierarchical Condition Category   **Coding Clinic**

● **W90 Exposure to other nonionizing radiation**

> **Excludes2** exposure to sunlight (X32)

> The appropriate 7th character is to be added to each code from category W90
>
> | | |
> |---|---|
> | A | initial encounter |
> | D | subsequent encounter |
> | S | sequela |

X ● **W90.0 Exposure to radiofrequency**
X ● **W90.1 Exposure to infrared radiation**
X ● **W90.2 Exposure to laser radiation**
X ● **W90.8 Exposure to other nonionizing radiation**

X ● **W92 Exposure to excessive heat of man-made origin**

> The appropriate 7th character is to be added to code W92
>
> | | |
> |---|---|
> | A | initial encounter |
> | D | subsequent encounter |
> | S | sequela |

● **W93 Exposure to excessive cold of man-made origin**

> The appropriate 7th character is to be added to each code from category W93
>
> | | |
> |---|---|
> | A | initial encounter |
> | D | subsequent encounter |
> | S | sequela |

● **W93.0 Contact with or inhalation of dry ice**
   X ● **W93.01 Contact with dry ice**
   X ● **W93.02 Inhalation of dry ice**
● **W93.1 Contact with or inhalation of liquid air**
   X ● **W93.11 Contact with liquid air**
     Contact with liquid hydrogen
     Contact with liquid nitrogen
   X ● **W93.12 Inhalation of liquid air**
     Inhalation of liquid hydrogen
     Inhalation of liquid nitrogen
X ● **W93.2 Prolonged exposure in deep freeze unit or refrigerator**
X ● **W93.8 Exposure to other excessive cold of man-made origin**

● **W94 Exposure to high and low air pressure and changes in air pressure**

> The appropriate 7th character is to be added to each code from category W94
>
> | | |
> |---|---|
> | A | initial encounter |
> | D | subsequent encounter |
> | S | sequela |

X ● **W94.0 Exposure to prolonged high air pressure**
● **W94.1 Exposure to prolonged low air pressure**
   X ● **W94.11 Exposure to residence or prolonged visit at high altitude**
   X ● **W94.12 Exposure to other prolonged low air pressure**
● **W94.2 Exposure to rapid changes in air pressure during ascent**
   X ● **W94.21 Exposure to reduction in atmospheric pressure while surfacing from deep-water diving**
   X ● **W94.22 Exposure to reduction in atmospheric pressure while surfacing from underground**
   X ● **W94.23 Exposure to sudden change in air pressure in aircraft during ascent**
   X ● **W94.29 Exposure to other rapid changes in air pressure during ascent**
● **W94.3 Exposure to rapid changes in air pressure during descent**
   X ● **W94.31 Exposure to sudden change in air pressure in aircraft during descent**
   X ● **W94.32 Exposure to high air pressure from rapid descent in water**
   X ● **W94.39 Exposure to other rapid changes in air pressure during descent**

X ● **W99 Exposure to other man-made environmental factors**

> The appropriate 7th character is to be added to code W99
>
> | | |
> |---|---|
> | A | initial encounter |
> | D | subsequent encounter |
> | S | sequela |

EXPOSURE TO SMOKE, FIRE AND FLAMES (X00-X08)

> **Excludes1** arson (X97)
>
> **Excludes2** explosions (W35-W40)
> lightning (T75.0-)
> transport accident (V01-V99)

● **X00 Exposure to uncontrolled fire in building or structure**

> **Includes** conflagration in building or structure
>
> *Code first any associated cataclysm*
>
> **Excludes2** exposure to ignition or melting of nightwear (X05)
> exposure to ignition or melting of other clothing and apparel (X06.-)
> exposure to other specified smoke, fire and flames (X08.-)

> The appropriate 7th character is to be added to each code from category X00
>
> | | |
> |---|---|
> | A | initial encounter |
> | D | subsequent encounter |
> | S | sequela |

X ● **X00.0 Exposure to flames in uncontrolled fire in building or structure**
   Coding Clinic: 2016, Q2, P5-6; 2015, Q1, P19
X ● **X00.1 Exposure to smoke in uncontrolled fire in building or structure**
X ● **X00.2 Injury due to collapse of burning building or structure in uncontrolled fire**
> **Excludes1** injury due to collapse of building not on fire (W20.1)
X ● **X00.3 Fall from burning building or structure in uncontrolled fire**
X ● **X00.4 Hit by object from burning building or structure in uncontrolled fire**
X ● **X00.5 Jump from burning building or structure in uncontrolled fire**
X ● **X00.8 Other exposure to uncontrolled fire in building or structure**

● **X01 Exposure to uncontrolled fire, not in building or structure**

> **Includes** exposure to forest fire

> The appropriate 7th character is to be added to each code from category X01
>
> | | |
> |---|---|
> | A | initial encounter |
> | D | subsequent encounter |
> | S | sequela |

X ● **X01.0 Exposure to flames in uncontrolled fire, not in building or structure**
X ● **X01.1 Exposure to smoke in uncontrolled fire, not in building or structure**
X ● **X01.3 Fall due to uncontrolled fire, not in building or structure**
X ● **X01.4 Hit by object due to uncontrolled fire, not in building or structure**
X ● **X01.8 Other exposure to uncontrolled fire, not in building or structure**

CHAPTER 20 (V00-Y99)

● X02   **Exposure to controlled fire in building or structure**

Includes   exposure to fire in fireplace exposure to fire in stove

The appropriate 7th character is to be added to each code from category X02

A	initial encounter
D	subsequent encounter
S	sequela

X ● **X02.0**   **Exposure to flames in controlled fire in building or structure**

X ● **X02.1**   **Exposure to smoke in controlled fire in building or structure**

X ● **X02.2**   **Injury due to collapse of burning building or structure in controlled fire**

Excludes1   injury due to collapse of building not on fire (W20.1)

X ● **X02.3**   **Fall from burning building or structure in controlled fire**

X ● **X02.4**   **Hit by object from burning building or structure in controlled fire**

X ● **X02.5**   **Jump from burning building or structure in controlled fire**

X ● **X02.8**   **Other exposure to controlled fire in building or structure**

● X03   **Exposure to controlled fire, not in building or structure**

Includes   exposure to bon fire exposure to camp fire exposure to trash fire

The appropriate 7th character is to be added to each code from category X03

A	initial encounter
D	subsequent encounter
S	sequela

X ● **X03.0**   **Exposure to flames in controlled fire, not in building or structure**
    Coding Clinic: 2015, Q1, P19

X ● **X03.1**   **Exposure to smoke in controlled fire, not in building or structure**

X ● **X03.3**   **Fall due to controlled fire, not in building or structure**

X ● **X03.4**   **Hit by object due to controlled fire, not in building or structure**

X ● **X03.8**   **Other exposure to controlled fire, not in building or structure**

X ● **X04**   **Exposure to ignition of highly flammable material**
Exposure to ignition of gasoline
Exposure to ignition of kerosene
Exposure to ignition of petrol

Excludes2   exposure to ignition or melting of nightwear (X05)
exposure to ignition or melting of other clothing and apparel (X06)

The appropriate 7th character is to be added to code X04

A	initial encounter
D	subsequent encounter
S	sequela

Coding Clinic: 2016, Q2, P4

X ● **X05**   **Exposure to ignition or melting of nightwear**

Excludes2   exposure to uncontrolled fire in building or structure (X00.-)
exposure to uncontrolled fire, not in building or structure (X01.-)
exposure to controlled fire in building or structure (X02.-)
exposure to controlled fire, not in building or structure (X03.-)
exposure to ignition of highly flammable materials (X04.-)

The appropriate 7th character is to be added to code X05

A	initial encounter
D	subsequent encounter
S	sequela

● X06   **Exposure to ignition or melting of other clothing and apparel**

Excludes2   exposure to uncontrolled fire in building or structure (X00.-)
exposure to uncontrolled fire, not in building or structure (X01.-)
exposure to controlled fire in building or structure (X02.-)
exposure to controlled fire, not in building or structure (X03.-)
exposure to ignition of highly flammable materials (X04.-)

The appropriate 7th character is to be added to each code from category X06

A	initial encounter
D	subsequent encounter
S	sequela

X ● **X06.0**   **Exposure to ignition of plastic jewelry**

X ● **X06.1**   **Exposure to melting of plastic jewelry**

X ● **X06.2**   **Exposure to ignition of other clothing and apparel**

X ● **X06.3**   **Exposure to melting of other clothing and apparel**

● X08   **Exposure to other specified smoke, fire and flames**

The appropriate 7th character is to be added to each code from category X08

A	initial encounter
D	subsequent encounter
S	sequela

● **X08.0**   **Exposure to bed fire**
Exposure to mattress fire

X ● **X08.00**   **Exposure to bed fire due to unspecified burning material**

X ● **X08.01**   **Exposure to bed fire due to burning cigarette**
    Coding Clinic: 2015, Q1, P19

X ● **X08.09**   **Exposure to bed fire due to other burning material**

● **X08.1**   **Exposure to sofa fire**

X ● **X08.10**   **Exposure to sofa fire due to unspecified burning material**

X ● **X08.11**   **Exposure to sofa fire due to burning cigarette**

X ● **X08.19**   **Exposure to sofa fire due to other burning material**

● **X08.2**   **Exposure to other furniture fire**

X ● **X08.20**   **Exposure to other furniture fire due to unspecified burning material**

X ● **X08.21**   **Exposure to other furniture fire due to burning cigarette**

X ● **X08.29**   **Exposure to other furniture fire due to other burning material**

X ● **X08.8**   **Exposure to other specified smoke, fire and flames**

▶ New   ⇒ Revised   ~~deleted~~ Deleted   Excludes 1   Excludes 2   Includes   Use additional   Code first   Code also   Key words
OGCR Official Guidelines   X Assign placeholder X   ● Use Additional Character(s)   ▌ Manifestation Code   Hierarchical Condition Category   Coding Clinic

CONTACT WITH HEAT AND HOT SUBSTANCES (X10-X19)

> **Excludes1**   exposure to excessive natural heat (X30)
> exposure to fire and flames (X00-X08)

● **X10**   **Contact with hot drinks, food, fats and cooking oils**

The appropriate 7th character is to be added to each code from category X10

A	initial encounter
D	subsequent encounter
S	sequela

X● **X10.0**   **Contact with hot drinks**

X● **X10.1**   **Contact with hot food**

X● **X10.2**   **Contact with fats and cooking oils**

● **X11**   **Contact with hot tap-water**

> **Includes**   contact with boiling tap-water
> contact with boiling water NOS

> **Excludes1**   contact with water heated on stove (X12)

The appropriate 7th character is to be added to each code from category X11

A	initial encounter
D	subsequent encounter
S	sequela

X● **X11.0**   **Contact with hot water in bath or tub**

> **Excludes1**   contact with running hot water in bath or tub (X11.1)

X● **X11.1**   **Contact with running hot water**
Contact with hot water running out of hose
Contact with hot water running out of tap

X● **X11.8**   **Contact with other hot tap-water**
Contact with hot water in bucket
Contact with hot tap-water NOS

X● **X12**   **Contact with other hot fluids**
Contact with water heated on stove

> **Excludes1**   hot (liquid) metals (X18)

The appropriate 7th character is to be added to code X12

A	initial encounter
D	subsequent encounter
S	sequela

● **X13**   **Contact with steam and other hot vapors**

The appropriate 7th character is to be added to each code from category X13

A	initial encounter
D	subsequent encounter
S	sequela

X● **X13.0**   **Inhalation of steam and other hot vapors**

X● **X13.1**   **Other contact with steam and other hot vapors**

● **X14**   **Contact with hot air and other hot gases**

The appropriate 7th character is to be added to each code from category X14

A	initial encounter
D	subsequent encounter
S	sequela

X● **X14.0**   **Inhalation of hot air and gases**

X● **X14.1**   **Other contact with hot air and other hot gases**

● **X15**   **Contact with hot household appliances**

> **Excludes1**   contact with heating appliances (X16)
> contact with powered household appliances (W29.-)
> exposure to controlled fire in building or structure due to household appliance (X02.8)
> exposure to household appliances electrical current (W86.0)

The appropriate 7th character is to be added to each code from category X15

A	initial encounter
D	subsequent encounter
S	sequela

X● **X15.0**   **Contact with hot stove (kitchen)**

X● **X15.1**   **Contact with hot toaster**

X● **X15.2**   **Contact with hotplate**

X● **X15.3**   **Contact with hot saucepan or skillet**
Contact with hot cooking pan
Contact with hot cooking pot

X● **X15.8**   **Contact with other hot household appliances**
Contact with cooker
Contact with kettle
Contact with light bulbs

X● **X16**   **Contact with hot heating appliances, radiators and pipes**

> **Excludes1**   contact with powered appliances (W29.-)
> exposure to controlled fire in building or structure due to appliance (X02.8)
> exposure to industrial appliances electrical current (W86.1)

The appropriate 7th character is to be added to code X16

A	initial encounter
D	subsequent encounter
S	sequela

X● **X17**   **Contact with hot engines, machinery and tools**

> **Excludes1**   contact with hot heating appliances, radiators and pipes (X16)
> contact with hot household appliances (X15)

The appropriate 7th character is to be added to code X17

A	initial encounter
D	subsequent encounter
S	sequela

X● **X18**   **Contact with other hot metals**
Contact with liquid metal

The appropriate 7th character is to be added to code X18

A	initial encounter
D	subsequent encounter
S	sequela

X● **X19**   **Contact with other heat and hot substances**

> **Excludes1**   objects that are not normally hot, e.g., an object made hot by a house fire (X00-X08)

The appropriate 7th character is to be added to code X19

A	initial encounter
D	subsequent encounter
S	sequela

EXPOSURE TO FORCES OF NATURE (X30-X39)

X ● X30   Exposure to excessive natural heat
Exposure to excessive heat as the cause of sunstroke
Exposure to heat NOS

   Excludes1   excessive heat of man-made origin (W92)
          exposure to man-made radiation (W89)
          exposure to sunlight (X32)
          exposure to tanning bed (W89)

The appropriate 7th character is to be added to code X30

A	initial encounter
D	subsequent encounter
S	sequela

X ● X31   Exposure to excessive natural cold
Excessive cold as the cause of chilblains NOS
Excessive cold as the cause of immersion foot or hand
Exposure to cold NOS
Exposure to weather conditions

   Excludes1   cold of man-made origin (W93.-)
          contact with or inhalation of dry ice (W93.-)
          contact with or inhalation of liquefied gas (W93.-)

The appropriate 7th character is to be added to code X31

A	initial encounter
D	subsequent encounter
S	sequela

X ● X32   Exposure to sunlight

   Excludes1   man-made radiation (tanning bed) (W89)

   Excludes2   radiation-related disorders of the skin and
          subcutaneous tissue (L55-L59)

The appropriate 7th character is to be added to code X32

A	initial encounter
D	subsequent encounter
S	sequela

X ● X34   Earthquake

   Excludes2   tidal wave (tsunami) due to earthquake (X37.41)

The appropriate 7th character is to be added to code X34

A	initial encounter
D	subsequent encounter
S	sequela

X ● X35   Volcanic eruption

   Excludes2   tidal wave (tsunami) due to volcanic eruption
          (X37.41)

The appropriate 7th character is to be added to code X35

A	initial encounter
D	subsequent encounter
S	sequela

● X36   Avalanche, landslide and other earth movements

   Includes   victim of mudslide of cataclysmic nature

   Excludes1   earthquake (X34)

   Excludes2   transport accident involving collision with
          avalanche or landslide not in motion
          (V01-V99)

The appropriate 7th character is to be added to each code from
   category X36

A	initial encounter
D	subsequent encounter
S	sequela

**X ● X36.0   Collapse of dam or man-made structure causing earth
movement**

X ● X36.1   Avalanche, landslide, or mudslide

● X37   Cataclysmic storm
The appropriate 7th character is to be added to each code from
   category X37

A	initial encounter
D	subsequent encounter
S	sequela

X ● X37.0   Hurricane
Storm surge   Typhoon

X ● X37.1   Tornado
Cyclone   Twister

X ● X37.2   Blizzard (snow) (ice)

X ● X37.3   Dust storm

● X37.4   Tidalwave

   **X ● X37.41   Tidal wave due to earthquake or volcanic
eruption**
Tidal wave NOS
Tsunami

   X ● X37.42   Tidal wave due to storm

   X ● X37.43   Tidal wave due to landslide

X ● X37.8   Other cataclysmic storms
Cloudburst
Torrential rain

   Excludes2   flood (X38)

X ● X37.9   Unspecified cataclysmic storm
Storm NOS

   Excludes1   collapse of dam or man-made structure
          causing earth movement (X36.0)

X ● X38   Flood
Flood arising from remote storm
Flood of cataclysmic nature arising from melting snow
Flood resulting directly from storm

   Excludes1   collapse of dam or man-made structure causing
          earth movement (X36.0)
          tidal wave NOS (X37.41)
          tidal wave caused by storm (X37.42)

The appropriate 7th character is to be added to code X38

A	initial encounter
D	subsequent encounter
S	sequela

● X39   Exposure to other forces of nature
The appropriate 7th character is to be added to each code from
   category X39

A	initial encounter
D	subsequent encounter
S	sequela

● X39.0   Exposure to natural radiation

   Excludes1   contact with and (suspected) exposure to
          radon and other naturally occurring
          radiation (Z77.123)
          exposure to man-made radiation
          (W88-W90)
          exposure to sunlight (X32)

   X ● X39.01   Exposure to radon

   X ● X39.08   Exposure to other natural radiation

X ● X39.8   Other exposure to forces of nature

OVEREXERTION AND STRENUOUS OR REPETITIVE MOVEMENTS (X50)

● **X50**   **Overexertion and strenuous or repetitive movements**

The appropriate 7th character is to be added to each code from category X50

A	initial encounter
D	subsequent encounter
S	sequela

Coding Clinic: 2016, Q4, P73-74

X● **X50.0**   **Overexertion from strenuous movement or load**
Lifting heavy objects
Lifting weights
Coding Clinic: 2016, Q4, P74

X● **X50.1**   **Overexertion from prolonged static or awkward postures**
Prolonged bending
Prolonged kneeling
Prolonged reaching
Prolonged sitting
Prolonged standing
Prolonged twisting
Static bending
Static kneeling
Static reaching
Static sitting
Static standing
Static twisting

X● **X50.3**   **Overexertion from repetitive movements**
Use of hand as hammer

Excludes2   Overuse from prolonged static or awkward postures (X50.1)

Coding Clinic: 2016, Q4, P74

X● **X50.9**   **Other and unspecified overexertion or strenuous movements or postures**
Contact pressure
Contact stress

ACCIDENTAL EXPOSURE TO OTHER SPECIFIED FACTORS (X52, X58)

X● **X52**   **Prolonged stay in weightless environment**
Weightlessness in spacecraft (simulator)

The appropriate 7th character is to be added to code X52

A	initial encounter
D	subsequent encounter
S	sequela

X● **X58**   **Exposure to other specified factors**
Accident NOS
Exposure NOS

The appropriate 7th character is to be added to code X58

A	initial encounter
D	subsequent encounter
S	sequela

INTENTIONAL SELF-HARM (X71-X83)

Purposely self-inflicted injury
Suicide (attempted)

● **X71**   **Intentional self-harm by drowning and submersion**

The appropriate 7th character is to be added to each code from category X71

A	initial encounter
D	subsequent encounter
S	sequela

X● **X71.0**   **Intentional self-harm by drowning and submersion while in bathtub A, D, S**

X● **X71.1**   **Intentional self-harm by drowning and submersion while in swimming pool A, D, S**

X● **X71.2**   **Intentional self-harm by drowning and submersion after jump into swimming pool A, D, S**

X● **X71.3**   **Intentional self-harm by drowning and submersion in natural water A, D, S**

X● **X71.8**   **Other intentional self-harm by drowning and submersion A, D, S**

X● **X71.9**   **Intentional self-harm by drowning and submersion, unspecified A, D, S**

X● **X72**   **Intentional self-harm by handgun discharge A, D, S**
Intentional self-harm by gun for single hand use
Intentional self-harm by pistol
Intentional self-harm by revolver

Excludes1   Very pistol (X74.8)

The appropriate 7th character is to be added to code X72

A	initial encounter
D	subsequent encounter
S	sequela

● **X73**   **Intentional self-harm by rifle, shotgun and larger firearm discharge**

Excludes1   airgun (X74.01)

The appropriate 7th character is to be added to each code from category X73

A	initial encounter
D	subsequent encounter
S	sequela

X● **X73.0**   **Intentional self-harm by shotgun discharge A, D, S**

X● **X73.1**   **Intentional self-harm by hunting rifle discharge A, D, S**

X● **X73.2**   **Intentional self-harm by machine gun discharge A, D, S**

X● **X73.8**   **Intentional self-harm by other larger firearm discharge A, D, S**

X● **X73.9**   **Intentional self-harm by unspecified larger firearm discharge A, D, S**

● **X74**   **Intentional self-harm by other and unspecified firearm and gun discharge**

The appropriate 7th character is to be added to each code from category X74

A	initial encounter
D	subsequent encounter
S	sequela

● **X74.0**   **Intentional self-harm by gas, air or spring-operated guns**

X● **X74.01**   **Intentional self-harm by airgun A, D, S**
Intentional self-harm by BB gun discharge
Intentional self-harm by pellet gun discharge

X● **X74.02**   **Intentional self-harm by paintball gun A, D, S**

X● **X74.09**   **Intentional self-harm by other gas, air or spring-operated gun A, D, S**

X● **X74.8**   **Intentional self-harm by other firearm discharge A, D, S**
Intentional self-harm by Very pistol [flare] discharge

X● **X74.9**   **Intentional self-harm by unspecified firearm discharge A, D, S**

X● **X75**   **Intentional self-harm by explosive material A, D, S**

The appropriate 7th character is to be added to code X75

A	initial encounter
D	subsequent encounter
S	sequela

X● **X76**   **Intentional self-harm by smoke, fire and flames A, D, S**

The appropriate 7th character is to be added to code X76

A	initial encounter
D	subsequent encounter
S	sequela

● **X77**   **Intentional self-harm by steam, hot vapors and hot objects**

The appropriate 7th character is to be added to each code from category X77

> A   initial encounter
> D   subsequent encounter
> S   sequela

X ● **X77.0**   Intentional self-harm by steam or hot vapors A, D, S ℞

X ● **X77.1**   Intentional self-harm by hot tap water A, D, S ℞

X ● **X77.2**   Intentional self-harm by other hot fluids A, D, S ℞

X ● **X77.3**   Intentional self-harm by hot household appliances A, D, S ℞

X ● **X77.8**   Intentional self-harm by other hot objects A, D, S ℞

X ● **X77.9**   Intentional self-harm by unspecified hot objects A, D, S ℞

● **X78**   **Intentional self-harm by sharp object**

The appropriate 7th character is to be added to each code from category X78

> A   initial encounter
> D   subsequent encounter
> S   sequela

X ● **X78.0**   Intentional self-harm by sharp glass A, D, S ℞

X ● **X78.1**   Intentional self-harm by knife A, D, S ℞

X ● **X78.2**   Intentional self-harm by sword or dagger A, D, S ℞

X ● **X78.8**   Intentional self-harm by other sharp object A, D, S ℞
Coding Clinic: 2022, Q1, P27

X ● **X78.9**   Intentional self-harm by unspecified sharp object A, D, S ℞

X ● **X79**   **Intentional self-harm by blunt object A, D, S ℞**

The appropriate 7th character is to be added to code X79

> A   initial encounter
> D   subsequent encounter
> S   sequela

X ● **X80**   **Intentional self-harm by jumping from a high place A, D, S ℞**
Intentional fall from one level to another

The appropriate 7th character is to be added to code X80

> A   initial encounter
> D   subsequent encounter
> S   sequela

● **X81**   **Intentional self-harm by jumping or lying in front of moving object**

The appropriate 7th character is to be added to each code from category X81

> A   initial encounter
> D   subsequent encounter
> S   sequela

X ● **X81.0**   Intentional self-harm by jumping or lying in front of motor vehicle A, D, S ℞

X ● **X81.1**   Intentional self-harm by jumping or lying in front of (subway) train A, D, S ℞

X ● **X81.8**   Intentional self-harm by jumping or lying in front of other moving object A, D, S ℞

● **X82**   **Intentional self-harm by crashing of motor vehicle**

The appropriate 7th character is to be added to each code from category X82

> A   initial encounter
> D   subsequent encounter
> S   sequela

X ● **X82.0**   Intentional collision of motor vehicle with other motor vehicle A, D, S ℞

X ● **X82.1**   Intentional collision of motor vehicle with train A, D, S ℞

X ● **X82.2**   Intentional collision of motor vehicle with tree A, D, S ℞

X ● **X82.8**   Other intentional self-harm by crashing of motor vehicle A, D, S ℞

● **X83**   **Intentional self-harm by other specified means**

> **Excludes1**   intentional self-harm by poisoning or contact with toxic substance - see Table of Drugs and Chemicals

The appropriate 7th character is to be added to each code from category X83

> A   initial encounter
> D   subsequent encounter
> S   sequela

X ● **X83.0**   Intentional self-harm by crashing of aircraft A, D, S ℞

X ● **X83.1**   Intentional self-harm by electrocution A, D, S ℞

X ● **X83.2**   Intentional self-harm by exposure to extremes of cold A, D, S ℞

X ● **X83.8**   Intentional self-harm by other specified means A, D, S ℞

ASSAULT (X92-Y09)

> **Includes**   homicide injuries inflicted by another person with intent to injure or kill, by any means

> **Excludes1**   injuries due to legal intervention (Y35.-)
> injuries due to operations of war (Y36.-)
> injuries due to terrorism (Y38.-)

● **X92**   **Assault by drowning and submersion**

The appropriate 7th character is to be added to each code from category X92

> A   initial encounter
> D   subsequent encounter
> S   sequela

X ● **X92.0**   Assault by drowning and submersion while in bathtub

X ● **X92.1**   Assault by drowning and submersion while in swimming pool

X ● **X92.2**   Assault by drowning and submersion after push into swimming pool

X ● **X92.3**   Assault by drowning and submersion in natural water

X ● **X92.8**   Other assault by drowning and submersion

X ● **X92.9**   Assault by drowning and submersion, unspecified

X ● **X93**   **Assault by handgun discharge**
Assault by discharge of gun for single hand use
Assault by discharge of pistol
Assault by discharge of revolver

> **Excludes1**   Very pistol (X95.8)

The appropriate 7th character is to be added to code X93

> A   initial encounter
> D   subsequent encounter
> S   sequela

● **X94**   **Assault by rifle, shotgun and larger firearm discharge**

> **Excludes1**   airgun (X95.01)

The appropriate 7th character is to be added to each code from category X94

> A   initial encounter
> D   subsequent encounter
> S   sequela

X ● **X94.0**   Assault by shotgun

X ● **X94.1**   Assault by hunting rifle

X ● **X94.2**   Assault by machine gun

X ● **X94.8**   Assault by other larger firearm discharge

X ● **X94.9**   Assault by unspecified larger firearm discharge

▶ New   ➡ Revised   ~~deleted~~ Deleted   Excludes 1   Excludes 2   Includes   Use additional   Code first   Code also   Key words

OGCR Official Guidelines   **X** Assign placeholder X   ● Use Additional Character(s)   Manifestation Code   ℞ Hierarchical Condition Category   **Coding Clinic**

● **X95**   **Assault by other and unspecified firearm and gun discharge**

The appropriate 7th character is to be added to each code from category X95

A	initial encounter
D	subsequent encounter
S	sequela

● **X95.0**   **Assault by gas, air or spring-operated guns**

X ● **X95.01**   **Assault by airgun discharge**
Assault by BB gun discharge
Assault by pellet gun discharge

X ● **X95.02**   **Assault by paintball gun discharge**

X ● **X95.09**   **Assault by other gas, air or spring-operated gun**

X ● **X95.8**   **Assault by other firearm discharge**
Assault by very pistol [flare] discharge

X ● **X95.9**   **Assault by unspecified firearm discharge**
Coding Clinic: 2025, Q1, P32; 2023, Q3, P8,12; 2016, Q3, P24

● **X96**   **Assault by explosive material**

Excludes1   incendiary device (X97)
terrorism involving explosive material (Y38.2-)

The appropriate 7th character is to be added to each code from category X96

A	initial encounter
D	subsequent encounter
S	sequela

X ● **X96.0**   **Assault by antipersonnel bomb**

Excludes1   antipersonnel bomb use in military or war (Y36.2-)

X ● **X96.1**   **Assault by gasoline bomb**

X ● **X96.2**   **Assault by letter bomb**

X ● **X96.3**   **Assault by fertilizer bomb**

X ● **X96.4**   **Assault by pipe bomb**

X ● **X96.8**   **Assault by other specified explosive**

X ● **X96.9**   **Assault by unspecified explosive**

X ● **X97**   **Assault by smoke, fire and flames**
Assault by arson
Assault by cigarettes
Assault by incendiary device

The appropriate 7th character is to be added to code X97

A	initial encounter
D	subsequent encounter
S	sequela

● **X98**   **Assault by steam, hot vapors and hot objects**

The appropriate 7th character is to be added to each code from category X98

A	initial encounter
D	subsequent encounter
S	sequela

X ● **X98.0**   **Assault by steam or hot vapors**

X ● **X98.1**   **Assault by hot tap water**

X ● **X98.2**   **Assault by hot fluids**

X ● **X98.3**   **Assault by hot household appliances**

X ● **X98.8**   **Assault by other hot objects**

X ● **X98.9**   **Assault by unspecified hot objects**

● **X99**   **Assault by sharp object**

Excludes1   assault by strike by sports equipment (Y08.0-)

The appropriate 7th character is to be added to each code from category X99

A	initial encounter
D	subsequent encounter
S	sequela

X ● **X99.0**   **Assault by sharp glass**

X ● **X99.1**   **Assault by knife**

X ● **X99.2**   **Assault by sword or dagger**

X ● **X99.8**   **Assault by other sharp object**

X ● **X99.9**   **Assault by unspecified sharp object**
Assault by stabbing NOS

X ● **Y00**   **Assault by blunt object**

Excludes1   assault by strike by sports equipment (Y08.0)

The appropriate 7th character is to be added to code Y00

A	initial encounter
D	subsequent encounter
S	sequela

X ● **Y01**   **Assault by pushing from high place**

The appropriate 7th character is to be added to code Y01

A	initial encounter
D	subsequent encounter
S	sequela

● **Y02**   **Assault by pushing or placing victim in front of moving object**

The appropriate 7th character is to be added to each code from category Y02

A	initial encounter
D	subsequent encounter
S	sequela

X ● **Y02.0**   **Assault by pushing or placing victim in front of motor vehicle**

X ● **Y02.1**   **Assault by pushing or placing victim in front of (subway) train**

X ● **Y02.8**   **Assault by pushing or placing victim in front of other moving object**

● **Y03**   **Assault by crashing of motor vehicle**

The appropriate 7th character is to be added to each code from category Y03

A	initial encounter
D	subsequent encounter
S	sequela

X ● **Y03.0**   **Assault by being hit or run over by motor vehicle**

X ● **Y03.8**   **Other assault by crashing of motor vehicle**

● **Y04**   **Assault by bodily force**

Excludes1   assault by:
submersion (X92.-)
use of weapon (X93-X95, X99, Y00)

The appropriate 7th character is to be added to each code from category Y04

A	initial encounter
D	subsequent encounter
S	sequela

X ● **Y04.0**   **Assault by unarmed brawl or fight**

X ● **Y04.1**   **Assault by human bite**

X ● **Y04.2**   **Assault by strike against or bumped into by another person**

X ● **Y04.8**   **Assault by other bodily force**
Assault by bodily force NOS

CHAPTER 20 (V00-Y99)

OGCR Section I.C.19.f.

Adult and child abuse, neglect and other maltreatment

Sequence first the appropriate code from categories T74 or T76 for abuse, neglect and other maltreatment, followed by any accompanying mental health or injury code(s).

If the documentation in the medical record states abuse or neglect it is coded as confirmed (T74.-). It is coded as suspected if it is documented as suspected (T76.-).

For cases of confirmed abuse or neglect an external cause code from the assault section (X92-Y09) should be added to identify the cause of any physical injuries. A perpetrator code (Y07) should be added when the perpetrator of the abuse is known. For suspected cases of abuse or neglect, do not report external cause or perpetrator code.

If a suspected case of abuse, neglect or mistreatment is ruled out during an encounter code Z04.71, Encounter for examination and observation following alleged physical adult abuse, ruled out, or code Z04.72, Encounter for examination and observation following alleged adult rape, should be used, not a code from T76.

If a suspected case of alleged rape or sexual abuse is ruled out during an encounter code Z04.41, Encounter for examination and observation following alleged adult rape or code Z04.42, Encounter for examination and observation following alleged child rape should be used, not a code from T76.

● Y07   Perpetrator of assault, maltreatment and neglect

    Note: Codes from this category are for use only in cases of confirmed abuse (T74.-)

        Selection of the correct perpetrator code is based on the relationship between the perpetrator and the victim

    Includes   perpetrator of abandonment
                   perpetrator of emotional neglect
                   perpetrator of mental cruelty
                   perpetrator of physical abuse
                   perpetrator of physical neglect
                   perpetrator of sexual abuse
                   perpetrator of torture

    Coding Clinic: 2016, Q4, P129

● Y07.0   Spouse or partner, perpetrator of maltreatment and neglect

        Spouse or partner, perpetrator of maltreatment and neglect against spouse or partner

    ● Y07.01   Husband, perpetrator of maltreatment and neglect

        Y07.010   Husband, current, perpetrator of maltreatment and neglect

        Y07.011   Husband, former, perpetrator of maltreatment and neglect

    ● Y07.02   Wife, perpetrator of maltreatment and neglect

        Y07.020   Wife, current, perpetrator of maltreatment and neglect

        Y07.021   Wife, former, perpetrator of maltreatment and neglect

    ● Y07.03   Male partner, perpetrator of maltreatment and neglect

        Male intimate or dating partner, perpetrator of maltreatment and neglect

        Y07.030   Male partner, current, perpetrator of maltreatment and neglect

        Y07.031   Male partner, former, perpetrator of maltreatment and neglect

    ● Y07.04   Female partner, perpetrator of maltreatment and neglect

        Female intimate or dating partner, perpetrator of maltreatment and neglect

        Y07.040   Female partner, current, perpetrator of maltreatment and neglect

        Y07.041   Female partner, former, perpetrator of maltreatment and neglect

● Y07.05   Non-binary partner, perpetrator of maltreatment and neglect

        Gender non-conforming partner, perpetrator of maltreatment and neglect

        Y07.050   Non-binary partner, current, perpetrator of maltreatment and neglect

        Y07.051   Non-binary partner, former, perpetrator of maltreatment and neglect

● Y07.1   Parent (adoptive) (biological), perpetrator of maltreatment and neglect

    Y07.11   **Biological father, perpetrator of maltreatment and neglect**

    Y07.12   **Biological mother, perpetrator of maltreatment and neglect**

    Y07.13   **Adoptive father, perpetrator of maltreatment and neglect**

    Y07.14   **Adoptive mother, perpetrator of maltreatment and neglect**

● Y07.4   Other family member, perpetrator of maltreatment and neglect

    ● Y07.41   Sibling, perpetrator of maltreatment and neglect

        Excludes1   stepsibling, perpetrator of maltreatment and neglect (Y07.435, Y07.436)

        Y07.410   **Brother, perpetrator of maltreatment and neglect**

        Y07.411   **Sister, perpetrator of maltreatment and neglect**

    ● Y07.42   Foster parent, perpetrator of maltreatment and neglect

        Y07.420   **Foster father, perpetrator of maltreatment and neglect**

        Y07.421   **Foster mother, perpetrator of maltreatment and neglect**

    ● Y07.43   Stepparent or stepsibling, perpetrator of maltreatment and neglect

        Y07.430   **Stepfather, perpetrator of maltreatment and neglect**

        Y07.432   **Male friend of parent (co-residing in household), perpetrator of maltreatment and neglect**

        Y07.433   **Stepmother, perpetrator of maltreatment and neglect**

        Y07.434   **Female friend of parent (co-residing in household), perpetrator of maltreatment and neglect**

        ➡ Y07.435   **Stepbrother, perpetrator of maltreatment and neglect**

        Y07.436   **Stepsister, perpetrator of maltreatment and neglect**

    ● Y07.44   Child, perpetrator of maltreatment and neglect

        Adopted child, perpetrator of maltreatment and neglect

        Biological child, perpetrator of maltreatment and neglect

        Daughter, perpetrator of maltreatment and neglect

        Foster child, perpetrator of maltreatment and neglect

        In-law child, perpetrator of maltreatment and neglect

        Non-binary child, perpetrator of maltreatment and neglect

        Son, perpetrator of maltreatment and neglect

        Stepchild, perpetrator of maltreatment and neglect

● **Y07.45 Grandchild, perpetrator of maltreatment and neglect**
  Adopted grandchild, perpetrator of maltreatment and neglect
  Biological grandchild, perpetrator of maltreatment and neglect
  Foster grandchild, perpetrator of maltreatment and neglect
  Granddaughter, perpetrator of maltreatment and neglect
  Grandson, perpetrator of maltreatment and neglect
  In-law grandchild, perpetrator of maltreatment and neglect
  Non-binary grandchild, perpetrator of maltreatment and neglect
  Step grandchild, perpetrator of maltreatment and neglect

● **Y07.46 Grandparent, perpetrator of maltreatment and neglect**
  Grandfather, perpetrator of maltreatment and neglect
  Grandmother, perpetrator of maltreatment and neglect
  Non-binary grandparent, perpetrator of maltreatment and neglect

● **Y07.47 Parental sibling, perpetrator of maltreatment and neglect**
  Aunt, perpetrator of maltreatment and neglect
  Non-binary parental sibling, perpetrator of maltreatment and neglect
  Uncle, perpetrator of maltreatment and neglect

● **Y07.49 Other family member, perpetrator of maltreatment and neglect**

  Y07.490 Male cousin, perpetrator of maltreatment and neglect

  Y07.491 Female cousin, perpetrator of maltreatment and neglect

  Y07.499 Other family member, perpetrator of maltreatment and neglect

● **Y07.5 Non-family member, perpetrator of maltreatment and neglect**

  Y07.50 Unspecified non-family member, perpetrator of maltreatment and neglect

● **Y07.51 Daycare provider, perpetrator of maltreatment and neglect**

  Y07.510 At-home childcare provider, perpetrator of maltreatment and neglect

  Y07.511 Daycare center childcare provider, perpetrator of maltreatment and neglect

  Y07.512 At-home adultcare provider, perpetrator of maltreatment and neglect

  Y07.513 Adultcare center provider, perpetrator of maltreatment and neglect

  Y07.519 Unspecified daycare provider, perpetrator of maltreatment and neglect

● **Y07.52 Healthcare provider, perpetrator of maltreatment and neglect**

  Y07.521 Mental health provider, perpetrator of maltreatment and neglect

  Y07.528 Other therapist or healthcare provider, perpetrator of maltreatment and neglect
    Nurse perpetrator of maltreatment and neglect
    Occupational therapist perpetrator of maltreatment and neglect
    Physical therapist perpetrator of maltreatment and neglect
    Speech therapist perpetrator of maltreatment and neglect

  Y07.529 Unspecified healthcare provider, perpetrator of maltreatment and neglect

  Y07.53 Teacher or instructor, perpetrator of maltreatment and neglect
    Coach, perpetrator of maltreatment and neglect

  Y07.54 Acquaintance or friend, perpetrator of maltreatment and neglect

  Y07.59 Other non-family member, perpetrator of maltreatment and neglect

  Y07.6 Multiple perpetrators of maltreatment and neglect

  Y07.9 Unspecified perpetrator of maltreatment and neglect

● **Y08 Assault by other specified means**
  The appropriate 7th character is to be added to each code from category Y08

A	initial encounter
D	subsequent encounter
S	sequela

● **Y08.0 Assault by strike by sport equipment**

  X● **Y08.01 Assault by strike by hockey stick**

  X● **Y08.02 Assault by strike by baseball bat**

  X● **Y08.09 Assault by strike by other specified type of sport equipment**

● **Y08.8 Assault by other specified means**

  X● **Y08.81 Assault by crashing of aircraft**

  X● **Y08.89 Assault by other specified means**

● **Y09 Assault by unspecified means**
  Assassination (attempted) NOS
  Homicide (attempted) NOS
  Manslaughter (attempted) NOS
  Murder (attempted) NOS

EVENT OF UNDETERMINED INTENT (Y21-Y33)

Undetermined intent is only for use when there is specific documentation in the record that the intent of the injury cannot be determined. If no such documentation is present, code to accidental (unintentional)

● **Y21 Drowning and submersion, undetermined intent**
  The appropriate 7th character is to be added to each code from category Y21

A	initial encounter
D	subsequent encounter
S	sequela

  X● **Y21.0 Drowning and submersion while in bathtub, undetermined intent**

  X● **Y21.1 Drowning and submersion after fall into bathtub, undetermined intent**

  X● **Y21.2 Drowning and submersion while in swimming pool, undetermined intent**

  X● **Y21.3 Drowning and submersion after fall into swimming pool, undetermined intent**

  X● **Y21.4 Drowning and submersion in natural water, undetermined intent**

  X● **Y21.8 Other drowning and submersion, undetermined intent**

  X● **Y21.9 Unspecified drowning and submersion, undetermined intent**

X● **Y22 Handgun discharge, undetermined intent**
  Discharge of gun for single hand use, undetermined intent
  Discharge of pistol, undetermined intent
  Discharge of revolver, undetermined intent

  Excludes2 very pistol (Y24.8)

  The appropriate 7th character is to be added to code Y22

A	initial encounter
D	subsequent encounter
S	sequela

CHAPTER 20 (V00–Y99)

● Y23 Rifle, shotgun and larger firearm discharge, undetermined intent

Excludes2 airgun (Y24.0)

The appropriate 7th character is to be added to each code from category Y23

A	initial encounter
D	subsequent encounter
S	sequela

- X● Y23.0 **Shotgun** discharge, undetermined intent
- X● Y23.1 **Hunting rifle** discharge, undetermined intent
- X● Y23.2 **Military firearm** discharge, undetermined intent
- X● Y23.3 **Machine gun** discharge, undetermined intent
- X● Y23.8 **Other larger firearm** discharge, undetermined intent
- X● Y23.9 **Unspecified** larger firearm discharge, undetermined intent

● Y24 Other and unspecified firearm discharge, undetermined intent

The appropriate 7th character is to be added to each code from category Y24

A	initial encounter
D	subsequent encounter
S	sequela

- X● Y24.0 **Airgun** discharge, undetermined intent
  BB gun discharge, undetermined intent
  Pellet gun discharge, undetermined intent
- X● Y24.8 **Other firearm** discharge, undetermined intent
  Paintball gun discharge, undetermined intent
  Very pistol [flare] discharge, undetermined intent
- X● Y24.9 **Unspecified** firearm discharge, undetermined intent

X● Y25 Contact with explosive material, undetermined intent

The appropriate 7th character is to be added to code Y25

A	initial encounter
D	subsequent encounter
S	sequela

X● Y26 Exposure to smoke, fire and flames, undetermined intent

The appropriate 7th character is to be added to code Y26

A	initial encounter
D	subsequent encounter
S	sequela

● Y27 Contact with steam, hot vapors and hot objects, undetermined intent

The appropriate 7th character is to be added to each code from category Y27

A	initial encounter
D	subsequent encounter
S	sequela

- X● Y27.0 Contact with **steam and hot vapors**, undetermined intent
- X● Y27.1 Contact with **hot tap water**, undetermined intent
- X● Y27.2 Contact with **hot fluids**, undetermined intent
- X● Y27.3 Contact with **hot household appliance**, undetermined intent
- X● Y27.8 Contact with **other hot objects**, undetermined intent
- X● Y27.9 Contact with **unspecified** hot objects, undetermined intent

● Y28 Contact with sharp object, undetermined intent

The appropriate 7th character is to be added to each code from category Y28

A	initial encounter
D	subsequent encounter
S	sequela

- X● Y28.0 Contact with **sharp glass**, undetermined intent
- X● Y28.1 Contact with **knife**, undetermined intent
- X● Y28.2 Contact with **sword or dagger**, undetermined intent
- X● Y28.8 Contact with **other sharp object**, undetermined intent
- X● Y28.9 Contact with **unspecified sharp object**, undetermined intent

X● Y29 Contact with blunt object, undetermined intent

The appropriate 7th character is to be added to code Y29

A	initial encounter
D	subsequent encounter
S	sequela

X● Y30 Falling, jumping or pushed from a high place, undetermined intent

Victim falling from one level to another, undetermined intent

The appropriate 7th character is to be added to code Y30

A	initial encounter
D	subsequent encounter
S	sequela

X● Y31 Falling, lying or running before or into moving object, undetermined intent

The appropriate 7th character is to be added to code Y31

A	initial encounter
D	subsequent encounter
S	sequela

X● Y32 Crashing of motor vehicle, undetermined intent

The appropriate 7th character is to be added to code Y32

A	initial encounter
D	subsequent encounter
S	sequela

X● Y33 Other specified events, undetermined intent

The appropriate 7th character is to be added to code Y33

A	initial encounter
D	subsequent encounter
S	sequela

LEGAL INTERVENTION, OPERATIONS OF WAR, MILITARY OPERATIONS, AND TERRORISM (Y35–Y38)

● Y35 Legal intervention

Includes any injury sustained as a result of an encounter with any law enforcement official, serving in any capacity at the time of the encounter, whether on-duty or off-duty. Includes: injury to law enforcement official, suspect and bystander

The appropriate 7th character is to be added to each code from category Y35

A	initial encounter
D	subsequent encounter
S	sequela

- ● Y35.0 **Legal intervention involving firearm discharge**
  - ● Y35.00 **Legal intervention involving unspecified firearm discharge**
    Legal intervention involving gunshot wound
    Legal intervention involving shot NOS
    - ● Y35.001 **Legal intervention involving unspecified firearm discharge, law enforcement official injured**
    - ● Y35.002 **Legal intervention involving unspecified firearm discharge, bystander injured**
    - ● Y35.003 **Legal intervention involving unspecified firearm discharge, suspect injured**

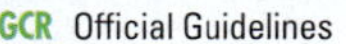 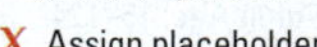 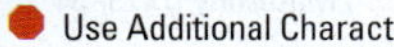 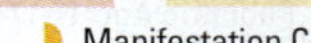 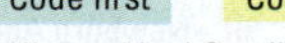

▶ New   ➡ Revised   ~~deleted~~ Deleted   Excludes 1   Excludes 2   Includes   Use additional   Code first   Code also   Key words

OGCR Official Guidelines   X Assign placeholder X   ● Use Additional Character(s)   ▌ Manifestation Code   Hierarchical Condition Category   **Coding Clinic**

● Y35.009   Legal intervention involving unspecified firearm discharge, unspecified person injured

● Y35.01   Legal intervention involving injury by machine gun
  ● Y35.011   Legal intervention involving injury by machine gun, law enforcement official injured
  ● Y35.012   Legal intervention involving injury by machine gun, bystander injured
  ● Y35.013   Legal intervention involving injury by machine gun, suspect injured
  ● Y35.019   Legal intervention involving injury by machine gun, unspecified person injured

● Y35.02   Legal intervention involving injury by handgun
  ● Y35.021   Legal intervention involving injury by handgun, law enforcement official injured
  ● Y35.022   Legal intervention involving injury by handgun, bystander injured
  ● Y35.023   Legal intervention involving injury by handgun, suspect injured
  ● Y35.029   Legal intervention involving injury by handgun, unspecified person injured

● Y35.03   Legal intervention involving injury by rifle pellet
  ● Y35.031   Legal intervention involving injury by rifle pellet, law enforcement official injured
  ● Y35.032   Legal intervention involving injury by rifle pellet, bystander injured
  ● Y35.033   Legal intervention involving injury by rifle pellet, suspect injured
  ● Y35.039   Legal intervention involving injury by rifle pellet, unspecified person injured

● Y35.04   Legal intervention involving injury by rubber bullet
  ● Y35.041   Legal intervention involving injury by rubber bullet, law enforcement official injured
  ● Y35.042   Legal intervention involving injury by rubber bullet, bystander injured
  ● Y35.043   Legal intervention involving injury by rubber bullet, suspect injured
  ● Y35.049   Legal intervention involving injury by rubber bullet, unspecified person injured

● Y35.09   Legal intervention involving other firearm discharge
  ● Y35.091   Legal intervention involving other firearm discharge, law enforcement official injured
  ● Y35.092   Legal intervention involving other firearm discharge, bystander injured
  ● Y35.093   Legal intervention involving other firearm discharge, suspect injured
  ● Y35.099   Legal intervention involving other firearm discharge, unspecified person injured

● Y35.1   Legal intervention involving explosives
  ● Y35.10   Legal intervention involving unspecified explosives
    ● Y35.101   Legal intervention involving unspecified explosives, law enforcement official injured
    ● Y35.102   Legal intervention involving unspecified explosives, bystander injured

● Y35.103   Legal intervention involving unspecified explosives, suspect injured
● Y35.109   Legal intervention involving unspecified explosives, unspecified person injured

● Y35.11   Legal intervention involving injury by dynamite
  ● Y35.111   Legal intervention involving injury by dynamite, law enforcement official injured
  ● Y35.112   Legal intervention involving injury by dynamite, bystander injured
  ● Y35.113   Legal intervention involving injury by dynamite, suspect injured
  ● Y35.119   Legal intervention involving injury by dynamite, unspecified person injured

● Y35.12   Legal intervention involving injury by explosive shell
  ● Y35.121   Legal intervention involving injury by explosive shell, law enforcement official injured
  ● Y35.122   Legal intervention involving injury by explosive shell, bystander injured
  ● Y35.123   Legal intervention involving injury by explosive shell, suspect injured
  ● Y35.129   Legal intervention involving other explosives, unspecified person injured

● Y35.19   Legal intervention involving other explosives
    Legal intervention involving injury by grenade
    Legal intervention involving injury by mortar bomb
  ● Y35.191   Legal intervention involving other explosives, law enforcement official injured
  ● Y35.192   Legal intervention involving other explosives, bystander injured
  ● Y35.193   Legal intervention involving other explosives, suspect injured
  ● Y35.199   Legal intervention involving other explosives, unspecified person injured

● Y35.2   Legal intervention involving gas
    Legal intervention involving asphyxiation by gas
    Legal intervention involving poisoning by gas
  ● Y35.20   Legal intervention involving unspecified gas
    ● Y35.201   Legal intervention involving unspecified gas, law enforcement official injured
    ● Y35.202   Legal intervention involving unspecified gas, bystander injured
    ● Y35.203   Legal intervention involving unspecified gas, suspect injured
    ● Y35.209   Legal intervention involving unspecified gas, unspecified person injured

  ● Y35.21   Legal intervention involving injury by tear gas
    ● Y35.211   Legal intervention involving injury by tear gas, law enforcement official injured
    ● Y35.212   Legal intervention involving injury by tear gas, bystander injured
    ● Y35.213   Legal intervention involving injury by tear gas, suspect injured
    ● Y35.219   Legal intervention involving injury by tear gas, unspecified person injured

● Y35.29   Legal intervention involving other gas
    ● Y35.291   Legal intervention involving other gas, law enforcement official injured
    ● Y35.292   Legal intervention involving other gas, bystander injured
    ● Y35.293   Legal intervention involving other gas, suspect injured
    ● Y35.299   Legal intervention involving other gas, unspecified person injured

● Y35.3   Legal intervention involving blunt objects
    Legal intervention involving being hit or struck by blunt object
   ● Y35.30   Legal intervention involving unspecified blunt objects
     ● Y35.301   Legal intervention involving unspecified blunt objects, law enforcement official injured
     ● Y35.302   Legal intervention involving unspecified blunt objects, bystander injured
     ● Y35.303   Legal intervention involving unspecified blunt objects, suspect injured
     ● Y35.309   Legal intervention involving unspecified blunt objects, unspecified person injured
   ● Y35.31   Legal intervention involving baton
     ● Y35.311   Legal intervention involving baton, law enforcement official injured
     ● Y35.312   Legal intervention involving baton, bystander injured
     ● Y35.313   Legal intervention involving baton, suspect injured
     ● Y35.319   Legal intervention involving baton, unspecified person injured
   ● Y35.39   Legal intervention involving other blunt objects
     ● Y35.391   Legal intervention involving other blunt objects, law enforcement official injured
     ● Y35.392   Legal intervention involving other blunt objects, bystander injured
     ● Y35.393   Legal intervention involving other blunt objects, suspect injured
     ● Y35.399   Legal intervention involving other blunt objects, unspecified person injured

● Y35.4   Legal intervention involving sharp objects
    Legal intervention involving being cut by sharp objects
    Legal intervention involving being stabbed by sharp objects
   ● Y35.40   Legal intervention involving unspecified sharp objects
     ● Y35.401   Legal intervention involving unspecified sharp objects, law enforcement official injured
     ● Y35.402   Legal intervention involving unspecified sharp objects, bystander injured
     ● Y35.403   Legal intervention involving unspecified sharp objects, suspect injured
     ● Y35.409   Legal intervention involving unspecified sharp objects, unspecified person injured
   ● Y35.41   Legal intervention involving bayonet
     ● Y35.411   Legal intervention involving bayonet, law enforcement official injured
     ● Y35.412   Legal intervention involving bayonet, bystander injured
     ● Y35.413   Legal intervention involving bayonet, suspect injured
     ● Y35.419   Legal intervention involving bayonet, unspecified person injured
   ● Y35.49   Legal intervention involving other sharp objects
     ● Y35.491   Legal intervention involving other sharp objects, law enforcement official injured
     ● Y35.492   Legal intervention involving other sharp objects, bystander injured
     ● Y35.493   Legal intervention involving other sharp objects, suspect injured
     ● Y35.499   Legal intervention involving other sharp objects, unspecified person injured

● Y35.8   Legal intervention involving other specified means
   ● Y35.81   Legal intervention involving manhandling
     ● Y35.811   Legal intervention involving manhandling, law enforcement official injured
     ● Y35.812   Legal intervention involving manhandling, bystander injured
     ● Y35.813   Legal intervention involving manhandling, suspect injured
     ● Y35.819   Legal intervention involving manhandling, unspecified person injured
   ● Y35.83   Legal intervention involving a conducted energy device
    Electroshock device (taser)
    Stun gun
     ● Y35.831   Legal intervention involving a conducted energy device, law enforcement official injured
     ● Y35.832   Legal intervention involving a conducted energy device, bystander injured
     ● Y35.833   Legal intervention involving a conducted energy device, suspect injured
     ● Y35.839   Legal intervention involving a conducted energy device, unspecified person injured
   ● Y35.89   Legal intervention involving other specified means
     ● Y35.891   Legal intervention involving other specified means, law enforcement official injured
     ● Y35.892   Legal intervention involving other specified means, bystander injured
     ● Y35.893   Legal intervention involving other specified means, suspect injured
      Coding Clinic: 2018, Q1, P5
     ● Y35.899   Legal intervention involving other specified means, unspecified person injured

● Y35.9   Legal intervention, means unspecified
   X ● Y35.91   Legal intervention, means unspecified, law enforcement official injured
   X ● Y35.92   Legal intervention, means unspecified, bystander injured
   X ● Y35.93   Legal intervention, means unspecified, suspect injured
   X ● Y35.99   Legal intervention, means unspecified, unspecified person injured

● **Y36**   **Operations of war**

> **Includes**   injuries to military personnel and civilians caused by war, civil insurrection, and peacekeeping missions
>
> **Excludes1**   injury to military personnel occurring during peacetime military operations (Y37.-)
> military vehicles involved in transport accidents with non-military vehicle during peacetime (V09.01, V09.21, V19.81, V29.818, V39.81, V49.81, V59.81, V69.81, V79.81)

The appropriate 7th character is to be added to each code from category Y36

> A   initial encounter
> D   subsequent encounter
> S   sequela

● **Y36.0**   **War operations involving explosion of marine weapons**
    Weapons and military watercraft

   ● **Y36.00**   **War operations involving explosion of unspecified marine weapon**
      War operations involving underwater blast NOS

     ● **Y36.000**   War operations involving explosion of unspecified marine weapon, **military personnel**

     ● **Y36.001**   War operations involving explosion of unspecified marine weapon, **civilian**

   ● **Y36.01**   **War operations involving explosion of depth-charge**

     ● **Y36.010**   War operations involving explosion of depth-charge, **military personnel**

     ● **Y36.011**   War operations involving explosion of depth-charge, **civilian**

   ● **Y36.02**   **War operations involving explosion of marine mine**
      War operations involving explosion of marine mine, at sea or in harbor

     ● **Y36.020**   War operations involving explosion of marine mine, **military personnel**

     ● **Y36.021**   War operations involving explosion of marine mine, **civilian**

   ● **Y36.03**   **War operations involving explosion of sea-based artillery shell**

     ● **Y36.030**   War operations involving explosion of sea-based artillery shell, **military personnel**

     ● **Y36.031**   War operations involving explosion of sea-based artillery shell, **civilian**

   ● **Y36.04**   **War operations involving explosion of torpedo**

     ● **Y36.040**   War operations involving explosion of torpedo, **military personnel**

     ● **Y36.041**   War operations involving explosion of torpedo, **civilian**

   ● **Y36.05**   **War operations involving accidental detonation of onboard marine weapons**

     ● **Y36.050**   War operations involving accidental detonation of onboard marine weapons, **military personnel**

     ● **Y36.051**   War operations involving accidental detonation of onboard marine weapons, **civilian**

   ● **Y36.09**   **War operations involving explosion of other marine weapons**

     ● **Y36.090**   War operations involving explosion of other marine weapons, **military personnel**

     ● **Y36.091**   War operations involving explosion of other marine weapons, **civilian**

● **Y36.1**   **War operations involving destruction of aircraft**

   ● **Y36.10**   **War operations involving unspecified destruction of aircraft**

     ● **Y36.100**   War operations involving unspecified destruction of aircraft, **military personnel**

     ● **Y36.101**   War operations involving unspecified destruction of aircraft, **civilian**

   ● **Y36.11**   **War operations involving destruction of aircraft due to enemy fire or explosives**
      War operations involving destruction of aircraft due to air to air missile
      War operations involving destruction of aircraft due to explosive placed on aircraft
      War operations involving destruction of aircraft due to rocket propelled grenade [RPG]
      War operations involving destruction of aircraft due to small arms fire
      War operations involving destruction of aircraft due to surface to air missile

     ● **Y36.110**   War operations involving destruction of aircraft due to enemy fire or explosives, **military personnel**

     ● **Y36.111**   War operations involving destruction of aircraft due to enemy fire or explosives, **civilian**

   ● **Y36.12**   **War operations involving destruction of aircraft due to collision with other aircraft**

     ● **Y36.120**   War operations involving destruction of aircraft due to collision with other aircraft, **military personnel**

     ● **Y36.121**   War operations involving destruction of aircraft due to collision with other aircraft, **civilian**

   ● **Y36.13**   **War operations involving destruction of aircraft due to onboard fire**

     ● **Y36.130**   War operations involving destruction of aircraft due to onboard fire, **military personnel**

     ● **Y36.131**   War operations involving destruction of aircraft due to onboard fire, **civilian**

   ● **Y36.14**   **War operations involving destruction of aircraft due to accidental detonation of onboard munitions and explosives**

     ● **Y36.140**   War operations involving destruction of aircraft due to accidental detonation of onboard munitions and explosives, **military personnel**

     ● **Y36.141**   War operations involving destruction of aircraft due to accidental detonation of onboard munitions and explosives, **civilian**

   ● **Y36.19**   **War operations involving other destruction of aircraft**

     ● **Y36.190**   War operations involving other destruction of aircraft, **military personnel**

     ● **Y36.191**   War operations involving other destruction of aircraft, **civilian**

● **Y36.2**   **War operations involving other explosions and fragments**

> **Excludes1**   war operations involving explosion of aircraft (Y36.1-)
> war operations involving explosion of marine weapons (Y36.0-)
> war operations involving explosion of nuclear weapons (Y36.5-)
> war operations involving explosion occurring after cessation of hostilities (Y36.8-)

● **Y36.20 War operations involving unspecified explosion and fragments**
   War operations involving air blast NOS
   War operations involving blast NOS
   War operations involving blast fragments NOS
   War operations involving blast wave NOS
   War operations involving blast wind NOS
   War operations involving explosion NOS
   War operations involving explosion of bomb NOS

● **Y36.200 War operations involving unspecified explosion and fragments, military personnel**

● **Y36.201 War operations involving unspecified explosion and fragments, civilian**

● **Y36.21 War operations involving explosion of aerial bomb**

● **Y36.210 War operations involving explosion of aerial bomb, military personnel**

● **Y36.211 War operations involving explosion of aerial bomb, civilian**

● **Y36.22 War operations involving explosion of guided missile**

● **Y36.220 War operations involving explosion of guided missile, military personnel**

● **Y36.221 War operations involving explosion of guided missile, civilian**

● **Y36.23 War operations involving explosion of improvised explosive device [IED]**
   War operations involving explosion of person-borne improvised explosive device [IED]
   War operations involving explosion of vehicle-borne improvised explosive device [IED]
   War operations involving explosion of roadside improvised explosive device [IED]

● **Y36.230 War operations involving explosion of improvised explosive device [IED], military personnel**

● **Y36.231 War operations involving explosion of improvised explosive device [IED], civilian**

● **Y36.24 War operations involving explosion due to accidental detonation and discharge of own munitions or munitions launch device**

● **Y36.240 War operations involving explosion due to accidental detonation and discharge of own munitions or munitions launch device, military personnel**

● **Y36.241 War operations involving explosion due to accidental detonation and discharge of own munitions or munitions launch device, civilian**

● **Y36.25 War operations involving fragments from munitions**

● **Y36.250 War operations involving fragments from munitions, military personnel**

● **Y36.251 War operations involving fragments from munitions, civilian**

● **Y36.26 War operations involving fragments of improvised explosive device [IED]**
   War operations involving fragments of person-borne improvised explosive device [IED]
   War operations involving fragments of vehicle-borne improvised explosive device [IED]
   War operations involving fragments of roadside improvised explosive device [IED]

● **Y36.260 War operations involving fragments of improvised explosive device [IED], military personnel**

● **Y36.261 War operations involving fragments of improvised explosive device [IED], civilian**

● **Y36.27 War operations involving fragments from weapons**

● **Y36.270 War operations involving fragments from weapons, military personnel**

● **Y36.271 War operations involving fragments from weapons, civilian**

● **Y36.29 War operations involving other explosions and fragments**
   War operations involving explosion of grenade
   War operations involving explosions of land mine
   War operations involving shrapnel NOS

● **Y36.290 War operations involving other explosions and fragments, military personnel**

● **Y36.291 War operations involving other explosions and fragments, civilian**

● **Y36.3 War operations involving fires, conflagrations and hot substances**
   War operations involving smoke, fumes, and heat from fires, conflagrations and hot substances

   Excludes 1 war operations involving fires and conflagrations aboard military aircraft (Y36.1-)
   war operations involving fires and conflagrations aboard military watercraft (Y36.0-)
   war operations involving fires and conflagrations caused indirectly by conventional weapons (Y36.2-)
   war operations involving fires and thermal effects of nuclear weapons (Y36.53-)

● **Y36.30 War operations involving unspecified fire, conflagration and hot substance**

● **Y36.300 War operations involving unspecified fire, conflagration and hot substance, military personnel**

● **Y36.301 War operations involving unspecified fire, conflagration and hot substance, civilian**

● **Y36.31 War operations involving gasoline bomb**
   War operations involving incendiary bomb
   War operations involving petrol bomb

● **Y36.310 War operations involving gasoline bomb, military personnel**

● **Y36.311 War operations involving gasoline bomb, civilian**

● **Y36.32 War operations involving incendiary bullet**

● **Y36.320 War operations involving incendiary bullet, military personnel**

● **Y36.321 War operations involving incendiary bullet, civilian**

● **Y36.33 War operations involving flamethrower**

● **Y36.330 War operations involving flamethrower, military personnel**

● **Y36.331 War operations involving flamethrower, civilian**

● **Y36.39 War operations involving other fires, conflagrations and hot substances**

● **Y36.390 War operations involving other fires, conflagrations and hot substances, military personnel**

● **Y36.391 War operations involving other fires, conflagrations and hot substances, civilian**

● **Y36.4 War operations involving firearm discharge and other forms of conventional warfare**

● **Y36.41 War operations involving rubber bullets**

● **Y36.410 War operations involving rubber bullets, military personnel**

● **Y36.411 War operations involving rubber bullets, civilian**

● **Y36.42** War operations involving firearms pellets
　● **Y36.42Ø** War operations involving firearms pellets, military personnel
　● **Y36.421** War operations involving firearms pellets, civilian
● **Y36.43** War operations involving other firearms discharge
　　War operations involving bullets NOS
　　Excludes1 war operations involving munitions fragments (Y36.25-)
　　war operations involving incendiary bullets (Y36.32-)
　● **Y36.43Ø** War operations involving other firearms discharge, military personnel
　● **Y36.431** War operations involving other firearms discharge, civilian
● **Y36.44** War operations involving unarmed hand to hand combat
　　Excludes1 war operations involving combat using blunt or piercing object (Y36.45-)
　　war operations involving intentional restriction of air and airway (Y36.46-)
　　war operations involving unintentional restriction of air and airway (Y36.47-)
　● **Y36.44Ø** War operations involving unarmed hand to hand combat, military personnel
　● **Y36.441** War operations involving unarmed hand to hand combat, civilian
● **Y36.45** War operations involving combat using blunt or piercing object
　● **Y36.45Ø** War operations involving combat using blunt or piercing object, military personnel
　● **Y36.451** War operations involving combat using blunt or piercing object, civilian
● **Y36.46** War operations involving intentional restriction of air and airway
　● **Y36.46Ø** War operations involving intentional restriction of air and airway, military personnel
　● **Y36.461** War operations involving intentional restriction of air and airway, civilian
● **Y36.47** War operations involving unintentional restriction of air and airway
　● **Y36.47Ø** War operations involving unintentional restriction of air and airway, military personnel
　● **Y36.471** War operations involving unintentional restriction of air and airway, civilian
● **Y36.49** War operations involving other forms of conventional warfare
　● **Y36.49Ø** War operations involving other forms of conventional warfare, military personnel
　● **Y36.491** War operations involving other forms of conventional warfare, civilian
● **Y36.5** War operations involving nuclear weapons
　　War operations involving dirty bomb NOS
　● **Y36.5Ø** War operations involving unspecified effect of nuclear weapon
　　● **Y36.5ØØ** War operations involving unspecified effect of nuclear weapon, military personnel
　　● **Y36.5Ø1** War operations involving unspecified effect of nuclear weapon, civilian

● **Y36.51** War operations involving direct blast effect of nuclear weapon
　　War operations involving blast pressure of nuclear weapon
　● **Y36.51Ø** War operations involving direct blast effect of nuclear weapon, military personnel
　● **Y36.511** War operations involving direct blast effect of nuclear weapon, civilian
● **Y36.52** War operations involving indirect blast effect of nuclear weapon
　　War operations involving being thrown by blast of nuclear weapon
　　War operations involving being struck or crushed by blast debris of nuclear weapon
　● **Y36.52Ø** War operations involving indirect blast effect of nuclear weapon, military personnel
　● **Y36.521** War operations involving indirect blast effect of nuclear weapon, civilian
● **Y36.53** War operations involving thermal radiation effect of nuclear weapon
　　War operations involving direct heat from nuclear weapon
　　War operation involving fireball effects from nuclear weapon
　● **Y36.53Ø** War operations involving thermal radiation effect of nuclear weapon, military personnel
　● **Y36.531** War operations involving thermal radiation effect of nuclear weapon, civilian
● **Y36.54** War operation involving nuclear radiation effects of nuclear weapon
　　War operation involving acute radiation exposure from nuclear weapon
　　War operation involving exposure to immediate ionizing radiation from nuclear weapon
　　War operation involving fallout exposure from nuclear weapon
　　War operation involving secondary effects of nuclear weapons
　● **Y36.54Ø** War operation involving nuclear radiation effects of nuclear weapon, military personnel
　● **Y36.541** War operation involving nuclear radiation effects of nuclear weapon, civilian
● **Y36.59** War operation involving other effects of nuclear weapons
　● **Y36.59Ø** War operation involving other effects of nuclear weapons, military personnel
　● **Y36.591** War operation involving other effects of nuclear weapons, civilian
● **Y36.6** War operations involving biological weapons
　● **Y36.6X** War operations involving biological weapons
　　● **Y36.6XØ** War operations involving biological weapons, military personnel
　　● **Y36.6X1** War operations involving biological weapons, civilian
● **Y36.7** War operations involving chemical weapons and other forms of unconventional warfare
　　Excludes1 war operations involving incendiary devices (Y36.3-, Y36.5-)
　● **Y36.7X** War operations involving chemical weapons and other forms of unconventional warfare
　　● **Y36.7XØ** War operations involving chemical weapons and other forms of unconventional warfare, military personnel

CHAPTER 2Ø (VØØ-Y99)

CHAPTER 20 (V00–Y99)

Y36.7X1   War operations involving chemical weapons and other forms of unconventional warfare, civilian

Y36.8   War operations occurring after cessation of hostilities
War operations classifiable to categories Y36.0–Y36.8 but occurring after cessation of hostilities

Y36.81   Explosion of mine placed during war operations but exploding after cessation of hostilities

Y36.810   Explosion of mine placed during war operations but exploding after cessation of hostilities, military personnel

Y36.811   Explosion of mine placed during war operations but exploding after cessation of hostilities, civilian

Y36.82   Explosion of bomb placed during war operations but exploding after cessation of hostilities

Y36.820   Explosion of bomb placed during war operations but exploding after cessation of hostilities, military personnel

Y36.821   Explosion of bomb placed during war operations but exploding after cessation of hostilities, civilian

Y36.88   Other war operations occurring after cessation of hostilities

Y36.880   Other war operations occurring after cessation of hostilities, military personnel

Y36.881   Other war operations occurring after cessation of hostilities, civilian

Y36.89   Unspecified war operations occurring after cessation of hostilities

Y36.890   Unspecified war operations occurring after cessation of hostilities, military personnel

Y36.891   Unspecified war operations occurring after cessation of hostilities, civilian

Y36.9   Other and unspecified war operations

X **Y36.90**   War operations, unspecified

X **Y36.91**   War operations involving unspecified weapon of mass destruction [WMD]

X **Y36.92**   War operations involving friendly fire

▶ **Y36.A**   Blast overpressure in war operations
▶ Code also type of explosive, if known
▶ accidental detonation of on board munitions (Y36.140)
▶ explosion of grenade (Y36.290)
▶ explosion of torpedo (Y36.040)
▶ improvised explosive device (Y36.230)

▶ X **Y36.A1**   Low level blast overpressure in war operations
▶ LLB overpressure in war operations
▶ Low level blast overpressure due to explosion in war operations

▶ X **Y36.A2**   High level blast overpressure in war operations
▶ High level blast overpressure due to explosion in war operations
▶ HLB overpressure in war operations

Y37   Military operations

Includes   Injuries to military personnel and civilians occurring during peacetime on military property and during routine military exercises and operations

Excludes1   military aircraft involved in aircraft accident with civilian aircraft (V97.81-)
military vehicles involved in transport accident with civilian vehicle (V09.01, V09.21, V19.81, V29.818, V39.81, V49.81, V59.81, V69.81, V79.81)
military watercraft involved in water transport accident with civilian watercraft (V94.81-)
war operations (Y36.-)

The appropriate 7th character is to be added to each code from category Y37

```
A   initial encounter
D   subsequent encounter
S   sequela
```

Y37.0   Military operations involving explosion of marine weapons

Y37.00   Military operations involving explosion of unspecified marine weapon
Military operations involving underwater blast NOS

Y37.000   Military operations involving explosion of unspecified marine weapon, military personnel

Y37.001   Military operations involving explosion of unspecified marine weapon, civilian

Y37.01   Military operations involving explosion of depth-charge

Y37.010   Military operations involving explosion of depth-charge, military personnel

Y37.011   Military operations involving explosion of depth-charge, civilian

Y37.02   Military operations involving explosion of marine mine
Military operations involving explosion of marine mine, at sea or in harbor

Y37.020   Military operations involving explosion of marine mine, military personnel

Y37.021   Military operations involving explosion of marine mine, civilian

Y37.03   Military operations involving explosion of sea-based artillery shell

Y37.030   Military operations involving explosion of sea-based artillery shell, military personnel

Y37.031   Military operations involving explosion of sea-based artillery shell, civilian

Y37.04   Military operations involving explosion of torpedo

Y37.040   Military operations involving explosion of torpedo, military personnel

Y37.041   Military operations involving explosion of torpedo, civilian

Y37.05   Military operations involving accidental detonation of onboard marine weapons

Y37.050   Military operations involving accidental detonation of onboard marine weapons, military personnel

Y37.051   Military operations involving accidental detonation of onboard marine weapons, civilian

▶ New   ▶ Revised   ~~deleted~~ Deleted   Excludes 1   Excludes 2   Includes   Use additional   Code first   Code also   Key words
OGCR Official Guidelines   X Assign placeholder X   ● Use Additional Character(s)   ▶ Manifestation Code   Hierarchical Condition Category   Coding Clinic

- **Y37.09** Military operations involving explosion of other marine weapons
  - **Y37.090** Military operations involving explosion of other marine weapons, military personnel
  - **Y37.091** Military operations involving explosion of other marine weapons, civilian
- **Y37.1** Military operations involving destruction of aircraft
  - **Y37.10** Military operations involving unspecified destruction of aircraft
    - **Y37.100** Military operations involving unspecified destruction of aircraft, military personnel
    - **Y37.101** Military operations involving unspecified destruction of aircraft, civilian
  - **Y37.11** Military operations involving destruction of aircraft due to enemy fire or explosives

    Military operations involving destruction of aircraft due to air to air missile

    Military operations involving destruction of aircraft due to explosive placed on aircraft

    Military operations involving destruction of aircraft due to rocket propelled grenade [RPG]

    Military operations involving destruction of aircraft due to small arms fire

    Military operations involving destruction of aircraft due to surface to air missile
    - **Y37.110** Military operations involving destruction of aircraft due to enemy fire or explosives, military personnel
    - **Y37.111** Military operations involving destruction of aircraft due to enemy fire or explosives, civilian
  - **Y37.12** Military operations involving destruction of aircraft due to collision with other aircraft
    - **Y37.120** Military operations involving destruction of aircraft due to collision with other aircraft, military personnel
    - **Y37.121** Military operations involving destruction of aircraft due to collision with other aircraft, civilian
  - **Y37.13** Military operations involving destruction of aircraft due to onboard fire
    - **Y37.130** Military operations involving destruction of aircraft due to onboard fire, military personnel
    - **Y37.131** Military operations involving destruction of aircraft due to onboard fire, civilian
  - **Y37.14** Military operations involving destruction of aircraft due to accidental detonation of onboard munitions and explosives
    - **Y37.140** Military operations involving destruction of aircraft due to accidental detonation of onboard munitions and explosives, military personnel
    - **Y37.141** Military operations involving destruction of aircraft due to accidental detonation of onboard munitions and explosives, civilian
  - **Y37.19** Military operations involving other destruction of aircraft
    - **Y37.190** Military operations involving other destruction of aircraft, military personnel
    - **Y37.191** Military operations involving other destruction of aircraft, civilian
- **Y37.2** Military operations involving other explosions and fragments
  - **Excludes1** military operations involving explosion of aircraft (Y37.1-)

    military operations involving explosion of marine weapons (Y37.0-)

    military operations involving explosion of nuclear weapons (Y37.5-)
  - **Y37.20** Military operations involving unspecified explosion and fragments

    Military operations involving air blast NOS

    Military operations involving blast NOS

    Military operations involving blast fragments NOS

    Military operations involving blast wave NOS

    Military operations involving blast wind NOS

    Military operations involving explosion NOS

    Military operations involving explosion of bomb NOS
    - **Y37.200** Military operations involving unspecified explosion and fragments, military personnel
    - **Y37.201** Military operations involving unspecified explosion and fragments, civilian
  - **Y37.21** Military operations involving explosion of aerial bomb
    - **Y37.210** Military operations involving explosion of aerial bomb, military personnel
    - **Y37.211** Military operations involving explosion of aerial bomb, civilian
  - **Y37.22** Military operations involving explosion of guided missile
    - **Y37.220** Military operations involving explosion of guided missile, military personnel
    - **Y37.221** Military operations involving explosion of guided missile, civilian
  - **Y37.23** Military operations involving explosion of improvised explosive device [IED]

    Military operations involving explosion of person-borne improvised explosive device [IED]

    Military operations involving explosion of vehicle-borne improvised explosive device [IED]

    Military operations involving explosion of roadside improvised explosive device [IED]
    - **Y37.230** Military operations involving explosion of improvised explosive device [IED], military personnel
    - **Y37.231** Military operations involving explosion of improvised explosive device [IED], civilian
  - **Y37.24** Military operations involving explosion due to accidental detonation and discharge of own munitions or munitions launch device
    - **Y37.240** Military operations involving explosion due to accidental detonation and discharge of own munitions or munitions launch device, military personnel
    - **Y37.241** Military operations involving explosion due to accidental detonation and discharge of own munitions or munitions launch device, civilian
  - **Y37.25** Military operations involving fragments from munitions
    - **Y37.250** Military operations involving fragments from munitions, military personnel
    - **Y37.251** Military operations involving fragments from munitions, civilian

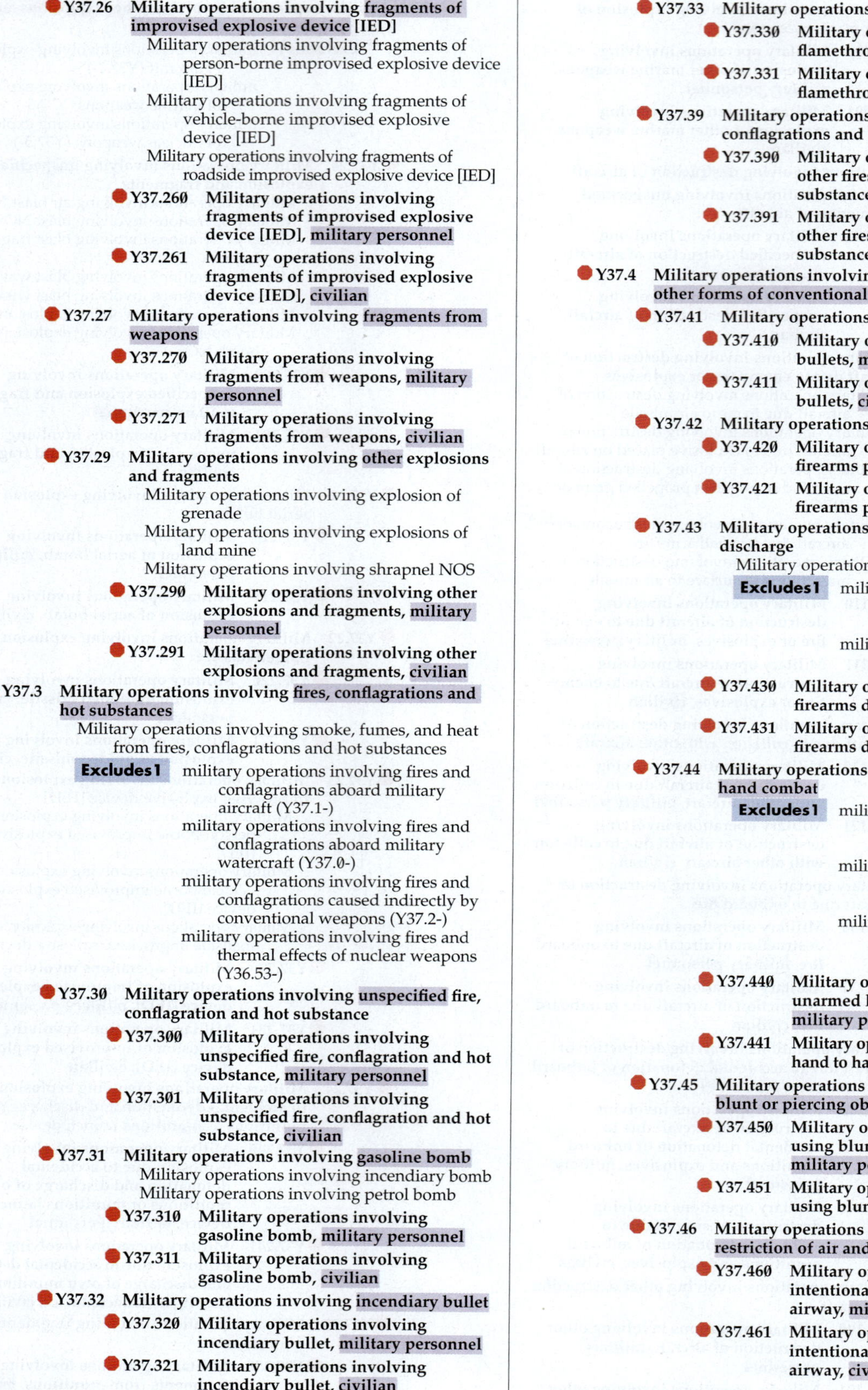

● **Y37.26 Military operations involving fragments of improvised explosive device [IED]**
Military operations involving fragments of person-borne improvised explosive device [IED]
Military operations involving fragments of vehicle-borne improvised explosive device [IED]
Military operations involving fragments of roadside improvised explosive device [IED]

   ● **Y37.260 Military operations involving fragments of improvised explosive device [IED], military personnel**

   ● **Y37.261 Military operations involving fragments of improvised explosive device [IED], civilian**

● **Y37.27 Military operations involving fragments from weapons**

   ● **Y37.270 Military operations involving fragments from weapons, military personnel**

   ● **Y37.271 Military operations involving fragments from weapons, civilian**

● **Y37.29 Military operations involving other explosions and fragments**
Military operations involving explosion of grenade
Military operations involving explosions of land mine
Military operations involving shrapnel NOS

   ● **Y37.290 Military operations involving other explosions and fragments, military personnel**

   ● **Y37.291 Military operations involving other explosions and fragments, civilian**

● **Y37.3 Military operations involving fires, conflagrations and hot substances**
Military operations involving smoke, fumes, and heat from fires, conflagrations and hot substances

   Excludes1   military operations involving fires and conflagrations aboard military aircraft (Y37.1-)
military operations involving fires and conflagrations aboard military watercraft (Y37.0-)
military operations involving fires and conflagrations caused indirectly by conventional weapons (Y37.2-)
military operations involving fires and thermal effects of nuclear weapons (Y36.53-)

   ● **Y37.30 Military operations involving unspecified fire, conflagration and hot substance**

     ● **Y37.300 Military operations involving unspecified fire, conflagration and hot substance, military personnel**

     ● **Y37.301 Military operations involving unspecified fire, conflagration and hot substance, civilian**

   ● **Y37.31 Military operations involving gasoline bomb**
Military operations involving incendiary bomb
Military operations involving petrol bomb

     ● **Y37.310 Military operations involving gasoline bomb, military personnel**

     ● **Y37.311 Military operations involving gasoline bomb, civilian**

   ● **Y37.32 Military operations involving incendiary bullet**

     ● **Y37.320 Military operations involving incendiary bullet, military personnel**

     ● **Y37.321 Military operations involving incendiary bullet, civilian**

● **Y37.33 Military operations involving flamethrower**

   ● **Y37.330 Military operations involving flamethrower, military personnel**

   ● **Y37.331 Military operations involving flamethrower, civilian**

● **Y37.39 Military operations involving other fires, conflagrations and hot substances**

   ● **Y37.390 Military operations involving other fires, conflagrations and hot substances, military personnel**

   ● **Y37.391 Military operations involving other fires, conflagrations and hot substances, civilian**

● **Y37.4 Military operations involving firearm discharge and other forms of conventional warfare**

   ● **Y37.41 Military operations involving rubber bullets**

     ● **Y37.410 Military operations involving rubber bullets, military personnel**

     ● **Y37.411 Military operations involving rubber bullets, civilian**

   ● **Y37.42 Military operations involving firearms pellets**

     ● **Y37.420 Military operations involving firearms pellets, military personnel**

     ● **Y37.421 Military operations involving firearms pellets, civilian**

   ● **Y37.43 Military operations involving other firearms discharge**
Military operations involving bullets NOS

     Excludes1   military operations involving munitions fragments (Y37.25-)
military operations involving incendiary bullets (Y37.32-)

     ● **Y37.430 Military operations involving other firearms discharge, military personnel**

     ● **Y37.431 Military operations involving other firearms discharge, civilian**

   ● **Y37.44 Military operations involving unarmed hand to hand combat**

     Excludes1   military operations involving combat using blunt or piercing object (Y37.45-)
military operations involving intentional restriction of air and airway (Y37.46-)
military operations involving unintentional restriction of air and airway (Y37.47-)

     ● **Y37.440 Military operations involving unarmed hand to hand combat, military personnel**

     ● **Y37.441 Military operations involving unarmed hand to hand combat, civilian**

   ● **Y37.45 Military operations involving combat using blunt or piercing object**

     ● **Y37.450 Military operations involving combat using blunt or piercing object, military personnel**

     ● **Y37.451 Military operations involving combat using blunt or piercing object, civilian**

   ● **Y37.46 Military operations involving intentional restriction of air and airway**

     ● **Y37.460 Military operations involving intentional restriction of air and airway, military personnel**

     ● **Y37.461 Military operations involving intentional restriction of air and airway, civilian**

- **Y37.47** Military operations involving unintentional restriction of air and airway
  - **Y37.470** Military operations involving unintentional restriction of air and airway, military personnel
  - **Y37.471** Military operations involving unintentional restriction of air and airway, civilian
- **Y37.49** Military operations involving other forms of conventional warfare
  - **Y37.490** Military operations involving other forms of conventional warfare, military personnel
  - **Y37.491** Military operations involving other forms of conventional warfare, civilian
- **Y37.5** Military operations involving nuclear weapons
  Military operation involving dirty bomb NOS
  - **Y37.50** Military operations involving unspecified effect of nuclear weapon
    - **Y37.500** Military operations involving unspecified effect of nuclear weapon, military personnel
    - **Y37.501** Military operations involving unspecified effect of nuclear weapon, civilian
  - **Y37.51** Military operations involving direct blast effect of nuclear weapon
    Military operations involving blast pressure of nuclear weapon
    - **Y37.510** Military operations involving direct blast effect of nuclear weapon, military personnel
    - **Y37.511** Military operations involving direct blast effect of nuclear weapon, civilian
  - **Y37.52** Military operations involving indirect blast effect of nuclear weapon
    Military operations involving being thrown by blast of nuclear weapon
    Military operations involving being struck or crushed by blast debris of nuclear weapon
    - **Y37.520** Military operations involving indirect blast effect of nuclear weapon, military personnel
    - **Y37.521** Military operations involving indirect blast effect of nuclear weapon, civilian
  - **Y37.53** Military operations involving thermal radiation effect of nuclear weapon
    Military operations involving direct heat from nuclear weapon
    Military operation involving fireball effects from nuclear weapon
    - **Y37.530** Military operations involving thermal radiation effect of nuclear weapon, military personnel
    - **Y37.531** Military operations involving thermal radiation effect of nuclear weapon, civilian
  - **Y37.54** Military operation involving nuclear radiation effects of nuclear weapon
    Military operation involving acute radiation exposure from nuclear weapon
    Military operation involving exposure to immediate ionizing radiation from nuclear weapon
    Military operation involving fallout exposure from nuclear weapon
    Military operation involving secondary effects of nuclear weapons
    - **Y37.540** Military operation involving nuclear radiation effects of nuclear weapon, military personnel
    - **Y37.541** Military operation involving nuclear radiation effects of nuclear weapon, civilian

- **Y37.59** Military operation involving other effects of nuclear weapons
  - **Y37.590** Military operation involving other effects of nuclear weapons, military personnel
  - **Y37.591** Military operation involving other effects of nuclear weapons, civilian
- **Y37.6** Military operations involving biological weapons
  - **Y37.6X** Military operations involving biological weapons
    - **Y37.6X0** Military operations involving biological weapons, military personnel
    - **Y37.6X1** Military operations involving biological weapons, civilian
- **Y37.7** Military operations involving chemical weapons and other forms of unconventional warfare

  Excludes1 military operations involving incendiary devices (Y36.3-, Y36.5-)
  - **Y37.7X** Military operations involving chemical weapons and other forms of unconventional warfare
    - **Y37.7X0** Military operations involving chemical weapons and other forms of unconventional warfare, military personnel
    - **Y37.7X1** Military operations involving chemical weapons and other forms of unconventional warfare, civilian
- **Y37.9** Other and unspecified military operations
  - **X Y37.90** Military operations, unspecified
  - **X Y37.91** Military operations involving unspecified weapon of mass destruction [WMD]
  - **X Y37.92** Military operations involving friendly fire
- **Y37.A** Blast overpressure in military operations
  - **Code also** type of explosive, if known
    - accidental detonation of on board munitions (Y37.140)
    - explosion of grenade (Y37.290)
    - explosion of torpedo (Y37.040)
    - improvised explosive device (Y37.230)
  - **X Y37.A1** Low level blast overpressure in military operations
    - LLB overpressure in military operations
    - Low level blast overpressure due to explosion in military operations
  - **X Y37.A2** High level blast overpressure in military operations
    - High level blast overpressure due to explosion in military operations
    - HLB overpressure in military operations
- **Y38 Terrorism**
  These codes are for use to identify injuries resulting from the unlawful use of force or violence against persons or property to intimidate or coerce a government, the civilian population, or any segment thereof, in furtherance of political or social objective

  Use additional code for place of occurrence (Y92.-)

  The appropriate 7th character is to be added to each code from category Y38

A	initial encounter
D	subsequent encounter
S	sequela

- **Y38.0** Terrorism involving explosion of marine weapons
  Terrorism involving depth-charge
  Terrorism involving marine mine
  Terrorism involving mine NOS, at sea or in harbor
  Terrorism involving sea-based artillery shell
  Terrorism involving torpedo
  Terrorism involving underwater blast

CHAPTER 20 (V00–Y99)

● **Y38.0X**   Terrorism involving explosion of marine weapons
    ● **Y38.0X1**   Terrorism involving explosion of marine weapons, public safety official injured
    ● **Y38.0X2**   Terrorism involving explosion of marine weapons, civilian injured
    ● **Y38.0X3**   Terrorism involving explosion of marine weapons, terrorist injured
● **Y38.1**   Terrorism involving destruction of aircraft
    Terrorism involving aircraft burned
    Terrorism involving aircraft exploded
    Terrorism involving aircraft being shot down
    Terrorism involving aircraft used as a weapon
    ● **Y38.1X**   Terrorism involving destruction of aircraft
       ● **Y38.1X1**   Terrorism involving destruction of aircraft, public safety official injured
       ● **Y38.1X2**   Terrorism involving destruction of aircraft, civilian injured
       ● **Y38.1X3**   Terrorism involving destruction of aircraft, terrorist injured
● **Y38.2**   Terrorism involving other explosions and fragments
    Terrorism involving antipersonnel (fragments) bomb
    Terrorism involving blast NOS
    Terrorism involving explosion NOS
    Terrorism involving explosion of breech block
    Terrorism involving explosion of cannon block
    Terrorism involving explosion (fragments) of artillery shell
    Terrorism involving explosion (fragments) of bomb
    Terrorism involving explosion (fragments) of grenade
    Terrorism involving explosion (fragments) of guided missile
    Terrorism involving explosion (fragments) of land mine
    Terrorism involving explosion of mortar bomb
    Terrorism involving explosion of munitions
    Terrorism involving explosion (fragments) of rocket
    Terrorism involving explosion (fragments) of shell
    Terrorism involving shrapnel
    Terrorism involving mine NOS, on land

> **Excludes1**   terrorism involving explosion of nuclear weapon (Y38.5)
> terrorism involving suicide bomber (Y38.81)

    ● **Y38.2X**   Terrorism involving other explosions and fragments
       ● **Y38.2X1**   Terrorism involving other explosions and fragments, public safety official injured
       ● **Y38.2X2**   Terrorism involving other explosions and fragments, civilian injured
       ● **Y38.2X3**   Terrorism involving other explosions and fragments, terrorist injured
● **Y38.3**   Terrorism involving fires, conflagration and hot substances
    Terrorism involving conflagration NOS
    Terrorism involving fire NOS
    Terrorism involving petrol bomb

> **Excludes1**   terrorism involving fire or heat of nuclear weapon (Y38.5)

    ● **Y38.3X**   Terrorism involving fires, conflagration and hot substances
       ● **Y38.3X1**   Terrorism involving fires, conflagration and hot substances, public safety official injured
       ● **Y38.3X2**   Terrorism involving fires, conflagration and hot substances, civilian injured
       ● **Y38.3X3**   Terrorism involving fires, conflagration and hot substances, terrorist injured

● **Y38.4**   Terrorism involving firearms
    Terrorism involving carbine bullet
    Terrorism involving machine gun bullet
    Terrorism involving pellets (shotgun)
    Terrorism involving pistol bullet
    Terrorism involving rifle bullet
    Terrorism involving rubber (rifle) bullet
    ● **Y38.4X**   Terrorism involving firearms
       ● **Y38.4X1**   Terrorism involving firearms, public safety official injured
       ● **Y38.4X2**   Terrorism involving firearms, civilian injured
       ● **Y38.4X3**   Terrorism involving firearms, terrorist injured
● **Y38.5**   Terrorism involving nuclear weapons
    Terrorism involving blast effects of nuclear weapon
    Terrorism involving exposure to ionizing radiation from nuclear weapon
    Terrorism involving fireball effect of nuclear weapon
    Terrorism involving heat from nuclear weapon
    ● **Y38.5X**   Terrorism involving nuclear weapons
       ● **Y38.5X1**   Terrorism involving nuclear weapons, public safety official injured
       ● **Y38.5X2**   Terrorism involving nuclear weapons, civilian injured
       ● **Y38.5X3**   Terrorism involving nuclear weapons, terrorist injured
● **Y38.6**   Terrorism involving biological weapons
    Terrorism involving anthrax
    Terrorism involving cholera
    A serious, often deadly, infectious disease of the small intestine
    Terrorism involving smallpox
    ● **Y38.6X**   Terrorism involving biological weapons
       ● **Y38.6X1**   Terrorism involving biological weapons, public safety official injured
       ● **Y38.6X2**   Terrorism involving biological weapons, civilian injured
       ● **Y38.6X3**   Terrorism involving biological weapons, terrorist injured
● **Y38.7**   Terrorism involving chemical weapons
    Terrorism involving gases, fumes, chemicals
    Terrorism involving hydrogen cyanide
    Terrorism involving phosgene
    Terrorism involving sarin
    ● **Y38.7X**   Terrorism involving chemical weapons
       ● **Y38.7X1**   Terrorism involving chemical weapons, public safety official injured
       ● **Y38.7X2**   Terrorism involving chemical weapons, civilian injured
       ● **Y38.7X3**   Terrorism involving chemical weapons, terrorist injured
● **Y38.8**   Terrorism involving other and unspecified means
    ● **Y38.80**   Terrorism involving unspecified means
       Terrorism NOS
    ● **Y38.81**   Terrorism involving suicide bomber
       ● **Y38.811**   Terrorism involving suicide bomber, public safety official injured
       ● **Y38.812**   Terrorism involving suicide bomber, civilian injured
    ● **Y38.89**   Terrorism involving other means
       Terrorism involving drowning and submersion
       Terrorism involving lasers
       Terrorism involving piercing or stabbing instruments
       ● **Y38.891**   Terrorism involving other means, public safety official injured
       ● **Y38.892**   Terrorism involving other means, civilian injured
       ● **Y38.893**   Terrorism involving other means, terrorist injured

● **Y38.9**   Terrorism, secondary effects

> **Note:** This code is for use to identify conditions occurring subsequent to a terrorist attack not those that are due to the initial terrorist attack.

   ● **Y38.9X**   Terrorism, secondary effects

     ● **Y38.9X1**   Terrorism, secondary effects, public safety official injured

     ● **Y38.9X2**   Terrorism, secondary effects, civilian injured categories

---

COMPLICATIONS OF MEDICAL AND SURGICAL CARE (Y62-Y84)

Includes   complications of medical devices surgical and medical procedures as the cause of abnormal reaction of the patient, or of later complication, without mention of misadventure at the time of the procedure

---

MISADVENTURES TO PATIENTS DURING SURGICAL AND MEDICAL CARE (Y62-Y69)

Excludes1   surgical and medical procedures as the cause of abnormal reaction of the patient, without mention of misadventure at the time of the procedure (Y83-Y84)

● **Y62**   Failure of sterile precautions during surgical and medical care

   Y62.0   Failure of sterile precautions during surgical operation

   Y62.1   Failure of sterile precautions during infusion or transfusion

   Y62.2   Failure of sterile precautions during kidney dialysis and other perfusion

   Y62.3   Failure of sterile precautions during injection or immunization

   Y62.4   Failure of sterile precautions during endoscopic examination

   Y62.5   Failure of sterile precautions during heart catheterization

   Y62.6   Failure of sterile precautions during aspiration, puncture and other catheterization

   Y62.8   Failure of sterile precautions during other surgical and medical care

   Y62.9   Failure of sterile precautions during unspecified surgical and medical care

● **Y63**   Failure in dosage during surgical and medical care

   Excludes2   accidental overdose of drug or wrong drug given in error (T36-T50)

   Y63.0   Excessive amount of blood or other fluid given during transfusion or infusion

   Y63.1   Incorrect dilution of fluid used during infusion

   Y63.2   Overdose of radiation given during therapy

   Y63.3   Inadvertent exposure of patient to radiation during medical care

   Y63.4   Failure in dosage in electroshock or insulin-shock therapy

   Y63.5   Inappropriate temperature in local application and packing

   Y63.6   Underdosing and nonadministration of necessary drug, medicament or biological substance

   Y63.8   Failure in dosage during other surgical and medical care

   Y63.9   Failure in dosage during unspecified surgical and medical care

● **Y64**   Contaminated medical or biological substances

   Y64.0   Contaminated medical or biological substance, transfused or infused

   Y64.1   Contaminated medical or biological substance, injected or used for immunization

   Y64.8   Contaminated medical or biological substance administered by other means

   Y64.9   Contaminated medical or biological substance administered by unspecified means

> Administered contaminated medical or biological substance NOS

● **Y65**   Other misadventures during surgical and medical care

   Y65.0   Mismatched blood in transfusion

   Y65.1   Wrong fluid used in infusion

   Y65.2   Failure in suture or ligature during surgical operation

   Y65.3   Endotracheal tube wrongly placed during anesthetic procedure

   Y65.4   Failure to introduce or to remove other tube or instrument

     Coding Clinic: 2025, Q2, P11

   ● **Y65.5**   Performance of wrong procedure (operation)

     ● **Y65.51**   Performance of wrong procedure (operation) on correct patient

       Wrong device implanted into correct surgical site

       Excludes1   performance of correct procedure (operation) on wrong side or body part (Y65.53)

     ● **Y65.52**   Performance of procedure (operation) on patient not scheduled for surgery

       Performance of procedure (operation) intended for another patient

       Performance of procedure (operation) on wrong patient

     ● **Y65.53**   Performance of correct procedure (operation) on wrong side or body part

       Performance of correct procedure (operation) on wrong side

       Performance of correct procedure (operation) on wrong site

   Y65.8   Other specified misadventures during surgical and medical care

     Coding Clinic: 2019, Q2, P24

Y66   Nonadministration of surgical and medical care

> Premature cessation of surgical and medical care

   Excludes1   DNR status (Z66)
> palliative care (Z51.5)

Y69   Unspecified misadventure during surgical and medical care

---

MEDICAL DEVICES ASSOCIATED WITH ADVERSE INCIDENTS IN DIAGNOSTIC AND THERAPEUTIC USE (Y70-Y82)

Includes   breakdown or malfunction of medical devices (during use) (after implantation) (ongoing use)

Excludes2   later complications following use of medical devices without breakdown or malfunctioning of device (Y83-Y84)

> misadventure to patients during surgical and medical care, classifiable to (Y62-Y69)

> surgical and other medical procedures as the cause of abnormal reaction of the patient, or of later complication, without mention of misadventure at the time of the procedure (Y83-Y84)

● **Y70**   Anesthesiology devices associated with adverse incidents

   Y70.0   Diagnostic and monitoring anesthesiology devices associated with adverse incidents

   Y70.1   Therapeutic (nonsurgical) and rehabilitative anesthesiology devices associated with adverse incidents

   Y70.2   Prosthetic and other implants, materials and accessory anesthesiology devices associated with adverse incidents

   Y70.3   Surgical instruments, materials and anesthesiology devices (including sutures) associated with adverse incidents

   Y70.8   Miscellaneous anesthesiology devices associated with adverse incidents, not elsewhere classified

● **Y71**   Cardiovascular devices associated with adverse incidents

---

CHAPTER 20 (VØØ-Y99)

Y71.Ø   **Diagnostic and monitoring** cardiovascular devices associated with adverse incidents

Y71.1   **Therapeutic (nonsurgical) and rehabilitative** cardiovascular devices associated with adverse incidents

Y71.2   **Prosthetic and other implants, materials and accessory** cardiovascular devices associated with adverse incidents

Y71.3   **Surgical instruments, materials** and cardiovascular devices (including sutures) associated with adverse incidents

Y71.8   **Miscellaneous** cardiovascular devices associated with adverse incidents, not elsewhere classified

● **Y72**   **Otorhinolaryngological** devices associated with adverse incidents

Y72.Ø   **Diagnostic and monitoring** otorhinolaryngological devices associated with adverse incidents

Y72.1   **Therapeutic (nonsurgical) and rehabilitative** otorhinolaryngological devices associated with adverse incidents

Y72.2   **Prosthetic and other implants, materials and accessory** otorhinolaryngological devices associated with adverse incidents

Y72.3   **Surgical instruments, materials** and otorhinolaryngological devices (including sutures) associated with adverse incidents

Y72.8   **Miscellaneous** otorhinolaryngological devices associated with adverse incidents, not elsewhere classified

● **Y73**   **Gastroenterology and urology** devices associated with adverse incidents

Y73.Ø   **Diagnostic and monitoring** gastroenterology and urology devices associated with adverse incidents

Y73.1   **Therapeutic (nonsurgical) and rehabilitative** gastroenterology and urology devices associated with adverse incidents

Y73.2   **Prosthetic and other implants, materials and accessory** gastroenterology and urology devices associated with adverse incidents

Y73.3   **Surgical instruments, materials** and gastroenterology and urology devices (including sutures) associated with adverse incidents

Y73.8   **Miscellaneous** gastroenterology and urology devices associated with adverse incidents, not elsewhere classified

● **Y74**   **General hospital and personal-use** devices associated with adverse incidents

Y74.Ø   **Diagnostic and monitoring** general hospital and personal-use devices associated with adverse incidents

Y74.1   **Therapeutic (nonsurgical) and rehabilitative** general hospital and personal-use devices associated with adverse incidents

Y74.2   **Prosthetic and other implants, materials and accessory** general hospital and personal-use devices associated with adverse incidents

Y74.3   **Surgical instruments, materials** and general hospital and personal-use devices (including sutures) associated with adverse incidents

Y74.8   **Miscellaneous** general hospital and personal-use devices associated with adverse incidents, not elsewhere classified

● **Y75**   **Neurological** devices associated with adverse incidents

Y75.Ø   **Diagnostic and monitoring** neurological devices associated with adverse incidents

Y75.1   **Therapeutic (nonsurgical) and rehabilitative** neurological devices associated with adverse incidents

Y75.2   **Prosthetic and other implants, materials and** neurological devices associated with adverse incidents

Y75.3   **Surgical instruments, materials** and neurological devices (including sutures) associated with adverse incidents

Y75.8   **Miscellaneous** neurological devices associated with adverse incidents, not elsewhere classified

● **Y76**   **Obstetric and gynecological** devices associated with adverse incidents

Y76.Ø   **Diagnostic and monitoring** obstetric and gynecological devices associated with adverse incidents

Y76.1   **Therapeutic (nonsurgical) and rehabilitative obstetric and gynecological** devices associated with adverse incidents

Y76.2   **Prosthetic and other implants, materials and accessory** obstetric and gynecological devices associated with adverse incidents

Y76.3   **Surgical instruments, materials** and obstetric and gynecological devices (including sutures) associated with adverse incidents

Y76.8   **Miscellaneous** obstetric and gynecological devices associated with adverse incidents, not elsewhere classified

● **Y77**   **Ophthalmic** devices associated with adverse incidents

Y77.Ø   **Diagnostic and monitoring** ophthalmic devices associated with adverse incidents

● Y77.1   **Therapeutic (nonsurgical) and rehabilitative ophthalmic** devices associated with adverse incidents

Y77.11   **Contact lens** associated with adverse incidents
Rigid gas permeable contact lens associated with adverse incidents
Soft (hydrophilic) contact lens associated with adverse incidents

Y77.19   **Other therapeutic (nonsurgical) and** rehabilitative ophthalmic devices associated with adverse incidents

Y77.2   **Prosthetic and other implants, materials and accessory** ophthalmic devices associated with adverse incidents

Y77.3   **Surgical instruments, materials** and ophthalmic devices (including sutures) associated with adverse incidents

Y77.8   **Miscellaneous** ophthalmic devices associated with adverse incidents, not elsewhere classified

● **Y78**   **Radiological** devices associated with adverse incidents

Y78.Ø   **Diagnostic and monitoring** radiological devices associated with adverse incidents

Y78.1   **Therapeutic (nonsurgical) and rehabilitative** radiological devices associated with adverse incidents

Y78.2   **Prosthetic and other implants, materials and accessory** radiological devices associated with adverse incidents

Y78.3   **Surgical instruments, materials** and radiological devices (including sutures) associated with adverse incidents

Y78.8   **Miscellaneous** radiological devices associated with adverse incidents, not elsewhere classified

● **Y79**   **Orthopedic** devices associated with adverse incidents

Y79.Ø   **Diagnostic and monitoring** orthopedic devices associated with adverse incidents

Y79.1   **Therapeutic (nonsurgical) and rehabilitative** orthopedic devices associated with adverse incidents

Y79.2   **Prosthetic and other implants, materials and accessory** orthopedic devices associated with adverse incidents

Y79.3   **Surgical instruments, materials** and orthopedic devices (including sutures) associated with adverse incidents

Y79.8   **Miscellaneous** orthopedic devices associated with adverse incidents, not elsewhere classified

● **Y8Ø**   **Physical medicine** devices associated with adverse incidents

Y8Ø.Ø   **Diagnostic and monitoring** physical medicine devices associated with adverse incidents

Y8Ø.1   **Therapeutic (nonsurgical) and rehabilitative** physical medicine devices associated with adverse incidents

Y8Ø.2   **Prosthetic and other implants, materials and accessory** physical medicine devices associated with adverse incidents

Y8Ø.3   **Surgical instruments, materials** and physical medicine devices (including sutures) associated with adverse incidents

Y8Ø.8   **Miscellaneous** physical medicine devices associated with adverse incidents, not elsewhere classified

▶ New   ➡ Revised   ~~deleted~~ Deleted   Excludes 1   Excludes 2   Includes   Use additional   Code first   Code also   Key words

OGCR Official Guidelines   X Assign placeholder X   ● Use Additional Character(s)   ▶ Manifestation Code   🔁 Hierarchical Condition Category   Coding Clinic

- **Y81** **General- and plastic-surgery** devices associated with adverse incidents
  - Y81.0 **Diagnostic and monitoring** general- and plastic-surgery devices associated with adverse incidents
  - Y81.1 **Therapeutic (nonsurgical)** and rehabilitative general- and plastic-surgery devices associated with adverse incidents
  - Y81.2 **Prosthetic and other implants, materials and accessory** general- and plastic-surgery devices associated with adverse incidents
  - Y81.3 **Surgical instruments, materials and general- and plastic-surgery devices (including sutures)** associated with adverse incidents
  - Y81.8 **Miscellaneous** general- and plastic-surgery devices associated with adverse incidents, not elsewhere classified
- **Y82** Other and unspecified medical devices associated with adverse incidents
  - Y82.8 **Other medical devices** associated with adverse incidents
  - Y82.9 **Unspecified medical devices** associated with adverse incidents

---

SURGICAL AND OTHER MEDICAL PROCEDURES AS THE CAUSE OF ABNORMAL REACTION OF THE PATIENT, OR OF LATER COMPLICATION, WITHOUT MENTION OF MISADVENTURE AT THE TIME OF THE PROCEDURE (Y83-Y84)

> **Excludes1**   misadventures to patients during surgical and medical care, classifiable to (Y62-Y69)
>
> **Excludes2**   breakdown or malfunctioning of medical device (after implantation) (during procedure) (ongoing use) (Y70-Y82)

- **Y83** **Surgical operation and other surgical** procedures as the cause of abnormal reaction of the patient, or of later complication, without mention of misadventure at the time of the procedure
  - Y83.0 Surgical operation with **transplant of whole organ** as the cause of abnormal reaction of the patient, or of later complication, without mention of misadventure at the time of the procedure
  - Y83.1 Surgical operation with **implant of artificial internal device** as the cause of abnormal reaction of the patient, or of later complication, without mention of misadventure at the time of the procedure
  - Y83.2 Surgical operation with **anastomosis, bypass or graft** as the cause of abnormal reaction of the patient, or of later complication, without mention of misadventure at the time of the procedure
  - Y83.3 Surgical operation with **formation of external stoma** as the cause of abnormal reaction of the patient, or of later complication, without mention of misadventure at the time of the procedure
  - Y83.4 **Other reconstructive surgery** as the cause of abnormal reaction of the patient, or of later complication, without mention of misadventure at the time of the procedure
  - Y83.5 **Amputation of limb(s)** as the cause of abnormal reaction of the patient, or of later complication, without mention of misadventure at the time of the procedure
  - Y83.6 **Removal of other organ (partial) (total)** as the cause of abnormal reaction of the patient, or of later complication, without mention of misadventure at the time of the procedure
  - Y83.8 **Other surgical procedures** as the cause of abnormal reaction of the patient, or of later complication, without mention of misadventure at the time of the procedure
    Coding Clinic: 2023, Q2, P14
  - Y83.9 Surgical procedure, **unspecified** as the cause of abnormal reaction of the patient, or of later complication, without mention of misadventure at the time of the procedure

- **Y84** **Other medical procedures** as the cause of abnormal reaction of the patient, or of later complication, without mention of misadventure at the time of the procedure
  - Y84.0 **Cardiac catheterization** as the cause of abnormal reaction of the patient, or of later complication, without mention of misadventure at the time of the procedure
  - Y84.1 **Kidney dialysis** as the cause of abnormal reaction of the patient, or of later complication, without mention of misadventure at the time of the procedure
  - Y84.2 **Radiological procedure and radiotherapy** as the cause of abnormal reaction of the patient, or of later complication, without mention of misadventure at the time of the procedure
    Coding Clinic: 2019, Q1, P21; 2017, Q1, P34
  - Y84.3 **Shock therapy** as the cause of abnormal reaction of the patient, or of later complication, without mention of misadventure at the time of the procedure
  - Y84.4 **Aspiration of fluid** as the cause of abnormal reaction of the patient, or of later complication, without mention of misadventure at the time of the procedure
  - Y84.5 **Insertion of gastric or duodenal sound** as the cause of abnormal reaction of the patient, or of later complication, without mention of misadventure at the time of the procedure
  - Y84.6 **Urinary catheterization** as the cause of abnormal reaction of the patient, or of later complication, without mention of misadventure at the time of the procedure
    Coding Clinic: 2025, Q2, P20
  - Y84.7 **Blood-sampling** as the cause of abnormal reaction of the patient, or of later complication, without mention of misadventure at the time of the procedure
  - Y84.8 **Other medical procedures** as the cause of abnormal reaction of the patient, or of later complication, without mention of misadventure at the time of the procedure
    Coding Clinic: 2024, Q1, P26; 2023, Q2, P28; 2021, Q1, P5
  - Y84.9 Medical procedure, **unspecified** as the cause of abnormal reaction of the patient, or of later complication, without mention of misadventure at the time of the procedure

---

SUPPLEMENTARY FACTORS RELATED TO CAUSES OF MORBIDITY CLASSIFIED ELSEWHERE (Y90-Y99)

Note: These categories may be used to provide supplementary information concerning causes of morbidity. They are not to be used for single-condition coding.

- **Y90** **Evidence of alcohol involvement determined by blood alcohol level**
    Code first any associated alcohol related disorders (F10)
    Coding Clinic: 2024, Q2, P10
  - Y90.0 Blood alcohol level of **less than 20 mg/100 ml**
  - Y90.1 Blood alcohol level of **20-39 mg/100 ml**
  - Y90.2 Blood alcohol level of **40-59 mg/100 ml**
  - Y90.3 Blood alcohol level of **60-79 mg/100 ml**
  - Y90.4 Blood alcohol level of **80-99 mg/100 ml**
  - Y90.5 Blood alcohol level of **100-119 mg/100 ml**
  - Y90.6 Blood alcohol level of **120-199 mg/100 ml**
  - Y90.7 Blood alcohol level of **200-239 mg/100 ml**
  - Y90.8 Blood alcohol level of **240 mg/100 ml or more**
  - Y90.9 **Presence** of alcohol in blood, **level not specified**

CHAPTER 20 (V00-Y99)

OGCR Section I.C.20.b.

Place of Occurrence Guideline

Codes from category Y92, Place of occurrence of the external cause, are secondary codes for use after other external cause codes to identify the location of the patient at the time of injury or other condition.

Generally, a place of occurrence code is assigned only once, at the initial encounter for treatment. However, in the rare instance that a new injury occurs during hospitalization, an additional place of occurrence code may be assigned. No 7th characters are used for Y92. Only one code from Y92 should be recorded on a medical record.

Do not use place of occurrence code Y92.9 if the place is not stated or is not applicable.

● Y92   **Place of occurrence of the external cause**

The following category is for use, when relevant, to identify the place of occurrence of the external cause. Use in conjunction with an activity code.

Place of occurrence should be recorded only at the initial encounter for treatment

● Y92.0   **Non-institutional (private) residence as the place of occurrence of the external cause**

     Excludes1   abandoned or derelict house (Y92.89)
                home under construction but not yet occupied (Y92.6-)
                institutional place of residence (Y92.1-)

● Y92.00   **Unspecified non-institutional (private) residence as the place of occurrence of the external cause**

   Y92.000   **Kitchen** of unspecified non-institutional (private) residence as the place of occurrence of the external cause

   Y92.001   **Dining room** of unspecified non-institutional (private) residence as the place of occurrence of the external cause

   Y92.002   **Bathroom** of unspecified non-institutional (private) residence as the place of occurrence of the external cause

   Y92.003   **Bedroom** of unspecified non-institutional (private) residence as the place of occurrence of the external cause

   Y92.007   **Garden or yard** of unspecified non-institutional (private) residence as the place of occurrence of the external cause

   Y92.008   **Other place** in unspecified non-institutional (private) residence as the place of occurrence of the external cause

   Y92.009   **Unspecified place** in unspecified non-institutional (private) residence as the place of occurrence of the external cause
          Home (NOS) as the place of occurrence of the external cause
          Coding Clinic: 2021, Q2, P5

● Y92.01   **Single-family non-institutional (private) house as the place of occurrence of the external cause**
     Farmhouse as the place of occurrence of the external cause

     Excludes1   barn (Y92.71)
                chicken coop or hen house (Y92.72)
                farm field (Y92.73)
                orchard (Y92.74)
                single family mobile home or trailer (Y92.02-)
                slaughter house (Y92.86)

   Y92.010   **Kitchen** of single-family (private) house as the place of occurrence of the external cause

   Y92.011   **Dining room** of single-family (private) house as the place of occurrence of the external cause

   Y92.012   **Bathroom** of single-family (private) house as the place of occurrence of the external cause

   Y92.013   **Bedroom** of single-family (private) house as the place of occurrence of the external cause

   Y92.014   **Private driveway** to single-family (private) house as the place of occurrence of the external cause

   Y92.015   **Private garage** of single-family (private) house as the place of occurrence of the external cause

   Y92.016   **Swimming pool** in single-family (private) house or garden as the place of occurrence of the external cause

   Y92.017   **Garden or yard** in single-family (private) house as the place of occurrence of the external cause

   Y92.018   **Other place** in single-family (private) house as the place of occurrence of the external cause

   Y92.019   **Unspecified** place in single-family (private) house as the place of occurrence of the external cause

● Y92.02   **Mobile home as the place of occurrence of the external cause**

   Y92.020   **Kitchen** in mobile home as the place of occurrence of the external cause

   Y92.021   **Dining room** in mobile home as the place of occurrence of the external cause

   Y92.022   **Bathroom** in mobile home as the place of occurrence of the external cause

   Y92.023   **Bedroom** in mobile home as the place of occurrence of the external cause

   Y92.024   **Driveway** of mobile home as the place of occurrence of the external cause

   Y92.025   **Garage** of mobile home as the place of occurrence of the external cause

   Y92.026   **Swimming pool** of mobile home as the place of occurrence of the external cause

   Y92.027   **Garden or yard** of mobile home as the place of occurrence of the external cause

   Y92.028   **Other place** in mobile home as the place of occurrence of the external cause

   Y92.029   **Unspecified** place in mobile home as the place of occurrence of the external cause

● Y92.03   **Apartment as the place of occurrence of the external cause**
     Condominium as the place of occurrence of the external cause
     Co-op apartment as the place of occurrence of the external cause

   Y92.030   **Kitchen** in apartment as the place of occurrence of the external cause

   Y92.031   **Bathroom** in apartment as the place of occurrence of the external cause

   Y92.032   **Bedroom** in apartment as the place of occurrence of the external cause

   Y92.038   **Other place** in apartment as the place of occurrence of the external cause

   Y92.039   **Unspecified** place in apartment as the place of occurrence of the external cause

---

▶ New   ➡ Revised   ~~deleted~~ Deleted   Excludes 1   Excludes 2   Includes   Use additional   Code first   Code also   Key words
OGCR Official Guidelines   **X** Assign placeholder X   ● Use Additional Character(s)   ▶ Manifestation Code   Hierarchical Condition Category   **Coding Clinic**

● **Y92.04**   **Boarding-house** as the place of occurrence of the external cause
    Y92.040   **Kitchen** in boarding-house as the place of occurrence of the external cause
    Y92.041   **Bathroom** in boarding-house as the place of occurrence of the external cause
    Y92.042   **Bedroom** in boarding-house as the place of occurrence of the external cause
    Y92.043   **Driveway** of boarding-house as the place of occurrence of the external cause
    Y92.044   **Garage** of boarding-house as the place of occurrence of the external cause
    Y92.045   **Swimming pool** of boarding-house as the place of occurrence of the external cause
    Y92.046   **Garden or yard** of boarding-house as the place of occurrence of the external cause
    Y92.048   **Other place** in boarding-house as the place of occurrence of the external cause
    Y92.049   **Unspecified** place in boarding-house as the place of occurrence of the external cause

● **Y92.09**   **Other non-institutional residence** as the place of occurrence of the external cause
    Y92.090   **Kitchen** in other non-institutional residence as the place of occurrence of the external cause
    Y92.091   **Bathroom** in other non-institutional residence as the place of occurrence of the external cause
    Y92.092   **Bedroom** in other non-institutional residence as the place of occurrence of the external cause
    Y92.093   **Driveway** of other non-institutional residence as the place of occurrence of the external cause
    Y92.094   **Garage** of other non-institutional residence as the place of occurrence of the external cause
    Y92.095   **Swimming pool** of other non-institutional residence as the place of occurrence of the external cause
    Y92.096   **Garden or yard** of other non-institutional residence as the place of occurrence of the external cause
    Y92.098   **Other place** in other non-institutional residence as the place of occurrence of the external cause
    Y92.099   **Unspecified** place in other non-institutional residence as the place of occurrence of the external cause
     Coding Clinic: 2017, Q2, P10

● **Y92.1**   **Institutional (nonprivate) residence** as the place of occurrence of the external cause
    Y92.10   **Unspecified** residential institution as the place of occurrence of the external cause
    ● Y92.11   **Children's home and orphanage** as the place of occurrence of the external cause
      Y92.110   **Kitchen** in children's home and orphanage as the place of occurrence of the external cause
      Y92.111   **Bathroom** in children's home and orphanage as the place of occurrence of the external cause
      Y92.112   **Bedroom** in children's home and orphanage as the place of occurrence of the external cause
      Y92.113   **Driveway** of children's home and orphanage as the place of occurrence of the external cause
      Y92.114   **Garage** of children's home and orphanage as the place of occurrence of the external cause
      Y92.115   **Swimming pool** of children's home and orphanage as the place of occurrence of the external cause
      Y92.116   **Garden or yard** of children's home and orphanage as the place of occurrence of the external cause
      Y92.118   **Other place** in children's home and orphanage as the place of occurrence of the external cause
      Y92.119   **Unspecified** place in children's home and orphanage as the place of occurrence of the external cause

● **Y92.12**   **Nursing home** as the place of occurrence of the external cause
    Home for the sick as the place of occurrence of the external cause
    Hospice as the place of occurrence of the external cause
    Y92.120   **Kitchen** in nursing home as the place of occurrence of the external cause
    Y92.121   **Bathroom** in nursing home as the place of occurrence of the external cause
    Y92.122   **Bedroom** in nursing home as the place of occurrence of the external cause
    Y92.123   **Driveway** of nursing home as the place of occurrence of the external cause
    Y92.124   **Garage** of nursing home as the place of occurrence of the external cause
    Y92.125   **Swimming pool** of nursing home as the place of occurrence of the external cause
    Y92.126   **Garden or yard** of nursing home as the place of occurrence of the external cause
    Y92.128   **Other place** in nursing home as the place of occurrence of the external cause
    Y92.129   **Unspecified** place in nursing home as the place of occurrence of the external cause
     Coding Clinic: 2017, Q2, P10

● **Y92.13**   **Military base** as the place of occurrence of the external cause
    Excludes1   military training grounds (Y92.83)
    Y92.130   **Kitchen** on military base as the place of occurrence of the external cause
    Y92.131   **Mess hall** on military base as the place of occurrence of the external cause
    Y92.133   **Barracks** on military base as the place of occurrence of the external cause
    Y92.135   **Garage** on military base as the place of occurrence of the external cause
    Y92.136   **Swimming pool** on military base as the place of occurrence of the external cause
    Y92.137   **Garden or yard** on military base as the place of occurrence of the external cause
    Y92.138   **Other place** on military base as the place of occurrence of the external cause
    Y92.139   **Unspecified** place military base as the place of occurrence of the external cause

CHAPTER 20 (V00-Y99)

● **Y92.14**   **Prison** as the place of occurrence of the external cause

   Y92.140   **Kitchen** in prison as the place of occurrence of the external cause

   Y92.141   **Dining room** in prison as the place of occurrence of the external cause

   Y92.142   **Bathroom** in prison as the place of occurrence of the external cause

   Y92.143   **Cell** of prison as the place of occurrence of the external cause

   Y92.146   **Swimming pool** of prison as the place of occurrence of the external cause

   Y92.147   **Courtyard** of prison as the place of occurrence of the external cause

   Y92.148   **Other place** in prison as the place of occurrence of the external cause

   Y92.149   **Unspecified** place in prison as the place of occurrence of the external cause

● **Y92.15**   **Reform school** as the place of occurrence of the external cause

   Y92.150   **Kitchen** in reform school as the place of occurrence of the external cause

   Y92.151   **Dining room** in reform school as the place of occurrence of the external cause

   Y92.152   **Bathroom** in reform school as the place of occurrence of the external cause

   Y92.153   **Bedroom** in reform school as the place of occurrence of the external cause

   Y92.154   **Driveway** of reform school as the place of occurrence of the external cause

   Y92.155   **Garage** of reform school as the place of occurrence of the external cause

   Y92.156   **Swimming pool** of reform school as the place of occurrence of the external cause

   Y92.157   **Garden or yard** of reform school as the place of occurrence of the external cause

   Y92.158   **Other place** in reform school as the place of occurrence of the external cause

   Y92.159   **Unspecified** place in reform school as the place of occurrence of the external cause

● **Y92.16**   **School dormitory** as the place of occurrence of the external cause

   Excludes1   reform school as the place of occurrence of the external cause (Y92.15-)
   school buildings and grounds as the place of occurrence of the external cause (Y92.2-)
   school sports and athletic areas as the place of occurrence of the external cause (Y92.3-)

   Y92.160   **Kitchen** in school dormitory as the place of occurrence of the external cause

   Y92.161   **Dining room** in school dormitory as the place of occurrence of the external cause

   Y92.162   **Bathroom** in school dormitory as the place of occurrence of the external cause

   Y92.163   **Bedroom** in school dormitory as the place of occurrence of the external cause

   Y92.168   **Other place** in school dormitory as the place of occurrence of the external cause

   Y92.169   **Unspecified** place in school dormitory as the place of occurrence of the external cause

● **Y92.19**   **Other specified residential institution** as the place of occurrence of the external cause

   Y92.190   **Kitchen** in other specified residential institution as the place of occurrence of the external cause

   Y92.191   **Dining room** in other specified residential institution as the place of occurrence of the external cause

   Y92.192   **Bathroom** in other specified residential institution as the place of occurrence of the external cause

   Y92.193   **Bedroom** in other specified residential institution as the place of occurrence of the external cause

   Y92.194   **Driveway** of other specified residential institution as the place of occurrence of the external cause

   Y92.195   **Garage** of other specified residential institution as the place of occurrence of the external cause

   Y92.196   **Pool** of other specified residential institution as the place of occurrence of the external cause

   Y92.197   **Garden or yard** of other specified residential institution as the place of occurrence of the external cause

   Y92.198   **Other place** in other specified residential institution as the place of occurrence of the external cause
   Coding Clinic: 2017, Q2, P11

   Y92.199   **Unspecified** place in other specified residential institution as the place of occurrence of the external cause
   Coding Clinic: 2017, Q2, P10

● **Y92.2**   **School, other institution and public administrative area** as the place of occurrence of the external cause
   Building and adjacent grounds used by the general public or by a particular group of the public

   Excludes1   building under construction as the place of occurrence of the external cause (Y92.6)
   residential institution as the place of occurrence of the external cause (Y92.1)
   school dormitory as the place of occurrence of the external cause (Y92.16-)
   sports and athletics area of schools as the place of occurrence of the external cause (Y92.3-)

● **Y92.21**   **School (private) (public) (state)** as the place of occurrence of the external cause

   Y92.210   **Daycare center** as the place of occurrence of the external cause

   Y92.211   **Elementary school** as the place of occurrence of the external cause
   Kindergarten as the place of occurrence of the external cause

   Y92.212   **Middle school** as the place of occurrence of the external cause

   Y92.213   **High school** as the place of occurrence of the external cause
   Coding Clinic: 2012, Q4, P108

   Y92.214   **College** as the place of occurrence of the external cause
   University as the place of occurrence of the external cause

   Y92.215   **Trade school** as the place of occurrence of the external cause

   Y92.218   **Other school** as the place of occurrence of the external cause

   Y92.219   **Unspecified** school as the place of occurrence of the external cause

Y92.22   **Religious institution** as the place of occurrence of the external cause
- Church as the place of occurrence of the external cause
- Mosque as the place of occurrence of the external cause
- Synagogue as the place of occurrence of the external cause

● Y92.23   **Hospital** as the place of occurrence of the external cause

    Excludes1   ambulatory (outpatient) health services establishments (Y92.53-)
         home for the sick as the place of occurrence of the external cause (Y92.12-)
         hospice as the place of occurrence of the external cause (Y92.12-)
         nursing home as the place of occurrence of the external cause (Y92.12-)

    Y92.230   **Patient room** in hospital as the place of occurrence of the external cause
    Y92.231   **Patient bathroom** in hospital as the place of occurrence of the external cause
    Y92.232   **Corridor** of hospital as the place of occurrence of the external cause
    Y92.233   **Cafeteria** of hospital as the place of occurrence of the external cause
    Y92.234   **Operating room** of hospital as the place of occurrence of the external cause
    Y92.238   **Other place** in hospital as the place of occurrence of the external cause
    Y92.239   **Unspecified** place in hospital as the place of occurrence of the external cause

● Y92.24   **Public administrative building** as the place of occurrence of the external cause
    Y92.240   **Courthouse** as the place of occurrence of the external cause
    Y92.241   **Library** as the place of occurrence of the external cause
    Y92.242   **Post office** as the place of occurrence of the external cause
    Y92.243   **City hall** as the place of occurrence of the external cause
    Y92.248   **Other public administrative building** as the place of occurrence of the external cause

● Y92.25   **Cultural building** as the place of occurrence of the external cause
    Y92.250   **Art gallery** as the place of occurrence of the external cause
    Y92.251   **Museum** as the place of occurrence of the external cause
    Y92.252   **Music hall** as the place of occurrence of the external cause
    Y92.253   **Opera house** as the place of occurrence of the external cause
    Y92.254   **Theater** (live) as the place of occurrence of the external cause
    Y92.258   **Other cultural public building** as the place of occurrence of the external cause

Y92.26   **Movie house or cinema** as the place of occurrence of the external cause

Y92.29   **Other specified public building** as the place of occurrence of the external cause
- Assembly hall as the place of occurrence of the external cause
- Clubhouse as the place of occurrence of the external cause

● Y92.3   **Sports and athletics area** as the place of occurrence of the external cause

● Y92.31   **Athletic court** as the place of occurrence of the external cause

    Excludes1   tennis court in private home or garden (Y92.09)

    Y92.310   **Basketball court** as the place of occurrence of the external cause
    Y92.311   **Squash court** as the place of occurrence of the external cause
    Y92.312   **Tennis court** as the place of occurrence of the external cause
    Y92.318   **Other athletic court** as the place of occurrence of the external cause

● Y92.32   **Athletic field** as the place of occurrence of the external cause
    Y92.320   **Baseball field** as the place of occurrence of the external cause
    Y92.321   **Football field** as the place of occurrence of the external cause
    Y92.322   **Soccer field** as the place of occurrence of the external cause
    Y92.328   **Other athletic field** as the place of occurrence of the external cause
         Cricket field as the place of occurrence of the external cause
         Hockey field as the place of occurrence of the external cause

● Y92.33   **Skating rink** as the place of occurrence of the external cause
    Y92.330   **Ice skating rink** (indoor) (outdoor) as the place of occurrence of the external cause
    Y92.331   **Roller skating rink** as the place of occurrence of the external cause

Y92.34   **Swimming pool** (public) as the place of occurrence of the external cause

    Excludes1   swimming pool in private home or garden (Y92.016)

Y92.39   **Other specified sports and athletic area** as the place of occurrence of the external cause
- Golf-course as the place of occurrence of the external cause
- Gymnasium as the place of occurrence of the external cause
- Riding-school as the place of occurrence of the external cause
- Stadium as the place of occurrence of the external cause

● Y92.4   **Street, highway and other paved roadways** as the place of occurrence of the external cause

    Excludes1   private driveway of residence (Y92.014, Y92.024, Y92.043, Y92.093, Y92.113, Y92.123, Y92.154, Y92.194)

● Y92.41   **Street and highway** as the place of occurrence of the external cause
    Y92.410   **Unspecified** street and highway as the place of occurrence of the external cause
         Road NOS as the place of occurrence of the external cause
    Y92.411   **Interstate highway** as the place of occurrence of the external cause
         Freeway as the place of occurrence of the external cause
         Motorway as the place of occurrence of the external cause
    Y92.412   **Parkway** as the place of occurrence of the external cause
    Y92.413   **State road** as the place of occurrence of the external cause

CHAPTER 20 (V00–Y99)

Y92.414 **Local residential or business street** as the place of occurrence of the external cause

Y92.415 **Exit ramp or entrance ramp** of street or highway as the place of occurrence of the external cause

● **Y92.48** **Other paved roadways** as the place of occurrence of the external cause

Y92.480 **Sidewalk** as the place of occurrence of the external cause

Y92.481 **Parking lot** as the place of occurrence of the external cause

Y92.482 **Bike path** as the place of occurrence of the external cause

Y92.488 **Other paved roadways** as the place of occurrence of the external cause

● **Y92.5** **Trade and service area** as the place of occurrence of the external cause

Excludes1 garage in private home (Y92.015)
schools and other public administration buildings (Y92.2-)

● **Y92.51** **Private commercial establishments** as the place of occurrence of the external cause

Y92.510 **Bank** as the place of occurrence of the external cause

Y92.511 **Restaurant or café** as the place of occurrence of the external cause

Y92.512 **Supermarket, store or market** as the place of occurrence of the external cause

Y92.513 **Shop (commercial)** as the place of occurrence of the external cause

● **Y92.52** **Service areas** as the place of occurrence of the external cause

Y92.520 **Airport** as the place of occurrence of the external cause

Y92.521 **Bus station** as the place of occurrence of the external cause

Y92.522 **Railway station** as the place of occurrence of the external cause

Y92.523 **Highway rest stop** as the place of occurrence of the external cause

Y92.524 **Gas station** as the place of occurrence of the external cause
Petroleum station as the place of occurrence of the external cause
Service station as the place of occurrence of the external cause

● **Y92.53** **Ambulatory health services establishments** as the place of occurrence of the external cause

Y92.530 **Ambulatory surgery center** as the place of occurrence of the external cause
Outpatient surgery center, including that connected with a hospital as the place of occurrence of the external cause
Same day surgery center, including that connected with a hospital as the place of occurrence of the external cause

Y92.531 **Health care provider office** as the place of occurrence of the external cause
Physician office as the place of occurrence of the external cause

Y92.532 **Urgent care center** as the place of occurrence of the external cause

Y92.538 **Other ambulatory health services establishments** as the place of occurrence of the external cause
Coding Clinic: 2019, Q1, P21

Y92.59 **Other trade areas** as the place of occurrence of the external cause
Office building as the place of occurrence of the external cause
Casino as the place of occurrence of the external cause
Garage (commercial) as the place of occurrence of the external cause
Hotel as the place of occurrence of the external cause
Radio or television station as the place of occurrence of the external cause
Shopping mall as the place of occurrence of the external cause
Warehouse as the place of occurrence of the external cause

● **Y92.6** **Industrial and construction area** as the place of occurrence of the external cause

Y92.61 **Building [any] under construction** as the place of occurrence of the external cause

Y92.62 **Dock or shipyard** as the place of occurrence of the external cause
Dockyard as the place of occurrence of the external cause
Dry dock as the place of occurrence of the external cause
Shipyard as the place of occurrence of the external cause

Y92.63 **Factory** as the place of occurrence of the external cause
Factory building as the place of occurrence of the external cause
Factory premises as the place of occurrence of the external cause
Industrial yard as the place of occurrence of the external cause

Y92.64 **Mine or pit** as the place of occurrence of the external cause
Mine as the place of occurrence of the external cause

Y92.65 **Oil rig** as the place of occurrence of the external cause
Pit (coal) (gravel) (sand) as the place of occurrence of the external cause

Y92.69 **Other specified industrial and construction area** as the place of occurrence of the external cause
Gasworks as the place of occurrence of the external cause
Power-station (coal) (nuclear) (oil) as the place of occurrence of the external cause
Tunnel under construction as the place of occurrence of the external cause
Workshop as the place of occurrence of the external cause

● **Y92.7** **Farm** as the place of occurrence of the external cause
Ranch as the place of occurrence of the external cause
Excludes1 farmhouse and home premises of farm (Y92.01-)

Y92.71 **Barn** as the place of occurrence of the external cause

Y92.72 **Chicken coop** as the place of occurrence of the external cause
Hen house as the place of occurrence of the external cause

Y92.73 **Farm field** as the place of occurrence of the external cause

Y92.74 **Orchard** as the place of occurrence of the external cause

Y92.79 **Other farm location** as the place of occurrence of the external cause

● **Y92.8** **Other places** as the place of occurrence of the external cause

  ● **Y92.81** **Transport vehicle** as the place of occurrence of the external cause

    Excludes1   transport accidents (V00-V99)

    Y92.810 **Car** as the place of occurrence of the external cause

    Y92.811 **Bus** as the place of occurrence of the external cause

    Y92.812 **Truck** as the place of occurrence of the external cause

    Y92.813 **Airplane** as the place of occurrence of the external cause

    Y92.814 **Boat** as the place of occurrence of the external cause

    Y92.815 **Train** as the place of occurrence of the external cause

    Y92.816 **Subway car** as the place of occurrence of the external cause

    Y92.818 **Other transport vehicle** as the place of occurrence of the external cause

  ● **Y92.82** **Wilderness area**

    Y92.820 **Desert** as the place of occurrence of the external cause

    Y92.821 **Forest** as the place of occurrence of the external cause

    Y92.828 **Other wilderness area** as the place of occurrence of the external cause

       Swamp as the place of occurrence of the external cause

       Mountain as the place of occurrence of the external cause

       Marsh as the place of occurrence of the external cause

       Prairie as the place of occurrence of the external cause

  ● **Y92.83** **Recreation area** as the place of occurrence of the external cause

    Y92.830 **Public park** as the place of occurrence of the external cause

    Y92.831 **Amusement park** as the place of occurrence of the external cause

    Y92.832 **Beach** as the place of occurrence of the external cause

       Seashore as the place of occurrence of the external cause

    Y92.833 **Campsite** as the place of occurrence of the external cause

    Y92.834 **Zoological garden** (zoo) as the place of occurrence of the external cause

    Y92.838 **Other recreation area** as the place of occurrence of the external cause

  ● **Y92.84** **Military training ground** as the place of occurrence of the external cause

  ● **Y92.85** **Railroad track** as the place of occurrence of the external cause

  ● **Y92.86** **Slaughter house** as the place of occurrence of the external cause

  ● **Y92.89** **Other specified places** as the place of occurrence of the external cause

       Derelict house as the place of occurrence of the external cause

Y92.9 **Unspecified place** or not applicable

● **Y93** **Activity codes**

  Note: Category Y93 is provided for use to indicate the activity of the person seeking healthcare for an injury or health condition, such as a heart attack while shoveling snow, which resulted from, or was contributed to, by the activity. These codes are appropriate for use for both acute injuries, such as those from Chapter 19, and conditions that are due to the long-term, cumulative effects of an activity, such as those from Chapter 13. They are also appropriate for use with external cause codes for cause and intent if identifying the activity provides additional information on the event. These codes should be used in conjunction with codes for external cause status (Y99) and place of occurrence (Y92).

  This section contains the following broad activity categories:

    Y93.0   Activities involving walking and running

    Y93.1   Activities involving water and water craft

    Y93.2   Activities involving ice and snow

    Y93.3   Activities involving climbing, rappelling, and jumping off

    Y93.4   Activities involving dancing and other rhythmic movement

    Y93.5   Activities involving other sports and athletics played individually

    Y93.6   Activities involving other sports and athletics played as a team or group

    Y93.7   Activities involving other specified sports and athletics

    Y93.8   Activities, other specified

    Y93.9   Activity, unspecified

    Y93.A   Activities involving other cardiorespiratory exercise

    Y93.B   Activities involving other muscle strengthening exercises

    Y93.C   Activities involving computer technology and electronic devices

    Y93.D   Activities involving arts and handcrafts

    Y93.E   Activities involving personal hygiene and interior property and clothing maintenance

    Y93.F   Activities involving caregiving

    Y93.G   Activities involving food preparation, cooking and grilling

    Y93.H   Activities involving exterior property and land maintenance, building and construction

    Y93.I   Activities involving roller coasters and other types of external motion

    Y93.J   Activities involving playing musical instrument

    Y93.K   Activities involving animal care

    ▶**Y93.L**   Other outdoor activity

● **Y93.0** **Activities involving walking and running**

    Excludes1   Activity, walking an animal (Y93.K1)

       Activity, walking or running on a treadmill (Y93.A1)

  Y93.01 **Activity, walking, marching and hiking**

     Activity, walking, marching and hiking on level or elevated terrain

    Excludes1   activity, mountain climbing (Y93.31)

  Y93.02 **Activity, running**

● **Y93.1** **Activities involving water and water craft**
    Excludes1   activities involving ice (Y93.2-)
    Y93.11   **Activity, swimming**
    Y93.12   **Activity, springboard and platform diving**
    Y93.13   **Activity, water polo**
    Y93.14   **Activity, water aerobics and water exercise**
    Y93.15   **Activity, underwater diving and snorkeling**
        Activity, SCUBA diving
    Y93.16   **Activity, rowing, canoeing, kayaking, rafting and tubing**
        Activity, canoeing, kayaking, rafting and tubing in calm and turbulent water
    Y93.17   **Activity, water skiing and wake boarding**
    Y93.18   **Activity, surfing, windsurfing and boogie boarding**
        Activity, water sliding
    Y93.19   **Activity, other involving water and watercraft**
        Activity involving water NOS
        Activity, parasailing
        Activity, water survival training and testing

● **Y93.2** **Activities involving ice and snow**
    Excludes1   activity, shoveling ice and snow (Y93.H1)
    Y93.21   **Activity, ice skating**
        Activity, figure skating (singles) (pairs)
        Activity, ice dancing
        Excludes1   activity, ice hockey (Y93.22)
    Y93.22   **Activity, ice hockey**
    Y93.23   **Activity, snow (alpine) (downhill) skiing, snowboarding, sledding, tobogganing and snow tubing**
        Excludes1   activity, cross country skiing (Y93.24)
    Y93.24   **Activity, cross country skiing**
        Activity, nordic skiing
    Y93.29   **Activity, other activity involving ice and snow**
        Activity, activity involving ice and snow NOS

● **Y93.3** **Activities involving climbing, rappelling and jumping off**
    Excludes1   activity, hiking on level or elevated terrain (Y93.01)
        activity, jumping rope (Y93.56)
        activity, trampoline jumping (Y93.44)
    Y93.31   **Activity, mountain climbing, rock climbing and wall climbing**
    Y93.32   **Activity, rappelling**
    Y93.33   **Activity, BASE jumping**
        Activity, building, Antenna, Span, Earth jumping
    Y93.34   **Activity, bungee jumping**
    Y93.35   **Activity, hang gliding**
    Y93.39   **Activity, other activity involving climbing, rappelling and jumping off**

● **Y93.4** **Activities involving dancing and other rhythmic movement**
    Excludes1   activity, martial arts (Y93.75)
    Y93.41   **Activity, dancing**
        Coding Clinic: 2012, Q4, P108
    Y93.42   **Activity, yoga**
    Y93.43   **Activity, gymnastics**
        Activity, rhythmic gymnastics
        Excludes1   activity, trampolining (Y93.44)
    Y93.44   **Activity, trampolining**
    Y93.45   **Activity, cheerleading**
    Y93.49   **Activity, other involving dancing and other rhythmic movements**

● **Y93.5** **Activities involving other sports and athletics played individually**
    Excludes1   activity, dancing (Y93.41)
        activity, gymnastic (Y93.43)
        activity, trampolining (Y93.44)
        activity, yoga (Y93.42)
    Y93.51   **Activity, roller skating (inline) and skateboarding**
    Y93.52   **Activity, horseback riding**
    Y93.53   **Activity, golf**
    Y93.54   **Activity, bowling**
    Y93.55   **Activity, bike riding**
    Y93.56   **Activity, jumping rope**
    Y93.57   **Activity, non-running track and field events**
        Excludes1   activity, running (any form) (Y93.02)
    Y93.59   **Activity, other involving other sports and athletics played individually**
        Excludes1   activities involving climbing, rappelling, and jumping (Y93.3-)
        activities involving ice and snow (Y93.2-)
        activities involving walking and running (Y93.0-)
        activities involving water and watercraft (Y93.1-)

● **Y93.6** **Activities involving other sports and athletics played as a team or group**
    Excludes1   activity, ice hockey (Y93.22)
        activity, water polo (Y93.13)
    Y93.61   **Activity, American tackle football**
        Activity, football NOS
    Y93.62   **Activity, American flag or touch football**
    Y93.63   **Activity, rugby**
    Y93.64   **Activity, baseball**
        Activity, softball
    Y93.65   **Activity, lacrosse and field hockey**
        Coding Clinic: 2015, Q1, P9
    Y93.66   **Activity, soccer**
    Y93.67   **Activity, basketball**
        Coding Clinic: 2019, Q4, P18
    Y93.68   **Activity, volleyball (beach) (court)**
    Y93.6A   **Activity, physical games generally associated with school recess, summer camp and children**
        Activity, capture the flag
        Activity, dodge ball
        Activity, four square
        Activity, kickball
    Y93.69   **Activity, other involving other sports and athletics played as a team or group**
        Cricket

● **Y93.7** **Activities involving other specified sports and athletics**
    Y93.71   **Activity, boxing**
    Y93.72   **Activity, wrestling**
    Y93.73   **Activity, racquet and hand sports**
        Activity, handball
        Activity, racquetball
        Activity, squash
        Activity, tennis
    Y93.74   **Activity, frisbee**
        Activity, ultimate frisbee
    Y93.75   **Activity, martial arts**
        Activity, combatives
    Y93.79   **Activity, other specified sports and athletics**
        Excludes1   sports and athletics activities specified in categories Y93.0-Y93.6

▶ New   ⇢ Revised   ~~deleted~~ Deleted   Excludes 1   Excludes 2   Includes   Use additional   Code first   Code also   Key words
OGCR Official Guidelines   X Assign placeholder X   ● Use Additional Character(s)   ▶ Manifestation Code   HCC Hierarchical Condition Category   Coding Clinic

● **Y93.8**   **Other activity**
     Coding Clinic: 2016, Q4, P74
    Y93.81   **Activity, refereeing a sports activity**
    Y93.82   **Activity, spectator at an event**
    Y93.83   **Activity, rough housing and horseplay**
     Coding Clinic: 2015, Q1, P8
    Y93.84   **Activity, sleeping**
    Y93.85   **Activity, choking game**
       Activity, blackout game
       Activity, fainting game
       Activity, pass out game
       Coding Clinic: 2016, Q4, P74-76
    Y93.89   **Activity, other specified**

OGCR   **See Section I.C.20.c.**

> Do not assign Y93.9, Unspecified activity, if the activity is not stated.

● **Y93.9**   **Activity, unspecified**
● **Y93.A**   **Activities involving other cardiorespiratory exercise**
      Activities involving physical training
    Y93.A1   **Activity, exercise machines primarily for cardiorespiratory conditioning**
       Activity, elliptical and stepper machines
       Activity, stationary bike
       Activity, treadmill
    Y93.A2   **Activity, calisthenics**
       Activity, jumping jacks
       Activity, warm up and cool down
    Y93.A3   **Activity, aerobic and step exercise**
    Y93.A4   **Activity, circuit training**
    Y93.A5   **Activity, obstacle course**
       Activity, challenge course
       Activity, confidence course
    Y93.A6   **Activity, grass drills**
       Activity, guerilla drills
    Y93.A9   **Activity, other involving other cardiorespiratory exercise**
      Excludes1   activities involving cardiorespiratory exercise specified in categories Y93.0-Y93.7

● **Y93.B**   **Activity involving other muscle strengthening exercises**
    Y93.B1   **Activity, exercise machines primarily for muscle strengthening**
    Y93.B2   **Activity, push-ups, pull-ups, sit-ups**
    Y93.B3   **Activity, free weights**
       Activity, barbells
       Activity, dumbbells
    Y93.B4   **Activity, pilates**
    Y93.B9   **Activity, other involving other muscle strengthening exercises**
      Excludes1   activities involving muscle strengthening specified in categories Y93.0-Y93.A

● **Y93.C**   **Activities involving computer technology and electronic devices**
      Excludes1   activity, electronic musical keyboard or instruments (Y93.J-)
    Y93.C1   **Activity, computer keyboarding**
       Activity, electronic game playing using keyboard or other stationary device
    Y93.C2   **Activity, hand held interactive electronic device**
       Activity, cellular telephone and communication device
       Activity, electronic game playing using interactive device
      Excludes1   activity, electronic game playing using keyboard or other stationary device (Y93.C1)
    Y93.C9   **Activity, other involving computer technology and electronic devices**

● **Y93.D**   **Activities involving arts and handcrafts**
      Excludes1   activities involving playing musical instrument (Y93.J-)
    Y93.D1   **Knitting and crocheting**
    Y93.D2   **Sewing**
    Y93.D3   **Furniture building and finishing**
       Furniture repair
    Y93.D9   **Activity, other involving arts and handcrafts**
● **Y93.E**   **Activities involving personal hygiene and interior property and clothing maintenance**
      Excludes1   activities involving cooking and grilling (Y93.G-)
         activities involving exterior property and land maintenance, building and construction (Y93.H-)
         activity involving caregiving (Y93.F-)
         activity, dishwashing (Y93.G1)
         activity, food preparation (Y93.G1)
         activity, gardening (Y93.H2)
    Y93.E1   **Activity, personal bathing and showering**
    Y93.E2   **Activity, laundry**
    Y93.E3   **Activity, vacuuming**
    Y93.E4   **Activity, ironing**
    Y93.E5   **Activity, floor mopping and cleaning**
    Y93.E6   **Activity, residential relocation**
       Activity, packing up and unpacking involved in moving to a new residence
    Y93.E8   **Activity, other personal hygiene activity**
    Y93.E9   **Activity, other household maintenance**
● **Y93.F**   **Activities involving person providing caregiving**
      Activity involving the provider of caregiving
    Y93.F1   **Activity, caregiving involving bathing**
    Y93.F2   **Activity, caregiving involving lifting**
      Coding Clinic: 2016, Q4, P74
    Y93.F9   **Activity, other caregiving**
● **Y93.G**   **Activities involving food preparation, cooking and grilling**
    Y93.G1   **Activity, food preparation and clean up**
       Activity, dishwashing
    Y93.G2   **Activity, grilling and smoking food**
    Y93.G3   **Activity, cooking and baking**
       Activity, use of stove, oven and microwave oven
    Y93.G9   **Activity, other activity involving cooking and grilling**
● **Y93.H**   **Activities involving property and land maintenance, building and construction**
    Y93.H1   **Activity, digging, shoveling and raking**
       Activity, dirt digging
       Activity, raking leaves
       Activity, snow shoveling
    Y93.H2   **Activity, gardening and landscaping**
       Activity, pruning, trimming shrubs, weeding
    Y93.H3   **Activity, building and construction**
    Y93.H9   **Activity, other activity involving property and land maintenance, building and construction**
● **Y93.I**   **Activities involving roller coasters and other types of external motion**
    Y93.I1   **Activity, rollercoaster riding**
    Y93.I9   **Activity, other involving external motion**
● **Y93.J**   **Activities involving playing musical instrument**
      Activity involving playing electric musical instrument
    Y93.J1   **Activity, piano playing**
       Activity, musical keyboard (electronic) playing
    Y93.J2   **Activity, drum and other percussion instrument playing**
    Y93.J3   **Activity, string instrument playing**
    Y93.J4   **Activity, winds and brass instrument playing**

CHAPTER 20 (V00-Y99)

● **Y93.K**   **Activities involving animal care**
     Excludes1   activity, horseback riding (Y93.52)
     Y93.K1   **Activity, walking an animal**
     Y93.K2   **Activity, milking an animal**
     Y93.K3   **Activity, grooming and shearing an animal**
     Y93.K9   **Activity, other activity involving animal care**
▶ ● **Y93.L**   **Other outdoor activity**
     ▶**Y93.L1**   **Activity, splitting wood**
     ▶**Y93.L9**   **Activity, other outdoor activity**

Y95   **Nosocomial condition**

● **Y99**   **External cause status**
     Note: A single code from category Y99 should be used in conjunction with the external cause code(s) assigned to a record to indicate the status of the person at the time the event occurred.
     Coding Clinic: 2016, Q4, P74
     Y99.0   **Civilian activity done for income or pay**
       Civilian activity done for financial or other compensation
       Excludes1   military activity (Y99.1)
           volunteer activity (Y99.2)
     Y99.1   **Military activity**
       Excludes1   activity of off duty military personnel (Y99.8)

     Y99.2   **Volunteer activity**
       Excludes1   activity of child or other family member assisting in compensated work of other family member (Y99.8)
     Y99.8   **Other external cause status**
       Activity NEC
       Activity of child or other family member assisting in compensated work of other family member
       Hobby not done for income
       Leisure activity
       Off-duty activity of military personnel
       Recreation or sport not for income or while a student
       Student activity
       Excludes1   civilian activity done for income or compensation (Y99.0)
           military activity (Y99.1)
     Coding Clinic: 2012, Q4, P108
     Y99.9   **Unspecified external cause status**

CHAPTER 21

FACTORS INFLUENCING HEALTH STATUS AND CONTACT WITH HEALTH SERVICES (Z00-Z99)

OGCR Chapter-Specific Coding Guidelines

21. Chapter 21: Factors influencing health status and contact with health services (Z00-Z99)
Note: The chapter specific guidelines provide additional information about the use of Z codes for specified encounters.

a. Use of Z codes in any healthcare setting
Z codes are for use in any healthcare setting. Z codes may be used as either a first-listed (principal diagnosis code in the inpatient setting) or secondary code, depending on the circumstances of the encounter. Certain Z codes may only be used as first-listed or principal diagnosis.

b. Z Codes indicate a reason for an encounter
Z codes are not procedure codes. A corresponding procedure code must accompany a Z code to describe any procedure performed.

c. Categories of Z Codes
1) Contact/Exposure
Category Z20 indicates contact with, and suspected exposure to, communicable diseases. These codes are for patients who do not show any sign or symptom of a disease but are suspected to have been exposed to it by close personal contact with an infected individual or are in an area where a disease is epidemic.

Category Z77, Other contact with and (suspected) exposures hazardous to health, indicates contact with and suspected exposures hazardous to health.

Contact/exposure codes may be used as a first-listed code to explain an encounter for testing, or, more commonly, as a secondary code to identify a potential risk.

2) Inoculations and vaccinations
Code Z23 is for encounters for inoculations and vaccinations. It indicates that a patient is being seen to receive a prophylactic inoculation against a disease. Procedure codes are required to identify the actual administration of the injection and the type(s) of immunizations given. Code Z23 may be used as a secondary code if the inoculation is given as a routine part of preventive health care, such as a well-baby visit.

3) Status
Status codes indicate that a patient is either a carrier of a disease or has the sequelae or residual of a past disease or condition. This includes such things as the presence of prosthetic or mechanical devices resulting from past treatment. A status code is informative, because the status may affect the course of treatment and its outcome. A status code is distinct from a history code. The history code indicates that the patient no longer has the condition.

A status code should not be used with a diagnosis code from one of the body system chapters, if the diagnosis code includes the information provided by the status code. For example, code Z94.1, Heart transplant status, should not be used with a code from subcategory T86.2, Complications of heart transplant. The status code does not provide additional information. The complication code indicates that the patient is a heart transplant patient.

For encounters for weaning from a mechanical ventilator, assign a code from subcategory J96.1, Chronic respiratory failure, followed by code Z99.11, Dependence on respirator [ventilator] status.

The status Z codes/categories are:

Z14	Genetic carrier
	Genetic carrier status indicates that a person carries a gene, associated with a particular disease, which may be passed to offspring who may develop that disease. The person does not have the disease and is not at risk of developing the disease.
Z15	Genetic susceptibility to disease Genetic susceptibility indicates that a person has a gene that increases the risk of that person developing the disease.

Codes from category Z15 should not be used as principal or first-listed codes. If the patient has the condition to which he/she is susceptible, and that condition is the reason for the encounter, the code for the current condition should be sequenced first. If the patient is being seen for follow-up after completed treatment for this condition, and the condition no longer exists, a follow-up code should be sequenced first, followed by the appropriate personal history and genetic susceptibility codes. If the purpose of the encounter is genetic counseling associated with procreative management, code Z31.5, Encounter for genetic counseling, should be assigned as the first-listed code, followed by a code from category Z15. Additional codes should be assigned for any applicable family or personal history.

Z16	Resistance to antimicrobial drugs This code indicates that a patient has a condition that is resistant to antimicrobial drug treatment. Sequence the infection code first.
Z17	Estrogen receptor status
Z18	Retained foreign body fragments
Z19	Hormone sensitivity malignancy status
Z21	Asymptomatic HIV infection status This code indicates that a patient has tested positive for HIV but has manifested no signs or symptoms of the disease.
Z22	Carrier of infectious disease Carrier status indicates that a person harbors the specific organisms of a disease without manifest symptoms and is capable of transmitting the infection.
Z28.3	Underimmunization status
Z33.1	Pregnant state, incidental This code is a secondary code only for use when the pregnancy is in no way complicating the reason for visit. Otherwise, a code from the obstetric chapter is required.
Z66	Do not resuscitate

This code may be used when it is documented by the provider that a patient is on do not resuscitate status at any time during the stay.

Z67	Blood type
Z68	Body mass index (BMI)
	BMI codes should only be assigned when the associated diagnosis (such as overweight or obesity) meets the definition of a reportable diagnosis (see Section III, Reporting Additional Diagnoses). Do not assign BMI codes during pregnancy. See Section I.B.14 for BMI documentation by clinicians other than the patient's provider.
Z74.01	Bed confinement status
Z76.82	Awaiting organ transplant status
Z78	Other specified health status

Code Z78.1, Physical restraint status, may be used when it is documented by the provider that a patient has been put in restraints during the current encounter. Please note that this code should not be reported when it is documented by the provider that a patient is temporarily restrained during a procedure.

Z79	Long-term (current) drug therapy

Codes from this category indicate a patient's continuous use of a prescribed drug (including such things as aspirin therapy) for the long-term treatment of a condition or for prophylactic use. It is not for use for patients who have addictions to drugs. This subcategory is not for use of medications for detoxification or maintenance programs to prevent withdrawal symptoms in patients with drug dependence (e.g., methadone maintenance for opiate dependence). Assign the appropriate code for the drug dependence instead.

Assign a code from Z79 if the patient is receiving a medication for an extended period as a prophylactic measure (such as for the prevention of deep vein thrombosis) or as treatment of a chronic condition (such as arthritis) or a disease requiring a lengthy course of treatment (such as cancer). Do not assign a code from category Z79 for medication being administered for a brief period of time to treat an acute illness or injury (such as a course of antibiotics to treat acute bronchitis).

Z88	Allergy status to drugs, medicaments and biological substances Except: Z88.9, Allergy status to unspecified drugs, medicaments and biological substances status
Z89	Acquired absence of limb
Z90	Acquired absence of organs, not elsewhere classified
Z91.0-	Allergy status, other than to drugs and biological substances
Z92.82	Status post administration of tPA (rtPA) in a different facility within the last 24 hours prior to admission to a current facility Assign code Z92.82, Status post administration of tPA (rtPA) in a different facility within the last 24 hours prior to admission to current

facility, as a secondary diagnosis when a patient is received by transfer into a facility and documentation indicates they were administered tissue plasminogen activator (tPA) within the last 24 hours prior to admission to the current facility. This guideline applies even if the patient is still receiving the tPA at the time they are received into the current facility. The appropriate code for the condition for which the tPA was administered (such as cerebrovascular disease or myocardial infarction) should be assigned first. Code Z92.82 is only applicable to the receiving facility record and not to the transferring facility record.

Z93	Artificial opening status
Z94	Transplanted organ and tissue status
Z95	Presence of cardiac and vascular implants and grafts
Z96	Presence of other functional implants
Z97	Presence of other devices
Z98	Other postprocedural states

Assign code Z98.85, Transplanted organ removal status, to indicate that a transplanted organ has been previously removed. This code should not be assigned for the encounter in which the transplanted organ is removed. The complication necessitating removal of the transplant organ should be assigned for that encounter.

See Section I.C.19. for information on the coding of organ transplant complications.

Z99	Dependence on enabling machines and devices, not elsewhere classified

Note: Categories Z89-Z90 and Z93-Z99 are for use only if there are no complications or malfunctions of the organ or tissue replaced, the amputation site or the equipment on which the patient is dependent.

4) History (of)

There are two types of history Z codes, personal and family. Personal history codes explain a patient's past medical condition that no longer exists and is not receiving any treatment, but that has the potential for recurrence, and therefore may require continued monitoring.

Family history codes are for use when a patient has a family member(s) who has had a particular disease that causes the patient to be at higher risk of also contracting the disease.

Personal history codes may be used in conjunction with follow-up codes and family history codes may be used in conjunction with screening codes to explain the need for a test or procedure. History codes are also acceptable on any medical record regardless of the reason for visit. A history of an illness, even if no longer present, is important information that may alter the type of treatment ordered.

The history Z code categories are:

Z80	Family history of primary malignant neoplasm
Z81	Family history of mental and behavioral disorders
Z82	Family history of certain disabilities and chronic diseases (leading to disablement)
Z83	Family history of other specific disorders
Z84	Family history of other conditions
Z85	Personal history of malignant neoplasm
Z86	Personal history of certain other diseases
Z87	Personal history of other diseases and conditions
Z91.4-	Personal history of psychological trauma, not elsewhere classified
Z91.5	Personal history of self-harm
Z91.81	History of falling
Z91.82	Personal history of military deployment
Z92	Personal history of medical treatment Except: Z92.0, Personal history of contraception Except: Z92.82, Status post administration of tPA (rtPA) in a different facility within the last 24 hours prior to admission to a current facility

5) Screening

Screening is the testing for disease or disease precursors in seemingly well individuals so that early detection and treatment can be provided for those who test positive for the disease (e.g., screening mammogram).

The testing of a person to rule out or confirm a suspected diagnosis because the patient has some sign or symptom is a diagnostic examination, not a screening. In these cases, the sign or symptom is used to explain the reason for the test.

A screening code may be a first-listed code if the reason for the visit is specifically the screening exam. It may also be used as an additional code if the screening is done during an office visit for other health problems. A screening code is not necessary if the screening is inherent to a routine examination, such as a pap smear done during a routine pelvic examination.

Should a condition be discovered during the screening then the code for the condition may be assigned as an additional diagnosis.

The Z code indicates that a screening exam is planned. A procedure code is required to confirm that the screening was performed.

The screening Z codes/categories:

Z11	Encounter for screening for infectious and parasitic diseases
Z12	Encounter for screening for malignant neoplasms
Z13	Encounter for screening for other diseases and disorders Except: Z13.9, Encounter for screening, unspecified
Z36	Encounter for antenatal screening for mother

6) Observation

There are three observation Z code categories. They are for use in very limited circumstances when a person is being observed for a suspected condition that is ruled out. The observation codes are not for use if an injury or illness or any signs or symptoms related to the suspected condition are present. In such cases the diagnosis/symptom code is used with the corresponding external cause code.

The observation codes are to be used as principal diagnosis only. The only exception to this is when the principal diagnosis is required to be a code from category Z38, Liveborn infants according to place of birth and type of delivery. Then a code from category Z05, Encounter for observation and evaluation of newborn for suspected diseases and conditions ruled out, is sequenced after the Z38 code. Additional codes may be used in addition to the observation code but only if they are unrelated to the suspected condition being observed.

Codes from subcategory Z03.7 Encounter for suspected maternal and fetal conditions ruled out, may either be used as a first-listed or as an additional code assignment depending on the case. They are for use in very limited circumstances on a maternal record when an encounter is for a suspected maternal or fetal condition that is ruled out during that encounter (for example, a maternal or fetal condition may be suspected due to an abnormal test result). These codes should not be used when the condition is confirmed. In those cases, the confirmed condition should be coded. In addition, these codes are not for use if an illness or any signs or symptoms related to the suspected condition or problem are present. In such cases the diagnosis/symptom code is used.

Additional codes may be used in addition to the code from subcategory Z03.7, but only if they are unrelated to the suspected condition being evaluated.

Codes from subcategory Z03.7 may not be used for encounters for antenatal screening of mother. *See Section I.C.21. Screening.*

For encounters for suspected fetal condition that are inconclusive following testing and evaluation, assign the appropriate code from category O35, O36, O40 or O41.

The observation Z code categories:

Z03	Encounter for medical observation for suspected diseases and conditions ruled out
Z04	Encounter for examination and observation for other reasons Except: Z04.9, Encounter for examination and observation for unspecified reason
Z05	Encounter for observation and evaluation of newborn for suspected diseases and conditions ruled out

7) Aftercare

Aftercare visit codes cover situations when the initial treatment of a disease has been performed and the patient requires continued care during the healing or recovery phase, or for the long-term consequences of the disease. The aftercare Z code should not be used if treatment is directed at a current, acute disease. The diagnosis code is to be used in these cases.

Exceptions to this rule are codes Z51.0, Encounter for antineoplastic radiation therapy, and codes from subcategory Z51.1, Encounter for antineoplastic chemotherapy and immunotherapy. These codes are to be first-listed, followed by the diagnosis code when a patient's encounter is solely to receive radiation therapy, chemotherapy, or immunotherapy for the treatment of a neoplasm. If the reason for the encounter is more than one type of antineoplastic therapy, code Z51.0 and a code from subcategory Z51.1 may be assigned together, in which case one of these codes would be reported as a secondary diagnosis.

The aftercare Z codes should also not be used for aftercare for injuries. For aftercare of an injury, assign the acute injury code with the appropriate 7th character (for subsequent encounter).

The aftercare codes are generally first-listed to explain the specific reason for the encounter. An aftercare code may be used as an additional code when some type of aftercare is provided in addition to the reason for admission and no diagnosis code is applicable. An example of this would be the closure of a colostomy during an encounter for treatment of another condition.

Aftercare codes should be used in conjunction with other aftercare codes or diagnosis codes to provide better detail on the specifics of an aftercare encounter visit, unless otherwise directed by the classification. Should a patient receive multiple types of antineoplastic therapy during the same encounter, code Z51.0, Encounter for antineoplastic radiation therapy, and codes from subcategory Z51.1, Encounter for antineoplastic chemotherapy and immunotherapy, may be used together on a record. The sequencing of multiple aftercare codes depends on the circumstances of the encounter.

Certain aftercare Z code categories need a secondary diagnosis code to describe the resolving condition or sequelae. For others, the condition is included in the code title.

Additional Z code aftercare category terms include fitting and adjustment, and attention to artificial openings.

Status Z codes may be used with aftercare Z codes to indicate the nature of the aftercare. For example code Z95.1, Presence of aortocoronary bypass graft, may be used with code Z48.812, Encounter for surgical aftercare following surgery on the circulatory system, to indicate the surgery for which the aftercare is being performed. A status code should not be used when the aftercare code indicates the type of status, such as using Z43.0, Encounter for attention to tracheostomy, with Z93.0, Tracheostomy status.

The aftercare Z category/codes:

Z42	Encounter for plastic and reconstructive surgery following medical procedure or healed injury
Z43	Encounter for attention to artificial openings
Z44	Encounter for fitting and adjustment of external prosthetic device
Z45	Encounter for adjustment and management of implanted device
Z46	Encounter for fitting and adjustment of other devices
Z47	Orthopedic aftercare
Z48	Encounter for other postprocedural aftercare
Z49	Encounter for care involving renal dialysis
Z51	Encounter for other aftercare and medical care

8) Follow-up

The follow-up codes are used to explain continuing surveillance following completed treatment of a disease, condition, or injury. They imply that the condition has been fully treated and no longer exists. They should not be confused with aftercare codes, or injury codes with a 7th character for subsequent encounter, that explain ongoing care of a healing condition or its sequelae. Follow-up codes may be used in conjunction with history codes to provide the full picture of the healed condition and its treatment. The follow-up code is sequenced first, followed by the history code.

A follow-up code may be used to explain multiple visits. Should a condition be found to have recurred on the follow-up visit, then the diagnosis code for the condition should be assigned in place of the follow-up code.

The follow-up Z code categories:

Z08	Encounter for follow-up examination after completed treatment for malignant neoplasm
Z09	Encounter for follow-up examination after completed treatment for conditions other than malignant neoplasm
Z39	Encounter for maternal postpartum care and examination

9) Donor

Codes in category Z52, Donors of organs and tissues, are used for living individuals who are donating blood or other body tissue.

These codes are only for individuals donating for others, not for self-donations. They are not used to identify cadaveric donations.

10) Counseling

Counseling Z codes are used when a patient or family member receives assistance in the aftermath of an illness or injury, or when support is required in coping with family or social problems.

The counseling Z codes/categories:

Z30.0-	Encounter for general counseling and advice on contraception
Z31.5	Encounter for procreative genetic counseling
Z31.6-	Encounter for general counseling and advice on procreation
Z32.2	Encounter for childbirth instruction
Z32.3	Encounter for childcare instruction
Z69	Encounter for mental health services for victim and perpetrator of abuse
Z70	Counseling related to sexual attitude, behavior and orientation
Z71	Persons encountering health services for other counseling and medical advice, not elsewhere classified
Z76.81	Expectant mother prebirth pediatrician visit

11) Encounters for Obstetrical and Reproductive Services

See Section I.C.15. Pregnancy, Childbirth, and the Puerperium, for further instruction on the use of these codes.

Z codes for pregnancy are for use in those circumstances when none of the problems or complications included in the codes from the Obstetrics chapter exist (a routine prenatal visit or postpartum care). Codes in category Z34, Encounter for supervision of normal pregnancy, are always first listed and are not to be used with any other code from the OB chapter.

Codes in category Z3A, Weeks of gestation, may be assigned to provide additional information about the pregnancy. Category Z3A codes should not be assigned for pregnancies with abortive outcomes (categories O00-O08), elective termination of pregnancy (code Z33.2), nor for postpartum conditions, as category Z3A is not applicable to these conditions. The date of the admission should be used to determine weeks of gestation for inpatient admissions that encompass more than one gestational week.

The outcome of delivery, category Z37, should be included on all maternal delivery records. It is always a secondary code. Codes in category Z37 should not be used on the newborn record.

Z codes for family planning (contraceptive) or procreative management and counseling should be included on an obstetric record either during the pregnancy or the postpartum stage, if applicable.

Z codes/categories for obstetrical and reproductive services:

Z30	Encounter for contraceptive management
Z31	Encounter for procreative management
Z32.2	Encounter for childbirth instruction
Z32.3	Encounter for childcare instruction
Z33	Pregnant state
Z34	Encounter for supervision of normal pregnancy
Z36	Encounter for antenatal screening of mother
Z3A	Weeks of gestation
Z37	Outcome of delivery
Z39	Encounter for maternal postpartum care and examination
Z76.81	Expectant mother prebirth pediatrician visit

12) Newborns and Infants

See Section I.C.16. Newborn (Perinatal) Guidelines, for further instruction on the use of these codes.

Newborn Z codes/categories:

Z76.1	Encounter for health supervision and care of foundling
Z00.1-	Encounter for routine child health examination
Z38	Liveborn infants according to place of birth and type of delivery

13) Routine and administrative examinations

The Z codes allow for the description of encounters for routine examinations, such as, a general check-up, or, examinations for administrative purposes, such as, a pre-employment physical. The codes are not to be used if the examination is for diagnosis of a suspected condition or for treatment purposes. In such cases the diagnosis code is used. During a routine exam, should a diagnosis or condition be discovered, it should be coded as an additional code. Pre-existing and chronic conditions and history codes may also be included as additional codes as long as the examination is for administrative purposes and not focused on any particular condition.

Some of the codes for routine health examinations distinguish between "with" and "without" abnormal findings. Code assignment depends on the information that is known at the time the encounter is being coded. For example, if no abnormal findings were found during the examination, but the encounter is being coded before test results are back, it is acceptable to assign the code for "without abnormal findings." When assigning a code for "with abnormal findings," additional code(s) should be assigned to identify the specific abnormal finding(s).

Pre-operative examination and pre-procedural laboratory examination Z codes are for use only in those situations when a patient is being cleared for a procedure or surgery and no treatment is given.

The Z codes/categories for routine and administrative examinations:

Z00	Encounter for general examination without complaint, suspected or reported diagnosis
Z01	Encounter for other special examination without complaint, suspected or reported diagnosis
Z02	Encounter for administrative examination Except: Z02.9, Encounter for administrative examinations, unspecified
Z32.0-	Encounter for pregnancy test

14) Miscellaneous Z codes

The miscellaneous Z codes capture a number of other health care encounters that do not fall into one of the other categories. Certain of these codes identify the reason for the encounter; others are for use as additional codes that provide useful information on circumstances that may affect a patient's care and treatment.

Prophylactic Organ Removal

For encounters specifically for prophylactic removal of an organ (such as prophylactic removal of breasts due to a genetic susceptibility to cancer or a family history of cancer), the principal or first-listed code should be a code from category Z40, Encounter for prophylactic surgery, followed by the appropriate codes to identify the associated risk factor (such as genetic susceptibility or family history).

If the patient has a malignancy of one site and is having prophylactic removal at another site to prevent either a new primary malignancy or metastatic disease, a code for the malignancy should also be assigned in addition to a code from subcategory Z40.0, Encounter for prophylactic surgery for risk factors related to malignant neoplasms. A Z40.0 code should not be assigned if the patient is having organ removal for treatment of a malignancy, such as the removal of the testes for the treatment of prostate cancer.

Miscellaneous Z codes/categories:

Z28	Immunization not carried out Except: Z28.3, Underimmunization status
Z29	Encounter for other prophylactic measures
Z40	Encounter for prophylactic surgery
Z41	Encounter for procedures for purposes other than remedying health state Except: Z41.9, Encounter for procedure for purposes other than remedying health state, unspecified
Z53	Persons encountering health services for specific procedures and treatment, not carried out
Z55	Problems related to education and literacy
Z56	Problems related to employment and unemployment
Z57	Occupational exposure to risk factors
Z58	Problems related to physical environment
Z59	Problems related to housing and economic circumstances
Z60	Problems related to social environment
Z62	Problems related to upbringing
Z63	Other problems related to primary support group, including family circumstances
Z64	Problems related to certain psychosocial circumstances
Z65	Problems related to other psychosocial circumstances
Z72	Problems related to lifestyle Note: These codes should be assigned only when the documentation specifies that the patient has an associated problem
Z73	Problems related to life management difficulty

Z74	Problems related to care provider dependency Except: Z74.01, Bed confinement status
Z75	Problems related to medical facilities and other health care
Z76.0	Encounter for issue of repeat prescription
Z76.3	Healthy person accompanying sick person
Z76.4	Other boarder to healthcare facility
Z76.5	Malingerer [conscious simulation]
Z91.1-	Patient's noncompliance with medical treatment and regimen
Z91.83	Wandering in diseases classified elsewhere
Z91.84-	Oral health risk factors
Z91.89	Other specified personal risk factors, not elsewhere classified

See Section I.B.14 for Z55-Z65 Persons with potential health hazards related to socioeconomic and psychosocial circumstances, documentation by clinicians other than the patient's provider.

15) Nonspecific Z codes

Certain Z codes are so non-specific, or potentially redundant with other codes in the classification, that there can be little justification for their use in the inpatient setting. Their use in the outpatient setting should be limited to those instances when there is no further documentation to permit more precise coding. Otherwise, any sign or symptom or any other reason for visit that is captured in another code should be used.

Nonspecific Z codes/categories:

Z02.9	Encounter for administrative examinations, unspecified
Z04.9	Encounter for examination and observation for unspecified reason
Z13.9	Encounter for screening, unspecified
Z41.9	Encounter for procedure for purposes other than remedying health state, unspecified
Z52.9	Donor of unspecified organ or tissue
Z86.59	Personal history of other mental and behavioral disorders
Z88.9	Allergy status to unspecified drugs, medicaments and biological substances status
Z92.0	Personal history of contraception

16) Z Codes That May Only Be Principal/First-Listed Diagnosis

The following Z codes/categories may only be reported as the principal/first-listed diagnosis, except when there are multiple encounters on the same day and the medical records for the encounters are combined:

Z00	Encounter for general examination without complaint, suspected or reported diagnosis Except: Z00.6
Z01	Encounter for other special examination without complaint, suspected or reported diagnosis
Z02	Encounter for administrative examination
Z03	Encounter for medical observation for suspected diseases and conditions ruled out
Z04	Encounter for examination and observation for other reasons
Z33.2	Encounter for elective termination of pregnancy
Z31.81	Encounter for male factor infertility in female patient
Z31.83	Encounter for assisted reproductive fertility procedure cycle
Z31.84	Encounter for fertility preservation procedure
Z34	Encounter for supervision of normal pregnancy
Z39	Encounter for maternal postpartum care and examination
Z38	Liveborn infants according to place of birth and type of delivery
Z40	Encounter for prophylactic surgery
Z42	Encounter for plastic and reconstructive surgery following medical procedure or healed injury
Z51.0	Encounter for antineoplastic radiation therapy
Z51.1-	Encounter for antineoplastic chemotherapy and immunotherapy
Z52	Donors of organs and tissues Except: Z52.9, Donor of unspecified organ or tissue
Z76.1	Encounter for health supervision and care of foundling
Z76.2	Encounter for health supervision and care of other healthy infant and child
Z99.12	Encounter for respirator [ventilator] dependence during power failure

CHAPTER 21

FACTORS INFLUENCING HEALTH STATUS AND CONTACT WITH HEALTH SERVICES (Z00-Z99)

Note: Z codes represent reasons for encounters. A corresponding procedure code must accompany a Z code if a procedure is performed. Categories Z00-Z99 are provided for occasions when circumstances other than a disease, injury or external cause classifiable to categories A00-Y89 are recorded as "diagnoses" or "problems." This can arise in two main ways:

(a) When a person who may or may not be sick encounters the health services for some specific purpose, such as to receive limited care or service for a current condition, to donate an organ or tissue, to receive prophylactic vaccination (immunization), or to discuss a problem which is in itself not a disease or injury.

(b) When some circumstance or problem is present which influences the person's health status but is not in itself a current illness or injury.

This chapter contains the following blocks:

Z00-Z13	Persons encountering health services for examination
Z14-Z15	Genetic carrier and genetic susceptibility to disease
Z16	Resistance to antimicrobial drugs
Z17	Estrogen, and other hormones and factors receptor status
Z18	Retained foreign body fragments
Z19	Hormone sensitivity malignancy status
Z20-Z29	Persons with potential health hazards related to communicable diseases
Z30-Z39	Persons encountering health services in circumstances related to reproduction
Z40-Z53	Encounters for other specific health care
Z55-Z65	Persons with potential health hazards related to socioeconomic and psychosocial circumstances
Z66	Do not resuscitate status
Z67	Blood type
Z68	Body mass index (BMI)
Z69-Z76	Persons encountering health services in other circumstances
Z77-Z99	Persons with potential health hazards related to family and personal history and certain conditions influencing health status

PERSONS ENCOUNTERING HEALTH SERVICES FOR EXAMINATIONS (Z00-Z13)

Note: Nonspecific abnormal findings disclosed at the time of these examinations are classified to categories R70-R94.

Excludes1 ~~examinations related to pregnancy and reproduction (Z30-Z36, Z39.-)~~

▶ **Excludes2** examinations related to pregnancy and reproduction (Z30-Z36, Z39.-)

● **Z00** **Encounter for general examination without complaint, suspected or reported diagnosis**

Excludes1 encounter for examination for administrative purposes (Z02.-)

Excludes2 encounter for pre-procedural examinations (Z01.81-)
special screening examinations (Z11-Z13)

● **Z00.0** **Encounter for general adult medical examination**
Encounter for adult periodic examination (annual) (physical) and any associated laboratory and radiologic examinations

Excludes1 encounter for examination of sign or symptom - code to sign or symptom
general health check-up of infant or child (Z00.12.-)

Coding Clinic: 2016, Q4, P131

Z00.00 **Encounter for general adult medical examination without abnormal findings** **A**
Encounter for adult health check-up NOS
Coding Clinic: 2017, Q4, P95; 2016, Q1, P37

Z00.01 **Encounter for general adult medical examination with abnormal findings** **A**
Use additional code to identify abnormal findings
Coding Clinic: 2016, Q1, P36

● **Z00.1** **Encounter for newborn, infant and child health examinations**

● **Z00.11** **Newborn health examination**
Health check for child under 29 days old
Use additional code to identify any abnormal findings

Excludes1 health check for child over 28 days old (Z00.12-)

Z00.110 **Health examination for newborn under 8 days old** **N**
Health check for newborn under 8 days old

Z00.111 **Health examination for newborn 8 to 28 days old** **N**
Health check for newborn 8 to 28 days old
Newborn weight check

● **Z00.12** **Encounter for routine child health examination**
Immunizations appropriate for age
Health check (routine) for child over 28 days old
Routine developmental screening of infant or child
Routine vision and hearing testing

Excludes1 health check for child under 29 days old (Z00.11-)
health supervision of foundling or other healthy infant or child (Z76.1-Z76.2)
newborn health examination (Z00.11-)

Z00.121 **Encounter for routine child health examination with abnormal findings** **P**
Use additional code to identify abnormal findings
Coding Clinic: 2024, Q4, P6; 2017, Q4, P95; 2016, Q1, P34-35

Z00.129 **Encounter for routine child health examination without abnormal findings** **P**
Encounter for routine child health examination NOS
Coding Clinic: 2016, Q1, P34

Z00.2 **Encounter for examination for period of rapid growth in childhood** **P**

Z00.3 **Encounter for examination for adolescent development state** **P**
Encounter for puberty development state

Z00.5 **Encounter for examination of potential donor of organ and tissue**

Z00.6 **Encounter for examination for normal comparison and control in clinical research program**
Examination of participant or control in clinical research program

● **Z00.7** **Encounter for examination for period of delayed growth in childhood**

Z00.70 **Encounter for examination for period of delayed growth in childhood without abnormal findings** **P**

Z00.71 **Encounter for examination for period of delayed growth in childhood with abnormal findings** **P**
Use additional code to identify abnormal findings

Z00.8 **Encounter for other general examination**
Encounter for health examination in population surveys

CHAPTER 21 (Z00-Z99)

● **Z01   Encounter for other special examination** without complaint, suspected or reported diagnosis

Includes   routine examination of specific system

Note: Codes from category Z01 represent the reason for the encounter. A separate procedure code is required to identify any examinations or procedures performed.

Excludes1   encounter for examination for administrative purposes (Z02.-)
encounter for examination for suspected conditions, proven not to exist (Z03.-)
~~encounter for laboratory and radiologic examinations as a component of general medical examinations (Z00.0-)~~
encounter for laboratory, radiologic and imaging examinations for sign(s) and symptom(s) - code to the sign(s) or symptom(s)

▶ **Excludes2**   encounter for laboratory and radiologic examinations as a component of general medical examinations (Z00.0-)
screening examinations (Z11-Z13)

● **Z01.0   Encounter for examination of eyes and vision**

Excludes1   examination for driving license (Z02.4)

Z01.00   Encounter for examination of eyes and vision without abnormal findings
Encounter for examination of eyes and vision NOS

Z01.01   Encounter for examination of eyes and vision with abnormal findings
Use additional code to identify abnormal findings
Coding Clinic: 2016, Q4, P21

● **Z01.02   Encounter for examination of eyes and vision following failed vision screening**

Excludes1   encounter for examination of eyes and vision with abnormal findings (Z01.01)
encounter for examination of eyes and vision without abnormal findings (Z01.00)

● **Z01.020   Encounter for examination of eyes and vision following failed vision screening without abnormal findings**

● **Z01.021   Encounter for examination of eyes and vision following failed vision screening with abnormal findings**
Use additional code to identify abnormal findings

● **Z01.1   Encounter for examination of ears and hearing**

Z01.10   Encounter for examination of ears and hearing without abnormal findings
Encounter for examination of ears and hearing NOS
Coding Clinic: 2016, Q4, P25

● **Z01.11   Encounter for examination of ears and hearing with abnormal findings**
Coding Clinic: 2016, Q3, P18

Z01.110   Encounter for hearing examination following failed hearing screening
Coding Clinic: 2016, Q3, P18-19

Z01.118   Encounter for examination of ears and hearing with other abnormal findings
Use additional code to identify abnormal findings
Coding Clinic: 2016, Q3, P17

Z01.12   Encounter for hearing conservation and treatment

● **Z01.2   Encounter for dental examination and cleaning**

Z01.20   Encounter for dental examination and cleaning without abnormal findings
Encounter for dental examination and cleaning NOS

Z01.21   Encounter for dental examination and cleaning with abnormal findings
Use additional code to identify abnormal findings

● **Z01.3   Encounter for examination of blood pressure**

Z01.30   Encounter for examination of blood pressure without abnormal findings
Encounter for examination of blood pressure NOS

Z01.31   Encounter for examination of blood pressure with abnormal findings
Use additional code to identify abnormal findings

● **Z01.4   Encounter for gynecological examination**

Excludes2   pregnancy examination or test (Z32.0-)
routine examination for contraceptive maintenance (Z30.4-)

● **Z01.41   Encounter for routine gynecological examination**
Encounter for general gynecological examination with or without cervical smear
Encounter for gynecological examination (general) (routine) NOS
Encounter for pelvic examination (annual) (periodic)

Use additional code:
for screening for human papillomavirus, if applicable (Z11.51)
for screening vaginal pap smear, if applicable (Z12.72)
to identify acquired absence of uterus, if applicable (Z90.71-)

Excludes1   gynecologic examination status-post hysterectomy for malignant condition (Z08)
screening cervical pap smear not a part of a routine gynecological examination (Z12.4)

Z01.411   Encounter for gynecological examination (general) (routine) with abnormal findings
Use additional code to identify any abnormal findings

Z01.419   Encounter for gynecological examination (general) (routine) without abnormal findings

Z01.42   Encounter for cervical smear to confirm findings of recent normal smear following initial abnormal smear

● **Z01.8   Encounter for other specified special examinations**

● **Z01.81   Encounter for preprocedural examinations**
Encounter for preoperative examinations
Encounter for radiological and imaging examinations as part of preprocedural examination

Z01.810   Encounter for preprocedural cardiovascular examination

Z01.811   Encounter for preprocedural respiratory examination

Z01.812   Encounter for preprocedural laboratory examination
Blood and urine tests prior to treatment or procedure
Coding Clinic: 2023, Q2, P4; 2021, Q1, P38

Z01.818   Encounter for other preprocedural examination
Encounter for preprocedural examination NOS
Encounter for examinations prior to antineoplastic chemotherapy

CHAPTER 21 (Z00-Z99)

▶ New   ⇒ Revised   ~~deleted~~ Deleted   Excludes 1   Excludes 2   Includes   Use additional   Code first   Code also   Key words
OGCR Official Guidelines   X Assign placeholder X   ● Use Additional Character(s)   ▸ Manifestation Code   ⬡ Hierarchical Condition Category   Coding Clinic

Z01.82   **Encounter for allergy testing**

      Excludes1   encounter for antibody response examination (Z01.84)

Z01.83   **Encounter for blood typing**

      Encounter for Rh typing

Z01.84   **Encounter for antibody response examination**

      Encounter for immunity status testing

      Excludes1   encounter for allergy testing (Z01.82)

Z01.89   **Encounter for other specified special examinations**

● **Z02** **Encounter for administrative examination**

Z02.0   **Encounter for examination for admission to educational institution**

      Encounter for examination for admission to preschool (education)

      Encounter for examination for re-admission to school following illness or medical treatment

Z02.1   **Encounter for pre-employment examination**

Z02.2   **Encounter for examination for admission to residential institution**

      Excludes1   examination for admission to prison (Z02.89)

Z02.3   **Encounter for examination for recruitment to armed forces**

Z02.4   **Encounter for examination for driving license**

Z02.5   **Encounter for examination for participation in sport**

      Excludes1   blood-alcohol and blood-drug test (Z02.83)

Z02.6   **Encounter for examination for insurance purposes**

● **Z02.7**   **Encounter for issue of medical certificate**

      Excludes1   encounter for general medical examination (Z00-Z01, Z02.0-Z02.6, Z02.8-Z02.9)

Z02.71   **Encounter for disability determination**

      Encounter for issue of medical certificate of incapacity

      Encounter for issue of medical certificate of invalidity

Z02.79   **Encounter for issue of other medical certificate**

● **Z02.8**   **Encounter for other administrative examinations**

Z02.81   **Encounter for paternity testing**

Z02.82   **Encounter for adoption services**

Z02.83   **Encounter for blood-alcohol and blood-drug test**

      Use additional code for findings of alcohol or drugs in blood (R78.-)

Z02.84   **Encounter for child welfare exam**

      Encounter for child welfare screening exam

      Excludes2   encounter for examination and observation for alleged child physical abuse(Z04.72)

               encounter for examination and observation for alleged child rape (Z04.42)

Z02.89   **Encounter for other administrative examinations**

      Encounter for examination for admission to prison

      Encounter for examination for admission to summer camp

      Encounter for immigration examination

      Encounter for naturalization examination

      Encounter for premarital examination

      Excludes1   health supervision of foundling or other healthy infant or child (Z76.1-Z76.2)

Z02.9   **Encounter for administrative examinations, unspecified**

● **Z03** **Encounter for medical observation for suspected diseases and conditions ruled out**

      This category is to be used when a person without a diagnosis is suspected of having an abnormal condition, without signs or symptoms, which requires study, but after examination and observation, is ruled out. This category is also for use for administrative and legal observation status.

      Excludes1   contact with and (suspected) exposures hazardous to health (Z77.-)

               encounter for observation and evaluation of newborn for suspected diseases and conditions ruled out (Z05.-)

               person with feared complaint in whom no diagnosis is made (Z71.1)

               signs or symptoms under study - code to signs or symptoms

Z03.6   **Encounter for observation for suspected toxic effect from ingested substance ruled out**

      Encounter for observation for suspected adverse effect from drug

      Encounter for observation for suspected poisoning

● **Z03.7** **Encounter for suspected maternal and fetal conditions ruled out**
Encounter for suspected maternal and fetal conditions not found
    Excludes1   known or suspected fetal anomalies affecting management of mother, not ruled out (O26.-, O35.-, O36.-, O40.-, O41.-)

    Z03.71 **Encounter for suspected problem with amniotic cavity and membrane ruled out**   M
Encounter for suspected oligohydramnios ruled out
Encounter for suspected polyhydramnios ruled out

    Z03.72 **Encounter for suspected placental problem ruled out**   M

    Z03.73 **Encounter for suspected fetal anomaly ruled out**   M
    Coding Clinic: 2016, Q4, P6

    Z03.74 **Encounter for suspected problem with fetal growth ruled out**   M

    Z03.75 **Encounter for suspected cervical shortening ruled out**   M

    Z03.79 **Encounter for other suspected maternal and fetal conditions ruled out**   M
    Coding Clinic: 2016, Q4, P7

● **Z03.8** **Encounter for observation for other suspected diseases and conditions ruled out**

    ● **Z03.81** **Encounter for observation for suspected exposure to biological agents ruled out**

       Z03.810 **Encounter for observation for suspected exposure to anthrax ruled out**

       Z03.818 **Encounter for observation for suspected exposure to other biological agents ruled out**

    ● **Z03.82** **Encounter for observation for suspected foreign body ruled out**
       Excludes1   retained foreign body (Z18.-)
retained foreign body in eyelid (H02.81)
residual foreign body in soft tissue (M79.5)

       Excludes2   confirmed foreign body ingestion or aspiration including:
foreign body in alimentary tract (T18)
foreign body in ear (T16)
foreign body on external eye (T15)
foreign body in respiratory tract (T17)

       Z03.821 **Encounter for observation for suspected ingested foreign body ruled out**

       Z03.822 **Encounter for observation for suspected aspirated (inhaled) foreign body ruled out**

       Z03.823 **Encounter for observation for suspected inserted (injected) foreign body ruled out**
Encounter for observation for suspected inserted (injected) foreign body in eye ruled out
Encounter for observation for suspected inserted (injected) foreign body in orifice ruled out
Encounter for observation for suspected inserted (injected) foreign body in skin ruled out

    Z03.83 **Encounter for observation for suspected conditions related to home physiologic monitoring device ruled out**
Encounter for observation for apnea alarm without findings
Encounter for observation for bradycardia alarm without findings
Encounter for observation for malfunction of home cardiorespiratory monitor
Encounter for observation for non-specific findings home physiologic monitoring device
Encounter for observation for pulse oximeter alarm without findings
    Excludes1   apnea NOS (R06.81)
neonatal bradycardia (P29.12)
newborn apnea (P28.4-)
primary sleep apnea of newborn (P28.3-)
sleep apnea (G47.3-)

    Z03.89 **Encounter for observation for other suspected diseases and conditions ruled out**

● **Z04** **Encounter for examination and observation for other reasons**
    Includes   encounter for examination for medicolegal reasons
This category is to be used when a person without a diagnosis is suspected of having an abnormal condition, without signs or symptoms, which requires study, but after examination and observation, is ruled-out. This category is also for use for administrative and legal observation status.

    Z04.1 **Encounter for examination and observation following transport accident**
    Excludes1   encounter for examination and observation following work accident (Z04.2)
    Coding Clinic: 2019, Q2, P11

    Z04.2 **Encounter for examination and observation following work accident**

    Z04.3 **Encounter for examination and observation following other accident**

    ● **Z04.4** **Encounter for examination and observation following alleged rape**
Encounter for examination and observation of victim following alleged rape
Encounter for examination and observation of victim following alleged sexual abuse
    Coding Clinic: 2016, Q4, P129

       Z04.41 **Encounter for examination and observation following alleged adult rape**   A
Suspected adult rape, ruled out
Suspected adult sexual abuse, ruled out

       Z04.42 **Encounter for examination and observation following alleged child rape**   P
Suspected child rape, ruled out
Suspected child sexual abuse, ruled out

    Z04.6 **Encounter for general psychiatric examination, requested by authority**

    ● **Z04.7** **Encounter for examination and observation following alleged physical abuse**

       Z04.71 **Encounter for examination and observation following alleged adult physical abuse**   A
Suspected adult physical abuse, ruled out
    Excludes1   confirmed case of adult physical abuse (T74.-)
encounter for examination and observation following alleged adult sexual abuse (Z04.41)
suspected case of adult physical abuse, not ruled out (T76.-)

Z04.72   **Encounter for examination and observation following alleged child physical abuse**   **P**
Suspected child physical abuse, ruled out
> **Excludes1**   confirmed case of child physical abuse (T74.-)
> encounter for examination and observation following alleged child sexual abuse (Z04.42)
> suspected case of child physical abuse, not ruled out (T76.-)

● **Z04.8**   **Encounter for examination and observation for other specified reasons**
Encounter for examination and observation for request for expert evidence

Z04.81   **Encounter for examination and observation of victim following forced sexual exploitation**

Z04.82   **Encounter for examination and observation of victim following forced labor exploitation**

Z04.89   **Encounter for examination and observation for other specified reasons**

Z04.9   **Encounter for examination and observation for unspecified reason**
Encounter for observation NOS

● **Z05**   **Encounter for observation and evaluation of newborn for suspected diseases and conditions ruled out**
This category is to be used for newborns, within the neonatal period (the first 28 days of life), who are suspected of having an abnormal condition, but without signs or symptoms, and which, after examination and observation, is ruled out.
Coding Clinic: 2022, Q1, P17-18; 2019, Q2, P11; 2016, Q4, P54, 77, 126-127, 130

Z05.0   **Observation and evaluation of newborn for suspected cardiac condition ruled out**   **N**

Z05.1   **Observation and evaluation of newborn for suspected infectious condition ruled out**   **N**
Coding Clinic: 2019, Q2, P11

Z05.2   **Observation and evaluation of newborn for suspected neurological condition ruled out**   **N**

Z05.3   **Observation and evaluation of newborn for suspected respiratory condition ruled out**   **N**

● **Z05.4**   **Observation and evaluation of newborn for suspected genetic, metabolic or immunologic condition ruled out**

Z05.41   **Observation and evaluation of newborn for suspected genetic condition ruled out**   **N**
Coding Clinic: 2016, Q4, P55

Z05.42   **Observation and evaluation of newborn for suspected metabolic condition ruled out**   **N**

Z05.43   **Observation and evaluation of newborn for suspected immunologic condition ruled out**   **N**

Z05.5   **Observation and evaluation of newborn for suspected gastrointestinal condition ruled out**   **N**

Z05.6   **Observation and evaluation of newborn for suspected genitourinary condition ruled out**   **N**

● **Z05.7**   **Observation and evaluation of newborn for suspected skin, subcutaneous, musculoskeletal and connective tissue condition ruled out**

Z05.71   **Observation and evaluation of newborn for suspected skin and subcutaneous tissue condition ruled out**   **N**

Z05.72   **Observation and evaluation of newborn for suspected musculoskeletal condition ruled out**   **N**

Z05.73   **Observation and evaluation of newborn for suspected connective tissue condition ruled out**   **N**

● **Z05.8**   **Observation and evaluation of newborn for other specified suspected condition ruled out**   **N**
Coding Clinic: 2022, Q1, P17-18

Z05.81   **Observation and evaluation of newborn for suspected condition related to home physiologic monitoring device ruled out**
Encounter for observation of newborn for apnea alarm without findings
Encounter for observation of newborn for bradycardia alarm without findings
Encounter for observation of newborn for malfunction of home cardiorespiratory monitor
Encounter for observation of newborn for non-specific findings home physiologic monitoring device
Encounter for observation of newborn for pulse oximeter alarm without findings
> **Excludes1**   encounter for observation for suspected conditions related to home physiologic monitoring device ruled out (Z03.83)
> neonatal bradycardia (P29.12)
> other newborn apnea (P28.4-)
> primary sleep apnea of newborn (P28.3-)

Z05.89   **Observation and evaluation of newborn for other specified suspected condition ruled out**

Z05.9   **Observation and evaluation of newborn for unspecified suspected condition ruled out**   **N**

OGCR   See Section II.C.21.c.8.

> The follow-up codes are used to explain continuing surveillance following completed treatment of a disease, condition, or injury. They imply that the condition has been fully treated and no longer exists. They should not be confused with aftercare codes, or injury codes with 7th character "D," that explain ongoing care of a healing condition or its sequelae. Follow-up codes may be used in conjunction with history codes to provide the full picture of the healed condition and its treatment. The follow-up code is sequenced first, followed by the history code.
>
> A follow-up code may be used to explain multiple visits. Should a condition be found to have recurred on the follow-up visit, then the diagnosis code for the condition should be assigned in place of the follow-up code.
>
> The follow-up Z code categories:
>
> Z08   Encounter for follow-up examination after completed treatment for malignant neoplasm
>
> Z09   Encounter for follow-up examination after completed treatment for conditions other than malignant neoplasm
>
> Z39   Encounter for maternal postpartum care and examination

Z08   **Encounter for follow-up examination after completed treatment for malignant neoplasm**
Medical surveillance following completed treatment
Use additional code to identify any acquired absence of organs (Z90.-)
Use additional code to identify the personal history of malignant neoplasm (Z85.-)
> **Excludes1**   aftercare following medical care (Z43-Z49, Z51)

Z09   **Encounter for follow-up examination after completed treatment for conditions other than malignant neoplasm**
Medical surveillance following completed treatment
Use additional code to identify any applicable history of disease code (Z86.-, Z87.-)
> **Excludes1**   aftercare following medical care (Z43-Z49, Z51)
> surveillance of contraception (Z30.4-)
> surveillance of prosthetic and other medical devices (Z44-Z46)
Coding Clinic: 2022, Q3, P4; 2021, Q1, P33; 2017, Q1, P9; 2015, Q1, P8

CHAPTER 21 (Z00-Z99)

OGCR Section II.C.21.c.5.

Screening

Screening is the testing for disease or disease precursors in seemingly well individuals so that early detection and treatment can be provided for those who test positive for the disease (e.g., screening mammogram).

The testing of a person to rule out or confirm a suspected diagnosis because the patient has some sign or symptom is a diagnostic examination, not a screening. In these cases, the sign or symptom is used to explain the reason for the test.

A screening code may be a first listed code if the reason for the visit is specifically the screening exam. It may also be used as an additional code if the screening is done during an office visit for other health problems. A screening code is not necessary if the screening is inherent to a routine examination, such as a pap smear done during a routine pelvic examination.

Should a condition be discovered during the screening then the code for the condition may be assigned as an additional diagnosis.

The Z code indicates that a screening exam is planned. A procedure code is required to confirm that the screening was performed.

The screening Z codes/categories:

Z11   Encounter for screening for infectious and parasitic diseases

Z12   Encounter for screening for malignant neoplasms

Z13   Encounter for screening for other diseases and disorders
       Except: Z13.9, Encounter for screening, unspecified

Z36   Encounter for antenatal screening for mother

● **Z11**   **Encounter for screening for infectious and parasitic diseases**
    Screening is the testing for disease or disease precursors in asymptomatic individuals so that early detection and treatment can be provided for those who test positive for the disease.

    Excludes1   encounter for diagnostic examination - code to sign or symptom

   Z11.0 **Encounter for screening for intestinal infectious diseases**
       Encounter for screening for active tuberculosis disease

   Z11.1 **Encounter for screening for respiratory tuberculosis**

   Z11.2 **Encounter for screening for other bacterial diseases**

   Z11.3 **Encounter for screening for infections with a predominantly sexual mode of transmission**

      Excludes2   encounter for screening for human immunodeficiency virus [HIV] (Z11.4)
                encounter for screening for human papillomavirus (Z11.51)

   Z11.4 **Encounter for screening for human immunodeficiency virus [HIV]**

●   **Z11.5** **Encounter for screening for other viral diseases**

      Excludes2   encounter for screening for viral intestinal disease (Z11.0)

    Z11.51 **Encounter for screening for human papillomavirus (HPV)**
         Coding Clinic: 2023, Q2, P3

    Z11.52 **Encounter for screening for COVID-19**
         Coding Clinic: 2023, Q2, P4; 2021, Q1, P37, 42

    Z11.59 **Encounter for screening for other viral diseases**
         Coding Clinic: 2021, Q1, P37

   Z11.6 **Encounter for screening for other protozoal diseases and helminthiases**
      Diseases or infestations caused by parasitic worms

      Excludes2   encounter for screening for protozoal intestinal disease (Z11.0)

   Z11.7 **Encounter for testing for latent tuberculosis infection**

   Z11.8 **Encounter for screening for other infectious and parasitic diseases**
       Encounter for screening for chlamydia
       Encounter for screening for rickettsial
       Encounter for screening for spirochetal
       Encounter for screening for mycoses

   Z11.9 **Encounter for screening for infectious and parasitic diseases, unspecified**

● **Z12**   **Encounter for screening for malignant neoplasms**
    Screening is the testing for disease or disease precursors in asymptomatic individuals so that early detection and treatment can be provided for those who test positive for the disease.

    Use additional code to identify any family history of malignant neoplasm (Z80.-)

    Excludes1   encounter for diagnostic examination - code to sign or symptom

   Z12.0 **Encounter for screening for malignant neoplasm of stomach**

●   **Z12.1** **Encounter for screening for malignant neoplasm of intestinal tract**

    Z12.10 **Encounter for screening for malignant neoplasm of intestinal tract, unspecified**

    Z12.11 **Encounter for screening for malignant neoplasm of colon**
        Encounter for screening colonoscopy NOS
        Coding Clinic: 2018, Q1, P7; 2017, Q1, P8-9

    Z12.12 **Encounter for screening for malignant neoplasm of rectum**

    Z12.13 **Encounter for screening for malignant neoplasm of small intestine**

   Z12.2 **Encounter for screening for malignant neoplasm of respiratory organs**

●   **Z12.3** **Encounter for screening for malignant neoplasm of breast**

    Z12.31 **Encounter for screening mammogram for malignant neoplasm of breast**

      Excludes1   inconclusive mammogram (R92.2)

      Coding Clinic: 2023, Q4, P44; 2015, Q1, P24

    Z12.39 **Encounter for other screening for malignant neoplasm of breast**

   Z12.4 **Encounter for screening for malignant neoplasm of cervix**
      Encounter for screening pap smear for malignant neoplasm of cervix

      Excludes1   when screening is part of general gynecological examination (Z01.4-)

      Excludes2   encounter for screening for human papillomavirus (Z11.51)

   Z12.5 **Encounter for screening for malignant neoplasm of prostate**

   Z12.6 **Encounter for screening for malignant neoplasm of bladder**

●   **Z12.7** **Encounter for screening for malignant neoplasm of other genitourinary organs**

    Z12.71 **Encounter for screening for malignant neoplasm of testis**

    Z12.72 **Encounter for screening for malignant neoplasm of vagina**
        Vaginal pap smear status - post hysterectomy for non-malignant condition

      Use additional code to identify acquired absence of uterus (Z90.71-)

      Excludes1   vaginal pap smear status - post hysterectomy for malignant conditions (Z08)

    Z12.73 **Encounter for screening for malignant neoplasm of ovary**

    Z12.79 **Encounter for screening for malignant neoplasm of other genitourinary organs**

●   **Z12.8** **Encounter for screening for malignant neoplasm of other sites**

    Z12.81 **Encounter for screening for malignant neoplasm of oral cavity**

    Z12.82 **Encounter for screening for malignant neoplasm of nervous system**

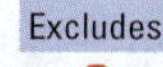

▶ New   ⇒ Revised   ~~deleted~~ Deleted   Excludes 1   Excludes 2   Includes   Use additional   Code first   Code also   Key words

OGCR Official Guidelines   X Assign placeholder X   ● Use Additional Character(s)   ▌ Manifestation Code   Hierarchical Condition Category   **Coding Clinic**

Z12.83　Encounter for screening for malignant neoplasm of **skin**

Z12.89　Encounter for screening for malignant neoplasm of **other sites**
Coding Clinic: 2021, Q1, P15

Z12.9　Encounter for screening for malignant neoplasm, site unspecified

● **Z13　Encounter for screening for other diseases and disorders**
Screening is the testing for disease or disease precursors in asymptomatic individuals so that early detection and treatment can be provided for those who test positive for the disease.

Excludes1　encounter for diagnostic examination - code to sign or symptom

Z13.0　**Encounter for screening for diseases of the blood and blood-forming organs and certain disorders involving the immune mechanism**

Z13.1　Encounter for screening for **diabetes mellitus**

● Z13.2　Encounter for screening for **nutritional, metabolic and other endocrine disorders**

　　Z13.21　Encounter for screening for **nutritional** disorder

● 　Z13.22　Encounter for screening for **metabolic disorder**

　　　　Z13.220　Encounter for screening for **lipoid disorders**
Encounter for screening for cholesterol level
Encounter for screening for hypercholesterolemia
Encounter for screening for hyperlipidemia

　　　　Z13.228　Encounter for screening for **other** metabolic disorders

　　Z13.29　Encounter for screening for **other** suspected endocrine disorder

Excludes2　encounter for screening for diabetes mellitus (Z13.1)

● Z13.3　Encounter for screening examination for mental health and behavioral disorders

　　Z13.30　Encounter for screening examination for mental health and behavioral disorders, unspecified

　　Z13.31　Encounter for screening for depression
Encounter for screening for depression, adult
Encounter for screening for depression for child or adolescent

　　Z13.32　Encounter for screening for maternal depression
Encounter for screening for perinatal depression

　　Z13.39　Encounter for screening examination for other mental health and behavioral disorders
Encounter for screening for alcoholism
Encounter for screening for intellectual disabilities

● Z13.4　Encounter for screening for certain **developmental disorders in childhood**　**P**
Encounter for development testing of infant or child
Encounter for screening for developmental handicaps in early childhood

Excludes2　encounter for routine child health examination (Z00.12-)

　　Z13.40　Encounter for screening for unspecified developmental delays

　　Z13.41　Encounter for autism screening

　　Z13.42　Encounter for screening for global developmental delays (milestones)
Encounter for screening for developmental handicaps in early childhood

　　Z13.49　Encounter for screening for other developmental delays

Z13.5　Encounter for screening for **eye and ear disorders**

Excludes2　encounter for general hearing examination (Z01.1-)
encounter for general vision examination (Z01.0-)
Coding Clinic: 2016, Q3, P17

Z13.6　Encounter for screening for **cardiovascular disorders**

● Z13.7　Encounter for screening for **genetic and chromosomal anomalies**

Excludes1　genetic testing for procreative management (Z31.4-)

　　Z13.71　Encounter for nonprocreative screening for genetic disease carrier status

　　Z13.79　Encounter for **other** screening for genetic and chromosomal anomalies

● Z13.8　Encounter for screening for **other specified** diseases and disorders

Excludes2　screening for malignant neoplasms (Z12.-)

● 　Z13.81　Encounter for screening for **digestive system** disorders

　　　　Z13.810　Encounter for screening for **upper** gastrointestinal disorder

　　　　Z13.811　Encounter for screening for **lower** gastrointestinal disorder

Excludes1　encounter for screening for intestinal infectious disease (Z11.0)

　　　　Z13.818　Encounter for screening for **other** digestive system disorders

● 　Z13.82　Encounter for screening for **musculoskeletal** disorder

　　　　Z13.820　Encounter for screening for **osteoporosis**

　　　　Z13.828　Encounter for screening for **other** musculoskeletal disorder

　　Z13.83　Encounter for screening for **respiratory** disorder NEC

Excludes1　encounter for screening for respiratory tuberculosis (Z11.1)

　　Z13.84　Encounter for screening for **dental disorders**

● 　Z13.85　Encounter for screening for **nervous system** disorders

　　　　Z13.850　Encounter for screening for **traumatic brain injury**

　　　　Z13.858　Encounter for screening for **other** nervous system disorders

　　Z13.88　Encounter for screening for disorder **due to exposure to contaminants**

Excludes1　those exposed to contaminants without suspected disorders (Z57-Z77.-)

　　Z13.89　Encounter for screening for **other** disorder
Encounter for screening for genitourinary disorders

Z13.9　Encounter for screening, **unspecified**

GENETIC CARRIER AND GENETIC SUSCEPTIBILITY TO DISEASE (Z14-Z15)

● Z14　Genetic carrier

● Z14.0　Hemophilia A carrier

　　Z14.01　Asymptomatic hemophilia A carrier

　　Z14.02　Symptomatic hemophilia A carrier

Z14.1　Cystic fibrosis carrier

Z14.8　Genetic carrier of other disease

CHAPTER 21 (Z00-Z99)

CHAPTER 21 (Z00-Z99)

● **Z15   Genetic susceptibility to disease**
> **Excludes1**   chromosomal anomalies (Q90-Q99)
> **Includes**   confirmed abnormal gene
> **Use additional** code, if applicable, for any associated family history of the disease (Z80-Z84)

● **Z15.0   Genetic susceptibility to malignant neoplasm**
> *Code first if applicable, any current malignant neoplasm (C00-C75, C81-C96)*
> **Use additional** code, if applicable, for any personal history of malignant neoplasm (Z85.-)

Z15.01   Genetic susceptibility to malignant neoplasm of breast

Z15.02   Genetic susceptibility to malignant neoplasm of ovary

Z15.03   Genetic susceptibility to malignant neoplasm of prostate

Z15.04   Genetic susceptibility to malignant neoplasm of endometrium

▶ **Z15.05   Genetic susceptibility to malignant neoplasm of fallopian tube(s)**

▶● **Z15.06   Genetic susceptibility to malignant neoplasm of digestive system**

▶ **Z15.060   Genetic susceptibility to colorectal cancer**

▶ **Z15.068   Genetic susceptibility to other malignant neoplasm of digestive system**
▶ Genetic susceptibility to biliary tract cancer
▶ Genetic susceptibility to gastric cancer
▶ Genetic susceptibility to pancreatic cancer
▶ Genetic susceptibility to small bowel cancer

▶ **Z15.07   Genetic susceptibility to malignant neoplasm of urinary tract**

Z15.09   Genetic susceptibility to other malignant neoplasm
> **Coding Clinic: 2021, Q1, P15**

Z15.1   Genetic susceptibility to epilepsy and neurodevelopmental disorders
> **Code also,** if applicable, related disorders such as:
> developmental and epileptic encephalopathy (G93.45)
> developmental disorder of speech and language (F80.-)
> developmental disorders of scholastic skills (F81.-)
> epilepsy, by specific type (G40.-)
> intellectual disabilities (F70-F79)
> other neurodevelopmental disorder (F88)
> pervasive developmental disorders (F84.-)

Z15.2   Genetic susceptibility to obesity
> **Code also,** if applicable, any associated manifestations, such as:
> other obesity (E66.8-)
> polyphagia (R63.2)
> **Use Additional** code to identify body mass index (BMI), if known (Z68.-)

▶ **Z15.3   Genetic susceptibility to kidney disease**
▶ **Code also,** if applicable, hypertension (I10-I1A)

● **Z15.8   Genetic susceptibility to other disease**

Z15.81   Genetic susceptibility to multiple endocrine neoplasia [MEN]
> **Excludes1**   multiple endocrine neoplasia [MEN] syndromes (E31.2-)

Z15.89   Genetic susceptibility to other disease

RESISTANCE TO ANTIMICROBIAL DRUGS (Z16)

● **Z16   Resistance to antimicrobial drugs**
> **Note:** The codes in this category are provided for use as additional codes to identify the resistance and non-responsiveness of a condition to antimicrobial drugs.
> *Code first the infection*
> **Excludes1**   Methicillin resistant Staphylococcus aureus infection (A49.02)
> Methicillin resistant Staphylococcus aureus pneumonia (J15.212)
> Sepsis due to Methicillin resistant Staphylococcus aureus (A41.02)

● **Z16.1   Resistance to beta lactam antibiotics**

Z16.10   Resistance to unspecified beta lactam antibiotics

Z16.11   Resistance to penicillins
> Resistance to amoxicillin
> Resistance to ampicillin

Z16.12   Extended spectrum beta lactamase (ESBL) resistance
> **Excludes2**   Methicillin resistant Staphylococcus aureus infection in diseases classified elsewhere (B95.62)

Z16.13   Resistance to carbapenem

Z16.19   Resistance to other specified beta lactam antibiotics
> Resistance to cephalosporins

● **Z16.2   Resistance to other antibiotics**

Z16.20   Resistance to unspecified antibiotic
> Resistance to antibiotics NOS

Z16.21   Resistance to vancomycin

Z16.22   Resistance to vancomycin related antibiotics

Z16.23   Resistance to quinolones and fluoroquinolones

Z16.24   Resistance to multiple antibiotics

Z16.29   Resistance to other single specified antibiotic
> Resistance to aminoglycosides
> Resistance to macrolides
> Resistance to sulfonamides
> Resistance to tetracyclines

● **Z16.3   Resistance to other antimicrobial drugs**
> **Excludes1**   resistance to antibiotics (Z16.1-, Z16.2-)

Z16.30   Resistance to unspecified antimicrobial drugs
> Drug resistance NOS

Z16.31   Resistance to antiparasitic drug(s)
> Resistance to quinine and related compounds

Z16.32   Resistance to antifungal drug(s)

Z16.33   Resistance to antiviral drug(s)

● **Z16.34   Resistance to antimycobacterial drug(s)**
> Resistance to tuberculostatics

Z16.341   Resistance to single antimycobacterial drug
> Resistance to antimycobacterial drug NOS

Z16.342   Resistance to multiple antimycobacterial drugs

Z16.35   Resistance to multiple antimicrobial drugs
> **Excludes1**   Resistance to multiple antibiotics only (Z16.24)

Z16.39   Resistance to other specified antimicrobial drug

▶ New   ➡ Revised   ~~deleted~~ Deleted   Excludes 1   Excludes 2   Includes   Use additional   Code first   Code also   Key words
OGCR Official Guidelines   **X** Assign placeholder X   ● Use Additional Character(s)   ▍ Manifestation Code   Ⓗ Hierarchical Condition Category   **Coding Clinic**

ESTROGEN, AND OTHER HORMONES AND FACTORS RECEPTOR STATUS (Z17)

● **Z17**   **Estrogen, and other hormones and factors receptor status**

Note: Use one code, as available, for each receptor: Z17.0, Z17.1, Z17.2-. Z17.3-

Code first malignant neoplasm of breast (C50.-)

Code first malignant neoplasm, such as: malignant neoplasm of ovary (C56.-)

Z17.0   **Estrogen receptor positive status [ER+]**
Coding Clinic: 2022, Q3, P15

Z17.1   **Estrogen receptor negative status [ER-]**

● **Z17.2**   **Progesterone receptor status**

     Z17.21   **Progesterone receptor positive status**
        PR+

     Z17.22   **Progesterone receptor negative status**
        PR-

● **Z17.3**   **Human epidermal growth factor 2 receptor**

     Z17.31   **Human epidermal growth factor receptor 2 positive status**
        HER2+

     Z17.32   **Human epidermal growth factor receptor 2 negative status**
        HER2-

● **Z17.4**   **Combined receptor status**

Note: Assign a code from subcategory Z17.4- when only a combined receptor status is documented

   ● **Z17.41**   **Hormone receptor positive**
        HR+

       Z17.410   **Hormone receptor positive with human epidermal growth factor receptor 2 positive status**
          HR+ with HER2+

       Z17.411 Hormone receptor positive with human epidermal growth factor receptor 2 negative status
          HR+ with HER2-

   ● **Z17.42**   **Hormone receptor negative**
        HR-

       Z17.420   **Hormone receptor negative with human epidermal growth factor receptor 2 positive status**
          HR- with HER2+

       Z17.421   **Hormone receptor negative with human epidermal growth factor receptor 2 negative status**
          HR- with HER2-
          TNBC
          Triple negative breast cancer

RETAINED FOREIGN BODY FRAGMENTS (Z18)

● **Z18**   **Retained foreign body fragments**

   Includes   embedded fragment (status)
          embedded splinter (status)
          retained foreign body status

   Excludes1   artificial joint prosthesis status (Z96.6-)
          foreign body accidentally left during a procedure (T81.5-)
          foreign body entering through orifice (T15-T19)
          in situ cardiac device (Z95.-)
          organ or tissue replaced by means other than transplant (Z96.-, Z97.-)
          organ or tissue replaced by transplant (Z94.-)
          personal history of retained foreign body fully removed Z87.821
          superficial foreign body (non-embedded splinter) - code to superficial foreign body, by site

● **Z18.0**   **Retained radioactive fragments**

     Z18.01   **Retained depleted uranium fragments**

     Z18.09   **Other retained radioactive fragments**
          Other retained depleted isotope fragments
          Retained nontherapeutic radioactive fragments

● **Z18.1**   **Retained metal fragments**

   Excludes1   retained radioactive metal fragments (Z18.01-Z18.09)

     Z18.10   **Retained metal fragments, unspecified**
          Retained metal fragment NOS

     Z18.11   **Retained magnetic metal fragments**

     Z18.12   **Retained nonmagnetic metal fragments**

     Z18.2   **Retained plastic fragments**
        Acrylics fragments
        Diethylhexylphthalates fragments
        Isocyanate fragments

● **Z18.3**   **Retained organic fragments**

     Z18.31   **Retained animal quills or spines**

     Z18.32   **Retained tooth**

     Z18.33   **Retained wood fragments**

     Z18.39   **Other retained organic fragments**

● **Z18.8**   **Other specified retained foreign body**

     Z18.81   **Retained glass fragments**

     Z18.83   **Retained stone or crystalline fragments**
          Retained concrete or cement fragments

     Z18.89   **Other specified retained foreign body fragments**
          Coding Clinic: 2016, Q3, P24

     Z18.9   **Retained foreign body fragments, unspecified material**

HORMONE SENSITIVITY MALIGNANCY STATUS (Z19)

● **Z19**   **Hormone sensitivity malignancy status**

Code first malignant neoplasm —*see* Table of Neoplasms, by site, malignant
Coding Clinic: 2016, Q4, P129

     Z19.1   **Hormone sensitive malignancy status**
        Coding Clinic: 2016, Q4, P76

     Z19.2   **Hormone resistant malignancy status**
        Castrate resistant prostate malignancy status
        Coding Clinic: 2016, Q4, P76

PERSONS WITH POTENTIAL HEALTH HAZARDS RELATED TO COMMUNICABLE DISEASES (Z20-Z29)

● **Z20**   **Contact with and (suspected) exposure to communicable diseases**

   Excludes1   carrier of infectious disease (Z22.-)
          diagnosed current infectious or parasitic disease - see Alphabetic Index

   Excludes2   personal history of infectious and parasitic diseases (Z86.1-)
   Coding Clinic: 2021, Q1, P37

● **Z20.0**   **Contact with and (suspected) exposure to intestinal infectious diseases**

     Z20.01   **Contact with and (suspected) exposure to intestinal infectious diseases due to Escherichia coli (E. coli)**

     Z20.09   **Contact with and (suspected) exposure to other intestinal infectious diseases**

     Z20.1   **Contact with and (suspected) exposure to tuberculosis**

     Z20.2   **Contact with and (suspected) exposure to infections with a predominantly sexual mode of transmission**

     Z20.3   **Contact with and (suspected) exposure to rabies**

     Z20.4   **Contact with and (suspected) exposure to rubella**

     Z20.5   **Contact with and (suspected) exposure to viral hepatitis**

     Z20.6   **Contact with and (suspected) exposure to human immunodeficiency virus [HIV]**

   Excludes1   asymptomatic human immunodeficiency virus [HIV]
          HIV infection status (Z21)

     Z20.7   **Contact with and (suspected) exposure to pediculosis, acariasis and other infestations**

● **Z20.8** **Contact with and (suspected) exposure to other communicable diseases**

  ● **Z20.81** **Contact with and (suspected) exposure to other bacterial communicable diseases**

    Z20.810 **Contact with and (suspected) exposure to anthrax**

    Z20.811 **Contact with and (suspected) exposure to meningococcus**

    Z20.818 **Contact with and (suspected) exposure to other bacterial communicable diseases**

  ● **Z20.82** **Contact with and (suspected) exposure to other viral communicable diseases**

    Z20.820 **Contact with and (suspected) exposure to varicella**

    Z20.821 **Contact with and (suspected) exposure to Zika virus**

    Z20.822 **Contact with and (suspected) exposure to COVID-19**

      Contact with and (suspected) exposure to SARS-CoV-2

      Coding Clinic: 2023, Q2, P3-4; 2022, Q2, P28,29; 2021, Q4, P109; 2021, Q1, P37-39, 42

    Z20.828 **Contact with and (suspected) exposure to other viral communicable diseases**

      Coding Clinic: 2022, Q3, P4; 2021, Q1, P37-39; 2016, Q4, P6-7, 121

  Z20.89 **Contact with and (suspected) exposure to other communicable diseases**

 Z20.9 **Contact with and (suspected) exposure to unspecified communicable disease**

Z21 **Asymptomatic human immunodeficiency virus [HIV] infection status** ℞𝒸

  HIV positive NOS

  Code first Human immunodeficiency virus [HIV] disease complicating pregnancy, childbirth and the puerperium, if applicable (O98.7-)

  Excludes1 acquired immunodeficiency syndrome (B20)
    contact with human immunodeficiency virus [HIV] (Z20.6)
    exposure to human immunodeficiency virus [HIV] (Z20.6)
    human immunodeficiency virus [HIV] disease (B20)
    inconclusive laboratory evidence of human immunodeficiency virus [HIV] (R75)

  Coding Clinic: 2022, Q1, P37; 2019, Q1, P10-11

● **Z22** **Carrier of infectious disease**

  Includes colonization status
    suspected carrier

  Excludes2 carrier of viral hepatitis (B18.-)

 Z22.0 **Carrier of typhoid**

 Z22.1 **Carrier of other intestinal infectious diseases**

 Z22.2 **Carrier of diphtheria**

 ● **Z22.3** **Carrier of other specified bacterial diseases**

  Z22.31 **Carrier of bacterial disease due to meningococci**

  ● **Z22.32** **Carrier of bacterial disease due to staphylococci**

    Z22.321 **Carrier or suspected carrier of Methicillin susceptible Staphylococcus aureus**
      MSSA colonization

    Z22.322 **Carrier or suspected carrier of Methicillin resistant Staphylococcus aureus**
      MRSA colonization

  ● **Z22.33** **Carrier of bacterial disease due to streptococci**

    Z22.330 **Carrier of Group B streptococcus**

      Excludes1 Carrier of streptococcus group B (GBS) complicating pregnancy, childbirth and the puerperium (O99.82-)

    Z22.338 **Carrier of other streptococcus**

  ● **Z22.34** **Carrier of Acinetobacter baumannii**

    Z22.340 **Carrier of carbapenem-resistant Acinetobacter baumannii**

    Z22.341 **Carrier of carbapenem-sensitive Acinetobacter baumannii**

    Z22.349 **Carrier of Acinetobacter baumannii, unspecified**

  ● **Z22.35** **Carrier of Enterobacterales**

    Carrier of E. coli
    Carrier of K. pneumoniae

    Z22.350 **Carrier of carbapenem-resistant Enterobacterales**

    Z22.358 **Carrier of other Enterobacterales**

      Carrier of carbapenem-sensitive Enterobacterales
      Carrier of ESBL-producing Enterobacterales
      Carrier of extended-spectrum beta-lactamase producing Enterobacterales

    Z22.359 **Carrier of Enterobacterales, unspecified**

  Z22.39 **Carrier of other specified bacterial diseases**

 Z22.4 **Carrier of infections with a predominantly sexual mode of transmission**

 Z22.6 **Carrier of human T-lymphotropic virus type-1 [HTLV-1] infection**

 Z22.7 **Latent tuberculosis**

  Latent tuberculosis infection (LTBI)

  Excludes1 nonspecific reaction to cell mediated immunity measurement of gamma interferon antigen response without active tuberculosis (R76.12)
    nonspecific reaction to tuberculin skin test without active tuberculosis (R76.11)

 Z22.8 **Carrier of other infectious diseases**

 Z22.9 **Carrier of infectious disease, unspecified**

Z23 **Encounter for immunization**

  Code first any routine childhood examination

  Note: Procedure codes are required to identify the types of immunizations given.

  Code also, if applicable, encounter for immunization safety counseling (Z71.85)

  Coding Clinic: 2024, Q4, P6

● **Z28** **Immunization not carried out and underimmunization status**

  Includes vaccination not carried out

  Code also, if applicable, encounter for immunization safety counseling (Z71.85)

 ● **Z28.0** **Immunization not carried out because of contraindication**

  Z28.01 **Immunization not carried out because of acute illness of patient**

  Z28.02 **Immunization not carried out because of chronic illness or condition of patient**

  Z28.03 **Immunization not carried out because of immune compromised state of patient**

  Z28.04 **Immunization not carried out because of patient allergy to vaccine or component**

  Z28.09 **Immunization not carried out because of other contraindication**

▶ New   ➡ Revised   ~~deleted~~ Deleted   Excludes 1   Excludes 2   Includes   Use additional   Code first   Code also   Key words

OGCR Official Guidelines   **X** Assign placeholder X   ● Use Additional Character(s)   ▶ Manifestation Code   ℞𝒸 Hierarchical Condition Category   **Coding Clinic**

Z28.1　Immunization not carried out because of patient decision for reasons of belief or group pressure
Immunization not carried out because of religious belief

● Z28.2　Immunization not carried out because of patient decision for other and unspecified reason

Z28.20　Immunization not carried out because of patient decision for unspecified reason

Z28.21　Immunization not carried out because of patient refusal

Z28.29　Immunization not carried out because of patient decision for other reason

Z28.3　Underimmunization status
Coding Clinic: 2021, Q4, P110
Use additional code, if applicable, to identify:
immunization not carried out because of contraindication (Z28.0-)
immunization not carried out because of patient decision for other and unspecified reason (Z28.2-)
immunization not carried out because of patient decision for reasons of belief or group pressure (Z28.1)
immunization not carried out for other reason (Z28.8-)

Z28.31　Underimmunization for COVID-19 status
Note: These codes should not be used for individuals who are not eligible for the COVID-19 vaccines, as determined by the healthcare provider.

Z28.310　Unvaccinated for COVID-19

Z28.311　Partially vaccinated for COVID-19

Z28.39　Other underimmunization status
Delinquent immunization status
Lapsed immunization schedule status

● Z28.8　Immunization not carried out for other reason

Z28.81　Immunization not carried out due to patient having had the disease

Z28.82　Immunization not carried out because of caregiver refusal
Immunization not carried out because of guardian refusal
Immunization not carried out because of parent refusal
Excludes1　immunization not carried out because of caregiver refusal because of religious belief (Z28.1)

Z28.83　Immunization not carried out due to unavailability of vaccine
Delay in delivery of vaccine
Lack of availability of vaccine
Manufacturer delay of vaccine

Z28.89　Immunization not carried out for other reason

Z28.9　Immunization not carried out for unspecified reason

● Z29　Encounter for other prophylactic measures
Excludes1　desensitization to allergens (Z51.6)
prophylactic surgery (Z40.-)
Coding Clinic: 2016, Q4, P130

● Z29.1　Encounter for prophylactic immunotherapy
Encounter for administration of immunoglobulin
Coding Clinic: 2016, Q4, P78-79

Z29.11　Encounter for prophylactic immunotherapy for respiratory syncytial virus (RSV)

Z29.12　Encounter for prophylactic antivenin

Z29.13　Encounter for prophylactic Rho(D) immune globulin
Coding Clinic: 2019, Q3, P5

Z29.14　Encounter for prophylactic rabies immune globin

Z29.3　Encounter for prophylactic fluoride administration
Coding Clinic: 2016, Q4, P79

● Z29.8　Encounter for other specified prophylactic measures
Coding Clinic: 2022, Q2, P27; 2016, Q4, P79

Z29.81　Encounter for HIV pre-exposure prophylaxis
Code also, if applicable, risk factors for HIV, such as:
contact with and (suspected) exposure to human immunodeficiency virus [HIV](Z20.6)
high risk sexual behavior (Z72.5-)

Z29.89　Encounter for other specified prophylactic measures

Z29.9　Encounter for prophylactic measures, unspecified
Coding Clinic: 2016, Q4, P79

PERSONS ENCOUNTERING HEALTH SERVICES IN CIRCUMSTANCES RELATED TO REPRODUCTION (Z30-Z39)

● Z30　Encounter for contraceptive management

● Z30.0　Encounter for general counseling and advice on contraception

● Z30.01　Encounter for initial prescription of contraceptives
Excludes1　encounter for surveillance of contraceptives (Z30.4-)

Z30.011　Encounter for initial prescription of contraceptive pills

Z30.012　Encounter for prescription of emergency contraception
Encounter for postcoital contraception

Z30.013　Encounter for initial prescription of injectable contraceptive

Z30.014　Encounter for initial prescription of intrauterine contraceptive device
Excludes1　encounter for insertion of intrauterine contraceptive device (Z30.430, Z30.432)

Z30.015　Encounter for initial prescription of vaginal ring hormonal contraceptive
Coding Clinic: 2016, Q4, P78

Z30.016　Encounter for initial prescription of transdermal patch hormonal contraceptive device
Coding Clinic: 2016, Q4, P78

Z30.017　Encounter for initial prescription of implantable subdermal contraceptive
Coding Clinic: 2016, Q4, P78

Z30.018　Encounter for initial prescription of other contraceptives
Encounter for initial prescription of barrier contraception
Encounter for initial prescription of diaphragm

Z30.019　Encounter for initial prescription of contraceptives, unspecified

Z30.02　Counseling and instruction in natural family planning to avoid pregnancy

Z30.09　Encounter for other general counseling and advice on contraception
Encounter for family planning advice NOS

Z30.2　Encounter for sterilization
Coding Clinic: 2021, Q3, P13

● Z30.4　Encounter for surveillance of contraceptives

Z30.40　Encounter for surveillance of contraceptives, unspecified

Z30.41　Encounter for surveillance of contraceptive pills
Encounter for repeat prescription for contraceptive pill

Z30.42　Encounter for surveillance of injectable contraceptive

CHAPTER 21 (Z00-Z99)

● **Z30.43**   **Encounter for surveillance of intrauterine contraceptive device**

    Z30.430   **Encounter for insertion of intrauterine contraceptive device**

    Z30.431   **Encounter for routine checking of intrauterine contraceptive device**

    Z30.432   **Encounter for removal of intrauterine contraceptive device**

    Z30.433   **Encounter for removal and reinsertion of intrauterine contraceptive device**
        Encounter for replacement of intrauterine contraceptive device

  Z30.44   **Encounter for surveillance of vaginal ring hormonal contraceptive device**
    Coding Clinic: 2016, Q4, P78

  Z30.45   **Encounter for surveillance of transdermal patch hormonal contraceptive device**
    Coding Clinic: 2016, Q4, P78

  Z30.46   **Encounter for surveillance of implantable subdermal contraceptive**
    Encounter for checking, reinsertion or removal of implantable subdermal contraceptive
    Coding Clinic: 2016, Q4, P78

  Z30.49   **Encounter for surveillance of other contraceptives**
    Encounter for surveillance of barrier contraception
    Encounter for surveillance of diaphragm

Z30.8   **Encounter for other contraceptive management**
  Encounter for postvasectomy sperm count
  Encounter for routine examination for contraceptive maintenance

  Excludes1   sperm count following sterilization reversal (Z31.42)
    sperm count for fertility testing (Z31.41)

Z30.9   **Encounter for contraceptive management, unspecified**

● **Z31**   **Encounter for procreative management**

  Excludes2   complications associated with artificial fertilization (N98.-)
    female infertility (N97.-)
    male infertility (N46.-)

Z31.0   **Encounter for reversal of previous sterilization**

● **Z31.4**   **Encounter for procreative investigation and testing**

  Excludes1   postvasectomy sperm count (Z30.8)

Z31.41   **Encounter for fertility testing**
  Encounter for fallopian tube patency testing
  Encounter for sperm count for fertility testing

Z31.42   **Aftercare following sterilization reversal**
  Sperm count following sterilization reversal

● **Z31.43**   **Encounter for genetic testing of female for procreative management**

  Use additional code for recurrent pregnancy loss, if applicable (N96, O26.2-)

  Excludes1   nonprocreative genetic testing (Z13.7-)

    Z31.430   **Encounter of female for testing for genetic disease carrier status for procreative management**

    Z31.438   **Encounter for other genetic testing of female for procreative management**

● **Z31.44**   **Encounter for genetic testing of male for procreative management**

  Excludes1   nonprocreative genetic testing (Z13.7-)

    Z31.440   **Encounter of male for testing for genetic disease carrier status for procreative management**

    Z31.441   **Encounter for testing of male partner of patient with recurrent pregnancy loss**   **A**

    Z31.448   **Encounter for other genetic testing of male for procreative management**   **A**

Z31.49   **Encounter for other procreative investigation and testing**

Z31.5   **Encounter for procreative genetic counseling**

● **Z31.6**   **Encounter for general counseling and advice on procreation**

  Z31.61   **Procreative counseling and advice using natural family planning**

  Z31.62   **Encounter for fertility preservation counseling**
    Encounter for fertility preservation counseling prior to cancer therapy
    Encounter for fertility preservation counseling prior to surgical removal of gonads

  Z31.69   **Encounter for other general counseling and advice on procreation**

Z31.7   **Encounter for procreative management and counseling for gestational carrier**

  Excludes1   pregnant state, gestational carrier (Z33.3)
  Coding Clinic: 2016, Q4, P78

● **Z31.8**   **Encounter for other procreative management**

  Z31.81   **Encounter for male factor infertility in female patient**

  Z31.82   **Encounter for Rh incompatibility status**
    Coding Clinic: 2015, Q3, P40

  Z31.83   **Encounter for assisted reproductive fertility procedure cycle**
    Patient undergoing in vitro fertilization cycle
    Use additional code to identify the type of infertility

    Excludes1   pre-cycle diagnosis and testing - code to reason for encounter
    Coding Clinic: 2022, Q2, P15,16

  Z31.84   **Encounter for fertility preservation procedure**
    Encounter for fertility preservation procedure prior to cancer therapy
    Encounter for fertility preservation procedure prior to surgical removal of gonads

  Z31.89   **Encounter for other procreative management**

Z31.9   **Encounter for procreative management, unspecified**

● **Z32**   **Encounter for pregnancy test and childbirth and childcare instruction**

● **Z32.0**   **Encounter for pregnancy test**

  Z32.00   **Encounter for pregnancy test, result unknown**
    Encounter for pregnancy test NOS

  Z32.01   **Encounter for pregnancy test, result positive**   **M**

  Z32.02   **Encounter for pregnancy test, result negative**

Z32.2   **Encounter for childbirth instruction**

Z32.3   **Encounter for childcare instruction**
  Encounter for prenatal or postpartum childcare instruction

● **Z33**   **Pregnant state**

Z33.1   **Pregnant state, incidental**   **M**
  Pregnancy NOS
  Pregnant state NOS

  Excludes1   complications of pregnancy (O00-O9A)
    pregnant state, gestational carrier (Z33.3)

Z33.2   **Encounter for elective termination of pregnancy**   **M**

  Excludes1   early fetal death with retention of dead fetus (O02.1)
    late fetal death (O36.4)
    spontaneous abortion (O03)
  Coding Clinic: 2023, Q2, P15; 2016, Q4, P130

Z33.3   **Pregnant state, gestational carrier**

  Excludes1   encounter for procreative management and counseling for gestational carrier (Z31.7)
  Coding Clinic: 2024, Q3, P9; 2016, Q4, P78

● **Z34**   **Encounter for supervision of normal pregnancy**

  Excludes1   any complication of pregnancy (O00-O9A)
    encounter for pregnancy test (Z32.0-)
    encounter for supervision of high risk pregnancy (O09.-)
  Coding Clinic: 2016, Q4, P6

▶ New   ⇥ Revised   ~~deleted~~ Deleted   Excludes 1   Excludes 2   Includes   Use additional   Code first   Code also   Key words

OGCR Official Guidelines   **X** Assign placeholder X   ● Use Additional Character(s)   ▸ Manifestation Code   Hierarchical Condition Category   **Coding Clinic**

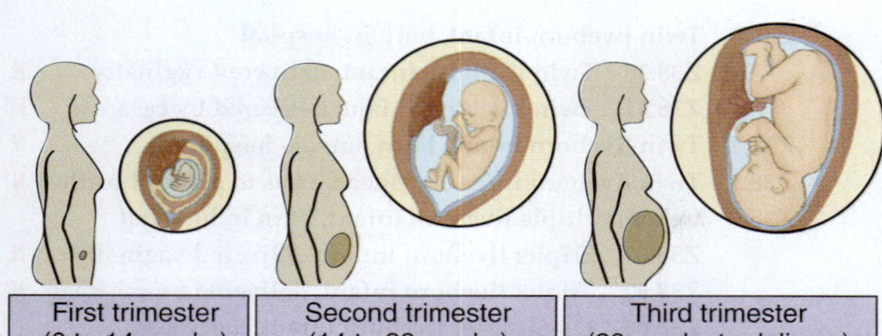

Figure 21-1   Trimesters. (From Shiland, Betsy J. Medical Terminology & Anatomy for ICD-10 Coding, ed 2, Mosby, 2015)

- ● **Z34.0   Encounter for supervision of normal first pregnancy**
    - **Z34.00   Encounter for supervision of normal first pregnancy, unspecified trimester**   M
    - **Z34.01   Encounter for supervision of normal first pregnancy, first trimester**   M
    - **Z34.02   Encounter for supervision of normal first pregnancy, second trimester**   M
    - **Z34.03   Encounter for supervision of normal first pregnancy, third trimester**   M
- ● **Z34.8   Encounter for supervision of other normal pregnancy**
    - **Z34.80   Encounter for supervision of other normal pregnancy, unspecified trimester**   M
    - **Z34.81   Encounter for supervision of other normal pregnancy, first trimester**   M
    - **Z34.82   Encounter for supervision of other normal pregnancy, second trimester**   M
    - **Z34.83   Encounter for supervision of other normal pregnancy, third trimester**   M
- ● **Z34.9   Encounter for supervision of normal pregnancy, unspecified**
    - **Z34.90   Encounter for supervision of normal pregnancy, unspecified, unspecified trimester**   M
    - **Z34.91   Encounter for supervision of normal pregnancy, unspecified, first trimester**   M
    - **Z34.92   Encounter for supervision of normal pregnancy, unspecified, second trimester**   M
    - **Z34.93   Encounter for supervision of normal pregnancy, unspecified, third trimester**   M
- ● **Z36   Encounter for antenatal screening of mother**
    - **Includes**   Encounter for placental sample (taken vaginally)
      Screening is the testing for disease or disease precursors in asymptomatic individuals so that early detection and treatment can be provided for those who test positive for the disease.
    - **Excludes1**   diagnostic examination - code to sign or symptom
      encounter for suspected maternal and fetal conditions ruled out (Z03.7-)
      suspected fetal condition affecting management of pregnancy - code to condition in Chapter 15
    - **Excludes2**   abnormal findings on antenatal screening of mother (O28.-)
      genetic counseling and testing (Z31.43-, Z31.5)
      routine prenatal care (Z34)
    - **Z36.0   Encounter for antenatal screening for chromosomal anomalies**   M
    - **Z36.1   Encounter for antenatal screening for raised alphafetoprotein level**   M
      Encounter for antenatal screening for elevated maternal serum alphafetoprotein level
    - **Z36.2   Encounter for other antenatal screening follow-up**   M
      Non-visualized anatomy on a previous scan
    - **Z36.3   Encounter for antenatal screening for malformations**   M
      Screening for a suspected anomaly

- **Z36.4   Encounter for antenatal screening for fetal growth retardation**   M
  Intrauterine growth restriction (IUGR)/small-for-dates
- **Z36.5   Encounter for antenatal screening for isoimmunization**   M
- ● **Z36.8   Encounter for other antenatal screening**
    - **Z36.81   Encounter for antenatal screening for hydrops fetalis**   M
    - **Z36.82   Encounter for antenatal screening for nuchal translucency**   M
    - **Z36.83   Encounter for fetal screening for congenital cardiac abnormalities**   M
    - **Z36.84   Encounter for antenatal screening for fetal lung maturity**   M
    - **Z36.85   Encounter for antenatal screening for Streptococcus B**   M
    - **Z36.86   Encounter for antenatal screening for cervical length**   M
      Screening for risk of pre-term labor
    - **Z36.87   Encounter for antenatal screening for uncertain dates**   M
    - **Z36.88   Encounter for antenatal screening for fetal macrosomia**   M
      Screening for large-for-dates
    - **Z36.89   Encounter for other specified antenatal screening**   M
    - **Z36.8A   Encounter for antenatal screening for other genetic defects**   M
- **Z36.9   Encounter for antenatal screening, unspecified**   M
- ● **Z3A   Weeks of gestation**
    - **Note:** Codes from category Z3A are for use, only on the maternal record, to indicate the weeks of gestation of the pregnancy, if known.
    - *Code first obstetric condition or encounter for delivery (O09-O60, O80-O82)*
    - **Coding Clinic: 2022, Q2, P3-4; 2016, Q4, P130; 2013, Q2, P33**
    - ● **Z3A.0   Weeks of gestation of pregnancy, unspecified or less than 10 weeks**
        - **Z3A.00   Weeks of gestation of pregnancy not specified**   M
        - **Z3A.01   Less than 8 weeks gestation of pregnancy**   M
        - **Z3A.08   8 weeks gestation of pregnancy**   M
        - **Z3A.09   9 weeks gestation of pregnancy**   M
    - ● **Z3A.1   Weeks of gestation of pregnancy, weeks 10-19**
        - **Z3A.10   10 weeks gestation of pregnancy**   M
        - **Z3A.11   11 weeks gestation of pregnancy**   M
        - **Z3A.12   12 weeks gestation of pregnancy**   M
        - **Z3A.13   13 weeks gestation of pregnancy**   M
        - **Z3A.14   14 weeks gestation of pregnancy**   M
        - **Z3A.15   15 weeks gestation of pregnancy**   M
        - **Z3A.16   16 weeks gestation of pregnancy**   M
          Coding Clinic: 2016, Q4, P5
        - **Z3A.17   17 weeks gestation of pregnancy**   M
        - **Z3A.18   18 weeks gestation of pregnancy**   M
          Coding Clinic: 2019, Q2, P11
        - **Z3A.19   19 weeks gestation of pregnancy**   M
    - ● **Z3A.2   Weeks of gestation of pregnancy, weeks 20-29**
        - **Z3A.20   20 weeks gestation of pregnancy**   M
          Coding Clinic: 2016, Q4, P6
        - **Z3A.21   21 weeks gestation of pregnancy**   M
        - **Z3A.22   22 weeks gestation of pregnancy**   M
          Coding Clinic: 2016, Q4, P6
        - **Z3A.23   23 weeks gestation of pregnancy**   M
        - **Z3A.24   24 weeks gestation of pregnancy**   M
        - **Z3A.25   25 weeks gestation of pregnancy**   M
        - **Z3A.26   26 weeks gestation of pregnancy**   M
        - **Z3A.27   27 weeks gestation of pregnancy**   M
        - **Z3A.28   28 weeks gestation of pregnancy**   M
        - **Z3A.29   29 weeks gestation of pregnancy**   M

CHAPTER 21 (Z00-Z99)

● **Z3A.3 Weeks of gestation of pregnancy, weeks 30-39**
- Z3A.30   30 weeks gestation of pregnancy   **M**
- Z3A.31   31 weeks gestation of pregnancy   **M**
- Z3A.32   32 weeks gestation of pregnancy   **M**
  - *Coding Clinic: 2016, Q4, P6*
- Z3A.33   33 weeks gestation of pregnancy   **M**
- Z3A.34   34 weeks gestation of pregnancy   **M**
- Z3A.35   35 weeks gestation of pregnancy   **M**
- Z3A.36   36 weeks gestation of pregnancy   **M**
- Z3A.37   37 weeks gestation of pregnancy   **M**
- Z3A.38   38 weeks gestation of pregnancy   **M**
  - *Coding Clinic: 2016, Q2, P34*
- Z3A.39   39 weeks gestation of pregnancy   **M**

● **Z3A.4 Weeks of gestation of pregnancy, weeks 40 or greater**
- Z3A.40   40 weeks gestation of pregnancy   **M**
- Z3A.41   41 weeks gestation of pregnancy   **M**
- Z3A.42   42 weeks gestation of pregnancy   **M**
- Z3A.49   Greater than 42 weeks gestation of pregnancy   **M**

● **Z37 Outcome of delivery**
This category is intended for use as an additional code to identify the outcome of delivery on the mother's record. It is not for use on the newborn record.

Excludes1   stillbirth (P95)

Z37.0 Single live birth   **M**
- *Coding Clinic: 2024, Q3, P9; 2016, Q2, P34*

Z37.1 Single stillbirth   **M**
Z37.2 Twins, both liveborn   **M**
Z37.3 Twins, one liveborn and one stillborn   **M**
Z37.4 Twins, both stillborn   **M**

● **Z37.5 Other multiple births, all liveborn**
- Z37.50   Multiple births, unspecified, all liveborn   **M**
- Z37.51   Triplets, all liveborn   **M**
- Z37.52   Quadruplets, all liveborn   **M**
- Z37.53   Quintuplets, all liveborn   **M**
- Z37.54   Sextuplets, all liveborn   **M**
- Z37.59   Other multiple births, all liveborn   **M**

● **Z37.6 Other multiple births, some liveborn**
- Z37.60   Multiple births, unspecified, some liveborn   **M**
- Z37.61   Triplets, some liveborn   **M**
- Z37.62   Quadruplets, some liveborn   **M**
- Z37.63   Quintuplets, some liveborn   **M**
- Z37.64   Sextuplets, some liveborn   **M**
- Z37.69   Other multiple births, some liveborn   **M**

Z37.7 Other multiple births, all stillborn   **M**
Z37.9 Outcome of delivery, unspecified   **M**
Multiple birth NOS
Single birth NOS

● **Z38 Liveborn infants according to place of birth and type of delivery**
This category is for use as the principal code on the initial record of a newborn baby. It is to be used for the initial birth record only. It is not to be used on the mother's record.
- *Coding Clinic: 2017, Q2, P6-7; 2016, Q4, P126-127, 130; 2015, Q2, P15*

● **Z38.0 Single liveborn infant, born in hospital**
Single liveborn infant, born in birthing center or other health care facility
- *Coding Clinic: 2017, Q2, P5-7*
- Z38.00   Single liveborn infant, delivered vaginally   **N**
  - *Coding Clinic: 2021, Q4, P23; 2018, Q4, P26; 2016, Q4, P7, 55*
- Z38.01   Single liveborn infant, delivered by cesarean   **N**
  - *Coding Clinic: 2017, Q2, P7; 2016, Q3, P18*

Z38.1 Single liveborn infant, born outside hospital   **N**
Z38.2 Single liveborn infant, unspecified as to place of birth   **N**
Single liveborn infant NOS

● **Z38.3 Twin liveborn infant, born in hospital**
- Z38.30   Twin liveborn infant, delivered vaginally   **N**
- Z38.31   Twin liveborn infant, delivered by cesarean   **N**

Z38.4 Twin liveborn infant, born outside hospital   **N**
Z38.5 Twin liveborn infant, unspecified as to place of birth   **N**

● **Z38.6 Other multiple liveborn infant, born in hospital**
- Z38.61   Triplet liveborn infant, delivered vaginally   **N**
- Z38.62   Triplet liveborn infant, delivered by cesarean   **N**
- Z38.63   Quadruplet liveborn infant, delivered vaginally   **N**
- Z38.64   Quadruplet liveborn infant, delivered by cesarean   **N**
- Z38.65   Quintuplet liveborn infant, delivered vaginally   **N**
- Z38.66   Quintuplet liveborn infant, delivered by cesarean   **N**
- Z38.68   Other multiple liveborn infant, delivered vaginally   **N**
- Z38.69   Other multiple liveborn infant, delivered by cesarean   **N**

Z38.7 Other multiple liveborn infant, born outside hospital   **N**
Z38.8 Other multiple liveborn infant, unspecified as to place of birth   **N**

● **Z39 Encounter for maternal postpartum care and examination**
Z39.0 Encounter for care and examination of mother immediately after delivery   **M**
Care and observation in uncomplicated cases when the delivery occurs outside a healthcare facility

Excludes1   care for postpartum complication - see Alphabetic index
- *Coding Clinic: 2021, Q3, P13*

Z39.1 Encounter for care and examination of lactating mother   **M**
Encounter for supervision of lactation

Excludes1   disorders of lactation (O92.-)

Z39.2 Encounter for routine postpartum follow-up   **M**

ENCOUNTERS FOR OTHER SPECIFIC HEALTH CARE (Z40-Z53)

Categories Z40-Z53 are intended for use to indicate a reason for care. They may be used for patients who have already been treated for a disease or injury, but who are receiving aftercare or prophylactic care, or care to consolidate the treatment, or to deal with a residual state

Excludes2   follow-up examination for medical surveillance after treatment (Z08-Z09)

● **Z40 Encounter for prophylactic surgery**
Excludes1   organ donations (Z52.-)
therapeutic organ removal - code to condition
- *Coding Clinic: 2016, Q4, P79*

● **Z40.0 Encounter for prophylactic surgery for risk factors related to malignant neoplasms**
Admission for prophylactic organ removal
➡ Use additional code to identify risk factor, such as genetic susceptibility to malignant neoplasm Z15.-

- Z40.00   Encounter for prophylactic removal of unspecified organ
- Z40.01   Encounter for prophylactic removal of breast
- Z40.02   Encounter for prophylactic removal of ovary(s)
  - ~~Encounter for prophylactic removal of ovary(s) and fallopian tube(s)~~
- Z40.03   Encounter for prophylactic removal of fallopian tube(s)
- Z40.09   Encounter for prophylactic removal of other organ

● **Z40.8   Encounter for other prophylactic surgery**
▶ **Z40.81   Encounter for prophylactic surgery for removal of ovary(s) for persons without known genetic/familial risk factors**
▶ Encounter for prophylactic oophorectomy for persons without known genetic/ familial risk factors
▶ **Z40.82   Encounter for prophylactic surgery for removal of fallopian tube(s) for persons without known genetic/familial risk factors**
▶ Encounter for prophylactic salpingectomy for persons without known genetic/familial risk factors
▶ Opportunistic salpingectomy
▶ **Z40.89   Encounter for other prophylactic surgery**
Z40.9   Encounter for prophylactic surgery, unspecified

● **Z41   Encounter for procedures for purposes other than remedying health state**
Z41.1   Encounter for cosmetic surgery
Encounter for cosmetic breast implant
Encounter for cosmetic procedure
Excludes1   encounter for plastic and reconstructive surgery following medical procedure or healed injury (Z42.-)
encounter for post-mastectomy breast implantation (Z42.1)
Z41.2   Encounter for routine and ritual male circumcision
Z41.3   Encounter for ear piercing
Z41.8   Encounter for other procedures for purposes other than remedying health state
Z41.9   Encounter for procedure for purposes other than remedying health state, unspecified

● **Z42   Encounter for plastic and reconstructive surgery following medical procedure or healed injury**
Excludes1   encounter for cosmetic plastic surgery (Z41.1)
encounter for plastic surgery for treatment of current injury - code to relevent injury
Z42.1   Encounter for breast reconstruction following mastectomy
Excludes1   deformity and disproportion of reconstructed breast (N65.1-)
Z42.8   Encounter for other plastic and reconstructive surgery following medical procedure or healed injury
Coding Clinic: 2017, Q1, P42

● **Z43   Encounter for attention to artificial openings**
Includes   closure of artificial openings
passage of sounds or bougies through artificial openings
reforming artificial openings
removal of catheter from artificial openings
toilet or cleansing of artificial openings
Excludes1   complications of external stoma (J95.0-, K94.-, N99.5-)
Excludes2   fitting and adjustment of prosthetic and other devices (Z44-Z46)
Z43.0   Encounter for attention to tracheostomy
Z43.1   Encounter for attention to gastrostomy
Excludes2   artificial opening status only, without need for care (Z93.-)
Z43.2   Encounter for attention to ileostomy
Coding Clinic: 2016, Q3, P5
Z43.3   Encounter for attention to colostomy
Z43.4   Encounter for attention to other artificial openings of digestive tract
Z43.5   Encounter for attention to cystostomy
Z43.6   Encounter for attention to other artificial openings of urinary tract
Encounter for attention to nephrostomy
Encounter for attention to ureterostomy
Encounter for attention to urethrostomy
Z43.7   Encounter for attention to artificial vagina

Z43.8   Encounter for attention to other artificial openings
Z43.9   Encounter for attention to unspecified artificial opening

● **Z44   Encounter for fitting and adjustment of external prosthetic device**
Includes   removal or replacement of external prosthetic device
Excludes1   malfunction or other complications of device - see Alphabetical Index presence of prosthetic device (Z97.-)
● **Z44.0   Encounter for fitting and adjustment of artificial arm**
● **Z44.00   Encounter for fitting and adjustment of unspecified artificial arm**
Z44.001   Encounter for fitting and adjustment of unspecified right artificial arm
Z44.002   Encounter for fitting and adjustment of unspecified left artificial arm
Z44.009   Encounter for fitting and adjustment of unspecified artificial arm, unspecified arm
● **Z44.01   Encounter for fitting and adjustment of complete artificial arm**
Z44.011   Encounter for fitting and adjustment of complete right artificial arm
Z44.012   Encounter for fitting and adjustment of complete left artificial arm
Z44.019   Encounter for fitting and adjustment of complete artificial arm, unspecified arm
● **Z44.02   Encounter for fitting and adjustment of partial artificial arm**
Z44.021   Encounter for fitting and adjustment of partial artificial right arm
Z44.022   Encounter for fitting and adjustment of partial artificial left arm
Z44.029   Encounter for fitting and adjustment of partial artificial arm, unspecified arm
● **Z44.1   Encounter for fitting and adjustment of artificial leg**
● **Z44.10   Encounter for fitting and adjustment of unspecified artificial leg**
Z44.101   Encounter for fitting and adjustment of unspecified right artificial leg
Z44.102   Encounter for fitting and adjustment of unspecified left artificial leg
Z44.109   Encounter for fitting and adjustment of unspecified artificial leg, unspecified leg
● **Z44.11   Encounter for fitting and adjustment of complete artificial leg**
Z44.111   Encounter for fitting and adjustment of complete right artificial leg
Z44.112   Encounter for fitting and adjustment of complete left artificial leg
Z44.119   Encounter for fitting and adjustment of complete artificial leg, unspecified leg
● **Z44.12   Encounter for fitting and adjustment of partial artificial leg**
Z44.121   Encounter for fitting and adjustment of partial artificial right leg
Z44.122   Encounter for fitting and adjustment of partial artificial left leg
Z44.129   Encounter for fitting and adjustment of partial artificial leg, unspecified leg
● **Z44.2   Encounter for fitting and adjustment of artificial eye**
Excludes1   mechanical complication of ocular prosthesis (T85.3)
Z44.20   Encounter for fitting and adjustment of artificial eye, unspecified
Z44.21   Encounter for fitting and adjustment of artificial right eye
Z44.22   Encounter for fitting and adjustment of artificial left eye

A

● **Z44.3 Encounter for fitting and adjustment of external breast prosthesis**

    Excludes1   complications of breast implant (T85.4-)
        encounter for adjustment or removal of breast implant (Z45.81-)
        encounter for initial breast implant insertion for cosmetic breast augmentation (Z41.1)
        encounter for breast reconstruction following mastectomy (Z42.1)

    Z44.30 Encounter for fitting and adjustment of external breast prosthesis, unspecified breast

    Z44.31 Encounter for fitting and adjustment of external right breast prosthesis

    Z44.32 Encounter for fitting and adjustment of external left breast prosthesis

  Z44.8 Encounter for fitting and adjustment of other external prosthetic devices

  Z44.9 Encounter for fitting and adjustment of unspecified external prosthetic device

● **Z45 Encounter for adjustment and management of implanted device**

    Includes   removal or replacement of implanted device
    Excludes1   malfunction or other complications of device - see Alphabetical Index
    Excludes2   encounter for fitting and adjustment of non-implanted device (Z46.-)

● **Z45.0 Encounter for adjustment and management of cardiac device**

● **Z45.01 Encounter for adjustment and management of cardiac pacemaker**

    Encounter for adjustment and management of cardiac resynchronization therapy pacemaker (CRT-P)

    Excludes1   encounter for adjustment and management of automatic implantable cardiac defibrillator with synchronous cardiac pacemaker (Z45.02)

    Z45.010 Encounter for checking and testing of cardiac pacemaker pulse generator [battery]
        Encounter for replacing cardiac pacemaker pulse generator [battery]

    Z45.018 Encounter for adjustment and management of other part of cardiac pacemaker

        Excludes1   presence of other part of cardiac pacemaker (Z95.0)

        Excludes2   presence of prosthetic and other devices (Z95.1-Z95.5, Z95.811-Z97)

  Z45.02 Encounter for adjustment and management of automatic implantable cardiac defibrillator
    Encounter for adjustment and management of automatic implantable cardiac defibrillator with synchronous cardiac pacemaker
    Encounter for adjustment and management of cardiac resynchronization therapy defibrillator (CRT-D)

    Coding Clinic: 2024, Q1, P22,23

  Z45.09 Encounter for adjustment and management of other cardiac device

  Z45.1 Encounter for adjustment and management of infusion pump

  Z45.2 Encounter for adjustment and management of vascular access device
    Encounter for adjustment and management of vascular catheters

    Excludes1   encounter for adjustment and management of renal dialysis catheter (Z49.01)

● **Z45.3 Encounter for adjustment and management of implanted devices of the special senses**

  Z45.31 Encounter for adjustment and management of implanted visual substitution device

● **Z45.32 Encounter for adjustment and management of implanted hearing device**

    Excludes1   encounter for fitting and adjustment of hearing aid (Z46.1)

    Z45.320 Encounter for adjustment and management of bone conduction device

    Z45.321 Encounter for adjustment and management of cochlear device

    Z45.328 Encounter for adjustment and management of other implanted hearing device

● **Z45.4 Encounter for adjustment and management of implanted nervous system device**

  Z45.41 Encounter for adjustment and management of cerebrospinal fluid drainage device
    Encounter for adjustment and management of cerebral ventricular (communicating) shunt

  Z45.42 Encounter for adjustment and management of neuropacemaker
    Encounter for adjustment and management of brain neurostimulator
    Encounter for adjustment and management of gastric neurostimulator
    Encounter for adjustment and management of peripheral nerve neurostimulator
    Encounter for adjustment and management of sacral nerve neurostimulator
    Encounter for adjustment and management of spinal cord neurostimulator
    Encounter for adjustment and management of vagus nerve neurostimulator

  Z45.49 Encounter for adjustment and management of other implanted nervous system device

● **Z45.8 Encounter for adjustment and management of other implanted devices**

● **Z45.81 Encounter for adjustment or removal of breast implant**
    Encounter for elective implant exchange (different material) (different size)
    Encounter for removal of tissue expander with or without synchronous insertion of permanent implant

    Excludes1   complications of breast implant (T85.4-)
        encounter for initial breast implant insertion for cosmetic breast augmentation (Z41.1)
        encounter for breast reconstruction following mastectomy (Z42.1)

    Z45.811 Encounter for adjustment or removal of right breast implant

    Z45.812 Encounter for adjustment or removal of left breast implant

    Z45.819 Encounter for adjustment or removal of unspecified breast implant

  Z45.82 Encounter for adjustment or removal of myringotomy device (stent) (tube)

  Z45.89 Encounter for adjustment and management of other implanted devices

  Z45.9 Encounter for adjustment and management of unspecified implanted device

▶ New   ➡ Revised   ~~deleted~~ Deleted   Excludes 1   Excludes 2   Includes   Use additional   Code first   Code also   Key words

OGCR Official Guidelines   **X** Assign placeholder X   ● Use Additional Character(s)   ▶ Manifestation Code   Hierarchical Condition Category   **Coding Clinic**

● **Z46   Encounter for fitting and adjustment of other devices**

Includes   removal or replacement of other device

Excludes1   malfunction or other complications of device - see Alphabetical Index

Excludes2   encounter for fitting and management of implanted devices (Z45.-)
issue of repeat prescription only (Z76.0)
presence of prosthetic and other devices (Z95-Z97)

Z46.0   Encounter for fitting and adjustment of spectacles and contact lenses

Z46.1   Encounter for fitting and adjustment of hearing aid

Excludes1   encounter for adjustment and management of implanted hearing device (Z45.32-)

Z46.2   Encounter for fitting and adjustment of other devices related to nervous system and special senses

Excludes2   encounter for adjustment and management of implanted nervous system device (Z45.4-)
encounter for adjustment and management of implanted visual substitution device (Z45.31)

Z46.3   Encounter for fitting and adjustment of dental prosthetic device

Encounter for fitting and adjustment of dentures

Z46.4   Encounter for fitting and adjustment of orthodontic device

● **Z46.5   Encounter for fitting and adjustment of other gastrointestinal appliance and device**

Excludes1   encounter for attention to artificial openings of digestive tract (Z43.1-Z43.4)

Z46.51   Encounter for fitting and adjustment of gastric lap band

Z46.59   Encounter for fitting and adjustment of other gastrointestinal appliance and device

Z46.6   Encounter for fitting and adjustment of urinary device

Excludes2   attention to artificial openings of urinary tract (Z43.5, Z43.6)

● **Z46.8   Encounter for fitting and adjustment of other specified devices**

Z46.81   Encounter for fitting and adjustment of insulin pump

Encounter for insulin pump instruction and training
Encounter for insulin pump titration

Z46.82   Encounter for fitting and adjustment of non-vascular catheter

Z46.89   Encounter for fitting and adjustment of other specified devices

Encounter for fitting and adjustment of wheelchair

Z46.9   Encounter for fitting and adjustment of unspecified device

● **Z47   Orthopedic aftercare**

Excludes1   aftercare for healing fracture - code to fracture with 7th character D

Z47.1   Aftercare following joint replacement surgery

Use additional code to identify the joint (Z96.6-)
Coding Clinic: 2020, Q1, P23-24

Z47.2   Encounter for removal of internal fixation device

Excludes1   encounter for adjustment of internal fixation device for fracture treatment - code to fracture with appropriate 7th character
encounter for removal of external fixation device - code to fracture with 7th character D
infection or inflammatory reaction to internal fixation device (T84.6-)
mechanical complication of internal fixation device (T84.1-)

● **Z47.3   Aftercare following explantation of joint prosthesis**

Aftercare following explantation of joint prosthesis, staged procedure
Encounter for joint prosthesis insertion following prior explantation of joint prosthesis
Coding Clinic: 2020, Q1, P23; 2015, Q1, P17

Z47.31   Aftercare following explantation of shoulder joint prosthesis

Excludes1   acquired absence of shoulder joint following prior explantation of shoulder joint prosthesis (Z89.23-)
shoulder joint prosthesis explantation status (Z89.23-)

Z47.32   Aftercare following explantation of hip joint prosthesis

Excludes1   acquired absence of hip joint following prior explantation of hip joint prosthesis (Z89.62-)
hip joint prosthesis explantation status (Z89.62-)
Coding Clinic: 2015, Q1, P17

Z47.33   Aftercare following explantation of knee joint prosthesis

Excludes1   acquired absence of knee joint following prior explantation of knee prosthesis (Z89.52-)
knee joint prosthesis explantation status (Z89.52-)

● **Z47.8   Encounter for other orthopedic aftercare**

Z47.81   Encounter for orthopedic aftercare following surgical amputation

Use additional code to identify the limb amputated (Z89.-)

Z47.82   Encounter for orthopedic aftercare following scoliosis surgery

Z47.89   Encounter for other orthopedic aftercare
Coding Clinic: 2015, Q1, P8

● **Z48   Encounter for other postprocedural aftercare**

Excludes1   encounter for aftercare following injury - code to Injury, by site, with appropriate 7th character for subsequent encounter
encounter for follow-up examination after completed treatment (Z08-Z09)

Excludes2   encounter for attention to artificial openings (Z43.-)
encounter for fitting and adjustment of prosthetic and other devices (Z44-Z46)

● **Z48.0   Encounter for attention to dressings, sutures and drains**

Excludes1   encounter for planned postprocedural wound closure (Z48.1)

Z48.00   Encounter for change or removal of nonsurgical wound dressing

Encounter for change or removal of wound dressing NOS

Z48.01   Encounter for change or removal of surgical wound dressing
Coding Clinic: 2019, Q2, P33; 2015, Q4, P38

Z48.02   Encounter for removal of sutures

Encounter for removal of staples
Coding Clinic: 2015, Q1, P6

Z48.03   Encounter for change or removal of drains

Z48.1   Encounter for planned postprocedural wound closure

Excludes1   encounter for attention to dressings and sutures (Z48.0-)

● **Z48.2   Encounter for aftercare following organ transplant**

Z48.21   Encounter for aftercare following heart transplant

Z48.22   Encounter for aftercare following kidney transplant

Z48.23   Encounter for aftercare following liver transplant

Z48.24   Encounter for aftercare following lung transplant

CHAPTER 21 (Z00-Z99)

● **Z48.28** **Encounter for aftercare following multiple organ transplant**

    Z48.280 Encounter for aftercare following heart-lung transplant 🅬

    Z48.288 Encounter for aftercare following multiple organ transplant

● **Z48.29** **Encounter for aftercare following other organ transplant**

    Z48.290 Encounter for aftercare following bone marrow transplant 🅬

    Z48.298 Encounter for aftercare following other organ transplant

Z48.3 **Aftercare following surgery for neoplasm**

    Use additional code to identify the neoplasm

● **Z48.8** **Encounter for other specified postprocedural aftercare**

  ● **Z48.81** **Encounter for surgical aftercare following surgery on specified body systems**

    These codes identify the body system requiring aftercare. They are for use in conjunction with other aftercare codes to fully explain the aftercare encounter. The condition treated should also be coded if still present.

       Excludes1   aftercare for injury - code the injury with 7th character D aftercare following surgery for neoplasm (Z48.3)

       Excludes2   aftercare following organ transplant (Z48.2-) orthopedic aftercare (Z47.-)

    Z48.810 Encounter for surgical aftercare following surgery on the sense organs

    Z48.811 Encounter for surgical aftercare following surgery on the nervous system

       Excludes2   encounter for surgical aftercare following surgery on the sense organs (Z48.810)

    Z48.812 Encounter for surgical aftercare following surgery on the circulatory system

       Coding Clinic: 2012, Q4, P96

    Z48.813 Encounter for surgical aftercare following surgery on the respiratory system

       Coding Clinic: 2019, Q2, P33

    Z48.814 Encounter for surgical aftercare following surgery on the teeth or oral cavity

    Z48.815 Encounter for surgical aftercare following surgery on the digestive system

       Coding Clinic: 2015, Q4, P38

    Z48.816 Encounter for surgical aftercare following surgery on the genitourinary system

       Excludes1   encounter for aftercare following sterilization reversal (Z31.42)

    Z48.817 Encounter for surgical aftercare following surgery on the skin and subcutaneous tissue

       Coding Clinic: 2015, Q1, P6

    Z48.89 **Encounter for other specified surgical aftercare**

● **Z49** **Encounter for care involving renal dialysis**

    Code also associated end stage renal disease (N18.6)

  ● **Z49.0** **Preparatory care for renal dialysis**

    Encounter for dialysis instruction and training

    Z49.01 **Encounter for fitting and adjustment of extracorporeal dialysis catheter** 🅬

       Removal or replacement of renal dialysis catheter

       Toilet or cleansing of renal dialysis catheter

    Z49.02 **Encounter for fitting and adjustment of peritoneal dialysis catheter** 🅬

  ● **Z49.3** **Encounter for adequacy testing for dialysis**

    Z49.31 **Encounter for adequacy testing for hemodialysis** 🅬

    Z49.32 **Encounter for adequacy testing for peritoneal dialysis** 🅬

       Encounter for peritoneal equilibration test

● **Z51** **Encounter for other aftercare and medical care**

    Code also condition requiring care

     Excludes1   follow-up examination after treatment (Z08-Z09)

    Coding Clinic: 2017, Q1, P49; 2016, Q4, P130

  Z51.0 **Encounter for antineoplastic radiation therapy**

    Coding Clinic: 2017, Q4, P103

  ● **Z51.1** **Encounter for antineoplastic chemotherapy and immunotherapy**

     Excludes2   encounter for chemotherapy and immunotherapy for nonneoplastic condition-code to condition

    Z51.11 **Encounter for antineoplastic chemotherapy**

       Coding Clinic: 2025, Q2, P16; 2022, Q1, P16; 2015, Q3, P19

    Z51.12 **Encounter for antineoplastic immunotherapy**

       Coding Clinic: 2024, Q1, P24

  Z51.5 **Encounter for palliative care**

    Coding Clinic: 2022, Q1, P19; 2017, Q1, P48-49

  Z51.6 **Encounter for desensitization to allergens**

    Coding Clinic: 2025, Q2, P16; 2016, Q4, P77-79

  ● **Z51.8** **Encounter for other specified aftercare**

     Excludes1   holiday relief care (Z75.5)

    Z51.81 **Encounter for therapeutic drug level monitoring**

       Code also any long-term (current) drug therapy (Z79.-)

       Excludes1   encounter for blood-drug test for administrative or medicolegal reasons (Z02.83)

    Z51.89 **Encounter for other specified aftercare**

       Coding Clinic: 2012, Q4, P96-97

  Z51.A **Encounter for sepsis aftercare**

● **Z52** **Donors of organs and tissues**

     Includes   autologous and other living donors

     Excludes1   cadaveric donor - omit code examination of potential donor (Z00.5)

    Coding Clinic: 2012, Q4, P100

  ● **Z52.0** **Blood donor**

    ● **Z52.00** **Unspecified blood donor**

      Z52.000 Unspecified donor, whole blood

      Z52.001 Unspecified donor, stem cells

      Z52.008 Unspecified donor, other blood

    ● **Z52.01** **Autologous blood donor**

      Z52.010 Autologous donor, whole blood

      Z52.011 Autologous donor, stem cells

      Z52.018 Autologous donor, other blood

    ● **Z52.09** **Other blood donor**

       Volunteer donor

      Z52.090 Other blood donor, whole blood

      Z52.091 Other blood donor, stem cells

      Z52.098 Other blood donor, other blood

▶ New   ⇨ Revised   ~~deleted~~ Deleted   Excludes 1   Excludes 2   Includes   Use additional   Code first   Code also   Key words

OGCR Official Guidelines   X Assign placeholder X   ● Use Additional Character(s)   ▌ Manifestation Code   🅬 Hierarchical Condition Category   Coding Clinic

● **Z52.1   Skin donor**
    Z52.10   Skin donor, unspecified
    Z52.11   Skin donor, autologous
    Z52.19   Skin donor, other
● **Z52.2   Bone donor**
    Z52.20   Bone donor, unspecified
    Z52.21   Bone donor, autologous
    Z52.29   Bone donor, other
  Z52.3   **Bone marrow donor**
  Z52.4   **Kidney donor**
  Z52.5   **Cornea donor**
  Z52.6   **Liver donor**
    Coding Clinic: 2012, Q4, P100
● **Z52.8   Donor of other specified organs or tissues**
  ● **Z52.81   Egg (Oocyte) donor**
    Z52.810   Egg (Oocyte) donor under age 35, anonymous recipient
        Egg donor under age 35 NOS
    Z52.811   Egg (Oocyte) donor under age 35, designated recipient
    Z52.812   Egg (Oocyte) donor age 35 and over, anonymous recipient
        Egg donor age 35 and over NOS
    Z52.813   Egg (Oocyte) donor age 35 and over, designated recipient
    Z52.819   Egg (Oocyte) donor, unspecified
    Z52.89   Donor of other specified organs or tissues
  Z52.9   **Donor of unspecified organ or tissue**
    Donor NOS
● **Z53   Persons encountering health services for specific procedures and treatment, not carried out**
  ● **Z53.0   Procedure and treatment not carried out because of contraindication**
    Z53.01   Procedure and treatment not carried out due to patient smoking
    Z53.09   Procedure and treatment not carried out because of other contraindication
  Z53.1   **Procedure and treatment not carried out because of patient's decision for reasons of belief and group pressure**
  ● **Z53.2   Procedure and treatment not carried out because of patient's decision for other and unspecified reasons**
    Z53.20   Procedure and treatment not carried out because of patient's decision for unspecified reasons
    Z53.21   Procedure and treatment not carried out due to patient leaving prior to being seen by health care provider
    Z53.29   Procedure and treatment not carried out because of patient's decision for other reasons
  ● **Z53.3   Procedure converted to open procedure**
    Coding Clinic: 2016, Q4, P79
    Z53.31   Laparoscopic surgical procedure converted to open procedure
        Coding Clinic: 2016, Q4, P100
    Z53.32   Thoracoscopic surgical procedure converted to open procedure
    Z53.33   Arthroscopic surgical procedure converted to open procedure
    Z53.39   Other specified procedure converted to open procedure
  Z53.8   **Procedure and treatment not carried out for other reasons**
  Z53.9   **Procedure and treatment not carried out, unspecified reason**

PERSONS WITH POTENTIAL HEALTH HAZARDS RELATED TO SOCIOECONOMIC AND PSYCHOSOCIAL CIRCUMSTANCES (Z55-Z65)

● **Z55   Problems related to education and literacy**
  Excludes1   disorders of psychological development (F80-F89)
  Z55.0   **Illiteracy and low-level literacy**
  Z55.1   **Schooling unavailable and unattainable**
  Z55.2   **Failed school examinations**
  Z55.3   **Underachievement in school**
  Z55.4   **Educational maladjustment and discord with teachers and classmates**
  Z55.5   **Less than a high school diploma**
    No general equivalence degree (GED)
  Z55.6   **Problems related to health literacy**
    Difficulty understanding health related information
    Difficulty understanding medication instructions
    Problem completing medical forms
  Z55.8   **Other problems related to education and literacy**
    Problems related to inadequate teaching
  Z55.9   **Problems related to education and literacy, unspecified**
    Academic problems NOS
● **Z56   Problems related to employment and unemployment**
  Excludes2   occupational exposure to risk factors (Z57.-)
        problems related to housing and economic circumstances (Z59.-)
  Z56.0   **Unemployment, unspecified**
  Z56.1   **Change of job**
  Z56.2   **Threat of job loss**
  Z56.3   **Stressful work schedule**
  Z56.4   **Discord with boss and workmates**
  Z56.5   **Uncongenial work environment**
    Difficult conditions at work
  Z56.6   **Other physical and mental strain related to work**
    ▶Workplace stress
  ● **Z56.8   Other problems related to employment**
    Z56.81   Sexual harassment on the job
    Z56.82   Military deployment status
        Individual (civilian or military) currently deployed in theater or in support of military war, peacekeeping and humanitarian operations
    Z56.89   Other problems related to employment
        ▶Furloughed
        ▶Underemployed
  Z56.9   **Unspecified problems related to employment**
    Occupational problems NOS
● **Z57   Occupational exposure to risk factors**
  Z57.0   **Occupational exposure to noise**
  Z57.1   **Occupational exposure to radiation**
  Z57.2   **Occupational exposure to dust**
  ● **Z57.3   Occupational exposure to other air contaminants**
    Z57.31   Occupational exposure to environmental tobacco smoke
        Excludes2   exposure to environmental tobacco smoke (Z77.22)
    Z57.39   Occupational exposure to other air contaminants
  Z57.4   **Occupational exposure to toxic agents in agriculture**
    Occupational exposure to solids, liquids, gases or vapors in agriculture
  Z57.5   **Occupational exposure to toxic agents in other industries**
    Occupational exposure to solids, liquids, gases or vapors in other industries
  Z57.6   **Occupational exposure to extreme temperature**
  Z57.7   **Occupational exposure to vibration**
  Z57.8   **Occupational exposure to other risk factors**
  Z57.9   **Occupational exposure to unspecified risk factor**

CHAPTER 21 (Z00-Z99)

- **Z58　Problems related to physical environment**
  - **Excludes2**　occupational exposure (Z57.-)
  - **Z58.6　Inadequate drinking-water supply**
    - Lack of safe drinking water
    - **Excludes2**　deprivation of water (T73.1)
  - **Z58.8　Other problems related to physical environment**
    - **Z58.81　Basic services unavailable in physical environment**
      - Unable to obtain internet service, due to unavailability in geographic area
      - Unable to obtain telephone service, due to unavailability in geographic area
      - Unable to obtain utilities, due to inadequate physical environment
    - **Z58.89　Other problems related to physical environment**

- **Z59　Problems related to housing and economic circumstances**
  - **Excludes2**　problems related to upbringing (Z62.-)
  - **Z59.0　Homelessness**
    - **Z59.00　Homelessness unspecified**
    - **Z59.01　Sheltered homelessness**
      - Doubled up
      - Living in a shelter such as: motel, scattered site housing, temporary or transitional living situation
    - **Z59.02　Unsheltered homelessness**
      - ▶Lives in a homeless encampment
      - Residing in place not meant for human habitation such as: abandoned buildings, cars, parks, sidewalk
      - Residing on the street
  - **Z59.1　Inadequate housing**
    - **Excludes1**　problems related to the natural and physical environment (Z77.1-)
    - **Z59.10　Inadequate housing, unspecified**
      - Inadequate housing NOS
    - **Z59.11　Inadequate housing environmental temperature**
      - Lack of air conditioning
      - Lack of heating
    - **Z59.12　Inadequate housing utilities**
      - Lack of electricity services
      - Lack of gas services
      - Lack of oil services
      - Lack of water services
      - **Excludes2**　basic services unavailable in physical environment (Z58.81)
        - ▶financial insecurity, difficulty paying for utilities (Z59.861)
        - lack of adequate food (Z59.4-)
        - other problems related to housing and economic circumstances (Z59.8-)
    - **Z59.19　Other inadequate housing**
      - Pest infestation
      - ▶Poor housing weatherization
      - Restriction of space
      - Technical defects in home preventing adequate care
      - Unsatisfactory surroundings
  - **Z59.2　Discord with neighbors, lodgers and landlord**
  - **Z59.3　Problems related to living in residential institution**
    - Boarding-school resident
    - **Excludes1**　institutional upbringing (Z62.22)
  - **Z59.4　Lack of adequate food**
    - **Excludes2**　deprivation of food (T73.0)
      - effects of hunger (T73.0)
      - inappropriate diet or eating habits (Z72.4)
      - malnutrition (E40-E46)
    - **Z59.41　Food insecurity**
    - **Z59.48　Other specified lack of adequate food**
      - Inadequate food
      - Lack of food

- **Z59.5　Extreme poverty**
- **Z59.6　Low income**
- **Z59.7　Insufficient social insurance and welfare support**
  - **Z59.71　Insufficient health insurance coverage**
    - Inadequate social insurance
    - Insufficient social insurance
    - No health insurance coverage
  - **Z59.72　Insufficient welfare support**
    - Inadequate welfare support
- **Z59.8　Other problems related to housing and economic circumstances**
  - **Z59.81　Housing instability, housed**
    - Foreclosure on home loan
    - Past due on rent or mortgage
    - Unwanted multiple moves in the last 12 months
    - **Z59.811　Housing instability, housed, with risk of homelessness**
      - Imminent risk of homelessness
    - **Z59.812　Housing instability, housed, homelessness in past 12 months**
    - **Z59.819　Housing instability, housed unspecified**
      - **Excludes2**　extreme poverty (Z59.5)
        - ▷financial insecurity (Z59.86-)
        - low income (Z59.6)
        - material hardship due to limited financial resources, not elsewhere classified (Z59.87)
  - **Z59.82　Transportation insecurity**
    - Excessive transportation time
    - Inaccessible transportation
    - Inadequate transportation
    - Lack of transportation
    - Unaffordable transportation
    - Unreliable transportation
    - Unsafe transportation
    - **Excludes2**　unavailability and inaccessibility of healthcare facilities (Z75.3)
  - **Z59.86　Financial insecurity**
    - ~~Bankruptcy~~
    - Burdensome debt
    - Economic strain
    - Financial strain
    - Money problems
    - Running out of money
    - Unable to make ends meet
    - **Excludes2**　extreme poverty (Z59.5)
      - low income (Z59.6)
      - material hardship, not elsewhere classified (Z59.87)
    - ▶**Z59.861　Financial insecurity, difficulty paying for utilities**
      - ▶Difficulty paying for electricity
      - ▶Difficulty paying for heat
      - ▶Difficulty paying for oil
      - ▶Difficulty paying water bill
      - ▶Utility disconnect notice due to inability to pay
      - ▶**Excludes2**　inadequate housing utilities (Z59.12)
    - ▶**Z59.868　Other specified financial insecurity**
      - ▶Bankruptcy
    - ▶**Z59.869　Financial insecurity, unspecified**

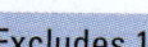

▶ New　　⇨ Revised　　~~deleted~~ Deleted　　Excludes 1　　Excludes 2　　Includes　　Use additional　　Code first　　Code also　　Key words
OGCR Official Guidelines　　X Assign placeholder X　　● Use Additional Character(s)　　▌Manifestation Code　　Hierarchical Condition Category　　Coding Clinic

Z59.87 **Material hardship due to limited financial resources, not elsewhere classified**
  Material deprivation due to limited financial resources
  Unable to obtain adequate childcare due to limited financial resources
  Unable to obtain adequate clothing due to limited financial resources
  Unable to obtain adequate utilities due to limited financial resources
  Unable to obtain basic needs due to limited financial resources
  Excludes2 extreme poverty (Z59.5)
    ➤financial insecurity, not elsewhere classified (Z59.86-)
    low income (Z59.6)

Z59.89 **Other problems related to housing and economic circumstances**
  Foreclosure on loan
  Isolated dwelling
  Problems with creditors

Z59.9 **Problem related to housing and economic circumstances, unspecified**

● **Z60** **Problems related to social environment**

Z60.0 **Problems of adjustment to life-cycle transitions**
  Empty nest syndrome
  Phase of life problem
  Problem with adjustment to retirement [pension]

Z60.2 **Problems related to living alone**

Z60.3 **Acculturation difficulty**
  Problem with migration
  Problem with social transplantation

Z60.4 **Social exclusion and rejection**
  Exclusion and rejection on the basis of personal characteristics, such as unusual physical appearance, illness or behavior.
  Social isolation
  Excludes1 target of adverse discrimination such as for racial or religious reasons (Z60.5)

Z60.5 **Target of (perceived) adverse discrimination and persecution**
  Excludes1 social exclusion and rejection (Z60.4)

Z60.8 **Other problems related to social environment**
  Inadequate social support
  Lack of emotional support

Z60.9 **Problem related to social environment, unspecified**

● **Z62** **Problems related to upbringing**
  Includes current and past negative life events in childhood
    current and past problems of a child related to upbringing
  Excludes2 maltreatment syndrome (T74.-)
    problems related to housing and economic circumstances (Z59.-)

Z62.0 **Inadequate parental supervision and control**

Z62.1 **Parental overprotection**

● **Z62.2** **Upbringing away from parents**
  Excludes1 problems with boarding school (Z59.3)

Z62.21 **Child in welfare custody** P
  Child in foster care
  Child in welfare guardianship

Z62.22 **Institutional upbringing**
  Child living in group home
  Child living in orphanage
  Code also, if applicable, child in welfare custody (Z62.21)

Z62.23 **Child in custody of non-parental relative**
  Child in care of non-parental family member
  Child in custody of grandparent
  Child in kinship care
  Guardianship by non-parental relative
  Code also, if applicable, child in welfare custody (Z62.21)

Z62.24 **Child in custody of non-relative guardian**
  Code also, if applicable, child in welfare custody (Z62.21)

Z62.29 **Other upbringing away from parents**

Z62.3 **Hostility towards and scapegoating of child** P

Z62.6 **Inappropriate (excessive) parental pressure**

● **Z62.8** **Other specified problems related to upbringing**
  Code also, if applicable:
  absence of family member (Z63.3-)
  disappearance and death of family member (Z63.4)
  disruption of family by separation and divorce (Z63.5)
  other specified problems related to primary support group (Z63.8)
  other stressful life events affecting family and household (Z63.7-)

● **Z62.81** **Personal history of abuse in childhood**
  Personal history of abuse in adolescence

Z62.810 **Personal history of physical and sexual abuse in childhood**
  Excludes1 current child physical abuse (T74.12, T76.12)
    current child sexual abuse (T74.22, T76.22)

Z62.811 **Personal history of psychological abuse in childhood**
  Excludes1 current child psychological abuse (T74.32, T76.32)

Z62.812 **Personal history of neglect in childhood**
  Excludes1 current child neglect (T74.02, T76.02)

Z62.813 **Personal history of forced labor or sexual exploitation in childhood**

Z62.814 **Personal history of child financial abuse**
  Excludes1 current child financial abuse (T74.A2)

Z62.815 **Personal history of intimate partner abuse in childhood**
  Excludes2 adult and child abuse, neglect and other maltreatment, confirmed (T74.-)

Z62.819 **Personal history of unspecified abuse in childhood**
  Excludes1 current child abuse NOS (T74.92, T76.92)

● **Z62.82** **Parent-child conflict**

Z62.820 **Parent-biological child conflict**
  Parent-child problem NOS

Z62.821 **Parent-adopted child conflict**

Z62.822 **Parent-foster child conflict**

Z62.823 **Parent-step child conflict**

CHAPTER 21 (Z00-Z99)

● Z62.83   **Non-parental relative or guardian-child conflict**

    Z62.831   **Non-parental relative-child conflict**
       Grandparent-child conflict
       Kinship-care child conflict
       Non-parental relative legal
         guardian-child conflict
       Other relative-child conflict

       Excludes1   group home staff-child
           conflict (Z62.833)

    Z62.832   **Non-relative guardian-child conflict**

       Excludes1   group home staff-child
           conflict (Z62.833)

    Z62.833   **Group home staff-child conflict**

● Z62.89   **Other specified problems related to upbringing**

    Z62.890   **Parent-child estrangement NEC**

    Z62.891   **Sibling rivalry**

    Z62.892   **Runaway [from current living environment]**
       Child leaving living situation
         without permission

    Z62.898   **Other specified problems related to upbringing**

Z62.9   **Problem related to upbringing, unspecified**

● Z63   **Other problems related to primary support group, including family circumstances**

    Excludes2   maltreatment syndrome (T74.-, T76)
       parent-child problems (Z62.-)
       problems related to negative life events in
         childhood (Z62.-)
       problems related to upbringing (Z62.-)

Z63.0   **Problems in relationship with spouse or partner**
    Relationship distress with spouse or intimate partner

    Excludes1   counseling for spousal or partner abuse
       problems (Z69.1)
       counseling related to sexual attitude,
       behavior, and orientation (Z70.-)

Z63.1   **Problems in relationship with in-laws**

● Z63.3   **Absence of family member**

    Excludes1   absence of family member due to
         disappearance and death (Z63.4)
       absence of family member due to
         separation and divorce (Z63.5)

    Z63.31   **Absence of family member due to military deployment**
       Individual or family affected by other family
         member being on military deployment

       Excludes1   family disruption due to return of
         family member from military
         deployment (Z63.71)

    Z63.32   **Other absence of family member**

Z63.4   **Disappearance and death of family member**
    Assumed death of family member
    Bereavement

Z63.5   **Disruption of family by separation and divorce**
    Marital estrangement

Z63.6   **Dependent relative needing care at home**

● Z63.7   **Other stressful life events affecting family and household**

    Z63.71   **Stress on family due to return of family member from military deployment**
       Individual or family affected by family
         member having returned from military
         deployment (current or past conflict)

    Z63.72   **Alcoholism and drug addiction in family**

    Z63.79   **Other stressful life events affecting family and household**
       Anxiety (normal) about sick person in family
       Health problems within family
       Ill or disturbed family member
       Isolated family

Z63.8   **Other specified problems related to primary support group**
    Family discord NOS
    Family estrangement NOS
    High expressed emotional level within family
    Inadequate family support NOS
    Inadequate or distorted communication within family

Z63.9   **Problem related to primary support group, unspecified**
    Relationship disorder NOS

● Z64   **Problems related to certain psychosocial circumstances**

Z64.0   **Problems related to unwanted pregnancy**

Z64.1   **Problems related to multiparity**

Z64.4   **Discord with counselors**
    Discord with probation officer
    Discord with social worker

● Z65   **Problems related to other psychosocial circumstances**

Z65.0   **Conviction in civil and criminal proceedings without imprisonment**

Z65.1   **Imprisonment and other incarceration**

Z65.2   **Problems related to release from prison**

Z65.3   **Problems related to other legal circumstances**
    Arrest
    Child custody or support proceedings
    Litigation
    Prosecution

Z65.4   **Victim of crime and terrorism**
    Victim of torture

Z65.5   **Exposure to disaster, war and other hostilities**

    Excludes1   target of perceived discrimination or
       persecution (Z60.5)

Z65.8   **Other specified problems related to psychosocial circumstances**
    At risk for feeling loneliness
    Religious or spiritual problem

Z65.9   **Problem related to unspecified psychosocial circumstances**

DO NOT RESUSCITATE STATUS (Z66)

Z66   **Do not resuscitate**
    DNR status

BLOOD TYPE (Z67)

● Z67   **Blood type**
    Coding Clinic: 2015, Q3, P40

    ● Z67.1   **Type A blood**

       Z67.10   **Type A blood, Rh positive**

       Z67.11   **Type A blood, Rh negative**

    ● Z67.2   **Type B blood**

       Z67.20   **Type B blood, Rh positive**

       Z67.21   **Type B blood, Rh negative**

    ● Z67.3   **Type AB blood**

       Z67.30   **Type AB blood, Rh positive**

       Z67.31   **Type AB blood, Rh negative**

    ● Z67.4   **Type O blood**

       Z67.40   **Type O blood, Rh positive**

       Z67.41   **Type O blood, Rh negative**

    ● Z67.9   **Unspecified blood type**

       Z67.90   **Unspecified blood type, Rh positive**

       Z67.91   **Unspecified blood type, Rh negative**
       Coding Clinic: 2015, Q3, P40

    Z67.A   **Duffy phenotype**

    Z67.A1   **Duffy null**
       Duffy phenotype Fy(a-b-)

    Z67.A2   **Duffy a positive**
       Duffy phenotype Fy(a+b-)

    Z67.A3   **Duffy b positive**
       Duffy phenotype Fy(a-b+)

    Z67.A4   **Duffy a and b positive**
       Duffy phenotype Fy(a+b+)

▶ New   ⇒ Revised   ~~deleted~~ Deleted   Excludes 1   Excludes 2   Includes   Use additional   Code first   Code also   Key words
OGCR Official Guidelines   X Assign placeholder X   ● Use Additional Character(s)   ▌ Manifestation Code   Hierarchical Condition Category   Coding Clinic

BODY MASS INDEX [BMI] (Z68)

OGCR Section I.B.14.

General Coding Guidelines

14. Documentation for BMI, Depth of Non-pressure ulcers, Pressure Ulcer Stages, Coma Scale, and NIH Stroke Scale

For the Body Mass Index (BMI), depth of non-pressure chronic ulcers, pressure ulcer stage, coma scale, and NIH stroke scale (NIHSS) codes, code assignment may be based on medical record documentation from clinicians who are not the patient's provider (i.e., physician or other qualified healthcare practitioner legally accountable for establishing the patient's diagnosis), since this information is typically documented by other clinicians involved in the care of the patient (e.g., a dietitian often documents the BMI, a nurse often documents the pressure ulcer stages, and an emergency medical technician often documents the coma scale). However, the associated diagnosis (such as overweight, obesity, acute stroke, or pressure ulcer) must be documented by the patient's provider. If there is conflicting medical record documentation, either from the same clinician or different clinicians, the patient's attending provider should be queried for clarification.

The BMI, coma scale, and NIHSS codes should only be reported as secondary diagnoses.

● **Z68**   **Body mass index [BMI]**
    Kilograms per meters squared
    Note: BMI adult codes are for use for persons 20 years of age or older.
       BMI pediatric codes are for use for persons 2-19 years of age.
       These percentiles are based on the growth charts published by the Centers for Disease Control and Prevention (CDC)
       Coding Clinic: 2018, Q4, P81; 2016, Q4, P129

   Z68.1   **Body mass index [BMI] 19.9 or less, adult**   A
       Coding Clinic: 2024, Q4, P14; 2017, Q1, P39

   ● **Z68.2**   **Body mass index [BMI] 20-29, adult**
     Z68.20   Body mass index [BMI] 20.0-20.9, adult   A
     Z68.21   Body mass index [BMI] 21.0-21.9, adult   A
     Z68.22   Body mass index [BMI] 22.0-22.9, adult   A
     Z68.23   Body mass index [BMI] 23.0-23.9, adult   A
     Z68.24   Body mass index [BMI] 24.0-24.9, adult   A
     Z68.25   Body mass index [BMI] 25.0-25.9, adult   A
     Z68.26   Body mass index [BMI] 26.0-26.9, adult   A
     Z68.27   Body mass index [BMI] 27.0-27.9, adult   A
     Z68.28   Body mass index [BMI] 28.0-28.9, adult   A
     Z68.29   Body mass index [BMI] 29.0-29.9, adult   A

   ● **Z68.3**   **Body mass index [BMI] 30-39, adult**
     Z68.30   Body mass index [BMI] 30.0-30.9, adult   A
     Z68.31   Body mass index [BMI] 31.0-31.9, adult   A
     Z68.32   Body mass index [BMI] 32.0-32.9, adult   A
     Z68.33   Body mass index [BMI] 33.0-33.9, adult   A
     Z68.34   Body mass index [BMI] 34.0-34.9, adult   A
     Z68.35   Body mass index [BMI] 35.0-35.9, adult   A
       Coding Clinic: 2022, Q3, P6
     Z68.36   Body mass index [BMI] 36.0-36.9, adult   A
     Z68.37   Body mass index [BMI] 37.0-37.9, adult   A
     Z68.38   Body mass index [BMI] 38.0-38.9, adult   A
     Z68.39   Body mass index [BMI] 39.0-39.9, adult   A

   ● **Z68.4**   **Body mass index [BMI] 40 or greater, adult**
     Z68.41   Body mass index [BMI] 40.0-44.9, adult   A
     Z68.42   Body mass index [BMI] 45.0-49.9, adult   A
     Z68.43   Body mass index [BMI] 50.0-59.9, adult   A
     Z68.44   Body mass index [BMI] 60.0-69.9, adult   A
     Z68.45   Body mass index [BMI] 70 or greater, adult   A

   ● **Z68.5**   **Body mass index [BMI] pediatric**
       Coding Clinic: 2018, Q4, P81
     Z68.51   Body mass index [BMI] pediatric, less than 5th percentile for age
       Coding Clinic: 2018, Q4, P82

     Z68.52   Body mass index [BMI] pediatric, 5th percentile to less than 85th percentile for age
     Z68.53   Body mass index [BMI] pediatric, 85th percentile to less than 95th percentile for age
     Z68.54   Body mass index [BMI] pediatric, 95th percentile for age to less than 120% of the 95th percentile for age
     Z68.55   Body mass index [BMI] pediatric, 120% of the 95th percentile for age to less than 140% of the 95th percentile for age
     Z68.56   Body mass index [BMI] pediatric, greater than or equal to 140% of the 95th percentile for age

PERSONS ENCOUNTERING HEALTH SERVICES IN OTHER CIRCUMSTANCES (Z69-Z76)

● **Z69**   **Encounter for mental health services for victim and perpetrator of abuse**
     Includes   counseling for victims and perpetrators of abuse

  ● **Z69.0**   **Encounter for mental health services for child abuse problems**

   ● **Z69.01**   **Encounter for mental health services for parental child abuse**

     Z69.010   **Encounter for mental health services for victim of parental child abuse**   P
       Encounter for mental health services for victim of child abuse by parent
       Encounter for mental health services for victim of child neglect by parent
       Encounter for mental health services for victim of child psychological abuse by parent
       Encounter for mental health services for victim of child sexual abuse by parent

     Z69.011   **Encounter for mental health services for perpetrator of parental child abuse**
       Encounter for mental health services for perpetrator of parental child neglect
       Encounter for mental health services for perpetrator of parental child psychological abuse
       Encounter for mental health services for perpetrator of parental child sexual abuse

     Excludes1   encounter for mental health services for non-parental child abuse (Z69.02-)

   ● **Z69.02**   **Encounter for mental health services for non-parental child abuse**

     Z69.020   **Encounter for mental health services for victim of non-parental child abuse** P
       Encounter for mental health services for victim of non-parental child neglect
       Encounter for mental health services for victim of non-parental child psychological abuse
       Encounter for mental health services for victim of non-parental child sexual abuse

     Z69.021   **Encounter for mental health services for perpetrator of non- parental child abuse**
       Encounter for mental health services for perpetrator of non-parental child neglect
       Encounter for mental health services for perpetrator of non-parental child psychological abuse
       Encounter for mental health services for perpetrator of non-parental child sexual abuse

CHAPTER 21 (Z00-Z99)

CHAPTER 21 (Z00–Z99)

● **Z69.1** **Encounter for mental health services for spousal or partner abuse problems**

     Z69.11 **Encounter for mental health services for victim of spousal or partner abuse**

       Encounter for mental health services for victim of spouse or partner neglect

       Encounter for mental health services for victim of spouse or partner psychological abuse

       Encounter for mental health services for victim of spouse or partner violence, physical

     Z69.12 **Encounter for mental health services for perpetrator of spousal or partner abuse**

       Encounter for mental health services for perpetrator of spouse or partner neglect

       Encounter for mental health services for perpetrator of spouse or partner psychological abuse

       Encounter for mental health services for perpetrator of spouse or partner violence, physical

       Encounter for mental health services for perpetrator of spouse or partner violence, sexual

● **Z69.8** **Encounter for mental health services for victim or perpetrator of other abuse**

     Z69.81 **Encounter for mental health services for victim of other abuse**

       Encounter for mental health services for victim of non-spousal adult abuse

       Encounter for mental health services for victim of spouse or partner violence, sexual

       Encounter for rape victim counseling

     Z69.82 **Encounter for mental health services for perpetrator of other abuse**

       Encounter for mental health services for perpetrator of non-spousal adult abuse

● **Z70** **Counseling related to sexual attitude, behavior and orientation**

     Includes   encounter for mental health services for sexual attitude, behavior and orientation

     Excludes2   contraceptive or procreative counseling (Z30-Z31)

     Z70.0 **Counseling related to sexual attitude**

     Z70.1 **Counseling related to patient's sexual behavior and orientation**

       Patient concerned regarding impotence

       Patient concerned regarding non-responsiveness

       Patient concerned regarding promiscuity

       Patient concerned regarding sexual orientation

     Z70.2 **Counseling related to sexual behavior and orientation of third party**

       Advice sought regarding sexual behavior and orientation of child

       Advice sought regarding sexual behavior and orientation of partner

       Advice sought regarding sexual behavior and orientation of spouse

     Z70.3 **Counseling related to combined concerns regarding sexual attitude, behavior and orientation**

     Z70.8 **Other sex counseling**

       Encounter for sex education

     Z70.9 **Sex counseling, unspecified**

● **Z71** **Persons encountering health services for other counseling and medical advice, not elsewhere classified**

     Excludes2   contraceptive or procreation counseling (Z30-Z31)

           sex counseling (Z70.-)

     Z71.0 **Person encountering health services to consult on behalf of another person**

       Person encountering health services to seek advice or treatment for non-attending third party

     Excludes2   anxiety (normal) about sick person in family (Z63.7)

           expectant (adoptive) parent(s) pre-birth pediatrician visit (Z76.81)

Z71.1 **Person with feared health complaint in whom no diagnosis is made**

     Person encountering health services with feared condition which was not demonstrated

     Person encountering health services in which problem was normal state

     "Worried well"

     Excludes1   medical observation for suspected diseases and conditions proven not to exist (Z03.-)

     Coding Clinic: 2016, Q4, P7

Z71.2 **Person consulting for explanation of examination or test findings**

Z71.3 **Dietary counseling and surveillance**

     Use additional code for any associated underlying medical condition

     Use additional code to identify body mass index (BMI), if known (Z68.-)

● **Z71.4** **Alcohol abuse counseling and surveillance**

     Use additional code for alcohol abuse or dependence (F10.-)

     Z71.41 **Alcohol abuse counseling and surveillance of alcoholic**

     Z71.42 **Counseling for family member of alcoholic**

       Counseling for significant other, partner, or friend of alcoholic

● **Z71.5** **Drug abuse counseling and surveillance**

     Use additional code for drug abuse or dependence (F11-F16, F18-F19)

     Z71.51 **Drug abuse counseling and surveillance of drug abuser**

     Z71.52 **Counseling for family member of drug abuser**

       Counseling for significant other, partner, or friend of drug abuser

Z71.6 **Tobacco abuse counseling**

     Use additional code for nicotine dependence (F17.-)

Z71.7 **Human immunodeficiency virus [HIV] counseling**

● **Z71.8** **Other specified counseling**

     Excludes2   counseling for contraception (Z30.0-)

     Z71.81 **Spiritual or religious counseling**

     Z71.82 **Exercise counseling**

     Z71.83 **Encounter for nonprocreative genetic counseling**

       Excludes1   counseling for procreative genetics (Z31.5)

                counseling for procreative management (Z31.6)

     Z71.84 **Encounter for health counseling related to travel**

       Encounter for health risk and safety counseling for (international) travel

       Code also, if applicable, encounter for immunization (Z23)

       Excludes2   encounter for administrative examination (Z02.-)

                encounter for other special examination without complaint, suspected or reported diagnosis (Z01.-)

     Z71.85 **Encounter for immunization safety counseling**

       Encounter for vaccine product safety counseling

       Code also, if applicable, encounter for immunization (Z23)

       Code also, if applicable, immunization not carried out (Z28.-)

       Excludes1   encounter for health counseling related to travel (Z71.84)

▶ New   ➡ Revised   ~~deleted~~ Deleted   Excludes 1   Excludes 2   Includes   Use additional   Code first   Code also   Key words

OGCR Official Guidelines   **X** Assign placeholder X   ● Use Additional Character(s)   ▶ Manifestation Code   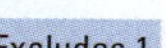 Hierarchical Condition Category   **Coding Clinic**

Z71.87 Encounter for pediatric-to-adult transition counseling
Code also chronic condition, if applicable, such as:
autism spectrum disorder (F84.0)
congenital malformations of the circulatory system (Q20-Q28)
cystic fibrosis (E84.-)
sickle-cell disorder (D57-)

Z71.88 Encounter for counseling for socioeconomic factors

Z71.89 Other specified counseling

Z71.9 Counseling, unspecified
Encounter for medical advice NOS

● **Z72 Problems related to lifestyle**
Excludes2   problems related to life-management difficulty (Z73.-)
problems related to socioeconomic and psychosocial circumstances (Z55-Z65)
Coding Clinic: 2016, Q4, P130

Z72.0 Tobacco use
Tobacco use NOS
Excludes1   history of tobacco dependence (Z87.891)
nicotine dependence (F17.2-)
tobacco dependence (F17.2-)
tobacco use during pregnancy (O99.33-)

Z72.3 Lack of physical exercise

Z72.4 Inappropriate diet and eating habits
Excludes1   behavioral eating disorders of infancy or childhood (F98.2.-F98.3)
eating disorders (F50.-)
lack of adequate food (Z59.48)
malnutrition and other nutritional deficiencies (E40-E64)

● **Z72.5 High risk sexual behavior**
Promiscuity
Excludes1   paraphilias (F65)

Z72.51 High risk heterosexual behavior

Z72.52 High risk homosexual behavior

Z72.53 High risk bisexual behavior

Z72.6 Gambling and betting
Excludes1   compulsive or pathological gambling (F63.0)

● **Z72.8 Other problems related to lifestyle**

● **Z72.81 Antisocial behavior**
Excludes1   conduct disorders (F91.-)

Z72.810 Child and adolescent antisocial behavior   P
Antisocial behavior (child) (adolescent) without manifest psychiatric disorder
Delinquency NOS
Group delinquency
Offenses in the context of gang membership
Stealing in company with others
Truancy from school

Z72.811 Adult antisocial behavior   A
Adult antisocial behavior without manifest psychiatric disorder

● **Z72.82 Problems related to sleep**

Z72.820 Sleep deprivation
Lack of adequate sleep
Excludes1   insomnia (G47.0-)

Z72.821 Inadequate sleep hygiene
Bad sleep habits
Irregular sleep habits
Unhealthy sleep wake schedule
Excludes1   insomnia (F51.0-, G47.0-)

Z72.823 Risk of suffocation (smothering) under another while sleeping
Child-caregiver co-sleeping
Infant bed-sharing

Z72.89 Other problems related to lifestyle
Self-damaging behavior

Z72.9 Problem related to lifestyle, unspecified

● **Z73 Problems related to life management difficulty**
Excludes2   problems related to socioeconomic and psychosocial circumstances (Z55-Z65)

Z73.0 Burn-out

Z73.1 Type A behavior pattern

Z73.2 Lack of relaxation and leisure

Z73.3 Stress, not elsewhere classified
Physical and mental strain NOS
Excludes1   stress related to employment or unemployment (Z56.-)

Z73.4 Inadequate social skills, not elsewhere classified

Z73.5 Social role conflict, not elsewhere classified

Z73.6 Limitation of activities due to disability
Excludes1   care-provider dependency (Z74.-)

● **Z73.8 Other problems related to life management difficulty**

● **Z73.81 Behavioral insomnia of childhood**

Z73.810 Behavioral insomnia of childhood, sleep-onset association type   P

Z73.811 Behavioral insomnia of childhood, limit setting type   P

Z73.812 Behavioral insomnia of childhood, combined type   P

Z73.819 Behavioral insomnia of childhood, unspecified type   P

Z73.82 Dual sensory impairment

Z73.89 Other problems related to life management difficulty

Z73.9 Problem related to life management difficulty, unspecified

● **Z74 Problems related to care provider dependency**
Excludes2   dependence on enabling machines or devices NEC (Z99.-)

● **Z74.0 Reduced mobility**

Z74.01 Bed confinement status
Bedridden

Z74.09 Other reduced mobility
Chairridden
Reduced mobility NOS
Excludes2   wheelchair dependence (Z99.3)

Z74.1 Need for assistance with personal care

Z74.2 Need for assistance at home and no other household member able to render care

Z74.3 Need for continuous supervision

Z74.8 Other problems related to care provider dependency

Z74.9 Problem related to care provider dependency, unspecified

● **Z75 Problems related to medical facilities and other health care**

Z75.0 Medical services not available in home
Excludes1   no other household member able to render care (Z74.2)

Z75.1 Person awaiting admission to adequate facility elsewhere

Z75.2 Other waiting period for investigation and treatment

Z75.3 Unavailability and inaccessibility of health care facilities
Excludes1   bed unavailable (Z75.1)

Z75.4 Unavailability and inaccessibility of other helping agencies

Z75.5 Holiday relief care

CHAPTER 21 (Z00-Z99)

CHAPTER 21 (Z00–Z99)

Z75.8 Other problems related to medical facilities and other health care

Z75.9 Unspecified problem related to medical facilities and other health care

● **Z76** Persons encountering health services in other circumstances

Z76.0 Encounter for issue of repeat prescription
Encounter for issue of repeat prescription for appliance
Encounter for issue of repeat prescription for medicaments
Encounter for issue of repeat prescription for spectacles

Excludes2 issue of medical certificate (Z02.7)
repeat prescription for contraceptive (Z30.4-)

Z76.1 Encounter for health supervision and care of foundling

Z76.2 Encounter for health supervision and care of other healthy infant and child   P
Encounter for medical or nursing care or supervision of healthy infant under circumstances such as adverse socioeconomic conditions at home
Encounter for medical or nursing care or supervision of healthy infant under circumstances such as awaiting foster or adoptive placement
Encounter for medical or nursing care or supervision of healthy infant under circumstances such as maternal illness
Encounter for medical or nursing care or supervision of healthy infant under circumstances such as number of children at home preventing or interfering with normal care

Z76.3 Healthy person accompanying sick person

Z76.4 Other boarder to healthcare facility

Excludes1 homelessness (Z59.0-)

Z76.5 Malingerer [conscious simulation]
Person feigning illness (with obvious motivation)

Excludes1 factitious disorder (F68.1-, F68.A)
peregrinating patient (F68.1-)

● **Z76.8** Persons encountering health services in other specified circumstances

Z76.81 Expectant parent(s) prebirth pediatrician visit
Pre-adoption pediatrician visit for adoptive parent(s)

Z76.82 Awaiting organ transplant status
Patient waiting for organ availability

Z76.89 Persons encountering health services in other specified circumstances
Persons encountering health services NOS
Coding Clinic:2022, Q3, P7

PERSONS WITH POTENTIAL HEALTH HAZARDS RELATED TO FAMILY AND PERSONAL HISTORY AND CERTAIN CONDITIONS INFLUENCING HEALTH STATUS (Z77-Z99)

Code also any follow-up examination (Z08-Z09)

● **Z77** Other contact with and (suspected) exposures hazardous to health

Includes contact with and (suspected) exposures to potential hazards to health

Excludes2 contact with and (suspected) exposure to communicable diseases (Z20.-)
exposure to (parental) (environmental) tobacco smoke in the perinatal period (P96.81)
newborn affected by noxious substances transmitted via placenta or breast milk (P04.-)
occupational exposure to risk factors (Z57.-)
retained foreign body (Z18.-)
retained foreign body fully removed (Z87.821)
toxic effects of substances chiefly nonmedicinal as to source (T51-T65)

● **Z77.0** Contact with and (suspected) exposure to hazardous, chiefly nonmedicinal, chemicals

● **Z77.01** Contact with and (suspected) exposure to hazardous metals

Z77.010 Contact with and (suspected) exposure to arsenic

Z77.011 Contact with and (suspected) exposure to lead

Z77.012 Contact with and (suspected) exposure to uranium

Excludes1 retained depleted uranium fragments (Z18.01)

Z77.018 Contact with and (suspected) exposure to other hazardous metals
Contact with and (suspected) exposure to chromium compounds
Contact with and (suspected) exposure to nickel dust

● **Z77.02** Contact with and (suspected) exposure to hazardous aromatic compounds

Z77.020 Contact with and (suspected) exposure to aromatic amines

Z77.021 Contact with and (suspected) exposure to benzene

Z77.028 Contact with and (suspected) exposure to other hazardous aromatic compounds
Aromatic dyes NOS
Polycyclic aromatic hydrocarbons

● **Z77.09** Contact with and (suspected) exposure to other hazardous, chiefly nonmedicinal, chemicals

Z77.090 Contact with and (suspected) exposure to asbestos

Z77.098 Contact with and (suspected) exposure to other hazardous, chiefly nonmedicinal, chemicals
Dyes NOS

● **Z77.1** Contact with and (suspected) exposure to environmental pollution and hazards in the physical environment

● **Z77.11** Contact with and (suspected) exposure to environmental pollution

Z77.110 Contact with and (suspected) exposure to air pollution

Z77.111 Contact with and (suspected) exposure to water pollution

Z77.112 Contact with and (suspected) exposure to soil pollution

Z77.118 Contact with and (suspected) exposure to other environmental pollution

● **Z77.12** Contact with and (suspected) exposure to hazards in the physical environment

Z77.120 Contact with and (suspected) exposure to mold (toxic)

Z77.121 Contact with and (suspected) exposure to harmful algae and algae toxins
Contact with and (suspected) exposure to (harmful) algae bloom NOS
Contact with and (suspected) exposure to blue-green algae bloom
Contact with and (suspected) exposure to brown tide
Contact with and (suspected) exposure to cyanobacteria bloom
Contact with and (suspected) exposure to Florida red tide
Contact with and (suspected) exposure to pfiesteria piscicida
Contact with and (suspected) exposure to red tide

▶ New   ➡ Revised   ~~deleted~~ Deleted   Excludes 1   Excludes 2   Includes   Use additional   Code first   Code also   Key words

OGCR Official Guidelines   **X** Assign placeholder X   ● Use Additional Character(s)   ▶ Manifestation Code   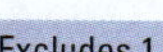 Hierarchical Condition Category   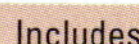 **Coding Clinic**

Z77.122   **Contact with and (suspected) exposure to** noise

Z77.123   **Contact with and (suspected) exposure to** radon and other naturally occurring radiation

   Excludes2   radiation exposure as the cause of a confirmed condition (W88-W90, X39.0-)
   radiation sickness NOS (T66)

Z77.128   **Contact with and (suspected) exposure to** other hazards in the physical environment

● **Z77.2   Contact with and (suspected) exposure to** other hazardous substances

Z77.21   **Contact with and (suspected) exposure to potentially** hazardous body fluids

Z77.22   **Contact with and (suspected) exposure to environmental** tobacco smoke (acute) (chronic)
   Exposure to second hand tobacco smoke (acute) (chronic)
   Passive smoking (acute) (chronic)

   Excludes1   nicotine dependence (F17.-)
   tobacco use (Z72.0)

   Excludes2   occupational exposure to environmental tobacco smoke (Z57.31)

Z77.29   **Contact with and (suspected) exposure to** other hazardous substances
   Coding Clinic: 2016, Q2, P34

▶ **Z77.3   Contact with and (suspected) exposure to war theater**

▶   **Z77.31   Contact with and (suspected) exposure to Gulf War theater**
   ▶ Contact with and (suspected) exposure to Persian Gulf War theater

▶   **Z77.39   Contact with and (suspected) exposure to other war theater**
   ▶ Agent Orange exposure

Z77.9   **Other contact with and (suspected) exposures hazardous to health**

● **Z78   Other specified health status**

   Excludes2   asymptomatic human immunodeficiency virus [HIV] infection status (Z21)
   postprocedural status (Z93-Z99)
   sex reassignment status (Z87.890)

Z78.0   **Asymptomatic menopausal state**   A
   Menopausal state NOS
   Postmenopausal status NOS

   Excludes2   symptomatic menopausal state (N95.1)

Z78.1   **Physical restraint status**

   Excludes1   physical restraint due to a procedure - omit code

Z78.9   **Other specified health status**

● **Z79   Long term (current) drug therapy**

   Includes   long term (current) drug use for prophylactic purposes

   Code also any therapeutic drug level monitoring (Z51.81)

   Excludes2   drug abuse and dependence (F11-F19)
   drug use complicating pregnancy, childbirth, and the puerperium (O99.32-)
   Coding Clinic: 2024, Q2, P26

● **Z79.0   Long term (current) use of anticoagulants and antithrombotics/antiplatelets**

   Excludes2   long term (current) use of aspirin (Z79.82)
   Coding Clinic: 2021, Q1, P12-13

Z79.01   **Long term (current) use of anticoagulants**
   Coding Clinic: 2023, Q2, P28; 2022, Q2, P17; 2021, Q1, P5

Z79.02   **Long term (current) use of antithrombotics/antiplatelets**

Z79.1   **Long term (current) use of** non-steroidal anti-inflammatories (NSAID)

   Excludes2   long term (current) use of aspirin (Z79.82)

Z79.2   **Long term (current) use of** antibiotics

Z79.3   **Long term (current) use of** hormonal contraceptives
   Long term (current) use of birth control pill or patch

Z79.4   **Long term (current) use of** insulin 🟣

   Excludes2   long-term (current) use of injectable non-insulin antidiabetic drugs (Z79.85)
   long term (current) use of oral hypoglycemic drugs (Z79.84)
   long term (current) use of oral antidiabetic drugs (Z79.84)

● **Z79.5   Long term (current) use of** steroids

Z79.51   **Long term (current) use of** inhaled steroids

Z79.52   **Long term (current) use of** systemic steroids
   Coding Clinic: 2024, Q3, P15

● **Z79.6   Long term (current) use of immunomodulators and immunosuppressants**

   Excludes2   long term (current) use of steroids (Z79.5-)
   long term (current) use of agents affecting estrogen receptors and estrogen levels (Z79.81-)

Z79.60   **Long term (current) use of unspecified immunomodulators and immunosuppressants**

Z79.61   **Long term (current) use of immunomodulator**
   Long term (current) use of apremilast
   Long term (current) use of immunomodulatory imide drug
   Long term (current) use of lenalidomide
   Long term (current) use of pomalidomide

● **Z79.62   Long term (current) use of immunosuppressant**

Z79.620   **Long term (current) use of immunosuppressive biologic**
   Long term (current) use of adalimumab
   Long term (current) use of etanercept
   Long term (current) use of infliximab
   Long term (current) use of monoclonal antibodies

Z79.621   **Long term (current) use of calcineurin inhibitor**
   Long term (current) use of cyclosporine
   Long term (current) use of tacrolimus

Z79.622   **Long term (current) use of Janus kinase inhibitor**
   Long term (current) use of tofacitinib

Z79.623   **Long term (current) use of mammalian target of rapamycin (mTOR) inhibitor**
   Long term (current) use of sirolimus

Z79.624   **Long term (current) use of inhibitors of nucleotide synthesis**
   Long term (current) use of azathioprine
   Long term (current) use mycophenolate
   Long term (current) use of purine synthesis (IMDH) inhibitors

CHAPTER 21 (Z00-Z99)

● **Z79.63** **Long term (current) use of chemotherapeutic agent**

     Z79.630 **Long term (current) use of alkylating agent**
         Long term (current) use of chlorambucil
         Long term (current) use of cisplatin
         Long term (current) use of cyclophosphamide

     Z79.631 **Long term (current) use of antimetabolite agent**
         Long term (current) use of 5-fluorouracil
         Long term (current) use of 6-mercaptopurine
         Long term (current) use of cytarabine
         Long term (current) use of methotrexate

     Z79.632 **Long term (current) use of antitumor antibiotic**
         Long term (current) use of bleomycin
         Long term (current) use of doxorubicin
         Long term (current) use of mitomycin C

     Z79.633 **Long term (current) use of mitotic inhibitor**
         Long term (current) use of paclitaxel
         Long term (current) use of plant alkaloids
         Long term (current) use of vinblastine
         Long term (current) use of vincristine

     Z79.634 **Long term (current) use of topoisomerase inhibitor**
         Long term (current) use of etoposide
         Long term (current) use of irinotecan
         Long term (current) use of topotecan

    Z79.64 **Long term (current) use of myelosuppressive agent**
         Long term (current) use of hydroxyurea

    Z79.69 **Long term (current) use of other immunomodulators and immunosuppressants**

● **Z79.8** **Other long term (current) drug therapy**

●   **Z79.81** **Long term (current) use of agents affecting estrogen receptors and estrogen levels**

Code first, if applicable:
     malignant neoplasm of breast (C50.-)
     malignant neoplasm of prostate (C61)

Use additional code, if applicable, to identify:
     estrogen receptor positive status (Z17.0)
     family history of breast cancer (Z80.3)
     genetic susceptibility to malignant neoplasm (cancer) (Z15.0-)
     personal history of breast cancer (Z85.3)
     personal history of prostate cancer (Z85.46)
     postmenopausal status (Z78.0)

     Excludes1   hormone replacement therapy (Z79.890)

     Z79.810 **Long term (current) use of selective estrogen receptor modulators (SERMs)**
         Long term (current) use of raloxifene (Evista)
         Long term (current) use of tamoxifen (Nolvadex)
         Long term (current) use of toremifene (Fareston)
         Coding Clinic: 2022, Q3, P15

     Z79.811 **Long term (current) use of aromatase inhibitors**
         Long term (current) use of anastrozole (Arimidex)
         Long term (current) use of exemestane (Aromasin)
         Long term (current) use of letrozole (Femara)

     Z79.818 **Long term (current) use of other agents affecting estrogen receptors and estrogen levels**
         Long term (current) use of estrogen receptor downregulators
         Long term (current) use of fulvestrant (Faslodex)
         Long term (current) use of gonadotropin-releasing hormone (GnRH) agonist
         Long term (current) use of goserelin acetate (Zoladex)
         Long term (current) use of leuprolide acetate (leuprorelin) (Lupron)
         Long term (current) use of megestrol acetate (Megace)

    Z79.82 **Long term (current) use of aspirin**

    Z79.83 **Long term (current) use of bisphosphonates**
         Coding Clinic: 2016, Q4, P42

    Z79.84 **Long term (current) use of oral hypoglycemic drugs**
         Long term (current) use of oral antidiabetic drugs

     Excludes2   long-term (current) use of injectable non-insulin antidiabetic drugs (Z79.85)
         long term (current) use of insulin (Z79.4)
         Coding Clinic: 2016, Q4, P76, 121-122, 126

    Z79.85 **Long-term (current) use of injectable non-insulin antidiabetic drugs**

     Excludes2   long term (current) use of insulin (Z79.4)
         long term (current) use of oral hypoglycemic drugs (Z79.84)

●   **Z79.89** **Other long term (current) drug therapy**

     Z79.890 **Hormone replacement therapy**

     Z79.891 **Long term (current) use of opiate analgesic**
         Long term (current) use of methadone for pain management

     Excludes1   methadone use NOS (F11.9-)
         use of methadone for treatment of heroin addiction (F11.2-)

     Z79.899 **Other long term (current) drug therapy**
         Coding Clinic: 2023, Q3, P17-18; 2015, Q4, P34, Q3, P21

● **Z80** **Family history of primary malignant neoplasm**

    Z80.0 **Family history of malignant neoplasm of digestive organs**
         Conditions classifiable to C15-C26
         Coding Clinic: 2018, Q1, P7

    Z80.1 **Family history of malignant neoplasm of trachea, bronchus and lung**
         Conditions classifiable to C33-C34

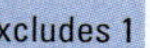

▶ New   ⇒ Revised   ~~deleted~~ Deleted   Excludes 1   Excludes 2   Includes   Use additional   Code first   Code also   Key words
OGCR Official Guidelines   **X** Assign placeholder X   ● Use Additional Character(s)   ▶ Manifestation Code   **HCC** Hierarchical Condition Category   **Coding Clinic**

Z80.2   **Family history of malignant neoplasm of other respiratory and intrathoracic organs**
Conditions classifiable to C30-C32, C37-C39

Z80.3   **Family history of malignant neoplasm of breast**
Conditions classifiable to C50.-

● Z80.4   **Family history of malignant neoplasm of genital organs**
Conditions classifiable to C51-C63

    Z80.41   Family history of malignant neoplasm of ovary

    Z80.42   Family history of malignant neoplasm of prostate

    Z80.43   Family history of malignant neoplasm of testis

▶   Z80.44   Family history of malignant neoplasm of fallopian tube(s)

    Z80.49   Family history of malignant neoplasm of other genital organs

● Z80.5   **Family history of malignant neoplasm of urinary tract**
Conditions classifiable to C64-C68

    Z80.51   Family history of malignant neoplasm of kidney

    Z80.52   Family history of malignant neoplasm of bladder

    Z80.59   Family history of malignant neoplasm of other urinary tract organ

Z80.6   **Family history of leukemia**
Conditions classifiable to C91-C95

Z80.7   **Family history of other malignant neoplasms of lymphoid, hematopoietic and related tissues**
Conditions classifiable to C81-C90, C96.-

Z80.8   **Family history of malignant neoplasm of other organs or systems**
Conditions classifiable to C00-C14, C40-C49, C69-C79

Z80.9   **Family history of malignant neoplasm, unspecified**
Conditions classifiable to C80.1

● **Z81   Family history of mental and behavioral disorders**

Z81.0   **Family history of intellectual disabilities**
Conditions classifiable to F70-F79

Z81.1   **Family history of alcohol abuse and dependence**
Conditions classifiable to F10.-

Z81.2   **Family history of tobacco abuse and dependence**
Conditions classifiable to F17.-

Z81.3   **Family history of other psychoactive substance abuse and dependence**
Conditions classifiable to F11-F16, F18-F19

Z81.4   **Family history of other substance abuse and dependence**
Conditions classifiable to F55

Z81.8   **Family history of other mental and behavioral disorders**
Conditions classifiable elsewhere in F01-F99

● **Z82   Family history of certain disabilities and chronic diseases (leading to disablement)**

Z82.0   **Family history of epilepsy and other diseases of the nervous system**
Conditions classifiable to G00-G99

Z82.1   **Family history of blindness and visual loss**
Conditions classifiable to H54.-

Z82.2   **Family history of deafness and hearing loss**
Conditions classifiable to H90-H91

Z82.3   **Family history of stroke**
Conditions classifiable to I60-I64

● Z82.4   **Family history of ischemic heart disease and other diseases of the circulatory system**
Conditions classifiable to I00-I5A, I65-I99

    Z82.41   Family history of sudden cardiac death

    Z82.49   Family history of ischemic heart disease and other diseases of the circulatory system

Z82.5   **Family history of asthma and other chronic lower respiratory diseases**
Conditions classifiable to J40-J47

    Excludes2   family history of other diseases of the respiratory system (Z83.6)

● Z82.6   **Family history of arthritis and other diseases of the musculoskeletal system and connective tissue**
Conditions classifiable to M00-M99

    Z82.61   Family history of arthritis

    Z82.62   Family history of osteoporosis

    Z82.69   Family history of other diseases of the musculoskeletal system and connective tissue

● Z82.7   **Family history of congenital malformations, deformations and chromosomal abnormalities**
Conditions classifiable to Q00-Q99

    Z82.71   Family history of polycystic kidney

    Z82.79   Family history of other congenital malformations, deformations and chromosomal abnormalities

Z82.8   **Family history of other disabilities and chronic diseases leading to disablement, not elsewhere classified**

● **Z83   Family history of other specific disorders**

    Excludes2   contact with and (suspected) exposure to communicable disease in the family (Z20.-)

Z83.0   **Family history of human immunodeficiency virus [HIV] disease**
Conditions classifiable to B20

Z83.1   **Family history of other infectious and parasitic diseases**
Conditions classifiable to A00-B19, B25-B94, B99

Z83.2   **Family history of diseases of the blood and blood-forming organs and certain disorders involving the immune mechanism**
Conditions classifiable to D50-D89

Z83.3   **Family history of diabetes mellitus**
Conditions classifiable to E08-E13

● Z83.4   **Family history of other endocrine, nutritional and metabolic diseases**
Conditions classifiable to E00-E07, E15-E88

    Z83.41   Family history of multiple endocrine neoplasia [MEN] syndrome

    Z83.42   Family history of familial hypercholesterolemia
        Coding Clinic: 2016, Q4, P77

●   Z83.43   Family history of other disorder of lipoprotein metabolism and other lipidemias

        Z83.430   Family history of elevated lipoprotein(a)
            Family history of elevated Lp(a)

        Z83.438   Family history of other disorder of lipoprotein metabolism and other lipidemia
            Family history of familial combined hyperlipidemia

    Z83.49   Family history of other endocrine, nutritional and metabolic diseases

● Z83.5   **Family history of eye and ear disorders**

●   Z83.51   Family history of eye disorders
Conditions classifiable to H00-H53, H55-H59

        Excludes2   family history of blindness and visual loss (Z82.1)

        Z83.511   Family history of glaucoma

        Z83.518   Family history of other specified eye disorder

    Z83.52   Family history of ear disorders
Conditions classifiable to H60-H83, H92-H95

        Excludes2   family history of deafness and hearing loss (Z82.2)

Z83.6   **Family history of other diseases of the respiratory system**
Conditions classifiable to J00-J39, J60-J99

    Excludes2   family history of asthma and other chronic lower respiratory diseases (Z82.5)

CHAPTER 21 (Z00-Z99)

● **Z83.7   Family history of diseases of the digestive system**
Conditions classifiable to D12, K00-K93

● **Z83.71   Family history of colonic polyps**
Excludes2   family history of malignant neoplasm of digestive organs (Z80.0)
Coding Clinic: 2021, Q1, P15

Z83.710   Family history of adenomatous and serrated polyps
Conditions classifiable to D12.-
Family history of tubular adenoma polyps
Family history of tubulovillous adenoma polyps
Family history of villous adenoma polyps

Z83.711   Family history of hyperplastic colon polyps

➡ **Z83.718   Family history of other colon polyps**
Family history of inflammatory colon polyps

Z83.719   Family history of colon polyps, unspecified
Family history of colon polyps NOS

Z83.72   Family history of familial adenomatous polyposis

Z83.79   Family history of other diseases of the digestive system

● **Z84   Family history of other conditions**

Z84.0   Family history of diseases of the skin and subcutaneous tissue
Conditions classifiable to L00-L99

● **Z84.1   Family history of disorders of kidney and ureter**
Conditions classifiable to N00-N29

▶ **Z84.11   Family history of APOL1-mediated kidney disease [AMKD]**

▶ **Z84.19   Family history of other disorders of kidney and ureter**

Z84.2   Family history of other diseases of the genitourinary system
Conditions classifiable to N30-N99
Coding Clinic: 2016, Q4, P77

Z84.3   Family history of consanguinity

● **Z84.8   Family history of other specified conditions**

Z84.81   Family history of carrier of genetic disease
Coding Clinic: 2021, Q1, P15

Z84.82   Family history of sudden infant death syndrome
Family history of SIDS

Z84.89   Family history of other specified conditions

▶ **Z84.A   Family history of exposure to diethylstilbestrol**
DES granddaughter or grandson
Family history of DES exposure
Third generation DES exposure

● **Z85   Personal history of malignant neoplasm**
Code first any follow-up examination after treatment of malignant neoplasm (Z08)
Use additional code to identify:
alcohol use and dependence (F10.-)
exposure to environmental tobacco smoke (Z77.22)
history of tobacco dependence (Z87.891)
occupational exposure to environmental tobacco smoke (Z57.31)
tobacco dependence (F17.-)
tobacco use (Z72.0)
Excludes2   personal history of benign neoplasm (Z86.01-)
personal history of carcinoma-in-situ (Z86.00-)
Coding Clinic: 2022, Q3, P28

● **Z85.0   Personal history of malignant neoplasm of digestive organs**

Z85.00   Personal history of malignant neoplasm of unspecified digestive organ

Z85.01   Personal history of malignant neoplasm of esophagus
Conditions classifiable to C15

● **Z85.02   Personal history of malignant neoplasm of stomach**

Z85.020   Personal history of malignant carcinoid tumor of stomach
Conditions classifiable to C7A.092

Z85.028   Personal history of other malignant neoplasm of stomach
Conditions classifiable to C16

● **Z85.03   Personal history of malignant neoplasm of large intestine**

Z85.030   Personal history of malignant carcinoid tumor of large intestine
Conditions classifiable to C7A.022-C7A.025, C7A.029

Z85.038   Personal history of other malignant neoplasm of large intestine
Conditions classifiable to C18

● **Z85.04   Personal history of malignant neoplasm of rectum, rectosigmoid junction, and anus**

Z85.040   Personal history of malignant carcinoid tumor of rectum
Conditions classifiable to C7A.026

Z85.048   Personal history of other malignant neoplasm of rectum, rectosigmoid junction, and anus
Conditions classifiable to C19-C21

Z85.05   Personal history of malignant neoplasm of liver
Conditions classifiable to C22

● **Z85.06   Personal history of malignant neoplasm of small intestine**

Z85.060   Personal history of malignant carcinoid tumor of small intestine
Conditions classifiable to C7A.01-

Z85.068   Personal history of other malignant neoplasm of small intestine
Conditions classifiable to C17

Z85.07   Personal history of malignant neoplasm of pancreas
Conditions classifiable to C25

Z85.09   Personal history of malignant neoplasm of other digestive organs

● **Z85.1   Personal history of malignant neoplasm of trachea, bronchus and lung**

● **Z85.11   Personal history of malignant neoplasm of bronchus and lung**

Z85.110   Personal history of malignant carcinoid tumor of bronchus and lung
Conditions classifiable to C7A.090

Z85.118   Personal history of other malignant neoplasm of bronchus and lung
Conditions classifiable to C34

Z85.12   Personal history of malignant neoplasm of trachea
Conditions classifiable to C33

● **Z85.2   Personal history of malignant neoplasm of other respiratory and intrathoracic organs**

Z85.20   Personal history of malignant neoplasm of unspecified respiratory organ

Z85.21   Personal history of malignant neoplasm of larynx
Conditions classifiable to C32

Z85.22   Personal history of malignant neoplasm of nasal cavities, middle ear, and accessory sinuses
Conditions classifiable to C30-C31

▶ New   ➡ Revised   ~~deleted~~ Deleted   Excludes 1   Excludes 2   Includes   Use additional   Code first   Code also   Key words
OGCR Official Guidelines   **X** Assign placeholder X   ● Use Additional Character(s)   ▌ Manifestation Code   Ⓗ Hierarchical Condition Category   **Coding Clinic**

● **Z85.23 Personal history of malignant neoplasm of thymus**

    Z85.230 Personal history of malignant carcinoid tumor of thymus
        Conditions classifiable to C7A.091

    Z85.238 Personal history of other malignant neoplasm of thymus
        Conditions classifiable to C37

    Z85.29 Personal history of malignant neoplasm of other respiratory and intrathoracic organs

Z85.3 Personal history of malignant neoplasm of breast
    Conditions classifiable to C50.-

● **Z85.4 Personal history of malignant neoplasm of genital organs**
    Conditions classifiable to C51-C63

    Z85.40 Personal history of malignant neoplasm of unspecified female genital organ

    Z85.41 Personal history of malignant neoplasm of cervix uteri

    Z85.42 Personal history of malignant neoplasm of other parts of uterus

    Z85.43 Personal history of malignant neoplasm of ovary

    Z85.44 Personal history of malignant neoplasm of other female genital organs
        Coding Clinic: 2024, Q2, P11,12

    Z85.45 Personal history of malignant neoplasm of unspecified male genital organ

    Z85.46 Personal history of malignant neoplasm of prostate
        Coding Clinic: 2023, Q2, P5

    Z85.47 Personal history of malignant neoplasm of testis

    Z85.48 Personal history of malignant neoplasm of epididymis

    Z85.49 Personal history of malignant neoplasm of other male genital organs

    ▶ **Z85.4A Personal history of malignant neoplasm of fallopian tube(s)**

● **Z85.5 Personal history of malignant neoplasm of urinary tract**
    Conditions classifiable to C64-C68

    Z85.50 Personal history of malignant neoplasm of unspecified urinary tract organ

    Z85.51 Personal history of malignant neoplasm of bladder

    ● **Z85.52 Personal history of malignant neoplasm of kidney**
        Excludes1   personal history of malignant neoplasm of renal pelvis (Z85.53)

        Z85.520 Personal history of malignant carcinoid tumor of kidney
           Conditions classifiable to C7A.093

        Z85.528 Personal history of other malignant neoplasm of kidney
           Conditions classifiable to C64

    Z85.53 Personal history of malignant neoplasm of renal pelvis

    Z85.54 Personal history of malignant neoplasm of ureter

    Z85.59 Personal history of malignant neoplasm of other urinary tract organ

Z85.6 Personal history of leukemia
    Conditions classifiable to C91-C95
    Excludes1   leukemia in remission C91.0-C95.9 with 5th character 1

● **Z85.7 Personal history of other malignant neoplasms of lymphoid, hematopoietic and related tissues**

    Z85.71 Personal history of Hodgkin lymphoma
        Conditions classifiable to C81

    Z85.72 Personal history of non-Hodgkin lymphomas
        Conditions classifiable to C82-C85
        Coding Clinic: 2022, Q3, P28

    Z85.79 Personal history of other malignant neoplasms of lymphoid, hematopoietic and related tissues
        Conditions classifiable to C88-C90, C96

        Excludes1   multiple myeloma in remission (C90.01)
            plasma cell leukemia in remission (C90.11)
            plasmacytoma in remission (C90.21)

● **Z85.8 Personal history of malignant neoplasms of other organs and systems**
    Conditions classifiable to C00-C14, C40-C49, C69-C75, C7A.098, C76-C79

    ● **Z85.81 Personal history of malignant neoplasm of lip, oral cavity, and pharynx**
        Conditions classifiable to C00-C14

        Z85.810 Personal history of malignant neoplasm of tongue

        Z85.818 Personal history of malignant neoplasm of other sites of lip, oral cavity, and pharynx

        Z85.819 Personal history of malignant neoplasm of unspecified site of lip, oral cavity, and pharynx

    ● **Z85.82 Personal history of malignant neoplasm of skin**

        Z85.820 Personal history of malignant melanoma of skin
           Conditions classifiable to C43
           Coding Clinic: 2022, Q3, P9

        Z85.821 Personal history of Merkel cell carcinoma
           Conditions classifiable to C4A

        Z85.828 Personal history of other malignant neoplasm of skin
           Conditions classifiable to C44

    ● **Z85.83 Personal history of malignant neoplasm of bone and soft tissue**
        Conditions classifiable to C40-C41; C45-C49

        Z85.830 Personal history of malignant neoplasm of bone

        Z85.831 Personal history of malignant neoplasm of soft tissue
           Excludes2   personal history of malignant neoplasm of skin (Z85.82-)

    ● **Z85.84 Personal history of malignant neoplasm of eye and nervous tissue**
        Conditions classifiable to C69-C72

        Z85.840 Personal history of malignant neoplasm of eye

        Z85.841 Personal history of malignant neoplasm of brain

        Z85.848 Personal history of malignant neoplasm of other parts of nervous tissue

    ● **Z85.85 Personal history of malignant neoplasm of endocrine glands**
        Conditions classifiable to C73-C75

        Z85.850 Personal history of malignant neoplasm of thyroid

        Z85.858 Personal history of malignant neoplasm of other endocrine glands
           Coding Clinic: 2024, Q2, P10

    Z85.89 Personal history of malignant neoplasm of other organs and systems
        Conditions classifiable to C7A.098, C76, C77-C79

Z85.9 Personal history of malignant neoplasm, unspecified
    Conditions classifiable to C7A.00, C80.1

CHAPTER 21 (Z00-Z99)

Z86 **Personal history of certain other diseases**
Code first any follow-up examination after treatment (Z09)

Z86.0 **Personal history of in-situ and benign neoplasms and neoplasms of uncertain behavior**

> **Excludes2** personal history of malignant neoplasms (Z85.-)

Z86.00 **Personal history of in-situ neoplasm**
Conditions classifiable to D00-D09

Z86.000 **Personal history of in-situ neoplasm of breast**
Conditions classifiable to D05

Z86.001 **Personal history of in-situ neoplasm of cervix uteri**
Conditions classifiable to D06
Personal history of cervical intraepithelial neoplasia III [CIN III]

Z86.002 **Personal history of in-situ neoplasm of other and unspecified genital organs**
Conditions classifiable to D07
Personal history of high-grade prostatic intraepithelial neoplasia III [HGPIN III]
Personal history of vaginal intraepithelial neoplasia III [VAIN III]
Personal history of vulvar intraepithelial neoplasia III [VIN III]

Z86.003 **Personal history of in-situ neoplasm of oral cavity, esophagus and stomach**
Conditions classifiable to D00

Z86.004 **Personal history of in-situ neoplasm of other and unspecified digestive organs**
Conditions classifiable to D01
Personal history of anal intraepithelial neoplasia (AIN III)

Z86.005 **Personal history of in-situ neoplasm of middle ear and respiratory system**
Conditions classifiable to D02

Z86.006 **Personal history of melanoma in-situ**
Conditions classifiable to D03

> **Excludes2** sites other than skin - code to personal history of in-situ neoplasm of the site

Z86.007 **Personal history of in-situ neoplasm of skin**
Conditions classifiable to D04
Personal history of carcinoma in situ of skin

Z86.008 **Personal history of in-situ neoplasm of other site**
Conditions classifiable to D09

▶ Z86.00A **Personal history of in-situ neoplasm of the fallopian tube(s)**

Z86.01 **Personal history of benign neoplasm**
Coding Clinic: 2017, Q1, P14

Z86.010 **Personal history of colon polyps**
Personal history of colorectal polyps
Personal history of rectal polyps
Coding Clinic: 2021, Q1, P15; 2017, Q1, P9, P14

Z86.0100 **Personal history of colon polyps, unspecified**
Personal history of colon polyps NOS

Z86.0101 **Personal history of adenomatous and serrated colon polyps**
Personal history of tubular adenoma polyps
Personal history of sessile adenomatous colon polyp
Personal history of sessile serrated colon polyp
Personal history of tubulovillous adenoma polyps
Personal history of villous adenoma polyps
Personal history of traditional serrated adenoma polyps

Z86.0102 **Personal history of hyperplastic colon polyps**

Z86.0109 **Personal history of other colon polyps**

Z86.011 **Personal history of benign neoplasm of the brain**

Z86.012 **Personal history of benign carcinoid tumor**

Z86.018 **Personal history of other benign neoplasm**
Coding Clinic: 2017, Q1, P14

Z86.03 **Personal history of neoplasm of uncertain behavior**

Z86.1 **Personal history of infectious and parasitic diseases**
Conditions classifiable to A00-B89, B99

> **Excludes1** personal history of infectious diseases specific to a body system sequelae of infectious and parasitic diseases (B90-B94)

Coding Clinic: 2016, Q4, P5

Z86.11 **Personal history of tuberculosis**

Z86.12 **Personal history of poliomyelitis**

Z86.13 **Personal history of malaria**

Z86.14 **Personal history of Methicillin resistant Staphylococcus aureus infection**
Personal history of MRSA infection

Z86.15 **Personal history of latent tuberculosis infection**

Z86.16 **Personal history of COVID-19**

> **Excludes1** post COVID-19 condition (U09.9)

Coding Clinic: 2022, Q3, P4; 2021, Q4, P103-105, 107-108; 2021, Q1, P34-35, 40-42, 44, 46

Z86.19 **Personal history of other infectious and parasitic diseases**
Coding Clinic: 2021, Q1, P34-35, 40-41

Z86.2 **Personal history of diseases of the blood and blood-forming organs and certain disorders involving the immune mechanism**
Conditions classifiable to D50-D89

Z86.3 **Personal history of endocrine, nutritional and metabolic diseases**
Conditions classifiable to E00-E88

Z86.31 **Personal history of diabetic foot ulcer**

> **Excludes2** current diabetic foot ulcer (E08.621, E09.621, E10.621, E11.621, E13.621)

Z86.32 **Personal history of gestational diabetes**
Personal history of conditions classifiable to O24.4-

> **Excludes1** gestational diabetes mellitus in current pregnancy (O24.4-)

Z86.39 **Personal history of other endocrine, nutritional and metabolic disease**
Coding Clinic: 2020, Q1, P13

- **Z86.5   Personal history of mental and behavioral disorders**
  Conditions classifiable to F40-F59
    - **Z86.51   Personal history of combat and operational stress reaction**   **A**
    - **Z86.59   Personal history of other mental and behavioral disorders**
- **Z86.6   Personal history of diseases of the nervous system and sense organs**
  Conditions classifiable to G00-G99, H00-H95
    - **Z86.61   Personal history of infections of the central nervous system**
      Personal history of encephalitis
      Personal history of meningitis
    - **Z86.69   Personal history of other diseases of the nervous system and sense organs**
      Coding Clinic: 2016, Q4, P25
- **Z86.7   Personal history of diseases of the circulatory system**
  Conditions classifiable to I00-I99
    Excludes2   old myocardial infarction (I25.2)
    personal history of anaphylactic shock (Z87.892)
    postmyocardial infarction syndrome (I24.1)
    - **Z86.71   Personal history of venous thrombosis and embolism**
        - **Z86.711   Personal history of pulmonary embolism**
        - **Z86.718   Personal history of other venous thrombosis and embolism**
    - **Z86.72   Personal history of thrombophlebitis**
    - **Z86.73   Personal history of transient ischemic attack (TIA), and cerebral infarction without residual deficits**
      Personal history of prolonged reversible ischemic neurological deficit (PRIND)
      Personal history of stroke NOS without residual deficits
        Excludes1   personal history of traumatic brain injury (Z87.820)
        sequelae of cerebrovascular disease (I69.-)
      Coding Clinic: 2023, Q1, P37; 2012, Q4, P3
    - **Z86.74   Personal history of sudden cardiac arrest**
      Personal history of sudden cardiac death successfully resuscitated
      Coding Clinic: 2024, Q1, P27
    - **Z86.79   Personal history of other diseases of the circulatory system**
      Coding Clinic: 2022, Q2, P15; 2020, Q1, P13
- **Z87   Personal history of other diseases and conditions**
  Code first any follow-up examination after treatment (Z09)
- **Z87.0   Personal history of diseases of the respiratory system**
  Conditions classifiable to J00-J99
    - **Z87.01   Personal history of pneumonia (recurrent)**
    - **Z87.09   Personal history of other diseases of the respiratory system**
- **Z87.1   Personal history of diseases of the digestive system**
  Conditions classifiable to K00-K93
    - **Z87.11   Personal history of peptic ulcer disease**
    - **Z87.19   Personal history of other diseases of the digestive system**
      Coding Clinic: 2017, Q1, P14
  - **Z87.2   Personal history of diseases of the skin and subcutaneous tissue**
    Conditions classifiable to L00-L99
      Excludes2   personal history of diabetic foot ulcer (Z86.31)
- **Z87.3   Personal history of diseases of the musculoskeletal system and connective tissue**
  Conditions classifiable to M00-M99
    Excludes2   personal history of (healed) traumatic fracture (Z87.81)

- **Z87.31   Personal history of (healed) nontraumatic fracture**
    - **Z87.310   Personal history of (healed) osteoporosis fracture**
      Personal history of (healed) fragility fracture
      Personal history of (healed) collapsed vertebra due to osteoporosis
    - **Z87.311   Personal history of (healed) other pathological fracture**
      Personal history of (healed) collapsed vertebra NOS
        Excludes2   personal history of osteoporosis fracture (Z87.310)
    - **Z87.312   Personal history of (healed) stress fracture**
      Personal history of (healed) fatigue fracture
    - **Z87.39   Personal history of other diseases of the musculoskeletal system and connective tissue**
- **Z87.4   Personal history of diseases of genitourinary system**
  Conditions classifiable to N00-N99
    - **Z87.41   Personal history of dysplasia of the female genital tract**
        Excludes1   personal history of intraepithelial neoplasia III of female genital tract (Z86.001, Z86.008, Z86.00A)
        personal history of malignant neoplasm of female genital tract (Z85.40-Z85.44, Z85.4A)
        - **Z87.410   Personal history of cervical dysplasia**
        - **Z87.411   Personal history of vaginal dysplasia**
        - **Z87.412   Personal history of vulvar dysplasia**
    - **Z87.42   Personal history of other diseases of the female genital tract**
    - **Z87.43   Personal history of diseases of male genital organs**
        - **Z87.430   Personal history of prostatic dysplasia**
            Excludes1   personal history of malignant neoplasm of prostate (Z85.46)
        - **Z87.438   Personal history of other diseases of male genital organs**
    - **Z87.44   Personal history of diseases of urinary system**
        Excludes1   personal history of malignant neoplasm of cervix uteri (Z85.41)
        - **Z87.440   Personal history of urinary (tract) infections**
        - **Z87.441   Personal history of nephrotic syndrome**
        - **Z87.442   Personal history of urinary calculi**
          Personal history of kidney stones
        - **Z87.448   Personal history of other diseases of urinary system**
- **Z87.5   Personal history of complications of pregnancy, childbirth and the puerperium**
  Conditions classifiable to O00-O9A
    Excludes2   recurrent pregnancy loss (N96)
    - **Z87.51   Personal history of pre-term labor**
        Excludes1   current pregnancy with history of pre-term labor (O09.21-)
    - **Z87.59   Personal history of other complications of pregnancy, childbirth and the puerperium**
      Personal history of trophoblastic disease

● **Z87.6** **Personal history of certain (corrected) conditions arising in the perinatal period**
Conditions classifiable to P00-P96

> **Excludes1** personal history of (corrected) congenital malformations (Z87.7-)

Z87.61 **Personal history of (corrected) necrotizing enterocolitis of newborn**

Z87.68 **Personal history of other (corrected) conditions arising in the perinatal period**

● **Z87.7** **Personal history of (corrected) congenital malformations**
Conditions classifiable to Q00-Q89 that have been repaired or corrected

> **Excludes1** congenital malformations that have been partially corrected or repair but which still require medical treatment - code to condition

> **Excludes2** other postprocedural states (Z98.-)
> personal history of medical treatment (Z92.-)
> presence of cardiac and vascular implants and grafts (Z95.-)
> presence of other devices (Z97.-)
> presence of other functional implants (Z96.-)
> transplanted organ and tissue status (Z94.-)

● **Z87.71** **Personal history of (corrected) congenital malformations of genitourinary system**

Z87.710 **Personal history of (corrected) hypospadias**

Z87.718 **Personal history of other specified (corrected) congenital malformations of genitourinary system**

● **Z87.72** **Personal history of (corrected) congenital malformations of nervous system and sense organs**

Z87.720 **Personal history of (corrected) congenital malformations of eye**

Z87.721 **Personal history of (corrected) congenital malformations of ear**

Z87.728 **Personal history of other specified (corrected) congenital malformations of nervous system and sense organs**

● **Z87.73** **Personal history of (corrected) congenital malformations of digestive system**

Z87.730 **Personal history of (corrected) cleft lip and palate**

Z87.731 **Personal history of (corrected) tracheoesophageal fistula or atresia**

Z87.732 **Personal history of (corrected) persistent cloaca or cloacal malformations**

Z87.738 **Personal history of other specified (corrected) congenital malformations of digestive system**

Z87.74 **Personal history of (corrected) congenital malformations of heart and circulatory system**

Z87.75 **Personal history of (corrected) congenital malformations of respiratory system**

● **Z87.76** **Personal history of (corrected) congenital malformations of integument, limbs and musculoskeletal system**

Z87.760 **Personal history of (corrected) congenital diaphragmatic hernia or other congenital diaphragm malformations**

Z87.761 **Personal history of (corrected) gastroschisis**

Z87.762 **Personal history of (corrected) prune belly malformation**

Z87.763 **Personal history of other (corrected) congenital abdominal wall malformations**

Z87.768 **Personal history of other specified (corrected) congenital malformations of integument, limbs and musculoskeletal system**

● **Z87.79** **Personal history of other (corrected) congenital malformations**

Z87.790 **Personal history of (corrected) congenital malformations of face and neck**

Z87.798 **Personal history of other (corrected) congenital malformations**

● **Z87.8** **Personal history of other specified conditions**

> **Excludes2** personal history of self harm (Z91.5-)

Z87.81 **Personal history of (healed) traumatic fracture**

> **Excludes2** personal history of (healed) nontraumatic fracture (Z87.31-)

● **Z87.82** **Personal history of other (healed) physical injury and trauma**
Conditions classifiable to S00-T88, except traumatic fractures

Z87.820 **Personal history of traumatic brain injury**

> **Excludes1** personal history of transient ischemic attack (TIA), and cerebral infarction without residual deficits (Z86.73)

Z87.821 **Personal history of retained foreign body fully removed**

Z87.828 **Personal history of other (healed) physical injury and trauma**

● **Z87.89** **Personal history of other specified conditions**

Z87.890 **Personal history of sex reassignment**

Z87.891 **Personal history of nicotine dependence**

> **Excludes1** current nicotine dependence (F17.2-)

Coding Clinic: 2017, Q2, P27

Z87.892 **Personal history of anaphylaxis**

Code also allergy status such as:
allergy status to drugs, medicaments and biological substances (Z88.-)
allergy status, other than to drugs and biological substances (Z91.0-)

Coding Clinic: 2025, Q2, P16

Z87.898 **Personal history of other specified conditions**

Coding Clinic: 2013, Q1, P21

● **Z88** **Allergy status to drugs, medicaments and biological substances**

> **Excludes2** allergy status, other than to drugs and biological substances (Z91.0-)

Z88.0 **Allergy status to penicillin**

Z88.1 **Allergy status to other antibiotic agents**

Z88.2 **Allergy status to sulfonamides**
Coding Clinic: 2015, Q3, P23

Z88.3 **Allergy status to other anti-infective agents**

Z88.4 **Allergy status to anesthetic agent**

Z88.5 **Allergy status to narcotic agent**

Z88.6 **Allergy status to analgesic agent**

Z88.7 **Allergy status to serum and vaccine**

Z88.8 **Allergy status to other drugs, medicaments and biological substances**

Z88.9 **Allergy status to unspecified drugs, medicaments and biological substances**

● **Z89 Acquired absence of limb**
  Includes amputation status
      postprocedural loss of limb
      post-traumatic loss of limb
  Excludes1 acquired deformities of limbs (M20-M21)
      congenital absence of limbs (Q71-Q73)
● **Z89.0 Acquired absence of thumb and other finger(s)**
 ● **Z89.01 Acquired absence of thumb**
  Z89.011 Acquired absence of right thumb
  Z89.012 Acquired absence of left thumb
  Z89.019 Acquired absence of unspecified thumb
 ● **Z89.02 Acquired absence of other finger(s)**
   Excludes2 acquired absence of thumb (Z89.01-)
  Z89.021 Acquired absence of right finger(s)
  Z89.022 Acquired absence of left finger(s)
  Z89.029 Acquired absence of unspecified finger(s)
● **Z89.1 Acquired absence of hand and wrist**
 ● **Z89.11 Acquired absence of hand**
  Z89.111 Acquired absence of right hand
  Z89.112 Acquired absence of left hand
  Z89.119 Acquired absence of unspecified hand
 ● **Z89.12 Acquired absence of wrist**
  Disarticulation at wrist
  Z89.121 Acquired absence of right wrist
  Z89.122 Acquired absence of left wrist
  Z89.129 Acquired absence of unspecified wrist
● **Z89.2 Acquired absence of upper limb above wrist**
 ● **Z89.20 Acquired absence of upper limb, unspecified level**
  Z89.201 Acquired absence of right upper limb, unspecified level
  Z89.202 Acquired absence of left upper limb, unspecified level
  Z89.209 Acquired absence of unspecified upper limb, unspecified level
    Acquired absence of arm NOS
 ● **Z89.21 Acquired absence of upper limb below elbow**
  Z89.211 Acquired absence of right upper limb below elbow
  Z89.212 Acquired absence of left upper limb below elbow
  Z89.219 Acquired absence of unspecified upper limb below elbow
 ● **Z89.22 Acquired absence of upper limb above elbow**
  Disarticulation at elbow
  Z89.221 Acquired absence of right upper limb above elbow
  Z89.222 Acquired absence of left upper limb above elbow
  Z89.229 Acquired absence of unspecified upper limb above elbow
 ● **Z89.23 Acquired absence of shoulder**
  Acquired absence of shoulder joint following explantation of shoulder joint prosthesis, with or without presence of antibiotic-impregnated cement spacer
  Z89.231 Acquired absence of right shoulder
  Z89.232 Acquired absence of left shoulder
  Z89.239 Acquired absence of unspecified shoulder
● **Z89.4 Acquired absence of toe(s), foot, and ankle**
 ● **Z89.41 Acquired absence of great toe**
  Z89.411 Acquired absence of right great toe
  Z89.412 Acquired absence of left great toe
  Z89.419 Acquired absence of unspecified great toe

● **Z89.42 Acquired absence of other toe(s)**
  Excludes2 acquired absence of great toe (Z89.41-)
  Z89.421 Acquired absence of other right toe(s)
  Z89.422 Acquired absence of other left toe(s)
  Z89.429 Acquired absence of other toe(s), unspecified side
● **Z89.43 Acquired absence of foot**
  Z89.431 Acquired absence of right foot
  Z89.432 Acquired absence of left foot
  Z89.439 Acquired absence of unspecified foot
● **Z89.44 Acquired absence of ankle**
  Disarticulation of ankle
  Z89.441 Acquired absence of right ankle
  Z89.442 Acquired absence of left ankle
  Z89.449 Acquired absence of unspecified ankle
● **Z89.5 Acquired absence of leg below knee**
 ● **Z89.51 Acquired absence of leg below knee**
  Z89.511 Acquired absence of right leg below knee
  Z89.512 Acquired absence of left leg below knee
  Z89.519 Acquired absence of unspecified leg below knee
 ● **Z89.52 Acquired absence of knee**
  Acquired absence of knee joint following explantation of knee joint prosthesis, with or without presence of antibiotic-impregnated cement spacer
  Z89.521 Acquired absence of right knee
  Z89.522 Acquired absence of left knee
  Z89.529 Acquired absence of unspecified knee
● **Z89.6 Acquired absence of leg above knee**
 ● **Z89.61 Acquired absence of leg above knee**
  Acquired absence of leg NOS
  Disarticulation at knee
  Z89.611 Acquired absence of right leg above knee
  Z89.612 Acquired absence of left leg above knee
  Z89.619 Acquired absence of unspecified leg above knee
 ● **Z89.62 Acquired absence of hip**
  Acquired absence of hip joint following explantation of hip joint prosthesis, with or without presence of antibiotic-impregnated cement spacer
  Disarticulation at hip
  Z89.621 Acquired absence of right hip joint
  Z89.622 Acquired absence of left hip joint
  Z89.629 Acquired absence of unspecified hip joint
 Z89.9 Acquired absence of limb, unspecified
● **Z90 Acquired absence of organs, not elsewhere classified**
  Includes postprocedural or post-traumatic loss of body part NEC
  Excludes1 congenital absence - see Alphabetical Index
  Excludes2 postprocedural absence of endocrine glands (E89.-)
● **Z90.0 Acquired absence of part of head and neck**
  Z90.01 Acquired absence of eye
  Z90.02 Acquired absence of larynx
  Z90.09 Acquired absence of other part of head and neck
    Acquired absence of nose
    Excludes2 teeth (K08.1)

● **Z90.1** Acquired absence of breast and nipple
     Z90.10 Acquired absence of unspecified breast and nipple
     Z90.11 Acquired absence of right breast and nipple
     Z90.12 Acquired absence of left breast and nipple
     Z90.13 Acquired absence of bilateral breasts and nipples
         Coding Clinic: 2022, Q3, P8
   Z90.2 Acquired absence of lung [part of]
   Z90.3 Acquired absence of stomach [part of]
● **Z90.4** Acquired absence of other specified parts of digestive tract
     ● **Z90.41** Acquired absence of pancreas
         Code also exocrine pancreatic insufficiency (K86.81)
         Use additional code to identify any associated: diabetes mellitus, postpancreatectomy (E13.-)
         insulin use (Z79.4)
         Z90.410 Acquired total absence of pancreas
             Acquired absence of pancreas NOS
         Z90.411 Acquired partial absence of pancreas
             Coding Clinic: 2024, Q2, P10
     Z90.49 Acquired absence of other specified parts of digestive tract
   Z90.5 Acquired absence of kidney
   Z90.6 Acquired absence of other parts of urinary tract
     Acquired absence of bladder
● **Z90.7** Acquired absence of genital organ(s)
     Excludes1 personal history of sex reassignment (Z87.890)
     Excludes2 female genital mutilation status (N90.81-)
     ● **Z90.71** Acquired absence of cervix and uterus
         Z90.710 Acquired absence of both cervix and uterus
             Acquired absence of uterus NOS
             Status post total hysterectomy
         Z90.711 Acquired absence of uterus with remaining cervical stump
             Status post partial hysterectomy with remaining cervical stump
         Z90.712 Acquired absence of cervix with remaining uterus
     ● **Z90.72** Acquired absence of ovaries
         Z90.721 Acquired absence of ovaries, unilateral
         Z90.722 Acquired absence of ovaries, bilateral
     Z90.79 Acquired absence of other genital organ(s)
         Coding Clinic: 2023, Q2, P5
● **Z90.8** Acquired absence of other organs
     Z90.81 Acquired absence of spleen
     Z90.89 Acquired absence of other organs
         Coding Clinic: 2023, Q3, P13

● **Z91** Personal risk factors, not elsewhere classified
     Excludes2 contact with and (suspected) exposures hazardous to health (Z77.-)
         exposure to pollution and other problems related to physical environment (Z77.1-)
         female genital mutilation status (N90.81-)
         occupational exposure to risk factors (Z57.-)
         personal history of physical injury and trauma (Z87.81, Z87.82-)
● **Z91.0** Allergy status, other than to drugs and biological substances
     Excludes2 allergy status to drugs, medicaments, and biological substances (Z88.-)
     ● **Z91.01** Food allergy status
         Excludes2 food additives allergy status (Z91.02)
         Z91.010 Allergy to peanuts

         Z91.011 Allergy to milk products
             Excludes1 lactose intolerance (E73.-)
         ▶ **Z91.0110** Allergy to milk products, unspecified
         ▶ **Z91.0111** Allergy to milk products with tolerance to baked milk
             ▶ **Excludes1** Allergy to milk products with reactivity to baked milk (Z91.0112)
         ▶ **Z91.0112** Allergy to milk products with reactivity to baked milk
             ▶ **Excludes1** Allergy to milk products with tolerance to baked milk (Z91.0111)
         Z91.012 Allergy to eggs
         ▶ **Z91.0120** Allergy to eggs, unspecified
         ▶ **Z91.0121** Allergy to eggs with tolerance to baked egg
             ▶ **Excludes1** Allergy to eggs with reactivity to baked egg (Z91.0122)
         ▶ **Z91.0122** Allergy to eggs with reactivity to baked egg
             ▶ **Excludes1** Allergy to egg with tolerance to baked egg (Z91.0121)
         Z91.013 Allergy to seafood
             Allergy to shellfish
             Allergy to octopus or squid ink
         Z91.014 Allergy to mammalian meats
             Allergy to beef
             Allergy to lamb
             Allergy to pork
             Allergy to red meats
         Z91.018 Allergy to other foods
             Allergy to nuts other than peanuts
     Z91.02 Food additives allergy status
     ● **Z91.03** Insect allergy status
         Z91.030 Bee allergy status
         Z91.038 Other insect allergy status
     ● **Z91.04** Nonmedicinal substance allergy status
         Z91.040 Latex allergy status
             Latex sensitivity status
         Z91.041 Radiographic dye allergy status
             Allergy status to contrast media used for diagnostic X-ray procedure
         Z91.048 Other nonmedicinal substance allergy status
     Z91.09 Other allergy status, other than to drugs and biological substances

▶ New   ➡ Revised   ~~deleted~~ Deleted   Excludes 1   Excludes 2   Includes   Use additional   Code first   Code also   Key words

OGCR Official Guidelines   **X** Assign placeholder X   ● Use Additional Character(s)   ▶ Manifestation Code   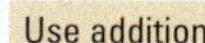 Hierarchical Condition Category   **Coding Clinic**

● **Z91.1   Patient's noncompliance with medical treatment and regimen**
  Code also, if applicable, to identify underdosing of specific drug (T36-T50 with final character 6)
  Excludes2   caregiver noncompliance with patient's medical treatment and regimen (Z91.A-)

● **Z91.11   Patient's noncompliance with dietary regimen**
  Code also, if applicable, food insecurity (Z59.4-)

  Z91.110   Patient's noncompliance with dietary regimen due to financial hardship

  Z91.118   Patient's noncompliance with dietary regimen for other reason
    Inability to comply with dietary regimen

  Z91.119   Patient's noncompliance with dietary regimen due to unspecified reason

● **Z91.12   Patient's intentional underdosing of medication regimen**
  Code first underdosing of medication (T36-T50) with fifth or sixth character 6
  Excludes1   poisoning (overdose) - code to poisoning

  Z91.120   Patient's intentional underdosing of medication regimen due to financial hardship

  Z91.128   Patient's intentional underdosing of medication regimen for other reason

● **Z91.13   Patient's unintentional underdosing of medication regimen**
  Code first underdosing of medication (T36-T50) with fifth or sixth character 6
  Excludes1   poisoning (overdose) - code to poisoning

  Z91.130   Patient's unintentional underdosing of medication regimen due to age-related debility

  Z91.138   Patient's unintentional underdosing of medication regimen for other reason

● **Z91.14   Patient's other noncompliance with medication regimen**
  Code first if applicable, adverse effect of underdosing (T36-T50)
  Patient's underdosing of medication NOS
  Coding Clinic: 2022, Q1, P36

  Z91.141   Patient's other noncompliance with medication regimen due to financial hardship

  Z91.148   Patient's other noncompliance with medication regimen for other reason

● **Z91.15   Patient's noncompliance with renal dialysis**

  Z91.151   Patient's noncompliance with renal dialysis due to financial hardship

  Z91.158   Patient's noncompliance with renal dialysis for other reason

● **Z91.19   Patient's noncompliance with other medical treatment and regimen**
  Patient's nonadherence to medical treatment

  Z91.190   Patient's noncompliance with other medical treatment and regimen due to financial hardship

  Z91.198   Patient's noncompliance with other medical treatment and regimen for other reason
  Coding Clinic: 2024, Q1, P24

  Z91.199   Patient's noncompliance with other medical treatment and regimen due to unspecified reason

● **Z91.4   Personal history of psychological trauma, not elsewhere classified**

● **Z91.41   Personal history of adult abuse**
  Excludes2   personal history of abuse in childhood (Z62.81-)

  Z91.410   Personal history of adult physical and sexual abuse   A
    Excludes1   current adult physical abuse (T74.11, T76.11)
      current adult sexual abuse (T74.21, T76.11)

  Z91.411   Personal history of adult psychological abuse   A

  Z91.412   Personal history of adult neglect   A
    Excludes1   current adult neglect (T74.01, T76.01)

  Z91.413   Personal history of adult financial abuse

  Z91.414   Personal history of adult intimate partner abuse

  Z91.419   Personal history of unspecified adult abuse   A

  Z91.42   Personal history of forced labor or sexual exploitation

  Z91.49   Other personal history of psychological trauma, not elsewhere classified

● **Z91.5   Personal history of self-harm**
  Code also mental health disorder, if known

  Z91.51   Personal history of suicidal behavior
    Personal history of parasuicide
    Personal history of self-poisoning
    Personal history of suicide attempt

  Z91.52   Personal history of nonsuicidal self-harm
    Personal history of nonsuicidal self-injury
    Personal history of self-inflicted injury without suicidal intent
    Personal history of self-mutilation

● **Z91.8   Other specified personal risk factors, not elsewhere classified**

  Z91.81   History of falling
    At risk for falling

  Z91.82   Personal history of military deployment   A
    Individual (civilian or military) with past history of military war, peacekeeping and humanitarian deployment (current or past conflict)
    Returned from military deployment
    Excludes2   personal history of military service (Z91.85)

  Z91.83   Wandering in diseases classified elsewhere
    Code first underlying disorder such as:
      Alzheimer's disease (G30.-)
      autism or pervasive developmental disorder (F84.-)
      intellectual disabilities (F70-F79)
      unspecified dementia with behavioral disturbance (F03.9-, F03.A-, F03.B-, F03.C-)

● **Z91.84   Oral health risk factors**

  Z91.841   Risk for dental caries, low

  Z91.842   Risk for dental caries, moderate

  Z91.843   Risk for dental caries, high

  Z91.849   Unspecified risk for dental caries

  Z91.85   Personal history of military service
    Excludes2   personal history of military deployment(Z91.82)
      personal history of serving in the armed forces
      personal history of veteran

CHAPTER 21 (Z00-Z99)

Z91.89 **Other specified personal risk factors, not elsewhere classified**
Increased risk for social isolation
Coding Clinic: 2017, Q1, P46

● **Z91.A** **Caregiver's noncompliance with patient's medical treatment and regimen**

● **Z91.A1** **Caregiver's noncompliance with patient's dietary regimen**
Caregiver's inability to comply with patient's dietary regimen
Code also, if applicable, food insecurity (Z59.4-)

Z91.A10 **Caregiver's noncompliance with patient's dietary regimen due to financial hardship**

Z91.A18 **Caregiver's noncompliance with patient's dietary regimen for other reason**

● **Z91.A2** **Caregiver's intentional underdosing of patient's medication regimen**
Code first underdosing of medication (T36-T50) with fifth or sixth character 6

Z91.A20 **Caregiver's intentional underdosing of patient's medication regimen due to financial hardship**

Z91.A28 **Caregiver's intentional underdosing of medication regimen for other reason**

Z91.A3 **Caregiver's unintentional underdosing of patient's medication regimen**
Code first underdosing of medication (T36-T50) with fifth or sixth character 6

● **Z91.A4** **Caregiver's other noncompliance with patient's medication regimen**
Caregiver's underdosing of patient's medication NOS

Z91.A41 **Caregiver's other noncompliance with patient's medication regimen due to financial hardship**

Z91.A48 **Caregiver's other noncompliance with patient's medication regimen for other reason**

● **Z91.A5** **Caregiver's noncompliance with patient's renal dialysis**

Z91.A51 **Caregiver's noncompliance with patient's renal dialysis due to financial hardship**

Z91.A58 **Caregiver's noncompliance with patient's renal dialysis for other reason**

● **Z91.A9** **Caregiver's noncompliance with patient's other medical treatment and regimen**
Caregiver's nonadherence to patient's medical treatment

Z91.A91 **Caregiver's noncompliance with patient's other medical treatment and regimen due to financial hardship**

Z91.A98 **Caregiver's noncompliance with patient's other medical treatment and regimen for other reason**

▶ **Z91.B** **Personal risk factor of exposure to diethylstilbestrol**
▶DES daughter or son
▶Personal risk factor of exposure to DES
▶Personal risk factor of exposure to DES in utero
▶Second generation DES exposure
▶*Code also*, associated conditions, such as:
▶conditions classifiable to C50.-
▶osteoporosis (M80.-)
▶premature menopause (E28.31-)

● **Z92** **Personal history of medical treatment**
Excludes2 postprocedural states (Z98.-)

Z92.0 **Personal history of contraception**
Excludes1 counseling or management of current contraceptive practices (Z30.-)
long term (current) use of contraception (Z79.3)
presence of (intrauterine) contraceptive device (Z97.5)

● **Z92.2** **Personal history of drug therapy**
Excludes2 long term (current) drug therapy (Z79.-)

Z92.21 **Personal history of antineoplastic chemotherapy**

Z92.22 **Personal history of monoclonal drug therapy**
Excludes2 personal history of immune checkpoint inhibitor therapy (Z92.26)

Z92.23 **Personal history of estrogen therapy**

● **Z92.24** **Personal history of steroid therapy**

Z92.240 **Personal history of inhaled steroid therapy**

Z92.241 **Personal history of systemic steroid therapy**
Personal history of steroid therapy NOS

Z92.25 **Personal history of immunosuppression therapy**
Excludes2 personal history of steroid therapy (Z92.24)

Z92.26 **Personal history of immune checkpoint inhibitor therapy**
Personal history of ICI drug therapy

Z92.29 **Personal history of other drug therapy**

Z92.3 **Personal history of irradiation**
Personal history of exposure to therapeutic radiation
Excludes1 exposure to radiation in the physical environment (Z77.12)
occupational exposure to radiation (Z57.1)

● **Z92.8** **Personal history of other medical treatment**
Coding Clinic: 2016, Q4, P72

Z92.81 **Personal history of extracorporeal membrane oxygenation (ECMO)**

Z92.82 **Status post administration of tPA (rtPA) in a different facility within the last 24 hours prior to admission to current facility**
Code first condition requiring tPA administration, such as:
acute cerebral infarction (I63.-)
acute myocardial infarction (I21.-, I22.-)

Z92.83 **Personal history of failed moderate sedation**
Personal history of failed conscious sedation
Excludes2 failed moderate sedation during procedure (T88.52)

Z92.84 **Personal history of unintended awareness under general anesthesia**
Excludes2 unintended awareness under general anesthesia during procedure (T88.53)
Coding Clinic: 2016, Q4, P72, 77

● **Z92.85** **Personal history of cellular therapy**
Excludes2 personal history of immune checkpoint inhibitor therapy (Z92.26)

Z92.850 **Personal history of Chimeric Antigen Receptor T-cell therapy**
Personal history of CAR T-cell therapy

Z92.858 **Personal history of other cellular therapy**

Z92.859 **Personal history of cellular therapy, unspecified**

Z92.86   **Personal history of gene therapy**
Z92.89   **Personal history of other medical treatment**
Coding Clinic: 2020, Q1, P18

● **Z93   Artificial opening status**
    Excludes1   artificial openings requiring attention or management (Z43.-)
        complications of external stoma (J95.0-, K94.-, N99.5-)

Z93.0   **Tracheostomy status**
Z93.1   **Gastrostomy status**
Z93.2   **Ileostomy status**
Z93.3   **Colostomy status**
    Ileal pouch status
    Kock pouch status
Z93.4   **Other artificial openings of gastrointestinal tract status**
● Z93.5   **Cystostomy status**
    Z93.50   **Unspecified cystostomy status**
    Z93.51   **Cutaneous-vesicostomy status**
    Z93.52   **Appendico-vesicostomy status**
    Z93.59   **Other cystostomy status**
Z93.6   **Other artificial openings of urinary tract status**
    Nephrostomy status
    Ureterostomy status
    Urethrostomy status
Z93.8   **Other artificial opening status**
Z93.9   **Artificial opening status, unspecified**

● **Z94   Transplanted organ and tissue status**
    Includes   organ or tissue replaced by heterogenous or homogenous transplant
    Excludes1   complications of transplanted organ or tissue - see Alphabetical Index
    Excludes2   presence of vascular grafts (Z95.-)

Z94.0   **Kidney transplant status**
Z94.1   **Heart transplant status**
    Excludes1   artificial heart status (Z95.812)
        heart-valve replacement status (Z95.2-Z95.4)
Z94.2   **Lung transplant status**
Z94.3   **Heart and lungs transplant status**
Z94.4   **Liver transplant status**
Z94.5   **Skin transplant status**
    Autogenous skin transplant status
Z94.6   **Bone transplant status**
Z94.7   **Corneal transplant status**
● Z94.8   **Other transplanted organ and tissue status**
    Z94.81   **Bone marrow transplant status**
    Z94.82   **Intestine transplant status**
    Z94.83   **Pancreas transplant status**
    Z94.84   **Stem cells transplant status**
    Z94.89   **Other transplanted organ and tissue status**
Z94.9   **Transplanted organ and tissue status, unspecified**

● **Z95   Presence of cardiac and vascular implants and grafts**
    Excludes2   complications of cardiac and vascular devices, implants and grafts (T82.-)

Z95.0   **Presence of cardiac pacemaker**
    Presence of cardiac resynchronization therapy (CRT-P) pacemaker
    Excludes1   adjustment or management of cardiac device (Z45.0-)
        adjustment or management of cardiac pacemaker (Z45.0)
        presence of automatic (implantable) cardiac defibrillator with synchronous cardiac pacemaker (Z95.810)
Coding Clinic: 2019, Q1, P33

Z95.1   **Presence of aortocoronary bypass graft**
    Presence of coronary artery bypass graft
Z95.2   **Presence of prosthetic heart valve**
    Presence of heart valve NOS
Z95.3   **Presence of xenogenic heart valve**
Z95.4   **Presence of other heart-valve replacement**
Z95.5   **Presence of coronary angioplasty implant and graft**
    Excludes1   coronary angioplasty status without implant and graft (Z98.61)
● Z95.8   **Presence of other cardiac and vascular implants and grafts**
    ● Z95.81   **Presence of other cardiac implants and grafts**
        Z95.810   **Presence of automatic (implantable) cardiac defibrillator**
            Presence of automatic (implantable) cardiac defibrillator with synchronous cardiac pacemaker
            Presence of cardiac resynchronization therapy defibrillator (CRT-D)
            Presence of cardioverter-defribrillator (ICD)
            Coding Clinic: 2022, Q2, P15
        Z95.811   **Presence of heart assist device**
        Z95.812   **Presence of fully implantable artificial heart**
        Z95.818   **Presence of other cardiac implants and grafts**
    ● Z95.82   **Presence of other vascular implants and grafts**
        Z95.820   **Peripheral vascular angioplasty status with implants and grafts**
            Excludes1   peripheral vascular angioplasty without implant and graft (Z98.62)
        Z95.828   **Presence of other vascular implants and grafts**
            Presence of intravascular prosthesis NEC
Z95.9   **Presence of cardiac and vascular implant and graft, unspecified**

● **Z96   Presence of other functional implants**
    Excludes2   complications of internal prosthetic devices, implants and grafts (T82-T85)
        fitting and adjustment of prosthetic and other devices (Z44-Z46)

Z96.0   **Presence of urogenital implants**
Z96.1   **Presence of intraocular lens**
    Presence of pseudophakia
● Z96.2   **Presence of otological and audiological implants**
    Z96.20   **Presence of otological and audiological implant, unspecified**
    Z96.21   **Cochlear implant status**
    Z96.22   **Myringotomy tube(s) status**
    Z96.29   **Presence of other otological and audiological implants**
        Presence of bone-conduction hearing device
        Presence of eustachian tube stent
        Stapes replacement
Z96.3   **Presence of artificial larynx**
● Z96.4   **Presence of endocrine implants**
    Z96.41   **Presence of insulin pump (external) (internal)**
    Z96.49   **Presence of other endocrine implants**
Z96.5   **Presence of tooth-root and mandibular implants**
● Z96.6   **Presence of orthopedic joint implants**
    Z96.60   **Presence of unspecified orthopedic joint implant**

CHAPTER 21 (Z00-Z99)

● **Z96.61　Presence of artificial shoulder joint**
　　Z96.611　Presence of right artificial shoulder joint
　　Z96.612　Presence of left artificial shoulder joint
　　Z96.619　Presence of unspecified artificial shoulder joint
● **Z96.62　Presence of artificial elbow joint**
　　Z96.621　Presence of right artificial elbow joint
　　Z96.622　Presence of left artificial elbow joint
　　Z96.629　Presence of unspecified artificial elbow joint
● **Z96.63　Presence of artificial wrist joint**
　　Z96.631　Presence of right artificial wrist joint
　　Z96.632　Presence of left artificial wrist joint
　　Z96.639　Presence of unspecified artificial wrist joint
● **Z96.64　Presence of artificial hip joint**
　　Hip-joint replacement (partial) (total)
　　Z96.641　Presence of right artificial hip joint
　　　　Coding Clinic: 2016, Q3, P17
　　Z96.642　Presence of left artificial hip joint
　　　　Coding Clinic: 2015, Q1, P16
　　Z96.643　Presence of artificial hip joint, bilateral
　　Z96.649　Presence of unspecified artificial hip joint
● **Z96.65　Presence of artificial knee joint**
　　Z96.651　Presence of right artificial knee joint
　　Z96.652　Presence of left artificial knee joint
　　　　Coding Clinic: 2019, Q3, P16
　　Z96.653　Presence of artificial knee joint, bilateral
　　Z96.659　Presence of unspecified artificial knee joint
● **Z96.66　Presence of artificial ankle joint**
　　Z96.661　Presence of right artificial ankle joint
　　Z96.662　Presence of left artificial ankle joint
　　Z96.669　Presence of unspecified artificial ankle joint
● **Z96.69　Presence of other orthopedic joint implants**
　　Z96.691　Finger-joint replacement of right hand
　　Z96.692　Finger-joint replacement of left hand
　　Z96.693　Finger-joint replacement, bilateral
　　Z96.698　Presence of other orthopedic joint implants
Z96.7　Presence of other bone and tendon implants
　　Presence of skull plate
● **Z96.8　Presence of other specified functional implants**
　　Z96.81　Presence of artificial skin
　　Z96.82　Presence of neurostimulator
　　　　Presence of brain neurostimulator
　　　　Presence of gastric neurostimulator
　　　　Presence of peripheral nerve neurostimulator
　　　　Presence of sacral nerve neurostimulator
　　　　Presence of spinal cord neurostimulator
　　　　Presence of vagus nerve neurostimulator
　　Z96.89　Presence of other specified functional implants
Z96.9　Presence of functional implant, unspecified

● **Z97　Presence of other devices**
　　Excludes2　fitting and adjustment of prosthetic and other devices (Z44-Z46)
　　　　presence of cerebrospinal fluid drainage device (Z98.2)
Z97.0　Presence of artificial eye
● **Z97.1　Presence of artificial limb (complete) (partial)**
　　Z97.10　Presence of artificial limb (complete) (partial), unspecified

　　Z97.11　Presence of artificial right arm (complete) (partial)
　　Z97.12　Presence of artificial left arm (complete) (partial)
　　Z97.13　Presence of artificial right leg (complete) (partial)
　　Z97.14　Presence of artificial left leg (complete) (partial)
　　Z97.15　Presence of artificial arms, bilateral (complete) (partial)
　　Z97.16　Presence of artificial legs, bilateral (complete) (partial)
Z97.2　Presence of dental prosthetic device (complete) (partial)
　　Presence of dentures (complete) (partial)
Z97.3　Presence of spectacles and contact lenses
Z97.4　Presence of external hearing-aid
Z97.5　Presence of (intrauterine) contraceptive device
　　Excludes1　checking, reinsertion or removal of implantable subdermal contraceptive (Z30.46)
　　　　checking, reinsertion or removal of intrauterine contraceptive device (Z30.43-)
Z97.8　Presence of other specified devices

● **Z98　Other postprocedural states**
　　Excludes2　aftercare (Z43-Z49, Z51)
　　　　follow-up medical care (Z08-Z09)
　　▶ fontan related circulation (I27.84-)
　　　　postprocedural complication - see Alphabetical Index
Z98.0　Intestinal bypass and anastomosis status
　　Excludes2　bariatric surgery status (Z98.84)
　　　　gastric bypass status (Z98.84)
　　　　obesity surgery status (Z98.84)
Z98.1　Arthrodesis status
Z98.2　Presence of cerebrospinal fluid drainage device
　　Presence of CSF shunt
Z98.3　Post therapeutic collapse of lung status
　　Code first underlying disease
● **Z98.4　Cataract extraction status**
　　Use additional code to identify intraocular lens implant status (Z96.1)
　　Excludes1　aphakia (H27.0)
　　Z98.41　Cataract extraction status, right eye
　　Z98.42　Cataract extraction status, left eye
　　Z98.49　Cataract extraction status, unspecified eye
● **Z98.5　Sterilization status**
　　Excludes1　female infertility (N97.-)
　　　　male infertility (N46.-)
　　Z98.51　Tubal ligation status
　　Z98.52　Vasectomy status
● **Z98.6　Angioplasty status**
　　Z98.61　Coronary angioplasty status
　　　　Excludes1　coronary angioplasty status with implant and graft (Z95.5)
　　　　Coding Clinic: 2022, Q4, P23
　　Z98.62　Peripheral vascular angioplasty status
　　　　Excludes1　peripheral vascular angioplasty status with implant and graft (Z95.820)
● **Z98.8　Other specified postprocedural states**
　　Coding Clinic: 2016, Q4, P76
　● Z98.81　Dental procedure status
　　　　Z98.810　Dental sealant status
　　　　Z98.811　Dental restoration status
　　　　　　Dental crown status
　　　　　　Dental fillings status
　　　　Z98.818　Other dental procedure status

▶ New　　⇨ Revised　　~~deleted~~ Deleted　　Excludes 1　　Excludes 2　　Includes　　Use additional　　Code first　　Code also　　Key words
OGCR Official Guidelines　　X Assign placeholder X　　● Use Additional Character(s)　　❘ Manifestation Code　　HCC Hierarchical Condition Category　　**Coding Clinic**

Z98.82 **Breast implant status**

  Excludes1 breast implant removal status (Z98.86)

  Coding Clinic: 2022, Q3, P8

Z98.83 **Filtering (vitreous) bleb after glaucoma surgery status**

  Excludes1 inflammation (infection) of postprocedural bleb (H59.4-)

Z98.84 **Bariatric surgery status**

  Gastric banding status
  Gastric bypass status for obesity
  Obesity surgery status

  Excludes1 bariatric surgery status complicating pregnancy, childbirth, or the puerperium (O99.84)

  Excludes2 intestinal bypass and anastomosis status (Z98.0)

  Coding Clinic: 2020, Q1, P12

Z98.85 **Transplanted organ removal status**

  Transplanted organ previously removed due to complication, failure, rejection or infection

  Excludes1 encounter for removal of transplanted organ - code to complication of transplanted organ (T86.-)

Z98.86 **Personal history of breast implant removal**

● **Z98.87** **Personal history of in utero procedure**

 Z98.870 **Personal history of in utero procedure during pregnancy**

  Excludes2 complications from in utero procedure for current pregnancy (O35.7)
  supervision of current pregnancy with history of in utero procedure during previous pregnancy (O09.82-)

 Z98.871 **Personal history of in utero procedure while a fetus**

● **Z98.89** **Other specified postprocedural states**

  Coding Clinic: 2016, Q4, P76

 Z98.890 **Other specified postprocedural states**

  Personal history of surgery, not elsewhere classified

  Coding Clinic: 2023, Q3, P13

 Z98.891 **History of uterine scar from previous surgery**

  Excludes1 Maternal care due to uterine scar from previous surgery (O34.2-)

  Coding Clinic: 2016, Q4, P52, P76

● **Z99** **Dependence on enabling machines and devices, not elsewhere classified**

 Coding Clinic: 2020, Q1, P11

● **Z99.0** **Dependence on aspirator**

● **Z99.1** **Dependence on respirator**

 Dependence on ventilator

 Z99.11 **Dependence on respirator [ventilator] status**

  ▶Ventilator status

  Coding Clinic: 2018, Q1, P14; 2015, Q1, P21

 Z99.12 **Encounter for respirator [ventilator] dependence during power failure**

  Excludes1 mechanical complication of respirator [ventilator] (J95.850)

● **Z99.2** **Dependence on renal dialysis**

 Hemodialysis status
 Peritoneal dialysis status
 Presence of arteriovenous shunt for dialysis
 Renal dialysis status NOS

  Excludes1 encounter for fitting and adjustment of dialysis catheter (Z49.0-)

  Excludes2 noncompliance with renal dialysis (Z91.15-)

 Coding Clinic: 2022, Q3, P16; 2016, Q1, P13

● **Z99.3** **Dependence on wheelchair**

 Wheelchair confinement status

 Code first cause of dependence, such as:
  muscular dystrophy (G71.0-)
  obesity (E66.-)

● **Z99.8** **Dependence on other enabling machines and devices**

● **Z99.81** **Dependence on supplemental oxygen**

  Dependence on long-term oxygen

 Z99.89 **Dependence on other enabling machines and devices**

  Dependence on machine or device NOS

  Coding Clinic: 2020, Q1, P11

CHAPTER 21 (Z00–Z99)

CHAPTER 22 (U00-U85)

CHAPTER 22

CODES FOR SPECIAL PURPOSES (U00-U85)

Note: Codes from this chapter are for use on newborn records only, never on maternal records.

This chapter contains the following blocks:

U00-U49	Provisional assignment of new diseases of uncertain etiology or emergency use

---

PROVISIONAL ASSIGNMENT OF NEW DISEASES OF UNCERTAIN ETIOLOGY OR EMERGENCY USE (U00-U49)

U07 Emergency use of U07

    U07.0 **Vaping-related disorder**

        Dabbing related lung damage
        Dabbing related lung injury
        E-cigarette, or vaping, product use associated lung injury [EVALI]
        Electronic cigarette related lung damage
        Electronic cigarette related lung injury

        Use additional code to identify manifestations, such as:
          abdominal pain (R10.84)
          acute respiratory distress syndrome (J80)
          diarrhea (R19.7)
          drug-induced interstitial lung disorder (J70.4)
          lipoid pneumonia (J69.1)
          weight loss (R63.4)

    U07.1 **COVID-19**

        Use additional code to identify pneumonia or other manifestations

        Use Additional code, if applicable, for associated conditions such as:
          COVID-19 associated coagulopathy (D68.8)
          disseminated intravascular coagulation (D65)
          hypercoagulable states (D68.69)
          thrombophilia (D68.69)

        Excludes1 coronavirus as the cause of diseases classified elsewhere (B97.2-)
          pneumonia due to SARS-associated coronavirus (J12.81)

        Coding Clinic: 2025, Q1, P34; 2022, Q2, P29; 2021, Q4, P109; 2021, Q1, P31-33, 36, 39-40, 47, 49

U09 Post COVID-19 condition

    U09.9 **Post COVID-19 condition, unspecified**

        Note: This code enables establishment of a link with COVID-19.

        This code is not to be used in cases that are still presenting with active COVID-19. However, an exception is made in cases of re-infection with COVID-19, occurring with a condition related to prior COVID-19.

        Post-acute sequela of COVID-19

        Code first the specific condition related to COVID-19 if known, such as:
          chronic respiratory failure (J96.1-)
          loss of smell (R43.8)
          loss of taste (R43.8)
          multisystem inflammatory syndrome (M35.81)
          pulmonary embolism (I26.-)
          pulmonary fibrosis (J84.10)

        Coding Clinic: 2021, Q4, P102-104,106

▶ New   ⇨ Revised   ~~deleted~~ Deleted   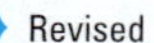 Excludes 1   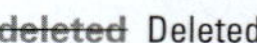 Excludes 2   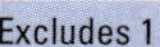 Includes   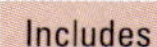 Use additional   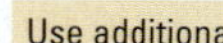 Code first   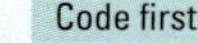 Code also   Key words

OGCR Official Guidelines   X Assign placeholder X   ● Use Additional Character(s)   ◗ Manifestation Code   Hierarchical Condition Category   Coding Clinic